Frank
Bauer
7/2012

CARDIAC SURGERY IN THE ADULT

NOTICE

Medicine is an ever-changing science. As new research and clinical experience broaden our knowledge, changes in treatment and drug therapy are required. The authors and the publisher of this work have checked with sources believed to be reliable in their efforts to provide information that is complete and generally in accord with the standards accepted at the time of publication. However, in view of the possibility of human error or changes in medical sciences, neither the authors nor the publisher nor any other party who has been involved in the preparation or publication of this work warrants that the information contained herein is in every respect accurate or complete, and they disclaim all responsibility for any errors or omissions or for the results obtained from use of the information contained in this work. Readers are encouraged to confirm the information contained herein with other sources. For example and in particular, readers are advised to check the product information sheet included in the package of each drug they plan to administer to be certain that the information contained in this work is accurate and that changes have not been made in the recommended dose or in the contraindications for administration. This recommendation is of particular importance in connection with new or infrequently used drugs.

CARDIAC SURGERY IN THE ADULT

Fourth Edition

Lawrence H. Cohn, MD

Virginia and James Hubbard Professor of Cardiac Surgery
Harvard Medical School
Division of Cardiac Surgery
Brigham and Women's Hospital
Boston, Massachusetts

McGraw Hill Medical

New York Chicago San Francisco Lisbon London Madrid Mexico City
Milan New Delhi San Juan Seoul Singapore Sydney Toronto

The McGraw-Hill Companies

Cardiac Surgery in the Adult, Fourth Edition

1 2 3 4 5 6 7 8 9 0 CTP/CTP 15 14 13 12 11

Set ISBN 978-0-07-163312-3; MHID 0-07-163312-X
Book ISBN 978-0-07-163310-9; MHID 0-07-163310-3
DVD ISBN 978-0-07-163311-6; MHID 0-07-163311-1

This book was set in Times Roman by Cenveo Publisher Services.
The editors were Brian Belval and Peter J. Boyle.
The production supervisor was Catherine H. Saggese.
Project management was provided by Vastavikta Sharma, Cenveo Publisher Services.
China Translation & Printing Services, Ltd. was the printer and binder.

Library of Congress Cataloging-in-Publication Data

Cardiac surgery in the adult. — 4th ed. / [edited by] Lawrence H. Cohn.
p. ; cm.
Includes bibliographical references and index.

Summary: "Cardiac Surgery in the Adult guides residents and practicing surgeons through diagnosis, treatment and management as well as operative strategy, decision-making, and technique in adult cardiac surgery. Developments in this field are constant and are in line with the surgical trends at large: less-invasive surgery with faster recovery times. Developments in this field include the use of robotic surgery, minimally invasive valve and coronary artery bypass surgery, stem-cell induced regenerative medicine, tissue engineering and more, all of which are discussed and completely updated. Trends also take into account the demographics of the patient with an eye toward cross-training the surgeon in endovascular skills by including topics such as percutaneous intervention and endovascular graft technology."—Provided by publisher.

ISBN 978-0-07-163312-3 (hardback : alk. paper)
I. Cohn, Lawrence H., 1937-
[DNLM: 1. Cardiac Surgical Procedures. 2. Adult. WG 169]
LC classification not assigned
617.4'12—dc23

2011031211

If I have seen further it is by standing on the shoulders of giants.
—Sir Isaac Newton

I dedicate this edition, to my mentors:
Norman E. Shumway, MD
Andrew Glenn Morrow, MD
Eugene Braunwald, MD
J. Englebert Dunphy, MD
Francis D. Moore, MD
John J. Collins, Jr., MD
John A. Mannick, MD

All who have influenced me in different ways to become the cardiac surgeon I am today.

CONTENTS

PART 1

FUNDAMENTALS

PART 2

PERIOPERATIVE/INTRAOPERATIVE CARE

PART 3

ISCHEMIC HEART DISEASE

PART 4 A

VALVULAR HEART DISEASE (AORTIC)

PART 4 B

VALVULAR HEART DISEASE (MITRAL)

PART 4 C

VALVULAR HEART DISEASE (OTHER)

PART 5

DISEASES OF THE GREAT VESSELS

PART 6

SURGERY FOR CARDIAC ARRHYTHMIAS

PART 7

OTHER CARDIAC OPERATIONS

PART 8

TRANSPLANT AND CARDIAC SUPPORT

CONTENTS OF DVD

CONTRIBUTORS

Michael A. Acker, MD
Professor, Department of Surgery, University of Pennsylvania School of Medicine, Philadelphia, Pennsylvania
Ischemic Mitral Regurgitation

Arvind K. Agnihotri, MD
Assistant Professor, Department of Surgery, Harvard Medical School, Boston, Massachusetts
Surgical Treatment of Complications of Acute Myocardial Infarction

Cary W. Akins, MD
Clinical Professor of Surgery, Department of Surgery, Harvard Medical School, Boston, Massachusetts
Myocardial Revascularization with Carotid Artery Disease

Jeremiah G. Allen, MD
Resident, Department of Surgery, Johns Hopkins Hospital, Baltimore, Maryland
Heart Transplantation

Robert H. Anderson, MD
Professor Emeritus, Institute of Child Health, University College, London, United Kingdom
Surgical Anatomy of the Heart

Mark P. Anstadt, MD
Associate Professor, Department of Surgery, Wright State University, Dayton, Ohio
Cardiopulmonary Resuscitation

Sary Aranki, MD
Associate Professor of Surgery, Harvard Medical School, Boston, Massachusetts
Mitral Valve Replacement

Pavan Atluri, MD
Assistant Professor of Surgery. Division of Cardiovascular Surgery, Department of Surgery, University of Pennsylvania, Philadelphia, Pennsylvania
Ischemic Mitral Regurgitation

Frank A. Baciewicz, Jr., MD
Professor of Cardiothoracic Surgery, Wayne State University, Detroit, Michigan
History of Cardiac Surgery

William A. Baumgartner, MD
Vincent L. Gott Professor, Division of Cardiac Surgery, Johns Hopkins Hospital, Baltimore, Maryland
Heart Transplantation

Joseph E. Bavaria, MD
Professor of Surgery, Department of Surgery, Hospital of the University of Pennsylvania, Philadelphia, Pennsylvania
Ascending Aortic Aneurysms

Shanda H. Blackmon, MD, MPH
Assistant Professor, Department of Surgery, Weill Cornell Medical College, Houston, Texas
Cardiac Neoplasms

Steven F. Bolling, MD
Professor of Cardiac Surgery, University of Michigan, Ann Arbor, Michigan
Nontransplant Surgical Options for Heart Failure

John Bozinovski, MD
Attending Cardiac Surgeon, Royal Jubilee Hospital, Victoria, BC, Canada
Extent II Thoracoabdominal Aortic Aneurysm Repair (DVD)

R. Morton Bolman, III, MD
Professor of Surgery, Harvard Medical School, Brigham and Women's Hospital, Boston, Massachusetts
Deep Hypothermic Circulatory Arrest

Morgan L. Brown, MD, PhD
Chief Resident, Department of Anesthesiology and Pain Medicine, University of Alberta, Edmonton, Alberta, Canada
Indications for Revascularization

Redmond P. Burke, MD
Professor of Pediatric Cardiac Surgery, Florida International University, Miami, Florida
Surgery for Adult Congenital Heart Disease

John G. Byrne, MD
William S. Stoney Professor of Cardiac Surgery, Vanderbilt Medical Center, Nashville, Tennessee
Reoperative Valve Surgery

Richard P. Cambria, MD
Professor of Surgery, Harvard Medical School, Boston, Massachusetts
Myocardial Revascularization with Carotid Artery Disease

Frederick Y. Chen, MD, PhD
Associate Professor of Surgery, Brigham and Women's Hospital, Harvard Medical School, Boston, Massachusetts
Computed Tomography of the Adult Cardiac Surgery Patient: Principles and Applications; Mitral Valve Repair

Albert T. Cheung, MD
Department of Anesthesiology and Critical Care, Hospital of the University of Pennsylvania, Philadelphia, Pennsylvania
Cardiac Anesthesia

W. Randolph Chitwood, Jr., MD, FRCS (Eng)
Professor of Cardiovascular Sciences, East Carolina University, Greenville, North Carolina
Minimally Invasive and Robotic Mitral Valve Surgery

George T. Christakis, MD, FRCS(C)
Professor of Surgery, University of Toronto, Toronto, Ontario, Canada
Bioprosthetic Aortic Valve Replacement: Stented Pericardial and Porcine Valves

Lawrence H. Cohn, MD
Virginia and James Hubbard Professor of Cardiac Surgery, Division of Cardiac Surgery, Harvard Medical School, Brigham and Women's Hospital, Boston, Massachusetts
Surgical Anatomy of the Heart; Minimally Invasive Aortic Valve Surgery; Mitral Valve Repair

William E. Cohn, MD
Associate Professor of Surgery, Transplant & Assist Devices Cardiothoracic Surgery, Baylor College of Medicine, Houston, Texas
Total Artificial Heart

John V. Conte, MD
Professor, Cardiac Surgery, Johns Hopkins University, Baltimore, Maryland
Heart Transplantation

Joseph S. Coselli, MD
Professor and Cullen Foundation Endowed Chair, Division of Cardiothoracic Surgery, Michael E. DeBakey Department of Surgery, Baylor College of Medicine, Houston, Texas
Descending and Thoracoabdominal Aortic Aneurysms

John M. Craig, MD
Chief Resident, Division of Cardiac Surgery, Massachusetts General Hospital, Boston, Massachusetts
Pericardial Disease

Willard M. Daggett, Jr., MD
Professor of Surgery Emeritus, Department of Surgery, Harvard Medical School, Boston, Massachusetts
Surgical Treatment of Complications of Acute Myocardial Infarction

Ralph J. Damiano, Jr., MD
Professor of Surgery, Department of Surgery, Washington University School of Medicine, St. Louis, Missouri
Surgery for Atrial Fibrillation

Tirone E. David, MD
Professor of Surgery, University of Toronto, Toronto, Ontario, Canada
Aortic Valve Repair and Aortic Valve-Sparing Operations; Surgical Treatment of Aortic Valve Endocarditis

William J. DeBois, MBA, CCP
Director, Cardiothoracic Surgery-Perioperative Services, Weill Cornell Medical College, New York, New York
Transfusion Therapy and Blood Conservation

Nimesh D. Desai, MD, PhD
Assistant Professor of Surgery, Department of Surgery, Hospital of the University of Pennsylvania, Philadelphia, Pennsylvania
Ascending Aortic Aneurysms

Verdi J. DiSesa, MD, MBA
Professor of Surgery, Temple University School of Medicine, Philadelphia, Pennsylvania
Valvular and Ischemic Heart Disease

Robert E. Eckart, DO
Director, Cardiac Arrhythmia Service, Department of Medicine, San Antonio Military Medical Center, San Antonio, Texas
Interventional Therapy for Atrial and Ventricular Arrhythmias

Fred H. Edwards, MD
Professor of Surgery, University of Florida, Jacksonville, Florida
Assessment of Cardiac Operations to Improve Performance

Samuel Edwards, MD
Clinical Fellow in Medicine, Beth Israel Deaconess Medical Center, Boston, Massachusetts
Pathophysiology of Aortic Valve Disease

Andrew W. El Bardissi, MD, MPH
Clinical Fellow of Surgery, Department of Surgery, Harvard Medical School, Brigham and Women's Hospital, Boston, Massachusetts
Deep Hypothermic Circulatory Arrest

Ann M. Emery, RN
Minneapolis, Minnesota
Aortic Valve Replacement with a Mechanical Cardiac Valve Prosthesis

Robert W. Emery, MD
Medical Director, Cardiovascular Surgery, St. Joseph's Hospital, St. Paul, Minnesota
Aortic Valve Replacement with a Mechanical Cardiac Valve Prosthesis

Maurice Enriquez-Sarano, MD
Professor, Mayo Clinic College of Medicine, Rochester, Minnesota
Principle and Practice of Echocardiography in Cardiac Surgery

Laurence M. Epstein, MD
Chief, Arrhythmia Service, Associate Professor of Medicine, Brigham and Women's Hospital, Harvard Medical School, Boston, Massachusetts
Interventional Therapy for Atrial and Ventricular Arrhythmias

Volkmar Falk, MD, PhD
Professor of Medicine Cardiovascular Surgery, University Hospital, Zurich, Switzerland
Minimally Invasive Myocardial Revascularization

James I. Fann, MD
Associate Professor of Cardiothoracic Surgery, Stanford University, Stanford, California
Pathophysiology of Mitral Valve Disease

Robert Saeid Farivar, MD, PhD
Assistant Professor, Cardiothoracic Surgery, University of Iowa, Iowa City, Iowa
Cardiac Surgical Physiology

Victor A. Ferraris, MD, PhD
Tyler Gill Professor of Surgery, Department of Surgery, University of Kentucky, Lexington, Kentucky
Assessment of Cardiac Operations to Improve Performance

O. Howard Frazier, MD
Professor of Surgery, Baylor College of Medicine and University of Texas Health Science Center, Houston, Texas
Total Artificial Heart

Robert P. Gallegos, MD, PhD
Cardiac Surgeon, Department of Cardiac Surgery, Brigham and Women's Hospital, Boston, Massachusetts
Mitral Valve Replacement

Isaac George, MD
Instructor in Surgery, Division of Cardiothoracic Surgery, Columbia University College of Physicians and Surgeons, New York Presbyterian Hospital, Columbia University Medical Center, New York, New York
Myocardial Revascularization after Acute Myocardial Infarction

A. Marc Gillinov, MD
Staff Cardiac Surgeon, Thoracic and Cardiovascular Surgery, Cleveland Clinic, Cleveland, Ohio
Pathophysiology of Aortic Valve Disease; Surgical Treatment of Mitral Valve Endocarditis

Donald D. Glower, MD
Professor of Surgery, Duke University Medical Center, Durham, North Carolina
Left Ventricular Aneurysm

G. V. Gonzalez-Stawinski, MD
Department of Thoracic and Cardiovascular Surgery, Cleveland Clinic, Cleveland, Ohio
Coronary Artery Reoperations

Joseph H. Gorman, III, MD
Professor of Surgery, University of Pennsylvania, Philadelphia, Pennsylvania
Ischemic Mitral Regurgitation

Robert C. Gorman, MD
Professor of Surgery, University of Pennsylvania, Philadelphia, Pennsylvania
Ischemic Mitral Regurgitation

Danielle Gottlieb, MD
Tissue Engineering for Cardiac Valve Surgery

Roberta A. Gottlieb, MD
Professor and Frederick G. Henry Chair in the Life Sciences, Biology Department, San Diego State University, San Diego, California
Myocardial Protection

Kevin L. Greason, MD
Assistant Professor, Division of Cardiovascular Surgery, Mayo Clinic, Rochester, Minnesota
Myocardial Revascularization with Cardiopulmonary Bypass

James P. Greelish, MD
Assistant Professor of Cardiac Surgery, Vanderbilt University, Nashville, Tennessee
Reoperative Valve Surgery

Igor D. Gregoric, MD
Associate Chief, Transplant Services; Director, Mechanical Circulatory Support; Clinical Associate Professor of Surgery; Department of Cardiothoracic and Vascular Surgery, Texas Heart Institute at St. Luke's Episcopal Hospital; The University of Texas Health and Science Center Houston and The University of MD Anderson Cancer Center, Houston, Texas
Total Artificial Heart

Randall B. Griepp, MD
Professor and Chairman Emeritus, Department of Cardiothoracic Surgery, Mount Sinai School of Medicine, New York, New York
Aneurysms of the Aortic Arch

Bartley P. Griffith, MD
Professor of Cardiac Surgery, University of Maryland, Baltimore, Maryland
Immunobiology of Heart and Heart-Lung Transplantation

Gary L. Grunkemeier, MD
Director, Medical Data Research Center, Providence Health & Services, Portland, Oregon
Statistical Treatment of Surgical Outcome Data

Tomas Gudbjartsson, MD, PhD
Professor of Surgery, Landspitali University Hospital, Department of Cardiothoracic Surgery, Faculty of Medicine, University of Iceland, Reykjavik, Iceland
Mitral Valve Replacement

Michael E. Halkos, MD
Assistant Professor of Cardiothoracic Surgery, Emory University School of Medicine, Atlanta, Georgia
Myocardial Revascularization without Cardiopulmonary Bypass

John W. Hammon, MD
Professor Emeritus of Surgery, Department of Cardiothoracic Surgery, Wake Forest University School of Medicine, Winston-Salem, North Carolina
Extracorporeal Circulation

Michael H. Hines, MD
Professor of Pediatric Surgery, Division of Cardiovascular Surgery, University of Texas Medical School at Houston, Houston, Texas
Extracorporeal Circulation

David M. Holzhey, MD
Consultant, Cardiac Surgery, University of Leipzig, Leipzig, Germany
Minimally Invasive Myocardial Revascularization

Jan Hommerding, RN, CNP
Heart Care Intervention NP, Heart Care, St. Joseph's Hospital, St. Paul, Minnesota
Aortic Valve Replacement with a Mechanical Cardiac Valve Prosthesis

Keith A. Horvath, MD
Director, Cardiothoracic Surgery Research Program, Chief, Cardiothoracic Surgery, National Heart, Lung and Blood Institute, National Institutes of Health, Bethesda, Maryland
Transmyocardial Laser Revascularization and Extravascular Angiogenetic Techniques to Increase Myocardial Blood Flow

Lynn C. Huffman, MD
Thoracic Resident, Cardiac Surgery, University of Michigan, Ann Arbor, Michigan
Nontransplant Surgical Options for Heart Failure

Joseph Huh, MD
Associate Professor of Cardiothoracic Surgery, Baylor College of Medicine, Houston, Texas
Descending and Thoracoabdominal Aortic Aneurysms

John S. Ikonomidis, MD, PhD, FRCS(C)
Horace G. Smithy Professor and Chief, Division of Cardiothoracic Surgery, Medical University of South Carolina, Charleston, South Carolina
Trauma to the Great Vessels

Neil B. Ingels, Jr., PhD
Consulting Professor, Cardiothoracic Surgery, Stanford University Medical Center Stanford, California
Pathophysiology of Mitral Valve Disease

O. Wayne Isom, MD
The Terry Allen Kramer Professor, Cardiothoracic Surgery, New York Presbyterian-Weill Cornell Medical Center, New York, New York
Transfusion Therapy and Blood Conservation

M. Salik Jahania, MD
Associate Professor of Surgery, Department of Surgery, Wayne State University School of Medicine, Detroit, Michigan
Myocardial Protection

Stuart W. Jamieson MD, FRCS
Endowed Chair and Distinguished Professor, Chief of Cardiovascular and Thoracic Surgery, Cardiovascular and Thoracic Surgery, University of California, San Diego, San Diego, California
Pulmonary Embolism and Pulmonary Thromboendarterectomy

Craig M. Jarrett, MD
Clinical Fellow in Surgery, Department of Surgery, Massachusetts General Hospital, Boston, Massachusetts
Pathophysiology of Aortic Valve Disease

Ruyun Jin, MD, MCR
Biostatistician, Medical Data Research Center, Providence Health & Services, Portland, Oregon
Statistical Treatment of Surgical Outcome Data

David L. Joyce, MD
Chief Resident, Cardiothoracic Surgery, Stanford University, Palo Alto, California
Lung Transplantation and Heart-Lung Transplantation

Zain I. Khalpey, MD, PhD, MRCS(Eng)
Cardiothoracic Surgery Fellow, Cardiac Surgery, Brigham and Women's Hospital, Harvard Medical School, Boston, Massachusetts
Postoperative Care of Cardiac Surgery Patients

Edward H. Kincaid, MD
Associate Professor of Cardiothoracic Surgery, Wake Forest University School of Medicine, Winston Salem, North Carolina
Aortic Valve Replacement with a Stentless Bioprosthetic Valve: Porcine or Pericardial

Neal D. Kon, MD
Howard Holt Bradshaw Professor and Chair, Cardiothoracic Surgery, Wake Forest School of Medicine, Winston-Salem, North Carolina
Aortic Valve Replacement with a Stentless Bioprosthetic Valve: Porcine or Pericardial

Karl H. Krieger, MD
Professor and Vice Chairman Philip Geier Professor of Cardiothoracic Surgery, CT Surgery, New York Presbyterian Hospital Cornell, New York, New York
Transfusion Therapy and Blood Conservation

Irving L. Kron, MD
S. Hurt Watts Professor and Chairman, Department of Surgery, University of Virginia Health System, Charlottesville, Virginia
Aortic Dissection

Jeremy D. Kukafka, MD
Assistant Professor, Anesthesiology and Critical Care, University of Pennsylvania School of Medicine, Philadelphia, Pennsylvania
Cardiac Anesthesia

Kanako K. Kumamaru, MD
Research Fellow, Radiology, Brigham and Women's Hospital, Boston, Massachusetts
Computed Tomography of the Adult Cardiac Surgery Patient: Principles and Applications

Leonard Y. Lee, MD
Associate Professor of Clinical Cardiothoracic Surgery, Department of Cardiothoracic Surgery, Weill Cornell Medical College of Cornell University, New York, New York
Transfusion Therapy and Blood Conservation

Eric J. Lehr, MD, PhD
Co-Director of Minimally Invasive and Robotic Cardiac Surgery, Director of Cardiac Surgery Research and Education, Swedish Medical Center, Seattle, Washington
Minimally Invasive and Robotic Mitral Valve Surgery

Scott A. LeMaire, MD
Professor and Director of Research, Division of Cardiothoracic Surgery, Michael E. DeBakey Department of Surgery, Baylor College of Medicine; Texas Heart Institute at St. Luke's Episcopal Hospital, Houston, Texas
Descending and Thoracoabdominal Aortic Aneurysms

Jerrold H. Levy, MD
Professor of Anesthesiology, Deputy Chair for Research, Co-Director Cardiothoracic Anesthesiology, Cardiothoracic Anesthesiology and Critical Care, Emory University School of Medicine, Atlanta, Georgia
Cardiac Surgical Pharmacology

James E. Lowe, MD
Professor of Surgery, Division of Cardiovascular and Thoracic Surgery, Duke University School of Medicine, Durham, North Carolina
Cardiopulmonary Resuscitation; Left Ventricular Aneurysm

Bruce W. Lytle, MD
Professor of Surgery, Department of Thoracic and Cardiovascular Surgery, Heart and Vascular Institute, Cleveland Clinic, Cleveland, Ohio
Coronary Artery Reoperations

Michael J. Mack, MD
Medical Director, Cardiovascular Surgery, Baylor Health Care System, Dallas, Texas
Percutaneous Catheter-Based Mitral Valve Repair

Michael M. Madani, MD
Professor of Cardiovascular and Thoracic Surgery, University of California–San Diego, San Diego, California
Pulmonary Embolism and Pulmonary Thromboendarterectomy

Joren C. Madsen, MD, DPhil
Professor of Surgery, Massachusetts General Hospital, Boston, Massachusetts
Surgical Treatment of Complications of Acute Myocardial Infarction

Hari R. Mallidi, MD
Assistant Professor, Department of Cardiothoracic Surgery, Stanford University, Stanford, California
Lung Transplantation and Heart-Lung Transplantation

Manu N. Mathur, MD
Consultant, Cardiothoracic Surgeon, Cardiothoracic Surgery, Royal North Shore Hospital, Sydney, Australia
Aneurysms of the Aortic Arch

John E. Mayer, Jr., MD
Professor of Surgery, Harvard Medical School, Boston, Massachusetts
Tissue Engineering for Cardiac Valve Surgery

Edwin C. McGee, Jr., MD
Associate Professor of Surgery, Northwestern University's Feinberg School of Medicine, Chicago, Illinois
Temporary Mechanical Circulatory Support

Spencer J. Melby, MD
Assistant Professor, Division of Cardiothoracic Surgery, University of Alabama at Birmingham, Birmingham, Alabama
Surgery for Atrial Fibrillation

Philippe Menasché, MD, PhD
Assistance Publique-Hôpitaux de Paris, Hôpital Européen Georges Pompidou, Department of Cardiovascular Surgery, Université Paris Descartes, Paris, France
Stem Cell–Induced Regeneration of Myocardium

Robert M. Mentzer, Jr., MD
Professor, Cardiothoracic Surgery and Physiology, Wayne State University School of Medicine, Detroit, Michigan
Myocardial Protection

Carlos M. Mery, MD, MPH
Cardiothoracic Surgery Fellow, Division of Thoracic and Cardiovascular Surgery
University of Virginia, Charlottesville, Virginia
Aortic Dissection

Hector I. Michelena, MD
Assistant Professor, Division of Cardiovascular Diseases, Mayo Clinic, Rochester, Minnesota
Echocardiography in Cardiac Surgery

Tomislav Mihaljevic, MD
Chief of Staff, Chair of Heart and Vascular Institute, Cleveland Clinic Abu Dhabi, United Arab Emirates
Pathophysiology of Aortic Valve Disease

Michael R. Mill, MD
Professor and Chief, Cardiothoracic Surgery, University of North Carolina at Chapel Hill, Chapel Hill, North Carolina
Surgical Anatomy of the Heart

D. Craig Miller, MD
Thelma and Henry Doelger Professor, Cardiovascular Surgery, Stanford University Medical Center, Stanford, California
Pathophysiology of Mitral Valve Disease

R. Scott Mitchell, MD
Professor, Cardiothoracic Surgery, Stanford University School of Medicine, Stanford, California
Endovascular Therapy for the Treatment of Thoracic Aortic Disease

Nader Moazami, MD
Attending Surgeon, Cardiothoracic Surgery, Minneapolis Heart Institute, Minneapolis, Minnesota
Temporary Mechanical Circulatory Support

Susan D. Moffatt-Bruce, MD, PhD
Associate Professor, Surgery, Ohio State University, Columbus, Ohio
Endovascular Therapy for the Treatment of Thoracic Aortic Disease

Friedrich W. Mohr, MD, PhD
Professor and Chief of the Department of Cardiac Surgery and Medical Director of the Heart Center Leipzig, Department of Cardiac Surgery, Heart Center Leipzig, University of Leipzig, Leipzig, Germany
Minimally Invasive Myocardial Revascularization

Yoshifumi Naka, MD, PhD
Associate Professor of Surgery, Columbia University College of Physicians and Surgeons, New York, New York
Long-term Mechanical Circulatory Support

Vuyisile T. Nkomo, MD, MPH
Assistant Professor, Cardiovascular Diseases and Internal Medicine, Mayo Clinic, Rochester, Minnesota
Echocardiography in Cardiac Surgery

Robert A. Oakes, MD
Resident, Department of Surgery, Division of Cardiac Surgery, Brigham and Women's Hospital, Boston, Massachusetts
Deep Hypothermic Circulatory Arrest

Patrick T. O'Gara, MD
Professor, Medicine, Harvard Medical School, Boston, Massachusetts
Preoperative Evaluation for Cardiac Surgery

Robert F. Padera, Jr. MD, PhD
Assistant Professor, Pathology, Harvard Medical School, Boston, Massachusetts
Cardiovascular Pathology

Steven M. Parnis, BS
Assistant Director, Center for Cardiac Support, Cardiovascular Sugery Research
Texas Heart Institute, Houston, Texas
Total Artificial Heart

Gosta B. Pettersson, MD, PhD
Vice Chair, Department of Thoracic and Cardiovascular Surgery, Cleveland Clinic, Cleveland, Ohio
Surgical Treatment of Mitral Valve Endocarditis

Karin Przyklenk, PhD
Director and Professor, Cardiovascular Research Institute, Wayne State University School of Medicine, Detroit, Michigan
Myocardial Protection

John D. Puskas, MD
Chief Cardiac Surgery, Associate Chief Cardiothoracic Surgery, Cardiothoracic Surgery Emory University Midtown, Atlanta, Georgia
Myocardial Revascularization without Cardiopulmonary Bypass

Goya Raikar, MD
Medical Director Oklahoma Heart Hospital, Cardiovascular Surgery, Oklahoma Heart Physicians, Oklahoma City, Oklahoma
Aortic Valve Replacement with a Mechanical Cardiac Valve Prosthesis

James G. Ramsay, MD
Professor, Chief of Service, Anesthesiology/Critical Care, Emory University, Atlanta, Georgia
Cardiac Surgical Pharmacology

Ardawan J Rastan, MD, PhD
Associate Professor, Department of Cardiac Surgery, University of Leipzig, Leipzig, Germany
Minimally Invasive Myocardial Revascularization

James D. Rawn, MD
Director, Cardiac Surgery Intensive Care Unit, Brigham and Women's Hospital, Boston, Massachusetts
Postoperative Care of Cardiac Surgery Patients

Michael J. Reardon, MD
Professor, Cardiovascular Surgery, The Methodist Hospital, Houston, Texas
Cardiac Neoplasms

T. Brett Reece, MD
Assistant Professor, Department of Surgery, Division of Cardiothoracic Surgery, University of Colorado, Aurora, Colorado
Aortic Dissection

Robert C. Robbins, MD
Professor, Cardiothoracic Surgery–Adult Cardiac Surgery, Chair, Department of Cardiothoracic Surgery , Director, Stanford Cardiovascular Institute, Stanford University School of Medicine, Stanford, California
Lung Transplantation and Heart-Lung Transplantation

Evelio Rodriguez, MD
Associate Professor, Cardiovascular Sciences and Pediatrics, East Carolina Heart Institute at East Carolina University, Greenville, North Carolina
Minimally Invasive and Robotic Mitral Valve Surgery

Jean Marie Ruddy, MD
Resident, Department of General Surgery, Medical University of South Carolina, Charleston, South Carolina
Trauma to the Great Vessels

Christian T. Ruff, MD, MPH
Instructor of Medicine, Associate Physician, Cardiovascular Division, Department of Medicine, Harvard Medical School and Brigham and Women's Hospital, Boston, Massachusetts
Preoperative Evaluation for Cardiac Surgery

Frank J. Rybicki, MD, PhD
Director, Applied Imaging Science Lab and Associate Professor, Department of Radiology, Brigham and Women's Hospital and Harvard Medical School, Boston, Massachusetts
Computed Tomography of the Adult Cardiac Surgery Patient: Principles and Applications

Edward B. Savage, MD
Clinical Associate Professor of Surgery, Florida International University, Miami, Florida
Cardiac Surgical Physiology

Joseph E. Savino, MD
Professor of Anesthesiology and Critical Care, Department of Anesthesiology and Critical Care, University of Pennsylvania School of Medicine, Philadelphia, Pennsylvania
Cardiac Anesthesia

Hartzell V. Schaff, MD
Stuart W. Harrington Professor of Surgery, Department of Surgery, Mayo Clinic, Rochester, Minnesota
Multiple Valve Disease

Jan D. Schmitto, MD, PhD
Cardiothoracic Surgeon, Department of Cardiac, Thoracic, Transplantation and Vascular Surgery, Hannover Medical School, Hannover, Germany
Postoperative Care of Cardiac Surgery Patients

Frederick J. Schoen, MD, PhD
Professor of Pathology and Health Sciences and Technology, Harvard Medical School, Executive Vice Chairman, Department of Pathology, Brigham and Women's Hospital, Director, Cardiac Pathology, Brigham and Women's Hospital, Boston, Massachusetts
Cardiovascular Pathology

Ashish S. Shah, MD
Assistant Professor of Surgery, Surgical Director, Lung Transplantation, Johns Hopkins Cardiac Surgery, Baltimore, Maryland
Heart Transplantation

David M. Shahian, MD
Professor of Surgery, Harvard Medical School, Boston, Massachusetts
Assessment of Cardiac Operations to Improve Performance

Ahmad Y. Sheikh, MD
Clinical Fellow, Cardiothoracic Surgery, Stanford University, Stanford, California
Lung Transplantation and Heart-Lung Transplantation

Prem S. Shekar MD, FRCSE
Assistant Professor of Surgery, Harvard Medical School, Boston, Massachusetts
Minimally Invasive Aortic Valve Surgery

Richard J. Shemin, MD
Robert and Kelly Day Chair of Cardiothoracic Surgery, Department of Surgery, David Geffen School of Medicine at UCLA, Los Angeles, California
Tricuspid Valve Disease

Tarang Sheth, MD, FRCPC
Director of Cardiac MR and CT, Diagnostic Imaging, Trillium Health Centre, Mississauga, Ontario, Canada
Computed Tomography of the Adult Cardiac Surgery Patient: Principles and Applications

David Spielvogel, MD
Professor, Department of Surgery, Division of Cardiothoracic Surgery, New York Medical College, Valhalla, New York
Aneurysms of the Aortic Arch

Henry M. Spotnitz, MD
George H. Humphreys, II, Professor of Surgery, Department of Surgery, Columbia University Medical Center, New York, New York
Surgical Implantation of Pacemakers and Automatic Defibrillators

Sotiris C. Stamou, MD, PhD
Assistant Professor of Surgery, Thoracic and Cardiovascular Surgery, Spectrum Health, Grand Rapids, Michigan
Surgical Treatment of Mitral Valve Endocarditis

Paul Stelzer, MD
Professor of Cardiothoracic Surgery, Mount Sinai Medical Center, New York, New York
Stentless Aortic Valve Replacement: Autograft/Homograft

Larry W. Stephenson, MD
Ford Webber Professor of Surgery and Chief, Division of Cardiothoracic Surgery, Wayne State University School of Medicine, Specialist-in-Chief, Cardiothoracic Surgery, Detroit Medical Center, Detroit, Michigan
History of Cardiac Surgery

Thoralf M. Sundt III, MD
Professor, Surgery, Harvard Medical School, Chief of Cardiac Surgery, Massachusetts General Hospital, Boston, Massachusetts
Indications for Revascularization; Myocardial Revascularization with Cardiopulmonary Bypass

Rakesh M. Suri, MD, DPhil
Associate Professor of Cardiovascular Surgery, Mayo Clinic, Rochester, Minnesota
Multiple Valve Disease

Lars G. Svensson, MD, PhD
Director Aorta Center; Marfan and CTD Clinic; Director Quality and Process, Improvement; Professor of Surgery, Department of Thoracic and Cardiovascular Surgery, Cleveland Clinic, Cleveland, Ohio
Percutaneous Treatment of Aortic Valve Disease

Hiroo Takayama, MD
Assistant Professor of Surgery, Columbia University, New York, New York
Long-term Mechanical Circulatory Support

Kenichi A. Tanaka, MD
Associate Professor, Department of Anesthesiology, Emory University, Atlanta, Georgia
Cardiac Surgical Pharmacology

Robin Varghese, MD
Instructor, Cardiothoracic Surgery, Mount Sinai Medical Center, New York, New York
Stentless Aortic Valve Replacement: Autograft/Homograft

William J. Vernick, MD
Assistant Professor, Department of Anesthesia and Critical Care, Hospital of the University of Pennsylvania, Philadelphia, Pennsylvania
Cardiac Anesthesia

Jennifer D. Walker, MD
Assistant Professor of Surgery, Surgery, Harvard Medical School, Boston, Massachusetts
Pericardial Disease

Scott A. Weldon, MA, CMI
Medical Illustration, Division of Cardiothoracic Surgery, Baylor College of Medicine, Houston, Texas
Extent II Thoracoabdominal Aortic Aneurysm Repair (DVD)

James T. Willerson, MD
President and Medical Director, Cardiology, Texas Heart Institute at St. Luke's Episcopal Hospital, Houston, Texas
Myocardial Revascularization with Percutaneous Devices

Mathew Williams, MD
Assistant Professor of Surgery and Medicine, Columbia University, New York, New York
Myocardial Revascularization after Acute Myocardial Infarction

James M. Wilson, MD
Director of Cardiology Education, Texas Heart Institute at St. Luke's Episcopal Hospital, Houston, Texas
Myocardial Revascularization with Percutaneous Devices

Berhane Worku, MD
Research Fellow, Cardiothoracic Surgery, Columbia University, New York, New York
Long-term Mechanical Circulatory Support

Bobby Yanagawa, MD, PhD
Division of Cardiac and Vascular Surgery, Schulich Heart Program, Sunnybrook Health Sciences Centre, Toronto, Ontario, Canada
Bioprosthetic Aortic Valve Replacement: Stented Pericardial and Porcine Valves

Yifu Zhou, MD
Staff Scientist, Cardiothoracic Surgery Research Program, National Heart, Lung and Blood Institute, National Institutes of Health, Bethesda, Maryland
Transmyocardial Laser Revascularization and Extravascular Angiogenetic Techniques to Increase Myocardial Blood Flow

FOREWORD

It is with a great deal of pleasure that I pen this foreword. This volume, first introduced in 1997 with L. Henry Edmunds, Jr., as editor, has evolved through three previous editions to become the must-have resource for adult cardiac surgeons around the world. Dr. Cohn, who was co-editor with Dr. Edmunds on the second edition and the sole editor for the third edition, has done a masterful job of keeping this text at the forefront of surgical thought and technique. I am certain that as this fourth edition reaches its audience, surgeons will agree that it will serve this purpose for many years to come. This is because Dr. Cohn's stated goals are "to publish information as quickly as possible" and "to cover the past, present, and future of cardiac surgery." Both are very worthy objectives.

By all preliminary indications, the fourth edition will carry on this tradition in spades. There are 70 chapters covering every conceivable topic in the field, and the list of authors reads like a *Who's Who* in world cardiac surgery. If you cannot find your topic here, chances are nothing has been written yet. This edition will also continue the innovative feature begun in the third edition of utilizing video clips to supplement the text descriptions of operations and procedures.

Mention should be made of the far-reaching decision some years ago by Dr. Cohn, when he began to bridge the gap between information printed on paper and information presented electronically. He led the initiative and personally helped fund the presentation of the third edition of *Cardiac Surgery in the Adult* as a free resource on CTSNet, making this valuable material available to thousands of surgeons around the world who would otherwise not be able to access the information it contains, and that they sorely need. This was truly a humanitarian act. We thank you, Dr. Cohn.

The pace of the information explosion is mirrored by the fact that the third edition was released in 2007, and the fourth edition will be in readers' hands toward the end of 2011—four short years. This stresses the need for getting new ideas and information out there ASAP, and the chapter contributors, whom I am sure Dr. Cohn gently badgered, his hard-working staff at the Brigham and Women's Hospital, the publishing group at McGraw-Hill, and, certainly most of all, editor Cohn, all deserve our deepest gratitude for another timely volume of up-to-date and factually correct information about this important branch of our specialty.

Enjoy!

Thomas B. Ferguson, MD
Professor Emeritus of Cardiothoracic Surgery
Washington University School of Medicine
St. Louis, Missouri

PREFACE

The fourth edition of *Cardiac Surgery in the Adult* is a collection of the most current knowledge and updated experiences of the world's leading cardiovascular experts treating adults with acquired, congenital, infectious, and traumatic diseases of the heart, including chapters from experts in the perioperative and postoperative management of patients.

Since the third edition, which was published in 2007, there have been many changes in the field of cardiovascular medicine. I believe this fourth edition will be a valuable tool to all in our specialty to help us understand the best treatment options available to our patients and how to master the skills to apply these therapies.

In addition, chapters on techniques long available to us for the treatment of all forms of adult acquired cardiac disease have been updated to re-emphasize the importance of the traditional approaches to heart disease. Video clip demonstrations of complex operative procedures, which we began in the third edition, continue in this edition and have increased in number.

I have dedicated this edition of *Cardiac Surgery in the Adult* to my surgical mentors. In this increasingly complex field of cardiovascular surgery I want to emphasize the importance of mentors in the training of surgical residents, fellows, and younger colleagues. In medical school Dr. Norman Shumway inspired me to be a heart surgeon and taught me how to become one. During my time at the National Heart Institute Dr. Andrew Glenn Morrow, along with his medical cohort Dr. Eugene Braunwald, taught me how to be an academic cardiothoracic surgeon. Dr. J. Englebert Dunphy from the University of California taught me a great deal when I first began my surgical training. And when I arrived at the Brigham and Women's Hospital in Boston I had the good fortune of working under Dr. Francis D. Moore, one of the all-time great academic surgeons. My friend and colleague, Dr. John J. Collins, Jr., gave me my first and only job as a cardiac surgeon, and we worked together for over 30 years to create one of the best cardiac surgery programs in the country. A more recent mentor is Dr. John A. Mannick, an outstanding leader and superb vascular surgeon. All of these men had a huge impact on my career. Without mentors we cannot learn the art and science of cardiovascular medicine to the highest level of excellence.

My thanks go to many individuals who have assisted in many ways to produce this volume. First and foremost, thanks to L. Henry "Hank" Edmunds, MD, for his initial inspiration for the first incarnation of *Cardiac Surgery in the Adult* and his trust in me to carry out his editorial expertise. Thank you to the editorial staff at McGraw-Hill, especially Mr. Brian Belval. A huge amount of gratitude goes to my executive assistant in the Division of Cardiac Surgery at the Brigham and Women's Hospital, Ann Maloney, who has been extremely helpful in the organization of the logistics and the publication minutia that is so important to a successful editorial process. A special thanks to Dr. Thomas Ferguson, a cardiac surgical pioneer and leader who has been president of both of the major American cardiothoracic surgical organizations, for writing an outstanding foreword to this edition.

Most importantly, we thank the chapter authors, who are some of the busiest physicians and surgeons in the world, for devoting their time and energy to produce superb chapters in every area in a timely fashion.

Finally, thanks to my family—Roberta, Leslie, Jennifer, Stephen, Carly, and Rachel—for their support, patience, and love through the production of *Cardiac Surgery in the Adult,* Fourth Edition.

Lawrence H. Cohn, MD
Boston, Massachusetts

PART 1

FUNDAMENTALS

CHAPTER 1

History of Cardiac Surgery

Larry W. Stephenson
Frank A. Baciewicz, Jr.

The development of major surgery was retarded for centuries by a lack of knowledge and technology. Significantly, the general anesthetics ether and chloroform were not developed until the middle of the nineteenth century. These agents made major surgical operations possible, which created an interest in repairing wounds to the heart, leading some investigators in Europe to conduct studies in the animal laboratory on the repair of heart wounds. The first simple operations in humans for heart wounds soon were reported in the medical literature.

HEART WOUNDS

On July 10, 1893, Dr. Daniel Hale Williams (Fig. 1-1), a surgeon from Chicago, successfully operated on a 24-year-old man who had been stabbed in the heart during a fight. The stab wound was slightly to the left of the sternum and dead center over the heart. Initially, the wound was thought to be superficial, but during the night the patient experienced persistent bleeding, pain, and pronounced symptoms of shock. Williams opened the patient's chest and tied off an artery and vein that had been injured inside the chest wall, likely causing the blood loss. Then he noticed a tear in the pericardium and a puncture wound to the heart "about one-tenth of an inch in length."[1]

The wound in the right ventricle was not bleeding, so Williams did not place a stitch through the heart wound. He did, however, stitch closed the hole in the pericardium. Williams reported this case 4 years later.[1] This operation, which is referred to frequently, is probably the first successful surgery involving a documented stab wound to the heart. At the time Williams' surgery was considered bold and daring, and although he did not actually place a stitch through the wound in the heart, his treatment seems to have been appropriate. Under the circumstances, he most likely saved the patient's life.

A few years after Williams' case, a couple of other surgeons actually sutured heart wounds, but the patients did not survive. Dr. Ludwig Rehn (Fig. 1-2), a surgeon in Frankfurt, Germany, performed what many consider the first successful heart operation.[2] On September 7, 1896, a 22-year-old man was stabbed in the heart and collapsed. The police found him pale, covered with cold sweat, and extremely short of breath. His pulse was irregular and his clothes were soaked with blood. By September 9, his condition was worsening, as shown in Dr. Rehn's case notes:

> Pulse weaker, increasing cardiac dullness on percussion, respiration 76, further deterioration during the day, diagnostic tap reveals dark blood. Patient appears moribund. Diagnosis: increasing hemothorax. I decided to operate entering the chest through the left fourth intercostal space, there is massive blood in the pleural cavity. The mammary artery is not injured. There is continuous bleeding from a hole in the pericardium. This opening is enlarged. The heart is exposed. Old blood and clots are emptied. There is a 1.5 cm gaping right ventricular wound. Bleeding is controlled with finger pressure. …
>
> I decided to suture the heart wound. I used a small intestinal needle and silk suture. The suture was tied in diastole. Bleeding diminished remarkably with the third suture, all bleeding was controlled. The pulse improved. The pleural cavity was irrigated. Pleura and pericardium were drained with iodoform gauze. The incision was approximated, heart rate and respiratory rate decreased and pulse improved postoperatively.
>
> … Today the patient is cured. He looks very good. His heart action is regular. I have not allowed him to work physically hard. This proves the feasibility of cardiac suture repair without a doubt! *I hope this will lead to more investigation regarding surgery of the heart. This may save many lives.*

Ten years after Rehn's initial repair, he had accumulated a series of 124 cases with a mortality of only 60%, quite a feat at that time.[3]

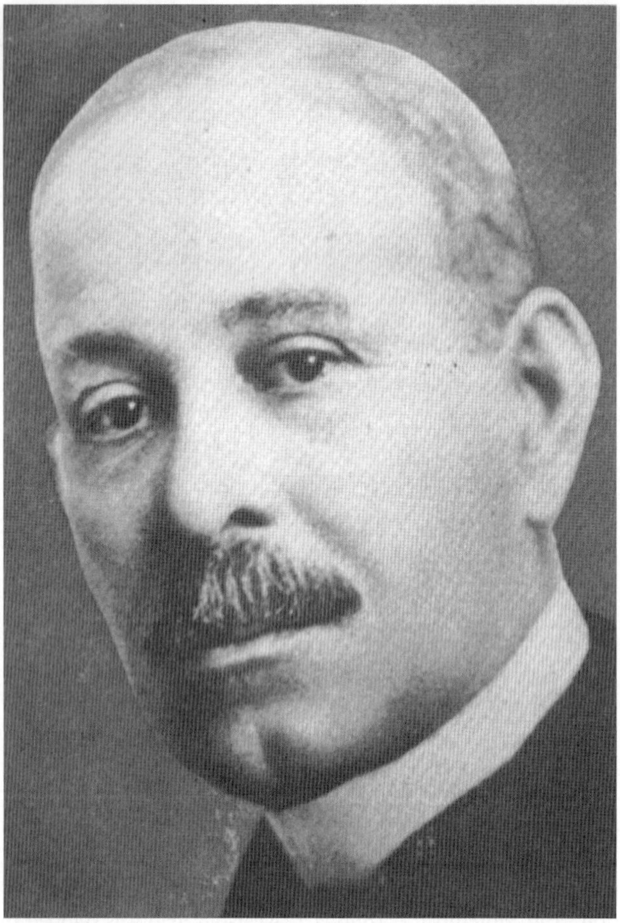

FIGURE 1-1 Daniel Hale Williams, a surgeon from Chicago, who successfully operated on a patient with a wound to the chest involving the pericardium and the heart. (*Reproduced with permission from Organ CH Jr, Kosiba MM: The Century of the Black Surgeons: A USA Experience. Norman, OK: Transcript Press, 1937; p 312*)

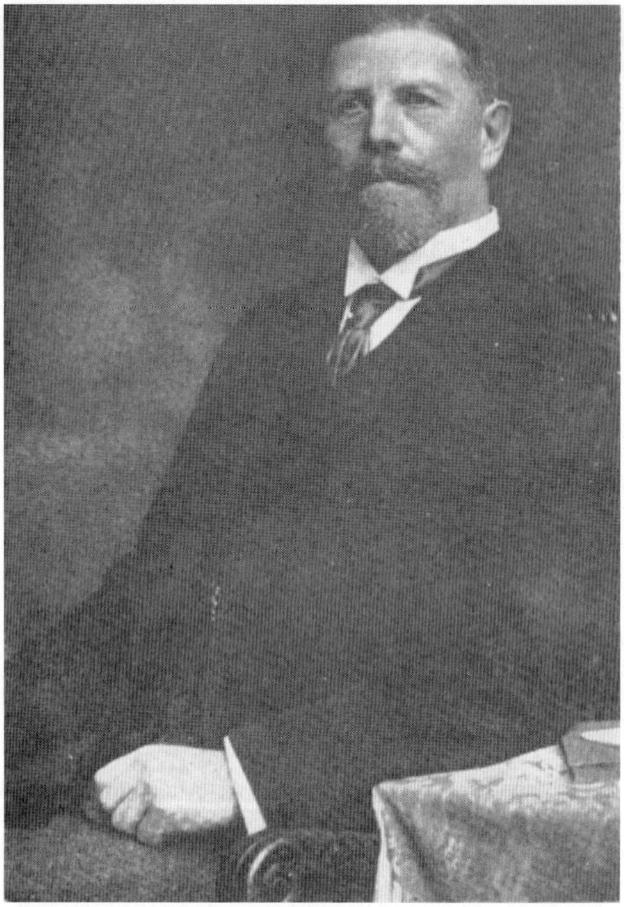

FIGURE 1-2 Ludwig Rehn, a surgeon from Frankfurt, Germany, who performed the first successful suture of a human heart wound. (*Reproduced with permission from Mead R: A History of Thoracic Surgery. Springfield, Charles C Thomas, 1961; p 887*)

Dr. Luther Hill was the first American to report the successful repair of a cardiac wound, in a 13-year-old boy who was a victim of multiple stab wounds.[4] When the first doctor arrived, the boy was in profound shock. The doctor remembered that Dr. Luther Hill had spoken on the subject of repair of cardiac wounds at a local medical society meeting in Montgomery, Alabama. With the consent of the boy's parents, Dr. Hill was summoned. He arrived sometime after midnight with six other physicians. One was his brother. The surgery took place on the patient's kitchen table in a rundown shack. Lighting was provided by two kerosene lamps borrowed from neighbors. One physician administered chloroform anesthesia. The boy was suffering from cardiac tamponade as a result of a stab wound to the left ventricle. The stab wound to the ventricle was repaired with two catgut sutures. Although the early postoperative course was stormy, the boy made a complete recovery. That patient, Henry Myrick, eventually moved to Chicago, where, in 1942, at the age of 53, he got into a heated argument and was stabbed in the heart again, very close to the original stab wound. This time, Henry was not as lucky and died from the wound.

Another milestone in cardiac surgery for trauma occurred during World War II when Dwight Harken, then a U.S. Army surgeon, removed 134 missiles from the mediastinum, including 55 from the pericardium and 13 from cardiac chambers, without a death.[5] It is hard to imagine this type of elective (and semielective) surgery taking place without sophisticated indwelling pulmonary artery catheters, blood banks, and electronic monitoring equipment. Rapid blood infusion consisted of pumping air into glass bottles of blood.

OPERATIVE MANAGEMENT OF PULMONARY EMBOLI

Martin Kirschner reported the first patient who recovered fully after undergoing pulmonary embolectomy in 1924.[6] In 1937, John Gibbon estimated that nine of 142 patients who had undergone the procedure worldwide left the hospital alive.[7] These dismal results were a stimulus for Gibbon to start work on a pump oxygenator that could maintain the circulation during pulmonary embolectomy. Sharp was the first to perform pulmonary embolectomy using cardiopulmonary bypass, in 1962.[8]

SURGERY OF THE PERICARDIUM

Pericardial resection was introduced independently by Rehn[9] and Sauerbruch.[10] Since Rehn's report, there have been few advances in the surgical treatment of constrictive pericarditis. Some operations are now performed with the aid of cardiopulmonary bypass. In certain situations, radical pericardiectomy that removes most of the pericardium posterior to the phrenic nerves is done.

CATHETERIZATION OF THE RIGHT SIDE OF THE HEART

Although cardiac catheterization is not considered heart surgery, it is an invasive procedure, and some catheter procedures have replaced heart operations. Werner Forssmann is credited with the first heart catheterization. He performed the procedure on himself and reported it in *Klrinische Wochenschrift*.[11] In 1956 Forssmann shared the Nobel Prize in Physiology or Medicine with Andre F. Cournand and Dickenson W. Richards, Jr. His 1929 paper states, "One often hesitates to use intercardiac injections promptly, and often, time is wasted with other measures. This is why I kept looking for a different, safer access to the cardiac chambers: the catheterization of the right heart via the venous system."

In this report by Forssmann, a photograph of the x-ray taken of Forssmann with the catheter in his own heart is presented. Forssmann, in that same report, goes on to present the first clinical application of the central venous catheter for a patient in shock with generalized peritonitis. Forssmann concludes his paper by stating, "I also want to mention that this method allows new options for metabolic studies and studies about cardiac physiology."

In a 1951 lecture Forssmann discussed the tremendous resistance he faced during his initial experiments.[12] "Such methods are good for a circus, but not for a respected hospital" was the answer to his request to pursue physiologic studies using cardiac catheterization. His progressive ideas pushed him into the position of an outsider with ideas too crazy to give him a clinical position. Klein applied cardiac catheterization for cardiac output determinations using the Fick method a half year after Forssmann's first report.[13] In 1930, Forssmann described his experiments with catheter cardiac angiography.[14] Further use of this new methodology had to wait until Cournand's work in the 1940s.

HEART VALVE SURGERY BEFORE THE ERA OF CARDIOPULMONARY BYPASS

The first clinical attempt to open a stenotic valve was carried out by Theodore Tuffier on July 13, 1912.[15] Tuffier used his finger to reach the stenotic aortic valve. He was able to dilate the valve supposedly by pushing the invaginated aortic wall through the stenotic valve. The patient recovered, but one must be skeptical as to what was accomplished. Russell Brock attempted to dilate calcified aortic valves in humans in the late 1940s by passing an instrument through the valve from the innominate or another artery.[16] His results were poor, and he abandoned the approach. During the next several years, Brock[17] and Bailey and colleagues[18] used different dilators and various approaches to dilate stenotic aortic valves in patients. Mortality for these procedures, which was often done in conjunction with mitral commissurotomy, was high.

Elliott Cutler worked for 2 years on a mitral valvulotomy procedure in the laboratory. His first patient underwent successful valvulotomy on May 20, 1923, using a tetrasomy knife.[19] Unfortunately, most of Cutler's subsequent patients died because he created too much regurgitation with his valvulotome, and he soon gave up the operation.

In Charles Bailey's 1949 paper entitled, "The Surgical Treatment of Mitral Stenosis," he states, "After 1929 no more surgical attempts [on mitral stenosis] were made until 1945. Dr. Dwight Harken, Dr. Horace Smithy, and the author recently made operative attempts to improve mitral stenosis. Our clinical experience with the surgery of the mitral valves has been five cases to date." He then describes his five patients, four of whom died and only one of whom lived a long life.[20]

A few days after Bailey's success, on June 16 in Boston, Dr. Dwight Harken successfully performed his first valvulotomy for mitral stenosis.[21]

The first successful pulmonary valvulotomy was performed by Thomas Holmes Sellers on December 4, 1947.[22]

Charles Hufnagel reported a series of 23 patients starting September 1952 who had this operation for aortic insufficiency.[23] There were four deaths among the first 10 patients and two deaths among the next 13. Hufnagel's caged-ball valve, which used multiple-point fixation rings to secure the apparatus to the descending aorta, was the only surgical treatment for aortic valvular incompetence until the advent of cardiopulmonary bypass and the development of heart valves that could be sewn into the aortic annulus position.

CONGENITAL CARDIAC SURGERY BEFORE THE HEART-LUNG MACHINE ERA

Congenital cardiac surgery began when John Streider at Massachusetts General Hospital first successfully interrupted a ductus on March 6, 1937. The patient was septic and died on the fourth postoperative day. At autopsy, vegetations filled the pulmonary artery down to the valve.[24] On August 16, 1938, Robert Gross, at Boston Children's Hospital, operated on a 7-year-old girl with dyspnea after moderate exercise.[25] The ductus was ligated and the patient made an uneventful recovery.

Modifications of the ductus operation soon followed. In 1944, Dr. Gross reported a technique for dividing the ductus successfully. The next major congenital lesion to be overcome was coarctation of the aorta. Dr. Clarence Crafoord, in Stockholm, Sweden, successfully resected a coarctation of the aorta in a 12-year-old boy on October 19, 1944.[26] Twelve days later he successfully resected the coarctation of a 27-year-old patient. Dr. Gross first operated on a 5-year-old boy with this condition on June 28, 1945.[27] After he excised the coarctation and rejoined the aorta, the patient's heart stopped suddenly. The patient died in the operating room. One week later, however, Dr. Gross operated on a second patient, a 12-year-old girl. This patient's operation was successful. Dr. Gross had been unaware of Dr. Crafoord's successful surgery several months previously, probably because of World War II.

In 1945, Dr. Gross reported the first successful case of surgical relief for tracheal obstruction from a vascular ring.[28] In the 5 years that followed Gross's first successful operation, he reported 40 more cases.

The famous Blalock-Taussig operation also was first reported in 1945. The first patient was a 15-month-old girl with a clinical diagnosis of tetralogy of Fallot with a severe pulmonary stenosis.[29] At age 8 months, the baby had her first cyanotic spell, which occurred after eating. Dr. Helen Taussig, the cardiologist, followed the child for 3 months, and during that time, cyanosis increased, and the child failed to gain weight. The operation was performed by Dr. Alfred Blalock at Johns Hopkins University on November 29, 1944. The left subclavian artery was anastomosed to the left pulmonary artery in an end-to-side fashion. The postoperative course was described as stormy; the patient was discharged 2 months postoperatively. Two additional successful cases were done within 3 months of that first patient.

Thus, within a 7-year period, three congenital cardiovascular defects, patent ductus arteriosus, coarctation of the aorta, and vascular ring, were attacked surgically and treated successfully. However, the introduction of the Blalock-Taussig shunt probably was the most powerful stimulus to the development of cardiac surgery because this operation palliated a complex intracardiac lesion and focused attention on the pathophysiology of cardiac disease.

Anomalous coronary artery in which the left coronary artery communicates with the pulmonary artery was the next surgical conquest. The surgery was performed on July 22, 1946, and was reported by Gunnar Biorck and Clarence Crafoord.[30] The anomalous coronary artery was identified and doubly ligated. The patient made an uneventful recovery.

Muller[31] reported successful surgical treatment of transposition of the pulmonary veins in 1951, but the operation addressed a partial form of the anomaly. Later in the 1950s, Gott, Varco, Lillehei, and Cooley reported successful operative variations for anomalous pulmonary veins.

Another of Gross's pioneering surgical procedures was surgical closure of an aortopulmonary window on May 22, 1948.[32] Cooley and colleagues[33] were the first to report on the use of cardiopulmonary bypass to repair this defect and converted a difficult and hazardous procedure into a relatively straightforward one.

Glenn[34] reported the first successful clinical application of the cavopulmonary anastomosis in the United States in 1958 for what has been termed the *Glenn shunt.* Similar work was done in Russia during the 1950s by several investigators. On January 3, 1957, Galankin,[35] a Russian surgeon, performed a cavopulmonary anastomosis in a 16-year-old patient with tetralogy of Fallot. The patient made a good recovery with significant improvement in exercise tolerance and cyanosis.

THE DEVELOPMENT OF CARDIOPULMONARY BYPASS

The development of the heart-lung machine made repair of intracardiac lesions possible. To bypass the heart, one needs a basic understanding of the physiology of the circulation, a method of preventing the blood from clotting, a mechanism to pump blood, and finally, a method to ventilate the blood.

One of the key requirements of the heart-lung machine was anticoagulation. Heparin was discovered in 1915 by a medical student, Jay McLean, working in the laboratory of Dr. William Howell, a physiologist at Johns Hopkins.[36]

John Gibbon contributed more to the success of the development of the heart-lung machine than anyone else.

Gibbon's work on the heart-lung machine took place over the next 20 years in laboratories at Massachusetts General Hospital, the University of Pennsylvania, and Thomas Jefferson University. In 1937, Gibbon reported the first successful demonstration that life could be maintained by an artificial heart and lung and that the native heart and lungs could resume function. Unfortunately, only three animals recovered adequate cardiorespiratory function after total pulmonary artery occlusion and bypass, and even they died a few hours later.[37] Gibbon's work was interrupted by World War II; afterward, he resumed his work at Thomas Jefferson Medical College in Philadelphia (Table 1-1).

Forest Dodrill and colleagues used the mechanical blood pump they developed with General Motors on a 41-year-old man[42] (Fig. 1-3). The machine was used to substitute for the left ventricle for 50 minutes while a surgical procedure was carried out to repair the mitral valve; the patient's own lungs were used to oxygenate the blood. This, the first clinically successful total left-sided heart bypass in a human, was performed on July 3, 1952, and followed from Dodrill's experimental work with a mechanical pump for univentricular, biventricular, or cardiopulmonary bypass. Although Dodrill and colleagues had used their pump with an oxygenator for total heart bypass in animals,[53] they felt that left-sided heart bypass was the most practical method for their first clinical case.

Later, on October 21, 1952, Dodrill and colleagues used their machine in a 16-year-old boy with congenital pulmonary stenosis to perform a pulmonary valvuloplasty under direct vision; this was the first successful right-sided heart bypass.[44] Between July 1952 and December 1954, Dodrill performed approximately 13 clinical operations on the heart and thoracic aorta using the Dodrill–General Motors machine, with at least five hospital survivors.[54] Although he used this machine with an oxygenator in the animal laboratory, he did not start using an oxygenator with the Dodrill–General Motors mechanical heart clinically until early 1955.

Hypothermia was another method to stop the heart and allow it to be opened.[91–93]

John Lewis closed an atrial septal defect in a 5-year-old girl on September 2, 1952 using a hypothermic technique.[43]

However, the use of systemic hypothermia for open intracardiac surgery was relatively short lived; after the heart-lung machine was introduced clinically, it appeared that deep hypothermia was obsolete. However, during the 1960s it became apparent that operative results in infants under 1 year of age using cardiopulmonary bypass were poor. In 1967, Hikasa and colleagues,[55] from Kyoto, Japan, published an article that reintroduced profound hypothermia for cardiac surgery in infants and used the heart-lung machine for rewarming. Their technique involved surface cooling to 20°C, cardiac surgery during

TABLE 1-1 Twilight Zone: Clinical Status of Open-Heart Surgery, 1951–1955

1951	*April 6:* Clarence Dennis at the University of Minnesota used a heart-lung machine to repair an ostium primum or AV canal defect in a 5-year-old girl. Patient could not be weaned from cardiopulmonary bypass.[38] *May 31:* Dennis attempted to close an atrial septal defect using heart-lung machine in a 2-year-old girl who died intraoperatively of a massive air embolus.[39]
1951	*August 7:* Achille Mario Digliotti at the University of Turino, Italy, used a heart-lung machine of his own design to partially support the circulation (flow at 1 L/min for 20 minutes) while he resected a large mediastinal tumor compressing the right side of the heart.[40] The cannulation was through the right axillary vein and artery. The patient survived. This was the first successful clinical use of a heart-lung machine, but the machine was not used as an adjunct to heart surgery.
1952	*February* (1952 or 1953 John Gibbon; see February 1953) *March:* John Gibbon used his heart-lung machine for right-sided heart bypass only while surgeon Frank Allbritten at Pennsylvania Hospital, Philadelphia, operated to remove a large clot or myxomatous tumor suspected by angiography.[41] No tumor or clot was found. The patient died of heart failure in the operating room shortly after discontinuing right-sided heart bypass.
1952	*July 3:* Dodrill used the Dodrill-GMR pump to bypass the left side of the heart while he repaired a mitral valve.[42] The patient survived. This was the first successful use of a mechanical pump for total substitution of the left ventricle in a human being. *September 2:* John Lewis, at the University of Minnesota, closed an atrial septal defect under direct vision in a 5-year-old girl. The patient survived. This was the first successful clinical heart surgery procedure using total-body hypothermia. A mechanical pump and oxygenator were not used. Others, including Dodrill, soon followed, using total-body hypothermia techniques to close atrial septal defects (ASDs) and perform pulmonary valvulotomies. By 1954, Lewis reported on 11 ASD closures using hypothermia with two hospital deaths.[43] He also operated on two patients with ventricular septal defect (VSD) in early 1954 using this technique. Both resulted in intraoperative deaths. *October 21:* Dodrill performed pulmonary valvulotomy under direct vision using Dodrill-GMR pump to bypass the right atrium, ventricle, and main pulmonary artery.[44] The patient survived. Although Dr. William Mustard in Toronto would describe a type of "corrective" surgical procedure for transposition of the great arteries (TGA) in 1964, which, in fact, for many years, would become the most popular form of surgical correction of TGA, his early results with this lesion were not good. In 1952 he used a mechanical pump coupled to the lung that had just been removed from a monkey to oxygenate the blood in seven children while attempts were made to correct their TGA defect.[45] There were no survivors.
1953	*February* (or 1952): Gibbon at Jefferson Hospital in Philadelphia operated to close an ASD. No ASD was found. The patient died intraoperatively. Autopsy showed a large patent ductus arteriosus.[46] *May 6:* Gibbon used his heart-lung machine to close an ASD in an 18-year-old woman with symptoms of heart failure.[46] The patient survived the operation and became the first patient to undergo successful open-heart surgery using a heart-lung machine. *July:* Gibbon used the heart-lung machine on two 5-year-old girls to close atrial septal defects.[46] Both died intraoperatively. Gibbon was extremely distressed and declared a moratorium on further cardiac surgery at Jefferson Medical School until more work could be done to solve problems related to heart-lung bypass. These were probably the last heart operation he performed using the heart-lung machine.
1954	*March 26:* C. Walton Lillehei and associates at the University of Minnesota closed a VSD under direct vision in a 15-month-old boy using a technique to support the circulation that they called *controlled cross-circulation.* An adult (usually a parent) with the same blood type was used more or less as the heart-lung machine. The adult's femoral artery and vein were connected with tubing and a pump to the patient's circulation. The adult's heart and lungs oxygenated and supported the circulation while the child's heart defect was corrected. The first patient died 11 days postoperatively from pneumonia, but six of their next seven patients survived.[47] Between March 1954 and the end of 1955, 45 heart operations were performed by Lillehei on children using this technique before it was phased out. Although controlled cross-circulation was a short-lived technique, it was an important stepping stone in the development of open-heart surgery. *July:* Clarence Crafoord and associates at the Karolinska Institute in Stockholm, Sweden, used a heart-lung machine of their own design coupled with total-body hypothermia (patient was initially submerged in an ice-water bath) to remove a large atrial myxoma in a 40-year-old woman.[48] She survived.

(*Continued*)

TABLE 1-1 Twilight Zone: Clinical Status of Open-Heart Surgery, 1951–1955 (*Continued*)

1955	*March 22:* John Kirklin at the Mayo Clinic used a heart-lung machine similar to Gibbon's, but with modifications his team had worked out over 2 years in the research laboratory, to successfully close a VSD in a 5-year-old patient. By May of 1955, they had operated on eight children with various types of VSDs, and four were hospital survivors. This was the first successful series of patients (ie, more than one) to undergo heart surgery using a heart-lung machine.[49]
	May 13: Lillehei and colleagues began using a heart-lung machine of their own design to correct intracardiac defects. By May of 1956, their series included 80 patients.[47] Initially they used their heart-lung machine for lower-risk patients and used controlled cross-circulation, with which they were more familiar, for the higher-risk patients. Starting in March 1955, they also tried other techniques in patients to oxygenate blood during heart surgery, such as canine lung, but with generally poor results.[47]
	Dodrill had been performing heart operations with the GM heart pump since 1952 and used the patient's own lungs to oxygenate the blood. Early in the year 1955, he attempted repairs of VSDs in two patients using the heart pump, but with a mechanical oxygenator of his team's design both died. On December 1, he closed a VSD in a 3-year-old girl using his heart-lung machine. She survived. In May 1956 at the annual meeting of the American Association for Thoracic Surgery, he reported on six children with VSDs, including one with tetralogy of Fallot, who had undergone open-heart surgery using his heart-lung machine. All survived at least 48 hours postoperatively.[50] Three were hospital survivors, including the patient with tetralogy of Fallot.
	June 30: Clarence Dennis, who had moved from the University of Minnesota to the State University of New York, successfully closed an ASD in a girl using a heart-lung machine of his own design.[51] Mustard successfully repaired a VSD and dilated the pulmonary valve in a 9-month-old with a diagnosis of tetralogy of Fallot using a mechanical pump and a monkey lung to oxygenate the blood.[52] He did not give the date in 1955, but the patient is listed as Human Case 7. Unfortunately, in the same report, cases 1–6 and 8–15 operated on between 1951 and the end of 1955 with various congenital heart defects did not survive the surgery using the pump and monkey lung, nor did another seven children in 1952, all with TGA (see timeline for 1952) using the same bypass technique.

Note: This list is not all-inclusive but likely includes most of the historically significant clinical open-heart events in which a blood pump was used to support the circulation during this period. (A twilight zone can mean an ill-defined area between two distinct conditions, such as the area between darkness and light.)

circulatory arrest for 15 to 75 minutes, and rewarming with cardiopulmonary bypass. At the same time, other groups reported using profound hypothermia with circulatory arrest in infants with the heart-lung machine for cooling and rewarming. Results were much improved, and subsequently the technique also was applied for resection of aortic arch aneurysms.

After World War II, John Gibbon resumed his research. He eventually met Thomas Watson, chairman of the board of the International Business Machines (IBM) Corporation. Watson was fascinated by Gibbon's research and promised help. Soon afterward, six IBM engineers arrived and built a machine that was similar to Gibbon's earlier machine, which contained a rotating vertical cylinder oxygenator and a modified DeBakey rotary pump. Gibbon operated on a 15-month-old girl with severe congestive heart failure (CHF). The preoperative diagnosis was atrial septal defect (ASD), but at operation, none was found. She died, and a huge patent ductus was found at autopsy. The next patient was an 18-year-old girl with CHF owing to an ASD. This defect was closed successfully on May 6, 1953, with the Gibbon-IBM heart-lung machine. The patient recovered, and several months later the defect was confirmed closed at cardiac catheterization.[56] Unfortunately, Gibbon's next two patients did not survive intracardiac procedures when the heart-lung machine was used. These failures distressed Dr. Gibbon, who declared a 1-year moratorium for the heart-lung machine until more work could be done to solve the problems causing the deaths.

During this period, C. Walton Lillehei and colleagues at the University of Minnesota studied a technique called *controlled cross-circulation*.[57] With this technique, the circulation of one dog was used temporarily to support that of a second dog while the second dog's heart was stopped temporarily and opened. After a simulated repair in the second dog, the animals were disconnected and allowed to recover.

Lillehei and colleagues[57] used their technique at the University of Minnesota to correct a VSD in a 12-month-old infant on March 26, 1954 (Fig. 1-4). Either a parent or a close relative with the same blood type was connected to the child's circulation. In Lillehei's first clinical case, the patient made an uneventful recovery until death on the eleventh postoperative day from a rapidly progressing tracheal bronchitis. At autopsy, the VSD was closed, and the respiratory infection was confirmed as the cause of death. Two weeks later, the second and third patients had VSDs closed by the same technique 3 days

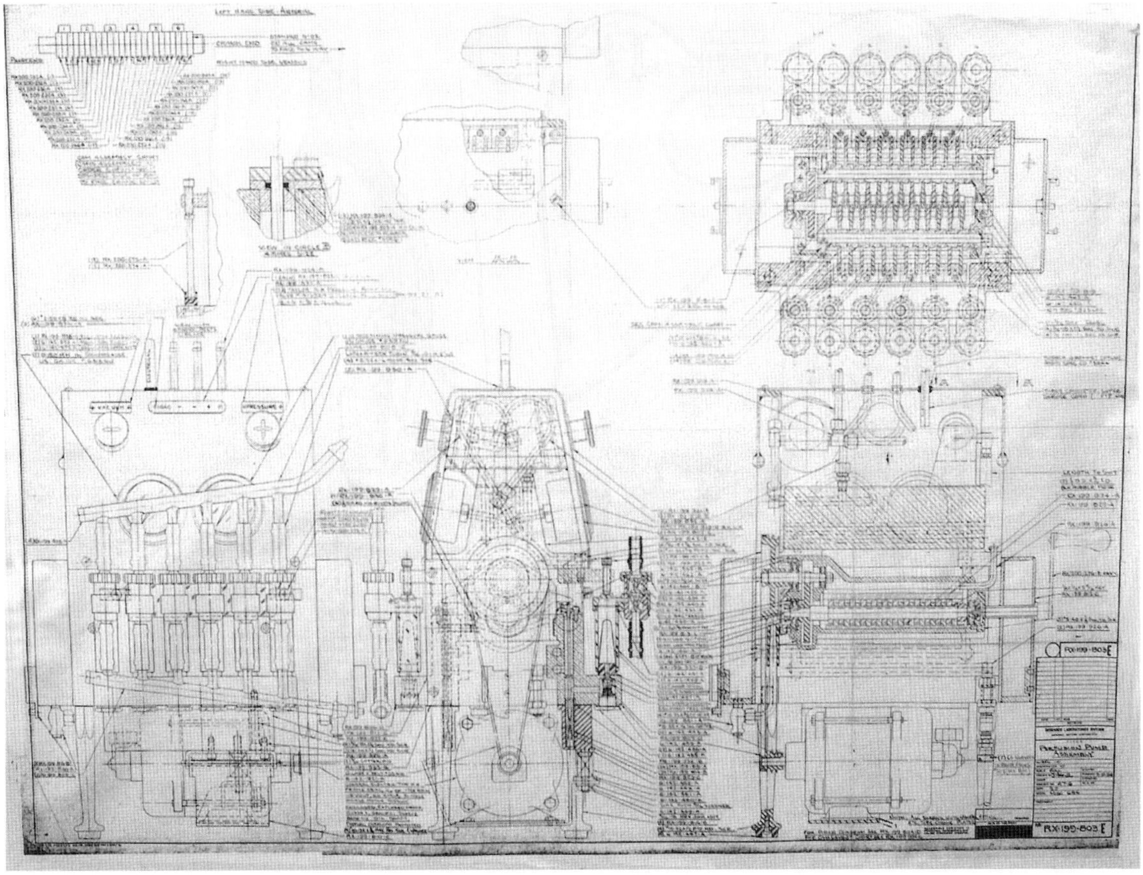

FIGURE 1-3 Blueprints by General Motors engineers of the Dodrill-GMR mechanical heart. (*Courtesy of Calvin Hughes.*)

apart. Both remained long-term survivors with normal hemodynamics confirmed by cardiac catheterization.

In 1955, Lillehei and colleagues[58] published a report of 32 patients that included repairs of VSDs, tetralogy of Fallot, and atrioventricularis communis defects. By May of 1955, the blood pump used for systemic cross-circulation by Lillehei and colleagues was coupled with a bubble oxygenator developed by Drs. DeWall and Lillehei, and cross-circulation was soon abandoned after use in 45 patients during 1954 and 1955. Although its clinical use was short-lived, cross-circulation was an important steppingstone in the development of cardiac surgery.

Meanwhile, at the Mayo Clinic only 90 miles away, John W. Kirklin and colleagues launched their open-heart program on March 5, 1955.[49] They used a heart-lung machine based on the Gibbon-IBM machine but with their own modifications. Kirklin wrote:[59]

> We investigated and visited the groups working intensively with the mechanical pump oxygenators. We visited Dr. Gibbon in his laboratories in Philadelphia, and Dr. Forest Dodrill in Detroit, among others. The Gibbon pump oxygenator had been developed and made by the International Business Machine Corporation and looked quite a bit like a computer. Dr. Dodrill's heart-lung machine had been developed and built for him by General Motors and it looked a great deal like a car engine. We came home, reflected and decided to try to persuade the Mayo Clinic to let us build a pump oxygenator similar to the Gibbon machine, but somewhat different. We already had had about a year's experience in the animal laboratory with David Donald using a simple pump and bubble oxygenator when we set about very early in 1953, the laborious task of building a Mayo-Gibbon pump oxygenator and continuing the laboratory research.
>
> Most people were very discouraged with the laboratory progress. The American Heart Association and the National Institutes of Health had stopped funding any projects for the study of heart-lung machines, because it was felt that the problem was physiologically insurmountable. David Donald and I undertook a series of laboratory experiments lasting about 1½ years during which time the engineering shops at the Mayo Clinic constructed a pump oxygenator based on the Gibbon model.
>
> … In the winter of 1954 and 1955 we had nine surviving dogs out of 10 cardiopulmonary bypass runs. With my wonderful colleague and pediatric cardiologist, Jim DuShane, we had earlier selected eight patients for intracardiac repair. Two had to be put off because two babies with very serious congenital heart disease came along and we decided to fit them into the schedule. We had determined to do all eight patients even if the first seven died. All of this was planned with the knowledge and approval of the governance of the Mayo Clinic. Our plan was then to return to the laboratory and spend the next 6 to 12 months

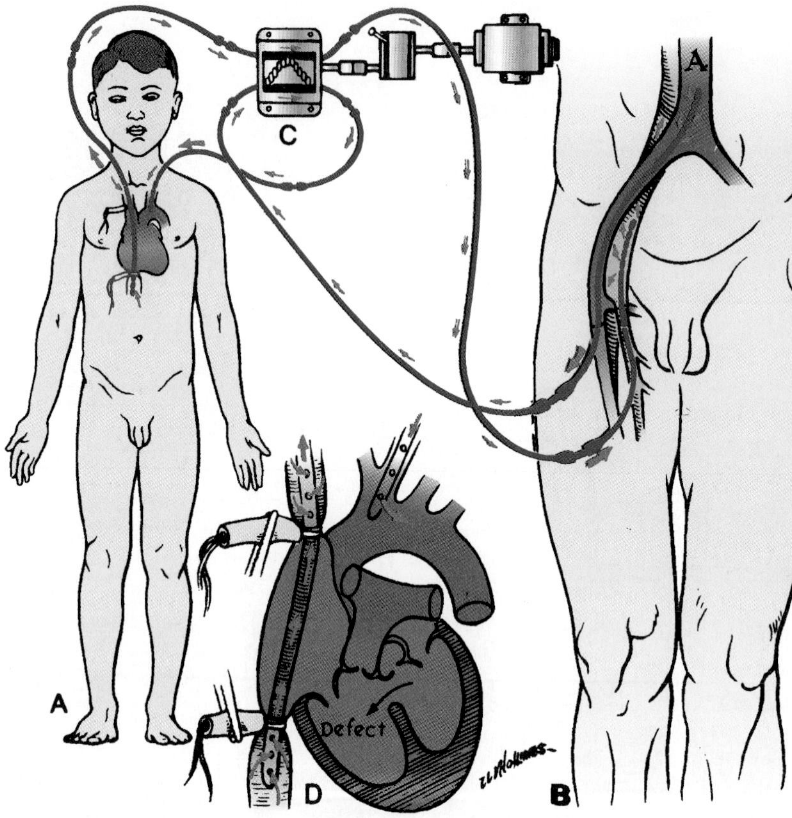

FIGURE 1-4 A depiction of the method of direct-vision intracardiac surgery using extracorporeal circulation by means of controlled cross-circulation. (A) The patient, showing sites of arterial and venous cannulations. (B) The donor, showing sites of arterial and venous (superficial femoral and great saphenous) cannulations. (C) The Sigma motor pump controlling precisely the reciprocal exchange of blood between the patient and donor. (D) Close-up of the patient's heart, showing the vena caval catheter positioned to draw venous blood from both the superior and inferior venae cavae during the cardiac bypass interval. The arterial blood from the donor circulated to the patient's body through the catheter that was inserted into the left subclavian artery. (*Reproduced with permission from Lillehei CW, Cohen M, Warden HE, et al: The results of direct vision closure of ventricular septal defects in eight patients by means of controlled cross circulation. Surg Gynecol Obstet 1955; 101:446. Copyright American College of Surgeons.*)

> solving the problems that had arisen in the first planned clinical trial of a pump oxygenator. … We did our first open-heart operation on a Tuesday in March 1955.

Kirklin continued:[59]

> Four of our first eight patients survived, but the press of the clinical work prevented our ever being able to return to the laboratory with the force that we had planned. By now, Walt Lillehei and I were on parallel, but intertwined paths.

By the end of 1956, many university groups around the world had launched into open-heart programs. Currently, it is estimated that more than 1 million cardiac operations are performed each year worldwide with use of the heart-lung machine. In most cases, the operative mortality is quite low, approaching 1% for some operations. Little thought is given to the courageous pioneers in the 1950s whose monumental contributions made all this possible.

Extracorporeal Life Support

Extracorporeal life support is an extension of cardiopulmonary bypass. Cardiopulmonary bypass was limited initially to no more than 6 hours. The development of membrane oxygenators in the 1960s permitted longer support. Donald Hill and colleagues in 1972 treated a 24-year-old man who developed shock lung after blunt trauma.[60] The patient was supported for 75 hours using a heart-lung machine with a membrane oxygenator, cannulated via the femoral vein and artery. The patient was weaned and recovered. Hill's second patient was supported for 5 days and recovered. This led to a randomized trial supported by the National Institutes of Health to determine the efficacy of this therapy for adults with respiratory failure. The study was conducted from 1972 to 1975 and showed no significant difference in survival between patients managed by extracorporeal life support (9.5%) and those who received conventional ventilatory therapy (8.3%).[61] Because of these results, most U.S. centers abandoned efforts to support adult patients using extracorporeal life support (ECLS), also known as *extracorporeal membrane oxygenation* (ECMO).

One participant in the adult trial decided to study neonates. The usual causes of neonatal respiratory failure have in common abnormal postnatal blood shunts known as *persistent fetal circulation* (PFC). This is a temporary, reversible phenomenon. In 1976, Bartlett and colleagues at the University of Michigan were the first to treat a neonate successfully using ECLS. More than 8000 neonatal patients have been treated using ECLS worldwide, with a survival rate of 82% (ELSO registry data).

MYOCARDIAL PROTECTION

Melrose and colleagues[62] in 1955 presented the first experimental study describing induced arrest by potassium-based cardioplegia. Blood cardioplegia was used "to preserve myocardial energy stores at the onset of cardiac ischemia." Unfortunately, the Melrose solution proved to be toxic to the myocardium, and as a result cardioplegia was not used widely for several years.

Gay and Ebert[63] and Tyres and colleagues[64] demonstrated that cardioplegia with lower potassium concentrations was safe. Studies by Kirsch and colleagues,[65] Bretschneider and colleagues,[66] and Hearse and colleagues[67] demonstrated the effectiveness of cardioplegia with other constituents and renewed interest in this technique. Gay and Ebert in 1973 demonstrated a significant reduction in myocardial oxygen consumption during potassium-induced arrest when compared with that of the fibrillating heart.[63] They also showed that the problems in the use of the Melrose solution in the early days of cardiac surgery probably were caused by its hyperosmolar properties and perhaps not the high potassium concentration.

In a 1978 publication by Follette and colleagues,[68] the technique of blood cardioplegia was reintroduced. In experimental and clinical studies, these authors demonstrated that hypothermic, intermittent blood cardioplegia provided better myocardial protection than normothermic, continuous coronary perfusion and/or hypothermic, intermittent blood perfusion without cardioplegia solution. The composition of the best cardioplegia solution remains controversial, and new formulations, methods of delivery, and recommended temperatures continue to evolve.

EVOLUTION OF CONGENITAL CARDIAC SURGERY DURING THE ERA OF CARDIOPULMONARY BYPASS

With the advent of cardiopulmonary bypass using either the cross-circulation technique of Lillehei and colleagues or the version of the mechanical heart-lung machine used by Kirklin and colleagues, the two groups led the way for intracardiac repairs for many of the commonly occurring congenital heart defects. Because of the morbidity associated with the heart-lung machine, palliative operations also were developed to improve circulatory physiology without directly addressing the anatomic pathology. These palliative operations included the Blalock-Taussig subclavian–pulmonary arterial shunt[28] with modifications by Potts and colleagues[69] and Waterston,[70] the Blalock-Hanlon operation to create an atrial septal defect,[71] and the Galankin-Glenn superior vena cava–right pulmonary arterial shunt.[34,35]

As the safety of cardiopulmonary bypass improved steadily, surgeons addressed more and more complex abnormalities of the heart in younger and younger patients. Some of the milestones in the development of operations to correct congenital heart defects using cardiopulmonary bypass appear in Table 1-2.

VALVULAR SURGERY: CARDIOPULMONARY BYPASS ERA

Cardiac valve repair or replacement under direct vision awaited the development of the heart-lung machine. The first successful aortic valve replacement (AVR) in the subcoronary position was performed by Dr. Dwight Harken and associates.[89] A caged-ball valve was used. Many of the techniques described in Harken's 1960 report are similar to those used today for AVR.

That same year, Starr and Edwards[90] successfully replaced the mitral valve using a caged-ball valve of their own design.

By 1967, nearly 2000 Starr-Edwards valves had been implanted, and the caged-ball-valve prosthesis was established as the standard against which all other mechanical prostheses would be compared.

In 1964, Starr and colleagues reported 13 patients who had undergone multiple valve replacement.[91] One patient had the aortic, mitral, and tricuspid valves replaced on February 21, 1963. Cartwright and colleagues, however, on November 1, 1961, were the first to replace both the aortic and mitral valves successfully with ball-valve prostheses that they had developed.[92] Knott-Craig and colleagues,[93] from the Mayo Clinic, successfully replaced all four heart valves in a patient with carcinoid involvement.

In 1961, Andrew Morrow and Edwin Brockenbrough[94] reported a treatment for idiopathic hypertrophic subaortic stenosis by resecting a portion of the thickened ventricular septum. They referred to this as *subaortic ventriculomyotomy.* They gave credit to William Cleland and H.H. Bentall in London, who had encountered this condition unexpectedly at operation and resected a small portion of the ventricular mass. The patient improved, but no postoperative hemodynamic studies had been reported. The subaortic ventriculomyotomy became the standard surgical treatment for this cardiac anomaly, although in some patients systolic anterior motion (SAM) of the anterior leaflet of the mitral valve necessitates mitral valve replacement with a low-profile mechanical valve.

An aortic homograft valve was used clinically for the first time by Heimbecker and colleagues in Toronto for replacement of the mitral valve in one patient and an aortic valve in another.[95] Survival was short, 1 day in one patient and 1 month in the other. Donald Ross reported on the first successful aortic valve placement with an aortic valve homograft.[96] He used a technique of subcoronary implantation developed in the laboratory by Carlos Duran and Alfred Gunning in Oxford.

The technique of AVR with a pulmonary autograft described initially by Ross in 1967 is advocated by some groups for younger patients who require AVR.[97] An aortic or pulmonary valve homograft is used to replace the pulmonary valve that has been transferred to the aortic position.

Other autogenous materials that have been used to manufacture valve prostheses include pericardium, fasciae latae, and dura mater. In the 1960s, Binet and colleagues[98] began to

TABLE 1-2 First Successful Intracardiac Repairs Using Cardiopulmonary Bypass or Cross-Circulation

Lesion	Year	Reference	Comment
Atrial septal defect	1953	Gibbon[56]	May 6, 1953
Ventricular septal defect	1954	Lillehei et al [57]	Cross-circulation
Complete atrioventricular canal	1954	Lillehei et al [58]	Cross-circulation
Tetralogy of Fallot	1954	Lillehei et al [57]	Cross-circulation
Tetralogy of Fallot	1955	Kirklin[49]	Cardiopulmonary bypass (CPB)
Total anomalous pulmonary veins	1956	Burroughs and Kirklin[72]	
Congenital aneurysm sinus of Valsalva	1956	McGoon et al[73]	
Congenital aortic stenosis	1956	Ellis and Kirklin[74]	First direct visual correction
Aortopulmonary window	1957	Cooley et al [75]	First closure using CPB
Double outlet right ventricle	1957	Kirklin et al [76]	Extemporarily devised correction
Corrected transposition great arteries	1957	Anderson et al[77]	
Transposition of great arteries: atrial switch	1959	Senning[78]	Physiologic total correction
Coronary arteriovenous fistula	1959	Swan et al[79]	
Ebstein's anomaly	1964	Hardy et al[80]	Repair of atrialized tricuspid valve
Tetralogy with pulmonary atresia	1966	Ross and Somerville[81]	Used aortic allograft
Truncus arteriosus	1967	McGoon et al[82]	Used aortic allograft
Tricuspid atresia	1968	Fontan and Baudet[83]	Physiologic correction
Single ventricle	1970	Horiuchi et al[84]	
Subaortic tunnel stenosis	1975	Konno et al[85]	
Transposition of great arteries: arterial switch	1975	Jatene et al[86]	Anatomic correction
Hypoplastic left heart syndrome	1983	Norwood et al[87]	Two-stage operation
Pediatric heart transplantation	1985	Bailey et al[88]	

develop and test tissue valves. In 1964, Duran and Gunning in England replaced an aortic valve in a patient using a xenograft porcine aortic valve. Early results with formaldehyde-fixed xenografts were good,[98] but in a few years these valves began to fail because of tissue degeneration and calcification.[99] Carpentier and colleagues revitalized interest in xenograft valves by fixating porcine valves with glutaraldehyde. Carpentier also mounted his valves on a stent to produce a bioprosthesis. Carpentier-Edwards porcine valves and Hancock and Angell-Shiley bioprostheses became popular and were implanted in large numbers of patients.[100,101]

With the development of cardiopulmonary bypass, valves could be approached under direct vision, and for the first time, mitral insufficiency could be attacked by reparative techniques. Techniques for mitral annuloplasty were described by Wooler and colleagues,[102] Reed and colleagues,[103] and Kay and colleagues.[104] The next step forward was development of annuloplasty rings by Carpentier and Duran. In the 1970s, few groups were involved in valve repairs. Slowly, techniques evolved, were tested clinically, and were followed over the years. Carpentier led the field by establishing the importance of careful analysis of valve pathology, describing in detail several techniques of valve repair, and reporting good results after early and late follow-up, especially with concomitant use of annuloplasty rings.[105]

From 1966 to 1968, a small epidemic of infective endocarditis in Detroit among heroin addicts broke out. Patients were dying of intractable gram-negative tricuspid valve endocarditis, often caused by *Pseudomonas aeruginosa.* Long-term antibiotic administration in combination with tricuspid valve replacement was 100% fatal. Starting in 1970, Arbulu operated on 55 patients; in 53, the tricuspid valve was removed without replacing it.[106,107] At 25 years, the actuarial survival is 61%.

CORONARY ARTERY SURGERY

Selective coronary angiography was developed by Sones and Shirey at the Cleveland Clinic and reported in their 1962 classic paper entitled, "Cine Coronary Arteriography."[108] They used a catheter to inject contrast material directly into the coronary artery ostia. This technique gave a major impetus to direct revascularization of obstructed coronary arteries.

From 1960 to 1967, several sporadic instances of coronary grafting were reported. All were isolated cases and, for uncertain reasons, were not reproduced. None had an impact on the development of coronary surgery. Dr. Robert H. Goetz performed what appears to be the first clearly documented coronary artery bypass operation in a human, which was successful. The surgery took place at Van Etten Hospital in New York City on May 2, 1960.[109] He operated on a 38-year-old man who was severely symptomatic and used a nonsuture technique to connect the right internal mammary artery to a right coronary artery. It took him 17 seconds to join the two arteries using a hollow metal tube. The right internal mammary artery–coronary artery connection was confirmed patent by angiography performed on the 14th postoperative day. The patient remained asymptomatic for about a year and then developed recurrent angina and died of a myocardial infarction on June 23, 1961. Goetz was severely criticized by his medical and surgical colleagues for this procedure, although he had performed it successfully many times in the animal laboratory. He never attempted another coronary bypass operation in a human.

Another example involved a case of autogenous saphenous vein bypass grafting performed on November 23, 1964, in a 42-year-old man who was scheduled to have endarterectomy of his left coronary artery.[110] Because the lesion involved the entire bifurcation, endarterectomy with venous patch graft was abandoned as too hazardous. The authors, Garrett, Dennis, and DeBakey, however, did not report this case until 1973. The patient was alive at that time, and angiograms showed the vein graft to be patent.

Shumaker[111] credits Longmire with the first internal mammary–coronary artery anastomosis. "It was almost surely Longmire, long-time chairman at UCLA, and his associate, Jack Cannon, who first performed an anastomosis between the internal mammary artery and a coronary branch, probably in early 1958."

The reference that Shumaker gives for this quotation from Longmire is a personal communication to Shumaker in 1990, which was 32 years after the fact!

As early as 1952, Vladimir Demikhov, the renowned Soviet surgeon, was anastomosing the internal mammary artery to the left coronary artery in dogs.[112] In 1967, at the height of the Cold War, a Soviet surgeon from Leningrad, V.I. Kolessov, reported his experience with mammary artery–coronary artery anastomoses for the treatment of angina pectoris in six patients in an American surgical journal.[113] The first patient in that series was done in 1964. Operations were performed through a left thoracotomy without extracorporeal circulation or preoperative coronary angiography. The following year, Green and colleagues[114] and Bailey and Hirose[115] separately published reports in which the internal mammary artery was used for coronary artery bypass in patients.

Rene Favalaro from the Cleveland Clinic used saphenous vein for bypassing coronary obstructions.[116] Favalaro's 1968 article focused on 15 patients, who were part of a larger series of 180 patients who had undergone the Vineberg procedure. In these 15 patients with occlusion of the proximal right coronary artery, an interpositional graft of saphenous vein also was placed between the ascending aorta and the right coronary artery distal to the blockage. The right coronary artery was divided, and the vein graft was anastomosed end to end. Favalaro states that this procedure was done because of the unfavorable results with pericardial patch reconstruction of the coronary artery. In an addendum to that paper, 55 patients were added, 52 for segmental occlusion of the right coronary and 3 others for circumflex disease.

The contributions by Favalaro, Kolessov, Green and colleagues, and Bailey and Hirose all were important, but arguably the official start of coronary bypass surgery as we know it today happened in 1969 when W. Dudley Johnson and coworkers from Milwaukee reported their series of 301 patients who had undergone various operations for coronary artery disease (CAD) since February of 1967.[117] In that report, the authors presented their results with direct coronary artery surgery during a 19-month period. They state:

> After two initial and successful patch grafts, the vein bypass technique has been used exclusively. Early results were so encouraging that last summer the vein graft technique was expanded and used to all major branches. Vein grafts to the left side of the arteries run from the aorta over the pulmonary artery and down to the appropriate coronary vessel. Right-sided grafts run along the atrioventricular groove and also attach directly to the aorta. There is almost no limit of potential (coronary) arteries to use. Veins can be sutured to the distal anterior descending or even to posterior marginal branches. Double vein grafts are now used in more than 40% of patients and can be used to any combination of arteries.

Johnson goes on to say:

> Our experience indicates that five factors are important to direct surgery. One: Do not limit grafts to proximal portions of large arteries. … Two: Do not work with diseased arteries. Vein grafts can be made as long as necessary and should be inserted into distal normal arteries. Three: Always do end-to-side anastomoses. … Four: Always work on a dry, quiet field. Consistently successful fine vessel anastomoses cannot be done on a moving, bloody target. … Five: Do not allow the hematocrit to fall below 35.

In discussing Dr. Johnson's presentation, Dr. Frank Spencer commented:

> I would like to congratulate Dr. Johnson very heartily. We may have heard a milestone in cardiac surgery today. Because for years, pathologists, cardiologists, and many surgeons have repeatedly stated that the pattern of coronary artery disease is so extensive that direct anastomosis can be done in only 5 to 7%

> of patients. If the exciting data by Dr. Johnson remain valid and the grafts remain patent over a long period of time, a total revision of thinking will be required regarding the feasibility of direct arterial surgery for CAD.[117]

The direct anastomosis between the internal mammary artery and the coronary artery was not as popular initially as the vein-graft technique; however, owing to the persistence of Drs. Green, Loop, Grondin, and others, internal mammary artery grafts eventually became the conduit of choice when their superior long-term patency became known.[118]

Denton Cooley and colleagues made two important contributions to the surgery for ischemic heart disease.[119] In 1956, with the use of cardiopulmonary bypass, they were the first to repair a ruptured interventricular septum following acute myocardial infarction. The patient did well initially but died of complications 6 weeks after the operation. Cooley and colleagues also were the first to report the resection of a left ventricular aneurysm with the use of cardiopulmonary bypass.[120]

ARRHYTHMIC SURGERY

Cobb and colleagues at Duke University developed the first successful surgical treatment for cardiac arrhythmias.[121] A 32-year-old fisherman was referred for symptomatic episodes of atrial tachycardia that caused CHF. On May 2, 1968, after epicardial mapping, a 5- to 6-cm cut was made extending from the base of the right atrial appendage to the right border of the right atrium during cardiopulmonary bypass. The incision transected the conduction pathway between the atrium and ventricle. Subsequent epicardial mapping indicated eradication of the pathway. Six weeks after the operation, heart size had decreased and lung fields had cleared. The patient eventually returned to work.

A year earlier, Dr. Dwight McGoon at the Mayo Clinic closed an ASD in a patient who also had Wolff-Parkinson-White (WPW) syndrome.[122] At operation, Dr. Birchell mapped the epicardium of the heart and localized the accessory pathway to the right atrioventricular groove. Lidocaine was injected into the site, and the delta wave disappeared immediately. Unfortunately, conduction across the pathway reappeared a few hours later. This probably was the first attempt to treat the WPW syndrome surgically. As a result of knowledge gained from the surgical treatment for WPW syndrome, more than 95% of all refractory clinical cases now are treated successfully by nonsurgical means.[122]

Ross and colleagues[123] in Sydney, Australia, and Cox and colleagues[124] in St. Louis, Missouri, used cryosurgical treatment of atrial ventricular node re-entry tachycardia. Subsequently, James L. Cox, after years of laboratory research, developed the Maze operation for atrial fibrillation.[125] That technique, with his subsequent modifications, is now known as the *Cox Maze procedure* and has become the world standard with which other techniques used to treat atrial fibrillation, either surgically or with catheters, are compared.[125]

Guiraudon and colleagues[126] from Paris, reported their results with an encircling endomyocardial ventriculotomy for the treatment of malignant ventricular arrhythmias. The following year, in 1979, Josephson and colleagues[127] described a more specific procedure for treatment of malignant ventricular arrhythmias. After endocardial mapping, the endocardial source of the arrhythmia was excised. Although the Guiraudon technique usually isolated the source of the arrhythmia, the incision also devascularized healthy myocardium and was associated with high mortality. Endocardial resection was safer and more efficacious and became the basis of all approaches for the treatment of ischemic ventricular tachycardia.[122]

Stimulated by the death of a close personal friend from ventricular arrhythmias, Dr. Mirowski developed a prototype defibrillator over a 3-month period in 1969. In 1980, Mirowski and colleagues described three successful cases using their implantable myocardial stimulator at Johns Hopkins.[128]

PACEMAKERS

In 1952 Paul Zoll applied electric shocks 2 ms in duration that were transmitted through the chest wall at frequencies from 25 to 60 per minute and increased the intensity of the shock until ventricular responses were observed. However, after 25 minutes of intermittent stimulation the patient died, although many subsequent patients recovered.[129] The next step came when Lillehei and colleagues reported a series of patients who had external pacing after open-heart surgery during the 1950s.[130] The field of open-heart surgery gave a major impetus to the development of pacemakers because there was a high incidence of heart block following many intracardiac repairs. The major difference between Zoll's pacing and that of Lillehei and colleagues was that Zoll used external electrodes placed on the chest wall, whereas Lillehei and colleagues attached electrodes directly to the heart at operation. Lillehei and colleagues used a relatively small external pacemaker to stimulate the heart and much less electric current. This form of heart pacing was better tolerated by the patient and was a more efficient way to stimulate the heart. The survival rate of Lillehei's patients with surgically induced heart block was improved significantly.

During this period, progress was made toward a totally implantable pacemaker. Elmquist and Senning[131] developed a pacer battery that was small enough for an epigastric pocket with electrodes connected to the heart. They implanted the unit in a patient with atrioventricular block in 1958. Just before implantation, the patient had 20 to 30 cardiac arrests a day. The first pacemaker that was implanted functioned only 8 hours; the second pacemaker implanted in the same patient had better success. The patient survived until January 2002 and had many additional pacemakers. Chardack and colleagues are perhaps better known for their development of the totally implantable pacemaker.[132] In 1961 they reported a series of 15 patients who had pacemakers that they had developed implanted.

Early implantable pacemakers were fixed-rate, asynchronous devices that delivered an impulse independent of the underlying cardiac rhythm. During the past 40 years, enormous progress has been made in the field of pacing technology. The number of individuals with artificial pacemakers is unknown; however, estimates indicate that approximately 500,000 Americans are living with a pacemaker and that each year another 100,000 or more patients require permanent pacemakers in the United States.

HEART, HEART-LUNG, AND LUNG TRANSPLANTATION

Alexis Carrel and Charles Guthrie reported transplantation of the heart and lungs while at the University of Chicago in 1905.[133] The heart of a small dog was transplanted into the neck of a larger one by anastomosing the caudad ends of the jugular vein and carotid artery to the aorta and pulmonary artery. The animal was not anticoagulated, and the experiment ended about 2 hours after circulation was established because of blood clot in the cavities of the transplanted heart.

Vladimir Demikhov, from Russia, described more than 20 different techniques for heart transplantation in 1950.[134] He also published various techniques for heart and lung transplantation. He was even able to perform an orthotopic heart transplant in a dog before the heart-lung machine was developed. This was accomplished by placing the donor heart above the dog's own heart, and then with a series of tubes and connections, he rerouted the blood from one heart to the other until he had the donor heart functioning in the appropriate position and the native heart removed. One of his dogs climbed the steps of the Kremlin on the sixth postoperative day but died shortly afterward of rejection.

Richard Lower and Norman Shumway established the technique for heart transplantation as it is performed today.[135] Preservation of the cuff of recipient left and right atria with part of the atrial septum was described earlier by Brock[136] in England and Demikhov[112] in Russia,[137] but it became popular only after Shumway and Lower reported it in their 1960 paper.

The first attempt at human heart transplantation was made by Hardy and colleagues[138] at the University of Mississippi. Because no human donor organ was available at the time, a large chimpanzee's heart was used; however, it was unable to support the circulation because of hyperacute rejection.

The first human-to-human heart transplant occurred December 3, 1967, in Capetown, South Africa.[139] The surgical team, headed by Christiaan Barnard, transplanted the heart of a donor who had been certified dead after the electrocardiogram showed no activity for 5 minutes into a 54-year-old man whose heart was irreparably damaged by repeated myocardial infarctions. The second human heart transplant using a human donor was performed on a child 3 days after the first on December 6, 1967, by Adrian Kantrowitz in Brooklyn, New York. Dr. Kantrowitz's patient died of a bleeding complication within the first 24 hours.[140] Barnard's patient, Lewis Washkansky, died on the 18th postoperative day. At autopsy, the heart appeared normal, and there was no evidence of chronic liver congestion, but bilateral pneumonia was present, possibly owing to severe myeloid depression from immunosuppression.[141]

On January 2, 1968, Barnard performed a second heart transplant on Phillip Blaiberg, 12 days after Washkansky's death.[142] Blaiberg was discharged from the hospital and became a celebrity during the several months he lived after the transplant. Blaiberg's procedure indicated that a heart transplant was an option for humans suffering from end-stage heart disease. Within a year of Barnard's first heart transplant, 99 heart transplants had been performed by cardiac surgeons around the world. However, by the end of 1968, most groups abandoned heart transplantation because of the extremely high mortality related to rejection. Shumway and Lower, Barnard, and a few others persevered both clinically and in the laboratory. Their efforts in discovering better drugs for immunosuppression eventually established heart transplantation as we know it today.

A clinical trial of heart-lung transplantation was commenced at Stanford University in 1981 by Reitz and colleagues.[143] Their first patient was treated with a combination of cyclosporine and azathioprine. The patient was discharged from the hospital in good condition and was well more than 5 years after the transplant.

The current success with heart, heart-lung, and lung transplantation is related in part to the discovery of cyclosporine by workers at the Sandoz Laboratory in Basel, Switzerland, in 1970. In December of 1980, cyclosporine was introduced at Stanford for cardiac transplantation. The incidence of rejection was not reduced, nor was the incidence of infection. However, these two major complications of cardiac transplantation were less severe when cyclosporine was used. Availability of cyclosporine stimulated many new programs across the United States in the mid-1980s.

The first human lung transplant was performed by Hardy and colleagues[144] at the University of Mississippi on June 11, 1964. The patient died on the 17th postoperative day. In 1971, a Belgian surgeon, Fritz Derom, achieved a 10-month survival in a patient with pulmonary silicosis.[145]

Much of the credit, however, for the success of lung transplantation belongs to the Toronto group, whose efforts were headed by Joel Cooper. Their successes were based on laboratory experimentation and the discovery of cyclosporine. After losing an early patient to bronchial anastomotic dehiscence in 1978, the group substituted cyclosporine for cortisone and wrapped the bronchial suture line with a pedicle of omentum. They also developed a comprehensive preoperative preparation program that increased the strength and nutritional status of the recipients. In 1986, Cooper and associates presented their first two successful patients, who had returned to normal activities and were alive 14 and 26 months after operation.[146]

HEART ASSIST AND ARTIFICIAL HEARTS

In 1963, Kantrowitz and colleagues reported the first use of the intra-aortic balloon pump (IABP) in three patients.[147] All were in cardiogenic shock but improved during balloon pumping. One survived to leave the hospital.

In 1963, Liotta and colleagues reported a 42-year-old man who had a stenotic aortic valve replaced but suffered a cardiac arrest the following morning.[148] The patient was resuscitated but developed severe ventricular failure. An artificial intrathoracic circulatory pump was implanted. The patient's pulmonary edema cleared, but he died 4 days later with the pump working continuously. In 1966, the same group used a newer intrathoracic pump to support another patient who could not be weaned from cardiopulmonary bypass. This pump maintained the circulation. The patient eventually died before the pump could be removed.[149] Later that year, the same group used a left ventricular assist device (LVAD) in a woman who could not be weaned from cardiopulmonary bypass after double valve replacement.[150] After 10 days of circulatory assistance, the patient was weaned successfully from the device and recovered. This woman was probably the first patient to be weaned from an assist device and leave the hospital.

The first human application of a totally artificial heart was by Denton Cooley and colleagues as a "bridge" to transplantation.[151] They implanted a totally artificial heart in a patient who could not be weaned from cardiopulmonary bypass. After 64 hours of artificial heart support, heart transplantation was performed, but the patient died of *Pseudomonas* pneumonia 32 hours after transplantation. The first two patients bridged successfully to transplantation were reported at almost the same time and in the same location by different groups. On September 5, 1984, in San Francisco,[152] Donald Hill implanted a Pierce-Donachy LVAD in a patient in cardiogenic shock. The patient received a successful transplant 2 days later and was discharged subsequently. The assist device used by Hill was developed at Pennsylvania State University by Pierce and Donachy. Phillip Oyer and colleagues at Stanford University placed an electrically driven Novacor LVAD in a patient in cardiogenic shock on September 7, 1984.[153] The patient was transplanted successfully and survived beyond 3 years. The device used by the Stanford group was developed by Peer Portner.

The first implantation of a permanent totally artificial heart (Jarvik-7) was performed by DeVries and colleagues at the University of Utah in 1982.[154] By 1985, they had implanted the Jarvik in four patients, and one survived for 620 days after implantation. This initial clinical experience was based heavily on the work of Kolff and colleagues.

THORACIC AORTA SURGERY

Alexis Carrel was responsible for one of the great surgical advances of the twentieth century: techniques for suturing and transplanting blood vessels.[155] Although Carrel initially developed his methods of blood vessel anastomosis in Lyon, France, his work with Charles Guthrie in Chicago led to many major advances in vascular, cardiac, and transplantation surgery. In a short period of time, these investigators perfected techniques for blood vessel anastomoses and transposition of arterial and venous segments using both fresh and frozen grafts. After leaving Chicago, Carrel continued to expand his work on blood vessels and organ transplantation and in 1912 received the Nobel Prize. Interestingly, Carrel's work did not receive immediate clinical application.

Rudolph Matas pioneered clinical vascular surgery. Matas' work took place before drugs were available to prevent blood clotting, before antibiotics, and without reliable blood vessel substitutes.[156] Matas performed 620 vascular operations between 1888 and 1940. Only 101 of these were attempts to repair arteries; most involved ligation. Matas developed three variations of his well-known endoaneurysmorrhaphy procedure. The most advanced was to reconstruct the wall of the blood vessel from within while using a rubber tube as a stent.

Vascular surgery advanced tentatively during World War II as traumatic injuries to major blood vessels were repaired in some soldiers with results significantly better than with the standard treatment of ligation.[157] The successful treatment of coarctation of the aorta by Crafoord and Gross added a major boost to the reconstructive surgery of arteries.

Shumaker reported the excision of a small descending thoracic aortic aneurysm with reanastomosis of the aorta in 1948.[158] Swan and colleagues[159] repaired a complex aneurysmal coarctation and used aortic homograft for reconstruction in 1950. Gross[160] reported a series of similar cases using homograft replacement. In 1951, DuBost and colleagues[161] in Paris resected an intra-abdominal aortic aneurysm with homograft replacement.

In 1953, Henry Bahnson,[162] from Johns Hopkins, successfully resected six saccular aneurysms of the aorta in eight patients. In the same year, DeBakey and Cooley[163] reported a 46-year-old man who had resection of a huge aneurysm of the descending thoracic aorta that measured approximately 20 cm in length and in greatest diameter. The aneurysm was resected and replaced with an aortic homograft approximately 15 cm in length.

During the Korean War, the arterial homograft and autogenous vein graft were used to reconstruct battlefield arterial injuries and reduce the overall amputation rate to 11.1%[164] compared with the rate of 49.6% reported in World War II. Although the vein autograft remains the first-choice peripheral vascular conduit today, the arterial homograft was superseded by the development of synthetic vascular grafts by Arthur Voorhees at Columbia University in 1952. Voorhees and colleagues developed Vinyon-N cloth tubes to substitute for diseased arterial segments.[165]

Another advance in aortic surgery appeared in 1955 when DeBakey and colleagues[166] reported six cases of aortic dissection treated by aggressive surgery. Because mortality of operation for acute dissections remained high, Myron Wheat Jr introduced medical therapy for the disease.[167]

During the late 1950s, the Houston group, consisting of Michael DeBakey, Denton Cooley, Stanley Crawford, and their other associates, systematically developed operations for resection and graft replacement of the ascending aorta,[168] descending aorta, and thoracoabdominal aorta.[169] Cardiopulmonary bypass was used for the ascending aortic resections. The high risk of paraplegia highlighted a major complication of thoracoabdominal aortic resections. The Houston group was the first to resect an aortic arch with the use of cardiopulmonary bypass in 1957 and replace the arch with a reconstituted aortic arch homograph.[170] More interesting is that Cooley and colleagues, using great ingenuity, resected a large aortic arch aneurysm that also involved a portion of the descending aorta in a 49-year-old patient on June 24, 1955. The surgery was done, without the use of cardiopulmonary bypass, by first sewing in a temporary graft from the ascending aorta to the distal descending aorta and sewing in two more temporary limbs off that graft, which were anastomosed to the left and right carotid arteries, while the aneurysm was resected and a permanent graft was placed.[171]

In 1968, Bentall and De Bono[172] introduced replacement of the ascending aorta and aortic valve with reanastomoses of the coronary ostia to the replacement graft. They described the composite-graft technique for replacement of the ascending aorta with reimplantation of the coronary arteries into the composite Dacron graft containing the prosthetic aortic valve. As mentioned, Cooley and DeBakey were first to replace the supracoronary ascending aorta in 1956. In 1963, Starr and colleagues[173] reported replacing the supracoronary ascending aorta and the aortic valve at the same sitting. The technique of fashioning "buttons" of aortic tissue adjacent to the coronary ostia and then incorporating these buttons into the aortic graft along with the aortic valve replacement was described by Wheat and colleagues[174] in 1964. Bentall and De Bono incorporated the aortic prosthesis into the tube graft and used the Wheat technique for implanting the coronary arteries into the composite graft.

Since the early 1990s, stents also have been used for the treatment of aneurysms in both the descending aorta and abdominal aorta.[175,176] The progress in this field is moving rapidly.

SUMMARY

The history of adult cardiac surgery continues to be written and will continue to evolve as long as acquired heart disease shortens lives. In the early days after the introduction of cardiopulmonary bypass, the pace of advance was torrid but, in a way, narrowly focused. Now hundreds of thousands of clinicians, scientists, and engineers are involved in a broad and deep effort to develop new and safer operations and procedures, new valves, new revascularization techniques, new biomaterials, new heart substitutes, new life-support systems, and new methods to control cardiac arrhythmias and ventricular remodeling after injury. This research and development is supported by a vigorous infrastructure of basic science in biology and medicine, chemistry and pharmacology, and engineering and computer technology. The history of cardiac surgery is only a prelude; the moving finger writes and having writ moves on to a bright, exciting future.

REFERENCES

1. Williams DH: Stab wound of the heart, pericardium—Suture of the pericardium—Recovery—Patient alive three years afterward. *Med Rec* 1897; 1.
2. Rehn L: On penetrating cardiac injuries and cardiac suturing. *Arch Klin Chir* 1897; 55:315.
3. Rehn L: Zur chirurgie des herzens und des herzbeutels. *Arch Klin Chir* 1907; 83:723. quoted from Beck CS: Wounds of the heart: the technic of suture. *Arch Surg* 1926; 13:212.
4. Hill LL: A report of a case of successful suturing of the heart, and table of thirty seven other cases of suturing by different operators with various terminations, and the conclusions drawn. *Med Rec* 1902; 2:846.
5. Harken DE: Foreign bodies in and in relation to the thoracic blood vessels and heart: I. Techniques for approaching and removing foreign bodies from the chambers of the heart. *Surg Gynecol Obstet* 1946; 83:117.
6. Kirschner M: Ein durch die Trendelenburgische operation geheiter fall von embolie der art. pulmonalis. *Arch Klin Chir* 1924; 133:312.
7. Gibbon JH: Artificial maintenance of circulation during experimental occlusion of pulmonary artery. *Arch Surg* 1937; 34:1105.
8. Sharp EH: Pulmonary embolectomy: successful removal of a massive pulmonary embolus with the support of cardiopulmonary bypass. Case report. *Ann Surg* 1962; 156:1.
9. Rehn I: Zur experimentellen pathologie des herzbeutels. *Verh Dtsch Ges Chir* 1913; 42:339.
10. Sauerbruch R: *Die Chirurgie der Brustorgane,* Vol. II. Berlin, 1925.
11. Forssmann W: Catheterization of the right heart. *Klin Wochenshr* 1929; 8:2085.
12. Forssmann W: 21 jahre herzkatheterung, rueckblick and ausschau. *Verh Dtsch Ges Kreislaufforschung* 1951; 17:1.
13. Klein O: Zur bestimmung des zirkulatorischen minutenvoumnens beim menschen nach dem fisckschen prinzip. *Meunsch Med Wochenschr* 1930; 77:1311.
14. Forssmann W: Ueber kontrastdarstellung der hoehlen des lebenden rechten herzens and der lungenschlagader. *Muensch Med Wochenschr* 1931; 78:489.
15. Tuffier T: Etat actuel de la chirurgie intrathoracique. *Trans Int Congr Med 1913* (London, 1914), 7; *Surgery* 1914; 2:249.
16. Brock RC: The arterial route to the aortic and pulmonary valves: the mitral route to the aortic valves. *Guys Hosp Rep* 1950; 99:236.
17. Brock, Sir Russell: Aortic subvalvular stenosis: surgical treatment. *Guys Hosp Rep* 1957; 106:221.
18. Bailey CP, Bolton HE, Nichols HT, et al: Commissurotomy for rheumatic aortic stenosis. *Circulation* 1954; 9:22.
19. Cutler EC, Levine SA: Cardiotomy and valvulotomy for mitral stenosis. *Boston Med Surg J* 1923; 188:1023.
20. Bailey CP: The surgical treatment of mitral stenosis. *Dis Chest* 1949; 15:377.
21. Naef AP: *The Story of Thoracic Surgery.* New York, Hogrefe & Huber, 1990.
22. Sellers TH: Surgery of pulmonary stenosis: a case in which the pulmonary valve was successfully divided. *Lancet* 1948; 1:988.
23. Hufnagel CA, Harvey WP, Rabil PJ, et al: Surgical correction of aortic insufficiency. *Surgery* 195435:673.
24. Graybiel A, Strieder JW, Boyer NH: An attempt to obliterate the patent ductus in a patient with subacute endarteritis. *Am Heart J* 1938; 15:621.
25. Gross RE, Hubbard JH: Surgical ligation of a patent ductus arteriosus: report of first successful case. *JAMA* 1939; 112:729.
26. Crafoord C, Nylin G: Congenital coarctation of the aorta and its surgical treatment. *J Thorac Cardiovasc Surg* 1945; 14:347.
27. Gross RE: Surgical correction for coarctation of the aorta. *Surgery* 1945; 18:673.
28. Gross RE: Surgical relief for tracheal obstruction from a vascular ring. *NEJM* 1945; 233:586.
29. Blalock A, Taussig HB: The surgical treatment of malformations of the heart in which there is pulmonary stenosis or pulmonary atresia. *JAMA* 1945; 128:189.
30. Biorck G, Crafoord C: Arteriovenous aneurysm on the pulmonary artery simulating patent ductus arteriosus botalli. *Thorax* 1947; 2:65.
31. Muller WH Jr: The surgical treatment of the transposition of the pulmonary veins. *Ann Surg* 1951; 134:683.
32. Gross RE: Surgical closure of an aortic septal defect. *Circulation* 1952; 5:858.
33. Cooley DA, McNamara DR, Latson JR: Aorticopulmonary septal defect: diagnosis and surgical treatment. *Surgery* 1957; 42:101.
34. Glenn WWL: Circulatory bypass of the right side of the hearts: IV. Shunt between superior vena cava and distal right pulmonary artery—report of clinical application. *NEJM* 1958; 259:117.
35. Galankin NK: Proposition and technique of cavo-pulmonary anastomosis. *Exp Biol (Russia)* 1957; 5:33.
36. Johnson SL: *The History of Cardiac Surgery, 1896–1955.* Baltimore, Johns Hopkins Press, 1970.
37. Gibbon JH Jr: Artificial maintenance of circulation during experimental occlusion of the pulmonary artery. *Arch Surg* 1937; 34:1105.
38. Dennis C, Spreng DS, Nelson GE, et al: Development of a pump oxygenator to replace the heart and lungs: an apparatus applicable to human patients, and application to one case. *Ann Surg* 1951; 134:709.
39. Miller CW: *King of Hearts: The True Story of the Maverick Who Pioneered Open Heart Surgery.* New York, Random House, 2000.
40. Digliotti AM: Clinical use of the artificial circulation with a note on intra-arterial transfusion. *Bull Johns Hopkins Hosp* 1952; 90:131.
41. Schumaker HB Jr: *A Dream of the Heart.* Santa Barbara, CA, Fithian Press, 1999.
42. Dodrill FD, Hill E, Gerisch RA: Temporary mechanical substitute for the left ventricle in man. *JAMA* 1952; 150:642.
43. Lewis FJ, Taufic M: Closure of atrial septal defects with the aid of hypothermia: experimental accomplishments and the report of one successful case. *Surgery* 1953; 33:52.
44. Dodrill FD, Hill E, Gerisch RA, Johnson A: Pulmonary valvuloplasty under direct vision using the mechanical heart for a complete bypass of the right heart in a patient with congenital pulmonary stenosis. *J Thorac Surg* 1953; 25:584.

45. Mustard WT, Chute AL, Keith JD, et al: A surgical approach to transposition of the great vessels with extracorporeal circuit. *Surgery* 1953; 6:39.
46. Romaine-Davis A: *John Gibbon and His Heart-Lung Machine.* Philadelphia, University of Pennsylvania Press, 1991.
47. Lillehei CW: Overview: Section III: Cardiopulmonary bypass and myocardial protection, in Stephenson LW, Ruggiero R (eds): *Heart Surgery Classics.* Boston, Adams Publishing Group, 1994; p 121.
48. Radegram K: The early history of open-heart surgery in Stockholm. *J Cardiac Surg* 2003; 18:564.
49. Kirklin JW, DuShane JW, Patrick RT, et al: Intracardiac surgery with the aid of a mechanical pump-oxygenator system (Gibbon type): report of eight cases. *Mayo Clin Proc* 1955; 30:201.
50. Dodrill FD, Marshall N, Nyboer J, et al: The use of the heart-lung apparatus in human cardiac surgery. *J Thorac Surg* 1957; 1:60.
51. Acierno LJ: *The History of Cardiology.* New York, Parthenon, 1994.
52. Mustard WT, Thomson JA: Clinical experience with the artificial heart lung preparation. *Can Med Assoc J* 1957; 76:265.
53. Dodrill FD, Hill E, Gerisch RA: Some physiologic aspects of the artificial heart problem. *J Thorac Surg* 1952; 24:134.
54. Stephenson LW: Forest Dewey Dodrill—Heart surgery pioneer, part II. *J Cardiac Surg* 2002; 17:247.
55. Hikasa Y, Shirotani H, Satomura K, et al: Open-heart surgery in infants with the aid of hypothermic anesthesia. *Arch Jpn Chir* 1967; 36:495.
56. Gibbon JH Jr: Application of a mechanical heart and lung apparatus to cardiac surgery. *Minn Med* 1954; 37:171.
57. Lillehei CW, Cohen M, Warden HE, et al: The results of direct vision closure of ventricular septal defects in eight patients by means of controlled cross circulation. *Surg Gynecol Obstet* 1955; 101:446.
58. Lillehei CW, Cohen M, Warden HE, et al: The direct vision intracardiac correction of congenital anomalies by controlled cross circulation. *Surgery* 1955; 38:11.
59. Kirklin JW: The middle 1950s and C. Walton Lillehei. *J Thorac Cardiovasc Surg* 1989; 98:822.
60. Hill JD, O'Brien TG, Murray JJ, et al: Prolonged extracorporeal oxygenation for acute posttraumatic respiratory failure (shock-lung syndrome): use of the Bramston membrane lung. *NEJM* 1972; 286:629.
61. Zapol WM, Snider MT, Hill JD, et al: Extracorporeal membrane oxygenation in severe acute respiratory failure: a randomized, prospective study. *JAMA* 1979; 242:2193.
62. Melrose DG, Dreyer B, Bentall MB, Baker JBE: Elective cardiac arrest. *Lancet* 1955; 2:21.
63. Gay WA Jr, Ebert PA: Functional, metabolic, and morphologic effects of potassium-induced cardioplegia. *Surgery* 1973; 74:284.
64. Tyers GFO, Todd GJ, Niebauer IM, et al: The mechanism of myocardial damage following potassium-induced (Melrose) cardioplegia. *Surgery* 1978; 78:45.
65. Kirsch U, Rodewald G, Kalmar P: Induced ischemic arrest. *J Thorac Cardiovasc Surg* 1972; 63:121.
66. Bretschneider HJ, Hubner G, Knoll D, et al: Myocardial resistance and tolerance to ischemia: physiological and biochemical basis. *J Cardiovasc Surg* 1975; 16:241.
67. Hearse DJ, Stewart DA, Braimbridge MV, et al: Cellular protection during myocardial ischemia. *Circulation* 1976; 16:241.
68. Follette DM, Mulder DG, Maloney JV, Buckberg GD: Advantages of blood cardioplegia over continuous coronary perfusion or intermittent ischemia. *J Thorac Cardiovasc Surg* 1978; 76:604.
69. Potts WJ, Smith S, Gibson S: Anastomosis of the aorta to a pulmonary artery. *JAMA* 1946; 132:627.
70. Waterston DJ: Treatment of Fallot's tetralogy in children under one year of age. *Rozhl Chir* 1962; 41:181.
71. Blalock A, Hanlon CR: The surgical treatment of complete transposition of the aorta and the pulmonary artery. *Surg Gynecol Obstet* 1950; 90:1.
72. Burroughs JT, Kirklin JW: Complete correction of total anomalous pulmonary venous correction: report of three cases. *Mayo Clin Proc* 1956; 31:182.
73. McGoon DC, Edwards JE, Kirklin JW: Surgical treatment of ruptured aneurysm of aortic sinus. *Ann Surg* 1958; 147:387.
74. Ellis FH Jr, Kirklin JW: Congenital valvular aortic stenosis: anatomic findings and surgical techniques. *J Thorac Cardiovasc Surg* 1962; 43:199.
75. Cooley DA, McNamara DG, Jatson JR: Aortico-pulmonary septal defect: diagnosis and surgical treatment. *Surgery* 1957; 42:101.
76. Kirklin JW, Harp RA, McGoon DC: Surgical treatment of origin of both vessels from right ventricle including cases of pulmonary stenosis. *J Thorac Cardiovasc Surg* 1964; 48:1026.
77. Anderson RC, Lillihei CW, Jester RG: Corrected transposition of the great vessels of the heart. *Pediatrics* 1957; 20:626.
78. Senning A: Surgical correction of transposition of the great vessels. *Surgery* 1959; 45:966.
79. Swan H, Wilson JH, Woodwork G, Blount SE: Surgical obliteration of a coronary artery fistula to the right ventricle. *Arch Surg* 1959; 79:820.
80. Hardy KL, May IA, Webster CA, Kimball KG: Ebstein's anomaly: a functional concept and successful definitive repair. *J Thorac Cardiovasc Surg* 1964; 48:927.
81. Ross DN, Somerville J: Correction of pulmonary atresia with a homograft aortic valve. *Lancet* 1966; 2:1446.
82. McGoon DC, Rastelli GC, Ongley PA: An operation for the correction of truncus arteriosus. *JAMA* 1968; 205:59.
83. Fontan F, Baudet E: Surgical repair of tricuspid atresia. *Thorax* 1971; 26:240.
84. Horiuchi T, Abe T, Okada Y, et al: Feasibility of total correction for single ventricle: a report of total correction in a six-year-old girl. *Jpn J Thorac Surg* 1970; 23:434 (in Japanese).
85. Konno S, Iami Y, Iida Y, et al: A new method for prosthetic valve replacement in congenital aortic stenosis associated with hypoplasia of the aortic valve ring. *J Thorac Cardiovasc Surg* 1975; 70:909.
86. Jatene AD, Fontes VF, Paulista PP, et al: Anatomic correction of transposition of the great vessel. *J Thorac Cardiovasc Surg* 1976; 72:364.
87. Norwood WI, Lang P, Hansen DD: Physiologic repair of aortic atresia-hypoplastic left heart syndrome. *NEJM* 1983; 308:23.
88. Bailey LL, Gundry SR, Razzouk AJ, et al: Bless the babies: one hundred fifteen late survivors of heart transplantation during the first year of life. *J Thorac Cardiovasc Surg* 1993; 105:805.
89. Harken DE, Soroff HS, Taylor WJ, et al: Partial and complete pros-theses in aortic insufficiency. *J Thorac Cardiovasc Surg* 1960; 40:744.
90. Starr A, Edwards ML: Mitral replacement: clinical experience with a ball-valve prosthesis. *Ann Surg* 1961; 154:726.
91. Starr A, Edwards LM, McCord CW, et al: Multiple valve replacement. *Circulation* 1964; 29:30.
92. Cartwright RS, Giacobine JW, Ratan RS, et al: Combined aortic and mitral valve replacement. *J Thorac Cardiovasc Surg* 1963; 45:35.
93. Knott-Craig CJ, Schaff HV, Mullany CJ, et al: Carcinoid disease of the heart: surgical management of ten patients. *J Thorac Cardiovasc Surg* 1992; 104:475.
94. Morrow AG, Brockenbrough EC: Surgical treatment of idiopathic hypertrophic subaortic stenosis: technic and hemodynamic results of subaortic ventriculomyotomy. *Ann Surg* 1961; 154:181.
95. Heimbecker RO, Baird RJ, Lajos RJ, et al: Homograft replacement of the human valve: a preliminary report. *Can Med Assoc J* 1962; 86:805.
96. Ross DN: Homograft replacement of the aortic valve. *Lancet* 1962; 2:487.
97. Ross DN: Replacement of aortic and mitral valves with a pulmonary autograft. *Lancet* 1967; 2:956.
98. Binet JP, Carpentier A, Langlois J, et al: Implantation de valves heterogenes dans le traitment des cardiopathies aortiques. *C R Acad Sci Paris* 1965; 261:5733.
99. Binet JP, Planche C, Weiss M: Heterograft replacement of the aortic valve, in Ionescu MI, Ross DN, Wooler GH (eds): *Biological Tissue in Heart Valve Replacement.* London, Butterworth, 1971; p 409.
100. Carpentier A: Principles of tissue valve transplantation, in Ionescu MI, Ross DN, Wooler GH (eds): *Biological Tissue in Heart Valve Replacement.* London, Butterworth, 1971; p 49.
101. Kaiser GA, Hancock WD, Lukban SB, Litwak RS: Clinical use of a new design stented xenograft heart valve prosthesis. *Surg Forum* 1969; 20:137.
102. Wooler GH, Nixon PG, Grimshaw VA, et al: Experiences with the repair of the mitral valve in mitral incompetence. *Thorax* 1962; 17:49.
103. Reed GE, Tice DA, Clause RH: A symmetric, exaggerated mitral annuloplasty: repair of mitral insufficiency with hemodynamic predictability. *J Thorac Cardiovasc Surg* 1965; 49:752.
104. Kay JH, Zubiate T, Mendez MA, et al: Mitral valve repair for significant mitral insufficiency. *Am Heart J* 1978; 96:243.
105. Carpentier A: Cardiac valve surgery: the French correction. *J Thorac Cardiovasc Surg* 1983; 86:23.
106. Arbulu A, Thoms NW, Chiscano A, Wilson RF: Total tricuspid valvulectomy without replacement in the treatment of *Pseudomonas* endocarditis. *Surg Forum* 1971; 22:162.
107. Arbulu A, Holmes RJ, Asfaw I: Surgical treatment of intractable right-sided infective endocarditis in drug addicts: 25 years' experience. *J Heart Valve Dis* 1993;2:129.
108. Sones FM, Shirey EK: Cine coronary arteriography. *Mod Concepts Cardiovasc Dis.* 1962;31:735.
109. Konstantinov IE: Robert H. Goetz: The surgeon who performed the first successful clinical coronary artery bypass operation. *Ann Thorac Surg* 2000;69:1966.

110. Garrett EH, Dennis EW, DeBakey ME: Aortocoronary bypass with saphenous vein grafts: seven-year follow-up. *JAMA* 1973; 223:792.
111. Shumaker HB Jr: *The Evolution of Cardiac Surgery.* Indianapolis, Indiana University Press, 1992.
112. Demikhov VP: *Experimental Transplantation of Vital Organs.* Authorized translation from the Russian by Basil Haigh. New York, Consultants Bureau, 1962.
113. Kolessov VI: Mammary artery–coronary artery anastomosis as a method of treatment for angina pectoris. *J Thorac Cardiovasc Surg* 1967; 54:535.
114. Green GE, Stertzer SH, Reppert EH: Coronary arterial bypass grafts. *Ann Thorac Surg* 1968; 5:443.
115. Bailey CP, Hirose T: Successful internal mammary–coronary arterial anastomosis using a minivascular suturing technic. *Int Surg* 1968; 49:416.
116. Favalaro RG: Saphenous vein autograft replacement of severe segmental coronary artery occlusion. *Ann Thorac Surg* 1968; 5:334.
117. Johnson WD, Flemma RJ, Lepley D Jr, Ellison EH: Extended treatment of severe coronary artery disease: a total surgical approach. *Ann Surg* 1969; 171:460.
118. Loop FD, Lytle BW, Cosgrove DM, et al: Influence of the internal-mammary-artery graft on 10-year survival and other cardiac events. *NEJM* 1986; 314:1.
119. Cooley DA, Belmonte BA, Zeis LB, Schnur S: Surgical repair of ruptured interventricular septum following acute myocardial infarction. *Surgery* 1957; 41:930.
120. Cooley DA, Henly WS, Amad KH, Chapman DW: Ventricular aneurysm following myocardial infarction: results of surgical treatment. *Ann Surg* 1959; 150:595.
121. Cobb FR, Blumenshein SD, Sealy WC, et al: Successful surgery interruption of the bundle of Kent in a patient with Wolff-Parkinson-White syndrome. *Circulation* 1968; 38:1018.
122. Cox JL: Arrhythmia surgery, in Stephenson LW, Ruggiero R (eds): *Heart Surgery Classics.* Boston, Adams, 1994; p 258.
123. Ross DL, Johnson DC, Denniss AR, et al: Curative surgery for atrioventricular junctional (AV node) reentrant tachycardia. *J Am Coll Cardiol* 1985; 6:1383.
124. Cox JL, Holman WL, Cain ME: Cryosurgical treatment of atrioventricular node reentrant tachycardia. *Circulation* 1987; 76:1329.
125. Cox JL: The surgical treatment of atrial fibrillation, IV surgical technique. *J Thorac Cardiovasc Surg* 1991; 101:584.
126. Guiraudon G, Fontaine G, Frank R, et al: Encircling endocardial ventriculotomy: a new surgical treatment for life-threatening ventricular tachycardias resistant to medical treatment following myocardial infarction. *Ann Thorac Surg* 1978; 26:438.
127. Josephson ME, Harken AH, Horowitz LN: Endocardial excision: A new surgical technique for the treatment of recurrent ventricular tachycardia. *Circulation* 1979; 60:1430.
128. Mirowski M, Reid PR, Mower MM, et al: Termination of malignant ventricular arrhythmias with an implanted automatic defibrillator in human beings. *NEJM* 1980; 303:322.
129. Zoll PM: Resuscitation of the heart in ventricular standstill by external electrical stimulation. *NEJM* 1952; 247:768.
130. Lillehei CW, Gott VL, Hodges PC Jr, et al: Transistor pacemaker for treatment of complete atrioventricular dissociation. *JAMA* 1960; 172:2006.
131. Elmquist R, Senning A: Implantable pacemaker for the heart, in Smyth CN (ed): *Medical Electronics: Proceedings of the Second International Conference on Medical Electronics, Paris, June, 1959.* London, Iliffe & Sons, 1960.
132. Chardack WM, Gage AA, Greatbatch W: Correction of complete heart block by a self-contained and subcutaneously implanted pacemaker: clinical experience with 15 patients. *J Thorac Cardiovasc Surg* 1961; 42:814.
133. Carrel A, Guthrie CC: The transplantation of vein and organs. *Am J Med* 1905; 10:101.
134. Demikhov VP: Experimental transplantation of an additional heart in the dog. *Bull Exp Biol Med (Russia)* 1950; 1:241.
135. Lower RR, Shumway NE: Studies on orthotopic homotransplantation of the canine heart. *Surg Forum* 1960; 11:18.
136. Brock R: Heart excision and replacement. *Guys Hosp Rep* 1959; 108:285.
137. Spencer F: Intellectual creativity in thoracic surgeons. *J Thorac Cardiovasc Surg* 1983; 86:172.
138. Hardy JD, Chavez CM, Hurrus FD, et al: Heart transplantation in man and report of a case. *JAMA* 1964; 188:1132.
139. Barnard CN: A human cardiac transplant: an interim report of a successful operation performed at Groote Schuur Hospital, Cape Town. *South Afr Med J* 1967; 41:1271.
140. Kantrowitz A: Heart, heart-lung and lung transplantation, in Stephenson LW, Ruggiero R (eds): *Heart Surgery Classics.* Boston, Adams, 1994; p 314.
141. Thomson G: Provisional report on the autopsy of LW. *South Afr Med J* 1967; 41:1277.
142. Ruggiero R: Commentary on Barnard CN: a human cardiac transplant: An interim report of a successful operation performed at Groote Schuur Hospital, Cape Town. *South Afr Med J* 1967; 41:1271; In Stephenson LW, Ruggiero R (eds): *Heart Surgery Classics.* Boston, Adams, 1994; p 327.
143. Reitz BA, Wallwork JL, Hunt SA, et al: Heart-lung transplantation: Successful therapy for patients with pulmonary vascular disease. *NEJM* 1982; 306:557.
144. Hardy JD, Webb WR, Dalton ML Jr, Walker GR Jr: Lung homotransplantation in man: report of the initial case. *JAMA* 1963; 286:1065.
145. Derom F, Barbier F, Ringoir S, et al: Ten-month survival after lung homotransplantation in man. *J Thorac Cardiovasc Surg* 1971; 61:835.
146. Cooper JD, Ginsberg RJ, Goldberg M, et al: Unilateral lung transplantation for pulmonary fibrosis. *NEJM* 1986; 314:1140.
147. Kantrowitz A, Tjonneland S, Freed PS, et al: Initial clinical experience with intra-aortic balloon pumping in cardiogenic shock. *JAMA* 1968; 203:135.
148. Liotta D, Hall W, Henly WS, et al: Prolonged assisted circulation during and after cardiac or aortic surgery: prolonged partial left ventricular bypass by means of intracorporeal circulation. *Am J Cardiol* 1963;1 2:399.
149. Shumaker HB Jr: *The Evolution of Cardiac Surgery.* Bloomington, University Press, 1992.
150. DeBakey ME: Left ventricular heart assist devices, in Stephenson LW, Ruggiero R (eds): *Heart Surgery Classics.* Boston, Adams, 1994.
151. Cooley DA, Liotta D, Hallman GL, et al: Orthotopic cardiac prosthesis for two-staged cardiac replacement. *Am J Cardiol* 1969; 24:723.
152. Hill JD, Farrar DJ, Hershon JJ, et al: Use of a prosthetic ventricle as a bridge to cardiac transplantation for postinfarction cardiogenic shock. *NEJM* 1986; 314:626.
153. Starnes VA, Ayer PE, Portner PM, et al: Isolated left ventricular assist as bridge to cardiac transplantation. *J Thorac Cardiovasc Surg* 1988; 96:62.
154. DeVries WC, Anderson JL, Joyce LD, et al: Clinical use of total artificial heart. *NEJM* 1984; 310:273.
155. Edwards WS, Edwards PD: *Alexis Carrel: Visionary Surgeon.* Springfield, IL, Charles C Thomas, 1974.
156. Acierno LJ: *The History of Cardiology.* New York, Parthenon, 1994.
157. DeBakey ME, Simeone FA: Battle injuries of the arteries in World War II. *Am J Surg* 1946; 123:534.
158. Shumaker HB: Surgical cure of innominate aneurysm: report of a case with comments on the applicability of surgical measures. *Surgery* 1947; 22:739.
159. Swan HC, Maaske M, Johnson M, Grover R: Arterial homografts: II. Resection of thoracic aneurysm using a stored human arterial transplant. *Arch Surg* 1950; 61:732.
160. Gross RE: Treatment of certain aortic coarctations by homologous grafts: a report of nineteen cases. *Ann Surg* 1951; 134:753.
161. DuBost C, Allary M, Oeconomos N: Resection of an aneurysm of the abdominal aorta: reestablishment of the continuity by a preserved human arterial graft, with results after five months. *Arch Surg* 1952; 62:405.
162. Bahnson HT: Definitive treatment of saccular aneurysms of the aorta with excision of sac and aortic suture. *Surg Gynecol Obstet* 1953; 96:383.
163. DeBakey ME, Cooley DA: Successful resection of aneurysm of thoracic aorta and replacement by graft. *JAMA* 1953; 152:673.
164. Hughes CW: Acute vascular trauma in Korean War casualties. *Surg Gynecol Obstet* 1954; 99:91.
165. Voorhees AB Jr, Janetzky A III, Blakemore AH: The use of tubes constructed from Vinyon-N cloth in bridging defects. *Ann Surg* 1952; 135:332.
166. DeBakey ME, Cooley DA, Creech O Jr: Surgical consideration of dissecting aneurysm of the aorta. *Ann Surg* 1955; 142:586.
167. Wheat MW Jr, Palmer RF, Bartley TD, Seelman RC: Treatment of dissecting aneurysms of the aorta without surgery. *J Thorac Cardiovasc Surg* 1965; 50:364.
168. Cooley DA, DeBakey ME: Resection of entire ascending aorta in fusiform aneurysm using cardiac bypass. *JAMA* 1956; 162:1158.
169. DeBakey ME, Creech O Jr, Morris GC Jr: Aneurysm of the thoracoabdominal aorta involving the celiac superior mesenteric, and renal arteries: report of four cases treated by resection and homo-graft replacement. *Ann Surg* 1956; 144:549.
170. DeBakey ME, Crawford ES, Cooley DA, Morris GC Jr: Successful resection of fusiform aneurysm of aortic arch with replacement by homograft. *Surg Gynecol Obstet* 1957; 105:657.
171. Cooley DA, Mahaffey DE, DeBakey ME: Total excision of the aortic arch for aneurysm. *Surg Gynecol Obstet* 1955; 101;667.

172. Bentall H, De Bono A: A technique for complete replacement of the ascending aorta. *Thorax* 1968; 23:338.
173. Starr A, Edwards WL, McCord MD, et al: Aortic replacement. *Circulation* 1963; 27:779.
174. Wheat MW Jr, Wilson JR, Bartley TD: Successful replacement of the entire ascending aorta and aortic valve. *JAMA* 1964; 188:717.
175. Miller C: Stent-grafts: avoiding major aortic surgery, in Stephenson LW, (ed): *State of the Heart: The Practical Guide to Your Heart and Heart Surgery* Fort Lauderdale, Write Stuff, 1999; p 230.
176. Parodi JC, Palmaz JC, Barone HD: Transfemoral intraluminal graft implantation for abdominal aortic aneurysms. *Ann Vasc Surg* 1991; 5:491.

CHAPTER 2

Surgical Anatomy of the Heart

Michael R. Mill
Robert H. Anderson
Lawrence H. Cohn

A thorough knowledge of the anatomy of the heart is a prerequisite for the successful completion of the myriad procedures performed by the cardiothoracic surgeon. This chapter describes the normal anatomy of the heart, including its position and relationship to other thoracic organs. It also describes the incisions used to expose the heart for various operations, and discusses in detail the cardiac chambers and valves, coronary arteries and veins, and the important but surgically invisible conduction tissues.

OVERVIEW

Location of the Heart Relative to Surrounding Structures

The overall shape of the heart is that of a three-sided pyramid located in the middle mediastinum (Fig. 2-1). When viewed from the heart's apex, the three sides of the ventricular mass are readily apparent (Fig. 2-2). Two of the edges are named. The *acute margin* lies inferiorly and describes a sharp angle between the sternocostal and diaphragmatic surfaces. The *obtuse margin* lies superiorly and is much more diffuse. The posterior margin is unnamed but is also diffuse in its transition.

One-third of the cardiac mass lies to the right of the midline and two-thirds to the left. The long axis of the heart is oriented from the left epigastrium to the right shoulder. The short axis, which corresponds to the plane of the atrioventricular groove, is oblique and is oriented closer to the vertical than the horizontal plane (see Fig. 2-1).

Anteriorly, the heart is covered by the sternum and the costal cartilages of the third, fourth, and fifth ribs. The lungs contact the lateral surfaces of the heart, whereas the heart abuts onto the pulmonary hila posteriorly. The right lung overlies the right surface of the heart and reaches to the midline. In contrast, the left lung retracts from the midline in the area of the cardiac notch. The heart has an extensive diaphragmatic surface inferiorly. Posteriorly, the heart lies on the esophagus and the tracheal bifurcation and bronchi that extend into the lung. The sternum lies anteriorly and provides rigid protection to the heart during blunt trauma and is aided by the cushioning effects of the lungs.

The Pericardium and Its Reflections

The heart lies within the pericardium, which is attached to the walls of the great vessels and the diaphragm. The pericardium can be visualized best as a bag into which the heart has been placed apex first. The inner layer, in direct contact with the heart, is the *visceral epicardium,* which encases the heart and extends several centimeters back onto the walls of the great vessels. The outer layer forms the *parietal pericardium,* which lines the inner surface of the tough fibrous pericardial sack. A thin film of lubricating fluid lies within the pericardial cavity between the two serous layers. Two identifiable recesses lie within the pericardium and are lined by the serous layer. The first is the *transverse sinus,* which is delineated anteriorly by the posterior surface of the aorta and pulmonary trunk and posteriorly by the anterior surface of the interatrial groove. The second is the *oblique sinus,* a cul-de-sac located behind the left atrium, delineated by serous pericardial reflections from the pulmonary veins and the inferior vena cava.

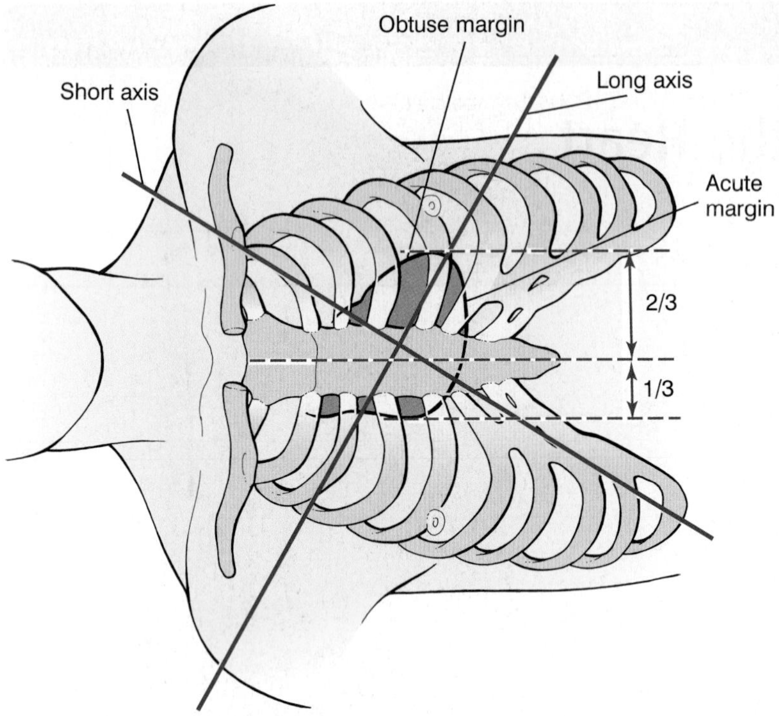

FIGURE 2-1 This diagram shows the heart within the middle mediastinum with the patient supine on the operating table. The long axis lies parallel to the interventricular septum, whereas the short axis is perpendicular to the long axis at the level of the atrioventricular valves.

Mediastinal Nerves and Their Relationships to the Heart

The vagus and phrenic nerves descend through the mediastinum in close relationship to the heart (Fig. 2-3). They enter through the thoracic inlet, with the phrenic nerve located anteriorly on the surface of the anterior scalene muscle and lying just posterior to the internal thoracic artery (internal mammary artery) at the thoracic inlet. In this position, the phrenic nerve is vulnerable to injury during dissection and preparation of the internal thoracic artery for use in coronary arterial bypass grafting. On the right side, the phrenic nerve courses on the lateral surface of the superior vena cava, again in harm's way

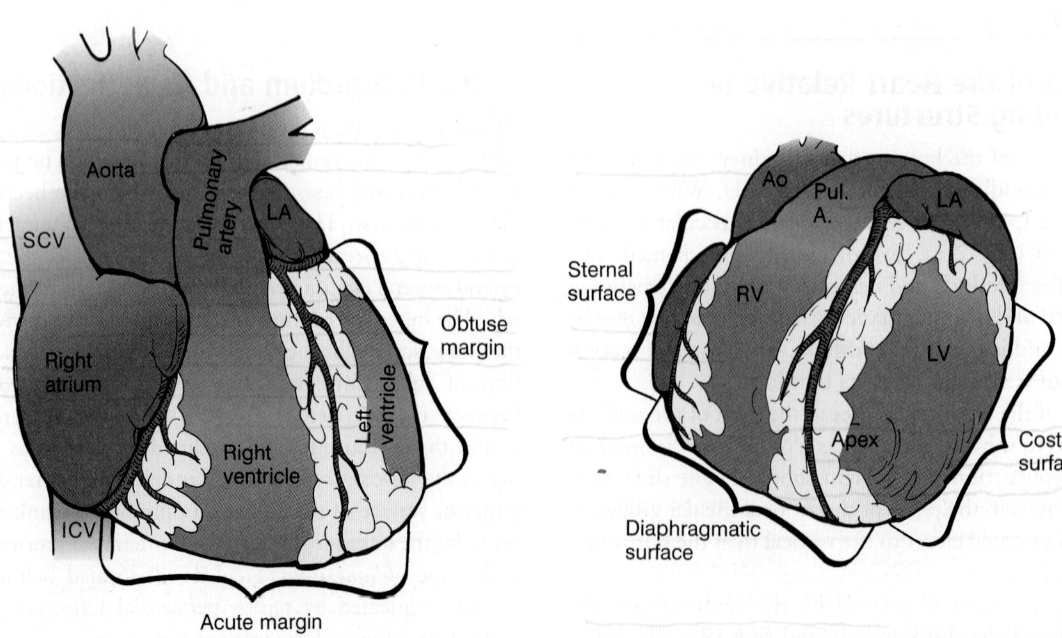

FIGURE 2-2 This diagram shows the surfaces and margins of the heart as viewed anteriorly with the patient supine on the operating table (*left*) and as viewed from the cardiac apex (*right*).

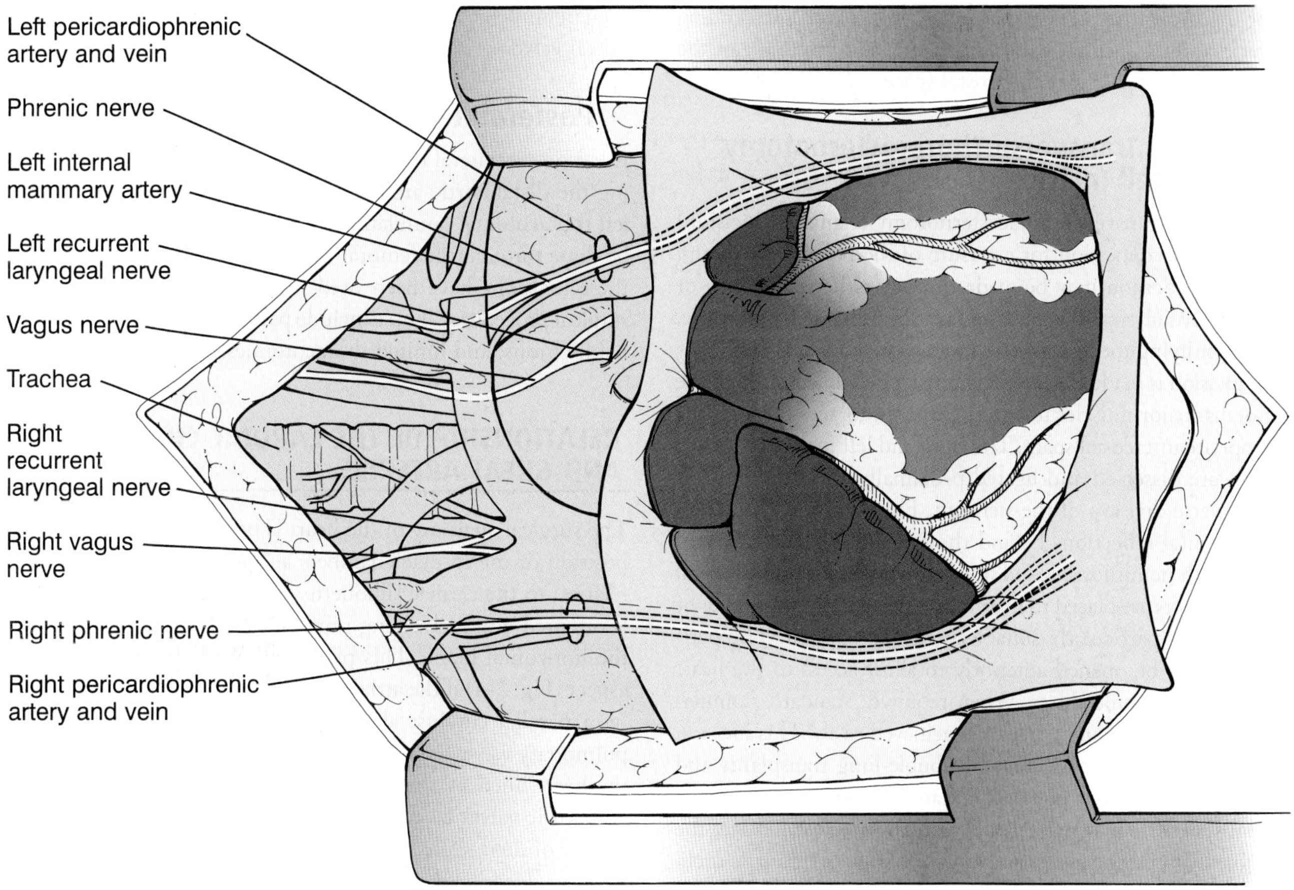

FIGURE 2-3 Diagram of the heart in relation to the vagus and phrenic nerves as viewed through a median sternotomy.

during dissection for venous cannulation for cardiopulmonary bypass. The nerve then descends anterior to the pulmonary hilum before reflecting onto the right diaphragm, where it branches to provide its innervation. In the presence of a left-sided superior vena cava, the left phrenic nerve is applied directly to its lateral surface. The nerve passes anterior to the pulmonary hilum and eventually branches on the surface of the diaphragm. The vagus nerves enter the thorax posterior to the phrenic nerves and course along the carotid arteries. On the right side, the vagus gives off the recurrent laryngeal nerve that passes around the right subclavian artery before ascending out of the thoracic cavity. The right vagus nerve continues posterior to the pulmonary hilum, gives off branches of the right pulmonary plexus, and exits the thorax along the esophagus. On the left, the vagus nerve crosses the aortic arch, where it gives off the recurrent laryngeal branch. The recurrent nerve passes around the arterial ligament before ascending in the tracheoesophageal groove. The vagus nerve continues posterior to the pulmonary hilum, gives rise to the left pulmonary plexus, and then continues inferiorly out of the thorax along the esophagus. A delicate nerve trunk known as the *subclavian loop* carries fibers from the stellate ganglion to the eye and head. This branch is located adjacent to the subclavian arteries bilaterally. Excessive dissection of the subclavian artery during shunt procedures may injure these nerve roots and cause Horner syndrome.

SURGICAL INCISIONS

Median Sternotomy

The most common approach for operations on the heart and aortic arch is the median sternotomy. The skin incision is made from the jugular notch to just below the xiphoid process. The subcutaneous tissues and presternal fascia are incised to expose the periostium of the sternum. The sternum is divided longitudinally in the midline. After placement of a sternal spreader, the thymic fat pad is divided up to the level of the brachiocephalic vein. An avascular midline plane is identified easily but is crossed by a few thymic veins that are divided between fine silk ties or hemoclips. Either the left or right or, occasionally, both lobes of the thymus gland are removed in infants and young children to improve exposure and minimize compression on extracardiac conduits. If a portion of the thymus gland is removed, excessive traction may result in injury to the phrenic nerve. The pericardium is opened anteriorly to expose the heart. Through this incision, operations within any chamber of the heart or on the surface of the heart and operations involving the proximal aorta, pulmonary trunk, and their primary branches can be performed. Extension of the superior extent of the incision into the neck along the anterior border of the right sternocleidomastoid muscle provides further exposure of the aortic arch and its branches for procedures involving these structures. Exposure of the proximal descending thoracic aorta is facilitated by a perpendicular extension of the incision through the third intercostal space.

Bilateral Transverse Thoracosternotomy (Clamshell Incision)

The bilateral transverse thoracosternotomy (clamshell incision) is an alternative incision for exposure of the pleural spaces and heart. This incision may be made through either the fourth or fifth intercostal space, depending on the intended procedure. After identifying the appropriate interspace, a bilateral submammary incision is made. The incision is extended down through the pectoralis major muscles to enter the hemithoraces through the appropriate intercostal space. The right and left internal thoracic arteries are dissected and ligated proximally and distally prior to transverse division of the sternum. Electrocautery dissection of the pleural reflections behind the sternum allows full exposure of both hemithoraces and the entire mediastinum. Bilateral chest spreaders are placed to maintain exposure. Morse or Haight retractors are particularly suitable with this incision. The pericardium may be opened anteriorly to allow access to the heart for intracardiac procedures. When required, standard cannulation for cardiopulmonary bypass is achieved easily. This incision is popular for bilateral sequential double-lung transplants and heart-lung transplants because of enhanced exposure of the apical pleural spaces. When made in the fourth intercostal space, the incision is useful for access to the ascending aorta, aortic arch, and descending thoracic aorta.

Anterolateral Thoracotomy

The right side of the heart can be exposed through a right anterolateral thoracotomy. The patient is positioned supine, with the right chest elevated to approximately 30 degrees by a roll beneath the shoulder. An anterolateral thoracotomy incision can be made that can be extended across the midline by transversely dividing the sternum if necessary. With the lung retracted posteriorly, the pericardium can be opened just anterior to the right phrenic nerve and pulmonary hilum to expose the right and left atria. The incision provides access to both the tricuspid and mitral valves and the right coronary artery. Cannulation may be performed in the ascending aorta and the superior and inferior venae cavae. Aortic cross-clamping, administration of cardioplegia, and removal of air from the heart after cardiotomy are difficult with this approach. This incision is particularly useful nonetheless for performance of the Blalock-Hanlon atrial septectomy or valve replacement after a previous procedure through a median sternotomy. A left anterolateral thoracotomy performed in a similar fashion to that on the right side may be used for isolated bypass grafting of the circumflex coronary artery or for left-sided exposure of the mitral valve.

Posterolateral Thoracotomy

A left posterolateral thoracotomy is used for procedures involving the distal aortic arch and descending thoracic aorta. With left thoracotomy, cannulation for cardiopulmonary bypass must be done through the femoral vessels. A number of variations of these incisions have been used for minimally invasive cardiac surgical procedures. These include partial sternotomies, parasternal incisions, and limited thoracotomies.

RELATIONSHIP OF THE CARDIAC CHAMBERS AND GREAT ARTERIES

The surgical anatomy of the heart is best understood when the position of the cardiac chambers and great vessels is known in relation to the cardiac silhouette. The atrioventricular junction is oriented obliquely, lying much closer to the vertical than to the horizontal plane. This plane can be viewed from its atrial aspect (Fig. 2-4) if the atrial mass and great arteries are removed by a parallel cut just above the junction. The tricuspid and pulmonary valves are widely separated by the inner curvature of the heart lined by the transverse sinus. Conversely, the mitral and aortic valves lie adjacent to one another, with fibrous continuity of their leaflets. The aortic valve occupies a central position, wedged between the tricuspid and pulmonary valves. Indeed, there is fibrous continuity between the leaflets of the aortic and tricuspid valves through the central fibrous body.

With careful study of this short axis, several basic rules of cardiac anatomy become apparent. First, the atrial chambers lie to the right of their corresponding ventricles. Second, the right atrium and ventricle lie anterior to their left-sided counterparts. The septal structures between them are obliquely oriented. Third, by virtue of its wedged position, the aortic valve is

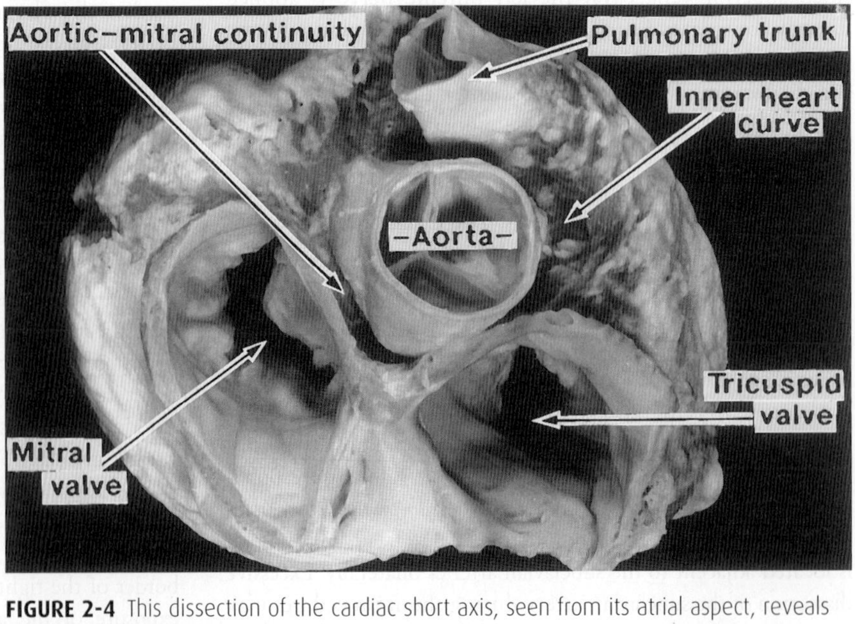

FIGURE 2-4 This dissection of the cardiac short axis, seen from its atrial aspect, reveals the relationships of the cardiac valves.

directly related to all the cardiac chambers. Several other significant features of cardiac anatomy can be learned from the short-axis section. The position of the aortic valve minimizes the area of septum where the mitral and tricuspid valves attach opposite each other. Because the tricuspid valve is attached to the septum further toward the ventricular apex than the mitral valve, a part of the septum is interposed between the right atrium and the left ventricle to produce the muscular atrioventricular septum. The central fibrous body, where the leaflets of the aortic, mitral, and tricuspid valves all converge, lies cephalad and anterior to the muscular atrioventricular septum. The central fibrous body is the main component of the fibrous skeleton of the heart and is made up in part by the right fibrous trigone, a thickening of the right side of the area of fibrous continuity between the aortic and mitral valves, and in part by the membranous septum, the fibrous partition between the left ventricular outflow tract and the right-sided heart chambers (Fig. 2-5). The membranous septum itself is divided into two parts by the septal leaflet of the tricuspid valve, which is directly attached across it (Fig. 2-6). Thus the membranous septum has an atrioventricular component between the right atrium and left ventricle, as well as an interventricular component. Removal of the noncoronary leaflet of the aortic valve demonstrates the significance of the wedged position of the left ventricular outflow tract in relation to the other cardiac chambers. The subaortic region separates the mitral orifice from the ventricular septum; this separation influences the position of the atrioventricular conduction tissues and the position of the leaflets and tension apparatus of the mitral valve (Fig. 2-7).

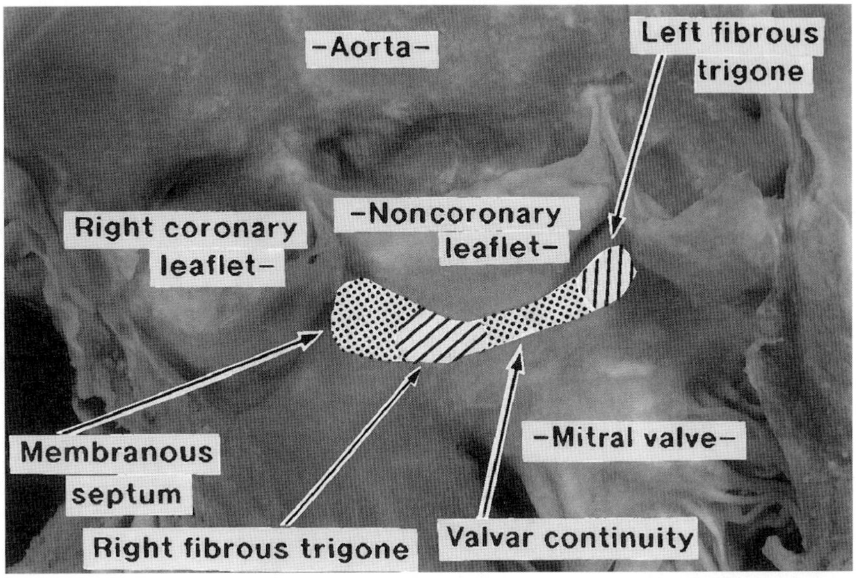

FIGURE 2-5 This view of the left ventricular outflow tract, as seen from the front in anatomical orientation, shows the limited extent of the fibrous skeleton of the heart.

THE RIGHT ATRIUM AND TRICUSPID VALVE

Appendage, Vestibule, and Venous Component

The right atrium has three basic parts: the appendage, the vestibule, and the venous component (Fig. 2-8). Externally, the right atrium is divided into the appendage and the venous component, which receives the systemic venous return. The junction of the appendage and the venous component is identified by a prominent groove, the *terminal groove.* This corresponds internally to the location of the terminal crest. The right atrial appendage has the shape of a blunt triangle, with a wide junction to the venous component across the terminal groove. The appendage also has an extensive junction with the vestibule of the right atrium; the latter structure is the smooth-walled atrial myocardium that inserts into the leaflets of the tricuspid valve. The most characteristic and constant feature of the morphology of the right atrium is that the pectinate muscles within

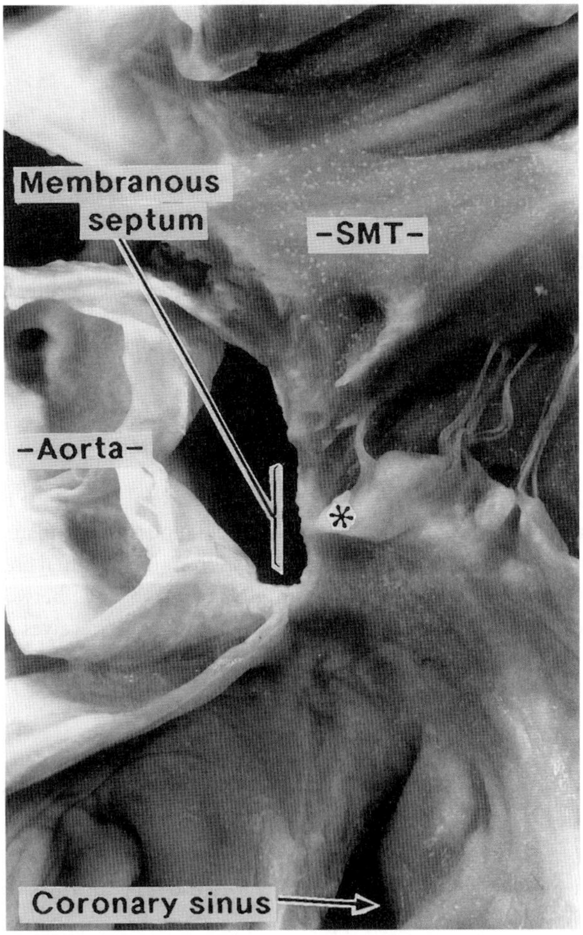

FIGURE 2-6 This dissection, made by removing the right coronary sinus of the aortic valve, shows how the septal leaflet of the tricuspid valve (*asterisk*) divides the membranous septum into its atrioventricular and interventricular components. SMT = septomarginal trabeculation.

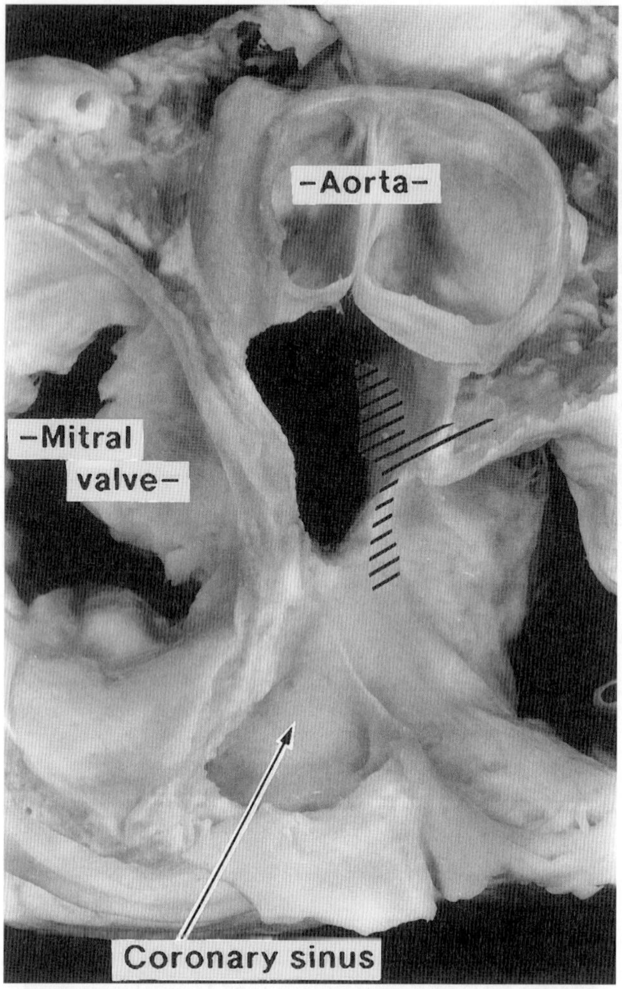

FIGURE 2-7 This dissection, made by removing the noncoronary aortic sinus (compare with Figs. 2-4 and 2-6), shows the approximate location of the atrioventricular conduction axis (*hatched area*) and the relationship of the mitral valve to the ventricular septum.

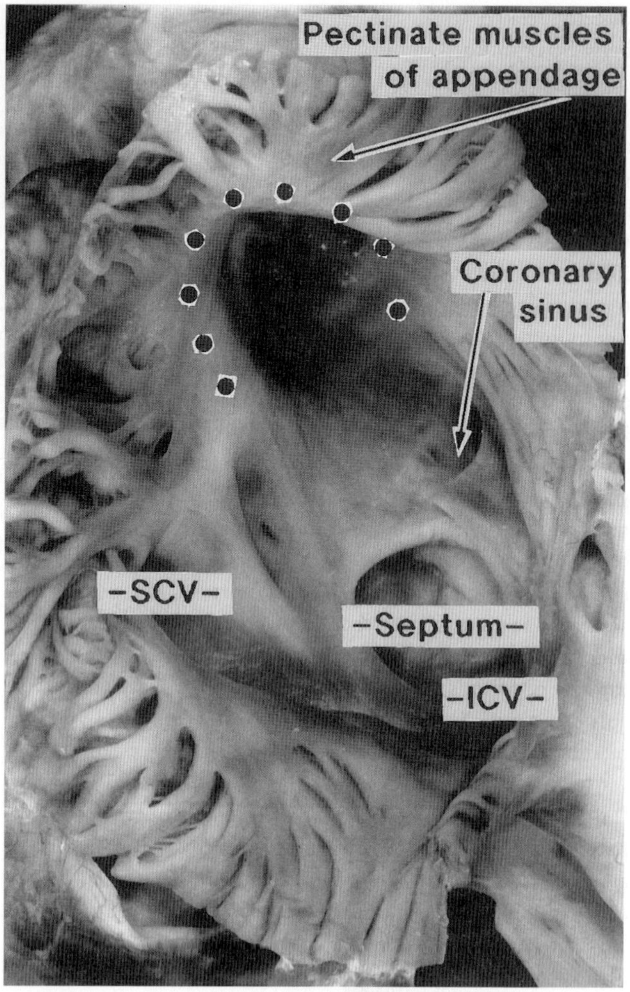

FIGURE 2-8 This view of the right atrium, seen in surgical orientation, shows the pectinate muscles lining the appendage, the smooth vestibule (*circles*) surrounding the orifice of the tricuspid valve, and the superior vena cava (SCV), inferior vena cava (ICV), and coronary sinus joining the smooth-walled venous component. Note the prominent rim enclosing the oval fossa, which is the true atrial septum (see Fig. 2-11).

the appendage extend around the entire parietal margin of the atrioventricular junction (Fig. 2-9). These muscles originate as parallel fibers that course at right angles from the terminal crest. The venous component of the right atrium extends between the terminal groove and the interatrial groove. It receives the superior and inferior venae cavae and the coronary sinus.

Sinus Node

The sinus node lies at the anterior and superior extent of the terminal groove, where the atrial appendage and the superior vena cava are juxtaposed. The node is a spindle-shaped structure that usually lies to the right or lateral to the superior cavoatrial junction (Fig. 2-10). In approximately 10% of cases, the node is draped across the cavoatrial junction in horseshoe fashion.[1]

The blood supply to the sinus node is from a prominent nodal artery that is a branch of the right coronary artery in approximately 55% of individuals and a branch of the circumflex artery in the remainder. Regardless of its artery of origin, the nodal artery usually courses along the anterior interatrial groove toward the superior cavoatrial junction, frequently within the atrial myocardium. At the cavoatrial junction, its course becomes variable and may circle either anteriorly or posteriorly or, rarely, both anteriorly and posteriorly around the cavoatrial junction to enter the node. Uncommonly, the artery arises more distally from the right coronary artery and courses laterally across the atrial appendage. This places it at risk of injury during a standard right atriotomy. The artery also may arise distally from the circumflex artery to cross the dome of the left atrium, where it is at risk of injury when using a superior approach to the mitral valve. Incisions in either the right or left atrial chambers always should be made with this anatomical variability in mind. In our experience, these vessels can be identified by careful gross inspection, and prompt modification of surgical incisions can be made accordingly.

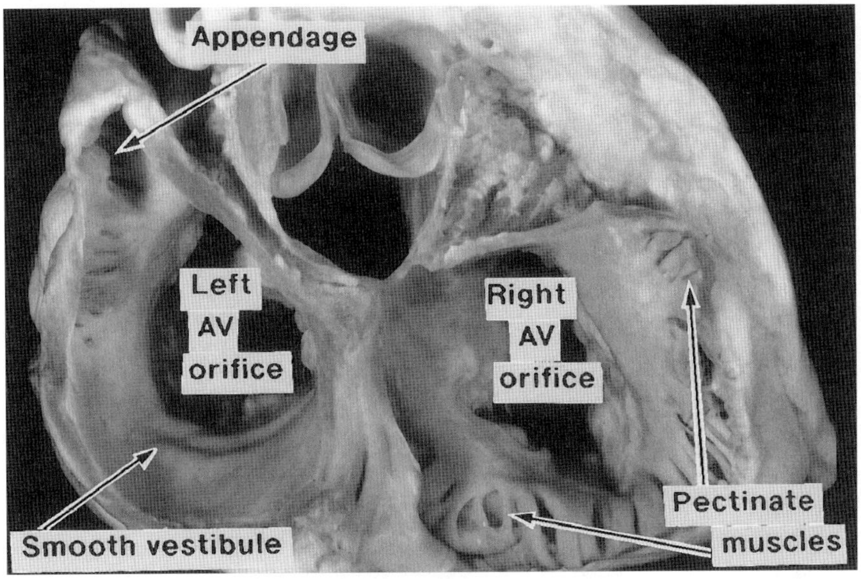

FIGURE 2-9 This dissection of the short axis of the heart (compare with Fig. 2-4) shows how the pectinate muscles extend around the parietal margin of the tricuspid valve. In the left atrium, the pectinate muscles are confined within the tubular left atrial appendage, leaving the smooth vestibule around the mitral valve confluent with the pulmonary venous component of the left atrium.

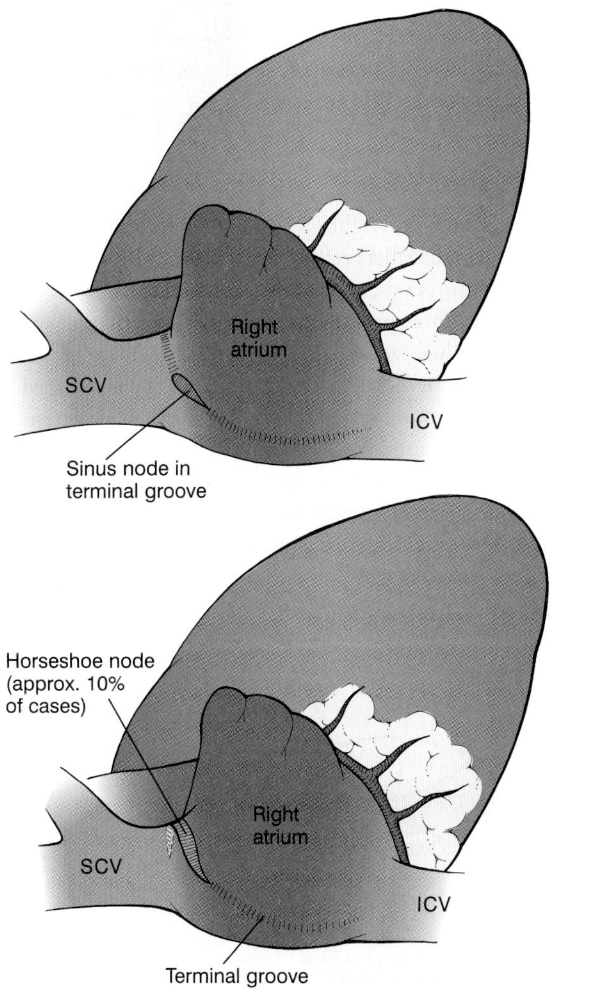

FIGURE 2-10 This diagram shows the location of the sinus node at the superior cavoatrial junction. The node usually lies to the right (*lateral*) side of the junction but may be draped in horseshoe fashion across the anterior aspect of the junction. ICV = inferior vena cava; SCV = superior vena cava.

Atrial Septum

The most common incision into the right atrium is made into the atrial appendage parallel and anterior to the terminal groove. Opening the atrium through this incision confirms that the terminal groove is the external marking of the prominent terminal crest. Anteriorly and superiorly, the crest curves in front of the orifice of the superior vena cava to become continuous with the so-called septum secundum, which, in reality, is the superior rim of the oval fossa. When the right atrium is inspected through this incision, there appears to be an extensive septal surface between the tricuspid valve and the orifices of the venae cavae. This septal surface includes the opening of the oval fossa and the orifice of the coronary sinus. The apparent extent of the septum is spurious because the true septum between the atrial chambers is virtually confined to the oval fossa[2,3] (Fig. 2-11). The superior rim of the fossa, although often referred to as the *septum secundum,* is an extensive infolding between the venous component of the right atrium and the right pulmonary veins. The inferior rim is directly continuous with the so-called sinus septum that separates the orifices of the inferior caval vein and the coronary sinus (Fig. 2-12).

The region around the coronary sinus is where the right atrial wall overlies the atrioventricular muscular septum. Removing the floor of the coronary sinus reveals the anterior extension of the atrioventricular groove in this region. Only a small part of the anterior rim of the oval fossa is a septal structure. The majority is made up of the anterior atrial wall overlying the aortic root. Thus dissection outside the limited margins of the oval fossa will penetrate the heart to the outside rather than provide access to the left atrium via the septum.

Atrioventricular Septum and Node: Triangle of Koch

In addition to the sinus node, another major area of surgical significance is occupied by the atrioventricular node. This structure lies within the triangle of Koch, which is demarcated

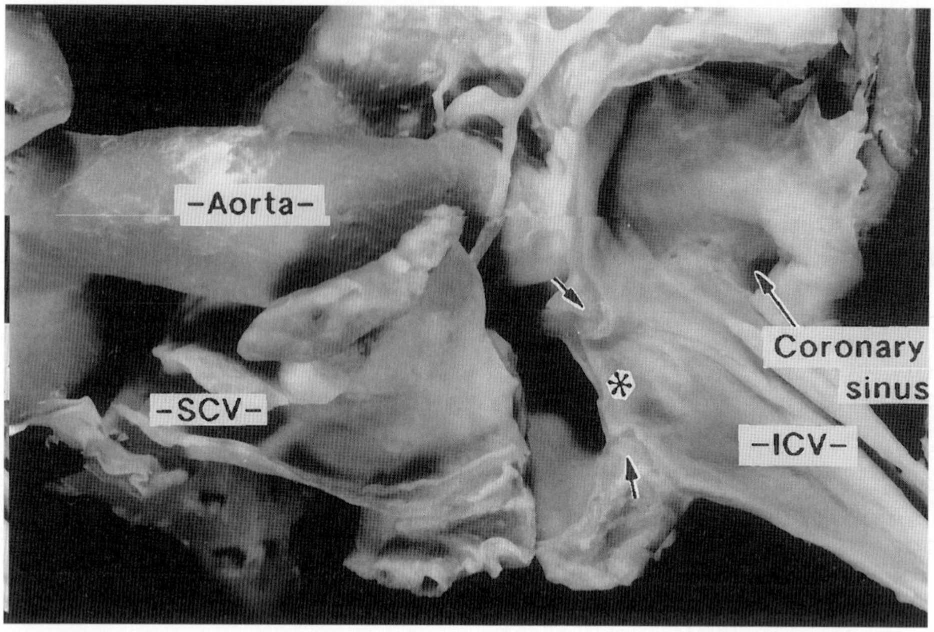

FIGURE 2-11 This transection across the middle of the oval fossa (*asterisk*) shows how the so-called septum secundum, the rim of the fossa, is made up of the infolded atrial walls (*arrows*). ICV = inferior vena cava; SCV = superior vena cava.

by the tendon of Todaro, the septal leaflet of the tricuspid valve, and the orifice of the coronary sinus (Fig. 2-13). The tendon of Todaro is a fibrous structure formed by the junction of the eustachian valve and thebesian valve (the valves of the inferior vena cava and the coronary sinus, respectively). The entire atrial component of the atrioventricular conduction tissues is contained within the triangle of Koch, which must be avoided to prevent surgical damage to atrioventricular conduction. The atrioventricular bundle (of His) penetrates directly at the apex of the triangle of Koch before it continues to branch on the crest of the ventricular septum (Fig. 2-14). The key to avoiding atrial arrhythmias is careful preservation of the sinus and atrioventricular nodes and their blood supply. No advantage is gained in attempting to preserve nonexistent tracts of specialized atrial conduction tissue, although it makes sense to avoid prominent muscle bundles where parallel orientation of atrial myocardial fibers favors preferential conduction (Fig. 2-15).

Tricuspid Valve

The vestibule of the right atrium converges into the tricuspid valve. The three leaflets reflect their anatomical location, being septal, anterosuperior, and inferior (or mural). The leaflets join together over three prominent zones of apposition; the peripheral ends of these zones usually are described as *commissures.* The leaflets are tethered at the commissures by fan-shaped cords arising from prominent papillary muscles. The anteroseptal commissure is supported by the medial papillary muscle. The major leaflets of the valve extend from this position in anterosuperior and septal directions. The third leaflet is less well defined. The anteroinferior commissure is usually supported by

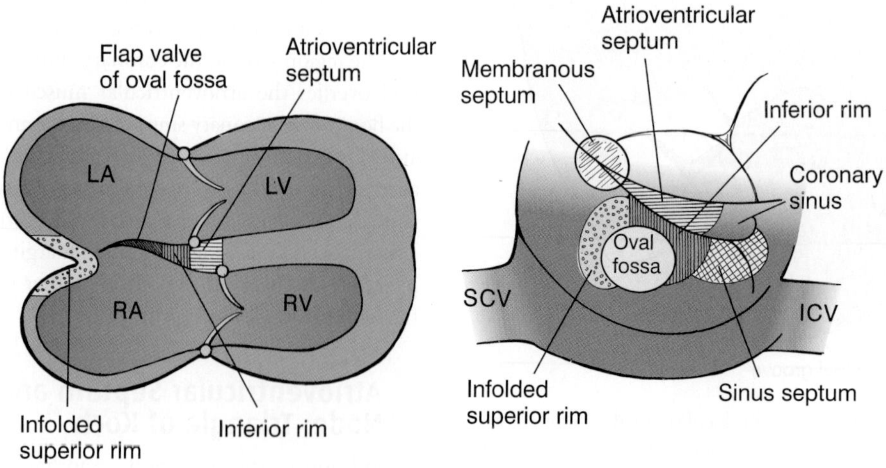

FIGURE 2-12 This diagram demonstrates the components of the atrial septum. The only true septum between the two atria is confined to the area of the oval fossa. ICV = inferior vena cava; SCV = superior vena cava.

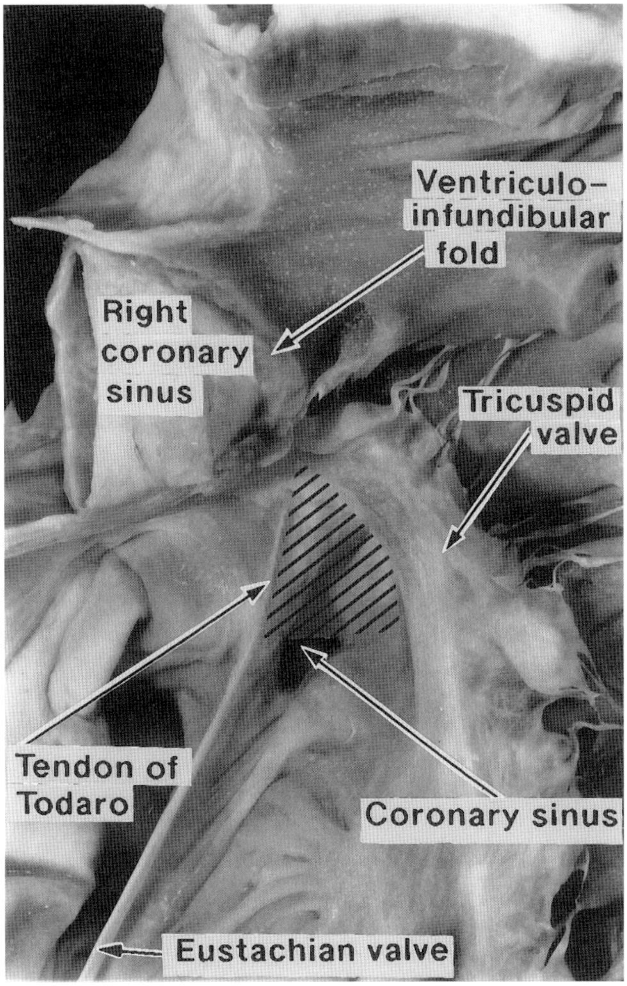

FIGURE 2-13 This dissection, made by removing part of the subpulmonary infundibulum, shows the location of the triangle of Koch (*shaded area*).

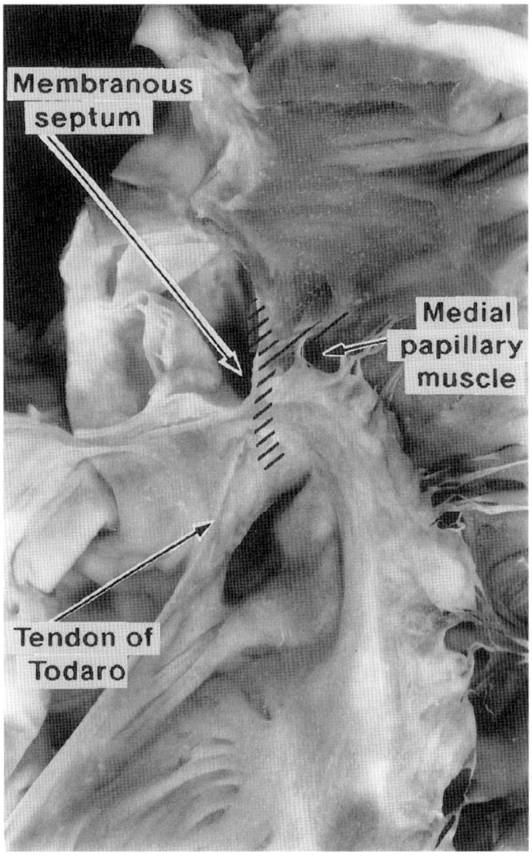

FIGURE 2-14 Further dissection of the heart shown in Fig. 2-13 reveals that a line joining the apex of the triangle of Koch to the medial papillary muscle marks the location of the atrioventricular conduction axis.

the prominent anterior papillary muscle. Often, however, it is not possible to identify a specific inferior papillary muscle supporting the inferoseptal commissure. Thus the inferior leaflet may seem duplicated. There is no well-formed collagenous annulus for the tricuspid valve. Instead, the atrioventricular groove more or less folds directly into the tricuspid valvar leaflets at the vestibule, and the atrial and ventricular myocardial masses are separated almost exclusively by the fibrofatty tissue of the groove. The entire parietal attachment of the tricuspid valve usually is encircled by the right coronary artery running within the atrioventricular groove.

THE LEFT ATRIUM AND MITRAL VALVE

Appendage, Vestibule, and Venous Component

Like the right atrium, the left atrium has three basic components: the appendage, the vestibule, and the venous component (Fig. 2-16). Unlike the right atrium, the venous component is considerably larger than the appendage and has a narrow junction with it that is not marked by a terminal groove or crest. There also is an important difference between the relationship of the appendage and vestibule between the left and right atria. As shown, the pectinate muscles within the right atrial appendage extend all around the parietal margin of the vestibule. In contrast, the left atrial appendage has a limited junction with the vestibule, and the pectinate muscles are located almost exclusively within the appendage (see Fig. 2-8). The larger part of the vestibule that supports and inserts directly into the mural leaflet of the mitral valve is directly continuous with the smooth atrial wall of the pulmonary venous component.

Because the left atrium is posterior to and tethered by the four pulmonary veins, the chamber is relatively inaccessible. Surgeons use several approaches to gain access. The most common is an incision just to the right of and parallel to the interatrial groove, anterior to the right pulmonary veins. This incision can be carried beneath both the superior and inferior venae cavae parallel to the interatrial groove to provide wide access to the left atrium. A second approach is through the dome of the left atrium. If the aorta is pulled anteriorly and to the left, an extensive trough may be seen between the right and left atrial appendages. An incision through this trough, between the pulmonary veins of the upper lobes, provides direct access to the left atrium. When this incision is made, it is important to remember the location of the sinus node artery, which may course along the roof of the left atrium if it arises from

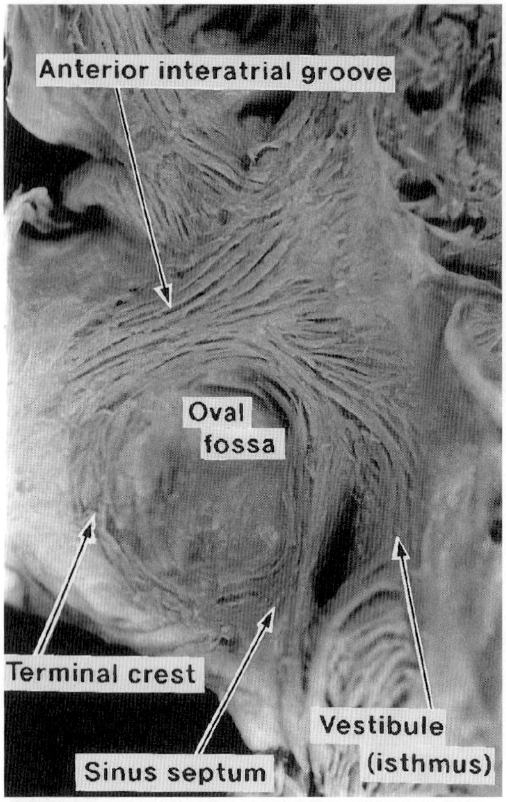

FIGURE 2-15 This dissection, made by careful removal of the right atrial endocardium, shows the ordered arrangement of myocardial fibers in the prominent muscle bundles that underscore preferential conduction. There are *no* insulated tracts running within the internodal atrial myocardium. (*Dissection made by Prof. Damian Sanchez-Quintana.*)

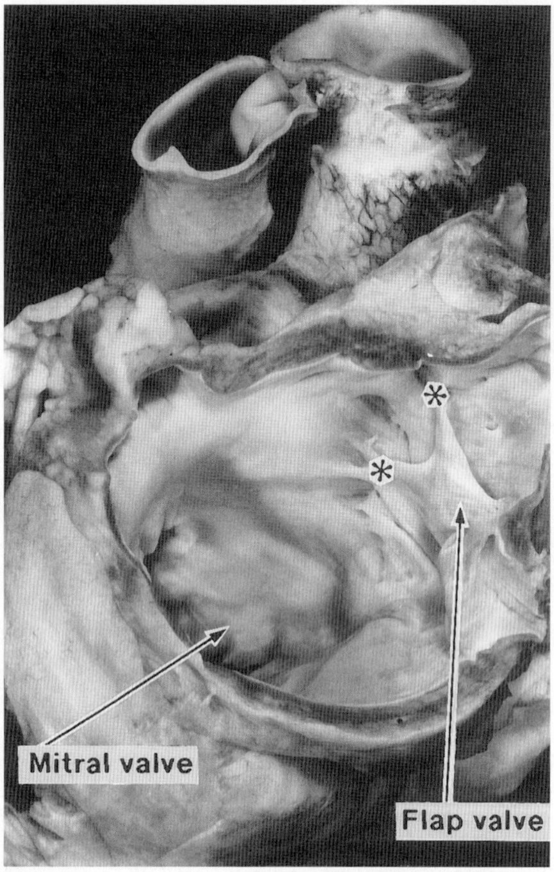

FIGURE 2-17 This view of the opened left atrium shows how the septal aspect is dominated by the flap valve, which is attached by its horns (*asterisks*) to the infolded atrial groove.

the circumflex artery. The left atrium also can be reached via a right atrial incision and an opening in the atrial septum.

When the interior of the left atrium is visualized, the small size of the mouth of the left atrial appendage is apparent. It lies to the left of the mitral orifice as viewed by the surgeon. The majority of the pulmonary venous atrium usually is located inferiorly away from the operative field. The vestibule of the mitral orifice dominates the operative view. The septal surface is located anteriorly, with the true septum relatively inferior (Fig. 2-17).

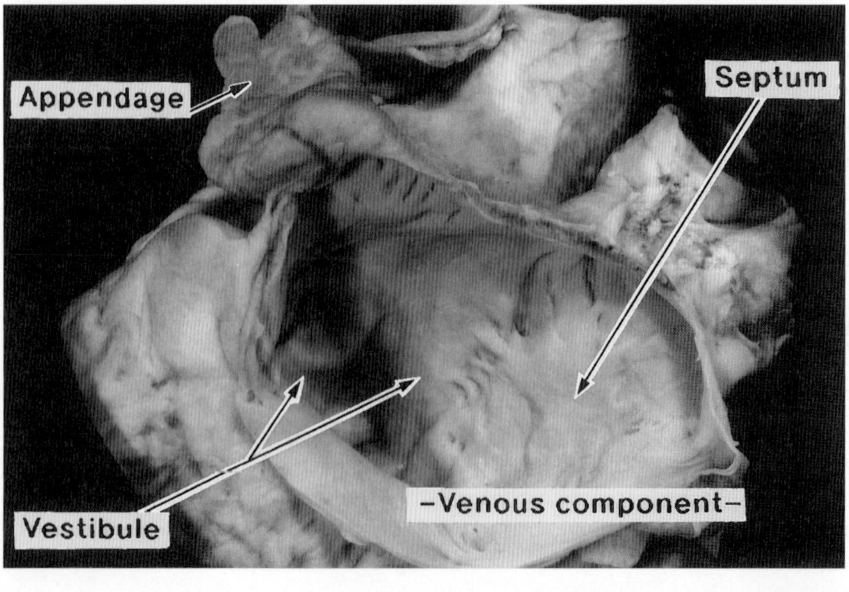

FIGURE 2-16 Like the right atrium, the left atrium (seen here in anatomical orientation) has an appendage, a venous component, and a vestibule. It is separated from the right atrium by the septum.

Mitral Valve

The mitral valve is supported by two prominent papillary muscles located in anterolateral and posteromedial positions. The two leaflets of the mitral valve have markedly different appearances (Fig. 2-18). The aortic (or anterior) leaflet is short, relatively square, and guards approximately one-third of the circumference of the valvar orifice. This leaflet is in fibrous continuity with the aortic valve and, because of this, is best referred to as the *aortic leaflet* because it is neither strictly anterior nor superior in position. The other leaflet is much shallower but guards approximately two-thirds of the circumference of the mitral orifice. Because it is connected to the parietal part of the atrioventricular junction, it is most accurately termed the *mural leaflet* but often is termed the *posterior leaflet.* It is divided into a number of subunits that fold against the aortic leaflet when the valve is closed. Although generally there are three, there may be as many as five or six scallops in the mural leaflet.

Unlike the tricuspid valve, the mitral valve leaflets are supported by a rather dense collagenous annulus, although it may take the form of a sheet rather than a cord. This annulus usually extends parietally from the fibrous trigones, the greatly thickened areas at either end of the area of fibrous continuity between the leaflets of the aortic and mitral valves (see Fig. 2-6). The area of the valvar orifice related to the right fibrous trigone and central fibrous body is most vulnerable with respect to the atrioventricular node and penetrating bundle (see Fig. 2-7). The midportion of the aortic leaflet of the mitral valve is related to the commissure between the noncoronary and left coronary cusps of the aortic valve. An incision through the atrial wall in this area may be extended into the subaortic outflow tract and may be useful for enlarging the aortic annulus during replacement of the aortic valve (Fig. 2-19). The circumflex coronary artery is adjacent to the left half of the mural leaflet, whereas the coronary sinus is adjacent to the right half of the mural leaflet (Fig. 2-20). These structures can be damaged during excessive dissection or by excessively deep placement of sutures during replacement or repair of the mitral valve. When the circumflex artery is dominant, the entire attachment of the mural leaflet may be intimately related to this artery (Fig. 2-21).

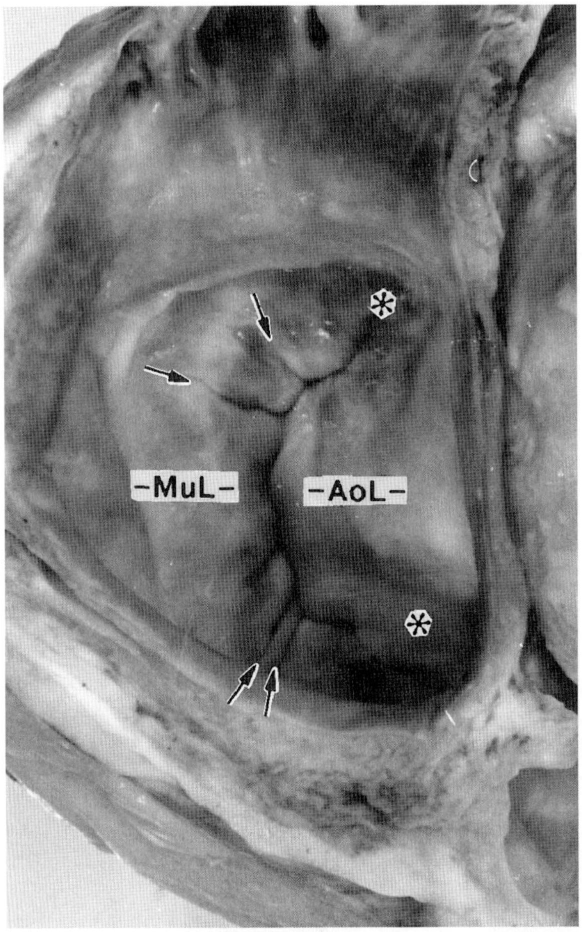

FIGURE 2-18 This view of the opened left atrium shows the leaflets of the mitral valve in closed position. There is a concave zone of apposition between them (*between asterisks*) with several slits seen in the mural leaflet (MuL). Note the limited extent of the aortic leaflet (AoL) in terms of its circumferential attachments.

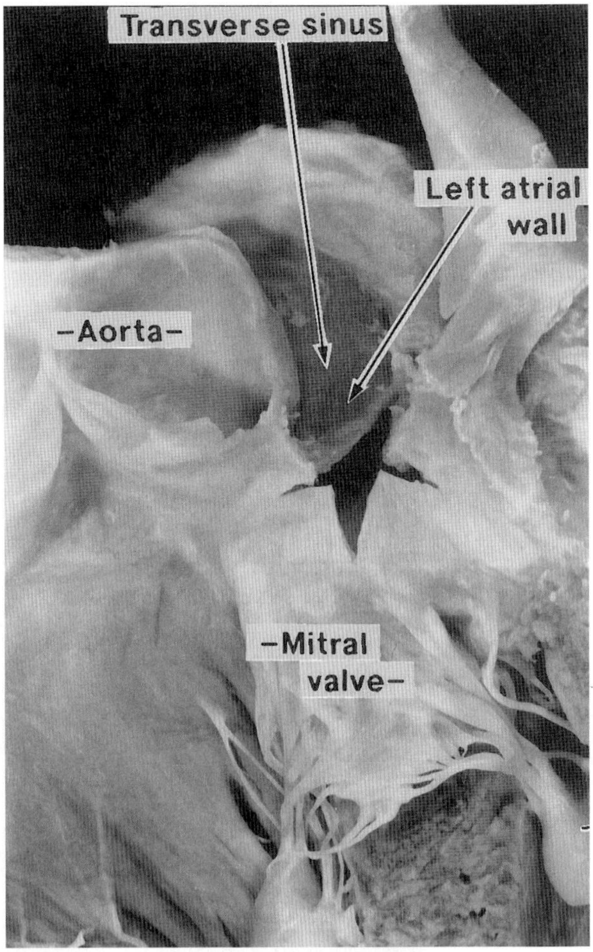

FIGURE 2-19 This dissection simulates the incision made through the aortic-mitral fibrous curtain to enlarge the orificial diameter of the subaortic outflow tract in a normal heart. (*Dissection made by Dr. Manisha Lal Trapasia.*)

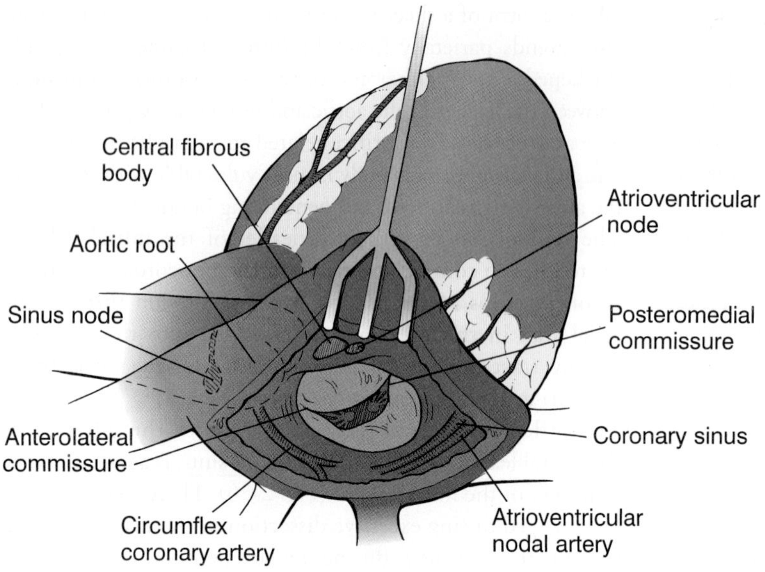

FIGURE 2-20 This diagram depicts the mitral valve in relationship to its surrounding structures as viewed through a left atriotomy.

THE RIGHT VENTRICLE AND PULMONARY VALVE

Inlet and Apical Trabecular Portions

The morphology of both the right and left ventricles can be understood best by subdividing the ventricles into three anatomically distinct components: the inlet, apical trabecular, and outlet portions.[2] This classification is more helpful than the traditional division of the right ventricle into the sinus and conus parts. The inlet portion of the right ventricle surrounds the tricuspid valve and its tension apparatus. A distinguishing feature of the tricuspid valve is the direct attachment of its septal leaflet. The apical trabecular portion of the right ventricle extends out to the apex. Here, the wall of the ventricle is quite thin and vulnerable to perforation by cardiac catheters and pacemaker electrodes.

Outlet Portion and Pulmonary Valve

The outlet portion of the right ventricle consists of the infundibulum, a circumferential muscular structure that supports the leaflets of the pulmonary valve. Because of the semilunar shape of the pulmonary valvar leaflets, this valve does not have an annulus in the traditional sense of a ringlike attachment. The leaflets have semilunar attachments that cross the musculoarterial junction in a corresponding semilunar

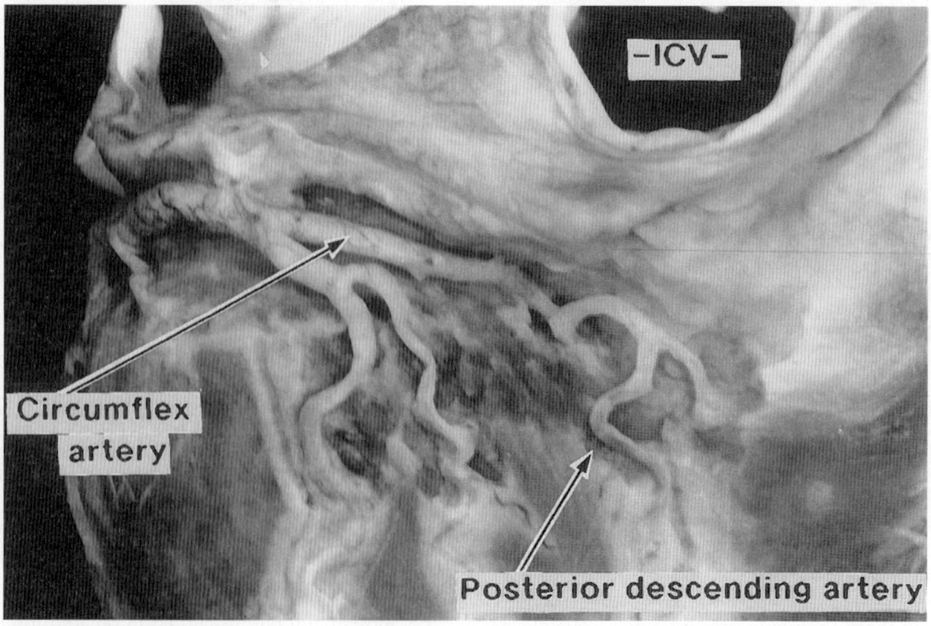

FIGURE 2-21 The extensive course of a dominant circumflex artery within the left atrioventricular groove shown in anatomic orientation. ICV = inferior vena cava.

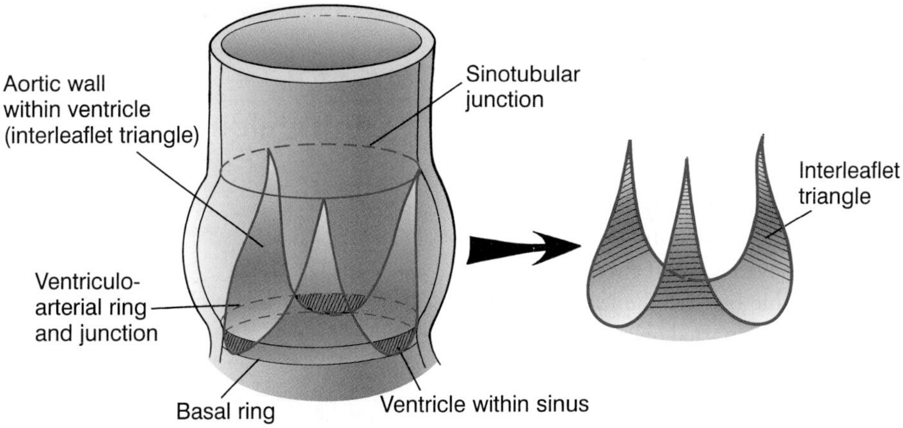

FIGURE 2-22 The semilunar valves do not have an annulus in the traditional sense. Rather, three rings can be identified anatomically, at the: (1) sinotubular junction, (2) musculoarterial junction, and (3) base of the sinuses within the ventricle.

fashion (Fig. 2-22). Therefore, instead of a single annulus, three rings can be distinguished anatomically in relation to the pulmonary valve. Superiorly, the sinotubular ridge of the pulmonary trunk marks the level of peripheral apposition of the leaflets (the commissures). A second ring exists at the ventriculoarterial junction. A third ring can be constructed by joining together the basal attachments of the three leaflets to the infundibular muscle. None of these rings, however, corresponds to the attachments of the leaflets, which must be semilunar to permit the valve to open and close competently. In fact, these semilunar attachments, which mark the hemodynamic ventriculoarterial junction, extend from the first ring, across the second, down to the third, and back in each cusp (Fig. 2-23).

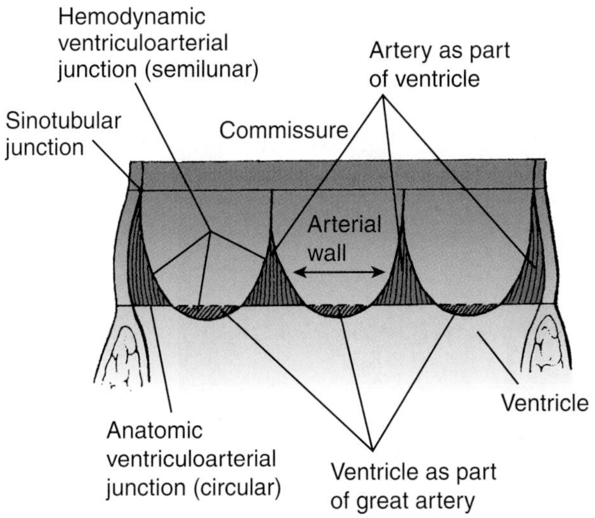

FIGURE 2-23 The hemodynamic ventriculoarterial junction of the semilunar valves extends from the sinotubular junction across the anatomical ventriculoarterial junction to the basal ring and back in each leaflet (see Fig. 2-22). This creates a portion of ventricle as part of the great artery in each sinus and a triangle of artery as part of the ventricle between each leaflet.

Supraventricular Crest and Pulmonary Infundibulum

A distinguishing feature of the right ventricle is a prominent muscular shelf, the supraventricular crest, which separates the tricuspid and pulmonary valves (Fig. 2-24). In reality, this

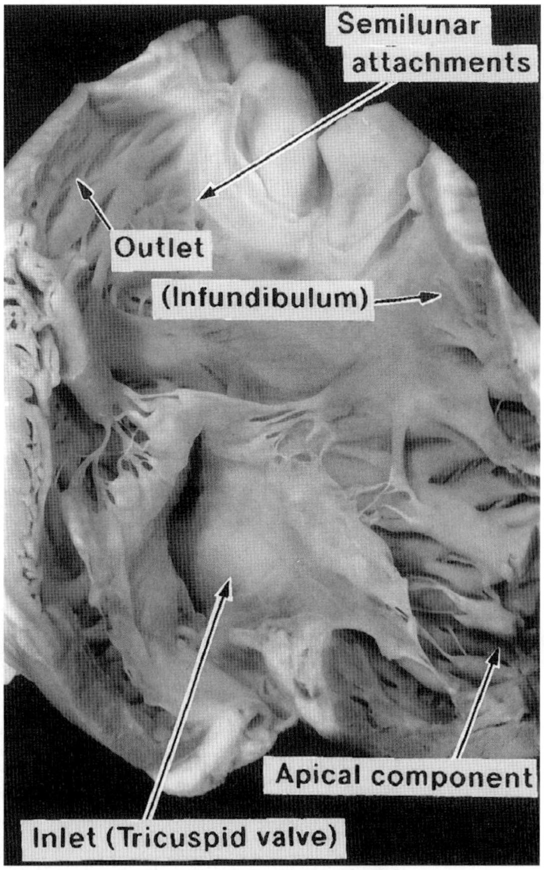

FIGURE 2-24 View of the opened right ventricle, in anatomical orientation, showing its three component parts and the semilunar attachments of the pulmonary valve. These are supported by the supraventricular crest.

muscular ridge is the posterior part of the subpulmonary muscular infundibulum that supports the leaflets of the pulmonary valve. In other words, it is part of the inner curve of the heart. Incisions through the supraventricular crest run into the transverse septum and may jeopardize the right coronary artery. Although this area is often considered the outlet component of the interventricular septum, in fact the entire subpulmonary infundibulum, including the ventriculoinfundibular fold, can be removed without entering the left ventricular cavity. This is possible because the leaflets of the pulmonary and aortic valves are supported on separate sleeves of right and left ventricular outlet muscle. There is an extensive external tissue plane between the walls of the aorta and the pulmonary trunk (Fig. 2-25), and the leaflets of the pulmonary and aortic valves have markedly different levels of attachments within their respective ventricles. This feature enables enucleation of the pulmonary valve, including its basal attachments within the infundibulum, during the Ross procedure without creating a ventricular septal defect. When the infundibulum is removed from the right ventricle, the insertion of the supraventricular crest between the limbs of the septomarginal trabeculation is visible (Fig. 2-26). This trabeculation is a prominent muscle column that divides superiorly into anterior and posterior limbs. The anterior limb runs superiorly into the infundibulum and supports the leaflets of the pulmonary valve. The posterior limb extends backward beneath the ventricular septum and runs into the inlet portion of the ventricle. The medial papillary muscle arises from this posterior limb. The body of the septomarginal trabeculation runs to the apex of the ventricle, where it divides into smaller trabeculations. Two of these trabeculations may be particularly prominent. One becomes the anterior papillary muscle, and the other crosses the ventricular cavity as the moderator band (Fig. 2-27).

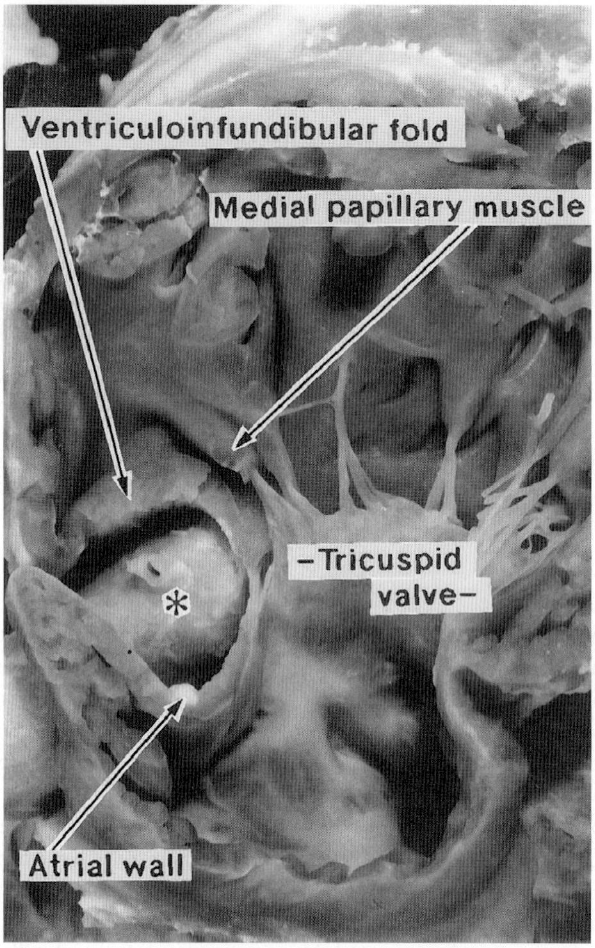

FIGURE 2-25 This dissection, viewed in surgical orientation, shows how the greater part of the supraventricular crest is formed by the freestanding subpulmonary infundibulum in relation to the right coronary aortic sinus (*asterisk*).

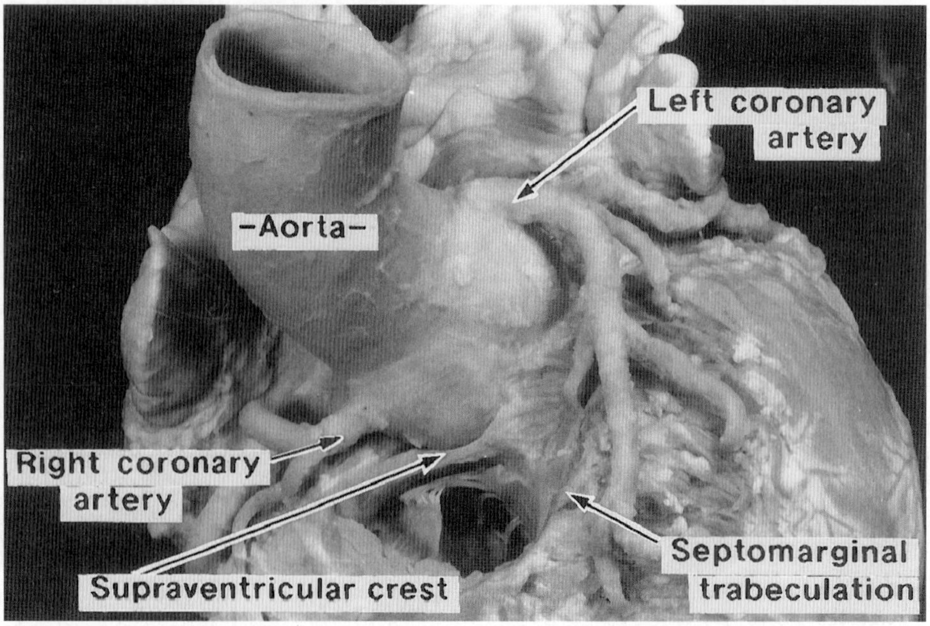

FIGURE 2-26 Removal of the freestanding subpulmonary infundibulum reveals the insertion of the supraventricular crest between the limbs of the septomarginal trabeculation and shows the aortic origin of the coronary arteries (anatomical orientation).

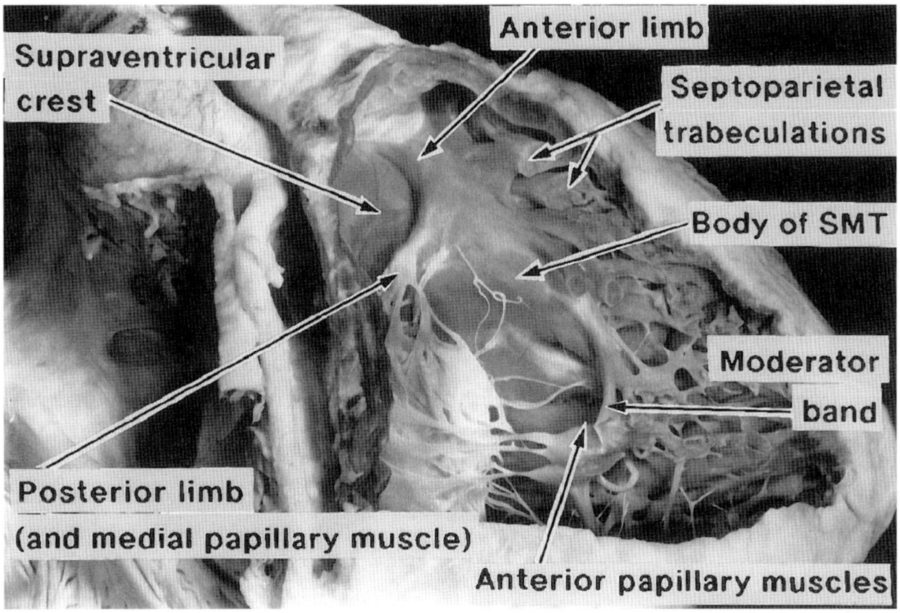

FIGURE 2-27 This dissection of the right ventricle, in anatomical orientation, shows the relations of supraventricular crest and septomarginal (SMT) and septoparietal trabeculations.

THE LEFT VENTRICLE AND AORTIC VALVE

Inlet and Apical Trabecular Portions

The left ventricle can be subdivided into three components, similar to the right ventricle. The inlet component surrounds and is limited by the mitral valve and its tension apparatus. The two papillary muscles occupy anterolateral and posteromedial positions and are positioned rather close to each other. The leaflets of the mitral valve have no direct septal attachments because the deep posterior diverticulum of the left ventricular outflow tract displaces the aortic leaflet away from the inlet septum. The apical trabecular component of the left ventricle extends to the apex, where the myocardium is surprisingly thin. The trabeculations of the left ventricle are quite fine compared with those of the right ventricle (Fig. 2-28). This characteristic is useful for defining ventricular morphology on diagnostic ventriculograms.

Outlet Portion

The outlet component supports the aortic valve and consists of both muscular and fibrous portions. This is in contrast to the

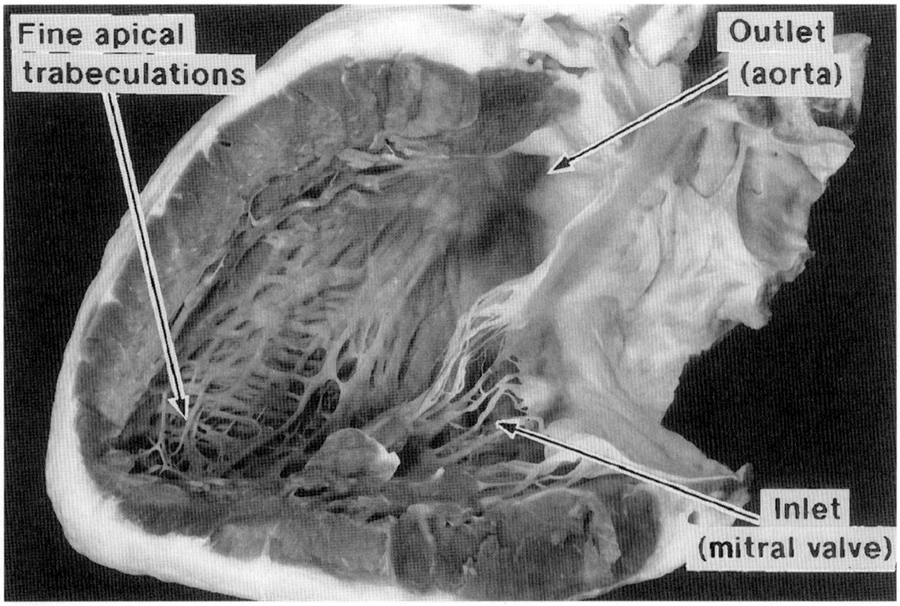

FIGURE 2-28 This dissection of the left ventricle shows its component parts and characteristically fine apical trabeculations (anatomical orientation).

infundibulum of the right ventricle, which consists entirely of muscle. The septal portion of the left ventricular outflow tract, although primarily muscular, also includes the membranous portion of the ventricular septum. The posterior quadrant of the outflow tract consists of an extensive fibrous curtain that extends from the fibrous skeleton of the heart across the aortic leaflet of the mitral valve and supports the leaflets of the aortic valve in the area of aortomitral continuity (see Fig. 2-5). The lateral quadrant of the outflow tract again is muscular and consists of the lateral margin of the inner curvature of the heart, delineated externally by the transverse sinus. The left bundle of the cardiac conduction system enters the left ventricular outflow tract posterior to the membranous septum and immediately beneath the commissure between the right and noncoronary leaflets of the aortic valve. After traveling a short distance down the septum, the left bundle divides into anterior, septal, and posterior divisions.

Aortic Valve

The aortic valve is a semilunar valve that is quite similar morphologically to the pulmonary valve. Likewise, it does not have a discrete annulus. Because of its central location, the aortic valve is related to each of the cardiac chambers and valves (see Fig. 2-4). A thorough knowledge of these relationships is essential to understanding aortic valve pathology and many congenital cardiac malformations.

The aortic valve consists primarily of three semilunar leaflets. As with the pulmonary valve, attachments of the leaflets extend across the ventriculoarterial junction in a curvilinear fashion. Each leaflet therefore has attachments to the aorta and within the left ventricle (Fig. 2-29). Behind each leaflet, the aortic wall bulges outward to form the sinuses of Valsalva. The leaflets themselves meet centrally along a line of coaptation, at the center of which is a thickened nodule called the *nodule of Arantius.* Peripherally, adjacent to the commissures, the line of coaptation is thinner and normally may contain small perforations. During systole the leaflets are thrust upward and away from the center of the aortic lumen, whereas during diastole they fall passively into the center of the aorta. With normal valvar morphology, all three leaflets meet along lines of coaptation and support the column of blood within the aorta to prevent regurgitation into the ventricle. Two of the three aortic sinuses give rise to coronary arteries, from which arise their designations as *right, left,* and *noncoronary sinuses.*

By sequentially following the line of attachment of each leaflet, the relationship of the aortic valve to its surrounding structures can be clearly understood. Beginning posteriorly, the commissure between the noncoronary and left coronary leaflets is positioned along the area of aortomitral valvar continuity. The fibrous subaortic curtain is beneath this commissure (see Fig. 2-29). To the right of this commissure, the noncoronary leaflet is attached above the posterior diverticulum of the left ventricular outflow tract. Here, the valve is related to the right atrial wall. As the attachment of the noncoronary leaflet ascends from its nadir toward the commissure between the noncoronary and right coronary leaflets, the line of attachment is directly above the portion of the atrial septum containing the atrioventricular node. The commissure between the noncoronary and right coronary leaflets is located directly above the penetrating atrioventricular bundle and the membranous ventricular septum (Fig. 2-30). The attachment of the right coronary leaflet then descends across the central fibrous body before ascending to the commissure between the right and left coronary leaflets. Immediately beneath this commissure, the wall of the aorta forms the uppermost part of the subaortic outflow. An incision through this area passes into the space between the facing surfaces of the aorta and pulmonary trunk (see Fig. 2-30). As the

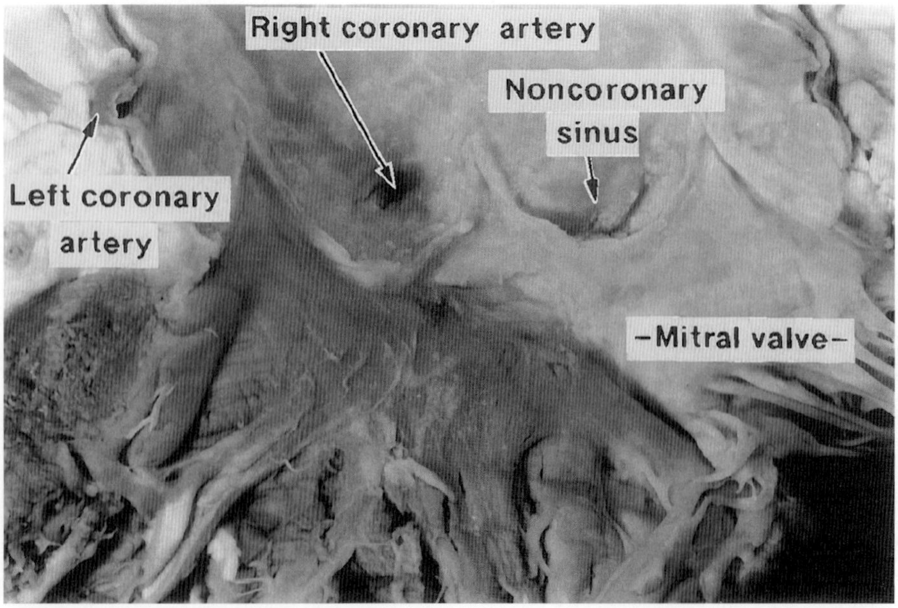

FIGURE 2-29 This dissection in anatomic orientation, made by removing the aortic valvar leaflets, emphasizes the semilunar nature of the hinge points (see Figs. 2-22 and 2-23). Note the relationship to the mitral valve (see Fig. 2-5).

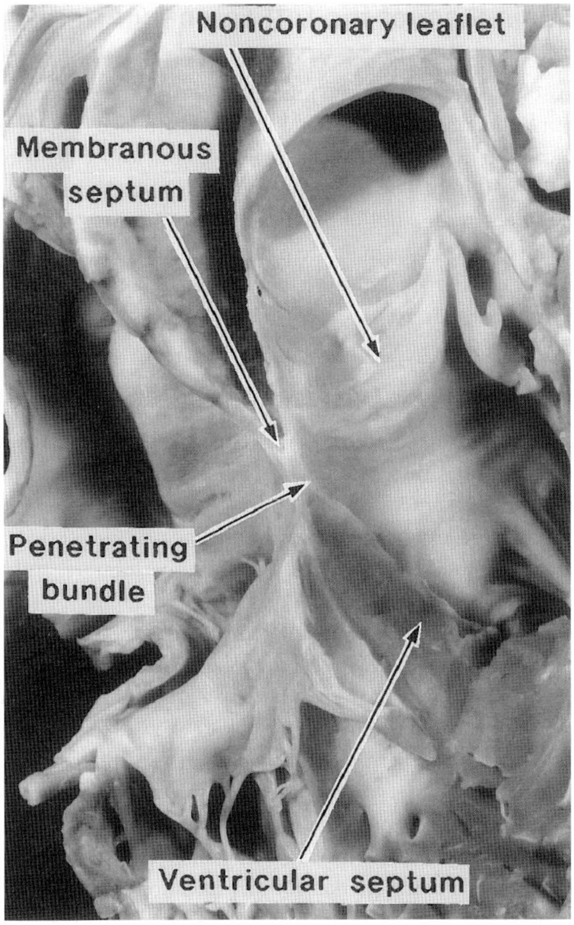

FIGURE 2-30 Dissection made by removing the right and part of the left aortic sinuses to show the relations of the fibrous triangle between the right and noncoronary aortic leaflets (anatomical orientation).

facing left and right leaflets descend from this commissure, they are attached to the outlet muscular component of the left ventricle. Only a small part of this area in the normal heart is a true outlet septum because both pulmonary and aortic valves are supported on their own sleeves of myocardium. Thus, although the outlet components of the right and left ventricles face each other, an incision below the aortic valve enters low into the infundibulum of the right ventricle. As the lateral part of the left coronary leaflet descends from the facing commissure to the base of the sinus, it becomes the only part of the aortic valve that is not intimately related to another cardiac chamber.

Knowledge of the anatomy of the aortic valve and its relationship to surrounding structures is important to successful replacement of the aortic valve, particularly when enlargement of the aortic root is required. The Konno-Rastan aortoventriculoplasty involves opening and enlarging the anterior portion of the subaortic region.[4,5] The incisions for this procedure begin with an anterior longitudinal aortotomy that extends through the commissure between the right and left coronary leaflets. Anteriorly, the incision is extended across the base of the infundibulum. The differential level of attachment of the aortic and pulmonary valve leaflets permits this incision without damage to the pulmonary valve (Fig. 2-31). Posteriorly, the incision extends through the most medial portion of the supraventricular crest into the left ventricular outflow tract. By closing the resulting ventricular septal defect with a patch, the aortic outflow tract is widened to allow implantation of a larger valve prosthesis. A second patch is used to close the defect in the right ventricular outflow tract.

Alternative methods to enlarge the aortic outflow tract involve incisions in the region of aortomitral continuity. In the Manouguian procedure (see Fig. 2-19), a curvilinear aortotomy is extended posteriorly through the commissure between the left and noncoronary leaflets down to and occasionally into the aortic leaflet of the mitral valve.[6] A patch is used to augment the incision posteriorly. When the posterior diverticulum of the outflow tract is fully developed, this incision can be made without entering other cardiac chambers, although not uncommonly the roof of the left atrium is opened. The Nicks procedure for enlargement of the aortic root involves an aortotomy that passes through the middle of the noncoronary leaflet into the fibrous subaortic curtain and may be extended into the aortic leaflet of the mitral valve.[7] This incision also may open the roof of the left atrium. When these techniques are used, any resulting defect in the left atrium must be closed carefully.

As discussed previously, the differential level of attachment of aortic and pulmonary valves, as well as the muscular nature of their support, allows the pulmonary valve to be harvested

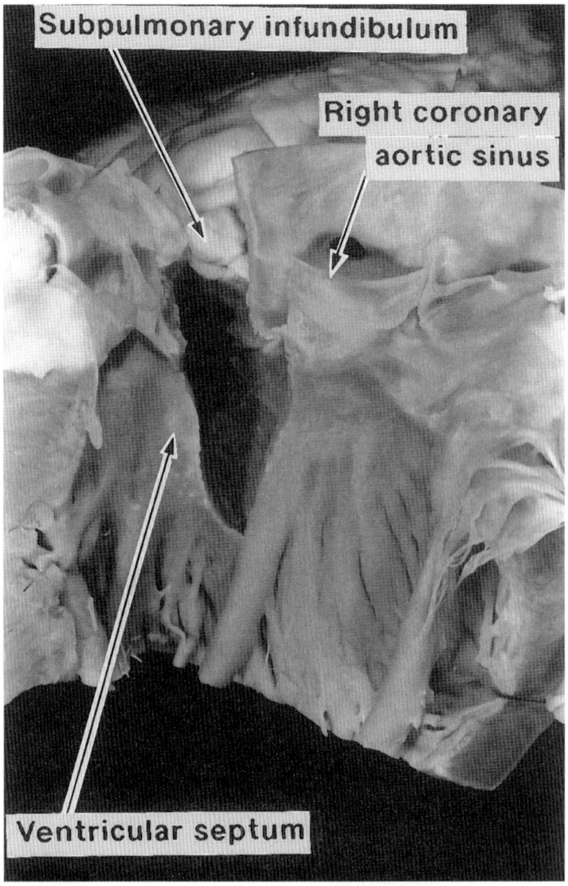

FIGURE 2-31 This incision, made in a normal heart, simulates the Konno-Rastan procedure for enlargement of the aortic root.

and used as a replacement for the aortic valve in the Ross procedure.[8,9] This procedure can be combined with the incisions of the Konno-Rastan aortoventriculoplasty to repair left ventricular outflow tract obstructions in young children with a viable autograft that has potential for growth and avoids the need for anticoagulation.

Accurate understanding of left ventricular outflow tract anatomy is also important in the treatment of aortic valvar endocarditis.[10,11] Because of the central position of the aortic valve relative to the other valves and cardiac chambers (see Fig. 2-4), abscess formation can produce fistulas between the aorta and any of the four chambers of the heart. Therefore, patients may present with findings of left-sided heart failure, left-to-right shunting, and/or complete heart block in addition to the usual signs of sepsis and systemic embolization.

THE CORONARY ARTERIES[12–14]

The right and left coronary arteries originate behind their respective aortic valvar leaflets (see Fig. 2-26). The orifices usually are located in the upper third of the sinuses of Valsalva, although individual hearts may vary markedly. Because of the oblique plane of the aortic valve, the orifice of the left coronary artery is superior and posterior to that of the right coronary artery. The coronary arterial tree is divided into three segments; two (the left anterior descending artery and the circumflex artery) arise from a common stem. The third segment is the right coronary artery. The dominance of the coronary circulation (right versus left) usually refers to the artery from which the posterior descending artery originates, not the absolute mass of myocardium perfused by the left or right coronary artery. Right dominance occurs in 85 to 90% of normal individuals. Left dominance occurs slightly more frequently in males than in females.

Main Stem of the Left Coronary Artery

The main stem of the left coronary artery courses from the left sinus of Valsalva anteriorly, inferiorly, and to the left between the pulmonary trunk and the left atrial appendage (Fig. 2-32). Typically, it is 10 to 20 mm in length, but can extend to a length of 40 mm. The left main stem can be absent, with separate orifices in the sinus of Valsalva for its two primary branches (1% of patients). The main stem divides into two major arteries of nearly equal diameter, the left anterior descending artery and the circumflex artery.

Left Anterior Descending Artery

The left anterior descending (or interventricular) coronary artery continues directly from the bifurcation of the left main stem, coursing anteriorly and inferiorly in the anterior interventricular groove to the apex of the heart (Fig. 2-33). Its branches include the diagonals, the septal perforators, and the right ventricular branches. The diagonals, which may be two to six in number, course along the anterolateral wall of the left ventricle and supply this portion of the myocardium. The first diagonal generally is the largest and may arise from the bifurcation of the left main stem (formerly known as the *intermediate artery*). The septal perforators branch perpendicularly into the ventricular septum. Typically, there are three to five septal perforators; the initial one is the largest and commonly originates just beyond the takeoff of the first diagonal. This perpendicular orientation is a useful marker for identification of the left anterior descending artery on coronary angiograms. The septal perforators supply blood to the anterior two-thirds of the ventricular septum. Right ventricular branches, which may not always be present, supply blood to the anterior surface of the right ventricle. In approximately 4% of hearts, the left anterior

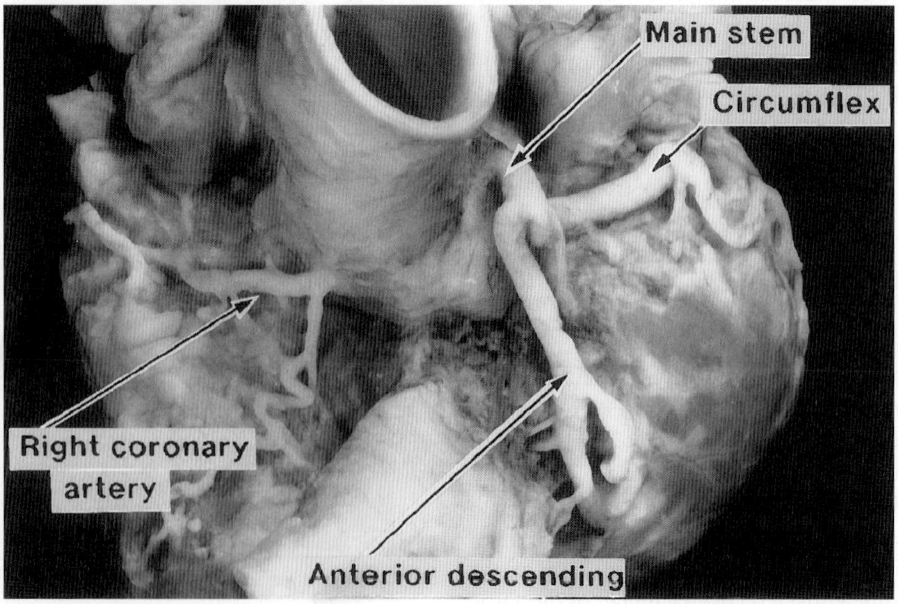

FIGURE 2-32 The short extent of the main stem of the left coronary artery is seen before it branches into the circumflex and anterior descending arteries. Note the small right coronary artery in this heart, in which the circumflex artery was dominant (see Fig. 2-21).

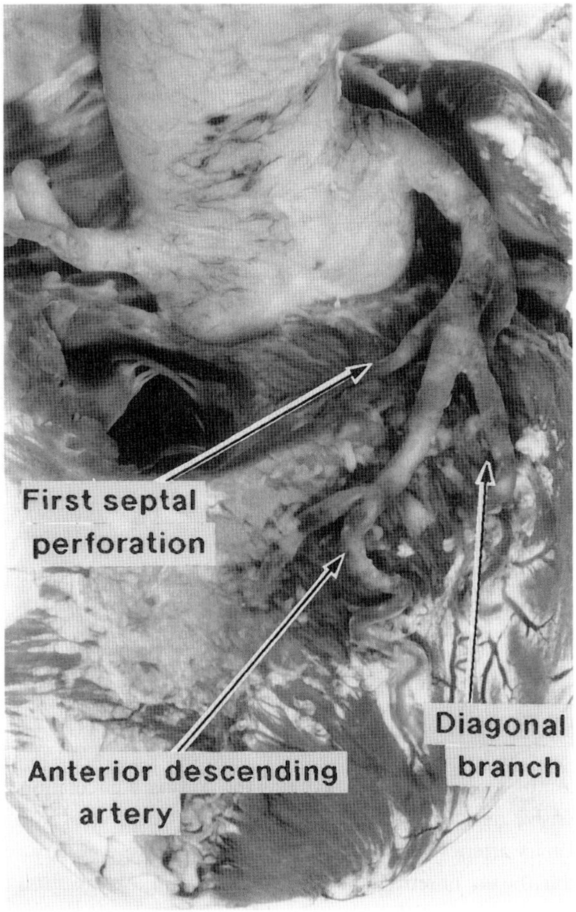

FIGURE 2-33 The important branches of the anterior descending artery are the first septal perforating and diagonal arteries.

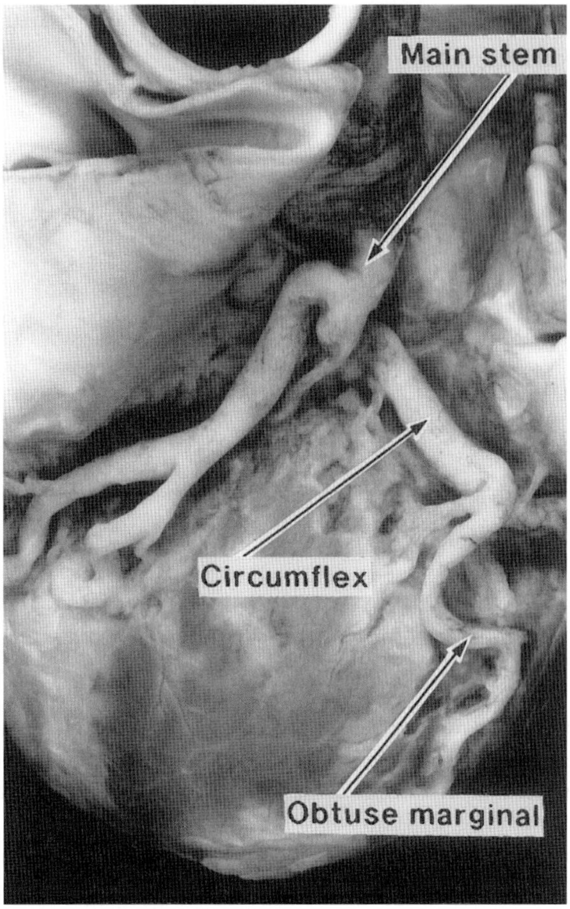

FIGURE 2-34 The important branches of the circumflex artery, seen in anatomical orientation.

descending artery bifurcates proximally and continues as two parallel vessels of approximately equal size down the anterior interventricular groove. Occasionally, the artery wraps around the apex of the left ventricle to feed the distal portion of the posterior interventricular groove. Rarely, it extends along the entire length of the posterior groove to replace the posterior descending artery.

Circumflex Artery

The left circumflex coronary artery arises from the left main coronary artery roughly at a right angle to the anterior interventricular branch. It courses along the left atrioventricular groove and in 85 to 95% of patients terminates near the obtuse margin of the left ventricle (Fig. 2-34). In 10 to 15% of patients, it continues around the atrioventricular groove to the crux of the heart to give rise to the posterior descending artery (left dominance; see Fig. 2-21). The primary branches of the left circumflex coronary artery are the obtuse marginals. They supply blood to the lateral aspect of the left ventricular myocardium, including the posteromedial papillary muscle. Additional branches supply blood to the left atrium and, in 40 to 50% of hearts, the sinus node. When the circumflex coronary artery supplies the posterior descending artery, it also supplies the atrioventricular node.

Right Coronary Artery

The right coronary artery courses from the aorta anteriorly and laterally before descending in the right atrioventricular groove and curving posteriorly at the acute margin of the right ventricle (Fig. 2-35). In 85 to 90% of hearts, the right coronary artery crosses the crux, where it makes a characteristic U-turn before bifurcating into the posterior descending artery and the right posterolateral artery. In 50 to 60% of hearts, the artery to the sinus node arises from the proximal portion of the right coronary artery. The blood supply to the atrioventricular node (in patients with right-dominant circulation) arises from the midportion of the U-shaped segment. The posterior descending artery runs along the posterior interventricular groove, extending for a variable distance toward the apex of the heart. It gives off perpendicular branches, the posterior septal perforators, that course anteriorly in the ventricular septum. Typically, these perforators supply the posterior one-third of the ventricular septal myocardium.

The right posterolateral artery gives rise to a variable number of branches that supply the posterior surface of the left ventricle. The circulation of the posteroinferior portion of the left ventricular myocardium is quite variable. It may consist of branches of the right coronary artery, the circumflex artery, or

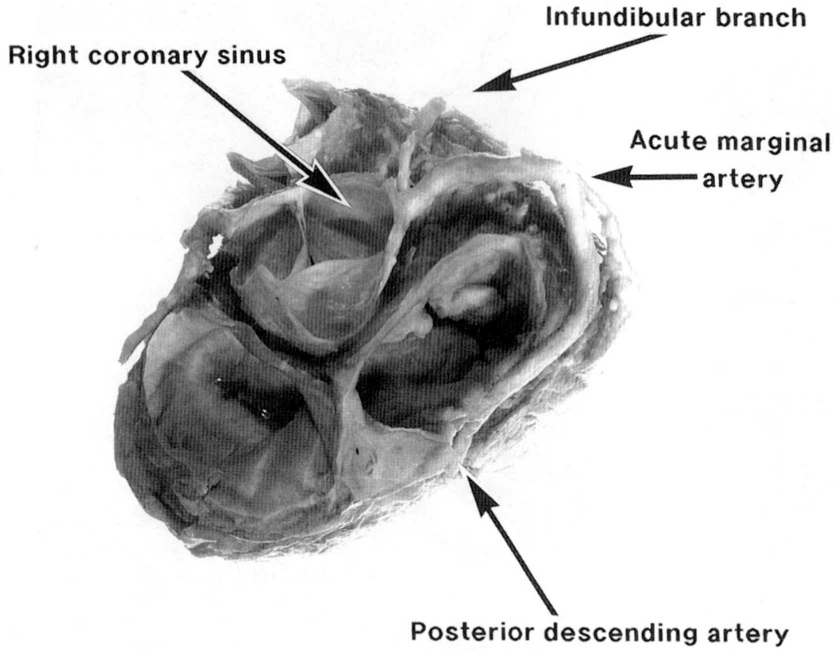

FIGURE 2-35 This dissection shows the relationships and branches of the right coronary artery.

both. The acute marginal arteries branch from the right coronary artery along the acute margin of the heart, before its bifurcation at the crux. These marginals supply the anterior free wall of the right ventricle. In 10 to 20% of hearts, one of these acute marginal arteries courses across the diaphragmatic surface of the right ventricle to reach the distal ventricular septum. The right coronary artery supplies important collaterals to the left anterior descending artery through its septal perforators. In addition, its infundibular (or conus) branch, which arises from the proximal portion of the right coronary artery, courses anteriorly over the base of the ventricular infundibulum and may serve as a collateral to the anterior descending artery. Kugel's artery is an anastomotic vessel between the proximal right coronary and the circumflex coronary artery that also can provide a branch that runs through the base of the atrial septum to the crux of the heart, where it supplies collateral circulation to the atrioventricular node.[15]

THE CORONARY VEINS[14]

A complex network of veins drains the coronary circulation. An extensive degree of collateralization among these veins and the coronary arteries and the paucity of valves within coronary veins enable the use of retrograde coronary sinus cardioplegia for intraoperative myocardial protection. The venous circulation can be divided into three systems: the coronary sinus and its tributaries, the anterior right ventricular veins, and the thebesian veins.

Coronary Sinus and Its Tributaries

The coronary sinus predominantly drains the left ventricle and receives approximately 85% of coronary venous blood. It lies within the posterior atrioventricular groove and empties into the right atrium at the lateral border of the triangle of Koch (Fig. 2-36). The orifice of the coronary sinus is guarded by the crescent-shaped

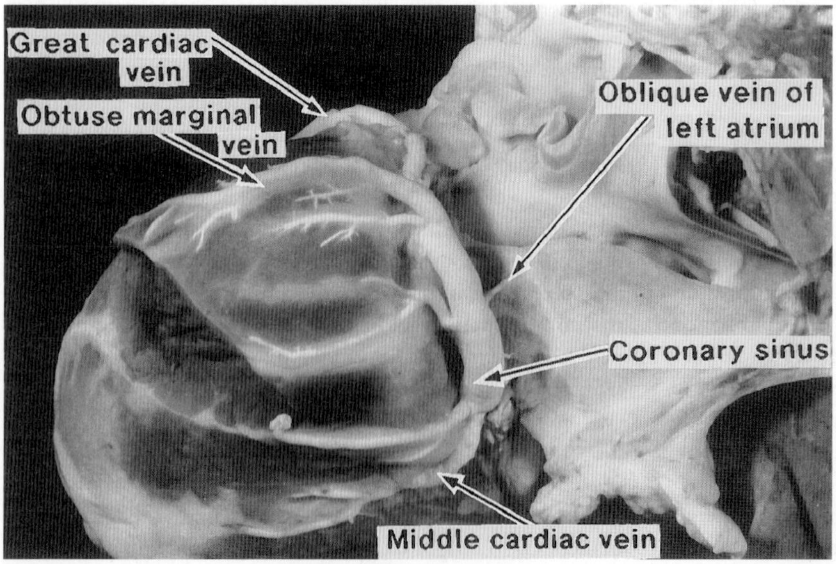

FIGURE 2-36 The coronary veins on the diaphragmatic surface of the heart, seen in anatomical orientation, have been emphasized by filling them with sealant. The tributaries of the coronary sinus are well demonstrated. Note that, strictly speaking, the sinus does not begin until the oblique vein enters the great cardiac vein.

thebesian valve. The named tributaries of the coronary sinus include the anterior interventricular vein, which courses parallel to the left anterior descending coronary artery. Adjacent to the bifurcation of the left main stem, the anterior interventricular vein courses leftward in the atrioventricular groove, where it is referred to as the *great cardiac vein.* It receives blood from the marginal and posterior left ventricular branches before becoming the coronary sinus at the origin of the oblique vein (of Marshall) at the posterior margin of the left atrium. The posterior interventricular vein, or *middle cardiac vein,* arises at the apex, courses parallel to the posterior descending coronary artery and extends proximally to the crux. Here, this vein drains either directly into the right atrium or into the coronary sinus just prior to its orifice. The *small cardiac vein* runs posteriorly through the right atrioventricular groove.

Anterior Right Ventricular Veins

The anterior right ventricular veins travel across the right ventricular surface to the right atrioventricular groove, where they either enter directly into the right atrium or coalesce to form the small cardiac vein. As indicated, this vein travels down the right atrioventricular groove, around the acute margin, and enters into the right atrium directly or joins the coronary sinus just proximal to its orifice.

Thebesian Veins

The thebesian veins are small venous tributaries that drain directly into the cardiac chambers. They exist primarily in the right atrium and right ventricle.

REFERENCES

1. Anderson KR, Ho SY, Anderson RH: The location and vascular supply of the sinus node in the human heart. *Br Heart J* 1979; 41:28.
2. Wilcox BR, Anderson RH: *Surgical Anatomy of the Heart.* New York, Raven Press, 1985.
3. Sweeney LJ, Rosenquist GC: The normal anatomy of the atrial septum in the human heart. *Am Heart J* 1979; 98:194.
4. Konno S, Imai Y, Iida Y, et al: A new method for prosthetic valve replacement in congenital aortic stenosis associated with hypoplasia of the aortic valve ring. *J Thorac Cardiovasc Surg* 1975; 70:909.
5. Rastan H, Koncz J: Aortoventriculoplasty: a new technique for the treatment of left ventricular outflow tract obstruction. *J Thorac Cardiovasc Surg* 1976; 71:920.
6. Manouguian S, Seybold-Epting W: Patch enlargement of the aortic valve ring by extending the aortic incision into the anterior mitral leaflet: new operative technique. *J Thorac Cardiovasc Surg* 1979; 78:402.
7. Nicks R, Cartmill T, Berstein L: Hypoplasia of the aortic root. *Thorax* 1970; 25:339.
8. Ross DN: Replacement of aortic and mitral valve with a pulmonary autograft. *Lancet* 1967; 2:956.
9. Oury JH, Angell WW, Eddy AC, Cleveland JC: Pulmonary autograft: past, present, and future. *J Heart Valve Dis* 1993; 2:365.
10. Wilcox BR, Murray GF, Starek PJK: The long-term outlook for valve replacement in active endocarditis. *J Thorac Cardiovasc Surg* 1977; 74:860.
11. Frantz PT, Murray GF, Wilcox BR: Surgical management of left ventricular-aortic discontinuity complicating bacterial endocarditis. *Ann Thorac Surg* 1980; 29:1.
12. Anderson RH, Becker AE: *Cardiac Anatomy.* London, Churchill Livingstone, 1980.
13. Kirklin JW, Barratt-Boyes BG: Anatomy, dimensions, and terminology, in Kirklin JW, Barratt-Boyes BG (eds): *Cardiac Surgery,* 2nd ed. New York, Churchill Livingstone, 1993; p 3.
14. Schlant RC, Silverman ME: Anatomy of the heart, in Hurst JW, Logue RB, Rachley CE, et al (eds): *The Heart,* 6th ed. New York, McGraw-Hill, 1986; p 16.
15. Kugel MA: Anatomical studies on the coronary arteries and their branches: 1. Arteria anastomotica auricularis magna. *Am Heart J* 1927; 3:260.

CHAPTER 3

Cardiac Surgical Physiology

Edward B. Savage
Robert Saeid Farivar

INTRODUCTION

A cardiac surgical procedure is the most acute application of basic dynamic physiology that exists in medical care. Basic physiologic concepts of electromechanical activation and association, loading conditions, inotropy, etc all affect a successful outcome. Working knowledge of these fundamental concepts is imperative to maintain and return a patient to normal function. The purpose of this chapter is to present a manageable outline of cardiac physiology that can be used in daily practice, as a framework against which pathologic processes can be measured, assessed, and treated.

CELLULAR COMPONENTS AND CELLULAR ACTIVATION

The heart beats are continuously based on the unique features of its component cells. A cardiac cycle begins when spontaneous depolarization of a pacemaker cell initiates an action potential. This electrical activity is transmitted to atrial muscle cells and the conduction system, which transmits the electrical activity to the ventricle. Activation is dependent on components of the cell membrane and cell, which induce and maintain the ion currents that promote and spread electrical activation.

The activity of cells in the heart is triggered by an *action potential.* An action potential is a cyclical activation of the cell comprised of a rapid change in the membrane potential (the electrical gradient across the cell membrane) and subsequent return to a resting membrane potential. This process is dependent on a selectively permeable cell membrane and proteins that actively and passively direct ion passage across the cell membrane. The specific components of the myocyte action potential are detailed in Fig. 3-3. The myocyte action potential is characterized by a rapid initial depolarization mediated by *fast channels* (sodium channels), then a plateau phase mediated by *slow channels* (calcium channels). Further details of this process are introduced as their components are described.

The Sarcolemma

The cardiac cell is surrounded by a membrane (*plasmalemma* or more specific to a muscle cell, *sarcolemma*). The structural components of the sarcolemma allow for the origination and then the conduction of an electrical signal through the heart with subsequent initiation of the *excitation-contraction coupling* process. The sarcolemma also participates in the regulation of excitation, contraction, and intracellular metabolism in response to neuronal and chemical stimulation.

The Phospholipid Bilayer

The sarcolemma is a *phospholipid bilayer* that provides a barrier between the extracellular compartment and the intracellular compartment or *cytosol.* The sarcolemma, which is only two molecules thick, consists of phospholipids and cholesterol aligned so that the lipid, or hydrophobic, portion of the molecule is on the inside of the membrane, and the hydrophilic portion of the molecule is on the outside (Fig. 3-1). The phospholipid bilayer provides a fluid barrier that is particularly *impermeable to diffusion of ions.* Small lipid-soluble molecules such as oxygen and carbon dioxide diffuse easily through the membrane. The water molecule, although insoluble in the membrane, is small enough that it diffuses easily through the membrane (or through pores in the membrane). Other, slightly larger molecules (sodium, chloride, potassium, calcium) cannot easily diffuse through the lipid bilayer and require specialized channels for transport.[1,2]

The specialized ion transport systems within the sarcolemma consist of *membrane-spanning proteins* that float in and penetrate through the lipid bilayer. These proteins are associated with three different types of ion transport: (1) diffusion

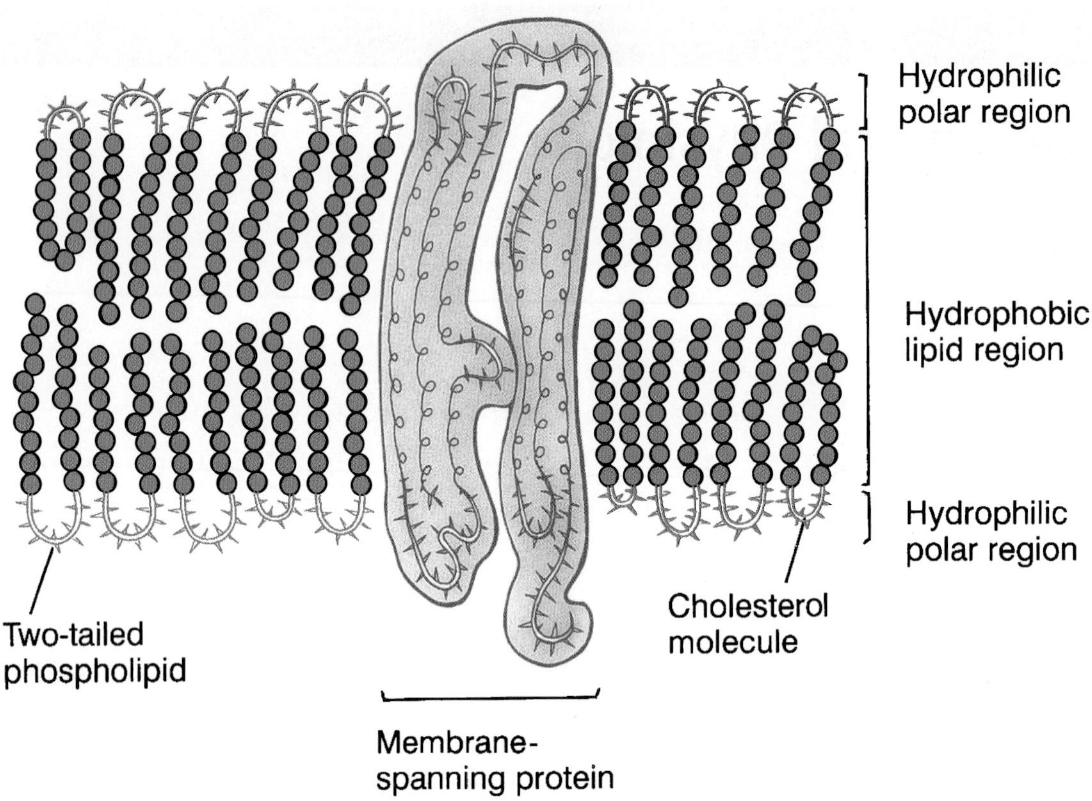

FIGURE 3-1 The sarcolemma is a bilayer in which phospholipid and cholesterol molecules are arranged with hydrophobic domains within the membrane and hydrophilic domains facing outward. The membrane-spanning protein shown here is similar to many ion channels, with six hydrophobic alpha-helices spanning the membrane and surrounding a central channel.

through transmembrane channels that can be opened or closed (gated) in response to electrical (voltage-gated) or chemical (ligand-gated) stimuli; (2) exchange of one ion for another by attachment to binding sites for transmission in response to an electrochemical gradient; and (3) active (energy-dependent) transport of ions against an electrochemical gradient.

Other proteins located in the sarcolemma serve as receptors for neuronal or chemical control of cellular processes.

Ion Channels

Most of the voltage-gated channels consist of four subunits that surround the water-filled pore through which ions cross the membrane. A schematic diagram of an ion channel is shown in Fig. 3-2. Each channel contains a selectivity filter that allows the passage of particular ions based upon pore size and electrical charge, and an activation gate regulated by conformational changes induced by either a voltage-sensitive or a ligand-binding region of the protein. Many channels also have an inactivation gate.[1,3]

Voltage-Gated Sodium Channels

The voltage-gated sodium channel is prominent in most electrically excitable muscle and nerve cells. Energy-dependent pumps and other ions create a large concentration gradient of positive sodium ions (142 mEq/L outside, 10 mEq/L inside) and a large electrical gradient (–70 to –90 mV outside to inside) across the cell membrane. Both gradients favor the influx of sodium. This passive influx is termed an *inward current.* The inward current of sodium ions begins to depolarize (reduce the electrical gradient) across the sarcolemma. When the membrane potential is raised to between –70 and –50 mV, the activation gate of the sodium channel opens. Sodium ions rapidly rush into the cell, depolarizing the sarcolemmal membrane. The inactivation gate of the sodium channel begins to close at the same voltage, with a built-in time delay, so the sodium channel is open for only a few milliseconds. Because these channels open and close so quickly, they are called *fast channels.* The inactivation gate of the sodium channel remains closed until the cell is repolarized to the resting negative membrane potential.[4,5]

Voltage-Gated Calcium Channels

There are two important calcium channels. The type T (transient)-calcium channels open as the membrane potential rises to –60 to –50 mV, and then close quickly. These T-calcium channels are important in early depolarization, especially in atrial pacemaker cells.

The second major calcium channel, type L (long-lasting) channel, a slow channel, leads to an inward (depolarizing) current that is slowly inactivated and therefore prolonged. These channels open at a less negative potential (–30 to –20 mV). Once open, the prolonged inward calcium current (Fig. 3-3) sustains the action potential. This increase in cytosolic calcium

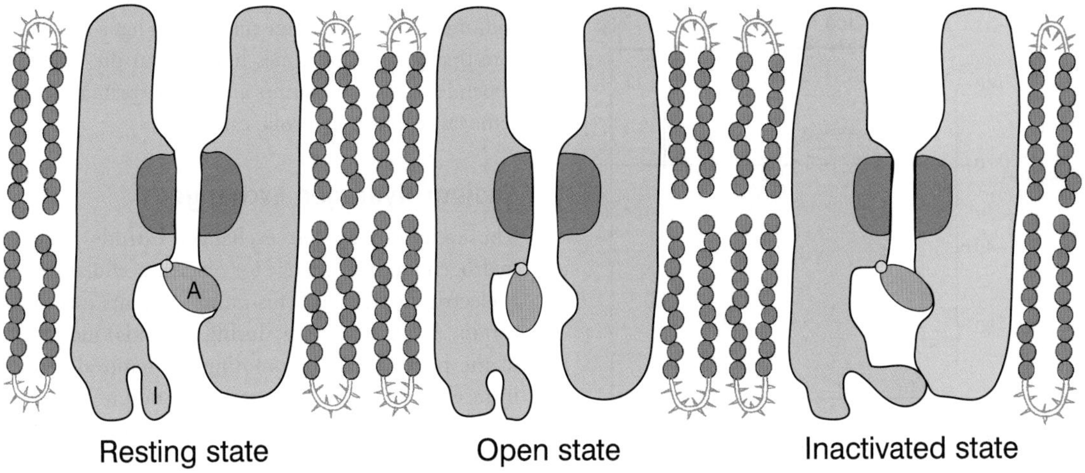

FIGURE 3-2 A voltage-gated sodium channel is schematically depicted. The shaded region is the selectivity filter. *A* represents the activation gate, and *I* represents the inactivation gate. At rest, the inactivation gate is open and the activation gate is closed. As the transmembrane potential rises from −80 to −60 mV, the activation gate opens, and sodium ions pass through the channel. Within a few milliseconds, the inactivation gate closes. Once the cell repolarizes, the resting ion channel returns to the resting state.

begins the excitation-contraction sequence. Beta-receptor stimulation induces conformational changes in the channel resulting in an increased influx of calcium ions and an associated increase in the strength of sarcomere contraction. This effect is attenuated by stimulation of acetylcholine and adenosine receptors.[6,7]

Potassium Channels

A variety of potassium channels both voltage- and ligand-gated are present in cardiac cells. Three voltage-gated potassium channels moderate the delayed rectifier current, which repolarizes the cell membrane (see Fig. 3-3).[8]

Several ligand-gated potassium channels have been identified. Acetylcholine and adenosine-activated potassium channels are time independent, and lead to hyperpolarization in pacemaker and nodal cells, thereby delaying spontaneous depolarization. A calcium-activated potassium channel opens in the presence of high levels of cytosolic calcium and probably enhances the delayed rectifier current, leading to early termination of the action potential. An ATP-sensitive potassium channel is closed in the metabolically normal myocyte, but is opened in the metabolically starved myocyte in which ATP stores have been depleted, leading to hyperpolarization of the cell, thereby retarding depolarization and contraction.

Energy-Dependent Ion Pumps

Sodium-Potassium ATP-Dependent Pump

The sodium-potassium pump uses the energy obtained from the hydrolysis of ATP to move three Na^+ ions out of the cell and two K^+ ions into the cell, each against its respective concentration gradient. Because there is a net outward current (three Na^+ ions for two K^+ ions), the pump contributes about 10 mV to the resting membrane potential. The activity of the pump is strongly stimulated by attachment of sodium to its binding site. The Na-K ATPase has a very high affinity for ATP, so that the pump continues to function even if ATP levels are reduced.

ATP-Dependent Calcium Pump

The ATP-dependent calcium pump transports calcium out of the cell against a strong concentration gradient. This action represents a net outward current, but the magnitude of this current is quite small because the bulk of calcium transferred out of the cell occurs with sodium-calcium exchange (described in the following). The cytosolic protein, *calmodulin,* can complex with calcium and facilitate the action of the pump; thus, increased intracellular calcium levels stimulate the pump.[9,10]

Ion Exchangers

Sodium-Calcium Exchanger

Multiple proteins that traverse the membrane allow ion exchanges using the potential energy of the electrochemical gradient, which favors the influx of sodium. The sodium-calcium exchanger exchanges three extracellular sodium ions for one intracellular calcium ion, leading to a net single positive charge transported into the cell with each exchange. The exchange system is sensitive to the concentration of sodium and calcium on both sides of the membrane, and to the membrane potential. If external sodium concentrations decrease, the driving force for removal of calcium from the cell is decreased, leading to an increase in cytosolic calcium (and a consequent increase in contraction). Thus hyponatremia can increase cardiac contractility. If the intracellular sodium concentration increases, as occurs with ischemia, the gradient for sodium influx is reduced, and the pump slows down or actually reverses, extruding sodium in exchange for an influx of calcium. This mechanism may be

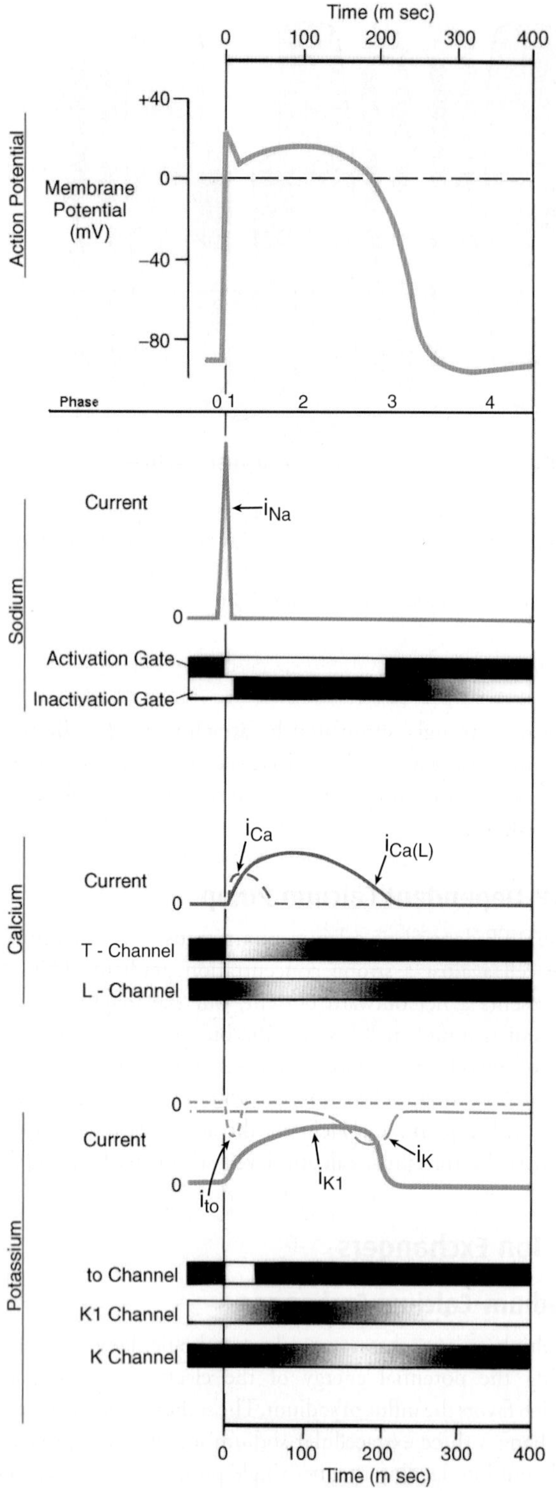

FIGURE 3-3 A typical ventricular myocyte action potential and the ion currents contributing to it are schematically represented. Inward (depolarizing) currents are depicted as positive, and outward (repolarizing) currents are depicted as negative. The horizontal filled bars show the state of the gate of the ion channel (white = open; black = closed; shaded = partially open). In the case of the sodium channel, both the activation and inactivation gates are shown (Ca – calcium; i = current; K = potassium; Na = sodium).

central to the accumulation of calcium during ischemia. The sodium-calcium exchange mechanism has a maximum exchange rate that is some 30 times higher than the sarcolemmal ATP-dependent calcium pump and is the primary mechanism for removal of excess cytosolic calcium.[7]

Sodium-Hydrogen Exchanger

The sodium-hydrogen exchanger extrudes one intracellular hydrogen ion in exchange for one extracellular sodium ion, and is electrically neutral. This pump prevents intracellular acidification. Acidification (eg, during ischemia) increases the affinity of the pump for H^+ promoting the removal of H^+ preserving intracellular pH at the expense of sodium accumulation. The accumulation of sodium ions may then trigger reversal of the sodium-calcium exchange pump to favor the accumulation of calcium within the cell. This is a possible mechanism underlying injury or cell death during ischemia-reperfusion.

Intracellular Communication Pathways

To allow concurrent activation of all the myofibrils in the muscle cell, the electrical activation signal must be rapidly and evenly spread through all portions of the cell. This is accomplished through the t-tubules, and the subsarcolemmal cistern and sarcotubular network of the sarcoplasmic reticulum.

Transverse Tubules (T-Tubules)

The basic contractile unit in a muscle cell is the sarcomere. Sarcomeres are joined together in the myofibril at the z-lines. A system of transverse tubules (t-tubules) extends the sarcolemma into the interior of the cardiac cell (Fig. 3-4). These tubules are perpendicular to the sarcomere, near the z-lines, extending the extracellular space close to the contractile proteins. The transverse tubules contain the calcium channels, which are in close relationship to the foot proteins of the subsarcolemmal cisternae.

Sarcoplasmic Reticulum

The sarcoplasmic reticulum is a membrane network within cytoplasm of the cell surrounding the myofibrils. The primary function of the sarcoplasmic reticulum is excitation-contraction coupling by sudden release of calcium to stimulate the contraction proteins and then rapid removal of this calcium to allow relaxation of the contractile elements. The subsarcolemmal cisternae and the sarcotubular network are the two portions of the sarcoplasmic reticulum that mediate this process.

The subsarcolemmal cisternae are near the sarcolemma and the t-tubules. Foot proteins are found in the membrane of the sarcoplasmic reticulum, with a large protein component extending into the gap between the subsarcolemmal cisternae and the sarcolemma of the t-tubule. The foot proteins respond to the release of calcium by opening a calcium channel, which allows the release of a much larger quantity of calcium from the subsarcolemmal cisternae. This is "calcium-triggered" calcium release, with calcium transported across the sarcolemma, leading to calcium release from the subsarcolemmal cisternae.

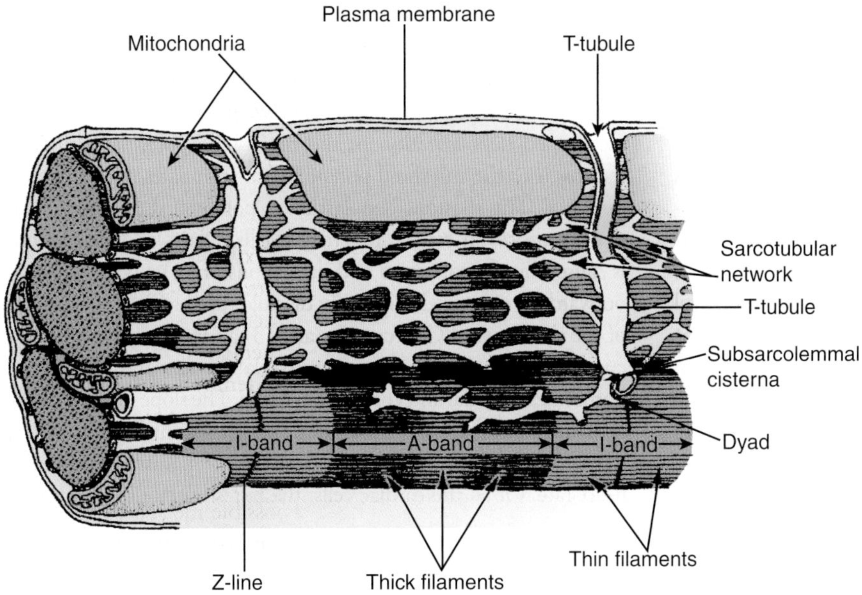

FIGURE 3-4 Myocyte anatomy. (*From Katz AM: Physiology of the Heart, 4th ed. Philadelphia, Lippincott Williams & Wilkins, 2006: p 21.*)

The magnitude of calcium release from the subsarcolemmal cisternae appears to be related to the magnitude of the trigger. The calcium channels then close and the calcium is returned to the sarcoplasmic reticulum by an ATP-dependent calcium pump located in the sarcotubular network.[1,10] The sarcotubular network is the portion of the sarcoplasmic reticulum that surrounds the contractile elements of the sarcomere.

Regulation of calcium transport by the cardiac sarcoplasmic reticulum occurs primarily at the site of the calcium pump. A calcium-calmodulin complex phosphorylates the pump to stimulate pump activity. Reduced ATP availability will slow pump function. Phospholamban inhibits the basal rate of calcium transport by the calcium pump. This inhibition is reversed when phospholamban is phosphorylated by a cyclic AMP- or calcium-calmodulin–dependent protein kinase. This is a very important mechanism for beta-adrenergic regulation; cyclic AMP levels increase with activation of the beta-adrenergic receptor. As phospholamban is phosphorylated, there is accelerated calcium turnover and increased sensitivity of the calcium pump, which facilitates uptake of calcium from the cytosol and relaxation of the heart. Phosphorylation of phospholamban does not affect the sarcolemmal calcium pump, thereby tending to favor retention of calcium within the cell (increasing the calcium content of the sarcoplasmic reticulum at the expense of calcium removed from the cell through the sarcolemma). This might lead to an increased pulse of calcium within the cell, thereby favoring increased contractility.[7,10] Phosphorylation of phospholamban, in the presence of intracellular calcium, stimulates calcium uptake to protect the heart from calcium overload.

In this ionic milieu, the importance of intracellular pH maintenance should be stressed. Regulation of intracellular pH is complex and beyond the scope of this text, but a few simple principles are important to review. Reduced intracellular pH diminishes the amount of calcium released from the sarcoplasmic reticulum and reduces the responsiveness of myofilaments to calcium. Elevation of the pH will have the opposite effect. The clinical relevance of this observation cannot be overstressed.

ELECTRICAL ACTIVATION OF THE HEART

Normal Cardiac Rhythm

The Resting Membrane Potential

The state of the cardiac cell is determined by a balance of forces based on electrical and chemical gradients. At rest (during diastole), the cardiac cell is polarized. The electrical potential across the sarcolemma is primarily determined by the concentration gradient of potassium across the membrane. This gradient is established by the sodium-potassium pump. However, once this pump shuts off, the steady state is determined by the balance of electrical and chemical forces. The sarcolemma is impermeable to some ions, permeable to others, and selectively permeable to others. Steady-state properties of a mixture of ions of variable permeabilities across a membrane are described by the *Gibbs-Donnan equilibrium*.[11] The sarcolemma prevents the diffusion of large anions (eg, proteins and organic phosphates). At rest, the sarcolemma is relatively permeable to potassium ions because of the open state of most potassium channels, but less permeable to sodium. The concentration gradient established by the sodium-potassium pump promotes the efflux of potassium ions across the sarcolemma. The outward flow of positive ions is counterbalanced by the increasing electronegativity of the interior of the cell owing to the impermeant anions. A Gibbs-Donnan equilibrium is established such that the electronegativity of the cell interior retards potassium ion efflux to the same degree that the concentration gradient favors K^+ efflux. At equilibrium, the forces balance with an intracellular potassium concentration of 135 mM and extracellular concentration of 4 mM and a predicted resting membrane potential of −94 mV. The actual resting membrane potential is measured at about −90 mV because of smaller contributions from the current of other less permeable ions (eg, sodium and calcium). However, the potassium current is the main determinant of the resting membrane potential.[12]

The Action Potential

The action potential represents the triggered response to a stimulus derived either internally (slow depolarizing ionic currents) or externally (depolarization of adjacent cells). A typical fast response action potential, which occurs in atrial and ventricular myocytes and special conduction fibers, is depicted in Fig. 3-3. As the transmembrane potential decreases to approximately –65 mV, the "fast" sodium channels open. These channels remain open for a few milliseconds when the inactivation gate of the "fast" sodium channel closes. The large gradient of sodium ions promotes rapid influx, depolarizing the cell to a slightly positive transmembrane potential: phase 0 of the action potential. A transient potassium current (i_{to}) causes a very early repolarization (phase 1) of the action potential, but this fast channel closes quickly. The plateau of the action potential (phase 2) is sustained at a neutral or slightly positive level by an inward flowing calcium current, first from the transient calcium channel and second through the long-lasting calcium channel. The plateau is also sustained by a decrease in the outward potassium current (i_{K1}). With time, the long-lasting calcium channels begin to close, and the repolarizing potassium current (i_K, the delayed rectifier current) leads to the initiation of phase 3 of the action potential. As repolarization progresses, the stronger first potassium current (i_{K1}) dominates, leading to full repolarization of the membrane to the resting negative potential. During the bulk of the depolarized interval (phase 4), the first potassium current predominates in myocytes.

Refractory Period

The sodium channels cannot respond to a second wave of depolarization until the inactivation gates are reopened (by repolarization during phase 3). As a result, the membrane is refractory to the propagation of a second impulse during this time interval, referred to as the absolute refractory period. As the membrane is repolarized during early phase 3 of the action potential, and some of the sodium channels have been reactivated, a short interval exists during which only very strong impulses can activate the cell, which is termed the *relative refractory period.* A drug that acts to speed up the inactivation gate will shorten both the absolute and the relative refractory periods.[1,13,14]

Spontaneous Depolarization

The action potential of the slow response cells of the nodal tissue (sinoatrial node, or SA node, and atrioventricular node, or AV node) differs from that in the fast response cells, as shown in Fig. 3-5. The rapid upstroke of phase 0 is less prominent due to the absence of fast Na^+ channels. Phase 1 is absent, as there is no rapid inward potassium current. In addition, the plateau phase (phase 2) is abbreviated because of the lack of a sustained active Na^+ inward current, and the lack of sustained calcium current. The repolarization phase (phase 3) leads to a resting phase (phase 4) that begins to depolarize again, as opposed to the relatively stable resting membrane potential of myocytes. The slowly depolarizing phase 4 resting potential is called the *diastolic depolarization current,* or the *pacemaker potential.* Continued depolarization of the membrane potential ultimately reduces it to the threshold potential that stimulates another action potential. This diastolic depolarization potential is the mechanism of *automaticity* in cardiac pacemaker cells. Diastolic depolarization is caused by the concerted and net actions of: (1) a decrease in the outward K^+ current during early diastole (phase 4); (2) persistence of the slow inward Ca^{2+} current; and (3) an increasing inward Na^+ current during diastole. The inward Na^+ current most likely predominates in nodal and conduction tissue. The slope of the diastolic depolarization determines the rate of action potential generation in the pacemaker cells, and is the primary mechanism determining heart rate. Of all the cardiac cells, the fastest rate of depolarization

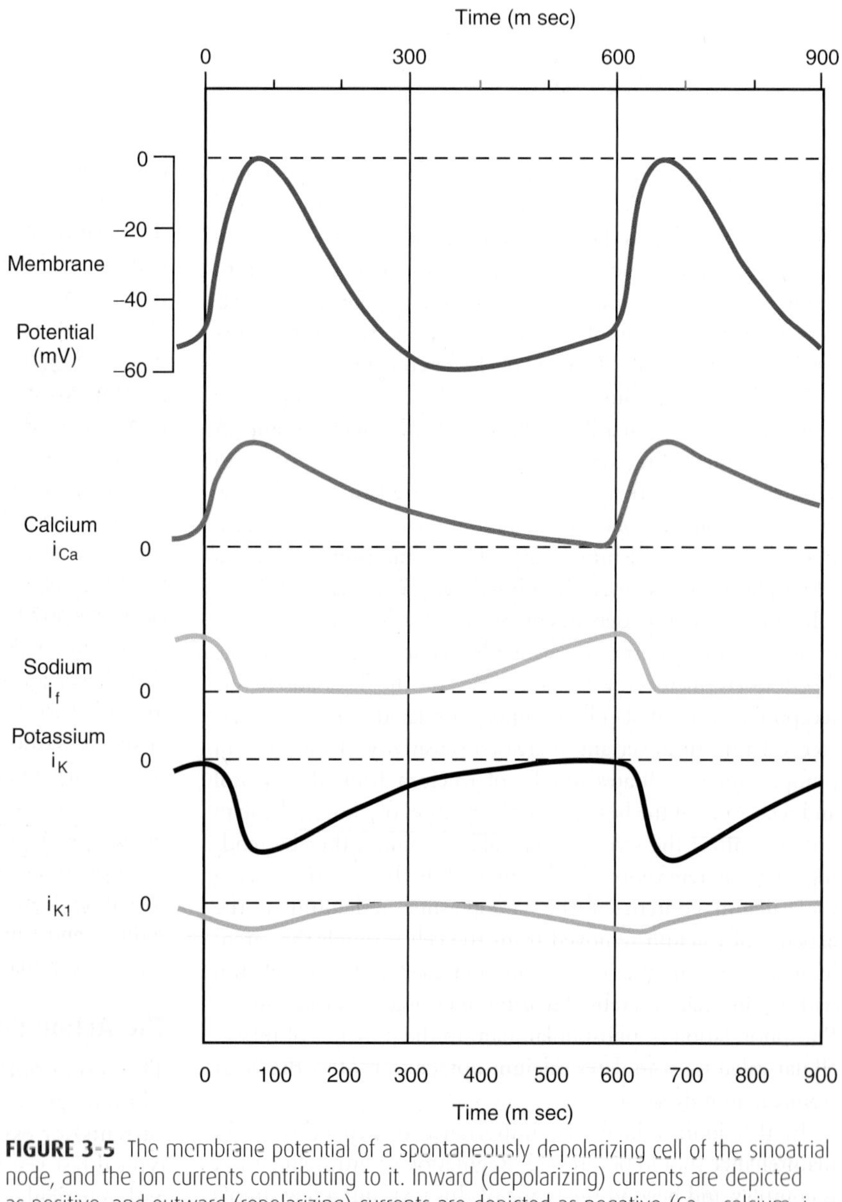

FIGURE 3-5 The membrane potential of a spontaneously depolarizing cell of the sinoatrial node, and the ion currents contributing to it. Inward (depolarizing) currents are depicted as positive, and outward (repolarizing) currents are depicted as negative (Ca = calcium; i = current; K = potassium; Na = sodium).

is in the SA node, and action potentials are generated at a rate of 70 to 80 per minute. The AV node is a slower rate of depolarization, at 40 to 60 times per minute. The ventricular myocytes are the slowest, at 30 to 40 times per minute. Once a depolarization is initiated in a pacemaker cell and propagated, it will depolarize the remainder of the heart in a synchronized and sequential manner. The heart rate can be altered by changing slope of the diastolic depolarization (eg, acetylcholine decreases the slope and heart rate; beta-adrenergic agonists increase the slope and heart rate). If the slope is unchanged, hyperpolarization (more negative resting potential) or raising the threshold potential will increase the time to reach threshold, thus decreasing the heart rate.

Propagation of the Action Potential

Each myocyte is mechanically anchored and electrically connected to the next myocyte by an intercalated disc at the end of the cell. These discs contain gap junctions that facilitate flow of charged molecules from one cell to the next. These pores are composed of a protein, connexin. Permeability through the cardiac gap junction is increased by both ATP- and cyclic AMP-dependent kinases. This allows the gap junctions to close if ATP levels fall, thereby reducing electrical and presumably mechanical activity, which is essential in limiting cell death when one region of the heart is damaged. It also allows conduction to increase when cyclic AMP increases in response to adrenergic stimulation.

After spontaneous depolarization occurs in the pacemaker cells of the SA node, the action potential is conducted throughout the heart. Special electrical pathways facilitate this conduction. Three internodal paths exist through the atrium between the SA node and the AV node. After traversing the AV node, the action potential is propagated rapidly through the bundle of His and into the Purkinje fibers located on the endocardium of the left and right ventricles. Rapid conduction through the atrium causes contraction of most of the atrial muscle synchronously (within 60 to 90 milliseconds). Similarly, the rapid conduction of the signal throughout the ventricle leads to synchronous contraction of the bulk of the ventricular myocardium (within 60 milliseconds). The delay in the propagation of the action potential through the AV node by 120 to 140 milliseconds allows the atria to complete contraction before the ventricles contract. Slow conduction in the AV node is related to a relatively higher internal resistance because of a small number of gap junctions between cells, and slowly rising action potentials.

Abnormal Cardiac Rhythm

Aberrant Pacemaker Foci

Normally the SA node spontaneously depolarizes first, such that the cardiac beat originates from this primary pacemaker site. If the SA node is damaged or slowed by vagal stimulation or drugs (eg, acetylcholine), pacemakers in the atrium, AV node, or the His-Purkinje system can take over. Occasionally, aberrant foci in the heart spontaneously depolarize, thereby leading to aberrant or "premature" contractions from the atrium or the ventricle. These contractions ordinarily do not interfere with the normal depolarization of the heart.

Re-entry Arrhythmias

Re-entry arrhythmias are perhaps the most common dangerous cardiac rhythm. Ordinarily, the action potential depolarizes the entire atrium or the entire ventricle in a short enough time interval so that all of the muscle is refractory to further stimulation at the same time. A re-entry arrhythmia is caused by propagation of an action potential through the heart in a "circus" movement. For re-entry to occur, there must be a unidirectional block (transient or permanent) to action potential propagation. Additionally, the effective refractory period of the reentered region must be shorter that the propagation time around the loop.[12] For example, if a portion of the previously depolarized myocardium has repolarized before the propagation of the action potential is completed throughout the atrium or ventricle, then that action potential can continue its propagation into this repolarized muscle. Such an event generally requires either dramatic slowing of conduction of the action potential, a long conduction pathway, or a shortened refractory period (Fig. 3-6). All of these situations occur clinically. Ischemia slows the sodium-potassium pump, which decreases the resting membrane potential and slows propagation of the action potential.

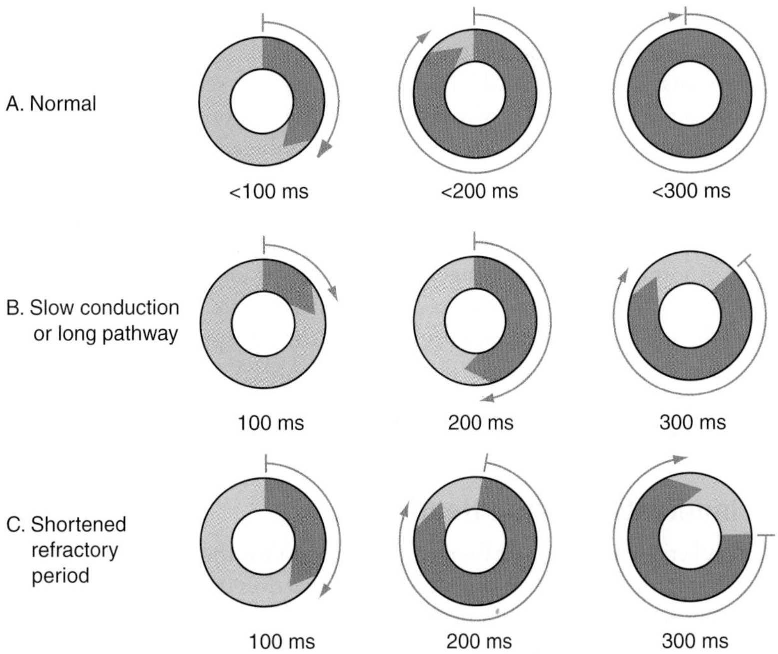

FIGURE 3-6 Three conditions predisposing to re-entry or "circus" pathways for action potential propagation are shown. Muscle that is refractory to action potential propagation is shown as black. Normally, as the action potential travels through the atrium or ventricle, all the muscle is depolarized sufficiently that the action potential encounters no more nonrefractory muscle and stops (*A*). If there is slowed conduction speed or a long pathway (*B*), the action potential may find repolarized (nonrefractory) muscle and continue in a circular path. Similarly, a shortened refractory period (*C*) may lead to rapid repolarization and predispose to a re-entry and continuation of the action potential.

Hyperkalemia decreases the resting membrane potential, which increases excitability and inactivates the sodium-potassium pump, slowing propagation of the action potential. Progressive atrial dilation creates a long conduction pathway around the atrium. Adrenergic stimulation shortens the refractory period.

A special type of reentry arrhythmia occurs in Wolff-Parkinson-White syndrome in which an accessory pathway electrically connects the atrium and the ventricle. This accessory pathway can complete a circular electrical pathway between the atrium and the ventricle. Conduction is unidirectional across the AV node and the accessory pathway creates a loop that has a propagation time that is greater than the AV node refractory period, resulting in supraventricular tachycardia. In an alternative situation, because the accessory pathway does not have the inherent delay and refractory period of the AV node, rapid atrial tachycardias can be conducted in a 1:1 manner across the accessory pathway, leading to ventricular rates as fast as 300 beats per minute.

REGULATION OF CELLULAR FUNCTION

Types of Receptors and Second Messengers

Numerous types of receptors are involved in regulating cardiovascular function. They include G-protein (GTP-binding proteins)–coupled receptors, enzyme-linked receptors, ion channel-linked receptors, and nuclear receptors. Other ligands, such as nitric oxide, bind directly to their intracellular target.[15] G-protein–coupled receptors are the most important. Ligand binding activates the synthesis of intracellular second messengers, protein kinases, and voltage-gated potassium channels.[16] The most important second messenger is cyclic AMP, which transmits the response to sympathetic stimulation. Cyclic AMP is produced from ATP by adenylyl cyclase and broken down to AMP by phosphodiesterases. Cyclic AMP production is promoted by sympathetic and inhibited by parasympathetic stimulation. Another second messenger, cyclic GMP is similarly produced, in response to nitric oxide and naturetic peptides, by guanylyl cyclase and broken down by phosphodiesterases and opposes the actions of cyclic AMP.[17] These and other second messengers activate signaling enzymes within the cell such as protein kinases.

Innervation of the Heart

Sympathetic fibers originate from the fourth and fifth thoracic spinal cord regions. Parasympathetic innervation derives through the vagus nerve connecting to the SA and AV nodes, atria, and blood vessels. Stretch receptors located in the atria and ventricles provide feedback to the central nervous system. Atrial natriuretic peptide (similar to B-type natriuretic peptide, which is clinically measured) is secreted by atrial myocytes in response to stretch and promotes natriuresis, diuresis, and smooth muscle relaxation. Stretch receptors on the posterior and inferior ventricular wall can trigger parasympathetic stimulation and inhibit sympathetic activity, leading to bradycardia and conduction block (von Bezold-Jarisch reflex).[18]

Parasympathetic Regulation

The parasympathetic nervous system is particularly important in control of the SA node. Acetylcholine released by the nerve endings of the parasympathetic system stimulates muscarinic receptors in the heart. The activated receptors produce an intracellular stimulatory G-protein that opens acetylcholine-gated potassium channels. An increased outward (repolarizing) flow of potassium leads to hyperpolarization of the SA node cells. Stimulation of the muscarinic receptors also inhibits the formation of cyclic AMP, inhibiting the opening of calcium channels. A decreased inward flow of calcium, combined with an increased outward flow of potassium, leads to slowing of the spontaneous diastolic depolarization of the SA node class (see Fig. 3-5). A similar effect in the AV node leads to slowing of conduction through the AV node.[1]

Sympathetic Stimulation and Blockade

Sympathetic or adrenergic receptors in the heart affect heart rate, contractility, conduction velocity, and automaticity; and in the peripheral vasculature they affect smooth muscle contraction and relaxation. Alpha-adrenergic receptors cause vasoconstriction. There are two types of beta-adrenergic receptors: the $beta_1$-adrenergic receptors, which predominate in the heart, and the $beta_2$-adrenergic receptors, which are present in blood vessels and promote relaxation. The number of beta receptors per unit area (receptor density) of the sarcolemma can be upregulated or downregulated in response to various stimuli. Receptor sensitivity can also change depending on ambient conditions and variable stimuli.[19] Cardiopulmonary bypass and ischemia cause downregulation of cardiac beta receptors. Acidemia causes desensitization of beta receptors. This is important in the perioperative period when acidemia can reduce cardiac contractility, systemic vascular tone, and the response to inotropic agents.

The $beta_1$-adrenergic receptor couples with adenylyl cyclase (Fig. 3-7). When the receptor site is occupied by an adrenergic agonist, a stimulatory G-protein is formed, which combines with GTP. This activated G-protein–GTP complex then promotes the activity of adenylyl cyclase, leading to the formation of cyclic AMP from ATP. The G-protein–GTP complex and the cyclic AMP actively promote calcium channel opening. The increased tendency for calcium channels to open during $beta_1$-receptor stimulation increases cytosolic calcium and leads to a number of physiologic effects: (1) A positive *chronotropic* (heart rate) effect whereby the heart rate, conduction, and contraction velocity increase and the action potential is shortened, leading to a shortening of systole; (2) a positive *dromotropic* (conduction velocity) effect of accelerated conduction through the AV node; and (3) a positive *inotropic* (contractility) effect. Increased activity of the sarcoplasmic reticulum calcium pump (more rapid calcium uptake) leads to more rapid relaxation, which facilitates ventricular filling; (4) a positive *lusitropic* (relaxation) effect.[20]

Two negative feedback systems diminish the response to beta agonists when stimulation is repetitive or persistent (tachyphylaxis). Increased cyclic AMP leads to: (1) increased phosphorylation of beta receptors leading to downregulation;

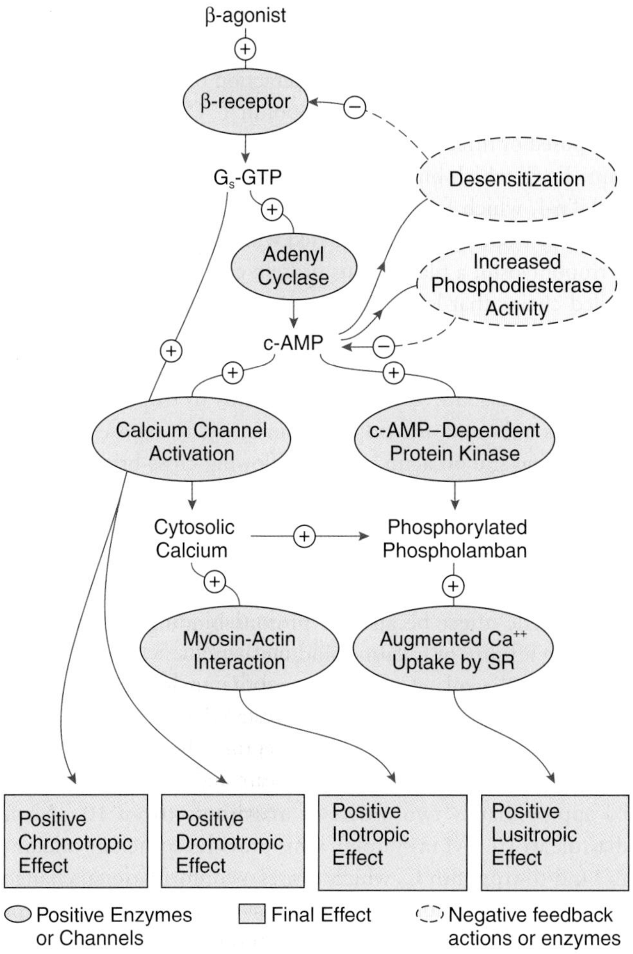

FIGURE 3-7 Adrenergic stimulation via the action of beta agonists on beta receptors leads to a cascade of events in the myocyte, some of which are shown here. Note that an increase in cyclic AMP causes the activation of two inhibitory pathways, retarding excessively sustained adrenergic stimulation (cyclic AMP = cyclic adenosine monophosphate; Gs = stimulatory G-protein; GTP = guanosine triphosphate; SR = sarcoplasmic reticulum).

and (2) increased activity of phosphodiesterase, the enzyme that degrades cyclic AMP. Acidosis will inhibit many steps in the sympathetic activation cascade, impairing contractility.

The activity spectrum of adrenergic receptors forms the basis of many therapeutic interventions; perioperatively to support cardiac function, and chronically to reduce mortality from myocardial infarction and treat congestive heart failure. The selectivity of the agonists and antagonists allows adaptation for various clinical scenarios. Some examples are detailed in Table 3-1.

Reduction in inotropy, lusitropy, chronotropy, and dromotropy by beta blockade will reduce myocardial oxygen consumption contributing to many of its beneficial effects. As beta blockade will lead to upregulation of sarcolemmal receptors, sudden cessation of beta blockade may cause a temporarily enhanced (and potentially dangerous) sensitivity to adrenergic stimulation.

Phosphodiesterase Inhibition

Cyclic AMP plays a central role in the regulation of the cardiac cell. Cytosolic levels of cyclic AMP are also increased by activation of receptors other than beta receptors (ie, for histamine, dopamine, glucagon), and are decreased by inhibitory G-proteins produced by stimulation of muscarinic receptors by acetylcholine and by stimulation of adenosine receptors. Referring to Fig. 3-7, one negative feedback response to the increase in cyclic AMP is an increase in phosphodiesterase, which breaks down cyclic AMP. Phosphodiesterase inhibitors (amrinone, milrinone) inhibit the breakdown of cyclic AMP and thereby increase its level in the cytosol. Their effect is synergistic to that of beta agonists. Because they do not stimulate the production of the G-protein–GTP complex, they have a lesser effect on calcium channel activation, and therefore less of the troublesome positive chronotropic and dromotropic effects of beta-adrenergic stimulation.[21]

TABLE 3-1 Adrenergic Agonists and Antagonists Correlating Selective Activity with Clinical Usage

	Drug	Alpha	Beta-1	Beta-2	Clinical Usage
Agonists	Epinephrine	Y	Y	Y	Low cardiac output, hypotension
	Norepinephrine	Y	Y		Hypotension
	Phenylephrine	Y			Hypotension
	Dobutamine		Y		Low cardiac output
	Dopamine	Y	Y		Low cardiac output, hypotension
	Isoproterenol		Y	Y	Bradycardia, low cardiac output, pulmonary hypertension
Antagonists (beta-blockers)	Metoprolol		Y		Tachycardia, hypertension, MI, angina
	Atenolol		Y		Tachycardia, hypertension, MI, angina
	Esmolol		Y		Tachycardia, hypertension, MI, angina
	Carvedilol	Y (alpha-1)	Y	Y	Congestive heart failure

Adenosine Receptors

There are four types of adenosine receptors. Adenosine receptors are linked to inhibitory and stimulatory G-proteins and various kinases. Activation of adenosine A_1 receptors leads to inhibition of cyclic AMP production, inhibition of the slow calcium channel, and opening of an adenosine-activated ATP-sensitive potassium (K_{ATP}) channel. This leads to hyperpolarization, which delays conduction through the AV node and slows the ventricular response to atrial tachycardia.[1,22] Pretreatment with adenosine confers a cardioprotective effect during ischemia and can inhibit the inflammatory responses initiated by ischemia and reperfusion.[22]

Other Regulators of Hemodynamic Function

Angiotensin II is a vasoconstrictor and reduces renal fluid excretion. It is the final effector of the renin-angiotensin-aldosterone system. Renin, secreted by the juxtaglomerular apparatus in the kidney, splits angiotensin I from angiotensinogen, produced by the liver. Angiotensin I is converted to angiotensin II by the angiotensin-converting enzyme (ACE or kininase II, the target of ACE inhibitors) mainly in the lungs. Angiotensin II acts by causing: 1) vasoconstriction to increase systemic vascular resistance; and (2) stimulation of the adrenal cortex to secrete aldosterone, which increases fluid volume and thus cardiac output. Through both actions, angiotensin II modifies blood pressure. Angiotensin II receptor blockers (ARBs) directly inhibit angiotensin II subtype IA receptors.

The endothelins (ETs) have multiple effects. When bound to ET-A receptors they cause vasoconstriction, increased contractility, and proliferation. When bound to ET-B receptors they stimulate the release of NO and prostacyclin and have a vasodilatory effect.[23]

Bradykinins, acting through their receptors, cause vasodilation. Arginine vasopressin promotes reabsorption of water by the kidney and has a vasoconstrictor effect. Naturetic peptides, released in response to atrial distention, promote diuresis and arteriolar dilatation. Nitric oxide at low concentrations causes vasodilation, reduces chronotropy, and has a positive inotropic effect.[24]

CONTRACTION OF CARDIAC MUSCLE

Molecular Level (The Sarcomere)

The primary contractile unit of all muscle cells is the sarcomere (see Fig. 3-4). Sarcomeres are connected end to end at the z-line to form myofibrils. The myocyte contains numerous myofibrils arranged in parallel. A portion of a sarcomere is schematically depicted in Fig. 3-8. Actin polymerizes to form the thin filaments that are anchored at the z-line. Myosin polymerizes to form the thick filaments of the sarcomere. Myosin consists of a tail of two "heavy" chains intertwined to form a helix, forming the rigid backbone of the thick filament. The globular head of myosin is attached to the heavy chain backbone by a mobile hinge and projects outward. The globular myosin head is an ATPase with a binding site for actin. Actin binds to the myosin globular head activating the myosin ATPase to hydrolyze ATP. This leads to a conformational change in the myosin that pulls the filament (Fig. 3-8B).

Two proteins modulate the interaction of actin and myosin; troponin and tropomyosin. Troponin ("T" in Fig. 3-8A) is composed of three units: Tn-C, the regulatory calcium binding unit; Tn-T, which binds the troponin complex to tropomyosin; and Tn-I, which facilitates interruption of actin-myosin interaction by tropomyosin. Associated with each troponin complex is tropomyosin; a filamentous protein composed of two tightly coiled chains that lays in the groove formed by the two intertwined filaments of actin. In the absence of calcium, Tn-I is tightly bound to actin so that tropomyosin blocks the binding of myosin to actin. When calcium binds to troponin C, Tn-I becomes unbound, the tropomyosin moves to expose the myosin binding site on actin, thereby allowing cross-bridge formation between actin and myosin. Tn-C has several regulatory sites that are affected by phosphorylation in response to hormonal and other stimuli, to alter the sensitivity and degree of force generation. Acidosis will reduce contractile force through an allosteric affect because of protons binding to Tn-I, and reducing affinity of calcium binding sites.[25]

During diastole, Ca^{2+} is unavailable to bind troponin C and the myosin binding site on actin is blocked. Depolarization leads to an influx of calcium ions and the subsequent "calcium-triggered, calcium release" increases the intracellular Ca^{2+} levels by approximately two orders of magnitude (from 10^{-7} M in diastole to 10^{-5} M in systole). This provides sufficient calcium to bind to troponin C, which causes a conformational change in the troponin molecule, removing the inhibitory effect of troponin I-tropomyosin, allowing actin-myosin cross-bridge formation (Fig. 3-8A). Cross-bridge formation activates the myosin ATPase and initiates the conformational change in the myosin "hinge" drawing the z-lines closer together (Fig. 3-8B). ADP and P_i are released. ATP binds to the myosin head, allowing dissociation from the actin and realigning the myosin globular head, preparing it to repeat the process. This process cycles until the end of muscular contraction is signaled by the reduction in intracellular calcium levels by sequestration into the sarcoplasmic reticulum.

The strength of the myocardial contraction is primarily mediated by the degree to which actin binding sites are exposed. This depends on the affinity of troponin for calcium and the availability of calcium ions. The initial calcium ion influx is altered by cyclic AMP, stimulatory and inhibitory G-proteins, and acetylcholine. The magnitude of the calcium trigger determines the magnitude of the cytosolic calcium release from the sarcoplasmic reticulum. The rate of uptake of calcium from the cytosol is altered by cyclic AMP (see Fig. 3-7). Cyclic AMP can phosphorylate a portion of the troponin molecule, facilitating the rapid release of calcium, increasing the rate of relaxation of the actin-myosin complex.[7,26]

The Cytoskeleton

Cytoskeletal elements include microfilaments composed of actin, intermediate filaments composed of desmin, and microtubules made of tubulin.[27] The cytoskeleton maintains cellular anatomy, transmits developed tension, and links adjacent

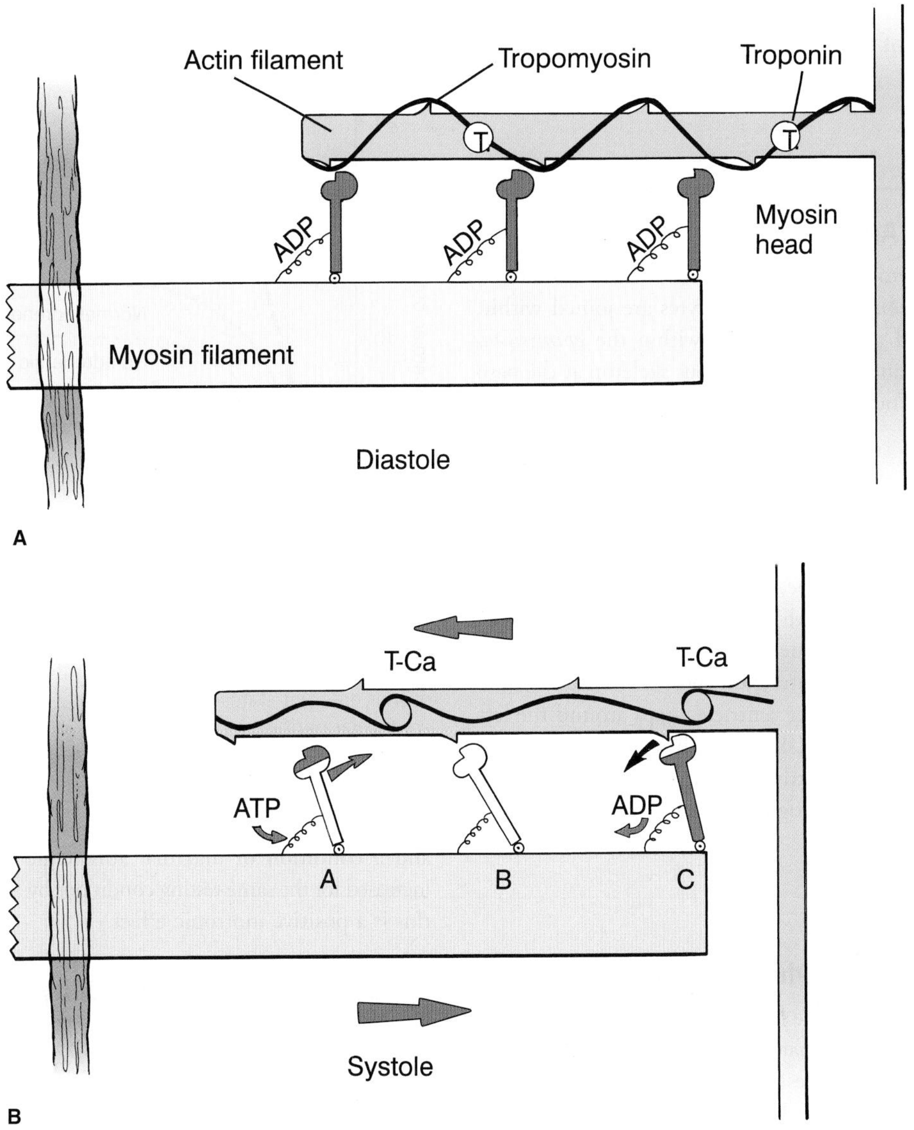

FIGURE 3-8 The interaction of actin and myosin filaments converts chemical energy into mechanical movement. In diastole, the active sites on the actin filament are covered by tropomyosin. When calcium combines with troponin, the tropomyosin is pulled away from the actin active sites, allowing the energized myosin heads (depicted in solid black and cocked at right angles to the filament) to engage and sweep the actin filament along. The myosin heads are de-energized in this process. Myosin ATPase re-cocks (re-energizes) the head by utilizing the energy derived from the hydrolysis of ATP. In systole, a de-energizing head (*C*), a de-energized head (*B*), and a re-energizing head (*A*) are shown.

myocytes. It also has a role in intracellular signaling. Cardiac myocytes are mechanically linked through the intercalated discs by the fascia adherens and desmosomes.[28] Sarcomere tension is transmitted through actin microfilaments to the fascia adherens of the intercalated discs. Intermediate filaments of adjacent cells are linked through desmosomes.

Regulation of the Strength of Contraction by Initial Sarcomere Length

In cardiac muscle, the strength of contraction is related to resting sarcomere length (see also the Frank-Starling relationship in the following). Maximal contraction force occurs when the resting sarcomere length is between 2 and 2.4 mm. At this length, there is optimal overlap of the actin and myosin maximizing the number of actin-myosin cross-bridges. Force declines at a greater sarcomere length, with decreased overlap of actin and myosin. In the heart, a decrease in contractility related to decreased overlap of the filaments does not seem to occur clinically, as the resting length of the cardiac sarcomere rarely exceeds 2.2 to 2.4 mm. Once this length is reached, a stiff parallel elastic element prevents further dilation. If chamber dilation does occur, it appears to be primarily through slippage of fibers or myofibers rather than stretching of sarcomeres.[1] Stretching the myocardium increases contractility by increasing the sensitivity of troponin C to calcium. This length-dependent sensitivity to calcium is an important part of the ascending limb of the Starling curve observed in the intact ventricle.

THE PUMP

Microscopic Architecture

Each myocyte is surrounded by a connective tissue framework called the *endomysium.* Groups of myocytes are joined within the *perimysium,* and the entire muscle within the *epimysium.* Muscle bundles are anchored in the fibrous skeleton at the base of the heart. Muscle bundles spiral around the cavity in overlapping patterns.

Macroscopic Architecture

The geometry of each ventricle is adapted to the function required of it. The left ventricle, which must eject against high pressure, is conical in shape with inlet and outlet adjacent at the base of the cone. Cavity volume is reduced during systole by a combination of concentric contraction and wall thickening, the latter predominating. The right ventricle wraps around the left ventricle, its cavity is crescent shaped with separated points of inflow and outflow. Cavity reduction is primarily a result of concentric contraction of the right ventricular free wall against the septum.

Mechanics

Clinically Measureable Physiologic Parameters

Cardiac surgeons can assess the function of the heart in a number of ways. Aortic, pulmonary artery, pulmonary capillary wedge, and central venous pressures can be measured directly. Cardiac output can be estimated using thermodilution or based on oxygen saturation measurements. From these direct measurements, other parameters can be derived—although less accurate because of the cumulative error of the measured parameters inherent in the calculation—such as pulmonary and systemic vascular resistance, and ventricular stroke work. Ejection fraction—defined as stroke volume/end-diastolic volume—can be estimated by echocardiography and ventriculography, but is subject to change based on loading conditions, heart rate, and degree of contractility. Although clinically useful, these parameters do not directly measure contractility.

The Frank-Starling Relationship

Within physiologic limits, the heart functions as a sump pump. The more the heart is filled during diastole, the greater the quantity of blood that will be pumped out of the heart during systole. Under normal circumstances, the heart pumps all the blood that comes back to it without excessive elevation of venous pressures. In the normal heart, as ventricular filling is increased, the strength of ventricular contraction increases. The influence of sarcomere length on the force of contraction is called the Frank-Starling relationship. This relationship for the left ventricle is depicted in Fig. 3-9. Also depicted in Fig. 3-9

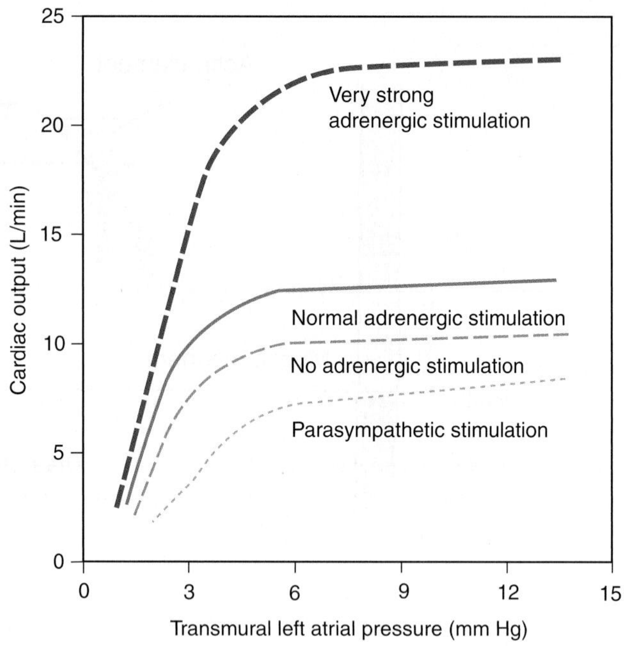

FIGURE 3-9 Starling curves for the left ventricle. The influence of four different states of neurohumoral stimulation on global ventricular performance is shown.

are two other states, a condition of normal adrenergic stimulation and a condition of maximal adrenergic stimulation. Force is increased for the same resting conditions by adrenergic stimulation; this is a positive inotropic effect.

Preload: Diastolic Distensibility and Compliance

Preload is the load placed on a resting muscle that stretches it to its functional length. In the heart, preload references the volume of blood in the cavity immediately prior to contraction (at end-diastole) because volume determines the degree of stretch imposed on the resting sarcomere. As volume cannot be easily assessed clinically, pressure is used as a surrogate; thus, the concept of preload is represented as the filling pressure of a chamber. The relationship between the end-diastolic pressure and the end-diastolic volume is complex. Several different diastolic pressure-volume relationships are shown in Fig. 3-11 (bold line). As end-diastolic volume increases, and the heart stretches, the end-diastolic pressure also increases. The compliance, or distensibility of the ventricle, is defined as the change in volume divided by the change in pressure. Conversely, the stiffness of the ventricle is the reciprocal of compliance, or the change in pressure divided by the change in volume.

A number of factors affect the diastolic pressure-volume relationship. A fibrotic heart, a hypertrophied heart, or an aging heart becomes increasingly stiff (Figs. 3-11C and 3-11E). In the case of fibrosis, this increasing stiffness is related to the development of a greater collagen network. In the case of hypertrophy, this increased stiffness is related both to stiffening of the noncontractile components of the heart and also to impaired relaxation of the heart. Relaxation is an active, energy-requiring process. This process is accelerated by catecholamine stimulation, but is impaired by ischemia, hypothyroidism, and chronic congestive heart failure. Examination of the diastolic pressure-volume curves in Fig. 3-11 reveals the importance of changes in diastolic distensibility in pathologic cardiac conditions.

Afterload: Vascular Impedance

The afterload of an isolated muscle is the tension against which it contracts. In simplest terms, for the heart, the afterload is determined by the pressure against which the ventricle must eject. The greater the afterload, the more mechanical energy that must be imparted to the blood mass (potential energy) to begin ejection. In addition to the potential energy imparted to the ejected blood by a change in pressure, the contracting left ventricle generates kinetic energy which overcomes the compliance of the distensible aorta and systemic arterial tree to move the blood into the arterial system. The energy necessary for this flow to occur is relatively small (potential energy >> kinetic energy). Resistance, which equals the change in pressure divided by cardiac output, reflects the potential energy imparted to blood. To accurately describe the forces overcome to eject blood from the ventricle, the compliance of the vascular system and kinetic energy imparted must also be considered: the impedance of the vascular system (commonly, but less accurately referred to as aortic impedance). Compliance reflects the capacity of the vascular system to accept the volume of ejected blood. When the vascular system is very compliant; resistance ≈ impedance. As compliance decreases (eg, with arteriosclerosis), resistance is less than impedance.[29] The interaction of resistance and compliance define the dicrotic notch, marking end-systole, closure of the aortic valve, on the aortic pressure tracing (Fig. 3-10).

The Cardiac Cycle

Multiple parameters of the cardiac cycle are represented in Fig. 3-10. By convention the cardiac cycle begins at end-diastole (ED), just prior to electrical activation of the ventricle. As the heart contracts, intracavitary pressure closes the mitral valve, then rapidly increases until the systemic diastolic pressure is reached (isovolumic contraction) and the aortic valve opens. Ejection begins and the intracavitary pressure continues to rise then fall as the ventricular volume decreases (ejection). When ejection ceases and the aortic valve closes, intracavitary pressure decreases rapidly until the mitral valve opens (isovolumic relaxation). Once the mitral valve opens, the ventricle fills rapidly, then more slowly as the intracavitary pressure slightly increases from distension prior to atrial systole (diastolic filling phase). The completion of atrial systole is the end of ventricular diastole. Atrial systole serves to increase the preload of the ventricle at a given systemic venous pressure.

A conceptual understanding of the venous pressure changes is important in diagnosing certain pathologic processes. The right atrial pressure is easily measured and pulmonary capillary wedge pressure is reflective of left atrial pressure. The "a" wave corresponds to atrial systole as pressure increases at end-diastole to complete ventricular filling. The "c" wave reflects pressure pushing the atrioventricular (AV) valve back into the atrium as the ventricular pressure rises then falls during systole. The "x" descent results from atrial relaxation and downward displacement

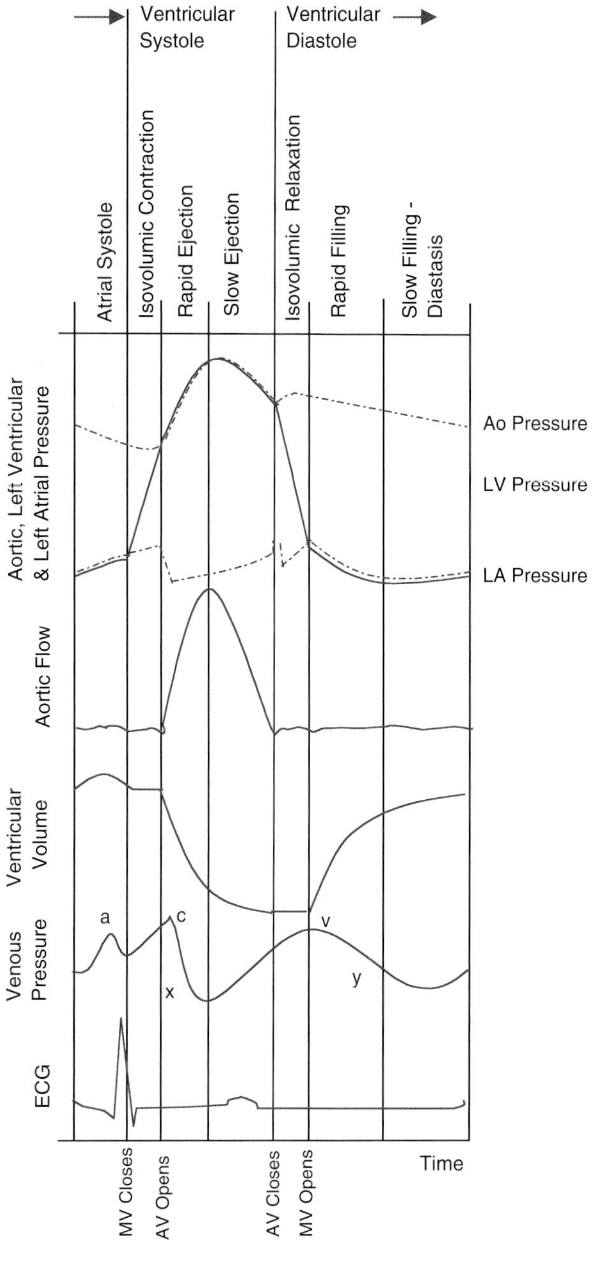

FIGURE 3-10 Temporal correlation of left atrial and ventricular, aortic, and systemic venous pressures, aortic flow, left ventricular volume and surface electrocardiogram.

of the AV valve with ventricular emptying. The "v" wave reflects the increasing atrial pressure from filling before the AV valve opens. The "y" descent is caused by rapid emptying of the atrium after the AV valve opens. Characteristic changes in these waveforms are used to diagnose and differentiate constrictive and restrictive processes, as discussed elsewhere in the text. A prominent left atrial "v" wave suggests mitral regurgitation.

Ventricular Pressure-Volume Relationships

The function of the heart can be described and quantified based on the relative intraventricular pressure and volume during the cardiac cycle (Fig. 3-11). Based on this relationship,

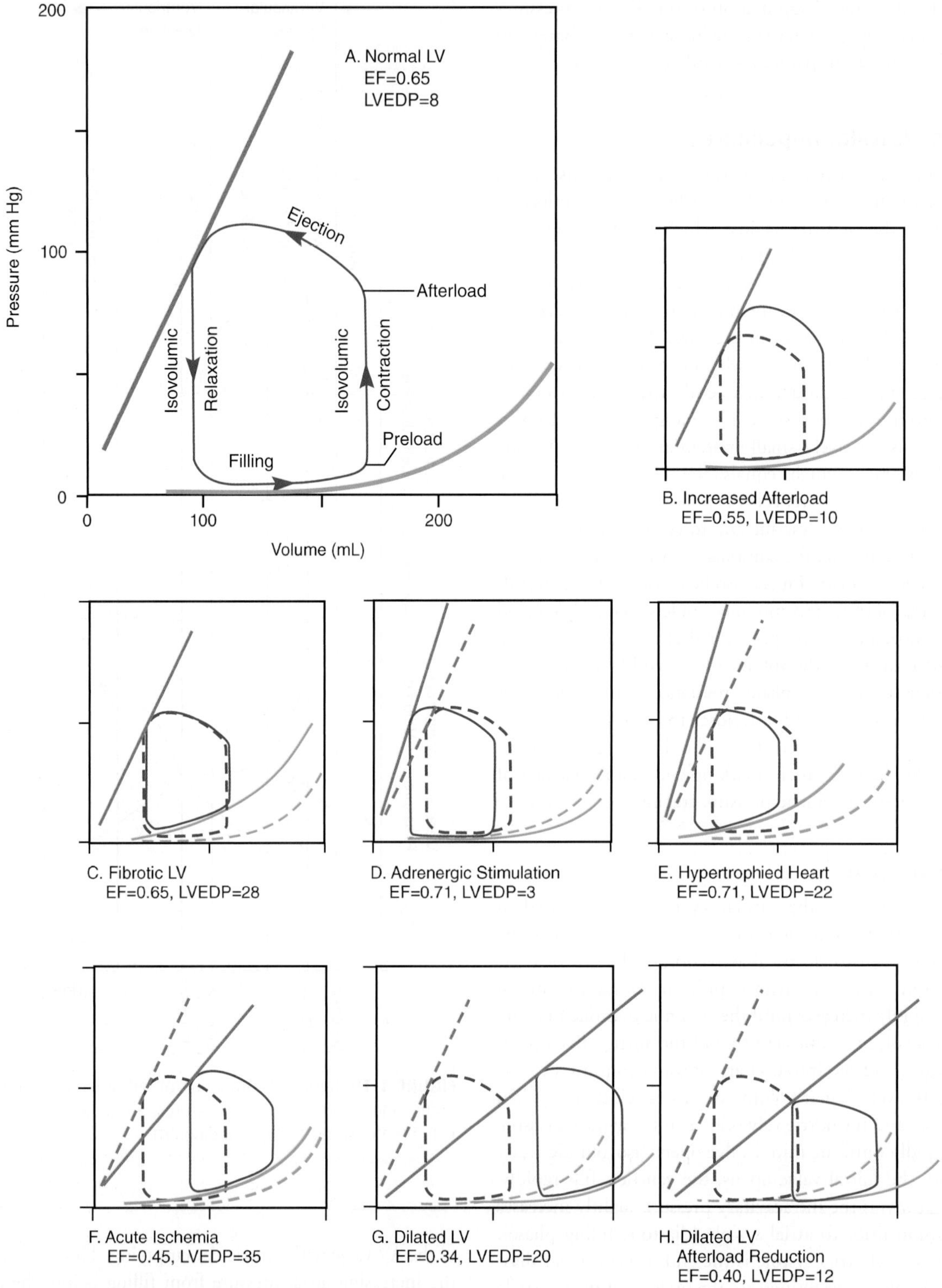

FIGURE 3-11 Left ventricular pressure-volume curves for various physiologic and pathologic conditions. (Detailed descriptions are in the text.) The bold curved line at the bottom of each loop series represents the diastolic pressure-volume relationship. The straight line located on the upper left side of each loop series is the end-systolic pressure-volume relationship. The stroke volume for each curve has been arbitrarily set at 75 mL. Systolic aortic pressure is 115 mm Hg in all curves except *B* (increased afterload, systolic pressure 140 mm Hg) and H (reduced afterload, systolic pressure 90 mm Hg) (EF = ejection fraction; LV = left ventricle; LVEDP = left ventricular end-diastolic pressure), in mm Hg.

various measures can be derived to assess cardiac performance. The ventricular pressure-volume relationship derives from the Frank-Starling relationship of sarcomere length and peak developed force: The force and extent of contraction (stroke volume) is a function of end-diastolic length (volume).

End-diastole (ED) is represented at the lower right corner of the loop in Fig. 3-11A. The pressure volume loop then successively tracks changes through isovolumic contraction (up to the upper right corner); ejection (left to the upper left corner, which represents end-systole [ES]); isovolumic relaxation (down to the bottom left corner); then filling (right to the lower right corner). Descriptive data to assess ventricular function are derived from the end-systolic pressure-volume point located in the upper left corner of the loop, and end-diastolic pressure-volume point located in the lower right corner of the loop. The area within the pressure-volume loop represents the internal work of the chamber.

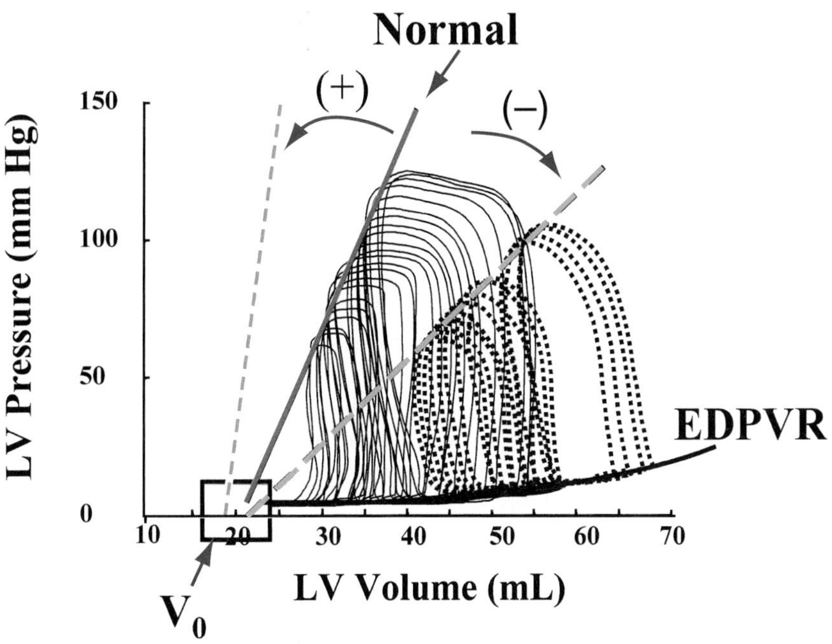

FIGURE 3-12 Two series of declining left ventricular pressure-volume loops generated during transient bicaval occlusion. Loops were generated in normal left ventricles (normal) and after 30 minutes of global normothermic ischemia and subsequent reperfusion (*dashed lines*). The end-systolic pressure-volume points from each series are connected by a line generated by linear regression. The end-diastolic pressure-volume relationship indicating chamber stiffness (inverse of compliance) is generated by fitting the end-diastolic point from each loop to an exponential curve. The volume axis intercept (V_0) is shown in the inset. A negative inotropic effect (ie, ischemia-reperfusion) is characterized by a decrease in the ESPVR slope, while a positive inotropic state is characterized by an increase in ESPVR slope. Notice that the V_0 for these conditions are in close proximity (*inset*). In some cases, a negative inotropic state is associated with a decrease in slope and an increase in V_0.

Contractility

The term *contractility* (inotropic state) refers to the intrinsic performance of the ventricle for a given preload, afterload, and heart rate. Otherwise stated, all the factors that impact cardiac performance independent of the acute effects of preload, afterload, and heart rate. In the purest sense, at a level of constant contractility, increased preload will increase cardiac output and stroke volume; increased afterload will decrease cardiac output and stroke volume; and increased heart rate (assuming adequate time for complete diastolic filling) will increase cardiac output without changing stroke volume. Although the inotropic state impacts cardiac output, it is difficult to quantify in clinically useful terms. For research purposes, the pressure-volume relationship can be used to quantify contractility by deriving the end-systolic pressure-volume relationship (ESPVR): Contractility is reflected in the slope (E_{ES}) and volume axis intercept (V_0) of the ESPVR (Fig. 3-12). Holding afterload and heart rate constant, a series of pressure-volume loops are inscribed during transient preload reduction induced by temporary vena caval occlusion; the area of the loops decreases and the loops are shifted to the left. The progressive pressure-volume points at end systole are then linearized to derive the ESPVR. Within a clinical range of systolic pressures (80 to 120 mm Hg), the end-systolic pressure-volume line is largely linear. An increase in inotropic state of the left ventricle is expressed as an increase in E_{ES} and sometimes a decrease in V_0. Conversely, a decrease in inotropic state is expressed as a decrease in E_{ES} and sometimes an increase in V_0 (see Fig. 3-12). As the ESPVR describes systolic function, the end-diastolic pressure volume relationship (EDPVR) (see Fig. 3-12) describes ventricular diastolic compliance (more specifically, the inverse of the slope of the EDPVR is compliance) a measure of lusitropy. The EDPVR is impacted by calcium uptake, ease of dissociation of contractile proteins, the cytoskeleton, ventricular wall thickness, and the pericardium.

Pressure-volume loops can be used to analyze various physiologic situations. Increased afterload (see Fig. 3-11B) moves the end-systolic pressure-volume point slightly upward and to the right. If stroke volume is maintained, end-diastolic volume must increase. Thus, though contractility is unchanged, ejection fraction is slightly decreased. Figure 3-11C shows the effect of a decrease in ventricular compliance (increased EDPVR) such as may result from hypertrophy, fibrosis, or cardiac tamponade. Systolic function is maintained (E_{ES} and V_0 are unchanged), and stroke volume and ejection fraction can be maintained but require an increased end-diastolic pressure. The positive inotropic (increased E_{ES}) and lusitropic (decreased EDPVR) effects of adrenergic stimulation (see Fig. 3-11D), at constant stroke volume, shift the pressure-volume loop to the left, and increase the ejection fraction. In the hypertrophied heart (see Fig. 3-11E), in contrast to Fig. 3-11C, diastolic compliance is decreased and systolic contractility is increased.

A constant stroke volume leads to an increase in end-diastolic filling pressure and decreased end-diastolic volume. The pressure-volume loop shifts to the left with an increase in ejection fraction. The ability of the hypertrophied heart to increase stroke volume is limited. Acute ischemia (see Fig. 3-11F) decreases diastolic compliance (increases EDPVR) and contractility. The pressure-volume loop shifts to the right and up to maintain stroke volume, consistent with the clinical observation of an acute decrease in ejection fraction and increase in left ventricular filling pressure. In the dilated heart of chronic congestive heart failure (see Fig. 3-11G) the pressure-volume loop is shifted to the right. Note that the slope of the diastolic pressure-volume curve (EDPVR) changes little, rather the curve shifts to the right. The end-diastolic pressure is not increased because of a change in compliance; instead, to maintain stroke volume, the pressure-volume loop has moved upward on the compliance curve. Contrast this with the fibrotic process discussed in the preceding. The effect of afterload reduction on the chronically failing heart from Fig. 3-11G is demonstrated in Fig. 3-11H. Note that the ESPVR, EDPVR, and stroke volume are unchanged. The pressure volume loop has moved back to the left, decreasing both the degree of chamber dilatation, end-diastolic pressure, and ejection fraction. A positive inotropic agent would shift the ESPVR line to the left (toward the dashed line), and the degree of dilatation would be reduced and both stroke volume and ejection fraction would be increased. It is important to remember that these relationships are idealized and may not completely reflect true clinical responses. For example, reduced diastolic dilatation from afterload reduction could return the ventricle to a state of improved intrinsic contractility. Despite these interactions, the pure concepts discussed here are very helpful in understanding the response of the heart to clinical interventions.

Another index of contractility, perhaps less influenced by other parameters, is the preload *recruitable stroke work* (PRSW) relationship. Stroke work is the area of the pressure-volume loop. For each pressure-volume loop derived by vena caval occlusion, the stroke work is plotted relative to its end-diastolic volume (Fig. 3-13).[30] The slope of the derived linear relationship is a measure of contractility independent (within physiologic ranges) of preload and afterload. The PRSW relationship reflects overall performance of the left ventricle, combining systolic and diastolic components.[31]

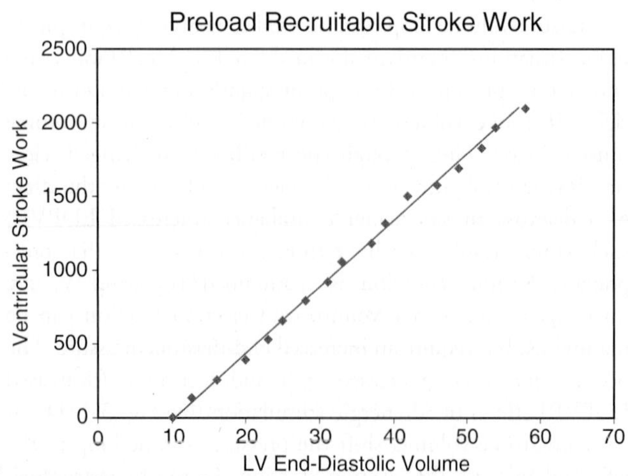

FIGURE 3-13 Plot of hypothetical measurement of preload recruitable stroke work.

Clinical Indices of Contractility

Clearly, from the preceding discussion, the degree of contractility can be assessed, but unlike blood pressure, an ideal number or range to describe it cannot be derived. Because ESPVR and PRSW are unique for each ventricle, these parameters more accurately measure changes in contractility. The greatest impediment to the clinical application of the ESPVR and PRSW is the difficulty measuring ventricular volume and inducing preload reduction to derive the pressure-volume loops. More easily measurable indices of contractility have been actively sought.

Ejection fraction is used by many clinicians as a measure of contractility. However, as noted in the discussion of Fig. 3-11, ejection fraction is influenced by preload and afterload alterations without any change in contractility. Depending on loading conditions, hearts with a lower ejection fraction can produce a greater cardiac output. Although roughly indicative of cardiac reserve, ejection fraction is an inconsistent marker for overall cardiac function perioperatively but is a useful, gross measure of cardiac reserve.

Myocardial Wall Stress

The left ventricle is a pressurized, irregularly shaped chamber. During systole, wall stress develops to overcome afterload and eject the blood. The pressure within the chamber and the geometry of the ventricle determine the tension in the wall. A model of the ventricle as a cylinder can be used to examine the effects of chamber size and wall thickness on wall stress. In this model, circumferential stress is based on the *law of LaPlace*

$$\sigma \propto \frac{Pr}{w}$$

where σ is wall stress ($\approx$ tension), P is transmural pressure, r is radius and w is wall thickness. This relationship has several important clinical implications. Wall tension must be balanced by the energy available. The only nutrient nearly completely extracted from the blood by the heart is oxygen and wall tension is the primary determinant of oxygen consumption. In one scenario, the heart can compensate for changes in wall stress. If systolic pressure within the ventricle is chronically increased (aortic stenosis or systemic hypertension), then compensatory hypertrophy or thickening of the ventricular wall can return systolic wall stress close to normal. However, as detailed in Fig. 3-11E, the price paid is that end-diastolic pressures must be higher.

In another scenario, the function of a heart that has dilated for other reasons is further compromised by the relationship between wall stress and oxygen consumption. As a result of or to compensate for systolic failure, the ventricle will dilate. The increased diastolic diameter proportionally increases wall stress and oxygen consumption. The ability of the heart to increase cardiac output in response to exercise will be limited, leading to symptoms.

ENERGETICS

Chemical Fuels

Nearly all chemical energy used by the heart is generated by oxidative phosphorylation. Anaerobic metabolism is very limited because anaerobic enzymes are not present in sufficient concentrations. The major fuels for the myocardium are carbohydrates (glucose and lactate) and free fatty acids. When sufficient oxygen is present, these fuels are used to generate ATP. Most of the ATP used by the heart (60 to 70%) is expended in the cyclic contraction of the muscle. Ten to fifteen percent is required for maintaining the concentration gradients across the cell membrane; the rest is used in the constant uptake and release of calcium by mitochondria, the breakdown and regeneration of glycogen, and the synthesis of triglycerides.

The heart is quite flexible in the aerobic state in its use of fuels. In the fasting state, lipids may account for 70% of the fuel used by the heart. When present in adequate amounts, fatty acids will inhibit use of glucose by the heart.[32] After a high carbohydrate meal, blood glucose and insulin levels are high and free fatty acids are low, and glucose accounts for close to 100% of the metabolism. During exercise, elevated lactate levels inhibit the uptake of free fatty acids and carbohydrates, mostly lactate, can account for up to 70% of the metabolism.[33]

Whatever the fuel source, oxygen is necessary for its efficient utilization. In the absence of oxygen, there are two mechanisms to provide ATP, glycolysis and conversion of phosphate stored in creatine phosphate, since free fatty acids and the by-products of glycolysis cannot be metabolized. Glycolysis is very inefficient—for 1 mole of glucose, 2 moles of ATP are produced by anaerobic glycolysis, compared with 38 moles of ATP with aerobic metabolism. Phosphate stored in creatine phosphate can convert ADP to ATP, but this is not stored in significant amounts.

The availability of ADP is the primary determinant of the rate of oxidative phosphorylation. With ischemia and hypoxia, ATP breaks down to ADP and subsequently to AMP, adenosine, and inosine. The nucleoside building blocks of ATP, adenosine, inosine, and hypoxanthine are lost from the ischemic myocardium. If oxygen is restored, ATP levels can be partially restored rapidly by salvage pathways with inosine, hypoxanthine, or inosine monophosphate. However, de novo synthesis of ATP is also required and can take hours or even days to restore significant ATP levels. Glycolysis becomes the primary, albeit inefficient source of ATP with ischemia; this leads to an increase in lactate. The increase in lactate and inorganic phosphate causes acidosis. Acidosis slows glycolysis by reducing the activity of 6-phosphofructo-1-kinase, the rate-limiting enzyme in the glycolytic pathway.[34] The excess protons compete with calcium-binding sites, interfering with contraction and relaxation. Nevertheless, ATP generated by glycolysis maintains cell viability. Glucose, insulin, and potassium support glycolysis and may be the source of the benefit of administering this combination after an ischemic insult.[35]

Determinants of Oxygen Consumption

Because nearly all the energy used by the heart is generated by oxidative metabolism, the rate of oxygen consumption ($M\dot{V}O_2$) is indicative of the metabolic rate of the heart:

$$M\dot{V}O_2 = \frac{CaO_2 - CvO_2}{CBF} \Big/ Mass$$

where $M\dot{V}O_2$ is myocardial oxygen consumption, CaO_2 is arterial oxygen content in mL O_2/100 mL blood, CvO_2 is coronary venous oxygen content in mL O_2/100 mL blood, *CBF* is coronary blood flow in mL/min. Because the bulk of the energy is expended on contraction, changes in the rate of oxygen consumption of the heart are directly related to changes in the contraction cycle and workload. Energy utilization can be increased by an increase in cardiac workload or a decrease in the efficiency of conversion of chemical to mechanical energy.

Minute work of the heart is the product of heart rate, stroke volume, and developed pressure. A change in each of these factors alters oxygen demand; however, minute work is not the direct determinant of oxygen consumption. The primary determinant of oxygen demand is the wall tension or stress developed in each cardiac cycle. Indeed, during the period of isovolumic contraction, energy is expended by the heart without the delivery of any kinetic energy to the blood.[36] The energetic cost of ejecting blood from the ventricular chamber is approximately 20 to 30% of that required for isovolumic contraction. To restate this simply, the principal determinant of the cardiac energy requirement is the pressure against which blood is ejected and the volume ejected at that pressure. An increase in afterload requires greater energy than an increase in volume ejected. Oxygen consumption is also increased as the heart dilates and begins ejection from a greater diastolic volume.

Cardiac efficiency relates oxygen consumption to cardiac work. Hence, cardiac efficiency = work/$M\dot{V}O_2$. The overall efficiency of the heart ranges from 5 to 40% depending on the type of work (pressure versus volume versus velocity) performed.[37–40] The low efficiency of the heart is caused by the expenditure of a predominant portion of the oxygen consumed in generating pressure and stretching internal elastic components of the myocardium during isovolumic systole (a form of internal work). The velocity of shortening, affected in part by inotropic state of the myocardium, also is not factored into the work equation, but contributes significantly to oxygen consumption. Dilation of the ventricle reduces efficiency because as cavity size increases the reduction in wall stress with ejection is decreased.

Following cardiac surgery, cardiac efficiency generally decreases because of the increase in $M\dot{V}O_2$ relative to the cardiac work performed. The additional oxygen consumed may result from an increase in basal metabolism and/or an increase in the cost of the excitation-contraction process, or inefficiencies of ATP production at the mitochondrial level.

A clear understanding of the role of wall tension and its relation to oxygen demand is essential in cardiac surgery. Excessive systemic pressure may place inordinate energy demands on a compromised ventricle. An intra-aortic balloon pump may shift the energy balance by reducing afterload and improving coronary blood flow. Ventricular distention during the weaning process after removal of the aortic cross-clamp, or with heart failure may create wall stress that outstrips the capacity to deliver oxygen to the myocardium. In the failing heart, where stroke volume is reduced, cardiac output is maintained by increasing heart rate, which increases the percentage of time that the myocardial wall stress is elevated, reduces the time when diastolic blood flow occurs, and creates an imbalance between oxygen demand and delivery.

FUNCTIONAL RESPONSES TO METABOLIC DEMANDS[41]

There are three distinct responses to altered metabolic demands. Two are responses to acute short-term alterations; the third is a response to chronic alterations in metabolic demands.

Acute Physiologic Responses

These responses consist of intrinsic physiologic adaptations to acute changes in hemodynamics and metabolic demands. Generally, these responses are regulated by changes in end-diastolic volume mediated by changes in preload and afterload. Beat-to-beat responses to changes in end-diastolic volume are important to equalizing the output of the ventricles.

Alterations of Biochemical Functions

Contractility (inotropy) and relaxation (lusitropy) change in response to altered metabolic demands. These are principally mediated by alterations in calcium fluxes in the myocyte.[42] The principal determinant of calcium concentration is the flux across the sarcoplasmic reticulum membrane. The fluxes are determined by the amount of calcium in the sarcoplasmic reticulum and the amount of calcium crossing the plasma membrane to stimulate calcium release. Reduced ATP levels inhibit calcium release and uptake. Enzymatic phosphorylation of myosin can increase the rate of cross-bridge cycling, and phosphorylation of troponin I facilitates relaxation.[43] Acidosis reduces contraction and relaxation by inhibiting many calcium pumps, channels, and exchangers.[44]

Altered Gene Expression

Chronic changes in metabolic demands will provoke proliferative responses leading to altered gene expression. These include changes in the types of myosin and actin and changes in the number of membrane channels and pumps.

CORONARY BLOOD FLOW

Normal Coronary Blood Flow

Resting coronary blood flow is slightly less than 1 mL per gram of heart muscle per minute. This blood flow is delivered to the heart through large epicardial conductance vessels and then into the myocardium by penetrating arteries leading to a plexus of capillaries. The bulk of the resistance to coronary flow is in the penetrating arterioles (20 to 120 μm in size). Because the heart is metabolically very active, there is a high density of capillaries such that there is approximately one capillary for every myocyte, with an intercapillary distance at rest of approximately 17 μm. Capillary density is greater in subendocardial myocardium compared with subepicardial tissue. When there is an increased myocardial oxygen demand, myocardial blood flow can increase to three or four times normal (coronary flow reserve). This is accomplished by vasodilation of the resistance vessels and recruitment of additional capillaries (many of which are closed in the resting state). Capillary recruitment is important in decreasing the intercapillary distance and the distance that oxygen and nutrients must diffuse through the myocardium.

The blood flow pattern from a coronary artery perfusing the left ventricle, measured by flow probe, is phasic in nature, with greater blood flow occurring in diastole than in systole.[45] The cyclic contraction and relaxation of the left ventricle produces this phasic blood flow pattern by extravascular compression of the arteries and intramyocardial microvessels during systole. There is a gradient in these systolic extravascular compressive forces, being greater or equal to intracavitary pressure in the subendocardial tissue, and decreasing toward the subepicardial tissue. Measurement of transmural blood flow distribution during systole shows that subepicardial vessels are preferentially perfused, whereas subendocardial vessels are significantly hypoperfused. Toward the end of systole, blood flow actually reverses in the epicardial surface vessels.[46] Hence, the subendocardial myocardium is perfused primarily during diastole, whereas subepicardial myocardium is perfused during both systole and diastole. A greater capillary density per square millimeter in the subendocardium compared with the subepicardial tissue facilitates the distribution of blood flow to the inner layer of myocardium.[47] The subendocardium is at greater risk of dysfunction, tissue injury, and necrosis during any reduction in perfusion. This is related to: (1) the greater systolic compressive forces; (2) the smaller flow reserve resulting from a greater degree of vasodilation; and (3) the greater regional oxygen demands owing to wall tension and segmental shortening. If end-diastolic pressure is elevated to 25, 30, or 35 mm Hg, then there is diastolic as well as systolic compression of the subendocardial vasculature. Flow to the subepicardium is effectively autoregulated as long as the pressure in the distal coronary artery is above approximately 40 mm Hg. Flow to the subendocardium, however, is effectively autoregulated only down to a mean distal coronary artery pressure of approximately 60 to 70 mm Hg. Below that level, local coronary flow reserve in the subendocardium is exhausted, and local blood flow decreases linearly with decreases in distal coronary artery pressure. Subendocardial perfusion is further compromised by pathologic processes that increase wall thickness and systolic and diastolic wall tension. Aortic regurgitation particularly threatens the subendocardium, because systemic diastolic arterial pressure is reduced and intraventricular systolic and diastolic pressures are elevated.[45,48]

In contrast to the phasic nature of blood flow in the left coronary artery, blood flow in the right coronary artery is relatively constant during the cardiac cycle. The constancy of blood flow is related to the lower intramural pressures and near absence of extravascular compressive forces in the right ventricle compared with the left ventricle.

Control of Coronary Blood Flow

Coronary blood flow is tightly coupled to the metabolic needs of the heart. Under normal conditions, 70% of the oxygen available in coronary arterial blood is extracted, near the physiologic maximum. Any increase in oxygen delivery comes mostly from an increase in blood flow. To maximize efficiency, local coronary blood flow is precisely controlled by a balance of vasodilator and vasoconstrictor mechanisms, including: (1) a *metabolic vasodilator system*; (2) a *neurogenic control system*; and (3) the *vascular endothelium*.[49] Blood flow is controlled by moment-to-moment adjustment of coronary tone of the resistance vessels, that is, arterioles and precapillary sphincters.

The metabolic vasodilator mechanism responds rapidly when local blood flow is insufficient to meet metabolic demand. The primary mediator is adenosine generated within the myocyte and released into the interstitial compartment. Adenosine relaxes arteriolar smooth muscle cells by activation of A_2 receptors. Adenosine is formed when the oxygen supply cannot sustain the rapid rephosphorylation of ADP to ATP. Once sufficient oxygen is supplied to the myocardium, less adenosine is formed. Adenosine is therefore the coupling agent between oxygen demand and supply. Other local vasodilators that influence coronary blood flow are carbon dioxide, lactic acid, and histamine.

The sympathetic nervous system acts through *alpha receptors* (vasoconstriction) and *beta receptors* (vasodilation). There is direct innervation of the large conductance vessels and lesser direct innervation of the smaller resistance vessels. Sympathetic receptors on the smooth muscle cells of the resistance vessels respond to humoral catecholamines. Alpha receptors predominate over beta receptors such that when norepinephrine is released from the sympathetic nerve endings, vasoconstriction ordinarily occurs.

Endothelium-dependent regulation of coronary artery blood flow is a dynamic balance between vasodilating and vasoconstricting factors. Vasodilators include nitric oxide (NO•) synthesized from L-arginine by endothelial nitric oxide synthase, and endothelially released adenosine. The principal vasoconstrictor is the endothelially derived constricting peptide endothelin-1. Other vasoconstrictors include angiotensin II and superoxide free radical.[50] NO• is dominant in local regulation of coronary arterial tone. NO• is released by the coronary vascular endothelium by both soluble factors (acetylcholine, adenosine, and ATP) and mechanical signals (shear stress and pulsatile stress secondary to increased intraluminal blood flow). If the endothelium is intact, acetylcholine from the sympathetic nerves causes vasodilation through generation of NO•. If the endothelium is not functionally intact, acetylcholine causes vasoconstriction by direct stimulation of the vascular smooth muscle. NO• is a potent inhibitor of platelet aggregation and neutrophil function (superoxide generation, adherence, and migration), which has implications in the anti-inflammatory response to ischemia-reperfusion and cardiopulmonary bypass.

Endothelin-1 interacts principally with specific endothelin receptors, ET_A, on vascular smooth muscle, and causes smooth muscle vasoconstriction. Endothelin-1 counteracts the vasodilator effects of endogenous adenosine, NO•, and prostacyclin (PGI_2). Endothelin-1 is rapidly synthesized in vascular endothelium, particularly during ischemia, hypoxia, and other stress conditions, where it acts in a paracrine fashion. ET-1 has a short half-life (4 to 7 minutes), which exceeds that of adenosine (8 to 12 seconds) and NO• (microseconds). However, the avid binding of ET-1 to ET_A receptors prolongs its effects beyond the half-life. Human coronary arteries demonstrate abundant endothelin-1 binding sites, suggesting that ET-1 has an important role in the control of coronary blood flow in humans.[51] The levels of ET-1 have been observed to increase with myocardial ischemia-reperfusion and after cardiac surgery.

Under ordinary circumstances the metabolic vasodilator system is the dominant force acting on the resistance vessels. For example, the increased metabolic activity caused by sympathetic stimulation leads to vasodilation of the coronary arterioles through the metabolic system, despite a direct vasoconstriction effect of norepinephrine.[52–54]

Coronary artery blood flow is also determined by perfusion pressure. However, in the coronary vasculature blood flow can remain constant over a range of perfusion pressures. The control mechanisms described allow *autoregulation* of blood flow adjusting vascular resistance to match blood flow requirements. The autoregulatory "plateau" occurs between approximately 60 and 120 mm Hg perfusion pressure. If distal coronary artery perfusion pressure is reduced by a critical stenosis or hypotension, vasodilator capacity will be exhausted and coronary blood flow will decrease, following a linear relationship with perfusion pressure. Because the subendocardial region of the left ventricle has a lower coronary vascular reserve, maximal dilation is reached in this region before the subepicardial tissue, and a preferential hypoperfusion of the subendocardial tissue results.

Hemodynamic Effect of Coronary Artery Stenosis

Surgically treatable atherosclerotic disease primarily affects the large conductance vessels of the heart. The hemodynamic effect of a stenosis is determined by *Poiseuille's law*, which describes the resistance of a viscous fluid to laminar flow through a cylindrical tube; specifically:

$$Q = \frac{\pi(\Delta P)}{8\eta} \cdot \frac{r^4}{l}$$

where Q is flow, ΔP is the pressure change, η is viscosity, r is radius, and l is length of the resistance segment. Resistance (pressure change/flow):

$$R = \frac{(\Delta P)}{Q} = \frac{8\eta}{\pi} \cdot \frac{l}{r^4}$$

is inversely proportional to the *fourth* power of the radius and directly proportional to the length of the narrowing. Therefore, a small change in diameter has a magnified effect on vascular resistance (Table 3-2). Conductance vessels are sufficiently large that a 50% reduction in the diameter of the vessel has minimal hemodynamic

TABLE 3-2 Effect of Degree and Length of Stenosis on Resistance to Flow Based on Poiseuille's Law

% Stenosis of a 1-cm-diameter Vessel	Radius in cm	Proportional Resistance for Various Segment Lengths (cm)		
		0.25 cm	1 cm	2 cm
0	0.5	[1]	4	8
50	0.25	16	64	128
60	0.2	39	156	313
70	0.15	123	494	988
80	0.1	625	2500	5000
90	0.05	10000	40000	80000
Proportional increase in resistance 80% versus 60% stenosis				16
Proportional increase in resistance 90% versus 60% stenosis				256

The value for a reference vessel of length 0.25 centimeters with 0% stenosis (in the box) is set to 1 for comparison.

effect. A 60% reduction in the diameter of the vessel has only a very small hemodynamic effect. As the stenosis progresses beyond 60% small decreases in diameter have significant effects on blood flow. For a given segment length, an 80% stenosis has a resistance that is 16 times greater a 60% stenosis. For a 90% stenosis, the resistance is 256 times greater than a 60% stenosis.[55] Furthermore, for successive stenoses in the same vessel the resistance is additive. An additional factor in resistance to flow is turbulence. Stenotic lesions can cause conversion from laminar to turbulent flow.[56] With laminar flow the pressure drop is proportional to flow rate Q; with turbulent flow pressure drop is proportional to (Q^2). For all of these reasons patients who have had a small progression in the degree of coronary stenosis may experience a rapid acceleration of symptoms.

Atherosclerosis also alters normal vascular regulatory mechanisms. The endothelium is often destroyed or damaged, so vasoconstrictor mechanisms are relatively unopposed by the impaired vasodilator mechanism; constriction is exaggerated and responses to stimuli that require dilatation are blunted.[57]

As noted, when a stenosis is less than 60%, little change is flow is noted. This is caused by compensation by the coronary flow reserve of the resistance vessels distal to the stenotic conductance vessel. As resistance to flow is additive, a decrease in distal resistance will balance an increase in proximal resistance and flow will be unchanged. As flow reserve decreases, any stimulus that increases myocardial oxygen demand (such as tachycardia, hypertension, or exercise) cannot be met by dilation of the distal vasculature, and myocardial ischemia results.[49]

In the human, coronary arterial vessels are end vessels with little collateral flow between major branches except in pathologic situations. With sudden coronary occlusion, although there is usually modest collateral flow through very small vessels (20 to 200 μm in size), this flow is generally insufficient to maintain cellular viability. Collateral flow gradually begins to increase over the next 8 to 24 hours, doubling by about the third day after total occlusion. Collateral blood flow development appears to be nearly complete after 1 month, restoring normal or nearly normal resting flow to the surviving myocardium in the ischemic region. Previous ischemic events or gradually developing stenoses can lead to larger pre-existing collaterals in the human heart. The presence of these pre-existing collaterals has been shown to be important in the prevention of ischemic damage if coronary occlusion should occur.[58]

Endothelial Dysfunction

As previously noted, nitric oxide, adenosine, and endothelin-1 are synthesized and released by the endothelium.[59,60] Ischemia-reperfusion, hypertension, diabetes, and hypercholesterolemia can impair generation of $NO^•$ and vasoconstriction may predominate, mediated by the relative overexpression of endothelin-1. Reperfusion after temporary myocardial ischemia is one situation in which $NO^•$ production may be impaired, leading to a vicious cycle in which the vasodilator reserve of the resistance vessels is reduced with a consequent and progressive "low-flow" or "no-flow" phenomenon. The coronary vascular $NO^•$ system may also be impaired in some cases after coronary artery bypass surgery.

The endothelium helps prevent cell-cell interactions between blood-borne inflammatory cells (ie, leukocytes and platelets) that initiate a local or systemic inflammatory reaction. Inflammatory cascades occur with sepsis, ischemia-reperfusion, and cardiopulmonary bypass. Under normal conditions, the vascular endothelium resists interaction with neutrophils and platelets by tonically releasing adenosine and NO•, which have potent antineutrophil and platelet inhibitory effects. Damage to the endothelium lowers the resistance to neutrophil adhesion. Neutrophils can damage the endothelium by adhesion to its surface, and subsequent release of oxygen radicals and proteases. This amplifies the inflammatory response and decreases the tonic generation and release of adenosine and NO•, which then permits further interaction with activated inflammatory cells. The products released by activated neutrophils have downstream physiologic consequences on other tissues, notably the heart, including increasing vascular permeability, creating blood flow defects (no-reflow phenomenon), and promoting the pathogenesis of necrosis and apoptosis.[61]

The triggers of these inflammatory reactions in the heart include cytokines (IL-1, IL-6, IL-8), complement fragments (C3a, C5a, membrane attack complex), oxygen radicals, and thrombin, which upregulate adhesion molecules expressed on both inflammatory cells (CD11a/CD18) and endothelium (P-selectin, E-selectin, and ICAM-1). The release of cytokines and complement fragments during cardiopulmonary bypass activates the vascular endothelium on a systemic basis, which contributes to the inflammatory response to cardiopulmonary bypass.[62] Both adenosine and NO• have been used therapeutically to reduce the inflammatory responses to cardiopulmonary bypass, and to reduce ischemic-reperfusion injury and endothelial damage.[63,64]

The Sequelae of Myocardial Hypoperfusion: Infarction, Myocardial Stunning, and Myocardial Hibernation

As oxygen delivery is reduced, contraction strength decreases rapidly (within 8 to 10 heartbeats). This is seen acutely in response to ischemia and is rapidly reversed with reperfusion. If the extent of reduction of coronary blood flow is severe, mild to moderate abnormalities in cellular homeostasis occur. Reduced cellular levels of ATP lead to a loss of adenine nucleotides from the cell. If the reduction in coronary flow is sustained, progressive loss of adenine nucleotides and the elevation of intracellular and intramitochondrial calcium may lead to cellular death and subsequent necrosis. Increased intramitochondrial calcium uncouples oxidative phosphorylation, creating a vicious cycle.[65] If the myocyte is reperfused before subcellular organelles are irreversibly damaged, the myocyte may slowly recover. A period of days is necessary for full recovery of myocyte ATP levels as adenine nucleotides must be resynthesized. During this time contractile processes are impaired. This impairment is related to reversible damage to the contractile proteins such that their responsiveness to cytosolic levels of calcium is diminished. The magnitude of the cytosolic pulse of calcium with each heartbeat appears to be nearly normal, but the magnitude of the consequent contraction is greatly reduced. Over a period of 1 to 2 weeks this myocardium gradually recovers. This viable but dysfunctional myocardium is called *stunned myocardium*.[66–68]

With chronic hypoperfusion, oxygen delivery is at a reduced level but above the level required for cell viability. This can cause a chronic hypocontractile state known as *hibernation*. Hibernation appears to be associated with a decrease in the magnitude of the pulse of calcium involved in the excitation-contraction process such that the calcium levels developed within the cytosol during each heartbeat are inadequate for effective contraction to occur. Histologic examination shows islets in the subendocardium where there is a loss of contractile proteins, sarcoplasmic reticulum, and alterations of other subcellular structures.[69,70] With reperfusion, hibernating myocardium can very quickly resume normal and effective contraction, though complete recovery may be delayed for several months.[66,71–73] This is of particular importance for patients with poor ventricular function but viable heart muscle.[74]

Reperfusion of acutely ischemic myocardium may cause further cellular damage and necrosis rather than lead to immediate recovery. The etiology of reperfusion injury is multifactorial. Damaged endothelium in the reperfused region fails to prevent adhesion and activation of leukocytes and platelets. Oxygen-free radicals are released. Derangement of the ATP-dependent sodium-potassium pump disrupts cell volume regulation with consequent leakage of water into the cell, explosive cell swelling, and rupture of the cell membrane. Techniques applied to reduce reperfusion injury, minimize adverse sequelae, and preserve myocytes include leukocyte depletion or inactivation, prevention of endothelial activation, free radical scavenging, reperfusion with solutions low in calcium content, and reperfusion with hyperosmolar solutions.[75,76] Both adenosine and low-dose NO• are potent cardioprotective agents that attenuate neutrophil-mediated damage, infarction, and apoptosis.[77]

The metabolic changes that occur with ischemia-reperfusion represent a complex system of adaptive mechanisms that allow the myocyte to survive despite a temporary reduction in oxygen delivery. These adaptive mechanisms may be triggered by a very brief coronary occlusion (as short as 5 minutes) such that the negative sequelae of a subsequent prolonged coronary occlusion are greatly minimized. This phenomenon has been called *ischemic preconditioning*. A coronary occlusion that might cause as much as 40% myocyte death in a region subjected to prolonged ischemia may be reduced to only 10% myocyte death if the prolonged period of ischemia is preceded by a 5-minute interval of "preconditioning" coronary occlusion.[75,78,79]

PHYSIOLOGY OF HEART FAILURE

Definition and Classification

Heart failure is the inability of the heart to deliver adequate blood to the tissues to meet end-organ metabolic needs at rest or during mild to moderate exercise. Processes that cause heart failure can impair systolic function (the ability to contract and empty) or diastolic function (the ability to relax and fill) or both. The acute and chronic stages of a myocardial infarction involving a large area of the left ventricle cause systolic heart failure. The acute loss of contractile function compromises the ability of the ventricle to maintain a normal stroke volume (Fig. 3-11F). As the infarction heals, the adaptive response of ventricular dilation reduces the heart's systolic functional reserve. Cardiomyopathies affect the myocardium globally leading to reduced systolic function. Long-standing valvular insufficiency alters ventricular geometry and muscular function leading to ventricular failure. In all these examples, the left ventricle dilates, which causes the pressure-volume relationship of the left ventricle to shift to the right (Fig. 3-11G). In these situations, the diastolic portion of the pressure-volume curves is not greatly changed. However, the global systolic performance of the heart (ie, the ability to pump blood) may be inadequate to meet even resting needs.[80,81]

Diastolic failure may occur without an impairment of systolic contractility if the myocardium becomes fibrotic or hypertrophied, or if there is an external constraint on filling such as with pericardial tamponade.[82] Increased stiffness of the left ventricular myocardium is associated with an excessive upward shift in the diastolic pressure-volume curve (Figs. 3-11C and 3-11E). The most common cause of increased myocardial stiffness is chronic hypertension with consequent left ventricular hypertrophy and diastolic stiffness (related both to myocyte hypertrophy and increased fibrosis of the ventricle).[83,84]

It should be noted from these examples that although one process may predominate, most patients with heart failure manifest both systolic and diastolic dysfunction.

Early Cardiac and Systemic Sequelae of Heart Failure

The adaptive homeostatic reactions of the body leading to heart failure depend on the duration of the ongoing pathologic process. When cardiac function acutely deteriorates and cardiac output diminishes, neurohumoral reflexes attempt to restore both cardiac output and blood pressure. Activation of the sympathetic adrenergic system in the heart and in the peripheral vasculature causes systemic vasoconstriction and increases heart rate and contractility. A variety of mediators formed during this adaptive stage, including norepinephrine, angiotensin II, vasopressin, B-type natriuretic peptic, and endothelin, not only promote renal retention of salt and water leading to volume expansion but also cause vasoconstriction. Aldosterone output is increased, conserving sodium. The concerted responses of the adrenergic system and the renin-angiotensin system alter the primary determinants of stroke volume and cardiac output—preload, afterload, and contractility. The heart responds to loss of systolic function by progressively dilating. This dilation leads to preservation of stroke volume by Frank-Starling mechanisms but increased stroke volume is achieved at the expense of ejection fraction, as shown in Fig. 3-11G as a right shift in the pressure-volume relationship of the left ventricle with an increase in end-diastolic volume (and pressure). In addition to a global dilation response, acute alterations in cardiac geometry may occur early after a large myocardial infarction, with thinning of the left ventricular wall in the region of the infarct as well as expansion of overall left ventricular cavity size. As volume expansion occurs, production of the cardiac atrial natriuretic peptide is increased, which tends to prevent excessive sodium retention and inhibit activation of the renin-angiotensin and aldosterone systems.[85–89]

Cardiac and Systemic Maladaptive Consequences of Chronic Heart Failure

The acute phase response is initially beneficial but becomes maladaptive and contributes to long-term problems in patients with heart failure (Fig. 3-14). In the latter stages of heart failure, the kidneys tend to retain sodium and become hyporesponsive to atrial natriuretic peptide and B-type natriuretic peptide.[86] Desensitization of beta-adrenergic receptors is a consequence of sustained stimulation with a reduced response to elevated circulating catecholamine levels.[19]

Left ventricular dilation is caused by hypertrophy of the myocytes as well as lengthening of the myocytes as sarcomeres are added. However, there is significant slippage of myofibrils leading to dilation without an increase in the number of myocytes. Progressive dilation of the heart leads to an increase in oxygen consumption during systole. Ventricular remodeling leads to progressive fibrosis.

Angiotensin and aldosterone stimulate collagen formulation and proliferation of fibroblasts in the heart, leading to an increase in the ratio of interstitial tissue to myocardial tissue in the noninfarcted regions of the heart.[90] The impact of aldosterone has been documented by the effectiveness of aldosterone receptor antagonists in improving the morbidity and mortality of patients with heart failure.[91] The progressive fibrosis leads to increased diastolic stiffness which limits diastolic filling and increases end-diastolic pressure. Fibrosis and increased ventricular size predispose to re-entry ventricular arrhythmias that are a common cause of death in the late stages of heart failure.[92] Hence, heart failure progresses as a result of a vicious cycle of left ventricular dilatation and remodeling, responses that decrease cardiac performance further.

Evidence has accumulated over the past decade that suggests endothelial dysfunction, release of cytokines, and apoptotic cell death may participate in the development of heart failure as a maladaptive reaction (see Fig. 3-14). Reduced availability of nitric oxide and increased production of vasoconstrictor agents such as endothelin and angiotensin II has been reported in failing hearts.[93] Heart failure is often accompanied by changes in the endogenous antioxidant defense mechanisms of the heart as well as evidence of oxidative injury to the myocardium. Cytokines, released from systemic and local inflammatory responses in the failing heart, directly activate inflammatory cells to release superoxide radicals and cause endothelial dysfunction by augmenting inflammatory cell–endothelial cell interactions. Cytokines may also directly induce necrotic and apoptotic myocyte cell death.[94]

Cardiac secretion of B-type natriuretic peptide (BNP) has been shown to be increased with heart failure. BNP is a cardiac neurohormone released as preproBNP that is enzymatically cleaved to N-terminal-proBNP and BNP upon ventricular

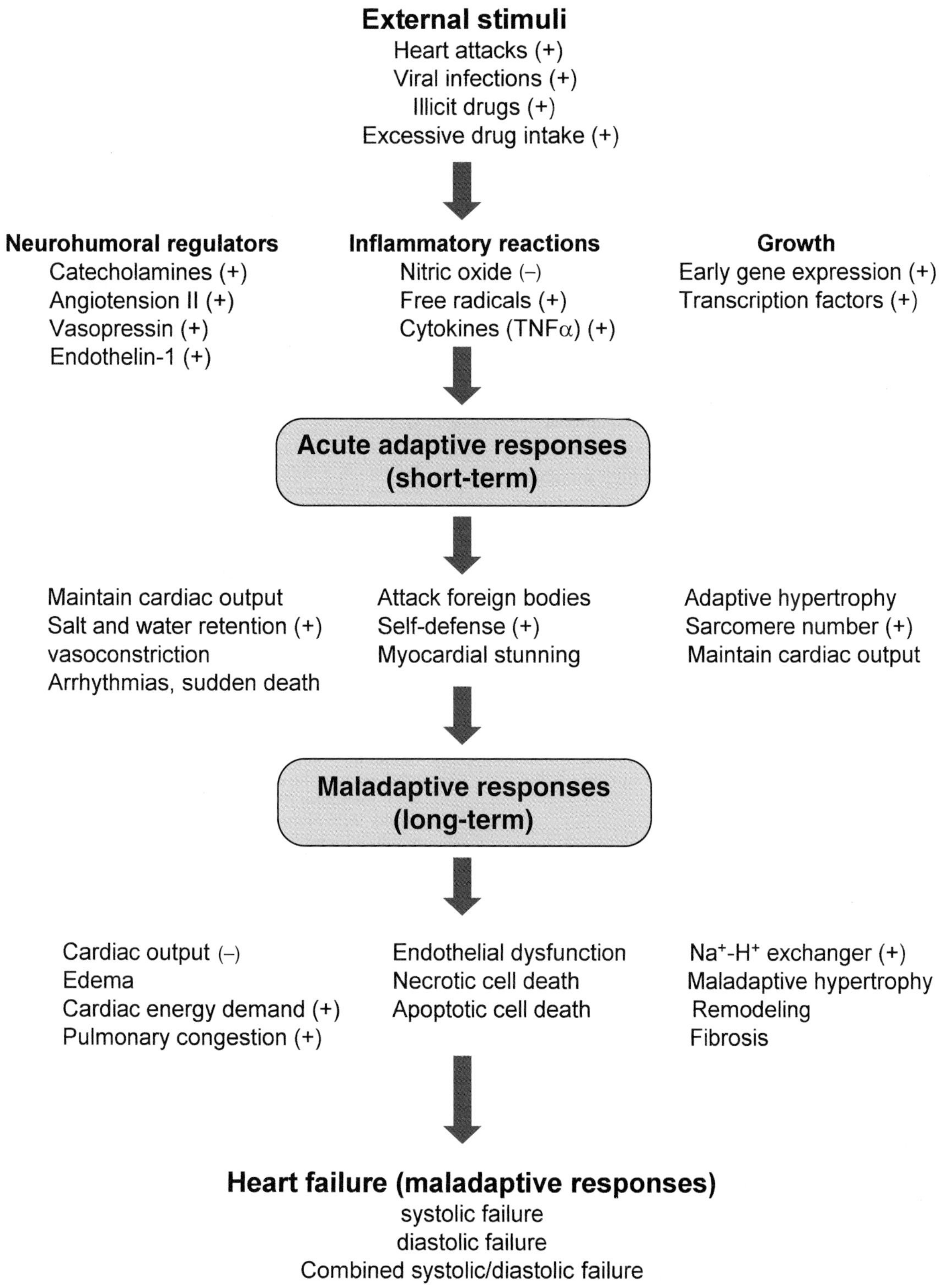

FIGURE 3-14 Pathophysiology of heart failure from stimulus (etiology) to acute adaptive and chronic maladaptive responses. (+) Indicates positive stimulation; (–) indicates negative factors that tend to reduce stimulation of heart failure.

myocyte stretch. The physiologic effects of BNP include natriuresis, vasodilation and neurohumoral changes. Measurement of plasma BNP is a useful and cost-effective marker for heart failure.[95] Other factors rather than stretch may stimulate BNP release including fibrosis, arrhythmias, ischemia, endothelial dysfunction, and cardiac hypertrophy.

ACKNOWLEDGMENTS

The authors would like to acknowledge the work of the authors of this chapter in the 2nd edition, Jakob Vinten-Johansen, Zhi-Qing Zhao, and Robert A. Guyton. The current revision was based on the solid foundation they had prepared.

KEY POINTS

- The myocardial cell is electrically active in a state of balance maintained by the flux of ions across a semipermeable membrane, tightly regulated by variable responses to external stimuli. The metabolic balance is maintained by voltage gated channels, energy-dependent pumps, and ion exchangers. Electrical stimulation is communicated efficiently through the cell and between cells to allow the release of calcium and coordinate contraction.
- The cardiac pump is designed to respond acutely to changes in preload and afterload and the response can be impacted by changes in intrinsic inotropy and lusitropy. This response is impacted by innervation, and paracrine and endocrine effects.
- The heart can use a number of different fuels, lipid or carbohydrates, but the rate-limiting step in cardiac energetics is the delivery of oxygen. Because of its high metabolic requirements, cardiac function quickly falters if oxidative phosphorylation is not possible.
- In the setting of reduced oxygen delivery the heart implements a number of acute and chronic adaptations that initially ensure continued function but eventually are maladaptive.
- Contractility is the intrinsic functional state of the heart at a constant preload, afterload, and heart rate. Indices of contractility are useful to understand and explain pathologic responses but difficult to measure in the clinical setting.
- Endothelial cell function is important for autoregulation of coronary blood flow and can be disrupted during cardiac surgical procedures.

REFERENCES

1. Opie LH: Fuels: carbohydrates and lipids, in Swynghedauw B, Taegtmeyer H, Ruegg JC, Carmeliet E (eds): *The Heart: Physiology and Metabolism.* New York, Raven Press, 1991; p 208.
2. Katz AM: Regulation of cardiac contraction and relaxation, in Willerson JT, Cohn JN (eds): *Cardiovascular Medicine.* New York, Churchill Livingstone, 1995; p 790.
3. Andersen OS, Koeppe RE: Molecular determinants of channel function. *Physiol Rev* 1992; 72:S89-158.
4. Catterall WA: Cellular and molecular biology of voltage-gated sodium channels. *Physiol Rev* 1992; 72:S15-48.
5. Levitan IB: Modulation of ion channels by protein phosphorylation and dephosphorylation. *Annu Rev Physiol* 1994; 56:193-212.
6. McDonald TF, Pelzer S, Trautwein, et al: Regulation and modulation of calcium channels in cardiac, skeletal, and smooth muscle cells. *Physiol Rev* 1994; 74:365-507.
7. Barry WH, Bridge JHB: Intracellular calcium homeostasis in cardiac myocytes. *Circulation* 1993; 87:1806-1815.
8. Pallotta BS, Wagoner PK: Voltage-dependent potassium channels since Hodgkin and Huxley. *Physiol Rev* 1992; 72:S49-67.
9. Horisberger JD, Lemas V, Kraehenbuhl JP, Rossier BC: Structure-function relationship of Na,K-ATPase. *Annu Rev Physiol* 1991; 53:565-584.
10. Pozzan T, Rizzuto R, Volpe P, Meldolesi J: Molecular and cellular physiology of intracellular calcium stores. *Physiol Rev* 1994; 74:595-636.
11. Kutchai HC: Ionic equalibria and resting membrane potentials, in Berne RM, Levy MV, Koeppen BM, Stanton BA (eds): *Physiology.* St. Louis, Mosby, 2004; pp 23-26.
12. Levy MN: Electrical activity of the heart, in Berne RM, Levy MV, Koeppen BM, Stanton BA (eds): *Physiology.* St. Louis, Mosby, 2004; pp 276-277.
13. Coraboeuf E, Nargeot J: Electrophysiology of human cardiac cells. *Cardiovasc Res* 1993; 27:1713-1725.
14. Naccarelli GV: Recognition and physiologic treatment of cardiac arrhythmias and conduction disturbances in Willerson JT, Cohn JN (eds): *Cardiovascular Medicine.* New York, Churchill Livingstone, 1995; p 1282.
15. Katz AM: *Physiology of the Heart,* 4th ed. Philadelphia, Lippincott Williams & Wilkins, 2006; p 217.
16. Katz AM: *Physiology of the Heart,* 4th ed. Philadelphia, Lippincott Williams & Wilkins, 2006; p 220.
17. Katz AM: *Physiology of the Heart,* 4th ed. Philadelphia, Lippincott Williams & Wilkins, 2006; p 227.
18. Katz AM: *Physiology of the Heart,* 4th ed. Philadelphia, Lippincott Williams & Wilkins, 2006; p 538.
19. Homcy CJ, Vatner ST, Vatner DE: Beta-adrenergic receptor regulation in the heart in pathophysiologic states: abnormal adrenergic responsiveness in cardiac disease. *Annu Rev Physiol* 1991; 53:137-159.
20. Feldman AM: Classification of positive inotropic agents. *J Am Coll Cardiol* 1993; 22:1223-1227.
21. Honerjager P: Pharmacology of bipyridine phosphodiesterase III inhibitors. *Am Heart J* 1991; 1939-1944.
22. Vinten-Johansen J, Zhao Z, Corvera JS, et al: Adenosine in myocardial protection in on-pump and off-pump cardiac surgery. *Ann Thorac Surg* 2003; 75:S691-699.
23. Hynynen MM, Khalil RA: The vascular endothelin system in hypertension. Recent patents and discoveries. *Recent Pat Cardiovasc Drug Discov* 2006; 1:95-108.
24. Katz AM: *Physiology of the Heart,* 4th ed. Philadelphia, Lippincott Williams & Wilkins, 2006; p 241.
25. Parsons B, Szczesna D, Zhao J, et al: The effect of pH on the Ca2+ affinity of the Ca+2 regulatory sites of skeletal and cardiac troponin C in skinned muscle fibres. *J Muscle Res Cell Motil* 1997; 18:599-609.
26. Ebashi S: Excitation-contraction coupling and the mechanism of muscle contraction. *Annu Rev Physiol* 1991; 53:1-16.
27. Katz AM: *Physiology of the Heart,* 4th ed. Philadelphia, Lippincott Williams & Wilkins, 2006; p 128.
28. Perriard JC, Hirschy A, Ehler E: Dilated cardiomyopathy: a disease of the intercalated disc? *Trends Cardiovasc Med* 2003; 13:30-38.
29. Briand M, Dumesnil JG, Kadem L, et al: Reduced systemic arterial compliance impacts significantly on left ventricular afterload and function in aortic stenosis: implications for diagnosis and treatment. *J Am Coll Cardiol* 2005; 46:291-298.
30. Glower DD, Spratt JA, Snow ND, et al: Linearity of the Frank-Starling relationship in the intact heart: the concept of preload recruitable stroke work. *Circulation* 1985; 71:994-1009.
31. Feneley MP, Skelton TN, Kisslo KB, et al: Comparison of preload recruitable stroke work, end-systolic pressure-volume and dP/dtmax-end-diastolic volume relations as indexes of left ventricular contractile performance in patients undergoing routine cardiac catheterization. *J Amer Coll Cardiol* 1992; 19:1522-1530.
32. Katz AM: *Physiology of the Heart,* 4th ed. Philadelphia, Lippincott Williams & Wilkins, 2006; p 74.
33. Taegtmeyer H: Myocardial metabolism, in Willerson JT, Cohn JN (eds): *Cardiovascular Medicine.* New York, Churchill Livingstone, 1995; p 752.
34. Hollidge-Horvat MG, Parolin ML, Wong D, Jones NL, Heigenhauser GJ: Effect of induced metabolic acidosis on human skeletal muscle metabolism during exercise. *Am J Physiol* 1999; 277:E647-658.
35. Apstein CS: The benefits of glucose-insulin-potassium for acute myocardial infarction (and some concerns). *J Am Coll Cardiol* 2003; 42:792-795.
36. Indolfi C, Ross J: The role of heart rate in myocardial ischemia and infarction: implications of myocardial perfusion-contraction matching. *Prog Cardiovasc Dis* 1993; 36:61-74.
37. Carden DL, Young JA, Granger DN: Pulmonary microvascular injury after intestinal ischemia-reperfusion: role of P-selectin. *J Appl Physiol* 1993; 75:2529-2534.
38. Luscinskas FW, Brock AF, Arnaout MA, Gimbrone MA: Endothelial-leukocyte adhesion molecule-1-dependent and leukocyte (CD11/CD18)-dependent mechanisms contribute to polymorphonuclear leukocyte adhesion to cytokine-activated human vascular endothelium. *J Immunol* 1989; 142:2257-2263.
39. Li J, Bukoski RD: Endothelium-dependent relaxation of hypertensive resistance arteries is not impaired under all conditions. *Circ Res* 1993; 72:290-296.
40. Johnston WE, Robertie PG, Dudas LM, Kon ND, Vinten-Johansen J: Heart rate-right ventricular stroke volume relation with myocardial revascularization. *Ann Thorac Surg* 1991; 52:797-804.
41. Katz AM: *Physiology of the Heart,* 4th ed. Philadelphia, Lippincott Williams & Wilkins, 2006; p 282.
42. Katz AM: *Physiology of the Heart,* 4th ed. Philadelphia, Lippincott Williams & Wilkins, 2006; p 297.
43. Katz AM: *Physiology of the Heart,* 4th ed. Philadelphia, Lippincott Williams & Wilkins, 2006; p 302.

44. Katz AM: *Physiology of the Heart,* 4th ed. Philadelphia, Lippincott Williams & Wilkins, 2006; p 304.
45. Beyar R: Myocardial mechanics and coronary flow dynamics, in Sideman S, Beyar R (eds): *Interactive Phenomena in the Cardiac System.* New York, Plenum Press, 1993; p 125.
46. Yamada H, Yoneyama F, Satoh K, et al: Comparison of the effects of the novel vasodilator FK409 with those of nitroglycerin in isolated coronary artery of the dog. *Br J Pharmacol* 1991; 103:1713-178.
47. Vinten-Johansen J, Weiss HR: Regional O_2 consumption in canine left ventricular myocardium in experimental acute aortic valvular insufficiency. *Cardiovasc Res* 1981; 15:305-312.
48. Guyton RA, McClenathan JH, Newman GE, Michaelis LL: Significance of subendocardial S-T segment elevation caused by coronary stenosis in the dog. Epicardial S-T segment depression, local ischemia and subsequent necrosis. *Am J Cardiol* 1977; 40:373-380.
49. Bradley AJ, Alpert JS: Coronary flow reserve. *Am Heart J* 1991; 1116-1128.
50. Stewart DJ, Pohl U, Bassenge E: Free radicals inhibit endothelium-dependent dilation in the coronary resistance bed. *Am J Physiol Heart Circ Physiol* 1988; 255:H765-H769.
51. Hou M, Chen Y, Traverse JH, Li Y, Barsoum M, Bache RJ: ET-A receptor activity restrains coronary blood flow in the failing heart. *J Cardiovasc Pharmacol* 2004; 43:764-769.
52. Umans JG, Levi R: Nitric oxide in the regulation of blood flow and arterial pressure. *Annu Rev Physiol* 1995; 57:771-790.
53. Gross SS, Wolin MS: Nitric oxide: pathophysiological mechanisms [review]. *Annu Rev Physiol* 1995; 57:737-769.
54. Highsmith RF, Blackburn K, Schmidt DJ: Endothelin and calcium dynamics in vascular smooth muscle. *Annu Rev Physiol* 1992; 54:257-277.
55. Katritsis D, Choi MJ, Webb-Peploe MM. Assessment of the hemodynamic significance of coronary artery stenosis: theoretical considerations and clinical measurements. *Prog Cardiovasc Dis* 1991; 34:69-88.
56. Levy MN: Hemodynamics, in Berne RM, Levy MV, Koeppen BM, Stanton BA (eds): *Physiology.* St. Louis, Mosby, 2004; pp 341-354.
57. Cohn PF: Mechanisms of myocardial ischemia. *Am J Cardiol* 1992; 70:14G-18G.
58. Charney R, Cohen M: The role of the coronary collateral circulation in limiting myocardial ischemia and infarct size. *Am Heart J* 1993; 126:937-945.
59. Meredith IT, Anderson TJ, Uehata A, et al: Role of endothelium in ischemic coronary syndromes. *Am J Cardiol* 1993; 72:27C-32C.
60. Harrison DG: Endothelial dysfunction in the coronary microcirculation: a new clinical entity or an experimental finding? [editorial; comment]. *J Clin Invest* 1993; 91:1-2.
61. Jordan JE, Zhao Z-Q, Vinten-Johansen J: The role of neutrophils in myocardial ischemia-reperfusion injury. *Cardiovasc Res* 1999; 43:860-878.
62. Boyle EM, Pohlman TH, Johnson MC, Verrier ED: Endothelial cell injury in cardiovascular surgery: the systemic inflammatory response. *Ann Thorac Surg* 1997; 63:277-284.
63. Vinten-Johansen J, Thourani VH, Ronson RS, et al: Broad spectrum cardioprotection with adenosine. *Ann Thorac Surg* 1999; 68:1942-1948.
64. Vinten-Johansen J, Sato H, Zhao Z-Q: The role of nitric oxide and NO-donor agents in myocardial protection from surgical ischemic-reperfusion injury. *Int J Cardiol* 1995; 50:273-281.
65. Katz AM: *Physiology of the Heart,* 4th ed. Philadelphia, Lippincott Williams & Wilkins, 2006; p 73.
66. Marban E: Myocardial stunning and hibernation: the physiology behind the colloquialisms [review]. *Circulation* 1991; 83:681-688.
67. Kusuoka H, Marban E: Cellular mechanisms of myocardial stunning [review]. *Annu Rev Physiol* 1992; 54:243-256.
68. Ross J: Left ventricular function after coronary artery reperfusion. *Am J Cardiol* 1993; 72:91G-97G.
69. Flemeng W, Suy R, Schwarz F, et al: Ultrastructural correlates of left ventricular contraction abnormalities in patients with chronic ischemic heart disease: determinants of reversible segmental asynergy postrevascularization surgery. *Am Heart J* 1981; 102:846-857.
70. Borgers M, Thoné F, Wouters L, et al: Structural correlates of regional myocardial dysfunction in patients with critical coronary artery stenosis: chronic hibernation? *Cardiovasc Pathol* 1993; 2:237-245.
71. Vanoverschelde JL, Melin JA, Depré C, et al: Time-course of functional recovery of hibernating myocardium after coronary revascularization. *Circulation* 1994; 90(Suppl):I-378.
72. Ross J: Myocardial perfusion-contraction matching implications for coronary heart disease and hibernation. *Circulation* 1991; 83:1076-1083.
73. Guth BD, Schulz R, Heusch G: Time course and mechanisms of contractile dysfunction during acute myocardial ischemia. *Circulation* 1993; 87:IV35-42.
74. Wijns W, Vatner SF, Camici PG: Hibernating myocardium. *NEJM* 1998; 339:173-181.
75. Granger DN, Korthuis RJ: Physiologic mechanisms of postischemic tissue injury. *Annu Rev Physiol* 1995; 57:311-332.
76. Vinten-Johansen J, Thourani VH: Myocardial protection: an overview. *J Extra Corpor Technol* 2000; 32:38-48.
77. Vinten-Johansen J, Zhao Z-Q, Sato H: Reduction in surgical ischemic-reperfusion injury with adenosine and nitric oxide therapy. *Ann Thorac Surg* 1995; 60:852-857.
78. Kloner RA, Yellon D: Does ischemic preconditioning occur in patients? *J Am Coll Cardiol* 1994; 24:1133-1142.
79. Carroll R, Yellon DM: Myocardial adaptation to ischemia—the preconditioning phenomenon. *Int J Cardiol* 1999; 68:S93-101.
80. Gaasch WH: Diagnosis and treatment of heart failure based on left ventricular systolic or diastolic dysfunction. *JAMA* 1994; 271:1276-1280.
81. Goldsmith SR, Dick C: Differentiating systolic from diastolic heart failure: pathophysiologic and therapeutic considerations. *Am J Med* 1993; 95:645-655.
82. Kass DA, Bronzwaer JG, Paulus WJ: What mechanisms underlie diastolic dysfunction in heart failure? *Circ Res* 2004; 94:1533-1542.
83. Litwin SE, Grossman W: Diastolic dysfunctions a cause of heart failure. *J Am Coll Cardiol* 1993; 22:49A-55A.
84. Bonow RO, Udelson JE: Left ventricular diastolic dysfunction as a cause of congestive heart failure. Mechanisms and management. *Ann Intern Med* 1992; 117:502-510.
85. Brandt RR, Wright RS, Redfield, Burnett JC: Atrial natriuretic in heart failure. *J Am Coll Cardiol* 1993; 22:86A-92A.
86. Floras JS: Clinical aspects of sympathetic activation and parasympathetic withdrawal in heart failure. *J Am Coll Cardiol* 1993; 22:72A-84A.
87. Pfeffer MA: Left ventricular remodeling after acute myocardial infarction. *Annu Rev Med* 1995; 46:455-466.
88. Komuro I, Yazaki I: Control of cardiac gene expression by mechanical stress. *Annu Rev Physiol* 1993; 55:55-75.
89. Schwartz K, Chassagne C, Boheler K: The molecular biology of heart failure. *J Am Coll Cardiol* 1993; 22:30A-33A.
90. Pfeffer JM, Fischer TA, Pfeffer MA: Angiotensin-converting enzyme inhibition and ventricular remodeling after myocardial infarction. *Annu Rev Physiol* 1995; 57:805-826.
91. Nolan PE: Integrating traditional and emerging treatment options in heart failure. *Am J Health Syst Pharm* 2004;61(Suppl 2):S14-22.
92. Weber KT, Brilla CG: Pathological hypertrophy and cardiac interstitium. Fibrosis and rennin-angiotensin-aldosterone system. *Circulation* 1991; 83:1849-1865.
93. Treasure CB, Alexander RW: The dysfunctional endothelium in heart failure. *J Am Coll Cardiol* 1993; 22:129A-134A.
94. Zhao Z-Q, Velez DA, Wang N-P, et al: Progressively developed myocardial apoptotic cell death during late phase of reperfusion. *Apoptosis* 2001; 6:279-290.
95. Gallagher MJ, McCullough PA: The emerging role of natriuretic peptides in the diagnosis and treatment of decompensated heart failure. *Curr Heart Fail Rep* 2004; 1:129-135.

CHAPTER 4

Cardiac Surgical Pharmacology

Jerrold H. Levy
Kenichi A. Tanaka
James G. Ramsay

INTRODUCTION

Clinical pharmacology associated with cardiac surgery is an important part of patient management. Patients in the perioperative period receive multiple agents that affect cardiovascular and pulmonary function. This chapter summarizes the pharmacology of the agents commonly used for treating the primary physiologic disturbances associated with cardiac surgery, hemodynamic instability, respiratory insufficiency, and alterations of hemostasis. For cardiovascular drugs, the common theme is that pharmacologic effects are produced by intracellular ion fluxes.

Several basic subcellular/molecular pathways are important in cardiovascular pharmacology, as shown in Fig. 4-1. The action potential in myocardial cells is a reflection of ion fluxes across the cell membrane, especially Na^+, K^+, and Ca^{2+}.[1,2] Numerous drugs used to control heart rate and rhythm act by altering Na^+ (eg, lidocaine and procainamide), K^+ (eg, amiodarone, ibutilide, and sotalol), or Ca^{2+} (eg, diltiazem) currents. Calcium also has a dominant effect on the inotropic state.[3,4]

Myocardial contractility is a manifestation of the interaction of actin and myosin, with conversion of chemical energy from ATP hydrolysis into mechanical energy. The interaction of actin and myosin in myocytes is inhibited by the associated protein tropomyosin. This inhibition is "disinhibited" by intracellular calcium. A similar situation occurs in vascular smooth muscle, where the interaction of actin and myosin (leading to vasoconstriction) is modulated by the protein calmodulin, which requires calcium as a cofactor. Thus intracellular calcium has a "tonic" effect in both the myocardium and vascular smooth muscle.

Numerous drugs used perioperatively alter intracellular calcium.[3,4]

Catecholamines (eg, norepinephrine, epinephrine, and dobutamine) with beta agonist activity regulate intramyocyte calcium levels via the nucleotide cyclic adenosine monophosphate (cyclic AMP) (Fig. 4-2). Beta agonists bind to receptors on the cell surface that are coupled to the intracellular enzyme adenylate cyclase via the stimulatory transmembrane GTP-binding protein. This leads to increased cyclic AMP synthesis, and cyclic AMP, in turn, acts as a second messenger for a series of intracellular reactions resulting in higher levels of intracellular calcium during systole. Less well known is that drugs with only alpha-adrenergic agonist activity also may increase intracellular Ca^{2+} levels, although by a different mechanism.[5,6] Although under investigation, the probable basis for the inotropic effect of alpha-adrenergic drugs is the stimulation of phospholipase C, which catalyzes hydrolysis of phosphatidyl inositol to diacylglycerol and inositol triphosphate (see Fig. 4-2). Both of these compounds increase the sensitivity of the myofilament to calcium, whereas inositol triphosphate stimulates the release of calcium from its intracellular storage site, the sarcoplasmic reticulum. There is still some debate about the mechanism for the inotropic effect of alpha-adrenergic agonists and its significance for the acute pharmacologic manipulation of contractility, but there is little debate about the importance of this mechanism in vascular smooth muscle, where the increase in intracellular calcium stimulated by alpha-adrenergic agonists can increase smooth muscle tone significantly. However, intracellular calcium in vascular smooth muscle is also controlled by cyclic nucleotides.[7,8] In contrast to the myocyte, in vascular smooth muscle, cyclic AMP has a primary effect of stimulating the uptake of calcium into intracellular storage sites, decreasing its availability (Fig. 4-3). Thus drugs that stimulate cyclic AMP production (beta agonists) or inhibit its

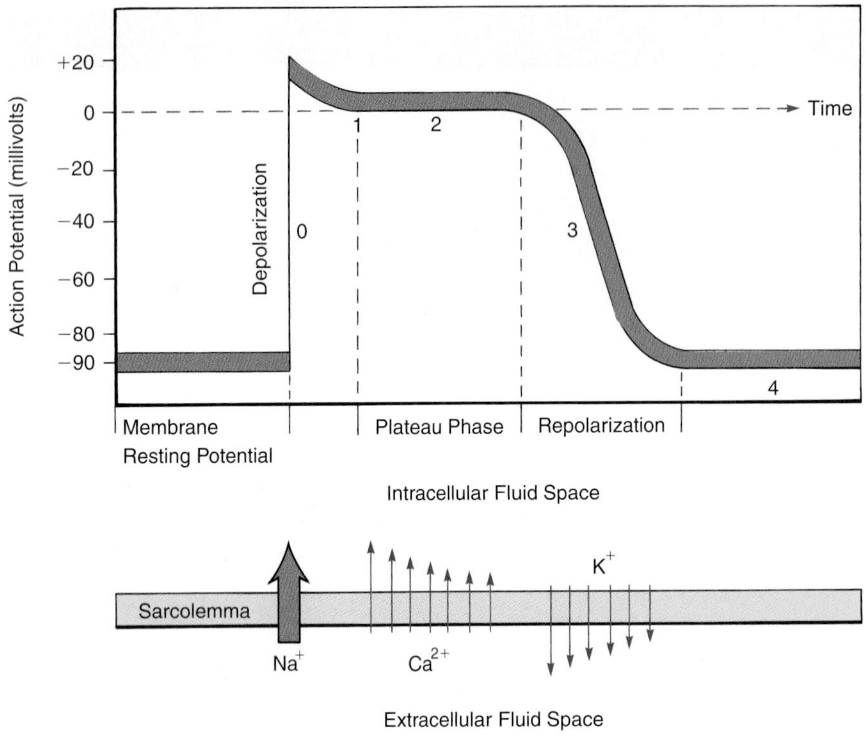

FIGURE 4-1 Cardiac ion fluxes and the action potential. The resting membrane potential is largely a reflection of the intercellular/intracellular potassium gradient. Depolarization of the membrane during phase 4 triggers an initial fast sodium channel with overshoot (phase 0) followed by recovery (phase 1) to a plateau (phase 2) maintained by an inward calcium flux and then repolarization owing to an outward potassium flux (phase 3).

breakdown (phosphodiesterase inhibitors) will cause vasodilation. In addition, cyclic guanosine monophosphate (cyclic GMP) also increases intracellular calcium storage (see Fig. 4-3), decreasing its availability for modulating the interaction of actin and myosin. Several commonly used pharmacologic agents act via cyclic GMP. For example, nitric oxide stimulates the enzyme guanylate cyclase, increasing cyclic GMP levels. Drugs such as nitroglycerin and sodium nitroprusside achieve their effect by producing nitric oxide as a metabolic product. Vasodilation is also produced by "cross-talk" between K^+ and Ca^{2+} fluxes. Decreased levels of ATP, acidosis, and elevated tissue lactate levels increase the permeability of the ATP-sensitive K^+ channel. This increased permeability results in hyperpolarization of the cell membrane that inhibits the entry of Ca^{2+} into the cell. This results in decreased vascular tone.

The simplistic overview of pathways of cardiac pharmacology as summarized in Figs. 4-1 through 4-3 also suggests the primary cause of difficulty in the clinical use of the drugs discussed in this chapter. The mechanisms of action for control of heart rate and rhythm, contractility, and vascular tone are interrelated. For example, beta-adrenergic agonists not only increase intracellular calcium to increase contractility, but they also alter K^+ currents, leading to tachycardia. Catecholamines not only have beta-adrenergic agonist activity, with inotropic and chronotropic effects, but they also possess alpha-agonist activity, leading to increased intracellular calcium in vascular smooth muscle and vasoconstriction. Phosphodiesterase inhibitors not only may increase contractility by increasing cyclic AMP in the myocyte, but they also may cause excessive vasodilation by increasing cyclic AMP in the vasculature. The interplay of the various mechanisms means the clinical art of cardiac surgical pharmacology lies as much in selecting drugs for their side effects as for their primary therapeutic effects.

ANTIARRHYTHMICS

Arrhythmias are common in the cardiac surgical period. A stable cardiac rhythm requires depolarization and repolarization in a spatially and temporally coordinated manner, and dysrhythmias may occur when this coordination is disturbed. The mechanisms for arrhythmias can be divided into abnormal impulse initiation, abnormal impulse conduction, and combinations of both.[9,10] Abnormal impulse initiation occurs as a result of increased automaticity (spontaneous depolarization of tissue that does not normally have pacemaking activity) or as a result of triggered activity from abnormal conduction after depolarizations during phase 3 or 4 of the action potential. Abnormal conduction often involves reentry phenomena, with recurrent depolarization around a circuit owing to unilateral conduction block in ischemic or damaged myocardium and retrograde activation by an alternate pathway through normal tissue. In this simplistic view, it is logical that dysrhythmias could be suppressed by slowing the conduction velocity of ectopic foci, allowing normal pacemaker cells to control heart rate, or by prolonging the action potential duration (and hence refractory period) to block conduction into a limb of a reentry circuit.

A scheme proposed originally by Vaughan Williams and modified subsequently[11,12] is used often to classify antidysrhythmic agents, and although alternative schemes describing specific channel-blocking characteristics have been proposed and may be more logical,[13] this discussion is organized using the Vaughan Williams system of four major drug categories. In this scheme, class I agents are those with local anesthetic properties that block Na^+ channels, class II drugs are beta-blocking agents, class III drugs prolong action potential duration, and class IV drugs are calcium entry blockers. Amiodarone is discussed in detail owing to its expanding role in treating

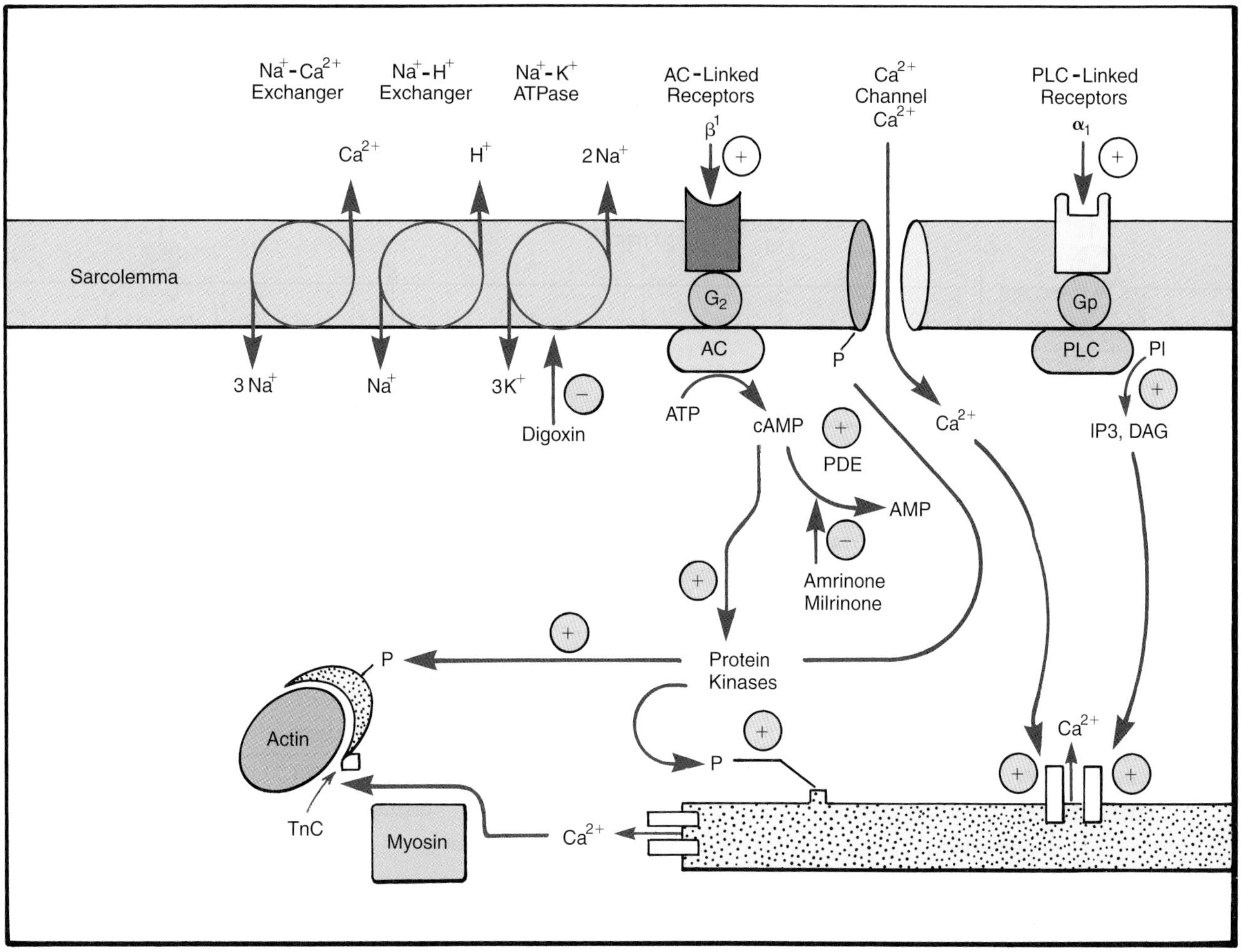

FIGURE 4-2 Mediators of cardiac contractility. Myocardial contractility is a manifestation of the interaction of actin and myosin, which is facilitated by the binding of calcium to troponin C (TnC). Intercellular calcium levels are controlled by direct flux across the membrane, by cyclic AMP, and by inositol triphosphate (IP_3) and diacylglycerol (DAG) produced by the action of phospholipase C (PLC). The synthesis of cyclic AMP is catalyzed by adenylate cyclase (AC), which is activated by binding of agonist to the beta-adrenergic receptor, and its breakdown is catalyzed by phosphodiesterase (PDE), which is inhibited by amrinone and milrinone. The action of PLC is activated by binding of agonist to the alpha-adrenergic receptor.

both supraventricular and ventricular arrhythmias and because its use has replaced many of the previously used agents. Because of the efficacy of intravenous amiodarone and its recommendations in Advanced Cardiac Life Support (ACLS) guidelines, many of the older drugs used in cardiac surgery have a historical perspective and are considered briefly.

CLASS I AGENTS

Although each of the class I agents blocks Na^+ channels, they may be subclassified based on electrophysiologic differences. These differences can be explained, to some extent, by consideration of the kinetics of the interaction of the drug and the Na^+ channel.[14,15] Class I drugs bind most avidly to open (phase 0 of the action potential; see Fig. 4-1) or inactivated (phase 2) Na^+ channels. Dissociation from the channel occurs during the resting (phase 4) state. If the time constant for dissociation is long in comparison with the diastolic interval (corresponding to phase 4), the drug will accumulate in the channel to reach a steady state, slowing conduction in normal tissue. This occurs with class Ia (eg, procainamide, quinidine, and disopyramide) and class Ic (eg, encainide, flecainide, and propafenone) drugs. In contrast, for the class Ib drugs (eg, lidocaine and mexiletine), the time constant for dissociation from the Na^+ channel is short, drug does not accumulate in the channel, and conduction velocity is affected minimally. However, in ischemic tissue, the depolarized state is more persistent, leading to greater accumulation of agent in the Na^+ channel and slowing of conduction in the damaged myocardium.

Procainamide is a class Ia drug that has various electrophysiologic effects.[16] Administration may be limited by the side effects of hypotension and decreased cardiac output.[17,18] The loading dose is 20 to 30 mg/min, up to 17 mg/kg, and should be followed by an intravenous infusion of 20 to 80 mg/kg per minute. Because procainamide prolongs action potential duration, widening of the QRS complex often heralds a potential

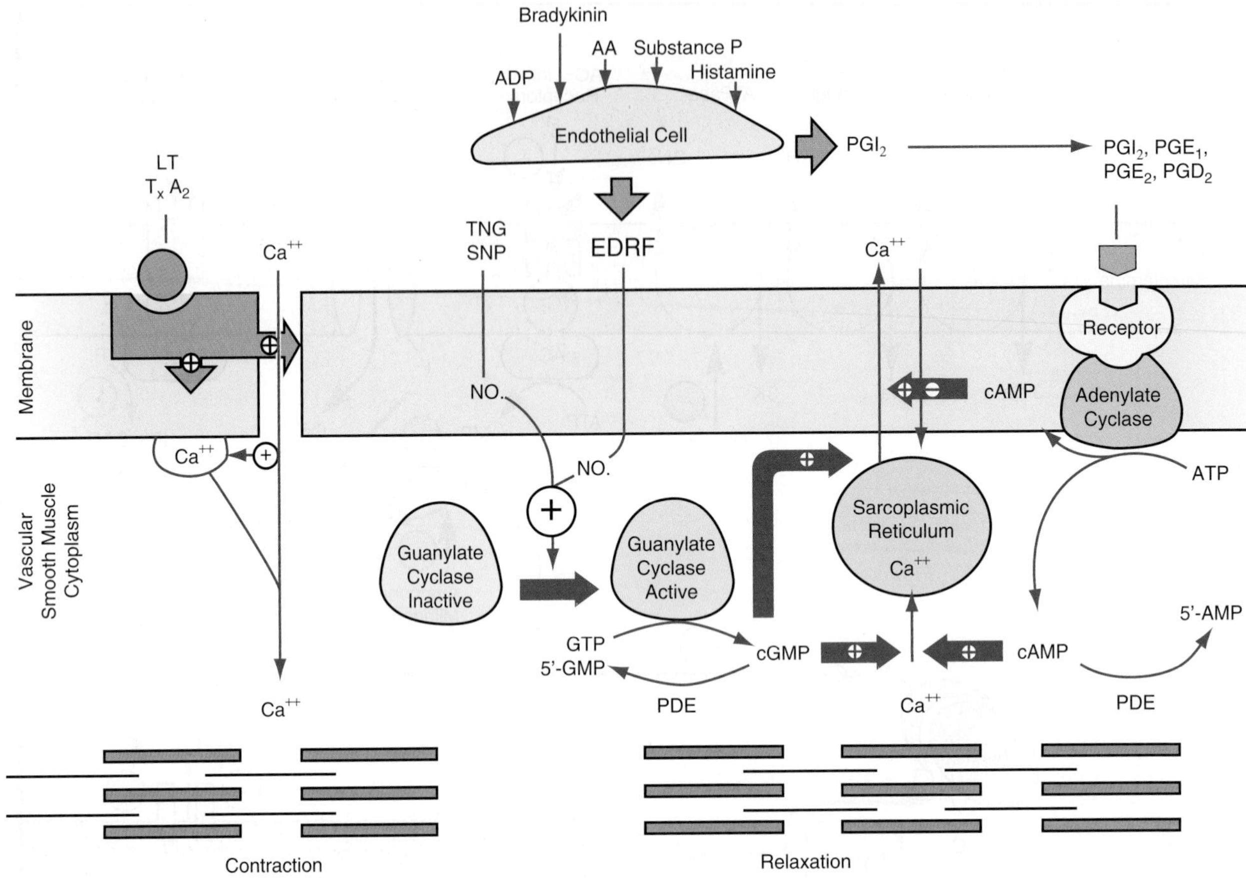

FIGURE 4-3. Mediators of vascular tone. Cyclic AMP and cyclic GMP increase the uptake of calcium into cellular storage sites in vascular smooth muscle, leading to vasodilation. The synthesis of cyclic GMP is catalyzed by guanylate cyclase, which is activated by nitric oxide (NO), which, in turn, is produced by nitroglycerin (NTG) and sodium nitroprusside (SNP). Excessive vasodilation often is a reflection of other endogenous mediators such as prostaglandins (PGI_2, PGE_1, PGE_2, and PGD_2) and thromboxane A_2 $_2(TxA_2)$. Several mediators, such as arachidonic acid (AA), bradykinin, histamine, and substance P, stimulate the release of endothelium-derived relaxing factor (EDRF), which is identified with NO. (*Reproduced with permission from Levy JH: Anaphylactic Reactions in Anesthesia and Intensive Care, 2nd ed. Boston, Butterworth-Heinemann, 1992.*)

overdose. The elimination of procainamide involves hepatic metabolism, acetylation to a metabolite with antiarrhythmic and toxic side effects, and renal elimination of this metabolite. Thus the infusion rate for patients with significant hepatic or renal disease should be at the lower end of this range.

Class Ib drugs include what is probably the best-known antiarrhythmic agent, lidocaine. As noted, lidocaine is a Na^+ channel blocker that has little effect on conduction velocity in normal tissue but slows conduction in ischemic myocardium.[14,15] Other electrophysiologic effects include a decrease in action potential duration but a small increase in the ratio of effective refractory period to action potential duration. The exact role of these electrophysiologic effects on arrhythmia suppression is unclear. Lidocaine has no significant effects on atrial tissue, and it is not recommended for therapy in shock-resistant ventricular tachycardia/fibrillation (VT/VF) in the recent *Guidelines for Emergency Cardiovascular Care.*[19] After an initial bolus dose of 1 to 1.5 mg/kg of lidocaine, plasma levels decrease rapidly owing to redistribution to muscle, fat, etc. Effective plasma concentrations are maintained only by following the bolus dose with an infusion of 20 to 50 mg/kg per minute.[20] Elimination occurs via hepatic metabolism to active metabolites that are cleared by the kidneys. Consequently, the dose should be reduced by approximately 50% in patients with liver or kidney disease. The primary toxic effects are associated with the central nervous system, and a lidocaine overdose may cause drowsiness, depressed level of consciousness, or seizures in very high doses. Negative inotropic or hypotensive effects are less pronounced than with most other antiarrhythmics. The other class Ib drugs likely to be encountered in the perioperative period are the oral agents tocainide and mexiletine, which have effects similar to lidocaine.[15]

The class Ic agents, including flecainide, encainide, and propafenone, markedly decrease conduction velocity.[20,21] The Cardiac Arrhythmia Suppression Trial (CAST) study[20,21] of moricizine found that although ventricular arrhythmias were suppressed, the incidence of sudden death was greater than with placebo with encainide and flecainide, and these drugs are not in wide use. Propafenone is available for oral use in the United States, but IV is available in Europe. The usual adult dose is 150 to 300 mg orally every 8 hours. It has beta-blocking (with resulting negative inotropic effects) as well as NA^+ channel-blocking activity; lengthens the PR, QRS, and QT duration; and may be used to treat both atrial and ventricular dysrhythmias.[15]

Class II Agents

Beta-receptor–blocking agents are another important group of antiarrhythmic (denoted class II in the Vaughan Williams scheme). However, because of their use as antihypertensive as well as antiarrhythmic agents, they are discussed elsewhere in this chapter, and we will move on to consider bretylium, amiodarone, and sotalol, the class III agents in the Vaughan Williams scheme. These drugs have a number of complex ion channel-blocking effects, but possibly the most important activity is K^+ channel blockade.[22] Because the flux of K^+ out of the myocyte is responsible for repolarization, an important electrophysiologic effect of class III drugs is prolongation of the action potential.[23]

Class III Agents

Ibutilide, dofetilide, sotalol, and bretylium are class III agents. Intravenous ibutilide and oral dofetilide are approved for the treatment of atrial fibrillation but carry the risk of torsades de pointes.[24,25] Sotalol is a nonselective beta-blocker that also has K^+ channel-blocking activity.[26] In the United States, it is now available for IV and previously for oral administration. The approved indication is for treating life-threatening ventricular arrhythmias, although it is effective against atrial arrhythmias as well. Bretylium is not used currently nor recommended in the most recent AHA *Guidelines for Emergency Cardiovascular Care*.[19]

Class IV Agents

Calcium entry blockers (class IV in the Vaughan Williams scheme), including verapamil and diltiazem, are antiarrhythmics. In sinoatrial and atrioventricular nodal tissue, Ca^{2+} channels contribute significantly to phase 0 depolarization, and the atrioventricular (AV) nodal refractory period is prolonged by Ca^{2+} entry blockade.[27,28]

This explains the effectiveness of verapamil and diltiazem in treating supraventricular arrhythmias. It is also clear why these drugs are negative inotropes. Both verapamil and diltiazem are effective in slowing the ventricular response to atrial fibrillation, flutter, and paroxysmal supraventricular tachycardia and in converting to sinus rhythm.[29–31] Verapamil has greater negative inotrope effects than diltiazem; therefore, it is used rarely for supraventricular arrhythmias. The intravenous dose of diltiazem is 0.25 mg/kg, with a second dose of 0.35 mg/kg if the response is inadequate after 15 minutes. The loading dose should be followed by an infusion of 5 to 15 mg/h. Intravenous diltiazem, although useful for rate control, has been replaced by intravenous amiodarone in clinical therapy of supraventricular tachycardia (SVT) and prophylaxis (see Amiodarone).

Other Drugs

One of the difficulties of classifying antiarrhythmics by the Vaughan Williams classification is that not all drugs can be incorporated into this scheme. Three examples are digoxin, adenosine, and magnesium, each of which has important uses in the perioperative period.

Digoxin inhibits the Na^+, K^+-ATPase pump, leading to decreased intracellular K^+, a less negative resting membrane potential, increased slope of phase 4 depolarization, and decreased conduction velocity. These direct effects, however, usually are dominated by indirect effects, including inhibition of reflex responses to congestive heart failure and a vagotonic effect.[10,32] The net effect is greatest at the AV node, where conduction is slowed and the refractory period is increased, explaining the effectiveness of digoxin in slowing the ventricular response to atrial fibrillation. The major disadvantages of digoxin are the relatively slow onset of action and many side effects, including proarrhythmia effects, and it is now used rarely for rate control in acute atrial fibrillation because of the advent of IV amiodarone and diltiazem.

Adenosine is an endogenous nucleoside that has an electrophysiologic effect similar to that of acetylcholine. Adenosine decreases AV node conductivity, and its primary antiarrhythmic effect is to break AV nodal reentrant tachycardia.[33] An intravenous dose of 100 to 200 μg/kg is the treatment of choice for paroxysmal supraventricular tachycardia. Adverse effects, such as bronchospasm, are short-lived because its plasma half-life is so short (1 to 2 seconds). This short half-life makes it ideal for treating reentry dysrhythmia, in which transient interruption can fully suppress the dysrhythmia.

Appropriate acid-base status and electrolyte balance are important because electrolyte imbalance can perturb the membrane potential, leading to arrhythmia generation, as can altered acid-base status, by effects on K^+ concentrations and sympathetic tone. Therapy for dysrhythmia should include correction of acid-base and electrolyte imbalances. Magnesium supplementation should be considered.[34] Magnesium deficiency is common in the perioperative period, and magnesium administration has been shown to decrease the incidence of postoperative dysrhythmia.[35]

AMIODARONE

Intravenous amiodarone has become one of the most administered intravenous antiarrhythmics used in cardiac surgery because of its broad spectrum of efficacy. Amiodarone was developed originally as an antianginal agent because of its vasodilating effects, including coronary vasodilation.[36] It has various ion channel-blocking activities.[10,29,36] The resulting electrophysiologic effects are complex, and there are differences in acute intravenous and chronic oral administration. Acute intravenous administration can produce decreases in heart rate and blood pressure, but there are minimal changes in QRS duration or QT interval. After chronic use, there may be significant bradycardia and increases in action potential duration in AV nodal and ventricular tissue, with increased QRS duration and QT interval.[37–39]

Pharmacokinetics

Amiodarone is a complex highly lipophilic drug that undergoes variable absorption (35 to 65%) after oral administration and is taken up extensively by multiple tissues with interindividual variation and complex pharmacokinetics.[38–40] The short initial context-sensitive half-life after intravenous administration represents drug redistribution. The true elimination half-life for amiodarone is extremely long, up to 40 to 60 days. Because of the huge volume of distribution (~60 L/kg) and a long duration of action, an active metabolite loading period of several months may be required before reaching steady-state tissue concentrations. Further, in life-threatening arrhythmias, intravenous loading often is starting to establish initial plasma levels. Measuring amiodarone plasma concentrations is not useful owing to the complex pharmacokinetics and the metabolites of the parent drug. Plasma concentrations greater than 2.5 mg/L have been associated with an increased risk of toxicity. The optimal dose of amiodarone has not been well characterized and may vary depending on the specific arrhythmias treated. Further, there may be differences in dose requirements for therapy of supraventricular and ventricular arrhythmias.[37–40]

Because of these distinctive pharmacokinetic properties, steady-state plasma levels are achieved slowly. Oral administration for a typical adult consists of a loading regimen of 80 to 1600 mg/d (in two or three doses) for 10 days, 600 to 800 mg/d for 4 to 6 weeks, and then maintenance doses of 200 to 600 mg/d. For intravenous loading, specific studies will be reviewed, but recommended dosing is 150 mg given over 10 minutes for acute therapy in an adult, followed first by a secondary loading infusion of 60 mg/h for 6 hours and then by a maintenance infusion of 30 mg/h to achieve a 1000 mg/d dosing.[37–40]

Electrophysiology

The electrophysiologic actions of amiodarone are complex and incompletely understood. Amiodarone produces all four effects according to the Vaughan Williams classification. It also has been shown to have use-dependent class I activity, inhibition of the inward sodium currents, and class II activity.[10] The antiadrenergic effect of amiodarone, however, is different from that of beta-blocker drugs because it is noncompetitive and additive to the effect of beta-blockers. Amiodarone depresses sinoatrial (SA) node automaticity, which slows the heart rate and conduction and increases refractoriness of the AV node, properties useful in managing supraventricular arrhythmia. Its class III activity results in increases in atrial and ventricular refractoriness and prolongation of the QTc interval. The effects of oral amiodarone on SA and AV nodal function are maximal within 2 weeks, whereas the effects on ventricular tachycardia (VT) and ventricular refractoriness emerge more gradually during oral therapy, becoming maximal after 10 weeks or more.

Indications

The primary indication for amiodarone is ventricular tachycardia or fibrillation.[40–48] It is also effective for the treatment of atrial dysrhythmias and in treating atrial fibrillation (see Atrial Fibrillation).

Side Effects

Although there are numerous adverse reactions to amiodarone, they occur with long-term oral administration and are rarely associated with acute intravenous administration. The most serious is pulmonary toxicity, which has not been reported with acute administration in a perioperative setting. Some case series have reported an increased risk of marked bradycardia and hypotension immediately after cardiac surgery in patients already on amiodarone at the time of surgery.[49,50] Other case-control studies, however, have not reproduced this finding.[51] None of the placebo-controlled trials of prophylactic amiodarone for perioperative atrial fibrillation prevention report adverse cardiovascular effects, although bradycardia and hypotension are known side effects.[52–56] Case reports and case series of postoperative acute pulmonary toxicity are similarly lacking in the rigor of randomized, controlled methodology.

PHARMACOLOGIC THERAPY OF SPECIFIC ARRHYTHMIAS

Ventricular Tachyarrhythmias

Intravenous amiodarone is approved for rapid control of recurrent VT or VF. Three randomized, controlled trials of patients with recurrent in-hospital, hemodynamically unstable VT or VF with two or more episodes within the past 24 hours who failed to respond to or were intolerant of lidocaine, procainamide, and (in two of the trials) bretylium have been reported.[42,44,46] Patients were critically ill with ischemic cardiovascular disease, 25% were on a mechanical ventilator or intra-aortic balloon pump before enrollment, and 10% were undergoing cardiopulmonary resuscitation at the time of enrollment. One study compared three doses of IV amiodarone: 525, 1050, and 2100 mg/d.[44] Because of the use of investigator-initiated intermittent open-label amiodarone boluses for recurrent VT, the actual mean amiodarone doses received by the three groups were 742, 1175, and 1921 mg/d. There was no statistically significant difference in the number of patients without VT/VF recurrence during the 1-day study period: 32 of 86 (41%), 36 of 92 (45%), and 42 of 92 (53%) for the low-, medium-, and high-dose groups, respectively. The number of supplemental 150-mg bolus infusions of amiodarone given by blinded investigators was statistically significantly less in those randomized to higher doses of amiodarone.

A wider range of amiodarone doses (125, 500, and 1000 mg/d) was evaluated by Sheinman and colleagues, including a low dose that was expected to be subtherapeutic.[46] This stronger study design, however, also was confounded by open-label bolus amiodarone injections given by study investigators. There was, however, a trend toward a relationship between intended amiodarone dose and VT/VF recurrence rate ($p = .067$). After adjustment for baseline imbalances, the median 24-hour recurrence rates of VT/VF, from lowest to highest doses, were 1.68, 0.96, and 0.48 events per 24 hours.

The third study compared two intravenous amiodarone doses (125 and 1000 mg/d) with bretylium (2500 mg/d).[42] Once again, the target amiodarone dose ratio of 8:1 was compressed to 1.8:1 because of open-label boluses. There was no significant difference in the primary outcome, which was median VT/VF recurrence rate over 24 hours. For low-dose amiodarone, high-dose amiodarone, and bretylium, these rates were 1.68, 0.48, and 0.96 events per 24 hours, respectively ($p = .237$). There was no difference between high-dose amiodarone and bretylium; however, more than 50% of patients had crossed over from bretylium to amiodarone by 16 hours.

The failure of these studies to provide clear evidence of amiodarone efficacy may be related to the "active-control study design" used, a lack of adequate statistical power, high rates of supplemental amiodarone boluses, and high crossover rates. Nonetheless, these studies provide some evidence that IV amiodarone (1 g/d) is moderately effective during a 24-hour period against VT and VF.

Sustained Monomorphic Ventricular Tachycardia and Wide QRS Tachycardia

Although the most effective and rapid treatment of any hemodynamically unstable sustained ventricular tachyarrhythmia is electrical cardioversion or defibrillation, intravenous antiarrhythmic drugs can be used for arrhythmia termination if the VT is hemodynamically stable. The *Guidelines for Emergency Cardiovascular Care*[19] has removed former recommendation of lidocaine and adenosine use in stable wide QRS tachycardia, now labeled as "acceptable" but not primarily recommended (lidocaine) or not recommended (adenosine). Intravenous procainamide and sotalol are effective, based on randomized but small studies;[10] amiodarone is also considered acceptable.[19]

Shock-Resistant Ventricular Fibrillation

The *Guidelines for Emergency Cardiovascular Care* recommends at least three shocks and epinephrine or vasopressin before any antiarrhythmic drug is administered.[10,19] No large-scale controlled, randomized studies have demonstrated efficacy for lidocaine, bretylium, or procainamide in shock-resistant VF,[10,19] and lidocaine and bretylium are no longer recommended in this setting.[19] Two pivotal studies have been reported recently studying the efficacy of agents in acute shock-resistant cardiac arrest.

The Amiodarone in the Out-of-Hospital Resuscitation of Refractory Sustained Ventricular Tachycardia (ARREST) study was randomized, double-blind, and placebo-controlled. The ARREST study in 504 patients showed that amiodarone 300 mg administered in a single intravenous bolus significantly improves survival to hospital admission in cardiac arrest still in VT or VF after three direct-current shocks (44% versus 34%; $p < .03$).[43] Although the highest survival rate to hospital admission (79%) was achieved when the amiodarone was given within 4 to 16 minutes of dispatch, there was no significant difference in the proportional improvement in the amiodarone group compared with the placebo group when drug administration was delayed (up to 55 minutes). Amiodarone also had the highest efficacy in patients (21% of all study patients) who had a return of spontaneous circulation before drug administration (survival to hospital admission increased to 64% from 41% in the placebo group). Among patients with no return of spontaneous circulation, amiodarone only slightly improved outcome (38% versus 33%).

Dorian performed a randomized trial comparing intravenous lidocaine with intravenous amiodarone as an adjunct to defibrillation in victims of out-of-hospital cardiac arrest.[48] Patients were enrolled if they had out-of-hospital ventricular fibrillation resistant to three shocks, intravenous epinephrine, and a further shock or if they had recurrent ventricular fibrillation after initially successful defibrillation. They were randomly assigned in a double-blind manner to receive intravenous amiodarone plus lidocaine placebo or intravenous lidocaine plus amiodarone placebo. The primary end point was the proportion of patients who survived to be admitted to the hospital. In total, 347 patients (mean age 67 ± 14 years) were enrolled. The mean interval between the time at which paramedics were dispatched to the scene of the cardiac arrest and the time of their arrival was 7 ± 3 minutes, and the mean interval from dispatch to drug administration was 25 ± 8 minutes. After treatment with amiodarone, 22.8% of 180 patients survived to hospital admission compared with 12.0% percent of 167 patients treated with lidocaine ($p = .009$). Among patients for whom the time from dispatch to the administration of the drug was equal to or less than the median time (24 minutes), 27.7% of those given amiodarone and 15.3% of those given lidocaine survived to hospital admission ($p = .05$). The authors concluded that compared with lidocaine, amiodarone leads to substantially higher rates of survival to hospital admission in patients with shock-resistant out-of-hospital ventricular fibrillation.

Supraventricular Arrhythmias

A supraventricular arrhythmia is any tachyarrhythmia that requires atrial or atrioventricular junctional tissue for initiation and maintenance. It may arise from reentry caused by unidirectional conduction block in one region of the heart and slow conduction in another, from enhanced automaticity akin to that seen in normal pacemaker cells of the sinus node and in latent pacemaker cells elsewhere in the heart, or from triggered activity, a novel type of abnormally enhanced impulse initiation caused by membrane currents that can be activated and inactivated by premature stimulation or rapid pacing.[56–58] Pharmacologic approaches to treating supraventricular arrhythmias, including atrial fibrillation, atrial flutter, atrial tachycardia, AV re-entrant tachycardia, and AV nodal re-entrant tachycardia, continue to evolve.[56–60] Because atrial fibrillation is perhaps the most common arrhythmia after cardiac surgery, this condition is emphasized in detail.

Atrial Fibrillation

Atrial fibrillation (AF) is a common complication of cardiac surgery that increases the length of stay in the hospital with resulting increases in health-care resource utilization.[56–61] Advanced age, previous AF, and valvular heart operations are the most consistently identified risk factors for this arrhythmia. Because efforts to terminate AF after its initiation are problematic, current interests are directed at therapies to prevent postoperative AF. Most studies suggest that prophylaxis with antiarrhythmic compounds can decrease the incidence of AF, length of hospital stay, and cost significantly. Class III antiarrhythmic drugs (eg, sotalol and ibutilide) also may be effective but potentially pose the risk of drug-induced polymorphic ventricular tachycardia (torsades de pointes). Newer promising intravenous agents including vernakalant are also being investigated. Defining which subpopulations benefit most from such therapy is important as older and more critically ill patients undergo surgery. Intravenous sotalol is currently available in the United States.

Amiodarone is also an effective approach for prophylactic therapy of AF. Intravenous amiodarone is an important consideration because loading with oral therapy is often not feasible in part owing to time required. There also may be added benefits of prophylactic therapies in high-risk patients, especially those prone to ventricular arrhythmias (ie, patients with preexisting heart failure).

Two studies deserve mention regarding prophylaxis with amiodarone. To determine if IV amiodarone would prevent atrial fibrillation and decrease hospital stay after cardiac surgery, Daoud and colleagues assessed preoperative prophylaxis in 124 patients who were given either oral amiodarone (64 patients) or placebo (60 patients) for a minimum of 7 days before elective cardiac surgery.[62] Therapy consisted of 600-mg amiodarone per day for 7 days and then 200 mg/d until the day of discharge from the hospital. The preoperative total dose of amiodarone was 4.8 ± 0.96 g over 13 ± 7 days. Postoperative atrial fibrillation occurred in 16 of the 64 patients in the amiodarone group (25%) and 32 of the 60 patients in the placebo group (53%). Patients in the amiodarone group were hospitalized for significantly fewer days than were patients in the placebo group (6.5 ± 2.6 versus 7.9 ± 4.3 days; $p = .04$). Total hospitalization costs were significantly less for the amiodarone group than for the placebo group ($18,375 ± $13,863 versus $26,491 ± $23,837; $p = .03$). Guarnieri and colleagues evaluated 300 patients randomized in a double-blind fashion to IV amiodarone (1 g/d for 2 days) versus placebo immediately after open-heart surgery.[54] The primary end points of the trial were incidence of atrial fibrillation and length of hospital stay. Atrial fibrillation occurred in 67 of 142 (47%) patients on placebo versus 56 of 158 (35%) on amiodarone ($p = .01$). Length of hospital stay for the placebo group was 8.2 ± 6.2 days, and 7.6 ± 5.9 days for the amiodarone group. Low-dose IV amiodarone was safe and effective in reducing the incidence of atrial fibrillation after heart surgery but did not significantly alter length of hospital stay.

In summary, AF is a frequent complication of cardiac surgery. Many cases can be prevented with appropriate prophylactic therapy. Beta-adrenergic blockers should be administered to most patients without contraindication. Prophylactic amiodarone should be considered in patients at high risk for postoperative AF. The lack of data on cost benefits and cost efficiency in some studies may reflect the lack of higher-risk patients in the study. Patients who are poor candidates for beta blockade may not tolerate sotalol, whereas amiodarone does not have this limitation. Additional studies also need to be performed to better assess the role of prophylactic therapy in off-pump cardiac surgery.

INOTROPIC AGENTS

Some depression of myocardial function is common after cardiac surgery.[63–65] The etiology is multifactorial—preexisting disease, incomplete repair or revascularization, myocardial edema, postischemic dysfunction, reperfusion injury, etc—and usually is reversible. Adequate cardiac output usually can be maintained by exploiting the Starling curve with higher preload, but often the cardiac function curve is flattened, and it is necessary to use inotropic agents to maintain adequate organ perfusion.

The molecular basis for the contractile property of the heart is the interaction of the proteins actin and myosin, in which chemical energy (in the form of ATP) is converted into mechanical energy. In the relaxed state (diastole), the interaction of actin and myosin is inhibited by tropomyosin, a protein associated with the actin-myosin complex. With the onset of systole, Ca^{2+} enters the myocyte (during phase 1 of the action potential). This influx of Ca^{2+} triggers the release of much larger amounts of Ca^{2+} from the sarcoplasmic reticulum. The binding of Ca^{2+} to the C subunit of the protein troponin interrupts inhibition of the actin-myosin interaction by tropomyosin, facilitating the hydrolysis of ATP with the generation of a mechanical force. With repolarization of the myocyte and completion of systole, Ca^{2+} is taken back up into the sarcoplasmic reticulum, allowing tropomyosin to again inhibit the interaction of actin and myosin with consequent relaxation of contractile force. Thus inotropic action is mediated by intracellular Ca^{2+}.[66] A novel drug, levosimendan, currently under clinical development in the United States but approved in several countries, increases the sensitivity of the contractile apparatus to Ca^{2+},[67] whereas the positive inotropic agents available for clinical use achieve their end by increasing intracellular Ca^{2+} levels.

The first drug to be considered is simply Ca^{2+} itself. In general, administration of calcium will increase the inotropic state of the myocardium when measured by load-independent methods, but it also will increase vascular tone (afterload) and impair diastolic function. In addition, the effects of calcium on myocardial performance depend on the plasma Ca^{2+} concentration. Ca^{2+} plays important roles in cellular function, and the intracellular Ca^{2+} concentration is highly regulated by membrane ion channels and intracellular organelles.[68,69] If the extracellular Ca^{2+} concentration is normal, administration of Ca^{2+} will have little effect on the intracellular level and less pronounced hemodynamic effects. On the other hand, if the ionized plasma calcium concentration is low, exogenous calcium administration may increase cardiac output and blood pressure.[70] It also should be realized that even with normal plasma Ca^{2+} concentrations, administration of Ca^{2+} may increase vascular tone, leading to increased blood pressure but no change in cardiac output. This increased afterload, as well as the deleterious effects on diastolic function, may be the basis of the observation that Ca^{2+} administration can blunt the response to epinephrine.[71] Routine use of Ca^{2+} at the end of bypass should be tempered by the realization that Ca^{2+} may have little effect on cardiac output while increasing systemic vascular resistance, although this in itself may be of importance. If there is evidence of myocardial ischemia, Ca^{2+} administration may be deleterious because it may exacerbate both coronary spasm and the pathways leading to cellular injury.[72,73]

Digoxin, although not effective as acute therapy for low-cardiac-output syndrome in the perioperative period, nevertheless well illustrates the role of intracellular Ca^{2+}. Digoxin functions by inhibiting Na^+, K^+-ATPase, which is responsible for the exchange of intracellular Na^+ with extracellular K^+.[3,4] It is thus responsible for maintaining the intracellular/extracellular K^+ and Na^+ gradients. When it is inhibited, intracellular Na^+ levels increase. The increased intracellular Na^+ is an increased chemical potential for driving the Ca^{2+}/Na^+ exchanger, an ion exchange mechanism in which intracellular Na^+ is removed from the cell in exchange for Ca^{2+}. The net effect is an increase in intracellular Ca^{2+} with an enhancement of the inotropic state.

The most commonly used positive inotropic agents are the beta-adrenergic agonists. The $beta_1$ receptor is part of a complex consisting of the receptor on the outer surface of the cell membrane and membrane-spanning G-proteins (so named because they bind GTP), which in turn stimulate adenylate cyclase on the inner surface of the membrane, catalyzing the formation cyclic adenosine monophosphate (cyclic AMP). The inotropic state is modulated by cyclic AMP via its catalysis of phosphorylation reactions by protein kinase A. These phosphorylation reactions "open" Ca^{2+} channels on the cell membrane and lead to greater release and uptake of Ca^{2+} from the sarcoplasmic reticulum.[3,4]

There are many drugs that stimulate $beta_1$ receptors and have a positive inotropic effect, including epinephrine, norepinephrine, dopamine, isoproterenol, and dobutamine, the most commonly used catecholamines in the perioperative period. Although there are differences in their binding at the $beta_1$ receptor, the most important differences between the various catecholamines are their relative effects on alpha- and $beta_2$-adrenergic receptors. In general, alpha stimulation of receptors on the peripheral vasculature causes vasoconstriction, whereas $beta_2$ stimulation leads to vasodilation (see the discussion elsewhere in this chapter). For some time it was believed that $beta_2$ and alpha receptors were found only in the peripheral vasculature, as well as a few other organs, but not in the myocardium. However, alpha receptors are found in the myocardium and mediate a positive inotropic effect.[5,6] The mechanism for this positive inotropic effect is probably the stimulation of phospholipase C, leading to hydrolysis of phosphatidyl inositol to diacylglycerol and inositol triphosphate, compounds that increase Ca^{2+} release from the sarcoplasmic reticulum and increase myofilament sensitivity to Ca^{2+}. It is also possible that alpha-adrenergic agents increase intracellular Ca^{2+} by prolonging action potential duration by inhibition of outward K^+ currents during repolarization or by activating the Na^+/H^+ exchange mechanism, increasing intracellular pH and increasing myofilament sensitivity to Ca^{2+}. Just as the exact mechanism is uncertain, the exact role of alpha-adrenergic stimulation in control of the inotropic state is unclear, although it is apparent that onset of the effect is slower than that of $beta_1$ stimulation.

Besides the discovery of alpha receptors in the myocardium, $beta_2$ receptors are present in the myocardium.[74] The fraction of $beta_2$ receptors (compared with $beta_1$ receptors) is increased in chronic heart failure, possibly explaining the efficacy of drugs with $beta_2$ activity in this setting. This phenomenon is part of the general observation of $beta_1$-receptor downregulation (decrease in receptor density) and desensitization (uncoupling of effect from receptor binding) that is observed in chronic heart failure.[75] Interestingly, it has been demonstrated in a dog model that this same phenomenon occurs with cardiopulmonary bypass (CPB).[76] In this situation, a newer class of drugs, the phosphodiesterase inhibitors, may be of benefit. These drugs, typified by the agents available in the United States, amrinone and milrinone, increase cyclic AMP levels independently of the beta receptor by selectively inhibiting the myocardial enzyme responsible for the breakdown of cyclic AMP.[3,4]

In clinical use, selection of a particular inotropic agent usually is based more on its side effects than its direct inotropic properties. Of the commonly used catecholamines, norepinephrine has alpha and $beta_1$ but little $beta_2$ activity and is both an inotrope and a vasopressor. Epinephrine and dopamine are mixed agonists with alpha, $beta_1$, and $beta_2$ activity. At lower doses, they are primarily inotropes and not vasopressors, although vasopressor effects become more pronounced at higher doses. This is especially true for dopamine, which achieves effects at higher doses by stimulating the release of norepinephrine.[77] Dobutamine is a more selective $beta_1$ agonist, in contrast to isoproterenol, which is a mixed beta agonist. Selection of a drug depends on the particular hemodynamic problem at hand. For example, a patient with depressed myocardial function in the presence of profound vasodilation may require a drug with both positive inotropic and vasopressor effects, whereas a patient who is vasoconstricted may benefit from some other choice. We recommend an empiric approach to selecting inotropic agents with careful monitoring of the response to the drug and selection of the agent that achieves the desired effect.

Clinical experience suggests that phosphodiesterase inhibitors can be effective when catecholamines do not produce an acceptable cardiac output.[78–80] There are few differences in the hemodynamic effects of the two drugs available for use in the United States, amrinone and milrinone. Both agents increase contractility with little effect on heart rate, and both are vasodilators. There is significant venodilation, as well as arteriodilation, and maintaining adequate preload is important in avoiding significant hypotension.[81,82] If amrinone is used, the bolus dose recommended in the product insert, 0.75 mg/mL, is inadequate to maintain therapeutic plasma levels, and a loading dose of 1.5 to 2.0 mg/mL should be used.[83] With either drug, administering the loading dose over 15 to 30 minutes may attenuate possible hypotension. Plasma levels drop rapidly after a loading dose because of redistribution, and the loading dose should be followed immediately by a continuous infusion.[83,84] Because of their longer half-lives, it is rather more difficult to readily titrate plasma levels than with catecholamines (which have plasma half-lives of a few minutes).

Phosphodiesterase inhibitors, specifically milrinone, facilitate separation from CPB with biventricular dysfunction and are used for treating low-cardiac-output syndrome after cardiac surgery.[82,85–87] Doolan and colleagues also demonstrated that milrinone, in comparison with placebo, significantly facilitated separation of high-risk patients from CPB.[88]

Levosimendan

Levosimendan is a class of drugs known as *calcium sensitizers.* The molecule is a pyridazinone-dinitrile derivative with additional action on adenosine triphosphate (ATP)–sensitive potassium channels.[67,89,90] Levosimendan is used intravenously for treating decompensated heart failure (HF) because it increases contractility and produces antistunning effects without increasing myocardial intracellular calcium concentrations or prolonging myocardial relaxation. Levosimendan also causes coronary and systemic vasodilation. In patients with HF, IV levosimendan reduced worsening HF or death significantly. IV levosimendan significantly also increased cardiac output and decreased filling pressure in decompensated HF in large, double-blind, randomized trials and after cardiac surgery in smaller trials. Levosimendan is well tolerated without arrhythmogenicity. In addition to sensitizing troponin to intracellular calcium, levosimendan inhibits phosphodiesterase III and open ATP-sensitive potassium channels (K_{ATP}), which may produce vasodilation. Unlike currently available intravenous inotropes, levosimendan does not increase myocardial oxygen use, and has been used effectively in beta-blocked patients. Levosimendan does not impair ventricular relaxation. Clinical studies have demonstrated short-term hemodynamic benefits of levosimendan over both placebo and dobutamine. Although large-scale, long-term morbidity and mortality data are scarce, the Levosimendan Infusion versus Dobutamine in Severe Low-Output Heart Failure (LIDO) study suggested a mortality benefit of levosimendan over dobutamine. Clinical studies comparing levosimendan with other positive inotropes, namely, milrinone, are lacking, and this agent is not available in North America.

Clinical Trials

Despite their common use after cardiac surgery, there have been relatively few comparative studies of inotropic agents in the perioperative period. In 1978, Steen and colleagues reported the hemodynamic effects of epinephrine, dobutamine, and epinephrine immediately after separation from CPB.[91] The largest mean increase in cardiac index was achieved with dopamine at 15 g/kg per minute. However, it should be noted that the only epinephrine dose studied was 0.04 g/kg per minute. In a later comparison of dopamine and dobutamine, Salomon and colleagues concluded that dobutamine produced more consistent increases in cardiac index, although the hemodynamic differences were small, and all patients had good cardiac indices at the onset of the study.[92] Fowler and colleagues also found insignificant differences in the hemodynamic effects of dobutamine and dopamine, although they reported that coronary flow increased more in proportion to myocardial oxygen consumption with dobutamine.[93] Although neither of these groups reported significant increases in heart rate for either dopamine or dobutamine, clinical experience has been otherwise. This is supported by a study by Sethna and colleagues, who found that the increase in cardiac index with dobutamine occurs simply because of increased heart rate, although they found that myocardial oxygen was maintained.[94] Butterworth and colleagues subsequently demonstrated that the older and much cheaper agent, epinephrine, effectively increased stroke volume without as great an increase in heart rate as dobutamine.[95] More recently, Feneck and colleagues compared dobutamine and milrinone and found them to be equally effective in treating low-cardiac-output syndrome after cardiac surgery.[96] This study was a comparison of two drugs, and the investigators emphasized that the most efficacious therapy is probably a combination of drugs. In particular, phosphodiesterase inhibitors require the synthesis of cyclic AMP to be effective, and thus use of a combination of a $beta_1$-adrenergic agonist and a phosphodiesterase inhibitor would be predicted to be more effective than either agent alone.

Finally, while global hemodynamic goals (ie, heart rate, blood pressure, filling pressures, and cardiac output) may be achieved with inotropic agents, this does not guarantee adequate regional perfusion, in particular renal and mesenteric perfusion. So far there have been few investigations of regional perfusion after cardiac surgery. There has been more interest in regional (especially mesenteric) perfusion in the critical care medicine literature, and some of the studies may be relevant to postoperative care of the cardiac surgical patient. Two studies have indicated that epinephrine may impair splanchnic perfusion, especially in comparison with combining norepinephrine and dobutamine.[97,98] Norepinephrine alone has variable effects on splanchnic blood flow in septic shock,[99] although adding dobutamine can improve splanchnic perfusion significantly when blood pressure is supported with norepinephrine.[98] Low-dose dopamine improves splanchnic blood flow,[100] but there is evidence that dopamine in higher doses impairs gastric perfusion.[101] The relevance of these studies of septic patients for the cardiac surgical patient is unclear, although there are similarities between the inflammatory responses to CPB and to sepsis.

VASOPRESSORS

CPB often is characterized by derangements of vascular tone. Sometimes CPB induces elevations in endogenous catecholamines, as well as other mediators, such as serotonin and arginine vasopressin (AVP), leading to vasoconstriction. However, often CPB is characterized by endothelial injury and a systemic inflammatory response, with a cascade of cytokine and inflammatory mediator release and profound vasodilation. The pathophysiology has a striking resemblance to that of sepsis or an anaphylactic reaction. Further, vasodilation after cardiac surgery may be exacerbated by the preoperative use of angiotensin-converting enzyme (ACE) inhibitors and post-CPB use of milrinone.

The mechanisms of vasodilatory shock have been reviewed recently.[102] Vascular tone is modulated by intracellular Ca^{2+}, which binds calmodulin. The Ca^{2+}-calmodulin complex activates myosin light-chain kinase, which catalyzes the phosphorylation of myosin to facilitate the interaction with actin. Conversely, intracellular cyclic GMP activates myosin phosphatase (also via a kinase-mediated phosphorylation of myosin phosphatase), which dephosphorylates myosin and inhibits the interaction of actin and myosin. A primary mediator of vasodilatory shock is nitric oxide (NO), which is induced by cytokine cascades. NO activates guanylate cyclase, with resulting loss of vascular tone. Another mechanism of vasodilation that may be particularly relevant to prolonged CPB is activation of ATP-sensitive potassium (K_{ATP}) channels. These channels are activated by decreases in cellular ATP or increases in hydrogen ion or lactate. All these could result from the abnormal perfusion associated with CPB and/or hypothermia. Increases in potassium channel conductance result in hyperpolarization of the vascular smooth muscle membrane, which decreases Ca^{2+} flux into the cell, leading to decreased vascular tone. A third mechanism of vasodilatory shock that also may be particularly relevant to cardiac surgery is deficiency of vasopressin. As noted earlier, CPB often induces the release of vasopressin, and this may contribute to the excessive vasoconstriction sometimes seen after CPB. However, it has been observed in several experimental models of shock that the initially high levels of vasopressin decrease as shock persists, leading some investigators to suggest that vasopressin stores are limited and are depleted by the initial response to hypotension.

Excessive vasodilation during shock usually is treated with catecholamines, most typically phenylephrine, dopamine, epinephrine, or norepinephrine.[103] Although catecholamines produce both alpha- and beta-adrenergic effects, alpha$_1$-adrenergic receptor stimulation produces vasoconstriction. As noted, stimulation of these receptors activates membrane phospholipase C, which in turn hydrolyzes phosphatidylinositol 4,55 diphosphate.[7] This leads to the subsequent generation of two second messengers, including diacyl glycerol and inositol triphosphate. Both these second messengers increase cytosolic Ca^{2+} by different mechanisms, which include facilitating release of calcium from the sarcoplasmic reticulum and potentially increasing the calcium sensitivity of the contractile proteins in vascular smooth muscle.

Mediator-induced vasodilation often is poorly responsive to catecholamines,[103] and the most potent pressor among catecholamines, norepinephrine, is required frequently. Some clinicians are concerned about renal, hepatic, and mesenteric function during norepinephrine administration. However, in septic patients, norepinephrine can improve renal function,[102–107] and there is evidence that it may improve mesenteric perfusion as well.[108] Given the hemodynamic similarities between septic patients and some patients at the end of CPB, these results often are extrapolated to the cardiac surgical patient but have not been confirmed by a systematic study. In some cases of profound vasodilatory shock, even norepinephrine is inadequate to restore systemic blood pressure. In this situation, low doses of vasopressin may be useful. Argenziano and colleagues[109] studied 40 patients with vasodilatory shock (defined as a mean arterial blood pressure of less than 70 mm Hg with a cardiac index greater than 2.5 L/m^2 per minute) after cardiac surgery. Arginine vasopressin levels were inappropriately low in this group of patients, and low-dose vasopressin infusion ($\leq$0.1 U/min) effectively restored blood pressure and reduced norepinephrine requirements without significantly changing cardiac index. These observations were similar to an earlier report of the use of vasopressin in vasodilatory septic shock.[110] Vasopressin also has been reported to be useful in treating milrinone-induced hypotension.[111] In this latter report, vasopressin was reported to increase urine output, presumably via glomerular efferent arteriole constriction. However, the overall effects on renal function are unclear. In addition, there are still important unanswered questions about vasopressin and mesenteric perfusion. Although vasopressin effectively may restore blood pressure in vasodilatory shock, it must be remembered that in physiologic concentrations it is a mesenteric vasoconstrictor, and mesenteric hypoperfusion may be a factor in developing sepsis and multiorgan dysfunction syndrome.

VASODILATORS

Different pharmacologic approaches are available to produce vasodilation (Table 4-1). Potential therapeutic approaches include: (1) blockade of alpha$_1$-adrenergic receptors, ganglionic transmission, and calcium channel receptors; (2) stimulation of central alpha$_2$-adrenergic receptors or vascular guanylate cyclase and adenylate cyclase; and (3) inhibition of phosphodiesterase enzymes and angiotensin-converting enzymes.[112] Adenosine in low concentrations is also a potent vasodilator with a short half-life, but it is used, as noted earlier, for its ability to inhibit atrioventricular conduction. Losartan, a novel angiotensin II (AII) antagonist, has just been released for treating hypertension but is not available for intravenous use.

Stimulation of Adenylate Cyclase (cyclic AMP)

Prostacyclin, prostaglandin E$_1$, and isoproterenol increase cyclic nucleotide formation (eg, adenosine-3′,5′-monophosphate and cyclic AMP) in vascular smooth muscle to produce calcium mobilization out of vascular smooth muscle. Inhibiting the breakdown of cyclic AMP by phosphodiesterase also will increase cyclic AMP.[112] Increasing cyclic AMP in vascular smooth muscle facilitates calcium uptake by intracellular storage sites, thus decreasing calcium available for contraction. The net effect of increasing calcium uptake is to produce vascular smooth muscle relaxation and hence vasodilation. However, most catecholamines with beta$_2$-adrenergic activity (eg, isoproterenol) and phosphodiesterase inhibitors have positive inotropic and other side effects that include tachycardia, glycogenolysis, and kaluresis.[113] Prostaglandins (ie, prostacyclin and prostaglandin E$_1$) are potent inhibitors of platelet aggregation and activation. Catecholamines with beta$_2$-adrenergic activity, phosphodiesterase inhibitors, and prostaglandin E$_1$ and prostacyclin have

TABLE 4-1 Vasodilators Used in the Treatment of Hypertension, Pulmonary Hypertension, and Heart Failure

Angiotensin-converting enzyme inhibitors
Angiotensin II antagonists
Alpha$_1$-adrenergic antagonists (prazosin)
Alpha$_2$-adrenergic agonists (clonidine)
Endothelin antagonists
Nitrates
Nitric oxide
Hydralazine
Phosphodiesterase inhibitors (milrinone, sildenafil)
Prostacyclin, PGE$_1$
Calcium channel blockers
Dihydropyridine agents (nifedipine, nicardipine, felodipine, amlodipine)

been used to vasodilate the pulmonary circulation in patients with pulmonary hypertension and right ventricular failure (see Table 4-1).[113]

Nitrates, Nitrovasodilators, and Stimulation of Guanylyl Cyclase (Cyclic GMP)

The vascular endothelium modulates vascular relaxation by releasing both nitric oxide and prostacyclin.[114–116] Inflammatory mediators also can stimulate the vascular endothelium to release excessive amounts of endothelium-derived relaxing factor (EDRF, or nitric oxide), which activates guanylyl cyclase to generate cyclic GMP.[89,90] Nitrates and sodium nitroprusside, however, generate nitric oxide directly, independent of vascular endothelium.[115,116] The active form of any nitrovasodilator is nitric oxide (NO), in which the nitrogen is in a +2 oxidation state. For any nitrovasodilator to be active, it first must be converted to NO. For nitroprusside, this is easily accomplished because nitrogen is in a +3 oxidation state, with the nitric oxide molecule bound to the charged iron molecule in an unstable manner, allowing nitroprusside to readily donate its nitric oxide moiety. For nitroglycerin, nitrogen molecules exist in a +5 oxidation state, and thus they must undergo significant metabolic transformations before they are converted to an active molecule. Nitroglycerin is a selective coronary vasodilator and does not produce coronary steal compared with nitroprusside because the small intracoronary resistance vessels, those less than 100 μm thick, lack whatever metabolic transformation pathway is required to convert nitroglycerin into its active form of nitric oxide.[115,116] Chronic nitrate therapy can produce tolerance through different mechanisms.[114–118] Sodium nitroprusside and nitroglycerin are effective vasodilators that produce venodilation that contributes significantly to the labile hemodynamic state.[114] Intravenous volume administration often is required with nitroprusside owing to the relative intravascular hypovolemia.

Dihydropyridine Calcium Channel Blockers

Dihydropyridine calcium channel blockers are direct arterial vasodilators.[119] Nifedipine was the first dihydropyridine calcium channel blocker, and intravenous forms studied in cardiac surgery include clevidipine, isradipine, and nicardipine. These agents are selective arterial vasodilators that have no effects on the vascular capacitance bed, atrioventricular nodal conduction, or negative inotropic effects.[120–125] Clevidipine and nicardipine are available in the United States, and offer novel and important therapeutic options to treat perioperative hypertension following cardiac surgery. Also, intravenous dihydropyridines can be used to treat acute hypertension that occurs during the perioperative period (ie, intubation, extubation, cardiopulmonary bypass–induced hypertension, and aortic cross-clamping) and postoperative hypertension.

Phosphodiesterase Inhibitors

The phosphodiesterase inhibitors currently available for use produce both positive inotropic effects and vasodilation.[126] When administered to patients with ventricular dysfunction, they increase cardiac output while decreasing pulmonary artery occlusion pressure, systemic vascular resistance, and pulmonary vascular resistance. Because of their unique mechanisms of vasodilation, they are especially useful for patients with acute pulmonary vasoconstriction and right ventricular dysfunction. Multiple forms of the drug are currently under investigation. The bipyridines (eg, amrinone and milrinone), imidazolones (eg, enoximone), and methylxanthines (eg, aminophylline) are the ones most widely available. Papaverine, a benzyl isoquinolinium derivative isolated from opium, is a nonspecific phosphodiesterase inhibitor and vasodilator used by cardiac surgeons for its ability to dilate the internal mammary artery.[126]

Angiotensin-Converting Enzyme Inhibitors

ACE inhibitors have growing use in managing heart failure, and more patients are receiving these drugs. The ACE inhibitors prevent the conversion of angiotensin I to angiotensin II by inhibiting an enzyme called *kininase* in the pulmonary and systemic vascular endothelium. This enzyme is also important for the metabolism of bradykinin, a potent endogenous vasodilator, and for release of EDRF. Although there are little data in the literature regarding the preoperative management of patients receiving these drugs, withholding them on the day of surgery has been our clinical practice based on their potential to produce excessive vasodilation during CPB. Although Tuman was unable to find any difference in blood pressure during CPB in patients receiving ACE inhibitors, contact activation during CPB has the ability to generate bradykinin and thus amplify the potential for vasodilation. The vasoconstrictor requirements were increased after bypass in his study.

Angiotensin II–Receptor Blockers

ACE inhibitors may not be tolerated in some patients owing to cough (common) and angioedema (rare). Inhibition of kininase II by ACE inhibitors leads to bradykinin accumulation in the lungs and vasculature, causing cough and vasodilation. Alternative treatment with angiotensin II–receptor blockers (ARBs) may be associated less frequently with these side effects because ARBs do not affect kinin metabolism. Six ARBs are currently available for antihypertensive therapy in the United States: losartan (Cozaar), valsartan (Diovan), irbesartan (Avapro), candesartan (Atacand), eprosartan (Teveten), and telmisartan (Micardis). Mortality in chronic heart failure is related to activation of the autonomic nervous and renin-angiotensin systems, and ACE inhibitor therapy seems to attenuate progression of myocardial dysfunction and remodeling. ACE inhibitors do not completely block angiotensin II (A-II) production,[127] and may even increase circulating A-II levels in patients with heart failure. It was thought initially that ARBs might offer advantages over ACE inhibitors for heart failure therapy in terms of tolerability and more complete A-II blockade. Although ARBs were better tolerated, all-cause mortality and the number of sudden deaths or resuscitated cardiac arrests were not different when losartan (Cozaar) and captopril (Capoten) were compared in patients (>60 years old, NYHA classes II to IV, LVEF < 40%).[128] Perioperative hypotension may be encountered in ARB-treated patients as well as ACE inhibitor–treated patients, and increased inotropic support may be required.

PHARMACOLOGIC MANIPULATION OF THE HEMOSTATIC SYSTEM DURING CARDIAC SURGERY

Numerous pharmacologic approaches to manipulate the hemostatic system in cardiac surgery include attenuating hemostatic system activation, preserving platelet function, and decreasing the need for transfusion of allogeneic blood products. Pharmacologic approaches to reduce bleeding and transfusion requirements in cardiac surgical patients are based on either preventing or reversing the defects associated with the CPB-induced coagulopathy.

BETA-ADRENERGIC RECEPTOR BLOCKERS

Not surprisingly, most of the effects observed after administration of a beta-adrenergic receptor blocker reflect the reduced responsiveness of tissues containing beta-adrenergic receptors to catecholamines present in the vicinity of those receptors. Hence the intensity of the effects of beta-blockers depends on both the dose of the blocker and the receptor concentrations of catecholamines, primarily epinephrine and norepinephrine. In fact, a purely competitive interaction of beta-blockers and catecholamines can be demonstrated in normal human volunteers as well as in isolated tissues studied in the laboratory. The presence of disease and other types of drugs modifies the responses to beta-blockers observed in patients, but the underlying competitive interaction is still operative. The key to successful use of beta-adrenergic receptor blockers is to titrate the dose to the desired degree of effect and to remember that excessive effects from larger than necessary doses of beta-adrenergic receptor blockers can be overcome by: (1) administering a catecholamine to compete at the blocked receptors; and/or (2) administering other types of drugs to reduce the activity of counterbalancing autonomic mechanisms that are unopposed in the presence of beta-receptor blockade. An example of the latter is propranolol-induced bradycardia, which reflects the increased dominance of the vagal cholinergic mechanism on cardiac nodal tissue. Excessive bradycardia may be relieved by administering atropine to block the cholinergic receptors, which are also located in the sinoatrial (SA) and atrioventricular (AV) nodes (see Table 4-2).

TABLE 4-2 Location and Actions of Beta-Adrenergic Receptors

Tissue	Receptor	Action	Opposing Actions
Heart			
Sinus and AV nodes	1	↑ Automaticity	Cholinergic receptors
Conduction pathways	1	↑ Conduction velocity	Cholinergic receptors
		↑ Automaticity	Cholinergic receptors
Myofibrils	1	↑ Contractility	—
		↑ Automaticity	—
Vascular smooth muscle (arterial, venous)	2	Vasodilation	Alpha-adrenergic receptors
Bronchial smooth muscle	2	Bronchodilation	Cholinergic receptors
Kidneys	1	↑ Renin release (juxtaglomerular cells)	$Alpha_1$-adrenergic receptors
Liver	2	↑ Glucose metabolism	$Alpha_1$-adrenergic receptors
		↑ Lipolysis	
Fat/adipose tissue	3	↑ Lipolysis	—
Skeletal muscle	2	↑ Potassium uptake glycogenolysis	—
Eye, ciliary muscle	2	Relaxation	Cholinergic receptors
GI tract	2	↑ Motility	Cholinergic receptors
Gallbladder	2	Relaxation	Cholinergic receptors
Urinary bladder detrusor muscle	2	Relaxation	Cholinergic receptors
Uterus	2	Relaxation	Oxytocin
Platelets	2	↓ Aggregation	$Alpha_2$-adrenergic receptors (aggregation)

Knowledge of the type, location, and action of beta receptor is fundamental to understanding and predicting effects of beta-adrenergic receptor–blocking drugs[129] (see Table 4-2). Beta-adrenergic receptor blockers are competitive inhibitors; hence, the intensity of blockade depends on both the dose of the drug and the receptor concentrations of catecholamines, primarily epinephrine and norepinephrine.

Beta-adrenergic receptor antagonists (blockers) include many drugs (Table 4-3) that typically are classified by their relative selectivity for $beta_1$ and $beta_2$ receptors (ie, cardioselective or nonselective), the presence or absence of agonistic activity, membrane-stabilizing properties, alpha-receptor–blocking efficacy, and various pharmacokinetic features (eg, lipid solubility, oral bioavailability, and elimination half-time).[129] The practitioner must realize that the selectivity of individual drugs for $beta_1$ and $beta_2$ receptors is relative, not absolute. For example, the risk of inducing bronchospasm with a $beta_1$-adrenergic (cardioselective) blocker (eg, esmolol or metoprolol) may be relatively less than with a nonselective blockers (eg, propranolol); however, the risk is still present.

TABLE 4-3 Beta-Adrenergic Receptors Blockers

Generic Name	Trade Name	Dosage Forms	$Beta_1$-Selective
Acebutolol	Sectral	PO	Yes
Atenolol	Tenormin	IV, PO	Yes
Betaxolol	Kerlone	PO	Yes
Bisoprolol	Zebeta	PO	Yes
Esmolol	Brevibloc	IV	Yes
Metoprolol	Lopressor, Toprol-XL	IV, PO	Yes
Carvedilol*	Coreg	PO	No
Carteolol	Cartrol	PO	No
Labetalol*	Normodyne, Trandate	IV, PO	No
Nadolol	Corgard	PO	No
Penbutolol	Levatol	PO	No
Pindolol	Visken	PO	No
Propranolol	Inderal	IV, PO	No
Sotalol	Betapace	PO	No
Timolol	Blocadren	PO	No

**$Alpha_1$: beta-adrenergic blocking ratio; carvedilol 1:10, labetalol 1:3 (oral)/1:7 (IV).*

Acute Myocardial Infarction

Earlier clinical trials of intravenous beta-adrenergic blockers in the early phases of acute myocardial infarction suggest they decrease mortality. Following myocardial infarction, chronic oral beta-blocking agents reduce the incidence of recurrent myocardial infarction (see Table 4-3).[130]

Supraventricular Tachycardias and Ventricular Dysrhythmias

Beta-adrenergic blocking agents are Vaughan Williams class II antidysrhythmics that primarily block cardiac responses to catecholamines. Propranolol (Inderal), esmolol (Brevibloc), and acebutolol (Sectral) are used commonly for this indication. Beta-blocking agents decrease spontaneous depolarization in the SA and AV nodes, decrease automaticity in Purkinje fibers, increase AV nodal refractoriness, increase threshold for fibrillation (but not for depolarization), and decrease ventricular slow responses that depend on catecholamines. Amiodarone, a class III agent, also exerts noncompetitive alpha- and beta-adrenergic blockade, which may contribute its antidysrhythmic and antihypertensive actions. Sotalol is another class III antidysrhythmic with nonselective beta-blocking action. There is evidence that beta-blocking agents also decrease intramyocardial conduction in ischemic tissue and reduce the risks of dysrhythmias to the extent that they decrease myocardial ischemia. Beta-adrenergic blockers are not particularly effective in controlling dysrhythmias that are not induced or maintained by catecholamines.[131]

Hypertension

Hypertension is a major risk factor for developing heart failure and other end-organ damage. Beta-blockers, along with diuretics, are considered to be the initial drug of choice for uncomplicated hypertension in patients aged less than 65 years.

During the early phases of therapy, there is a decrease in cardiac output, a rise in systemic vascular resistance (SVR), and relatively little change in mean arterial blood pressure. Within hours to days, SVR normalizes, and blood pressure declines. In addition, the release of renin from the juxtaglomerular apparatus in the kidney is inhibited ($beta_1$ blockade). Beta-blocking agents with intrinsic agonistic activity reduce systemic vascular resistance below pretreatment levels presumably by activating $beta_2$ receptors in vascular smooth muscle. Most beta-adrenergic blockers are used with other agents in treating chronic hypertension. When combined with a vasodilator, beta-blockers limit reflex tachycardia. For example, when propranolol is combined with intravenous nitroprusside (a potent arterial dilator), it prevents reflex release of renin and reflex tachycardia induced by nitroprusside.[132]

Acute Dissecting Aortic Aneurysm

The primary goal in managing dissecting aneurysms is to reduce stress on the dissected aortic wall by reducing the systolic acceleration of blood flow. Beta-blockers reduce cardiac inotropy and ventricular ejection fraction. Beta-blockers also may limit reflex sympathetic responses to vasodilators that are used to control systemic arterial pressure.

Pheochromocytoma

The presence of catecholamine-secreting tissue is tantamount to the continuous or intermittent infusion of a varying mixture of norepinephrine and epinephrine. It is absolutely essential that virtually complete alpha-adrenergic receptor blockade be established prior to administering the beta-blocker to prevent exacerbation of hypertensive episodes by unopposed alpha-adrenergic receptor activity in vascular smooth muscle.

Chronic Heart Failure

It is now understood that activation of the autonomic nervous system (ANS) and renin-angiotensin system (RAS) as compensatory mechanisms for the failing heart actually may contribute to deterioration of myocardial function. Mortality in chronic heart failure seems related to activation of ANS and RAS. Progression of myocardial dysfunction and remodeling may be attenuated by the use of beta-blocking agents and ACE inhibitors. Carvedilol (Coreg) is a beta-blocker approved by the FDA to treat patients with heart failure. It has an $alpha_1$- and nonselective beta-blocking activity (alpha:beta = 1:10). It is contraindicated in severe decompensated heart failure and asthma. In patients with atrial fibrillation and left-sided heart failure treated with carvedilol, improved ejection fraction, and a trend toward a decreased incidence of death and chronic heart failure hospitalization were observed in a retrospective analysis of a U.S. carvedilol study. There are several ongoing clinical trials with carvedilol, metoprolol (Toprol), and bisoprolol (Zebeta). The results of these studies may provide answers as to which beta-blocking agent would be most successful in the treatment of specific patient populations.

Other Indications

The other clinical applications of beta-adrenergic receptor blockers listed in Table 4-4 are based on largely symptomatic treatment or empirical trials of beta-adrenergic antagonists.

Side Effects and Toxicity

The most obvious and immediate signs of a toxic overdose of a beta-adrenergic receptor blocker are hypotension, bradycardia, congestive heart failure, decreased AV conduction, and a widened QRS complex on the electrocardiogram. Treatment is aimed at blocking the cholinergic receptor responses to vagal nerve activity (eg, atropine) and administering a sympathomimetic to compete with the beta-blockers at adrenergic receptors. In patients with asthma and chronic obstructive pulmonary disease (COPD), beta-blockers may cause bronchospasm. Beta blockers may increase levels of plasma triglycerides and reduce levels of high-density lipoprotein (HDL) cholesterol. Rarely, beta-blockers may mask the symptoms of hypoglycemia in diabetic patients. Other side effects include mental depression, physical fatigue, altered sleep patterns, sexual dysfunction, and gastrointestinal symptoms, including indigestion, constipation, and diarrhea (see Table 4-4).

TABLE 4-4 Clinical Applications of Beta-Adrenergic Receptor Blockers

Angina pectoris
Acute myocardial infarction (prophylaxis)
Supraventricular tachycardia
Ventricular dysrhythmias
Hypertension (usually in combination with other drugs)
Pheochromocytoma (after alpha-receptor blockade is established)
Acute dissecting aortic aneurysm
Hyperthyroidism
Hypertrophic obstructive cardiomyopathy (IHSS)
Dilated cardiomyopathy (selected patients)
Migraine prophylaxis
Acute panic attack
Alcohol withdrawal syndrome
Glaucoma (topically)

Drug Interactions

Pharmacokinetic drug interactions include reduced gastrointestinal absorption of the beta-blocker (eg, aluminum-containing antacids and cholestyramine), increased biotrans-formation of the beta-blocker (eg, phenytoin, phenobarbital, rifampin, and smoking), and increased bioavailability owing to decreased biotransformation (eg, cimetidine and hydralazine). Pharmacodynamic interactions include an additive effect with calcium channel blockers to decrease conduction in the heart and a reduced antihypertensive effect of beta-blockers when administered with some of the nonsteroidal anti-inflammatory drugs (NSAIDs).

DIURETICS

Diuretics are drugs that act directly on the kidneys to increase urine volume and produce a net loss of solute (principally sodium and other electrolytes) and water. Diuretics and beta-blockers are initial drugs of choice for uncomplicated hypertension in patients younger than 65 years.[132] The currently available diuretic drugs have a number of other uses in medicine (eg, glaucoma and increased intracranial pressure). The principal indications for the use of diuretics by intravenous administration in the perioperative period are to: (1) increase urine flow in oliguria; (2) reduce intravascular volume in patients at risk for acute heart failure from excessive fluid administration or acute heart failure; and (3) mobilize edema.

Renal function depends on adequate renal perfusion to maintain the integrity of renal cells and provide the hydrostatic pressure that produces glomerular filtration. There are no drugs that act directly on the renal glomerulus to affect glomerular filtration rate (GFR). In the normal adult human of average size, GFR averages 125 mL/min, and urine production approximates 1 mL/min. In other words, 99% of the glomerular filtrate is reabsorbed. Diuretics act primarily on specific segments of the renal tubule to alter reabsorption of electrolytes, principally sodium, and water.

There are two basic mechanisms behind the renal tubular reabsorption of sodium. First, sodium is extruded from the tubular cell into peritubular fluid primarily by active transport of the sodium ion, which reflects the action of the Na^+, K^+-ATPase pump as well as the bicarbonate reabsorption mechanism (see the following). This extrusion of sodium creates an electrochemical gradient that causes diffusion of sodium from the tubular lumen into the tubular cell. Second, sodium moves from the glomerular filtrate in the tubular fluid into the peritubular fluid by several different mechanisms. The most important quantitatively is the sodium electrochemical gradient created by the active extrusion of sodium from the tubular cell into the peritubular fluid. In addition, sodium is coupled with organic solutes and phosphate ions, exchanged for hydrogen ions diffusing from the tubular cell into the tubular lumen, and coupled to the transfer of a chloride ion or a combination of potassium and two chloride ions (Na^+-K^+-$2Cl^-$ cotransport) from the tubular fluid into the tubular cell. Diuretics are classified by their principal site of action in the nephron and by the primary mechanism of their naturetic effect (Table 4-5).

Osmotic Diuretics

Mannitol is the principal example of this type of diuretic, which is used for two primary indications: (1) prophylaxis and early treatment of acute renal failure that is characterized by a decrease in GFR leading to a decreased urine volume and an increase in the concentration of toxic substances in the renal tubular fluid; and (2) enhancing the actions of other diuretics by retaining water and solutes in the tubular lumen, thereby providing the substrate for the action of other types of diuretics. Normally, 80% of the glomerular filtrate is reabsorbed isosmotically in the proximal tubules. By its osmotic effect, mannitol limits the reabsorption of water and dilutes the proximal tubular fluid. This reduces the electrochemical gradient for sodium and limits its reabsorption so that more is delivered to the distal portions of the nephron. Mannitol produces a prostaglandin-mediated increase in renal blood flow that partially washes out the medullary hypertonicity, which is essential for the countercurrent mechanism promoting the reabsorption of water in the late distal tubules and collecting system under the influence of antidiuretic hormone (ADH). Mannitol is used often (25 to 50 g) as part of the priming solution of cardiopulmonary bypass for the above-mentioned indications. The principal toxicity of mannitol is acute expansion of the extracellular fluid volume leading to HF in the patient with compromised cardiac function (see Table 4-5).

High-Ceiling (Loop) Diuretics

Furosemide (Lasix), bumetanide (Bumex), and ethacrynic acid (Edecrin) are three chemically dissimilar compounds that have the same primary diuretic mechanism of action. They act on the tubular epithelial cell in the thick ascending loop of Henle to inhibit the Na^+-K^+-$2Cl^-$ cotransport mechanism. Their peak diuretic effect is far greater than that of the other diuretics currently available. Administered intravenously, they have a rapid onset and relatively short duration of action, the latter reflecting both the pharmacokinetics of the drugs and the body's compensatory mechanisms to the consequences of diuresis.

TABLE 4-5 Classification of Diuretics

Site of Action	Mechanism	
Osmotic	Proximal convoluted and late proximal for NA^+ diffusion from tubular fluid into tubular cell	↓ Electrochemical gradient
	Late proximal tubule	↓ Gradient for Cl^- (accompanying NA^+ diffusion)
	Thick ascending loop of Henle	↓ Na^+-K^+-$2Cl^-$ cotransport
Carbonic	Proximal convoluted tubule anhydrase inhibitors	↓ Na^+-H^+ exchange$^+$
Thiazides	Distal convoluted tubule	↓ Na^+-Cl^- cotransport
High-ceiling loop diuretics	Thick ascending loop of Henle	↓ Na^+-K^+-$2Cl^-$ cotransport
Potassium-sparing diuretics	Late distal tubule and collecting duct	↓ Electrogenic Na^+ entry into cells (driving force for K^+ secretion)

These three diuretics increase renal blood flow without increasing GFR and redistribute blood flow from the medulla to the cortex and within the renal cortex. These changes in renal blood flow are also short-lived, reflecting the reduced extracellular fluid volume resulting from diuresis. Minor actions, including carbonic anhydrase inhibition by furosemide and bumetanide and actions on the proximal tubule and on sites distal to the ascending limb, remain controversial. All three of the loop diuretics increase the release of renin and prostaglandin, and indomethacin blunts the release as well as the augmentation in renal blood flow and natruresis. All three of the loop diuretics produce an acute increase in venous capacitance for a brief period of time after the first intravenous dose is administered, and this effect is also blocked by indomethacin.

Potassium, magnesium, and calcium excretion is increased in proportion to the increase in sodium excretion. In addition, there is augmentation of titratable acid and ammonia excretion by the distal tubules leading to metabolic alkalosis, which is also produced by contraction of the extracellular volume. Hyperuricemia can occur but usually is of little physiologic significance. The nephrotoxicity of cephaloridine, and possibly other cephalosporins, is increased. A rare but serious side effect of the loop diuretics is deafness, which may reflect electrolyte changes in the endolymph.

Because of their high degree of efficacy, prompt onset, and relatively short duration of action, the high-ceiling or loop diuretics are favored for intravenous administration in the perioperative period to treat the three principal problems cited earlier. Dosage requirements vary considerably among patients. Some may only require furosemide 3 to 5 mg IV to produce a good diuresis. And for some patients, the less potent benzothiazides may be sufficient.

Benzothiazides

Hydrochlorothiazide (HCTZ) is the prototype of more than a dozen currently available diuretics in this class. Although the drugs differ in potency, they all act by the same mechanism of action and have the same maximum efficacy. All are actively secreted into the tubular lumen by tubular cells and act in the early distal tubules to decrease the electroneutral Na^+-Cl^- cotransport reabsorption of sodium. Their moderate efficacy probably reflects the fact that more than 90% of the filtrated sodium is reabsorbed before reaching the distal tubules. Their action is enhanced by their combined administration with an osmotic diuretic such as mannitol. The benziothiazides increase urine volume and the excretion of sodium, chloride, and potassium. The decreased reabsorption of potassium reflects the higher rate of urine flow through the distal tubule (diminished reabsorption time).

This class of diuretics produces the least disturbance of extracellular fluid composition, reflecting their moderate efficacy as diuretics and perhaps suggesting their usefulness when a moderate degree of diuretic effect is indicated. Their principal side effects include hyperuricemia, decreased calcium excretion, and enhanced magnesium loss. Hyperglycemia can occur and reflects multiple variables. With prolonged use and development of a contracted extracellular fluid volume, urine formation decreases (ie, tolerance develops to their diuretic actions). These agents also have a direct action on the renal vasculature to decrease GFR.

Carbonic Anhydrase Inhibitors

Acetazolamide (Diamox) is the only diuretic of this class available for intravenous administration. Its use is directed primarily toward alkalinization of urine in the presence of metabolic alkalosis, which is a common consequence of prolonged diuretic therapy. It acts in the proximal convoluted tubule to inhibit carbonic anhydrase in the brush border of the tubular epithelium, thereby reducing the destruction of bicarbonate ions (ie, conversion to CO_2 that diffuses into the tubular cell). The carbonic anhydrase enzyme in the cytoplasm of the tubular cell is also inhibited, and as a consequence, conversion of CO_2 to carbonic acid is reduced markedly, as is the availability of hydrogen ions for the Na-H exchange mechanism. Hence the reabsorption of both sodium and bicarbonate in the proximal tubules is diminished. However, more than half the bicarbonate is reabsorbed in more distal segments of the nephron, thereby limiting the overall efficacy of this class of diuretics.

Potassium-Sparing Diuretics

Spironolactone (Aldactone) is a competitive antagonist of aldosterone. Spironolactone binds to the cytoplasmic aldosterone receptor and prevents its conformational change to the active form, thereby aborting the synthesis of active transport proteins in the late distal tubules and collecting system in which the reabsorption of sodium and secretion of potassium are reduced.

Triamterene (Dyrenium) and amiloride (Midamor) are potassium-sparing diuretics with a mechanism of action independent of the mineralocorticoids. They have a moderate natriuretic effect leading to an increased excretion of sodium and chloride with little change or a slight increase in potassium excretion when the latter is low. When potassium secretion is high, they produce a sharp reduction in the electrogenic entry of sodium ions into the distal tubular cells and thereby reduce the electrical potential that is the driving force for potassium secretion.

Both types of potassium-sparing diuretics are used primarily in combination with other diuretics to reduce potassium loss. Their principal side effect is hyperkalemia. It is appropriate to limit the intake of potassium when using this type of diuretic. It is also appropriate to use this type of diuretic cautiously in patients taking ACE inhibitors, which decrease aldosterone formation and consequently increase serum potassium concentrations.

Other Measures to Enhance Urine Output and Mobilization of Edema Fluid

The infusion of albumin (5 to 25% solutions) or other plasma volume expanders (eg, hetastarch) is often employed in an attempt to draw water and its accompanying electrolytes (ie, edema fluid) osmotically from the tissues into the circulating blood and thereby enhance their delivery to the kidneys for excretion. In the presence of a reduced circulating blood volume, this approach seems to be a logical method to increase the circulating blood volume and renal perfusion. The limiting feature of this approach to enhancing diuresis relates to the fact that the osmotic effect of albumin and plasma expanders is transient because they can diffuse (at a rate slower than water) from blood through capillary membranes into tissue. The albumin or plasma expander then tends to hold water and its accompanying electrolytes in tissue (ie, rebound edema). The same limiting feature applies to osmotic diuretics such as mannitol, which may transiently draw water and its accompanying electrolytes from tissues into the circulating blood for delivery to the kidneys, where the mannitol passes through the glomerulus and delays the reabsorption of water and its accompanying electrolytes from the proximal tubular fluid. Although this mechanism may enhance the actions of other diuretics, it is a transient effect that is limited by the diffusion of mannitol from blood into tissues with the production of rebound edema.

Dopamine, at doses from 1 to 3 μg/kg per minute, has been used conventionally to support mesenteric and renal perfusion. Its vascular action is mediated via vascular dopamine 1 (D_1) receptors in coronary, mesenteric, and renal vascular beds. By activating adenyl cyclase and raising intracellular concentrations of cyclic AMP, D_1-receptor agonists cause vasodilatation. There are also dopamine 2 (D_2) receptors that antagonize D_1-receptor stimulation. Fenoldopam (Corlopam), a parenteral D_1-receptor–specific agonist, was approved by the FDA recently. The Joint National Commissions VII recommendations include this drug for hypertensive emergencies.[132,133] Infusion of fenoldopam (0.1 to 0.3 μg/kg per minute) causes an increase in GFR, renal blood flow, and Na^+ excretion.

Clinical trials of dopamine failed to show improvement in renal function, which probably is a result of the nonspecificity of dopamine. As a catecholamine and a precursor in the metabolic synthesis of norepinephrine and epinephrine, dopamine has inotropic and chronotropic effects on the heart. The inotropic effect is mediated by $beta_1$-adrenergic receptors and usually requires infusion rates higher than those able to produce enhanced renal perfusion and diuresis. However, there are varied pharmacokinetic responses to dopamine infusion even in healthy subjects; therefore, the use of a "renal dose" dopamine regimen may not always result in the desirable effects. Stimulation of catecholamine receptors and D_2 receptors antagonizes the effects of D_1-receptor stimulation. Current data do not consistently demonstrate improved renal outcomes with use of the D_1-receptor–specific agonist fenoldopam.

HERBAL MEDICINE

A large number of Americans take herbal remedies for their health. Most of these herbal therapies are not supported by clear scientific evidence and are not under rigorous control by the FDA.[134–136] Patients who take alternative remedies may not necessarily disclose this information to their physicians.[135] There are increasing concerns regarding serious drug interactions between herbal therapy and prescribed medication. Some of the most common herbal remedies and drug interactions are summarized in Table 4-6.

Airway Management

Airway management in cardiovascular surgical patients is important because patients often present with coexisting conditions that may complicate endotracheal intubation. For example, a patient with morbid obesity and sleep apnea may require awake intubation with a fiberoptic bronchoscope, or a history of smoking and COPD may make the patient susceptible to rapid desaturation and/or bronchospasm. Airway management in the perioperative period is a primary responsibility of the anesthesiologist, but the surgeon becomes involved in the absence of the anesthesiologist or in assisting the anesthesiologist in difficult situations. Airway management involves instrumentation and mechanics (not discussed here) and employs pharmacologic approaches to overcome pathophysiologic problems contributing to airway obstruction and to facilitate manipulation and instrumentation of the airway. Pharmacologic agents are considered at the end of this section.

Five major challenges may be encountered in airway management. Each of these is described succinctly below to facilitate understanding of the roles that drugs play in meeting the challenges. The five challenges are (1) overcoming airway obstruction, (2) preventing pulmonary aspiration, (3) performing endotracheal intubation, (4) maintaining intermittent positive-pressure ventilation (IPPV), and (5) reestablishing spontaneous ventilation and airway protective reflexes.

Airway Obstruction

Obstruction to gas flow can occur from the entry of a foreign object (including food) into the airway and as a result of pathophysiologic processes involving airway structures (eg, trauma and edema). In the anesthetized or comatose patient, the loss of muscle tone can allow otherwise normal tissues (eg, tongue and epiglottis) to collapse into the airway and cause obstruction. The first measure in relieving such obstructions involves manipulation of the head and jaw, insertion of an artificial nasal or oral airway device, and evacuation of obstructing objects and substances (eg, blood, secretions, or food particles). Except for drugs used to facilitate endotracheal intubation (see the following), the only drug useful to improve gas flow through a narrowed airway is a mixture of helium and oxygen (Heliox), which has a much reduced viscosity resulting in reduced resistance to gas flow.

Aspiration

The upper airway (above the larynx/epiglottis) is a shared porthole to the lungs (gas exchange) and gastrointestinal tract (fluids and nutrition). Passive regurgitation or active vomiting resulting in accumulation of gastric contents in the pharynx places the patient at risk of pulmonary aspiration, especially under circumstances in which airway reflexes (eg, glottic closure and coughing) and voluntary avoidance maneuvers are suppressed (eg, anesthesia or coma). Particulate matter can obstruct the tracheobronchial tree, and acidic fluid ($pH < 2.5$) can injure the lung parenchyma. The resulting pneumonitis can cause significant morbidity (eg, acute respiratory distress syndrome) and has a high mortality rate. Preoperative restriction of fluids and food

TABLE 4-6 Commonly Used Herbal Remedies

Name	Common Uses	Side Effects/Drug Interactions
Cayenne (paprika)	Muscle spasm, GI disorders	Skin ulcers/blistering Hypothermia
Echinacea	Common cold antitussive urinary tract infections	May cause hepatotoxicity May decrease effects of steroids and cyclosporine
Ephedra (Ma-huang)	Antitussive, bacteriostatic	Enhanced sympathomimetic effects with guanethidine or monoamine oxidase inhibitor (MAOI) Arrhythmias with halothane or digoxin Hypertension with oxytocin
Feverfew	Migraine, antipyretic	Platelet inhibition, rebound headache, aphthous ulcers, GI irritation
Garlic	Lipid-lowering, antihypertensive antithrombotic	May potentiate warfarin
Ginger	Antinauseant antispasmodic	May potentiate aspirin and warfarin
Ginkgo	Improve circulation	May potentiate aspirin and warfarin
Ginseng	Adaptogenic enhance energy level, antioxidant	Ginseng abuse syndrome: sleepiness, hypertonia, edema May cause mania in patients on phenelzine May decrease effects of warfarin Postmenopausal bleeding Mastalgia
Goldenseal	Diuretic, anti-inflammatory, laxative hemostatic	Overdose may cause paralysis; aquaretic (no sodium excretion); may worsen edema/hypertension
Kava-kava	Anxiolytic	Potentiates barbiturates and benzodiazepines Potentiates ethanol May increase suicide risk in depression
Licorice	Antitussive gastric ulcers	High blood pressure, hypokalemia, and edema
Saw palmetto	Benign prostatic hypertrophy, antiandrogenic	Additive effects with other hormone replacement therapy (eg, HRT)
St. John's wort	Antidepressant, anxiolytic	Possible interaction with MAOIs Decreases metabolism of fentanyl and ondansetron
Valerian	Mild sedative, anxiolytic	Potentiates barbiturates and benzodiazepines

(NPO status) does not guarantee the absence of aspiration risks. Similarly, the advance placement of a nasogastric or orogastric tube may serve to reduce intragastric pressure but does not guarantee complete removal of gastric contents. Nevertheless, both NPO orders and the insertion of a nasogastric or orogastric tube under some circumstances are worthwhile measures to reduce the risks of pulmonary aspiration. In some circumstances, the deliberate induction of vomiting in a conscious patient may be indicated, but this is done rarely and almost never involves the use of an emetic drug. In fact, more often antiemetic drugs are employed to reduce the risks of vomiting during airway manipulation and induction of anesthesia.

Drug therapy to reduce the risks of pulmonary aspiration is focused on decreasing the quantity and acidity of gastric contents and on facilitating endotracheal intubation (see the following). Nonparticulate antacids (eg, sodium citrate [Bicitra]) are used to neutralize the acidity of gastric fluids. Drugs to reduce gastric acid production include H_2-receptor blockers (eg, cimetidine [Tagamet], ranitidine [Zantac], famotidine [Pepcid]) and inhibitors of gastric parietal cell hydrogen-potassium ATPase (proton pump inhibitors, eg, omeprazole [Prilosec], lansoprazole [Prevacid], and esomeprazole [Nexium]). Metoclopramide [Reglan] enhances gastric emptying and increases gastroesophageal sphincter tone. Cisapride [Propulsid] also increases gastrointestinal motility via the release of acetylcholine at the myenteric plexus.

Antiemetic drugs are used more commonly in the postoperative period and include several different drug classes: anticholinergics (eg, scopolamine [Transderm Scop]), antihistamines (eg, hydroxyzine [Vistaril] and, promethazine [Phenergan]), and antidopaminergics (eg, droperidol [Inapsine] and prochlorperazine [Compazine]). Antidopaminergic agents may cause extrapyramidal side effects in elderly patients. More costly but effective alternatives include the use of antiserotinergics (eg, ondansetron [Zofran] and dolasetron [Anzemet]).

Endotracheal Intubation

Drugs are employed for three purposes in facilitating endotracheal intubation: (1) to improve visualization of the larynx during laryngoscopy; (2) to prevent closure of the larynx; and (3) to facilitate manipulation of the head and jaw.

For bronchoscopy, laryngoscopy, or fiberoptic endotracheal intubation, the reflex responses to airway manipulation can be suppressed by several different methods alone or in combination. Topical anesthesia (2 or 4% lidocaine spray) can be used to anesthetize the mucosal surfaces of the nose, oral cavity, pharynx, and epiglottis. Atomized local anesthetic can be inhaled to anesthetize the mucosa below the vocal cords. The subglottic mucosa also can be anesthetized topically by injecting local anesthetic into the tracheal lumen through the cricothyroid membrane. A bilateral superior laryngeal nerve block eliminates sensory input from mechanical contact or irritation of the larynx above the vocal cords. It must be remembered that anesthesia of the mucosal surfaces to obtund airway reflexes compromises the reflex protective mechanisms of the airway and increases the patient's vulnerability to aspiration of substances from the pharynx. Improvement of visualization of the larynx includes decreasing salivation and tracheal bronchial secretions by administration of an anticholinergic drug (eg, glycopyrrolate), reducing mucosal swelling by topical administration of a vasoconstrictor (eg, phenylephrine), and minimizing bleeding owing to mucosal erosion by instrumentation, which also is minimized by topical vasoconstrictors. The use of steroids in minimizing acute inflammatory responses in the airway may have some delayed benefit, but steroids usually are not indicated just before intubation.

Systemic drugs, usually administered intravenously, can be used to obtund the cough reflex. Intravenous lidocaine (1 to 2 mg/kg) transiently obtunds the cough reflex without affecting spontaneous ventilation to any significant degree. The risks of central nervous system (CNS) stimulation and seizure-like activity have to be kept in mind and can be reduced by the prior administration of an intravenous barbiturate or benzodiazepine in small doses. Intravenous opioids are effective in suppressing cough reflexes, but the doses required impair spontaneous ventilation to the point of apnea. A combination of an intravenous opioid and a major tranquilizer (eg, neuroleptic analgesia) allows the patient to tolerate an endotracheal tube with much smaller doses of the opioid and less embarrassment of spontaneous ventilation. Small doses of opioids are also useful in obtunding airway reflexes during general anesthesia provided either by intravenous (eg, thiopental) or inhaled anesthetics (eg, isoflurane). Not only do the opioids obtund the cough reflex that results in closure of the larynx, but they also are useful in limiting the autonomic sympathetic response to endotracheal intubation that typically leads to hypertension and tachycardia.

Skeletal muscle relaxants are used most commonly in conjunction with a general anesthetic to allow manipulation of the head and jaw and prevent reflex closure of the larynx. Of course, they also render the patient apneic, and two procedures are used commonly to maintain oxygenation of the patient's blood. First, the patient breathes 100% oxygen by mask while still awake to eliminate nitrogen from the lungs, and then a rapid-sequence administration of an intravenous anesthetic (eg, thiopental) is followed immediately by a rapid-acting neuromuscular blocker [eg, succinylcholine or rocuronium], and cricoid pressure is applied (Sellick maneuver). As soon as the muscle relaxation is apparent (30 to 90 seconds), laryngoscopy is performed, an endotracheal tube is inserted, the tracheal tube cuff is inflated, and the position of the tube in the trachea is verified. Second, when there is minimal risk of pulmonary aspiration (eg, presumed empty stomach); the patient is anesthetized and paralyzed while ventilation is supported by intermittent positive pressure delivered via a face mask. At the appropriate time, laryngoscopy is performed, and the endotracheal tube is inserted.

Normalizing Pulmonary Function during Positive-Pressure Ventilation

Once an endotracheal tube is in place, it is common practice in the operating room to maintain general anesthesia and partial muscular paralysis in order to facilitate positive-pressure ventilation and continued toleration of the endotracheal tube by the patient. Postoperatively, in the post-anesthesia care unit (PACU) and intensive care unit (ICU), general anesthesia and partial muscular paralysis may be continued if prolonged positive-pressure ventilation is anticipated, or sedatives may be administered by intravenous infusion to allow toleration of the endotracheal tube in anticipation of recovery of spontaneous ventilation and tracheal extubation.

Three other problems are encountered in the patient whose ventilation is supported mechanically by an endotracheal tube: (1) poor ventilatory compliance; (2) bronchoconstriction; and (3) impaired gas exchange. Poor ventilatory compliance can reflect limited compliance of the chest wall and diaphragm, limited compliance of the lungs per se, or both. Deepening general anesthesia and administration of a skeletal muscle relaxant can be used to reduce intercostal and diaphragmatic muscle tone, but they obviously cannot improve the chest cavity compliance that is fixed by disease (eg, scoliosis or emphysema).

Poor lung compliance may reflect pulmonary interstitial edema, consolidation, bronchial obstruction (eg, mucus plugs), bronchoconstriction, or compression of the lung by intrathoracic substances (eg, pneumothorax, hemothorax, or tumor mass). Treatment of these involves drug therapy of heart failure and infection and procedures such as bronchoscopy, thoracentesis, etc.

Bronchoconstriction may exist chronically (eg, asthma or reactive airways disease), and these conditions can be exacerbated by the collection of tracheobronchial secretions in the presence of an endotracheal tube, which reduces the effectiveness of coughing in clearing the airway. Occasionally bronchoconstriction can be induced by mechanical stimulation of the airway by an endotracheal tube or other object in an otherwise normal patient. Drug treatment is focused on reducing bronchial smooth muscle tone (eg, $beta_2$ sympathomimetic or anticholinergic agents), minimizing tracheal bronchial secretions, and decreasing sensory input from the tracheal bronchial tree (eg, topical anesthetic, deeper general anesthesia, intravenous lidocaine, or an opioid). Acute treatment of bronchoconstriction may involve any combination of the following: (1) an aerosolized beta$_2$ sympathomimetic and/or anticholinergic agent; and (2) systemic intravenous administration of a beta$_2$ sympathomimetic agent, a phosphodiesterase inhibitor (eg, theophylline salts [aminophylline]), and/or an anticholinergic agent.

Intravenous steroids are indicated in severe bronchoconstriction, especially in asthmatic patients, for whom they have been effective in the past. With the administration of 100% oxygen, blood oxygenation usually is not the main problem in patients with bronchoconstriction; it is the progressive development of hypercarbia and the trapping of air in lung parenchyma that reduces ventilatory compliance and increase intrathoracic pressure. These, in turn, reduce venous return and may cause a tamponade-like impairment of cardiac function.

Impaired alveolar-capillary membrane gas exchange can result from alveolar pulmonary edema (treated by diuretics, inotropes, and vasodilators), decreased pulmonary perfusion (treated by inotropes and vasodilators), and lung consolidation (antibiotic therapy for infection).

Restoration of Spontaneous Ventilation and Airway Protective Mechanisms

The anesthesiologist attempts to tailor the anesthetic plan according to postoperative expectations for the patient. In the relatively healthy patient for whom tracheal extubation can be anticipated in the operating room, the goal is to have the patient breathing spontaneously with airway reflexes intact and the patient arousable to command immediately on completion of the operation. The challenge for the anesthesiologist is to maintain satisfactory general anesthesia through the entire course of the operation and yet have the patient sufficiently recovered from anesthetic drugs, including hypnotics and opioids, shortly after conclusion of the operation. If this is not possible, then the patient is transferred to the PACU to allow additional time for elimination of drugs that depress spontaneous ventilation and cough reflexes. Another possibility is to administer antagonists to opioids (eg, naloxone) and benzodiazepines (eg, flumazenil), but this approach risks sudden awakening, pain, and uncontrolled autonomic sympathetic activity leading to undesirable hemodynamic changes. And there is the risk of recurrent ventilatory depression because it is difficult to match the doses of the antagonists to the residual amounts of anesthetic drugs. On the other hand, it is fairly routine for the effects of neuromuscular blockers to be antagonized by administration of an anticholinesterase (eg, neostigmine) in combination with an anticholinergic agent (eg, atropine) to limit the autonomic cholinergic side effects of the anticholinesterase.

When the expectation is for maintenance of mechanical ventilation for some time in the postoperative period, then the patient's tolerance of the endotracheal tube is facilitated by the persistent effect of residual anesthetic drugs subsequently supplemented by administration of intravenous hypnotics (eg, propofol) and opioids (eg, fentanyl or morphine). These agents can be associated with side effects, including respiratory depression, especially when they are used concurrently. Dexmedetomidine (Precedex), an alpha$_2$-adrenergic agonist, may offer advantages for sedation during weaning from mechanical ventilation because it provides sedation, pain relief, anxiety reduction, stable respiratory rates, and predictable cardiovascular responses. Dexmedetomidine facilitates patient comfort, compliance, and comprehension by offering sedation with the ability to rouse patients. This "arousability" allows patients to remain sedated yet communicate with health-care workers.

When the appropriate time comes to have the patient take over his or her own ventilation completely, these sedative and analgesic drugs are weaned to a level allowing satisfactory maintenance of blood oxygenation and carbon dioxide removal, easy arousal of the patient, and at least partial restoration of airway reflex mechanisms.

Pharmacology Related to Airway and Lung Management

Cardiac surgical patients are usually kept intubated and ventilated at the end of surgery, and ventilator support is withdrawn in the intensive care unit. Sedative drugs are required to facilitate this transfer from operating room to intensive care, and while the patient is ventilated. Some patients require continued ventilation because of primary pulmonary disease, underlying cardiac disease and/or perioperative complications. Others may require medications to treat bronchospasm or airway obstruction, or to facilitate re-intubation if they develop respiratory failure once extubated.

Sedative Medications to Facilitate Mechanical Ventilation

Propofol

The medications used in cardiac surgery patients are the same as those used in other mechanically ventilated patients. A common approach is to use propofol, an intravenous anesthetic/sedative agent that is rapidly eliminated by the liver and therefore facilitates rapid awakening. This drug is not water soluble so is supplied in a lipid emulsion; for short-term infusions (less than a day or two) lipid accumulation is not an issue, but triglyceride levels should be measured if the drug is given in high doses, especially at the same time as intravenous feeding. The hemodynamic effects of propofol are mostly a result of vasodilation, both arterial and venous, as well as the usual "withdrawal of sympathetic tone," which occurs when anxious, stressed patients are sedated. In addition there is a mild bradycardia and blunted heart rate response to hypotension, and a mild negative inotropic effect usually not relevant at clinical doses. The clinical dose range for sedation is 25 to 75 ug/kg per minute.

Benzodiazepines

Benzodiazepines are also used to facilitate mechanical ventilation, commonly midazolam (Versed) or lorazepam (Ativan). These drugs do not have the vasodilating effects of propofol, are good amnestic agents, but have a major disadvantage in that awakening is less predictable and more often prolonged, especially with lorazepam. In addition, these drugs appear to be more associated with postoperative delirium than other sedative drugs. Despite these problems, benzodiazepines are useful in the sedation of severely hypotensive patients requiring vasoconstrictor support. They have minimal if any direct cardiovascular effects, but withdrawal of sympathetic tone can lead to hypotension. Midazolam is usually administered as a continuous infusion of 1 to 4 mg/h, while lorazepam is most often given by intermittent dosing of 1 to 2 mg every 4 to 6 hours.

Dexmedetomidine

A relatively new addition to the sedative drug family is dexmedetomidine (Precedex), a centrally acting alpha$_2$ agonist. This drug is the same class as clonidine, but has a much greater affinity for the alpha receptor. Not surprisingly, the most common hemodynamic effect, which sometimes limits its use, is bradycardia and hypotension. This drug can be used as a single agent to facilitate transfer from the OR to the ICU and the period of ventilator weaning and extubation. The major advantage of dexmedetomidine is that it does not affect ventilatory drive and patients can usually be aroused while receiving the drug. It also has a significant analgesic component, different from propofol or the benzodiazepines. The usual infusion rate of dexmedetomidine is 0.2 to 0.7 ug/kg per hour, preceded by a loading dose of 1 ug/kg over 20 to 30 minutes. The loading dose can be reduced or not given if hemodynamics warrant.

Opioids

The main reason patients need sedation during mechanical ventilation is to tolerate the presence of a transoral tracheal tube. In addition to general discomfort, there is continuous airway stimulation by the foreign object. To blunt airway reflexes as well as to treat postoperative pain, it is useful to add an opioid drug to whichever sedative agent the patient is receiving. For early postoperative awakening (ie, in the first hours) this is less of an issue as there is usually residual opioid effect from drugs given intraoperatively; however, patients will need additional opioid as they awaken and experience pain. For patients ventilated overnight or longer, use of opioid drugs will have these same benefits and likely result in a reduced need for the sedative drug. Fentanyl is a commonly used drug in this setting, partly because it has a rapid onset of action and relatively rapid recovery if dosing is not prolonged. Infusions of 1 to 4 ug/kg per hour are used. Alternatively intermittent dosing with 1 to 4 mg of morphine or 0.5- to 1-mg hydromorphone (Dilaudid) every 1 to 4 hours may be employed.

Medications Used to Facilitate Urgent Tracheal Intubation

Patients in extremis (eg, during cardiac or respiratory arrest) rarely require medications to facilitate intubation. In decompensating patients who are fully or partially conscious, challenges may include agitation, resistance to opening the mouth, and/or closed vocal cords when intubation is attempted. In some patients small doses of sedative/opioid medications with a rapid onset such as midazolam and fentanyl, respectively, are adequate; in others an anesthetic induction agent such as propofol or etomidate can be used, with or without a paralytic drug. The disadvantage to propofol is hypotension caused by vasodilation, as referred to in the preceding. This drug should be used in incremental doses, 10 to 20 mg at time, until a dose of 1 to 2 mg/kg has been given. Etomidate has no direct cardiovascular effects and is usually given in a dose of 0.15 to 0.3 mg/kg. This drug has an unusual side effect of impairing steroid synthesis and has been associated with adrenal insufficiency in critically ill patients when given by infusion. In addition, many patients experience unusual movements as this drug is administered. In general, the use of paralytic drugs is discouraged unless there is an anesthesiology provider or someone skilled in the use of these drugs and airway management present.

Succinylcholine is the most rapidly acting paralytic agent with an onset of 30 to 60 seconds, and is given in a dose of 1 mg/kg. This depolarizing agent causes potassium release and must be avoided in hyperkalemic patients. It causes stimulation of muscarinic and nicotinic receptors, an increase in serum catecholamines, and many different, usually mild dysrhythmias have been reported. Alternatively, rocuronium in a dose of 0.5 mg/kg can be given, but 60 to 90 seconds are required for adequate paralysis. Rocuronium in this dose has no cardiovascular effect. If an anesthetic induction agent and/or paralytic drug are being considered, an important issue is the possibility of aspiration of stomach contents. In an urgent situation the risk of this is reduced if the drugs are administered in rapid sequence with an assistant providing cricoid pressure (to occlude the esophagus), and manual ventilation is minimized until the tube is in place.

Drugs to Treat Airway Pathology: Stridor/Edema, Bronchospasm, Secretions

Fluid overload, prolonged positioning with the head dependent, or superior vena cava obstruction may all lead to edema of the upper airway. Alternatively, trauma from intubation or other devices in the oropharynx (eg, TEE probe) may cause glottis edema. There may be edema below the cords resulting from presence of the endotracheal tube/cuff. The common treatments for airway narrowing resulting from edema are: (1) use of a mixture of helium/oxygen; (2) inhaled racemic epinephrine; (3) diuretics and head-up position; and (4) a brief course of dexamethasone (IV).

Helium/Oxygen. Helium with oxygen (Heliox) is supplied as an 80%:20% mix. Helium is less dense than nitrogen, facilitating laminar rather than turbulent flow through a narrowed airway. If a patient can not tolerate the relatively low concentration of oxygen (20%), then additional oxygen will need to be administered. Although the greatest benefit is provided by 80% helium, concentrations of 40 to 50% provide some benefit.

Racemic Epinephrine. Racemic epinephrine is supplied as 1% solution and administered through an aerosol mask in a dose of 2.5 mL to cause vasoconstriction and reduced airway edema. Absorption of epinephrine can cause tachycardia and hypertension.

Diuretics and Dexamethasone. Specific diuretic drugs are discussed in the preceding; when a rapid effect is desired then

TABLE 4-7 Inhaled Bronchodilators and Mucolytics

	Drug	Mechanism	Dosage	Frequency
Bronchodilators	Albuterol	$Beta_2$ agonist	2.5 mg/3 mL	Q 4–6 h*
	Levalbuterol	$Beta_2$ agonist	0.63–1.25 mg/3 mL	Q 6 h
	Ipratropium	Anticholinergic	0.5 mg/3 mL	Q 4–6 h
Mucolytic	Dornase alpha	cleaves DNA	2.5 mg/3 cc	Q 12 h

*May be given more frequently.

usually a loop diuretic such as furosemide is employed. Although this may not specifically treat airway edema, the combination of elevated head and diuresis will reduce edema in the upper body. Dexamethasone is used as part of the "steroids for anything that swells" philosophy. There is little evidence of efficacy of corticosteroids in this setting; dexamethasone is used to avoid the mineralocorticoid effect of other potent intravenous steroid preparations. The usual dose is 8 mg followed by 4 mg every 6 hours for four to eight doses.

Bronchodilators and Mucolytics. A summary of bronchodilator and mucolytic drugs is given in Table 4-7. In the cardiac surgical patient, wheezing is more likely because of fluid overload or left ventricular failure than primary bronchospastic disease, but inhaled bronchodilators may give some relief while treatment of the primary disorder is being instituted (eg, diuresis or administration of an inotropic drug). In order of preference, inhaled beta agonists, anticholinergic agents, and intravenous steroids are used.[137] All three may be indicated. Beta agonists relax smooth muscle in the airways and usually have the most rapid therapeutic effect. In the acute setting aerosolized drug via a facemask is more effective than metered-dose inhalers. It should be noted that management of chronic asthma focuses on inhaled anti-inflammatory agents, but these drugs are not helpful in the acute setting such as postoperatively. The presence of tenacious secretions should prompt consideration of an inhaled mucolytic such as dornase/DNAse (Pulmozyme). N-acetylcysteine (Mucomyst) is another mucolytic but may cause airway irritation so should not be given in the setting of acute bronchospasm. See the table for dosages of these drugs (see Table 4-7).

REFERENCES

1. Lynch C III: Cellular electrophysiology of the heart, in Lynch C III (ed): *Cellular Cardiac Electrophysiology: Perioperative Considerations.* Philadelphia, Lippincott, 1994; p 1.
2. Katz AM: Cardiac ion channels. *NEJM* 1993; 328:1244.
3. Colucci WS, Wright RF, Braunwald E: New positive inotropic agents in the treatment of heart failure, part I. *NEJM* 1986; 314:290.
4. Colucci WS, Wright RF, Braunwald E: New positive inotropic agents in the treatment of heart failure, part II. *NEJM* 1986; 314:349.
5. Terzic A, Puceat M, Vassort G, Vogel SM: Cardiac $alpha_1$ adrenoreceptors: an overview. *Pharmacol Rev* 1993; 45:147.
6. Berridge MJ: Inositol lipids and calcium signaling. *Proc R Soc Lond (Biol)* 1988; 234:359.
7. Lucchesi BR: Role of calcium on excitation-coupling in cardiac and vascular smooth muscle. *Circulation* 1978; 8:IV-1.
8. Kukovertz WR, Poch G, Holzmann S: Cyclic nucleotides and relaxation of vascular smooth muscle, in Vanhoutte PM, Leusen I (eds): *Vasodilation.* New York, Raven Press, 1981; p 339.
9. Singh BN, Sarma JS: Mechanisms of action of antiarrhythmic drugs relative to the origin and perpetuation of cardiac arrhythmias. *J Cardiovasc Pharmacol Ther* 2001; 6:69.
10. Pinter A, Dorian P: Intravenous antiarrhythmic agents. *Curr Opin Cardiol* 2001; 16:17.
11. Roden DM: Antiarrhythmic drugs: from mechanisms to clinical practice. *Heart* 2000; 84:339.
12. Vaughan Williams EM: A classification of antiarrhythmic agents reassessed after a decade of new drugs. *J Clin Pharmacol* 1984; 24:129.
13. The Task Force of the Working Group on Arrhythmias of the European Society of Cardiology: The "Sicilian gambit": a new approach to the classification of antiarrhythmic drugs based on their actions on arrhythmic mechanisms. *Eur Heart J* 1991; 12:1112.
14. Hondeghem LM: Antiarrhythmic agents: modulated receptor applications. *Circulation* 1987; 75:514.
15. Zipes DP, Camm AJ, Borggrefe M, et al: ACC/AHA/ESC 2006 Guidelines for Management of Patients With Ventricular Arrhythmias and the Prevention of Sudden Cardiac Death: a report of the American College of Cardiology/American Heart Association Task Force and the European Society of Cardiology Committee for Practice Guidelines (writing committee to develop Guidelines for Management of Patients With Ventricular Arrhythmias and the Prevention of Sudden Cardiac Death): developed in collaboration with the European Heart Rhythm Association and the Heart Rhythm Society. *Circulation* 2006; 114:e385.
16. Hoffman BF, Rosen MR, Wit AL: Electrophysiology and pharmacology of cardiac arrhythmias: VII. Cardiac effects of quinidine and procainamide. *Am Heart J* 1975; 90:117.
17. Giardenia EG, Heissenbuttel RH, Bigger JT Jr: Intermittent intravenous procaine amide to treat ventricular arrhythmias: correlation of plasma concentration with effect on arrhythmia, electrocardiogram, and blood pressure. *Ann Intern Med* 1973; 78:183.
18. Stiell IG, Wells GA, Field B, et al: Advanced cardiac life support in out-of-hospital cardiac arrest. *NEJM* 2004; 351:647.
19. The 2005 American Heart Association Guidelines for Cardiopulmonary Resuscitation and Emergency Cardiovascular Care. *Circulation* 2005; 112:IV1-203.
20. Cardiac Arrhythmia Suppression Trial (CAST) Investigators: Preliminary report, effect of encainide and flecainide on mortality in a randomized trial of arrhythmia suppression after myocardial infarction. *NEJM* 1989; 321:406.
21. Echt DS, Liebson PR, Mitchell LB, et al: Mortality and morbidity in patients receiving encainide, flecainide or placebo: The Cardiac Arrhythmia Suppression Trial. *NEJM* 1991; 324:781.
22. Escande D, Henry P: Potassium channels as pharmacologic targets in cardiovascular medicine. *Eur Heart J* 1993; 14:2.
23. Singh BN: Arrhythmia control by prolonging repolarization: the concept and its potential therapeutic impact. *Eur Heart J* 1993; 14:14.
24. Kudenchuk PJ: Advanced cardiac life support antiarrhythmic drugs. *Cardiol Clin* 2002; 20:79.
25. Balser JR: Perioperative arrhythmias: incidence, risk assessment, evaluation, and management. *Card Electrophysiol Rev* 2002; 6:96.
26. Mahmarian JJ, Verani MS, Pratt CM: Hemodynamic effects of intravenous and oral sotalol. *Am J Cardiol* 1990; 65:28A.
27. Levy JH, Huraux C, Nordlander M: Treatment of perioperative hypertension, in Epstein M (ed): *Calcium Antagonists in Clinical Medicine.* Philadelphia, Hanley and Belfus, 1997; p 345.

28. Conti VR, Ware DL: Cardiac arrhythmias in cardiothoracic surgery. *Chest Surg Clin North Am* 2002; 12:439.
29. Waxman HL, Myerburg RJ, Appel R, Sung RJ: Verapamil for control of ventricular rate in paroxysmal supraventricular tachycardia and atrial fibrillation or flutter: a double-blind randomized cross-over study. *Ann Intern Med* 1981; 94:1.
30. Salerno DM, Dias VC, Kleiger RE, et al: Efficacy and safety of intravenous diltiazem for treatment of atrial fibrillation and atrial flutter: the Diltiazem-Atrial Fibrillation/Flutter Study Group. *Am J Cardiol* 1989; 63:1046.
31. Ellenbogen KA, Dias VC, Plumb VJ, et al: A placebo-controlled trial of continuous intravenous diltiazem infusion for 24-hour heart rate control during atrial fibrillation and atrial flutter: a multi-center study. *J Am Coll Cardiol* 1991; 18:891.
32. Smith TW, Antman EM, Friedman PL, et al: Digitalis glycosides: mechanisms and manifestations of toxicity, part I. *Prog Cardiovasc Dis* 1984; 26:413.
33. DiMarco JP, Sellers TD, Berne RM, et al: Adenosine: electrophysiological effects and therapeutic use for terminating paroxysmal supraventricular tachycardia. *Circulation* 1983; 68:1254.
34. Hollifield JW: Potassium and magnesium abnormalities: diuretics and arrhythmias in hypertension. *Am J Med* 1984; 77:28.
35. England MR, Gordon G, Salem M, Chernow B: Magnesium administration and dysrhythmia after cardiac surgery: a placebo-controlled, double-blind, randomized trial. *JAMA* 1992; 268:2395.
36. Singh BN, Vaughan Williams EM: The effect of amiodarone, a new antianginal drug, on cardiac muscle. *Br J Pharmacol* 1970; 39:657.
37. Connolly SJ: Evidence-based analysis of amiodarone efficacy and safety. *Circulation* 1999; 100:2025.
38. Chow MS: Intravenous amiodarone: pharmacology, pharmacokinetics, and clinical use. *Ann Pharmacother* 1996; 30:637.
39. Mitchell LB, Wyse G, Gillis AM, Duff HJ: Electropharmacology of amiodarone therapy initiation. *Circulation* 1989; 80:34.
40. Holt DW, Tucker GT, Jackson PR, Storey GCA: Amiodarone pharmacokinetics. *Am Heart J* 1983; 106:840.
41. Fogoros RN, Anderson KP, Winkle RA, et al: Amiodarone: clinical efficacy and toxicity in 96 patients with recurrent, drug-refractory arrhythmias. *Circulation* 1983; 68:88.
42. Kowey PR, Levine JH, Herre JM, et al: Randomized, double-blind comparison of intravenous amiodarone and bretylium in the treatment of patients with recurrent, hemodynamically destabilizing ventricular tachycardia or fibrillation. *Circulation* 1995; 92:3255.
43. Kudenchuk PJ, Cobb LA, Copass MK, et al: Amiodarone for resuscitation after out-of-hospital cardiac arrest due to ventricular fibrillation. *NEJM* 1999; 341:871.
44. Levine JH, Massumi A, Scheinman MM, et al: Intravenous amiodarone for recurrent sustained hypotensive ventricular tachyarrhythmias. Intravenous Amiodarone Multicenter Trial Group. *J Am Coll Cardiol* 1996; 27:67.
45. Morady F, Sauve MJ, Malone P, et al: Long-term efficacy and toxicity of high-dose amiodarone therapy for ventricular tachycardia or ventricular fibrillation. *Am J Cardiol* 1983; 52:975.
46. Scheinman MM, Levine JH, Cannom DS, et al: Dose-ranging study of intravenous amiodarone in patients with life-threatening ventricular tachyarrhythmias. *Circulation* 1995; 92:3264.
47. Scheinman MM, Winkle RA, Platia EV, et al: Intravenous amiodarone for recurrent sustained hypotensive ventricular tachyarrhythmias. *J Am Coll Cardiol* 1996; 27:67.
48. Dorian P, Cass D, Schwartz B, et al: Amiodarone as compared with lidocaine for shock-resistant ventricular fibrillation. *NEJM* 2002; 346:884.
49. Kupferschmid JP, Rosengart TK, McIntosh CL, et al: Amiodarone-induced complications after cardiac operation for obstructive hypertrophic cardiomyopathy. *Ann Thorac Surg* 1989; 48:359.
50. Rady MY, Ryan T, Starr NJ: Preoperative therapy with amiodarone and the incidence of acute organ dysfunction after cardiac surgery. *Anesth Analg* 1997; 85:489.
51. Daoud EG, Strickberger SA, Man KC, et al: Preoperative amiodarone as prophylaxis against atrial fibrillation after heart surgery. *NEJM* 1997; 337:1785.
52. Dorge H, Schoendube FA, Schoberer M, et al: Intraoperative amiodarone as prophylaxis against atrial fibrillation after coronary operations. *Ann Thorac Surg* 2000; 69:1358.
53. Giri S, White CM, Dunn AB, et al: Oral amiodarone for prevention of atrial fibrillation after open-heart surgery, the Atrial Fibrillation Suppression Trial (AFIST): a randomised, placebo-controlled trial. *Lancet* 2001; 357:830.
54. Guarnieri T, Nolan S, Gottlieb SO, et al: Intravenous amiodarone for the prevention of atrial fibrillation after open-heart surgery: The Amiodarone Reduction in Coronary Heart (ARCH) trial. *J Am Coll Cardiol* 1999; 34:343.
55. Lee SH, Chang CM, Lu MJ, et al: Intravenous amiodarone for prevention of atrial fibrillation after coronary artery bypass grafting. *Ann Thorac Surg* 2000; 70:157.
56. Carlson MD: How to manage atrial fibrillation: an update on recent clinical trials. *Cardiol Rev* 2001; 9:60.
57. Fuster V, Ryden LE, Asinger RN, et al: ACC/AHA/ESC guidelines for the management of patients with atrial fibrillation: executive summary. *Circulation* 2001; 104:2118.
58. Maisel WH, Rawn JD, Stevenson WG: Atrial fibrillation after cardiac surgery. *Ann Intern Med* 2001; 135:1061.
59. Hogue CW Jr, Hyder ML: Atrial fibrillation after cardiac operation: risks, mechanisms, and treatment. *Ann Thorac Surg* 2000; 69:300.
60. Reddy P, Richerson M, Freeman-Bosco L, et al: Cost-effectiveness of amiodarone for prophylaxis of atrial fibrillation in coronary artery bypass surgery. *Am J Health Syst Pharm* 1999; 56:2211.
61. Reiffel JA: Drug choices in the treatment of atrial fibrillation. *Am J Cardiol* 2000; 85:12D.
62. Daoud EG, Strickberger SA, Man KC, et al: Preoperative amiodarone as prophylaxis against atrial fibrillation after heart surgery. *NEJM* 1997; 337:1785.
63. Gray R, Maddahi J, Berman D, et al: Scintigraphic and hemodynamic demonstration of transient left ventricular dysfunction immediately after uncomplicated coronary artery bypass grafting. *J Thorac Cardiovasc Surg* 1979; 77:504.
64. Mangano DT: Biventricular function after myocardial revascularization in humans: deterioration and recovery patterns during the first 24 hours. *Anesthesiology* 1985; 62:571.
65. Breisblatt WM, Stein K, Wolfe CJ, et al: Acute myocardial dysfunction and recovery: a common occurrence after coronary bypass surgery. *J Am Coll Cardiol* 1990; 15:1261.
66. Fabiato A, Fabiato F: Calcium and cardiac excitation-contraction coupling. *Ann Rev Physiol* 1979; 41:473.
67. Figgitt DP, Gillies PS, Goa KL: Levosimendan. *Drugs* 2001; 61:613.
68. Doggrell SA, Brown L: Present and future pharmacotherapy for heart failure. *Exp Opin Pharmacother* 2002; 3:915.
69. Endoh M: Mechanism of action of Ca^2 sensitizers—update 2001. *Cardiovasc Drugs Ther* 2001; 15:397.
70. Drop LJ, Geffin GA, O'Keefe DD, et al: Relation between ionized calcium concentration and ventricular pump performance in the dog under hemodynamically controlled conditions. *Am J Cardiol* 1981; 47:1041.
71. Zaloga GP, Strickland RA, Butterworth JF, et al: Calcium attenuates epinephrine's β-adrenergic effects in postoperative heart surgery patients. *Circulation* 1990; 81:196.
72. Engelman RM, Hadji-Rousou I, Breyer RH, et al: Rebound vasospasm after coronary revascularization in association with calcium antagonist withdrawal. *Ann Thorac Surg* 1984; 37:469.
73. Cheung JY, Bonventre JV, Malis CD, Leaf A: Calcium and ischemic injury. *NEJM* 1986; 314:1670.
74. Del Monte F, Kaumann AJ, Poole-Wilson PA, et al: Coexistence of functioning β_1 and β_2-adrenoreceptors in single myocytes from human ventricle. *Circulation* 1993; 88:854.
75. Bristow MR, Ginsburg R, Minobe W, et al: Decreased catecholamine sensitivity and β-adrenergic receptor density in failing human hearts. *NEJM* 1982; 307:205.
76. Schwinn DA, Leone BJ, Spahn DR, et al: Desensitization of myocardial β-adrenergic receptors during cardiopulmonary bypass: evidence for early uncoupling and late down-regulation. *Circulation* 1991; 84:2559.
77. Port JD, Gilbert EM, Larabee P, et al: Neurotransmitter depletion compromises the ability of indirect acting amines to provide inotropic support in the failing human heart. *Circulation* 1990; 81:929.
78. Goenen M, Pedemonte O, Baele P, Col J: Amrinone in the management of low cardiac output after open-heart surgery. *Am J Cardiol* 1985; 56:33B.
79. Robinson RJS, Tchervenkov C: Treatment of low cardiac output after aortocoronary surgery using a combination of norepinephrine and amrinone. *J Cardiothorac Anesth* 1987; 3:229.
80. Prielipp RC, Butterworth JF 4th, Zaloga GP, et al: Effects of amrinone on cardiac index, venous oxygen saturation and venous admixture in patients recovering from cardiac surgery. *Chest* 1991; 99:820.
81. Levy JH, Bailey JM: Amrinone: its effects on vascular resistance and capacitance in human subjects. *Chest* 1994; 105:62.
82. Levy JH, Bailey JM, Deeb GM: Intravenous milrinone in cardiac surgery. *Ann Thorac Surg* 2002; 73:325.
83. Bailey JM, Levy JH, Rogers G, et al: Pharmacokinetics of amrinone during cardiac surgery. *Anesthesiology* 1991; 75:961.
84. Bailey JM, Levy JH, Kikura M, et al: Pharmacokinetics of intravenous milrinone in patients undergoing cardiac surgery. *Anesthesiology* 1994; 81:616.

85. Feneck RO: Effects of variable dose in patients with low cardiac output after cardiac surgery. European Multicenter Trial Group. *Am Heart J* 1991; 121:1995.
86. Kikura M, Levy JH, Michelsen LG, et al: The effect of milrinone on hemodynamics and left ventricular function after emergence from cardiopulmonary bypass. *Anesth Analg* 1997; 85:16.
87. Butterworth JF 4th, Hines RL, Royster RL, James RL: A pharmacokinetic and pharmacodynamic evaluation of milrinone in adults undergoing cardiac surgery. *Anesth Analg* 1995; 81:783.
88. Doolan LA, Jones EF, Kalman J, et al: A placebo-controlled trial verifying the efficacy of milrinone in weaning high-risk patients from cardiopulmonary bypass. *J Cardiothorac Vasc Anesth* 1997; 11:37.
89. Follath F, Cleland JG, Just H, et al: Efficacy and safety of intravenous levosimendan compared with dobutamine in severe low-output heart failure (the LIDO study): a randomised double-blind trial. *Lancet* 2002; 360:196.
90. Slawsky MT, Colucci WS, Gottlieb SS, et al: Acute hemodynamic and clinical effects of levosimendan in patients with severe heart failure. *Circulation* 2000; 102:2222.
91. Steen H, Tinker JH, Pluth JR, et al: Efficacy of dopamine, dobutamine, and epinephrine during emergence from cardiopulmonary bypass in man. *Circulation* 1978; 57:378.
92. Salomon NW, Plachetka JR, Copeland JG: Comparison of dopamine and dobutamine following coronary artery bypass grafting. *Ann Thorac Surg* 1981; 3:48.
93. Fowler MB, Alderman EL, Oesterle SN, et al: Dobutamine and dopamine after cardiac surgery: greater augmentation of myocardial blood flow with dobutamine. *Circulation* 1984; 70:1103.
94. Sethna DH, Gray RJ, Moffit EA, et al: Dobutamine and cardiac oxygen balance in patients following myocardial revascularization. *Anesth Analg* 1982; 61:917.
95. Butterworth JF 4th, Prielipp RC, Royster RL, et al: Dobutamine increases heart rate more than epinephrine in patients recovering from aortocoronary bypass surgery. *J Cardiothorac Vasc Anesth* 1992; 6:535.
96. Feneck RO, Sherry KM, Withington S, et al: Comparison of the hemodynamic effects of milrinone with dobutamine in patients after cardiac surgery. *J Cardiothorac Vasc Anesth* 2001; 15:306.
97. Meier-Hellmann A, Reinhart K, Bredle DL, et al: Epinephrine impairs splanchnic perfusion in septic shock. *Crit Care Med* 1997; 25:399.
98. Levy B, Bollaert PE, Charpentier C, et al: Comparison of norepinephrine and dobutamine to epinephrine for hemodynamics, lactate metabolism, and gastric tonometric variables in septic shock: a prospective, randomized study. *Intensive Care Med* 1997; 23:282.
99. Ruokonen E, Takala J, Kari A, et al: Regional blood flow and oxygen transport in septic shock. *Crit Care Med* 1993; 21:1296.
100. Meier-Hellmann A, Bredle DL, Specht M, et al: The effects of low-dose dopamine on splanchnic blood flow and oxygen utilization in patients with septic shock. *Intensive Care Med* 1997; 23:31.
101. Marik PE, Mohedin M: The contrasting effects of dopamine and norepinephrine on systemic and splanchnic oxygen utilization in hyperdynamic sepsis. *JAMA* 1994; 272:1354.
102. Landry DW, Oliver JA: The pathogenesis of vasodilatory shock. *NEJM* 2001; 345:588.
103. Levy JH: *Anaphylactic Reactions in Anesthesia and Intensive Care,* 2nd ed. Boston, Butterworth-Heinemann, 1992.
104. Desjars P, Pinaud M, Potel G, et al: A reappraisal of norepinephrine in human septic shock. *Crit Care Med* 1987; 15:134.
105. Meadows D, Edwards JD, Wilkins RG, Nightingale P: Reversal of intractable septic shock with norepinephrine therapy. *Crit Care Med* 1998; 16:663.
106. Hesselvik JF, Broden B: Low dose norepinephrine in patient with septic shock and oliguria: effects on afterload, urine flow, and oxygen transport. *Crit Care Med* 1989; 17:179.
107. Martin C, Eon B, Saux P, et al: Renal effects of norepinephrine used to treat septic shock patients. *Crit Care Med* 1990; 18:282.
108. Marik PE, Mohedin M: The contrasting effects of dopamine and norepinephrine on systemic and splanchnic oxygen utilization in hyperdynamic sepsis. *JAMA* 1994; 272:1354.
109. Argenziano M, Chen JM, Choudhri AF, et al: Management of vasodilatory shock after cardiac surgery: identification of predisposing factors and use of a novel pressor agent. *J Thorac Cardiovasc Surg* 1998; 116:973.
110. Landry DW, Levin HR, Gallant EM, et al: Vasopressin deficiency in vasodilatory septic shock. *Crit Care Med* 1997; 25:1279.
111. Gold JA, Cullinane S, Chen J, et al: Vasopressin as an alternative to norepinephrine in the treatment of milrinone-induced hypotension. *Crit Care Med* 2000; 28:249.
112. Levy JH: The ideal agent for perioperative hypertension. *Acta Anaesth Scand* 1993; 37:20.
113. Huraux C, Makita T, Montes F, Szlam F: A comparative evaluation of the effects of multiple vasodilators on human internal mammary artery. *Anesthesiology* 1998; 88:1654.
114. Harrison DG, Bates JN: The nitrovasodilators: new ideas about old drugs. *Circulation* 1993; 87:1461.
115. Anderson TJ, Meredith IT, Ganz P, et al: Nitric oxide and nitrovasodilators: similarities, differences and potential interactions. *J Am Coll Cardiol* 1994; 24:555.
116. Harrison DG, Kurz MA, Quillen JE, et al: Normal and pathophysiologic considerations of endothelial regulation of vascular tone and their relevance to nitrate therapy. *Am J Cardiol* 1992; 70:11B.
117. Munzel T, Giaid A, Kurz S, Harrison DG: Evidence for a role of endothelin 1 and protein kinase C in nitrate tolerance. *Proc Natl Acad Sci USA* 1995; 92:5244.
118. Munzel T, Sayegh H, Freeman, Harrison DG: Evidence for enhanced vascular superoxide anion production in tolerance: a novel mechanism underlying tolerance and cross-tolerance. *J Clin Invest* 1995; 95:187.
119. Fleckenstein A: Specific pharmacology of calcium in the myocardium, cardiac pacemakers and vascular smooth muscle. *Annu Rev Pharmacol* 1977; 17:149.
120. Begon C, Dartayet B, Edouard A, et al: Intravenous nicardipine for treatment of intraoperative hypertension during abdominal surgery. *J Cardiothorac Anesth* 1989; 3:707.
121. Cheung DG, Gasster JL, Neutel JM, Weber MA: Acute pharmacokinetic and hemodynamic effects of intravenous bolus dosing of nicardipine. *Am Heart J* 1990; 119:438.
122. David D, Dubois C, Loria Y: Comparison of nicardipine and sodium nitroprusside in the treatment of paroxysmal hypertension following aortocoronary bypass surgery. *J Cardiothorac Vasc Anesth* 1991; 5:357.
123. Lambert CR, Grady T, Hashimi W, et al: Hemodynamic and angiographic comparison of intravenous nitroglycerin and nicardipine mainly in subjects without coronary artery disease. *Am J Cardiol* 1993; 71:420.
124. Singh BN, Josephson MA: Clinical pharmacology, pharmacokinetics, and hemodynamic effects of nicardipine. *Am Heart J* 1990; 119:427A.
125. Leslie J, Brister N, Levy JH, et al: Treatment of postoperative hypertension after coronary artery bypass surgery: double-blind comparison of intravenous isradipine and sodium nitroprusside. *Circulation*1994; 90:II256.
126. Huraux C, Makita T, Montes F, et al: A comparative evaluation of the effects of multiple vasodilators on human internal mammary artery. *Anesthesiology* 1998; 88:1654.
127. Dzau VJ, Sasamura H, Hein L: Heterogeneity of angiotensin synthetic pathways and receptor subtypes: physiological and pharmacological implications. *J Hypertens* 1993; 11:S13.
128. Granger CB, Ertl G, Kuch J, et al: Randomized trial of candesartan cilexetil in the treatment of patients with congestive heart failure and a history of intolerance to angiotensin-converting enzyme inhibitors. *Am Heart J* 2000; 139:609.
129. Lefkowitz RH, Hoffman BB, Taylor P: Neurotransmission: The autonomic and somatic motor nervous system, in Hardman JL, Molinoff PB, Ruddon RW, Gilman AG (eds): *The Pharmacological Basis of Therapeutics.* New York, McGraw-Hill, 1996; p 110.
130. Fleisher LA, Beckman JA, Brown KA, et al: 2009 ACCF/AHA focused update on perioperative beta blockade incorporated into the ACC/AHA 2007 guidelines on perioperative cardiovascular evaluation and care for noncardiac surgery: a report of the American college of cardiology foundation/American Heart Association task force on practice guidelines. *Circulation* 2009; 120:e169-276.
131. Antiarry review bizarre.
132. Volpe M, Tocci G: 2007 ESH/ESC Guidelines for the management of hypertension, from theory to practice: global cardiovascular risk concept. *J Hypertens* 2009; 27(Suppl 3):S3.
133. Moser M: From JNC I to JNC 7—what have we learned? *Prog Cardiovasc Dis* 2006; 48:303-315
134 8. Eisenberg DM, Davis RB, Ettner SL, et al: Trends in alternative medicine use in the United States, 1990–1997: results of a follow-up national survey. *JAMA* 1998; 280:1569.
135 9. Ang-Lee MK, Moss J, Yuan CS: Herbal medicines and perioperative care. *JAMA* 2001; 286:208.
136. American Society of Anesthesiologists: *What You Should Know About Your Patients' Use of Herbal Medicines.* Available at: www.asahq.org/ ProfInfo/ herb/herbbro.html.
137. National Heart Blood and Lung Institute, Expert Panel Report 3 (EPR3): *Guidelines for the Diagnosis and Management of Asthma.* http://www.nhlbi.nih.gov/guidelines/asthma/gdln.htm; 2007, pp 248-249.

CHAPTER 5

Cardiovascular Pathology

Frederick J. Schoen
Robert F. Padera

INTRODUCTION

In the past several decades, cardiovascular pathology has been launched into the forefront of high-quality patient care as a direct result of the virtual explosion in the number and scope of cardiovascular surgical and interventional diagnostic and therapeutic procedures and devices. Cardiovascular pathology informs the practice of cardiovascular surgery and medicine through defining the pathologic anatomy in individual patients and patient cohorts, and in developing and testing procedures and prosthetic devices that facilitate evidence-based choices among surgical or catheter-based interventional options and optimize short- and long-term patient management. Importantly, beyond implicit clinical benefit for individual patients, the discipline of cardiovascular pathology is a cornerstone of modern cardiovascular research and the preclinical development and clinical implementation of innovative drugs, devices, and other therapeutic options.

This chapter summarizes pathologic considerations most relevant to surgery and catheter-based interventions used to diagnose and treat the major forms of acquired cardiovascular disease. It emphasizes pathologic anatomy, clinico-pathologic correlations, and pathophysiologic mechanisms in the various forms of structural heart disease. In view of space limitations, several important areas (eg, aortic disease) are necessarily omitted from discussion and others (eg, cardiac assist and replacement devices) are abbreviated, as they are discussed in greater detail elsewhere in this book. Moreover, although we have not included the key pathologic considerations herein, we are mindful that the number of adults with congenital heart disease is increasing rapidly and that they have unique and important clinical and pathologic concerns.[1,2]

MYOCARDIAL RESPONSE TO INCREASED WORK AND MYOCARDIAL DISEASE

Myocardial Hypertrophy

Hypertrophy is the compensatory response of the cardiac muscle (the *myocardium*), to increased work (Fig. 5-1).[3] This structural and functional adaptation accompanies nearly all forms of heart disease, and its consequences often dominate the clinical picture. Hypertrophy induces an increase in the overall mass and size of the heart that reflects increased size of individual myocytes largely through addition of contractile elements (*sarcomeres*) and associated cell and tissue elements. Functionally beneficial augmentation of myocyte number (*hyperplasia*) in response to stress or injury has not been demonstrated in the adult heart.

The pattern of hypertrophy reflects the nature of the stimulus (see Fig. 5-1B). Pressure overload (eg, in systemic hypertension or aortic stenosis) induces *concentric hypertrophy* with an increased ventricular mass, increased wall thickness, and increased ratio of wall thickness to cavity radius without dilation. In contrast, volume-overload (eg, in aortic or mitral regurgitation, myocardial infarction, or dilated cardiomyopathy) promotes hypertrophy accompanied by chamber dilation, in which both ventricular radius and total mass are increased (sometimes called *eccentric hypertrophy*). In myocardial infarction, where there is regional myocyte necrosis and loss, hypertrophy occurs only in noninfarcted regions of myocardium (termed *compensatory hypertrophy*).

In contrast, the chamber wall is affected globally by the increased chamber pressure of hypertension, the pressure or volume overload of valvular heart disease, and in dilated cardiomyopathy. The constellation of regional changes that occurs in

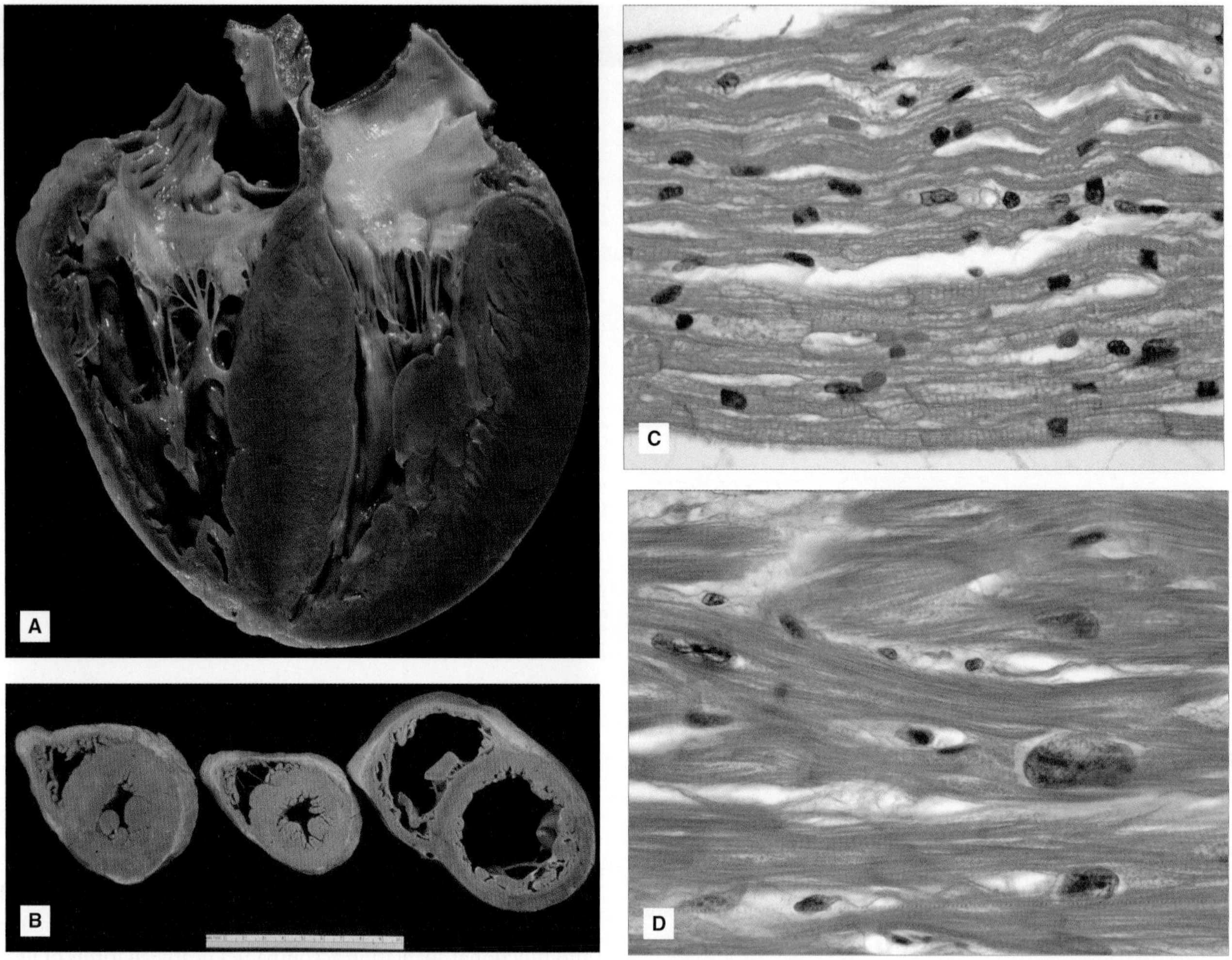

FIGURE 5-1 Summary of the gross and microscopic changes in cardiac hypertrophy. (**A**) Gross photo of heart with hypertrophy caused by aortic stenosis. The wall of the left ventricle is thick and the chamber is not dilated. The left ventricle is on the lower right in this apical four-chamber view of the heart. (**B**) Altered cardiac configuration in left ventricular hypertrophy without and with dilation, viewed in transverse heart sections. Compared with a normal heart (*center of this panel*), a pressure overloaded heart, caused for example by aortic valve stenosis (*left* in [B]), has increased mass and a thick left ventricular wall, whereas a volume overloaded heart, caused for example by mitral valve regurgitation, is both hypertrophied and dilated (*right*), having increased mass with a near normal or diminished wall thickness. (**C**) Photomicrograph of normal myocardium. (**D**) Photomicrograph of hypertrophied myocardium, showing large cells with enlarged. (*[B] Reproduced with permission from Edwards WD: Cardiac anatomy and examination of cardiac specimens, in Emmanouilides GC, Riemenschneider TA, Allen HD, et al [eds]: Moss and Adams Heart Disease in Infants, Children, and Adolescents: Including the Fetus and Young Adults, 5th ed. Philadelphia, Williams & Wilkins, 1995; p 86. [C and D] Reproduced with permission from Schoen FJ, Mitchell RN: The heart, in Kumar V, Fausto N, Abbas A, et al [eds]: Robbins/Cotran Pathologic Basis of Disease, 8th ed. Philadelphia, WB Saunders, 2010; pp 529-687.*)

both infarcted and noninfarcted myocardium or more globally in pressure and volume overload is called *ventricular remodeling*.[4] At a cell level, pressure overload promotes augmentation of cell width via parallel addition of sarcomeres; in contrast, volume overload and/or dilation stimulate augmentation of both cell width and length via both parallel and series addition of sarcomeres.

The changes in the heart described in the preceding initially increase the efficiency of the heart, enhance function, and are thereby adaptive. However, when these changes are excessive and prolonged, they may ultimately become deleterious and contribute to cardiac failure. This can occur via several mechanisms. Because the vasculature does not proliferate commensurate with increased cardiac mass, hypertrophied myocardium is usually relatively deficient in blood vessels and thereby particularly vulnerable to ischemic damage. Moreover, myocardial fibrous tissue is often increased. Also important are the molecular changes that accompany and likely mediate enhanced function in hypertrophied hearts, and which may subsequently promote development of heart failure. For example, hypertrophy induces a gene expression profile in cardiac myocytes that is generally similar to that of proliferating cells generally and particularly that of fetal cardiac myocytes during development. Differentially expressed proteins may be less functional and/or more or less abundant than normal. Hypertrophied and/or failing myocardium also may have mechanical disadvantage, reduced adrenergic responsiveness, decreased calcium availability, impaired mitochondrial function, and microcirculatory spasm. Apoptosis of cardiac myocytes may also contribute to heart failure. Novel therapeutic strategies for heart failure treatment based on molecular mechanisms are under investigation.[5–7]

Thus, owing to the totality of the changes described above, cardiac hypertrophy comprises a tenuous balance. The adaptive changes may be overwhelmed by potentially deleterious structural, functional, and biochemical/molecular alterations, including quantitative or qualitative alterations in cardiac configuration, metabolic requirements of an enlarged muscle mass, protein synthesis, decreased capillary/myocyte ratio, fibrosis, microvascular spasm, and impaired contractile mechanisms. Hypertrophy also decreases myocardial compliance and may thereby hinder diastolic filling. In addition, left ventricular hypertrophy is an independent risk factor for cardiac mortality and morbidity, especially sudden death.[8]

Heart failure can occur with pressure or volume overload of many causes, owing to both regional and global lesions (Fig. 5-2). Although left ventricular hypertrophy regresses in many cases following removal of the stimulus, the extent of resolution in an individual is unpredictable. Moreover, progressive cardiac failure may ensue following cardiac surgery and despite revascularization or hemodynamic adjustment, for example, by valve replacement or repair (see Fig. 5-2B). In addition, markedly increased cardiac muscle mass may compromise intraoperative myocardial preservation.

Cardiomyopathies

Cardiomyopathies are diseases in which the primary cardiovascular abnormality is in the myocardium. A *primary cardiomyopathy* comprises a condition solely or predominantly confined to heart muscle, whereas a *secondary cardiomyopathy* (often called *specific heart muscle disease*) implies myocardial involvement as a feature of a generalized systemic or multisystem disorder, such as amyloidosis, hemochromatosis, other infiltrative and storage diseases, drug and other toxic reactions, sarcoidosis, various autoimmune and collagen vascular diseases, or neuromuscular/neurologic disorders (eg, Duchenne-Becker muscular dystrophy). Primary cardiomyopathies are subdivided into genetic, mixed, and acquired categories, underscoring the role of recently elucidated molecular and genetic mechanisms.[9] Genetic causes of primary cardiomyopathy include hypertrophic cardiomyopathy, arrhythmogenic right ventricular cardiomyopathy, left ventricular noncompaction, the ion channel disorders (eg, long QT and Brugada syndromes), and some cases of dilated cardiomyopathy. Acquired causes of primary cardiomyopathy include myocarditis (inflammatory cardiomyopathy), and stress-provoked (tako-tsubo), tachycardia-induced, and peripartum cardiomyopathy. The terms *ischemic heart disease, valvular heart disease,* and *hypertensive heart disease* are preferred over the terms *ischemic cardiomyopathy, valvular cardiomyopathy,* and *hypertensive cardiomyopathy,* because these conditions more likely reflect compensatory and remodeling changes induced by another cardiovascular abnormality. The epicardial coronary arteries are usually free of significant obstructions in patients with cardiomyopathies.

In some cases (eg, myocarditis, sarcoidosis, amyloidosis, and hemochromatosis) the cause of a cardiomyopathy may be revealed by light and/or electron microscopic examination of an endomyocardial biopsy specimen, and other conditions such as arrhythmogenic right ventricular cardiomyopathy and hypertrophic cardiomyopathy have characteristic gross and microscopic features demonstrable upon evaluation of the heart at the time of transplantation or autopsy. In endomyocardial biopsy, also used in the management of the ongoing surveillance of cardiac transplant recipients,[10] a bioptome is inserted into the

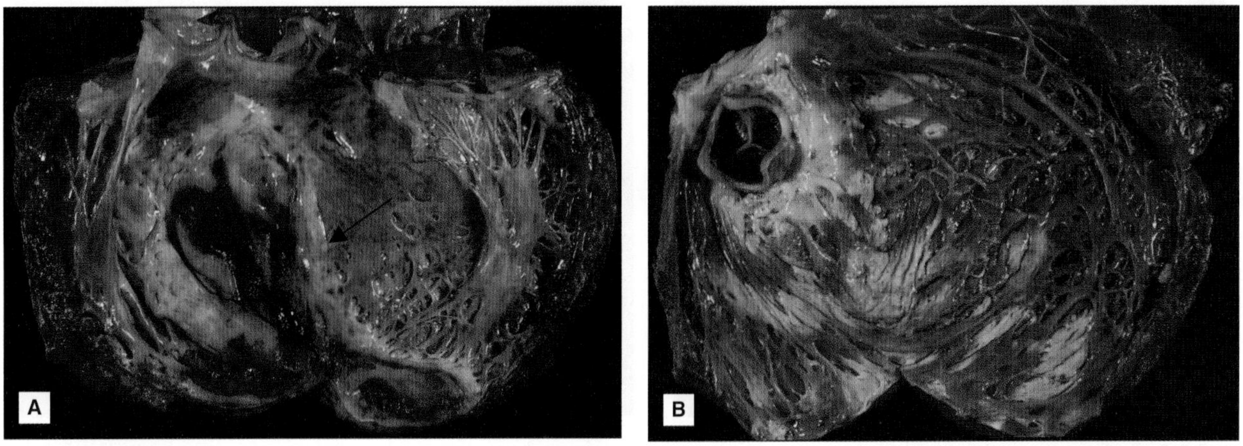

FIGURE 5-2 Cardiac failure necessitating heart transplantation. (A) Ischemic heart disease, with a large anteroapical-septal myocardial infarct (with mural thrombus) noted to the left of center of the photo (*arrow*). (B) Four years following mitral valve replacement with a porcine bioprosthesis for congenital deformity causing mitral regurgitation. (*[A] Reproduced with permission from Schoen FJ: Interventional and Surgical Cardiovascular Pathology: Clinical Correlations and Basic Principles. Philadelphia, WB Saunders, 1989.*)

right internal jugular or femoral vein and advanced under fluoroscopic or echocardiographic guidance through the tricuspid valve, to the apical half of the right side of the ventricular septum, yielding 1- to 3-mm fragments of myocardium. Correlation between right- and left-sided findings generally is good in most myocardial diseases and transplant rejection.

Common variants of primary cardiomyopathy are illustrated in Fig. 5-3.

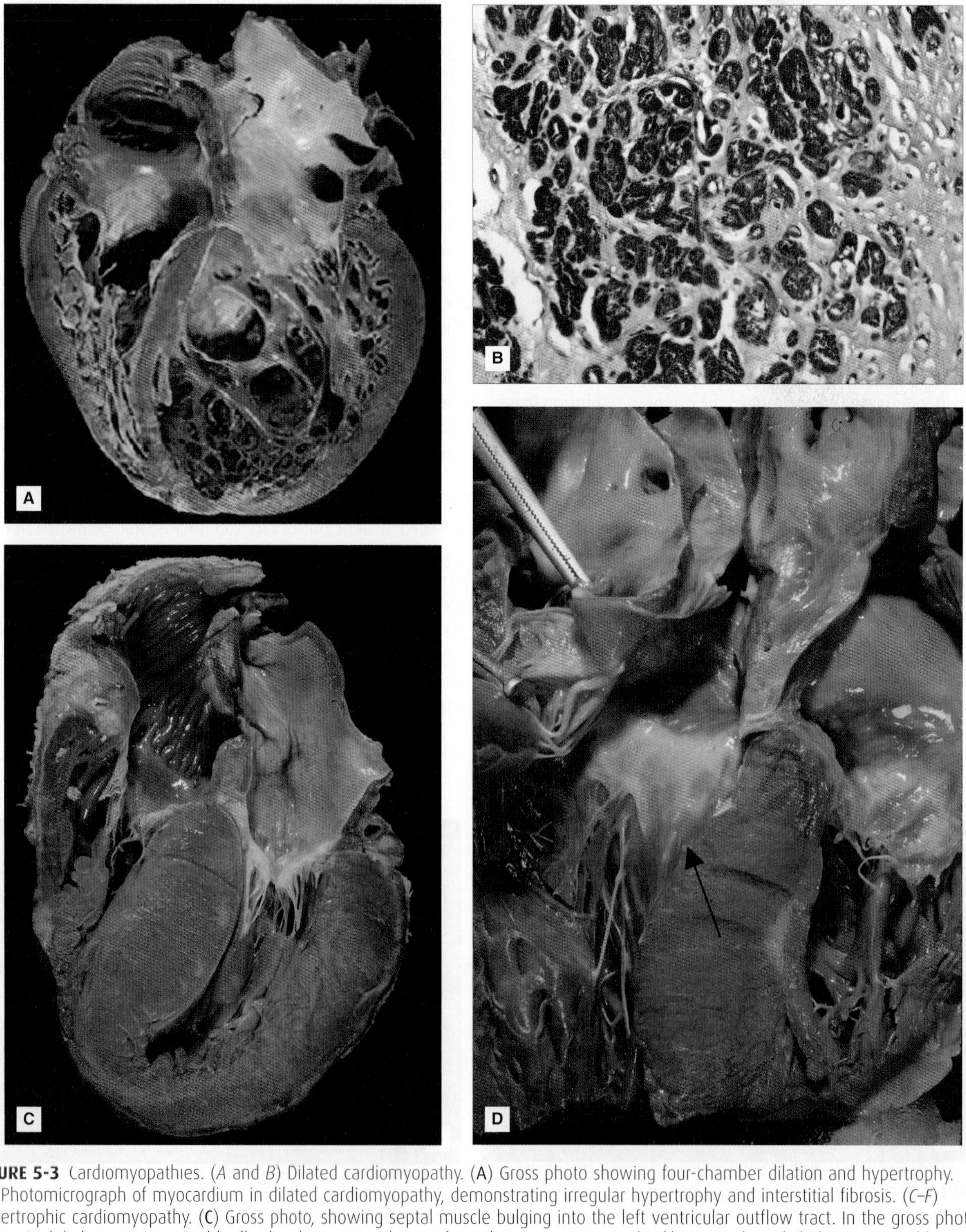

FIGURE 5-3 Cardiomyopathies. (*A* and *B*) Dilated cardiomyopathy. (**A**) Gross photo showing four-chamber dilation and hypertrophy. (**B**) Photomicrograph of myocardium in dilated cardiomyopathy, demonstrating irregular hypertrophy and interstitial fibrosis. (*C–F*) Hypertrophic cardiomyopathy. (**C**) Gross photo, showing septal muscle bulging into the left ventricular outflow tract. In the gross photo shown in (**D**) the anterior mitral leaflet has been moved away from the septum to reveal a fibrous endocardial plaque, caused by systolic anterior motion (see text). In (A) and (C), the LV is on the right side of the photo; in (D) the LV is on the left.

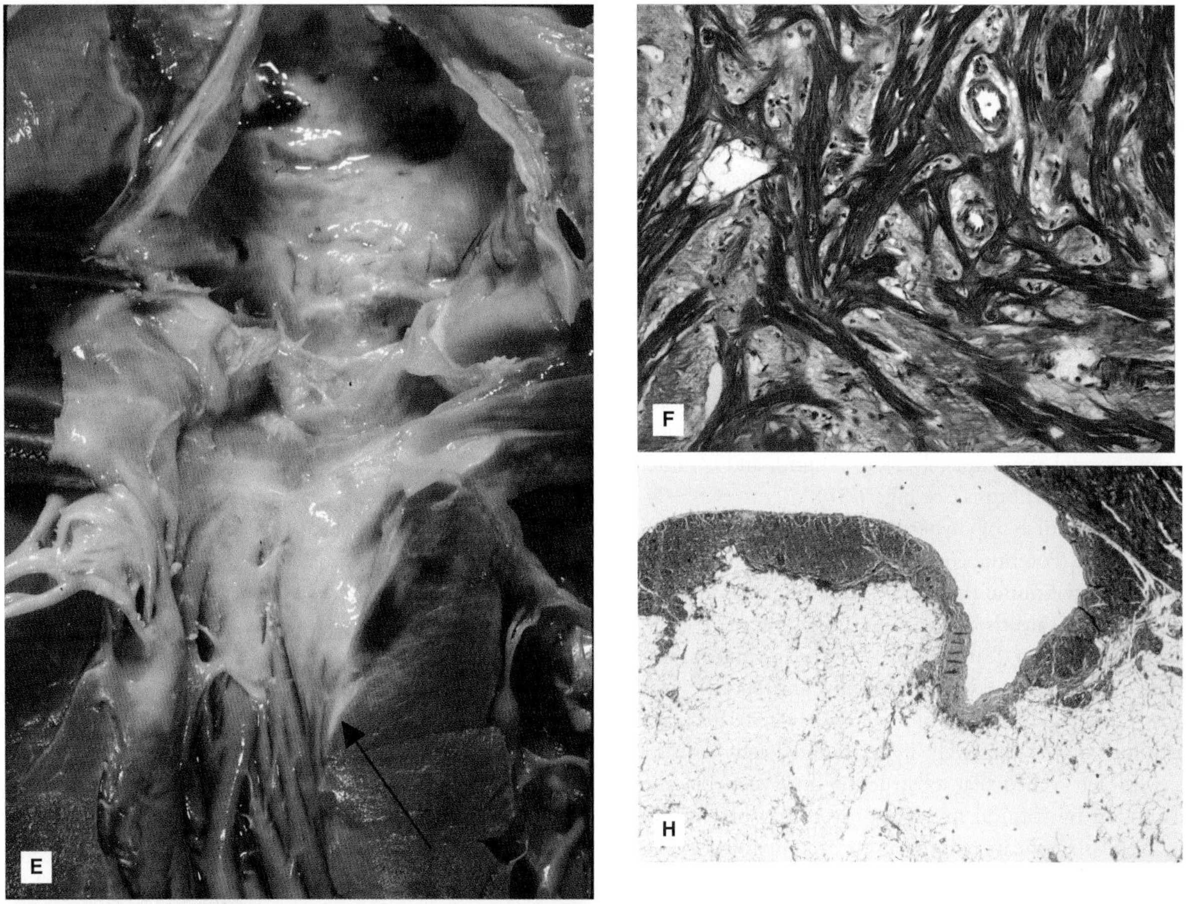

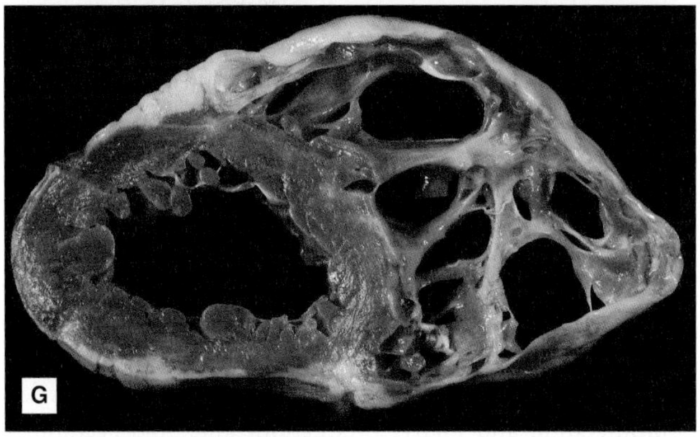

FIGURE 5-3 (*Continued*). Cardiomyopathies. (E) Gross photo of left ventricular outflow tract of patient with extensive fibrosis owing to remote surgical septal myotomy/myectomy. (F) Photomicrograph of myocardium in hypertrophic cardiomyopathy demonstrating myofiber disarray, with marked hypertrophy, abnormal branching of myocytes, and interstitial fibrosis. (*G* and *H*) Arrhythmogenic right ventricular cardiomyopathy. (G) Gross photograph, showing dilation of the right ventricle (on the right) and near transmural replacement of the right ventricular free-wall myocardium by fat and fibrosis. (H) Photomicrograph of the right ventricular free wall in arrythmogenic right ventricular cardiomyopathy, demonstrating focal transmural replacement of myocardium by fibrosis and fat. Fibrosis (collagen) is blue in the Masson trichrome stain in parts (*B*), (*F*), and (*H*).

Dilated Cardiomyopathy

Dilated cardiomyopathy is characterized by cardiomegaly usually to two to three times normal weight, and four-chamber dilation (see Fig. 5-3A).[11] The primary functional abnormality in dilated cardiomyopathy is impairment of left ventricular systolic function. Mural thrombi are sometimes present, predominantly in the left ventricle and are a potential source of thromboemboli. The histologic changes in dilated cardiomyopathy, comprising myocyte hypertrophy and interstitial fibrosis, are nonspecific and indistinguishable from those in failing muscle in ischemic or valvular heart disease (see Fig. 5-3B). Moreover, the severity of the morphologic changes does not necessarily correlate with the severity of dysfunction or the patient's prognosis.

Dilated cardiomyopathy has a genetic and often familial basis in approximately 30 to 50% of cases, with autosomal dominant (most common), autosomal recessive, X-linked and mitochondrial inheritance reported. Mutations most commonly involve genes encoding proteins of the cardiac myocyte cytoskeleton. Secondary cardiomyopathies yielding a dilated phenotype also occur as a result of alcoholism and pregnancy-associated nutritional deficiency or immunologic reaction.[12]

Hypertrophic Cardiomyopathy

Hypertrophic cardiomyopathy is characterized macroscopically by massive myocardial hypertrophy without dilation (see Fig. 5-3C), often with disproportionate thickening of the ventricular septum relative to the free wall of the left ventricle (ratio >1.3) (termed *asymmetric septal hypertrophy*). In some patients, the basal septum is markedly thickened at the level of the mitral valve, and the outflow of the left ventricle may be narrowed during systole, yielding left ventricular outflow tract obstruction. In such cases, contact between the left ventricular outflow tract and the anterior mitral leaflet during ventricular systole (observed by echocardiography as systolic anterior motion of the mitral valve) results in LV outflow tract endocardial thickening, in a configuration that mirrors the anterior leaflet of the mitral valve. The most important microscopic features in hypertrophic cardiomyopathy include: (1) disorganized myocytes and contractile elements within cells (*myofiber disarray*) typically involving 10 to 50% of the septum; (2) extreme myocyte hypertrophy, with myocyte diameters frequently more than 40 μm (normal approximately 15 to 20 μm); and (3) interstitial and replacement fibrosis (see Fig. 5-3F).

The clinical course of hypertrophic cardiomyopathy is extremely variable. Potential complications include atrial fibrillation with potential mural thrombus formation and embolization, infective endocarditis of the mitral valve, intractable cardiac failure, and sudden death. Sudden death is common, with risk related to the degree of hypertrophy and specific gene mutations.[13] Reduced stroke volume results from decreased diastolic filling of the massively hypertrophied left ventricle. Patients with left ventricular obstruction may benefit from septal reduction by surgical myotomy/myectomy or chemical ablation.[14] End-stage heart failure can be accompanied by cardiac dilation.

Hypertrophic cardiomyopathy has a genetic basis in virtually all cases.[15] In many patients the disease is familial, with autosomal dominant transmission and variable expression; remaining cases are sporadic. Hundreds of mutations have been identified in 11 genes; almost all genes are for sarcomeric proteins, most commonly β-myosin heavy chain. Nevertheless, the mechanism by which defective sarcomeric proteins produce the phenotype of hypertrophic cardiomyopathy is yet incompletely defined.

Restrictive Cardiomyopathy

Restrictive cardiomyopathy is characterized by impeded diastolic relaxation and left ventricular filling, often with preserved systolic function (called *diastolic dysfunction*). Any disorder that interferes with ventricular filling can cause restrictive cardiomyopathy (eg, eosinophilic endomyocardial disease, amyloidosis, storage diseases, or postirradiation fibrosis) or mimic it (eg, constrictive pericarditis or hypertrophic cardiomyopathy). In restrictive cardiomyopathy, biatrial dilation but not ventricular dilation may be prominent. Distinct morphologic patterns may be revealed by endomyocardial biopsy, particularly in deposition processes such as amyloid or Fabry's disease.[16]

Arrhythmogenic Right Ventricular Cardiomyopathy

Arrhythmogenic right ventricular cardiomyopathy is characterized by a dilated right ventricular chamber and severely thinned right ventricular wall, with extensive fatty infiltration, loss of myocytes with compensatory myocyte hypertrophy, and interstitial fibrosis (see Fig. 5-3G–H).[17] Clinical features include right-sided heart failure and arrhythmias. Arrhythmias are often brought on by exertion, and this condition is associated with sudden death in athletes. Right ventricular cardiomyopathy is associated with mutations in several genes involved in cell-cell adhesion, including plakoglobin, desmoplakin, plakophilin-2, and desmoglein-2.

CORONARY ARTERY AND ISCHEMIC HEART DISEASE

Myocardial ischemia is a physiologic condition that occurs when perfusion via coronary flow is inadequate to meet metabolic needs, thus interfering with the cellular delivery of oxygen and nutrients to cardiac myocytes, and removal of waste products. Myocardial ischemia is most often caused by diminished perfusion of the myocardium resulting from obstruction or narrowing of a coronary artery secondary to atherosclerosis. Nonatherosclerotic epicardial coronary artery obstructions can also occur in autoimmune diseases (eg, systemic lupus erythematosus and rheumatoid arthritis), progressive systemic sclerosis (scleroderma), vasculitis (eg, Buerger disease and Kawasaki disease), fibromuscular dysplasia, and as a result of dissection, spasm, or embolism. Obstruction of the small intramural coronary arteries occurs in diabetes, the Fabry disease, and amyloidosis and in cardiac allografts (see later). Decreased coronary flow leading to global hypoperfusion and myocardial ischemia can also occur as a result of systemic hypotension and during cardiopulmonary bypass. Ischemia can also result from increased cardiac demand secondary to exercise, tachycardia, hyperthyroidism, or ventricular hypertrophy and/or dilation. Moreover, the effects of ischemia are potentiated when oxygen supply is decreased secondary to anemia, hypoxia, or cardiac failure.

Atherosclerosis

Atherosclerosis is a chronic, progressive, multifocal disease of the vessel wall, beginning in the intima, whose characteristic lesion is the atheroma or plaque that forms through intimal thickening (mediated predominantly by smooth muscle cell proliferation and matrix production) and lipid accumulation (mediated primarily by insudation of lipid into the arterial wall followed by monocyte/macrophage phagocytosis).[18] Atherosclerosis primarily affects the large elastic arteries and large- and medium-sized muscular arteries of the systemic circulation, particularly near branches, sharp curvatures, and bifurcations. Coronary arterial atherosclerosis involves especially the epicardial branches of the left anterior descending (LAD) and circumflex arteries, and the right coronary diffusely, but generally not their intramural branches. Most atheromas in the coronary arteries are segmental and eccentric, with plaque-free segments longitudinal and circumferentially. In early lesions, the plaque bulges outward at the expense of the media with the arterial lumen remaining circular in cross-section at essentially the same original diameter (ie, the vessel wall outer diameter enlarges, a process termed *vascular remodeling*).[19]

Although veins are usually spared from atherosclerosis, venous bypass grafts interposed within branches of the arterial system (such as saphenous vein grafts) frequently develop intimal thickening and ultimately atherosclerotic obstructions. Paradoxically, some arteries used as arterial grafts, including the internal mammary artery, are largely spared.

Pathogenesis

The prevailing theory of lesion formation in atherosclerosis centers on interactions among arterial wall endothelial and vascular smooth muscle cells, circulating monocytes, platelets, and plasma lipoproteins. A key contributor to atherosclerosis is endothelial cell injury induced by chronic hypercholesterolemia, homocystinemia, chemicals in cigarette smoke, viruses, localized hemodynamic forces, systemic hypertension, hyperglycemia, or the local effects of cytokines. These factors cause phenotypic and hence functional changes in endothelial cells, called *endothelial dysfunction.*[20] Endothelial dysfunction causes: (1) vasoconstriction owing to decreased production of the vasodilator nitric oxide; (2) increased permeability to lipoproteins; (3) expression of tissue factor leading to thrombosis; and (4) expression of certain injury-induced adhesion molecules leading to adherence of platelets and inflammatory cells.

Progression from an early, subendothelial lesion (called a *fatty streak*) to a complex atheromatous plaque involves the following processes: (1) monocytes adhere to endothelial cells, migrate into the subendothelial space, and transform into tissue macrophages; (2) smooth muscle cells migrate from the media into the intima, proliferate, and secrete collagen and other extracellular matrix constituents; (3) lipids accumulate via phagocytosis in macrophages (forming foam cells) and smooth muscle cells, as well as extracellularly; (4) lipoproteins are oxidized in the vessel wall leading to generation of potent biologic stimuli such as chemoattractants and cytotoxins; (5) persistent chronic inflammation; (6) cellular necrosis with release of intracellular lipids (mostly cholesterol esters); and often (7) calcification. Mature atherosclerotic plaques consist of a central core of lipid, cholesterol crystals, macrophages, smooth muscle cells, foam cells, and lymphocytes along with necrotic debris, separated from the lumen by a fibrous cap rich in collagen.

Clinical manifestations of advanced coronary arterial atherosclerosis occur through encroachment of the lumen leading to progressive stenosis, or to acute plaque disruption with thrombosis (see the following). In the absence of significant coronary blockages, myocardial perfusion is adequate at rest, and compensatory vasodilation provides flow reserve that is more than sufficient to accommodate increased metabolic demand during vigorous exertion. When the coronary luminal cross-sectional area is decreased by approximately 75%, blood flow becomes limited during exertion; with 90% reduction, coronary flow may be inadequate at rest. However, occlusions that develop slowly may stimulate the formation of collateral vessels that protect against distal myocardial ischemia. Aneurysms may form secondary to atherosclerosis as a result of destruction of the media beneath a plaque, a process most common in the aorta and other large vessels (where plaque does not easily cause obstruction). The natural history, morphologic features, key pathogenetic events, and clinical complications of atherosclerosis are summarized in Figs. 5-4 and 5-5.

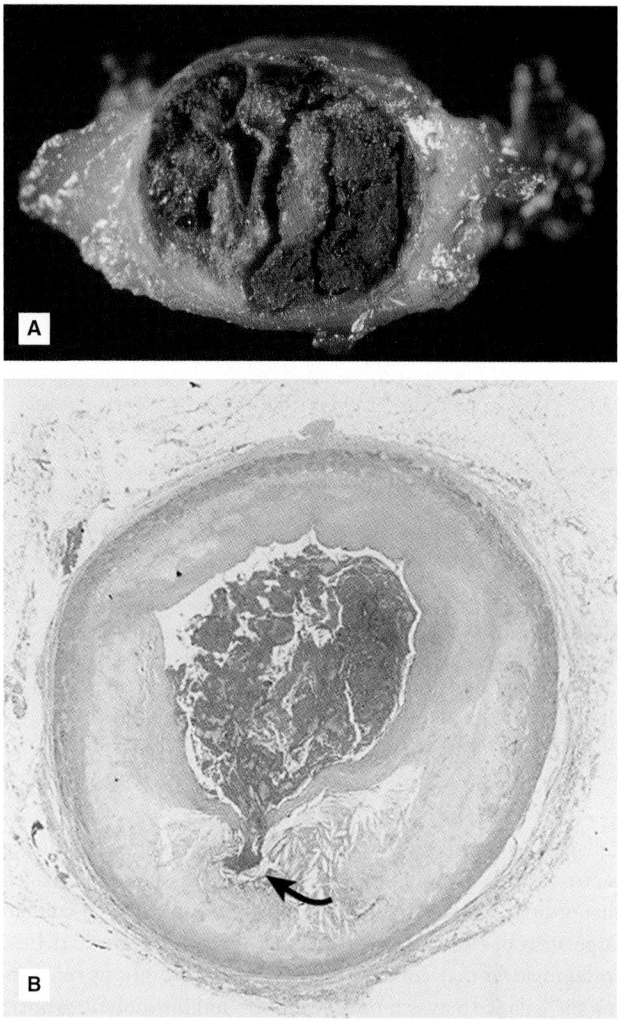

FIGURE 5-4 Acute plaque rupture with superimposed thrombus complicating coronary arterial atherosclerosis and triggering fatal myocardial infarction. (A) Gross photo. (B) Photomicrograph. (The arrow demonstrates the site of plaque rupture.) (*[B] Reproduced with permission from Schoen FJ: Interventional and Surgical Cardiovascular Pathology: Clinical Correlations and Basic Principles. Philadelphia, WB Saunders, 1989.*)

Role of Acute Plaque Change

The onset and prognosis of ischemic heart disease are not well predicted by the angiographically determined extent and severity of luminal obstructions.[21] The conversion of chronic stable angina or an asymptomatic state to an *acute coronary syndrome* (ie, myocardial infarction, unstable angina, and sudden coronary death) is dependent on dynamic vascular changes, such as fracture or rupture of the fibrous cap, exposing deep plaque constituents. Less commonly, the change is fissuring, and/or ulceration of the fibrous cap, which results in flow disruption and exposure of the luminal blood to highly thrombogenic surfaces, thereby setting the stage for platelet aggregation and mural or total thrombosis.[22]

Plaques having a high propensity to rupture are known as *vulnerable plaques.* Such lesions: (1) have a thin collagenous fibrous cap and few smooth muscle cells (the cells that produce

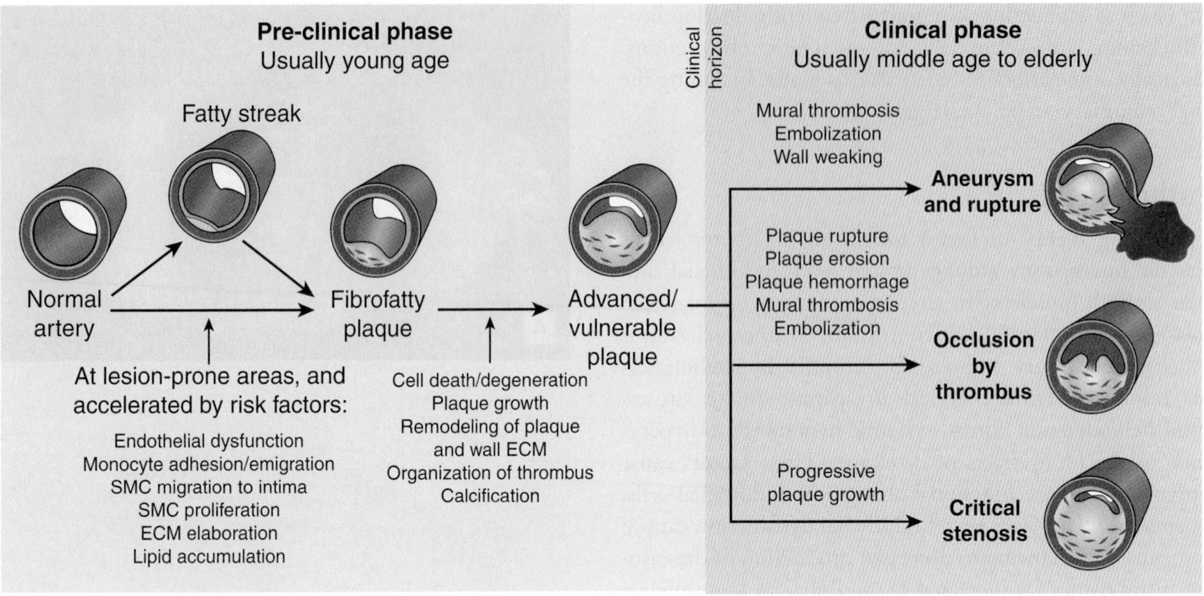

FIGURE 5-5 Schematic diagram summarizing the morphology, pathogenesis, and complications of atherosclerosis. Plaques usually develop slowly and insidiously over many years, beginning in childhood or shortly thereafter and exerting clinical effect in middle age or later. As described in the text, lesions may progress from a fatty streak to a fibrous plaque and then to plaque complications that lead to disease. ECM = extracellular matrix; SMC = smooth muscle cell. (*Reproduced with permission from Mitchell RN, Schoen FJ: Blood vessels, in Kumar V, Fausto N, Abbas A, et al [eds]: Robbins/Cotran Pathologic Basis of Disease, 8th ed. Philadelphia, WB Saunders, 2010; pp 487-528.*)

collagenous matrix); (2) contain many macrophages producing matrix metalloproteinases (enzymes that degrade the collagen that ordinarily lends strength to the fibrous cap); and (3) contain large areas of foam cells, extracellular lipid and necrotic debris. Inflammation may contribute to coronary thrombosis by altering the balance between prothrombotic and fibrinolytic properties of the endothelium. There is evidence that lipid lowering by diet or drugs such as statins (HMG CoA reductase inhibitors) reduces accumulation of macrophages expressing matrix-degrading enzymes and thereby stabilizes plaque by increasing the thickness and strength of the fibrous cap.[23]

Vulnerable plaques are not necessarily significantly obstructive. Indeed, pathologic and clinical studies show that plaques that rupture and lead to coronary occlusion often produced only mild to moderate luminal stenosis (and often no symptoms) prior to acute plaque change. Thus, there is great interest in identifying vulnerable plaques in individuals at a potentially therapeutic stage. Calcification of the coronary arteries detected noninvasively by electron beam computed tomography predicts the extent of atherosclerotic disease overall but does not predict plaque instability. The most relevant features of plaque structure can be evaluated using intravascular ultrasound, optical coherence tomography (OCT), and potentially noninvasive molecular imaging.[24,25]

The events that trigger abrupt changes in plaque configuration and superimposed thrombosis and the efficacy and safety of interventional therapies depend on influences both intrinsic (eg, structure and composition, as described in the preceding) and extrinsic (eg, blood pressure, vasospasm, and platelet reactivity) to the plaque.[26,27] Potential outcomes for ruptured plaques include progression to thrombotic occlusion, nonocclusive thrombosis, healing at the site of plaque erosion, atheroembolization or thromboembolization, organization of mural thrombus (plaque progression), and organization of the occlusive mass with recanalization.

Ischemic Myocardial Injury

The clinical manifestations of ischemic heart disease most frequently reflect the downstream effects of a complex and dynamic interaction among fixed atherosclerotic narrowing of the epicardial coronary arteries, intraluminal thrombosis overlying a ruptured or fissured atherosclerotic plaque, platelet aggregation, vasospasm, and the responses of the myocardium to ischemia.

Progression of Injury

The changes in the myocardium following the onset of myocardial ischemia are sequential and the cellular consequences are primarily determined by the severity and duration of flow deprivation (Table 5-1). Within seconds of onset, ischemia induces a transition from aerobic metabolism to anaerobic glycolysis in cardiac myocytes, leading to inadequate production of high-energy phosphates such as ATP, and the accumulation of metabolites such as lactic acid, causing intracellular acidosis. Myocardial function is exquisitely sensitive to these biochemical consequences, with total loss of contraction within 2 minutes in severe ischemia. Nevertheless, ischemic changes in an individual cell are not immediately lethal, and injury is potentially reversible if the duration of ischemia is short (<20 minutes). Irreversible injury of cardiac myocytes marked by cell membrane structural defects occurs only after 20 to 40 minutes within the most severely ischemic area (Fig. 5-6). Lethal injury to groups of cells owing to severe prolonged ischemia causes *myocardial infarction*.

TABLE 5-1 Approximate Time of Onset and Recognition of Key Features of Ischemic Myocardial Injury

Event/process	Time of onset
Onset of anerobic metabolism	Within seconds
Loss of contractility	<2 min
ATP* reduced to 50% of normal to 10% of normal	 10 min 40 min
Irreversible cell injury	20–40 min
Microvascular injury	>1 h
Pathologic feature	**Time of recognition**
Ultrastructural features of reversible injury	5–10 min
Ultrastructural features of irreversible damage	20–40 min
Wavy fibers Staining defect with tetrazolium dye Classic histologic features of necrosis	1–3 h 2–3 h 6–12 h
Gross alterations	12–24 h

**ATP = adenosine triphosphate.*

Within the region of myocardium vulnerable to die if ischemia is not relieved in a timely manner (termed the *area at risk*), loss of perfusion is not uniform, and not all cells in the area at risk are equally affected. The most severely affected myocytes, and therefore the first to become necrotic, reside in the subendocardium and in the papillary muscles furthest from lateral regions of adequate perfusion. If uninterrupted ischemia progresses, there is a *wavefront* of cell death outward from the mid-subendocardial region toward, eventually encompassing the lateral borders and less severely ischemic subepicardial and peripheral regions of the area at risk. In myocardial infarction, approximately 50% of the area at risk becomes necrotic in approximately 3 to 4 hours. The final transmural extent of an infarct is generally established within 6 to 12 hours. The key principle is that if perfusion is restored prior to the onset of irreversible changes, cell death can be prevented. Thus, restoration of flow to a severely ischemic area via therapeutic intervention can alter the outcome, depending on the interval between the onset of ischemia and restoration of blood flow (*reperfusion*).[28]

Neither reversible ischemia nor necrosis existing less than 6 or more hours before patient death are visible by routine gross or microscopic pathologic analysis of a cardiac specimen at autopsy. However, in a patient who died at least 2 to 3 hours following the onset of infarction, the presence of a necrotic region may be detected as a staining defect with triphenyl tetrazolium chloride (TTC), a dye that turns viable myocardium a brick-red color on reaction of the dye with intact myocardial dehydrogenases.[29] The earliest observable microscopic features of infarction are intense eosinophilia, nuclear pyknosis, and loss of myocytes in clusters; some may be stretched and wavy. Short-term ischemia insufficient to cause frank necrosis cannot be reliably demonstrated by pathologic examination.

Tissue Repair Following Myocardial Infarction. The inflammation and repair sequence in response to myocardial

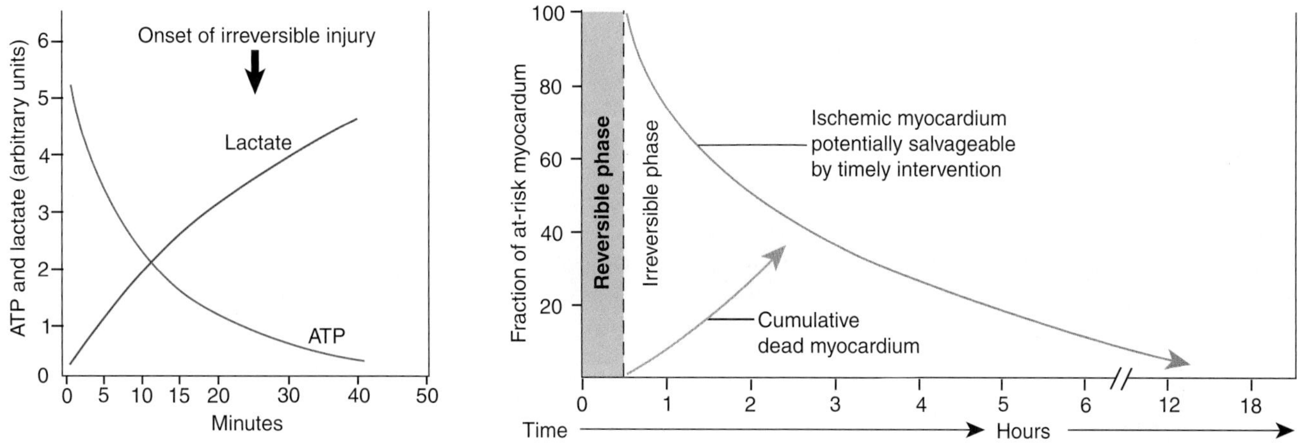

FIGURE 5-6 Temporal sequence of early biochemical findings and progression of necrosis after onset of severe myocardial ischemia. *Left panel:* Early changes include loss of ATP and accumulation of lactate. *Right panel:* Myocardial injury is potentially reversible for approximately 20 minutes after the onset of even the most severe ischemia. Thereafter, progressive loss of viability occurs, which is complete by 6 to 12 hours. The benefits of reperfusion are greatest when it is achieved early; progressively smaller benefit is accrued when reperfusion is delayed. (*Reproduced with permission from Schoen FJ, Mitchell RN: The heart, in Kumar V, Fausto N, Abbas A, et al [eds]: Robbins/Cotran Pathologic Basis of Disease, 8th Ed. Philadelphia, WB Saunders, 2010; pp 529-687.*)

cell death follows a largely stereotyped sequence similar to tissue repair following injury at extracardiac sites. The inflammatory reaction is characterized by early exudation of polymorphonuclear leukocytes, seen after 6 to 12 hours and maximal within 1 to 3 days. Subsequently (3 to 5 days), the infiltrate consists predominantly of macrophages that remove the necrotic tissue and set the stage for collagen production by fibroblasts accompanied by neovascularization beginning approximately 7 to 10 days at the margins of preserved tissue. The gross appearance reflects the progressive microscopic changes (Fig. 5-7). Ultimately, the infarcted tissue is replaced by dense collagenous scar, which is fully mature by about 6 to 8 weeks. Healing of myocardial infarction may be altered by reperfusion (see the following), mechanical stress, gender, and neurohumoral and other factors.[30]

Although cardiac myocytes are traditionally thought incapable of regeneration, a growing body of evidence suggests that regeneration of cardiac myocytes can occur under certain circumstances, including at the viable borders of myocardial infarcts.[31] Whether this capacity for renewal can be harnessed to therapeutic advantage is not yet known (discussed later in this chapter).

Effects of Reperfusion

Reperfusion of an ischemic zone can alter the progression of myocardial ischemic injury, in both jeopardized and already necrotic myocardium. Reperfusion occurring before the onset of irreversible injury prevents infarction altogether. Reperfusion later (ie, following some cell death) may limit infarct size through salvage of myocytes located outside the leading edge of the "wavefront," provided that these myocytes are only reversibly injured at the time reperfusion occurs.[32] Thus, the potential for recovery of viable tissue decreases with increasing severity and duration of ischemia (see Fig. 5-6). Owing to the typical progression of ischemic injury, reperfusion 3 to 4 hours following onset of ischemia is considered the practical limit for significant myocardial salvage.

Reperfused previously ischemic myocardium may have hemorrhage (owing to microvascular damage; see the following) and necrotic myocytes with transverse eosinophilic lines (called *contraction bands*) that represent hypercontracted sarcomeres (Fig. 5-8) caused by ischemic cell membrane damage followed by a massive cellular influx of calcium derived from the restored blood flow. In reperfusion after especially severe global ischemia, the left ventricle may undergo a massive tetanic contraction (*stone heart syndrome*).[33]

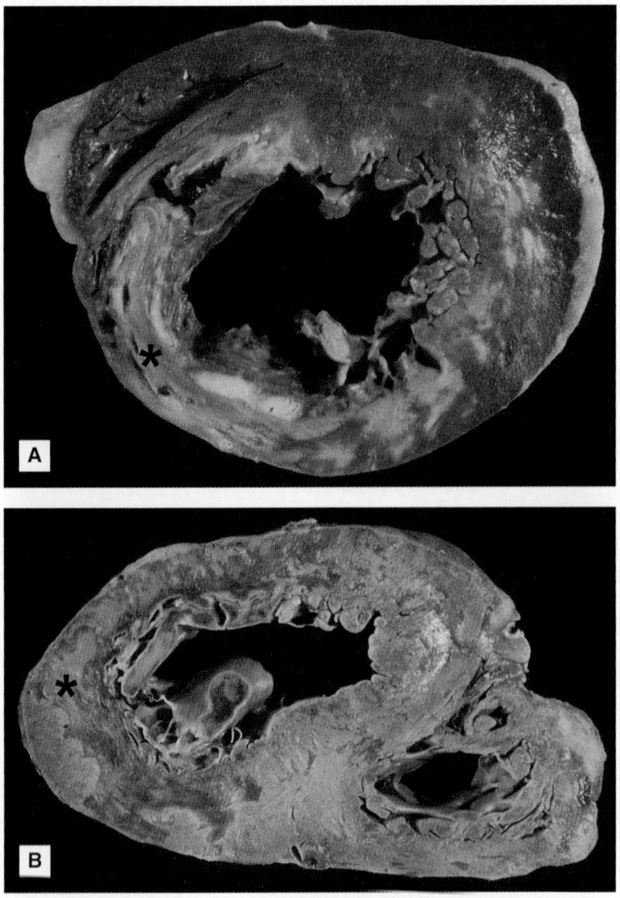

FIGURE 5-7 Gross photos of healing myocardial infarcts (A) approximately 3 to 4 days, (B) approximately 2 weeks. Asterisk highlights area of damage in each case.

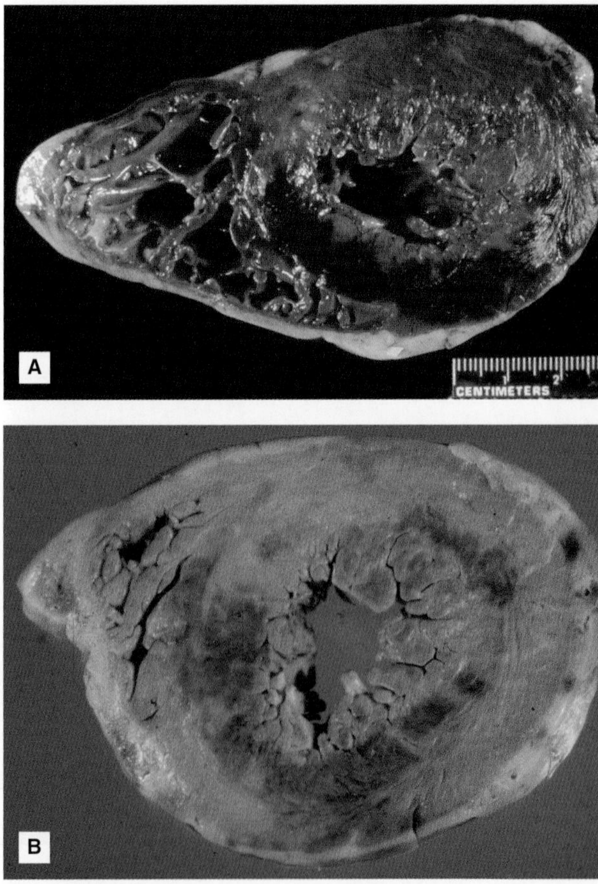

FIGURE 5-8 Reperfusion following severe myocardial ischemia. (A) Large, densely hemorrhagic anteroseptal acute myocardial infarct from patient treated by intracoronary thrombolysis for left anterior descending (LAD) artery thrombus, approximately 4 hours following onset. (B) Subendocardial circumferential hemorrhagic acute myocardial necrosis occurring perioperatively in cardiac valve replacement.

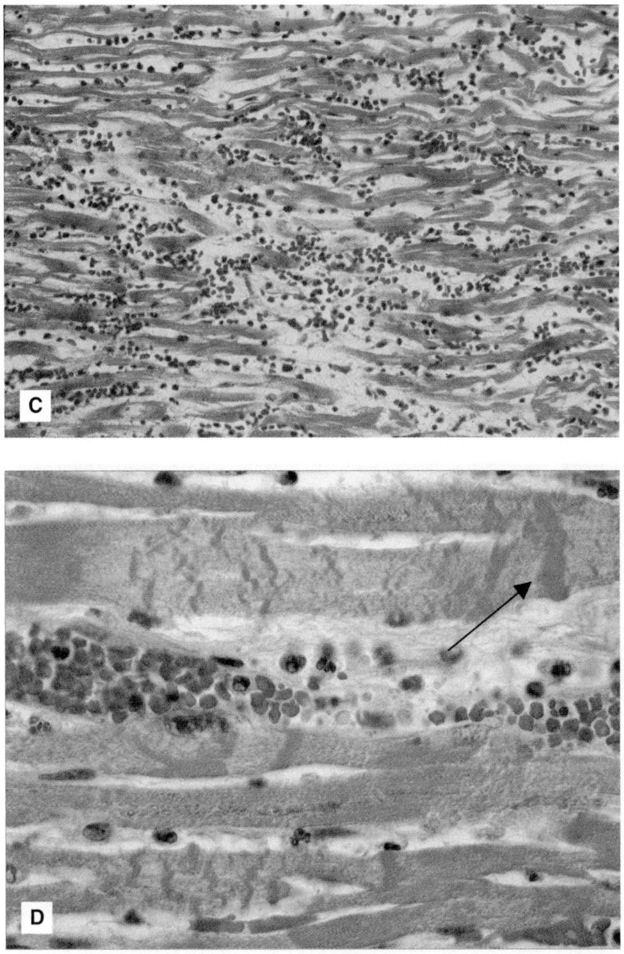

FIGURE 5-8 (*Continued*). Reperfusion following severe myocardial ischemia. (C) Photomicrograph of hemorrhagic myocardial necrosis. (D) High-power photomicrograph demonstrating contraction bands (*arrow*). Hematoxylin and eosin 375×.

Microvascular injury can follow myocyte injury in severe, prolonged myocardial ischemia, eventuating in hemorrhage during reperfusion, visible grossly and microscopically (resulting from vascular wall incompetence), and/or occlusion (resulting from endothelial or interstitial edema and/or plugging by platelet or neutrophil aggregates). Microvascular occlusions may inhibit the reperfusion of damaged regions (*no-reflow phenomenon*).[34] Moreover, reperfusion may damage some of the ischemic but still viable myocytes that were not irreversibly injured (called *reperfusion injury*). Arrhythmias may occur after reperfusion, possibly secondary to myocyte damage by oxygen free radicals and/or increased intracellular calcium.

Myocardial Stunning, Hibernation, and Preconditioning. Although reperfusion may salvage ischemic but not necrotic myocardium, metabolic and functional recovery is usually not instantaneous; indeed, reversible postischemic myocardial dysfunction (*myocardial stunning*) may persist for hours to days following brief periods of ischemia.[35] Myocardial stunning may occur after percutaneous coronary intervention, cardiopulmonary bypass, or ischemia related to unstable angina or stress.

Regions of viable myocardium with chronically impaired function may exist in the setting of chronically reduced coronary blood flow (termed *hibernating myocardium*).[36] Myocardial hibernation is characterized by: (1) persistent wall motion abnormality; (2) low myocardial blood flow; and (3) evidence of viability in at least some of the affected areas. Contractile function of hibernating myocardium can improve if blood flow returns toward normal or if oxygen demand is reduced. Correction of this abnormality is likely responsible for the reversal of longstanding defects in ventricular wall motion observed following coronary bypass graft surgery or percutaneous coronary intervention. Morphologically, sublethal chronic ischemic injury often manifests as myocyte vacuolization, particularly in the subendocardium.[37]

Adaptation to short-term transient ischemia (ie, duration insufficient to cause cell death) may induce tolerance against subsequent, more severe ischemic insults (*ischemic preconditioning*).[38] Thus, short (5-minute) periods of cardiac ischemia followed by reperfusion can protect myocardium against injury during a prolonged period of subsequent ischemia. Understanding the yet uncertain mechanisms of this protection could lead to targets for "pre-emptive" pharmacologic stimulation of these pathways.

Myocardial Infarction and Its Complications

Coronary atherosclerosis with acute plaque rupture and superimposed thrombosis often results in a *transmural* (Q-wave) myocardial infarct, in which ischemic necrosis involves at least half and usually a nearly full thickness of the ventricular wall in the distribution of the involved artery. In contrast, a *subendocardial* (nontransmural, non–Q wave) infarct constitutes an area of ischemic necrosis that is limited to the inner third to half of the ventricular wall, which can occur in the setting of episodic hypotension, global ischemia, or hypoxemia, or from interruption by reperfusion of the evolution of a transmural infarct. Subendocardial infarction can be multifocal, often extending laterally beyond the perfusion territory of a single coronary artery, especially when associated with diffuse stenosing coronary atherosclerosis without acute plaque rupture or thrombosis.

The short-term mortality rate from acute myocardial infarction has declined from 30% in the 1960s to 7 to 10% or less today, especially for patients who receive aggressive reperfusion/revascularization and pharmacologic therapy. However, half of all deaths from myocardial infarction occur within the first hour after the onset of symptoms, often before the victims can reach the hospital. Poor prognostic factors include advanced age, female gender, diabetes mellitus, and a previous myocardial infarction. Left ventricular function and the extent of obstructive lesions in vessels perfusing viable myocardium are the most important prognostic factors.

Important complications of myocardial infarction include ventricular dysfunction, cardiogenic shock, arrhythmias, cardiac rupture, infarct extension and expansion, papillary muscle dysfunction, right ventricular involvement, ventricular aneurysm, pericarditis, and systemic arterial embolism; the cardiac rupture syndromes and ventricular aneurysm are illustrated in Fig. 5-9. Outcome after myocardial infarction is dependent on infarct size, location, and transmurality. Patients with transmural anterior infarcts are at greatest risk for regional dilation and mural thrombi and have a worse clinical course than those with inferior-posterior infarcts. In contrast, inferior-posterior infarcts are more likely to have serious conduction blocks and right ventricular involvement.

Myocardial infarcts produce functional abnormalities approximately proportional to their size. Large infarcts have a higher probability of cardiogenic shock and congestive heart failure. Nonfunctional scar tissue resulting from previous infarcts and areas of stunned or hibernating myocardium may also contribute to overall ventricular dysfunction. Cardiogenic shock following myocardial infarction is generally indicative of a large infarct (often >40% of the left ventricle). The high mortality of myocardial dysfunction and cardiogenic shock has been alleviated somewhat in recent years by the use of intra-aortic balloon pumps and ventricular assist devices to bridge patients through phases of prolonged reversible ischemic dysfunction.

Although many patients have cardiac rhythm abnormalities following myocardial infarction, the conduction system is

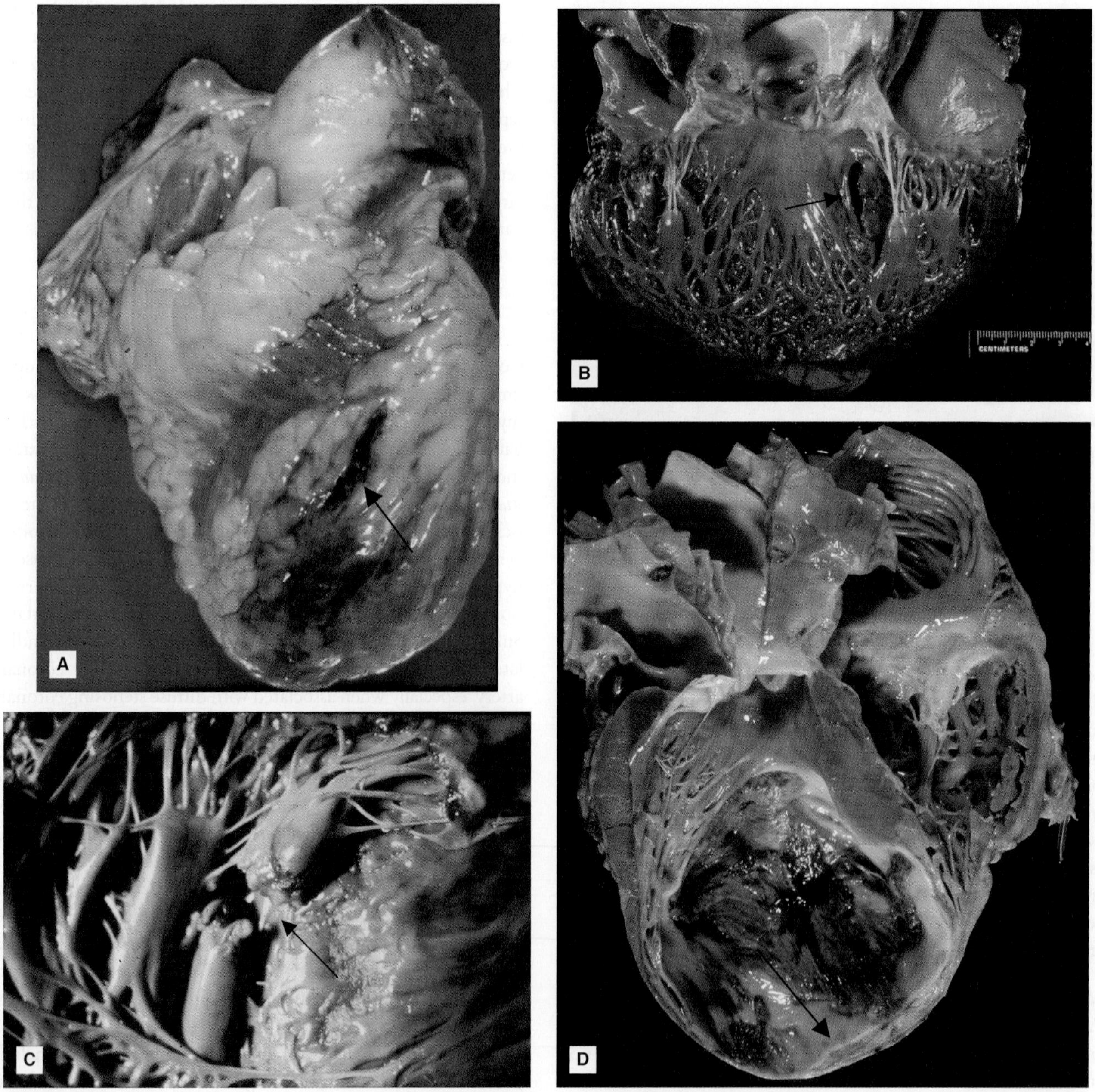

FIGURE 5-9 Cardiac rupture syndromes and ventricular aneurysm following myocardial infarction. (A) Anterior myocardial rupture (*arrow*). (B) Rupture of the ventricular septum (*arrow*). (C) Rupture of a necrotic papillary muscle (*arrow*). (D) Large left ventricular aneurysm, with thin fibrotic wall (*arrow*) and mural thrombus. (*[A–C] Reproduced with permission from Schoen FJ, Mitchell RN. The heart, in Kumar V, Fausto N, Abbas A, et al [eds]: Robbins/Cotran Pathologic Basis of Disease, 8th ed. Philadelphia, WB Saunders, 2010; p 529.*)

involved by necrosis only in a minority, and heart block following myocardial infarction usually is transient. Tachyarrhythmias usually originate in areas of severely ischemic or necrotic myocardium, owing to electrically unstable ischemic myocardium, often at the edge of an infarct. Ischemia without frank infarction can lead directly to lethal arrhythmias owing to myocardial irritability; indeed, autopsy studies of sudden death victims and clinical studies of resuscitated survivors of cardiac arrest show that only a minority of patients with ischemia-induced malignant ventricular arrhythmias develop a full-blown acute myocardial infarction.

Cardiac rupture syndromes comprise three entities (see Fig. 5-9 A–C): (1) rupture of the ventricular free wall (most common), usually with hemopericardium and cardiac tamponade; (2) rupture of the ventricular septum (less common), leading to an acquired ventricular septal defect with a left-to-right shunt; and (3) papillary muscle rupture (least common), resulting in the acute onset of severe mitral regurgitation. Acute free-wall ruptures usually are rapidly fatal and are the cause of death in 8 to 10% of patients with fatal acute transmural myocardial infarcts; repair is rarely possible.[39] Ruptures tend to occur relatively early following infarction with as many as 25% presenting within 24 hours (mean interval 4 to 5 days), most commonly through the lateral free wall. A pericardial adhesion that arrests the rapidly moving blood front and aborts a rupture may result in a contained rupture with a hematoma communicating with the ventricular cavity (*false aneurysm*); half of false aneurysms eventually rupture.

Postinfarction septal ruptures with acute ventricular septal defect complicate 1 to 2% of infarcts. They are of two types: (1) single or multiple sharply localized, jagged, linear passageways that connect the ventricular chambers (simple type), usually involving the anteroapical aspect of the septum; and (2) defects that tunnel serpiginously through the septum to a somewhat distant opening on the right side (complex type), usually involving the basal inferoseptal wall.[40] In complex lesions, the tract may extend into regions remote from the site of the infarct, such as the right ventricular free wall. Without surgery, the prognosis is poor for patients with infarct-related ventricular septal defects.

Papillary muscles are particularly vulnerable to ischemic injury and rupture, particularly the posterior medial papillary muscle. Papillary muscle rupture can occur later than other rupture syndromes (as late as 1 month after MI). Because tendinous cords arise from the heads of the papillary muscles and provide continuity with each of the valve leaflets, interference with the structure or function of either papillary muscle can result in dysfunction of both mitral valve leaflets.

Isolated right ventricular infarction is rare, but involvement of the right ventricle by extension of an inferoseptal infarct occurs in approximately 10% of transmural infarcts and can have important functional consequences, including right ventricular failure with or without tricuspid regurgitation and arrhythmias.

Infarct *extension* is characterized by incremental new or recurrent necrosis in the same distribution as a completed recent infarct. Extension most often occurs between 2 and 10 days after the original infarction, forms along the lateral and subepicardial borders of a recent infarct, and histologically appears younger than the previously necrotic myocardium. In contrast, infarct *expansion* is a disproportionate thinning and dilation of the infarcted region occurring through a combination of: (1) slippage between muscle bundles, reducing the number of myocytes across the infarct wall; (2) disruption of myocardial cells; and (3) tissue loss within the necrotic zone. Infarct expansion does not lead to additional necrotic myocardium per se, but may promote intracardiac mural thrombus formation. The increase in ventricular volume caused by regional dilation increases the wall stress and thereby the workload of noninfarcted myocardium. Infarct expansion is often the substrate for late aneurysm formation. Occurring in approximately 30% of transmural infarcts, infarct expansion increases morbidity and mortality.

Ventricular aneurysms are large scars that paradoxically bulge during ventricular systole and often result from a large transmural infarct that undergoes expansion (see Fig. 5-9D).[41] Although frequently as thin as 1 mm, ventricular aneurysms rarely rupture owing to their walls of tough fibrous or fibrocalcific tissue. Hypertrophied myocardial remnants as well as necrotic but inadequately healed myocardium often are present in aneurysm walls and mural thrombus is common. Some pharmacologic approaches to limiting infarct size, such as steroids and other anti-inflammatory agents, could exacerbate infarct expansion and aneurysm formation.

Ventricular remodeling comprises the collective structural changes that occur both in the necrotic zone and uninvolved areas of the heart, including left ventricular dilation, wall thinning by infarct expansion, compensatory hypertrophy of noninfarcted myocardium, and potentially late aneurysm formation.[42] Congestive heart failure secondary to coronary artery disease occurs when the overall function of viable myocardium can no longer maintain an adequate cardiac output or regions of hyperfunctioning residual myocardium suffer additional ischemic episodes.

Revascularization

The rationale for revascularization in early acute myocardial infarction is as follows: (1) prolonged thrombotic occlusion of a coronary artery causes transmural infarction; (2) the extent of necrosis during an evolving myocardial infarction progresses as a wavefront and becomes complete only 6 to 12 hours or more following coronary occlusion (see Fig. 5-6); (3) both early- and long-term mortality following acute myocardial infarction correlate strongly with the amount of residual functioning myocardium; and (4) early reperfusion rescues some jeopardized myocardium.[43] Thus, the benefits of thrombolytic therapy or early percutaneous coronary intervention depend on and are assessed by the amount of myocardium salvaged, recovery of left ventricular function, and resultant reduction in mortality. These clinical endpoints are largely determined by the time interval between onset of symptoms and a successful intervention adequacy of early coronary reflow, and the degree of residual stenosis of the infarct vessel. Spontaneous recanalization via endogenous thrombolysis can be beneficial to left ventricular function but occurs in fewer than 10% of patients within the critical interval.

Percutaneous Coronary Intervention

Percutaneous coronary intervention (PCI) is used in patients with stable angina, unstable angina, or acute myocardial infarction to restore blood flow through a diseased portion of the coronary circulation obstructed by atherosclerotic plaque and/or thrombotic deposits, and in obstructions in saphenous vein grafts, internal mammary artery grafts, and occasionally coronary arteries in transplanted hearts.

Percutaneous Transluminal Coronary Angioplasty. In percutaneous transluminal coronary angioplasty (PTCA), the plaque splits at its weakest point and enlargement of the lumen and increased blood flow occurs by plaque fracture (the predominant mechanism), and by embolization, compression, redistribution of the plaque contents, and overall mechanical expansion of the vessel wall.[44] The split extends at least to the intimal-medial border and often into the media, is accompanied by variable circumferential and longitudinal medial dissection, and can induce a flap that impinges on the lumen. These changes result in local flow abnormalities and generation of new, thrombogenic blood-contacting surfaces (to some extent similar to what is observed with spontaneously disrupted plaque). These changes contribute to the propensity for acute thrombotic closure that occurs in up to 5% of patients.

The long-term success of PTCA is limited by the development of progressive restenosis, which occurs in 30 to 50% of patients, most frequently within the first 4 to 6 months.[45] Although vessel wall recoil and organization of thrombus likely contribute, the major process leading to restenosis is excessive medial smooth muscle migration to the intima, proliferation and secretion of abundant extracellular matrix as an exaggerated response to angioplasty-induced injury.

Coronary atherectomy of primary or restenosis lesions mechanically removes obstructive tissue by excision. Deep arterial resection, including medial and even adventitial elements, occurs frequently but has not been associated with acute symptomatic complications. The morphology of arterial vessel healing after directional or rotational atherectomy is similar to that following angioplasty.

Stents. Stents are expandable tubes of metallic or polymeric mesh that are used to splint open the vessel wall at the site of balloon angioplasty and thereby mitigate the negative sequelae of PTCA.[46] Stents preserve luminal patency and provide a larger and more regular lumen by acting as a scaffold to support the disrupted vascular wall and minimize flow disruption and flow disruption and thrombus formation. Stenting has been shown to be superior to angioplasty alone in vessels greater than 3 mm in diameter, chronic total occlusions, stenotic vein grafts, restenotic lesions after angioplasty alone, and patients with myocardial infarction.[47]

Stent technology has undergone a rapid evolution, including sequentially: (1) bare-metal stents (BMS); and (2) drug-eluting stents (DES), both used extensively in clinical interventional cardiology; and more recently, (3) completely resorbable/biodegradable stents (RBS), which are presently in preclinical development and clinical trials. Bare-metal stents for coronary implantation are short tubular segments of metal mesh composed of balloon-expandable 316L stainless steel or nickel-titanium alloy (Nitinol) that range from approximately 2.5 to 3.5 mm in diameter and approximately 1 to 3 cm in length. Development has focused on permitting stents to become more flexible and more easily delivered and deployed, allowing the treatment of a greater number and variety of lesions.

Key stent complications are thrombosis, usually occurring early, and late proliferative restenosis (Fig. 5-10). Thrombotic occlusion, occurring in 1 to 3% of patients within 7 to 10 days of the procedure (see Fig. 5-10A), has largely been overcome by aggressive multidrug treatment with antiplatelet agents such as clopidogrel, aspirin, and glycoprotein IIb/IIIa inhibitors. The major long-term complication of bare-metal stenting is in-stent

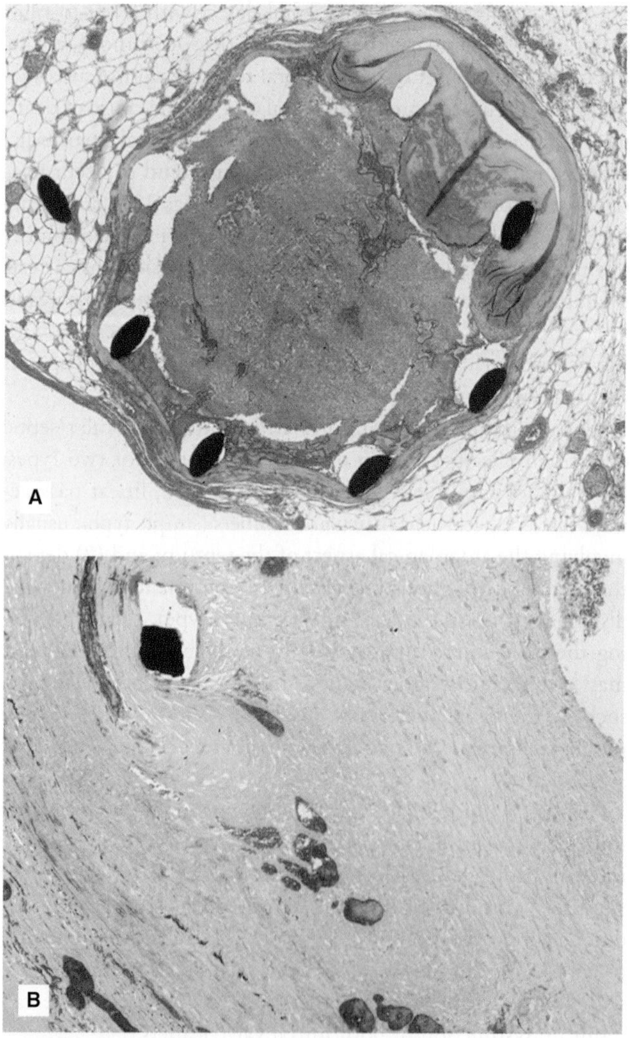

FIGURE 5-10 Stent pathology. (A) Thrombosis. H & E stain. (B) Thickened proliferative neointima separating the stent wires (*black structure*) from the lumen, with bare metal coronary artery stent implanted long term. Movat stain. (*[B] Reproduced with permission from Schoen FJ, Edwards WD: Pathology of cardiovascular interventions including endovascular therapies, revascularization, vascular replacement, cardiac assist/replacement, arrhythmia control, and repaired congenital heart disease, in Silver MD, Gotlieb AI, Schoen FJ [eds]: Cardiovascular Pathology, 3rd ed. Philadelphia, Churchill Livingstone, 2001; p 678.*)

restenosis, which occurs in 50% of patients within 6 months.[48] The causes of stent thrombosis and restenosis are complex and are largely owing to stent-tissue interactions, including inflammation, which may interfere with healing and re-endothelialization.[49] Damage to the endothelial lining and stretching of the vessel wall stimulate adherence and accumulation of platelets, fibrin, and leukocytes. Stent wires may eventually become completely embedded in an endothelium-lined intimal fibrosis layer composed of smooth muscle cells in a collagen matrix (see Fig. 5-10B). This tissue may thicken secondary to the release of growth factors, chemotactic factors, and inflammatory mediators from platelets and other inflammatory cells that result in increased migration and proliferation of smooth muscle cells, and increased production of extracellular matrix molecules, narrowing the lumen and resulting in restenosis.

DES effectively inhibit in-stent restenosis.[50,51] The drugs used most widely are rapamycin (sirolimus)[52] and paclitaxel[53] in the Cypher (Cordis) and Taxus (Boston Scientific) stents, respectively. Rapamycin, a drug used for immunosuppression in solid organ transplant recipients, inhibits proliferation, migration, and growth of smooth muscle cells and extracellular matrix synthesis. Paclitaxel, a drug used in the chemotherapeutic regimens for several types of cancer, also has similar anti–smooth muscle cell activities. These drugs are embedded in a polymer matrix (such as a copolymer of poly-*n*-butyl methacrylate and polyethylene–vinyl acetate or a gelatin-chondroitin sulfate coacervate film) that is coated onto the stent.

Data from recent studies suggest a small but significant increased risk of late (>1 year postimplantation) stent thrombosis causing myocardial infarction and/or sudden death in patients who have DES.[54] The significance and causes of later stent thrombosis are subjects of active controversy and investigation. However, animal studies and some clinical data suggest that late stent thrombosis may be related to DES-induced inhibition of stent endothelialization.

RBS ultimately resorb and facilitate removal of foreign material that may potentiate a thrombotic event, permit more versatility in subsequent therapies, and do not interfere with the diagnostic evaluation by noninvasive imaging such as cardiac magnetic resonance and CT. Several RBS are in development or in clinical trials. The key challenge is to achieve an optimal practical balance among biocompatibility, and control the kinetics of stent degradation at a rate appropriate to maintain mechanical strength to limit recoil.[55]

Coronary Artery Bypass Graft Surgery

Coronary artery bypass graft (CABG) surgery improves survival in patients with significant left main coronary artery disease, three-vessel (and possibly two-vessel) disease, or reduced ventricular function, and prolongs and improves the quality of life in patients with left main equivalent disease (proximal left anterior descending and proximal left circumflex), but does not protect them from the risk of subsequent myocardial infarction.[56] The principal mechanism for these benefits is thought to be the restoration of blood flow to hibernating myocardium.

The hospital mortality rate for CABG surgery is approximately 1% in low-risk patients, with fewer than 3% of patients suffering perioperative myocardial infarction. The most consistent predictors of mortality after CABG are urgency of operation, age, prior cardiac surgery, female gender, low left ventricular ejection fraction, degree of left main stenosis, and number of vessels with significant stenoses. The most common mode of early death after CABG is acute cardiac failure leading to low output or arrhythmias, owing to myocardial necrosis (often with features of reperfusion described in the preceding), postischemic dysfunction of viable myocardium, or a metabolic cause, such as hypokalemia. As in cardiac surgery in general, the risk of perioperative myocardial infarction increases with the degree of cardiomegaly, and in patients who have had preoperative infarction.

Early thrombotic occlusion of the graft vessel may occur, usually potentiated by inadequate distal run-off from extremely small and/or atherosclerotic distal native coronaries. Additional factors may include dissection of blood into the graft or native vessel at the anastomotic site, atherosclerosis or arterial branching at the anastomotic site, or distortion of a graft that is too short or too long for the intended bypass. In some cases, thrombosis occurring early postoperatively involves only the distal portion of the graft, suggesting that early graft thrombosis was initiated at the distal anastomosis. Most patients who die early after CABG have patent grafts.

The patency of saphenous vein grafts is reported as 60% at 10 years; occlusion results from (with increasing postoperative interval) thrombosis, progressive intimal thickening, and/or obstructive atherosclerosis.[57] Between 1 month and approximately 1 year, graft stenosis is usually caused by intimal hyperplasia with excessive smooth muscle proliferation and extracellular matrix production (similar to that seen in restenosis following angioplasty and stenting). Atherosclerosis becomes the predominant mechanism in graft occlusion beyond 1 to 3 years after CABG, and earliest in those patients with the most significant atherosclerotic risk factors. Plaques in grafts often have poorly developed fibrous caps with large necrotic cores, and can develop secondary dystrophic calcific deposits that extend to the lumen (Fig. 5-11); thus, the potential for disruption, aneurysmal dilation and embolization of atherosclerotic lesions in vein grafts exceeds that for native coronary atherosclerotic lesions, and balloon angioplasty, stenting or intraoperative manipulation of grafts may potentiate atheroembolism.

In contrast to saphenous vein grafts, internal mammary artery (IMA) grafts have greater than 90% patency at 10 years (Fig. 5-12).[58] Multiple factors likely contribute to the remarkably higher long-term patency of IMA grafts compared with vein grafts. Although free saphenous vein grafts sustain disruption of their vasa vasora and nerves, endothelial damage, medial ischemia, and acutely increased internal pressure, an internal mammary artery graft generally has minimal preexisting atherosclerosis and requires minimal surgical manipulation, maintains its nutrient blood supply, is adapted to arterial pressures, needs no proximal anastomosis, and has an artery-to-artery distal anastomosis. Graft and recipient vessel have comparable sizes with the internal mammary artery but are disparate (graft

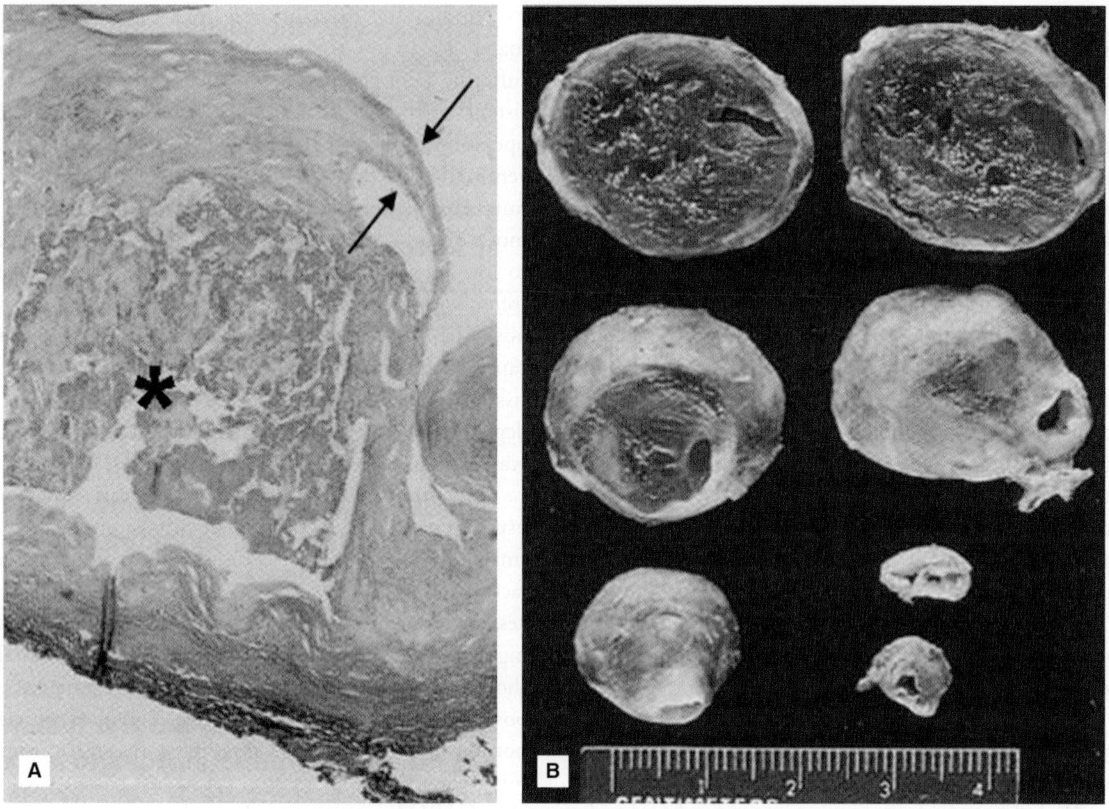

FIGURE 5-11 Atherosclerosis of saphenous vein bypass graft. (A) Fibrous cap (*between arrows*) is attenuated over the necrotic core (*large asterisk*). Lumen is at upper right. (B) Saphenous vein graft aneurysm. Hematoxylin and eosin (A) 100×; Gross photo. ([*A*] *Reproduced with permission from Schoen FJ: Interventional and Surgical Cardiovascular Pathology: Clinical Correlations and Basic Principles. Philadelphia, WB Saunders, 1989.*) Verhoff von Giesen stain (for elastin) 10×. ([*B*] *Reproduced with permission from Liang BT, Antman EM, Taus R, et al [eds]: Atherosclerotic aneurysms of aortocoronary vein grafts. Am J Cardiol 1988; 61:185.*)

substantially larger) with saphenous vein. Radial and gastroepiploic arteries are occasionally used successfully. The advent of off-pump and minimally invasive coronary artery bypass grafting has stimulated efforts to facilitate sutureless anastomosis of the graft to the aorta.[59]

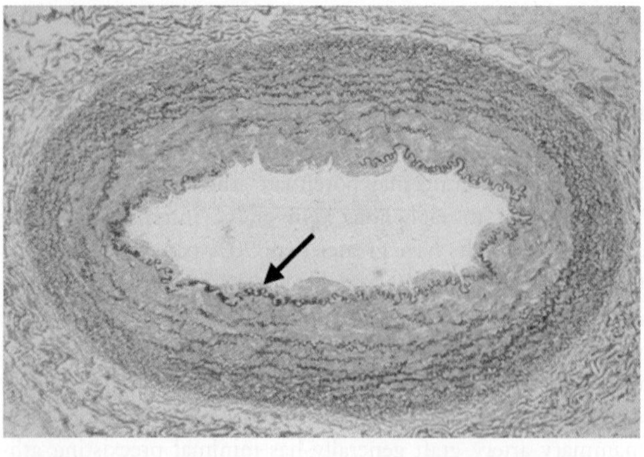

FIGURE 5-12 Internal mammary artery as coronary artery bypass graft removed 13 years following surgery, demonstrating near-normal morphology, including an intact internal elastic lamina (*arrow*) Verhoff von Giesen stain (for elastin, *black*) 60×. (*Reproduced with permission from Schoen FJ: Interventional and Surgical Cardiovascular Pathology: Clinical Correlations and Basic Principles. Philadelphia, WB Saunders, 1989.*)

VALVULAR HEART DISEASE

Structure-Function Correlations in Normal Valves

Normal valve function requires structural integrity and coordinated interactions among multiple anatomical components. For the atrioventricular valves (mitral and tricuspid), these elements include leaflets, commissures, annulus, tendinous cords (chordae tendineae), papillary muscles, and the atrial and ventricular myocardium. For the semilunar valves (aortic and pulmonary), the key structures are the cusps, commissures, and their respective supporting structures in the aortic and pulmonary roots.

The anatomy of the mitral and aortic valves is illustrated in Fig. 5-13.

Mitral Valve

Of the two leaflets of the mitral valve (see Fig. 5-13A), the anterior (also called septal, or aortic) leaflet is roughly triangular and deep, with the base inserting on approximately one-third of the annulus. The posterior (also called mural, or ventricular) leaflet, although more shallow, is attached to about two-thirds of the annulus and typically has a scalloped appearance. The mitral leaflets have a combined area approximately twice that of the annulus; they meet during systole with apposition to approximately 50% of the depth of the posterior leaflet and

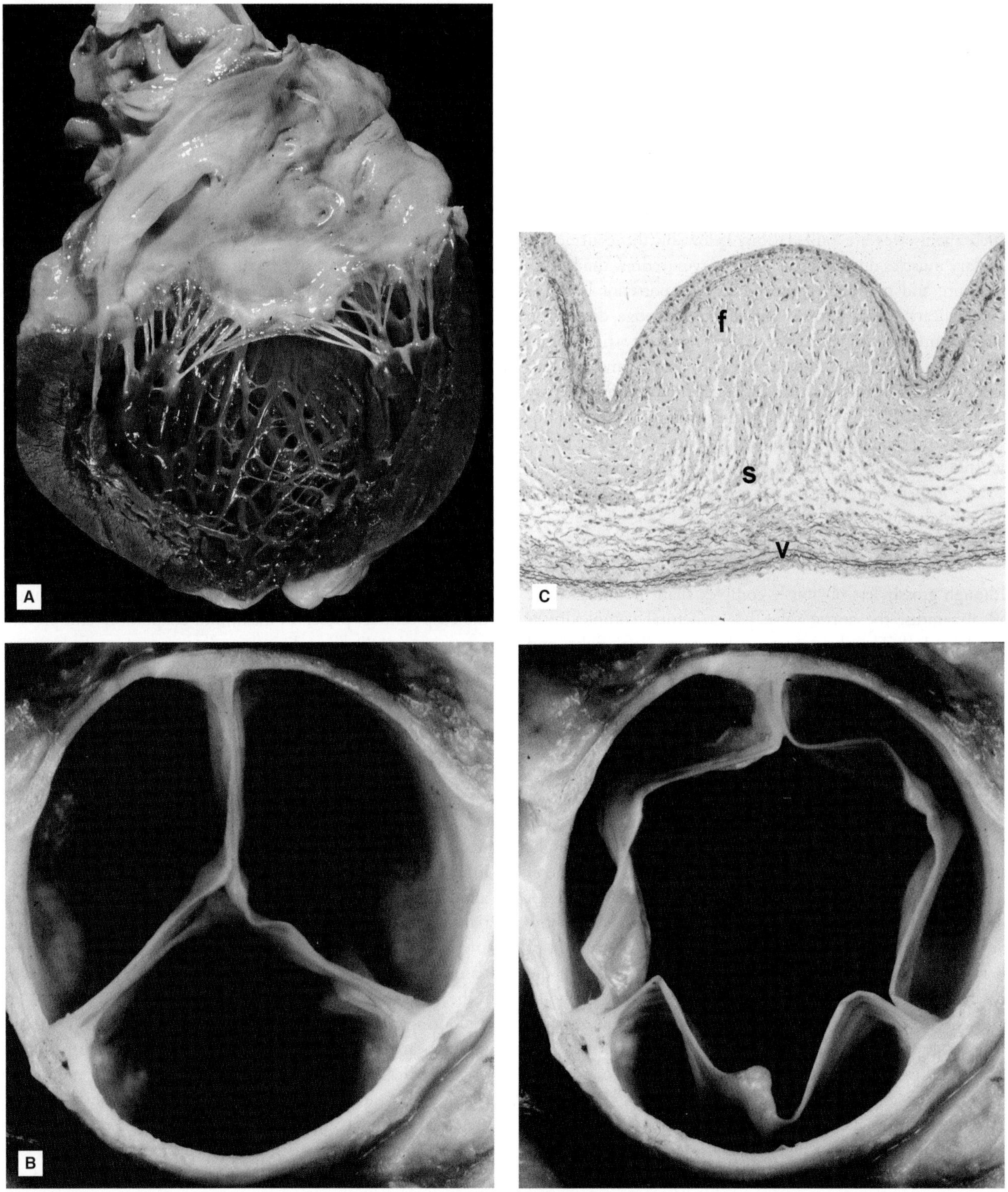

FIGURE 5-13 Normal mitral and aortic valves. In (A), opened left ventricle of the normal heart, demonstrating mitral valve and components of the mitral apparatus. (B) Aortic valve viewed from distal aspect in open (*right*) and closed (*left*) phases. (C) Normal aortic valve histology, demonstrating layered structure, including the fibrosa (f) spongiosa (s), and ventricularis (*v*) layers. The inflow surface is at bottom. Verhoeff van Giesen (stain for elastin, *black*) 150×. (*[A] Reproduced with permission from Schoen FJ: Interventional and Surgical Cardiovascular Pathology: Clinical Correlations and Basic Principles. Philadelphia, WB Saunders, 1989. [B and C] Reproduced with permission from Schoen FJ, Edwards WD: Valvular heart disease: general principles and stenosis, in Silver MD, Gotlieb AI, Schoen FJ [eds]: Cardiovascular Pathology, 3rd ed. New York, Churchill Livingstone, 2001; p 402.*)

30% that of the anterior leaflet. Each leaflet receives tendinous cords from both anterior and posterior papillary muscles. The mitral valve orifice is D-shaped, with the flat anteromedial portion comprising the attachment of the anterior mitral leaflet in the subaortic region. This part of the annulus is fibrous and noncontractile; the posterolateral portion of the annulus is muscular and contracts during systole to asymmetrically reduce the area of the orifice. The edges of the mitral leaflets are held in or below the plane of the orifice by the tendinous cords, which themselves are pulled from below by the contracting papillary muscles during systole. This serves to draw the leaflets to closure and maintain competence. The posterior leaflet is more delicate, has a shorter annulus-to-free-edge dimension than the anterior, and is therefore more prone to postinflammatory fibrous retraction and deformation owing to myxomatous degeneration. The posterior leaflet has distinct scallops that are designated P1, P2, P3, respectively, beginning from the anterolateral toward the posteromedial commissure. The orifice of the tricuspid valve is larger and less distinct than that of the mitral; its three leaflets (anterior, posterior, and septal) are larger and thinner than those of the mitral valve.

Aortic Valve

Although grossly less obviously complex than the mitral valve and apparatus, the aortic valve has structural complexity at several levels.[60] The three aortic valve cusps (left, right, and noncoronary) attach to the aortic wall in a semilunar fashion, ascending to the commissures and descending to the base of each cusp (see Fig. 5-13B). Commissures are spaced approximately 120 degrees apart and occupy the three points of the annular crown, representing the site of separation between adjacent cusps. Behind the valve cusps are dilated pockets of aortic root, called the sinuses of Valsalva. The right and left coronary arteries arise from individual orifices behind the right and left cusps, respectively. At the midpoint of the free edge of each cusp is a fibrous nodule called the nodule of Arantius. A thin, crescent-shaped portion of the cusp on either side of the nodule, termed the lunula, defines the surface of apposition of the cusps when the valve is closed (approximately 40% of the cuspal area). Fenestrations (holes) near the free edges commonly occur as a developmental or degenerative abnormality, are generally small (<2 mm in diameter), and have no functional significance, because the lunular tissue does not contribute to separate aortic from ventricular blood during diastole. In contrast, defects in the portion of the cusp below the lunula are associated with functional incompetence; such holes also suggest previous or active infection. When the aortic valve is closed during diastole, there is a back pressure on the cusps of approximately 80 mm Hg. The pulmonary valve cusps and surrounding tissues have architectural similarity to but are more delicate than those of the corresponding aortic components, and lack coronary arterial origins.

All four cardiac valves essentially have the same microscopically inhomogeneous architecture, consisting of well-defined tissue layers, covered by endothelium. Using the aortic valve as the paradigm (see Fig. 5-13C), the *ventricularis* faces the left ventricular chamber, and is enriched in radially aligned elastic fibers, which enable the cusps to have minimal surface area when the valve is open but stretch during diastole to form a large coaptation area. The *spongiosa* is centrally located and is composed of loosely arranged collagen and abundant proteoglycans. This layer has negligible structural strength, but accommodates relative movement between layers during the cardiac cycle and absorbs shock during closure. The *fibrosa* provides structural integrity and mechanical stability through a dense aggregate of circumferentially aligned, densely packed collagen fibers, largely arranged parallel to the cuspal free edge. Normal human aortic and pulmonary valve cusps have few blood vessels; they are sufficiently thin to be perfused from the surrounding blood. In contrast, the mitral and tricuspid leaflets contain a few capillaries in their most basal thirds.

With specializations that include crimp of collagen fibers along their length, bundles of collagen in the fibrous layer oriented toward the commissures, and grossly visible corrugations, cusps are extremely soft and pliable when unloaded, but taut and stiff during the closed phase. Moreover, the orientation of connective tissue and other architectural elements is nonrandom in the plane of the cusp, yielding greater compliance in the radial than circumferential direction. The fibrous network within the cusps effectively transfers the stresses of the closed phase to the annulus and aortic wall. This minimizes sagging of the cusp centers, preserves maximum coaptation, and prevents regurgitation. During diastole, adjacent cusps of the aortic valve coapt over a substantial area (as much as one-third of the cuspal area). For the mitral valve, the subvalvular apparatus including tendinous cords and papillary muscles is the critical mechanism of valve competency.

Valvular Cell Biology

Recent studies have fostered an emerging picture of how valves form embryologically, mature in the fetus, and function, adapt, maintain homeostasis, and change throughout life. These essential relationships facilitate an understanding of valve pathology and mechanisms of disease, foster the development of improved tissue heart valve substitutes, and inform innovative approaches to heart valve repair and regeneration.[61]

During normal development of the heart, the heart tube undergoes looping, following which the valve cusps/leaflets originate from mesenchymal outgrowths known as endocardial cushions.[62] A subset of endothelial cells in the cushion-forming area, driven by a complex array of signals from the underlying myocardium, changes their phenotype to mesenchymal cells and migrates into the acellular extracellular matrix called cardiac jelly. Likely regulated by TGFβ and VEGF, the transformation of endocardial cells to mesenchymal cells is termed transdifferentiation or endothelial-to-mesenchymal transformation (EMT).

Subsequent to morphogenesis, embryonic fetal valves possess a dynamic structure composed of a nascent ECM and cells with characteristics of myofibroblasts.[63] Changes in cell phenotype and ECM remodeling continue throughout human fetal and postnatal development, and throughout life, leading to ongoing changes in properties, as evidenced by increasing valve stiffness with increasing age.[64]

Two types of cells are present in the fully formed aortic valve: endothelial cells located superficially and interstitial cells located deep to the surface. Aortic valve endothelial cells (VEC) have a different phenotype than those in the adjacent aorta and elsewhere,[65,66] but the implications of these differences are not yet known. The second cell type comprises the valvular interstitial cells (VICs). VICs have variable properties of fibroblasts, smooth muscle cells, and myofibroblasts; they maintain the valvular extracellular matrix, the key determinant of valve durability. To maintain integrity and pliability throughout life, the valve cusps and leaflets must undergo ongoing physiologic remodeling that entails synthesis, degradation and reorganization of its ECM, which depends on matrix degrading enzymes such as matrix metalloproteinases (MMPs). Although VIC are predominantly fibroblast-like in normal valves, VIC can become activated when exposed to environmental (ie, mechanical and chemical) stimulation. Activated VIC assume a myofibroblast-like phenotype and mediate connective tissue remodeling.

Pathologic Anatomy of Valvular Heart Disease

Cardiac valve operations utilizing replacement or repair usually are undertaken for dysfunction caused by calcification, fibrosis, fusion, retraction, perforation, rupture, stretching, infection, dilation, or congenital malformations of the valve leaflets/cusps or associated structures. Valvular stenosis, defined as inhibition of forward flow secondary to obstruction caused by failure of a valve to open completely, is almost always caused by a primary cuspal abnormality and is caused by a chronic disease process. In contrast, valvular insufficiency, defined as reverse flow caused by failure of a valve to close completely, may result from either intrinsic disease of the valve cusps or from damage to or distortion of the supporting structures (eg, the aorta, mitral annulus, chordae tendineae, papillary muscles, and ventricular free wall) without primary cuspal pathology. Regurgitation may appear either acutely, as with rupture of cords, or chronically, as with leaflet scarring and retraction. Both stenosis and insufficiency can coexist in a single valve. The most commonly encountered types of valvular heart disease are illustrated in Figs. 5-14 and 5-15.

Calcific Aortic Valve Stenosis

Calcific aortic stenosis (AS), the most frequent valvular abnormality requiring surgery, is usually the consequence of calcium phosphate deposition in either an anatomically normal aortic valve or in a congenitally bicuspid valve (see Fig. 5-14A,B).[67] Stenotic, previously normal tricuspid valves present primarily in the seventh to ninth decades of life, while bicuspid valves with superimposed calcification generally become symptomatic earlier (usually sixth to seventh decades).[68]

Calcific aortic stenosis is characterized by heaped-up, calcified masses initiated in the cuspal fibrosa at the points of maximal cusp flexion (the margins of attachment); they protrude distally from the aortic aspect into the sinuses of Valsalva, inhibiting cuspal opening. However, although the ventricular surfaces of the cusps usually remain smooth, the calfic depoosits often extend close to ventricular surface (see Fig. 5-14C). The calcification process generally does not involve the free cuspal edges, appreciable commissural fusion is absent, and the mitral valve generally is uninvolved. Calcified material resembling bone is often present (see Fig. 5-14D). Aortic valve *sclerosis* comprises a common, earlier, and hemodynamically less significant stage of the calcification process. Nevertheless, aortic sclerosis is associated with an increase of approximately 50% in the risk of death from cardiovascular causes and the risk of myocardial infarction, even in the absence of hemodynamically significant obstruction of left ventricular outflow.[69]

Aortic stenosis induces a pressure gradient across the valve, which may reach 75 to 100 mg Hg in severe cases, necessitating a left ventricular pressure of 200 mg Hg or more to expel blood. Cardiac output is maintained by the development of concentric

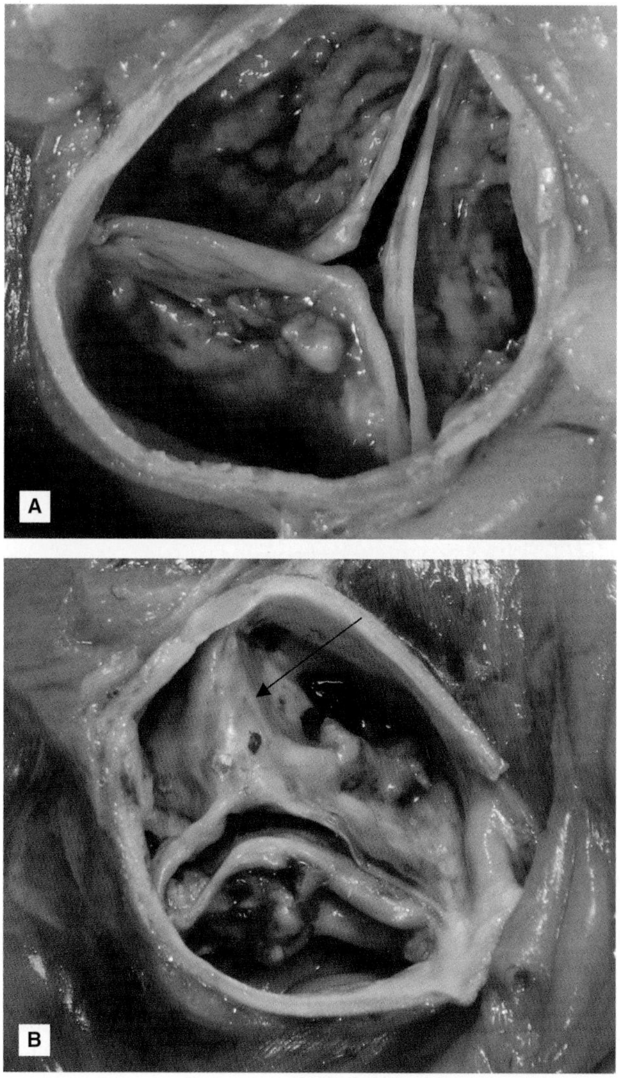

FIGURE 5-14 Calcific aortic valve stenosis. (A) Calcific aortic valve disease causing aortic stenosis in an elderly patient, characterized by mineral deposits at basal aspect of cusps. (B) Calcification of congenitally bicuspid aortic valve, having two unequal cusps, the larger with a central raphe (*arrow*). (C and *D*) Photomicrographs of calcific deposits in calcific aortic valve disease. Hematoxylin and eosin 15×.

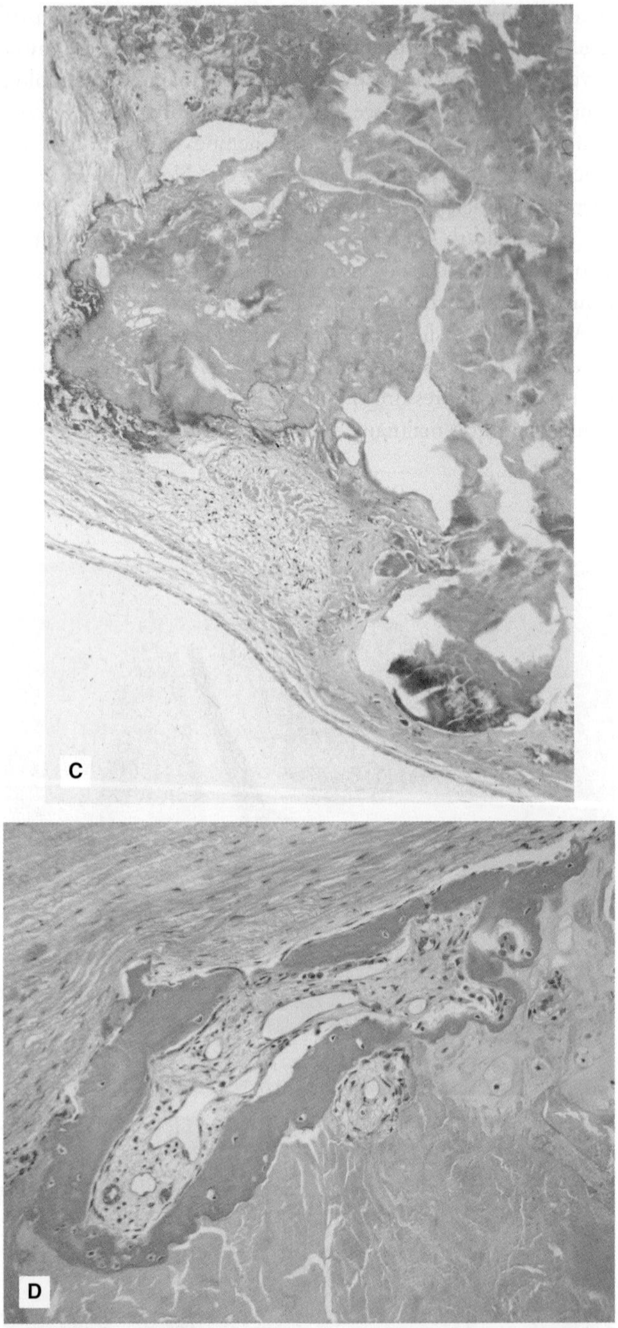

FIGURE 5-14 (*Continued*). Calcific aortic valve stenosis. (**C**) Nearly transmural deposits with only thin uninvolved cusp on inflow surface (at bottom). (**D**) Bone formation (osseous metaplasia).

left ventricular hypertrophy secondary to the pressure overload. The onset of symptoms such as angina, syncope, or heart failure in aortic stenosis heralds the exhaustion of compensatory cardiac hyperfunction, and carries a poor prognosis if not treated by aortic valve replacement. Other complications of calcific aortic stenosis include embolization that may occur spontaneously or during interventional procedures, hemolysis, infective endocarditis, and extension of the calcific deposits into the ventricular septum causing conduction abnormalities.

Aortic valve calcification has been traditionally considered a degenerative, dystrophic, and passive process. However, recent studies suggest active regulation of calcification in aortic valves similar in some respects to that in the atherosclerotic process in arteries, with mechanisms that include inflammation, lipid infiltration, and phenotypic modulation of VIC to an osteoblastic phenotype,[70] and overlapping risk factors. Similarities to atherosclerosis have stimulated interest in the possibility that statin drugs may decrease the rate of aortic stenosis progression; however, benefit of statins for AS has not been supported by clinical studies.[71]

Congenitally Bicuspid Aortic Valve

With a prevalence of approximately 1%, bicuspid aortic valve (BAV) is a frequent abnormality.[72] The two cusps are typically of unequal size, with the larger (conjoined) cusp having a midline raphe, representing an incomplete separation or congenital fusion of two cusps. Less frequently, the cusps are of equal size (see Fig. 5-14B). Neither stenotic nor symptomatic at birth or throughout early life, BAV are predisposed to accelerated calcification; ultimately, almost all become stenotic. Aortic pathology, including dilation and/or dissection, commonly accompanies BAV. BAV and other congenital valve abnormalities underlie over two-thirds of aortic stenosis in children and almost 50% in adults. Infrequently, they become purely incompetent, or complicated by infective endocarditis, even when the valve is hemodynamically normal. Only rarely is an uncomplicated BAV encountered incidentally at autopsy.

Recent studies have confirmed previous reports of familial clustering of BAV and left ventricular outflow tract obstruction malformations, and their association with other cardiovascular malformations.[73] For example, mutations in the signaling and transcriptional regulator NOTCH1 caused a spectrum of developmental aortic valve abnormalities and severe calcification in two families with nonsyndromic familial aortic valve disease.[74]

Mitral Annular Calcification

Calcific deposits also can develop in the ring (annulus) of the mitral valve of elderly individuals, especially women. Although generally asymptomatic, the calcific nodules may lead to regurgitation by interference with systolic contraction of the mitral valve ring or, very rarely, stenosis by impairing mobility of the mitral leaflets during opening. Occasionally, the calcium deposits may penetrate sufficiently deeply to impinge on the atrioventricular conduction system to produce arrhythmias (and rarely sudden death). Patients with mitral annular calcification have an increased risk of stroke, and the calcific nodules, especially if ulcerated, can be the nidus for thrombotic deposits or infective endocarditis.

Rheumatic Heart Disease

Rheumatic fever is an acute, often recurrent, inflammatory disease that generally follows a pharyngeal infection with group A beta-hemolytic streptococci, principally in children. In the past several decades, rheumatic fever and rheumatic heart disease have declined markedly but not disappeared in the United States and other developed countries. Evidence strongly suggests that rheumatic fever is the result of an immune response to streptococcal antigens, inciting either a cross-reaction to tissue antigens, or a streptococcal-induced autoimmune reaction to normal tissue antigens.[75]

Chronic rheumatic heart disease most frequently affects the mitral and to a lesser extent the aortic and/or the tricuspid

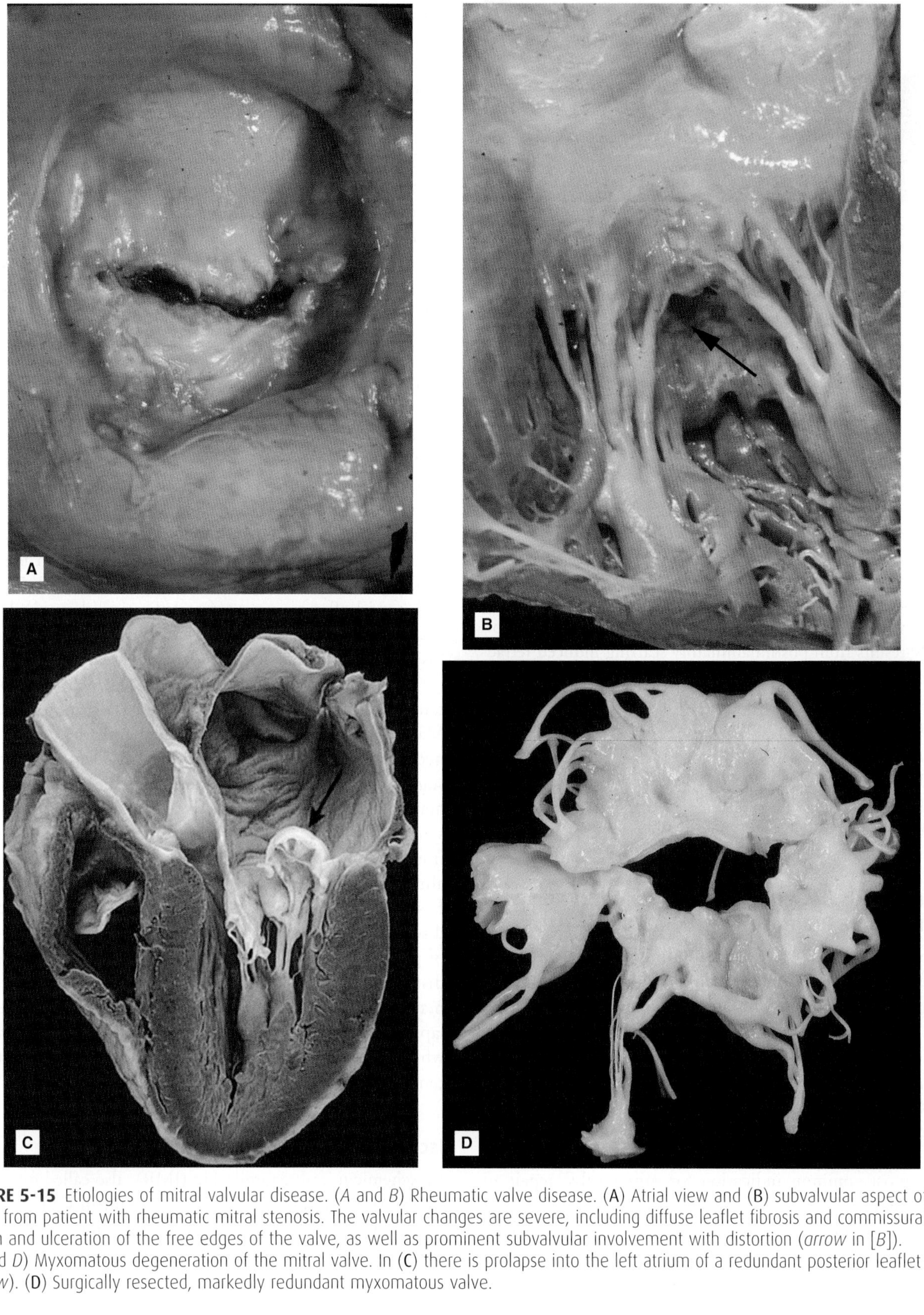

FIGURE 5-15 Etiologies of mitral valvular disease. (*A* and *B*) Rheumatic valve disease. (A) Atrial view and (B) subvalvular aspect of valve from patient with rheumatic mitral stenosis. The valvular changes are severe, including diffuse leaflet fibrosis and commissural fusion and ulceration of the free edges of the valve, as well as prominent subvalvular involvement with distortion (*arrow* in [*B*]). (*C* and *D*) Myxomatous degeneration of the mitral valve. In (C) there is prolapse into the left atrium of a redundant posterior leaflet (*arrow*). (D) Surgically resected, markedly redundant myxomatous valve.

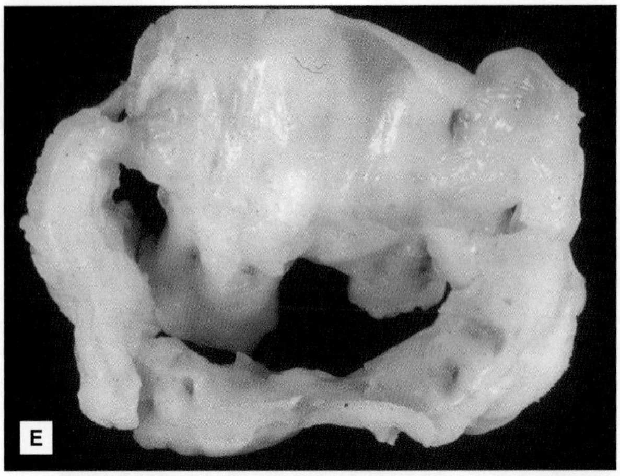

FIGURE 5-15 *(Continued)*. Etiologies of mitral valvular disease. (E) Mitral valve lesion associated with the diet medication Phen-Fen. *([A and B] Reproduced with permission from Schoen FJ: Interventional and Surgical Cardiovascular Pathology: Clinical Correlations and Basic Principles. Philadelphia, WB Saunders, 1989. [E] Reproduced with permission from Schoen FJ, Edwards WD: Valvular heart disease: general principles and stenosis, in Silver MD, Gotlieb AI, Schoen FJ [eds]: Cardiovascular Pathology, 3rd ed. New York, Churchill Livingstone, 2001; p 402.)*

valves. Usually dominated by mitral stenosis,[76] chronic rheumatic valve disease is characterized by fibrous or fibrocalcific thickening of leaflets and tendinous cords, and commissural and chordal fusion (see Fig. 5-15A and B). Stenosis results from leaflet and chordal fibrous thickening and commissural fusion, with or without secondary calcification. Regurgitation usually results from postinflammatory scarring-induced retraction of cords and leaflets. Combinations of lesions may yield valves that are both stenotic and regurgitant. Although considered the pathognomonic inflammatory myocardial lesions in acute rheumatic fever, Aschoff nodules are found infrequently in myocardium sampled at autopsy or at valve replacement surgery, most likely reflecting the extended interval from acute disease to critical functional impairment.

Myxomatous Degeneration of the Mitral Valve (Mitral Valve Prolapse)

Myxomatous mitral valve disease (mitral valve prolapse) causes chronic, pure, isolated mitral regurgitation.[77] Owing to improved imaging technology and large community studies, a prevalence of mitral valve prolapse of approximately 2% has been established with a rate of the serious complications, including heart failure, mitral regurgitation, infective endocarditis, stroke, or other manifestation of thromboembolism, progressive congestive heart failure, sudden death, or atrial fibrillation of approximately 3%. Mitral valve prolapse is the most common indication for mitral valve repair or replacement.

In mitral valve prolapse (MVP), one or both mitral leaflets are enlarged, redundant, or floppy and will prolapse, or balloon back into the left atrium during ventricular systole (see Fig. 5-15C). The three characteristic anatomic changes in mitral valve prolapse are: (1) intercordal ballooning (hooding) of the mitral leaflets or portions thereof (most frequently involving the posterior leaflet), sometimes accompanied by elongated, thinned, or ruptured cords; (2) rubbery diffuse leaflet thickening that hinders adequate coaptation and interdigitation of leaflet tissue during valve closure; and (3) annular dilation, with diameters and circumferences that may exceed 3.5 and 11.0 cm, respectively (see Fig. 5-15D). Pathologic mitral annular enlargement predominates in and may be confined to the posterior leaflet, because the anterior leaflet is firmly anchored by the fibrous tissue at the aortic valve and is far less distensible. The key microscopic changes in myxomatous degeneration are attenuation or focal disruption of the fibrous layer of the valve, on which the structural integrity of the leaflet depends, and focal or diffuse thickening of the spongy layer by proteoglycan deposition (which gives the tissue an edematous, blue appearance on microscopy called *myxomatous* by pathologists).[78] These changes in tissue structure and composition weaken the leaflet. Concomitant involvement of the tricuspid valve is present in 20 to 40% of cases, and the aortic and pulmonary valves also may be affected.

Secondary changes may occur, including: (1) fibrous thickening along both surfaces of the valve leaflets; (2) linear thickening of the subjacent mural endocardium of the left ventricle as a consequence of friction-induced injury by cordal hamstringing of the prolapsing leaflets; (3) thrombi on the atrial surfaces of the leaflets, particularly in the recesses behind the ballooned leaflet segments; (4) calcification along the base of the posterior mitral leaflet; and (5) cordal thickening and fusion that can resemble postrheumatic disease.

The pathogenesis of myxomatous degeneration is uncertain, but this valvular abnormality is a common feature of Marfan's syndrome and occasionally other hereditary connective tissue disorders such as Ehlers-Danlos syndrome, suggesting an analogous connective tissue defect. In these heritable disorders of connective tissue, including Marfan's syndrome, MVP is usually associated with mutations in fibrillin-1 (FBN-1); recent evidence also has implicated abnormal TGF-β signaling (similar to the aortic abnormalities in the pathogenesis of Marfan's syndrome and related disorders).[79] Although it is unlikely that more than 1 to 2% of patients with MVP have an identifiable connective tissue disorder, studies utilizing genetic linkage analysis have mapped families with autosomal dominant mitral valve prolapse to specific chromosomal abnormalities, several of which involve genes that could be involved in valvular tissue remodeling.

Ischemic Mitral Regurgitation

In ischemic mitral regurgitation (IMR), also called functional mitral regurgitation, the leaflets are intrinsically normal, whereas myocardial structure and function are altered by ischemic injury.[80] Present in 10 to 20% of patients with coronary artery disease, IMR worsens prognosis following myocardial infarction, with reduced survival directly related to the severity of the regurgitation. Mechanisms of IMR include an ischemic papillary muscle that fails to tighten the cords during systole, and fibrotic, shortened papillary muscle that fixes the chordae deeply within the ventricle. Nevertheless, papillary muscle dysfunction alone is generally insufficient to produce IMR, and regional dysfunction and dilation with an increasing spherical shape of the LV, which pulls the papillary muscles down and away from the center of the chamber, usually contributes. There is substantial interest in developing surgical and/or percutaneous approaches to the repair of ischemic mitral regurgitation.[81]

Carcinoid and Drug-Induced Valve Disease

Patients with the carcinoid syndrome often develop plaquelike intimal thickenings of the endocardium of the tricuspid valve, right ventricular outflow tract, and pulmonary valve superimposed on otherwise unaltered endocardium.[82] The left side of the heart is usually unaffected. These lesions are related to elaboration by carcinoid tumors (most often primarily in the gut) of bioactive products, including serotonin, which cause valvular endothelial cell proliferation but are inactivated by passage through the lung.

Left-sided but similar valve lesions, have been reported to complicate the administration of fenfluramine and phentermine (fen-phen), appetite suppressants used for the treatment of obesity, which may affect systemic serotonin metabolism (see Fig. 5-15E).[83] Typical diet drug-associated plaques have proliferation of myofibroblast-like cells in a myxoid stroma. Similar left-sided plaques may be found in patients who receive methysergide or ergotamine therapy for migraine headaches; these serotonin analogs are metabolized to serotonin as they pass through the pulmonary vasculature. Moreover, drug-related valve disease has been reported in patients taking pergolide mesylate, an ergot-derived dopamine receptor agonist used to treat Parkinson's disease and restless leg syndrome.[84]

Infective Endocarditis

Infective endocarditis is characterized by colonization or invasion of the heart valves, mural endocardium, aorta, aneurysmal sacs, or other blood vessels, by a microbiologic agent, leading to the formation of friable vegetations laden with organisms (Fig. 5-16).[85] Although virtually any type of microbiologic agent can cause infective endocarditis, most cases are bacterial.

The clinical classification into acute and subacute forms is based on the range of severity of the disease and its tempo, on the virulence of the infecting microorganism, and presence of underlying cardiac disease. *Acute endocarditis* is a destructive infection by a highly virulent organism, often involving a previously normal heart valve and leading to death within days to weeks in more than 50% of patients if left untreated. In contrast, in a more indolent lesion, called *subacute endocarditis,* organisms of low virulence cause infection on previously deformed valves; in this situation, the infection may pursue a protracted course of weeks to months during which the infection may be undetected and untreated.

The modified Duke criteria provide a standardized assessment of patients with suspected infective endocarditis that integrates factors predisposing patients to the development of infective endocarditis, blood-culture evidence of infection, echocardiographic findings, and clinical and laboratory information.[86] The previously important clinical findings of petechiae, subungual hemorrhages, Janeway's lesions, Osler's nodes, and Roth's spots in the eyes (secondary to retinal microemboli) have now become uncommon owing to the shortened clinical course of the disease as a result of antibiotic therapy.

Vegetations composed of fibrin, inflammatory cells, and organisms are the hallmark of endocarditis. *Staphylococcus*

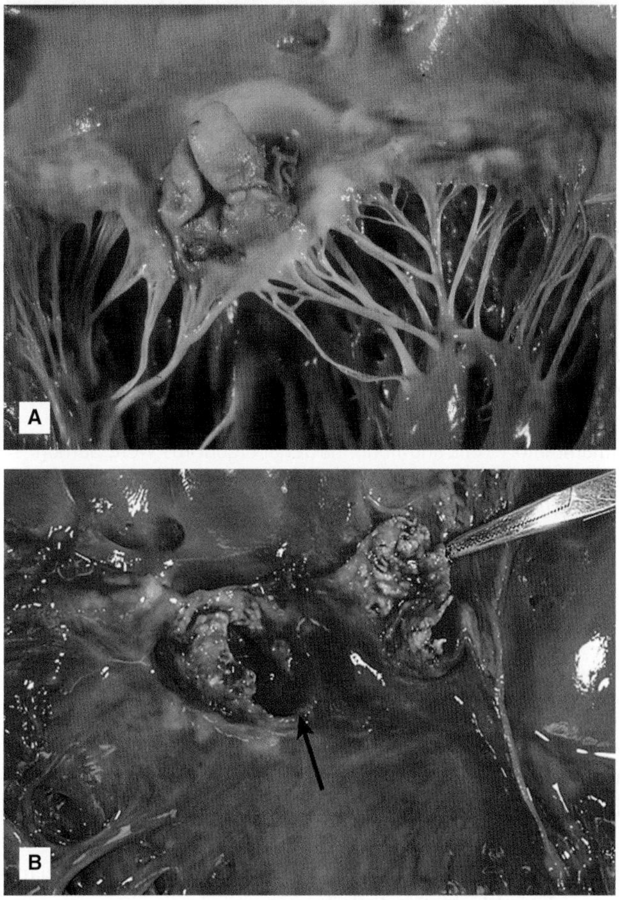

FIGURE 5-16 Infective (bacterial) endocarditis. (A) Endocarditis of mitral valve with damage to the anterior mitral leaflet. (B) Acute endocarditis of congenitally bicuspid aortic valve (caused by *Staphylococcus aureus*), with large vegetation, causing extensive cuspal destruction and ring abscess (*arrow*). (*[B] Reproduced with permission from Schoen FJ: Interventional and Surgical Cardiovascular Pathology: Clinical Correlations and Basic Principles. Philadelphia, WB Saunders, 1989.*)

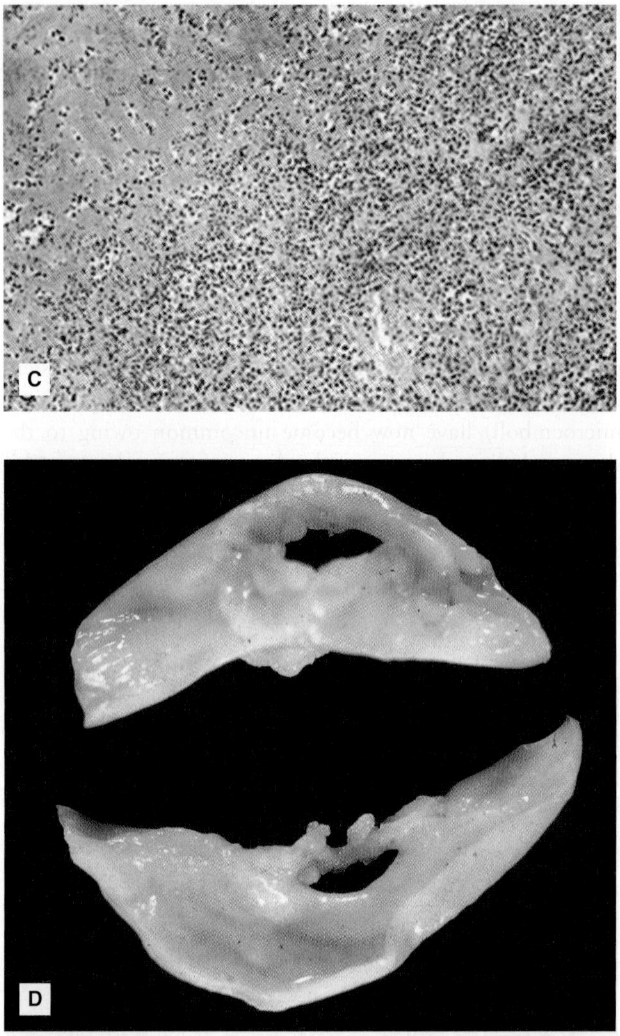

FIGURE 5-16 (*Continued*). Infective (bacterial) endocarditis. (**C**) Photomicrograph of vegetation, showing extensive acute inflammatory cells and fibrin. Bacterial organisms were demonstrated by tissue Gram stain. (*[C] Reproduced with permission from Schoen FJ. Surgical pathology of removed natural and prosthetic heart valves. Human Pathol 1987; 18:558.*) (**D**) Healed endocarditis, demonstrating aortic valvular destruction but no active vegetations on a congenitally bicuspid aortic valve.

aureus is the leading cause of acute endocarditis and produces necrotizing, ulcerative, invasive, and highly destructive valvular infections. The subacute form is usually caused by *Streptococcus viridans.* Cardiac abnormalities, such as chronic rheumatic heart disease, congenital heart disease (particularly anomalies that have small shunts or tight stenoses creating high-velocity jet streams), myxomatous mitral valves, bicuspid aortic valves, and artificial valves and their sewing rings predispose to endocarditis. In intravenous drug abusers, left-sided lesions predominate, but right-sided valves are commonly affected. In about 5 to 20% of all cases of endocarditis, no organism can be isolated from the blood (*culture-negative endocarditis*), often because of prior antibiotic therapy or organisms difficult to culture.[87]

The complications of endocarditis include valvular insufficiency (rarely stenosis), abscess of the valve annulus (*ring abscess*), suppurative pericarditis, and embolization. With appropriate antibiotic therapy, vegetations may undergo healing, with progressive sterilization, organization, fibrosis, and occasionally calcification. Cusp or leaflet perforation, cordal rupture, or fistula formation from a ring abscess into an adjacent cardiac chamber or great vessel can cause regurgitation. Ring abscesses are generally associated with virulent organisms, and a relatively high mortality rate.

Valve Reconstruction and Repair

Reconstructive procedures to repair mitral insufficiency of various etiologies and to minimize the severity of rheumatic mitral stenosis are now highly effective and commonplace. A recent survey of practice in the United States showed that 69% of mitral valve operations for mitral regurgitation currently use repairs.[88] Reconstructive therapy of selected patients with aortic insufficiency and aortic dilation may also be done occasionally, but repair of aortic stenosis has been notably less successful. The major advantage of repair over replacement relates to the elimination of both prosthesis-related complications and the need for chronic anticoagulation therapy. Other reported advantages include a lower hospital mortality, better long-term function owing to the ability to maintain the continuity of the mitral apparatus, and a lower rate of postoperative endocarditis. Figures 5-17 and 5-18 illustrate the pathologic anatomy of various open and catheter-based mitral valve reconstruction procedures. Figure 5-19 illustrates the difficulty of surgical repairs for aortic stenosis.

Percutaneous endovascular repair approaches to valvular heart disease include balloon valvuloplasty, percutaneous placement of a mitral annular constraint device in the coronary sinus, and double-orifice edge-to-edge mitral valve repair without cardiopulmonary bypass for the treatment of mitral regurgitation. Catheter-based endovascular valve repair is most likely to be used in patients with severe disease deemed inoperable and in patients with early-stage regurgitant lesions in whom valve repair may prevent progressive ventricular dilation. Percutaneous transluminal balloon dilation of stenotic valves has been used successfully to relieve some congenital and acquired stenoses of native pulmonary, aortic, and mitral valves, and stenotic right-sided porcine bioprosthetic valves.

Mitral Stenosis

Commissurotomy may be employed in the operative repair of some stenotic mitral valves in which fibrosis and shortening of both cords and leaflets have markedly decreased leaflet mobility and area. Factors that compromise the late functional results of or technically prevent mitral commissurotomy and thereby necessitate valve replacement include: (1) left ventricular dysfunction; (2) pulmonary venous hypertension and right-sided cardiac factors, including right ventricular failure, tricuspid regurgitation, or a combination of these; (3) systemic embolization; (4) coexistent cardiac disorders, such as coronary artery or aortic valve diseases; (5) residual or progressive mitral valve disease, including valve restenosis, residual (unrelieved) stenosis,

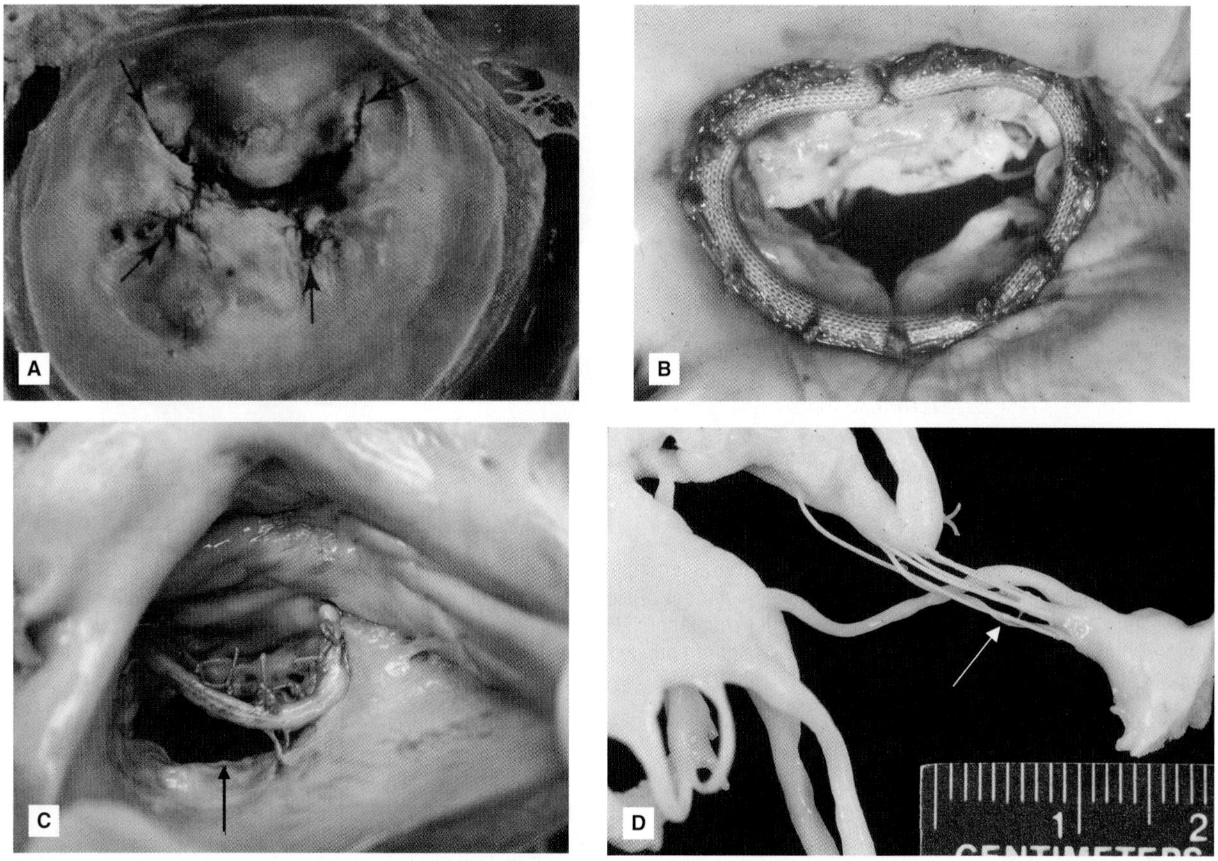

FIGURE 5-17 Open surgical reconstructive procedures for mitral valve disease. (A) Mitral commissurotomy in mitral stenosis; incised commissures are indicated by arrows. (B) Mitral valve repair with annuloplasty ring. (C) Dehiscence of mitral annuloplasty ring (*arrow*). (D) ePTFE suture replacement (*arrow*) of ruptured cord in myxomatous mitral valve. (*[A] Reproduced with permission from Schoen FJ, St. John Sutton M: Contemporary issues in the pathology of valvular heart disease. Hum Pathol 1987; 18:568. Copyright WB Saunders, 1987. [C] Courtesy of William A. Muller, MD, PhD, Northwestern University School of Medicine, Chicago. [D] Reproduced with permission from Schoen FJ, Edwards WD: Valvular heart disease: general principles and stenosis, in Silver MD, Gotlieb AI, Schoen FJ [eds]: Cardiovascular Pathology, 3rd ed. Churchill Livingstone, 2001; p 402.*)

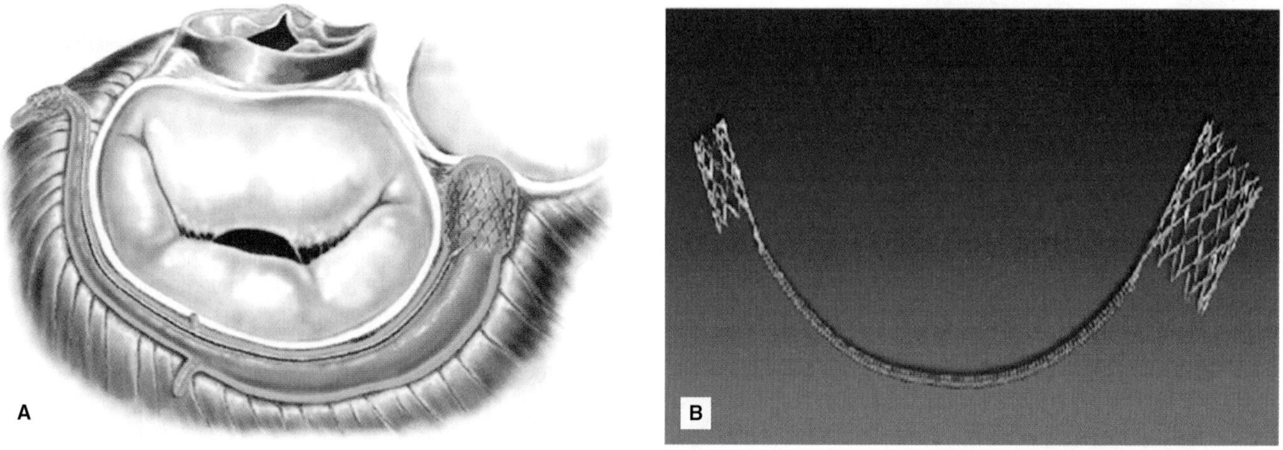

FIGURE 5-18 Percutaneous correction of mitral regurgitation. (A) Schematic approach utilizing the proximity of the coronary sinus to the posterior mitral annulus to effect a simulated annuloplasty. Diagram showing the relationship of the coronary sinus and the posterior leaflet of the mitral valve. A remodeling device is seen within the coronary sinus. (B) The Monarc device consists of two anchoring stents with a bridge connector that shortens approximately 25% over the space of weeks with the intention of reducing the dimensions of the mitral annulus.

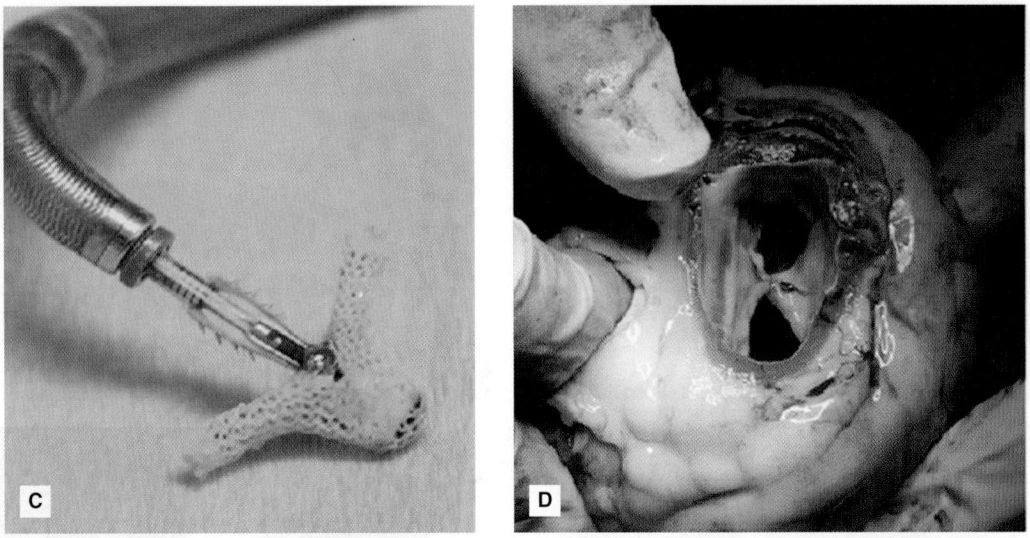

FIGURE 5-18 (*Continued*). Percutaneous correction of mitral regurgitation. (**C** and **D**) Edge-to-edge approximation of the anterior and posterior leaflets of the mitral valve is achieved by deployment of clip (Evalve mitral clip device) that is analogous to an Alfieri stitch, thereby creating a double orifice with improved leaflet coaptation. (*Reproduced with permission from Schoen FJ, Webb JG: Prosthetics and the heart, in McManus BM, Braunwald E [eds]: Atlas of Cardiovascular Pathology for the Clinician. Philadelphia, Current Medicine, 2008; pp 241-256.*)

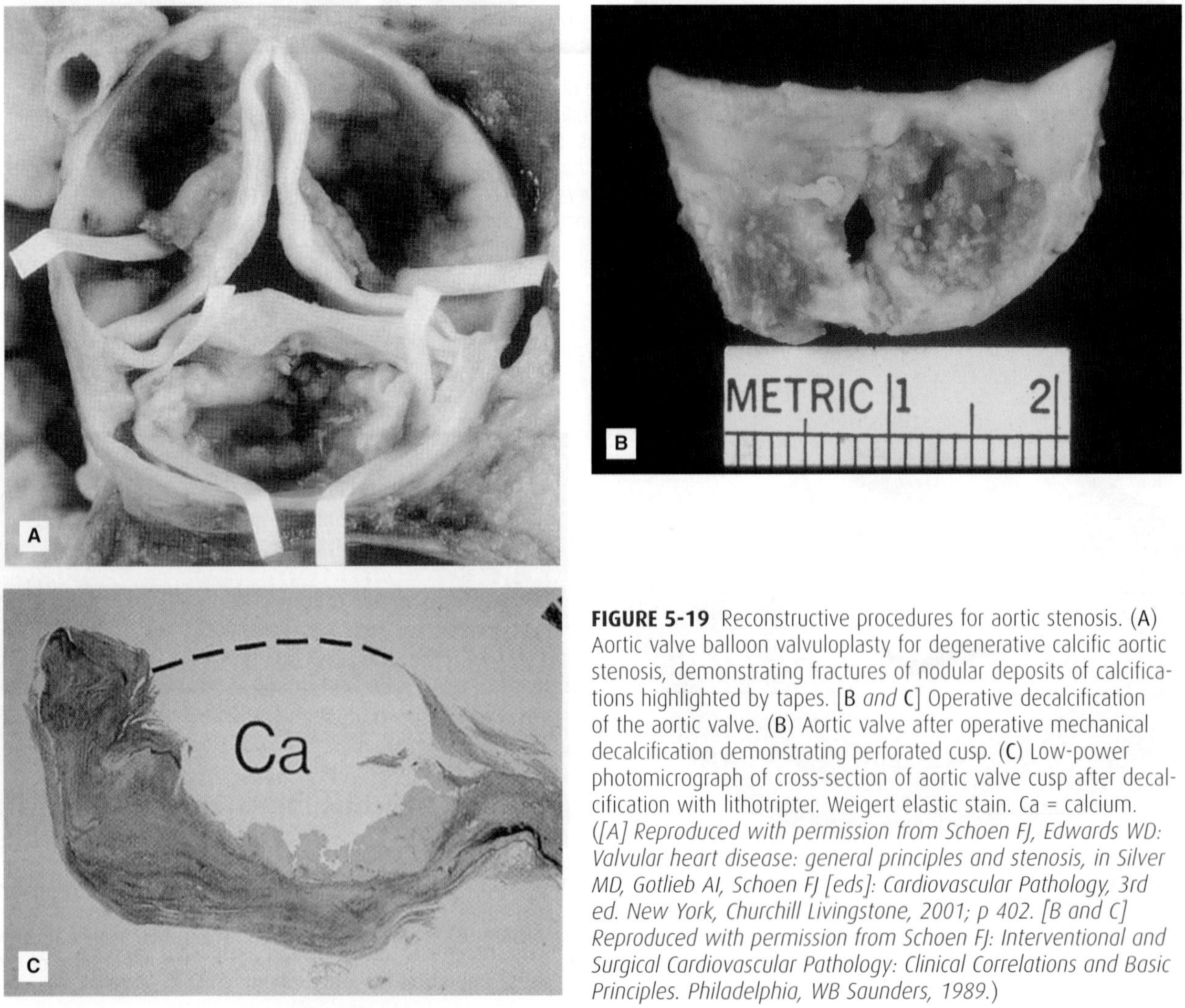

FIGURE 5-19 Reconstructive procedures for aortic stenosis. (**A**) Aortic valve balloon valvuloplasty for degenerative calcific aortic stenosis, demonstrating fractures of nodular deposits of calcifications highlighted by tapes. [**B** *and* **C**] Operative decalcification of the aortic valve. (**B**) Aortic valve after operative mechanical decalcification demonstrating perforated cusp. (**C**) Low-power photomicrograph of cross-section of aortic valve cusp after decalcification with lithotripter. Weigert elastic stain. Ca = calcium. (*[A] Reproduced with permission from Schoen FJ, Edwards WD: Valvular heart disease: general principles and stenosis, in Silver MD, Gotlieb AI, Schoen FJ [eds]: Cardiovascular Pathology, 3rd ed. New York, Churchill Livingstone, 2001; p 402. [B and C] Reproduced with permission from Schoen FJ: Interventional and Surgical Cardiovascular Pathology: Clinical Correlations and Basic Principles. Philadelphia, WB Saunders, 1989.*)

or regurgitation induced at operation; (6) advanced leaflet (especially commissural) calcification; (7) subvalvar (predominantly chordal) fibrotic changes; and (8) significant regurgitation owing to retraction.

Percutaneous balloon mitral valvuloplasty has been used to treat mitral stenosis for over two decades, with excellent success in patients with suitable valvular and subvalvular morphology.[89] However, because balloon valvuloplasty largely involves separation of the fused leaflets at the commissures, this procedure is also unlikely to provide significant benefit to patients with the valve features summarized in the preceding obviating surgical commissurotomy.

Mitral Regurgitation

Reconstructive techniques are widely used to repair mitral valves with nonrheumatic mitral regurgitation.[90–92] Structural defects responsible for chronic mitral regurgitation include: (1) dilation of the mitral annulus; (2) leaflet prolapse into the left atrium with or without elongation or rupture of chordae tendineae; (3) redundancy and deformity of leaflets; (4) leaflet perforations or defects; and (5) restricted leaflet motion as a result of commissural fusion in an opened position, and leaflet retraction, or chordal shortening or thickening.

Following surgical resection of excess anterior or posterior leaflet tissue in valves with redundancy, annuloplasty with or without a prosthetic ring is used to reduce the annulus dimension to correspond to the amount of leaflet tissue available. Edge-to-edge (Alfieri stitch) mitral valve repair has also been used.[93] Tissue substitutes such as glutaraldehyde-pretreated xenograft or autologous pericardium can be used to repair or enlarge leaflets. Ruptured or elongated cords may be repaired by shortening or replacement with pericardial tissue or thick suture material.

Percutaneous approaches currently being evaluated for mitral regurgitation attempt to emulate one or more of the components of surgical mitral valve repair, including annular reduction and edge-to-edge mitral leaflet apposition.[94] However, leaflet resection and cordal modification cannot be easily done via catheter, and there is considerable anatomical variability of the coronary sinus.[95] Percutaneous approaches in various stages of development and clinical evaluation include implantation of a device in the coronary sinus, left atrium (or both), or by device placement behind the posterolateral leaflet of the mitral valve (see Fig. 5-18A and B). The goal is to plicate or straighten the posterior mitral annulus. Additional annuloplasty approaches, presently in preclinical testing, include a suture annuloplasty from the ventricular side of the mitral annulus, thermal modification of the annulus to obtain shrinkage, and a percutaneous ventricular restraint system that attempts to reshape the left ventricle. Another catheter-based approach uses an edge-to-edge clip prosthesis simulating the edge-to-edge surgical (Alfieri stitch) repair in which the midportions of the anterior and posterior mitral leaflets are clipped together (see Fig. 5-18C and D).

Aortic Stenosis

In balloon dilation of calcific aortic stenosis, individual functional responses vary considerably and data suggest a modest early incremental benefit, high early mortality, and high restenosis rate. Improvement derives from commissural separation, fracture of calcific deposits, and stretching of the valve cusps (see Fig. 5-19A). The major complications include cerebrovascular accident secondary to embolism, massive regurgitation owing to valve trauma, and cardiac perforation with tamponade. Fractured calcific nodules can themselves prove dangerous.[96] In pediatric cases in which the cusps are generally pliable, cuspal stretching, tearing, or avulsion may also occur.

In calcific aortic stenosis the calcific deposits arise deep in the valve fibrous layer (see Fig. 5-14C). Their removal by sharp dissection or ultrasonic debridement generally removes a considerable fraction of the valve substance, resulting in severe compromise of mechanical integrity (see Fig. 5-19B and C).[97]

Valve Replacement

Severe symptomatic valvular heart disease other than pure mitral stenosis or incompetence is most frequently treated by excision of the diseased valve(s) and replacement by a functional substitute. Five key factors determine the results of valve replacement in an individual patient: (1) technical aspects of the procedure; (2) intraoperative myocardial ischemic injury; (3) irreversible and chronic structural alterations in the heart and lungs secondary to the valvular abnormality; (4) coexistent obstructive coronary artery disease; and (5) valve prosthesis reliability and host-tissue interactions.

Valve Types and Prognostic Considerations

Cardiac valvular substitutes are of two types, mechanical and biologic tissue (Fig. 5-20 and Table 5-2).[98,99] Prostheses function passively, responding to pressure and flow changes within the heart. Mechanical valves are composed of nonphysiologic biomaterials and employ a rigid, mobile occluder (composed of pyrolytic carbon in contemporary valves), in a metallic cage (cobalt-chrome or titanium alloy) as in the Bjork-Shiley, Hall-Medtronic, or Omniscience valves, or two carbon hemidisks in a carbon housing (as in the St. Jude Medical, CarboMedics CPHV, and On-X prostheses). Pyrolytic carbon has high strength and fatigue and wear resistance and good thromboresistance. Tissue valves resemble natural semilunar valves, with pseudoanatomical central flow and biological material. In the past decade, innovations in tissue valve technologies and design have expanded indications for their use. Contemporary utilization of bioprosthetic tissue valves is estimated to be about 80% of all aortic and 69% of all mitral substitute heart valves.[99–101] Most tissue valves are bioprosthetic xenografts fabricated from porcine aortic valve or bovine pericardium, which have been preserved in a dilute glutaraldehyde solution, and a small percentage are cryopreserved allografts.

In a recent compilation of risk models of isolated valve surgery by the Society for Thoracic Surgeons, the overall mortality was 3.4% (3.2% aortic and 5.7% mitral) and varied strongly with case mix.[102] The majority of early deaths are caused by hemorrhage, pulmonary failure, low cardiac output, and sudden death with or without myocardial necrosis or documented arrhythmias. Potential

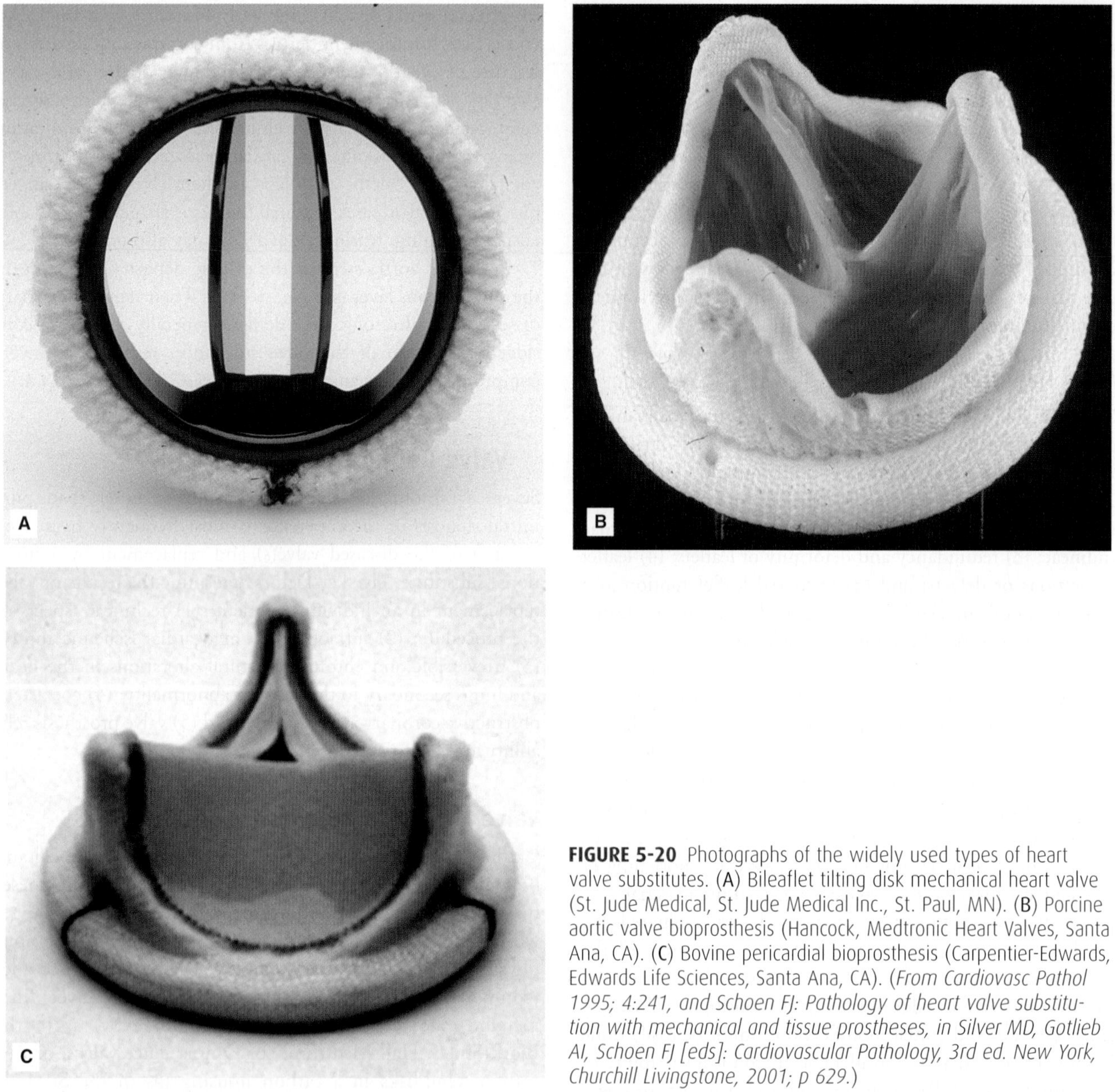

FIGURE 5-20 Photographs of the widely used types of heart valve substitutes. (A) Bileaflet tilting disk mechanical heart valve (St. Jude Medical, St. Jude Medical Inc., St. Paul, MN). (B) Porcine aortic valve bioprosthesis (Hancock, Medtronic Heart Valves, Santa Ana, CA). (C) Bovine pericardial bioprosthesis (Carpentier-Edwards, Edwards Life Sciences, Santa Ana, CA). *(From Cardiovasc Pathol 1995; 4:241, and Schoen FJ: Pathology of heart valve substitution with mechanical and tissue prostheses, in Silver MD, Gotlieb AI, Schoen FJ [eds]: Cardiovascular Pathology, 3rd ed. New York, Churchill Livingstone, 2001; p 629.)*

complications related to mitral valve insertion include hemorrhagic disruption and dissection of the atrioventricular groove, perforation or entrapment of the left circumflex coronary artery by a suture, and pseudoaneurysm or rupture of the left ventricular free wall.

Improvement in late outcome has occurred predominantly from earlier referral of patients for valve replacement, decreased intraoperative myocardial damage, improved surgical technique and enhanced valve prostheses. Following valve replacement with currently used devices, the probability of 5-year survival is about 80% and of 10-year survival about 70%, depending on overall functional state, preoperative left ventricular function, left ventricular and left atrial size, and extent and severity of coronary artery disease.

Valve-Related Complications

Although early prosthetic valve–associated complications are unusual, prosthetic valve–associated pathology becomes an important consideration beyond the early postoperative period. Late death following valve replacement results predominantly from either cardiovascular pathology unrelated to the substitute valve or prosthesis-associated complications. In the few randomized studies of mechanical prosthetic and bioprosthetic valves (comprising Bjork-Shiley mechanical and porcine aortic bioprosthetic valves), approximately 60% or more patients had an important device-related complication within 10 years postoperatively. Moreover, long-term survival was better among patients with a mechanical valve, but with an increased risk of bleeding.[103,104] Valve-related complications frequently necessitate reoperation, now accounting for approximately 10 to 15% of all valve procedures, and they may cause death. Four categories of valve-related complications are most important: thromboembolism and related problems, infection, structural dysfunction (ie, failure or degeneration of the biomaterials comprising a prosthesis), and nonstructural dysfunction (ie, miscellaneous

TABLE 5-2 Types and Characteristics of Commonly Used Substitute Heart Valves*

Valve type	Model(s)	Hemodynamics	Freedom from thrombosis/ thromboembolism	Durability
Mechanical				
Caged ball	Starr-Edwards	+§	+	+++
Single tilting disk	Bjork-Shiley Hall-Medtronic Omnicarbon	++	++	+++†
Bileaflet tilting disk	St. Jude Medical Carbomedics Edwards-Duromedics	+++	+++	+++‡
Tissue				
Heterograft/xenograft bioprostheses	Carpentier-Edwards (porcine and bovine pericardial) Hancock (porcine) Ionescu-Shiley (bovine pericardial) Mitroflow (bovine pericardial)	++	+++	++
Homograft/allograft	Cryopreserved human aortic/pulmonary valve	++++	++++	++

*Presently or previously.
†Except Bjork-Shiley 60°/70° convexo-concave valve (see text).
‡Except previous model of Edwards-Duromedics valve (see text).
§Performance criteria: + = least favorable to ++++ = most favorable.
Source: Data adapted from Vongpatanasin et al.[189]

complications and modes of failure not encompassed in the previous groups) (Table 5-3).[105]

Thrombosis and Thromboembolism. *Thromboembolic complications* are the major valve-related cause of mortality and morbidity after replacement with mechanical valves, and patients receiving them require lifetime chronic therapeutic anticoagulation with warfarin derivatives.[106,107] Thrombotic deposits on a prosthetic valve can immobilize the occluder(s) or cusps, or shed emboli (Fig. 5-21). Owing to their biologic material that comprises the cusps and central flow, tissue valves are less thrombogenic than mechanical valves; their recipients generally do not require long-term anticoagulation in the absence of another specific indication, such as atrial fibrillation. Nevertheless, the rate of thromboembolism in patients with mechanical valves on anticoagulation is not widely different from that in patients with bioprosthetic valves without anticoagulation (2 to 4% per year). Chronic oral anticoagulation also carries a risk of hemorrhage. Anticoagulation is particularly difficult to manage in pregnant women.[108] The risk of thromboembolism is potentiated by preoperative or postoperative cardiac functional impairment.

"Virchow's triad" of factors promoting thrombosis (surface thrombogenicity, hypercoagulability, and locally static blood flow) largely predicts the relative propensity toward and locations of thrombotic deposits.[109] For example, with caged-ball prostheses, thrombi form distal to the poppet at the cage apex. Tilting disk prostheses are particularly susceptible to total

TABLE 5-3 Complications of Substitute Heart Valves

Generic	Specific
Thrombotic limitations	Thrombosis Thromboembolism Anticoagulation-related hemorrhage
Infection	Prosthetic valve endocarditis
Structural dysfunction (intrinsic)	Wear Fracture Poppet escape Cuspal tear Calcification Commisural region dehiscence
Nonstructural dysfunction (most extrinsic)	Pannus (tissue overgrowth) Entrapment by suture or tissue Paravalvular leak Disproportion Hemolytic anemia Noise

Source: Modified with permission from Schoen FJ, Levy RJ, Piehler HR: Pathological considerations in replacement cardiac valves. Cardiovasc Pathol 1992; 1:29

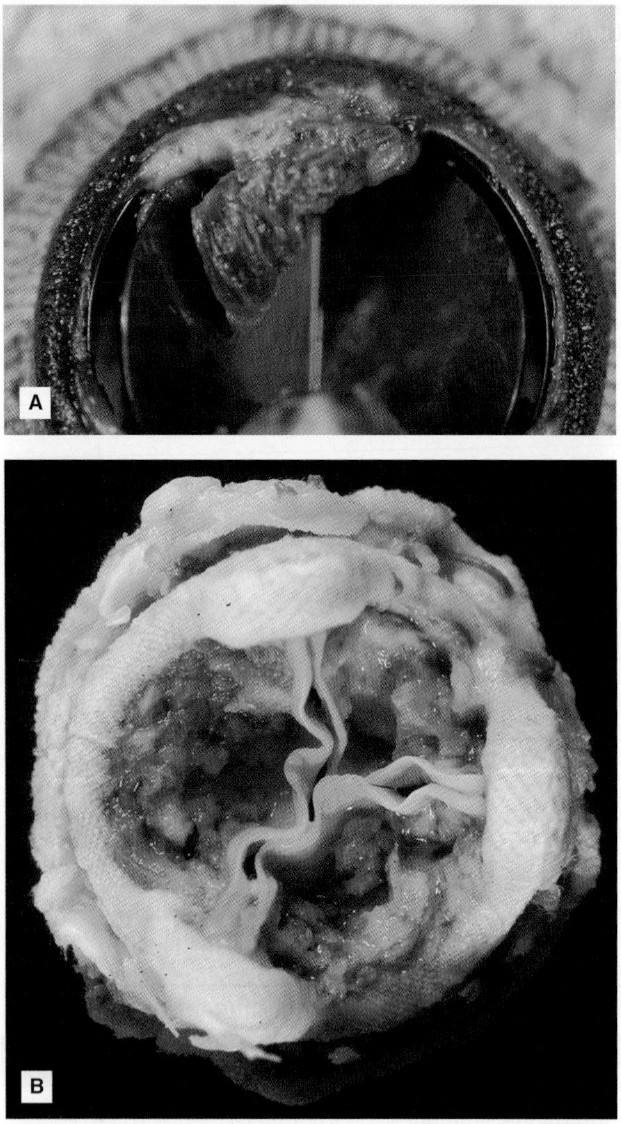

FIGURE 5-21 Thrombotic occlusion of substitute heart valves. (A) Bileaflet tilting disk prosthesis, with thrombus initiated in the region of the pivot guard, causing near-total occluder immobility. (B) Porcine bioprosthesis, with thrombus filling the bioprosthetic sinuses of Valsalva. (*[A] Reproduced with permission from Anderson JM, Schoen FJ: Interactions of blood with artificial surfaces, in Buchart EG, Bodnar E [eds]: Thrombosis, Embolism, and Bleeding. London, ICR Publishers, 1992; p 160. [B] Reproduced with permission from Schoen FJ, Hobson CE: Anatomic analysis of removed prosthetic heart valves: causes of failure of 33 mechanical valves and 58 bioprostheses, 1980 to 1983. Hum Pathol 1985; 16:549.*)

thrombotic occlusion or shedding emboli from small thrombi, with the thrombotic deposits generally initiated in a flow stagnation zone in the minor orifice of the outflow region of the prosthesis. In contrast, bileaflet tilting disk valves are most vulnerable to thrombus formation near the hinges where the leaflets insert into the housing (see Fig. 5-21A). Late thrombosis of a bioprosthetic valve is marked by large thrombotic deposits in one or more of the prosthetic sinuses of Valsalva (see Fig. 5-21B), and no causal underlying cuspal pathology can usually be demonstrated by pathologic studies. Some valve thromboemboli, especially early postoperatively with any valve type, can be initiated at the valve sewing cuff before it is healed, thus providing the rationale for early antithrombotic therapy for all types.

As with other devices in which nonphysiologic artificial surfaces are exposed to blood at high fluid shear stresses, platelet deposition dominates initial blood-surface interaction, and prosthetic valve thromboembolism correlates strongly with altered platelet function. Nevertheless, although platelet-suppressive drugs largely normalize indices of platelet formation and partially reduce the frequency of thromboembolic complications in patients with mechanical prosthetic valves, antiplatelet therapy alone is generally considered insufficient to adequately prevent thromboembolism. The lack of vascular tissue adjacent to thrombi that form on bioprosthetic or mechanical valves retards their histologic organization and may prolong the susceptibility to embolization as well as render the age of such thrombi difficult to determine microscopically. Nevertheless, this feature may allow thrombolytic therapy to be an option in some cases.[110]

Prosthetic Valve Endocarditis. *Prosthetic valve infective endocarditis* (Fig. 5-22) occurs in 3 to 6% of recipients of substitute valves.[111] Infection can occur early (<60 days postoperative) or late. The microbial etiology of early prosthetic valve endocarditis is dominated by the staphylococcal species, *Staphylococcus epidermidis* and *S. aureus,* even though prophylactic regimens used today target these microorganisms. The clinical course of early prosthetic valve endocarditis tends to be fulminant, and accompanied by valvular or annular destruction or persistent bacteremia. In the generally less virulent late endocarditis, a source of infection and/or bacteremia can often be found; the most frequent initiators are dental procedures, urologic infections and interventions, and indwelling catheters. The most common organisms in these late infections are *S. epidermidis, S. aureus, S. viridans,* and enterococci. Rates of infection of bioprostheses and mechanical valves are similar, and previous endocarditis on a natural or substitute valve markedly increases the risk.

Infections associated with mechanical prosthetic valves and some with bioprosthetic valves are localized to the prosthesis-tissue junction at the sewing ring, and accompanied by tissue destruction around the prosthesis (see Fig. 5-22A). This comprises a ring abscess, with potential paraprosthetic leak, dehiscence, fistula formation, or heart block caused by conduction system damage. Bioprosthetic valve infections may involve, and are occasionally limited to, the cuspal tissue, sometimes causing secondary cuspal tearing or perforation with valve incompetence or obstruction (see Fig. 5-22B and C). Surgical reintervention usually is indicated for large highly mobile vegetations or cerebral thromboembolic episodes, or persistent ring abscess.

Structural Valve Dysfunction. *Prosthetic valve dysfunction* owing to materials degradation can necessitate reoperation or cause prosthesis-associated death (Fig. 5-23). Durability considerations vary widely for mechanical valves and bioprostheses, specific types of each, different models of a particular prosthesis (utilizing different materials or having different design features), and even for the same model prosthesis placed in the aortic rather than the mitral site. Mechanical valve structural failure is often catastrophic and may be life threatening; in

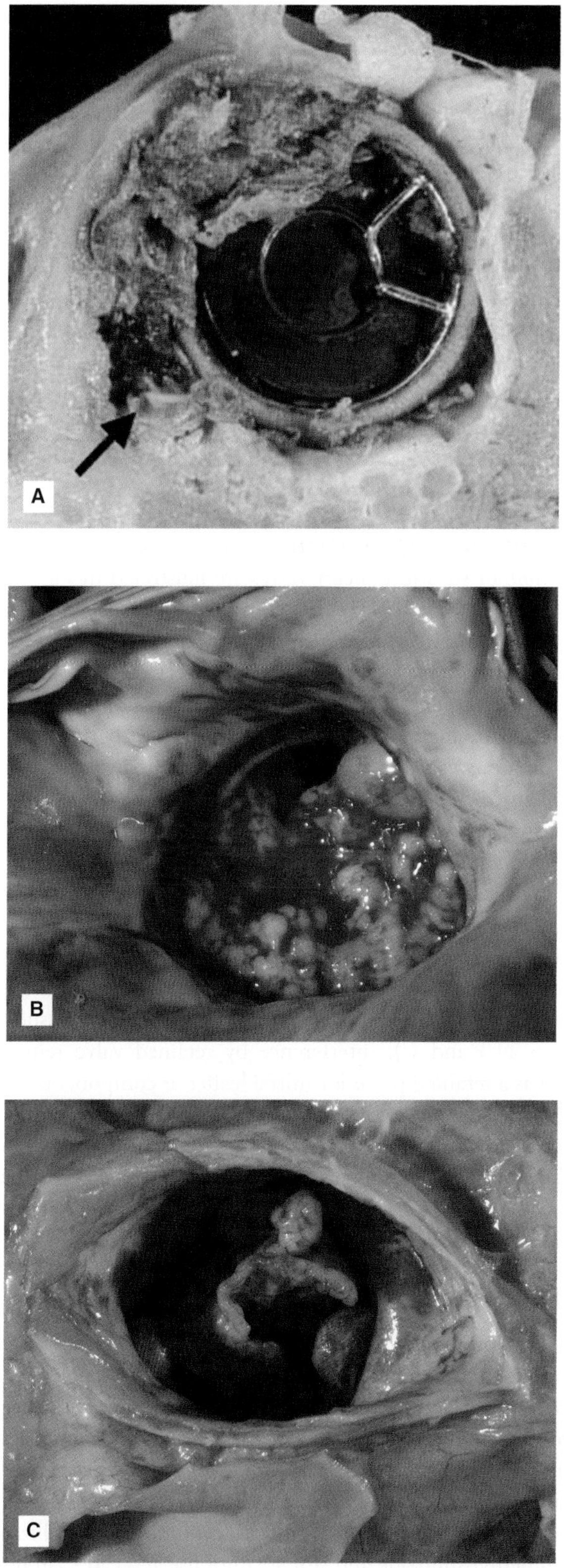

FIGURE 5-22 Prosthetic valve endocarditis. (A) Endocarditis with large ring abscess (*arrow*) observed from ventricular surface of aortic Bjork-Shiley tilting disk prosthesis in patient who died suddenly. Ring abscess impinged on proximal atrioventricular conduction system. (*B* and *C*) Bioprosthetic valve endocarditis viewed from inflow (B) and outflow (C) aspects. (*[A] Reproduced with permission from Schoen FJ: Cardiac valve prostheses: pathological and bioengineering considerations. J Cardiac Surg 1987; 2:65.*)

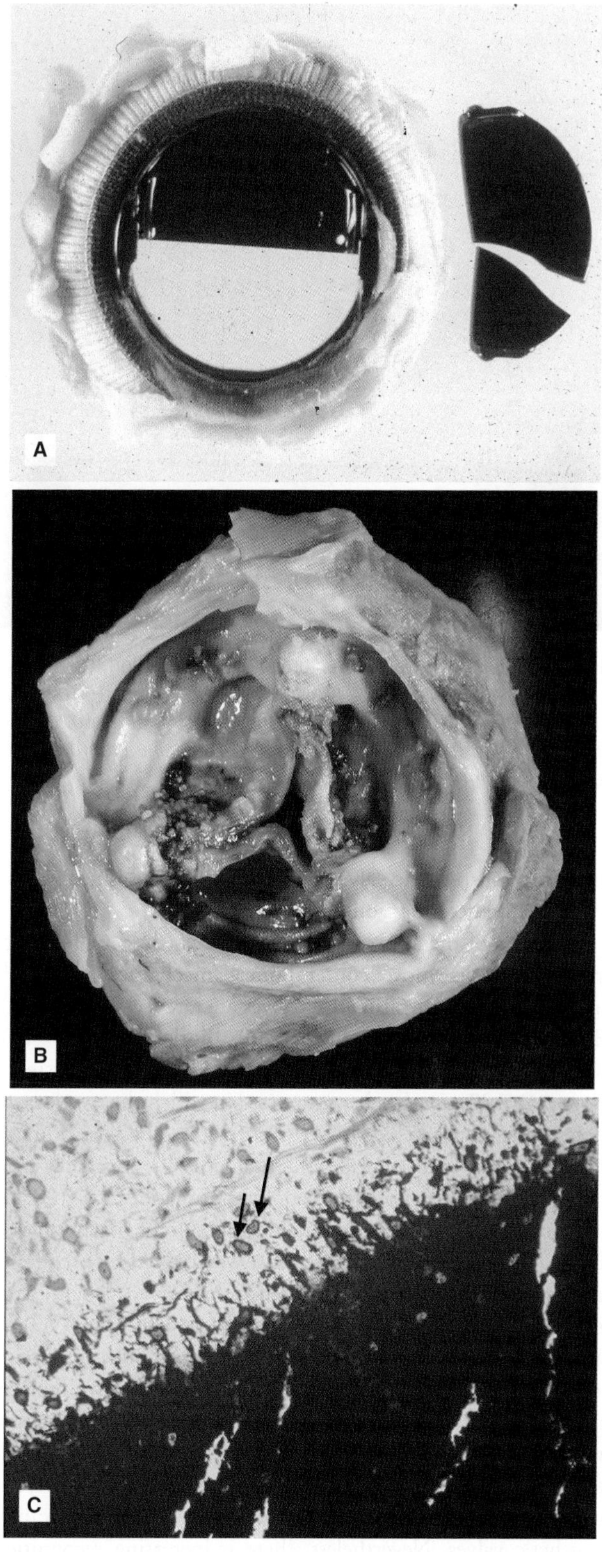

FIGURE 5-23 Structural valve dysfunction. (A) Disk fracture and escape in a Hemex-Duramedics heart valve prosthesis. (*B* and *C*) Porcine valve primary tissue failure owing to calcification with severe stenosis. (B) Gross photograph. (C) Photomicrograph demonstrating predominant site of calcification in cells of the residual porcine valve matrix (*arrows*). (*[A] Reproduced with permission from Schoen FJ, et al: Pathological considerations in substitute heart valves. Cardiovasc Pathol 1992; 1:29. Hum Pathol 1985; 16:549. [C] Reproduced from Schoen FJ: Pathology of heart valve substitution with mechanical and tissue prostheses, in Silver MD, Gotlieb AI, Schoen FJ [eds]: Cardiovascular Pathology, 3rd ed. New York, Churchill Livingtone, p. 629.*)

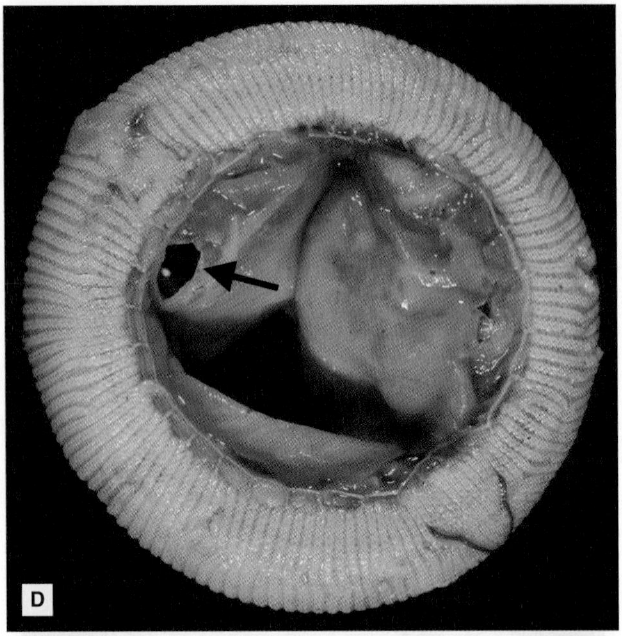

FIGURE 5-23 *(Continued)*. Structural valve dysfunction. (**D**) Clinical porcine bioprosthesis with noncalcific tear of one cusp (*arrow*). *([B] Reproduced with permission from Schoen FJ, et al: Long-term failure rate and morphologic correlations in porcine bioprosthetic heart valves. Am J Cardiol 1983; 51:957.)*

contrast, bioprosthetic valve failure generally causes progressive symptomatic deterioration.

Fractures of metallic carbon components (disks or housing) are unusual in most contemporary mechanical valves.[112] Fractures of bileaflet tilting disk valves are rare (see Fig. 5-23A). However, of approximately 86,000 Bjork-Shiley 60- and 70-degree Convexo-Concave heart valves implanted, a cluster of more than 500 cases has been reported in which the two attachment points of the welded outlet strut fractured because of metal fatigue, leading to disk escape and often death.[113] Single leg strut fractures have been noted at a presymptomatic stage in some patients.[114] In contrast, structural dysfunction of tissue valves is the major cause of failure of the most widely used bioprostheses (flexible-stent-mounted, glutaraldehyde-preserved porcine aortic valves, and bovine pericardial valves) (see Fig. 5-23B–D).[115] Within 15 years following implantation, 30 to 50% of porcine aortic valves implanted as either mitral or aortic valve replacements require replacement because of structural dysfunction manifested as primary tissue failure. Cuspal mineralization is the key mechanism with regurgitation through secondary tears, the most frequent failure mode, particularly in porcine aortic bioprosthetic valves. Nevertheless, there is increasing recognition that noncalcific structural damage owing to collagen fiber disruption (independent of calcification) contributes to bioprosthetic heart valve failure.[116] Pure stenosis owing to calcific cuspal stiffening occurs less frequently. Calcific deposits are usually localized to cuspal tissue (*intrinsic calcification*), but calcific deposits extrinsic to the cusps may occur in thrombi or endocarditic vegetations. Calcification is markedly accelerated in younger patients, with children and adolescents having an especially accelerated course. Bovine pericardial valves can also suffer tearing and calcification with abrasion of the pericardial tissue an important contributing factor in some designs.[117]

The morphology and determinants of calcification of bioprosthetic valve tissue have been widely studied in experimental models. The process is initiated primarily within residual membranes and organelles of the nonviable connective tissue cells that have been devitalized by glutaraldehyde pretreatment procedures, and involves reaction of calcium-containing extracellular fluid with membrane-associated phosphorus. The pathologic changes in bioprosthetic valves that occur following implantation are largely rationalized on the basis of changes induced by the preservation and manufacture of a bioprosthesis, including: (1) denudation of surface cells, including endothelial cells in porcine aortic valves, and mesothelial cells in bovine pericardium; (2) loss of viability of the interstitial cells; and (3) locking of the cuspal microstructure in a static geometry.

Nonstructural Dysfunction. *Extrinsic (nonstructural) complications* of substitute heart valves are illustrated in Fig. 5-24. Paravalvular defects may be clinically inconsequential may aggravate hemolysis or may cause heart failure through regurgitation. Early paravalvular leaks may be related to suture knot failure, inadequate suture placement, or separation of sutures from a pathologic annulus in endocarditis with ring abscess, myxomatous valvular degeneration, or calcified valvular annulus as in calcific aortic stenosis or mitral annular calcification. Late small paravalvular leaks usually are caused by anomalous tissue retraction from the sewing ring between sutures during healing. Paravalvular defects tend to be small and difficult to locate by surgical or pathologic examination (see Fig. 5-24A).

Extrinsic factors can mediate late prosthetic valve stenosis or regurgitation, including a large mitral annular calcific nodule, septal hypertrophy, exuberant overgrowth of fibrous tissue (see Fig. 5-24B and C), interference by retained valve remnants (such as a retained posterior mitral leaflet or components of the submitral apparatus; Fig. 5-24D), or unraveled, long, or looped sutures or knots (see Fig. 5-24E). With bioprosthetic valves, cuspal motion can be restricted by sutures looped around stents, and suture ends cut too long may erode into or perforate a bioprosthetic valve cusp.

Valvular Allografts/Homografts

Aortic or pulmonary valves (with or without associated vascular conduits) transplanted from one individual to another have exceptionally good hemodynamic profiles, a low incidence of thromboembolic complications without chronic anticoagulation, and a low reinfection rate following valve replacement for endocarditis.[118] Contemporary cryopreserved allografts, in which freezing is performed with protection from crystallization by dimethyl-sulfoxide and storage until use at −196°C in liquid nitrogen, have demonstrated freedom from degeneration and durability equal to or better than those of conventional porcine bioprosthetic valves (approximately 50 to 90% valve survival at 10 to 15 years compared with 40 to 60% for bioprostheses).

Morphologic changes are summarized in Fig. 5-25. Cryopreserved human allograft heart valves/conduits show gross changes of conduit calcification and cuspal stretching (see Figs. 5-25A and B). Microscopically, there is progressive loss of

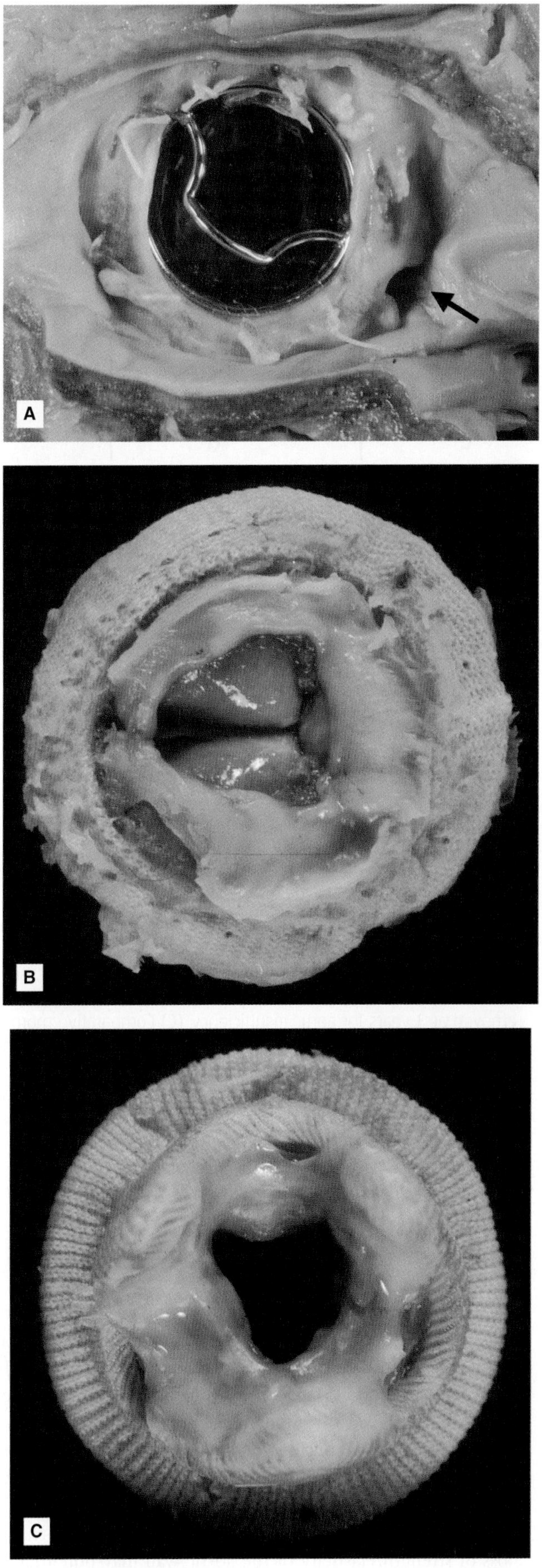

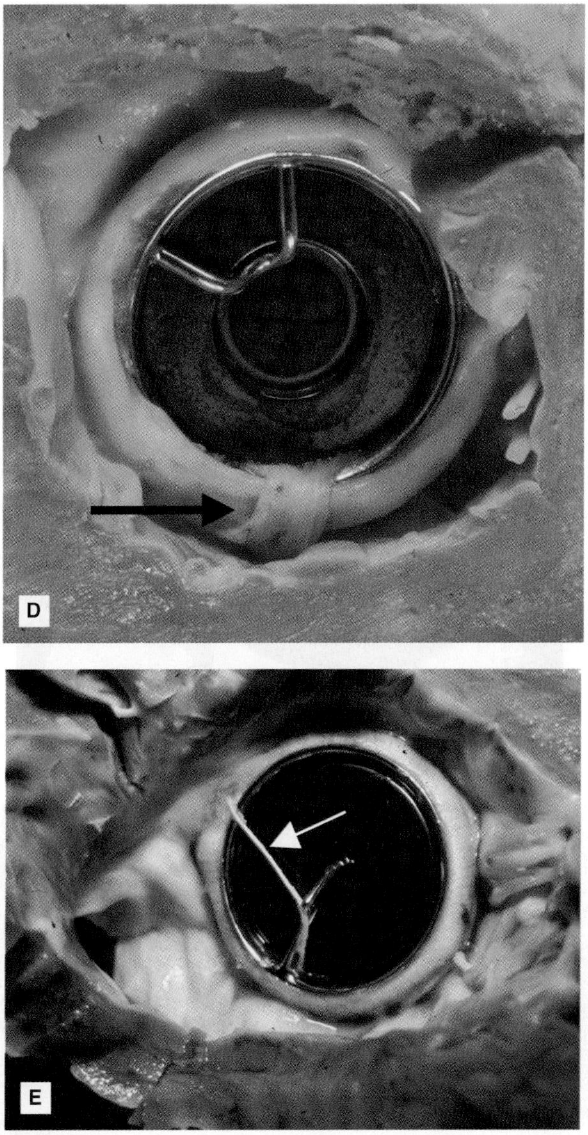

FIGURE 5-24 Nonstructural dysfunction of prosthetic heart valves. (A) Paravalvular leak adjacent to mitral valve prosthesis (*arrow*). (B) Tissue overgrowth compromising inflow orifice of porcine bioprosthesis. (C) Tissue overgrowth incorporating and resultant retraction and obliteration of bioprosthetic valve cusps. (D) Immobility of tilting disk leaflet by impingement of retained component of submitral apparatus (*arrow*) that had moved through orifice late following mitral valve replacement surgery. (E) Suture (*arrow*) looped around central strut of a Hall-Medtronic tilting disk valve causing disk immobility. (*[A and C] Reproduced with permission from Schoen FJ: Pathologic considerations in replacement heart valves and other cardiovascular prosthetic devices, in Schoen FJ, Gimbrone MA [eds]: Cardiovascular Pathology: Clinicopathologic Correlations and Pathogenetic Mechanisms. Philadelphia, Williams & Wilkins, 1995; p 194. [B] Reproduced with permission from Schoen FJ, et al: Pathologic considerations in substitute heart valves. Cardiovasc Pathol 1992; 1:29. [D] Reproduced with permission from Schoen FJ: Pathology of cardiac valve replacement, in Morse D, Steiner RM, Fernandez J [eds]: Guide to Prosthetic Cardiac Valves. New York, Springer-Verlag, 1985; p 209.* Nonstructural dysfunction of prosthetic heart valves. *[E] Photo courtesy of Office of the Chief Medical Examiner, New York City.*)

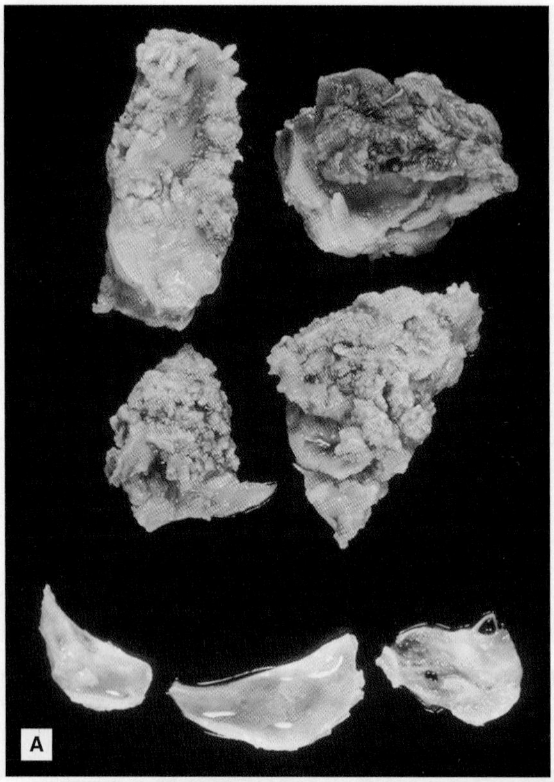

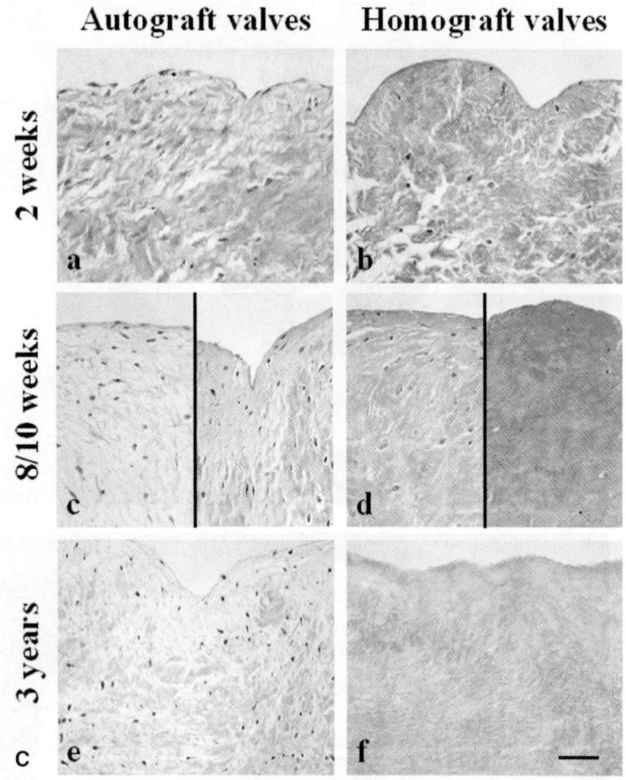

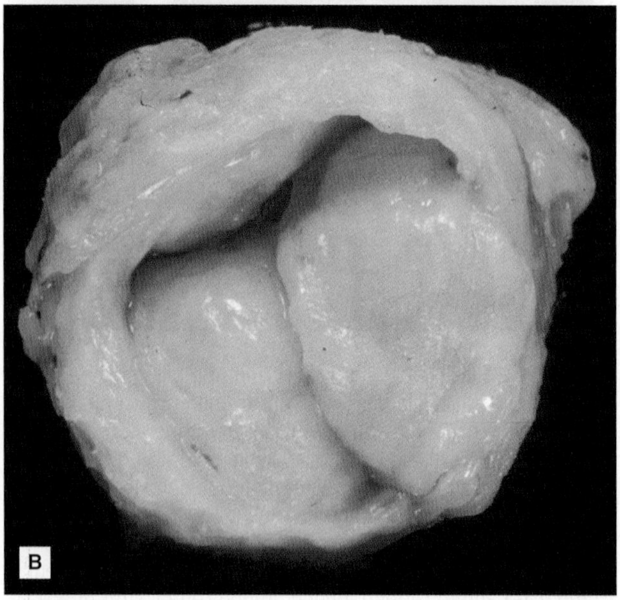

FIGURE 5-25 Morphology of valve allografts (homografts) valve and pulmonary valve autografts. (**A**) Gross photograph of pulmonary valve allograft removed following 7 years for conduit stenosis in a child. The pulmonary arterial wall is heavily calcified but the cusps are not. (**B**) Gross appearance of cryopreserved aortic valve allograft removed at 3 years for aortic insufficiency. (**C**) Comparative morphologic features of autografts and homografts obtained from the same patients. Autograft valves had near-normal structure and cellular population (**a**, **c**, **e**), in contrast, homografts from the same patients (**b**, **d**, **f**) had a progressive collagen hyalinization and loss of cellularity. Bar = 200 μm. × 400. (*[C] Reproduced with permission from Rabkin-Aikawa E, Aikawa M, Farber M, et al: Clinical pulmonary autograft valves: pathological evidence of adaptive remodeling in the aortic site. J Thorac Cardiovasc Surg 2004; 128:552-562.*)

normal structural demarcations and cells beginning in days. Long-term explants are devoid of both surface endothelium and deep connective tissue cells; they have minimal inflammatory cellularity (Fig. 5-25C).[119]

Pulmonary Valvular Autografts

Often called the *Ross operation* in recognition of its originator, Sir Donald Ross, pulmonary autograft replacement of the aortic valve yields excellent hemodynamic performance, avoids anticoagulation, and carries a low risk of thromboembolism.[120]

Explanted pulmonary autograft cusps show: (1) near-normal trilaminar structure; (2) near-normal collagen architecture; (3) viable endothelium and interstitial cells; (4) usual outflow surface corrugations; (5) sparse inflammatory cells; and (6) absence of calcification and thrombus (see Fig. 5-25).[121] However, the arterial walls show considerable transmural damage (probably perioperative ischemic injury caused by disruption of vasa vasorum) with scaring and loss of medial smooth muscle cells and elastin. The early necrosis and healing with probable resultant loss of strength/elasticity of the aortic wall may potentiate late aortic root dilation.[122,123]

Stentless Porcine Aortic Valve Bioprostheses

Nonstented (stentless) porcine aortic valve bioprostheses consist of glutaraldehyde-pretreated pig aortic root and valve cusps that have no supporting stent.[124] The most widely used models, St. Jude Medical Toronto SPV (St. Jude Medical Inc., St. Paul, MN), Medtronic Freestyle (Medtronic Heart Valves, Santa Ana, CA) and Edwards Prima (Edwards Life Sciences, Irvine, CA), bioprostheses differ slightly in overall configuration, details of glutaraldehyde fixation conditions, and anticalcification pretreatment. The principal advantage of a stentless porcine aortic valve is that it generally allows for the implantation of a larger bioprosthesis (than stented) in any given aortic root, which is hypothesized to enhance hemodynamics and thereby regression of hypertrophy and patient survival.[125]

The available evidence suggests that the durability of stentless bioprostheses is comparable with that of contemporary stented bioprostheses. However, nonstented porcine aortic valves have greater portions of aortic wall exposed to blood than in currently used stented valves, and calcification of the aortic wall and inflammation at the junction of aortic wall within the recipient's tissue, are potentially deleterious, owing to the large area of this interface. Calcification of the wall portion of a stentless valve could stiffen the root, cause nodular calcific obstruction potentiate wall rupture, or provide a nidus for emboli. Analyses of explanted nonstented valves show pannus and tissue degeneration, manifest as tears and cuspal calcification, but not substantial aortic wall calcification.[126,127]

Catheter-Based Valve Replacement

New catheter techniques for inserting foldable prosthetic valves within stenotic aortic and pulmonary valves, and for emulating surgical repair of regurgitant mitral valves are in various stages of preclinical development and early clinical use.[128,129] Presently, catheter-based, often percutaneous valve replacement is most widely used in patients with severe aortic stenosis disease deemed otherwise inoperable as a bridge to valve replacement in patients in whom surgery needs to be delayed, and in congenital heart disease, in which percutaneous pulmonary valve replacement may find a distinct niche to obviate the morbidity of reoperation to replace malfunctioning pulmonary conduits.

Catheter-based valve replacement uses a device which has two components: (1) an outer stentlike structure and (2) leaflets; these two components together constitute a functioning valvular prosthesis. Representative designs are illustrated in Fig. 5-26. The stent holds open a valve annulus or segment of a prosthetic conduit and resists the tendency of a vessel, valve annulus and diseased native leaflets to recoil following balloon dilation, supports the valve leaflets, and provides the means for seating of the prosthesis in the annulus or vessel.

The devices generally consist of biologic tissue such as bovine, equine, or porcine pericardium and bovine jugular venous valves mounted within a collapsable stent. The stents can be made from self-expandable or shape-memory materials such as nickel-titanium alloys (eg, Nitinol), or from balloon-expandable materials such as stainless steel, platinum-iridium, or other alloys. For a balloon-expandable device the delivery strategy involves collapsing the device over a balloon and placing it within a catheter-based sheath. The catheter containing the device can be inserted into the femoral artery (or vein) using essentially the same technique for deployment of coronary artery stents. In aortic stenosis, the device is passed from the femoral artery retrograde up the aorta to the aortic valve and deployed between the cusps of the calcified aortic valve, pushing the diseased cusps out of the way. Alternatively, the device can be deployed in an antegrade fashion through a minimally

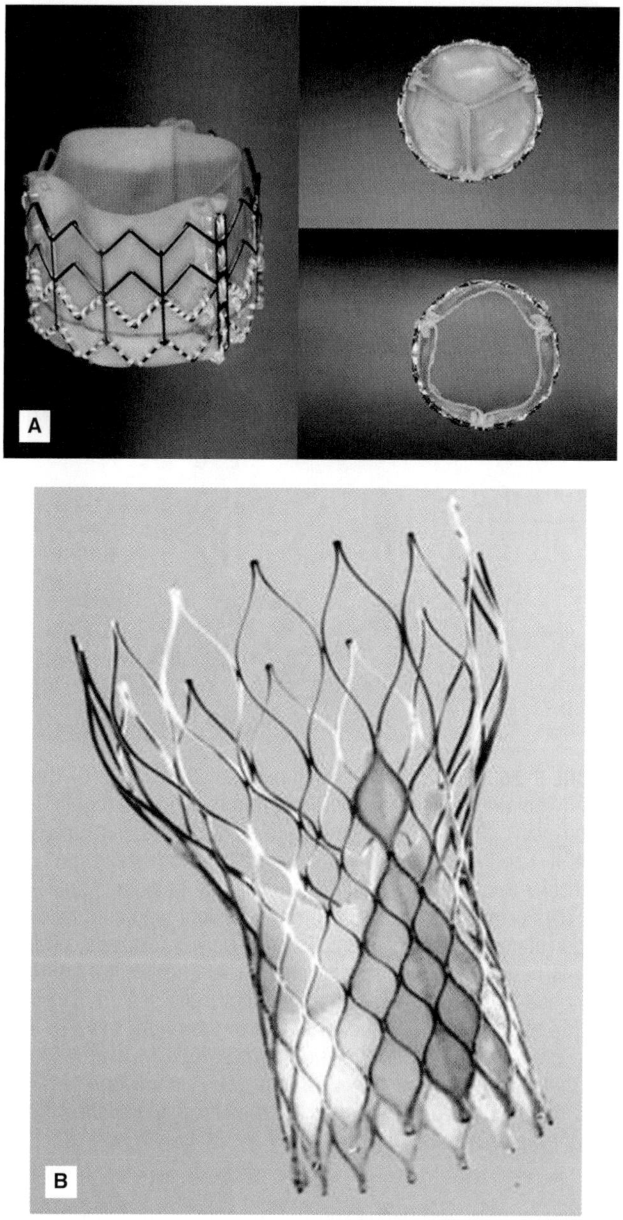

FIGURE 5-26 Percutaneous valve devices. (A) The Cribier-Edwards/Sapien valve consists of three equine pericardial leaflets fixed to a balloon-expandable steel stent. It is hand crimped over a delivery balloon prior to deployment. (B) The Corevalve system is constructed of porcine or bovine pericardium attached to a self-expanding nickel-titanium alloy (nitinol) stent. The ventricular portion has a high radial force to compress the native valve. The midportion is tapered to avoid interference with the coronary arteries. The aortic portion is flared to provide additional fixation against the wall of the ascending aorta.

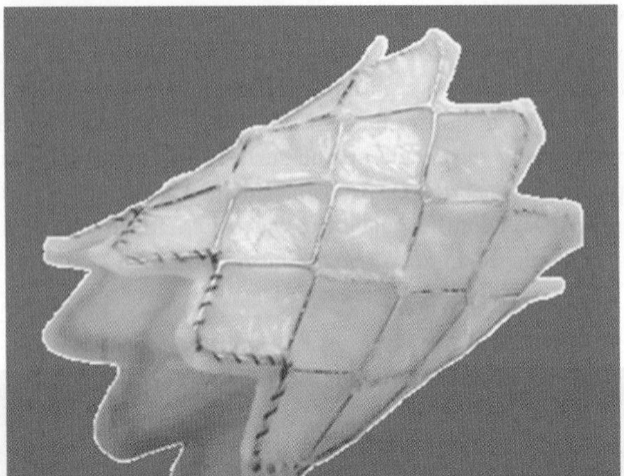

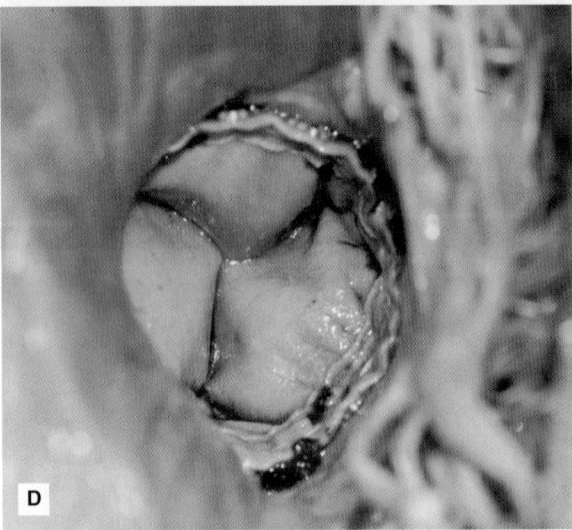

FIGURE 5-26 (*Continued*). Percutaneous valve devices. (**C**) The Melody pulmonary valve is constructed from a bovine jugular venous valve attached with sutures to a platinum-iridium alloy stent. Its use is primarily in failed surgically constructed right ventricular to pulmonary artery conduits in the pediatric population. (**D**) Postmortem photograph from a patient who died following percutaneous valve implantation. The valve prosthesis can be seen to be fully expanded within the left ventricular outflow tract with good leaflet coaptation. The interventricular septum can be seen to the left and the anterior leaflet of the mitral valve to the right. (*Reproduced with permission from Schoen FJ, Webb JG: Prosthetics and the heart, in McManus BM, Braunwald E [eds.]: Atlas of Cardiovascular Pathology for the Clinician. Philadelphia, Current Medicine, 2008; pp 241.*)

invasive surgical approach exposing the apex of the left ventricle. The transapical approach is favored in patients with significant atherosclerotic disease of the femoral artery and aorta. These devices may also play a role in the treatment of surgically implanted bioprosthetic valves that are failing because of stenosis or regurgitation in a so-called "valve-in-valve" application, in which a new valve is placed via catheter into the lumen of the existing valve.

Several devices are currently in various stages of development and clinical use in the aortic and pulmonary position. The two transcatheter aortic valves with the largest clinical experience are the Edwards SAPIEN device and the CoreValve system.[130,131] The SAPIEN device is composed of a balloon expandable stainless steel stent that houses a bovine pericardial valve. The stent has a low profile and is designed to be placed in the subcoronary position. There is a polymer skirt circumferentially attached to the stent to reduce paravalvular leaks. The CoreValve device is composed of a self-expandable Nitinol stent that houses a porcine pericardial trileaflet valve. The CoreValve stent is longer and is meant to be placed in the left ventricular outflow tract extending into the aortic root. These devices have been used in approximately 4000 patients worldwide, the first-in-man experience was reported in 2002, and clinical trials are ongoing. The Medtronic Melody transcatheter pulmonary valve is composed of a balloon expandable platinum-iridium alloy stent which houses a segment of bovine jugular vein containing its native venous valve. The Melody was designed to be used in children or young adults with congenital heart disease who have received surgically implanted right ventricular outflow tract conduits that are failing either because of stenosis or regurgitation.

Catheter-based stent-mounted prosthetic valves present novel challenges. Valved stents are significantly larger than most existing percutaneous cardiac catheters and devices, and are presently on the order of 22 to 24 Fr. In the aortic position, there is the potential to impede coronary flow, or interfere with anterior mitral leaflet mobility or the conduction system or the native diseased leaflets. Stent architecture may also preclude future catheter access to the coronaries for possible interventions. Secure seating within the aortic annulus or a pulmonary conduit and long-term durability of both the stent and the valve tissue are also major considerations.

CARDIAC REPLACEMENT AND ASSIST

Cardiac Transplantation

Cardiac transplantation provides long-term survival and improved quality of life for many individuals with end-stage cardiac failure.[132] Overall predicted 1-year survival is presently approximately 86% and 5-year survival is about 70%.[133] The most common indications for cardiac transplantation, accounting for 90% of the patients, are idiopathic cardiomyopathy and end-stage ischemic heart disease; other recipients have congenital, other myocardial, or valvular heart disease.

Hearts explanted at the time of transplantation may also have previously undiagnosed conditions and unexpected findings.[134] Most frequent is eosinophilic or hypersensitivity myocarditis, seen in 7 to 20% of explants and characterized by a focal or diffuse mixed inflammatory infiltrate, rich in eosinophils, and generally associated with minimal myocyte necrosis. In virtually all cases, the hypersensitivity is a response to one or more of the many heart failure medications taken by transplant candidates, including dobutamine. Several diseases responsible for the original cardiac failure can recur in and cause dysfunction of the allograft, including amyloidosis, sarcoidosis, giant-cell myocarditis, acute rheumatic carditis, and Chagas' disease.

Recipients of heart transplants undergo surveillance endomyocardial biopsies on an institution-specific schedule, which typically evolves from weekly during the early postoperative period, to biweekly until 3 to 6 months, and then approximately one to four times annually, or at any time when there is a change in clinical state. Histologic findings of rejection frequently precede clinical signs and symptoms of acute rejection. Optimal biopsy interpretation requires four or more pieces of myocardial tissue; descriptions of technical details and potential tissue artifacts are available.[135]

The major sources of mortality and morbidity following cardiac transplantation are perioperative ischemic injury, infection, allograft rejection, lymphoproliferative disease, and obstructive graft vasculopathy.

Early Ischemic Injury

Ischemic injury can originate from the ischemia that accompanies procurement and implantation of the donor heart. Several time intervals are potentially important: (1) the donor interval between brain death and heart removal, perhaps partially related to terminal administration of pressor agents or the release of norepinephrine and cytokines associated with brain death; (2) the interval of warm ischemia between donor cardiectomy to cold storage; (3) the interval during cold transport; and (4) the interval during rewarming, trimming, and implantation. Hypertrophy and coronary obstructions tend to promote ischemia, whereas decreased tissue temperature and cardioplegic arrest mitigate against ischemic injury. As in other situations of transient myocardial ischemia, frank necrosis, or prolonged ischemic dysfunction of viable myocardium or both may be present. Myocardial injury can cause low cardiac output in the perioperative period.

Perioperative myocardial ischemic injury may be detectable in endomyocardial biopsies. Owing to the anti-inflammatory effects of immunosuppressive therapy, the histologic progression of healing of myocardial necrosis in transplanted hearts may be delayed (Fig. 5-27). Therefore, the repair phase of perioperative myocardial necrosis frequently confounds the diagnosis of rejection in the first postoperative month, and in some cases, for as long as 6 weeks. Late ischemic necrosis suggests occlusive graft vasculopathy (see the following).

Rejection

Improved immunosuppressive regimens in heart transplant patients have substantially decreased the incidence and severity of rejection episodes. Hyperacute rejection occurs rarely, most often when a major blood group incompatibility exists between donor and recipient, and acute rejection is unusual earlier than 2 to 4 weeks postoperatively. Although acute rejection episodes occur largely in the first several months after transplantation, rejection can occur years postoperatively, rationalizing the practice of many transplant centers to continue late surveillance biopsies at late but widely spaced intervals.

Acute cellular rejection is characterized histologically by an inflammatory cell infiltrate, with or without damage to cardiac myocytes; in late stages, vascular injury may become prominent (Fig. 5-28). Until recently, the International Society for Heart and Lung Transplantation (ISHLT) working formulation from 1990 was the most widely accepted and used to guide immunosuppressive therapy in heart transplant recipients.[136] In 2004, the grading system was revised as follows (with the "R" reflecting the revised system): Grade 0R—no rejection (no change from 1990), Grade 1R—mild rejection (1990 grades 1A, 1B, and 2), Grade 2R—moderate rejection (1990 grade 3A), and Grade 3R—severe rejection (1990 grades 3B and 4). The 1990 and 2004 formulations are compared in Table 5-4.

Acute antibody-mediated rejection (AMR) remains a controversial entity with a highly varied incidence among transplant centers without consensus on recognition, diagnosis either by histopathologic or immunologic testing, and clinical impact. AMR is diagnosed by nonspecific clinicopathologic findings, including: (1) cardiac dysfunction in the absence of cellular rejection or ischemic injury; (2) histologic features of interstitial edema, endothelial cell swelling, and intravascular macrophages on endomyocardial biopsy; (3) positive immunoperoxidase staining for C4d; and (4) the presence of circulating antidonor antibodies. AMR most often is diagnosed in sensitized patients (including those with previous transplantation, transfusion or pregnancy, and previous ventricular assist device use) and is associated with worse graft survival.

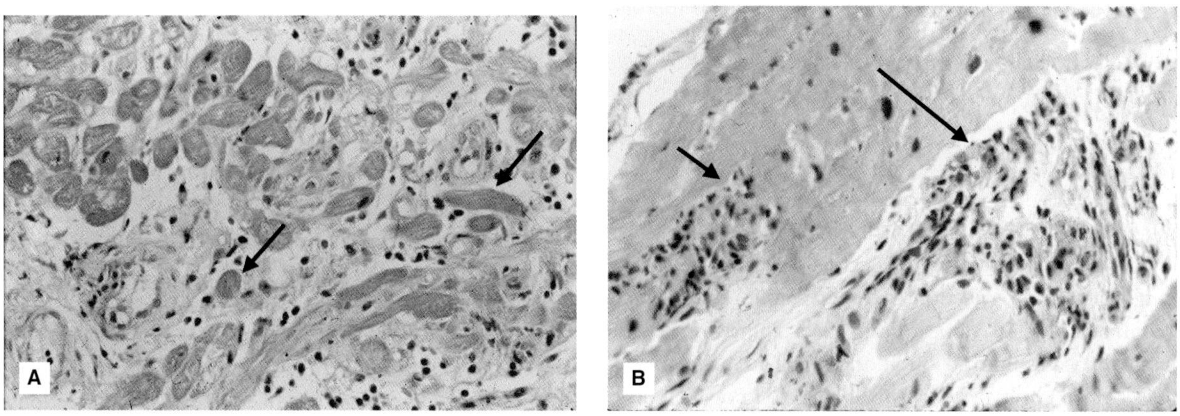

FIGURE 5-27 Perioperative ischemic myocardial injury demonstrated on endomyocardial biopsy. (A) Coagulative myocyte necrosis (*arrows*). (B) Healing perioperative ischemic injury with predominantly interstitial inflammatory response (*arrows*), not encroaching on and clearly separated from adjacent viable myocytes. The infiltrate consists of a mixture of polymorphonuclear leukocytes, macrophages, lymphocytes, and plasma cells. Hematoxylin and eosin, 200×.

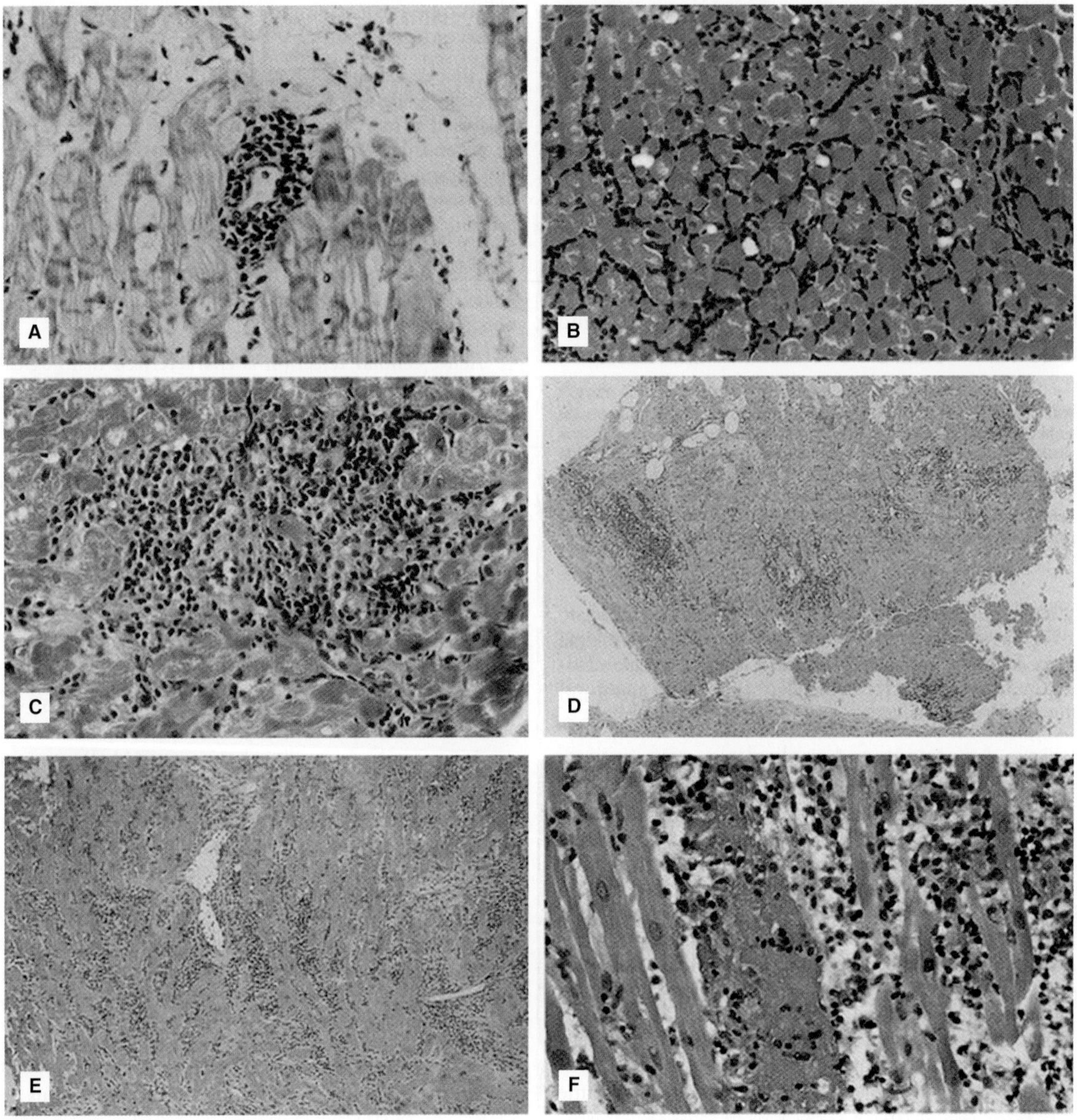

FIGURE 5-28 Histologic features of cardiac transplant rejection, designated as International Society for Heart and Lung Transplantation (ISHLT), 2004 Formulation, grades of rejection. (**A–C**) Grade 1R (mild). Focal perivascular lymphocytic and diffuse interstitial lymphocytic infiltrate without damage to adjacent myocytes, and up to one focus of dense lymphocytic infiltrate with associated myocyte damage, respectively. (**D**) Grade 2R (moderate). Multiple foci of dense lymphocytic infiltrates with associated myocyte damage and intervening areas of uninvolved myocardium. (**E and F**) Grade 3R (severe). Diffuse infiltrate with associated myocyte damage and polymorphous infiltrate with extensive myocyte damage, edema, and hemorrhage, respectively. (H&E stain). (*Reproduced with permission from Winters GL, Schoen FJ: Pathology of cardiac transplantation, in Silver MD, Gotlieb AI, Schoen FJ [eds]: Cardiovascular Pathology, 3rd ed. Philadelphia, WB Saunders, 2001; pp 725.*)

The contribution of AMR to allograft coronary disease is unknown. Some transplant centers treat AMR with plasmapheresis.

Findings in surveillance endomyocardial biopsies that must be distinguished from rejection include lymphoid infiltrates either confined to the endocardium or extending into the underlying myocardium and often accompanied by myocyte damage (so-called Quilty lesions, which have no known clinical significance), old biopsy sites, and healing ischemic injury either in the perioperative period or resulting from graft vasculopathy. Lymphoproliferative disorders and infections also may be seen in biopsies.

Infection

The immunosuppressive therapy required in all heart transplant recipients confers an increased risk of infection with bacterial, fungal, protozoan, and viral pathogens, with cytomegalovirus (CMV) and *Toxoplasma gondii* remaining common opportunistic infections in this setting. Prophylaxis is typically given to patients at high risk of primary CMV infection (donor seropositive, recipient seronegative). Viral and parasitic infections can present a challenge in endomyocardial biopsies as the multifocal lymphocytic infiltrates with occasional necrosis seen with these infections can mimic rejection.

TABLE 5-4 ISHLT Standardized Cardiac Biopsy Grading of Acute Cellular Rejection: Clinicopathologic Comparison of 1990 and 2004 Formulations

Rejection level	Histologic findings	Rejection grade 1990	Rejection grade 2004	Clinical response
None	Normal	0	0R	No change
Mild	Lymphocytic inflammation ± one focus of myocyte damage	1A, 1B, 2	1R	No/minimal change to chronic immunosuppressive regimen
Moderate	Lymphocytic inflammation + multiple foci of myocyte damage	3A	2R	Steroid bolus ± change in chronic immunosuppressive regimen
Severe	Lymphocytic inflammation + diffuse myocyte damage ± vascular injury	3B, 4	3R	Aggressive therapy (eg, steroids ± monoclonal antibodies [OKT3])

ISHLT = International Society for Heart and Lung Transplantation.

Graft Vasculopathy (Graft Coronary Arteriosclerosis)

Graft vasculopathy is the major limitation to long-term graft and recipient survival following heart transplantation.[137] Up to 50% of recipients have angiographically evident disease 5 years after transplantation, whereas intravascular ultrasound identifies graft vasculopathy in 75% of patients at 3 years posttransplant. However, graft vasculopathy may become significant at any time and can progress at variable rates. We have encountered graft coronary disease in several patients as early as 6 to 12 months postoperatively at the Brigham and Women's Hospital.

Graft vasculopathy (Fig. 5-29) occurs diffusely and ultimately involves both intramyocardial and epicardial allograft vessels, potentially leading to myocardial infarction, arrhythmias, congestive heart failure, or sudden death. Although this process has been called accelerated atherosclerosis, the morphology of the obstructive lesion of graft vasculopathy is distinct from that of typical atherosclerosis (Table 5-5).

The vessels involved have concentric occlusions characterized by marked intimal proliferation of myofibroblasts and smooth muscle cells with deposition of collagen, ECM, and lipid (see Fig. 5-29A and B). Lymphocytic infiltration varies from almost none to quite prominent. The internal elastic lamina often is almost completely intact, with only focal fragmentation. The resulting myocardial pathology includes subendocardial myocyte vacuolization (indicative of sublethal ischemic

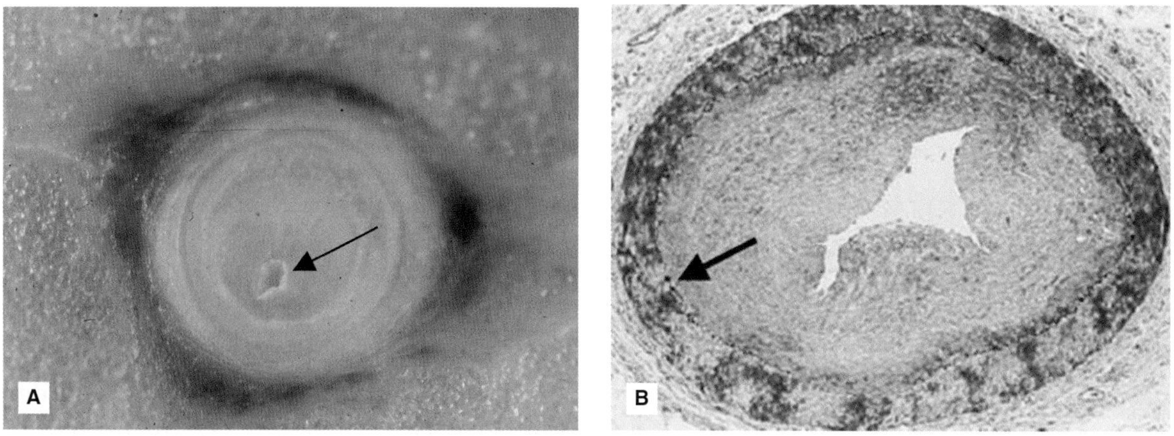

FIGURE 5-29 Gross and microscopic features of graft coronary disease and graft arteriosclerosis–induced myocardial pathology in heart transplant recipients. (A) Gross photograph of transverse cross-section of heart from patient who died of graft arteriosclerosis. Severe concentric stenosis of an epicardial coronary is apparent with only a pinhole lumen (*arrow*). (B) Histologic appearance of graft arteriosclerosis as low-power photomicrograph of vessel cross-section, demonstrating severe, near-complete, and predominantly concentric intimal proliferation with nearly intact internal elastic lamina (*arrow*). Verhoff-van Gieson stain (for elastin) 60×. (*[B] Reproduced with permission from Salomon RN, Hughes CWH, Schoen FJ, et al: Human coronary transplantation-associated arteriosclerosis: evidence for a chronic immune reaction to activated graft endothelial cells. Am J Pathol 1991; 138:791.*)

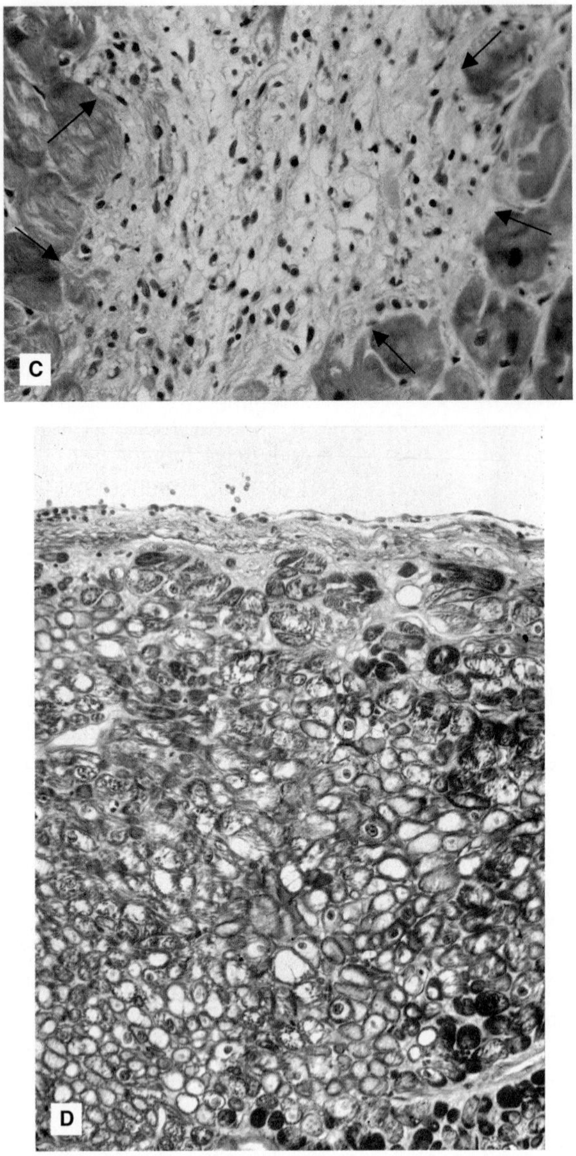

FIGURE 5-29 (*Continued*). Gross and microscopic features of graft coronary disease and graft arteriosclerosis–induced myocardial pathology in heart transplant recipients. (**C**) Myocardial microinfarct indicative of disease of small intramural arteries (*outlined by arrows*) Hematoxylin and eosin. and (**D**) subendocardial myocyte vacuolization indicative of severe chronic ischemia. Trichrome stain, 375×.

injury) and myocardial coagulation necrosis (indicative of infarction).

Although the precise mechanisms of graft vasculopathy are not definitely established, there is mounting evidence that chronic allogenic immune response to the transplant and nonimmunologic factors contribute to the vascular injury. Hyperlipidemia, advanced donor age, CMV infection, perioperative graft ischemia, diabetes, and hyperhomocysteinemia have been associated with graft vasculopathy, but their roles in the evolution of the disease remain uncertain. There is no apparent difference in the frequency with which graft vasculopathy develops in patients who were transplanted for end-stage coronary artery disease and those operated for idiopathic cardiomyopathy.

TABLE 5-5 Characteristics of Graft Arteriosclerosis versus Typical Atherosclerosis

Graft arteriosclerosis	Typical atherosclerosis
Rapid onset (months to years)	Slow onset (many years)
Risk factors uncertain	Hypertension, lipids, smoking, etc
Usually silent/congestive heart failure, sudden death	Chest pain, etc
Diffuse	Focal
Epicardial/intramural	Epicardial
Concentric	Eccentric
Lesions rarely complicated	Lesions often complicated
Smooth muscle cells, macrophages, lymphocytes	Smooth muscle cells, macrophages, foam cells
Primary immunologic mechanism(s)	Complicated stimuli
Difficult to treat; retransplant usually only option	Revascularization by angioplasty, stents, aortocoronary bypass

Source: Reproduced with permission from Schoen FJ, Libby P: Cardiac transplant graft arteriosclerosis. Trends Cardiovasc Med 1991; 1:216.

Early diagnosis of graft vasculopathy is limited by the lack of clinical symptoms of ischemia in the denervated allograft, by the relative insensitivity of coronary angiography, which frequently underestimates the extent and severity of this diffuse disease, and by the exclusive or predominant involvement of small intramyocardial vessels. Histologic changes of chronic ischemia such as subendothelial myocyte vacuolization can be seen on surveillance biopsies as evidence of myocardial ischemia and may suggest graft vasculopathy (see Fig. 5-29C and D). Obstructive vascular lesions are not usually amenable to PCI or coronary artery bypass grafting because of their diffuse distribution. For most cases, retransplantation is the only effective therapy for established graft atherosclerosis.

Posttransplant Lymphoproliferative Disorders

Posttransplant lymphoproliferative disorders (PTLDs) are a well-recognized and serious complication of the high-intensity long-term immunosuppressive therapy required to prevent rejection in cardiac allografts. Several factors increase the risk of PTLD, including pretransplant Epstein-Barr virus (EBV) seronegativity (10- to 75-fold increase), young recipient age, and CMV infection or mismatching (donor-positive, recipient-negative).[138]

PTLDs can present as an infectious mononucleosis-like illness or with localized solid tumor masses, especially in extranodal sites (eg, heart, lungs, gastrointestinal tract). The vast majority (>90%) of PTLDs derive from the B-cell lineage and are associated with EBV infection, although T- or NK-cell origin and late-arising EBV-negative lymphoid malignancies have been described. There is strong evidence that the lesions progress from polyclonal B-cell hyperplasias (early lesions) to lymphomas (monomorphic PTLDs) in a short period of time, in association with the appearance of cytogenetic abnormalities. Therapy centers on a stepwise approach of antiviral treatment and reduction in immunosuppression, and then progression to lymphoma chemotherapy.

Cardiac Assist Devices and Total Artificial Hearts

Continuing and increasing discrepancy between the number of available donor hearts and therefore transplants performed (<2300 annually in the United States, and declining) and the number of patients in the terminal phase of heart failure and refractory to medical management (estimated at 250,000 to 500,000 in the United States, and rising) has prompted efforts in the development of ventricular assist devices (VADs), total artificial hearts, and other therapies.

Mechanical cardiac assist devices and artificial hearts have traditionally been used in two settings: for ventricular augmentation sufficient to permit a patient to survive postcardiotomy or postinfarction cardiogenic shock while ventricular recovery is occurring, and as a bridge to transplantation when ventricular recovery is not expected and the goal is hemodynamic support until a suitable donor organ is located. More recently, left ventricular assist devices (LVADs) have been shown to provide long-term cardiac support with survival and quality-of-life improvement over optimal medical therapy in patients with end-stage congestive heart failure who are not candidates for transplantation. LVADs are also being investigated as a "bridge-to-recovery" in patients with congestive heart failure to induce reverse ventricular remodeling leading to an improvement in cardiac function that would eventually allow device removal. Many types of pumps are currently under development or in clinical use as ventricular assist devices.[139] Mechanical devices that entirely replace the native heart are currently in use or under development as bridge to transplant (eg, CardioWest Total Artificial Heart)[140] or as destination therapy (eg, AbioCor).[141]

The major complications of cardiac assist devices are hemorrhage, thrombosis/thromboembolism, infection, and durability limitations (Fig. 5-30). Hemorrhage continues to be a problem in device recipients, although the risk of major hemorrhage has been decreasing with improved devices, therapies, and methods. Many factors predispose to perioperative hemorrhage, including: (1) coagulopathy secondary to hepatic dysfunction, poor nutritional status, and antibiotic therapy; (2) platelet dysfunction and thrombocytopenia secondary to cardiopulmonary bypass; and (3) the extensive nature of the required surgery.

Nonthrombogenic blood-contacting surfaces are essential for a clinically useful cardiac assist device or artificial heart. Indeed, thromboembolism occurred in most patients having long-term implantation of the Jarvik-7 artificial heart and is a major design consideration for current devices. Thrombi form primarily in association with crevices and voids, especially in areas of disturbed blood flow such as near connections of conduits and other components to each other and the natural heart (see Fig. 5-30A). Most pulsatile pumps have used smooth polymeric pumping bladders; these are frequently associated with thromboembolic complications. One approach to the design of the blood pump is the use of textured polyurethane and titanium surfaces, which accumulate a limited platelet/fibrin pseudointimal membrane that is resistant to thrombosis, allowing only antiplatelet therapy for anticoagulation in most device recipients (HeartMate I, Thoratec). Newer, continuous-flow VADs are carefully designed to minimize thrombosis, but anticoagulation therapy is typically required.

Accounting for significant morbidity and mortality following the prolonged use of cardiac assist devices, infection can occur either within the device or associated with percutaneous drive lines (see Fig. 5-30B). Susceptibility to infection is potentiated by not only the usual prosthesis-associated factors (see later), but also by the multisystem organ damage from the underlying disease, the periprosthetic culture medium provided by postoperative hemorrhage, and by prolonged hospitalization with the associated risk of nosocomial infections. Assist device–associated infections are often resistant to antibiotic therapy and host defenses, but are generally considered not an absolute contraindication to subsequent cardiac transplantation. Novel device designs, including alternative sites for driveline placement and the elimination of the driveline altogether with transcutaneous energy transmission technology, may play a role in further decreasing infection.

Other complications include hemolysis, pannus formation around anastomotic sites, calcification, and device malfunction.[142] Device failure can result from fracture or tear of one of the prosthetic valves within the device conduits in pulsatile VADs, as this application provides a particularly severe test of valve durability (see Fig. 5-30C), or secondary to damage or dehiscence to the pumping bladder (see Fig. 5-30D). There is evidence that patients on VAD are more likely to develop allosensitization, which can pose a significant risk to post-transplantation outcome in the bridge-to-transplant patients.[143] These complications not only have significant morbidity and can be fatal, but they may make a previously suitable patient ineligible for future transplantation.

Long-term LVADs are primarily used as a bridge to transplantation because cardiac transplantation currently offers a better long-term outlook for most patients. In a subset of patients, support by LVAD sporadically results in improved cardiac function, with heart transplantation no longer necessary even after removal of the LVAD (bridge to recovery). Left ventricular assist device support is now recognized to offer potential for myocardial recovery, a favorable outcome that is further enhanced by combination with pharmacologic therapy. LVADs lead to lowered cardiac pressure and volume overload in the myocardium followed by decreased ventricular wall tension, reduced cardiomyocyte hypertrophy, improved coronary perfusion, and decreased chronic ischemia.

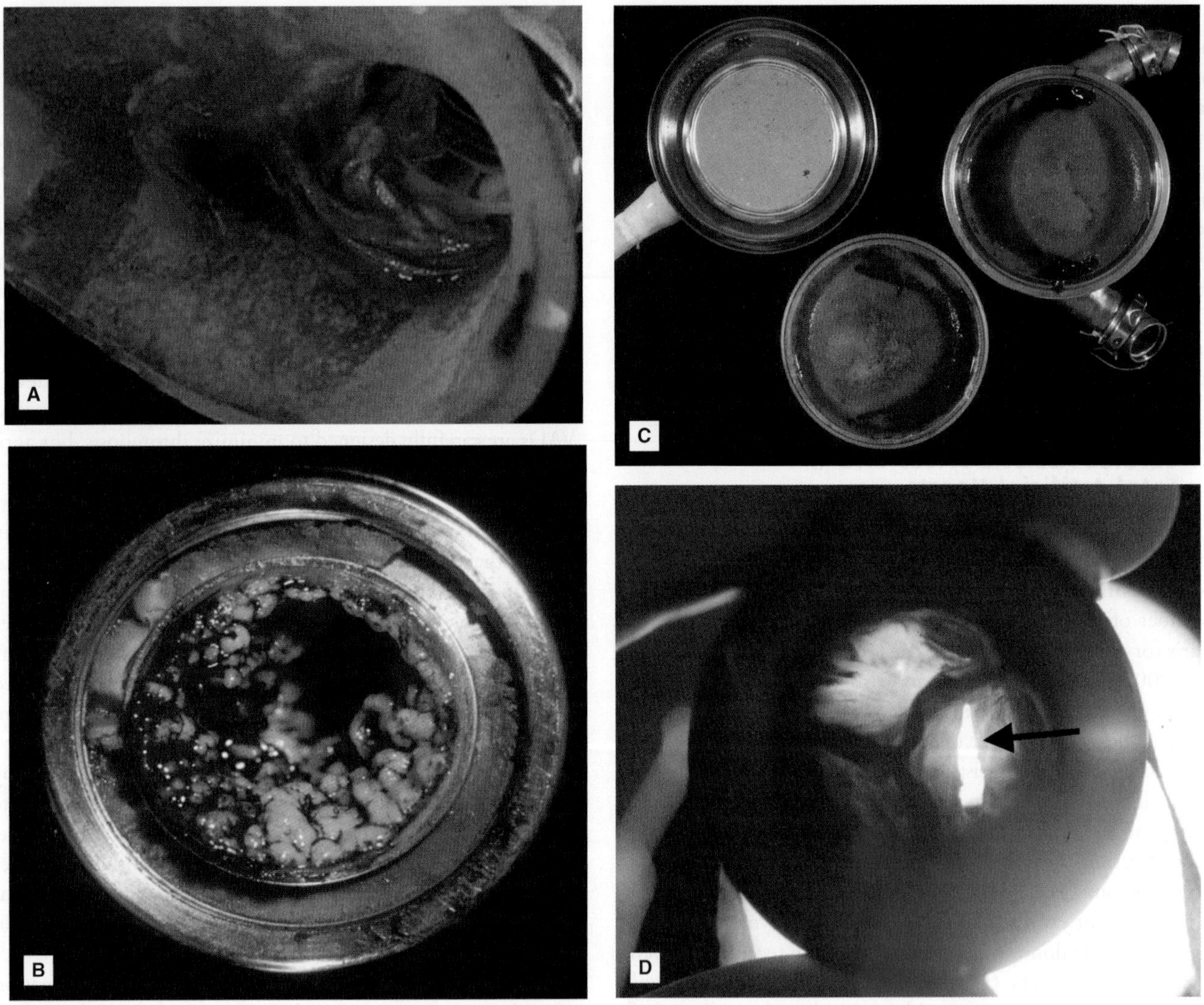

FIGURE 5-30 Complications of left ventricular assist devices (LVADs). (A) Thrombotic deposits at the pump outflow/housing junction, respectively. (B) Fungal infection in LVAD outflow graft. (C) Dehiscence of the bladder of a left ventricular assist device. (D) Cuspal tear in inflow valve of LVAD. This patient was not a transplant candidate and had been on the LVAD as destination therapy for about 12 months before the tear occurred causing regurgitation. The valve was replaced without incident. (*[A] Reproduced with permission from Fyfe B, Schoen FJ: Pathologic analysis of 34 explanted Symbion ventricular assist devices and 10 explanted Jarvik-7 total artificial hearts. Cardiovasc Pathol 1993; 2:187. [B–C] Reproduced with permission from Schoen FJ, Edwards WD: Pathology of cardiovascular interventions, including endovascular therapies, revascularization, vascular replacement, cardiac assist/replacement, arrhythmia control and repaired congenital heart disease, in Silver MD, Gotlieb AI, Schoen FJ [eds]: Cardiovascular Pathology, 3rd ed. Philadelphia, WB Saunders, 2001; p 678.*)

To what extent recovery of myocardial function can occur during VAD implantation is uncertain. Many pathophysiologic changes occur during the progression to end-stage heart failure, ranging from the subcellular (eg, abnormal mitochondrial function and calcium metabolism) to the organ and system level (eg, ventricular dilation, decreased ejection fraction, and neurohormonal changes), leading to the signs and symptoms of congestive failure. Implantation of an LVAD can reverse many of these changes (*reverse remodeling*), leading to increased cardiac output, decreased ventricular end-diastolic volume, and normalization of neurohormonal status such that a small fraction of patients can be weaned from the device without the need for subsequent cardiac transplantation. Current research focuses on the mechanisms of cardiac recovery, identification of patients who could achieve recovery, and specifics such as the timing and duration of therapy; a key goal is to identify potential predictors and novel therapeutic targets capable of enhancing myocardial repair.[144]

ARRHYTHMIAS

Arrhythmias generally occur as a result of disorders of electrical impulse formation, disorders of electrical impulse conduction, or a combination of the two. The underlying anatomic substrates for arrhythmogenesis are many. Many of the primary cardiomyopathies can present with arrhythmias, including the genetic (eg, hypertrophic cardiomyopathy, arrhythmogenic right ventricular cardiomyopathy, and the ion channelopathies), mixed (eg, dilated cardiomyopathy), and acquired (eg, myocarditis) groups. Many secondary cardiomyopathies also may have arrhythmias as a predominant feature (eg, sarcoidosis). A common cause of arrhythmias and sudden death (especially in the older adult population) is ischemic heart disease, both in patients with and without a prior myocardial infarction. Myocardial hypertrophy and fibrosis of any etiology (eg, secondary to valvular heart disease, hypertension, or a remote infarction) also can provide the anatomical and functional substrate for the development of an arrhythmia. These underlying processes and pathologic anatomy increase the risk of spontaneous lethal arrhythmias in the setting of acute initiating events such as acute ischemia, neurohormonal activation, changes in electrolytes, and other metabolic stressors.[145]

Treatments for arrhythmias and their complications include pharmacologic therapy, and device therapy[146] (eg, pacemakers, defibrillators), and ablation therapy.

Pacemakers and Implantable Cardioverter-Defibrillators

Modern cardiac pacing is achieved by a system of interconnected components consisting of: (1) a pulse generator that includes a power source and electric circuitry to initiate the electric stimulus and to sense normal activity; (2) one or more electrically insulated conductors leading from the pulse generator to the heart, with a bipolar electrode at the distal end of each; and (3) a tissue, or blood and tissue, interface between electrode and adjacent stimulatable myocardial cells, which is of critical importance in the proper functioning of the pacemaker. Typically, a layer of nonexcitable fibrous tissue forms around the tip of the electrode. This fibrosis may be induced by the electrode itself or may result from myocardial scarring from some other cause, most commonly a healed myocardial infarction. The thickness of this nonexcitable tissue between the electrode and excitable tissue determines the stimulus threshold, or the strength of the pacing stimulus required to initiate myocyte depolarization, and thus the amount of energy required from the pacemaker. Attempts to reduce the thickness of this layer (thereby extending battery life) include improved lead designs[147] with active fixation and the use of slow, local release of corticosteroids from the lead tip. Implantable cardioverter-defibrillators (ICDs) are used in the treatment of patients who have life-threatening ventricular arrhythmias that are refractory to medical management and unsuitable for other surgical or ablative therapy, and have similar components to the pacemaker described in the preceding. These devices sense arrhythmias that can lead to sudden death and deliver therapy in the form of rapid ventricular pacing and/or a defibrillation current to terminate the dysrhythmic episode. ICDs also must overcome the barrier posed by the interfacial fibrosis at the electrode tip.

Complications from the use of pacemakers include lead displacement, vascular or cardiac perforation leading to hemothorax, pneumothorax or tamponade, lead entrapment, infection, erosion of the device into adjacent tissues owing to pressure necrosis, rotation of the device within the pocket, thrombosis and/or thromboembolism, and lead fracture, in addition to malfunction of the device itself. If the lead needs to be extracted for chronic infection or device-related defects, damage to the myocardium and/or tricuspid valve may occur secondary to encasement of the lead in fibrous tissue. Similar complications affect ICDs, with additional considerations being the consequences of repeated defibrillations on the myocardium and vascular structures, including myocardial necrosis, and the risk of oversensing (with resultant unnecessary shocks) or undersensing (with resultant sudden death). Increased attention has been paid of late to malfunctioning ICDs because of electrical flaws in a specific model that resulted in failure to terminate fatal arrhythmias.[148]

Ablation

Ablation involves the directed destruction of arrhythmogenic myocardium, accessory pathways, or conduction system structures to control or cure a variety of arrhythmias, including atrial flutter and fibrillation, ventricular tachycardias, and paroxysmal supraventricular tachycardias that are refractory to medical management.[149,150] Ablation can be carried out as part of a surgical procedure, or through percutaneous catheter means. Electrophysiologic (EP) studies can be used to (1) provide information on the type of rhythm disturbance, (2) terminate a tachycardia by electrical stimulation, (3) evaluate the effects of therapy, (4) ablate myocardium involved in the tachycardia, and (5) identify patients at risk for sudden cardiac death.

Radiofrequency ablation acutely produces coagulation necrosis within the myocardium directly underneath the source tip, eliminating the source or pathway of the arrhythmia. The characteristic histologic changes include loss of myocyte striations, loss or pyknosis of nuclei, hypereosinophilia, and contraction bands. The edge of the fresh lesion is often hemorrhagic with interstitial edema (Fig. 5-31) and inflammation. The area undergoes the usual progression of healing similar to that in an infarct, with an early neutrophilic infiltrate, followed by macrophages to handle the necrotic debris, followed by granulation tissue formation and eventual scarring. Through

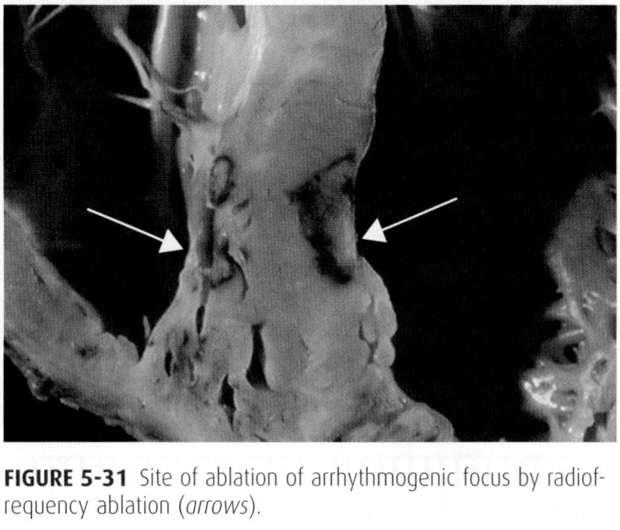

FIGURE 5-31 Site of ablation of arrhythmogenic focus by radiofrequency ablation (*arrows*).

the use of irrigated, cooled catheters, the lesions can penetrate deeply into the myocardium. Techniques using other forms of energy, including cryoablation, microwave, and lasers, have been used to create lesions in the myocardium for the treatment of arrhythmias.

NEOPLASTIC HEART DISEASE

Although metastatic tumors to the heart are present in 1 to 3% of patients dying of cancer, primary tumors of the heart are unusual.[151,152] The most common tumors, in descending order of frequency, are: myxomas, lipomas, papillary fibroelastomas, angiomas, fibromas, and rhabdomyomas, all benign and accounting for approximately 80% of primary tumors of the adult heart. The remaining 20% are malignant tumors, including angiosarcomas, other sarcomas, and lymphomas. Many cardiac tumors have a genetic basis.

The most frequent cardiac tumors are illustrated in Fig. 5-32.

Myxoma

Myxomas are the most common primary tumor of the heart in adults, accounting for about 50% of all benign cardiac tumors. They typically arise in the left atrium (80%) along the interatrial septum near the fossa ovalis. Occasionally, myxomas arise in the right atrium (15%), the ventricles (3 to 4%), or valves. These tumors arise more frequently in women and usually present between the ages of 50 and 70 years. Sporadic cases of myxoma are almost always single, whereas familial cases can be multiple and present at an earlier age.

Myxomas range from small (<1 cm) to large (up to 10 cm) and form sessile or pedunculated masses that vary from globular and hard lesions mottled with hemorrhage to soft, translucent, papillary, or villous lesions having a myxoid and friable appearance (see Fig. 5-32A). The pedunculated form frequently is sufficiently mobile to move into or sometimes through the ipsilateral atrioventricular valve annulus during ventricular diastole, causing intermittent and often position-dependent obstruction. Sometimes, such mobility exerts a wrecking ball effect, causing damage to and secondary fibrotic thickening of the valve leaflets.

Clinical manifestations are most often determined by tumor size and location; some myxomas are incidentally detected in patients undergoing echocardiography for other indications, whereas others may present with sudden death. Symptoms are generally a consequence of valvular obstruction, obstruction of pulmonary or systemic venous return, embolization, or a syndrome of constitutional symptoms. Intracardiac obstruction may

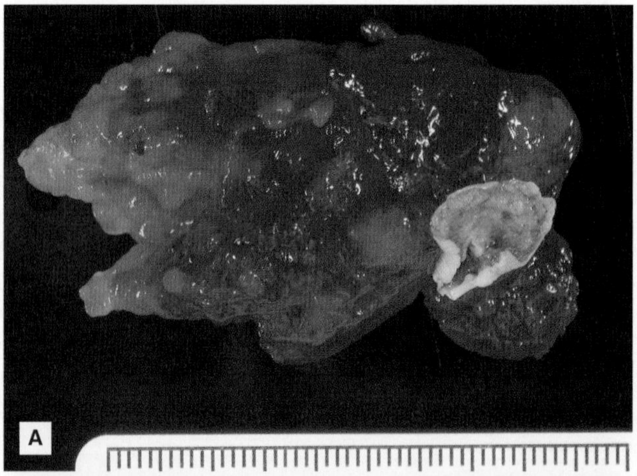

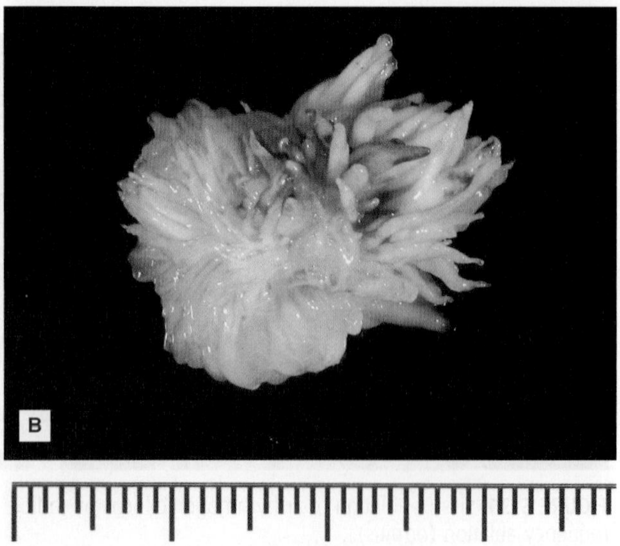

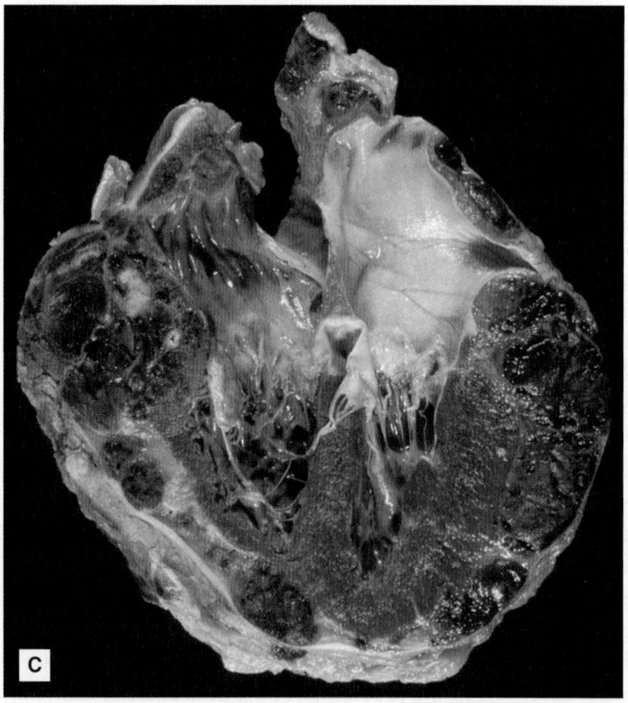

FIGURE 5-32 Gross features of primary cardiac tumors. (A) Resected left atrial myxoma, as Irregular polypoid, gelatinous friable mass. The resection margin that surrounds the proximal portion of the stalk is at right. (B) Papillary fibroelastoma. Gross photograph demonstrating resemblance of this lesion to sea anemone, with papillary fronds. (C) Massive pericardial angiosarcoma, subepicardial and with deep myocardial invasion at multiple sites. (*[C] Reproduced with permission from Schoen FJ: Interventional and Surgical Cardiovascular Pathology: Clinical Correlations and Basic Principles. Philadelphia, WB Saunders, 1989.*)

mimic the presentation of mitral or tricuspid stenosis with dyspnea, pulmonary edema, and right-sided heart failure. Fragmentation of a left-sided tumor with embolization may mimic the presentation of infective endocarditis with transient ischemic attacks, strokes, and cutaneous lesions; emboli from right-sided lesions may present as pulmonary hypertension. Constitutional symptoms such as fever, erythematous rash, weight loss, and arthralgias may result from the release of the acute-phase reactant interleukin-6 from the tumor leading to these inflammatory and autoimmune manifestations. Echocardiography, including transesophageal echocardiography, provides a means to noninvasively identify the masses and their location, attachment, and mobility. Surgical removal usually is curative with excellent short- and long-term prognosis. Rarely, the neoplasm recurs months to years later, usually secondary to incomplete removal of the stalk.

The Carney complex is a multiple neoplasia syndrome featuring cardiac and cutaneous myxomas, endocrine and neural tumors, as well as pigmented skin and mucosal lesions. Previously described cardiac myxoma syndromes such as LAMB (lentigines, atrial myxoma, mucocutaneous myxomas, and blue nevi) and NAME (nevi, atrial myxomas, mucinosis of the skin, and endocrine overactivity) are now encompassed by the Carney complex. The Carney complex is inherited as an autosomal dominant trait, and is associated with mutations in the PRKAR1 gene encoding the R1 regulatory subunit of cyclic AMP–dependent protein kinase A.

Histologically, myxomas are composed of stellate or globular cells (myxoma cells), often in formed structures that variably resemble poorly formed glands or vessels, endothelial cells, macrophages, mature or immature smooth muscle cells, and a variety of intermediate forms embedded within an abundant acid mucopolysaccharide matrix and covered by endothelium. Although it had long been questioned whether cardiac myxomas were neoplasms, hamartomas, or organized thrombi, it is now widely believed that they represent benign neoplasia. These tumors are thought to arise from remnants of subendocardial vasoformative reserve cells or multipotential primitive mesenchymal cells, which can differentiate along multiple lineages, giving rise to the mixture of cells present within these tumors.

Other Cardiac Tumors and Tumor-like Conditions

Cardiac lipomas are discrete masses that are typically epicardial, but may occur anywhere within the myocardium or pericardium. Most are clinically silent, but some may cause symptoms secondary to arrhythmias, pericardial effusion, intracardiac obstruction, or compression of coronary arteries. Magnetic resonance imaging is useful in the diagnosis of adipocytic lesions because of its ability to identify fatty tissues. Histologically, these tumors are composed of mature adipocytes, identical to lipomas elsewhere. A separate, non-neoplastic condition called lipomatous hypertrophy of the interatrial septum is characterized by accumulation of unencapsulated adipose tissue in the interatrial septum that can lead to arrhythmias. Histologically, this tissue is composed of a mixture of mature and immature adipose tissue and cardiac myocytes, in contrast to the pure mature adipose tissue of a proper lipoma.

Papillary fibroelastomas[153] are usually solitary and located on the valves, particularly the ventricular surfaces of semilunar valves and the atrial surfaces of atrioventricular valves. The most common site is the aortic valve, followed by the mitral valve. They constitute a distinctive "sea anemone" cluster of hairlike projections up to 1 cm or more in length, and can mimic valvular vegetations echocardiographically (see Fig. 5-32B).[154] Histologically, they are composed of a dense core of irregular elastic fibers, coated with myxoid connective tissue, and lined by endothelium. They may contain focal platelet-fibrin thrombus and serve as a source for embolization, commonly to cerebral or coronary arteries. Surgical excision is recommended to eliminate these embolic events. Although classified with neoplasms, fibroelastomas may represent organized thrombi, similar to the much smaller, usually trivial, whisker-like Lambl's excrescences that are frequently found on the aortic valves of older individuals.

Rhabdomyomas comprise the most frequent primary tumor of the heart in infants and children.[155] They are usually multiple and involve the ventricular myocardium on either side of the heart. They consist of gray-white myocardial masses up to several centimeters in diameter that may protrude into the ventricular or atrial chambers, causing functional obstruction. These tumors tend to spontaneously regress, so surgery is usually reserved for patients with severe hemodynamic disturbances or arrhythmias refractory to medical management. Most cardiac rhabdomyomas occur in patients with tuberous sclerosis, the clinical features of which also include infantile spasms, skin lesions (hypopigmentation, shagreen patch, subcutaneous nodules), retinal lesions, and angiomyolipomas. This disease, in its familial form, exhibits autosomal dominant inheritance, but about half the cases are sporadic owing to new mutations. Histologically, rhabdomyomas contain characteristic "spider cells," which are large, myofibril-containing, rounded or polygonal cells with numerous glycogen-laden vacuoles separated by strands of cytoplasm running from the plasma membrane to the centrally located nucleus.

Cardiac fibromas, although also occurring predominantly in children and presenting with heart failure or arrhythmias, or incidentally, differ from rhabdomyomas in being solitary lesions that may show calcification on a routine chest radiograph.[156] Fibromas are white, whorled masses that are typically ventricular. There is an increased risk of cardiac fibromas in patients with Gorlin's syndrome (nevoid basal cell carcinoma syndrome),[157] an autosomal dominant disorder characterized by skin lesions, odontogenic keratocysts of the jaw, and skeletal abnormalities. Histologically, fibromas consist of fibroblasts showing minimal atypia and collagen with the degree of cellularity decreasing with increasing age of the patient at presentation. Although they are grossly well circumscribed, there is usually an infiltrating margin histologically. Calcification and elastin fibers are not uncommon in these lesions.

Sarcomas, with angiosarcomas, undifferentiated sarcomas, and rhabdomyosarcomas being the most common, are not distinctive from their counterparts in other locations. They tend to involve the right side of the heart, especially the right atrioventricular groove (see Fig. 5-32C). The clinical course is rapidly progressive as a result of local infiltration with intracavity obstruction and early metastatic events.

Peculiar microscopic-sized cellular tissue fragments have been noted incidentally as part of endomyocardial biopsy or surgically removed tissue specimens, either free-floating or loosely attached to a valvular or endocardial mass.[158] Termed mesothelial/monocytic incidental cardiac excrescences (MICE), they appear histologically largely as clusters and ribbons of mesothelial cells and entrapped erythrocytes and leukocytes, embedded within a fibrin mesh. These "masses" are considered artifacts of no clinical significance formed by compaction of mesothelial strips (likely from the pericardium) or other tissue debris and fibrin, which are transported via catheters or around an operative site on a cardiotomy suction tip.

BIOMATERIALS AND TISSUE ENGINEERING

Biomaterials are synthetic or modified biologic materials that are used in implanted or extracorporeal medical devices to augment or replace body structures and functions.[159,160] Biomaterials include polymers, metals, ceramics, carbons, processed collagen, and chemically treated animal or human tissues, the latter exemplified by glutaraldehyde-preserved heart valves and pericardium. Biomaterials in medical devices interact with the surrounding tissues. The first generation of biomedical materials (eg, metals used for early valve substitutes) was generally designed to be inert; the goal was to reduce the host inflammatory responses to the implanted material. By the mid-1980s, a second generation of technology, comprising *bioactive* biomaterials, was emerging that could interact with the host in a beneficial manner (eg, biodegradable polymer sutures, drug delivery systems, textured bladder surfaces in ventricular assist devices). In the recent past, with a greater understanding of material-tissue interactions at the cellular and molecular levels, *regenerative* materials are being designed to stimulate specific cellular and tissue responses at the molecular level.[161,162]

Biomaterial-tissue interactions comprise effects of both the implant on the host tissues and the host on the implant, and are important in mediating prosthetic device complications (Fig. 5-33).[163] These interactions have local and potentially systemic consequences. Complications of cardiovascular medical devices, irrespective of anatomical site of implantation, can be grouped into six major categories: (1) thrombosis and thromboembolism; (2) device-associated infection; (3) exuberant or defective healing; (4) biomaterials failure (eg, degeneration, fracture); (5) adverse local tissue interaction (eg, toxicity, hemolysis); and (6) adverse effects distant from the intended site of the device (eg, biomaterials/device migration, systemic hypersensitivity).

Blood-Surface Interaction

Thromboembolic complications of cardiovascular devices cause significant mortality and morbidity. Thrombotic deposits can impede the function of a prosthetic heart valve, vascular graft, or blood pump, or cause distal emboli. As in the cardiovascular system in general, surface thrombogenicity, hypercoagulability, and locally static blood flow (called *Virchow's triad*), present individually or in combination, determine both the relative propensity toward thrombus formation and the location of

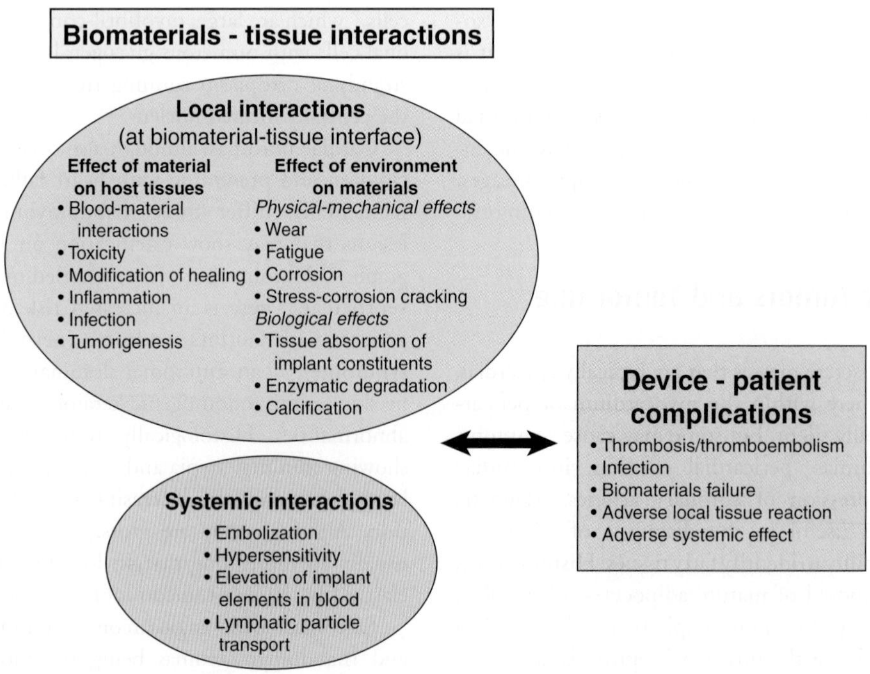

FIGURE 5-33 Overview of potential interactions of biomaterials with tissue, comprising local, distant, and systemic effects of the biomaterial on the host tissue, as well as the physical and biologic effects of the environment on the materials and the device. These interactions comprise the pathophysiologic basis for device complications and failure modes. (*Modified with permission from Schoen FJ: Introduction to host reactions to biomaterials and their evaluation, in Ratner BD, Hoffman AS, Schoen FJ, Lemons JE [eds]: Biomaterials Science: An Introduction to Materials in Medicine, 2nd ed. Orlando, Elsevier, 2004; p 293.*)

thrombotic deposits with specific devices. No known synthetic or modified biologic surface is as thromboresistant as the normal, unperturbed endothelium. Like a blood vessel denuded of endothelium, foreign materials on contact with blood spontaneously and rapidly (within seconds) absorb a film of plasma components, primarily protein, followed by platelet adhesion.[164] If conditions of relatively static flow are present, macroscopic thrombus can ensue. Considerable evidence implicates a primary role for blood platelets in the thrombogenic response to artificial surfaces.[165] The specific physical and chemical characteristics of materials that regulate the outcomes of blood-surface interaction are incompletely understood.

Coagulation proteins, complement products, other proteins, and platelets are activated, damaged, and consumed by blood-material interactions. The clinical approach to control of thrombosis in cardiovascular devices is generally through systemic anticoagulants, particularly Coumadin (warfarin) or antiplatelet agents. Coumadin inhibits thrombin formation but does not inhibit platelet-mediated thrombosis.

Hemolysis (damage to red blood cells) in implants and extracorporeal circulatory systems results from both cell-surface contact and turbulence-induced shear forces. Erythrocytes have reduced survival following cardiopulmonary bypass. Also, with earlier model heart valve prostheses, renal tubular hemosiderosis or cholelithiasis occurred in many patients, indicative of chronic hemolysis. Implantation of synthetic vascular grafts has been demonstrated to lower platelet survival, a defect that is largely alleviated by antiplatelet therapy. Also, late following implantation, platelet survival in recipients of such grafts is largely restored; possibly as a result of graft surface "passivation" by adsorbed protein.

Tissue-Biomaterials Interaction

Synthetic biomaterials elicit a *foreign body reaction,* a special form of nonimmune inflammatory response with an infiltrate predominantly composed of macrophages.[166,167] For most biomaterials implanted into solid tissue, encapsulation by a relatively thin fibrous tissue capsule (composed of collagen and fibroblasts) resembling a scar ultimately occurs, often with a fine capillary network at its junction with normal tissue. Ongoing mild chronic inflammation associated with this fibrous capsule is common with clinical implants; however, a substantial inflammatory infiltrate consisting of monocytes/macrophages and multinucleated foreign body giant cells in the vicinity of a foreign body generally suggests persistent tissue irritation. Although immunologic reactions have been proposed rarely for synthetic biomaterial-tissue interactions,[168] and antibodies can be elicited by implantation of some materials in finely pulverized form, proven clinical cardiovascular device failure owing to immunologic reactivity is rare.

Healing of a Vascular Graft, Heart Valve Sewing Cuff, or Endovascular Stent

Healing of a vascular graft, heart valve sewing cuff, or endovascular stent derives principally from overgrowth from the host vessel across anastomotic sites; this tissue is called *pannus.* Grafts, fabrics, and stents used as cardiovascular implants heal primarily by ingrowth of endothelium and smooth muscle cells from the cut edges of the adjacent artery, and contact points with vessels and/or myocardium; here endothelium is present, and the tissue is called a *neointima.* Two additional potential mechanisms of endothelialization exist: (1) tissue ingrowth through the fabric of a graft with interstices large enough to permit ingrowth of fibrovascular elements arising from capillaries extending from outside to inside the graft, which may permit endothelial cells to migrate to the luminal surface at a large distance from the anastomosis; and (2) deposition of functional endothelial cell progenitors from the circulating blood.[169]

Exuberant fibrous tissue can occur at a vascular anastomosis as an overactive but physiologic repair response (Fig. 5-34). Synthetic and biologic vascular grafts often fail because of generalized or anastomotic narrowing mediated by connective tissue proliferation in the intima, and heart valve prostheses can have excessive pannus that occludes the orifice. Intimal hyperplasia results primarily from smooth muscle cell migration, proliferation, and extracellular matrix elaboration following and possibly mediated by acute or ongoing endothelial cell injury. Important contributing factors include: (1) surface thrombogenesis; (2) delayed or incomplete endothelialization of the fabric; (3) disturbed flow across the anastomosis; and (4) mechanical "mismatch" at the junction of implant and host tissues.

Diminished healing also is clinically important in certain circumstances, such as periprosthetic leak associated with heart valve prostheses. Moreover, markedly diminished endothelialization owing to toxicity of the cytostatic agents, paclitaxel and sirolimus, has been implicated in late thrombosis of drug-eluting coronary stents. For uncertain reasons, humans have a limited ability to completely endothelialize cardiovascular prostheses, and full endothelialization of clinical grafts (yielding an intact *neointima*) usually does not occur. Endothelial cell coverage generally is restricted to a zone near an anastomosis, typically 10 to 15 mm, thereby allowing healing of intracardiac fabric patches and prosthetic valve sewing rings, but not long vascular grafts. Thus, except adjacent to an anastomosis of a vascular graft, a compacted platelet-fibrin aggregate (*pseudointima*) comprises the inner lining, even after long-term implantation. Because firm adherence of such linings to the underlying graft may be impossible, dislodgment of the lining and formation of a flap-valve can occur and cause obstruction.[170] Current research focuses on novel vascular graft materials that enhance endothelial cell attachment, grafts, and other implants preseeded with unmodified or genetically engineered endothelial cells, attempts to block smooth muscle cell proliferation, and engineered tissue vascular grafts (see the following).[171]

Infection

Infection is a common complication of implanted prosthetic devices and a frequent source of morbidity and mortality.[172,173] Early implant infections (<1 to 2 months postoperatively) most likely result from intraoperative contamination or early postoperative wound infection. In contrast, late infections generally occur by a hematogenous route, and can be initiated by bacteremia

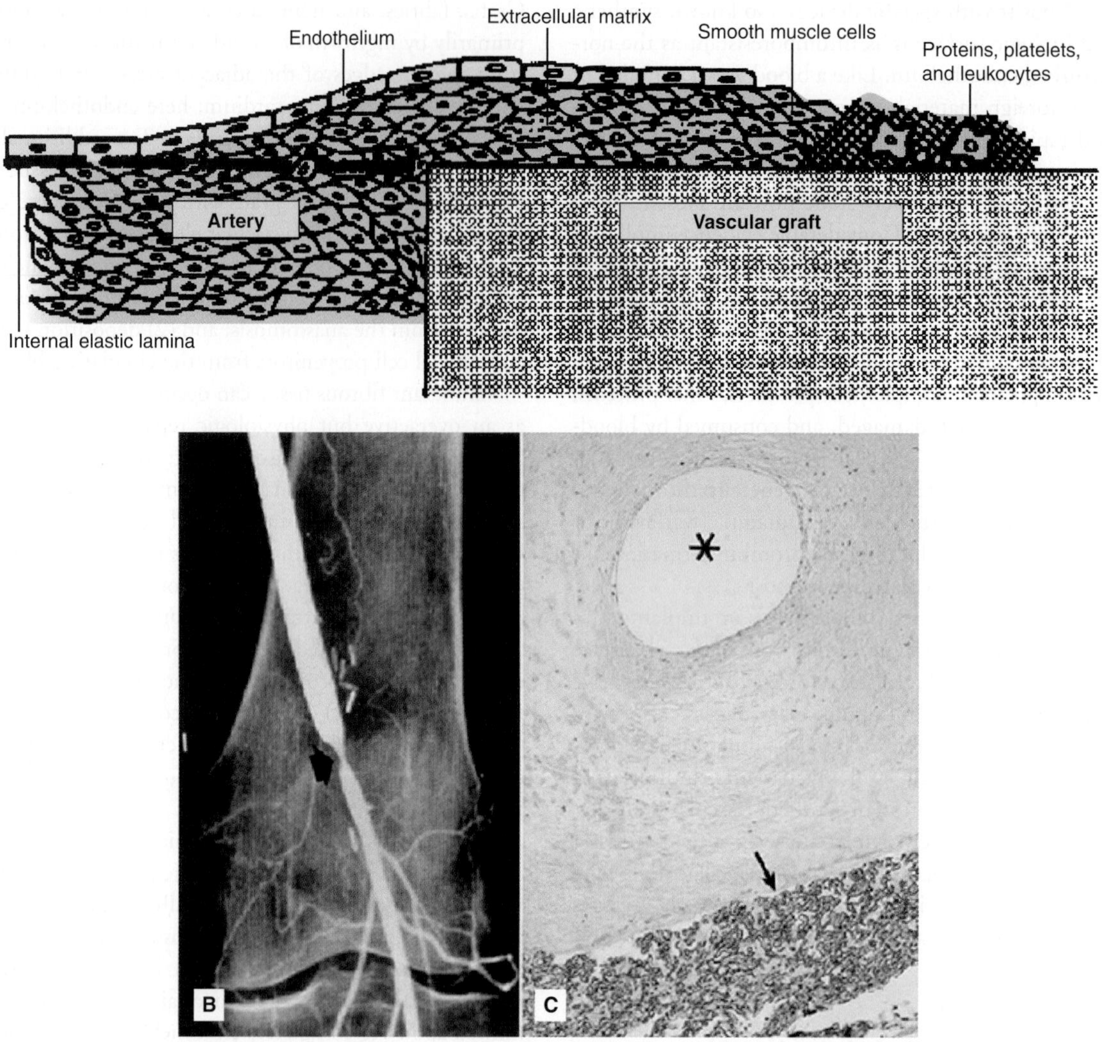

FIGURE 5-34 Vascular graft healing. (A) Schematic diagram of pannus formation, the major mode of graft healing with currently available vascular grafts. Smooth muscle cells migrate from the media to the intima of the adjacent artery and extend over and proliferate on the graft surface. The thin smooth muscle cell layer is covered by a proliferating layer of endothelial cells. (*B* and *C*) Anastomotic hyperplasia at the distal anastomosis of synthetic femoropopliteal graft. (B) Angiogram demonstrating constriction of distal graft anastomosis (*arrow*). (C) Photomicrograph demonstrating Gore-Tex graft (*arrow*) with prominent intimal proliferation and very small residual lumen (*asterisk*). (*Reproduced with permission from Schoen FJ: Interventional and Surgical Cardiovascular Pathology: Clinical Correlations and Basic Principles. Philadelphia, WB Saunders, 1989; p 7.*)

induced by therapeutic dental, gastrointestinal, or genitourinary procedures. Antibiotics given prophylactically at the time of device implantation and shortly before subsequent diagnostic and therapeutic procedures may protect against implant infection.

The presence of a foreign body potentiates infection in several ways. Microorganisms may inadvertently be introduced into deep tissue locations by contamination at device implantation, bypassing natural barriers against infection. Some devices, such as many of the current left ventricular assist devices, require a percutaneous driveline, providing a continuous potential means of entry for microorganisms. The production of a *biofilm* (ie, a multicellular consortium of microbial cells that is irreversibly associated with a material surface and enclosed in a self-produced extracellular matrix composed primarily of polysaccharides) by the organisms is protective against the humoral and cellular immune response of the host.[174] Infections associated with medical devices are characterized microbiologically by a high prevalence of organisms capable of forming protective biofilms,[175] including gram-positive bacteria such as *S. epidermidis, S. aureus, Enterococcus faecalis,* and *S. viridans,* gram-negative bacteria such as *Escherichia coli* and *Pseudomonas aeruginosa,* and fungi such as *Candida albicans.* Some of these organisms, especially *S. epidermidis* and *S. viridans,* are of relatively low virulence in the absence of a foreign body, but are frequent causes of medical device infection. Biofilm inhibits the penetration and effectiveness of opsonizing antibodies, inflammatory cells, and antibiotics. Moreover, vasculature may be diminished and there may be necrotic tissue in the vicinity of an implant. Consequently, an implant-associated infection often persists until the device is removed.

Tissue Engineering and Cardiovascular Regeneration

Tissue engineering comprises therapeutic approaches that use living cells together with natural materials or synthetic polymers to develop or regenerate functional tissues.[176–178] In the most widely used generic strategy to engineering tissues, the first step involves the seeding of cells on a synthetic polymer scaffold (usually a bioresorbable polymer in a porous configuration) or natural material (such as collagen or chemically treated tissue), each in the desired geometry for the engineered tissue, and a tissue is matured in vitro. The cells may be either fully differentiated or stem cells. The in vitro phase is done in a metabolically and mechanically supportive environment with growth media (a *bioreactor*), the cells proliferate, and an elaborate extracellular matrix is created in the form of a "new" tissue (the *construct*). In the second step, the construct is implanted in vivo into the appropriate anatomical location. Remodeling of the construct in vivo following implantation is intended to recapitulate normal functional architecture of an organ or tissue. Another collection of methods uses the in vivo environment as the bioreactor and thereby aims to recruit endogenous cells to build tissues from within. Key processes occurring during the in vitro and in vivo phases of tissue formation and maturation are: (1) cell proliferation, sorting, and differentiation; (2) extracellular matrix production and organization; (3) degradation of the scaffold; and (4) remodeling and potentially growth of the tissue.

Active research yielding progress has occurred with tissue-engineered vascular grafts, myocardium, and heart valves, as discussed in the following.

Engineered Vascular Grafts

Because of the failure of small-diameter synthetic vascular grafts, engineered blood vessels of small caliber are actively being investigated.[179,180] Vascular cells have been applied onto tubular resorbable polymer scaffolds matured in vitro in a bioreactor prior to in vivo implantation.[181] Exposure to pulsatile physical forces generally enhances graft properties; pulsed grafts are thicker, have greater suture retention, and higher cell and collagen density than nonpulsed engineered grafts, and have a histologic appearance similar to that of native arteries. Other investigators have fabricated mechanically sound engineered tissue vascular grafts by constructing a cohesive cellular sheet of smooth muscle cells, rolling this sheet to form the vessel media, analogous to a jelly roll, wrapping a sheet of human fibroblasts around the media to serve as an adventitia, and seeding endothelial cells in the lumen.[182] Vessel "equivalents" composed of collagen and cultured bovine fibroblasts, and smooth muscle and endothelial cells have been investigated, but despite reinforcement with a Dacron mesh, such grafts have been unable to withstand burst strengths for in vivo applications.[183] Another approach to vascular graft engineering utilizes naturally derived matrices with or without cell repopulation prior to implantation.[184] Vascular grafts fabricated from small intestine submucosa used as experimental vascular grafts in dogs were reported to be completely endothelialized and histologically similar to arteries.[185]

Another approach to vascular engineering extends the concept of Sparks' silicone mandril-grown graft used clinically in the 1970s, in which a collagenous tube was formed as the fibrous capsule reactive to an implanted foreign body (silicone mandril) adjacent to a diseased vessel; the mandril was subsequently removed yielding an autologous tissue tube.[186] However, owing to the variability of the quality of tissue generated in older patients in areas of circulatory insufficiency, such vascular replacements developed aneurysms when used clinically. Grafts grown as the reactive tissue that forms around silicone tubing inserted into the peritoneal cavity of rats, rabbits, and dogs, everted (so that mesothelial cells become the blood-contacting surface), and grafted into the carotid artery of the same animal remained patent up to 4 months.[187]

Clinical series of tissue engineered blood vessels as pulmonary artery segments and hemodialysis access grafts have been reported.[188,189] Clinically employed conventional ePTFE vascular grafts have been seeded with endothelial cells at the time of implantation.[190]

Regeneration of Cardiac Tissue

The classical view is that the adult heart responds to mechanical overload by hypertrophy (increase in cell size) and to severe ischemic or other injury by cell death (see earlier). Functional increase in cardiac myocyte number by cell regeneration or hyperplasia has generally not been considered possible. Nevertheless, several lines of research raise enthusiasm that clinically important cardiac regeneration may indeed be possible.

Recent evidence that myocyte regeneration and death occur physiologically, and that these cellular processes are enhanced in pathologic states, has challenged the view of the heart as a postmitotic organ. Heart homeostasis may be regulated by a stem cell compartment in the heart characterized by multipotent cardiac stem cells that possess the ability to acquire the distinct cell lineages of the myocardium. They are capable of regenerating myocytes and coronary vessels throughout life and have the capacity to adapt to increases in pressure and volume loads.[191] Moreover, adult bone marrow cells may be able to differentiate into cells beyond their own tissue boundary and create cardiomyocytes and coronary vessels. Myocardial tissue generated from cells, scaffolds, and bioreactors has been encouraging with respect to construct survival, vascularization, and integration, but significant functional improvement has yet to be demonstrated.[192,193] Application of cyclic mechanical stretch and electrical signals have been shown to enhance cell differentiation and force of contraction.[194]

Animal experiments and some early-phase clinical trials lend credence to the notion that cell-based cardiac repair may be an achievable therapeutic target, including: (1) the possibility that the heart may have endogenous mechanisms of repair; (2) cell-based therapies in which fetal or adult cardiomyocytes, skeletal myoblasts or non–muscle stem or differentiated cells are injected into the heart; and (3) experimental generation of functional myocardium by cell-scaffold-bioreactor tissue engineering approaches yielding a prosthetic myocardial patch.[195–197] Clinical trials have used cells derived from skeletal muscle and bone marrow, and basic researchers are investigating sources of new cardiomyocytes, such as resident myocardial progenitors and embryonic stem cells to achieve structural and functional integration of the graft with the host myocardium. Nevertheless, the most appropriate form of cellular therapy for myocardial injury remains to be identified, and it is unclear at present whether the beneficial effects observed in some studies are a result of functional and electrically integrated myocytes (the ideal), enhancement of angiogenesis owing to a local and non-specific inflammatory reaction at the site of injection, or a "paracrine" effect, whereby transplanted cells produce growth factors, cytokines, and other local signaling molecules that are beneficial to the infarct through neovascularization and/or scar remodeling.

Engineered Heart Valves

Recent scientific and technological progress has stimulated the goal of generating a living valve replacement device that would obviate the complications of conventional valve replacement, adapt to changing environmental conditions in the recipient, and potentially grow with a growing patient.[198–200] Innovative work toward this objective is active in many laboratories, and may eventually lead to clinical application. The long-term success of a tissue engineered (living) valve replacement will depend on the ability of its living cellular components (particularly VIC) to assume normal function with the capacity to repair structural injury, remodel the ECM, and potentially grow.

Tissue engineered heart valves (TEHV) grown as valved conduits from autologous cells (either vascular wall cells or bone marrow–derived mesenchymal stem cells) seeded on biodegradable synthetic polymers grown in vitro have functioned in the pulmonary circulation of growing lambs for up to 5 months.[201,202] These grafts evolved in vivo to a specialized layered structure that resembled that of native semilunar valve. A recent study has shown that pulmonary vascular walls fabricated from vascular wall cells and biodegradable polymer and implanted into very young lambs enlarged proportionally to overall animal growth over a 2-year period.[203]

To eliminate the need for in vitro cell seeding and culture steps, an alternative tissue engineering strategy has used either a scaffold of a decellularized naturally derived biomaterial (such as animal or human allograft valve, or decellularized sheep intestinal submucosa [SIS]) implanted without prior seeding but with the intent of harnessing intrinsic circulating cells to populate and potentially remodel the scaffold.[204] Tissue-derived scaffolds must possess desirable three-dimensional architecture, mechanical properties, and potential adhesion/migration sites for cell attachment and ingrowth. Decellularized porcine valves implanted in humans had a strong inflammatory response and suffered structural failure.[205]

Translation of heart valve tissue engineering and regenerative medicine from the laboratory to the clinical realm has exciting potential but also formidable challenges and uncertainties. Key hurdles include selection and validation of suitable animal models, development of guidelines for characterization and assurance of the quality of an in vitro fabricated tissue engineered heart valve for human implantation, and strategies to understand, monitor, and potentially control patient variability in wound healing and tissue remodeling in vivo.

DISCLOSURE

Frederick J. Schoen is or has been a consultant to Celxcel, Corazon, Cordis, Direct Flow Medical, Ethicon, Edwards Lifesciences, Medtronic, Pi-R-Square, Sadra Medical, Sorin Medical, St. Jude Medical, and Sulzer Carbomedics, in the past 5 years.
Robert Padera is or has been a consultant to Atria, Direct Flow, Du Pont, Medtronic, Mitral Solutions, Mitralign, Sadra, Sorin, St. Jude, and Transmedics.

REFERENCES

1. Williams RG, Pearson GD, Barst RJ, et al: Report of the National Heart, Lung, and Blood Institute Working Group on research in adult congenital heart disease. *J Am Coll Cardiol* 2006; 47:701.
2. Schoen FJ, Edwards WD: Pathology of cardiovascular interventions, including endovascular therapies, revascularization, vascular replacement, cardiac assist/replacement, arrhythmia control and repaired congenital heart disease, in Silver MD, Gotlieb AI, Schoen FJ (eds): *Cardiovascular Pathology*. 3rd Ed. Philadelphia, Churchill Livingstone, 2001; p 678.
3. Schoen FJ, Mitchell RN: The heart, in Kumar V, Abbas A, Fausto N, Aster J (eds): *Robbins and Cotran Pathologic Basis of Disease,* 8th ed. Philadelphia, WB Saunders, 2010; p 529.
4. Opie LH, Commerford PJ, Gersh BJ, Pfeffer MA: Controversies in ventricular remodeling. *Lancet* 2006; 367:356.
5. Diwan A, Dorn GW 2nd: Decompensation of cardiac hypertrophy. Cellular mechanisms and novel therapeutic targets. *Physiology* 2007; 22:56.
6. Vinge LE, Raake PW, Koch WJ: Gene therapy in heart failure. *Circ Res* 2008; 102:1458.
7. Van Rooij E, Marshall WS, Olson EN: Toward microRNA-based therapeutics for heart disease. The sense in antisense. *Circ Res* 2008; 103:919.
8. Gosse P: Left ventricular hypertrophy as a predictor of cardiovascular risk. *J Hypertens Suppl* 2005; 23:S37.
9. Ashrafian H, Watkins H: Reviews of translational medicine and genomics in cardiovascular disease. New disease taxonomy and therapeutic implications of cardiomyopathies. Therapeutics based on molecular phenotype. *J Am Coll Cardiol* 2007; 49:1251.
10. Cunningham KS, Veinot JP, Butany J: An approach to endomyocardial biopsy interpretation. *J Clin Pathol* 2006; 59:121.
11. Burkett EL, Hershberger RE: Clinical and genetic issues in familial dilated cardiomyopathy. *J Am Coll Cardiol* 2005; 45:969.
12. Cooper LT Jr: Myocarditis. *NEJM* 2009; 360:1526.
13. Spirito P, Bellone P, Harris KM, et al: Magnitude of left ventricular hypertrophy predicts the risk of sudden death in hypertrophic cardiomyopathy. *NEJM* 2000; 342:1778.
14. Hess OM, Sigwart U: New treatment strageties for hypertrophic obstructive cardiomyopathy. Alcohol ablation of the septum. The new gold standard? *J Am Coll Cardiol* 2004; 44:2054.
15. Bos JM, Towbin JA, Ackerman MJ: Diagnostic, prognostic, and therapeutic implications of genetic testing for hypertrophic cardiomyopathy. *J Am Coll Cardiol* 2009; 54:201.
16. Aurigemma GP, Gaasch WH: Clinical practice. Diastolic heart failure. *NEJM* 2004; 351:1097.
17. Basso C, Corrado D, Marcus FL, et al: Arrhythmogenic right ventricular cardiomyopathy. *Lancet* 2009; 373:1289.
18. Libby P, Theroux P: Pathophysiology of coronary artery disease. *Circulation* 2005; 111:3481.
19. Schoenhagen P, Ziada KM, Vince DG, et al: Arterial remodeling and coronary artery disease. The concept of "dilated" versus "obstructive" coronary atherosclerosis. *J Am Coll Cardiol* 2001; 38:297.
20. Mitchell RN, Schoen FJ: Blood vessels, in Kumar V, Abbas A, Fausto N, Aster J (eds): *Robbins and Cotran Pathologic Basis of Disease,* 8th ed. Philadelphia, WB Saunders, 2010; p 487.
21. Naghavi M, Libby P, Falk E, et al: From vulnerable plaque to vulnerable patient. A call for new definitions and risk management strategies. Parts 1 and 2. *Circulation* 2003; 108: 1664 and 1772.
22. Fuster V, Moreno PR, Fayad ZA, et al: Atherothrombosis and high-risk plaque. Part I. evolving concepts. *J Am Coll Cardiol* 2005; 46:947.
23. Aikawa M, Libby P: The vulnerable atherosclerotic plaque. Pathogenesis and therapeutic approach. *Cardiovasc Pathol* 2004; 13:125.

24. McVeigh ER: Emerging imaging techniques. *Circ Res* 2006; 98:879.
25. Jaffer FA, Libby P, Weissleder R: Molecular and cellular imaging of atherosclerosis. Emerging applications. *J Am Coll Cardiol* 2006; 47:1328.
26. Slager CJ, Wentzel JJ, Gijsen FJ, et al: The role of shear stress in the generation of rupture-prone vulnerable plaques. *Nat Clin Pract Cardiovasc Med* 2005; 2:401.
27. Kolodgie FD, Burke AP, Farb A: The thin-cap fibroatheroma. A type of vulnerable plaque. the major precursor lesion to acute coronary syndromes. *Curr Opin Cardiol* 2001; 16:285.
28. Yellon DM, Hausenloy DJ: Myocardial reperfusion injury. *NEJM* 2007; 357:1121.
29. Vargas SO, Sampson BA, Schoen FJ: Pathologic detection of early myocardial infarction. A critical review of the evolution and usefulness of modern techniques. *Mod Pathol* 1999; 12:635.
30. Ertl G, Frantz S: Healing after myocardial infarction. *Cardiovasc Res* 2005; 66:22.
31. Beltrami AP, Urbanek K, Kajstura J, et al: Evidence that cardiac myocytes divide after myocardial infarction. *NEJM* 2001; 344:1750.
32. Faxon DP. Early reperfusion strategies after acute ST-segment elevation myocardial infarction. The importance of timing. *Nat Clin Pract Cardiovasc Med* 2005; 2:22.
33. Hutchins GM, Silverman KJ: Pathology of the stone heart syndrome. Massive myocardial contraction band necrosis and widely patent coronary arteries. *Am J Pathol* 1979; 95:745.
34. Alfayoumi F, Srinivasan V, Geller M, Gradman A: The no-reflow phenomenon. Epidemiology, pathophysiology, and therapeutic approach. *Rev Cardiovasc Med* 2005; 6:72.
35. Camici PG, Prasad SK, Rimoldi OE: Stunning, hibernation, and assessment of myocardial viability. *Circulation* 2008; 117:103.
36. Slezak J, Tribulova N, Okruhlicova L, et al: Hibernating myocardium. Pathophysiology, diagnosis, and treatment. *Can J Physiol Pharmacol* 2009; 87:252.
37. Winters GL, Schoen FJ: Graft arteriosclerosis-induced myocardial pathology in heart transplant recipients. Predictive value of endomyocardial biopsy. *J Heart Lung Transplant* 1997; 16:985.
38. Kharbanda RK, Nielsen TT, Redington AN: Translation of remote ischaemic preconditioning into clinical practice. *Lancet* 2009; 374:1557.
39. McMullan MH, Maples MD, Kilgore TL Jr, et al: Surgical experience with left ventricular free wall rupture. *Ann Thorac Surg* 2001; 71:1894.
40. Birnbaum Y, Fishbein MC, Blanche C, et al: Ventricular septal rupture after acute myocardial infarction. *NEJM* 2002; 347:1426.
41. Antunes MJ, Antunes PE: Left-ventricular aneurysms. From disease to repair. *Expert Rev Cardiovasc Ther* 2005; 3:285.
42. Cohn JN, Ferrari R, Sharpe N. Cardiac remodeling—concepts and clinical implications. a consensus paper from an international forum on cardiac remodeling. *J Am Coll Cardiol* 2000; 35:569.
43. Antman EM, Braunwald E: ST-Elevation myocardial infarction. Pathology, pathophysiological and clinical feature, in Libby P, Bonow RD, Mann DL, Zipes DD (eds): *Braunwald's Heart Disease. A Textbook of Cardiovascular Medicine*, 8th ed. Philadelphia, WB Saunders, 2008; p 1207.
44. Landau C, Lange RA, Hillis LD: Percutaneous transluminal coronary angioplasty. *NEJM* 1994; 330:981.
45. Haudenschild CC: Pathobiology of restenosis after angioplasty. *Am J Med* 1993; 94(Suppl):40.
46. Daemen J, Serruys PW: Drug-eluting stent update 2007: Part I. A survey of current and future generation drug-eluting stents: meaningful advances or more of the same? Part II: Unsettled issues. *Circulation* 2007; 116:316 and 961.
47. Agostoni P, Valgimigli M, Biondi-Zoccai GG, et al: Clinical effectiveness of bare-metal stenting compared with balloon angioplasty in total coronary occlusions: insights from a systematic overview of randomized trials in light of the drug-eluting stent era. *Am Heart J* 2006; 151:682
48. Farb A, Sangiorgi G, Carter AJ, et al: Pathology of acute and chronic coronary stenting in humans. *Circulation* 1999; 99:44.
49. Welt FG, Rogers C: Inflammation and restenosis in the stent era. *Arterioscler Thromb Vasc Biol* 2002; 22:1769.
50. Nakazawa G, Finn AV, Kolodgie FD, Virmani R: A review of current devices and a look at new technology. Drug eluting stents. *Expert Rev Med Dev* 2009; 6:33.
51. Kukreja N, Onuma Y, Daemen J, Serruys PW: The future of drug-eluting stents. *Pharmacol Res* 2008; 57:171.
52. Sousa JE, Costa MA, Sousa AG, et al: Two-year angiographic and intravascular ultrasound follow-up after implantation of sirolimus-eluting stents in human coronary arteries. *Circulation* 2003; 107:381.
53. Ong AT, Serruys PW: An overview of research in drug-eluting stents. *Nat Clin Pract Cardiovasc Med* 2005; 2:647.
54. Holmes DR, Kereiakes DJ, Laskey WK, et al: Thrombosis and drug-eluting stents: an objective appraisal. *J Am Coll Cardiol* 2007; 50:109.
55. Ramcharitar S, Serruys PW: Fully biodegradable coronary stents: progress to date. *Am J Cardiovasc Drugs* 2008; 8:305
56. Opie LH, Commerford PJ, Gersh BJ: Controversies in stable coronary artery disease. *Lancet* 2006; 367:69.
57. Schachner T: Pharmacologic inhibition of vein graft neointimal hyperplasia. *J Thorac Cardiovasc Surg* 2006; 131:1065.
58. Loop FD, Lytle BW, Cosgrove DM, et al: Influence of the internal-mammary-artery graft on 10-year survival and other cardiac events. *NEJM* 1986; 314:1.
59. Falk V, Walther T, Gummert JF: Anastomotic devices for coronary artery bypass grafting. *Expert Rev Med Dev* 2005; 2:223.
60. Ho SY: Structure and anatomy of the aortic root. *Eur J Echocardiogr* 2009; 10:i3.
61. Schoen FJ: Evolving concepts of cardiac valve dynamics. The continuum of development, functional structure, pathology and tissue engineering. *Circulation* 2008; 118:1864.
62. Combs MD, Yutzey KE: Heart valve development. Regulatory networks in development and disease. *Circ Res* 2009; 105:408.
63. Aikawa E, Whittaker P, Farber M, et al: Human semilumar cardiac valve remodeling by activated cells from fetus to adult. *Circulation* 2006; 113:1344.
64. Christie GW, Barratt-Boyes BG: Age-dependent changes in the radial stretch of human aortic valve leaflets determined by biaxial testing. *Ann Thorac Surg* 1995; 60 (S1):156.
65. Davies PF, Passerini AG, Simmons GA: Aortic valve. Turning over a new leaf(let) in endothelial phenotypic heterogeneity. *Arterioscler Thromb Vasc Biol* 2004; 24:1331.
66. Simmons CA, Grant GR, Manduchi E, Davies PF: Spatial heterogeneity of endothelial phenotypes correlates with side-specific vulnerability to calcification in normal porcine aortic valves. *Circ Res* 2005; 96:792.
67. Carabello BA, Paulus WJ: Aortic stenosis. *Lancet* 2009; 363:956.
68. Roberts WC, Ko JM: Frequency by decades of unicuspid, bicuspid, and tricuspid aortic valves in adults having isolated aortic valve replacement for aortic stenosis, with or without associated aortic regurgitation. *Circulation* 2005; 111:920.
69. Otto CM, Lind BK, Kitzman DW, et al: Association of aortic-valve sclerosis with cardiovascular mortality and morbidity in the elderly. *NEJM* 1999; 341:142.
70. O'Brien KD: Pathogenesis of calcific aortic valve disease. A disease process comes of age (and a good deal more). *Arterioscler Thromb Vasc Biol* 2006; 26:1721.
71. Rajamannan NM: Calcific aortic stenosis. Lessons learned from experimental and clinical studies. *Arterioscler Thromb Vasc Biol* 2009; 29:162.
72. Fedak PW, Verma S, David TE, et al: Clinical and pathophysiological implications of a bicuspid aortic valve. *Circulation* 2002; 106:900.
73. Cripe L, Andelfinger G, Martin LJ, et al: Bicuspid aortic valve is heritable. *J Am Coll Cardiol* 2004; 44:138.
74. Garg V, Muth AN, Ransom JF, et al: Mutations in NOTCH1 cause aortic valve disease. *Nature* 2005; 437:270.
75. Bryant PA, Robins-Browne R, Carapetis JR, Curtis N: Some of the people, some of the time. Susceptibility to acute rheumatic fever. *Circulation* 2009; 119:742.
76. Chandrashekhar Y, Westaby S, Narula J: Mitral stenosis. *Lancet* 2009; 374:1271.
77. Hayek E, Gring CN, Griffin BP: Mitral valve prolapse. *Lancet* 2005; 365:507.
78. Rabkin E, Aikawa M, Stone JR, et al: Activated interstitial myofibroblasts express catabolic enzymes and mediate matrix remodeling in myxomatous heart valves. *Circulation* 2001; 104:2525.
79. Gelb BD: Marfan's Syndrome and related disorders—more tightly connected than we thought. *NEJM* 2006; 355:841.
80. Badiwala MV, Verma S, Rao V: Surgical management of ischemic mitral regurgitation. *Circulation* 2009; 120:1287.
81. Marwick TH, Lancellotti P, Pierard L: Ischemic mitral regurgitation. Mechanisms and diagnosis. *Heart* 2009; 95:1711.
82. Fox DJ, Khattar RS: Carcinoid heart disease. Presentation, diagnosis, and management. *Heart* 2004; 90:1224.
83. Bhattacharyya S, Schapira AH, Mikhailidis DP, Davar J: Drug-induced fibrotic valvular heart disease. *Lancet* 2009; 374:577.
84. Zadikoff C, Rochon P, Lang A: Cardiac valvulopathy associated with pergolide use. *Can J Neurol Sci* 2006; 33:27.
85. Haldar SM, O'Gara PT: Infective endocarditis: diagnosis and management. *Nat Clin Pract Cardiovasc Med* 2006; 3:310.
86. Bashore TM, Cabell C, Fowler V Jr: Update on infective endocarditis. *Curr Probl Cardiol* 2006; 31:274.

87. Werner M, Andersson R, Olaison L, Hogevik H: A clinical study of culture-negative endocarditis. *Medicine* 2003; 82:263.
88. Gammie JS, Sheng S, Griffith BP, et al: Trends in mitral valve surgery in the United States: Results from the Society of Thoracic Surgeons Adult Cardiac Surgery Database. *Ann Thorac Surg* 2009; 87:1431.
89. Nobuyoshi M, Arita T, Shirai S, et al: Percutaneous balloon mitral valvuloplasty : a review. *Circulation* 2009; 119:e211.
90. Carabello BA: The current therapy for mitral regurgitation. *J Am Coll Cardiol* 2008; 52:319.
91. Enriquez-Sarano M, Akins CW, Vahanian A: Mitral regurgitation. *Lancet* 2009; 373:1382.
92. Bouma W, van der Horst IC, Wijdh-den Hamer IJ, et al: Chronic ischaemic mitral regurgitation: current treatment results and new mechanism-based surgical approaches. *Eur J Cardiothorac Surg* 2010; 37:170.
93. Kherani AR, Cheema FH, Casher J, et al: Edge-to-edge mitral valve repair. The Columbia Presbyterian experience. *Ann Thorac Surg* 2004; 78:73.
94. Mack M: Percutaneous mitral valve therapy. When? Which patients? *Curr Opin Cardiol* 2009 24:125.
95. Maselli D, Guarracino F, Chiaramonti F, et al: Percutaneous mitral annuloplasty. An anatomic study of human coronary sinus and its relation with mitral valve annulus and coronary arteries. *Circulation* 2006; 114:377.
96. Treasure CB, Schoen FJ, Treseler PA, et al: Leaflet entrapment causing acute severe aortic insufficiency during balloon aortic valvuloplasty. *Clin Cardiol* 1989; 12:405.
97. Schoen FJ, Edwards WD: Valvular heart disease. General principles and stenosis, in Silver MD, Gotlieb AI, Schoen FJ (eds): *Cardiovascular Pathology*, 3rd ed. Philadelphia, WB Saunders, 2001; p 402.
98. Huh J, Bakaeen F: Heart valve replacement: which valve for which patient? *Curr Cardiol Rep* 2006; 8:109.
99. Kidane AG, Burriesci G, Cornejo P, et al: Current developments and future prospects for heart valve replacement therapy. *J Biomed Mater Res B Appl Biomater* 2009; 88:290.
100. Brown JM, O'Brien SM, Wu C, et al: Isolated aortic valve replacement in North America comprising 108,687 patients in 10 years: changes in risks, valve types, and outcomes in the Society of Thoracic Surgeons National Database. *J Thorac Cardiovasc Surg* 2009; 137:82.
101. Gammie JS, Sheng S, Griffith BP, et al: Trends in mitral valve surgery in the United States: results from the Society of Thoracic Surgeons Adult Cardiac Surgery Database. *Ann Thorac Surg* 2009; 87:1431.
102. O'Brien SM, Shahian DM, Filardo G, et al: The Society of Thoracic Surgeons 2008 cardiac surgery risk models: Part 2—isolated valve surgery. *Ann Thorac Surg* 2009; 88:S23.
103. Hammermeister KE, Sethi GK, Henderson WG, et al: Outcomes 15 years after valve replacement with a mechanical versus a bioprosthetic valve. Final report of the Veterans Affairs randomized trial. *J Am Coll Cardiol* 2000; 36:1152.
104. Oxenham H, Bloomfield P, Wheatley DJ, et al: Twenty year comparison of a Bjork-Shiley mechanical heart valve with porcine bioprostheses. *Heart* 2003; 89:715.
105. Akins CW, Miller DC, urina MI, et al: Guidelines for reporting morality and morbidity after cardiac valve interventions. *Ann Thorac Surg* 2008; 85:1490.
106. Sun JC, Davidson MJ, Lamy A, Eikelboom JW: Antithrombotic management of patients with prosthetic heart valves: current evidence and future trends. *Lancet* 2009; 374:565.
107. Butchart EG. Antithrombotic management in patients with prosthetic valve: a comparison of American and European guidelines. *Heart* 2009; 95:430.
108. Elkayam U, Bitar F: Valvular heart disease and pregnancy. Part II: prosthetic valves. *J Am Coll Cardiol* 2005; 46:403.
109. Bennett PC, Silverman SH, Gill PS, Lip GY: Peripheral arterial disease and Virchow's triad. *Thromb Haemost* 2009; 101:1032.
110. Lengyel M, Horstkotte D, Voller H, et al: Recommendations for the management of prosthetic valve thrombosis. *J Heart Valve Dis.* 2005; 14:567.
111. Habib G, Thuny F, Avierinos JF: Prosthetic valve endocarditis: current approach and therapeutic options. *Prog Cardiovasc Dis* 2008; 50:274.
112. Odell JA, Durandt J, Shama DM, Vythilingum S: Spontaneous embolization of a St. Jude prosthetic mitral valve leaflet. *Ann Thorac Surg* 1985; 39:569.
113. Blot WJ, Ibrahim MA, Ivey TD, et al: Twenty-five–year experience with the Björk-Shiley convexoconcave heart valve. A continuing clinical concern. *Circulation* 2005; 111:2850.
114. O'Neill WW, Chandler JG, Gordon RE, et al: Radiographic detection of strut separations in Bjork-Shiley convexo-concave mitral valves. *NEJM* 1995; 333:414.
115. Schoen FJ, Levy RJ: Calcification of tissue heart valve substitutes. Progress toward understanding and prevention. *Ann Thorac Surg* 2005; 79:1072.
116. Sacks MS, Schoen FJ: Collagen fiber disruption occurs independent of calcification in clinically explanted bioprosthetic heart valves. *J Biomed Mater Res* 2002; 62:359.
117. Hilbert SL, Ferrans VJ, McAllister HA, et al: Ionescu-Shiley bovine pericardial bioprostheses. Histologic and ultrastructural studies. *Am J Pathol* 1992; 140:1195.
118. O'Brien MF, Harrocks S, Stafford EG, et al: The homograft aortic valve. A 29-year, 99.3% follow up of 1,022 valve replacements. *J Heart Valve Dis* 2001; 10:334.
119. Mitchell RN, Jonas RA, Schoen FJ: Pathology of explanted cryopreserved allograft heart valves. Comparison with aortic valves from orthotopic heart transplants. *J Thorac Cardiovasc Surg* 1998; 115:118.
120. Botha CA: The Ross operation. Utilization of the patient's own pulmonary valve as a replacement device for the diseased aortic valve. *Expert Rev Cardiovasc Ther* 2005; 3:1017.
121. Rabkin-Aikawa E, Aikawa M, Farber M, et al: Clinical pulmonary autograft valves. Pathologic evidence of adaptive remodeling in the aortic site. *J Thorac Cardiovasc Surg* 2004; 128:552.
122. Elkins RC, Thompson DM, Lane MM, et al: Ross operation: 16-year experience. *J Thoracic Cardiovasc Surg* 2008; 136:623.
123. Takkenberg JJ, Klieverik LM, Schoof PH, et al: The Ross Procedure: a systematic review and meta-analysis. *Circulation* 2009; 119:222.
124. Luciani GB, Santini F, Mazzucco A: Autografts, homografts, and xenografts: overview of stentless aortic valve surgery. *J Cardiovasc Med* 2007; 8:91.
125. Borger MA, Carson SM, Ivanov J, et al: Stentless aortic valves are hemodynamically superior to stented valves during mid-term follow-up. A large retrospective study. *Ann Thorac Surg* 2005; 80:2180.
126. Fyfe BS, Schoen FJ: Pathologic analysis of non-stented FreestyleTM aortic root bioprostheses treated with amino oleic acid (AOA). *Sem Thorac Cardiovasc Surg* 1999; 11:151.
127. Butany J, Collins MJ, Nair V, et al: Morphological findings in explanted Toronto stentless porcine valves. *Cardiovasc Pathol* 2006; 15:41.
128. Vahanian A, Alfieri OR, Al-Attar N, et al: Transcatheter valve implantation for patients with aortic stenosis: a position statement from the European Association of Cardio-Thoracic Surgery (EACTS) and the European Society of Cardiology (ESC), in collaboration with the European Association of percutaneous Cardiovascular Interventions (EAPCI). *Eur J Cardiothorac Surg* 2008; 34:1.
129. Rahimtoola SH: The year in valvular heart disease. *J Am Coll Cardol* 2009; 53:1894.
130. Zajarias A, Cribier AG: Outcomes and safety of percutaneous aortic valve replacement. *J Am Coll Cardiol* 2009; 53:1829.
131. Webb JG, Altwegg L, Boone RH, et al: Transcatheter aortic valve implantation. Impact on clinical and valve-related outcomes. *Circulation* 2009; 119:3009.
132. Hunt SA, Haddad F: The changing face of heart transplantation. *J Am Coll Cardiol* 2008; 52:587.
133. Taylor DO, Stehlik J, Edwards LB, et al: Registry of the international society for heart and lung transplantation: twenty-six official adult heart transplant report—2009. *J Heart Lung Transplant* 2009; 28:1007.
134. Winters GL, Schoen FJ: Pathology of cardiac transplantation, in Silver MD, Gotlieb AI, Schoen FJ (eds): *Cardiovascular Pathology.* 3rd ed., Philadelphia, Churchill Livingstone, 2001; p 725.
135. Stewart S, Winters GL, Fishbein MC, et al: Revision of the 1990 working formulation for the standardization of nomenclature in the diagnosis of heart rejection. *J Heart Lung Transplant* 2005; 24:1710.
136. Billingham ME, Cary NRB, Hammond ME, et al: A working formulation for the standardization of nomenclature in the diagnosis of heart and lung rejection. Heart rejection study group. *J Heart Transplant* 1990; 9:587.
137. Mitchell RN: Graft vascular disease: immune response meets the vessel wall. *Ann Rev Pathol* 2009; 4:19.
138. Nalesnik MA: The diverse pathology of post-transplant lymphoproliferative disorders. The importance of a standardized approach. *Transpl Infect Dis* 2001; 3:88.
139. Patel SM, Throckmorton AL, Untaroiu A, et al: The status of failure and reliability testing of artificial blood pumps. *ASAIO J* 2005; 51:440.
140. Copeland JG, Smith RG, Arabia FA, et al: Cardiac replacement with a total artificial heart as a bridge to transplantation. *NEJM* 2004; 351:859.
141. Samuels LE, Dowling R: Total artificial heart. Destination therapy. *Cardiol Clin* 2003; 21:115.
142. Horton SC, Khodaverdian R, Powers A, et al: Left ventricular assist device malfunction. A systematic approach to diagnosis. *J Am Coll Cardiol* 2004; 43:1574.

143. Itescu S, John R: Interactions between the recipient immune system and the left ventricular assist device surface. Immunological and clinical implications. *Ann Thorac Surg* 2003; 75:S58.
144. Felkin LE, Lara-Pezzi E, George R, et al: Expression of extracellular matrix genes during myocardial recovery from heart failure after left ventricular assist device support. *J Heart Lung Transplant* 2009; 28:117.
145. Saffitz JE: The pathology of sudden cardiac death in patients with ischemic heart disease—arrhythmology for anatomic pathologists. *Cardiovasc Pathol* 2005; 14:195.
146. Kusumoto FM, Goldschlager N: Device therapy for cardiac arrhythmias. *JAMA* 2002; 287:1848.
147. Kistler PM, Liew G, Mond HG: Long-term performance of active-fixation pacing leads. A prospective study. *Pacing Clin Electrophysiol* 2006; 29:226.
148. Steinbrook R: The controversy over Guidant's implantable defibrillators. *NEJM* 2005; 353:221.
149. Kirkpatrick JN, Burke MC, Knight BP: Postmortem analysis and retrieval of implantable pacemakers and defibrillators. *NEJM* 2006; 354:1649.
150. Myerburg RJ, Feigal DW, Lindsay BD: Life-threatening malfunction of implantable cardiac devices. *NEJM* 2006; 354:2309.
151. Sabatine MS, Colucci WS, Schoen FJ: Primary tumors of the heart, in Zipes DD, Libby P, Bonow RD, Braunwald E (eds): *Braunwald's Heart Disease. A Textbook of Cardiovascular Medicine,* 7th ed. Philadelphia, WB Saunders, 2004; p 1807.
152. Reardon MJ, Walkes JC, Benjamin R: Therapy insight: malignant primary cardiac tumors. *Nat Clin Pract Cardiovasc Med* 2006; 3:548.
153. Gowda RM, Khan IA, Nair CK, et al: Cardiac papillary fibroelastoma. A comprehensive analysis of 725 cases. *Am Heart J* 2003; 146:404.
154. Howard RA, Aldea GS, Shapira OM, et al: Papillary fibroelastoma. Increasing recognition of a surgical disease. *Ann Thorac Surg* 1999; 68:1881.
155. Isaacs H Jr: Fetal and neonatal cardiac tumors. *Pediatr Cardiol* 2004; 25:252.
156. Cho JM, Danielson GK, Puga FJ, et al: Surgical resection of ventricular cardiac fibromas. Early and late results. *Ann Thorac Surg* 2003; 76:1929.
157. Bossert T, Walther T, Vondrys D, et al: Cardiac fibroma as an inherited manifestation of nevoid basal-cell carcinoma syndrome. *Tex Heart Inst J* 2006; 33:88.
158. Lin CY, Tsai FC, Fang BR: Mesothelial/monocytic incidental cardiac excrescences of the heart. Case report and literature review. *Int J Clin Pract Suppl* 2005; 147:23.
159. Ratner BD, Hoffman S, Schoen FJ, et al: *Biomaterials Science. An Introduction to Materials in Medicine,* 2nd ed. San Diego, Academic Press, 2004.
160. Langer R, Tirrell DA: Designing materials for biology and medicine. *Nature* 2004; 428:487.
161. Hench LL, Polak JM: Third-generation biomedical materials. *Science* 2002; 295:1014.
162. Lutolf MP, Hubbell JA: Synthetic biomaterials as instructive extracellular microenvironments for morphogenesis in tissue engineering. *Nat Biotechnol* 2005; 23:47.
163. Schoen FJ: Introduction to host reactions to biomaterials and their evaluation, in Ratner BD, Hoffman AS, Schoen FJ, et al (eds): *Biomaterials Science. An Introduction to Materials in Medicine,* 2nd ed. San Diego, Academic Press, 2004; p 293.
164. Hanson SR: Blood coagulation and blood-materials interactions, in Ratner BD, Hoffman AS, Schoen FJ, Lemons JE (eds): *Biomaterials Science. An Introduction to Materials in Medicine,* 2nd ed. Orlando, Academic Press, 2004; p 332.
165. Anderson JM, Schoen FJ: Interactions of blood with artificial surfaces, in Butchart EG, Bodnar E (eds): *Current Issues in Heart Valve Disease. Thrombosis, Embolism and Bleeding.* London, ICR Publishers, 1992; p 160.
166. Anderson JM: Inflammation, wound healing and the foreign body response. Perspectives and possibilities in biomaterials science, in Ratner BD, Hoffman AS, Schoen FJ (eds): *Biomaterials Science. An Introduction to Materials in Medicine,* 2nd ed. Orlando, Academic Press, 2004; p 296.
167. Tang L, Hu W: Molecular determinants of biocompatibility. *Expert Rev Med Dev* 2005; 2:493.
168. Mitchell RN: Innate and adaptive immunity. The immune response to foreign materials. Perspectives and possibilities in biomaterials science. In. Ratner BD, Hoffman AS, Schoen FJ, Lemons JE (eds): *Biomaterials Science. An Introduction to Materials in Medicine,* 2nd ed. Orlando, Academic Press, 2004; 304.
169. Sata M: Role of circulating vascular progenitors in angiogenesis, vascular healing, and pulmonary hypertension: lessons from animal models. *Arterioscler Thromb Vasc Biol* 2006; 26:1008.
170. DiDonato RM, Danielson GK, McGoon DC, et al: Left ventricle-aortic conduits in pediatric patients. *J Thorac Cardiovasc Surg* 1984; 88:82.
171. Xue L, Greisler HP: Biomaterials in the development and future of vascular grafts. *J Vasc Surg* 2003; 37:472.
172. Darouiche RO: Treatment of infections associated with surgical implants. *NEJM* 2004; 350:1422.
173. Vinh DC, Embil JM: Device related infections: a review. *J Long Term Eff Med Implants* 2005; 15:467.
174. Conlan RM, Costerson JW: Biofilms. Survival mechanisms of clinically relevant microorganisms. *Clin Microbiol Rev* 2002; 15:167.
175. Costerson JW, Cook G, Shirtliff M, et al: Biofilms, biomaterials and device-related infections, in Ratner BD, Hoffman AS, Schoen FJ, et al (eds): *Biomaterials Science. An Introduction to Materials in Medicine,* 2nd ed. San Diego, Elsevier Academic Press, 2004; p 345.
176. Vacanti JP, Langer R: Tissue engineering. The design and fabrication of living replacement devices for surgical reconstruction and transplantation. *Lancet* 1999; 354:SI32.
177. Fuchs JR, Nasseri BA, Vacanti JP: Tissue engineering. A 21st century solution to surgical reconstruction. *Ann Thorac Surg* 2001; 72:577.
178. Rabkin E, Schoen FJ: Cardiovascular tissue engineering. *Cardiovasc Pathol* 2002; 11:305.
179. Nerem RM, Ensley AE: The tissue engineering of blood vessels and the heart. *Am J Transplant* 2004; 4:36.
180. Isenberg BC, Williams C, Tranquillo RT: Small-diameter artificial arteries engineered in vitro. *Circ Res* 2006; 98:25.
181. Gong Z, NIklason LE: Blood vessels engineered from human cells. *Trends Cardiovasc Med* 2006; 16:153.
182. L'Heureux N, Paquet S, Labbe R, et al: A completely biological tissue-engineered human blood vessel. *FASEB J* 1998; 12:447.
183. Weinberg CB, Bell E: A blood vessel model constructed from collagen and cultured vascular cells. *Science* 1986; 231:397.
184. Kaushall S, Amiel GE, Gulesarian KJ, et al: Functional small diameter neovessels using endothelial progenitor cells expanded ex-vivo. *Nature Med* 2001; 7:1035.
185. Lantz GC, Badylak SF, Hiles MC, et al: Small intestine submucosa as a vascular graft. A review. *J Invest Surg* 1993; 3:297.
186. Sparks CH: Silicone mandril method for growing reinforced autogenous femoro-popliteal artery graft in situ. *Ann Surg* 1973; 177:293.
187. Hoenig MR, Campbell GR, Rolfe BE, Campbell JH: Tissue-engineered blood vessels. Alternative to autologous grafts? *Arterioscler Thromb Vasc Biol* 2005; 25:1128.
188. Shin'oka T, Imai Y, Ikada Y: Transplantation of a tissue-engineered pulmonary artery. *NEJM* 2001; 344:532.
189. McAllister MC, Maruszewski M, Garrido SA, et al: Effectiveness of haemodialysis access with an autologous tissue-engineered vascular graft: a multicentre cohort study. *Lancet* 2009; 373:1440.
190. Meinhart JG, Deutsch M, Fischlein T, et al: Clinical autologous in vitro endothelialization of 153 infrainguinal ePTFE grafts. *Ann Thorac Surg* 2001; 71:S327.
191. Anversa P, Leri A, Kajstura J: Cardiac regeneration. *J Am Coll Cardiol* 2006; 47:1769.
192. Cohen S, Leor J: Rebuilding broken hearts. Biologists and engineers working together in the fledgling field of tissue engineering are within reach of one of their greatest goals. Constructing a living human heart patch. *Sci Am* 2004; 291:44.
193. Zimmerman WH, Didie M, Doker S, et al: Heart muscle engineering. An update on cardiac muscle replacement therapy. *Cardiovasc Res* 2006; 71:419.
194. Radisic M, Park H, Shing H, et al: Functional assembly of engineered myocardium by electrical stimulation of cardiac myocytes cultured on scaffolds. *Proc Natl Acad Sci USA* 2004; 101:18129.
195. Dimmeler S, Zeiher AM, Schneider MD: Unchain my heart. The scientific foundations of cardiac repair. *J Clin Invest* 2005; 115:572.
196. Laflamme MA, Murry CE: Regenerating the heart. *Nat Biotechnol* 2005; 23:845.
197. Fukuda K, Yuasa S: Stem cells as a source of regenerative cardiomyocytes. *Circ Res* 2006; 98:1002.
198. Mendelson KA, Schoen FJ: Heart valve tissue engineering. Concepts, approaches, progress, and challenges. *Ann Biomed Eng* 2006; 34:1799.
199. Sacks MS, Schoen FJ, Mayer JE: Bioengineering challenges for heart valve tissue engineering. *Ann Rev Biomed Engin* 2009; 11:289.
200. Schoen FJ: Heart valve tissue engineering: quo vadis? *Curr Opin Biotechnol* 2011 [Epub ahead of print].
201. Hoerstrup SP, Sodian R, Daebritz S, et al: Functional living trileaflet heart valves grown in-vitro. *Circulation* 2000; 102:III-44.

202. Rabkin E, Hoerstrup SP, Aikawa M, et al: Evolution of cell phenotype and extracellular matrix in tissue-engineered heart valves during in-vitro maturation and in-vivo remodeling. *J Heart Valve Dis* 2002; 11:1.
203. Hoerstrup SP, Cummings I, Lachat M, et al: Functional growth in tissue engineered living vascular grafts. Follow up at 100 weeks in a large animal model. *Circulation* 2006; 114:159.
204. Matheny RG, Hutchison ML, Dryden PE, et al: Porcine small intestine submucosa as a pulmonary valve leaflet substitute. *J Heart Valve Dis* 2000; 9:769.
205. Simon P, Kasimir MT, Seebacher G, et al: Early failure of the tissue engineered porcine heart valve SYNERGRAFT in pediatric patients. *Eur J Cardiothorac Surg* 2003; 23:1002.

CHAPTER 6

Computed Tomography of the Adult Cardiac Surgery Patient: Principles and Applications

Frank J. Rybicki
Tarang Sheth
Kanako K. Kumamaru
Frederick Y. Chen

OVERVIEW

Over the last decade, advances in computed tomography (CT) technology have revolutionized the diagnosis of cardiovascular disease. As illustrated in this chapter, CT has dramatically reduced, and for some clinical indications eliminated, the need for diagnostic arterial catheterization. In the process, CT has become invaluable in cardiac diagnosis and surgical planning.

CT is based on a source of x-rays and a system to detect those x-rays that pass though the patient. The x-ray source and detector are mounted on the "CT gantry" that rotates around the patient. As detailed below, two major technology advances have enabled CT to image the beating heart. The first is the speed at which the CT gantry rotates. The second is the incorporation of an increasing number of detectors that can resolve small anatomic detail. One of the great promises of modern CT is the ability to noninvasively exclude coronary artery disease in as little as one heartbeat (Fig. 6-1). However, the role of CT extends far beyond the coronary arteries alone. Using the same CT acquisition, native coronary imaging can be extended to coronary bypass grafts, the beating myocardium, valve motion, ventricular outflow tracks, and cardiac lesions.

In order to understand the clinical contribution of CT and to avoid pitfalls in image interpretation, it is essential for the surgeon to appreciate the basic principles of CT used in cardiac imaging. This chapter is divided into two sections. The first section describes the technical considerations for cardiac CT. By understanding each component, the surgeon will be better able to distinguish image artifacts from pathology. The second section reviews those CT examinations that are most frequently performed in the noninvasive cardiovascular imaging program at Brigham and Women's Hospital (BWH), detailing the strengths and limitations of each exam.

Section A

Cardiac CT Protocols

INTRODUCTION

Most advances in cardiac CT, for example in coronary CT angiography (CTA), have focused on the development of protocols consistent with the rapid incremental improvements in the technology. One of the major technological advances has been the incorporation of multiple elements into the CT detector system, called Multi-Detector CT (MDCT). MDCT is synonymous with multi-slice CT. Data from each of the detectors is used to reconstruct an axial slice perpendicular to the long axis, or z-axis, of the patient. The width of the detectors determines the slice thickness and thus the ability to resolve small anatomic detail (spatial resolution) of the scanner. Thinner slices yield superior spatial resolution; however, comparing two scanners that produce the same number of slices, the scanner with thinner slices will have less z-axis (ie, craniocaudal)

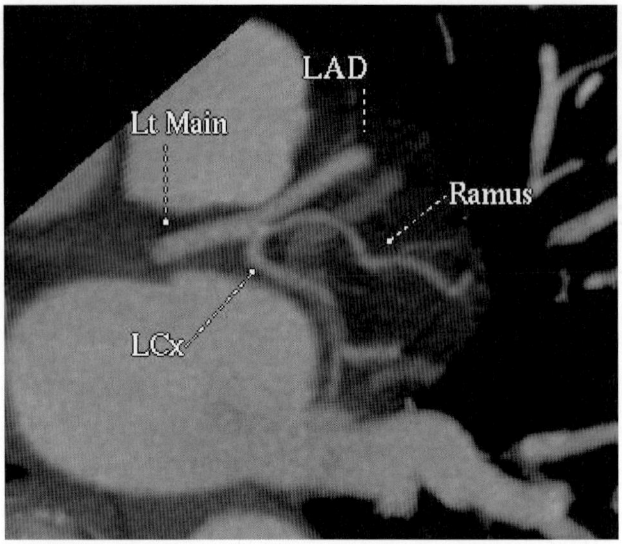

FIGURE 6-1 Selected coronary computed tomography angiography (*CTA*) image of the proximal left coronary arterial system in a patient scheduled for isolated mitral valve surgery. Using the protocol detailed in this chapter, CT demonstrated normal coronary arteries in this patient, eliminating the need for arterial catheterization.

coverage per gantry rotation and thus will have a longer scan time. To date, the minimum detector width and largest number of detector rows is 0.5 mm and 320, respectively.[1] This yields 16 cm (0.5 mm × 320) z-axis coverage per gantry rotation, and thus the entire heart can be imaged with data acquired over a single R-R interval.

TEMPORAL RESOLUTION

Successful cardiac imaging by any modality relies on the ability of the hardware to produce motion-free images or, in other words, to image faster than the heart beats. Because it requires that the gantry be rotated around the patient, CT is inherently slower than digital subtraction angiography (DSA) where each frame corresponds to a single projection image. As described below, CT has recently become much faster and thus cardiac CT can now be routinely performed.

Temporal resolution is the metric that measures imaging speed. For a CT scanner with a single photon source, the temporal resolution is one half of the CT gantry rotation time. This is because image reconstruction requires CT data acquired from one half (180 degrees) of a complete gantry rotation. All manufacturers have gantry rotation times less than or equal to 350 milliseconds. Using this gantry rotation time as an example, an ECG-gated cardiac image can be reconstructed (using single-segment reconstruction, described below) with CT data acquired over 175 milliseconds of the cardiac cycle. Thus, the reconstructed images inherently display the average of the cardiac motion over the 175 milliseconds during which the data was acquired. This is how ECG gating enables cardiac CT. Without gating, cardiac images are nondiagnostic because the reconstruction "averages" the motion over the entire R-R interval, for example over 1000 milliseconds for a patient with a heart rate of 60 beats per minute.

There are additional strategies to improve temporal resolution. The first uses two independent x-ray CT sources and two independent (64-slice) detector systems built into the CT gantry. The second x-ray source is positioned 90 degrees from the first x-ray source, and the second detection system is positioned 90 degrees from the first detection system. With respect to temporal resolution, the practical consequence of this CT configuration is that 180 degrees of gantry rotation can be achieved in half the time (eg, 82.5 ms as opposed to 165 ms). This halves the temporal resolution (to 82.5 ms), and thus for this "dual-source" CT configuration, motion is averaged over only 82.5 ms. Another strategy uses both x-ray CT source-detector systems to sample the entire heart within a single R-R interval by rapidly moving the patient through the scanner.[2] Both implementations of such systems have technical advantages and disadvantages that are beyond the scope of this chapter.

For single-source scanners, temporal resolution can be improved by adopting a so-called "multisegment" image reconstruction. The difference between single-segment and multisegment reconstruction is that in the former, 180 degrees of data are acquired from a single heartbeat, whereas multisegment reconstruction uses several heartbeats to obtain the one half gantry CT data. For example, in a two-segment reconstruction, two heartbeats are used to generate a single axial slice, and thus the temporal resolution is halved. Similarly, if four heat beats are used (four segment reconstruction), only 45 degrees of data are used from each heartbeat. This yields a fourfold reduction in the effective temporal resolution, making it theoretically possible to perform high spatial resolution cardiac CT in patients with a rapid (eg, >70 beats per minute) heart rate. However, because multiple heartbeats are used to fill the 180 degrees of gantry rotation necessary for the reconstruction, stable periodicity of the heart is essential. When beat-to-beat variations in heart rate occur, image quality is degraded significantly. In our experience, multisegment reconstruction works well in patients with high heart rates who are being studied for clinical indications where the highest image quality may not be required (studies of graft patency, pericardial calcification, etc.). For more demanding applications (eg, native coronary CT angiography) we still routinely employ beta-blockade for heart rates greater than 60 beats per minute.

BETA-BLOCKADE FOR HEART RATE CONTROL

As suggested above, beta blockade is an important component of most cardiac CT examinations. As the temporal resolution of cardiac CT improves, the dependence on lowering the heart rate will naturally be mitigated. However, the speed of all CT scanners is inferior to coronary catheterization, and thus beta-blockade is recommended for the large majority of patients in whom it is safe. In our experience, many surgical patients have standing orders for beta-blockers as part of their medical therapy, and image quality is excellent. When this is not the case, either oral and/or IV metoprolol is routinely administered.

ECG GATING

ECG gating refers to the simultaneous acquisition of both the patient's electrocardiogram (ECG) tracing and CT data. By acquiring both pieces of information, CT images can be reconstructed using only a short temporal segment of the R-R interval. Each segment is named by its "phase" in the cardiac cycle; the common nomenclature is to name the percentage of a specific phase with respect to its position in the R-R interval. For example, reconstruction of 20 (equally spaced) phases would be named as 0%, 5%, 10%...95%. The period in which the heart has the least motion is usually (but not always) in mid diastole, near 75%. Thus, the CT exposure (and subsequent patient radiation level) can be lowered by limiting the exposure to a small part of the R-R interval where coronary motion is expected to be a minimum. This is termed "prospective" ECG gating because the reconstruction phase and width is determined prospectively. The disadvantage of this approach is that cine loops of the entire R-R interval cannot be reconstruction because there is no complete data set throughout the R-R interval. If this is desired, so-called "retrospective" ECG gating can be used, at the expense of high radiation levels.

For patients who require imaging of bypass grafts, it is important to note that periodic displacement of both saphenous vein grafts (SVG), radial grafts, and internal mammary artery (IMA) grafts is far less than the motion of the native coronary arteries. Thus, for these vessels, a single reconstruction at mid-diastole is usually sufficient (Fig. 6-2), and prospective ECG gating is routinely used. However, the benefits of lower radiation in this population are relatively moot, because the latent period for a radiation-induced malignancy is roughly a decade for blood tumors and significantly longer for solid tumors. Patients under consideration for repeat bypass surgery typically have a shorter life expectancy based on cardiac status. Thus, it is *essential* that the surgeon not only recognizes that motion has degraded image quality, but also realizes that additional reconstructions, and even repeat imaging, *can and should* be performed. If the entire course of the graft is not clear to the surgeon at a single cardiac phase, it is almost always the case that another phase will yield motion-free depiction of the graft

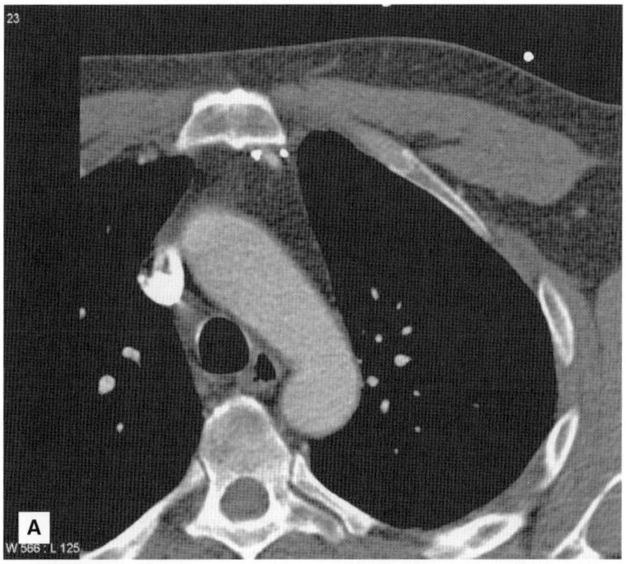

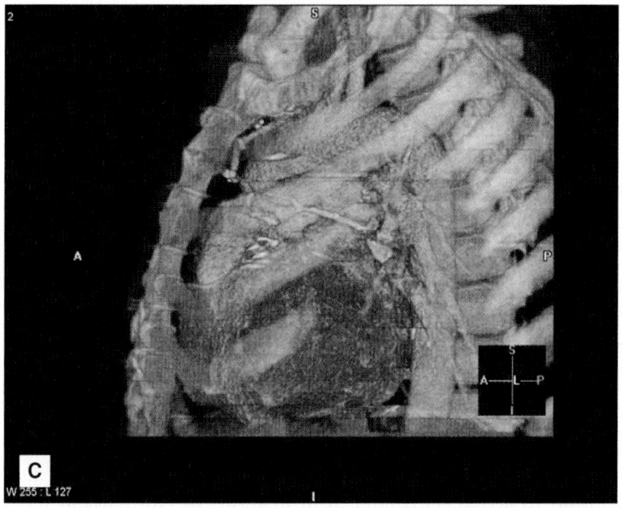

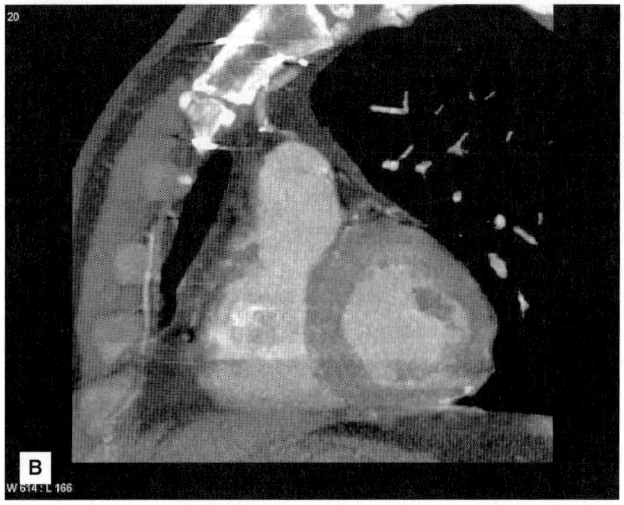

FIGURE 6-2 ECG-gated CT images from a single reconstruction at middiastole for a patient scheduled for redo CABG. The patient is status post LIMA to LAD coronary bypass grafting. (**A**) Axial image demonstrates the LIMA graft coursing between two staples and adherent to the posterior table of the sternum. (**B**) Multiplanar reformatting is now performed routinely to detect and illustrate cases where repeat thoracotomy through the sternal incision is likely to damage a patent LIMA graft. An alternate surgical approach was required for this patient. (**C**) Selected image from a three-dimensional (3D) volume rendering again demonstrates the course of the graft. Volume rendering fully surveys the thoracic landmarks and is useful for spatial relationships and the communication of important findings

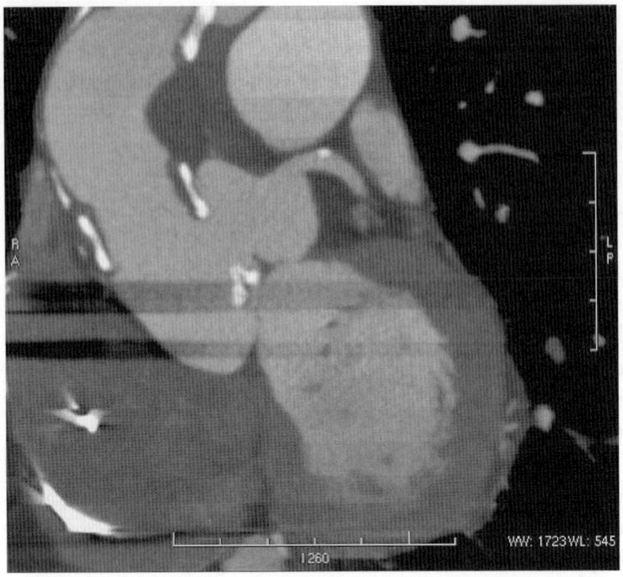

FIGURE 6-3 ECG-gated CT image through the left ventricle and the aortic valve in a patient status post aortic root repair. Note the pacemaker (*right heart wires*); magnetic resonance imaging (MRI) was contraindicated. The repair is well visualized and without complication, with only mild aortic valve calcification (cine images showed a tricuspid valve with no significant stenosis). This image also demonstrates a punctate calcified plaque along the superior course of the proximal left main coronary artery, without a significant stenosis.

segment that was poorly seen. At BWH, open communication between the radiologist and surgeon for every case has eliminated this pitfall and ensures that the maximum amount of imaging data is incorporated into presurgical planning.

In cine CT, such as imaging the aortic valve over the entire R-R interval, images are acquired with retrospective ECG gating and subsequently reconstructed throughout the cardiac cycle and then played, in cine mode, to demonstrate function. Each individual image (Fig. 6-3) offers an outstanding assessment of the aortic valve and root structure. Cine CT can also be used to assess ventricular-wall motion. In comparison with magnetic resonance imaging (MRI), the gold standard for global- and regional-wall motion abnormalities, CT often has inferior temporal resolution. However, it is important to emphasize that cine CT does not require a separate image acquisition. The entire CT data set (coronary, valve, myocardium, pericardium) is acquired in a single breath hold; cine CT is simply part of the image postprocessing.

For surgical patients, CT has the distinct advantage over MRI in that it is by far the best imaging modality to identify and quantify calcification. Also, the most common contraindications for cardiac CT (eg, impaired renal function as measured by glomerular filtration rate or alternatively by serum creatinine) differ from those for MRI (pacemaker), and thus CT can often be used for patients who cannot have MRI. Single heartbeat cardiac CT is now a clinical reality, with an entire cardiac acquisition in approximately one second.[3] In addition to the fact that patient radiation is decreased, multiple scans can be performed with the same injection of iodinated contrast material, creating the opportunity for a host of additional studies (eg, myocardial perfusion)[4,5] that are, at present, largely in the domain of cardiac MRI and nuclear cardiology.

PATIENT IRRADIATION

Because ECG gating is required, ascending aorta and cardiac CT delivers more patient irradiation than CT of any other body part. Although details regarding cardiac CT dosimetry are beyond the scope of this chapter, discussions regarding CT dose must be based on sound principles. The radiation risk most commonly quoted relates to the probability that the CT scan will result in the development of a fatal radiation-induced neoplasm. Human data for radiation at this low level (the level delivered in ECG gated cardiac CT) is very sparse; all anecdotal reports support a long latency period as described above. For this reason, patients should be separated into two groups: those with a life expectancy of roughly 10 to 15 years or less, and those with a longer life expectancy. In the former group, the only dose consideration is whether the radiation could cause a skin burn (the only short-term complication of any consequence). X-ray skin burns are extremely uncommon, particularly in CT (even for ECG-gated studies), and typically result from multiple exams repeated at short-term intervals. Thus, for this subset of patients, *radiation dose should not be a consideration* in determining a modality for coronary imaging. For those patients for whom radiation is an important consideration, prospective ECG gating should be used. For cine evaluations in these younger patients, x-ray current modulation is a strategy to lower the radiation dose. The tube current (expressed as the mA) is modulated over the course of the cardiac cycle so that the desired (high) diagnostic current is delivered only in diastole. The patient dose is decreased because the tube current is reduced for the remainder of the cardiac cycle. Although current modulation is helpful in many cases (eg, pediatric patients), the decision to use it should be made after consultation between surgeon and radiologist because the potential drawbacks are significant. Most importantly, when current modulation is used, images reconstructed during phases with low tube current are relatively noisy because less tube current is used to generate them.

SCANNING PARAMETERS

The *scan time* refers to the time required to complete the CT acquisition along the z-axis of the patient. As described above, better temporal resolution decreases the scan time, not only decreasing cardiac motion, but also enabling breath hold CT. This is important in cardiac CT because in comparison with nongated CT, ECG gating not only increases patient radiation but also increases the scan time.

In practical terms, a 64-slice ECG-gated cardiac CT scan (craniocaudal, or z-axis imaging over ~15 cm) can be performed in roughly 10 seconds, versus 20 to 25 seconds with a 16-slice scanner. One great benefit of wide area detector CT is faster (single heartbeat) scans. If this option is not available, increasing the thickness of the detectors increases the z-axis coverage per rotation and thus decreases the scan time. For example, in a patient who cannot perform the breath hold, using thicker detector widths (eg, 1mm thickness as opposed to 0.5mm thickness) will decrease the scan time by providing more z-axis coverage per rotation. However, routinely increasing the width of the detectors for cardiac applications is undesirable because it degrades the *spatial resolution* of the examination. In general, spatial resolution refers to the ability to differentiate small detail in an image. This is an essential component to coronary imaging because the diameter of the proximal coronary arteries are on the order or 3 to 4 mm. Substitution of 0.5mm reconstructed images with 1mm images thus impacts the ability to see detail that may be required for accurate diagnoses. Routine consultation between the surgeon and radiologist is essential to best understand and optimize the tradeoff between scan time and slice thickness. For example, imaging of the myocardium and ascending aorta almost never requires submillimeter slices, because the pathology is larger. Thus, for dyspneic patients who require only imaging of the ascending aorta, thicker slices are used to cut the scan time.

The scanning parameters that primarily determine the number of photons used to create a CT image are termed "mAs," or milliamperes-seconds and "kV," or kilovolts. The former represents the x-ray tube current; the latter refers to the voltage applied within the tube. For the surgeon, choosing the best numbers (typical values are 550 to 700 effective mAs, 120 kV) is far less important than understanding the fact that modern cardiac CT pushes the limits of technology, and thus creates tradeoffs with respect to the x-ray CT source. The source generates photons that are either attenuated by the patient or reach the detectors. When more photons reach the detectors, the image quality is higher because there is less noise. The decision to image with thinner slices (eg, 0.5mm as opposed to 1mm) means that fewer photons reach the detector; thus, thinner slices have more noise. This is especially important in obese patients because their increased body mass absorbs more photons than thin patients. For the same effective mAs and kV, images of obese patients can be dramatically degraded by greater image noise.

If there were no limit to the number of photons that an x-ray CT source could produce, the solution would be to simply increase the number of photons (and the radiation dose) until image noise was satisfactory. Unfortunately, because the x-ray CT tube heats excessively when pushed to its maximum, there is a limit to the number of photons that can be produced. This is why image noise becomes problematic with thin slice imaging of obese patients. When this is the case, consultation between surgeon and radiologist is important because diagnostic images can often be obtained by increasing the image thickness, scanning a smaller z-axis field of view (FOV), or both. The latter can be particularly useful if the exam can be tailored to the most important structure. Scanning a smaller z-axis means that more photons can be generated and used before the x-ray CT tube reaches its heat limit.

On the other hand, whenever possible, the z-axis FOV should be generous, as unexpected pathology can extend both cranially and caudally. For example, an ECG-gated cardiac and ascending aorta exam to evaluate extension of the intimal flap into the coronary arteries can reveal extension into the great vessels. Also, scanning must allow for variations in the FOV induced by breath holding. As a general rule, for scanning the native coronaries alone, the superior border of the FOV is set at the axial slice corresponding to the top of the carina. This is typically 2 to 3 cm superior to the origin of the left main. The inferior border should scan through the entire inferior wall of the heart and should include several slices of the liver to account for cardiac displacement during breath holding. For bypass graft imaging, the superior border of the field of view must include the subclavian arteries and the origin of both IMAs.

CONTRAST MATERIAL

With the exception of scans performed solely for the assessment of cardiac and aortic calcification, CT examinations are performed with iodinated contrast material. Effective communication between surgeon and radiologist is important in optimizing the use of contrast material, particularly in the decision of whether to use a single or a dual injection system. A single system injects only contrast, whereas a dual system has two reservoirs to inject contrast followed by saline. Dual injection is essential for many applications, and it is routine in coronary imaging. The contrast and saline delivery are timed so that the left heart, aorta, and coronary arteries are enhanced with contrast while the right heart is filled with saline. The use and the timing of the saline are essential parts of the exam because artifacts that limit interpretation of the right coronary artery (RCA) will be induced if the right heart and central veins are densely enhanced with contrast (as opposed to saline). However, for patients in whom imaging requires enhancement of both the left and right heart (eg, assessment of both the mitral and tricuspid valves), saline cannot be used and less dense contrast material may be chosen to lessen potential artifacts.

SUMMARY

Advances in technology such as submillimeter spatial resolution, up to 320 detector rows, and rapid gantry rotation times with dual x-ray CT source and detector systems have enabled ECG-gated CT to make a positive contribution to the care of cardiac surgery patients. The surgeon must recognize that cardiac protocols push the limit of technology, and thus CT of the heart is more complicated than a scan of any other body part. Consequently, routine and effective communication between the surgeon and the radiologist will result in the best possible patient outcomes.

Section B

Applications in Cardiac Surgical Patients

NATIVE CORONARY CTA

One of the most common clinical indications for cardiac CT is to evaluate the native coronary arteries for stenosis (Figs. 6-4 to 6-7). Numerous validation studies have evaluated cardiac CT for this

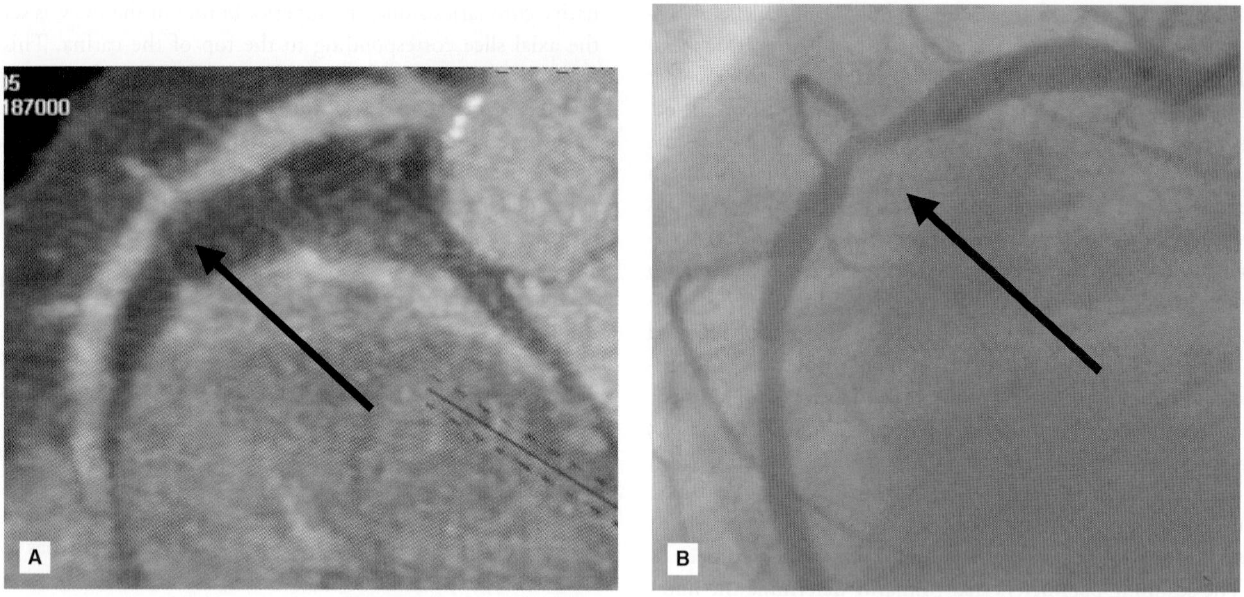

FIGURE 6-4 Proximal RCA 50% stenosis diagnosed by coronary CT angiography and confirmed by conventional angiography. Double oblique maximum intensity projection image (4 mm thick) through proximal RCA (**A**) and LAO projection still image from conventional angiogram (**B**) demonstrate a segment of approximately 50% stenosis (arrows).

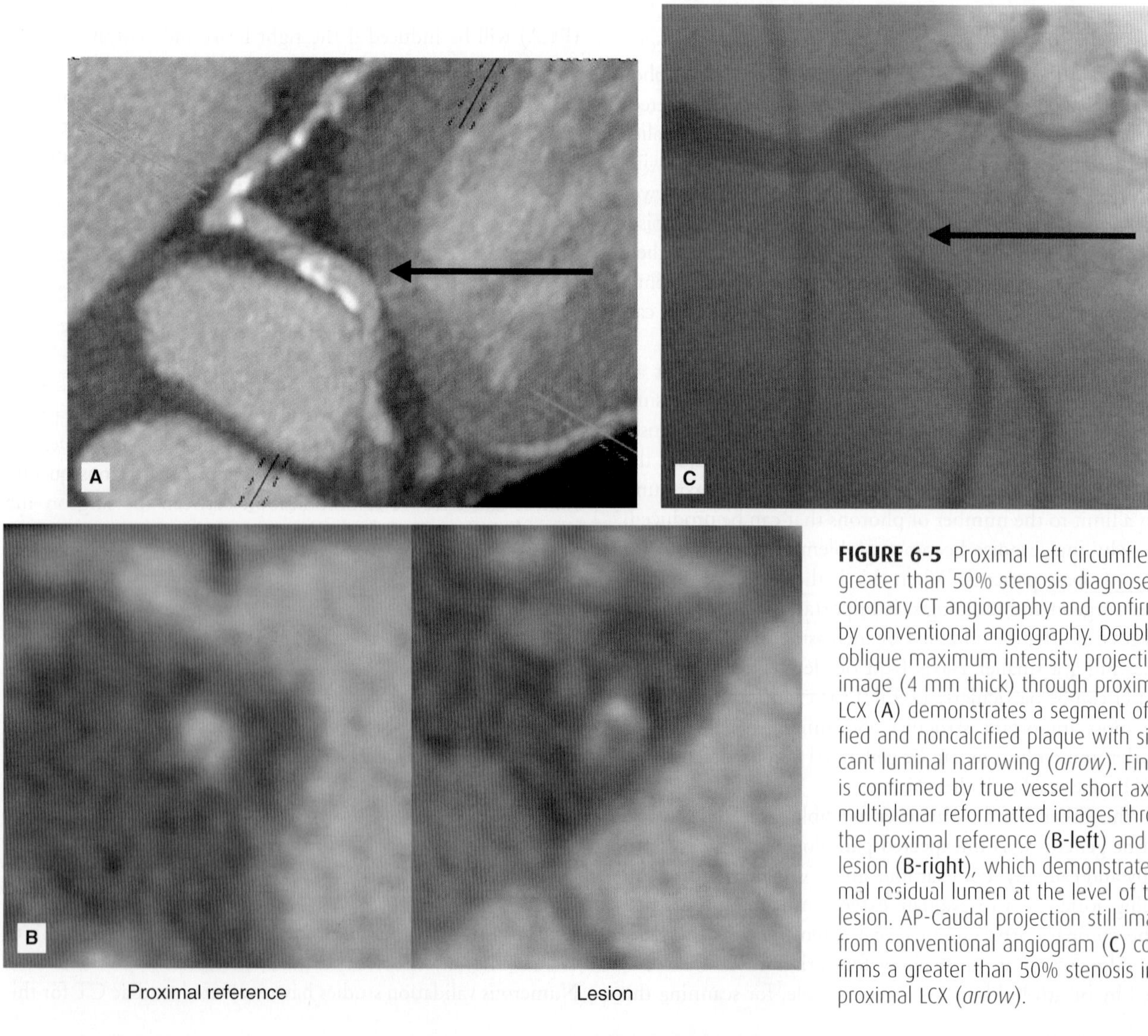

FIGURE 6-5 Proximal left circumflex greater than 50% stenosis diagnosed by coronary CT angiography and confirmed by conventional angiography. Double oblique maximum intensity projection image (4 mm thick) through proximal LCX (**A**) demonstrates a segment of calcified and noncalcified plaque with significant luminal narrowing (*arrow*). Finding is confirmed by true vessel short axis multiplanar reformatted images through the proximal reference (**B-left**) and the lesion (**B-right**), which demonstrate minimal residual lumen at the level of the lesion. AP-Caudal projection still image from conventional angiogram (**C**) confirms a greater than 50% stenosis in the proximal LCX (*arrow*).

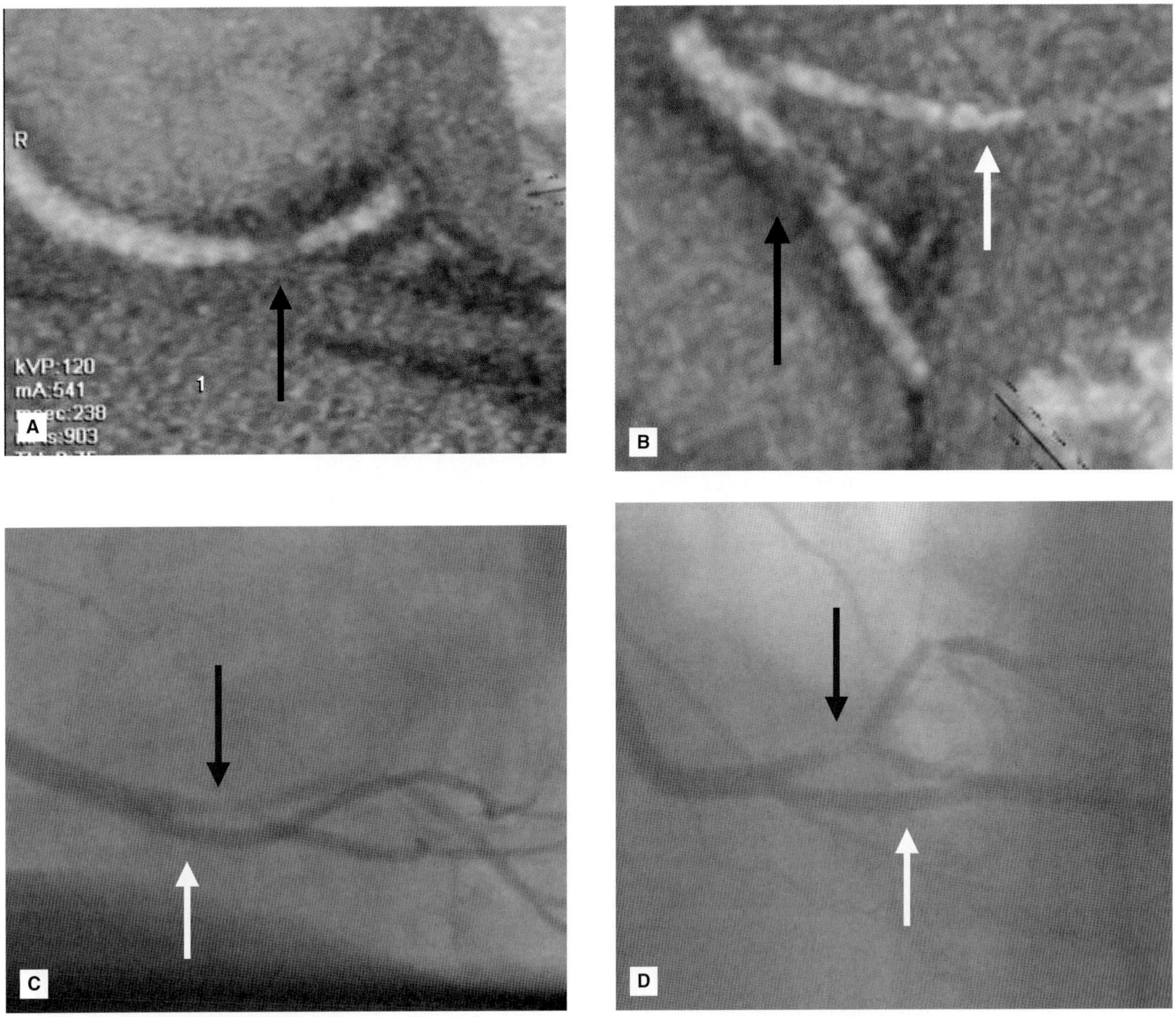

FIGURE 6-6 Right coronary artery greater than 50% stenosis diagnosed by CT and confirmed by conventional angiography. Double oblique maximum intensity projection images (4 mm thick) through ongoing RCA at 90 degree angles (**A**, **B**) demonstrate a segment of noncalcified plaque with nonvisualization of lumen (black arrow). The PIV is also partially demonstrated (*white arrow*). Finding is confirmed by LAO (**C**) and AP-cranial (**D**) projection still images conventional angiogram (*black arrow*). The PIV is also seen (*white arrow*).

purpose.[6–19] In these studies, data are typically reported on a per coronary artery segment basis, comparing CTA and DSA. A significant stenosis is generally defined as greater than 50%, determined by quantitative coronary angiography. Data are also analyzed on a per patient basis regarding the value of CTA in ruling-in or excluding CAD. Literature to date reports on patient populations with a relatively high prevalence of CAD (ie, patients already scheduled for DSA.

1. Nonevaluable coronary segments were included as being positive for a significant coronary stenosis.
2. Sensitivity and specificity were not calculated separately for 16-slice and 64-slice scanner.
3. Percentage of nonevaluable "patients"
4. Sensitivity and specificity were calculated on "vessel"-based analysis.
5. CT images were interpreted independently by two radiologists with unequal experience in reading coronary CTA.

Table 6-1 summarizes published data. Among the most consistent findings is a very high negative predictive value (NPV) of coronary CTA when performed with 64- or greater detector row scanners. The data and our experience suggest a very high NPV, effectively arguing that cardiac CTA can effectively exclude CAD in patients with low to intermediate pretest probability of disease. Consequently, CTA has become increasingly useful for the cardiac surgeon in managing patients scheduled for noncoronary cardiac surgery. If the clinical suspicion is low, but not insignificant, CTA affords the surgeon a method of assessing coronary disease without subjecting the patient to femoral arterial puncture with its known complications. For example, patients undergoing isolated mitral valve surgery for degenerative, myxomatous disease have a low prevalence of CAD, making CTA an ideal alternative to conventional angiography to exclude significant CAD. When the CT protocol described in Section A is followed, high-quality

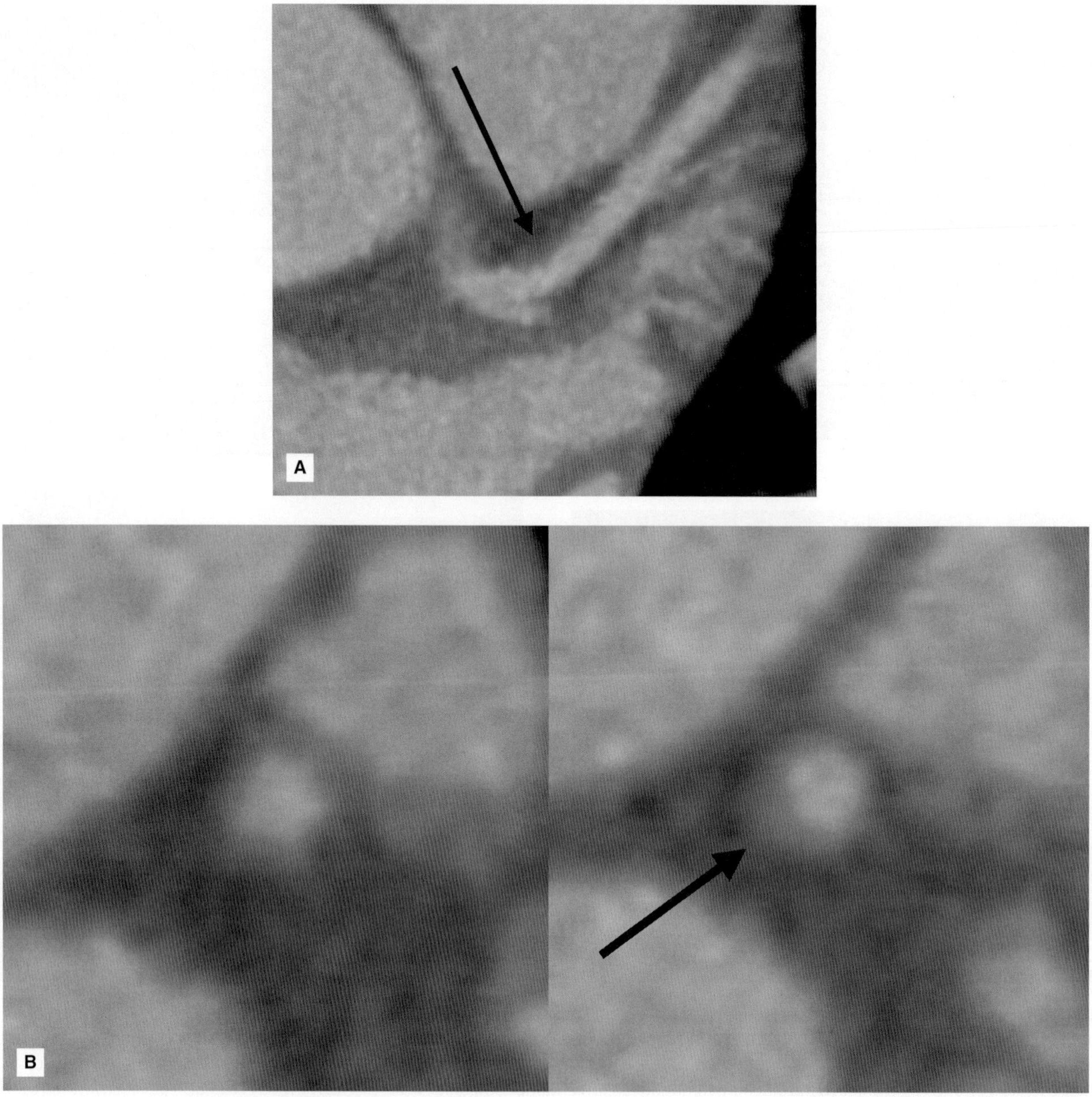

FIGURE 6-7 Proximal LAD less than 50% stenosis diagnosed by coronary CT angiography. Double oblique maximum intensity projection image (4 mm thick) through proximal LAD (**A**) demonstrates a segment of noncalcified plaque that is not associated with any significant luminal narrowing (*arrow*). True vessel short-axis multiplanar reformatted images through the lesion (**B-right**) and through proximal reference segment (**B-left**) confirm minimal luminal narrowing. Low-density (ie, noncalcified) plaque with positive vessel remodeling is seen (*arrow*). This case highlights the ability of CTA to detect early stages of subclinical atherosclerosis. This lesion would presumably not have been detected at a conventional angiogram.

imaging is *routine*, and when CTA excludes CAD, surgeons have increased confidence in using CTA alone. Follow-up with DSA can be reserved for those patients who might benefit from catheter-based intervention.

CORONARY ARTERY BYPASS GRAFT CTA

Cardiac CT provides the cardiac surgeon with a non-invasive method to assess graft patency after CABG. Studies using early 16-detector row CT scanners suggest 100% sensitivity and specificity for identifying occluded versus patent grafts[20–22] with benefits from advanced image postprocessing tools.[23] In clinical practice, this application is of value in the evaluation of the symptomatic patient in the early postoperative period in whom graft failure is being considered (Fig. 6-8). It is particularly useful for the demonstration of patent grafts in patients with a remote surgical history and unknown graft anatomy prior to DSA, and in patients in whom conventional angiography fails

TABLE 6-1 Summary of Data for Native coronary Arteries for Stenosis

Author	MDCT	Study	N	Sens by Seg	Spec by Seg	Not Eval Seg	NPV by Patient
Hoffman[6]	16	JAMA 2005 All segments >1.5 mm	103	95%	98%	6.4%	95%
Garcia[7]	16	JAMA 2006 All segments >2 mm	187	85%	91%	29%	87%
Turkvatan[8]	16	Acta Radiol 2008 All segments >1.5 mm	153	85%	97%	20%	94%
Hausleiter[9]	16	Eur Heart J 2007 All segments >2 mm	129	93%	87%	11%*	99%
	64		114	92%	92%	7.4%*	99%
Marano[10]	16	Eur Radiol 2009 All segments	284	70%†	96%†	22%	91%
	64		66			21%	89%
Shabestari[11]	64	Am J Cardiol 2007 All segments >1.5 mm	143	92%	97%	1.2%	83%
Cademartiri[12]	64	Radiol Med 2008 All segments	134	76%	87%	12%‡	94%
Budoff[13]	64	JACC 2008 All segments	230	84%§	90%§	n/a	99%
Miller[14]	64	NEJM 2008 All segments >1.5 mm	291	75%§	93%§	1%	83%
Meijboom [15]	64	JACC 2008 All segments	360	88%	90%	n/a*	97%
Bettencourt[16]	64	Circ Cardiovasc Imaging 2009 All segments	237	89%	97%	n/a*	99%
Gouya[17]	64	Radiology 2009 All segments > 1.5 mm	114	66,73%‖	94,95%‖	1%	89,100%‖
Maffei[18]	64	Radiol Med 2009 All segments	1372	94%	95%	n/a	99%
Dewey[19]	320	Circulation 2009 All segments	30	78%	98%	0%	100%

Eval = evaluable; NPV = negative predictive value; Seg = segment; Sens = sensitivity; Spec = specificity

to demonstrate a known graft (Fig. 6-9). In the reoperative setting, such data has virtually revolutionized surgical decision-making and planning prior to surgery in patients who have already undergone CABG.

Patients with recurrent angina after bypass surgery may have developed stenosis or occlusion in bypass grafts, or may have progression of native coronary disease. In these patients, CTA can be more limited. For example, exclusion of significant stenosis in a graft may be problematic because of metallic surgical clips that cause artifact (Fig. 6-10). Moreover, native CAD in these patients is often advanced and heavily calcified. A large volume of calcium may result in an uninterpretable study for

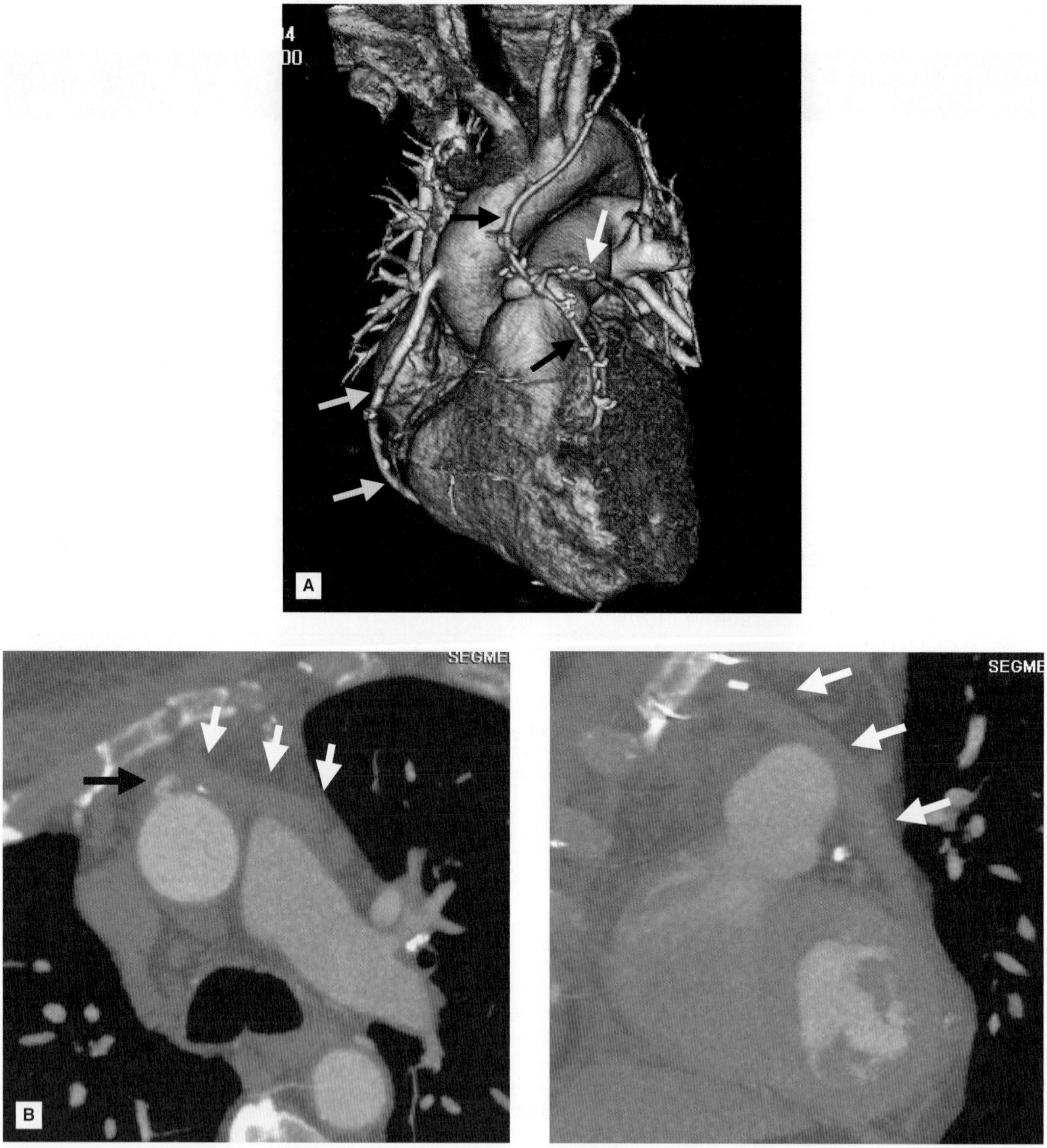

FIGURE 6-8 (A) Postoperative cardiac CT performed for evaluation of graft patency. Three-dimensional volume-rendered image demonstrates patent LIMA to LAD (*black arrows*), T-graft RIMA to obtuse marginal (*white arrow*), and SVG to RCA (*grey arrows*). This study was obtained in a patient 1 day after off-pump coronary artery bypass grafting. The patient had developed recurrent chest pain and an elevated troponin. Cardiac CT ruled out early graft failure as a cause for the patient's presentation. (B) Companion case in a different patient. Oblique multiplanar reformatted images demonstrate an acutely occluded saphenous vein graft to obtuse marginal. Note the patent graft stump (*black arrow*) and thrombosed graft body (*white arrows*).

many segments of the native coronaries (Fig. 6-11). CTA for plaque assessment in such patients may not be definitive; consequently conventional angiography may be preferred in this population.[24] Obviously, the less calcification and metal artifact present, the more useful CTA is.

In the research context, graft patency is an important outcome in the evaluation of different surgical techniques. Randomized controlled trials utilizing conventional angiography for assessment of graft patency typically demonstrate a 10 to 20% rate of noncompliance. This noncompliance is at least

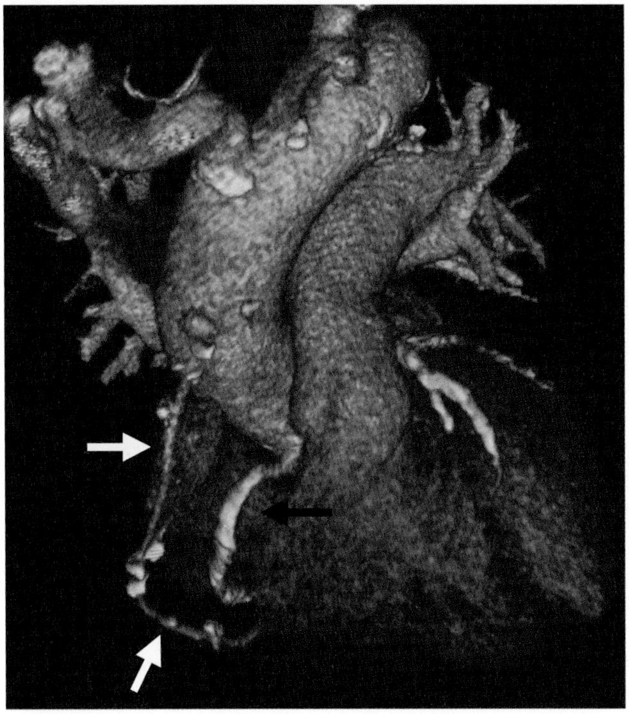

FIGURE 6-9 Cardiac CT performed to evaluate possible radial graft occlusion. The patient had surgery 1 month prior and presented with recurrent angina. The radial to RCA graft could not be selective catheterized at conventional angiography and was also not seen at aortic root injection. Three-dimensional volume-rendered image demonstrates patent radial graft (*white arrows*) to RCA (*black arrow*). The anastomosis is not seen on this orientation.

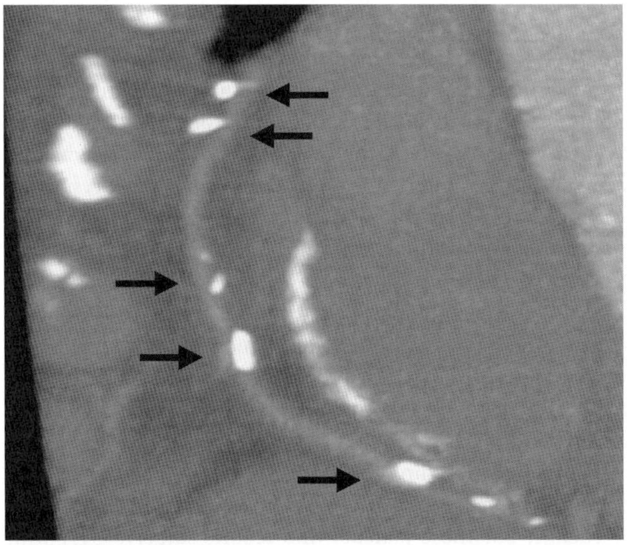

FIGURE 6-10 Surgical clip artifacts can limit cardiac CT evaluation of coronary bypass grafts. Double oblique maximum intensity projection image (10 mm thick) demonstrates multiple surgical clips placed along the length of a radial to PIV graft (*black arrows*). Artifact from these metallic clips can partially or completely obscure the adjacent vessel lumen, precluding evaluation of these segments for the presence or absence of stenosis. Although CT can unequivocally demonstrate graft patency based on the delivery of contrast throughout the entire course of the graft, surgical clip artifact usually does not allow complete graft evaluation to rule out graft stenosis.

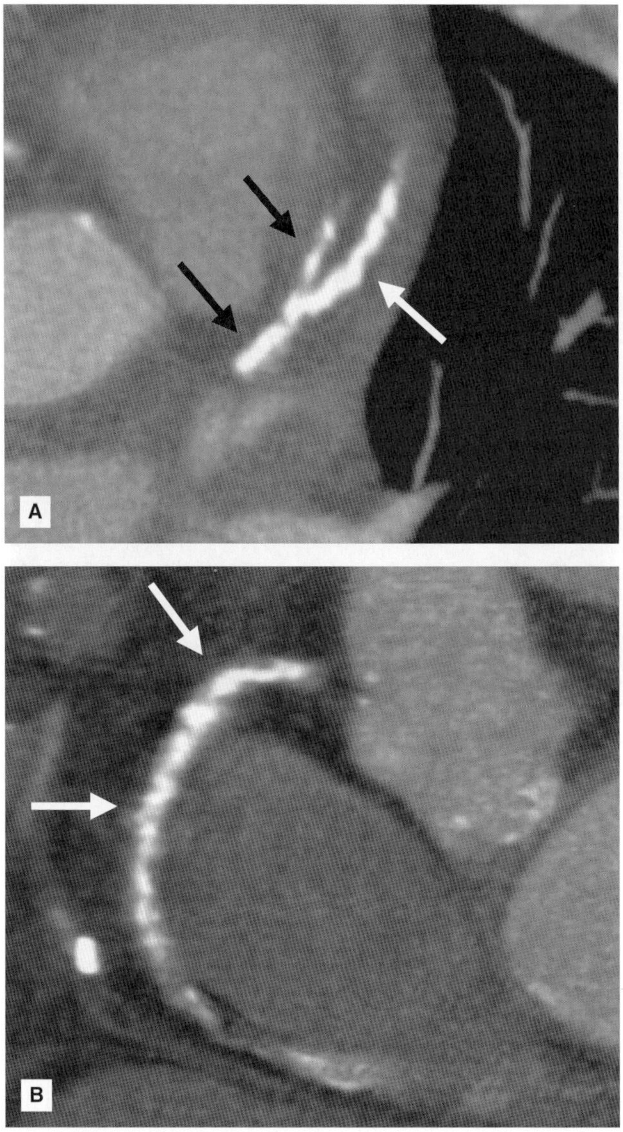

FIGURE 6-11 Cardiac CT is often limited in its evaluation of native coronary arteries in the postcoronary artery bypass graft patient because of the presence of advanced and heavily calcified coronary atherosclerosis. Double oblique maximum intensity projection image (4 mm) demonstrates (A) the proximal LAD (*black arrows*) and a large first diagonal branch (*white arrow*) and (B) the proximal right coronary artery (*white arrows*). The white areas are very high attenuation and represent calcification. All vessel segments demonstrated are heavily calcified. The extent of calcification completely obscures the vessel lumen and presence or absence of stenosis cannot be reliably assessed.

partly attributable to the invasive nature of the test. [25–27] Cardiac CT is an attractive, noninvasive, and very accurate method to assess graft patency for clinical trials, again obviating a traditional arterial puncture with its risks and known complications. Cardiac CT may also be used for routine postoperative control of grafts following implementation of a new surgical technique in a local center practice (Fig. 6-12).

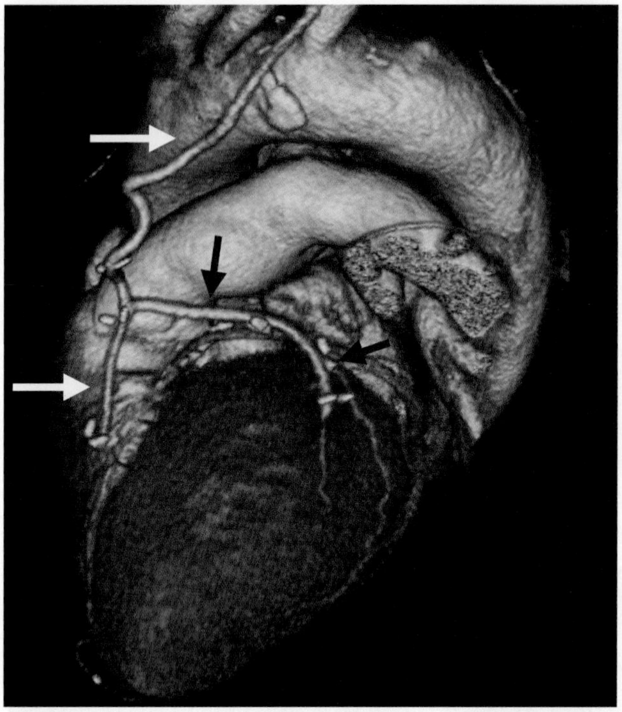

FIGURE 6-12 Cardiac CT obtained for postoperative graft control in a patient who underwent MVST. Three-dimensional volume-rendered image demonstrates patent LIMA to LAD (*white arrows*) and radial T-graft to obtuse marginal (*black arrows*).

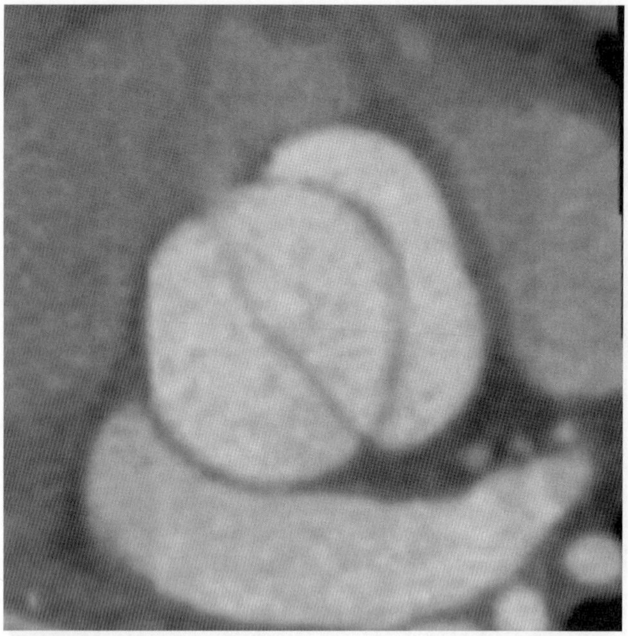

FIGURE 6-13 Demonstration of aortic root and aortic valve. Axial oblique multiplanar reformatted image from a systolic dataset demonstrates an open bicuspid aortic valve. Note the precise definition of the aortic wall, free from the cardiac motion related artifacts that are present at conventional thoracic CT scanning. Aortic root size measurements are highly accurate because of lack of motion artifacts and the high spatial resolution of the cardiac CT scanning (<0.5 mm).

THE AORTA: THE ROOT, THE ASCENDING AORTA, THE ARCH, AND THE DESCENDING AORTA

Surgery of the aortic root, the ascending aorta, the arch, and the descending aorta is becoming increasingly commonplace as the population ages. CT has been used for many years to assess the thoracic aorta. Non–ECG-gated CT is highly accurate in the assessment of the aortic arch and descending thoracic aorta because they are not subject to significant cardiac motion. However, ECG-gated cardiac CT adds motion-free imaging of the aortic root and ascending aorta. Without question, any aorta surgery involving the aorta (whether the root, the arch, the ascending, or the descending portion) requires preoperative CTA for surgical decision-making. The superior imaging of ECG-gated CTA better defines the pathology and hence facilitates the preoperative planning. For example, CTA is by far the best imaging modality to clearly define aortic calcification.

If portions of the aorta are calcified on CTA, then aortic cross clamping and cannulation for cardiopulmonary bypass at those sites are contraindicated in order to avoid embolic phenomenon and stroke. Thus, preoperative cardiopulmonary bypass strategy and myocardial protection are often critically altered by preoperative CTA.

As with calcification, CT is the most accurate modality to evaluate the aortic root, with both 2D and 3D visualization (Fig. 6-13). Not only can the aortic root be sized from multiple imaging planes, but also the exact location of the aneurismal pathology with respect to the valve and sinotubular junction can often be defined.[28] This assessment is critical for preoperative decision making and surgical planning. In patients with ascending aortic aneurysm, if the aortic root is determined to be aneurysmal near the coronary ostia, surgical decision making changes from a simple tube graft repair for the aneurysm to a much more complex composite root repair with coronary reimplantation. In addition, motion-free images obtained with ECG gating allow for definitive exclusion of type A dissection (Fig. 6-14). Three-dimensional volume rendering optimally depicts other aortic root pathologies such as coronary anomalies or a sinus of valsalva aneurysm (Fig. 6-15). In patients with a sinus of valsalva aneurysm, as opposed to a root aneurysm, CT alters surgical strategy for repair.

For known ascending aortic aneurysms that do not meet size criteria for surgery, CTA is excellent to periodically assess size or change. For those patients who require surgery, CTA with 3D volume-rendered images provides the surgeon with preoperative visualization of aneurysm size and extent. The extension of an ascending aortic aneurysm into the arch can be demonstrated and, as mentioned above, the expected location of aortic cross-clamping can be determined preoperatively (Fig. 6-16). The location of normal aorta distally and the extent of arch involvement will preoperatively determine the arterial cardiopulmonary bypass cannulation site as well as the need for concomitant arch repair, circulatory arrest, or selective antegrade

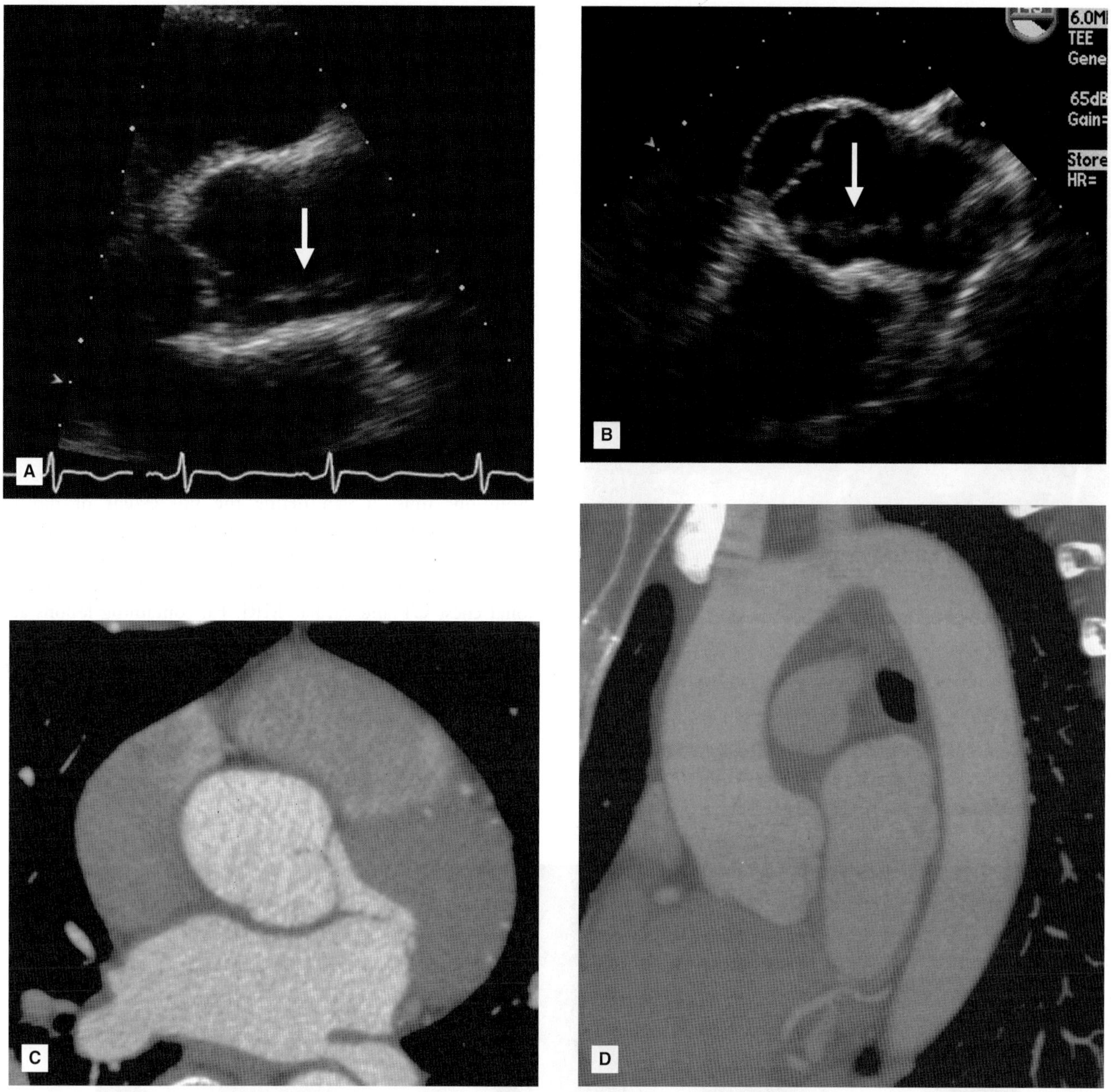

FIGURE 6-14 Although multiple modalities may be used for evaluation of the aortic root, cardiac CT is the gold standard for all pathology of the aorta, including the exclusion and characterization of type A dissection. Parasternal long-axis image from trans-thoracic echocardiogram (A) demonstrates a linear area of echogenicity (white arrow) above the noncoronary cusp of the aortic valve concerning for an intimal flap. The finding was detected incidentally in a patient with recent stroke and possible patent foramen ovale (PFO). Subsequent transesophageal echocardiogram (B) again demonstrated the finding. Axial image from cardiac CT scan (C) provides excellent visualization of the aortic root and definitively excludes the present of an intimal flap. Sagittal oblique maximum intensity projection image (D) demonstrates aortic root and ascending aorta to be normal. No further evaluation is needed. Echocardiographic findings were presumed to be from artifact.

perfusion. Selective antegrade cerebral perfusion itself is dependent on intact right axillary and innominate arteries, and CTA is optimal for defining this anatomy. Because the success of a procedure can be compromised by unexpected intraoperative findings, CT has contributed enormously to surgical planning by defining anatomy that would not be preoperatively visualized with any other imaging modality.

In patients with aortic dissection, CTA allows the surgeon to understand the extent of the intimal flap. In particular, ECG-gated CT offers information regarding dissection of the ascending aorta (the proximal extent of the dissection flap and its relationship to the coronary arteries and the aortic valve) that was not available before gating was routinely performed. The location of the true and false lumen is critical in the preoperative

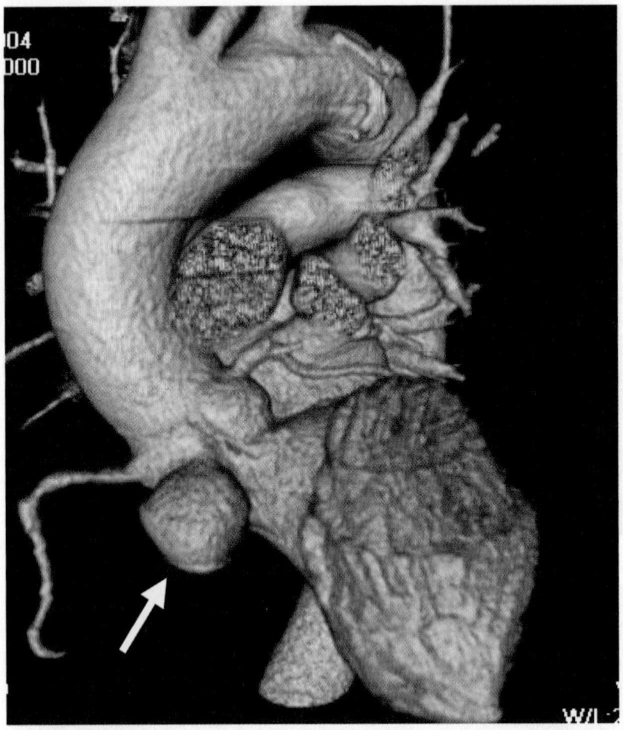

FIGURE 6-15 Cardiac CT provides optimal visualization of complex aortic root pathology. Prior echocardiogram suggested the entire aortic root to be aneurysmal at greater than 4.5 cm. Three-dimensional volume-rendered image from cardiac CT demonstrates a 2.6 cm sinus of Valsalva aneurysm arising off of the right coronary sinus (*white arrow*). The remainder of the aortic root is normal.

planning, the operative sequence, and the extent of repair. For example, in dissection of the descending aorta, end-organ perfusion is assessed by demonstrating contrast enhancement of individual organs and related compromise of the celiac, superior mesenteric, inferior mesenteric or renal arteries. As is the case for a nonsurgical aneurysm, if a descending thoracic aortic dissection is stable and to be followed expectantly, CTA remains the gold standard for periodic assessment.

CARDIAC MASSES

Cardiac MRI is the modality most commonly used for high spatial resolution cross-sectional imaging to evaluate cardiac and pericardial masses. However, CT may be preferred if the mass is known to extend into the mediastinum, chest wall, or lung, or if the patient has a contraindication to MRI. CT also evaluates extracardiac thoracic structures with high spatial resolution; thus, it can define the full extent of disease (Fig. 6-17). CT is also useful as a single follow-up examination in patients with metastases to the heart and lungs because it avoids the need for periodic assessment with both conventional chest CT and cardiac MRI. Fat-containing lesions are very amenable to evaluation by CT, because lesions have a characteristic appearance, appearing black relative to water (Fig. 6-18).

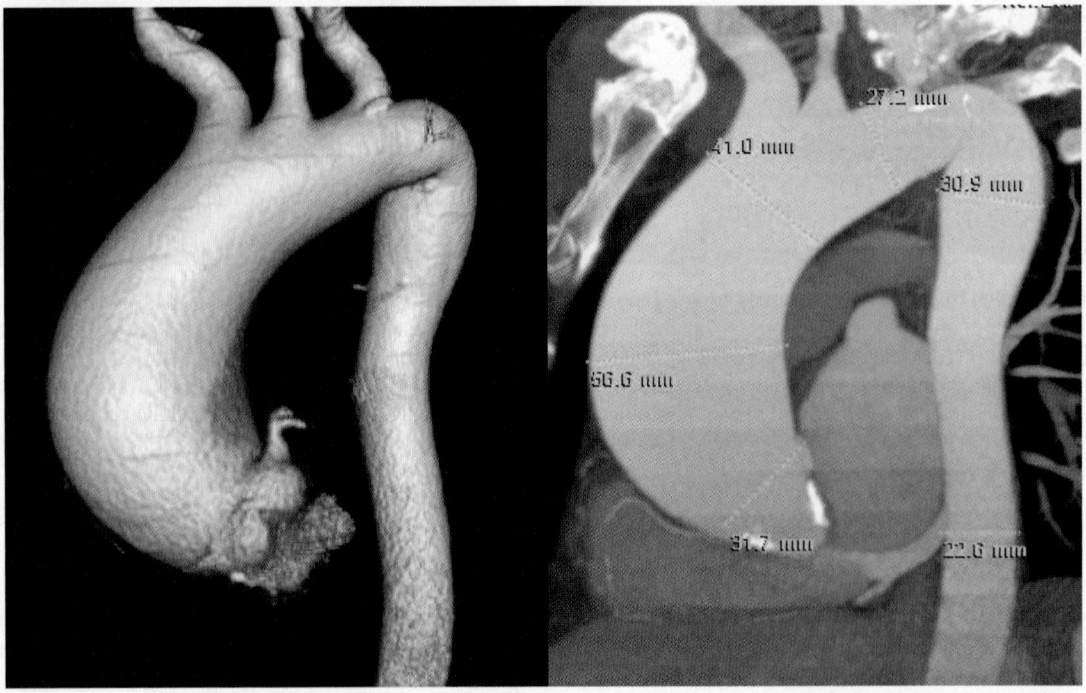

FIGURE 6-16 Comprehensive evaluation of ascending aortic aneurysm for preoperative planning. On the left, 3D volume-rendered image demonstrates an aneurysmal ascending aorta. Sagittal oblique maximum intensity projection image (20 mm thick) can be used to demonstrate aortic size measurements. The aneurysm can be seen to extend into the aortic arch. As the entire ascending aorta and proximal arch needed to be replaced, cross clamping could not occur proximal to the innominate in this patient and would have to occur in the middistal arch altering the surgical risk of the procedure.

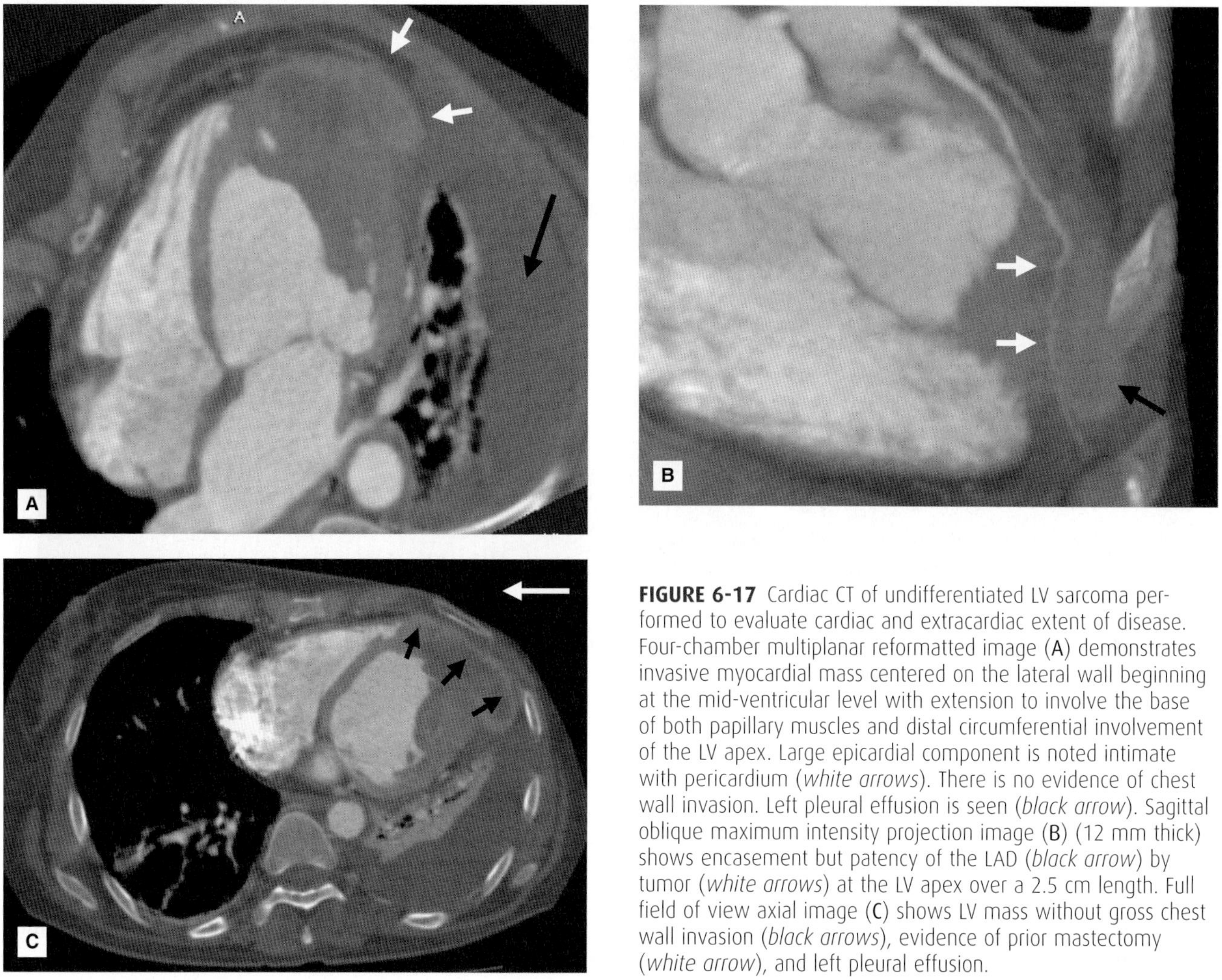

FIGURE 6-17 Cardiac CT of undifferentiated LV sarcoma performed to evaluate cardiac and extracardiac extent of disease. Four-chamber multiplanar reformatted image (A) demonstrates invasive myocardial mass centered on the lateral wall beginning at the mid-ventricular level with extension to involve the base of both papillary muscles and distal circumferential involvement of the LV apex. Large epicardial component is noted intimate with pericardium (*white arrows*). There is no evidence of chest wall invasion. Left pleural effusion is seen (*black arrow*). Sagittal oblique maximum intensity projection image (B) (12 mm thick) shows encasement but patency of the LAD (*black arrow*) by tumor (*white arrows*) at the LV apex over a 2.5 cm length. Full field of view axial image (C) shows LV mass without gross chest wall invasion (*black arrows*), evidence of prior mastectomy (*white arrow*), and left pleural effusion.

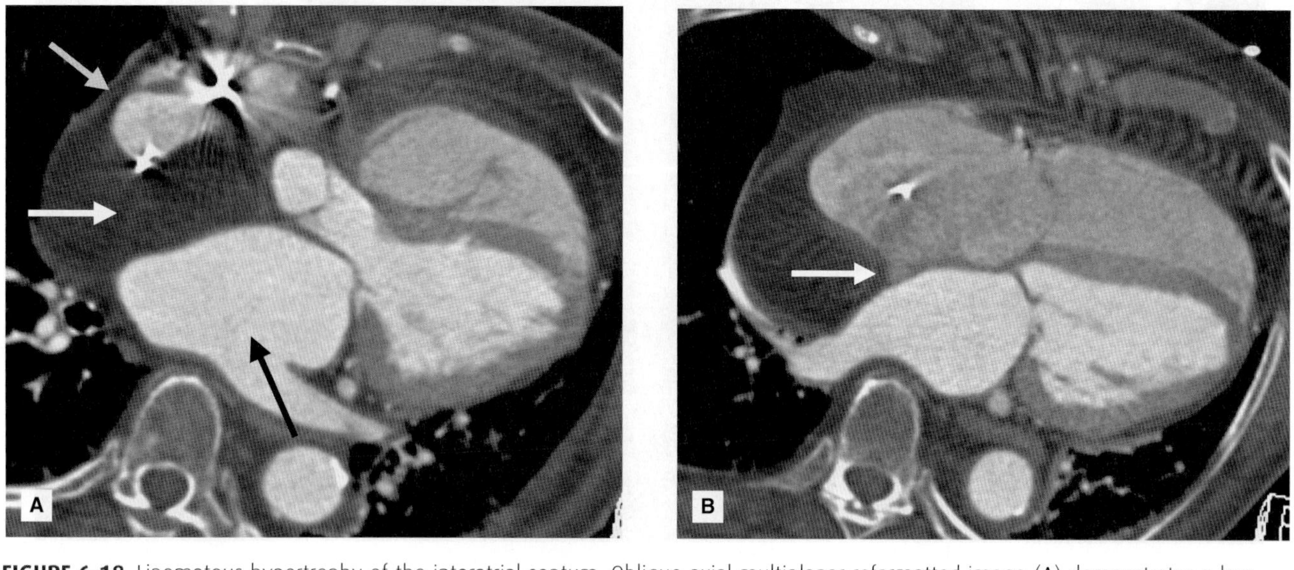

FIGURE 6-18 Lipomatous hypertrophy of the interatrial septum. Oblique axial multiplanar reformatted image (A) demonstrates a low attenuation mass (*white arrow*) insinuated between SVC (*grey arrow*) and left atrium (*black arrow*). Second more caudal image (B) demonstrates characteristic sparing of the fossa ovalis (*white arrow*). This lesion is nonencapsulated and can be quite extensive as in this case. Note presence of leads from pacemaker that precluded an MR study.

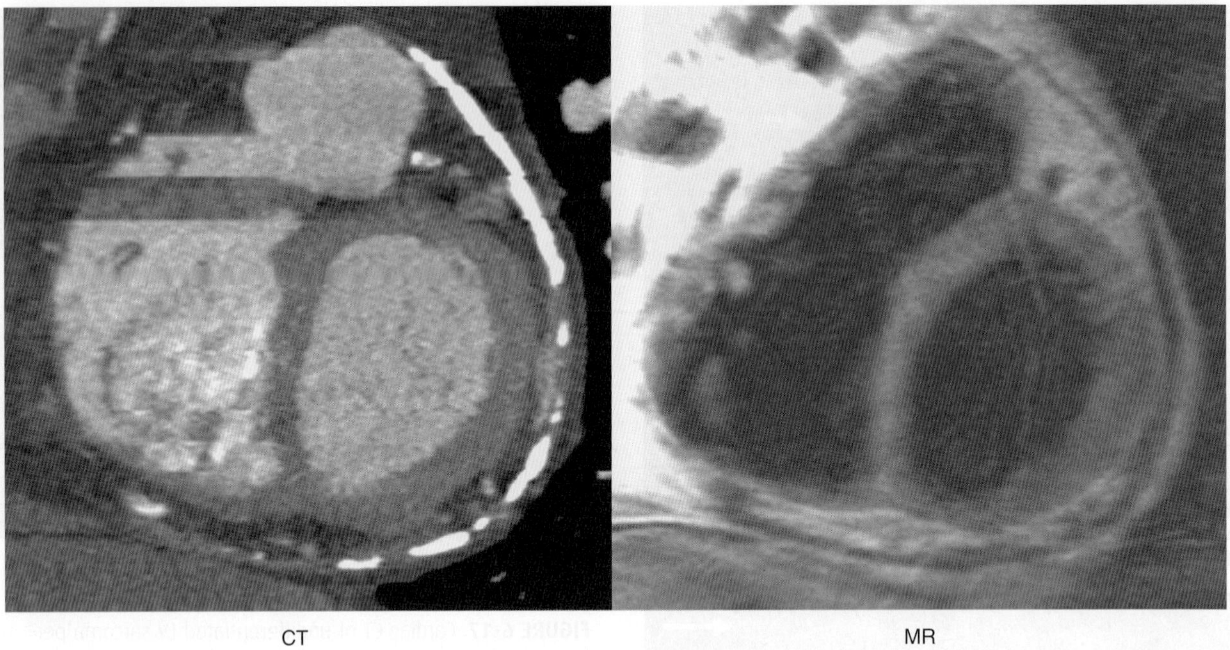

FIGURE 6-19 Calcific constrictive pericarditis. Short axis multiplanar reformatted image from cardiac CT demonstrates extensive thickening and calcification involving left-sided pericardium. In the appropriate clinical setting, these findings would support the diagnosis of constrictive pericarditis. Short axis double inversion recovery fast spin echo image from cardiac MR in the same patient also shows abnormal pericardial thickening, but is insensitive to calcification.

IMAGING OF THE PERICARDIUM

In patients with clinically suspected constrictive pericarditis, cardiac MRI or CT can be used to confirm and measure pericardial thickening. In comparison with MRI, CT far better demonstrates the presence and extent of calcification. This may be of value in confirming chronic calcific pericardial thickening, supporting the diagnosis of constrictive pericarditis (Fig. 6-19). In these cases, 3D volume rendering to illustrate regional localization of pericardial abnormality functions as an outstanding preoperative planning tool prior to pericardial stripping (Fig. 6-20).

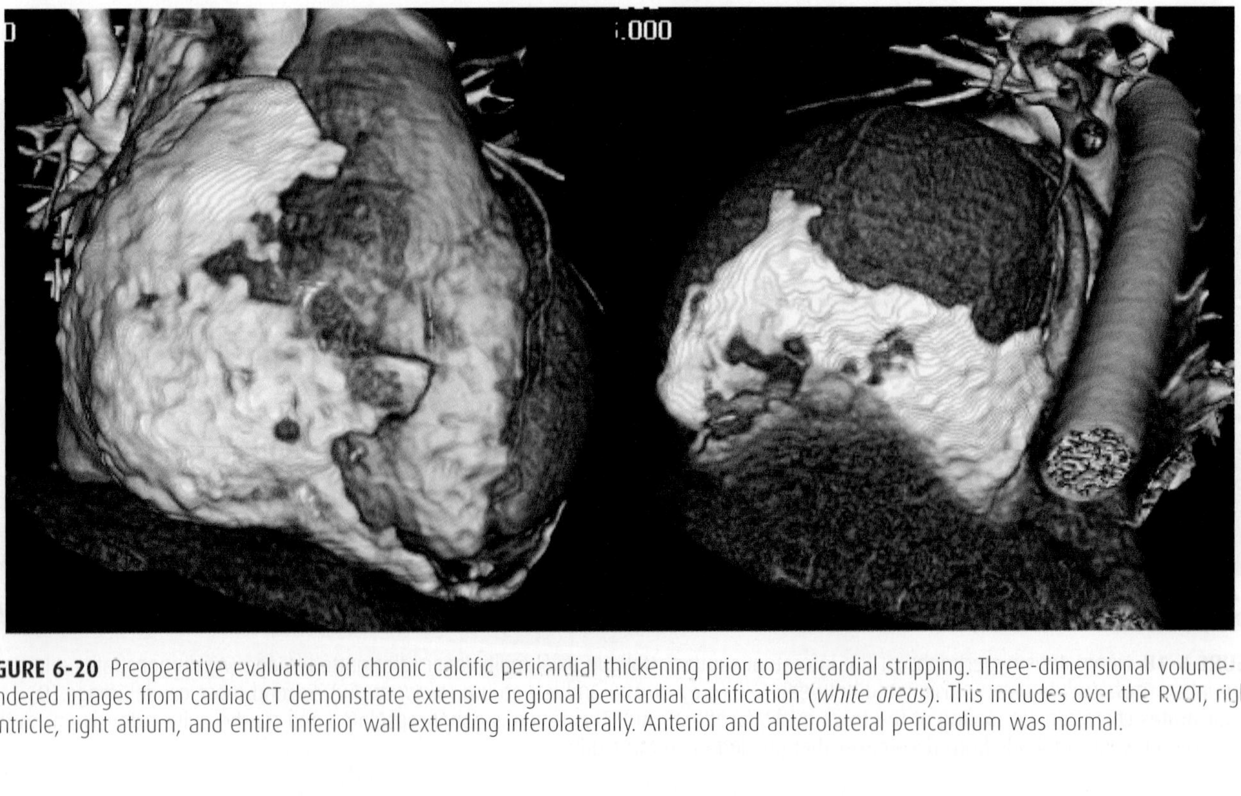

FIGURE 6-20 Preoperative evaluation of chronic calcific pericardial thickening prior to pericardial stripping. Three-dimensional volume-rendered images from cardiac CT demonstrate extensive regional pericardial calcification (*white areas*). This includes over the RVOT, right ventricle, right atrium, and entire inferior wall extending inferolaterally. Anterior and anterolateral pericardium was normal.

VALVE IMAGING

In patients with suspected valve dysfunction based on echocardiography, cine CT from retrospective ECG gating as described in Section A provides valuable additional data. As noted earlier, reconstruction is performed for all phases of the cardiac cycle, and the reformatted data can be played in a cine loop. This has relevance in assessment in native, bioprosthetic, and mechanical aortic valves. Recent experience suggests an excellent correlation between planimetric valves areas obtained by CT, MRI, and TEE (transesophageal echocardiography).[29] Consequently, CT can be used as an alternate modality for evaluation of aortic valve area. This is relevant if transthoracic echocardiography is of poor technical quality or discrepant with a clinically expected result. Because patients may be evaluated with CT for concomitant aortic aneurysm or coronary artery disease prior to aortic valve surgery, valve area may be obtained from CT with no additional scanning and only a small amount of image post-processing. CT can be used in correlation with valve area as determined with echocardiography (Fig. 6-21).

Postoperative evaluation of bioprosthetic valves may also be conducted using CT scanning. Although echocardiographically determined transvalvular gradients are the reference standard for determination of "effective" orifice area, CT provides a useful correlative modality—particularly when the echo is technically challenging or discordant with clinical findings. In patients with unexpectedly high gradients post valve implantation, increasing use of CT will provide more information to guide management (Fig. 6-22). In patients with suspected bioprosthetic valve endocarditis, CT can be an invaluable modality to delineate paravalvular and valvular sequela of the infection (Fig. 6-23).

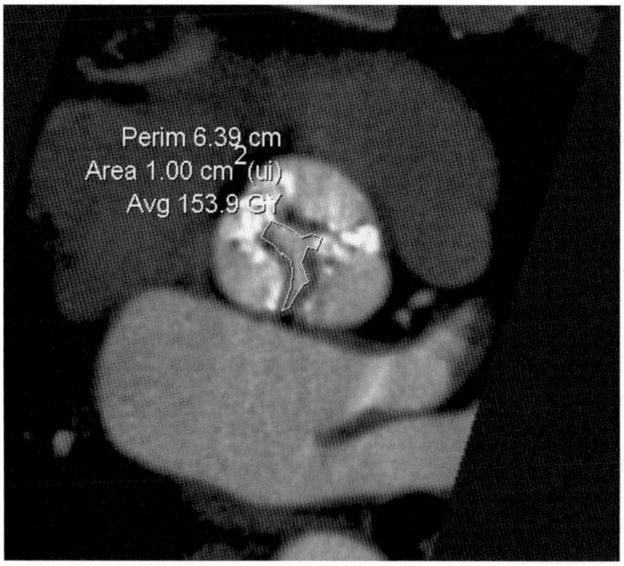

FIGURE 6-21 Reformatted CT angiography through the aortic valve shows calcification and stenosis with a valve area of 1 cm^2 measured by direct planimetry.

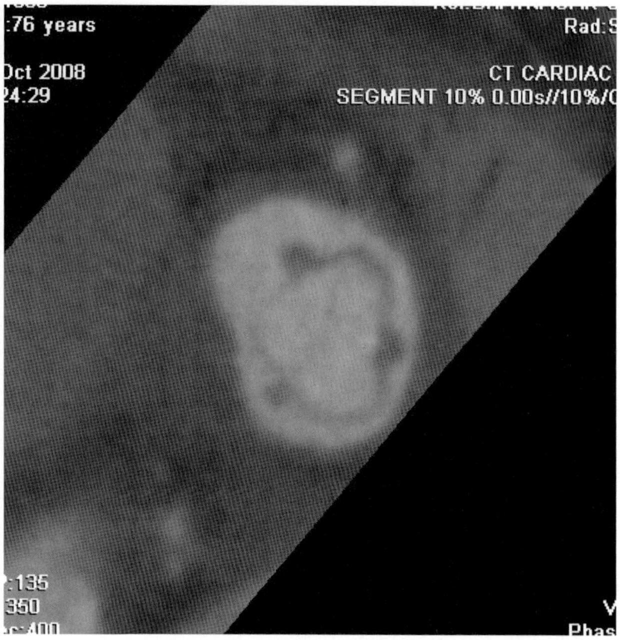

FIGURE 6-22 Seventy-seven year old man with a #23 Medtronic Mosaic valve. The patient developed shortness of breath approximately 1 year following surgery. Echocardiography, which demonstrated a peak gradient of 78 mm Hg; the effective orifice area was reported at 0.9cm^2. Subsequent cardiac CT showed a normal valve area of 1.7 cm^2, providing reassurance to both patient and surgeon.

Cardiac CT also permits high resolution functional evaluation of mechanical aortic valve prostheses without artifact (Fig. 6-24). CT can be readily incorporated to evaluate valve dysfunction, measure opening angles, and to elucidate the underlying cause of valve failure. Fig. 6-25 illustrates correlation between CT and surgical specimen in a mechanical aortic valve patient with restricted opening angle and elevated gradients. CT readily made the preoperative diagnosis of pannus ingrowth.

PREOPERATIVE PLANNING AND SURGICAL GUIDANCE

Reoperative Surgery

Reoperative cardiac surgery with live coronary grafts after previous CABG represents one of the most difficult problems in cardiac surgery. Reoperative sternotomy is challenging secondary to adhesions, loss of tissue planes, and the potential for injury to patent grafts, the aorta, and the right ventricle. Injury to a patent left internal thoracic artery graft to the LAD is associated with a mortality of 50%.[30,31] Cardiac CT has been revolutionary in precisely defining the relationship of important structures (e.g, the aorta, right ventricle, or live grafts) to the midline and sternum for reentry planning (Fig. 6-26). At BWH, every reoperative surgery includes a preoperative CTA with z-axis coverage to include all grafts

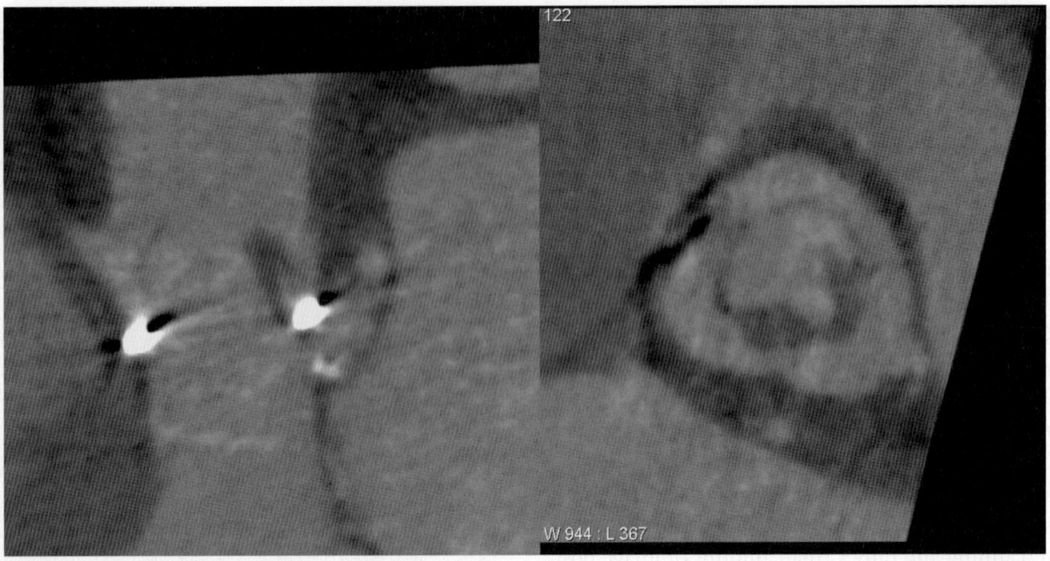

FIGURE 6-23 Patient with clinically suspected bioprosthetic valve endocarditis. Left image shows a pseudoaneurysm originating below the aortic valve ring and exerting mass effect on the adjacent left atrial wall. The right image shows nodular thickening of the aortic valve leaflets consistent with vegetations

and the entire course of the IMAs. Preoperative identification of all structures at risk is mandatory, and different, specific operative approaches always remain in consideration.[32] Experience suggests that preoperative cardiac CT will lead to a modification in surgical strategy for 1 in 5 patients undergoing redo cardiac surgery.[23] For example, if CT demonstrates a patent left internal mammary artery (LIMA) is close to the midline or a right ventricle directly adherent to the posterior table of the sternum, cardiopulmonary bypass is instituted prior to reentry. Definition of live grafts with respect to their proximal placement of the aorta is instrumental in determining, *before the operation,* the precise manner in which those grafts will be handled. For example, in reoperative surgery for aortic valve replacement (AVR) in the setting of live grafts, CTA allows the surgeon to plan preoperatively whether or not those grafts will have to be divided in carrying out the aortotomy for the AVR. As described above, CT also allows the cardiac surgeon to preoperatively plan the precise location of the aortotomy itself.

Minimally Invasive Surgery Coronary Artery Bypass Grafting

Minimally invasive coronary artery bypass surgery is becoming an alternative to open surgery. With limited intraoperative access for direct visualization, aspects of coronary artery anatomy such as vessel diameter, extent of calcification, and the presence of intramyocardial segments become even more important to define preoperatively (Fig. 6-27). In addition, 3D models that combine visualization of a partially transparent thoracic cage over mediastinal structures allow the surgeon to obtain detailed preoperative understanding of the patient's cardiothoracic anatomy (Fig. 6-28). Preoperative CT has demonstrated usefulness for MIDCAB[33] and totally endoscopic coronary artery bypass surgery.[34] CT is also expected to become invaluable for procedures such as multivessel small thoracotomy coronary revascularization.

CT VERSUS MRI OF THE HEART

Throughout this chapter, comparisons between CT and MRI have illustrated the strengths and limitations of each. Both modalities give the surgeon valuable pre- and postoperative information. Although the modality best suited for specific clinical indications evolves with the technology, at present certain generalizations can be made. Cardiac CT is invaluable in reoperative cardiac surgery because it offers higher quality noninvasive angiography of native coronary arteries and bypass grafts. Because 3D volume rendering with CT has higher quality and better spatial resolution, it is preferred for preoperative planning for reoperative CABG or minimally invasive cardiac surgery. All calcification is poorly seen on MRI and superbly seen with CT, and thus CT is far superior in demonstrating coronary, myocardial, pericardial, and valvular calcification. The same is true for mechanical valve prostheses; because of large areas of artifact on MR images, functional evaluation is only possible with CT. Finally, all patients with a surgical problem of the aorta require evaluation with CT.

The strengths of MRI include high temporal resolution, greater blood-myocardial image contrast, multiparametric functional evaluation, and techniques for myocardial tissue characterization. In addition, cardiac MRI is invaluable in assessing myocardial function, contractility, and actual tissue perfusion and viability. For these reasons, MRI remains the gold standard to assess biventricular volumes, function, and myocardial mass. A variety of MRI pulse sequences can accurately delineate areas of chronic myocardial infarction, identify

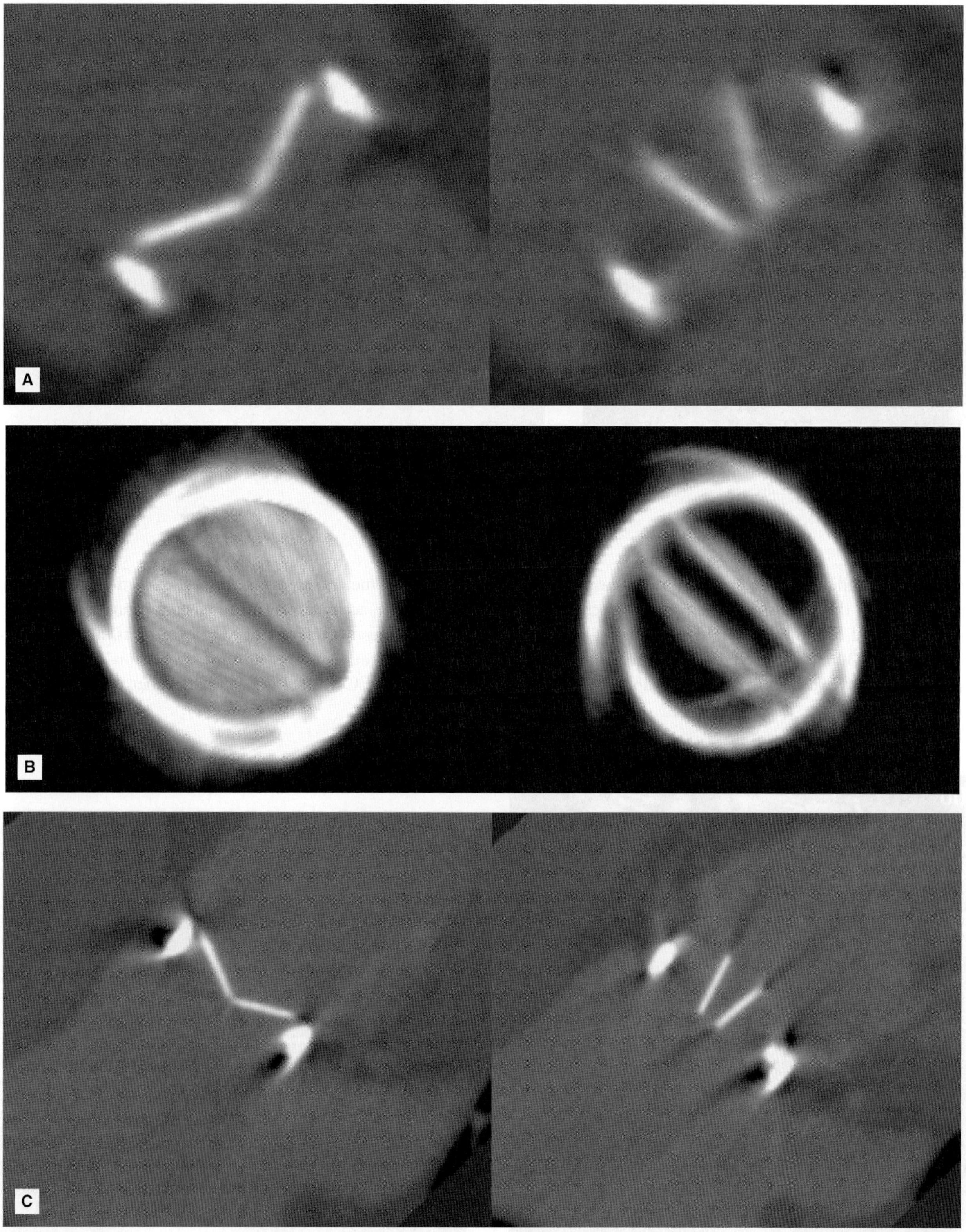

FIGURE 6-24 Evaluation of mechanical valve function with cardiac CT. Coronal oblique multiplanar reformatted images (A) demonstrate closed and open positions of mechanical AVR in a patient with suspected valve dysfunction based on echo-Doppler. Axial oblique slab maximum intensity projection images (B) demonstrate closed and open position of mechanical AVR in a patient in atrial fibrillation at the time of cardiac CT. Although image quality is degraded by arrhythmia, optimization of the dataset with ECG-editing can result in diagnostic quality images. Four-chamber oblique multiplanar reformatted images (C) demonstrate closed and open positions of a mechanical MVR. Images can be generated over the cardiac cycle and displayed in a cine movie format to allow dynamic evaluation of valve function. Because the study is performed with contrast, thrombus or perivalvular abscess can also be identified if present.

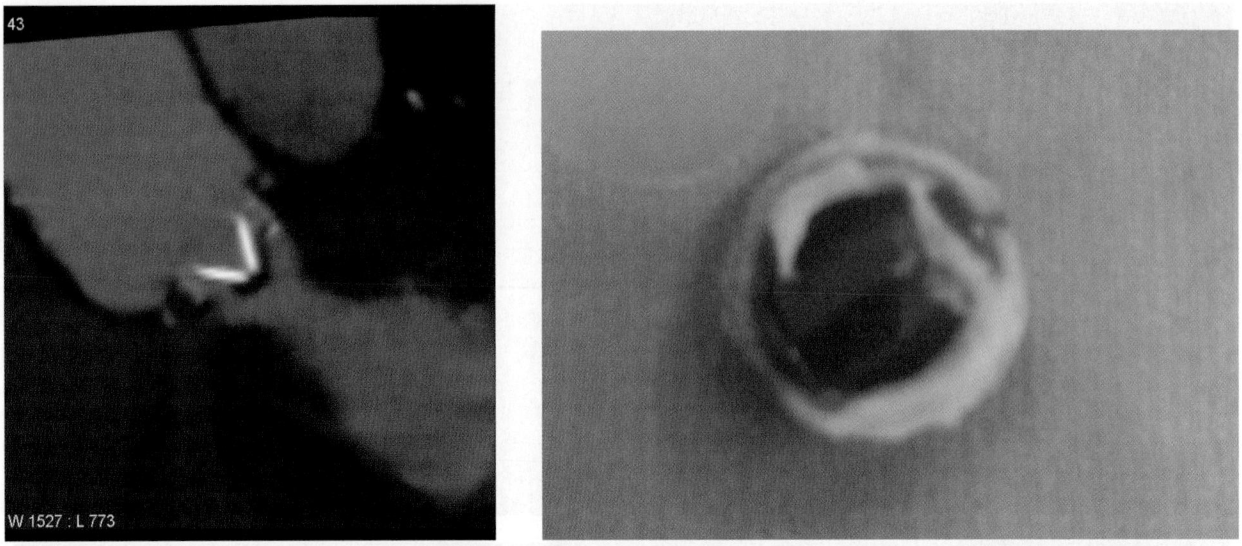

FIGURE 6-25 Patient with mechanical aortic valve. Low density material restricting leaflet opening on the undersurface of the valve is suspicious for pannus ingrowth causing restricted opening angle (*left*). Photograph of explant (*right*) demonstrates the pannus with high correlation with presurgical imaging.

certain specific cardiomyopathies, and confirm the presence of neoplasm. With the use of parallel imaging techniques to increase the speed of the MRI acquisition, very high temporal resolution (20 to 30 milliseconds) can be obtained to study bioprosthetic and native valve function. In addition, measurements of flow parameters through a vessel cross-section can be used to, for example, accurately quantify valvular regurgitant lesions.

One distinct advantage of MRI over CT is that MRI delivers no patient radiation. As detailed in Section A, the radiation exposure in ECG-gated CT is higher than that for CT of any

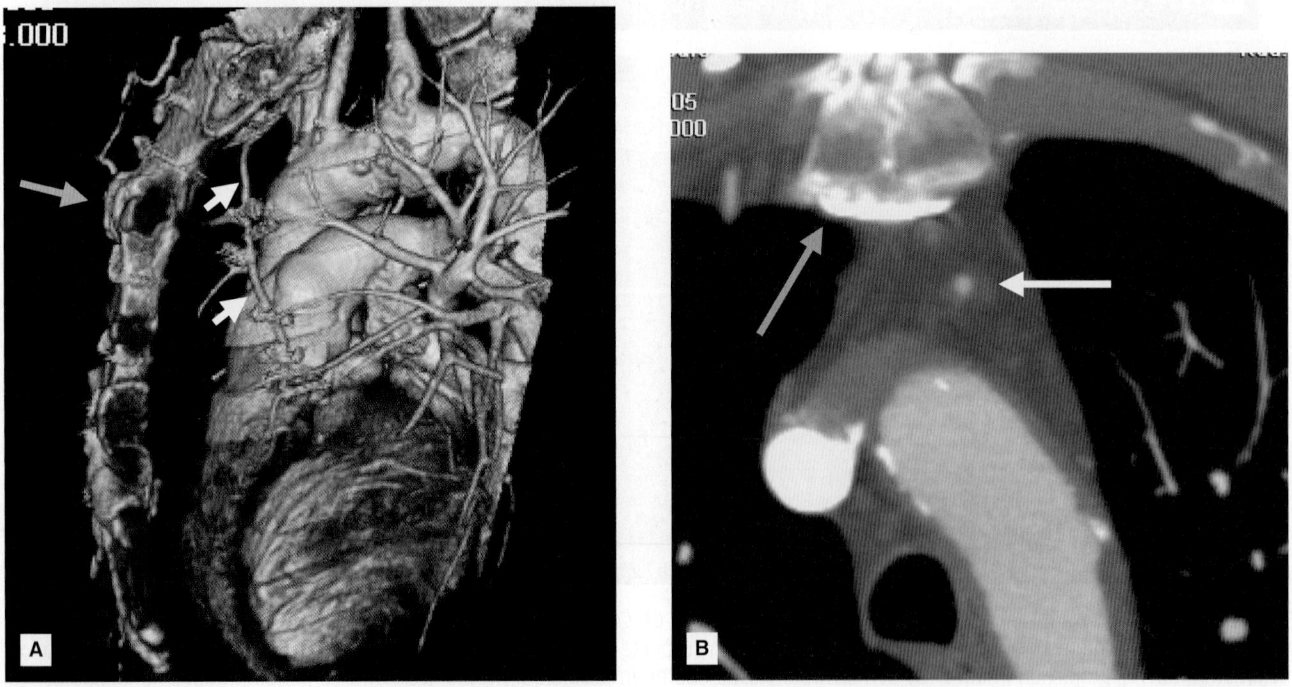

FIGURE 6-26 Planning for re-operative coronary artery bypass grafting. Laterally orientated 3D volume-rendered image (A) from a patient who had previously undergone left internal mammary artery (LIMA) coronary bypass grafting. The LIMA (*white arrows*) is grafted to the left anterior descending coronary artery. Note the relatively large distance between the grafted LIMA and the sternum (grey arrow). Axial image (B) clearly shows the LIMA graft (*white arrow*) to be clear of midline and well posterior to the sternum (*grey arrow*). Because the most common surgical approach in a redo CABG is repeat thoracotomy through the sternal incision, this study demonstrates that surgical revascularization through sternal re-entry has no significant risk of damage to the patent LIMA graft.

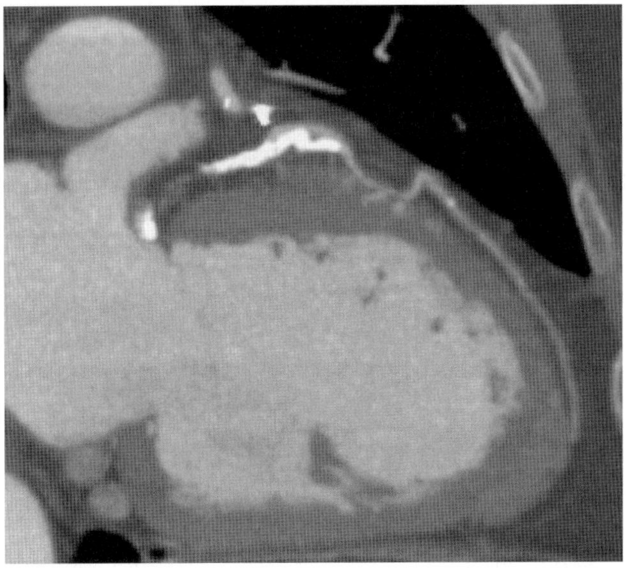

FIGURE 6-27 Preoperative planning for minimally invasive cardiac surgery (MIDCAB). Two- chamber plane maximum intensity projection image (6 mm thick) demonstrates the LAD. A segment of heavy calcification is identified in the proximal vessel (*black arrow*), this corresponds to the site of the stenotic lesion. No significant calcification is present in the remainder of the vessel. Immediately beyond the calcified segment an intramyocardial segment is present (*white arrows*).

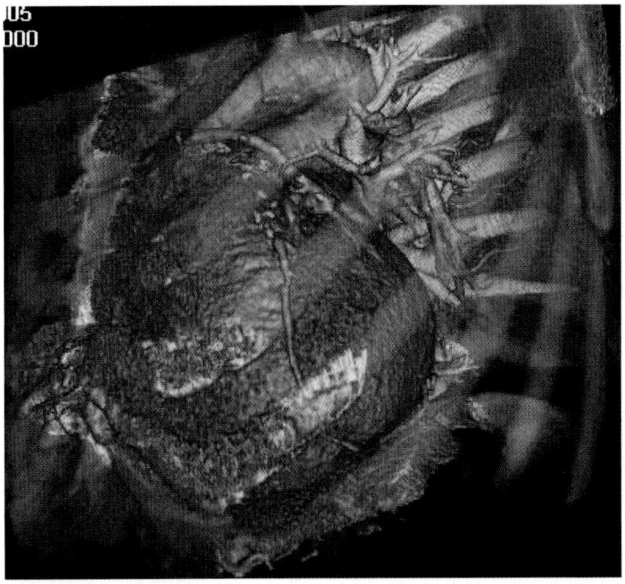

FIGURE 6-28 Preoperative planning for minimally invasive cardiac surgery (MIDCAB). Specialized display protocols for 3D volume-rendered images can be used to provide combined visualization of a semi-transparent thoracic cage and underlying cardiac and mediastinal structures. These models can be rotated and viewed from any angle or degree of magnification. With cardiac CT, 3D localization of target vessels, accessibility from proposed incision site, and position of LV apex with respect to chest wall can all be understood preoperatively.

other body part. In younger patients, who typically have less comorbid disease and may require multiple follow-up examinations over years or decades, MRI should be used when possible.

SUMMARY

Dramatic progress in CT technology has enabled advanced cardiac imaging for cardiac surgery patients. As the newest cardiac imaging modality to enter clinical practice, cardiac CT has rapidly demonstrated broad ranging applicability, and in particular CT has revolutionized the preoperative assessment of patients for reoperative surgery. Understanding the technical considerations will allow the surgeon to appreciate the inherent strengths and weaknesses of cardiac CT and to optimally communicate with the radiologist. This, in turn, will result in the best quality diagnostic examination in the vast majority of cardiac surgery patients.

REFERENCES

1. Steigner ML, et al: Narrowing the phase window width in prospectively ECG-gated single heart beat 320-detector row coronary CT angiography. *Int J Cardiovasc Imaging* 2009; 25(1):85-90.
2. Achenbach S et al: High-pitch spiral acquisition: a new scan mode for coronary CT angiography. *J Cardiovasc Comput Tomogr* 2009; 3(2):117-121.
3. Rybicki FJ et al: Initial evaluation of coronary images from 320-detector row computed tomography. *Int J Cardiovasc Imaging* 2008; 24(5):535-546.
4. George RT et al: Adenosine stress 64- and 256-row detector computed tomography angiography and perfusion imaging: a pilot study evaluating the transmural extent of perfusion abnormalities to predict atherosclerosis causing myocardial ischemia. *Circ Cardiovasc Imaging* 2009; 2(3):174-182.
5. Blankstein R et al: Cardiac myocardial perfusion imaging using dual source computed tomography. *Int J Cardiovasc Imaging* 2009; 25:209-216.
6. Hoffmann MH et al: Noninvasive coronary angiography with multislice computed tomography. *JAMA* 2005; 293(20):2471-2478.
7. Garcia MJ, Lessick J, Hoffmann MH: Accuracy of 16-row multidetector computed tomography for the assessment of coronary artery stenosis. *JAMA* 2006; 296(4):403-411.
8. Turkvatan A et al: Clinical value of 16-slice multidetector computed tomography in symptomatic patients with suspected coronary artery disease. *Acta Radiol* 2008; 49(4):400-408.
9. Hausleiter J et al: Non-invasive coronary computed tomographic angiography for patients with suspected coronary artery disease: the Coronary Angiography by Computed Tomography with the Use of a Submillimeter resolution (CACTUS) trial. *Eur Heart J* 2007; 28(24):3034-3041.
10. Marano R et al: Italian multicenter, prospective study to evaluate the negative predictive value of 16- and 64-slice MDCT imaging in patients scheduled for coronary angiography (NIMISCAD-Non Invasive Multicenter Italian Study for Coronary Artery Disease). *Eur Radiol* 2009; 19(5): 1114-1123.
11. Shabestari AA et al: Diagnostic performance of 64-channel multislice computed tomography in assessment of significant coronary artery disease in symptomatic subjects. *Am J Cardiol* 2007; 99(12):1656-1661.
12. Cademartiri F et al: 64-slice computed tomography coronary angiography: diagnostic accuracy in the real world. *Radiol Med* 2008; 113(2):163-180.
13. Budoff MJ et al: Diagnostic performance of 64-multidetector row coronary computed tomographic angiography for evaluation of coronary artery stenosis in individuals without known coronary artery disease: results from the prospective multicenter ACCURACY (Assessment by Coronary Computed Tomographic Angiography of Individuals Undergoing Invasive Coronary Angiography) trial. *J Am Coll Cardiol* 2008; 52(21):1724-1732.
14. Miller JM et al: Diagnostic performance of coronary angiography by 64-row CT. *NEJM* 2008; 359(22):2324-2336.
15. Meijboom WB et al: Diagnostic accuracy of 64-slice computed tomography coronary angiography: a prospective, multicenter, multivendor study. *J Am Coll Cardiol* 2008; 52(25):2135-2144.
16. Bettencourt N et al.: Multislice computed tomography in the exclusion of coronary artery disease in patients with presurgical valve disease. *Circ Cardiovasc Imaging* 2009; 2(4):306-313.

17. Gouya H et al: Coronary artery stenosis in high-risk patients: 64-section CT and coronary angiography–prospective study and analysis of discordance. *Radiology* 2009; 252(2):377-385.
18. Maffei E et al: Diagnostic accuracy of 64-slice computed tomography coronary angiography in a large population of patients without revascularisation: registry data and review of multicentre trials. *Radiol Med* 2010; 115(3):368-384.
19. Dewey M et al: Noninvasive coronary angiography by 320-row computed tomography with lower radiation exposure and maintained diagnostic accuracy: comparison of results with cardiac catheterization in a head-to-head pilot investigation. *Circulation* 2009; 120(10):867-875.
20. Schlosser, T., et al: Noninvasive visualization of coronary artery bypass grafts using 16-detector row computed tomography. *J Am Coll Cardiol* 2004; 44(6):1224-1229.
21. Martuscelli E et al: Evaluation of venous and arterial conduit patency by 16-slice spiral computed tomography. *Circulation* 2004; 110(20): 3234-3238.
22. Chiurlia E et al: Follow-up of coronary artery bypass graft patency by multislice computed tomography. *Am J Cardio.* 2005; 95(9):1094-1097.
23. Gasparovic H et al: Three dimensional computed tomographic imaging in planning the surgical approach for redo cardiac surgery after coronary revascularization. *Eur J Cardiothorac Surg* 2005; 28(2):244-249.
24. Mollet NR, Cademartiri F: Computed tomography assessment of coronary bypass grafts: ready to replace conventional angiography? *Int J Cardiovasc Imaging* 2005; 21(4):453-454.
25. Puskas JD et al.: Off-pump vs conventional coronary artery bypass grafting: early and 1-year graft patency, cost, and quality-of-life outcomes: a randomized trial. *JAMA* 2004; 291(15):1841-1849.
26. Khan NE et al: A randomized comparison of off-pump and on-pump multivessel coronary-artery bypass surgery. *NEJM* 2004; 350(1):21-28.
27. Collins P et al: Radial artery versus saphenous vein patency randomized trial: five-year angiographic follow-up. *Circulation* 2008; 117(22):2859-2864.
28. Buckley O et al.: Imaging features of intramural hematoma of the aorta. *Int J Cardiovasc Imaging* 2010; 26(1):65-76.
29. Pouleur AC et al: Aortic valve area assessment: multidetector CT compared with cine MR imaging and transthoracic and transesophageal echocardiography. *Radiology* 2007; 244(3):745-754.
30. Elami A, Laks H, Merin G: Technique for reoperative median sternotomy in the presence of a patent left internal mammary artery graft. *J Card Surg* 1994; 9(2):123-127.
31. Steimle CN, Bolling SF: Outcome of reoperative valve surgery via right thoracotomy. *Circulation* 1996; 94(9 Suppl):II126-II128.
32. Aviram G et al: Modification of surgical planning based on cardiac multidetector computed tomography in reoperative heart surgery. *Ann Thorac Surg* 2005; 79(2):589-595.
33. Caimmi PP et al: Cardiac angio-CT scan for planning MIDCAB. *Heart Surg Forum* 2004; 7(2):E113-E116.
34. Herzog C et al: Multi-detector row CT versus coronary angiography: preoperative evaluation before totally endoscopic coronary artery bypass grafting. *Radiology* 2003; 229(1):200-208.

CHAPTER 7

Assessment of Cardiac Operations to Improve Performance

Victor A. Ferraris
Fred H. Edwards
David M. Shahian

ASSESSING CARDIAC OPERATIONS—AN OVERVIEW

Historical—Hunter, Nightingale, Codman, and Cochrane

> It may seem a strange principle to enunciate as the very first requirement in a Hospital that it should do the sick no harm. It is quite necessary, nevertheless, to lay down such a principle, because the actual mortality in hospitals…is very much higher than…the mortality of the same class of diseases among patients treated out of hospital…
>
> Florence Nightingale, 1863

Surgeons often assume that performance improvement is a new concept arising from the complexities of modern medicine and surgery. Assessing risk to improve outcomes is not a new principle. The formal assessment of patient care had its beginnings in the mid-1800s.One of the earliest advocates of analyzing outcome data was Florence Nightingale, who was troubled by observations that hospitalized patients died at higher rates than those treated out of hospital.[1] She also noted a vast difference in mortality rates among different English hospitals, with London hospitals having as high as a 90% mortality rate, whereas smaller rural hospitals had a much lower mortality rate (12 to15%). Although England tracked hospital mortality rates since the 1600s, the analysis of these rates was in its infancy. Nightingale made the important observation that raw mortality rates were not an accurate reflection of outcome, because some patients were sicker when they presented to the hospital and, therefore, would be expected to have a higher mortality. Nightingale translated these observations into a highly successful improvement plan by suggesting simple measures such as better sanitation, less crowding, and location of hospitals distant from crowded urban areas. Her observations and action plans likely represent the beginning of risk adjustment to implement performance improvement.

Earlier contributions to performance improvement came from John Hunter in the 1700s. Hunter was relatively uneducated by the standards of the time but he had two qualities that allowed him to become the pre-eminent surgeon of the time and the father of modern surgery.[2] He had great technical skill and a belief that disease was caused by anatomic abnormalities. More importantly, he was unwilling to accept hypothetical abstract explanations of illness like "humors" or "spirits." He required that he verified causes of illness himself and that he could explain them on the basis of anatomy. For example, treatment of venereal disease was an important part of a physician's practice in the mid-1700s.Hunter was outspoken about the failure of the majority of medications claiming to cure gonorrhea. He said that "gonorrhea could be cured by the most ignorant, because gonorrhea mostly cures itself." He even performed an ingenious test by treating some of his patients with pills made of bread. He recorded the results and almost all of the patients had resolution of gonorrhea. This was one of the first trials documenting the *placebo effect.* John Hunter's friends and patients included Benjamin Franklin, Edward Jenner, Lord Byron, Casanova, and Adam Smith. His list of enemies was probably equally as distinguished. What is clear is that the assessment of outcomes of illness could not advance without understanding the basic anatomic disease substrate that John Hunter proposed.

Ernest Amory Codman, a Boston surgeon, was an early advocate of outcome analysis and scrutiny of results. Codman was a classmate of Harvey Cushing and became interested in the issues of outcome analysis after a friendly bet with Cushing about who had the lowest complication rate with the delivery of anesthesia. This effort not only represented the first intraoperative patient records, but also served as a foundation for Codman's later interest (almost passion) for documentation of outcomes. Codman actually paid a publisher to disseminate the results obtained in his privately owned Boston hospital.[3] Codman was perhaps the first advocate of searching for a cause of all complications. He felt that most bad outcomes were ultimately the result of physician errors or omissions and completely ignored any contribution from hospital-based and process-related factors. His efforts were not well received by his peers, and eventually his private hospital closed because of lack of referrals.

Further definition of outcome assessment occurred in the mid-1900s.As more and more therapeutic options became available to treat the diseases that predominated in the early twentieth century, a need arose to determine the best alternative of multiple therapies. Randomized trials were first used in the 1940sto test hypotheses. One of the earliest randomized trials was conducted to determine whether streptomycin was effective against tuberculosis.[4] Although the trial proved the effectiveness of streptomycin against tuberculosis, it stimulated a great deal of controversy. After World War II, several clinicians advocated the use of randomized, controlled trials (RCTs) to better identify the optimal treatment to provide the best outcome. Foremost among these was Archie Cochrane (Fig. 7-1).Cochrane lived during an exciting time. He lobbied for a national health service in Great Britain but this advocacy was tempered by 4 years as a prisoner of war in multiple WWII German POW camps. He saw soldiers die from tuberculosis and he was never sure what the best treatment was. He could choose between collapse therapy, bed rest, supplemental nutrition, or even high-dose vitamin therapy. A quote from his book sums up his frustration.[5]

> I had considerable freedom of clinical choice of therapy: my trouble was that I did not know which to use and when. I would gladly have sacrificed my freedom for a little knowledge.
>
> Cochrane, 1971

His experience with the uncertainty about the best treatment for TB and other chest diseases continued after the war, when he became a patron of randomized controlled trials (or RCTs as he liked to refer to them) to test important medical hypotheses. In 1987, the year before Cochrane died, he referred to a systematic review of RCTs of care during pregnancy and childbirth as "a real milestone in the history of randomized trials and in the evaluation of care. "He suggested that other specialties should copy the methods used. This led to the opening of the first Cochrane center (in Oxford, UK) in 1992 and the founding of the *Cochrane Collaboration* in 1993.Today the Cochrane Collaboration is a repository of RCTs, both disease-specific and specialty-specific (http://www.cochrane.org).The ascendancy of RCTs represents a major step forward in outcome assessment to improve surgical operations.

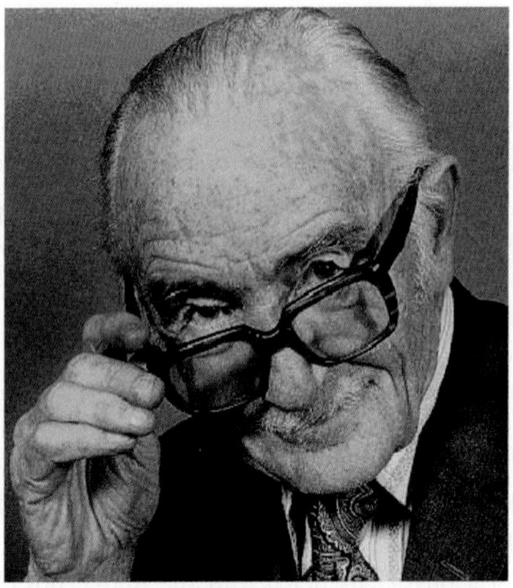

1934-36: Medical student, University College Hospital, London.
1936: International Brigade, Spanish Civil War.
1939-46: Captain, Royal Army Medical Corps.
1941: Taken prisoner of war in June 1941 in Crete; POW medical officer in Salonica (Greece) and Hildburghausen, Elsterhorst, and Wittenberg-am-Elbe (Germany).
1947-48: Studied the epidemiology of tuberculosis at Henry Phipps Institute, Philadelphia, USA.
1948-60: Member, Medical Research Council Pneumoconiosis Research Unit, Penarth, Wales.
1960-69: David Davies Professor of Tuberculosis and Chest Diseases, Welsh National School of Medicine, Cardiff, Wales.
1960-74: Director, Medical Research Council Epidemiology Research Unit, Cardiff, Wales.
1972: Publication by the Nuffield Provincial Hospitals Trust of his book *Effectiveness and Efficiency – Random Reflections on Health Services*.

FIGURE 7-1 Portrait of Archie Cochrane with brief biography. (*Used with permission from the Cochrane Collaboration.*)

Measures of Successful Operations

Performance Measures—Outcomes, Structure, and Process

In the early 1960s Donabedian suggested that quality in health care is defined as improvement in patient status after accounting for the patient's severity of illness, presence of comorbidity, and the medical services received.[6] He further proposed that quality could best be measured by considering three domains: structure, process, and outcome. Only recently has the notion of measuring healthcare quality using this Donabedian framework been accepted and implemented. In 2000, the Institute of Medicine (IOM) issued a report that was highly critical of the U.S. health-care system, suggesting that between 50,000 and 90,000 unnecessary deaths occur yearly because of errors in the health-care system.[7] The Institute of Medicine reports created a heightened awareness of more global aspects of quality. For most of the history of cardiac surgery, quality was equated with operative mortality (ie, *outcome measure*).After the IOM report appeared, a distinct change in the landscape of quality assessment occurred, and other aspects of Donabedian's framework were utilized. The narrow focus on operative mortality gave way to a broader analysis that also included additional outcome measures falling under the general category of *operative morbidity*. The emphasis on such outcomes measures expanded to include the processes of surgical care delivery. *Process measures* monitor provider compliance with desirable, often evidence-based, processes and systems of care. These measures typically include the choice of medication, timing of antibiotic administration, use of surgical techniques such as the internal thoracic artery graft, and other interventions considered appropriate for optimal care. Finally, *structural measures* such as the use of health information technology, physical plant design, participation in systematic clinical registries, and procedural volume are also considered important elements in this more global model of medical quality and performance. All these measures fall under the general rubric of *performance measures.* Birkmeyer and coworkers enumerated certain advantages and disadvantages associated with each specific type of performance measure.[8] For example, the fact that structural measures can be readily tabulated in an inexpensive manner using administrative data is a distinct advantage. On the other hand, many structural measures do not lend themselves to alteration. Particularly in smaller hospitals, there may simply be no way to increase procedural volume or to introduce costly design changes in an attempt to improve their performance on structural measures. Attempts to alter structure might even have adverse consequences (eg, unnecessary operations, costly and unnecessary new beds). Process measures are often linked to health-care quality and they are usually actionable on a practical level. Their major disadvantage lies in the fact that process measures may not be generally applicable to all patients undergoing a given procedure, and their linkage to outcomes may be weak. Outcomes measures are the most important endpoint for patients, but accurate assessment of outcomes is often limited by inadequate sample size and lack of appropriate risk adjustment.

The following definitions are adapted from those proposed by the Joint Commission on Accreditation of Healthcare Organizations (formerly JCAHO now officially called The Joint Commission):

- **Performance measure:** A quantitative entity that provides an indication of an organization's performance in relation to a specified process or outcome
- **Outcome measure:** A measure that indicates the results of process measures. Examples are operative mortality, the frequency of postoperative mediastinitis, renal failure, myocardial infarction, etc.
- **Process measure:** A measure that focuses on a process leading to a certain outcome. Intrinsic in this definition is a scientific basis for believing that the process will increase the probability of achieving a desired outcome. Examples include the rate of IMA (CABG) patients or the fraction of CABG patients placed on beta-blocking agents postoperatively.
- **Structural measure:** A measure that assesses whether an appropriate number, type, and distribution of medical personnel, equipment, and/or facilities are in place to deliver optimal health care. Examples include enrollment in a national database or procedural volume.

Although there are numerous proposed criteria for an ideal performance measure, the following are generally accepted attributes:

- The measure must be clearly linked to quality of care.
- The measure must be objective, evidence-based, and risk-adjusted if possible.
- The physician must have the ability to influence the measure in a clinical setting.
- The measure must be sufficiently well defined to permit practical measurement.

Several national organizations are specifically devoted to the rigorous development and evaluation of performance measures. Perhaps the most visible of these is the National Quality Forum (NQF), a public-private collaborative organization that uses a process of exhaustive, evidence-based scrutiny of candidate measures to determine their relevance to both patients and health-care providers. The NQF considers whether candidate measures can be measured accurately and whether actionable interventions can improve performance for candidate measures. Having gone through this "trial by fire," NQF-endorsed measures have a high level of national credibility not otherwise possible.

Patient Satisfaction

Other outcomes following cardiac procedures, such as patient satisfaction and health-related quality of life, are less well studied but extremely important in the assessment of performance. Meeting or exceeding patients' expectations is a major goal of the health-care system. The growing importance of patient-reported outcomes also reflects the increasing prevalence of chronic disease in our aging population. The goal of therapeutic interventions is often to relieve symptoms and improve quality of life, rather than cure a disease and prolong survival. This is especially important in selecting elderly patients for cardiac operations. One early report from the United Kingdom suggested that as many as one third of patients over the age of 70 had no improvement in their disability and overall sense of well-being after cardiac surgery.[9] More recent studies suggest that CABG results in excellent health-related quality of life 10 to 15 years after surgery in most patients,[10] and that this benefit extends to those patients older than 80 years of age.[11] Future research into patient-perceived performance assessment is inevitable given the aging of populations in the developed countries.

RISK STRATIFICATION AND COMORBIDITY—LEVELING THE PLAYING FIELD

Risk Stratification and Risk Models

Essential for the assessment of the success of cardiac operations is the ability to arrange patients according to their severity of illness. Viewed simplistically, patients who are sicker before operation have a greater chance of a poor outcome. Various risk-adjustment systems assess and adjust for the incremental risk associated with specific preoperative factors variously known as risk factors, risk predictors, comorbidities, or covariates. These are discussed in detail in Chapter 8. Table 7-1 is a partial listing of some of the severity measures commonly used in risk assessment of patients undergoing cardiac procedures. The risk stratification systems listed in Table 7-1 are in constant evolution, and the descriptions in the table may not reflect current or future versions of these systems. For example, in 2009 the Society of Thoracic Surgeons published the most extensive, comprehensive set of cardiac surgery risk models yet available. Twenty-seven risk models encompassed nine endpoints for each of three major groups of cardiac procedures (isolated CABG, isolated valve, and valve + CABG).[12-14]

TABLE 7-1 Examples of Risk Stratification Systems Used for Patients Undergoing Cardiac Surgical Procedures

Severity System	Data Source	Classification Approach	Outcomes Measured
APACHE III	Values of 17 physiologic parameters and other clinical information	Integer scores from 0 to 299 measured within 24 hours of ICU admission	In-hospital death
Pennsylvania	Clinical findings collected at time of admission	Probability of in-hospital death ranging from 0 to 1 based on logistic regression model and MediQual's Atlas admission severity score	In-hospital death and cost of procedure
New York	Condition-specific clinical variables from discharge record	Probability of in-hospital death ranging from 0 to 1 based on logistic regression model	In-hospital death
Society for Thoracic Surgeons	Condition-specific clinical variables from discharge record	Originally used Bayesian algorithm to assign patient to risk interval (percent mortality interval).More recently used logistic and hierarchical regression methods.	In-hospital death and morbidity
EuroSCORE	Condition specific clinical variables from discharge record	Additive logistic regression model with scores based on presence or absence of important risk factors	30-day and in-hospital mortality
Veterans Administration	Condition-specific clinical variables measured 30 days after operation	Logistic regression model used to assign patient to risk interval (percent mortality interval)	In-hospital death and morbidity
Parsonnet	Condition specific clinical variables from discharge record	Additive multiple regression model with scores between 0 and 158 based on 14 weighted risk factors	Death within 30 days of operation
Canadian	Condition specific clinical variables entered at time of referral for cardiac surgery	Range of scores from 0 to 16 based on logistic regression odds ratio for six key risk factors	In-hospital mortality, ICU stay and postoperative length of stay
Northern New England	Condition specific clinical variables and comorbidity index entered from discharge record	Scoring system based on logistic regression coefficients used to calculate probability of operative mortality from 7 clinical variables and 1 comorbidity index	In-hospital mortality
Cleveland Clinic	Condition specific clinical variables from discharge record	Range of scores from 0 to 33 based on univariate odds ratio for each of 13 risk factors	In-hospital death or death within 30 days of operation

Canadian = Ontario Ministry of Health Provincial Adult Cardiac Care Network; Cleveland Clinic = Cleveland Clinic Foundation Risk Stratification System; New York = New York State Department of Health Cardiac Surgery Reporting System; Northern New England = Northern New England Cardiovascular Disease Study Group; Parsonnet = Parsonnet risk stratification model; Pennsylvania = Pennsylvania Cost Containment Committee for Cardiac Surgery; Society for Thoracic Surgeons = Society of Thoracic Surgeons Risk Stratification System; Veteran's Administration = Veteran's Administration Cardiac Surgery Risk Assessment Program.

Most risk-adjustment algorithms share several common features. First, the risk factors or covariates in the model are associated with a specific outcome. Second, if the goal is to measure provider performance, the risk factors include only patient characteristics (not hospital, physician, or regional characteristics) present prior to surgery, not factors that might be influenced by the health-care provider (eg, what type of cardioplegia was used).[15] Third, a sufficient number of patients must have the risk factor, and a sufficient number must experience the adverse outcome, in order to construct the risk models. Finally, it is necessary to define the period of observation for the outcomes of interest (eg, in-hospital or 30-day mortality).

The severity indices listed in Table 7-1 define severity predominantly based on clinical measures (eg, risk of death or other adverse clinical outcome).At least, two of the severity measures shown in Table 7-1 (MedisGroups used in the Pennsylvania Cardiac Surgery Reporting System and the Canadian Provincial Adult Cardiac Care Network of Ontario) assess severity based on resource use (eg, hospital length-of-stay, cost) as well as on clinical measures.[16,17] Of the nine severity measures listed in Table 7-1, only one, the APACHE III system, computes a risk score independent of patient diagnosis.[18] All of the others in the table are diagnosis-specific systems that use only patients with particular diagnoses in computing severity scores.

Once developed from a reference population, each of the risk stratification measures shown in Table 7-1 are validated against a different set of patients to assure that they are adequate predictors of the population risk of operative mortality or other outcomes. Although useful, these risk models are imperfect.[19] There are too many individual patient and procedural differences, many of them unknown or unmeasured, to allow completely accurate preoperative risk assessment. Dupuis and coworkers suggest that risk stratification and risk models are good predictors of population risk but not of individual patient risk.[19] The most important reason that risk-adjustment methods fail to completely predict individual outcomes is that the data set used to derive the risk score comes from retrospective, observational data that contain inherent selection bias (ie, patients were given a certain treatment that resulted in a particular outcome because a clinician had a selection bias about what treatment that particular patient should receive.)In *observational datasets*, patients are not allocated to a given treatment in a randomized manner. In addition, clinician bias is not always founded in evidence-based data. Methods are available that attempt to overcome some of these limitations of observational data. These methods include use of instrumental variables and propensity scores.[20,21] Observational datasets are much more readily available and represent "real-world" treatment and outcomes compared with RCTs.An excellent review of the subtleties of evaluating the performance of risk-adjustment methods is given in the book by Iezzoni, and this reference is recommended to the interested reader.[22]

Ideally, differences in risk-adjusted outcomes result from differences in quality of care, but this is not necessarily the case. One study simulated the mortality experience for a hypothetical set of hospitals assuming perfect risk adjustment and with prior perfect knowledge of poor quality providers.[23] These authors used various simulation models, including Monte Carlo simulation, and found that under all reasonable assumptions, sensitivity for determining poor quality was less than 20% and the predictive error for determining high outliers was greater than 50%.Much of the observed mortality rate differences between high outliers and nonoutliers were attributable to random variation. Park and coauthors suggest that providers identified as high outliers using conventional risk adjustment methods do not provide lower quality care than do nonoutliers.[24]

Comorbidities as Risk Factors

Comorbidities are coexisting diagnoses that are indirectly related to the principal surgical diagnosis but that may alter the outcome of operations. These are vitally important because physicians or hospitals that care for patients with a higher prevalence of serious comorbid conditions are at significant disadvantage in unadjusted comparisons. Comorbid illness in patients with cardiac disease is common. In one series of patients with myocardial infarction, 26% also had diabetes, 30% had arthritis, 6%had chronic lung problems and 12% had gastrointestinal disorders.[25]

Several generic indices of comorbidity are available for general medical and surgical diagnoses, although none are as specific or detailed as the risk models used in cardiac surgery. Table 7-2 compares 13 commonly used comorbidity measures. The Charlson Index, the CIRS, the ICED, and the Kaplan Index are valid and reliable measures of comorbidity as measured in certain specific patient populations, but not in patients undergoing cardiac operations.[26] The other nine comorbidity measures in Table 7-2 do not have sufficient data to assess their validity and reliability and are probably less useful than the four validated measures. There are many limitations of comorbidity indices, and they are not applied widely in studies of efficacy or medical effectiveness for cardiac operations.

Perhaps the most serious drawback of comorbidity scoring systems is the imprecision of the data used to form the indices. Most of the data used to construct the indices comes from two sources:(1) *administrative databases* in the form of computerized discharge abstract data and (2) out-of-hospital follow-up reports including *questionnaires* and medical chart reviews. Administrative data in the form of discharge abstracts include clinical diagnoses that are often assigned by nonphysicians not involved in the care of the patient. Inaccuracies in discharge coding, and in administrative databases in general, are common.[27,28] Less serious diagnoses are often not coded for in the most seriously ill patients. Additionally, the accuracy of out-of-hospital follow-up studies is hard to validate and these studies may contain significant inaccuracies. Despite their shortcomings, analyses that compare physician or hospital outcomes and that do not provide some adjustment, albeit imperfect, for patient comorbidity will likely discriminate against providers or hospitals that treat disproportionate numbers of elderly patients with multiple comorbid conditions.

The Performance of Risk Models

Many risk models for cardiac operations are used to assess surgical performance (Table 7-3).Before a risk model and its component risk factors are used to evaluate provider performance,

TABLE 7-2 Characteristics and Study Populations of Commonly Used Comorbidity Indices

Comorbidity Index	Variables in the Index	Weights Used to Compute Index	Final Index Score	Population Used to Derive Index
Charlson Index	19 comorbid conditions	Relative risk for each comorbid condition derived from logistic regression of mortality	Sum of weights	Cancer patients, heart disease, pneumonia, elective noncardiac operations, amputees
CIRS	13 body systems	Score from 0 to 4 for each body system	Sum of weights	Elderly patients, many institutionalized for long-term care
ICED	14 disease categories and 10 functional categories	Score of 1 to 5 for disease categories and1 to3 for functional categories	Scoring algorithm that sums up disease and functional scores to arrive at values from 1 to 4	Total hip replacements and nursing home patients
Kaplan Index	Two categories—vascular or nonvascular disease	Graded 0 thru 3 for each category.	Most severe condition. Two grade 2 are ranked as grade 3	Diabetes and breast cancer
BOD Index	59 diseases	0 thru 4 for each disease	Sum of weights	Long-stay nursing home patients
Cornoni-Huntley Index	3 categories	1—No comorbidity 2—Impaired hearing or vision. 3—Heart disease, stroke, or diabetes 4—Both 2 and 3	Graded 1 through 4	Hypertensive population and age greater than 75 years
Disease count	Number of diseases present based on ICD-9 codes	Sum number of diseases	Maximum score based on number of diseases	Breast cancer, MI, HIV, asthma, appendicitis, low back pain, pneumonia, diabetes, abdominal hernia
DUSOI Index	Every health problem rated on four domains: 1—Symptoms 2—Complications 3—Prognosis 4—Prognosis with treatment	0 to 5 for each health problem	Scoring algorithm leading to scores between 0 and 100	Primary care patients.

Hallstrom Index	10 chronic diseases and 6 cardiac symptoms	Number of chronic diseases and number of cardiac symptoms	Score = 1.67 × number of chronic diseases × number of cardiac symptoms	Out of hospital ventricular fibrillation
Hurwitz Index	Assessment of three categories:	No comorbidity Nondisabling comorbidity Disabling comorbidity	Status of comorbidity	Low back pain
Incalzi Index	52 diseases	Relative risk based on logistic regression of mortality	Sum of relative risks	Geriatric and general medicine population.
Liu Index	38 comorbidities	0 to 5 severity for each comorbidity	Sum of scores for each comorbidity	Stroke population
Shwartz Index	21 comorbidities	Relative risks from model that predicts medical costs	Sum of relative risks for each comorbidity.	Stroke, lung disease, heart disease, prostate cancer, hip fracture, and low back pain

Adapted from de Groot and coworkers[26]

TABLE 7-3 Recently Published Risk Variables Used in Models to Predict Coronary Bypass Surgical Mortality (adapted from the Annals of Thoracic Surgery13,147)

Risk Model	STS	NYS	Canada	USA	Emory	VA	Australia	Canada	Cleveland	Israel	Duke	NNE	Stroke	Parsonnet	
Number of patients	774,881	174,210	57,187	50,357	17,128	13,368	12,712	12,003	7491	4918	4835	3654	3055	2152	
No. ofrisk factors	29	29	16	13	7	6	9	5	9	7	9	9	10	8	Sum
Age	X	X	X		X	X	X	X	X	X	X	X	X	X	13
Gender	X	X	X	X	X	X		X	X		X		X		10
Surgical urgency	X	X		X		X	X		X		X	X	X		9
Ejection fraction	X	X	X			X		X	X		X	X	X		9
Renal dysfunction/	X	X	X	X	X						X	X		X	8
Creatinine	X														
Previous CABG	X	X		X	X				X			X	X		7
NYHA class		X	X	X	X		X				X				6
Left main disease	X	X	X						X		X	X	X		7
Diseased coronary vessels	X	X	X			X			X		X		X		7
Peripheral vascular disease	X	X		X			X		X	X					6
Diabetes mellitus	X	X	X			X					X			X	6
Cerebrovascular disease	X	X		X	X		X								5
Intraop/postop variables				X				X		X				X	4
Myocardial infarction	X	X	X	X	X										5
Body size	X	X	X										X		4
Preoperative IABP	X	X	X				X								4
Cardiogenic shock/unstable	X	X	X									X			4
COPD	X	X	X												3
PTCA	X	X		X											3
Angina	X		X					X							3

Intravenous nitrates		X			X						2
Arrhythmias		X					X				2
History of heart operation	X		X		X						3
Hemodynamic instability	X	X								X	3
Charlson comorbidity score								X	X		2
Dialysis dependence	X	X	X								3
Valvular heart disease	X										11
Pulmonary hypertension		X								X	2
Diuretics		X			X						2
Systemic hypertension	X					X					2
Serum albumin							X				1
Race	X	X									2
Previous CHF	X							X			2
Myocardial infarction timing	X	X									2
Cardiac index							X				1
LV end-diastolic pressure									X		1
CVA timing	X	X									2
Liver disease				X							1
Neoplasia/Metastatic disease				X							1
Ventricular aneurysm				X							1
Steroids	X	X									2
Digitalis		X									1
Thrombolytic therapy										X	1
Arterial bicarbonate							X				1
Calcified ascending aorta										X	1

these models are tested for accuracy. Many patient variables are candidate risk factors for operative mortality following coronary revascularization. Examples include serum BUN, cachexia, oxygen delivery, HIV, case volume, low hematocrit on bypass, the diameter of the coronary artery, and resident involvement in the operation. On the surface, these variables seem like valid risk factors, but many are not. All putative risk factors should be subjected to rigorous scrutiny like those variables listed in Table 7-3. The regression diagnostics (eg, receiver operating characteristics (ROC) curves and cross-validation studies) performed on the models included in Tables 7-1 and 7-3 suggest that the models are good, but not perfect, at predicting outcomes. In statistical terms this means that all of the variability in operative mortality is not explained by the set of risk factors included in the regression models. Hence, it is possible that inclusion of new putative risk factors in the regression equations may improve the validity and precision of the models. New regression models, and new risk factors, must be scrutinized and tested using cross-validation methods and other regression diagnostics before acceptance.

It is uncertain whether inclusion of many more risk factors will significantly improve the quality and predictive ability of regression models, and there is an ongoing tension between parsimonious models and those that contain many variables. For example, the Society for Thoracic Surgeons (STS) risk stratification model, described in Tables 7-1 and 7-3, includes many predictor variables, whereas the Toronto risk adjustment scheme includes only five predictor variables (see Table 7-3).Yet the regression diagnostics for these two models are similar, suggesting that both models have equal precision and predictive capabilities. Studies show that much of the predictive ability of risk models is contained in a relatively few number of risk factors.[29,30] Other studies suggest that the limiting factor in the accuracy of current risk models may be failure to understand and account for all the important factors related to risk.[31] Additionally, risk models are useful for predicting the average outcome for a population of patients with specific risk factors, but not necessarily accurate for predicting the outcome for a specific patient. Further work needs to be done, both to explain the differences in risk factors seen among the various risk stratification models and to determine which models are best suited for studies of quality improvement and performance assessment.

Occasionally negative studies appear that suggest that a particular patient variable is **not** a risk factor for a particular patient outcome. Care must be exercised in interpreting negative results.[32] Many putative risk factors labeled as "no different from control" in studies using inadequate samples have not received a fair test. For example, Burns and associates studied preoperative template bleeding times in 43 patients undergoing elective CABG.[33] They found no increased postoperative blood loss in patients with prolonged skin bleeding times. Their study reports five patients whose bleeding times were prolonged greater than 8 minutes. In this small sample size there was a trend toward more units of blood transfused, but differences between high and low bleeding time groups were reported as "not significant" by the authors at the $\alpha = 5\%$ level (ie, $p = 0.05$). Using the author's data, it is possible to compute a β error for this negative observation of less than 0.5.This means that there is as much as a 50% chance that the negative finding is really a false-negative result. This high false-negative rate occurs because of the small sample size and the wide variation in the bleeding time values. We have found elevated bleeding time (>10 minutes) to be a significant multivariate risk factor for excessive blood transfusion after CABG in two different studies.[34,35] Although there is controversy about the value of bleeding time as a screening test,[36] it is possible that disregarding the bleeding time after an inconclusive negative trial, such as that of Burns and coworkers, may ignore a potentially important risk factor. Care must be taken in the interpretation of a negative finding, especially in a small study group. Freiman and coauthors sounded a similar cautionary note after reviewing the medical literature over a ten-year period.[37] These authors found that 50 of 71 "negative" randomized controlled trials could have missed a 50% therapeutic improvement from intervention because the sample size studied was too small.[37] Their conclusions were that many therapies discarded as ineffective after inconclusive negative trials may still have a clinically important effect. Today journal editors and authors are much more aware of the relationships among sample size, statistical power, and negative test results compared with the earlier report of Freiman and coauthors. Nonetheless, negative findings in a literature report require scrutiny and an understanding of type II statistical errors.[38] Finally, some risk factors may not appear to improve the discrimination of a particular model, but they may still be very important predictors of outcome if present in a particular patient.[39]

GOALS OF CARDIAC SURGICAL PERFORMANCE ASSESSMENT

Assessing Quality of Care—Underuse, Misuse, and Overuse

Assessing the quality of cardiac care is a worthy goal of measuring performance. However, this goal is elusive and a little bit like trying to define "pornography"—everyone knows it when they see it, but it is very hard to define. A major problem arises in attaining this goal because uniform definitions of quality of care are not available. Performance measures are a means of assessing cardiac surgical performance. Providers who do not meet the performance standards outlined by these measures are guilty of *misuse* of health care resources. But there are other indices of health-care quality not covered by these measures, including appropriateness of care and disparities in care (eg, women and minorities receiving worse care).Inappropriate use of procedures is often referred to as *overuse*, and failure to provide indicated care as *underuse*. Both are found in treatment of cardiovascular diseases. For example, there is substantial geographic variation in the rates at which patients with cardiovascular diseases undergo diagnostic procedures, with little, if any, evidence that these variations are related to survival or improved outcome. In one study, coronary angiography was performed in 45% of patients after acute myocardial infarction for patients in Texas compared with 30 for patients in New York State ($p < 0.001$ for comparison between states).[40] Another study showed large variations in care delivered to patients having cardiac operations.[41] Among six institutions that treated very similar patients (Veteran's Administration Medical Centers), there were large differences in the percentage of elective, urgent, and emergent cases at each institution, ranging from 58to 96% elective, 3 to 31% urgent, and 1 to 8% emergent.[41] There was also a tenfold difference in the preoperative use of intra-aortic balloon counterpulsation for control of unstable angina, varying from 0.8 to 10.6%.[41] Similar variations in physician-specific practices exist for mitral valve procedures, carotid end arterectomy, and blood transfusion during cardiac procedures.[42-44] This variation in clinical practice may reflect uncertainty about the efficacy of available interventions, or differences in practitioners' clinical judgment.

Although wide differences in use of cardiac interventions initially fueled charges of overuse in certain areas,[45] recent evaluations suggest that underuse of indicated cardiac interventions (either PTCA or CABG) may be a cause of this variation.[46,47] Whether caused by underuse or overuse of cardiovascular services, regional variations in resource utilization suggest that a rigorous definition of the "correct" treatment of acute myocardial infarction, as in other cardiovascular disease states, is elusive and the definition of quality of care for such patients is imperfect. Regional variations in cardiovascular care delivery are only a few of the examples of unclear best practices. Age, gender, race, community size, and hospital characteristics influence utilization of diagnostic and operative interventions without much evidence that these factors should direct the appropriate treatment for various cardiac disorders.[48,49] Although performance measures that define performance assessment may be a way to judge quality of care among providers, much more work needs to be done to define best practices and to limit practice variations before performance measures reflect quality of care.

Improving Quality of Care (Expert Guidelines)

Recognizing the difficulties in defining "best practices" for a given illness, professional organizations opted to promote practice guidelines or "suggested therapy" for given diseases.[50,51] These practice guidelines represent a compilation of available published evidence, including randomized trials and risk-adjusted observational studies, as well as consensus among panels of experts proficient at treating a given disease. For example, the practice guideline for coronary artery bypass grafting is available for both practitioners and the lay public on the Internet (http://www.acc.org/qualityandscience/clinical/guidelines/CABG/index.pdf).Guidelines are a list of recommendations that have varying support in the literature. The strength of a guideline recommendation is often graded by class and by level of evidence used to support the class of recommendation. A typical rating scheme used by the Society of Thoracic Surgeons Evidence Based Workforce and by the Joint American College of Cardiology/American Heart Association Task Force on Practice Guidelines has three classes of recommendations as follows:

- Class I—Conditions for which there is evidence and/or general agreement that a given procedure or treatment is beneficial, useful, and effective.
- Class II—Conditions for which there is conflicting evidence and/or a divergence of opinion about the usefulness/efficacy of a procedure or treatment.
    - Class IIa—Weight of evidence/opinion is in favor of usefulness/efficacy.
    - Class IIb—Usefulness/efficacy is less well established by evidence/opinion.
- Class III—Conditions for which there is evidence and/or general agreement that a procedure/treatment is not useful/effective and in some cases may be harmful.

Evidence supporting the various classes of recommendations ranges from high quality randomized controlled trials to consensus opinion of experts. Three categories describe the level of evidence used to arrive at the class of recommendation:

Level A—Data derived from multiple randomized clinical trials or meta-analyses
Level B—Data derived from a single randomized trial, or nonrandomized studies
Level C—Consensus opinion of experts, case studies, or standard-of-care

Guidelines provide surgeons with accepted evidence-based standards of care that most would agree on, with an ultimate goal of limiting deviations from accepted standards. Guideline development represents a work in progress, and the best approach has yet to be determined. Many recommendations that appear in professional guidelines are developed from lower levels of evidence including expert consensus.[52] Many published guidelines do not adhere to currently accepted standards for developing guidelines,[53] and barriers to acceptance of practice guidelines exist.[54] For example, guidelines for the management of bleeding during cardiac procedures are available but are relatively unsuccessful in limiting nonautologous blood transfusion.[55] There is still marked variability in transfusion practices and blood conservation interventions.[56] These limitations of the effectiveness of guidelines in altering physician practices are a drawback of the guideline efforts, and the most important aspect of practice guideline development is their implementation in real-world practice.

Efficacy Studies (RCTs) versus Effectiveness (Observational) Studies

There are many efficacy studies relating to cardiothoracic surgery. These studies attempt to isolate one procedure or device as beneficial for patient outcome. The study population in efficacy studies is specifically chosen to contain as uniform a group as possible. Typical examples of efficacy studies include randomized, prospective, clinical trials (RCTs) comparing use of a procedure or device in a well-defined population compared with an equally well-defined control population. Efficacy studies are different than effectiveness studies.[5] The latter deal with whole populations and attempt to determine the best treatment option that provides optimal outcome in a population that would typically be treated by a practicing surgeon. An example of an *effectiveness study* is a retrospective study of outcome in a large population treated with a particular intervention (eg, heart valve or blood conservation measure).Risk stratification is capable of isolating associations between outcome and risk factors. Methodological enhancements in risk adjustment, such as propensity matching,[57] are capable of reducing biases inherent in population-based, retrospective studies but can never eliminate all confounding biases in observational studies.

One reasonable strategy for using risk stratification to improve patient care is to isolate high-risk subsets from population-based, retrospective studies (ie, effectiveness studies) and then to test interventions to improve outcome in high-risk subsets using RCTs. This is a strategy that should ultimately lead to the desired goal of improved patient care. For example, a population-based study on postoperative blood transfusion revealed that the following factors were significantly associated with excessive blood transfusion (defined as more than 4 units of blood products after CABG):(1) template bleeding time, (2) red blood cell volume, (3) cardiopulmonary bypass time, and (4) advanced age.[35] Based on these retrospective effectiveness studies, investigators hypothesized that interventions aimed at reducing blood transfusion after CABG would most likely benefit patients with prolonged bleeding time and low red blood cell volume. A prospective clinical trial tested this hypothesis using two blood conservation techniques, platelet-rich plasma saving and normovolemic hemodilution of whole blood, in patients undergoing CABG. Results showed that blood conservation interventions reduced bleeding and blood transfusion only in the high-risk subset of patients.[34] These studies imply that more costly interventions such as use of platelet-rich plasma savers are more efficacious in high-risk patients, with the high-risk subset defined by risk stratification methodologies.

Other Goals of Outcome Analysis: Cost Containment and Altering Physician Practices

Financial factors are a major force behind health care reform. America's health care costs amount to 15 to 20% of the gross national product and this figure is rising at an unsustainable rate of 6% annually. Institutions that pay for health care are demanding change, and these demands are fueled by studies that suggest that 20 to 30% of care is inappropriate with services both underused and overused compared with evidence-based practice standards.[58] This resulted in a shift in emphasis, with health-care costs being emphasized on equal footing with clinical outcomes of care. Sometimes the two are combined into one number, *value*, which is quality divided by cost.

As noted previously, variations in physician practice distort the allocation of health-care funds in an inappropriate way. Research suggests that there is a 17-year lag time between medical discovery and when most patients benefit from the discovery.[59] The failure on the part of some surgeons to implement innovation has a huge cost in terms of morbidity and mortality.[60] Solutions to this problem involve altering physician practice patterns to be consistent with best available evidence, something that has been extremely difficult to do.[61] How can physician practice patterns be changed in order to improve outcome? Evidence suggests that the typical process of outcome assessment, the case-by-case review (traditionally done in the morbidity and mortality [M and M] conference format), may not be cost-effective, may not change surgeon practice patterns, and may not improve quality.[62] Health care experts suggest that the M and M conference should be replaced by external accountability using profiles of practice patterns at institutional, regional, or national levels. One alternative model for quality improvement involves oversight that emphasizes the appropriate balance between internal mechanisms for quality assessment and improvement and external accountability.[62] Risk adjustment is an essential element particularly for the latter approach so that surgeons who operate on high-risk patients are not penalized for their potentially higher rate of adverse outcomes. Accurate risk assessment is essential for fairness and to assure acceptance by all stakeholders.

Rewarding High Performers ("Pay for Performance")

Performance measures are regarded as the cornerstone of quality assessment. Identifying performance measures and undertaking steps to comply with these measures involves a management philosophy that seeks to integrate organizational functions (eg, technical aspects of care delivery and customer service)in order to meet customer needs. Beginning a quality initiative of this sort typically employs the following steps:

- A patient population is specified.
- Process measures are developed to serve as quality metrics for this population.
- The process measures are collected.
- Compliance with performance measures is tracked for participating centers.
- Aggregate results are used to establish norms and benchmarks.
- Participating centers receive data feedback compared with benchmarks.
- Participating centers are evaluated for their adherence to performance measures.

It becomes immediately apparent that the validity of this approach is primarily dependent on the validity of the performance measures. This recognition led to the emergence of several national organizations specifically devoted to the rigorous development of performance measures, most notably the National Quality Forum (NQF).

The NQF, with the assistance of the Society of Thoracic Surgeons, played a central role in developing national consensus standards for adult cardiac surgery. This process yielded 20 NQF-endorsed measures (Table 7-4).These measures constitute a unique set of nationally accepted tools that can be used to determine the quality of care in cardiac surgical programs. Prior to their development, there was no general agreement on the specific parameters linked to "quality" in cardiac surgery. NQF measures provide the "toolbox" for quality measurement in cardiac surgery and are used by payors to determine quality and guide resources to high performers.

The STS Database provides benchmark values for all of the performance measures in Table 7-4. In the most direct application of NQF measures, an institution simply compares its values against the benchmark values. This process allows providers to pinpoint opportunities for improvement so that resources can

TABLE 7-4 NQF Endorsed National Standards for Cardiac Surgery

1. Participation in a systematic database for cardiac surgery
2. Surgical volume for CABG, valve surgery, and CABG + valve surgery
3. Timing of prophylactic antibiotic administration
4. Selection of prophylactic antibiotic
5. Preoperative beta blockade
6. Use of internal mammary artery
7. Duration of prophylactic antibiotic
8. Prolonged intubation (<24 hours postoperatively)
9. Deep sternal wound infection rate
10. Stroke/cerebrovascular accident
11. Postoperative renal insufficiency
12. Surgical re-exploration
13. Anti-platelet medications at discharge
14. Beta blockade at discharge
15. Anti-lipid treatment at discharge
16. Risk-adjusted operative mortality for CABG
17. Risk-adjusted operative mortality for aortic valve replacement (AVR)
18. Risk-adjusted operative mortality for mitral valve replacement (MVR)
19. Risk-adjusted operative mortality for MVR + CABG
20. Risk-adjusted operative mortality for AVR + CABG

be specifically directed to areas of greatest need with the expectation that payors will provide increased resources to those institutions that meet the standards.

More sophisticated approaches to performance assessment involve combining process, structural, and outcome measures into a composite measure,[63] one of the most important recent trends in performance measurement.Composite models are strongly endorsed by the Institute of Medicine. They provide a much more comprehensive assessment of provider quality than any single measure, and they demonstrate relative quality comparisons between an institution and a national benchmark. Composite models are preferred, because it is possible to excel in one specific area of performance but not in another. For example, it is possible to have low operative mortality but have infrequent use of internal mammary artery bypass in patients undergoing CABG, and the latter adversely impacts a patient's long-term outcome. A composite measure accounts for both of these domains of performance.

Many believe that additional incentives for quality improvement can be obtained by linking quality scores to reimbursement.[64] This concept, commonly called *pay-for-performance* (P4P) or *value-based purchasing*, is supported by a variety of organizations. Effective performance-based payments show positive results in private industrial applications and, in spite of the absence of convincing evidence, there is widespread belief that similar results can be obtained in medicine.P4P is particularly popular amongst third-party payers. Historically payment was based on the number and the complexity of services provided to patients, but with P4P, some portion of payment is determined by the quality rather than the quantity of services. It remains to be seen whether reimbursement incentives will lead to meaningful improvements in quality of care.

There are several reimbursement models associated with P4P, the most common of which is the *tournament model.* In the tournament approach, there are unequivocal winners and losers. Top performers get bonuses which come from reduced payments to the lower performers. Although popular because of its simplicity, this budget-neutral approach in which one "robs Peter to pay Paul," penalizes precisely the group which most needs financial resources for improvement.[65] Regardless of the mode of implementation, it is obvious that *performance measures* are destined to be an important and intrinsic part of the surgical milieu in upcoming years.

TYPES OF ASSESSMENT OF CARDIAC PROCEDURES

Assessment Using Operative Mortality

By far, the bulk of available experience with outcome assessment in cardiothoracic surgery deals with operative mortality, particularly in patients undergoing coronary revascularization. Table 7-3 is a list of risk models used to assess operative mortality in patients undergoing coronary revascularization. Many of the risk stratification analyses shown in Table 7-1 and Table 7-3 are used to evaluate mortality outcomes in CABG patients, because mortality is such an unequivocal endpoint of greatest interest to patients and is recorded with high accuracy. For the diagnosis of ischemic heart disease, Table 7-3 lists the significant risk factors found to be important for a spectrum of the risk stratification systems. The definition of operative mortality varies among the different systems (either 30-day mortality and/or in-hospital mortality), but the risk factors identified by each of the stratification schemes in Table 7-3 show many similarities. Some variables are risk factors in almost all stratification systems; some variables are only rarely significant risk factors. Separate data sets validated each of the models; hence, there is some justification in using any of the risk stratification methods both in preoperative assessment of patients undergoing coronary artery bypass grafting (CABG) and in assessing provider performance (either physicians or hospitals).Validation and assessment of surgeons and hospitals using the risk models in Table 7-3 must be done with caution, because, as described previously, risk models are imperfect. Results indicating that a provider is a statistical outlier should always be corroborated by clinical review.

There are many critical features of any risk-adjustment algorithm that must be considered when determining its suitability for profiling provider performance. Daley provides a summary of the key features that are necessary to validate any risk adjustment model.[66] Differences in risk-adjusted mortalities across providers may not necessarily reflect differences in the process and structure of care,[67] an issue that needs further study.

Assessment Using Postoperative Morbidity and Resource Utilization

Patients with nonfatal outcomes following operations for ischemic heart disease make up more than 95% of the pool of patients undergoing operation. Obviously all non-fatal operative results are not equivalent. Patients who experience renal failure requiring lifelong dialysis, or a serious sternal wound infection, have not had the same result as a patient who leaves the hospital with no major complications, as occurs in about 85% of patients entered in the STS Database. The complications occurring in surviving patients range from serious organ system dysfunction to minor limitation or dissatisfaction with lifestyle, and account for a significant fraction of the cost of the procedures. We estimate that as much as 40% of the yearly hospital costs for CABG are consumed by 10 to 15% of the patients who have serious complications after operation.[68] This is an example of a statistical principle called the *Pareto principle* and also suggests that reducing morbidity in high risk cardiac surgical patients has significant impact on cost reduction.

A great deal of information exists on nonfatal complications after cardiac operations. Several large databases identify risk factors for both nonfatal morbidity and increased resource utilization. Table 7-5 is a summary of some of the risk factors identified by available risk stratification models that are associated with either serious postoperative morbidity or increased resource utilization as measures of undesirable outcomes.

STS Risk Models for Postoperative Morbidity

For many years, operative mortality was the sole criterion for a successful CABG procedure. This concept gave way to a broader focus on the entire hospitalization associated with CABG. There is universal agreement that nonfatal complications play a central role in the assessment of CABG quality, but many morbidity outcomes are relatively difficult to define and track. Risk adjustment is particularly difficult because of the fact that risk factors for most complications are not well established. The low frequency of some complications also creates statistical challenges.

Shroyer and coworkers used part of the large national experience captured in the *Society of Thoracic Surgeons Database* to examine five important postoperative CABG complications: stroke, renal failure, reoperation within 24 hours after CABG, prolonged (>24 hours) postoperative ventilation, and mediastinitis.[69] Revised morbidity models using contemporary statistical approaches followed this landmark study by Shroyer and coworkers.[12-14] In 2009, the STS morbidity risk models were updated using data from 2002 to2006, with specific models for isolated CABG, isolated valve, and combined CABG + valve procedures. Given the contemporary data and large reference populations (eg, 774,881 patients for isolated CABG model), these are the most comprehensive, nationally representative, and thoroughly documented morbidity risk models currently available. These risk models will undoubtedly play an important role in future attempts at performance assessment.

Patient Satisfaction as an Outcome

Patients' assessment of surgical outcome is an alternate means of judging performance.There are several difficulties with measurement of patient-reported outcomes, and consequently cardiothoracic surgeons are not deeply involved with systematic measurements of patient satisfaction after operation. One problem is that patient-reported outcomes may be dependent on the type of patient who is reporting them and not on the type of care received. For example, younger Caucasian patients with better education and higher income are more likely to give less favorable ratings of physician care.[70]

Considerable research deals with instruments that are available to measure patient satisfaction. At least two of these instruments, the *Short-Form Health Survey or SF-36*[71] and the *San Jose Medical Group's Patient Satisfaction Measure,*[72] are used to monitor patient satisfaction over time. The current status of these and other measures of patient satisfaction does not allow accurate comparisons among providers, because the quality of the data generated by these measures is poor. These instruments are characterized by low response rates, inadequate sampling, infrequent use, and unavailability of satisfactory benchmarks. Nonetheless, available evidence indicates that feedback on patient satisfaction data to physicians may impact physician practices.[73] It is likely that managed care organizations and hospitals will use patient-reported outcome measures to make comparisons between institutions and between individual providers.

Risk stratification methodology can identify patients who are optimal candidates for revascularization based on quality of life and functional status considerations .Multivariate risk factors associated with unimproved postoperative quality of life after CABG include female gender,[74] patients with anxiety and depressive disorders,[75,76] and operations complicated by sternal wound infection.[77] Interestingly, patients who have CABG are likely to have equivalent mid-term health-related quality of life compared with patients undergoing percutaneous coronary interventions.[78] One comparative study found no difference between patients older than 65 years and those younger than or equal to 65 with regard to quality of life outcomes (symptoms, cardiac functional class, activities of daily living and emotional and social functioning).[79] This study identified a direct relationship between clinical severity and quality of life indicators, because patients with less comorbid conditions and better preoperative functional status had better quality of life indicators six months after operation than those with significant comorbidities.In contrast, Rumsfeld and coworkers found that improvement in the self-reported quality of life (from Form

TABLE 7-5 Risk Factors Associated with Increased Length of Stay (L),Increased Incidence of Organ Failure Morbidity (M), or Both (L/M) Following Coronary Revascularization

Risk Factor	STS[69]	STS Updated[13]	Boston[148]	Albany[68]	VA[149]	Canada[17]
Demographics						
Advanced age.	M	M	L		M	L
Low preoperative red blood cell volume.	M			L/M		
Race		M				
Female gender.	M	M				L
Disease-specific diagnoses						
CHF	M	M	L	L/M	M	
Concomitant valve disease	M	M			M	L
Reoperation	M	M			M	L
LV dysfunction (ejection fraction)	M	M				L
Surgical priority	M	M			M	L
3-vessel disease		M				
IABP preop	M	M	L			
Active endocarditis					M	
Left-main disease		M				
Preoperative atrial fibrillation		M				
Comorbid conditions						
Obesity		M	L			
Renal dysfunction	M	M	L	L	M	
Diabetes		M				
Peripheral vascular disease	M	M		L	M	
Chronic obstructive lung disease	M	M		L		
Cerebrovascular disease	M	M		L/M		
Hypertension	M	M		L/M		
Immunosuppression		M				

CHF = congestive heart failure; IABP = intraaortic balloon counterpulsation; LV = left ventricular.

SF-36) was more likely in patients who had relatively poor health status before CABG compared with those who had relatively good preoperative health status.[80] Interestingly, these same authors found that poor preoperative self-reported quality of life indicator was an independent predictor of operative mortality following CABG.[81] These findings suggest that the risks of patient dissatisfaction after CABG are poorly understood but may be dependent on preoperative comorbid factors as well as on the indications for, and technical complexities of, the operation itself. At present there is no well-established risk model to identify patients who are likely to report dissatisfaction with operative intervention following CABG.

Composite Performance Measures for CABG

Recently, performance assessment expanded to include nonfatal adverse outcomes. In developing a set of performance measures for cardiac surgery, the NQF included five major complications (stroke, reoperation, prolonged ventilation, renal failure, and sternal infection) as important outcomes to measure. They also added a number of process measures, including use of the internal thoracic artery and a number of evidence-based perioperative medications (preoperative beta-blockade; discharge beta-blockade, lipid-lowering agents, and aspirin). Participation in a systematic data registry and procedural volume were included as structural measures of quality. In 2005, the STS embarked on development of a *composite measure* of CABG quality that incorporated many of these NQF individual measures. The Institute of Medicine and the NQF advocate composite measures of healthcare quality because composite scores provide a much more comprehensive view of quality compared with a single measure alone. Furthermore, the additional endpoints provide an increased number of observations and allow increased discrimination among providers. In a series of 2007 publications, the STS described the development of a composite measure that consists of 11 individual outcomes and process endpoints within four quality domains (risk-adjusted operative mortality, risk-adjusted major morbidity, use of the internal mammary artery for revascularization and use of NQF-endorsed cardiac medications).[63,82] Using this framework and based on their composite score, providers are rated one, two, or three stars depending on whether there is a 99% Bayesian probability that their performance is below, at, or superior to the national STS average performance. This composite scoring methodology is gaining acceptance by health care providers and is the most widely used national system for assessing CABG provider quality. Furthermore, the feedback reports to providers from this composite scoring system are designed to show areas of strength and weakness to guide their internal performance improvement activities.

USING DATA TO IMPROVE PERFORMANCE—CASE STUDIES

STS Database and Quality Improvement

The Society of Thoracic Surgeons recognized a compelling need for a national standard in cardiac surgery as early as 1986 when a formal STS committee was formed to develop a national database of cardiac surgery. This committee gathered and analyzed in order to establish a national standard of care in cardiac surgery. The *STS Database* is a voluntary registry that currently collects perioperative patient data from more than 90 % of cardiac centers in the United States. Individual participant sites enter extensive clinical data on each patient undergoing cardiac surgery. This information is harvested quarterly and aggregated at the Duke Clinical Research Institute (DCRI).The data are analyzed and reports, which include benchmark data and risk-adjusted outcomes, are provided to each site. This reporting process allows sites to pinpoint areas in need of improvement so that tailored quality assessment and performance improvement programs can be developed. The database has numerous important practical applications that allow performance assessment and document workload.

The STS database allows accurate determination of thoracic surgeons' workload.To paraphrase Winston Churchill, never have so many physicians and other health care professionals owed so much to so few. The "few" in this case are the 29 members of the *American Medical Association/Specialty Society Relative Value Scale Update Committee, or* RUC (rhymes with "truck") for short. The RUC's recommendations to the Centers for Medicare and Medicaid Services (CMS) significantly influence the relative values assigned to physician services and, as a result, how much physicians are paid. STS data allows monitoring of trends in the patient profile of cardiac surgery patients over the years. This kind of information impacts negotiations with RUC. Deliberations with the RUC were traditionally based on small surveys but the use of STS data allowed a more accurate presentation of objective information that provides a truly fair and meaningful workload analysis.[83]

The STS database reporting and feedback process to individual sites produced impressive performance improvements in surgical outcomes. Database information showed a progressive increase in CABG operative risk from 1993 to 2008.In spite of that risk, however, the observed operative mortality steadily declined from over 4% to approximately 2% during this period.

The database plays a central role in the current national quality initiatives. Information from the database allows one to monitor and analyze all of the *National Quality Forum* (NQF) performance measures specified in Table 7-4. Specific NQF-based reports allow STS database participants to focus directly on the national measures chosen to reflect cardiac surgical quality. In addition, composite measures are available from the STS database. These composite measures (see previous) determine the net impact of all CABG performance measures (structural, process, and outcome measures) generated from the STS database.[13] Composite scores are likely better indicators of performance than any single performance measure.

There is a groundswell of public demand for *provider report cards* and other hospital/surgeon ranking systems. The advantages and disadvantages of such reporting systems are addressed elsewhere in this chapter, but it should be mentioned that numerous third party payers are in the process of developing these scorecard protocols. In order to pre-empt the development of ill-advised and simplistic scorecards, STS experts developed a fair and meaningful quality rating system based on objective information from the STS Database.[13]

The STS Database presently contains records of approximately three million patients, thereby making it the largest cardiac surgery database in the world. This clinical database is an exceptionally valuable resource for cardiac surgeons and its risk assessment algorithms are generally accepted as standard quality assessment tools in cardiac surgery. The database has numerous important practical applications including performance assessment, workload documentation, provider benchmarking and documentation of national performance measures. These applications serve to promote quality improvement and ensure that the specialty is well represented in national regulatory programs.

Management Philosophy and Performance Assessment

American health care made almost unbelievable strides in the last 100 years. We are at the brink of being able to treat disease at the genotypic molecular level. Further, cardiac surgeons treat patients considered inoperable as recently as a decade ago. Yet almost no one is happy with the health-care system. It costs too much, excludes many, is inefficient, and is ignorant about its own effectiveness. A similar state of confusion existed with Japanese industry after World War II. Out of the confusion and crisis of post-World War II, Japan became a monolith of efficiency. Two major architects of this transformation were an American statistician, W. Edwards Deming, and a Romanian-American theoretician, J.M. Juran. They led the way in establishing and implementing certain principles of management and efficiency based on quality. Their efforts are recognized in Japan by the annual awarding of the Deming Prizes in recognition of achievements in attaining high quality. Deming's and Juran's books are some of the classics of quality management in industry.[84,85]

Deming's and Juran's management philosophy are sometimes referred to as *total quality management* or TQM. The amazing turnaround in Japanese industry led many organizations to embrace and modify the principles of TQM, including organizations involved in delivery and assessment of health care. Table 7-6 outlines the key features of TQM. An example of the application of the principles of TQM to health care delivery is described in the book by Berwick and coworkers.[86]

TABLE 7-6 Principles of Total Quality Management (TQM) Applied to Health Care

Principle	Explanation
Health care delivery is a process.	The purpose of a process is to add value to the input of the process. Each person in an organization is part of one or more processes.
Quality defects arise from problems with the process.	Former reliance on quotas, numerical goals, and discipline of workers is unlikely to improve quality, because these measures imply that workers are at fault and that quality will get better if workers do better. The problem is with the process not with the worker. Quality improvement involves "driving out fear" on the part of the worker, and breaking down barriers between departments so that everyone may work effectively as a team for the organization.
Customer–supplier relationships are the most important aspect of quality.	A customer is anyone who depends on the organization. The goal of quality improvement is to improve constantly and to establish a long-term relationship of loyalty and trust between customer (patient) and supplier (health care organization) and, thereby, meet the needs of the patient. The competitive advantage for an organization that can better meet the needs of the customer is obvious. The organization will gain market share, reduce costs, and waste less effort in activities that do not add value for patients.
Understand the causes of variability.	Failure to understand variation in critical processes within the organization is the cause of many serious quality problems. Unpredictable processes are flawed and are difficult to study and assess. Managers must understand the difference between random (or common-cause) variation and special variation in a given outcome.
Develop new organizational structures	Managers are leaders not enforcers. Eliminate management by objective numerical goals. Remove barriers that rob workers of their right to pride of workmanship. Empower everybody in the organization to achieve the transformation to a quality product.
Focus on the most 'vital few' processes.	This is known as the *Pareto principle* (first applied by Juran) and states that whenever a number of individual factors contribute to an outcome, relatively few of those items account for the bulk of the effect. By focusing on the "vital few," the greatest reward for effort will occur.
Quality reduces cost.	Poor quality is costly. Malpractice suits, excessive use of costly laboratory tests, and unnecessarily long hospital stay, are examples of costly poor quality. The premise that it is too costly to implement quality control is incorrect.
Statistics and scientific thinking are the foundation of quality.	Managers must make decisions based on accurate data, using scientific methods. Not only managers, but all members of the organization, utilize the scientific method for improving processes as part of their normal daily activity.

These authors recount the experiences of the National Demonstration Project on Quality Improvement in Health Care in applying principles of TQM to solve a broad spectrum of health care problems. Twenty-one health care organizations throughout the United States participated in an experiment to learn and implement TQM principles at every level within an institution. This effort produced improvement in customer-supplier throughput (improvement in the patient care process) to a variable extent.

The development and success of TQM stimulated creation of other similar quality management philosophies. Some examples include the Six-Sigma approach developed by Motorola, the Toyota Production System, Lean Manufacturing, the Disney Way Management System, Change Management systems, and the Theory of Constraints. These management programs are characterized by a desire to reduce waste and error through careful analysis of processes and bottlenecks in the throughput. They often use statistical quality control whenever applicable. They emphasize standardization, reduction of output variance, and focus on systems approaches to problems rather than blaming individuals. Some, but not all, of these management principles have applications in health care, and they have been extensively and successfully applied at the Virginia Mason Clinic in Seattle.

Total Quality Management is the management philosophy often used for healthcare applications. A TQM project starts from critical observations. For example, excessive blood transfusion after operation may result in increased morbidity, including disease transmission, increased infection risk, and increased cost. Tools such as flow diagrams that document all of the steps in the process are used in a TQM project (eg, steps involved in the blood transfusion process after CABG).A logical starting point for efforts to improve the quality of the blood transfusion process would be to focus on a high-risk subset of patients who consume a disproportionate amount of blood resources. An Italian economist, named Pareto, made the observation that a few factors account for the majority of the outcomes of a complex process, and this has been termed the *Pareto principle.* Juran was one of the first to apply this principle to manufacturing in the United States and Japan.[85] A graphical method of identifying the spectrum of outcomes in a process is included in most statistics programs, and is termed a Pareto diagram. Figure 7-2 is an example of a Pareto diagram for blood product transfusion. Figure 7-2 suggests that about 20% of the patients consume 80% of the blood products transfused following cardiac procedures. Substantial savings in cost and possibly other morbidity will result by decreasing the amount of blood transfusion in these 20% of "high-end" users. For TQM purposes, strategies can be devised and tested to decrease blood product consumption in the high-risk subset, and ultimately, monitors are set up to measure the effectiveness of the new strategies. Other tools of TQM such as data sampling strategies and use of control charts play an important role in the process.

Northern New England TQM Project

A superb example of a TQM-based approach to improving cardiac surgery quality is the Northern New England Cardiovascular Study Group (NNECVDSG).Founded in 1987, this voluntary consortium of clinicians, scientists, and administrators represents cardiac surgery programs in Northern New England. Its mission is to study and improve the quality of cardiovascular care provided to patients through the use of systematic data collection and feedback. Shortly after its formation, this group developed and validated a logistic risk model to account for case mix differences across its member institutions,[87] Using this model, the group analyzed CABG outcomes for 3055 patients operated on at five medical centers in Maine, New Hampshire, and Vermont between July 1987 and April 1989.[88] Overall unadjusted CABG mortality was 4.3% but this varied substantially among centers (3.1 to6.3%).Even after case-mix adjustment, significant variability persisted among medical centers (p = 0.021) and surgeons (p = 0.025).In 1990, the NNECVDSG initiated a regional intervention aimed at reducing both absolute CABG mortality and inter-institutional variability.[89] The three major components of this TQM approach included feedback of outcomes data, training in continuous quality improvement techniques, and site visits to each program. During the latter, visitors from each discipline

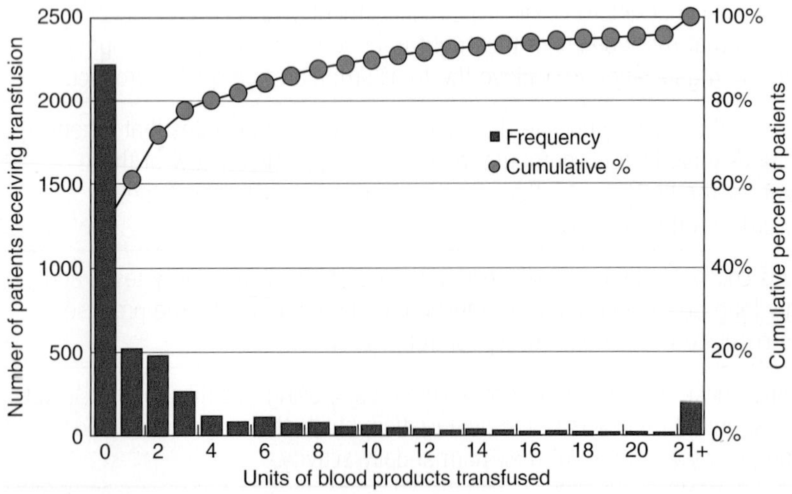

FIGURE 7-2 Pareto diagram of blood transfusion in 4457 patients undergoing cardiac procedures at Albany Medical Center Hospital over a 4 year period. *(Reprinted with permission from Ferraris, et al, Annals of Thoracic Surgery[50])*

focused on the practice of their counterparts at the host institutions. Numerous changes were implemented as a result of these site visits including technical aspects, processes of care, personnel organization and training, decision-making, and methods of evaluating care. Following these interventions, observed mortality declined to less than expected in all categories of patient acuity.

Subsequent to these landmark papers, the consortium continued to grow in size, and the registry forms the basis for numerous publications aimed at improving the care of cardiac surgical patients. Their publications cover a wide range of topics including the impact of preoperative variables on hospital and long-term mortality, the optimal conduct of cardiopulmonary perfusion, the prevention of specific postoperative complications, on-pump vs. off-pump CABG surgery, and modes of death following CABG.[90-92] Over two decades since its inception, the NNECVDSG remains at the forefront of efforts to improve cardiac surgery quality through voluntary, confidential, and collaborative TQM.

CONTROVERSIES IN THE ASSESSMENT OF PERFORMANCE

Dangers of Outcome Assessment—Risk Aversion

After the introduction of provider report cards in NY and Pennsylvania in the early 1990s, studies emerged suggesting that providers were changing their practice patterns in response. The release of risk-adjusted data may alienate providers and result in the sickest patients having less accessibility to care. This may have already happened in New York State[93–95] and in other regions where risk-adjusted mortality and cost data were released to the public. Of even more concern is the selection bias that may exist in managed care HMO enrollment. Morgan and coworkers suggest that Medicare HMOs benefit from the selective enrollment of healthier Medicare recipients and the dis-enrollment or outright rejection of sicker beneficiaries.[96] This form of separation of patients into unfavorable or favorable risk categories is a direct result of risk assessment and may be an unintended consequence of performance assessment methodology. This type of discrimination undermines the effectiveness and appropriateness of care. Omoigui and colleagues addressed this issue in a report about the effect of publication of surgeon-specific report cards in NY state.[94] These authors concluded that surgeons in that state were less willing to operate on high risk patients. Patients in NY state were subsequently transferred in disproportionately large numbers to the Cleveland Clinic, where both their expected and observed adverse outcomes exceeded those of other referral areas without report cards. Although this "outmigration" phenomenon was challenged by some, additional studies in NY and Pennsylvania suggest that the concept of risk aversion may have some validity.[97–100] With the increasing use of percutaneous coronary interventions, a similar phenomenon was observed, with evidence of risk aversion in states with public reporting.[101–104] Clearly there is some degree of risk aversion in public reporting environments, and this could result in denial of care to the high-risk patients that might benefit most from intervention. Others suggest that it may redirect such patients to the most experienced providers, which could be a more positive result.[100,105] To mitigate the problem of risk aversion, some suggested not reporting or separately reporting the results of the most seriously ill patients, some of whom have risk factors that are difficult to adequately model with available risk models like those in Table 7-3. It is also important to review patients turned down for high-risk CABG or PCI to be certain that report cards are not having the unintended negative consequence of denial of appropriate care.

Validity and Reliability of Assessment Methods

Accuracy of Databases

Perhaps the most important tool of any outcome assessment endeavor is a database that is made up of a representative sample of the study group of interest. The accuracy of the data elements in any such database cannot be overemphasized.[106] Factors such as the source of data, the outcome of interest, the methods used for data collection, standardized definitions of the data elements, data reliability checking, and the time frame of data collection are essential features that must be considered when either constructing a new database or deciding about using an existing database.[106]

Data obtained from claims or administrative databases are less reliable than those obtained from clinical databases. Because claims data are generated for the collection of bills, their clinical accuracy is inadequate and it is likely that these databases overestimate complications for billing purposes. They may incorrectly classify some surgical procedures, and this in turn may result in erroneous and misleading outcomes results.[107] Furthermore, claims data underestimate the effects of comorbid illness and contain major deficiencies in important prognostic variables for CABG, such as left ventricular function and number of diseased vessels. The Duke Databank for Cardiovascular Disease found major discrepancies between clinical and claims databases, with claims data failing to identify more than half of the patients with important comorbid conditions such as CHF, cerebrovascular disease and angina.[22,108] The Health Care Financing Administration (HCFA) used claims data to evaluate variations in the mortality rates in hospitals treating Medicare patients. After an initially disastrous effort at risk adjustment from claims data,[109,110] HCFA developed new search and analysis algorithms. Despite these advances, the HCFA administration halted release of the 1993 Medicare hospital mortality report because of concerns about the database and fears that the figures would unfairly punish inner-city public facilities.[111] The quality of databases used to generate comparisons cannot be overemphasized.

Logistic Regression and Hierarchical Regression Models

One of the most common yet controversial applications of logistic regression models is provider profiling, sometimes mandated by governmental organizations,[112,113] in which case the results are usually published as report cards and made available to the public. The statistical methodology previously used to develop most such report cards is straightforward. The probability of mortality for each of a provider's patients during a given time period is estimated using logistic regression or some other multivariate method based on a large database containing multiple surgeons' patients. These probabilities are aggregated to determine a particular provider's expected mortality, or *E*. The observed mortality, *O*, is simply the counted number of operative deaths. An *O/E ratio* has a value close to one if the performance is what would be predicted from the model. Ratios significantly greater than one imply worse than expected performance, and ratios significantly less than one suggest better than expected performance. Often, the O/E ratios are multiplied by the population unadjusted mortality rate to obtain the *risk-adjusted mortality ratio* (RAMR) also called a *standardized mortality ratio* (SMR).

Statisticians realize that this intuitively appealing approach, aggregating patient-level data to make inferences about providers using logistic regression, is not ideal.[114] Assessing operative mortality among hospitals and among surgeons is inherently multilevel. Multiple levels exist that may alter operative mortality, including surgeons, hospitals, referring physicians, etc. In such situations simply aggregating between levels may lead to erroneous conclusions. This was long ago recognized in education, where the analogous situation would be the inappropriate aggregation of pupil test scores to evaluate teacher performance. Multilevel or hierarchical models are available for such situations, and these models address most of the major concerns regarding the use of standard models that assess multilevel processes involving multiple surgeons and multiple hospitals. For example, the sample sizes from various providers often differ substantially. In the latter situation, the observed estimates of observed mortality are a much less accurate reflection of their true but unobserved future mortality. Hierarchical models "shrink" the observed mortality rates of lower volume providers toward the mean of the overall population of providers, a way of borrowing strength or pooling the data from multiple levels of hospitals and providers. The resulting estimates are more accurate and stable. Standard logistic models do not accurately partition the multiple levels of variability (between and within providers), which is one of the central questions to be answered by profiling. Hierarchical models correctly partition this variability and account for sample size variation and compensate for multiple comparisons. Numerous studies investigated the difference in the results of provider profiling obtained from traditional logistic regression versus hierarchical modeling. For example, Goldstein and Spiegelhalter, using a hierarchical model of operative mortality of surgeons in New York state, reduced the number of surgeon outliers from three to one.[115] A logical objection to the use of hierarchical models is that, by reducing the chance of false outlier identification, it may also reduce the sensitivity to detect true outliers. Ultimately, this tradeoff is a health policy and regulatory decision.[112] Hierarchical models are complex and require not only extensive computer resources but also close planning and oversight by a statistician experienced in these methods. Most investigators regard them as the best model for multilevel comparisons, and hierarchical modeling is used both by the state of Massachusetts and by the Society of Thoracic Surgeons for the development of provider profiles.

The Downside of Performance Assessment

Cost and Imperfection

Collecting risk-adjusted data and implementing performance enhancement adds to the administrative costs of the health care system. It is estimated that 20% of health care costs ($150 billion to $180 billion/year) are spent on the administration of health care.[116] The logistical costs of implementing a risk-adjustment system are substantial. Additional costs are incurred in implementing quality measures that are suggested by risk-stratification methodology. A disturbing notion is that the costs of performance assessment may outweigh the payers' willingness to pay for these benefits. For example, Iowa hospitals estimated that they spent $2.5 million annually to gather MedisGroups severity data that was mandated by the state. Because of the cost, the state abandoned this mandate and concluded that neither consumers nor purchasers used the data anyway.[117] Similarly, one report suggests that public release of quality indicators did not significantly improve composite hospital performance.[118] It is possible that quality improvement may cost rather than save money; although one of the principles of TQM (often quoted by Deming) is that the least expensive means to accomplish a task (eg, deliver health care) is the means that employs the highest quality in the process. Ultimately, improved quality will be cost-efficient, but start-up costs may be daunting. In order to be cost-effective, any cost savings realized from performance assessment must be factored into the total costs of gathering risk-adjusted data and implementing quality improvement. Further, given the substantial costs of a single serious complication such as stroke, dialysis-dependent renal failure, or a sternal infection, the cost savings of performance assessment and quality improvement programs may be substantial.

Interpretation of Risk Adjusted Outcomes

One of the least well understood aspects of performance report cards is the correct interpretation of risk-adjusted or risk-standardized outcomes, which are derived by comparing observed outcomes with those predicted by statistical risk models. There is a tendency by the public, by insurance companies and by government officials to regard Risk-Adjusted Mortality Ratios (eg, O/E ratios) and Risk-adjusted or Standardized Mortality Rates as the ultimate metric of provider performance. Compared with unadjusted rates these are certainly superior approaches, but their limitations must be recognized. First, all risk models are only approximations of reality, and they cannot adjust for all possible combinations of risk factors. These models are useful for predicting population average outcomes given a particular patient mix, but they are less useful for predicting the outcome for specific patients. Second, even if there were perfect risk adjustment, the results for a particular provider must be correctly interpreted. The risk-standardized or risk-adjusted mortality for a hospital reflects its performance for its specific patient case mix, compared with what would have been expected had these same patients been cared for by an average provider in the reference population. Because *indirect* rather than *direct* standardization is used for virtually all risk models used in profiling, it is not appropriate to directly compare the risk-adjusted results of one institution with those of another. The risk-adjusted mortality of a small community hospital is based largely on a low-risk population. Even though it is adjusted, it cannot be compared directly to the risk-adjusted rate of a quaternary referral center, which is based largely on a population of patients that the community program rarely if ever sees. In this extreme example, these two hospitals may have virtually no types of patients in common, and even though their rates are adjusted they should not be directly compared with one another.

Ranking Providers—League Tables versus Funnel Plots

There is a problem with report cards of provider results that appear in the lay press and on the Internet. Most report cards rank providers in the form of league tables, similar to tables used in sports to rank teams or individuals. League tables always have someone on top and someone on the bottom. In general, the public does not understand that there is no meaningful difference for the vast majority of names published in league tables of cardiac surgeons' performance.[119] The limited sample size of any individual surgeon or hospital leads to wide fluctuation in outcomes over time. Reporting of one surgeon as being better (ie, higher in the league table) than another is inaccurate and probably unethical. Spiegelhalter addressed this concern and suggested better options for reporting surgeons' and hospitals' results.[120] He advocated funnel plots as a far better alternative to league tables to report provider outcomes. A funnel plot is a plot of individual surgeons' volume (x-axis) versus risk-adjusted mortality (y-axis) with population confidence intervals. The plot allows immediate identification of outliers (ie, providers outside the confidence intervals) and gives the viewer an estimate of the larger uncertainties (ie, increased confidence intervals) of risk-adjusted mortality of low-volume providers compared with high-volume providers. The limits of uncertainty (ie, control limits) form a funnel around the provider outcome. The United Kingdom Central Cardiac Audit Database (http://www.ic.nhs.uk/services/national-clinical-audit-support-programme-ncasp/heart-disease/adult-cardiac-surgery) and the STS Congenital Heart Surgery Database Report use funnel plots to identify outliers.[119]

FUTURE DIRECTIONS

Effectiveness and Appropriateness of Care

Since the Institute of Medicine report on medical errors that appeared in 2000,[7] reducing medical errors both by physicians and by hospitals garnered significant resources. Since then, several authors suggested that the culture of safety in hospitals is unchanged.[121,122] Brennan and coauthors point out that the IOM distinguishes safety from effectiveness. Effectiveness is defined as an intervention based on available evidence that improves quality, whereas safety encompasses a much narrower definition of limiting accidental injury.[121] These authors suggest redirection of health care goals toward effectiveness interventions and away from accident reduction interventions. An important advantage of focus on effectiveness is the ease with which effectiveness outcomes can be measured compared with safety outcomes. There is some evidence that focus on evidence-based interventions (eg, providing aspirin to cardiac patients when they leave the hospital) improves the effectiveness of treatment with secondary benefit of reducing errors.[123] Furthermore, there is still a reluctance to deal transparently with medical mistakes. Health care providers did not spend significantly increased resources on safety and error management largely because the return on this type of investment is very hard to measure. On the other hand, quality improvement efforts based on evidence of effectiveness are likely to be more readily embraced and may save more lives than will safety-related interventions that lack an evidence base.[121]

Practice guidelines present evidence-based recommendations regarding cardiovascular interventions.[50] It is reasonable to ask how successful these practice guidelines are in altering practice. Most studies suggest that implementation of practice guidelines is difficult and changes in practice related to guideline recommendations are rare.[54,124] Professional societies addressed this difficulty by introducing *appropriateness criteria*. Appropriateness criteria are lists of appropriate indications for interventions in common clinical scenarios. They document indications for drug or device intervention with a scale metric. For example, the AHA/ACC/STS Joint Task Force generated appropriateness criteria for coronary revascularization that used a scale of 1 to 10.[125] Values of 7 through 10 indicated that coronary revascularization is appropriate for patients with a particular scenario. Scores of 1 to 3 indicate revascularization is inappropriate and unlikely to improve health outcomes or survival. The mid range scores (4 to 6) suggests that improvement in survival or other health care outcomes with coronary revascularization is uncertain. The aim of appropriateness criteria is to guide physician decision making toward use of evidence based interventions. It is likely that expansion of the appropriateness criteria concept will occur.

Decision Analysis, Machine Learning, and Neural Networks

Development of risk models to predict outcomes from cardiac surgical interventions (eg, Tables 7-1 and 7-3) consumes a great deal of effort. Although the models are fairly accurate at predicting outcomes for populations of patients undergoing operations, they still have distinct limitations. The biggest drawback of these risk models is their mediocre performance at predicting outcomes for individual patients.[19] Consequently, risk-adjustment to predict individual outcomes is difficult to apply at the bedside and is often inaccurate. For patient-specific needs, risk stratification and outcomes assessment are in their infancy.

Better patient-specific predictors of outcome are needed for clinical decision making. The decision to operate for coronary artery diseases is extremely complex because there are more than two alternative treatments, more than two outcomes, and many intervening events that may occur to alter outcomes. As mentioned above, there are enormous variations in the way that surgeons practice. These variations can increase cost, cause harm, and confuse patients. Other global enhancements are available to direct surgeons toward evidence based care. These include decision analysis systems, artificial intelligence, and computer intensive risk modeling. The tools of *decision analysis*, similar to how airline pilots make decisions about complicated flight problems, were applied to the area of physician decision making in an effort to eliminate practice variations and to provide accurate and effective decisions at the patient bedside.[126,127] Decision models generated to address surgical outcomes typically employ the familiar decision tree. An important part of creating the decision tree is to estimate the probabilities of each of the various outcomes for a given set of interventions. This part of the decision analysis tree relies heavily on the results of risk stratification and regression modeling, especially computer-intensive methods such as Bayesian models, to arrive at a probability of risk for a particular outcome. All of the diverse pieces of evidence used to form consensus guidelines, including meta-analyses, expert opinions, unpublished sources, randomized trials, and observational studies are employed to arrive at probabilities of outcome and intervening events. For example, Gage et al. performed a cost-effectiveness analysis of aspirin and warfarin for stroke prophylaxis in patients with nonvalvular atrial fibrillation.[128] They used information from published meta-analyses of individual-level data from five randomized trials of antithrombotic therapy in atrial fibrillation to estimate the rates of stroke without therapy, the percentage reduction in the risk of stroke in users of warfarin, and the percentage of mild, moderate, or severe intracranial hemorrhages following anticoagulation. Their decision tree suggests that in 65-year-old patients with nonvalvular atrial fibrillation but no other risk factors for stroke, prescribing warfarin instead of aspirin would affect quality-adjusted survival minimally but increase costs significantly. Application of decision analysis methods to clinical decision making can standardize care and decrease risks of therapy but these methods are in the early developmental phase and much more work needs to be done before ready acceptance by surgeons.

The quantum increase in computational power that evolved over the past decade led to an entirely new "culture" of modeling called *machine learning* or algorithmic models.[20,129] Rather than using classical statistical models with their specific assumptions and limitations, algorithmic modeling is focused more on predictive accuracy and less on trying to constrain nature to a particular parametric equation set of input variables. Examples of such algorithmic techniques include neural networks, decision and regression trees, and support vector machines. Because these models often do not provide an easily understood relationship between predictor and outcome variables, some have pejoratively referred to them as "black boxes,"[129] However, despite this criticism, such models may, in many instances, provide superior predictive accuracy, even though the mechanism behind the relationship may be less transparent. Furthermore, in machine learning techniques, the numbers of predictors that can enter the model are not limited as they are in standard regression.

It was postulated over a decade ago that machine learning or artificial intelligence methods such as *neural networks* would provide the next major advance in predictive modeling for cardiac surgery. However, a large study to test this postulate was conducted by Lippmann and Shahian at the MIT Lincoln Laboratory using data from the 1993 Society of Thoracic Surgeons database of 80,606 patients who underwent CABG.[31] A two-layer neural network did not provide any substantial improvement compared with standard logistic regression, and this neural network also underestimated risk in the highest risk groups. Somewhat improved performance was obtained by combining the results of the neural network with those of logistic regression; however, the absolute improvement in ROC curve area was relatively small. The failure of neural networks to improve predictive accuracy is likely a reflection of the imperfect and limited information presented to these models, which is the same information used to develop and evaluate traditional statistical models. No modeling technique is better than the information presented to it for training, and neural networks are no exception. It may well be that if presented with a more comprehensive set of predictor variables, some of which are not even recognized today as being significant, these machine learning techniques may prove to be more accurate. More work in this area is likely to proceed in the future.

Volume/Outcome Relationship and Targeted Regionalization

At least 10 large studies addressed the notion that hospitals performing small numbers of CABG operations have higher operative mortality (http://www.nap.edu/catalog/10005.html). Seven of these ten studies found increased operative mortality in low volume providers. In three other large studies there was no such association. In general, the volume-outcome association for CABG is weaker compared with that of other complex and much less frequently performed procedures such as esophagectomy and pancreatectomy.[130–132] The Institute of Medicine summarized the relationship between higher-volume and better outcome and concluded that procedure or patient volume is an imprecise indicator of quality even though a majority of the studies reviewed showed some association between higher procedure volume and better outcome. Many other risk factors are more important determinants of outcome than provider volume in the STS database.[133,134] Furthermore, the volume-outcome association applies only to average performance for certain provider volume categories. Some individual low-volume programs have superb performance, whereas some high-volume programs have inferior performance. The real problem with low-volume programs is that it is very hard to accurately measure their performance in a reasonably short time-frame because their sample sizes are too small. Strategies that improve the performance measurement and the actual outcomes of low-volume providers may prove helpful.[132] Nallamothu and coauthors advocate a role for "selective regionalization" of higher risk patients, because they found that low risk patients did equally well in high volume or low volume hospitals.[135] Other authors point out that a policy of regionalized referrals for CABG might have unintended adverse effects on health care including increased cost, decreased patient satisfaction, overcrowding of referral centers, and reduced availability of surgical services in remote or rural locations.[136] Furthermore, there is no clear cut proof that a policy of regionalization would have the desired effects. Peterson and co-authors reviewed the STS National Cardiac Database to evaluate the relationship of CABG volume to outcome.[133] They found almost no potential benefit in closing low-volume centers. The wide variability in risk-adjusted mortality among hospitals with similar volume precluded the ability of hospital volume to discriminate those centers with significantly better or worse mortality. They suggested that procedural volume is not an adequate marker of quality for CABG surgery. Other authors reached similar conclusions regarding the limited ability of regionalization to impact outcomes.[137,138] Other more important process and structural variables are principle determinants of outcomes in CABG patients.

Human Factors Research and Performance Assessment

Surgeons make errors in the operating room. The causes of these errors and their ultimate impact on outcomes are an important measure of performance. Structured observation of surgeons by experts in human factor analysis can provide performance assessment and improve outcomes.[139] The airline industry had success in limiting errors by instituting human factor analysis of pilots during simulated flight. This industry is used as a model of successful implementation of error avoidance behavior and process improvement.[140] de Leval and co-authors applied these same principles of human factors analysis to pediatric cardiac surgery with some success.[141] They employed self-assessment questionnaires and human factors researchers who observed behavior in the operating room, an approach similar to the quality improvement steps used in the airline industry. Their study highlighted the important role of human factors in adverse surgical outcomes. More importantly, they found that appropriate behavioral responses in the operating room can mitigate potentially harmful events during operation. Such studies emphasize that human factors are associated with outcomes, both good and bad. Behavior modification and process improvement that involves human factor analysis hold great promise for future error reduction in cardiac surgery.

Public Reporting and Provider Accountability

Today there is an unprecedented call for accountability and public reporting. That call comes from consumer groups and insurers as it has in the past, but today it is coming from governmental organizations including the U.S. Congress as well. There is now federal legislative force mandating the collection and the release of this information. The Centers for Medicare and Medicaid Services (CMS), for example, made it quite clear that their upcoming "pay for performance" programs will include mandated public reporting of data.

The World Wide Web provides ready access to a wide variety of medical facts, particularly concerning cardiothoracic surgery. Simple Internet searches provide the public with literature reviews of particular procedures, the results of randomized trials, new innovations, and surgeon and hospital-specific outcomes. This ready public access will undoubtedly increase. There is limited external scrutiny or validation of many of the information sources. Most information available on these sites is accepted at face value by the public and quality control of the information sources is limited to self-imposed efforts on the part of the website authors. The *Agency for Healthcare Research and Quality* (AHRQ) attempted to empower the public to critically evaluate the various web-based sources of health care information in order to limit the spread of misinformation. The success of the AHRQ efforts is uncertain but becomes extremely critical as the amount of healthcare information available on the web skyrockets.

Despite shortcomings associated with web-based public information sources, the national cry for public reporting continues unabated. Recognizing the inevitability of this national movement, the Society of Thoracic Surgeons initiated a project to develop a public reporting format that contains clinical data that is meaningful, audited, totally transparent and clinically relevant both for physicians and for the public. In collaboration with *Consumers Union*, the well respected consumer rating organization, the STS began publishing the composite CABG results for those program participants that agreed to do so. This type of partnership may well become the paradigm for other professional organizations as they manage public reporting.

Information Management: Electronic Medical Records

Medical records are an invaluable source of information about patient risk factors and outcomes. Inevitably computer applications are applied to medical records. Pilot studies assessed the importance of computerized medical records in a variety of clinical situations. Perhaps the most important example of successful implementation of computerized medical records lies within the Veteran's Health Affairs (VHA) medical system in the United States.[142] Over a 20-year period the VHA system of hospitals completed a dramatic conversion from sub-standard care to a nationally recognized superb health care delivery system.[142] This transformation was aided, if not completely caused by, the implementation of a costly but highly successful computerized medical record system. Iezzoni pointed out the difficulties with computerized medical records and suggests that they may not adequately reflect the importance of chronic disability while at the same time prolonging the time that physicians spend documenting care into the computer system.[143] Yet the advantages of reduced medical errors, improved efficiency, and expanded access to medical information all overshadow most objections to implementation of an electronic information system.

Legislation likely to be passed by Congress allocates health care reforms that include an investment of $50 billion to promote health information technology.[144] Further, in its economic recovery package, the Obama administration plans to spend $19 billion to accelerate the use of computerized medical records in doctors' offices (http://www.nytimes.com/2009/03/01/business/01unbox.html).Medical experts agree that electronic patient records, when used wisely, can help curb costs and improve care. Pending legislation indicates that physicians will be paid a bonus only for the "meaningful use" of digital records, although the government has not yet defined that term precisely. The new legislation also calls for creation of "regional health I.T. extension centers" to help doctors in small office practices use electronic records.It is apparent that the need for data about large groups of patients exists, especially for managed care and capitation initiatives. It is reasonable to expect that efforts to computerize medical records will expand. Applications of electronic medical records that may be available in the future for cardiothoracic surgeons include monitoring of patient outcomes, supporting clinical decision making, and real-time tracking of resource utilization.

Computer applications were applied to the electronic medical record in hopes of minimizing physician errors in ordering. Computerized physician order entry (CPOE) is one of these applications that monitors and offers suggestions when physicians' orders do not meet a pre-designed computer algorithm. CPOE is viewed as a quality indicator and private employer-based organizations used the presence of CPOE to judge whether hospitals should be part of their preferred network (http://www.leapfroggroup.org/).One of these private groups is the Leapfrog Group and an initial survey by this Group in 2001 found that only 3.3% of responding hospitals currently had CPOE systems in place (http://www.ctsnet.org/reuters/reutersarticle.cfm?article=19325).In New York State, several large corporations and health-care insurers agreed to pay hospitals that meet the CPOE standards a bonus on all healthcare billings submitted. Other computer-based safety initiatives that involve the electronic medical record are likely to surface in the future. The impact of these innovations on the quality of health care is untested and any benefit remains to be proven.

The success of information technology used to reduce medical errors is mixed. Innovations that employ monitoring of electronic medical records may reduce errors.[145] However, with the increasing implementation of commercial CPOE systems in various settings of care evidence suggests that some implementation approaches may not achieve previously published results or may actually cause new errors or even harm.[146] Much work needs to be done before computer-aided methods lead to medical error reduction but the future will see more efforts of this type made. The increasing role of CPOE systems in health care invites much more scrutiny about the effectiveness of these systems in actual practice.

SUMMARY

Performance assessment and public reporting are here to stay, and they are likely to revolutionize the practice of medicine. Adequate risk adjustment is essential for outcomes analysis so that providers are not penalized when they care for severely ill patients. Composite performance measures, encompassing a broad spectrum of quality metrics, will be increasingly used. Cardiothoracic surgeons have been at the forefront of all these activities and innovations, but much work remains to be done. The ultimate goal of performance assessment is to improve patient care and to maintain the highest possible professional standards.

REFERENCES

1. Cohen IB: Florence Nightingale. *Sci Am*1984;250:128-137.
2. Moore W: *The Knife Man: The Extraordinary Life and Times of John Hunter, Father of Modern Surgery.* New York,Broadway Books,2005.
3. Codman E: *A Study in Hospital Efficiency as Demonstrated by the Case Report of the First Five Years of a Private Hospital.* Boston, Thomas Todd Company, 1917.
4. Daniels M, Hill A: Chemotherapy of pulmonary tuberculosis in young adults.An analysis of the combinedresults of three Medical Research Council trials. *Br Med J* 1952;1:1162.
5. Cochrane A: *Effectiveness & Efficiency.Random Reflections on Health Services.* London, Royal Society of Medicine Press Limited, 1971.
6. Donabedian A, Bashshur R: *An Introduction to Quality Assurance in Health Care.* New York, Oxford University Press, 2003.
7. Kohn LT, Corrigan J, Donaldson MS, Institute of Medicine (U.S.). Committee on Quality of Health Care in America: *To Err is Human: Building a Safer Health System.* Washington, DC, National Academy Press, 2000.
8. Birkmeyer JD, Dimick JB, Birkmeyer NJ: Measuring the quality of surgical care: structure, process, or outcomes? *J Am Coll Surg* 2004;198:626-632.
9. Kallis P, Unsworth-White J, Munsch C, et al: Disability and distress following cardiac surgery in patients over 70 years of age. *Eur J Cardiothorac Surg* 1993;7:306-311; discussion 312.
10. Herlitz J, Brandrup-Wognsen G, Evander MH, et al: Quality of life 15 years after coronary artery bypass grafting. *Coron Artery Dis* 2009; 20:363-369.
11. Krane M, Bauernschmitt R, Hiebinger A, et al: Cardiac reoperation in patients aged 80 years and older. *Ann Thorac Surg* 2009;87:1379-1385.
12. O'Brien SM, Shahian DM, Filardo G, et al: The Society of Thoracic Surgeons 2008 cardiac surgery risk models: part 2–isolated valve surgery. *Ann Thorac Surg* 2009;88:S23-42.
13. Shahian DM, O'Brien SM, Filardo G, et al: The Society of Thoracic Surgeons 2008 cardiac surgery risk models: part 1–coronary artery bypass grafting surgery. *Ann Thorac Surg* 2009;88:S2-22.
14. Shahian DM, O'Brien SM, Filardo G, et al: The Society of Thoracic Surgeons 2008 cardiac surgery risk models: part 3—valve plus coronary artery bypass grafting surgery. *Ann Thorac Surg* 2009;88:S43-62.
15. Kozower BD, Ailawadi G, Jones DR, et al: Predicted risk of mortality models: surgeons need to understand limitations of the University HealthSystem Consortium models. *J Am Coll Surg* 2009;209:551-556.
16. Steen PM, Brewster AC, Bradbury RC, Estabrook E, Young JA: Predicted probabilities of hospital death as a measure of admission severity of illness. *Inquiry* 1993;30:128-141.
17. Tu JV, Jaglal SB, Naylor CD: Multicenter validation of a risk index for mortality, intensive care unit stay, and overall hospital length of stay after cardiac surgery. Steering Committee of the Provincial Adult Cardiac Care Network of Ontario. *Circulation* 1995;91:677-684.
18. Knaus WA, Wagner DP, Draper EA, et al: The APACHE III prognostic system. Risk prediction of hospital mortality for critically ill hospitalized adults. *Chest* 1991;100:1619-1636.
19. Dupuis JY: Predicting outcomes in cardiac surgery: risk stratification matters? *Curr Opin Cardiol* 2008;23:560-567.
20. Blackstone EH: Breaking down barriers: helpful breakthrough statistical methods you need to understand better. *J Thorac Cardiovasc Surg* 2001;122:430-439.
21. Koch CG, Khandwala F, Nussmeier N, Blackstone EH: Gender and outcomes after coronary artery bypass grafting: a propensity-matched comparison. *J Thorac Cardiovasc Surg* 2003;126:2032-2043.
22. Iezzoni LI: *Risk adjustment for measuring health care outcomes,* 3rd ed. Chicago, Health Administration Press, 2003.
23. Zalkind DL, Eastaugh SR: Mortality rates as an indicator of hospital quality. *Hosp Health Serv Adm* 1997;42:3-415.
24. Park RE, Brook RH, Kosecoff J, et al: Explaining variations in hospital death rates. Randomness, severity of illness, quality of care. *JAMA* 1990;264:484-490.
25. Stewart AL, Greenfield S, Hays RD, et al: Functional status and well-being of patients with chronic conditions. Results from the Medical Outcomes Study. *JAMA*1989;262:907-913.
26. de Groot V, Beckerman H, Lankhorst GJ, Bouter LM: How to measure comorbidity: a critical review of available methods. *Journal of Clinical Epidemiology* 2003;56:221-229.

27. Woodworth GF, Baird CJ, Garces-Ambrossi G, Tonascia J, Tamargo RJ: Inaccuracy of the administrative database: comparative analysis of two databases for the diagnosis and treatment of intracranial aneurysms. *Neurosurgery* 2009;65:251-256; discussion 256-257.
28. Iezzoni LI, Daley J, Heeren T, et al: Using administrative data to screen hospitals for high complication rates. *Inquiry* 2000;31:40-55.
29. Tu JV, Sykora K, Naylor CD: Assessing the outcomes of coronary artery bypass graft surgery: how many risk factors are enough? Steering Committee of the Cardiac Care Network of Ontario. *J Am Coll Cardiol* 1997;30:1317-1323.
30. Jones RH, Hannan EL, Hammermeister KE, et al: Identification of preoperative variables needed for risk adjustment of short-term mortality after coronary artery bypass graft surgery. The Working Group Panel on the Cooperative CABG Database Project.*J Am Coll Cardiol* 1996; 28:1478-1487.
31. Lippmann RP, Shahian DM: Coronary artery bypass risk prediction using neural networks. *Ann Thorac Surg* 1997;63:1635-1643.
32. Ferraris VA, Ferraris SP: Assessing the medical literature: let the buyer beware. *Ann Thorac Surg* 2003;76:4-11.
33. Burns ER, Billett HH, Frater RW, Sisto DA: The preoperative bleeding time as a predictor of postoperative hemorrhage after cardiopulmonary bypass. *J Thorac Cardiovasc Surg* 1986;92:310-312.
34. Ferraris VA, Berry WR, Klingman RR: Comparison of blood reinfusion techniques used during coronary artery bypass grafting. *Ann Thorac Surg* 1993;56:433-439; discussion 440.
35. Ferraris VA, Gildengorin V: Predictors of excessive blood use after coronary artery bypass grafting. A multivariate analysis. *J Thorac Cardiovasc Surg* 1989;98:492-497.
36. Gewirtz AS, Miller ML, Keys TF: The clinical usefulness of the preoperative bleeding time. *Arch Patho lLab Med* 1996;120:353-356.
37. Freiman JA, Chalmers TC, Smith HJ, Kuebler RR: The importance of Beta, the type II error, and sample size in the design and interpretation of the randomized controlled trial.in Bailar JC, Mosteller F (eds):*Medical Uses of Statistics*. Boston, NEJM Books, 1992; pp 357-373.
38. Ferraris VA, Ferraris SP: Risk stratification and comorbidity,in Cohn LH, Edmunds LH (eds):*Cardiac Surgery in the Adult*. New York,McGraw-Hill, 2003, pp 187-224.
39. Cook NR: Use and misuse of the receiver operating characteristic curve in risk prediction. *Circulation* 2007;115:928-935.
40. Guadagnoli E, Hauptman PJ, Ayanian JZ, et al: Variation in the use of cardiac procedures after acute myocardial infarction. *NEJM* 1995;333: 573-578.
41. Tobler HG, Sethi GK, Grover FL, et al: Variations in processes and structures of cardiac surgery practice. *Medical Care* 1995;33:OS43-58.
42. Maddux FW, Dickinson TA, Rilla D, et al: Institutional variability of intraoperative red blood cell utilization in coronary artery bypass graft surgery. *Am J Med Qual* 2009;24:403-411.
43. Magner D, Mirocha J, Gewertz BL: Regional variation in the utilization of carotid endarterectomy. *J Vasc Surg* 2009;49:893-901; discussion 901.
44. Harris KM, Pastorius CA, Duval S, et al: Practice variation among cardiovascular physicians in management of patients with mitral regurgitation. *Am J Cardiol* 2009;103:255-261.
45. Schneider EC, Leape LL, Weissman JS, et al: Racial differences in cardiac revascularization rates: does "overuse" explain higher rates among white patients? *AnnIntern Med* 2001;135:328-337.
46. Philbin EF, McCullough PA, DiSalvo TG, et al: Underuse of invasive procedures among Medicaid patients with acute myocardial infarction. *Am J Public Health* 2001;91:1082-1088.
47. Filardo G, Maggioni AP, Mura G, et al: The consequences of under-use of coronary revascularization; results of a cohort study in Northern Italy. *Eur Heart J* 2001;22:654-662.
48. Alter DA, Austin PC, Tu JV: Community factors, hospital characteristics and inter-regional outcome variations following acute myocardial infarction in Canada. *Can J Cardiol* 2005;21:247-255.
49. Sonel AF, Good CB, Mulgund J, et al: Racial variations in treatment and outcomes of black and white patients with high-risk non-ST-elevation acute coronary syndromes: insights from CRUSADE (Can Rapid Risk Stratification of Unstable Angina Patients Suppress Adverse Outcomes With Early Implementation of the ACC/AHA Guidelines?). *Circulation* 2005;111:1225-1232.
50. Ferraris VA, Ferraris SP, Saha SP, et al: Perioperative blood transfusion and blood conservation in cardiac surgery: the Society of Thoracic Surgeons and The Society of Cardiovascular Anesthesiologists clinical practice guideline. *Ann Thorac Surg* 2007;83:S27-86.
51. Eagle KA, Guyton RA, Davidoff R, et al: ACC/AHA 2004 guideline update for coronary artery bypass graft surgery: summary article. A report of the American College of Cardiology/American Heart Association Task Force on Practice Guidelines (Committee to Update the 1999 Guidelines for Coronary Artery Bypass Graft Surgery). *J Am Coll Cardiol* 2004; 44:e213-310.
52. Tricoci P, Allen JM, Kramer JM, Califf RM, Smith SC, Jr.: Scientific evidence underlying the ACC/AHA clinical practice guidelines. *JAMA* 2009;301:831-841.
53. Shaneyfelt TM, Mayo-Smith MF, Rothwangl J: Are guidelines following guidelines? The methodological quality of clinical practice guidelines in the peer-reviewed medical literature. *JAMA*1999;281: 1900-1905.
54. Enhancing the use of clinical guidelines: a social norms perspective. *J Am Coll Surg* 2006;202:826-836.
55. Goodnough LT, Despotis GJ: Establishing practice guidelines for surgical blood management. *Am J Surg* 1995;170:16S-20S.
56. Stover EP, Siegel LC, Body SC, et al: Institutional variability in red blood cell conservation practices for coronary artery bypass graft surgery. Institutions of the MultiCenter Study of Perioperative Ischemia Research Group. *J Cardiothorac Vasc Anesth* 2000;14:171-176.
57. Austin PC: The relative ability of different propensity score methods to balance measured covariates between treated and untreated subjects in observational studies. *Med Decis Making* 2009;29:661-677.
58. Barbour G: The role of outcomes data in health care reform. *Ann Thorac Surg* 1994;58:1881-1884.
59. Albanese M, Mejicano G, Xakellis G, Kokotailo P: Physician practice change I: a critical review and description of an Integrated Systems Model. *Acad Med* 2009;84:1043-1055.
60. Lenfant C: Shattuck lecture—clinical research to clinical practice—lost in translation? *NEJM* 2003;349:868-874.
61. Heffner JE: Altering physician behavior to improve clinical performance. *Top Health Inf Manage* 2001;22:1-9.
62. Anonymous: The oversight of medical care: a proposal for reform. American College of Physicians. *Ann Intern Med* 1994;120:423-431.
63. Shahian DM, Edwards FH, Ferraris VA, et al: Quality measurement in adult cardiac surgery: part 1—Conceptual framework and measure selection. *Ann Thorac Surg* 2007;83:S3-12.
64. Casale AS, Paulus RA, Selna MJ, et al: "ProvenCareSM": a provider-driven pay-for-performance program for acute episodic cardiac surgical care. *Ann Surg* 2007;246:613-621; discussion 621-613.
65. Karve AM, Ou FS, Lytle BL, Peterson ED: Potential unintended financial consequences of pay-for-performance on the quality of care for minority patients. *Am Heart J* 2008;155:571-576.
66. Daley J: Criteria by which to evaluate risk-adjusted outcomes programs in cardiac surgery. *Ann Thorac Surg* 1994;58:1827-1835.
67. Daley J: Validity of risk-adjustment methods,in Iezzoni LI (ed):*Risk Adjustment for Measuring Healthcare Outcomes*. Chicago, Health Administration Press, 1997; pp 331-363.
68. Ferraris VA, Ferraris SP: Risk factors for postoperative morbidity. *J Thorac Cardiovasc Surg* 1996;111:731-738;discussion 738-741.
69. Shroyer ALW, Coombs LP, Peterson ED, et al: The Society of Thoracic Surgeons: 30-day operative mortality and morbidity risk models. *Ann Thorac Surg* 2003;75:1856-1864; discussion 1864-1855.
70. Lee TH, Shammash JB, Ribeiro JP: Estimation of maximum oxygen uptake from clinical data: performance of the Specific Activity Scale. *Am Heart J* 1988;115:203-204.
71. Ware JE, Sherbourne CD: The MOS 36-item short-form health survey (SF-36). I. Conceptual framework and item selection. *Med Care* 1992;30:473-483.
72. Lee TH, American College of Cardiology. Private Sector Relations Committee: *Evaluating the Quality of Cardiovascular Care: a Primer*. Bethesda, MD, American College of Cardiology, 1995.
73. Cope DW, Linn LS, Leake BD, Barrett PA: Modification of residents' behavior by preceptor feedback of patient satisfaction. *J Gen Intern Med* 1986;1:394-398.
74. Peric V, Borzanovic M, Stolic R, et al: Quality of life in patients related to gender differences before and after coronary artery bypass surgery. *Interact Cardiovasc ThoracSurg* 2010; 10:232-238.
75. Lee GA: Determinants of quality of life five years after coronary artery bypass graft surgery. *Heart Lung* 2009;38:91-99.
76. Tully PJ, Baker RA, Turnbull DA, et al: Negative emotions and quality of life six months after cardiac surgery: the dominant role of depression not anxiety symptoms. *J Behav Med* 2009; 32:510-522.
77. Jideus L, Liss A, Stahle E: Patients with sternal wound infection after cardiac surgery do not improve their quality of life. *Scand Cardiovasc J* 2009;43:194-200.
78. Loponen P, Luther M, Korpilahti K, et al: HRQoL after coronary artery bypass grafting and percutaneous coronary intervention for stable angina. *Scand Cardiovasc J* 2009;43:94-99.

79. Guadagnoli E, Ayanian JZ, Cleary PD: Comparison of patient-reported outcomes after elective coronary artery bypass grafting in patients aged greater than or equal to and less than 65 years. *Am J Cardiol* 1992; 70:60-64.
80. Rumsfeld JS, Magid DJ, O'Brien M, et al.: Changes in health-related quality of life following coronary artery bypass graft surgery. *Annals of Thoracic Surgery.* 2001;72:2026-2032.
81. Rumsfeld JS, MaWhinney S, McCarthy M, et al: Health-related quality of life as a predictor of mortality following coronary artery bypass graft surgery. Participants of the Department of Veterans Affairs Cooperative Study Group on Processes, Structures, and Outcomes of Care in Cardiac Surgery. *JAMA*1999;281:1298-1303.
82. O'Brien SM, Shahian DM, DeLong ER, et al: Quality measurement in adult cardiac surgery: part 2—Statistical considerations in composite measure scoring and provider rating. *Ann Thorac Surg* 2007;83:S13-26.
83. Smith PK, Mayer JE, Jr., Kanter KR, et al: Physician payment for 2007: a description of the process by which major changes in valuation of cardiothoracic surgical procedures occurred. *Ann Thorac Surg* 2007; 83:12-20.
84. Deming WE: *Out of the Crisis.* Cambridge, MA, Massachusetts Institute of Technology Center for Advanced Engineering Study, 1986.
85. Juran JM: *A History of Managing for Quality: The Evolution, Trends, and Future Directions of Managing for Quality.* Milwaukee, WI, ASQC Quality Press, 1995.
86. Berwick DM, Godfrey AB, Roessner J, National Demonstration Project on Quality Improvement in Health Care: *Curing Health Care: New Strategies for Quality Improvement.* San Francisco, Jossey-Bass, 1990.
87. O'Connor GT, Plume SK, Olmstead EM, et al: Multivariate prediction of in-hospital mortality associated with coronary artery bypass graft surgery. Northern New England Cardiovascular Disease Study Group. *Circulation* 1992;85:2110-2118.
88. O'Connor GT, Plume SK, Olmstead EM, et al: A regional prospective study of in-hospital mortality associated with coronary artery bypass grafting. The Northern New England Cardiovascular Disease Study Group. *JAMA*1991;266:803-809.
89. O'Connor GT, Plume SK, Olmstead EM, et al: A regional intervention to improve the hospital mortality associated with coronary artery bypass graft surgery. The Northern New England Cardiovascular Disease Study Group. *JAMA*1996;275:841-846.
90. Birkmeyer NJ, Charlesworth DC, Hernandez F, et al: Obesity and risk of adverse outcomes associated with coronary artery bypass surgery. Northern New England Cardiovascular Disease Study Group. *Circulation* 1998;97:1689-1694.
91. Braxton JH, Marrin CA, McGrath PD, et al: 10-year follow-up of patients with and without mediastinitis. *Semin Thorac Cardiovasc Surg* 2004;16:70-76.
92. Hernandez F, Cohn WE, Baribeau YR, et al: In-hospital outcomes of off-pump versus on-pump coronary artery bypass procedures: a multicenter experience. *Ann Thorac Surg* 2001;72:1528-1533; discussion 1533-1524.
93. Green J, Wintfeld N: Report Cards on Cardiac-Surgeons—Assessing New-York States Approach. *NEJM* 1995;332:1229-1232.
94. Omoigui N, Annan K, Brown K, et al: Potential explanation for decreased CABG-related mortality in NewYorkState: outmigration to Ohio. *Circulation* 1994;90:93.
95. Ferraris VA: The dangers of gathering data. *J Thorac Cardiovasc Surg* 1992;104:212-213.
96. Morgan RO, Virnig BA, DeVito CA, Persily NA: The Medicare-HMO revolving door—the healthy go in and the sick go out. *NEJM* 1997;337:169-175.
97. Schneider EC, Epstein AM: Use of public performance reports: a survey of patients undergoing cardiac surgery. *JAMA* 1998;279:1638-1642.
98. Schneider EC, Epstein AM: Influence of cardiac-surgery performance reports on referral practices and access to care. A survey of cardiovascular specialists. *NEJM* 1996;335:251-256.
99. Burack JH, Impellizzeri P, Homel P, Cunningham JN, Jr: Public reporting of surgical mortality: a survey of New York State cardiothoracic surgeons. *Ann Thorac Surg* 1999;68:1195-1200; discussion 1201-1192.
100. Dranove D, Kessler D, McClellan M, Satterthwaite M: Is more information better? The effects of 'report cards' on health care providers. *JPolitical Economy* 2003;111:555-588.
101. Moscucci M, Eagle KA, Share D, et al: Public reporting and case selection for percutaneous coronary interventions: an analysis from two large multicenter percutaneous coronary intervention databases. *J Am Coll Cardiol* 2005;45:1759-1765.
102. Apolito RA, Greenberg MA, Menegus MA, et al: Impact of the New York State Cardiac Surgery and Percutaneous Coronary Intervention Reporting System on the management of patients with acute myocardial infarction complicated by cardiogenic shock. *Am Heart J* 2008;155:267-273.
103. Resnic FS, Welt FG: The public health hazards of risk avoidance associated with public reporting of risk-adjusted outcomes in coronary intervention. *J Am Coll Cardiol* 2009;53:825-830.
104. Narins CR, Dozier AM, Ling FS, Zareba W: The influence of public reporting of outcome data on medical decision making by physicians. *Arch Intern Med* 2005;165:83-87.
105. Glance LG, Dick A, Mukamel DB, et al: Are high-quality cardiac surgeons less likely to operate on high-risk patients compared to low-quality surgeons? Evidence from New York State. *Health Serv Res* 2008;43:300-312.
106. Daley J: Validity of risk-adjustment methods,in Iezzoni L (ed):*Risk Adjustment for Measuring Health Care Outcomes.* Ann Arbor, MI, Health Administration Press, 1994; p 239.
107. Shahian DM, Silverstein T, Lovett AF: Comparison of clinical and administrative data sources for hospital coronary artery bypass graft surgery report cards. *Circulation* 2007;115:1518-1527.
108. Jollis JG, Ancukiewicz M, DeLong ER: Discordance of databases designed for claims payment versus clinical information systems. Implications for outcomes research. *Ann Intern Med* 1993;119:844-850.
109. Blumberg MS: Comments on HCFA hospital death rate statistical outliers. Health Care Financing Administration. *Health Serv Res* 1987; 21:715-739.
110. Dubois RW: Hospital mortality as an indicator of quality,in Goldfield N, Nash DB (eds):*Providing Quality Care.* Philadelphia, American College of Physicians, 1989; pp 107-131.
111. Podolsky D, Beddingfield KT: America's best hospitals. *U.S. News and World Report* 1993;115:66.
112. Shahian DM, Torchiana DF, Normand SL: Implementation of a cardiac surgery report card: lessons from the Massachusetts experience. *Ann Thorac Surg* 2005;80:1146-1150.
113. Hannan EL, Kumar D, Racz M, Siu AL, Chassin MR: New York State's Cardiac Surgery Reporting System: four years later. *Ann Thorac Surg.* 1994;58:1852-1857.
114. Shahian DM, Torchiana DF, Shemin RJ, Rawn JD, Normand SL: Massachusetts cardiac surgery report card: implications of statistical methodology. *Ann Thorac Surg* 2005;80:2106-2113.
115. Goldstein H, Spiegelhalter DJ: League tables and their limitations:statistical issues in comparisons of institutional performance (with discussion). *J R Stat Soc (Series A)* 1996;159:385-443.
116. Woolhandler S, Himmelstein DU: Costs of care and administration at for-profit and other hospitals in the United States. *NEJM* 1997;336:769-774.
117. Anonymous: Iowa:Classic test of a future concept. *Medical Outcomes & Guidelines Alert* 1995:8.
118. Tu JV, Donovan LR, Lee DS, et al: Effectiveness of public report cards for improving the quality of cardiac care: the EFFECT study: a randomized trial. *JAMA* 2009;302:2330-2337.
119. Jacobs JP, Cerfolio RJ, Sade RM: The ethics of transparency: publication of cardiothoracic surgical outcomes in the lay press. *Ann Thorac Surg* 2009;87:679-686.
120. Spiegelhalter DJ: Funnel plots for comparing institutional performance. *Stat Med* 2005;24:1185-1202.
121. Brennan TA, Gawande A, Thomas E, Studdert D: Accidental deaths, saved lives, and improved quality. *NEJM* 2005;353:1405-1409.
122. Leape LL, Berwick DM: Five years after To Err Is Human: what have we learned? *JAMA*2005;293:2384-2390.
123. Kolata G: Program Coaxes Hospitals to See Treatments Under Their Noses *New York Times on the web.* New York.December 25, 2004.
124. Leape LL, Weissman JS, Schneider EC, et al: Adherence to practice guidelines: the role of specialty society guidelines. *Am Heart J* 2003;145:19-26.
125. Patel MR, Dehmer GJ, Hirshfeld JW, Smith PK, Spertus JA: ACCF/SCAI/STS/AATS/AHA/ASNC 2009 Appropriateness Criteria for Coronary Revascularization: a report by the American College of Cardiology Foundation Appropriateness Criteria Task Force, Society for Cardiovascular Angiography and Interventions, Society of Thoracic Surgeons, American Association for Thoracic Surgery, American Heart Association, and the American Society of Nuclear Cardiology endorsed by the American Society of Echocardiography, the Heart Failure Society of America, and the Society of Cardiovascular Computed Tomography. *J Am Coll Cardiol* 2009;53:530-553.
126. Petitti D: *Meta-Analysis, Decision Analysis, and Cost-Effectiveness Analysis.* Vol 31, 2nd ed. New York, Oxford University Press, 2000.
127. Hunink MG: In search of tools to aid logical thinking and communicating about medical decision making. *Med Decis Making* 2001;21:267-277.
128. Gage BF, Cardinalli AB, Albers GW, Owens DK: Cost-effectiveness of warfarin and aspirin for prophylaxis of stroke in patients with nonvalvular atrial fibrillation. *JAMA*1995;274:1839-1845.

129. Breiman L: Statistical modeling: the two cultures. *Stat Sci* 2001;16:199-231.
130. Shahian DM: Improving cardiac surgery quality—volume, outcome, process? *JAMA* 2004;291:246-248.
131. Shahian DM, Normand SL: The volume-outcome relationship: from Luft to Leapfrog. *Ann Thorac Surg* 2003;75:1048-1058.
132. Shahian DM, Normand SL: Low-volume coronary artery bypass surgery: measuring and optimizing performance. *J Thorac Cardiovasc Surg* 2008;135:1202-1209.
133. Peterson ED, Coombs LP, DeLong ER, Haan CK, Ferguson TB: Procedural volume as a marker of quality for CABG surgery. *JAMA* 2004;291:195-201.
134. Zacharias A, Schwann TA, Riordan CJ, et al: Is hospital procedure volume a reliable marker of quality for coronary artery bypass surgery? A comparison of risk and propensity adjusted operative and midterm outcomes. *Ann Thorac Surg* 2005;79:1961-1969.
135. Nallamothu BK, Saint S, Ramsey SD, et al: The role of hospital volume in coronary artery bypass grafting: Is more always better? *J Am Coll Cardiol* 2001;38:1923-1930.
136. Nallamothu BK, Eagle KA, Ferraris VA, Sade RM: Should coronary artery bypass grafting be regionalized? *Ann Thorac Surg* 2005;80:1572-1581.
137. Rathore SS, Epstein AJ, Volpp KG, Krumholz HM: Hospital coronary artery bypass graft surgery volume and patient mortality, 1998-2000. *Ann Surg* 2004;239:110-117.
138. Hannan EL: Workshop summary,in Hewitt M, America CoQoHCi, Board NCP (eds):*Interpreting the Volume-Outcome Relationship in the Context of Health Care Quality: Workshop Summary.* Washington, DC, Institute of Medicine, 2000; p 11.
139. Carthey J: The role of structured observational research in health care. *Qual Saf Health Care* 2003;12 Suppl 2:ii13-16.
140. Richardson WC, Berwick DM, Bisgard JC, et al: The Institute of Medicine Report on Medical Errors: misunderstanding can do harm. Quality of Health Care in America Committee. 2000:E42.
141. de-Leval MR, Carthey J, Wright DJ, Farewell VT, Reason JT: Human factors and cardiac surgery: a multicenter study. *J Thorac Cardiovasc Surg* 2000;119:661-672.
142. Longman P: *Best care anywhere: why VA health care is better than yours.* Sausalito, CA, PoliPointPress,Distributed by Publishers Group West, 2007.
143. Iezzoni L: Measuring the severity of illness and case mix,in Goldfield ND (ed):*Providing Quality Care: The Challenge to Clinicians.* Philadelphia, American College of Physicians, 1989:70-105.
144. D'Avolio LW: Electronic medical records at a crossroads: impetus for change or missed opportunity? *JAMA* 2009;302:1109-1111.
145. Langdorf MI, Fox JC, Marwah RS, Montague BJ, Hart MM: Physician versus computer knowledge of potential drug interactions in the emergency department. *Acad Emerg Med* 2000;7:1321-1329.
146. Classen DC, Avery AJ, Bates DW: Evaluation and certification of computerized provider order entry systems. *J Am Med Inform Assoc* 2007; 14:48-55.
147. Grunkemeier GL, Zerr KJ, Jin R: Cardiac surgery report cards:making the grade. *Ann Thorac Surg* 2001;72:1845-1848.
148. Lahey SJ, Borlase BC, Lavin PT, Levitsky S: Preoperative risk factors that predict hospital length of stay in coronary artery bypass patients > 60 years old. *Circulation* 1992;86:II181-185.
149. Hammermeister KE, Johnson R, Marshall G, Grover FL: Continuous assessment and improvement in quality of care. A model from the Department of Veterans Affairs Cardiac Surgery. *Ann Surg* 1994;219: 281-290.

CHAPTER 8

Statistical Treatment of Surgical Outcome Data

Ruyun Jin
Gary L. Grunkemeier

INTRODUCTION

The results (outcome) of cardiac surgery can be measured in several ways. The type of variable used as the measure of a particular outcome determines the statistical methods that should be used for its analysis. For example, some administrative outcomes are captured by continuous variables, such as hospital charges (in dollars) or length of stay (in days). Other outcomes are collected as categorical variables, such as discharge destination (eg, acute-care facility, specialized nursing facility, or home). Health-related quality of life is another kind of outcome, which is often measured by the Medical Outcome Study (MOS) 36-Item Short-Form Health Survey (SF-36),[1] the Sickness Impact Profile,[2] or disease-specific quality-of-life measures, and can be transferred to quality-adjusted life years (QALYs).[3] Economic endpoints have been used increasingly, such as cost-effective ratio.[4]

However, the major outcomes of interest to clinicians are described by variables that indicate the occurrence of (usually adverse) events, such as death, stroke, infection, reoperation, etc. Statistically, we must differentiate between two fundamentally different types of events based on their timing: *early (one-time) events* and *late (time-related) events*. Different types of analyses are used for these two types of events. We divide the areas of statistical inquiry into three major categories based on the goals of the analysis: *summarize*, *compare*, and *model*. This chapter will describe and illustrate the statistical methods used most often in each situation.

EVENT TYPES

Early, One-Time Events

In cardiac surgery, early events are those occurring within 30 days of surgery or before hospital discharge, whichever is later. By the time of the analysis, the early outcome of every patient presumably is known. Thus, every patient has a "yes" or "no" value for the event being studied, and an estimate of the probability of the event can be determined by the ratio of patients with the event to total patients, usually multiplied by 100 and expressed as a percentage.

Late, Time-Related Events

Late events are those that occur after discharge and more than 30 days after surgery. The analysis of these events is complicated by two considerations. First, the time of occurrence must be taken into account because, for example, a death at 6 months will have a different effect on the analysis than a death at 6 years. Second, in the usual ongoing analysis, some patients will have experienced a late event, whereas others will not have experienced an event but are still alive and at risk for the event and may have it in the future. Their event status is termed *censored*, which means that it is known not to have occurred by the time of the latest follow-up. For example, a patient in the study who had surgery 5 years ago and is still alive has a time of death that is not yet known. But we have partial information about his or her survival time, namely, that it exceeds, or is *censored* at, 5 years. When dealing with censored data, it is necessary to use special statistical methods. It is not appropriate, for example, to summarize late mortality by a simple percentage such as the number of late deaths divided by the number of patients. Mortality varies over, and must be related to, postoperative time. The simple "late mortality" percentage in any series of patients will be 100% if the investigator waits long enough.

ANALYSIS GOALS

Statistics are derived for many purposes of varying complexity. The most common ones used for evaluating cardiac surgery are (1) to *summarize* the results from a single series, (2) to *compare* the results between two or more series or subgroups of the same series based on a single discriminating variable or risk factor, and (3) to construct a multivariable *model* that considers the simultaneous effect of many risk factors.

Summarize

A study usually includes series of patients, and rather than listing a particular variable of interest for each individual, the first use of statistics is to summarize the variable for the entire group with a single, representative number (statistic). The sample *average*, or *mean value*, and the *median* (50th percentile) provide a measure of central tendency; the *standard deviation* and the *interquartile range* measure the dispersion of the individual values. A single-valued estimate such as this is called a *point estimate*, but, acknowledging the imprecision of a single estimated value, a range of estimate values should also be given. The *standard error* (SE) is a measure of the precision of an estimate, and a *confidence interval* (CI), a range of values for the estimate that is consistent with the observed data, can be constructed using its SE or in other, often better ways.

Compare

A study often consists of evaluating subgroups of patients who received different treatments. Thus, in addition to summarizing the outcomes from the subgroups, we are interested in comparing their summary statistics. To do so, we typically compute another statistic that combines data from both groups and that follows (often approximately) some known statistical reference distribution, such as a *normal* (bell-shaped) or other (*chi-square*, *t*, etc) distribution. We then see how extreme or improbable the value computed from our data would be in that reference distribution if there were in fact no difference between the two groups we are comparing. This probability is called the *p-value*, and when it is smaller than .05 (5%), the difference we have observed is said to be *statistically significant*. This value (.05) is a completely arbitrary number, although in practice it is applied almost universally. Note that the level of significance is inversely related to the sample size. A given difference, no matter how small, will be statistically significant ($p < .05$) if the sample size is large enough. Conversely, a large different will not be significant if the sample size is too small. Thus, the *clinical importance* of a given difference is more important than the *statistical significance* of that difference.

A different paradigm for making comparisons and constructing CIs that has gained much prominence with the availability of computing power and specific software is the *bootstrapping* technique.[5] Instead of using an assumed statistical distribution, it generates many repeated random samples from the data themselves to produce the reference distribution.

Model: Multivariable Regression

Comparing the outcomes between two groups based on a single factor, as described in the preceding section, is called *univariable* (or sometimes *bivariable*) *analysis*, to distinguish it from *multivariable analysis*, in which several characteristics of each subgroup are considered simultaneously. Most clinical studies are based on observational data collected in the normal delivery of care, and the patient subgroups may differ with regard to several influential characteristics. A multiple regression analysis can determine the influence of the treatment under study on the outcome variable after simultaneously adjusting for these potential patient differences. The result is a statistical model that consists of the group of factors that significantly affects the outcome and which may or may not ultimately include the treatment being studied. Each factor is assigned a coefficient that indicates the amount of weight given to that factor in the model. The model hopefully gives us a fuller understanding of the interrelationship among the treatment being studied, the outcome variable, and other important risk factors. One can compute the expected outcome for any patient using these weights applied to the values of that patient's particular set of risk factors.

MATERIALS AND METHODS

Clinical Material

To describe and illustrate the statistical methods used most frequently in the cardiac surgical literature, we will use a historical data set of mitral valve replacements with Starr-Edwards (S-E) heart valves. Dr. Albert Starr and his group at the Oregon Health Sciences University and Providence St. Vincent Medical Center in Portland, Oregon, implanted 1255 S-E mitral valves in adult patients (age >20 years old) from 1965 to 1994.[6] A prospective lifetime follow-up service was implemented for every patient. The total follow-up through 2002 was 11,621 patient-years, with a maximum of 37 years. (*Note:* In all figures in this chapter, we have plotted the curves only up the time where more than 20 patients were at risk because the estimates beyond that time are imprecisely determined.) Table 8-1 contains a summary of the selected four variables (*Disclaimer:* More variables ordinarily would be considered in a real study than in this simple expository exercise. The data set used in this chapter was chosen only to illustrate the statistical methods.) Several valve models are represented in this group: "FINAL S-E valve model" refers to the Model 6120 valve, which is the most recently used model of the S-E valve; "PREVIOUS S-E valve model" refers to all the other models, which were discontinued. Patients in the FINAL valve model group have a higher mean age, more valve re-replacement surgery, and more concomitant coronary artery bypass grafting (CABG).

Statistical Software

Most of the statistical methods described in this chapter are available in the commonly used statistical software package. The statistical analyses and graphics in this chapter were done using PASW Statistics 17 (SPSS, Inc., Chicago, IL), Stata 10.1 (Stata Corp., College Station, TX), S-PLUS 6.2 (Insightful Corp., Seattle, WA), and the open-source program R version 2.10.0 (R Foundation for Statistical Computing, Vienna, Austria, www.R-project.org).

TABLE 8-1 Mitral Valve Clinical Material and Univariable Comparison of Early Mortality by Valve Model

	Previous	Final
Clinical material		
Number of patients	543	712
Mean age ± S.D. (years)	53.0 ± 10.8	60.3 ± 11.3
Female (%)	60.6	61.8
Re-replacement (%)	4.6	6.9
Concomitant CABG (%)	10.1	20.2
Early mortality		
Number of deaths	25	58
Point estimate (%)	4.6	8.1
Standard error (%)	0.9	1.0
95% confidence interval (%)		
Normal approximation	(2.8, 6.4)	(6.4, 10.2)
Exact binomial	(3.0, 6.7)	(6.2, 10.4)
Comparison statistics	*p*-value (2-sided)	
Pearson chi-square	0.012	
With continuity correction	0.017	
Fisher's exact test	0.016	

The only functionality not found in standard statistical packages is cumulative incidence ("Actual") analysis. Cumulative incidence in the presence of competing events is implemented in the Stata ado file *stcompet*.[7] In addition, Stata version 11 has just included *stcurve* and *stcrreg* for computing and comparing cumulative curves.

Cumulative incidence is also available for S-PLUS and R with the package *cmprsk*.[8] Finally, the NCSS Statistical Analysis System (NCSS, Kaysville, UT) does implement this function directly.

EARLY EVENTS

We will use operative deaths to illustrate the statistical treatment of early events.

Summarize

The *mean* (point estimate) operative mortality is computed as the number of operative deaths divided by the number of patients. Multiplying by 100 converts this decimal to a percentage (P). The SE of a proportion P based on N patients equals the square root of $P(1 - P)/N$. Thus, as shown in Table 8-1, the percentages of patients with early death are 4.6% (SE = 0.9%) and 8.1% (SE = 1.0%) for the PREVIOUS and the FINAL valve model groups, respectively. Table 8-1 also contains the 95% CI, computed by two popular methods. The first method is the simple (asymptotic) method based on the fact that the *binomial* distribution, which governs proportions, can be approximated by the normal (bell-shaped) distribution as the sample size increases.[9] This CI is computed easily as the point estimate plus and minus twice the SE. A second method uses the (exact) binomial distribution directly.[10] Although the "exact" method sounds like it obviously would be the most desirable, there are other methods that may have better statistical properties.[11]

Compare

To demonstrate a *univariable* comparison, operative mortality between the two valve model groups was used. This does not seem very interesting clinically because valve model should have little to do with operative mortality; nevertheless, many valve comparison papers attempt to draw clinical conclusions from just such questionable comparisons. Comparing two proportions gives rise to a matrix with two rows (for the two valve groups) and two columns (for the two possible outcomes) called a *two-by-two contingency table.* Several methods have been used to assess the significance of such tables.[12] The most common method for extracting a *p*-value from such a matrix is the *(Pearson) chi-square test.* This test has an alternative, more conservative form using a *continuity correction.* Validity of the chi-square test depends on having an adequate sample size (technically, each cell of the table should have an expected size of at least 5), and when this is not the case, the *Fisher's exact test* is often used. All three tests find that the FINAL valve model has significantly higher operative mortality because the *p*-values are smaller than .05 (see Table 8-1).

Model

Logistic Regression

The simple comparison above showed that operative mortality with the FINAL valve model was significantly higher than with the PREVIOUS valve model. But patients with the FINAL valve model were older and had more concomitant CABG and re-replacement operations (see Table 8-1). Could the apparent difference in operative mortality between valve models be a result of these patient characteristics, instead of the valve itself? We explore this possibility using a multivariable analysis.

For binary (dichotomous) outcomes such as operative mortality, the most common method for developing a multivariable model is *logistic regression.*[13] In this model, operative death is the outcome (*dependent variable*), and patient characteristics, plus valve model, are the potential risk factors (*independent variables*). For technical reasons, logistic regression does not use the probability (p) of death directly as the dependent variable in the model. Instead, it uses the logarithm of the *odds* $p/(1 - p)$

of death. To facilitate interpretation of a regression coefficient (B) from such a model, the coefficient can be converted into an *odds ratio* (OR) by using the exponential function. Most statistical programs do this automatically, and the ORs are sometimes labeled exp(B). The 95% CI for the OR is computed as the exponential of the normal approximation CI (mean plus and minus twice the SE) for the coefficient itself.

A stepwise regression program begins with a univariable test of each potential risk factor,[13] using a model with a single variable to get the OR and p-value associated with that variable. If the OR is greater than 1, that variable is a risk factor (meaning that it adds to the risk). If the OR is less than 1, it is a protective factor. For the heart valve example (Table 8-2), age, concomitant CABG, and valve model are statistically significant (their p-values are less than .05). These variables, plus any others showing a trend toward association with operative mortality (usually $p < .2$), would be included in the next step of the stepwise logistic regression. In the final regression model, only age and concomitant CABG are still significant (see Table 8-2). After those effects are accounted for, the effect of valve model is no longer significant ($p = .515$). Thus, by this analysis, the apparent increase in operative mortality in the FINAL valve model group seems to be an artifact; FINAL valve model is apparently a surrogate for older age and more bypass surgery, which themselves are primarily responsible for the increased mortality. There are no doubt other clinical variables to consider in this model, but because we used the data only for demonstration purposes, not all possible variables were included. As a rule of thumb, 10 events can support one risk factor considered in a risk model.[14] In our data set, there are 83 operative deaths, so we would have been justified in considering about eight risk factors. In practice, researchers would reference the published models and study their own data to select more variables for consideration.

The OR of a binary variable such as concomitant CABG (2.76 in Table 8-2) means that the odds of mortality for a patient having concomitant CABG are 2.76 times those of a patient not undergoing concomitant CABG. This is the point estimate; the interval estimate (see Table 8-2) ranges from 1.69 to 4.52. When the lower limit of the 95% CI is greater than 1 (as it is for concomitant CABG, ie, 1.69), the OR will be significantly greater than 1. For a continuous variable such as age, the OR of 1.04 means that for each year of age, the odds of an operative death are multiplied by 1.04.

Evaluating the Risk Model

Discrimination: Receiver Operating Characteristic(ROC) Curve. The discrimination of a risk model is the ability to separate those who will have an event from those who will not. Traditionally, the discrimination is evaluated by the c-index, which is the area under the receiver operating characteristic (ROC) curve,[15] This is the probability that a death will have a higher risk score than a survivor. Generally, a c-index between 0.7 and 0.8 is considered acceptable discrimination, a c-index between 0.8 and 0.9 is considered excellent discrimination, and a c-index greater than 0.9 is considered outstanding discrimination.[16]

Calibration: Hosmer-Lemeshow Statistics. Calibration is the measure of how close the predictions are to reality. For example, if 100 patients had risks of 5% from a well-calibrated model, then 5 of them would be expected to die. Calibration is evaluated by the Hosmer-Lemeshow (H-L) statistic, which computes the significance of the difference between the observed and expected events.[17] If the H-L statistic is significant ($p < .05$), it may be a sign of poor calibration. For our final model in Table 8-2, the c-index is 0.710 (95% CI 0.653–0.767) and the H-L statistic is $p = .365$. These values can be considered optimistic, however, because the data used to generate the model also were used to test it. Ideally, one would use a different data set, or bootstrap resampling of the original data, to test the model.[18] There are some technical issues with the H-L statistic.[19-21] Accordingly, in the next section we introduce a visual, continuous analog of the H-L test using the CUSUM methodology.

Using the Model for Risk-Adjusted Provider Comparisons

O/E Ratio. The predicted (expected) mortality from logistic regression can be used to compare the risk-adjusted performance between groups of patients, eg, to compare different surgical techniques or different providers. If the ratio of observed (O) to expected (E) mortality, the *O/E ratio*, is greater than 1, then there are more deaths than expected by the model, and if the *O/E* ratio is less than 1, there are fewer deaths than expected. The CI of the *O/E* ratio can be calculated by using a normal approximation method, which, as usual, gives a symmetric interval around the point estimate, or by using a logarithmic transformation, which provides a more appropriate

TABLE 8-2 Univariable and Multivariable (Logistic Regression) Modeling of Early Mortality

	Univariable		Multivariable			
Variable	p-value	Odds Ratio	Coefficient	SE	p-value	Odds Ratio (95% CI)
Age	<.001	1.05	0.045	0.012	<.001	1.04 (1.02, 1.07)
Concomitant CABG	<.001	3.78	1.016	0.251	<.001	2.76 (1.69, 4.52)
FINAL valve model	.014	1.84			(.515)	
Female gender	.361	0.81				
Re-replacement	.314	1.52				

TABLE 8-3 Ratio of Observed to Expected Early Mortality (O/E ratio)

Valve Model	Previous	Final
Observed mortality	25/543 = 4.6%	58/712 = 8.1%
Expected mortality	27.5/543 = 5.1%	55.5/712 = 7.8%
O/E ratio	0.91	1.05
95% confidence interval		
Normal approximation	(0.55, 1.27)	(0.80, 1.29)
Log transformation	(0.61, 1.35)	(0.83, 1.32)
Odds ratio	0.90	1.05
95% confidence interval	(0.60, 1.35)	(0.80, 1.38)

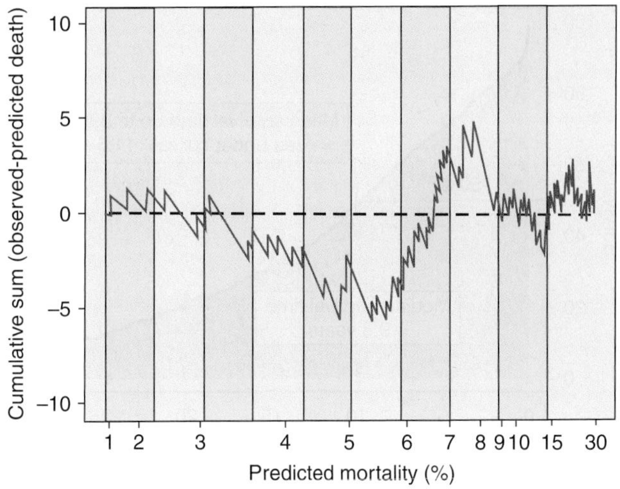

FIGURE 8-1 CUSUM plot of operative death. Vertical axis is the cumulative sum of observed deaths minus predicted deaths by the logistic regression model in Table 8-2. The horizontal axis is scaled in number of patients (ordered by the predicted risk), so it is nonlinear in predicted risk of death. The blue/white bars each contain 10% of the patients.

asymmetric interval.[22,23] Table 8-3 contains these values for our heart valve example. The CIs for the *O*/*E* ratios for both groups include 1, which means that their risk-adjusted mortalities are not different from those predicted by the model.

Odds Ratio (OR). Another method to compare the risk-adjusted performance between groups is using OR, which is technically more suitable. The OR is the ratio of the odds of observed O/(1-O) to the odds of the expected E/(1-E). An OR of 1 indicates that the observed death is equally likely to occur as predicted; an OR greater than 1 indicates that the observed death is more likely to occur than predicted; an OR less than 1 indicates that the observed death is less likely to occur as predicted. The CI of the OR can be calculated by using a likelihood-based method or, more easily, as an output from the logistic regression.[24]

CUSUM Techniques. *Cumulative sum* (CUSUM) analysis methods are often used to examine the performance of a provider across time, by plotting the cumulative sum of observed minus expected events as a function of surgery date.[25] For a data set whose observed mortality exactly fits the expected, the line would lie along the horizontal line y = 0. When the CUSUM lies below the y = 0 line, it means fewer deaths were observed than were expected, and when the CUSUM lies above the y = 0 line, it means more deaths were observed than were expected. When the CUSUM is going up, it means the performance is getting worse than expected; When the CUSUM is going down, it means the performance is getting better than expected. Thus CUSUM can be used to detect a learning curve.[26] The 95% prediction limits (point-wise 95% confidence intervals) account for the excursions from y = 0 that could be expected to happen by chance.[27]

CUSUM can be used for other purposes when using different variables for the x-axis. When the dependent (outcome) variable is dichotomous (death), it is difficult to appreciate its relationship to a continuous risk factor, eg, age, graphically. The CUSUM[25] can be used to overcome this difficulty by plotting the CUSUM against age to give us a graphic view. This technique can also be used to examine the fit of a model, by plotting the cumulative sum of observed minus predicted deaths as a function of predicted mortality (Fig. 8-1). For a model whose observed mortality exactly fit the expected, the line would lie along the horizontal line y = 0. When the horizontal axis equals the predicted risk, the CUSUM could be thought of as a continuous version of the H-L test of model calibration, which is based on the differences in observed minus expected deaths in each of the 10 deciles of risk, shown by shaded vertical bars in Fig. 8-1.

TIME-RELATED EVENTS

We use both death and thromboembolism (TE) to illustrate methods for the analysis of time-related events.

Summarize

Survival Curve

A single percentage is adequate to summarize mortality at a single point in time, such as the operative period (see preceding). To express the pattern of late survival, however, requires a different estimate at virtually every postoperative time, ie, a survivorship function, whose plot is the familiar survival curve. The most common way to estimate a survival curve is the *Kaplan-Meier* (KM) *method,*[28] called *nonparametric* or *distribution-free,* because it does not presuppose any particular underlying statistical distribution. If all the patients in a given series were dead, the survival curve would be very simple to construct,

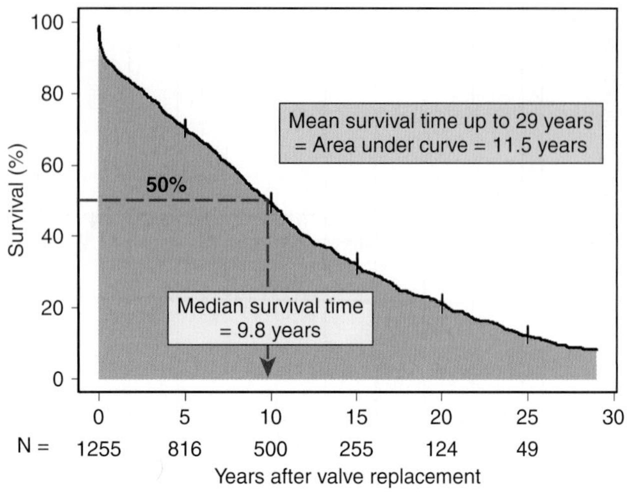

FIGURE 8-2 Kaplan-Meier survival curve. Vertical lines at 5-year intervals indicate the 95% CIs of the survival percentages. Numbers below the horizontal axis indicate the number of patients remaining at risk.

as the percentage that had lived until each point in time. The KM method allows these percentages to be estimated before all the patients have died in an ongoing series, using the assumption that patients who are still alive (whose survival time is censored) will have the same risk of future death as those who have already died. Figure 8-2 shows the KM survival curve for the mitral valve patients, with the 95% CI at 5-year intervals using the greenwood method.[29] The median survival time can be calculated as the survival time at which the survival curve crosses 50% (blue line in Fig. 8-2). The mean survival time can be calculated as the area under the completed survival curve. If the observation is not completed, the survival curve could be fitted with a suitable distribution, such as a Gompertz distribution, that could be extrapolated to estimate the uncompleted part, or reported as a conditional mean as we did in Fig. 8-2 (blue area).

Hazard Function

Besides survival curves, there are several other statistical functions that can characterize the distribution of a time-related event. Survival curves are the easiest to interpret and apply to a patient or a population because they integrate the possibly varying risks over time and produce the probability of being alive at each point in time. The *hazard function* $h(t)$ can be considered the fundamental building block of the other functions. The instantaneous hazard measures the risk of the event at each moment for an individual who is so far event-free. For technical reasons, the *instantaneous hazard* is difficult to measure directly, but its integral, the *cumulative hazard function,* is easy to produce either by taking the negative logarithm of the KM estimate[30] or by computing it directly using the *Nelson-Aalen method.*[31] This latter estimate can be derived from the two basic curves in the upper panel of Fig. 8-3. In the modern *counting process* formulation of survival analysis,[32,33] these two curves are

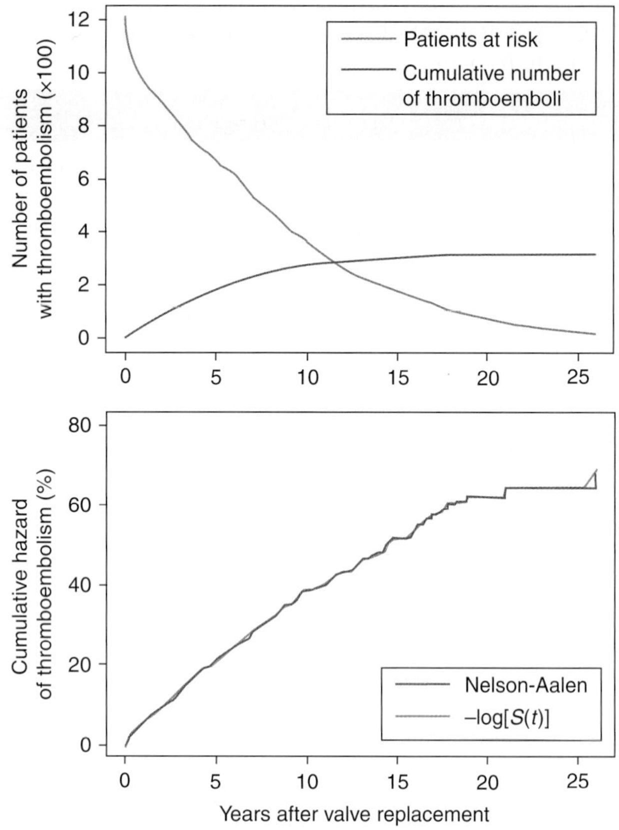

FIGURE 8-3 Cumulative hazard function of late thromboembolism (TE). The upper panel shows the two basic curves used to create the cumulative hazard function by the Nelson-Aalen method. The lower panel shows that the cumulative hazard function created by two methods are almost identical.

the fundamental survival processes. The red curve counts the number of patients still at risk at time t and is called the *at-risk process* $Y(t)$. The blue curve counts the number of events that have happened by time t and is called the *event counting process.* The blue curve rises 1 unit when each event occurs. The cumulative hazard function is similar to the blue curve, except that it rises $1/Y(t)$ each time an event occurs. The lower panel of Fig. 8-3 shows the cumulative hazard function estimated this way and also as the negative logarithm of the KM curve, $-\log[S(t)]$.

Linearized Rate

One property of the cumulative hazard function is that it will be a straight line when the event hazard is constant. It is this property that gave rise to the name used in the cardiac literature to measure event rates that are presumed to be constant over time. If the (instantaneous) hazard is a constant λ, then the cumulative hazard function $H(t)$ is a linear function of postoperative time t with slope λ: $H(t) = \lambda t$. In the cardiac literature, this constant risk parameter is called a *linearized rate.* For a given event in a series of patients, the maximum-likelihood estimate of this rate is the number of events (E) divided by the total follow-up time (T) in patient-years: E/T. Multiplying this

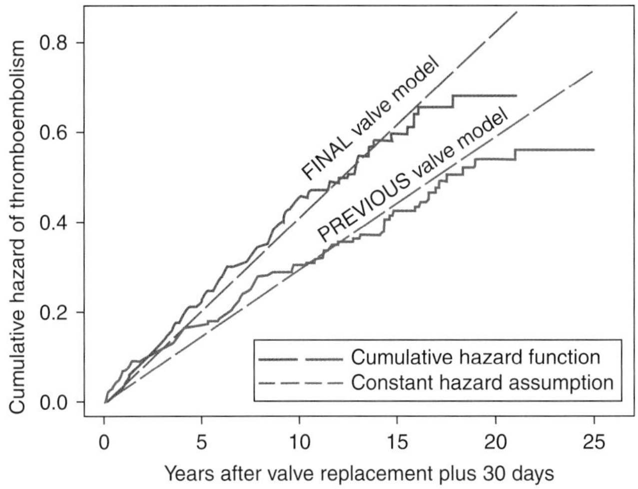

FIGURE 8-4 Cumulative hazard functions of late thromboembolism (TE) by valve model group. The straight lines depict the constant-hazard assumption. The total follow-up time is 4604 years and 4341 years for the FINAL and PREVIOUS valve models, respectively.

by 100 converts it to "events per 100 patient-years," often abbreviated as *percent per patient-year* or *percent per year.* The SE is the square root of *E,* divided by *T.* Early events are usually not included in the calculation because the risk of most events is higher after operation, so the assumption of a constant hazard would not hold. Figure 8-4 shows that the cumulative hazard functions for two valve groups fit the constant hazard assumption fairly well, with a slight decline in the slope after about 10 years.

Table 8-4 contains the linearized late TE rates by valve model based on the number of late TEs and late follow-up (patient-years beyond 30 days). The normal approximation (the mean plus and minus two times the SE) yields approximate 95% CIs. A preferred approximation is based on a suggestion owing to Cox,[34] which was recommended after a comparison of several methods.[35] In this method, the upper and lower 95% confidence limits are given by the 0.025 and 0.975 quantiles, respectively, of the chi-square distribution with $2E + 1$ degrees of freedom divided by $2T$. Another general technique for producing CI that usually is found to have very good properties is the *likelihood-ratio method.*[36] In our example, the CIs given by these three methods agree well, differing from each other only in the second decimal place. Note that the Cox limits and the likelihood-ratio limits are not symmetric around the point estimate, as the normal approximation limits are. (Cox's method also coincides with the probability interval produced by *Bayesian analysis*[37] using a noninformative prior.)

"Actual" Analysis

The KM method is often used for events other than death. Figure 8-5 contains a KM TE-free curve for the mitral valve patients. When used for events such as TE that are not necessarily fatal, KM estimates the probability of being event-free given the unrealistic condition that death does not occur. But patients do, in fact, die before such an event has happened to them, so the KM event-free estimate is lower than the real ("actual") event-free percentage. Another method, called *cumulative incidence* in the statistical literature[38] and *"actual" analysis* in the cardiac literature, provides a mortality-adjusted event-free percentage.[39–42] The CI of the "actual" curve can be calculated by *Gray's method.*[43,44] The "actual" TE-free curve for this mitral valve series is much higher than the KM TE-free curve (see Fig. 8-5). Besides providing an unrealistic estimate of the probability of TE, there is another, more technical problem with using the KM method in this situation. Its use is justified only if the risk of future TE for patients who died TE-free would have been the same as for those who actually had a TE. But this assumption cannot be proven from the data, so that the KM TE estimate generally is regarded as statistically inappropriate.[45]

Compare

The log-rank statistic is chosen most often to compare survival (or event free) curves.[46] Figure 8-6 shows the survival curves for the PREVIOUS and FINAL valve models, including all deaths, early and late. The PREVIOUS model has significantly better survival according to this univariable comparison (log-rank test $p = .042$). But the difference is mostly because of early deaths; if we only consider late deaths, there is no significant difference between the two groups (log-rank test $p = .172$).

Comparing late TEs using linearized rates (see Fig. 8-4) also shows identical levels of statistical significance using three different methods of testing: a normal-approximation method, a

TABLE 8-4 Summary and Univariable Comparison of Linearized Rates of Late Thromboembolisms by Valve Model

Valve Model	Previous	Final	*p*-value (2-sided)
Summarize			
Number of late thromboembolisms	129	191	
Late follow-up (patient-years)	4341	4604	
Linearized rate			
Point estimate (%/year)	2.97	4.15	
Standard error (%/year)	0.26	0.29	
95% confidence interval (%/year)			
Normal approximation	(2.47, 3.48)	(3.57, 4.72)	.003
Cox's method	(2.49, 3.52)	(3.59, 4.77)	.003
Likelihood ratio	(2.49, 3.50)	(3.58, 4.78)	.003

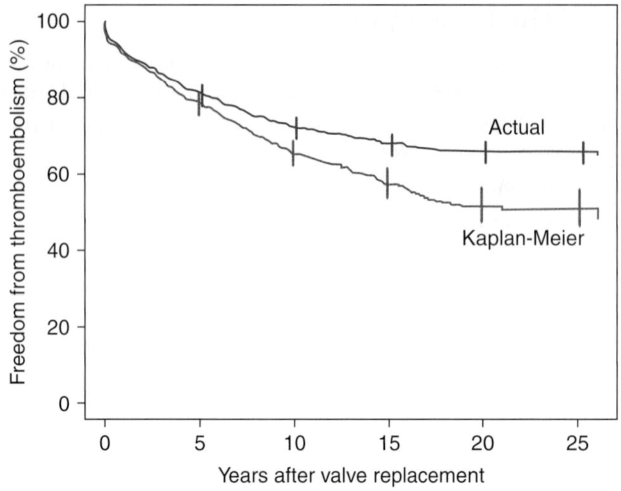

FIGURE 8-5 Thromboembolism-free curves constructed by the Kaplan-Meier method and the "actual" (complement of the cumulative incidence) method. Vertical lines at 5-year intervals indicate the 95% CIs of the event-free percentages.

method recommended by Cox,[34] and a likelihood-ratio method[47] (see Table 8-4).

Comparison of cumulative incidence curves, or their complement, the "actual" event-free curves, can be accomplished using special techniques.[44]

Model

Cox Regression

Analogous to logistic regression, which provides multivariable analysis of the simple percentages associated with operative mortality, there is a widely used method for assessing multivariable influences on late survival: *Cox proportional hazards regression.*[14] This method assumes that the *hazard ratio* (HR) for all risk factors is constant over time. Table 8-5 shows the result of this regression as applied to the valve data for late survival. The univariable comparisons show three variables (ie, age, concomitant CABG, and female gender) to be significant. The final Cox model includes all five variables, although FINAL valve model and re-replacement were not significant by univariable analysis. This latter finding demonstrates that the practice of allowing only significant (by univariable analysis) variables to enter a stepwise regression may eliminate important risk factors.

The HRs for female and FINAL valve model are less than 1; this means that they are protective factors rather than risk factors. For each significant factor ($p < .05$) in the model, whether a risk or protective factor, the 95% CI does not include 1. *Note:* The univariable log-rank test shows no significant difference between the survival of PREVIOUS and FINAL valve models ($p = .172$); the multivariable Cox regression shows that FINAL valve model has a lower risk of death (HR = 0.85, $p = .030$). Thus, the univariable log-rank test and multivariable Cox regression give opposite results. This tells us that if the groups are not compatible, as in this example, a multivariable comparison should be preferred. When the groups are compatible, such as in a randomized clinical trial, univariable comparisons may be appropriate.

An analog of the Cox regression model can be used for regression analysis of cumulative incidence and "actual" event-free curves.[43]

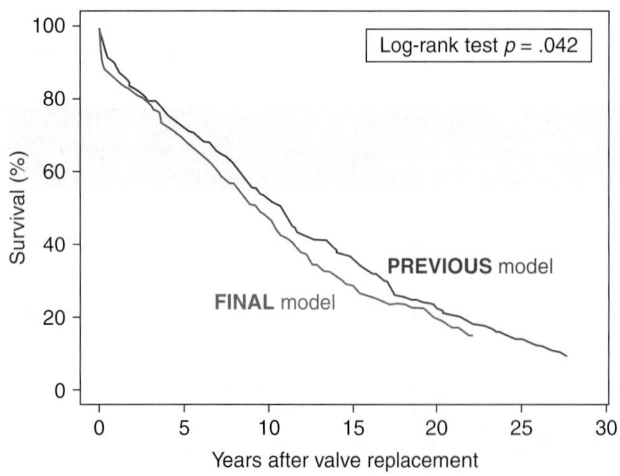

FIGURE 8-6 Survival by valve model. Overall survival significantly favors the PREVIOUS valve model based on this Univariable analysis that includes the higher mortality risk of the patients with the FINAL valve model.

Parametric Regression

The preceding sections discussed nonparametric methods and nonparametric or semiparametric regression models to describe the survival data, such as KM curves and Cox regression, which do not make any assumptions about the underlying distribution of the survival or hazard functions. Another way to deal with survival data is to use a *parametric method.* A family of distributions is chosen, and the data are used to select the best-fitting member of that family by estimating the parameters that define the distribution. Three popular distributions used in cardiac surgery research are the *exponential, Weibull,* and *Gompertz distributions.* There are several functions that can be used to characterize a survival distribution. We have already discussed three of them: the *hazard function* $h(t)$, the *cumulative hazard function* $H(t)$, and the *survival function* $S(t)$. The hazard function can be considered the fundamental quantity from which the others are derived. It is the risk of the event at each instant of time t for a patient who is so far event-free. The cumulative hazard is the mathematical integral of the (instantaneous) hazard function. And the survival function is the exponential of the negative cumulative hazard: $S(t) = \exp[-H(t)]$.

Figure 8-7 shows typical plots of these three functions for the *exponential, Weibull,* and *Gompertz distributions,* with a selection of values for their parameters. The upper row of plots contains the hazard functions $h(t)$, the second row is the cumulative hazard functions $H(t)$, and the third row is the survival functions $S(t)$. Table 8-6 contains the formulas used for these functions. The exponential is the simplest lifetime distribution,

TABLE 8-5 Multivariable Modeling of Late Survival by Cox Regression and Gompertz Regression

	Univariable		Multivarible Cox Regression		Multivarible Gompertz Regression*	
Variable	*p*-value	Hazard Ratio	*p*-value	Hazard Ratio (95% CI)	*p*-value	Hazard Ratio (95% CI)
Age	<.001	1.04	<.001	1.05 (1.04, 1.05)	<.001	1.05 (1.04, 1.05)
Concomitant CABG	<.001	1.65	.052	1.23 (1.00, 1.50)	.049	1.23 (1.00, 1.50)
FINAL valve model	.172	1.1	.03	0.85 (0.73, 0.98)	.03	0.85 (0.73, 0.98)
Female gender	.005	0.82	.005	0.81 (0.70, 0.94)	.004	0.81 (0.70, 0.94)
Re-replacement	.135	1.25	.036	1.37 (1.02, 1.83)	.036	1.37 (1.02, 1.83)

*Additional parameters in the Gompertz regression: scale constant = −5.412, shape = 0.055.

having only a single parameter λ called the *scale parameter*, which is the (constant) hazard ("linearized") rate. The Weibull distribution is a natural generalization of the exponential distribution that adds a second parameter α called the *shape parameter* to accommodate an increasing ($\alpha > 1$) or decreasing ($\alpha < 1$) risk. The cumulative hazard reduces to the exponential distribution (constant risk) when $\alpha = 1$. The Weibull distribution is used commonly for time to failure and is employed in the cardiac literature to model structural deterioration of prosthetic heart valves. A Gompertz distribution[48] has a scale parameter λ and a shape parameter α. Its hazard function is an exponential function of time. The Gompertz distribution is widely used to model survival, especially in older age groups. Figure 8-8 uses the late death information from the heart valve data to show the fits derived from these three distributions. The data fits the Gompertz distribution very well.

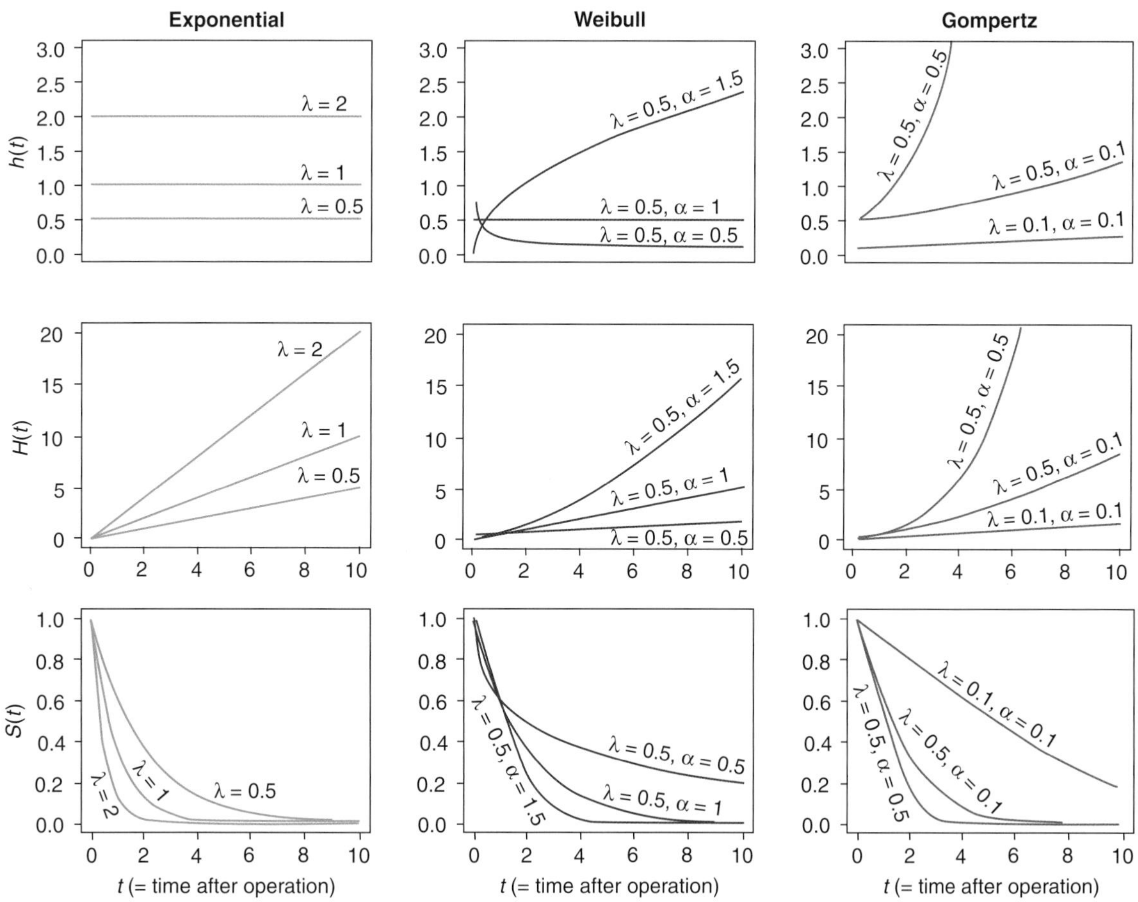

FIGURE 8-7 Hazard (top row), cumulative hazard (middle row), and survival function (bottom row) for the exponential, Weibull, and Gompertz distributions with various parameters.

TABLE 8-6 Formulas for the Hazard, Cumulative Hazard, and Survival Functions for Three Commonly Used Statistical Distributions

	Exponential	Weibull	Gompertz
Hazard function $h(t)$	λ	$\alpha\lambda t^{\alpha-1}$	$\lambda e^{\alpha t}$
Cumulative hazard $H(t)$	λt	λt^{α}	$\lambda(e^{\alpha t-1})/\alpha$
Survival function $S(t)$	$\exp(-\lambda t)$	$\exp(-\lambda t^{\alpha})$	$\exp[\lambda(1-e^{\alpha t})/\alpha]$
Mean time to event	$1/\lambda$	$\Gamma(1+1/\alpha)/\lambda$	$\int S(t)dt$
Median time to event	$\log(2)/\lambda = 0.693/\lambda$	$(\log(2)/\lambda)^{1/\alpha} = (0.693/\lambda)^{1/\alpha}$	$\text{Log}(1+\log(2)\alpha/\lambda)/\alpha$

Notes: $\Gamma()$ is the gamma function.
There is not a simple formula for the mean time to event of the Gompertz distribution.

Some of the advantages of the parametric method (over nonparametric or semiparametric methods) are:

- The hazard function itself can be portrayed easily, which otherwise requires many data points and a complicated smoothing technique.
- The survival curve can be extrapolated into the future (beyond the maximum follow-up time).
- The median time to failure can be given, which otherwise cannot be estimated until the event-free curve reaches 50%.
- The mean time to failure can be given, which otherwise cannot be estimated until the event-free curve reaches 0%.
- The resulting curves may reproduce the underlying mortality process, which is no doubt smooth over time, more faithfully unlike the random roughness of the original observed data points, which results in graphic peculiarities.
- The entire survival experience can be summarized with a small number of parameters.

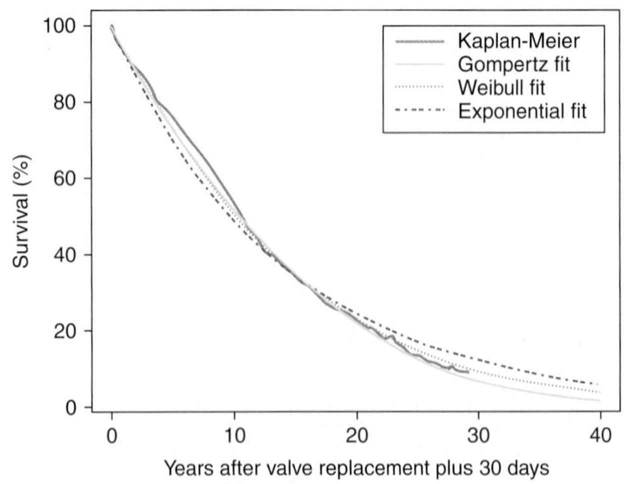

FIGURE 8-8 Three parametric distributions used to fit the Kaplan-Meier survival curve. The exponential (constant hazard) is that the least good fit. The Weibull, with an increasing (power function) hazard, fits the curve better than the exponential. The best fit is the Gompertz model, which has an exponentially increasing hazard.

A final and important advantage of fitting parametric models is that there may be a theoretical basis for the model that helps us understand the physical process rather than just describe it. The Weibull distribution has such a theoretical interpretation as the time to failure of a physical system that depends on very many parts (sites) for integrity. Thus, the Weibull distribution is a commonly used distribution for failure analysis and is employed in the cardiac literature to model the structural deterioration of prosthetic heart valves. The Gompertz distribution is used widely to model for human mortality, especially for older populations, based on the assumption that the "average exhaustion of a man's power to avoid death to be such that at the end of equal infinitely small intervals of time he lost equal portions of his remaining power to oppose destruction which he had at the commencement of these intervals."[49]

These parametric distributions also can be used as the basis for regression models; usually the scale parameter is expanded to contain the risk factors. For the mitral valve data, a Gompertz regression produced hazard ratios identical to those of the Cox regression (see Table 8-5).

CONCLUSIONS

1. Different analytical methods must be used for outcome events after surgery depending on whether they are one-time (operative) or time-related (late) events.
2. Factors found significant on Univariable analysis often are overturned by multivariable ate analysis because they are surrogates for other more clinically fundamental variables. This was the case with valve model in both the early and overall analysis of mortality. The converse also can happen; re-replacement was not significant for overall mortality by itself but became so in concert with other risk factors. Multivariable analysis, adjusting with the other risk factor, always should be the first choice.
3. The hazard and cumulative hazard functions measure the instantaneous and cumulative risks of an event, respectively. The cumulative hazard is easier to obtain. The survival curve converts their risks into probabilities of experiencing the events.

4. Linearized rates provide a convenient single-parameter summary of late-event rates but should not be used unless the hazard function is approximately constant.
5. Kaplan-Meier analysis estimates survival probabilities as a function of time after surgery. When used for events that are not necessarily fatal, KM estimates probabilities as if death were eliminated, whereas "actual" analysis gives a true mortality-adjusted estimate of the event probabilities.
6. Parametric regression is a useful tool to analyze long-term outcome. Usually, the Gompertz distribution is good for survival, and the Weibull distribution fits tissue and structural valve deterioration very well.

REFERENCES

1. Ware JE, Jr., Sherbourne CD: The MOS 36-item short-form health survey (SF-36). I. Conceptual framework and item selection. *Med Care* 1992; 30(6):473-483.
2. Gilson BS, Gilson JS, Bergner M, et al: The sickness impact profile. Development of an outcome measure of health care. *Am J Public Health* 1975; 65(12):1304-1310.
3. Miller TR: Valuing nonfatal quality of life losses with quality-adjusted life years: the health economist's meow. *J Forensic Econ* 2000; 13(2):145-167.
4. Hlatky MA, Boothroyd DB, Johnstone IM: Economic evaluation in long-term clinical trials. *Stat Med* 2002; 21(19):2879-2888.
5. Efron B, Tibshirani R: Bootstrap methods for standard errors, confidence intervals, and other measures of statistical accuracy. *Stat Sci* 1986; 1(1):54-75.
6. Gao G, Wu Y, Grunkemeier GL, Furnary AP, Starr A: Forty-year survival with the Starr-Edwards heart valve prosthesis. *J Heart Valve Dis* 2004; 13(1):91-96.
7. Coviello E: STCOMPET: Stata module to generate cumulative incidence in presence of competing events. http://econpapers.repec.org/software/bocbocode/s431301.htm. Accessed December 4, 2009.
8. Gray RJ: cmprsk R package http://biowww.dfci.harvard.edu/~gray/. Accessed December 4, 2009.
9. Vollset SE: Confidence intervals for a binomial proportion. *Stat Med* 1993; 12:809-824.
10. Ling RF: Just say no to binomial (and other discrete distributions) tables. *Am Statistician* 1992; 46:53-54.
11. Agresti A, Coull BA: Approximate is better than 'exact' for interval estimation of binomial proportions. *Am Statistician* 1998; 52:119-126.
12. Fleiss JL, Levin B, Paik MC: Assessing significance in a fourfold table, in Balding DJ, Cressie NA, Fisher NI (eds): *Statistical Methods for Rates and Proportions*, 3rd ed. Hoboken, Wiley, 2003; 50-63.
13. Hosmer DW, Lemeshow S: *Applied Survival Analysis*, 2nd ed. New York, Wiley, 2000.
14. Harrell FE, Jr, Lee KL, Mark DB: Multivariable prognostic models: issues in developing models, evaluating assumptions and adequacy, and measuring and reducing errors. *Stat Med* 1996; 15:361-387.
15. Hanley JA, McNeil BJ: The meaning and use of the area under a receiver operating characteristic (ROC) curve. *Radiology* 1982; 143:29-36.
16. Hosmer DW, Lemeshow S: Area under the ROC curve, in Cressie NAC, Fisher NI, Johnstone IM, et al (eds): *Applied Logistic Regression*, 2nd ed. New York, Wiley, 2000; pp 160-164.
17. Hosmer DW, Lemeshow S: A goodness-of-fit test for the multiple regression model. *Commun Stat* 1980; A10:1043-1069.
18. Harrell FE, Jr: General aspects of fitting regression models. *Regression Modeling Strategies: With Applications to Linear Models, Logistic Regression, and Survival analysis.* New York, Springer, 2001; pp 11-40.
19. Hosmer DW, Hosmer T, Cessie L, Lemeshow S: A Comparison of Goodness-of-Fit Tests for the Logistic Regression Model. *Stat Med* 1997; 16:965-980.
20. le Cessie S, van Houwelingen HC: Testing the fit of a regression model via score tests in random effects models. *Biometrics* 1995; 51(2):600-614.
21. Van Houwelingen JC, Le Cessie S: Predictive value of statistical models. *Stat Med* 1990; 9(11):1303-1325.
22. Hosmer DW, Lemeshow S: Confidence interval estimates of an index of quality performance based on logistic regression models. *Stat Med* 1995; 14(19):2161-2172.
23. Smith DW: Evaluating risk adjustment by partitioning variation in hospital mortality rates. *Stat Med* 1994; 13(10):1001-1013.
24. Grunkemeier GL, Wu Y: What are the odds? *Ann Thorac Surg* 2007; 83(4):1240-1244.
25. Royston P: The use of CUSUMs and other techniques in modelling continuous covariates in logistic regression. *Stat Med* 1992; 11(8):1115-1129.
26. Novick RJ, Fox SA, Stitt LW, et al: Assessing the learning curve in off-pump coronary artery surgery via CUSUM failure analysis. *Ann Thorac Surg* 2002; 73(1):S358-362.
27. Grunkemeier GL, Jin R, Wu Y: Cumulative sum curves and their prediction limits. *Ann Thorac Surg* 2009; 87(2):361-364.
28. Kaplan EL, Meier P: Nonparametric estimation from incomplete observations. *J Am Stat Assoc* 1958; 53:457-481.
29. Greenwood M, Jr: A report on the natural duration of cancer. *Reports on Public Health and Medical Subjects,* Vol 33. London, His Majesty's Stationery Office, 1926; pp 1-26.
30. Peterson AV, Jr: Expressing the Kaplan-Meier estimator as a function of empirical subsurvival functions. *J Am Stat Assoc* 1977; 72:854-858.
31. Aalen O: Nonparametric inference for a family of counting processes. *Ann Statist* 1978; 6(4):701-726.
32. Andersen PK, Borgan O, Gill RD, Keiding N: *Statistical Models Based on Counting Processes (Springer Series in Statistics).* New York, Springer, 1996.
33. Fleming TR, Harrington DP: *Counting Processes and Survival Analysis.* New York, Wiley, 1991.
34. Cox DR: Some simple approximate test for Poisson variates. *Biometrika* 1953; 40:354-360.
35. Grunkemeier GL, Anderson WN, Jr.: Clinical evaluation and analysis of heart valve substitutes. *J Heart Valve Dis* 1998; 7(2):163-169.
36. Kalbfleisch JD, Prentice RL: Exponential sampling illustration, in Balding DJ, Bloomfield P, Cressie NAC (eds): *The Statistical Analysis of Failure Time Data,* 2nd ed. Hoboken, Wiley, 2002; pp 62-65.
37. Martz HF, Waller RA: *Bayesian Reliability Analysis.* New York, Wiley, 1982.
38. Kalbfleisch JD, Prentice RL: Representation of competing risk failure rates, in Balding DJ, Bloomfield P, Cressie NAC (eds): *The Statistical Analysis of Failure Time Data.* 2nd ed. Hoboken, Wiley, 2002; pp 251-254.
39. Grunkemeier GL, Anderson RP, Miller DC, Starr A: Time-related analysis of nonfatal heart valve complications: cumulative incidence (actual) versus Kaplan-Meier (actuarial). *Circulation* 1997; 96(9 Suppl):II-70-75.
40. Grunkemeier GL, Jamieson WR, Miller DC, Starr A: Actuarial versus actual risk of porcine structural valve deterioration. *J Thorac Cardiovasc Surg* 1994; 108(4):709-718.
41. Miller CC, 3rd, Safi HJ, Winnerkvist A, Baldwin JC: Actual versus actuarial analysis for cardiac valve complications: the problem of competing risks. *Curr Opin Cardiol* 1999; 14(2):79-83.
42. Akins CW, Hilgenberg AD, Vlahakes GJ, et al: Late results of combined carotid and coronary surgery using actual versus actuarial methodology. *Ann Thorac Surg* 2005; 80(6):2091-2097.
43. Fine JP, Gray RJ: A proportional hazards model for the subdistribution of a competing risk. *J Am Stat Assoc* 1999; 94:496-509.
44. Gray RJ: A class of K-sample tests for comparing the cumulative incidence of a competing risk. *Ann Statist* 1988; 16(3):1141-1154.
45. Grunkemeier GL, Jin R, Eijkemans MJ, Takkenberg JJ: Actual and actuarial probabilities of competing risks: apples and lemons. *Ann Thorac Surg* 2007; 83(5):1586-1592.
46. Peto R, Pike MC, Armitage P, et al: Design and analysis of randomized clinical trials requiring prolonged observation of each patient. II. analysis and examples. *Br J Cancer* 1977; 35(1):1-39.
47. Kalbfleisch JD, Prentice RL: Comparisons of two exponemtial samples, in Balding DJ, Bloomfield P, Cressie NAC (eds): *The Statistical Analysis of Failure Time Data,* 2nd ed. Hoboken, Wiley, 2002; pp 66-68.
48. Gompertz B. On the nature of the function expressive of the law of human mortality and on the new mode of determining the value of life contingencies. *Phil Trans R Soc A* 1825; 115:513-580.
49. Johnson NL, Kotz S, Blakrishnan N: *Continuous Univariate Distributions: Volumne II,* 2nd ed. New York, Wiley, 1995.

PART 2
PERIOPERATIVE/INTRAOPERATIVE CARE

CHAPTER 9

Preoperative Evaluation for Cardiac Surgery

Christian T. Ruff
Patrick T. O'Gara

INTRODUCTION

Improved outcomes and advances in surgical techniques have enabled the application of cardiac surgery in patient populations previously considered ineligible for an intervention of this magnitude. During the previous decade, the in-hospital mortality rate for coronary artery bypass surgery (CABG), the most common surgical procedure in the world, declined from 2.8 to 1.6% (43% relative reduction) despite an older and sicker patient population.[1,2] Thorough preoperative risk assessment by the medical and surgical team is of critical importance in minimizing perioperative and long-term morbidity and mortality. It also enables physicians to counsel patients and families on what they can expect postoperatively, thus allowing them to make informed decisions regarding the treatment options available to them. This chapter reviews the essential information that the cardiologist and surgeon must collect and review to evaluate a patient for cardiac surgery. This information includes patient and disease characteristics, medications, and surgical considerations that can be integrated into scoring systems to provide a semiquantitative risk assessment (Table 9-1).

RISK ASSESSMENT

Patient Characteristics and Conditions

Age

The volume of cardiac surgical procedures in elderly people continues to increase as life expectancy improves and benefits outweigh risks. Although perioperative mortality does not vary significantly by age, 1-year mortality is greater in patients greater than 75 years of age.[3] Octogenarians have nearly double the mortality rate compared with younger patients (4.1 versus 2.3%) and more than 60% have at least one nonfatal postoperative complication.[4,5] The most prevalent complications include prolonged ventilation in intensive care units, reoperation for bleeding, and pneumonia—all of which result in longer hospital stays.[5] A higher proportion of complications occur in elderly patients with low body weight (BMI <23).[6] There is evidence that off-pump (OP) surgery using only arterial conduits may confer a survival benefit and improve long-term quality of life.[7,8] With improved surgical techniques and careful patient selection, nonagenarians can safely undergo cardiac surgery with a 95% 30-day survival and 93% survival to hospital discharge.[9]

Gender

Some but not all epidemiologic studies suggest that female gender is an independent predictor of postoperative morbidity and mortality.[10–12] Gender differences are present in both traditional CABG and off-pump surgery.[13] Several large retrospective cohort studies of patients undergoing CABG found that women had higher mortality rates than men, even after adjusting for comorbidities and confounding factors, including BSA.[10,11] Possible explanations for worse outcomes in women include smaller coronary arteries (which might enhance the difficulty of performing anastomoses and limit graft flow), differences in referral for surgery (ie, women being referred at later disease stages), and gender differences in self-reported outcomes.[14] Data suggest that benefit in terms of quality of life after cardiac surgery is similar for men and women.[15]

Race

Although crude post-CABG mortality rates differ significantly by race, data suggest that after controlling for patient and hospital variables, these differences are small.[16,17] However, in the

TABLE 9-1 Preoperative Risk Assessment Checklist

Patient Characteristics and Conditions
Age
Gender
Race
Diabetes
Renal function
Pulmonary function
Hematologic (HIT)
Atrial fibrillation
Surgical Considerations
Emergency
Reoperation
Prior radiation
Surgical complexity (CABG, valve, aorta, combined)
Technique (minimally invasive, off-pump, hybrid)
Medications
Antiplatelet/anticoagulant
Beta blockers
ACE inhibitors and ARBs
Statins
Risk Scores
EuroSCORE
Society of Thoracic Surgeons Score (STS)
Northern New England (NNE)

ACE = angiotensin-converting enzyme; ARBs = angiotensin-II receptor blockers; CABG = coronary artery bypass graft surgery; HIT = heparin-induced thrombocytopenia type II.

United States, self-described black race is associated with an increased risk of postoperative complications, including prolonged ventilatory support, length of stay, reoperation for bleeding, and postoperative renal failure.[18]

Diabetes

Patients with diabetes have significantly worse outcomes following cardiac surgery.[19–21] Studies have shown diabetes to be an independent predictor of in-hospital mortality after CABG although emerging evidence indicates that the severity of diabetes, specifically target organ damage, may be important in risk stratification.[22,23] Postoperative mortality does not differ significantly between nondiabetic and diabetic patients without diabetic sequelae, although diabetic patients with vascular disease and/or renal failure have an increased risk of mortality.[23] Insulin-dependent type II diabetics in particular are at increased risk of major postoperative complications including renal failure, deep sternal wound infection, and prolonged hospital stay.[24,25] Strict perioperative glucose control has been shown to lower operative mortality and the incidence of mediastinits.[26,27] Off-pump surgery also appears to decrease postoperative morbidity in diabetic patients.[28]

Renal Function

Renal dysfunction is common in patients undergoing cardiac surgery. Approximately half of patients undergoing CABG have at least mild renal dysfunction and one-fourth have at least moderate renal dysfunction.[29] There is a graded increase in operative mortality and morbidity with worsening preoperative renal function.[29–31] Renal insufficiency is associated with greater risk of both 30-day (OR = 3.7) and 1-year mortality (OR = 4.6).[32] Even mild renal dysfunction (serum creatinine 1.47 to 2.25 mg/dL) is associated with increased rates of operative and long-term mortality, need for postoperative dialysis, and postoperative stroke.[33]

Renoprotective drugs, such as fenoldopam and *N*-acetylcysteine, have no effect on the deterioration of renal function in high-risk patients.[34,35] Off-pump CABG is associated with a lower prevalence of the need for postoperative renal replacement therapy; larger studies are needed to determine if this correlates with improved outcomes.[36]

Pulmonary Function

It is well established that patients with compromised pulmonary function, predominantly owing to chronic obstructive pulmonary disease (COPD), have a higher mortality and increased incidence of postoperative complications including arrhythmias, reintubation, pneumonia, prolonged ICU duration, and increased hospital length of stay.[37,38] Postoperative respiratory failure is a common complication (14.8% in a New York State database) with a higher incidence (14.8%) in combined CABG and valve operations.[39] Optimizing respiratory status prior to surgery, including smoking cessation, antibiotics for pneumonia, and treatment of COPD flares with bronchodilator therapy and steroids is a critical part of preoperative management.[40] There is evidence that intensive inspiratory muscle training prevents postoperative pulmonary complications in high-risk patients.[41]

Hematologic

The most important hematologic consideration in patients undergoing cardiac surgery is heparin-induced thrombocytopenia type II (HIT). HIT is an immune-mediated, potentially life-threatening thrombotic condition characterized by the formation of antibodies against the heparin-platelet factor 4 (PF4) complex.[42] A diagnosis of HIT should be suspected in patients begun on heparin therapy within the preceding 5 to 10 days who have unexplained thrombocytopenia, venous or arterial thrombosis, or a platelet count that has fallen 50% or more from baseline even if absolute thrombocytopenia is not present.[42] HIT can occur earlier in patients recently exposed to heparin. HIT can also be caused by exposure to low molecular weight heparin (LMWH), but the incidence is much lower.[43] Although the prevalence of HIT antibodies is relatively common preoperatively (4.3%) and postoperatively (22.4%), the occurrence of thrombotic events occurs only in a minority of patients (6.3%) who have a positive antibody.[42] CABG patients with HIT have a dramatically increased risk of vein graft occlusion (68% versus 20%); however, they do not appear to have an increased rate of internal mammary graft occlusion.[44]

There is emerging consensus regarding anticoagulant management of patients with HIT.[42] Repeat heparin exposure during CBP is an option for patients with a previous history of HIT if repeat antibody testing is negative on two consecutive daily samples, although it is prudent to use alternative antithrombotic agents for preoperative and postoperative anticoagulation. Patients with prior HIT and detectable antibodies are at higher risk with reexposure and should only be administered heparin if platelet activation assays (ie, serotonin release assay) are negative. For patients with acute HIT, it is recommended to delay surgery if possible. If surgery must proceed, bivalirudin is an alternative, although attention must be given to its several unique pharmacologic properties.[42]

It is difficult to manage the competing risks of thrombosis and bleeding in patients with hypercoagulable disorders. Aggressive prophylaxis with unfractionated heparin or LMWH is indicated for patients not on chronic anticoagulation.[45,46] Special considerations should be given to patients with antiphospholipid syndrome owing to their high risk of thrombotic events and the difficulty in interpreting coagulation parameters.[47,48]

Atrial Fibrillation

Preexisting AF in patients undergoing CABG is not associated with increased in-hospital mortality or major morbidity but is a risk factor for reduced 5-year survival.[49] However, postoperative AF (POAF) is associated with increased in-hospital and long-term mortality, stroke, hemodynamic compromise, renal failure, longer length of stay, and greater hospitalization costs.[50,51] AF is common after cardiac surgery, occurring in up to 40% of CABG patients, 50% of patients undergoing valve surgery and as many of 60% of patients after combined CABG and valve operation.[50,52–54] The pathophysiology of postoperative AF is likely related to the age-related degenerative changes in the atrial myocardium coupled with inflammation, bleeding into the pericardial space, and perioperative electrophysiologic abnormalities in atrial refractoriness, conduction velocity, and transmembrane potentials.[55] Evaluation of the risk for POAF is an important part of preoperative evaluation because prophylactic therapy can substantially reduce the incidence of AF.

Established risk factors for the development of POAF include history of AF, male gender, decreased left ventricular ejection fraction (LVEF), left atrial enlargement, valvular heart surgery, COPD, diabetes, chronic renal failure, rheumatic heart disease, and withdrawal from beta blocker and angiotensin 1 converting enzyme inhibitor (ACE inhibitor) therapy.[50,56]

A large Cochrane Database meta-analysis reviewed 58 randomized trials of more than 8500 patients and determined that beta blockers (OR 0.35), sotalol (OR 0.36), amiodarone (0.54), and atrial pacing (OR 0.57) were all highly effective in reducing postoperative AF.[57] Overall, prophylactic therapy was associated with a nonsignificant 24% reduction in stroke. In a meta-analysis of randomized trials and risk-adjusted observational studies, off-pump (OP) CABG was associated with significant reductions in postoperative AF (41 and 22%, respectively).[58]

Practical recommendations include the continued use of beta blockers through the perioperative period because they are effective and safe in most patients.[56] Amiodarone can be added to high-risk patients but should be a second-line agent because of its short- and long-term safety profile. There are limited but emerging data suggesting that the addition of magnesium, statins, N-3 polyunsaturated fatty acids, nitroprusside, and corticosteroids might be of additional benefit.[56] Although prophylaxis is effective, it is still controversial whether preventing POAF translates into a reduction in stroke and postoperative complications.

Surgical Considerations

Reoperation

Hospital mortality among patients undergoing reoperative cardiac surgery has traditionally been higher than among patients undergoing primary operation.[59–61] This is likely due to the higher risk profile of patients undergoing reoperation (older, more extensive vascular and coronary disease, multiple comorbidities) and the demanding surgical aspects including sternal reentry, pericardial adhesions, in situ arterial grafts, and diseased saphenous vein grafts.[62]

Despite these factors, hospital mortality associated with coronary reoperation has decreased with greater surgical experience and now approaches that of primary CABG.[62,63] With careful preoperative risk evaluation and surgical management, reoperation can be performed safely.

Prior Radiation

Patients receiving thoracic radiation for treatment of malignancies before cardiac surgery have poorer short- and long-term outcomes.[64,65] Thoracic radiation exposure is heterogeneous with respect to different malignancies and there is a gradient of risk.

A study dividing patients undergoing cardiac surgery into three levels of radiation exposure: extensive (Hodgkin's disease, thymoma, and testicular cancer), variable (non-Hodgkin's lymphoma and lung cancer), and tangential (breast cancer), demonstrated that patients with extensive radiation exposure had longer radiation-to-operation interval, poorer pulmonary function and more severe aortic regurgitation, diastolic dysfunction, and left main coronary stenosis.[66] Hospital deaths (13 versus 8.6 versus 2.4%) and respiratory complications (24 versus 20 versus 9.6%) were higher after more extensive radiation, and 4-year survival was poorer (64 versus 57 versus 80%).

Surgical Complexity and Technique

It is important to consider the type of cardiac surgical procedure (CABG, valve, or combined) as well as the surgical technique (on-pump, off-pump, minimally invasive, robotic, and hybrid) when providing preoperative risk assessment as mortality and morbidity risk may vary.

Valve surgeries generally have a higher complication rate than isolated CABG and combined surgeries have the highest

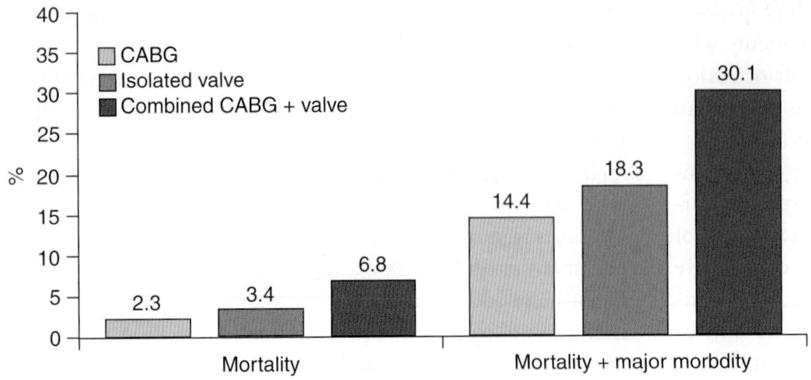

FIGURE 9-1 Thirty-day mortality and a composite end point of mortality and major in-hospital morbidity (stroke, renal failure, prolonged ventilation, deep sternal wound infection, and reoperation) from the Society of Thoracic Surgeons National Adult Cardiac Surgery Database (STS NCD).[67–69] CABG = coronary artery bypass graft surgery.

risk (Fig. 9-1). Participants in the Society of Thoracic Surgeons National Adult Cardiac Surgery Database (STS NCD) collected data from 2002 and 2006 on more than 3.6 million procedures.[67–69] They reported 30-day mortality and a composite end point of mortality and major in-hospital morbidity, including stroke, renal failure, prolonged ventilation, deep sternal wound infection, and reoperation. CABG mortality was 2.3%, with a 14.4% rate for the combined end point of mortality and major morbidity.[67] Isolated valve procedures had a higher mortality rate of 3.4% (aortic valve replacement [AVR] 3.2%, mitral valve replacement [MVR] 5.7%, and mitral valve prolapse [MVP] 1.6%).[68] Combined mortality and major morbidity was also higher at 18.3% (AVR 17.4%, MVR 26.7%, MVP 12.7%). Combined CABG and valve procedures had the highest mortality rate at 6.8% (AVR + CABG 5.6%, MVR + CABG 11.6%, and MVP + CABG 7.4%) with combined mortality and major morbidity of 30.1% (AVR + CABG 26.3%, MVR + CABG 43.2%, and MVP + CABG 33.5%).[69]

Minimally invasive surgical techniques can be divided by approach and use of cardiopulmonary bypass (CBP). The use of alternatives to standard median sternotomy has become increasingly adopted in surgical centers for both CABG and valve surgeries. The potential benefits of minimally invasive surgery are earlier extubation, reduced incisional and thoracic discomfort, lower rates of wound infection, less blood loss, and shorter recovery times.[70]

Off-pump CABG (OP CABG) is performed with small skin incisions and stabilization devices to reduce motion of target vessels while anastomoses are performed without CBP. Current surgical approaches to valve surgery require cardiopulmonary bypass and cardioplegic arrest. Meta-analyses of observational and randomized trials of OP CABG versus CBP have not demonstrated a clear advantage of OP CABG over CBP with respect to mortality or morbidity.[58,71] Compared with on-pump surgery, OP CABG generally shows consistent reductions in postoperative AF, blood loss, wound infections, and myocardial injury, with nonsignificant trends toward lower death, MI, and stroke.[58,72,73] The benefits of OP CABG are particularly notable in elderly patients and those with heavily calcified (porcelain) aortas.[72]

There have been steady technologic advancements in optics, instrumentation, and perfusion technology that have facilitated use of totally endoscopic robotic cardiac surgery.[74] This technology has been applied to many cardiac surgical procedures, in particular mitral valve repair (MVP) and totally endoscopic coronary artery bypass (TECAB) grafting. Short-term results are promising but long-term studies are lacking.

Simultaneous "hybrid" percutaneous coronary intervention and minimally invasive surgical bypass grafting procedures in a single, specially designed operating suite are also gaining more widespread acceptance. Hybrid procedures require close cooperation between surgical and interventional teams. Although there are limited data available, hybrid patients have similar angiographic vessel patency and major adverse cardiac events (MACE) at 6 months with shorter hospital length of stay, intubation times, and less blood loss despite aggressive antiplatelet therapy.[75]

MEDICATIONS

Patients undergoing cardiac surgery are frequently on several medications for their preexisting cardiovascular conditions including aspirin, clopidogrel, beta blockers, ACE inhibitors, and statins. Perioperative medical therapy has been demonstrated to improve outcomes in patients undergoing cardiac surgery; however, these medications are probably underutilized because of concern for postoperative complications. Careful review of a patient's medication record with an assessment of the potential risks and benefits of continuing each medication is an important component of preoperative evaluation.

Antiplatelet Therapy

Aspirin

Aspirin (ASA) is a common medication in patients undergoing cardiac surgery. There are conflicting data regarding the benefits and risks of preoperative (predominantly CABG) ASA. Preoperative ASA has been demonstrated to reduce in-hospital mortality in several observational and case control studies.[76–78] A large retrospective study in patients undergoing CABG found a 66% mortality reduction.[76] The concern for excess bleeding, however, limits the use of preoperative ASA. Early studies indicated that preoperative ASA increased the rates of postoperative bleeding and need for transfusions, although this was not seen in subsequent studies.[76,77,79,80]

There are several guideline statements that provide slightly different recommendations regarding the use of preoperative ASA. The 2007 focused update of the 2004 ACC/AHA guidelines for the management of patients with ST-elevation MI (STEMI) recommends that ASA should not be withheld before either elective or nonelective CABG.[81] The 2008 American College of Chest Physicians (ACCP) guideline on the primary and secondary prevention of CAD and the 2005 Society of Thoracic Surgeons practice guideline on antiplatelet drugs during CABG in stable patients recommend that it is reasonable to withhold ASA prior to elective CABG but that it should be resumed in the early postoperative period if there are no contraindications.[82,83]

Clopidogrel

Preoperative clopidogrel is associated with increased postoperative bleeding, transfusions, and reoperation.[84,85] The 2004 ACC/AHA CABG guideline and the 2008 American College of Chest Physicians (ACCP) guideline on the primary and secondary prevention of CAD recommend stopping clopidogrel 5 to 7 days before surgery.[19,83] This approach is reasonable for patients with planned elective stenting or in patients with STEMI (less than 1% proceed to CABG), but is problematic for individuals presenting with non-ST elevation ACS where the decision between PCI and CABG is not known until angiography. Because early clopidogrel therapy is critical to reduce the devastating complication of stent thrombosis, it is reasonable to give clopidogrel in this setting and accept the risk of bleeding in the minority of patients who proceed to surgical revascularization. Similar considerations are likely needed for new third-generation thienopyridines.[86,87] One such agent, prasugrel, has recently become available and has demonstrated more potent platelet inhibition than clopidogrel at a cost of increased bleeding.[86]

Beta Blockers

Beta blockers are a cornerstone of treatment for patients with ischemic heart disease and heart failure.[88,89] Beta blockade has been shown to reduce the rate of cardiovascular events in high-risk patients undergoing noncardiac surgery.[90,91] Only 60% of cardiac surgical patients receive preoperative beta blockers; however, because of the concern for postoperative vasoplegia and exacerbation of reactive airway disease.[92,93] A large North American observational analysis demonstrated preoperative administration of beta blockers was associated with a survival benefit with the exception of patients with a severely depressed left ventricular ejection fraction (<30%).[94] Beta blockers are also highly effective in reducing the incidence and duration of postoperative AF (see atrial fibrillation section).

ACE Inhibitors

ACE inhibitors decrease mortality and cardiovascular events in patients with hypertensive and ischemic heart disease.[95] Preoperative treatment with ACE inhibitors is controversial. ACE inhibitors and angiotensin II receptor blockers (ARBs) have been shown to reduce the incidence of postoperative AF.[50,96] The withdrawal of chronic ACE inhibition can cause rebound hypertension and an increase in ischemia-related events.[97,98] However, preoperative administration of ACE inhibitors or ARBs has been associated with postoperative vasoplegia and an increased requirement for vasopressor drug administration.[92,99]

Statins

Preoperative statin therapy is associated with a 38 to 43% reduction in mortality.[100,101] Beneficial reductions are also observed with stroke and the incidence of postoperative AF.[101] Statin pretreatment (atorvastatin 40 mg daily) initiated 7 days prior to surgery is associated with shorter hospital length of stay.[102] The effects are lipid-independent and are likely mediated through anti-inflammatory and other pleiotropic effects.[103,104] It is recommended that all patients undergoing cardiac surgery (especially CABG) receive preoperative statin therapy unless contraindicated.[19]

RISK SCORES

Preoperative risk assessment has important implications not only for individual patient well-being, but also as a qualitative tool to serve as a reference standard to compare outcomes among surgeons, institutions, or assessment of new procedures and techniques. There are numerous risk stratification scores and systems that have been developed from large databases to quantity the mortality and morbidity risks of cardiac surgery. Both patient and surgical factors are considered preoperatively and assessed for their ability to predict postoperative complications. This section focuses on three of the most widely used risk scoring systems: EuroSCORE, the Society of Thoracic Surgeons Score, and the Northern New England Score (Table 9-2).

All of these risk models share important limitations. Preoperative risk factors included in the model can change significantly over time, leading to substantial underestimation or overestimation of postoperative risk.[105] Caution should also be used when interpreting the results of a model with respect to an individual patient's risk. The models are derived from large databases and do not include important considerations for an individual's specific risk profile such as surgeon experience and comorbidities not incorporated in the model's derivation.

The European System for Cardiac Operative Risk Evaluation (EuroSCORE)

The EuroSCORE, initially published in 1999, is the most rigorously evaluated scoring system in cardiac surgery.[106] The score is calculated by assessing 17 risk factors (patient, cardiac, and operation) known to affect outcome. There are two available methods: the original additive model and more recent logistic model.[107,108] Studies have indicated that the additive model overestimates mortality in low-risk patients and underestimates mortality in high-risk patients.[108–110] The logistic model was designed to address these issues but there is still concern that this model overestimates mortality in many risk groups.[108] The logistic EuroSCORE is more accurate at predicting mortality in combined CABG and valve surgery.[111] The EuroSCORE can be calculated online (www.euroscore.org).

Society of Thoracic Surgeons Score (STS)

The STS has an extensive database that includes more than 2 million procedures since 1997. Similar to the EuroSCORE, an online calculator is available (www.sts.org), although there is

TABLE 9-2 Comparison of Preoperative Risk Factors for Risk Stratification Models

Preoperative Risk Factor	EuroSCORE	STS	NNE (CABG Only)
Age	X	X	X
Gender	X	X	X
Race	X	X	
Weight/BSA		X	X
IABP/inotropes		X	X
LV function	X	X	X
Renal disease	X	X	X
Lung disease	X	X	X
PVD	X	X	X
Diabetes		X	X
Neurologic dysfunction	X	X	X
Active endocarditis	X		
UA or recent MI	X		X
Previous cardiac surgery	X	X	X
Combined surgery	X	X	X
Aortic involvement	X	X	X
Valve surgery	X	X	X
Emergency surgery	X	X	X

BSA = body surface area; CABG = coronary artery bypass graft surgery; EuroSCORE = European System for Cardiac Operative Risk Evaluation; IABP = intraaortic balloon pump; LV = left ventricle; MI = myocardial infarction; NNE = Northern New England; PVD = peripheral vascular disease; STS = Society of Thoracic Surgery; UA = unstable angina.
Adapted from Granton J, Cheng D: Risk stratification models for cardiac surgery. Semin Cardiothoracic Vasc Anesthes 2008; 12(3):167-174.

more extensive data entry required to calculate a score. Models have been developed and revised for CABG, valve surgery, and combined procedures.[67–69] These models include mortality as well as multiple morbidity end points, including stroke, renal failure, prolonged ventilation, deep sternal wound infection, and prolonged postoperative stay at 30 days. Unfortunately the STS score was not included in the most comprehensive analysis comparing 19 different scoring systems, but other studies demonstrate that STS showed similar discriminative capability and predictive performance with EuroSCORE and other risk algorithms.[112,113]

Northern New England Score (NNE)

The Northern New England scoring system was initially published in 1992 with data collected in the United States from 1987 to 1989.[114] The initial model only predicted CABG mortality, but the Northern New England Cardiovascular Disease Study Group developed a second scoring system based on data between 1996 and 1998 that included the incidence of neurologic events and mediastinitis as additional end points. This scoring system was adopted by the ACC/AHA guideline committee on CABG and is often referred to as the ACC/AHA model.[19,113] The model has reasonable predictive capabilities compared with other systems.[115] There are now additional models available specifically for aortic and mitral valve surgery.[116] All models are available online (www.nnecdsg.org).

STROKE AND NEUROCOGNITIVE DECLINE

Stroke

Atherosclerosis is a polyvascular problem. The incidence of coexisting coronary and carotid artery disease varies between 2 and 14%.[117,118] In patients undergoing CABG, 17 to 22% of patients have a carotid artery stenosis greater than 50%, and 6 to 12% have a stenosis greater than 80%.[119,120] Stroke is a feared and devastating complication of cardiac surgery, with a reported incidence ranging from 0.8 to 7%.[40] Approximately 30% of postoperative strokes are caused by significant carotid artery stenosis, with increasing risk correlated with the severity of the stenosis, even in asymptomatic patients.[19,21] Other predictors of stroke include advanced age, type of surgery, aortic atheroma, and duration of CBP (Table 9-3).[21,121]

Because patients with a perioperative stroke have a threefold increased risk of death compared with patients without stroke and many are left with significant disability, carotid revascularization as a combined or staged procedure with CABG can be considered.[122] Current ACC/AHA guidelines recommend (Class IIa; Level of Evidence C) that carotid endarterectomy (CEA) before or concomitant with CABG in patients with symptomatic carotid stenosis or in asymptomatic patients with a unilateral or bilateral internal carotid stenosis of 80%.[123] Carotid artery stenting is a less invasive alternative.

The optimal management of these patients remains controversial. A systematic review of 97 studies involving 8972 operative outcomes after staged and synchronous CEA and CABG revealed a 10 to 12% incidence of death, stroke, and myocardial infarction.[124] Carotid artery stenting has been suggested as a possible less risky alternative; however, pooled analysis of studies demonstrate a similarly elevated risk.[117] These results suggest that the presence of carotid stenosis is a marker of advanced atherosclerotic disease and risk that might persist despite revascularization.[117] Observational studies suggest

TABLE 9-3 Risk Factors for Neurologic Complications

Predictor	Beta Coefficient	Odds Ratio	95% CI
Previous neurologic events	1.88	6.8	4.2-12.8
Age >70 years	1.46	4.5	1.2-7.8
Preoperative anemia	1.22	4.2	2.8-6.6
Aortic atheroma	1.45	3.7	2.0-5.8
Duration of myocardial ischemia	1.12	2.8	1.8-3.2
Number of bypasses	1.06	2.3	1.5-2.3
LVEF <35%	1.01	2.2	1.2-1.5
IDDM	0.9	1.5	1.3-2.5
Duration of ECC	0.48	1.4	1.0-2.2
Reoperation	0.48	1.4	0.9-2.4
Emergency operation	0.46	1.2	0.7-2.0

CI = confidence interval; ECC = extracorporeal circulation; IDDM = insulin dependent diabetes mellitus; LVEF = left ventricle ejection fraction.

Source: Boeken et al: Neurological complications after cardiac surgery: risk factors and correlation to the surgical procedure. Thorac Cardiovasc Surg 2005; 53(1):33-36.

that high-risk patients may have reduced cerebral complication rates with OP CABG.[125–127] Systemic hypothermia reduces the cerebral metabolic rate and may provide protection against transient periods of cerebral ischemia, although randomized trials comparing the safety of normothermic and hypothermic CPB have produce conflicting results.[128,129] As a consequence, the ACC/AHA guidelines state that selective carotid screening should only be considered in the following high-risk patient groups: older than 65 years, left main coronary artery stenosis, carotid bruit on examination, PVD, history of smoking, and history of transient ischemic attack or stroke.[123]

Neurocognitive Decline

Disturbances in memory, executive function, motor speed, attention, and other cognitive functions can be detected in up to 80% of patients in the first several weeks after CABG when formal neuropsychiatric testing is performed.[130–132] The severity can range from subtle deficits to profound delirium and disability. Cerebral microemboli have been implicated as a potential causative mechanism.[133] Postoperative hyperthermia has also been associated with greater neurocognitive dysfunction.[134] Deficits usually resolve gradually in most patients.

CONCLUSIONS

Preoperative risk assessment is critical to minimize perioperative and long-term morbidity and mortality. Risk assessment incorporates important patient and surgical information that can be integrated into several validated scoring systems, although an individualized approach is necessary to optimize the perioperative care of the patient. Importantly, it also allows physicians to provide patients and families realistic expectations of the potential risks and benefits of surgery, enabling them to make informed decisions about their health care.

REFERENCES

1. Peterson ED: Innovation and comparative-effectiveness research in cardiac surgery. *NEJM* 2009; 361(19):1897-1899.
2. Lloyd-Jones D, Adams R, Carnethon M, et al: Heart disease and stroke statistics—2009 update: A report from the American Heart Association Statistics Committee and Stroke Statistics Subcommittee. *Circulation* 2009; 119(3):480-486.
3. Conaway DG, House J, Bandt K, et al: The elderly: health status benefits and recovery of function one year after coronary artery bypass surgery. *J Am Coll Cardiol* 2003; 42(8):1421-1426.
4. Weissman C: Pulmonary complications after cardiac surgery. *Semin Cardiothorac Vasc Anesth* 2004; 8(3):185-211.
5. Barnett SD, Halpin LS, Speir AM, et al: Postoperative complications among octogenarians after cardiovascular surgery. *Ann Thorac Surg* 2003; 76(3):726-731.
6. Maurer MS, Luchsinger JA, Wellner R, Kukuy E, Edwards NM: The effect of body mass index on complications from cardiac surgery in the oldest old. *J Am Geriatr Soc* 2002; 50(6):988-994.
7. Kurlansky PA, Williams DB, Traad EA, et al: Arterial grafting results in reduced operative mortality and enhanced long-term quality of life in octogenarians. *Ann Thorac Surg* 2003; 76(2):418-426; discussion 427.
8. Matsuura K, Kobayashi J, Tagusari O, et al: Off-pump coronary artery bypass grafting using only arterial grafts in elderly patients. *Ann Thorac Surg* 2005; 80(1):144-148.
9. Bacchetta MD, Ko W, Girardi LN, et al: Outcomes of cardiac surgery in nonagenarians: a 10-year experience. *Ann Thorac Surg* 2003; 75(4): 1215-1220.
10. Guru V, Fremes SE, Austin PC, Blackstone EH, Tu JV: Gender differences in outcomes after hospital discharge from coronary artery bypass grafting. *Circulation* 2006; 113(4):507-516.
11. Blankstein R, Ward RP, Arnsdorf M, et al: Female gender is an independent predictor of operative mortality after coronary artery bypass graft surgery: contemporary analysis of 31 midwestern hospitals. *Circulation* 2005; 112(9_suppl):I-323-327.
12. Toumpoulis IK, Anagnostopoulos CE, Balaram SK, et al: Assessment of independent predictors for long-term mortality between women and men after coronary artery bypass grafting: are women different from men? *J Thorac Cardiovasc Surg* 2006; 131(2):343-351.
13. Emmert MY, Salzberg SP, Seifert B, et al: Despite modern off-pump coronary artery bypass grafting women fare worse than men. *Interact Cardiovasc Thorac Surg* 2010; 10(5):737-741.
14. Vaccarino V, Lin ZQ, Kasl SV, et al: Sex differences in health status after coronary artery bypass surgery. *Circulation* 2003; 108(21):2642-2647.
15. Falcoz PE, Chocron S, Laluc F, et al: Gender analysis after elective open heart surgery: a two-year comparative study of quality of life. *Ann Thorac Surg* 2006; 81(5):1637-1643.
16. Lucas FL, Stukel TA, Morris AM, Siewers AE, Birkmeyer JD: Race and surgical mortality in the United States. *Ann Surg* 2006; 243(2):281-286.
17. Zacharias A, Schwann TA, Riordan CJ, et al: Operative and late coronary artery bypass grafting outcomes in matched African-American versus Caucasian patients: evidence of a late survival-Medicaid association. *J Am Coll Cardiol* 2005; 46(8):1526-1535.
18. Taylor NE, O'Brien S, Edwards FH, Peterson ED, Bridges CR: Relationship between race and mortality and morbidity after valve replacement surgery. *Circulation* 2005; 111(10):1305-1312.
19. Eagle KA, Guyton RA, Davidoff R, et al: ACC/AHA 2004 guideline update for coronary artery bypass graft surgery: a report of the American College of Cardiology/American Heart Association Task Force on Practice Guidelines (Committee to Update the 1999 Guidelines for Coronary Artery Bypass Graft Surgery). *Circulation* 2004; 110(14):e340-437.

20. Mangano CM, Diamondstone LS, Ramsay JG, et al: Renal dysfunction after myocardial revascularization: risk factors, adverse outcomes, and hospital resource utilization. The Multicenter Study of Perioperative Ischemia Research Group. *Ann Intern Med* 1998; 128(3):194-203.
21. Charlesworth DC, Likosky DS, Marrin CA, et al: Development and validation of a prediction model for strokes after coronary artery bypass grafting. *Ann Thorac Surg* 2003; 76(2):436-443.
22. Clough RA, Leavitt BJ, Morton JR, et al: The effect of comorbid illness on mortality outcomes in cardiac surgery. *Arch Surg* 2002; 137(4):428-432; discussion 432-433.
23. Leavitt BJ, Sheppard L, Maloney C, et al: Effect of diabetes and associated conditions on long-term survival after coronary artery bypass graft surgery. *Circulation* 2004; 110(11 Suppl 1):II41-44.
24. Luciani N, Nasso G, Gaudino M, et al: Coronary artery bypass grafting in type II diabetic patients: a comparison between insulin-dependent and non-insulin-dependent patients at short- and mid-term follow-up. *Ann Thorac Surg* 2003; 76(4):1149-1154.
25. Kubal C, Srinivasan AK, Grayson AD, Fabri BM, Chalmers JA: Effect of risk-adjusted diabetes on mortality and morbidity after coronary artery bypass surgery. *Ann Thorac Surg* 2005; 79(5):1570-1576.
26. Furnary AP, Gao G, Grunkemeier GL, et al: Continuous insulin infusion reduces mortality in patients with diabetes undergoing coronary artery bypass grafting. *J Thorac Cardiovasc Surg* 2003; 125(5):1007-1021.
27. Furnary AP, Zerr KJ, Grunkemeier GL, Starr A: Continuous intravenous insulin infusion reduces the incidence of deep sternal wound infection in diabetic patients after cardiac surgical procedures. *Ann Thorac Surg* 1999; 67(2):352-360; discussion 360-362.
28. Srinivasan AK, Grayson AD, Fabri BM: On-pump versus off-pump coronary artery bypass grafting in diabetic patients: a propensity score analysis. *Ann Thorac Surg* 2004; 78(5):1604-1609.
29. Cooper WA, O'Brien SM, Thourani VH, et al: Impact of renal dysfunction on outcomes of coronary artery bypass surgery: results from the Society of Thoracic Surgeons National Adult Cardiac Database. *Circulation* 2006; 113(8):1063-1070.
30. Wang F, Dupuis JY, Nathan H, Williams K: An analysis of the association between preoperative renal dysfunction and outcome in cardiac surgery: estimated creatinine clearance or plasma creatinine level as measures of renal function. *Chest* 2003; 124(5):1852-1862.
31. Hillis GS, Zehr KJ, Williams AW, et al: Outcome of patients with low ejection fraction undergoing coronary artery bypass grafting: renal function and mortality after 3.8 years. *Circulation* 2006; 114(1 Suppl):I414-419.
32. Lok CE, Austin PC, Wang H, Tu JV: Impact of renal insufficiency on short- and long-term outcomes after cardiac surgery. *Am Heart J* 2004; 148(3):430-438.
33. Zakeri R, Freemantle N, Barnett V, et al: Relation between mild renal dysfunction and outcomes after coronary artery bypass grafting. *Circulation* 2005; 112(9 Suppl):I270-275.
34. Bove T, Landoni G, Calabro MG, et al: Renoprotective action of fenoldopam in high-risk patients undergoing cardiac surgery: a prospective, double-blind, randomized clinical trial. *Circulation* 2005; 111(24): 3230-3235.
35. Burns KE, Chu MW, Novick RJ, et al: Perioperative N-acetylcysteine to prevent renal dysfunction in high-risk patients undergoing CABG surgery: a randomized controlled trial. *JAMA* 2005; 294(3):342-350.
36. Bucerius J, Gummert JF, Walther T, et al: On-pump versus off-pump coronary artery bypass grafting: impact on postoperative renal failure requiring renal replacement therapy. *Ann Thorac Surg* 2004; 77(4): 1250-1256.
37. Cohen A, Katz M, Katz R, Hauptman E, Schachner A: Chronic obstructive pulmonary disease in patients undergoing coronary artery bypass grafting. *J Thorac Cardiovasc Surg* 1995; 109(3):574-581.
38. Fuster RG, Argudo JA, Albarova OG, et al: Prognostic value of chronic obstructive pulmonary disease in coronary artery bypass grafting. *Eur J Cardiothorac Surg* 2006; 29(2):202-209.
39. Filsoufi F, Rahmanian PB, Castillo JG, Chikwe J, Adams DH: Predictors and early and late outcomes of respiratory failure in contemporary cardiac surgery. *Chest* 2008; 133(3):713-721.
40. Weisberg AD, Weisberg EL, Wilson JM, Collard CD: Preoperative evaluation and preparation of the patient for cardiac surgery. *Med Clin North Am* 2009; 93(5):979-994.
41. Hulzebos EH, Helders PJ, Favie NJ, et al: Preoperative intensive inspiratory muscle training to prevent postoperative pulmonary complications in high-risk patients undergoing CABG surgery: a randomized clinical trial. *JAMA* 2006; 296(15):1851-1857.
42. Warkentin TE, Greinacher A, Koster A, Lincoff AM, American College of Chest Physicians: Treatment and prevention of heparin-induced thrombocytopenia: American College of Chest Physicians Evidence-Based Clinical Practice Guidelines (8th ed). *Chest* 2008; 133(6 Suppl): 340S-380S.
43. Martel N, Lee J, Wells PS: Risk for heparin-induced thrombocytopenia with unfractionated and low-molecular-weight heparin thromboprophylaxis: a meta-analysis. *Blood* 2005; 106(8):2710-2715.
44. Liu JC, Lewis BE, Steen LH, et al: Patency of coronary artery bypass grafts in patients with heparin-induced thrombocytopenia. *Am J Cardiol* 2002; 89(8):979-981.
45. Clagett GP, Anderson FA, Jr, Geerts W, et al: Prevention of venous thromboembolism. *Chest* 1998; 114(5 Suppl):531S-560S.
46. Kearon C, Crowther M, Hirsh J: Management of patients with hereditary hypercoagulable disorders. *Annu Rev Med* 2000; 51:169-185.
47. Massoudy P, Cetin SM, Thielmann M, et al: Antiphospholipid syndrome in cardiac surgery: an underestimated coagulation disorder? *Eur J Cardiothorac Surg* 2005; 28(1):133-137.
48. Hogan WJ, McBane RD, Santrach PJ, et al: Antiphospholipid syndrome and perioperative hemostatic management of cardiac valvular surgery. *Mayo Clin Proc* 2000; 75(9):971-976.
49. Rogers CA, Angelini GD, Culliford LA, Capoun R, Ascione R: Coronary surgery in patients with preexisting chronic atrial fibrillation: early and midterm clinical outcome. *Ann Thorac Surg* 2006; 81(5):1676-1682.
50. Mathew JP, Fontes ML, Tudor IC, et al: A multicenter risk index for atrial fibrillation after cardiac surgery. *JAMA* 2004; 291(14):1720-1729.
51. Almassi GH, Schowalter T, Nicolosi AC, et al: Atrial fibrillation after cardiac surgery: a major morbid event? *Ann Surg* 1997; 226(4):501-511; discussion 511-513.
52. Maisel WH, Rawn JD, Stevenson WG: Atrial fibrillation after cardiac surgery. *Ann Intern Med* 2001; 135(12):1061-1073.
53. Villareal RP, Hariharan R, Liu BC, et al: Postoperative atrial fibrillation and mortality after coronary artery bypass surgery. *J Am Coll Cardiol* 2004; 43(5):742-748.
54. Creswell LL, Schuessler RB, Rosenbloom M, Cox JL: Hazards of postoperative atrial arrhythmias. *Ann Thorac Surg* 1993; 56(3):539-549.
55. Cox JL: A perspective of postoperative atrial fibrillation in cardiac operations. *Ann Thorac Surg* 1993; 56(3):405-409.
56. Echahidi N, Pibarot P, O'Hara G, Mathieu P: Mechanisms, prevention, and treatment of atrial fibrillation after cardiac surgery. *J Am Coll Cardiol* 2008; 51(8):793-801.
57. Crystal E, Garfinkle MS, Connolly SS, et al: Interventions for preventing post-operative atrial fibrillation in patients undergoing heart surgery. *Cochrane Database Syst Rev* 2004; (4):CD003611.
58. Wijeysundera DN, Beattie WS, Djaiani G, et al: Off-pump coronary artery surgery for reducing mortality and morbidity: meta-analysis of randomized and observational studies. *J Am Coll Cardiol* 2005; 46(5):872-882.
59. Edwards FH, Clark RE, Schwartz M: Coronary artery bypass grafting: The Society of Thoracic Surgeons National Database Experience. *Ann Thorac Surg* 1994; 57(1):12-19.
60. He GW, Acuff TE, Ryan WH, He YH, Mack MJ: Determinants of operative mortality in reoperative coronary artery bypass grafting. *J Thorac Cardiovasc Surg* 1995; 110(4 Pt 1):971-978.
61. Noyez L, van Eck FM: Long-term cardiac survival after reoperative coronary artery bypass grafting. *Eur J Cardiothorac Surg* 2004; 25(1):59-64.
62. Sabik III JF, Blackstone EH, Houghtaling PL, Walts PA, Lytle BW: Is reoperation still a risk factor in coronary artery bypass surgery? *Ann Thorac Surg* 2005; 80(5):1719-1727.
63. Davierwala PM, Maganti M, Yau TM: Decreasing significance of left ventricular dysfunction and reoperative surgery in predicting coronary artery bypass grafting-associated mortality: a twelve-year study. *J Thorac Cardiovasc Surg* 2003; 126(5):1335-1344.
64. Handa N, McGregor CG, Danielson GK, et al: Valvular heart operation in patients with previous mediastinal radiation therapy. *Ann Thorac Surg* 2001; 71(6):1880-1884.
65. Handa N, McGregor CG, Danielson GK, et al: Coronary artery bypass grafting in patients with previous mediastinal radiation therapy. *J Thorac Cardiovasc Surg* 1999; 117(6):1136-1142.
66. Chang ASY, Smedira NG, Chang CL, et al: Cardiac surgery after mediastinal radiation: extent of exposure influences outcome. *J Thorac Cardiovasc Surg* 2007; 133(2):404-413.e3.
67. Shahian DM, O'Brien SM, Filardo G, et al: The society of thoracic surgeons 2008 cardiac surgery risk models: Part 1—Coronary artery bypass grafting surgery. *Ann Thorac Surg* 2009; 88(1 Suppl 1):S2-S22.
68. O'Brien SM, Shahian DM, Filardo G, et al: The society of thoracic surgeons 2008 cardiac surgery risk models: Part 2—Isolated valve surgery. *Ann Thorac Surg* 2009; 88(1 Suppl 1):S23-S42.
69. Shahian DM, O'Brien SM, Filardo G, et al: The society of thoracic surgeons 2008 cardiac surgery risk models: Part 3—Valve plus coronary artery bypass grafting surgery. *Ann Thorac Surg* 2009; 88(1 Suppl 1):S43-S62.

70. Verma S, Fedak PW, Weisel RD, et al: Off-pump coronary artery bypass surgery: fundamentals for the clinical cardiologist. *Circulation* 2004; 109(10):1206-1211.
71. Parolari A, Alamanni F, Polvani G, et al: Meta-analysis of randomized trials comparing off-pump with on-pump coronary artery bypass graft patency. *Ann Thorac Surg* 2005; 80(6):2121-2125.
72. Sellke FW, DiMaio JM, Caplan LR, et al: Comparing on-pump and off-pump coronary artery bypass grafting: numerous studies but few conclusions. A scientific statement from the American Heart Association Council on Cardiovascular Surgery and Anesthesia in collaboration with the Interdisciplinary Working Group on Quality of Care and Outcomes Research. *Circulation* 2005; 111(21):2858-2864.
73. Puskas JD, Williams WH, Duke PG, et al: Off-pump coronary artery bypass grafting provides complete revascularization with reduced myocardial injury, transfusion requirements, and length of stay: a prospective randomized comparison of two hundred unselected patients undergoing off-pump versus conventional coronary artery bypass grafting. *J Thorac Cardiovasc Surg* 2003; 125(4):797-808.
74. Modi P, Rodriguez E, Chitwood WR, Jr: Robot-assisted cardiac surgery. *Interact Cardiovasc Thorac Surg* 2009; 9(3):500-505.
75. Reicher B, Poston RS, Mehra MR, et al: Simultaneous "hybrid" percutaneous coronary intervention and minimally invasive surgical bypass grafting: feasibility, safety, and clinical outcomes. *Am Heart J* 2008; 155(4): 661-667.
76. Bybee KA, Powell BD, Valeti U, et al: Preoperative aspirin therapy is associated with improved postoperative outcomes in patients undergoing coronary artery bypass grafting. *Circulation* 2005; 112(9 Suppl): I286-292.
77. Dacey LJ, Munoz JJ, Johnson ER, et al: Effect of preoperative aspirin use on mortality in coronary artery bypass grafting patients. *Ann Thorac Surg* 2000; 70(6):1986-1990.
78. Sun JC, Crowther MA, Warkentin TE, Lamy A, Teoh KH: Should aspirin be discontinued before coronary artery bypass surgery? *Circulation* 2005; 112(7):e85-90.
79. Goldman S, Copeland J, Moritz T, et al: Starting aspirin therapy after operation. Effects on early graft patency. Department of Veterans Affairs Cooperative Study Group. *Circulation* 1991; 84(2):520-526.
80. Sethi GK, Copeland JG, Goldman S, et al: Implications of preoperative administration of aspirin in patients undergoing coronary artery bypass grafting. Department of Veterans Affairs Cooperative Study on Antiplatelet Therapy. *J Am Coll Cardiol* 1990; 15(1):15-20.
81. Antman EM, Hand M, Armstrong PW, et al: 2007 Focused Update of the ACC/AHA 2004 Guidelines for the Management of Patients with ST-Elevation Myocardial Infarction: a report of the American College of Cardiology/American Heart Association Task Force on Practice Guidelines. Developed in collaboration with the Canadian Cardiovascular Society: endorsed by the American Academy of Family Physicians: 2007 Writing Group to Review New Evidence and Update the ACC/AHA 2004 Guidelines for the Management of Patients with ST-Elevation Myocardial Infarction, writing on behalf of the 2004 Writing Committee. *Circulation* 2008; 117(2):296-329.
82. Ferraris VA, Ferraris SP, Moliterno DJ, et al: The society of thoracic surgeons practice guideline series: Aspirin and other antiplatelet agents during operative coronary revascularization (executive summary). *Ann Thorac Surg* 2005; 79(4):1454-1461.
83. Becker RC, Meade TW, Berger PB, et al: The primary and secondary prevention of coronary artery disease: American college of chest physicians evidence-based clinical practice guidelines (8th edition). *Chest* 2008; 133(6 Suppl):776S-814S.
84. Hongo RH, Ley J, Dick SE, Yee RR: The effect of clopidogrel in combination with aspirin when given before coronary artery bypass grafting. *J Am Coll Cardiol* 2002; 40(2):231-237.
85. Kapetanakis EI, Medlam DA, Petro KR, et al: Effect of clopidogrel premedication in off-pump cardiac surgery: are we forfeiting the benefits of reduced hemorrhagic sequelae? *Circulation* 2006; 113(13):1667-1674.
86. Wiviott SD, Braunwald E, McCabe CH, et al: Prasugrel versus clopidogrel in patients with acute coronary syndromes. *NEJM* 2007; 357(20): 2001-2015.
87. Wallentin L, Becker RC, Budaj A, et al: Ticagrelor versus clopidogrel in patients with acute coronary syndromes. *NEJM* 2009; 361(11):1045-1057.
88. Anderson JL, Adams CD, Antman EM, et al: ACC/AHA 2007 Guidelines for the Management of Patients with Unstable Angina/non ST-Elevation Myocardial Infarction: a report of the American College of Cardiology/American Heart Association Task Force on Practice Guidelines (Writing Committee to Revise the 2002 Guidelines for the Management of Patients with Unstable Angina/Non ST-Elevation Myocardial Infarction): developed in collaboration with the American College of Emergency Physicians, the Society for Cardiovascular Angiography and Interventions, and the Society of Thoracic Surgeons: endorsed by the American Association of Cardiovascular and Pulmonary Rehabilitation and the Society for Academic Emergency Medicine. *Circulation* 2007; 116(7):e148-304.
89. Hunt SA, Abraham WT, Chin MH, et al: ACC/AHA 2005 guideline update for the diagnosis and management of chronic heart failure in the adult: a report of the American College of Cardiology/American Heart Association Task Force on Practice Guidelines (Writing Committee to Update the 2001 Guidelines for the Evaluation and Management of Heart Failure): developed in collaboration with the American College of Chest Physicians and the International Society for Heart and Lung Transplantation: endorsed by the Heart Rhythm Society. *Circulation* 2005; 112(12):e154-235.
90. Mangano DT, Layug EL, Wallace A, Tateo I: Effect of atenolol on mortality and cardiovascular morbidity after noncardiac surgery: multicenter study of perioperative ischemia research group. *NEJM* 1996; 335(23): 1713-1720.
91. Boersma E, Poldermans D, Bax JJ, et al: Predictors of cardiac events after major vascular surgery: role of clinical characteristics, dobutamine echocardiography, and beta-blocker therapy. *JAMA* 2001; 285(14):1865-1873.
92. Levin MA, Lin H, Castillo JG, et al: Early on-cardiopulmonary bypass hypotension and other factors associated with vasoplegic syndrome. *Circulation* 2009; 120(17):1664-1671.
93. Gottlieb SS, McCarter RJ, Vogel RA: Effect of beta-blockade on mortality among high-risk and low-risk patients after myocardial infarction. *NEJM* 1998; 339(8):489-497.
94. Ferguson TB, Jr, Coombs LP, Peterson ED, Society of Thoracic Surgeons National Adult Cardiac Surgery Database: Preoperative beta-blocker use and mortality and morbidity following CABG surgery in North America. *JAMA* 2002; 287(17):2221-2227.
95. Garg R, Yusuf S: Overview of randomized trials of angiotensin-converting enzyme inhibitors on mortality and morbidity in patients with heart failure. Collaborative Group on ACE Inhibitor Trials. *JAMA* 1995; 273(18): 1450-1456.
96. White CM, Kluger J, Lertsburapa K, Faheem O, Coleman CI: Effect of preoperative angiotensin converting enzyme inhibitor or angiotensin receptor blocker use on the frequency of atrial fibrillation after cardiac surgery: a cohort study from the atrial fibrillation suppression trials II and III. *Eur J Cardiothorac Surg* 2007; 31(5):817-820.
97. Hasija S, Makhija N, Chowdhury M, et al: Prophylactic vasopressin in patients receiving the angiotensin-converting enzyme inhibitor ramipril undergoing coronary artery bypass graft surgery. *J Cardiothorac Vasc Anesth* 2010; 24(2):230-238.
98. Konstam MA, Rousseau MF, Kronenberg MW, et al: Effects of the angiotensin converting enzyme inhibitor enalapril on the long-term progression of left ventricular dysfunction in patients with heart failure. SOLVD Investigators. *Circulation* 1992; 86(2):431-438.
99. Raja SG, Fida N: Should angiotensin converting enzyme inhibitors/angiotensin II receptor antagonists be omitted before cardiac surgery to avoid postoperative vasodilation? *Interact Cardiovasc Thorac Surg* 2008; 7(3):470-475.
100. Hindler K, Shaw AD, Samuels J, et al: Improved postoperative outcomes associated with preoperative statin therapy. *Anesthesiology* 2006; 105(6): 1260-1272; quiz 1289-1290.
101. Liakopoulos OJ, Choi YH, Haldenwang PL, et al: Impact of preoperative statin therapy on adverse postoperative outcomes in patients undergoing cardiac surgery: a meta-analysis of over 30,000 patients. *Eur Heart J* 2008; 29(12):1548-1559.
102. Patti G, Chello M, Candura D, et al: Randomized trial of atorvastatin for reduction of postoperative atrial fibrillation in patients undergoing cardiac surgery: results of the ARMYDA-3 (Atorvastatin for Reduction of MYocardial Dysrhythmia After cardiac surgery) study. *Circulation* 2006; 114(14):1455-1461.
103. Ray KK, Cannon CP: The potential relevance of the multiple lipid-independent (pleiotropic) effects of statins in the management of acute coronary syndromes. *J Am Coll Cardiol* 2005; 46(8):1425-1433.
104. Le Manach Y, Coriat P, Collard CD, Riedel B: Statin therapy within the perioperative period. *Anesthesiology* 2008; 108(6):1141-1146.
105. Gao D, Grunwald GK, Rumsfeld JS, et al: Time-varying risk factors for long-term mortality after coronary artery bypass graft surgery. *Ann Thorac Surg* 2006; 81(3):793-799.
106. Nashef SA, Roques F, Michel P, et al: European system for cardiac operative risk evaluation (EuroSCORE). *Eur J Cardiothorac Surg* 1999; 16(1):9-13.
107. Roques F, Michel P, Goldstone AR, Nashef SA: The logistic EuroSCORE. *Eur Heart J* 2003; 24(9):881-882.

108. Bhatti F, Grayson AD, Grotte G, et al: The logistic EuroSCORE in cardiac surgery: how well does it predict operative risk? *Heart* 2006; 92(12): 1817-1820.
109. Zingone B, Pappalardo A, Dreas L: Logistic versus additive EuroSCORE. A comparative assessment of the two models in an independent population sample. *Eur J Cardiothorac Surg* 2004; 26(6):1134-1140.
110. Keogh BE: Logistic, additive or historical: is EuroSCORE an appropriate model for comparing individual surgeons' performance? *Heart* 2006; 92(12):1715-1716.
111. Karthik S, Srinivasan AK, Grayson AD, et al: Limitations of additive EuroSCORE for measuring risk stratified mortality in combined coronary and valve surgery. *Eur J Cardiothorac Surg* 2004; 26(2):318-322.
112. Nilsson J, Algotsson L, Hoglund P, Luhrs C, Brandt J: Early mortality in coronary bypass surgery: the EuroSCORE versus the society of thoracic surgeons risk algorithm. *Ann Thorac Surg* 2004; 77(4):1235-1239; discussion 1239-1240.
113. Granton J, Cheng D: Risk stratification models for cardiac surgery. *Semin Cardiothorac Vasc Anesth* 2008; 12(3):167-174.
114. O'Connor GT, Plume SK, Olmstead EM, et al: Multivariate prediction of in-hospital mortality associated with coronary artery bypass graft surgery. Northern New England Cardiovascular Disease Study Group. *Circulation* 1992; 85(6):2110-2118.
115. Nilsson J, Algotsson L, Hoglund P, Luhrs C, Brandt J: Comparison of 19 pre-operative risk stratification models in open-heart surgery. *Eur Heart J* 2006; 27(7):867-874.
116. Nowicki ER, Birkmeyer NJ, Weintraub RW, et al: Multivariable prediction of in-hospital mortality associated with aortic and mitral valve surgery in Northern New England. *Ann Thorac Surg* 2004; 77(6):1966-1977.
117. Guzman LA, Costa MA, Angiolillo DJ, et al: A systematic review of outcomes in patients with staged carotid artery stenting and coronary artery bypass graft surgery. *Stroke* 2008; 39(2):361-365.
118. Huh J, Wall MJ, Jr, Soltero ER: Treatment of combined coronary and carotid artery disease. *Curr Opin Cardiol* 2003; 18(6):447-453.
119. Schwartz LB, Bridgman AH, Kieffer RW, et al: Asymptomatic carotid artery stenosis and stroke in patients undergoing cardiopulmonary bypass. *J Vasc Surg* 1995; 21(1):146-153.
120. Berens ES, Kouchoukos NT, Murphy SF, Wareing TH: Preoperative carotid artery screening in elderly patients undergoing cardiac surgery. *J Vasc Surg* 1992; 15(2):313-321; discussion 322-323.
121. Boeken U, Litmathe J, Feindt P, Gams E: Neurological complications after cardiac surgery: risk factors and correlation to the surgical procedure. *Thorac Cardiovasc Surg* 2005; 53(1):33-36.
122. Dacey LJ, Likosky DS, Leavitt BJ, et al: Perioperative stroke and long-term survival after coronary bypass graft surgery. *Ann Thorac Surg* 2005; 79(2):532-536; discussion 537.
123. Eagle KA, Guyton RA, Davidoff R, et al: ACC/AHA 2004 guideline update for coronary artery bypass graft surgery: summary article: a report of the American College of Cardiology/American Heart Association Task Force on Practice Guidelines (Committee to Update the 1999 Guidelines for Coronary Artery Bypass Graft Surgery). *Circulation* 2004; 110(9): 1168-1176.
124. Naylor AR, Cuffe RL, Rothwell PM, Bell PR: A systematic review of outcomes following staged and synchronous carotid endarterectomy and coronary artery bypass. *Eur J Vasc Endovasc Surg* 2003; 25(5):380-389.
125. Zamvar V, Williams D, Hall J, et al: Assessment of neurocognitive impairment after off-pump and on-pump techniques for coronary artery bypass graft surgery: prospective randomised controlled trial. *BMJ* 2002; 325(7375):1268.
126. Sharony R, Bizekis CS, Kanchuger M, et al: Off-pump coronary artery bypass grafting reduces mortality and stroke in patients with atheromatous aortas: a case control study. *Circulation* 2003; 108(Suppl 1): II15-20.
127. Karthik S, Musleh G, Grayson AD, et al: Coronary surgery in patients with peripheral vascular disease: effect of avoiding cardiopulmonary bypass. *Ann Thorac Surg* 2004; 77(4):1245-1249.
128. Randomised trial of normothermic versus hypothermic coronary bypass surgery. The Warm Heart Investigators. *Lancet* 1994; 343(8897):559-563.
129. Martin TD, Craver JM, Gott JP, et al: Prospective, randomized trial of retrograde warm blood cardioplegia: myocardial benefit and neurologic threat. *Ann Thorac Surg* 1994; 57(2):298-302; discussion 302-304.
130. Van Dijk D, Jansen EW, Hijman R, et al: Cognitive outcome after off-pump and on-pump coronary artery bypass graft surgery: a randomized trial. *JAMA* 2002; 287(11):1405-1412.
131. van Dijk D, Keizer AM, Diephuis JC, et al: Neurocognitive dysfunction after coronary artery bypass surgery: a systematic review. *J Thorac Cardiovasc Surg* 2000; 120(4):632-639.
132. Selnes OA, McKhann GM: Neurocognitive complications after coronary artery bypass surgery. *Ann Neurol* 2005; 57(5):615-621.
133. Clark RE, Brillman J, Davis DA, et al: Microemboli during coronary artery bypass grafting. Genesis and effect on outcome. *J Thorac Cardiovasc Surg* 1995; 109(2):249-257; discussion 257-258.
134. Grocott HP, Mackensen GB, Grigore AM, et al: Postoperative hyperthermia is associated with cognitive dysfunction after coronary artery bypass graft surgery. *Stroke* 2002; 33(2):537-541.

CHAPTER 10

Cardiac Anesthesia

William J. Vernick
Albert T. Cheung
Jeremy D. Kukafka
Joseph S. Savino

INTRODUCTION

The cardiac anesthesiologist is challenged with the requirements of maintaining general anesthesia while also serving as the patient's intensivist and diagnostician, facilitating the surgery and maintaining vital organ function. The objectives of a general anesthetic are analgesia, amnesia, and unconsciousness while supporting vital physiologic function and creating satisfactory operating conditions. An effective general anesthetic blunts the physiologic responses to surgical trauma and hemodynamic perturbations while permitting recovery at a predictable time after the operation. To accomplish this, the anesthesiologist must act as the patient's medical intensivist: support life with mechanical ventilation; control the circulation; and diagnose and treat acute emergencies that may occur during surgical incision, rapid changes in body temperature, extracorporeal circulation, and acute shifts in intravascular volume. The cardiac anesthesiologist must provide complex diagnostics in order to facilitate surgery by determining the competency of heart reconstructive procedures and measuring the cardiovascular response to altered cardiac anatomy and physiology. The task in cardiac surgery is unique because of the nature of the operations and the narrow tolerance for hemodynamic alterations in patients with critical cardiac disease. Anesthetic management of the cardiac surgical patient is intimately related to the planned operative procedure and the anticipated timing of intraoperative events.

PREOPERATIVE EVALUATION

The preoperative visit by the anesthesiologist is aimed at the formulation of an anesthetic plan based on the patient's surgical illness, scheduled operation, and concomitant medical problems. The medical history is elicited by questioning the patient and reviewing the medical records. The anesthesiologist must know the status of the cardiovascular system, related morbidity, and concurrent medications to design the anesthetic safely for a patient undergoing heart surgery. All anesthetic drugs have a direct effect on cardiac function, vascular tone, and/or the autonomic nervous system. The American Society of Anesthesiologists (ASA) has developed a physical status classification as a general measure of the patient's severity of illness (Table 10-1).[1]

In addition to contributing to postoperative morbidity, concurrent medical illness often defines an acceptable range for monitored parameters that are controlled during cardiac surgery. Acceptable intraoperative blood pressure may be altered based on several preoperative findings. The brain of a patient with long-standing severe hypertension may perfuse inadequately if the blood pressure during surgery is maintained only within what is typically considered a "normal" range because of a "rightward shift" of the cerebral autoregulation curve over time. History of a previous stroke often suggests intrinsic cerebrovascular disease that also may dictate alteration of blood pressure and blood product administration management. The response to bronchodilators in patients with chronic obstructive pulmonary disease may permit guided management of perioperative bronchospasm to ensure adequate respiration. A history of a difficult intubation or an adverse response to a specific drug is also highly relevant to the anesthesia plan.

Although a focused medical history pertaining to the patient's cardiac disease often takes priority, there are additional items in the history that are important to the cardiac anesthesiologist that might not be as pertinent in the realm of noncardiac surgery. For

TABLE 10-1 American Society of Anesthesiologists, Physical Status Classification

Class 1: Normal healthy patient
Class 2: Systemic disease without end-organ dysfunction
Class 3: Systemic disease with end-organ dysfunction that is not incapacitating (eg, diabetes mellitus with abnormal renal function)
Class 4: Systemic disease with end-organ dysfunction that is incapacitating (eg, diabetes mellitus with renal failure and ketoacidosis)
Class 5: Moribund patient unexpected to survive beyond 24 yours (eg, diabetes mellitus with renal failure, ketoacidosis, and infarcted bowel requiring vasopressor support)
E*: Emergency surgery

*The E is added to the classification number.

example, the presence of esophageal pathology could contraindicate the placement of a transesophageal echocardiography (TEE) probe (Table 10-2). A history of previous venous thrombosis or pulmonary embolism might make one consider avoiding antifibrinolytic medications. The presence of Reynaud's disease may complicate radial arterial catheterization.

The anesthesiologist is responsible for informing the patient of the conduct of the planned anesthetic and associated risks while obtaining consent for the anesthesia and related procedures. The exchange of information between patient and physician is often a balance between providing sufficient insight regarding possible complications without producing harmful anxiety. An outline of upcoming events accompanied by an informative discussion of risks and options typically leads to informed consent.

The preoperative ordering of tests evaluating cardiac function before noncardiac surgery, such as stress testing, echocardiography, and cardiac catheterization, are the focus of much debate and have generated an extensive literature.[3,4] However, in cardiac surgery, these tests are part of routine cardiac surgical evaluation for operative planning. Although the decision to order these preoperative tests is not applicable to the cardiac anesthesiologist, the importance of their review is critical. Not only are these tests used in formulating an anesthetic plan but are also used to focus the intraoperative TEE examinations and as a basis for comparison to the operative TEE findings.

Laboratory tests are ordered to complement findings of the medical history and physical examination. Routine preoperative laboratory tests include a complete blood with platelet count; electrolyte battery with blood glucose, serum creatinine, and blood urea nitrogen levels; and prothrombin time and partial thromboplastin times. Other laboratory tests may be ordered based on patient-specific disease. A chest radiograph, electrocardiogram (ECG), and urinalysis complete routine testing. Pulmonary function tests are not routinely ordered and their usefulness in cardiac surgery is debatable except in lung transplantation. Outside of lung resection during thoracic surgery, they have not been found to be predictive of postoperative pulmonary complications.[5,6] The review of chest computed axial tomography (CT) scans may have important implications for the cardiac anesthesiologist in patients with aortic disease such as aortic aneurysmal compression of the esophagus or major branches of the pulmonary arterial and main bronchial trees.

Most concurrent medications are continued until right up to the operation, including most cardiovascular medications. Oral medications can be taken according to schedule on the day of surgery with a small sip of water. Although increase in mortality after acute beta-blocker withdrawal have been more clearly shown in vascular surgery[7,8] than in cardiac surgery, withdrawal in cardiac surgery has been linked to an increased incidence of postoperative supraventricular arrhythmias.[9,10] Concern also exists with the preoperative discontinuation of vasodilators leading to perioperative vasoconstriction. The preoperative continuation of ACE inhibitors remains controversial given reports of postanesthesia induction hypotension and decreased perioperative renal perfusion.[11–14] Although from a retrospective observational cohort study, its preoperative continuation has also recently been linked to an increased incidence of mortality, renal failure, and the necessity of inotropic support after cardiac surgery.[15] For patients scheduled for late afternoon surgery and not receiving maintenance intravenous fluids, preoperative diuretics may be withheld to avoid preoperative dehydration. Finally, a potential for acute withdrawal must be considered after sudden cessation of chronic opioid or benzodiazepines use.

In contrast to antihypertensives, most anticoagulants are discontinued before surgery. Warfarin is generally stopped 5 days before the operation. In patients with mechanical heart valves, heparin bridge therapy is utilized. The oral antiplatelet drug, clopidogrel, is typically stopped for at least 5 days in order to allow the generation of new functioning platelets. When intravenous heparin is administered for unstable angina pectoris, it may be unwise to discontinue it preoperatively.

TABLE 10-2 Contraindications to Transesophageal Echocardiography[2]

Absolute	Esophageal stricture	Esophageal Diverticula	Esophageal Tumor	Recent upper GI suture line	Esophageal interruption
Relative	Symptomatic hiatal hernia	Esophagitis	Coagulopathy	Esophageal varices	Unexplained upper GI bleed

The physical examination includes measurement of height, weight, and vital signs as well as a comprehensive assessment of the heart, lungs, peripheral vasculature, and nervous system. The exam is often focused in order to quickly identify signs suggestive of circulatory deficiency, such as the lack of equal and bilateral pulses, lower extremity edema, ascites, distended neck veins, or the inability to lie flat. No anesthesiologist's exam is complete without a thorough examination of the airway. Samsoon's modification of the Mallampati classification used to predict a difficult airway is based on the examiner's ability to view intraoral structures:[16,17]

Class 1: Soft palate, tonsillar fauces, tonsillar pillars, and uvula
Class 2: Soft palate, tonsillar fauces, and uvula
Class 3: Soft palate and base of uvula
Class 4: Soft palate not visualized

Classes 1 and 2 represent airway anatomy associated with minimal difficulty with tracheal intubation. Classes 3 and 4 are more likely associated with an inability to intubate the trachea using conventional direct laryngoscopy. Other features associated with difficult intubations include a recessed chin, small mouth, large tongue, and inability to sublux the mandible.

Before the patient enters the operating room, the anesthesiologist formulates a plan to control the circulatory response to anesthesia, secure the airway, and maintain body homeostasis. Emergency operations are incompatible with leisurely preparation but instead are dictated by a sense of urgency. Rarely, however, is there any opportunity to provide reassurance to the patient or to prepare for the anesthetic and operation meticulously. The multidisciplinary nature of cardiac surgery requires precise communication between the anesthesiologist and the surgeon. Frank and open communication between all members of the operative team has been identified as an important element in the current effort to promote patient safety.

MONITORING PHYSIOLOGIC FUNCTIONS DURING ANESTHESIA

Extensive physiologic monitoring is employed during cardiac operations because virtually every major physiologic system required for life is affected. The reasons for physiologic monitoring are (1) to ensure patient safety in the absence of protective reflexes made ineffective by anesthetic drugs, (2) to enable pharmacologic and mechanical control of vital function, and (3) to diagnose acute emergencies that require immediate treatment. For example, morbidity as a consequence of breathing circuit disconnects, loss of oxygen from the hospital's central supply, or unrecognized esophageal or main stem endotracheal intubations can be prevented by capnography, pulse oximetry, airway pressure monitors, oxygen analyzers, and a stethoscope.

The senses of touch, hearing, and sight are the basic monitors. Electronic monitors are vigilance aids that supplement the anesthesiologist's perceptions. The selection of monitors is dictated by the utility of the data generated, expense, and risk. Routine or essential monitors that have been deemed cost-effective with low risk:benefit ratios include pulse oximetry, noninvasive blood pressure, capnography, temperature, ECG, precordial or esophageal stethoscope, and oxygen analyzers. These have been defined by the American Society of Anesthesiologists (House of Delegates, 1989) as essential monitors to be used in all surgical patients requiring anesthesia unless there are contraindications (eg, esophageal stethoscope during esophageal surgery) (Table 10-3). Other noninvasive and invasive monitors are used only with clear indication.

The growth in monitoring technology and sophistication is paralleled by an equal growth in cost. The balance between cost and enhancement of patient safety must be considered when additional monitoring is selected. It is difficult to justify a monitor that provides data that does not influence medical or surgical management.

TABLE 10-3 Physiologic Monitors

Organ System	ASA Standard Operating Room Monitors	Additional Monitoring for Cardiac Surgery
Cardiovascular	ECG Noninvasive blood pressure	Invasive blood pressure CVP PAP/PAOP Cardiac output SvO_2 TEE Vascular ultrasound
Pulmonary	Capnography Pulse oximeter Airway pressure Stethoscope Oxygen analyzer	Arterial blood gases Anesthetic gas concentrations Spirometry
Nervous system		EEG SSEP MEP Transcranial Doppler CSF pressure Bispectral index Cerebral oximetry
Metabolic	Temperature Urine output	Serum electrolytes Acid-base Glucose Serum osmolarity
Hematopoietic		Hematocrit Activated coagulation time aPTT, TT heparin concentration Platelet count Platelet function TEG SvO_2, rSO_2

Measurement of Blood Pressure

Blood pressure is the most commonly measured index of cardiovascular stability in the perioperative period. Anesthetics and surgery cause changes in blood pressure that are often rapid and may be great enough to cause harm unless anticipated and treated. However, a change in blood pressure that alters perfusion pressure may not change organ blood flow. This is because most vital organs can autoregulate blood flow in response to changes in mean arterial blood pressure, permitting constant blood flow over a range of perfusion pressures.[18] In chronically hypertensive patients, the boundaries for autoregulation are shifted so that significant decreases in organ perfusion may occur with blood pressures in the considered "normal" range. Both the type and dose of anesthetic medications can affect the relationship between vital organ perfusion and blood pressure. For example, volatile anesthetics are potent vasodilators that tend to disrupt cerebral autoregulation in a dose-dependent manner to render blood flow more linearly dependent on blood pressure (Fig. 10-1).

Although noninvasive blood pressure monitoring suffices for most patients during routine noncardiac surgery, direct measure of arterial blood pressure with an indwelling arterial catheter is necessary for cardiac surgery in order to detect changes quickly, to measure nonpulsatile blood pressure during cardiopulmonary bypass, and to facilitate arterial blood sampling for laboratory analysis. The measuring system includes an intra-arterial catheter and low-compliance saline-filled tubing connected to a transducer with a pressure-sensing diaphragm. The transducer has a strain gauge that converts the mechanical energy (displacement of the diaphragm by a change in pressure) into an electric signal that typically is displayed as a pressure waveform with numeric outputs for systolic, diastolic, and mean pressures. The mean blood pressure is determined by calculating the area under several pulse waveforms and averaging over time. This represents a more accurate measure of mean arterial blood pressure than weighted averages of systolic and diastolic pressures.

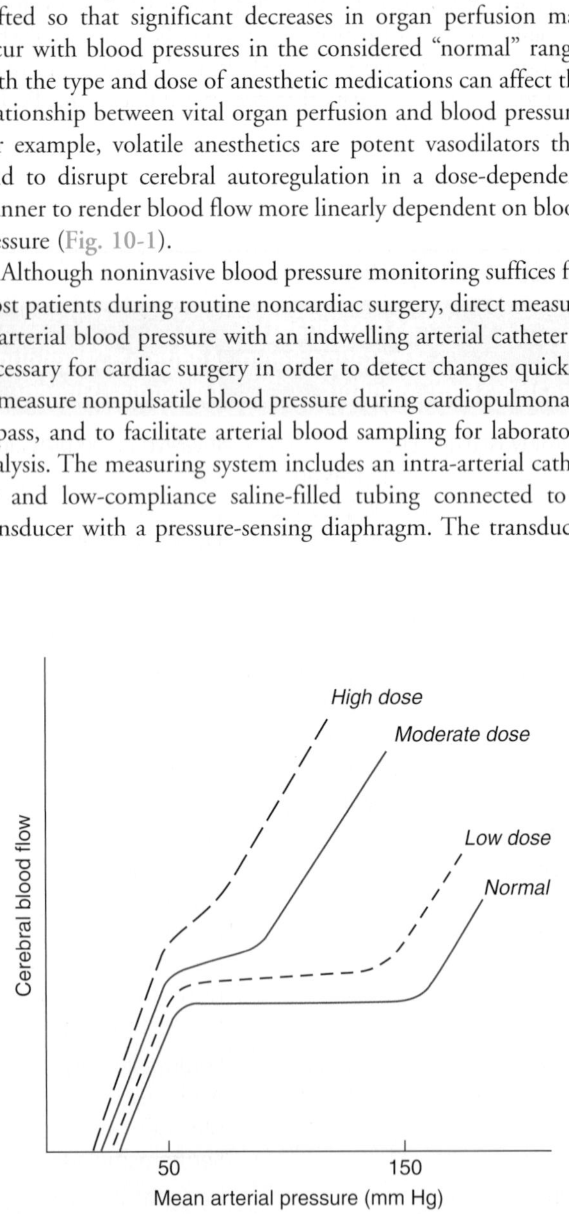

FIGURE 10-1 Autoregulation maintains a constant cerebral blood flow between mean arterial blood pressures of 50 to 150 mm Hg in the conscious,unanesthetized state. Increasing doses of potent inhalation anesthetics produce a dose-dependent disruption of autoregulation owing to cerebral vasodilatation. (*Modified with permission from Shapiro H: Anesthesia effects upon cerebral blood flow, cerebral metabolism, electroencephalogram and evoked potentials, in Miller RD [ed]: Anesthesia, 2nd ed. New York, Churchill-Livingstone, 1986; p 1249.*)

The transducer requires a zero reference at the level of the right atrium. Any movement of the patient or the transducer that changes the vertical distance between the transducer and the right atrium affects the value of the blood pressure measured. If the transducer is lowered, the pressure diaphragm senses arterial blood pressure plus hydrostatic pressure generated from the vertical column of fluid contained in the tubing and displays a falsely high blood pressure. A transducer elevated above the zero reference level decreases the displayed blood pressure. A 1-cm column of water (blood) exerts a hydrostatic pressure equal to 0.74 mm Hg. Small changes in patient or transducer position have a relatively insignificant effect on arterial blood pressure measurements but have a more important effect on lower-amplitude pressure measurements, such as central venous, pulmonary artery, and pulmonary artery occlusion pressures.

The radial artery is the most common site for insertion of an intra-arterial catheter. Twenty-gauge catheters are preferred when the radial artery is used because larger catheters are more likely to cause thrombosis. The wrist is chosen for arterial cannulation most often because of dual blood supply to the hand, preventing ischemia in the setting of a catheter related thrombosis. A patent palmar arch allows the hand to remain perfused despite a potential thrombosis of either the radial or ulnar artery assuming adequate flow through the other vessel. Distal embolization remains a risk though. The radial is the more superficial vessel and generally considered easier to cannulate. The Allen's test was designed to assess ulnar and palmar arch blood flow during abrupt occlusion of the radial artery, but its value to predict morbidity with radial artery cannulation is equivocal.[19] Other sites selected for the insertion of an intra-arterial catheterization include the brachial, axillary, and femoral arteries.

The contour of the arterial pressure waveform is different in central and peripheral arteries. The propagating pressure waveform loses energy and momentum with a corresponding delay in transmission, loss of high-frequency components such as anacrotic and dicrotic notches, lower systolic and pulse pressures, and decreased mean pressure.[20] The changes in the pulse waveform can be attributed to damping, blood viscosity, vessel diameter, vessel elastance, and the effects of reflectance of the incident arterial waveform by the artery-arteriolar junction.[21,22] The blood pressure waveform measured in the ascending aorta is minimally affected by reflected waves in contrast to measurement of blood pressure in the dorsalis pedis or radial artery.

The contour of the pressure waveform can also be affected by the physical construction of the monitoring system. A hyper-resonant response to a change in pressure, or ringing, occurs when the frequency response of the monitoring system (ie, extension tubing, catheter, and stopcocks) is close to the frequency of the pressure waveform.[20] The natural or resonant frequency f_n of a monitoring system is defined by

$$f_n = \frac{1}{2\pi}\sqrt{\frac{\pi D^2}{4pL \cdot C}}$$

where C is compliance of the measuring system, L is the length of the tubing, D is the diameter of the catheter extension tubing, and p is the density of the solution.

To prevent ringing, the natural frequency of the monitoring system f_n must be greater than the frequencies of the pulse waveform. Any process that decreases f_n, such as narrow, long, compliant tubing, may cause *ringing*.[23] Ringing increases the value of the systolic blood pressure and decreases the value of the diastolic blood pressure but generally does not affect the value of the mean arterial pressure.

Damping is the tendency of the measuring system, through frictional losses, to blunt the peaks and troughs in a signal.[24] Kinks in the pressure tubing or catheter, stopcocks, and air bubbles contribute to damping. Overdamped systems underestimate systolic blood pressure and overestimate diastolic blood pressure. When long lengths of tubing are necessary, deliberate damping may improve the fidelity of the arterial waveform.

Testing a measuring system for ringing and damping ensures that an arterial contour is reproduced faithfully. A simple test involves a brief flush of the high-pressure saline-filled catheter extension assembly. Flush and release should produce a rapid return of the pressure waveform to baseline with minimal oscillations. A gradual return to baseline and loss of higher-frequency components of the waveform suggests overdamping. A rapid return to baseline followed by sustained oscillations suggests ringing.

Electrocardiogram

The intraoperative ECG monitor has evolved from the fading-ball oscilloscope to a sophisticated microprocessor analog display. ECG signals are filtered digitally to eliminate electrical artifact produced by high-frequency (60-Hz) electrical power lines, electrocautery, patient movement, and baseline drift. The bandwidth filter modes are diagnostic, monitor, and filter. The diagnostic mode has the widest bandwidths (least filtered signal) and is preferred for detecting ST-segment changes caused by myocardial ischemia. Monitor and filter modes have progressively narrower bandwidths that effectively eliminate high-frequency interference and baseline drift but decrease the sensitivity of detecting ST-segment changes and decrease the specificity of ST-segment change to diagnose myocardial ischemia. Abnormal ST-segment depression (>1 mV) can occur from excessive low-frequency filtering and result in the misdiagnosis of myocardial ischemia. Filter modes are useful for detecting P waves and changes in cardiac rhythm in the presence of high-frequency interference.

The ECG is the most sensitive and practical monitor for the detection and diagnosis of disorders of cardiac rhythm and conduction and myocardial ischemia and infarction. Continuous monitoring of leads II and V_5 is common (Fig. 10-2). Together

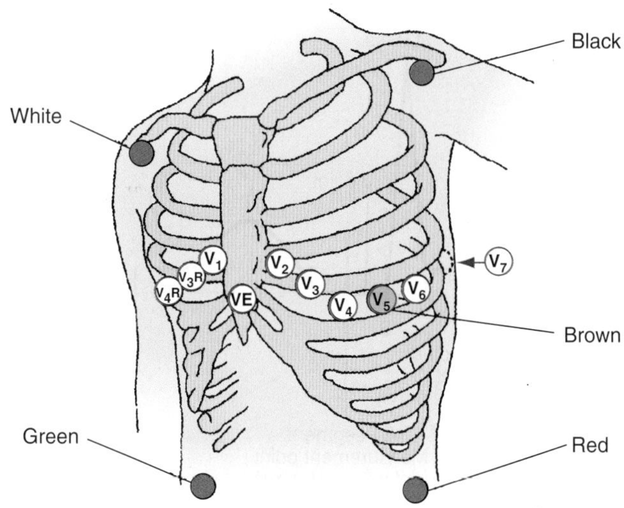

FIGURE 10-2 Standard intraoperative electrocardiogram (ECG) lead placement. Typically, leads II and V_5 are monitored continuously.

these leads detect greater than 90% of ischemic episodes in patients with coronary artery disease who have noncardiac surgery.[25]

Diagnostic criteria for myocardial ischemia based on the ECG are (1) acute ST-segment depression greater than 0.1 mV 60 ms beyond the J point or (2) acute ST-segment elevation greater than 0.2 mV 60 ms beyond the J point[26] (Fig. 10-3). The normal ST-segment curves smoothly into the T wave. Flat ST segments that form an acute angle with the T wave or downsloping ST segments are worrisome for subendocardial ischemia. ST-segment elevation occurs with transmural myocardial injury but also may occur after direct current (dc) cardioversion and in normal adults. The lack of specificity of ST-T-wave changes for myocardial ischemia is a major limitation of intraoperative ECG monitoring. Pericarditis, myocarditis, mitral valve prolapse, stroke, and digitalis therapy may produce changes in the ST segment that mimic myocardial ischemia.

Digital signal processing handles much larger quantities of information than the unaided eye and may increase the ability to detect ischemic episodes. ST-segment position analyzers automatically measure the displacement of the ST segment from a predetermined reference and enhance the ability to quantify changes in ST-segment position. Appropriate application requires accurate identification of the various loci in the P-QRS-T-wave complex. The operator defines the baseline and the J point of a reference QRS complex by movement of a cursor. New QRS-T-wave complexes are superimposed onto a predefined mean reference complex. Vertical ST-segment displacement is measured in millivolts and displayed graphically in 1-mV increments (Fig. 10-3). Because the accuracy of automated ST-segment monitoring is vulnerable to baseline drift and dependent on appropriate identification of the PR and ST segments, the diagnosis of myocardial ischemia is always verified by inspecting the actual ECG tracing.

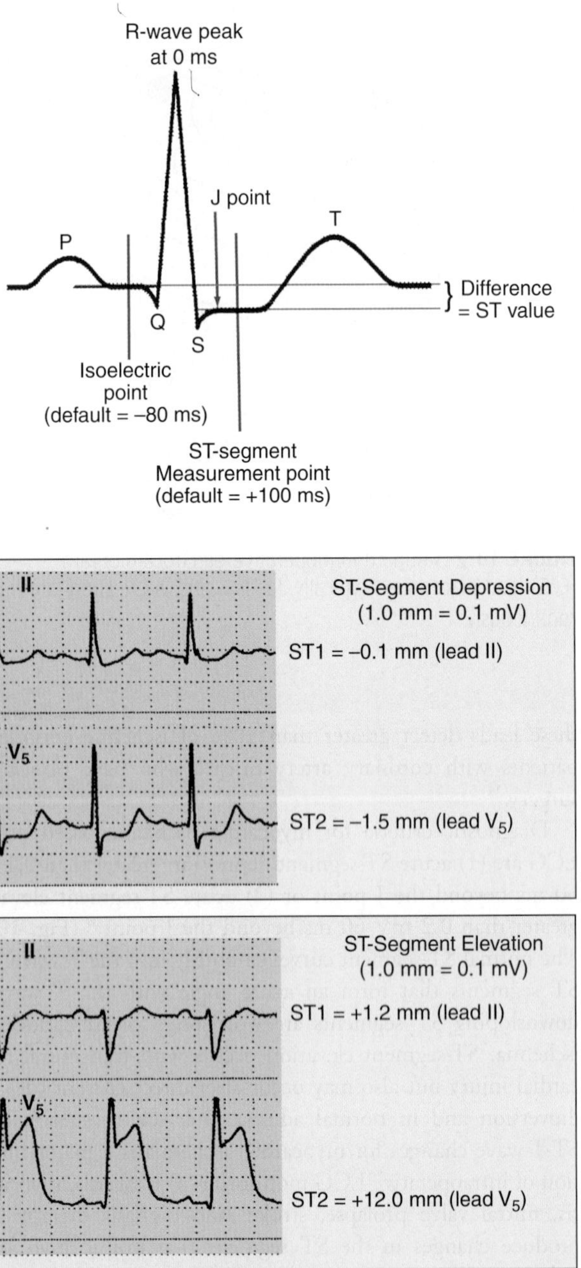

FIGURE 10-3 Automated ST-segment monitoring of the ECG can be used to detect intraoperative myocardial ischemia. General criteria for myocardial ischemia are ST-segment depression greater than 0.1 mV or ST-segment elevation greater than 0.4 mV that persists for longer than 1 minute. At fast heart rates, the ST-segment measurement point may occur on the upslope of the T wave, causing erroneous indication of ST-segment elevation.

Disturbances of rhythm and conduction are common during anesthesia and especially during cardiac surgery. Instrumentation of the heart, hypothermia, electrolyte abnormalities, myocardial reperfusion, myocardial ischemia, and mechanical factors such as surgical manipulation of the heart affect normal propagation of the cardiac action potential. Heart rate is measured by averaging several RR intervals of the ECG. The ECG may not sense the R wave of the selected lead if the electrical vector is isoelectric. A prominent T wave or pacemaker spike may be miscounted as an R wave by the ECG and artifactually double the rate. Usually, heart rate is best monitored by selecting the lead with an upright R wave and adjusting the sensitivity.

The QT interval can be measured only on hard copy. A normal QT interval is less than half the RR interval, but the QT interval must be corrected for heart rates higher than 90 or lower than 65 beats per minute. A prolonged QT interval increases the risk of reentrant ventricular tachydysrhythmias and may occur from hypokalemia, hypothermia, and drug effect (eg, quinidine or procainamide).

The ECG is monitored to confirm the electrical dormancy of the heart during aortic cross-clamping and perfusion with cold cardioplegia. Hypothermia decreases action potential conduction velocity, and high-dose potassium decreases the transcellular membrane potassium concentration gradient to prevent depolarization of cardiac muscle. During cardiopulmonary bypass and aortic cross-clamping, the loss and persistent absence of electromechanical activity suggest that myocardial oxygen consumption is maintained at a minimum.

Monitoring the ECG is most valuable when it begins before induction of general anesthesia. A hard copy of the pertinent leads permits comparison should a change be detected. An abnormal or marginal finding is less worrisome if it was present in the preoperative ECG and remains unchanged during the perioperative period. However, new-onset ST-T-wave changes or disturbances in rhythm and conduction suggest an ongoing active process that usually requires immediate attention.

Capnography

Capnometry is the measure of carbon dioxide (CO_2) concentration in a gas. The capnogram is the continuous graphic display of airway carbon dioxide partial pressure (Fig. 10-4). The capnogram is the single most effective monitor for detecting esophageal intubation, apnea, breathing circuit disconnects, accidental extubation of the trachea, and airway obstruction. Tracheal intubation is verified by detection of physiologic carbon dioxide concentrations in the exhaled gas. Changes in its contour reflect disorders of ventilation, carbon dioxide production, or carbon dioxide transport to the lungs. A steep increase in the phase 3 slope of the exhaled CO_2 concentration suggests partial airway obstruction, either mechanical (eg, tube kinking) or physiologic (eg, bronchospasm). A progressive decrease in

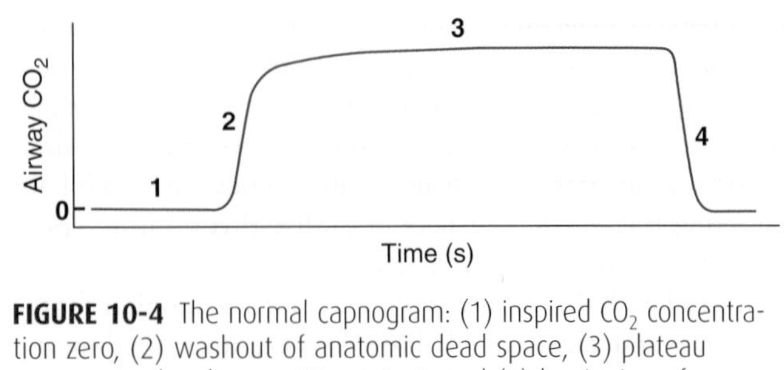

FIGURE 10-4 The normal capnogram: (1) inspired CO_2 concentration zero, (2) washout of anatomic dead space, (3) plateau represents alveolar gas CO_2 content, and (4) beginning of inhalation.

exhaled carbon dioxide concentration occurs with decreased CO_2 production (eg, hypothermia), increased minute ventilation, or increases in physiologic dead space ventilation such as pulmonary embolus or a drop in cardiac output. A progressive increase in exhaled carbon dioxide concentration occurs with hypoventilation, increased CO_2 production (eg, malignant hyperthermia), or increased delivery of CO_2 to the lungs (eg, during weaning off bypass with an increase in pulmonary blood flow). Despite the complex interplay of mechanical and physiologic factors that affect the shape of the capnogram, with any abrupt change in contour, an acute change in the patient's cardiovascular, pulmonary, or metabolic state should be considered.

Anesthetic Gas Monitors

Inhaled volatile anesthetics are different from other parenteral medications. They are delivered as a vapor through the breathing circuit. The clinical effect is determined by the partial pressure of this vapor in the brain, which is in equilibrium with the blood and the alveoli. Measuring the partial pressure of the volatile anesthetic at end expiration approximates the partial pressure in the alveoli and therefore the brain. Monitoring the end-tidal gas mixture adds precision to the administration of inhaled anesthetics and guards against inadvertent overdose.

The concentration of anesthetic gases is displayed as a percentage of the partial pressure of the anesthetic vapor to atmospheric pressure. This concentration can be measured using a variety of techniques, including mass spectroscopy, infrared spectroscopy, Raman spectroscopy, electrochemical and polarographic sensors, and piezoelectric absorption.[27]

Pulse Oximetry

Pulse oximeters were adopted universally into the practice of anesthesia almost immediately after their introduction despite the lack of published data demonstrating improved outcome with their use. The pulse oximeter is reusable, inexpensive, and noninvasive while providing continuous online data regarding the arterial hemoglobin saturation and pulse rate. The pulse oximeter can detect a decrease in oxyhemoglobin saturation even before changes in the color of the patient's skin or blood are evident.[28] Its major limitations include a subjectivity to electrical interference and motion artifact as well as a high failure rate during periods of low flow or inadequate perfusion. In addition, pulsatile flow is required for proper function.[29]

The pulse oximeter is able to measure the percentage of oxyhemoglobin in arterial blood because of differences in the optical absorption properties of oxy- and deoxyhemoglobin. Using transillumination, oximetry emits wavelengths of 660 and 940 nanometers (nm). Oxyhemoglobin has a higher optical absorption in the infrared spectrum (940 nm), whereas reduced hemoglobin absorbs more light in the red band (660 nm). The ratio R of light absorbance at the two wavelengths is a function of the relative proportions of the two forms of hemoglobin. Rapid signal processing then permits reliable and rapid determination of the relative proportion of oxy- and deoxyhemoglobin. Calculation of arterial hemoglobin saturation is based on calibration algorithms derived from R ratios in healthy volunteers.

Arterial oxyhemoglobin saturation is distinguished from venous through the use of photoplethysmography by isolating the pulsatile component of the absorbed signal. The peaks and troughs in the blood volume pulse of the site being transilluminated produces a corresponding pulsatile effect on light absorption, rendering the calculated oxyhemoglobin saturation independent of nonpulsatile venous blood and soft tissue. Because the R values were determined in healthy volunteers, they are less accurate at oxyhemoglobin saturations below 70%. Motion artifact produces a high absorption of light at both wavelengths and an R value of approximately 1, which corresponds to an oxyhemoglobin saturation of approximately 85%.

Measurement of Temperature

Profound changes in body temperature during cardiac surgery are common, often deliberate, and affect vital organ function (Fig. 10-5). Anesthetized patients are poikilothermic. Intrinsic temperature regulation normally controlled by the hypothalamus fails during general anesthesia. Hypothermia occurs by passive and active heat loss. Passive mechanisms of cooling include radiation, evaporation, convection, and conduction. Active cooling usually occurs with extracorporeal circulation and with the use of cold or iced solutions poured into the chest cavity. Deliberate hypothermia during cardiac surgery is designed to arrest and cool the heart, decrease systemic oxygen consumption, and protect organs from hypoperfusion. Hyperthermia may result from preexisting fever, bacteremia,

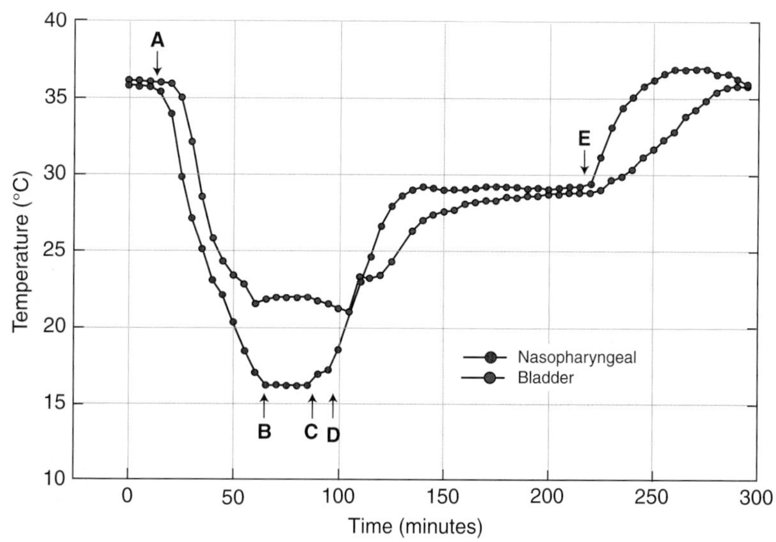

FIGURE 10-5 Time course of changes in nasopharyngeal (*black*) and bladder (*blue*) temperature during a cardiac operation performed on cardiopulmonary bypass employing deliberate hypothermia and deep hypothermic circulatory arrest (DHCA). Marked events: A = onset of deliberate hypothermia, B = onset of DHCA, C = end of DHCA, D = rewarming to 29°C, E = rewarming to normothermia.

malignant hyperthermia, or overzealous rewarming during cardiopulmonary bypass. The monitoring and control of systemic temperature is important because either unintentional hypothermia or hyperthermia can be deleterious to the patient.

Hypothermia after cardiopulmonary bypass is the result of ineffective or most commonly insufficient rewarming. Cold operating rooms; cold, wet surgical drapes; a large surgical incision; and administration of cold intravenous fluids also contribute. Hypothermia exacerbates dysrhythmias and coagulopathy, potentiates the effects of anesthetic drugs and neuromuscular blockers, increases vascular resistance, decreases the availability of oxygen, and contributes to postoperative shivering. The elderly are especially susceptible because of limited compensatory reserve. Although there is evidence to support the efficacy of mild therapeutic hypothermia for brain protection after cardiac arrest and subsequent resuscitation,[30] the optimal target temperature of induced hypothermia for neuro-protection during cardiopulmonary bypass, or even the need for hypothermia at all remains highly contentious in cardiac surgery currently.[31,32]

Temperature typically is monitored from several sites during cardiac surgery. Blood temperature can be measured from the tip of a pulmonary artery catheter and within the cardiopulmonary bypass circuit (typically venous and arterial lines). Blood temperature is the first to change in response to deliberate hypothermia or active rewarming during cardiopulmonary bypass. Nasopharyngeal and tympanic temperatures reflect the temperature of the brain and closely track blood temperature because these sites are highly perfused. Rectal and bladder temperatures provide a measure of core temperature only at equilibrium. Esophageal temperature often underestimates core temperature because of the cooling effects of ventilation in the adjacent trachea. Axillary and inguinal temperatures are shell measurements and are impractical. The possibility of an increased gradient between the measured nasopharyngeal and actual brain temperature should be considered and careful attention should be made to prevent cerebral hyperthermia.[33] Arterial inflow temperatures during rewarming should be limited to a maximum of 37 to 37.5°C to help prevent a large gradient between the inflow temperature and the brain temperature. Post operative hyperthermia has been associated with a worsened neurologic outcome.[33]

The degree and site of temperature changes are important indicators of an intact circulatory system. A persistent discrepancy in temperature between two sites may be a sign of malperfusion. Rewarming during cardiopulmonary bypass normally is associated with an increase in nasopharyngeal or tympanic temperature accompanied by a more gradual increase in temperature in organs with low perfusion. A persistently cold nasopharynx with a normal rate of increase in rectal temperature may be a result of aortic dissection and hypoperfusion of the head.

Measurement of Cardiac Output and Central Venous and Pulmonary Artery Pressures

Cannulation of the central venous circulation permits central administration of drugs, rapid administration of fluids through short, large-bore cannulas, and the measure of central venous pressure. The most commonly used site for central venous access is the internal jugular vein because of reliable insertion, ease of access from the head of the table, decreased risk of pneumothorax, and decreased risk of catheter kinking during sternal retraction. The subclavian vein is the preferred site for insertion of a central venous catheter for long-term intravenous total parenteral nutrition because of a decreased risk of blood-borne infection.[34] The most important complication of internal jugular vein cannulation is inadvertent puncture or cannulation of the carotid or subclavian artery. Cannulation of the central venous circulation is confirmed by manometry, either electrical or mechanical, before insertion of a large-bore catheter. Ultrasound-guided cannulation of the internal jugular vein renders the procedure less dependent on anatomic landmarks and is associated with a decrease in the number of unsuccessful cannulation attempts[35] (Fig. 10-6). With the advent and wide availability of portable ultrasound imaging devices, ultrasound-guided central venous cannulation is becoming commonplace to increase the success rate and decrease the risk of complications.[36] TEE can be used to verify the presence of a wire in the right atrium or superior vena cava (SVC). It can also be used to verify correct placement of the central venous or pulmonary artery catheter tip.[37]

Central venous pressure (CVP) can be measured via the central venous catheter or a proximal port in a Swan-Ganz catheter. The pressure is best measured at end exhalation to exclude the transmission of intrathoracic pressure. The CVP tracing is normally composed of five waves. The A and C waves represent atrial contraction and isovolumetric right ventricular contraction. The X descent occurs with right ventricle ejection as the tricuspid annulus descends. The V and Y waves represent right atrial filling, first during late ventricular contraction and then during early diastole with tricuspid valve opening.

The CVP is traditional thought of as a measure of the overall volume status of a patient, with normovolemia represented by a CVP of 6 to 10 mm Hg during positive pressure ventilation.

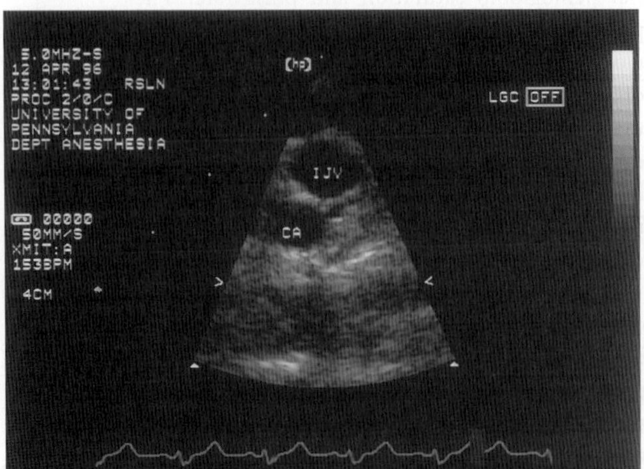

FIGURE 10-6 A two-dimensional short-axis image of the internal jugular vein (IJV) and carotid artery (CA) using a handheld ultrasound transducer.

However, studies have consistently shown that the CVP does not correlate with measured circulated blood volume or fluid challenge responsiveness.[38–41] The CVP value is dependent on the interaction between cardiac function and venous return. Venous return can be affected not only by the mean circulatory filling pressure (the equalization of pressure throughout the entire vascular system if heart was theoretically stopped temporarily) and the cardiac function but also by changes in venous tone. For example, after the induction of general anesthesia, a drop in CVP often represents anesthetic induced venodilation, not acute hypovolemia. The sensitivity of the CVP as a measure of volume status is affected by the body's advanced compensatory mechanisms designed to maintain homeostasis, and these significant changes in blood volume may not be associated with a change in the CVP. A 10% loss of blood volume can easily be compensated for by an auto-transfusion of volume from venous capacitance vessels without a change in the CVP and significant volume loading can occur without a concomitant rise in CVP as fluid accumulates in the same splanchnic venous beds.

Using the CVP as a measure of volume status is further complicated by the differences between intramural and transmural pressure. The pressure measured by an intravascular catheter represents the intramural pressure. The transmural pressure is the difference between the intramural pressure and the pressure surrounding the vascular structures. This difference represents the driving pressure for venous return whereas the measured intramural pressure may not. Increases in intrathoracic and intra-abdominal pressure as well as pericardial pressure will be transmitted to the intravascular space, increasing the CVP without increasing transmural pressure and thus without increasing venous return or indicating a degree of hypervolemia.

Beyond simply measuring pressure, the contour of the CVP waveform can provide other important clinical information. The presence of cannon A waves can confirm the diagnosis of a junctional rhythm in situations wherein the ECG is difficult to discern (also seen with tricuspid stenosis or right ventricular diastolic dysfunction). Large V waves during ventricular systole occur with significant tricuspid regurgitation. Deep X and Y descents can be seen during right sided volume overload, often in conjunction with tricuspid regurgitation. Right ventricular diastolic dysfunction can be suggested by a flattening of the Y descent.

Pulmonary artery catheters (PAC) are inserted via the central venous circulation through the right side of the heart with the catheter tip positioned just downstream of the pulmonic valve. The PAC can measure pulmonary artery pressure, pulmonary artery occlusion pressure, cardiac output, and mixed venous oxygen saturation and also permits the calculation of the derived values of systemic and pulmonary vascular resistance. The pulmonary artery occlusion pressure can be used as an index of left ventricular preload in the absence of mitral stenosis. However, the use of this pressure measurement to estimate preload is limited because of variability in left ventricular size and compliance. Pulmonary artery occlusion pressures (PAOP) can be affected by myocardial compliance, mode of ventilation, and ventricular afterload. Similar to the CVP, the PAOP can also be affected by increases in intrathoracic, intra-abdominal, and pericardial pressure. Increases in PA pressures or PAOP may often indicate myocardial dysfunction or myocardial ischemia (Fig. 10-7). Hemodynamic parameters derived from the pulmonary artery catheter have been shown not to be as sensitive or as specific for detecting myocardial ischemia as the ECG.[42]

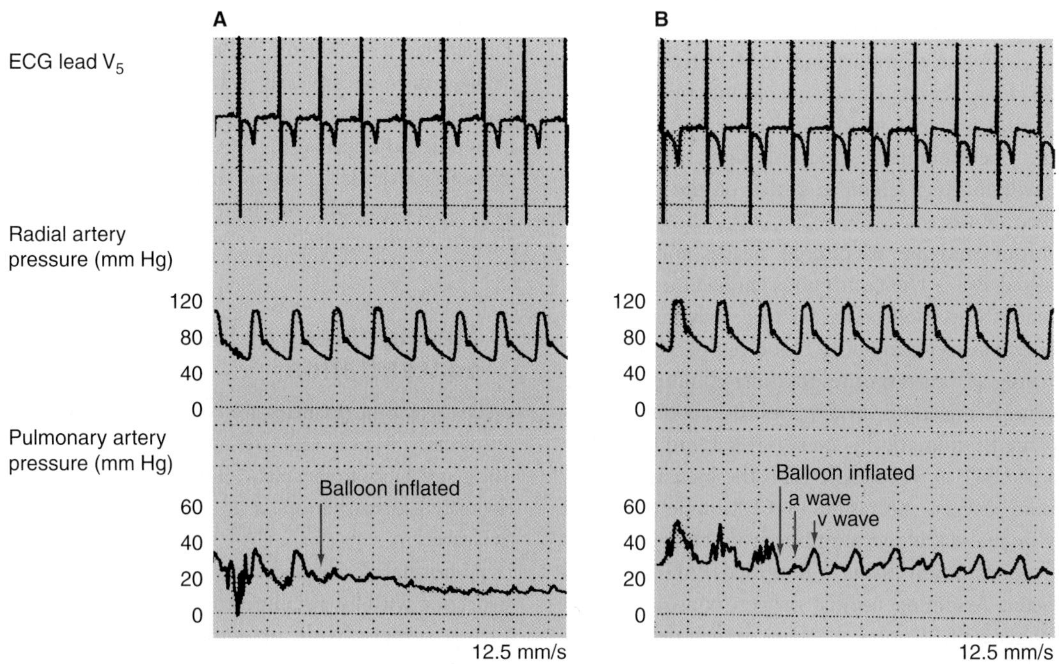

FIGURE 10-7 Pulmonary artery occlusion pressure tracing at two time points. The acute onset of myocardial ischemia (*B*) was associated with ST-segment depression in ECG lead V_5, increased pulmonary artery pressures, and a prominent *v* wave.

Complications associated with insertion of a PAC include infection, dislodgment of endocardial pacemaker wires, dislodgement of right atrial or ventricular clot or tumor, atrial and ventricular arrhythmias, pulmonary infarction, pulmonary artery rupture, perforation of the right atrium or ventricle, catheter entrapment, and heart block. The incidence of right bundle-branch block (RBBB) from catheter insertion is approximately 3% and may lead to complete heart block in patients with a preexisting left bundle-branch block (LBBB).[43] Most PACs are now heparin-bonded to decrease the incidence of thrombus formation.[44] Chronic indwelling PACs are associated with a progressive thrombocytopenia.[45]

Multiport pulmonary artery catheters equipped with a tip thermistor permit the measurement of pulmonary blood flow or cardiac output by thermodilution. Thermodilution cardiac output uses an indicator-dilution technique. The indicator, a known volume of cold saline, is injected rapidly into a proximal port in the right atrium. Cardiac output (CO) is calculated from the rate of change in blood temperature at the PAC catheter tip over time using the Stewart-Hamilton equation:[46,47]

$$\mathrm{CO} = \frac{V(T_B - T_1)K_1K_2}{\int_0^\infty \Delta T_B(t)dt}$$

where CO is cardiac output, V is the volume of the injectate, T_B is the blood temperature at time 0, T_1 is the injectate temperature at time 0, $\Delta T_B(t)$ is the change in blood temperature at time t, K_1 is the density factor, and K_2 is the computation factor.

Thermodilution measures the degree of mixing that occurs between the cold injectate and blood. More mixing implies increased flow. Complete mixing of 10 mL of cold injectate with a circulating blood volume produces a small decrease in temperature at the catheter tip. Poor mixing, suggestive of slow, sluggish flow, produces a large decrease in temperature as the injectate bolus passes the thermistor. The derived value for cardiac output is inversely proportional to the area under the thermodilution curve. Rapid infusion of cold intravenous fluids at the time of measurement may falsely increase the derived cardiac output. Thermodilution measures right-sided cardiac output, which will not equal left-sided cardiac output in patients with intracardiac shunts.

Cardiac output may be monitored nearly continuously using a specialized PAC. The continuous cardiac output catheter intermittently heats blood adjacent to a proximal portion of the catheter and senses changes in blood temperature at the catheter tip using a fast-response thermistor. The method requires no manual injections, and values are acquired, averaged, and updated automatically every several minutes. The only true disadvantage to these catheters is the increased cost.

Mixed venous oxygen saturation ($S\bar{v}O_2$)can be measured intermittently by manual blood sampling from the pulmonary artery port or continuously using a modified PAC equipped with an oximeter. Assuming normal oxygen consumption, a normal ($S\bar{v}O_2$) generally denotes adequate oxygen delivery but does not provide information about the adequacy of perfusion to specific organs. A normal ($S\bar{v}O_2$) may not reflect adequate tissue perfusion in patients with intracardiac shunts, sepsis, or liver failure. Oxygen consumption may change significantly during or after cardiac surgery as patients are warmed or as they begin to emerge from anesthesia, leading to a drop in ($S\bar{v}O_2$). However, a significant decrease in ($S\bar{v}O_2$) often signifies a decrement in oxygen delivery representing compromised cardiac output, anemia, or hypoxia.

($S\bar{v}O_2$) provides an alternative method to calculate cardiac output if oxygen consumption is assumed based on a nomogram derived from resting awake subjects. By the Fick equation, cardiac output is equal to the rate of systemic oxygen consumption divided by the arterial-venous oxygen content difference:

$$\begin{aligned}
O_2 \text{ delivery} &= \mathrm{CO} \times \mathrm{Ca}o_2 \\
O_2 \text{ delivery} &= \bar{\mathrm{V}}o_2 + (\mathrm{CO} \times \mathrm{C}\bar{\mathrm{V}}o_2) \\
\mathrm{CO} \times \mathrm{Ca}o_2 &= \bar{\mathrm{V}}o_2 + (\mathrm{CO} \times \mathrm{C}\bar{\mathrm{V}}o_2) \\
\mathrm{CO}\,(\mathrm{Ca}o_2 - \mathrm{C}\bar{\mathrm{V}}O_2) &= \bar{\mathrm{V}}o_2
\end{aligned}$$

$$\mathrm{CO} = \frac{\bar{\mathrm{V}}o_2}{\mathrm{Ca}o_2 - \mathrm{C}\bar{v}O_2}$$

where Vo_2 is oxygen consumption, CO is cardiac output, Cao_2 is the oxygen content in arterial blood, and CvO_2 is the oxygen content in mixed venous blood. Errors may occur when oxygen consumption is well below the assumed nomogram in sedated, hypothermic, or anesthetized patients, with an overestimation of cardiac output.

Although routine use of a pulmonary artery catheter for monitoring patients during cardiac operation is debated, it does provide clinical information that is used to direct therapy in high-risk patients (Figs. 10-8 and 10-9). The pulmonary artery catheter appears to demonstrate continued utility in the care of patients with pulmonary hypertension and right ventricular dysfunction.[48] Because an insidious decrease in ($S\bar{v}O_2$) may be an early warning of impending circulatory insufficiency, ventricular dysfunction, ongoing bleeding, or impending tamponade, ($S\bar{v}O_2$) pulmonary artery catheters may be particularly useful in the intensive care unit, where early deterioration can be detected and treated before an adverse event occurs.

Measurement of Electrolyte Concentration

Electrolyte abnormalities are common during and after cardiopulmonary bypass and are measured intermittently, typically using stat laboratory tests.[49] The capability to detect and treat electrolyte disturbances is an important aspect of intraoperative care.

Abnormalities in sodium and water homeostasis are often associated with heart failure and compounded by hemodilution during surgery with or without cardiopulmonary bypass. Nonosmotic secretion of arginine vasopressin provoked by surgical stress, pain, hypotension, or nonpulsatile perfusion contributes to the development of hyponatremia by stimulating

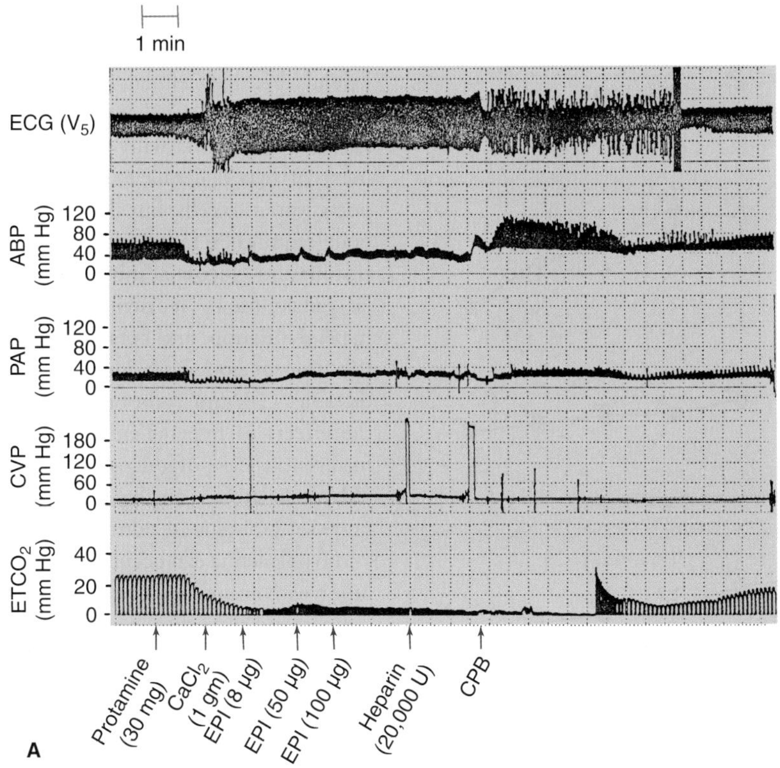

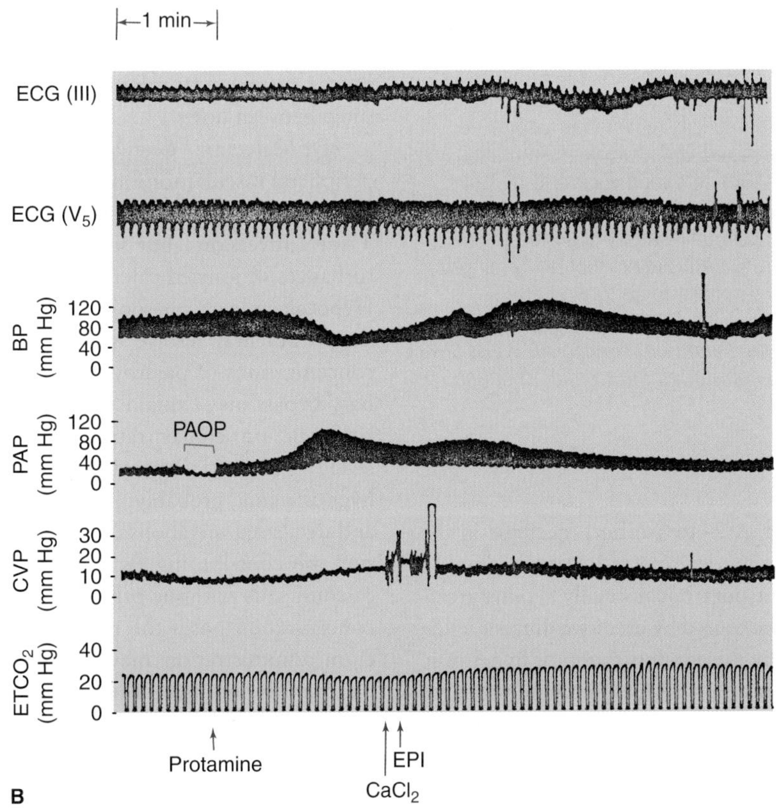

FIGURE 10-8 Intraoperative hemodynamic recordings showing the time sequence of systemic severe vasodilation (A) and catastrophic pulmonary vasoconstriction-type (B) protamine reactions during the reversal of heparin anticoagulation in patients undergoing heart operation. Arterial blood pressure (ABP) and pulmonary artery pressure (PAP) decrease in parallel during systemic vasodilation. In contrast, an increase in PAP and central venous pressure (CVP) precedes the decrease in ABP during the pulmonary vasoconstriction-type reaction. The decreases in end-tidal carbon dioxide concentration ($ETCO_2$) during the protamine reactions reflect the decrease in blood flow through the lungs.

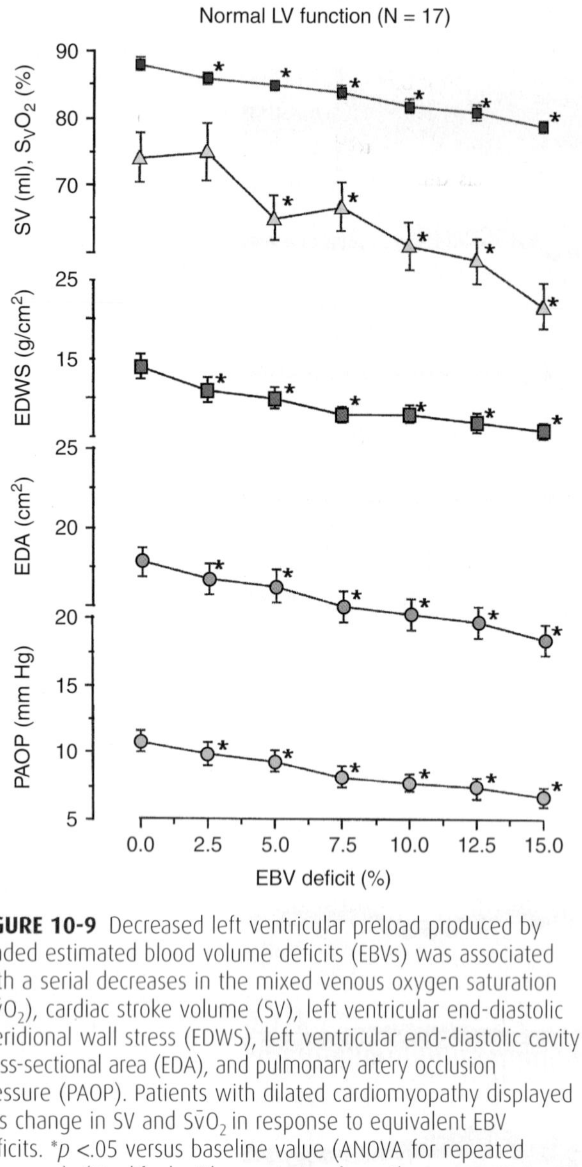

FIGURE 10-9 Decreased left ventricular preload produced by graded estimated blood volume deficits (EBVs) was associated with a serial decreases in the mixed venous oxygen saturation ($S\bar{v}O_2$), cardiac stroke volume (SV), left ventricular end-diastolic meridional wall stress (EDWS), left ventricular end-diastolic cavity cross-sectional area (EDA), and pulmonary artery occlusion pressure (PAOP). Patients with dilated cardiomyopathy displayed less change in SV and $S\bar{v}O_2$ in response to equivalent EBV deficits. *$p < .05$ versus baseline value (ANOVA for repeated measures). (*Modified with permission from Cheung AT, Weiss SJ, Savino JS: Protamine-induced right-to-left intracardiac shunting. Anesthesiology 1991; 75:904.*)

renal retention of free water. A 2- to 5-mEq/L decrease in the plasma sodium concentration is expected after beginning cardiopulmonary bypass but does not normally require treatment. Hypernatremia may be caused by excessive diuresis without free-water repletion or by the administration of hypertonic sodium bicarbonate solutions. An 8.4% sodium bicarbonate solution has an osmolality of 2000 mOsm/l or 6.9 times the osmolality of plasma. Hyperkalemia is common because of high-potassium cardioplegic solutions that are distributed into the systemic circulation. Hyperkalemia during cardiac surgery also may be caused by hemolysis, acidosis, massive depolarization of muscle, and tissue cell death. Increasing serum potassium concentration is manifested by peaked T waves, a widened QRS complex, disappearance of the P wave, heart block, and conduction abnormalities that may be life threatening. Very high concentrations of potassium used to provide cardioplegia inhibit spontaneous depolarization and produce asystole. Patients with diabetes mellitus are at increased risk for hyperkalemia because cellular uptake of potassium is mediated by insulin. Impaired renal excretion of potassium enhances hyperkalemia in patients with renal insufficiency. The initial treatment of hyperkalemia is aimed at redistributing extracellular potassium into cells, but the elimination of potassium from the body requires excretion by the kidneys or gastrointestinal tract. Insulin and glucose administration rapidly decrease extracellular potassium by redistributing the ion into cells. Alkalosis, hyperventilation, and beta-adrenergic agonists also favor redistribution of potassium into cells, but the response is less predictable. Calcium carbonate and calcium chloride antagonize the effects of hyperkalemia at the cell membrane. A typical intravenous dose of glucose and insulin for the acute treatment of hyperkalemia is 1 g/kg of glucose and 1 unit of regular insulin per 4 g of glucose administered.

Hypokalemia can occur during cardiac surgery from hemodilution with nonpotassium priming solutions, diuresis, or increased sympathetic tone during nonpulsatile perfusion. Intraoperative hypokalemia is exacerbated by preoperative potassium depletion from chronic diuretic therapy. Routine insulin administration for hyperglycemia and the frequent use of beta$_2$-adrenergic agonists stimulate cellular uptake of potassium, also contributing to the frequent occurrence of hypokalemia in cardiac surgical patients. Hypokalemia predisposes to atrial arrhythmias, ventricular ectopy, digitalis toxicity, and prolonged response to neuromuscular blocking drugs. Hypokalemia is treated by slow administration of KCl in increments of 10 mEq, with potassium concentrations measured between doses.

Hypocalcemia decreases myocardial contractility and peripheral vascular tone and is associated with tachycardia.[50,51] Hypocalcemia produces prolongation of the QT interval and T wave inversions, but significant arrhythmias owing to disturbances in ionized calcium concentration are not common. Hypocalcemia occurs soon after the onset of cardiopulmonary bypass but may resolve without treatment. Increasing serum concentrations of parathyroid hormone during cardiopulmonary bypass may explain, in part, the gradual increase in ionized calcium concentration to precardiopulmonary bypass levels.[52] The etiology of cardiopulmonary bypass–induced hypocalcemia probably is multifactorial, but hemodilution and decreased metabolism of citrate after rapid blood transfusion are contributing factors. The routine administration of calcium salts without prior measurement of ionized calcium concentration poses the risk of hypercalcemia. Excessive calcium administration may increase the risk of postoperative pancreatitis and myocardial reperfusion injury.[53]

Magnesium deficiency is common in cardiac surgical patients, and acute magnesium supplementation decreases the incidence of postoperative cardiac dysrhythmias and overall morbidity after cardiac operations.[54,55] However, measuring total plasma magnesium concentration has questionable clinical significance because the value primarily reflects the concentration of protein-bound magnesium and not physiologically active, ionized magnesium.[56]

Blood glucose control for cardiac surgery is controversial. Most would agree that treatment of severe hyperglycemia is warranted. Hyperglycemia has been shown to increase morbidity and mortality in nonsurgical patients after stroke and myocardial infarction as well as in patients after cardiac surgery.[57–59] However, there are conflicting data regarding support for an aggressive treatment strategy designed at normalizing blood glucose. In a mixed surgical critical care population, intensive insulin therapy to maintain glucose ≤110 mg/dL reduced morbidity and mortality but with an increased incidence of hypoglycemia.[60] In a meta-analysis of randomized clinical trials conducted in intensive care units, evidence suggested that intensive insulin therapy significantly increased the risk of hypoglycemia and offered no overall mortality benefit.[61–63] Thus far, the literature has only focused on glucose control in the intensive care units. The benefit, if any, of glucose control *during* cardiac surgery currently remains unknown. No evidence exists supporting or refuting aggressive control. The stress of cardiac surgery, acute changes in catecholamine levels, large swings in body temperature, administration of steroids, and large volumes of intravenous fluids all affect blood glucose. The efficacy of intravenous insulin to reduce blood glucose is further complicated by hypothermia when insulin degradation is slowed as is insulin's ability to induce cells to increase glucose uptake (ie, insulin resistance). Over simplistic protocols that do not take into account the increased half life of intravenous insulin and its decreased effectiveness during cold conditions may result in patients receiving progressively increasing doses of insulin with little immediate effect. The slowly metabolized insulin will linger during hypothermia. With systemic rewarming, the large depots of insulin could produce severe hypoglycemia as well as clinically significant hypokalemia. Regardless of glucose management strategy, rapid and frequent measurement of blood glucose is essential.

Monitoring the Nervous System

Neurologic complications, including stroke, paralysis, cognitive dysfunction, blindness, and peripheral nerve injury, are second only to heart failure as the major cause of morbidity and mortality after cardiac surgery.[64] Because a full neurologic examination is not possible during general anesthesia, the objective of intraoperative neurophysiologic monitoring is to provide a means for early detection of neurologic injury or impending injury to permit early intervention in an effort to restore function before the injury becomes permanent.

Electroencephalography (EEG)

EEG is a measure of spontaneous electrical brain activity recorded from electrodes placed in standard patterns on the scalp. Electrical activity of individual electrodes is amplified and then recorded as continuous wavelets that have different frequencies and amplitudes. These data can be displayed as raw EEG or broken down into basic components of frequency and amplitude and displayed as a spectral analysis. A change in EEG activity from baseline during a procedure may indicate ischemia of the cerebral cortex as a consequence of hypoperfusion. Intraoperative EEG can also detect seizure activity masked by general anesthetics or electrocortical silence induced by deliberate hypothermia.

Intraoperative application of EEG can be justified for any cardiac operation where there is a risk for cerebral hypoperfusion such as combined cardiac and carotid endarterectomy procedures. EEG is very sensitive for detecting cerebral malperfusion and can be used to detect malperfusion of the aortic arch branch vessels during aortic dissection repair.[65] Hypothermia produces dose-dependent slowing of the EEG. The predictable actions of hypothermia on EEG activity have made EEG a useful monitor and surrogate for brain temperature in order to determine the adequacy of deliberate hypothermia for circulatory arrest procedures.[66] When performing intraoperative EEG, it is important to recognize that anesthetic agents can attenuate EEG amplitude and frequencies. Marking the EEG in the event of bolus sedative hypnotic administration or when the inhaled anesthetic concentration is changed will help to distinguish EEG changes caused by general anesthetics from changes as a consequence of neurologic injury.

Bispectral Index

The occurrence of awareness under anesthesia is a rare, approximately 0.2% with general anesthesia.[67] In patients at high risk for awareness, the incidence may be near 1%.[68,69] Cardiac surgery is associated with an increased risk of intraoperative awareness.[69–73] The American Society of Anesthesiologists published a "practice advisory" intended to assist decision making pertaining to this issue.[74] The consequences of anesthetic awareness can be significant, leading to long-term psychologic distress including post-traumatic stress disorder. This is caused by several factors, such as hemodilution of intravenous anesthetics from the bypass circuit, hemodynamic instability leading to the decrease or discontinuation of anesthetics, and the inability to measure end-tidal concentrations of inhaled anesthetics if used during bypass. There are several devices commercially available for monitoring anesthetic depth. The bispectral index or BIS monitor (Aspect Medical Systems) is the most widely used of these devices. By using a pad placed directly on the scalp, a frontal electroencephalogram signal is processed in order to calculate a dimensionless value of the patient's level of consciousness. The BIS values range between 0 and 100 with below 40 indicating a deep level of consciousness and between 40 and 60 considered adequate for most general anesthetics.[75] It's clinical utility in preventing anesthetic awareness or reducing over-administration of anesthetics has been studied in several randomized trials with mixed results.[67,75,76]

Near Infrared Cerebral Oximetry

Although the technology has been in existence for over 25 years,[77] only within the last 5 to 10 years has the use of continuous noninvasive cerebral oxygen saturation monitoring expanded. The device is based, like pulse oximetry, on the different absorption characteristics of oxygenated and deoxygenated hemoglobin when exposed to near infrared spectrum light (NIRS). Applied on each temple are two pads that each emits a near-infrared light signal that penetrates all tissues in the cranium using the transillumination characteristics of the skull. Signal contamination from extracerebral tissue saturations such as the bone and soft tissue are prevented from mixing with those from the brain and cerebral vasculature by using the concept of spatial resolution. Each pad employs two separate signal detectors at predetermined distances from the original light source. Signals from shallow tissues (extracerebral) return to the detector closer to the original light source and thus can be separated from the interpretation of signals from the deeper target tissues (intracerebral) that take a longer path.[78] The sample size of the brain tissue monitored, however, is small and represents only approximately 1 ml of brain.[79]

The cerebral oximeter provides a continuous measurement of the percentage of oxygenated hemoglobin residing in the tested intracerebral tissue. Because the ratio of arterial to venous blood is 15:85,[80] the cerebral saturation measured primarily reflects cerebral venous saturation, ie, the balance between oxygen supply and demand. The only cerebral oximeter approved for use in the United States currently is the INVOS 4100 and 5100 (Somanetics Corp, Troy MI).

A major critique of the system is that there is no established normative range or threshold for pathologic change. In a study of healthy elderly noncardiac surgical patients, the mean baseline value was 63+/−8%.[81] However, a wide range of interpatient variability has been found.[82] Other factors that can lead to variability include hemoglobin concentration of the measured site and pad positioning. A 20% decline from baseline values is the most commonly used indicator of pathologic change. It is based mostly on the findings of neurologic change after carotid artery occlusion during carotid endarterectomy.[83,84]

Another dilemma facing practitioners is what to do when faced with low starting baseline cerebral saturations and how to determine when pathologic changes occur in these patients. It has been estimated that 7% of patients have baseline saturations below 50%.[82]

The most validated use of cerebral oximetry in cardiac surgery is as a predictor of postoperative neurocognitive dysfunction and extended hospitalization in those patients who have prolonged cerebral desaturations in the operating room.[85–87] Reports on the diagnosis and treatment of cerebral desaturation and presumed hypoperfusion during cardiac surgery include a diverse list of causes such as anemia, hypocapnia, extreme neck turning, SVC occlusion, and low perfusion pressure.[79,88,89] There is also a growing list of reports of its utilization in guiding length of cooling and conduct of antegrade cerebral perfusion during aortic arch repair and circulatory arrest (Fig. 10-10).[90–93] Although cerebral oximetry represents an exciting tool to monitor the adequacy of brain perfusion, issues with sensitivity and specificity remain, likely preventing a more widespread adoption currently. Embolic events to regions beyond the small sample sizes of brain will clearly be missed. To date there is only on randomized prospective study evaluating cerebral oximetry monitoring with a defined treatment algorithm.[87]

Motor and Somatosensory Evoked Potentials

The most common application of somatosensory evoked potential (SSEP) or motor evoked potential (MEP) monitoring

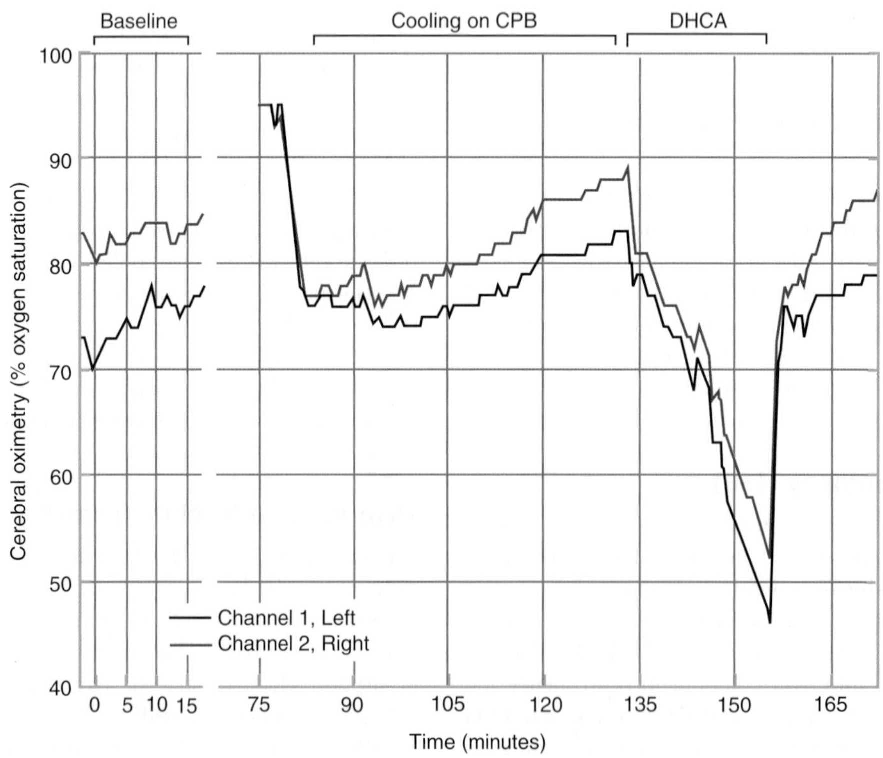

FIGURE 10-10 Changes in left hemispheric (Channel 1) and right hemispheric (Channel 2) cerebral oxygen saturation prior to general anesthesia (baseline), deliberate hypothermia on cardiopulmonary bypass (cooling on CPB), deep hypothermic circulatory arrest (DHCA), and restoration of antegrade cerebral perfusion (after DHCA). Cerebral oxygen saturation was measured by near infrared spectroscopy using percutaneous sensors positioned on both sides of the forehead.

in cardiothoracic surgery is for the detection of spinal cord ischemia during open or endovascular repair of the descending thoracic or thoracoabdominal aorta (Fig. 10-11).[94–96] During these operations decreases in lower extremity SSEP or MEP amplitudes, indicating spinal cord ischemia, can be used to prompt interventions to increase arterial pressure, decrease lumbar CSF pressure, or reimplant segmental arterial branches in an effort to increase spinal cord perfusion to prevent paraplegia. The detection of reversible spinal cord ischemia by intraoperative MEP or SSEP monitoring may also identify patients who may be at risk for delayed postoperative paraplegia. Decreased SSEP and MEP amplitude have been shown to correlate with spinal cord ischemia, but the sensitivity and specificity of these techniques for detecting and reducing the incidence of spinal cord ischemia remains to be verified.[97] Conditions other than spinal cord ischemia may produce MEP or SSEP changes.[94]

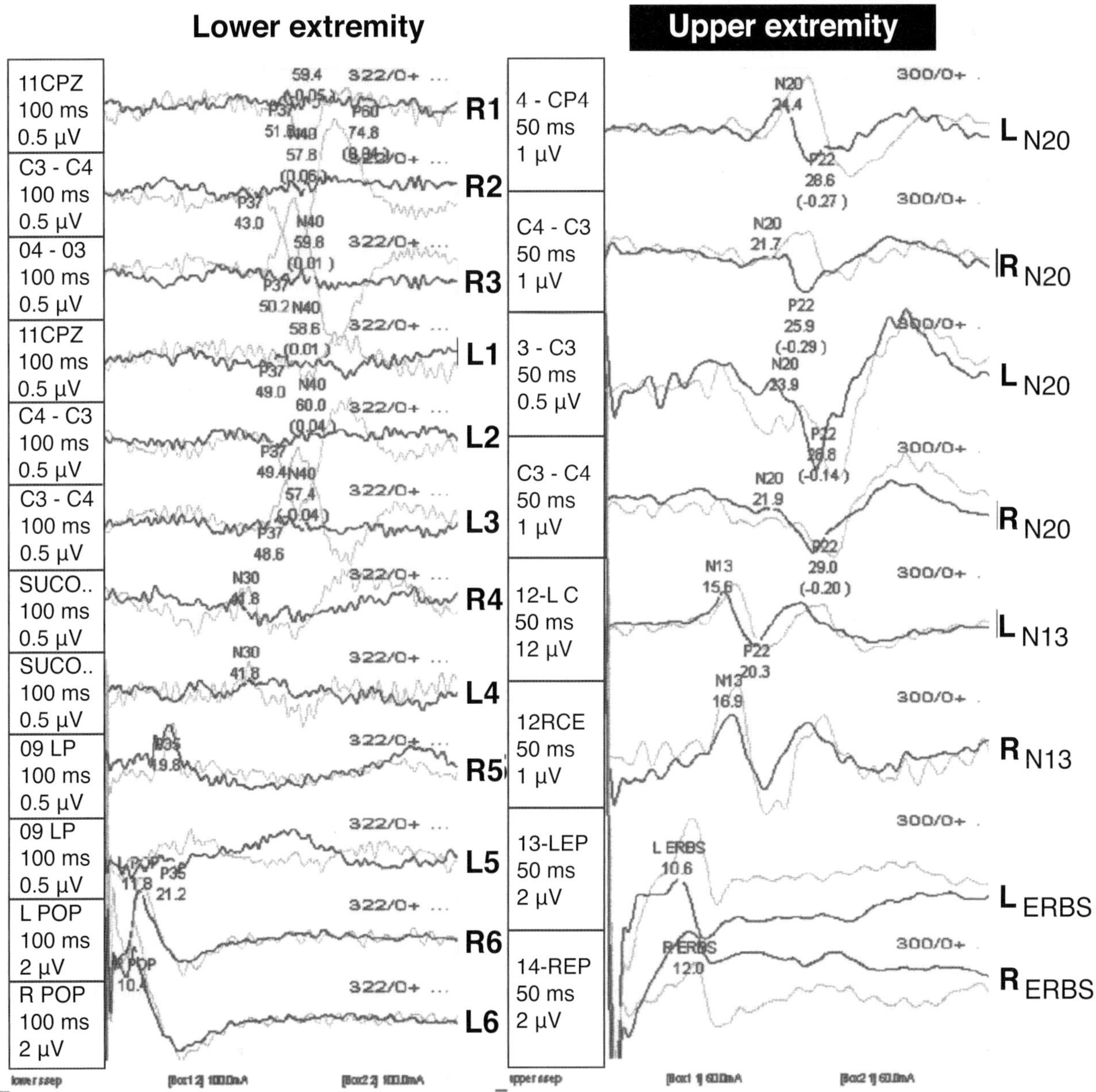

FIGURE 10-11 Intraoperative somatosensory evoked potential (SSEP) recordings from the lower (*left panel*) and upper (*right panel*) extremities that demonstrated intraoperative spinal cord ischemia during thoracoabdominal aortic aneurysm repair. Lower extremity SSEPs were generated by stimulation of the anterior tibial nerves at the ankles (*left panel*). Upper extremity SSEPs were generated by stimulation of the median nerves at the wrists (*right panel*). Bilateral disappearance of SSEP signals from the right (R) and left (L) lower extremities recorded at the cortex (R1, R2, R3, L1, L2, L3) and spine (R4, L4) with preservation of SSEP signals from the lumbar plexus (R5, L5) and popliteal nerves (R6, L6) indicated the acute onset of spinal cord ischemia. Upper extremity SSEP signals from the right (R) and left (L) brachial plexus (ERBS), cervical spine (N13), and cortex (N20) were maintained during the episode. The light grey tracings were the baseline SSEP signals used for comparison.

Intraoperative monitoring of SSEP is performed by placing stimulating electrodes on the skin adjacent to peripheral nerves in the arms or legs. Electrical stimulation of the peripheral nerves in the limbs generates action potentials that can be measured from recording electrodes over the lumbar plexus, brachial plexus, spine, brainstem, thalamus, and cerebral cortex. Motor evoked potentials (MEPs) are generated by transcortical electrical stimulation of the motor cortex that produces myogenic potentials that can be recorded in skeletal muscle. In theory, monitoring MEP should be more sensitive and specific than SSEP to detect spinal cord ischemia in the territory supplied by the anterior spinal artery. An advantage of SSEP monitoring is that it is relatively reliable and easy to interpret during general anesthesia without a contraindication to neuromuscular blockade. Although high concentrations of inhaled anesthetics, thiopental, or propofol can attenuate cortical SEP signals, a balanced general anesthetic with inhaled anesthetics maintained at a concentration of 0.5 MAC provide consistent conditions for monitoring intraoperative SSEP.

Detection of Cerebral Embolization

Intraoperative TEE, epiaortic ultrasound, and transcranial Doppler (TCD) are instruments that can be used to assess the risk and detect arterial embolic events (Fig. 10-12). The embolic burden to the cerebral circulation measured by quantitative TCD correlates with the incidence of intraoperative surgical manipulation and postoperative neurologic deficits.[98] Intraoperative TEE can be applied to detect right-to-left intracardiac shunting through an atrial septal defect,[99,100] intracardiac masses,[101,102] or residual air within the cardiac chambers.[103] Routine epiaortic ultrasonography or TEE to assess the degree of aortic atherosclerosis and guide the insertion of the aortic cannula and application of the aortic cross-clamp has been recommended for decreasing the risk of neurologic injury during CPB.[104]

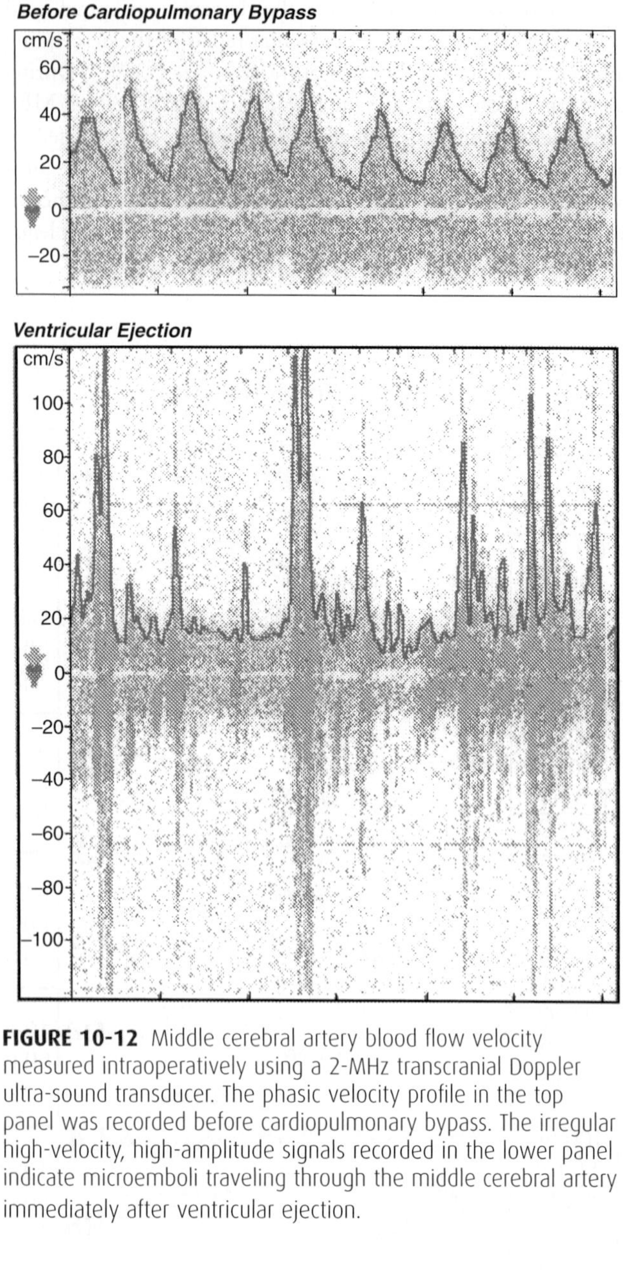

FIGURE 10-12 Middle cerebral artery blood flow velocity measured intraoperatively using a 2-MHz transcranial Doppler ultra-sound transducer. The phasic velocity profile in the top panel was recorded before cardiopulmonary bypass. The irregular high-velocity, high-amplitude signals recorded in the lower panel indicate microemboli traveling through the middle cerebral artery immediately after ventricular ejection.

ANESTHETICS AND NEUROMUSCULAR BLOCKERS

Inhaled Anesthetics

Inhaled anesthetics alone produce all the conditions necessary for operation.[105] The unit of concentration used clinically is termed minimum alveolar concentration, or MAC, which is defined as the concentration of volatile agent that produces immobility in 50% of people in response to a painful stimuli.[106] The most commonly used inhaled anesthetics are isoflurane, sevoflurane, and desflurane. Isoflurane is older, less expensive, with a longer onset and recovery time. Desflurane has a short onset and a rapid recovery time but is pungent and can stimulate airway and sympathetic reflexes. Sevoflurane offers a lack of airway reactivity, a nonpungent odor, and minimal cardiovascular and respiratory side effects.[107,108] The accumulation of compound A, a potential renal toxin and byproduct of sevoflurane use, has been associated only with low fresh gas flow (<1 L/min).

All inhaled anesthetics cause circulatory depression at concentrations necessary to produce general anesthesia. When ventilation is controlled, the circulatory actions of the inhaled anesthetics are what usually limit the anesthetic dose that can be tolerated, particularly in patients with cardiovascular disease. For this reason, lower doses of inhaled anesthetics usually are combined with other anesthetics, such as opioids, to produce a balanced general anesthetic for cardiac operations. The decrease in blood pressure caused by volatile anesthetics is a direct result of vasodilation and depression of myocardial contractility and an indirect result of attenuation of sympathetic nervous system activity. The decrease in blood pressure is so predictable that it is often used as a sign for assessing the depth of anesthesia. Overdose with inhaled anesthetics is manifested by hypotension, arrhythmias, and bradycardia that, if unrecognized, may lead to circulatory shock.

The inhaled anesthetics decrease myocardial contractility based on both experimental and clinical studies (Fig. 10-13).[109–111] Inhalation anesthetics produce a dose-dependent decrease in

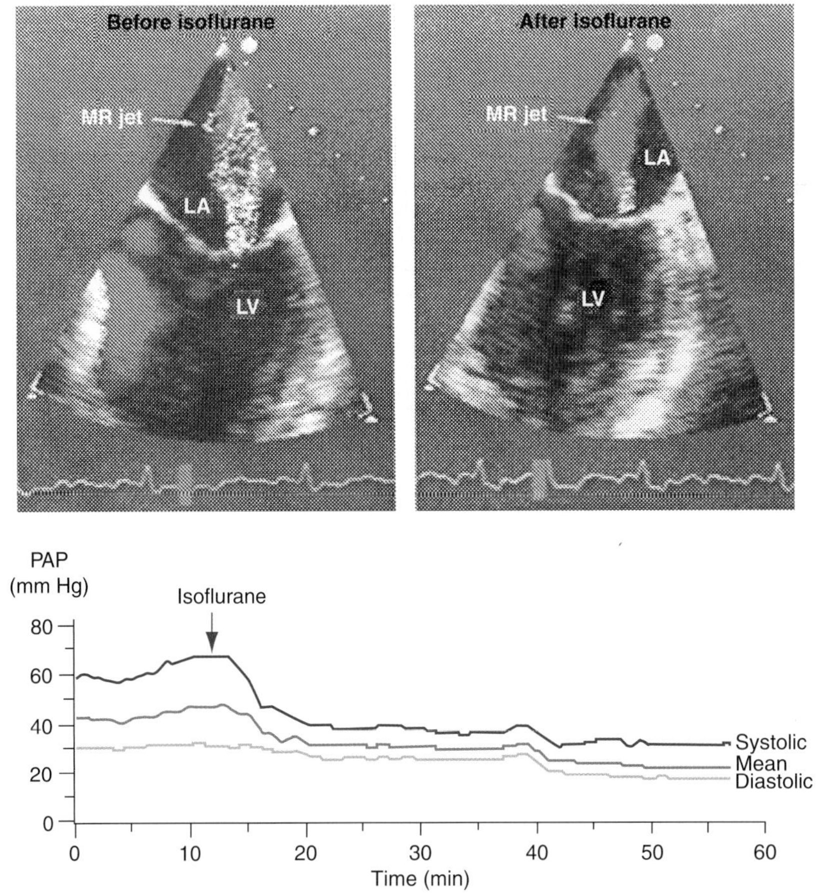

FIGURE 10-13 The relationship of increasing doses of isoflurane to the magnitude of mitral regurgitation and pulmonary artery pressures. The systemic unloading effects of isoflurane decreased mitral regurgitation from moderate to mild and decreased pulmonary artery pressures almost to normal.

profound ventricular dysfunction may not tolerate the cardiovascular depressant effects of inhaled anesthetics given in concentrations that are needed to produce anesthesia. Volatile anesthetics have a proportionally greater negative inotropic effect on diseased myocardium than on normal myocardium.

The administration of inhaled anesthetics in patients with preexisting cardiovascular diseases has potential advantages. The myocardial depressant and arterial vasodilatory actions of inhaled anesthetics decrease afterload and myocardial oxygen consumption, which benefits patients with coronary insufficiency creating a more favorable myocardial oxygen balance. In addition inhaled anesthetics are potent coronary vasodilators. Isoflurane causes endothelium-dependent inhibition of the contractile response of canine coronary arteries.[117] However, anesthetic-induced hypotension may reduce coronary perfusion pressure and coronary blood flow.

Regional blood flow to other vital organs may be modified by inhaled anesthetics because of their effects on metabolic demands and autoregulation. The normal circulatory response to hypotension and low cardiac output is redistribution of blood flow to vital organs (ie, brain, heart, and kidneys) and a decrease in blood flow to skin, muscle, and the gastrointestinal system. Volatile inhalation anesthetics impair this protective response because of nonspecific vasodilation and can compromise vital organ

mean maximal velocity of circumferential myocardial shortening, mean maximal developed force, and dP/dt.[112–114] Isoflurane, desflurane, and sevoflurane decrease global left ventricular systolic function at any given left ventricular loading condition or at any given degree of underlying sympathetic tone (Fig. 10-14). Experimental studies suggest these agents cause minimal changes in left ventricular diastolic compliance but impair left ventricular diastolic relaxation in a dose-dependent manner.[115] The effects of each individual inhaled anesthetic on cardiovascular function depend on selective dose-dependent effects of the drug on myocyte contraction and relaxation, vascular smooth muscle tone, and sympathetic nervous system reflexes; as well as the underlying disease state, intravascular volume status, surgical stimulation, temperature, mode of ventilation, and acid-base status. Despite a decrease in myocardial contractility, cardiac output generally is unchanged at 1.0 MAC of isoflurane because of direct arterial vasodilation and preservation of baroceptor reflexes, with a resulting decrease in ventricular afterload and increase in heart rate and stroke volume (Fig. 10-15).[116]

Although sympathetic nervous system activation owing to nociception may often mask clinical signs of circulatory depression caused by inhaled anesthetics, patients in shock or with

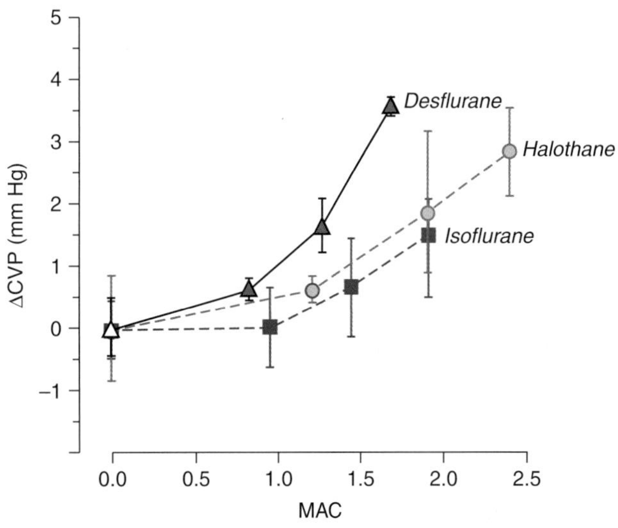

FIGURE 10-14 Dose-dependent changes in central venous pressure produced by halothane, isoflurane, and desflurane in normocarbic adults. (*Data from Weiskopf RB, Cahalan MK, Eger EI 2nd, et al: Cardiovascular actions of desflurane in normocarbic volunteers. Anesth Analg 1991; 73:143. Used with permission.*)

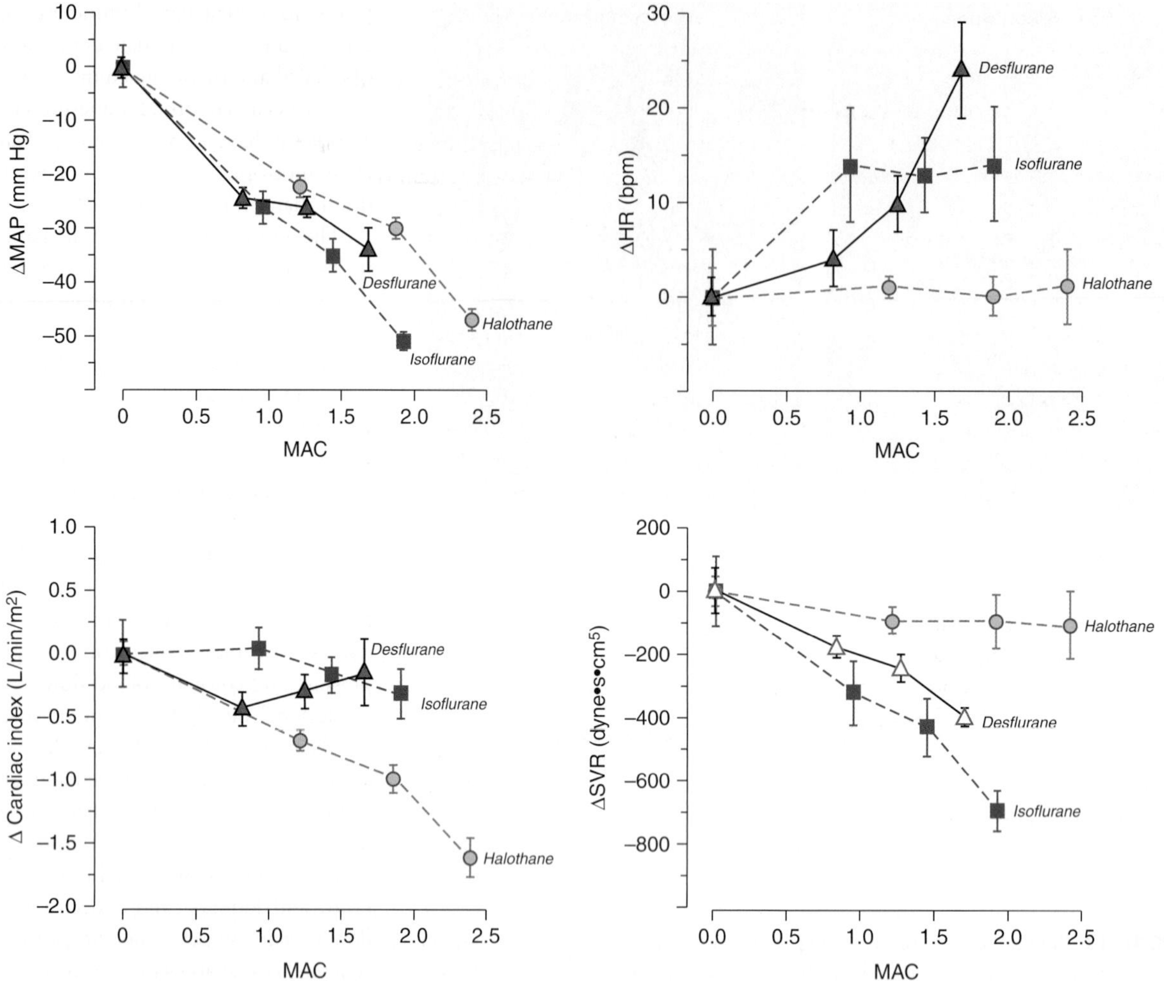

FIGURE 10-15 Dose-dependent changes in mean arterial pressure, heart rate, cardiac index, and systemic vascular resistance produced by halothane, isoflurane, and desflurane in normocarbic adults. Despite the myocardial depressant effects of isoflurane and desflurane, cardiac output is maintained during anesthesia with these agents in part because of a decrease in left ventricular afterload and increase in heart rate. (*Data from Weiskopf RB, Cahalan MK, Eger EI 2nd, et al: Cardiovascular actions of desflurane in normocarbic volunteers. Anesth Analg 1991; 73:143. Used with permission.*)

perfusion if administered in high doses during periods of circulatory shock.

In general, carefully conducted clinical trials suggest that almost any inhaled anesthetic can be administered safely to patients with cardiovascular disease if the hemodynamic condition of the patient is optimally controlled.[118]

Sedative-Hypnotics

Sedative-hypnotics describe a broad class of anesthetic drugs that includes barbiturates, benzodiazepines, etomidate, propofol, and ketamine. They are used for preoperative sedation, can produce immediate loss of consciousness during intravenous induction of general anesthesia, supplement the actions of the inhaled anesthetics, and provide sedation in the immediate postoperative period. The circulatory effects of individual agents are an important consideration for patients with cardiovascular disease. The sedative-hypnotics can have direct effects on cardiac contractility and vascular tone, in addition to indirect effects on autonomic tone.

The barbiturates, such as thiopental or methohexital, are negative inotropic agents. They produce dose-dependent decreases in ventricular dP/dt and the force-velocity relationship of ventricular muscle.[119] Induction of general anesthesia with a barbiturate is associated with a decrease in blood pressure and cardiac output. In comparison with barbiturates, propofol appears to cause less myocardial depression.[120,121] The decrease in arterial pressure after propofol administration is attributed primarily to arterial and venous dilatation.[122,123] Propofol is well suited for continuous intravenous infusion for sedation because it has a short duration of action and can be titrated to effect. Propofol given intravenously for sedation in a nonintubated patient requires the presence of an anesthesiologist because respiratory depression is common. Etomidate can be administered for rapid induction of general anesthesia in patients with preexisting hemodynamic compromise because it generally causes little or no change in circulatory parameters,[124] except when patients are critically relying on elevated sympathetic tone. This agent is particularly useful for unstable patients undergoing emergency operation. Etomidate has virtually no effect on myocardial contractility even in diseased ventricular muscle.[125,126] However, etomidate inhibits adrenal synthesis of cortisol by blocking beta-hydroxylase. This adrenal suppression effect has mostly been ignored when the drug is limited to short-term uses, such as an intravenous anesthetic induction. Newer data suggest this adrenal insufficiency may occur even following a single induction dose.[127] The clinical relevance of this insufficiency remains to be determined.[128]

Ketamine often increases heart rate and blood pressure after anesthetic induction because it maintains sympathetic tone.[129] The direct negative inotropic and vasodilating effects of ketamine can be unmasked when it is administered to critically ill patients with catecholamine depletion.[130] Ketamine is not used routinely because it may cause postoperative delirium, especially if it is administered in the absence of other sedative-hypnotics.

Narcotic Anesthetics

Narcotics remain an important adjunct for cardiac anesthesia. Analgesic actions are mediated by direct activation of opioid receptors in the central nervous system, spinal cord, and periphery. Narcotic-based anesthetics offer the advantages of profound analgesia, attenuation of sympathetically-mediated cardiovascular reflexes in response to pain, and virtually no direct effects on myocardial contractility or vasomotor tone. Narcotics may be administered intravenously, intrathecally, or into the lumbar or thoracic epidural space. Even though narcotics have little direct action on the cardiovascular system, they may cause profound hemodynamic changes indirectly by attenuating sympathetic tone. Narcotics decrease serum catecholamine levels and produce cardiovascular depression indirectly, especially in a patient who are critically ill and dependent on endogenous catecholamines (eg, those with severe hypovolemia or cardiac tamponade). Morphine sulfate may decrease blood pressure by provoking the release of histamine.

Problems encountered with narcotic-based anesthetics include difficulty estimating the dose required because of patient variability, predicting the duration of postoperative narcotic-induced respiratory depression, and ensuring hypnosis during the operation. Rapid administration of narcotics is associated with muscle rigidity that may impede the ability to ventilate the patient immediately after the induction of general anesthesia.[131] The rigidity usually affects the thoracic and abdominal musculature and is observed commonly with the larger doses of narcotic used in cardiac anesthesia. Myoclonic activity often associated with muscle rigidity easily can be mistaken for grand mal seizures. There is no evidence that opioids induce seizures when there is adequate oxygenation and ventilation.[132] Opioid-induced muscle rigidity is readily reversed by the administration of neuromuscular blockers.

Opioid tolerance is represented by a decrease in response (both analgesia and respiratory depression) to a narcotic owing to prior exposure. Tachyphylaxis is the rapid development of drug tolerance without necessarily prior exposure. Drug dependence is a patient condition or disorder that occurs as a consequence of sustained exposure to a drug such that withdrawal or antagonism of the drug prohibits normal function.[133] Perioperative exposure to morphine and synthetic narcotics is unlikely to produce the downregulation and desensitization of opioid receptors believed necessary for narcotic dependence.[134] Cardiac surgical patients receiving narcotic infusions in the intensive-care unit often develop tachyphylaxis and require increasing doses to sustain the desired effect.[135]

Ultra–short-acting narcotics (eg, remifentanil) may have a unique niche in cardiac anesthesia because their effect is terminated almost immediately after discontinuing the drug infusion owing to rapid in vivo ester hydrolysis.[136] Remifentanil successfully attenuates the sympathetic response to painful stimuli in cardiac surgery.[137] Profound intraoperative analgesia can be provided while facilitating early resumption of respiration, consciousness, and extubation. Remifentanil can also be used to facilitate the use of motor evoked potentials to in order to monitor spinal motor pathways during thoracic aortic surgery.[138]

Neuromuscular Blocking Drugs

Neuromuscular blocking drugs are administered to facilitate intubation of the trachea, prevent patient movement during operation, improve surgical exposure of the operating field, and attenuate metabolic demands caused by potential shivering during hypothermia. Except for succinylcholine, the neuromuscular blocking drugs used in clinical practice are typically nondepolarizing competitive antagonists of acetylcholine at the nicotinic acetylcholine receptor of the motor end plate. Succinylcholine is an acetylcholine agonist that produces rapid, short-acting muscle paralysis by depolarizing the motor end plate.

Muscle relaxants are chosen based on the desired speed of onset, duration of action, route of elimination, spectrum of cardiovascular side effects, and cost (Table 10-4). The newer neuromuscular blocking drugs such as vecuronium and rocuronium have virtually no cardiovascular side effects and do not depend primarily on renal function for elimination. *Cis*-atracurium degrades spontaneously by pH- and temperature-dependent Hofmann elimination and is independent of both renal and liver function. Succinylcholine has the most rapid onset of action (90 seconds) but produces unpredictable changes in heart rate; increases serum potassium concentration by approximately 0.5 mEq/L; may cause life-threatening hyperkalemia in patients with denervation, burn, or compression injuries; and can trigger malignant hyperthermia in susceptible individuals. Pancuronium increases blood pressure and heart rate by blocking muscarinic acetylcholine receptors in the sinoatrial node, increases sympathetic activity via antimuscarinic actions, and inhibits reuptake of catecholamines.

Discontinuing general anesthesia or sedation before complete recovery from neuromuscular blockade is very distressing for patients because the awake, alert, and paralyzed patient has no means to communicate discomfort. Discontinuing mechanical ventilatory support in patients with residual neuromuscular blockade may cause acute or delayed respiratory failure. Even mild residual neuromuscular blockade contributes to pulmonary insufficiency by compromising mechanics of breathing and decreasing negative inspiratory force, vital capacity, tidal volume, and the ability to generate an effective cough. Muscle fatigue may produce airway obstruction by decreasing muscle

TABLE 10-4 Neuromuscular Blocking Drugs

Drug	ED_{95} (mg/kg)	Dose (mg/kg)	Onset (min)	Duration (min)	Effects of Drug On: HR	BP	CO	Histamine Release	Renal Elimination
Succinylcholine	0.25	1.5	1–1.5	12–15	(+)	(+)	(0)	(+)	0%
D-Tubocurarine	0.51	0.6	3–5	180–240	(+)	(–)	(–)	(+++)	60%
Pancuronium	0.07	0.1	3–5	180–240	(++)	(+)	(+)	(0)	70%
Vecuronium	0.06	0.1	2–3	75–120	(0)	(0)	(0)	(0)	15%
Cis-atracurium	0.05	0.2	2–3	60–90	(0)	(0)	(0)	(0)	<5%
Rocuronium	0.3	0.6	1–2	45–90	(0)	(0)	(0)	(0)	0%
Mivacurium	0.1	0.2	2–3	40–60	(0)	(0)	(0)	(+)	<5%

BP = arterial pressure; CO = cardiac output; dose = initial dose required for intubation of the trachea; duration = time after injection required for recovery to 95% of baseline function; ED_{95} = dose required to produce 95% suppression of muscle twitch in response to nerve stimulation; HR = heart rate; histamine release = drug-induced histamine release; onset = time required to achieve conditions required for tracheal intubation; renal elimination = percentage of injected dose that is dependent on renal function for excretion; (+) = increase; (–) = decrease; (0) = no effect.

tone in the oropharynx. Recovery from nondepolarizing neuromuscular blockade may be hastened by administering an acetylcholinesterase inhibitor such as neostigmine or edrophonium that decreases degradation of acetylcholine at the neuromuscular junction and thereby increases the concentration of the neurotransmitter at the motor end plate. The undesirable systemic effects of acetylcholine-esterase inhibitors are bronchospasm, bradycardia, and hypersalivation, which can be minimized by simultaneous administration of anticholinergic agents such as atropine or glycopyrrolate. Severe bradycardia has been described in heart transplant patients after reversal of neuromuscular blockade, possibly owing to the nonantagonized parasympathetic activity associated with acetylcholinesterase inhibitors in the denervated heart.[139] Reliable reversal of neuromuscular blockade with cholinesterase inhibitors usually is achieved only after muscle strength has recovered spontaneously to approximately 25% of baseline levels. Recovery of neuromuscular function is usually measured by a transcutaneous nerve stimulator applied over the ulnar nerve just proximal to the hand with monitoring of thumb twitch strength.

Local Anesthetics

Local anesthetic drugs inhibit the propagation of action potentials in electrically excitable tissue by blocking sodium channels. Common local anesthetics used during anesthesia and surgery include lidocaine, bupivacaine, and ropivacaine. Lidocaine has a quick onset of action but a shorter duration of analgesia than the other two. Local anesthetics can be delivered by topical application to mucosa, infiltration into tissues, injection into the region of a peripheral nerve, infusion into the epidural space, or injection intrathecally into cerebrospinal fluid. Regional nerve blocks can be used to supplement a general anesthetic or to provide postoperative analgesia. Epinephrine often is added to local anesthetic solutions to prolong the anesthetic duration but may cause tachycardia or cardiac arrhythmias when absorbed into the systemic circulation.

Local anesthetic toxicity can occur because of systemic absorption of the injected drug or because of inadvertent direct intravascular injection. It can result in both neurologic and cardiovascular toxicity. The spectrum of neurologic symptoms extend from simply minor auditory and visual disturbances, progressing to motor twitching, and finally to grand mal seizures depending on the rise of local anesthetic blood levels. The blood concentration needed to produce neurologic symptoms can be low, particularly with a rapid injection, because of the high arterial supply of the brain. Most often neurologic symptoms are short lived as the drug is rapidly cleared, again because of high cerebral arterial flow. At higher drug blood levels, excitatory neurologic symptoms dissipate and central nervous system depression is seen, typically in conjunction with cardiovascular toxicity.

Cardiovascular toxicity is manifested by hypotension, cardiac arrhythmia, and myocardial depression, which may progress to complete cardiovascular collapse with electrical standstill. Bupivacaine has been noted to block cardiac sodium channels and thus conduction at blood levels just above that of seen with neurologic toxicity.[140] Because of this, it is widely considered to have a higher degree of specific cardiac toxicity than ropivacaine. Bupivacaine has a slower disassociation from inactivated sodium channels then lidocaine, which likely contributes to its enhanced cardiotoxicity.[140] Some authors, however, believe the increased cardiac toxicity to merely be related to a lower potency of ropivacaine versus bupivacaine and not to any intrinsic properties of bupivacaine.[141] Treatment of local anesthetic toxicity includes traditional Advanced Cardiac Life Support (ACLS) including epinephrine but may necessitate brief cardiopulmonary bypass to allow for recovery. A novel therapy has recently been described with the use of lipid emulsion. Although the precise mechanism of action remains unknown, there have been numerous reports of miraculous recovery with its intravenous administration.[142–144]

SPECIAL ANESTHETIC TECHNIQUES

Emergency Airway Management

Establishing a patent and secure airway is essential for the conduct of general anesthesia and is the first step in emergency life support for cardiovascular resuscitation. Tracheal intubation for airway protection and mechanical ventilation can be challenging in a patient with cardiovascular disease. General anesthesia is typically employed to facilitate tracheal intubation; however, the effects of general anesthetics produce respiratory depression and usually apnea in addition to vasodilation and cardiac depression. Difficultly with the establishment of an airway can create hypoxia and hypercarbia, and could potentially lead to cardiovascular collapse. The aspiration of gastric contents from an unprotected airway in an anesthetized or unarousable patient may also lead to pneumonitis. Inadequate anesthesia during tracheal intubation may provoke myocardial ischemia or tachyarrhythmias in susceptible patients. The American Society of Anesthesiologists has established practice guidelines for the emergency management of the difficult airway.[145] The difficult airway (eg, Mallampati class 4) often can be intubated using fiberoptic bronchoscopy. This technique requires time and special equipment. The risk of hypertension, tachycardia, and discomfort during tracheal intubation in an awake patient can be offset partially by topical anesthesia and as well as light sedation. Fiberoptic intubation can also be achieved with the patient asleep, when mask ventilation is assumed to be acceptable, although the possibility that the establishment of an airway will be unsuccessful must be considered in this scenario.

Single-Lung Ventilation

Single-lung ventilation, or the ability to collapse one lung and selectively ventilate the contralateral lung, is necessary for operative exposure when the heart or great vessels are approached through a lateral thoracotomy incision. Selective lung ventilation is integral in the intraoperative management of patients undergoing minimally invasive direct coronary artery bypass (MIDCAB) procedures. Adequate surgical exposure with minithoracotomy for coronary revascularization without cardiopulmonary bypass requires deflation of the left lung. Single-lung ventilation is also used in patients undergoing thoracoscopic procedures, lung transplantation, open thoracic aortic operations, aortic or mitral valve surgery through a right thoracotomy, closure of large bronchopleural fistulas, intrathoracic robotic surgery, or life-threatening hemoptysis. Single-lung ventilation may be achieved using double-lumen endobronchial tubes (Fig. 10-16) or bronchial blockers (Fig. 10-17).

Wire-guided bronchial blocker kits often contain an adapter for use with a standard endotracheal tube and include ports for the bronchial blocker and fiberoptic bronchoscope.

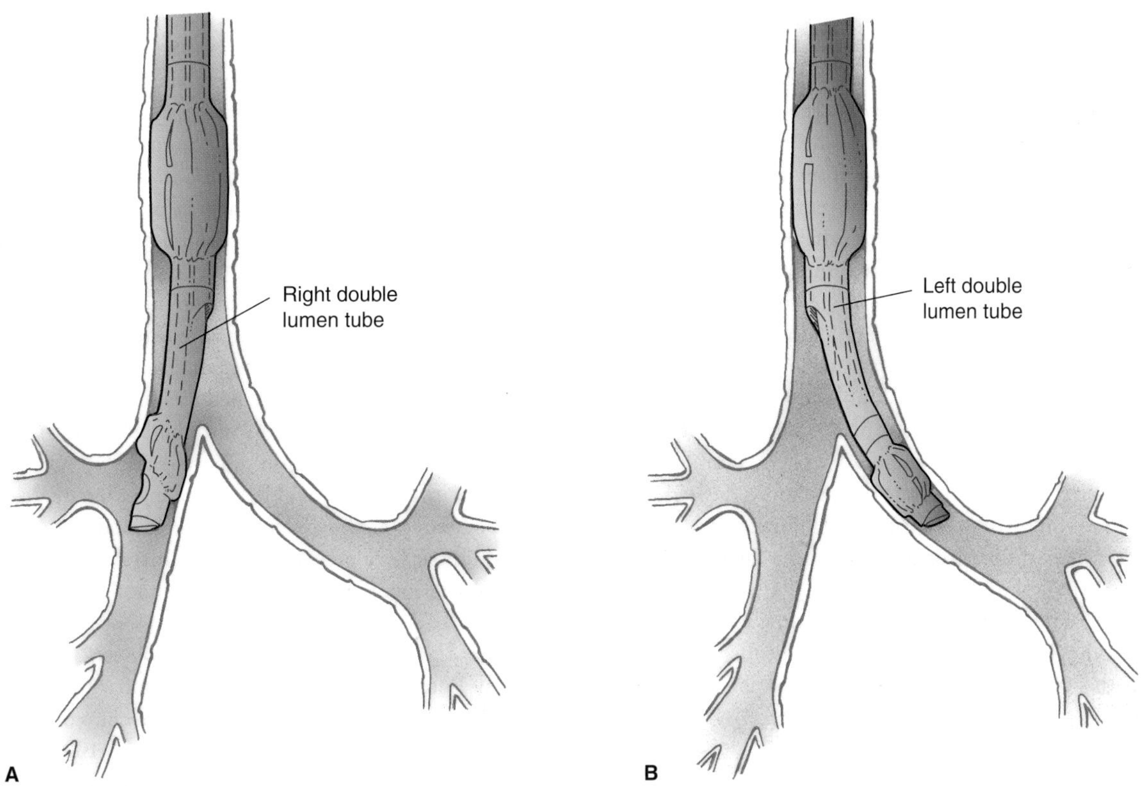

FIGURE 10-16 (A) Right-sided double-lumen endobronchial tube positioned such that Murphy's eye is aligned with the orifice of the right upper lobe bronchus. Indications for a right-sided tube are surgery involving the left main stem bronchus; patients with a prior left pneumonectomy, stenosis, compression, or mass in the left main stem bronchus; and circumstances in which the trachea needs to be protected from soilage from contents in the right lung (eg, abscess). (B) Left-sided double-lumenen dobronchial tube.

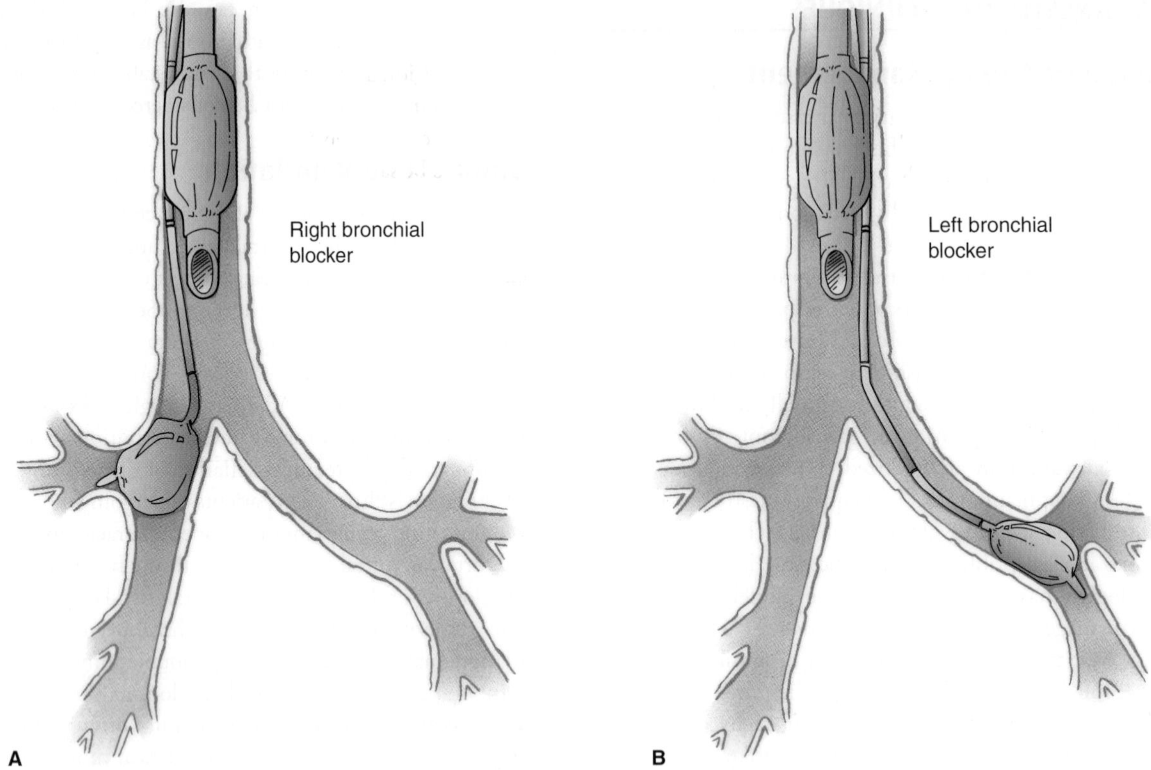

FIGURE 10-17 Bronchial blockers permit single-lung ventilation but do not permit suctioning or rapid deflation of the nonventilated lung. Position of the bronchial blocker is less stable compared with a double-lumen endobronchial tube.

A central lumen for the blocker contains a monofilament loop that passes out the end of the catheter. Placement of the loop over a fiberoptic bronchoscope permits the bronchial blocker to be guided directly into position using the bronchoscope. Removal of the monofilament loop from the central lumen provides a port for venting the nonventilated lung. Other styled blockers have a steerable tip that can be visualized through the bronchoscope and manipulated into a main bronchi. Bronchial blockers for lung isolation are preferred when the larynx is too small to accommodate a double-lumen endobronchial tube or in a patient with an anticipated difficult airway. This is because the larger double-lumen endobronchial tube is often more challenging to place than a smaller single lumen tube. Also, because of the design of the double lumen tube, adjunctive intubation strategies are more difficult than with a single lumen tube. A bronchial blocker may also be chosen when it is difficult or dangerous to change an in situ endotracheal single lumen tube, or when the trachea or main stem bronchus are distorted by a mediastinal mass or aortic aneurysm. The routine use of fiberoptic bronchoscopy has decreased the complication rate and uncertainty regarding positioning of these devices in the airway.

Controlling Lumbar Cerebrospinal Fluid Pressure

Spinal fluid drainage may improve neurologic outcome from spinal cord ischemia during thoracic and thoracoabdominal aortic operations.[146–148] Based on evidence from meta-analysis of randomized and nonrandomized clinical trials, lumbar CSF drainage is recommended as part of a multimodal approach to prevent paraplegia after thoracoabdominal aortic surgery.[149,150] The physiologic rational of lumbar CSF drainage is to improve spinal cord perfusion pressure, which is approximated by the difference between the mean arterial pressure and the CSF pressure.[151] Based on this principle, successful application of CSF drainage also requires interventions to increase arterial pressure and to decrease the central venous pressure.[151,152] CSF drainage is achieved by aseptic insertion of a subarachnoid catheter through a Tuohy needle positioned in a lower lumbar vertebral interspace. The insertion of a CSF drain before anticoagulation for extracorporeal circulation appears safe.[151,153] The catheter typically is inserted the night before an operation or 1 to 2 hours before systemic anticoagulation. CSF is drained passively to reduce lumbar CSF pressure to approximately 10 to 12 mm Hg during operation. CSF drainage is continued typically for 24 to 48 hours after an operation. In the absence of spinal cord ischemia, the catheter is capped for another 24 hours before removal. Emergent implementation of lumbar CSF drainage to a target lumbar CSF pressure of 10 mm Hg, combined with augmentation of the mean arterial pressure to 100 mm Hg, has been reported to be effective for the treatment of delayed-onset paraplegia or paraparesis after thoracic and thoracoabdominal aortic reconstruction.[151] Complications associated with lumbar CSF catheters include meningitis, persistent CSF leak, breakage and retention of catheter fragments, and hemorrhage.[154–156]

Intracranial hypotension is an important complication of lumbar CSF drainage and is believed to contribute to the risk of subdural hematoma.[157] The risk of intracranial hypotension can be managed by continuously monitoring CSF pressure and the volume of CSF drained. The risk of hemorrhagic complications can be managed by ensuring adequate platelet and coagulation function during both the insertion and removal of the lumbar CSF drain.

Regional Anesthesia and Analgesia

Epidural or intrathecal (neuraxial) administration of local anesthetics and narcotics can provide profound postoperative analgesia after cardiac surgical operations with less sedation or respiratory depression than parenteral narcotic analgesia.[158–160] A continuous infusion or intermittent bolus technique can be used. Patient-controlled epidural analgesia (PCEA) can also be triggered by patient demand with a predetermined maximum lockout to help prevent overdose. PCEA is an effective method to titrate the dose of epidural local anesthetic and/or narcotic based on clinical need. The potential clinical advantages of epidural or intrathecal analgesia are less postoperative pain, decreased duration of postoperative ventilatory support, attenuation of the surgical stress responses, and improved pulmonary function.[161]

The most common side effect of neuraxial analgesia is hypotension caused by local anesthetic blockade of the preganglionic vasomotor efferents of the sympathetic nervous system and loss of compensatory vasoconstriction. The potency of this side effect can be lessened by decreasing the concentration of the local anesthetic used. Respiratory depression can occur with systemic absorption of epidural narcotics or the rostral rise in the CSF with intrathecal administration. The onset of respiratory depression can be unpredictable and can sometimes be quite delayed. Nausea and pruritus are also common side effects of epidural or intrathecal narcotics. Epidural hematoma formation leading to spinal cord compression is a rare but potentially catastrophic complication of epidural and intrathecal analgesia, with an estimated frequency of 1 in 150,000 patients.[162] Instrumentation of the epidural space during the performance of neuraxial anesthesia or the removal of a catheter is contraindicated in anticoagulated or coagulopathic patients.[163,164]

Epidural or intrathecal catheters are most often inserted before the operation, typically before the induction of anesthesia. This theoretically allows the conscious, but usually sedated patient, to report pain associated with needle and/or catheter-induced paresthesias or with drug administration, which could represent intraneural injection. Pain during needle placement or with the injection of local anesthetic has been associated with neurologic injury during regional anesthesia.[165,166] The performance of neuraxial anesthesia before induction allows for maximizing the time between needle placement and systemic heparinization, which must be at least 1 hour. In some centers, epidural or intrathecal catheters are placed the night before surgery when full dose anticoagulation is employed for cardiopulmonary bypass to increase the safety margin.

As alluded to above, concern for epidural hematoma leading to spinal cord compression and possibly permanent paralysis during or after cardiopulmonary bypass in patients who receive full systemic heparinization remains paramount. The American Society of Regional Anesthesia, in their 2002 consensus statement, determined that although neuraxial anesthesia in patients who subsequently receive low-dose heparin in vascular surgery has proved to be safe, the safety in patients receiving full systemic heparinization for cardiac surgery requires further study.[167] There are an increasing number of recent reports describing the successful use of both spinal and epidural anesthesia for cardiac surgery.[168–170] This evidence, in addition to data from the successful use of CSF catheters in cardiac surgery, would suggest that the incidence of epidural hematoma formation in carefully selected patients is low. However, currently, there still is insufficient evidence to properly characterize the risks and especially the benefits of neuraxial anesthesia compared with more conventional anesthetic techniques and this has continued to preclude the widespread acceptance of neuraxial anesthesia in cardiac surgery.[171]

Minimal Invasive Cardiac Surgery

The widespread adoption and expansion of minimally invasive cardiac surgery has presented the cardiac anesthesiologist with many new challenges. Because of a limited exposure to the heart and great vessels, the cardiac surgeon relies heavily on the cardiac anesthesiologist to assist in these cases. It is common for the anesthesiologist to be requested to pericutaneously place cannulas that are traditional placed directly in the surgical field. Examples include large venous drainage cannula (14 to 21 French) placed in the right internal jugular vein (IJV) to provide venous inflow to the bypass circuit, retrograde cardioplegia cannula (EndoPlege Sinus Catheter, Edwards Lifesciences LLC, Cardiovations) advanced into the coronary sinus from the right IJV (Fig. 10-18), a pulmonary artery vent to decompress the

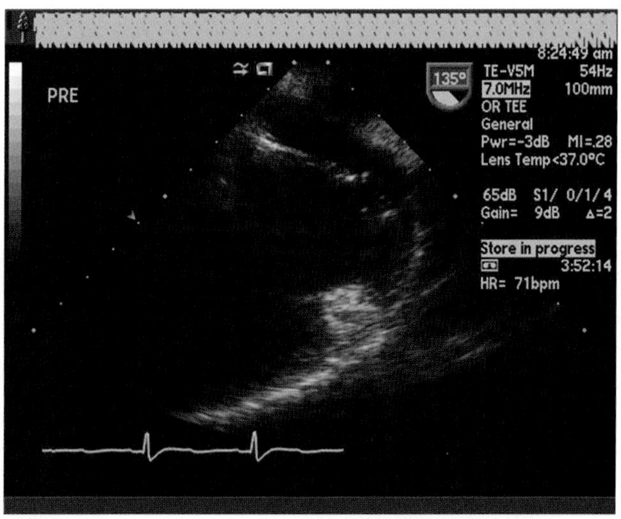

FIGURE 10-18 Percutaneously inserted retrograde coronary sinus catheter (EndoPlege Sinus Catheter, Edwards Lifesciences LLC, Cardiovations) shown entering the right atrium and directed into the coronary sinus, guided by transesophageal echocardiography.

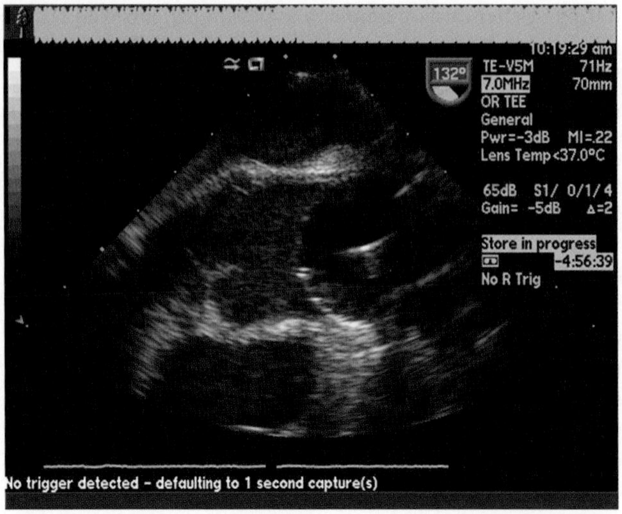

FIGURE 10-19 Endo-aortic balloon (EndoClamp Aortic Catheter, Edwards Lifesciences LLC, Cardiovations) shown inflated inside the proximal ascending aorta just downstream (distal) to the aortic root, providing internal occlusion of the aorta for open chamber cardiac surgery, venting of the aortic root, and antegrade cardioplegia through the coronary ostia.

left heart during bypass, and pacing wires advanced through a specialized pulmonary artery catheter. Lung isolation is also typically requested during surgery involving a thoracotomy incision. In addition to performing new specialized procedures, minimally invasive cardiac surgery also requires intensive TEE examinations. Not only is it important because of the limited ability for direct surgical inspection of the heart and great vessels, TEE is critical for the placement and/or confirmation of most of the surgical cannulas used during minimally invasive cardiac surgery. The use of an endoaortic balloon (EndoClamp Aortic Catheter, Edwards Lifesciences LLC, Cardiovations) also mandates TEE guidance for proper positioning in the ascending aorta (Fig. 10-19).

THE CONDUCT OF ANESTHESIA, SURGERY, NURSING, AND PERFUSION

Cardiac surgery is conducted in an interdisciplinary environment among surgeon, anesthesiologist, perfusionist, and nursing staff. Since the release of the Institute of Medicine report *To Err is Human* in 1999, there has been an increased awareness of the impact of medical errors on health care.[172] The use of crew resource management has been identified as an important component to reduce medical errors in the surgical arena.[173] The cardiac anesthesiologist is in a unique position to take on a leadership role in such patient safety activities, including pre- and postoperative briefing-debriefing sessions and patient safety "time outs."

The anesthetic begins before the patient arrives in the operating room. The patient's identification and scheduled procedure are verified immediately before and again after arrival in the operating room. The physical condition of the patient is assessed clinically, and medical events that occurred over the previous 12 to 24 hours are reviewed. For elective surgery, the patient should have fasted for a minimum of 8 hours before induction of general anesthesia, although it has become debatable whether 8 hours is necessary. Patients are often premedicated with a sedative-hypnotic (eg, a benzodiazepine) and/or an analgesic (eg, fentanyl) unless the associated mild degree of respiratory depression would be considered dangerous.

The patient is escorted into the operating room and placed onto the operating table. The operating room requires a minimum of 800 ft^2 to comfortably accommodate the patient, health-care providers, standard operating room equipment, intraoperative cell salvage machine, heart-lung machine, and assist devices, if needed.[174] The required square footage may be greater for the higher-technology procedures such as robotic surgery. Routine noninvasive monitors are applied and prophylactic antibiotics are administered with the goal of antibiotic completion in adequate time before incision. An arterial catheter is inserted, most often in the radial artery. A blood sample is acquired for laboratory analysis, and a blood type and crossmatch are requested, if not done already. A central venous catheter is always indicated, although in many patients it can be inserted after the induction of general anesthesia. A pulmonary artery catheter is used commonly to provide measures of cardiac output and estimates of ventricular filling pressures.[175] Large-bore intravenous catheters are often inserted for patients, particularly in those who are undergoing reoperation because of the possibility of rapid blood loss during sternotomy. The immediate availability of typed and cross-matched blood is verified before skin incision. External defibrillation pads are applied to patients undergoing reoperation or in procedures in which access to the heart with internal paddles would not be readily available.

Induction of general anesthesia is achieved by intravenous administration of sedative-hypnotics, inhalation of volatile potent anesthetics, or both, most often in conjunction with opioids. Inhalation inductions permit maintenance of spontaneous ventilation and a controlled titration of anesthetic dose but prolong the excitatory phase of anesthesia when the patient is prone to cough, move, develop laryngospasm, or vomit and aspirate. Inhalation inductions are not commonly used in adults. Intravenous induction produces rapid apnea that requires immediate ventilatory support. Administration of neuromuscular-blocking drugs produces profound muscle paralysis and facilitates laryngoscopy and tracheal intubation. Vasoactive drugs are titrated, if necessary, to counteract the cardiovascular effects of anesthetics and loss of sympathetic tone. Laryngoscopy is extremely stimulating and, if the patient is inadequately anesthetized, may cause hypertension, tachycardia, or stimulate vasovagal reflexes. Most adult patients can be intubated with an 8.0-mm internal-diameter polyvinyl chloride endotracheal tube that accommodates an adult flexible bronchoscope. The tip of the tracheal tube is secured above the carina by documenting breath sounds bilaterally.

The patient is positioned before surgical preparation and draping, typically with the arms tucked at the side and a shoulder roll under the scapula. Regions susceptible to pressure injuries are protected and padded, and the patient is positioned to decrease pressure on the postcondylar groove of the humerus.[176] ECG wires, tubes, and lines are not run under the arm. The incorporation of a simple examination of extremity nerve function during the postoperative visit provides a means to detect peripheral nerve injury.

Maintenance of general anesthesia is achieved by continuous or intermittent administration of anesthetic drugs titrated to effect while monitoring the conduct of the operation and vital physiologic functions. Anesthetics are chosen based on the patient's preoperative cardiovascular function, drug pharmacokinetics, and the dose-dependent pharmacologic actions. Surgical incision in the presence of inadequate concentrations of a volatile or intravenous anesthetic produces hypertension, tachycardia, tachypnea, and movement. In the absence of stimulation, the same anesthetic produces cardiovascular depression, hypotension, and apnea. The anesthesiologist titrates the anesthetic to a measurable end point by monitoring effects. As anesthetics are increasingly tailored for rapid emergence, lower doses and shorter acting medications are often employed that may predispose to intraoperative awareness if patient response is not closely monitored. Decisions to administer benzodiazepines prophylactically may be prudent in selected patients, such as those with a history of drug resistance or tolerance and young age. High doses of benzodiazepines may preclude early emergence.

Short-acting vasoactive agents with rapid onset of action usually are preferred for controlling hemodynamics because conditions can change rapidly. Vasopressors and inotropic agents sometimes are required to support the circulation in response to anesthetic-induced vasodilation and cardiac depression. Using nitroglycerin to modify venous capacitance permits buffering acute changes in intravascular volume. Heart rate can be controlled by short-acting cardioselective beta-adrenergic agonists and antagonists, vagolytic agents, or chronotropic drugs or, alternatively, by direct cardiac pacing. The urgency to control hemodynamic parameters with pharmacologic therapy must be tempered by recognizing the risk of drug overdose from overzealous treatment. Intraoperative events associated with acute increases in anesthetic requirements are sternotomy, chest wall retraction, manipulation and cannulation of the aorta, rewarming during cardiopulmonary bypass, and sternal wiring. Intraoperative awareness from insufficient anesthesia may occur during cardiac surgery, especially if a greater emphasis is placed on avoiding cardiovascular actions of anesthetic agents than on providing sufficient anesthesia.

Initiation of cardiopulmonary bypass acutely changes circulating drug concentrations. The addition of 2 L of pump prime has a negligible effect on plasma concentrations of lipophilic drugs with a large volume of distribution but significantly decreases the concentration of drugs distributed primarily in the intravascular space. Despite measurable decreases in blood anesthetic concentrations during cardiopulmonary bypass, the anesthetic level may not change because systemic hypothermia decreases anesthetic requirements, potentiates the effects of neuromuscular blocking drugs, and increases the solubility of volatile anesthetics in blood. Rewarming returns anesthetic requirements to baseline levels and predisposes to inadequate anesthesia if therapeutic drug concentrations are not maintained. The judicious use of sedative-hypnotics, analgesics, and amnestic agents during rewarming decreases the incidence of recall but does not guarantee unconsciousness. Volatile inhalation anesthetics can be given during cardiopulmonary bypass by adding them to the oxygen-rich gas mixture ventilating the pump oxygenator. This use of volatile anesthetics requires an effective scavenging system to prevent accumulation of anesthetic gases in ambient air.

Separation from cardiopulmonary bypass requires effective communication among members of the intraoperative team. Similar to an airline pilot preparing to land, the cardiac anesthesiologist has a checklist that ensures that all systems are in working order (Table 10-5).

The importance of a check list cannot be overstated, because many tasks must be incorporated into a successful separation from cardiopulmonary bypass and in the difficult cases it may be easy for a distraction to lead one to forget a critically important component. Beyond ensuring adequate anesthesia, careful management of the patient's hemodynamics is necessary. Anesthetic induced changes in vascular tone and cardiac function are now often superimposed on post cardiopulmonary bypass systemic inflammation and myocardial stunning. A TEE examination is usually performed to assess the adequacy of cardiac filling, contractility, and valvular function, as well as confirming a successful surgical result. Occasionally, findings

TABLE 10-5 Checklist for Preparation to Separate from Cardiopulmonary Bypass

1. Stable rhythm preferably with a synchronized atrial contraction
2. Pacemaker and cables available
3. Positive inotropes available (eg, epinephrine, dopamine)
4. Vasodilators available (eg, nitroglycerine, nitroprusside)
5. Vasopressors available (eg, phenylephrine, norepinephrine)
6. Adequate levels of anesthesia and paralysis
7. Normothermia: nasopharyngeal temperature = 37°C, rectal or bladder temperature = 35°C
8. Normal serum electrolyte concentrations: K^+, Ca^{+2}
9. Normal serum glucose
10. Normal blood acid-base status
11. No systemic oxygen debt: oxygen saturation in cardiopulmonary bypass venous inflow >70%
12. Acceptable O_2-carrying capacity: hemoglobin concentration
13. Normal systemic vascular resistance
14. Recalibration of pressure transducers
15. ECG in diagnostic mode
16. Clearance of air by TEE
17. Hemothorax evacuated
18. Ventilation with 100% oxygen and atelectatic lungs reexpanded

from the TEE exam will necessitate a return to cardiopulmonary bypass and further surgical intervention. An arterial blood sample is obtained following protamine administration to ensure adequate heparin reversal and for arterial blood gas analysis. Continued bleeding after heparin neutralization indicates the need for further surgical hemostasis or the administration of the platelet concentrates, coagulation factors, or anti-fibrinolytics. After the sternum is reapproximated and the wounds closed and dressed, the patient is prepared for transport. Before departing the operating suite for the intensive care unit (ICU), pertinent patient information should be communicated to the critical care unit team about to accept the patient in order to facilitate transfer of care on arrival.

ANESTHESIA IN THE IMMEDIATE POSTOPERATIVE PERIOD

Continuous visual inspection of the patient and continuous monitoring of pulse oximetry, blood pressure, and ECG during transport to the postoperative ICU is standard. Meticulous attention is necessary from all members of the operating team even though the operation is completed, because the transition from operating room to ICU is fraught with risk. Transport usually entails a decrease in monitoring compared to the controlled setting of a cardiac OR. Smaller, sometimes less reliable, transport monitors replace the large screens with multichannel leads and pressure waveforms. Capnography is not typically monitored during transport. Occult bleeding into the chest with the chest tubes off suction may manifest itself during transport and early signs may be nonspecific and limited to hypotension, respiratory variations in the blood pressure tracing, or passive drainage of blood into the chest tubes. The discontinuation of anesthetic gases without supplementation with intravenous agents may result in an early, unanticipated emergence from general anesthesia. Intravenous sedative-hypnotic or analgesic drugs administered in the immediate postoperative period to treat surgical manipulation may contribute to hypotension during transport as stimulation has decreased. Conversion from the anesthesia machine ventilator to a hand-bag assembly for controlled ventilation (eg, Mapleson system) often results in hypoventilation. Careful attention must also remain on the patient's intrinsic rhythm and temporary pacemaker function.

Anesthesia is often extended into the early postoperative period because of the need for mechanical ventilatory support, treatment of hypothermia, and management of pain. Hypertension and tachycardia occur in the setting of tracheal intubation if abrupt emergence occurs. Several hours may be needed to achieve criteria required for tracheal extubation (eg, minimal bleeding, cardiovascular stability, and systemic rewarming). Vasodilation and increased cutaneous blood flow with active rewarming typically occurs after arrival into the intensive care unit. Postoperative positive-pressure ventilation is often quite different with the chest closed. Tidal volumes may be decreased, especially in the setting of an in situ internal mammary graft, because the expanding lung can impinge on the pedicle graft and place tension on the fresh suture lines. Arrival in the intensive-care unit triggers a battery of laboratory tests designed to assess rapid changes in vital organ function and prompt corrective therapy. These tests include a chest radiograph, ECG, complete blood and platelet count, chemistry battery with blood urea nitrogen and serum creatinine determinations, a serum glucose determination, prothrombin time and partial thromboplastin time, and arterial blood gas determination.

Preemptive patient management during the operation and in the early postoperative period can decrease intensive-care-unit and hospital length of stay after cardiac surgery.[177] Traditionally, high-dose narcotic anesthesia provided profound analgesia, sympathetic blockade, and a gradual emergence that was managed over a time course of 8 to 12 hours. With high-dose narcotic anesthesia, patient recovery often was determined by the duration of action of the anesthetic given in the operating room. The time required for recovery from general anesthesia may be decreased by short-acting sedative-hypnotics (eg, propofol) or analgesics administered by infusion that continues into the postoperative period and permits recovery according to the patient's condition rather than the anesthetic. Implementation of protocol-based care plans designed to expedite patient recovery after cardiac operations requires a coordinated effort and mutual understanding between the anesthesiologist, surgeon, and critical care team.

REFERENCES

1. Owens WD, Felts JA, Spitznagel EL, Jr: ASA physical status classifications: a study of consistency of ratings. *Anesthesiology* 1978; 49:239-243.
2. Kahn R, Shernan S, Konstadt S: Intraoperative echocardiography, in Kaplan J (ed): *Kaplan's Cardiac Anesthesia,* 5th ed. Philadelphia, Saunders, 2006; pp 437-488.
3. Eagle KA, Berger PB, Calkins H, et al: ACC/AHA Guideline Update for Perioperative Cardiovascular Evaluation for Noncardiac Surgery—Executive Summary. A report of the American College of Cardiology/American Heart Association Task Force on Practice Guidelines (Committee to Update the 1996 Guidelines on Perioperative Cardiovascular Evaluation for Noncardiac Surgery). *Anesth Analg* 2002; 94:1052-1064.
4. Fleisher LA, Eagle KA: Guidelines on perioperative cardiovascular evaluation: what have we learned over the past 6 years to warrant an update? *Anesth Analg* 2002; 94:1378-1379.
5. Greillier L, Thomas P, Loundou A, et al: Pulmonary function tests as a predictor of quantitative and qualitative outcomes after thoracic surgery for lung cancer. *Clin Lung Cancer* 2007; 8:554-561.
6. Smetana GW, Lawrence VA, Cornell JE: Preoperative pulmonary risk stratification for noncardiothoracic surgery: systematic review for the American College of Physicians. *Ann Intern Med* 2006; 144:581-595.
7. Hoeks SE, Scholte Op Reimer WJ, van Urk H, et al: Increase of 1-year mortality after perioperative beta-blocker withdrawal in endovascular and vascular surgery patients. *Eur J Vasc Endovasc Surg* 2007; 33:13-19.
8. Shammash JB, Trost JC, Gold JM, et al: Perioperative beta-blocker withdrawal and mortality in vascular surgical patients. *Am Heart J* 2001; 141:148-153.
9. Booth JV, Ward EE, Colgan KC, et al: Metoprolol and coronary artery bypass grafting surgery: does intraoperative metoprolol attenuate acute beta-adrenergic receptor desensitization during cardiac surgery? *Anesth Analg* 2004; 98:1224-1231, table of contents.
10. Myhre ES, Sorlie D, Aarbakke J, Hals PA, Straume B: Effects of low dose propranolol after coronary bypass surgery. *J Cardiovasc Surg* (Torino) 1984; 25:348-352.
11. Tuman KJ, McCarthy RJ, O'Connor CJ, Holm WE, Ivankovich AD: Angiotensin-converting enzyme inhibitors increase vasoconstrictor requirements after cardiopulmonary bypass. *Anesth Analg* 1995; 80:473-479.
12. Carrel T, Englberger L, Mohacsi P, Neidhart P, Schmidli J: Low systemic vascular resistance after cardiopulmonary bypass: incidence, etiology, and clinical importance. *J Card Surg* 2000; 15:347-353.
13. Argenziano M, Chen JM, Choudhri AF, et al: Management of vasodilatory shock after cardiac surgery: identification of predisposing factors and use of a novel pressor agent. *J Thorac Cardiovasc Surg* 1998; 116:973-980.

14. Arora P, Rajagopalam S, Ranjan R, et al: Preoperative use of angiotensin-converting enzyme inhibitors/angiotensin receptor blockers is associated with increased risk for acute kidney injury after cardiovascular surgery. *Clin J Am Soc Nephrol* 2008; 3:1266-1273.
15. Miceli A, Capoun R, Fino C, et al: Effects of angiotensin-converting enzyme inhibitor therapy on clinical outcome in patients undergoing coronary artery bypass grafting. *J Am Coll Cardiol* 2009; 54:1778-1784.
16. Samsoon GL, Young JR: Difficult tracheal intubation: a retrospective study. *Anaesthesia* 1987; 42:487-490.
17. Mallampati SR, Gatt SP, Gugino LD, et al: A clinical sign to predict difficult tracheal intubation: a prospective study. *Can Anaesth Soc J* 1985; 32:429-434.
18. Strandgaard S, Olesen J, Skinhoj E, Lassen NA: Autoregulation of brain circulation in severe arterial hypertension. *Br Med J* 1973; 1:507-510.
19. Cheng EY, Lauer KK, Stommel KA, Guenther NR: Evaluation of the palmar circulation by pulse oximetry. *J Clin Monit* 1989; 5:1-3.
20. Bedford RF, Shah N: Blood pressure monitoring, in Blitt CD, Hines RL (eds): *Invasive and Noninvasive Monitoring in Anesthesia and Critical Care Medicine*, 3rd ed. New York, Churchill Livingstone, 1995; p 95.
21. O'Rourke MF: Pressure and flow waves in systemic arteries and the anatomical design of the arterial system. *J Appl Physiol* 1967; 23:139-149.
22. Bruner JM, Krenis LJ, Kunsman JM, Sherman AP: Comparison of direct and indirect methods of measuring arterial blood pressure, part III. *Med Instrum* 1981; 15:182-188.
23. Boutros A, Albert S: Effect of the dynamic response of transducer-tubing system on accuracy of direct blood pressure measurement in patients. *Crit Care Med* 1983; 11:124-127.
24. Prys-Roberts C: Measurement of intravascular pressure, in Saidman LJ, Smith NT (eds): *Monitoring in Anesthesia.* New York, Churchill Livingstone, .
25. London MJ, Hollenberg M, Wong MG, et al: Intraoperative myocardial ischemia: localization by continuous 12-lead electrocardiography. *Anesthesiology* 1988; 69:232-241.
26. Mangano DT, Browner WS, Hollenberg M, et al: Association of perioperative myocardial ischemia with cardiac morbidity and mortality in men undergoing noncardiac surgery. The Study of Perioperative Ischemia Research Group. *NEJM* 1990; 323:1781-1788.
27. Philip JH, Feinstein DM, Raemer DB: Monitoring anesthetic and respiratory gases, in Blitt CD, Hines RL (eds): *Monitoring in Anesthesia and Critical Care.* New York, Churchill Livingstone, ; p 363.
28. Moller JT, Johannessen NW, Espersen K, et al: Randomized evaluation of pulse oximetry in 20,802 patients: II. Perioperative events and postoperative complications. *Anesthesiology* 1993; 78:445-453.
29. Pan PH, Gravenstein N: Intraoperative pulse oximetry: frequency and distribution of discrepant data. *J Clin Anesth* 1994; 6:491-495.
30. Bernard SA, Gray TW, Buist MD, et al: Treatment of comatose survivors of out-of-hospital cardiac arrest with induced hypothermia. *NEJM* 2002; 346:557-563.
31. Martin TD, Craver JM, Gott JP, et al: Prospective, randomized trial of retrograde warm blood cardioplegia: myocardial benefit and neurologic threat. *Ann Thorac Surg* 1994; 57:298-302; discussion 302-304.
32. Grech ED, Baines M, Steyn R, et al: Normothermic versus hypothermic coronary bypass surgery. *Lancet* 1994; 343:1155-1156.
33. Grigore AM, Murray CF, Ramakrishna H, Djaiani G: A core review of temperature regimens and neuroprotection during cardiopulmonary bypass: does rewarming rate matter? *Anesth Analg* 2009; 109: 1741-1751.
34. Reed CR, Sessler CN, Glauser FL, Phelan BA: Central venous catheter infections: concepts and controversies. *Intensive Care Med* 1995; 21:177-183.
35. Troianos CA, Jobes DR, Ellison N: Ultrasound-guided cannulation of the internal jugular vein. A prospective, randomized study. *Anesth Analg* 1991; 72:823-826.
36. Randolph AG, Cook DJ, Gonzales CA, Pribble CG: Ultrasound guidance for placement of central venous catheters: a meta-analysis of the literature. *Crit Care Med* 1996; 24:2053-2058.
37. Mahmood F, Sundar S, Khabbaz K: Misplacement of a guidewire diagnosed by transesophageal echocardiography. *J Cardiothorac Vasc Anesth* 2007; 21:420-421.
38. Gelman S: Venous function and central venous pressure: a physiologic story. *Anesthesiology* 2008; 108:735-748.
39. Wiesenack C, Fiegl C, Keyser A, Prasser C, Keyl C: Assessment of fluid responsiveness in mechanically ventilated cardiac surgical patients. *Eur J Anaesthesiol* 2005; 22:658-665.
40. Rex S, Brose S, Metzelder S, et al: Prediction of fluid responsiveness in patients during cardiac surgery. *Br J Anaesth* 2004; 93:782-788.
41. Pinsky MR, Teboul JL: Assessment of indices of preload and volume responsiveness. *Curr Opin Crit Care* 2005; 11:235-239.
42. van Daele ME, Sutherland GR, Mitchell MM, et al: Do changes in pulmonary capillary wedge pressure adequately reflect myocardial ischemia during anesthesia? A correlative preoperative hemodynamic, electrocardiographic, and transesophageal echocardiographic study. *Circulation* 1990; 81:865-871.
43. Sprung CL, Elser B, Schein RM, Marcial EH, Schrager BR: Risk of right bundle-branch block and complete heart block during pulmonary artery catheterization. *Crit Care Med* 1989; 17:1-3.
44. Mangano DT: Heparin bonding and long-term protection against thrombogenesis. *NEJM* 1982; 307:894-895.
45. Kim YL, Richman KA, Marshall BE: Thrombocytopenia associated with Swan-Ganz catheterization in patients. *Anesthesiology* 1980; 53:261-262.
46. Swan HJ, Ganz W, Forrester J, et al: Catheterization of the heart in man with use of a flow-directed balloon-tipped catheter. *NEJM* 1970; 283: 447-451.
47. Kozak M, Robertson BJ, Chambers CE: Cardiac catheterization laboratory: Diagnostic and therapeutic procedures in the adult patient, in Kaplan JA (ed): *Kaplan's Cardiac Anesthesia*, 5th ed. Philadelphia, Saunders, 2006; p 299.
48. Shure D: Pulmonary-artery catheters—peace at last? *NEJM* 2006; 354: 2273-2274.
49. Cheung A, Chernow B: Perioperative electrolyte disorders, in Benumof JL, Saidman LJ (eds): *Anesthesia and Perioperative Complications.* St Louis, Mosby-Year Book, 1991; p 466.
50. Drop LJ: Ionized calcium, the heart, and hemodynamic function. *Anesth Analg* 1985; 64:432-451.
51. Bronsky B, Dubin A, Waldstein SS: Calcium and the electrocardiogram: Electrocardiographic manifestations of hypoparathyroidism. *Am J Cardiol* 1961; 7:823.
52. Robertie PG, Butterworth JFt, Royster RL, et al: Normal parathyroid hormone responses to hypocalcemia during cardiopulmonary bypass. *Anesthesiology* 1991; 75:43-48.
53. Fernandez-del Castillo C, Harringer W, Warshaw AL, et al: Risk factors for pancreatic cellular injury after cardiopulmonary bypass. *NEJM* 1991; 325:382-387.
54. Aglio LS, Stanford GG, Maddi R, et al: Hypomagnesemia is common following cardiac surgery. *J Cardiothorac Vasc Anesth* 1991; 5:201-208.
55. England MR, Gordon G, Salem M, Chernow B: Magnesium administration and dysrhythmias after cardiac surgery. A placebo-controlled, double-blind, randomized trial. *JAMA* 1992; 268:2395-2402.
56. Vyvyan HA, Mayne PN, Cutfield GR: Magnesium flux and cardiac surgery. A study of the relationship between magnesium exchange, serum magnesium levels and postoperative arrhythmias. *Anaesthesia* 1994; 49:245-249.
57. Ouattara A, Lecomte P, Le Manach Y, et al: Poor intraoperative blood glucose control is associated with a worsened hospital outcome after cardiac surgery in diabetic patients. *Anesthesiology* 2005; 103:687-694.
58. Capes SE, Hunt D, Malmberg K, Pathak P, Gerstein HC: Stress hyperglycemia and prognosis of stroke in nondiabetic and diabetic patients: a systematic overview. *Stroke* 2001; 32:2426-432.
59. Egi M, Bellomo R, Stachowski E, French CJ, Hart G: Variability of blood glucose concentration and short-term mortality in critically ill patients. *Anesthesiology* 2006; 105:244-252.
60. van den Berghe G, Wouters P, Weekers F, et al: Intensive insulin therapy in the critically ill patients. *NEJM* 2001; 345:1359-1367.
61. Griesdale DE, de Souza RJ, van Dam RM, et al: Intensive insulin therapy and mortality among critically ill patients: a meta-analysis including NICE-SUGAR study data. *CMAJ* 2009; 180:821-827.
62. Wiener RS, Wiener DC, Larson RJ: Benefits and risks of tight glucose control in critically ill adults: a meta-analysis. *JAMA* 2008; 300:933-944.
63. Finfer S, Chittock DR, Su SY, et al: Intensive versus conventional glucose control in critically ill patients. *NEJM* 2009; 360:1283-1297.
64. Floyd TF, Cheung AT, Stecker MM: Postoperative neurologic assessment and management of the cardiac surgical patient. *Semin Thorac Cardiovasc Surg* 2000; 12:337-348.
65. Bavaria JE, Brinster DR, Gorman RC, et al: Advances in the treatment of acute type A dissection: an integrated approach. *Ann Thorac Surg* 2002; 74:S1848-1852; discussion S1857-1863.
66. Stecker MM, Cheung AT, Pochettino A, et al: Deep hypothermic circulatory arrest: II. Changes in electroencephalogram and evoked potentials during rewarming. *Ann Thorac Surg* 2001; 71:22-28.
67. Sebel PS, Bowdle TA, Ghoneim MM, et al: The incidence of awareness during anesthesia: a multicenter United States study. *Anesth Analg* 2004; 99:833-839, table of contents.
68. Ranta S, Jussila J, Hynynen M: Recall of awareness during cardiac anaesthesia: influence of feedback information to the anaesthesiologist. *Acta Anaesthesiol Scand* 1996; 40:554-560.

69. Phillips AA, McLean RF, Devitt JH, Harrington EM: Recall of intraoperative events after general anaesthesia and cardiopulmonary bypass. *Can J Anaesth* 1993; 40:922-926.
70. Adams DC, Hilton HJ, Madigan JD, et al: Evidence for unconscious memory processing during elective cardiac surgery. *Circulation* 1998; 98:II289-292; discussion II292-293.
71. Gilron I, Solomon P, Plourde G: Unintentional intraoperative awareness during sufentanil anaesthesia for cardiac surgery. *Can J Anaesth* 1996; 43:295-298.
72. Goldmann L, Shah MV, Hebden MW: Memory of cardiac anaesthesia. Psychological sequelae in cardiac patients of intra-operative suggestion and operating room conversation. *Anaesthesia* 1987; 42:596-603.
73. Ranta SO, Herranen P, Hynynen M: Patients' conscious recollections from cardiac anesthesia. *J Cardiothorac Vasc Anesth* 2002; 16:426-430.
74. Practice advisory for intraoperative awareness and brain function monitoring: a report by the American Society of Anesthesiologists Task Force on Intraoperative Awareness. *Anesthesiology* 2006; 104:847-864.
75. Avidan MS, Zhang L, Burnside BA, et al: Anesthesia awareness and the bispectral index. *NEJM* 2008; 358:1097-1108.
76. Myles PS, Leslie K, McNeil J, Forbes A, Chan MT: Bispectral index monitoring to prevent awareness during anaesthesia: the B-Aware randomised controlled trial. *Lancet* 2004; 363:1757-1763.
77. Jobsis FF: Noninvasive, infrared monitoring of cerebral and myocardial oxygen sufficiency and circulatory parameters. *Science* 1977; 198:1264-1267.
78. Casati A, Spreafico E, Putzu M, Fanelli G: New technology for noninvasive brain monitoring: continuous cerebral oximetry. *Minerva Anestesiol* 2006; 72:605-625.
79. Murkin JM: Applied neuromonitoring and improving central nervous system outcomes. *Artif Organs* 2008; 32:851-855.
80. Plachky J, Hofer S, Volkmann M, et al: Regional cerebral oxygen saturation is a sensitive marker of cerebral hypoperfusion during orthotopic liver transplantation. *Anesth Analg* 2004; 99:344-349, table of contents.
81. Casati A, Fanelli G, Pietopaoli P, Proietti R, Montanini S: In a population of elderly patients undergoing elective non-cardiac surgery, cerebral oxygen desaturation is associated with prolonged length of stay. *Anesthesiology* 2003; 99:.
82. Kim MB, Ward DS, Cartwright CR, et al: Estimation of jugular venous O2 saturation from cerebral oximetry or arterial O2 saturation during isocapnic hypoxia. *J Clin Monit Comput* 2000; 16:191-199.
83. Cho H, Nemoto EM, Yonas H, Balzer J, Sclabassi RJ: Cerebral monitoring by means of oximetry and somatosensory evoked potentials during carotid endarterectomy. *J Neurosurg* 1998; 89:533-538.
84. Samra SK, Dy EA, Welch K, et al: Evaluation of a cerebral oximeter as a monitor of cerebral ischemia during carotid endarterectomy. *Anesthesiology* 2000; 93:964-970.
85. Slater JP, Guarino T, Stack J, et al: Cerebral oxygen desaturation predicts cognitive decline and longer hospital stay after cardiac surgery. *Ann Thorac Surg* 2009; 87:36-44; discussion 44-45.
86. Yao FS, Tseng CC, Ho CY, Levin SK, Illner P: Cerebral oxygen desaturation is associated with early postoperative neuropsychological dysfunction in patients undergoing cardiac surgery. *J Cardiothorac Vasc Anesth* 2004; 18:552-558.
87. Murkin JM, Adams SJ, Novick RJ, et al: Monitoring brain oxygen saturation during coronary bypass surgery: a randomized, prospective study. *Anesth Analg* 2007; 104:51-58.
88. Edmonds HL, Jr: Multi-modality neurophysiologic monitoring for cardiac surgery. *Heart Surg Forum* 2002; 5:225-228.
89. Edmonds HL, Jr, Ganzel BL, Austin EH, 3rd: Cerebral oximetry for cardiac and vascular surgery. *Semin Cardiothorac Vasc Anesth* 2004; 8:147-166.
90. Rubio A, Hakami L, Munch F, et al: Noninvasive control of adequate cerebral oxygenation during low-flow antegrade selective cerebral perfusion on adults and infants in the aortic arch surgery. *J Card Surg* 2008; 23:474-479.
91. Cheng HW, Chang HH, Chen YJ, et al: Clinical value of application of cerebral oximetry in total replacement of the aortic arch and concomitant vessels. *Acta Anaesthesiol Taiwan* 2008; 46:178-183.
92. Tobias JD, Russo P, Russo J: Changes in near infrared spectroscopy during deep hypothermic circulatory arrest. *Ann Card Anaesth* 2009; 12:17-21.
93. Mascio CE, Myers JA, Edmonds HL, Austin EH, 3rd: Near-infrared spectroscopy as a guide for an intermittent cerebral perfusion strategy during neonatal circulatory arrest. *ASAIO J* 2009; 55:287-290.
94. Guerit JM, Witdoeckt C, Verhelst R, et al: Sensitivity, specificity, and surgical impact of somatosensory evoked potentials in descending aorta surgery. *Ann Thorac Surg* 1999; 67:1943-1946; discussion 1953-1958.
95. Jacobs MJ, Elenbaas TW, Schurink GW, Mess WH, Mochtar B: Assessment of spinal cord integrity during thoracoabdominal aortic aneurysm repair. *Ann Thorac Surg* 2002; 74:S1864-1866; discussion S1892-1898.
96. Shine TS, Harrison BA, De Ruyter ML, et al: Motor and somatosensory evoked potentials: their role in predicting spinal cord ischemia in patients undergoing thoracoabdominal aortic aneurysm repair with regional lumbar epidural cooling. *Anesthesiology* 2008; 108:580-587.
97. Keyhani K, Miller CC, 3rd, Estrera AL, et al: Analysis of motor and somatosensory evoked potentials during thoracic and thoracoabdominal aortic aneurysm repair. *J Vasc Surg* 2009; 49:36-41.
98. Clark RE, Brillman J, Davis DA, et al: Microemboli during coronary artery bypass grafting. Genesis and effect on outcome. *J Thorac Cardiovasc Surg* 1995; 109:249-257; discussion 257-258.
99. Cheung AT, Weiss SJ, Savino JS: Protamine-induced right-to-left intracardiac shunting. *Anesthesiology* 1991; 75:904-907.
100. Weiss SJ, Cheung AT, Stecker MM, et al: Fatal paradoxical cerebral embolization during bilateral knee arthroplasty. *Anesthesiology* 1996; 84:721-723.
101. Pearson AC, Labovitz AJ, Tatineni S, Gomez CR: Superiority of transesophageal echocardiography in detecting cardiac source of embolism in patients with cerebral ischemia of uncertain etiology. *J Am Coll Cardiol* 1991; 17:66-72.
102. Cheung AT, Levin SK, Weiss SJ, Acker MA, Stenach N: Intracardiac thrombus: a risk of incomplete anticoagulation for cardiac operations. *Ann Thorac Surg* 1994; 58:541-542.
103. Savino JS, Weiss SJ: Images in clinical medicine. Right atrial tumor. *NEJM* 1995; 333:1608.
104. Shann KG, Likosky DS, Murkin JM, et al: An evidence-based review of the practice of cardiopulmonary bypass in adults: a focus on neurologic injury, glycemic control, hemodilution, and the inflammatory response. *J Thorac Cardiovasc Surg* 2006; 132:283-290.
105. Longnecker DE, Cheung AT: Pharmacology of inhalational anesthetics, in Longnecker DE, Tinker JH, Morgan GE (eds): *Principles and Practices of Anesthesiology*, 2nd ed. St Louis, Mosby, 1998; p 1123.
106. Quasha AL, Eger EI, 2nd, Tinker JH: Determination and applications of MAC. *Anesthesiology* 1980; 53:315-334.
107. Varadarajan SG, An J, Novalija E, Stowe DF: Sevoflurane before or after ischemia improves contractile and metabolic function while reducing myoplasmic Ca(2+) loading in intact hearts. *Anesthesiology* 2002; 96:125-133.
108. Loeckinger A, Keller C, Lindner KH, Kleinsasser A: Pulmonary gas exchange in coronary artery surgery patients during sevoflurane and isoflurane anesthesia. *Anesth Analg* 2002; 94:1107-1112, table of contents.
109. Kikura M, Ikeda K: Comparison of effects of sevoflurane/nitrous oxide and enflurane/nitrous oxide on myocardial contractility in humans. Load-independent and noninvasive assessment with transesophageal echocardiography. *Anesthesiology* 1993; 79:235-243.
110. Pagel PS, Kampine JP, Schmeling WT, Warltier DC: Comparison of the systemic and coronary hemodynamic actions of desflurane, isoflurane, halothane, and enflurane in the chronically instrumented dog. *Anesthesiology* 1991; 74:539-551.
111. Stowe DF, Monroe SM, Marijic J, Bosnjak ZJ, Kampine JP: Comparison of halothane, enflurane, and isoflurane with nitrous oxide on contractility and oxygen supply and demand in isolated hearts. *Anesthesiology* 1991; 75:1062-1074.
112. Kemmotsu O, Hashimoto Y, Shimosato S: Inotropic effects of isoflurane on mechanics of contraction in isolated cat papillary muscles from normal and failing hearts. *Anesthesiology* 1973; 39:470-477.
113. Brown BR, Jr, Crout JR: A comparative study of the effects of five general anesthetics on myocardial contractility. I. Isometric conditions. *Anesthesiology* 1971; 34:236-245.
114. Van Trigt P, Christian CC, Fagraeus L, et al: Myocardial depression by anesthetic agents (halothane, enflurane and nitrous oxide): quantitation based on end-systolic pressure-dimension relations. *Am J Cardiol* 1984; 53:243-247.
115. Pagel PS, Kampine JP, Schmeling WT, Warltier DC: Alteration of left ventricular diastolic function by desflurane, isoflurane, and halothane in the chronically instrumented dog with autonomic nervous system blockade. *Anesthesiology* 1991; 74:1103-1114.
116. Kotrly KJ, Ebert TJ, Vucins EJ, Roerig DL, Kampine JP: Baroreceptor reflex control of heart rate during morphine sulfate, diazepam, N2O/O2 anesthesia in humans. *Anesthesiology* 1984; 61:558-563.
117. Blaise G, Sill JC, Nugent M, Van Dyke RA, Vanhoutte PM: Isoflurane causes endothelium-dependent inhibition of contractile responses of canine coronary arteries. *Anesthesiology* 1987; 67:513-517.
118. Slogoff S, Keats AS: Randomized trial of primary anesthetic agents on outcome of coronary artery bypass operations. *Anesthesiology* 1989; 70:179-188.

119. Stowe DF, Bosnjak ZJ, Kampine JP: Comparison of etomidate, ketamine, midazolam, propofol, and thiopental on function and metabolism of isolated hearts. *Anesth Analg* 1992; 74:547-558.
120. Park WK, Lynch C, 3rd: Propofol and thiopental depression of myocardial contractility. A comparative study of mechanical and electrophysiologic effects in isolated guinea pig ventricular muscle. *Anesth Analg* 1992; 74:395-405.
121. Lepage JY, Pinaud ML, Helias JH, et al: Left ventricular performance during propofol or methohexital anesthesia: isotopic and invasive cardiac monitoring. *Anesth Analg* 1991; 73:3-9.
122. Muzi M, Berens RA, Kampine JP, Ebert TJ: Venodilation contributes to propofol-mediated hypotension in humans. *Anesth Analg* 1992; 74: 877-883.
123. Rouby JJ, Andreev A, Leger P, et al: Peripheral vascular effects of thiopental and propofol in humans with artificial hearts. *Anesthesiology* 1991; 75:32-42.
124. Gooding JM, Corssen G: Effect of etomidate on the cardiovascular system. *Anesth Analg* 1977; 56:717-719.
125. Riou B, Lecarpentier Y, Chemla D, Viars P: In vitro effects of etomidate on intrinsic myocardial contractility in the rat. *Anesthesiology* 1990; 72: 330-340.
126. Riou B, Lecarpentier Y, Viars P: Effects of etomidate on the cardiac papillary muscle of normal hamsters and those with cardiomyopathy. *Anesthesiology* 1993; 78:83-90.
127. Vinclair M, Broux C, Faure P, et al: Duration of adrenal inhibition following a single dose of etomidate in critically ill patients. *Intensive Care Med* 2008; 34:714-719.
128. Jabre P, Combes X, Lapostolle F, et al: Etomidate versus ketamine for rapid sequence intubation in acutely ill patients: a multicentre randomised controlled trial. *Lancet* 2009; 374:293-300.
129. White PF, Way WL, Trevor AJ: Ketamine—its pharmacology and therapeutic uses. *Anesthesiology* 1982; 56:119-136.
130. Waxman K, Shoemaker WC, Lippmann M: Cardiovascular effects of anesthetic induction with ketamine. *Anesth Analg* 1980; 59:355-358.
131. Benthuysen JL, Smith NT, Sanford TJ, Head N, Dec-Silver H: Physiology of alfentanil-induced rigidity. *Anesthesiology* 1986; 64:440-446.
132. Smith NT, Benthuysen JL, Bickford RG, et al: Seizures during opioid anesthetic induction—are they opioid-induced rigidity? *Anesthesiology* 1989; 71:852-862.
133. Bailey PL, Clark NJ, Pace NL, Isern M, Stanley TH: Failure of nalbuphine to antagonize morphine: a double-blind comparison with naloxone. *Anesth Analg* 1986; 65:605-611.
134. Puttfarcken PS, Cox BM: Morphine-induced desensitization and down-regulation at mu-receptors in 7315C pituitary tumor cells. *Life Sci* 1989; 45:1937-1942.
135. Shafer A, White PF, Schuttler J, Rosenthal MH: Use of a fentanyl infusion in the intensive care unit: tolerance to its anesthetic effects? *Anesthesiology* 1983; 59:245-248.
136. Egan TD, Lemmens HJ, Fiset P, et al: The pharmacokinetics of the new short-acting opioid remifentanil (GI87084B) in healthy adult male volunteers. *Anesthesiology* 1993; 79:881-892.
137. Steinlechner B, Dworschak M, Birkenberg B, et al: Low-dose remifentanil to suppress haemodynamic responses to noxious stimuli in cardiac surgery: a dose-finding study. *Br J Anaesth* 2007; 98:598-603.
138. Macdonald DB: Intraoperative motor evoked potential monitoring: overview and update. *J Clin Monit Comput* 2006; 20:347-377.
139. Backman SB, Stein RD, Ralley FE, Fox GS: Neostigmine-induced bradycardia following recent vs remote cardiac transplantation in the same patient. *Can J Anaesth* 1996; 43:394-398.
140. Clarkson CW, Hondeghem LM: Mechanism for bupivacaine depression of cardiac conduction: fast block of sodium channels during the action potential with slow recovery from block during diastole. *Anesthesiology* 1985; 62:396-405.
141. Polley LS, Columb MO, Naughton NN, Wagner DS, van de Ven CJ: Relative analgesic potencies of ropivacaine and bupivacaine for epidural analgesia in labor: implications for therapeutic indexes. *Anesthesiology* 1999; 90:944-950.
142. Litz RJ, Roessel T, Heller AR, Stehr SN: Reversal of central nervous system and cardiac toxicity after local anesthetic intoxication by lipid emulsion injection. *Anesth Analg* 2008; 106:1575-1577, table of contents.
143. Rosenblatt MA, Abel M, Fischer GW, Itzkovich CJ, Eisenkraft JB: Successful use of a 20% lipid emulsion to resuscitate a patient after a presumed bupivacaine-related cardiac arrest. *Anesthesiology* 2006; 105: 217-218.
144. Litz RJ, Popp M, Stehr SN, Koch T: Successful resuscitation of a patient with ropivacaine-induced asystole after axillary plexus block using lipid infusion. *Anaesthesia* 2006; 61:800-801.
145. Practice Guidelines for Management of the Difficult Airway. A report by the American Society of Anesthesiologists Task Force on Management of the Difficult Airway. *Anesthesiology* 1993; 78:597-602.
146. Blaisdell FW, Cooley DA: The mechanism of paraplegia after temporary thoracic aortic occlusion and its relationship to spinal fluid pressure. *Surgery* 1962; 51:351-355.
147. Svensson LG, Von Ritter CM, Groeneveld HT, et al: Cross-clamping of the thoracic aorta. Influence of aortic shunts, laminectomy, papaverine, calcium channel blocker, allopurinol, and superoxide dismutase on spinal cord blood flow and paraplegia in baboons. *Ann Surg* 1986; 204:38-47.
148. Khan SN, Stansby G: Cerebrospinal fluid drainage for thoracic and thoracoabdominal aortic aneurysm surgery. *Cochrane Database Syst Rev* 2004; CD003635.
149. Cina CS, Abouzahr L, Arena GO, et al: Cerebrospinal fluid drainage to prevent paraplegia during thoracic and thoracoabdominal aortic aneurysm surgery: a systematic review and meta-analysis. *J Vasc Surg* 2004; 40:36-44.
150. Bower TC, Murray MJ, Gloviczki P, et al: Effects of thoracic aortic occlusion and cerebrospinal fluid drainage on regional spinal cord blood flow in dogs: correlation with neurologic outcome. *J Vasc Surg* 1989; 9:135-144.
151. Cheung AT, Weiss SJ, McGarvey ML, et al: Interventions for reversing delayed-onset postoperative paraplegia after thoracic aortic reconstruction. *Ann Thorac Surg* 2002; 74:413-419; discussion 420-421.
152. Etz CD, Luehr M, Kari FA, et al: Paraplegia after extensive thoracic and thoracoabdominal aortic aneurysm repair: does critical spinal cord ischemia occur postoperatively? *J Thorac Cardiovasc Surg* 2008; 135:324-330.
153. Cheung AT, Pochettino A, McGarvey ML, et al: Strategies to manage paraplegia risk after endovascular stent repair of descending thoracic aortic aneurysms. *Ann Thorac Surg* 2005; 80:1280-1288; discussion 1288-1289.
154. Cheung AT, Pochettino A, Guvakov DV, et al: Safety of lumbar drains in thoracic aortic operations performed with extracorporeal circulation. *Ann Thorac Surg* 2003; 76:1190-1196; discussion 1196-1197.
155. Wynn MM, Mell MW, Tefera G, Hoch JR, Acher CW: Complications of spinal fluid drainage in thoracoabdominal aortic aneurysm repair: a report of 486 patients treated from 1987 to 2008. *J Vasc Surg* 2009; 49: 29-34; discussion 34-35.
156. Estrera AL, Sheinbaum R, Miller CC, et al: Cerebrospinal fluid drainage during thoracic aortic repair: safety and current management. *Ann Thorac Surg* 2009; 88:9-15; discussion 15.
157. Dardik A, Perler BA, Roseborough GS, Williams GM: Subdural hematoma after thoracoabdominal aortic aneurysm repair: an underreported complication of spinal fluid drainage? *J Vasc Surg* 2002; 36:47-50.
158. Swenson JD, Hullander RM, Wingler K, Leivers D: Early extubation after cardiac surgery using combined intrathecal sufentanil and morphine. *J Cardiothorac Vasc Anesth* 1994; 8:509-514.
159. Fitzpatrick GJ, Moriarty DC: Intrathecal morphine in the management of pain following cardiac surgery. A comparison with morphine i.v. *Br J Anaesth* 1988; 60:639-644.
160. Aun C, Thomas D, St John-Jones L, et al: Intrathecal morphine in cardiac surgery. *Eur J Anaesthesiol* 1985; 2:419-426.
161. Scott NB, Turfrey DJ, Ray DA, et al: A prospective randomized study of the potential benefits of thoracic epidural anesthesia and analgesia in patients undergoing coronary artery bypass grafting. *Anesth Analg* 2001; 93:528-535.
162. Practice Guidelines for Acute Pain Management in the Perioperative Setting: an updated report by the American Society of Anesthesiologists Task Force on Acute Pain Management. *Anesthesiology* 2004; 100:1573-1581.
163. Moore R, Follette DM, Berkoff HA: Poststernotomy fractures and pain management in open cardiac surgery. *Chest* 1994; 106:1339-1342.
164. Robinson RJ, Brister S, Jones E, Quigly M: Epidural meperidine analgesia after cardiac surgery. *Can Anaesth Soc J* 1986; 33:550-555.
165. Auroy Y, Benhamou D, Bargues L, et al: Major complications of regional anesthesia in France: The SOS Regional Anesthesia Hotline Service. *Anesthesiology* 2002; 97:1274-1280.
166. Cheney FW, Domino KB, Caplan RA, Posner KL: Nerve injury associated with anesthesia: a closed claims analysis. *Anesthesiology* 1999; 90: 1062-1069.
167. Horlocker TT, Wedel DJ, Benzon H, et al: Regional anesthesia in the anticoagulated patient: defining the risks (the second ASRA Consensus Conference on Neuraxial Anesthesia and Anticoagulation). *Reg Anesth Pain Med* 2003; 28:172-197.
168. Hemmerling TM, Djaiani G, Babb P, Williams JP: The use of epidural analgesia in cardiac surgery should be encouraged. *Anesth Analg* 2006; 103:1592; author reply 1592-1593.
169. Pastor MC, Sanchez MJ, Casas MA, Mateu J, Bataller ML: Thoracic epidural analgesia in coronary artery bypass graft surgery: seven years' experience. *J Cardiothorac Vasc Anesth* 2003; 17:154-159.

170. Byhahn C, Meininger D, Kessler P: [Coronary artery bypass grafting in conscious patients: a procedure with a perspective?]. *Anaesthesist* 2008; 57:1144-1154.
171. Vandermeulen EP, Van Aken H, Vermylen J: Anticoagulants and spinal-epidural anesthesia. *Anesth Analg* 1994; 79:1165-1177.
172. Kohn LT, Corrigan JM, Donaldson MS: *To Err Is Human: Building a Safer Health System.* National Academy Press, Washington, DC, 1999.
173. Grogan EL, Stiles RA, France DJ, et al: The impact of aviation-based teamwork training on the attitudes of health-care professionals. *J Am Coll Surg* 2004; 199:843-848.
174. ACC/AHA Guidelines and Indications for Coronary Artery Bypass Graft Surgery. A report of the American College of Cardiology/American Heart Association Task Force on Assessment of Diagnostic and Therapeutic Cardiovascular Procedures (Subcommittee on Coronary Artery Bypass Graft Surgery). *Circulation* 1991; 83:1125-1173.
175. Practice Guidelines for Pulmonary Artery Catheterization. A report by the American Society of Anesthesiologists Task Force on Pulmonary Artery Catheterization. *Anesthesiology* 1993; 78:380-394.
176. Practice Advisory for the Prevention of Perioperative Peripheral Neuropathies: a report by the American Society of Anesthesiologists Task Force on Prevention of Perioperative Peripheral Neuropathies. *Anesthesiology* 2000; 92:1168-1182.
177. Ramsay JG, DeLima LG, Wynands JE, et al: Pure opioid versus opioid-volatile anesthesia for coronary artery bypass graft surgery: a prospective, randomized, double-blind study. *Anesth Analg* 1994; 78: 867-875.

CHAPTER 11

Echocardiography in Cardiac Surgery

Maurice Enriquez-Sarano
Vuyisile T. Nkomo
Hector I. Michelena

INTRODUCTION

Echocardiography has become the major imaging and diagnostic modality of cardiac disease, so all cardiac specialists, cardiologists or surgeons, need to understand basic principles, approaches, indications, physiologic determinants, pitfalls, and expected results in order to make appropriate interpretations. Beyond the physical principles affecting imaging results, Doppler-echocardiography is, like all complex testing modalities, subject to operator dependence and Bayesian interpretation of results. Hence, quality of imaging and congruence of reported results should be critically challenged by clinician "consumers." The present summary of Doppler-echocardiographic principles provides basic to advanced knowledge for major cardiac conditions mostly acquired, to ensure proper functioning of the team echocardiographer-cardiac surgeon.

PRINCIPLES OF ECHOCARDIOGRAPHY FOR THE CARDIAC SURGEON: A PRIMER

Echocardiography uses high-frequency ultrasound (2.0 to 7.5 MHz) to image the heart and measure blood flow velocity. It is important to understand some principles of ultrasound for proper interpretation. *Imaging* is produced by reflection of ultrasound (produced by crystals contained in the transducer) on cardiac walls. To achieve reflection, ultrasound first has to penetrate body tissues. Penetration of ultrasonic energy is excellent in water (blood), mediocre in fat, and minimal through air and bones because they are such strong reflectors that no energy is left to progress within the cardiac tissues. Therefore, echocardiographers use *windows* (between the ribs, sternum, and lungs) such as parasternal, apical, subcostal, suprasternal, transesophageal, or intracardiac to ensure good penetration of ultrasound. Ultrasonic imaging is not photography, and images of cardiac structures (eg, aortic walls) are generated by a "scan-converter" counting the time between emission of ultrasound and return of the reflected wave to the same crystal and calculating the distance from transducer to reflective structure assuming a constant speed of ultrasonic progression in blood. This mostly true assumption ensures excellent measurement of depth, but lateral resolution is less precise because strong reflectors tend to diffract ultrasounds, which rebound not only toward the original crystal, but also adjoining ones. Thus, a point is well defined in depth but appears fattened laterally (lateral lobes). Clinically, this lateral "thickening" of echoes tends to minimize apparent size of cavities. Strong reflectors (eg, calcified walls) also reflect so much ultrasonic energy that travels back to the transducer, to the wall again, and transducer again that artifact at double depth may be generated. Single crystal imaging is M-mode echo, whereas two-dimensional (2D) echo is produced by a series of crystals. 2D echo is a tomography that slices the heart and requires comprehensive imaging to mentally reconstruct the heart. Newly developed three-dimensional (3D) imaging produces an ultrasonic cone reflecting the true 3D heart structure, but diffraction of ultrasound waves and computational issues degrade imaging definition. Hopefully future development will provide high resolution and 3D imaging.

Intracardiac velocity is measured based on the Doppler effect; that is, a moving target changes the wavelength of the reflected sound. The frequency change (Doppler shift) magnitude is proportional to the velocity of the moving target and its direction indicates the direction of the moving target (toward or away from the transducer). Velocity measurement is very precise if ultrasound beam and moving target directions are

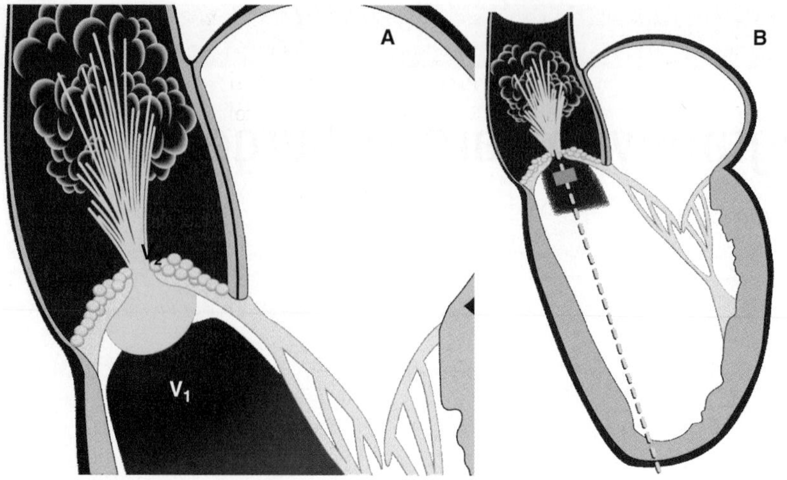

FIGURE 11-1 Flow through a restrictive orifice and measures by Doppler. (A) A restrictive orifice creates a pattern of flow convergence proximal to the orifice with acceleration of flow through the narrowest portion of the orifice (vena contracta) and expansion with deceleration beyond the orifice. (B) The necessary alignment of ultrasound beam and flow is shown to measure accurately velocity. The small box proximal to the jet represents a sample volume of pulsed-wave Doppler. (*Figure courtesy of FA Miller.*)

identical (Fig. 11-1). With angulation of these directions measured velocity decreases with the cosine of the angle (Cosine 90 degrees = 0, no signal). Thus, to measure blood velocity, appropriate alignment is required. As alignment is uncertain; a multiwindow search of peak velocity (indicating alignment) is indispensable. Blood and tissue velocities can be measured depending on filters. Two types of Doppler ultrasound can be used, pulsed Doppler (velocity is measured through a small gate), precisely locating the measure but limited in peak velocity measurement, and continuous wave Doppler, which does not discriminate location on the ultrasonic beam but allows measurement of high velocity (ie, gradients). Indeed, a small orifice (stenosis) forces blood (incompressible fluid) to accelerate (constant flow, smaller orifice means higher velocity). Velocity (V) allows one to calculate gradients usually with the simplified Bernoulli equation (gradient = $4V^2$), which ignores some components (viscous, inertia), but is generally accurate for clinical purposes. It should be noted that compared with catheterization, gradient may be underestimated because of angulation, but can also be slightly overestimated because of pressure recovery. This phenomenon is caused by energy conservation (constant through a stenotic orifice), so that when kinetic energy (velocity) is maximal at the stenotic orifice, potential energy (pressure) is lowest, but after the orifice, when blood decelerates, potential energy (pressure) increases. Thus, slightly downstream from the orifice, where catheters are usually placed, pressure is higher and the gradient lower than at the valve orifice itself. This phenomenon is usually minimal, but can be clinically relevant with some prostheses or small aortas. Color flow imaging is based on velocity measurement by Doppler and is coded yellow for flows toward the transducer and blue away. Color flow imaging does not measure volumetric flow, but indicates displacement of red blood cells. It cannot show flows at a 90-degree angle to the ultrasonic beam (which appear black), and displays high velocities as "aliasing," in which when the maximum blue color is reached the color switches to yellow for higher velocity (and so on) giving high-velocity jets their mosaic appearance. Jet imaging is a major application of color flow. Jet extent is influenced by technical, physiologic, and physical factors. For example, a lower color scale will detect lower velocities and artificially increase the jet area. Physiologically, jet extent is determined by jet momentum, that is, the product of flow by velocity. Thus, very small jets must have very low flow, but larger jets can be caused by higher jet velocity (eg, higher ventricular pressure enlarges MR jet despite unchanged flow). Physically, jets are constrained by cavity size so that larger cavities contain larger jets but also jets directed on a wall are constrained irrespective of their flow. Thus, interpretation of jet extent should be made with awareness of these pitfalls.

MODALITIES OF DOPPLER-ECHOCARDIOGRAPHY

Echocardiography provides essential information for most adult cardiovascular diseases requiring cardiac surgery, regarding cardiac structure, function, and hemodynamics, and is crucial for indicating and planning surgery and anesthesia, intraoperative management, and postoperative monitoring to ensure the best possible outcome. However, multiple echocardiographic modalities respond to different clinical questions that should be clearly defined by the managing team for optimal utilization.

Transthoracic Echocardiography

Transthoracic echocardiography (TTE) is completely noninvasive and safe. It is crucial that all different windows and views be used with multiple tomographic slices to obtain high-resolution assessment of anatomy and function of the heart and great vessels,[1] with several submodalities available:

- *Standard TTE* includes 2D morphologic assessment and 2D-derived M-mode measurement of cardiac dimensions with pulsed wave and continuous wave Doppler. Color-flow imaging verifies normalcy of valve function and intracardiac flows. Visual assessment of ejection fraction is often appropriate and can be combined with M-mode measurements. Using continuous wave Doppler (CWD), tricuspid regurgitation allows estimation of right ventricular systolic pressure.[2]
- *TTE with advanced hemodynamics* is indicated for most patients with valve diseases or poor hemodynamics. Doppler-echocardiography calculates stroke volume, cardiac output, and index. Flow across an orifice is the product of cross-sectional area (CSA, often assumed circular, where area = πr^2) by flow velocity and stroke volume (SV) sums flow over the cardiac cycle (product of cross-sectional area and summed velocities, called time velocity integral ($SV = CSA \times TVI$). Cardiac output is SV multiplied by hear rate and cardiac index, the ratio of output to body surface area. These principles are simple, but pitfalls have to be recognized: The SV is consistently measurable on the aortic orifice, because it is circular and the flow profile is usually flat (meaning that velocities are identical throughout the orifice). SV measurement is more difficult on the mitral valve and quasi-impossible on the tricuspid. Even aortic SV can be underestimated if the diameter (squared in calculation of CSA) is underestimated. Continuous wave Doppler (CWD) measures velocity and pressure gradients for stenotic valves with the simplified but accurate Bernoulli equation (gradient = $4V^2$).[3,4] Note that catheterization peak to peak gradient (not recommended) is not the peak gradient but is closer to the mean gradient. Mean gradient obtained by Doppler correlates extremely well with catheterization. Velocity decay through a diastolic orifice (mitral stenosis or aortic regurgitation) is faster with a larger orifice and allows assessment of the severity of the disease.[5] Another important principle in advanced Doppler hemodynamics is the conservation of mass. Blood is incompressible, and when passing through a stenotic orifice, blood flow remains constant through increase in flow velocity (smaller area, higher velocity). This principle, which is also the basis of Gorlin's formulas, is the foundation of stenotic[6] and regurgitant[7] effective area measurement by Doppler, whereby orifice area equals flow/velocity. The flow measurement can be deduced from stroke volumes, or for regurgitant valves can be measured by the proximal isovelocity surface area (PISA) method. In this method the flow convergence proximal to a regurgitant orifice (ie, blood converges toward the orifice) is analyzed by color flow imaging, which provides speed of blood and size of flow convergence allowing calculation of flow (flow = $2 \pi r^2 Vr$, where r is the radius of the flow convergence and Vr the blood velocity indicated by the machine as aliasing velocity) and regurgitant volume. Thus, comprehensive hemodynamic assessment should provide cardiac index, pulmonary pressures, valve lesion severity (orifice area regurgitant or stenotic), and overload severity (gradient or regurgitant volume).[8]
- *TTE with advanced cardiac size and function assessment* involves ventricular and atrial characterization. Left ventricular (LV) size is usually characterized as end-diastolic and end-systolic diameters. These dimensions are useful but have important limitations in that they poorly estimate LV dilatation and are biased versus women, who with smaller body size have smaller LV dimensions. Measurement of LV volumes has been codified by the American Society of Echocardiography.[9] One limitation of LV volume measurement is underestimation of true volumes because of LV trabeculations and echo lateral lobes, which can be addressed by using contrast agents that pass in the left heart. These agents allow visualization of the entire LV and accurate measurement of LV volumes and stroke volume with minimal interobserver and intraobserver variability and their use should be generalized for patients with LV overload or enlargement.[10] LV diastolic function is critical information to obtain in many diseases. Although the reference standard is LV filling pressure obtained by high-fidelity catheters, routine LV diastolic function can be obtained by Doppler-echo, by compounding Doppler signals of mitral inflow, LV myocardial velocity, and pulmonary venous inflow.[11] Assessment of right ventricular size and function is mostly qualitative, and much progress remains to be made.

  Left atrial (LA) dimension from parasternal views is a useful measure of LA enlargement but usually underestimates LA posterior development. The American Society of Echocardiography preferred measure of LA size is the LA volume by area length method from two orthogonal views. This measure is simple, reproducible, and LA volume indexed to body surface area greater than or equal to 40 cm/m^2 is considered marked LA enlargement. Information on right atrial size is limited, and volume measurements are possible.[9]
- *TTE with respirometer study* is used when pericardial versus restrictive myocardial disease are suspected.[12] It allows characterization of the excessive flow changes with respiration observed in pericardial diseases with cardiac compression (tamponade, constriction). Pericardial effusion is readily visible by echo, but 2D signs of tamponade are insensitive. Pericardial thickening is difficult to measure by echocardiography. Observation of excess LV septal displacement with respiration, mitral inflow increase with expiration and reduction with inspiration and the opposite changes of tricuspid inflow are helpful in diagnosing pericardial compressions.
- *Stress with TTE* is used much more than with TEE and mostly in myocardial diseases.[13,14] Several goals can be achieved. First, diagnosis of ischemia is based on maximum stress with either exercise (preferred) or dobutamine in patients who have a noncardiac impairment to exercise.[14] Rarely, other stressors have been used. Second, myocardial viability can be assessed in patients with reduced LV function by low-dose dobutamine, which stimulates function of viable myocardium and biphasic response (improved contraction at low dose, then ischemia with reduced contraction at high dose) is suggestive of viability. Third, hemodynamic stress is usually performed on a recumbent bike with continuous imaging.[15] It is particularly useful

in mitral stenosis to characterize the exertional increase in gradient and pulmonary pressure. It has also been used in patients with mitral regurgitation to measure a dynamic increase of regurgitation with stress.[15]

- *TTE with three-dimensional (3D) imaging* was recently added to our armamentarium. Although the ability to display the 3D structure is certainly interesting, the current tradeoff is a loss of resolution that results in increased apparent thickness of tissue and increased complexity of lesion definition.[16]
- *Interventional Echocardiography: Echo guided interventions.* Echocardiography plays an essential role in guiding interventions. The most direct is guidance of pericardiocentesis by TTE, which ensures safe access to the pericardium for drainage of compressive (including postoperative) effusions.[17] Echo guidance by TTE is also essential in mitral balloon valvuloplasty success and is bound to have a growing role with the promises or percutaneous and periapical insertion of sutureless prostheses or percutaneous mitral repair procedures. The role of TEE versus TTE remains uncertain.

Transesophageal Echocardiography

TEE provides superior quality in imaging the heart and great vessels owing to excellent ultrasound penetration from the esophagus allowing use of higher ultrasonic frequency providing higher resolution. TEE allows multiplane 2D imaging (Fig. 11-2) with color, pulsed, and continuous wave Doppler and is the test of choice with difficult or nonfeasible (eg, during surgery) TTE images or for detection with superior sensitivity of vegetations, abscesses, mitral ruptured chords, intra-atrial (particularly appendage) thrombi, pulmonary venous abnormalities, interatrial shunt, aortic dissection, or severe atherosclerosis.

The risks attached to TEE are extremely low, but not absent. In a multicenter survey of 15 European institutions, among 10,218 successful TEE, one patient with previous esophageal pathology died (mortality 0.01%).[18] Overall complications are approximately 0.2%,[18,19] and odynophagia occurs in 0.1%.[20] There is no known esophageal damage resulting from thermal or barometric injury with TEE, but poor perfusion, descending thoracic aortic aneurysms, previous prolonged use of steroids, previous thoracic irradiation, large left atria, and advanced age[21,22] predispose to esophageal injury. Carefully ruling out esophageal disease is essential before TEE and continuous cardiopulmonary monitoring of blood pressure, heart rate, respirations, and oxygen saturation is necessary. Esophageal perforation should be suspected in the presence of pneumothorax, pleural effusion, sepsis, and/or respiratory distress in the early postoperative period[21] and should lead to prompt contrast swallow study with Gastrografin.

Drawbacks and limitations of TEE are related to: (1) the hemodynamic effect of conscious sedation or anesthesia, which affects the evaluation of cardiac diseases, particularly valve regurgitations; (2) the limited ability to modify the position of the transducer so that hemodynamic assessment by TEE is usually

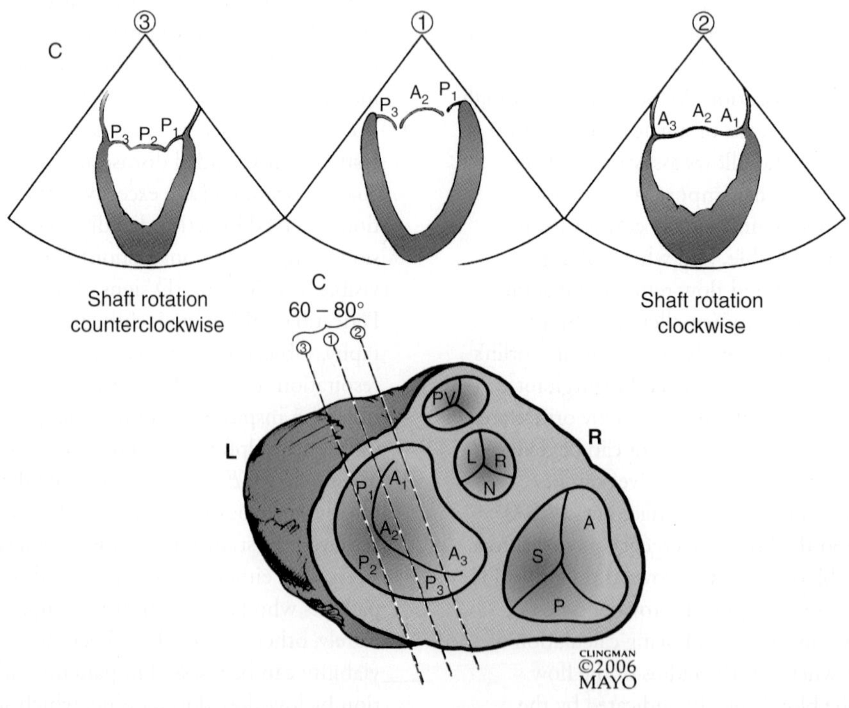

FIGURE 11-2 Imaging of the mitral valve by transesophageal echocardiography. This schematic description shows the four-chamber cut (*C*), and the segment of the mitral valve observed by clockwise and counterclockwise rotation of the probe (*shaft*). The heart is seen from a posterior view, with the planes of imaging in the lower part (numbered 1, 2, and 3), represented as two-dimensional views above. A_1, A_2, A_3 = segments of anterior mitral leaflet; A, S, P = anterior, septal, and posterior leaflets of the tricuspid valve; L = left; R, right; L, R, N = left-, right-, and noncoronary cusps of the aortic valve; P_1, P_2, P_3 = scallops of the posterior leaflet; PV = pulmonary valve.

limited; (3) the loss of image quality in the distant field so that LV apical abnormalities are most often better defined by TTE. Multiplane TEE transducers are now the rule and rotation of 180 degrees allows recording of most imaging planes. Standard views with transducer in midesophagus (about 25 to 30 cm from incisors), distal esophagus (about 30 to 35 cm from incisors), and stomach fundus (about 35 to 40 cm from incisors) allow complete cardiac morphologic and functional assessment. Intraoperative (IO) echocardiography detects unexpected findings, confirms morphologic findings, and monitors LV performance[23] and surgical results.[24] Unsuspected findings reported in 12 to 15% of cases[25] lead to alteration of the surgical plan in 8 to 14% of patients (Fig. 11-3). Postcardiopulmonary bypass findings of significance are noted in 5 to 6% of patients and may lead to second pump runs, the indication of which depend on original surgical indication and hemodynamic instability.[25,26] Thus, IO-TEE is cost effective and avoids later reoperations. IO-TEE also detects residual air in cardiac cavities post-cardiopulmonary bypass, which is indicative of more thorough de-airing maneuvers.[27] Aortic atheroma detected by TEE contributes to postoperative embolisms and strokes. The suggestion that altered handling of the aorta may reduce strokes[28] should be further evaluated. Postoperatively, IO-TEE may be helpful in patients with poor hemodynamics. Markedly reduced LV function or regional wall motion abnormalities may reveal ischemia, particularly those caused by bypass graft dysfunction of air embolism. Dysfunction of the implanted device or repaired valve or vessel should also be carefully sought to discuss revision. Unexpected complications such as aortic dissection or hematoma may require urgent correction. Finally, in patients in whom an intra-aortic balloon pump is required, examination of the aorta may reveal atheroma with floating debris that may lead to thromboembolic complications. Overall, IO-TEE has been shown to be an essential addition to intraoperative monitoring.[25,29,30]

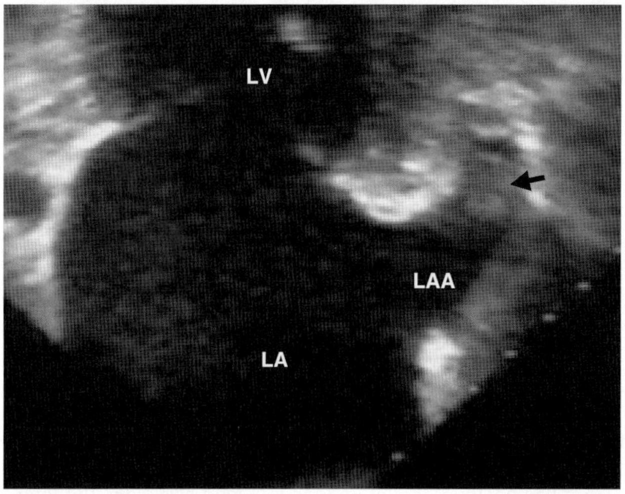

FIGURE 11-3 Transesophageal echocardiography of a patient with a thrombus (*arrow*) in the left atrial appendage (LAA). LA = left atrium; LV = left ventricle.

Utilization of Echocardiography in Cardiac Surgery

Echocardiography is used before, during, and after cardiac surgery to ensure appropriate indication for surgery, verify the results of the intervention, diagnose complications, and assess long-term results of surgery. Preoperatively, echocardiography defines the morphology of cardiac lesions and thereby often the etiology and mechanism of disease, but also provides hemodynamic information, characterizes disease severity, and often defines markers of poor outcome. This role is most usually that of TTE, which records patients' status under routine hemodynamic conditions reflective of daily living circumstances. Intraoperative assessment is mostly performed by TEE to detect unexpected findings, verify preoperative assessment, and assess postoperative results when hemodynamic conditions are restored (and possible use of second bypass runs). Postoperatively TTE detects early complication and defines the early and long-term quality of result of the operation and of LV function.

ECHOCARDIOGRAPHY IN SPECIFIC CARDIAC DISEASES TREATED BY CARDIAC SURGERY

The diagnostic value of echocardiography pre-, intra-, and postoperatively depends on the type of cardiac disease.

Valve Diseases

Native Valve Disease

Preoperatively, it is essential that echocardiography reports sequentially valvular disease etiology, specific mechanism, and valve dysfunction type and severity (eg, rheumatic disease with valvular retraction, mixed mitral valve disease with severe MR and mild MS), but also the associated ventricular and atrial alterations that may affect outcome and management.

Mitral Valve Diseases. Mitral valve diseases are now dominated by mitral regurgitation caused by degenerative diseases and functional regurgitation caused by primary LV disease; they are approached quite differently clinically.

Organic Mitral Valve Regurgitation.

- *Preoperative assessment: etiology and mechanism.* Organic MR results from diseases affecting valve leaflets or supporting structures resulting in improper coaptation. Etiology and mechanism are important to define, as these determine reparability, which is an essential determinant of improved outcome.[31] TTE can usually determine organic MR etiology (Fig. 11-4), the most frequent of which is degenerative with myxomatous mitral valve diseases with prolapse (± flail segment) or fibroelastic degeneration of the mitral leaflets, which is generally associated with primary flail leaflet or annular (± valvular) calcification.[32] Distinction between the diffusely myxomatous valve and fibroelastic degeneration is not accepted by all investigators, but echocardiographic presentation is usually strikingly different with diffuse valve thickening and excess tissue (hooding) in the former,

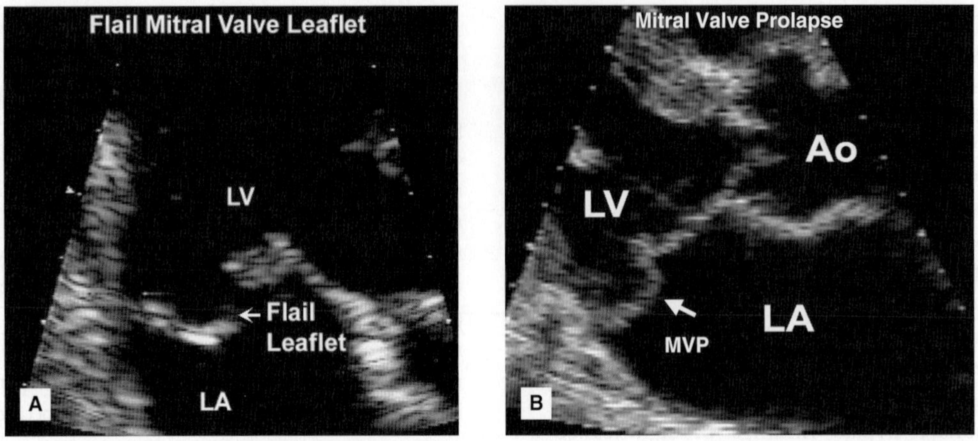

FIGURE 11-4 Examples of morphologic examination of organic mitral regurgitation in transthoracic echocardiography. (A) The patient has a flail segment of the posterior leaflet with marked gap between anterior and posterior leaflet during systole and tip of posterior leaflet in the left atrium. (B) The simple mitral valve prolapse (or billowing mitral valve) shows posterior movement of the leaflet in the left atrium but no gap between leaflets and the tip of the posterior leaflet remains in the left ventricle in systole. Ao = Aorta; LA = left atrium; LV = left ventricle; MVP = mitral valve prolapse.

whereas the latter is characterized by a normal-appearing leaflet apart from in the flail segment. Rheumatic valves are echocardiographically characterized by thickening (with distal predominance) and valve retraction leading to shortened (sometimes absent) coaptation with limited mobility of leaflets (particularly posterior). Rheumatic lesions are difficult to distinguish from those caused by lupus, anticardiolipin syndrome, radiation, or drugs (diet pills or ergot). Endocarditis creates destructive lesions with, in addition to vegetations, ruptured chordae, or perforations. Cleft anterior leaflets are rare and easily recognized in the short axis, but smaller posterior leaflet clefts may be missed. In analyzing MR mechanisms, Carpentier's classification[33] simplified description into three basic types based on leaflet motion—type 1, normal; type 2, excessive; and type 3, restricted motion—and on anatomic localization (two commissures and three segments by leaflet starting with A_1 and P_1 for the anterior and posterior leaflets close to the external commissure). Beyond these important and useful classifications, detailed description should be provided by echocardiography (eg, for an endocarditic etiology, mechanisms can be type 1, perforation, located on A_2 for example versus mechanism type 2, ruptured chordae located on P_3, for example). Complete etiology and mechanism description is usually obtained by TTE (85 to 90% in our institution) and is supported by jet direction, but may require TEE (Fig. 11-5). In operated patients, TEE is currently widely used (preoperatively or intraoperatively) so that the echo-anatomical correspondence is important to memorize. In the midesophageal position, the electronic dial 180-degree inspection arc allows complete anatomical mitral valve examination.[34] Evaluation of the mitral valve with the transgastric short axis is difficult, but may confirm the location of defects. Color flow imaging, by showing where the flow convergence is located and the initial direction of the jet is useful to confirm MR mechanism. This complete etiologic and mechanistic analysis is particularly important for each surgeon to define the probability of valve repair in view of the lesions. Degenerative lesions, unless extensive annular calcification is present, are particularly prone to repair, which provides the best postoperative outcome.[32]

- *Preoperative assessment: valve dysfunction severity.* Color Doppler alerts to MR presence (Figs. 11-6 and 11-7),[35]

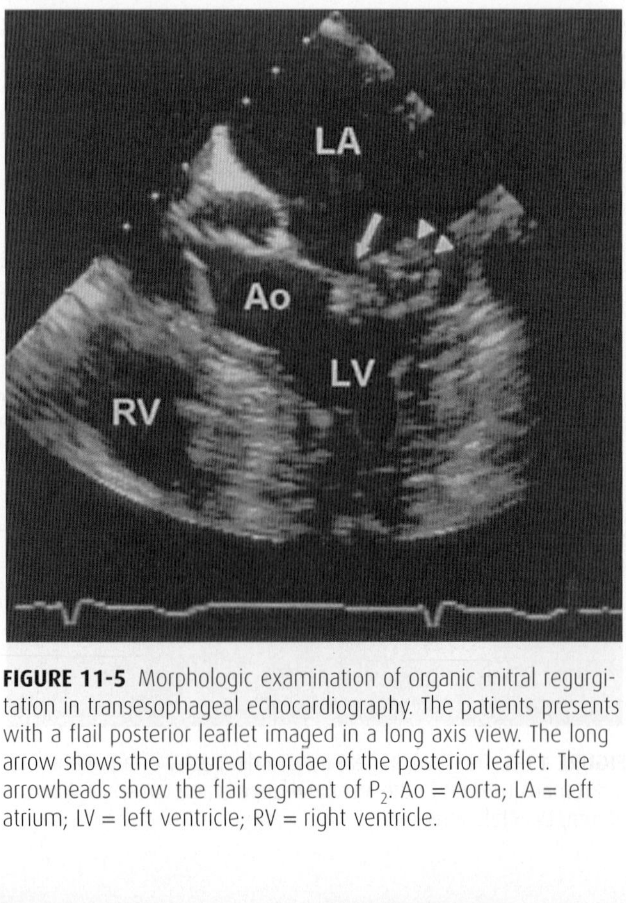

FIGURE 11-5 Morphologic examination of organic mitral regurgitation in transesophageal echocardiography. The patients presents with a flail posterior leaflet imaged in a long axis view. The long arrow shows the ruptured chordae of the posterior leaflet. The arrowheads show the flail segment of P_2. Ao = Aorta; LA = left atrium; LV = left ventricle; RV = right ventricle.

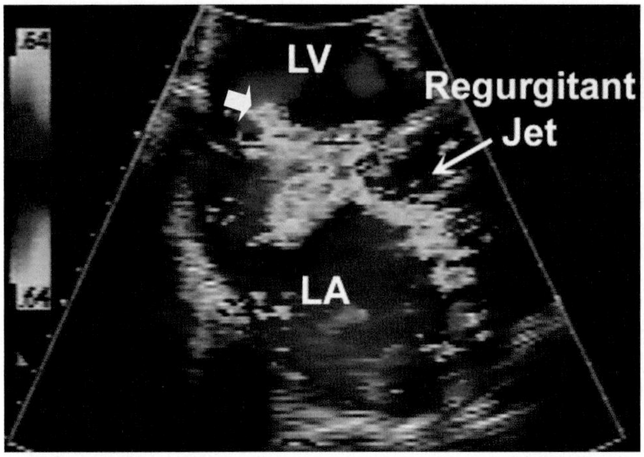

FIGURE 11-6 Eccentric jet of mitral regurgitation (MR) seen a thin layer of color with aliasing appearing as a mosaic color in the left atrium (LA). The MR severity is often underestimated with this type of jet, but visualization of a large flow convergence (*large arrow*) in the left ventricle (LV) suggests severe MR.

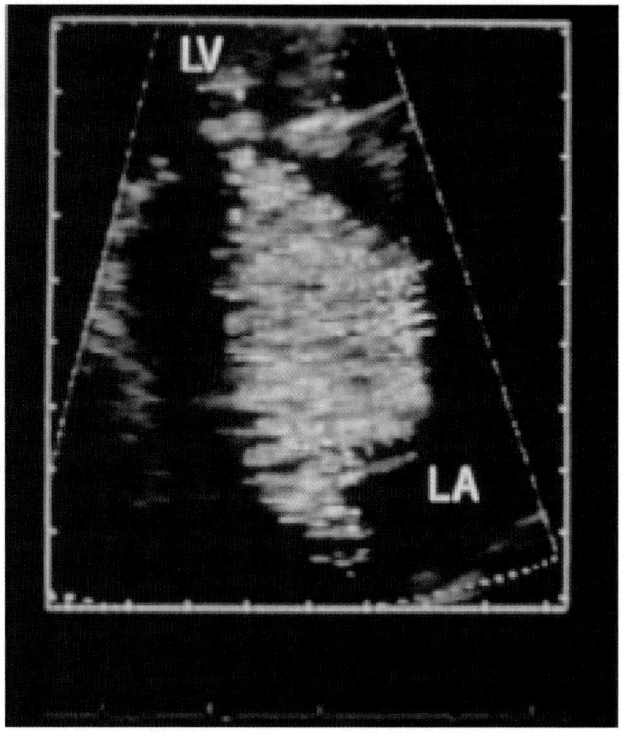

FIGURE 11-7 Central jet of mitral regurgitation (MR) seen as a large area of mosaic flow in the left atrium (LA). The MR severity is often overestimated with this type of jet. LV = Left ventricle.

but estimation of MR severity should rely on comprehensive assessment (Fig. 11-8) based on American Society of Echocardiography criteria,[8] and not just on jet extent in the LA, because jet constraints by the LA wall make this measurement unreliable.[36] The signs of severe MR are classified as (Table 11-1) specific (eg, flail, large flow convergence, large vena contracta, pulmonary flow reversal), supportive (eg, dense jet, high E velocity, enlarged LV, and LA), and quantitative (regurgitant volume greater than or equal to 60 mL, effective regurgitant orifice greater than or equal to 40 mm^2). It is important to note that pulmonary venous flow systolic blunting is not interchangeable with reversal; blunting can be seen in all grades of MR and has a very low predictive value for the severity of MR.[37,38] The suboptimal sensitivity of PV flow reversal is another

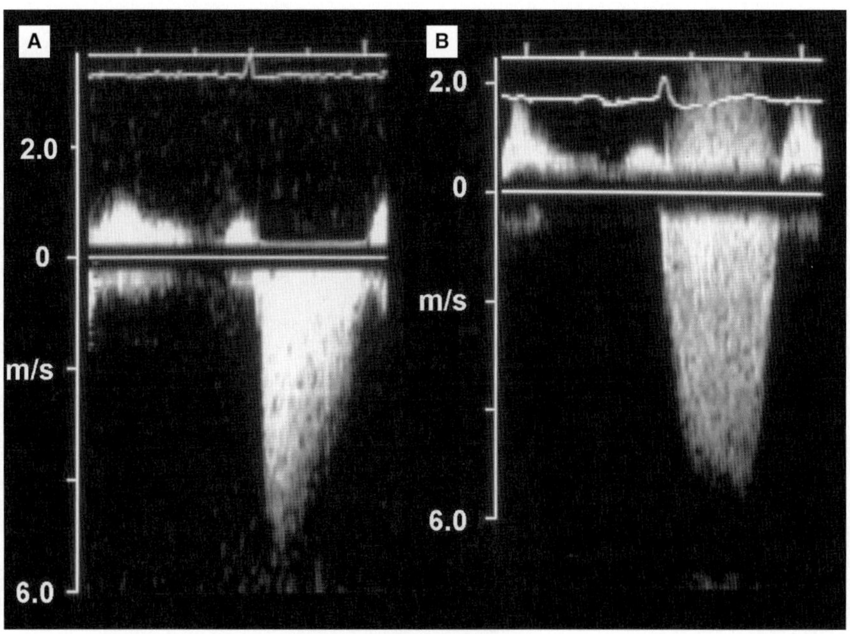

FIGURE 11-8 Continuous wave Doppler of mitral regurgitant (MR) jets. (A) The jet is holosystolic, but the peak velocity is reached during the first half of systole suggesting the existence of a large V wave on the left atrial pressure that leads to rapid equalization of pressure between ventricle and atrium. This type of jet is often seen in acute MR. (B) the jet is also holosystolic, but the peak velocity is reached in mid-late systole without late effacement of velocity. This type of jet is often seen in patients with chronic MR without a large V wave.

TABLE 11-1 Qualitative Signs of Severe Valve Regurgitation

	AR	MR	TR
Specific signs	Central jets of width ≥65% of LVOT Vena contracta >0.6 cm	Vena contracta ≥0.7 cm with large central jet or swirling eccentric jet Large flow convergence Systolic reversal in pulmonary veins Flail leaflet or ruptured papillary muscle	Flail, incomplete coaptation Central jet with area ≥10 cm^2 Vena contracta >0.7 cm Systolic reversal in hepatic veins
Supportive signs	PHT <200 ms Holodiastolic aortic reversal ≥Moderate LV enlargement	Dense triangular jet by CWD E-wave–dominant Enlarged LV and LA	Dense triangular jet by CWD Large flow convergence Enlarged RV

CWD = Continuous wave Doppler; LA = left atrium; LV = left ventricle; LVOT = left ventricular outflow tract; PHT = pressure half time; RV = right ventricle

reason that highlights the importance of quantifying MR (Fig. 11-9).[38] Quantitative methods derived from PISA, quantitative Doppler (Fig. 11-10), or quantitative 2D (LV volumes) have been extensively validated in mitral regurgitation.[7,39,40] Although surgery is mostly reserved for patients with severe MR (Fig. 11-11), severity of the regurgitation is a continuum best quantified than categorized (Table 11-2). MR severity tends to progress by 5 and 7 mL/beat of regurgitant volume per year,[41] so that patients who are not immediately operated should be regularly monitored. As indicated in the guidelines, acquiring proficiency in quantification of MR degree in an important step in developing advanced valve centers.

- *Preoperative assessment: prognostic indicators. Assessment of LV* is usually performed by measuring LV diameters and ejection fraction.[42] End-systolic diameter greater than or equal to 40 to 45 mm[43,44] and ejection fraction less than 60%[45,46] are markers of poor outcome. These characteristics are considered class I indications for surgery but the postoperative outcome when these characteristics are observed[45] is not optimal, so these markers should be considered as advanced signs indicating a rescue surgery. *LA diameter*

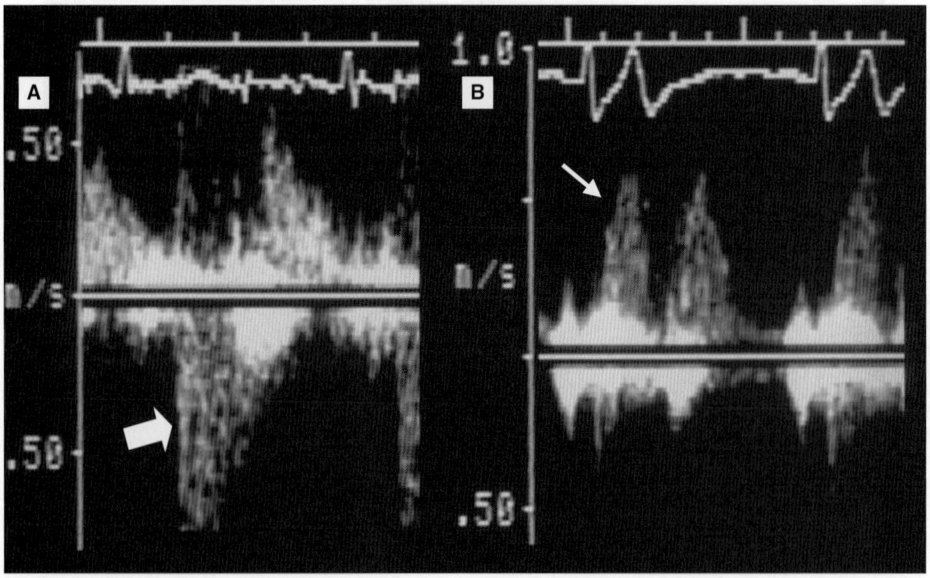

FIGURE 11-9 Pulsed-wave Doppler of pulmonary venous flow in two cases of mitral regurgitation. (A) There a systolic flow reversal (negative flow in systole—*large arrow*) consistent with severe mitral regurgitation (MR) and large V wave on the left atrial pressure. (B) There is a normal forward flow (positive flow in systole—*thin arrow*) suggestive of the absence of V wave. The systolic pulmonary venous flow reversal is a specific sign with high positive predictive value but of low sensitivity for severe MR.

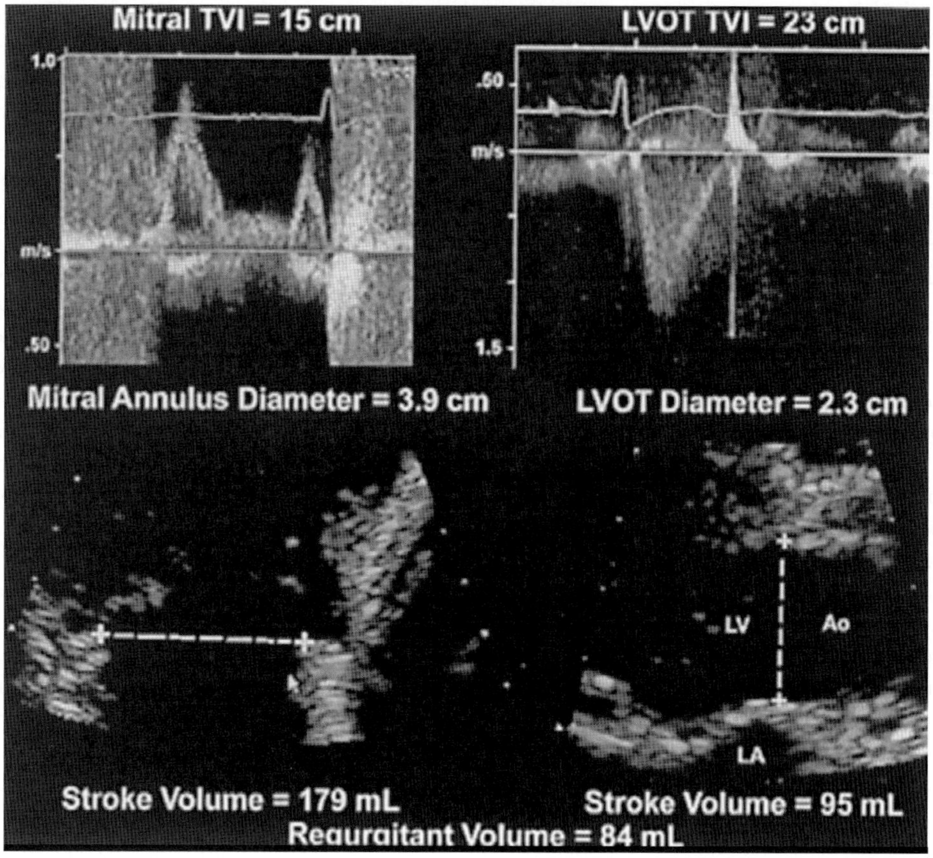

FIGURE 11-10 Quantitative Doppler assessment of mitral regurgitation (MR) based on stroke volume measurement using the annular diameter to calculate the annular area and its product with the pulsed wave Doppler as the stroke volume traversing the specific annular area. The left part of the figure measures the mitral stroke volume (179 mL/beat) while the right side measures the aortic stroke volume (95 mL/beat). Thus, the regurgitant volume is calculated as the difference between mitral and aortic stroke volume or 84 mL/beat.

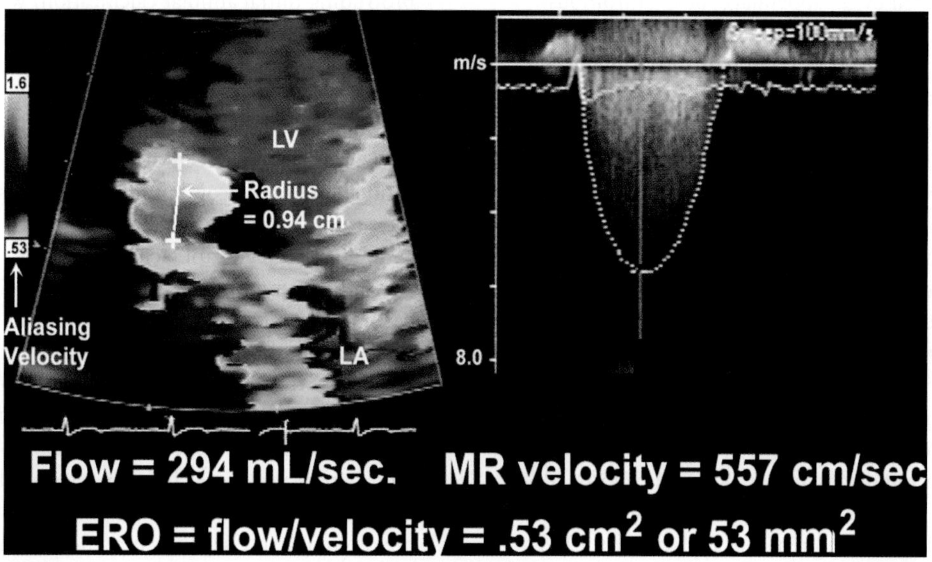

FIGURE 11-11 Proximal isovelocity surface area (PISA) method of quantifying mitral regurgitation (MR). The left side of the figure shows the flow convergence zone with color baseline shift. This allows to measure the flow convergence radius (R = 0.94 cm) and using the aliasing velocity (Vr = 53 cm/s) to calculate the regurgitant flow (flow = $6.28 \times R^2 \times Vr$) at 294 mL or cc/s. The right side of the figure shows the velocity of MR measured by continuous wave Doppler. The ratio of flow by velocity is the effective regurgitant orifice, 0.53 cm^2.

TABLE 11-2 Quantitative Thresholds for Severe Regurgitation

	AR	Organic MR	Functional MR	TR
ERO	≥0.30 cm^2	≥0.40 cm^2	≥0.20 cm^2	≥0.40 cm^2
RVol	≥60 mL	≥60 mL	≥30 mL	≥45 mL

greater than or equal to 50 mm is associated with a high risk of subsequent atrial fibrillation under medical management,[47] but also after successful surgery.[48] Therefore, LA dilatation should alert early for the need of surgery. Pulmonary hypertension is considered as a marker of poorly tolerated MR, although its association to subsequent prognosis is uncertain.[42] *MR severity assessment* is essential for prognosis.[49] Although MR assessment may be qualitative, quantitation provides stronger prognostic information.[50] In asymptomatic patients with organic, holosystolic MR,[50] the risk of death under medical management increased by 18% for each 10 mm^2 ERO increment. ERO was the strongest echocardiographic predictor of outcome. With ERO greater than or equal to 40 mm^2 the risk of death is multiplied by 5 and that of cardiac events by 8 compared with mild MR and excess mortality is observed as compared to the general population. Importantly, surgery restores life expectancy in these asymptomatic patients. Therefore, echocardiographic data participate importantly in the indication of surgery.

- *Intraoperative assessment.* Before cardiopulmonary bypass TEE confirms the mitral lesions[32,51] but also identifies associated conditions that may benefit from surgical therapy (eg, patent foramen ovale, appendage, or LA thrombus). Whether the valve is amenable to repair should be resolved preoperatively,[32,52] and surprises are rare regarding extent or type of lesions that may lead to change in strategy. After cardiopulmonary bypass, intraoperative TEE assesses mitral repair results,[53] and the need for a second pump run is based on the presence of residual MR. Timing of evaluation is crucial. Postbypass TEE performed too early with inappropriate loading conditions results in faulty assessment of residual MR. Insufficient preload and low ventricular pressure minimize regurgitant orifices with residual MR underestimation. Adequately performed postbypass TEE correlates well with predischarge assessment of residual MR.[54] It is essential not to tolerate MR postbypass, unless very trivial, as residual MR initially judged acceptable often requires reoperation during follow-up.[55] Thus post-CPB IO-TEE serves as a tool in deciding which patient should return to CPB for a second repair or replacement. Over time, surgical management of anterior leaflet pathology and bileaflet prolapse has evolved,[56,57] and new techniques emerged that provide better results. IO-TEE still plays a pivotal role in identification of mechanisms and anatomic location of disease as well as post-CPB evaluation of results.

After mitral valve repair, major repair failures are three-fold: insufficient correction of the mitral lesion with residual MR (eg, residual prolapse), LV outflow tract obstruction, or stenotic repair. Severe residual MR obviously is rare but requires immediate correction. Observation of milder residual MR by IO-TEE immediately after repair with "less than echo-perfect" result, leads to higher long-term reoperation risk for MR.[55] IO-TEE must define mechanism and anatomic location of the defect causing residual MR to determine correction strategy and possibility of re-repair. LV outflow tract obstruction is caused by systolic anterior motion of the mitral valve with contact to the LV septum, to which contribute excess or deformed mitral tissue, small LV size, and hyperdynamic LV function.[58] LV outflow tract obstruction occurs in 1 to 4% of mitral valve repairs[59,60] and is diagnosed by visualization of the systolic motion combined with increased velocity through the LV outflow tract. LV outflow tract obstruction results generally in notable residual MR caused by the deformation of the mitral valve in systole, and it is essential in patients with residual MR to rule out LV outflow tract obstruction before recommending a second pump run.[53] Most usually increase LV filling, reducing or discontinuing inotropic drugs, and in some cases of beta-blocker administration, resulting in elimination of LV obstruction.[53] If the obstruction persists, consideration should be given to a second CPB run for sliding valvuloplasty, although the systolic anterior motion tends to improve over time,[59] and most patients can be managed medically. Prevention of LV outflow tract obstruction is based on careful examination of excess tissue on pre-bypass IO-TEE to select the patients who may benefit from specific repair techniques such as sliding annuloplasty.[60,61] Markedly restrictive repairs with stenosis result from combination of anatomical alterations (diseased, rigid leaflets, commissural fusion, markedly protruding mitral annular calcification) with excessive repairs (rings too small and/or large edge to edge sutures). Diagnosis is based on high transvalvular gradients greater than or equal to 8 to 10 mm Hg by Doppler. Normal postrepair gradients (3 to 6 mm Hg) may be exacerbated by high output and tachycardia with reduced diastolic filling period. It is thus prudent before a second pump run to reassess mitral gradient after cardiac output has stabilized and after administration of beta blockers to control tachycardia.

- The most common immediate complications after mitral valve replacement are periprosthetic leaks and mechanical dysfunction of the prosthesis owing to interaction of tissue remnants with the mobile elements of a prosthesis.[62] In contrast to TTE, TEE has no shadowing from the mitral prosthesis, so periprosthetic MR should be carefully sought after bypass and those clinically relevant distinguished from the minor paravalvular[63] or intravalvular[64] leaks that are often noted. Diagnosis is accurate and should lead to prompt consideration of a second pump run, particularly if the paravalvular leak persists after protamine administration. The location and severity of the leak are critical to evaluate in multiple planes and enhance the probability of a simple repair, thus avoiding prosthesis dismounting. Mobile prosthetic elements can be impinged upon by suture or valve material, leading to obstruction or most often regurgitation, which sometimes varies beat to beat because of variable interaction. Thus it is important to examine the prosthesis for a sufficient time to ensure consistent and appropriate function.

- *Postoperative assessment: valvular result.* Postoperative assessment is performed consistently at predischarge and yearly, as well as often 3 to 6 months postoperatively in our practice. Although the IO-TEE is quite accurate in assessing residual valve dysfunction, changes in loading conditions and remodeling may reveal valvular dysfunction. The MR recurrence rate after valve repair is 5 to 10% at 10 years[55,56] and in two-thirds of cases results from new valve lesions (eg, new ruptured chordae), whereas in one-third it results from defective repair (eg, insufficiently corrected prolapse of anterior leaflet in bileaflet prolapse). TTE provides the mechanism and location of the MR and allows discussion of re-repair. It also allows assessment of MR severity. MR qualitative assessment is even more difficult after than before repair, and quantitative techniques (particularly the PISA method) are of particular importance. We rarely refer patients with moderate regurgitant volumes (30 to 60 mL/beat) for reoperation. Development of stenotic repair is rare and is observed mostly with rheumatic or rigid leaflets, sometimes after edge-to-edge repair. Standard repair represents a mild stenosis, which combined with enlarged LA may lead to new atrial fibrillation,[48] and thrombus formation with possible stroke, for which TEE allows thorough examination of the LA appendage. New dysfunction of a mitral prosthesis often requires TEE examination, particularly for detection of prosthetic thrombosis or tissue degeneration.

  Left ventricular assessment. After surgical correction of MR, preload is decreased with decline of end-diastolic volume, but end-systolic indices are little changed so that ejection fraction falls by an average of 10%.[44] However, this response shows large individual variation and LV reverse remodeling may affect the long-term LV function achieved. There are no definite predictors of reverse remodeling and LV end-systolic indices need to be monitored closely during the first postoperative year.[43] The value of medical therapies, shown to result in reverse remodeling in patients with primary LV dysfunction (beta blockers, angiotensin-enzyme inhibitors) is not established, but early diagnosis may lead to early intervention. Irrespective, residual postoperative LV ejection fraction is an important predictor of postoperative survival and should be monitored. The result seen early after surgery is usually stable, unless marked LV dilatation results in further dysfunction or coronary disease leads to intrinsic myocardial deterioration.

Functional Mitral Valve Regurgitation. Functional MR occurs on structurally normal valves caused by primary LV alteration (coronary disease, cardiomyopathy, myocarditis or transient LV dysfunction). Although the primary disease is myocardial, functional MR diagnosed by angiography[65] or echocardiography[66,67] exerts an important influence on outcome, but major controversy persists regarding the role of mitral surgery in these patients.[68,69]

- *Preoperative assessment.* Functional MR diagnosis is based on: (1) The presence of LV dysfunction (generalized most often but sometimes localized requiring a thorough regional assessment); and (2) a structurally "normal" mitral valve with normal tissue or at most minor degenerative calcifications (Fig. 11-12). It is also important to demonstrate the deformation of the mitral valve leading to functional MR. Apical and posterior displacement of papillary muscles applies traction through the inextensible chordae on both leaflets, resulting in apical displacement of the leaflet bodies, leading to altered coaptation.[70,71] This deformation of normal leaflets called "tenting" directly determines functional MR severity (Fig. 11-13). The mechanism of MR is usually a central gap in coaptation, which is worse during isovolumic contraction and relaxation, when the LV exerts a low pressure on the leaflets. With ischemic LV dysfunction the MR may originate from the medial commissure in which the traction may be predominant, but apart from scars of myocardial infarction there are no specific sign of ischemic versus myopathic MR. Traction of chords on the leaflets may be inhomogeneous and predominate on one leaflet.[72] In such cases an "overshoot" of the other (less tethered) leaflet behind the most tethered leaflet is observed, should not be mistaken for a prolapse and may cause unusual eccentric jets. Therefore, functional MR mechanism is not just the frequent annular dilatation but is more complex involving a combination of annular and

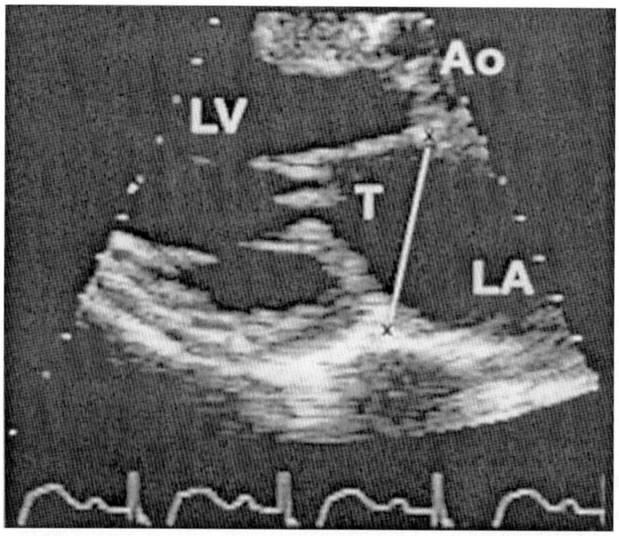

FIGURE 11-12 Two-dimensional echocardiography showing the parasternal long-axis view of a patient with functional mitral regurgitation (MR). Note the protrusion of mitral leaflets toward the left ventricle (LV), resulting in a large tenting area (T) between leaflets and annulus (white line with x marking the mitral annulus) and in insufficient coaptation surface available on each leaflet to prevent MR. Ao = Aorta; LA = left atrium. (*Reproduced with authorization of the American Heart Association.*)

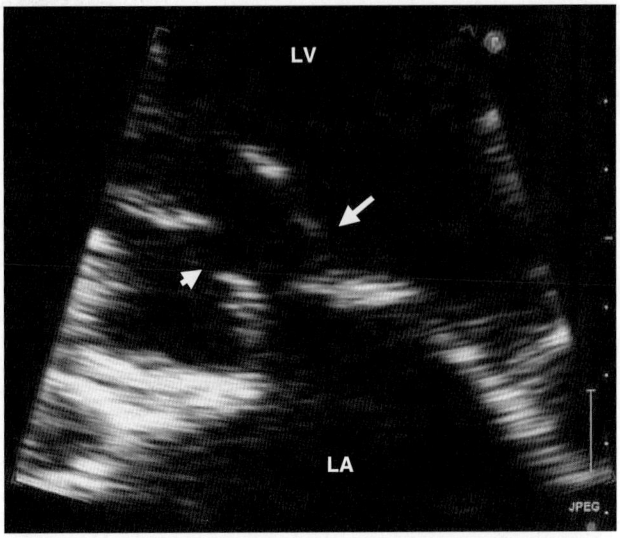

FIGURE 11-13 Two-dimensional echocardiography showing an apical view of a patient with functional mitral regurgitation (MR). The view shows the posterior papillary muscle within the left ventricle (LV), and the chordae attached to the anterior leaflet (*long arrow*) and to the posterior leaflet (*short arrow*) tethering the leaflets within the ventricle as cause to leaflet tenting. LA = Left atrium.

leaflet tethering alterations (Fig. 11-14). MR severity assessment is particularly crucial in view of the notable surgical risk. MR jets that are central tend to be overestimated, and diastolic function alterations may mimic the tall E wave

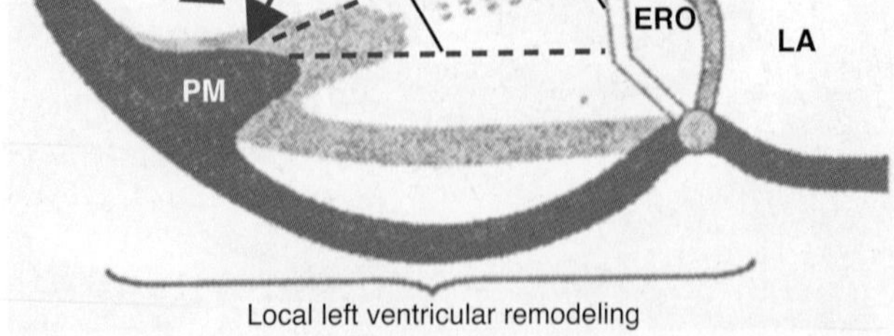

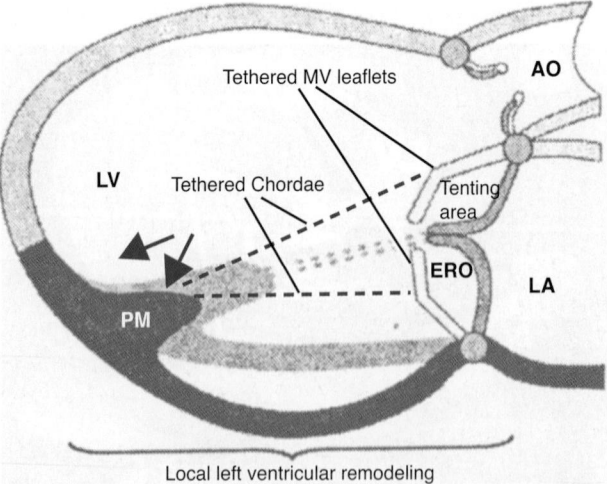

FIGURE 11-14 Schematic representation of the mechanism of functional mitral regurgitation (MR). In light gray is represented the normal position of the papillary muscle (PM) chordae (*dashed lines*) and mitral leaflets shown with adequate coaptation surface. With local left ventricular (LV) remodeling the papillary muscle is repositioned apically and posteriorly (*dark gray*) and exerts traction through the non-distensible chordae on the leaflets. Traction on the strut chords (inserted on the mid-portion of each leaflet) is most manifest, leading to deformation of the mitral leaflet, tenting, reduced coaptation, and creation of an effective regurgitant orifice (ERO). Ao = Aorta; LA = left atrium.

and low systolic venous flow, which is usually suggestive of severe MR. Thus, it is essential to quantify the MR but two essential issues need to be examined. First, functional MR is prominent during isovolumic contraction and relaxation, but as these phases involve little regurgitant driving force their contribution to the regurgitant volume is small and it is essential with the PISA method to quantify MR in mid-systole. Second, the grading of MR has been established in organic MR, but recent data[15,66,73] suggest that thresholds of effective regurgitant orifice (ERO) associated with poor outcome are lower in functional than organic MR. Thus, pending further confirmation patients with functional MR and ERO greater than or equal to 20 mm^2 should be considered as having severe MR; and this prognostic effect comes in addition to ejection fraction and left atrial volume.[74] Functional MR is dynamic. ERO often increases during exercise, which may have important functional[75] and outcome[15] implications, but uniformly decreases during dobutamine echocardiography, making this test useless for the assessment of functional MR. Although the role of imaging during exercise in defining the surgical indications needs further evaluation, a dynamic ERO may also decrease with interventions such as vasodilatation or beta-blockade. Not surprisingly, sedation or anesthesia necessary for TEE may minimize MR and lead to its underestimation[76] compared with habitual life conditions. Preoperative assessment of functional MR should also focus on other components of the disease, namely LV remodeling, systolic dysfunction, and diastolic dysfunction because severe LV remodeling may be a marker for poor response to valve repair.[77]

- *Intraoperative assessment.* Before bypass it is essential to confirm the structurally normal mitral leaflet and to avoid in the MR assessment the pitfall of reduced loading caused by anesthesia. Thus, if the degree of MR is in doubt, assessment with increasing loading conditions similar to those of outpatient evaluation should be performed by a loading challenge, but this does not replace an appropriate outpatient evaluation. Post-bypass, IO-TEE evaluates residual MR. After repair, reduced loading conditions may lead to major underestimation of residual functional MR, emphasizing the importance of adjusting preload and afterload. Functional MR is particularly prone to recurring after surgical correction because of continued LV remodeling, continued displacement of papillary muscles and mitral valve tenting,[78] despite a repair judged as adequate intraoperatively. Thus, post-bypass assessment is difficult and may be overly optimistic; therefore, a careful judgment of residual tenting and valve deformation is essential. Contrary to organic MR, the most advanced subsets of patients benefit as much from bioprosthetic replacement as they do from repair.[79] Thus doubts on repair quality should be pursued aggressively to decide if a new pump run and valve replacement should be recommended.
- *Postoperative assessment* focuses on potential recurrence of MR and its mechanism if present (increased tenting versus insufficient annular restriction).[68,78] Postoperative MR should also be quantified if more than mild. Beyond MR,

echocardiography focuses on the assessment of LV dysfunction, its systolic and diastolic components, and its consequences on LA and pulmonary pressures. Active prevention of further LV remodeling is recommended and should be monitored by echocardiography.

Mitral Valve Stenosis. Mitral stenosis is currently treated preferentially by balloon valvuloplasty,[80] so surgery's role is relatively limited. However, some patients may benefit from surgery rather than balloon valvuloplasty, and the role of echo in defining these subsets should be carefully examined.

- *Preoperative evaluation.* The classical mitral valve stenosis (MS) invariably is caused by rheumatic disease, and its features are characteristic (immobile posterior leaflet, fused commissures with reduced orifice area, and hockey stick deformation of the anterior leaflet in diastole (Fig. 11-15). Other causes of stenosis are lupus or anticardiolipin diseases (which produce very similar lesions), ergot heart disease, and other iatrogenic valve diseases (which thicken leaflets without fusing commissures), and protruding annular calcifications (which restrict the orifice without commissural fusion). Anatomical analysis is essential because balloon valvuloplasty is the most widely used procedure to treat MS and produces a commissurotomy identical to closed commissurotomy (hemi-commissurotomy in most cases). Therefore, balloon valvuloplasty is not indicated with: (1) Mitral obstructions without commissural fusion; (2) heavily calcified mitral valve; (3) MS with nodular calcification of both commissures (high risk of splitting the leaflet and not the commissures)[81]; and (4) MS associated with more than mild MR. In such cases, the best treatment is surgery with valve replacement. Thus, an essential component of MS echo assessment is the short-axis view to ascertain commissural fusion as well as severity and location of calcifications.[81] Another decision-making component is the alteration of subvalvular apparatus.[82] Very short chordae or direct insertion of papillary muscle on leaflets may lead to poor results of balloon valvuloplasty, but may allow good surgical commissurotomy, splitting commissures, and papillary muscles. MS severity is assessed using two variables, the transvalvular gradient representing the pressure overload to the LA and pulmonary circulation and the mitral valve area (MVA) (Fig. 11-16). The gradient measured is the mean

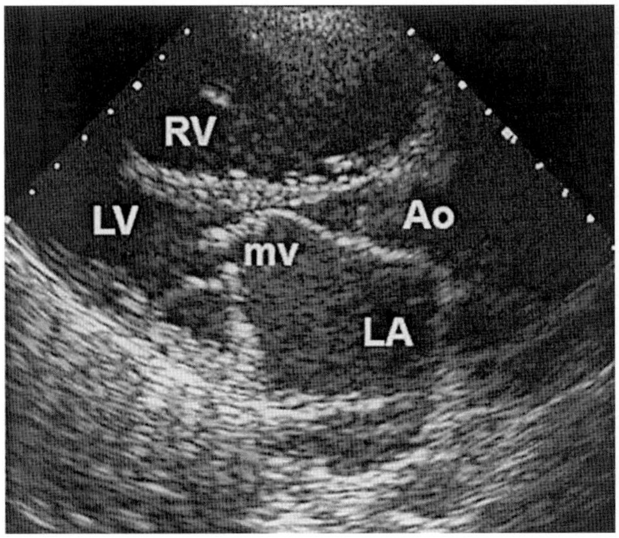

FIGURE 11-15 Parasternal long axis view of a patient with mitral stenosis. Note the thickening and hockey-stick deformation of the anterior leaflet of the mitral valve (mv) and the protrusion of the posterior leaflet. Note also the normal left ventricle (LV) contrasting with the enlarged left atrium (LA) and right ventricle (RV). Ao = Aorta.

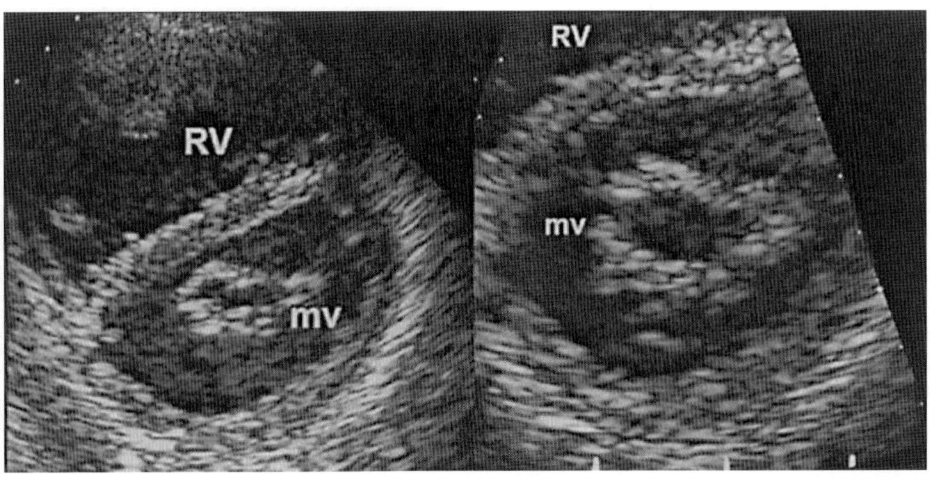

FIGURE 11-16 Mitral valve (mv) area of a patients with mitral stenosis (MS) before (*A*) and after (*B*) commissurotomy. Note in (*A*) the narrow orifice and in (*B*) the large orifice with wide opening of the medial commissure. Note also in (*A*) the right ventricular (RV) enlargement with signs of pulmonary hypertension manifested by a flat septum and D-shaped left ventricle. In (*B*) the position of the septum and the shape of the left ventricle have normalized.

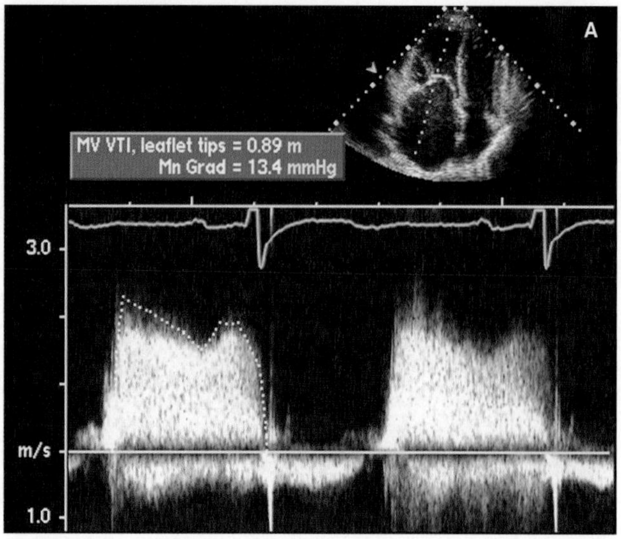

FIGURE 11-17 Continuous wave Doppler recording of the mitral gradient in a patient with severe mitral stenosis (MS). Note the high velocity greater than or equal to 2m/s with mean gradient greater than 13 mm Hg. Note also the flat slope of deceleration of the early diastolic velocity consistent with severe MS.

gradient (Fig. 11-17), which is affected by severity of the stenosis, and increased by tachycardia and amplified transvalvular flow (anemia, pregnancy, hyperthyroidism, associated MR), and decreased by bradycardia and low cardiac output. Mild MS is associated with a resting mean diastolic Doppler (measured by continuous wave Doppler) gradient less than or equal to 5 mm Hg, moderate with a gradient 5 to 10 mm Hg, and severe with a gradient greater than or equal to 10 mm Hg. The normal MVA is 4 to 6 cm^2 and guidelines for MS severity suggest thresholds of 2.0 cm^2 for mild MS, 1.5 cm^2 for moderate MS, and 1.0 for severe MS. However, most patients undergoing interventions for MS are in the range of 1 to 1.2 cm^2 and symptomatic, so that in our institution MVA less than 1.5 cm^2 are considered severe MS. MS severity assessment involves also LA enlargement and elevation of pulmonary pressure and in time may also involve right heart enlargement and failure and tricuspid regurgitation, whereas LV remains normal sized, but may show reduced ejection fraction. MVA measurement can be obtained through several methods that are combined because all methods have limitations and averaging reduces the risk of error. The pressure half-time (PHT) method is the simplest, measured from the Doppler mitral signal using the deceleration from the peak early velocity and calculates MVA using the empiric formula 220/PHT.[83] However, this method may not be accurate with changes in LV or LA compliance and has a wide range of error with short diastole.[84] Other methods of MVA measurement are: (1) Direct orifice planimetry in short-axis view (technically demanding); (2) continuity equation in which MVA is calculated as the ratio of flow measured on the aortic valve to mitral velocity (false if MR or AR); and (3) the PISA method, imaging the mitral inflow with color using baseline shift (requires an angle correction for the funnel shape of the mitral valve with potential for error).[85,86] Important issues in MS severity assessment are: (1) The essential combination of methods of MVA assessment to minimize the potential for error; and (2) the need for exercise hemodynamic (with bike allowing continuous hemodynamic monitoring) assessment in patients who present with low gradient and doubt on the MS severity. Thus, TTE provides assessment of MS severity and in most cases the procedure most suited for treatment. Outpatient TEE is systematic in patients considered for balloon valvuloplasty to assess presence of LA thrombus and MR.

- *Intraoperative assessment* in patients with MS is most often that of mitral replacement, but in patients suited for open commissurotomy, provides anatomical and MR reassessment before bypass and repair assessment postoperatively. A high gradient or moderate MR may lead to consideration of a second pump run after mitral repair. Mobile element dysfunction or periprosthetic regurgitation suggests consideration for further correction after valve replacement. Although decisions with regard to repair of tricuspid regurgitation should be made preoperatively, IO-TEE allows reassessment, rarely discovery of organic tricuspid lesions, and consideration of repair of associated moderate or severe regurgitation.
- *Postprocedure assessment* follows the usual post-dismissal and 1-year assessment (Fig. 11-18). Mitral stenosis remains a progressive lesion even after valve repair and there is potential for recurrence of severe MS and also for progressive scarring and retraction of the mitral valve leading to MR progression. Depending on the severity of the mitral lesions, age and MR a notable proportion of patients need reoperation between 5 and 10 years after the original intervention (balloon valvuloplasty or valve repair). Patients should be carefully monitored to avoid progressive heart failure and pulmonary hypertension. After surgery, pulmonary

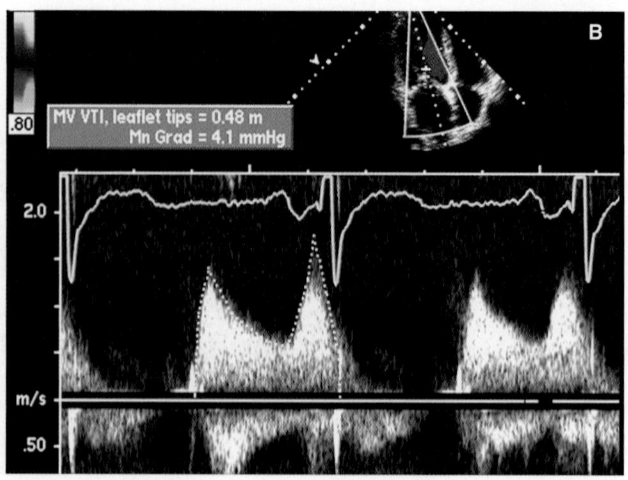

FIGURE 11-18 Continuous wave Doppler in the same patient as Fig. 11-16 after commissurotomy. The mean gradient is now low with rapid deceleration of early diastolic velocity consistent with mild MS.

hypertension caused by MS regress almost uniformly unless chronic pulmonary disease had developed, LV dysfunction most usually normalizes with normalization of preload unless coronary disease was present, but LA enlargement persists and patients with atrial fibrillation remain at substantial risk for stroke.

Mixed Mitral Valve Disease. Mixed mitral valve diseases have substantial component of stenosis and regurgitation and most result from rheumatic disease, a situation now rare in western countries but prevalent in developing countries.

- *Preoperative assessment* recognizes the rheumatic valve lesions and the combination of stenosis and regurgitation precluding the possibility of valve repair. The major challenge is the evaluation of the severity of the mitral valve disease. Often the stenosis and regurgitation are both moderate, and criteria for severe valve diseases are difficult to establish. Transvalvular gradient higher than expected on the basis of MVA alone, reflects the severity of the combined disease.
- *Intraoperative assessment* shows rheumatic features and absence of postoperative complications. Tricuspid regurgitation is frequent in mixed valve disease and often requires associated repair.
- *Postoperative assessment* is important, not only to monitor the mitral prosthesis but also to assess LV function. LV dysfunction is a frequent complication of the MR of mixed mitral valve diseases so that aggressive detection and treatment of this complication is essential to obtain the best outcome.

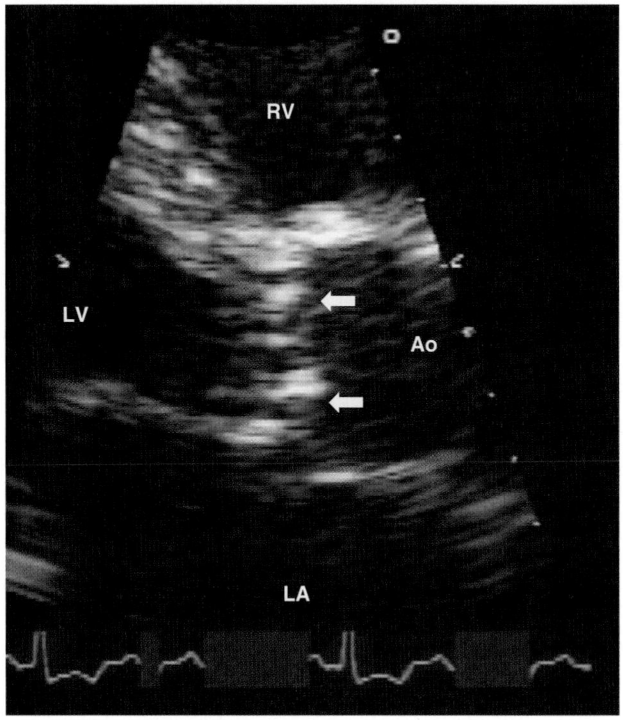

FIGURE 11-19 Two-dimensional echocardiography of a patient with aortic stenosis (AS). The aortic valve (*arrows*) is heavily calcified (*dense nodules*). Ao = Aorta; LA = left atrium; LV = left ventricle; RV = right ventricle.

Aortic Valve Diseases. Aortic valve diseases are now dominated by aortic stenosis. The aortic valve is normally formed by three cusps and is bicuspid in 1 to 2% of the population, but the physiology of the aortic valve is poorly understood irrespective of the cusp number.

Aortic Stenosis.

- *Preoperative assessment* focuses on etiology and mechanism, although assessment is usually simplified compared with the mitral valve. Most aortic stenoses (AS) are caused by degenerative disease irrespective of the number of cusps. Recent data emphasized the atherosclerotic mechanism of AS with initial cholesterol deposition and lipid oxidization, but bicuspid valves tend to calcify more frequently than tricuspid valve for unknown reasons. Rheumatic aortic stenosis is now rare and is characterized by commissural fusion, whereas commissures are open in degenerative diseases. However, clinically the various etiologies of AS in the adult are difficult to recognize, because valves are uniformly calcified in advanced AS. Therefore, morphologically 2D echo recognizes valvular calcification associated with AS in the adult (Fig. 11-19). Absence of aortic valve calcification makes AS unlikely and makes a systolic gradient most likely to originate from subvalvular or supravalvular region. In children, calcification is inconsistent and not indispensable to AS diagnosis. Valvular calcification is difficult to analyze by echocardiography[87] and is more precisely measured with high-resolution computed tomography.[88] The volume or score of calcification is linked to AS severity in a nonlinear manner so that both measures are complementary in assessing AS.[88] The fact that most AS are caused by valve rigidity caused by calcification and not to commissural fusion explains the lack of efficacy of balloon valvuloplasty in AS. The LV responds to pressure overload by increasing wall thickness and LV mass, but this response is variable and its absence does not rule out severe AS. LV hypertrophy regresses after aortic valve replacement, the only approved treatment of AS currently available.[42] Recently developed percutaneous aortic valve replacement offer an option for inoperable patients,[89] and is currently evaluated. Poststenotic aortic dilatation is frequent but rarely requires repair.

Assessment of AS severity is the major goal of TTE. The opening of even just one aortic leaflet to the aortic wall is usually a marker for nonsevere AS, but the AS severity should be assessed quantitatively by measuring mean systolic gradient[3] as marker of pressure overload and aortic valve area (AVA) to assess lesion severity.[6] Normal aortic valve opening area is 2.5 to 4.5 cm^2, AS is considered present with AVA less than or equal to 2 cm^2 and with a pressure gradient developing across the aortic valve and AS is considered severe (Fig. 11-20) with AVA less than or equal to 1.0 cm^2 (using the continuity equation) and mean gradient greater than or equal to 40 mm Hg (using the Doppler velocity).[42] Other criteria of AS are peak velocity greater than or equal to 4 m/sec[90,91] and velocity ratio (LV outflow tract to jet) less than or equal to 0.25.[6] Indeed, in patients with LV outflow tract obstruction AVA may not be

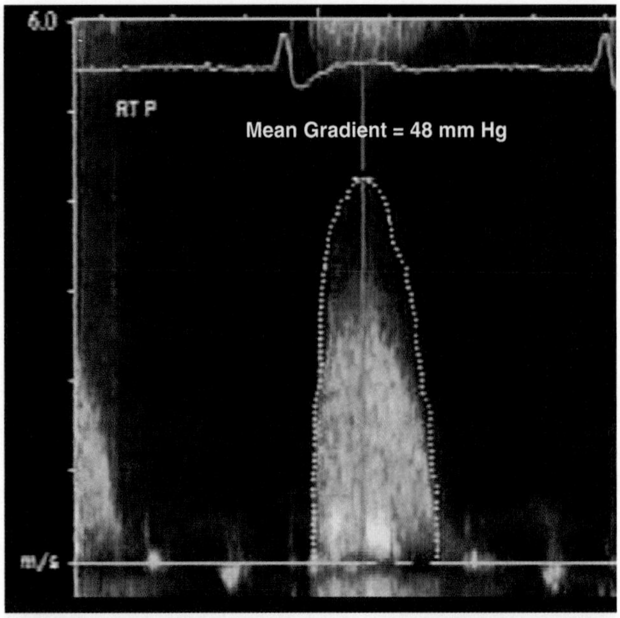

FIGURE 11-20 Continuous wave Doppler obtained from the right parasternal window (RTP) in a patient with severe aortic stenosis (AS). The peak velocity is greater than 4 m/s and the mean gradient is 48 mm Hg.

measurable and velocity may be the only available criterion to diagnose severe AS (Fig. 11-21). AS is progressive because of progressive calcium deposition, with gradient progression by 5 to 7 mm Hg per year and AVA decline by 0.1 cm^2 per year.[92,93] The major pitfall of gradient measurement is underestimation resulting from excessive flow-ultrasonic beam angle, so that systematic multi-window Doppler is the key to appropriate assessment of AS severity.

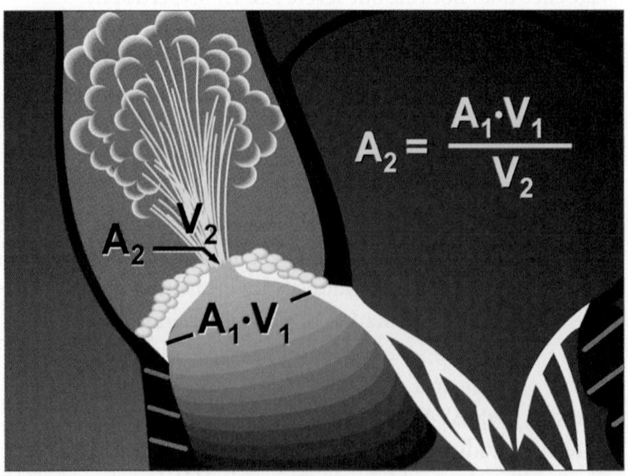

FIGURE 11-21 Schematics of the measurement of aortic valve area in aortic stenosis (AS). Because blood is incompressible flow is constant through the left ventricular outflow tract (*area A_1*) through the aortic orifice (*area A_2*). Thus the aortic stenosis manifested itself by increased velocity ($V_2 > V_1$). Flow is equal to area multiplied by velocity aortic valve area $A_2 = (A_1 \times V_1)/V_2$. (*Reproduced by the courtesy of FA Miller.*)

Another pitfall is the underestimation of the LV outflow tract diameter necessary to the measurement of stroke volume and valve area. Such underestimation leads to underestimation of valve area. Thus, the triad of normal LV function, low gradient, and low AVA warrants ruling out inadequate echo measurements with comprehensive reassessment in a reference laboratory. Nevertheless, recent data suggest that severe AS with low gradient resulting from low stroke volume despite normal EF is a real entity associated with poor prognosis.[94] Conversely, severe AS with low gradient is more logical in patients with reduced LV function,[95–97] but the differential includes low AVA caused by insufficiently forceful ejection to overcome the inertia of a mildly stenotic valve. Diagnosis of severe AS with low gradient requires confirmation, obtained by high-resolution computed tomography measuring high calcium load[88] and/or dobutamine echocardiography that increases myocardial contraction and aortic flow in patients with low EF. The classic response is an increased gradient with severe AS (Fig. 11-22) and an increased AVA with cardiomyopathy and mild AS.[95,97] However, this test may not be conclusive in patients lacking contractile response[96] who may benefit from AVR if the AS is severe.[98]

Although classically asymptomatic severe AS was considered well tolerated, recent data demonstrated excess mortality during follow-up and noted that a large proportion of patients were never offered surgery.[90] Therefore, surgery in asymptomatic patients based on echocardiographic criteria is debated. Asymptomatic patients with rapid decline in AVA and large calcification load display poor clinical outcomes under medical management[87,88] and may be considered for surgery, whereas those with reduced LV function are definitely at high risk and should be offered prompt surgery if the AS is severe.[99]

- *Intraoperative assessment* examines the valve morphology, confirms the large calcification load, and can measure the orifice area by direct planimetry before institution of

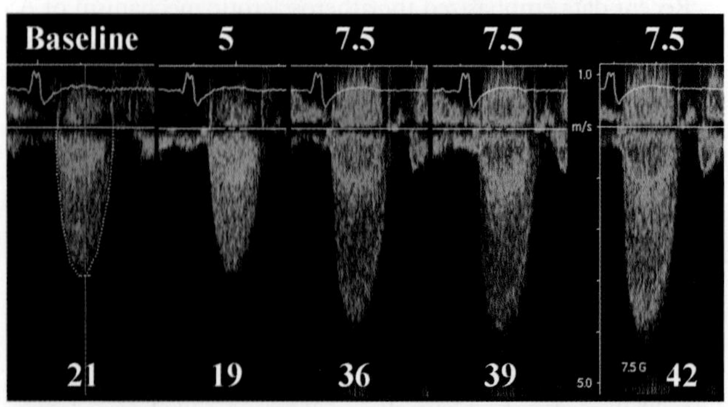

FIGURE 11-22 Measurement of aortic velocity by continuous wave Doppler in a patient with severe aortic stenosis, low ejection fraction, low output, and low gradient. The baseline (*left panel*) mean gradient was 21 mm Hg and increased (*bottom line*) with increasing doses of Dobutamine (*top line*). The peak dose was 7.5 μg/min and the mean gradient reached was 42 mm Hg. (*Reproduced by the courtesy of D Messika-Zeitoun.*)

bypass. AVA measurement by 2D is difficult, because one has to ascertain measurement at the leaflet tip and cannot replace an appropriate Doppler hemodynamic measurement before surgery. Determination of the aortic annulus size may be helpful for early surgical sizing of allografts destined for the aortic position or homograft and may play a role in preventing patient–prosthesis mismatch, which is a cause of postoperative mortality and morbidity,[100,101] and may be prevented by sizing, taking into account the patient body surface area. Another important goal of IO-TEE is examination of ascending aorta and for patients with aneurysmal dilatation, consideration of ascending aortic repair. IO-TEE in patients undergoing aortic valve replacement for severe AS may alter the planned surgical procedure in approximately 10% for unexpected severe MR, PFO, mass, or thrombus. Post-bypass, specific issues examined are lack of signs of dysfunction of prostheses and potential changes in LV function and functional MR. In patients with prominent LV hypertrophy, LV outflow tract obstruction may occur after AVR and should be detected by color imaging or Doppler and verified by simultaneous intraventricular pressure measurement. Myectomy associated with valve replacement may prevent or treat the LV outflow obstruction. Attempts at measuring prosthetic gradient using transgastric approach are of uncertain reliability and lack of patient–prosthesis mismatch cannot be ascertained by intraoperative Doppler-echo currently.

- *Postoperative assessment* focuses on prosthetic, LV, and aortic evaluation. Prosthetic function is not entirely predictable on the basis of patient and prosthesis size and the postoperative Doppler-echo is essential in detecting obstruction, particularly thrombosis, and after mismatch. Reoperation, considered in limited cases for mismatch,[100] is the mainstay of treatment for prosthetic thrombosis or pannus formation, all manifested by prosthetic obstruction.[102] In the diagnosis of prosthetic obstruction, it is important to consider the role of pressure recovery, which may lead to (usually slight) gradient overestimation by Doppler. The 2D examination rarely discriminates between causes of obstruction for which the context of occurrence is more specific. Degeneration of bioprostheses is rarely observed in elderly patients currently affected by AS, but is part of the yearly prosthetic monitoring. LV function is usually maintained after valve replacement for AS. Changes are observed in two circumstances. First, patients with LV dysfunction owing to critical AS generally display improvement in ejection fraction and sometimes normalization after AVR.[103] Even small improvements have important beneficial effects on outcome, but persistence of LV dysfunction requires active medical therapy. Second, patients with associated coronary disease may display postoperatively decline in LV function owing to the coronary disease despite successful aortic valve surgery. Such patients also need active echocardiographic follow-up to ensure appropriate medical treatment.[104] Ascending aortic dilatation generally stabilizes postoperatively, but the rare possibility of continued enlargement and need for repair also require regular echocardiographic follow-up.

A particularly difficult group of patients for follow-up is those with postradiation heart disease,[105] in whom cardiac disease is only part of postradiation lesions that affect the lungs with frequent persistence of postoperative symptoms. The valve disease is only part of the cardiac disease often involving coronary lesions, conduction abnormalities, pericardial constriction, and myocardial fibrosis. These complex lesions often lead to complex follow-up.

Aortic Regurgitation.

- *Preoperative assessment* focuses on the etiology and mechanism in that it determines the possibility of repair.[106] Most frequently aortic regurgitation in western countries is caused by degenerative diseases.[107,108] Minor calcifications may be noted, but rarely with thickened myxomatous tissue. The AR is caused by annular enlargement and sometimes to valve prolapse. Bicuspid aortic valve is the second cause of AR and leads to regurgitation by mal-coaptation and sometimes prolapse of the largest cusp. Aortic root disease involves annuloaortic ectasia more often than Marfan's syndrome or aortitis (eg, syphilis). Rheumatic AR is recognized by the retraction of leaflet, leaving a central regurgitant orifice, and is rarely repairable. Endocarditis is recognized by echo when vegetations are present and may require TEE (Fig. 11-23). Repair is predictable with detection of a perforation, but is not possible with calcified or retracted leaflet. Repair is also particularly feasible with a prolapsed leaflet, especially if the valve is bicuspid or with dystrophic leaflets and moderate AR, in which resuspension of commissures may be sufficient. Therefore, morphologic assessment should be focused on clearly defining the AR mechanism.

AR results in both volume and pressure overload of the LV, which adapts by both concentric and eccentric remodeling until a point of afterload mismatch when LV systolic function fails. Assessment of LV size and systolic function

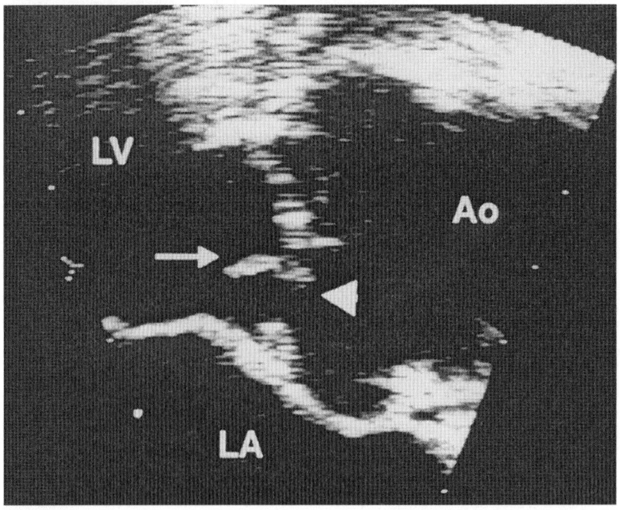

FIGURE 11-23 Imaging of the aortic valve in a patient with endocarditic aortic regurgitation (AR). The long arrow denotes vegetation, whereas the arrowhead denotes a perforation of the noncoronary cusp. Ao = Aorta; LA = left atrium; LV = left ventricle.

by echo is essential. The recommended approach is M-mode 2D-guided, but with increasing frequency LV volumes are calculated, particularly with use of contrast injection. Moderate LV dysfunction defined as EF less than or equal to 50% and severe LV dysfunction (EF ≤35%) justify rescue surgery, but result in decreased postoperative survival.[108] No lower limit of EF contraindicates firmly surgery. Even patients with EF less than or equal to 35% may benefit from valve replacement. EF less than 55% is associated with reduced survival under medical treatment and should be strong consideration for surgery before LV dysfunction affects postoperative survival. Marked LV enlargement is another indication for surgery and is uncovered by LV dimensions greater than or equal to 75 mm (end-diastolic) or greater than or equal to 55 mm (end-systolic)[109] or better greater than or equal to 25 mm/m^2 (end-systolic adjusted to body surface area)[107] as women with smaller body sizes almost never reach absolute LV sizes comparable to men.[110] These differences lead to worse postoperative outcomes in women, emphasizing adjustment of LV measures to body size.[110] Exercise changes in LV function may be helpful, but monitoring of complex variables such as wall stress limit applicability.[111]

Assessment of AR severity is vital to the surgical indication and should be based on comprehensive integration of all signs.[8] Among qualitative approaches, color Doppler (Fig. 11-24) detects the presence of aortic regurgitation and provides simple measures of AR severity (Fig. 11-25). Vena contracta greater than or equal to 0.6 cm and ratio of jet width/left ventricular outflow tract width greater than or equal to 65% in parasternal long axis view suggest severe AR (Fig. 11-26), but jet length does not correlate with AR severity.[112] Color Doppler has many limitations when assessing AR severity and is used as a gross estimation.

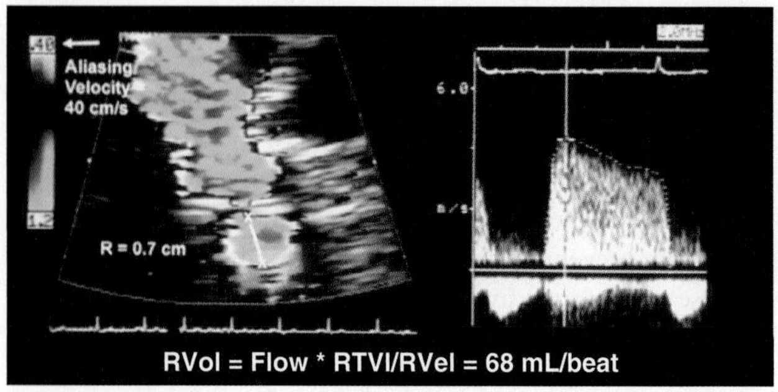

FIGURE 11-25 Quantitation of aortic regurgitation (AR) using the proximal isovelocity surface area (PISA) method. Note that the color baseline is shifted upward. On the left panel analysis of the flow convergence allows measurement of the regurgitant flow and on the left panel, AR velocity is measured using continuous wave Doppler to calculate the regurgitant volume (RVol) as flow multiplied by the ratio of regurgitant time velocity integral (RTVI) to regurgitant velocity (RVel).

Eccentric jet direction leads to underestimation of AR and jets arising from the entire coaptation line of bicuspid valves may be overestimated. Holodiastolic flow reversal in the abdominal or descending thoracic aorta is consistent with severe AR (Fig. 11-27). Maximum AR velocity (measured by CW Doppler) deceleration suggest severe AR with fast pressure half-time (<200 ms, Fig. 11-28). However, AR velocity deceleration is also influenced by LV compliance and reflects elevated LV end-diastolic pressure. Quantitative AR assessment is essential for patients with moderate or severe AR.[8] Regurgitant volume and ERO can be calculated by PISA,[113] quantitative Doppler (mitral and aortic stroke volumes) or LV volumetric method.[40] Although regurgitant volume greater than or equal to 60 mL/beat,

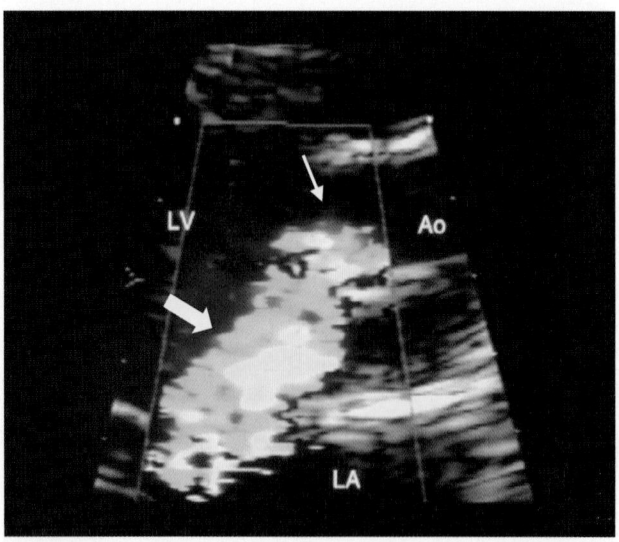

FIGURE 11-24 Parasternal view of aortic regurgitation (AR) using color flow imaging. The flow convergence (*thin arrow*) and jet (*thick arrow*) are well seen. Note the limited expansion of the jet resulting from its eccentricity.

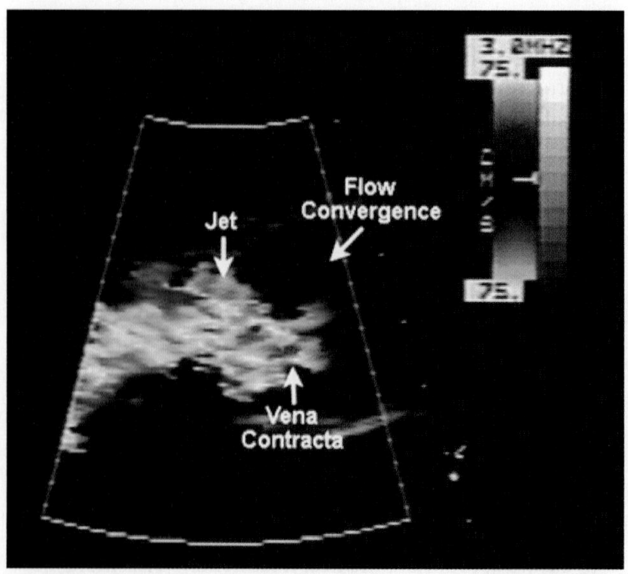

FIGURE 11-26 Parasternal view of aortic regurgitant flow used to delineate and measure the vena contracta (narrow neck) of the aortic regurgitation.

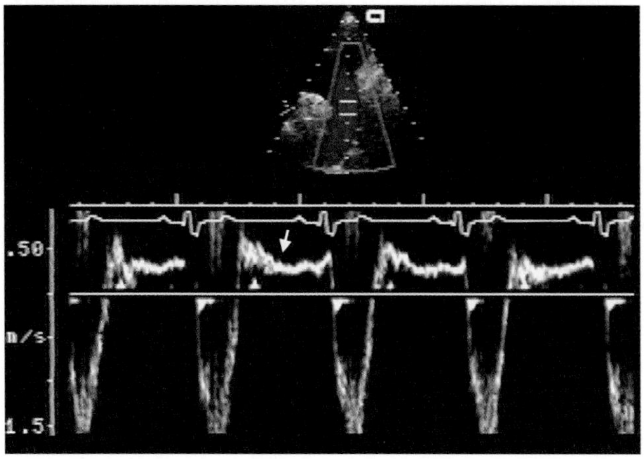

FIGURE 11-27 Recording of pulsed-wave Doppler in the high descending aorta in a patient with severe aortic regurgitation. Note a holodiastolic reversal of flow with high velocity (*arrow*) during diastole.

similarly to MR is consistent with severe regurgitation, smaller ERO (≥ 30 mm^2) than in MR is consistent with severe AR because the longer diastolic than systolic time allows larger volume overload for smaller orifice size.[8] Quantitative methods are not as consistently applicable in AR than in MR, but have relatively few limitations and should be used in clinical practice similarly to MR.[113]

- *Intraoperative assessment.* Pre-bypass, IO-TEE verifies the aortic valve lesions and the extent of aortic aneurysmal dilatation. Aortic valve repair is a safe alternative to valve replacement in selected patients with AR and requires detailed assessment of the AR mechanism.[106] Assessment of the AR mechanism by IO-TEE is accurate and reliable compared with surgical findings. Rarely, IO-TEE notes aortic dissection or wall hematoma not previously diagnosed, and IO-TEE can assist in identifying patients likely to benefit from aortic valve repair.[114] AR quantitation is challenging by TEE, and although deep transgastric views may show the AR flow convergence, imaging is usually poor using this view. A broad jet width on color-flow in central AR is suggestive of severe regurgitation but a simple and more reliable method is measurement of the vena contracta width by TEE, a surrogate measure of the ERO.[115] Vena contracta assessment by TEE is feasible and has been validated for AR.

  Post-bypass IO-TEE verifies the functional result anatomically and for residual AR. This early assessment is important because aortic valve repair is a technique in progress, and results that appear mediocre should lead to consideration of a second pump run. Mismatch is unusual after valve replacement for AR because the annulus is generally dilated with AR and often allows insertion of a sufficiently sized prosthesis. Residual periprosthetic regurgitation is a notable problem in patients with endocarditis, particularly when recent, and these patients should be actively evaluated with appropriate loading conditions.
- *Postoperative assessment* focuses on prosthetic or repair function. In patients with allograft replacement of the aortic valve and homograft replacement of the pulmonary valve, calcification of the pulmonary homograft may develop and requires a systematic examination of the pulmonary outflow tract. Valve repair failure most often involves recurrent prolapse, and timely diagnosis requires regular echo follow-up.[106,116] Patients with AR are younger than those with AS, and bioprosthetic or homograft aortic valve replacement are associated with notable rates of primary failure depending on age. In patients with dystrophic aortic valves, late aortic dissection may develop and requires careful examination of the aorta and progressive aortic dilatation should lead to consider TEE or computed tomography. LV function is of particular concern if patients were operated with EF less than 50%.[108] In general, because of the high preoperative wall stress, aortic valve replacement is associated with improvement in LV function, but the effect is usually modest and the need for vasoactive treatment aimed at improving LV function and clinical outcome should be assessed postoperatively.

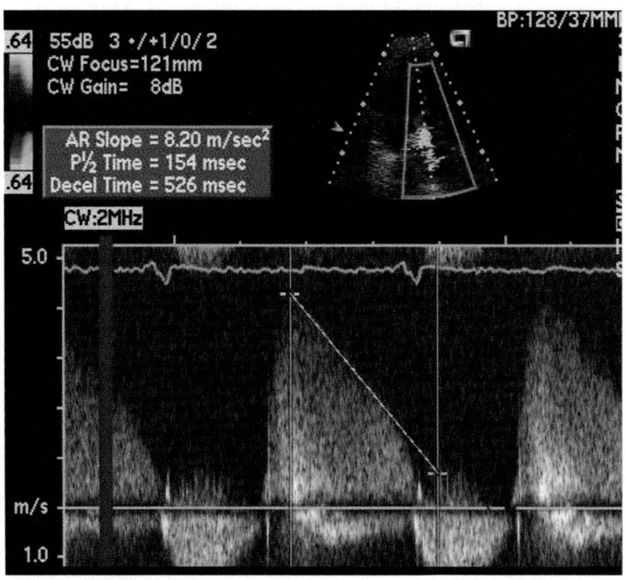

FIGURE 11-28 Continuous wave Doppler recording in a patient with endocarditic aortic regurgitation (AR). The rapid deceleration of AR velocity in diastole is quite different from that noted in Fig. 11-25 and is consistent with acute and severe AR revealing low end-diastolic gradient between the low aortic diastolic pressure and the high left ventricular end-diastolic pressure. The pressure half-time of 154 ms is shorter than the 200 threshold for severe AR.

Mixed Aortic Valve Disease. Mixed aortic valve disease is often rheumatic or associated with aortic valve calcifications precluding valve repair. The essential step in preoperative evaluation is severity assessment of the valve disease. A composite of moderate AS (with valve area >1.0 cm^2) and moderate AR (with regurgitant volume <60 mL) may represent severe valve disease and is diagnosed by a higher mean gradient than the AS severity would justify. IO-TEE and postoperative monitoring are similar to those of AS and AR.

Tricuspid Valve Diseases. Tricuspid valve diseases are dominated by functional tricuspid regurgitation. However, the numerous etiologies that may result in notable tricuspid disease and the frequency with which these lesions may be ignored are salient issues.

Tricuspid Valve Stenosis. Tricuspid valve stenosis is mostly rheumatic, associated with mitral stenosis, and rarely pure. It is difficult to diagnose as there are no absolute morphologic criteria. The essential diagnostic step is to perform a continuous wave Doppler examination of the tricuspid valve when the morphology is unusual. Mean gradients greater than or equal to 5 mm Hg are significant for the tricuspid valve, and the degree of inferior vena cava dilatation reflects the hemodynamic consequences of the stenosis. IO-TEE can also examine the obstruction of tricuspid valve if the preoperative hemodynamic assessment was insufficient. Tricuspid valve replacement is usually required and postoperative echo focuses on the appropriate function of the prosthesis. Other causes of organic tricuspid valve disease, such as carcinoid heart disease, produce in general mixed tricuspid valve disease with dominant regurgitation.

Tricuspid Valve Regurgitation.

- *Preoperative assessment.* Tricuspid regurgitation (TR) is called functional when the valve is structurally normal and regurgitation ensues from incomplete coaptation. Functional TR is the usual consequence of right ventricular dilatation owing to pulmonary hypertension of left-sided heart disease or pulmonary disease, but can also be caused by primary right ventricular dysfunction or primary atrial and annular dilatation seen in chronic atrial fibrillation. Organic causes of TR include myxomatous valve degeneration with or without ruptured chordae.[117] TR caused by excessive valve movement can also result from endocarditis with destructive lesions, blunt chest trauma with chordal or papillary muscle rupture, and iatrogenic trauma postmyocardial biopsy. Echocardiography establishes the mechanism more definitely than the etiology of these types of TRs, but is essential in planning valve repair, which is often highly successful.[117] Organic TR with restricted valve motion includes serotoninergic lesions such as carcinoid heart disease, diet drug valve diseases, ergot valve disease, postradiation valve disease rarely, or more frequently leaflet impingement (or perforation) by pacemaker or defibrillator leads.[118] The degree of valve thickening or rigidity is an essential guide in predicting repair versus replacement. Congenital causes such as Ebstein's anomaly are uncommonly diagnosed in adulthood but may cause severe TR and may be easily missed by a cursory echocardiography.

  There is growing appreciation of tricuspid valve regurgitation as an independent predictor of long-term outcome irrespective of the original cause of this heterogeneous valve disease.[117,119] The important consequence of this recognition is that surgery for isolated TR is more common, that in left-sided valve disease the coexistence of TR should not be ignored because simultaneous correction is often required and that high-quality echocardiographic assessment of TR severity is warranted as the clinical signs of TR are often ignored. Assessment of TR severity uses mainly: (1) The size of the jet in the right atrium (larger is more severe), but with the usual limitation of jets (underestimated with eccentricity and overestimated with high ventricular pressure); (2) vena contracta width greater than or equal to 7 mm as a sign of severe TR,[120] useful but limited by lateral resolution issues; (3) the presence of systolic flow reversal in hepatic veins, specific for severe TR but not sensitive; and (4) quantitation of TR by the PISA method.[121,122] For TR quantitation, as right- versus left-sided circulatory system is a lower pressure system, thresholds for severe TR compared with MR are similar for ERO ($\geq$0.40 cm^2), but lower for regurgitant volume ($\geq$45 mL/beat).[122] Severe TR can lead to right-sided volume overload with right ventricular and right atrial enlargement, and right ventricular systolic dysfunction.[117] There are no quantitative criteria to assess these changes yet, but qualitative assessment provides useful information. With right ventricular volume overload, the septum may display paradoxic motion and affect LV function and ultimately exercise capacity. With advanced cases, inferior vena cava and hepatic veins dilatation reflect elevated right atrial pressure.
- *Intraoperative assessment.* TR is often overlooked and should be assessed without sedation in the outpatient setting.[123] IO-TEE before initiation of bypass requires restoration of preload conditions to assess TR. Quantitative assessment of TR by TEE has limitations and cannot replace preoperative assessment. Annular enlargement is important to assess because it is associated with recurrence of TR,[124] or even development of severe TR in patients with no or mild TR preoperatively.[124] Annulus diameter greater than 70 mm has been considered as markedly enlarged,[124] but there is no consensus on specific annular diameters (absolute or adjusted for body size) that should indicate tricuspid repair. After bypass it is important to assess residual TR, although its absence is not invariably synonymous with operative success. Persistent right ventricular enlargement and dysfunction tend to improve later. IO-TEE in patients in whom tricuspid surgery is considered results in alteration of surgical plan in approximately 10% of cases. Rarely is surgery converted to tricuspid replacement as is considered a predictor of worse survival.
- *Postoperative assessment* focuses mostly on relatively frequent recurrent TR. TR recurrence depends on surgical techniques used, such as lack of ring annuloplasty,[125] lesions (leaflet tethering or thickening),[126] severe TR at baseline,[125,126] IO residual TR, and persistence of pulmonary hypertension of left-sided disease. Right ventricular enlargement and dysfunction improve but often incompletely, particularly if pressure or volume overload persists.

Pulmonary Valve Diseases. Pulmonary valve diseases are mostly congenital but can also be acquired, owing to carcinoid heart disease (now exceptionally rheumatic heart disease) and endocarditis.

- *Preoperative assessment* requires the proactive examination of the pulmonary valve as the usual examination tends to record few views of the valve and TEE may be particularly helpful. Knowledge of a disease susceptible to affect the pulmonary valve is essential in focusing attention to this valve.[127] The valve morphology is difficult to analyze and requires unusual views, elongating the subvalvular, valvular, and supravalvular region. Thickening can be observed and more rarely prolapse, retraction, or vegetation. Morphologically, pulmonary annulus can be constricted in carcinoid disease in association to intrinsic valve thickening.[128] Dilatation of pulmonary artery is important to assess and may require TEE. Hemodynamic assessment is somewhat simpler. Continuous wave Doppler assesses appropriately pulmonary stenosis. Mild pulmonary regurgitation is frequent in normal individuals. Severe pulmonary regurgitation is rare, detected by color Doppler, but ascertaining severe regurgitation is difficult because the jet may be of limited extent and duration owing to equalization of pulmonary and right ventricular pressure. In such cases, rapid deceleration of regurgitant jet is suggestive of severe regurgitation.

- *IO assessment.* As pulmonary stenosis is most usually treated by balloon valvuloplasty, operative treatment is reserved for regurgitant or mixed lesions. Measurement of pulmonary annulus and assessment of subvalvular or supravalvular stenosis is important to operative management. Postoperative assessment of pulmonary regurgitation intends to avoid more than moderate residual regurgitation but is more difficult than outpatient evaluation as restoration of normal hemodynamic condition is inconsistent. Careful examination of color and continuous wave Doppler is important in that regard.
- *Postoperative assessment* focuses on assessing function of native repaired or prosthetic pulmonary valve. Degeneration, stenosis, and regurgitation may develop over time and should be diagnosed early with a combination of color and continuous wave Doppler. Right ventricular dilatation and dysfunction may persist after surgery or recur with dysfunction of the treated pulmonary valve.[129]

Bacterial Endocarditis

The incidence of bacterial endocarditis has remained unchanged despite the decline in rheumatic valve disease, and effective antibiotics continue to carry considerable mortality and morbidity. As the risk associated with endocarditis drops precipitously with therapy, prompt diagnosis and treatment are essential to improve diagnosis.

- *Preoperative assessment* is centered on diagnosis and assessment of complications. Echocardiography aids in the rapid diagnosis of endocarditis provides one of two major Duke diagnostic criteria by demonstrating presence of typical vegetations.[130] Less typical but suspicious lesions represent a minor diagnostic criterion. Vegetations vary in size or shape and are mobile masses attached to endocardium or implanted material and frequently showing high-frequency oscillations. Vegetations are made of fibrin and are of low density when recent, but there are no definitive criteria to differentiate them from thrombi, particularly on foreign material, or from Lamb's excrescences when small.[131] Therefore, diagnosis of vegetation implies contextual interpretation. TEE is superior to TTE in detecting vegetations (sensitivity 95% versus 65 to 80%, respectively), especially in prosthetic valve endocarditis, in which TTE may miss vegetations because of shadowing. Right-sided vegetations are usually bigger than left-sided and TEE does not improve diagnostic accuracy.

  Apart from diagnosis, TTE and TEE evaluate the presence and severity of endocarditic lesions. Endocarditis is destructive to valves and cardiac tissue, and may lead to abscess formation. Valve lesions are perforations or ruptures of supportive structures. Perforations are voids that are often difficult to visualize directly by TTE or TEE, but color observation of regurgitating flow with flow convergence in the center of a valve leaflet is strongly supportive of a perforation.[58] Ruptures of chordae have nonspecific features unless a vegetation is attached to their tip. Aortic valve prolapse may result from destruction of the central coaptation zone or supporting commissural area. Abscesses may involve any region of the myocardium, but often involve the fibrosa between mitral and aortic annulus. Expansion of annular abscesses may lead to conduction abnormalities or cavity (aneurysm) formation when the abscess ruptures in a cardiac cavity, most often the LV, with sometimes secondary rupture and fistula formation. These complex lesions are better identified by TEE than TTE.[132] Of note, abscess cavities are rarely seen around the mitral and tricuspid annuli and abscesses are more prone to be present in patients with prosthetic valve endocarditis. Nevertheless, in all cases of endocarditis comprehensive assessment of all possible abscesses and fistulous tracts is indispensable. Assessment of severity of valve lesions is particularly difficult, because regurgitations resulting from destructive valve lesions form and progress acutely by sudden tissue loss. Thus, clinical signs of regurgitation, particularly murmur intensity and color flow jets, may not be impressive because of rapid equalization of pressure (eg, in acute endocarditic AR, LV diastolic pressure is markedly elevated and early in diastole equalizes the aortic pressure so that murmur and jet are brief and of low energy). This acuteness makes quantitation of regurgitation, particularly measure of effective regurgitant orifice, essential in assessing regurgitation severity.[8] Also heart failure may rapidly progress because of valve regurgitation, particularly in patients with acute endocarditic AR, and surgery may be urgently indicated. In patients with MR or TR, heart failure may be controllable with medical treatment and may offer some opportunity for sufficient antibiotic therapy.[133] Nevertheless, even in clinically stable endocarditis it is essential to monitor lesions and valvular regurgitation severity by regular echocardiography. Rarely, vegetations can be complicated by accumulation and valvular obstruction, and more frequently by embolism. Characteristics of vegetations, such as size (>10 mm) and marked mobility, are predictors of the risk of embolism,[134] which led to the controversy regarding intervention for ablation of vegetations. Although this controversy is unresolved, the precipitous decline in vegetation size with antibiotic treatment and the risk of embolism associated with surgery should be taken into account in this discussion.[134] Over time endocarditic lesions become chronic and vegetations heal, leaving fibrotic lesions offering more solid suturing possibilities.

- *Intraoperative assessment* confirms the lesions, assesses the possibility of silent progression and an unexpected abscess cavity or fistulous tract, and reassesses regurgitations that may have appeared moderate on preoperative assessment. Careful examination is particularly important in moderate lesions that may require interventional treatment simultaneously with severe lesions.

  Post-bypass, it is essential to examine the surgical correction of complex abscesses and fistulous tracts. Also, examination of all reparative procedures and seating of prosthetic valves is particularly important, because recently infected valvular and annular tissue may not offer a solid basis for suturing.
- *Postoperative assessment* usually demonstrates that acute LV dysfunction is reversible. Recurrence of endocarditis is rare with appropriate antibiotic treatment, and development of echocardiographic signs may be delayed, in contrast to fever and positive blood cultures. A possible complication is the occurrence of aseptic perivalvular regurgitation developing with some delay after the intervention. Low-intensity murmurs may contrast with symptoms, and early detection is paramount by systematic TTE and sometimes TEE in order to provide appropriate care. Repeated prosthetic dehiscence owing to tissue friability is not uncommon and makes such situations difficult to manage.

Prosthetic Valves

Prosthetic valves require specific approaches, and comparison with early postoperative assessment is essential to detect dysfunction.

Echocardiography of Prosthetic Valves. Although valve repair is generally preferred, valve replacement remains the leading way to correct severe valvular disease. Echocardiography is currently the best approach to evaluate prosthetic valves, but has limitations for appropriate interpretation. All prostheses are responsible for acoustic shadowing behind them, so examination of all aspects of a prosthesis often requires both TTE and TEE. Morphologically, specific characteristics influence the imaging of mechanical prostheses. For example, in a ball-cage prosthesis, the ball transmits ultrasound slower than blood, so its distal limit appears beyond the prosthetic seating. In bileaflet prostheses, leaflets may be placed with an angle to the thoracic wall, thereby preventing visualization. Struts of bioprostheses may prevent imaging of leaflets. With Doppler, the presence of a restrictive orifice may create pressure recovery, so gradients may be somewhat overestimated, particularly with small aortas. In prostheses that have no clinical signs of dysfunction, it is important to obtain early and serial hemodynamic assessment to serving as a reference if the clinical issue of dysfunction arises. Each prosthesis is characterized by its gradient, effective orifice area, and physiologic regurgitation. The gradient is measured by continuous wave Doppler, from apical views for mitral and tricuspid prostheses and multiple views for aortic prostheses. Mean and peak gradient are measured using the same $4V^2$ formula used in native valves. Each type and size of prosthesis has a range of expected gradient that should be used as a guide to assessment of normal function. Effective orifice area (EOA) is measurable for aortic prostheses, similarly to the valve area of AS, as the ratio of stroke volume (LV outflow tract) to time velocity integral of prosthetic jet velocity. For mitral and tricuspid prostheses measuring orifice area relies on aortic stroke volume, which is not adequate if AR or prosthetic regurgitation is present. Lack of mitral or tricuspid prosthetic stenosis beyond the normal range is defined by a rapidly declining velocity (and gradient) in early diastole. Physiologic regurgitation of prostheses is common and constant in appearance in mechanical prostheses but rare in bioprostheses. It is readily visible for aortic prostheses, but more difficult to detect with TTE for mitral or tricuspid prostheses because of prosthetic shadowing, and may be only observable by color with TEE. However, physiologic regurgitation is detectable by continuous wave Doppler and is usually brief, faint, and central. TEE is not necessary in normally functioning prostheses clinically and by TTE unless other lesions (eg, aortic dilatation or aneurysm) are suspected.

Mechanical Prosthesis Dysfunction. There is no primary failure of mechanical prostheses components because the ball variance of Starr-Edwards prostheses and strut ruptures of Bjork-Shiley prostheses have been eliminated. The mechanism of failure of mechanical prostheses is rarely by tissue interposition or more frequently by obstruction owing to thrombosis or its chronic equivalent, pannus formation, or periprosthetic regurgitation. Tissue interposition is usually detected early and characterized mostly by regurgitation because of lack of closure of the mobile element, but can have a component of stenosis. Incomplete movement of the mobile element can be detected by TTE, TEE, or fluoroscopy with angle of movement measurement. Hemodynamic dysfunction is detected by Doppler. Increased flow velocities beyond normal range (and beyond previous measurement) suggest increased pressure gradients and prosthetic obstruction. However, with increased flow (pregnancy, anemia, hyperthyroidism, sepsis) gradients may increase so that stenosis should be characterized if possible by measuring the effective orifice area using continuity equations.[135] A ratio of valvular to subvalvular velocity greater than or equal to 3 suggests aortic prosthesis stenosis, whereas a slow decline in diastolic velocity suggests mitral or tricuspid prosthesis stenosis.[136] A stenotic prosthesis should rule out patient–prosthesis mismatch by confrontation with prosthetic size and previous measurements.[101] Sudden obstruction suggests acute thrombosis, whereas progressive obstruction suggests pannus formation, but the mechanism of obstruction is rarely directly defined by echocardiography, although a thrombus may be seen by TEE in acute thrombosis. Thrombus size affects the potential efficacy of thrombolysis.[137] If thrombolysis is elected as a treatment because the prosthesis is in a tricuspid location or reoperation is high risk, monitoring of the prolonged thrombolysis administration requires daily echocardiography with subsequent frequent measurements because recurrence is common, affecting approximately half of successfully treated patients.[138] Pannus obstruction is organized and not affected by thrombolysis.[102] Postoperatively recurrence of prosthetic thrombosis should be monitored by Doppler. If large enough, periprosthetic regurgitation is usually associated with hemolysis and heart failure or progression of symptoms, but inconsistently with a murmur.

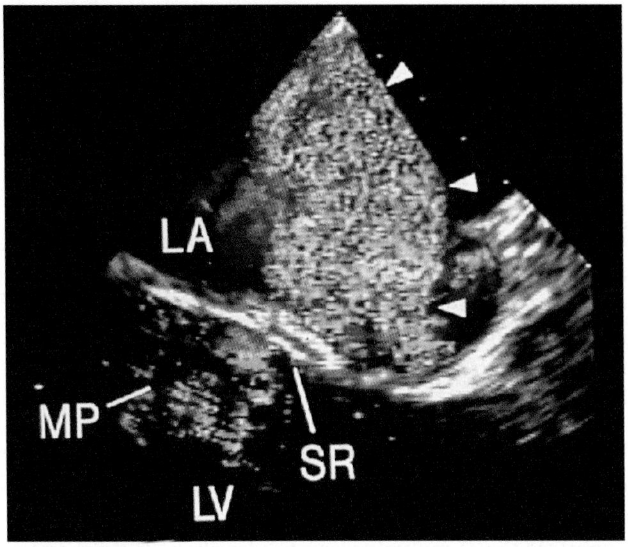

FIGURE 11-29 Transesophageal imaging of severe periprosthetic regurgitation (*arrowheads*) around the sewing ring (SR) of a mitral prosthesis (MP). LA = Left atrium; LV = left ventricle.

TTE detects easily the regurgitant jet on aortic prostheses and jet origin determination requires complete prosthesis scanning to observe periannular flow (Fig. 11-29). Shadowing often prevents TTE from recording the color jet for mitral and tricuspid prostheses, but detection of periprosthetic regurgitation is possible by continuous wave Doppler, leading to TEE for assessing regurgitation severity (Fig. 11-30).

Biological Prosthesis Dysfunction. Although thrombus (exceedingly rare) and periprosthetic regurgitation (rare) may occur on bioprostheses, primary tissue failure is the most frequent failure mode.[139] The specific mechanism can be early, because of tears, which are often close to struts, or late, because of calcification or rupture of cups. The diagnosis of valve stenosis caused by calcification is based on standard Doppler criteria of excessive gradient, decreased effective orifice area, persistence of end-diastolic high velocity in mitral and tricuspid prostheses, and direct visualization of calcifications by TTE or TEE if necessary. The diagnosis of tissue failure with regurgitation is suspected by murmur and confirmed by color imaging, but severity is often difficult to confirm because of eccentric jets (even by TEE). In this circumstance, observations of a severe lesion such as a torn cusp and a large flow convergence proximal to the intraprosthetic regurgitant orifice are important clues to a severe regurgitation. With primary tissue failure it is important to exclude prosthetic endocarditis by blood cultures and searching for vegetations by TEE.

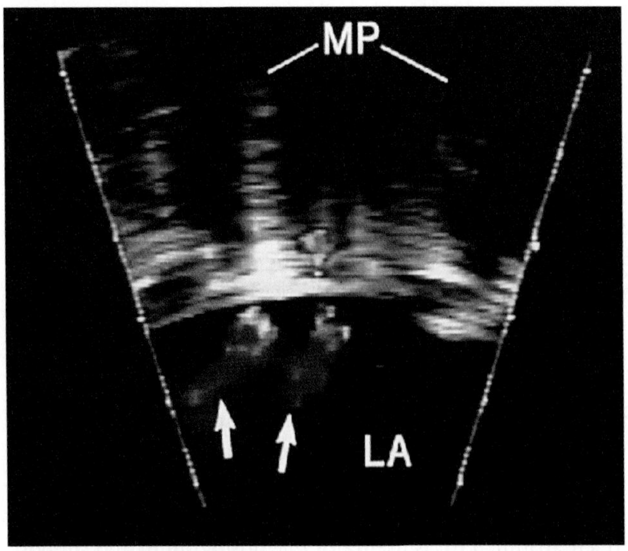

FIGURE 11-30 Physiologic regurgitation (*arrows*) on a St. Jude mitral prosthesis (MP).

Coronary Diseases

Coronary artery disease is the most frequent indication for cardiac surgery. Echocardiography does not allow direct observation of coronary lesions unless intravascular ultrasound is used for proximal coronary segments, but observes consequences of coronary disease. Echocardiography is pivotal to suspect coronary disease on the basis of stress-induced ischemia, assess myocardial viability, and diagnose myocardial infarction and its complications requiring surgical intervention.[13]

Diagnosis of Coronary Diseases

Echocardiography uses multiple tomographic planes to assess regional wall motion.[13] The American Society of Echocardiography recommends 16-segment analysis of LV for regional wall motion evaluation. Wall thickness increase in systole greater than or equal to 40% characterizes normal LV contractility, whereas reduced contractility (hypokinetic) is less than 30% and absent (akinetic) is less than 10%. Myocardial segment outward motion during systole (dyskinesis) is usually associated with thinning, whereas aneurysm is permanent wall outward bulging with or without dyskinesis. LV segments are scored from 1 to 5—with 1, normal; 2, hypokinetic; 3, akinetic; 4, dyskinetic; 5, aneurysmal—and the wall motion score index is the sum of scores divided by the number of segments visualized.[13] A wall motion score index of 1 is normal and greater than or equal to 2 is associated with poor outcome after myocardial infarction. Resting scar (wall akinetic, dyskinetic, or aneurysmal and dense with thinning) is a resting abnormality diagnostic of myocardial infarction and coronary disease (wall motion abnormalities without scar are seen in cardiomyopathies). Stress echo can identify coronary disease by inducing new regional wall motion abnormalities.[14] There are many stress modalities, including exercise treadmill or bicycle, pharmacologic with dobutamine, adenosine, or dipyridamole, and rarely TEE atrial pacing.[140] Pharmacologic or pacing stress testing is reserved for patients who are unable to exercise enough to reach maximum effort. With stress, normal LV response is hyperdynamic with increased ejection fraction and decreased LV end-systolic dimension. Resting regional wall motion abnormalities unchanged with stress are consistent with coronary disease (previous myocardial infarction) but without ischemia. Increased LV end-systolic dimension or decreased ejection fraction with stress suggest severe coronary artery disease. The diagnostic value of stress echo is imperfect, with acceptable sensitivity but mediocre specificity similar to other stress modalities. The indication of stress echo for diagnosing coronary disease should be weighed according to the pretest probability of disease and is most contributive in the intermediate probability range. The prognostic value of stress echo is considerable in patients presenting with chest pain, justifying its widespread use.[141] In evaluating chest pain, echo may reveal resting regional wall motion abnormalities consistent with acute coronary syndrome, but is usually associated with a good prognosis if normal. Stress echo is safe in patients with no sign of myocardial infarction or ischemia and normal baseline echo. In overt acute coronary syndromes, a wall motion score index greater than or equal to 1.7 suggests a large area at risk. Postoperatively, stress echo is most useful when chest pain is moderate or atypical to weigh the indication of repeat coronary angiogram. The localizing value of regional abnormalities for a specific coronary bed is mediocre and cannot imply that a specific graft may be dysfunctioning.

Myocardial Viability

Myocardial contraction declines when greater than or equal to 20% of myocardial wall is ischemic or infracted. Resting hypokinesis or akinesis does not rule out viability (myocardial hibernation) and may improve with revascularization. Dobutamine stress echo is the preferred stress method to assess viability in patients with LV dysfunction (with or without regional abnormalities).[142] With increasing infusion rates of dobutamine, initial improved contractility of an akinetic segment at low dose suggests viability, and worsening with higher doses (biphasic response) suggests ischemia. This biphasic pattern suggests viable myocardium and improvement potential with revascularization. Functional recovery after revascularization is frequent when sustained improvement with dobutamine (monophasic response) is observed, but is rare with scarred or unresponsive myocardium. Strain rate imaging with low-dose dobutamine may be useful to detect viability.

Complications of Coronary Diseases

Heart failure with cardiogenic shock complicating acute myocardial infarction is the leading cause of hospital death caused by myocardial infarction and may be caused by various mechanisms demanding specific interventions. Echocardiography identifies mechanisms of circulatory failure and also high-risk patients with LV dysfunction, particularly with markedly reduced ejection fraction or MR greater than or equal to moderate.[143]

Free Wall Rupture. Free wall rupture is an important cause of death. There are no predictive echocardiographic features defining a high risk of rupture, but echocardiography provides early and rapid diagnosis in patients with this fatal complication. In hemodynamically unstable patients, free wall rupture should be suspected with pericardial effusion, particularly a gelatinous-appearing pericardial clot and with thin-walled myocardium.[144] An incomplete free wall rupture results in a "subepicardial aneurysm" contained by the epicardial layer. The pericardial effusion, even if compressive and with signs of tamponade, should not be taped for evacuation because this may precipitate catastrophic rupture, but minimal echo-guided tap to confirm blood presence may help the surgical decision. Rarely, color Doppler detects flow in the pericardial cavity, but absence of such flow does not rule out rupture. Intramyocardial hematoma is consistent with impending rupture. A pseudoaneurysm is a contained rupture bordered by an organized clot, and is diagnosed on the basis of a narrow neck with to and fro flow and carries a considerable risk of delayed rupture. Detection of early free wall rupture allows surgical repair. Postoperatively, as the infarct is often limited in size, excellent long-term result can be obtained.

Ventricular Septal Rupture. Ventricular septal rupture complicating myocardial infarction occurs in the first weeks of infarction. Echo shows the ventricular septal defect, but it is important to use multiple views to identify it, as those associated with inferior infarction may be elusive. The defect borders are ragged, different from those of congenital defect and fall of myocardial eschars tend to increase the defect size progressively. Color Doppler is critical to diagnosis by demonstrating directly left-to-right shunt at the ventricular level, and TEE is rarely needed. Surgery is preferable before hemodynamic compromise is intractable but shunt may recur postsurgery because of progressive septal necrosis, which should be monitored. Closure by endovascular devices is possible but entails the possibility of a recurrent shunt postprocedure.

Papillary Muscle Rupture. MR associated with acute myocardial infarction may be functional or organic because of papillary muscle rupture, but both are often silent, so MR is frequently revealed by echo, which is indicated by hemodynamic compromise or pulmonary edema. Rupture of papillary muscle may be incomplete (one head partially separated but remaining attached to papillary muscle) or complete (head detachment from papillary muscle resulting in a flail leaflet). The morphologic abnormality is diagnosed by TTE, but TEE may be necessary.[145] Color flow imaging detects MR, but may underestimate MR because of rapid and severe increase in LA pressure. Confirmation by echo of papillary muscle rupture leads to prompt surgical correction. Repair is often feasible with IO-TEE monitoring and MR rarely recurs postoperatively.

Right Ventricular Myocardial Infarction. Right ventricular myocardial infarction is typically associated with an inferior infarct, but rarely is isolated. Patients present with elevated jugular venous pressure contrasting with clear lungs, or may present with hypotension or shock. TTE provides rapid diagnosis, showing an enlarged and hypokinetic right ventricle, commonly associated with LV inferior wall motion abnormalities. Color Doppler reveals TR with normal pulmonary pressure and low peak velocity. High right atrial pressure may lead to right-to-left shunting via a patent foramen ovale, clinically manifest as hypoxemia and diagnosed by agitated saline contrast injection showing the shunt as contrast passing from right to left atrium. TEE is useful for diagnosing shunt and supporting closure of patent foramen ovale percutaneously and resulting in marked clinical improvement. The right ventricular function almost universally improves over time, but residual TR may be observed and may require surgical correction.

Pericardial, Endocardial, and Myocardial Diseases

Pericardial effusion was the first clinical application of echocardiography and remains, with other pericardial diseases, one of the most important indications of the test.

Pericardial Effusion

Pericardial effusion is an echo-free space around the heart after anatomical landmarks of the pericardium, covering both ventricles and most of the right atrium, whereas a small portion of the LA wall is surrounded by pericardium. Pericardial effusion should be differentiated from left pleural effusion, an echo-free space extending posteriorly to the descending aorta and from increased pericardial fat content, of typical granular appearance that does not deserve medical attention. Pericardial effusion is often compressive if large (with a swinging heart within the effusion), but tamponade may occur in small acute effusions. Diagnosis of tamponade relies on inferior vena cava dilatation, invagination of right atrial wall in diastole, expiratory collapse of right ventricle, and marked respiratory variability (of opposite timing) of mitral and tricuspid inflows.[146] Although classically large effusions required surgical drainage, an echo-directed pericardial tap with prolonged catheter drainage is now the mainstay and is particularly useful in postoperative effusions. Approaches are most often para-apical and rarely subcostal. Effusions of aortic dissection or myocardial infarction should not be drained percutaneously because full rupture may ensue. Other indications of surgical drainage are purulent effusions, pericardial thrombi, and loculated effusions that cannot be safely reached. Postoperatively echo monitors recurrence of effusions and possible occurrence of constriction.[147]

Pericardial Constriction

These can occur while fluid remains in the pericardium, but are mostly caused by a thickened rigid pericardium.[148] Classical tuberculosis pericarditis is now rare and most constrictive pericarditis is idiopathic, postoperative, and rarely results from hemopericardium, purulent pericarditis, radiation, or inflammatory disease of the pericardium. The diagnosis should be suspected when heart failure with dilatation of inferior vena cava is associated with normal LV function. Echo-Doppler signs specific of pericardial constriction are increased pericardial thickness (which is difficult to measure), ventricular interaction indicating fixed intrapericardial space diagnosed by leftward septal shift, decreased mitral inflow and pulmonary venous flow, and increased tricuspid inflow during inspiration, atrial interaction with diastolic hepatic venous flow reversal with expiration,[149] and isolation from thoracic pressure changes with stable superior vena caval flow with respiration. Pericardial constriction should be differentiated from restrictive cardiomyopathy, which is not associated with ventricular interaction and displays reduced myocardial velocity by tissue Doppler (which is normal in pericardial constriction). Pericardial constriction and chronic obstructive pulmonary disease share the respiratory variation of flow, but subtle differences allow diagnosis. Thus, Doppler is the mainstay of preoperative diagnosis of constriction. IO-TEE shows the thickened pericardium and monitors the sudden hemodynamic changes post-pericardectomy. Postoperatively echo monitors the persistence of constrictive signs that may result from severe epicarditis or insufficient pericardectomy.

Endomyocardial Fibrosis

Endomyocardial fibrosis starts as endomyocarditis with thrombosis, which becomes organized and fibrotic, resulting in elevated filling pressures. Images show the apical obliterative thrombosis early, which invades the region below the posterior mitral leaflet and encases it. Eosinophilia is generally observed. Fibrosis ensues and results in mitral and tricuspid regurgitation. IO-TEE allows monitoring of potential aggravation of valve regurgitations during endomyocardectomy. Postoperative persistence of signs of elevated pressures is common.

Cardiomyopathies

Cardiomyopathies are usually easily diagnosed when presenting with congestion owing to LV dysfunction. Regional wall motion abnormalities may be present and are not synonymous with coronary diseases. It is not possible to rule out myocarditis by echo. IO-TEE during cardiac transplantation excludes dysfunction of the donor heart and monitors tolerance of frequent residual pulmonary hypertension. Posttransplantation assessment notes atrial enlargement, a feature of the atrial connection, with dual atrial activity. Over time, myocardial biopsy may result in severing of tricuspid chordae and flail tricuspid valve and require tricuspid repair. Restrictive cardiomyopathy is exemplified by amyloidosis, which characteristically displays wall thickening of LV and RV, mild valvular regurgitation, pericardial effusion, and restrictive LV filling. Occurrence of LV systolic dysfunction or irreversible diastolic dysfunction is associated with poor prognosis. Rarely these patients undergo cardiac transplantation. Hypertrophic cardiomyopathy may be mostly basal and obstructive. LV outflow tract obstruction results from the characteristic septal bulge with systolic anterior motion of the mitral valve and is diagnosed by late peaking systolic acceleration by Doppler. These patients benefit from myectomy guided by measures of depth and thickness of the septal bulge to be removed by IO-TEE.[150] Elimination of the obstruction and MR are the IO measures of success as well as absence of iatrogenic ventricular septal defect. Midventricular and apical hypertrophic cardiomyopathy can be easily missed and have complex intracardiac flows but rarely require surgery.

Diseases of the Aorta

The entire thoracic aorta can be visualized by combined TTE and TEE,[151] but TEE provides complete and detailed imaging of the aorta and should be preferred if a disease of the aorta is suspected.

Aortic Dissection

Aortic dissection can be diagnosed by TTE, despite limited view, which may be sufficient to direct patients to the operating room where TEE is performed, but TEE should be performed when the diagnosis is uncertain. TTE has limited sensitivity (79%) compared with TEE (99%) in diagnosing aortic dissection, and a negative TTE should be followed by TEE when aortic dissection is suspected.[152] Aortic dissection is seen as an undulating intimal flap and should be distinguished from artifacts often seen in the aorta, particularly using color flow imaging. Proximally, the extent of the dissection, dislocation of the Valsalva sinuses intima, prolapse or aortic cusp, and presence and severity of AR should be defined, but should not delay surgery in type A dissection. Involvement of coronary ostia (particularly right) may cause myocardial infarction but is not easily defined, even by TEE. Pericardial effusion may cause tamponade, is particularly concerning for imminent aortic rupture and should lead to prompt surgery. IO-TEE helps define extent of residual dissection of thoracic aorta and presence of pleural effusion. Postoperatively, TEE evaluates residual AR if the aortic valve has been preserved, and LV function if myocardial infarction is suspected and there is progression of residual aortic dissection.

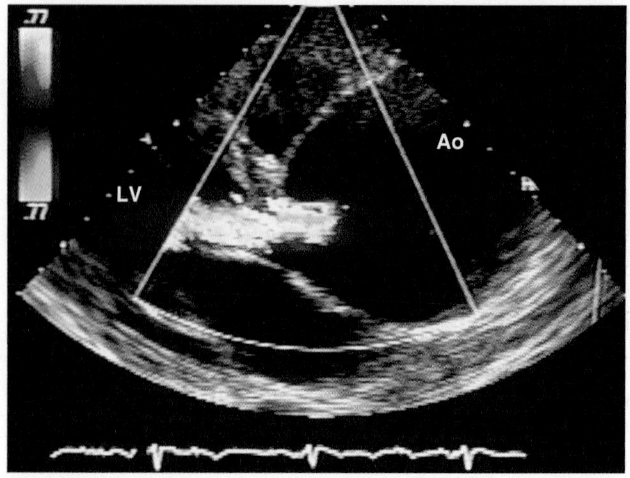

FIGURE 11-31 Annulo-aortic ectasia associated with aortic regurgitation diagnosed by transthoracic echocardiography. Ao = Aorta; LV = left ventricle.

Aortic Hematoma and Rupture

Intramural hematoma precedes aortic dissection in 15 to 20% of cases.[151,153] It results from blood collection between intima and adventitia and appears as increased echo density along the aortic wall visible by TEE but usually not by TTE. Aortic perforation can be caused by aortic ulcers complicating atherosclerosis. Diagnosis is raised in older patients with upper chest (and back) pain but is difficult even using TEE. Aortic rupture complicates deceleration injury and can be diagnosed by TEE. Despite the trauma, TEE is feasible in most patients, rarely complicated, and sensitive to detect isthmic rupture. Pseudoaneurysm resulting from containment of rupture by surrounding tissue can be differentiated from true aneurysm by sharply demarcated rupture site and narrow communication between aorta and pseudoaneurysm.

Aortic Aneurysms

Aortic aneurysms are visualized and measurable by TTE and TEE, but complete extent is determined better by TEE (Fig. 11-31). Rupture rates increase with aneurysm size, considerable if greater than or equal to 6 cm but are also notable between 5.5 and 6 cm. Smaller aneurysms can be followed serially with echo. Patients with Marfan's syndrome and those with bicuspid aortic valve are at risk of aortic dilatation and potentially dissection. Sinus of Valsalva aneurysm is best assessed from parasternal long and short axis views and may cause compression of adjacent structures or may rupture into the cardiac chambers, most commonly the right atrium or right ventricle.[154]

Aortic Atherosclerosis

Aortic atherosclerosis causes plaques and debris within the aorta, particularly in older people. Plaques of higher thickness, irregular surface (ulceration), and with mobile components have higher embolic potential.[155] Intraoperatively, the presence of severe aortic plaques is of particular importance when an intra-aortic balloon pump is considered. The role of cholesterol embolism in postoperative strokes and decline in renal function is uncertain.

Aortic Coarctation

Aortic coarctation can be diagnosed by TTE with suprasternal imaging and Doppler gradient measured at rest and with exercise. TEE shows the narrowed descending thoracic aorta and both the frequently associated bicuspid aortic valve. Postoperatively echo follows the residual stenosis and the progression of aortic valve dysfunction and of ascending aortic enlargement.

REFERENCES

1. Tajik AJ, Seward JB, Hagler DJ, Mair DD, Lie JT: Two-dimensional real-time ultrasonic imaging of the heart and great vessels. Technique, image orientation, structure identification, and validation. *Mayo Clin Proc* 1978; 53:271-303.
2. Currie PJ, Seward JB, Chan KL, et al: Continuous wave Doppler determination of right ventricular pressure: a simultaneous Doppler-catheterization study in 127 patients. *J Am Coll Cardiol* 1985; 6: 750-756.
3. Hatle L, Angelsen BA, Tromsdal A: Non-invasive assessment of aortic stenosis by Doppler ultrasound. *Br Heart J* 1980; 43:284-292.
4. Currie PJ, Hagler DJ, Seward JB, et al: Instantaneous pressure gradient: a simultaneous Doppler and dual catheter correlative study. *J Am Coll Cardiol* 1986; 7:800-806.
5. Hatle L, Brubakk A, Tromsdal A, Angelsen B: Noninvasive assessment of pressure drop in mitral stenosis by Doppler ultrasound. *Br Heart J* 1978; 40:131-140.
6. Oh JK, Taliercio CP, Holmes DR Jr, et al: Prediction of the severity of aortic stenosis by Doppler aortic valve area determination: prospective Doppler-catheterization correlation in 100 patients. *J Am Coll Cardiol* 1988; 11:1227-1234.
7. Enriquez-Sarano M, Seward JB, Bailey KR, Tajik AJ: Effective regurgitant orifice area: a noninvasive Doppler development of an old hemodynamic concept. *J Am Coll Cardiol* 1994; 23:443-451.
8. Zoghbi WA, Enriquez-Sarano M, Foster E, et al: Recommendations for evaluation of the severity of native valvular regurgitation with two-dimensional and Doppler echocardiography. *J Am Soc Echocardiogr* 2003; 16:777-802.

9. Lang RM, Bierig M, Devereux RB, et al: Recommendations for chamber quantification: a report from the American Society of Echocardiography's Guidelines and Standards Committee and the Chamber Quantification Writing Group, developed in conjunction with the European Association of Echocardiography, a branch of the European Society of Cardiology. *J Am Soc Echocardiogr* 2005; 18:1440-1463.
10. Thomson HL, Basmadjian AJ, Rainbird AJ, et al: Contrast echocardiography improves the accuracy and reproducibility of left ventricular remodeling measurements: a prospective, randomly assigned, blinded study. *J Am Coll Cardiol* 2001; 38:867-875.
11. Nishimura RA, Tajik AJ: Evaluation of diastolic filling of left ventricle in health and disease: Doppler echocardiography is the clinician's Rosetta Stone. *J Am Coll Cardiol* 1997; 30:8-18.
12. Oh JK, Hatle LK, Seward JB, et al: Diagnostic role of Doppler echocardiography in constrictive pericarditis. *J Am Coll Cardiol* 1994; 23:154-162.
13. Armstrong WF, Pellikka PA, Ryan T, Crouse L, Zoghbi WA: Stress echocardiography: recommendations for performance and interpretation of stress echocardiography. Stress Echocardiography Task Force of the Nomenclature and Standards Committee of the American Society of Echocardiography. *J Am Soc Echocardiogr* 1998; 11:97-104.
14. Pellikka PA: Stress echocardiography in the evaluation of chest pain and accuracy in the diagnosis of coronary artery disease. *Prog Cardiovasc Dis.* 1997; 39:523-532.
15. Lancellotti P, Troisfontaines P, Toussaint AC, Pierard LA : Prognostic importance of exercise-induced changes in mitral regurgitation in patients with chronic ischemic left ventricular dysfunction. *Circulation* 2003; 108:1713-1717.
16. Watanabe N, Ogasawara Y, Yamaura Y, et al: Mitral annulus flattens in ischemic mitral regurgitation: geometric differences between inferior and anterior myocardial infarction: a real-time 3-dimensional echocardiographic study. *Circulation* 2005; 112:I458-462.
17. Tsang TS, Enriquez-Sarano M, Freeman WK, et al: Consecutive 1127 therapeutic echocardiographically guided pericardiocenteses: clinical profile, practice patterns, and outcomes spanning 21 years. *Mayo Clin Proc* 2002; 77:429-436.
18. Daniel WG, Erbel R, Kasper W, et al: Safety of transesophageal echocardiography. A multicenter survey of 10,419 examinations. *Circulation* 1991; 83:817-821.
19. Kallmeyer IJ, Collard CD, Fox JA, Body SC, Shernan SK: The safety of intraoperative transesophageal echocardiography: a case series of 7200 cardiac surgical patients. *Anesth Analg* 2001; 92:1126-1130.
20. Rousou JA, Tighe DA, Garb JL, et al: Risk of dysphagia after transesophageal echocardiography during cardiac operations. *Ann Thorac Surg* 2000; 69:486-489; discussion 489-490.
21. Brinkman WT, Shanewise JS, Clements SD, Mansour KA: Transesophageal echocardiography: not an innocuous procedure. *Ann Thorac Surg* 2001; 72:1725-1726.
22. Zalunardo MP, Bimmler D, Grob UC, et al: Late oesophageal perforation after intraoperative transoesophageal echocardiography. *Br J Anaesth* 2002; 88:595-597.
23. Matsumoto M, Oka Y, Strom J, et al: Application of transesophageal echocardiography to continuous intraoperative monitoring of left ventricular performance. *Am J Cardiol* 1980; 46:95-105.
24. Shanewise JS, Cheung AT, Aronson S, et al: ASE/SCA guidelines for performing a comprehensive intraoperative multiplane transesophageal echocardiography examination: recommendations of the American Society of Echocardiography Council for Intraoperative Echocardiography and the Society of Cardiovascular Anesthesiologists Task Force for Certification in Perioperative Transesophageal Echocardiography. *J Am Soc Echocardiogr* 1999; 12:884-900.
25. Couture P, Denault AY, McKenty S, et al: Impact of routine use of intraoperative transesophageal echocardiography during cardiac surgery. *Can J Anaesth* 2000; 47:20-26.
26. Qaddoura FE, Abel MD, Mecklenburg KL, et al: Role of intraoperative transesophageal echocardiography in patients having coronary artery bypass graft surgery. *Ann Thorac Surg* 2004; 78:1586-1590.
27. Schoenburg M, Kraus B, Muehling A, et al: The dynamic air bubble trap reduces cerebral microembolism during cardiopulmonary bypass. *J Thorac Cardiovasc Surg* 2003; 126:1455-1460.
28. Gold JP, Torres KE, Maldarelli W, et al: Improving outcomes in coronary surgery: the impact of echo-directed aortic cannulation and perioperative hemodynamic management in 500 patients. *Ann Thorac Surg* 2004; 78: 1579-1585.
29. Chaliki HP, Click RL, Abel MD: Comparison of intraoperative transesophageal echocardiographic examinations with the operative findings: prospective review of 1918 cases. *J Am Soc Echocardiogr* 1999; 12:237-240.
30. Gillinov A, Cosgrove D, Blackstone E, et al: Durability of mitral valve repair for degenerative disease. *J Thorac Cardiovasc Surg* 1998; 116:734-743.
31. Enriquez-Sarano M, Schaff HV, Orszulak TA, et al: Valve repair improves the outcome of surgery for mitral regurgitation. A multivariate analysis. *Circulation* 1995; 91:1022-1028.
32. Enriquez-Sarano M, Freeman WK, Tribouilloy CM, et al: Functional anatomy of mitral regurgitation: accuracy and outcome implications of transesophageal echocardiography. *J Am Coll Cardiol* 1999; 34: 1129-1136.
33. Carpentier A: Cardiac valve surgery—the "French correction." *J Thorac Cardiovasc Surg* 1983; 86:323-337.
34. Foster GP, Isselbacher EM, Rose GA, et al: Accurate localization of mitral regurgitant defects using multiplane transesophageal echocardiography. *Ann Thorac Surg* 1998; 65:1025-1031.
35. Helmcke F, Nanda N, Hsiung M, et al: Color Doppler assessment of mitral regurgitation with orthogonal planes. *Circulation* 1987; 75:175-183.
36. Enriquez-Sarano M, Tajik A, Bailey K, Seward J: Color flow imaging compared with quantitative Doppler assessment of severity of mitral regurgitation: influence of eccentricity of jet and mechanism of regurgitation. *J Am Coll Cardiol* 1993; 21:1211-1219.
37. Pu M, Griffin BP, Vandervoort PM, et al: The value of assessing pulmonary venous flow velocity for predicting severity of mitral regurgitation: a quantitative assessment integrating left ventricular function. *J Am Soc Echocardiogr* 1999; 12:736-743.
38. Enriquez-Sarano M, Dujardin KS, Tribouilloy CM, et al: Determinants of pulmonary venous flow reversal in mitral regurgitation and its usefulness in determining the severity of regurgitation. *Am J Cardiol* 1999; 83: 535-541.
39. Enriquez-Sarano M, Miller FA Jr, Hayes SN, et al: Effective mitral regurgitant orifice area: clinical use and pitfalls of the proximal isovelocity surface area method. *J Am Coll Cardiol* 1995; 25:703-709.
40. Enriquez-Sarano M, Bailey KR, Seward JB, et al: Quantitative Doppler assessment of valvular regurgitation. *Circulation* 1993; 87: 841-848.
41. Enriquez-Sarano M, Basmadjian AJ, Rossi A, et al: Progression of mitral regurgitation: a prospective Doppler echocardiographic study. *J Am Coll Cardiol* 1999; 34:1137-1144.
42. Bonow RO, Carabello BA, Kanu C, et al: ACC/AHA 2006 Guidelines for the Management of Patients with Valvular Heart Disease: a report of the American College of Cardiology/American Heart Association Task Force on Practice Guidelines (writing committee to revise the 1998 Guidelines for the Management of Patients With Valvular Heart Disease): developed in collaboration with the Society of Cardiovascular Anesthesiologists: endorsed by the Society for Cardiovascular Angiography and Interventions and the Society of Thoracic Surgeons. *Circulation* 2006; 114:e84-231.
43. Matsumura T, Ohtaki E, Tanaka K, et al: Echocardiographic prediction of left ventricular dysfunction after mitral valve repair for mitral regurgitation as an indicator to decide the optimal timing of repair. *J Am Coll Cardiol* 2003; 42:458-463.
44. Enriquez-Sarano M, Tajik A, Schaff H, et al: Echocardiographic prediction of left ventricular function after correction of mitral regurgitation: results and clinical implications. *J Am Coll Cardiol* 1994; 24: 1536-1543.
45. Enriquez-Sarano M, Tajik A, Schaff H, et al: Echocardiographic prediction of survival after surgical correction of organic mitral regurgitation. *Circulation* 1994; 90:830-837.
46. Ling H, Enriquez-Sarano M, Seward J, et al: Clinical outcome of mitral regurgitation due to flail leaflets. *NEJM* 1996; 335: 1417-1423.
47. Grigioni F, Avierinos JF, Ling LH, et al: Atrial fibrillation complicating the course of degenerative mitral regurgitation. Determinants and long-term outcome. *J Am Coll Cardiol* 2002; 40:84-92.
48. Kernis SJ, Nkomo VT, Messika-Zeitoun D, et al: Atrial fibrillation after surgical correction of mitral regurgitation in sinus rhythm: incidence, outcome, and determinants. *Circulation* 2004; 110:2320-2325.
49. Avierinos JF, Gersh BJ, Melton LJ 3rd, et al: Natural history of asymptomatic mitral valve prolapse in the community. *Circulation* 2002; 106: 1355-1361.
50. Enriquez-Sarano M, Avierinos JF, Messika-Zeitoun D, et al: Quantitative determinants of the outcome of asymptomatic mitral regurgitation. *NEJM* 2005; 352:875-883.
51. Himelman RB, Kusumoto F, Oken K, et al: The flail mitral valve: echocardiographic findings by precordial and transesophageal imaging and Doppler color flow mapping. *J Am Coll Cardiol* 1991; 17:272-279.
52. Monin JL, Dehant P, Roiron C, et al: Functional assessment of mitral regurgitation by transthoracic echocardiography using standardized imaging planes diagnostic accuracy and outcome implications. *J Am Coll Cardiol* 2005; 46:302-309.

53. Freeman WK, Schaff HV, Khandheria BK, et al: Intraoperative evaluation of mitral valve regurgitation and repair by transesophageal echocardiography: incidence and significance of systolic anterior motion. *J Am Coll Cardiol* 1992; 20:599-609.
54. Saiki Y, Kasegawa H, Kawase M, Osada H, Ootaki E: Intraoperative TEE during mitral valve repair: does it predict early and late postoperative mitral valve dysfunction? *Ann Thorac Surg* 1998; 66:1277-1281.
55. Mohty D, Orszulak TA, Schaff HV, et al: Very long-term survival and durability of mitral valve repair for mitral valve prolapse. *Circulation* 2001; 104:I1-I7.
56. Smedira NG, Selman R, Cosgrove DM, et al: Repair of anterior leaflet prolapse: chordal transfer is superior to chordal shortening. *J Thorac Cardiovasc Surg* 1996; 112:287-291; discussion 291-282.
57. Salati M, Moriggia S, Scrofani R, Santoli C: Chordal transposition for anterior mitral prolapse: early and long-term results. *Eur J Cardiothorac Surg* 1997; 11:268-273.
58. Agricola E, Oppizzi M, De Bonis M, et al: Multiplane transesophageal echocardiography performed according to the guidelines of the American Society of Echocardiography in patients with mitral valve prolapse, flail, and endocarditis: diagnostic accuracy in the identification of mitral regurgitant defects by correlation with surgical findings. *J Am Soc Echocardiogr* 2003; 16:61-66.
59. Grossi EA, Galloway AC, Parish MA, et al: Experience with twenty-eight cases of systolic anterior motion after mitral valve reconstruction by the Carpentier technique. *J Thorac Cardiovasc Surg* 1992; 103:466-470.
60. Mascagni R, Al Attar N, Lamarra M, et al: Edge-to-edge technique to treat post-mitral valve repair systolic anterior motion and left ventricular outflow tract obstruction. *Ann Thorac Surg* 2005; 79:471-473; discussion 474.
61. Jebara VA, Mihaileanu S, Acar C, et al: Left ventricular outflow tract obstruction after mitral valve repair. Results of the sliding leaflet technique. *Circulation* 1993; 88:II30-34.
62. Jaggers J, Chetham PM, Kinnard TL, Fullerton DA: Intraoperative prosthetic valve dysfunction: detection by transesophageal echocardiography. *Ann Thorac Surg* 1995; 59:755-757.
63. Ionescu A, Fraser AG, Butchart EG: Prevalence and clinical significance of incidental paraprosthetic valvar regurgitation: a prospective study using transoesophageal echocardiography. *Heart* 2003; 89:1316-1321.
64. Meloni L, Aru G, Abbruzzese PA, et al: Regurgitant flow of mitral valve prostheses: an intraoperative transesophageal echocardiographic study. *J Am Soc Echocardiogr* 1994; 7:36-46.
65. Lamas G, Mitchell G, Flaker G, et al: Clinical significance of mitral regurgitation after acute myocardial infarction. *Circulation* 1997; 96: 827-833.
66. Grigioni F, Enriquez-Sarano M, Zehr KJ, Bailey KR, Tajik AJ: Ischemic mitral regurgitation: long-term outcome and prognostic implications with quantitative Doppler assessment. *Circulation* 2001; 103:1759-1764.
67. Bursi F, Enriquez-Sarano M, Nkomo VT, et al: Heart failure and death after myocardial infarction in the community: the emerging role of mitral regurgitation. *Circulation* 2005; 111:295-301.
68. Bax JJ, Braun J, Somer ST, et al: Restrictive annuloplasty and coronary revascularization in ischemic mitral regurgitation results in reverse left ventricular remodeling. *Circulation* 2004; 110:II103-108.
69. Wu AH, Aaronson KD, Bolling SF, et al: Impact of mitral valve annuloplasty on mortality risk in patients with mitral regurgitation and left ventricular systolic dysfunction. *J Am Coll Cardiol* 2005; 45:381-387.
70. Yiu S, Enriquez-Sarano M, Tribouilloy C, Seward J, Tajik A: Determinants of the degree of functional mitral regurgitation in patients with systolic left ventricular dysfunction: a quantitative clinical study. *Circulation* 2000; 102:1400-1406.
71. Otsuji Y, Handschumacher MD, Schwammenthal E, et al: Insights from three-dimensional echocardiography into the mechanism of functional mitral regurgitation: direct in vivo demonstration of altered leaflet tethering geometry. *Circulation* 1997; 96:1999-2008.
72. Kumanohoso T, Otsuji Y, Yoshifuku S, et al: Mechanism of higher incidence of ischemic mitral regurgitation in patients with inferior myocardial infarction: quantitative analysis of left ventricular and mitral valve geometry in 103 patients with prior myocardial infarction. *J Thorac Cardiovasc Surg* 2003; 125:135-143.
73. Grigioni F, Detaint D, Avierinos JF, et al: Contribution of ischemic mitral regurgitation to congestive heart failure after myocardial infarction. *J Am Coll Cardiol* 2005; 45:260-267.
74. Rossi A, Cicoira M, Zanolla L, et al: Determinants and prognostic value of left atrial volume in patients with dilated cardiomyopathy. *J Am Coll Cardiol* 2002; 40:1425.
75. Pierard LA, Lancellotti P: The role of ischemic mitral regurgitation in the pathogenesis of acute pulmonary edema. *NEJM* 2004; 351:1627-1634.
76. Aklog L, Filsoufi F, Flores KQ, et al: Does coronary artery bypass grafting alone correct moderate ischemic mitral regurgitation? *Circulation* 2001; 104:I68-75.
77. Braun J, Bax JJ, Versteegh MI, et al: Preoperative left ventricular dimensions predict reverse remodeling following restrictive mitral annuloplasty in ischemic mitral regurgitation. *Eur J Cardiothorac Surg* 2005; 27: 847-853.
78. Hung J, Papakostas L, Tahta SA, et al: Mechanism of recurrent ischemic mitral regurgitation after annuloplasty: continued LV remodeling as a moving target. *Circulation* 2004; 110:II85-90.
79. Gillinov AM, Wierup PN, Blackstone EH, et al: Is repair preferable to replacement for ischemic mitral regurgitation? *J Thorac Cardiovasc Surg* 2001; 122:1125-1141.
80. Ben Farhat M, Ayari M, Maatouk F, et al: Percutaneous balloon versus surgical closed and open mitral commissurotomy: seven-year follow-up results of a randomized trial. *Circulation* 1998; 97:245-250.
81. Cannan CR, Nishimura RA, Reeder GS, et al: Echocardiographic assessment of commissural calcium: a simple predictor of outcome after percutaneous mitral balloon valvotomy. *J Am Coll Cardiol* 1997; 29:175-180.
82. Abascal VM, Wilkins GT, Choong CY, et al: Echocardiographic evaluation of mitral valve structure and function in patients followed for at least 6 months after percutaneous balloon mitral valvuloplasty. *J Am Coll Cardiol* 1988; 12:606-615.
83. Hatle L, Angelsen B, Tromsdal A: Noninvasive assessment of atrioventricular pressure half-time by Doppler ultrasound. *Circulation* 1979; 60: 1096-1104.
84. Thomas JD, Wilkins GT, Choong CY, et al: Inaccuracy of mitral pressure half-time immediately after percutaneous mitral valvotomy. Dependence on transmitral gradient and left atrial and ventricular compliance. *Circulation* 1988; 78:980-993.
85. Rodriguez L, Thomas JD, Monterroso V, et al: Validation of the proximal flow convergence method. Calculation of orifice area in patients with mitral stenosis. *Circulation* 1993; 88:1157-1165.
86. Messika-Zeitoun D, Cachier A, Brochet E, et al: Evaluation of mitral valve area by the proximal isovelocity surface area method in mitral stenosis: Could it be simplified? *Eur J Echocardiogr* 2007; 8(2):116-121.
87. Rosenhek R, Binder T, Porenta G, et al: Predictors of outcome in severe, asymptomatic aortic stenosis. *NEJM* 2000; 343: 611-617.
88. Messika-Zeitoun D, Aubry MC, Detaint D, et al: Evaluation and clinical implications of aortic valve calcification measured by electron-beam computed tomography. *Circulation* 2004; 110: 356-362.
89. Cribier A, Eltchaninoff H, Bash A, et al: Percutaneous transcatheter implantation of an aortic valve prosthesis for calcific aortic stenosis: first human case description. *Circulation* 2002; 106:3006-3008.
90. Pellikka PA, Sarano ME, Nishimura RA, et al: Outcome of 622 adults with asymptomatic, hemodynamically significant aortic stenosis during prolonged follow-up. *Circulation* 2005; 111:3290-3295.
91. Otto CM, Burwash IG, Legget ME, et al: Prospective study of asymptomatic valvular aortic stenosis. Clinical, echocardiographic, and exercise predictors of outcome. *Circulation* 1997; 95:2262-2270.
92. Brener SJ, Duffy CI, Thomas JD, Stewart WJ: Progression of aortic stenosis in 394 patients: relation to changes in myocardial and mitral valve dysfunction. *J Am Coll Cardiol* 1995; 25:305-310.
93. Bellamy MF, Pellikka PA, Klarich KW, Tajik AJ, Enriquez-Sarano M: Association of cholesterol levels, hydroxymethylglutaryl coenzyme-A reductase inhibitor treatment, and progression of aortic stenosis in the community. *J Am Coll Cardiol* 2002; 40:1723-1730.
94. Hachicha Z, Dumesnil JG, Bogaty P, Pibarot P: Paradoxical low-flow, low-gradient severe aortic stenosis despite preserved ejection fraction is associated with higher afterload and reduced survival. *Circulation* 2007; 115:2856-2864.
95. Monin JL, Monchi M, Gest V, et al: Aortic stenosis with severe left ventricular dysfunction and low transvalvular pressure gradients: risk stratification by low-dose dobutamine echocardiography. *J Am Coll Cardiol* 2001; 37:2101-2107.
96. Monin JL, Quere JP, Monchi M, et al: Low-gradient aortic stenosis: operative risk stratification and predictors for long-term outcome: a multicenter study using dobutamine stress hemodynamics. *Circulation* 2003; 108:319-324.
97. Nishimura RA, Grantham JA, Connolly HM, et al: Low-output, low-gradient aortic stenosis in patients with depressed left ventricular systolic function: the clinical utility of the dobutamine challenge in the catheterization laboratory. *Circulation* 2002; 106:809-813.
98. Tribouilloy C, Levy F, Rusinaru D, et al: Outcome after aortic valve replacement for low-flow/low-gradient aortic stenosis without contractile reserve on dobutamine stress echocardiography. *J Am Coll Cardiol* 2009; 53:1865-1873.

99. Lund O, Flo C, Jensen FT, et al: Left ventricular systolic and diastolic function in aortic stenosis. Prognostic value after valve replacement and underlying mechanisms. *Eur Heart J* 1997; 18:1977-1987.
100. Mohty-Echahidi D, Malouf JF, Girard SE, et al: Impact of prosthesis-patient mismatch on long-term survival in patients with small St Jude Medical mechanical prostheses in the aortic position. *Circulation* 2006; 113:420-426.
101. Tasca G, Mhagna Z, Perotti S, et al: Impact of prosthesis-patient mismatch on cardiac events and midterm mortality after aortic valve replacement in patients with pure aortic stenosis. *Circulation* 2006; 113:570-576.
102. Roudaut R, Roques X, Lafitte S, et al: Surgery for prosthetic valve obstruction. A single center study of 136 patients. *Eur J Cardiothorac Surg* 2003; 24:868-872.
103. Connolly HM, Oh JK, Orszulak TA, et al: Aortic valve replacement for aortic stenosis with severe left ventricular dysfunction. Prognostic indicators. *Circulation* 1997; 95:2395-2400.
104. Connolly HM, Oh JK, Schaff HV, et al: Severe aortic stenosis with low transvalvular gradient and severe left ventricular dysfunction: result of aortic valve replacement in 52 patients. *Circulation* 2000; 101:1940-1946.
105. Handa N, McGregor CG, Danielson GK, et al: Valvular heart operation in patients with previous mediastinal radiation therapy. *Ann Thorac Surg* 2001; 71:1880-1884.
106. Minakata K, Schaff HV, Zehr KJ, et al: Is repair of aortic valve regurgitation a safe alternative to valve replacement? *J Thorac Cardiovasc Surg* 2004; 127:645-653.
107. Dujardin KS, Enriquez-Sarano M, Schaff HV, et al: Mortality and morbidity of aortic regurgitation in clinical practice. A long-term follow-up study. *Circulation* 1999; 99:1851-1857.
108. Chaliki HP, Mohty D, Avierinos JF, et al: Outcomes following aortic valve replacement in patients with severe aortic regurgitation and markedly reduced left ventricular function. *Circulation* 2002; 106:2687-2693.
109. Bonow RO, Rosing DR, McIntosh C, et al: The natural history of asymptomatic patients with aortic regurgitation and normal ventricular function. *Circulation* 1983; 68:509-517.
110. Klodas E, Enriquez-Sarano M, Tajik AJ, et al: Surgery for aortic regurgitation in women. Contrasting indications and outcomes compared with men. *Circulation* 1996; 94:2472-2478.
111. Borer J, Hochreiter C, Herrold E, et al: Prediction of indication for valve replacement among asymptomatic or minimally symptomatic patients with chronic aortic regurgitation and normal left ventricular performance. *Circulation* 1998; 97:525-534.
112. Tribouilloy CM, Enriquez-Sarano M, Bailey KR, Seward JB, Tajik AJ: Assessment of severity of aortic regurgitation using the width of the vena contracta: a clinical color Doppler imaging study. *Circulation* 2000; 102: 558-564.
113. Tribouilloy CM, Enriquez-Sarano M, Fett SL, et al: Application of the proximal flow convergence method to calculate the effective regurgitant orifice area in aortic regurgitation. *J Am Coll Cardiol* 1998; 32: 1032-1039.
114. Movsowitz HD, Levine RA, Hilgenberg AD, Isselbacher EM: Transesophageal echocardiographic description of the mechanisms of aortic regurgitation in acute type A aortic dissection: implications for aortic valve repair. *J Am Coll Cardiol* 2000; 36:884-890.
115. Enriquez-Sarano M, Tajik AJ: Clinical practice. Aortic regurgitation. *NEJM* 2004; 351:1539-1546.
116. Haydar HS, He GW, Hovaguimian H, et al: Valve repair for aortic insufficiency: surgical classification and techniques. *Eur J Cardiothorac Surg* 1997; 11:258-265.
117. Messika-Zeitoun D, Thomson H, Bellamy M, et al: Medical and surgical outcome of tricuspid regurgitation caused by flail leaflets. *J Thorac Cardiovasc Surg* 2004; 128:296-302.
118. Lin G, Nishimura RA, Connolly HM, et al: Severe symptomatic tricuspid valve regurgitation due to permanent pacemaker or implantable cardioverter-defibrillator leads. *J Am Coll Cardiol* 2005; 45:1672-1675.
119. Nath J, Foster E, Heidenreich PA: Impact of tricuspid regurgitation on long-term survival. *J Am Coll Cardiol* 2004; 43:405-409.
120. Tribouilloy CM, Enriquez-Sarano M, Bailey KR, Tajik AJ, Seward JB: Quantification of tricuspid regurgitation by measuring the width of the vena contracta with Doppler color flow imaging: a clinical study. *J Am Coll Cardiol* 2000; 36:472-478.
121. Rivera JM, Mele D, Vandervoort PM, et al: Effective regurgitant orifice area in tricuspid regurgitation: clinical implementation and follow-up study. *Am Heart J* 1994; 128:927-933.
122. Tribouilloy CM, Enriquez-Sarano M, Capps MA, Bailey KR, Tajik AJ: Contrasting effect of similar effective regurgitant orifice area in mitral and tricuspid regurgitation: a quantitative Doppler echocardiographic study. *J Am Soc Echocardiogr* 2002; 15:958-965.
123. Anderson CA, Shernan SK, Leacche M, et al: Severity of intraoperative tricuspid regurgitation predicts poor late survival following cardiac transplantation. *Ann Thorac Surg* 2004; 78: 1635-1642.
124. Dreyfus GD, Corbi PJ, Chan KM, Bahrami T: Secondary tricuspid regurgitation or dilatation: which should be the criteria for surgical repair? *Ann Thorac Surg* 2005; 79:127-132.
125. McCarthy PM, Bhudia SK, Rajeswaran J, et al: Tricuspid valve repair: durability and risk factors for failure. *J Thorac Cardiovasc Surg* 2004; 127: 674-685.
126. Fukuda S, Song JM, Gillinov AM, et al: Tricuspid valve tethering predicts residual tricuspid regurgitation after tricuspid annuloplasty. *Circulation* 2005; 111:975-979.
127. Bouzas B, Kilner PJ, Gatzoulis MA: Pulmonary regurgitation: not a benign lesion. *Eur Heart J* 2005; 26:433-439.
128. Pellikka P, Tajik A, Khandheria B, et al: Carcinoid heart disease. Clinical and echocardiographic spectrum in 74 patients. *Circulation* 1993; 87: 1188-1196.
129. Connolly HM, Schaff HV, Mullany CJ, Abel MD, Pellikka PA: Carcinoid heart disease: impact of pulmonary valve replacement in right ventricular function and remodeling. *Circulation* 2002; 106:I51-I56.
130. Durack DT, Lukes AS, Bright DK: New criteria for diagnosis of infective endocarditis: utilization of specific echocardiographic findings. Duke Endocarditis Service. *Am J Med* 1994; 96:200-209.
131. Reynolds HR, Jagen MA, Tunick PA, Kronzon I: Sensitivity of transthoracic versus transesophageal echocardiography for the detection of native valve vegetations in the modern era. *J Am Soc Echocardiogr* 2003; 16: 67-70.
132. Karalis DG, Bansal RC, Hauck AJ, et al: Transesophageal echocardiographic recognition of subaortic complications in aortic valve endocarditis. Clinical and surgical implications. *Circulation* 1992; 86: 353-362.
133. Wallace SM, Walton BI, Kharbanda RK, et al: Mortality from infective endocarditis: clinical predictors of outcome. *Heart* 2002; 88:53-60.
134. Sanfilippo AJ, Picard MH, Newell JB, et al: Echocardiographic assessment of patients with infectious endocarditis: prediction of risk for complications. *J Am Coll Cardiol* 1991; 18:1191-1199.
135. Dumesnil JG, Honos GN, Lemieux M, Beauchemin J: Validation and applications of mitral prosthetic valvular areas calculated by Doppler echocardiography. *Am J Cardiol* 1990; 65:1443-1448.
136. Stewart SF, Nast EP, Arabia FA, et al: Errors in pressure gradient measurement by continuous wave Doppler ultrasound: type, size and age effects in bioprosthetic aortic valves. *J Am Coll Cardiol* 1991; 18:769-779.
137. Tong AT, Roudaut R, Ozkan M, et al: Transesophageal echocardiography improves risk assessment of thrombolysis of prosthetic valve thrombosis: results of the international PRO-TEE registry. *J Am Coll Cardiol* 2004; 43:77-84.
138. Roudaut R, Labbe T, Lorient-Roudaut MF, et al: Mechanical cardiac valve thrombosis. Is fibrinolysis justified? *Circulation* 1992; 86:II8-15.
139. Cohn LH, Collins JJ Jr, Rizzo RJ, et al: Twenty-year follow-up of the Hancock modified orifice porcine aortic valve. *Ann Thorac Surg* 1998; 66:S30-34.
140. Pellikka PA, Roger VL, Oh JK, et al: Stress echocardiography. Part II. Dobutamine stress echocardiography: techniques, implementation, clinical applications, and correlations. *Mayo Clin Proc* 1995; 70:16-27.
141. Arruda-Olson AM, Juracan EM, Mahoney DW, et al: Prognostic value of exercise echocardiography in 5,798 patients: is there a gender difference? *J Am Coll Cardiol* 2002; 39:625-631.
142. Rizzello V, Poldermans D, Schinkel AF, et al: Long term prognostic value of myocardial viability and ischaemia during dobutamine stress echocardiography in patients with ischaemic cardiomyopathy undergoing coronary revascularisation. *Heart* 2006; 92:239-244.
143. Picard MH, Davidoff R, Sleeper LA, et al: Echocardiographic predictors of survival and response to early revascularization in cardiogenic shock. *Circulation* 2003; 107:279-284.
144. Purcaro A, Costantini C, Ciampani N, et al: Diagnostic criteria and management of subacute ventricular free wall rupture complicating acute myocardial infarction. *Am J Cardiol* 1997; 80:397-405.
145. Moursi MH, Bhatnagar SK, Vilacosta I, et al: Transesophageal echocardiographic assessment of papillary muscle rupture. *Circulation* 1996; 94: 1003-1009.
146. Tsang TS, Oh JK, Seward JB, Tajik AJ: Diagnostic value of echocardiography in cardiac tamponade. *Herz* 2000; 25:734-740.
147. Pepi M, Muratori M, Barbier P, et al: Pericardial effusion after cardiac surgery: incidence, site, size, and haemodynamic consequences. *Br Heart J* 1994; 72:327-331.
148. Ling LH, Oh JK, Breen JF, et al: Calcific constrictive pericarditis: is it still with us? *Ann Intern Med* 2000; 132:444-450.
149. Hurrell DG, Nishimura RA, Higano ST, et al: Value of dynamic respiratory changes in left and right ventricular pressures for the diagnosis of constrictive pericarditis. *Circulation* 1996; 93: 2007-2013.

150. Ommen SR, Maron BJ, Olivotto I, et al: Long-term effects of surgical septal myectomy on survival in patients with obstructive hypertrophic cardiomyopathy. *J Am Coll Cardiol* 2005; 46: 470-476.
151. Bansal RC, Chandrasekaran K, Ayala K, Smith DC: Frequency and explanation of false negative diagnosis of aortic dissection by aortography and transesophageal echocardiography. *J Am Coll Cardiol* 1995; 25:1393-1401.
152. Sommer T, Fehske W, Holzknecht N, et al: Aortic dissection: a comparative study of diagnosis with spiral CT, multiplanar transesophageal echocardiography, and MR imaging. *Radiology* 1996; 199:347-352.
153. Nienaber CA, von Kodolitsch Y, Petersen B, et al: Intramural hemorrhage of the thoracic aorta. Diagnostic and therapeutic implications. *Circulation* 1995; 92:1465-1472.
154. Katz ES, Cziner DG, Rosenzweig BP, et al: Multifaceted echocardiographic approach to the diagnosis of a ruptured sinus of Valsalva aneurysm. *J Am Soc Echocardiogr* 1991; 4:494-498.
155. Katz ES, Tunick PA, Rusinek H, et al: Protruding aortic atheromas predict stroke in elderly patients undergoing cardiopulmonary bypass: experience with intraoperative transesophageal echocardiography. *J Am Coll Cardiol* 1992; 20:70-77.

CHAPTER 12

Extracorporeal Circulation

John W. Hammon
Michael H. Hines

INTRODUCTION

Cardiopulmonary bypass for support during cardiac surgery is unique because blood exposed to foreign, nonendothelial cell surfaces is collected and continuously recirculated throughout the body. This contact with synthetic surfaces within the perfusion circuit, as well as open tissue surfaces within the wound triggers a defense reaction that involves at least five plasma protein systems and five types of circulating blood cells. This inflammatory response to cardiopulmonary bypass initiates a powerful thrombotic stimulus and the production, release, and circulation of vasoactive and cytotoxic substances that affect every organ and tissue within the body. Because of this, open-heart surgery using cardiopulmonary bypass is essentially not possible without anticoagulation, usually with heparin; thus the inflammatory response to cardiopulmonary bypass involves the consequences of exposing *heparinized* blood to foreign surfaces, not lined with endothelial cells.

Although the inflammatory response has been well characterized, the development of a nonthrombogenic artificial surface that would allow heparin-free circulatory support has not yet occurred. This chapter summarizes the application of extracorporeal circulation in adult cardiac surgery, and is divided into three sections. The first section describes the components and operation of perfusion systems and related special topics. The issues of thrombosis and bleeding are addressed in the second section, whereas the humoral response to cardiopulmonary bypass, including the reaction of blood elements and the inflammatory response are presented later in this chapter. The final section, deals with organ damage as a consequences of extracorporeal perfusion.

Section A

Perfusion Systems

COMPONENTS

During cardiopulmonary bypass (CPB) for cardiac surgery, blood is typically drained by gravity into the venous reservoir of the heart-lung machine via cannulas placed in the superior and inferior vena cavae or a single cannula placed in the right atrium. Specialized cannulas can also be placed into the lower IVC through a femoral approach. Blood from the reservoir is then pumped through a hollow fiber oxygenator, and after appropriate gas exchange takes place, into the systemic arterial system through a cannula placed in the distal ascending aorta, the femoral artery, or the axillary artery (Fig. 12-1). This basic extracorporeal perfusion system can be adapted to provide partial or total circulatory and respiratory support or partial support for the left or right heart or for the lungs separately.

The complete heart-lung machine includes many additional components (Fig. 12-2).[1] Most manufacturers consolidate a *hollow-fiber oxygenator, venous reservoir,* and *heat exchanger* into a single unit. A *microfilter-bubble trap* is added to the arterial outflow. Depending on the operation, various suction systems can be used to return blood from the surgical field, cardiac chambers, and/or the aorta, directly back into the cardiotomy reservoir, through a *microfilter and then into* the venous reservoir. Increasing evidence of the potential harmful effects of returning fat and lipid particles from the field into directly into the circulation, have increasingly led surgeons to preferentially

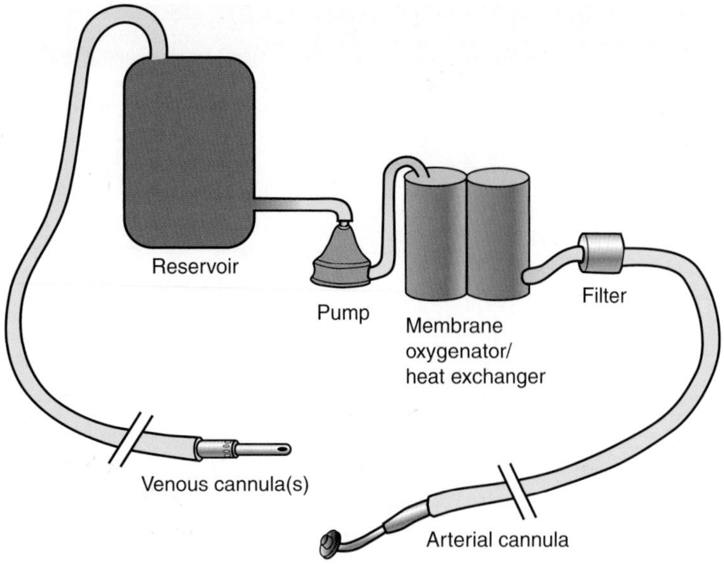

FIGURE 12-1 Basic cardiopulmonary bypass circuit with membrane oxygenator and centrifugal pump.

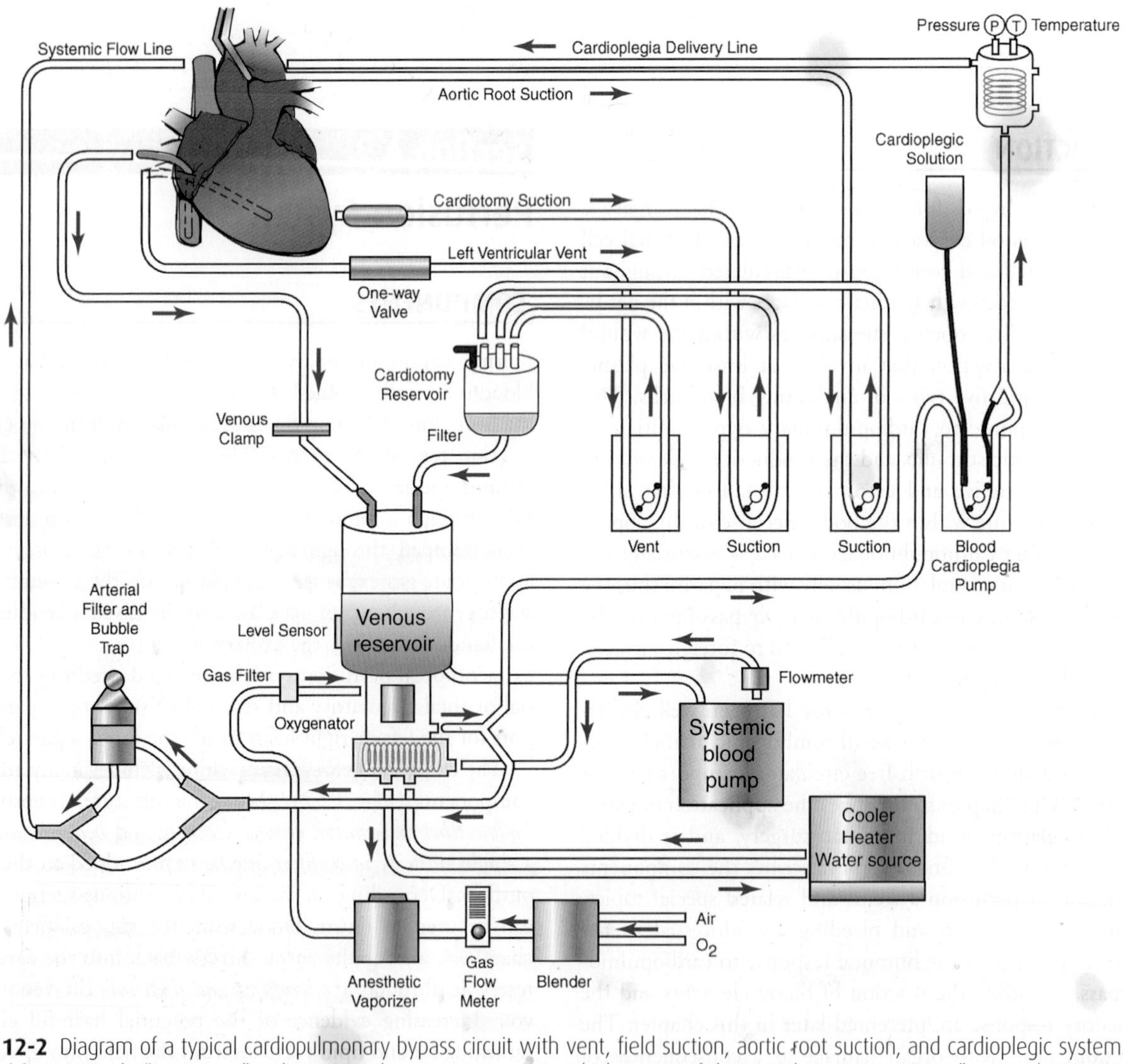

FIGURE 12-2 Diagram of a typical cardiopulmonary bypass circuit with vent, field suction, aortic root suction, and cardioplegic system. Blood is drained from a single "two-stage" catheter into the venous reservoir, which is part of the membrane oxygenator/heat exchanger unit. Venous blood exits the unit and is pumped through the heat exchanger and then the oxygenator. Arterialized blood exits the oxygenator and passes through a filter/bubble trap to the aortic cannula, which is usually placed in the ascending aorta. Blood aspirated from vents and suction systems enters a separate cardiotomy reservoir, which contains a microfilter, before entering the venous reservoir. The cardioplegic system is fed by a spur from the arterial line to which the cardioplegic solution is added and is pumped through a separate heat exchanger into the antegrade or retrograde catheters. Oxygenator gases and water for the heat exchanger are supplied by independent sources.

use a *cell saver system to collect and wash shed blood within the surgical field,* and return the blood to the patient or circuit as packed red cells. In addition to adjusting pump flow, partially occluding *clamps* on venous and arterial lines allow additional regulation of venous drainage and flow. Access ports for sampling and *sensors* for monitoring pressures, temperatures, oxygen saturation, blood gases, and pH are included within most CPB systems. A separate pump and circuit for the administration of *cardioplegic* solutions at controlled composition, rate, and temperature is usually included in the system. An untrafilter can be easily added within the circuit for the removal of excess fluid, electrolytes, and some inflamatory mediators, or simply for hemoconcentration.

Venous Cannulation and Drainage

Principles of Venous Drainage

Venous blood usually enters the circuit by gravity or siphonage into a venous reservoir placed 40 to 70 cm below the level of the heart. The amount of drainage is determined by central venous pressure, the height differential and any resistance within the system (cannulas, tubing, and connectors). Successful drainage is dependent on a continuous column of blood or fluid and the absence of air within the system. Central venous pressure is determined by intravascular volume and venous compliance, which is influenced by medications, sympathetic tone, and anesthesia. Inadequate blood volume or excessive siphon pressure may cause compliant venous or atrial walls to collapse against cannular intake openings to produce "chattering" or "fluttering." This phenomenon is corrected by adding volume to the system (circuit and/or patient), or partially occludding the venous line near the inlet to decrease the negative pressure.

Venous Cannulas and Cannulation

Most venous cannulas are made out of flexible plastic, which may be stiffened with wire reinforcement to prevent kinking. Cannula tips may be straight or angled and often are constructed of thin, rigid plastic or metal. Cannula sizes are selected based on patient size and weight, anticipated flow rate, and an index of catheter flow characteristics and resistance (provided by the manufacturer), as well as size of the vessel to be cannulated. For an average adult with 60-cm negative siphon pressure, a 30-French cannula in the superior vena cava (SVC), and 34 French in the IVC or a single 42-French cavoatrial catheter almost always provides excellent venous drainage. Thin metal tipped right angle cannulas allow placement of smaller diameter cannulas with equal flow characterisitcs, and assist with insertion directly into the vena cavae. Catheters are typically inserted through pursestring guarded incisions in the right atrial appendage, lateral atrial wall, or directly in the SVC and IVC.

Three basic approaches for central venous cannulation are used: bicaval, single atrial, or cavoatrial ("two-stage") (Fig. 12-3). *Bicaval cannulation* and caval tourniquets are necessary to prevent bleeding into the field, and air entry into the system when the right heart is entered during CPB. Because of coronary sinus return, caval tourniquets should not be tightened without decompressing the right atrium if the heart is not still ejecting. Bicaval cannulation without caval snares is sometimes preferred to facilitate venous return during exposure of the left atrium and mitral valve.

Single venous cannulation is adequate for most aortic valve and coronary artery surgery; however, usually a cavo-atrial cannula ("two-stage") is employed (Fig. 12-3B). Introduced via the right atrial appendage, the narrowed distal end is guided into the IVC, leaving the wider proximal portion with multiple side

How do you Air lock venous line

1/4 inch arterial + venous lines

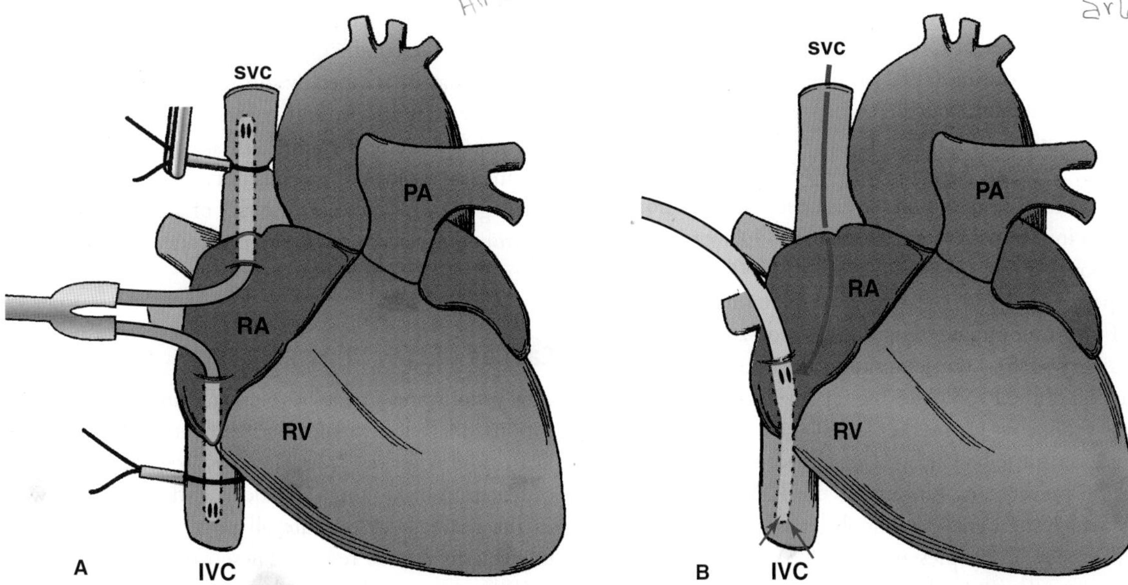

FIGURE 12-3 Placement of venous cannulas. (A) Cannulation of both cavae from incisions in the right atrium. (B) Cannulation using the "two-stage cannula." Blood in the right atrium is captured by vents in the expanded shoulder several inches from the narrower IVC catheter tip.

holes to rest within the mid-right atrium. This tends to provide better venous drainage than a single cannula; however, proper positioning is critical.[2] Care must be taken with both a single and two-stage cannula as elevation of the heart may kink the superior cavoatrial junction, decreasing venous return, and potentially, and more importantly, impeding venous outflow from the cerebral circulation.

Venous cannulation can also be accomplished via the femoral or iliac veins through an open or percutaneous technique. This technique is frequently employed in emergency situations, where central venous cannulation may be difficult (as in complex redo sternotomies[3]) or for cardiopulmonary support when a thoracotomy is the approach of choice, as in descending aortic procedures, or redo mitral valve operations. It is also valuable in the support of critically ill or unstable patients prior to the induction of anesthesia, and for applications of CPB that do not require a chest incision. Adequate venous drainage requires the use of larger cannulas (up to 28 French), with the drainage ports either within the intrahepatic IVC or in the right atrium. Transesophageal echocardiography (TEE) can be particularly helpful in assuring proper placement of these cannulas. Specially designed commercially manufactured long, ultrathin, wire-reinforced catheters are available for this purpose.

Persistent Left Superior Vena Cava

A persistent left superior vena cava (PLSVC) is present in 0.3 to 0.5% of the general population and usually drains into the coronary sinus; however, in about 10% of cases it drains into the left atrium.[4] Although more common in association with other congenital defects, it can be seen as an isolated anomaly, and should be suspected when the (left) innominate vein is small or absent, or when a large coronary sinus (or the PLSVC itself) is seen on baseline TEE.[5]

A PLSVC may complicate the delivery of retrograde cardioplegia or entry into the right heart.[6] If an adequate-sized innominate vein is present (30% of patients), the PLSVC can simply be occluded during CPB, assuming the ostium of the coronary sinus is present, and the coronary venous drainage is not dependent on the PLSVC.[7] If the right SVC is absent (approximately 20% of patients with PLSVC), the left cava cannot be occluded and should be drained. With a normal RSVC, but an innominate vein that is absent (40% of patients) or small (about 33%), occlusion of the PLSVC may cause venous hypertension and possible cerebral injury. Although division of the innominate vein during redo-sternotomy or complex surgery such as transplantation has been shown to be safe, occlussion of the PLSVC during CPB relies on drainage of the cerebral venous return by the contralateral system, and so special attention must be paid to assure adequate RSVC cannula size, and prevent any kinking of the RSVC. In circumstances in which retrograde cardioplegia is required (severe aortic insufficiency) in the presence of a PLSVC, the retrograde cardioplegia cannula can be directly inserted into the coronary sinus and secured with a pursestring around the orifice of the coronary sinus, and with temporary snaring of the PLSVC, successful retrograde cardioplegia can be delivered.

Augmented or Assisted Venous Return

Negative pressure can be applied to the venous line to provide assisted venous drainage using either a roller or a centrifugal pump system,[8] or by applying a regulated vacuum to a closed hard-shell venous reservoir (vacuum-assisted venous drainage, VAVD).[9] This may permit use of smaller diameter catheters[10] and may be helpful when long, peripheral catheters are used. However augmented negative pressure in the venous line increases the risk of aspirating gross or microscopic air and causing cerebral injury,[11,12] hemolysis, or aspiration of air into the blood phase of hollow fiber oxygenators. Conversely, positive pressure in the venous reservoir can cause air to enter the venous lines and the right heart.[13] These potential complications require special safety monitors and devices and adherence to detailed protocols when using assisted venous drainage techniques.[13,14]

Complications Associated with Venous Cannulation and Drainage

Atrial arrhythmias, bleeding from atrial or vena caval tears, air embolization, venous injury, or obstruction owing to catheter malposition, reversing arterial and venous lines, and unexpected decannulation can all occur during the conduct of cannulation for CPB. Encircling the vena cavae for snaring may lacerate branches or nearby vessels (eg, right pulmonary artery), or injure the vena cava itself. All of these injuries are more likely in the presence of previous surgey, and need to be recognized and corrected early to assure the proper conduct of CPB and minimize additional complications.

Either before or after CPB, cannulas still in place may compromise venous return to the right atrium. The venous cannulas in the SVC, or the superior caval tape may displace or compromise central venous or pulmonary arterial monitoring catheters. Conversely, monitoring catheters may compromise the function of caval tapes, allowing air to enter the venous lines between the cannulas and the catheters or sheaths.

During the conduct of the operation itself, any intracardiac catheter may be trapped by sutures, which may impede removal before or after the wound is closed. Any connection between the atmosphere and cannula intake ports may entrain air to produce an air lock or gaseous microembolism. Assisted venous drainage (AVD) increases the risk of air entrainment.[15] Finally, improperly placed pursestring sutures may obstruct a cava when tied, particularly in the SVC.[16]

Causes of Low Venous Return

Low venous pressure, hypovolemia, drug- or anesthetic-induced venous dilatation, inadequate differential height between the heart and the reservoir, inadequate cannula size, cannula obstruction or kinking, "air-lock," and excessive flow resistance in the drainage system are all possible causes of impaired or inadequate venous return. These can usually be prevented or quickly corrected through close attention to detail, keeping the venous lines visible within the field when possible, and perhaps most importantly, frequent and detailed communication between surgeon and perfusionist. In addition to contributing to inadequate antegrade flow from the pump, partial obstruction of the venous line may lead to right ventricular distention and impair contractility off CPB.

Arterial Cannulation

Arterial Cannulas

The tip of the arterial cannula is usually the narrowest part of the perfusion system and may produce high pressure differentials, jets, turbulence, and cavitation at the required flows for CPB, particularly if the arterial catheters are small. Most arterial catheters are rated by a performance index, which relates external diameter, flow, and pressure differential.[17] High-velocity jets may damage the aortic wall, dislodge atheroemboli, produce dissections, disturb flow to nearby vessels, and cause cavitation and hemolysis. Pressure differences that exceed 100 mm Hg cause excessive hemolysis and protein denaturation.[18] Weinstein[19] attributed a predominance of left-sided stroke after cardiac surgery to the "sand-blasting" effect of end-hole aortic cannulas directing debris into the left carotid artery. Available aortic catheters with only side ports[20] are designed to minimize jet effects and better distribute arch vessel perfusion and pressure[21] and may be associated with fewer strokes.[19]

Recently a dual-stream aortic perfusion catheter has been developed that features an inflatable horizontal streaming baffle that is designed to protect the arch vessels from atherosclerotic and other emboli and permits selective cerebral hypothermia.[22] Another novel aortic cannula features a side port that deploys a 120-μm mesh filter to remove particulate emboli beyond the ascending aorta.[23] Although this catheter may increase the pressure gradient by 50%,[24] it has been shown to remove an average of eight emboli in 99% of 243 patients studied, and reduce the incidence of cerebral injuries below an expected rate.[25]

Connection to the Patient

Anatomical sites available for arterial inflow include the proximal aorta, innominate artery and distal arch, femoral, external iliac, axillary, and subclavian arteries. Cannulation can be direct by arterial puncture within a pursestring, through a side graft anastomosed to an arterial vessel, or percutaneous, although usually only in emergency situations. The choice is influenced by the planned operation[26] and distribution of atherosclerotic disease.[27]

Atherosclerosis of the Ascending Aorta

Dislodgement of atheromatous debris from the aortic wall from manipulation,[28] cross-clamping, or the sand-blasting effect of the cannula jet is a major cause of perioperative stroke[29] as well as a risk factor for aortic dissection[30] and postoperative renal dysfunction.[31] Simple palpation has been shown to be sensitive and accurate for detecting severe atherosclerosis than epiaortic ultrasonic scanning.[28,32] Although some have advocated for its use, even transesophageal echocardiolgraphy (TEE) views of the middle and distal ascending aorta are often inadequate.[32,33] Epiaortic scanning is now the preferred method of screening in all patients with a history of transient ischemic attack, stroke, severe peripheral vascular disease, palpable calcification in the ascending aorta, calcified aortic knob on chest radiograph, age older than 50 to 60 years, or TEE findings of moderate aortic atherosclerosis.[28] A calcified aorta ("porcelain aorta"), which occurs in 1.2 to 4.3% of patients,[34] is another indication for relocation of the aortic cannula.[35] Alternative sites include the distal aortic arch[34] along with the innominate, axillary-subclavian, or femoral arteries.

Ascending Aortic Cannulation

The distal ascending aorta is the the most common cannulation site because of easy access, and few complications. The cannula is usually placed through a small stab wound within one or two concentric pursestring sutures, that are then snared to secure the cannula and provide hemostasis. Risk of dissection may be reduced by avoiding cannulation into the hypertensive aorta, and many surgeons choose to transiently reduce the systemic pressure below 100 mm Hg. The observation of pulsatile back bleeding into the cannula confirms that the tip is within the lumen of the aorta, and then the cannula should be positioned to direct flow to the mid-transverse aorta. The use of a long catheter with the tip placed beyond the left subclavian artery has also been reported.[36] Proper cannula placement is critical[21] and is confirmed by noting pulsatile pressure in the aortic line monitor and equivalent pressure in the radial artery. The cannula must be properly secured in place to prevent inadvertant dislodgement during the conduct of the operation.

Complications include difficult insertion; bleeding; tearing of the aortic wall; intramural or malposition of the cannula tip (in or against the aortic wall, toward the valve, or in an arch vessel)[37]; atheromatous emboli; failure to remove all air from the arterial line after connection; injury to the aortic back wall; high line pressure, indicating obstruction to flow; inadequate or excessive cerebral perfusion[38]; inadvertent decannulation; and aortic dissection.[39] It is essential to monitor aortic line and radial artery pressures and carefully observe the aorta for possible cannula-related complications particularly during the initiation of CPB as well as during the placement of aortic clamps. Asymmetric cooling of the face or neck may suggest a problem with cerebral perfusion. Late bleeding and infected or noninfected false aneurysms are delayed complications of aortic cannulation.

Aortic dissection occurs in 0.01 to 0.09% of aortic cannulations[30,40] and is more common in patients with aortic root disease. Early signs of aortic dissection include discoloration beneath the adventia near the cannulation site, an increase in arterial line pressure, or a sharp reduction in return to the venous reservoir. TEE may be helpful in confirming the diagnosis,[41] but prompt action is necessary to limit the dissection and maintain perfusion. The cannula must be promptly transferred to a peripheral artery or uninvolved distal aorta. Blood pressure should be controlled pharmacologically and perfusion cooling to temperatures less than 20°C initiated. During hypothermic circulatory arrest, the aorta is opened at the original site of cannulation and repaired by direct suture, patch, or circumferential graft.[40] When recognized early, survival rates range from 66 to 85%, but when undiscovered until late during of after the operation, survival is approximately 50%.

Cannulation of the Femoral or Iliac Artery

These vessels are usually the first alternative to aortic cannulation, but may be the primary choice for rapid initiation of cardiopulmonary bypass for severe bleeding, cardiac arrest, acute intraoperative dissection, or severe shock. It is also a common first choice for limited access cardiac surgery, as well as in selected reoperative patients.[3] Femoral or iliac cannulation limits cannula size but the retrograde distribution of blood flow is similar to antegrade flow.[42] Percutaneous cannulation kits are available for emergency femoral access, and many surgeons also use these long wire reinforced peripheral arterial cannulas with an open Seldinger technique, inserting the cannula through a pursestring in the femoral or iliac vessel by direct cutdown. This may reduce some of the complications of open insertion of large short cannluas, and simplifies cannula removal and arterial repair. Femoral cannulation may be associated with many complications,[3] including tears, dissection, late stenosis or thrombosis, bleeding, lymphatic collection or drainage, groin infection, and cerebral and coronary atheroembolism. In patients with prior aortic dissections, retrograde femoral perfusion may create a malperfusion situation; thus, some surgeons recommend alternative cannulation sites for these patients.[43] Ischemic complications of the distal leg may occur during prolonged (3- to 6-hour) retrograde perfusions,[44,45] unless perfusion is provided to the distal vessel. This may be provided by a small Y catheter in the distal vessel[45] or a side graft sutured to the artery.[46]

Retrograde arterial dissection is the most serious complication of femoral or iliac arterial cannulation and may extend to the aortic root or cause retroperitoneal hemorrhage with an incidence of around 1% or less,[47] and is associated with a mortality of about 50%. This complication is more common in patients greater than 40 years, and in those with significantly diseased arteries. The diagnosis is similar to an aortic cannula dissection and may be confirmed by TEE of the descending thoracic aorta.[41] Antegrade perfusion in the true lumen must be immediately resumed by either the heart itself or cannulation in the distal aorta or axillary-subclavian artery. It is not always necessary to repair the dissected ascending aorta unless it progresses proximally to involve the aortic root.[47]

Other Sites for Arterial Cannulation

The axillary-subclavian artery has been increasingly used for cannulation.[48,49] Advantages include freedom from atherosclerosis, antegrade flow into the arch vessels, and protection of the arm and hand by collateral flow. Because of these advantages and the dangers of retrograde perfusion in patients with aortic dissection, some surgeons prefer this cannulation site over femoral access for these patients.[49] Brachial plexus injury and axillary artery thrombosis are reported complications.[48] The axillary artery is approached through a subclavicular incision, whereas the intrathoracic subclavian artery may be cannulated through a thoracotomy.[50]

Occasionally the innominate artery may be cannulated through a pursestring suture without obstructing flow to the right carotid artery by using a 7- or 8-French cannula.[26] The ascending aorta can also be cannulated by passing a cannula through the aortic valve from the left ventricular apex.[51] Coselli and Crawford[52] also describe retrograde perfusion through a graft sewn to the abdominal aorta.

Venous Reservoir

The venous reservoir serves as volume reservoir during cardiopulmonary bypass and particularly with the body exsanguination of deep hypothermic circulatory arrest. It is placed immediately before the arterial pump when a membrane oxygenator is used (see Fig. 12-1). This reservoir serves as a high-capacitance (ie, low-pressure) receiving chamber for venous return, facilitates gravity drainage, is a venous bubble trap, provides access for drugs, fluids, or blood, and increases the storage capacity for the perfusion system. As much as 1 to 3 L of blood may be translocated from patient to circuit when full CPB is initiated. The venous reservoir also provides several seconds of reaction time if venous return is suddenly decreased or interrupted.

Reservoirs may be rigid (hard) plastic canisters ("open" types) or soft, collapsible plastic bags ("closed" types). The rigid canisters facilitate volume measurements and management of venous air, often have larger capacity, are easier to prime, permit suction for vacuum-assisted venous drainage, and may be less expensive. Some hard-shell venous reservoirs incorporate macrofilters and microfilters and can serve as cardiotomy reservoirs to receive vented blood.

Disadvantages include the use of silicon antifoam compounds, which may produce microemboli,[53] and increased activation of blood elements.[54] Soft bag reservoirs eliminate the blood-gas interface and by collapsing reduce the risk of pumping massive air emboli if venous return is suddenly interrupted.

Oxygenators

Membrane oxygenators imitate the natural lung by interspersing a thin membrane of microporous polypropylene or polymethylpentene (0.3- to 0.8-μm pores), or silicone rubber between the gas and blood phases. Compared with previously used bubble oxygenators, membrane oxygenators are safer, produce less particulate and gaseous microemboli,[55] are less reactive to blood elements, and allow superior control of blood gases.[56] With microporous membranes, plasma-filled pores prevent gas entering blood, but facilitate transfer of both oxygen and CO_2. Because oxygen is poorly diffusible in plasma, blood must be spread as a thin film (approximately 100 μm) over a large area with high differential gas pressures between compartments to achieve oxygenation. Areas of turbulence and secondary flow enhance diffusion of oxygen within blood and thereby improve oxyhemoglobin saturation.[57] Carbon dioxide is highly diffusible in plasma and easily exits the blood compartment despite small differential pressures across the membrane.

The most popular design uses sheaves of hollow fibers (120 to 200 μm) connected to inlet and outlet manifolds within a hard-shell jacket (Fig. 12-4). The most efficient configuration creates turbulence by passing blood between fibers and oxygen within fibers. Arterial PCO_2 is controlled by gas flow rate, and PO_2 is controlled by the fraction of inspired oxygen

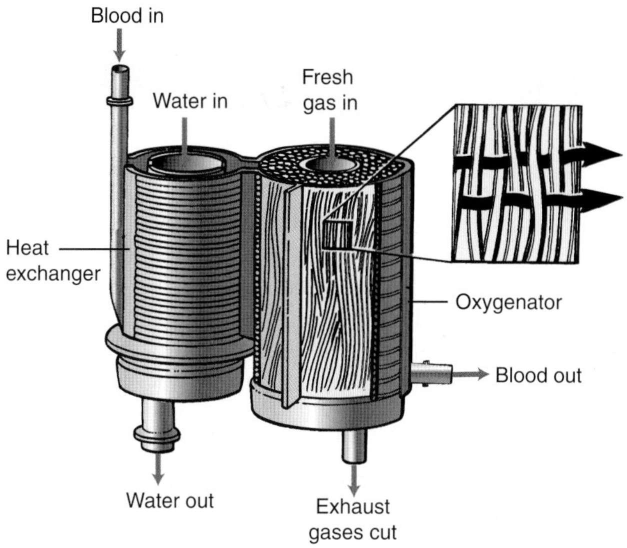

FIGURE 12-4 Diagram of a hollow fiber membrane oxygenator and heat exchanger unit. Blood enters the heat exchanger first and flows over water-cooled or water-warmed coils and then enters the oxygenator to pass between woven strands of hollow fibers. Oxygen enters one end of the bundles of hollow fibers and exits at the opposite end. The hollow fiber bundles are potted at each end to separate the blood and gas compartments. Oxygen and carbon dioxide diffuse in opposite directions across the aggregate large surface of the hollow fibers.

(FIO_2) produced by an air-oxygen blender. Modern membrane oxygenators add up to 470 mL of O_2 and remove up to 350 mL CO_2 per minute at 1 to 7 L of flow with priming volumes of 220 to 560 mL and resistances of 12 to 15 mm Hg per liter blood flow. Most units combine a venous reservoir, heat exchanger, and hollow fiber membrane oxygenator into one compact unit.

Oxygen and CO_2 diffuse across thin silicone membranes, which are made into envelopes and wound around a spool to produce a spiral coil oxygenator. Gas passes through the envelope and blood passes between the coil windings. Because of protein leakage that frequently ccurs with hollow fiber membranes after 8 to 12 hours of use, these spiral coil silicone membranes have been preferred for the prolonged perfusions (days) used in long-term respiratory and cardiac support of extracorporeal membrane oxygenation or "ECMO" systems. More recently, however, the development of polymethylpentene oxygenators have combined the benefit of efficient small surface area hollow fiber oxygenators without the detrimental plasma leakage seen with polypropylene, and have allowed these membranes to be used with both CPB and ECMO.

Other membranes feature a very thin (0.05 μm), solid membrane on the blood side of a highly porous support matrix. This membrane reduces the risk of gas emboli and plasma leakage during prolonged CPB, but may impair transfer of volatile anesthetics.[58]

Flow regulators, flow meters, gas blender, oxygen analyzer, gas filter, and moisture trap are parts of the oxygenator gas supply system used to control the ventilating gases within membrane oxygenators. Often an anesthetic vaporizer is added, but care must be taken to prevent volatile anesthetic liquids from destroying plastic components of the perfusion circuit.

Bubble oxygenators are obsolete in the United States, but may still be used elsewhere for short-term CPB because of low cost and efficiency. Because each bubble presents a new foreign surface to which blood elements react, bubble oxygenators cause progressive injury to blood elements and entrain more gaseous microemboli.[59] In bubble oxygenators, venous blood drains directly into a chamber into which oxygen is infused through a diffusion plate (sparger). The sparger produces thousands of small (approximately 36-μm) oxygen bubbles within blood. Gas exchange occurs across a thin film at the blood-gas interface around each bubble. Carbon dioxide diffuses into the bubble and oxygen diffuses outward into blood. Small bubbles improve oxygen exchange by effectively increasing the surface area of the gas-blood interface,[60] but are difficult to remove. Large bubbles facilitate CO_2 removal. Bubbles and blood are separated by settling, filtration, and defoaming surfactants in a reservoir. Bubble oxygenators add 350 to 400 mL oxygen to blood and remove 300 to 330 mL CO_2 per minute at flow rates from 1 to 7 L/min.[56] Priming volumes are less than 500 mL. Commercial bubble oxygenators incorporate a reservoir and heat exchanger within the same unit and are placed upstream to the arterial pump.

Oxygenator malfunction requiring change during CPB occurs in 0.02 to 0.26% of cases,[61–63] but the incidence varies between membrane oxygenator designs.[64] Development of abnormal resistant areas in the blood path is the most common cause,[63] but other problems include leaks, loss of gas supply, rupture of connections, failure of the blender, and deteriorating gas exchange. Blood gases need to be monitored to ensure adequate CO_2 removal and oxygenation. Heparin coating may reduce development of abnormally high resistance areas.[62]

Heat Exchangers

Heat exchangers control body temperature by heating or cooling blood passing through the perfusion circuit. Hypothermia is frequently used during cardiac surgery to reduce oxygen demand or facilitate operative exposure with brief periods of circulatory arrest. Because gases are more soluble in cold than in warm blood, rapid rewarming of cold blood within the circuit or the body may cause formation of bubble emboli.[65] Most membrane oxygenator units incorporate a heat exchanger upstream to the oxygenator to minimize this potential problem. Blood should not be heated above 40°C to prevent denaturation of plasma proteins, and the temperature gradient between the body and the perfusion circuit remain within 10°C to prevent bubble emboli. The heat exchanger may be supplied by hot and cold tap water, but separate heater/cooler units with convenient temperature-regulating controls are preferred. Leakage of water into the blood path can cause hemolysis and malfunction of heater/cooler units may occur.[61]

Separate heat exchangers are needed for cardioplegia. The simplest system uses bags of precooled cardioplegia solution; however, commonly cardioplegia fluid is circulated through through a dedicated heat exchanger or tubing coils placed in an ice or warm water bath.

TABLE 12-1 Roller Versus Centrifugal Pump

	Roller Pump	Centrifugal Pump
Description	Nearly occlusive Afterload independent	Nonocclusive Afterload sensitive
Advantages	Low prime volume Low cost No potential for backflow Shallow sine-wave pulse	Portable, position insensitive Safe positive and negative pressure Adapts to venous return Superior for right or left heart bypass Preferred for long-term bypass Protects against massive air embolism
Disadvantages	Excessive positive and negative pressure Spallation Tubing rupture Potential for massive air embolism Necessary occlusion adjustments Requires close supervision	Large priming volume Requires flowmeter Potential passive backward flow Higher cost

Pumps

Most heart-lung machines use two types of pumps, although roller pumps can be used exclusively (Table 12-1). Centrifugal pumps are usually used for the primary perfusion circuit for safety reasons and for a possible reduction in injury to blood elements, although this remains controversial and unproved.[66]

Centrifugal pumps (Fig. 12-5) consist of a vaned impeller or nested, smooth plastic cones, which when rotated rapidly, propel blood by centrifugal force.[67] An arterial flowmeter is required to determine forward blood flow, which varies with the speed of rotation and the afterload of the arterial line. Unless a check valve is used,[68] the arterial line must be clamped to prevent backward flow when the pump is off. Centrifugal blood pumps generate up to 900 mm Hg of forward pressure, but only 400 to 500 mm Hg of negative pressure and, therefore, less cavitation and fewer gaseous microemboli. They can pump small amounts of air, but become "deprimed" if more than 30 to 50 mL of air enters the blood chamber. Centrifugal pumps are probably superior for temporary extracorporeal cardiac assist devices and left heart bypass, and for generating pump-augmented venous return.

Roller pumps consist of a length of 1/4- to 5/8-inch (internal diameter) polyvinyl, silicone, or latex tubing, which is compressed by two rollers 180 degrees apart, inside a circular raceway. Forward flow is generated by roller compression and flow rate depends upon the diameter of the tubing, rate of rotation (RPM), the length of the compression raceway, and completeness of compression or "occlusion." Compression is adjusted before use to be barely nonocclusive against a standing column of fluid that produces 45 to 75 mm Hg back pressure.[69] Hemolysis and tubing wear are minimal at this degree of compression.[69] Flow rate is determined from calibration curves for each pump for different tubing sizes and rates of rotation. Roller pumps are inexpensive, reliable, safe, insensitive to afterload, and have small priming volumes, but can produce high negative pressures and microparticles shed from compressed tubing (spallation).[70] Roller pumps are vulnerable to careless operation that results in: propelling air; inaccurate flow calibration; backflow when not in use if rollers are not sufficiently occlusive; excessive pressure with rupture of connections if arterial inflow is obstructed; tears in tubing; and changing roller compression settings during operation. In general roller pumps rather than centrifugal pumps are used for sucker systems and for delivering cardioplegic solutions.

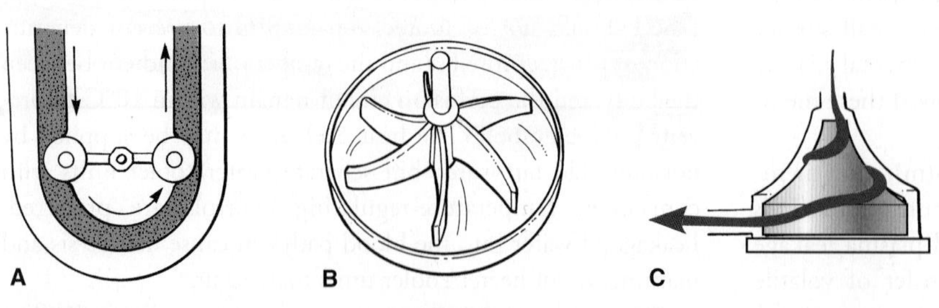

FIGURE 12-5 Diagrams of blood pumps. (A) Roller pump with two rollers, 180 degrees apart. The compression of the rollers against the raceway is adjustable and is set to be barely nonocclusive. Blood is propelled in the direction of rotation. (B) The impeller pump uses vanes mounted on a rotating central shaft. (C) The centrifugal pump uses three rapidly rotated, concentric cones to propel blood forward by centrifugal force.

Centrifugal pumps produce pulseless blood flow and standard roller pumps produce a sine wave pulse around 5 mm Hg. The arterial cannula dampens the pulse of pulsatile pumps, and it is difficult to generate pulse pressures above 20 mm Hg within the body during full CPB.[71] To date no one has conclusively demonstrated the need for pulsatile perfusion during short- or long-term CPB or circulatory assistance.[72]

Complications that may occur during operation of either type of pump include loss of electricity; loss of the ability to control pump speed, which produces "runaway pump" or "pump creep" when turned off; loss of the flow meter or RPM indicator; rupture of tubing in the roller pump raceway; and reversal of flow by improper tubing in the raceway. A means to manually provide pumping in case of electrical failure should always be available.

Filters and Bubble Traps

Microemboli

During clinical cardiac surgery with CPB the wound and the perfusion circuit generate gaseous and biologic and nonbiologic particulate microemboli (<500 μM diameter).[23,73,74] Microemboli produce much of the morbidity associated with cardiac operations using CPB (see section 'Organ Damage' later in this chapter). Gaseous emboli contain oxygen or nitrogen and may enter the perfusate from multiple sources and pass through other components of the system.[12,15] Potential sources of gas entry include stopcocks, sampling and injection sites,[74] priming solutions, priming procedures, intravenous fluids, vents, the cardiotomy reservoir, tears or breaks in the perfusion circuit, loose pursestring sutures (especially during augmented venous return),[12] rapid warming of cold blood,[65] cavitation, oxygenators, venous reservoirs with low perfusate levels,[15] and the heart and great vessels. Bubble oxygenators produce many gaseous emboli; membrane oxygenators produce very few.[55,56] Aside from technical errors (open stopcocks, empty venous reservoir, air in the heart) the cardiotomy reservoir is the largest source of gaseous emboli in membrane oxygenator perfusion systems.

Blood produces a large number of particulate emboli related to thrombus formation (clots), fibrin, platelet and platelet-leukocyte aggregation, hemolyzed red cells, cellular debris, and generation of chylomicrons, fat particles, and denatured proteins.[75] Stored donor blood is also an important source of blood-generated particles.[76] Other biologic emboli include atherosclerotic debris and cholesterol crystals and calcium particles dislodged by cannulation, manipulation for exposure, or the surgery itself. Both biologic and nonbiologic particulate emboli are aspirated from the wound. Bits of muscle, bone, and fat are mixed with suture material, talc, glue, and dust and aspirated into the cardiotomy reservoir.[76,77] Materials used in manufacture, spallated material, and dust may also enter the perfusate from the perfusion circuit[76] if it is not first rinsed by recirculating saline through a prebypass microfilter, which is discarded.

In vivo microemboli larger than 100 microns are detected by transcranial Doppler ultrasound,[78] fluorescein angiography,[55] TEE, and retinal inspection. In the circuit, microemboli are monitored by arterial line ultrasound[79] or monitoring screen filtration pressure. Microfilter weights and examination, histology of autopsy tissues, and electron particle size counters of blood samples[76] verify microemboli beyond the circuit.

Prevention and Control of Microemboli

Table 12-2 outlines sources of microemboli. Major methods include using a membrane oxygenator and cardiotomy reservoir filter; minimizing and washing blood aspirated from the field[80]; and preventing air entry into the circuit and using left ventricular vents when the heart is opened.[81,82]

TABLE 12-2 Major Sources of Microemboli

Gas	Foreign	Blood
Bubble oxygenators	Atherosclerotic debris	Fibrin
Air entry into the circuit	Fat, fat droplets	Free fat
Residual air in the heart	Fibrin clot	Aggregated chylomicrons
Loose purse-string sutures	Cholesterol crystals	Denatured proteins
Cardiotomy reservoir	Calcium particles	Platelet aggregates
Rapid rewarming	Muscle fragments	Platelet-leukocyte aggregates
Cavitation	Tubing debris, dust	Hemolyzed red cells
	Bone wax, talc	Transfused blood
	Silicone antifoam	
	Glue, Surgicel	
	Cotton sponge fiber	

The brain receives 14% of the cardiac output and is the most sensitive organ for microembolic injury.[83] Strategies to selectively reduce microembolism to the brain include reducing $PaCO_2$ to cause cerebral vasoconstriction[84]; hypothermia[85]; placing aortic cannulas downstream to the cerebral vessel[36,74]; and using special aortic cannulas with[22,23,30] or without[19] special baffles or screens designed to prevent cannula-produced cerebral atherosclerotic emboli.

Two types of blood microfilters are available for use within the perfusion circuit: depth and screen.[86,87] Depth filters consist of packed fibers or porous foam, have no defined pore size, present a large, tortuous, wetted surface, and remove microemboli by impaction and absorption. Screen filters are usually made of woven polyester or nylon thread, have a defined pore size, and filter by interception. Screen filters vary in pore size and configuration and block most air emboli; however, as pore size decreases, resistance increases. As compared with no filter, studies indicate that all commercial filters effectively remove gaseous and particulate emboli.[88,89] Most investigations find that the Dacron wool depth filter is most effective, particularly in removing microscopic and macroscopic air. Pressure differences across filters vary between 24 and 36 mm Hg at 5 L/min flow. Filters cause slight hemolysis and tend to trap some platelets; nylon filters may also activate complement.[86]

The need for microfilters in the cardiotomy suction reservoir is universally accepted,[77] and most commercial units contain an integrated micropore filter. The need for a filter in the cardioplegia delivery system, however, remains debatable,[90] and although almost always used, the requirement of an arterial line filter is unsettled.[87] In vitro studies demonstrate that an arterial filter reduces circulating microemboli[89] and clinical studies are confirmatory.[89] However, these filters do not remove all microemboli generated by the extracorporeal circuit.[12,74,77] When bubble oxygenators are used, studies show equivocal or modest reductions in microemboli[55,91] and neurologic outcome markers.[91] In contrast, membrane oxygenators produce far fewer microemboli and when used without an arterial filter, the numbers of microemboli are similar to those found with bubble oxygenators plus arterial line filters.[87]

Although the efficacy of arterial line microfilters remains unsettled, their use is almost universal;[92] and although they are effective bubble traps, they do increase cost, occasionally obstruct during use, are difficult to de-air during priming, and require a small bypass line and valved purge line to remove any air.

Other sources of biologic microemboli may be more important. Cerebral microemboli are most numerous during aortic cannulation,[93,94] application and release of aortic clamps,[94] and at the beginning of cardiac ejection after open heart procedures.[95] Furthermore, as compared with perfusion microemboli, surgically induced emboli are more likely to cause postoperative neurologic deficits.[96]

Leukocyte-Depleting Filters

Leukocyte depleting filters are discussed later in this chapter and have been recently reviewed.[97] These filters reduce circulating leukocyte counts in most studies,[98] but fail to produce convincing evidence of clinical benefit.[99]

Tubing and Connectors

The various components of the heart-lung machine are connected by polyvinyl tubing and fluted polycarbonate connectors. Medical grade polyvinyl chloride (PVC) tubing is universally used because it is flexible, compatible with blood, inert, nontoxic, smooth, nonwettable, tough, transparent, resistant to kinking and collapse, and can be heat sterilized. To reduce priming volume, tubing connections should be short. To reduce turbulence, cavitation, and stagnant areas, the flow path should be smooth and uniform without areas of constriction or expansion. Wide tubing improves rheology, but also increases priming volume. In practice 1/2- to 5/8-inch (internal diameter) tubing is used for most adults, but until a compact, integrated, complete heart-lung machine can be designed and produced as a unit, the flow path will produce some turbulence. Loose tubing connections can be sources of air intake or blood leakage and so all connections must be secure. For convenience and safety, most tubing and connectors are prepackaged and disposable.

Heparin-Coated Circuits

Heparin can be bound to blood surfaces of all components of the extracorporeal circuit by ionic or covalent bonds. The Duraflo II heparin coating ionically attaches heparin to a quaternary ammonium carrier (alkylbenzyl dimethyl-ammonium chloride), which binds to plastic surfaces (Edwards Lifesciences, Irvine, CA). Covalent attachment is produced by first depositing a polyethylenimine polymer spacer onto the plastic surface, to which heparin fragments bind (Carmeda Bioactive Surface, Medtronic, Inc., Minneapolis, MN). Ionic-bound heparin slowly leaches, but this is irrelevant in clinical cardiac surgery. The use of heparin-coated circuits during CPB has spawned an enormous literature[100–102] and remains controversial largely because studies are contaminated by patient selection, reduced doses of systemic heparin, and washing or discarding field-aspirated blood.[102] There is no credible evidence that heparin-coated perfusion circuits reduce the need for systemic heparin or reduce bleeding or thrombotic problems associated with CPB. Although the majority of studies indicate that heparin coatings reduce concentrations of C3a and C5b-9,[103] the inflammatory response to CPB is not reduced and the evidence for clinical benefit is not convincing.[104]

Other surface modifications and coatings in development[101] include a phosphorylcholine coating,[105] surface-modifying additives,[107] and a trillium biopassive surface.[106]

Cardiotomy Reservoir and Field Suction

Blood aspirated from the surgical wound may be directed to the cardiotomy reservoir for defoaming, filtration, and storage before it is added directly to the perfusate. A sponge impregnated with a surfactant removes bubbles by reducing surface tension at the blood interface and macro, micro, or combined filters remove particulate emboli. Negative pressure is generated by either a roller pump or vacuum applied to the rigid outer shell of the reservoir. The degree of negative pressure and blood level must be monitored to avoid excessive suction or introducing air into the perfusate.

The cardiotomy suction and reservoir are major sources of hemolysis, particulate and gaseous microemboli, fat globules, cellular aggregates, platelet injury and loss, thrombin generation, and fibrinolysis.[73,77,108] Air aspirated with wound blood contributes to blood activation and destruction and is difficult to remove because of the high proportion of nitrogen, which is poorly soluble in blood. High suction volumes and admixture of air are particularly destructive of platelets and red cells.[108] Commercial reservoirs are designed to minimize air entrainment and excessive injury to blood elements. Air and microemboli removal are also facilitated by allowing aspirated blood to settle within the reservoir before it is added to the perfusate.

An alternative method for recovering field-aspirated blood is to dilute the blood with saline and then remove the saline to return only packed red cells to the perfusate. Two types of centrifugal cell washers automate the process. Intermittant centrifugation (eg, Haemonetics Cell Saver, Meomonetics Corp., Braintree, MA) removes air, thrombin, and many biologic and nonbiologic microemboli from the aspirate at the cost of discarding plasma. Continuous centrifugation (eg, Fresenius/Terumo CATS, Elkton, MD) in addition removes fat and activated leukocytes.[109] A third alternative is to discard all field-aspirated blood, although most surgeons would find this practice unacceptible if it increased allogeneic blood transfusion. Increasingly, field-aspirated blood is recognized as a major contributor to the thrombotic, bleeding, and inflammatory complications of CPB.

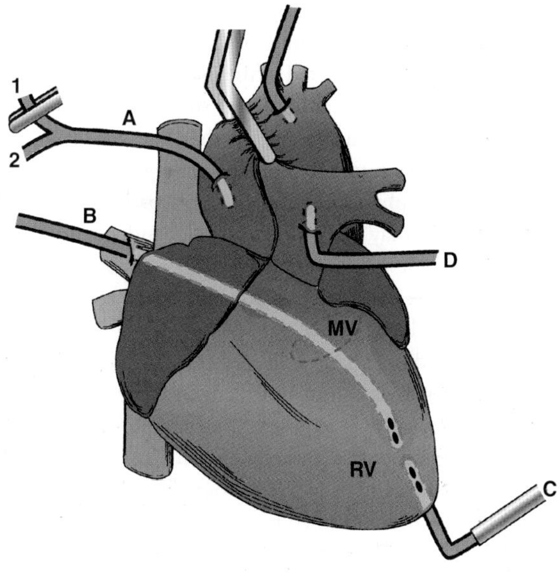

FIGURE 12-6 Diagram shows locations used to vent (decompress the heart). (A) Aortic root vent, which can also be used to administer cardioplegic solution after the ascending aorta is clamped. (B) A catheter placed in the right superior pulmonary vein/left atrial junction can be passed through the mitral valve into the left ventricle. (C) Direct venting of the left ventricle at the apex. (D) Venting the main pulmonary artery, which decompresses the left atrium because pulmonary veins lack valves.

Venting the Heart

If the heart is unable to contract, distention of either ventricle is detrimental to subsequent contractility.[110] Right ventricular distention during cardiac arrest or ventricular fibrillation is rarely a problem, but left ventricular distention can be insidious in that blood can enter the flaccid, thick-walled chamber from multiple sources during this period. During CPB, blood escaping atrial or venous cannulas and from the coronary sinus and thebesian veins may pass through the unopened right heart into the pulmonary circulation. This blood plus bronchial arterial and venous blood, blood regurgitating through the aortic valve, and blood from undiagnosed abnormal sources (patent foramen ovale, patent ductus, etc.) may distend the left ventricle unless a vent catheter is used (Fig. 12-6). During CPB bronchial blood and noncoronary collateral flow average approximately 140 ± 182 and 48 ± 74 mL/min, respectively.[111]

There are several methods for venting the left heart during cardiac arrest. Although it was used commonly in the past, few surgeons in the modern era vent the left ventricular apex directly because of inconvenience and myocardial injury. Most often a multihole, soft-tip catheter (8 to 10 French) is inserted into the junction of the right superior pulmonary vein and left atrium (see Fig. 12-6) or left atrial appendage and may or may not be passed into the left ventricle. Others prefer to place a small suction catheter into the pulmonary artery.[112] The ventricle can also be vented by passing a catheter retrograde across the aortic valve when working on the mitral valve. Vent catheters are drained to the cardiotomy reservoir by a roller pump, vacuum source, or gravity drainage,[113] but must be carefully monitored for malfunction. If connected to a roller pump, the system should be carefully tested before use to ensure proper operation. Although inspection and palpation may detect ventricular distention, TEE monitoring or direct measurements of left atrial or pulmonary arterial pressures are more reliable. The heart is no longer vented for most myocardial revascularization operations, but the ventricle must be protected from distention.[114] If the heart cannot remain decompressed during distal anastomoses, a vent should be inserted. Often the cardioplegia line inserted into the aortic root is used for venting when not used for cardioplegia.[115]

The most common and serious complication of left heart venting is residual air when the heart is filled and begins to contract. De-airing maneuvers and TEE are important methods for ensuring removal of all residual air. In addition, many surgeons aspirate the ascending aorta via a small metal or plastic cannula to detect and remove any escaping air as the heart begins to eject.[116] Bleeding, atrial perforation, mitral valve injury, and direct injury to the myocardium are other complications associated with left ventricular vents.

Cardioplegia Delivery Systems

Cardioplegic solutions contain 8 to 20 mEq/L potassium, magnesium, and often other components that are infused into the aortic root proximal to the aortic cross clamp, or retrograde into the coronary sinus to arrest the heart in diastole. The carrier may be crystalloid or blood and is infused at temperatures around 4 or 37°C, depending upon surgeon's preference. Normothermic cardioplegia must be delivered almost continuously to keep the heart arrested while cold cardioplegia may be infused intermittently. Cardioplegic solutions are delivered through a separate perfusion system that includes a reservoir, heat exchanger, roller pump, bubble trap, and perhaps microfilter (see Fig. 12-2). Temperature and infusion pressure are monitored. The system may be completely independent of the main perfusion circuit or it may branch from the arterial line. The system also may be configured to vent the aortic root when not delivering cardioplegia.

Antegrade cardioplegia is delivered through a small cannula in the aortic root or via cannulas directly into the coronary ostia when the aortic valve is exposed. Retrograde cardioplegia is delivered through a cuffed catheter inserted into the coronary sinus.[117] Proper placement of the retrograde catheter is critical, but not difficult, and is verified by palpation, TEE, color of the aspirated blood, or pressure waveform of a catheter pressure sensor.[118] Complications of retrograde cardioplegia include rupture or perforation of the sinus, hematoma, and rupture of the catheter cuff.[119]

Hemoconcentrators (Hemofiltration/Ultrafiltration)

Hemoconcentrators, like oxygenators, contain one of several available semipermeable membranes (typically hollow fibers) that transfer water, electrolytes (eg, potassium), and molecules up to 20 kDa out of the blood compartment.[120] Hemoconcentrators may be connected to either venous or arterial lines or a reservoir in the main perfusion circuit, but require high pressure in the blood compartment to effect fluid removal. Thus a roller pump is needed unless connected to the arterial line. Suction may or may not be applied to the air side of the membrane to facilitate filtration. Up to 180 mL/min of fluid can be removed at flows of 500 mL/min.[121] Hemoconcentrators conserve platelets and most plasma proteins as compared with centrifugal cell washers, and may allow greater control of potassium concentrations than diuretics.[122] Aside from cost, disadvantages are few and adverse effects are rare.[121]

Perfusion Monitors and Safety Devices

Table 12-3 lists monitors and safety devices that are commonly used during CPB. *Pressure in the arterial line* between pump and arterial line filter is monitored continuously to instantly detect any increased resistance to arterial inflow into the patient. This pressure should be higher than radial arterial pressure because of resistance of the filter (if used) and cannula. The arterial pressure monitor may be connected to an audible alarm or the pump switch to alert the perfusionist to dangerous increases in the arterial line pressure.

An *arterial line flowmeter* is essential for centrifugal pumps and may be desirable to confirm flow calculations with roller pumps as well.

In-line devices are available to continuously measure *blood gases, hemoglobin/hematocrit,* and *some electrolytes.*[123] Placed within the venous line, these devices permit continuous assessment of oxygen supply and demand.[124] In the arterial line the devices offer better control of blood gases.[125] The need for these devices is unproved and because reliability is still uncertain, use may distract operative personnel and spawn unnecessary laboratory measurements.[126] The use of automated analyzers by the perfusion team in the operating room is an alternative if frequent

TABLE 12-3 Safety Devices and Procedures

Device or Procedure	Usage (%)*
Low venous blood level alarm With pump cut-off	60–100 34–80
High arterial line pressure alarm With pump cut-off	84–94 35–75
Macrobubble detector With pump cut-off	42–88 62–63
Arterial line filter	44–99
Pre-bypass recirculation/filtration	75–81
Oxygen supply filter	81–95
In-line venous oxygen saturation	75–76
In-line arterial oxygen saturation	12–13
Oxygenator gas supply oxygen analyzer	43–53
One-way valved intracardiac vent lines	18–73
Batteries in heart-lung machine	29–85
Alternate dedicated power supply	36
Electrical generator	28
Back-up arterial pump head	80
Back-up heater-cooler	97
Back-up oxygen supply	88–91
Emergency lighting	62–91
Pre-bypass activated clotting time	74–99
Activated clotting time during cardiopulmonary bypass	83
Pre-bypass check list	74–95
Written protocols	49–75
Log of perfusion incidents	46
Log of device failures	52

Usage data represent ranges from various surveys, in references 94, 151, 354, 363, and 364.

measurement of blood gases, hematocrit, and electrolytes is desirable.[123]

The *flow and concentration of oxygen* entering the oxygenator should be monitored.[127] Some teams also monitor exit gases to indirectly estimate metabolic activity and depth of anesthesia.[127] Some manufacturers recommend monitoring the *pressure gradient across membrane oxygenators,* which may be an early indication of oxygenator failure, although it is a rare event.[62–64]

Temperatures of the water entering heat exchangers must be monitored and carefully controlled to prevent blood protein denaturation and gaseous microemboli.[65] During operations using deep hypothermia, changes in venous line temperatures reflect rates of temperature change in the patient, and monitoring arterial inflow temperature helps prevent brain hyperthermia during rewarming.

A *low-level sensor* with alarms on the venous reservoir and a bubble detector on the arterial line are additional safety devices sometimes used. A *one-way valve* is recommended in the purge line between an arterial filter/bubble trap and cardiotomy reservoir to prevent air embolism. Ultrasound transducers imbedded in the arterial perfusion tubing distal to the filter are now available to monitor low-level air entry into the circulation. Valves in the venous and vent lines protect against retrograde air entry into the circulation or in the arterial line to prevent inadvertent exsanguination.[68]

Automatic data collection systems are available for preoperative calculations and to process and store data during CPB.[128] Computer systems for operating CPB are in development.[129]

CONDUCT OF CARDIOPULMONARY BYPASS

The Perfusion Team

Although the surgeon is directly responsible for the outcome of the operation, he or she needs a close working relationship with both the anesthesiologist and the perfusionist. These three principals must communicate freely, often, and candidly. Their overlapping and independent responsibilities relevant to CPB are best defined by written policies that include protocols for various types of operations and emergencies and by periodic multidisciplinary conferences. This teamwork is not unlike the communication advocated for the cockpit crew of commercial and military aircraft.

The surgeon determines the planned operation, target perfusion temperatures, methods of cardioplegia, cannulations, and anticipated special procedures. During operation the surgeon communicates the procedural steps involved in connecting and disconnecting the patient to CPB and interacts with the other principals to coordinate perfusion management with surgical exposure and working conditions. The perfusionist is responsible for setting up and priming the heart-lung machine, performing safety checks, operating the heart-lung machine, monitoring the conduct of bypass, monitoring anticoagulation, adding prescribed drugs, and maintaining a written perfusion record.

The anesthesiologist monitors the operative field, anesthetic state and ventilation of the patient, the patient's physiology, and conduct of perfusion. A vigilant anesthesiologist is the safety officer and often "troubleshooter" of these complex procedures and along with the surgeon is in the best position to anticipate, detect, and correct deviations from desired conditions. In addition the anesthesiologist provides TEE observations before, during, and immediately after bypass.

Assembly of Heart-Lung Machine

The perfusionist is responsible for setting up and preparing the heart-lung machine and all associated components necessary for the proposed operation. Most perfusionists use commercial, sterile, pre-prepared customized tubing packs that are connected to the various components that constitute the heart-lung machine. This dry assembly takes about 10 to 15 minutes, and a dry system can be kept in standby for up to 7 days. Once the system is primed with fluid, which takes about 15 minutes, it should be used within 8 hours to prevent malfunction of the oxygenator. After assembly, the perfusionist conducts a safety inspection and completes a written pre-bypass checklist.

Priming

Traditional adult extracorporeal perfusion circuits require 1.5 to 2.0 L of balanced electrolyte solution such as lactated Ringer's solution, Normosol-A, or Plasma-Lyte. Before connections are made to the patient, the prime is recirculated through a micropore filter to remove any residual particulate matter or air. In the average-sized adult, the priming volume represents approximately 30 to 35% of the patient's blood volume and reduces the hematocrit to about two-thirds of the preoperative value. In smaller patients or in the presence of peroperative anemia, banked blood may be added to the prime volume to raise the hematocrit to a predetermined minimum (eg, 25% or more), to achieve an acceptable resultant hemotocrit once CPB has been initiated. There is no consensus regarding the optimal hematocrit during CPB; most perfusates have hematocrits between 20 and 25% when used with moderate hypothermia (25 to 32°C). Dilution reduces perfusate viscosity, which is not a problem during clinical CPB, but also reduces oxygen-carrying capacity; mixed venous oxygen saturations less than 60% usually prompt either transfusion or increased pump flow.[124] Sometimes 12.5 to 50 g of mannitol is added to stimulate diuresis and possibly minimize postoperative renal dysfunction.

Efforts to avoid the use of autologous blood include reducing the priming requirement of the machine by using smaller-diameter and shorter tubing lengths and operating the machine with minimal perfusate in the venous and cardiotomy reservoirs. This latter practice increases the risk of air embolism, the risk of which can be reduced by using collapsible reservoirs and reservoir level sensors that stop the pump. In recent years, smaller, more compact circuits have been designed to reduce the prime volume and subsequent hemodilution, reducing transfusion requirements and platelet consumption.[130] Many of these circuits have totally removed the venous reservoir and used a variety of coated surfaces in an attempt to reduce hemodilution, avoid points of stasis and minimize activation of inflammation and coagulation cascades. A typical such mini-circuit is pictured in Fig. 12-7.

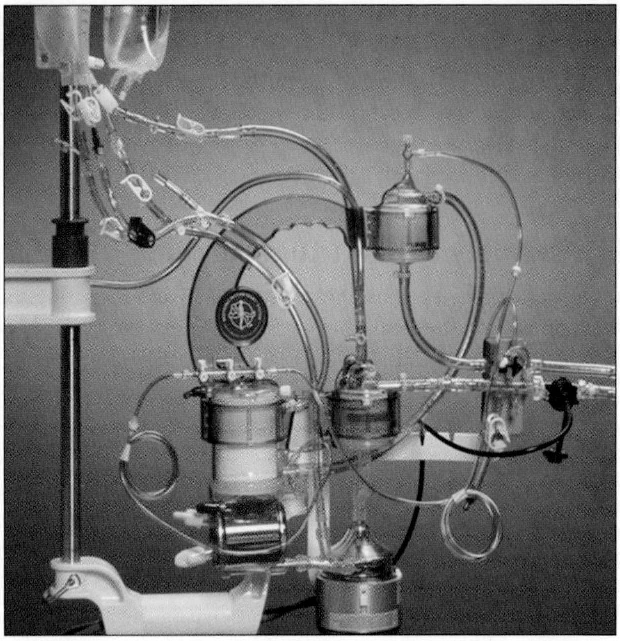

FIGURE 12-7 Typical miniature closed cardiopulmonary bypass circuit that uses coated surfaces to reduce coagulation and inflammation and removes the venous reservior and excess tubing to reduce hemodilution.

Autologous blood prime is another technique to minimize hemodilution, which displaces and then removes crystalloid prime by draining blood volume from the patient into the circuit just before beginning CPB.[131] This method reduces perfusate volume, but phenylephrine may be required to maintain stable hemodynamics.[131] The method reduces transfusions and does not affect clinical outcome.

The use of colloids (albumin, gelatins, dextrans, and hetastarches) in the priming volume is controversial.[132] Although their use clearly minimizes the decrease in colloid osmotic pressure[133] and may reduce the amount of fluid entering the extracellular space, any impact on clinical outcome remains unproved. Prospective clinical studies have failed to document significant clinical benefits with albumin,[133] which is expensive and may have adverse effects.[134] Hetastarch may contribute to postoperative bleeding.[135] McKnight et al. found no influence of prime composition on postoperative nitrogen balance.[136] Because of possible adverse effects, including neurologic deficits, the addition of glucose and/or lactate to the prime is generally avoided.[137,138]

Anticoagulation and Reversal

Porcine heparin (300 to 400 units/kg IV) is administered before arterial or venous cannulas are inserted, and CPB is not started until anticoagulation is confirmed by either an activated clotting time (ACT) or the Hepcon test. Although widely used, bovine heparin is more antigenic in inducing antiplatelet IgG antibodies than is porcine heparin.[139] Although the distribution of intravenously administered heparin has been shown to be extremely rapid,[140] in general, the anticoagulation effect is measured about 3 minutes after heparin administration. However, groups differ in the minimum ACT that is considered safe for CPB. The generally accepted minimum for ACT before initiation of CPB is greater than or equal to 400 seconds; however, many groups recommend 480 seconds[141] because heparin only partially inhibits thrombin formation during CPB. More recently, in an attempt to reduce surgical bleeding, some centers have advocated accepting lower ACTs in the 300 range. Although early unpublished results may suggest that this can be done safely, it is still not generally accepted. Outside the United States, where aprotinin is still available, it is important to measure ACT with kaolin as opposed to celite, because celite may artifactually and erroneously increases the ACT. Failure to achieve a satisfactory ACT may result from either inadequate heparin dosage or low concentrations of antithrombin. If a total of 500 units/kg of heparin fails to adequately prolong ACT, antithrombin III should be administered to the patient either as fresh-frozen plasma or as recombinant antithrombin III when available[142] to increase antithrombin concentrations to overcome "heparin resistance." Antithrombin III is a necessary cofactor that binds circulating thrombin; heparin accelerates this reaction a thousandfold. See Thrombosis and Bleeding for mangagement of patients with suspected or proved heparin-induced antiplatelet IgG antibodies and alternative anticoagulants to heparin.

During CPB, ACT or the Hepcon test is measured every 30 minutes. If ACT goes below the target level, more heparin is given. As a general rule, one-third of the initial total heparin bolus required for adequate anticoagulation is given every hour even when the ACT is within the normal range. The Hepcon test titrates the heparin concentration and is more reproducible than ACT, but ACT provides satisfactory monitoring of anticoagulation. Although excessively high concentrations of heparin (ACT >1000 s) may cause remote bleeding away from operative sites, low concentrations increase circulating thrombin concentrations and risk clotting within the extracorporeal perfusion circuit.

After the patient has successfully weaned from CPB and remains stable, 1 mg of protamine is given for each 100 units of heparin given in the initial bolus dose, but not to exceed 3 mg/kg. The heparin–protamine complex activates complement and may causes acute hypotension, which may be attenuated by the administration of calcium (2 mg/1 mg protamine). Once the administration of protamine has begun, it is generally recommended that the use of cardiotomy suction into the reservoir is discontinued because of the risk of generating clot within the circuit and losing the potential for emergency support should the patient become unstable. Rarely, protamine may cause an anaphylactic reaction in patients with antibodies to protamine insulin.[143] This severe reaction may require urgently placing the patient back on CPB, although it may also be treating with resuscitation using epinephrine and immediate discontinuation of the protamine infusion. Neutralization of heparin is usually confirmed by an ACT or Hepcon test and more protamine (50 mg) is given if either test remains prolonged and bleeding is a problem. *Heparin rebound* is a term used to describe a delayed heparin effect because of release of tissue heparin after protamine is cleared from the circulation, particularly from heparin deposited in adipose tissues, and seen more often in obese patients. Although protamine is a mild anticoagulant at higher doses, one or two supplemental 25- to 50-mg doses can be given empirically if heparin rebound is suspected, or if the ACT remains elevated. It is also noted that the ACT can be elevated in the presence of significant thrombocytopenia, despite the full reversal of heparin. As a rule, the heart-lung machine should be available for unexpected decompensation and the need for urgent return to CPB until the wound is closed, the drapes are removed, and at many centers until the patient leaves the operating room.

Initiation of Cardiopulmonary Bypass

Once the appropriate cannulation has occurred and adequate anticoagulation has been confirmed, CPB is initiated at the surgeon's request with concurrence of the anesthesiologist and perfusionist. As the venous return enters the machine, the perfusionist progressively increases arterial flow while monitoring the patient's blood pressure and volume levels in all reservoirs. Six observations are critical:

1. Is venous drainage adequate for the desired flow?
2. Is pressure in the arterial line acceptable?
3. Is arterial blood adequately oxygenated?
4. Is systemic arterial pressure acceptable?
5. Is systemic venous pressure acceptable?
6. Is the heart adequately decompressed?

Once full stable cardiopulmonary bypass is established for at least 2 minutes, lung ventilation is discontinued, perfusion cooling may begin, and the aorta may be clamped for arresting the heart. Just as is seen with initiation of dialysis, it is not uncommon to see some vasodilation and early hypotension as the patient is first exposed to the artificial surfaces, particularly the oxygenator. This can usually be managed by the perfusionist with increased flows until the vasodilation resolves, although occassionally vasopressors such as neosynephrine may be transiently required.

Cardioplegia

Antegrade blood or crystalloid cardioplegia is administered directly into the aortic root at 60 to 100 mm Hg pressure proximal to the aortic cross-clamp by a dedicated cardioplegia roller pump (see Fig. 12-2). Blood entering the right atrium from the coronary sinus is captured by the right atrial or unsnared caval catheters. If the caval snares are tightened, the right atrium should be vented to prevent right ventricular distention. Many surgeons choose to monitor myocardial temperature and administer cardioplegia to cool the myocardium to a specific temperature range. Others deliver a specific amount of cardioplegia, or moniter the electrical activity to determine the delivered volume. With appropriate delivery of antegrade cardioplegia, the heart should usually arrest within 30 to 60 seconds, and failure to do so may indicate problems with delivery of the solution or unrecognized aortic regurgitation. Some surgeons monitor myocardial temperature or pH via direct needle sensors.[144]

The usual flow of retrograde cardioplegia is 200 to 400 mL/min at coronary sinus pressures between 30 and 50 mm Hg.[145] Higher pressures may injure the coronary venous system[119]; low pressures usually indicate inadequate delivery owing to malposition of the catheter or leakage around the catheter cuff, but may also indicate a tear in the coronary sinus. Induction of electrical arrest is slower (2 to 4 minutes) than with antegrade delivery, and retrograde cardioplegia may provide incomplete protection of the right ventricle.[117]

Key Determinants of Safe Perfusion

The following offers rational guidelines for management of CPB, which uses manipulation of temperature, hematocrit, pressure, and flow rate to adequately support cellular metabolism during nonphysiologic conditions.

Blood Flow Rate

Under normal circumstances, basal cardiac output is determined by oxygen consumption, which is approximately 250 mL/min. It is impractical to measure oxygen consumption while on CPB, so a generally accepted flow rate at 35 to 37°C with a hematocrit of 25% is approximately 2.4 L/min/m^2 in deeply anesthetized and muscle-relaxed patients. Hemodilution reduces blood oxygen content from approximately 20 to 10 to 12 mL/dL; consequently, flow rate must increase over resting normal cardiac output or oxygen demand must decrease. The resistance of venous catheters, turbulence, and loss of physiologic controls of the vasculature may also effect venous return and limit maximum pump flow.

Hypothermia reduces oxygen consumption by a factor of 0.5 for every 10°C decrease in temperature. However, at both normothermia and hypothermia maximal oxygen consumption falls with decreasing flow as described in the following equation:

$$V_{O_2} = 0.44\,(Q - 62.7) + 71.6$$

This relationship at various temperatures is depicted in Figure 12-8. For this reason Kirklin and Barratt-Boyes[146]

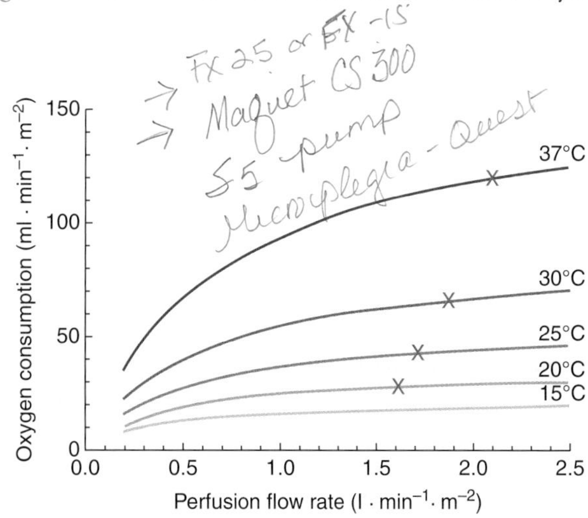

FIGURE 12-8 Nomogram relating oxygen consumption to perfusion flow rate and temperature. The small xs indicate clinical flow rates used by Kirklin and Barratt-Boyes. (*Reproduced with permission from Kirklin JW, Barratt-Boyes BG: Hypothermia, circulatory arrest, and cardiopulmonary bypass, in Kirklin JW, Barratt-Boyes BG [eds]: Cardiac Surgery, 2nd ed. New York, Churchill Livingstone, 1993, p 91.*)

recommend that flows be reduced only to levels that permit at least 85% of maximal oxygen consumption. At 30°C this flow rate in adults is approximately 1.8 L/min/m^2; at 25°C, 1.6 L/min/m^2; and at 18°C, 1.0 L/min/m^2.

As long as mean arterial pressure remains above 50 to 60 mm Hg (ie, above the autoregulatory range), cerebral blood flow is preserved even if systemic flow is less than normal. However, there is a hierarchal reduction of flow to other organs as total systemic flow is progressively reduced. First skeletal muscle flow falls, then abdominal viscera and bowel, and finally renal blood flow.

Pulsatile Flow

Theoretical benefits of pulsatile blood flow include increased transmission of energy to the microcirculation, which reduces critical capillary closing pressure, augments lymph flow, and improves tissue perfusion and cellular metabolism. Theoretically, pulsatile flow reduces vasocontrictive reflexes and neuroendocrine responses and may increase oxygen consumption, reduce acidosis, and improve organ perfusion. However, despite extensive investigation no one has convincingly demonstrated a benefit of pulsatile blood flow over nonpulsatile blood flow for short- or long-term CPB.[71,147] Two studies reported the association of pulsatile flow with lower rates of mortality, myocardial infarction, and low cardiac output syndrome,[148] but others failed to detect clinical benefits.[149]

Pulsatile CPB can reproduce the normal pulse pressure within the body, but is expensive, complicated, and requires a large-diameter aortic cannula. Higher nozzle velocities increase trauma to blood elements,[150] and pulsations may damage micromembrane oxygenators.[151] Thus for clinical CPB, nonpulsatile blood flow is an acceptable, nonphysiologic compromise with few disadvantages.

Arterial Pressure

Systemic arterial blood pressure is a function of flow rate, blood viscosity (hematocrit), and vascular tone. Perfusion of the brain is normally protected by autoregulation, but autoregulation appears to be lost somewhere between 55 and 60 mm Hg during CPB at moderate hypothermia and a hematocrit of 24%.[84,152] Cerebral blood flow may still be adequate at lower arterial pressures,[153] but the only prospective randomized study found a lower combined major morbidity/mortality rate when mean arterial pressure was maintained near 70 mm Hg (average 69 ± 7) rather than below 60 (average 52).[154] In older patients, who may have vascular disease[155] and/or hypertension, mean arterial blood pressure is generally maintained between 70 and 80 mm Hg at 37°C. Higher pressures are undesirable because collateral blood flow to the heart and lungs increases blood in the operative field.

Hypotension during CPB may be the result of low pump flow, aortic dissection, measurement error, or vasodilatation. Phenylephrine is most often used to elevate blood pressure, but arginine vasopressin (0.05 to 0.1 unit/min) has more recently been introduced. If anesthesia is adequate, hypertension can be treated with nitroprusside, an arterial dilator, or nitroglycerin, which predominantly dilates veins and pulmonary vessels.

Hematocrit

The ideal hematocrit during CPB remains controversial. Low hematocrits reduce blood viscosity and hemolysis, reduce oxygen-carrying capacity, and reduce the need for autologous blood transfusion. In general, viscosity remains stable when percent hematocrit and blood temperature (in degrees Celsius) are equal (ie, viscosity is constant at hematocrit 37%, temperature 37°C, or at hematocrit 20%, temperature 20°C). Hypothermia reduces oxygen consumption and permits perfusion at 26°C to 28°C with hematocrits between 18 and 22%, but at higher temperatures limits on pump flow may not satisfy oxygen demand.[156,157] Hill[158] found that hematocrit during CPB did not affect either hospital mortality or neurologic outcome, but DeFoe observed[159] increasing hospital mortality with hematocrits below 23% during CPB; thus the issue remains unresolved.[160] However, higher hematocrits (25 to 30%) during CPB appear justified[157] in view of the increasing safety of autologous blood transfusion, improved neurologic outcomes with higher hematocrits in infant cardiac surgery,[161] and more frequent operations near normothermia in older sicker patients.

Temperature

The ideal temperature for uncomplicated adult cardiac surgery is also an unsettled question.[157] Until recently nearly all operations reduced body temperature to 25 to 30°C during CPB to protect the brain, support hypothermic cardioplegia, permit perfusion at lower flows and hematocrits, and increase the safe duration of circulatory arrest in case of emergency. Hypothermia, however, interferes with enzyme and organ function, aggravates bleeding, increases systemic vascular resistance, delays cardiac recovery, lengthens duration of bypass, increases the risk of cerebral hyperthermia, and is associated with higher levels of depression and anxiety postoperatively.[162] Because the embolic risk of cerebral injury often is greater than perfusion risk, perfusion at higher temperatures (33 to 35°C), or "tepid" CPB, is recommended, in part because detrimental high blood temperatures are avoided during rewarming.[163] Increasingly, efforts are made to avoid cerebral hyperthermia during and after operation, and one study suggests improved neuropsychometric outcomes if patients are rewarmed to only 34°C.[164]

pH/P_{CO_2} Management

There are two strategies for managing pH/P_{CO_2} during hypothermia: pH stat and alpha stat. During deep hypothermia and circulatory arrest (see the following) there is increasing evidence that pH-stat management may produce better neurologic outcomes during pediatric cardiac surgery.[161] Alpha stat may be better in adults.[165] pH stat maintains temperature-corrected pH 7.40 at all temperatures and requires the addition of CC_2 as the patient is cooled. Alpha stat allows the pH to increase during cooling so that blood becomes alkalotic. Cerebral blood flow is higher, and pressure is passive and uncoupled from cerebral oxygen demand with pH stat. With alpha stat, cerebral blood flow is lower, autoregulated, and coupled to cerebral oxygen demand.[166]

Arterial $Pa{O_2}$

PaO_2 should probably be kept above 150 mm Hg to assure complete arterial saturation. Whether or not high levels (ie, >200 mm Hg) are detrimental has not yet been determined.

Glucose

Although Hill[158] found no relationship between blood glucose concentrations during CPB and adverse neurologic outcome, others have been concerned that hyperglycemia (>180 mg/dL) aggravates neurologic injury[138] and other morbidity/mortality,[167] and recently many studies have documented the importance of tight glucose control in the prevention of infection, neurologic injury, renal and cardiac complications, as well as a reduction in ICU length of stay and overall mortality.[168]

Patient Monitors

Systemic arterial pressure is typically monitored by radial, brachial, or femoral arterial catheter. Central venous pressure is routinely monitored by a jugular venous catheter. Routine use of a Swan-Ganz pulmonary arterial catheter is controversial and not necessary for uncomplicated operations in low-risk patients.[169] During CPB the pulmonary artery catheter should be withdrawn into the main pulmonary artery to prevent lung perforation and suture ensnarement.

Transesophageal Echocardiography

A comprehensive transesophageal echocardiography (TEE) examination[170] is an important monitor during most applications of CPB[171] to assess catheter and vent insertion and location[117,172,173]; severity of regional atherosclerosis[33]; myocardial injury, infarction, dilatation, contractility, thrombi, and residual air; undiagnosed anatomic abnormalities[170]; valve function after repair or replacement; diagnosis of dissection[41,174]; and adequacy of de-airing at the end of CPB.[175]

Temperature

Bladder or rectal temperature is usually used to estimate temperature of the main body mass, but does not reflect brain temperature.[176] Esophageal and pulmonary artery temperatures may be affected by local cooling associated with cardioplegia. The jugular venous bulb temperature is considered the best surrogate for brain temperature, but is more cumbersome to obtain.[177] Nasopharyngeal or tympanic membrane temperatures are more commonly used, but tend to underestimate jugular venous bulb temperature during rewarming by 3 to 5°C.[178] During rewarming, arterial line temperature correlates best with jugular venous bulb temperature.[179]

Neurophysiologic Monitoring

The efficacy of neurophysiologic monitoring during CPB is under investigation and not yet established as necessary. Techniques being investigated include jugular venous bulb temperature and saturation, transcranial Doppler ultrasound, near-infrared transcranial reflectance spectroscopy (NIRS), and the raw or processed electroencephalogram (EEG).[180]

Adequacy of Perfusion

During CPB oxygen consumption (VO_2) equals pump flow rate multiplied by the difference in arterial (CaO_2) and venous oxygen content (CVO_2). For a given temperature, maintaining VO_2 at 85% predicted maximum during CPB assures adequate oxygen delivery (see Fig. 12-8).[146] Oxygen delivery (DO_2) equals pump flow multiplied by CaO_2 and should be greater than 250 mL/min/m^2 during normothermic perfusion.[156] Mixed venous oxygen saturation (SVO_2) assesses the relationship between DO_2 and VO_2; values less than 60% indicate inadequate oxygen delivery. Because of differences in regional vascular tone, higher SVO_2 does not assure adequate oxygen delivery to all vascular beds.[181] Metabolic acidosis (base deficit) or elevated lactic acid levels may indicate inadequate perfusion, even in the face of "normal" SVO_2 measurements.

Urine Output

Urine output is usually monitored but varies with renal perfusion, temperature, composition of the pump prime, diuretics, absence of pulsatility, and hemoconcentration. Urine production is reassuring during CPB and oliguria requires investigation.

Gastric Tonometry and Mucosal Flow

These Doppler and laser measurements gauge splanchnic perfusion but are rarely used clinically.

Weaning from Cardiopulmonary Bypass

Before stopping CPB the patient is rewarmed to 34 to 36°C, the heart is defibrillated if necessary, and the lungs are reexpanded and ventilated. The cardiac rhythm is monitored, and hematocrit, blood gases, acid-base status, and plasma electrolytes are reviewed. If the heart has been opened, TEE is recommended for detection and removal of trapped air before the heart is allowed to eject. Caval catheters are adjusted to ensure unobstructed venous return to the heart. If the need for inotropic drugs is anticipated, these are started at low flow rates. Vent catheters are removed, although sometimes an aortic root vent is placed on gentle suction to remove undiscovered air.

Once preparations are completed, the surgeon, anesthesiologist, and perfusionist begin to wean the patient off CPB. The perfusionist gradually occludes the venous line to allow filling of the right heart and ejection through the lungs to the left side, while simultaneously reducing pump input as cardiac rate and rhythm, arterial pressure and pulse, and central venous pressure are monitored and adjusted. Initially blood volume within the pump is kept constant, but as pump flow approaches zero, volume is added or removed from the patient to produce arterial and venous pressures within the physiologic ranges. During weaning, cardiac filling and contractility is often monitored by TEE, and intracardiac repairs and regional myocardial contractility are assessed. Pulse oximetry saturation near 100%, end-tidal CO_2 greather than 25 mm Hg, and mixed venous oxygen saturation higher than 65% confirm satisfactory ventilation and circulation. When cardiac performance is satisfactory and stable, all catheters and cannulas are removed, protamine is given to reverse the heparin, and blood return from the surgical field is discontinued.

Once the patient is hemodynamically stable, as determined by surgeon and anesthesiologist, and after starting wound closure, the perfusate may be returned to the patient in several ways. The entire perfusate may be washed and returned as packed cells, excess fluid may be removed by a hemoconcentrator, or the perfusate, which still contains heparin, can be gradually pumped into the patient for hemoconcentration by the kidneys. Occasionally some of the perfusate must be bagged and given later. The heart-lung machine should not be completely disassembled until the chest is closed and the patient is ready to leave the operating room.

SPECIAL TOPICS

Special Applications of Extracorporeal Perfusion

Reoperations, surgery of the descending thoracic aorta, and minimally invasive procedures may be facilitated by surgical incisions other than midline sternotomy. These alternative incisions often require alternative methods for connecting the patient to the heart-lung machine. Some alternative applications of CPB are presented in the following.

Right Thoracotomy

Anterolateral incisions through the fourth or fifth interspaces provide easy access to the cavae and right atrium, adequate access to the ascending aorta, as well as exposure to the left atrium and mitral valve, but no direct access to the left ventricle. Adequate exposure of the ascending aorta is available for cross-clamping, aortotomy, and administration of cardioplegia by retracting the right atrial appendage. De-airing the left ventricle (eg, after mitral valve repair) is more difficult. External pads facilitate defibrillation.

Left Thoracotomy

Lateral or posterolateral incisions in the left chest are used for a variety of operations. Venous return may be captured by cannulating the pulmonary artery via a stab wound in the right ventricle, or by retrograde cannulation of the left pulmonary artery or cannulation of the left iliac or femoral vein. With iliac or femoral cannulation, venous return may be augmented by threading the cannula into the right atrium using TEE guidance.[182] The descending thoracic aorta or left subclavian, iliac, or femoral arteries are accessible for arterial cannulation.

Left Heart Bypass

Left heart bypass uses the beating right heart to pump blood through the lungs to provide gas exchange.[183] An oxygenator is not used and intake cannulation sites are exposed through a left thoracotomy. The left superior pulmonary vein–left atrial junction is an excellent cannulation site for capturing blood. The left atrial appendage can also be used, but may be more friable and therefore more difficult with which to work. The apex of the left ventricle is infrequently used because of the potential for myocardial injury. The tip of the intake catheter must be free in the left atrium and careful technique is required to avoid air entry during cannulation and perfusion. The extracorporeal circuit typically consists only of tubing and a centrifugal pump and does not include a reservoir, heat exchanger, or bubble trap. This reduces the thrombin burden and may permit reduced or no heparin if anticoagulation poses an additional risk (eg, in acute head injury). Otherwise, full heparin doses are recommended. The reduced perfusion circuit precludes the ability to add or sequester fluid, adjust temperature, or intercept systemic air emboli. Intravenous volume expanders may be needed to maintain adequate flows; temperature usually can be maintained without a heat exchanger.[184]

Full left heart bypass may be employed for left-sided coronary artery surgery by draining all of the pulmonary venous return out of the left atrium and leaving no blood for left ventricular ejection. If the heart fibrillates, blood can still passively pass through the right heart and lungs, but often an elevated central venous pressure is required.[185]

Partial left heart bypass is identical in configuration and cannulation to full left heart bypass and is used to facilitate surgery on the descending thoracic aorta. This accomplishes two goals by providing perfusion to the lower body beyond the aortic clamps, as well as allowing the perfusionist to remove preload as needed by increasing the flow, thereby controlling the perfusion pressure in the proximal aorta, preventing both hypotension, as well as hypertension and potential LV strain. The patient's left ventricle supplies blood to the aorta proximal to aortic clamps, and the circuit supplies blood to the distal body. Typically about two-thirds normal basal cardiac output (ie, 1.6 L/min/m^2) is pumped to the lower body. Arterial pressure is monitored proximal (radial or brachial) and distal (right femoral, pedal) to the aortic clamps. Blood volume in the body and circuit is assessed by central venous pressure and TEE monitoring of chamber dimensions. Management is more complicated because of the single venous circulation and separated arterial circulations.[183]

Partial Cardiopulmonary Bypass

Partial CPB with an oxygenator is also used to facilitate surgery of the descending thoracic aorta. After left thoracotomy, systemic venous and arterial cannulas are placed as described in the preceding. The perfusion circuit includes a reservoir, pump, oxygenator, heat exchanger, and bubble trap. The beating left ventricle supplies the upper body and heart, so lungs must be ventilated and upper body oxygen saturation should be independently monitored. Blood flow to the separate upper and lower circulations must be balanced as described for partial left heart bypass.

Full Cardiopulmonary Bypass

Full CPB with peripheral cannulation is used when access to the chest is dangerous because of proximity of the heart, vital vessels (eg, mammary arterial graft), or pathologic condition (eg, ascending aortic mycotic aneurysm) abutting the anterior chest wall.[3] The patient is supine and a complete extracorporeal perfusion circuit is prepared and primed. Venous cannulas may be inserted into the right atrium via the iliac or femoral vessels and/or the right jugular vein. The iliac, femoral, or axillary-subclavian arteries may be used for arterial cannulation. Initiation of CPB decompresses the heart, but profound cooling is usually deferred to keep the heart beating and decompressed until the surgeon can insert a vent catheter, unless the conduct and complexity of the operation dictate deep hypothermic circulatory arrest prior to dividing the sternum.

Femoral Vein to Femoral Artery Bypass

Femoral vein to femoral artery bypass with full CPB is used to initiate bypass outside the operating room for emergency circulatory assistance,[3] supportive angioplasty,[186] intentional (aneurysm repair) or accidental hypothermia. Femoral vessel cannulation is occasionally used during other operations to facilitate control of bleeding (eg, cranial aneurysm, tumor invading the inferior vena cava) or ensure oxygenation (eg, lung transplantation, upper airway reconstruction).

Cannulation for Minimally Invasive (Limited Access) Surgery

Off-pump coronary artery bypass (OP-CAB) describes construction of coronary arterial bypass grafts on the beating heart without CPB. Minimally invasive direct coronary artery bypass (MID-CAB) refers to coronary arterial bypass grafting with or without CPB through small, strategically placed incisions. Peripheral cannulation sites, described above, may be used, but often central cannulation of the aorta, atrium, or central veins is accomplished using specially designed or smaller cannulas placed through the operative incision or through a separate small incisions in the chest wall.[187] Venous return may be augmented by applying negative pressure (see discussion of venous cannulation above); often soft tipped arterial catheters are used to minimize arterial wall trauma.[20]

The Port-Access System provides a means for full CPB, cardioplegia administration, and aortic cross-clamping without exposing the heart and can be used for both valvular and coronary arterial operations.[173] Through the right internal jugular vein separate transcutaneous catheters are inserted into the coronary sinus for retrograde cardioplegia and the pulmonary artery for left heart venting. A multilumen catheter is inserted through the femoral artery and using TEE and/or fluoroscopy is positioned in the ascending aorta for arterial pump inflow, for balloon occlusion of the ascending aorta, and administration of antegrade cardioplegia into the aortic root. Venous return is captured by a femoral venous catheter advanced into the right atrium. The system allows placement of small skin incisions directly over the parts of the heart that require surgical attention.

Minimally invasive surgery using CPB is associated with potential complications that include perforation of vessels or cardiac chambers, aortic dissection, incomplete de-airing, systemic air embolism, and failure of the balloon aortic clamp.

Because CO_2 is heavier than air and more soluble in blood, the surgical field is sometimes flooded with CO_2 at 5- to 10-L/min flow to displace air when the heart is open. The intra-aortic balloon occluder can leak, prolapse through the aortic valve, or move distally to occlude arch vessels. For safety the position of the occluding balloon is closely monitored by TEE, bilateral radial arterial pressures, and one of the following: transcranial Doppler ultrasound, cerebral near-infrared spectroscopy, or electroencephalogram.[188]

Deep Hypothermic Circulatory Arrest

Deep hypothermic circulatory arrest (DHCA) is commonly used for operations involving the aortic arch, a heavily calcified or porcelain aorta, thoracoabdominal aneurysms, pulmonary thromboendarterectomy, selected uncommon cardiovascular and neurologic procedures,[189] and certain complex congenital heart procedures. The technology involves reducing body temperature to less than 20°C, arresting the circulation for a short period, and then rewarming to 37°C. Deep hypothermia reduces cerebral oxygen consumption (Fig. 12-9), and attenuates release of toxic neurotransmitters and reactive oxidants during ischemia and reperfusion.[190]

Because perfusion cooling produces differential temperatures within both the body and brain,[176] more than one temperature is customarily monitored. Bladder, pulmonary artery, esophageal, or rectal temperatures are used to estimate body temperature. Nasopharyngeal and tympanic membrane temperatures are imperfect surrogates for mean brain temperature. Most surgical teams cool to either EEG silence, jugular venous saturation greater than 95%, or for at least 30 minutes before stopping circulation at nasopharyngeal or tympanic membrane temperatures below 20°C. Caloric exchange is proportional to body mass, rate of perfusion, and temperature differences

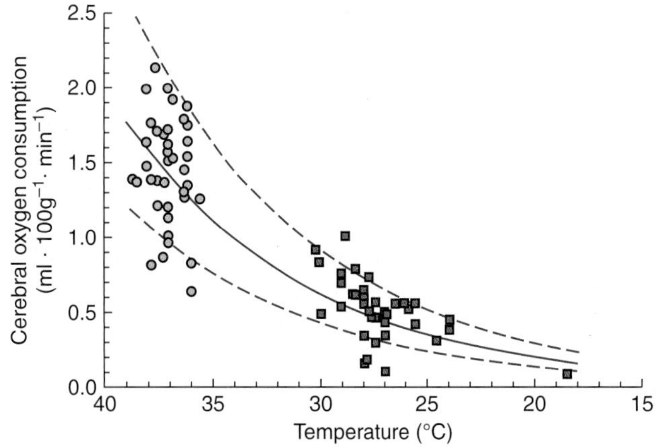

FIGURE 12-9 Relation between cerebral oxygen consumption and nasopharyngeal temperature during CPB at 2 L/min/m². (*Reproduced with permission from Kirklin JW, Barratt-Boyes BG: Hypothermia, circulatory arrest, and cardiopulmonary bypass, in Kirklin JW, Barratt-Boyes BG [eds]: Cardiac Surgery, 2nd ed. New York, Churchill Livingstone, 1993, p 91.*)

between patient and perfusate; however, rates of perfusion cooling and rewarming are restricted (see the section on heat exchangers). Perfusion cooling is usually supplemented by surface cooling using hypothermia blankets and/or packing the head in ice. Hyperthermia is avoided by keeping arterial inflow temperature below 37°C during rewarming, and by avoiding gradients greater than 10° between the inflow blood temperature and the lowest monitored body temperature.

Changes in temperature affect acid-base balance, which must be monitored and managed during deep hypothermia. The pH-stat protocol (CO_2 is added to maintain temperature corrected blood pH at 7.4) may be preferred over the alpha-stat protocol, which allows cold blood to become alkalotic. Compared with alpha-stat, pH-stat increases the rate and uniformity of brain cooling,[191,192] slows the rate of brain oxygen consumption by 30 to 40% at 17°C,[192] and improves neurologic outcomes in animal models[161,193] and in infants,[194] but not necessarily in adults.[195] Hyperglycemia appears to increase brain injury and is avoided during deep hypothermia.[196] The value of high-dose corticosteroids or barbiturates remains unproved.

The safe duration of circulatory arrest during deep hypothermia is unknown. In adults arrest times as short as 25 minutes are associated with poor performance on neuropsychologic tests of fine motor function and memory.[197] Ergin[198] found duration of arrest was a predictor of temporary neurologic dysfunction, which correlated with long-term neuropsychologic deficits.[199] At 18°C, cerebral metabolism and oxygen consumption are 17 to 40% of normothermia[200] and abnormal encephalographic patterns and cerebrovascular responses can be detected after 30 minutes of circulatory arrest.[200] Most investigators,[201] but not all[202] report increased mortality and adverse neurologic outcomes after 40 to 65 minutes of circulatory arrest in adults. Most surgeons try to keep the period of arrest at less than 45 minutes and, if the operation allows, many perfuse for 10 to 15 minutes between serial arrest periods of 10 to 20 minutes. (For more details on DHCA, see Chapter 14.)

Antegrade and Retrograde Cerebral Perfusion

Antegrade cerebral perfusion is used in lieu of DHCA or as a supplement. Once the body has been appropriately cooled as for DHCA, the cerebral vessels can be cannulated separately and perfused together by a single pump[203] or perfused collectively after a graft with a side branch is sewn to the top of the aortic arch from which the innominate, left carotid, and left subclavian arteries originate. Separate perfusion of separately cannulated vessels is rarely done. Perfusion is usually provided by a separate roller pump that receives blood from the arterial line. Line pressure is monitored and a microfilter may or may not be used. The cerebral vessels are collectively perfused with cold blood between 10 and 18°C and at approximate flows of 10 mL/kg/min; perfusion pressures are usually restricted to 30 to 70 mm Hg, though individual protocols vary widely.[204] The adequacy of cerebral perfusion can be assessed by monitoring jugular venous saturation or near-infrared spectroscopy. Selective antegrade cerebral perfusion risks dislodging atheromatous emboli or causing air embolism, cerebral edema, or injury from excessive perfusion pressure.

Retrograde cerebral perfusion (RCP) was initially introduced in 1980 as emergency treatment for massive air embolism.[205] Later, Ueda introduced continuous RCP for cerebral protection as an adjunct to deep hypothermic circulatory arrest during aortic surgery.[206] During RCP and DHCA the superior vena cava is perfused at pressures usually between 25 and 40 mm Hg, temperatures between 8 and 18°C, and flows between 250 and 400 mL/min from a sideport off the arterial line, which is clamped downstream from the sideport. Some surgeons advocate much higher pressures and flows to compensate for runoff and have not shown detrimental effects.[207] A snare is usually placed around the superior caval catheter cephalad to the azygous vein to reduce runoff. The IVC may or may not be occluded.[208]

Retrograde cerebral perfusion has been widely and safely used,[207,209] but its effectiveness in protecting the brain is not clear.[210] The method can wash out some particulate emboli entering from arteries, which is a major cause of brain injury after aortic surgery.[211] However, it is not clear how adequately and completely all regions of the brain are perfused.[210] Lin[209] found cortical flows to be only 10% of control values. RCP slows but does not arrest the decrease in cerebral oxygen saturation[203,207] and the decay in amplitude of somatosensory evoked potentials.[212] Other clinical and animal studies have suggested RCP provides some cerebral protection over DHCA alone.[207,209] A few studies report that antegrade cerebral perfusion provides better protection than the retrograde technique.[203]

Complications and Risk Management

Life-threatening incidents can occur in 0.4 to 2.7% of operations with CPB and the incidence of serious injury or death is between 0.06 and 0.08% (Table 12-4).[61,92] Massive air embolism, aortic dissection, dislodgement of cannulas, and clotting within the circuit during perfusion are the principal causes of serious injury or death. Malfunctions of the heat exchanger, oxygenator, pumps, and electrical supply are the most common threatening incidents related to equipment. Others include premature takedown or clotting within the perfusion circuit.

Massive Air Embolism

The incidence of massive air embolism is between 0.003 to 0.007% with 50% of outcomes adverse.[61,92] Air can enter any component of the perfusion circuit at any time during an operation if the integrity of the circuit is broken.[213] Stopcocks, connections, vent catheters, empty reservoirs, pursestring sutures, cardioplegia infusion catheters, and unremoved air in opened cardiac chambers are the most common sources of air emboli. Uncommon sources include oxygenator membrane leaks, residual air in the circuit after priming, reversal of flow in venous, vent or arterial lines, and unexpected inspiration by the patient during cannula removal.

Massive air embolism during perfusion is a catastrophe, and management guidelines are evolving.[14,205,213] Perfusion should

TABLE 12-4 Adverse Incidents Involving Cardiopulmonary Bypass

	Incidence (Events/1000)	Death or Serious Injury (%)*
Protamine reaction	1.3	10.5
Thrombosis during cardiopulmonary bypass	0.3–0.4	2.6–5.2
Aortic dissection	0.4–0.8	14.3–33.1
Dislodgment of cannula	0.2–1.6	4.2–7.1
Rupture of arterial connection	0.2–0.6	0–3.1
Gas embolism	0.2–1.3	0.2–8.7
Massive systemic gas embolism	0.03–0.07	50–52
Electrical power failure	0.2–1.8	0–0.6
Pump failure	0.4–0.9	0–3.5
Heater-cooler problems	0.5–3	0
Replace oxygenator during cardiopulmonary bypass	0.2–1.3	0–0.7
Other oxygenator problems	0.2–0.9	0
Urgent resetup after takedown	2.9	13
Early unplanned cessation of cardiopulmonary bypass	0.2	0–0.7

Percentage of incidents that resulted in death or serious injury. Data derived from references 94 and 151.

stop immediately and clamps should be placed on both venous and arterial lines. Air in the circuit should be rapidly removed by recirculation and entrapment of all air in a reservoir or bubble trap. The patient should be immediately placed in steep Trendelenburg position and blood and air at the site of entry should be aspirated until no air is retrieved. TEE should be rapidly employed to search for air, but perfusion must resume promptly depending upon body temperature to prevent ischemic brain damage. Cooling to deep hypothermia should be considered to protect the brain and other organs while air is located and removed. As soon as possible, retrograde perfusion of the brain should be undertaken while the aortic arch is simultaneously aspirated with the patient in steep Trendelenburg position. Corticosteroids and/or barbiturates may be considered. Depending upon circumstances and availability, hyperbaric oxygen therapy may be helpful if patients can be treated within 5 hours of operation.[214]

Risk Management

Minimizing risks of extracorporeal perfusion requires strict attention to personnel training, preparation and training for emergencies, equipment function, and record keeping.[14] All members of the operative team must be trained, certified, and recertified in their respective roles and participate in continuing education programs. A policy manual for the perfusion team and written protocols should be developed and continuously updated for various types of operations and emergencies. Emergency kits are prepared for out-of-operating-room (OR) crises. Adequate supplies are stocked in designated locations with sufficient inventory to support any operation or emergency for a specified period. An inventory of supplies is taken and recorded at regular intervals. Checklists are prepared and used for setting up the perfusion system and connecting to the patient. Equipment is inspected at regular intervals; worn, loose, or outdated parts are replaced; and preventive maintenance is provided and documented. New equipment is thoroughly checked before use and instructions are thoroughly digested by all user personnel. Safety alarms are optional; none replace the vigilance and attention of all OR personnel during an operation. Complete, signed written records are required for every perfusion; adverse events are recorded in a separate log and reviewed by the entire OR team. A continuous quality assurance program is desirable.[215]

During the procedure communication must be open among the surgeon, anesthetist, and perfusionist to coordinate activites. Statements are verbally acknowledged. Distractive conversations are discouraged. The entire OR team is committed to a zero-error policy, which can only be achieved by discipline and attention to details.[216]

Section B

Response of Humoral and Cellular Elements of Blood to Extracorporeal Circulation

Within the body the endothelial cell, the only surface in contact with circulating blood, simultaneously maintains the fluidity of blood and the integrity of the vascular system. This remarkable cell maintains a dynamic equilibrium by producing anticoagulants to maintain blood in a fluid state and generating procoagulant substances to enhance gel formation when perturbed. Blood proteins circulate as inert zymogens, which convert to active enzymes when stimulated. Likewise, blood cells remain quiescent until activated to express surface receptors and release proteins and enzymes involved in coagulation and inflammation. The continuous exposure of heparinized blood to the perfusion circuit and to cell tissues and fluid constituents of the wound during clinical cardiac surgery produces an intense thrombotic stimulus that involves both the tissue factor pathway (extrinsic coagulation pathway) in the wound and the contact and intrinsic coagulation pathways in the perfusion circuit. Thrombin is continuously generated and circulated despite massive doses of heparin in all applications of extracorporeal perfusion.[217] This powerful enzyme along with tissue factor from the wound and many other cytokines also activate an inflammatory reaction, which can damage tissues and ultimately produce cell death by necrosis or apoptosis.

THROMBOSIS AND BLEEDING

Initial Reactions in the Perfusion Circuit

When heparinized blood contacts any biomaterial, plasma proteins are instantly adsorbed (<1 second) onto the surface to form a *monolayer* of selected proteins.[218] Different biomaterials have different intrinsic surface activities for each plasma protein. The physical and chemical composition of the *biomaterial surface* determine the intrinsic surface activity of the biomaterial. Thus intrinsic surface activity differs among biomaterial surfaces, plasma proteins, and different bulk concentrations of plasma proteins. The composition of the protein monolayer is specific for the biomaterial and various concentrations of proteins in the plasma, but the topography of the adsorbed protein layer may not be uniform across the surface of the biomaterial.[219] Thus it is not possible to predict the "thrombogenicity" of any biomaterial except by trial and error.

On most biomaterial surfaces fibrinogen is selectively adsorbed, but the adsorbed concentration of fibrinogen and other proteins may change over time.[220] The complexity of blood–biomaterial interactions is further compounded by the fact that adsorbed proteins often undergo limited conformational changes[221] that may expose "receptor" amino acid sequences that are recognized by specific blood cells or bulk plasma proteins.

Thus heparinized blood does not directly contact biomaterial surfaces in extracorporeal perfusion circuits, but contacts

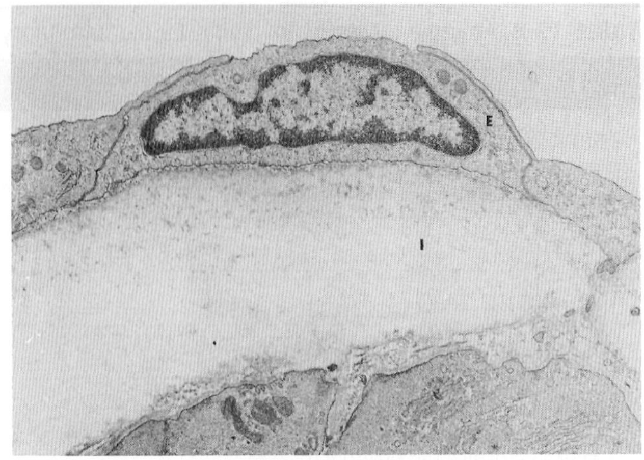

FIGURE 12-10 Electron micrograph of a rabbit endothelial cell (*E*), the only known nonthrombogenic surface. Note the overlapping junctions with neighboring endothelial cells. Endothelial cells rest on the internal elastic lamina (*I*), which abut medial smooth muscle cells. The vessel lumen is at the top. (*Reproduced with permission from Stemerman MB: Anatomy of the blood vessel wall, in Colman RW, Hirsh J, Marder VJ, Salzman E [eds]: Hemostasis and Thrombosis: Basic Principles and Clinical Practice, 2nd ed. Philadelphia, JB Lippincott, 1987, p 775.*)

monolayers of densely packed, immobile plasma proteins arranged in undefined mosaics that differ between locations and possibly across time. All biomaterial surfaces, including heparin-coated surfaces, are *procoagulant*[222]; only the endothelial cell is truly nonthrombogenic (Fig. 12-10).

Anticoagulation

ECP and cardiopulmonary bypass (CPB) are not possible without anticoagulation; the large procoagulant surface quickly overwhelms natural circulating anticoagulants—antithrombin, proteins C and S, tissue factor pathway inhibitor, and plasmin—to produce thrombin and thrombosis within the circuit. Thrombin is produced in extracorporeal perfusion systems with small surface areas and high-velocity flow,[223] but thrombosis may not be apparent if other procoagulants (eg, addition of blood from wounds) are absent. Generation of thrombin varies widely between applications of extracorporeal technology, but this powerful and potentially dangerous enzyme is produced whenever blood contacts a nonendothelial cell surface (Fig. 12-11).

During CPB and open heart surgery (OHS) high concentrations of heparin (3 to 4 mg/kg, initial dose) are needed to maintain the fluidity of blood. Heparin has both advantages and disadvantages; the most notable advantages are parenteral use, immediate onset of action, and rapid reversal by protamine or recombinant platelet factor 4.[224] Heparin does not directly inhibit coagulation, but acts by accelerating the actions of the natural protease, antithrombin.[225] Heparin-catalyzed antithrombin, however, does not inhibit thrombin bound to fibrin[226] or factor Xa bound to platelets within clots[227]; thus, heparin only partially inhibits thrombin in vivo. Antithrombin

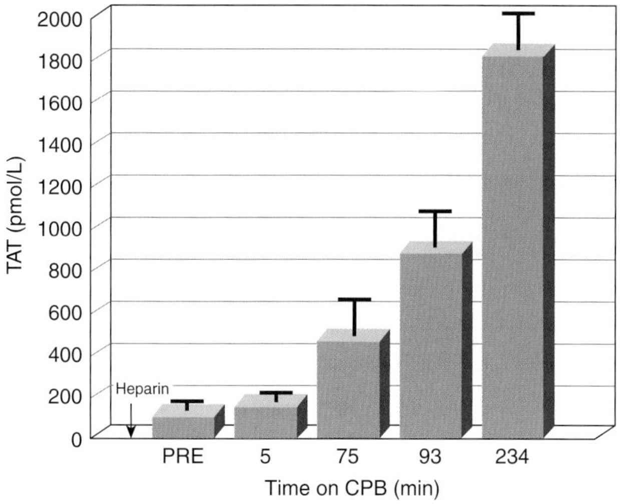

FIGURE 12-11 Plasma thrombin-antithrombin (TAT) measurements of thrombin generation during CPB and clinical cardiac surgery of varying duration. *(Data from Brister SJ, Ofosu FA, Buchanan MR: Thrombin generation during cardiac surgery: is heparin the ideal anticoagulant? Thromb Haemost 1993; 70:259.)*

primarily binds thrombin; its action on factors Xa and IXa is much slower. Heparin inhibits coagulation at the end of the cascade after nearly all other coagulation proteins have been converted to active enzymes. In addition, heparin to varying degrees activates several blood constituents: platelets,[228] factor XII,[229] complement, neutrophils, and monocytes.[230] Thrombin concentrations cannot be measured in real time and only insensitive, indirect methods are available to regulate heparin anticoagulation in the operating room.[231]

Heparin is also associated with some clinical idiosyncrasies. In some patients recent, prolonged parenteral heparin may reduce antithrombin concentrations and produce *heparin resistance.*[232] Insufficient antithrombin may also occur because of insufficient synthesis or increased consumption in cachectic patients and patients with advanced liver or renal disease. The deficiency in antithrombin prevents heparin from prolonging activated clotting times to therapeutic levels. In these patients fresh-frozen plasma or recombinant antithhrombin is needed to increase plasma antithrombin concentrations to inhibit thrombin. *Heparin rebound* is a delayed anticoagulant effect after protamine neutralization because of the rapid metabolism of protamine and delayed seepage of heparin into the circulation from lymphatic tissues and other deposits. Heparin is also associated with an allergic response in some patients that produces heparin-induced thrombocytopenia (HIT) with or without thrombosis (HITT). Lastly, heparin only partially suppresses thrombin formation during CPB and all applications of extracorporeal perfusion and mechanical circulatory and respiratory assistance despite doses two to three times those used for other indications (see Fig. 12-11).[217]

Potential alternatives for heparin during ECP include low molecular weight heparin, danaparoid (Organan), recombinant hirudin (Lepirudin), and the organic chemical, argatroban (Texas Biotechnology Corp.). All have important drawbacks and are approved for use in heparin-induced thrombocytopenia and in patients with circulating IgG anti-heparin–PF4 complex antibodies (see the following). Low molecular weight heparins have long half-lives in plasma (4 to 8 hours), require antithrombin as a cofactor, primarily inhibit factor Xa, and are not reversible by protamine.[233] Danaparoid is a mixture of heparin sulfate, dermatan sulfate, and chrondroitin sulfate that catalyzes antithrombin to inhibit thrombin and factor Xa. The anticoagulant effect is long lasting (plasma half-life 4.3 hours)[234] and is not reversed by protamine.

Recombinant hirudin (Lepirudin) is a direct inhibitor of thrombin, is effective rapidly, does not have an effective antidote, is monitored by the partial thromboplastin time, is cleared by the kidney, and has a relatively short half-life in plasma (40 minutes).[235] This drug has been successfully used during CPB and open heart surgery, but in many instances bleeding after bypass has been troublesome and substantial. A newer drug is a semisynthetic bivalent thrombin inhibitor composed of 12 amino acids from hirudin.[236] This drug, bivalirudin (Angiomax), has a shorter half-life than hirudin and therefore may be safer. Argatroban is also a direct thrombin inhibitor with rapid onset of action and short plasma half-life (40 to 50 minutes).[237] Argatroban is metabolized in the liver and is without an antidote, but can be monitored with partial thromboplastin times or activated clotting times. At present there growing experience with the use of argatroban as an alternative anticoagulant when heparin cannot be used.[238]

Heparin-Associated Thrombocytopenia, Heparin-Induced Thrombocytopenia, and Heparin-Induced Thrombocytopenia and Thrombosis

Heparin-associated thrombocytopenia (HAT) is a benign, nonimmune, 5 to 15% decrease in platelet count that occurs within a few hours to 3 days after heparin exposure. Heparin-induced thrombocytopenia (HIT) and heparin-induced thrombocytopenia and thrombosis (HITT) are different manifestations of the same immune disease. Heparin binds to platelets in the absence of an antibody and releases small amounts of platelet factor 4 (as occurs in HAT). PF4 avidly binds heparin to form a heparin-PF4 (H-PF4) complex, which is antigenic in some people. In these individuals IgG antibodies to the *H-PF4 complex* are produced within 5 to 15 days after exposure to heparin and continue to circulate for approximately 3 to 6 months.[239] *IgG-anti-H-PF4 antibodies* plus *H-PF4 complexes* form *HIT complexes,* which unite IgG Fc terminals to platelet Fc receptors (Fig. 12-12). This binding strongly stimulates platelets to release more PF4.[240] A self-perpetuating, accelerating cascade of platelet activation, release, and aggregation ensues. Since platelet granules contain several procoagulatory proteins (eg, thrombin, fibronectin, factor V, fibrinogen, von Willebrand factor), release also activates coagulation proteins to generate thrombin.

The intensity of the immune reaction varies between patients, but also varies by the indications for heparin use. Patients who do not have conditions that activate platelets have a low incidence of HIT after administration of heparin, because few PF4 molecules are available to form H-PF4 complexes.

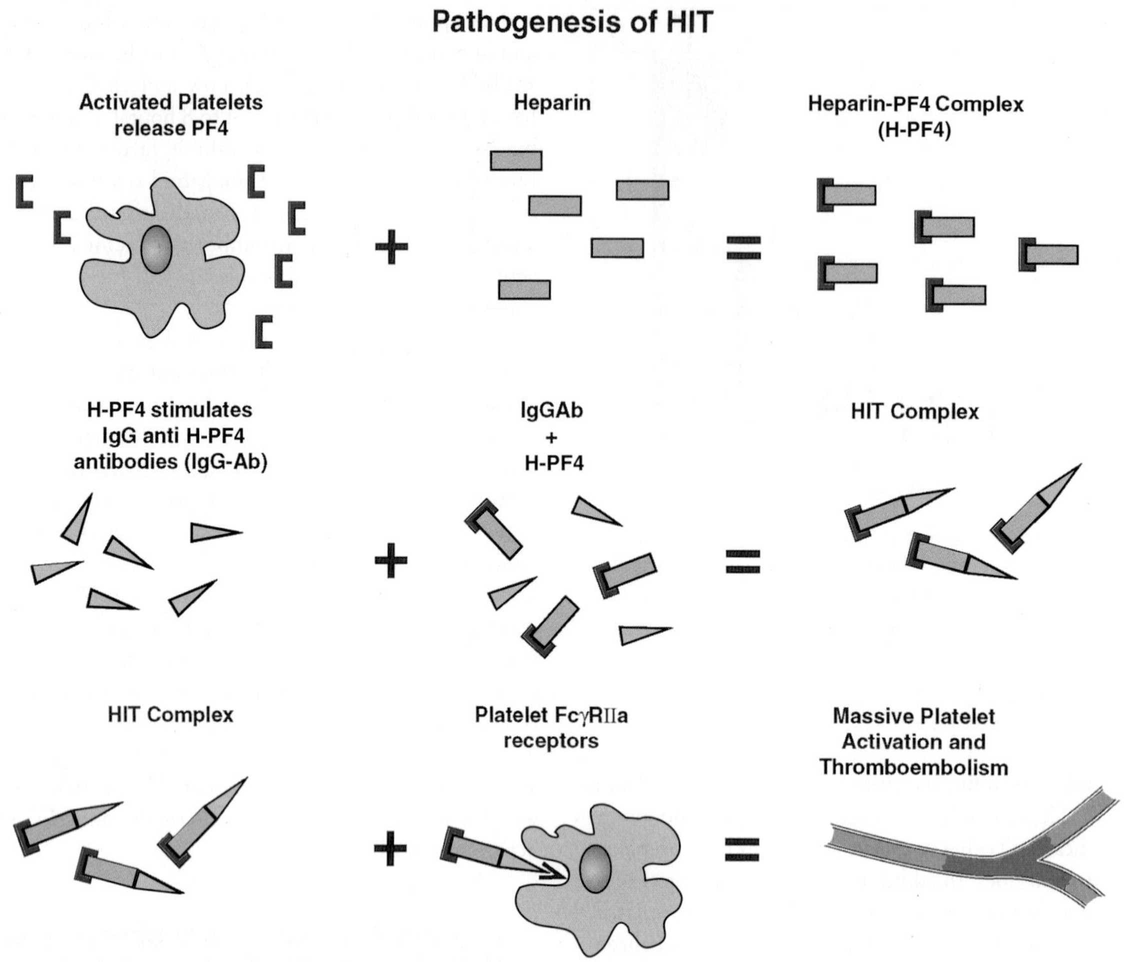

FIGURE 12-12 The generation of HIT complexes. Read each horizontal group of three left to right beginning at top left. See text for full explanation.

Large doses of heparin are given and huge numbers of platelets are activated during CPB. Thus after CPB, 50% of patients have IgG anti-H-PF4 antibodies; 2% have immune heparin-induced thrombocytopenia; and approximately 1% develop HITT.[241] Because IgG antibodies are transient, a second heparin exposure 6 months after HIT is not likely to produce HIT or HITT,[239] but will stimulate production of new IgG antibodies to the H-PF4 complex. The danger is a second heparin exposure when IgG anti-H-PF4 antibodies are still circulating.

IgG anti-H-PF4 antibodies are detected in two ways. The serotonin release test detects the release of radioactive serotonin from normal platelets washed by the patient's serum.[242] An enzyme immunoassay measures IgG anti-H-PF4 antibodies directly. Both assays are equally sensitive in patients with clinical HIT, but the enzyme immunoassay is more sensitive in detecting IgG anti-H-PF4 antibodies in patients without other evidence of the disease.[243]

The clinical presentation of HIT may be insidious. If the platelet count was originally normal, the earliest sign is an abrupt decrease of at least 50% in platelet count (to <150,000/μL) in a patient who has had exposure to heparin within the past 5 to 15 days. This event is a preoperative stop sign for elective cardiac operations. After CPB, platelet counts less than 80,000/μL should trigger an order to stop all heparin, including heparin flushes, and obtain daily platelet counts. The patient should be thoroughly examined for deep vein thrombosis, extremity ischemia, stroke, myocardial infarction, or any evidence of intravascular thrombosis using ultrasound and appropriate radiographic technology. Any evidence of vascular thrombosis should prompt a plasma sample for IgG anti-H-PF4 antibodies. A positive antibody test confirms the diagnosis of HIT in patients with thrombocytopenia and HITT in those with either venous or arterial thrombosis or both. It is important to stress that HIT or HITT is a clinical diagnosis, and a positive antibody test is *not* required before stopping heparin.

Once the diagnosis of HIT or HITT is suspected, management must focus on prevention of further intravascular thrombosis. Bleeding is rarely the problem; intravascular thrombosis is. Neither heparin nor platelet transfusions should be given; platelet transfusions only add more PF4 if heparin and IgG anti-H-PF4 antibodies are still circulating. If heparin is proven absent from the circulation, platelet transfusions may be used very cautiously if the patient has significant nonsurgical bleeding. Surgical measures to reopen thrombosed large arteries are usually futile because the platelet-rich thrombus (white clot) often extends into small arteries and arterioles.

Modern management also includes full anticoagulation with recombinant hirudin (Lepirudin), argatroban, or possibly bivalirudin to prevent further extension of thrombosis or development of clinical intravascular thrombosis. This may occur in 40 to 50% of patients with HIT who are treated only with heparin cessation.[244] At present there is little experience with argatroban in cardiac surgical patients with HITT, but the drug is a direct thrombin inhibitor, has attractive pharmokinetics, and is approved for patients with HITT.[245] Full anticoagulation with hirudin in fresh postoperative cardiac surgical patients is recommended, but the safety zone between bleeding and thrombosis is narrow. The patient must be carefully monitored for pericardial tamponade and signs of hidden bleeding. Hirudin is monitored by aPTT and the range used is similar to that with intravenous heparin. Dose must be reduced in patients with renal failure because the kidney clears the drug. Argatroban is sometimes a better choice, but it should be remembered that it is difficult to manage in the presence of liver disease because it is metabolized in that organ. In most patients oral anticoagulation with warfarin is started at the same time as intravenous hirudin.

Emergency or urgent open heart surgery with CPB using hirudin is possible in patients with circulating IgG anti-HPF4 antibodies. The therapeutic level of drug should be between 3.5 and 4.5 µg/mL during CPB.[246] Greinacher recommends bolus doses of 0.25 mg/kg IV and 0.2 mg/kg in the priming volume followed by an infusion of 0.5 mg/min until 15 minutes before stopping CPB. At that time 5 mg of hirudin is added to the perfusate to prevent clotting within the heart-lung machine.

Coagulation and Extracorporeal Perfusion: Thrombin Generation

Generation of thrombin during cardiopulmonary bypass and other applications of extracorporeal circulatory technology is the cause of the thrombotic and bleeding complications associated with ECP. Theoretically, if thrombin formation could be completely inhibited during ECP, the consumptive coagulopathy, which consumes coagulation proteins and platelets and causes bleeding complications, would not occur.

Thrombin generation and the fibrinolytic response primarily involve the extrinsic and intrinsic coagulation pathways, the contact and fibrinolytic plasma protein systems, and platelets, monocytes, and endothelial cells.

Contact System

The contact system includes four primary plasma proteins—factor XII, prekallikrein, high molecular weight kininogen (HMWK), and C-1 inhibitor and is activated during CPB and clinical cardiac surgery.[247] This system is involved in complement and neutrophil activation and the inflammatory response to ECP, but is not involved in thrombin formation in vivo.

Intrinsic Coagulation Pathway

The intrinsic coagulation pathway probably does not generate thrombin in vivo, but does initiate thrombin formation when blood contacts nonendothelial cell surfaces such as perfusion circuits.[248]

Extrinsic (Tissue Factor) Coagulation Pathway

The extrinsic coagulation pathway is the major coagulation pathway in vivo and is a major source of thrombin generation during CPB and clinical cardiac surgery.[249,250] Exposure of blood to tissue factor by direct contact in the wound or by wound blood aspirated into the ECP circuit initiates the extrinsic coagulation pathway.[251] Tissue factor (TF) is a cell-bound glycoprotein that is constitutively expressed on the cellular surfaces of fat, muscle, bone, epicardium, adventia, injured endothelial cells, and many other cells except pericardium.[252] Plasma TF associated with wound monocytes is a second source of TF and may be an important source during CPB and clinical cardiac surgery.[253]

Common Coagulation Pathway

Factor Xa is the gateway protein of the common coagulation pathway. Factor Xa slowly cleaves prothrombin to α-thrombin, the active enzyme, and a fragment, F1.2, and is the major pathway producing thrombin.[251] F1.2 is a useful marker of the reaction.

Thrombin

Thrombin is a powerful enzyme that accelerates its own formation by several feedback loops.[254] Thrombin is the major activator of factor XI and the exclusive activator of factor VIII in the intrinsic pathway. Thrombin is a secondary activator of factor VII, but once formed may be the most important activator in the wound.

Thrombin has both procoagulant and anticoagulant properties.[254] Thrombin is the enzyme that cleaves fibrinogen to fibrin and in the process creates two fragments, fibrinopeptides A and B. Thrombin activates platelets via the platelet thrombin receptor and thus may be the major agonist for platelets both in the wound and in the perfusion circuit. Thrombin also activates factor XIII to cross-link fibrin to an insoluble form and attenuate fibrinolysis.

Thrombin also stimulates the production of anticoagulants. Surface glycosaminoglycans, such as heparan sulfate, inhibit thrombin and coagulation via antithrombin. Thrombin stimulates endothelial cells to produce tissue plasminogen activator, t-PA, which is the major enzyme that cleaves plasminogen to plasmin, and initiates fibrinolysis.

Thrombin Generation during Extracorporeal Perfusion

All applications of extracorporeal perfusion and exposure of blood to nonendothelial cell surfaces generate thrombin.[217] F1.2 is a protein fragment that is formed when prothrombin is cleaved to thrombin; thus F1.2 is a measure of thrombin generation but not of thrombin activity. F1.2 and thrombin-antithrombin (TAT) complex increase progressively during clinical cardiac surgery with CPB, during applications of circulatory assist devices[255] and during extracorporeal life support (ECLS) (Fig. 12-13). The amount of thrombin produced seems to vary with the intensity of the stimuli for thrombin production and may vary with age, comorbid disease, and clinical health of the patient. Complex cardiac surgery that requires several hours of

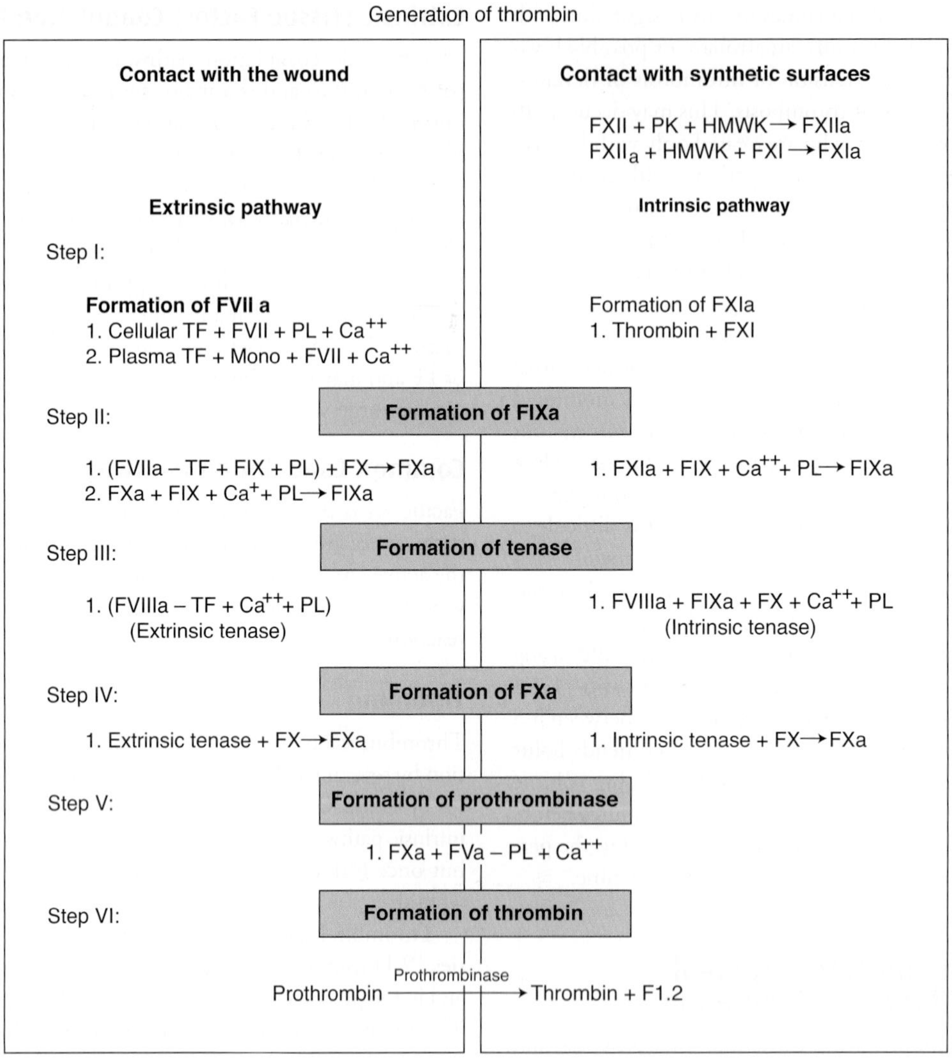

FIGURE 12-13 Steps in the generation of thrombin in the wound and in the perfusion circuit via the extrinsic, intrinsic, and common coagulation pathways. PK, prekallikrein; HMWK, high molecular weight kininogen; Ca^{2+}, calcium ion; PL, cellular phospholipid surface; TF, tissue factor; mono, monocyte. Activated coagulation proteins are indicated by the suffix -a.

CPB produces more F1.2 than short procedures with minimal exposure of circulating blood to the wound.[256] Thrombin generation varies with the amount and type of anticoagulant used; surface area of the blood–biomaterial interface; duration of exposure to the surface; turbulence, stagnation, and cavitation within perfusion circuits; and to a lesser degree temperature and the "thromboresistant" characteristics of biomaterial surfaces.[257]

For many years blood contact with the biomaterials of the perfusion circuit was thought to be the major stimulus to thrombin formation during CPB and OHS. Increasing evidence indicates that the wound is the major source of thrombin generation during CPB and clinical cardiac surgery. This understanding has encouraged development of strategies to reduce the amounts of circulating thrombin during clinical cardiac surgery by either discarding wound blood[258] or exclusively salvaging red cells by centrifugation and washing in a cell saver. The reduced thrombin formation in the perfusion circuit has also supported strategies for reducing the systemic heparin dose during first-time coronary revascularization procedures using heparin-bonded circuits.[259] Although there is no good evidence that heparin-bonded circuits reduce thrombin generation, there is strong evidence that discarding wound plasma or limiting exposure of circulating blood to the wound (eg, less bleeding in the wound) does reduce the circulating thrombin burden.[260]

Cellular Procoagulants and Anticoagulants

Platelets

Platelets are activated by thrombin, contact with the surface of nonendothelial cells, heparin, and platelet-activating factor produced by a variety of cells during all applications of extracorporeal perfusion and/or recirculation of anticoagulated blood that has been exposed to a wound. Circulating thrombin and platelet contact with surface-adsorbed fibrinogen in the perfusion circuit are probably the earliest and strongest agonists. Circulating thrombin, although rapidly inhibited by antithrombin, is a powerful agonist and binds avidly to two specific thrombin receptors on platelets: PAR-1 and GPIbα.[261] As CPB continues, complement, plasmin, hypothermia, epinephrine, and other agonists also activate platelets and contribute to their loss and dysfunction.

The initial platelet reaction to agonists is shape change. Circulating discoid platelets extend pseudopods, centralize granules, express GPIb and GPIIb/IIIa receptors,[262] and secrete soluble and bound P selectin receptors from alpha granules.[263] GPIIb/IIIa ($\alpha_{IIb}\beta3$) receptors almost instantaneously bind platelets to exposed binding sites on the α- and γ-chains on surface-adsorbed fibrinogen (Fig. 12-14),[264] but the rough surfaces accumulate more platelets than smooth surfaces. Platelet adhesion and aggregate formation reduce the circulating platelet count, which is already reduced by dilution with pump priming solutions.

Plasma fibrinogen forms bridges between platelets expressing GPIIb/IIIa receptors to produce circulating platelet aggregates. Platelet bound P-selectin binds platelets to monocytes and neutrophils to form aggregates.[265] During ECP the circulating platelet pool is reduced by dilution, adhesion, aggregation, destruction, and consumption. The platelet mass consists of a reduced number of morphologically normal platelets, platelets with pseudopod formation, new and larger platelets released from megakaryocytes, partially and completely degranulated platelets. Most of the circulating platelets appear structurally normal, but bleeding times increase and remain prolonged for several hours after protamine.[266] The functional state of the circulating intact platelet during and early after CPB is reduced, but it is not clear whether this functional defect is intrinsic or extrinsic to the platelet. Flow cytometry studies of circulating intact platelets show little change in platelet membrane receptors.[267]

Monocytes

In the wound with calcium present, monocytes associate with plasma tissue factor to rapidly accelerate the conversion of factor VII to factor VIIa.[268] This association is specific for monocytes as the reaction is essentially nil for platelets, neutrophils, and lymphocytes—and does not occur if monocytes, plasma tissue factor, or factor VII is not present. The major sources of tissue factor in the wound are the combination of monocytes, plasma tissue factor, and cell-bound tissue factor.

Endothelial Cells

Endothelial cells, charged with maintaining the fluidity of circulating blood and the integrity of the vascular system, are activated during CPB and clinical cardiac surgery by thrombin, C5a, IL-1, and TNF-α.[269] Endothelial cells produce both procoagulants and anticoagulants. Procoagulant activities of endothelial cells include expression of tissue factor and production of a host of procoagulant proteins.[270] Anticoagulant activities of endothelial cells include the production of tissue plasminogen activator (t-PA), heparin sulfate, tissue factor inhibitor protein, prostacyclin, nitric oxide, and adenosine.[271]

Fibrinolysis

Circulating thrombin activates endothelial cells to produce tissue plasminogen activator (t-PA), which binds avidly to fibrin.[272] Endothelial cells are the principal source of t-PA.[273] The combination of t-PA, fibrin, and plasminogen cleaves plasminogen to plasmin; plasmin cleaves fibrin. This reaction produces the protein fragment, D-dimer, which is a useful marker of fibrinolysis, and a marker of thrombin activity because fibrin is cleaved from fibrinogen by thrombin.[274]

Fibrinolysis is controlled by native protease inhibitors, α2-antiplasmin, α2-macroglobulin, and plasminogen activator inhibitor-1.[274] Alpha 2-antiplasmin rapidly inhibits unbound plasmin, preventing the enzyme from circulating, but poorly inhibits plasmin bound to fibrin.

Consumptive Coagulopathy

Simultaneous and ongoing thrombin formation and fibrinolysis is by definition a consumptive coagulopathy[275] and is present

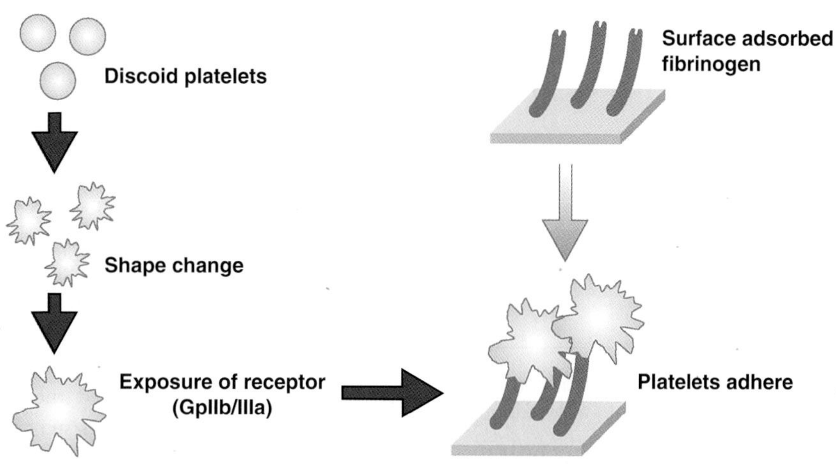

FIGURE 12-14 Adhesion of activated platelets binding to surface-adsorbed fibrinogen via GPIIb/IIIa ($\alpha_{IIb}\beta3$) receptors. The same receptors bind plasma fibrinogen molecules to form platelet aggregates.

in all applications of ECP. In the normal state the fluidity of blood and the integrity of the vascular system are established and maintained by an equilibrium between procoagulants favoring clot and anticoagulants favoring liquidity (Fig. 12-15A). Blood contact with ECP systems and the wound disrupts this equilibrium to produce a massive procoagulant stimulus that overwhelms natural anticoagulants; therefore, an exogenous anticoagulant, heparin, is required for nearly all applications of ECP (Fig. 12-15B). Exceptions are only possible in applications that produce a relatively weak procoagulant stimulus and a minimal thrombin burden that can be contained by natural anticoagulants. Surgeons must realize that any blood exposure to nonendothelial cell surfaces, including prosthetic heart valves, produces a procoagulant stimulus whether or not a clot is produced. Except for the healthy endothelial cell, no nonthrombogenic surface exists.

This concept of an equilibrium between procoagulants and anticoagulants is helpful in managing the thrombotic and bleeding complications associated with all applications of ECP. During ECP procoagulant stimuli, manifested by thrombin formation that is not measurable in real time, must be balanced by *either* increased anticoagulation or a reduction in the thrombin burden to maintain equilibrium. After ECP, anticoagulants must be inhibited to avoid excessive bleeding. During consumptive coagulopathy, coagulation proteins and platelets are consumed and may become too deficient to generate thrombin and fibrin-platelet clots. In cardiac surgical patients many additional variables affect the coagulation equilibrium and impact the availability of coagulation proteins and functional platelets. These variables include the quantity of blood in contact with the wound; surface area of the perfusion system; duration of perfusion; circulating anticoagulants; and to lesser degrees temperature and the rheology and biomaterials of the perfusion system. Patient factors also affect the coagulation equilibrium; these include age, infection, history or presence of cardiogenic shock, massive blood losses and transfusions, platelet coagulation deficiencies, fibrinolysis, liver disease, cachexia, reoperation, and hypothermia.

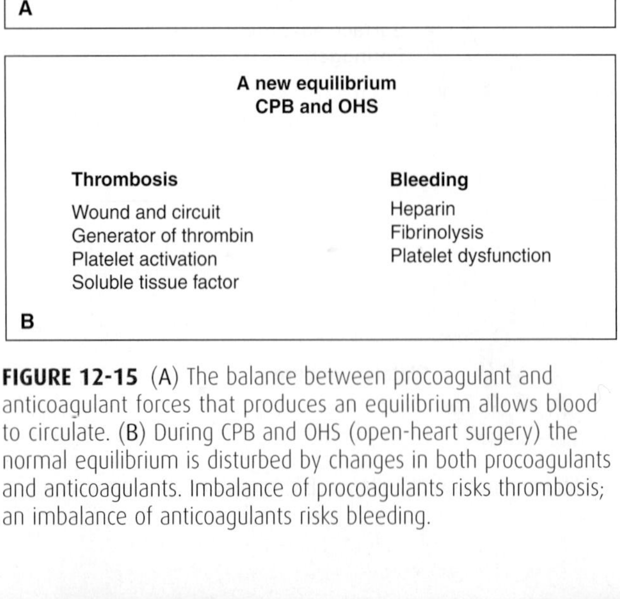

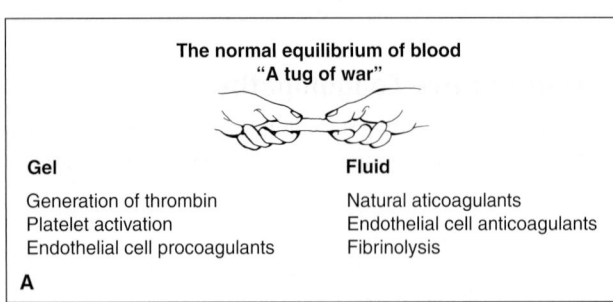

FIGURE 12-15 (A) The balance between procoagulant and anticoagulant forces that produces an equilibrium allows blood to circulate. (B) During CPB and OHS (open-heart surgery) the normal equilibrium is disturbed by changes in both procoagulants and anticoagulants. Imbalance of procoagulants risks thrombosis; an imbalance of anticoagulants risks bleeding.

Management of Bleeding

The cornerstone of bleeding management is meticulous surgical hemostasis during all phases of an operation. The surgical techniques, topical agents, and customary drugs used do not need reiteration for trained surgeons. Most cardiac surgical operations involving CPB are accompanied by net blood losses between 200 to 600 mL. Reoperations; complex procedures; prolonged (>3 hours) cardiopulmonary bypass; and patient factors listed above may be associated with excessive and ongoing blood losses. Most surgeons use an antifibrinolytic, such as tranexamic acid or epsilon amino caproic acid, to reduce fibrinolysis in prolonged or complex operations. Problem patients who bleed excessively after heparin neutralization require an attempt to rebalance procoagulants and anticoagulants to near normal, pre–CPB concentrations.

The most useful tests in the operating room are an activated clotting time or a protamine titration test to assess the presence of heparin; prothrombin time to uncover deficiency in the extrinsic coagulation pathway; and platelet count. If heparin is neutralized, the partial thromboplastin time may be measured to assess possible deficiency of coagulation proteins. Other tests such as measurements of fibrinogen, template bleeding time, and the thromboelastograph are controversial and/or difficult to obtain. Platelet counts below 80,000 to 100,000/μL should initiate platelet transfusions in bleeding patients, except those with IgG anti-H-PF4 antibodies, to add functioning platelets to the mass of partially dysfunctional platelets.

Measurements of F1.2 and D-dimer are two tests that can be very helpful and probably should be made available on an emergency basis in hospitals that perform complex procedures and offer mechanical circulatory and respiratory assistance. F1.2 measures thrombin formation by factor Xa, and if absent or low, there may be a deficiency in the concentrations of coagulation proteins; fresh-frozen plasma is needed. If F1.2 and D-dimer (a measurement of fibrinolytic activity) are both elevated, thrombin is being formed and an antifibrinolytic (Tranexamic acid or epsilon amino caproic acid) is needed to neutralize plasmin. If both markers or F1.2 remain elevated after the antifibrinolytic drug, this indicates continuing thrombin generation, and the cause (eg, infection usually) should be aggressively treated with antibiotics. Some thrombin is needed to stop bleeding, but excessive thrombin production feeds the consumptive coagulopathy. As with diffuse intravascular coagulopathy,[275] no guaranteed therapeutic recipe is known; success requires patience, persistence, and judicious use of platelets, antifibrinolytics, specific clotting factors, and replacement transfusions to rebalance the coagulation equilibrium at near normal concentrations of the constituents.

THE INFLAMMATORY RESPONSE

Primary Blood Constituents

Complement

The complement system constitutes a group of more than 30 plasma proteins that interact to produce powerful vasoactive anaphylatoxins, C3a, C4a, and C5a, and the terminal complement cytotoxic complex, C5b-9.[276] Complement is activated by three pathways, but only the classical and alternative pathways are involved in cardiopulmonary bypass. Direct contact between heparinized blood and the synthetic surfaces of the extracorporeal perfusion circuit activates the contact plasma proteins and the classical complement pathway. Activation of C1, possibly by activated factor XIIa, sequentially activates C2 and C4 to form C4b2a (classical C3 convertase) that cleaves C3 to form C3a and C3b (Fig. 12-16).

Generation of C3b activates the alternative pathway, which involves factors B and D in the formation of C3bBb, which is the alternative pathway C3 convertase that cleaves C3 to form C3a and C3b (see Fig. 12-16). Whereas the classical pathway proceeds in sequential steps, the alternative pathway contains a feedback loop that greatly amplifies cleavage of C3 by membrane-bound C3 convertase to membrane-bound C3b and C3a. During CPB complement is largely activated by the alternative pathway.[277]

The complement system is activated at three different times during CPB and cardiac surgery: during blood contact with nonendothelial cell surfaces[278] and wound exudate–containing tissue factor[279]; after protamine administration and formation of the protamine–heparin complex[280]; and after reperfusion of the ischemic, arrested heart.[281] CPB and myocardial reperfusion activate complement by both the classical and alternative pathways; the heparin-protamine complex activates complement by the classical pathway.

The two C3 convertases effectively merge the two complement pathways by producing C3b, which activates C5 to C5a and C5b (see Fig. 12-16). C3a and C5a are potent vasoactive anaphylatoxins. C5a, which avidly binds to neutrophils and therefore is difficult to detect in plasma, is the major agonist. C3b acts as an opsonin, which binds target cell hydroxyl groups and renders them susceptible to phagocytic cells expressing specific receptors for C3b.[282,283] C5b is the first component of the terminal pathway that ultimately leads to formation of the membrane attack complex, C5b-9. In prokaryotic cells like erythrocytes, C5b-9 creates transmembrane pores, which cause death by intracellular swelling after loss of the intracellular/interstitial osmotic gradient. In eukaryotic cells, deposits of C5b-9 may not be immediately lethal but may eventually cause injury mediated by release of arachidonic acid metabolites (thromboxane A2, leukotrienes) and oxygen free radicals by macrophages and neutrophils, respectively.[284]

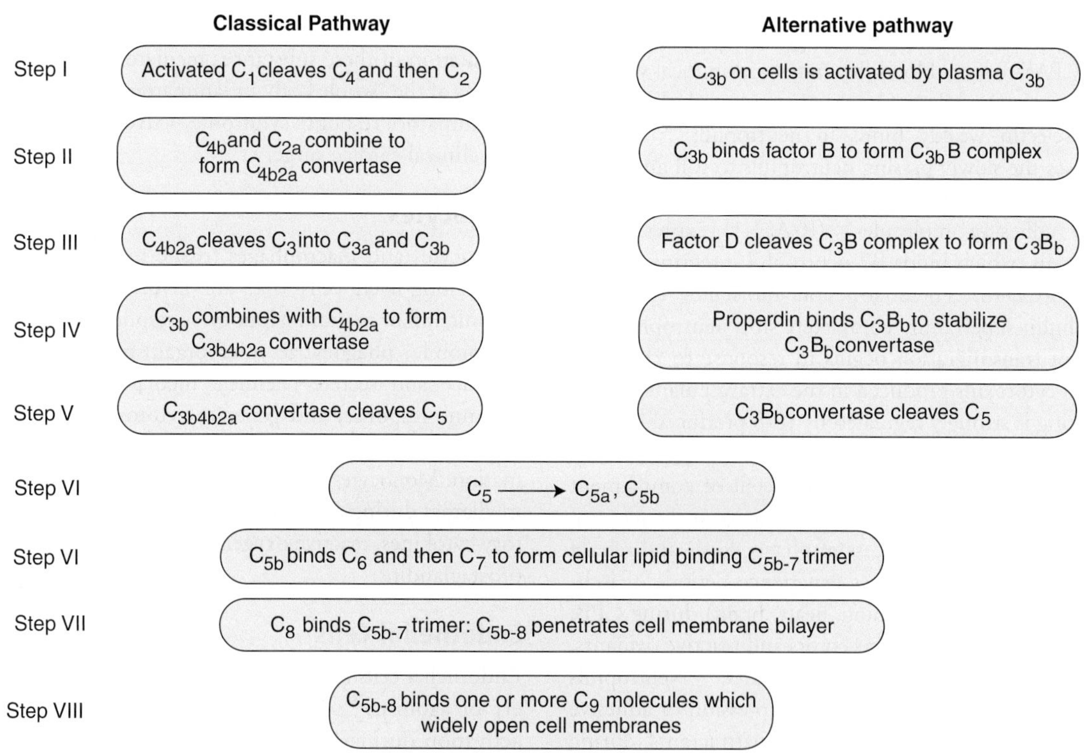

Classical Pathway
Alternative pathway
Step I
Activated C_1 cleaves C_4 and then C_2
C_{3b} on cells is activated by plasma C_{3b}
Step II
C_{4b} and C_{2a} combine to form C_{4b2a} convertase
C_{3b} binds factor B to form C_{3b}B complex
Step III
C_{4b2a} cleaves C_3 into C_{3a} and C_{3b}
Factor D cleaves C_3B complex to form C_3B_b
Step IV
C_{3b} combines with C_{4b2a} to form C_{3b4b2a} convertase
Properdin binds C_3B_b to stabilize C_3B_b convertase
Step V
C_{3b4b2a} convertase cleaves C_5
C_3B_b convertase cleaves C_5
Step VI
$C_5 \longrightarrow C_{5a}, C_{5b}$
Step VI
C_{5b} binds C_6 and then C_7 to form cellular lipid binding $C_{5b\text{-}7}$ trimer
Step VII
C_8 binds $C_{5b\text{-}7}$ trimer: $C_{5b\text{-}8}$ penetrates cell membrane bilayer
Step VIII
$C_{5b\text{-}8}$ binds one or more C_9 molecules which widely open cell membranes

FIGURE 12-16 Steps in activation of the classical and alternative complement pathways and formation of the membrane attack complex, C5b-9. (*Adapted with permission from Walport MJ: Complement. NEJM 2001; 344:1058; and Plumb ME, Sadetz JM: Proteins of the membrane attack complex, in Volkankis JE, Frank ME [eds]: The Human Complement System in Health and Disease. New York, Marcel Dekker, 1998, p 119.*)

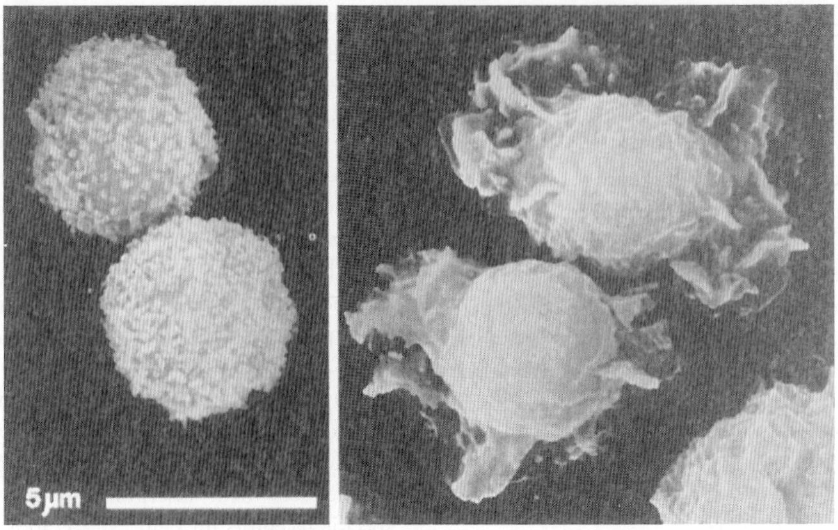

FIGURE 12-17 Scanning electron micrographs of resting neutrophils (*left*) and 5 seconds after exposure to a chemoattractant. (*Reproduced with permission from Baggiolini M: Chemokines and leukocyte traffic. Nature 1998; 392:565.*)

Neutrophils

Neutrophils are strongly activated during cardiopulmonary bypass (Fig. 12-17).[285] The principal agonists are kallikrein and C5a produced by the contact and complement systems. Neutrophils are recruited to localized areas of injury or inflammation by chemokines, complement proteins (C5a), IL-1β, TNF-α, and adhesion molecules. During CPB thrombin stimulates endothelial cell production of platelet activating factor (PAF).[286] Thrombin and PAF cause rapid expression of P-selectin by endothelial cells.[287] Regional vasoconstriction mediated by PAF reduces blood flow rates within local vascular beds to allow neutrophils to marginate near endothelial cell surfaces. P-selectin weakly binds to neutrophils[288]; selectin binding causes the slowly passing neutrophils to roll and eventually stop (Fig. 12-18).[289] Stronger adherence is produced by intracellular adhesion molecule-1 (ICAM-1) expressed on endothelial cells, which binds β2 neutrophil integrins, principally CD11b/CD18. These adhesion molecules from the immunoglobulin superfamily completely stop neutrophils and the process of transmigration begins in response to chemoattractants and cytotoxins produced in the extravascular space.[290] This trafficking is strongly regulated by IL-8 produced by neutrophils, macrophages, and other cells.[291]

Using pseudopods and following the scent of complement proteins (C5a, C3b) and IL-8, neutrophils arrive at the scene of inflammation to begin the process of phagocytosis and release of cytotoxins. Organs and tissues experience periods of ischemia followed by reperfusion (lung, heart, brain) during CPB, and as a result express adhesion receptors and reactive oxidants, and are sources of neutrophil chemoattractants.[292] Neutrophils vary considerably among individuals in expression of adhesive receptors[293] and responsiveness to chemoattractants during CPB. The presence of diabetes, oxidative stress, and perhaps genetic factors (see the following) influences expression of cellular and soluble adhesive receptors and cytokines, which affect neutrophil adhesion and release of granule contents. Neutrophils contain a potent arsenal of proteolytic and cytotoxic substances. Azurophilic granules contain lysozyme, myeloperoxidase, cationic proteins, elastase, and collagenases.[294] Activated neutrophils, in a "respiratory burst," also produce cytotoxic reactive oxygen and nitrogen intermediates including superoxide anion, hydrogen peroxide, hydroxyl radicals, singlet oxygen molecules. Finally, neutrophils produce arachidonate metabolites, prostaglandins, leukotrienes, and platelet-activating factor. During CPB these vasoactive and cytotoxic substances are produced and released into the extracellular environment and circulation. Circulation of these substances mediates many of the manifestations of the "whole body inflammatory response" or "systemic inflammatory response syndrome" (SIRS) associated with CPB and clinical cardiac surgery.[295]

Monocytes

Monocytes and macrophages (tissue monocytes) are relatively large, long-lived cells that are involved in both acute and chronic inflammation. Monocytes respond to chemical signals, are mobile, phagocytize microorganisms and cell fragments, produce and secrete chemical mediators, participate in the immune response, and generate cytotoxins.[296] Monocytes are activated during CPB and have a major role in thrombin formation. Monocytes also produce and release many inflammatory mediators during acute inflammation, including proinflammatory cytokines, reactive oxygen and nitrogen intermediates, and prostaglandins.

Endothelial Cells

Endothelial cells are activated during CPB and OHS by a variety of agonists.[297] The principal agonists for endothelial cell activation during CPB are thrombin, C5a, and the cytokines IL-1β and TNF-α. IL-1β and TNF-α induce the early expression of P-selectin and the later synthesis and expression of E-selectin, which are involved in the initial stages of neutrophil and monocyte adhesion. The two cytokines also induce expression

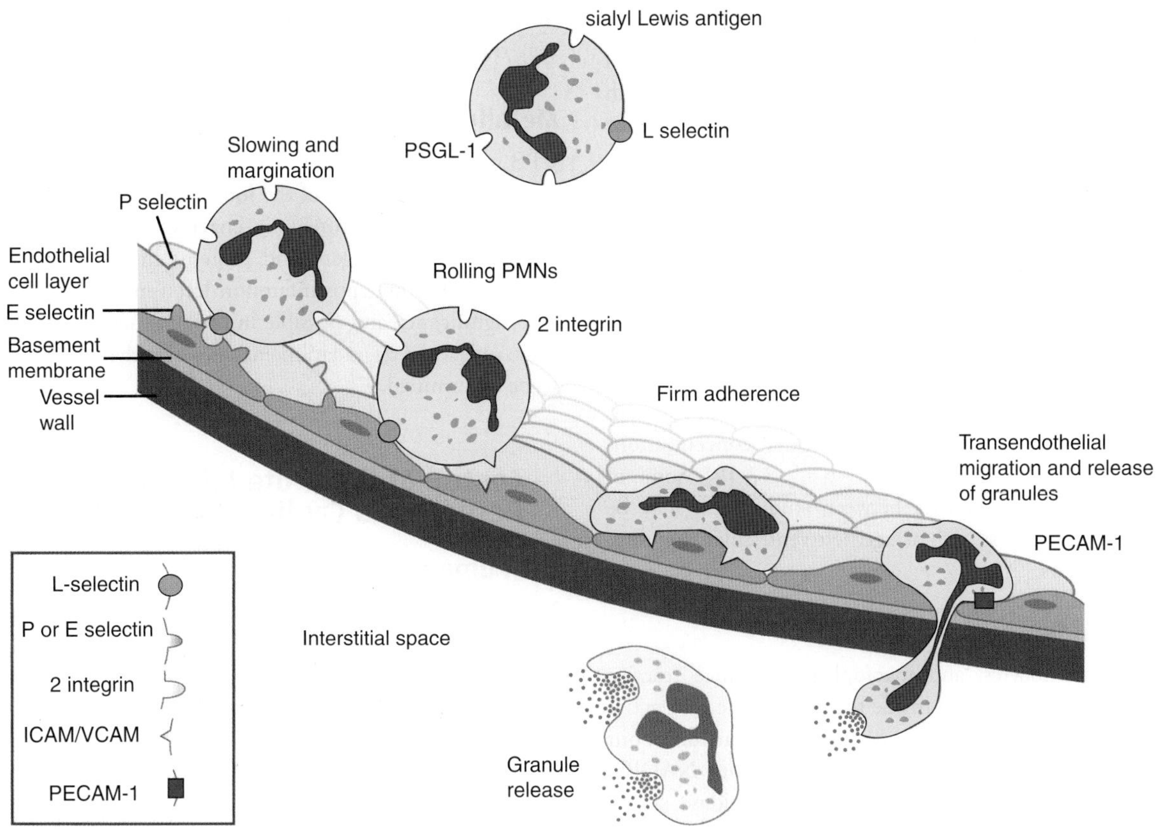

FIGURE 12-18 Mechanism of arrest and transmigration of neutrophils into the interstitial space. Neutrophils constitutively express L-selectin, which binds to endothelial cell glycoprotein ligands. Simultaneously, early response cytokines stimulate endothelial cells to rapidly express P-selectin and later E-selectin receptors, which weakly bind neutrophil PSGL-1 ligands. Marginated neutrophils, which are slowed by local vasoconstriction and reduced blood flow, lightly adhere to endothelial cells via selectin expression and begin to roll. Neutrophils activated by C5a, kallikrein, and early response cytokines express β2 CD11b and c receptors, which bind firmly to cytokine-activated endothelial cell intergrins, ICAM-1 and VCAM-1. Once arrested, L-selectins are shed and PECAM receptors on endothelial cell surfaces mediate neutrophil transmigration through endothelial cell junctions, led by chemoattractants into the interstitial space.

of ICAM-1 and VCAM-1, which firmly bind neutrophils and monocytes to the endothelium and initiate leukocyte trafficking to the extravascular space (see Fig. 12-18). Experimentally ICAM-1 is upregulated during CPB in pulmonary vessels[298] and there is evidence that selectins are upregulated during CPB and in myocardial ischemia-reperfusion sequences. IL-1β and TNF-α induce endothelial cell production of the chemotactic proteins IL-8 and MCP-1, and induce production of PGI2 (prostacyclin) by the cyclooxygenase pathway and NO by NO synthase. These two vasodilators reduce shear stress and increase vascular permeability and therefore enhance leukocyte adhesion and transmigration.

Platelets

Platelets are probably initially activated during CPB by thrombin, which is the most potent platelet agonist. Plasma epinephrine, PAF, vasopressin, from other cells, and internally generated thromboxane A2 contribute to activation as CPB continues. Platelets possess several protease-activated receptors to most of these agonists and to collagen, which has an important role in adhesion and thrombus formation. Platelets contribute to the inflammatory response by synthesis and release of eicosanoids[299]; serotonin from dense granules; chemokines, and other proteins.[300] Platelets also produce and release acid hydrolases from membrane-bound lysozymes. Platelet-secreted cytokines may be particularly involved in the inflammatory response to CPB because of strong activation of platelets in both the wound and perfusion circuit.

Other Mediators of Inflammation

Anaphylatoxins

The anaphylatoxins C3a, C4a, and C5a are bioactive protein fragments released by cleavage of complement proteins C3, C4, and C5. These fragments have potent proinflammatory and immunoregulatory functions and contract smooth muscle cells, increase vascular permeability, serve as chemoattractants, and in the case of C5a, activate neutrophils and monocytes.[301] Anaphylatoxins contribute to increased pulmonary vascular resistance, edema, and neutrophil sequestration and an increase in extravascular water during CPB. The duration of postoperative ventilation directly correlates with plasma C3a concentrations.[302] C3a and C5a are important mediators in ischemia/reperfusion injuries.

Cytokines

Cytokines are small, cell-signaling peptides produced and released into blood or the extravascular environment by both blood and tissue cells. Cytokines stimulate specific receptors on other cells to initiate a response in that cell. All blood leukocytes and endothelium produce cytokines, but many tissue cells including fibroblasts, smooth muscle cells and cardiac monocytes also produce cytokines.[303] IL-1β and TNF-α are early response cytokines that are produced by macrophages. These proteins stimulate surrounding cells to produce chemokines. The main anti-inflammatory cytokine observed during CPB is IL-10, which inhibits the production of chemokines from leukocytes.[304] Proinflammatory cytokines increase during and after cardiac surgery using CPB with peak concentrations occurring 12 to 24 hours after CPB[305] (Fig. 12-19). Some of the variation in measurements between studies also may be caused by patient factors such as age, left ventricular function, and genetic factors.[306]

Reactive Oxidants

Neutrophils, monocytes, and macrophages produce reactive oxidants, which are cytotoxic inside the phagosome, but act as cytotoxic mediators of acute inflammation outside. Four enzymes generate a large menu of reactive oxidants: NADPH (nicotinamide adenine dinucleotide phosphate) oxidase, superoxide dismutase, nitric oxide synthase, and myeloperoxidase.[307] The four products produced by these enzymes, O_2, H_2O_2, NO, and HOCL, generate all reactive oxidants from nonenzymatic reactions with other molecules or ions.

Endotoxins

Endotoxins, including lipopolysaccharides, and fragments of bacteria that are powerful agonists for complement, neutrophils, monocytes, and other leukocytes.[308] Endotoxins have been detected during CPB and after aortic cross-clamping.[309] Sources include contaminants within sterilized infusion solutions, the bypass circuit, and possibly the gastrointestinal tract owing to changes in microvascular intestinal perfusion, which may translocate bacteria.[310]

Metalloproteinases

CPB induces the synthesis and release of matrix metalloproteinases, [311] which are one of the four major classes of mammalian proteinases. These proteolytic enzymes have a major role in degradation of collagens and proteins in the pathogenesis of atherosclerosis and postinfarction left ventricular remodeling. The significance and possible injury produced by activation of these interstitial degradation enzymes over the long term remain to be determined.

Control of the Acute Inflammatory Response to Cardiopulmonary Bypass

Off-Pump Cardiac Surgery

Myocardial revascularization without either CPB or cardioplegia reduces the acute inflammatory response, but does not prevent it.[312] The response to surgical trauma, myocardial ischemia, manipulation of the heart, pericardial suction, heparin, protamine, other drugs, and anesthesia activates the extrinsic clotting system and produces an increase in the markers of acute inflammation, C3a, C5b-9, proinflammatory cytokines (TNF-α, il-6, IL-9), neutrophil elastase, and reactive oxidants, but the magnitude of the response is significantly less than that observed with CPB.[313] Although it has not been shown that the attenuated acute inflammatory response directly reduces organ dysfunction, elderly patients, and those with reduced renal and pulmonary function often tolerate off-pump surgery with less morbidity and mortality than patients created with CPB.[314]

Perfusion Temperature

Release of mediators of inflammation is temperature sensitive. Normothermic CPB increases the release of cytokines and other cellular and soluble mediators of inflammation,[312]

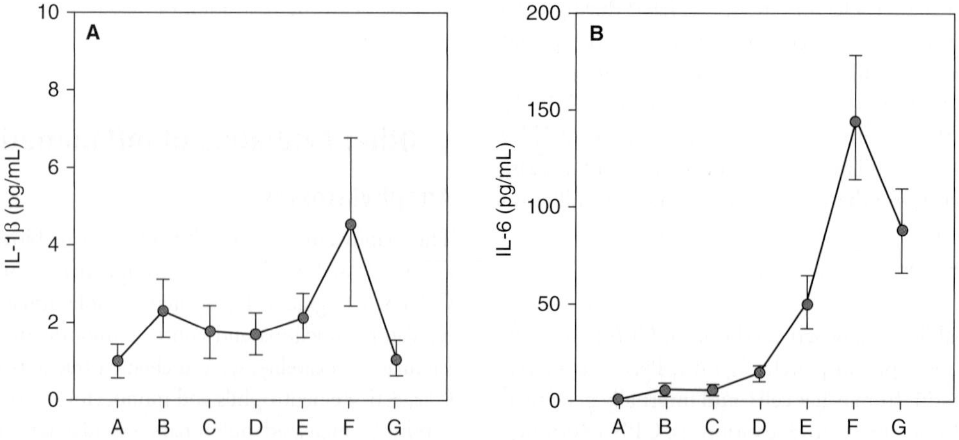

FIGURE 12-19 Changes in IL-1β (A) and IL-6 (B) in 30 patients who had elective first-time myocardial revascularization. Letters on x-axis represent the following events: (*A*) induction of anesthesia; (*B*) 5 minutes after heparin; (*C*) 10 minutes after starting CPB; (*D*) end of CPB; (*E*) 20 minutes after protamine; (*F*) 3 hours after CPB; (*G*) 24 hours after CPB. (*Redrawn from Steinberg JB, Kapelanski DP, Olson JD, Weiler JM: Cytokine and complement levels in patients undergoing cardiopulmonary bypass. J Thorac Cardiovasc Surg 1993; 106:1008.*)

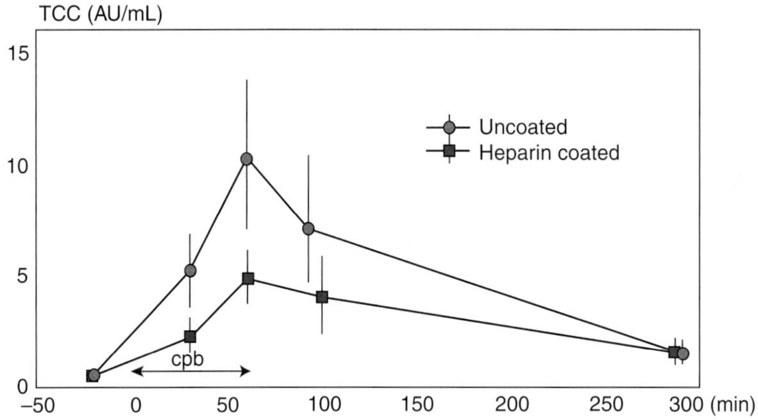

FIGURE 12-20 Changes in C5b-9 (TCC) terminal complement complex in heparin coated (n = 15) and uncoated (n = 14) perfusion circuits during myocardial revascularization. The two curves are significantly different by ANOVA (p = .004). (*Reproduced with permission from Videm V, Mollnes TE, Fosse E, et al: Heparin-coated cardiopulmonary bypass equipment, I: biocompatibility markers and development of complications in a high-risk population. J Thorac Cardiovasc Surg 1999; 117:794.*)

whereas hypothermia reduces production and release of these mediators until rewarming begins.[315] Perfusion at tepid temperatures between 32 and 34°C is a reasonable compromise for many operations requiring 1 to 2 hours of CPB.[316]

Perfusion Circuit Coatings

Ionic- or covalent-bonded heparin perfusion circuits are the most widely used surface coatings and are often combined with reduced doses of systemic heparin in first-time myocardial revascularization patients.[317] It is well established that heparin is an agonist for platelets, complement, factor XII, and leukocytes, but there is no reproducible evidence that heparin coating either produces a nonthrombogenic surface or reduces activation of the clotting cascade. [318] Clinical trials that have combined heparin-coated circuits with reduced systemic heparin and exclusion of field-aspirated blood from the perfusion circuit have demonstrated significant clinical benefits[319] (Fig. 12-20). New surface coatings are being developed or undergoing clinical studies.[320] In clinical trials these surface coatings significantly reduced platelet loss and granule release, and reduced markers of thrombin generation.[320,321] PMEA (poly-2- methylethylacrylate) is another manufactured surface coating designed to reduce surface adsorption of plasma proteins. Laboratory studies show reduced surface adsorption of fibrinogen and reduced bradykinin and thrombin generation in pigs.[321] Clinical studies show significant reductions in C3a, C4D, and neutrophil elastase, but ambivalent effects on IL-6 and platelets.[322]

Modified Ultrafiltration

Modified ultrafiltration to remove intravascular (and extravascular) water and inflammatory substances has produced improved results in adults and children.[323,324] Dialysis during CPB in adults may be beneficial in removing water, potassium, and protein wastes in patients with renal insufficiency.

Complement Inhibitors

The sequential activation cascade with convergence of the classical and alternative pathways at C3 offers many opportunities for inhabitation by recombinant proteins. Using a humanized, recombinant antibody to C5 (h5G1.1-scFv), Fitch et al. demonstrated that generation of C5b-9 was completely blocked in a dose-response manner (Fig. 12-21) and that neutrophil and monocyte CD11b/CD18 expression was attenuated in patients during and for several hours after clinical cardiac surgery using CPB.[325] Large scale clinical trials that have followed have shown significant improvements in morbidity and mortality.[326]

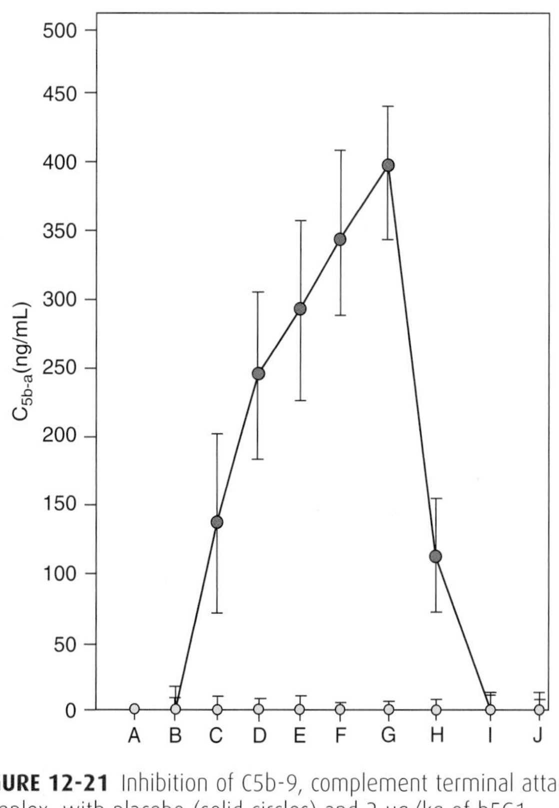

FIGURE 12-21 Inhibition of C5b-9, complement terminal attack complex, with placebo (solid circles) and 2 μg/kg of h5G1. 1-scFv (open circles) during clinical cardiac surgery with CPB. Letters on x-axis represent the following events: (*A*) before heparin; (*B*) 5 minutes after drug; (*C*) 5 minutes after cooling to 28°C; (*D*) after beginning rewarming; (*E*) 5 minutes after reaching 32°C; (*F*) 5 minutes after reaching 37°C; (*G*) 5 minutes after CPB; (*H*) 2 hours after CPB; (*I*) 12 hours after CPB; (*J*) 24 hours after CPB. HcG1.1-scFv completely inhibited formation of the C5b-9 terminal attack complex. (*Data redrawn from Fitch JCK, Rollins S, Matis L, et al: Pharmacology and biological efficacy of a recombinant, humanized, single-chain antibody C5 complement inhibitor in patients undergoing coronary artery bypass graft surgery with cardiopulmonary bypass. Circulation 1999; 100:2499.*)

Other complement recombinant protein inhibitors have been developed and are under active investigation because of the importance of this plasma protein system in CPB, ischemia/reperfusion, and injuries that summon the acute inflammatory response. Although any effective and safe inhibitor is welcome, C3 may be a better target for inhibition because both activation pathways are blocked at the point of convergence and because C3 concentrations in plasma are 15 times greater than C5.[327]

Glucocorticoids

Many investigators have used glucocorticoids to suppress the acute inflammatory response to CPB and clinical cardiac surgery, but beneficial effects in adult patients have been inconsistent.[328] Steroids reduce release of rapid-response cytokines, TNF-α, and IL-1β from macrophages, enhance release of IL-10, and suppress expression of endothelial cell selectins and neutrophil integrins.[329] Clinical results from a few randomized trials are conflicting: One study observed earlier extubation and reduced shivering,[330] but another found increased blood glucose levels and delayed extubation.[331] A recent large meta-analysis found that low-dose corticosteroids reduced atrial fibrillation incidence, and decreased ICU and hospital length of stay without increasing infectious complications.[332]

Section C

Organ Damage

Cardiopulmonary bypass can preempt normal reflex and chemoreceptor control of the circulation, initiate coagulation, activate blood cells, release circulating cell-signaling proteins, generate vasoactive and cytotoxic substances, and produce a variety of microemboli. Venous pressure can be elevated, plasma colloid osmotic pressure is reduced, flow is nonpulsatile, and temperature is manipulated. Tissues and organs may suffer from regional malperfusion that is independent of physiologic controls, and is caused by microemboli, increased interstitial water, and perfusion with a variable amount of cytotoxic substances. Reversible and irreversible cell injury may occur, but damage is diffusely distributed throughout the entire body as individual cells or small groups of cells are affected. Ischemia-reperfusion injury augments damage to the heart and on occasion to other organs. Amazingly, the body is able to withstand and for the most part repair the cellular damage, although some abnormalities may appear later. This section summarizes the reversible and permanent organ damage produced by cardiopulmonary bypass (CPB) and complements the preceding two sections of this chapter and the chapter on ischemia and reperfusion (see Chapter 3).

Mechanisms

Cardiac output during CPB is carefully monitored and synchronized with temperature and hemoglobin concentration to ensure that the entire body is adequately supplied with oxygen (see earlier section on extracorporeal perfusion systems). Excessive hemodilution reduces oxygen delivery,[333] and hemoglobin concentrations significantly below 8 g/L cause organ dysfunction at temperatures above 30°C.[334] However, regional hypoperfusion is not monitored; is independent of reflex and chemoreceptor controls; and is influenced by the inflammatory response, which produces circulating vasoactive substances. Regional perfusion is also influenced by acid-base relationships during cooling and may affect postoperative organ function. Alpha-stat management (pH increases during cooling) decreases cerebral perfusion during hypothermia; pH stat (pH 7.40 is maintained by adding CO_2) improves organ perfusion but may increase embolic injury.[335] Temperature differences within the body and within organs produce regional temperature-perfusion mismatch,[336] which can precipitate regional hypoperfusion and acidosis caused by inadequate oxygen delivery.

The inflammatory response produces the cytotoxic compounds and activated neutrophils and monocytes that can and do destroy organ and tissue cells. These agents directly access the specialized cells of every organ by passing between endothelial cell junctions to reach the interstitial compartment. Reduced plasma colloid osmotic pressure, elevated venous pressure, and widened endothelial cell junctions[337] increase the volume of the interstitial space during CPB in proportion to the duration of bypass, magnitude of the dissection, transfusions, and other factors. In prolonged complicated perfusions the interstitial compartment may increase 18 to 33%,[338] but intracellular water does not increase during CPB.

Microemboli are defined as particles less than 500 microns in diameter. They enter the circulation during CPB from a variety of sources.[339] Table 12-2 summarizes sources of gas, foreign, and blood-generated microemboli, which are more fully discussed earlier. Air entry into the perfusion circuit produces the most dangerous gas emboli because nitrogen is poorly soluble in blood and is not a metabolite. Carbon dioxide is rapidly soluble in blood and is sometimes used to flood the surgical field to displace air. Foreign emboli, largely generated in the surgical wound, reach the circulation from the surgical field via the cardiotomy reservoir. The cardiotomy reservoir is the primary source of foreign emboli and the major source of blood-generated emboli, particularly fat emboli.[340] Extensive activation and physical damage to blood elements produce a wide variety of emboli, which tend to increase with the duration of perfusion.[335]

Strategies for Reducing Microemboli

Although discussed in earlier sections, the principal methods for reducing circulating microemboli deserve emphasis and include the following: adequate anticoagulation; membrane oxygenator; washing blood aspirated from the surgical wound[341]; filtering the cardiotomy reservoir; secure pursestring sutures around cannulas; strict control of all air entry sites within the perfusion circuit; removal of residual air from the heart and great vessels; avoidance of atherosclerotic emboli; and selective filtration of cerebral vessels (Table 12-5).[342,343]

Many intraoperative strategies are available to reduce cerebral atherosclerotic embolization. These include routine epicardial

TABLE 12-5 Minimizing Microemboli

Membrane oxygenator, centrifugal arterial pump
Cardiotomy reservoir filter (≤40 μm)
Arterial line filter/bubble trap (≤40 μm)
Keep temperature differentials <8–10°C
Prime with carbon dioxide flush; recirculate with saline and filter (5 μm)
Prevent air entry into the circuit Snug purse-string sutures Three-way stopcocks on all sampling ports Meticulous syringe management Adequate cardiotomy reservoir volume (for debubbling) Avoid excessive suction on vents One-way valved purge lines for bubble traps Use transesophageal echocardiography to locate trapped intracardiac air; de-air thoroughly
Wash blood aspirated from the surgical field
Prevent thrombus formation with adequate anticoagulation
Assess inflow cannulation site by epiaortic ultrasound imaging
Cannulate distal aorta or axillary artery
Consider use of special aortic cannulas

echocardiography of the ascending aorta to detect both anterior and posterior atherosclerotic plaques and find sites free of atherosclerosis for placing the aortic cannula.[344] Recently, special catheters with or without baffles or screens have been developed to reduce the number of atherosclerotic emboli that reach the cerebral circulation.[345] In patients with moderate or severe ascending aortic atherosclerosis a single application of the aortic clamp as opposed to partial or multiple applications is strongly recommended and has been shown to reduce postoperative neuronal and neurocognitive deficits in a large clinical series.[346] Retrograde cardioplegia is preferred over antegrade cardioplegia in these patients to avoid a sandblasting effect of the cardioplegic solution.[347] No aortic clamp may be safe or even possible in some patients with severe atherosclerosis or porcelain aorta. If intracardiac surgery is required in these patients, deep hypothermia may be used with or without graft replacement of the ascending aorta. If only revascularization is needed, pedicled single or sequential arterial grafts,[348] T or Y grafts from a pedicled mammary artery,[349] or vein grafts anastomosed to arch vessels can be used.

In-depth or screen filters are essential for cardiotomy reservoirs and are usually used in arterial lines. The efficacy of arterial line filters is controversial because screen filters with a pore size less than 20 microns cannot be used because of flow resistance across the filter. However, air and fat emboli can pass through filters although 20 micron screen filters more effectivly trap microemboli than larger sizes.[350]

Cardiac Injury

It is difficult to separate postoperative cardiac dysfunction from injury owing to CPB, ischemia/reperfusion, direct surgical trauma, the disease being treated, and maladjustment of preload and afterload to myocardial contractile function. The heart, like all organs and tissues, is subject to microemboli, protease and chemical cytotoxins, activated neutrophils and monocytes, and regional hypoperfusion during CPB before and after cardioplegia or fibrillatory arrest. However, the heart is protected from CPB for at least one half of the case when the aorta is cross-clamped. Some degree of myocardial "stunning" during the period coronary blood flow is interrupted is inevitable,[351] as is some degree of reperfusion injury after ischemia. Both myocardial edema and distention of the flaccid cardioplegic heart during aortic cross-clamping[352] reduce myocardial contractility. Lastly, if myocardial contractility is weak, excessive preload or high afterload during weaning from CPB increases ventricular end-diastolic volume, myocardial wall stress, and oxygen consumption. Thus postoperative performance of the heart depends upon many variables and not just the injuries produced by CPB.

Neurologic Injury

The brain is the effecter organ for all behavior, innate and learned. It is the monarch of blood flow and will shut down all other vascular systems to preserve its own supply. Conversely, dysfunction in other organs can adversely affect brain function. It monitors other organ systems and is acutely sensitive and responsive to both the external and internal environment. Thus, even small injuries to the brain may produce symptomatic, functional losses that would not be detectable or important in other organs. Regional hypoperfusion, edema, microemboli, circulating cytotoxins or subtle changes in blood glucose, insulin, or calcium may result in changes in cognitive function, ranging from subtle to profound. A small 2-mm infarct may cause a disruption of behavioral patterns, physiologic and physical function changes can pass unnoticed, be accepted, and dismissed, or profoundly compromise the patient's quality of life. Move the lesion half a centimeter and the same volume lesion may result in a catastrophic stroke. Thus the brain is the most sensitive organ exposed to damage by CPB and also the organ that, with the heart, is most important to protect.

Assessment

Routine assessment of neurologic injury that occurs in the setting of cardiac surgery is not done for most patients because of the priority of the cardiac lesion as well as costs in time and money. General neurologic examinations by members of the surgical team or individuals lacking specialized training are not adequate to rule out subtle neurologic injuries, and this is the principal reason that the incidence of stroke, or neurologic or neuropsychological injury varies widely in the surgical literature.[353]

The most obvious neurologic abnormalities are paresis, loss of vital brain functions such as speech, vision, comprehension, or coma. These are commonly lumped under the general heading of stroke. Disorders of awareness or consciousness can include coma, delirium, and confusion, but transitory episodes of delirium and confusion are often dismissed as caused by anesthesia or medications. More subtle losses are determined by comparison of preoperative and postoperative performances using a standard battery of neuropsychological tests prepared by a group of neuropsychologists. A neuropsychological examination is basically an extension of the neurologic examination with a much greater emphasis on higher cortical function. Dysfunction is objectively defined as a deviation from the expected, relative to a large population. For example, although performing at a 95 IQ level is in the normal range, it is low for a physician, and a search for a neurologic impairment would be triggered by such a poor performance. A 20% decline in two or more of these tests, compared with the patient's own baseline, suggests a neuropsychological deficit that should be followed until resolved or not resolved.[354] In studies involving long-term follow-up the inclusion of a control group of unoperated patients with the same disease and similar demographics helps define the causes of neuropsychological decline that occurs later than 3 to 6 months after surgery.[355]

Computed axial tomograms (CAT) or magnetic resonance imaging (MRI) scans are essential for the definitive diagnosis of stroke, delirium, or coma. Preoperative imaging is usually not necessary when new techniques such as diffusion-weighted MRI imaging, MRI spectroscopy, or MRI angiography are used to assess possible new lesions after operation.[356] Biochemical markers of neurologic injury after cardiac surgery are relatively nonspecific and inconclusive. Neuron-specific enolase (NSE) is an intracellular enzyme found in neurons, normal neuroendocrine cells, platelets, and erythrocytes.[357] S-100 is an acidic calcium-binding protein found in the brain.[358] The beta dimer resides in glial and Schwann cells. Both S-100 and NSE increase in spinal fluid with neuronal death and may correlate with stroke or spinal cord injury after CPB.[359] However, plasma levels are contaminated by aspiration of wound blood into the pump and hemolysis and are often elevated after prolonged CPB in patients without otherwise detectable neurologic injury.[360] Newer blood-borne biochemical markers such as Tau have been identified, but as of yet have not been shown to be diagnostic for subtle neurologic injury.

Populations at Risk

Advancing age increases the risk of stroke or cognitive impairment in the general population, and surgery, regardless of type, increases the risk still higher.[361] In 1986 Gardner and colleagues reported the risk of stroke during CABG surgery to be directly related to age.[362] A European study compared 321 elderly patients without surgery to 1218 patients who had noncardiac surgery and found a 26% incidence of cognitive dysfunction 1 week after operation and a 10% incidence at 3 months.[363] Between 1974 and 1990 the number of patients undergoing cardiac surgery over age 60 and over age 70 increased twofold and sevenfold, respectively[364] (Fig. 12-22). Genetic factors also influence the incidence of cognitive dysfunction after cardiac surgery.[365] The incidence of cognitive dysfunction at 1 week after cardiac surgery is approximately double that of noncardiac surgery.

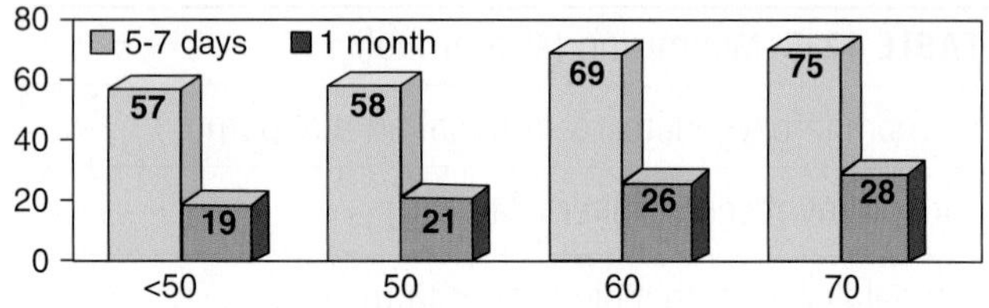

FIGURE 12-22 Effect of age by decade on neuropsychologic outcome after CABG. Abnormal neuropsychologic outcomes at 1 week and 1 month postoperative are more common with advancing age. Percentages of patients with deficits on two or more tests are shown ($n = 374$). *(Reproduced with permission from Hammon JW, Stump DA, Kon ND, et al: Risk factors and solutions for the development of neurobehavioral changes after coronary artery bypass grafting. Ann Thorac Surg 1998: 63:1613.)*

As the age of cardiac surgical patients' increases, the number with multiple risk factors for neurologic injury also increases. Hypertension and diabetes occur in approximately 55 and 25% of cardiac surgical patients, respectively.[366] Fifteen percent have carotid stenosis of 50% or greater, and up to 13% have had a transient ischemic attack or prior stroke. The total number of MRI atherosclerotic lesions in the brachiocephalic vessels adds to the risk of stroke or cognitive dysfunction,[367] as does the severity of atherosclerosis in the ascending aorta as detected by epiaortic ultrasound scanning.[368] Palpable ascending aortic atherosclerotic plaques markedly increase the risk of right carotid arterial emboli as detected by Doppler ultrasound.[369] The incidence of severe aortic atherosclerosis is 1% in cardiac surgical patients less than 50 years old and is 10% in those aged 75 to 80.[370]

Mechanisms of Injury

The three major causes of neurologic dysfunction and injury during cardiac surgery are microemboli, hypoperfusion, and a generalized inflammatory reaction, which can occur in the same patient at the same time for different reasons. The vast majority of intraoperative strokes are caused by the embolization of atherosclerotic material from the aorta and brachiocephalic vessels. This occurs as a result of manipulation of the heart and major thoracic vasculature as well as dislodgement of atheromata from shearing forces directed at the walls of vessels from inflow cardiopulmonary bypass cannulae.[371] Microemboli are distributed in proportion to blood flow[20]; thus reduced cerebral blood flow reduces microembolic injury but increases the risk of hypoperfusion.[372] During CPB both alpha-stat acid-base management and phenylephrine reduce cerebral injury in adults, probably by causing cerebral vessel vasoconstriction and reducing the number of microemboli.[373] Air, atherosclerotic debris, and fat are the major types of microemboli causing brain

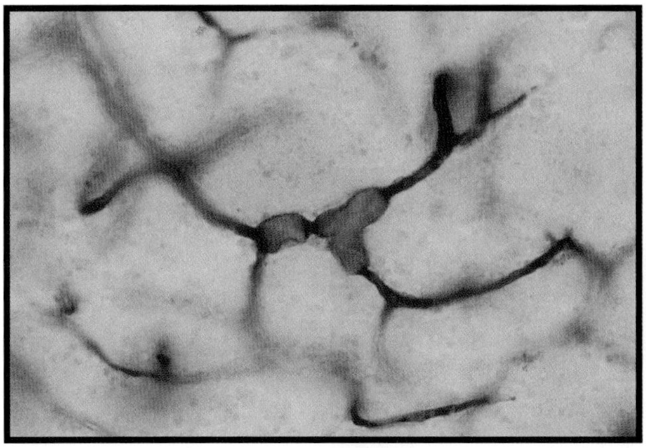

FIGURE 12-23 Small capillary and arterial dilatations (SCADs) in cerebral vessels in a patient who expired 48 hours after CABG using cardiopulmonary bypass. (Alkaline phosphatase-stained celloidin section, 100 μm thick: × 100.)

injury in clinical practice, and all cause neuronal necrosis by blocking cerebral vessels.[374] Massive air embolism causes a large ischemic injury, but gaseous cerebral microemboli may directly damage endothelium in addition to blocking blood flow.[375] The identification of unique small capillary arteriolar dilatations (SCADs) in the brain associated with fat emboli[376] (Fig. 12-23) raises the possibility that these emboli not only block small vessels, but also release cytotoxic free radicals, which may significantly increase the damage to lipid-rich neurons.

Anemia and elevated cerebral temperature increase cerebral blood flow but may cause inadequate oxygen delivery to the brain,[377] however, these conditions are easily avoided during clinical cardiac surgery. Although some investigators speculate that normothermic and/or hyperthermic CPB cause cerebral hypoperfusion,[378] experimental studies indicate that cerebral blood flow increases with temperature. Brain injuries associated with this practice are more likely due to increased cerebral microemboli, which produce larger lesions at higher cerebral temperatures.[376]

Neuroprotective Strategies

Recommended conditions for protecting the brain during CPB include mild hypothermia (32 to 34°C) and hematocrit above 25%.[161] Temporary increases in cerebral venous pressure caused by superior vena cava obstruction and excessive rewarming above blood temperatures of 37°C should be avoided.[379] A randomized study in which patients were mildly rewarmed to 35°C core temperature demonstrated improved neurocognitive outcomes over patients rewarmed to 37°C. Either jugular venous bulb oxygen saturation or near-infrared cerebral oximetry are recommended for monitoring cerebral perfusion in patients who may be at high risk for cerebral injury.[380]

Barbiturates reduce cerebral metabolism by decreasing spontaneous synaptic activity and provide a definite neuroprotective effect during clinical cardiac surgery using CPB.[381] Unfortunately, these agents delay emergence from anesthesia and prolong intensive care unit stays. NMDA (*N*-methyl-D-aspartate) antagonists, which are effective in animals, provide mild protection compared with control patients, but have a high incidence of neurologic side effects.[382] A small study demonstrated a neuroprotective effect of lidocaine, but this beneficial effect has not been reproduced.[383] Thus corticosteroids are the only drugs with potential neuroprotective effects that have significant evidence for a positive effect on outcomes.[332]

Off-pump myocardial revascularization theoretically avoids many of the causes of cerebral injury owing to CPB, but, as noted, many causes of neuronal injury are independent of CPB and related to atherosclerosis and air entry sites into the circulation. Nonrandomized measurements of carotid emboli by Doppler ultrasound indicate fewer emboli and slightly improved neurocognitive outcomes in high-risk patients who have off-pump surgery.[384] Clinical trials of off-pump versus on-pump patients failed to show a significant difference in neurologic outcomes among methods.[385]

Prognosis

Patients with intraoperative stroke or those who develop stroke symptoms in the first week after surgery often improve in direct relation to the lesion size and location on imaging studies. Neuropsychologic deficits that are present after 3 months are almost always permanent.[386] Assessments after that time are confounded by development of new deficits, particularly in aged patients.[387,388]

The difficulty of separating intraoperative brain injury from that which occurs in the early or late postoperative period has been recently addressed by a reanalysis of data published earlier. The authors tracked specific neuropsychological deficits that persisted unchanged for 6 months (persistent deficits) and separated them from new deficits that appeared after surgery[389] (Fig. 12-24). Using this technique it is possible to accurately measure surgical brain injury and design techniques to eliminate this important cause of morbidity. Late follow-up studies should include a control group with similar risk factors but not having cardiac operations.[390] This technique demonstrated similar outcomes in surgical and nonsurgical controls at 3 years, putting to rest the previous fear that surgical patients had recurrent neurocognitive deficits and were thus at greater risk for poor long-term outcomes. In a recent study, a group of surgical patients who were evaluated with preoperative and postoperative neuropsychological studies had rigid control of cardiovascular risk factors.[391] They demonstrated no delayed or late cognitive decline offering hope that aggressive medical therapy can compliment skillful surgery in preventing neurological injury.

Lung Injury

Patient factors and the separate effects of operation and CPB combine to compromise lung function early after operation. Chronic smoking and emphysema are the most common patient factors, but muscular weakness, chronic bronchitis, occult pneumonia, preoperative pulmonary edema, and unrelated respiratory disease are other contributors to postoperative pulmonary dysfunction. Incisional pain, lack of movement, shallow respiratory sighs, increased work of breathing, reduced pulmonary compliance, weak cough, increased pulmonary arterial-venous

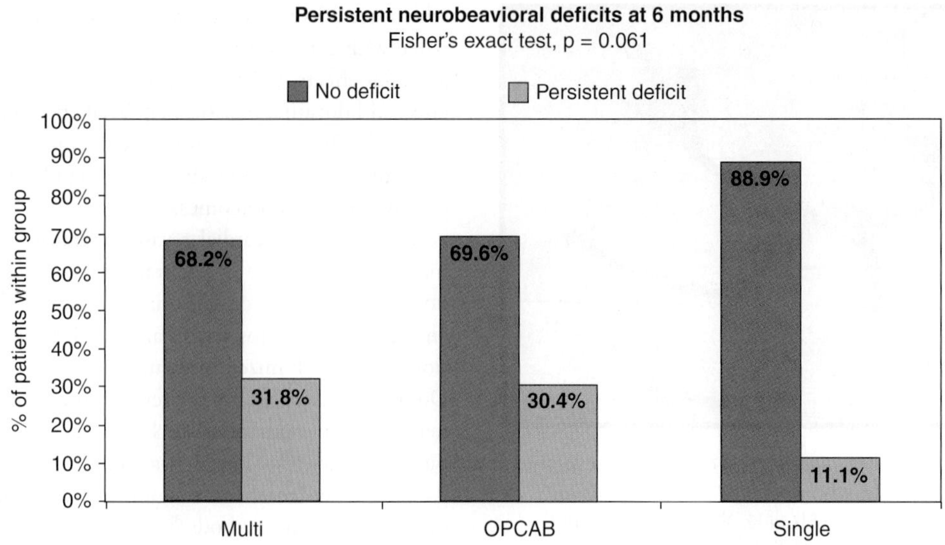

FIGURE 12-24 Neurobehavioral deficits at 6 months after coronary artery bypass surgery. Note that an intraoperative strategy utilizing a single cross clamp results in fewer persistent neuropsyscological deficits than multiple cross clamp or off pump coronary artery bypass (OPCAB). (*Reproduced with permission from Hammon JW, Stump DA, Butterworth JF, et al: Coronary artery bypass grafting with single cross clamp results in fewer persistent neuropsychological deficits than multiple clamp or off-pump coronary artery bypass grafting. Ann Thorac Surg 2007; 84:1174.*)

shunting, and interstitial edema, to some degree, are consequences of anesthesia and any operation. CPB significantly adds to this injury.

During CPB the lungs are supplied by the bronchial arteries and pulmonary arterial blood flow may be absent or minimal. Whether or not alveolar cells suffer an ischemic/reperfusion injury is unclear, but the lungs are subject to many insults that combine to increase pulmonary capillary permeability and interstitial lung water. Hemodilution, reduced plasma oncotic pressure, and temporary elevation of left atrial or pulmonary venous pressure during CPB or during weaning from CPB increase extravascular lung water.[392] Microemboli and circulating cellular, vasoactive, and cytotoxic mediators of the inflammatory response reach the lung via bronchial arteries during CPB and with resumption of the pulmonary circulation during weaning.[393,394] These agents increase pulmonary capillary permeability, perivascular edema, and bronchial secretions, and perhaps cause observed changes in alveolar surfactant.[395] The combination of increased interstitial lung water and bronchial secretions, altered surfactant, patient factors, and the consequences of operation reduces pulmonary compliance and functional residual capacity and increases the work of breathing.[396] All of these changes combine to enhance regional atelectasis, increase susceptibility to infection, and increase the physiologic arterial-venous shunt, which reduces systemic arterial PaO_2.

Postoperative respiratory care is based on restoring normal pulmonary capillary permeability and interstitial lung volume; preventing atelectasis; reinflating atelectatic segments; maintaining normal arterial blood gases; and preventing infection and facilitating removal of bronchial mucus. Improved postoperative respiratory care, an understanding of the mechanisms of lung injury during CPB, and efforts to prevent or control the causes of injury[397] have markedly reduced the incidence of pulmonary complications in recent years. (See Chapter 16 for a more detailed discussion of postoperative care.)

Acute respiratory distress syndrome (ARDS) is a rare complication of lung injury during cardiopulmonary bypass and is usually caused by intrabronchial bleeding from traumatic injury by the endotracheal tube or pulmonary artery catheter or to extravasation of blood into alveoli from acute increases in pulmonary venous pressure or severe pulmonary capillary toxic injury.[398]

Renal Injury

As with other organs, the preoperative health of the kidneys is a major factor in the ability of that organ to withstand the microembolic, cellular, and regional malperfusion injuries caused by extracorporeal circulation. Risk factors include previous renal injury, increased age, and complex disease or cardiac operation.[399] The incidence of acute renal failure requiring dialysis after CPB is remarkably low, averaging 1%; however, the incidence increases to 5% with complex operations.

Some degree of renal injury is inevitable during CPB and postperfusion proteinuria occurs in all patients.[400] Renal blood and plasma flow, creatinine clearance, free water clearance, and urine volume decrease without hemodilution.[401] Hemodilution attenuates most of these functional changes and also reduces the risk of hemoglobin precipitation in renal tubules if plasma-binding proteins become saturated with free hemoglobin during extracorporeal perfusion. Hemoglobin is toxic to renal tubules and precipitation can block both blood and urine flow to the tubules. Hemodilution dilutes plasma hemoglobin; improves flow to the outer renal cortex; improves total renal blood flow; increases creatinine, electrolyte, and water clearance; and increases glomerular filtration and urine volume.[402]

Perioperative periods of low cardiac output and/or hypotension added to the microembolic, cellular, and cytotoxic injuries of CPB and to any preoperative renal disease are the major cause of postoperative renal failure.[403] Low cardiac output reduces renal perfusion pressure and causes angiotensin II production and renin release, which further decrease renal blood flow. Kidneys, already compromised by preoperative disease and the CPB injury, are particularly sensitive to ischemic injury secondary to low cardiac output and hypotension. Thus perioperative management includes efforts to maximize cardiac output using dopamine or dobutamine if necessary, avoiding renal arterial vasoconstrictive drugs, providing adequate crystalloid infusions to maintain urine volume, and alkalinizing urine to minimize precipitation of tubular hemoglobin if excessive hemolysis has occurred.

If perioperative low cardiac output and hypotension do not occur, the normal kidney has sufficient functional reserve to provide adequate renal function during and after operation. The appearance of oliguric renal failure is ominous and usually requires dialysis, which is generally permanent if required for more than 2 weeks. Oliguric renal failure markedly increases morbidity and mortality by approximately eightfold.

Injury to the Liver and Gastrointestinal Organs

Although subjected to microemboli, cytotoxins, and regional malperfusion during CPB, the enormous functional reserve and reparative processes of the normal liver nearly always overcome the injury without consequences. Often liver enzymes are mildly elevated, and 10 to 20% of patients are mildly jaundiced. Persistent and rising bilirubin 2 or more days after CPB may precede development of liver failure and is associated with increased morbidity and mortality.[404] Catastrophic liver failure, however, occurs in patients with overwhelming sepsis, oliguric renal failure, anesthetic or drug toxicity, or after a prolonged period of low cardiac output or an episode of hemorrhagic shock and multiple blood transfusions and is uniformly fatal. The liver usually is involved in patients who develop multiorgan failure and is often presaged by sudden hypoglycemia.

Pancreatic Injury

Less than 1% of patients develop clinical pancreatitis after CPB, but approximately 30% develop a transitory, asymptomatic increase in plasma amylase and/or lipase.[405] A history of recurrent pancreatitis, perioperative circulatory shock or hypotension, excessively prolonged CPB, and continuous, high doses of inotropic agents are risk factors for developing postoperative pancreatitis.[406] Experimentally and clinically, high doses of calcium increase intracellular trypsinogen activation and histologic evidence of pancreatitis.[407] Fulminant pancreatits is very rare, but is often fatal.

Stomach and Gut Injury

CPB at adequate flow rates does not decrease splanchnic blood flow.[408] Risk factors for gastrointestinal complications include advanced age, emergency surgery, prolonged CPB, postoperative low cardiac output or shock, prolonged vasopressor therapy, and elevated preoperative systemic venous pressure.[409]

CPB decreases gastric pH, which declines further after operation. Before the advent of H2 blockers and regular use of antacids, duodenal and/or gastric erosion, ulcer, and bleeding were frequent complications after clinical cardiac surgery and were associated with mortality that approached 33 to 50%.[410] These complications are now uncommon.

Several days to 1 week after operation very elderly patients rarely may develop mesenteric vasculitis or severe mesenteric vasoconstriction in response to vasopressors that proceeds to small bowel ischemia and/or infarction. New onset abdominal pain with a silent, rigid abdomen and abrupt rise in white count may be the only signs of this catastrophic complication, which is frequently fatal. If suspected before infarction, infusion of papaverine or alternative vasodilators directly into the mesenteric arteries may prevent or limit subsequent infarction.

The role of CPB in the etiology of gastrointestinal complications is not completely known. If the complications listed in the preceding develop, an increase in the morbidity and mortality may be expected.[411]

REFERENCES

1. Gravlee GP, Davis RF, Kurusz M, Utley JR: *Cardiopulmonary Bypass: Principles and Practice,* 2nd ed. Philadelphia, Lippincott Williams & Wilkins, 2000.
2. Arom KV, Ellestad C, Grover FL, Trinkle JK: Objective evaluation of the efficacy of various venous cannulas. *J Thorac Cardiovasc Surg* 1981; 81:464.
3. Merin O, Silberman S, Brauner R, et al: Femoro-femoral bypass for repeat open-heart surgery. *Perfusion* 1998; 13:455.
4. Winter FS: Persistent left superior vena cava: survey of world literature and report of thirty additional cases. *Angiology* 1954; 5:90.
5. Hasel R, Barash PG: Dilated coronary sinus on pre-bypass echocardiography. *J Cardiothorac Vasc Anesth* 1996; 10:430.
6. Shahian DM: Retrograde coronary sinus cardioplegia in the presence of persistent left superior vena cava. *Ann Thorac Surg* 1992; 54:1214.
7. Yokota M, Kyoku I, Kitano M, et al: Atresia of the coronary sinus orifice: fatal outcome after intraoperative division of the drainage left superior vena cava. *J Thorac Cardiovasc Surg* 1989; 98:30.
8. Toomasian JM, McCarthy JP: Total extrathoracic cardiopulmonary support with kinetic assisted venous drainage: experience in 50 patients. *Perfusion* 1998; 13:137.
9. Taketani S, Sawa Y, Massai T, et al: A novel technique for cardiopulmonary bypass using vacuum system for venous drainage with pressure relief valve: an experimental study. *Artif Organs* 1998; 22:337.
10. Humphries K, Sistino JJ: Laboratory evaluation of the pressure flow characteristics of venous cannulas during vaccum-assisted venous drainage. *J Extracorp Tech* 2002; 34:111.
11. Willcox TW, Mitchell SJ, Gorman DF: Venous air in the bypass circuit: a source of arterial line emboli exacerbated by vacuum-assisted venous drainage. *Ann Thorac Surg* 1999; 68:1285.
12. Willcox TW: Vacuum-assisted venous drainage: to air or not to air, that is the question: has the bubble burst? *J Extracorp Tech* 2002; 34:24.
13. Davila RM, Rawles T, Mack MJ: Venoarterial air embolus: a complication of vacuum-assisted venous drainage. *Ann Thorac Surg* 2001; 71:1369.
14. Hessel EA II: Cardiopulmonary bypass equipment, in Estafanous FG, Barash PG, Reves JG (eds): *Cardiac Anesthesia: Principles and Clinical Practice,* 2nd ed. Philadelphia, Lippincott Williams & Wilkins, 2001, p 335.
15. Jones TJ, Deal DD, Vernon JC, et al: How effective are cardiopulmonary bypass circuits at removing gaseous microemboli? *J Extracorp Tech* 2002; 34:34.
16. Ambesh SP, Singh SK, Dubey DK, Kaushik S: Inadvertent closure of the superior vena cava after decannulation: a potentially catastrophic complication after termination of bypass [letter]. *J Cardiothorac Vasc Anesth* 1998; 12:723.

17. Brodman R, Siegel H, Lesser M, Frater R: A comparison of flow gradients across disposable arterial perfusion cannulas. *Ann Thorac Surg* 1985; 39:225.
18. Galletti PM, Brecher GA: *Heart-lung Bypass*. New York, Grune & Stratton, 1962.
19. Weinstein GS: Left hemispheric strokes in coronary surgery: implication for end-hole aortic cannulas. *Ann Thorac Surg* 2001; 71:128.
20. Muehrcke DD, Cornhill JF, Thomas JD, Cosgrove DM: Flow characteristics of aortic cannulae. *J Card Surg* 1995; 10:514.
21. Joubert-Hubner E, Gerdes A, Klarproth P, et al: An in-vitro evaluation of aortic arch vessel perfusion characteristics comparing single versus multiple stream aortic cannulae. *Eur J Cardiothorac Surg* 1999; 15:359.
22. Cook DJ, Zehr KJ, Orszulak TA, Slater JM: Profound reduction in brain embolization using an endoaortic baffle during bypass in swine. *Ann Thorac Surg* 2002; 73:198.
23. Reichenspurner H, Navia JA, Benny G, et al: Particulate embolic capture by an intra-aortic filter device during cardiac surgery. *J Thorac Cardiovasc Surg* 2000; 119:233.
24. Gerdes A, Hanke T, Sievers H-H: In vivo hydrodynamics of the Embol-X cannula. *Perfusion* 2002; 17:153.
25. Harringer W: Capture of a particulate embolic during cardiac procedures in which aortic cross-clamp is used. *Ann Thorac Surg* 2000; 70:1119.
26. Banbury MK, Cosgrove DM 3rd: Arterial cannulation of the innominate artery. *Ann Thorac Surg* 2000; 69:957.
27. Mills NL, Everson CT: Atherosclerosis of the ascending aorta and coronary artery bypass: pathology, clinical correlates, and operative management. *J Thorac Cardiovasc Surg* 1991; 102:546.
28. Beique FA, Joffe D, Tousignant G, Konstadt S: Echocardiographic-based assessment and management of atherosclerotic disease of the thoracic aorta. *J Cardiothorac Vasc Anesth* 1998; 12:206.
29. Blauth CI, Cosgrove DM, Webb BW, et al: Atheroembolism from the ascending aorta. *J Thorac Cardiovasc Surg* 1992; 103:1104.
30. Murphy DA, Craver JM, Jones EL, et al: Recognition and management of ascending aortic dissection complicating cardiac surgical operations. *J Thorac Cardiovasc Surg* 1983; 85:247.
31. Davila-Roman VG, Kouchoukos NT, Schechtman KB, Barzilai B: Atherosclerosis of the ascending aorta is a predictor of renal dysfunction after cardiac operations. *J Thorac Cardiovasc Surg* 1999; 117:111.
32. Davila-Roman V, Phillips K, Davila R, et al: Intraoperative transesophageal echocardiography and epiaortic ultrasound for assessment of atherosclerosis of the thoracic aorta. *J Am Coll Cardiol* 1996; 28:942.
33. Konstadt SN, Reich DL, Quintana C, Levy M: The ascending aorta: how much does transesophageal echocardiography see? *Anesth Analg* 1994; 78:240.
34. Gaudino M, Glieca F, Alessandrini F, et al: The unclampable ascending aorta in coronary artery bypass patients: a surgical challenge of increasing frequency. *Circulation* 2000; 102:1497.
35. Byrne JG, Aranki SF, Cohn LH: Aortic valve operations under deep hypothermic circulatory arrest for the porcelain aorta: "no-touch" technique. *Ann Thorac Surg* 1998; 65:1313.
36. Grossi EA, Kanchuger MS, Schwartz DS, et al: Effect of cannula length on aortic arch flow: protection of the atheromatous aortic arch. *Ann Thorac Surg* 1995; 59:710.
37. McLeskey CH, Cheney FW: A correctable complication of cardiopulmonary bypass. *Anesthesiology* 1982; 56:214.
38. Watson BG: Unilateral cold neck. *Anaesthesia* 1983; 38:659.
39. Magner JB: Complications of aortic cannulation for open-heart surgery. *Thorax* 1971; 26:172.
40. Gott JP, Cohen CL, Jones EL: Management of ascending aortic dissections and aneurysms early and late following cardiac operations. *J Card Surg* 1990; 5:2.
41. Troianos CA, Savino JS, Weiss RL: Transesophageal echocardiographic diagnosis of aortic dissection during cardiac surgery. *Anesthesiology* 1991; 75:149.
42. Lees MH, Herr RH, Hill JD, et al: Distribution of systemic blood flow of the rhesus monkey during cardiopulmonary bypass. *J Thorac Cardiovasc Surg* 1971; 61:570.
43. Svensson LG: Editorial comment: autopsies in acute Type A aortic dissection, surgical implications. *Circulation* 1998; 98:II-302.
44. Hendrickson SC, Glower DD: A method for perfusion of the leg during cardiopulmonary bypass via femoral cannulation. *Ann Thorac Surg* 1998; 65:1807.
45. Gates JD, Bichell DP, Rizzu RJ, et al: Thigh ischemia complicating femoral vessel cannulation for cardiopulmonary bypass. *Ann Thorac Surg* 1996; 61:730.
46. Van derSalm TJ: Prevention of lower extremity ischemia during cardiopulmonary bypass via femoral cannulation. *Ann Thorac Surg* 1997; 63:251.
47. Carey JS, Skow JR, Scott C: Retrograde aortic dissection during cardiopulmonary bypass: "nonoperative" management. *Ann Thorac Surg* 1977; 24:44.
48. Sabik JF, Lytle BW, McCarthy PM, Cosgrove DM: Axillary artery: an alternative site of arterial cannulation for patients with extensive and peripheral vascular disease. *J Thorac Cardiovasc Surg* 1995; 109:885.
49. Neri E, Massetti M, Capannini G, et al: Axillary artery cannulation in type A aortic dissection operations. *J Thorac Cardiovasc Surg* 1999; 118:324.
50. Whitlark JD, Sutter FP: Intrathoracic subclavian artery cannulation as an alternative to the femoral or axillary artery cannulation [letter]. *Ann Thorac Surg* 1998; 66:296.
51. Golding LAR: New cannulation technique for the severely calcified ascending aorta. *J Thorac Cardiovasc Surg* 1985; 90:626.
52. Coselli JS, Crawford ES: Femoral artery perfusion for cardiopulmonary bypass in patients with aortoiliac artery obstruction. *Ann Thorac Surg* 1987; 43:437.
53. Orenstein JM, Sato N, Arron B, et al: Microemboli observed in deaths following cardiopulmonary bypass surgery: silicone antifoam agents and polyvinyl chloride tubing as source of emboli. *Hum Pathol* 1982; 13:1082.
54. Schonberger JPAM, Everts PAM, Hoffman JJ: Systemic blood activation with open and closed venous reservoirs. *Ann Thorac Surg* 1995; 59:1549.
55. Blauth CI, Smith PL, Arnold JV, et al: Influence of oxygenator type on the prevalence and extent of micro-emboli retinal ischemia during cardiopulmonary bypass: assessment by digital image analysis. *J Thorac Cardiovasc Surg* 1990; 99:61.
56. Pearson DT: Gas exchange; bubble and membrane oxygenators. *Semin Thorac Cardiovasc Surg* 1990; 2:313.
57. Drinker PA, Bartlett RH, Bialer RM, Noyes BS Jr: Augmentation of membrane gas transfer by induced secondary flows. *Surgery* 1969; 66:775.
58. Wiesenack C, Wiesner G, Keyl C, et al: In vivo uptake and elimination of isoflurane by different membrane oxygenators during cardiopulmonary bypass. *Anesthesiology* 2002; 97:133.
59. Clark RE, Beauchamp RA, Magrath RA, et al: Comparison of bubble and membrane oxygenators in short and long term perfusions. *J Thorac Cardiovasc Surg* 1979; 78:655.
60. Hammond GL, Bowley WW: Bubble mechanics and oxygen transfer. *J Thorac Cardiovasc Surg* 1976; 71:422.
61. Jenkins OF, Morris R, Simpson JM: Australasian perfusion incident survey. *Perfusion* 1997; 12:279.
62. Wahba A, Philipp A, Behr R, Birnbaum DE: Heparin-coated equipment reduces the risk of oxygenator failure. *Ann Thorac Surg* 1998; 65:1310.
63. Fisher AR: The incidence and cause of emergency oxygenator changeovers. *Perfusion* 1999; 14:207.
64. Svenmarker S, Haggmark S, Jansson E, et al: The relative safety of an oxygenator. *Perfusion* 1997; 12:289.
65. Geissler HJ, Allen JS, Mehlhorn U, et al: Cooling gradients and formation of gaseous microemboli with cardiopulmonary bypass: an echocardiographic study. *Ann Thorac Surg* 1997; 64:100.
66. Moen O, Fosse E, Broten J, et al: Difference in blood activation related to roller/centrifugal pumps and heparin coated/uncoated surfaces in a cardiopulmonary bypass model circuit. *Perfusion* 1996; 11:113.
67. Leschinsky BM, Zimin NK: Centrifugal blood pumps—a brief analysis: development of new designs. *Perfusion* 1991; 6:115.
68. Kolff J, McClurken JB, Alpern JB: Beware centrifugal pumps: not a one-way street, but a dangerous siphon! *Perfusion* 1990; 5:225.
69. Bernstein EF, Gleason LR: Factors influencing hemolysis with roller pumps. *Surgery* 1967; 61:432.
70. Uretzky G, Landsburg G, Cohn D, et al: Analysis of microembolic particles originating in extracorporeal circuits. *Perfusion* 1987; 2:9.
71. Wright G: Hemodynamic analysis could resolve the pulsatile blood flow controversy [current review]. *Ann Thorac Surg* 1994; 58:1199.
72. Edmunds LH Jr: Pulseless cardiopulmonary bypass. *J Thorac Cardiovasc Surg* 1982; 84:800.
73. Pearson DT: Micro-emboli: gaseous and particulate, in Taylor KM (ed): *Cardiopulmonary Bypass: Principles and Management*. Baltimore, Williams & Wilkins, 1986, p 313.
74. Borger MA, Feindel CM: Cerebral emboli during cardiopulmonary bypass: effect of perfusionist interventions and aortic cannulas. *J Extracorp Tech* 2002; 34:29.
75. Lee WH Jr, Krumhaar D, Fonkalsrud EW, et al: Denaturation of plasma proteins as a cause of morbidity and death after intracardiac operations. *Surgery* 1961; 50:1025.
76. Liu J-F, Su Z-F, Ding W-X: Quantitation of particle microemboli during cardiopulmonary bypass: experimental and clinical studies. *Ann Thorac Surg* 1992; 54:1196.

77. Brooker RF, Brown WR, Moody DM, et al: Cardiotomy suction: a major source of brain lipid emboli during cardiopulmonary bypass. *Ann Thorac Surg* 1998; 65:1651.
78. Ringelstein EB, Droste DW, Babikian VL, et al: Consensus on microembolus detection by TCD. *Stroke* 1998; 29:725.
79. Wright G, Furness A, Haigh S: Integral pulse frequency modulated ultrasound for the detection and quantification of gas microbubbles in flowing blood. *Perfusion* 1987; 2:131.
80. Kincaid E, Jones T, Stump D, et al: Processing scavenged blood with a cell saver reduces cerebral lipid microembolization. *Ann Thorac Surg* 2000; 70:1296.
81. Hammon JW, Stump DA, Hines M, et al: Prevention of embolic events during coronary artery bypass graft surgery. *Perfusion* 1994; 9:412.
82. Hammon JW, Stump DA, Kon ND, et al: Risk factors and solutions for the development of neurobehavioral changes after coronary artery bypass grafting. *Ann Thorac Surg* 1997; 63:1613.
83. Edmunds LH Jr: Thromboembolic complications of current cardiac valvular prostheses. *Ann Thorac Surg* 1982; 34:96.
84. Plochl W, Cook DJ: Quantification and distribution of cerebral emboli during cardiopulmonary bypass in the swine: the impact of $PaCO_2$. *Anesthesiology* 1999; 90:183.
85. Cook DJ, Plochl W, Orszulak TA: Effect of temperature and PaCO2 on cerebral embolization during cardiopulmonary bypass in swine. *Ann Thorac Surg* 2000; 69:415.
86. Berman L, Marin F: Micropore filtration during cardiopulmonary bypass, in Taylor KM (ed): *Cardiopulmonary Bypass: Principles and Management.* Baltimore, Williams & Wilkins, 1986, p 355.
87. Joffe D, Silvay G: The use of microfilters in cardiopulmonary bypass. *J Cardiothorac Vasc Anesth* 1994, 8:685.
88. Ware JA, Scott MA, Horak JK, Solis RT: Platelet aggregation during and after cardiopulmonary bypass: effect of two different cardiotomy filters. *Ann Thorac Surg* 1982; 34:204.
89. Gourlay T: The role of arterial line filters in perfusion safety. *Perfusion* 1988; 3:195.
90. Munsch C, Rosenfeldt F, Chang V: Absence of particle-induced coronary vasoconstriction during cardioplegic infusion: is it desirable to use a microfilter in the infusion line? *J Thorac Cardiovasc Surg* 1991; 101:473.
91. Pugsley W, Klinger L, Paschalie C, et al: The impact of micro-emboli during cardiopulmonary bypass on neurological functioning. *Stroke* 1994; 25:1393.
92. Mejak BL, Stammers A, Raush E, et al: A retrospective study of perfusion incidents and safety devices. *Perfusion* 2000; 15:51.
93. Sylivris S, Levi C, Matalanis G, et al: Pattern and significance of cerebral microemboli during coronary artery bypass grafting. *Ann Thorac Surg* 1998; 66:1674.
94. Grocott HP, Croughwell ND, Amory DW, et al: Cerebral emboli and serum S-100-B during cardiac operation. *Ann Thorac Surg* 1998; 65:1645.
95. Milsom FP, Mitchell SJ: A dual-vent left heart de-airing technique markedly reduces carotid artery microemboli. *Ann Thorac Surg* 1998; 66:785.
96. Clark RE, Brillman J, Davis DA, et al: Microemboli during coronary artery bypass grafting: genesis and effects on outcome. *J Thorac Cardiovasc Surg* 1995; 109:249.
97. Morris SJ: Leucocyte reduction in cardiovascular surgery. *Perfusion* 2001; 11:371.
98. Gu YJ, deVries AJ, Voa P, et al: Leukocyte depletion during cardiac operations: a new approach through the venous bypass circuit. *Ann Thorac Surg* 1999; 67:604.
99. Hurst T, Johnson D, Cujec B, et al: Depletion of activated neutrophils by a filter during cardiac valve surgery. *Can J Anaesth* 1997; 44:131.
100. Mahoney CB: Heparin-bonded circuits: clinical outcome and costs. *Perfusion* 1998; 13:1892.
101. Hsu L-C: Heparin-coated CPB circuits: current status. *Perfusion* 2001; 16:417.
102. Edmunds LH Jr, Stenach N: The blood-surface interface, in Gravlee GP, Davis RF, Kurusz M, Utley JR (eds): *Cardiopulmonary Bypass: Principles and Practice,* 2nd ed. Media, PA, Williams & Wilkins, 2000; p 149.
103. Videm V, Mollnes TE, Fosse E, et al: Heparin-coated cardiopulmonary bypass equipment, I: biocompatibility markers and development of complications in a high-risk population. *J Thorac Cardiovasc Surg* 1999; 117:794.
104. Wildevuur CRH, Jansen DGM, Bezemer PD, et al: Clinical evaluation of Duraflo II heparin treated extracorporeal circuits. *Eur J Cardiothorac Surg* 1997; 11:616.
105. DeSomer F, VanBelleghem Y, Cases F, et al: Phosphorylcholine coating offers natural platelet preservation during CPB. *Perfusion* 2002; 17:39.
106. Ereth MH, Nuttall GA, Clarke SH, et al: Biocompatibility of trillium biopassive surface-coated oxygenator versus un-coated oxygenator during CPB. *J Cardiothorac Vasc Anesth* 2001; 15:545.
107. Gu YJ, Boonstra PW, Rijnsburger AA, et al: Cardiopulmonary bypass circuit treated with surface-modifying additives: a clinical evaluation of blood compatibility. *Ann* Thorac Surg 1998; 65:1343.
108. Edmunds LH Jr, Saxena NH, Hillyer P, Wilson TJ: Relationship between platelet count and cardiotomy suction return. *Ann Thorac Surg* 1978; 25:306.
109. Kincaid EH, Jones TJ, Stump DA, et al: Processing scavinged blood with a cell saver reduces cerebral lipid microembolism. *Ann Thorac Surg* 2000; 70(4):1296.
110. Downing SW, Edmunds LH Jr: Release of vasoactive substances during cardiopulmonary bypass. *Ann Thor Surg* 1992; 54:1236.
111. Baile EM, Ling IT, Heyworth JR, et al: Bronchopulmonary anastomotic and noncoronary collateral blood flow in humans during cardiopulmonary bypass. *Chest* 1985; 87:749.
112. Little AG, Lin CY, Wernley JA, et al: Use of the pulmonary artery for left ventricular venting during cardiac operations. *J Thorac Cardiovasc Surg* 1984; 87:532.
113. Casha AR: A simple method of aortic root venting for CABG [letter]. *Ann Thorac Surg* 1998; 66:608.
114. Olinger GM, Bonchek LI: Ventricular venting during coronary revascularization: assessment of benefit by intraoperative ventricular function curves. *Ann Thorac Surg* 1978; 26:525.
115. Salomon NW, Copeland JG: Single catheter technique for cardioplegia and venting during coronary artery bypass grafting. *Ann Thorac Surg* 1980; 29:88.
116. Marco JD, Barner HB: Aortic venting: comparison of vent effectiveness. *J Thorac Cardiovasc Surg* 1977; 73:287.
117. Clements F, Wright SJ, deBruijn N: Coronary sinus catheterization made easy for port-access minimally invasive cardiac surgery. *J Cardiothorac Vasc Anesth* 1998; 12:96.
118. Aldea GS, Connelly G, Fonger JD, et al: Directed atraumatic coronary sinus cannulation for retrograde cardioplegia administration. *Ann Thorac Surg* 1992; 54:789.
119. Panos AL, Ali IS, Birnbaum PL, et al: Coronary sinus injuries during retrograde continuous normothermic blood cardioplegia. *Ann Thorac Surg* 1992; 54:1132.
120. Journois D, Israel-Biet E, Pouard P, et al: High volume, zero-balance hemofiltration to reduce delayed inflammatory response to cardiopulmonary bypass in children. *Anesthesiology* 1996; 85:965.
121. Boldt J, Zickmann B, Fedderson B, et al: Six different hemofiltration devices for blood conservation in cardiac surgery. *Ann Thorac Surg* 1991; 51:747.
122. High KM, Williams DR, Kurusz M: Cardiopulmonary bypass circuits and design, in Hensley FA Jr, Martin DE (eds): *A Practical Approach to Cardiac Anesthesia,* 2nd ed. Boston, Little, Brown, 1995, p 465.
123. Stammers AH: Monitoring controversies during cardiopulmonary bypass: how far have we come? *Perfusion* 1998; 13:35.
124. Baraka A, Barody M, Harous S, et al: Continuous venous oximetry during cardiopulmonary bypass: influence of temperature changes, perfusion flow and hematocrit level. *J Cardiothorac Anesth* 1990; 4:35.
125. Pearson DT: Blood gas control during cardiopulmonary bypass. *Perfusion* 1988; 31:113.
126. Mark JB, Fitzgerald D, Fenton T, et al: Continuous arterial and venous blood gas monitoring during cardiopulmonary bypass. *J Thorac Cardiovasc Surg* 1991; 102:431.
127. Kirson LE, Goldman JM: A system for monitoring the delivery of ventilating gas to the oxygenator during cardiopulmonary bypass. *J Cardiothorac Vasc Anesth* 1994; 8:51.
128. Berg E, Knudsen N: Automatic data collection for cardiopulmonary bypass. *Perfusion* 1988; 3:263.
129. Beppu T, Imai Y, Fukui Y: A computerized control system for cardiopulmonary bypass. *J Thorac Cardiovasc Surg* 1995; 109:428.
130. Castiglioni A, Verzini A, Pappalardo F, et al: Minimally invasive closed circuit versus standard extracorporeal circulation for aortic valve replacement. *Ann Thorac Surg* 2007; 83:586-91.
131. Rosengart T, DeBois W, O'Hara M, et al: Retrograde autologous priming for cardiopulmonary bypass: a safe and effective means of decreasing hemodilution and transfusion requirements. *J Thorac Cardiovasc Surg* 1998; 115:426.
132. Boldt J: Volume therapy in cardiac surgery: does the kind of fluid matter? *J Cardiothorac Vasc Anesth* 1999; 13:752.
133. Hoeft A, Korb H, Mehlhorn U, et al: Priming of CPB with human albumin or ringer lactate: effect on colloid osmotic pressure and extravascular lung water. *Br J Anaesth* 1991; 66:77.

134. Cochrane Injuries Group Albumin Reviews: Human albumin administration in critically ill patients: systemic review of randomized controlled trials. *BMJ* 1998; 317:235.
135. Wilkes MM, Navickis RJ, Sibbald WJ: Albumin versus hydroxyethyl starch in CPB surgery: a meta-analysis of post-operative bleeding. *Ann Thorac Surg* 2001; 72:527.
136. McKnight CK, Elliott MJ, et al: The cardiopulmonary bypass pump priming fluid and nitrogen balance after open heart surgery in adults. *Perfusion* 1986; 1:47.
137. McKnight CK, Elliott MJ, Pearson DT, et al: The effect of four different crystalloid bypass pump priming fluids upon the metabolic response to cardiac operations. *J Thorac Cardiovasc Surg* 1985; 90:97.
138. Lanier WL: Glucose management during cardiopulmonary bypass: cardiovascular and neurologic implications. *Anesth Analg* 1991; 72:423.
139. Francis JL, Palmer GJ III, Moroose R, Drexler A: Comparison of bovine and porcine heparin in heparin antibody formation after cardiac surgery. *Ann Thorac Surg* 2003; 75(1):15-16.
140. Heres EK, Speight K, Benckart D, et al: The clinical onset of heparin is rapid. *Anesth Analg* 2001; 92:1391-1395.
141. Bull BS, Huse WM, Brauer FS, et al: Heparin therapy during extracorporeal circulation: the use of a drug response curve to individualize heparin and protamine dosage. *J Thorac Cardiovasc Surg* 1975; 69:685.
142. Levy JH, Despotis GJ, Szlam F, et al: Recombinant human transgenic antithrombin in cardiac surgery: a dose finding study. *Anesthesiology* 2002; 96:1095.
143. Weiss ME, Nyhan D, Peng Z, et al: Association of protamine IgE and IgG antibodies with life-threatening reactions to intravenous protamine. *NEJM* 1989; 320:886.
144. Khabbaz KR, Zankoul F, Warner KG: Intraoperative metabolic monitoring of the heart, II: online measurement of myocardial tissue pH. *Ann Thorac Surg* 2001; 72:S2227.
145. Ikonomidis JS, Yau IM, Weisel RD, et al: Optimal flow rates for retrograde warm cardioplegia. *J Thorac Cardiovasc Surg* 1994; 107:510.
146. Kirklin JW, Barrett-Boyes BE: *Cardiac Surgery*, 2nd ed. New York, Wiley, 1993, Ch. 2.
147. Taylor KM, Bain WH, Maxted KJ, et al: Comparative studies of pulsatile and nonpulsatile bypass, I: pulsatile system employed and its hematologic effects. *J Thorac Cardiovasc Surg* 1978; 75:569.
148. Taylor KM, Bain WH, Davidson KG, Turner MA: Comparative clinical study of pulsatile and non-pulsatile perfusion in 350 consecutive patients. *Thorax* 1982; 37:324.
149. Shaw PJ, Bates D, Cartlige NEF: Analysis of factors predisposing to neurological injury in patients undergoing coronary bypass operations. *QJM* 1989; 72:633.
150. Rees W, Schiessler A, Schulz F, et al: Pulsatile extra-corporeal circulation: fluid-mechanic considerations. *Perfusion* 1993; 8:459.
151. Gourlay T, Taylor KM: Pulsatile flow and membrane oxygenators. *Perfusion* 1994; 9:189.
152. Sugurtekin H, Boston US, Cook DJ: Bypass flow, mean arterial pressure, and cerebral perfusion during cardiopulmonary bypass in dogs. *J Cardiothorac Vasc Anesth* 2000; 14:25.
153. Hill SE, van Wermeskerken GK, Lardenoye J-WH, et al: Intraoperative physiologic variables and outcome in cardiac surgery, part I: in-hospital mortality. *Ann Thorac Surg* 2000; 69:1070.
154. Gold JP, Charlson MR, Williams-Russa P, et al: Improvements of outcomes after coronary artery bypass: a randomized trial comparing intraoperative high versus low mean arterial pressure. *J Thorac Cardiovasc Surg* 1995; 110:1302.
155. Hartman GS, Yao F-S, Bruefach M, et al: Severity of aortic atheromatous disease diagnosed by transesophageal echocardiography predicts stroke and other outcomes associated with coronary artery surgery: a prospective study. *Analg Anesth* 1996; 83:701.
156. Liam B-L, Plöchl W, Cook DJ, et al: Hemodilution and whole body oxygen balance during normothermic cardiopulmonary bypass in dogs. *J Thorac Cardiovasc Surg* 1998; 115:1203.
157. Cook DJ: Optimal conditions for cardiopulmonary bypass. *Semin Cardiothorac Vasc Anesth* 2001; 5:265.
158. Hill SE, VanWermesker, Ken GK, et al: Intraoperative physiologic variables and outcome in cardiac surgery, part I: in-hospital mortality. *Ann Thorac Surg* 2000; 69:1070.
159. DeFoe GR, Ross CS, Olmstead EM, et al: Lowest hematocrit on bypass and adverse outcomes associated with coronary artery bypass grafting. *Ann Thorac Surg* 2001; 71:769.
160. Groom RC: High or low hematocrits during cardiopulmonary bypass for patients undergoing coronary artery bypass graft surgery? An evidence-based approach to the question. *Perfusion* 2002; 17:99.
161. Jonas RA: Optimal pH strategy for hypothermic circulatory arrest [editorial]. *J Thorac Cardiovasc Surg* 2001; 121:204.
162. Khatri P, Babyak M, Croughwell ND, et al: Temperature during coronary artery bypass surgery affects quality of life. *Ann Thorac Surg* 2001; 71:110.
163. Engleman RM, Pleet AB, Hicks R, et al: Is there a relationship between systemic perfusion temperature during coronary artery bypass grafting and extent of intraoperative ischemic central nervous system injury? *J Thorac Cardiovasc Surg* 2000; 119:230.
164. Nathan HJ, Wells GA, Munson JL, Wozny D: Neuroprotective effect of mild hypothermia in patients undergoing coronary artery surgery with cardiopulmonary bypass. A randomized trial. *Circulation* 2001; 104(suppl I):I-85.
165. Stephan H, Weyland A, Kazmaier S, et al: Acid-base management during hypothermic cardiopulmonary bypass does not affect cerebral metabolism but does affect blood flow and neurologic outcome. *Br J Anaesth* 1992; 69:51.
166. Murkin JM, Farrar JK, Tweed WA, et al: Cerebral autoregulation and flow/metabolism coupling during cardiopulmonary bypass: rhe influence of $PaCO_2$. *Anesth Analg* 1987; 66:825.
167. Van den Berghe G, Wouters P, Weekers, et al: Intensive insulin therapy in critically ill patients. *NEJM* 2001; 345:1359.
168. Shine TS, Uchikado M, Crawford CC, Murray MJ: Importance of perioperative blood glucose management in cardiac surgical patients. *Asian Cardiovasc Thorac Annals* 2007; 15:534-538.
169. Bernard GR, Sopko G, Cerra F, et al: National Heart Lung and Blood Institute and Food and Drug Administration Workshop Report: Pulmonary Artery Catheterization and Clinical Outcomes (PACC). *JAMA* 2000; 283:2568.
170. Shanewise JS, Cheung AT, Aronson S, et al: ASE/SCA guidelines for performing a comprehensive intraoperative multiplane transesophageal echocardiography examination: recommendation of the American Society of Echocardiography council for intraoperative echocardiography and the Society of Cardiovascular Anesthesiologists task force for certification in perioperative echocardiography. *Anesth Analg* 1999; 99:870.
171. Lucina MG, Savage RM, Hearm C, Kraenzler EJ: The role of transesophageal echocardiography on perfusion management. *Semin Cardiothorac Vasc Anesth* 2001; 5:321.
172. Paul D, Hartman GS: Foley balloon occlusion of the atheromatous ascending aorta: the role of transesophageal echocardiography. *J Cardiothorac Vasc Anesth* 1998; 12:61.
173. Siegel LC, St Goar FG, Stevens JH, et al: Monitoring considerations for Port-Access cardiac surgery. *Circulation* 1997; 96:562.
174. Yamada E, Matsumura M, Kimura S, et al: Usefulness of transesophageal echocardiography in detecting changes in flow dynamics responsible for malperfusion phenomena observed during surgery of aortic dissection. *Am J Cardiol* 1997; 79:1149.
175. Tingleff J, Joyce FS, Pettersson G: Intraoperative echocardiographic study of air embolism during cardiac operations. *Ann Thorac Surg* 1995; 60:673.
176. Stone JG, Young WL, Smith CR, et al: Do standard monitoring sites reflect true brain temperature when profound hypothermia is rapidly induced and reversed? *Anesthesiology* 1995; 82:344.
177. Rumana CS, Gopinath SP, Uzura M, et al: Brain temperature exceeds systemic temperature in head-injured patients. *Crit Care Med* 1998; 26:562.
178. Johnson RZ, Fox MA, Grayson A, et al: Should we rely on nasopharyngeal temperature during cardiopulmonary bypass? *Perfusion* 2002; 17:145.
179. Nussmeier NA, personal communication, 2002.
180. Stump DA, Jones JJ, Rorie KD: Neurophysiologic monitoring and outcomes in cardiovascular surgery [review article]. *J Cardiothorac Vasc Anesth* 1999; 13:600.
181. McDaniel LB, Zwischenberger JM, Vertrees RA, et al: Mixed venous oxygen saturation during cardiopulmonary bypass poorly predicts regional venous saturation. *Anesth Analg* 1994; 80:466.
182. Wenger R, Bavaria JE, Ratcliffe M, Edmunds LH Jr: Flow dynamics of peripheral venous catheters during extracorporeal membrane oxygenator (ECMO) with a centrifugal pump. *J Thorac Cardiovasc Surg* 1988; 96:478.
183. Hessel EA II: Bypass techniques for descending thoracic aortic surgery. *Semin Cardiothorac Vasc Anesth* 2001; 5:293.
184. Ireland KW, Follette DM, Iguidbashian J, et al: Use of a heat exchanger to prevent hypothermia during thoracic and thoracoabdominal aneurysm repairs. *Ann Thorac Surg* 1993; 55:534.
185. Edmunds LH Jr, Austen WG, Shaw RS, Kosminski S: Clinical and physiologic considerations of left heart bypass during cardiac arrest. *J Thorac Cardiovasc Surg* 1961; 41:356.

186. Hedlund KD, Dattilo R: Supportive angioplasty [letter]. *Perfusion* 1990; 5:297.
187. Toomasian JM: Cardiopulmonary bypass for less invasive procedures. *Perfusion* 1999; 14:279.
188. Grocott HP, Smith MS, Glower DC, Clements FM: Endovascular aortic balloon clamp malposition during minimally invasive cardiac surgery. *Anesthesiology* 1998; 88:1396.
189. Young WL, Lawton MT, Gupta DF, Hashimoto T: Anesthetic management of deep hypothermic circulatory arrest for cerebral aneurysm surgery. *Anesthesiology* 2002; 96:497.
190. Soong WAL, Uysal S, Reich DL: Cerebral protection during surgery of the aortic arch. *Semin Cardiothorac Vasc Anesth* 2001; 5:286.
191. Hiramatsu T, Miura T, Forbess JM, et al: pH strategies and cerebral energetics before and after circulatory arrest. *J Thorac Cardiovasc Surg* 1995; 109:948.
192. Kurth CD, O'Rourke MM, O'Hara IB: Comparison of pH-stat and alpha stat cardiopulmonary bypass on cerebral oxygenation and blood flow in relation to hypothermic circulatory arrest in piglets. *Anesthesiology* 1998; 98:110.
193. Sakamoto T, Zurakowski D, Duebener LF, et al: Combination of alpha-stat strategy and hemodilution exacerbates neurologic injury in a survival piglet model with deep hypothermic circulatory arrest. *Ann Thorac Surg* 2002; 73:180.
194. Jonas RA, Bellinger DC, Rappaport LA et al: Relation of pH-strategy and development outcome after hypothermic circulatory arrest. *J Thorac Cardiovasc Surg* 1993; 106:362.
195. Hindman BJ: Choice of α-stat or ph-stat management and neurologic outcomes after cardiac surgery: it depends. *Anesthesiology* 1998; 98:5.
196. Ekroth R, Thompson RJ, Lincoln C, et al: Elective deep hypothermia with total circulatory arrest: changes in plasma creatine kinase BB, blood glucose, and clinical variables. *J Thorac Cardiovasc Surg* 1989; 97:30.
197. Reich DL, Uysal S, Sliwinski M, et al: Neuropsychological outcome following deep hypothermia circulatory arrest in adults. *J Thorac Cardiovasc Surg* 1999; 117:156.
198. Ergin MA, Galla JD, Lansman SL, et al: Hypothermic circulatory arrest in operations on the thoracic aorta. *J Thorac Cardiovasc Surg* 1994; 107:788.
199. Ergin MA, Uysal S, Reich DL, et al: Temporary neurological dysfunction after deep hypothermic circulatory arrest: a clinical marker of long term functional deficit. *Ann Thorac Surg* 1999; 67:1886.
200. Mezrow CK, Midulla PS, Sadeghi AM, et al: Quantitative electroencephalography: a method to assess cerebral injury after hypothermic circulatory arrest. *J Thorac Cardiovasc Surg* 1995; 109:925.
201. Newberger JW, Jonas RA, Wernovsky G, et al: A comparison on the perioperative neurologic defect of hypothermic circulatory arrest versus low flow cardiopulmonary in infant heart surgery. *NEJM* 1993; 329:1057.
202. Grabenwoger M, Ehrlich M, Cartes-Zumelzu F, et al: Surgical treatment of aortic arch aneurysms in profound hypothermia and circulatory arrest. *Ann Thorac Surg* 1997; 64:1067.
203. Higami T, Kozawa S, Asada T, et al: Retrograde cerebral perfusion versus selective cerebral perfusion as evaluated by cerebral oxygen saturation during aortic arch reconstruction. *Ann Thorac Surg* 1999; 67:1091.
204. Kazui T, Kimura N, Yamada O, Komatsu S: Surgical outcome of aortic arch aneurysms using selective cerebral perfusion. *Ann Thorac Surg* 1994; 57:904.
205. Mills NL, Ochsner JL: Massive air embolism during cardiopulmonary bypass: causes, prevention, and management. *J Thorac Cardiovasc Surg* 1980; 80:708.
206. Ueda Y, Miki S, Kusuhara K, et al: Surgical treatment of aneurysm or dissection involving the ascending aorta and aortic arch, utilizing circulatory arrest and retrograde cerebral perfusion. *J Cardiovasc Surg* 1990; 31:553.
207. Ganzel BL, Edmonds HL Jr, Pank JR, Goldsmith LJ: Neurophysiologic monitoring to assure delivery of retrograde cerebral perfusion. *J Thorac Cardiovasc Surg* 1997; 113:748.
208. DeBrux J-L, Subayi J-B, Pegis J-D, Dillet J: Retrograde cerebral perfusion: anatomic study of the distribution of blood to the brain. *Ann Thorac Surg* 1995; 60:1294.
209. Lin PJ, Chang GH, Tan PPC, et al: Prolonged circulatory arrest in moderate hypothermia with retrograde cerebral perfusion: is brain ischemic? *Circulation* 1996; 95 (suppl II):II-166.
210. Murkin JM: Retrograde cerebral perfusion: is the brain really being perfused? [editorial]. *J Cardiothorac Vasc Anesth* 1998; 12:249.
211. Kouchoukos NT: Adjuncts to reduce the incidence of embolic brain injury during operations on the aortic arch. *Ann Thorac Surg* 1994; 57:243.
212. Cheung AT, Bavaria JE, Weiss SJ, et al: Neurophysiologic effects of retrograde cerebral perfusion used for aortic reconstruction. *J Cardiothorac Vasc Anesth* 1998; 12:252.
213. Kurusz M, Butler BD, Katz J, Conti VR: Air embolism during cardiopulmonary bypass. *Perfusion* 1995; 10:361.
214. Ziser A, Adir Y, Lavon H, Shupof A: Hyperbaric oxygen therapy for massive arterial air embolism during cardiac operations. *J Thorac Cardiovasc Surg* 1999; 117:818.
215. Pedersen T, Kaargen AL, Benze S: An approach toward total quality assurance in cardiopulmonary bypass: which data to register and how to assess perfusion quality. *Perfusion* 1996; 11:39.
216. Palanzo DA: Perfusion safety: past present and future. *J Cardiothorac Vasc Anesth* 1997; 11:383.
217. Brister SJ, Ofosu FA, Buchanan MR: Thrombin generation during cardiac surgery: is heparin the ideal anticoagulant? *Thromb Haemost* 1993; 70:259.
218. Uniyal S, Brash JL: Patterns of adsorption of proteins from human plasma onto foreign surfaces. *Thromb Haemost* 1982; 47:285.
219. Horbett TA: Proteins: structure, properties, and adsorption to surfaces, in Ratner BD, Hoffman AS, Schoen FJ, and Lemons JE (eds): *Biomaterials Science: An Introduction to Materials in Medicine.* San Diego, Academic Press, 1996, p 133.
220. Horbett TA: Principles underlying the role of adsorbed plsma proteins in blood interactions with foreign materials. *Cardiovasc Pathol* 1993; 2:137S.
221. Brash JL, Scott CF, ten Hove P, et al: Mechansim of transient adsorption of fibrinogen from plasma to solid surfaces: role of the contact and fibrinolytic systems. *Blood* 1988; 71:932.
222. Edmunds LH Jr, Stenach N: The blood-surface interface, in Gravlee GP, Davis RF, Kurusz M, Utley JR (eds): *Cardiopulmonary Bypass: Principles and Practice,* 2nd ed. Media, PA, Williams & Wilkins, 2000, p 149.
223. Edmunds LH Jr: Blood activation in mechanical circulatory assist devices. *J Congestive Heart Failure Circ* 2000; 1(supp l):141.
224. Bernabei AF, Gikakis N, Maione T, et al: Reversal of heparin anticoagulation by recombinant platelet factor 4 and protamine sulfate in baboons during cardiopulmonary bypass. *J Thorac Cardiovasc Surg* 1995; 109:765.
225. Rosenberg RD, Edelberg M, Zhang L: The heparin-antithrombin system: a natural anticoagulant mechanism, in Colman RW, Hirsh J, Marder VJ, et al (eds): *Hemostasis and Thrombosis: Basic Principles and Clinical Practice.* Philadelphia, JB Lippincott, 2001, p 711.
226. Weitz JI, Hudoba M, Massel D, et al: Clot-bound thrombin is protected from inhibition by heparin- antithrombin III-independent inhibitors. *J Clin Invest* 1990; 86:385.
227. Eisenberg PR, Siegel JE, Abendschein DR, Miletich JP: Importance of factor Xa in determining the procoagulant activity of whole-blood clots. *J Clin Invest* 1993; 91:1877.
228. Khuri S, Valeri CR, Loscalzo J, et al: Heparin causes platelet dysfunction and increases fibrinolysis before the institution of cardiopulmonary bypass. *Ann Thorac Surg* 1995; 60:1008.
229. Sobel M, McNeill PM, Carlson PL, et al: Heparin inhibition of von Willebrand factor-dependent platelet function in vitro and in vivo. *J Clin Invest* 1991; 87:1878.
230. Kirklin JK, Chenoweth DE, Naftel DC, et al: Effects of protamine administration after cardiopulmonary bypass on complement, blood elements, and the hemodynamic state. *Ann Thorac Surg* 1986; 41:193.
231. Shore-Lesserson L, Gravlee GP: Anticoagulation for cardiopulmonary bypass, in Gravlee GP, Davis RF, Kurusz M, Utley JR (eds): *Cardiopulmonary Bypass: Principles and Practice.* Philadelphia, Lippincott Williams & Wilkins, 2000, p 435.
232. Dietrich W, Spannagl M, Schramm W, et al: The influence of preoperative anticoagulation on heparin response during cardiopulmonary bypass. *J Thorac Cardiovasc Surg* 1991; 102:505.
233. Hirsh J, Levine MN: Low molecular weight heparin. *Blood* 1992; 79:1.
234. Danhof M, de Boer A, Magnani HN, Stiekema JC: Pharmacokinetic considerations on Orgaran (Org 10172) therapy. *Haemostasis* 1992; 22:73.
235. Stringer KA, Lindenfeld J: Hirudins: antithrombin anticoagulants. *Ann Pharmacother* 1992; 26:1535.
236. Gladwell TD: Bivalirudin: a direct thrombin inhibitor. *Clin Ther* 2002; 1:38.
237. Swan SK, St Perer JV, Lanbrecht LJ, Hursting MJ: Comparison of anticoagulant effects and safety of argatroban and heparin in healthy subjects. *Pharmacotherapy* 2000; 20:756.
238. Beiderlinden M, Treschan TA, Gorlinger K, et al: Argatroban anticoagulation in critically ill patients. *Ann Pharmacother* 2007; 42:421.
239. Warkentin TE, Kelton JG: Temporal aspects of heparin-induced thrombocytopenia. *NEJM* 2001; 344:1286.

240. Horne DK: Nonimmune heparin-platelet interactions: implications for the pathogenesis of hearin-induced thrombocytopenia, in Warkentin TE, Greinacher A (eds): *Heparin-Induced Thrombocytopenia.* New York, Marcel Dekker, 2001, p 137.
241. Lee DH, Warkentin TE: Frequency of heparin-induced thrombocytopenia, in Warkentin TE, Greinacher A (eds): *Heparin-Induced Thrombocytopenia.* New York, Marcel Dekker, 2001, p 87.
242. Warkentin TE, Greinacher A: Laboratory testing for heparin-induced thrombocytopenia, in Warkentin TE, Greinacher A (eds): *Heparin-Induced Thrombocytopenia.* New York, Marcel Dekker, 2001, p 231.
243. Warkentin TE, Greinacher A: Laboratory testing for heparin-induced thrombocytopenia, in Warkentin TE, Greinacher A (eds): *Heparin-Induced Thrombocytopenia.* New York, Marcel Dekker, 2001, p 231.
244. Wallis DE, Workman KL, Lewis BE, et al: Failure of early heparin cessation as treatment for heparin-induced thrombocytopenia. *Am J Med* 1999; 106:629.
245. Nuttall GA, Oliver WJ Jr, Santrach PJ, et al: Patients with a history of type II heparin-induced thrombocytopenia with thrombosis requiring cardiac surgery with cardiopulmonary bypass: A prospective observational case series. *Anesth Analg* 2003; 96:344.
246. Greinacher A: Recombinant hirudin for the treatment of heparin-induced thrombocytopenia, in Warkentin TE, Greinacher A (eds): *Heparin-Induced Thrombocytopenia.* New York, Marcel Dekker, 2001, p 349.
247. Colman RW: Contact activation pathway: inflammatory, fibrinolytic, anticoagulant, antiadhesive and antiangiogenic activities, in Colman RW, Hirsh J, Marder VJ, et al (eds): *Hemostasis and Thrombosis: Basic Principles and Practice.* Philadelphia, Lippincott Williams & Wilkins, 2001, p 103.
248. Sundaram S, Gikakis N, Hack CE, et al: Nafamostat mesilate, a broad spectrum protease inhibitor, modulates cellular and humoral activation in simulated extracorporeal circulation. *Thromb Haemost* 1996; 75:76.
249. Boisclair MD, Lane DA, Philippou H, et al: Mechanisms of thrombin generation during surgery and cardiopulmonary bypass. *Blood* 1993; 82:3350.
250. Chung JH, Gikakis N, Rao AK, et al: Pericardial blood activates the extrinsic coagulation pathway during clinical cardiopulmonary bypass. *Circulation* 1996; 93:2014.
251. Jenny NS, Mann KG: Thrombin, in Colman RW, Hirsh J, Marder VJ, et al (eds): *Hemostasis and Thrombosis: Basic Principles and Practice.* Philadelphia, Lippincott Williams & Wilkins, 2001, p 171.
252. Drake TA, Morrissey JH, Edgington TS: Selective cellular expression of tissue factor in human tissues. *Am J Pathol* 1989; 134:1087.
253. Hattori T, Khan MMH, Coleman RW, Edmunds LH: Plasma tissue factor plus activated peripheral mononuclear cells activate Factors VII and X in cardiac surgical wounds. *JACC* 2005; 46(4):707.
254. Hirsh J, Colman RW, Marder VJ, et al: Overview of thrombosis and its treatment, in Colman RW, Hirsh J, Marder VJ, et al (eds): *Hemostasis and Thrombosis: Basic Principles and Practice.* Philadelphia, Lippincott Williams & Wilkins, 2001, p 1071.
255. Spanier T, Oz M, Levin H, Weinberg A, et al: Activation of coagulation and fibrinolytic pathways in patients with left ventricular assist devices. *J Thorac Cardiovasc Surg* 1996; 112:1090.
256. Ovrum E, Holen EA, Tangen G, et al: Completely heparinized cardiopulmonary bypass and reduced systemic heparin: clinical and hemostatic effects. *Ann Thorac Surg* 1995; 60:365.
257. Rubens FD, Labow RS, Lavallee GR, et al: Hematologic evaluation of cardiopulmonary bypass circuits prepared with a novel block copolymer. *Ann Thorac Surg* 1999; 67:696.
258. Aldea GS, O'Gara P, Shapira OM, et al: Effect of anticoagulation protocol on outcome in patients undergoing CABG with heparin-bonded cardiopulmonary bypass circuits. *Ann Thorac Surg* 1998; 65:425.
259. Despotis GJ, Joist JH, Hogue CW, et al: More effective suppression of hemostatic system activation in patients undergoing cardiac surgery by heparin dosing based on heparin blood concentrations rather than ACT. *Thromb Haemost* 1996; 76:902.
260. Tabuchi N, Haan J, Boonstra PW, van Oeveren W: Activation of fibrinolysis in the pericardial cavity during cardiopulmonary bypass. *J Thorac Cardiovasc Surg* 1993; 106:828.
261. Coughlin SR, Vu T-K H, Hung DT, Wheaton VI: Characterization of a functional thrombin receptor. *J Clin Invest* 1992; 89:351.
262. Michelson AD, MacGregor H, Barnard MR, et al: Reversible inhibition of human platelet activation by hypothermia in vivo and in vitro. *Thromb Haemost* 1994; 71:633.
263. Weerasinghe A, Taylor KM: The platelet in cardiopulmonary bypass. *Ann Thorac Surg* 1998; 66:2145.
264. Rinder CS, Bonnert J, Rinder HM, et al: Platelet activation and aggregation during cardiopulmonary bypass. *Anesthesiology* 1991; 74:388.
265. Gluszko P, Rucinski B, Musial J, et al: Fibrinogen receptors in platelet adhesion to surfaces of extracorporeal circuit. *Am J Physiol* 1987; 252:H615.
266. Zilla P, Fasol R, Groscurth P, et al: Blood platelets in cardiopulmonary bypass operations. *J Thorac Cardiovasc Surg* 1989; 97:379.
267. Kestin AS, Valeri CR, Khuri SF, et al: The platelet function defect of cardiopulmonary bypass. *Blood* 1993; 82:107.
268. Khan MMH, Hattori T, Niewiarowski S, Edmunds LH, Coleman RW: Truncated and microparticle-free soluble tissue factor bound to peripheral monocytes preferentially activate factor VII. *Thromb Haemost* 2006; 95:462.
269. Steinberg JB, Kapelanski DP, Olson JD, Weiler JM: Cytokine and complement levels in patients undergoing cardiopulmonary bypass. *J Thorac Cardiovasc Surg* 1993; 106:1008.
270. Saadi S, Platt JL: Endothelial cell responses to complement activation, in Volankis JE, Frank MM (eds): *The Human Complement System in Health and Disease.* New York, Marcel Dekker, 1998, p 335.
271. Vane JR, Anggard EE, Botting RM: Regulatory functions of the vascular endothelium. *NEJM* 1990; 323:27.
272. Levin EG, Marzec U, Anderson J, et al: Thrombin stimulates tissue plasminogen activator from cultured human endothelial cells. *J Clin Invest* 1984; 74:1988.
273. Francis CW, Marder VJ: Physiologic regulation and pathologic disorders of fibrinolysis, in Colman RW, Hirsh J, Marder VJ, et al: *Hemostasis and Thrombosis: Basic Principles and Practice.* Philadelphia, Lippincott Williams & Wilkins, 2001, p 975.
274. Bachmann F: Plasminogen-plasmin enzyme system, in Colman RW, Hirsh J, Marder VJ, et al: *Hemostasis and Thrombosis: Basic Principles and Practice.* Philadelphia, Lippincott Williams & Wilkins, 2001, p 275.
275. Feinstein DI, Marder VJ, Colman RW: Consumptive thrombohemorrhagic disorders, in Colman RW, Hirsh J, Marder VJ, et al: *Hemostasis and Thrombosis: Basic Principles and Practice.* Philadelphia, Lippincott Williams & Wilkins, 2001, p 1197.
276. Walport MJ: Complement. *NEJM* 2001; 344:1058.
277. Fung M, Loubser PG, Ündar A, et al: Inhibition of complement, neutrophil, and platelet activation by an anti-factor D monoclonal antibody in simulated cardiopulmonary bypass circuits. *J Thorac Cardiovasc Surg* 2001; 122:113.
278. van Oeveren W, Kazatchkine MD, Descamps-Latscha B, et al: Deleterious effects of cardiopulmonary bypass: a prospective study of bubble versus membrane oxygenation. *J Thorac Cardiovasc Surg* 1985; 89:888.
279. Chenoweth DE, Cooper SW, Hugli TE, et al: Complement activation during cardiopulmonary bypass: evidence for generation of C3a and C5a anaphylactoxins. *NEJM* 1981; 304:497.
280. Cavarocchi NC, Schaff HV, Orszulak TA, et al: Evidence for complement activation by protamine-heparin interaction after cardiopulmonary bypass. *Surgery* 1985; 98:525.
281. Weisman HF, Bartow T, Leppo MK, et al: Recombinant soluble CR1 suppressed complement activation, inflammation, and necrosis associated with reperfusion of ischemic myocardium. *Trans Assoc Am Phys* 1990; 103:64.
282. Walport MJ: Complement. *NEJM* 2001; 344:1058.
283. Moat NE, Shore DF, Evans TW: Organ dysfunction and cardiopulmonary bypass: the role of complement and complement regulatory proteins. *Eur J Cardiothorac Surg* 1993; 7:563.
284. Moat NE, Shore DF, Evans TW: Organ dysfunction and cardiopulmonary bypass: the role of complement and complement regulatory proteins. *Eur J Cardiothorac Surg* 1993; 7:563.
285. Dreyer WJ, Smith CW, Entman ML: Neutrophil activation during cardiopulmonary bypass. *J Thorac Cardiovasc Surg* 1993; 105:763.
286. Fantone JC: Cytokines and neutrophils: neutrophil-derived cytokines and the inflammatory response, in Remick DG, Friedland JS (eds): *Cytokines in Health and Disease,* 2nd ed. New York, Marcel Dekker, 1997, p 373.
287. Warren JS, Ward PA: The inflammatory response, in Beutler E, Coller BS, Lichtman MA, et al: *Williams Hematology,* 6th ed. New York, McGraw-Hill, 2001, p 67.
288. Yang J, Furie BC, Furie B: The biology of P-selectin glycoprotein ligand-1: its role as a selectin counterreceptor in leukocyte-endothelial and leukocyte-platelet interaction. *Thromb Haemost* 1999; 81:1.
289. Springer TA: Traffic signals for lymphocyte circulation and leukocyte migration: the multistep paradigm. *Cell* 1994; 76:301.
290. Asimakopoulos G, Taylor KM: Effects of cardiopulmonary bypass on leukocyte and endothelial adhesion molecules. *Ann Thorac Surg* 1998; 66:2135.
291. Smith WB, Gamble JR, Clarklewis I, Vadas MA: Chemotactic desensitization of neutrophils demonstrates interleukin-8 (IL-8)-dependent and IL-8-independent mechanisms of transmigration through cytokine-activated endothelium. *Immunology* 1993; 78:491.

292. Hayashi Y, Sawa Y, Ohtake S, et al: Peroxynitrite formation from human myocardium after ischemia-reperfusion during open heart operation. *Ann Thorac Surg* 2001; 72:571.
293. Ilton MK, Langton PE, Taylor ML, et al: Differential expression of neutrophil adhesion molecules during coronary artery surgery with cardiopulmonary bypass. *J Thorac Cardiovasc Surg* 1999; 118:930.
294. Borregaard N, Cowland JB: Granules of the human neutrophilic polymorphonuclear leukocyte. *Blood* 1997; 89:3503.
295. Blackstone EH, Kirklin JW, Stewart RW, et al: The damaging effects of cardiopulmonary bypass, in Wu KK, Roxy EC (eds): *Prostaglandins in Clinical Medicine: Cardiovascular and Thrombotic Disorders.* Chicago, Yearbook Medical Publishers, 1982, p 355.
296. Chung JH, Gikakis N, Drake TA, et al: Pericardial blood activates the extrinsic coagulation pathway during clinical cardiopulmonary bypass. *Circulation* 1996; 93:2014.
297. Vane JR, Anggard EE, Botting RM: Regulatory functions of the vascular endothelium. *NEJM* 1990; 323:27.
298. Dreyer WJ, Burns AR, Phillips SC, et al: Intercellular adhesion molecule-1 regulation in the canine lung after cardiopulmonary bypass. *J Thorac Cardiovasc Surg* 1998; 115:689.
299. Funk CD: Platelet eicosanoids, in Colman RW, Hirsh J, Marder VJ, et al (eds): *Hemostasis and Thrombosis: Basic Principles and Practice.* Philadelphia, Lippincott Williams & Wilkins, 2001, p 533.
300. Fukami MH, Holmsen H, Kowalska A, Niewiarowski S: Platelet secretion, in Colman RW, Hirsh J, Marder VJ, et al (eds): *Hemostasis and Thrombosis: Basic Principles and Practice.* Philadelphia, Lippincott Williams & Wilkins, 2001, p 559.
301. Ember JA, Jagels MA, Hugli TE: Characterization of complement anaphylatoxins and their biological responses, in Volankis JE, Frank MM (eds): *The Human Complement System in Health and Disease.* New York, Marcel Dekker, 1998, p 241.
302. Steinberg JB, Kapelanski DP, Olson JD, Weiler JM: Cytokine and complement levels in patients undergoing cardiopulmonary bypass. *J Thorac Cardiovasc Surg* 1993; 106:1008.
303. Pizzo SV, Wu SM: a-Macroglobulins and kinins, in Colman RW, Hirsh J, Marder VJ, et al (eds): *Hemostasis and Thrombosis: Basic Principles and Practice.* Philadelphia, Lippincott Williams & Wilkins, 2001, p 367.
304. Powrie F, Bean A, Moore KW: Interleukin-10, in Remick DG, Friedland JS (eds): *Cytokines in Health and Disease,* 2nd ed. New York, Marcel Dekker, 1997, p 143.
305. Frering B, Philip I, Dehoux M, et al: Circulating cytokines in patients undergoing normothermic cardiopulmonary bypass. *J Thorac Cardiovasc Surg* 1994; 108:636.
306. Drabe N, Zünd G, Grünenfelder J, et al: Genetic predisposition in patients undergoing cardiopulmonary bypass surgery is associated with an increase of inflammatory cytokines. *Eur J Cardiothorac Surg* 2001; 20:609.
307. Babior BM. Phagocytes and oxidative stress. *Am J Med* 2000; 109:33.
308. Kharazmi A, Andersen LW, Baek L, et al: Endotoxemia and enhanced generation of oxygen radicals by neutrophils from patients undergoing cardiopulmonary bypass. *J Thorac Cardiovasc Surg* 1989; 98:381.
309. Nilsson L, Kulander L, Nystrom S-O, Eriksson O: Endotoxins in cardiopulmonary bypass. *J Thorac Cardiovasc Surg* 1990; 100:777.
310. Neuhof C, Wendling J, Friedhelm D, et al: Endotoxemia and cytokine generation in cardiac surgery in relation to flow mode and duration of cardiopulmonary bypass. *Shock* 2001; 16:39.
311. Smith EEJ, Naftel DC, Blackstone EH, Kirklin JW: Microvascular permeability after cardiopulmonary bypass. *J Thorac Cardiovasc Surg* 1987; 94:225.
312. Menasché PH: The systemic factor: The comparative roles of cardiopulmonary bypass and off-pump surgery in the genesis of patient injury during and following cardiac surgery. *Ann Thorac Surg* 2001; 72: S2260.
313. Ascione R, Lloyd CT, Underwood MJ: Inflammatory response after coronary revascularization with and without cardiopulmonary bypass. *Ann Thorac Surg* 2000; 69:1198.
314. Cleveland JC Jr, Shroyer LW, Chen AY, et al: Off-pump coronary artery bypass grafting decreases risk-adjusted mortality and morbidity. *Ann Thorac Surg* 2001; 72:1282.
315. Menasché P, Peynet J, Heffner-Cavaillon N, et al: Influence of temperature on neutrophil trafficking during clinical cardiopulmonary bypass. *Circulation* 1995; 92(suppl II): II-334.
316. Menasché P: The inflammatory response to cardiopulmonary bypass and its impact on postoperative myocardial function. *Curr Opin Cardiol* 1995; 10:597.
317. Øvrum E, Tangen G, Øystese R, et al: Comparison of two heparin-coated extracorporeal circuits with reduced systemic anticoagulation in routine coronary artery bypass operations. *J Thorac Cardiovasc Surg* 2001; 121:324.
318. Gorman RC, Ziats NP, Gikakis N, et al: Surface-bound heparin fails to reduce thrombin formation during clinical cardiopulmonary bypass. *J Thorac Cardiovasc Surg* 1996; 111:1.
319. Aldea GS, O'Gara P, Shapira OM, et al: Effect of anticoagulation protocol on outcome in patients undergoing CABG with heparin-bonded cardiopulmonary bypass circuits. *Ann Thorac Surg* 1998; 65:425.
320. Wendel HP, Ziemer G: Coating-techniques to improve the hemocompatibility of artificial devices used for extracorporeal circulation. *Eur J Cardiothorac Surg* 1999; 16:342.
321. Gunaydin S, Farsak B, Kocakulak M, et al: Clinical performance and biocompatibility of poly (2-methoxyethylacrylate) coated extracorporeal circuits. *Ann Thorac Surg* 2002; 74:819.
322. Ninomiya M, Miyaji K, Takamoto S: Poly (2-methoxyethy-lacrylate)-coated bypass circuits reduce perioperative inflammatory response. *Ann Thorac Surg* 2003; 75:913.
323. Naik SK, Knight A, Elliot M: A prospective randomized study of a modified technique of ultrafiltration during pediatric open-heart surgery. *Circulation* 1991; 84(suppl III): III-422.
324. Luciani GB, Menon T, Vecchi B, et al: Modified ultrafiltration reduces morbidity after adult cardiac operations: a prospective, randomized clinical trial. *Circulation* 2001; 104(suppl I): I-253.
325. Fitch JCK, Rollins S, Matis L, et al: Pharmacology and biological efficacy of a recombinant, humanized, single-chain antibody C5 complement inhibitor in patients undergoing coronary artery bypass graft surgery with cardiopulmonary bypass. *Circulation* 1999; 100:2499.
326. Carrier M, Menasche P, Levy M, et al: Inhibition of Complement activation by pexelizumab reduces death in patients undergoing combined valve replacement and coronary bypass surgery. *J Thorac Cardiovasc Surg* 2006; 131:352.
327. Chai PJ, Nassar R, Oakeley AE, et al: Soluble complement receptor-1 protects heart, lung, and cardiac myofilament function from cardiopulmonary bypass damage. *Circulation* 2000; 101:541.
328. Paparella D, Yau TM, Young E: Cardiopulmonary bypass induced inflammaion: pathophysiology and treatment update. *Eur J Cardiothorac Surg* 2002; 21:232.
329. Cronstein BN, Kimmel SC, Levin RI, et al: A mechanism for the antiinflammatory effects of corticosteroids: the glucocorticoid receptor regulates leukocyte adhesion to endothelial cells and expression of endothelial-leukocyte adhesion molecule 1 and intercellular adhesion molecule 1. *Proc Natl Acad Sci USA* 1992; 89:9991.
330. Harig F, Hohenstein B, von der Emde J, Weyand M: Modulating IL-6 and IL-10 levels by pharmacologic strategies and the impact of different extracorporeal circulation parameters during cardiac surgery. *Shock* 2001; 16:33.
331. Yared JP, Starr NJ, Torres FK, et al: Effects of single dose, postinduction dexamethasone on recovery after cardiac surgery. *Ann Thorac Surg* 2000; 69:1420.
332. Ho KM, Tan JA. Benefits and risks of corticoid prophylaxis in adult cardiac surgery. *Circulation* 2009; 119:1853.
333. Levy JH, Hug CC: Use of cardiopulmonary bypass in studies of the circulation. *Br J Anaesth* 1988; 60:35S.
334. Carson JL, Poses RM, Spence RK, et al: Severity of anaemia and operative mortality and morbidity. *Lancet* 1988; 1:727.
335. Stump DA, Brown WR, Moody DM, et al: Microemboli and neurologic dysfunction after cardiovascular surgery. *Semin Cardiothorac Vascular Anesth* 1999; 3:47.
336. Stone JG, Young WL, Smith CR, et al: Do standard monitoring sites reflect true brain temperature when profound hypothermia is rapidly induced and reversed? *Anesthesiology* 1995; 82:344.
337. Smith EEJ, Naftel DC, Blackstone EH, Kirklin JW: Microvascular permeability after cardiopulmonary bypass. *J Thorac Cardiovasc Surg* 1987; 94:225.
338. Pacifico AD, Digerness S, Kirklin JW: Acute alterations of body composition after open intracardiac operations. *Circulation* 1970; 41:331.
339. Edmunds LH Jr, Williams W: Microemboli and the use of filters during cardiopulmonary bypass, in Utley JR (ed): *Pathophysiology and Techniques of Cardiopulmonary Bypass,* vol II. Baltimore, Williams & Wilkins, 1983, p 101.
340. Brooker RF, Brown WR, Moody DM, et al: Cardiotomy suction: a major source of brain lipid emboli during cardiopulmonary bypass. *Ann Thorac Surg* 1998; 65:1651.
341. Kincaid EH, Jones TJ, Stump DA, et al: Processing scavenged blood with a cell saver reduces cerebral lipid microembolization. *Ann Thorac Surg* 2000; 70:1296.
342. Reichenspurner H, Navia JA, Benny G et al: Particulate embolic capture by an intra-aortic filter device during cardiac surgery. *J Thorac Cardiovasc Surg* 2000; 119:233.

343. Cook DJ, Zehr KJ, Orszulak TA, Slater JM: Profound reduction in brain embolization using an endoaortic baffle during bypass in swine. *Ann Thorac Surg* 2002; 73: 198.
344. Barzilai B, Marshall WG Jr, Saffitz Je, et al: Avoidance of embolic complications by ultrasonic characterization of the ascending aorta. *Circulation* 1989; 80:1275.
345. Reichenspurner H, Navia JA, Benny G, et al: Particulate embolic capture by an intra-aortic filter device during cardiac surgery. *J Thorac Cardiovasc Surg* 2000; 119:233.
346. Hammon JW, Stump DA, Butterworth JE,et. al: Single cross clamp improves six month cognitive outcome in high risk coronary bypass patients. *J Thorac Cardiovasc Surg* 2006; 131:114.
347. Loop FD, Higgins TL, Panda R, et al: Myocardial protection during cardiac operations: decreased morbidity and lower cost with blood cardioplegia and coronary sinus perfusion. *J Cardiovasc Surg* 1992; 104:608.
348. Sundt TM, Barner HB, Camillo CJ, et al: Total arterial revascularization with an internal thoracic artery and radial artery T graft. *Ann Thorac Surg* 1999; 68:399.
349. Tector AJ, Amundsen S, Schmahl TM, et al: Total revascularization with T grafts. *Ann Thorac Surg* 1994; 57:33.
350. Jones TJ, Deal DD, Vernon JC, et al: The propagation of entrained air during cardiopulmonary bypass is affected by circuit design but not by vacuum assisted venous drainage. *Anesth Analg* 2000; 90:39.
351. Braunwald E, Kloner RA: The stunned myocardium: prolonged, postischemic ventricular dysfunction. *Circulation* 1982; 66:1146.
352. Downing SW, Savage EB, Streicher JS, et al: The stretched ventricle: myocardial creep and contractile dysfunction after acute nonischemic ventricular distention. *J Thorac Cardiovasc Surg* 1992; 104:996.
353. Newman S: The incidence and nature of neuropsychological morbidity following cardiac surgery. *Perfusion* 1989; 4:93.
354. Murkin JM, Stump DA, Blumenthal JA, et al: Defining dysfunction: group means versus incidence analysis-a statement of consensus. *Ann Thorac Surg* 1997; 64:904.
355. Selnes OA, Grega MA, Bailey MM, et al: Neurocognitive outcomes 3 years after coronary artery bypass graft surgery: a controlled study. *Ann Thorac Surg* 2007; 84:1885.
356. Baird A, Benfield A, Schlaug G, et al: Enlargement of human cerebral ischemic lesion volumes measured by diffusion-weighted magnetic resonance imaging. *Ann Neurol* 1997; 41:581.
357. Maragos PJ, Schmechel DE: Neuron-specific enolase, a clinically useful marker for neurons and neuroendocrine cells. *Annu Rev Neurol Sci* 1987; 10:269.
358. Zimmer DB, Cornwall EH, Landar A, Song W: The S-100 protein family: history, function, and expression. *Brain Res Bull* 1995; 37: 417.
359. Johnsson P, Blomquist S, Luhrs C, et al: Neuron-specific enolase increases in plasma during and immediately after extracorporeal circulation. *Ann Thorac Surg* 2000; 69:750.
360. Anderson RE, Hansson LO, Liska J, et al: The effect of cardiotomy suction on the brain injury marker S100 beta after cardiopulmonary bypass. *Ann Thorac Surg* 2000; 69:847.
361. Shaw PJ, Bates D, Cartlidge NE, et al: Neurologic and neuropsychological morbidity following: major surgery: comparison of coronary artery bypass and peripheral vascular surgery. *Stroke* 1987; 18:700.
362. Gardner TJ, Horneffer PJ, Manolio TA, et al: Stroke following coronary artery bypass surgery: a ten year study. *Ann Thorac Surg* 1985; 40:574.
363. Moller JT, Cluitmans P, Rasmussen LS, et al: Long-term postoperative cognitive dysfunction in the elderly ISPOCD study. ISPOCD investigators, International Study of Post-Operative Cognitive Dysfunction. *Lancet* 1998; 351:857.
364. Jones EL, Weintraub WS, Craver JM, et al: Coronary bypass surgery: is the operation different today? *J Thorac Cardiovasc Surg* 1991; 101:108.
365. Tardiff BE, Newman MF, Saunders AM, et al: Preliminary report of a genetic basis for cognitive decline after cardiac operations. *Ann Thorac Surg* 1997; 64:715.
366. Weintraub WS, Wenger NK, Jones EL, et al: Changing clinical characteristics of coronary surgery patients: differences between men and women. *Circulation* 1993; 88:79.
367. Goto T, Baba T, Yoshitake A, et al: Craniocervical and aortic atherosclerosis as neurologic risk factors in coronary surgery. *Ann Thorac Surg* 2000; 69:834.
368. Wareing TH, Davila-Roman VG, Daily BB, et al: Strategy for the reduction of stroke incidence in cardiac surgical patients. *Ann Thorac Surg* 1993; 55:1400.
369. Stump DA, Kon NA, Rogers AT, et al: Emboli and neuropsychologic outcome following cardiopulmary bypass. *Echocardiography* 1996; 13:555.
370. Tuman KJ, McCarthy RJ, Najafi H, et al: Differential effects of advanced age on neurologic and cardiac risks of coronary operations. *J Thorac Cardiovasc Surg* 1992; 104:1510.
371. Lata A, Stump D, Deal D, et al: Cannula design reduces particulate and gaseous emboli during cardiopulmonary bypas for coronary artery bypass grafting. *J Cardiac Surg* (in press).
372. Jones TJ, Stump DA, Deal D, et al: Hypothermia protects the brain from embolization by reducing and redirecting the embolic load. *Ann Thorac Surg* 1999; 68:1465.
373. Murkin JM, Farrar JK, Tweed WA, et al: Cerebral autoregulation and flow/metabolism coupling during cardiopulmonary bypass: the role of $PaCO_2$. *Anesth Analg* 1987; 66:665.
374. Stump DA, Brown WR, Moody DM, et al: Microemboli and neurologic dysfunction after cardiovascular surgery. *Semin Cardiothorac Vascular Anesth* 1999; 3:47.
375. Helps SC, Parsons DW, Reilly PL, et al: The effect of gas emboli on rabbit cerebral blood flow. *Stroke* 1990; 21:94.
376. Moody DM, Brown WR, Challa VR, et al: Efforts to characterize the nature and chronicle the occurrence of brain emboli during cardiopulmonary bypass. *Perfusion* 1995; 9:316.
377. Cook DJ, Oliver WC, Orsulak TA, et al: Cardiopulmonary bypass temperature, hematocrit, and cerebral oxygen delivery in humans. *Ann Thorac Surg* 1995; 60:1671.
378. Martin TC, Craver JM, Gott MP, et al: Prospective, randomized trial of retrograde warm-blood cardioplegia: myocardial benefit and neurological threat. *Ann Thorac Surg* 1994; 59:298.
379. Nathan HJ, Wells GA, Munson JL, Wozny D: Neuroprotective effect of mild hypothermia in patients undergoing coronary artery surgery with cardiopulmonary bypass. *Circulation* 2001; 104(suppl I):I-85.
380. Brown R, Wright G, Royston D: A comparison of two systems for assessing cerebral venous oxyhaemoglobin saturation during cardiopulmonary bypass in humans. *Anesthesia* 1993; 48:697.
381. Nussmeier N, Arlund C, Slogoff S: Neuropsychiatric complications after cardiopulmonary bypass: cerebral protection by a barbiturate. *Anesthesiology* 1986; 64:165.
382. Arrowsmith JE, Harrison MJG, Newman SP, et al: Neuroprotection of the brain during cardiopulmonary bypass: a randomized trial of remacemide during coronary artery bypass in 171 patients. *Stroke* 1998; 29:2357.
383. Mitchell SJ, Pellet O, Gorman DF, et al: Cerebral protection by lidocaine during cardiac operations. *Ann Thorac Surg* 1999; 67:1117.
384. Diegeler A, Hirsch R, Schneider F, et al: Neuromonitoring and neurocognitive outcome in off-pump versus conventional coronary bypass operation. *Ann Thorac Surg* 2000; 69:1162.
385. Puskas J, Cheng D, Knight J, et al: Off-pump versus conventional coronary artery bypass grafting: a meta-analysis and consensus statement from the 2004 ISMICS consensus conference. *Innovat Cardiothorac Surg* 2005; 1:3-27.
386. Newman MF, Kirchner JL, Phillips-Bute B, et al: Longitudinal assessment of neurocognitive function after coronary artery bypass grafting. *NEJM* 2001; 344:395-402.
387. Sotaniemi KA: Cerebral outcome after extracorporeal circulation: comparison between prospective and retrospective evaluations. *Arch Neurol* 1983; 40:75.
388. Vermeer SE, Longstreth Jr WT, Koudstaal PJ: Silent brain infarcts: a systematic review. *Lancet Neurol* 2007; 6:611.
389. Hammon JW, Stump DA, Butterworth JE, et al: CABG with single cross clamp results in fewer persistent neuropsychologicl deficits than multiple clamp or OPCAB. *Ann Thorac Surg* 84: 1174.
390. Selnes OA, Grega MA, Borowicz LM, et al: Cognitive outcomes three years after coronary bypass surgery: a comparison of on-pump coronary bypass surgery and nonsurgical controls. *Ann Thorac Surg* 2005; 79: 1201.
391. Mullges W, Babin-Ebell J, Reents W, Toyka KV. Cognitive performance after coronary bypass grafting: a follow-up study. *Neurology* 2002; 59: 741.
392. Maggart M, Stewart S: The mechanisms and management of non-cardiogenic pulmonary edema following cardiopulmonary bypass. *Ann Thorac Surg* 1987; 43:231.
393. Allardyce D, Yoshida S, Ashmore P: The importance of microembolism in the pathogenesis of organ dysfunction caused by prolonged use of the pump oxygenator. *J Thorac Cardiovasc Surg* 1966; 52:706.
394 Tonz M, Mihaljevic T, von Segesser LK, et al: Acute lung injury during cardiopulmonary bypas: are the neutrophils responsible? *Chest* 1995; 108:1551.
395. McGowan FX, del Nido PJ, Kurland G, et al: Cardiopulmonary bypass significantly impairs surfactant activity in children. *J Thorac Cardiovasc Surg* 1993; 106:968.
396. Oster JB, Sladen RN, Berkowitz DE: Cardiopulmonary bypass and the lung, in Gravlee GP, Davis RF, Kurusz M, Utley JR (eds): *Cardiopulmonary Bypass: Principles and Practice.* Philadelphia, Lippincott Williams & Wilkins, 2000, p 367.

397. Cogliati AA, Menichetti A, Tritapepe L, et al: Effects of three techniques of lung management on pulmonary function during cardiopulmonary bypass. *Acta Anaesth Belg* 1996; 47:73.
398. Sirivella A, Gielchinsky I, Parsonnet V: Management of catheter-induced pulmonary artery perforation: a rare complication in cardiovascular operations. *Ann Thorac Surg* 2001; 72:2056.
399. Zanardo G, et al: Acute renal failure in the patient undergoing cardiac operation: prevalence, mortality rate, and main risk factors. *J Thorac Cardiovasc Surg* 1994; 107:1489.
400. Utley JR: Renal function and fluid balance with cardiopulmonary bypass, in Gravlee GP, Davis RF, Utley JR (eds): *Cardiopulmonary Bypass: Principles and Practice.* Baltimore, Williams & Wilkins, 1993, p 488.
401. Clyne DH, Kant KS, Pesce AJ, et al: Nephrotoxicity of low molecular weight serum proteins: physicochemical interactions between myoglobin, hemoglobin, Bence Jones proteins and Tamm-Horsfall mucoprotein. *Curr Prob Clin Biochem* 1979; 9:299.
402. Abel, RM, Buckley, MJ, Austen, WG, et al: Etiology, incidence and prognosis of renal failure following cardiac operations: results of a prospective analysis of 500 consecutive patients. *J Thorac Cardiovasc Surg* 1976; 71:32.
403. Mangano C, et al: Renal dysfunction after myocardial revascularization: risk factors, adverse outcomes and hospital resource utilization. The Multicenter Study of Perioperative Ischemia Research Group. *Anesth Analg* 1998; 1:3.
404. Ryan TA, Rady MY, Bashour CA, et al: Predictors of outcome in cardiac surgical patients with prolonged intensive care stay. *Chest* 1997; 112:1035.
405. Rattner DW, Gu Z-Y, Vlahakes GJ, et al: Hyperamylasemia after cardiac surgery. *Ann Surg* 1989; 209:279.
406. Fernandez-del Castillo C, Harringer W, Warshaw AL, et al: Risk factors for pancreatic celular injury after cardiopulmonary bypass. *NEJM* 1991; 325:382.
407. Mithofer K, Fernandes-del Castillo C, Frick TW, et al: Acute hypercalcemia causes acute pancreatitis and ectopic trypsinogen activation in the rat. *Gastroenterology* 1995; 109:239.
408. Mori A, Watanabe K, Onoe M, et al: Regional blood flow in the liver, pancreas and kidney during pulsatile and nonpulsatile perfusion under profound hypothermia. *Jpn Circ J* 1988; 52:219.
409. Shangraw RE: Splanchnic, hepatic and visceral effects, in Gravlee GP, Davis RF, Utley JR (eds): *Cardiopulmonary Bypass: Principles and Practice.* Baltimore, Williams & Wilkins, 1993, p 391.
410. Fiddian-Green RG, Baker S: Predictive value of the stomach wall pH for complications after cardiac operations: comparison with other monitoring. *Crit Care Med* 1987, 15:153.
411. Diaz-Gomez JL, Nutter B, Xu M, et al: The effect of postoperative gastrointestinal complications in patients undergoing coronary bypass surgery. *Ann Thorac Surg* 2010; 90:109.

CHAPTER 13

Transfusion Therapy and Blood Conservation

Leonard Y. Lee
William J. DeBois
Karl H. Krieger
O. Wayne Isom

INTRODUCTION

With the development of cardiac surgery in the 1950s to correct congenital heart defects came the need for large-volume blood transfusions. In the 1960s and 1970s, the introduction of valve prostheses and direct grafting of coronary arteries made the correction of acquired heart disease a possibility. These landmarks, along with the liberal use of homologous blood transfusion therapy, led to rapid growth of the field. Commensurate with the growth of cardiac surgery as a field was an increasing incidence of transfusion-transmitted hepatitis in the 1970s, ultimately alerting the public and treating physicians to the concept of blood conservation. The emergence of infection by human immunodeficiency virus (HIV) greater heightened the interest in this area, leading to the current practices of blood conservation therapy in cardiac surgery.

Historically, open-heart surgery has been associated with a high usage of blood transfusion. Some reports suggest that up to 70% of this patient population requires blood transfusions, resulting in an average of two to four donor exposures per patient.[1,2] It has been reported that 10% of all red blood cell units transfused in the United States are administered during coronary bypass surgery.[3] Almost all patients received blood transfusion in the early days of cardiac surgery. However, with an increased awareness of blood-borne infectious diseases, lack of donors, great cost to both the patient and the institution, allergic reaction, blood-type mismatch, and the needs of special populations such as Jehovah's Witnesses, a greater effort has been made to perform open-heart procedures without blood transfusions even in high-risk patients. Advances in perioperative medications that minimize blood loss; greater tolerance of lower hematocrits, especially on bypass; and improvements in surgical techniques resulting in shorter operative times have allowed for these extensive procedures to be performed without significant blood loss.

The high transfusion rates associated with cardiac surgery have been well characterized and are likely caused by the coagulopathy, platelet dysfunction, and red cell hemolysis that occur as a result of the cardiopulmonary bypass circuit.[4–6] The introduction of hemodilution using crystalloid pump-priming solution rather than whole blood dramatically reduced the transfusion requirements seen during coronary artery bypass grafting (CABG) procedures.[7] Although this technique has reduced the amount of blood transfused during cardiopulmonary bypass (CPB), the resulting hemodilution contributes to the risk of low intraoperative and postoperative hematocrit, especially in patients who weigh less than 70 kg, thereby posing a new risk for transfusion.

Efforts at reducing the use of homologous blood in cardiac surgery began almost 40 years ago. The efforts to decrease allogeneic blood exposures have been a topic of constant review and attention because of the desires of both patients and their physicians to conserve blood during the perioperative period. These joint efforts have affected virtually every aspect of the manner in which heart surgery and CPB are performed. Our experience combined with the experiences of others has led to the development of an integrated, comprehensive blood conservation program that makes the goal of bloodless heart surgery possible.

PAST EXPERIENCE: A REVIEW OF THE LITERATURE

Since the earlier edition of this chapter, aprotinin has been discontinued; however, we still include information on it for historical perspective. Also transfusion-related acute lung injury (TRALI) has become highly investigated. Review of our practice indicates that the timing of transfusion, or when packed red blood cells are given to treat anemia is of importance in cardiac surgery outcomes. We have also noticed that in our patient population, an academic medical center setting, baseline hematocrit has trended lower over the past several years. Conservation of blood products becomes even more critical as both transfusion risk and product demand increases.

Prediction of Bleeding

Avoidance of transfusion is desired for cardiac surgery patients. There are, however, many factors that cause patients to be either anemic or have excessive postsurgical bleeding requiring homologous blood transfusion. These mechanisms for bleeding include inherited and acquired disorders, including platelet dysfunction, coagulation factor deficiency, excessive fibrinolysis, and other induced alterations related to hypothermia or medications.[8]

Even with anemic preoperative patients we have been able to successfully avoid transfusion. This can be accomplished by reducing hemodilution via use of low prime perfusion circuitry and avoidance of excessive crystalloid infusion perioperatively. Current prime volume can safely be reduced to 700 mL. Retrograde autologous priming of the entire circuit further reduces perfusion-related hemodilution to negligible levels.

There have been several reports of minimizing the use of blood and blood products both intraoperatively and postoperatively. Although most of these studies have focused on the use of one particular modality or pharmacologic agent, these techniques were applied in the context of an entire set of blood conservation measures. Collectively the results of these reports provide an important body of information that can be used as an aid to evaluate the relative effectiveness of various combinations of the presently available blood conservation techniques.[9–11]

Later groups took advantage of pharmacologic developments such as serine protease inhibitors, antifibrinolytics, and erythropoietin. By the early 1990s, these pharmacologic adjuncts to blood conservation had become readily available and could be categorized as agents useful in perioperative stimulation of bone marrow for red blood cell production (eg, erythropoietin) and agents useful in reducing postoperative bleeding (eg, serine protease inhibitors and antifibrinolytics).

In 1990, Ovrum and colleagues confirmed the effectiveness of the simple "core" approach to blood conservation.[11] In 121 consecutive elective CABG patients, the authors achieved a transfusion rate of 4.1% and 0.06 unit per patient. In 1991, Ovrum applied these same principles to 500 elective CABG patients and obtained similar low rates of transfusion (2.4% of patients).[12] The authors found this six-step blood conservation program to be simple, safe, and cost effective.

By the 1990s, there also were some technical advances in CPB designed to minimize the need for transfusions as well as for hemodilution. With better oxygenators came a reduction in the volume of the CPB circuit, accompanied by a reduction in the amount of hemodilution that occurred.[13] Circuit volume could be further reduced by replacing as much of the crystalloid circuit prime as possible with autologous blood drained from the arterial cannula into the circuit immediately prior to CPB, called *retrograde autologous priming* (RAP), as well as displacing the venous side of the crystalloid prime when first initiating CPB.[14] These relatively simple maneuvers can reduce the crystalloid prime to a volume of roughly 200 mL. In addition, technical advances such as leukocyte filters and heparin-bonded circuits reduced the inflammatory response of the body to the blood interface with the CPB circuit, which ultimately can lead to less homologous blood requirement.[15,16]

The addition of newer pharmacologic and technologic advances to the proven "core" conservation measures as established by Cosgrove and Ovrum had the potential to markedly reduce and even eliminate the need for transfusion even in the face of the more difficult patient characteristics increasingly being encountered. This then became the goal of blood conservation programs.

PREOPERATIVE MANAGEMENT

Identification of Patients at Risk

The coagulopathy associated with CPB is related primarily to the interaction of blood components with the artificial surfaces of the CPB circuit, which results in derangements in platelet function, abnormal functioning of the coagulation cascades, and excessive fibrinolysis. The administration of high-dose heparin to prevent coagulation within the CPB circuit and hypothermia achieved during bypass further contribute to hemostatic derangements. Finally, although the use of asanguineous crystalloid prime rather than the whole-blood pump prime used historically has reduced the amount of blood transfused during CPB dramatically, the resulting hemodilution contributes to the risk of low intraoperative and postoperative hematocrit, which can be independent risk factors for transfusion in the postoperative period. Other risk factors can be assessed in the preoperative state that can identify those patients who may be at high risk of bleeding or who have a low red cell mass, both of which may require autologous blood transfusions.

One of the most important predictors of postoperative bleeding in the surgical patient is a personal or family history of any excessive bleeding or documented bleeding disorders. Many disorders can be confirmed with simple laboratory tests demonstrating some level of coagulation derangement. However, in the cardiothoracic patient population, medications and acquired medical diseases and their associated hemostatic defects are likely to be the most common risk for bleeding. Notably, the use of aspirin alone or included in other medications intended for pain relief or treatment of other ailments is very common. The prevalence among patients undergoing unplanned surgery may be as high as 50%, and this may be even higher among patients with previously diagnosed coronary artery disease.[17–19] The currently published data suggest that this does not represent a significant bleeding risk, and there is little evidence to suggest that bleeding times correlate with operative blood loss in these patients.[20] Heparin will inhibit factors II and X, and may lead to immune-mediated thrombocytopenia. Coumadin can block gamma-carboxylation and lead to multiple factor deficiency.

Herbal Extracts for Cardiovascular Health

The use of herbal extracts and complementary medicine has become popular in the prevention of arterial thrombotic disease. In 1997, an estimated $21 billion was spent in the United States on complementary and alternative therapies.[21,22] Herbs such as thyme and rosemary have been shown to have a direct inhibitory effect on platelets.[23]

Despite the increased potassium contained in fruits and nuts, menu planning for patients on warfarin can include a healthy diet of these foods without compromising the stability of their oral anticoagulation therapy because most fruits are not important sources of vitamin K, with the exception of some berries, green fruits, and prunes.[24] In a case report regarding fish oil supplementation, it was demonstrated that additional anticoagulation could have resulted from an interaction with warfarin therapy. This case reveals that a significant rise in the international normalization ratio (INR) occurred after the dose of concomitant fish oil was doubled. Fish oil, an omega-3 polyunsaturated fatty acid, consists of eicosapentaenoic acid and docosahexaenoic acid. This fatty acid may affect platelet aggregation and/or vitamin K–dependent coagulation factors. Omega-3 fatty acids may lower thromboxane A_2 supplies within the platelet, as well as decrease factor VII levels.[25]

The popularity of herbal additives can be evidenced by the more than $700 million spent annually and the continued expected spending on such products.[26] Despite the potential benefits of many herbs with regard to improved well-being, many adverse risks exist. Primarily there is an increased cardiovascular risk among the more commonly used supplements, herbs such as garlic, ginger, and gingko are associated with platelet dysfunction–derived bleeding, whereas supplements such as ginseng and licorice may lead to elevated blood pressure.[27]

Health-care workers can play a crucial role in identifying possible drug interactions by asking patients taking warfarin about herbal and other alternative medicine product use. Furthermore, the clinical importance of herb–drug interactions depends on many factors associated with the particular herb, drug, and patient. Herbs should be labeled appropriately to alert consumers to potential interactions when used concomitantly with drugs and should recommend a consultation with one's general practitioner.

Autologous Blood Donation

One of the primary concerns in blood conservation is the patient's size and preoperative red blood cell volume. Two early reports by Cosgrove and Utley demonstrated these factors in addition to preoperative anemia as independent risk factors for blood transfusion.[28,29] As discussed later in this chapter, there are several relatively simple manipulations to the CPB circuit that can be made to reduce the amount of hemodilution that the patient experiences while on bypass to reduce the overall risk of transfusions.

Preoperative autologous donation (PAD) is a recognized strategy to reduce the risk of homologous blood transfusion in the perioperative period. Although this technique has been in practice since the 1960s, its use in cardiac surgery did not achieve widespread acceptance until the 1980s, with the advent of HIV, as an effort to reduce homologous blood exposures. Unfortunately, in cardiac surgery, the acuteness of the operations and dealing with an older and sicker patient population often preclude PAD because there must be enough preoperative time for autologous collection as well as red blood cell mass regeneration before arriving in the operating room.

Several preoperative characteristics can identify the cardiac patient who is eligible for PAD. The first criterion is that the patient be able to wait the required time for donation and red blood cell regeneration. This length of time typically varies depending on the type of surgical procedure planned (larger operative procedures likely requiring a larger amount of blood) and patient characteristics (eg, body size, blood volume, and hematocrit). In general, this time is a minimum of 2 weeks per unit of blood donated to allow for red blood cell regeneration. The second criterion is that the patient be healthy enough to undergo donation. This criterion would preclude patients with severe left main stem stenosis, critical aortic stenosis, congestive heart failure, and idiopathic hypertrophic subaortic stenosis, as well as patients with severe coronary artery disease and ongoing ischemia, given that many of these patients would have been screening failures for the first criterion. The third criterion is that the patients not have active endocarditis. The time between donation and receiving the PAD unit is ample time for bacteria to replicate in the donated unit with resulting bacteremia, which is potentially life threatening. The fourth criterion is that the patient has an adequate hematocrit and red blood cell mass. A preoperative hematocrit of less than 33% regardless of red blood cell mass is a contraindication to PAD according to the American Association of Blood Banks (AABB) guidelines. A patient with a hematocrit of greater than 33% may be eligible provided that other criteria are met.

Several options exist for patients who historically were not eligible for PAD. Recombinant erythropoietin can be used to accelerate red blood cell production in anemic patients; this strategy is used commonly in Jehovah's Witness patients to increase their red blood cell mass before surgery.[30] However, this can be quite costly; as a result, it is usually reserved for patients who are unable to tolerate homologous blood transfusions whether for religious reasons or because they have a rare blood type. An alternative strategy is to stimulate the body to increase the release of endogenous erythropoietin by allowing patients with hematocrits below the traditional cutoff to undergo PAD. The resulting anemia experienced by the patient in the postdonation period is a strong stimulant for endogenous erythropoietin production, ultimately leading to an increase in red blood cell mass.[30]

Red blood cell mass is related to patient body size.[31] A traditional cutoff of 110 lb had been used for PAD. However, the AABB does make specific allowances for PAD in smaller patients. The current recommendation is that no more than 15% of the patient's effective blood volume should be removed at any given time, which takes into account smaller patient body size. PAD should be pursued aggressively for these small patients with low red blood cell mass and hematocrit because they are at highest risk of receiving a blood transfusion at some time during their hospital stay. The mean rate of red blood cell generation of the studies that provided adequate data is 0.46 units per week, or slightly less than 1 unit every 2 weeks.[32] In conjunction with PAD, oral iron therapy should be initiated at the time of first donation to ensure adequate iron stores for red blood cell regeneration.

Owing to the relatively acute illness of the population, rarely is there sufficient time for PAD in the cardiothoracic surgical patient.[33] In addition, PAD has been supplanted largely by intraoperative blood salvage techniques for reasons of cost-effectiveness (ie, blood withdrawal, preparation, storage, and potential erythropoietin therapy add to costs) and advances in intraoperative blood salvage techniques such as intraoperative autologous donation (IAD; discussed later in this chapter), retrograde autologous prime of the CPB circuit, use of cell salvage, and regular use of cardiotomy suction.

PHARMACOLOGIC STRATEGIES FOR BLOOD CONSERVATION

A number of drugs have been used to decrease blood loss and the use of blood transfusion associated with cardiac surgery. Interest has been renewed recently in antifibrinolytics, a relatively old class of drug. Currently, three such medications are used clinically; two are synthetic antifibrinolytics (ie, epsilon-aminocaproic acid and tranexamic acid), and one is naturally occurring (ie, aprotinin derived from bovine lung). Linked with the resurgence of interest in these drugs is interest in diminishing homologous blood transfusions related to cardiac surgery.

Epsilon-Aminocaproic Acid

Epsilon-aminocaproic acid (EACA) is a synthetic antifibrinolytic agent first described in 1959 that derives its effect by forming reversible complexes with either plasminogen or plasmin, saturating the lysine-binding sites and thus displacing plasminogen and therefore plasmin from the surface of fibrin. This blockage of plasminogen binding to fibrin blocks plasminogen activation and therefore fibrinolysis. The overall effect is to block the dissolution of the fibrin clot.

Several studies have demonstrated the efficacy of EACA in reducing bleeding after open heart surgery. Although EACA was first used in situations in which excessive bleeding was encountered, Lambert and colleagues used EACA in 1979 to successfully treat patients with coagulation disorders, who comprise 20% of total primary coronary bypass patients.[34] Del Rossi used EACA in 1989 as a prophylactic tool to reduce blood loss in 350 patients undergoing CPB, having an impact on both blood loss and transfusion of autologous blood and blood products.[35]

Tranexamic Acid

The mechanism of action of tranexamic acid (TA) is similar to that of EACA. The significant difference between EACA and TA is that TA is roughly 10 times more potent than EACA. As with EACA, postoperative bleeding and homologous blood requirements were similarly decreased with the use of TA, as shown by Horrow in 1990 in 38 patients undergoing CPB.[36]

Aprotinin

Aprotinin is a serine protease inhibitor with antithrombotic, antifibrinolytic, and anti-inflammatory effects. It was recently removed from the market. We include it for historical perspective. It was effective in reducing bleeding and the need for blood transfusions after cardiac surgery with cardiopulmonary bypass. Additional benefits, such as cerebral protection, were hypothesized but not yet thoroughly substantiated.

Aprotinin is a low-molecular-weight serine-protease inhibitor with a lysine residue occupying its active center. It is a naturally occurring polypeptide isolated from bovine lung. Reversible enzyme–inhibitor complexes with various proteases are formed that display activity against trypsin, plasmin, streptokinase–plasma complex, tissue kallikrein, and plasma kallikrein. Because aprotinin is a nonspecific serine antiprotease, it intervenes in the coagulation cascade in multiple loci, working to decrease bleeding in CPB patients by its antiplasmin and antikallikrein effects.

Aprotinin was first used in cardiac surgery by Tice and colleagues, who described the administration of 10,000 to 20,000 kallikrein inhibitory units (KIU), resulting in rapid establishment of hemostasis in five patients who had undergone CPB; they also demonstrated increased bleeding and increased fibrinolytic activity.[37] The currently accepted regimen of high-dose aprotinin (5 to 6 million unit average total dose) is reflective of the experiences of the Hammersmith group, which serendipitously saw a reduction in bleeding in patients receiving aprotinin to reduce kallikrein-mediated lung inflammation during CPB.[38] Since this report, multiple reports have emerged citing the efficacy of aprotinin as compared with other antifibrinolytics and controls in reducing bleeding complications, homologous blood transfusions, and inflammation primarily in the reoperative setting.[39–41] Despite these advantages, Mangano and colleagues reported that aprotinin use was associated with an increased risk of renal failure, myocardial infarction, and stroke.[42] In this nonrandomized observational trial of 4374 patients undergoing revascularization, the group concluded that aprotinin use was not prudent in comparison with less expensive alternatives such as aminocaproic acid and TA. Limitations to this study include nonblinded randomization and a significantly higher operative risk in the aprotinin study group that required complicated propensity adjustment to statistically match groups.

In October 2007, the Blood Conservation Using Antifibrinolytics in a Randomized Trial (BART) study was stopped prematurely after preliminary data from 2163 patients demonstrated a trend toward an increase in all-cause 30-day mortality in patients receiving aprotinin. Based on this preliminary finding, the marketing and distribution of aprotinin was suspended.[43]

Recombinant Activated Factor VII

The use of recombinant factor VII has been shown to induce hemostasis in patients with severe hemophilia A or B with factor specific inhibitors.[44] Recombinant activated factor VII complexes with all available tissue factor to activate factor X directly and induce thrombin generation. This leads to the formation of a tight and stable fibrin plug that is resistant to early fibrinolysis.[45]

Off-label use in cardiac surgery has been indicated when all efforts at conventional hemostasis have been exhausted. These include non–red blood cell product support (eg, fresh-frozen plasma, platelets, and cryoprecipitate), topical agents, desmopressin, and antifibrinolytics. When hemostasis is still not satisfactory, we have given a recombinant factor VIIa (rFVIIa) dose of between 75 and 100 μg/kg. Efficacy is variable with rFVIIa use, ranging from no difference from standard therapy to causing mortal thrombosis. Bruckner reported evidence of thrombosis during support with left ventricular assist when giving high doses for patients requiring higher doses (30 to 70 μg/kg) had a dramatically higher incidence of serious thromboembolic events.[46]

Heymann and colleagues reported in a retrospective analysis that rFVIIa was safe with regard to risk of thrombosis, but blood loss and transfusion rates were similar. High mortality rates were seen in both groups in house and at 6 months (approximately 30 and 50%, respectively).[47] Conversely, Raivio reported in a retrospective series that rFVIIa was significantly more effective in restoring hemostasis; however, severe postoperative thromboembolic complications occurred in 25% of the patients.[48] The rFVIIa doses in these two studies ranged from 60 to 80 μg/kg and from 24 to 192 μg/kg, respectively.

Diprose and colleagues compared rFVIIa to placebo in a randomized, double-blind study following complex non–coronary artery cardiac surgery. The group found in this 20-patient study that homologous transfusions were significantly fewer in the study group cohort. There were no differences in regard to adverse events, but this pilot study had limitations that include being underpowered and prone to type I error.[49] Despite the effectiveness that has been demonstrated in single-patient case reports and small-scale studies, we recommend caution when using this product until more prospective, randomized studies are available to determine safety and effectiveness.

TOPICAL HEMOSTATIC AGENTS

The limited efficacy of topical agents such as oxidized cellulose and microfibrillar collagen has led to the development of new products with novel applicator systems that are direct activators of the clotting cascade. Additionally, pericardial lavage with aprotinin or EACA has been shown to be ineffective at reducing transfusion requirements and may enhance mediastinal adhesion formation.[50–52] As a result of the limitations of more traditional agents, the new-generation topical agents have gained appeal owing to their inherent effectiveness as well as their ease of use.

BioGlue (CryoLife, Inc., Kennesaw, GA) is a biologic glue approved initially for use in the repair of aortic dissection. This product is composed of purified bovine serum, albumin, and glutaraldehyde. The action is almost instantaneous because glutaraldehyde exposure leads to the tenuous binding of lysine molecules, proteins, and tissue surfaces. Raanani described the use of BioGlue as an aid in aortic reconstructive surgery, avoiding the use of stiff Teflon felt strips.[53]

Tisseel VH (Baxter Healthcare Corp., Glendale, CA) is a topical protein solution sealer that is sprayed onto hemorrhagic surfaces. This fibrin sealant contains fibrinogen, thrombin, calcium chloride, and aprotinin. When the protein and thrombin solutions are mixed and sprayed topically, a viscous solution that sets rapidly into an elastic coagulum is produced. A study by Rousou demonstrated that fibrin sealant was safe with regard to viral transmission and highly effective in controlling localized bleeding in cardiac operations.[54]

The gelatin-based hemostatic sealant FloSeal (Fusion Medical Technologies, Inc., Mountain View, CA) activates the clotting cascade and simultaneously forms a nondisplacing hemostatic plug. A FloSeal kit contains a bovine-derived gelatin matrix, a bovine-derived thrombin component, and a syringe applicator. The gelatinous matrix is biocompatible and reabsorbed in 6 to 8 weeks. In a series of patients undergoing open heart procedures, the Fusion Matrix Group studied FloSeal versus Gelfoam-Thrombin in procedures in which standard surgical means were ineffective at controlling bleeding.[55] FloSeal stopped bleeding in a significantly higher number of patients than did standard therapy with no differences in adverse events; however, there was no mention of each product's effect on transfusion rates.

PLATELET INHIBITORS AND THEIR EFFECT ON BLOOD USAGE

The two groups of platelet inhibitors are GP IIb/IIIa blocking agents and the adenosine diphosphate (ADP) receptor site blockers. The first group acts via inhibition with the glycoprotein (GP) IIb/IIIa receptor antagonists, which has greatly reduced the need for emergent CABG in patients undergoing angioplasty or coronary stenting procedures. Other adjuncts include the adenosine diphosphate (ADP) receptor blockers. These agents pose new challenges in terms of bleeding risk for the cardiac surgical team for patients exposed to these agents who are subsequently referred for surgery.

GP IIb/IIIa Inhibitors

The final common pathway of platelet aggregation leading to coronary artery occlusion is the cross-linking of receptor GP IIb/IIIa on adjacent platelets by adhesive plasma proteins (fibrinogen). As a result, receptor blockade of GP IIb/IIIa results in blocking platelet aggregation and subsequent thrombus formation. A population of patients with ischemic heart disease who may be expected to require CABG despite maximal therapy with GP IIb/IIIa inhibitors still remains. Currently, there are no controlled studies of the effect of GP IIb/IIIa inhibitors on patients undergoing CABG. However, the use of

TABLE 13-1 Antiplatelet Agents

Drug	Binding	Mechanism	Half-life
Glycoprotein IIb/IIIa Inhibitors			
Abciximab (ReoPro)	Noncompetitive	GP IIb/IIIa inhibition	30 minutes
Tirofiban (Aggrastat)	Reversible	GP IIb/IIIa inhibition	2.2 hours
Eptifibatide (Integrilin)	Reversible	GP IIb/IIIa inhibition	2.5 hours
Adenosine Diphosphate (ADP) Inhibition			
Clopidogrel (Plavix)	Irreversible	ADP-mediated platelet aggregation	8 hours
Prasugrel (Effient)	Irreversible	ADP-mediated platelet aggregation	4 hours
Ticagrelor (Brilinta)	Reversible	ADP-mediated platelet aggregation	12 hours
Congrelor (intravenous)	Reversible	ADP-mediated platelet aggregation	3–5 minutes

these inhibitors may enhance the risk of bleeding compared with elective procedures in patients not receiving these agents. The currently used agents are summarized in Table 13-1.

Guidelines for GP IIb/IIIa inhibitor Patients Requiring Cardiac Surgery

1. Stop the GP IIb/IIIa inhibitor.
2. Delay surgery (if possible, if the patient remains stable) for up to 12 hours if abciximab, tirofiban, or eptifibatide is used, and up to 7 days if clopidogrel is used.
3. Maintain standard heparin dosing despite elevated bleeding times.
4. Use ultrafiltration via the zero-balance technique while on CPB.
5. Transfuse platelets as needed as opposed to prophylactically, preferably once off CPB and after protamine administration.[56]

Guidelines for Adenosine Diphosphate (ADP) Inhibitor Patients Requiring Cardiac Surgery

Adenosine Diphosphate (ADP) Inhibition

Clopidogrel has become an essential component of therapy in patients with acute coronary syndrome because it significantly improves patient outcomes.

However, there are drawbacks to this therapy, which include delayed onset of action, large interindividual variability in platelet response (as high as 30% nonresponders), and irreversibility of its inhibitory effect on platelets.[57–59] Some of the new ADP inhibitors have the advantages of reversible receptor blockade as well as shorter half-lives, which may offer the cardiac surgical team the luxury of offering shorter waiting times with potentially less bleeding complications and ultimately safer operations for the patients who are referred for surgery.

Several companies have developed assays to assess platelet function (platelet aggregation) in the face of using these platelet inhibitors. It is our recommendation to use these studies because they may be cost effective ways of determining the patient's readiness for surgery as a routine part of the standard coagulation profile.

Heparin-Induced Thrombocytopenia and Cardiac Surgery

Heparin-induced thrombocytopenia and thrombosis (HITT) is a serious complication of heparin therapy. This immunologic response develops in approximately 1 to 3% of patients treated with unfractionated heparin (UFH) for 5 to 10 days.[60,61] HITT is a severe prothrombotic condition, with affected individuals having a 20 to 50% risk of developing new thromboembolic events. The mortality rate is approximately 20%; in addition, approximately 10% of patients require amputations or suffer other major morbidity.[62,63] Although there is no best way to anticoagulate these patients, when surgical delay is unavoidable, few options exist. Most reports, however, are limited single case reports with significant morbidity and mortality.

Currently, direct thrombin inhibitors (DTIs) are recommended for HITT (Table 13-2). Limitations of these agents include the lack of a reversal agent and route of clearance.[64]

These agents have several advantages over UFH. Because they do not rely on antithrombin III levels and do not bind to plasma proteins, the anticoagulant effect is more predictable. Also, DTIs inhibit fibrin-bound thrombin as well as fluid-phase thrombin, leading to a greater antithrombotic effect.

Specific recommendations on how to treat patients with HITT cannot be given at this time. Diagnosis of HITT is difficult because assays vary in both specificity and sensitivity. Second, and vital to this dilemma, are the lack of randomized trials. Most data available for treating these patients are derived from single case reports and small retrospective trials. Dosing of the available anticoagulation agents is not fully understood, and there is no reversal agent. Because drug elimination varies for these agents, renal or liver function must be fully assessed.

TABLE 13-2 Direct Thrombin Inhibitors for HITT

Drug	Monitored	Excretion	Half-life
Lepirudin (Refludan)	APTT 1.5–2.5 times baseline	Kidney	40–60 min
Argatroban	APTT 1.5–3 times baseline	Liver	45 min
Bivalirudin (Angiomax)	APTT or ACT 1.5–3 times baseline	Kidney	25 min

INTRAOPERATIVE AND POSTOPERATIVE MANAGEMENT

Intraoperative Period

Intraoperative autologous donation (IAD) of whole blood has many advantages over PAD. IAD does not require a delay in surgery; it can be performed efficiently and with minimal additional cost. In addition, the blood product obtained by IAD is whole blood, which is transfused within 2 to 3 hours of collection and therefore contains active platelets and factors. The resulting advantages are the avoidance of coagulopathy frequently seen after CPB and the addition of red blood cell mass capable of oxygen transport. The storage process limits the amount of blood loss during surgery via lap pads and discard suction. Additionally this technique spares the damaging effects of the heart-lung machine, which include contact activation of platelets and complement as well as red blood cell hemolysis. Because IAD serves to decrease red blood cell requirements in a volume-dependent manner, the maximum amount of blood should be removed from each individual patient so as to optimize blood conservation efforts. The amount of blood that an individual patient is capable of donating via IAD depends strictly on the patient's own physiologic parameters, estimated blood volume (based on height-weight nomogram), pre-IAD hematocrit, and pre-CPB hematocrit.[65] In Fig. 13-1 is our nomogram for allowable IAD blood drainage. It conservatively estimates the volume of blood

Preop Hematocrit% in OR			IAD Removal Volume mL								
Weight kg	30%	32%	34%	36%	38%	40%	42%	44%	46%	48%	50%
40	338	361	384	406	429	451	474	496	519	541	564
45	418	446	474	502	530	558	585	613	641	669	697
50	498	531	564	598	631	664	697	730	764	797	830
55	578	616	655	693	732	770	809	847	886	924	963
60	658	701	745	789	833	877	921	964	1008	1052	1096
65	737	787	836	885	934	983	1032	1082	1131	1180	1229
70	817	872	926	981	1035	1090	1144	1199	1253	1308	1362
75	897	957	1017	1076	1136	1196	1256	1316	1375	1435	1495
80	977	1042	1107	1172	1237	1302	1368	1433	1498	1563	1628
85	1057	1127	1197	1268	1338	1409	1479	1550	1620	1691	1761
90	1136	1212	1288	1364	1439	1515	1591	1667	1742	1818	1894
95	1216	1297	1378	1459	1541	1622	1703	1784	1865	1946	2000
100	1296	1382	1469	1555	1642	1728	1814	1901	1987	2000	2000
105	1376	1468	1559	1651	1743	1834	1926	2000	2000	2000	2000
110	1456	1553	1650	1747	1844	1941	2000	2000	2000	2000	2000
115	1535	1638	1740	1842	1945	2000	2000	2000	2000	2000	2000
120	1615	1723	1831	1938	2000	2000	2000	2000	2000	2000	2000
125	1695	1808	1921	2000	2000	2000	2000	2000	2000	2000	2000
130	1775	1893	2000	2000	2000	2000	2000	2000	2000	2000	2000
135	1855	1978	2000	2000	2000	2000	2000	2000	2000	2000	2000
140	1934	2000	2000	2000	2000	2000	2000	2000	2000	2000	2000
145	2000	2000	2000	2000	2000	2000	2000	2000	2000	2000	2000
150	2000	2000	2000	2000	2000	2000	2000	2000	2000	2000	2000
	Legend						Based on 70 mL/kg BV, RAP, 1000 mL Dilution and 24% CPBhct				
	0 BAG	No IAD									
	I BAG	500 mL									
	2 BAGS	1000 mL									
	3 BAGS	1500 mL									
	4 BAGS	2000 mL									

FIGURE 13-1 Intraoperative autologous donation nomogram.

that can be removed to achieve a hematocrit of 24% or greater (based on a 1000-mL CPB prime volume).

Minimal hemodilution by red blood cell priming of the CPB circuit with the patient's own blood is a useful technique in avoiding transfusions. Techniques include low-prime circuitry and retrograde autologous prime (RAP).[66,67] Up to 90% of the crystalloid prime of the CPB circuit can be displaced with autologous blood using RAP. This technique involves partial priming of the bypass circuit with the patient's own blood from the arterial cannula just before instituting CPB. In addition, the venous loop also can be primed in a similar manner when first instituting CPB, displacing the crystalloid prime in the venous loop. The result is the replacement of virtually all the crystalloid prime with autologous blood, thereby reducing the amount of hemodilution the patient experiences on CPB. Available low prime circuitry (<1000 mL) allows for complete autologous priming of the CPB circuit and less hemodynamic alteration during RAP.

TRANSFUSION TRIGGERS

The literature indicates that the anesthetized patient on full CPB at moderate hypothermia can safely tolerate a hematocrit as low as 15%, with the exception of patients at risk for decreased cerebral oxygen delivery, namely, those with a history of cerebrovascular accident (CVA), diabetes, or cerebrovascular disease.[68] These latter patients can tolerate a hematocrit as low as 18% when using moderate hypothermia.[69] Once the patient is warm and being weaned from CPB, these percentage points are raised by 2% each (17 and 20%, respectively) because the relative protective effects of the hypothermia are no longer present. In our institution, once the patient is off CPB, our practice has been to retransfuse all or as much as possible remaining blood in the CPB circuit to the patient and then give all available cell salvage blood, including any blood remaining in the CPB circuit that was not initially given back to the patient, then any IAD blood, and then finally PAD blood if available. Then and only then, if the hematocrit remains unsatisfactorily low, does the patient receive homologous blood.

Once the patient leaves the operating room, we use a transfusion trigger corresponding to a hematocrit of 22% in asymptomatic patients. In patients older than 80 years of age, a trigger of 24% is used. These numbers are meant to serve as guidelines; if a patient is at all symptomatic (ie, tachycardic, hypotensive, ischemic, or showing any evidence of end-organ hypoperfusion), he or she will receive homologous blood transfusion therapy. To apply minimum transfusion standards safely and appropriately, the cardiac surgeon or anesthesiologist must have an understanding of the lowest safe level of anemia under the variety of conditions encountered by the cardiac surgical patient. This understanding then can be combined with an assessment of the patient's clinical status to determine the true need for red blood cell transfusion.

CONCLUSION

Blood conservation is an important component to improving health care. This process has the ability to improve patient outcome, reduce cost, and increase the availability of such an important commodity.[70] The reduction of transfusions has been shown in many studies to improve surgical results and even eliminate certain complications.[71–73] As cardiac surgery patients present with higher acuity it becomes ever more challenging to reduce exposure to banked blood products. Arora demonstrated that patients with a preoperative hemoglobin of 12 g/dL or less had a significant risk for transfusion.[78] Other risk factors for transfusion most notably were emergent procedure and renal failure at time of surgery.

Our group reviewed the use of heparin-coated CPB circuits and the effect on blood usage and pulmonary function in 200 patients. As seen in Table 13-3 coated circuitry reduced overall blood usage and resulted in reduced ventilator time and time to ambulation. An interesting finding was that patients who were not transfused postoperatively had improved outcomes as well, regardless of whether they had coated circuitry or not. One explanation is that if blood transfusion occurs on bypass, the lungs are not immediately exposed to the transfused blood because the homologous blood is given into the arterial rather than the venous system, thus avoiding a first-pass effect. Typically if a transfusion is given postoperatively it is infused

TABLE 13-3 Effect of Post CPB Transfusion on Patients Undergoing Bypass Procedures Utilizing Noncoated Versus Coated Circuitry

	Transfused PostCPB	$RBC\text{-}CPB_{units}$	$RBC\text{-}Post\ CPB_{units}$	Vent-hr	TIME to walk hr
Coated Circuit $n = 100$	No	0.6	0.0	6.7**	36.7
	Yes	2.0	1.7	9.7	39.9
NonCoated Circuit $n = 100$	No	0.7	0.0	8.6	40.4
	Yes	1.6	2.2	12.0**	65.1**

CPB = Cardiopulmonary bypass; RBC = red blood cells, Vent-hr = ventilator time in hours, * = significantly lower than group, **significantly higher than group, $p < 0.05$.

TABLE 13-4 Lowest Hematocrit on CPB and Postoperative Complications

	Demographics					Risk Preop %		Postoperative Complications %			
Group Lowest HCT CPB	Weight kg	Preop HCT %	PreCPB HCT %	RBC-units CPB	RBC-units LOS	Renal Insufficiency	CHF	Death	Respiratory Failure	Renal Failure	Discharged to Home
HCT 25% n = 30	91	41	34	3%	18%	3%	6%	0%	0%	0%	91%
HCT 20% n = 30	75	35	28	66%	100%	12%	36%	3%	10%	12%	60%
HCT < 18% n = 30	70	34	27	85%	100%	12%	39%	0%	20%	12%	50%

CPB = Cardiopulmonary bypass; Hct = hematocrit; RBC = red blood cells.

into a central vein, thereby having almost immediate exposure to the lungs. Thus the timing of blood transfusion may be important.

If we review the "two-hit" lung injury model of transfusion-related acute lung injury (TRALI), transfusion immediately post-CPB may be a similar scenario.[74,75] The "first hit" is usually described as an underlying illness that primes the pulmonary endothelial cells and leukocytes or an inflammatory response incited by an event such as cardiopulmonary bypass itself. The "second hit" is delivered by the transfusion of red blood cells into the venous system. If we look at this model of TRALI, the optimal timing of blood transfusion for the typical patient undergoing a procedure utilizing cardiopulmonary bypass may be before separating from bypass to avoid the first-pass effect and thereby the "second hit." Further studies will be required to substantiate this assumption, however.

Intuitively the smaller patient with a low preoperative hematocrit is at high risk of transfusion. We reviewed our data related to this and found that all patients less than or equal to 70 kg were transfused during their length of stay (Table 13-4). These patients also had the highest incidence of respiratory failure and the need for rehabilitation therapy. This has led us to change our transfusion practice whereby we attempt to transfuse all red cells on cardiopulmonary bypass. Initially we started this practice for patients less than or equal to 70 kg with hematocrits of 28% or less. With the use of lower prime perfusion circuitry (<1000 mL) we have reduce the threshold to 25% or less for when we will blood prime. These values and thresholds will change as we continue to optimize the perfusion circuitry.

There is no question that some aspects of the blood conservation approach are more costly than others. However, when taken in the context of the cost of blood products, their use, the potential reduction in the risk of reexplorations, and the reduction or elimination of the risks of homologous blood exposures, these costs may seem a little more reasonable. Overutilization of blood products leads to increased direct and indirect costs. The cost for a unit of red blood cells is over $1400.[76] This includes approximately $600 for the direct product cost and more than $800 for the adverse event cost related to transfusion. Other implications of transfusion include increased mortality and morbidity when "older blood" that is greater than 14 days old is transfused.[77]

As patients present with even higher levels of risk the cardiac surgeon will appreciate any options that may reduce blood exposure. The typical patient is anemic and has many risk factors for significant bleeding because of exposure to platelet inhibition. Fortunately cardiac surgery groups can take advantage of techniques that reduce hemodilution and preserve hematologic function of coagulation. These options include retrograde autologous priming, intraoperative autologous donation, and coated-reduced prime perfusion circuitry.

Historically, cardiac surgery has been associated with a high incidence of blood transfusion, with up to 70% of these patients receiving homologous blood transfusions at some point during their hospital stay. However, with improving technology, awareness of blood conservation techniques, and better pharmacologic agents, a multidisciplinary approach to blood conservation can make "bloodless heart surgery" entirely possible. For the purely elective patient, these techniques are initiated preoperatively with PAD, whereas other patients are eligible for one or all of the remainder of the in-hospital techniques described. Using a team approach that both optimizes and integrates the use of each of these measures, the use of homologous blood can be markedly reduced in a majority of cardiac surgical patients.

KEY POINTS

- Blood conservation should be approached in a multidisciplinary fashion. This team should include members from departments of surgery, anesthesiology, nursing, perfusion, transfusion therapy, and quality.
- Blood usage data should be collected, reviewed, and discussed at monthly meetings
- Intraoperative autologous donation should be maximized using the blood removal nomogram. This blood product must be labeled and checked as if it were a homologous transfusion.
- The anesthesiologist should minimize hemodilution with judicious maintenance of fluid balance (using vasopressor and fluid).
- The surgeon should minimize blood loss via meticulous technique and minimal lap pads and sponges.
- The perfusionist should minimize hemodilution to negligible levels by optimizing retrograde autologous priming techniques and reduce pump prime.
- The operating room nurses and technicians should be diligent in avoiding blood loss at the operative field and aiding in the availability of blood products when needed.
- Red blood cells should be transfused during cardiopulmonary bypass when needed, rather than waiting until later when they can increase the risk of lung injury.

REFERENCES

1. Belisle S, Hardy JF: Hemorrhage and the use of blood products after adult cardiac operations: myths and realities. *Ann Thorac Surg* 1996; 62:1908.
2. Goodnough LT, Despostis GJ, Hohue CW, et al: On the need for improved transfusion indicators in cardiac surgery. *Ann Thorac Surg* 1995; 60:473.
3. Surgenor DM, Wallace EL, Churchill WH, et al: Red cell transfusion in coronary artery bypass surgery. *Transfusion* 1992; 32:458.
4. Boyle EM, Verrier VD, Spiess BD: The procoagulant response to injury. *Ann Thorac Surg* 1997; 64:S16.
5. Hunt BJ, Parratt RN, Segal HC, et al: Activation of coagulation and fibrinolysis during cardiothoracic operations. *Ann Thorac Surg* 1998; 65:712.
6. Woodman RC, Harker LA: Bleeding complications associated with cardiopulmonary bypass. *Blood* 1990; 76:1680.
7. Cooley DA, Beall AC, Grondin P: Open-heart operations with disposable oxygenators, 5% dextrose prime, and normothermia. *Surgery* 1962; 52:713.
8. Despotis G, Avidan M, Eby C: Prediction and management of bleeding in cardiac surgery. *J Throm Haemost* 2009; 7(Suppl 1):111-117.
9. Eyjolfsson A, Scicluna S, Johnsson P, Petersson F, Jönsson H: Characterization of lipid particles in shed mediastinal blood. *Ann Thorac Surg* 2008; 85:978-981.
10. Cosgrove DM, Thurer RL, Lytle BW, et al: Blood conservation during myocardial revascularization. *Ann Thorac Surg* 1979; 28:184.
11. Ovrum E, Holen EA, Linstein MA: Elective coronary artery bypass without homologous blood transfusion. *Scand J Thorac Cardiovasc Surg* 1991; 25:13.

12. Ovrum E, Holen EA, Abdelnoor M, et al: Conventional blood conservation techniques in 500 consecutive coronary artery bypass operations. *Ann Thorac Surg* 1991; 51:500.
13. DeBois WJ, Sukhram Y, McVey J, et al: Reduction in homologous transfusion using a low prime circuit. *J Extracorpor Technol* 1996; 28:58.
14. Rosengart TR, DeBois WJ, O'Hara M, et al: Retrograde autologous priming for cardiopulmonary bypass: a safe and effective means of decreasing hemodilution and transfusion requirements. *J Thorac Cardiovasc Surg* 1998; 115:426.
15. Lilly KJ, O'Gara PJ, Treanor PR, et al: Heparin-bonded circuits without a cardiotomy: A description of a minimally invasive technique of cardiopulmonary bypass. *Perfusion* 2002; 7:95.
16. Hamada Y, Kawachi K, Nakata T, et al: Antiinflammatory effect of heparin-coated circuits with leukocyte-depleting filters in coronary bypass surgery. *Artif Organs* 2001; 25:1004.
17. Ferraris VA, Swanson E: Aspirin usage and perioperative blood loss in patients undergoing unexpected operations. *Surg Gynecol Obstet* 1983; 156:439.
18. Ferraris VA, Gildengorin VJ: Predictors of excessive blood use after coronary artery bypass grafting: a multivariate analysis. *Thorac Cardiovasc Surg* 1989; 98:492.
19. Bashein G, Nessly ML, Rice AL, et al: Preoperative aspirin therapy and reoperation for bleeding after coronary artery bypass surgery. *Arch Intern Med* 1991; 151:89.
20. Rodgers RP, Levin J: A critical reappraisal of the bleeding time. *Semin Thromb Hemost* 1990; 16:1.
21. Eisenberg DM, Kessler RC, Foster C, et al: Unconventional medicine in the United States. *NEJM* 1993; 328:246.
22. Eisenberg DM, Davis RB, Ettner SL, et al: Trends in alternative medicine use in the United States, 1990–1997: results of follow-up national survey. *JAMA* 1998; 280:1569.
23. Junichiro Y, Path FRC, Yamada K, et al: Testing various herbs for antithrombotic effect. *Nutrition* 2005; 21:580.
24. Dismore ML, Haytowitz DB, Gebhardt SE, et al: Vitamin K content of nuts and fruits in the US diet. *J Am Diet Assoc* 2003; 103:1650.
25. Buckley MS, Goff AD, Knapp WE: Fish oil interaction with warfarin. *Ann Pharmacother* 2004; 38:50.
26. Winter G: FDA warns food companies about herbal additives. *New York Times,* June 7, 2001; p C1.
27. Valli G, Giardina E: Benefits, adverse effects and drug interactions of herbal therapies with cardiovascular effects. *J Am Coll Cardiol* 2002; 39:1083.
28. Cosgrove DM, Loop FD, Lytle BW, et al: Determinants of blood utilization during myocardial revascularization. *Ann Thorac Surg* 1985; 40:380.
29. Utley JR, Wallace DJ, Thomason ME, et al: Correlates of preoperative hematocrit value in patients undergoing coronary artery bypass. *J Thorac Cardiovasc Surg* 1989; 98:451.
30. Rosengart TK, Helm RE, DeBois WJ, et al: Open heart operations without transfusion using a multimodality blood conservation strategy in 50 Jehovah's Witness patients: Implications for a "bloodless" surgical technique. *J Am Coll Surg* 1997; 184:618.
31. Sandrelli L, Pardini A, Lorusso R, et al: Impact of autologous blood predonation on a comprehensive blood conservation program. *Ann Thorac Surg* 1995; 59:730.
32. Goodnough LT, Verbrugge D, Marcus RE, et al: The effect of patient size and dose of recombinant human erythropoietin therapy on red blood cell volume expansion in autologous blood donors for elective orthopedic operation. *J Am Coll Surg* 1994; 179:171.
33. Owings DV, Kruskall MS, Thurer RL, et al: Autologous blood donations prior to elective cardiac surgery: safety and effect on subsequent blood use. *JAMA* 1989; 262:1963.
34. Lambert CJ, Marengo-Rowe AJ, Leveson JE, et al: The treatment of postperfusion bleeding using epsilon-aminocaproic acid, cryoprecipitate, fresh-frozen plasma, and protamine sulfate. *Ann Thorac Surg* 1979; 28:440.
35. DelRossi AJ, Cernaianu AC, Botros S, et al: Prophylactic treatment of postperfusion bleeding using EACA. *Chest* 1989; 96:27.
36. Horrow JC, Hlavacek J, Strong MD, et al: Prophylactic tranexamic acid decreases bleeding after cardiac operations. *J Thorac Cardiovasc Surg* 1990; 99:70.
37. Tice DA, Worth MH Jr: Recognition and treatment of postoperative bleeding associated with open-heart surgery. *Ann NY Acad Sci* 1968; 146:745.
38. Royston D: The serine antiprotease aprotinin (Trasylol): a novel approach to reducing postoperative bleeding. *Blood Coagul Fibrinol* 1990; 1:55.
39. Barrons RW, Jahr JS: A review of post-cardiopulmonary bypass bleeding, aminocaproic acid, tranexamic acid, and aprotinin. *Am J Ther* 1996; 3:821.
40. Casati V, Guzzon D, Oppizzi M, et al: Hemostatic effects of aprotinin, tranexamic acid and epsilon-aminocaproic acid in primary cardiac surgery. *Ann Thorac Surg* 1999; 68:2252.
41. Laupacis A, Fergusson D: Drugs to minimize perioperative blood loss in cardiac surgery: meta-analyses using perioperative blood transfusion as the outcome. The International Study of Peri-operative Transfusion (ISPOT) investigators. *Anesth Analg* 1997; 85:1258.
42. Mangano DT, Tudor IC, Dietzel C: The risk associated with aprotinin in cardiac surgery. *NEJM* 2006; 354:353.
43. Mangano DT, Miao Y, Vuylsteke A, et al: Mortality associated with aprotinin during 5 years following coronary artery bypass graft surgery. *JAMA* 2007; 297:471-479.
44. Hedner U, Glazer S, Pingel K, et al: Successful use of recombinant factor VIIa in patient with severe hemophilia A during synovectomy. *Lancet* 1988; 2:1193.
45. Hedner U: Recombinant factor VIIa (rFVIIa) as a hemostatic agent. *Semin Hematol* 2001; 38:43.
46. Bruckner BA, DiBardino DJ, Ning Q, et al: High incidence of thromboembolic events in left ventricular assist device patients treated with recombinant activated factor VII. *J Heart Lung Transplant* 2009; 28(8):785.
47. Heymann C, Redlich U, Jain U, et al: Recombinant activated factor VII for refractory bleeding after cardiac surgery: a retrospective analysis of safety and efficacy. *Crit Care Med* 2005; 33:2241.
48. Raivio P, Suojaranta-Ylinen R, Kuitunen A: Recombinant factor VIIa in the treatment of postoperative hemorrhage after cardiac surgery. *Ann Thorac Surg* 2005; 80:66.
49. Diprose P, Herbertson MJ, O'Shaughnessy B, et al: Activated recombinant factor VII after cardiopulmonary bypass reduces allogeneic transfusion in complex noncoronary cardiac surgery: randomized, double-blinded, placebo-controlled pilot study. *Br J Anaesth* 2005; 95:596.
50. De Bonis M, Cavaliere F, Alessandrini F, et al: Topical use of tranexamic acid in coronary artery bypass operations: a double-blind, prospective, randomized, placebo-controlled study. *Thorac Cardiovasc Surg* 2000; 119:575.
51. Cicek S, Theodoro DA: Topical aprotinin in cardiac operations: a note of caution. *Ann Thorac Surg* 1996; 61:1039.
52. O'Regan DJ, Giannopoulos N, Mediratta N, et al: Topical aprotinin in cardiac operations. *Ann Thorac Surg* 1994; 58:778.
53. Raanani E, Latter DA, Errett LE, et al: Use of BioGlue in aortic surgical repair. *Ann Thorac Surg* 2001; 72:638.
54. Rousou J, Levitsky S, Gonzalez-Lavin L, et al: Randomized clinical trial of fibrin sealant in patients undergoing resternotomy or reoperation after cardiac operations: a multicenter study. *J Thorac Cardiovasc Surg* 1989; 97:194.
55. Oz MC, Cosgrove DM III, Badduke BR, et al: Controlled clinical trial of a novel hemostatic agent in cardiac surgery. The Fusion Matrix Study Group. *Ann Thorac Surg* 2000; 69:1376.
56. Lee LY, DeBois W, Krieger KH, et al: The effects of platelet inhibitors on blood use in cardiac surgery. *Perfusion* 2002; 17:33.
57. Schömig A: Is there need for a new player in the antiplatelet-therapy field? *NEJM* 2009; 361;11.
58. Malinin A, Pokov A, Spergling M, et al: Monitoring platelet inhibition after clopidogrel with the VerifyNow-P2Y12 rapid analyzer: the verify thrombosis risk assessment (VERITAS) study. *Thromb Res* 2007; 119(3):277.
59. Serebruany, VL: Variability in platelet responsiveness to clopidogrel among 544 Individuals. *J Am Coll Cardiol* 2005; 45:246.
60. Schmitt BP, Adelman B: Heparin-associated thrombocytopenia: a critical review and pooled analysis. *Am J Med Sci* 1993; 305:208.
61. Warkentin TE, Greinacher A: Heparin-induced thrombocytopenia and cardiac surgery. *Ann Thorac Surg* 2003; 76:2121.
62. Warkentin TE, Levine MN, Hirsh J, et al: Heparin-induced thrombocytopenia in patients treated with low-molecular-weight heparin or unfractionated heparin. *NEJM* 1995; 332:1330.
63. Nand S, Wong W, Yuen B, et al: Heparin-induced thrombocytopenia with thrombosis: incidence, analysis of risk factors, and clinical outcomes in 108 consecutive patients treated at a single institution. *Am J Hematol* 1997; 56:12.
64. Spiess BD, DeAnda A, McCarthy HL, et al: Off-pump coronary artery bypass graft surgery anticoagulation with bivalirudin: a patient with HITT syndrome type II and renal failure. *J Cardiothorac Vasc Anesth* 2006; 20:106.
65. Helm RE, Klemperer JD, Rosengart TK, et al: Intraoperative autologous blood donation preserves red cell mass but does not decrease postoperative bleeding. *Ann Thorac Surg* 1996; 62:1431.
66. Rosengart TK, DeBois W, O'Hara M, et al: Retrograde autologous priming for cardiopulmonary bypass: a safe and effective means of decreasing hemodilution and transfusion requirements. *J Thorac Cardiovasc Surg* 1998; 115:426.

67. Shapira OM, Aldea GS, Treanor PR, et al: Reduction of allogeneic blood transfusions after open heart operations by lowering cardiopulmonary bypass prime volume. *Ann Thorac Surg* 1998; 65:724.
68. Fang WC, Helm RE, Krieger KH, et al: Impact of minimum hematocrit during cardiopulmonary bypass on mortality in patients undergoing coronary artery surgery. *Circulation* 1997; 96:II194.
69. Beall AC Jr, Yow EM Jr, Bloodwell RD, et al: Open heart surgery without blood transfusion. *Arch Surg* 1967; 94:567.
70. Rosengart TK, Helm RE, DeBois WJ, et al: Open heart operations without transfusion using a multimodality blood conservation strategy in 50 Jehovah's Witness patients: implications for a "bloodless" surgical technique. *J Am Coll Surg* 1997; 184:618.
71. Rousou JA, Engelman RM, Flack JE 3rd, et al: The "primeless pump": a novel technique for intraoperative blood conservation. *Cardiovasc Surg* 1999; 7:228.
72. Karkouti K, Cohen MM, McCluskey SA, Sher GD: A multivariable model for predicting the need for blood transfusion in patients undergoing first-time elective coronary bypass graft surgery. *Transfusion* 2001; 41:1193.
73. Takai H, Eishi K, Yamachika S, et al: The efficacy of low prime volume completely closed cardiopulmonary bypass in coronary artery revasularization. *Ann Thorac Cardiovasc Surg* 2004; 10:178.
74. Silliman CC, Ambruso DR, Boshkov LK: Transfusion-related acute lung injury. *Blood* 2005; 105:2266.
75. Sheppard CA, Logdberg LE, Zimring JC, et al: Transfusion-related acute lung injury. *Hematol Oncol Clin North Am* 2007; 21:163.
76. DeAnda A Jr, Baker KM, Roseff SD, et al: Developing a blood conservation program in cardiac surgery. *Am J Med Qual* 2006; 21(4):230.
77. Koch CG, Li L, Sessler DI, et al: Duration of red-cell storage and complications after cardiac surgery. *NEJM* 2008; 358:1229.
78. Arora RC, Légare J, Buth KJ, et al: Identifying patients at risk of intraoperative and postoperative transfusion in isolated CABG: toward selective conservation strategies. *Ann Thorac Surg* 2004; 78:1547.

CHAPTER 14

Deep Hypothermic Circulatory Arrest

Andrew W. El Bardissi
Robert A. Oakes
R. Morton Bolman III

HISTORY AND CURRENT APPLICATIONS

Deep hypothermic circulatory arrest (DHCA) came about as an extension and unification of the work being done in the 1950s in cardiopulmonary bypass (Gibbon), systemic hypothermia (Bigelow), and aortic surgery (Debakey, Cooley, Crawford). Successful intracardiac surgery was based on the use of cardiopulmonary bypass (CPB); however, some procedures (eg, aortic arch surgery) could not be performed with standard CPB cannulation because of an inability to perfuse the cerebrum. Bigelow's work in the animal lab demonstrated that moderate hypothermia could be protective in cases in which CPB was halted for up to 10 minutes.[1] The earliest use of DHCA in adult cardiac surgery has been accredited to Niazi and Lewis in 1958.[2] Initially, DHCA was performed topically without the assistance of CPB; however, it soon became apparent that at hypothermic temperatures the heart would fibrillate or slow to a stop. Rewarming also proved to be quite difficult because of poor circulatory function during hypothermia. Many of these issues were improved on with the coordination of CPB with DHCA by the physiologist Gollan and the continued development and improvement of pump oxygenators and heat exchangers.[3] Extensive work on the metabolic aspects of DHCA were studied and put into clinical practice by Griepp and others in the 1970s, leading to safe and reliable techniques that have been adopted by many into general practice.

Currently, DHCA in adult cardiac surgery is used in ascending aortic and aortic arch replacements for aneurysmal disease, dissections, and extensive aortic calcifications (porcelain aorta). Circulatory arrest has also been described for resection of complex inferior vena cava (IVC) and cardiac tumors and pulmonary thromboendarterectomies, and has been widely adopted in congenital heart surgery for the repair of complex congenital lesions.

NECESSITY OF DEEP HYPOTHERMIC CIRCULATORY ARREST

The adult human brain is the organ most susceptible to ischemic injury. Under normal conditions, cerebral autoregulation matches cerebral blood flow (CBF) to cerebral oxygen consumption and cerebral metabolic activity ($CMRO_2$) under a wide range of cerebral perfusion pressures.[4] Yet, despite the effectiveness of cerebral autoregulation at normal physiologic perfusion pressures, the duration of cerebral ischemic tolerance at normothermia is approximately 5 minutes, making irreversible damage imminent unless adjunct perfusion methodologies or alternative strategies are employed to decrease the cerebral metabolic requirement.

The brain consumes 20% of the total body oxygen consumption, with 40% of its energy used in the preservation of cellular integrity and 60% in the transmission of nerve impulses.[5] Because the brain does not have the ability to store oxygen, $CMRO_2$ is a true index of brain metabolic activity and has been the variable of interest in studies attempting to determine the effectiveness of hypothermia in providing cerebral protection. For example, studies have demonstrated that a 10°C reduction in body temperature reduces $CMRO_2$ by a factor of four[4] (Fig. 14-1). This exponential decrease in metabolic rate differs from the linear reduction in CBF that occurs with hypothermia[6]; a discrepancy that results in the uncoupling between cerebral blood flow and cerebral metabolism occurring at approximately 22°C.[4]

Clinically, the reduction in cerebral metabolic function at hypothermic temperatures translates into periods of "safety" during circulatory arrest. Human studies have found a reasonable duration of DHCA with a low risk of neurocognitive insult to be no greater than 29 minutes at 13°C[7]; however, common

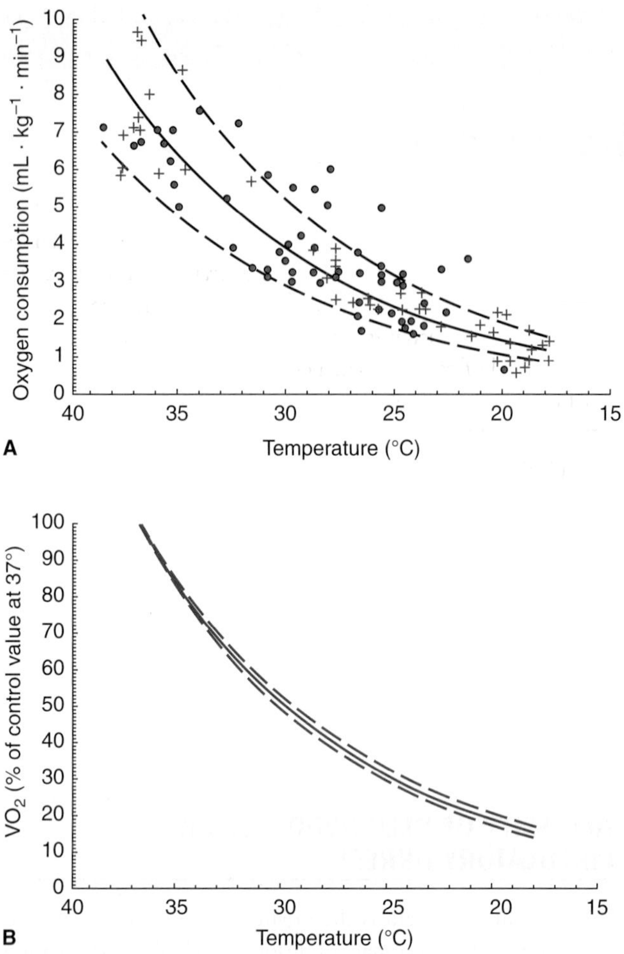

FIGURE 14-1 Relationship of temperature and oxygen consumption. (*Reproduced with permission from Kouchoukos NT, Karp RB, Blackstone EH, Doty DB, Hanley FL [eds]: Kirklin/Baratt-Boyes Cardiac Surgery, 3rd ed. New York, Churchill Livingstone, 2003, Figure 2-1.*)

clinical practice has pushed the limits of DHCA. It is not uncommon for DHCA to be performed at 18 to 20°C and prolonged for greater than 30 minutes; however, there continues to be controversy regarding optimal DHCA guidelines secondary to a lack of data in the current scientific literature.

NEUROCOGNITIVE EVENTS IN DHCA

During DHCA, the types of neurologic events are generally grouped into three different etiologies. These include focal cerebrovascular events, which are most often caused by thromboembolism; global cerebral necrosis, which occurs because of a failure to maintain the minimum oxygen and metabolic requirements during DHCA; and apoptosis, which occurs in specific regions of the brain and may also occur under oxygen/metabolic stress.

Focal Cerebrovascular Events

The occurrence of focal cerebrovascular events or stroke, which is not unique to DHCA but noteworthy in all instances of cardiac surgery, warrants special discussion caused by the high-risk population undergoing aortic arch surgery. The etiology of stroke in this subset of patients is not caused by a mismatch between the cerebral metabolic requirement and oxygen delivery, but rather is the consequence of an embolic event. Previous studies have found ascending aortic atherosclerosis to be an independent risk factor in the occurrence of early stroke and is likely caused by fragmentation of existing debris.[8] Strategies that may prevent these intraoperative events include epiaortic scanning, which may assist in alteration of cannulation strategy.[9] Furthermore, by assisting in flushing of debris from the cerebral vasculature, the adjunctive use of retrograde cerebral perfusion may be successful in reducing the incidence of focal cerebrovascular events that are caused by embolic events.

Global Cerebral Necrosis

Global cerebral necrosis occurs in those situations when the minimum oxygen and cerebral metabolic requirements are not met during DHCA. As such, the occurrence of frank cerebral necrosis is rare assuming adequate hypothermia with cerebral electrical suppression has been achieved, and the duration of circulatory arrest does not deplete the neuron's ability to maintain basic cellular processes. In instances of profound ischemia in which these requirements are not met, adenosine triphosphate (ATP) molecules are depleted and the cell reverts to anaerobic metabolism of glycolytic substrates,[10] which in turn yields an inadequate amount of ATP. The depletion of ATP is the primary insult that leads to the irreversible failure of basic cellular ionic pumps and redistribution of cellular ions.[10] Failure of the Na^+-K^+ ATPase pump results in an influx of Na^+ and Cl^- ions, which causes cellular swelling and neuronal depolarization,[11] thereby resulting in accumulation of intracellular calcium.

The accumulation of intracellular calcium is the central and direct mediator of irreversible ischemic cellular injury.[12] High intracellular concentrations of calcium causes the activation of phospholipases A and C, resulting in hydrolysis of membrane phospholipids and disruption of organelle structure and function.[12] In summary, although DHCA provides adequate cerebral protection by minimizing the neuronal metabolic requirement, irreversible ischemia and frank necrosis may still occur if guidelines are not adhered to that are designed to minimize the cerebral metabolic requirement while maintaining adequate oxygen delivery.

Activation of Programmed Cerebral Death

In situations of low, but not depleted levels of ATP, the release of calcium into the cytoplasm initiates programmed cellular death, rather than uncontrolled and frank necrosis. This second mechanism of cellular death after DHCA is termed *apoptosis,* and occurs in the context of adequate cellular metabolism and energy stores. Apoptosis occurs after a highly specific activation of genes, receptors, and enzymes, and results in the destruction of cellular structure in a programmed and predictable manner.[13] Cerebral apoptosis occurs principally via two intracellular pathways that are centered on caspases 3 and 8, a family of proteases that activate a series of biochemical cellular reactions that result in nuclear karyorrhexis and margination of the nuclear chromatin in the absence of inflammation.[14] The prolonged inability of the neuron to restore calcium homeostasis and ensure the turnover of cytostructure proteins is responsible for a progressive loss of cellular function and eventual death.[15] As a result, apoptosis is a progressive and active energy-dependent process characterized by the breakdown and phagocytosis of neurons.

Neuronal death in the setting of DHCA can also be accelerated secondary to excessive neuronal stimulation and hyperactivity,[15] thereby causing an energetic mismatch and inducing the release of toxic neurotransmitters. *Excitotoxicity* is a term applied to the death of cells caused by overstimulation of excitatory amino acids (primarily glutamate), and is believed to be a fundamental process involved in postischemic neuronal cell damage.[16] With partially depleted energetic stores, glutamate, the principal excitatory neurotransmitter, has been shown to have potent neurotoxic activities,[17] ultimately catalyzing and accelerating neuronal cell death.

Studies have demonstrated that these apoptotic pathways, although common to all cells, occur more commonly in certain regions of the brain after DHCA.[18] This concept, termed *selective vulnerability*, does not appear to be caused by uneven cooling[19]; rather, it is caused by regional cellular vulnerability.[20] In the adult brain, neurons in the hippocampus, cerebellum, striatum, amygdala, lateral thalamic nucleus, and third to fifth layers of the neocortex are the primary regions in which programmed cellular death occurs.[15] Cellular death via these apoptotic mechanisms begins as soon as 1 hour after reperfusion,[15] and continues for several days thereafter. Clinically, patients may demonstrate neurologic deficits consistent with regions of selective apoptosis.[21] These symptoms may include memory impairment, poor cognition, labile emotional state, and altered motor function. Interestingly, although clinical neurologic function continues to progressively improve throughout the postoperative period,[21] ongoing cellular death may occur up to 1 week after DHCA.

CURRENT APPLICATION OF DEEP HYPOTHERMIC CIRCULATORY ARREST

Cooling

There is wide institution and surgeon variability in the methodologies of cooling during the application of DHCA. Once CPB is commenced at normothermia, the heat exchanger is used to create a temperature gradient not exceeding 7 to 10°C between pump inflow and outflow.[22] The time interval required to attain equilibration of temperature between blood and tissue is directly related to the temperature gradient (between perfusate and organs), blood flow, and tissue-specific coefficients of temperature exchange. In general, standard parameters suggest that cooling should generally occupy at least 30 minutes, with some evidence suggesting that cooling times of at least 75 minutes[4,23] may be necessary to ensure even and adequate cooling. A short duration of cooling results in wide variation in temperature between organs, within organs themselves, as well as a rapid increase in the rate at which core body temperature drifts upward once circulatory arrest has been achieved.

Certain factors should alter cooling strategy; occlusive vascular disease and altered vascular reactivity may reduce cerebral perfusion significantly and delay temperature equilibration. Thus, to enhance and complement deep cooling in these situations, topical cerebral cooling should be performed by placing ice packs around the head. Topical cooling assists in the maintenance of cortical and subcortical temperature while reducing heat conduction across the skull.[24] Special attention should also be given to obese patients, as they often require a substantially longer period of cooling to achieve and maintain hypothermia.

Although the goal of DHCA is to obtain and maximize a period of minimal cerebral metabolism, there are little data to suggest optimal parameters for interrupting antegrade flow and commencing with circulatory arrest. Generally accepted parameters include jugular venous saturation greater than 95%, the complete absence of SSEPs and/or EEG silence, and cooling for at least 30 minutes.[7] These are discussed in depth later in this chapter.

CEREBRAL PERFUSION DURING DEEP HYPOTHERMIC CIRCULATORY ARREST

In complex aortic reconstructions requiring prolonged periods (>40 minutes) of circulatory arrest, DHCA alone may not provide adequate cerebral protection. In these situations, adjunct methodologies to DHCA, such as selective antegrade cerebral perfusion and retrograde cerebral perfusion, have been employed and have gained widespread adoption.

Selective Antegrade Cerebral Perfusion

Kazui et al. described the first use of selective antegrade cerebral perfusion in which perfusion was administered through both the innominate and left common carotid arteries.[25] Since that time, selective antegrade cerebral perfusion has gained widespread popularity as a modality to provide optimal cerebral protection during complex ascending and transverse aortic reconstructions. Antegrade perfusion of the brain during DHCA is typically administered through a cannula inserted in the right axillary artery (Fig. 14-2). The axillary artery has become the artery of choice caused by its size, accessibility, and resistance to atherosclerotic disease burden. The right axillary artery is generally approached through an infraclavicular or deltopectoral groove incision. A 6-, 8-, or 10-mm Dacron graft is anastomosed in an end-to-side fashion to provide adequate flow and to ensure adequate perfusion of the right upper extremity. Direct cannulation of the axillary artery is avoided caused by the risk of inducing trauma, which may lead to dissection. The innominate artery is subsequently isolated proximal to takeoff of the right subclavian artery and perfusate temperature is usually set at 18°C with a flow between 10 and 20 mL/kg per minute and adjusted to maintain a pressure of between 40 and 50 mm Hg in the right radial artery.

The need to cannulate relatively small and often diseased arch arteries and the presence of additional cannulas in the operating field constitute the main drawbacks of the technique. Direct cannulation of the common carotid or axillary arteries

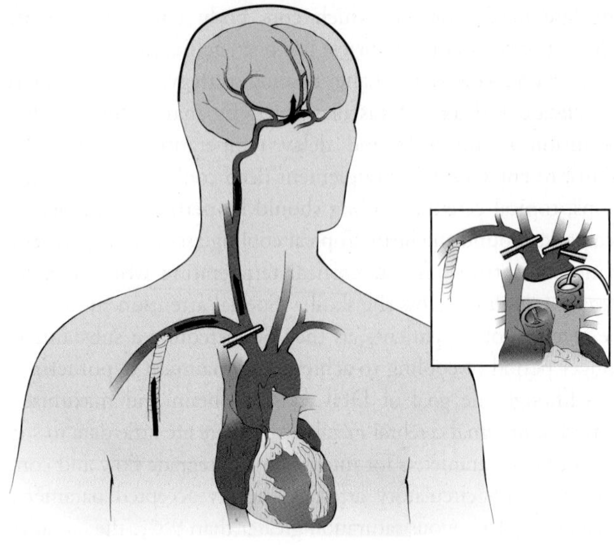

FIGURE 14-2 Schematic of right axillary artery cannulation for antegrade cerebral perfusion (ACP). Insert shows open aortic arch and ACP with occlusion of arch vessels to ensure perfusion of Circle of Willis.

can result in dissection of the arterial wall and embolism of atheromatous plaque material or air. Furthermore, arterial flow depends on proper positioning of the cannula tip within the vessel. For these reasons, some surgeons rely on a unilateral perfusion of the brain with sole cannulation and perfusion of the right subclavian artery. In these situations, the right vertebral and right common carotid artery territories are perfused in an antegrade fashion. The blood reaches the left cerebral hemisphere through the circle of Willis and, to a lesser extent, through cervicofacial connections. Therefore, it is important that the take-offs of the left common carotid and left subclavian arteries be occluded to avoid a steal of blood down these arteries. Occlusion (usually with an inflatable balloon) of the descending aorta is also a useful maneuver to improve overall body perfusion. Effective somatic perfusion (including the abdominal organs, spinal cord, and lower limb musculature) has been documented with this maneuver.[26] The presence of an aberrant right subclavian artery (*arteria lusoria*) is a clear contraindication to the use of this perfusion method. The aberrant origin of the artery usually is identified readily by computed tomographic scanning or magnetic resonance imaging. The burst of blood from the descending aorta during opening of the aortic arch should alert the surgeon to this anatomical variation and prompt a direct cannulation of the ostium of the right and left common carotid arteries.

Sequential perfusion of the cerebral arteries provides additional safety to unilateral cerebral perfusion and avoids cannulation of small or diseased arch arteries.[27] The right subclavian artery remains perfused during the whole procedure. A vascular graft is sewn immediately to a common patch of aortic wall including all the arch vessels,[28] or the second branch of a multiple-arm prosthesis is anastomosed to the left common carotid artery. Perfusion then is instituted through this additional graft and enhances cerebral perfusion.

Retrograde Cerebral Perfusion

Retrograde cerebral perfusion (RCP) is performed by isolation and perfusion through the superior vena cava shortly after the interruption of antegrade arterial flow. The superior vena cava (SVC) is typically snared below the azygous vein to provide retrograde cerebral blood flow and blood flow to the anterior spinal plexus and, to a small degree, the remainder of the visceral organs (Fig. 14-3). Alternatively, the SVC is directly cannulated for bypass, the cannula snared, and arterial flow directed into the SVC from the cardiopulmonary bypass circuit after clamping the IVC cannula. Pressurization of the venous system to 20 to 25mm Hg allows for blood flow into the upper extremities, jugular veins, and spinal channels, eventually crossing the capillary bed into the arterial system and finally draining into the open aortic arch. The proposed benefits of RCP are to maintain cerebral hypothermia, flush out embolic debris and air, provide metabolic support, and allow for the removal of toxic metabolites and waste products.[29]

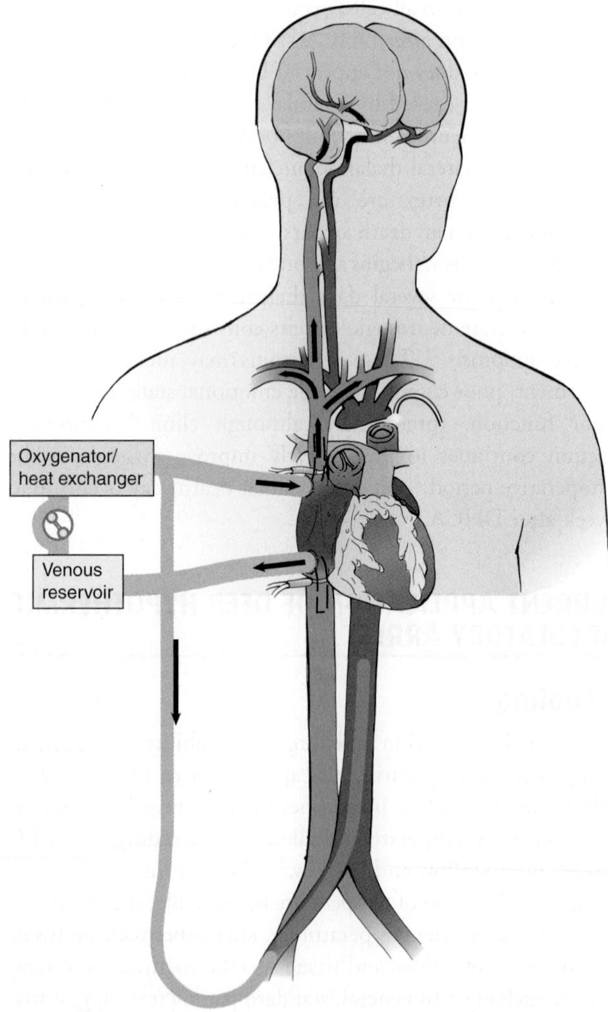

FIGURE 14-3 Schematic of retrograde cerebral perfusion (RCP). Arterial blood is perfused via the superior vena cava, with a target CVP of 25 mm Hg. Flow can be monitored through the open aortic arch. Balloon occlusion catheter can be employed to increase perfusion to body.

The initial report that described the use of RCP to assist in brain protection during circulatory arrest created considerable controversy.[30] Investigators questioned whether perfusion of the brain via the cerebral venous system offered any metabolic delivery to the brain, whereas others felt that high venous cerebral pressure may cause edema. Based on the subsequent results of clinical and experimental studies, it is now generally accepted that RCP produces deep and homogeneous cooling of the brain hemispheres and the expulsion of solid particles or gaseous bubbles from the arch arteries.[31] Although there is generally excellent backflow with RCP and an open aortic arch, occlusion of the inferior vena cava to decrease the pressure gradient between the two venous territories effectively reduces the amount of stolen blood.[32] Interstitial edema is a rare but potential complication of retrograde perfusion and can lead to cerebral edema and hypertension when the perfusion pressure is set above 25 mm Hg.[33]

Because RCP is nonphysiologic, it is critical that the conduct of administering RCP is performed correctly. For venous-to-arterial blood flow to occur, the aortic arch must be wide open during RCP, thereby minimizing the pressure gradient between the venous and arterial vasculature. Any arterial occlusion, including severe atherosclerotic cerebrovascular disease, may impede cerebral perfusion, and may result in cerebral edema in cases of high venous pressure. Furthermore, contrary to common practice, patients should only be partially exsanguinated at the onset of circulatory arrest to assure that full venous capacitance is obtained. RCP in these situations is most likely to contribute to optimal retrograde cerebral blood flow and exceptional results when performed correctly.[34]

Rewarming after DHCA

Rewarming represents a critical time period during which any additional harm to neurons might induce permanent injury or death. Providing a favorable hematologic environment, ensuring optimal hemodynamic conditions, and avoiding cerebral hyperactivity should provide optimal conditions for recovery of the energy-depleted brain.[14] It is crucial to begin reperfusion slowly after circulatory arrest. An initial period of "cold blood low-pressure reperfusion" washes out accumulated metabolites, buffers free radicals, and provides substrates for regeneration of high-energy molecules before the resumption of cerebral electrical activity. Furthermore, an adequate hematocrit during this reperfusion period is attractive not only because of its oxygen-carrying[4] capacity, but also because of its buffer, redox, and free-radical scavenging capacity. Glycemia should be monitored closely and treated aggressively, because hyperglycemia, which is stimulated by the release of endogenous catecholamines, increases intracellular acidosis and can prevent or delay the restitution of metabolic homeostasis.[35] During rewarming, cerebral vascular resistance and energetic metabolism are impaired in proportion to the severity of ischemia.[36] Cerebral perfusion is reduced and glucose is derived in part from the less efficient anaerobic pathway, with oxygen coupling during oxidative phosphorylation being partially interrupted.[37] This vulnerable period can last for 6 to 8 hours after initiation of reperfusion.[21] During this time, an abnormally high extraction of oxygen and glucose is necessary to sustain the cerebral metabolic rate.[38] Jugular venous oxygen saturation is often below 40% during this recovery period and cerebral autoregulation may not compensate for reduction in oxygen delivery, which could occur with postoperative events such as acute hypotension, hypoxemia, and anemia.

The temperature of the perfusate during the rewarming phase should be managed carefully. Detection of increased cerebral activity should prompt immediate therapeutic action, which includes deep anesthesia, appropriate sedation, and reduction of temperature. Monitoring cerebral electrical activity during the rewarming phase (and thereafter if circulatory arrest has exceeded the safe ischemic period or if signs of abnormal electrical activity are present) could help to limit the extent of secondary damage to the brain. The perfusate temperature should not exceed 37°C because a relative hypothermia may prove to be beneficial for optimal brain recovery. It is our practice to maintain perfusate temperature at 37°C for a period of at least 20 minutes when a patient has achieved normothermia to minimize a downward hypothermic trend. Electrical hyperactivity of the brain can trigger overwhelmingly destructive reactions. The disorder is not uncommon after prolonged circulatory arrest and actually is considered a sign of ischemic injury.[39]

Outcomes after DHCA, RCP, and SACP

Clinical neurologic deficits after DHCA encompass a variety of disorders ranging from deep coma to subtle, barely perceptible alterations in cognitive functions, to focal deficiencies and behavioral changes. In the immediate postoperative period, the return of sophisticated neurologic function is often obscured by the administration of sedative and analgesic agents. A focal deficit is caused by interruption of blood in a terminal vascular territory, usually secondary to embolism, and is often the consequence of atheromatous burden. The clinical expression, typically, is a motor-sensory deficit, aphasia, or cortical blindness. Computed tomographic scanning and magnetic resonance imaging are able to detect a sharply demarcated area of necrosis in the cerebral cortex. The prevalence of a focal deficit in clinical series ranges from 5 to 10% after elective aortic surgery with the use of deep hypothermic circulatory arrest. Age, atherosclerosis, and manipulation of aorta are more potent risk factors than the duration of circulatory arrest.[24] Retrograde perfusion of the aorta during cardiopulmonary bypass (with the arterial cannula inserted into the femoral or iliac artery) also has been associated with an increased risk of focal deficit because retrograde flow can dislodge floating atheromatous plaques and thrombi loosely attached to the walls of thoracic aortic aneurysms.[40]

Diffuse neurologic deficits are caused by global cerebral ischemia that produces various levels of cellular dysfunction. In its mildest forms, the neurons are viable but temporarily unable to function properly. The clinical spectrum of neuropsychological disorders ranges from benign and reversible conditions such as transient confusion, stupor, delirium, and agitation to more serious and debilitating conditions such as seizures, parkinsonism, and coma. Imaging studies are often normal, although in the most severe forms, scattered areas of necrosis may appear. The wide range of incidences (from 3 to 30%) of diffuse deficits after circulatory arrest quoted in the literature reflects the subtle and often unrecognized nature of most deficits. Scrupulous postoperative evaluation of neurologic function discloses a frequency of between 10 and 20%.[41,42] Age, conduct of cardiopulmonary bypass, and prolonged duration of circulatory arrest are recognized risk factors for the occurrence of diffuse deficits. Disorders that impair vascular reactivity and cerebral autoregulation, such as diabetes and hypertension, have also been associated with an increased incidence of diffuse deficits.[43]

With refinement in neurologic evaluation, including behavioral and cognitive testing, it appears that subtle deficits occur in a much larger proportion of patients after relatively short ischemic times. Transient neurologic dysfunction, a condition once not considered a deficit, and postoperative electroencephalographic hyperactivity appear now as definitive markers of long-lasting cerebral injury.[33,41] One-fourth of patients with transient deficits perform poorly on postoperative neuropsychological testing, and the deficit, affecting mainly memory and fine motor function, persists in many of them after hospital discharge. The risk of transient neurologic deficit starts when deep hypothermic circulatory arrest exceeds 25 minutes.[24] The risk initially is linearly related to the duration of circulatory arrest and rises more steeply after 50 minutes of ischemia[24] (Fig. 14-4).

Based on these findings and accumulated experience, it appears that the majority of patients can support unharmed a circulatory arrest of 30 minutes at 18°C (Fig. 14-5), provided that electrocerebral silence has been obtained. No deficit, or only a transient neurologic dysfunction, is expected when the ischemic period extends to 40 minutes, provided that rewarming is performed correctly and hemodynamic stability is maintained postoperatively. With an arrest time of more than 40 minutes, neurologic deficit is prone to occur, particularly in high-risk patients, such as those presenting with diabetes, hypertension, or old age. Further cooling of the brain to 13 to 15°C reduces the risk and makes a deficit again less likely if the arrest time does not exceed 40 minutes, and renders it no more severe than a transient dysfunction if it lasts 50 minutes. In these cases, careful rewarming with close monitoring of cerebral activity, deep anesthesia, and hemodynamic stability are critical for a favorable outcome.

Outcomes after Selective Antegrade Cerebral Perfusion

Evaluating the benefit of SACP is a difficult task because most studies in the literature are limited by selection bias. The primary benefit of SACP is not to reduce the incidence of embolic events, but rather to increase the safe duration of hypothermic circulatory arrest and allow for the application of circulatory arrest under moderate temperatures.[28,44] Thus, it is not surprising that the majority of clinical studies have demonstrated no reduction in the incidence of permanent stroke.[27,45–49] Overall, permanent stroke incidences after SACP in the literature range from 1 to 16%,[50,51] likely reflecting the diversity and complexity of the patient population in which SACP is used. Generally, however, permanent stroke after elective aortic surgery with SACP occurs in 2.5 to 5% of patients.[50,52] The incidence of global neurologic dysfunction, which is caused by failure to appropriately protect the cerebrum, is reduced in patients who undergo SACP compared with DHCA alone.[52] Furthermore, because SACP does not require deep hypothermia, other postoperative complications such as reintubation, renal failure, and ventilator times may also be reduced.[52] There is also evidence that SACP may improve long-term survival, although the exact mechanism is not completely clear.[52] Although prospective studies are lacking, it appears that SACP may be primarily advantageous in those situations in which a prolonged period of circulatory arrest is anticipated. These may include complex Type I aortic dissections and aortic arch reconstructions.

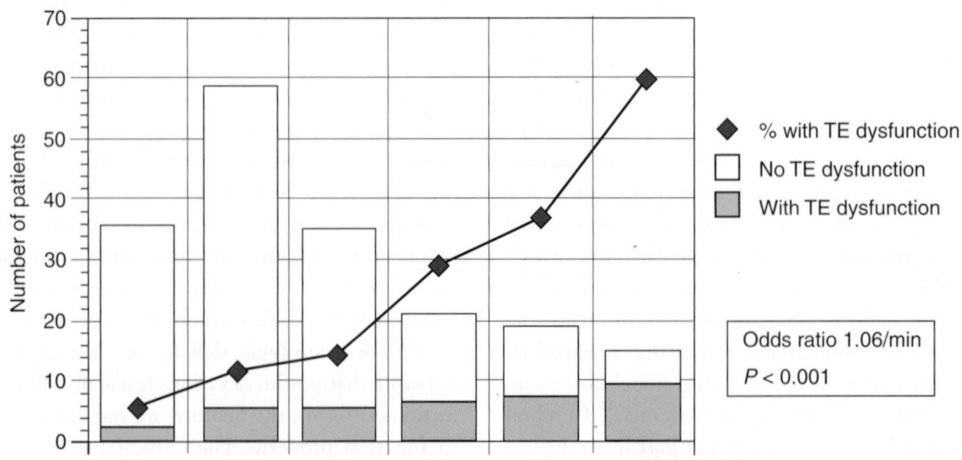

FIGURE 14-4 Prevalence of temporary (TE) neurologic dysfunction as a function of duration of circulatory arrest time. (*Reproduced with permission from Kouchoukos NT, Karp RB, Blackstone EH, Doty DB, Hanley FL [eds]: Kirklin/Baratt-Boyes Cardiac Surgery, 3rd ed. New York, Churchill Livingstone, 2003, Figure 2-2.*)

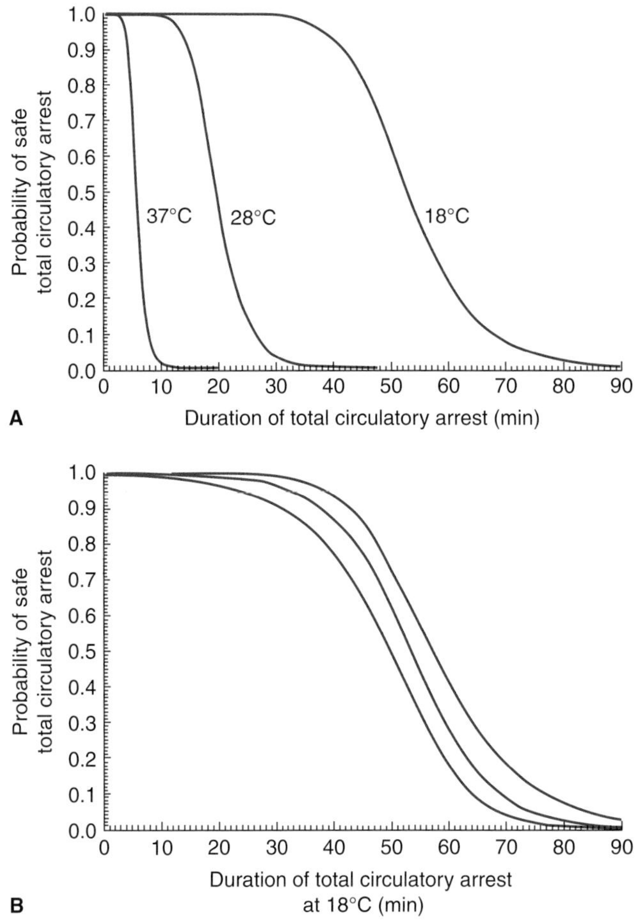

FIGURE 14-5 Probability of safe (absence of structural or functional damage) circulatory arrest according to duration. A. Estimate at nasopharyngeal temperatures of 37d, 28d, and 18d C. B. Estimate at 18d C with dashed lines representing 70% confidence limits. At 30 minutes, safe arrest is likely, and at 45 minutes, it is probable. Other data suggest that, at 45 minutes, damage will probably be only structural and without evident functional sequelae. (*Reproduced with permission from Kouchoukos NT, Karp RB, Blackstone EH, Doty DB, Hanley FL [eds]: Kirklin/Baratt-Boyes Cardiac Surgery, 3rd ed. New York, Churchill Livingstone, 2003, Figure 2-9A, B.*)

Outcomes after Retrograde Cerebral Perfusion

Recent clinical research using RCP has demonstrated encouraging results. A reduction in both mortality and neurologic damage has been documented regularly with the adjunctive use of retrograde cerebral perfusion compared with classic deep hypothermia alone.[53–57] Some studies confirmed the limited capacity of retrograde perfusion to sustain cerebral metabolism.[58,59] Yet, the inability of RCP to meet cerebral requirements does not indicate that it is ineffective as an adjunctive means of cerebral perfusion, because RCP has proved extremely effective at maintaining cerebral hypothermia as well as preventing intracellular acidosis, which may contribute to apoptosis and in turn result in temporary and/or permanent neurologic dysfunction.[60]

Most surgeons acknowledge the potential capacity of retrograde cerebral perfusion to prolong the period of safe circulatory arrest; however, it is generally not an adjunctive modality that is used for complex repairs in which a period of circulatory arrest of greater than 50 minutes is anticipated. This method should be viewed as a valuable but not an alternative adjunct to conventional methods when longer periods of circulatory arrest are anticipated. Some have found alternative uses of RCP that may prove to be beneficial. For example, at the Brigham and Women's Hospital we have recently adopted the use of DHCA with RCP for patients who undergo ascending aortic aneurysm repair to facilitate the creation of an open distal anastomosis, thereby allowing for the resection of all aneurysmal ascending aortic tissue. A recent study has demonstrated no overall difference in the incidence of neurologic events or mortality when compared with the standard aortic cross-clamp, closed distal anastomosis approach.[61]

TEMPERATURE MANAGEMENT DURING DEEP HYPOTHERMIC CIRCULATORY ARREST

Accurate temperature monitoring is vital to the prevention of cerebral injury during DHCA. There have been a number of peripheral sites used to assess body temperature, yet it has been well documented that peripheral temperature differs from core cerebral temperature[62]; a differential that becomes more pronounced during rapid warming or cooling. Although possible, during complex cardiovascular surgical procedures, it is simply not feasible to directly monitor cerebral temperature. As such, it becomes important to understand the limitations of temperature measurement at peripheral sites, including rectal, bladder, nasopharyngeal, and jugular venous sites. Most institutions have adopted nasopharyngeal monitoring because it appears to be the most reliable approximate of cerebral temperature. There is no single nasopharyngeal temperature that results in electrocerebral silence. In one large study, the minimal nasopharyngeal temperature necessary to obtain electrocerebral silence in all patients was 12.5°C; at the classic 18°C, 40% of patients still exhibited electrical activity.[63]

Accurate monitoring of temperature serves not only to assure that adequate hypothermia is achieved during circulatory arrest, but it also assists in the prevention of hyperthermia during the warming phase of CPB. Although there is a high correlation between nasopharyngeal and brain temperature during cooling, nasopharyngeal temperature underestimates brain temperature during rewarming by 2 to 3°C.[64] This discrepancy is important because hyperthermia during rewarming exacerbates cerebral activity and disturbs cellular metabolism after circulatory arrest.

pH MANAGEMENT

Arterial carbon dioxide tension is a major regulatory factor that impacts cerebral blood flow during CPB and DHCA. Two strategies for blood gas monitoring have been proposed for management during hypothermia. Alpha-stat management aims to maintain a normal pH and $PaCO_2$ (a pH of 7.40 and a $PaCO_2$ of 40 mm Hg) in warmed (37°C) blood. In vivo, under hypothermic conditions, when using alpha-stat management, blood becomes alkaline and hypocapnic. The second management strategy, pH-stat, aims to maintain a pH of 7.40 and $PaCO_2$ of 40 mm Hg under hypothermic conditions. Consequently, under pH-stat management, when rewarmed to 37°C, blood becomes acidotic and hypercapnic.

Alpha-stat management preserves autoregulation of brain perfusion and optimizes cellular enzyme activity. Caused by blood alkalosis at hypothermic conditions, the curve of oxyhemoglobin dissociation is shifted to the right, corresponding to an increased affinity of oxygen for hemoglobin. With a corresponding further shift of oxyhemoglobin to the right owing to hypothermia, the availability of oxygen carried by the hemoglobin molecule becomes reduced. At deep hypothermic temperatures, oxygen dissolved in blood represents the major source of oxygen to tissues. Comparatively, the pH-stat strategy, results in a powerful and sustained dilatation of the cerebral vessels. Autoregulation of brain perfusion is lost and cerebral blood flow is increased. The time for temperature equilibration between blood and brain is shortened, resulting in quick and homogeneous cooling of the brain. Hypercapnia shifts the oxyhemoglobin dissociation curve to the left and results in an increased availability of oxygen to tissues.

There are conflicting data regarding the optimal strategy for pH management. Theoretically, both strategies are capable of maintaining energy balance and cellular hemostasis during long periods of hypothermia. Studies in the adult cardiac surgery literature have provided evidence that the alpha-stat management technique provides optimal neurological outcomes.[65–67] Yet, amid animal study findings, and suspicion that infant physiology may require a different pH management strategy, retrospective[68,69] and prospective studies[18,70] have indicated that pH-stat management yields a decrease in patient morbidity in neonates and infants. The superiority of the pH-stat strategy has not been confirmed in adults. In fact, prospective studies in the adult cardiac surgery literature have found no difference[71] and even inferior neuropsychological outcomes.[65]

Because the alpha-stat strategy maintains a physiologic coupling between cerebral blood flow and metabolism, it appears to result in better outcomes in adults where the risk of underperfusion or overperfusion within the brain is substantial.[72] Cerebral edema which can be a consequence of cerebral overperfusion, is less likely to occur with alpha-stat management. The preservation of cerebral autoregulation may attenuate the homogeneous distribution of blood that is prone to occur in adult patients with underlying vasculopathic risk factors such as atherosclerosis, hypertension, and diabetes. Comparatively, the underlying etiology of the neonatal brain damage in patients undergoing DHCA is most often caused by hypoperfusion during periods of low systemic flow. Under pH-stat conditions cerebral oxygen supply is enhanced, thereby indicating why there may be a significant improvement in neurologic outcome compared to alpha-stat[70] in this population.

GLYCEMIC MANAGEMENT DURING DHCA

The relationship between intraoperative hyperglycemia and adverse postoperative outcomes has been well established in the cardiac surgery literature.[73] There are two main mechanisms of morbidity that can be the result of intraoperative hyperglycemia, especially in the context of circulatory arrest. Hyperglycemia results in the anaerobic conversion of glucose to lactate, thereby worsening intracellular acidosis and limiting cellular metabolism, which ultimately increases the likelihood of apoptosis.[74] Additionally, hyperglycemia increases the release of excitatory amino acids, which can have profoundly negative effects during periods of cerebral ischemia.[75] For these reasons, aggressive management of hyperglycemia with intravenous insulin administration should be pursued in patients who undergo DHCA. Although the data are sparse regarding the optimal glycemic range during DHCA, it appears that the risk of adverse neurologic events increases significantly at blood glucose levels greater than 180 mg/dL.[76]

HEMATOCRIT MONITORING

Since the inception of DHCA, it has been widely accepted that a deleterious and potential fatal consequence of deep hypothermia is increased cellular rigidity and viscosity, which may increase the risk of end organ ischemic events.[77] Conversely, however, hemodilution reduces the oxygen carrying capacity of the blood and in conjunction with the left-shift of the oxyhemoglobin curve, may predispose to organ damage (particularly cerebral) secondary to limited oxygen delivery. These conflicting findings have led to variability in hematocrit manipulation during DCHA with a range of post-prime CPB hematocrit values between 10 and 30%.[78,79] Subsequent animal investigations have found that during DHCA, hemoglobin acts as a reservoir during the arrest period,[80] with lower hematocrit levels predisposing to a higher incidence of cerebral necrosis. Previous studies have found that the optimal hematocrit that provides adequate oxygen delivery during a 60-minute course of DHCA to be approximately 30%.[80]

The majority of the evidence examining optimal hematocrit levels has been in the setting of CPB only, however, many of these findings have been applied to conditions of DHCA as well. For example, human studies have found that low intraoperative hematocrit levels with CPB may be independently associated with an increased risk of mortality[81] with one study identifying that an intraoperative hematocrit less than 22% to be independently associated with the risk of stroke.[82] Although these findings are likely generalizable to DHCA, there are other factors under manipulation during hypothermia that affect the interpretability of such data. As previously discussed, pH, temperature, and hematocrit are all intricately and independently associated with oxygen delivery during hypothermia as a result of oxyhemoglobin dissociation. Each of these parameters can encompass a wide range of values based on institutional practices, anesthesia preferences, and/or surgeon preferences. Yet, taking the interaction of these factors into account, studies have demonstrated that a hematocrit level of 30% or greater has the potential to significantly improve neurologic outcomes irrespective of other perfusion conditions.[83]

ELECTROENCEPHALOGRAPHIC AND SOMATOSENSORY EVOKED POTENTIAL MONITORING

Electroencephalographic (EEG) monitoring during DHCA has been a useful adjunct to the assessment of cerebral function. Current EEG monitors use between 4 and 16 channels and require placement of electrodes at specific cortical sites by trained technicians. Although it has been found to be a very sensitive and clinically relevant predictor of postoperative cerebral dysfunction, EEG monitoring has poor specificity[84] and often requires a dedicated technician to place electrodes and interpret tracings. As such, many centers have strayed away from continuous monitoring in lieu of other technologies that provide simpler, yet suitable alternatives to the evaluation of cerebral electrical activity and or metabolism.

Newer devices, such as the Bispectral Index (BIS) monitor, uses Fourier transformation and bispectral analysis of a one-channel processed EEG pattern to produce a single number index, which is strongly correlated with cerebral electrical activity.[85] A BIS index ranges from 0 (flat line EEG) to 100 (awake state) and provides the operator with an accurate assessment of cerebral electrical activity. At the Brigham and Women's Hospital, it is currently our practice to use BIS monitoring during all circulatory arrest cases caused by its simplicity and reliability.

Somatosensory evoked potential monitoring (SSEP) is an alternative neuromonitoring technology that has also been used as a substitute to EEG. SSEP detects neural activity at the median nerves, which serve as a surrogate for cerebral activity. SSEP monitoring is generally easier to assess and interpret, because there is less electric noise interference and electrical activity is not significantly influenced by anesthetic drugs. The sensitivity and specificity of SSEP monitoring in determining the occurrence of early postoperative neurologic events approaches 100%,[86] making it an extremely useful and simple modality for determining and maintaining the optimal level of hypothermia.

JUGULAR VENOUS BULB SATURATION

Jugular venous bulb saturation is viewed by some to be one of the most critical aspects of monitoring during DHCA. By assessing the SvO_2, use of this modality allows the surgical team to infer the rate of cerebral oxygen uptake, and consequently ongoing cerebral metabolism. Guidelines suggest that SvO_2 should exceed 95% to ensure that maximal cerebral metabolic suppression has been attained.[87] Ongoing continuous oxygen extraction suggests active cerebral metabolic activity and may predispose to energy depletion and subsequent neurologic events. Studies have shown that use of a jugular venous bulb catheter is associated with lower central temperatures,[88] yet their use has not been shown to be independently associated with an improvement in neurologic outcome.[88] A unique advantage to the jugular venous bulb catheter is the ability to obtain a near-direct measurement of cerebral temperature, thus allowing for two modes of critical measurement, which may increase the likelihood of a safe operation.

It should be noted that the modalities that aim to assess neural cell arrest (temperature, EEG/SSEP, and jugular venous bulb saturation) each have varying levels of specificity and often produce differing results. For example, under conditions of EEG/SSEP arrest, some have found low jugular venous bulb oxygen saturation levels,[89] suggesting that even in the setting of electrocerebral silence there is continuous metabolic activity. In the clinical setting, electrocerebral silence (as assessed by electroencephalography) is generally obtained at a mean nasopharyngeal temperature of 17.5°C[63]; however, this is not universally true, as some studies have reported continuous phasic activity at this temperature,[90] which may be caused by individual patient characteristics and/or methodologies of cooling. These variations are also confounded by the fact that the brain temperature is not measured directly and can differ markedly among sites of temperature measurement. In summary, complete suppression of cerebral metabolic activity should be the goal when undergoing DHCA; however, it must often be surmised by a number of clinically relevant variables. As such, multimodality monitoring is the safest approach to assessing cerebral metabolic suppression.[91]

TRANSCRANIAL NONINVASIVE CEREBRAL OXIMETRY

Transcranial noninvasive cerebral oximetry is a relatively new technology that uses an infrared light source contained in an adhesive patch placed on the patient's forehead. This light source transmits photons to the outer cortical layer and uses a near infrared spectroscopy to measure both arterial and venous hemoglobin (rSO_2) concentration. Cerebral oximetry is primarily used through the duration of DHCA and functions to assess major changes in cerebral oxyhemoglobin concentrations that suggest an increase in cerebral metabolism that may predispose the occurrence of cerebral ischemia.

The use of rSO_2 has been validated as an appropriate measure of cerebral oxygen concentration when compared with standard approaches such as SvO_2.[92] Yet, because this technology is new, there are still concerns about the interpretability of the data and intervention threshold. Commonly accepted interventional thresholds include a relative desaturation of 10 scale units below the baseline reading or an absolute value less than 50.[93]

PHARMACOLOGIC ADJUNCTS

Barbiturates

Barbiturates have been found to decrease the energy required for synaptic transmission, thereby allowing oxygen under conditions of hypothermic circulatory arrest to be used exclusively for cellular metabolism.[94] In addition to providing global cerebral protection, barbiturates appear to also be beneficial in cases of focal ischemia[95] by reducing the extent and severity of cerebral infarction by mechanisms that are not completely understood. The first human study that demonstrated the neuroprotective effect of barbiturates in cardiac surgery was performed by administering thiopentone during the periods of time most likely to result in embolism; cannulating and weaning from CPB.[96] There was a significant decrease in the incidence and extent of neuropsychiatric deficits in the thiopentone group. The neuroprotective benefit of barbiturates is not without risk, because the greatest benefit is appreciated at high doses, which are associated with a negative inotropic effect and may induce sedation that would prolong time to extubation. Studies using lower doses of barbiturates (thiopental at 15 to 30 mg/kg) have found that cerebral metabolism is in fact minimized,[97] yet few prospective randomized clinical studies have demonstrated an appreciable effect on the reduction of neuropsychiatric events after DHCA.[97] As such, widespread adoption in the use of thiopental during DHCA has not yet been appreciated.

Volatile Anesthetics

Volatile anesthetics—including halothane, isoflurane, desflurane, and sevoflurane—confer global cerebral protection at minimum alveolar concentration. Mechanistically, they provide protection via inhibition of excitotoxicity, depression of metabolic demand, and improvement of cerebral oxygenation.[98] These protective effects are primarily mediated by inhibiting glutamate release, binding to *N*-methyl-d-aspartate and alpha-amino-3-hydroxyl-5-methyl-4-isozazole propionate receptors while upregulating GABA-aminobutyric acid receptors.[99] In contrast with barbiturates, volatile anesthetics are capable of producing an isoelectric EEG with minimal effect on cardiac output and hemodynamics.[100] Most of the promising data suggesting a beneficial effect of volatile anesthetics have been performed on animal models with isoflurane and have demonstrated a reduction in brain injury after permanent or transient cerebral ischemic events.[101,102] However, the scarcity of clinical information makes it difficult to infer the role of these volatile anesthetics in patients who undergo DHCA.

Corticosteroids

CPB causes a systemic inflammatory response that increases capillary permeability as well as impacts vascular tone, fluid distribution, and organ function and has been implicated in postoperative cerebral dysfunction.[103]Many have hypothesized that this inflammatory response may exacerbate the oxidative stress that the brain experiences during periods of hypothermia and circulatory arrest, leading some to suggest the use of anti-inflammatory medications. The use of high-dose steroids has been linked to a reduction in cytokines and TNF-alpha[104] and has demonstrated a survival benefit when employed during cardiac surgery and CPB likely caused by the prevention of capillary leak syndrome and decreasing cardiac output.[105] Capillary leak may be particularly detrimental in the setting of DHCA since increased permeability of the blood brain barriers is associated with a higher frequency of apoptosis caused by activation of caspases.[106]

Corticosteroids appear to provide unique benefits when used during DHCA. In addition to their antiapoptotic properties, studies have found that steroid pretreatment is associated with a significant improvement in pulmonary function[104] as well as superior cerebral oxygen metabolism and recovery of cerebral blood flow after DHCA.[106] Yet, although some studies have demonstrated a neuroprotective advantage in patients who received corticosteroid pretreatment,[107] others have demonstrated no appreciable clinical advantage.[108] This discrepancy is likely caused by variable treatment algorithms, including dose, timing, and safe duration of DHCA making future studies necessary before widespread application is adopted.

CAN'T MISS PEARLS

- DHCA allows for the performance of complex ascending aortic and arch reconstructions by minimizing cerebral metabolism.
- When performed correctly, DHCA at a systemic temperature of 18°C, allows for a "safe" operative period of approximately 30 to 40 minutes.
- In cases in which a prolonged period of circulatory arrest is anticipated, selective antegrade cerebral perfusion, employed either alone or supplemented with retrograde cerebral perfusion, provides additional cerebral protection, and prolongs the "safe period" of DHCA.
- Aggressive monitoring and intraoperative management of temperature, glycemia, hematocrit, pH, and cerebral activity (via EEG, SSEPs, or transcranial Doppler monitoring) is critical to the safety of DHCA.
- Pharmacologic adjuncts such as barbiturates, corticosteroids, and the use of volatile anesthetics provide optimal cerebral protection during DHCA.

REFERENCES

1. Bigelow WG, Lindsay WK, Greenwood WF: Hypothermia; its possible role in cardiac surgery: an investigation of factors governing survival in dogs at low body temperatures. *Ann Surg.* Nov 1950; 132(5):849-866.
2. Niazi SA, Lewis FJ: Profound hypothermia in man; report of a case. *Ann Surg* 1958; 147(2):264-266.
3. Griepp RB, Stinson EB, Hollingsworth JF, Buehler D: Prosthetic replacement of the aortic arch. *J Thorac Cardiovasc Surg* 1975; 70(6): 1051-1063.
4. Greeley WJ, Kern FH, Ungerleider RM, et al: The effect of hypothermic cardiopulmonary bypass and total circulatory arrest on cerebral metabolism in neonates, infants, and children. *J Thorac Cardiovasc Surg* 1991; 101(5):783-794.
5. Michenfelder JD, Theye RA: Cerebral protection by thiopental during hypoxia. *Anesthesiology* 1973; 39(5):510-517.
6. Mezrow CK, Midulla PS, Sadeghi AM, et al: Evaluation of cerebral metabolism and quantitative electroencephalography after hypothermic circulatory arrest and low-flow cardiopulmonary bypass at different temperatures. *J Thorac Cardiovasc Surg* 1994; 107(4):1006-1019.
7. McCullough JN, Zhang N, Reich DL, et al: Cerebral metabolic suppression during hypothermic circulatory arrest in humans. *Ann Thorac Surg* 1999; 67(6):1895-1899; discussion 1919-1821.
8. Blauth CI, Cosgrove DM, Webb BW, et al: Atheroembolism from the ascending aorta. An emerging problem in cardiac surgery. *J Thorac Cardiovasc Surg* 1992; 103(6):1104-1111; discussion 1111-1102.
9. Davila-Roman VG, Barzilai B, Wareing TH, Murphy SF, Kouchoukos NT: Intraoperative ultrasonographic evaluation of the ascending aorta in 100 consecutive patients undergoing cardiac surgery. *Circulation* 1991; 84(5 Suppl):III47-53.
10. Siesjo BK: Cerebral circulation and metabolism. *J Neurosurg* 1984; 60(5):883-908.
11. Kuwashima J, Fujitani B, Nakamura K, Kadokawa T, Yoshida K: Biochemical changes in unilateral brain injury in the rat: s possible role of free fatty acid accumulation. *Brain Res* 1976; 110(3):547-557.
12. Meyer FB, Sundt TM Jr, Yanagihara T, Anderson RE: Focal cerebral ischemia: pathophysiologic mechanisms and rationale for future avenues of treatment. *Mayo Clin Proc* 1987; 62(1):35-55.
13. Thompson CB: Apoptosis in the pathogenesis and treatment of disease. *Science* 1995; 267(5203):1456-1462.
14. Amir G, Ramamoorthy C, Riemer RK, Reddy VM, Hanley FL: Neonatal brain protection and deep hypothermic circulatory arrest: pathophysiology of ischemic neuronal injury and protective strategies. *Ann Thorac Surg* 2005; 80(5):1955-1964.
15. Ditsworth D, Priestley MA, Loepke AW, et al: Apoptotic neuronal death following deep hypothermic circulatory arrest in piglets. *Anesthesiology* 2003; 98(5):1119-1127.

16. Baumgartner WA, Walinsky PL, Salazar JD, et al: Assessing the impact of cerebral injury after cardiac surgery: will determining the mechanism reduce this injury? *Ann Thorac Surg* 1999; 67(6):1871-1873; discussion 1874-1891.
17. Lipton SA, Rosenberg PA: Excitatory amino acids as a final common pathway for neurologic disorders. *NEJM* 1994; 330(9):613-622.
18. Bellinger DC, Jonas RA, Rappaport LA, et al: Developmental and neurologic status of children after heart surgery with hypothermic circulatory arrest or low-flow cardiopulmonary bypass. *NEJM* 1995; 332(9):549-555.
19. Kurth CD, O'Rourke MM, O'Hara IB, Uher B: Brain cooling efficiency with pH-stat and alpha-stat cardiopulmonary bypass in newborn pigs. *Circulation* 1997; 96(9 Suppl):II-358-363.
20. Bottiger BW, Schmitz B, Wicssner C, Vogel P, Hossmann KA: Neuronal stress response and neuronal cell damage after cardiocirculatory arrest in rats. *J Cereb Blood Flow Metab* 1998; 18(10):1077-1087.
21. Kurth CD, Priestley M, Golden J, McCann J, Raghupathi R: Regional patterns of neuronal death after deep hypothermic circulatory arrest in newborn pigs. *J Thorac Cardiovasc Surg* 1999; 118(6):1068-1077.
22. Griepp RB, Galla JD, Apaydin AZ, Ergin MA: Cerebral protection in aortic surgery. *Adv Card Surg* 2000; 12:1-22.
23. Harrington DK, Fragomeni F, Bonser RS: Cerebral perfusion. *Ann Thorac Surg* 2007; 83(2):S799-804; discussion S731-824.
24. Ergin MA, Griepp EB, Lansman SL, et al: Hypothermic circulatory arrest and other methods of cerebral protection during operations on the thoracic aorta. *J Cardiac Surg* 1994; 9(5):525-537.
25. Kazui T, Inoue N, Komatsu S: Surgical treatment of aneurysms of the transverse aortic arch. *J Cardiac Surg* 1989; 30(3):402-406.
26. Pigula FA, Gandhi SK, Siewers RD, et al: Regional low-flow perfusion provides somatic circulatory support during neonatal aortic arch surgery. *Ann Thorac Surg* Aug 2001; 72(2):401-406; discussion 406-407.
27. Hagl C, Ergin MA, Galla JD, et al: Neurologic outcome after ascending aorta-aortic arch operations: effect of brain protection technique in high-risk patients. *J Thorac Cardiovasc Surg* 2001; 121(6):1107-1121.
28. Hagl C, Khaladj N, Karck M, et al: Hypothermic circulatory arrest during ascending and aortic arch surgery: the theoretical impact of different cerebral perfusion techniques and other methods of cerebral protection. *Eur J Cardiothorac Surg* 2003; 24(3):371-378.
29. Wong CH, Bonser RS: Retrograde cerebral perfusion: clinical and experimental aspects. *Perfusion* 1999; 14(4):247-256.
30. Ueda Y, Miki S, Kusuhara K, et al: Surgical treatment of aneurysm or dissection involving the ascending aorta and aortic arch, utilizing circulatory arrest and retrograde cerebral perfusion. *J Cardiovasc Surg (Torino)* 1990; 31(5):553-558.
31. Pagano D, Boivin CM, Faroqui MH, Bonser RS: Retrograde perfusion through the superior vena cava perfuses the brain in human beings. *J Thorac Cardiovasc Surg* 1996; 111(1):270-272.
32. Juvonen T, Weisz DJ, Wolfe D, et al: Can retrograde perfusion mitigate cerebral injury after particulate embolization? A study in a chronic porcine model. *J Thorac Cardiovasc Surg* 1998; 115(5):1142-1159.
33. Reich DL, Uysal S, Ergin MA, et al: Retrograde cerebral perfusion during thoracic aortic surgery and late neuropsychological dysfunction. *Eur J Cardiothorac Surg* 2001; 19(5):594-600.
34. Pochettino A, Cheung AT. Pro: Retrograde cerebral perfusion is useful for deep hypothermic circulatory arrest. *J Cadiovasc Vasc Anesthesia* 2003; 17(6):764-767.
35. Anderson RV, Siegman MG, Balaban RS, Ceckler TL, Swain JA: Hyperglycemia increases cerebral intracellular acidosis during circulatory arrest. *Ann Thorac Surg* 1992; 54(6):1126-1130.
36. van der Linden J, Astudillo R, Ekroth R, Scallan M, Lincoln C: Cerebral lactate release after circulatory arrest but not after low flow in pediatric heart operations. *Ann Thorac Surg* 1993; 56(6):1485-1489.
37. Siesjo BK, Siesjo P: Mechanisms of secondary brain injury. *Eur J Anaethesiol* 1996; 13(3):247-268.
38. Mezrow CK, Sadeghi AM, Gandsas A, et al: Cerebral effects of low-flow cardiopulmonary bypass and hypothermic circulatory arrest. *Ann Thorac Surg* 1994; 57(3):532-539; discussion 539.
39. Newburger JW, Jonas RA, Wernovsky G, et al: A comparison of the perioperative neurologic effects of hypothermic circulatory arrest versus low-flow cardiopulmonary bypass in infant heart surgery. *NEJM* 1993; 329(15):1057-1064.
40. Tenenbaum A, Motro M, Shapira I, et al: Retrograde embolism and atherosclerosis development in the human thoracic aorta: are the fluid dynamics explanations valid? *Med Hypotheses* 2001; 57(5):642-647.
41. Reich DL, Uysal S, Sliwinski M, et al: Neuropsychologic outcome after deep hypothermic circulatory arrest in adults. *J Thorac Cardiovasc Surg* 1999; 117(1):156-163.
42. Bellinger DC, Wypij D, duPlessis AJ, et al: Neurodevelopmental status at eight years in children with dextro-transposition of the great arteries: the Boston Circulatory Arrest Trial. *J Thorac Cardiovasc Surg* 2003; 126(5):1385-1396.
43. Kumral E, Yuksel M, Buket S, et al: Neurologic complications after deep hypothermic circulatory arrest: types, predictors, and timing. *Texas Heart Inst J* 2001; 28(2):83-88.
44. Kamiya H, Hagl C, Kropivnitskaya I, et al: The safety of moderate hypothermic lower body circulatory arrest with selective cerebral perfusion: a propensity score analysis. *J Thorac Cardiovasc Surg* 2007; 133(2):501-509.
45. Di Eusanio M, Schepens MA, Morshuis WJ, et al: Antegrade selective cerebral perfusion during operations on the thoracic aorta: factors influencing survival and neurologic outcome in 413 patients. *J Thorac Cardiovasc Surg* 2002; 124(6):1080-1086.
46. Strauch JT, Spielvogel D, Lauten A, et al: Axillary artery cannulation: routine use in ascending aorta and aortic arch replacement. *Ann Thorac Surg* 2004; 78(1):103-108; discussion 103-108.
47. Bavaria JE, Pochettino A, Brinster DR, et al: New paradigms and improved results for the surgical treatment of acute type A dissection. *Ann Surg* 2001; 234(3):336-342; discussion 342-333.
48. Khaladj N, Shrestha M, Meck S, et al: Hypothermic circulatory arrest with selective antegrade cerebral perfusion in ascending aortic and aortic arch surgery: a risk factor analysis for adverse outcome in 501 patients. *J Thorac Cardiovasc Surg* 2008; 135(4):908-914.
49. Appoo JJ, Augoustides JG, Pochettino A, et al: Perioperative outcome in adults undergoing elective deep hypothermic circulatory arrest with retrograde cerebral perfusion in proximal aortic arch repair: evaluation of protocol-based care. *J Cardiothorasc Vasc Anesthesia* 2006; 20(1):3-7.
50. Immer FF, Moser B, Krahenbuhl ES, et al: Arterial access through the right subclavian artery in surgery of the aortic arch improves neurologic outcome and mid-term quality of life. *Ann Thorac Surg* 2008; 85(5):1614-1618; discussion 1618.
51. Budde JM, Serna DL Jr, Osborne SC, Steele MA, Chen EP: Axillary cannulation for proximal aortic surgery is as safe in the emergent setting as in elective cases. *Ann Thorac Surg* 2006; 82(6):2154-2159; discussion 2159-2160.
52. Halkos ME, Kerendi F, Myung R, et al: Selective antegrade cerebral perfusion via right axillary artery cannulation reduces morbidity and mortality after proximal aortic surgery. *J Thorac Cardiovasc Surg* 2009; 138(5):1081-1089.
53. Okita Y, Minatoya K, Tagusari O, et al: Prospective comparative study of brain protection in total aortic arch replacement: deep hypothermic circulatory arrest with retrograde cerebral perfusion or selective antegrade cerebral perfusion. *Ann Thorac Surg* 2001; 72(1):72-79.
54. Coselli JS: Retrograde cerebral perfusion via a superior vena caval cannula for aortic arch aneurysm operations. *Ann Thorac Surg* 1994; 57(6):1668-1669.
55. Bavaria JE, Woo YJ, Hall RA, Carpenter JP, Gardner TJ: Retrograde cerebral and distal aortic perfusion during ascending and thoracoabdominal aortic operations. *Ann Thorac Surg* 1995; 60(2):345-352; discussion 352-343.
56. Kitamura M, Hashimoto A, Aomi S, Imamaki M, Koyanagi H: Medium-term results after surgery for aortic arch aneurysm with hypothermic cerebral perfusion. *Eur J Cardiothorac Surg* 1995;9(12):697-700.
57. Safi HJ, Brien HW, Winter JN, et al: Brain protection via cerebral retrograde perfusion during aortic arch aneurysm repair. *Ann Thorac Surg* 1993; 56(2):270-276.
58. Ye J, Yang L, Del Bigio MR, et al: Retrograde cerebral perfusion provides limited distribution of blood to the brain: a study in pigs. *J Thorac Cardiovasc Surg* 1997; 114(4):660-665.
59. de Brux JL, Subayi JB, Pegis JD, Pillet J: Retrograde cerebral perfusion: anatomic study of the distribution of blood to the brain. *Ann Thorac Surg* 1995; 60(5):1294-1298.
60. Cheung AT, Bavaria JE, Weiss SJ, Patterson T, Stecker MM: Neurophysiologic effects of retrograde cerebral perfusion used for aortic reconstruction. *J Cardiothorac Vasc Anesthesia* 1998; 12(3):252-259.
61. El Bardissi A, Bolman RM: Routine hypothermia with circulatory arrest and retrograde cerebral perfusion for ascending aortic reconstruction. *J Thorac Cardiovasc Surg* 2010; under review.
62. Severinghaus JW: Temperature gradients during hypothermia. *Ann NY Acad Sci* 1959; 80:515-521.
63. Stecker MM, Cheung AT, Pochettino A, et al: Deep hypothermic circulatory arrest: I. Effects of cooling on electroencephalogram and evoked potentials. *Ann Thorac Surg* 2001; 71(1):14-21.
64. Kaukuntla H, Harrington D, Bilkoo I, et al: Temperature monitoring during cardiopulmonary bypass—do we undercool or overheat the brain? *Eur J Cardiothorac Surg* 2004; 26(3):580-585.
65. Patel RL, Turtle MR, Chambers DJ, et al: Alpha-stat acid-base regulation during cardiopulmonary bypass improves neuropsychologic outcome in patients undergoing coronary artery bypass grafting. *J Thorac Cardiovasc Surg* 1996; 111(6):1267-1279.

66. Stephan H, Weyland A, Kazmaier S, et al: Acid-base management during hypothermic cardiopulmonary bypass does not affect cerebral metabolism but does affect blood flow and neurological outcome. *Br J anaesthesia* 1992; 69(1):51-57.
67. Murkin JM, Martzke JS, Buchan AM, Bentley C, Wong CJ: A randomized study of the influence of perfusion technique and pH management strategy in 316 patients undergoing coronary artery bypass surgery. I. Mortality and cardiovascular morbidity. *J Thorac Cardiovasc Surg* 1995; 110(2):340-348.
68. Hiramatsu T, Miura T, Forbess JM, et al: pH strategies and cerebral energetics before and after circulatory arrest. *J Thorac Cardiovasc Surg* 1995; 109(5):948-957; discussion 957-948.
69. Wong PC, Barlow CF, Hickey PR, et al: Factors associated with choreoathetosis after cardiopulmonary bypass in children with congenital heart disease. *Circulation* 1992; 86(5 Suppl):II118-126.
70. du Plessis AJ, Jonas RA, Wypij D, et al: Perioperative effects of alpha-stat versus pH-stat strategies for deep hypothermic cardiopulmonary bypass in infants. *J Thorac Cardiovasc Surg* 1997; 114(6):991-1000; discussion 1000-1001.
71. Bashein G, Townes BD, Nessly ML, et al: A randomized study of carbon dioxide management during hypothermic cardiopulmonary bypass. *Anesthesiology* 1990; 72(1):7-15.
72. Halstead JC, Spielvogel D, Meier DM, et al: Optimal pH strategy for selective cerebral perfusion. *Eur J Cardiothorac Surg* 2005; 28(2):266-273; discussion 273.
73. Gandhi GY, Nuttall GA, Abel MD, et al: Intraoperative hyperglycemia and perioperative outcomes in cardiac surgery patients. *Mayo Clin Proc* 2005; 80(7):862-866.
74. Dietrich WD, Alonso O, Busto R: Moderate hyperglycemia worsens acute blood-brain barrier injury after forebrain ischemia in rats. *Stroke* 1993; 24(1):111-116.
75. Siesjo BK: Acidosis and ischemic brain damage. *Neurochem Pathol* 1988; 9:31-88.
76. Lam AM, Winn HR, Cullen BF, Sundling N: Hyperglycemia and neurological outcome in patients with head injury. *J Neurosurg* 1991; 75(4):545-551.
77. Bjork VO, Sternlieb JJ, Davenport C: From the spinning disc to the membrane oxygenator for open-heart surgery. *Scand J Thorac Cardiovasc Surg* 1985; 19(3):207-216.
78. Eke CC, Gundry SR, Baum MF, et al: Neurologic sequelae of deep hypothermic circulatory arrest in cardiac transplant infants. *Ann Thorac Surg* 1996; 61(3):783-788.
79. Nicolas F, Daniel JP, Bruniaux J, et al: Conventional cardiopulmonary bypass in neonates. A physiological approach—10 years of experience at Marie-Lannelongue Hospital. *Perfusion* 1994; 9(1):41-48.
80. Shin'oka T, Shum-Tim D, Jonas RA, et al: Higher hematocrit improves cerebral outcome after deep hypothermic circulatory arrest. *J Thorac Cardiovasc Surg* 1996; 112(6):1610-1620; discussion 1620-1611.
81. Fang WC, Helm RE, Krieger KH, et al: Impact of minimum hematocrit during cardiopulmonary bypass on mortality in patients undergoing coronary artery surgery. *Circulation* 1997; 96(9 Suppl):II-194-199.
82. Habib RH, Zacharias A, Schwann TA, et al: Adverse effects of low hematocrit during cardiopulmonary bypass in the adult: should current practice be changed? *J Thorac Cardiovasc Surg* 2003; 125(6):1438-1450.
83. Sakamoto T, Zurakowski D, Duebener LF, et al: Interaction of temperature with hematocrit level and pH determines safe duration of hypothermic circulatory arrest. *J Thorac Cardiovasc Surg* 2004; 128(2):220-232.
84. Witoszka MM, Tamura H, Indeglia R, Hopkins RW, Simeone FA: Electroencephalographic changes and cerebral complications in open-heart surgery. *J Thorac Cardiovasc Surg* 1973; 66(6):855-864.
85. Sigl JC, Chamoun NG: An introduction to bispectral analysis for the electroencephalogram. *J Clin Monit* 1994; 10(6):392-404.
86. Ghariani S, Spaey J, Liard L, et al: [Sensitivity, specificity, and impact on the surgical strategy of the perioperative neuromonitoring of somatic evoked potentials in vascular surgery performed with circulatory arrest under deep hypothermia]. *Neurophysiol Clin* 1998; 28(4):335-341.
87. Apostolakis E, Akinosoglou K: The methodologies of hypothermic circulatory arrest and of antegrade and retrograde cerebral perfusion for aortic arch surgery. *Ann Thorac Cardiovasc Surg* 2008; 14(3):138-148.
88. Reich DL, Horn LM, Hossain S, Uysal S: Using jugular bulb oxyhemoglobin saturation to guide onset of deep hypothermic circulatory arrest does not affect post-operative neuropsychological function. *Eur J Cardiothorac Surg* 2004; 25(3):401-406; discussion 406-408.
89. Strauch JT, Spielvogel D, Lauten A, et al: Optimal temperature for selective cerebral perfusion. *J Thorac Cardiovasc Surg* 2005; 130(1):74-82.
90. Harden A, Pampiglione G, Waterston DJ: Circulatory arrest during hypothermia in cardiac surgery: an E.E.G. study in children. *BMJ* 1966; 2(5522):1105-1108.
91. Edmonds HL Jr: Multi-modality neurophysiologic monitoring for cardiac surgery. *Heart Surg Forum* 2002; 5(3):225-228.
92. Daubeney PE, Pilkington SN, Janke E, et al: Cerebral oxygenation measured by near-infrared spectroscopy: comparison with jugular bulb oximetry. *Ann Thorac Surg* 1996; 61(3):930-934.
93. Cho H, Nemoto EM, Yonas H, Balzer J, Sclabassi RJ: Cerebral monitoring by means of oximetry and somatosensory evoked potentials during carotid endarterectomy. *J Neurosurg* 1998; 89(4):533-538.
94. Michenfelder JD: A valid demonstration of barbiturate-induced brain protection in man—at last. *Anesthesiology* 1986; 64(2):140-142.
95. Hoff JT, Smith AL, Hankinson HL, Nielsen SL: Barbiturate protection from cerebral infarction in primates. *Stroke* 1975; 6(1):28-33.
96. Nussmeier NA, Arlund C, Slogoff S: Neuropsychiatric complications after cardiopulmonary bypass: cerebral protection by a barbiturate. *Anesthesiology* 1986; 64(2):165-170.
97. Steyn RS, Jeffrey RR: An adjunct to cerebral protection during circulatory arrest. *Eur J Cardiothorac Surg* 1993; 7(8):443-444.
98. Miura Y, Grocott HP, Bart RD, et al: Differential effects of anesthetic agents on outcome from near-complete but not incomplete global ischemia in the rat. *Anesthesiology* 1998; 89(2):391-400.
99. Harada H, Kelly PJ, Cole DJ, Drummond JC, Patel PM: Isoflurane reduces N-methyl-D-aspartate toxicity in vivo in the rat cerebral cortex. *Anesthesia and Analgesia* 1999; 89(6):1442-1447.
100. Stevens WC, Cromwell TH, Halsey MJ, et al: The cardiovascular effects of a new inhalation anesthetic, Forane, in human volunteers at constant arterial carbon dioxide tension. *Anesthesiology* 1971; 35(1):8-16.
101. Blanck TJ, Haile M, Xu F, et al: Isoflurane pretreatment ameliorates postischemic neurologic dysfunction and preserves hippocampal Ca2+/calmodulin-dependent protein kinase in a canine cardiac arrest model. *Anesthesiology* 2000; 93(5):1285-1293.
102. Zheng S, Zuo Z: Isoflurane preconditioning induces neuroprotection against ischemia via activation of P38 mitogen-activated protein kinases. *Mol Pharmacol* 2004; 65(5):1172-1180.
103. Finn A, Naik S, Klein N, et al: Interleukin-8 release and neutrophil degranulation after pediatric cardiopulmonary bypass. *J Thorac Cardiovasc Surg* 1993; 105(2):234-241.
104. Bronicki RA, Backer CL, Baden HP, et al: Dexamethasone reduces the inflammatory response to cardiopulmonary bypass in children. *Ann Thorac Surg* 2000; 69(5):1490-1495.
105. Shum-Tim D, Tchervenkov CI, Jamal AM, et al: Systemic steroid pretreatment improves cerebral protection after circulatory arrest. *Ann Thorac Surg* 2001; 72(5):1465-1471; discussion 1471-1462.
106. Shum-Tim D, Nagashima M, Shinoka T, et al: Postischemic hyperthermia exacerbates neurologic injury after deep hypothermic circulatory arrest. *J Thorac Cardiovasc Surg* 1998; 116(5):780-792.
107. Langley SM, Chai PJ, Jaggers JJ, Ungerleider RM: Preoperative high dose methylprednisolone attenuates the cerebral response to deep hypothermic circulatory arrest. *Eur J Cardiothorac Surg* 2000; 17(3):279-286.
108. Schubert S, Stoltenburg-Didinger G, Wehsack A, et al: Large-dose pretreatment with methylprednisolone fails to attenuate neuronal injury after deep hypothermic circulatory arrest in a neonatal piglet model. *Anesthesia Analgesia* 2005; 101(5):1311-1318.

CHAPTER 15

Myocardial Protection

Robert M. Mentzer, Jr.
Roberta A. Gottlieb
Karin Przyklenk
M. Salik Jahania

INTRODUCTION

In the setting of heart surgery, myocardial protection refers to strategies and methodologies used in the operating room to attenuate or prevent perioperative infarction and/or postischemic ventricular dysfunction. This is in contrast to the instance in which a patient presents with an acute myocardial infarction (MI). Here the objective is to reduce infarct size at reperfusion. The underlying pathophysiology in both settings, however, relates to the etiology and consequences of ischemia-reperfusion injury. After surgery the injury manifests by low cardiac output, hypotension, and a need for postoperative inotropic support. The damage may be reversible or irreversible and is differentiated by the presence of electrocardiographic abnormalities, elevations in the levels of specific plasma enzymes or proteins such as creatine kinase and troponin I or T, and/or the presence of regional or global echocardiographic wall motion abnormalities. Depending on the criteria, the incidence of postoperative MI after CABG surgery ranges between 3% and 18%. The incidence of severe ventricular dysfunction, heart failure, and death, despite advances in surgical techniques, ranges between 2 and 15%; the higher mortality rates are associated with high-risk patients with minimal cardiac reserve.

These complications have an enormous impact on both families and society. From an economic standpoint alone, revascularization procedures are costly. In 2004 cardiovascular disease was responsible for more than 1 million hospital stays; it was the most expensive condition treated, with a total cost of more than $44 billion. More than half of the hospitalizations for coronary atherosclerosis were for patients who received percutaneous coronary intervention (PCI) or coronary artery bypass graft (CABG) surgery.[1] With respect to CABG surgery alone, the initial hospital cost is approximately $10 billion annually; the complications after CABG consume an additional $2 billion in U.S. health care resources each year.[2–5] A reduction in perioperative complications associated with heart surgery could have a significant impact on resource utilization and overall operative costs. Because one cause of morbidity and mortality after heart surgery is ischemia-reperfusion injury, the purpose of this chapter is to review its underlying mechanisms, review the history of myocardial protection, update the reader regarding the current protective techniques, and discuss new strategies under investigation.

ISCHEMIA-REPERFUSION INJURY

The etiologies of perioperative myocardial necrosis and postischemic myocardial dysfunction after cardiac surgery are multifactorial. Myocardial necrosis and associated cardiac biomarkers may arise as a result of ischemia caused by intrinsic coronary disease not amenable to revascularization, anesthetic factors, atrial cannulation, aortic cross-clamping, suturing of heart muscle, plaque and platelet embolism, and graft spasm or thrombosis. Despite the considerable progress made to date, high-risk heart surgery patients including those with unstable angina, poor ventricular function, diabetes, repeat CABG, and advanced age continue to experience postoperative complications such as low cardiac output, perioperative myocardial infarction, and heart failure requiring prolonged intensive care. In many of these patients these complications are caused by ischemia-reperfusion injury and inadequate myocardial protection. Thus there is a compelling unmet need to develop new methods to protect the heart during surgery.

Deleterious Sequelae of Ischemia-Reperfusion

Myocardial ischemia-reperfusion injury can manifest as postischemic "stunning," which is reversible and/or apoptosis or myocardial infarction, which are irreversible. Myocardial stunning is an injury that lasts for hours to days despite the restoration of normal blood flow. Typically, these patients require some form of temporary inotropic support in the immediate postoperative period in order to maintain an adequate cardiac output. Stunned cardiomyocytes exhibit minimal ultrastructural damage that resolves within hours to days following relief of ischemia. Apoptosis, or programmed cell death, is a pattern of cell death that affects single cells. It is characterized by retention of an intact cell membrane, cell shrinkage, chromatin condensation, and phagocytosis without inflammation.[6,7] Apoptotic cell death caused by ischemia-reperfusion contributes significantly to the development of infarction as well as the loss of cells surrounding the infarct area. A large fraction of dying cells may exhibit features of both apoptosis and necrosis, ie, both nuclear condensation and plasma membrane damage. Ultimately, after prolonged ischemia, irreversible cellular injury is characterized by a broad spectrum of reperfusion-related pathologies including membrane destruction, cell swelling, ultra-structural changes of mitochondria, DNA degradation, cytolysis, and the induction of an inflammatory response.[8–10]

Long-Term Clinical Consequences

Although the consequences of inadequate myocardial protection usually are apparent in the immediate postoperative period, eg, low cardiac output syndrome, the full impact of inadequate protection may not be appreciated for months to years. Klatte and colleagues reported that patients with increased peak creatine kinase-myocardial band (CK-MB) enzyme ratios after CABG surgery exhibited a greater 6-month mortality.[11] The 6-month mortality rates were 3.4%, 5.8%, 7.8%, and 20% for patients with peak CK-MB ratios <5, 5-10, 11-20, and >20-fold greater than the upper limits of normal (UNL), respectively. Conversely, the cumulative 6-month survival was inversely related to the peak CK-MB ratio.

In another study, Costa[12] and colleagues reported that normal postoperative CK-MB levels were observed in only 38.1% of 496 patients who underwent CABG surgery. When the CK-MB levels were stratified, the incidence of death at 30 days was 0.0%, 0.5%, 5.4%, and 7.0% when the enzyme levels were normal, 1–3, 4–5, and >5-fold higher than ULN, respectively. The one year mortality for these groups was 1.1%, 0.5%, 5.4%, and 10.5%, respectively. The peak postoperative cardiac enzyme level correlated significantly with worse clinical outcome. Thus, although CK-MB elevations are often dismissed as inconsequential in the setting of multivessel CABG surgery, they occur frequently and are associated with significant increases in both repeat myocardial infarction and death beyond the immediate perioperative period. Consistent with this is the evidence by Steuer [13] and associates in which they examined postoperative serum aspartate aminotransferase and CK-MB levels and their relationship to early cardiac-related death and late survival in 4911 patients who underwent CABG consecutively during a 6-year period. They reported that elevated enzyme levels on the first postoperative day greatly increased the risk of early cardiac death and were associated with a 40 to 50% increased risk in late mortality at 7 years.

Finally, in a retrospective analysis Brener et al. showed that CK-MB elevation was common after both percutaneous and surgical revascularization.[14] The incidence of CK-MB elevation above the normal range was 90% for CABG surgery and 38% for PCI. The elevations exceeded 10× ULN for 6% of the CABG patients and 5% of the PCI patients. After 3 years average follow-up, the cumulative mortality was 8% for CABG surgery, and 10% for PCI. Thus, even relatively small CK-MB elevations after interventions are associated with increased mortality over time. Similar observations were made when troponin release was used as a biomarker of myocardial injury. Lehrke et al. reported in a series of 204 patients that a serum troponin-T concentration of 0.46 μg/L or more 48 hours after surgery was associated with a 4.9-fold increase in long-term risk of death.[15] In short, it appears that biomarkers are frequently increased after CABG surgery, and they are associated with a decrease in short-, medium-, and long-term survival. Although the greater enzyme release may reflect underlying pathology, ie, a heart that is more vulnerable to injury, it is also reasonable to suggest that limiting myocardial necrosis will have a beneficial effect on survival. Therefore, a better understanding of the mechanisms underlying ischemia-reperfusion injury is needed. An appreciation of current techniques and development of new approaches are warranted in order to reduce long-term morbidity and mortality.

Cellular Mediators

The primary mediators of ischemia-reperfusion injury include intracellular Ca^{2+} overload and oxidative stress induced by reactive oxygen species (ROS) generated at the onset of reperfusion (Fig. 15-1).[16] The molecule nitric oxide (NO) also can interact with molecules derived from superoxide (O_2^-) or peroxides to generate reactive nitrogen species that are capable of inducing injury as well.[17] In addition, metabolic alterations occurring during ischemia can contribute directly and indirectly to Ca^{2+} overload and ROS formation. For example, decreased cytosolic phosphorylation potential, ie, $[ATP]/([ADP] \times [P_i])$, results in less free energy from ATP hydrolysis than is necessary to drive the energy-dependent pumps (sarcoplasmic reticulum Ca^{2+}-ATPase, the sarcolemmal Ca^{2+}-ATPase) that maintain intracellular calcium homeostasis. [18] With the onset of ischemia and the fall in intracellular pH, there is a concomitant activation of the Na^+-H^+ exchanger. This results in an accumulation of intracellular Na^+. At the onset of reperfusion there is a reversal of the Na^+-Ca^{++} exchanger, which in turn exacerbates intracellular calcium accumulation that leads to injury of the sarcoplasmic reticulum, opening of the mitochondrial permeability transition pore (mPTP), and lethal injury of the myofibrillar contractile elements.[19]

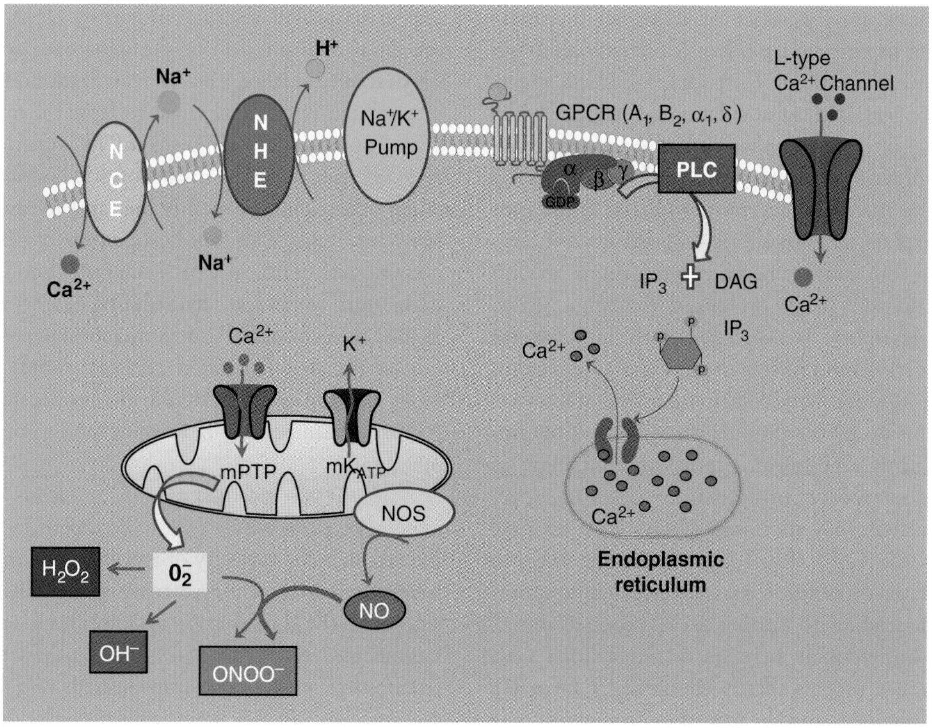

FIGURE 15.1 Myocardial alterations associated with ischemia-reperfusion injury. Intracellular Ca^{2+} overload and the formation of reactive oxygen species are the two primary causes of ischemia-reperfusion injury. With the onset of ischemia, glycolysis increases and the intracellular pH rapidly falls. This results in activation of the NHE, inhibition of the Na/K ATPase, and an increase in the $[Na^+]_i$. Other causes of intracellular calcium accumulation include: (a) reversal in the direction of the Na^+/Ca^{2+} exchanger; and (b) activation of various GPCRs, which activate PLC and generate IP_3—the latter causing Ca^{2+} release from intracellular stores including the ER. Simultaneously, ROS and RNS production occurs; the source may involve complex I and III of the mitochondrial respiratory chain. Ischemia may also induce an opening of mitoK_{ATP} channels and serve as a protective mechanism. At the onset of RP, exacerbation of intracellular calcium accumulation can lead to intracellular calcium overload. The mitochondrial Ca^{2+} uniporter can buffer increases in cytosolic Ca^{2+}, but increased mitochondrial Ca^{2+} can induce excess ROS formation. This is accompanied by the release of a burst in ROS production that leads to thiol oxidation, peroxidation of phospholipids, further disruption of ion pumps, accumulation of mitochondrial calcium, and a reduction in contractile protein Ca^{2+} sensitivity. It is hypothesized that RP-induced oxidative stress and the increase in $[Ca^{2+}]_m$ ultimately result in the opening of pores in the inner mitochondrial membrane (mPTP). Pore opening leads to uncoupling of oxidative phosphorylation, activation of degradative enzymes such as phospholipases, nucleases, and proteases, and the release of cytochrome *c*. Together these result in both apoptotic and necrotic cell death. Ca^{2+} = calcium; $[Ca^{2+}]_i$ = intracellular calcium concentration; $[Ca^{2+}]_m$ = intramitochondrial calcium concentration; DAG = diacylglycerol; ER = endoplasmic reticulum; GPCR = G-protein coupled receptor; IP_3 = inositol trisphosphate; mK_{ATP} channel = mitochondrial ATP-sensitive potassium channel; mPTP = mitochondrial permeability transition pore; Na+ = sodium; $[Na+]_i$ = intracellular sodium concentration; NHE = sodium-hydrogen exchanger; NO = nitric oxide; PLC = phospholipase C; RP = reperfusion; NCE = sodium-calcium exchanger; NOS = nitric oxide synthase.

The metabolic changes that occur during ischemia also reduce the endogenous antioxidant defense systems of cardiac myocytes. The first line of defense against mitochondrial ROS formation and its deleterious effects is the GSH (reduced glutathione)/GSSG (oxidized glutathione) system, which is directly linked to the NADPH:$NADP^+$ ratio via the enzyme glutathione reductase. The depletion of glutathione levels increases ROS formation, oxidative stress, and $[Ca^{2+}]_i$.[20,21] Because NADPH is not formed during ischemia, the normal metabolic mechanism for regenerating the reduced glutathione does not function. Thus, the formation of ROS during reperfusion occurs at a time when the myocyte's endogenous defense mechanisms are depressed. The NADPH:$NADP^+$ ratio is a primary determinant of the redox state of the cell, and there is evidence that redox state plays a key role in determining the bioactivity and redox state of NO.[17,22] In addition, there are several reports that in the absence of normal levels of its cofactors, nitric oxide synthase (NOS) itself can generate superoxide anion.[23] Although systolic intracellular calcium $[Ca^{2+}]_i$ may return to normal early in the reperfused stunned myocardium, transient increases in $[Ca^{2+}]_i$ can activate Ca^{2+}-dependent isoforms of protein kinase C (PKC), proteases such as calpain, and endonucleases.[24] Calpain activation and its subsequent action on contractile proteins have been implicated in the reduction of myofilament Ca^{2+} sensitivity observed in stunned myocardium.[25]

Similarly, there is considerable evidence that ROS are involved in mediating myocardial stunning. Various spin-trap agents and chemical probes have demonstrated the rapid release of ROS into the vascular space during reperfusion after brief ischemia in vivo.[26] It is also now recognized that mitochondria are a primary source of intracellular ROS in cardiac myocytes.[27,28] There is no question that scavengers of ROS and antioxidants, when administered before the onset of ischemia, attenuate myocardial stunning in vitro and in vivo. Moreover, although the evidence is equivocal, efficacy is in some instances maintained when scavengers and antioxidants are administered before or at the onset of reperfusion.[16,29] It has been shown that ROS can attack thiol residues of numerous proteins such as the SR Ca^{2+}-ATPase, the ryanodine receptor, and contractile proteins.[30] This may explain why myofibrils isolated from in vivo reperfused stunned but not ischemic myocardium exhibit reduced Ca^{2+} sensitivity.[31] More prolonged ischemia, which produces irreversible injury, is associated with more severe intracellular Ca^{2+} overload and further depletion of endogenous antioxidants, conditions that both contribute to and are exacerbated during reperfusion by the production of ROS. The production of ROS during reperfusion appears to contribute to Ca^{2+} overload because exposure of normal myocytes to exogenous ROS is associated with increased L-type Ca^{2+} channel current and increased $[Ca^{2+}]_i$.[21,32,33] Conversely, increases in $[Ca^{2+}]_i$ during ischemia-reperfusion may adversely affect mitochondrial function, leading to further ROS production.[33,34] Mitochondria can buffer small increases in intracellular Ca^{2+} via the Ca uniporter, a process that is energetically favorable owing to the $[Ca^{2+}]$ gradient and the mitochondrial membrane potential. During reperfusion, the increase in cytosolic Ca^{2+} enhances mitochondrial Ca^{2+} uptake. Because excess cytosolic Ca^{2+} has been associated with the loss of myocyte viability, mitochondrial Ca^{2+} buffering is initially cardioprotective.[35] However, continued mitochondrial Ca^{2+} buffering in the face of decreased antioxidant reserves and excess ROS formation sets up a cycle that ultimately may lead to the total collapse of mitochondrial membrane potential and cell death. The synergistic interactions between Ca^{2+} overload and ROS formation during conditions of decreased antioxidant reserves also may provide an explanation of why ROS scavengers are not very effective at reducing irreversible injury when administered at reperfusion.[36]

Broadening the Spectrum of Ischemia-Reperfusion Injury

Historically, myocardial ischemia-reperfusion injury has been characterized as either reversible or irreversible based on staining techniques, enzyme release, and histology. There is now increasing evidence that this injury represents a transition from reversible to irreversible injury and that it occurs as a continuum, not as an all-or-none phenomenon. For example, apoptosis occurs before severe depletion in ATP and loss of membrane integrity but ultimately leads to cell death.[37,38] The phenomenon of apoptosis appears to commence during reperfusion with the formation of intracellular ROS and/or intracellular calcium overload[39,40] (Fig. 15-2). This process is initiated by translocation of the proapoptotic proteins Bad and Bax from the cytosol to the mitochondrial membrane. Heterodimerization of Bad or Bax with the antiapoptotic Bcl-2 or Bcl-xl can lead to the release of cytochrome *c* from mitochondria into the cytosol.[40–42] Formation of a cytosolic complex consisting of cytochrome *c*, apoptosis activating factor 1 (APAF-1), and caspase-9 leads to activation of caspase 3 and the cleavage of poly(ADP)-ribose polymerase (PARP) protein. Activation of PARP is the final step in apoptosis, activated in part by DNA fragmentation and the rapid consumption of the remaining adenine nucleotides. As described earlier, the increased intracellular ROS and/or intracellular calcium overload collapse the mitochondrial membrane potential, leading to mPTP opening, which, if not reversed, can result in mitochondrial swelling, rupture of the outer mitochondrial membrane, and release of cytochrome *c*. However, more commonly, opening of the mPTP leads to necrotic cell death, in which the mitochondrial F_0F_1 ATP synthase runs in reverse, hydrolyzing ATP in a futile effort to restore mitochondrial inner membrane potential. The depletion of the already-limited cytosolic supplies of ATP compromises the ability to maintain ion homeostasis via the Na^+/K^+ ATPase, culminating in swelling and rupture of the plasma membrane.

The physiologic relevance of apoptosis during myocardial ischemia-reperfusion has yet to be determined. This is owing to the fact that the majority of reports on apoptosis in this setting have been based on measurements of DNA fragmentation and laddering, the final steps in apoptotic cell death. Once DNA is fragmented, the cell's ability to synthesize new proteins to repair itself is severely compromised, and these cells, even if they survive a first ischemic episode, may die at an accelerated rate during subsequent stress or ischemia. However, studies conducted in other tissues and in isolated cells including cardiomyocytes indicate that the apoptotic program can be detected much earlier. One of the earliest signs of apoptosis is the translocation of phosphatidylserine from the inner face of the plasma membrane to the cell surface, a process that can be detected by annexin V, which has a strong affinity for phosphatidylserine.[43] Apoptosis in cardiac myocytes can be demonstrated with fluorescein isothiocyanate (FITC)-conjugated annexin V staining of the plasma membrane much earlier than DNA fragmentation (via the TUNEL assay and DNA laddering).[44] There are also reports that this early stage of apoptosis does not irreversibly commit cells to programmed cell death in noncardiac tissue; a significant proportion of myocytes, when subjected to simulated ischemia-reperfusion, exhibit signs of early apoptosis (positive annexin-FITC staining, intact membrane cell death, decreased cell width, and increased mitochondrial $[Ca^{2+}]$).[45,46] In the setting of ischemia-reperfusion injury, it appears that mPTP opening and necrotic cell death contribute more to myocardial injury than apoptosis, and interventions to prevent apoptosis (eg, with caspase inhibitors) have been disappointing.

Thus, it appears that ischemia-reperfusion injury, ie, myocardial stunning, apoptosis, and infarction, manifests in a variety of interrelated ways. Apoptosis may proceed to necrosis when mitochondria are no longer able to withstand the intracellular Ca^{2+} overload and oxidative stress induced by ROS and when oxidative phosphorylation is unable to keep pace with energy demands. Because of the resulting decrease in the myocardial phosphorylation potential, energy-dependent ion pumps cannot maintain normal ion gradients. This results in cell swelling and, ultimately, loss of membrane integrity. These disturbances can be further exacerbated by the influx of macrophages and leukocytes, complement activation, and endothelial plugging by platelets and neutrophils. If cell death in ischemic

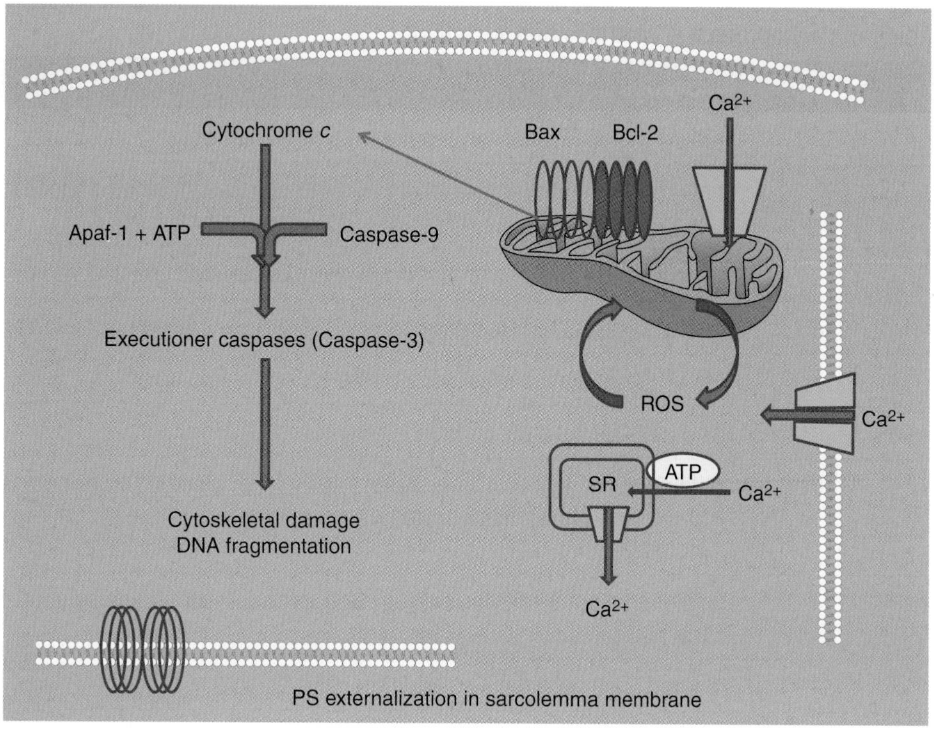

FIGURE 15.2 Proposed mechanisms of cardiomyocyte apoptosis following ischemia-reperfusion injury. Intracellular Ca^{2+} overload during ischemia and reperfusion and reactive oxygen species (ROS) formation during reperfusion are thought to be the primary mediators of the intrinsic pathway of apoptosis. The mechanisms of Ca^{2+} overload and ROS formation are described in detail in the text. Ischemia-reperfusion-associated effects on metabolism and decreased levels of the endogenous antioxidant glutathione lead to excess electron leak from the mitochondrial electron transport chain generating mitochondrial ROS. The mitochondrial Ca^{2+} uniporter can buffer increases in cytosolic Ca^{2+}, but increased mitochondrial Ca^{2+} can induce excess ROS formation. Likewise, ROS formation can induce intracellular Ca^{2+} overload. Through mechanisms that are not well defined, two families of closely related proteins (Bcl-2 and Bax) modulate the cell's response to apoptotic stimuli. Bcl-2 is an antiapoptotic protein that appears to be capable of inhibiting cytochrome *c* release either directly or by forming a complex with and inhibiting the proapoptotic family of proteins (Bax). Bax is thought to translocate from the cytosol to the mitochondrial membrane during the apoptotic process. Two early events in apoptosis are the externalization of phosphatidylserine (PS) residues in the sarcolemma and the release of cytochrome *c* from the mitochondria. PS externalization can be detected with fluorescently tagged annexin-5, thus permitting the detection of the early stages of apoptosis; it is thought to mark the apoptosis cell for ingestion by professional phagocytes. Cytochrome *c* released from the mitochondria complexes with an apoptotic protease-activating factor 1 (Apaf-1) and procaspase 9. In the presence of ATP, procaspase 9 is cleaved into the active caspase 9 with the resulting activation of the cytosolic protease caspase 3, often referred to as the *executioner caspase*. Caspase 3 protease activity leads to irreversible damage to cell morphology and DNA fragmentation and laddering. Apaf-1 = apoptotic protease activating factor 1; Bax = proapoptotic family of proteins; Bcl-2 = antiapoptotic protein; Ca^{2+} = calcium; PS = phosphatidylserine; ROS = reactive oxygen species; SR = sarcoplasmic reticulum.

reperfused myocardium progresses from apoptosis to necrosis, and if early apoptosis is indeed reversible, then one therapeutic approach for the treatment or prevention of ischemia-reperfusion injury would be to target the early events in apoptosis. Regardless of which stage is being addressed, current cardioprotection strategies are designed to reduce cellular and subcellular ROS formation and oxidative stress, to enhance the heart's endogenous antioxidant defense mechanisms, and to prevent intracellular Ca^{2+} overload.

CARDIOPROTECTION: HISTORICAL PERSPECTIVES

In 1883, Ringer described the antagonistic effects of calcium and potassium ions on cardiac contraction. In 1929, Hooker reported the successful resuscitation of dogs with potassium in which ventricular fibrillation was induced by electric shock.[47,48] In 1930, Wiggers reported that injections of potassium chloride were capable of abrogating ventricular fibrillation and arrested the heart in diastole. He also demonstrated that revival of the heart was possible using calcium chloride and massage.[49] The work by Wiggers led Beck, a thoracic surgeon, to successfully apply defibrillation therapy and save a human life using this method.[50] This resulted in a surge in basic and clinical research in the field of fibrillation and defibrillation with the principles applied to cardiac surgery.

With the advent of cardiopulmonary bypass, there was a need to refine techniques to protect the heart and create a quiescent and bloodless field for the unhurried repair of intracardiac defects. Over the next 50 years, a variety of cardioprotective methods and techniques were introduced (Table 15-1). One of the first methodologies evolved from the concept of shielding

TABLE 15-1 Evolution of Cardioprotective Methods and Techniques

Reference	Year	Innovation
Bigelow WG et al[51]	1950	Studied the application of hypothermia to cardiac surgery in canines
Swan H et al[66]	1953	Showed that hypothermic arrest (26°C) in humans provided a bloodless field for operating
Melrose DG et al[52]	1955	Introduced the concept of reversible chemical cardiac arrest in canines
Lillehei CW et al[67]	1956	Heart was protected by retrograde coronary sinus infusion of oxygenated blood
Lam CR et al[68]	1957	One of the earliest known uses of the term "cardioplegia"
Gerbode F, Melrose D[69]	1958	Used potassium citrate to induce cardiac arrest in humans
McFarland JA[70]	1960	Challenged the safety of the Melrose technique; changed from potassium arrest to intermittent aortic occlusion or coronary artery perfusion for myocardial protection
Bretschneider HJ et al[56]	1964	Developed a sodium-poor, calcium-free, procaine-containing solution to arrest the heart
Sondergaard KT[71,72]	1964	Adopted Bretschneider's solution for clinical use
Gay WA, Ebert PA[59]	1973	Credited with revival of potassium-induced cardioplegia; demonstrated that potassium solution could arrest a canine heart for 60 minutes without cellular damage
Roe BB et al[60]	1973	Demonstrated that "the modalities of cardioplegia, hypothermia, and capillary washout" provided effective myocardial protection
Tyres GF[53]	1974	Demonstrated in preclinical studies that an infusion of cold blood to maintain myocardial temperature <4°C provided 90 minutes of protection
Hearse DJ et al[57]	1975	Emphasized preischemic infusions to negate ischemic injuries in rats; this formula became known as St. Thomas solution no. 1
Braimbridge MV et al[58]	1975	One of the first to use St. Thomas solution no. 1 clinically
Effler DB et al[73]	1976	Simple aortic clamping at room temperatures recommended
Buckberg GD[62]	1979	Blood is an effective vehicle for infusing potassium into coronary arteries
Akins CW[74]	1984	Hypothermic fibrillatory arrest for coronary revascularization without cardioplegia
Murry CE et al[75]	1986	First to report that brief periods of ischemia (preconditioning) and reperfusion enable the heart to withstand longer periods of ischemia
Lichtenstein SV et al[76] Salerno TA et al[77]	1991	Reported warm antegrade and retrograde blood cardioplegia safe
Ikonomidis JS et al[78]	1995	Combined normothermic continuous retrograde cardioplegia with intermittent antegrade infusions
Teoh LK et al[79]	2002	Introduced concept that intermittent cross-clamp fibrillation in CABG surgery patients confers cardioprotection via ischemic preconditioning and adenosine receptor activation
Quinn DW et al[80]	2006	Phase II human trial demonstrated efficacy of cardioprotective effects of systemic glucose-insulin-potassium (GIK) when administered perioperatively
Mentzer RM et al[81]	2008	Phase III myocardial protection trial in humans demonstrated proof of concept that perioperative MI can be reduced with intravenous infusion of a pharmacologic agent in CABG surgery patients

the heart from perioperative insult using hypothermia. Bigelow and colleagues suggested using hypothermia "as a form of anesthetic" to expand the scope of surgery. The technique "might permit surgeons to operate upon the 'bloodless heart' without recourse to extra corporal pumps, and perhaps allow transplantation of organs."[51]

Five years later, Melrose and colleagues reported another way to stop and restart the human heart reliably by injecting potassium citrate into the root of the aorta at both normal and reduced body temperatures.[52] Soon thereafter, the clinical application of potassium citrate arrest was adopted by many centers. Interest in using the Melrose technique waned, however, with subsequent reports that potassium citrate arrest was associated with myocardial injury and necrosis. Within a short time, many cardiac surgeons shifted from using potassium-induced arrest to normothermic cardiac ischemia (ie, normothermic heart surgery performed with the aorta occluded while the patient was on cardiopulmonary bypass), intermittent aortic occlusion, or coronary artery perfusion. Experimental and clinical evidence showed, however, that normothermic cardiac ischemia was associated with metabolic acidosis, hypotension, and low cardiac output.[53–55]

As a consequence, there was a renewed interest in discovering ways to arrest the heart. Bretschneider published the principle of arresting the heart with a low-sodium, calcium-free solution.[56] It was Hearse and colleagues, however, who studied the various components of cardioplegic solutions, which led to the development and use of St. Thomas solution.[57] The components of this crystalloid solution were based on Ringer's solution with its normal concentrations of sodium and calcium with the addition of potassium chloride (16 mmol/L) and magnesium chloride (16 mmol/L) to arrest the heart instantly. The latter component was shown by Hearse to provide an additional cardioprotective benefit. In 1975, Braimbridge and colleagues introduced this crystalloid solution into clinical practice at St. Thomas Hospital.[58]

Gay and Ebert showed experimentally that lower concentrations of potassium chloride could achieve the same degree of chemical arrest and myocardial protection afforded by the Melrose solution without the associated myocardial necrosis reported earlier.[58,59] Shortly thereafter, Roe and colleagues reported an operative mortality of 5.4% for patients who underwent cardiac surgery with potassium-induced arrest as the primary form of myocardial protection.[60] In 1977, Tyers and colleagues demonstrated that potassium cardioplegia provided satisfactory protection in over 100 consecutive cardiac patients.[61]

By the 1980s, normothermic aortic occlusion had been replaced for the most part by cardioplegia to protect the heart during cardiac surgery. The major controversy at the time was not whether cardioplegic solutions should be used, but what was the ideal composition. The chief variants consisted of (1) the Bretschneider solution, containing primarily sodium, magnesium, and procaine; (2) the St. Thomas solution, consisting of potassium, magnesium, and procaine added to Ringer's solution; and (3) potassium-enriched solutions containing no magnesium or procaine (Table 15-2). Coincident with this controversy, another variant of cardioplegia was introduced, ie, the use of potassium-enriched blood cardioplegia.[62,63] Theoretically, blood cardioplegia would be a superior delivery vehicle based on its oxygenating and buffering capacity. Ironically, Melrose and colleagues initially used blood as the vehicle to deliver high concentrations of potassium citrate more than 20 years earlier.

Although hypothermia and potassium infusions remain the cornerstone of myocardial protection today, a variety of cardioprotective techniques and solutions are used that allow patients to undergo heart operations with excellent 30-day outcomes.[64,65]

CARDIOPLEGIC SURGERY

Cardioplegic surgery techniques utilize solutions containing a variety of chemical agents that are designed to arrest the heart rapidly in diastole, create a quiescent operating field, and provide reliable protection against ischemia-reperfusion injury. Although contemporary cardiac surgery in low-risk patients is relatively safe, patient characteristics have been changing over the past decade. In addition to coronary heart disease and poor ventricular function, patients are presenting with more comorbidities such as obesity, renal dysfunction, peripheral vascular disease, and emphysema. Despite ongoing improvements in cardioplegic techniques, low cardiac output syndrome (LCOS) frequently occurs after surgery and is a major factor associated with poor outcomes. In the absence of technical complications, the most common cause of postoperative LCOS is inadequate myocardial preservation. For this reason, there is a real need to develop more effective strategies and novel additives to existing cardioplegic solutions. Currently there are two types of cardioplegic solutions that are used: *crystalloid cardioplegia* and *blood cardioplegia*. These solutions are administered most frequently under hypothermic conditions.

Crystalloid Cardioplegia

One of the first cardioplegic solutions used to protect the heart during surgery consisted of a cold crystalloid formulation. It was developed on the premise that its administration would protect the heart by reducing its metabolism and aid the surgeon by providing a bloodless field. Over the years a number of crystalloid cardioplegic solutions have been developed that contain different ingredients. The rationale for these ingredients has been based on the need to: (1) induce a rapid cardiac arrest using potassium or magnesium; (2) reduce energy demand and conserve ATP reserves; (3) maintain intracellular ionic and metabolic homeostasis; (4) lower myocardial oxygen consumption; (5) enhance anaerobic and aerobic energy production utilizing glucose and amino acids; (6) stabilize the pH using bicarbonate, phosphate, or histidine buffers; (7) stabilize cellular membranes by using steroids, oxygen free radical scavengers such as glutathione, calcium antagonists, and/or procaine; (8) avoid intracellular calcium overload by providing a hypocalcemic environment and adding magnesium; and (9) prevent cellular edema by the addition of colloids such as mannitol to maintain normal oncotic pressures.

TABLE 15-2 Components of Various Cardioplegic Solutions

Solution	Composition*							
Intracellular Crystalloid CP	Sodium	Potassium	Magnesium	Calcium	Buffer	pH	Osmolarity (mOsm/L)	Other Components
Bretschneider's no. 3	12.0	10.0	4.0	0	Histidine	7.4	320	Procaine; mannitol
Bretschneider's HTK	15.0	9.0	4.0	0	Histidine	7.3	310	α-ketoglutarate; tryptophan; mannitol
Roe's	27.0	20.0	3.0	0	Tham	7.6	347	Glucose
Extracellular Crystalloid CP								
St. Thomas no. 1	144.0	20.0	32.0	4.8	None	5.5	285	Procaine
St. Thomas no. 2	110.0	16.0	32.0	1.2	Bicarbonate	7.8	324	None
Tyer's	138.0	25.0	3.0	1.0	Bicarbonate	7.8	275	Acetate; gluconate
Blood CP†								
Cold Induction	118.0	18.0	1.6	0.3-0.5	± Tham	7.6-7.8	320-340	Glucose; oxygen
Warm Induction	122.0	25.0	1.6	0.15-0.25	± Tham	7.5-7.6	340-360	Glucose; oxygen; glutamate; aspartate

*Values are expressed in milliequivalents per liter unless otherwise note.
†The blood cardioplegia composition when delivered in a blood to crystalloid solution ratio of 4:1.
CP = Cardioplegia.

There are basically two types of crystalloid cardioplegic solutions: the intracellular type and the extracellular type.[82] Both types can be used as preservation solutions for organ transplantation. The intracellular types are characterized by absent or low concentrations of sodium and calcium. The extracellular types contain relatively higher concentrations of sodium, calcium, and magnesium. Both types avoid concentrations of potassium >40 mmol/L (typical range is 10 to 40 mmol/L), contain bicarbonate for buffering, and are osmotically balanced. Examples of various crystalloid cardioplegic solutions are shown in Table 15-2.

Operative Procedure

Although the degree of core cooling varies from center to center, patients undergoing cardiac surgery are placed on cardiopulmonary bypass (CPB) and often cooled to between 33 and 28°C. To initiate immediate chemical arrest, the solution is infused after cross-clamping the aorta through a cardioplegic catheter inserted into the aorta proximal to the cross-clamp. The catheter may or may not be accompanied by a separate vent cannula. The cold hyperkalemic crystalloid solution then is infused (antegrade) at a volume that generally does not exceed 1000 mL. One or more infusions of 300 to 500 mL of the cardioplegic solution may be administered if there is evidence of electrical heart activity resumption or if a prolonged ischemic time is anticipated. If myocardial revascularization is being performed, the aortic cross-clamp can be removed after completing the distal anastomoses, and the heart reperfused while the proximal anastomoses are completed using a partial occlusion clamp. Alternatively, the proximal grafts can be performed after the distal grafts have been completed with the cross-clamp still in place (the single-clamp technique). Another approach is to perform the proximal aortic grafts first and then to cross-clamp the aorta and infuse the cardioplegic solution. When valve repair or replacement is being performed, the crystalloid cardioplegia can be administered directly into the coronary arteries via cannulation of the coronary ostia. Crystalloid cardioplegia also can be administered retrograde via a coronary sinus catheter with or without a self-inflating silicone cuff.

Outcomes

Although there is a concern that crystalloid cardioplegia lacks blood components and therefore has a limited oxygen-carrying capacity, this has not been shown to be clinically relevant. Likewise, although there is preclinical evidence that hyperkalemic crystalloid cardioplegia may damage coronary vascular endothelium and impair the ability of endothelial cells to replicate and produce endothelial-derived factors, this has not been shown to be of clinical significance.[83,84] In fact, there are numerous clinical studies that demonstrate that crystalloid cardioplegia is as effective as blood cardioplegia, particularly in centers where it is the primary form of protection.[85,86]

Cold Blood Cardioplegia

Cold blood cardioplegia, widely employed throughout the world, is the cardioplegic technique used most often in the United States. The rationale for using blood as a vehicle for hypothermic potassium-induced cardiac arrest is that it: (1) provides an oxygenated environment and a method for intermittent reoxygenation of the heart during arrest; (2) limits hemodilution when large volumes of cardioplegic solution are used; (3) affords an excellent buffering capacity and osmotic properties; (4) allows for electrolyte composition and pH that are physiologic; (5) offers a number of endogenous antioxidants and free-radical scavengers; and (6) is less complex than other solutions to prepare.

Although there are a variety of formulations, it is usually prepared by combining autologous blood obtained from the extracorporeal circuit while the patient is on cardiopulmonary bypass with a crystalloid cardioplegic solution that consists of citrate-phosphate-dextrose (CPD), tris-hydroxymethylaminomethane (tham), or bicarbonate (buffers), and potassium chloride. The CPD is used to lower the ionic calcium; the buffer is used to maintain an alkaline pH at approximately 7.8. The final concentration of potassium used to arrest the heart is approximately 20 to 25 mEq/L. After the initial induction dose for rapid arrest, subsequent administrations may be intermittent or continuous and utilize a concentration of 8 to 10 mEq/L (the low concentration maintenance dose)[87,88] (Table 15-2).

Before administering blood cardioplegia, the temperature of the solution usually is lowered with a heat-exchanging coil to between 12 and 4°C. The ratio of blood to crystalloid varies among centers, with the most common ratios being 8:1, 4:1, and 2:1. This, in turn, affects the final hematocrit of the blood cardioplegia infused. For example, if the hematocrit of the autologous blood obtained from the extracorporeal circuit is 30, these ratios would result in a blood cardioplegia with a hematocrit of approximately 27, 24, and 20, respectively.

The use of undiluted blood cardioplegia, or "miniplegia" (using a minimum amount of crystalloid additives), also has been reported to be effective. Petrucci et al. studied the use of all blood miniplegia in a clinically relevant swine preparation and compared miniplegia with crystalloid cardioplegia. They concluded that the use of all blood miniplegia was effective or superior in the acutely ischemic heart.[89] Velez and colleagues tested the hypothesis that an all-blood cardioplegia in an acute ischemia-reperfusion canine preparation (66:1 blood:crystalloid ratio) would provide superior protection compared with a 4:1 blood cardioplegia delivered in a continuous retrograde fashion.[90] They found very little difference between the animal groups with respect to infarct size or postischemic recovery of function. This is consistent with the findings by Rousou and colleagues years earlier that it is the level of hypothermia that is important in blood cardioplegia, not necessarily the hematocrit.[91]

With respect to efficacy, there are numerous preclinical studies and nonrandomized and randomized clinical trials that demonstrate cold blood cardioplegia is an effective way to provide excellent myocardial protection. Many of these same studies have suggested that cold blood cardioplegia is superior to cold crystalloid cardioplegia. It is important to note that other investigators have shown crystalloid cardioplegia to be as cardioprotective and cost-effective, if not more so. Unfortunately, even the most contemporary clinical trials comparing the efficacy of blood cardioplegia with crystalloid cardioplegia have involved single-center studies, enrolled a limited number of patients, focused on a specific subset of patients, and/or omitted details regarding clinical management. In 2006, Guru et al. reported the results of a meta-analysis of 34 clinical trials that compared blood cardioplegia to crystalloid cardioplegia. A lower incidence of low cardiac output syndrome and CK-MB release was observed in patients administered blood cardioplegia. No difference however was observed in the incidence of perioperative myocardial infarction or mortality.[92] Jacob et al. analyzed clinical data from 15 randomized trials. Although eight of the trials reported statistically significant outcomes favoring blood cardioplegia, and five showed statistically significant differences in enzyme release, the bulk of the evidence favoring one over the other was inconclusive.[86]

Warm Blood Cardioplegia

The concept of using warm (normothermic) blood cardioplegia as a cardioprotective strategy dates back to the 1980s. In 1982 Rosenkranz and colleagues reported that warm induction with normothermic blood cardioplegia, with multidose cold blood cardioplegia maintenance of arrest, resulted in better recovery of function in canines than a similar protocol using cold blood induction.[93] In 1986, Teoh and colleagues provided experimental evidence that a terminal infusion of warm blood cardioplegia before removing the cross-clamp (a "hot shot") accelerated myocardial metabolic recovery.[94] This was followed by a report in 1991 by Lichtenstein and colleagues that normothermic blood cardioplegia in humans is an effective cardio-protective approach.[76] They compared the results of 121 consecutive patients undergoing CABG surgery who received antegrade normothermic blood cardioplegia operations to an historical group of 133 patients who received antegrade hypothermic blood cardioplegia. The operative mortality in the warm cardioplegic group was 0.9% compared with 2.2% for the historical controls.

Despite these encouraging reports, there are concerns that for any given patient, it is difficult to determine how long a warm heart can tolerate an ischemic insult if the infusion is interrupted or flow rates are reduced owing to an obscured surgical field or a maldistribution of the cardioplegic solution. Another concern is the report by Martin and colleagues that warm cardioplegia is associated with an increased incidence of neurologic deficits.[43] In a prospective, randomized study conducted in more than 1000 patients, the efficacies of continuous warm blood cardioplegia with systemic normothermia (≥35°C) were compared with intermittent cold oxygenated crystalloid cardioplegia and moderate systemic hypothermia (≤28°C). Although operative mortalities were similar (1.0 versus 1.6%, respectively), the incidence of permanent neurologic deficits was threefold greater in the warm blood group (3.1 versus 1.0%). In this study, it appears that warm blood cardioplegia offered no distinct advantage over cold crystalloid cardioplegia, and it may be suboptimal if its delivery is interrupted for any reason. Subsequent studies have indicated however that appropriately designed protocols using intermittent antegrade warm blood cardioplegia provide clinically acceptable myocardial protection.[95–97]

Tepid Blood Cardioplegia

Both cold blood (4 to 10°C) and warm blood cardioplegic solutions (37°C) have temperature-related advantages and disadvantages. As a consequence, a number of studies were performed in the 1990s to determine the optimal temperature. Hayashida and colleagues were one of the first groups to study specifically the efficacy of tepid blood (29°C) cardioplegia.[98] In this study, 72 patients undergoing CABG were randomized to receive cold (8°C) antegrade or retrograde, tepid (29°C) antegrade or retrograde, or warm (37°C) ante-grade or retrograde blood cardioplegia. Although protection was adequate for all three, the tepid antegrade cardioplegia was the most effective in reducing anaerobic lactate acid release during the arrest period. These authors reported similar findings when the tepid solution was delivered continuously retrograde and intermittently antegrade.[99] In contrast, Baretti et al. reported in anesthetized open-chest swine placed on cardiopulmonary bypass that tepid normokalemic continuous antegrade blood cardioplegia was associated with an increased incidence of intermittent fibrillation.[100]

Subsequent to this report, Mallidi et al. analyzed the effects of cold blood and warm or tepid blood cardioplegia on early and late outcomes after CABG surgery. Warm blood cardioplegia was used in 4532 patients; cold blood cardioplegia was used in 1532 patients. Actuarial survival at five years was 91.1% in the warm blood cardioplegia group, and 89.9% in the cold blood cardioplegia group (p = 0.09). They concluded that warm or tepid blood cardioplegia may be associated with better early and late event-free survivals. For the most part, however, although tepid blood cardioplegia may be safe and effective, the majority of studies have been single-center studies conducted in relatively small cohorts of patients. Whether tepid cardioplegia confers superior protection over other current methodologies remains to be determined.[101]

Methods of Delivery

In addition to a variety of formulations and temperatures, there are also many different ways of administering the cardioplegic solutions (Fig. 15-3). As one might expect with so many options, the optimal delivery method also remains controversial.

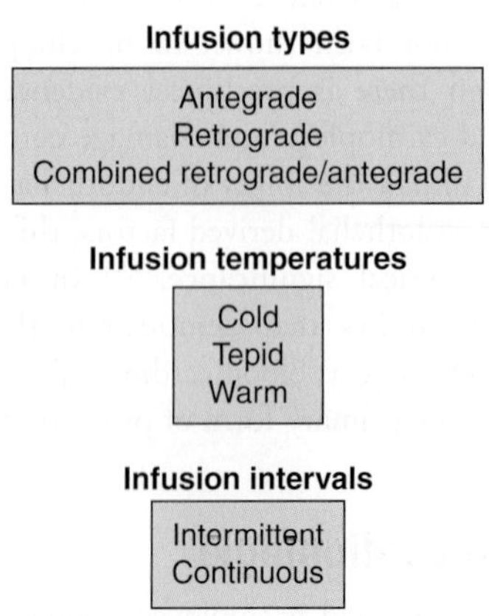

FIGURE 15.3 Methods for delivering cardioplegic solutions.

The various methods include intermittent antegrade, antegrade via the graft, continuous antegrade, continuous retrograde, intermittent retrograde, antegrade followed by retrograde, and simultaneous antegrade and retrograde infusions. Although all methods generally are good, comparisons are difficult because there are numerous confounding factors such as (1) the composition of the solution, (2) the temperature of the solution, (3) the duration of the infusion, (4) the infusion pressure, (5) the type and complexity of the operation, (6) the need for surgical exposure, and (7) the expected versus actual cross-clamp time.

Antegrade Cardioplegia

The most widely used method of delivering cardioplegic solutions entails the injection of the solution into the aortic root while the ascending aorta is cross-clamped, the antegrade method. After the initiation of cardiopulmonary bypass (CPB), chemical arrest can be achieved quickly with the infusion of the solution through a catheter inserted into the aorta proximal to the cross-clamp (close to the aortic root). The catheter may or may not be accompanied by a separate vent cannula. The induction dose usually has a higher concentration of potassium than subsequent maintenance doses, and is infused at a rate of 250 to 300 mL per minute to ensure aortic valve closure. The induction rate of infusion ranges between 10 mL/kg and 15 mL/kg body weight. The typical aortic root perfusion pressure is maintained between 60 mm Hg and 80 mm Hg. Adjustments in rates of administration are made to accommodate patients with hypertrophied ventricles. Intermittent maintenance doses of 300 to 500 mL of low-dose cardioplegia are administered every 15 to 20 minutes or earlier if there is evidence of resumption of electrical activity. During CABG surgery, in order to minimize cold ischemia and aortic cross-clamp time, the heart can be reperfused earlier by removal of the aortic cross-clamp as soon as the distal anastomoses are completed; the proximal anastomoses can be performed using a partial occlusion clamp. Alternatively, the proximal grafts can be performed after the distal grafts have been completed with the cross-clamp still in place (the single-clamp technique).

The administration of antegrade cardioplegia depends on a competent aortic valve and hence is liable to be ineffective and relatively contraindicated in patients with significant aortic valve incompetence. In such cases, antegrade cardioplegia can be administered directly into the coronary arteries via cannulation of the individual coronary ostium. This technique is used in cases requiring the opening of the ascending aorta, such as in aortic valve replacement, ascending aortic aneurysm repair, and aortic root replacement procedures. Coronary ostial infusion may be necessary for induction in patients with severe aortic incompetence in the presence of coronary sinus pacing leads. Potential complications using this approach include coronary dissection, unintentional selective delivery into left anterior descending or left circumflex artery because of a short left main coronary artery and the late occurrence of coronary ostial stenosis.[102]

Retrograde Cardioplegia

Retrograde cardioplegia entails placement of a coronary sinus catheter with or without a self-inflating silicone cuff and infusion of the cardioplegic solution either for induction or for maintenance of cardioplegia. This approach originated with a concept developed by Pratt in 1898, who suggested that oxygenated blood could be supplied to the ischemic heart via the coronary venous system.[103] Sixty years later, Lillehei and colleagues used retrograde coronary sinus perfusion to protect the heart during aortic valve surgery.[67] Today, it is an accepted method for delivering a cardioplegic solution and is used frequently as an adjunct to antegrade cardioplegia. Placement of the catheter is often facilitated by the use of catheters that are precurved and the simultaneous use of TEE imaging to guide placement. Care must be taken to avoid rupture of the coronary sinus, an uncommon but real and potentially fatal complication. This can be prevented by infusing the solution at a rate that ensures that the coronary sinus profusion pressure does not exceed 45 to 50 mm Hg. The retrograde approach can be used for continuous or intermittent delivery of blood or crystalloid cardioplegia as well. In situations where the native coronary arteries are severely stenotic or totally occluded, the antegrade approach may result in an uneven distributed in the myocardium. In this situation retrograde infusion or infusion via the vein grafts as they are completed can be complementary. Although most routine on-pump cardiac procedures can be done with good outcomes when only the antegrade technique is used, patients with poor ventricular function, high-risk patients requiring long aortic cross clamp times, and those with occlusive coronary disease may benefit from a dual approach, ie, both antegrade and retrograde techniques are used.

Another advantage to the retrograde technique is that it may be effective in reducing the risk of embolization from saphenous vein grafts that could occur during antegrade perfusion for reoperative coronary artery bypass surgery. The retrograde approach also has the theoretical advantage of ensuring a more homogeneous distribution of the cardioplegic solution to regions of the heart that are poorly collateralized.

Despite these advantages, retrograde cardioplegia is not without its limitations. Numerous experimental and clinical studies have shown that cardioplegia administered via the coronary sinus can result in a poor distribution of the solution to the right ventricle. This may be related to the variable venous anatomy of the heart and drainage via the Thebesian veins. The anterior region of the right ventricle is poorly drained by the coronary sinus, and it is not uncommon for the heart to have a number of coronary sinus anomalies. Thus, the retrograde approach may result in the heterogeneous distribution of cardioplegia. Nevertheless, it is felt that coronary sinus retroperfusion facilitates right ventricular hypothermia as the effluent travels through conductance vessels. The hypothermia may counteract the potentially decreased cardioplegic nutritive supply because of the shunting of blood via Thebesian veins. Because hypothermia is an important element of cardioprotection afforded the right ventricle by retrograde cardioplegia, it is unlikely that warm or tepid retrograde cardioplegia would confer similar protection to this region of the heart.

To address these concerns, a technique for simultaneously delivering cardioplegia both antegrade and retrograde is available. The feasibility and safety of this approach was first reported in 1984.[104] Subsequently, Cohen and coworkers used sonicated albumen and transesophageal echocardiography (TEE) intraoperatively to assess the effects of delivering a cardioplegic solution antegrade and retrograde simultaneously.[105] They reported that perfusion of the left and right anterior ventricles was most consistently achieved using the simultaneous approach. They noted, however, that antegrade infusion was associated with superior perfusion of the left ventricle when compared with retrograde delivery alone and that right ventricular perfusion was inconsistent with both antegrade and retrograde delivery. Thus, it is still unclear when the simultaneous use of both methods is most appropriate.

Continuous Cardioplegia versus Intermittent Cardioplegia

Cardioplegic surgery with aortic cross clamping may necessitate interruption of coronary flow for variable lengths of time. Logically, continuous cold blood cardioplegia would seem to be the better technique to use to address this problem. The major advantage of using intermittent cardioplegia is the ability to achieve and sustain a dry, quiescent operative field. Although a continuous infusion, especially if it is oxygenated, has the theoretical advantage of minimizing ischemia, from a practical standpoint, it is unlikely that this can be achieved reliably. Whether one uses continuous retrograde infusion via the coronary sinus, or handheld coronary ostial infusion in the open aortic root, with few exceptions, both necessitate interruption of the surgical steps while the infusion is delivered.

Many attempts have been made to sort out the clinical superiority of continuous infusion. One such study compared the efficacy of continuous versus intermittent cold blood cardioplegia administered in a retrograde fashion. Seventy patients undergoing CABG surgery for three-vessel coronary artery disease were prospectively randomized to receive retrograde cold blood cardioplegia either intermittently or in a continuous fashion. Ventricular performance was assessed by left and right ventricular stroke work index, and cardiac output. Degree of myocardial injury was assessed by measuring release of the biomarkers lactate and hypoxanthine. The investigators found continuous delivery of retrograde cold blood cardioplegia to be superior in preserving ventricular performance and minimizing myocardial injury.[106] A limitation of the study was the relatively small number of patients studied.

In conclusion, there is still controversy regarding superiority of blood versus crystalloid cardioplegia, the ideal temperature, and best method of delivery. A recent survey of practice patterns in the United Kingdom, in 2004, showed that 56% of all cardioplegia on-pump surgery was performed with cold blood cardioplegia, whereas warm blood cardioplegia was used in 14% of cases. In the same survey 14% of surgeons used crystalloid cardioplegia, 21% used retrograde cardioplegia, and 16% did not use any cardioplegia, preferring to use cross-clamp fibrillation only. Based on these observations and experiences in the United States, it appears that most surgeons favor cold intermittent blood cardioplegia. Nevertheless, a wide spectrum of variation exists among heart centers; there is no international consensus regarding the ideal cardioplegic solution or its use.[107] Awareness of the options allows the surgeon to utilize the best approach that meets the individual needs of the patient.

NONCARDIOPLEGIC SURGERY

Intermittent cross-clamping with fibrillation (ICCF) and systemic hypothermia with intermittent elective fibrillatory arrest are the most common forms of noncardioplegic heart surgery used today. The objective is to provide a relatively quiescent surgical field without having to arrest the heart with a cardioplegic solution.

Intermittent Aortic Cross-Clamping with Fibrillation

This technique is the earliest method developed to protect the heart during surgery and is still used at many centers. The patient is placed on cardiopulmonary bypass, the ascending aorta is cannulated, and generally a dual-stage single venous cannula is used. Often the patient is cooled to between 30 and 32°C. This technique allows the surgeon to operate in a relatively quiet field during ventricular fibrillation. In the setting of CABG surgery, the aortic cross-clamp is removed intermittently after the completion of each graft. The duration of fibrillation is determined by how long it takes to perform the distal anastomosis. After completion of the revascularization, the heart is defibrillated and the proximal anastomoses is performed on the beating heart using an aortic partial occlusion clamp. This technique is particularly useful in patients with cold agglutinin disease, an autoimmune phenomenon in which antibody directly agglutinates human red cells at low temperatures. In these patients, open-heart operations with hypothermia carry the risk of red cell agglutination and may result in hemolysis, myocardial infarction, renal insufficiency and cerebral damage.

As a result of increasing pressures to reduce cost and yet maintain acceptable levels of cardioprotection, there is an interest in using this approach. There are a number of reports that indicate that satisfactory protection can be conferred using this technique. In 1992, Bonchek et al. reported a large clinical series in which the advantages and safety of this technique were meticulously analyzed.[108] In this study, the authors reviewed the outcomes of the first 3000 patients at their institution who underwent primary CABG using the ICCF technique. Preoperative risk factors, eg, age, gender, left ventricular dysfunction, preoperative use of the intra-aortic balloon pump (IABP), the urgency of operation, and operative deaths were analyzed. In this series, 29% of the patients were older than 70 years of age, 27% were females, 9.7% had an ejection fraction of less than 0.30, 13% had an MI less than 1 week preoperatively, and 31% had preinfarction angina in the hospital. Only 26% underwent purely elective operations. Using the noncardioplegic cardioprotective technique, the authors reported an elective operative mortality rate of 0.5%, an urgent mortality rate of 1.7%, and an emergency rate of 2.3%. Postoperatively, inotropic support was needed in only 6.6% of the patients, and only 1% required insertion of the IABP. It is important to note, however, that this was a retrospective, single-center institutional experience. The findings would have been enhanced if the analysis had included a similarly matched group of patients at the same institution in which cardioplegic arrest had been employed. Nevertheless, the findings do suggest that noncardioplegic strategies can provide satisfactory myocardial protection even in high-risk patients.

In 2002, Raco and colleagues reported their experience in 800 consecutive CABG operations performed by a single surgeon using ICCF in both elective and nonelective settings. The patients were divided into three cohorts: (1) elective, (2) urgent, and (3) emergent. The mean age, number of distal grafts, and mortality among the three groups were comparable. The mortality rate in the elective, urgent, and emergent groups were 0.6%, 3.1%, and 5.6%, respectively, and consistent with outcomes associated with cardioplegic surgery. Because this report reflects the experience of a single surgeon, there is the concern that the technique may not be generally applicable. Regardless, the findings do support the notion that ICCF is a safe technique for both elective and nonelective patients undergoing CABG surgery.[109–111] In 2003, Bonchek et al. reported their experience in 8300 patients who underwent CABG surgery without cardioplegia. The unadjusted mortality rates in elective, urgent, and emergent patients was 0.9%, 1.5%, and 4.0%, respectively. The overall mortality was 1.7%, a rate considerably lower than the 3.27% predicted based on the Society of Thoracic Surgeons National Database model.[112] This experience represented the work of five surgeons, three of whom had not been trained in noncardioplegic surgery; it provides additional evidence that ICCF is an effective form of cardioprotection. Evidence that the cardioprotective effects of ischemic preconditioning (IPC) may contribute to the efficacy of ICCF in the human heart and have resulted in a resurgence of interest in using this method of protection, especially in the United Kingdom. Results in animal studies indicate that the protective effect of ICCF is blocked by protein kinase C inhibitors and K_{ATP} channel antagonists, both of which have been implicated in the signaling pathways involved in IPC.[113] Regardless of the mechanism, there are numerous reports that indicate that noncardioplegic strategies, such as ICCF, can provide satisfactory myocardial protection even in high-risk patients.[114]

Systemic Hypothermia and Elective Fibrillatory Arrest

Elective fibrillatory arrest is another safe approach to protect the heart during noncardioplegic heart surgery. The use of systemic hypothermia (26 to 30°C) and maintenance of systemic perfusion pressure between 80 and 100 mm Hg are key elements. This approach is particularly applicable in the setting of the severely calcified "porcelain aorta," where clamping the aorta may be associated with increased risk of stroke and aortic dissection. Under these circumstances the distal anastomoses are performed locally, occluding the coronary artery using vascular clamps or sutures. The proximal anastomoses can be completed during short periods of hypothermic circulatory arrest. Alternatively, the proximal anastomoses can be based entirely on an in situ internal thoracic artery. Using this approach one can avoid manipulation of the aorta altogether.

Akins, in 1984, reported a low incidence of perioperative MI and a low hospital mortality rate in 500 consecutive patients using this technique.[74] In 1987, Akins and Carroll assessed that late results of hypothermic fibrillatory arrest in 1000 consecutive patients undergoing nonemergent CABG surgery using hypothermic fibrillatory arrest. They concluded that the technique is effective for myocardial preservation and yields excellent event-free survival. Potential disadvantages with this approach include: (1) the surgical field may be obscured as a result of existing collateral circulation; (2) ventricular fibrillation may be associated with increased muscular tone and thus compromise the surgeon's ability to position the heart for optimal exposure; (3) aortic valvular regurgitation may be exacerbated; and (4) it is generally not applicable for intracardiac procedures. An advantage with the technique is that it can be used when aortic occlusion or cardioplegic arrest is not desirable, eg, in the setting of a calcified ascending aorta.

This approach can also be used in patients undergoing mitral valve surgery.[115] Imanaka et al., in 2003, published a retrospective observational study in which mitral valve surgery was performed in 27 patients with ischemic mitral regurgitation using perfused ventricular fibrillation. Concomitant procedures included CABG in 23 patients and the Dor procedure in 5 patients. Surgery was performed using moderate hypothermia (~28°C) and fibrillatory arrest; flow rates on bypass were maintained at 2.4 L/min/m^2 and the perfusion pressure was 70 mm Hg. Among these select patients, the mortality rate was 3.7%. The authors concluded that extended periods of ventricular fibrillation during hypothermic surgery can be well tolerated without excessive morbidity and mortality and is appropriate in patients in whom aortic cross-clamping is unsuitable or the duration of cross-clamping is expected to be long.[116]

NOVEL PRECLINICAL STRATEGIES FOR CARDIOPROTECTION

There are a number of physiologic processes and pharmacologic agents known to confer protection against ischemia-reperfusion injury in the experimental setting. Although the current evidence in support of the efficacy of these novel approaches is largely limited to preclinical studies, several trials are underway to determine the clinical relevance of these new approaches. The purpose of this section is to review emerging cardioprotective strategies that hold the most promise.

Physiologic Processes

Ischemic Preconditioning

"Precondition with ischemia" is an endogenous adaptive phenomenon whereby the heart becomes more tolerant to a period of prolonged ischemia if first exposed to brief episodes of coronary artery occlusion. This adaptation to ischemia was first described by Murry and colleagues and is referred to as *classic, first window,* or *early phase* ischemic preconditioning (IPC).[75] IPC is associated with a reduction in infarct size, apoptosis, and reperfusion-associated arrhythmias.[117] IPC has been demonstrated in every animal species studied and appears to persist as long as 1 to 2 hours after the ischemic preconditioning stimulus.[118,119] It becomes ineffective when the sustained ischemic insult exceeds 3 hours. This suggests that the protection is conferred only when prolonged ischemia is followed by timely reperfusion.

Subsequent studies have revealed that this endogenous defense mechanism can manifest itself in multiple ways. After the acute phase of preconditioning disappears, a second phase of protection appears 24 hours later and is sustained for up to 72 hours. This has been referred to as the *second window of protection, late-phase preconditioning,* or *delayed preconditioning.* Unlike classic IPC, which protects only against infarction, the late phase protects against both infarction and myocardial stunning.[120,121]

Cellular Mechanisms of IPC. These reports of adaptation to ischemia have resulted in major investigative efforts to elucidate the intracellular mechanism(s) that underlie the heart's endogenous defenses against ischemia-reperfusion injury. The assumption is that a better understanding of these mechanism(s) could lead to the development of potent new therapeutic modalities that are more effective in treating or preventing the deleterious consequences of ischemia-reperfusion injury. One of the earliest hypotheses was that stimulation of cardiomyocyte adenosine A_1 and/or A_3 receptors was the primary mediator of acute ischemic preconditioning.[119,122] Subsequent studies have revealed that in addition to adenosine, there are multiple guanine nucleotide-binding (G) protein–coupled receptors (GPCRs) that, once activated, can mimic the infarct-reducing effect of ischemic preconditioning, eg, bradykinin, endothelin, and α_1-adrenergic, muscarinic, angiotensin II, and delta-opioid receptors (Fig. 15-4). The infusion of exogenous agents that mimic ischemic preconditioning is referred to as *pharmacologic preconditioning.* Exactly which of these receptors is the most important in mediating endogenous preconditioning is unknown because there appear to be species differences and redundant signaling pathways. Regardless, it is now thought that these

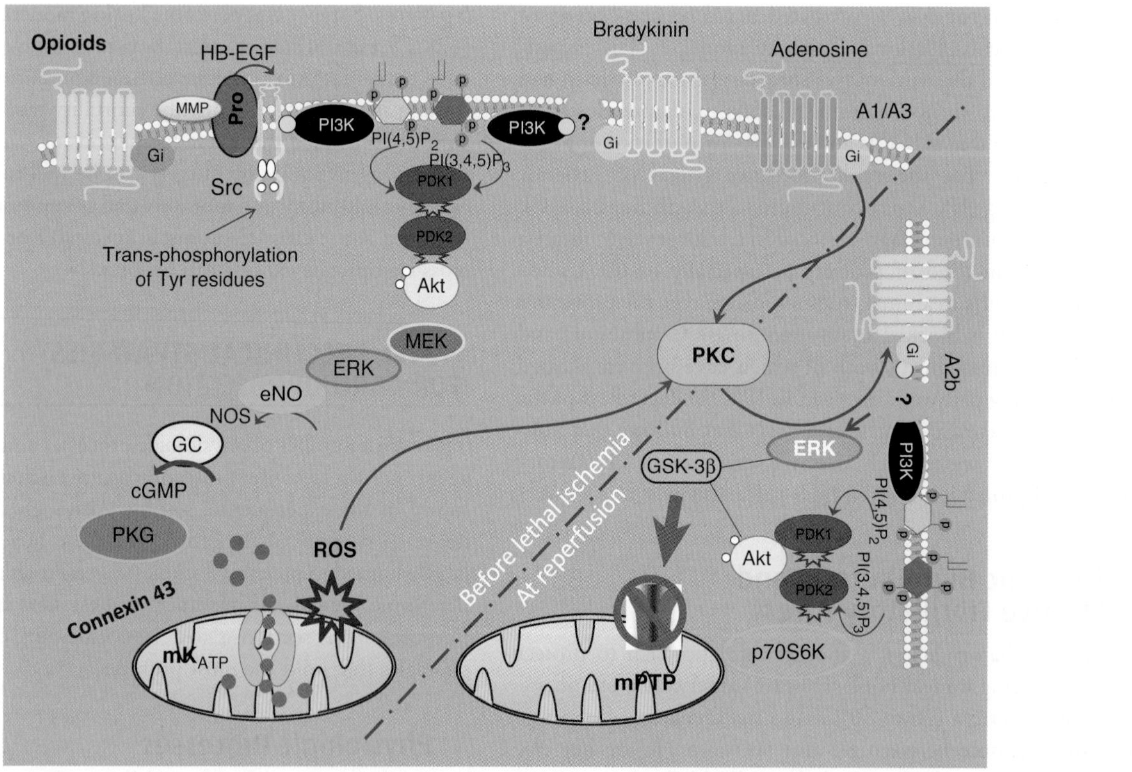

FIGURE 15.4 Signaling pathways of ischemic preconditioning. Numerous triggers (opioids, bradykinin, and adenosine) and intracellular signaling pathways are involved in the cardioprotection conferred by IPC. The signal transduction pathways are complex, interactive, and include the HB-EGF receptor, PI3K, Akt, ERK1/2, eNOS, PKG, the opening of the mK_{ATP} channel, ROS production, PKC activation, p70 S6 kinase, and GSK-3β. Possible end effectors of IPC include the opening of the mK_{ATP} channel and inhibition of the mitochondrial permeability transition pore opening. If only a few mitochondria are affected, cytochrome *c* may be released and induce apoptosis and cause cell death at a later time. Recent evidence suggests a unique role for the adenosine A2b receptor when activated at the time of reperfusion. Although the process of autophagy has been implicated in IPC induced cardioprotection, where and how this process interacts with the signaling pathways remains to be determined. eNOS = endothelial NOS; ERK = extracellular-signal regulated kinase; GC = guanylyl cyclase; GSK-3β = glycogen synthase kinase; HB-EGF = heparin-binding epidermal growth factor; IPC = ischemic preconditioning; MEK = mitogen activated protein kinase; mK_{ATP} = mitochondrial ATP-dependent potassium channel; MMP = matrix metalloproteinases; mPTP = mitochondrial permeability transition pore; NO = nitric oxide; NOS = NO synthase; PDK = phosphoinositide-dependent kinase; PI3 = phosphatidylinositol 3-kinase; $PI_{4,5}P_2$ = phosphatidylinositol bisphosphate; $PI_{3,4,5}P_3$ = phosphatidylinositol trisphosphate; PKC = protein kinase C; Pro = Pro-HB-EGF; PKG = protein kinase G; P70S6K = p70S6 kinase; ROS = reactive oxygen species;. (*Adapted from: Cohen MV, Downey JM: Adenosine: trigger and mediator of cardioprotection. Basic Res Cardiol 2008; 103[3]:203-215. Epub 2007 Nov 12. Review. PubMed PMID:17999026.*)

triggers of IPC result in alterations in certain enzymes, such as tyrosine kinases, isoforms of PKC, and mitogen-activated protein kinases (p38 and extracellular signal regulated kinase [ERK]) that, in turn, confer protection against irreversible injury before the onset of prolonged ischemia.

Interestingly, IPC-induced cardioprotection appears to require repopulation of receptors and activation (or, in some instances, reactivation) of "prosurvival" kinases upon relief of sustained ischemia. In this regard, Hausenloy and Yellon introduced the term *Reperfusion Injury Salvage Kinase (RISK)* pathway to represent the PI3K–Akt and ERK 1/2 pro-survival kinases activated at the time of reperfusion and proposed that manipulation and upregulation of the RISK pathway may represent another approach to myocardial protection.[123]

Although the identity of the end effector(s) of IPC remain speculative, significant evidence has accumulated indicating that the cardiomyocyte mitochondria are key targets of conditioning-induced protection (Fig. 15-4).[124,125] Specifically, inhibition of mPTP and the opening of the mitochondrial K_{ATP} (mK_{ATP}) channel have been implicated as the effectors of IPC.[126,127] Under normal conditions the mitochondrial inner membrane is impermeable to most metabolites and ions and the mPTP is closed. Although the molecular structure of the pore has yet to be determined, it is characterized by the formation of a large conductance megachannel that is regulated by cyclophilin D in the matrix. Although early investigations implicated the voltage-dependent anion channel in the outer mitochondrial membrane and the adenine nucleotide translocator (ANT) in the inner membrane in addition to cyclophilin D, genetic studies have refuted that model. Mouse models in which all ANT isoforms were deleted still exhibited mPTP opening; this was also the case for deletion of VDAC isoforms. However, deletion of cyclophilin resulted in hearts that were much more resistant to I/R injury, and further studies revealed that although the threshold for mPTP opening was greatly increased, it was still possible to trigger pore opening. It was concluded that cyclophilin D plays an important regulatory role in mPTP opening, but the molecular composition remains uncertain. Under conditions of stress, the mPTP may open, resulting in depolarization of the inner mitochondrial membrane and an influx of water and ions into the matrix because of its high oncotic pressure. Matrix swelling expands the highly folded inner membrane, but ultimately ruptures the outer membrane, resulting in release of cytochrome *c* and other pro-apoptotic factors. Even in the absence of the outer membrane rupture, loss of mitochondrial membrane potential results in ATP hydrolysis by the F_0F_1 ATP synthase in an effort to restore membrane potential. This futile cycling accelerates energy depletion.

An ATP-sensitive potassium channel in the mitochondrial inner membrane (mK_{ATP}) has been implicated on the basis of pharmacologic effects of diazoxide and pinacidil (channel openers) and 5-hydroxydecanoate and glibenclamide (channel closers). Many pharmacologic studies have demonstrated a protective role for the putative mK_{ATP}, although its molecular composition remains unknown. Garg and Hu have proposed that PKC activation enhances the import of plasma membrane K_{ATP} channels into mitochondria. This was based on their observation that in COS-7 cells, Kir6.2 protein (a subunit of K_{ATP} channels) and channel activity increased in mitochondria after PMA treatment, and this increase was inhibited by the selective PKC inhibitor chelerythrine. Pharmacologically triggered opening of the mK_{ATP} channel has been shown to reduce calcium overload, mitochondrial free-radical production, and swelling and to preserve ATP levels after ischemia/reperfusion.[128]

Although early-phase preconditioning shares many of the same signaling mechanisms with late-phase preconditioning, the most obvious difference between the two is the apparent requirement for protein synthesis in the latter. Late-phase IPC has been shown to be associated with the upregulation of various proteins, including, but not limited to, heat-shock proteins, inducible NOS (iNOS), cyclooxygenase 2, heme oxygenase, and manganese superoxide dismutase.[129,130] There are, however, conflicting reports on what specific proteins are upregulated during late-phase preconditioning, which may be because of species differences as well as stimulus-specific responses.

Clinical Relevance. There is considerable circumstantial evidence that ischemic preconditioning occurs in the human. Investigators have reported that patients experiencing angina before an MI have a better in-hospital prognosis and a reduced incidence of cardiogenic shock, fewer and less severe episodes of congestive heart failure, and smaller infarcts as assessed by cardiac enzyme release.[131] Moreover, follow-up studies suggest that patients who have had angina before an infarct have better long-term survival rates.[132–134] There are also a myriad of reports that patients who undergo percutaneous coronary interventions (PCI) have an enhanced tolerance to ischemia after the first balloon inflation, provided that the first balloon inflation exceeds 60 to 90 seconds.[118] Chest pain severity, regional wall motion abnormalities, ST-segment elevation, QT dispersion, lactate production, and CKMB release all have been reported to be attenuated in this setting as well.[135,136]

In patients undergoing PCI, a preconditioning-like effect has been mimicked by the administration of a variety of pharmacologic agents that are known to induce preconditioning in animal studies. For example, the administration of adenosine before PCI has been reported to attenuate myocardial ischemic indices during the first balloon inflation.[137] Administration of other agents, such as bradykinin and nicorandil (a K_{ATP} channel opener), also have been reported to produce similar effects.[138,139] Conversely, the administration of aminophylline (a nonselective adenosine receptor antagonist), glibenclamide (a K_{ATP} channel blocker), or naloxone (an opioid receptor blocker) reportedly abolishes the effects of ischemic preconditioning during PCI.[140,141] Additional studies provide evidence of delayed pharmacologic preconditioning in the clinical setting. Leesar and colleagues reported that a 4-hour intravenous infusion of nitroglycerin (an NO donor) 24 hours before PCI decreased ST-segment changes and reduced chest pain during the first balloon occlusion compared with patients treated with saline vehicle.[142] An earlier report by this same group indicated that delayed preconditioning with nitroglycerin decreased exercise-induced ST-segment changes and improved exercise tolerance. Thus, there are observational studies that support the hypothesis that myocardial protection conferred by ischemic preconditioning and its possible mediators in animal studies is translatable to humans. It is important to note, however, that classic or early ischemic preconditioning observed in animals is associated with a reduction in infarct size, but not protection against stunning, and that many of the clinical studies are either retrospective in nature or have used surrogate markers of injury as end points.

With respect to a role for IPC during cardiac surgery, numerous small trials have been conducted.[143] One of the first studies was conducted by Yellon and colleagues in patients undergoing CABG surgery.[144] Patients were subjected to a protocol that involved two cycles of 3 minutes of global ischemia. The aorta was cross-clamped intermittently and the heart was paced at 90 beats per minute to induce ischemia. This was followed by 2 minutes of reperfusion before a 10-minute period of global ischemia and ventricular fibrillation. Myocardial biopsies were obtained during the 10-minute period of global ischemia, and ATP tissue content was measured. The results showed that the ATP levels in the biopsies obtained from patients subjected to the preconditioning-like protocol were higher. However, because ATP content is not a marker of necrosis, a follow-up study was performed, and troponin T serum levels were measured. In this study, the investigators reported that troponin release was attenuated in the patients subjected to the preconditioning protocol. In 2002, Teoh and colleagues reported that IPC conferred myocardial protection beyond that provided by intermittent cross-clamp fibrillation in patients undergoing CABG.[79] Other investigators have reported similar findings.

Thus, a number of cardiac surgical studies suggest IPC may be effective in the setting of aortic cross-clamping and administration of cardioplegia. It is important to note, however, that to date the total number of patients studied has been relatively small, and the outcomes have been limited to surrogate markers of myocardial necrosis, viz., CK-MB levels and troponin release, and not clinical endpoints. This explains in part why IPC has not been adopted as an adjuvant approach among the myocardial protection techniques employed to date. A more promising strategy may be to develop a better understanding of the intracellular events and effectors that confer protection and then design the appropriate pharmacologic agent to mimic the phenomenon.

Postconditioning. The phenomenon of ischemic postconditioning (PostCond) was first reported by Zhao et al. in the canine model.[145] The term refers to rapid intermittent interruptions of blood flow in the early phase of reperfusion, ie, relief of ischemia in a stuttered or staccato manner. Although the cellular mechanisms underlying PostCond are poorly defined, they appear to involve many of the same signal transduction pathways that are involved in IPC, including cell surface receptor signaling, pro-survival kinases, the mPTP, and the mK_{ATP} channel. Although the duration and frequency of reperfusion may be variable, for the most part, the cycles that induce PostCond are measured in seconds in smaller species, and slightly longer in larger animals and humans, justifying the name *stuttering reperfusion.* The reduction in infarct size appears to be comparable with that observed with IPC. Preclinical studies conducted in multiple models and species (including dog, rat, rabbit, mouse, and pig) have demonstrated a reduction in infarct size that ranges from 20 to 70%. The restoration of blood flow in a stuttering manner during early reperfusion is of major interest to clinicians because it holds particular promise for patients presenting with an acute MI. In the surgical setting, PostCond could be applied in the operating room after release of the aortic cross-clamp.

Evidence that PostCond exists in humans was first reported in patients undergoing PCI. Patients receiving brief balloon inflations/deflations in the initial minutes of reperfusion during PCI exhibited smaller ST-segment changes and lower levels of total creatine kinase release compared with patients that were not subjected to stuttering reperfusion. More recently, Darling et al. conducted a retrospective chart review in patients undergoing emergent cardiac catheterization for ST-segment elevation MI (STEMI).[146] The hypothesis was that outcome would be better in patients undergoing multiple balloon inflations after primary angioplasty. Patients were divided into two cohorts: those who, at the discretion of the interventional cardiologist, received one to three balloon inflations, and those in whom four or more inflations were applied. In this retrospective analysis, peak CK release was less in patients requiring ≥four inflations. In a separate study by Lønborg et al., the cardioprotective effects of PostCond in patients treated with PCI was evaluated using MRI.[147] These investigators reported that mechanical PostCond appeared to be independent of the size of myocardium at risk. The findings were consistent with the concept that stuttering reperfusion confers cardioprotection during percutaneous interventions.

In the context of heart surgery, Luo reported a beneficial effect of surgical PostCond in 24 patients undergoing repair for Tetralogy of Fallot (TOF) at the time of aortic declamping. The postconditioning protocol consisted of aortic reclamping for 30 seconds and declamping for 30 seconds. The process was repeated twice. The intervention was reported to reduce perioperative troponin T and CK-MB release and decreased the need for inotropic support after surgery.[148] A similar finding was reported by the same investigator in a study of adult patients undergoing valve surgery and children undergoing corrective surgery using cardioplegia.

Thus, there is evidence that a PostCond protocol may be of benefit to patients undergoing heart surgery. Although PostCond may offer more promise than IPC in terms of clinical application, it is important to note that both are invasive in nature. Ultimately, the elucidation of mechanisms underlying PostCond may hold the most promise for development of new therapeutic approaches to cardioprotection.

Remote Ischemic Preconditioning. Remote ischemic preconditioning is a phenomenon whereby brief ischemia of one organ or tissue confers protection on a distant naive organ or tissue against a sustained ischemia-reperfusion injury. Remote ischemic preconditioning (RIPC) was first described by Przyklenk and colleagues in 1993.[149] In the original study, the investigators questioned whether IPC protected only the heart cells exposed to brief coronary artery occlusions or was it possible for repetitive or stuttering occlusions in a remote naive vascular bed to reduce infarct size in the area subjected to prolonged ischemia. They used a canine preparation in which a branch of the circumflex coronary artery was subjected to four episodes of 5-minute occlusion and reperfusion; this was followed by 1 hour occlusion of the left anterior descending (LAD) coronary artery. After 4.5 hours of reflow, infarct size in the distribution of the LAD was measured. A marked reduction in infarct size was observed. Since then, numerous other investigators have confirmed these findings, and the phenomenon has been observed in various species and with different organs. Brief occlusions of the renal and mesenteric arteries and brief restriction of blood flow to the skeletal muscle of the lower limb have been shown to reduce myocardial infarct size by up to 65%.[150] As a consequence, RIPC is now also referred to as interorgan preconditioning.

Not surprisingly, multiple mechanisms have been implicated to play a role in triggering and mediating remote preconditioning, including both humoral factors (such as adenosine, bradykinin, and calcitonin gene-related peptide), and neuronal factors, followed by activation of one or more kinases (including p38MAPK, ERK1/2 and JNK). To date the mechanism(s) underlying RIPC remain largely speculative. As with many other cardioprotective interventions, lack of a clear understanding of the molecular basis of the phenomenon has not dampened enthusiasm to apply the approach clinically as a possible new approach to cardioprotection in humans.

One of the first studies involving patients was conducted in 17 children undergoing congenital heart surgery with cardiopulmonary bypass.[151] Brief intermittent lower limb ischemia was associated with attenuated troponin release and a reduction in the need for postoperative inotropic support. Other investigators have reported similar findings in patients undergoing both adult heart surgery and resection of abdominal aortic aneurysms. For example, in one study involving 23 adult patients undergoing on-pump CABG surgery in which cold blood cardioplegia was used, RIPC was associated with a 42% reduction in total troponin T release. RIPC was induced by three 5-minute cycles of right forearm ischemia by inflating a blood pressure cuff on the upper arm to 200 mm Hg with an intervening 5-minute reperfusion period. The control group had a deflated cuff placed on the upper arm for 30 minutes. The outcome was similar to another study by Hausenloy et al., in which 57 patients undergoing elective CABG surgery were randomly assigned to RIPC or control groups. During the CABG operation, either intermittent cross-clamping or cardioplegia was used. RIPC was associated with a reduction in perioperative troponin T release by 43%.[152] Whether this mode of cardioprotection will become a standard of care will depend on whether or not RIPC can be shown to have a salutary effect on more robust clinical endpoints such as perioperative MI, stroke, and death.

Autophagy. Autophagy is the process whereby a double-membrane structure called the autophagosome sequesters cytoplasmic components such as ubiquitinated protein aggregates or organelles including mitochondria, peroxisomes, and endoplasmic reticulum. It is involved in degradation of long-lived proteins and the removal of excess or damaged organelles. The outer autophagosomal membrane fuses with a lysosomal membrane to deliver its contents into an autophagolysosome where the cargo is degraded by lysosomal hydrolases and the resulting macromolecules recycled[153] (Fig. 15-5).

One of the first studies to suggest autophagy is an adaptive process responsive to stress in the heart was the report by Decker et al. in which they described an association between the formation of autophagosomes and an increase in degenerating mitochondria in rabbit hearts exposed to hypoxia and reperfusion. Reperfusion restored contractility and injured myocytes underwent a cellular repair process that involved a marked increase in lysosomal autophagy. These investigators concluded that this process is important in the efforts to repair cardiac cells during and after hypoxia.[154]

Autophagy has now been reported to be upregulated in isolated cells subjected to simulated ischemia and reperfusion and rodent models of ex vivo and in vivo ischemia reperfusion injury. Shimomura showed that upregulation of autophagy in HL-1 myocytes protected against cell death induced by simulated ischemia reperfusion (sI/R) whereas inhibition of autophagy enhanced cell death.[155] Dosenko et al. was one of the first to report a more direct linkage between autophagy and cytoprotection and observed that autophagy may have a protective effect during anoxia-reoxygenation.[156] Subsequently, upregulation of autophagy induced by sI/R in HL-1 myocytes was reported to be protective, whereas inhibition of autophagy enhanced cell death. Hamacher-Brady and colleagues subjected HL-1 cells to sI/R as an in vitro model of ischemia reperfusion. Using three-dimensional high-resolution fluorescence imaging, they analyzed the autophagic response to sI/R. They observed that autophagy is an important underlying protective response against sI/R injury.[157] Matsui et al. found that glucose deprivation increased the number of autophagosomes in neonatal cardiac myocytes, and that inhibiting autophagy with 3-methyladenine (3-MA) enhanced cell death induced by glucose deprivation.[158] Yan et al. reported that cardiac myocytes with enhanced autophagy were negative for apoptosis, whereas apoptotic cells were negative for autophagy in a porcine model of chronic myocardial ischemia and hibernating myocardium.[159]

Gurusamy et al. investigated the role of autophagy during ischemia-reperfusion injury and reported that increased BAG-1 expression in the heart correlated with the onset of protection in an in vivo model of myocardial stunning.[160] Collectively, these studies suggest that upregulation of autophagy promotes survival during stress such as ischemia-reperfusion.

There is now direct evidence that autophagy plays an important role in mediating ischemic and pharmacologic preconditioning. Yitzhaki et al. investigated the effect of the adenosine preconditioning agent 2-chloro-N(6)-cyclopentyladenosine (CCPA) on autophagy and cell survival after sI/R and GFP-LC3 infected HL-1 cells and neonatal rat cardiomyocytes. Autophagy was induced within 10 minutes of adenosine treatment and increased autophagy was evident when examined 24 hours later. Inhibition of autophagy resulted in significant loss of both immediate and delayed cytoprotection against sI/R as measured by release of lactate dehydrogenase. To assess autophagy in vivo, transgenic mice expressing the red fluorescent autophagy marker mCherry-LC3 were treated with CCPA. Treated hearts

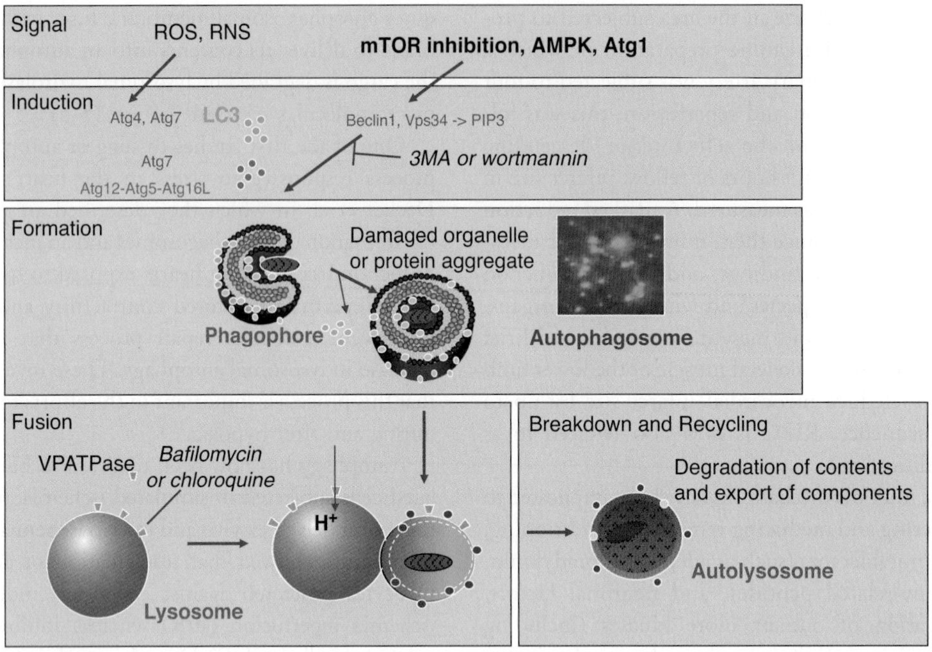

FIGURE 15.5 Cellular process of autophagy. Autophagy is a dynamic adaptive process in the setting of I/R injury. The process involves the synthesis of a cup-shaped pre-autophagosomal double-membrane structure that surrounds cytoplasmic material and closes to form an autophagosome. This process is regulated by the autophagy proteins Atg 4, Atg7, LC3, and the complex of Atg12-Atg5-Atg16L. The process is activated by a number of stimuli including ROS or RNS. Induction by Beclin1 and Vps34 in conjunction with other Atg proteins results in the formation of an isolation membrane to which Atg proteins are recruited. Atg12-Atg5 and LC3 proteins are involved in the expansion of the membrane. This allows the phagophore to surround and engulf damaged organelles or protein aggregates that may accumulate as a result of I/R injury. The result is the formation of an autophagosome. The green insert shows autophagosomes (*green puncta*). This photo was obtained in a cell expressing a fusion protein of green fluorescent protein (GFP) fused to the N-terminus of LC3; the GFP-LC3 was incorporated into the double membrane structure of the phagophore. Wortmannin and 3 MA are agents that can inhibit the initiation phase of autophagy; bafilomycin and chloroquine can inhibit the degradation phase. AMPK = AMP-activated protein kinase ; Atg1,Atg4, Atg7, Atg12, Atg16L = autophagy regulating proteins; I/R = ischemia/reperfusion; LC3 = light chain 3; mTOR = mammalian target of rapamycin; PIP3 = phosphatidylinositol 3,4,5-trisphosphate; 3MA = 3-methyladenine; RNS = reactive nitrogen species; ROS = reactive oxygen species; Vps34 = a class III PI3 kinase involved in vesicular trafficking, nutrient signaling, and autophagy. (*Adapted from Gottlieb RA, Finley KD, Mentzer RM Jr: Cardioprotection requires taking out the trash. Basic Res Cardiol 2009; 104:169-180.*)

revealed a large increase in the number of autophagosomes. Subsequent ex vivo and in vivo studies examining the role of autophagy in pharmacologic and ischemic preconditioning have provided strong evidence that autophagy is required for the protective effect. Based on these findings, it appears that autophagy may serve as an important mediator of protection of the preconditioning agent CCPA.[161] A more detailed understanding of the role of autophagy in myocardial protection may lead to a new therapeutic approach to the management and treatment of ischemia-reperfusion injury.

Pharmacologic Agents

Considerable progress has been made towards limiting myocardial ischemia-reperfusion injury in the setting of global ischemia associated with surgical procedures. Despite considerable efforts to translate promising experimental results into clinical therapies, interventions to date have yielded few successes with the exceptions of adenosine and glucose-insulin-potassium. These disappointments led the National Heart Lung and Blood Institute to convene a working group to discuss the reasons for the failure to translate potential therapies for protecting the heart from ischemia and reperfusion. The working group concluded that cardioprotection in the setting of acute myocardial infarction, cardiac surgery, and cardiac arrest requires more relevant animal models corresponding to the human conditions of atherosclerosis, hypercholesterolemia, hypertension, diabetes, and advanced age, all of which are increasingly recognized to interfere with cardioprotective strategies.[162] At the same time, a number of recent studies provided a sense of optimism regarding the encouraging clinical data for the following cardioprotective interventions.

Adenosine

There is considerable experimental evidence that activation of various adenosine receptor subtypes results in cardioprotection similar to that induced by IPC. Preischemic administration of the nucleoside adenosine retards the rate of ischemia-induced ATP depletion, prolongs the time to onset of ischemic contracture, attenuates myocardial stunning, enhances postischemic myocardial energetics, and reduces infarct size.[163]

There are at least four distinct adenosine receptor subtypes, which are designated A_1, A_{2a}, A_{2b}, and A_3. They couple to a variety of guanine nucleotide-binding (G) proteins (G_o, $G_{i\alpha2}$, $G_{i\alpha3}$, G_q, and G_s) depending on the receptor subtype and tissue studied. There is definitive evidence that two, and possibly three, of these receptors are expressed in the adult human heart. Recent preclinical reports suggest that an adenosine A_{2b} receptor agonist confers cardioprotection when administered before the onset of ischemia (preconditioning) and at reperfusion (postconditioning).[164]

With respect to cardiac surgery, there have been a limited number of clinical trials performed. Fremes and colleagues reported the results of an open-label, nonrandomized CABG surgery study in which adenosine administration was combined with antegrade warm blood cardioplegia. The adenosine concentrations studied were 15, 20, and 25 mol/L. These investigators reported that adenosine could be added safely as a supplement to cardioplegic solutions, but it had no effect on myocardial function at the doses studied.[165]

Cohen and colleagues observed a similar lack of efficacy in a phase II double-blind, placebo-controlled trial performed in patients undergoing CABG surgery. Patients were treated with placebo (saline) or warm blood cardioplegia supplemented with 15, 50, or 100 μM adenosine. These investigators found that adenosine had no effect on survival, the incidence of MI or the incidence of low cardiac output syndrome. A limitation of this study was the use of low concentrations of adenosine in the setting of warm blood cardioplegia. The nucleoside is metabolized rapidly to inosine and hypoxanthine, and the half-life in blood is measured in seconds, thus limiting its potential effect.[166]

Mentzer and colleagues reported a beneficial effect in an open-label, single-center study in which the safety, tolerance, and efficacy of high doses of adenosine were studied when added to cold blood cardioplegia in CABG surgery patients. Sixty one patients were randomized to receive standard cold blood cardioplegia or cold blood cardioplegia containing one of five adenosine doses ranging between 100 μM and 2 mM. Invasive and noninvasive studies of myocardial function were obtained sequentially after bypass. Parameters included the recording of inotropic utilization rates for the postoperative treatment of low cardiac output. Blood samples were collected for the measurement of nucleoside levels. High-dose adenosine treatment was associated with a 249-fold increase in the plasma adenosine concentration and was associated with a reduction in postbypass inotropic drug utilization, improved regional wall motion, and global function measured by transthoracic echocardiography.[167]

Subsequently, Mentzer and colleagues examined the effects of high-dose adenosine treatment in 253 patients randomized to one of three treatment arms. This was a double-blind, placebo-controlled multicenter trial using cold blood cardioplegia; adenosine was administered in three different concentrations and rates. Invasive and noninvasive measurements of ventricular performance were obtained before, during, and after surgery. The results of this study revealed a trend toward a decrease in high-dose inotropic agent utilization rates and a lower incidence of perioperative MI. A posthoc composite outcome analysis revealed that patients who received the high-dose adenosine were less likely to experience high-dose dopamine and epinephrine use, insertion of an intra aortic balloon pump, MI, or death.[168]

In summary, there is preclinical and clinical evidence that adenosine is a cardioprotective agent. Its clinical use is limited because large doses are associated with marked hypotension in patients not on cardiopulmonary bypass. The identification of a selective adenosine receptor subtype, eg, an adenosine A_{2b} agonist that confers protection without systemic hypotension could lead to the development of a drug that is effective in preventing perioperative MI and stunning similar to that observed with late-phase preconditioning.

Acadesine

This agent is a member of a class of drugs referred to as adenosine regulating agents. It is a purine nucleoside analog that purportedly raises adenosine tissue levels selectively during ischemic conditions.[169] The mechanism by which this agent regulates adenosine levels during ATP catabolism has not been fully established. Early preclinical studies have indicated that acadesine treatment: (1) improves left ventricular wall motion after intermittent ischemia, (2) attenuates frequency of ventricular arrhythmias, and (3) attenuates myocardial stunning and preserves myocardial function after cardiac arrest and cold cardioplegia. The observations led to five large-scale clinical trials in CABG surgery patients in the 1990s. The findings, however, were inconclusive due in part to the fact they were powered to detect only effect sizes of 50% or more.

As a consequence, Mangano combined the data from all five trials and performed a meta-analysis approach. The entire clinical experience of acadesine in more than 4000 CABG patients were analyzed to determine the effects of this agent on prespecified perioperative outcomes of MI, stroke, and cardiac death. The results of the meta-analysis indicated that acadesine given intravenously before and during surgery along with a fixed concentration in cardioplegia solution was effective in reducing perioperative MI, cardiac death, and combined adverse cardiovascular outcomes.[170]

Subsequently, Mangano et al. examined the two-year all-cause mortality after perioperative MI in a follow-up of the Acadesine 1024 Trial. Although the primary outcome was negative, the findings at two years among patients experiencing postreperfusion MI indicated a significant four-fold reduction in mortality (15/54 patients versus 3/46 patients).[171] Based on these findings, a large scale Phase III study was initiated in 2010 (RED CABG). This study was stopped after 30% enrollment, however, due to futility. Whether the apparent lack of efficacy was due to clinical trial design, the characteristics of this class of drugs, or properties unique to agent itself, is unknown. It is important to note, however, that the salutary effects of this agent may not be apparent immediately after the operation.

Sodium-Hydrogen Exchanger Inhibitors

The sodium-hydrogen exchangers (NHEs) are a family of membrane proteins with nine isoforms that are involved in the transport of hydrogen ions in exchange for sodium ions. NHE-1 is the isoform that is expressed in the heart and may play a minor role in the normal excitation-contraction coupling process; however, it has been implicated in the etiology of arrhythmias, stunning, apoptosis, necrosis associated with acute myocardial ischemia-reperfusion injury, postinfarction ventricular remodeling, and heart failure.

The driving forces for Na^+/H^+ exchange are the relative transmembrane N^+ and H^+ gradients. The activity of the exchanger is regulated by the interaction of the H^+ with a sensor site on the exchanger protein and can be additionally modulated by phosphorylation.[172] During ischemia, cytoplasmic pH falls as low as 6.6 because of increased production of H^+ from anaerobic glycolysis, but upon reperfusion, NHE-1 is activated to restore intracellular pH by exchange of intracellular protons for extracellular sodium. The resulting accumulation of intracellular Na^+ is further exacerbated by diminished activity of Na^+/K^+ ATPase as a result of ischemia and lowered ATP availability. The increased intracellular Na^+ competes for sites on the Na^+/Ca^{++} exchanger and can actually drive it to run in reverse, resulting in cytosolic calcium overload. As noted earlier, calcium overload has numerous adverse consequences including activation of calcium-dependent proteases and phospholipases, gap junction dysfunction, and triggering of the mPTP culminating in membrane rupture and cell death (see Fig. 15-1).

The EXPEDITION trial was initiated to address the safety and efficacy of NHE-1 inhibition by cariporide in the prevention of death or MI in patients undergoing CABG surgery. High-risk CABG patients (n = 5,770) were randomized to receive either intravenous cariporide or placebo. The composite endpoint was assessed at 5 days, and patients were followed for up to 6 months. The results revealed an 18.3% relative risk reduction (RRR) in the incidence of death or MI at 5 days (p = 0 .0002). The RRR for death or MI at day 30 and month 6 was 16.1% (p = 0.0009) and 15.7% (p = 0.0006), respectively. When analyzed separately, the RRR in the incidence of MI alone at 5 days was 23.8% (p = 0.000005) and at month 6 was 25.6% (p = 0.000001). The mortality rate, however, increased at 5 days from 1.5% in the placebo group to 2.2% in the group with cariporide. This was associated with an overall increase in the incidence of cerebrovascular events. Thus, although cariporide treatment was effective in reducing the incidence of nonfatal MI, its efficacy was associated with toxicity, and the overall assessment of benefits and risks associated with cariporide indicated that the imbalances in the safety profile outweighed the reduction in the observed MI rate. Thus, it is unlikely that cariporide will be used clinically. The importance of the study, however, is that myocardial necrosis after CABG is higher than previously appreciated and it suggested NHE-1 inhibitors represent a new class of drugs that hold promise for reduction of myocardial infarction associated with ischemia-reperfusion injury.[81]

Glucose-Insulin-Potassium

There are numerous studies that suggest glucose-insulin-potassium (GIK) infusions are effective in reducing perioperative MIs, postischemic myocardial dysfunction, and atrial fibrillation in patients undergoing heart surgery.[173] The rationale for this form of treatment is based on the concept that insulin stimulates potassium reuptake through stimulation of the Na^+,K^+-ATPase while it stimulates glucose uptake for glycolytic energy production. High glucose, insulin, and an increased glycolytic flux also increase pyruvate generation and in turn preserve the citric acid cycle. Additionally, glycolytic ATP protects membranes, drives uptake of Ca^{2+} by the sarcoplasmic reticulum, and improves sodium homeostasis of ischemic myocardium.

Despite a strong rationale for its application in surgery, the efficacy of GIK in heart surgery remains controversial. This is due in part to the mixed results with the use of GIK to treat patients with acute myocardial infarction. In 1997, Fath-Ordoubadi and Beatt showed a benefit of treatment in a meta-analysis of patients who received GIK reperfusion therapy for acute myocardial infarction.[174] Van der Horst reported a benefit of GIK in 940 randomized STEMI patients treated by PCI. It was only in the subgroup of 156 patients without heart failure, however, that a significant reduction in mortality was seen.[175] In a follow-up report, Timmer et al. were unable to demonstrate a therapeutic benefit in patients without signs of heart failure. Thus, a role for GIK in the treatment of acute myocardial infarction (STEMI) is yet to be determined.[176]

With respect to cardiac surgery, Lazar et al. conducted a study to determine whether tight perioperative glycemic control in diabetic CABG patients with a modified GIK solution would optimize myocardial metabolism and improve perioperative outcomes. Patients (n = 141) were randomized to receive GIK or no GIK. The preoperative patient profiles were similar in age, sex, ejection fraction, urgency of surgery, or the type of diabetes. Although the 30-day survival was comparable in both groups, the GIK-treated patients had significantly higher cardiac indices and less need for inotropic support. There was also a lower incidence of atrial fibrillation. Follow-up data two years after surgery were available in 60 of 70 (83.3% GIK) and 60 of 69 (86.9% GIK) patients. Survival was better in the patients who received GIK; the investigators attributed this to long-lasting benefits from perioperative GIK treatment.[177]

In another single-center study, Quinn et al. reported their results with a prospective, randomized, double-blind, placebo-controlled trial in 280 nondiabetic CABG surgery patients. They found that GIK treatment was associated with fewer episodes of low cardiac output, less inotropic support postoperatively, and a reduction in serum cardiac troponin I levels. The authors concluded that GIK is an effective, inexpensive, and safe adjunctive cardioprotective technique.[80]

In contrast, S. Bruemmer-Smith et al. reported that GIK infusion during surgery failed to reduce myocardial cellular damage as measured by cTnI levels six hours after cardiopulmonary bypass. It was associated with increased hyperglycemia. In this study, only 42 patients were enrolled although it was a randomized, prospective, double-blinded study in patients undergoing elective CABG surgery. The patients received either GIK or placebo administered via a central line. The groups were well-matched for aged and number of bypassed vessels.[178] In another study, Lell et al. reported on 46 patients undergoing elective off-pump CABG surgery; the patients received either normal saline or a GIK infusion for 12 hours. These investigators were unable to demonstrate a beneficial effect on cardiac performance using the clinical measurements of cardiac index and inotropic requirements. They did report the finding of a persistent hyperglycemia, however, despite the use of supplemental insulin.[179] Finally, Barcellos et al. reported their experience with 24 patients with type-2 diabetes mellitus who underwent CABG surgery. Patients were administered GIK or subcutaneous insulin from the onset of anesthesia until 12 hours postoperatively. The use of GIK neither improved the cardiac index nor reduced the use inotropic agents albeit it did improve glucose control.[180]

Thus, the evidence supporting the efficacy of GIK in the setting of heart surgery is still controversial. Although a meta-analysis of randomized studies using GIK suggests that it may improve postoperative recovery of contractile function and reduce atrial arrhythmias, the individual studies have involved small numbers of patients and, therefore, insufficiently powered to detect efficacy. Until a large randomized, multicenter clinical trial has been performed, the use of GIK as a form of myocardial protection will remain controversial.

MYOCARDIAL PROTECTION DURING BEATING HEART SURGERY

In an effort to minimize complications associated with cardiopulmonary bypass, such as stroke and a systemic inflammatory response, the number of coronary artery bypass graft operations performed without cardiopulmonary bypass (off-pump: OPCAB). The assumption is that avoidance of aortic cross-clamping will be associated with a lower incidence of cerebrovascular complications and perioperative MI, lower rates of renal and respiratory failure, less postoperative bleeding, less pain, and shorter hospitalization. There is a concern, however, that OPCAB may be associated with incomplete revascularization, a higher incidence of perioperative myocardial infarction, and a reduction in long-term graft patency.[181–183] Although the relative benefits of OPCAB versus on-pump CABG surgery remain to be determined, as many as 20% of CABG patients undergo the procedure off-pump. Thus it is important to appreciate the principles and methods of myocardial protection as it relates to beating heart surgery.

The acceptance of OPCAB is due in part to the development and refinement of a myriad of surgical aids that allow for stabilization and local immobilization of the heart during grafting. Techniques include the temporary occlusion of the coronary artery or shunting of blood during sustained coronary artery occlusion. Because temporary occlusion of an already diseased artery may aggravate ongoing ischemia, pharmacologic agents and nonpharmacologic maneuvers are used to protect the heart during displacement required to access lateral and inferior wall vessels. Many of these interventions are designed to reduce myocardial oxygen demand at a time when supply is limited.

Ischemia during temporary occlusion of a coronary artery during OPCAB may last from 6 to 25 minutes based on the surgeon's experience, quality and size of the vessel, and adequacy of the exposure. Most patients with preexisting severe coronary heart disease have experienced self-limiting episodes of ischemia during daily life and may have imparted a certain degree of tolerance to the surgically induced ischemia. This tolerance has been documented using ECGs, transesophageal echocardiography, and continuous SVO_2 monitoring. In order to better understand the differences between OPCAB and on-pump surgery, Chowdhury et al. investigated the release pattern of various cardiac biomarkers in 50 patients undergoing cardioplegic and noncardioplegic coronary artery bypass surgery. The various markers included cardiac troponin I, heart-type fatty acid-binding protein, CK-MB, high-sensitivity C-reactive protein and myoglobin. Measurements were obtained at baseline and then at hourly intervals up to 72 hours after completion of the last anastomosis in the noncardioplegic OPCAB group, and after release of aortic cross clamp in the cardioplegic group. They observed a greater release of cardiac troponin I, high-sensitivity C-reactive protein, and heart-type fatty acid-binding protein in the cardioplegic group. They concluded that OPCAB surgery is associated with less injury.[184] It is important to note, however, that efficacy was measured using surrogate markers of protection and the actual incidence of perioperative death and MI were similar in both groups of patients. Finally, whether or not OPCAB surgery is associated with less injury, patients undergoing this form or revascularization are still at risk of ischemic injury.

One approach to minimizing the risk of injury is to reduce myocardial oxygen demand. Pharmacologic beta-blockade is frequently instituted to reduce inotropy and achieve negative chronotropy using ultra-short-acting beta blockers such as esmolol and labetalol. Another approach is to optimize the systemic mean blood pressures while reducing afterload. Calcium channel blockers, such as diltiazem, have been used to afford an effective reduction in blood pressure while minimizing a depression in myocardial contractility that may occur with beta blockers. Patients who become hypertensive during the operation may benefit from intravenous nitrates, which allows for coronary vasodilation and increased blood flow via collaterals. Gentle core cooling, by allowing the body temperature to drift to 35–36°C and deepening the level of anesthesia are concurrent measures that can also be employed.

Ischemic preconditioning is another approach that has been used to impart tolerance to ischemia-reperfusion injury. Although its efficacy has yet to be established in the context of meaningful clinical outcomes, it may be a reasonable approach given the findings by Shroyer et al. These investigators analyzed both short-term and long-term outcomes in 2203 patients randomized to undergo either on-pump or off-pump surgery. The primary endpoints included mortality and complications such as reoperation, need for new mechanical support, cardiac arrest, coma, stroke or renal failure before discharge or within 30 days of surgery. The long-term outcome consisted of the composite endpoint of death from any cause, repeat revascularization procedure, or a nonfatal myocardial infarction within one year. Secondary endpoints included graft patency and neurologic outcomes. Although there were no differences at 30 days, they observed that OPCAB patients had a higher incidence of death from cardiac causes within one year, tended to have lower graft patency and had fewer arteries bypassed. The incidence of stroke or resource utilization was similar for both on-pump and off-pump procedures.[185] Although OPCAB can be performed safely, the advantages over on-pump procedures remain to be elucidated. Moreover, the survival findings suggest that this approach to myocardial revascularization does not obviate the need to develop new methods to prevent complications associated with ischemia-reperfusion injury.

CONCLUSION

Although considerable progress has been made in the field of cardioprotection, the ideal solution, technique, or delivery method has yet to be discovered. This is due, in part, to the complex nature of ischemia-reperfusion injury and our limited understanding of the endogenous mechanisms that exist. Likewise, effective cardioprotection in the operating room can no longer be evaluated in the context of 30-day mortality, as we now know that the injurious consequences of inadequate myocardial protection may not be manifest for months to years after the heart operation.

ACKNOWLEDGMENTS

Mrs. Kristyn Hagood provided research support and was an active participant in the preparation of this manuscript.

REFERENCES

1. Lloyd-Jones D et al: Heart disease and stroke statistics—2009 update: a report from the American Heart Association Statistics Committee and Stroke Statistics Subcommittee. *Circulation* 2009; 119(3):e21-181.
2. Mangano DT: Cardiovascular morbidity and CABG surgery—a perspective: epidemiology, costs, and potential therapeutic solutions. *J Card Surg* 1995; 10(4 Suppl):366-368.
3. Eagle KA et al: ACC/AHA 2004 guideline update for coronary artery bypass graft surgery: summary article. A report of the American College of Cardiology/American Heart Association Task Force on Practice Guidelines (Committee to Update the 1999 Guidelines for Coronary Artery Bypass Graft Surgery). *J Am Coll Cardiol* 2004; 44(5):e213-310.
4. Nagle PC, Smith AW: Review of recent US cost estimates of revascularization. *Am J Manag Care* 2004; 10(11 Suppl):S370-376.
5. Smith PK et al: Cost analysis of aprotinin for coronary artery bypass patients: analysis of the randomized trials. *Ann Thorac Surg* 2004; 77(2):635-642; discussion 642-643.
6. Abbate A et al: Electron microscopy characterization of cardiomyocyte apoptosis in ischemic heart disease. *Int J Cardiol* 2007; 114(1):118-120.
7. Eefting F et al: Role of apoptosis in reperfusion injury. *Cardiovasc Res* 2004; 61(3):414-426.
8. Verma S et al: Fundamentals of reperfusion injury for the clinical cardiologist. *Circulation* 2002; 105(20):2332-2336.
9. Buja LM, Weerasinghe P: Unresolved issues in myocardial reperfusion injury. *Cardiovasc Pathol* 2010; 19(1):29-35.
10. Yellon DM, Hausenloy DJ: Myocardial reperfusion injury. *NEJM* 2007; 357(11):1121-1135.
11. Klatte K et al: Increased mortality after coronary artery bypass graft surgery is associated with increased levels of postoperative creatine kinase-myocardial band isoenzyme release: results from the GUARDIAN trial. *J Am Coll Cardiol* 2001; 38(4):1070-1077.
12. Costa MA et al: Incidence, predictors, and significance of abnormal cardiac enzyme rise in patients treated with bypass surgery in the arterial revascularization therapies study (ARTS). *Circulation* 2001; 104(22): 2689-2693.
13. Steuer J et al: Impact of perioperative myocardial injury on early and long-term outcome after coronary artery bypass grafting. *Eur Heart J* 2002; 23(15):1219-1227.
14. Brener SJ et al: Association between CK-MB elevation after percutaneous or surgical revascularization and three-year mortality. *J Am Coll Cardiol* 2002; 40(11):1961-1967.
15. Lehrke S et al: Cardiac troponin T for prediction of short- and long-term morbidity and mortality after elective open heart surgery. *Clin Chem* 2004; 50(9):1560-1567.
16. Bolli R, Marban E: Molecular and cellular mechanisms of myocardial stunning. *Physiol Rev* 1999; 79(2):609-634.
17. Droge W: Free radicals in the physiological control of cell function. *Physiol Rev* 2002; 82(1):47-95.
18. Mallet RT, Bunger R: Energetic modulation of cardiac inotropism and sarcoplasmic reticular Ca2+ uptake. *Biochim Biophys Acta* 1994; 1224(1): 22-32.
19. Halestrap AP, Pasdois P: The role of the mitochondrial permeability transition pore in heart disease. *Biochim Biophys Acta* 2009; 1787(11): 1402-1415.
20. Verbunt RJ, Van der Laarse A: Glutathione metabolism in non-ischemic and postischemic rat hearts in response to an exogenous prooxidant. *Mol Cell Biochem* 1997; 167(1-2):127-134.
21. Sharikabad MN et al: Effect of calcium on reactive oxygen species in isolated rat cardiomyocytes during hypoxia and reoxygenation. *J Mol Cell Cardiol* 2000; 32(3):441-452.
22. Gow AJ, Ischiropoulos H: Nitric oxide chemistry and cellular signaling. *J Cell Physiol* 2001; 187(3):277-282.
23. Xia Y et al: Superoxide generation from endothelial nitric-oxide synthase. A Ca2+/calmodulin-dependent and tetrahydrobiopterin regulatory process. *J Biol Chem* 1998; 273(40):25804-25808.
24. Matsumura Y et al: Intracellular calcium level required for calpain activation in a single myocardial cell. *J Mol Cell Cardiol* 2001; 33(6): 1133-1142.
25. Tsuji T et al: Rat cardiac contractile dysfunction induced by Ca2+ overload: possible link to the proteolysis of alpha-fodrin. *Am J Physiol Heart Circ Physiol* 2001; 281(3):H1286-1294.
26. Sekili S et al: Direct evidence that the hydroxyl radical plays a pathogenetic role in myocardial "stunning" in the conscious dog and demonstration that stunning can be markedly attenuated without subsequent adverse effects. *Circ Res* 1993; 73(4):705-723.
27. Vanden Hoek TL et al: Mitochondrial electron transport can become a significant source of oxidative injury in cardiomyocytes. *J Mol Cell Cardiol* 1997; 29(9):2441-2450.
28. Sun JZ et al: Evidence for an essential role of reactive oxygen species in the genesis of late preconditioning against myocardial stunning in conscious pigs. *J Clin Invest* 1996; 97(2):562-576.
29. Li Q et al: Gene therapy with extracellular superoxide dismutase attenuates myocardial stunning in conscious rabbits. *Circulation* 1998; 98(14): 1438-1448.
30. Xu KY, Zweier JL, Becker LC: Hydroxyl radical inhibits sarcoplasmic reticulum Ca(2+)-ATPase function by direct attack on the ATP binding site. *Circ Res* 1997; 80(1):76-81.
31. Kawakami M, Okabe E: Superoxide anion radical-triggered Ca2+ release from cardiac sarcoplasmic reticulum through ryanodine receptor Ca2+ channel. *Mol Pharmacol* 1998; 53(3):497-503.
32. Josephson RA et al: Study of the mechanisms of hydrogen peroxide and hydroxyl free radical-induced cellular injury and calcium overload in cardiac myocytes. *J Biol Chem* 1991; 266(4):2354-2361.
33. Thomas GP et al: Hydrogen peroxide-induced stimulation of L-type calcium current in guinea pig ventricular myocytes and its inhibition by adenosine A1 receptor activation. *J Pharmacol Exp Ther* 1998; 286(3): 1208-1214.
34. Halestrap AP et al: Elucidating the molecular mechanism of the permeability transition pore and its role in reperfusion injury of the heart. *Biochim Biophys Acta* 1998: 1366(1-2):79-94.
35. Delcamp TJ et al: Intramitochondrial [Ca2+] and membrane potential in ventricular myocytes exposed to anoxia-reoxygenation. *Am J Physiol* 1998; 275(2 Pt 2):H484-494.
36. Tanaka M et al: Superoxide dismutase plus catalase therapy delays neither cell death nor the loss of the TTC reaction in experimental myocardial infarction in dogs. *J Mol Cell Cardiol* 1993; 25(4):367-378.
37. Gill C, Mestril R, Samali A: Losing heart: the role of apoptosis in heart disease—a novel therapeutic target? *FASEB J* 2002; 16(2):135-146.
38. Elsasser A et al: The role of apoptosis in myocardial ischemia: a critical appraisal. *Basic Res Cardiol* 2001; 96(3):219-226.
39. Maulik N, Yoshida T, Das DK: Oxidative stress developed during the reperfusion of ischemic myocardium induces apoptosis. *Free Radic Biol Med* 1998; 24(5):869-875.
40. Freude B et al: Apoptosis is initiated by myocardial ischemia and executed during reperfusion. *J Mol Cell Cardiol* 2000; 32(2):197-208.
41. Kirshenbaum LA, de Moissac D: The bcl-2 gene product prevents programmed cell death of ventricular myocytes. *Circulation* 1997; 96(5): 1580-1585.
42. Kluck RM et al: The release of cytochrome *c* from mitochondria: a primary site for Bcl-2 regulation of apoptosis. *Science* 1997; 275(5303): 1132-1136.

43. Martin SJ et al: Early redistribution of plasma membrane phosphatidylserine is a general feature of apoptosis regardless of the initiating stimulus: inhibition by overexpression of Bcl-2 and Abl. *J Exp Med* 1995; 182(5): 1545-1556.
44. Rucker-Martin C et al: Early redistribution of plasma membrane phosphatidylserine during apoptosis of adult rat ventricular myocytes in vitro. *Basic Res Cardiol* 1999; 94(3):171-179.
45. Narayan P, Mentzer RM Jr, Lasley RD: Annexin V staining during reperfusion detects cardiomyocytes with unique properties. *Am J Physiol Heart Circ Physiol* 2001; 281(5):H1931-H1937.
46. Hammill AK, Uhr JW, Scheuermann RH: Annexin V staining due to loss of membrane asymmetry can be reversible and precede commitment to apoptotic death. *Exp Cell Res* 1999; 251(1):16-21.
47. Ringer S: A further contribution regarding the influence of the different constituents of the blood on the contraction of the heart. *J Physiol* 1883; 4(1):29-42.
48. Hooker D: On the recovery of the heart in electric shock. *Am J Physiol* 1929-1930; 91:305-328.
49. Wiggers C: Studies on ventricular fibrillation produced by electric shock. *Am J Physiol* 1929; 93(1):197-212.
50. Beck CS, Pritchard WH, Feil HS: Ventricular fibrillation of long duration abolished by electric shock. *J Am Med Assoc* 1947; 135(15):985.
51. Bigelow WG, Lindsay WK, Greenwood WF: Hypothermia; its possible role in cardiac surgery: an investigation of factors governing survival in dogs at low body temperatures. *Ann Surg* 1950; 132(5):849-866.
52. Melrose DG et al: Elective cardiac arrest. *Lancet* 1955; 269(6879): 21-22.
53. Tyers GF et al: Protection from ischemic cardiac arrest by coronary perfusion with cold Ringer's lactate solution. *J Thorac Cardiovasc Surg* 1974; 67(3):411-418.
54. Colapinto ND, Silver MD: Prosthetic heart valve replacement. Causes of early postoperative death. *J Thorac Cardiovasc Surg* 1971; 61(6):938-944.
55. Iyengar SR et al: An experimental study of subendocardial hemorrhagic necrosis after anoxic cardiac arrest. *Ann Thorac Surg* 1972; 13(3):214-224.
56. Bretschneider HJ et al: Myocardial resistance and tolerance to ischemia: physiological and biochemical basis. *J Cardiovasc Surg (Torino)* 1975; 16(3):241-260.
57. Hearse DJ, Stewart DA, Braimbridge MV: Cellular protection during myocardial ischemia: the development and characterization of a procedure for the induction of reversible ischemic arrest. *Circulation* 1976; 54(2):193-202.
58. Braimbridge MV et al: Cold cardioplegia or continuous coronary perfusion? Report on preliminary clinical experience as assessed cytochemically. *J Thorac Cardiovasc Surg* 1977; 74(6): 900-906.
59. Gay WA Jr, Ebert PA: Functional, metabolic, and morphologic effects of potassium-induced cardioplegia. *Surgery* 1973; 74(2):284-290.
60. Roe BB et al: Myocardial protection with cold, ischemic, potassium-induced cardioplegia. *J Thorac Cardiovasc Surg* 1977; 73(3):366-374.
61. Tyers GF et al: Preliminary clinical experience with isotonic hypothermic potassium-induced arrest. *J Thorac Cardiovasc Surg* 1977; 74(5): 674-681.
62. Buckberg GD: A proposed "solution" to the cardioplegic controversy. *J Thorac Cardiovasc Surg* 1979; 77(6):803-815.
63. Follette DM et al: Advantages of blood cardioplegia over continuous coronary perfusion or intermittent ischemia. Experimental and clinical study. *J Thorac Cardiovasc Surg* 1978; 76(5):604-619.
64. Ferguson TB Jr et al: A decade of change—risk profiles and outcomes for isolated coronary artery bypass grafting procedures, 1990-1999: a report from the STS National Database Committee and the Duke Clinical Research Institute. Society of Thoracic Surgeons. *Ann Thorac Surg* 2002; 73(2):480-489; discussion 489-490.
65. Mentzer RM Jr: Does size matter? What is your infarct rate after coronary artery bypass grafting? *J Thorac Cardiovasc Surg* 2003; 126(2):326-328.
66. Swan H et al: Hypothermia in surgery; analysis of 100 clinical cases. *Ann Surg* 1955; 142(3):382-400.
67. Lillehei CW et al: The direct vision correction of calcific aortic stenosis by means of a pump-oxygenator and retrograde coronary sinus perfusion. *Dis Chest* 1956; 30(2):123-132.
68. Lam CR et al: Clinical experiences with induced cardiac arrest during intracardiac surgical procedures. *Ann Surg* 1957; 146(3):439-449.
69. Gerbode F, Melrose D: The use of potassium arrest in open cardiac surgery. *Am J Surg* 1958; 96(2):221-227.
70. McFarland J: Myocardial necrosis following elective cardiac arrest induced with potassium citrate. *J Thorac Cardiovasc Surg* 1960; 64:833-839.
71. Sondergaard T et al: Cardioplegic cardiac arrest in aortic surgery. *J Cardiovasc Surg (Torino)* 1975; 16(3):288-290.
72. Sondergaard T, Senn A: [109. Clinical experience with cardioplegia according to Bretschneider]. *Langenbecks Arch Chir* 1967; 319:661-665.
73. Effler DB (editorial): The mystique of myocardial preservation. *J Thorac Cardiovasc Surg* 1976; 72(3):468-470.
74. Akins CW: Noncardioplegic myocardial preservation for coronary revascularization. *J Thorac Cardiovasc Surg* 1984; 88(2):174-181.
75. Murry CE, Jennings RB, Reimer KA: Preconditioning with ischemia: a delay of lethal cell injury in ischemic myocardium. *Circulation* 1986; 74(5):1124-1136.
76. Lichtenstein SV et al: Warm heart surgery. *J Thorac Cardiovasc Surg* 1991; 101(2):269-274.
77. Salerno TA et al: Retrograde continuous warm blood cardioplegia: a new concept in myocardial protection. *Ann Thorac Surg* 1991; 51(2): 245-247.
78. Ikonomidis JS et al: Myocardial protection for coronary bypass grafting: the Toronto Hospital perspective. *Ann Thorac Surg* 1995; 60(3):824-832.
79. Teoh LK et al: The effect of preconditioning (ischemic and pharmacological) on myocardial necrosis following coronary artery bypass graft surgery. *Cardiovasc Res* 2002; 53(1):175-180.
80. Quinn DW et al: Improved myocardial protection during coronary artery surgery with glucose-insulin-potassium: a randomized controlled trial. *J Thorac Cardiovasc Surg* 2006; 131(1):34-42.
81. Mentzer RM Jr et al: Sodium-hydrogen exchange inhibition by cariporide to reduce the risk of ischemic cardiac events in patients undergoing coronary artery bypass grafting: results of the EXPEDITION study. *Ann Thorac Surg* 2008; 85(4):1261-1270.
82. Sunderdiek U, Feindt P, Gams E: Aortocoronary bypass grafting: a comparison of HTK cardioplegia vs. intermittent aortic cross-clamping. *Eur J Cardiothorac Surg* 2000; 18(4):393-399.
83. Parolari A et al: Endothelial damage during myocardial preservation and storage. *Ann Thorac Surg* 2002; 73(2):682-690.
84. Yang Q, He GW: Effect of cardioplegic and organ preservation solutions and their components on coronary endothelium-derived relaxing factors. *Ann Thorac Surg* 2005; 80(2):757-767.
85. Ovrum E et al: Cold blood versus cold crystalloid cardioplegia: a prospective randomised study of 345 aortic valve patients. *Eur J Cardiothorac Surg* 2010; 38(6):745-749.
86. Jacob S et al: Is blood cardioplegia superior to crystalloid cardioplegia? *Interact Cardiovasc Thorac Surg* 2008; 7(3):491-498.
87. Allen BS, Buckberg GD: Myocardial management in arterial revascularization, in He G-W (ed): *Arterial Grafts for Coronary Artery Bypass Surgery.* Singapore, Springer, 1999; pp 83-105.
88. Hayashi Y et al: "Initial, continuous and intermittent bolus" administration of minimally-diluted blood cardioplegia supplemented with potassium and magnesium for hypertrophied hearts. *Heart Lung Circ* 2006; 15(5):325-331.
89. Petrucci O et al: Use of (all-blood) miniplegia versus crystalloid cardioplegia in an experimental model of acute myocardial ischemia. *J Card Surg* 2008; 23(4):361-365.
90. Velez DA et al: All-blood (miniplegia) versus dilute cardioplegia in experimental surgical revascularization of evolving infarction. *Circulation* 2001; 104(12 Suppl 1):I296-302.
91. Rousou JA et al: The effect of temperature and hematocrit level of oxygenated cardioplegic solutions on myocardial preservation. *J Thorac Cardiovasc Surg* 1988; 95(4):625-630.
92. Guru V et al: Is blood superior to crystalloid cardioplegia? A meta-analysis of randomized clinical trials. *Circulation* 2006; 114(1 Suppl): I331-1338.
93. Rosenkranz ER et al: Benefits of normothermic induction of blood cardioplegia in energy-depleted hearts, with maintenance of arrest by multidose cold blood cardioplegic infusions. *J Thorac Cardiovasc Surg* 1982; 84(5):667-677.
94. Teoh KH et al: Accelerated myocardial metabolic recovery with terminal warm blood cardioplegia. *J Thorac Cardiovasc Surg* 1986; 91(6): 888-895.
95. Minatoya K et al: Intermittent antegrade warm blood cardioplegia for CABG: extended interval of cardioplegia. *Ann Thorac Surg* 2000; 69(1): 74-76.
96. Franke UF et al: Intermittent antegrade warm myocardial protection compared to intermittent cold blood cardioplegia in elective coronary surgery—do we have to change? *Eur J Cardiothorac Surg* 2003; 23(3): 341-346.
97. Casalino S et al: The efficacy and safety of extending the ischemic time with a modified cardioplegic technique for coronary artery surgery. *J Card Surg* 2008; 23(5):444-449.
98. Hayashida N et al: The optimal cardioplegic temperature. *Ann Thorac Surg* 1994; 58(4):961-971.
99. Hayashida N et al: Minimally diluted tepid blood cardioplegia. *Ann Thorac Surg* 1998; 65(3):615-621.

100. Baretti R et al: Continuous antegrade blood cardioplegia: cold vs. tepid. *Thorac Cardiovasc Surg* 2002; 50(1):25-30.
101. Mallidi HR et al: The short-term and long-term effects of warm or tepid cardioplegia. *J Thorac Cardiovasc Surg* 2003; 125(3):711-720.
102. Onorati F et al: Does antegrade blood cardioplegia alone provide adequate myocardial protection in patients with left main stem disease? *J Thorac Cardiovasc Surg* 2003; 126(5):1345-1351.
103. Pratt FH: The nutrition of the heart through the vessels of Thebesius and the coronary veins. *Am J Physiol,* 1898; 1:86.
104. Ihnken K et al: The safety of simultaneous arterial and coronary sinus perfusion: experimental background and initial clinical results. *J Card Surg* 1994; 9(1):15-25.
105. Cohen G et al: Intraoperative myocardial protection: current trends and future perspectives. *Ann Thorac Surg* 1999; 68(5):1995-2001.
106. Louagie YA et al: Continuous cold blood cardioplegia improves myocardial protection: a prospective randomized study. *Ann Thorac Surg,* 2004; 77(2):664-671.
107. Karthik S et al: A survey of current myocardial protection practices during coronary artery bypass grafting. *Ann R Coll Surg Engl* 2004; 86(6): 413-415.
108. Bonchek LI et al: Applicability of noncardioplegic coronary bypass to high-risk patients. Selection of patients, technique, and clinical experience in 3000 patients. *J Thorac Cardiovasc Surg* 1992; 103(2):230-237.
109. Raco L, Mills E, Millner RJ: Isolated myocardial revascularization with intermittent aortic cross-clamping: experience with 800 cases. *Ann Thorac Surg* 2002; 73(5):1436-1439; discussion 1439-1440.
110. Boethig D et al: Intermittent aortic cross-clamping for isolated CABG can save lives and money: experience with 15307 patients. *Thorac Cardiovasc Surg* 2004; 52(3):147-151.
111. Korbmacher B et al: Intermittent aortic cross-clamping for coronary artery bypass grafting: a review of a safe, fast, simple, and successful technique. *J Cardiovasc Surg (Torino)* 2004; 45(6):535-543.
112. Bonchek LI: Non-cardioplegic coronary bypass is effective, teachable, and still widely used: letter 1. *Ann Thorac Surg* 2003; 76(2):660-661; author reply 661-662.
113. Fujii M, Chambers DJ: Myocardial protection with intermittent cross-clamp fibrillation: does preconditioning play a role? *Eur J Cardiothorac Surg* 2005; 28(6):821-831.
114. Scarci M et al: Does intermittent cross-clamp fibrillation provide equivalent myocardial protection compared to cardioplegia in patients undergoing bypass graft revascularisation? *Interact Cardiovasc Thorac Surg* 2009; 9(5):872-878.
115. Imanaka K et al: Mitral valve surgery under perfused ventricular fibrillation with moderate hypothermia. *Circ J* 2002; 66(5):450-452.
116. Imanaka K et al: Noncardioplegic surgery for ischemic mitral regurgitation. *Circ J* 2003; 67(1):31-34.
117. Raphael J: Physiology and pharmacology of myocardial preconditioning. *Semin Cardiothorac Vasc Anesth* 2010; 14(1):54-59.
118. Kloner RA, Jennings RB: Consequences of brief ischemia: stunning, preconditioning, and their clinical implications: part 2. *Circulation* 2001; 104(25):3158-3167.
119. Cohen MV, Baines CP, Downey JM: Ischemic preconditioning: from adenosine receptor to KATP channel. *Annu Rev Physiol* 2000; 62:79-109.
120. Bolli R: The early and late phases of preconditioning against myocardial stunning and the essential role of oxyradicals in the late phase: an overview. *Basic Res Cardiol* 1996; 91(1):57-63.
121. Bolli R: The late phase of preconditioning. *Circ Res* 2000; 87(11): 972-983.
122. Kin H et al: Postconditioning attenuates myocardial ischemia-reperfusion injury by inhibiting events in the early minutes of reperfusion. *Cardiovasc Res* 2004; 62(1):74-85.
123. Hausenloy DJ, Yellon DM: New directions for protecting the heart against ischaemia-reperfusion injury: targeting the Reperfusion Injury Salvage Kinase (RISK)-pathway. *Cardiovasc Res* 2004; 61(3): 448-460.
124. O'Rourke B: Evidence for mitochondrial K+ channels and their role in cardioprotection. *Circ Res* 2004; 94(4):420-432.
125. Gomez L et al: Inhibition of mitochondrial permeability transition pore opening: translation to patients. *Cardiovasc Res* 2009; 83(2):226-233.
126. Heusch G, Boengler K, Schulz R: Inhibition of mitochondrial permeability transition pore opening: the Holy Grail of cardioprotection. *Basic Res Cardiol* 2010; 105(2):151-154.
127. Gross GJ, Peart JN: KATP channels and myocardial preconditioning: an update. *Am J Physiol Heart Circ Physiol* 2003; 285(3):H921-930.
128. Garg V, Hu K: Protein kinase C isoform-dependent modulation of ATP-sensitive K+ channels in mitochondrial inner membrane. *Am J Physiol Heart Circ Physiol* 2007; 293(1):H322-332.
129. Przyklenk K et al: Cardioprotection 'outside the box'—the evolving paradigm of remote preconditioning. *Basic Res Cardiol* 2003; 98(3): 149-157.
130. Guo Y et al: Evidence for an essential role of cyclooxygenase-2 as a mediator of the late phase of ischemic preconditioning in mice. *Basic Res Cardiol* 2000; 95(6):479-484.
131. Kloner RA et al: Previous angina alters in-hospital outcome in TIMI 4. A clinical correlate to preconditioning? *Circulation* 1995; 91(1):37-45.
132. Anzai T et al: Preinfarction angina as a major predictor of left ventricular function and long-term prognosis after a first Q wave myocardial infarction. *J Am Coll Cardiol* 1995; 26(2):319-327.
133. Ottani F et al: Prodromal angina limits infarct size. A role for ischemic preconditioning. *Circulation* 1995; 91(2):291-297.
134. Tamura K et al: Association of preceding angina with in-hospital life-threatening ventricular tachyarrhythmias and late potentials in patients with a first acute myocardial infarction. *Am Heart J* 1997; 133(3):297-301.
135. Ishihara M et al: Implications of prodromal angina pectoris in anterior wall acute myocardial infarction: acute angiographic findings and long-term prognosis. *J Am Coll Cardiol* 1997; 30(4):970-975.
136. Kloner RA et al: Prospective temporal analysis of the onset of preinfarction angina versus outcome: an ancillary study in TIMI-9B. *Circulation* 1998; 97(11):1042-1045.
137. Leesar MA et al: Nonelectrocardiographic evidence that both ischemic preconditioning and adenosine preconditioning exist in humans. *J Am Coll Cardiol* 2003; 42(3):437-445.
138. Leesar MA et al: Bradykinin-induced preconditioning in patients undergoing coronary angioplasty. *J Am Coll Cardiol* 1999; 34(3):639-650.
139. Ishii H et al: Impact of a single intravenous administration of nicorandil before reperfusion in patients with ST-segment-elevation myocardial infarction. *Circulation* 2005; 112(9):1284-1288.
140. Tomai F et al: Ischemic preconditioning during coronary angioplasty is prevented by glibenclamide, a selective ATP-sensitive K+ channel blocker. *Circulation* 1994; 90(2):700-705.
141. Tomai F et al: Effects of naloxone on myocardial ischemic preconditioning in humans. *J Am Coll Cardiol* 1999; 33(7):1863-1869.
142. Leesar MA et al: Delayed preconditioning-mimetic action of nitroglycerin in patients undergoing coronary angioplasty. *Circulation* 2001; 103(24):2935-2941.
143. Walsh SR et al: Ischaemic preconditioning during cardiac surgery: systematic review and meta-analysis of perioperative outcomes in randomised clinical trials. *Eur J Cardiothorac Surg* 2008; 34(5):985-994.
144. Yellon DM, Alkhulaifi AM, Pugsley WB: Preconditioning the human myocardium. *Lancet* 1993; 342(8866):276-277.
145. Zhao ZQ et al: Inhibition of myocardial injury by ischemic postconditioning during reperfusion: comparison with ischemic preconditioning. *Am J Physiol Heart Circ Physiol* 2003; 285(2):H579-588.
146. Darling CE et al: 'Postconditioning' the human heart: multiple balloon inflations during primary angioplasty may confer cardioprotection. *Basic Res Cardiol* 2007; 102(3): 274-278.
147. Lonborg J et al: Cardioprotective effects of ischemic postconditioning in patients treated with primary percutaneous coronary intervention, evaluated by magnetic resonance. *Circ Cardiovasc Interv* 2010; 3(1):34-41.
148. Luo W et al: Postconditioning in cardiac surgery for tetralogy of Fallot. *J Thorac Cardiovasc Surg* 2007; 133(5):1373-1374.
149. Przyklenk K et al: Regional ischemic 'preconditioning' protects remote virgin myocardium from subsequent sustained coronary occlusion. *Circulation* 1993; 87(3):893-899.
150. Hausenloy DJ, Yellon DM: Remote ischaemic preconditioning: underlying mechanisms and clinical application. *Cardiovasc Res* 2008; 79(3): 377-386.
151. Cheung MM et al: Randomized controlled trial of the effects of remote ischemic preconditioning on children undergoing cardiac surgery: first clinical application in humans. *J Am Coll Cardiol* 2006; 47(11): 2277-2282.
152. Hausenloy DJ et al: Effect of remote ischaemic preconditioning on myocardial injury in patients undergoing coronary artery bypass graft surgery: a randomised controlled trial. *Lancet* 2007; 370(9587):575-579.
153. Gustafsson AB, Gottlieb RA: Autophagy in ischemic heart disease. *Circ Res* 2009; 104(2):150-158.
154. Decker RS, Wildenthal K: Lysosomal alterations in hypoxic and reoxygenated hearts. I. Ultrastructural and cytochemical changes. *Am J Pathol* 1980; 98(2):425-444.
155. Shimomura H et al: Autophagic degeneration as a possible mechanism of myocardial cell death in dilated cardiomyopathy. *Jpn Circ J* 2001; 65(11):965-968.
156. Dosenko VE et al: Protective effect of autophagy in anoxia-reoxygenation of isolated cardiomyocyte? *Autophagy* 2006; 2(4):305-306.

157. Hamacher-Brady A, Brady NR, Gottlieb RA: Enhancing macroautophagy protects against ischemia/reperfusion injury in cardiac myocytes. *J Biol Chem* 2006; 281(40):29776-29787.
158. Matsui Y et al: Distinct roles of autophagy in the heart during ischemia and reperfusion: roles of AMP-activated protein kinase and Beclin 1 in mediating autophagy. *Circ Res* 2007; 100(6):914-922.
159. Yan L et al: Autophagy in chronically ischemic myocardium. *Proc Natl Acad Sci USA* 2005; 102(39):13807-13812.
160. Gurusamy N et al: Cardioprotection by adaptation to ischaemia augments autophagy in association with BAG-1 protein. *J Cell Mol Med* 2009; 13(2):373-387.
161. Yitzhaki S et al: Autophagy is required for preconditioning by the adenosine A1 receptor-selective agonist CCPA. *Basic Res Cardiol* 2009; 104(2):157-167.
162. Bolli R et al: Myocardial protection at a crossroads: the need for translation into clinical therapy. *Circ Res* 2004; 95(2):125-134.
163. Sommerschild HT, Kirkeboen KA: Adenosine and cardioprotection during ischaemia and reperfusion–an overview. *Acta Anaesthesiol Scand* 2000; 44(9):1038-1055.
164. Cohen MV, Downey JM: Adenosine: trigger and mediator of cardioprotection. *Basic Res Cardiol* 2008; 103(3):203-215.
165. Fremes SE et al: Phase 1 human trial of adenosine-potassium cardioplegia. *Circulation* 1996; 94(9 Suppl):II370-375.
166. Cohen G et al: Phase 2 studies of adenosine cardioplegia. *Circulation* 1998; 98(19 Suppl): II225-233.
167. Mentzer RM Jr et al: Safety, tolerance, and efficacy of adenosine as an additive to blood cardioplegia in humans during coronary artery bypass surgery. *Am J Cardiol* 1997; 79(12A):38-43.
168. Mentzer RM Jr et al: Adenosine myocardial protection: preliminary results of a phase II clinical trial. *Ann Surg* 1999; 229(5):643-649; discussion 649-650.
169. Mullane K: Acadesine: the prototype adenosine regulating agent for reducing myocardial ischaemic injury. *Cardiovasc Res* 1993; 27(1):43-47.
170. Mangano DT: Effects of acadesine on myocardial infarction, stroke, and death following surgery. A meta-analysis of the 5 international randomized trials. The Multicenter Study of Perioperative Ischemia (McSPI) Research Group. *JAMA* 1997; 277(4):325-332.
171. Mangano DT et al: Post-reperfusion myocardial infarction: long-term survival improvement using adenosine regulation with acadesine. *J Am Coll Cardiol* 2006; 48(1):206-214.
172. Avkiran M, Marber MS: Na(+)/H(+) exchange inhibitors for cardioprotective therapy: progress, problems and prospects. *J Am Coll Cardiol* 2002; 39(5):747-753.
173. Bothe W et al: Glucose-insulin-potassium in cardiac surgery: a meta-analysis. *Ann Thorac Surg* 2004; 78(5):1650-1657.
174. Fath-Ordoubadi F, Beatt KJ: Glucose-insulin-potassium therapy for treatment of acute myocardial infarction: an overview of randomized placebo-controlled trials. *Circulation* 1997; 96(4):1152-1156.
175. van der Horst IC et al: Glucose-insulin-potassium infusion inpatients treated with primary angioplasty for acute myocardial infarction: the glucose-insulin-potassium study: a randomized trial. *J Am Coll Cardiol* 2003; 42(5):784-791.
176. Timmer JR et al: Glucose-insulin-potassium infusion in patients with acute myocardial infarction without signs of heart failure: the Glucose-Insulin-Potassium Study (GIPS)-II. *J Am Coll Cardiol* 2006; 47(8): 1730-1731.
177. Lazar HL et al: Tight glycemic control in diabetic coronary artery bypass graft patients improves perioperative outcomes and decreases recurrent ischemic events. *Circulation* 2004; 109(12):1497-1502.
178. Bruemmer-Smith S et al: Glucose, insulin and potassium for heart protection during cardiac surgery. *Br J Anaesth* 2002; 88(4):489-495.
179. Lell WA et al: Glucose-insulin-potassium infusion for myocardial protection during off-pump coronary artery surgery. *Ann Thorac Surg* 2002; 73(4):1246-1251; discussion 1251-1252.
180. Barcellos Cda S, Wender OC, Azambuja PC: Clinical and hemodynamic outcome following coronary artery bypass surgery in diabetic patients using glucose-insulin-potassium (GIK) solution: a randomized clinical trial. *Rev Bras Cir Cardiovasc* 2007; 22(3):275-284.
181. Caputo M et al: Incomplete revascularization during OPCAB surgery is associated with reduced mid-term event-free survival. *Ann Thorac Surg* 2005; 80(6):2141-2147.
182. Gill IS et al: Early and follow-up angiography in minimally invasive coronary bypass without mechanical stabilization. *Ann Thorac Surg* 2000; 69(1):56-60.
183. Balacumaraswami L et al: Does off-pump total arterial grafting increase the incidence of intraoperative graft failure? *J Thorac Cardiovasc Surg* 2004; 128(2):238-244.
184. Chowdhury UK et al: Myocardial injury in coronary artery bypass grafting: on-pump versus off-pump comparison by measuring high-sensitivity C-reactive protein, cardiac troponin I, heart-type fatty acid-binding protein, creatine kinase-MB, and myoglobin release. *J Thorac Cardiovasc Surg* 2008; 135(5):1110-1119, 1119 e1-10.
185. Shroyer AL et al: On-pump versus off-pump coronary-artery bypass surgery. *NEJM* 2009; 361(19):1827-1837.

CHAPTER 16

Postoperative Care of Cardiac Surgery Patients

Zain I. Khalpey
Jan D. Schmitto
James D. Rawn

INTRODUCTION

Mortality and morbidity in cardiac surgery have continued to decline despite increases in patient age, comorbid conditions, and procedure complexity. Much of this success can be attributed to advances in critical care. This chapter outlines strategies and principles of modern postoperative care.

CARDIOVASCULAR CARE

Hemodynamic Assessment

Assessment and optimization of hemodynamics are generally the principal focus of care after cardiac surgery. Appropriate management requires knowledge of preoperative cardiac function and an appreciation of the impact of intraoperative events. The goal of postoperative hemodynamic management is the maintenance of adequate oxygen delivery to vital tissues in a way that avoids unnecessary demands on a heart recovering from the stress of cardiopulmonary bypass, ischemia, and surgery.

A basic initial hemodynamic assessment includes a review of current medications, heart rate and rhythm, mean arterial pressure, central venous pressure, and EKG analysis to exclude ischemia and conduction abnormalities. The presence of a pulmonary artery catheter enables the measurement of pulmonary artery pressures, left-sided filling pressures (pulmonary capillary wedge pressure, PCWP), and mixed venous oxygen saturation (MVO_2). Cardiac output, as well as pulmonary and systemic vascular resistances can also be calculated when a PA catheter is present. Cardiac output is determined using thermodilution or by using Fick equation. Cardiac output (CO), blood pressure (BP), and systemic vascular resistance (SVR) are related to each other using Ohm's law (Table 16-1). Reasonable minimum goals for most patients include an MVO_2 of about 60%, mean arterial pressure (MAP) greater than 65 mm Hg, and a cardiac index (CI) greater than 2 L/min/m^2. Goals should be individualized. Patients with a history of hypertension or significant peripheral vascular disease will probably benefit from higher blood pressure; patients who are bleeding or have suture lines in fragile tissue are best served with tighter control. Strategies designed to produce a supranormal cardiac index or MVO_2 have failed to demonstrate a survival advantage.[1]

Failure to achieve adequate cardiac output and end-organ oxygen delivery can be caused by many, often codependent factors. These include volume status (preload), peripheral vascular tone (afterload), cardiac pump function, heart rate and rhythm, and blood oxygen–carrying capacity.

Volume status is readily determined by invasive monitoring. Central venous pressure (CVP), unless it is very low, is an unreliable indicator of left ventricular end-diastolic volume (LVEDV). (An elevated central venous pressure can be seen in volume overload, right heart failure, tricuspid and mitral regurgitation, pulmonary hypertension, cardiac tamponade, tension pneumothorax, and pulmonary embolism.) Pulmonary artery diastolic pressure correlates with left-sided filling pressures when pulmonary vascular resistance (PVR) is normal (low). PCWP (or left atrial pressure if this is being directly measured) provides the most accurate assessment of left-sided filling pressures, and its correlation with pulmonary artery diastolic pressure should be noted to enable a more continuous assessment of left-sided pressures. Determination of optimum filling pressures is generally empiric where a wedge pressure of 15 mm Hg is generally adequate, but many patients require significantly higher pressures. Most patients arrive from the

TABLE 16-1 Common Intensive Care Values and Formulae

Early Postoperative Hemodynamic Parameters	Expected Values
Mean arterial pressure (MAP)	60–90 mm Hg
Systolic blood pressure (sBP)	90–140 mm Hg
Right arterial pressure (RAP)	5–15 mm Hg
Cardiac index (CI)	2.2–4.4 L/min/m^2
Pulmonary artery wedge pressure (PAWP)	10–15 mm Hg
Systemic vascular resistance (SVR)	1400–2800 dyn-s/cm^5
Common Hemodynamic Formulae	**Normal Values**
$CO = SV \times HR$ $CI = CO/BSA$ CO = cardiac output; HR = heart rate; SV = stroke volume; BSA = body surface area	4–8 L/min 2.2–4.0 L/min/m^2
$SV = \frac{CO\ (L/min) \times 1000\ (mL/L)}{HR}$	60–100 mL/beat (1 mL/kg/beat)
$SVI = SV \div BSA$ SVI = Stroke volume index	33–47 mL/beat/m^2
$MAP = DP + \frac{(SP - DP)}{3}$	70–100 mm Hg
$SVR = \frac{MAP - CVP \times 80}{CO}$ CVP = central venous pressure; Ohm's law: Voltage (V) = Current (I) × Resistance (R); Resistance is directly proportional to viscosity (hematocrit) and inversely proportional to the radius to the 4th power	800–1200 dyn-s/cm^5
$PVR = \frac{PAP - PCWP \times 80}{CO}$ PAP = mean pulmonary arterial pressure, PCWP = pulmonary capillary wedge pressure, PVR = pulmonary vascular resistance	50–250 dyn-s/cm^5
$LVSWI = SVI \times (MAP - PCWP) \times 0.0136$ LVSWI = left ventricular stroke work index	45–75 mg-M/beat/m^2
O_2 delivery = CO (Hb × %sat) (1.39) + (Pao_2) (0.0031) 1.39 is milliliters of oxygen transported per gram of serum hemoglobin (Hb); 0.0032 is solubility coefficient of oxygen dissolved in solution (mL/torr of Pao_2)	60–80%
A-V O_2 Difference = (1.34) (Hb) × ($Sao_2 - Svo_2$) $\text{Fick cardiac output} = \frac{\text{estimated } O_2 \text{ consumption}}{\text{A-V } O_2 \text{ difference}}$ A-V = arteriovenous oxygen difference. Oxygen consumption is measured from a nomogram based on age, sex, height, weight; Hb = serum hemoglobin (g/dL), Sao_2 = arterial oxygen saturation (%) in arterial blood, Svo_2 = mixed venous oxygen saturation (%) from the pulmonary artery in the absence of a shunt or calculated MVO_2 = (3 × SVC saturation + IVC saturation) ÷ 4, if a left-right shunt is present; 1.34 = mL O_2/g of Hb, 10 dL/L	Normal Pvo_2 = 40 torr and Svo_2 = 75% Normal Pao_2 = 100 torr and Sao_2 = 99%
$\text{Shunt fraction} = \frac{Qp}{Qs} = \frac{(Sao_2 - MVO_2)}{(Pvo_2 - Pao_2)}$ Qp = pulmonary flow (L/min); Qs = systemic flow (L/min)	Normal <5%

TABLE 16-1 Common Intensive Care Values and Formulae (*Continued*)

$EF\ (\%) = \dfrac{\text{end-diastolic volume} - \text{end-systolic volume}}{\text{end-diastolic volume}}$ EF = ejection fraction (an index of ventricular activity)	60–70%	
Respiratory Formulae	**Normal Values**	
$D(A - a)O_2 = (FIO_2) \times (713) - PaO_2 - (PaO_2 \div 0.8)$ $D(A - a)O_2$ = alveolar-arterial oxygen difference, taking FIO_2 (inspired oxygen into consideration); a sensitive index of efficiency of gas exchange	Suboptimal oxygenation >350 on 100% oxygen Or $PaO_2 < 500$ torr on 100% oxygenation	
Renal and Metabolic Values and Formulae		
$C_{CR} = \dfrac{(140 - \text{age}) \times \text{wt (kg)}}{72 \times Cr} \times 0.8$ (for females) Cockroft and Gault equation for creatinine clearance (C_{CR}) (an approximation to glomerular filtration rate, GFR) Or more precisely with 24- or 2-h urine specimen: $C_{CR} = (U_{CR} \div P_{CR}) \times$ (volume/1440 min, or 120 min) U_{CR} and P_{CR} = urinary and plasma creatinine concentrations	$C_{CR} < 55$ mL/min threshold below which surgical risk increases[98]	
Evaluating Oliguria	**Prerenal**	**Renal**
BUN/Cr	>20:1	<10:1
U/P creatinine	>40	<20
U_{osm}	>500	<400
U/P osmolality	>1.3	<1.1
Urine specific gravity	>1.020	1.010
U_{Na} (mEq/L)	<20	>40
FE_{Na}	<1%	>2%
Urinary sediment	Hyaline casts	Tubular epithelial casts; granular casts
BUN = urea nitrogen, serum (7–18 mg/dL)		
$FE_{Na} = \dfrac{U_{Na} \times P_{CR}}{P_{Na} \times U_{CR}} \times 100$ FE_{Na} = Fractional excretion of sodium; U and P are urinary and plasma concentrations of sodium and creatinine, respectively	Normal, 1–3%	
Anion gap = $(Na^+) - ([Cl^-] + [HCO_3^-])$ Elevated by: ethanol, uremia (chronic renal failure), diabetic ketoacidosis, paraldehyde, phenformin, iron tablets, isoniazide, lactic acidosis (CN^-, CO, shock), ethanol, ethylene glycol, salicylates	Normal = 8–12	
$C_{H_2O} = V - C_{osm}$ $C_{osm} = U_{usm} \times V/P_{osm}$ C_{H_2O} = Free water clearance; V = urine flow rate; P_{osm} and U_{osm} = plasma and urine osmolarity, respectively	P_{osm} = 275–295 mOsmol/kg	

(*Continued*)

TABLE 16-1 Common Intensive Care Values and Formulae (*Continued*)

Capillary Fluid Exchange (Starling Forces)	Edema
Net Filtration Pressure = P_{net} = ([P_c − P_{i0} − [π_c − π_i]) K_f = filtration constant (capillary permeability) Net fluid flow = (P_{net}) (K_f) P_c = capillary pressure—tends to move fluid out of capillary P_i = interstitial fluid pressure—tends to move fluid into capillary π_c = plasma colloid oncotic pressure—tends to cause osmosis of fluid into capillary π_I = interstitial fluid colloid osmotic pressure—tends to cause osmosis of fluid out of capillary	1. High P_c; heart failure 2. Low π_c; nephritic syndrome 3. High K_f; toxins, sepsis, inflammatory cytokines 4. High π_i; lymphatic blockage

Prosthetic Heart Valves: Current Anticoagulation Regimens (Adapted from Nagaranjan, 2004)[99]	Coumadin Target INR/Aspirin 81 mg
AVR mechanical	2.5–3.0/yes, if high risk
AVR bioprosthetic (tissue)	2.5–3.0 (3 months) or none if aspirin used/yes
MVR mechanical	2.5–3.5 (indefinitely)/yes, if high risk
MVR bioprosthetic or MV repair	2.5–3.0 (3 months; continue 1 year if history of embolism; indefinitely if AF and LA thrombus at time of surgery)/ yes, after 3 months
AVR and MVR mechanical	2.5–3.0 (indefinitely)/yes
AVR and MVT bioprosthetic (tissue)	2.5–3.0 (3 months)/yes, after 3 months
Atrial fibrillation (with any of the above)	2.5–3.0 (indefinitely)/yes

AF = atrial fibrillation; AVR = aortic valve replacement; MVR = mitral valve replacement; high risk = AF, myocardial infarction, enlarged left atrium (LA), endocardial damage, low EF, history of systemic emobolism despite adequate anticoagulation.

operating room with a significant net fluid gain, but much of this excess volume is extravascular owing to third space and pleural cavity accumulation. Vasoplegia is often created by a systemic inflammatory response to cardiopulmonary bypass (CPB), and it is common to have a significant continuous volume requirement in the immediate postoperative period. Urine output and bleeding are common sources of ongoing fluid loss. Hypothermia promotes vasoconstriction. As patients rewarm, changes in peripheral vascular tone contribute to labile hemodynamics, which are often best treated with volume replacement.

Peripheral vascular tone needs to be sufficient to provide the patient with adequate blood pressure; excess vasoconstriction can increase the systemic vascular resistance tremendously, therefore creating dangerous levels of hypertension and decrease cardiac output. Decreased afterload can be caused, in part, by medications (sedative, anesthetic agents, and preoperative ACE inhibitors), increased temperature, and a systemic inflammatory response to cardiopulmonary bypass, whereas increases in afterload can be caused by medications, hypothermia, or increased sympathetic output (including pain and anxiety), or may be secondary to hypovolemia or pump failure.

Left ventricular pump function can be influenced by levels of exogenous or endogenous inotropes, postoperative stunning, ischemia or infarction, valve function, acidosis, electrolyte abnormalities, hypoxia, or cardiac tamponade. Bradycardia, arrhythmias, and conduction defects can also adversely affect cardiac output.

The oxygen-carrying capacity of blood is a function of hematocrit and oxygenation. A hematocrit of 23% and oxygen saturation greater than 92% is usually adequate for a stable postoperative patient.

It is important not to allow the evaluation of the patient to become obscured by too many numbers or theories, and an overall assessment of the patient is always more important than any single parameter. Trends in hemodynamic parameters are usually more important than isolated values. Patients generally do well if they have warm, well-perfused extremities, a normal mental status and good urine output (greater than 0.5 cc/kg/min). Acute changes in hemodynamic status are common postoperatively, and vigilant monitoring enables care to be more preemptive than reactive.

Hemodynamic Management

Fluid Management

As emphasized, the goal of postoperative hemodynamic management is the maintenance of adequate end-organ perfusion without taxing the heart unnecessarily. Assessment and optimization of intravascular volume status are generally the first steps in this process. Most patients have ongoing fluid requirements in the immediate postoperative period that can be caused by persistent third spacing, warming, diuresis, vasodilation, and bleeding. Careful monitoring of fluid balances and filling pressures should guide volume resuscitation. Starling curves are highly variable; it is helpful to correlate cardiac output and MVO_2 with changes in volume status. Patients with ventricular hypertrophy (eg, those with a history of hypertension or aortic stenosis) or diastolic dysfunction usually need higher filling pressures. Patients with persistently low filling pressures despite aggressive fluid administration are usually either bleeding or vasodilated. Calculation of CO and SVR can often help sort this out. In the case of significant vasodilation, judicious use of a pressor agent can help to decrease fluid requirements. Inotropic agents should not be administered for the treatment of hypovolemia. Fluid requirements can often be reduced after extubation; decreased intrathoracic pressure improves venous return.

The choice of an optimal resuscitation fluid is unresolved. In the acute setting, colloid infusions achieve comparable hemodynamic effects with less volume when compared with crystalloid solutions. After 1 hour, 80% of 1000 cc of 5% albumin solution is retained intravascularly. In situations characterized by loss of vascular endothelial integrity (ie, after CPB), albumin may redistribute into the interstitial space and increase third space fluid accumulation. One study has shown that the accumulation of extravascular pulmonary water is unaffected by the prime type or the type of fluid administered postoperatively.[2] The largest prospective randomized controlled study comparing colloid with crystalloid has been unable to demonstrate a difference in outcomes.[3] Albumin and hetastarch provide comparable hemodynamic benefits, although hetastarch should be avoided in bleeding or coagulopathic patients or in those with renal impairment.

Although unusual in the immediate postoperative period, volume overload is a common problem in the days after surgery. If patients have normal cardiac function, they often diurese appropriately without intervention. Conversely, volume overload is a common cause of postoperative heart failure. Diuretics and vasodilators are frequently required in patients with impaired pump function before or after surgery, or in those who received large volumes of fluid perioperatively. Patients with impaired renal function may require renal replacement therapy (ultrafiltration, continuous veno-venous hemofiltration, or hemodialysis) to become euvolemic. Rapid diuresis accompanied by inadequate electrolyte repletion is frequently arrhythmogenic.

Pharmacologic Support

Medications are used perioperatively to provide vasoconstriction, venous and arterial vasodilation, inotropic support, and treatment of arrhythmias. As summarized in Table 16-2, many of the medications commonly used have multiple actions. Selection of appropriate agents depends on accurate hemodynamic assessment.

Pressors are indicated for vasodilated patients who have normal pump function and are unresponsive to volume. These agents include alpha agents (neosynephrine) and vasopressin. Methylene blue has demonstrated efficacy in vasopressor-resistant hypotension. Pressors can contribute to peripheral ischemia and vasospasm of coronary arteries and arterial conduits. Careful monitoring of extremity perfusion and electrocardiographic changes is required when using these agents.

Vasodilators are indicated for hypertensive patients and for patients who are normotensive with poor pump function. Nitroglycerin and sodium nitroprusside are commonly used in the immediate postoperative period. Both have the advantage of being short-acting and easy to titrate. Both can cause hypoxia by inhibiting pulmonary arterial hypoxic vasoconstriction and increasing blood flow through poorly oxygenated lung. Nitroglycerin is a stronger venodilator than an arterial dilator, and can increase intercoronary collateral blood flow, but patients can quickly become tachyphylactic. Prolonged nitroprusside use can lead to cyanide toxicity, and methemaglobin levels must be monitored. Nicardipine is a calcium channel blocker with minimal effects on contractility or AV nodal conduction; it appears to have the efficacy of nipride without its toxicity. Nesiritide, or brain naturetic peptide, promotes diuresis in addition to vasodilation and may have beneficial lusitropic effects in patients with diastolic dysfunction.

Hypertension can also be treated with beta blockers. These agents work by decreasing heart rate and contractility. Esmolol is useful in the presence of labile blood pressure because of its short half-life. Labetolol combines beta- and alpha-adrenergic blockade. Patients whose pump function is inotrope dependent should not receive beta blockers.

Inotropic agents are indicated when low cardiac output persists despite optimization of fluid status (preload) and vascular tone (afterload). These agents include beta-adrenergic agents (dobutamine) and cyclic nucleotide phosphodiesterase inhibitors (milrinone). Both of these agents increase cardiac output by increasing myocardial contractility and reducing afterload through peripheral vasodilation. Dobutamine is shorter-acting and easier to titrate; milrinone achieves increases in cardiac output with lower myocardial oxygen consumption. Both are arrhythmogenic and can exacerbate coronary ischemia. Both epinephrine and norepinephrine combine beta- and alpha-adrenergic agonist effects; they are pressors in addition to positive inotropes. Dopamine in low doses causes splanchnic and renal vasodilation. Because perioperative beta-blockade has been shown to improve mortality and morbidity after cardiac surgery, it seems reasonable to avoid the gratuitous use of inotropes,

TABLE 16-2 Common ICU Scenarios and Management Strategies

Cardiac Output Syndromes					
MAP	**CVP**	**CO**	**PCW**	**SVR**	**Strategy**
Normotensive	High	Low	High	Normal/high	Venodilator/diuretic/inotrope
Hypertension	High	Normal	High	High	Vasodilator/iNO/iPGI$_2$
Hypotension	Low	Low	Low	Normal	Volume
Hypotension	High	Low	High	High	Inotrope/IABP/vasodilator
Hypotension	Normal/low	Normal/high	Normal/low	Low	alpha-agent

CO = cardiac output; CVP = central venous pressure; iNO = inhaled nitric oxide; iPGI$_2$ = inhaled prostacyclin; SVR = systemic vascular resistance.

Commonly Used Vasoactive Drugs and Hemodynamic Effects						
Pharmacologic Agent	**HR**	**PCW**	**CI**	**SVR**	**MAP**	**MVO$_2$**
Inotropic Agents						
Dobutamine	↑↑	↓	↑	↓	↑↓	↑↔
Milrinone	↑	↓	↑	↓↓	↓	↑↓
Mixed Vasoactive Agents						
Epinephrine	↑↑	↑↓	↑	↑	↑	↑
Norepinephrine	↑↑	↑↑	↑	↑↑	↑↑	↑
Dopamine	↑↑	↑↓	↑	↑↓	↑↓	↑
Vasopressor Agents						
Phenylephrine	↔	↑	↔	↑↑	↑↑	↑↔
Vasopressin	↔	↔	↔	↑↑	↑↑	↑↔
Methylene blue	↔	↔	↔	↑	↑	↑
Vasodilating Agents						
Nitroglycerine	↑	↓↔	↔	↓	↓	↔↓
Nitroprusside	↑↑	↓↔	↔	↓↓	↓↓	↔↓
Nicardipine	↔	↔	↔	↓↓	↓↓	↔
Nesiritide	↔	↓↔	↔	↓	↓	↔

CI = Cardiac index; HR = heart rate; MAP = mean arterial pressure; MVO$_2$ = mixed venous oxygen saturation; PCW = pulmonary capillary wedge; SVR = systemic vascular resistance.

NASPE/BPEG Pacemaker Identification Codes[100]

Code Positions				
I	*II*	*III*	*IV*	*V*
Chamber Paced	**Chamber Sensed**	**Response to Sensing**	**Programmable Functions**	**Antitachyarrhythmia Functions**
V—ventricle	**V**—ventricle	**T**—triggers pacing	**P**—programmable rate and/or output	**P**—antitachyarrhythmia
A—atrium	**A**—atrium	**I**—inhibits pacing	**M**—multiprogrammable	**S**—shock
D—double	**D**—double	**D**—triggers and inhibits pacing	**C**—communicating functions (telemetry)	**D**—dual (pacer and shock)
O—none	**O**—none	**O**—none	**R**—rate modulation	**O**—none
S—single chamber	**S**—single chamber	—	**O**—none	—

TABLE 16-2 Common ICU Scenarios and Management Strategies (*Continued*)

Postoperative Mediastinal Bleeding

Bleeding Scenario	Diagnosis	Strategy
<50 cc/h Stable BP, coagulopathy	Post-CPB	Observation
100 cc/h		
Hypothermic	Hypothermia (see above)	Rewarming strategies
Acute hypotension (MAP<50 mm Hg)		Fluid resuscitation (aim MAP 60–65 mm Hg)
Diffuse bloody ooze	Borderline coagulopathy	
Coagulopathy:		PEEP trial (5–10 cm H_2O),
1. High PTT, PT	Rebound heparin effect	Coagulation screen
2. INR >1.4	Deficient clotting factors	Heparin level; protamine
3. Low fibrinogen	Deficient clotting factors	Fresh-frozen plasma
4. Platelets $<10^5/\mu L$	Thrombocytopenia	Fresh-frozen plasma
5. Platelets $>10^5/\mu L$	Platelet dysfunction	Platelet pool
6. Bleeding >10 min	Fibrinolysis	DDAVP
7. Bleeding >30 min (High D-dimers, evidence of fibrinolysis)	Fibrinolysis	Tranexamic acid, ε-aminocaproic acid, aprotinin
>200–300 cc/h **>200 cc/h for 4 h** **>300 cc/h for 2–3 h** **>400 cc/h for 1 h**	Surgical bleeding	Surgical reexploration

BP = Blood pressure; CPB = cardiopulmonary bypass; DDAVP = desmopressin (synthetic vasopressin); FDP = fibrin and fibrinogen degradation products; PEEP = positive end-expiratory pressure; PT = prothrombin time; PTT = activated partial thromboplastin time.

and efforts should be made to rapidly wean these agents when they are no longer required.

Heart Rate and Rhythm Management

Deviations from normal sinus rhythm can cause significant clinical deterioration and optimization of heart rate, and rhythm is frequently an effective way to improve hemodynamic status.

Pacing

Within normal rate ranges, cardiac output increases linearly with heart rate, and pacing is often very helpful (see Table 16-2). However, it is important to carefully monitor the response to pacing. For example, sinus bradycardia is often more effective than ventricular pacing at a more normal rate. Ventricular pacing can cause ventricular dysfunction and dys-synchrony, and the loss of consistent filling from atrial contraction can lead to clinical deterioration. If possible, atrial pacing is preferred to AV pacing, which is preferred to ventricular pacing. Pacing too rapidly can adversely affect cardiac performance by decreasing filling time or inducing ischemia. Internal pacemakers can often be reprogrammed to improve output.

Heart block can occur after aortic, mitral, and tricuspid valve surgery. It is also associated with inferior myocardial infarction and can be secondary to medications (eg, digoxin, amiodarone, calcium channel blockers, and beta blockers). If a bi-atrial trans-septal approach to the mitral valve is employed, the sinus rhythm is can be lost owing to the division of the sinoatrial node.[4] Heart block is frequently transient. If the ventricular escape rate is absent or insufficient, pacing wire thresholds need to be carefully monitored and backup pacing methods employed (by transvenous wire or pacing pulmonary artery catheter, external pacing pads) if needed while waiting for placement of a permanent pacemaker.

Ventricular Arrhythmias

Nonsustained ventricular tachycardia (VT) is common after cardiac surgery and typically a reflection of perioperative ischemia/reperfusion injury, electrolyte abnormalities (typically hypokalemia and hypomagnesemia), or an increase in exogenous or endogenous sympathetic stimulation. Generally, nonsustained VT is more important as a symptom of an underlying cause requiring diagnosis and correction than as a cause of hemodynamic instability.

Sustained VT persisting for more than 30 seconds or associated with significant hemodynamic compromise requires more aggressive treatment. Ongoing ischemia should be ruled out (coronary angiography is necessary), electrolytes should be replaced, and inotropes should be minimized. Beta blockers, amiodarone, and lidocaine are useful therapies. Electrocardioversion should be employed if sustained VT causes significant compromise.

Atrial Fibrillation and Flutter

Background. The incidence of postoperative atrial fibrillation (POAF) after cardiothoracic surgery is 30 to 50%,[5] and has been shown to be higher in the elderly (age ≥ 75 years), renally impaired and COPD patients.[6] This is associated with an increased risk of stroke, longer hospitalization, higher cost, and greater risk of long-term mortality.[7]

Prophylaxis. The incidence of POAF is 20 to 40% in CABG patients, but it is generally even more common in those undergoing valve and combined procedures. POAF is typically a transient reversible phenomenon that may develop in patients who possess an electrophysiologic substrate for the arrhythmia that is present before or as a result of surgery. Numerous studies support the efficacy of beta blockers in POAF prevention; they are currently the most common medication used in POAF prophylaxis. Therefore, beta blockers should be started or resumed as soon as they can be safely tolerated after cardiac surgery. Inotropic support, hemodynamic compromise, COPD, and AV block (PR interval greater than 0.24 millisecond, or second- or third-degree block) are contraindications. Beta blockers appear to provide more effective prophylaxis when they are dosed with high frequency and titrated to produce an effect on heart rate and blood pressure. Sotalol and amiodarone are also effective for prophylaxis but not superior. Beta blockers also confer benefits other than atrial fibrillation prophylaxis, are easy to titrate, and do not have the toxicities associated with amiodarone. Although beta blockers and amiodarone are known to reduce the incidence of postoperative AF after cardiac surgery, the postinflammatory milieu after cardiothoracic surgery may also be involved in the pathogenesis of postoperative arrythmias. For example, IL6 and CRP elevation postoperatively and AF have been linked. Although statin treatment appeared to lower the risk of postoperative AF in some initial observational studies, no benefit was noted in a recent, well-conducted cohort study of more than 4000 patients. In the only randomized clinical trial in this arena Atorvastatin started 7 days before cardiac surgery was associated with a greater than 60% reduction in the incidence of postoperative AF among 200 patients undergoing coronary artery bypass graft (CABG) surgery. However, the extraordinarily high AF rate (approximately 60%) in the control group of this study was not representative of the experience at most centers. Furthermore, beta blockers, which unequivocally reduce postoperative AF, were not administered routinely after surgery and the number of patients undergoing concomitant valve surgery was small (n = 41). Although in patients treated with postoperative beta blockers, statin treatment reduces the incidence of POAF; when used at higher dosages, there is not enough evidence that statin treatment prevents AF among patients receiving postoperative beta blockers. Our group has shown that statin therapy in the elderly and renally impaired patients undergoing noncoronary cardiac surgery may be renoprotective. The recently started SPAR Trial (an international, prospective multicenter trial) will investigate perioperative high-dose use of statins (greater than 40 mg simvastatin, 3-hydroxy-3-methylglutaryl-coenzyme A [HMG-CoA] reductase inhibitors) to reduce the postinflammatory milieu after cardiac surgery and therefore might decrease the incidence of POAF.

Treatment. There are many treatment strategies for the management of atrial fibrillation. We have found that the use of a guideline reduces the incidence of atrial fibrillation and decreases the disruption and anxiety that it creates (see Fig. 16-1). The principal premise of this strategy is the recognition that for most patients with new-onset atrial fibrillation, the arrhythmia is self-limited (90% of patients are in sinus rhythm within 6 to 8 weeks independent of treatment approach). The pursuit of a rate control and anticoagulation strategy usually produces outcomes comparable to a rhythm control strategy. Our prophylactic regimen begins with metoprolol 12.5 to 25 mg PO qid and is titrated upward as tolerated.

RACE II. Guidelines recommend strict rate control in patients with permanent atrial fibrillation (AF), but this is still not based on clinical evidence. RACE II (Rate Control Efficacy in Permanent Atrial Fibrillation: a Comparison between Lenient versus Strict Rate Control II) was a prospective, multicenter, randomized, open-label, noninferiority trial designed to compare two rate-control strategies in patients with permanent AF (Fig. 16-2). Six hundred fourteen patients were assigned to undergo a lenient rate-control strategy (resting heart rate 110 beats per minute) or a strict rate-control strategy (resting heart rate 80 beats per minute and heart rate during moderate exercise 110 beats per minute). The primary outcome was a composite of death from any cause, hospitalization for heart failure, stroke, systemic embolism, bleeding, and life-threatening arrhythmic events. To achieve the target heart rates patients were given beta blockers, calcium channel blockers, and/or digoxin. During follow-up ranging from 2 to 3 years, the primary outcome occurred in 12.9% of patients in the lenient-control group, as compared with 14.9% of patients in the strict-control group (p = .0001 for the prespecified noninferiority margin; see Fig. 16-1). More patients in the lenient-control group met the heart rate targets (97.7 versus 67.0% in the strict-control group; p = .001) with fewer total visits (75 versus 684; p = .001). In conclusion, lenient rate control was noninferior to strict rate control in the prevention of major cardiovascular events in patients with permanent AF. Furthermore, for both patients and health care providers, lenient rate control is more convenient, because fewer outpatient visits and examinations are needed. The clinical implications of RACE II are that lenient rate control may be adopted as a first-choice rate-control strategy in patients with permanent AF. Nevertheless, because the study was relatively small, large-scale studies have to reveal the long-term effect of lenient rate versus strict control in patients with AF in more detail.

1. **Initial assessment:** The management of atrial fibrillation should be guided by the answers to the after three questions:
   a. **Is the patient symptomatic?** Atrial fibrillation is generally well tolerated, and overly aggressive management can cause significant morbidity. Nonetheless, the

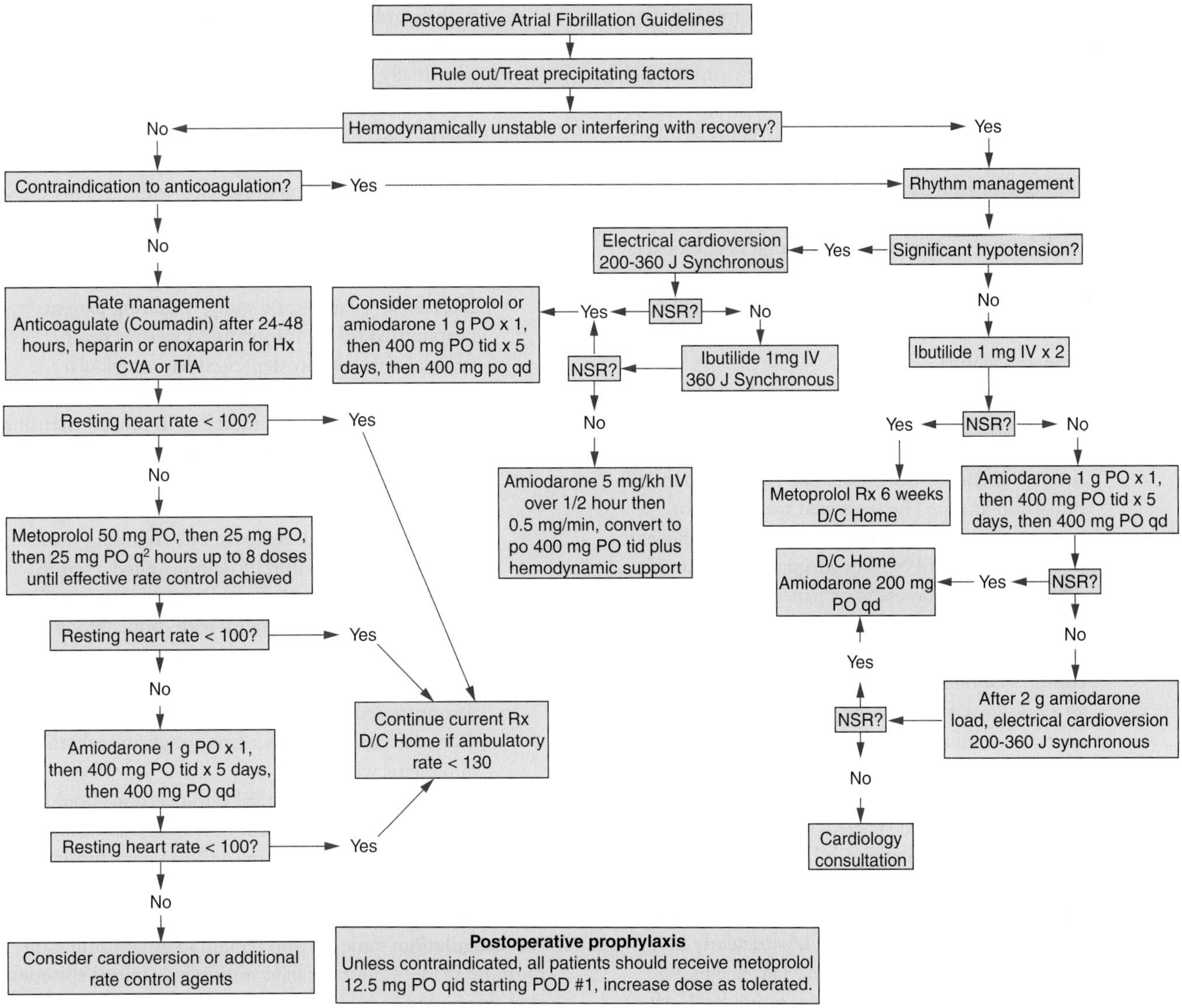
Postoperative Atrial Fibrillation Guidelines
Rule out/Treat precipitating factors
Hemodynamically unstable or interfering with recovery?
No
Yes
Contraindication to anticoagulation?
Yes
Rhythm management
No
Rate management Anticoagulate (Coumadin) after 24-48 hours, heparin or enoxaparin for Hx CVA or TIA
Resting heart rate < 100?
Yes
No
Metoprolol 50 mg PO, then 25 mg PO, then 25 mg PO q2 hours up to 8 doses until effective rate control achieved
Resting heart rate < 100?
Yes
No
Amiodarone 1 g PO x 1, then 400 mg PO tid x 5 days, then 400 mg PO qd
Resting heart rate < 100?
Yes
No
Consider cardioversion or additional rate control agents
Continue current Rx D/C Home if ambulatory rate < 130
Consider metoprolol or amiodarone 1 g PO x 1, then 400 mg PO tid x 5 days, then 400 mg po qd
Electrical cardioversion 200-360 J Synchronous
Yes
Significant hypotension?
NSR?
Yes
No
Ibutilide 1mg IV 360 J Synchronous
NSR?
No
Amiodarone 5 mg/kh IV over 1/2 hour then 0.5 mg/min, convert to po 400 mg PO tid plus hemodynamic support
No
Ibutilide 1 mg IV x 2
NSR?
Yes
No
Metoprolol Rx 6 weeks D/C Home
Amiodarone 1 g PO x 1, then 400 mg PO tid x 5 days, then 400 mg PO qd
D/C Home Amiodarone 200 mg PO qd
Yes
NSR?
No
Yes
NSR?
After 2 g amiodarone load, electrical cardioversion 200-360 J synchronous
No
Cardiology consultation
Postoperative prophylaxis
Unless contraindicated, all patients should receive metoprolol 12.5 mg PO qid starting POD #1, increase dose as tolerated.

FIGURE 16-1 Postoperative atrial fibrillation guidelines. *(Adapted with permission from Maisel WH, Rawn JD, Stevenson WG: Atrial fibrillation after cardiac surgery. Ann Intern Med 2001; 135:1061.)*

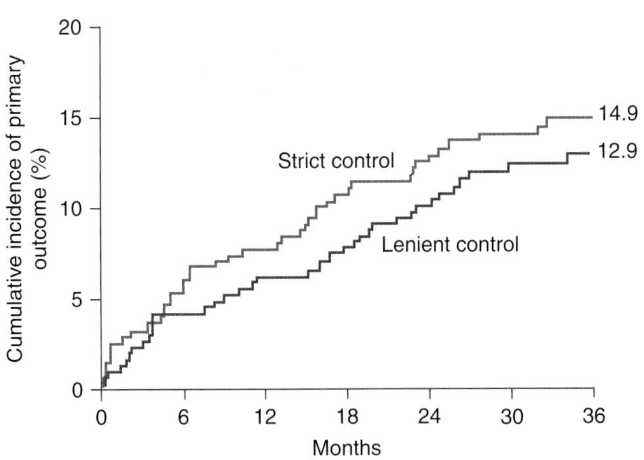
Cumulative incidence of primary outcome (%)
20
15
10
5
0
Strict control
Lenient control
14.9
12.9
0
6
12
18
24
30
36
Months

FIGURE 16-2 RACE II. Kaplan-Meier estimates of the cumulative incidence of the primary outcome, according to treatment group. The numbers at the end of the Kaplan-Meier curves is the estimated cumulative incidence of the primary outcome at 3 years.

first step in the management of atrial fibrillation is an assessment of its hemodynamic significance. Significant symptoms may respond to rate control alone or may require chemical or electrical cardioversion. Evidence of compromise include hypotension, changes in mental status, decreased urine output, impaired peripheral perfusion, angina pectoris symptoms, and decreased cardiac output or increased filling pressures.

b. **What are the precipitating factors?** Appropriate management of atrial fibrillation requires identification and treatment of potential risk factors. Atrial fibrillation can result from ischemia, atrial distention, increased sympathetic tone, electrolyte imbalances (particularly hypokalemia and hypomagnesemia precipitated by diuresis), acid-base disturbances, sympathomimetic medications (inotropes, bronchodilators), beta-blocker withdrawal, pneumonia, atelectasis, and pulmonary embolism.

c. **What are the goals of therapy?** Hemodynamic stability is the primary goal. For most patients, rate control is sufficient because 90% of patients with new-onset atrial fibrillation after cardiac surgery will be in normal sinus rhythm in 6 weeks. Evidence of hemodynamic compromise or interference with recovery should prompt chemical or electrical cardioversion.

2. **Drug therapy:** Agents can be conveniently divided into rate control and rhythm control agents, although beta blockers are also effective in converting atrial fibrillation postoperatively. Mono drug therapy is generally better than poly drug therapy.
   a. **Rate control agents:**
      (1) **Beta blockers.** Metoprolol should be first-line therapy in most patients and can be given per os (PO) or intravenously. Metoprolol should be titrated to effect with a heart rate goal less than 100 beats/min at rest. The suggested treatment for new-onset atrial fibrillation is 50 mg PO, followed by 25 mg PO until NSR or adequate rate control is achieved, up to 8 doses. Some patients may require over 400 mg/day PO.
      (2) **Calcium channel blockers.** Diltiazem is the agent of choice. It should be initiated as a bolus at 0.25 mg/kg IV, followed by 0.35 mg/kg IV, followed by a continuous infusion 5 to 15 mg.
      (3) **Digoxin** can be considered in patients with contraindications to beta blockers, in particular those with poor ejection fraction. There is some evidence that it increases atrial automaticity. It has a half-life of 38 to 48 hours in patients with normal renal function, significant potential toxicity, and a narrow therapeutic range. Levels must be monitored, particularly in patients with renal insufficiency. Many agents, including amiodarone, increase its serum level. After chemical cardioversion, attempts should be made to minimize the number of rate control agents used.
   b. **Antiarrhythmics**
      (1) **Metoprolol** (± diltiazem)
      (2) **Ibutilide** is given as a 1-mg intravenous bolus and repeated once if cardioversion fails to occur. Patients need to be monitored for a small but significant incidence of torsades de pointes, which may be increased if given in conjunction with amiodarone.
      (3) **Amiodarone** can cause myocardial depression and heart block; significant hypotension is most commonly associated with rapid bolus infusion. Significant toxicity is associated with prolonged use of amiodarone, and consideration should be given to discontinuing the drug within 6 weeks of surgery.
      (4) **Adenosine** is helpful in the treatment of supraventricular tachycardia (SVT). (It should be avoided in transplant recipients, partially revascularized patients and those with atrial flutter.)
      (5) **Dronedarone** is an amiodarone analog without iodine moiety in its structure, and is similar to amiodarone with regard to its structural and electrophysiologic properties.[8] Dronedarone is largely denuded of the potentially life-threatening adverse effects of antiarrhythmics. Major clinical studies have demonstrated both rhythm and rate-controlling efficacy of dronedarone compared to placebo without any serious adverse effects in patients with AF. However, the ANDROMEDA trial (The Antiarrhythmic-Trial with Dronedarone in Moderate-to-Severe Congestive Heart Failure Evaluating Morbidity Decrease),[9] a large-scale study, including patients hospitalized for symptomatic congestive heart failure (with severely depressed left ventricular systolic functions), was prematurely terminated because of the increased mortality in the dronedarone arm compared with placebo, indicating a lack of safety in this group of patients. Conversely, the recently published ATHENA study (including more than 4600 high-risk patients, but excluding those with severe heart failure)[10] demonstrated a significant reduction in cardiovascular hospitalizations and cardiovascular mortality with dronedarone compared with placebo. In contrast, the DIONYSOS study, comparing dronedarone with amiodarone, demonstrated better safety but lower efficacy of dronedarone for the maintenance of sinus rhythm in patients with AF.[11]

3. **Electrical cardioversion:** Electrical cardioversion should be used emergently for the treatment of hemodynamically unstable atrial fibrillation, starting at 200 J (synchronous). Sedation should be used. Overdrive pacing can be attempted in patients with atrial wires who are in atrial flutter.
4. **Anticoagulation:** Patients who remain in atrial fibrillation for more than 24 hours or have multiple sustained episodes over this period should be started on Coumadin in the absence of contraindications. Heparin (IV or low molecular weight SQ) should be considered after 48 hours in patients with a history of stroke or TIAs or who have a low ejection fraction. Coumadin should not be initiated in patients who may require permanent pacer placement.

Postoperative Ischemia and Infarction

Postoperative ischemia and infarction can be caused by inadequate intraoperative myocardial protection, kinked, spasmed, or thrombosed conduits, thrombosed endarterectomized vessels, or embolization by air or atherosclerotic debris. It should be suspected in the presence of otherwise unexplained poor pump function, ST changes, new bundle branch block or complete heart block, ventricular arrhythmias, or enzyme elevation. Electrocardiographic changes should be correlated with the anatomy of known atherosclerotic or revascularized territories. Air embolism preferentially involves the right coronary artery, and inferior ST changes are generally present in the operating room. It typically resolves within hours. It is worth noting that nonspecific ST changes are common postoperatively and usually benign. Pericardial changes are generally characterized by diffuse concave ST elevations, accompanied by a pericardial rub and delayed in onset by at least 12 hours after surgery.

New wall motion abnormalities or mitral regurgitation diagnosed echocardiographically can help determine the hemodynamic significance of suspected ischemia or infarction. Knowledge of the quality of conduits, anastamoses, and target vessels is critical in planning management strategy (eg, there may be little to gain and much to lose in attempting to improve flow to a small, highly diseased posterior descending artery with poor run-off). On the other hand, if the patient appears to be at risk for significant myocardium, a timely trip to the operating room or cardiac catheterization laboratory can dramatically improve outcomes. Ongoing ischemia should prompt consideration of standard strategies, including anticoagulation, beta blockade, and nitroglycerin as tolerated. Intra-aortic balloon placement should be considered to minimize inotropc requirements, decrease myocardial oxygen requirements, and/or minimize infarct size.

Right Ventricular Failure and Pulmonary Hypertension

Right ventricular failure can be a particularly difficult postoperative problem. It can be caused by perioperative ischemia or infarction or acute increases in pulmonary vascular resistance (PVR). Preexisting pulmonary hypertension is commonly caused by left-sided heart failure, aortic stenosis, mitral valve disease, and pulmonary disease. Chronic pulmonary hypertension is characterized by abnormal increased vasoconstriction and vascular remodeling.[12] Acute increases in PVR are commonly caused by acute left ventricular dysfunction, mitral valve insufficiency or stenosis, volume overload, pulmonary edema, atelectasis, hypoxia, or acidosis. Pulmonary embolism should also be considered, but it is rare in the immediate postoperative period. As the right heart fails it becomes distended, central venous pressure increases, tricuspid regurgitation may develop, and pulmonary artery pressures and left-sided filling pressures become inadequate. Strategies for reversing this potentially fatal process begin with identifying potentially reversible etiologies. Volume status and left-sided function should be optimized. The right ventricle has its own Starling curve, and although the failing RV often needs more volume to ensure adequate left-sided filling, overdistention will worsen function. Judicious use of PEEP to recruit atelectatic lung and hyperventilation can decrease the impact of pulmonary vasoconstriction mediated by hypoxia and hypercapnia. Use of intravenous vasodilators (commonly nitroprusside, nitroglycerin, tolazoline [PGI_2], hydralazine, prostacyclin, adenosine, and nicardipine) to reduce PVR is frequently limited by systemic hypotension. Inotropes (typically milrinone, which also provides vasodilation) can be beneficial. Because no intravenous vasodilator is selective for the pulmonary vasculature, topical administration can be significantly more effective in reducing PVR without causing systemic hypotension. Inhaled NO and PGI_2 have comparable efficacy. They can also improve oxygenation by shunting blood to ventilated lung.

Valve Diseases: Special Postoperative Considerations

Aortic Valve Replacement

The different pathophysiologies associated with aortic stenosis (primarily a pressure overload phenomenon) versus aortic insufficiency (volume overload) can result in significantly different postoperative courses.

Aortic Stenosis. Aortic stenosis can lead to the development of a hypertrophied, noncompliant left ventricle. For some patients, replacement of a stenotic valve allows a ventricle conditioned to pumping against abnormally high afterload to easily achieve supranormal levels of cardiac output and blood pressure postoperatively. Meticulous blood pressure control is frequently required to avoid disrupting fresh suture lines. In some patients, the degree of ventricular hypertrophy can lead to dynamic outflow obstruction; the condition is most effectively treated with volume, beta blockers, and afterload augmentation. Even without dynamic outflow obstruction, reduced compliance (diastolic dysfunction) can create significant hemodynamic compromise if the patient becomes hypovolemic or loses normal sinus rhythm. (Up to 30% of stroke volume can be dependent on synchrony between atria and ventricle.) The placement of atrial wires in addition to ventricular wires can provide significant advantages in the event that the patient is bradycardic or experiences heart block postoperatively.

Aortic Regurgitation. The left ventricle in a patient with aortic regurgitation is frequently dilated without significant hypertrophy and often functions poorly postoperatively. Optimization of volume, afterload, inotropy, and rhythm in these patients is often challenging.

Mitral Valve Repair/Replacement

Mitral Regurgitation. After repair or replacement of an incompetent mitral valve, increased afterload and consequent greater wall stress unmask LV dysfunction. Frequently inotropic support and systemic vasodilation is required to reduce the afterload mismatch seen after surgery. Occasionally LV dysfunction can be the result of inadvertent suture placement over the circumflex coronary artery.

Mitral Stenosis. Unlike patients with mitral regurgitation, patients with mitral stenosis typically have preserved LV function. Exacerbation of preexisting pulmonary hypertension is common, however. Postoperative strategies focus on optimizing right ventricular function and decreasing pulmonary vascular resistance.

BLEEDING, THROMBOSIS, AND TRANSFUSION STRATEGIES

One of the principal challenges of cardiac surgery is to achieve sufficient anticoagulation while supported on cardiopulmonary bypass without experiencing excessive bleeding postoperatively. Not surprisingly, patients undergoing off-pump CABG experience a significant reduction in postoperative bleeding and blood product transfusion requirements.[13] Excessive bleeding and its complications, including blood product transfusions, cause significant morbidity and mortality.

Preoperative Evaluation

Preoperative evaluation includes documenting a history of abnormal bleeding or thrombosis, and obtaining basic coagulation studies, a hematocrit and platelet count. A history of recent heparin exposure associated with thrombocytopenia, should suggest a diagnosis of heparin induced thrombocytopenia (HIT). Confirmation of the presence of IgG directed against platelet factor 4 (the prevalence of these antibodies in patients with previous heparin exposure can be up to 35%)[14] requires either a delay in surgery until the assay is negative (usually 3 months), or if surgery is more urgently required, an alternative anticoagulation strategy is mandated. Recent experience with the direct thrombin inhibitor bivalirudin appears promising in this scenario.

Preoperative medications that can increase bleeding risk are common. Aspirin inhibits cyclooxygenase, reduces the synthesis of thromboxane-A_2 (TXA_2), and decreases platelet aggregation. Preoperative aspirin use modestly increases postoperative bleeding, but preoperative and early postoperative use (ie, within 6 hours) is beneficial to outcome and ultimate survival.[15] Other antiplatelet agents have more profound impacts on platelet function. The glycoprotein IIb/IIIa inhibitors eptifibatide (Integrilin) and tirofiban (Aggrastat) are sufficiently short-acting that surgery can be safely conducted despite recent exposure. Abciximab (Reopro) usually requires a 24- to 48-hour delay in surgery, if feasible, to avoid catastrophic bleeding. Clopidogrel (Plavix) is a thienopyridine derivative that blocks platelet ADP P_2Y_{12} receptors, inhibiting platelet activation by preventing ADP-mediated responses, decreasing alpha-granule release, lowering TXA_2 and P-selectin expression with some anti-inflammatory effects. Cessation of clopidogrel is preferred 5 days preoperatively, but is not advisable in patients with drug eluting coronary artery stents. Customarily, Coumadin (which inhibits the vitamin-dependent clotting factors II, VII, IX, and X) is discontinued 4 to 7 days preoperatively to allow gradual correction of the INR.

Intraoperative Strategies

Multiple intraoperative strategies have evolved to prevent unnecessary bleeding blood product transfusion. Antithrombolytics ε-aminocaproic acid (Amicar) and Tranexamic acid (Cyclokapron) inhibit plasminogen activation and limit fibrinolysis. Topical use of tranexamic acid intraoperatively before closure may be a simple and effective way to reduce postoperative bleeding,[16] particularly in patients with friable tissue who are having reoperations or have had previous exposure to chest irradiation. Aprotinin (Trasylol), a serine protease inhibitor and activates factor XII (Hageman factor), has antifibrinolytic properties (main hemostatic effect) and protection of platelets. The drug is used primarily for patients who are at high risk for postoperative bleeding. A recent retrospective study has questioned aprotinin's safety.[17]

Retrograde autologous priming of the CPB circuit involves displacing circuit prime at the initiation of CPB with the patient's blood draining both antegrade through the venous cannula and retrograde through the arterial cannula.[18] This strategy has been shown to significantly decrease the requirement for blood transfusion after CABG. The use of heparin-bonded circuitry has enabled the safe use of lower anticoagulation targets while on bypass. Careful attention to hemostasis intraoperatively and avoidance of excessive use of the cell saver (which depletes platelets and clotting factors) pays dividends postoperatively.

Postoperative Bleeding

Strategies for avoiding postoperative hypothermia are also very important. Hypothermia (less than or equal to 35°C) on arrival to the ICU is associated with delayed extubation, shivering, and increased peripheral O_2 consumption, hemodynamic instability, atrial and ventricular arrhythmias, increased systemic vascular resistance, and coagulopathy.

Most patients are mildly coagulopathic postoperatively, but only a minority bleeds excessively. Postoperative coagulopathy can be caused by residual or rebound heparin effects after CPB, thrombocytopenia (qualitative and quantitative), clotting factor depletion, hypothermia, and hemodilution. Chest tube outputs persistently greater than 50 to 100 cc per hour or other clinical evidence of bleeding demand attention.

The treatment of postoperative bleeding depends initially on making a judgment: Is bleeding surgical, coagulopathic, or both? Surgical bleeding is treated as soon as possible by reexploration, whereas coagulopathies are corrected in the ICU. Coagulopathic patients rarely have significant clot formation in their chest tubes. Standard maneuvers include warming the patient, controlling blood pressure, extra PEEP, additional ε-amino caproic acid, calcium gluconate, and blood products. In general, blood products should not be used to correct coagulation abnormalities unless the patient is bleeding significantly. All allogeneic blood products can contribute to transfusion-related lung injury and have other adverse effects. Protamine is rarely indicated and can increase bleeding. Desmopressin (DDAVP) is a synthetic vasopressin analog that acts by increasing the concentration of von Willebrand factor, an important mediator of platelet adhesion. It is beneficial in patients with von Willebrand disease and those with severe platelet dysfunction secondary to uremia anitplatelet agents.

Recombinant factor VIIa (rFVIIa) is a drug approved for use in hemophiliacs that has been used successfully in arresting bleeding in patients with life-threatening hemorrhage after cardiac surgery. On combination with tissue factor, it activates the extrinsic coagulation system via factor X, resulting in thrombin generation and prompt correction of the PT with no evidence of systemic thrombosis.[19]

Mediastinal Reexploration

Reexploration should be considered when CT outputs are greater than 400 mL/h for 1 hour, greater than 300 mL/h for 2 to 3 hours, and 200 mL/h for 4 hours (see Table 16-2)[20] or if signs of tamponade or hemodynamic instability develop. Tamponade should be considered in the presence of hypotension, tachycardia, elevated filling pressures, increasing inotrope requirements, pulsus paradoxus, and/or equalization of right and left atrial pressures. An echocardiogram can be useful in this situation but cannot rule out tamponade. Chest x-rays are a necessary element of the evaluation for bleeding; look for widening of the mediastinum or evidence of hemothorax. Chest x-rays should be repeated on all patients with initial high chest tube output that later subsides to ensure that chest tubes have not clotted.

Autotransfusion

Autotransfusion of shed mediastinal blood remains controversial. Red blood cell viability in unwashed shed mediastinal blood is comparable to that of autologous whole blood.[21] Additionally, there is evidence indicating no apparent clinical coagulopathy (low fibrinogen levels, but normal coagulation times at 1 and 24 hours) after reinfusion of shed blood.[22] This method of blood salvage is without allogeneic transfusion risks and is possibly immunostimulatory.

Blood Transfusions

Blood transfusions can both benefit and harm. Despite meticulous preoperative planning, correcting drug-induced coagulopathies and intraoperative cell saving techniques with "bloodless" fields bleeding postoperatively is inevitable. The Canadian Critical Care Trials group restricted transfusion for hemoglobin to less than 7.0 g/dL versus 10.8 g/dL, with no change in mortality rate.[23] An NIH consensus conference concluded that patients with a hemoglobin level greater than 10.9 g/dL do not require blood, whereas those with less than 7.0 g/dL benefited from blood.[24] Tissue perfusion is dependent on cardiac output and the hemoglobin level. A safe lower limit for the hematocrit in the stable postoperative patient after cardiac surgery is 22 to 24%.[25] A marginal MVO_2 or evidence of ischemia provides a rationale for increasing hematocrit.

To inform decisions about blood transfusion, Murphy and coworkers aimed to quantify associations of transfusion with clinical outcomes and cost in patients having cardiac surgery.[26] Therefore, the authors linked clinical, hematology, and blood transfusion databases with the UK population register. Murphy found that transfusion was associated with increased relative cost of admission (any transfusion 1.42 times [95% CI, 1.37 to 1.46], varying from 1.11 for 1 U to 3.35 for 9 U). The author revealed also that transfused patients, at any time after their operations, were less likely to have been discharged from hospital (hazard ratio [HR], 0.63; 95% CI, 0.60 to 0.67) and were more likely to have died (0 to 30 days: HR, 6.69; 95% CI, 3.66 to 15.1; 31 days to 1 year: HR, 2.59; 95% CI, 1.68 to 4.17; 1 year: HR, 1.32; 95% CI, 1.08 to 1.64). Murphy concluded that red blood cell transfusion in patients having cardiac surgery is strongly associated with both infection and ischemic postoperative morbidity, hospital stay, increased early and late mortality, and hospital costs.

Immunomodulation

It has become evident that blood transfusions have immunomodulating effects (by either alloimmunization or tolerance induction) that may increase the risk of nosocomial infections, transfusion-associated graft versus host disease (TAGVHD), transfusion-related lung injury (TRALI), cancer recurrence, and the possible development of autoimmune diseases later in life. Furthermore, the risk of "newer" transfusion-transmitted diseases has become recognized. Proinflammatory mediators and cytokines have been associated with an increased risk of wound infection, sepsis, pulmonary, and renal insufficiency.[27]

RESPIRATORY CARE

Postoperative Pulmonary Pathophysiology

After the introduction of cardiopulmonary bypass nearly 50 years ago pulmonary complications were recognized and attributed to pulmonary vascular overload. "Pump lung" ranges from a mild to severe pulmonary dysfunction secondary to the inflammatory response provoked by the bypass circuit. Increases are seen in the A-a gradient, pulmonary shunt fraction, and pulmonary edema, with a resultant decrease in compliance. Many inflammatory mediators have been implicated. Complement is activated (C3a, C5b-C9) and can directly damage pulmonary endothelium as well as sequester neutrophils. When activated, these neutrophils release oxygen-free radicals and proteases, furthering injury. Macrophage cytokine production and platelet degranulation have also been demonstrated in models of bypass-induced lung injury.[28] Transfusion-related lung injury may also exacerbate lung dysfunction.

In spite of increased knowledge of the mechanisms of injury, to date there have been no interventions with clear clinical benefit. To the contrary, administration of methylprednisolone in a randomized double-blinded study significantly increased A-a gradient and shunt fraction, decreased both static and dynamic compliance and delayed early extubation in a dose-dependent manner.

Assessment on Arrival

On arrival to the intensive care unit, auscultation of the lungs should be performed to ensure equal breath sounds and absence of bronchospasm. Ventilator settings are usually a mandatory mode such as SIMV or AC, with FIO_2 100%, rate 12 to 18, TV 6 to 10 cc/kg, PEEP 5 cm H_2O, and PS 8 to 10 cm H_2O if IMV. A review of the initial postoperative CXR review confirms proper endotracheal tube position 2 to 3 cm above the carina, and proper nasogastric tube and intravenous line placement. Clinicians should be alert for pneumothoraces, hemothoraces, and a widened mediastinum. Arterial blood gas should confirm adequate oxygenation, and absence of hypercapnea or metabolic acidosis. Arterial blood gas results should be correlated with pulse oximetry and minute ventilation.

Troubleshooting Hypoxia

As discussed, oxygenation in all patients will be diminished compared with the baseline. However, the inability to wean FIO_2 below 50% within the first few postoperative hours should prompt a reevaluation, because many causes can be treated.

Sometimes simply replacing the pulse oximeter probe onto another finger or an earlobe will improve the reported oxygen saturation. This is particularly true in patients with peripheral vasoconstriction, and more frequent ABGs may be necessary for correlation. The use of hemodynamic drips such as nitroglycerin, milrinone, and particularly sodium nitroprusside can increase shunt fraction (by abrogating hypoxic pulmonary vasoconstriction) enough to require a high FIO_2 to maintain adequate oxygenation. Increasing PEEP to improve alveolar recruitment may help or changing agents may be necessary.[29] Nebulizer treatments may be necessary for bronchospasm, and repeat CXR may demonstrate pneumothorax, retained hemothorax, retained mediastinal hematoma, atelectasis, or a new infiltrate representing aspiration.

Atelectasis, particularly in the left lower lobe, is present to some degree in nearly all patients. Bibasilar atelectasis is believed to be the combined product of the prolonged supine position, and intraoperative muscle relaxation, allowing upward displacement of abdominal contents and the diaphragm. This reduces functional reserve capacity (FRC) by up to 1 L. On the left, this is compounded by pleurotomy for internal mammary artery take-down, compression of the left lung, and decreased ventilatory tidal volumes to clear the field for IMA dissection. Left lower lobar atelectasis caused by phrenic nerve injury is not likely to resolve acutely with bronchoscopic aspiration. However, lobar atelectasis in general, especially when associated with mucus plugging, is improved by bronchoscopic aspiration in approximately 80% of cases.[30] A prospective study comparing bronchoscopy with aggressive chest physiotherapy found the two techniques to be equally effective,[31] but only if one adheres to the chest physiotherapy regimen.

Sedation

Sedation and pain relief in cardiac surgery "fast-tracking" relies on short-acting agents, including propofol, fentanyl, and midazolam. Dexmedetomidine is a highly selective $alpha_2$-adrenoreceptor agonist and has anxiolytic, sympatholytic, and analgesic effects without contributing to respiratory depression, oversedation, or delirium. It may provide myocardial protection.[32] Hypotension and bradycardia can occur.

Early Extubation

Stable patients with a normal mental status can often be extubated either in the operating room or within a few hours of arrival in the intensive care unit. Once an arterial blood gas has confirmed adequate oxygenation and ventilation, pulse oximetry and monitoring of minute ventilation can guide extubation, often without the need for subsequent blood gases.

Patients usually excluded from planning for early extubation include those with: (1) preoperative pulmonary failure requiring intubation; (2) uncompensated congestive heart failure with pulmonary edema; (3) severe pulmonary hypertension or right heart failure requiring hyperventilation or nitric oxide; (4) cardiogenic shock (including requirement of intra-aortic balloon counterpulsion); (5) deep hypothermic circulatory arrest; (6) persistent hypothermia less than 35.5°C; (7) persistent hypoxia PAO_2:FIO_2 less than 200; (8) persistent acidosis with pH less than 7.30; (9) persistent mediastinal bleeding; or (10) cerebrovascular accident or reduced mental status (inability to follow commands or protect airway).

Weaning and Extubation

For patients unable to wean from the vent immediately after surgery, a spontaneous breathing trial (30 minutes of spontaneous breathing with 5 cm H_2O of pressure support or unassisted breathing through a T-tube) has been shown to be the most accurate predictor of a successful extubation. Breathing trials are typically discontinued for signs of distress such as respiratory frequency greater than 35/minute, O_2 saturation less than 90%, HR greater than 140 bpm, SBP greater than 180 or less than 90 mm Hg, agitation, diaphoresis, or anxiety[33] introduced the concept of a rapid-shallow breathing index (RSBI; f/VT; breaths/minute/liter). In their study of medical patients, the RSBI was calculated over one minute of unassisted spontaneous breathing through a T-tube. A RSBI of greater than 105 indicated a 95% likelihood that a subsequent weaning trial would not lead to successful extubation, and an RSBI less than 105 indicated an 80% likelihood of subsequent success. The minute ventilation V_E and MIP were significantly less predictive.

The strategy of daily or intermittent spontaneous breathing trials (SBT) was also directly compared with weaning strategies based on stepwise reduction in the frequency of intermittent mandatory ventilation (IMV), or stepwise reduction in the level of pressure-support ventilation (PSV). Daily or intermittent SBTs lead to successful extubation two to three times earlier than either IMV or PSV weans.[33]

In a prospective series of ICU patients, the 20% false-positive predictive value of a RSBI less than 105 is overwhelmingly caused by newly acquired problems,[34] with only 7% of failures being referable to the process that initially required intubation. No direct study of the outcome of these strategies exists in the cardiac surgery population, but they are in broad clinical use, and we recommend at least daily SBTs.

The decision to extubate must take into account the combined factors of mechanics as described in the preceding, as well as estimation of the patient's ability to manage secretions and protect his or her airway.[35]

Extubation Failure

Overall, approximately 5% of cardiothoracic patients require reintubation.[36] Patients with COPD have a 14% incidence,[37] whereas those with a past history of stroke have a 10% incidence.[38] Other risk factors include: NYHA class IV functional status, renal failure, need for intra-aortic balloon counterpulsion, reduced PO_2:FIO_2, reduced vital capacity, longer operating room time, longer CPB run and longer initial ventilatory requirement.[39] Unfortunately in ICU patients overall reintubation is an ominous predictor of increased length of stay and increased mortality.

Chronic Ventilation and Tracheotomy

In the early 1960s, translaryngeal intubation was associated with a prohibitively high rate of tracheal stenosis. As a result, a consensus existed that tracheotomy should be performed for patients requiring mechanical ventilation for longer than 3 days.[40] Low-pressure cuffs and soft tubes have since muddled this question of timing. A consensus subsequently evolved in that patients who continue to require mechanical ventilation at 2 weeks should undergo tracheotomy. Data surrounding this practice has been soft. Several trials suggest earlier discontinuation of mechanical ventilation and reduced complications associated with earlier tracheotomy.[40,41] Causation is not clear, but compelling arguments for reduced dead-space and airway resistance, as well as facilitated pulmonary toilet is made in favor of early tracheotomy. It is also strongly suggested that clinician behavior is positively affected by the presence of a tracheostomy tube. Namely, more aggressive attempts at weaning and discontinuation of mechanical support are made because reconnecting the ventilator is easy.[41]

Percutaneous dilatational tracheotomy (PDT) performed in the ICU is increasingly becoming recognized as a safe procedure. A recent randomized prospective study of medical patients projected to require more than 14 days of mechanical ventilation[42] compared two groups: PDT within 48 hours and 14 to 16 days. One hundred twenty patients were enrolled. In the early PDT group, there was a strongly significant reduction in duration of mechanical ventilation (7.6 ± 4.0 versus 17.4 ± 5.3 days, $p < .001$), incidence of pneumonia (5 versus 25%, $p < .005$), and mortality (31.7 versus 61.7 %, $p < .005$). There was no difference in incidence or severity of tracheal stenosis identified in-hospital and at 10 weeks. With hope and with increasing evidence, early tracheotomy will come to be viewed more widely as beneficial to patient recovery rather than as an admission of defeat.

Pleural Effusion

Accumulation of fluid in the pleural space is common after cardiac surgery, particularly on the left side, and usually resolves with time and diuresis. The specific cause is often unknown, but a combination of factors can contribute, including fluid overload, hypoalbuminemia, pericardial and pleural inflammation (postpericardiotomy syndrome), atelectasis, pneumonia, or pulmonary embolism. Pleural effusion can cause chest pain or heaviness, shortness of breath, or hypoxia, or be implicated in leukocytosis. Symptomatic effusions should be tapped, and usually thoracentesis does not have to be repeated. Nonsteroidal anti-inflammatory agents are used to treat postperiocardotomy syndrome. Occasionally, tube thoracostomy drainage may be necessary until resolution of the inciting process. In contrast, retained hemothorax should be evacuated to avoid delayed developent of fibrothorax requiring decortication.

Pneumonia

Nosocomial pneumonias have high associated mortality and the incidence of ventilator-associated pneumonia increases approximately 1% per day.[43] Clinical diagnosis involves identification of a new or progressive infiltrate on CXR, change in character of sputum, leukocytosis, and fever.[44] Expectorated sputum cultures are considered to be very inaccurate, and directed bronchosopic sampling is preferred. Proper bronchoalveolar lavage requires large volumes of irrigant (greater than 100 cc) and is infrequently performed. More commonly tracheobronchial aspiration is performed using several cc of normal saline. Gram stain containing greater than 25 squamous epithelial cells per LPF indicates oral contamination. More than 25 neutrophils per LPF suggest infection. Quantitative culture of 10^5 to 10^6 cfu/cc ("moderate to numerous," "3 to 4+") is indicative of infection, whereas less than or equal to 10^4 cfu/cc ("rare to few," "1 to 2+") is more suggestive of colonization. Gram-negative organisms are the most common, and should be the target of first-line empiric antibiotic coverage. Specific patient factors and culture results and sensitivities will further refine antibiotic therapy.[45]

The important role of pulmonary toilet in both the prevention and treatment of nosocomial pneumonias cannot be overemphasized. All patients should be encouraged to get out of bed and ambulate (even if attached to a ventilator), turn, cough, and deep breathe with chest physiotherapy and bronchodilators. Sterile in-line suctioning should be performed in ventilated patients to aid in secretion clearance. Nasotracheal suctioning is extremely effective in unintubated patients in that the procedure stimulates very strong coughing and secretion clearance. Therapeutic fiberoptic bronchoscopy can also be performed.

Pulmonary Embolism

Deep vein thrombosis (DVT) and pulmonary thromboembolism (PE) are considered uncommon in the cardiac surgery population. Reported incidence of PE ranges from 0.5 to 3.5%, accounting for only 0.3 to 1.7% of perioperative deaths. This is believed to result from large intraoperative doses of heparin, both a quantitative and qualitative thrombocytopenia post-CPB, and increased use of antiplatelet agents and anticoagulants, as well as early ambulation. A recent autopsy study demonstrated a 52% incidence of DVT and that 20% of deceased patients have minor PE,[46] and that PE is identified as the cause of death in 7%. Unfortunately, risks of bleeding and heparin-induced thrombocytopenia make the choice of heparin DVT prophylaxis problematic. Intermittent pneumatic compression devices are effective if patients and staff are compliant with their use.

The diagnosis of PE requires a high index of suspicion, and should be considered in any patient who postoperatively acquires a newly increased PaO_2:FIO_2 gradient, shortness of breath, or reduced exercise tolerance, particularly in the setting of a clear or unchanged CXR. Diagnosis is fairly reliably obtained by PE-protocol thin-cut high-speed helical computed tomography of the chest,[47] although accuracy is still influenced by pretest probability.[48]

RENAL AND METABOLIC SUPPORT

Perioperative Renal Dysfunction/ Insufficiency

The new onset of renal dysfunction after cardiac surgery is correlated with significant morbidity and mortality. The incidence of ARF in CABG patients in the 1997 STS database was 3.14%, and 0.87% of these patients required dialysis.[49]

Chertow studied 43,642 VA patients undergoing CABG or valve surgery.[50] The overall risk of acute renal failure requiring dialysis was 1.1%. The mortality rate in this group was 63.7% compared with 4.3% in patients without ARF. Decreased myocardial function and advanced atherosclerosis were independent risk factors for the development of dialysis-dependent renal failure.

Patients with preoperative renal dysfunction (serum creatinine greater than 1.5 mg/dL) have a higher incidence of stroke, bleeding complications, dialysis, prolonged mechanical ventilation, length of stay, and death. Chertow found that preoperative renal function correlated with postoperative renal failure. The risk of ARF was 0.5, 0.8, 1.8, and 4.9%, with baseline serum creatinine concentrations of less than 1 mg/dL, 1.0 to 1.4 mg/dL, 1.5 to 1.9 mg/dL, and 2.0 to 2.9 mg/dL, respectively. Chronic dialysis patients undergoing cardiac surgery have an 11.4% operative mortality rate, a 73% complication rate, and a 32% 5-year actuarial survival rate.[51] Cardiac surgery after renal transplantation has an associated operative mortality rate of 8.8%.[52]

Patients with recent or long-standing hypertension should undergo renal angiography at the time of catheterization to assess renal artery stenosis, which if significant, can be treated preoperatively in hope of improving postoperative renal function. To optimize preoperative renal function, contrast loads should be minimized and patients should be well hydrated and receive renoprotective agents (eg, *N*-acetylcysteine).

Effects of Cardiopulmonary Bypass on Renal Function

Operative considerations include limiting the duration of CPB and maintenance of mean arterial pressures greater than 60 mm Hg. Additional effects of CPB include trauma to the blood constituents, especially erythrocytes, with increased free hemoglobin levels and microparticle embolic insults to the kidneys. Hypothermia (during rewarming, vasodilation, and hyperemia of tissue beds result in third spacing of fluid), hemodilution (reduces viscosity of blood and plasma oncotic pressure), and ischemia reperfusion injury can influence renal function. Additionally, CPB leads to an increased release of catecholomines, hormones (rennin, aldosterone, angiotensin II, vasopressin, atrial natriuretic peptide, urodilan)[53] and inflammatory cytokines (kallikrein, bradykinin), which also affect renal function adversely. These adverse stimuli cause low renal blood flow, decreased glomerular filtration rate (GFR), and an increase in renal vascular resistance. Hypotension and pressor agents accentuate this response. Ultrafiltration is used in long pump runs to decrease volume overload in patients with renal dysfunction.

Independent of preoperative renal function, the primary postoperative goal is the maintenance of adequate renal perfusion pressure and a urine output greater than the 0.5 cc/kg/h. Brisk diuresis (greater than 200 to 300 cc/h) is common after CPB. Volume replacement and maintenance of adequate blood pressure and cardiac output are required for adequate renal perfusion. The best measure of kidney perfusion is adequate urine output independent of diuretics. Beyond optimizing hemodynamics and avoiding nephrotoxic medications, there is no convincing evidence that treatment with diuretics, mannitol, dopamine, fenoldapam, nesiritide, or any other agent is renoprotective. This is not to say, however, that these agents are not beneficial in promoting diuresis and avoiding renal replacement therapies in the event of renal dysfunction.

Electrolyte Disturbances

Calcium

Levels of ionized calcium (normal, 1.1 to 1.3 mmol/L) are critical for myocardial performance and are involved in reperfusion injury. Hypocalcemia causes a prolonged QT interval. Postoperatively hypocalcemia is common after CPB or an episode of hemodilution, sepsis, or citrated blood transfusions. The concentration of calcium ion is greatest in the intracellular space, with small amounts in the extracellular fluid (ECF). Calcium levels bound to albumin change with the levels of serum albumin, whereas ionized levels remain unchanged.

Potassium

Potassium fluxes during cardiac surgery can be significant and affect cardiac automaticity and conduction. Cardioplegia, decreased urine output, decreased insulin levels, and RBC hemolysis all contribute to hyperkalemia.[54] Brisk diuresis, insulin, and alkalosis can cause hypokalemia.[55] Aggressive treatment of hypokalemia decreases the incidence of perioperative arrhythmias. Serum potassium levels and replacement protocols are integral parts of the early postoperative management. Serum potassium rises logarithmically with replacement; larger quantities are required to treat significant hypokalemia.

Magnesium

Magnesium (normal, 1.5 to 2 mEq/L) is the second most common intracellular cation after potassium. It is involved in endothelial cell homeostasis,[56] cardiac excitability, and muscle contraction through its role as an ATP cofactor and calcium antagonist, it is also closely involved in the regulation of intracellular potassium.[57] After hemodilution and CPB, hypomagnesaemia is common (greater than 70% of patients), and is associated with an increased risk of atrial fibrillation and torsades de pointes.[58]

Endocrine Dysfunction

Diabetes Mellitus

Up to 30% of patients have diabetes (type I or II) in the cardiac surgery population. After CPB the hormonal stress response (increased growth hormone, catecholomines, and cortisol) causes hyperglycemia (even in nondiabetics) with a decrease in insulin production; this may persist for up to 24 hours postoperatively and is exacerbated by exogenous catecholamine administration. Tight control of blood glucose levels with continuous insulin infusions has been shown to reduce the incidence of sternal wound infection by an order of magnitude. Recently, a more aggressive approach aimed at maintaining blood glucose levels at or below 110 mg/dL in critically ill patients resulted in a reduction in mortality rate from 8.0 to 4.6% at 12 months.[59]

NICE-Sugar Study. The NICE-Sugar Study was performed to determine the optimal target range for blood glucose in critically ill patients.[60] Therefore, the study investigators investigated in 6104 patients intensive glucose control within 24 hours after admission to an intensive care unit (ICU). Adults who were expected to require treatment in the ICU on three or more consecutive days were randomly assigned to undergo either intensive glucose control, with a target blood glucose range of 81 to 108 mg/dL (4.5 to 6.0 mmol/L), or conventional glucose control, with a target of less than or equal to 180 mg/dL (less than or equal to 10.0 mmol/L). Both groups had similar characteristics at baseline. A total of 829 patients (27.5%) in the intensive-control group and 751 (24.9%) in the conventional-control group died (odds ratio for intensive control, 1.14; 95% confidence interval, 1.02 to 1.28; $p = .02$). The treatment effect did not differ significantly between operative (surgical) patients and nonoperative (medical) patients (odds ratio for death in the intensive-control group, 1.31 and 1.07, respectively; $p = .10$). Severe hypoglycemia (blood glucose level, p, 1.31 and 1.07, respectimmol per liter]) was reported in 206 of 3016 patients (6.8%) in the intensive-control group and 15 of 3014 (0.5%) in the conventional-control group ($p < .001$). There was no significant difference between the two treatment groups in the median number of days in the ICU ($p = .84$) or hospital ($p = .86$) or the median number of days of mechanical ventilation ($p = .56$) or renal-replacement therapy ($p = .39$).

In conclusion, the study investigators of the NICE-Sugar Study summarize that intensive glucose control leads to an increase of mortality among adults in the ICU; a blood glucose target of less than or equal to 180 mg/dL resulted in lower mortality than did a target of 81 to 108 mg/dL.

Adrenal Dysfunction

The strain of cardiac surgery activates the hypothalamic-pituitary-adrenal (HPA) axis and increases plasma ACTH and cortisol levels. Subclinical adrenal insufficiency is present in up to 20% of the elderly population and can be unmasked by the stress of surgery. Any patient taking exogenous steroids within 6 months of surgery should receive stress-dose steroids perioperatively. Any patient exhibiting prolonged, unexplained vasodilatory shock should be suspected of having adrenal insufficiency. A cosyntropin stimulation test should be performed for diagnosis. In the interim, dexamethasone may be administered IV without interfering with the test.

RELEVANT POSTOPERATIVE COMPLICATIONS

Neurologic

Central Nervous System

The incidence of stroke after cardiac surgery is procedure specific and varies between 1 to 4%. Ricotta and colleagues associated carotid stenosis (greater than 50%), redo heart surgery, valve surgery, and prior stroke with increased postoperative neurologic risk.[61] John and colleagues reviewed 19,224 patients in New York state.[62] The stroke rate was 1.4% after CABG, with a 24.8% mortality rate in that group. Multivariable logistic regression identified the after predictor variables: calcified aorta, prior stroke, age, carotid artery disease, duration of CPB, renal failure, peripheral vascular disease, smoking, and diabetes. Intraoperative factors that may cause postoperative neurologic deficits include particulate macroembolization of air, debris, or thrombus, microembolization of white blood cells, platelets, or fibrin,[63] duration of CPB,[64] cerebral hypoperfusion during nonpulsatile CPB, and hypothermic circulatory arrest.[65]

Neuropsychiatric deficits (neurocognitive dysfunction, delirium, seizures) are very common, occurring in up to 50 to 70% of patients after cardiac surgery. The cause of these neuropsychiatric disorders is uncertain and remains controversial. Although the dysfunction remains unclear, patients remain at risk for long-term cognitive decline. Van Dijk and colleagues[66] reviewed 12 cohort studies; a pooled analysis of six comparable studies showed 22.5% of patients to have a cognitive deficit at 2 months after operation. However, this may be related to progression of underlying cerebrovascular disease rather than CABG or cardiopulmonary bypass.[67]

Up to 50% of cardiac surgery patients experience delirium, particularly those with preexisting organic mental disorders, significant prior alcohol consumption, advanced age, or intracranial cerebral artery disease.[68] Perioperative opiate, anesthetic, and sedative administrations are a significant contributing factor. Right-sided parietal lobe lesions may present as delirium. Other causes of postoperative delirium in the cardiac intensive care patient include renal failure, hepatic failure, and thyroid abnormalities. EEGs on these patients are usually abnormal, whereas in primary psychiatric diseases they are normal. Treatment involves correcting metabolic abnormalities, establishing a normal sleep-wake cycle, and minimizing medications likely to cause delirium.

Brachial Plexus Injury/Peripheral Nerve Injury

Excessive sternal retraction during a median sternotomy may cause a brachial plexus injury, as the first rib may impinge the lower trunk and branches.[69] IMA harvesting may also cause damage to the brachial plexus with serious consequences.[70] Malpositioning of the upper limbs during surgery may result in a neuropraxia because of compression of the ulnar nerve.[71] Palsy or plegia of dorsiflexion and eversion of the foot can be caused by common peroneal nerve stretch or compression at the level of the head of the fibula.[72] Saphenous neuropathy (sensory changes on the medial side of the calf to the great toe) after open vein graft harvesting (less so with endoscopic harvest) is also a potential complication secondary to the avulsion of pretibial or infrapatellar branches of the nerve.[73]

Gastrointestinal

Mesenteric ischemia after cardiac surgery is infrequent but usually catastrophic.[74] Risk factors include duration of bypass (hypoperfusion), use of pressor support (sympathetic vascoconstriction), use of the IABP or other sources of atherosclerotic embolism, atrial fibrillation, peripheral vascular disease, and heparin-induced thrombocytopenia. Early surgical intervention (less than 6 hours) is associated with a 48% mortality rate, and this rises to 99% with delays (greater than 6 hours) in surgical intervention. Gastrointestinal bleeding is common and can cause significant morbidity. The incidence of gastrointestinal bleeding can be reduced with the use of H_2-inhibitors, proton pump inhibitors and sucralfate.[75] Other pertinent complications affecting the gastrointestinal system include pancreatitis (hyperamylasemia, 35 to 65% leads to 0.4 to 3% with overt pancreatitis)[76] occasionally seen after CPB (etiology unknown), acute acalculous cholecystitis (2 to 15% of all acute cholecystitis cases, likely owing to hypoperfusion, narcotics or parenteral nutrition that promote biliary stasis),[77] swallowing dysfunction, oropharyngeal dysphasia secondary to tracheal intubation or perioperative use of TEE,[78] or small or large bowel ileus. (Olgilvie's syndrome is associated with long-term ventilation.)[79] Preoperative liver dysfunction (noncardiac cirrhosis) is associated with a high incidence of postoperative morbidity and mortality (Child class A cirrhosis: 20% morbidity, 0% mortality; Child class B cirrhosis: 80% morbidity, 100% mortality). Although 20% of patients develop a transient hyperbilirubinemia, fewer than 1% have significant hepatocellular damage that progresses to chronic hepatitis or liver failure.[80]

Infections

Nosocomial Infections

Ten to twenty percent of cardiac surgery patients develop a nosocomial infection. Infections may be related to the surgical wound, lung, urinary tract, invasive lines or devices, or the gastrointestinal tract. Prolonged mechanical ventilation is associated with nosocomial pneumonia. These are second only to urinary tract infection in frequency and carry the highest mortality rate.[44] Smokers and COPD patients are most likely to be colonized preoperatively and have a higher incidence of pneumonia (15.3 versus 3.6% in controls).[81]

Catheter-related infections (ie, bladder and vascular related) are common in the ICU. The most common pathogens are *Staphylococcus aureus* (12%), coagulase-negative staphylococci (11%), *Candida albicans* (11%), *Pseudomonas aeruginosa* (10%), and *Enterococcus* sp.[82]

Fever

Fevers are common in the intensive care setting, but are a poor indicator of postoperative bacteremia (3.2% incidence in 835 febrile CABG patients).[83] The yield of true positive bacteremia ranges from 4 to 5%, with a contamination rate ranging from 32 to 47%.[84] Noninfectious causes of fever relative to cardiac surgery include myocardial infarction, postpericardiotomy syndrome, and drug fever. Infectious causes include wound infection, UTI, pneumonia, catheter sepsis, and loculated areas of contaminated blood accumulation (eg, pericardial, pleural, retroperitoneal, and leg wound spaces).

Sepsis/Septic Shock

Septic shock after cardiac surgery can have devastating consequences. Pathophysiologic features of sepsis include systemic inflammation, coagulation changes, impaired fibrinolysis, and subsequent target organ failure, with overall multiorgan failure, irreversible shock, and death (20 to 50%).[85] Mixed venous oxygen saturation can be abnormally high secondary to shunting and a failure to extract oxygen at the cellular level. In vasodilatory shock the maintenance of end-organ tissue perfusion is critical; this includes aggressive fluid management and vasopressin.[86] Methylene blue (which inhibits NO synthesis) has been used successfully in refractory hypotension. Bernard and colleagues[87] for the PROWESS study group showed a distinct survival advantage in the treatment of severe sepsis utilizing drotrecogin alfa (activated) or recombinant human activated protein C (Zigris). The mechanism of action is a modulation of the systemic inflammatory, procoagulant, and fibrinolytic reaction to infection. In a randomized study of 1690 patients the mortality rate was 30.8% in the placebo group versus 24.7% in the treatment group.

Wounds

Delayed Sternal Closure/Sternal Infection. Complicated operations with persistent bleeding and hemodynamic instability (owing to tissue edema) may preclude primary sternal closure. Delayed sternal closure allows hemodynamic stabilization, and diuresis.[88] Anderson and colleagues[89] outlined the recent Brigham and Women's Hospital experience; 1.7% (87 of 5177) open chests were managed with a hospital survival rate of 76%. Complications included deep sternal infection ($n = 4$), stroke ($n = 8$), and dialysis ($n = 13$). Multivariate analysis revealed mechanical ventricular assistance and reoperation for bleeding as independent predictors of in-hospital mortality.

Superficial and Deep Sternal Wounds. Superficial and deep sternal wound infections are significant complications of cardiac surgery. Deep sternal infection with associated mediastinitis occurs in 1 to 2% of cardiac operations, with a resultant mortality rate approaching 10%.[90] Common organisms are *Staphylococcus epidermidis, Staphylococcus* (including methicillin-resistant *Staphylococcus aureus* [MRSA]), *Corynebacterium*, and enteric gram-negative bacilli.[91] Patients predisposed to sternal infections include those with significant comorbidities (eg, obesity, diabetes, COPD, renal dysfunction, low serum albumin), prolonged CPB, reoperations, diabetics with bilateral IMA harvests,[92] and patients with hyperglycemia.[93] Simple preoperative measures such as clipping of chest hair, using Hibiclens washes, administration of adequate prophylactic antibiotics before skin incision, ensuring good intraoperative hemostasis without the use of bone wax, and closure with subcuticular sutures and Dermabond (topical adhesive) rather than skin staples; additionally, tight glucose control during surgery and in the days after surgery have a significantly lower sternal wound infection rate.

Minor infections frequently respond to intravenous antibiotics, opening of the wound, and local wound care. Deeper infections require intravenous antibiotics (6 weeks); initial empiric therapy should consist of broad coverage against gram-positive cocci and gram-negative bacilli with the regimen adjusted when cultures (blood, mediastinal, or deep sternal wound drainage) have been speciated. The mainstay of treatment is surgical exploration and extensive debridement, which may require removal of the sternum with primary or secondary closure with muscle or an omental flap.[94] Postoperative vacuum-assisted closure (VAC)[95] of mediastinal wounds improves wound healing and reduces hospital length of stay.

Nutrition

Preoperative debilitated or cachectic patients (ie, more than 10% weight loss over 6 months) with albumin levels of less than 3.5 g/dL[96] are exceptionally prone to complications such as infections after surgery. There is no evidence to support a role for preoperative hyperalimentation. BMI (a good nutritional index) of less than 15 kg/m^2 is associated with increased in morbidity. Postoperative patients have accelerated catabolic protein loss, usually requiring 25 to 40 Kcal/kg/day. Advances in immunonutritional pharmacology (arginine, glutamine, and n-3 fatty acids) in complex postoperative cardiac surgery patients may have a defined role in the future.[97]

REFERENCES

1. Kreter B, Woods M: Antibiotic prophylaxis for cardiothoracic operations. Meta-analysis of thirty years of clinical trials. *J Thorac Cardiovasc Surg* 1992; 104(3):590-599.
2. Gallagher JD, Moore RA, Kerns D, et al: Effects of colloid or crystalloid administration on pulmonary extravascular water in the postoperative period after coronary artery bypass grafting. *Anesth Analg* 1985; 64(8):753-758.
3. Finfer S, Bellomo R, Boyce N, et al: A comparison of albumin and saline for fluid resuscitation in the intensive care unit. *NEJM* 2004; 350(22): 2247-2256.
4. Garcia-Villarreal OA, Gonzalez-Oviedo R, Rodriguez-Gonzalez H, et al: Superior septal approach for mitral valve surgery: a word of caution. *Eur J Cardiothorac Surg* 2003; 24(6):862-867.
5. Echahidi N, Pibarot P, O'Hara G, Mathieu P: Mechanisms, prevention and treatment of atrial fibrillation after cardiac surgery. *J Am Coll Cardiol* 2008, 51:793-801.
6. Nisanoglu V, Erdil N, Aldemir M, et al: Atrial fibrillation after coronary artery bypass grafting in elderly patients: incidence and risk factor analysis. *Thorac Cardiovasc Surg* 2007; 55(1): 32-38.
7. Villareal RP, Hariharan R, Liu BC, et al: Postoperative atrial fibrillation and mortality after coronary artery bypass surgery. *J Am Coll Cardiol* 2004; 43:742-748.
8. Yalta K, Turgut OO, Yilmaz MB, Yilmaz A, Tandogan I: Dronedarone: a promising alternative for the management of atrial fibrillation. *Cardiovasc Drugs Ther* 2009; 23(5):385-393.
9. Betteridge J, Gibson M, on behalf of the ANDROMEDA study investigators: Effect of rosuvastatin and atorvastatin on LDL-C and CRP levels in patients with type 2 diabetes: results of the ANDROMEDA study. Poster presentation at: the 74th European Atherosclerosis Society Congress; April 17-21, 2004; Seville, Spain.
10. Hohnloser SH: New pharmacological options for patients with atrial fibrillation: the ATHENA trial. *Rev Esp Cardiol* 2009; 62, 479; 481.
11. Cook GE, Sasich LD, Sukkari SR: DIONYSOS study comparing dronedarone with amiodarone. *BMJ* 2010;340:c285, doi: 10.1136/bmj.c285 (published 19 January 2010).
12. Martin KB, Klinger JR, Rounds SI: Pulmonary arterial hypertension: new insights and new hope. *Respirology* 2006; 11(1):6-17.
13. Puskas JD, Williams WH, Duke PG, et al: Off-pump coronary artery bypass grafting provides complete revascularization with reduced myocardial injury, transfusion requirements, and length of stay: a prospective randomized comparison of two hundred unselected patients undergoing off-pump versus conventional coronary artery bypass grafting. *J Thorac Cardiovasc Surg* 2003; 125(4):797-808.
14. Bauer TL, Arepally G, Konkle BA, et al: Prevalence of heparin-associated antibodies without thrombosis in patients undergoing cardiopulmonary bypass surgery. *Circulation* 1997; 95(5):1242-1246.
15. Mangano DT: Aspirin and mortality from coronary bypass surgery. *NEJM* 2002; 347(17):1309-1317.
16. Abul-Azm A, Abdullah KM: Effect of topical tranexamic acid in open heart surgery. *Eur J Anaesthesiol* 2006; 23(5):1-5.
17. Mangano DT, Tudor IC, Dietzel C: The risk associated with aprotinin in cardiac surgery. *NEJM* 2006; 354(4):353-365.
18. Rosengart TK, Helm RE, DeBois WJ, et al: Open heart operations without transfusion using multimodality blood conservation strategy in 50 Jehovah's Witness patients: implications for a "bloodless" surgical technique. *J Am Coll Surg* 1997; 184(6):618-629.
19. Murkin JM: A novel hemostatic agent: the potential role of recombinant activated factor VII (rFVIIa) in anesthetic practice. *Can J Anaesth* 2002; 49(10):S21-26.
20. Bojar RM: *Manual of Perioperative Care in Adult Cardiac Surgery*, 4th ed. Malden, Blackwell, 2005.
21. Murphy GJ, Allen SM, Unsworth-White J, et al: Safety and efficacy of perioperative cell salvage and autotransfusion after coronary artery bypass grafting: a randomized trial. *Ann Thorac Surg* 2004; 77(5):1553-1559.
22. Munoz M, Garcia-Vallejo JJ, Ruiz MD, et al: Transfusion of post-operative shed blood: laboratory characteristics and clinical utility. *Eur Spine J* 2004; 13(Suppl 1):S107-113.
23. Hebert PC, Wells G, Blajchman MA, et al: A multicenter, randomized, controlled clinical trial of transfusion requirements in critical care. Transfusion Requirements in Critical Care Investigators, Canadian Critical Care Trials Group. *NEJM* 1999; 340(6):409-417.
24. Consensus conference. Perioperative red blood cell transfusion. *JAMA* 1988; 260(18):2700-2703.
25. Doak GJ, Hall RI: Does hemoglobin concentration affect perioperative myocardial lactate flux in patients undergoing coronary artery bypass surgery? *Anesth Analg* 1995; 80(5):910-916.
26. Murphy GJ, Reeves BC, Rogers CA, et al: Increased mortality, postoperative morbidity, and cost after red blood cell transfusion in patients having cardiac surgery. *Circulation* 2007; 116(22): 2544-2552.
27. Chelemer SB, Prato BS, Cox PM Jr, et al: Association of bacterial infection and red blood cell transfusion after coronary artery bypass surgery. *Ann Thorac Surg* 2002; 73(1):138-142.
28. Ng CS, Wan S, Yim AP, et al: Pulmonary dysfunction after cardiac surgery. *Chest* 2002; 121(4):1269-1277.
29. Berthelsen P SHO, Husum B, et al: PEEP reverses nitroglycerin-induced hypoxemia after coronary artery bypass surgery. *Acta Anaesthesiol Scand* 1986; 30:243-246.
30. Kreider ME LD: Bronchoscopy for atelectasis in the ICU. *Chest* 2003; 124:344-350.
31. Marini JJ PD, Hudson LD: Acute lobar attelectasis: a prospective comparison of fiberoptic bronchoscopy and respiratory therapy. *Am Rev Respir Dis* 1979; 119:971-978.
32. Stevens RD, Burri H, Tramer MR: Pharmacologic myocardial protection in patients undergoing noncardiac surgery: a quantitative systematic review. *Anesth Analg* 2003; 97(3):623-633.
33. Esteban A, Frutos F, Tobin MJ, et al: A comparison of four methods of weaning patients from mechanical ventilation. Spanish Lung Failure Collaborative Group. *NEJM* 1995; 332(6):345-350.
34. Epstein SK: Etiology of extubation failure and the predictive value of the rapid shallow breathing index. *Am J Respir Crit Care Med* 1995; 152(2): 545-549.
35. Epstein SK. Decision to extubate. *Intensive Care Med* 2002; 28(5): 535-546.
36. Engoren M, Buderer NF, Zacharias A, et al: Variables predicting reintubation after cardiac surgical procedures. *Ann Thorac Surg* 1999; 67(3):661-665.
37. Cohen A, Katz M, Katz R, et al: Chronic obstructive pulmonary disease in patients undergoing coronary artery bypasses grafting. *J Thorac Cardiovasc Surg* 1995; 109(3):574-581.
38. Redmond JM, Greene PS, Goldsborough MA, et al: Neurologic injury in cardiac surgical patients with a history of stroke. *Ann Thorac Surg* 1996; 61(1):42-47.
39. Heffner JE: Timing tracheotomy: calendar watching or individualization of care? *Chest* 1998; 114(2):361-363.
40. Maziak DE, Meade MO, Todd TR: The timing of tracheotomy: a systematic review. *Chest* 1998; 114(2):605-609.
41. Pierson DJ: Tracheostomy and weaning. *Respir Care* 2005; 50(4): 526-533.
42. Rumbak MJ, Newton M, Truncale T, et al: A prospective, randomized, study comparing early percutaneous dilational tracheotomy to prolonged translaryngeal intubation (delayed tracheotomy) in critically ill medical patients. *Crit Care Med* 2004; 32(8):1689-1694.
43. Fagon JY, Chastre J, Domart Y, et al: Nosocomial pneumonia in patients receiving continuous mechanical ventilation. Prospective analysis of 52 episodes with use of a protected specimen brush and quantitative culture techniques. *Am Rev Respir Dis* 1989; 139(4):877-884.

44. Beck KD, Gastmeier P: Clinical or epidemiologic diagnosis of nosocomial pneumonia: is there any difference? *Am J Infect Control* 2003; 31(6): 331-335.
45. Baselski VS, Wunderink RG: Bronchoscopic diagnosis of pneumonia. *Clin Microbiol Rev* 1994; 7(4):533-558.
46. Rastan AJ, Gummert JF, Lachmann N, et al: Significant value of autopsy for quality management in cardiac surgery. *J Thorac Cardiovasc Surg* 2005; 129(6):1292-1300.
47. Schoepf UJ, Savino G, Lake DR, et al: The age of CT pulmonary angiography. *J Thorac Imaging* 2005; 20(4):273-279.
48. Roy PM, Colombet I, Durieux P, et al: Systematic review and meta-analysis of strategies for the diagnosis of suspected pulmonary embolism. *BMJ* 2005; 331(7511):259.
49. Bahar I, Akgul A, Ozatik MA, et al: Acute renal failure after open heart surgery: risk factors and prognosis. *Perfusion* 2005; 20(6):317-322.
50. Chertow GM, Lazarus JM, Christiansen CL, et al: Preoperative renal risk stratification. *Circulation* 1997; 95(4):878-884.
51. Franga DL, Kratz JM, Crumbley AJ, et al: Early and long-term results of coronary artery bypass grafting in dialysis patients. *Ann Thorac Surg* 2000; 70(3):813-818; discussion 819.
52. Dresler C, Uthoff K, Wahlers T, et al: Open heart operations after renal transplantation. *Ann Thorac Surg* 1997; 63(1):143-146.
53. Sehested J, Wacker B, Forssmann WG, et al: Natriuresis after cardiopulmonary bypass: relationship to urodilatin, atrial natriuretic factor, antidiuretic hormone, and aldosterone. *J Thorac Cardiovasc Surg* 1997; 114(4): 666-671.
54. Weber DO, Yarnoz MD: Hyperkalemia complicating cardiopulmonary bypass: analysis of risk factors. *Ann Thorac Surg* 1982; 34(4):439-445.
55. Gennari FJ: Hypokalemia. *NEJM* 1998; 339(7):451-458.
56. Shechter M, Sharir M, Labrador MJ, et al: Oral magnesium therapy improves endothelial function in patients with coronary artery disease. *Circulation* 2000; 102(19):2353-2358.
57. Agus ZS, Morad M: Modulation of cardiac ion channels by magnesium. *Annu Rev Physiol* 1991; 53:299-307.
58. England MR, Gordon G, Salem M, et al: Magnesium administration and dysrhythmias after cardiac surgery. A placebo-controlled, double-blind, randomized trial. *JAMA* 1992; 268(17):2395-2402.
59. Van den Berghe G, Wouters P, Weekers F, et al: Intensive insulin therapy in the critically ill patients. *NEJM* 2001; 345(19):1359-1367.
60. The NICE-SUGAR Study Investigators: Intensive versus conventional glucose control in critically ill patients. *NEJM* 2009; 360(13):1283-1297.
61. Ricotta JJ, Faggioli GL, Castilone A, et al: Risk factors for stroke after cardiac surgery: Buffalo Cardiac-Cerebral Study Group. *J Vasc Surg* 1995; 21(2):359-363; discussion 364.
62. John R, Choudhri AF, Weinberg AD, et al: Multicenter review of preoperative risk factors for stroke after coronary artery bypass grafting. *Ann Thorac Surg* 2000; 69(1):30-35; discussion 35-36.
63. Borger MA, Ivanov J, Weisel RD, et al: Stroke during coronary bypass surgery: principal role of cerebral macroemboli. *Eur J Cardiothorac Surg* 2001; 19(5):627-632.
64. Brown WR, Moody DM, Challa VR, et al: Longer duration of cardiopulmonary bypass is associated with greater numbers of cerebral microemboli. *Stroke* 2000; 31(3):707-713.
65. Hickey PR: Neurologic sequelae associated with deep hypothermic circulatory arrest. *Ann Thorac Surg* 1998; 65(6 Suppl):S65-69; discussion S69-70, S74-66.
66. van Dijk D, Keizer AM, Diephuis JC, et al: Neurocognitive dysfunction after coronary artery bypasses surgery: a systematic review. *J Thorac Cardiovasc Surg* 2000; 120(4):632-639.
67. McKhann GM: Neurocognitive complications after coronary artery bypass surgery. *Ann Neurol* 2005; 57(5):615-621.
68. Smith LW, Dimsdale JE. Postcardiotomy delirium: conclusions after 25 years? *Am J Psychiatry* 1989; 146(4):452-458.
69. Vander Salm TJ, Cutler BS, Okike ON: Brachial plexus injury after median sternotomy. Part II. *J Thorac Cardiovasc Surg* 1982; 83(6):914-917.
70. Vahl CF, Carl I, Muller-Vahl H, et al: Brachial plexus injury after cardiac surgery. The role of internal mammary artery preparation: a prospective study on 1000 consecutive patients. *J Thorac Cardiovasc Surg* 1991; 102(5):724-729.
71. Morin JE, Long R, Elleker MG, et al: Upper extremity neuropathies after median sternotomy. *Ann Thorac Surg* 1982; 34(2):181-185.
72. Vazquez-Jimenez JF, Krebs G, Schiefer J, et al: Injury of the common peroneal nerve after cardiothoracic operations. *Ann Thorac Surg* 2002;73(1):119-122.
73. Sharma AD, Parmley CL, Sreeram G, et al: Peripheral nerve injuries during cardiac surgery: risk factors, diagnosis, prognosis, and prevention. *Anesth Analg* 2000; 91(6):1358-1369.
74. Klotz S, Vestring T, Rotker J, et al: Diagnosis and treatment of nonocclusive mesenteric ischemia after open heart surgery. *Ann Thorac Surg* 2001; 72(5):1583-1586.
75. Cook DJ, Reeve BK, Guyatt GH, et al: Stress ulcer prophylaxis in critically ill patients. Resolving discordant meta-analyses. *JAMA* 24-31 1996; 275(4):308-314.
76. Ihaya A, Muraoka R, Chiba Y, et al: Hyperamylasemia and subclinical pancreatitis after cardiac surgery. *World J Surg* 2001; 25(7):862-864.
77. Rady MY, Kodavatiganti R, Ryan T. Perioperative predictors of acute cholecystitis after cardiovascular surgery. *Chest* 1998; 114(1):76-84.
78. Hogue CW Jr, Lappas GD, Creswell LL, et al: Swallowing dysfunction after cardiac operations. Associated adverse outcomes and risk factors including intraoperative transesophageal echocardiography. *J Thorac Cardiovasc Surg* 1995; 110(2):517-522.
79. Geller A, Petersen BT, Gostout CJ: Endoscopic decompression for acute colonic pseudo-obstruction. *Gastrointest Endosc* 1996; 44(2):144-150.
80. Raman JS, Kochi K, Morimatsu H, et al: Severe ischemic early liver injury after cardiac surgery. *Ann Thorac Surg* 2002; 74(5):1601-1606.
81. Carrel TP, Eisinger E, Vogt M, et al: Pneumonia after cardiac surgery is predictable by tracheal aspirates but cannot be prevented by prolonged antibiotic prophylaxis. *Ann Thorac Surg* 2001; 72(1):143-148.
82. Gordon SM, Serkey JM, Keys TF, et al: Secular trends in nosocomial bloodstream infections in a 55-bed cardiothoracic intensive care unit. *Ann Thorac Surg* 1998; 65(1):95-100.
83. Kohman LJ, Coleman MJ, Parker FB Jr: Bacteremia and sternal infection after coronary artery bypass grafting. *Ann Thorac Surg* 1990; 49(3): 454-457.
84. Badillo AT, Sarani B, Evans SR: Optimizing the use of blood cultures in the febrile postoperative patient. *J Am Coll Surg* 2002; 194(4):477-487; quiz 554-476.
85. Sands KE, Bates DW, Lanken PN, et al: Epidemiology of sepsis syndrome in 8 academic medical centers. *JAMA* 1997; 278(3):234-240.
86. Jochberger S, Mayr VD, Luckner G, et al: Serum vasopressin concentrations in critically ill patients. *Crit Care Med* 2006; 34(2):293-299.
87. Bernard GR, Vincent JL, Laterre PF, et al: Efficacy and safety of recombinant human activated protein C for severe sepsis. *NEJM* 2001; 344(10):699-709.
88. Donatelli F, Triggiani M, Benussi S, et al: Advantages of delayed sternal closure in cardiac-compromised adult patients. *J Card Surg* 1995; 10(6): 632-636.
89. Anderson CA, Filsoufi F, Aklog L, et al: Liberal use of delayed sternal closure for postcardiotomy hemodynamic instability. *Ann Thorac Surg* 2002; 73(5):1484-1488.
90. Gottlieb LJ, Beahm EK, Krizek TJ, et al: Approaches to sternal wound infections. *Adv Card Surg* 1996; 7:147-162.
91. Olsson C, Tammelin A, Thelin S: *Staphylococcus aureus* bloodstream infection after cardiac surgery: risk factors and outcome. *Infect Control Hosp Epidemiol* 2006; 27(1):83-85.
92. Lev-Ran O, Mohr R, Amir K, et al: Bilateral internal thoracic artery grafting in insulin-treated diabetics: should it be avoided? *Ann Thorac Surg* 2003; 75(6):1872-1877.
93. Latham R, Lancaster AD, Covington JF, et al: The association of diabetes and glucose control with surgical-site infections among cardiothoracic surgery patients. *Infect Control Hosp Epidemiol* 2001; 22(10):607-612.
94. Sjogren J, Gustafsson R, Nilsson J, et al: Clinical outcome after poststernotomy mediastinitis: vacuum-assisted closure versus conventional treatment. *Ann Thorac Surg* 2005; 79(6):2049-2055.
95. Rich MW, Keller AJ, Schechtman KB, et al: Increased complications and prolonged hospital stay in elderly cardiac surgical patients with low serum albumin. *Am J Cardiol* 1989; 63(11):714-718.
96. Carney DE, Meguid MM: Current concepts in nutritional assessment. *Arch Surg* 2002; 137(1):42-45.
97. Heyland DK, Novak F, Drover JW, et al: should immunonutrition become routine in critically ill patients? A systematic review of the evidence. *JAMA* 2001; 286(8):944-953.
98. Walter J, Mortasawi A, Arnrich B, et al: Creatinine clearance versus serum creatinine as a risk factor in cardiac surgery. *BMC Surg* 2003; 3:4.
99. Nagaranjan DV, Lewis PS, Botha P, Dunning J: Is addition of anti-platelet therapy to warfarin beneficial to patients with prosthetic heart valves? *Int Cardiovasc Thorac Surg* 2004; 3:450-455.
100. Bernstein AD, Daubert JC, Fletcher RD, et al: The Revised NASPE/BPEG generic code for antibradycardia, adaptive-rate, and multisite pacing. *Pacing Clin Electrophysiol* 2000; 25:260-264.

CHAPTER 17

Cardiopulmonary Resuscitation

Mark P. Anstadt
James E. Lowe

INTRODUCTION

Cardiovascular disease remains the leading cause of death in the United States.[1,2] Acute myocardial infarctions associated with ischemic heart disease accounts for the majority of sudden deaths.[3]

Sudden cardiac death is the unexpected, nontraumatic, abrupt cessation of effective cardiac function associated with absent or acute symptoms of less than 1 hour.[4,5] Prodromes such as chest pain, palpitations, or fatigue may occur within the preceding 24 hours.[4] The majority of deaths occur within 2 hours of the onset of symptoms.[1,2,6–8] Most victims die before reaching a hospital.[1,2]

Cardiopulmonary resuscitation (CPR) describes the emergency measures used to restore cardiovascular and respiratory function. Notably, cardiocerebral resuscitation represents preferable terminology as it conveys more appropriate emphasis on neurologic recovery. Clinical interventions have been formulated as Advanced Cardiac Life Support (ACLS) guidelines[9] based on scientific data established by the American Heart Association (AHA) and International Liaison Committee on Resuscitation.[10]

CPR and/or ACLS are performed in 1 to 2% of patients admitted to teaching hospitals (including approximately 30% of patients who die).[11,12] The goals are to restore spontaneous circulation (ROSC), and ultimately, survive. Early defibrillation is the single most effective means for ROSC. Otherwise, ROSC depends on improving myocardial perfusion and treating underlying disorders. Mechanical circulatory support devices and therapeutic hypothermia represent treatment interventions that may improve these life-saving endeavors. Overall survival rates remain low (Table 17-1), and successful resuscitation frequently results in neurologic impairment.[13–15,129] The clinical integration of rapid response, early defibrillation, circulatory support devices, hypothermia, and neuroprotective agents should improve future outcomes.

PHARMACOLOGIC THERAPY DURING CPR

Peripheral venous access is preferred for speed, and avoiding CPR interruption. Drugs take 1 to 2 minutes to reach the central circulation during CPR. Administration should be by bolus followed by flushes and extremity elevation. Peak drug concentrations are lower with peripheral versus central injection. Central access should be considered when responses to peripheral administration are absent. Internal jugular and supraclavicular sites are preferred to the femoral because return to the inferior vena cava is impaired during CPR. Long femoral lines may overcome this problem. Routine fluid administration is not indicated without evidence of hypovolemia as this may adversely affect coronary pressure by raising right atrial pressure.

When venous access is not possible, drugs may be administered via an endotracheal tube. Medications are given via a catheter passed beyond the tube's tip using twice the IV dose diluted in saline or water. Water provides better absorption but results in more adverse effects on PaO_2. Rapid insufflations are given after each bolus for drug dispersion. Intracardiac injection is not recommended during routine CPR. It may be used for epinephrine during open chest cardiac massage (OCM), or if no other access is obtainable. Intracardiac injection can result in complications including: cardiac injury, tamponade, and pneumothorax.

The principal agents recommended for ACLS are adrenergic agonists and antiarrhythmics. Alpha-adrenergic agonists have been the only drugs that definitively improved outcome in

TABLE 17-1 Published Reports of Clinical Outcomes after Cardiac Arrest

			Hospital Discharge		Long-Term Survival (%)									CPC Neurologic Outcomes (%)‡					
Author, year	Rhythm	No. Cases	No.	(%)	30 Days	3 Mo	6 Mo	8 Mo	1 Year	2 Years	3 Years	4 Years	5 Years	1) Intact	2) Moderate	3) Severe	4) Coma	5)Brain Dead	Hospital Setting
Abramson, 1982[142]	All*	NR§	100	NR	33	29								36					In and out
Brindley, 2002[39]	All	247	55	22.4															In
Bunch, 2003[40]	VF†	200	80	40									99	40					Out
Cobb, 1978[144]	VF	406	383	94					26	36									Out
Cohn, 2004[47]	All	105	22	21	21									73	20	7	0	0	In
Dorian, 2002[25]	VF	347	14	4															Out
Earnest, 1980[14]	NR	117	38	32							25			57		7			Out
Eisenburg, 1982[126]	All	1567	302	19			81		76	66	55	49							Out
Gudjonsson,1982[125]	All	222	21	9										81					Out
Herlitz, 2005[38]	All	13,453	NR	NR	4														Out
Liberthson, 1974[124]	VF	301	42	14										60	28	12			In and out
Lund, 1973[143]	All	1263	94	7				81		81					21				Out
Nichol, 2008[147]	All	11,898	954	8															Out
Peberdy, 2003[41]	All	14,720	2502	17										86					In
Rockswold, 1979[127]	All	514	83	16					15	50				59	41				Out
Sandroni, 2004[42]	All	114	37	32			24	26						57		14			In
Snyder, 1980[146]	All	63	25	40										64	32	4			In
Wernberg, 1979[145]	All	1686	72	4											18	6			In and out
Wik, 2005[32]	All	176	6	3										83	17				Out

*ALL = Cardiac arrest, PEA, VT/VF = respiratory arrest.
†NR = Nct reported; VF = ventricular fibrillation.
‡CPC = Cerebral performance categories (1 to 5).
§NR = not reported.
Neurologic outcome expressed as percent patients with designated cerebral perfusion categories as defined in Cohn AC, Wilson WM, Yan B, et al: Analysis of clinical outcomes following in-hospital adult cardiac arrest. Intern Med J 2004; 34:398-402.

CPR. Their primary benefit is vasoconstriction. Increased peripheral resistance results in elevated aortic pressure, improving coronary perfusion. The minimum coronary perfusion pressure and blood flow needed for successful defibrillation are 15 mm Hg and 15 to 20 mL/min/100 g, respectively. CPR rarely achieves these minimums without pressors. Epinephrine has this beneficial effect. Its beta-adrenergic effect may improve the treatment of cardiac arrest. One milligram is recommended every 3 to 5 minutes during resuscitation attempts.[10] Epinephrine improves ROSC and survival in animal models of cardiac arrest. Clinical trials using higher epinephrine doses demonstrated higher rates of ROSC, but no survival advantage.[16,17] One trial found high-dose epinephrine had more adverse effects, which may be partly explained by increased oxygen demands.

Other nonadrenergic vasoconstrictive agents have been studied as alternatives to epinephrine. Vasopressin acts on unique receptors and may be beneficial for treating cardiac arrest refractory to epinephrine. Laboratory and clinical data indicate vasopressin may be preferable to epinephrine.[18,19] A recent meta-analyses of five randomized clinical trials comparing vasopressin to epinephrine during cardiac arrest[20] found no evidence to support the use of one drug over the other. Epinephrine is less expensive. However, vasopressin continues to be an acceptable alternative for treating cardiac arrest.

Vasopressin also mediates adrenocorticotropin release during CPR.[21] The hypothalamic-pituitary-adrenal axis is suppressed in cardiac arrest victims,[21–23] and low serum cortisol levels have been identified as a poor prognostic factor for ROSC.[22,23] Adrenal function in patients who have ROSC may also be insufficient for survival.[24] Further clinical trials are needed to determine if administration of corticosteroids during CPR and/or following ROSC may benefit outcome.

The effectiveness of antiarrhythmics in sudden death has not been well substantiated. Randomized clinical trials have demonstrated amiodarone effectiveness in treating cardiac arrest.[25–29] Amiodarone significantly improved survival to hospital admission compared with placebo for VF/VT.[28] The most recent randomized clinical trial found amiodarone significantly increased survival to hospital admission compared to lidocaine when used to treat sudden death.[25] Survival to discharge was observed, but did not reach statistical significance. Amiodarone is recommended for the treatment of persistent VT and/or VF. Lidocaine is an acceptable alternative.

Magnesium sulfate should be administered for suspected hypomagnesemia or torsades de pointes. It is recommended for refractory VF/VT. Hypomagnesemia is associated with ventricular arrhythmias and sudden cardiac death and may hinder potassium replenishment in hypokalemic patients. Hypermagnesemia can cause flaccid paralysis and cardiorespiratory arrest.

Atropine enhances atrioventricular node conduction and sinus node automaticity. It is indicated for symptomatic bradycardia and asystolic arrest. Asystole from prolonged ischemia is usually fatal. Atropine is unlikely to benefit, but is not harmful in such circumstances. Adverse effects include tachycardia and anticholinergic effects.

Judicious use of $NaHCO_3$ may be appropriate for correcting severe acidosis during cardiac arrest. Notably, $NaHCO_3$ increases CO_2, which may accumulate rapidly, leading to a hypercarbic venous acidemia. Diffusion of CO_2 across cell membranes may result in paradoxic intracellular acidosis and decrease the likelihood of successful resuscitation. Hypocarbic arterial alkalemia or the so-called venoarterial paradox may develop. Therefore, $NaHCO_3$ may increase CO_2 levels, worsen the venoarterial paradox, and exacerbate intracellular acidosis. Other potential adverse effects include alkalemia with leftward shifts in the oxyhemoglobin desaturation curve, hyperosmolality, hypernatremia, and hypotension. Finally, $NaHCO_3$ has not been shown to improve results in cardiac arrest and is only recommended for severe acidosis, hyperkalemia, tricyclic antidepressant overdose, or prolonged CPR.[9]

TECHNIQUES IN CARDIOPULMONARY RESUSCITATION

Basic life support (BLS) defines the methods used to sustain ventilation and blood flow until ACLS can restore spontaneous circulation. Airway, breathing, circulation, defibrillation (ABCD) algorithms describe these standardized approaches (Fig. 17-1).[3]

Airway Management

Initial management of unresponsive patients is ensuring a patent airway.[9] The airway is open using the head-tilt–chin-lift

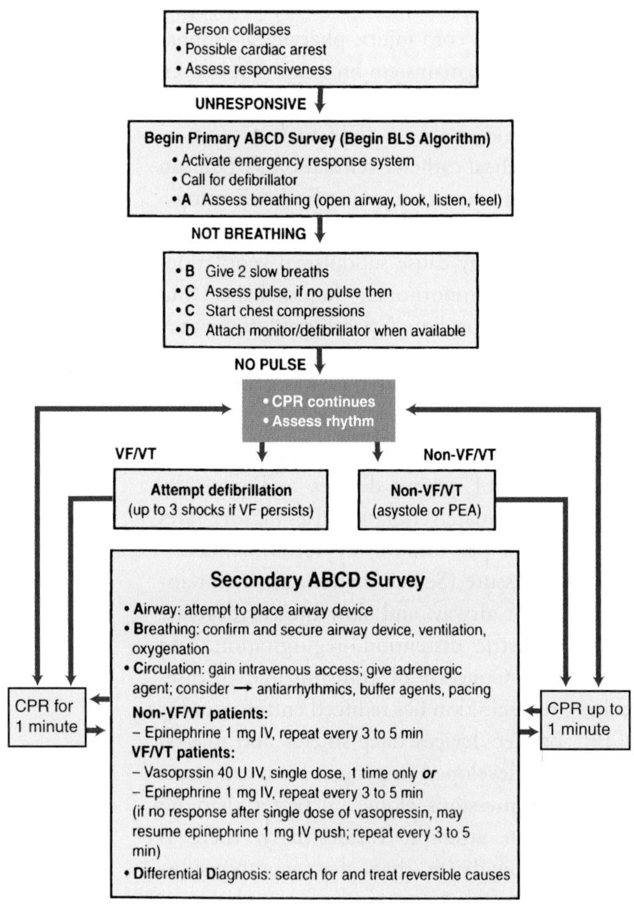

FIGURE 17-1 Universal treatment algorithm for adult emergency cardiac care.

maneuver. The jaw-thrust technique is an alternative for suspected neck trauma; however, it is more difficult to perform. Both relieve posterior displacement of the tongue, which is a common cause of airway obstruction. Difficult ventilation should be addressed by repositioning and considering foreign body obstruction. The Heimlich maneuver, or *subdiaphragmatic abdominal thrust,* is recommended for relieving obstruction from foreign bodies. Rapid thrusts to the subxiphoid region can dislodge a foreign body by increasing expiratory pressure. Chest thrusts are more appropriate for obese patients and women in late stages of pregnancy. Magill forceps can be used to retrieve foreign bodies when necessary.

Masks, and oral and nasal airways may be used with mouth-to-mask ventilation or bag-valve devices. Bag-valve devices reduce exposure to potential infection, but require two rescuers.[10] Nasopharyngeal airways are considered for nonintubated patients. Oropharyngeal airways can be used in unconscious patients but add risk for laryngospasm and regurgitation.[10]

Endotracheal intubation (ETT) is the preferred method of airway management. ETT maintains an open airway, decreases risk of gastric distention and aspiration, and is an alternative drug administration route. Orotracheal intubation is ideal unless a neck injury is suspected, in which case nasotracheal intubation is recommended. ETT can be complicated by esophageal intubation, oral trauma, pharyngeal laceration, vocal cord injury, pharyngeal-esophageal perforation, mainstem bronchus intubation, and aspiration. Esophageal intubation is likely with a low end-tidal CO_2 ($ETCO_2$).

Transtracheal catheter ventilation (TTC) can be instituted when routine methods fail using a catheter passed across the cricothyroid membrane. TTC may cause suboptimal ventilation, including pneumothorax, hemorrhage, and esophageal perforation. Cricothyroidotomy may also be considered for difficult airways. Otherwise, tracheostomy is indicated when ventilation cannot be achieved.

Mouth-to-mouth ventilation/nasal is used in the absence of airway devices and generally results in adequate ventilation. Respiratory rates of 10 to 12 per minute are recommended.[10] Cricoid pressure (Sellick maneuver), maintaining a patent airway, and slow breaths decrease risk for gastric distention, regurgitation, and aspiration. Concern of transmissible diseases during resuscitation has reduced enthusiasm for CPR. Barrier devices (face shields and masks) have been developed to protect from exposure. Chest compressions alone are better than no resuscitation attempt. Interestingly, there is increasing evidence that chest compressions alone may result in survival rates and neurologic outcomes comparable to CPR with ventilation.[29,30,128]

Closed Chest Cardiac Massage

Closed chest cardiac massage (CCM) is the principal means of restoring blood flow during CPR. CCM is best when the victim is supine on a firm surface (Fig. 17-2). Compressions are given to the lower sternum at 100/min, with a rate of 30 compressions: 2 breaths. Compressions of 4 to 6 cm should occupy 50% of the cycle. At best, CCM creates minimal perfusion to vital organs and is unable to sustain life.[31–34] Survival becomes exceedingly low with more than 30 minutes of CCM. ROSC is dependent on proper CCM techniques,[33] but studies have demonstrated these techniques are frequently suboptimal.[31,32]

Discontinuation of CPR

Discontinuation of CPR remains controversial, with no clearly defined criteria. Determining the adequacy of CCM is subjective

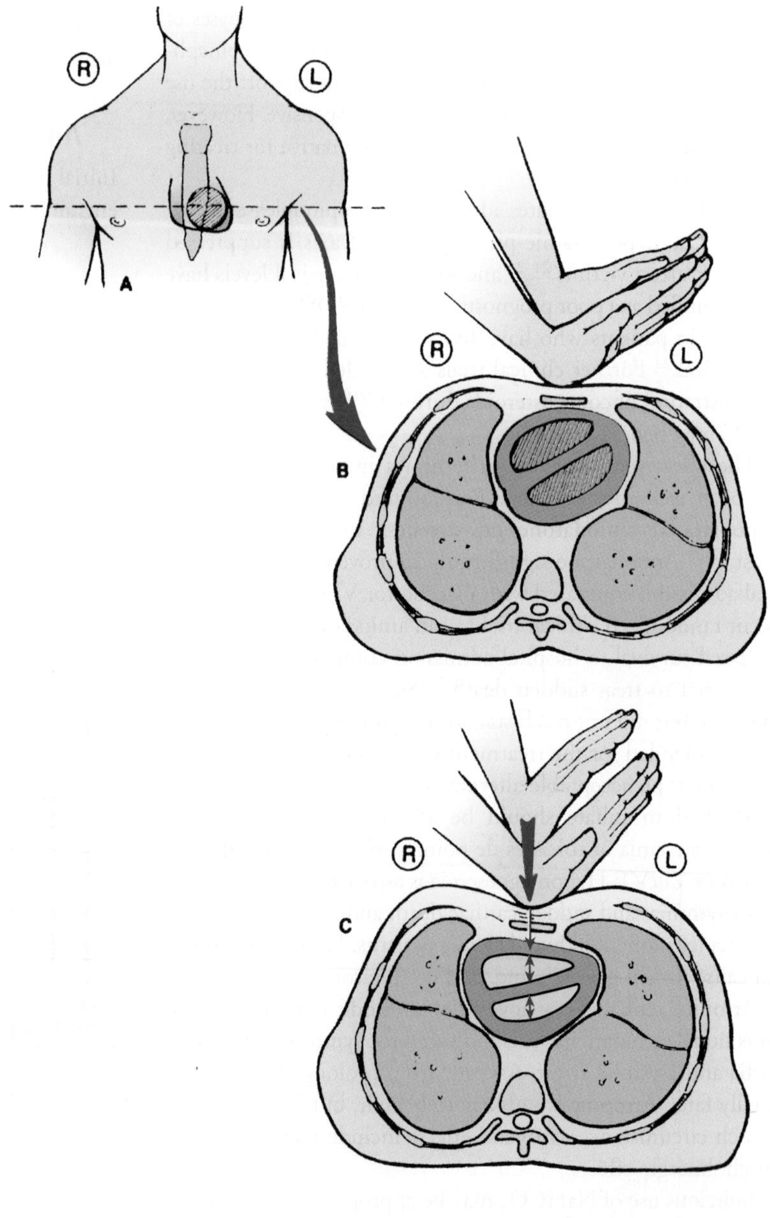

FIGURE 17-2 Cross-sectional view of closed chest cardiac massage. Compressions are delivered with high velocity and moderate force, resulting in cardiac compression.

because palpable pulses do not signify forward flow. Reactive pupils and/or spontaneous respirations indicate some cerebral perfusion, but correlate poorly with outcome. Aortic diastolic pressure may be the best measure of CPR effectiveness[35] but is usually not available.

Alternatively, $ETCO_2$ can provide useful information and predict ROSC.[36,37] Low $ETCO_2$ suggests poor perfusion, esophageal intubation, airway obstruction, massive pulmonary embolus, or hypothermia.

Successful ROSC and survival are influenced by many factors. Ventricular fibrillation (VF), early defibrillation, rapid onset of CPR or ACLS, witnessed arrest, and early age all have favorable implications.[38,39–41,42] These factors, should all be considered before abandoning resuscitation.

Complications of CPR

Common complications associated with CCM are rib and sternal fractures.[43] Others include aspiration, gastric dilatation, anterior mediastinal hemorrhage, epicardial hematoma, hemopericardium, myocardial contusion, pneumothorax, air embolus, hemothorax, lung contusion, and oral/dental injuries.[43–45] The liver and spleen are the most commonly injured intra-abdominal organs, reported in 1 to 2% of cases.[43] Significant injuries can involve the trachea, esophagus, stomach, cervical spine, vena cava, retroperitoneum, and myocardium.[43]

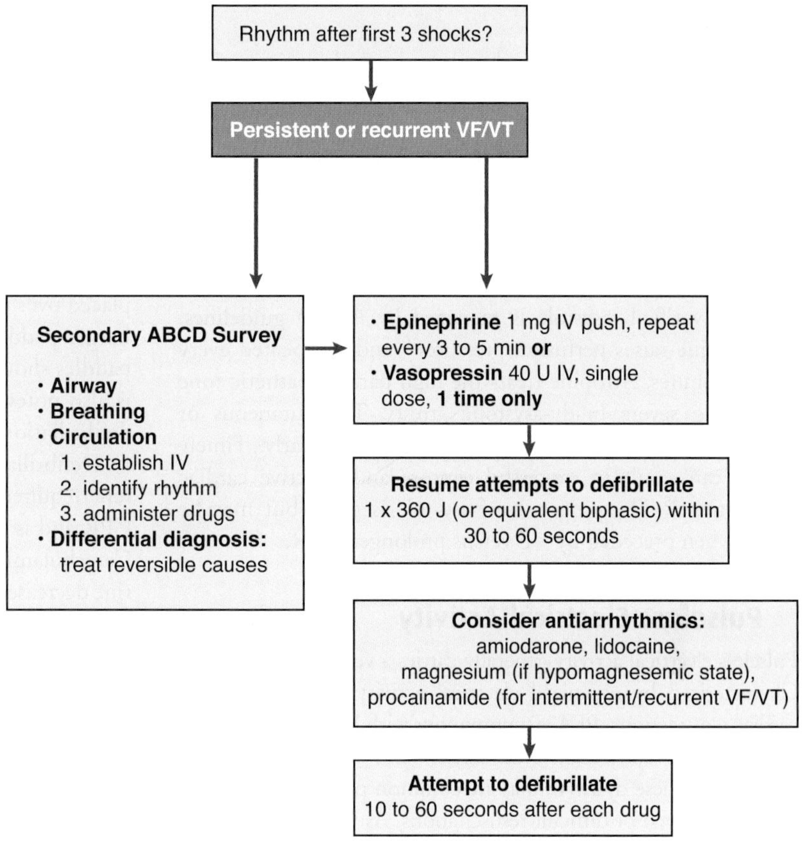

FIGURE 17-3 Treatment algorithm for persistent ventricular fibrillation and pulseless ventricular tachycardia (VF/VT).

SUDDEN DEATH TREATMENT CONSIDERATIONS

Sudden death generally presents as ventricular fibrillation/tachycardia (VF/VT), asystole, or electromechanical dissociation (EMD), also called pulseless electrical activity (PEA). VF may continue after defibrillation attempts (*shock-resistant*) or persist despite other therapeutic interventions (*persistent* or *refractory*). Also, successfully treated VF may recur (*recurrent*). These patterns are felt to have different etiologies, priorities of treatment, and prognoses. Early identification of the underlying rhythm is important for selecting the recommended treatment algorithm (see Fig. 17-1).

Ventricular Tachycardia

Ventricular tachycardia (VT) is an arrhythmia characterized by premature ventricular depolarizations (>100/min). Cardiac arrest occurs with rapid, sustained VT. VF is uncoordinated, continuous contraction of the ventricles. More than 80% of monitored cardiac arrests originate with VF/VT.[46] Most survivors have VF/VT as the initial rhythm.[38,41,47] Rapid defibrillation is the key determinant for survival[38,48,49] and should precede all other therapy if immediately available.[9,10] Delay negatively impacts successful defibrillation.[50] Mortality increases 4 to 10% for every minute preceding defibrillation attempts.[48] Survival rates approach zero when countershocks are attempted more than 10 to 12 minutes after arrest.[51] Current guidelines therefore emphasize early defibrillation and use of automated external defibrillation systems.[10]

Optimal treatment VF or pulseless VT begins with immediate defibrillation, when possible. Energy for initial defibrillation is 200 J. If VF continues, a second shock (200 to 300 J) is given immediately. A third countershock (360 J) is given if the second fails. It is vital that three consecutive shocks are given without delay for other interventions. CPR is performed whenever defibrillation attempts fail. Figure 17-3 outlines treatment algorithms for persistent VF/VT. Epinephrine or vasopressin is given IV or via the endotracheal tube. Vasopressin should only be given once, and subsequent defibrillation attempted (360 J). Epinephrine is given every 3 to 5 minutes. Refractory VF is treated with antiarrhythmics. Amiodarone may be the most efficacious in this setting.[25–27,52] Lidocaine is also acceptable for recurrent VF or pulseless VT; however, it is not recommended over amiodarone.[38] Defibrillation should be attempted 30 to 60 seconds after each drug.[10]

Prognosis for VF or pulseless VT is better than for asystole or PEA. Up to 30% of patients with witnessed VF/VT arrest are successfully resuscitated.[41,47,53,54] Failure of initial defibrillation attempts is a poor prognostic sign.

Asystole

Asystole is absence of electrical and mechanical cardiac activity and frequently indicates a terminal event. ACLS is indicated while other treatable causes are considered. Priorities include effective CPR and rhythm confirmation. Low-amplitude VF may occasionally masquerade as asystole. Incorrect lead placement or equipment malfunction should be considered. Countershocks do not benefit *true* asystole, and may induce parasympathetic discharge diminishing the chance of ROSC.

Once verified, asystole is managed by ABCD guidelines. Epinephrine raises perfusion pressures[10] and is repeated every 3 to 5 minutes. Atropine treats the high parasympathetic tone underlying severe brady-asystolic arrests. Transcutaneous or transvenous pacing may be effective if applied early. Timely pacing can result in successful capture and effective cardiac contraction.[55] The prognosis of asystole is grim, but may be better when preceded by VF versus prolonged CPR.

Pulseless Electrical Activity

Pulseless electrical activity generally carries a very poor prognosis. Characterized by organized electrical activity without effective cardiac contractions, PEA is synonymous with EMD and includes pulseless idioventricular, bradycardia, and ventricular escape rhythms.[10] These dysrhythmias are common proximate causes of death in delayed or difficult resuscitations. As with asystole, PEA mandates assessment for reversible causes. Rapid, narrow-complex activity may indicate a treatable condition. Associated trauma may be an indication for emergency thoracotomy[56] to address cardiac tamponade of cardiovascular injury. Thoracotomy allows cardiac massage and aortic occlusion, which may be lifesaving. PEA following open heart surgery is a clinical scenario in which chest reopening is generally recommended.[57]

Cardioversion

Cardioversion is the *only* effective treatment for VF. Defibrillation depolarizes and results in temporary asystole.[58] Pacemaker cells then restore myocardial activation. Myocardial contraction resumes if high-energy phosphates depleted by CPR are sufficient. The probability of successful defibrillation is best immediately after witnessed arrests. Success rates decline rapidly during CPR, which only slows the deteriorating state. Once available, a defibrillator should be positioned with quick-look paddles for rhythm evaluation. VF or pulseless VT is treated immediately. Blind defibrillation is rarely indicated. Asynchronous shocks are given for VF or pulseless VT. Synchronous shocks are given for stable rhythms (eg, atrial fib/flutter, monomorphic VT)[10] to avoid impinging on the relative refractory period.

Energy levels for cardioversion impact success. Low currents may be ineffective and excessive energy levels cause myocardial injury.[59,60] The lowest energy for defibrillation is desired. A prospective study demonstrated that 175 and 320 J were equally effective for initial defibrillation attempts;[61] therefore, 200 J is recommended for initial defibrillation attempts.[10] The range for second countershocks is 200 to 360 J.

Body size impacts defibrillation energy requirements.[10] The optimal current for defibrillation is 30 to 40 A.[62] Adult transthoracic impedance is 70 to 80 gV, requiring a 200-J countershock for a 30-A current.[63] However, impedance varies significantly depending on energy delivery, chest size, electrode size, interelectrode distance, paddle-skin coupling, respiration, and antecedent countershocks.[62] Keep one electrode positioned on the right parasternal border below the clavicle, and the other in the left midaxillary line, level with the nipple.[10] Electrodes must not touch so the currents pass through the heart. During open chest resuscitation, one paddle is placed over the right ventricle, and the other behind the apex. Larger paddles are preferred for their lower resistance. Small paddles should only be used if required to fit in the chest.[64] It is also noteworthy that compression of the heart reduces the defibrillation threshold.[65]

Defibrillation threshold (DFT) describes the amount of current required to defibrillate the heart. DFT increases during CPR and is primarily affected by coronary perfusion pressure. Catecholamines decrease the DFT.[66] It was thought epinephrine decreased the DFT through beta-adrenergic effects; instead, this is owing to alpha-adrenergic increases in systemic pressure. Time-dependent increases in DFT observed during CPR are not completely understood. Adenosine may act through A_1 receptors to increase DFT over time.[67] Aminophylline, an adenosine receptor antagonist, decreases DFTs.

The presence of pacemakers and automatic internal cardio defibrillators (AICDs) impact defibrillation management. Paddles should not be placed directly over pacemaker generators,[68] and these devices should be interrogated to reassess pacing thresholds after defibrillation. AICDs are not a contraindication to external defibrillation for VF/VT,[130] and are shielded to withstand countershocks. AICD patches may increase transthoracic resistance.[69] Therefore, paddle orientation should be changed if initial countershocks fail. After defibrillation, the AICD unit should be tested.

Automated external defibrillators (AED) are increasingly common. AEDs analyze ECG pattern, sounds an alarm and discharges when VF is detected. They require less training and are more rapid at administering countershocks.[51] AEDs have equivalent survival compared with manual defibrillators.[70] Clinical trials have confirmed AEDs can be used safely and effectively by the lay person.[71]

Current-controlled defibrillators may improve the success of defibrillation.[72] These devices enhance delivery of energy and reduce risk of excessive energy delivery. The delivery of biphasic (bidirectional) or multipulse, multipathway shocks are methods used for internal defibrillators,[63] but efficacy for external defibrillation has not been established.[73]

A precordial thump may achieve defibrillation and be used when a defibrillator is not immediately available. It may be successful in 11 to 25% during VT. Unfortunately, precordial thumps may result in VF, asystole, or EMD, and are less unlikely to convert VF.[74]

Chest compressions must be temporarily discontinued to avoid electrical shock of those performing CPR. This hands-off interval is also used for rhythm analysis before defibrillation. Prolonging the hands-off period can significantly reduce the probability of successful cardioversion, and be kept as short as possible.[74]

PHYSIOLOGY OF CARDIOPULMONARY RESUSCITATION

Mechanisms generating forward blood flow during CPR have been a subject of significant controversy. Investigations have demonstrated chest compressions translate directly to the heart.[75] However, other mechanisms have been elucidated.

At least two other mechanisms appear responsible for blood flow during CPR. The thoracic pump was discovered by observing that coughing during cardiac arrest generated forward flow. Chest compressions also cause a rise in thoracic pressures capable of forcing blood into the systemic circulation.[34] The heart in this circumstance merely functions as a conduit. Many studies have validated the thoracic pump mechanism during CPR.[31,76]

Another mechanism for blood flow generated during CPR is the abdominal pump. This emphasizes effects of abdominal compressions, which are now advocated for CPR.[77] The abdominal pump operates through arterial and venous components. The arterial component reflects compression of the abdominal aorta, forcing blood into the peripheral circulation. The aortic valve remains closed during abdominal compression and resists retrograde arterial flow. Simultaneously, the venous component fills the heart from venous pressure. Both contribute hemodynamic benefits during abdominal compressions in CPR.

Clearly, the cardiac, thoracic, and abdominal pump mechanisms are important concepts of CPR physiology. The technique(s) employed during CPR dictates which mechanism predominates. Other factors that can influence effectiveness of these pump mechanisms include: cycle rates, compression durations, body habitus, cardiac size, chest wall stiffness, and the presence of pulmonary disease, as well as the duration of the resuscitation effort. Understanding these mechanisms has led to improved CPR techniques and adjunctive devices, which are directed towards improved vital organ perfusion.

CPR TECHNIQUE AND MECHANICAL ADJUNCTS

The high mortality rates associated with cardiac arrest are in part attributed to inadequate perfusion generated by CCM. Therefore a number of adjunctive devices have been developed to enhance the effectiveness of CCM.

Active Compression-Decompression

Active compression-decompression (ACD) is one means for improving the effectiveness of CCM. Originating from successful resuscitation with a plunger, a device consisting of a handheld suction cup with a central piston was developed (Fig. 17-4). ACD-CPR can increase aortic pressures resulting in improved cerebral, coronary, and renal blood flow.[78] Ventricular filling and venous return are augmented by negative intrathoracic pressure during the active decompression phase. Two studies

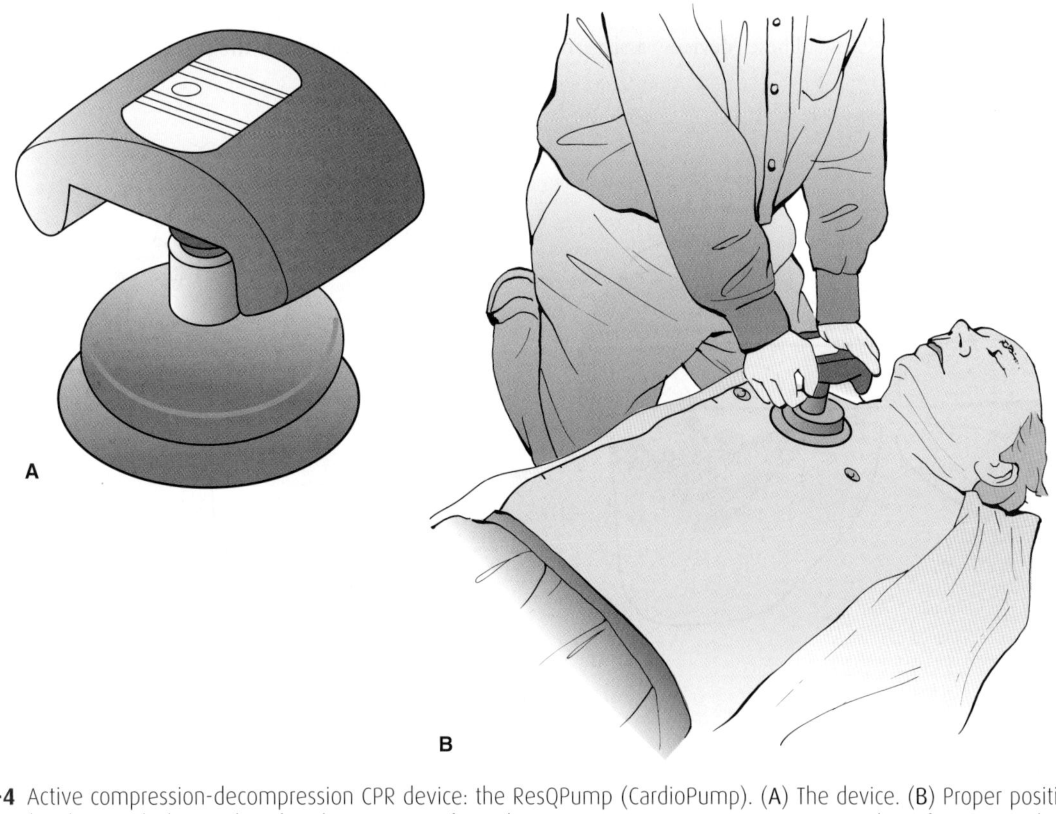

FIGURE 17-4 Active compression-decompression CPR device: the ResQPump (CardioPump). (A) The device. (B) Proper position of the ResQPumpTM (CardioPump). (*Reproduced with permission from the American Heart Association: ACLS—the reference textbook, in Cummins RO (ed). ACLS: Principles and Practice. CPR: Assessment, Adjuncts, and Alternatives. 2003; p 190*).

reported increased ROSC and 24-hour survival with the ACD device. Survival to discharge was higher with ACD in both studies but did not reach statistical significance.[79,80] Data from 2866 patients using the ACD device were subsequently combined.[81] ACD improved 1-hour survival, but long-term outcome was not significantly different from standard CPR. A randomized clinical trial demonstrated significantly improved 1-year survival following ACD compared with standard CPR.[82] Notably, a prospective trial found that combining ACD with controlled ventilation using an inspiratory impedance threshold device improved short-term survival when compared with standard CPR.[83]

Synchronizing chest and abdominal pumping techniques within the same compression cycle is another means for improving the effectiveness of CCM. Termed, "phased thoracic abdominal compression-decompression CPR" (PTACD-CPR), this technique employs abdominal compression during the relaxation phase of chest compression. Simplified applications involve compressing the chest and abdomen at equal durations. Initial clinical studies using PTACD-CPR yielded improvements in outcome measures.[84] Return of spontaneous circulation and survival to discharge were both significantly improved using PTACD-CPR for inpatient cardiac arrests.[84–86] A hand-held device has been developed that allows single rescuer PTACD-CPR combined with compression-decompression mechanics (Fig. 17-5). The method was deemed safe and effective by investigators.[54] Further studies are warranted to determine its potential impact on survival rates.

Noninvasive Mechanical Devices

Noninvasive mechanical devices have been developed to enhance the ergonomics of CPR. These devices assist in improving CPRs performance effectiveness, which can minimize the fatigue associated with performing CPR.

Fatigue becomes a particularly significant problem when attempting to perform ACD-CPR for extended periods of time. This led to developing an automatic chest compression device. Clinical applications have found its use feasible for out-of-hospital CPR.[87] Preliminary trials indicated the device improves the 30-day survival of patients suffering witnessed cardiac arrest.[88]

The pneumatic vest is another noninvasive mechanical device that alternates pressures around the thoracic cage (Vest-CPR). Vest-CPR utilizes a pneumatic bladder tailored to fit the chest wall. Air is forced into and out of the vest by a pneumatic drive. Clinical trials demonstrated improved outcomes with an increased rate of ROSC.[89] Another device has been described that employs a constricting band.[90] This portable device is currently available that provides mechanical vest-CPR (Fig. 17-6). Further trials are needed to determine the impact of vest-CPR devices on clinical outcomes.

Open Chest Cardiac Massage

Open chest cardiac massage is a valuable resuscitative method that is effective at returning blood flow during cardiac arrest. OCM was popularized by surgeons for resuscitation before 1960. The technique is currently advocated for specific circumstances such as cardiac arrest from penetrating chest trauma. Precluding effective CPR, OCM should also be considered for cardiac arrest resulting from hypothermia, massive pulmonary embolism, pericardial tamponade, intrathoracic hemorrhage, postcardiotomy arrest, and chest deformity. OCM is usually performed via a left lateral thoracotomy except after recent cardiac surgery for which the prior sternotomy is reentered. A

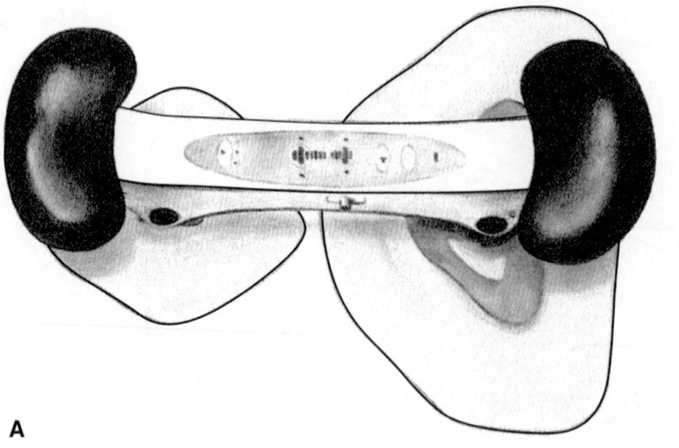
A

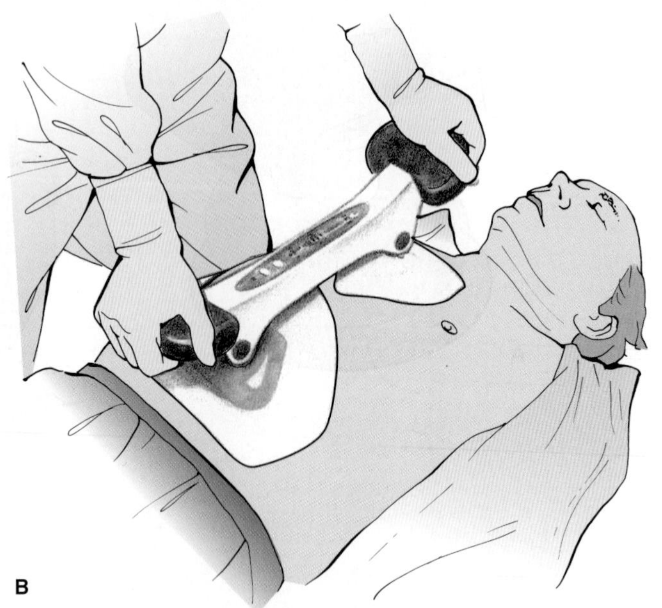
B

FIGURE 17-5 Device for phased thoracic-abdominal compression-decompression CPR (PTACD-CPR). The hand-held device alternates chest compression and abdominal decompression with chest decompression and abdominal compression. (A) The device. (B) Proper position of the device for clinical use. (*Reproduced with permission from the American Heart Association: ACLS—the reference textbook, in Cummins RO (ed). ACLS: Principles and Practice. CPR: Assessment, Adjuncts, and Alternatives. 2003; p 193*).

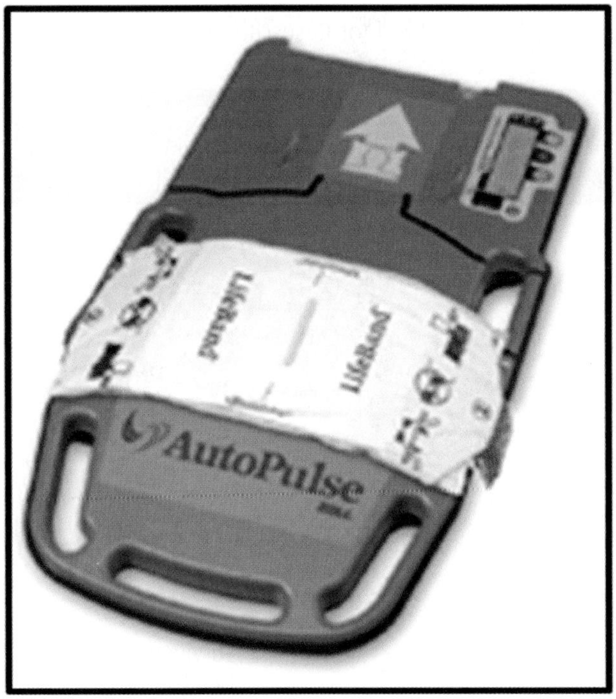

FIGURE 17-6 Autopulse Noninvasive Cardiac Support Pump by ZOLL Medical Corporation. The device delivers vest-CPR without interruptions or fatigue. (*Reproduced with permission from ZOLL Medical Corp, Chelmsford, MA.*)

left thoracotomy is performed at approximately the fifth intercostal space. The pericardium is entered anterior to the phrenic nerve and the heart compressed between both hands. Alternatively, one-hand massage may be performed while using the other to control bleeding or occlude the descending thoracic aorta (Fig. 17-7).

Numerous studies have demonstrated superior hemodynamics during OCM compared with CCM.[91,92] Notable are increased diastolic pressures and reduced central venous pressures,[57] which favorably impacts coronary perfusion compared with CCM. Cardiac output and cerebral blood flow are higher during OCM,[92] explaining how OCM can successfully ROSC after failed efforts with CCM. However, outcomes cannot be expected to improve when OCM follows prolonged CPR.[93] Laboratory studies suggest that OCM can improve outcomes if applied after relatively short durations of ineffective CCM. A prospective, nonrandomized clinical trial illustrated the importance of instituting OCM earlier to improve outcome.[94] Patients who received OCM had improved outcomes, which declined as the duration of CCM before OCM increased.

Timely application of OCM can improve survival in a variety of clinical scenarios. One setting in which OCM has been used routinely is in the postcardiotomy ICU. One review strongly confirmed the benefit of open chest massage in patients suffering cardiac arrest following open heart surgery.[57] The study found that reopening the chest in this setting has the greatest potential benefit in patients arresting within 24 hours of surgery and performed within 10 minutes of cardiac arrest.

Potential complications of OCM include right ventricular perforation, hemorrhage, lung laceration, phrenic nerve injury, esophageal and aortic injury, cardiac lacerations, and empyema. Infection is surprisingly low (5%) given the nature of the procedure, and related limitations on sterile technique.

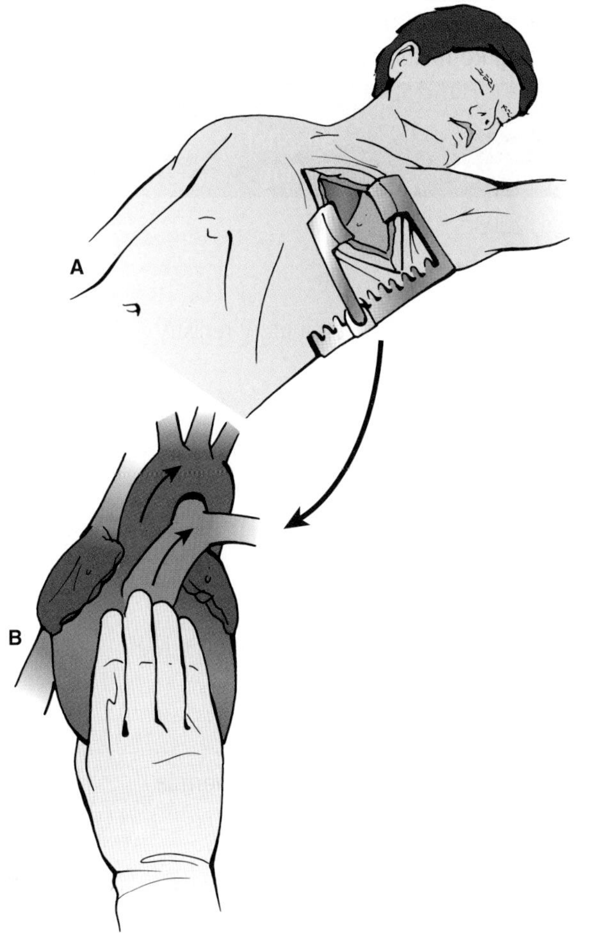

FIGURE 17-7 Technique of open chest cardiac massage. The heart is exposed via an anterolateral thoracotomy through the fifth intercostal space. The pericardium is opened if there is evidence of pericardial tamponade; otherwise, it is left intact. The heart is massaged at a rate of 60 to 80 beats per minute.

The intra-aortic balloon pump improves hemodynamics during CPR. However, its value in this setting appears limited.

Cardiopulmonary Bypass

Cardiopulmonary bypass (CPB) has seen increased use for treating refractory cardiac arrest.[95] Hemodynamics, survival, and neurologic function are improved in experimental models of cardiac arrest treated with CPB versus standard CCM. Although clinical reports are uncontrolled, and frequently anecdotal, the growing body of evidence demonstrates CPB is efficacious for the treatment of not only cardiogenic shock,[131] but also cardiac arrest. It is noteworthy that several studies have demonstrated improved survival with good neurologic outcomes using CPB after prolonged periods of CPR. CPR efforts and patient selection are important considerations when interpreting these clinical results. Patients have been successfully bridged to transplantation utilizing CPB after cardiac arrest.[96–98]

TABLE 17-2 Published Clinical Series in which Cardiopulmonary Bypass Was Utilized for Resuscitation of Patients Suffering Refractory Cardiac Arrest

Author, Year	Hospital Setting	No. Treated	No. (%) ROSC	No. (%) Survival	CPR Duration (min) Median (Range) or Mean ± SD
Chen, 2003[99]	In	57	38 (67)	18 (32)	47 ± 13
Chen, 2008[149]	In	59	55 (93)	17 (29)	53 ± 37
Conrad, 2004[137]	Voluntary registry	43	NR*	9 (21)	NR
Kurose, 1995[138]	In	9	2 (22)	2 (22)	80 (35–130)
Mair, 1996[139]	ER	5 (cannulated 7)	4 (57)	3 (43)	20–60
Martin, 1998[98]	ER & witnessed Out	10 (cannulated 13)	6 (46)	0 (0)	32 ± 13.6
Massetti, 2005[97]	In and out	40	18 (45)	8 (20)	105 ± 44
Raithel, 1989[140]	In	29	NR	6 (21)	NR
Rousou, 1994[141]	Cardiac surgical ICU	16	NR	9 (56)	Survivors: 50 ± 7 Deaths: 51 ± 6
Schwarz, 2003[96]	In and out	17 (cannulated 21)	9 (43)	3 (14)	NR
Silfvast, 2003[104]	Out, hypothermia	23	NR	14 (61)	67.25 (43.75–109)
Sung, 2006[148]	In	22	NR	9 (41)	Survivors:43 ± 20
Younger, 1999[136]	ER and in	21 (cannulated 25)	14 (57)	9 (36)	Survivors: 21 ± 16 Deaths: 43 ± 32

*NR = Not reported.
Outcomes represented as percent of patients in which cannulation was attempted.

Most impressive are the improved outcomes when CPB was used to treat refractory cardiac arrest.[95,132,148] Because of the heterogeneity among these studies, it is difficult to arrive at objective selection criteria. There is also a paucity of reported complications. Therefore, future studies need to better define patient selection criteria and related risk/benefit considerations to guide CPB use (Table 17-2). Prognostic factors that are felt to be important include age, treatable conditions, adequacy of CPR, and timely intervention. Generally, CPB should be instituted within 30 to 45 minutes of witnessed arrests after more extended periods of CCM has been documented.[97,99] Clearly, CPB can result in successful resuscitation following prolonged periods of CPR in pediatric cases[100,101] and hypothermic cardiac arrests.

Hypothermic cardiac arrest is a unique category in which survival can follow prolonged cardiac arrest. CPB has a unique capability for rewarming during resuscitative circulatory support.[102,103] The largest experience in adults treated for hypothermia was reported from Finland.[104] Findings indicated that age and arterial pH at presentation had significant prognostic implications. The duration of CPR did not affect the likelihood of survival in these cases.

Direct Mechanical Ventricular Actuation

Direct mechanical ventricular actuation (DMVA) is a unique non–blood contacting device that provides systolic *and* diastolic actuation of the ventricular myocardium (Fig. 17-8). DMVA is pneumatically regulated with an atraumatic vacuum attachment. Rapid application is performed within minutes through a thoracotomy or sternotomy, which results in physiologic, pulsatile blood flow.[105,133] Pulsatile reperfusion probably best explains the improved neurologic outcome following resuscitative circulatory support using DMVA versus CPB in animals.[106–108] Lack of blood contact also circumvents the need for anticoagulants and reduces thromboembolic complications. DMVA has been used successfully in humans for bridge to transplantation, postcardiotomy support, and recovery from severe myocarditis.[105,134] Recent studies have demonstrated DMVA's favorable effect on maladaptive cell signaling when supporting the severely failing heart.[109,110] Myocardial strain analysis has demonstrated myocardial function improves within 10 minutes of DMVA resuscitative circulatory support.[111] Particularly notable are the findings of improved neurologic function following resuscitative support with DMVA versus CPB. DMVA's unique ability to provide

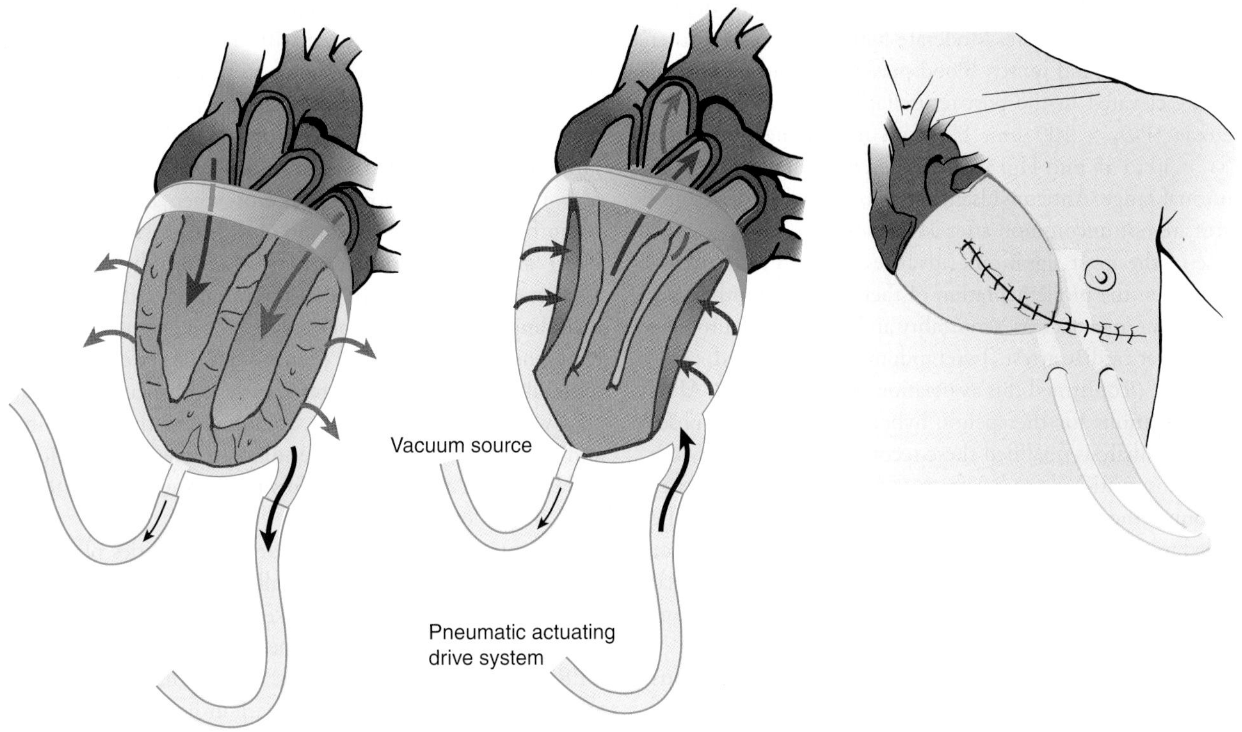

FIGURE 17-8 Direct mechanical ventricular actuation (DMVA). The ventricles are encompassed by a pneumatically driven device that is vacuum attached to the arrested heart.

immediate pulsatile reperfusion may best explain its beneficial impact on cerebral resuscitation.

CEREBRAL PROTECTION/RESUSCITATION

The goal of CPR is to provide sufficient blood flow to vital organs until definitive intervention. The brain is the organ most vulnerable to ischemia during cardiac arrest. Consciousness is lost in seconds, high-energy phosphates and glycogen stores are depleted in minutes with lactic acid accumulation causing secondary cytotoxic effects. Limited cerebral blood flow actually may exacerbate the sequelae by allowing anaerobic metabolism. These circumstances help explain why CPR out-of-hospital cardiac arrest results in so few neurologically intact survivors.[112]

Given the importance of cerebral resuscitation, it has been suggested that current CPR protocols put too much emphasis on ventilation. Cardiocerebral resuscitation appears to convey more appropriate emphasis on the brain and fosters the development of new treatment paradigms.[113] Recent examples include recommended techniques when performing basic CPR. The reluctance to perform mouth-to-mouth ventilation has led to guidelines for cardiac only resuscitation (chest compressions only). Data from multicenter trials have found cardiac only resuscitation may lead to improved survival and neurologic outcome.[30] The findings are best explained by improvements in cerebral blood flow. Specifically, chest compressions are used to initiate CPR and are not interrupted for ventilation.

CCM generates limited blood flow. During CPR, only venous valves can prevent transmission of high, intrathoracic pressures to the jugular venous system. Cerebral blood flow is kept at 50 mL/min/100 g by autoregulation when cerebral perfusion pressures are in the normal physiologic range.[114] CPR results in low cerebral perfusion pressures, seldom exceeding 40 mm Hg.[115] Cerebral flow is only 10 to 15% of normal, which may be more harmful than no flow at all.

Mechanical circulatory support is an obvious means for improving cerebral blood flow during CPR. This is supported by the growing body of clinical evidence indicating the implementation of CPB after failed CPR attempts improves outcomes. Laboratory investigations have demonstrated pulsatile flow is superior to nonpulsatile flow with regard to cerebral resuscitation. Pulsatile reperfusion results in favorable flow to the gray matter,[106] which correlates with increased postresuscitation cerebral high energy phosphate content.[107] Cerebral function and histopathology are significantly improved following pulsatile versus nonpulsatile reperfusion.[108,135]

There are other critical aspects related to cerebral resuscitation, which deserve further consideration. Neurons function for up to 60 minutes during ischemia. However, reperfusion can cause neuronal damage that is multifactorial in origin. Calcium overload, free-radical injury, and no-reflow phenomenon may all contribute to reperfusion injury.[114] No-reflow describes states of hypoperfusion that follow cerebral ischemia. Platelet aggregation, altered calcium flux, vasoconstriction, and pericapillary edema are all presumed causative factors. Intracranial pressure may not be as important because it commonly returns to normal after cardiac arrest except after cerebral trauma. Cerebral blood flow remains depressed for 18 to 24 hours after a severe ischemic insult. Subsequent hypoperfusion is believed secondary to calcium-induced precapillary vasoconstriction.

Cerebral blood flow after ischemic injury is critically dependent on perfusion pressure. Moderate hypotension can further cerebral ischemia and injury. Blood pressure should be normal or mildly elevated in the post-resuscitation period. Moderate hyperoxia (PO_2 = 100 mm Hg) and mild hyperventilation ($PaCO_2$ = 30 to 35 mm Hg) are desirable. Arterial pH is kept in the normal range. Anticonvulsants are given as needed, because seizures are not uncommon after ischemic brain injury.

One of the most significant advances in cerebral resuscitation has been the implementation of therapeutic hypothermia. Mild hypothermia decreases mortality and improves neurologic recovery after cardiac arrest. Two randomized, controlled, clinical trials[116,117] confirmed this association. This led to new AHA recommendations for therapeutic hypothermia.[118] The subsequent meta-analysis qualified these recommendations.[119] More recently, observational studies from growing clinical databases have found the safety and efficacy of hypothermia can be extended to routine clinical practice.[120,121] A new clinical device is now available to selectively chill the brain using intra-nasal cooling (Fig. 17-9). Further trials will be needed to demonstrate its effectiveness.

Other considerations after ROSC include continuous hemodynamic monitoring, and use of supplemental oxygen. Antiarrhythmics are continued as arrhythmias commonly occur from increased circulating catecholamines. Beta-adrenergic blockade should be instituted, unless bradycardia is a problem. Bradycardia requires airway and ventilation be carefully assessed. Atropine, epinephrine, and/or pacing are indicated if hypotension accompanies bradyarrhythias.

Antiarrhythmics, pacemakers, and automatic internal cardiodefibrillators are also important considerations for patients surviving sudden death. Clinical studies have shown survival can be significantly improved with these interventions.[72,122,123] Amiodarone has also been shown to be effective in this regard.

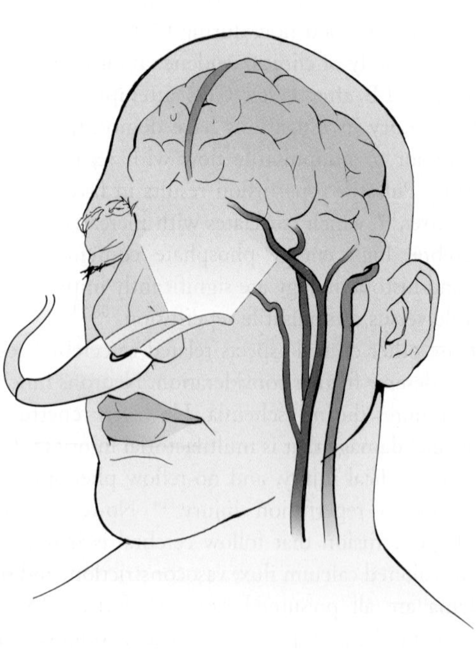

FIGURE 17-9 The RhinoChill delivers an intra-nasal agent to selectively cool the brain. (*Reproduced with permission from BeneChill, Inc., San Diego, CA.*)

Predicting which patients will survive resuscitation efforts remains elusive. Patients presenting in VF/VT have a better prognosis compared with asystole or PEA.[11,41,47] Advanced age may not be a prognostic indicator when considering other comorbidities.[11,12,42,47] Location of the arrest (ICU versus non-ICU) also impacts outcome.[11,12] Comorbid conditions are associated with more than 95% of mortalities after cardiac arrest including renal failure, metastatic cancer, pneumonia, sepsis, hypotension, stroke, and homebound lifestyle.[11] Survival is more likely for witnessed arrests, early defibrillation CPR initiated within 5 minutes, CPR durations less than 15 minutes, and postresuscitation hypothermia is implemented. Mortality increases from 44% for CPR less than 15 minutes to 95% for CPR that is longer in duration.[11,42]

In contrast to inpatients, where comorbidities play a major role, delayed therapy outweighs all other prognostic factors for out-of-hospital arrests. Other key determinants for survival include the initial rhythm, witnessed arrest, downtime before CPR, and any delay in treatment. Early definitive care is associated with improved outcome. As with in-hospital arrest, VF/VT has the best prognosis, and bystander CPR is strongly associated with improved survival rates.[118] Decreased mortality from bystander CPR is primarily from reduced postresuscitation anoxic encephalopathy. Return of consciousness within 24 to 48 hours of arrest is a favorable prognostic sign.[11] Therapeutic hypothermia has significantly enhanced the likelihood of neurologic recovery and survival.

Long-term survival in patients discharged after an out-of-hospital arrest is very reasonable. Reported 1-year survival rate ranges from 75 to 85%, and approximately 50% are still alive at four years (see Table 17-1). The majority of these patients ultimately die of cardiac causes.[14,124] Positive predictors for long-term survival are: cardiac arrest associated with acute myocardial infarction (MI), no prior history of MI, and also short-time intervals between arrest, CPR, and definitive care.[125] Primary antiarrhythmic events, congestive heart failure, impaired left ventricular function, extensive coronary artery disease, and complex premature ventricular depolarizations are less likely to result in long-term survival after discharge.

Unfortunately, not all patients who survive sudden death have a subsequent good quality of life.[126] Depression is a common problem following discharge, but usually resolves within a few months.[11] The incidence and characteristics of mental impairment in those who survive is variable. Significant neurologic impairment usually results in death before hospital discharge. While neurologic deficits can be very disabling,[127,134] many survivors of sudden death retain normal neurologic function.

ETHICAL CONSIDERATIONS

Resuscitation efforts should be discontinued when ACLS efforts do not result in ROSC. Discontinuation is based on clinical judgment. Although several studies have shown that CPR for longer than 30 minutes is unlikely to result in long-term survival. There are many growing reports of neurologically intact survivors after prolonged resuscitation.[11] This is particularly evident when examining the use of mechanical circulatory support. Considerations for discontinuing ACLS should also include underlying medical conditions.

CONCLUSION

Early defibrillation, effective BLS, and timely ACLS measures represent the major theme in the treatment of cardiac arrest. Unfortunately, survival rates have remained disappointingly low. A more appropriate focus on cerebral resuscitation should substantially improve future clinical outcomes. The use of circulatory support in patients that fail initial ACLS efforts has clearly demonstrated promise when initial resuscitation efforts fail. Defining qualified selection criteria and treatment protocols will require further study. Additionally, it will be important to implement those therapies that improve neurologic recovery. Therapeutic hypothermia has clearly had one of the greatest recent impacts in this regard. Integrating hypothermia, resuscitative circulatory support devices, and cerebroprotective agents has compelling potential. They can justify and help guide future clinical trials. New paradigms and treatment protocols for CPR may evolve from these critically needed investigations.

REFERENCES

1. American Heart Association: *Heart Disease and Stroke Statistics—2004 Update.* Dallas, TX: American Heart Association; 2003.
2. Roger WJ, Canto JG, Lambrew CT, et al: Temporal trends in the treatment of over 1.5 million patients with myocardial infarction in the US from 1990 through 1999: the National Registry of Myocardial Infarction 1, 2 and 3. *J Am Coll Cardiol* 2000; 36:2056-2063.
3. Antman EM, Anbe DT, Armstrong PW, et al: ACC/AHA guidelines for the management of patients with ST-Elevation myocardial infarction-executive summary. *J Am Coll Cardiol* 2004; 44:671-719.
4. Myerburg RJ, Castellanos A: Cardiac arrest and sudden death, in Braunwald E (ed): *Heart Disease.* Philadelphia, WB Saunders, 1992; p 756.
5. Eisenberg MS, Bergner L, Hallstrom A: Survivors of out-of-hospital cardiac arrest: morbidity and long-term survival. *Am J Emerg Med* 1984; 2:189.
6. Kannel WB, Doyle JT, McNamara PM, et al: Precursors of sudden coronary death: factors related to the incidence of sudden death. *Circulation* 1975; 51:606.
7. Kuller L, Lilienfeld A, Fisher R: Epidemiologic study of sudden and unexpected deaths due to arteriosclerotic heart disease. *Circulation* 1966; 34:1056.
8. Girdon T, Kannel WB: Premature mortality from coronary heart disease: the Framingham study. *JAMA* 1971; 215:1617.
9. Emergency Cardiac Care Committee and Subcommittees, American Heart Association: 2005 American Heart Association Guidelines for Cardiopulmonary Resuscitation and Emergency Cardiovascular Care. *Circulation* 2005; 112(Suppl I):IV-1-IV-203.
10. American Heart Association in Collaboration with International Liaison Committee on Resuscitation Guidelines 2000, for Cardiopulmonary Resuscitation and Emergency Cardiovascular Care: Introduction to the International Guidelines 2000, for CPR and ECC: A Consensus on Science. *Circulation* 2000; 102(Suppl I):I-1-I-11.
11. Bedell SE, Delbanco TL, Cook EF, et al: Survival after cardiopulmonary resuscitation in the hospital. *NEJM* 1983; 309:569.
12. DeBard ML: Cardiopulmonary resuscitation: analysis of six years experience and review of the literature. *Ann Emerg Med* 1981; 10:408.
13. Longstreth WT Jr, Inui TS, Cobb LA, et al: Neurologic recovery after out-of-hospital cardiac arrest. *Ann Intern Med* 1983; 98:588.
14. Earnest MP, Yarnell PR, Merrill SL, et al: Long-term survival and neurologic status after resuscitation from out-of-hospital cardiac arrest. *Neurology* 1980; 30(12):1298-1302.
15. Plaisance P, Lurie KG, Vicaut E, et al: A comparison of standard cardiopulmonary resuscitation and active compression-decompression resuscitation for out-of-hospital cardiac arrest. *NEJM* 1999; 341:1569.
16. Brown CG, Martin DR, Pepe PE, et al: A comparison of standard dose and high dose epinephrine in cardiac arrest outside the hospital. The Multicenter High-Dose Epinephrine Study Group. *NEJM* 1992; 327:1051.
17. Marwick TH, Case C, Siskind V, et al: Adverse effect of early high-dose adrenaline on outcome of ventricular fibrillation. *Lancet* 1988; II:66.
18. Lindner KH, Prengel AW, Pfenninger EG, et al: Vasopressin improves vital organ blood flow during closed-chest CPR in pigs. *Circulation* 1995; 91:215.
19. Lindner KH, Dirks B, Strohmenger HU, et al: Randomized comparison of epinephrine and vasopressin in patients with out-of-hospital ventricular fibrillation. *Lancet* 1997; 349:535.
20. Aung K, Htay T: Vasopressin for cardiac arrest. A systematic review and meta-analysis. *Arch Intern Med* 2005; 165:17-24.
21. Kornberger E, Prengel AW, Krismer A, et al: Vasopressin-mediated adrenocorticotropin release increases plasma cortisol concentrations during cardiopulmonary resuscitation. *Crit Care Med* 2000; 28:3517-3521.
22. Hekimian G, Baugnon T, Thuong M, et al: Cortisol levels and adrenal reserve after successful cardiac arrest resuscitation. *Shock* 2004; 22:116-119.
23. Ito T, Saitoh D, Takasu A, et al: Serum cortisol as a predictive marker of the outcome in patients resuscitated after cardiopulmonary arrest. *Resuscitation* 2004; 62:55-60.
24. Pene F, Hyvernat H, Mallet V, et al: Prognostic value of relative adrenal insufficiency after out-of-hospital cardiac arrest. *Intern Care Med* 2005; 31:627-633.
25. Dorian P, Cass D, Schwartz B, et al: Amiodarone as compared with lidocaine for shock-resistant ventricular fibrillation. *NEJM* 2002; 346(12): 884-890.
26. Sceinman MM, Levine JH, Cannom DS, et al: For the Intravenous Amiodarone Multicenter Investigators Group: dose-ranging study of intravenous amiodarone in patients with life-threatening ventricular tachyarrhythmias. *Circulation* 1995; 92:3264.
27. Kowey PR, Levine JH, Herre JM, et al: For the Intravenous Amiodarone Multicenter Investigators Group. Randomized, double-blind comparison of intravenous amiodarone and bretylium in the treatment of patients with recurrent, hemodynamically destabilizing ventricular tachycardia or fibrillation. *Circulation* 1995; 92:3255.
28. Kudenchuk PJ, Cobb LA, Copass MK, et al: Amiodarone for resuscitation after out-of-hospital cardiac arrest due to ventricular fibrillation. *NEJM* 1999; 341:871.
29. Hullston A: Cardiopulmonary resuscitation by chest compression alone or with mouth-to-mouth ventilation. *NEJM* 2000; 342:1546.
30. SOS-KANTO study group: Cardiopulmonary resuscitation by bystanders with chest compression only (SOS-KANTO): an observational study. *Lancet* 2007; 369:920-926.
31. Abella BS, Alvarado JP, Myklebust H, et al: Quality of cardiopulmonary resuscitation during in-hospital cardiac arrest. *JAMA* 2005; 293:305-310.
32. Wik L, Kramer-Johansen J, Myklebust H, et al: Quality of cardiopulmonary resuscitation during out-of-hospital cardiac arrest. *JAMA* 2005; 293:299-304.
33. Abella BS, Sandbo N, Vassilatos P, et al: Chest compression rates during cardiopulmonary resuscitation are suboptimal: a prospective study during in-hospital cardiac arrest. *Circulation* 2005; 111(4):428-434.
34. Maier GW, Tyson GS, Olsen CO, et al: The physiology of external cardiac massage: high-impulse cardiopulmonary resuscitation. *Circulation* 1984; 70:86.
35. Niemann JT, Criley JM, Rosborough JP, et al: Predictive indices of successful cardiac resuscitation after prolonged arrest and experimental cardiopulmonary resuscitation. *Ann Emerg Med* 1985; 14:521.
36. Garnett AR, Ornato JP, Gonzalez ER, et al: End-tidal carbon dioxide measurement during cardiopulmonary resuscitation. *JAMA* 1987; 257:512.
37. Sanders AB, Kern KB, Otto CW, et al: End-tidal carbon dioxide monitoring during cardiopulmonary resuscitation: a prognostic indicator for survival. *JAMA* 1989; 262:1347.
38. Herlitz J, Engdahl J, Svensson L, et al: Factors associated with an increased chance of survival among patients suffering from an out-of-hospital cardiac arrest in a national perspective in Sweden. *Am Heart J* 2005; 149:61-66.
39. Brindley PG, Markland DM, Mayers I, et al: Predictors of survival following in-hospital adult cardiopulmonary resuscitation. *CMAJ* 2002; 167(4):343.
40. Bunch TJ, White RD, Gersh BJ, et al: Long-term outcomes of out-of-hospital cardiac arrest after successful early defibrillation. *NEJM* 2003; 348(26):2626-2633.
41. Peberdy MA, Kaye W, Ornato JP, et al: Cardiopulmonary resuscitation of adults in the hospital: a report of 14720 cardiac arrests from the National Registry of Cardiopulmonary Resuscitation. *Resuscitation* 2003; 58:297-308.

42. Sandroni C, Ferro G, Santangelo S, et al: In-hospital cardiac arrest: survival depends mainly on the effectiveness of the emergency response. *Resuscitation* 2004; 62:291-297.
43. Krischer JP, Fine EG, Davis JH, et al: Complications of cardiac resuscitation. *Chest* 1987; 92:287.
44. Bedell SE, Fulton EJ: Unexpected findings and complications at autopsy after cardiopulmonary resuscitation (CPR). *Arch Intern Med* 1986; 146:1725.
45. Powner DJ, Holcombe PA, Mello LA: Cardiopulmonary resuscitation-related injuries. *Crit Care Med* 1984; 12:54.
46. DeLuna AB, Coumel P, Leclerq JF: Ambulatory sudden cardiac death: mechanism of production of fatal arrhythmia on the basis of data from 157 cases. *Am Heart J* 1989; 117:151.
47. Cohn AC, Wilson WM, Yan B, et al: Analysis of clinical outcomes following in-hospital adult cardiac arrest. *Intern Med J* 2004; 34:398-402.
48. Weaver WD, Cobb LA, Hallstrom AP, et al: Factors influencing survival after out-of-hospital cardiac arrest. *J Am Coll Cardiol* 1986; 7:752.
49. Stiell IG, Wells GA, Field BJ, et al: Improve out-of-hospital cardiac arrest survival through the inexpensive optimization of an existing defibrillation program. OPALS Study Phase II. *JAMA* 1999; 281:1175.
50. Winkle RA, Mead RH, Ruder MA, et al: Effect of duration of ventricular fibrillation on defibrillation efficacy in humans. *Circulation* 1990; 81:1477.
51. Cummins RO: From concept to standard of care? Review of the clinical experience with automated external defibrillators. *Ann Emerg Med* 1989; 18:1270.
52. Levine JH, Massumi A, Scheinman MM, et al: Intravenous amiodarone for recurrent sustained hypotensive ventricular tachyarrhythmias. *J Am Coll Cardiol* 1996; 27:67.
53. Marwick TH, Case CC, Siskind V, et al: Prediction of survival from resuscitation: a prognostic index derived from multivariate logistic model analysis. *Resuscitation* 1991; 22:129.
54. Arntz HR, Agrawal R, Richter H, et al: Phased chest and abdominal compression-decompression versus conventional cardiopulmonary resuscitation in out-of-hospital cardiac arrest. *Circulation* 2001; 104(7):768-72.
55. Cummins R, Graves J, Horan S, et al: Pre-hospital transcutaneous pacing for asystolic arrest. *Ann Emerg Med* 1990; 19:239.
56. Ivatury RR, Rohman M: Emergency department thoracotomy for trauma: a collective review. *Resuscitation* 1987; 15:23.
57. Mackay JH, Powell SJ, Osgathorp J, et al: Six-year prospective audit of chest reopening after cardiac arrest. *Eur J Cardiothorac Surg* 2002; 22(3): 421-425.
58. Eysmann SB, Marchlinski FE, Buxton A, et al: Electrocardiographic changes after cardioversion of ventricular arrhythmias. *Circulation* 1986; 73:73.
59. Ewy GA, Taren D, Banert J, et al: Comparison of myocardial damage from defibrillator discharge at various dosages. *Med Instrum* 1980; 14:9.
60. Warner ED, Dahl AAJ, Webb SW, et al: Myocardial injury from transthoracic countershock. *Arch Pathol Lab Med* 1975; 99:55.
61. Weaver WD, Cobb LA, Copass MK, et al: Ventricular fibrillation: a comparative trial using 175-J and 320-J shocks. *NEJM* 1982; 307:1101.
62. Kerber RE, Martins JB, Kienzle MG, et al: Energy, current, and success in defibrillation and cardioversion: clinical studies using an automated impedance-based method of energy adjustment. *Circulation* 1988; 77:1038.
63. Kerber RE: Electrical treatment of cardiac arrhythmias: defibrillation and cardioversion. *Ann Emerg Med* 1993; 22:296.
64. Atkins DL, Sirna S, Kieso R, et al: Pediatric defibrillation: importance of paddle size in determining transthoracic impedance. *Pediatrics* 1988; 82:914.
65. Idriss SF, Anstadt M, Anstadt GL, et al: The effect of cardiac compression on defibrillation efficacy and the upper limit of vulnerability. *J Cardiovasc Electrophysiol* 1995; 6:368.
66. Rattes MF, Sharma AD, Klein GJ, et al: Adrenergic effects on internal cardiac defibrillation threshold. *Am J Physiol* 1987; 253:H500.
67. Lerman BB, Engelstein ED: Metabolic determinants of defibrillation: role of adenosine. *Circulation* 1995; 91:838.
68. Levine PA, Barold SS, Fletcher RD, et al: Adverse acute and chronic effects of electrical defibrillation on implanted unipolar cardiac pacing systems. *J Am Coll Cardiol* 1983; 1:1413.
69. Walls JT, Schuder JC, Curtis JJ, et al: Adverse effects of permanent cardiac internal defibrillator patches on external defibrillation. *Am J Cardiol* 1989; 64:1144.
70. Cummins RO, Eisenberg MS, Litwin PE, et al: Automatic external defibrillators used by emergency medical technicians: a controlled clinical trial. *JAMA* 1987; 257:1605.
71. Public Access Defibrillation Trial Investigators: Public-access defibrillation and survival after out-of-hospital cardiac arrest. *NEJM* 2004; 351:637-646.
72. Bigger JT, Whang W, Rottman JN, et al: Mechanisms of death in the CABG Patch Trial: a randomized trial of implantable cardiac defibrillator prophylaxis in patients at high risk of death after coronary artery bypass graft surgery. *Circulation* 1999; 99:1419.
73. Kerber RE, Bourland JD, Kallok MJ, et al: Transthoracic defibrillation using sequential and simultaneous dual shock pathways: experimental studies. *PACE* 1990; 13:207.
74. Eftestøl T, Sunde K, Steen PA: Effects of interrupting precordial compressions on the calculated probability of defibrillation success during out-of-hospital cardiac arrest. *Circulation* 2002; 105:2270-2273.
75. Newton JR, Glower DD, Wolfe JA, et al: A physiologic comparison of external cardiac massage techniques. *J Thorac Cardiovasc Surg* 1988; 95:892.
76. Niemann JT, Rosborough JP, Hausknecht M, et al: Pressure synchronized cineangiography during experimental cardiopulmonary resuscitation. *Circulation* 1981; 64:985.
77. Beyar R, Kishon Y, Kimmel E, et al: Intrathoracic and abdominal pressure variations as an efficient method for cardiopulmonary resuscitation: studies in dogs compared with computer model results. *Cardiovasc Res* 1985; 19:335.
78. Schultz JJ, Coffeen P, Sweeney M, et al: Evaluation of standard and active compression-decompression CPR in an acute human model of ventricular fibrillation. *Circulation* 1994; 89:684.
79. Cohen TJ, Goldner BG, Maccaro PC, et al: A comparison of active compression-decompression cardiopulmonary resuscitation with standard cardiopulmonary resuscitation for cardiac arrests occurring in the hospital. *NEJM* 1993; 329:1918.
80. Tucker KJ, Galli F, Savitt MA, et al: Active compression-decompression resuscitation: effects on initial return of circulation and survival after in-hospital cardiac arrest. *Circulation* 1993; 88(Suppl I):I-10.
81. Mauer DK, Nolan J, Plaisance P, et al: Effect of active compression-decompression resuscitation (ACD-CPR) on survival: a combined analysis of individual patient data. *Resuscitation* 1999; 41:249.
82. Plaisance P, and the French Active Compression-Decompression Cardiopulmonary Resuscitation Study Group (Lariboisiere University, Paris, France): A comparison of standard cardiopulmonary resuscitation and active compression-decompression resuscitation for out-of-hospital cardiac arrest. *Ann Emerg Med* 2000; 341:569.
83. Wolcke BB, Mauer DK, Schoefmann MF, et al: Comparison of standard cardiopulmonary resuscitation versus the combination of active compression-decompression cardiopulmonary resuscitation and an inspiratory impedance threshold device for out-of-hospital cardiac arrest. *Circulation* 2003; 108(18):2201-2205.
84. Sack JB, Kesselbrenner MB, Bergman D: Survival from in-hospital cardiac arrest with interposed abdominal compression during cardiopulmonary resuscitation. *JAMA* 1992; 267:379.
85. Mateer JR, Stueven HA, Thompson BM, et al: Pre-hospital IAC-CPR versus standard CPR: paramedic resuscitation of cardiac arrest. *Am J Emerg Med* 1985; 3:143.
86. Sack JB, Kesselbrenner MB, Jarrad A: Interposed abdominal compression-cardiopulmonary resuscitation and resuscitation outcome during asystole and electromechanical dissociation. *Circulation* 1992; 86:192.
87. Wik L, Kiil S: Use of an automatic mechanical chest compression device (LUCAS) as a bridge to establishing cardiopulmonary bypass for a patient with hypothermic cardiac arrest. *Resuscitation* 2005; 66(3):391-394.
88. Steen S, Sjoberg T, Olsson P, et al: Treatment of out-of-hospital cardiac arrest with LUCAS, a new device for automatic mechanical compression and active decompression resuscitation. *Resuscitation* 2005; 67(1):25-30.
89. Weston CFM, de Latorre FJ, Dick W, et al: VEST-CPR system: results of a multicenter randomized pilot study. *J Am Coll Cardiol* 1998; 31(Suppl A): A-403.
90. Halperin HR, Berger R, Chandra N, et al: Cardiopulmonary resuscitation with a hydraulic-pneumatic band. *Crit Care Med* 2000; 28(11): 203-206.
91. Alifimoff JK: Open versus closed chest cardiac massage in nontraumatic cardiac arrest. *Resuscitation* 1987; 15:13.
92. Bircher N, Safar P: Cerebral preservation during cardiopulmonary resuscitation in dogs. *Crit Care Med* 1985; 13:135.
93. Geehr EC, Lewis FR, Auerbach PS: Failure of open-chest massage to improve survival after prehospital nontraumatic cardiac arrest. *NEJM* 1986; 314:1189.
94. Takino M, Okada Y: Optimum timing of resuscitation thoracotomy for non-traumatic out-of-hospital cardiac arrest. *Resuscitation* 1993; 26:69.
95. Nichol G, Karmy-Jones R, Salerno, et al: Systematic review of percutaneous cardiopulmonary bypass for cardiac arrest or cardiogenic shock states. *Resuscitation* 2006; 70:381-394.
96. Schwarz B, Mair P, Margreiter J, et al: Experience with percutaneous venoarterial cardiopulmonary bypass for emergency circulatory support. *Crit Care Med* 2003; 31(3):758-764.

97. Massetti M, Tasle M, LePage O, et al: Back from Irreversibility: extracorporeal life support for prolonged cardiac arrest. *Ann Thorac Surg* 2005; 79:178-184.
98. Martin GB, Rivers EP, Paradis NA, et al: Emergency department cardiopulmonary bypass in the treatment of human cardiac arrest. *Chest* 1998; 113:743-751.
99. Chen YS, Chao A, Yu HY, et al: Analysis and results of prolonged resuscitation in cardiac arrest patients rescued by extracorporeal membrane oxygenation. *J Am Coll Cardiol* 2003; 41(2):197-203.
100. Kelly RB, Porter PA, Meier AH, et al: Duration of cardiopulmonary resuscitation before extracorporeal rescue: how long is not long enough? *ASAIO J* 2005; 51:665-667.
101. Morris MC, Wernovsky G, Nadkarni VM: Survival outcomes after extracorporeal cardiopulmonary resuscitation instituted during active chest compressions following refractory in-hospital pediatric cardiac arrest. *Pediatr Crit Care Med* 2004; 5:440-446.
102. Wollenek G, Honarwar N, Golej J, et al: Cold water submersion and cardiac arrest in treatment of severe hypothermia with cardiopulmonary bypass. *Resuscitation* 2002; 52:255.
103. Farstad M, Andersen KS, Koller ME, et al: Rewarming from accidental hypothermia by extracorporeal circulation: a retrospective study. *Eur J Cardiothorac Surg* 2001; 20:58.
104. Silfvast T, Pettila V: Outcome from severe accidental hypothermia in Southern Finland: a 10-year review. *Resuscitation* 2003; 59(3):285-290.
105. Lowe JE, Hughes C, Biswass SS: Non-blood contacting biventricular support: direct mechanical ventricular actuation. *Operative Tech Thorac Cardiovasc Surg* 1999; 4:345.
106. Anstadt MP, Tedder M, Hegde SS, et al: Pulsatile reperfusion improves cerebral blood flow compared to nonpulsatile reperfusion following cardiac arrest. *Ann Thorac Surg* 1993; 56(3):453-461.
107. Anstadt MP, Tedder M, Banit DM, et al: Pulsatile flow attenuates cerebral reperfusion injury. *Circulation* 1993; 88(4)(Suppl I):I-170.
108. Anstadt MP, Stonnington MJ, Tedder M, et al: Pulsatile reperfusion after cardiac arrest improves neurologic outcome. *Ann Surg* 1991; 214(4): 478-490.
109. Franga DL, Wicker DL, White S, et al: Direct cardiac compression attenuates myocardial stress and injury in the acutely failing heart. *J Am Coll Surg* 2003; 197(3):S25.
110. Anstadt MP, Kerns S, Wozniak CJ, et al: Direct mechanical ventricular actuation of the acutely failing heart attenuates maladaptive cell signaling. *Circulation* 2009; 120:S1490.
111. Anstadt MP, Budharaju S, Darner RJ, et al: Ventricular actuation improves systolic and diastolic myocardial function in the small failing heart. *Ann Thorac Surg* 2009; 88:1982-1988.
112. Eckstein M, Stratton SJ, Chan LS: Cardiac arrest resuscitation evaluation in Los Angeles: CARE-LA. *Ann Emerg Med* 2005; 45:504-509.
113. Ewy GA, Kern KB, Sanders AB, et al: Cardiocerebral resuscitation for cardiac arrest. *Am J Med* 2006; 119:6-9.
114. Safar P: Cerebral resuscitation after cardiac arrest: research initiatives and future directions. *Ann Emerg Med* 1993; 22:324.
115. Brown CB, Schlifer J, Jenkins J, et al: Effect of direct mechanical ventricular assistance on myocardial hemodynamics during ventricular fibrillation. *Crit Care Med* 1989; 17:1175.
116. The Hypothermia after Cardiac Arrest Study Group: Mild therapeutic hypothermia to improve the neurologic outcome after cardiac arrest. *NEJM* 2002; 346:549-556.
117. Bernard SA, Gray TW, Buist MD, et al: Treatment of comatose survivors of out-of-hospital cardiac arrest with induced hypothermia. *NEJM* 2002; 346:557-563.
118. Nolan JP, Morley PT, Vanden Hoek TL, et al: Therapeutic hypothermia after cardiac arrest. an advisory statement by the advanced life support task force of the international liaison committee on resuscitation. *Circulation* 2003; 108:118-121.
119. Holzer M, Bernard SA, Hachimi-Idrissi S, et al: Hypothermia for neuroprotection after cardiac arrest: systematic review and individual patient data meta-analysis. *Crit Care Med* 2005; 33:414-418.
120. Arrich J: The European Resuscitation Council Hypothermia After Cardiac Arrest Registry Study Group. Clinical application of mild therapeutic hypothermia after cardiac arrest. *Crit Care Med* 2007; 35:1041-1047.
121. Rittenberger JC, Guyette FX, Tisherman SA, et al: Outcomes of a hospital-wide plan to improve care of comatose survivors of cardiac arrest. *Resuscitation* 2008; 79(2):198-204.
122. Bigger JT, for the CABG Patch Trial Investigators: Prophylactic use of implanted cardiac defibrillators in patients at high risk for ventricular arrhythmias after coronary artery bypass graft surgery. *NEJM* 1997; 337:1569.
123. Buxton AE, Lee KL, Fisher JD, et al: A randomized study of the prevention of sudden death in patients with coronary artery disease. *NEJM* 1999; 341:1882.
124. Liberthson RR, Nagel EL, Hirschman JC, et al: Pre-hospital ventricular defibrillation: prognosis and follow-up course. *NEJM* 1974; 291(7):317.
125. Gudjonsson H, Baldvinsson E, Oddsson G, et al: Results of attempted cardiopulmonary resuscitation of patients dying suddenly outside the hospital in Reykjavik and the surrounding area 1976-79. *Acta Med Scand* 1982; 212:247.
126. Eisenberg MS, Hallstrom A, Bergner L: Long-term survival after out-of-hospital cardiac arrest. *NEJM* 1982; 306(22):1340-1343.
127. Rockswold G, Sharma B, Ruiz E, et al: Follow-up of 514 consecutive patients with cardiac arrest outside the hospital. *JACEP* 1979; 8(6):216-220.
128. Hallstrom A, Cobb L, Johnson E, et al: Cardiopulmonary resuscitation by chest compression alone or with mouth-to-mouth ventilation. *NEJM* 2000; 342:1546.
129. Kudenchuk PJ, Cobb LA, Copass MK, et al: Amiodarone for resuscitation after out-of-hospital cardiac arrest due to ventricular fibrillation. *NEJM* 1993; 341:871.
130. Cummins RO: *Textbook of Advanced Cardiac Life Support*. Dallas, American Heart Association, 1994.
131. Sunami H, Fujita Y, Okada T, et al: Successful resuscitation from prolonged ventricular fibrillation using a portable percutaneous cardiopulmonary support system. *Anesthesiology* 2003; 99(5):1227-1229.
132. Sergeant P, Meyns B, Wouters P, et al: Long-term outcome after coronary artery bypass grafting in cardiogenic shock or cardiopulmonary resuscitation. *J Thorac Cardiovasc Surg* 2003; 126(5):1279-1286.
133. Anstadt MP, Hendry PJ, Plunkett MD, et al: Mechanical cardiac actuation achieves hemodynamics similar to cardiopulmonary bypass. *Surgery* 1990; 108:442.
134. Lowe JE, Anstadt MP, VanTright P, et al: First successful bridge to cardiac transplantation using direct mechanical ventricular actuation. *Ann Thorac Surg* 1991; 52:1237.
135. Snyder BD, Hauser WA, Loewenson RB, et al: Neurologic prognosis after cardiopulmonary arrest, III: seizure activity. *Neurology* 1980; 30:1292.
136. Younger JG, Schreiner RJ, Swaniker F, et al: Extracorporeal resuscitation of cardiac arrest. *Acad Emerg Med* 1999; 6:700-707.
137. Conrad AD, Rycus PT, Dalton H: Extracorporeal Life Support Registry Report. *ASAIO J* 2005; 51:4-10.
138. Kurose M, Okamoto K, Sato T, et al: The determinant of severe cerebral dysfunction in patients undergoing emergency extracorporeal life support following cardiopulmonary resuscitation. *Resuscitation* 1995; 30:15-20.
139. Mair P, Hoermann C, Moertl M, et al: Percutaneous venoarterial extracorporeal membrane oxygenation for emergency mechanical circulatory support. *Resuscitation* 1996; 33:29-34.
140. Raithel SC, Swartz MT, Braun PR, et al: Experience with an emergency resuscitation system. *ASAIO Transactions* 1989; 35:475-477.
141. Rousou JA, Engelman RM, Flack Je 3rd, et al: Emergency cardiopulmonary bypass in the cardiac surgical unit can be a lifesaving measure in postoperative cardiac arrest. *Circulation* 1994; 90(Suppl II): II-280-I-284.
142. Abramson N, Safar P, Detre K: Neurologic function in CPR survivors. *Circulation* 1982; 66(Suppl II):II-350;1400.
143. Lund I, Skulberg A: Resuscitation of cardiac arrest outside hospitals: experiences with a mobile intensive care unit in Oslo. *Acta Anaesthesiol Scand* 1973; (Suppl 53):13-16.
144. Cobb L, Hallstrom A, Weaver D, et al: Prognostic factors in patients resuscitated from sudden cardiac death, in Wilhelmsen L, Hjalmarson A (eds): *Acute and Long-Term Management of Myocardial Ischemia*. Molndal, Sweden, Lindgren and Soner, 1978; p 106.
145. Wernberg M, Thomassen A: Prognosis after cardiac arrest occurring outside intensive care and coronary units. *Acta Anaesthesiol Scand* 1979; 23(1):69-77.
146. Snyder BD, Loewenson RB, Gumnit RJ, et al: Neurologic prognosis after cardiopulmonary arrest: II. Level of consciousness. *Neurology* 1980; 30(1):52-58.
147. Nichol G, Thomas E, Callaway W: Regional variation in out-of hospital cardiac arrest incidence and outcome. *JAMA* 2008; 300(12):1423-1431.
148. Sung K, Lee YT, Park PW: Improved survival after cardiac arrest using emergent autopriming percutaneous cardiopulmonary support. *Ann Thorac Surg* 2006; 82:651-656.
149. Chen YS, Lin JW, Yu HY, et al: Cardiopulmonary resuscitation with assisted extracorporeal life-support versus conventional cardiopulmonary resuscitation in adults with in-hospital cardiac arrest: an observational study and propensity analysis. *Lancet* 2008; 372:554-561.

CHAPTER 18

Temporary Mechanical Circulatory Support

Edwin C. McGee, Jr.
Nader Moazami

INTRODUCTION

A number of ventricular assist devices (VADs) are available for acute circulatory support. As opposed to long-term VADs, which are designed for bridge to transplantation or long-term support in the nontransplant patient, temporary VADs are designed to reestablish adequate organ perfusion rapidly. Patients in cardiogenic shock require early aggressive therapy. Despite relief of ischemia, inotropic drugs, and control of cardiac rhythm, some patients remain hemodynamically unstable and require some type of mechanical circulatory support in order to restore a normal cardiac output. Cardiogenic shock occurs in 2.4 to 12% of patients with acute myocardial infarction (AMI).[1] The Should We Emergently Revascularize Occluded Coronaries for Cardiogenic Shock (SHOCK) trial demonstrated mortality of greater than 50% despite revascularization.[2] If instituted promptly, temporary mechanical support potentially leads to improved survival in this group of patients.[3] The need for circulatory support in the postcardiotomy period is relatively low and has been estimated to be in the range of 0.2 to 0.6%,[4] but when it occurs, it needs to be managed effectively if the patient is to be salvaged. Additional indications for acute VADs are in chronic heart failure patients who suffer cardiovascular collapse, and severe cases of myocarditis and postpartum cardiomyopathy.

All practicing cardiac surgeons should have an understanding of current devices, and have at least one of these support systems available. Studies show that even smaller facilities that do not have advanced heart failure programs can have improved patient survival if a device can be implemented rapidly and the patient is transferred to a tertiary care facility with expanded capabilities.[5]

This chapter describes the devices currently available, indications for support, patient management, and the overall morbidity and mortality associated with temporary mechanical support. In addition, it describes some of the more promising devices that have just received approval or are currently undergoing trial. The goal of all temporary assist devices is to alleviate shock and establish an environment in which the native heart and end organs can recover. If recovery is unlikely, then a bridge to a long-term device, typically for bridging to a transplant (see Chapters 64 and 66), may be the best strategy. Rarely should individuals be supported directly to heart transplantation from an acute support device, because the newer generations of long-term devices typically provide more reliable support and allow for better rehabilitation in an out-of-hospital setting (see Chapter 66). In select patients, it may be possible to bridge a patient who is not a transplant candidate to a long-term device.

COUNTERPULSATION

Historical Notes

Intra-aortic balloon pumps (IABPs) are often the first line of mechanical assistance utilized for patients in cardiogenic shock. The concept of increasing coronary blood flow by counterpulsation was demonstrated by Kantrowitz and Kantrowitz in 1953 in a canine preparation and again by Kantrowitz and McKinnon in 1958 using an electrically stimulated muscle wrap around the descending thoracic aorta to increase diastolic aortic pressure.[6] In 1961, Clauss and colleagues used an external counterpulsation system synchronized to the heartbeat to withdraw blood from the femoral artery during systole and reinfuse it during diastole.[7,8] One year later, Moulopoulos and colleagues produced an inflatable latex balloon that was inserted into the descending thoracic aorta through the femoral artery and inflated with carbon dioxide.[8] Inflation and deflation were synchronized to the electrocardiogram to produce counterpulsation that reduced end-systolic arterial pressure and increased diastolic pressure. In 1968, Kantrowitz reported survival of one of three patients with postinfarction cardiogenic shock refractory to medical therapy using an intra-aortic balloon pump.[9] These pioneering studies introduced the concept of supporting the failing circulation by mechanical means. Currently, intra-aortic balloon counterpulsation is used in an estimated 70,000 patients annually.[6]

Physiology

The major physiologic effects of the IABP are a concomitant reduction in left ventricular afterload along with an increase in coronary perfusion pressure secondary to an increase in aortic diastolic pressure.[10] Important related effects include reduction in left ventricular systolic wall tension and oxygen consumption, reduction in left ventricular end-systolic and end-diastolic volumes, reduced preload, and an increase in coronary artery and collateral vessel blood flow.[11] Cardiac output increases because of improved myocardial contractility owing to increased coronary blood flow and the reduced afterload and preload, but the IABP does not directly move or significantly redistribute blood flow.[12] Intra-aortic balloon pump counterpulsation reduces peak systolic wall stress (afterload) by 14 to 19% and left ventricular systolic pressure by approximately 15%.[12] Because peak systolic wall stress is related directly to myocardial oxygen consumption, myocardial oxygen requirements are reduced proportionately. As measured by echocardiography and color-flow Doppler mapping, peak diastolic flow velocity increases by 117% and the coronary flow velocity integral increases by 87% with counterpulsation.[13] Experimentally, collateral blood flow to ischemic areas increases up to 21% at mean arterial pressures greater than 90 mm Hg.[14]

Several variables affect the physiologic performance of the IABP. The position of the balloon should be just downstream of the left subclavian artery (Fig. 18-1). Diastolic augmentation of coronary blood flow increases with proximity to the aortic valve.[15] The balloon should fit the aorta so that inflation nearly occludes the vessel. Experimental work indicates that for adults, balloon volumes of 30 or 40 mL significantly improve both left ventricular unloading and diastolic coronary perfusion pressure when compared with smaller volumes. Inflation should be timed to coincide with closure of the aortic valve, which for clinical purposes occurs at the dicrotic notch of the aortic blood pressure trace (Fig. 18-2). Early inflation reduces stroke volume, increases ventricular end-systolic and -diastolic volumes, and increases both afterload and preload. Diastolic counterpulsation is visualized easily as a pressure curve in the arterial waveform and indicates increased diastolic perfusion of the coronary vessels (and/or bypass grafts).[16] Deflation should occur as late as possible to maintain the duration of the augmented diastolic blood pressure but before the aortic valve opens and the ventricle ejects. For practical purposes, deflation is timed to occur with the onset of the electrocardiographic R wave. Active deflation of the balloon creates a suction effect

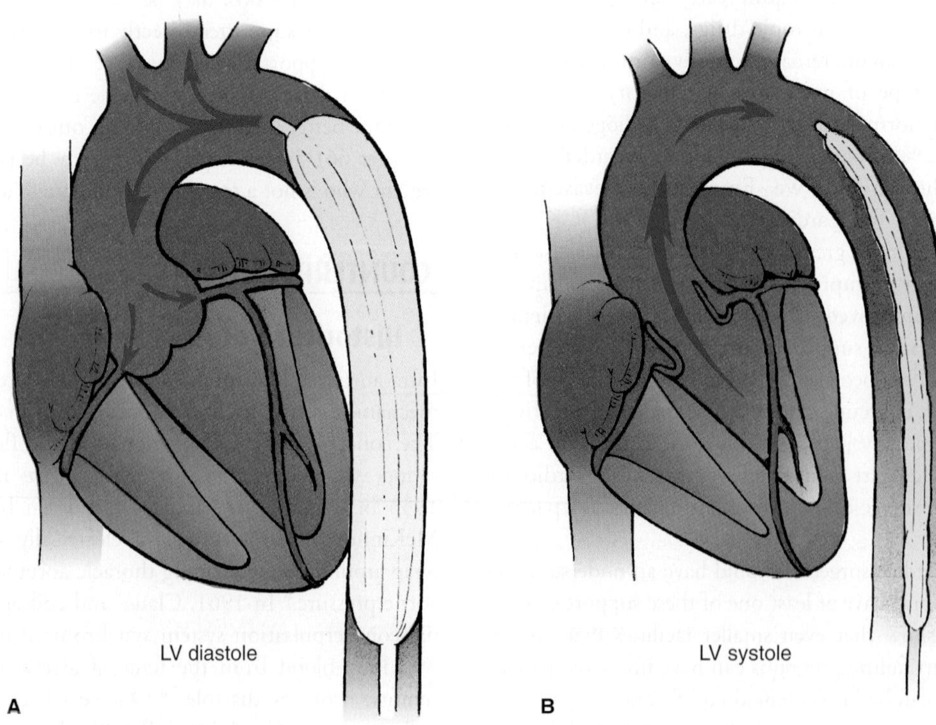

FIGURE 18-1 (A) Balloon inflation during left ventricular (LV) diastole occludes the descending thoracic aorta, closes the aortic valve, and increases proximal coronary and cerebral perfusion. (B) Balloon deflation during LV systole decreases LV afterload and myocardial oxygen demand.

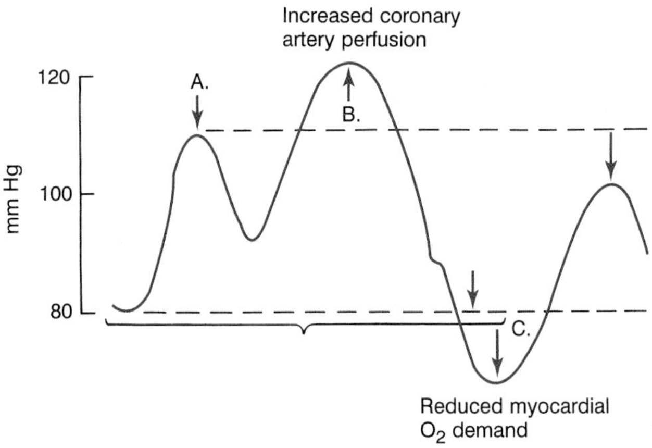

FIGURE 18-2 Illustration showing the effect of the intra-aortic balloon on aortic pressure. After ejection produces the pulse (**A**), inflation of the balloon increases aortic diastolic pressure (**B**). At end diastole, sudden deflation reduces aortic end-diastolic pressure (**C**) below that of an unassisted beat and reduces afterload and myocardial oxygen demand.

that acts to decrease left ventricular afterload (and therefore myocardial oxygen consumption).

Biologic factors that influence the in situ hemodynamic performance of the IABP include heart rate and rhythm, mean arterial diastolic pressure, competence of the aortic valve, and compliance of the aortic wall. Severe aortic regurgitation is a contraindication to use of the IABP as a very low mean aortic diastolic pressures reduce aortic root pressure augmentation and coronary blood flow. A calcified, noncompliant aorta increases diastolic pressure augmentation but risks injury to the aortic wall. On the other hand, young patients with a highly elastic, compliant aorta may manifest decreased diastolic pressure augmentation.

By far the most important biologic variables are heart rate and rhythm. Optimal performance requires a regular heart rate with an easily identified R wave or a good arterial pulse tracing with a discrete aortic dicrotic notch. Current balloon pumps trigger off the electrocardiographic R wave or the arterial pressure tracing. Both inflation and deflation are adjustable, and operators attempt to time inflation to coincide with closure of the aortic valve and descent of the R wave. During tachycardia, the IABP usually is timed to inflate every other beat; during chaotic rhythms, the device is timed to inflate in an asynchronous fixed mode that may or may not produce a mean decrease in afterload and an increase in preload. In unstable patients, every effort is made to establish a regular rhythm, including a paced rhythm, so that the IABP can be timed properly. The newer-generation IABP consoles come with algorithms that select the most appropriate trigger mode and time inflation and deflation automatically.

Indications

The traditional indications for insertion of the IABP are cardiogenic shock, uncontrolled myocardial ischemic pain, and postcardiotomy low cardiac output.[17] In recent years, indications for IABP have broadened to include patients with high-grade left main coronary artery stenosis, high-risk or failed percutaneous transluminal coronary angioplasty, atherectomy, or stents; patients with poorly controlled ventricular arrhythmias before or after operation; and patients with postinfarction ventricular septal defect (VSD) or acute mitral insufficiency after myocardial infarction (MI).[18] In addition, the IABP occasionally is used prophylactically in high-risk patients with poor left ventricular function (LVF) with either mitral regurgitation or preoperative low cardiac output owing to hibernating or stunned myocardium. These patients may benefit from temporary afterload reduction during weaning from cardiopulmonary bypass, particularly if myocardial contractility is not improved immediately by revascularization. In some institutions, a femoral artery catheter is inserted in anticipation of IABP use in patients undergoing complex procedures who have myocardial dysfunction. Some groups routinely insert an IABP before insertion of more long-term left ventricular assist systems to optimize perfusion and right ventricular function.

Techniques of Insertion

The IABP usually is inserted into the common femoral artery either by the percutaneous technique or surgical cut down. A cut down is used most often during cardiopulmonary bypass when the pulse is absent. The superficial femoral artery is avoided because of its smaller size and increased possibility of leg ischemia. For patients with small vessels, a 7-French catheter without a sheath is recommended to lessen the possibility of leg ischemia. The iliac and axillary arteries and, very rarely, the abdominal aorta are infrequently used alternate sites.[19,20] Direct insertion into the ascending aorta is used intraoperatively in patients with severe aortoiliac or femoral occlusive disease that prevents passage of the balloon catheter.[21,22]

An IABP is inserted using Seldinger's technique. Although percutaneous insertion was associated with a higher incidence of leg ischemia in the past, this is no longer true. In the catheterization laboratory, both the guidewire and balloon are monitored by fluoroscopy, but this is not essential if not readily available. In the operating room, the guidewire and balloon are typically placed and positioned under echocardiographic guidance.[23] The catheter can be inserted without the sheath in some instances.[24] The balloon catheter usually fits snugly in the arterial wound, so a pursestring suture is not needed. If bleeding is present around the entrance site, sutures are used for control.

The timing of inflation and deflation of the balloon must be monitored closely during counterpulsation. This usually is done easily by observing the continuously displayed arterial pressure tracing; a second systolic pulse should appear with every heartbeat and begin just after the smaller first pulse begins to decay. Timing the balloon for irregular rhythms is difficult, and the circulatory support provided by the balloon is compromised. In these patients, attempts are made to convert the patient to a sinus or paced rhythm or to slow (80 to 90 beats per minute) atrial fibrillation using appropriate drugs or cardioversion. For tachycardias greater than 110 to 120 beats per minute, the balloon is timed to provide inflation on alternate beats if the machine is not able to follow each beat reliably. Generally, patients are not given heparin for the IABP, but the practice varies from center to center. The exit site of the catheter must be kept clean with antiseptics and covered in an effort to prevent local infection or septicemia.

A percutaneous IABP can be removed without exposing the femoral puncture site. The exit site is prepped and securing sutures are cut. The balloon catheter is disconnected from the pump and completely deflated using a 50-mL syringe. The balloon is removed, and retrograde bleeding is allowed from the femoral artery, which theoretically flushes any distal clot into the wound. The femoral artery then is compressed, and antegrade flushing then is allowed. Finally, steady nonocclusive pressure is held over the femoral puncture site. Pressure is maintained over the puncture site for 30 minutes to ensure that thrombus closes the hole. If the balloon is inserted via a cut down, the balloon preferably is removed in the operating room. The puncture site is closed with sutures. If blood flow to the lower limb is impaired after removal, a local thromboembolectomy using Fogarty catheters and potentially an angioplasty procedure with a vein patch are done to restore full flow to the limb.

If the percutaneous needle punctures the iliac artery above the inguinal ligament intentionally or inadvertently in obese individuals, removal should be done through a surgical incision in the operating room because the backward slope of the pelvis makes pressure difficult to maintain after withdrawal, and substantial occult retroperitoneal bleeding may occur.

If the common femoral or iliac arteries cannot be used because of occlusive disease or inability to advance the guidewire, the axillary artery usually is exposed below the middle third of the clavicle for insertion.[19,20] This vessel is smaller than the femoral artery but generally more compliant. Fluoroscopy or transesophageal echocardiography is recommended to ensure that the guidewire does not advance into the ascending aorta.

Transaortic insertion of an IABP can be done for postcardiotomy patients who have severe peripheral vascular or aortoiliac disease that precludes femoral insertion. A more effective strategy in such patients would be direct placement of a direct support VAD.

Complications

Reported complication rates of the IABP vary between 12.9 and 29% and average approximately 20%.[25] Life-threatening complications are rare. Leg ischemia is by far the most common complication (incidence 9 to 25%); other complications include balloon rupture, thrombosis within the balloon, septicemia, infection at the insertion site, bleeding, false aneurysm formation, lymph fistula, lymphocele, and femoral neuropathy.[26] There is no significant difference in limb ischemia in the different types of IABPs clinically available.[25,27]

Balloon rupture occurs in approximately 1.7% of patients and usually is manifested by the appearance of blood within the balloon catheter and only occasionally by the pump alarm. Rupture may be slightly more common with transaortic insertion. Although helium usually is used to inflate the balloon, gas embolism has not been a problem. If rupture occurs, the balloon should be deflated forcibly to minimize thrombus formation within the balloon and should be promptly removed. If the patient is IABP-dependent, a guidewire is introduced through the ruptured balloon, the original balloon is removed, and a second balloon catheter is inserted over the wire. If the ruptured balloon is not removed easily, a second balloon is inserted via the opposite femoral or iliac artery or through the axillary artery to maintain circulatory support.

Removal of a kinked or thrombosed ruptured balloon that cannot be withdrawn easily requires operation because it can severely lacerate the iliac or femoral artery upon removal and lead to uncontrollable hemorrhage. The catheter should be withdrawn as far as possible until resistance is met. The location of the tip should be determined by x-ray or ultrasound, and an incision should be planned to expose that segment of the vascular system. The trapped balloon is removed through an arteriotomy after control of the vascular segment is obtained.

Although the incidence of clinically significant lower leg ischemia varies in from 9 to 25% of patients, up to 47% have evidence of ischemia during the time the IABP is used.[26] Thus, the preinsertion status of the pedal pulses should be determined and recorded before the IABP is inserted in every patient. After insertion, the circulation of the foot is followed hourly by palpating pulses or Doppler ultrasound. Foot color, mottling, temperature, and capillary refill are observed. The appearance of pain, decreased sensation, and compromised circulation indicates severe ischemia that requires restoration of the circulation to the extremity as soon as possible. There are three alternatives. If the patient is not balloon-dependent, the balloon is removed immediately. In the majority of patients, this relieves the distal ischemia; a few patients require surgical exploration of the puncture site, removal of thrombus and/or emboli, and reconstruction of the femoral artery. If the patient is balloon-dependent, a second balloon catheter can be introduced into the opposite femoral or iliac artery and the first removed. Several risk factors for development of leg ischemia have emerged. Female gender, peripheral vascular disease, diabetes, cigarette smoking, advanced age, obesity, and cardiogenic shock are reported to increase the risk of ischemic complications after IABP. Because the IABP is inserted for compelling indications, identification of risk factors does not influence management, except to encourage removal of the device as soon as the cardiac status of the patient allows. In some series, longer duration of IABP counterpulsation is associated with an increased risk of complications.[26] Although most ischemic complications are the result of impairment of arterial inflow, severe atherosclerotic diseases of the descending thoracic aorta may produce embolization of atherosclerotic material. Approximately 1% of patients develop false aneurysms at the femoral puncture site either in the hospital or shortly after discharge, and rare patients develop an arteriovenous fistula. Both conditions are confirmed readily by duplex scanning.

Results

Very few complications of IABP cause death. Rare instances of bleeding (retroperitoneal or aortic), septicemia, central nervous system injury, or aortic dissection may cause or contribute to a patient's death. Mortality is higher in patients with ischemic leg complications than in those without this complication.

Without revascularization, IABP produces a marginal increase in survival, but with revascularization, both short- and long-term survival as well as quality of life have been shown to be improved.[28] However, mortality is high in patients who receive an IABP because of the cardiac problems that led to the need for the device. Overall hospital mortality ranges from 26 to 50%.[29,30] Risk factors for hospital mortality include advanced age, female gender, high New York Heart Association (NYHA) class, preoperative nitroglycerin, operative or postoperative insertion, and transaortic insertion in one study and age and diabetes mellitus in another. A third study correlates hospital death with AMI, ejection fraction of less than 30%, NYHA class IV, and prolonged aortic cross-clamp and bypass times.[30] Time of insertion affects hospital mortality. Preoperative insertion is associated with a mortality of 18.8 to 19.6%.[17] Mortality for intraoperative insertion is 27.6 to 32.3%.[17] Postoperative insertion produces a mortality of 39 to 40.5%. Mortality is highest at 68% for patients with pump failure, lowest at 34% for patients with coronary ischemia, and 48% for patients who had a cardiac operation. Long-term survival varies with the type of operation and is highest in patients who had cardiac transplantation or myocardial revascularization.[17] Patients who received an IABP and required valve surgery with or without revascularization have a poorer prognosis. Creswell and colleagues found 58.8% of all patients alive at 1 year and 47.2% alive at 5 years. Naunheim and associates found that nearly all survivors were in NYHA class I or II.[31] Approximately 18% of hospital survivors have some symptoms of lower extremity ischemia.

Given the overall ease of IABP insertion, excellent physiologic augmentation of coronary blood flow and left ventricular unloading, this form of therapy should be considered as the first line of mechanical support in patients who do not have significant peripheral vascular disease. There is some suggestion that preoperative prophylactic IABP insertion in high-risk patients (eg, left ventricular ejection fraction [LVEF] of less than 40%, unstable angina, left main stenosis of greater than 70%, or redo coronary artery bypass grafting [CABG]) can improve cardiac index, length of intensive care unit (ICU) stay, and reduce mortality.[32] However, with meticulous myocardial protection and the judicious use of inotropes, such as epinephrine and milrinone, most groups experienced in dealing with such high-risk patients do not find routine IABP insertion helpful. When an IABP is used, it is important to understand that it is not the final therapy in terms of mechanical support for the failing heart. If the shock state persists, as evidence by a depressed cardiac index, then some form of direct mechanical support must be implemented so as to restore adequate end-organ perfusion. Failure to adequately treat a patient in cardiogenic shock will most assuredly result in the patient's demise.

DIRECT CIRCULATORY SUPPORT

Background

The need for acute cardiac support beyond cardiopulmonary bypass was clear from the early days of cardiac surgery. Spencer and colleagues reported the first successful clinical use of a temporary device in 1965 after four patients were placed on femoral-femoral cardiopulmonary bypass. Only one patient survived to discharge. Subsequently, in 1966, the first successful use of a left ventricular assist device was reported after a double-valve operation.[33] DeBakey used an assist device that was implanted in an extracorporeal location between the left atrium and the axillary artery, marking the first use of an extracorporeal temporary device support system. The patient survived for 10 days on the pump, eventually was discharged home, and became a long-term survivor.

The excitement surrounding these events prompted the formation of the Artificial Heart Program in 1964 and propelled the National Heart Institute to support and encourage the development of mechanical circulatory support systems. One of the objectives of this program was to promote the development of a support system that would be used in cases of acute hemodynamic collapse.

Ideal Device

Despite recent advances in biotechnology, recognition of many of the problems and complications associated with extracorporeal circulation has delineated the limitations of these devices. The components of an ideal device must overcome some of the existing problems.

An ideal device should be capable of supporting adequate flow, maximizing hemodynamics, and unloading the ventricle for patients of all sizes. Current devices have addressed the problem associated with variations in patient size by being designed as extracorporeal systems. Therefore, by virtue of having small-diameter cannulae transversing the chest, the pumps can support patients with varying body surface area. The disadvantage of such a system is the potential for driveline and mediastinal infections. In addition, the length of the cannula between the heart and the device, particularly the inflow cannula, predisposes to areas of stasis and potential thrombus generation. All current pumps require anticoagulation, which increases the ever-present threat of early postoperative bleeding. In addition, requirements for transfusion of large amounts of coagulation factors and platelets enhance the inflammatory response that is induced by surgery and is further perpetuated by the circuit. Activation of the contact and complement systems and the release of cytokines by leukocytes, endothelial cells, and macrophages further increase the potential negative and detrimental effects of use of temporary assist devices.[34,35] The ensuing inflammatory cascade and volume overload can have detrimental effects on the pulmonary vascular resistance and lead to right ventricular overload, often necessitating the addition of a right ventricular assist device.

Current temporary assist devices all have the capability of biventricular support as needed, provided that the lungs can support oxygenation and ventilation. In cases of acute lung injury superimposed on circulatory failure, extracorporeal life support (ECLS) can be configured with conventional or the more recent centrifugal pumps.

The multitude of clinical scenarios that often lead to the need for mechanical support all require that support be instituted in an expeditious manner. Therefore, all current devices

TABLE 18-1 Characteristics of an Ideal Temporary Support Device

Accommodates patients of all sizes, regardless of body surface area
Easy to insert
Maximizes hemodynamics while unloading the heart to allow for myocardial recovery
Is adaptable for patients who require biventricular support
Supports the use of an oxygenator as needed, particularly in the group of patients with acute lung injury
Requires minimal anticoagulation
Has a biocompatible surface that does not promote thrombus generation
Causes minimal destruction of blood or plasma components
Allows for ambulation and physical rehabilitation
Converts easily to a long-term implantable device

must be easily implantable. In the postcardiotomy setting with access to the great vessels, the cannulae should allow the versatility of choosing any inflow or outflow site that is clinically indicated (see the following). In an active resuscitative setting, such as cardiac arrest in the catheterization laboratory, in which time is critical and transport to the operating room often impractical, percutaneous cannulation must be an option.

Table 18-1 summarizes some of the components of an ideal temporary support device. At present, no single device is inclusive of all the components. Until the rapid innovations in this field lead to the development of an ideal device, the currently available technology must be tailored to the specific requirements of each patient, taking into consideration the duration of support needed.

Indications for Support and Patient Selection

A wide range of indications exist for acute mechanical support, the primary goal of all being rapid restoration of the circulation and stabilization of hemodynamics. The routine use of transesophageal echocardiography (TEE) has helped greatly in assessing the etiology of cardiogenic shock by allowing evaluation of ventricular function, regional wall motion abnormalities, and valvular mechanics. In a patient with mechanical complications secondary to MI such as acute rupture with tamponade, acute papillary muscle rupture, or postinfarction VSD, emergent surgical correction may obviate the need for device support. Similarly, in the postcardiotomy setting with failure to separate from cardiopulmonary bypass, TEE may direct the surgeon to the need for additional revascularization and reparative valve surgery and successful weaning from bypass.

If echocardiography fails to reveal a surgically correctable cause for cardiogenic shock, most surgeons use hemodynamic data to consider the need for mechanical assistance. These criteria include a cardiac index of less than 2.2 L/min/m^2, systolic blood pressure of less than 90 mm Hg, mean pulmonary capillary wedge pressure or central venous pressure of greater than 20 mm Hg, and concomitant use of high doses of at least two inotropic agents.[36] These situations may be associated clinically with arrhythmias, pulmonary edema, and oliguria. In such circumstances, use of an IABP may be considered as the first step. In the postcardiotomy setting, the preceding hemodynamic criteria, in absence of mechanical support, are associated with a greater than 50% chance of mortality.[29] In this setting, some believe that earlier implantation of an assist device capable of supporting higher flows and allowing the heart to rest may improve results and allow for recovery of stunned myocardium.[37] Furthermore, new pharmacologic agents such as the phosphodiesterase inhibitor milrinone, nitric oxide, and vasopressin have helped to optimize hemodynamics during this critical initial period, reducing the need for concomitant right ventricular support.[38,39]

Once mechanical assistance has been instituted, the stabilized patient can undergo periodic evaluation to assess native heart recovery, end-organ function, and neurologic status. If appropriate, evaluation for cardiac transplantation ensues. Patients without malignancy, severe untreated infection, or neurologic deficit and who are not at an advanced age are selected for cardiac transplantation if all other criteria are met, and there is no sign of cardiac recovery. In this subgroup, we generally transition to a chronic ventricular assist device until an organ becomes available. In patients with gradual improvement in myocardial pump function, the devices may be weaned and removed.

DEVICES

Devices currently approved by the Food and Drug Administration (FDA) for temporary support include centrifugal pumps, roller pumps, venoarterial extracorporeal membrane oxygenation (ECLS, ECMO), the ABIOMED blood pumps and Impella devices, the Thoratec paracorporeal pump (PVAD), CentriMag (Levitronix, LLC), and the TandemHeart system (CardiacAssist, Inc). A number of other devices are undergoing investigation for short-term support.

Continuous-Flow Pumps

Two types of pumps are available commercially for extracorporeal circulation: roller pumps and centrifugal pumps. In adults, roller pumps are used rarely, if ever, for temporary circulatory support beyond routine cardiopulmonary bypass applications because of important disadvantages. Although inexpensive, roller pumps are insensitive to line pressure and require unobstructed inflow. Additionally, roller pumps may cause spallation of tubing particles and are subject to tubing failure at unpredictable times. These systems require constant vigilance and are difficult to operate for extended periods. Use of roller pumps beyond 4 to 5 hours is associated with hemolysis and, for this reason, is inappropriate for mechanical assistance that may involve several days to weeks of support.[40] Axial flow pumps, in which the pump rotor is parallel to the blood path, have entered the field of temporary support with the introduction of the Impella devices,[41] but most of the experience with temporary support devices has been with centrifugal pumps.

Centrifugal Pumps

Centrifugal pumps are familiar assist systems because of their routine use in cardiopulmonary bypass. In these devices, the blood path is perpendicular to rotor. Although many different pump-head designs are available, they all work on the principle of generating a rotary motion by virtue of moving blades, impellers, or concentric cones. These pumps generally can provide high flow rates with relatively modest increases in pressure. They require priming and deairing prior to use in the circuit, and the amount of flow generated is sensitive to outflow resistance and filling pressures. The differences in design of the various commercially available pump heads are in the numbers of impellers, the shape and angle of the blades, and the priming volume. The only exception is the Medtronic Bio-Pump (Medtronic Bio-Medicus, Inc., Eden Prairie, MN), which is based on two concentric cones generating the rotary motion. The pump heads are disposable, relatively cheap to manufacture, and mounted on a magnetic motorized unit that generates the power. Despite design differences, in vitro and in vivo testing has shown no clear superiority of one pump over the other.[40,42] Although earlier designs caused mechanical trauma to the blood elements leading to excessive hemolysis, the newly engineered pumps are less traumatic and can be used for longer periods.

Complications. Complications with temporary mechanical assistance are high and are very similar for patients on centrifugal pump support or ECLS. The major complications reported by a voluntary registry for temporary circulatory assistance using primarily left ventricular, right ventricular, and biventricular assist devices (LVADs, RVADs, and BVADs) are bleeding, persistent shock, renal failure, infection, neurologic deficits, thrombosis and emboli, hemolysis, and technical problems. The incidence of these complications in 1279 reported patients differed significantly between continuous perfusion systems and pneumatically driven systems (see the following) with respect to bleeding, renal failure, infection, and hemolysis. Neurologic deficits occurred in approximately 12% of patients, and in Golding's experience, noncerebral emboli occurred equally often.[43] Golding also found that 13% of patients also developed hepatic failure. An autopsy study found anatomical evidence of embolization in 63% of patients, even though none had emboli detected clinically.[44]

Results. Although a meaningful comparison of results of centrifugal support from different institutions is not possible, in general, overall survival has been in the range of 21 to 41%. The voluntary registry reported the experience with 604 LVADs, 168 RVADs, and 507 BVADs; approximately 70% were with continuous-flow pumps and the remainder with pulsatile pumps.[45] There were no significant differences in the percentage of patients weaned from circulatory assistance or the percentage discharged from the hospital according to the type of perfusion circuitry. Overall, 45.7% of patients were weaned, and 25.3% were discharged from the hospital.[45] The registry also reports that long-term survival of patients weaned from circulatory support is 46% at 5 years.[45] Most of the mortality occurs in the hospital before discharge or within 5 months of discharge.

Golding reported an identical hospital survival rate for 91 patients in 1992 using only centrifugal pumps, and Noon reported that 21% of 129 patients were discharged.[43,46] Patients who received pulsatile circulatory assistance were supported significantly longer than those supported by centrifugal pumps, but there were no differences in the percentage of patients weaned or discharged. Survivors were supported an average of 3.1 days using continuous-flow pumps. Patients supported for AMI did poorly; only 11.5% survived to be discharged. Joyce reports that 42% of patients supported by Sarns impeller pumps eventually were discharged.[47]

Extracorporeal Life Support (ECLS/ECMO)

By the 1960s, it was clear that cardiopulmonary bypass was not suitable for patients requiring circulatory support for several days to weeks. The development of ECLS as a temporary assist device (also referred to as *extracorporeal membrane oxygenation* [ECMO]) is a direct extension of the principles of cardiopulmonary bypass and follows the pioneering efforts of Bartlett and colleagues in demonstrating the efficacy of this technology in neonatal respiratory distress syndrome.[48]

There are a number of key differences between cardiopulmonary bypass and ECLS. The most obvious difference is the duration of required support. Whereas cardiopulmonary bypass typically is employed for several hours during cardiac surgery, ECLS is designed for longer duration of support. With ECLS, lower doses of heparin are used, and reversal of heparin is not an issue. Because a continuous circuit is used, areas of stasis, such as the cardiotomy suction and venous reservoir, are not present. These differences are thought to reduce the inflammatory response and the more pronounced coagulopathy that can be seen with cardiopulmonary bypass,[49] although there is generally a rapid rise of inflammatory cytokines with initiation of ECLS support.[50]

A typical ECLS circuit is demonstrated in Fig. 18-3. The system consists of the following:

1. *Hollow-fiber membrane oxygenator with an integrated heat-exchange system.* The microporous membrane provides the necessary gas-transfer capability via the micropores where there is direct blood-gas interface with minimal resistance to diffusion. By virtue of the membranes being close to each other, the diffusion distance has been reduced without a significant pressure drop across the system.[51] Control of oxygenation and ventilation is relatively easy. Increasing the total gas flow rate increases CO_2 removal (increasing the "sweep") by reducing the gas-phase CO_2 partial pressure and promoting diffusion. Blood oxygenation is controlled simply by changing the fraction of O_2 in the gas supplied to the oxygenator.
2. *Centrifugal pump.* These pumps are totally nonocclusive and afterload-dependent. An increase in downstream resistance, such as significant hypertension, will decrease forward flow to the body. Therefore, flow is not determined

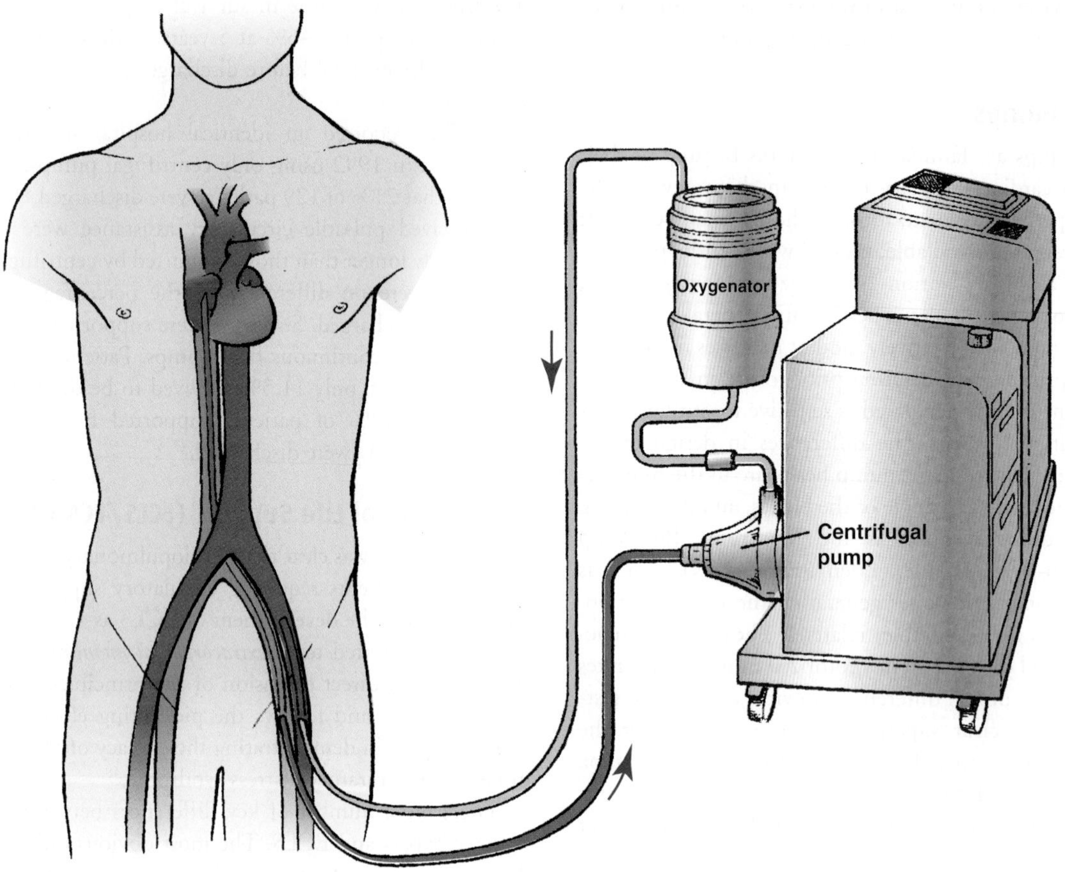

FIGURE 18-3 Percutaneous ECMO support is attained via femoral vessel access. Right atrial blood is drained via a catheter inserted into the femoral vein and advanced into the right atrium. Oxygenated blood is perfused retrograde via the femoral artery. Distal femoral artery perfusion is not illustrated.

by rotational flow alone, and a flowmeter needs to be incorporated in the arterial outflow to quantitate the actual pump output. If the pump outflow should become occluded, the pump will not generate excessive pressure and will not rupture the arterial line. Similarly, the pump will not generate significant negative pressure if the inflow becomes occluded. This protects against cavitation and microembolus formation. The newer generation magnetically levitated centrifugal pumps have been also used recently in the ECLS circuit and may have less traumatic effect on the blood elements.[52]

3. *Heat exchanger.* This allows for control of blood temperature as it passes through the extracorporeal circuit. Generally, the transfer of energy occurs by circulating nonsterile water in a countercurrent fashion against the circulating blood. Use of water as the heat-exchange medium provides an even temperature across the surface of the heat exchanger without localized hot spots. The use of a heat exchanger allows for maintenance of normothermia given the potential heal loss that can occur through the long circuit.
4. *Circuitry interfaced between the patient and the system.* The need for systemic anticoagulation on ECLS and the complications associated with massive coagulopathy and persistent bleeding during the postcardiotomy period led to the development of biocompatible heparin-bonded bypass circuits. In 1991, the Carmeda Corporation in Stockholm, Sweden, released a heparin-coating process that could be used to produce an antithrombotic surface.[51] This process was applied to extracorporeal tubing and the hollow-fiber microporous oxygenator surface.[53] Initial experience suggested that the need for systemic anticoagulation had been eliminated. In addition, heparin coating has been associated with a decrease in the inflammatory response with reduced granulocyte[54] and complement activation.[55] Bindslev and colleagues[56] and Mottaghy and colleagues[57] reported excellent hemodynamic support with minimal postoperative blood loss in experimental animals for up to 5 days. Magovern and Aranki reported similar excellent results with clinical application.[58,59]

Although these heparin-bonded circuits were initially thought to completely eliminate the need for heparinization, thrombus formation without anticoagulation remains a persistent problem. In a study of 30 adult patients with cardiogenic shock who underwent ECLS using the heparin-bonded circuits and no systemic anticoagulation, 20% of patients developed left ventricular thrombus by transesophageal echocardiography, and an additional 6% had a visible clot in the pump head.[60]

Protamine administration after starting ECLS can precipitate intracardiac clot. If the left ventricle does not eject and blood remains static within the ventricle, clot formation is more likely. Intracavitary clot is more likely in patients with MI owing to expression of tissue factor by the injured cells. Protamine may bind to the heparinized coating of the new circuit and negate an anticoagulant effect.[61]

Cannulation. The main difference between the centrifugal pump and ECLS is the presence of an in-line oxygenator. As a result, ECLS can be used for biventricular support by using central or peripheral cannulation. Intraoperatively, the most common application of ECLS has been for patients who cannot be weaned from cardiopulmonary bypass after heart surgery. In these cases, the existing right atrial and aortic cannulas can be used. An alternative strategy is to convert the system to peripheral cannulas, which potentially permits later decannulation without opening the chest.[62]

Cannulation is accomplished by surgical cut down or percutaneous insertion. The entire vessel does not need to be mobilized, and exposure of the anterior surface of the vessels typically suffices. A pursestring suture is placed over the anterior surface of the vessel. The largest cannula that the vessel can accommodate is selected. Typically, arterial cannulae of 16 to 20 French and venous cannulae of 18 to 28 French are used. The cannulation is performed under direct vision using Seldinger's technique. A stab incision is made in the skin with a no. 11 blade knife, a needle is inserted through the stab incision into the vessel, and a guidewire is advanced gently. Dilators then are passed sequentially to gently dilate the tract and the insertion point in the vessel. The cannulae then are inserted, the guidewire is removed, and a clamp is applied. For venous drainage, a long venous cannula is directed into the femoral vein to the level of the right atrium under transesophageal echocardiographic guidance.

To minimize limb complications from ischemia, one strategy is to place an 8- to 10-French perfusion cannula in the superficial femoral artery distal to the primary arterial inflow cannula to perfuse the leg (Fig. 18-4). This cannula is connected to a tubing circuit that is spliced into the arterial circuit with a Y-connector. The distal cannula directs continuous flow into the leg and significantly reduces the incidence of leg ischemia. It should be noted, however, that limb ischemia associated with long-term peripheral cannulation relates not just to arterial perfusion, but also to the relative venous obstruction that can occur with large venous lines. In such circumstances distal venous drainage can be established by splicing another small venous cannula into the circuit.

An alternative strategy is to completely mobilize the common femoral artery and sew a 8- or 10-mm short Dacron graft to its anterior surface as a "chimney." The graft serves as the conduit for the arterial cannula, and no obstruction to distal flow exists. This strategy also allows for a more secure connection and avoids problems with inadvertent dislodgement of the cannulae because of loosening of the pursestrings. In general, complete percutaneous placement of arterial cannulae is avoided to prevent iatrogenic injury during insertion and ensure proper positioning of the cannula. However, when venovenous bypass

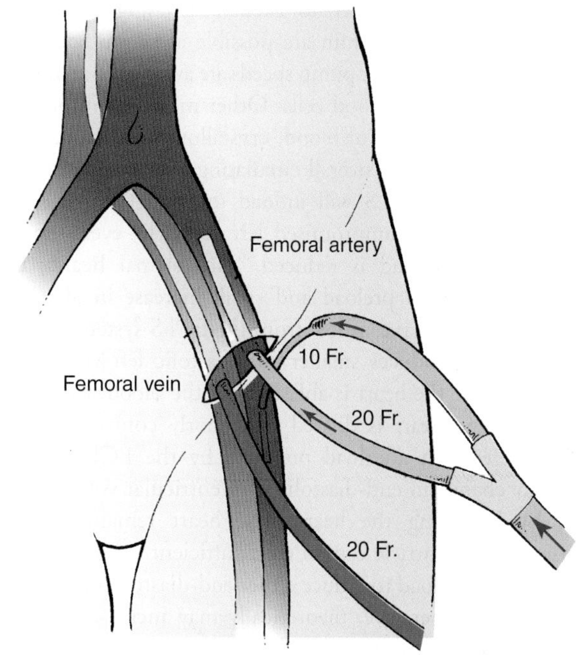

FIGURE 18-4 Surgical exposure of the femoral vessels facilitates cannulation for ECMO. A small 10-French cannula is used to perfuse the distal femoral artery.

is the only mode of support needed, percutaneous cannulation is performed. Surgical exposure is not necessary, and bleeding is less with this technique. Although traditionally the perfusion circuit involves atrial drainage and femoral reinfusion (aortofemoral flow), a recent prospective study has shown the reverse circuit (femoroatrial flow) to provide higher maximal extracorporeal flow and higher pulmonary arterial mixed venous oxygenation.[63]

Central cannulation sometimes is indicated because of either severe peripheral vascular disease or the desire to deliver the highly oxygenated blood directly to the coronary arteries and cerebral circulation. In patients with an open chest, aortic and right atrial cannulae are used. Reinforcing pursestring sutures are placed and tied over rubber chokers and buttons for later tying at decannulation. The catheters are brought through the chest wall through separate stab wounds, and after bleeding is secured, the chest is covered, but not closed, over mediastinal drainage tubes.[64]

An alternative central cannulation site is the axillary artery. Direct cannulation of this artery has been associated with progressive edema of the arm.[65] Therefore, the best strategy to maintain arm perfusion is to expose the axillary artery and sew a 8- or 10-mm graft to the vessel as a "chimney." The cannula then is placed in the graft and tied securely with several circumferential umbilical tapes.

Once instituted, the system is simple enough to be monitored by trained ICU nurses and maintained by a perfusionist on a daily basis. Evidence of clots in the pump head requires a change. Leakage of plasma across the membrane from the blood phase to the gas phase may be a problem, gradually decreasing the efficiency of the oxygenator and increasing resistance to flow and necessitating oxygenator exchanges. Using this system, ECLS flows of 4 to 6 L/min are possible at pump speeds of 3000 to 3200 rpm. Higher pump speeds are avoided to minimize mechanical trauma to blood cells. Other means of improving flow include transfusion of blood, crystalloid, or other colloid solutions to increase the overall circulating volume.

Physiologically, ECLS will unload the right ventricle but will not unload the compromised left ventricle, even though left ventricular preload is reduced.[59] In normal hearts, the marked reduction in preload and small increase in afterload produced by the arterial inflow from the ECLS system reduces wall stress and produces smaller end-diastolic left ventricular volumes because the heart is able to eject the blood it receives. However, if the heart is dilated and poorly contracting, the marked increase in afterload provided by the ECLS system offsets any change in end-diastolic left ventricular volume produced by bypassing the heart. The heart remains dilated because the left ventricle cannot eject sufficient volume against the increased afterload to reduce either end-diastolic or -systolic volume. ECLS, therefore, theoretically may increase left ventricular wall stress and myocardial oxygen consumption unless an IABP or other means is used to unload the left ventricle mechanically and reduce left ventricular wall stress.[59]

As mentioned, the versatility of ECLS is that it allows rapid restoration of circulation by peripheral cannulation during active resuscitation in the setting of acute cardiac arrest, acute pulmonary embolism, or patients in cardiogenic shock who cannot be moved safely to the operating room.

An isolated RVAD is rarely indicated in the postcardiotomy setting because, in general, these patients have global biventricular dysfunction. ECLS as an RVAD (with outflow to the pulmonary artery) may be used only in patients with good function of the left ventricle who manifest right ventricular failure and hypoxia.

Complications. The experience in adults with ECLS for postoperative cardiogenic shock is associated with high rates of bleeding. Surgical bleeding from the chest is exacerbated by anticoagulation and the consumptive coagulopathy caused by the ECLS circuit.[66] Pennington reported massive bleeding in six of six adults supported by ECLS after cardiac surgery. Even without the chest wound, bleeding was the major complication in a large study of long-term ECLS for acute respiratory insufficiency.[67] Muehrcke reported experience with ECLS using heparin-coated circuitry with no or minimal heparin.[68] The incidence of reexploration was 52% in the Cleveland Clinic experience; transfusions averaged 43 units of packed cells, 59 units of platelets, 51 units of cryoprecipitate, and 10 units of fresh-frozen plasma. Magovern reported somewhat less use of blood products, but treated persistent bleeding by replacement therapy and did not observe evidence of intravascular clots; two patients developed stroke after perfusion stopped. Other important complications associated with ECLS using heparin-coated circuits included renal failure requiring dialysis (47%), bacteremia or mediastinitis (23%), stroke (10%), leg ischemia (70%), oxygenator failure requiring change (43%), and pump change (13%).[69] Nine of 21 patients with leg ischemia required thrombectomy and one amputation. Half the patients developed marked left ventricular dilatation, and six patients developed intracardiac clot detected by TEE. Intracardiac thrombus may form within a poorly contracting, nonejecting left ventricle or atrium because little blood reaches the left atrium with good right atrial drainage. We have observed intracardiac thrombus in heparinized patients and those perfused with pulsatile devices and a left atrial drainage cannula. Therefore, the problem is not unique to ECLS or the location of the left-sided drainage catheter, but is related to left ventricular dysfunction and stagnant flow. In patients on temporary VADs in whom LV clot forms, the clot is removed at the time of permanent VAD implantation.

Results. Magovern reported improved results in 14 patients supported by a heparin-coated ECLS circuit after operations for myocardial revascularization.[59] Eleven of 14 patients (79%) with revascularization survived, but none of three patients with mitral valve surgery and none of four patients who underwent elective circulatory arrest survived. Overall, 52% of the whole group survived, but two patients developed postperfusion strokes that probably were the result of thrombi produced during perfusion. Although the Cleveland Clinic experience with heparin-coated ECLS circuits produced a survival rate of 30%, the patient population was more diversified and represented only 0.38% of cardiac operations done during the same time period.[60]

The Cleveland Clinic reported their results looking at 202 adults with cardiac failure.[34] With an extended follow-up up of 7.5 years (mean 3.8 years), survival was reported to be 76% at 3 days, 38% at 30 days, and 24% at 5 years. Patients surviving 30 days had a 63% chance of being alive at 5 years, demonstrating that the high early mortality remains the Achilles heal of this technology. Interestingly, patients who were weaned or bridged to transplantation had a higher overall survival (40 and 45%, respectively). Failure to wean or bridge was secondary to end-organ dysfunction and included renal and hepatic failure and occurrence of a neurologic event while on support.[34] Another report from the Cleveland Clinic looking at 19,985 patients undergoing cardiac operations found that 107 (0.5%) required ECLS for postcardiotomy failure.[4] Younger age, number of reoperations, emergency operations, higher creatinine concentration, greater left ventricular dysfunction (LVD), and history of MI were significant predictors of the need for mechanical support. Although overall survival was 35%, in the subgroup bridged to a chronic implantable device, survival was 72%.

Newer Devices

TandemHeart. The TandemHeart PTVA (percutaneous ventricular assist) System (CardiacAssist, Inc., Pittsburgh, PA) has 510k FDA approval for short-term (<6 hours) mechanical support. It was envisioned for the short-term support of high-risk percutaneous interventions in the catheterization lab.[70] The device is powered by a small hydrodynamic centrifugal pump that resides in a paracorporeal location. The rotor of the pump is suspended and lubricated by a fluid interface of heparinized saline. Cannulas are introduced from the femoral vessels by either percutaneous or direct insertion techniques. Pump inflow is achieved by a novel, proprietary 21-French cannula delivered across the atrial septum. Outflow typically is directed into the common femoral artery (Fig. 18-5). Position is facilitated and confirmed by fluoroscopy and intracardiac ultrasound (ICE).[71]

As opposed to an ECLS circuit, excellent left atrial decompression is achieved as long as the inflow cannula is appropriately positioned. The device can be introduced either in the catheterization laboratory using fluoroscopy or directly in the operating room using TEE guidance. Most of the experience with the device has been in the catheterization laboratory, where it has been used extensively to facilitate high-risk percutaneous interventions.[72] Flows of up to 4 L are typical. With surgically implanted larger cannulae flows up to 8 L are possible.

The TandemHeart can be configured in many ways to achieve effective mechanical support. The inlet and outlet connectors to the pump are 3/8 – 3/8 connectors, and as such can be connected to any of a number of commercially available percutaneous or surgically implanted cannulae.

Patients with this device are typically kept in bed, given that the device is inserted through the femoral vessels. An ACT of 200s is targeted while the patients are on support. The TandemHeart is a very versatile system that can be deployed and discontinued rapidly. One beneficial aspect for postcardiotomy support is that the entire device can be removed in the ICU without reopening the patient's chest. RVAD configurations with right atrial inflow and outflow to the main pulmonary artery are possible in both open[73] and percutaneous configurations.[74] With a percutaneous approach the 21-French transeptal cannula is directed into the main pulmonary artery under flouroscopy.[74]

Complete percutaneous biventricular support is also possible, but is somewhat cumbersome given the vascular access requirements. When faced with a patient that needs biventricular support, most groups are splicing an oxygenator into the circuit and using right atrial or biatrial drainage. In essence such a configuration converts the assist system to ECLS circuit.[75] With transeptal drainage the issues of left-sided congestion, which sometimes plague ECLS patients, are nonexistent. Gregoric and the group from Texas Heart Institute reported on the outcomes of nine patients with refractory shock, supported by the TandemHeart. Eight patients had an IABP and three were undergoing active chest compressions. Once neurologic and end-organ recovery ensued, the patients were transitioned to permanent continuous-flow VADs. Three patients were ultimately transplanted and 1-year survival for the entire group was 100%.[76] The Texas Heart Group has also had extensive

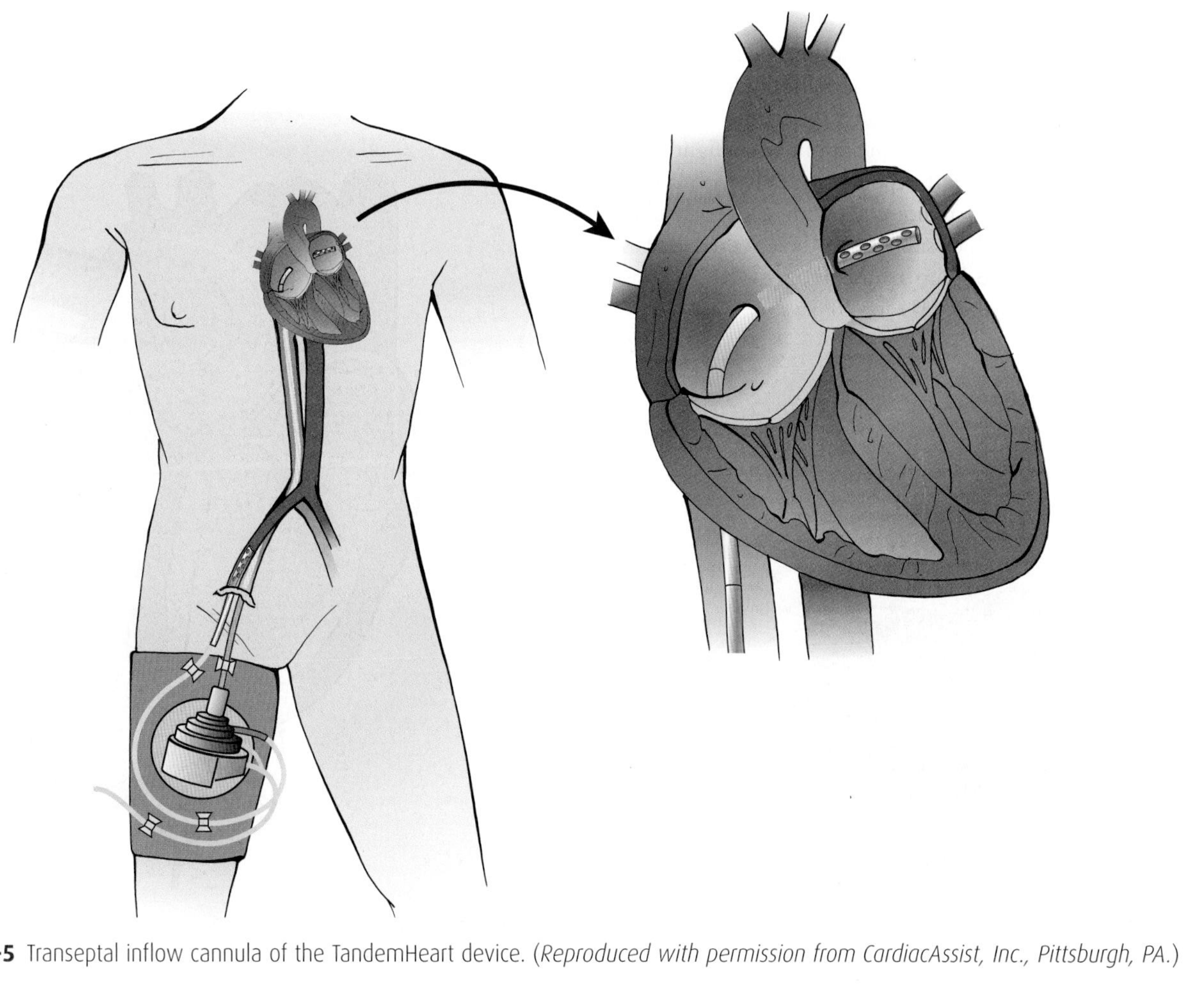

FIGURE 18-5 Transeptal inflow cannula of the TandemHeart device. (*Reproduced with permission from CardiacAssist, Inc., Pittsburgh, PA.*)

experience with using to the TandemHeart to support conventional surgery and recently reported the outcomes of eight patients in shock secondary to critical aortic stenosis supported with preoperative TandemHeart. Five were receiving chest compressions at the time of TandemHeart Insertion. All underwent conventional aortic valve replacement after a mean duration of support of 6 days. One patient died of postoperative sepsis. The other seven patients were discharged from the hospital and were all alive at the time of the report.[76]

Brinkman and the group at Medical City Dallas reported on the outcomes of 22 patients supported with the TandemHeart device. Mean duration of support was 6.8 days with no pump failures or pump related neurologic events. Three patients developed bleeding and two patients had lower extremity ischemic complications. In 11 patients who were neurologically intact at the time of TandemHeart Insertion, five went on to receive transplants while on TandemHeart support, three went on to permanent LVAD placement, and two recovered. Of 11 patients with indeterminate neurologic status or multiorgan failure, seven died, two went on to receive permanent LVADs, one was transplanted, and one recovered.[77] It should be noted that use of a TandemHeart beyond 6 hours and use with an oxygenator are off-label uses of the device. It is important to remember that when placing a long-term VAD in a patient on Tandem Support, it is necessary to repair the atrial septum. Failure to do so can lead to hypoxia caused by entrainment of unoxygenated blood across the atrial septal defect created by the TandemHeart inlet cannula.

Levitronix CentriMag. The Levitronix CentriMag pump is a centrifugal pump with a fully magnetically levitated impeller (Fig. 18-6).[78] Very little friction is generated and it requires only a very small priming volume. It can be configured for both right- and left-sided heart support, typically with central cannulation via median sternotomy. With good cannula placement, more than 9 L of support can be achieved. It has FDA 510K approval for 6 hours of use as an LVAD and has FDA approval for use as an RVAD for 30 days.

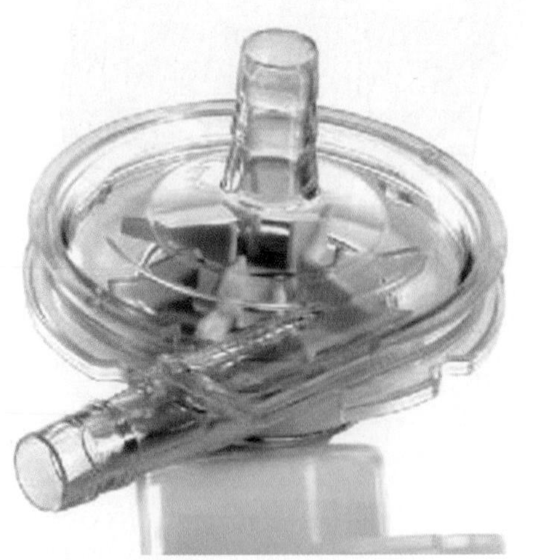

FIGURE 18-6 Levitronix CentriMag. (*Reproduced with permission from Levitronix, Waltham, MA.*)

The group at the University of Minnesota reported the outcomes of 12 patients supported with CentriMag BiVADs.[3] Of 12 patients who presented in cardiogenic shock, eight went on to receive long-term implantable VADs, two recovered, and two died. Thirty-day survival was 75% and 1-year survival was 63%.[3]

The group at the University of Pittsburgh recently reported the results of using CentriMag as a temporary RVAD. The indication for RV support was postcardiotomy RV failure in seven (24%), RV failure postcardiac transplant in 10 (35%), and RV failure post-LVAD placement in 12 (41%) patients. The RVAD was able to be weaned in 43% of postcardiotomy patients, 70% of transplant patients, and 58% of LVAD patients after a mean duration of support of 8 days. The authors concluded that the CentriMag was easy to implant, provided effective support, and was easy to wean,[79] with low overall morbidity.

As with similar pumps, the CentriMag can be configured with an oxygenator to create an ECLS circuit.[80]

Axial Flow Pumps

Impella. The Impella pump has been acquired by ABIOMED, Inc. and is being marketed as the Impella Recover system. The device is a microaxial pump, with both peripheral and central cannulation configurations available. In either case, the pump is directed across the aortic valve into the left ventricle (Fig. 18-7). The cannula portion of the device, which sits across the aortic valve, is contiguous with the integrated motor that comprises the largest-diameter section of the catheter (see Fig. 18-7). The

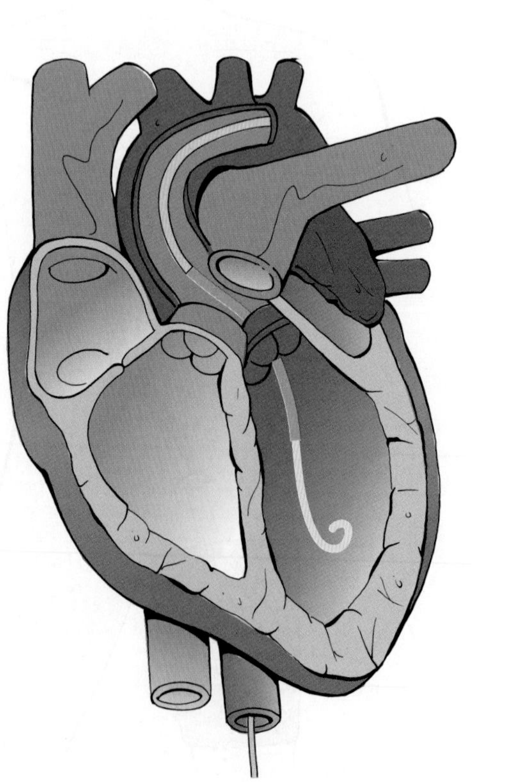

FIGURE 18-7 Impella device. (*Reproduced with permission from ABIOMED, Danvers, MA.*)

small diameter of the cannula is designed to allow easy coaptation of the aortic valve leaflets around it, resulting in minimal aortic valve insufficiency. Its hemodynamic support results from the design feature that provides active forward flow that increases net cardiac output, and its ability to address the needs for myocardial protection stems from simultaneously unloading work from the ventricle (decreasing myocardial oxygen demand) and augmenting coronary flow (increasing oxygen supply).[81–83]

The device comes in two sizes depending on indication for use and desired flow. The smaller Impella 2.5 is capable of generating flows up to 2.5 L/min. Experience with Impella 2.5 is largely with high-risk percutaneous interventions in which the device maintains hemodynamic stability during balloon inflation and stent deployment. In addition, in cases of myocardial infarction it may help in reducing infarct size. In a recent prospective randomized trial 20 patients underwent high-risk percutaneous coronary intervention while being supported with the Impella 2.5. All patients had poor left ventricular function and had interventions on the left main or the last remaining patent conduit. Patients with recent ST-segment elevation myocardial infarction or cardiogenic shock were excluded. The primary safety end point was the incidence of major adverse cardiac events at 30 days. The primary efficacy end point was freedom from hemodynamic compromise during intervention. The Impella 2.5 device was implanted successfully in all patients. The mean duration of circulatory support was 1.7 ± 0.6 hours (range, 0.4 to 2.5 hours). Mean pump flow during PCI was 2.2 ± 0.3 L/min. At 30 days, the incidence of major adverse cardiac events was 20%. (Two patients had a periprocedural myocardial infarction, and two patients died at days 12 and 14.) There was no evidence of aortic valve injury, cardiac perforation, or limb ischemia. Two patients (10%) developed mild, transient hemolysis without clinical sequelae. None of the patients developed hemodynamic compromise during PCI.[84]

The larger-size Impella 5.0 is designed to generate flows of up to 5 L/min and is more appropriate for hemodynamic support for cardiogenic shock. The device can be inserted percutaneously or directly through the aorta in the operating room. As with all left ventricular assist devices, the actual flow depends on adequacy of blood return to the left side on the heart, which in return depends on right ventricular function, pulmonary vascular resistance, and adequate blood volume. Although the device provides superior hemodynamic support compared with IABP, a recent meta-analysis suggested that early survival is not necessarily improved.[85]

The results of this limited study likely have to do more with the acuteness and duration of hemodynamic collapse in the patients than the efficacy of restoring circulatory flow. Several isolated reports suggest the novel ways that patients can be supported using this technology, including one as a bridge to a more long-term device, and another for support of primary graft failure status post-heart transplant.[86]

A right ventricular support device also has been developed and reported.[87] The development and implementation of this kind of device can be particularly useful in patients in need of chronic LVAD therapy. Theoretically, a percutaneously implanted device can support the right heart during the critical days after LVAD implantation to allow for recovery of the right ventricle and the gradual reduction in pulmonary vascular resistance. This kind of device will significantly facilitate patient management and reduce the need for high doses of inotropic support.[88]

Pulsatile Pumps

ABIOMED BVS 5000/AB5000

The ABIOMED BVS 5000 blood pump is an extracorporeal device designed to provide pulsatile univentricular or biventricular support. In 1992, it became the first such device to receive FDA approval. It has been used in thousands of patients in Europe and the United States for the purpose of postcardiotomy pump failure. The system is widely utilized for postcardiotomy support and is available in over 450 centers in the United States. The pump is configured as a dual-chamber device containing both an atrial chamber and a ventricular chamber that pumps the blood pneumatically to the outflow cannula (Fig. 18-8). The two chambers and the outflow tract are divided by trileaflet polyurethane valves that allow for unidirectional blood flow.

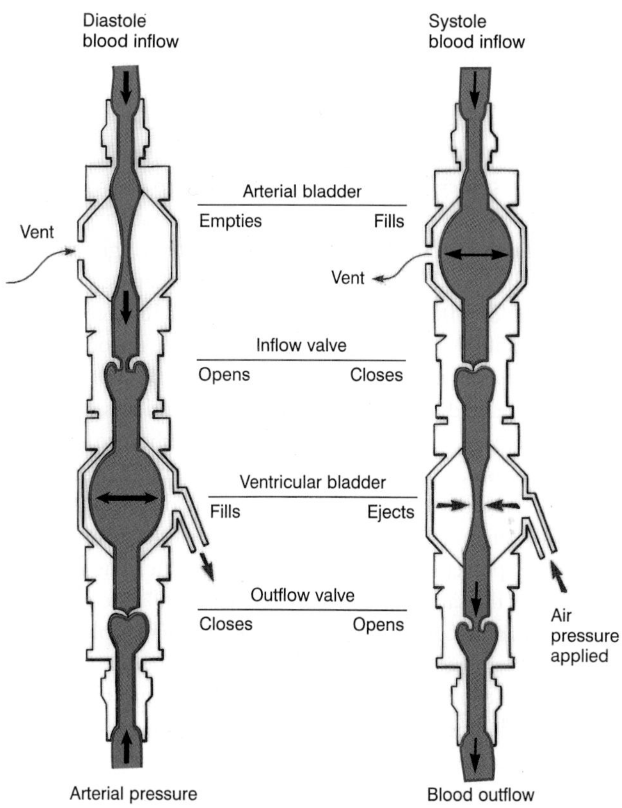

FIGURE 18-8 The ABIOMED BVS 5000. (*Left*) The atrial chamber empties through a one-way valve into the ventricular chamber (diastole). (*Right*) The pneumatically driven pump compresses the ventricular chamber, and blood flows through a one-way valve into the patient (systole). During pump systole, the atrial chamber fills by gravity.

The pump chamber itself consists of a collapsible polyurethane bladder with a capacity of 100 mL. With the BVS 5000 and BVS 5000i consoles, filling of the atrial chamber depends on gravity (the height of the chamber relative to the patient's atrium), the central venous pressure (preload), and the central venous capacitance. The atrial bladder operates in a fill-to-empty mode and therefore can be affected by changes in the height of the pump relative to the patient or the volume status of the patient. The pump usually is set approximately 25 cm below the bed. The adequacy of filling can be assessed visually because the pump is transparent. The passive filling (absence of negative-pressure generation) is designed to prevent atrial collapse with each pump cycle as well as to prevent entrainment of air into the circuitry.

The ventricular chamber requires active pulsatile pumping by a pneumatic driveline. Compressed air is delivered to the chamber, causing bladder collapse and forcing blood out of the pump to the patient. During diastole, air is vented to the atmosphere, allowing refilling of the chamber during the next cycle. The rate of pumping and the duration of pump systole and diastole are adjusted by the pump microprocessor that operates asynchronous to the native heart rate. The pump makes adjustments automatically to account for preload and afterload changes and delivers a constant stroke volume of approximately 80 mL. The maximum output is approximately 5 to 6 L/min with the BVS 5000i console. This design requires minimal input by personnel except during periods of weaning. Medical management should include optimizing the patient's hydration status and outflow resistance because the pump's performance depends on these parameters.

The device has not demonstrated any significant hemolysis, and provides excellent ventricular decompression if a proper cannulation strategy is employed. As opposed to the centrifugal pump and ECLS, patients can be extubated and have limited mobility, such as transfer from bed to chair or dangling of the legs from the bed. The BVS 5000 blood pump can be driven by both the BVS 5000 console and the newer AB5000 console.

The AB5000 circulatory support system, introduced in 2004, consists of the pneumatically driven AB5000 ventricle and the updated AB5000 console, which utilizes vacuum-assisted drainage. The ventricle is designed for short to intermediate (<3-month) support and incorporates many of the features of the ABIOCOR total artificial heart. It is driven pneumatically with valves that are constructed of Angioflex, Abiombed's proprietary polyether-based polyurethane plastic. The AB5000 system uses the same cannulae as the BVS 5000 system. Inflow cannulae can be configured for atrial or ventricular placement. Perhaps the most attractive aspect of the upgraded system is that bedside conversion from the BVS 5000 pump to the ventricle is made possible by quick-connect attachments. As such, patients implanted with a BVS 5000 system at an outlying hospital can be converted to the more long-term ventricle at the receiving institution without reopening the patient's chest or going on bypass. However, the combination of the high vacuum setting and smaller cannula size can lead to hemolysis.[89] Optimal cannula placement without chamber collapse or a high-velocity jet at the inflow cannula tip must be confirmed by transesophageal echocardiography before leaving the operating room. Anticoagulation to an activated clotting time (ACT) of 200 seconds is recommended.

Cannulation. ABIOMED cannulae are constructed from polyvinyl chloride and have a velour body sleeve that is tunneled subcutaneously. Three sizes of wire-reinforced inflow cannulas are available commercially. These include malleable 32-, 36-, and 42-French cannulas. Arterial cannulas have a precoated Dacron graft attached and are available in two sizes: a 10-mm graft for anastomosis to the smaller and lower-resistance pulmonary artery and a 12-mm graft for anastomosis to the ascending aorta.

Careful cannula insertion is important for optimal performance. Venous inflow must be unimpeded, and outflow grafts must not be kinked. In addition, careful consideration must be given to cannula position when bypass grafts cross the epicardial surface of the heart. Depending on the location of these grafts, these cannulae must be placed such that graft compression cannot occur. The three-dimensional layout of this geometry must be visualized and thought out in advance, particularly if chest closure is planned. Any graft compression will make recovery unlikely.

It is technically much easier to use cardiopulmonary bypass for placement of these cannulas, although off-pump insertion is possible and may be preferable in certain clinical situations, particularly for isolated right-sided support. A side-biting clamp typically is used on the aorta to perform the outflow anastomosis. If the patient is on cardiopulmonary bypass, the pulmonary artery anastomosis can be done without the need of a partial cross-clamp. The length of the graft is measured from the anticipated skin exit site to the site of anastomosis, and the preclotted Dacron graft is cut to an appropriate length such that there is no excessive tension or any kinking. The cutaneous exit site is planned so that approximately 2 cm of the velour cuff extends from the skin and the remainder is in the subcutaneous tunnel. The cannula is not tunneled subcutaneously until after completion of the anastomosis. For the aortic anastomosis, incorporation of a Teflon or pericardial strip helps to control suture-line bleeding. If an off pump insertion is planned, cannulae must be tunneled before anastomosis.

For atrial cannulation, a double-pledgeted pursestring suture using 3-0 polypropylene is placed concentrically. Tourniquets must be secured firmly to prevent inadvertent loosening of the pursestring suture and bleeding from the insertion sites. In addition, the heart generally is volume loaded to prevent air embolism during insertion.

For pump inflow, the 36-French malleable cannula is typically used because it provides versatility to accommodate variations in anatomy and clinical conditions. Left atrial cannulation can be achieved via the interatrial groove, the dome of the left atrium, or the left atrial appendage. The right atrial appendage provides the most hemostatic way to cannulate the right atrium because securing ligatures can be placed about the appendage and cannula to afford hemostasis. Alternatively, the body of the right ventricle or left ventricular apex may be cannulated. In the absence of left ventricular clot, the cannula can be introduced through a cruciate-shaped ventriculotomy. Ventricular cannulation offers the advantages of excellent ventricular decompression, which may enhance ventricular recovery. Bleeding in the setting of a recent MI is a consideration, but usually is not a problem if careful reinforced sutures are placed. A purse string of 00 polypropylene suture passed through a collar of bovine pericardium is a helpful hemostatic adjunct in particularly friable ventricles. Additionally, a hand-made or preordered chimney made from a preclotted graft sewn to a felt collar facilitates ventricular cannulation. A "top-hat" type conduit is constructed and with the "brim" sewn to the left ventricle using mattress sutures. A ventriculotomy is made and a cannula is introduced through the conduit. If recovery occurs, the graft can be stapled to achieve hemostasis. It is simply removed and the site closed or converted to a more formal inlet cannulation if a long-term device must be used.

The consoles for the ABIOMED device are relatively simple to operate. The control system automatically adjusts the duration of pump diastole and systole primarily in response to changes in preload. Pump rate and flow are visible on the display monitor. With the AB5000, console vacuum is adjusted to the lowest possible setting that provides adequate flow.

Complications. As with all patients who require postcardiotomy mechanical support, complications are frequent. Guyton reported 75% bleeding complications, 54% respiratory failure, 52% renal failure, and 26% permanent neurologic deficit.[90] Infection occurred in 13 patients (28%) while on the device, but only three cases were considered device-related. Other complications included embolism in 13% and hemolysis in 17% and mechanical problems related to the atrial cannula site in 13% of patients. No major changes in platelet count or blood chemistries occur during the period of circulatory support.

Jett reported on 55 patients supported on the ABIOMED for a variety of indications, including postcardiotomy failure (28), failed transplant allograft (8), AMI (2), and myocarditis (1).[37] They reported a 40% incidence of bleeding, 50% respiratory complications, and 25% neurologic complications. Marelli and colleagues also reported a similar incidence of complications in 19 status I patients, with three developing renal failure, nine reexplored for bleeding, and three dying of sepsis and multisystem organ failure.[91] As with all acute mechanical support systems, these relatively high complication rates are a reflection of the significant preexisting hemodynamic insult necessitating implementation of mechanical support. Early device insertion should be considered and may improve overall outcome.[36]

Results. The ABIOMED system is available in more than 500 U.S centers, with more than 6000 patients supported to date. Results from several reports have been summarized in Table 18-2 In a multicenter study, Guyton and colleagues reported that 55% of postcardiotomy patients were weaned from support and 29% were discharged from the hospital.[90] However, 47% of patients who had not experienced cardiac arrest before being placed on circulatory support were discharged. Of 14 patients who had experienced cardiac arrest, only one (7%) was discharged. In another report of 500 patients treated with the BVS 5000 system that included 265 (53%) who could not be weaned from cardiopulmonary bypass, 27% of patients were discharged from the hospital.[92] Recent data using this device in a wide range of clinical situations, including postcardiotomy failure, have indicated successful wean in 83% and discharge to home in 45% of patients. These excellent results are also reported by Marelli and colleagues in 14 of 19 patients who were weaned or transplanted with a 1-year survival of 79%.[91] Korfer also reported 50% hospital discharge in 50 postcardiotomy patients supported with the ABIOMED and 7 of 14 patients transplanted with a 1-year survival of 86%.[93] The ABIOMED worldwide registry experience suggests that better results can be expected from experienced centers with heart transplant programs.[37]

A more recent report by Anderson and colleagues looked at the outcomes of patients transferred on the BVS 5000 at "spoke" centers and converted to the AB 5000 at "hubs."[94] Fifty patients were studied over a 2-year period with a survival to either recovery, transplant, or destination VAD of 42%.[94]

TABLE 18-2 Clinical Experience with ABIOMED Support for Postcardiotomy Cardiogenic Shock

Reference	Patients (no.)	Biventricular Support (%)	Mean Duration of Support (Days)	Weaned, no. (%)	Discharged, no. (%)
Guyton	31	52	4.7	17 (55)	9 (29)
Minami	26	31	NR	16 (62)	3 (50)
Körfer	55	NR	5.7 ± 6.9	33 (60)	27 (49)
ABIOMED postmarket surveillance study registry*	876	50	5	NR	271 (31)

**Voluntary ABIOMED Registry.*
NR = not reported.
Source: ABIOMED postmarket surveillance study data courtesy of Diane Walsh, ABIOM ED, Inc., Danvers, MA.

Thoratec Ventricular Assist Device

The Thoratec paracorporeal (PVAD) (Thoratec Laboratories Corp., Pleasanton, CA) was introduced clinically in 1976 under an investigational device exemption (IDE) and was approved for bridge to heart transplantation in 1995 and postcardiotomy support in 1998, respectively.

The device is a pneumatically driven pulsatile pump that contains two seamless polyurethane bladders within a rigid housing.[95] The inlet and outlet ports contain mono-strut tilting-disk valves to provide unidirectional flow. The effective stroke volume of each prosthetic ventricle is 65 mL. The pneumatic drive console applies alternating negative and positive pressures to fill and empty each prosthetic bladder. Multiple settings can be adjusted to potentially optimize pump filling to provide univentricular (LVAD or RVAD) or biventricular support (BiVAD).

Thoratec pumps reside on the upper abdominal wall and are connected to the heart with large wire reinforced cannula. The Dual Drive Console (DDC) is a large, wheeled pneumatic controller that is used early in the patient's course to optimize VAD parameters. The TLC-II driver is smaller and is approved for out-of-hospital use.

Cannulation. Device implantation typically is performed on cardiopulmonary bypass. It is important to select the cannula position and cutaneous exit sites carefully. The pump should be planned to rest on the anterior abdominal wall. Lateral placement may lead to excessive tension at the skin exit sites and prevent formation of a seal. Approximately 1.5 to 2 cm of the felt covering of the cannulas must extend beyond the skin exit site, with the remainder in the subcutaneous tunnel to promote ingrowth of tissue and create a seal. The distance between the inlet and outlet portion of the pump is 4 cm, and the distance between the inlet and outlet cannulas of the pump should be planned accordingly. The cannulae must be long enough to allow for pump connection but should be trimmed to prevent the pump from kinking when the patient sits.

The arterial cannulas are available with a 14-mm graft (for the pulmonary artery) or an 18-mm graft (for the aorta) and must be cut to length after the appropriate exit site has been selected. They come in two lengths, 15 and 18 cm, which again are selected based on the patient's anatomy and the planned exit site. The graft is generally sewn on the aorta or pulmonary artery after applying a partial-occluding clamp and sewn with 4-0 polypropylene suture with or without a strip of pericardium or Teflon felt for reinforcement. Inflow can be accomplished by cannulation of the atria or the ventricles.[96] All cannulations generally are reinforced with a double layer of pledgeted concentric pursestring sutures. For atrial cannulation, a 51-French right-angled cannula is available in two lengths, 25 and 30 cm. For the left atrium, the cannula is inserted through the atrial appendage, the interatrial groove, or the superior dome of the left atrium. For right atrial cannulation, the cannula is inserted ideally into the right atrial appendage and directed toward the inferior vena cava.

Inflow cannulation of the left ventricle is preferred over left atrial cannulation,[96] because it provides better drainage, higher flows, and perhaps improves the chance of myocardial recovery. Left ventricular cannulation also decreases the amount of stasis in the LV in the poorly contractile heart, which decreases thrombus formation. Atrially cannulated patients who develop thrombus are at high risk for thromboembolic complication because the ventricle usually continues to eject. Left ventricular cannulation is achieved by placing a concentric layer of pledgeted horizontal mattress sutures at the apex of the left ventricle or the acute margin of the right ventricle (superior to the posterior descending artery). The previously placed sutures are passed sequentially through the cuff, the apex of the heart is elevated, the left ventricle cored, and the cannula seated. The cannula then is inserted and secured by tying the sutures. The free end can then be directed out through the previously planned cutaneous exit site, and a tubing clamp placed to maintain hemostasis until the pump is connected. Connecting the cannulae to the pump is difficult and must be done with care. The connections to the pump have a sharp, beveled edge that should be directed carefully under gentle pressure to fit the cannulas without damaging the inner surface of the tube. In addition, if this tip bends, it may provide a nidus for thrombus formation. Gentle hand pumping can be performed to ensure complete air evacuation using an aortic vent. Deairing of PVADs is best achieved by keeping the heart full and keeping the pumps full at all time.

Complications. The complications reported for patients bridged to transplantation are similar to those reported for postcardiotomy patients. In a multicenter trial, the most common complications were bleeding in 42%, renal failure in 36%, infection in 36%, neurologic events in 22%, and multisystem organ failure in 16% of patients.[95] Similar complications have been reported from other centers.[97,98]

Results. Most contemporary usage of the Thoratec PVADs has been for smaller individuals needing mechanical support or for those needing biventricular support as a bridge to transplant. Especially in cases of postpartum cardiomyopathy or myocarditis, recovering of adequate native heart function has been reported.[99] PVADs can also be used for postcardiotomy and post–MI shock patients, as well as for graft failure posttransplant. After cardiotomy, results are similar to those obtained with ECLS and the ABIOMED BVS 5000. In a review of 145 patients with nonbridge use of the Thoratec device, 37% were weaned and 21% were discharged. More experienced centers have achieved hospital survival rates of greater than 40%.[97,98]

The Thoratec premarket approval experience for the treatment of 53 patients with postcardiotomy heart failure had an in-hospital survival of 28%. The majority of these patients were supported with a BiVAD. The Bad Oeynhausen group, however, has reported a 60% survival for postcardiotomy patients supported with the Thoratec device.[97] Clearly the greatest advantage that the Thoratec device offers is that it can be applied for longer duration of support than any other temporary device mentioned previously. This feature may be uniquely advantageous, particularly because the duration of support necessary is usually unclear in advance. All other devices mentioned have an increasing complication rate with longer duration of support. Furthermore, the Thoratec device allows for physical rehabilitation, ambulation, and home discharge. The durability advantage of the PVAD must be weighed against the ease with which the newer generation of acute support devices can be inserted and then easily be transitioned to newer-generation chronic devices with improved complication profiles.

BRIDGE-TO-BRIDGE STRATEGY

The *bridge-to-bridge strategy* refers to the use of one of the temporary support systems in an attempt to stabilize a moribund patient to allow for the institution of a more long-term support device if short-term stabilization occurs and more meaningful recovery is anticipated.

The clinical scenarios in which the bridge-to-bridge strategy is entertained include patients who remain in cardiogenic shock despite inotropic support and IABP counterpulsation, chronic heart failure patients with acute decompensation, and patients with cardiac arrest. Improved results with implantable ventricular assist devices have prompted implementation of strategies using acute support devices as a means to rapidly establish circulatory support to maintain hemodynamics as transplant evaluation is initiated and neurologic status is determined. This strategy is aimed at maximizing patient survival and limiting the duration of support with temporary assist devices by early transition to a chronic ventricular assist device that allow patient rehabilitation and eventual transplantation. Furthermore, operative and perioperative costs of implanting the more permanent LVADs are avoided in patients who already may have suffered irreversible sequelae of multisystem organ failure.[100]

Historically ECLS has been the device of choice as full cardiopulmonary support can be established rapidly by peripheral cannulation. Pagani and colleagues reported the results of 33 patients with primary cardiac failure who were placed on ECLS.[101] The etiology was ischemic in 58%, nonischemic in 30%, and postcardiotomy in 12%. Overall, 73% of these patients were in cardiac arrest or had experienced a cardiac arrest within 15 to 30 minutes of initiation of ECLS. Ten patients who were transplant candidates and could not be weaned from ECLS were bridged to an LVAD. Six patients were transplanted and discharged, two were alive on the LVAD awaiting transplantation, and two died. Overall, ECLS was discontinued in 27% of patients because of absolute contraindications to transplantation, primarily because of neurologic injury. However, 80% of patients transitioned to an LVAD survived. This aggressive strategy and remarkable survival are secondary to the selection of patients who are most likely to survive at the expense of more initial deaths on ECLS. If the entire group of patients in this study is considered, only 36% survived to discharge. Interestingly, the need for RVAD support in the group of patients with ECLS as a bridge strategy was 40%, significantly higher than the 10% reported for patients who receive an LVAD as the initial device. This may be secondary to the inflammatory response to ECLS and associated increase in pulmonary vascular resistance.[102,103] On the other hand, an increased frequency of multisystem organ failure may lead to a greater need for perioperative BiVAD support.[104–106]

More recently a number of centers are using the TandemHeart [77,107] and CentriMag[3] for bridging to long-term devices, as has been described in earlier sections of this chapter. As the field of temporary circulatory support advances, devices such as the TandemHeart and Impella, which can be placed percutaneously, offer a distinct advantage because they can be placed in the catheterization lab without major operative intervention. It is worthwhile to note that in a recent series from the Texas Heart Institute, five of eight patients were undergoing chest compressions when the TandemHeart was implanted.[76]

Device Selection

To date, insufficient data exist to recommend one device over another for patients who require temporary mechanical support. Use of a particular device often is based on availability rather than science.

For centers with multiple devices, patient presentation and cardiopulmonary status determine the device selected. Patients undergoing cardiopulmonary resuscitation are best served by urgent femoral cannulation. This avoids the time delay of transportation and sternotomy. Patients with severe hypoxia and lung injury either from aspiration or pulmonary edema benefit from the oxygenation and lung rest provided with ECLS. In all ECLS patients it is important to adequately lower the left atrial pressure, because hypoxia secondary to continued pulmonary venous congestion precludes weaning of the ECLS circuit.

For postcardiotomy support, typically patients are supported for 48 to 72 hours while transplant evaluation is completed. Then they are transitioned to a more long-term device if myocardial recovery has failed. This approach avoids high-risk emergency heart transplantation and provides the time necessary for improved organ function.

Biventricular support is often required for fulminant myocarditis. Recovery may be possible, but often requires long-term support with a chronic device.

The TandemHeart with percutaneous transseptal left atrial drainage is a very attractive option for patients sustaining arrest in the catheterization laboratory. The Impella 5.0 also has a role to play in this patient population.

Patient Management

The ultimate goal is to maintain optimal perfusion of all end organs, to allow time for recovery from an acute hemodynamic insult and prevent further deterioration of organ function. Ideally, pump flow would achieve a mixed venous saturation of greater than 70%. Low-flow states can often be corrected by intravascular volume expansion. With centrifugal pumps, speed can be adjusted to control flow and allow some degree of cardiac ejection to decrease the likelihood of stasis and intracardiac thrombus formation. Increasing flow rates by using excessive pump speeds can also cause significant hemolysis. Fluid administration to expand intravascular volume is the best way to increase flow. However, right-sided heart failure also may manifest as a low-flow state in the presence of low pulmonary artery pressures. This condition usually requires the institution of right-sided circulatory support and is associated with a lower overall survival.

Ventilatory Support

Peak inspiratory pressures are maintained below 35-cm H_2O. Inspired oxygen is set initially at 100% with a positive end-expiratory pressure of 5-cm H_2O. Fractional inspired oxygen then is decreased gradually to less than 50%, with partial pressure of oxygen maintained at between 85 and 100 mm Hg. These measures are instituted to diminish the deleterious effect of barotrauma and oxygen toxicity in the setting of lung injury.

Bleeding/Anticoagulation

Anticoagulation should be done judiciously to weigh the balance of excessive risk of bleeding against clot formation in the pump. Platelet counts decrease within the first 24 hours of support; therefore, counts are monitored every 8 hours, and platelets are transfused to maintain counts above 50,000/mm^3 during routine support and above 100,000/mm^3 if bleeding is present. Fresh-frozen plasma and cryoprecipitate are given to control coagulopathy and maintain the fibrinogen concentration at greater than 250 mg/dL and also replace other coagulation factors consumed by the circuit. Anticoagulation is achieved by systemic heparinization with a continuous infusion starting at 8 to 10 μg/kg per hour and titrated to maintain the partial thromboplastin time (PTT) at between 45 and 55 seconds once hemostasis is achieved. In most cases, heparin infusion is started within 24 hours if used in the postcardiotomy setting, but sooner in patients without a sternotomy. One must be constantly vigilant for the signs of tamponade, which is heralded by falling pump flows, falling mixed venous saturation, rising filling pressures, and falling hemoglobin. Every effort must be made to alleviate tamponade and achieve hemostasis before transferring a patient. An ambulance is far less suited to the management of tamponade or ongoing hemorrhage than is the operating room. In reality bleeding is far more of a lethal problem in the first days of support than is thromboembolism, and anticoagulation should be used judiciously.

Fluid Management

Patients are diuresed aggressively while on support to minimize third-space fluid accumulations. If response to diuretic therapy is suboptimal, we use continuous ultrafiltration or continuous venovenous hemodialysis (CVVHD). This system permits control over fluid balance that can be adjusted for volume removal and also allows for dialysis as needed.

Neurologic Monitoring

Patients are sedated with fentanyl or propofol infusion to maintain comfort. Muscle paralysis is used as needed to decrease the energy expenditure and chest wall stiffness to allow for optimal adjustment of the ventilation parameters. All patients are assessed periodically off sedation to establish neurologic function. Response to simple commands, ability to move all extremities, and spontaneous eye movements are used as gross indications of intact sensorium. A low threshold of obtaining computed tomographic (CT) scans of the head is exercised if any change is noted or index of suspicion is high.

Weaning

A weaning trial is usually attempted after 48 to 72 hours of support. It is critical not to rush weaning and to allow time for myocardial as well as end-organ recovery. The principle of weaning is common to all devices, and all have various controls available that allow reduction in flow, thereby enabling more work to be performed by the heart. Flow is reduced gradually at increments of 0.5 to 1 L/min. Adequate anticoagulation is critical during this low-flow phase to prevent pump thrombosis, and, in general, it is not recommended to reduce flow to less than 2.0 L/min for a prolonged period. We add additional heparin during this period to maintain an ACT of more than 300 seconds. With optimal pharmacologic support and continuous TEE evaluation of ventricular function, flows are reduced while monitoring systemic blood pressure, cardiac index, pulmonary pressures, and ventricular size. Maintenance of cardiac index and low pulmonary pressures with preserved LVF by echocardiography suggests that weaning is likely. A weaning failure manifests as a falling systemic blood pressure along with a drop in cardiac output and rising pulmonary artery pressures. A failed attempt at weaning should result in resumption of full flow. Absence of ventricular recovery after several weaning attempts is a poor prognostic sign. Patients who are transplant candidates undergo a full evaluation and subsequently are staged to a long-term ventricular assist device as a bridge to cardiac transplantation. We and others have found that early conversion to chronic ventricular support is beneficial and improves the low survival that is associated with cardiogenic shock, particularly in the postcardiotomy setting.[4,66,108]

CONCLUSION

Currently a number of options exist for temporary circulatory support, and with advances in technology, the number of devices will expand. Each device has advantages and disadvantages, and to date, none satisfies all the requirements of an ideal device. We have clearly learned many lessons that should direct the development of systems and strategies that maximize survival and reduce complications. In this arena, better understanding of the host inflammatory response, appreciation of the induced derangement in the coagulation cascade, and development of systems that do not require anticoagulation should improve overall outcomes. In addition, development of therapies that alter reperfusion injury and preserve organ function is important.

Risk analysis also has taught us that patients requiring postcardiotomy support generally fit into a particular profile. Specifically, these are patients who require emergency operations, have poor ventricular reserve, are older, and have extensive atherosclerotic coronary disease and preexisting renal dysfunction. Preoperative awareness should prompt maximization of medical pharmacologic support and a readiness to implement mechanical devices early in the face of cardiac pump failure.

Use of the standard centrifugal pump gradually has fallen out of favor. Use of the Thoratec PVAD has also waned with the emergence of less morbid and more patient-friendly long-term pumps. Traditional ECLS support has fallen out of favor in centers that are experienced with newer acute support devices such as the TandemHeart and CentriMag. It will be interesting to see if devices such as the Impella, which can be placed percutaneously without advanced techniques such as transeptal puncture, will provide adequate support in patients with profound shock. Traditionally transplantation has been the only therapy available for patients supported with acute support devices who have not manifested recovery. Recently improved results have been reported with the use of a continuous-flow pump in stage D heart failure patients who are not transplant candidates.[109] Historically salvage rates for patients in cardiogenic shock, transitioned to destination VADs have been dismal.[110] Hopefully earlier use of more effective and less morbid acute support devices can improve results in this population.

KEY POINTS

1. Be familiar with and have available at least on of the available temporary support systems.
2. Be able to recognize cardiogenic shock in the preoperative and postoperative patient.
3. Initiate pharmacologic and first-line mechanical support (IABP) in the shock patient.
4. Attempt to treat the causative issue.
5. If conservative methods fail, act quickly to implement direct cardiac support to decompress the heart and restore adequate end-organ perfusion.
6. Initiate discussions with a center at which advanced heart failure therapies (transplant/long-term VAD) are possible.
7. Stabilize the patient and initiate transfer to a tertiary center for definitive therapy/weaning.

REFERENCES

1. Goldberg RJ, Gore JM, Alpert JS, et al: Cardiogenic shock after acute myocardial infarction. Incidence and mortality from a community-wide perspective, 1975 to 1988. *N Engl J Med* 1991; 325(16):1117-1122.
2. Hochman JS, Sleeper LA, Webb JG, et al: Early revascularization in acute myocardial infarction complicated by cardiogenic shock. SHOCK Investigators. Should we emergently revascularize occluded coronaries for cardiogenic shock? *N Engl J Med* 1999; 341(9):625-634.
3. John R, Liao K, Lietz K, et al: Experience with the Levitronix CentriMag circulatory support system as a bridge to decision in patients with refractory acute cardiogenic shock and multisystem organ failure. *J Thorac Cardiovasc Surg* 2007; 134(2):351-358.
4. Smedira NG, Blackstone EH: Postcardiotomy mechanical support: risk factors and outcomes. *Ann Thorac Surg* 2001; 71(3 Suppl):S60-66; discussion S82-5.
5. Helman DN, Morales DL, Edwards NM, et al: Left ventricular assist device bridge-to-transplant network improves survival after failed cardiotomy. *Ann Thorac Surg* 1999; 68(4):1187-1194.
6. Kantrowitz A: Origins of intraaortic balloon pumping. *Ann Thorac Surg* 1990; 50(4):672-674.
7. Clauss RH, Birtwell WC, Albertal G, et al: Assisted circulation. I. The arterial counterpulsator. *J Thorac Cardiovasc Surg* 1961; 41:447-458.
8. Moulopoulos SD, Topaz S, Kolff WJ: Diastolic balloon pumping (with carbon dioxide) in the aorta—a mechanical assistance to the failing circulation. *Am Heart J* 1962; 63:669-675.
9. Kantrowitz A, Tjonneland S, Freed PS, et al: Initial clinical experience with intraaortic balloon pumping in cardiogenic shock. *JAMA* 1968; 203(2):113-118.
10. Powell WJ Jr, Daggett WM, Magro AE, et al: Effects of intra-aortic balloon counterpulsation on cardiac performance, oxygen consumption, and coronary blood flow in dogs. *Circ Res* 1970; 26(6):753-764.
11. Dunkman WB, Leinbach RC, Buckley MJ, et al: Clinical and hemodynamic results of intraaortic balloon pumping and surgery for cardiogenic shock. *Circulation* 1972; 46(3):465-477.
12. Buckley MJ, Leinbach RC, Kastor JA, et al: Hemodynamic evaluation of intra-aortic balloon pumping in man. *Circulation* 1970; 41(5 Suppl): II130-136.
13. Katz ES, Tunick PA, Kronzon I: Observations of coronary flow augmentation and balloon function during intraaortic balloon counterpulsation using transesophageal echocardiography. *Am J Cardiol* 1992; 69(19): 1635-1639.
14. Weber KT, Janicki JS: Coronary collateral flow and intra-aortic balloon counterpulsation. *Trans Am Soc Artif Intern Organs* 1973; 19:395-401.
15. Weber KT, Janicki JS, Walker AA: Intra-aortic balloon pumping: an analysis of several variables affecting balloon performance. *Trans Am Soc Artif Intern Organs* 1972; 18(0):486-492.
16. Kern MJ, Aguirre FV, Tatineni S, et al: Enhanced coronary blood flow velocity during intraaortic balloon counterpulsation in critically ill patients. *J Am Coll Cardiol* 1993; 21(2):359-368.
17. Creswell LL, Rosenbloom M, Cox JL, et al: Intraaortic balloon counterpulsation: patterns of usage and outcome in cardiac surgery patients. *Ann Thorac Surg* 1992; 54(1):11-18; discussion 18-20.
18. O'Murchu B, Foreman RD, Shaw RE, et al: Role of intraaortic balloon pump counterpulsation in high risk coronary rotational atherectomy. *J Am Coll Cardiol* 1995; 26(5):1270-1275.
19. McBride LR, Miller LW, Naunheim KS, Pennington DG: Axillary artery insertion of an intraaortic balloon pump. *Ann Thorac Surg* 1989; 48(6): 874-875.
20. Blythe D: Percutaneous axillary artery insertion of an intra-aortic balloon pump. *Anaesth Intensive Care* 1995; 23(3):406-407.
21. Hazelrigg SR, Auer JE, Seifert PE: Experience in 100 transthoracic balloon pumps. *Ann Thorac Surg* 1992; 54(3):528-532.
22. Pinkard J, Utley JR, Leyland SA, Morgan M, Johnson H: Relative risk of aortic and femoral insertion of intraaortic balloon pump after coronary artery bypass grafting procedures. *J Thorac Cardiovasc Surg* 1993; 105(4): 721-728.
23. Tatar H, Cicek S, Demirkilic U, et al: Exact positioning of intra-aortic balloon catheter. *Eur J Cardiothorac Surg* 1993; 7(1): 52-53.
24. Phillips SJ, Tannenbaum M, Zeff RH, et al: Sheathless insertion of the percutaneous intraaortic balloon pump: an alternate method. *Ann Thorac Surg* 1992; 53(1):162-162.
25. Patel JJ, Kopisyansky C, Boston B, et al: Prospective evaluation of complications associated with percutaneous intraaortic balloon counterpulsation. *Am J Cardiol* 1995; 76(16):1205-1207.
26. Alle KM, White GH, Harris JP, May J, Baird D: Iatrogenic vascular trauma associated with intra-aortic balloon pumping: identification of risk factors. *Am Surg* 1993; 59(12):813-817.
27. Nishida H, Koyanagi H, Abe T, et al: Comparative study of five types of IABP balloons in terms of incidence of balloon rupture and other complications: a multi-institutional study. *Artif Organs* 1994; 18(10): 746-751.
28. O'Rourke MF, Norris RM, Campbell TJ, Chang VP, Sammel NL: Randomized controlled trial of intraaortic balloon counterpulsation in early myocardial infarction with acute heart failure. *Am J Cardiol* 1981; 47(4):815-820.
29. Baldwin RT, Slogoff S, Noon GP, et al: A model to predict survival at time of postcardiotomy intraaortic balloon pump insertion. *Ann Thorac Surg* 1993; 55(4):908-913.
30. Pi K, Block PC, Warner MG, Diethrich EB: Major determinants of survival and nonsurvival of intraaortic balloon pumping. *Am Heart J* 1995; 130(4):849-853.
31. Naunheim KS, Swartz MT, Pennington DG, et al: Intraaortic balloon pumping in patients requiring cardiac operations. Risk analysis and long-term follow-up. *J Thorac Cardiovasc Surg* 1992; 104(6): 1654-1660.
32. Christenson JT, Schmuziger M, Simonet F: Effective surgical management of high-risk coronary patients using preoperative intra-aortic balloon counterpulsation therapy. *Cardiovasc Surg* 2001; 9(4):383-390.
33. DeBakey ME: Left ventricular bypass pump for cardiac assistance. Clinical experience. *Am J Cardiol* 1971; 27(1):3-11.
34. Smedira NG, Moazami N, Golding CM, et al: Clinical experience with 202 adults receiving extracorporeal membrane oxygenation for cardiac failure: survival at five years. *J Thorac Cardiovasc Surg* 2001; 122(1): 92-9102.
35. Peek GJ, Scott R, Killer HM, et al: A porcine model of prolonged closed chest venovenous extracorporeal membrane oxygenation. *ASAIO J* 1999; 45(5):488-495.

36. Samuels LE, Kaufman MS, Thomas MP, et al: Pharmacological criteria for ventricular assist device insertion following postcardiotomy shock: experience with the Abiomed BVS system. *J Cardiol Surg* 1999; 14(4):288-293.
37. Jett GK: Postcardiotomy support with ventricular assist devices: selection of recipients. *Semin Thorac Cardiovasc Surg* 1994; 6(3):136-139.
38. Argenziano M, Choudhri AF, Moazami N, et al: Randomized, double-blind trial of inhaled nitric oxide in LVAD recipients with pulmonary hypertension. *Ann Thorac Surg* 1998; 65(2):340-345.
39. Argenziano M, Choudhri AF, Oz MC, et al: A prospective randomized trial of arginine vasopressin in the treatment of vasodilatory shock after left ventricular assist device placement. *Circulation* 1997; 96(9 Suppl):II-286-290.
40. Curtis JJ, Walls JT, Schmaltz RA, et al: Use of centrifugal pumps for postcardiotomy ventricular failure: technique and anticoagulation. *Ann Thorac Surg* 1996; 61(1):296-300.
41. Siess T, Nix C, Menzler F: From a lab type to a product: a retrospective view on Impella's assist technology. *Artif Organs* 2001; 25(5):414-421.
42. Magovern GJ Jr: The Bio-Pump and postoperative circulatory support. *Ann Thorac Surg* 1993; 55(1):245-249.
43. Golding LA, Crouch RD, Stewart RW, et al: Postcardiotomy centrifugal mechanical ventricular support. *Ann Thorac Surg* 1992; 54(6): 1059-1063.
44. Curtis JJ, Walls JT, Boley TM, Schmaltz RA, Demmy TL: Autopsy findings in patients on postcardiotomy centrifugal ventricular assist. *ASAIO J* 1992; 38(3):M688-690.
45. Mehta SM, Aufiero TX, Pae WE Jr, Miller CA, Pierce WS: Results of mechanical ventricular assistance for the treatment of post cardiotomy cardiogenic shock. *ASAIO J* 1996; 42(3):211-218.
46. Noon GP, Ball JW, Short HD: Bio-Medicus centrifugal ventricular support for postcardiotomy cardiac failure: a review of 129 cases. *Ann Thorac Surg* 1996; 61(1):291-295.
47. Joyce LD, Kiser JC, Eales F, et al: Experience with generally accepted centrifugal pumps: personal and collective experience. *Ann Thorac Surg* 1996; 61(1):287-290.
48. Bartlett RH, Roloff DW, Custer JR, Younger JG, Hirschl RB: Extracorporeal life support: the University of Michigan experience. *JAMA* 2000; 283(7):904-908.
49. Peek GJ, Firmin RK: The inflammatory and coagulative response to prolonged extracorporeal membrane oxygenation. *ASAIO J* 1999; 45(4): 250-263.
50. McIlwain IRB, Timpa JG, Kurundkar AR, et al: Plasma concentrations of inflammatory cytokines rise rapidly during ECMO-related SIRS due to the release of preformed stores in the intestine. *Lab Invest* 2008; 90(1): 128-139.
51. Larm O, Larsson R, Olsson P: A new non-thrombogenic surface prepared by selective covalent binding of heparin via a modified reducing terminal residue. *Biomater Med Devices Artif Organs* 1983; 11(2-3):161-173.
52. Aziz TA, Singh G, Popjes E, et al: Initial experience with CentriMag extracorporal membrane oxygenation for support of critically ill patients with refractory cardiogenic shock. *J Heart Lung Transplant* 2010; 29(1): 66-71.
53. Videm V, Mollnes TE, Garred P, Svennevig JL: Biocompatibility of extracorporeal circulation. In vitro comparison of heparin-coated and uncoated oxygenator circuits. *J Thorac Cardiovasc Surg* 1991; 101(4):654-660.
54. Redmond JM, Gillinov AM, Stuart RS, et al: Heparin-coated bypass circuits reduce pulmonary injury. *Ann Thorac Surg* 1993; 56(3):474-478; discussion 479.
55. Videm V, Svennevig JL, Fosse E, et al: Reduced complement activation with heparin-coated oxygenator and tubings in coronary bypass operations. *J Thorac Cardiovasc Surg* 1992; 103(4): 806-813.
56. Bindslev L, Gouda I, Inacio J, et al: Extracorporeal elimination of carbon dioxide using a surface-heparinized veno-venous bypass system. *ASAIO Trans* 1986; 32(1):530-533.
57. Mottaghy K, Oedekoven B, Poppel K, et al: Heparin free long-term extracorporeal circulation using bioactive surfaces. *ASAIO Trans* 1989; 35(3):635-637.
58. Aranki SF, Adams DH, Rizzo RJ, et al: Femoral veno-arterial extracorporeal life support with minimal or no heparin. *Ann Thorac Surg* 1993; 56(1):149-155.
59. Magovern GJ, Magovern JA, Benckart DH, et al: Extracorporeal membrane oxygenation: preliminary results in patients with postcardiotomy cardiogenic shock. *Ann Thorac Surg* 1994; 57(6):1462-1468.
60. Muehrcke DD, McCarthy PM, Stewart RW, et al: Complications of extracorporeal life support systems using heparin-bound surfaces. The risk of intracardiac clot formation. *J Thorac Cardiovasc Surg* 1995; 110(3): 843-851.
61. von Segesser LK, Gyurech DD, Schilling JJ, Marquardt K, Turina MI: Can protamine be used during perfusion with heparin surface coated equipment? *ASAIO J* 1993; 39(3):M190-194.
62. Scherer M, Moritz A, Martens S: The use of extracorporeal membrane oxygenation in patients with therapy refractory cardiogenic shock as a bridge to implantable left ventricular assist device and perioperative right heart support. *J Artif Organs* 2009; 12(3):160-165.
63. Rich PB, Awad SS, Crotti S, et al: A prospective comparison of atrio-femoral and femoro-atrial flow in adult venovenous extracorporeal life support. *J Thorac Cardiovasc Surg* 1998; 116(4): 628-632.
64. Curtis JJ: Centrifugal mechanical assist for postcardiotomy ventricular failure. *Semin Thorac Cardiovasc Surg* 1994; 6(3):140-146.
65. Edmunds LH, Herrmann HC, DiSesa VJ, et al: Left ventricular assist without thoracotomy: clinical experience with the Dennis method. *Ann Thorac Surg* 1994; 57(4):880-885.
66. Pennington DG, Merjavy JP, Codd JE, et al: Extracorporeal membrane oxygenation for patients with cardiogenic shock. *Circulation* 1984; 70(3 Pt 2):I130-137.
67. Zapol WM, Snider MT, Hill JD, et al: Extracorporeal membrane oxygenation in severe acute respiratory failure. A randomized prospective study. *JAMA* 1979; 242(20):2193-2196.
68. Muehrcke DD, McCarthy PM, Stewart RW, et al: Extracorporeal membrane oxygenation for postcardiotomy cardiogenic shock. *Ann Thorac Surg* 1996; 61(2):684-691.
69. Kolobow T, Rossi F, Borelli M, Foti G: Long-term closed chest partial and total cardiopulmonary bypass by peripheral cannulation for severe right and/or left ventricular failure, including ventricular fibrillation. The use of a percutaneous spring in the pulmonary artery position to decompress the left heart. *ASAIO Trans* 1988; 34(3):485-489.
70. Vranckx P, Foley DP, de Feijter PJ, et al: Clinical introduction of the TandemHeart, a percutaneous left ventricular assist device, for circulatory support during high-risk percutaneous coronary intervention. *Int J Cardiovasc Intervent* 2003; 5(1):35-39.
71. Kar B, Adkins LE, Civitello AB, et al: Clinical experience with the TandemHeart percutaneous ventricular assist device. *Tex Heart Inst J* 2006; 33(2):111-115.
72. Giombolini C, Notaristefano S, Santucci S, et al: Percutaneous left ventricular assist device, TandemHeart, for high-risk percutaneous coronary revascularization. A single centre experience. *Acute Card Care* 2006; 8(1): 35-40.
73. Takagaki M, Wurzer C, Wade R, et al: Successful conversion of TandemHeart left ventricular assist device to right ventricular assist device after implantation of a HeartMate XVE. *Ann Thorac Surg* 2008; 86(5): 1677-1679.
74. Prutkin JM, Strote JA, Stout KK: Percutaneous right ventricular assist device as support for cardiogenic shock due to right ventricular infarction. *J Invasive Cardiol* 2008; 20(7):E215-216.
75. Herlihy JP, Loyalka P, Jayaraman G, Kar B, Gregoric ID: Extracorporeal membrane oxygenation using the TandemHeart System's catheters. *Tex Heart Inst J* 2009; 36(4):337-341.
76. Gregoric ID, Loyalka P, Radovancevic R, et al: TandemHeart as a rescue therapy for patients with critical aortic valve stenosis. *Ann Thorac Surg* Dec 2009; 88(6):1822-1826.
77. Brinkman WT, Rosenthal JE, Eichhorn E, et al: Role of a percutaneous ventricular assist device in decision making for a cardiac transplant program. *Ann Thorac Surg* 2009; 88(5):1462-1466.
78. De Robertis F, Birks EJ, Rogers P, et al: Clinical performance with the Levitronix CentriMag short-term ventricular assist device. *J Heart Lung Transplant* 2006; 25(2):181-186.
79. Bhama JK, Kormos RL, Toyoda Y, et al: Clinical experience using the Levitronix CentriMag system for temporary right ventricular mechanical circulatory support. *J Heart Lung Transplant* 2009; 28(9):971-976.
80. Khan NU, Al-Aloul M, Shah R, Yonan N: Early experience with the Levitronix CentriMag device for extra-corporeal membrane oxygenation following lung transplantation. *Eur J Cardiothorac Surg* 2008; 34(6): 1262-1264.
81. Burzotta F, Paloscia L, Trani C, et al: Feasibility and long-term safety of elective Impella-assisted high-risk percutaneous coronary intervention: a pilot two-centre study. *J Cardiovasc Med (Hagerstown)* 2008; 9(10): 1004-1010.
82. Jurmann MJ, Siniawski H, Erb M, Drews T, Hetzer R: Initial experience with miniature axial flow ventricular assist devices for postcardiotomy heart failure. *Ann Thorac Surg* 2004; 77(5):1642-1647.
83. Meyns B, Dens J, Sergeant P, et al: Initial experiences with the Impella device in patients with cardiogenic shock. Impella support for cardiogenic shock. *Thorac Cardiovasc Surg* 2003; 51(6):312-317.

84. Dixon SR, Henriques JP, Mauri L, et al: A prospective feasibility trial investigating the use of the Impella 2.5 system in patients undergoing high-risk percutaneous coronary intervention (The PROTECT I Trial): initial U.S. experience. *JACC Cardiovasc Interv* 2009; 2(2):91-96.
85. Cheng JM, den Uil CA, Hoeks SE, et al: Percutaneous left ventricular assist devices vs. intra-aortic balloon pump counterpulsation for treatment of cardiogenic shock: a meta-analysis of controlled trials. *Eur Heart J* 2009; 30(17):2102-2108.
86. Samoukovic G, Rosu C, Giannetti N, Cecere R: The Impella LP 5.0 as a bridge to long-term circulatory support. *Interact Cardiovasc Thorac Surg* 2009; 8(6):682-683.
87. Sugiki H, Nakashima K, Vermes E, Loisance D, Kirsch M: Temporary right ventricular support with Impella Recover RD axial flow pump. *Asian Cardiovasc Thorac Ann* 2009; 17(4):395-400.
88. Martin J, Benk C, Yerebakan C, et al: The new "Impella" intracardiac microaxial pump for treatment of right heart failure after orthotopic heart transplantation. *Transplant Proc* 2001; 33(7-8): 3549-3550.
89. Samuels LE, Holmes EC, Garwood P, Ferdinand F: Initial experience with the Abiomed AB5000 ventricular assist device system. *Ann Thorac Surg* 2005; 80(1):309-312.
90. Guyton RA, Schonberger JP, Everts PA, et al: Postcardiotomy shock: clinical evaluation of the BVS 5000 Biventricular Support System. *Ann Thorac Surg* 1993; 56(2):346-356.
91. Marelli D, Laks H, Fazio D, et al: Mechanical assist strategy using the BVS 5000i for patients with heart failure. *Ann Thorac Surg* 2000; 70(1):59-66.
92. Jett GK: ABIOMED BVS 5000: experience and potential advantages. *Ann Thorac Surg* 1996; 61(1):301-304; discussion 311-303.
93. Korfer R, El-Banayosy A, Arusoglu L, et al: Temporary pulsatile ventricular assist devices and biventricular assist devices. *Ann Thorac Surg* 1999; 68(2):678-683.
94. Anderson MB, Gratz E, Wong RK, Benali K, Kung RT: Improving outcomes in patients with ventricular assist devices transferred from outlying to tertiary care hospitals. *J Extra Corpor Technol* 2007; 39(1):43-48.
95. Farrar DJ, Hill JD: Univentricular and biventricular Thoratec VAD support as a bridge to transplantation. *Ann Thorac Surg* 1993; 55(1): 276-282.
96. Arabia FA, Paramesh V, Toporoff B, et al: Biventricular cannulation for the Thoratec ventricular assist device. *Ann Thorac Surg* 1998; 66(6): 2119-2120.
97. Korfer R, el-Banayosy A, Posival H, et al: Mechanical circulatory support with the Thoratec assist device in patients with postcardiotomy cardiogenic shock. *Ann Thorac Surg* 1996; 61(1):314-316.
98. Pennington DG, McBride LR, Swartz MT, et al: Use of the Pierce-Donachy ventricular assist device in patients with cardiogenic shock after cardiac operations. *Ann Thorac Surg* 1989; 47(1):130-135.
99. Holman WL, Bourge RC, Kirklin JK: Case report: circulatory support for seventy days with resolution of acute heart failure. *J Thorac Cardiovasc Surg* 1991; 102(6):932-934.
100. Oz MC, Goldstein DJ, Pepino P, et al: Screening scale predicts patients successfully receiving long-term implantable left ventricular assist devices. *Circulation* 1995; 92(9 Suppl):II169-173.
101. Pagani FD, Aaronson KD, Swaniker F, Bartlett RH: The use of extracorporeal life support in adult patients with primary cardiac failure as a bridge to implantable left ventricular assist device. *Ann Thorac Surg* 2001; 71(3 Suppl):S77-81; discussion S82-75.
102. Plotz FB, van Oeveren W, Bartlett RH, Wildevuur CR: Blood activation during neonatal extracorporeal life support. *J Thorac Cardiovasc Surg* 1993; 105(5):823-832.
103. Jamadar DA, Kazerooni EA, Cascade PN, et al: Extracorporeal membrane oxygenation in adults: radiographic findings and correlation of lung opacity with patient mortality. *Radiology* 1996; 198(3):693-698.
104. Reinhartz O, Farrar DJ, Hershon JH, et al: Importance of preoperative liver function as a predictor of survival in patients supported with Thoratec ventricular assist devices as a bridge to transplantation. *J Thorac Cardiovasc Surg* 1998; 116(4):633-640.
105. Farrar DJ, Hill JD, Pennington DG, et al: Preoperative and postoperative comparison of patients with univentricular and biventricular support with the Thoratec ventricular assist device as a bridge to cardiac transplantation. *J Thorac Cardiovasc Surg* 1997; 113(1):202-209.
106. Kormos RL, Gasior TA, Kawai A, et al: Transplant candidate's clinical status rather than right ventricular function defines need for univentricular versus biventricular support. *J Thorac Cardiovasc Surg* 1996; 111(4): 773-782.
107. Gregoric ID, Jacob LP, La Francesca S, et al: The TandemHeart as a bridge to a long-term axial-flow left ventricular assist device (bridge to bridge). *Tex Heart Inst J* 2008; 35(2):125-129.
108. DeRose JJ, Umana JP, Argenziano M, et al: Improved results for postcardiotomy cardiogenic shock with the use of implantable left ventricular assist devices. *Ann Thorac Surg* 1997; 64(6):1757-1762.
109. Slaughter MS, Rogers JG, Milano CA, et al: Advanced heart failure treated with continuous-flow left ventricular assist device. *N Engl J Med* 2009; 361(23):2241-2251.
110. Lietz K, Long JW, Kfoury AG, et al: Outcomes of left ventricular assist device implantation as destination therapy in the post-REMATCH era: implications for patient selection. *Circulation* 2007; 116(5):497-505.

PART 3

ISCHEMIC HEART DISEASE

CHAPTER 19

Indications for Revascularization

Morgan L. Brown
Thoralf M. Sundt III

INTRODUCTION

Coronary artery disease remains the most common pathology with which cardiologists and cardiac surgeons are faced. Accordingly, the practicing cardiac surgeon is confronted with no clinical question more often than, "Is coronary bypass indicated in this patient?" It is the aim of this chapter to provide a practical overview of the current indications for myocardial revascularization with sufficient reference to the relevant studies on which they are based to afford the reader an appreciation for the strengths and limitations of their conclusions.

CLINICAL AND LABORATORY ASSESSMENT OF CORONARY ARTERY DISEASE

A surgeon's first introduction to a patient with coronary artery disease is frequently an angiogram. In addition to the coronary anatomy, however, the clinical presentation and results of noninvasive studies of myocardial perfusion and function are necessary to characterize the pathophysiologic implications of the angiographic disease and its impact on prognosis and, therefore, to make a clinically appropriate recommendation. In the technological era in which we practice, the importance of the clinical history bears emphasis—particularly in an aging population. Because one of the objectives of surgery is to improve symptoms and quality of life, a thorough appreciation of the patient's functional status is a prerequisite in selecting the optimal therapeutic strategy.

The system proposed by the Canadian Cardiovascular Society for grading the clinical severity of angina pectoris is widely accepted (Table 19-1). Unfortunately, angina is a highly subjective phenomenon for both patient and physician, and prospective evaluation of the assessment of functional classification by the CCS criteria has demonstrated a reproducibility of only 73%.[1] Furthermore, there may be a strikingly poor correlation between the severity of symptoms and the magnitude of ischemia, as is notoriously the case among diabetic patients with asymptomatic "silent ischemia."

Electrocardiography (ECG), if abnormal, is helpful in assessing ischemic burden. Unfortunately, it demonstrates no pathognomonic signs in half of patients with chronic stable angina. Still the monitoring of an ECG under stress conditions is simple and inexpensive, and is therefore useful as a screening examination. Among patients with anatomically defined disease, stress ECG provides additional information about the severity of ischemia and the prognosis of the disease. The sensitivity of the test increases with age, with the severity of the patient's disease, and with the magnitude of observed ST-segment shift.[2] If ST-segment depression is greater than 1 mm, stress ECG has a predictive value of 90%, whereas a 2-mm shift with accompanying angina is virtually diagnostic.[3] Early onset of ST-segment depression and prolonged depression after the discontinuation of exercise are strongly associated with significant multivessel disease. Unfortunately, many patients cannot achieve their target heart rates owing to beta blockade or a limitation to their exercise tolerance caused by coexisting disease, decreasing the usefulness of this test in these often high-risk patients. Resting abnormalities in the ECG may also limit the predictive accuracy of the test.

Perfusion imaging with thallium-201 or a technetium-99m–based tracer may be particularly useful in patients with abnormalities on their baseline ECG. Reversible defects demonstrated by comparison of images obtained after injection of the tracer at peak stress with rest images is indicative of ischemia, and hence viability. An irreversible defect indicates a nonviable scar. The results obtained with both tracers are similar, with the

TABLE 19-1 Canadian Cardiovascular Society Angina Classification

Canadian Cardiovascular Society
Angina Classification
0 = No angina
1 = Angina only with strenuous or prolonged exertion
2 = Angina with walking at a rapid pace on the level, on a grade, or upstairs (slight limitation of normal activities)
3 = Angina with walking at a normal pace less than 2 blocks or one flight of stairs (marked limitation)
4 = Angina with even mild activity

average sensitivity around 90% and specificity of approximately 75%.[4] For patients unable to exercise, pharmacologic vasodilators such as adenosine or dipyridamole may be used with similar sensitivity.[5]

Echocardiographic imaging during exercise or pharmacologic stress has gained increasing popularity among cardiologists. Comparative studies have demonstrated accuracy similar to that of nuclear studies with sensitivity and specificity both around 85%.[4] Patients unable to exercise may be stressed with high-dose dipyridamole, or more commonly dobutamine at doses from 5 to 40 μg/kg/min. An initial augmentation of contractility followed by loss or "drop out" is diagnostic of ischemia (and accordingly viability), whereas failure to augment contractility at low dose suggest scar. Additionally, information regarding concomitant valvular disease may be obtained during the examination.[6]

GUIDELINES FOR REVASCUARLIZATION

The guidelines for surgical revascularization established by the American College of Cardiology and American Heart Association are shown in Table 19-2.[7] The basis for these guidelines resides in the large body of literature comparing medical therapy with surgical revascularization and, more recently, percutaneous coronary interventions (PCI).

Before reviewing the results of the seminal trials of CABG versus medical therapy performed in the 1970s and those of newer prospectively randomized trials comparing the results of surgery with PCI and medical therapy, some limitations of these trials must be recognized. First, in retrospective or registry studies, it is difficult to ensure comparable patient populations by virtue of the extraordinary anatomical and physiologic complexity of coronary artery disease as well as the heterogeneity of the patient substrate. Differences in ventricular function and comorbidities such as age, diabetes, peripheral vascular disease, and pulmonary disease may have a profound impact on outcomes such as survival or quality of life. For example, caution must be exercised in interpreting the results of nonrandomized and registry reports of PCI versus surgery, because the patients subjected to the former more often have single- or double-vessel disease,[8,9] whereas the latter commonly have triple-vessel or left main disease.[8,9] Attempts to correct for selection bias with statistical techniques such as propensity matching are only as valid as the parameters entered into the model. Data less tangible than gender or chronologic age, such as socioeconomic status or "physiologic age," are not easily accounted for in such analyses and yet may be a critical determinant of outcomes. Despite this limitation, retrospective and registry data provide a better glimpse of the real world of coronary artery disease. Most prospective randomized trials include only a fraction of the total population undergoing revascularization by virtue of strict entry criteria. For example, the Bypass Angioplasty Revascularization Investigators (BARI) trial entered only 5% of total patients screened.[10] Therefore, although the prospectively randomized studies do provide objective data directly applicable to the specific patient subset represented in the study, extrapolation of the results to the more heterogeneous populations seen clinically can only be made if the implicit caveats are clearly understood. We must be mindful of the inescapable tradeoff between selection bias in registry studies and entry bias in randomized studies.

Second, as a consequence of the overrepresentation of patients at lowest risk of death in randomized trials, most are statistically underpowered with respect to survival analysis. For example, given current survival statistics, we would need approximately 2000 patients in each arm of a study to detect a 30% difference in mortality. The problem is compounded by the exclusion of the very patients for whom one would anticipate a survival advantage with adequate revascularization, such as those with depressed ventricular function. Randomized studies frequently employ softer end points such as angina or quality of life, or create composites of qualitatively different end points, such as death, stroke, and myocardial infarction (MI). Meaningful analysis is further complicated by relatively short-term follow-up in most studies. Events such as the need for subsequent revascularization and recurrence of angina characteristically occur at different time intervals after these therapies (restenosis after PCI versus graft occlusion after CABG), and an 8- to 10-year follow-up period is needed to adequately compare long-term results. Patients themselves are also generally interested in outcomes measured in years, not months.

Significant improvements in each of the treatment strategies for coronary artery disease are occurring constantly. Examples include the use of antiplatelet agents, angiotensin-converting enzyme inhibitors, lipid-lowering therapy, internal thoracic aortic (ITA) grafts, intravascular stents, and the development of drug eluting stents. These advances, along with aggressive secondary prevention after revascularization, have steadily reduced the morbidity and mortality of coronary artery disease in all patients, making differences in the hard end point of survival difficult to demonstrate for any therapy.[11] This trend will likely increase as the beneficial effect of secondary prevention becomes more widely appreciated.

TABLE 19-2 AHA/ACC Guidelines for CABG*

Asymptomatic/Mild Angina

Class I
1. Left main stenosis
2. Left main equivalent (proximal LAD and proximal circumflex)
3. Three-vessel disease

Class IIa
1. Proximal LAD stenosis and one- or two-vessel disease

Class IIb
1. One- or two-vessel disease not involving proximal LAD
If a large territory at risk on noninvasive studies or LVEF <50%, IIa and IIb become class I indications

Stable Angina

Class I
1. Left main stenosis
2. Left main equivalent (proximal LAD and proximal circumflex)
3. Three-vessel disease
4. Two-vessel disease with proximal LAD stenosis and EF <50% or demonstrable ischemia
5. One- or two-vessel disease without proximal LAD stenosis but with a large territory at risk and high-risk criteria on noninvasive testing
6. Disabling angina refractory to medical therapy

Class IIa
1. Proximal LAD stenosis with one-vessel disease
2. One- or two-vessel disease without proximal LAD stenosis, but with a moderate territory at risk and demonstrable ischemia

Unstable Angina/Non–ST-Segment Elevation MI (NSTEMI)

Class I
1. Left main
2. Left main equivalent
3. Ongoing ischemia not responsive to maximal nonsurgical therapy

Class IIa
1. Proximal LAD stenosis with one- or two-vessel disease

Class IIb
1. One- or two-vessel disease without proximal LAD stenosis when PCI not possible (becomes class I if high-risk criteria on noninvasive testing)

ST-Segment Elevation (Q wave) MI

Class I
1. Failed PCI with persistent pain or shock and anatomically feasible
2. Persistent or recurrent ischemia refractory to medical treatment with acceptable anatomy who have a significant territory at risk and not a candidate for PCI
3. Requires surgical repair of post-infarct ventricular septal rupture or mitral valve insufficiency
4. Cardiogenic shock in patients <75 years of age who have ST elevation, LBBB, or a posterior MI within 18 hours of onset
5. Life-threatening ventricular arrhythmias in the presence of ≥50% left main stenosis or three-vessel disease

Class IIa
1. Primary reperfusion in patients who have failed fibrinolytics or PCI and are in the early stages (6–12 h) of an evolving STEMI
2. Mortality with CABG is elevated the first 3–7 days after STEMI/NSTEMI. After 7 days, criteria for revascularization in previous sections apply.

(Continued)

TABLE 19-2 AHA/ACC Guidelines for CABG* (*Continued*)

Poor LV Function

Class I

1. Left main stenosis
2. Left main equivalent
3. Proximal LAD stenosis and two- to three-vessel disease

Class IIa

1. Significant viable territory and noncontractile myocardium

Life-Threatening Ventricular Arrhythmias

Class I

1. Left main disease
2. Three-vessel disease

Class IIa

1. Bypassable one- or two-vessel disease
2. Proximal LAD disease and one- or two-vessel disease
   These become class I indications if arrhythmia is resuscitated cardiac death or sustained ventricular tachycardia.

Failed PCI

Class I

1. Ongoing ischemia with significant territory at risk
2. Shock

Class IIa

1. Foreign body in critical position
2. Shock with coagulopathy and no previous sternotomy

Class IIb

1. Shock with coagulopathy and previous sternotomy

Previous CABG

Class I

1. Disabling angina refractory to medical therapy
2. Nonpatent previous bypass grafts, but with class I indications for native CAD

Class IIa

1. Large territory at risk
2. Vein grafts supplying LAD or large territory are >50% stenosed

Class I: Conditions for which there is evidence and/or general agreement that a given procedure or treatment is useful and effective.
Class II: Conditions for which there is conflicting evidence and/or a divergence of opinion about the usefulness or efficacy of a procedure.
Class IIa: Weight of evidence/opinion is in favor of usefulness/efficacy.
Class IIb: Usefulness/efficacy is less well established by evidence/opinion.
Class III: Conditions for which there is evidence and/or general agreement that the procedure/treatment is not useful/effective and in some cases may be harmful.
ACC = American College of Cardiology; AHA = American Heart Association; CABG = coronary artery bypass grafting; EF = ejection fraction; LAD = left anterior descending; LITA = left internal thoracic artery; LVEF = left ventricular ejection fraction; PCI = percutaneous transluminal coronary angioplasty.

COMPARATIVE TRIALS OF REVASCULARIZATION VERSUS MEDICAL THERAPY IN STABLE ANGINA

Medical Therapy

In the decades since coronary artery bypass (CABG) surgery was popularized and coronary angioplasty introduced, an enormous volume of data on the results of invasive revascularization has been collected. Remarkably, almost from the outset many of these studies have been prospectively randomized. Yet in the current era there is a dearth of data concerning pharmacologic therapies for chronic coronary artery disease despite remarkable recent drug development. For example, although nitrates are unquestionably effective in relieving symptoms, the impact of long-acting nitrates on clinical outcomes has never been rigorously tested. Furthermore, there has been only one trial of beta-blocker therapy in the treatment of angina, the Atenolol Silent Ischemia Study (ASIST), which demonstrated benefit for patients with mild effort induced angina or silent ischemia.[12] A handful of studies of combination therapy with beta blockers and calcium channel blockers have also demonstrated antianginal benefit.[13–15]

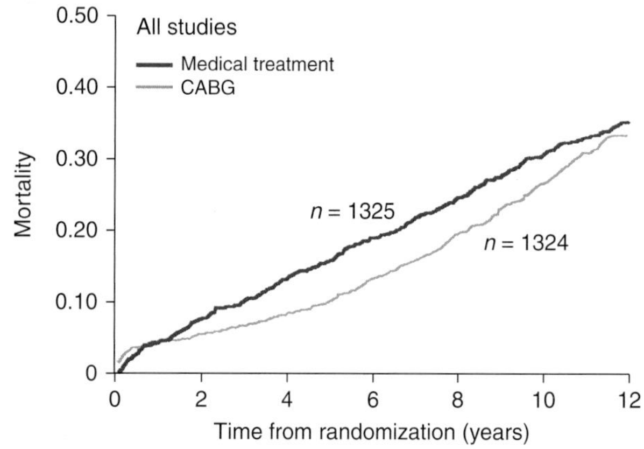

FIGURE 19-1 Survival (mortality) curves for all medically and surgically treated patients with chronic stable angina enrolled in seven prospective randomized controlled trials. (*Reproduced with permission from Yusuf S, Zucker D, Peduzzi P, et al: Effect of coronary artery bypass graft surgery on survival: overview of 10-year results from randomized trials by the Coronary Artery Bypass Graft Surgery Trial: 1st collaboration. Lancet 1994; 344:563.*)

Surgical versus Medical Therapy

Three major randomized studies, the Coronary Artery Surgery Study (CASS),[16] the Veterans Administration Cooperative Study Group (VA),[17,18] and the European Coronary Surgery Study (ECSS),[19,20] as well as several other smaller randomized trials,[21–23] conducted between 1972 and 1984, provide the foundation for comparing the outcomes of medical and surgical therapy. Despite the limitations noted in the preceding, these studies are remarkably consistent in their major findings, and the qualitative conclusions drawn from them continue to be generalizable to current practice.

The central message from all of these studies is that the relative benefits of bypass surgery over medical therapy on survival are greatest in those patients at highest risk as defined by the severity of angina and/or ischemia, the number of diseased vessels, and the presence of left ventricular dysfunction.[24] For example, thus far, no study has shown survival benefit for CABG over medical therapy for patients with single-vessel disease. It should be emphasized, however, that these trials involved primarily patients with moderate chronic stable angina. These conclusions may, therefore, not necessarily apply to patients with unstable angina or to those with more severe degrees of chronic stable angina.

A meta-analysis of the seven randomized trials cited in the preceding demonstrated a statistically enhanced survival at 5, 7, and 10 years, for surgically treated patients at highest risk (4.8% annual mortality) and moderate risk (2.5% annual mortality), but no evidence of a survival benefit for those patients at lowest risk.[24] The overall survival benefit at 12 years for the three large and four smaller randomized studies is shown in Fig. 19-1. Nonrandomized studies have also demonstrated a beneficial effect of surgery on survival of patients with multivessel disease and severe ischemia regardless of left ventricular function.[25–28]

There have been three recent randomized controlled trials of invasive revascularization by PCI or CABG versus medical therapy. Their results make an even stronger case for revascularization. In the Asymptomatic Cardiac Ischemia Pilot (ACIP) trial, patients with anatomy amenable to CABG were randomized to angina-directed anti-ischemic therapy, drug therapy guided by noninvasive measures of ischemia, or revascularization by CABG or PCI.[29] At 2 years, there was a statistically significant difference in mortality of 6.6% in the angina-guided group, 4.4% in the ischemia-guided group, and 1.1% in the revascularization group. The rates of death or MI were also statistically different at 12.1%, 8.8%, and 4.7%, respectively. The Medicine, Angioplasty, or Surgery Study (MASS-II) trial randomized patients with multivessel disease among medical therapy, PCI, and CABG. Although survival at 1 year was equivalent, freedom from additional intervention was 99.5% for surgical patients and 93.7% for medically treated patients. Reintervention was, incidentally, even higher in the PCI group than the medical group, with 86.7% free of additional intervention. Angina was superior in the CABG group (88%) than in the PCI group (79%) or medical therapy group (46%).[30]

In the Trial of Invasive versus Medical Therapy in Elderly Patients with Chronic Symptomatic Coronary-Artery Disease (TIME) study, elderly patients were studied with chronic angina. This failed to demonstrate a difference between optimized medical therapy and an invasive revascularization strategy (PCI or CABG) in terms of symptoms, quality of life, and death or nonfatal myocardial infarction (20% versus 17%, $p = .71$). However, medically treated patients were at higher risk because of major clinical events (64% versus 26% for invasive, $p < .001$), which were mainly attributable to rehospitalization and revascularization.[31] In this trial of severely symptomatic elderly patients, it was encouraging that the price of an initially conservative strategy, followed by crossover to revascularization in approximately

50% of patients, was not paid for in terms of death or myocardial infarction.[31]

Early concern over a prohibitive operative mortality among patients with impaired ventricular function has been superseded by the recognition that the survival of these patients on medical therapy was much worse than their survival with revascularization. This, coupled with ever-improving surgical techniques, such as advances in myocardial preservation and perioperative support, has made this specific subgroup the one in which the relative survival benefit of surgical therapy is the greatest. Accordingly, left ventricular dysfunction in patients with documented ischemia is now considered an important indication—rather than contraindication—for surgical revascularization.[16,24,25,32] Recent evidence that ischemic, viable, hypokinetic myocardium (hibernating or stunned) regains stronger contractile function after effective revascularization, has prompted expansion of the indications for surgical revascularization among patients with severe left ventricular dysfunction to include patients who would otherwise be considered candidates for cardiac transplantation. This subject is discussed in more detail in the following.

In summary, in regard to chronic stable angina, a survival advantage is demonstrable for surgical revascularization over medical therapy in patients with: left main disease;[33] triple-vessel disease and left ventricular dysfunction;[34,35] two-vessel disease and proximal LAD disease;[36] and severe ischemia and multivessel disease (Fig. 19-2).[37,38] Those survival advantages have not been demonstrable among patients with single-vessel disease.[39–41]

Apart from affording a survival benefit, CABG is indicated for the relief of angina pectoris and improvement in the quality of life. Between 80 and 90% of patients who are symptomatic on medical therapy become symptom-free after CABG. This benefit extends to low-risk patients for whom survival benefit from surgery is not likely.[24] Relief of symptoms appears to relate to both the completeness of revascularization and maintenance of graft patency, with the benefit of CABG diminishing with time. Recurrence of angina following CABG surgery occurs at rates of 3 to 20% per year. Although enhanced survival is reported when an ITA graft is used to the LAD, there is no significant difference in postoperative freedom from angina.[41] This may be because of vein graft occlusion or progression of native disease in grafted or ungrafted vessels.[17]

Unfortunately, few patients experience an advantage in work rehabilitation with surgery as compared with medical management. Generally, employment declines in both groups and is determined nearly as much by socioeconomic factors as age, preoperative unemployment, and type of job as by type of therapy or clinical factors such as postoperative angina. Notably, surgical revascularization has not been shown to reduce the incidence of nonfatal events such as myocardial infarction (MI), although this may be because of perioperative infarctions that offset the lower incidence of infarction in each study follow-up.[26,42]

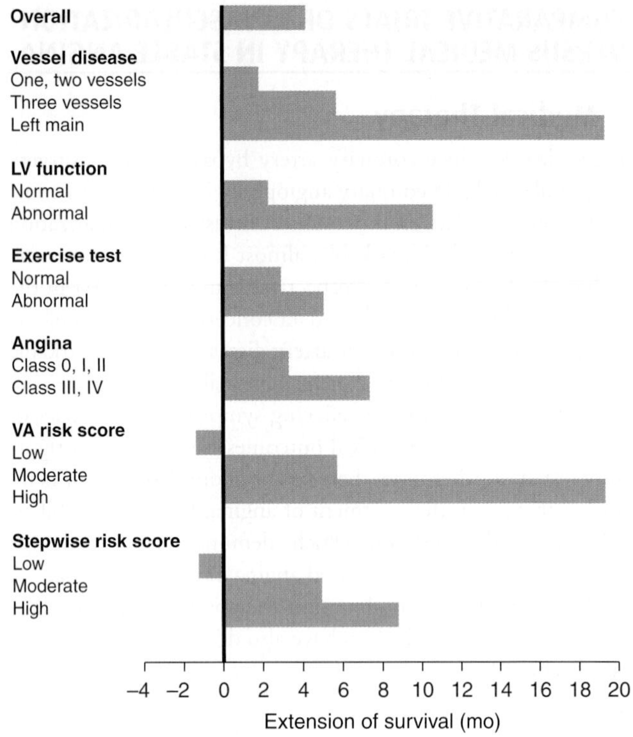

FIGURE 19-2 Extension of survival in months for various subgroups of patients with chronic stable angina treated by surgery as compared with those treated by medicine in seven prospective randomized controlled trials. (*Reproduced with permission from Yusuf S, Zucker D, Peduzzi P, et al: Effect of coronary artery bypass graft surgery on survival: overview of 10-year results from randomized trials by the Coronary Artery Bypass Graft Surgery Trial: 1st collaboration. Lancet 1994; 344:563.*)

PCI versus Medical Therapy

Despite the increasing application of catheter-based technology to multivessel disease, the majority of interventions have historically been in single-vessel disease. Accordingly, most of the data comparing angioplasty with medical therapy are derived from studies comprised principally or exclusively of patients with a limited extent of obstructive disease, although most people with angiographically detectable stenosis in one vessel have more extensive atherosclerotic changes throughout most of their coronary vessels. Many of these trials also antedate the use of IIb/IIIa inhibitors, clopidogrel, and stents. Although angiographic success rates of 85 to 90% are commonplace, no study to date has ever shown a benefit in survival or subsequent MI for PCI over medical therapy in patients with stable angina pectoris. However, the results of several recent studies have demonstrated improvement in symptoms and exercise tolerance.

In the ACME (A Comparison of angioplasty with MEdical therapy)–I study, 212 patients with documented ischemia and a single coronary artery stenosis greater than 70% were randomly assigned to medical therapy or angioplasty.[43] After 6 months, there was no mortality difference in either treatment group; however, PCI provided more complete angina relief with fewer medications and better quality of life scores, as well as longer exercise duration on stress testing than medical therapy.[43] This benefit came at some cost, however; among the 100 angioplasty patients, 19 underwent repeat PCI and seven underwent CABG during the first 6 months, compared with 11 angioplasty procedures and no CABG surgery in the patients randomized to medical therapy.[43] Moreover, nearly half of all patients assigned to initial medical therapy were asymptomatic at 6 months. Because this modest symptomatic benefit was achieved at such a large procedural and financial cost, patients who are either asymptomatic or have mild symptoms should have objective evidence of ischemia before PCI.[44] In a follow-up study by the same investigators, 101 patients with stable angina and two-vessel disease were randomized to PCI or medical therapy.[45] At 6 months, both groups had similar improvement in exercise duration, freedom from angina, and overall quality of life. These studies together suggest that, in many patients, an initial trial of medical therapy is appropriate.

Several other studies have included patients with multivessel disease. In the Randomized Intervention Treatment of Angina (RITA)–2, of 1018 patients with stable angina randomized to medicine or PCI, one-third had two-vessel disease and 7% had three-vessel disease.[46] Perhaps surprisingly, at a median follow-up of 2.7 years, the primary end points of death or MI had occurred twice as often in the PCI group (6.3 versus 3.3%, $p < .02$). Surgical revascularization was required during the follow-up interval in 7.9% of the PCI group and repeat angioplasty was required in 11%. In the medical group, 23% of patients required revascularization. Angina relief and exercise tolerance were improved to a greater degree in the angioplasty group early, but this difference disappeared by 3 years. These results are echoed in the MASS-II trial, in which angina relief was superior with PCI, but rates of intervention/reintervention were actually higher in the PCI group.[30] Again, this supports an initial strategy of medical therapy.

A comparison of PCI versus medicine as initial strategy among patients with hyperlipidemia was examined in the Atorvastatin versus REvascularization Trial (AVERT).[47] Among 341 patients with one- or two-vessel disease, ischemic events were actually less common in the medical than PCI groups (13% versus 21%, $p < .05$). Although criticized for employing outdated angioplasty technology and other issues, the results of this study are consonant with the demonstration that lipid-lowering agents may have a powerful impact on ischemic events.[48] In some respects, the lower use of aggressive lipid-lowering agents in the PCI arm biased the results in favor of medical therapy.

The most recently published trial, COURAGE, randomized 2287 patients with stable angina and objective evidence of ischemia to best medical therapy or PCI and medical management. All patients received long-acting metoprolol, amlodipine, and/or isosorbide mononitrate, as well as lisinopril or losartan. Patients had aggressive antilipid therapy and appropriate antiplatelet therapy. The primary finding of this trial was a lack of benefit of PCI over best medical therapy for death, myocardial infarction, or other major cardiovascular events.[49] Although this result has caused much controversy in the cardiology community, it is consistent with older studies.

A meta-analysis of percutaneous interventions versus medical management was published in 2005.[50] In patients with stable coronary artery disease, no benefit was found for invasive therapy in terms of death, MI, or need for subsequent revascularization. These studies provide compelling evidence that, thanks to substantial improvements in medical management, all patients should have a trial of optimized medical therapy before invasive intervention.

PCI versus CABG

Randomized Studies

A number of studies comparing an initial strategy of angioplasty versus early surgery have been carried out, all with similar results. It is important to recognize that these studies are comparisons of treatment strategies and not head-to-head comparisons of revascularization techniques. Accordingly, crossover is permitted and end points are selected to determine adverse consequences of the algorithm on an "intention to treat" basis.

A single-center Swiss study of 134 patients with isolated LAD disease was reported in 1994.[51] At 2.5 years of follow-up there was no significant difference in combined outcomes of MI and cardiac death between treatment groups. There was, however, a greater need for surgical revascularization in the initial PCI treatment group, with 25% requiring a second revascularization procedure compared with only 4.4% in the initial CABG group. Although the PCI patients were taking significantly more antianginal medication, clinical impairment level, stress test performance, and quality-of-life indices did not differ at 2 years. These findings held up at 5 years[52] with no difference between groups with respect to mortality or functional outcome despite repeat procedures in the PCI group.

The Medicine, Angioplasty or Surgery Study (MASS) from Brazil compared medical therapy, PCI, and CABG using an ITA bypass at a single center in 214 patients with stable angina, normal left ventricular function, and proximal stenosis of the left anterior descending coronary artery.[53] In this relatively small but nonetheless important randomized trial, the combined end point of cardiac death, MI, or refractory angina requiring revascularization was statistically significantly less in surgically treated patients. Moreover, there was no significant difference between patients treated medically or with PCI. In comparison with medical therapy, however, both PCI and CABG surgery were shown to provide improved relief of severe symptoms of angina pectoris and a lower frequency of inducible ischemia on treadmill exercise testing. There was no difference among the three strategies with respect to mortality or late MI at 1 year. Similar findings were obtained at 5-year follow-up.[54]

The results of the second MASS trial, which enrolled 611 patients with multivessel disease, reported 1-year outcomes as noted in the preceding.[39] Although technology is a moving target, this trial has the advantage that approximately 70% of PCI patients had stents placed. Despite this, the results were remarkably similar to MASS, with a lower incidence of adverse events in the medical group than PCI group. Surgical therapy provided the best angina relief and lowest incidence of adverse events. All therapies had similar survival rates.

A number of larger prospectively randomized studies comparing PCI with CABG have been reported in recent years. All share the limitation that, in general, only a very small minority of patients undergoing revascularization at any center were entered into these trials.[55,56] Accordingly, the populations included in the trials may not be generally reflective of clinical practice. For instance, few patients in these studies had significant LV dysfunction and most randomized patients had only one- or two-vessel disease. In the RITA trial, approximately one-third of patients had single-vessel disease.[57] Among clinically eligible patients in the Bypass Angioplasty Reperfusion Investigation (BARI)[39] and Emory Angioplasty versus Surgery Trial (EAST)[40] trials, approximately two-thirds of patients were excluded on angiographic grounds that included chronic total occlusion, left main coronary artery stenosis, diffuse disease, or other anatomical factors making PCI potentially dangerous. Consequently these randomized trials contain only a portion of the spectrum of patients with coronary artery disease encountered clinically. Entry bias has a significant impact on the likelihood of observing an outcome difference among therapies. Because a high proportion of the randomized patients are in the low-risk group, it is possible that any potential survival benefit of CABG surgery over PCI in high- and moderate-risk groups may be masked.[56]

A second consideration in evaluating these studies is that the success of revascularization procedures depends not only on the criteria employed to define success, but also on the interpretation of those criteria by both patient and physician. In the 1985 to 1986 National Heart, Lung, and Blood Institute PCI Registry, 99% of patients were discharged alive from hospital, and 92% did not sustain a MI or require CABG surgery.[58] In the BARI trial, 99% of patients survived hospitalization and 88.6% of PCI-treated patients did not have MI or require repeat revascularization by angioplasty or surgery during the initial hospitalization.[39] Employing event-free criteria (death, MI, CABG) for the initial hospitalization, PCI can be judged successful. However, if a repeat revascularization procedure within 5 years is regarded as a negative outcome, then far fewer patients are treated successfully. Regardless, the lack of differences in mortality or MI rates permits individuals to select one or the other procedure as initial therapy without the likelihood that they will pay a price with their health.

In the BARI, EAST, RITA, CABRI, and GABI multivessel PCI versus CABG surgery trials,[39,40,57,59,60] mortality was similar between 1 and 5 years of follow-up in both the PCI and CABG treatment groups. Mortality ranged from 3% in the CABRI trial at 1 year follow-up[59] and 3.4% in the RITA trial at 2.5 years[57] to 13% in the BARI trial at 5 years.[61] A slightly higher incidence of MI was noted in some of these trials.

The incidence of repeat revascularization is higher among patients treated with angioplasty than surgery in all trials carried out to date, ranging from 36.5% in the CABRI trial at 1 year follow-up to 62% in the EAST trial at 3 years. Repeat revascularization in the EAST trial for angioplasty-treated patients was much higher than that in the BARI, CABRI, and RITA trials. In contrast with PCI, repeat revascularization is less common after CABG in these same studies. The incidence of repeat revascularization procedures in multivessel patients randomized to CABG surgery ranged from 3.5% in the CABRI trial to 13.5% in the EAST trial.[40,59] Generally, repeat revascularization procedures were required five to eight times more often in patients with multivessel disease initially treated with angioplasty as compared with those randomized to initial CABG surgery. The incidence of angina at follow-up also was generally greater in the PCI-treated patients.

In the BARI trial at 5 years, 54.5% of patients initially assigned to PCI had undergone a repeat revascularization procedure, including repeat PCI in 23.2%, CABG in 20.5%, and both in 10.8%.[61] Among angina-free patients at 5 years, only 48% of the angioplasty-treated patients compared with 94% of the CABG surgery patients had not had an additional revascularization procedure after their initial procedure. An important subgroup analysis of the BARI trial demonstrated a marked survival benefit with surgery for patients with insulin-dependent diabetes receiving an ITA.

Several more recent studies of PCI versus surgery have confirmed these findings. The Argentine Randomized Trial of Coronary Angioplasty versus Bypass Surgery in Multi-vessel Disease (ERACI) trial conducted between 1998 and 1990 demonstrated no difference in death or MI, but superior event-free survival in the CABG group at 1 and 3 years.[62,63] In the French Monocentric Study, 152 patients with multivessel disease underwent PCI or CABG.[64] Again, superior event-free survival was seen in the surgical group, driven predominantly by a lesser need for subsequent revascularization.

The impact of advanced stent technology on the comparative results of PCI and CABG has been recently investigated as well. In the Arterial Revascularization Therapy Study (ARTS), 1205 patients with multivessel disease underwent CABG or PCI with bare-metal stents.[65] No significant differences in the primary end point of freedom from death, stroke, or MI at 1 year were observed, although the need for revascularization remained higher in the angioplasty than surgery groups. Similarly the second Argentine Randomized Trial of Coronary Angioplasty versus Bypass Surgery in multivessel disease (ERACI II) study group[66] demonstrated that, even with the use of stents, repeat revascularization was more common in the PCI group, particularly among diabetics in whom repeat revascularization was required in 22.3% versus 3.1% in the CABG group. Of note, in this study, the 30-day mortality was higher in the CABG than PCI group, as was the incidence of Q wave MI. Despite a high operative mortality rate (5.7%) in the surgery group that raised many questions, at 5 years, there was no difference in survival and again, CABG patients had a lower incidence of revascularization. The Surgery Or Stent (SOS study), which compared outcomes in almost 1000 patients with multivessel disease, demonstrated similar all-cause mortality among surgical compared to angioplasty patients and confirmed higher rates of repeat revascularization after angioplasty and lower freedom from angina pectoris in both patients with and without a recent acute coronary syndrome.[67] Of interest in this study, the reintervention rate, while still higher than after surgery, was far below that previously reported for angioplasty at only 17%. Mercado et al. performed a meta-analysis of the ARTS, ERATSII, MASSII, and SOS trials that demonstrated similar rates of death, MI, or stroke at 1 year and higher repeat revascularization rates with PCI.[68] A meta-analysis of 5-year data was also recently published, confirming the 1-year results with repeat revascularization more frequent after PCI than CABG (29% versus 7.9%, $p < .001$) (Fig. 30-3).[69]

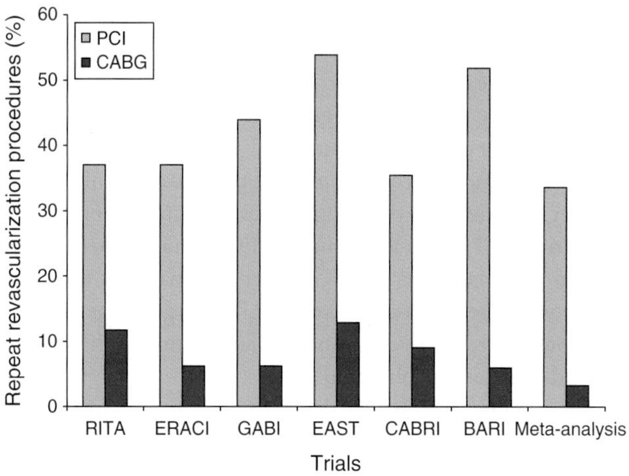

FIGURE 19-3 Risk of repeat revascularization in six randomized trials of PCI versus CABG surgery and a meta-analysis.[74] See references 58, 59, 76–78, and 80 for an explanation of acronyms.

The most recent trial, the Synergy between PCI with Taxus and Cardiac Surgery (SYNTAX) trial, assessed the optimal revascularization strategy for patients with three-vessel or left main coronary artery disease by randomizing 1800 patients to either CABG or drug-eluting stents.[70] At 12 months, the rates of myocardial infarction and death were similar between groups, but stroke was significantly more common in the CABG patients (2.2% versus 0.6% at 1 year). It should be noted that the CABG group had much less aggressive medical management postoperatively, including fewer patients on antiplatelet medications, which may account for some of the increase in stroke risk. Despite the use of DES, the rates of reintervention were still significantly higher (13.5% versus 5.9%) in the PCI group than the CABG group. Because of the lack of difference in early mortality and myocardial infarction, some cardiologists have begun to suggest that left main should no longer be an indication for CABG.[71] However, others maintain that the evidence for PCI is still inadequate and that the greater freedom from reintervention with CABG suggests that CABG remains the treatment of choice for patients with left main disease.[72]

In conclusion, the randomized trials of PCI versus CABG are useful, but only if results are interpreted in a context of patients entering or eligible to enter these trials.[55,56] PCI is a reasonable alternative to CABG surgery, and for many patients it is the preferred initial approach, provided the patient understands that there may be a higher incidence of recurrent angina and need for repeat revascularization procedures, as well as a year-long commitment to use of clopidogrel because of concern regarding catastrophic late stent thrombosis. For most patients similar to those included in these published trials, it is reassuring that a nonsurgical revascularization procedure does not place them at increased risk of MI or death in comparison with the outcomes of surgical therapy. To extrapolate these results to patients who would not have met entry criteria, however, it is intellectually flawed and potentially misleading.

Nonrandomized Database Comparisons

The information provided by randomized studies is complemented by information gleaned from large, prospectively managed, nonrandomized database studies. Such registries provide insight into the management of the sizeable population of patients who would not have been eligible for randomization. The Duke Cardiovascular Disease Databank followed 9263 patients undergoing clinically indicated coronary angiography between 1984 and 1990 for a mean of 5 years after nonrandomized treatment by CABG, PCI, or medical therapy.[9] Patients with valvular disease, prior revascularization, significant (>75%) left main disease, and congenital and nonischemic cardiomyopathy were excluded. Overall, 39% of the patients had one-vessel disease, 31% two-vessel disease, and 30% three-vessel disease. Initial therapy was medical in 3053 patients, PCI in 2788 patients, and CABG in 3422 patients. To correct for baseline differences among treatment groups, a standard covariate adjustment was performed that included all identified prognostic factors in a multivariate survival model. Complete follow-up was obtained in 97% of patients. The 5-year survival was 91%, remarkably similar to that reported from Emory, which showed an overall adjusted 5-year survival rate of 93% in both groups.[32] The mortality hazard ratios derived from the Cox regression model to evaluate relative survival differences in this database study are shown for medicine versus CABG surgery in Fig. 19-4, PCI versus medicine in Fig. 19-5, and PCI versus CABG in Fig. 19-6.[9]

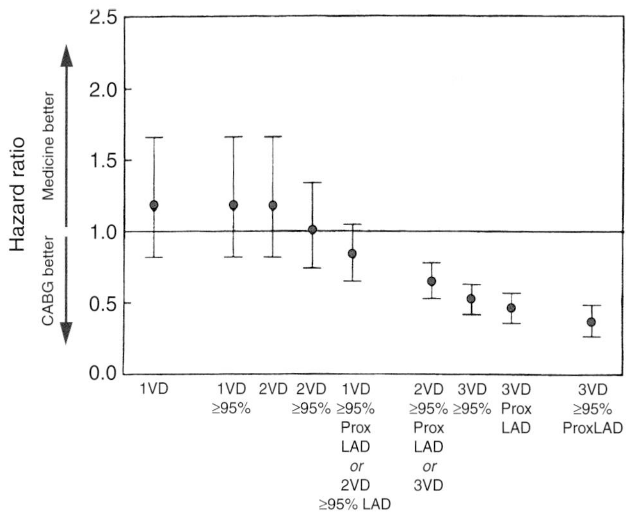

FIGURE 19-4 Hazard (mortality) ratios for CABG surgery versus medicine calculated from the Cox regression model to evaluate relative survival differences. Points indicate hazard ratios for each level of a weighted (0 to 100), hierarchical, prognostic coronary artery disease index. Bars indicate 99% confidence intervals. Horizontal line at 1.0 indicates point of prognostic equivalence between treatments. Hazard ratios below this line favor CABG; those above the line favor medicine. Prox LAD = Proximal left anterior descending coronary artery; VD = vessel disease. *(Reproduced with permission from Mark DB, Nelson CL, Califf RM, et al: Continuing evolution of therapy for coronary artery disease: initial results from the era of coronary angioplasty. Circulation 1994; 89:2015.)*

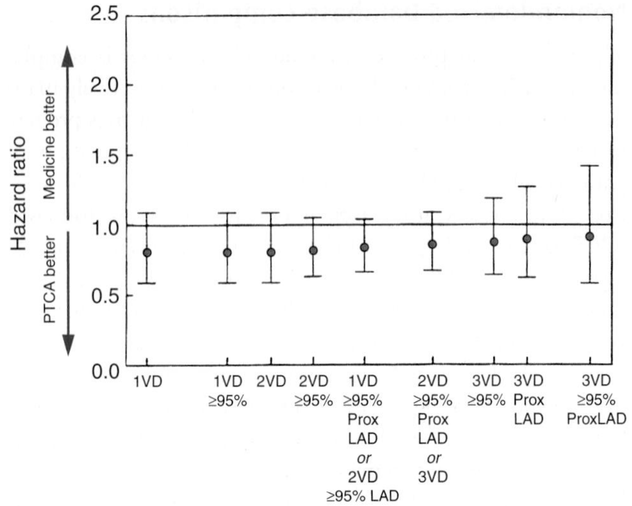

FIGURE 19-5 Hazard ratios for PCI versus medicine. See Fig. 19-4 for explanation. Points below the horizontal line favor PCI. (*Reproduced with permission from Mark DB, Nelson CL, Califf RM, et al: Continuing evolution of therapy for coronary artery disease: initial results from the era of coronary angioplasty. Circulation 1994; 89:2015.*)

From a practical standpoint, in this database study and in the randomized trials, the effect of revascularization on survival depended largely on the extent of the coronary artery disease and is an example of the concept of benefit in relationship to a "gradient of risk." For the least severe (one-vessel) disease, there were no survival advantages of revascularization over medical therapy in up to 5 years of follow-up.[9] For intermediate levels of coronary artery disease severity (ie, two-vessel disease), there was a higher 5-year survival rate for patients undergoing revascularization than for those treated medically. For patients with the most-severe coronary artery disease (ie, three-vessel disease), CABG surgery provided a significant and consistent survival advantage over medical therapy. PCI appeared prognostically equivalent to medical therapy in these patients, but only a small number of patients in this subgroup underwent angioplasty. In comparing PCI with CABG surgery, PCI demonstrated a small survival advantage over CABG surgery for patients with less-severe two-vessel disease, whereas CABG surgery was superior for more severe two-vessel disease (ie, proximal left anterior descending artery involvement).[9]

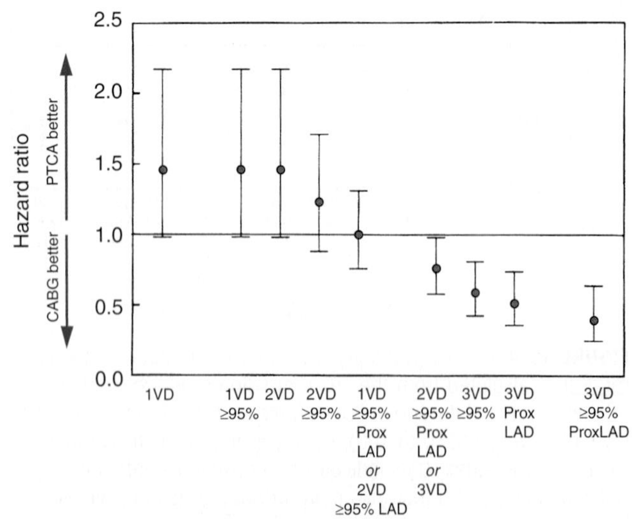

FIGURE 19-6 Hazard ratios for CABG surgery versus PCI. See Fig. 19-4 for explanation. Points below the horizontal line favor CABG. (*Reproduced with permission from Mark DB, Nelson CL, Califf RM, et al: Continuing evolution of therapy for coronary artery disease: initial results from the era of coronary angioplasty. Circulation 1994; 89:2015.*)

These important findings have been confirmed in the current era of PCI with stent implantation using the New York State Database published in 1999 using cases from 1993 to 1995.[73] In this study, a survival benefit was observed with angioplasty at 3 years for those patients with single-vessel disease not involving the LAD, whereas those with LAD or three-vessel disease had superior outcomes with surgery. In the more recent study of patients with multivessel disease who received PCI, survival was higher among the 37,212 patients who underwent CABG than among the 22,102 patients who underwent stent placement after adjustment for known risk factors. The adjusted hazard ratio for the long-term risk of death after CABG relative to stents was 0.64 (0.56 to 0.74) for three-vessel disease and proximal LAD disease. This hazard ratio increased to 0.76 (0.60 to 0.96) for patients with two-vessel disease and LAD involvement[74] (Fig. 19-7). This study has limitations of being a nonrandomized study and subject to bias; however, the surprising finding of a survival advantage apparent as early as 3 years postprocedure suggests that improvements in cardiac surgical anesthetic care, myocardial protection, and intensive care management have at least matched if not surpassed advances in percutaneous technology. It is important to note that PCI targets the culprit lesion. In contrast, CABG surgery targets both the culprit lesion and potential future culprit lesions by bypassing the diseased vessel. This in part may explain the apparent mortality benefit derived with CABG (Fig. 19-8).[75]

SPECIAL CIRCUMSTANCES

Acute Coronary Syndromes

The acute coronary syndromes (ACS) cover a wide spectrum from ST-segment elevation MI with underlying coronary obstruction to Prinzmetal's or variant angina in patients with coronary vasospasm in the absence of significant underlying obstruction. The term non–ST-segment elevation ACS encompasses the entities of unstable angina, non–Q wave MI, and postinfarction angina. They denote acute, symptomatic imbalances of the myocardial oxygen supply-demand ratio over a short time span. Prinzmetal angina, or coronary vasospasm, is diagnosed definitively by electrocardiograms obtained during the episode of pain and is treated medically. Unstable angina is not a uniform clinical entity, but comprises the spectrum of myocardial ischemia between chronic stable angina and MI, and is defined as a recent change in the severity, character, or trigger threshold of chronic stable angina or new-onset angina.

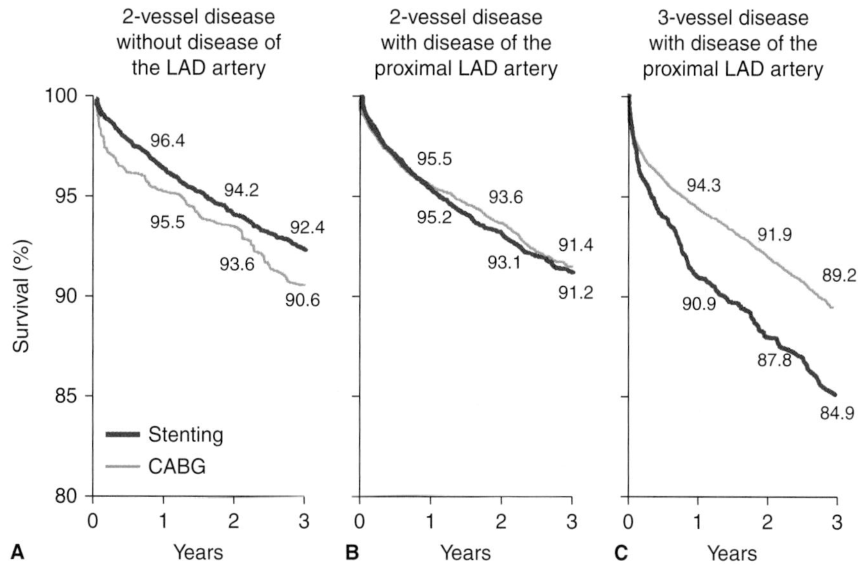

FIGURE 19-7 Unadjusted Kaplein-Meier survival curves in patients with two-vessel disease without involvement of the LAD artery (A), patients with two-vessel disease with involvement of the proximal LAD artery (B), and patients with three-vessel disease with involvement of the proximal LAD artery (C). (*Reproduced with permission from Hannan E, Racz M, Walford G, et al: Long-term outcomes of coronary-artery bypass grafting versus stent implantation. NEJM 2005; 352:2174.*)

Approximately 5.6 million Americans have chronic angina, and about 350,000 develop new-onset angina each year. Unstable angina develops in approximately 750,000 Americans each year and is associated with subsequent MI in approximately 10%. Postinfarction angina is defined as the presence of angina or other evidence of myocardial ischemia in a patient with a recent (1- to 2-week) Q wave or non–Q wave MI.

The initial approach to the patient with non–ST-segment elevation ACS (NSTEMI) is pharmacologic stabilization followed by risk stratification. The latter is based on multiple clinical, demographic, and ECG variables in addition to the use of serum biomarkers. In institutions with facilities for early angiography, patients at intermediate or high risk (the majority) undergo early angiography with a view to revascularization. In many parts of the world, however, angiographic facilities are limited and an alternative approach based upon pharmacologic stabilization followed by mobilization and risk stratification using stress testing is employed.

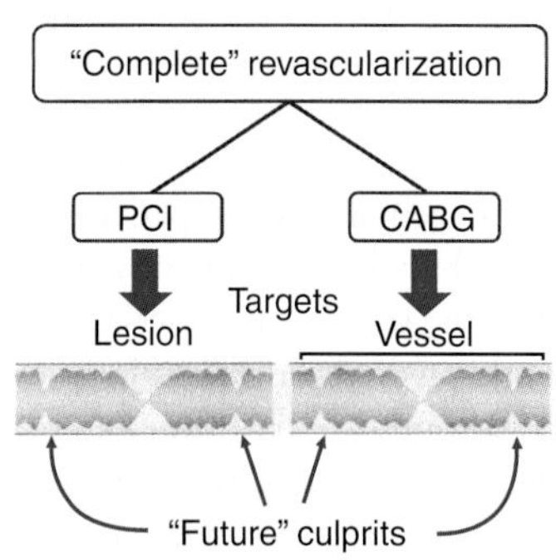

FIGURE 19-8 PCI is directed against specific culprit lesions. By bypassing diseased vessels, CABG surgery treats both culprit lesions and future culprit lesions. (*Reproduced with permission from Opie LH, Commerford PJ, Gersh BJ: Controversies in stable coronary artery disease. Lancet 2006; 367;69.*)

The most recent randomized controlled trials of aggressive versus conservative approaches to non–ST-segment elevation ACS are the FRISC II, TACTICS, and VINO trials.[76–78] Despite differences between these trials, the results favor an aggressive strategy with a view toward revascularization in the majority of the patients shown to be at high risk (eg, older patients, diabetics, those with ST-segment depression on ECG, and those with elevated CPK-MB or serum troponins).

CABG versus Medical Therapy in ACS

The technical advances in PCI in the setting of ACS have relegated CABG largely to a secondary position in most cases. The special circumstances of postinfarction mechanical complications of papillary muscle rupture, ventricular septal defect, and shock are addressed specifically in other chapters of this text. It should be noted here, however, that two multicenter trials and one single-center randomized trial involving a total of 823 patients have evaluated the relative merits of CABG surgery and medical therapy in unstable angina, excluding left main disease, poor left ventricular function (ejection fraction <30%), and age greater than 70 years during the 1970s.[79–81] The VA cooperative study demonstrated improved survival and a lower rate of recurrent angina with surgery, and at both 5 and 8 years there were fewer subsequent hospitalizations for cardiac reasons in the surgical group.[79] Interestingly, there was no difference in progression to Q wave MI between medical and surgical groups. Like the VA study, the National Cooperative Study Group Trial[80] showed no difference in progression to Q wave MI, but less severe subsequent angina with operation. Unlike the VA trial, however, there was no survival difference at 2 years

(90% in both groups). Of note, 32% of the medical group crossed over to surgery by 24 months. As current medical therapy was not available to these patients, there is significant difficulty in extrapolating the results of these trials to current clinical practice. Finally, Bertolasi and colleagues reported a single-center study of 113 patients, which demonstrated less subsequent angina, fewer infarctions, and a survival benefit for surgery in short-term follow-up.[81]

In the TIMI-IIIB trial of medical management followed by early PCI or CABG, 6-week mortality and nonfatal MI rates were 2.1 and 6.1% among 1473 patients with unstable angina or non–Q wave MI (NQWMI).[82] This study compared the results of a strategy of initial stabilization followed by aggressive treatment involving routine angiography followed by revascularization in the presence of suitable anatomy with a conservative arm reserving angiography for those with recurrent angina or a positive stress test. At 42 days and 1 year follow-up there was no difference in death or MI between the two groups. Subsequent subset analyses have demonstrated a trend in favor of an aggressive approach to revascularization over medical therapy in patients at higher risk as characterized by an elevated CPK-MB fraction (NQWMI).[82] In the end, revascularization rates were similar, with only the timing of that revascularization event being different.

The Veterans Affairs non–Q wave infarcts and strategies in hospitals (VANQUISH) trial[83] was a similar design to TIMI-IIIB. A higher early mortality rate was observed in the invasive group than in the medical group, possibly because of the extraordinarily high perioperative mortality rate of 7.7% in the CABG group. The opposite result was found in the second Fragmin and Fast Revascularization during Instability in Coronary Artery Disease trial (FRISC II).[76] These investigators found a benefit with early revascularization, particularly among patients with elevated troponins. The reason for such different results among these studies is likely owing to differences in patient populations studied. It is likely that higher-risk patients benefit from an aggressive approach, whereas lower-risk patients have less to gain and so are more likely to suffer adverse consequences.

The Angina With Extremely Serious Operative Mortality Evaluation (AWESOME) trial was reported in 2004,[84] comparing results from PCI and CABG among patients with more than one of the following risk factors: prior CABG; ACS within 7 days; LVEF less than 35%; age greater than 70 years; or intra-aortic balloon pump. The results suggested that PCI and CABG have similar outcomes for acute coronary syndromes in these patients even in the presence of low ejection fractions.

PCI for Acute MI

Because of the rapidity with which vessel patency can be restored using percutaneous techniques, PCI has all but replaced CABG in the setting of acute ST elevation MI (STEMI). Both thrombolytic therapy and direct or primary angioplasty can restore coronary artery patency and flow during acute STEMI. In the absence of hemorrhagic concerns, however, thrombolytic therapy is more widely available and is standard early therapy for acute transmural MI when immediate angioplasty is unavailable.

In the few instances in which surgical revascularization must be undertaken following thrombolysis or acute angioplasty, perioperative bleeding is increased. Bleeding has been shown not to be excessive if glycoprotein IIb/IIa inhibitors are discontinued at least 2 hours preoperatively[85] or if a platelet transfusion is provided in the presence of abciximab.[86] Clopidogrel should be held for 5 days before surgery if possible.[87]

Several early myocardial reperfusion trials have assessed the role of routine adjunctive angioplasty given that not all arteries can be reopened by thrombolysis, reocclusion occurs in some arteries initially opened, and reocclusion is associated with increased morbidity and mortality.[88,89] In these studies, the addition of routine angioplasty to thrombolytic therapy did not enhance patency, improve left ventricular function, or reduce early mortality in comparison with a more conservative approach of ischemia-driven angiography, but did increase expense and vascular bleeding problems.[90,91] A meta-analysis of adjunctive PCI and thrombolysis versus thrombolysis only showed no early benefit of PCI except in patients who have clinical indications for early revascularization (eg, postinfarction angina).[92] These studies were performed in an early phase of PCI, however, and the addition of stents as well as IIb/IIIa inhibitors and new lytics have more recently renewed interest in a combined strategy.

Asymptomatic Coronary Artery Disease

The role of revascularization either by PCI or CABG versus medical therapy in the setting of asymptomatic coronary artery disease has been studied in the Asymptomatic Cardiac Ischemia Pilot (ACIP) trial.[93] Of 558 patients with coronary artery disease and medically controlled angina, treatment was randomized to either revascularization or medical therapy directed toward eliminating angina or eliminating ischemia during ambulatory ECG. Revascularization was more effective than medical therapy in relieving ischemia, and CABG was superior to PCI (70% freedom from ischemia versus 46%, $p < .002$). Mortality at 1 and 2 years was superior for revascularization as compared with angina-directed medical therapy, but not superior to ischemia directed medical therapy.[29,93] The greatest benefit was among those patients with the most severe disease. Importantly, many of these patients with "silent ischemia" on ambulatory ECG monitoring did have symptomatic angina at other times and thus were not truly asymptomatic.

The documentation of ischemia, however, is critical. Several studies emphasize the flaws in the assumption that one can identify future culprit lesions in the absence of symptoms or documentation of ischemia. Among patients undergoing serial coronary arteriography who subsequently developed acute MI or unstable angina, the severity of stenosis at the time of initial angiogram is poorly predictive of the culprit lesion causing the acute ischemic syndrome.[94,95] In most cases the severity of the lesion responsible for subsequent ischemia was less than 50%, and in many patients it was not present at all on the initial angiogram, raising concern regarding the number of asymptomatic or minimally symptomatic patients undergoing angioplasty without stress testing.[96] Bech and associates have demonstrated that fractional flow reserve exceeded 0.75 in 91 of 325 patients planned for PCI without noninvasive evaluation of ischemia, and that among those patients, angioplasty had no impact on event-free survival or angina.[97]

Drug-Eluting Stents

Recent progress in stent technology, particularly the introduction of drug-eluting stents (DESs), promises to further reduce the incidence of restenosis. The use of stents has reduced adverse remodeling, and stents eluting medications such as sirolimus or paclitaxel, are having a profound effect on the patterns of interventions for CAD. When compared with bare-metal stents, DESs have not been shown to convey any advantage in terms of MI or mortality, but do demonstrate decreased rates of angiographic restenosis in a meta-analysis of 11 randomized trials.[98] In an observational study of 1680 patients who had CABG or PCI with a DES, CABG provided a benefit in terms of major cardiac events for patients with two- or three-vessel disease, as well as diabetic patients.[99] In another cohort of patients with multivessel disease, CABG was associated with lower rates of death, myocardial infarction, and target-vessel revascularization than drug-eluting stents. Thus, although DES may have some advantage over bare-metal stents, the indications for PCI and CABG have not changed.[100]

Left Main Disease

Significant left main disease has been considered an indication for CABG rather than PCI for many years, but recently studies have begun to question this. In a matched cohort of more than 1100 patients with unprotected left main disease, there was no difference in the rates of death or the composite outcome of death, Q wave myocardial infarction, or stroke between patients undergoing CABG or PCI despite a greater rate of target-vessel revascularization in the PCI group, including the patients who received DES.[101] Another single-center observational study focused on octogenarians reported no significant differences in cardiac death, myocardial infarction, or major adverse cardiac events between CABG and PCI at a mean follow-up of 2 years.[102] Recently, a randomized study enrolled 105 patients with unprotected left main coronary artery disease. The study had the unusual primary end point of the change in left ventricular ejection fraction after 1 year. The authors found that there was a significant increase in ejection fraction only in the PCI group (3.3%) compared with the CABG group (0.5%). There was no difference in survival at 1 year or in major cardiac adverse events. However, it should be noted that of the patients who received CABG, only 72% received a LIMA graft, which would generally not be reflective of current surgical practice.

Severe Left Ventricular Dysfunction

Left ventricular dysfunction is a predictor of increased operative risk for most cardiac surgical procedures, and in the early days of coronary revascularization these patients were not offered CABG. Like age, however, it is also a strong predictor of poor outcome with medical therapy. Accordingly, more recently significant LV dysfunction has been considered an indication rather than contraindication to surgical revascularization. In some patients, LV function has been shown to improve—sometimes dramatically so—after revascularization, leading to the concept of "hibernating" or "stunned" myocardium.[103–105] The identification of viable myocardium, which is potentially recoverable, depends on the identification of preserved metabolic activity by positron emission tomography (PET), cell membrane integrity by thallium-201 or technetium-99m SPECT, or dobutamine stress echocardiography.[106]

The only randomized trial in patients with severe LV dysfunction, the Surgical Treatment for Ischemic Heart Failure (STICH) trial, compared medical versus surgical therapy. The results from this hypothesis have not yet been published. However, a number of retrospective analyses of the impact of revascularization on outcome in patients with LV dysfunction with or without demonstrable viability have been reported (Fig. 19-9).[107] Allman and colleagues reported the results of a meta-analysis of these studies[108] demonstrating a 79.6% reduction in annual mortality (16% versus 3.2%, $p < .0001$) among patients with severe three-vessel disease, severely depressed LV function, and evidence of viability undergoing surgery versus medical therapy. Among those patients without demonstrable viability, the mortality rates were similar (7.7% versus 6.2%, $p =$ NS). This study is subject to all of the limitations of a retrospective surgical series, however, including perhaps most importantly the unaccountable effect of clinical judgment employed in selecting patients for one therapy versus another.

The relative roles of CABG and PCI in this population are not clearly defined despite the number of randomized trials of angioplasty versus surgery, largely because these patients were excluded from trial entry. In a multicenter study of patients with left ventricular dysfunction (ejection fraction <40%), slightly more than one-fourth of the patients were dead in the 2 years following multivessel angioplasty.[109] Similar results have been reported from other studies of PCI in patients with multivessel disease and left ventricular dysfunction. Overall, the outcome with PCI appears less favorable than that obtained after CABG surgery,[32] possibly as a function of more complete revascularization in surgical patients.[110]

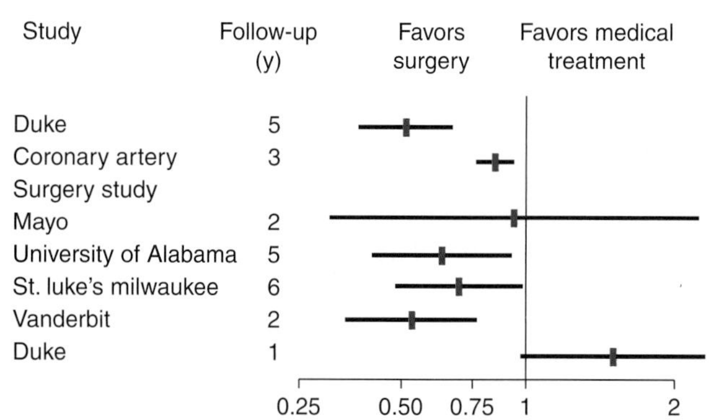

FIGURE 19-9 Relative risk of mortality for coronary artery bypass grafting compared with medical therapy in moderate-to-severe left ventricular systolic dysfunction, ranked in order of study quality. (*Reproduced with permission from Chareonthaitawee P, Gersch BJ, Araoz PA, et al: Revascularization in severe left ventricular dysfunction: the role of viability testing. J Am Coll Cardiol 2005; 46;567.*)

Completeness of revascularization may be particularly important in patients with left ventricular dysfunction. An analysis of data from the CASS registry demonstrated that, among patients with triple-vessel disease, 4-year survival was dependent on the number of vessels bypassed, particularly among those with more severe angina and those with worse ventricular function.[110] For PCI, complete of revascularization of target arteries ranged from 57 to 61% in the prospective randomized trials in which complete revascularization was not a protocol requirement (BARI, EAST, CABRI). In the GABI and RITA trials complete revascularization by PCI was targeted and was achieved in 86% in GABI and in 81 and 63% of patients with two- or three-vessel disease in RITA.[59,60]

Total Occlusion

In most patients with chronic, totally occluded coronary arteries, revascularization is not possible, although the advent of stent technology has offered some improvement in this area. In the randomized trials of multivessel PCI versus CABG, 35 to 37% of the patients excluded were disqualified because of the presence of a chronic total occlusion of a coronary artery serving viable myocardium. Thus the high proportion of trial patients with less than three-vessel disease, well-preserved ventricular function, and absence of chronically occluded arteries produces a study population that favors a higher incidence of complete revascularization by PCI and attenuated consequences of incomplete revascularization than expected in community practices. Among patients with severe angina, triple-vessel disease, and ventricular dysfunction, survival is greater in those with three or more coronary arteries bypassed than in those with only two vessels bypassed.[24,109] CABG surgery improves survival in patients with three- and two-vessel disease with left ventricular dysfunction compared with medical therapy. Although angioplasty may have a similar survival benefit, its influence on this high-risk subgroup has not been fully tested or reported.

The Elderly

Age is a predictor of operative risk in most models, but is also a predictor of poor outcome with medical therapy in the presence of coronary artery disease. The Swiss Multicenter Trial of invasive versus medical therapy in the elderly (TIME) trial briefly noted in the preceding, examined 301 patients greater the age of 75 with chronic angina were randomized to medical therapy with or without invasive evaluation.[31] Of those undergoing angiography, two-thirds had revascularization. At the 1-year follow-up interval, there was no statistical difference in death or nonfatal myocardial infarction rates. Symptoms and quality of life were also similar. However, there was a substantial increased risk of rehospitalization with revascularization in those who had medical treatment. These data suggest that invasive evaluation should be offered to elderly people who are symptomatic only after adequate medical therapy.

The choice of mode of revascularization will be particularly impacted in this group of patients by the presence of comorbidities that may increase the risk of surgical intervention, such as cerebrovascular disease, renal dysfunction, and pulmonary disease. The impact of a reduction in operative morbidity through "off-pump" coronary bypass (OPCAB) on this choice is as yet unclear. There are an increasing number of studies to suggest that it is in just this group of patients with comorbid conditions that "off-pump" surgery offers its greatest advantage over conventional surgery. The majority of these studies are not randomized, however, making their results less conclusive than one would hope. There are two retrospective and nonrandomized trials reviewing elderly patients who underwent OPCAB. There were more grafts in the standard CABG for both studies, but there were fewer strokes, incidences of prolonged respiratory failure, bleeding, transfusions in the OPCAB group, and both ICU and hospital length of stay were reduced. Reoperation for bleeding, MI, renal failure, wound infections, and operative mortality were not significantly different.[111,112] Among the randomized trials, there has been no consistent advantage to OPCAB with respect to neurocognitive outcomes, a particularly important end point in elderly people.[113] A meta-analysis of both randomized and observational studies of OPCAB and standard "on-pump" CABG in diverse populations[113,114] has failed to demonstrate any difference except for a reduction in atrial fibrillation in the OPCAB group (OR 0.59 [0.46–0.77]). The impact, therefore, of newer technologies on modifying the indications for CABG in elderly people is as yet unclear.

Diabetes Mellitus

It has been recognized for many years that patients with diabetes mellitus are at higher risk following percutaneous[115,116] or surgical[117] revascularization. The BARI trial was the first trial large enough to identify significant differences in outcome between diabetic and nondiabetic patients. In this study, which included 353 diabetic patients, a survival benefit was observed among insulin-dependent patients undergoing CABG with an ITA, as compared with those undergoing PCI. The explanation for this is not entirely clear, although an intriguing observation is that while the incidence of subsequent MI is similar between groups, survival after MI is superior among those who have undergone surgical revascularization.[118] In fact, diabetics suffering spontaneous Q wave MI were more than 10 times as likely to die with their infarction if they had been treated with PCI as compared with CABG. No such protective effect was seen among nondiabetic patients either with or without Q wave MI. This survival difference was even more pronounced at 7 years with 76.4% of diabetics in the surgical arm alive as compared with 55.7% in the angioplasty arm.[119]

The physiologic basis for this difference remains a matter of speculation, although the completeness of revascularization may be a factor. Because of the significant incidence of restenosis after PCI in diabetics, Van Belle and colleagues[120] analyzed ejection fraction at 6 months and long-term cardiac mortality and morbidity among 513 diabetic patients stratified according to the presence of occlusive restenosis ($n = 94$), nonocclusive restenosis ($n = 257$), and no restenosis ($n = 162$). The mortality rose with restenosis (24% without restenosis, 35% with nonocclusive restenosis, and 59% with occlusion), and ejection fraction fell with occlusion (decrease of 4.8% ± 12.6%).

Coronary occlusion was strongly predicted by coronary occlusion by multivariate analysis.

The results of the BARI trial prompted retrospective post hoc analyses of several earlier trials. The results have been variable. An analysis of diabetic patients from the CABRI trial at 8 years demonstrated a mortality rate of 3.5% for CABG patients versus 15.6% for PCI.[121] There was also a nonsignificant trend for better survival among diabetic patients treated surgically in the EAST trial.[122] A meta-analysis of pooled data pertaining to diabetic patients from CABRI, EAST, and RITA, however, found similar 5-year mortality rates following CABG or PCI.[123]

The follow-up study to BARI, BARI-2D, has recently been reported.[124] A total of 2368 patients with diabetes mellitus and stable coronary artery disease were randomized to receive either intensive medical therapy or intensive medical therapy and prompt revascularization (CABG or PCI left to clinical judgment). At 5 years there was no different in survival or freedom from major cardiovascular events (myocardial infarction or stroke) between medical therapy and revascularization groups. This trial was not designed to compare CABG and PCI in diabetes, but rather to examine a strategy of intensive medical therapy compared with revascularization. However, in the stratum of patients who received CABG, there were fewer major cardiovascular events when compared with medical therapy (22.4 versus 30.5%, $p = .002$). In the stratum of patients who received PCI, there was no difference in major cardiovascular events when compared with medical therapy.

Several other data bank studies have also been conducted. The Northern New England Cardiovascular Disease Study Group evaluated survival 5 years after treatment among 7159 diabetic patients with multivessel disease who were treated with CABG or PCI between 1992 and 1996.[125] Of this group, 38.6% of patients were clinically and angiographically similar to those randomized in BARI. Patients were treated according to physician preference. Those undergoing CABG were more likely to have three-vessel disease and tended to be older with greater degrees of ventricular impairment and obstructive lung disease. There were more women and more urgent interventions in the PCI group. After adjusting for these variables, PCI was associated with a significantly greater mortality rate at 5 years (risk ratio 1.49, 95% confidence interval 1.02 to 2.17, $p = .037$) and particularly among diabetics with three-vessel disease (hazard ratio 2.01, confidence interval 1.04 to 3.91, $p = .038$).

Diabetes is a condition characterized biologically by an inflammatory, proliferative, and prothrombotic state. This may account in part for the increased risk of restenosis and occlusion. Because diabetics tend to have more diffuse disease, the importance of complete revascularization, which is more often achieved surgically that percutaneously, may be enhanced. Another explanation may have more to do with patient selection than vascular biology. It has long been recognized from the previously cited studies that the survival advantage of CABG over medical therapy is greater the more extensive the coronary disease; and more recent studies of PCI versus CABG have demonstrated similar trends. Diabetic patients tend to have more extensive disease, and in BARI diabetics had a higher frequency of three-vessel disease, diffuse disease, proximal LAD disease, and left ventricular dysfunction.

In this respect, it is interesting to note that in community studies[126] and the BARI Registry, although diabetics have a poorer outcome with both PCI and CABG in comparison with nondiabetics, there were no significant differences in outcomes between these therapies in the diabetic subgroup. It must be emphasized that in these nonrandomized trials in which the selection of therapy was at the discretion of the physician and the patient, a very clear trend was noted. The "sicker" patients with left ventricular dysfunction and triple-vessel disease were far more likely to undergo CABG in contrast with patients with double-vessel disease and preserved left ventricular function. Therefore, these registry studies suggest that although the differences between bypass surgery and PCI in diabetics may be caused by altered vascular biology, these differences are magnified by the process of randomization in which patients who probably would have been treated with CABG in clinical practice were randomized to PCI.

From a clinical standpoint in regard to patient selection for coronary revascularization and the method of revascularization, the assessment of diabetics should be made on standard principles, namely, the severity and extent of coronary disease, the potential for complete revascularization, the presence or absence of left ventricular dysfunction, and the technical suitability of the lesions for PCI. The results of the aforementioned studies suggest that a preference for surgical over percutaneous revascularization is, at this time, appropriate among diabetics—at least those with extensive disease and/or ventricular dysfunction. This recommendation may change if new technologies such as drug-eluting stents and antiplatelet agents are successful in reducing the risk of restenosis and occlusion. DES are being used with greater frequency due to subset analysis of the TAXUS IV and SIRIUS trials showing a significant decrease in restenosis. However, these studies were not powered to determine restenosis rates in diabetics and there is significant risk of a type I error.[127–129] Furthermore, the potential impact of risk factor reduction may alter the risk:benefit balance in future in this important and increasing subset of patients presenting with coronary artery disease. Current data suggest that the decreased incidence of repeat revascularization, cardiac rehospitilization, and recurrent angina can be reduced to the level of nondiabetics if diabetics maintain optimal glycemic control (HbA1c ≤ 7%).[130] Irrespective of the mode of therapy, an aggressive approach to risk factor modification is required.

End-Stage Renal Disease

End-stage renal disease (ESRD) is a growing problem. Cardiovascular disease is the most common cause of death among those with ESRD; therefore, there will likely be high rates of revascularization required in these patients in the future. Comorbidities complicating surgical or percutaneous revascularization, such as diabetes, hypertension, and calcified vessels, are more common in patients with ESRD, increasing the risk of intervention. A study conducted by the Northern New England Consortium found dialysis-dependent patients with renal failure to be 3.1 times more likely to die after CABG after adjusting for known risk factors (OR 3.1, [2.1 to 3.7], $p < .001$).[131] They also found significantly increased rates of mediastinitis (3.6% versus 1.2%)

as well as postoperative stroke (4.3% versus 1.7%).[157] The long-term survival was also decreased with renal failure, which was found to be a highly significant predictor of mortality after adjustment.[132] Despite these risks, the prognosis without surgical correction of coronary artery disease is poor. Revascularization in patients with ESRD is associated with improved survival compared with medical management.[133]

REFERENCES

1. Goldman L, Hashimoto B, Cook EF, et al: Comparative reproducibly and validity of systems for assessing cardiovascular functional class: advantage of a new activity scale. *Circulation* 1976; 54:522.
2. Chang JA, Froelicher VF: Clinical and exercise test markers of prognosis in patients with stable coronary artery disease. *Curr Probl Cardiol* 1994; 19:533.
3. Ribisl PM, Morris CK, Kawaguchi T, et al: Angiographic patterns and severe coronary artery disease. Exercise test correlates. *Arch Intern Med* 1992; 152:1618.
4. Gibbons RJ, Chatterjee K, Daley J, et al: ACC/AHA/ACP-ASIM guidelines for the management of patients with chronic stable angina: a report for the American College of Cardiology/American Heart Association Task Force on Practice Guidelines. *J Am Coll Cardiol* 1999; 33:2092.
5. Ritchie JL, Bateman TM, Bonow RO, et al: Guidelines for clinical use of cardiac radionuclide imaging. Report of the American College of Cardiology/American Heart Association Task Force on Assessment of Diagnostic and Therapeutic Cardiovascular Procedures (Committee on Radionuclide Imaging), developed in collaboration with the American Society of Nuclear Cardiology. *J Am Coll Cardiol* 1995; 25:521.
6. Cheitlin MD, Alpert JS, Armstrong WF, et al: ACC/AHA Guidelines for the Clinical Application of Echocardiography. A report of the American College of Cardiology/American Heart Association Task Force on Practice Guidelines (Committee on Clinical Application of Echocardiography). Developed in collaboration with the American Society of Echocardiography. *Circulation* 1997; 95:1686.
7. Eagle KA, Guyton RA, Davidoff R, et al: ACC/AHA 2004 Guideline update for coronary artery bypass graft surgery: a report of the American College of Cardiology/American Heart Association Task Force on Practice Guidelines (Committee to Revise the 1999 Guidelines for Coronary Artery Bypass Graft Surgery). *Circulation* 2004; 110:e340.
8. Lenzen MJ, Boersma E, Sholte OP, et al: Management and outcome of patients with established coronary artery disease: the Euro Heart Survey on coronary revascularization. *Eur Heart J* 2005; 26:1169.
9. Mark DB, Nelson CL, Califf RM, et al: Continuing evolution of therapy for coronary artery disease. Initial results from the era of coronary angioplasty. *Circulation* 1994; 89:2015.
10. Serruys PW, Unger F, Sousa JE, et al: Comparison of coronary-artery bypass surgery and stenting for the treatment of multivessel disease. *NEJM* 2001; 344:1117.
11. Pearson T, Rapaport E, Criqui M, et al: Optimal risk factor management in the patient after coronary revascularization: a statement for healthcare professions; from an American Heart Association Writing Group. *Circulation* 1994; 90:3125.
12. Pepine C, Cohn PF, Deedwania C, et al: Effects of treatment on outcome in mildly asymptomatic patients with ischemia during daily life. The Atenolol Silent Ischemia Study (ASIST). *Circulation* 1994; 90:762.
13. Detry JM, Lichtlen PR, Magnani B, et al: Amlodipine reduces transient myocardial ischemia in patients with coronary artery disease: double-blind Circadian Anti-Ischemia Program in Europe (CAPE trial). *J Am Coll Cardiol* 1994; 24:1460.
14. Savonitto S, Ardissiono D, Egstrup K, et al: Combination therapy with metoprolol and nifedipine versus monotherapy in patients with stable angina pectoris. Results of the International Multicenter Angina Exercise (IMAGE) study. *J Am Coll Cardiol* 1996; 27:311-316.
15. Von Arnim T, for the TIBBS Investigators: Prognostic significance of transient ischemic episodes: Response to treatment shows improved prognosis. Results of the Total Ischemic Burden Bisoprolol Study (TIBBs) Follow-up. *J Am Coll Cardiol* 1996; 28:20-24.
16. CASS Principal Investigators and Their Associates: Coronary Artery Surgery Study (CASS): a randomized trial of coronary artery bypass surgery; survival data. *Circulation* 1983; 68:939.
17 Veterans Administration Coronary Artery Bypass Surgery Cooperative Study Group: Eleven-year survival in the Veterans Administration Randomized Trial of Coronary Bypass Surgery for Stable Angina. *NEJM* 1984; 311:1333.
18. Murphy ML, Hultgren HN, Detre K, et al: Treatment of chronic stable angina: a preliminary report of survival data of the randomized Veterans Administration Cooperative Study. *NEJM* 1977; 1297:621.
19. Varnauskas E: European Coronary Surgery Study Group: Twelve-year follow-up of survival in the randomized European Coronary Surgery Study. *NEJM* 1988; 319:332.
20. European Coronary Surgery Study Group: Prospective randomized study of coronary artery bypass surgery in stable angina pectoris: second interim report. *Lancet* 1980; 2:491.
21. Norris RM, Agnew TM, Brandt PWT, et al: Coronary surgery after recurrent myocardial infarction: progress of a trial comparing surgical and nonsurgical management for asymptomatic patients with advanced coronary disease. *Circulation* 1981; 63:788.
22. Mathur VS, Guinn GA: Prospective randomized study of the surgical therapy of stable angina. *Cardiovasc Clin* 1977; 8:131.
23. Kloster FE, Kremkau EL, Ritzman LW, et al: Coronary bypass for stable angina. *NEJM* 1979; 300:149.
24. Yusuf S, Zucker D, Peduzzi P, et al: Effect of coronary artery bypass graft surgery on survival: overview of ten-year results from randomized trials by the Coronary Artery Bypass Graft Surgery Trialist Collaboration. *Lancet* 1994; 344:563.
25. Kaiser GC, Davis KB, Fisher LD, et al: Survival following coronary artery bypass grafting in patients with severe angina pectoris (CASS): an observational study. *J Thorac Cardiovasc Surg* 1985; 89:513.
26. Myers WO, Schaff HV, Fisher LD, et al: Time to first new myocardial infarction in patients with severe angina and three-vessel disease comparing medical and early surgical therapy: a CASS Registry study of survival. *J Thorac Cardiovasc Surg* 1988; 95:382.
27. Mock MB, Ringqvist I, Fisher LD, et al: Survival of medically treated patients in the Coronary Artery Surgery Study (CASS) registry. *Circulation* 1982; 66:562.
28. Harris PJ, Harrell FE Jr, Lee KL, et al: Survival in medically treated coronary artery disease. *Circulation* 1979; 60:1259.
29. Davies RF, Goldberg AD, Forman S, et al: Asymptomatic Cardiac Ischemia Pilot (ACIP) study two-year follow-up: outcomes of patients randomized to initial strategies of medical therapy versus revascularization. *Circulation* 1997; 95:2037.
30. Hueb W, Soares PR, Gersh BJ, et al: The medicine, angioplasty, or surgery study (MASS-II): a randomized, controlled clinical trial of three therapeutic strategies for multivessel coronary artery disease: one-year results. *J Am Coll Cardiol* 2004; 43:1743.
31. The TIME investigators: Trial of invasive versus medical therapy in elderly patients with chronic symptomatic coronary-artery disease (TIME): a randomized trial. *Lancet* 2001; 358:951-957.
32. Kirklin JW, Naftel DC, Blackstone EH, et al: Summary of a consensus concerning death and ischemic events after coronary artery bypass grafting. *Circulation* 1989; 79 (suppl I):I-81.
33. Takaro T, Hultgren HN, Lipton MJ, et al: The VA Cooperative Randomized Study of Surgery for Coronary Arterial Occlusive Disease. II. Subgroup with significant left main lesions. *Circulation* 1976; 51(suppl III):III-107.
34. Passamani E, Davis KB, Gillespie MJ, et al: A randomized trial of coronary artery bypass surgery: survival of patients with a low ejection fraction. *NEJM* 1985; 312:1665.
35. Peduzzi P, Hultgren HN: Effect of medical vs surgical treatment on symptoms in stable angina pectoris: the Veterans Administration Cooperative Study of Surgery for Coronary Arterial Occlusive Disease. *Circulation* 1979; 60:888.
36. European Coronary Surgery Study Group: Long-term results of prospective randomized study of coronary artery bypass surgery in stable angina pectoris. *Lancet* 1982; 2:1173.
37. Mock MB, Fisher LD, Holmes DR Jr, et al: Comparison of effects of medical and surgical therapy on survival in severe angina pectoris and 2 vessel coronary artery disease with and without left ventricular dysfunction: a Coronary Artery Surgery Study Registry study. *Am J Cardiol* 1988; 61:1198.
38. Weiner DA, Ryan TJ, McCabe CH, et al: The role of exercise testing in identifying patients with improved survival after coronary artery bypass surgery. *J Am Coll Cardiol* 1986; 8:741.
39. The Bypass Angioplasty Revascularization Investigation (BARI) Investigators: a clinical trial comparing coronary bypass surgery with angioplasty in patients with multivessel disease. *NEJM* 1996; 335:217.
40. King SB 3rd, Barnhart HX, Kosinski AS, et al: Angioplasty or surgery for multivessel coronary artery disease: comparison of eligible registry and randomized patients in the EAST trial and influence of treatment selections on outcomes. Emory Angioplasty versus Surgery Trial Investigators. *Am J Cardiol* 1997; 79:1453.

41. Loop FD, Lytle BW, Cosgrove DM, et al: Influence of the internal-mammary-artery graft on 10-year survival and other cardiac events. *NEJM* 1986; 314:1.
42. The VA Coronary Artery Bypass Surgery Cooperative Study Group: Eighteen-year follow-up in the Veterans Affairs Cooperative Study of Coronary Artery Bypass Surgery for stable angina. *Circulation* 1992; 86:121.
43. Parisi AF, Folland ED, Hartigan P (on behalf of the Veterans Affairs ACME Investigators): a comparison of angioplasty with medical therapy in the treatment of single-vessel coronary artery disease. *NEJM* 1992; 326:10.
44. Ryan TJ, Bauman WB, Kennedy J, et al: ACC/AHA task force report: Guidelines for percutaneous transluminal coronary angioplasty. A report of the American College of Cardiology/American Heart Association Task Force on Assessment of Diagnostic and Therapeutic Cardiovascular Procedures (Committee on Percutaneous Transluminal Angioplasty). *J Am Coll Cardiol* 1993; 22:2033.
45. Folland ED, Hartigan PM, Parisi AF, for the Veterans Affairs ACME Investigators: Percutaneous transluminal coronary angioplasty versus medical therapy for stable angina pectoris: outcomes for patients with double-vessel versus single-vessel coronary artery disease in a Veterans Affairs cooperative randomized trial. *J Am Coll Cardiol* 1997; 29:1505.
46. Pocock SJ, Henderson RA, Clayton T, et al: Quality of life after coronary angioplasty or continued medical treatment for angina: three-year follow-up in the RITA-2 trial. Randomized Intervention Treatment of Angina. *J Am Coll Cardiol* 2000; 35:907-914.
47. Scandinavian Simvastatin Survival Study Group. Randomized trial of cholesterol lowering in 4444 patients with coronary heart disease: the Scandinavian Simvastatin Survival Study (4S). *Lancet* 1994; 344: 1383-1389.
48. Sacks FM, Pfeffer MA, Moye LA, et al: The effect of pravastatin on coronary events after myocardial infarction in patients with average cholesterol levels. *NEJM* 1996; 335:1001-1009.
49. Boden WE, O'Rourke RA, Teo KK, et al: Optimal medical therapy with or without PCI for stable coronary disease. *NEJM* 2007; 356:1.
50. Katritsis DG, Ioannidis JP: Percutaneous coronary intervention versus conservative therapy in nonacute coronary artery disease: a meta-analysis. *Circulation* 2005; 111:2906.
51. Goy JJ, Eeckhout E, Burnand B, et al: Coronary angioplasty versus left internal mammary artery grafting for isolated proximal left anterior descending artery stenosis. *Lancet* 1994; 343:1449.
52. Goy JJ, Eeckhout E, Moret C, et al: Five-year outcome in patients with isolated proximal left anterior descending coronary artery stenosis treated by angioplasty or left internal mammary artery grafting. A prospective trial. *Circulation* 1999; 99(25):3255-3259.
53. Hueb WA, Bellotti G, de Oliveira SA, et al: The Medicine, Angioplasty, or Surgery Study (MASS): A prospective, randomized trial of medical therapy, balloon angioplasty, or bypass surgery for single proximal left anterior descending artery stenoses. *J Am Coll Cardiol* 1995; 26:1600.
54. Hueb WA, Soares PR, Almeida De Oliveira S, et al: Five-year follow-up of the Medicine, Angioplasty, or Surgery Study (MASS): a prospective, randomized trial of medical therapy, balloon angioplasty, or bypass surgery for single proximal left anterior descending coronary artery stenosis. *Circulation* 1999; 100(19 Suppl):II107-113.
55. Pocock SJ, Henderson RA, Rickards AF, et al: Meta-analysis of randomized trials comparing coronary angioplasty with bypass surgery. *Lancet* 1995; 346:1184.
56. Sim I, Gupta M, McDonald K, et al: A meta-analysis of randomized trials comparing coronary artery bypass grafting with percutaneous transluminal coronary angioplasty in multivessel coronary artery disease. *Am J Cardiol* 1995; 76:1025.
57. RITA Trial Participants: Coronary angioplasty versus coronary artery bypass surgery: the Randomized Intervention Treatment of Angina (RITA) trial. *Lancet* 1993; 341:573.
58. Detre K, Holubkov R, Kelsey S, et al: Percutaneous transluminal coronary angioplasty in 1985–1986 and 1977–1981: The National Heart, Lung and Blood Institute Registry. *NEJM* 1988; 318:265.
59. CABRI trial participants: First-year results of CABRI (Coronary Angioplasty versus Bypass Revascularization Investigation). *Lancet* 1995; 346:1179.
60. Hamm CW, Reimers J, Ischinger T, et al, for the German Angioplasty Bypass Surgery Investigation: A randomized study of coronary angioplasty compared with bypass surgery in patients with symptomatic multivessel coronary disease. *NEJM* 1994; 331:1037.
61. The BARI Investigators: Influence of diabetes on 5-year mortality and morbidity in a randomized trial comparing CABG and PTCA in patients with multivessel disease: the Bypass Angioplasty Revascularization Investigation (BARI) *Circulation* 1997; 96:1761.
62. Rodriguez A, Boullon F, Perez-Balino N, et al, on behalf of the ERACI Group: Argentine randomized trial of percutaneous transluminal coronary angioplasty versus coronary artery bypass surgery in multivessel disease (ERACI): in-hospital results and 1-year follow-up. *J Am Coll Cardiol* 1993; 22:1060.
63. Rodriguez A, Mele E, Peyregne E, et al: Three-year follow-up of the Argentine Randomized Trial of Percutaneous Transluminal Coronary Angioplasty Versus Coronary Artery Bypass Surgery in Multivessel Disease (ERACI). *J Am Coll Cardiol* 1996; 27:1178.
64. Carrie Dm Elbaz M, Puel J, et al: Five-year outcome after coronary angioplasty versus bypass surgery in multivessel coronary artery disease: results from the French Monocentric Study. *Circulation* 1997; 96(9 Suppl): II-1-6.
65. Serruys PW, Unger F, Sousa JE, et al: Arterial Revascularization Therapies Study Group. Comparison of coronary-artery bypass surgery and stenting for the treatment of multivessel disease. *NEJM* 2001; 344(15):1117-1124.
66. Rodriguez A, Bernardi V, Navia J, et al: Argentine Randomized Study: Coronary Angioplasty with Stenting versus Coronary Bypass Surgery in patients with Multiple-Vessel Disease (ERACI II): 30-day and one-year follow-up results. ERACI II Investigators. *J Am Coll Cardiol* 2001; 37:51-58.
67. Zhang Z, Pertus JA, Mahoney EM, et al: The impact of acute coronary syndrome on clinical, economic, and cardiac-specific health status after coronary artery bypass surgery versus stent-assisted percutaneous coronary intervention: 1-year results from the stent or surgery (SoS) trial. *Am Heart J* 2005; 140:175.
68. Mercado N, Wijns W, Serruys PW, et al: One-year outcomes of coronary artery bypass graft surgery versus percutaneous coronary intervention with multiple stenting for multisystem disease: a meta-analysis of individual patient data from randomized clinical trials. *J Thorac Cardiovasc Surg* 2005; 130:512.
69. Daemen J, Boersma E, Flather M, et al: Long-term safety and efficacy of percutaneous coronary intervention with stenting and coronary artery bypass surgery for multivessel coronary artery disease: a meta-analysis with 5-year patient-level data from the ARTS, ERACI-II, MASS-II, and SoS Trials. *Circulation* 2008; 118:1146.
70. Serruys PW, Morice MC, Kappetein P, et al: Percutaneous coronary intervention versus coronary-artery bypass grafting for severe coronary artery disease. *NEJM* 2009; 360:962.
71. Moses JW, Leon MB, Stone GW: Left main percutaneous coronary intervention crossing the threshold: time for a guidelines revision! *J Am Coll Cardiol* 2009; 54:1512.
72. Taggart DP, Kaul S, Boden WE, et al: Revascularization for unprotected left main stem coronary artery stenosis: stenting or surgery. *J Am Coll Cardiol* 2008; 51:885.
73. Hannan EL, Racz MJ, McCallister BD, et al: A comparison of three-year survival after coronary artery bypass graft surgery and percutaneous transluminal coronary angioplasty. *J Am Coll Cardiol* 1999; 33:63.
74. Hannan EL, Racz MJ, Walford G, et al: Long-term outcomes of coronary-artery bypass grafting versus stent implantation. *NEJM* 2005; 352:2174.
75. Opie LH, Commerford PJ, Gersh BJ: Controversies in stable coronary artery disease. *Lancet* 2006; 367;69.
76. Lagerqvist B, Husted S, Kontny F, et al: Fast Revascularization during InStability in Coronary artery disease II Investigators. A long term perspective on the protective effects of an early invasive strategy on unstable coronary artery disease: two-year follow-up of the FRISC-II invasive study. *J Am Coll Cardiol* 2002; 40;1902.
77. Cannon CP, Wientraub WS, Demopoous LA, et al: Comparison of early invasive and conservative strategies in patients with unstable coronary syndromes treated with the glycoprotein IIb/IIIa inhibitor tirofiban. *NEJM* 2001; 344:1879-1887.
78. Spacek R, Widimsky P, Straka Z, et al: Value of first day angiography/angioplasty in evolving non-ST segment elevation myocardial infarction: an open multicenter randomized trial. The VINO study. *Eur Heart J* 2002; 23:230-238.
79. Luchi RJ, Scott SM, Deupree RH, et al: Comparison of medical and surgical treatment for unstable angina pectoris: results of a Veterans Administration cooperative study. *NEJM* 1987; 316:977.
80. National Cooperative Study Group: Unstable angina pectoris: National cooperative study group to compare surgical and medical therapy: II. In-hospital experience and initial follow-up results in patients with one, two and three vessel disease. *Am J Cardiol* 1978; 42:839.
81. Bertolasi CA, Tronge JE, Riccitelli MA, et al: Natural history of unstable angina with medical or surgical therapy. *Chest* 1976; 70:596.

82. Anderson HV, Cannon CP, Stone PH, et al: One-year results of the Thrombolysis in Myocardial Ischemia (TIMI) IIIB clinical trial. A randomized comparison of tissue-type plasminogen activator versus placebo and early invasive versus early conservative strategies in unstable angina and non–Q wave myocardial infarction. *J Am Coll Cardiol* 1995; 26:1643.
83. Boden WE, O'Rourke RA, Crawford MH, et al: Outcomes in patients with acute non-Q wave myocardial infarction randomly assigned to an invasive as compared with a conservative management strategy. Veterans Affairs Non-Q wave Infarction Strategies in Hospital (VANQWISH) Trial Investigators. *NEJM* 1998; 338(25):1785-1792.
84. Sedlis SP, Ramanathan KB, Morrison DA, et al: Outcome of percutaneous coronary intervention versus coronary bypass grafting for patients with low left ventricular ejection fractions, unstable angina pectoris, and the risk factors for adverse outcomes with bypass (the AWESOME Randomized Trial and Registry). *J Am Coll Cardiol* 2004; 94:118.
85. Dyke CM, Bhatia D, Lorenz TJ, et al: Immediate coronary artery bypass surgery after platelet inhibition with eptifibatide: results from PURSUIT. Platelet glycoprotein IIb/IIIa in unstable angina: receptor suppression using Integrilin therapy. *Ann Thorac Surg* 2000; 70: 866.
86. Singh M, Nuttal GA, Ballman KV, et al: Effect of abciximab on the outcome of emergency coronary artery bypass grafting after failed percutaneous coronary intervention. *Mayo Clin Proc* 2001; 76:784.
87. Yusuf S, Zhao F, Mehta SR, et al: Effects of Clopidogrel in addition to aspirin in patients with acute coronary syndromes with ST-segment elevation. *NEJM* 2001; 345:494.
88. Grines CL, Browne KF, Marco J, et al: A comparison of immediate angioplasty with thrombolytic therapy in acute myocardial infarction. *NEJM* 1993; 328:673.
89. Gibbons RJ, Holmes DR, Reeder GS, et al: Immediate angioplasty compared with the administration of a thrombolytic agent followed by conservative treatment for myocardial infarction. *NEJM* 1993; 328:685.
90. Simons ML, Betriu A, Col J, et al: Thrombolysis with tissue plasminogen activator in acute myocardial infarction: no additional benefit from immediate percutaneous coronary angioplasty. *Lancet* 1988; 1:197.
91. Rogers WJ, Baim DS, Gore JM, et al: Comparison of immediate invasive, delayed invasive, and conservative strategies after tissue-type plasminogen activator: results of the thrombolysis in myocardial infarction (TIMI) phase II-A trial. *Circulation* 1990; 81:1457.
92. Michels KB, Yusuf S: Does PCI in acute myocardial infarction affect mortality and reinfarction rates? *Circulation* 1995; 91:476.
93. Rogers WJ, Bourassa MG, Andrews TC, et al: Asymptomatic Cardiac Ischemia Pilot (ACIP) Study: outcome at 1 year for patients with asymptomatic cardiac ischemia randomized to medical therapy or revascularization. *J Am Coll Cardiol* 1995; 26:594.
94. Giroud D, Li JM, Urban P, et al: Relation of the site of acute myocardial infarction to the most severe coronary arterial stenosis at prior angiography. *Am J Cardiol* 1992; 69:729.
95. Little WC, Constantinescu M, Applegate RJ, et al: Can coronary angiography predict the site of a subsequent myocardial infarction in patients with mild to moderate coronary artery disease? *Circulation* 1988; 78:1157.
96. Topol EJ, Ellis SG, Cosgrove DM, et al: Analysis of coronary angioplasty practice in the United States with an insurance-claims data base. *Circulation* 1993; 87:1489.
97. Bech GJ, De Bruyne B, Pijls NH, et al: Fractional flow reserve to determine the appropriateness of angioplasty in moderate coronary stenosis: a randomized trial. *Circulation* 2001; 103:2928.
98. Babapulle MN, Joseph L, Belisle P, et al: A hierarchical Bayesian meta-analysis of randomized clinical trials of drug-eluting stents. *Lancet* 2004; 364:583.
99. Javaid A, Steinberg DH, Buch AN, et al: Percutaneous coronary intervention with drug-eluting stents for patients with multivessel coronary artery disease. *Circulation* 2007; 116:I-200.
100. Li Y, Zheng Z, Xu B, et al: Comparison of drug-eluting stents and coronary artery bypass surgery for the treatment of multivessel coronary disease three-year follow-up results from a single institution. *Circulation* 2009; 119:2040.
101. Seung KB, Park DW, Kim YH: Stents versus coronary-artery bypass grafting for left main coronary artery disease. *NEJM* 2008; 358:1781.
102. Rodes-Cabau J, DeBlois J, Bertrand OF, et al: Nonrandomized comparison of coronary artery bypass surgery and percutaneous coronary intervention for the treatment of unprotected left main coronary artery disease in octogenarians. *Circulation* 2008; 188:2374.
103. Braunwald E, Rutherford JD: Reversible ischemic left ventricular dysfunction: Evidence for 'hibernating' myocardium. *J Am Coll Cardiol* 1986; 8:1467.
104. Ross J Jr: Myocardial perfusion-contraction matching: Implications for coronary artery disease and hibernation. *Circulation* 1991; 83:1076.
105. Dilsizian V, Bonow RO: Current diagnostic techniques of assessing myocardial viability in hibernating and stunned myocardium. *Circulation* 1993; 87:1.
106. Bax JJ, Wijns W, Cornel JH, et al: Accuracy of currently available techniques for prediction of functional recovery after revascularization on patients with left ventricular dysfunction due to coronary artery disease: comparison of pooled data. *J Am Coll Cardiol* 1997; 30:1451-1460.
107. Chareonthaitawee P, Gersch BJ, Araoz PA, et al: Revascularization in severe left ventricular dysfunction: the role of viability testing. *J Am Coll Cardiol* 2005; 46;567.
108. Allman KC, Shaw LJ, Hachamovitch R, et al: Myocardial viability testing and impact of revascularization on prognosis in patients with coronary artery disease and left ventricular dysfunction: a meta-analysis. *J Am Coll Cardiol* 2002; 39:1151.
109. Ellis SG, Cowley MJ, DiSciascio G, et al: Determinants of 2-year outcome after coronary angioplasty in patients with multivessel disease on the basis of comprehensive procedural evaluation: implications for patient selection. *Circulation* 1991; 83:1905.
110. Bell MR, Gersh BJ, Schaff HV, et al: Effect of completeness of revascularization on long-term outcome of patients with three-vessel disease undergoing coronary artery bypass surgery. A report from the Coronary Artery Surgery Study (CASS) Registry. *Circulation* 1992; 86:446-457.
111. Hoff SJ, Ball SK, Coltharp WH, et al: Coronary artery bypass in patients 80 years and over: is off-pump the operation of choice? *Ann Thorac Surg* 2002; 74:S1340.
112. Hirose H, Amano A, Takhashi A: Off-pump coronary artery bypass grafting for elderly patients. *Ann Thorac Surg* 2001; 72:2013.
113. Hogue CW Jr, Sundt TM 3rd, Goldberg M, et al: Neurological complications of cardiac surgery: the need for new paradigms in prevention and treatment. *Semin Thorac Cardiovasc Surg* 1999; 2:105.
114. Wijeysundera DN, Beattie WS, Djainai G, et al: Off-pump coronary artery surgery for reducing mortality and morbidity: meta-analysis of randomized and observational studies. *J Am Coll Cardiol* 2005; 46:872.
115. Kip KE, Faxon DP, Detre RM, et al: Coronary angioplasty in diabetic patients: The National Heart, Lung and Blood Institute Percutaneous Transluminal Coronary Angioplasty Registry. *Circulation* 1996; 94:1818.
116. Stein B, Weintraub WS, Gebhart SSP, et al: Influence of diabetes mellitus on early and late outcome after percutaneous transluminal coronary angioplasty. *Circulation* 1995; 91:979.
117. Salomon NW, Page US, Okies JE, et al: Diabetes mellitus and coronary artery bypass: short-term risk and long-term prognosis. *J Thorac Cardiovasc Surg* 1983; 85:264.
118. Detre KM, Lombardero MS, Brooks MM, et al: The effect of previous coronary-artery bypass surgery on the prognosis of patients with diabetes who have acute myocardial infarction. Bypass Angioplasty Revascularization Investigation Investigators. *NEJM* 2000; 342(14):989-997.
119. BARI Investigators: Seven-year outcome in the Bypass Angioplasty Revascularization Investigation (BARI) by treatment and diabetic status. *J Am Coll Cardiol* 2000; 35:1122-1129.
120. Van Belle E, Ketelers R, Bauters C, et al: Patency of percutaneous transluminal angiographic follow-up: the key determinant of survival in diabetics after coronary balloon angioplasty. *Circulation* 2001; 103: 1185-1187.
121. Bertrand M: Long-term follow-up of European revascularization trials. Presented at the 68th Scientific Sessions, Plenary Session XII, American Heart Association, Anaheim, CA, November, 1995.
122. King SB 3rd, Kosinski AS, Guyton RA, et al: Eight-year mortality in the Emory Angioplasty versus Surgery Trial (EAST). *J Am Coll Cardiol* 2002;35(5):1116-1121.
123. Ellis SG, Nairns CR: Problem of angioplasty in diabetics. *Circulation* 1997; 96:1707-1710.
124. The BARI 2D Study Group: A randomized trial of therapies for type 2 diabetes and coronary artery disease. *NEJM* 2009; 360:2503.
125. Niles NW, McGrath PD, Malenka D, et al: Survival of patients with diabetes and multivessel coronary artery disease after surgical or percutaneous coronary revascularization: results of a large regional prospective study. *J Am Coll Cardiol* 2001; 37:1008-1015.
126. Barsness GW, Peterson ED, Ohman EM, et al: Relationship between diabetes mellitus and long-term survival after coronary bypass and angioplasty. *Circulation* 1997; 96:2551.
127. Hermiller JB, Raizner A, Cannon L, et al: TAXUS-IV Investigators. Outcomes with the polymer-based paclitaxel-eluting TAXUS stent in patients with diabetes mellitus: the TAXUS-IV trial. *J Am Coll Cardiol* 2005; 45:1172.

128. Moussa I, Leon MB, Baim DS, et al: Impact of sirolimus-eluting stents on outcome in diabetic patients: a SIRIUS (SIRolImUS-coated Bx velocity balloon-expandable stent in the treatment of patients with de novo coronary artery lesions) substudy. *Circulation* 2004; 199:2273.
129. Finn AV, Palacious IF, Kastrati A, et al: Drug-eluting stents for diabetes mellitus: a rush to judgment? *J Am Coll Cardiol* 2005; 45:479.
130. Corpus RA, Georg PB, House JA, et al: Optimal glycemic control is associated with a lower rate of target vessel revascularization in treated type II diabetic patients undergoing elective percutaneous coronary intervention. *J Am Coll Cardiol* 2004; 43:8.
131. Dacey LJ, Liu JY, Braxton JH, et al: Northern New England Cardiovascular Disease Study Group. Long-term survival of dialysis patients after coronary bypass grafting. *Ann Thorac Surg* 2002; 72:458.
132. Liu JY, Birkmeye NJ, Sanders JH, et al: Risks of morbidity and mortality in dialysis patients undergoing coronary artery bypass surgery. Northern New England Cardiovascular Disease Study Group. *Circulation* 2000; 102:2973.
133. McCullough PA: Evaluation and treatment of coronary artery disease in patients with end-stage renal disease. *Kidney Int Suppl* 2005; 95:S51.

CHAPTER 20

Myocardial Revascularization with Percutaneous Devices

James M. Wilson
James T. Willerson

INTRODUCTION

At its height, the popularity of surgical coronary revascularization spurred improvement in catheter-based technology—first for imaging quality and later for attempted therapy. In 1974, Andreas Gruentzig completed development of the double-lumen balloon catheter that was miniaturized for use in coronary arteries. Soon afterward, techniques for percutaneous transluminal coronary angioplasty (PTCA) expanded as technical breakthroughs were applied to subselective catheters, devices, guidewires, balloon materials, and lastly, coronary stents. Presently trial evidence attests that percutaneous therapy is useful as a treatment in patients with unacceptably controlled angina whose anatomy does not imply a survival benefit from revascularization or for patients with uncontrollable, unstable symptoms. However, surgical and percutaneous revascularization cannot be considered equivalent.[1]

BALLOON ANGIOPLASTY

Principles

In the early balloon angioplasty era, several technical limitations restricted percutaneous techniques to low-risk patients with proximal, discrete coronary artery stenoses, and procedural outcomes lacked predictability. As advances in tools and techniques were developed, higher-risk patients became candidates for percutaneous therapy. Over time, several principles for safety and success were recognized (Table 20-1).

Tools

Guiding Catheters

Guiding catheters differ from diagnostic catheters in that a wire-braid supports a thin catheter wall, allowing for a larger central lumen and providing enough rigidity to support the advance of subselective catheters to the distal regions of the coronary bed. The anatomy of the ascending aorta and the origin of the treated coronary artery determine the shape of the guiding catheter that will provide the most secure positioning (Fig. 20-1). The choice of guiding catheter often is the deciding factor for success when approaching challenging anatomy or when complications increase procedural difficulty. Guiding catheter manipulation is a common cause of procedural complications that necessitate urgent transition to coronary artery bypass surgery.

Guidewires

When the guiding catheter position remains secure, the guidewire allows control of the distal vessel. Different wires vary in stiffness, coatings, diameter, and design of the distal steering tip. For most procedures, the chosen wire is a 190- to 300-cm monofilament that is 0.0254 to 0.0356 cm in diameter, with either a graded tapering segment welded to the tip or a gradual taper of the monofilament. The central wire core at the tip is "plastic," or malleable, and may be shaped by the operator. In many wire designs, a wire coil wrapped around the central filament projects a blunter, less traumatic tip to the vessel that it

TABLE 20-1 Principles of Percutaneous Coronary Intervention

1. The patient's outcome is a function of age and comorbidity.
2. The procedure's outcome is a function of anatomy and proper planning (ie, sequence and equipment choices, such as guidewires and device).
3. Proximal and distal control of the treated vessel must be maintained. a. Choose proper guide catheter support. b. Maintain distal wire position. c. Keep the guide, device, and distal wire tip visible during any movement of any device.
4. Needs and limits to treatment options such as devices, adjuvant medical therapy, contrast use, and circulatory support are determined by a. Vascular access b. Clinical setting (eg, stable angina or acute myocardial infarction) c. Ventricular function d. Comorbidities: diabetes mellitus, renal insufficiency
5. The following factors can lead to failure: a. Incomplete understanding of the three-dimensional anatomy of the course to be taken and lesion to be treated b. Unrealistic interpretation of i. The capacity of available techniques to achieve success ii. The allowance of specific anatomy to accept percutaneous manipulation iii. Ignorance or inattention to technique in subselective device movement c. Inattention to anticoagulation d. Inattention to catheter hygiene (minimizing blood and contrast stagnation within the guiding catheter or other devices)

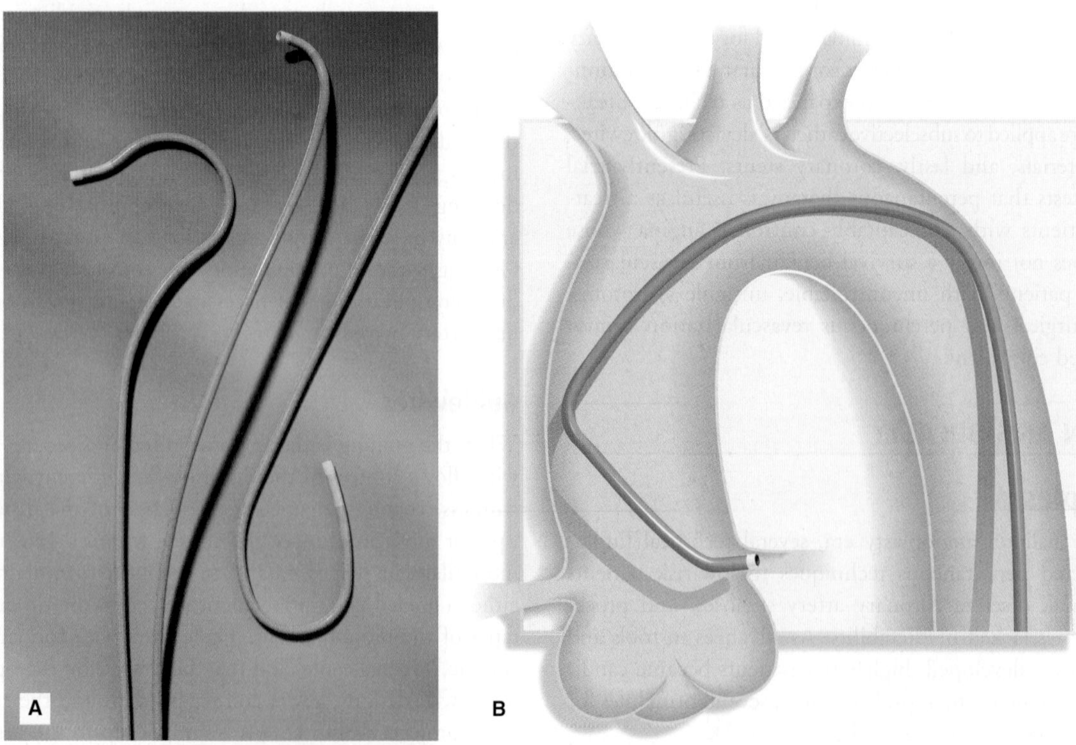

FIGURE 20-1 Commonly used guiding catheters are shown in the relaxed state (A) and as engaged with the coronary ostia in preparation for PCI: left Judkins (B), left Amplatz (C), XB (extra backup) (D), right Judkins (E), right Amplatz (F), and left coronary bypass (G). (*Reprinted with permission from Cordis Corporation, a Johnson & Johnson company.*)

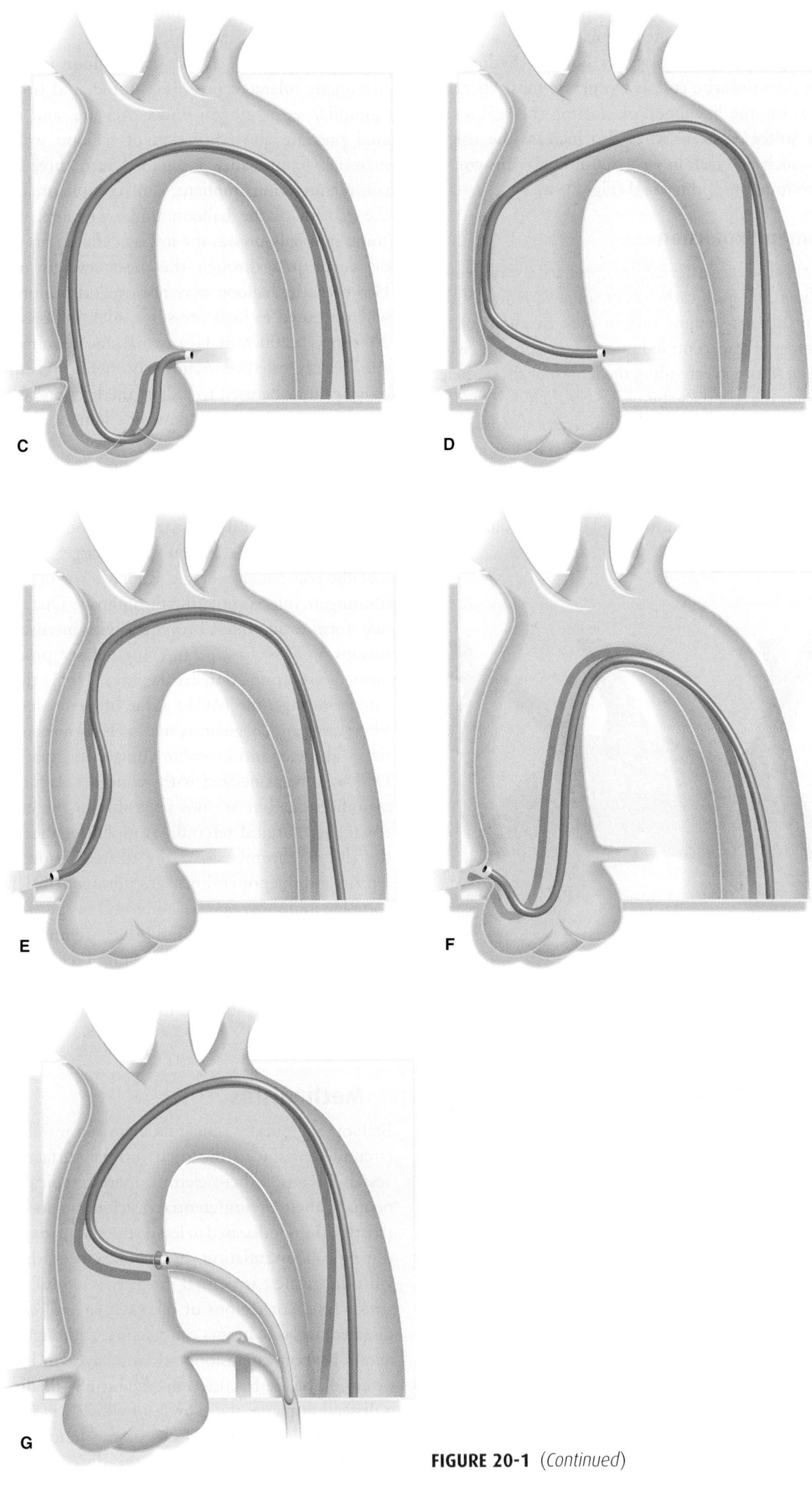

FIGURE 20-1 *(Continued)*

must traverse. Generally, the softest tip is the safest tip. However, in certain situations, such as treatment of a chronic total occlusion, a stiffer wire tip with a bonded, hydrophilic coating, rather than the wire coil, is frequently most effective. Although increasing the likelihood of crossing the lesion successfully, these stiffer, "slicker" wires also increase the risk of complications, such as creation of a subintimal wire course, dissection or perforation of the vessel (Fig. 20-2).

Tools for Lumen Expansion

The vast bulk of subselective devices for coronary artery manipulation are balloon inflation catheters or some variation of this theme. Balloon catheter designs vary in the placement of the proximal opening of the central lumen. The "on the wire" design has a central lumen extending the length of the catheter. This design affords the best trackability and capability for maneuvering through difficult anatomy but requires an assistant to manipulate the wire during device advance. The "monorail" design has a central lumen extending only through the distal balloon shaft of the catheter. The remaining catheter shaft communicates only with the balloon lumen. This design, although less trackable, allows the procedure to be performed without the need for an assistant.

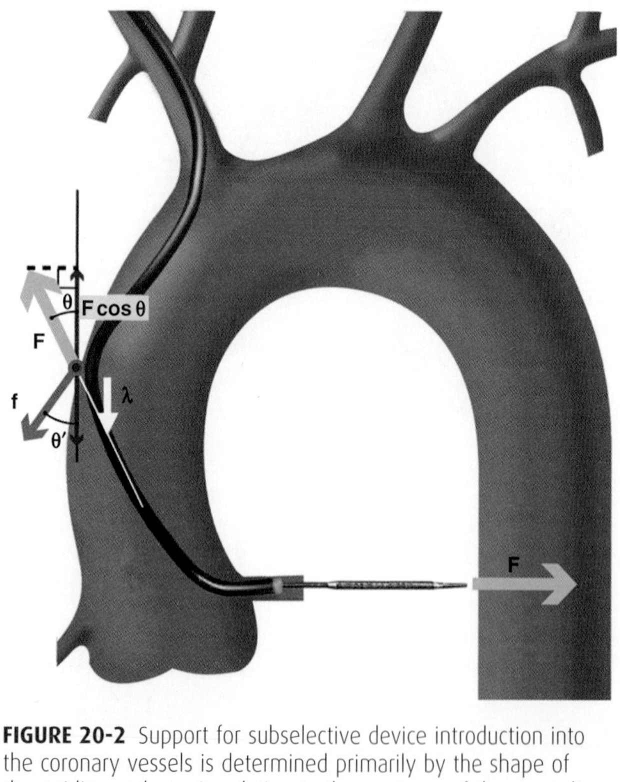

FIGURE 20-2 Support for subselective device introduction into the coronary vessels is determined primarily by the shape of the guiding catheter in relation to the anatomy of the ascending aorta and origin of the left main coronary artery. Shown graphically, advance of the device forces the catheter backward. This movement is opposed by the alignment of the catheter with the coronary artery and by friction developing through contact between the primary curve of the catheter and the opposing wall of the aorta. (*Reprinted with permission from Ikari Y, Nagaoka M, Kim JY, et al: The physics of guiding catheters for the left coronary artery in transfemoral and transradial interventions. J Invas Cardiol 2005; 17:636.*)

Properties of the angioplasty balloon include compliance, maximally tolerated pressure, profile, and friction coefficient. Compliance, or growth under pressure, and maximally tolerated pressure are a function of balloon wall thickness and material. Compliance is divided into three categories: noncompliant, semicompliant, and compliant, depending upon the growth of the balloon under pressure. The thin-walled, compliant balloon has the lowest deflated profile, allowing the device to pass through the most severely occluded vessels. However, the balloon may not expand uniformly or lengthen when exposed to high pressures, such as pressures in excess of 20 atm (15,200 mm Hg), which are required to dilate hard and heavily calcified stenoses or stents. A variety of balloon coatings may be used to reduce the friction coefficient or protect from abrasion (as in passing a stent).

Antithrombotic Therapy

During an angioplasty procedure, blood may stagnate in the guiding catheter or near the treated lesion when a wire or device is placed within the lumen of the target lesion. In addition, metallic components of the guidewire or other devices attract fibrinogen, thus stimulating thrombosis. Therefore, a thrombus may form easily unless prevented with intense anticoagulation therapy (Table 20-2). Most angioplasty procedures are performed with unfractionated heparin (UFH) titrated to an activated clotting time (ACT) value of more than 300 seconds.[2] Alternative anticoagulants, such as low-molecular-weight heparins and direct antithrombin antagonists, may be used.[3–7] The DTI may be associated with reduced risk for major bleeding complications but are not reversible in the event of need for emergency surgical referral.[8] Antiplatelet therapy also reduces the risk of thrombosis at the treated lesion. In addition to aspirin and thienopyridines, glycoprotein IIb/IIIa (GP IIb/IIIa) complex inhibitors may be employed in specific circumstances. The GP IIb/IIIa complex inhibitors are unique in their ability to impair platelet–platelet aggregation, regardless of the type or intensity of stimulus. Anticoagulation is titrated to a lower intensity (an ACT of 200 to 250 seconds) when GP IIb/IIIa inhibitors are used.

Mechanisms

Balloon angioplasty transmits increased intraluminal pressures circumferentially to the rigid intimal surface of the diseased vessel. Because atherosclerotic lesions typically are heterogeneous in their circumferential distribution and physical characteristics, the nondiseased or less diseased wall may be overstretched during balloon inflation. In most instances, the lesion segment with the greatest structural integrity is a focal point for applied stress. Adjacent regions of the vascular wall can shift, and the diseased, inelastic intima can fracture. Although this mechanism allows balloon expansion and an increase in luminal diameter, extension of the fracture into the intima–media border creates a dissection plane, the growth of which will be determined by the mechanical characteristics of the lesion and the amount of force applied. If growth of the dissection plane results in

TABLE 20-2 Adjunctive Pharmacologic Therapy for PCI

	Use	Setting	Dose	Duration of Effect	Duration of Therapy	Complication
Aspirin	Antiplatelet	All PCI	81 mg	5–7 d	Permanent	GI bleeding
Clopidogrel	Antiplatelet	All PCI	600 mg 6 h before PCI; 75 mg/d	5–7 d	1 y	Bleeding TTP (rare)
Abciximab	Antiplatelet	ACS	0.25 µg/kg + 0.125 g/kg/min	72 h	12 h	Bleeding Thrombocytopenia
Prasugrel	Antiplatelet	All PCI	60 mg bolus; 10 mg/d	5–7 d	1 y	Bleeding
Eptifibatide	Antiplatelet	ACS	180 µg/kg bolus; repeat after 10 min + infusion 2 µg/kg/min	4 h	12–72 h	Bleeding
Tirofiban	Antiplatelet	ACS	0.4 µg/kg/min for 30 min 0.1 µg/kg/min	4 h	12–72 h	Bleeding
Heparin	Anticoagulation	All PCI	100 IU/kg 60 IU/kg*	6 h	During procedure	Bleeding Thrombocytopenia Thrombosis
Bivalirudin	Anticoagulation	UFH alternative	1 mg/kg bolus + 2.5 mg/kg/h for 4 h	2 h	During procedure + 4–6 h if no clopidogrel bolus	Bleeding
Argatroban	Anticoagulation	UFH alternative	350 µg/kg bolus + 25 µg/kg/min	2 h	During procedure + 4–6 h if no clopidogrel bolus	Bleeding
Enoxaparin	Anticoagulation	UFH alternative	1 mg/kg 0.7 mg/kg*	6 h	During procedure	Bleeding
Dalteparin	Anticoagulation	UFH alternative	100 IU/kg 70 IU/kg*	6 h	During procedure	Bleeding
Acetylcysteine	Contrast nephropathy prophylaxis	GFR <60 ML/min	600 mg every 12 h	Unknown	Begin 12 h before and continue for 12 h afterward	None
Verapamil/diltiazem/ nicardipine	Vasodilator	No/slow-reflow	0.1–0.5 mg IC	20–30 min	As needed	Hypotension Bradycardia
Nitroprusside	Vasodilator	No/slow-reflow	30 µcg IC	30–60 s	As needed	Hypotension
Adenosine	Vasodilator	No/slow-reflow	50 µcg IC	30 s	As needed	Bradycardia

*Recommended dose in conjunction with glycoprotein IIb/IIIa inhibitor therapy.
ACS = Acute coronary syndrome; GFR = glomerular filtration rate; GI = gastrointestinal; IC = intracoronary; PCI = percutaneous coronary intervention; TTP = thrombotic thrombocytopenic purpura; UFH = unfractionated heparin.

significant displacement of the diseased intima, the vessel will close. This event, termed *abrupt* or *acute occlusion,* complicates about 10% of balloon angioplasty procedures. Overstretching the minimally diseased or nondiseased wall without creating plaque fracture typically results in early recoil of the treated lesion to its original state.

After balloon deflation, a small amount of thrombus accumulates, providing the stimulus and framework for colonization by inflammatory cells and myofibroblasts and the eventual, local synthesis of temporary (intimal hyperplasia) and permanent (collagen-rich) connective tissue. In addition, mechanical injury to the media and adventitia results in scar formation. The scar's contracture may reduce vessel cross-sectional area—a phenomenon termed *negative remodeling.*[9,10] During vascular healing, the encroaching intimal hyperplasia that peaks in volume at about 3 months, combined with negative remodeling, results in restenosis after 40% to 50% of balloon angioplasty procedures.[11–13]

Outcomes

In approximately 2 to 10% of balloon angioplasty procedures, intimal dissection, thrombosis, and perhaps medial smooth muscle spasm combine to produce abrupt closure.[14,15] Abrupt closure may be treated successfully with repeat balloon inflation but is treated more commonly with stent implantation.[16] The specter of abrupt closure and myocardial infarction (MI) or emergency bypass surgery and its complications historically has limited the application of balloon angioplasty.

In patients with stable angina, mortality from a balloon angioplasty procedure is 1% at 1 month.[17] About half the deaths are the result of a procedural complication, and most are related to low cardiac output (Table 20-3).[18] Although the incidence of restenosis (>50% diameter stenosis during follow-up) is 40 to 50% within 6 to 9 months of a PTCA procedure,[11,13,19] only 25% of patients report recurrent angina that warrants further investigation.[20] Patients with restenosis have an increased risk of MI and coronary artery bypass surgery.[21]

TABLE 20-3 Causes of Death after PTCA[18]

Low-output failure	66.1%
Ventricular arrhythmias	10.7%
Stroke	4.1%
Preexisting renal failure	4.1%
Bleeding	2.5%
Ventricular rupture	2.5%
Respiratory failure	2.5%
Pulmonary embolism	1.7%
Infection	1.7%

PTCA = Percutaneous transluminal coronary angioplasty.

DEVICE-ASSISTED ANGIOPLASTY

Stents

The two failure modes of balloon angioplasty, abrupt closure and restenosis, have stimulated development of myriad devices, all with the goal of reducing the risk of the procedure, the risk of restenosis, or both. Only coronary stents have been shown to be advantageous over balloon angioplasty, except in cases of severely calcified lesions (Table 20-4). There are numerous coronary stent designs, but the majority of those in current use consist of a stainless steel (or alloy, such as cobalt chromium) cylinder that has been "carved," creating a so-called slotted-tube design. Stent expansion creates a series of interlocking cells, resembling a cylindrical meshwork (Fig. 20-3). Stents are thus deformable, but when expanded, they maintain sufficient rigidity to act as scaffolding after deflation of the angioplasty balloon. Intimal disruption is contained and far less likely to propagate and occlude the treated vessel. In addition, the rigid framework left behind becomes part of the vessel wall, addressing the issue of remodeling, which is one of the mechanisms of restenosis.

Stents allow safe expansion of the vessel beyond that typically achieved with PTCA at the time of balloon expansion; however, stent use increases thrombotic and inflammatory responses of the vessel wall. The increased injury and a foreign-body response to stent struts result in a more intense and prolonged local inflammatory response.[22] As a result, stent placement paradoxically exacerbates intimal hyperplasia.[23,24] Using the late (6- or 9-month) loss in lumen diameter after stent implantation as a measure of intimal hyperplasia, even the most modern stent designs fall within a range of about 0.8 mm, more than twice the loss incurred after PTCA (0.32 mm). As a result, when examining restenosis after angioplasty, the impact of stent for percutaneous coronary revascularization (PCR) is rather small in comparison with that of PTCA.[23,24] The bulk of intimal hyperplasia and risk of restenosis are functions of the size of the treated lumen on completion of the procedure, length of the treated lesion, and presence of unstable angina, hypertension, and diabetes mellitus (Table 20-5).[25–27] Long-term follow-up studies suggest that a stent that does not reocclude during the first 6 to 9 months after implantation is not subject to late, rapid disease progression.[28–32]

By reducing the likelihood of both abrupt closure requiring emergency coronary artery bypass surgery and restenosis, stent-assisted angioplasty is more effective than routine balloon angioplasty for virtually any type of coronary artery lesion. Registry data describe a risk for emergency surgery of only 0.3 to 1.1%, and a procedural mortality of less than 1%.[33–36] The likelihood of procedural complications may be estimated on the basis of lesion characteristics (Table 20-6).[37] Depending on lesion characteristics and the number of lesions treated, after 1 year, 5 to 10% of patients require coronary artery bypass surgery, and 15 to 20% undergo a second PTCR procedure.[38–41] After 5 years, 10 to 15% of patients require another revascularization procedure because of the development of severe stenosis at an

TABLE 20-4 Devices Used for Coronary Angioplasty

	Experience	Ease of Use	Complications	Efficacy	Lesion Type
POBA	++++	++++	+	+++	Any
Cutting balloon	+	++	++	+++	Calcified lesion, ISR, bifurcation
Rotational atherectomy	+++	+	+++	+++	Heavily calcified, nondilatable ISR
Directional atherectomy	+	+	+++	+	Bifurcation, ostial lesion
Laser atherectomy	++	++	++	++	Calcification, ISR, thrombus
Aspiration (mechanical)	++	+	+	++	Thrombus
Aspiration (manual)	+	+++	+	++	Thrombus

ISR = In-stent restenosis; POBA = plain old balloon angioplasty.

untreated site.[32] Diabetes increases the risk for adverse outcomes by increasing the risk of restenosis and disease progression at untreated sites.

As noted in the description of the guidewire, iron components of stent struts attract fibrinogen and offer a site for platelet attachment and thrombosis. The increased risk of thrombosis at the treated site persists until endothelialization is complete. As a result, more intense antithrombotic therapy is required during the procedure and for up to 1 year afterward.[42,43]

Stents may be used as a drug-delivery system. However, rather than simply applying a drug to the stent surface, from which it will dissipate quickly, drug delivery is controlled by using a surface polymer or by altering the design or the material used to construct the stent.[44] This method of drug delivery, called a *drug-eluting stent* (DES), allows the drug to be applied at high concentrations at the site of interest and reduces the probability of systemic toxicity.

Drug-eluting stents reduce the primary determinant of restenosis by 50 to 100%, as determined by quantitation of late lumen loss after angioplasty (Fig. 20-4). Studies examining the efficacy of the DES introduced new nomenclature to the follow-up end points. The most useful follow-up end point is

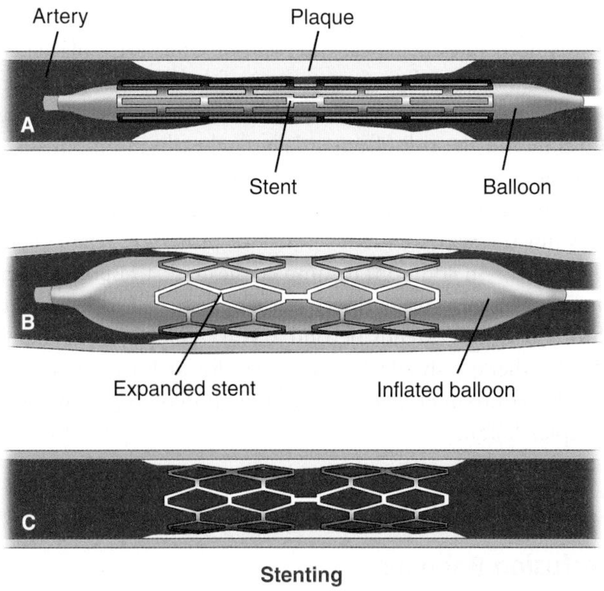

FIGURE 20-3 The coronary stent is a metallic "meshwork" that increases its rigidity when cold-worked by balloon expansion. Buttressing of the vascular wall, propagation of dissection, and early vascular recoil are reduced significantly. (*Reprinted by permission from Texas Heart Institute, www.texasheart.org.*)

TABLE 20-5 Approximate Risk of Restenosis Based on Final Lumen Diameter and Stent Length

	Final Lumen Diameter (mm)				
	2.0	2.5	3.0	3.5	4.0
Stent Length (mm)	Percent Risk				
15	32%	22%	14%	8%	4%
30	42%	30%	20%	11%	7%
45	52%	39%	28%	15%	10%
60	60%	47%	35%	20%	13%

Summarized and modified from de Feyter PJ, Kay P, Disco C, Serruys PW: Reference chart derived from post-stent-implantation intravascular ultrasound predictors of 6-month expected restenosis on quantitative coronary angiography. Circulation 1999;100(17):1777-1783.

TABLE 20-6 Risk Factors for Ischemic Events after Stent Placement[37]

Strongest correlates		
Nonchronic total occlusion		
Degenerated SVG		
Moderately strong correlates		
Length ≥ 10 mm		
Lumen irregularity		
Large filling defect		
Calcium + angle ≥45		
Eccentric		
Severe calcification		
SVG age ≥10 years		
	Outcomes	
Group	**Definition**	**Death/MI Emergency CABG**
Highest risk	Either of the strongest correlates	12.7%
High risk	≥3 moderate correlates	8.2%
Moderate risk	1-2 moderate correlates	3.4%
Low risk	No risk factors	2.1%

CABG = Coronary artery bypass graft surgery; MI = myocardial infarction; SVG = saphenous vein graft.

termed *target vessel failure* (TVF), signified by cardiac death, MI, or repeat revascularization of the treated vessel. One year after the procedure, TVF is reduced from 19.4 to 21% with a bare-metal stent (BMS) to 8.8 to 10% with a paclitaxel or sirolimus DES.[38,41]

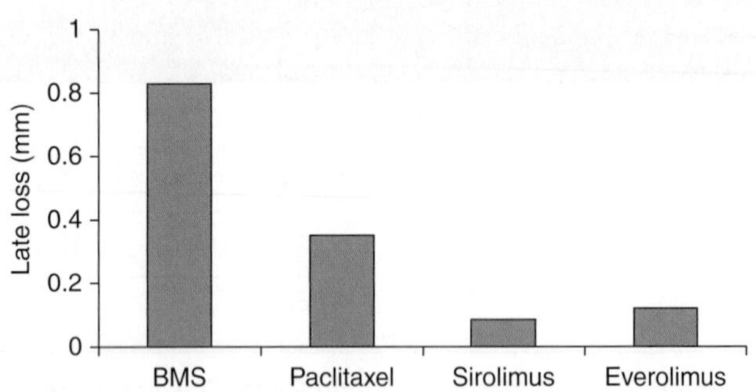

FIGURE 20-4 The effect of various stents on intimal hyperplasia in randomized trials is shown. A bare-metal stent's intimal hyperplasia thickness, or late loss, shown on the left, is compared with the late loss of drug-eluting stents shown at the right. BMS = Bare-metal stent.

Reduced rates of repeat intervention after DES placement have been reported for every type of lesion studied, except bifurcation lesions, in which the risk of restenosis remains significant, and the risk of potentially fatal early thrombosis is as high as 3.5% (Table 20-7).[38,45–52] However, the impact of DESs on failure of long-term treatment and repeat procedures does not translate to a reduced risk of procedure-related complications.[53] In addition, incomplete healing, a response to the eluting polymer, or both, confer an increased risk of stent thrombosis that extends beyond 1 year. As a result, dual antiplatelet therapy should be continued for at least 1 year after the procedure in all patients and indefinitely in patients with complex lesions.

Other Devices

Perfusion Balloons

Before the routine use of coronary stents, abrupt closure owing to dissection could be treated with repeat balloon inflation and, if unsuccessful, coronary artery bypass surgery. Prolonged balloon inflation generally was necessary for successful restoration of patency, but in the event of failure, transport for emergency

TABLE 20-7 The Clinical Impact of Drug-Eluting Stents

Population	End Point	BMS (%)	DES (%)
Total[38,41]	TVF	20-24.1	9.9-10.8
Diabetes mellitus[117]	MACE 9 mo	27.2-36.3	11.3-15
Insulin-treated[118]	MACE 9 mo	31.5	19.6
Myocardial infarction[119]	TVR 8 mo	32	18
"Complex" lesions[120]	TLR 12 mo	29.8	2.4
Long lesion small vessel[121-123]	MACE 9 mo	18.3-22.6	4-8
Small vessel[45]	MACE 8 mo	31.3	9.3
Bifurcation[46,124-126]	TVR 6 mos.	13.3-38	8.6-19
Restenosis[127]	TVR 6 mos.	33	8-19
Saphenous vein graft lesion[47]	MACE 6 mos.	28.1	11.5

BMS = Bare-metal stent; DES = drug-eluting stent; MACE = major adverse cardiac event; TLR = target lesion revascularization; TVF = target vessel failure; TVR = target vessel revascularization.

surgery often was accompanied by severe ischemia of the treated territory. As a result, balloon catheters with a short third-lumen opening just proximal and distal to the balloon were developed. These catheters, or "perfusion balloons," allowed for prolonged balloon inflation with far less ischemia and could be used to ameliorate the severity of ischemia during transport for surgery after an unsuccessful procedure. Since the introduction of the coronary stent, perfusion balloons rarely are used.

Atherectomy

When introduced, the concept of reducing the bulk of the obstructing atheroma was quite attractive. The idea was to reduce vessel wall thickness or "debulk," allowing for balloon expansion at a lower pressure. With less force applied for lumen expansion, theoretically the likelihood of abrupt closure would be reduced, as would the degree of arterial injury at the time of treatment. Several devices used for debulking have been developed and studied, including directional coronary atherectomy, percutaneous transluminal rotational ablation, and laser ablation. Unfortunately, when subjected to rigorous examination, debulking devices provide no incremental gain over plain balloon angioplasty in achieving procedural success or avoiding restenosis.[54–57] Although each device has developed a specific niche (see Table 20-4), their routine use generally is associated with an increased risk of procedural complications, including perforation and MI.[57–59]

Rotational atherectomy requires additional discussion because, unlike the other types of atherectomy, it is still commonly used. The Rotablator (Boston Scientific Corporation, Natick, MA) is an olive-shaped device that is coated with diamond chips. It is attached to an electrical motor, which causes the device to rotate at high speeds. The device is designed to abrade a rigid atherosclerotic intima, creating microemboli that are small enough to pass through the coronary microcirculation without incident. It is also useful as an initial treatment method for very rigid, heavily calcified lesions. However, the concept is not without failings. Microembolization is likely to exacerbate ischemia and therefore is contraindicated when there are thrombotic lesions, if there is impaired microcirculatory flow associated with a recent MI, or if the treated vessel is the last remaining patent vessel. Use of this device is also associated with an increased risk of perforation in highly angulated lesions.

Aspiration Devices

A number of coronary aspiration devices are available to reduce the risk of distal embolization and diminish the local concentration of prothrombotic and vasoactive substances. These devices range from a simple end-hole catheter attached to a syringe to a complex suction catheter with or without an associated mechanical disrupter. These devices forcibly extract components of the thrombus or atheroma.[60] Their use may improve flow after treatment of thrombus-laden lesions or saphenous vein grafts (Fig. 20-5).[61]

Embolic Protection Devices

During balloon angioplasty, mechanical dissolution of thrombus, if present, may result in macroembolization and distal vessel occlusion. The high-pressure manipulation of an atheromatous lesion also may free cholesterol crystals and other components of the lesion, resulting in distal microembolization, thrombosis, and slow- or no-reflow phenomenon. Several devices have been developed to reduce the frequency or impact of distal

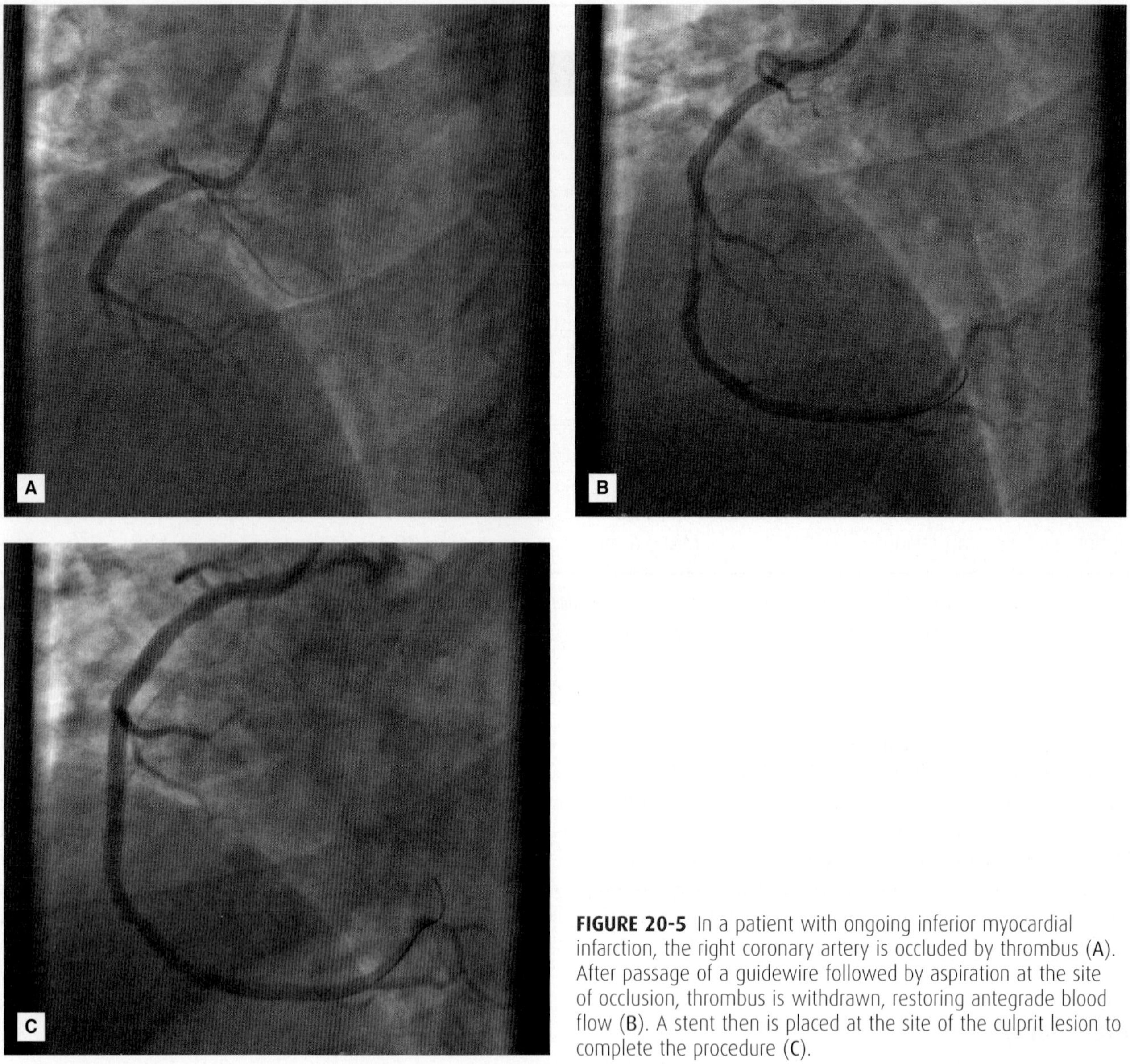

FIGURE 20-5 In a patient with ongoing inferior myocardial infarction, the right coronary artery is occluded by thrombus (**A**). After passage of a guidewire followed by aspiration at the site of occlusion, thrombus is withdrawn, restoring antegrade blood flow (**B**). A stent then is placed at the site of the culprit lesion to complete the procedure (**C**).

embolization. These devices may be placed distal or proximal to the treated lesion. Distal devices are mounted on the guidewire and use either a suspended micropore filter to trap particulate matter of 100 to 150 μm or larger or balloon occlusion of the treated vessel with posttreatment aspiration to capture embolized material. Proximally placed devices temporarily interrupt flow and aspirate the treated vessel. The PercuSurge GuardWire Plus (Medtronic, Minneapolis, MN) is a balloon occlusion and aspiration device that underwent testing in vein grafts in the Saphenous Vein Graft Angioplasty Free of Emboli Randomized (SAFER) trial.[62] The trial demonstrated a 42% reduction in creatine kinase (CK) elevations and more than a 50% reduction in the no-reflow phenomenon.[62] Unfortunately, these results did not apply to patients with MI.[63]

Imaging Devices

Angiographic imaging allows imaging of the coronary lumen but may be unreliable in the setting of severe calcification, difficult branching patterns, or previously placed coronary stents. Furthermore, a thrombus that may increase the risk of PCR may go undetected by standard angiographic imaging. Therefore, a number of alternative imaging methods have been developed to improve diagnosis, plan revascularization efforts, and evaluate the success of such efforts. Angioscopy or fiberoptic imaging requires occlusion of the imaged vessel and perfusion with saline. Although a useful tool to investigate the presence or components of thrombus within coronary vessels, angioscopy has not been a useful adjunct to PCR. In contrast, intracoronary ultrasound imaging has proved especially useful. Ultrasound imaging allows accurate determination of vessel size, luminal reduction, lesion components, and progress associated with revascularization attempts. Ultrasound guidance for stent implantation is associated with a greater than 30% reduction in the need for repeat procedures.[64] Of equal importance, intracoronary ultrasound is an invaluable research tool used to investigate the accuracy of contrast angiography and the impact of mural lesion components on complications and outcomes after angioplasty.

Devices That Measure Lesion Severity

The hemodynamic significance of coronary lesions, the appropriateness of a treatment, and the success of treatment may be determined by the following two means: a guidewire that measures the velocity of blood flow within coronary arteries or a calculation that measures pressure distal to a coronary lesion.

A miniaturized Doppler-equipped guidewire with a 12-MHz transducer uses a pulsed interrogation that samples 5.2 mm beyond the guidewire tip at an angle of 14 degrees on either side. Assuming that the cross-sectional area of the interrogated vessel remains constant during all measurements, the ratio of velocities measured reflects the ratio of blood flow between any two measurements. The most important and reliable parameter that a flow probe measures is the ratio of resting flow to vasodilated coronary flow, a value known as *coronary flow reserve.* When measured using the Doppler probe, the value is termed *coronary velocity reserve* (CVR). As a coronary lesion becomes flow limiting, attempts to normalize tissue perfusion by autoregulation result in arteriolar dilatation at rest. Therefore, the administration of an arteriolar vasodilator such as adenosine will have little additional effect on flow velocity. The absence of an appropriate increase in velocity during adenosine- or dipyridamole-induced arteriolar vasodilation produces abnormal flow reserve. A CVR less than 2.0 indicates hemodynamically significant lesions.

CVR measurement reflects changes in flow relative to an assumed normal baseline state but is subject to error when baseline flow is abnormal. Examples of abnormal states include left ventricular (LV) hypertrophy, fibrosis, and perhaps anemia. In addition, abnormally large or small driving pressure gradients may fall outside the range of normal coronary autoregulation, altering the basal-to-hyperemic ratio. Failure to achieve arteriolar dilatation in response to adenosine or dipyridamole will produce an abnormal calculated flow reserve. Examples that affect arteriolar dilatation include diabetes mellitus, amyloidosis, and recent caffeine or theophylline ingestion.

An alternative to flow measurement is pressure measurement, proximally and distally to the lesion in question. Under normal conditions, epicardial vessels present little detectable resistance to flow. Therefore, driving pressure (P_{Ao}) and arteriolar resistance pressure (P_{RA}) determine maximal coronary blood flow. The presence of a flow-limiting coronary lesion will cause some of the driving pressure to be lost, so maximal flow will depend on the distal coronary pressure (P_d)-to-P_{RA} gradient and arteriolar resistance. Therefore, the fraction of maximal basal flow that remains possible in the presence of the lesion is

$$\dot{O}_{\text{lesion}}/\dot{O}_{\text{no lesion}} = (P_d - P_{RA}/R_{\text{basal}})/\text{–}(P_{Ao} - P_{RA}/R_{\text{basal}})$$

Canceling resistance and assuming that right atrial pressure remains constant results in a very simple relationship:

$$\dot{O}_{\text{lesion}}/\dot{O}_{\text{no lesion}} = P_d/P_{Ao}$$

This ratio, called the myocardial *fractional flow reserve* (FFR), is obtained after the administration of adenosine. An FFR of 0.75 or less identifies a hemodynamically significant lesion. Routine use of FFR to ensure the necessity of PCI reduces the risk of adverse events both immediately and at 1 year.[65]

BRACHYTHERAPY

Before the advent of DESs, restenosis after angioplasty or stent implantation could be treated by medical therapy, repeat angioplasty, or coronary artery bypass surgery. The frequency of restenosis led to a large population of patients with multiple treatment failures, intractable symptoms, and prohibitive risks for surgical treatment. Because a proportion of the cell population colonizing a treated lesion and contributing to restenosis arose from the media of the treated lesion, radiation therapy to prevent cell replication was proposed. The well-recognized dangers of high-dose, external-beam radiation limited dosing to local application, but this therapy still was seen as a substantial risk. Although a source of increased adverse events when used as a treatment for de novo coronary lesions, radiation brachytherapy for the treatment of refractory in-stent restenosis has met with limited success.[66,67]

CIRCULATORY SUPPORT

Performance of a percutaneous revascularization procedure includes an obligatory period of ischemia in the treated region. The duration of ischemia may be prolonged in the event of abrupt closure or distal embolization, and recovery may be incomplete or delayed for a period of days, as in the treatment of acute MI. For patients with depressed LV systolic function or those in whom the treated territory is large, there is a risk for developing cardiogenic shock during and after the procedure. This risk substantially increases the possibility of acute renal failure, stroke, and death. The likelihood of shock complicating an angioplasty procedure may be predicted by using a scoring method that incorporates the extent and severity of systolic dysfunction present before the procedure and the extent that can be expected as a result of the procedure (Table 20-8).[37]

TABLE 20-8 A Score Predicting the Need for Circulatory Support[128]

Six Arterial Segments	LAD, D_1, S_1, OM, PLV, PDA
Score 1	Target lesion or any additional lesion >70% diameter stenosis
Score 0.5	Subtended region is hypokinetic but has no stenosis
For a score >3	Consider IABP

D_1 = First diagonal branch; IABP = intra-aortic balloon pump; LAD = left anterior descending artery; OM = obtuse marginal branch; PDA = posterior descending artery; PLV = posterior left ventricular artery; S_1 = first septal branch.

Elective placement of an intra-aortic balloon pump (IABP) is associated with a reduced risk of hypotension and major complications.[68]

The percutaneous left ventricular assist device (PLVAD) is a miniaturized axial-flow pump that is being used increasingly for support of patients in shock or during high-risk angioplasty procedures.[69] The PLVAD is capable of providing up to 4 L of additional blood flow per minute. Although it can provide superior circulatory support, the PLVAD has not shown any survival advantage when compared with the IABP, and vascular access-site complications are more frequent with the PLVAD.[70]

COMPLICATIONS OF PCR

In addition to abrupt closure and restenosis, there are several other potential complications of PCR that may influence the risk:benefit ratio for an individual patient. These complications include bleeding, vascular access–site complications, stroke, radiocontrast nephropathy, and MI owing to distal embolization.

Hemorrhage

Bleeding that requires transfusion or results in hemodynamic instability occurs in 0.5 to 4% of PCR procedures, depending on patient variables (eg, age, gender, and presence of peripheral vascular disease), procedural variables (eg, location of femoral arteriotomy and duration), and pharmacologic variables (eg, intensity of antithrombotic therapy).[2] A number of devices have been designed to improve femoral hemostasis after sheath removal, but none has proved superior to standard compression hemostasis.[71] With the availability of lower-profile equipment, the radial artery is being used with greater frequency, which results in a reduction in bleeding and access-site complications.[72]

Ischemia

Stroke complicates approximately 0.18% of PCR procedures.[73] Its occurrence is associated with increased age, depressed left ventricular ejection fraction (LVEF), diabetes mellitus, saphenous vein graft intervention, and complicated or prolonged procedures requiring the placement of an intra-aortic balloon pump.[74]

Myocardial infarction complicates 5 to 30% of PCR procedures, depending on the definition of infarction.[75] Using a definition of new Q wave, the incidence is 1%.[76] When any elevation of the MB fraction of CK (CK-MB) is used as the definition, as many as 38% of patients have a periprocedural MI.[75] Use of more stringent definitions of infarction, such as greater than three or 10 times the upper limit of normal, reduces the reported values to 11% to 18% or 5%, respectively.[76–78] Actually, any elevation carries prognostic significance, but elevation above three times the upper limit of normal is accepted as a definition of periprocedural MI.

Elevated markers of myocardial injury may be seen after apparently uncomplicated procedures.[75] One mechanism for such events is microscopic distal embolization. When severe, microscopic distal embolization of a coronary artery creates the angiographic appearance of slow vessel filling, it is termed *no-* or *slow-reflow*. No-reflow is seen most often in the setting of saphenous vein graft angioplasty, but also may complicate rotational atherectomy and primary PCR for acute MI. Methods of quantifying abnormal flow after PCR include a subjective estimation of flow velocity, the Thrombolysis in Myocardial Infarction (TIMI) flow rate (III, normal; II, slow; I, minimal contrast material flow beyond the treated site; and 0, no flow), and the more objective method of corrected TIMI frame count. Individual frames of the angiographic image are counted from the time of contrast material entry into the treated vessel until a predetermined distal landmark is reached. No-reflow may be a brief and self-limiting phenomenon, but when prolonged, it is associated with increased mortality.[79] Pharmacologic manipulations, including intracoronary verapamil, adenosine, and nitroprusside, may be used in an attempt to prevent or treat no-reflow phenomenon (see Table 20-2).

Perforation of the coronary artery complicates 0.5% of angioplasty procedures,[80] and its frequency increases almost 10-fold when ablation devices are used (1.3% for ablation versus 0.1% for PTCA; $p < .001$). Coronary artery perforation occurs more frequently in elderly and female patients (Table 20-9).[80,81]

TABLE 20-9 Coronary Artery Perforations Classified by Severity

Type	Incidence (%)	Treatment	Mortality
I: A visible extraluminal crater without extravasation*	26	Nonsurgical 95% of the time	Rarely fatal
II: Pericardial or myocardial blushing (Fig. 20-6)*	50	Require surgery 10% of the time	13%
III: 1-mm diameter perforation with contrast material streaming	26	Require surgery or covered stent	63%

*Typically a result of improper guidewire manipulation or placement.

Summarized and modified from Ellis SG, Ajluni S, Arnold AZ, et al: Increased coronary perforation in the new device era. Incidence, classification, management, and outcome. Circulation 1994; 90(6):2725-2730.

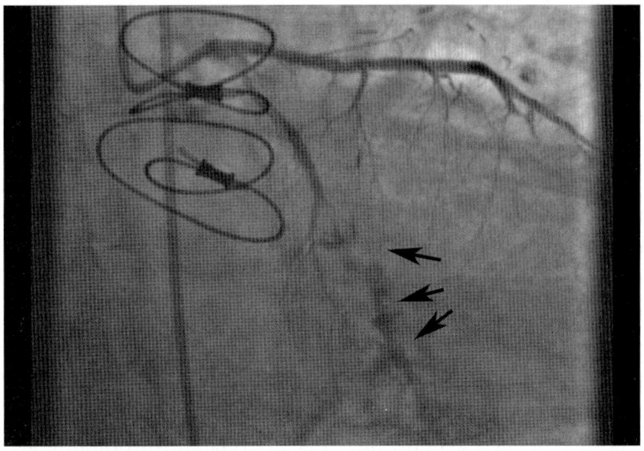

FIGURE 20-6 In the setting of early saphenous vein graft closure with myocardial infarction and postinfarction angina, attempts to access the culprit native vessel with a stiff guidewire have led to coronary perforation. Shown in this injection of the left coronary artery are occlusions of the left anterior descending and left circumflex coronary arteries. Staining is seen (*arrows*) in the region of the attempted recanalization of the left circumflex coronary artery identifying perforation (type II). The patient was treated successfully with reversal of anticoagulation and temporary occlusion of the circumflex using the PTCA balloon. PTCA = Percutaneous transluminal coronary angioplasty.

Pericardial tamponade is frequently but not invariably associated with coronary artery perforation. The overall incidence of tamponade after PCI is 0.12% and doubles when ablation devices are used. PCI-associated tamponade is recognized 55%[82] of the time during or after the procedure while the patient is still in the catheterization laboratory and 45% of the time after the patient leaves the laboratory. A minority of episodes of late tamponade (13%) are associated with recognized coronary artery perforation. Tamponade requires surgical treatment in 39% of patients, is closely associated with MI complicating PCR, and carries a mortality rate of 42%.[82]

The covered stent that was developed for, but failed to reduce the risk of, saphenous vein graft restenosis[83] presently is used as a rescue device after coronary artery perforation or for the treatment of coronary or saphenous vein graft aneurysms (Fig. 20-7).[84] When a covered stent is used for the treatment of coronary artery perforation, the need for emergency surgery is reduced, and the outcome of coronary artery perforation is improved. A small number of patients, however, still will require surgery.[85]

Toxicity

Acute renal failure after exposure to radiocontrast material, or *radiocontrast nephropathy* (RCN), is poorly understood. Its occurrence is a function of age, congestive heart failure, hemodynamic instability, diabetes mellitus, preexisting renal insufficiency, anemia, peripheral vascular disease, and the amount of contrast material administered.[86–88] The incidence of RCN after coronary angiography is 5 to 6%, with the nadir of renal function occurring 3 to 5 days after the procedure.[89] Even a transient decline in renal function leads to an increased risk of ischemic cardiovascular events during follow-up, and renal failure requiring hemodialysis is seen in about 10% of patients with RCN, increasing both short- and long-term mortality.[86,87,90]

The only methods for reducing the risk of RCN are the use of iso-osmolar contrast, volume expansion, and, perhaps, acetylcysteine administration. Iodixanol, an iso-osmolar nonionic contrast agent, reduced the incidence of RCN after noncardiac angiography.[91] Giving four oral doses (600 mg each of *N*-acetylcysteine; two doses on the day before and two on the day of the procedure) has met with varied outcomes in several studies but appears to be beneficial.[92,93] Administering crystalloid solution in volumes sufficient to maintain brisk urine flow, perhaps aided by alkalinization of urine pH, is the most effective intervention to ensure an adequate volume state.[94]

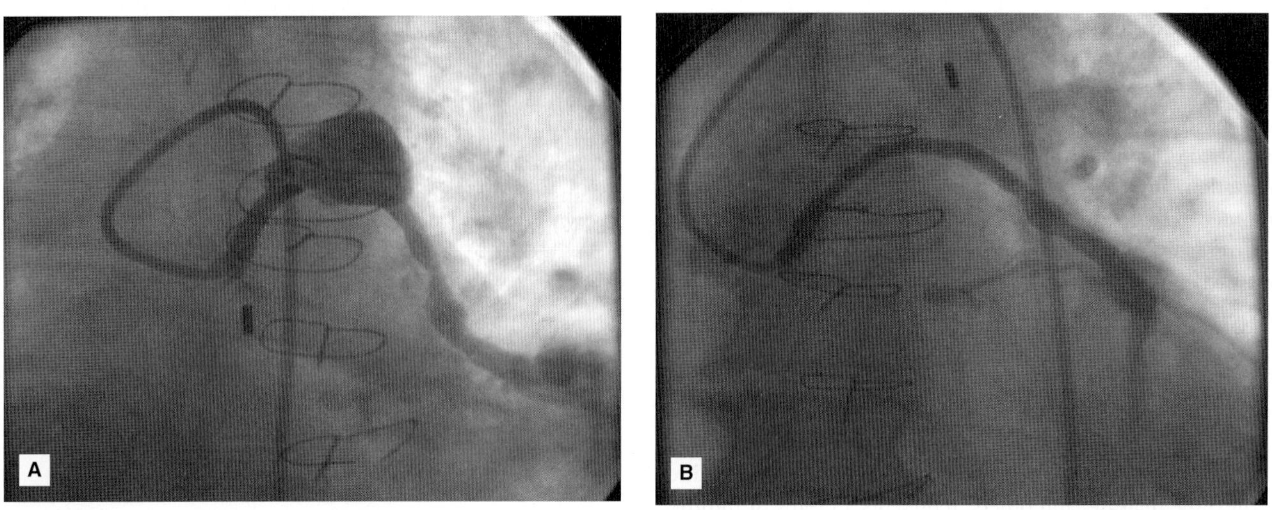

FIGURE 20-7 A large saphenous vein graft aneurysm (A) is treated with a covered stent (B).

SPECIAL CIRCUMSTANCES

Acute Coronary Syndromes (ACS)

Successful PTCA and stent implantation (in most instances) within the first 6 hours of ST-segment elevation MI is at least as effective as, and perhaps more effective than, thrombolytic agents in limiting myocardial damage and improving in-hospital survival.[95–97] The routine use of coronary stents for acute MI is associated with a restenosis rate of 17% and a 6-month event-free survival of 83 to 95%[98–101] The use of DESs reduces the risk of any adverse event from 17 to 9.4% at 300 days.[49] After failed attempts at thrombolysis or for patients with cardiogenic shock who received thrombolysis, stent revascularization increases myocardial salvage and reduces the risk of death, heart failure, or reinfarction.[102–105]

Previous Coronary Artery Bypass

Stent implantation with the assistance of embolic protection devices is the preferred method for percutaneous treatment of saphenous vein grafts.[62,103] The use of distal embolic protection reduces the risk of periprocedural MI from 14.7 to 8.6%.[62] Unfortunately, diseased grafts have a high probability of developing new lesions, reducing long-term event-free survival. After stent implantation, overall survival is 79% at 4 years, but survival free of MI or another revascularization procedure is only 29%.[106–110] Drug-eluting stents reduce the risk of restenosis after saphenous vein graft PCR but will not affect the likelihood of progression elsewhere in the diseased graft.[47]

THE FUTURE

The future of interventional cardiology lies in reducing procedural risk and extending treatment durability. For many patients, the goal of providing durable treatment success has been very nearly achieved with the introduction of DESs, an approach that has yet to be fully explored. However, a DES does not reduce procedural risk, and problems remain for patients with diffuse atherosclerosis, diabetes mellitus, bifurcation lesions, and acute coronary syndromes. The suggestion that poor outcomes may be expected after PCI and that surgical revascularization may be more appropriate have been recognized and can be measured objectively using the SYNTAX score.[111] Its adoption, utilization, and regular refinement will be difficult but necessary in order to match the right patient to the right treatment.[112]

Ironically, the goal of reducing procedural risk has been pursued most effectively for saphenous vein graft revascularization with the development of distal embolic protection devices. However, for native-vessel interventions, particularly during acute coronary syndromes, further advances likely will be pharmacologic rather than technical. Drawing on observations made in ischemic preconditioning, modification of myocardial energy metabolism with drugs, such as ranolazine, perhexiline maleate, and others, represents a means of improving the heart's ability to withstand ischemia, thus temporizing the impact of temporary vascular occlusion and macroembolization or microembolization.[113–115] In addition, inhibitors of the protein kinase family of enzymes, central to intracellular signaling, also may improve the heart's ability to withstand ischemia and reduce the severity of reperfusion injury.

Local drug delivery has met with great success in reducing the problem of restenosis. However, there are numerous methods of modifying the physiology driving intimal hyperplasia after stent implantation. New DES platforms offer the alternative of eluting multiple drugs at different rates, reducing the need for systemic medical therapy, such as prolonged dual antiplatelet therapy. In addition, complex molecules that can be absorbed by the body are being developed as stent platforms. The use of such a stent, one that delivers antithrombotic and antiproliferative drug therapy, could conceivably allow PCR protection from acute closure, recoil, thrombosis, and restenosis, without contributing to vessel rigidity that increases the difficulty of subsequent procedures.

A growing number of patients who are surviving longer with severe multivessel coronary artery disease remain hampered by severe angina pectoris. In many instances, years of slow, steady disease progression have left extensive collateral vessels that prevent infarction and the near or complete loss of major branch vessels. These patients currently have no option for percutaneous or surgical revascularization. For this population, the use of stem cells, perhaps the most efficient producers of cytokines and growth factors in their proper sequence, has met with early success. Direct injection of stem cells into regions of ischemic myocardium improves walking time and reduces the frequency of angina attacks.[116]

KEY POINTS

1. Percutaneous revascularization is best used as a treatment for unacceptable symptom control in patients who do not have anatomic indications for revascularization for prolonging survival.
2. Stent implantation substantially improves the safety of PCI, and the use of drug-eluting stents reduces the likelihood of long-term treatment failure. However, the use of drug-eluting stents requires that patients be candidates for long-term, dual antiplatelet drug therapy.
3. Measurement of the fractional flow reserve (FFR) is crucial for determining the necessity of PCI. Its routine use for the evaluation of moderate lesions results in a reduced risk of major complications of intervention compared with angiographic analysis alone.
4. When possible, all saphenous vein graft interventions should be performed with distal protection devices in place.
5. In patients who, for clinical reasons, can be treated by percutaneous or surgical means, the SYNTAX score should be used to ensure objective measurement of the most appropriate therapy.

ACKNOWLEDGMENT

Chrissie Chambers provided editorial support for this chapter.

REFERENCES

1. Boden WE, O'Rourke RA, Teo KK, et al: Optimal medical therapy with or without PCI for stable coronary disease. *NEJM* 2007; 356(15):1503-1516.
2. Hillegass WB, Brott BC, Chapman GD, et al: Relationship between activated clotting time during percutaneous intervention and subsequent bleeding complications. *Am Heart J* 2002; 144(3):501-507.
3. Ferguson JJ, Califf RM, Antman EM, et al: Enoxaparin vs unfractionated heparin in high-risk patients with non-ST-segment elevation acute coronary syndromes managed with an intended early invasive strategy: primary results of the SYNERGY randomized trial. *JAMA* 2004; 292(1): 45-54.
4. Lincoff AM, Bittl JA, Kleiman NS, et al: Comparison of bivalirudin versus heparin during percutaneous coronary intervention (the Randomized Evaluation of PCI Linking Angiomax to Reduced Clinical Events [REPLACE]-1 trial). *Am J Cardiol* 2004; 93(9):1092-1096.
5. Lincoff AM, Kleiman NS, Kereiakes DJ, et al: Long-term efficacy of bivalirudin and provisional glycoprotein IIb/IIIa blockade vs heparin and planned glycoprotein IIb/IIIa blockade during percutaneous coronary revascularization: REPLACE-2 randomized trial. *JAMA* 2004; 292(6): 696-703.
6. Madan M, Radhakrishnan S, Reis M, et al: Comparison of enoxaparin versus heparin during elective percutaneous coronary intervention performed with either eptifibatide or tirofiban (the ACTION Trial). *Am J Cardiol* 2005; 95(11):1295-1301.
7. Matthai WH, Jr. Use of argatroban during percutaneous coronary interventions in patients with heparin-induced thrombocytopenia. *Semin Thromb Hemost* 1999; 25(Suppl 1):57-60.
8. Stone GW, McLaurin BT, Cox DA, et al: Bivalirudin for patients with acute coronary syndromes. *NEJM* 2006; 355(21):2203-2216.
9. Liu MW, Roubin GS, King SB 3rd: Restenosis after coronary angioplasty. Potential biologic determinants and role of intimal hyperplasia. *Circulation* 1989; 79(6):1374-1387.
10. Schwartz RS, Edwards WD, Huber KC, et al: Coronary restenosis: prospects for solution and new perspectives from a porcine model. *Mayo Clin Proc* 1993; 68(1):54-62.
11. Nobuyoshi M, Kimura T, Nosaka H, et al: Restenosis after successful percutaneous transluminal coronary angioplasty: serial angiographic follow-up of 229 patients. *J Am Coll Cardiol* 1988; 12(3):616-623.
12. Schwartz RS, Holmes DR Jr, Topol EJ: The restenosis paradigm revisited: an alternative proposal for cellular mechanisms. *J Am Coll Cardiol* 1992; 20(5):1284-1293.
13. Serruys PW, Luijten HE, Beatt KJ, et al: Incidence of restenosis after successful coronary angioplasty: a time-related phenomenon. A quantitative angiographic study in 342 consecutive patients at 1, 2, 3, and 4 months. *Circulation* 1988; 77(2):361-371.
14. Detre KM, Holmes DR Jr, Holubkov R, et al: Incidence and consequences of periprocedural occlusion. The 1985-1986 National Heart, Lung, and Blood Institute Percutaneous Transluminal Coronary Angioplasty Registry. *Circulation* 1990; 82(3):739-750.
15. Sinclair IN, McCabe CH, Sipperly ME, Baim DS: Predictors, therapeutic options and long-term outcome of abrupt reclosure. *Am J Cardiol* 1988; 61(14):61G-66G.
16. George BS, Voorhees WD 3rd, Roubin GS, et al: Multicenter investigation of coronary stenting to treat acute or threatened closure after percutaneous transluminal coronary angioplasty: clinical and angiographic outcomes. *J Am Coll Cardiol* 1993; 22(1):135-143.
17. Kadel C, Vallbracht C, Buss F, et al: Long-term follow-up after percutaneous transluminal coronary angioplasty in patients with single-vessel disease. *Am Heart J* 1992; 124(5):1159-1169.
18. Malenka DJ, O'Rourke D, Miller MA, et al: Cause of in-hospital death in 12,232 consecutive patients undergoing percutaneous transluminal coronary angioplasty. The Northern New England Cardiovascular Disease Study Group. *Am Heart J* 1999; 137(4 Pt 1):632-638.
19. Holmes DR Jr, Vlietstra RE, Smith HC, et al: Restenosis after percutaneous transluminal coronary angioplasty (PTCA): a report from the PTCA Registry of the National Heart, Lung, and Blood Institute. *Am J Cardiol* 1984; 53(12):77C-81C.
20. Berger PB, Bell MR, Garratt KN, et al: Initial results and long-term outcome of coronary angioplasty in chronic mild angina pectoris. *Am J Cardiol* 1993; 71(16):1396-1401.
21. Weintraub WS, Ghazzal ZM, Douglas JS Jr, et al: Long-term clinical follow-up in patients with angiographic restudy after successful angioplasty. *Circulation* 1993; 87(3):831-840.
22. Farb A, Sangiorgi G, Carter AJ, et al: Pathology of acute and chronic coronary stenting in humans. *Circulation* 1999; 99(1):44-52.
23. Fischman DL, Leon MB, Baim DS, et al: A randomized comparison of coronary-stent placement and balloon angioplasty in the treatment of coronary artery disease. Stent Restenosis Study Investigators. *NEJM* 1994; 331(8):496-501.
24. Serruys PW, de Jaegere P, Kiemeneij F, et al: A comparison of balloon-expandable-stent implantation with balloon angioplasty in patients with coronary artery disease. Benestent Study Group. *NEJM* 1994; 331(8): 489-495.
25. Cutlip DE, Chauhan MS, Baim DS, et al: Clinical restenosis after coronary stenting: perspectives from multicenter clinical trials. *J Am Coll Cardiol* 2002; 40(12):2082-2089.
26. de Feyter PJ, Kay P, Disco C, Serruys PW: Reference chart derived from post-stent-implantation intravascular ultrasound predictors of 6-month expected restenosis on quantitative coronary angiography. *Circulation* 1999;100(17):1777-1783.
27. Serruys PW, Kay IP, Disco C, et al: Periprocedural quantitative coronary angiography after Palmaz-Schatz stent implantation predicts the restenosis rate at six months: results of a meta-analysis of the BElgian NEtherlands Stent study (BENESTENT) I, BENESTENT II Pilot, BENESTENT II and MUSIC trials. Multicenter Ultrasound Stent In Coronaries. *J Am Coll Cardiol* 1999; 34(4):1067-1074.
28. Choussat R, Klersy C, Black AJ, et al: Long-term (≥8 years) outcome after Palmaz-Schatz stent implantation. *Am J Cardiol* 2001;88(1):10-16.
29. Karam C, Fajadet J, Beauchet A, et al: Nine-year follow-up of balloon-expandable Palmaz-Schatz stent in patients with single-vessel disease. *Catheter Cardiovasc Interv* 2000; 50(2):170-174.
30. Kiemeneij F, Serruys PW, Macaya C, et al: Continued benefit of coronary stenting versus balloon angioplasty: five-year clinical follow-up of Benestent-I trial. *J Am Coll Cardiol* 2001; 37(6):1598-1603.
31. Kimura T, Yokoi H, Nakagawa Y, et al: Three-year follow-up after implantation of metallic coronary-artery stents. *NEJM* 1996; 334(9): 561-566.
32. Laham RJ, Carrozza JP, Berger C, et al: Long-term (4- to 6-year) outcome of Palmaz-Schatz stenting: paucity of late clinical stent-related problems. *J Am Coll Cardiol* 1996; 28(4):820-826.
33. Di Sciascio G, Patti G, D'Ambrosio A, Nusca A: Coronary stenting in patients with depressed left ventricular function: acute and long-term results in a selected population. *Catheter Cardiovasc Interv* 2003; 59(4): 429-433.
34. Kornowski R, Mehran R, Satler LF, et al: Procedural results and late clinical outcomes following multivessel coronary stenting. *J Am Coll Cardiol* 1999; 33(2):420-426.
35. McGrath PD, Malenka DJ, Wennberg DE, et al: Changing outcomes in percutaneous coronary interventions: a study of 34,752 procedures in northern New England, 1990 to 1997. Northern New England Cardiovascular Disease Study Group. *J Am Coll Cardiol* 1999; 34(3): 674-680.
36. Villareal RP, Lee VV, Elayda MA, Wilson JM: Coronary artery bypass surgery versus coronary stenting: risk-adjusted survival rates in 5,619 patients. *Tex Heart Inst J* 2002; 29(1):3-9.
37. Ellis SG, Guetta V, Miller D, et al: Relation between lesion characteristics and risk with percutaneous intervention in the stent and glycoprotein IIb/IIIa era: An analysis of results from 10,907 lesions and proposal for new classification scheme. *Circulation* 1999; 100(19):1971-1976.
38. Holmes DR Jr, Leon MB, Moses JW, et al: Analysis of 1-year clinical outcomes in the SIRIUS trial: a randomized trial of a sirolimus-eluting stent versus a standard stent in patients at high risk for coronary restenosis. *Circulation* 2004; 109(5):634-640.
39. Macaya C, Serruys PW, Ruygrok P, et al: Continued benefit of coronary stenting versus balloon angioplasty: one-year clinical follow-up of Benestent trial. Benestent Study Group. *J Am Coll Cardiol* 1996; 27(2):255-261.
40. Serruys PW, Unger F, Sousa JE, et al: Comparison of coronary-artery bypass surgery and stenting for the treatment of multivessel disease. *NEJM* 2001; 344(15):1117-1124.
41. Stone GW, Ellis SG, Cox DA, et al: One-year clinical results with the slow-release, polymer-based, paclitaxel-eluting TAXUS stent: the TAXUS-IV trial. *Circulation* 2004; 109(16):1942-1947.
42. Mehta SR, Yusuf S, Peters RJ, et al: Effects of pretreatment with clopidogrel and aspirin followed by long-term therapy in patients undergoing percutaneous coronary intervention: the PCI-CURE study. *Lancet* 2001; 358(9281):527-533.
43. Steinhubl SR, Berger PB, Mann JT 3rd, et al: Early and sustained dual oral antiplatelet therapy following percutaneous coronary intervention: a randomized controlled trial. *JAMA* 2002; 288(19):2411-2420.
44. Finkelstein A, McClean D, Kar S, et al: Local drug delivery via a coronary stent with programmable release pharmacokinetics. *Circulation* 2003; 107(5):777-784.

45. Ardissino D, Cavallini C, Bramucci E, et al: Sirolimus-eluting vs uncoated stents for prevention of restenosis in small coronary arteries: a randomized trial. *JAMA* 2004; 292(22):2727-2734.
46. Colombo A, Moses JW, Morice MC, et al: Randomized study to evaluate sirolimus-eluting stents implanted at coronary bifurcation lesions. *Circulation* 2004; 109(10):1244-1249.
47. Ge L, Iakovou I, Sangiorgi GM, et al: Treatment of saphenous vein graft lesions with drug-eluting stents: immediate and midterm outcome. *J Am Coll Cardiol* 2005; 45(7):989-994.
48. Iakovou I, Schmidt T, Bonizzoni E, et al: Incidence, predictors, and outcome of thrombosis after successful implantation of drug-eluting stents. *JAMA* 2005; 293(17):2126-2130.
49. Lemos PA, Saia F, Hofma SH, et al: Short- and long-term clinical benefit of sirolimus-eluting stents compared to conventional bare stents for patients with acute myocardial infarction. *J Am Coll Cardiol* 2004; 43(4):704-708.
50. Moussa I, Leon MB, Baim DS, et al: Impact of sirolimus-eluting stents on outcome in diabetic patients: a SIRIUS (SIRolImUS-coated Bx Velocity balloon-expandable stent in the treatment of patients with de novo coronary artery lesions) substudy. *Circulation* 2004; 109(19):2273-2278.
51. Nakamura S, Muthusamy TS, Bae JH, et al: Impact of sirolimus-eluting stent on the outcome of patients with chronic total occlusions. *Am J Cardiol* 2005; 95(2):161-166.
52. Stone GW, Ellis SG, Cannon L, et al: Comparison of a polymer-based paclitaxel-eluting stent with a bare metal stent in patients with complex coronary artery disease: a randomized controlled trial. *JAMA* 2005; 294(10):1215-1223.
53. Babapulle MN, Joseph L, Belisle P, et al: A hierarchical Bayesian meta-analysis of randomised clinical trials of drug-eluting stents. *Lancet* 2004; 364(9434):583-591.
54. Adelman AG, Cohen EA, Kimball BP, et al: A comparison of directional atherectomy with balloon angioplasty for lesions of the left anterior descending coronary artery. *NEJM* 1993; 329(4):228-233.
55. Appelman YE, Piek JJ, Strikwerda S, et al: Randomised trial of excimer laser angioplasty versus balloon angioplasty for treatment of obstructive coronary artery disease. *Lancet* 1996; 347(8994):79-84.
56. Foley DP, Melkert R, Umans VA, et al: Differences in restenosis propensity of devices for transluminal coronary intervention. A quantitative angiographic comparison of balloon angioplasty, directional atherectomy, stent implantation and excimer laser angioplasty. CARPORT, MERCATOR, MARCATOR, PARK, and BENESTENT Trial Groups. *Eur Heart J* 1995; 16(10):1331-1346.
57. Topol EJ, Leya F, Pinkerton CA, et al: A comparison of directional atherectomy with coronary angioplasty in patients with coronary artery disease. The CAVEAT Study Group. *NEJM* 1993; 329(4):221-227.
58. Bittl JA, Chew DP, Topol EJ, et al: Meta-analysis of randomized trials of percutaneous transluminal coronary angioplasty versus atherectomy, cutting balloon atherotomy, or laser angioplasty. *J Am Coll Cardiol* 2004; 43(6):936-942.
59. Feld H, Schulhoff N, Lichstein E, et al: Coronary atherectomy versus angioplasty: the CAVA Study. *Am Heart J* 1993; 126(1):31-38.
60. Beran G, Lang I, Schreiber W, et al: Intracoronary thrombectomy with the X-sizer catheter system improves epicardial flow and accelerates ST-segment resolution in patients with acute coronary syndrome: a prospective, randomized, controlled study. *Circulation* 2002; 105(20):2355-2360.
61. Stone GW, Cox DA, Low R, et al: Safety and efficacy of a novel device for treatment of thrombotic and atherosclerotic lesions in native coronary arteries and saphenous vein grafts: results from the multicenter X-Sizer for treatment of thrombus and atherosclerosis in coronary applications trial (X-TRACT) study. *Catheter Cardiovasc Interv* 2003; 58(4):419-427.
62. Baim DS, Wahr D, George B, et al: Randomized trial of a distal embolic protection device during percutaneous intervention of saphenous vein aorto-coronary bypass grafts. *Circulation* 2002; 105(11):1285-1290.
63. Stone GW, Webb J, Cox DA, et al: Distal microcirculatory protection during percutaneous coronary intervention in acute ST-segment elevation myocardial infarction: a randomized controlled trial. *JAMA* 2005; 293(9):1063-1072.
64. Casella G, Klauss V, Ottani F, et al: Impact of intravascular ultrasound-guided stenting on long-term clinical outcome: a meta-analysis of available studies comparing intravascular ultrasound-guided and angiographically guided stenting. *Catheter Cardiovasc Interv* 2003; 59(3):314-321.
65. Tonino PA, De Bruyne B, Pijls NH, et al: Fractional flow reserve versus angiography for guiding percutaneous coronary intervention. *NEJM* 2009; 360(3):213-224.
66. Leon MB, Teirstein PS, Moses JW, et al: Localized intracoronary gamma-radiation therapy to inhibit the recurrence of restenosis after stenting. *NEJM* 2001; 344(4):250-256.
67. Waksman R, Bhargava B, White RL, et al: Intracoronary radiation for patients with refractory in-stent restenosis: an analysis from the WRIST-Crossover Trial. Washington Radiation for In-stent Restenosis Trial. *Cardiovasc Radiat Med* 1999; 1(4):317-322.
68. Briguori C, Sarais C, Pagnotta P, et al: Elective versus provisional intra-aortic balloon pumping in high-risk percutaneous transluminal coronary angioplasty. *Am Heart J* 2003; 145(4):700-707.
69. Thiele H, Lauer B, Hambrecht R, et al: Reversal of cardiogenic shock by percutaneous left atrial-to-femoral arterial bypass assistance. *Circulation* 2001; 104(24):2917-2922.
70. Thiele H, Sick P, Boudriot E, et al: Randomized comparison of intra-aortic balloon support with a percutaneous left ventricular assist device in patients with revascularized acute myocardial infarction complicated by cardiogenic shock. *Eur Heart J* 2005; 26(13):1276-1283.
71. Nikolsky E, Mehran R, Halkin A, et al: Vascular complications associated with arteriotomy closure devices in patients undergoing percutaneous coronary procedures: a meta-analysis. *J Am Coll Cardiol* 2004; 44(6):1200-1209.
72. Mann T, Cowper PA, Peterson ED, et al: Transradial coronary stenting: comparison with femoral access closed with an arterial suture device. *Catheter Cardiovasc Interv* 2000; 49(2):150-156.
73. Wong SC, Minutello R, Hong MK. Neurological complications following percutaneous coronary interventions (a report from the 2000-2001 New York State Angioplasty Registry). *Am J Cardiol* 2005; 96(9):1248-1250.
74. Fuchs S, Stabile E, Kinnaird TD, et al: Stroke complicating percutaneous coronary interventions: incidence, predictors, and prognostic implications. *Circulation* 2002; 106(1):86-91.
75. Califf RM, Abdelmeguid AE, Kuntz RE, et al: Myonecrosis after revascularization procedures. *J Am Coll Cardiol* 1998; 31(2):241-251.
76. Stone GW, Mehran R, Dangas G, et al: Differential impact on survival of electrocardiographic Q-wave versus enzymatic myocardial infarction after percutaneous intervention: a device-specific analysis of 7147 patients. *Circulation* 2001; 104(6):642-647.
77. Brener SJ, Lytle BW, Schneider JP, et al: Association between CK-MB elevation after percutaneous or surgical revascularization and three-year mortality. *J Am Coll Cardiol* 2002; 40(11):1961-1967.
78. Briguori C, Colombo A, Airoldi F, et al: Statin administration before percutaneous coronary intervention: impact on periprocedural myocardial infarction. *Eur Heart J* 2004; 25(20):1822-1828.
79. Lee CH, Wong HB, Tan HC, et al: Impact of reversibility of no reflow phenomenon on 30-day mortality following percutaneous revascularization for acute myocardial infarction-insights from a 1,328 patient registry. *J Interv Cardiol* 2005; 18(4):261-266.
80. Ellis SG, Ajluni S, Arnold AZ, et al: Increased coronary perforation in the new device era. Incidence, classification, management, and outcome. *Circulation* 1994; 90(6):2725-2730.
81. Fasseas P, Orford JL, Panetta CJ, et al: Incidence, correlates, management, and clinical outcome of coronary perforation: analysis of 16,298 procedures. *Am Heart J* 2004; 147(1):140-145.
82. Fejka M, Dixon SR, Safian RD, et al: Diagnosis, management, and clinical outcome of cardiac tamponade complicating percutaneous coronary intervention. *Am J Cardiol* 2002; 90(11):1183-1186.
83. Schachinger V, Hamm CW, Munzel T, et al: A randomized trial of polytetrafluoroethylene-membrane-covered stents compared with conventional stents in aortocoronary saphenous vein grafts. *J Am Coll Cardiol* 2003; 42(8):1360-1369.
84. Ly H, Awaida JP, Lesperance J, Bilodeau L: Angiographic and clinical outcomes of polytetrafluoroethylene-covered stent use in significant coronary perforations. *Am J Cardiol* 2005; 95(2):244-246.
85. Briguori C, Nishida T, Anzuini A, et al: Emergency polytetrafluoroethylene-covered stent implantation to treat coronary ruptures. *Circulation* 2000; 102(25):3028-3031.
86. Freeman RV, O'Donnell M, Share D, et al: Nephropathy requiring dialysis after percutaneous coronary intervention and the critical role of an adjusted contrast dose. *Am J Cardiol* 2002; 90(10):1068-1073.
87. Marenzi G, Lauri G, Assanelli E, et al: Contrast-induced nephropathy in patients undergoing primary angioplasty for acute myocardial infarction. *J Am Coll Cardiol* 2004; 44(9):1780-1785.
88. Mehran R, Aymong ED, Nikolsky E, et al: A simple risk score for prediction of contrast-induced nephropathy after percutaneous coronary intervention: development and initial validation. *J Am Coll Cardiol* 2004; 44(7):1393-1399.
89. Mueller C, Buerkle G, Buettner HJ, et al: Prevention of contrast media associated nephropathy: randomized comparison of 2 hydration regimens in 1620 patients undergoing coronary angioplasty. *Arch Intern Med* 2002; 162(3):329-336.

90. Lindsay J, Apple S, Pinnow EE, et al: Percutaneous coronary intervention-associated nephropathy foreshadows increased risk of late adverse events in patients with normal baseline serum creatinine. *Catheter Cardiovasc Interv* 2003; 59(3):338-343.
91. Aspelin P, Aubry P, Fransson SG, et al: Nephrotoxic effects in high-risk patients undergoing angiography. *NEJM* 2003; 348(6):491-499.
92. Misra D, Leibowitz K, Gowda RM, et al: Role of N-acetylcysteine in prevention of contrast-induced nephropathy after cardiovascular procedures: a meta-analysis. *Clin Cardiol* 2004; 27(11):607-610.
93. Tepel M, van der Giet M, Schwarzfeld C, et al: Prevention of radiographic-contrast-agent-induced reductions in renal function by acetylcysteine. *NEJM* 2000; 343(3):180-184.
94. Kagan A, Sheikh-Hamad D: Contrast-induced kidney injury: focus on modifiable risk factors and prophylactic strategies. *Clin Cardiol* 2010; 33(2):62-66.
95. Andersen HR, Nielsen TT, Rasmussen K, et al: A comparison of coronary angioplasty with fibrinolytic therapy in acute myocardial infarction. *NEJM* 2003; 349(8):733-742.
96. Ribichini F, Steffenino G, Dellavalle A, et al: Comparison of thrombolytic therapy and primary coronary angioplasty with liberal stenting for inferior myocardial infarction with precordial ST-segment depression: immediate and long-term results of a randomized study. *J Am Coll Cardiol* 1998; 32(6):1687-1694.
97. Schomig A, Kastrati A, Dirschinger J, et al: Coronary stenting plus platelet glycoprotein IIb/IIIa blockade compared with tissue plasminogen activator in acute myocardial infarction. Stent versus Thrombolysis for Occluded Coronary Arteries in Patients with Acute Myocardial Infarction Study Investigators. *NEJM* 2000; 343(6):385-391.
98. Antoniucci D, Santoro GM, Bolognese L, et al: A clinical trial comparing primary stenting of the infarct-related artery with optimal primary angioplasty for acute myocardial infarction: results from the Florence Randomized Elective Stenting in Acute Coronary Occlusions (FRESCO) trial. *J Am Coll Cardiol* 1998; 31(6):1234-1239.
99. Mahdi NA, Lopez J, Leon M, et al: Comparison of primary coronary stenting to primary balloon angioplasty with stent bailout for the treatment of patients with acute myocardial infarction. *Am J Cardiol* 1998; 81(8):957-963.
100. Neumann FJ, Kastrati A, Schmitt C, et al: Effect of glycoprotein IIb/IIIa receptor blockade with abciximab on clinical and angiographic restenosis rate after the placement of coronary stents following acute myocardial infarction. *J Am Coll Cardiol* 2000; 35(4):915-921.
101. Rodriguez A, Bernardi V, Fernandez M, et al: In-hospital and late results of coronary stents versus conventional balloon angioplasty in acute myocardial infarction (GRAMI trial). Gianturco-Roubin in Acute Myocardial Infarction. *Am J Cardiol* 1998; 81(11):1286-1291.
102. Berger PB, Holmes DR Jr, Stebbins AL, et al: Impact of an aggressive invasive catheterization and revascularization strategy on mortality in patients with cardiogenic shock in the Global Utilization of Streptokinase and Tissue Plasminogen Activator for Occluded Coronary Arteries (GUSTO-I) trial. An observational study. *Circulation* 1997; 96(1): 122-127.
103. Giugliano GR, Kuntz RE, Popma JJ, et al: Determinants of 30-day adverse events following saphenous vein graft intervention with and without a distal occlusion embolic protection device. *Am J Cardiol* 2005; 95(2): 173-177.
104. Schomig A, Ndrepepa G, Mehilli J, et al: A randomized trial of coronary stenting versus balloon angioplasty as a rescue intervention after failed thrombolysis in patients with acute myocardial infarction. *J Am Coll Cardiol* 2004; 44(10):2073-2079.
105. Sutton AG, Campbell PG, Graham R, et al: A randomized trial of rescue angioplasty versus a conservative approach for failed fibrinolysis in ST-segment elevation myocardial infarction: the Middlesbrough Early Revascularization to Limit INfarction (MERLIN) trial. *J Am Coll Cardiol* 2004; 44(2):287-296.
106. Brener SJ, Ellis SG, Apperson-Hansen C, et al: Comparison of stenting and balloon angioplasty for narrowings in aortocoronary saphenous vein conduits in place for more than five years. *Am J Cardiol* 1997; 79(1):13-18.
107. Eeckhout E, Goy JJ, Stauffer JC, et al: Endoluminal stenting of narrowed saphenous vein grafts: long-term clinical and angiographic follow-up. *Cathet Cardiovasc Diagn* 1994; 32(2):139-146.
108. Frimerman A, Rechavia E, Eigler N, et al: Long-term follow-up of a high risk cohort after stent implantation in saphenous vein grafts. *J Am Coll Cardiol* 1997; 30(5):1277-1283.
109. Piana RN, Moscucci M, Cohen DJ, et al: Palmaz-Schatz stenting for treatment of focal vein graft stenosis: immediate results and long-term outcome. *J Am Coll Cardiol* 1994; 23(6):1296-1304.
110. Wong SC, Baim DS, Schatz RA, et al: Immediate results and late outcomes after stent implantation in saphenous vein graft lesions: the multicenter U.S. Palmaz-Schatz stent experience. The Palmaz-Schatz Stent Study Group. *J Am Coll Cardiol* 1995; 26(3):704-712.
111. Sianos G, Morel MA, Kappetein AP, et al: The SYNTAX Score: an angiographic tool grading the complexity of coronary artery disease. *EuroIntervention* 2005; 1(2):219-227.
112. Valgimigli M, Serruys PW, Tsuchida K, et al: Cyphering the complexity of coronary artery disease using the syntax score to predict clinical outcome in patients with three-vessel lumen obstruction undergoing percutaneous coronary intervention. *Am J Cardiol* 2007; 99(8):1072-1081.
113. Kennedy JA, Kiosoglous AJ, Murphy GA, et al: Effect of perhexiline and oxfenicine on myocardial function and metabolism during low-flow ischemia/reperfusion in the isolated rat heart. *J Cardiovasc Pharmacol* 2000; 36(6):794-801.
114. Morrow DA, Givertz MM. Modulation of myocardial energetics: emerging evidence for a therapeutic target in cardiovascular disease. *Circulation* 2005; 112(21):3218-3221.
115. Tracey WR, Treadway JL, Magee WP, et al: Cardioprotective effects of ingliforib, a novel glycogen phosphorylase inhibitor. *Am J Physiol Heart Circ Physiol* 2004; 286(3):H1177-1184.
116. Perin EC, Dohmann HF, Borojevic R, et al: Improved exercise capacity and ischemia 6 and 12 months after transendocardial injection of autologous bone marrow mononuclear cells for ischemic cardiomyopathy. *Circulation* 2004; 110(11 Suppl 1):II213-218.
117. Sabaté M. Diabetes and Sirolimus-Eluting Stent (DIABETES) Trial. *Transcatheter Therapeutics*, 2004; Washington, DC.
118. Hermiller JB, Raizner A, Cannon L, et al: Outcomes with the polymer-based paclitaxel-eluting TAXUS stent in patients with diabetes mellitus: the TAXUS-IV trial. *J Am Coll Cardiol* 2005; 45(8):1172-1179.
119. Valgimigli M, Percoco G, Malagutti P, et al: Tirofiban and sirolimus-eluting stent vs abciximab and bare-metal stent for acute myocardial infarction: a randomized trial. *JAMA* 2005; 293(17):2109-2117.
120. Kelbaeck H, editor. Stenting of Coronary Arteries in Non-Stress/BENESTENT Disease (SCANDSTENT). American College of Cardiology 2005 Scientific Sessions; 2005; Orlando, FL.
121. Degertekin M, Arampatzis CA, Lemos PA, et al: Very long sirolimus-eluting stent implantation for de novo coronary lesions. *Am J Cardiol* 2004; 93(7):826-829.
122. Schampaert E, Cohen EA, Schluter M, et al: The Canadian study of the sirolimus-eluting stent in the treatment of patients with long de novo lesions in small native coronary arteries (C-SIRIUS). *J Am Coll Cardiol* 2004; 43(6):1110-1115.
123. Schofer J, Schluter M, Gershlick AH, et al: Sirolimus-eluting stents for treatment of patients with long atherosclerotic lesions in small coronary arteries: double-blind, randomised controlled trial (E-SIRIUS). *Lancet* 2003; 362(9390):1093-1099.
124. Cervinka P, Stasek J, Pleskot M, Maly J. Treatment of coronary bifurcation lesions by stent implantation only in parent vessel and angioplasty in sidebranch: immediate and long-term outcome. *J Invasive Cardiol* 2002; 14(12):735-740.
125. Tanabe K, Hoye A, Lemos PA, et al: Restenosis rates following bifurcation stenting with sirolimus-eluting stents for de novo narrowings. *Am J Cardiol* 2004; 94(1):115-118.
126. Yamashita T, Nishida T, Adamian MG, et al: Bifurcation lesions: two stents versus one stent—immediate and follow-up results. *J Am Coll Cardiol* 2000; 35(5):1145-1151.
127. Kastrati A, Mehilli J, von Beckerath N, et al: Sirolimus-eluting stent or paclitaxel-eluting stent vs balloon angioplasty for prevention of recurrences in patients with coronary in-stent restenosis: a randomized controlled trial. *JAMA* 2005; 293(2):165-171.
128. Ellis SG, Myler RK, King SB 3rd, et al: Causes and correlates of death after unsupported coronary angioplasty: implications for use of angioplasty and advanced support techniques in high-risk settings. *Am J Cardiol* 1991; 68(15):1447-1451.

CHAPTER 21

Myocardial Revascularization with Cardiopulmonary Bypass

Kevin L. Greason
Thoralf M. Sundt III

INTRODUCTION

Coronary artery disease (CAD) remains the single largest killer of Americans, accounting for almost half a million deaths per year. It imposes a particular burden on the elderly, with more than 80% of all CAD deaths occurring in those over age 65.[1] The magnitude of this impact takes on great significance because it is expected that the number of Americans older than 65 years of age will double over the next two decades.[2] If you add to this aging population the anticipated increase in the prevalence of important risk factors for CAD such as diabetes mellitus and obesity, the population at risk for CAD can only be expected to increase.

Myocardial revascularization represents an effective treatment strategy shown to prolong survival. Techniques of revascularization include percutaneous coronary intervention (PCI) and coronary artery bypass graft surgery (CABG), which can be performed with or without cardiopulmonary bypass. Current techniques for CABG can be carried out with low perioperative morbidity and mortality, with excellent long-term outcomes despite an increasing risk profile.[3] Coronary artery bypass graft surgery with cardiopulmonary bypass remains the standard by which the other techniques (ie, PCI, off-pump CABG) are measured.[4,5] It is expected that it will continue to be a cornerstone in the management of CAD in the foreseeable future.

HISTORY OF CORONARY ARTERY BYPASS GRAFTING

The modern era of myocardial revascularization with cardiopulmonary bypass began in 1954 when Dr. John Gibbon reported the development of the cardiopulmonary bypass machine.[6] An additional seminal advance occurred with the development of coronary angiography by Mason Sones at the Cleveland Clinic in 1957, which opened the door to the elective treatment of coronary atherosclerosis by means of direct revascularization.[7] Initial reports by Rene Favaloro and Donald B. Effler on their techniques to treat clinical events associated with stenotic lesions of the coronary arteries culminated in the first large series of aorto-to-coronary artery venous grafts reported in 1969.[8] Simultaneously Dudley Johnson of Milwaukee published a series of 301 patients in 1969.[9] The success of these techniques was soon demonstrated in larger series initiating the modern era of coronary artery surgery.

INDICATIONS FOR SURGICAL CORONARY REVASCULARIZATION

The indications for CABG are reviewed in detail in Chapter 19. In brief, the indications established by the American Heart Association and American College of Cardiology (AHA/ACC) consensus panel are based predominantly on the results of trials comparing surgical revascularization with medical therapy for patients with chronic stable angina.[10] Three major trials, the Coronary Artery Surgery Study (CASS), the Veterans Administration Coronary Artery Bypass Cooperative Study Group, and the European Coronary Surgery Study (ECSS), demonstrated the greatest survival benefit of revascularization to be among those patients at highest risk of death from the disease itself as defined by the severity of angina and/or ischemia, the number of diseased vessels, and the presence of left ventricular dysfunction.[11–13]

PREDICTION OF OPERATIVE RISK

Prediction of risk-adjusted outcomes permits both the surgeon and the patient to weigh the potential benefits of operation against risks of perioperative morbidity and/or mortality. The patient's comprehension of benefit versus risk is paramount to informed consent before coronary artery bypass surgery. Accurate risk-adjusted prediction of postoperative morbidity and mortality also provides an important quality improvement tool to understand and examine the variability in institutional and individual surgeon performance.

A number of cardiac surgery databases have been used to develop risk models for predicting operative morbidity and mortality in patients undergoing CABG.[10] One of the more user-friendly risk assessment tools is that provided by the STS Risk Calculator (http://www.sts.org/quality-research-patient-safety/quality/risk-calculator-and-models/risk-calculator), which provides an assessment of individual patient operative risk derived using the Society of Thoracic Surgeons (STS) database (Table 21-1). The STS risk algorithm is proprietary and is based on data voluntarily submitted by participating centers on 503,478 patients undergoing isolated CABG in the United States from 1997 to 1999; the application is available for public use.

Overall, the average risks of 30-day operative death and major complication for patients reported to the STS database undergoing CABG from 1997 to 1999 were 3.05 and 13.4%, respectively. Specific complications included stroke (1.6%), renal failure (3.5%), reoperation (5.2%), prolonged ventilation (5.9%), and sternal infection (0.63%). Risk models were developed using multivariate analysis to stratify the strength of the association from among 30 potential preoperative risk factors for mortality and major complications as shown in Tables 21-2 and 21-3. Except for deep sternal wound infection, the development of any of these complications correlated with an increased risk-adjusted operative mortality.[14]

A preliminary sense of operative mortality can be derived simply from an understanding of the core variables most predictive of risk in the aforementioned data sets. The strongest predictors of operative mortality include nonelective surgery, low ejection fraction, and prior heart surgery. Chronic comorbidities are also associated with an increased operative mortality after coronary bypass, including treated diabetes, peripheral vascular occlusive disease, chronic renal insufficiency, and chronic obstructive pulmonary disease (COPD).[10]

PREOPERATIVE ASSESSMENT

Patient Evaluation

Regardless of the risk model applied, there is no substitute for clinical evaluation of the patient. Unfortunately, all too often the assessment focuses disproportionately on coronary anatomy and insufficiently on the nature, duration, and severity of ischemic symptoms, as well as signs and symptoms of congestive heart failure (CHF). In addition, history of or coexisting cerebrovascular and/or peripheral vascular disease, malignancy, sternal radiation, COPD, diabetes mellitus, or renal and/or hepatic insufficiency can have major impact on the operative morbidity and even mortality, not all of which are captured in risk models.

Current medications and dosages with special attention to antiplatelet agents such as clopidogrel must be reviewed. Operation in the setting of recent clopidogrel use is associated

TABLE 21-1 Independent Variables Associated with Mortality after Isolated Coronary Artery Bypass Graft Surgery

Variable	Odds Ratio	95% Confidence Interval
Multiple reoperations	4.19	3.61–4.86
First reoperation	2.76	2.62–2.91
Shock	2.04	1.90–2.19
Surgery status	1.96	1.88–2.05
Renal failure/dialysis	1.88	1.80–1.96
Immunosuppressants	1.75	1.57–1.95
Insulin-dependent diabetes mellitus	1.5	1.42–1.58
Intra-aortic balloon pump use	1.46	1.37–1.55
Chronic lung disease	1.41	1.35–1.48
Percutaneous transluminal coronary angioplasty, 6 hours	1.32	1.18–1.48

Data were collected from 503,478 patients undergoing isolated CABG in the U.S. from 1997 to 1999 from Society of Thoracic Surgeons' database. Variables are listed in decreasing order of importance.

Source: Data from Shroyer AL, Coombs LP, Peterson ED, et al: The Society of Thoracic Surgeons: 30-day operative mortality and morbidity risk models. Ann Thorac Surg 2003; 75:1856.

TABLE 21-2 Variables Associated with Development of a Major Complication after Isolated Coronary Artery Bypass Graft Surgery

Variable	Odds Ratio	95% Confidence Interval
Renal failure/dialysis	2.49	2.41–2.58
Multiple reoperations	2.13	1.92–2.36
Shock	1.86	1.78–1.95
Intra-aortic balloon pump use	1.78	1.72–1.84
First reoperation	1.75	1.70–1.81
Insulin-dependent diabetes mellitus	1.59	1.54–1.64
Surgery status	1.58	1.53–1.63
Chronic lung disease	1.41	1.38–1.45
Immunosuppressants	1.34	1.26–1.43
Percutaneous transluminal coronary angioplasty <6 hours	1.33	1.23–1.43

Any major complication is defined as the composite outcome of stroke, renal failure, prolonged ventilation, mediastinitis, or reoperation. Data collected from 503,478 patients undergoing isolated CABG in the U.S. from 1997 to 1999 from the Society of Thoracic Surgeons' database. Variables are listed in decreasing order of importance.
Source: Data from Shroyer AL, Coombs LP, Peterson ED, et al: The Society of Thoracic Surgeons: 30-day operative mortality and morbidity risk models. Ann Thorac Surg 2003; 75:1856.

TABLE 21-3 Variables Associated with Development of a Specific Postoperative Complication

Stroke	Renal Failure	Prolonged Ventilation	Mediastinitis	Reoperation
Variable, Odds Ratio (95% Confidence Interval)				
PVD/CVD, 1.5(1.44–1.56)	Renal failure/dialysis, 4.3 (4.09–4.52)	Multiple reoperations, 2.3 (2.01–2.64)	IDDM, 2.74 (2.47–3.03)	Multiple reoperations, 1.69 (1.49–1.97)
Renal failure/dialysis, 1.49 (1.37–1.62)	IDDM, 2.26 (2.16–2.37)	IABP, 2.26 (2.17–2.36)	Chronic lung disease, 1.62 (1.47–1.78)	Shock, 1.46 (1.37–1.56)
IDDM, 1.48 (1.37–1.59)	Shock, 1.6 (1.48–1.72)	First reoperation, 1.97 (1.89–2.05)	NIDDM, 1.53 (1.38–1.70)	First reoperation, 1.40 (1.33–1.47)
Previous CVA, 1.43 (1.33–1.53)	Multiple reoperations, 1.6 (1.33–1.92)	Renal failure/dialysis, 1.95 (1.86–2.04)	Immunosuppressants, 1.49 (1.18–1.89)	PTCA <6 hours, 1.42 (1.28–1.58)
Surgery status, 1.38 (1.29–1.48)	First reoperation, 1.55 (1.46–1.64)	Shock, 1.95 (1.85–2.06)	IABP, 1.43 (1.25–1.64)	Renal failure/dialysis, 1.38 (1.33–1.44)
Shock, 1.36 (1.21–1.52)	IABP, 1.54 (1.45–1.64)	Chronic lung disease, 1.67 (1.61–1.73)	Mitral insufficiency, 1.39 (1.17–1.65)	IABP, 1.36 (1.29–1.43)
NIDDM, 1.36 (1.28–1.45)	Ilmmunosuppressants, 1.48 (1.33–1.64)	IDDM, 1.53 (1.47–1.59)	Obese female, 1.38 (1.35–1.42)	Chronic lung disease, 1.32 (1.27–1.37)
HTN, 1.30 (1.22–1.38)	PTCA <6 hours, 1.46 (1.29–1.66)	Surgery status, 1.46 (1.41–1.52)	Renal failure/dialysis, 1.27 (1.14–1.41)	Mitral insufficiency, 1.31 (1.23–1.40)

Data collected from 503,478 patients undergoing isolated CABG in the U.S. from 1997 to 1999 from the Society of Thoracic Surgeons' database. Variables are listed in decreasing order of importance.
CVA = cerebrovascular accident; HTN = history of hypertension; IABP = intra-aortic balloon pump; IDDM = insulin-dependent diabetes mellitus; NIDDM = non-insulin-dependent diabetes mellitus; PTCA = percutaneous transluminal coronary angioplasty; PVD/CVD = peripheral vascular disease/cardiovascular disease.
Source: Data from Shroyer AL, Coombs LP, Peterson ED, et al: The Society of Thoracic Surgeons: 30-day operative mortality and morbidity risk models. Ann Thorac Surg 2003; 75:1856.

with excessive bleeding and need for reoperation.[15] Most surgeons recommend 5 days from the last administered dose of clopidogrel before undertaking CABG with cardiopulmonary bypass.

Physical examination of the lungs and heart should focus on the stigma of ischemic and valvular heart disease. Cardiac murmurs warrant further evaluation. Additionally, the adequacy of presternal soft tissues to permit wound closure should be considered and evidence of venous varicosities or prior vein stripping may impact plans for conduit harvest. Peripheral pulses should be documented as their presence or absence may impact from which leg to harvest the vein or place an intra-aortic balloon pump. A detailed neurologic examination of the ulnar, radial, and median nerves should be document in the case of planned radial artery harvest.

Diagnostic evaluation should be directed by the clinical assessment, but at a minimum should include a renal panel (creatinine), complete blood count, and chest x-ray. The ECG should be reviewed for evidence of previous myocardial infarction and conduction abnormalities. Radiologic evaluation should rule out concomitant neoplasm, active pulmonary infection, and/or ascending aorta calcification; the latter should be further assessed with a noncontrast CT scan because it will impact the location for arterial cannulation and aortic cross-clamp placement.

Hemodynamically significant coronary artery lesions on angiography are conventionally defined as those lesions with a 50% loss of arterial diameter, which is sufficient to impair coronary blood flow reserve and distal coronary pressure.[10] An assessment should be made of left ventricular function and regional wall motion abnormalities as well as the presence and degree of valvular abnormalities, including aortic stenosis and mitral regurgitation either with left heart catheterization or echocardiography (our preferred method).

It is in the surgeon's best interest to develop a good relationship with the patient and his or her significant others. Specifics including the risks, benefits, and alternatives to surgery need to be discussed to permit an informed decision. Ideally, this discussion is held in the presence of the patient's significant others, because patients often have difficulty absorbing the details of the discussion at the time related to the stress of the situation. Should the patient experience a major complication or mortality, it is often the patient's significant others with whom the surgeon will most often interact. Additionally, anticipated need for postoperative rehabilitation, as well as the tempo and time course of recovery is also of interest to all parties. A clear understanding of the expectations for the perioperative period will reduce everyone's anxiety about surgery and may promote early patient recovery. Good rapport with patients and their significant others is also the physician's best protection from litigation should untoward events occur.

BYPASS CONDUITS

Internal Thoracic Artery

The left internal thoracic artery (ITA) as a bypass graft to the left anterior descending coronary artery has been proven to provide superior early and late survival and better event-free survival after CABG.[24] The unparalleled long-term patency and better clinical outcomes associated with the use of the ITA make it the conduit of first choice for anastomosis to the left anterior descending coronary artery in almost all patients regardless of age, and establish an argument to use the right ITA as conduit to other targets as well.

Characteristics

The ITA demonstrates remarkable resistance to development of atherosclerosis, which may be in part attributable to a greater resistance of its endothelium to harvest injury as compared with the saphenous vein. Under electron microscopy examination thrombogenic intimal defects are essentially nonexistent in the ITA but are commonly detected in venous grafts.[16] Perhaps more significantly, however, is the nonfenestrated internal elastic lamina of the ITA that may inhibit cellular migration, thereby preventing initiation of intimal hyperplasia. In addition, the medial layer of the ITA is thin, with fewer smooth muscle cells and a lesser proliferative response to known mitogens such as platelet-derived growth factor and pulsatile mechanical stretch.[17,18]

The endothelium of the ITA is itself unique as well. With a significantly higher basal production of the vasodilators nitric oxide and prostacyclin, the ITA demonstrates a favorable response to pharmacologic agents commonly used in the postoperative period. For instance, the ITA shows vasodilation in response to milrinone and yet does not vasoconstrict in response to norepinephrine.[19] Furthermore, nitroglycerin causes vasodilation in the ITA, but not in the saphenous vein.[20] The endogenous secretion of such vasodilators may also have a "downstream" effect on the coronary vasculature, explaining the common observation that the native coronary vessel itself often appears relatively protected from progressive atherosclerotic disease distal to the anastomosis. Finally, the ITA exhibits remarkable remodeling over time, adapting to the demand for increased flow by often increasing in diameter over time as observed on late postoperative angiograms, a phenomenon mediated by the endothelium.[21]

Surgical Anatomy of the Internal Thoracic Artery

The ITA arises from the undersurface of the first portion of the subclavian artery opposite the thyrocervical trunk. The left ITA originates as a single artery in 70% of patients and as a common trunk with other arteries in 30%. In contrast, the right ITA originates as a single artery in 95% of cases.[22] At the level of the clavicle and the first rib, the ITA passes at first downward and medially behind the subclavian vein and lateral to the innominate vein. In this area, the phrenic nerve crosses the ITA from its lateral to its medial side, before contacting the pericardium. The phrenic nerve crosses anterior to the ITA 66% of the time on the left and 74% of the time on the right.[22] It is important to keep these relations in mind to avoid phrenic nerve injury during proximal ITA harvest.

Below the first costal cartilage the ITA descends almost vertically and slightly laterally at a short distance from the margin of the sternum. The ITA lies posterior to the cartilages of the upper six ribs and the intervening internal intercostal muscles.

In the upper chest there is a bare area of variable length where the ITA is covered only by the endothoracic fascia and parietal pleura. Below this level the transversus thoracis muscle covers the posterior surface of the ITA. The mean distance of the left ITA from the sternal margin at the level of the first intercostal space is 10.5 ± 3.2 mm, whereas at the level of the sixth intercostal space the distance increases to 20.0 ± 6.7 mm. The right ITA is slightly closer to the sternal margin than the left ITA. At the level of the sixth rib the ITA bifurcates into its terminal branches: the musculophrenic and superior epigastric arteries. The length of the ITA in situ ranges from 15 to 26 cm, with a mean of 20.4 ± 2.1 cm; the left ITA is slightly longer than the right.[22] A pair of internal mammary veins accompanies the ITA; at the most superior portion these veins form a single vessel, which runs medial to the artery and drains into the innominate vein.

Pedicled Harvest Technique

After the sternum is divided, the left ITA is harvested using an internal mammary retractor to expose of the internal mammary bed (Fig. 21-1). Excessive distraction of the sternal leaves can cause costal fractures or dislocation of the costosternal joints, resulting in severe postoperative pain as well as brachial plexus injury. The parietal pleura and loose connective tissue with accompanying fat is dissected away from the chest wall. It is our preference to enter the left pleural space to allow easier exposure of the ITA, especially in its most proximal aspect, and to permit the ITA to fall into a more lateral and posterior path upon wound closure. Slightly rotating the operating table to the patient's left and decreasing the patient's tidal volume can aid in the visualization.

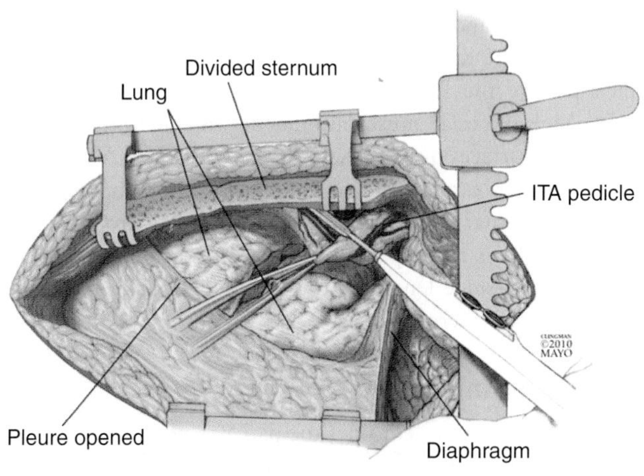

FIGURE 21-1 Internal thoracic artery (ITA) harvest. A self-retaining mammary retractor is used for exposure of the ITA bed. The left pleura is dissected away from the mammary pedicle and opened along the course of the ITA. The endothoracic fascia is incised medial and lateral to the ITA pedicle. The pedicle is carefully separated with blunt dissection from the underside of the rib. Gentle traction on the pedicle exposes arterial and venous branches at the level of the intercostal spaces; vessels are clipped on the ITA side and cauterized or clipped on the chest wall side. The proximal dissection is carried to the inferior border of the subclavian vein; the distal dissection is then carried to the level of the ITA bifurcation. The transversus thoracis muscle must be divided to expose the ITA bifurcation. The ITA is divided after full heparinization, either at the end of harvest or just before grafting of the left anterior descending (LAD) artery. *(Copyrighted and used with permission of Mayo Foundation for Medical Education and Research, all rights reserved.)*

The ITA is identified lateral to the border of the sternum by inspection of the bare area or by palpation in the area of artery covered by muscle. It can be harvested using either a pedicled, semiskeletonized, or a skeletonized technique. When taken as a pedicle, the dissection plane can be started in the bare area of the ITA at the level of the third or fourth rib or at the level of the lower sternum. The intercostal space is avoided as the initial point of exposure because it contains the branch vessels. The endothoracic fascia is incised medially for a distance of about 4 cm using the Bovey electrocautery at low setting (ie, 20). The pedicle is carefully separated from the chest wall using gentle blunt dissection with the Bovey electrocautery tip. Exposure can be enhanced by pushing the pedicle away with closed forceps or by gently grasping the fascia. The ITA is a fragile vessel and the conduit should never be grasped with the forceps. Gentle posterior traction on the pedicle allows exposure of arterial and venous branches, which should be clipped and divided.

After the pedicle has been freed for about 4 cm, the endothoracic fascia is incised laterally, allowing the pedicle to fall away from the chest wall. Dissection is continued proximally and distally to the level of the subclavian vein and ITA bifurcation. Attention should be given to avoid injury to the phrenic nerve during the proximal exposure. Once the dissection is completed, the patient is heparinized and the pedicle sprayed with a papaverine solution (1 cc [30 mg] of papaverine added to 9 cc of saline). Three minutes after heparinization, the distal ITA is doubly clipped just proximal to the bifurcation and the artery divided. An atraumatic bulldog clamp is applied to the distal end of the artery. Alternatively, the pedicle may be left in situ and transected just before using the conduit.

Skeletonization of the Internal Thoracic Artery

Sternal blood flow decreases significantly after pedicled ITA harvest. Skeletonized harvest, however, reduces the degree of sternal ischemia. Two prospective randomized studies assessing sternal blood supply using bone scan with single photon emission computed tomography after skeletonized and pedicled harvest have demonstrated significant reduction in sternal vascularity after pedicled harvest, whereas skeletonized harvest resulted in minimal change in sternal blood supply. Multivariate analysis found harvesting technique to be the only factor responsible for postoperative sternal ischemia.[23,24]

Low rates of sternal wound infection have been reported using skeletonized bilateral ITA harvest. Matsa and associates observed a deep sternal wound infection rate of 1.7% among 765 patients undergoing bilateral skeletonized ITA harvest. Of note, sternal complications occurred in only 2.6% of 231 diabetic patients in this study, which was not significantly different from that of the nondiabetic patients.[25] In Calafiore and coworkers' review of 842 patients undergoing bilateral skeletonized ITA harvest compared with a historical nonskeletonized bilateral ITA control group, skeletonized harvest was associated with a reduced incidence of sternal wound complications (4.5%) versus pedicle harvest (1.7%). Diabetic patients in the study derived the greatest benefit from skeletonized harvest with respect to sternal wound complications: 10% in the pedicle harvest versus 2.2% in the skeletonized harvest groups.[26]

Using the skeletonized harvest technique, only the artery is mobilized, leaving the internal thoracic venous plexus intact. Although skeletonization is a technically more demanding and time-consuming procedure, it increases luminal diameter and free flow compared with a pedicled graft, and also provides a longer conduit.[26] Some surgeons have expressed concerns regarding functional integrity, vasoreactive profile, and early and long-term patency; however several investigators have shown no difference in endothelial integrity, endothelial-dependent or neurogenic-dependent vasoreactivity between the techniques of pedicle or skeletonized harvest.[27–29] Furthermore, there does not appear to be any difference with respect to early and midterm patency.[30,31]

Patency

The superior late patency of an ITA graft to the left anterior descending coronary artery compared to a saphenous vein graft (SVG) was initially demonstrated by Barner and colleagues in the 1985.[32] Superior patency translates into improved 10-year survival (LITA-to-LAD artery 82.6% versus SVG-to-LAD artery 71%) with less incidence of myocardial infarction (MI), hospitalization for cardiac events, and cardiac reoperations.[33] The superior performance of ITA grafts appears to persist in the current era despite the use of agents to improve vein graft performance. In the BARI trial the patency rates at 1 and 4 years for ITA grafts were 98 and 91% compared with vein grafts, which were 87 and 83%, respectively.[34,35] The superior patency of the ITA becomes even more prominent with longer follow-up. In an angiographic study of 1408 symptomatic post-CABG patients, patency rates for the LITA at 10 and 15 years were 95 and 88%, respectively, whereas SVG patencies were 61 and 32% at the same time intervals.[36]

Radial Artery

The use of the radial artery (RA) as a conduit for coronary bypass was originally described by Carpentier and associates in 1973. Spasm of the artery was common during surgery and was managed by mechanical dilation. The initial results were disappointing with 32% of grafts occluded at 2 years.[37] Accordingly, the RA was abandoned as a conduit for CABG. Acar and colleagues revived the use of the RA after several grafts, angiographically demonstrated to be "occluded" early postoperatively, were patent during restudy 15 years later. Acar postulated that harvest injury was responsible for the spasm/graft occlusion.[38] Proponents of the RA as a conduit have demonstrated encouraging mid- and long-term results with a pedicled harvesting technique and pharmacologic manipulation to prevent radial artery vasospasm[39] As a result, this conduit has enjoyed a remarkable resurgence of interest as a supplementary arterial conduit for coronary revascularization.

Characteristics

Histologically, the RA has a fenestrated internal elastic lamina and a thicker wall than the ITA with a higher density of myocytes in its media.[40] The RA is also more likely to have atherosclerotic changes at the time of harvest than the ITA, with 28% of RAs having some degree of demonstrable atherosclerosis, as compared with only 6% of ITAs. Whether these differences indicate that the RA will prove more susceptible to graft atherosclerosis with reduced patency is unknown.[41]

Physiologically, the RA is equally sensitive to norepinephrine as the ITA; however, given its greater muscle mass, it generates a higher force of contraction, accounting for its well-recognized propensity for spasm.[42] Fortunately, the RA also readily responds to a variety of vasodilators, including calcium channel blockers, papaverine, nitrates, and milrinone. In vitro, nitroglycerine appears to be the most effective agent for inhibiting and reversing RA spasm.[43] Additionally, nitroglycerin has been shown to be better tolerated clinically, equally effective, and less expensive than diltiazem in prophylaxis of RA spasm after CABG in a prospective randomized trial.[44]

Surgical Anatomy of the Radial Artery

The RA originates from the brachial artery just proximal to the biceps tendon. In the proximal forearm the RA courses underneath the brachioradialis muscle. As it courses distally, it emerges from the lower surface of the muscle, becoming more superficial, and runs beneath the antebrachial fascia between the tendon of the brachioradialis muscle and the flexor carpi radialis muscle and anterior to the radius and pronator quadratus muscle. The recurrent radial artery originates from the lateral aspect of the RA soon after its origin from the brachial artery. Multiple small muscular branches emerge from the deep and lateral surfaces of the artery. At the wrist the RA gives rise to the palmar carpal branch, the dorsal carpal branch, the superficial palmar branch, and the deep palm.[45] Throughout its course the RA is accompanied by a rich plexus of venae comitantes. The average length of the RA ranges between 18 and 22 cm with an internal diameter of 2 to 3 mm.[46]

Harvest Technique

It is most common to consider the patient's nondominant arm for harvest, partially out of concern for the impact of even subtle neurologic changes, and partially given the convenience of harvesting the left radial artery simultaneously with the left ITA. The extremity of interest must have adequate ulnar collateral circulation to ensure viability of the hand. Assessment of collateral circulation is best performed via noninvasive duplex ultrasonography.[47] The RA of the dominant hand can also be harvested if needed. Tatoulis and associates reported 261 patients undergoing bilateral RA harvesting with safe functional outcomes of both extremities.[48]

The arm is prepped circumferentially and the hand wrapped in a sterile fashion. The upper extremity is place on an arm board perpendicular to the long axis of the operating table. As shown in Fig. 21-2, a medially curved incision is made on the skin overlying the RA from a point 2 cm proximal to the styloid process of the radius to a point 2 cm distal to the elbow

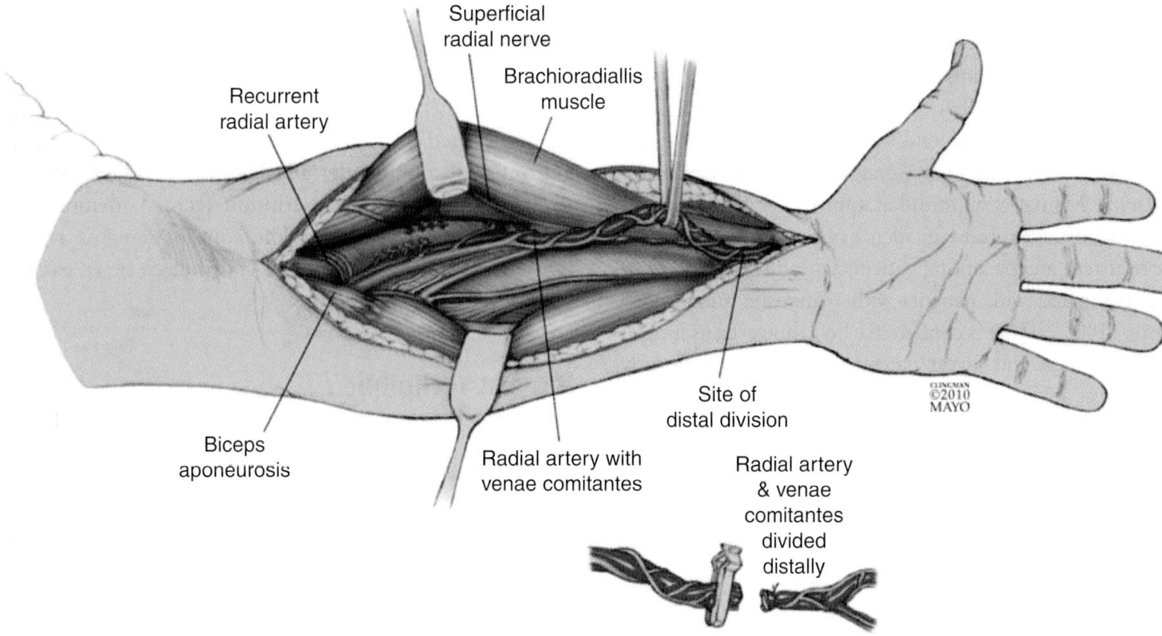

FIGURE 21-2 Radial artery harvest. A medially curved incision is made on the forearm over the artery. The deep fascia of the forearm is incised directly over the artery. The brachioradialis muscle is retracted laterally. Dissection is begun at the distal end and the satellite veins are divided. The RA is harvested as a pedicle with minimal manipulation. The proximal end of the dissection is marked by the radial recurrent branch, which is left intact. After the pedicle is free and heparin has been given, the artery is divided proximally and distally and stored in a room temperature solution of lactate, nitroglycerin, and papaverine. Hemostasis of the operative field is obtained and the arm is closed in multiple layers. A closed suction drain is placed. (*Copyrighted and used with permission of Mayo Foundation for Medical Education and Research, all rights reserved.*)

crease and 1 cm medial to the biceps tendon. The subcutaneous tissue is divided with the cautery. The dissection can be initiated at either end depending on the surgeons' preference. The deep fascia of the forearm is incised directly over the RA.

The RA is harvested as a pedicle with minimal manipulation using sharp dissection, diathermy, or the harmonic scalpel (our preferred method). There are data to suggest that early graft flow is superior when the harmonic scalpel is used.[49] On the proximal half of the forearm, gentle lateral retraction of the brachioradialis muscle aids exposure. At the distal end of the dissection the satellite veins are identified and divided. The proximal end of the dissection is marked by the radial recurrent artery branch and a large venous plexus in the medial aspect of the RA. It is our routine to leave the recurrent radial branch intact. The artery is divided proximally and distally and stored in a room temperature solution of lactate, nitroglycerin, and papaverine.

After the RA is removed from the forearm, hemostasis of the operative field is obtained and the arm is closed in multiple layers. A closed suction drain is placed, which we feel helps reduce postoperative seroma formation. A circumferential elastic wrap is applied. The arm is then abducted and secured to the table. Reports of endoscopic RA harvest are beginning to emerge with good functional and cosmetic results; nonetheless the impact of the technique on graft patency is unknown.[50] We have not adopted the technique.

Two cutaneous nerves are of importance to note during RA dissection. The lateral antebrachial cutaneous nerve lies superficial to the belly of the brachioradialis muscle and runs close to its medial border. Placing the skin incision medial to the edge of the brachioradialis prevents potential injury. Damage to this nerve will produce paresthesias and numbness of the radial aspect of the volar forearm. The superficial branch of the radial nerve lies under the brachioradialis muscle and in the proximal two-thirds of the forearm runs parallel to the RA. Injury to this nerve will result in paresthesias and numbness of the thumb and the dorsum of the hand. The nerve can best be protected by avoiding excessive lateral retraction on the brachioradialis muscle.[45,51] Transient paresthesias, numbness, and thumb weakness are common and are reported by almost a third of patients after RA harvest; fortunately, the symptoms gradually resolve with time so that after 1 year only 10% of patients have residual complaints with only 1% reporting their symptoms as severe.[52–54]

Patency

Acar and associates in 1992 reported on 122 radial grafts with a 100% patency rate at 2 weeks and 93% patency at 9 months.[55] The results appear durable with reported patencies at 48 months of 89%. Several factors may affect RA graft patency, however, including both target artery runoff and competitive flow. In the prospective, randomized Radial Artery Patency Study, more severe target coronary artery stenosis was associated with lower rate of occlusion (>90% stenosis = 5.9% versus 70 to 89% stenosis = 11.8%).[56] The graft failure rate is highest if the target vessel is the right coronary artery system, but this may be related more to the coronary artery than the bypass conduit; one study showed equal patency of radial artery and saphenous vein bypass grafts to the right coronary artery.[57–59]

The proximal radial artery can be sutured to the ITA as a T- or Y-graft (composite), sutured directly to the ascending aorta, or sutured to the proximal portion or hood of a separate vein graft. In addition, a segment of vein can be interposed between the aorta and proximal radial artery in an end-to-end fashion. Comparisons have been made between the T- or Y-graft and direct aortic anastomosis methods. Maniar et al. found at approximately 30 months follow-up, a significantly greater incidence of postoperative angiography for recurrent angina among patients with direct aortic anastomosis as compared with patients with composite anastomosis (19% versus 11%).[59] There is controversy here, however, as Jung et al. found that 1-, 2-, and 5-year patency rates were significantly better with direct aortic anastomosis as compared with composite anastomosis.[60] Importantly, it appears that the overall patency of radial artery grafts to ideal targets may be superior to that of saphenous vein bypass grafts at 5 years, 98% versus 86%.[61]

Other Arterial Conduits

A variety of arterial conduits have been used in patients in whom no other conduits are available. The gastroepiploic artery (GEA) for the most part is utilized as an alternative conduit or as part of an all-arterial revascularization strategy. Despite the enthusiastic support of a small cohort of surgeons, the widespread use of the GEA as a coronary conduit has not been adopted, perhaps because of the increased operative time and relative difficulty required to harvest the conduit, the potential for perioperative and long-term abdominal complications, and the lack of consensus on the long-term benefit for total arterial revascularization. Anecdotal use of the ulnar, left gastric, splenic, thoracodorsal, lateral femoral circumflex and inferior epigastric arteries as coronary graft conduits has been reported in the literature. The popularity of the RA, however, has in large measure superseded these options.

Greater Saphenous Vein

The saphenous vein continues to be one of the most commonly used conduits in coronary bypass grafting. Characteristics that have solidified the greater saphenous vein as a coronary artery bypass conduit include its ease of harvest, ready availability, versatility, resistance to spasm, and thoroughly studied long-term results. Unfortunately there is a loss of clinical benefit after CABG because of time-related attrition. Accordingly, there is interest in pharmacologic strategies to maximize early and late venous graft patency.

Prospective randomized trials have shown that early aspirin administration reduces mortality after CABG. Aspirin within 48 hours after CABG also reduces early postoperative complications, including mortality, myocardial infarction, stroke, renal failure, and bowel infarction.[62] More recently, it has been recognized that lipid-lowering agents reduce the progression of graft atherosclerosis.[63,64] Aggressive use of statins to achieve a low-density lipoprotein cholesterol <100 mg/dL decrease by one-third the number of grafts affected with atherosclerosis at angiographic follow-up and also decreased the need for repeat revascularization.[63] With clear documentation of improved outcomes with these two pharmacologic strategies, systematic approaches to ensure their universal application are needed.[10]

Finally, in the future, gene therapy may allow modification of the venous vascular endothelium to avert development of intimal hyperplasia. Unfortunately, the PREVENT IV trial, testing whether short-term angiographic vein graft failure could be diminished with treatment of the saphenous vein before grafting with edifoligide (an oligonucleotide decoy that binds to and inhibits E2F transcription factors), demonstrated no impact of the treatment.[65] The concept remains a valid one, however, and gene therapy will continue to be an exciting area of investigation in the future.

Harvest Technique

Saphenous vein harvest can be performed with an open or endoscopic technique. Open-vein harvest can be performed with a completely opened technique or bridged technique. In the completely open technique an extensile skin incision provides the best exposure of the vein and may allow for harvest with the least amount of surgical trauma, but that advantage comes at the risk of higher rates of wound complications and postoperative pain. Bridged skin incisions may decrease pain and wound complications but may also increase surgical manipulation of the vein conduit.

Open-vein dissection can be started either in the upper thigh, above the knee, or at the ankle (Fig. 21-3). Some surgeons prefer to harvest vein from the lower leg because of a more appropriate vein caliber and wall thickness, as well as greater distance from the perineum (a potential source of infection). Others prefer to harvest vein from the thigh, arguing improved wound healing, particularly among patients with distal peripheral arterial occlusive disease. We are not aware of any data supporting one location over another. Because of the greater amount of adipose tissue present in the thigh area, wound breakdown in that location may prove more of a nuisance to treat. The fundamentals of vein harvest are to procure the conduit with a minimal amount of trauma to the vein. Specifically, the vein should not be grasped with forceps, stretched, or overdistended, because patency rates may be related to endothelial damage induced during harvest and preparation of the conduit. Identification of the vein is easiest at the ankle, just lateral to the medial malleolus.

In the completely open technique, a skin incision directly over the trajectory of the vein is made, taking care not to create skin flaps. Purposeful, directed, sharp dissection is used to free the vein from the surrounding tissue. Side branches on the vein can initially be left long. Once dissection is completed, the vein is ligated and divided proximally and distally. A blunt-tipped vein cannula is inserted into the distal end of the vein and the vein gently flushed and dilated with a room temperature solution of plasmalyte. The side branches can be clipped flush with the vein at this time, taking care to avoid narrowing of the conduit lumen.

When using a bridged technique, several step incisions are performed over the course of the vein. Dissection of the vein is otherwise carried out in a similar fashion as describe above. Exposure of the vein with the bridge technique may be less than optimal. Caution is necessary here to avoid excessive tension or manipulation of the conduit as an adjunct to deal with less than adequate exposure of those segments of the vein covered by a skin

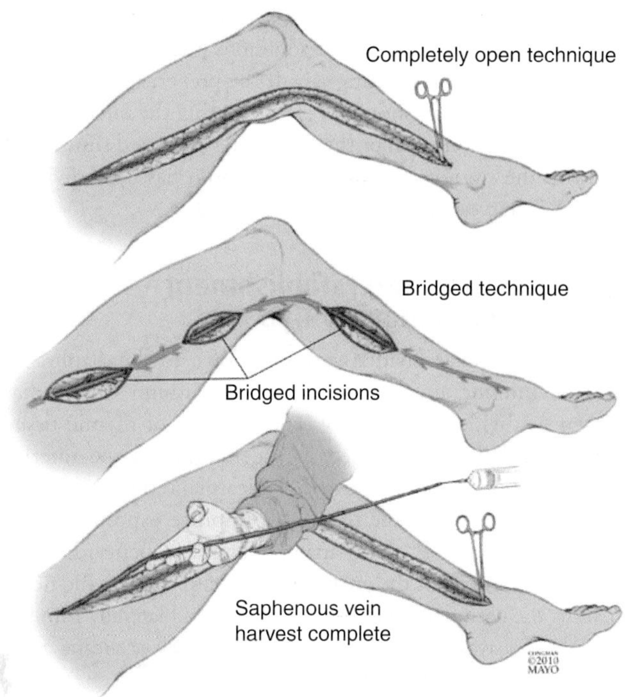

FIGURE 21-3 Saphenous vein harvest: open and bridged technique. Open technique (*top*): Dissection can be started in the upper thigh, above the knee, or at the ankle. Identification of the vein is easiest at the ankle, just above the medial malleolus. An incision is made overlying the vein and extended directly over its trajectory. The vein is dissected and all venous tributaries are ligated and divided in situ. Bridged technique (*middle*): Two- or three-step incisions are performed over the course of the vein. Dissection of the vein is carried in a similar fashion as the opened technique except that branches are divided in situ and ligated once the vein is explanted. Completed dissection (*bottom*): Once dissection is completed, the vein is ligated and divided proximally and distally. Stumps of side branches on the vein are left long and then are ligated flush with the vein, avoiding narrowing of the conduit. The vein is then gently flushed and stored in a solution of room temperature plasmalyte. The skin incisions are closed and the leg is wrapped with an elastic bandage. (*Copyrighted and used with permission of Mayo Foundation for Medical Education and Research, all rights reserved.*)

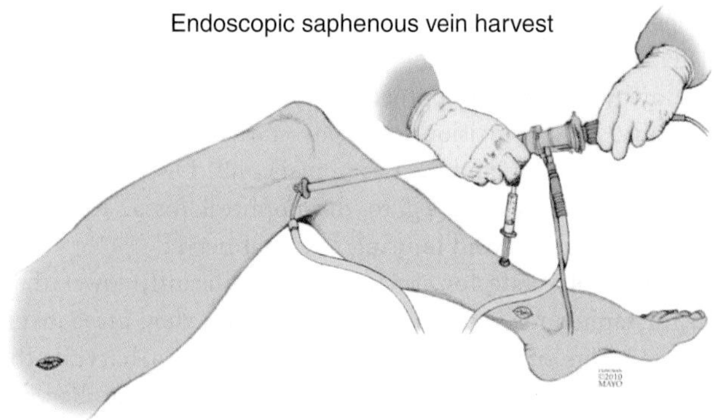

FIGURE 21-4 Endoscopic saphenous vein harvest. A 2.0-cm skin incision is made in the medial aspect of the knee. CO_2 insufflation is established. Harvesting is directed toward the groin region as far proximally as possible. Side branches are divided by using bipolar cauterizing scissors. Once dissection is completed, a small puncture is made in the groin directly over the vein and the vein is exteriorized under endoscopic guidance. After removing the vein from the leg, side branches are clipped. If any branches have been avulsed, the vein is repaired with interrupted 7-0 polypropylene sutures. (*Copyrighted and used with permission of Mayo Foundation for Medical Education and Research, all rights reserved.*)

bridge. For all techniques of vein harvest located in the lower thigh and more distal, care should be taken to avoid trauma to the saphenous nerve, which is in close proximity to the vein. Injury to the nerve can result in debilitating postoperative neuralgia.

Endoscopic vein harvest starts with a 1.5- to 2.0-cm skin incision in the medial aspect of the extremity above the knee (Fig. 21-4). Carbon dioxide insufflation for visualization and dissection is established. Dissection is directed toward the groin region as far proximally as possible and then distally as far as needed to obtain the required length of conduit. Side branches are divided by using bipolar cauterizing scissors. Once dissection is completed, small skin punctures are made at the limits of the dissection and the vein exteriorized, ligated, and divided. The vein is removed and otherwise prepared in the standard fashion. Following skin closure, the leg is wrapped with a circumferential elastic bandage.

Patency

Minimally invasive harvest of the saphenous vein using an endoscopic technique is gaining popularity because it greatly reduces the wound morbidity associated with the open harvest techniques. Endoscopic harvest decreases wound complication rates and produces an improved cosmetic result, although the operative time devoted to harvest is increased as are the number of defects to the harvested conduit requiring suture repair. Initial reports showed no detrimental effects of harvest technique on vein morphology, endothelial structure or function, or graft patency.[66,67] However, in recent report of 3000 patients treated with CABG, endovascular vein harvest was associated with higher rates of vein-graft failure, death, myocardial infarction, and repeat revascularization.[68]

The polar opposite to endoscopic vein harvest is the "no-touch" technique in which the vein is removed with a pedicle of surrounding tissue. The harvested vein is not distended and it is stored in heparinized blood. In a randomized study of 104 patients using this technique, the angiographic patency at 18 months was 89% for conventional versus 95% for no-touch grafts. At 8.5 years, patency rates were 76% for the conventional group versus 90% for the no-touch group. Multivariate analysis showed that the most important surgical factors for graft patency were the technique of harvesting the conduit and the vein quality. By comparison, the patency of internal thoracic artery grafts was 90% in the study.[69]

Other Venous Conduits

Alternative venous conduits such as the lesser saphenous and/or upper extremity cephalic veins are usually secondary choices for conduit. If it is planned to use either of these veins, preoperative vein mapping can help guide conduit harvest. The lesser saphenous vein can be harvested in a supine position through a lateral approach by flexing the hip and medially rotating the knee or by an inferior approach with straight elevation of the extremity. A skin incision is usually started midway between the Achilles tendon and the lateral malleolus. Dissection is carried proximally up the leg to the popliteal fossa. Attention should be paid to avoid injuring the sural nerve.

The patency rate for arm veins is significantly lower than that of saphenous veins and for that reason they are considered conduits of last resort.[70] For cephalic vein harvest, the arm is prepared and positioned as during radial artery harvest. Incisions are placed along the medial and superior aspect of the arm. The cephalic vein is relatively thin-walled in comparison with the greater saphenous vein and is predisposed to aneurysmal dilatation.

CONDUCT OF OPERATION

Procedures are done under general anesthesia with central venous access, radial arterial lines, and pulmonary artery catheters. Transesophageal echocardiography may be helpful for identifying unsuspected intracardiac lesions or aortic atherosclerosis, and for evaluating ventricular function at the end of the procedure. If ventricular function is poor, a femoral arterial line will facilitate later placement of an intra-aortic balloon pump (IABP). We routinely use a temperature-monitoring urinary catheter. The patient is positioned in the supine position with arms tucked at the side. Care should be taken to avoid peripheral nerve complications caused by pressure injury. The lower extremities are positioned with a slight external rotation and flexion of the knees. The patient is prepared and draped to include the lower neck, the chest, and abdomen between the anterior axillary lines, and the lower extremities circumferentially.

Incisions

By far the most common approach for CABG is via median sternotomy. Cannulation for cardiopulmonary bypass, managing aortic valve insufficiency, monitoring the left ventricle for distention, and evacuating air all are easier with the midline approach. The skin incision extends from a point midway between the angle of Louis and the sternal notch to just below the tip of the xiphoid process. The scalpel is used to extend the incision through the subcutaneous tissues down to the sternum. Extensive Bovey cautery to the subcutaneous tissues should be avoided because tissue destruction here may result in increased risk of wound complication. Charcoal does not bleed, but neither does it heal.

Special attention should be devoted to identifying the middle of the sternum. The middle of the sternal periosteum is noted and marked with cautery, although we avoid scoring the periosteum continuously from notch to xiphoid as this devascularizes the periosteum unless the saw passes exactly down the line. The interclavicular ligament is divided in the sternal notch, allowing palpation of the posterior aspect of the sternal manubrium. The xiphoid process is identified and divided in the midline with heavy scissors and the midline diaphragmatic muscle attachments divided. A finger should be inserted under the sternum to document a free space anterior to the pericardium. If there are no significant adhesions present, the sternum is divided with the oscillating saw. If the prepericardial space is adhered, the sternum should be divided using the microsagittal saw. The saphenous vein or the RA can be harvested simultaneous with the sternotomy. Once the sternum has been divided, the ITA is harvested as previously described.

Cannulation and Establishment of Cardiopulmonary Bypass

The pericardium is divided vertically down to the diaphragm and the inferior attachment of the pericardium to the diaphragm is divided transversely. The remnant of thymic tissue and pericardial fat is divided in the midline to the inferior aspect of the left innominate vein. Pericardial retraction sutures create a pericardial cradle or well to improve exposure of the ascending aorta and right atrium. The left pericardium is divided at the level of the great vessels toward the phrenic nerve to allow the completed ITA bypass graft to fall laterally into the pleural space away from the sternum. The distal ascending aorta is inspected and palpated for soft nonatherosclerotic areas suitable for arterial cannulation, root ventilation, proximal graft anastomoses, and aortic cross-clamp placement (Fig. 21-5). In

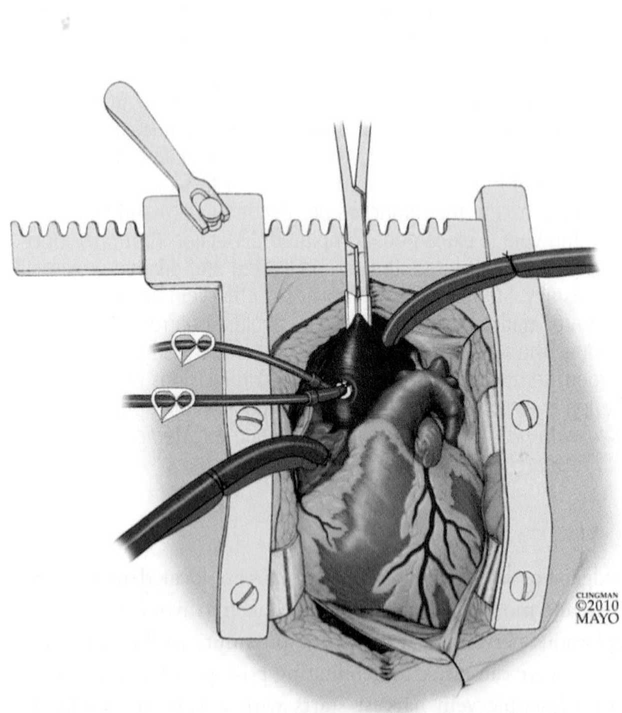

FIGURE 21-5 Cannulation. After full systemic heparinization, cannulation of the distal ascending aorta is performed with an appropriately sized curved or straight tip aortic cannula. A two-stage venous cannula is used for access to the right atrium, usually through the right atrial appendage. An aortic root cardioplegia/vent is placed. A retrograde cardioplegia cannula may be placed at the discretion of the surgeon. Patients with significant aortic regurgitation will benefit from placement of a left ventricle vent (placed via the right superior pulmonary) to avoid distention of the left ventricle during infusion of cardioplegia into the aortic root. *(Copyrighted and used with permission of Mayo Foundation for Medical Education and Research, all rights reserved.)*

some institutions epicardial ultrasound of the ascending aorta is performed. Now is the time to redirect the conduct of the operation should the aorta harbor areas of significant calcification, a topic of later discussion.

Systemic anticoagulation is achieved with the intravenous administration of 300 U/kg of unfractionated heparin and the adequacy of anticoagulation documented by an activated clotting time (ACT) over 450 seconds. In anticipation of aortic cannulation the systolic blood pressure should be reduced to about 100 mm Hg to minimize the risk of aortic dissection. Two partial-thickness concentric diamond-shaped purse-string sutures using 2-0 Ethibond suture are placed in the distal ascending aorta or proximal aortic arch, leaving enough room on the ascending aorta for all necessary proximal aortic work. The size of the purse strings should be large enough to accept the aortic cannula tip, usually 20-22 French. The ends of the sutures are passed through tourniquets that will be used for tightening the purse strings. The aortic adventitia within the purse strings is divided in preparation for aortotomy. The adventitia just superior to the planned aortotomy is grasped with a forceps and an aortotomy equal in size to the cannula tip is created with a no. 11 scalpel blade. Bleeding is easily controlled with slight inferior traction of the forceps on the adventitia. The aortic cannula is inserted and properly positioned, and the purse strings are tightened. The tourniquets are secured to the aortic cannula with a heavy silk tie and then the cannula is secured to the skin.

Placement of the aortic cannula can result in acute aortic dissection. Intraluminal positioning of the cannula is confirmed by watching for the cannula to fill with arterial blood. The aortic cannula is de-aired and connected to the arterial end of the pump tubing. An additional method to asses for the presence of aortic dissection is to have the perfusionist check the wave form and pressure of the arterial cannula pulse and to deliver a test infusion of 50 to 100 mL of fluid through the cannula. If an aortic dissection is present, often the test infusion will result in an increase in arterial cannula pressure.

Venous cannulation is accomplished with a two-stage venous cannula inserted in the right atrial appendage. A 2-0 Ethibond purse-string suture is placed around the tip of the right atrial appendage. The purse string should be wide enough for easy access of the selected venous cannula. An atriotomy is made with scissors at the tip of the appendage. Small bridging fibers of muscle are divided with scissors to permit easy entry of the cannula. The venous cannula is cautiously inserted, the tip of which should lie in the inferior vena cava. The purse-string suture is tightened and the tourniquet secured to the venous cannula with a heavy silk tie. The venous line is connected to the pump tubing.

An aortic root cannula is placed in the ascending aorta and retrograde cardioplegia cannula placed in the coronary sinus via the right atrium. The patient is placed on cardiopulmonary bypass at 2.4 L/min/m^2 and may be perfused at normothermia or may be cooled to 34°C. Once the patient is on full bypass, flow ventilation is stopped. A left ventricle vent may be placed via the right superior pulmonary vein at this time if there is significant aortic regurgitation. Target vessels are easier to identify before cardioplegic arrest while they are fully distended in their native state. The locations of planned distal anastomoses are marked with a scalpel. The pump flow is turned down temporarily and the aortic cross-clamp applied just proximal to the arterial cannula and bypass flow returned to normal.

Cold blood cardioplegia (10 mL/kg) is administered and may be delivered antegrade, retrograde, or both, with special attention given during this time to look for evidence of aortic regurgitation such as a flaccid aorta and/or left ventricle distention. Two available options to treat significant aortic regurgitation include completion of the procedure using only retrograde cardioplegia or placement of a left ventricle vent via the right superior pulmonary vein (our preferred method). Rarely is aortic valve replacement required. Additional doses of cardioplegia (5 mL/kg) are given via the antegrade and retrograde catheters approximately every 20 minutes throughout the remainder of the cross-clamp period.

DISTAL ANASTOMOSES

Location of Targets and Sequence of Anastomoses

Arteriotomy sites should be chosen proximal enough to offer the largest-sized coronary target but distal enough to avoid areas of obstruction or significant atherosclerotic disease. Arteriotomies at bifurcations should be avoided. Diseased vessels with an intramyocardial course can often be localized by noting epicardial indentation, accompanying epicardial veins, or a whitish streak within the myocardium. Sharp dissection of overlying tissue is required to identify the desired target site. Often a very diseased vessel will be less diseased in the intramyocardial segment.

The LAD coronary artery can be particularly difficult to identify when it has an intramyocardial course. It can be relatively easy to inadvertently enter the right ventricular cavity while dissecting in the interventricular fat plane. If such a ventriculotomy is small, it can be closed with fine 6-0 polypropylene sutures, keeping in mind that the right ventricle is a low-pressure chamber and deep bites of myocardium are not necessary. However, if the right ventricle has been opened for a distance, it is best repaired using interrupted, pledgetted 2-0 Prolene suture (MH needle) in a horizontal mattress fashion, passing the needle under the ITA-LAD anastomosis. If difficulty is encountered in identifying an LAD artery, a fine probe may be passed retrograde via a small transverse arteriotomy into the LAD artery at the apex of the heart. The tip of the probe can be palpated in the proximal portion of the artery and cut down on appropriately. The distal arteriotomy is repaired with interrupted fine suture (7-0 or 8-0 Prolene). The repair can be done with or without a small vein patch.

The distribution of cardioplegia is usually relatively uniform; however, the sequence of anastomoses may be planned based on ischemic regions if myocardial protection is a particular concern. Grafting the most ischemic area first, using a distal-proximal routine, will permit early antegrade delivery of cardioplegia through the graft to the area of myocardial ischemia. Alternatively, the sequence of anastomoses may be dictated by the quality of the conduit itself, matching the best conduit to the most important territories. It is customary to perform the left internal thoracic artery-to-LAD artery anastomosis last to avoid tension and potential disruption of the anastomosis.

Arteriotomy

The choice of the site of arteriotomy is critical. Opening into a plaque may force endarterectomy, whereas injury to the posterior wall with the knife transforms a straightforward anastomosis into a complex repair. Silastic tapes placed proximally and distally around the coronary artery may help to stabilize the vessel, a technique often employed when grafting the distal right coronary artery or when there is significant back bleeding from the opened vessel. The arteriotomy is performed with a fine scalpel blade and extended with fine Pott's scissors proximally and distally. The arteriotomy should match the conduit diameter, and should be at least 1.5 times the luminal diameter of the distal coronary artery (Fig. 21-6).

Anastomotic Technique

The goal of the anastomosis is to join the conduit and the target vessel with precise endothelial approximation affording minimal resistance to flow. The wall of the vessel should be handled with care, avoiding endothelial injury to prevent thrombotic complications. Coronary anastomoses are typically constructed with continuous 7-0 polypropylene suture. Sutures should be evenly spaced to prevent leaks at the conclusion of the anastomosis. In order to increase anastomotic area, we prefer to bevel the conduits at approximately 30 degrees and notch them at the heel. Anastomoses are performed with continuous suture. We prefer a continuous, parachuting technique initiated at the heel for virtually all anastomoses regardless of their configuration (ie, end-to-side versus side-to-side sequential anastomosis).

Venous conduit is brought onto the field with a mosquito clamp on the adventitia at the toe of the conduit. An end-to-side anastomosis is accomplished with continuous sutures (Fig. 21-7). Starting at the 3 o'clock position on the right side of the vessel, the suture is passed outside-in on the conduit and then inside-out at the corresponding location of the target coronary vessel. Two more sutures are taken before the heel (2 and 1 o-clock positions), one directly in the heel (12 o'clock), and then two more on the left side (11 and 10 o'clock positions) of the anastomosis before parachuting the conduit down to the target vessel.

The anastomosis is continued by placing additional sutures moving in a counterclockwise fashion around the anastomosis until the other thread is encountered. The technique encourages one to move out of the heel and toe areas of the anastomosis, minimizing the risk of narrowing the outflow. Care must be taken to prevent suturing the back wall of the coronary, and the proper amount of tension on the follow-through must be provided to avoid both leakage and a purse-string effect. Just before completion of the anastomosis, a 1-mm probe is passed proximally

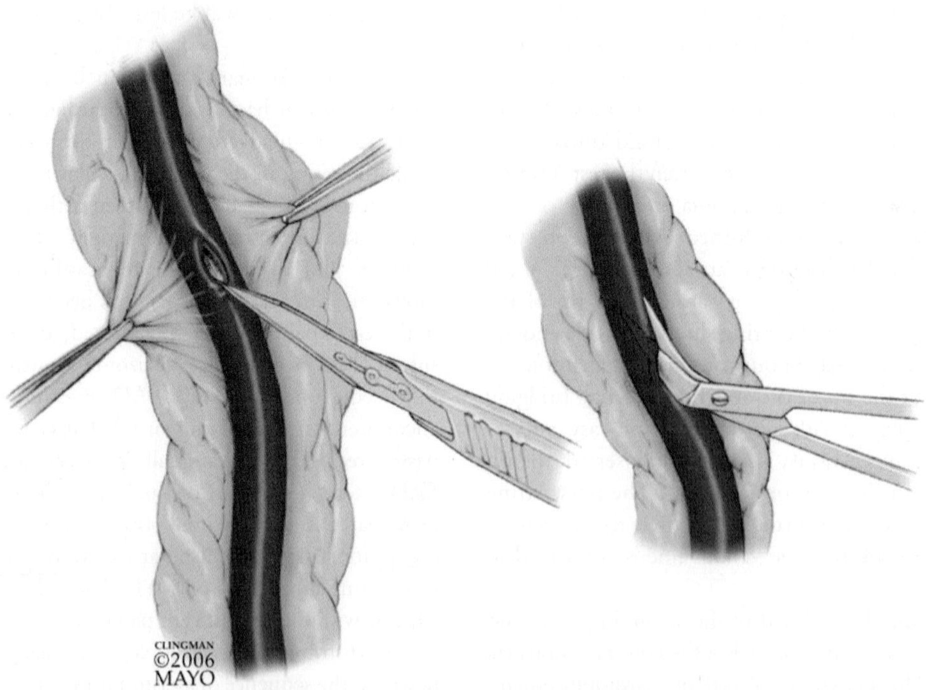

FIGURE 21-6 Distal anastomosis: Arteriotomy. Arteriotomy sites should be proximal enough to offer the largest-sized coronary target, and just distal enough to avoid the area of obstruction. Intramyocardial vessels can often be localized by noting epicardial indentation, accompanying epicardial veins, or a whitish streak within the myocardium. Sharp dissection of overlying tissue is then required to identify the desired target site. The arteriotomy is then performed with a no. 11 blade. The arteriotomy is extended with fine Pott's scissors proximally and distally. The arteriotomy should match the conduit diameter, and should be at least 1.5 times the diameter of the distal coronary. *(Copyrighted and used with permission of Mayo Foundation for Medical Education and Research, all rights reserved.)*

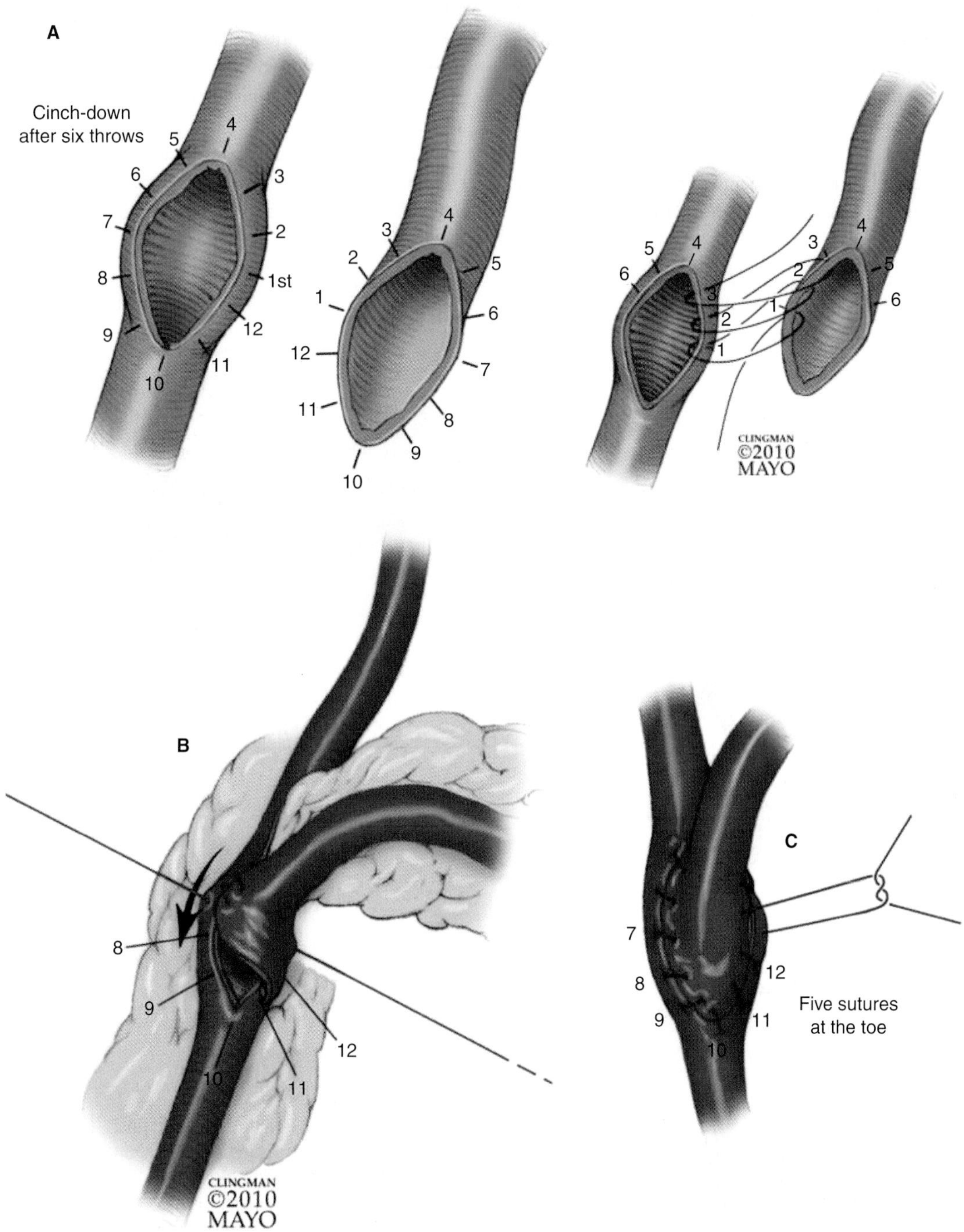

FIGURE 21-7 Distal anastomosis suture technique. (A) The conduit is beveled at 30 degrees and notched at the heel. We use a continuous, parachuting technique with 7-0 or 8-0 polypropylene suture. The conduit is brought onto the field with a mosquito clamp on the adventitia at the toe of the conduit. An end-to-side anastomosis is accomplished with 12 sutures. Starting at 3 o'clock on the right side of the vessel, the suture is passed outside-in on the conduit and then inside-out at the corresponding location of the target vessel. (B) Two more stitches are taken before the heel, one directly in the heel, and then two more on the left side of the anastomosis before parachuting the conduit down to the target vessel. (C) The anastomosis is then completed by placing another six stitches evenly spaced in the same manner for the toe. (*Copyrighted and used with permission of Mayo Foundation for Medical Education and Research, all rights reserved.*)

and distally to ensure patency. To prevent anastomotic tension and torsion, pedicled conduits (ie, left ITA) can be suture-fixated to the adjacent epicardium.

Sequential grafting permits efficient use of conduit and has the potential for increased flow in the conduit. When planning sequential anastomoses, the most distal anastomosis should be to the largest target vessel with the greatest outflow potential. If the reverse situation is created, the most distal anastomosis is at increased risk for failure, given the likelihood of preferential flow to the larger more proximal anastomosis.[71,72] A clear disadvantage of sequential grafting is the reliance of two or more distal targets on a single conduit and proximal anastomosis, placing a potentially larger region of myocardium at jeopardy.[72]

Some surgeons avoid using the ITA for sequential grafting or as a donor for composite T- or Y-grafting of other conduits because of concerns of compromising critical ITA-to-LAD flow. However, several series have demonstrated successful use of the ITA for sequential grafting of stenotic diagonal coronary arteries with excellent results.[73,74] The left ITA has also been used for multiple sequential anastomoses to the circumflex territory with grafting of the right ITA to the LAD artery.[75] Sequential grafting has also been performed with the right GEA as well as the RA.[76,77]

When constructing a sequential anastomosis, it is our preference to complete the distal anastomosis first and move proximally (Fig. 21-8). We feel that this facilitates determination of

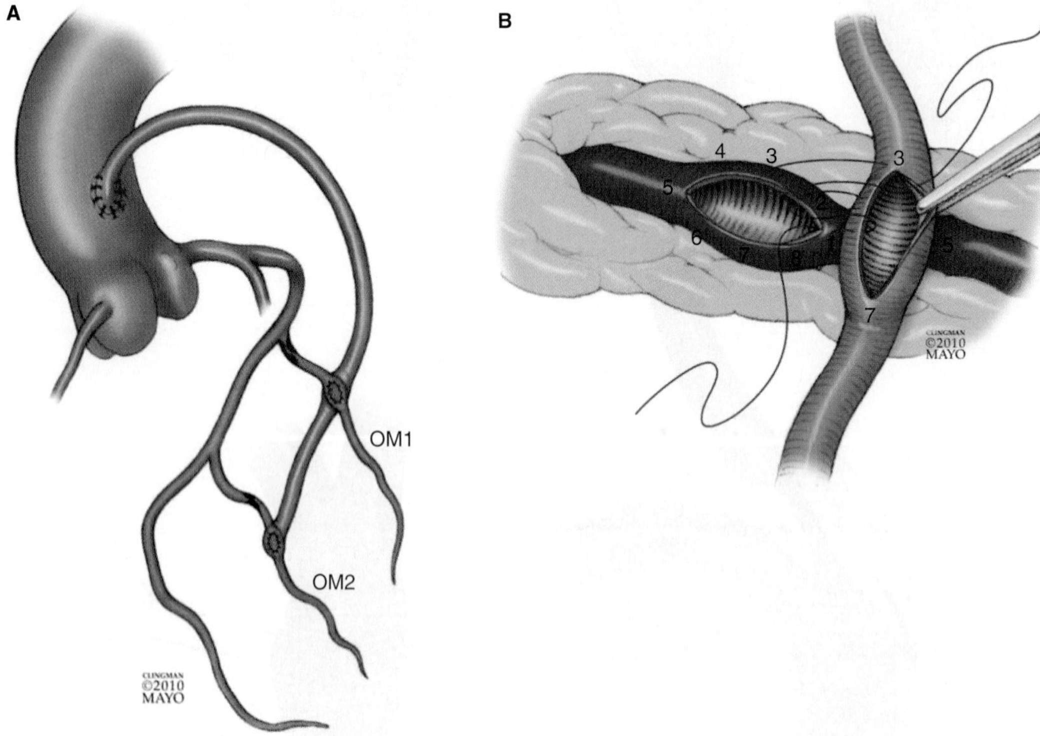

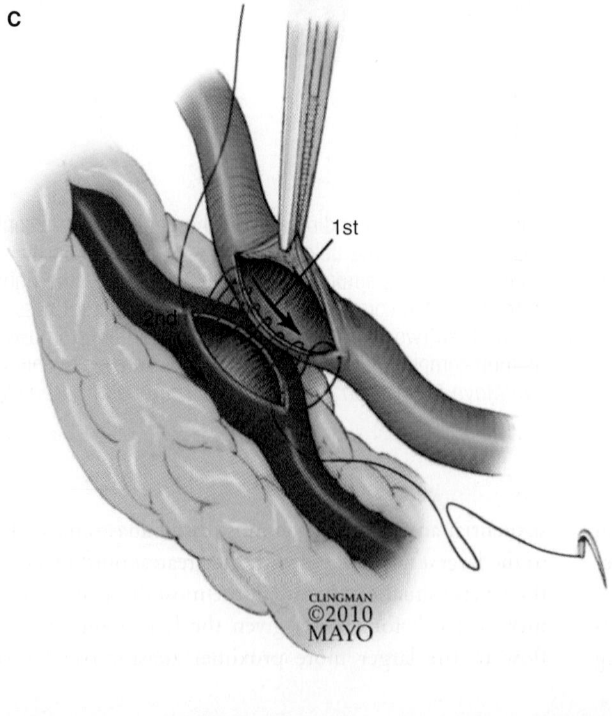

FIGURE 21-8 Sequential anastomosis. (A) Order of anastomoses: The order in which sequential anastomoses are performed is important to facilitate optimal inter graft spacing and avoid kinking. The distal anastomosis is completed first and the more proximal sequential anastomosis is performed second, except for an LAD-diagonal graft, in which the diagonal is performed first followed by the LAD. (B) Perpendicular sequential side-to-side anastomosis: Arteriotomies are made in the direction of the long axis of the coronary and the conduit. Care must be taken not to make the arteriotomies too long, because there is risk of creating a "gull-wing"deformity. The two incisions are aligned perpendicular to one another. The suture is passed starting inside-out at the apex of the target coronary and then outside-in at the mid-portion the conduit. An eight-stitch anastomosis is completed creating a diamond-shaped anastomosis. (C) Longitudinal sequential side-to-side anastomosis: The arteriotomy for longitudinal anastomosis may be made as long as necessary without risk of distorting the conduit. The anastomosis is begun at the heel and the far wall is completed open. It is then parachuted down and the front wall completed. (*Copyrighted and used with permission of Mayo Foundation for Medical Education and Research, all rights reserved.*)

optimal inter graft spacing. In the case of the LAD-diagonal graft, however, it is easier to move from proximal to distal, performing the diagonal anastomosis first. Sequential side-to-side anastomoses may be perpendicular or longitudinal. When constructing perpendicular anastomoses care must be taken not to make the arteriotomies too long, as there is risk of creating a "gull-wing" deformity and placing the graft at jeopardy. Arteriotomies in both the conduit and target are made in the direction of the long axis of the vessel. The two incisions are then aligned perpendicular to one another and the anastomosis completed, creating a diamond-shaped anastomosis. The arteriotomy for longitudinal anastomosis may be made as long as necessary without risk of distorting the conduit. Typically, the longitudinal anastomosis is begun at the heel as previously described.

CORONARY ENDARTERECTOMY

Coronary endarterectomy predated CABG as a direct surgical approach to relieving coronary occlusive disease. Coronary endarterectomy has been relegated to a position of secondary importance, however, thanks to the reliable and reproducible results obtained with CABG. Recently there has been increased interest in endarterectomy techniques, because the patient population coming to CABG has a greater atherosclerotic burden owing to diabetes, hyperlipidemia, and advanced age.[78] Most commonly, the need for endarterectomy arises intraoperatively when no soft site can be identified for arteriotomy or a vessel has been inadvertently opened in an extensively diseased area not amenable to grafting. Occasionally, endarterectomy is undertaken electively in patients with diffuse and extensive coronary disease with no other choices except transplantation.

The perioperative risk of CABG with endarterectomy is higher than that for CABG alone in most studies. In a retrospective study of 1478 patients, the reported mortality rate with endarterectomy was 3.2%, which was higher than for CABG alone (2.2%). Perioperative MI rate was also higher in the endarterectomy group, 4.2% versus 3.4%. The risk of mortality appears to increase when multiple vessels require endarterectomy: single-vessel endarterectomy mortality = 1.8% versus multiple-vessel endarterectomy mortality = 5.5%.[79,80] There has been controversy regarding the risk of endarterectomy of the LAD, with some studies showing increased risk whereas others demonstrate no increased risk.[79–81]

The late results of endarterectomy are inferior to those of routine CABG, with reported 3-year patency for ITA grafts to endarterectomized LAD targets ranging from 74 to 80%.[82,83] Despite this, angina relief is remarkably good initially. Unfortunately, the rate of recurrent angina is somewhat higher than after uncomplicated CABG; reported recurrence of angina is 25% at 5 years after endarterectomy.[79,84] The reported 5-year survival following coronary endarterectomy ranges from 76 to 83%.[79,84] Among patients in whom bypass to more distal non-diseased segments is not possible, coronary endarterectomy with subsequent bypass offers a viable alternative to leaving a territory ungrafted.

Technique

The technique of endarterectomy requires that the central core be extracted adequately in order to relieve obstruction of the branch vessels. Patency of a graft to the endarterectomized vessel depends upon the adequacy of runoff and therefore the distal endpoints of the endarterectomy core must be smoothly tapered. If the core fractures leaving behind disease in side branches, distal counter-incisions may be needed to obtain a satisfactory result.

The RCA is the vessel most often endarterectomized, usually at the level of its bifurcation. A manual eversion endarterectomy is performed after entering at the vessel approximately 1 cm proximal to the crux. A circumferential plane of dissection between the core and the adventitia is developed with a fine coronary spatula. The core is transected proximally and gently grasped with DeBakey forceps while the spatula is used to tease the adventitia away from the core. The core is regrasped hand over hand as distally as possible to avoid fracture. When the crux is reached, the posterior descending artery and the left ventricular branch are endarterectomized separately. If endarterectomy of the proximal segment of the RCA is needed, we prefer to use an open technique because it is difficult to obtain nice tapering of the core at the takeoff of the acute marginal branches with a retrograde eversion endarterectomy. The vessel wall is then reconstructed with a long hood created with the bypass conduit of choice.

We prefer open extended technique when the LAD is endarterectomized (Fig. 21-9). The vessel is opened as far proximal as possible if endarterectomy is anticipated. If the vessel has been opened in its mid-portion before it is apparent that endarterectomy is necessary, we extend the incision in the adventitia proximally before developing the endarterectomy plane. Retrograde eversion endarterectomy is dangerous because branch vessels will not be opened. Once the core is separated from the adventitia, it is transected proximally at the heel and the vessel is opened beyond the takeoff of the major diagonals to permit individual eversion endarterectomy of each of the branches. The segment is reconstructed with a long hood of the conduit of choice or a vein patch into which the ITA is anastomosed. The circumflex artery is the most infrequently endarterectomized vessel. Its rapid branching pattern makes satisfactory endarterectomy difficult. We tend to begin with an eversion technique, focusing our efforts on opening the largest distal branches as much as possible.

PROXIMAL ANASTOMOSES

Proximal anastomoses of saphenous vein or RA to the aorta are performed after the distal anastomoses under the same cross-clamp clamp. Our preferred technique is to complete each respective bypass graft in a distal anastomosis-proximal anastomosis fashion. Completion of the each respective bypass graft allows antegrade cardioplegia down the completed graft, aiding in myocardial protection. The single cross-clamp technique results in longer cross-clamp times than with the partial occlusion clamp method. However, the partial occlusion clamp technique requires additional aortic manipulation and has been

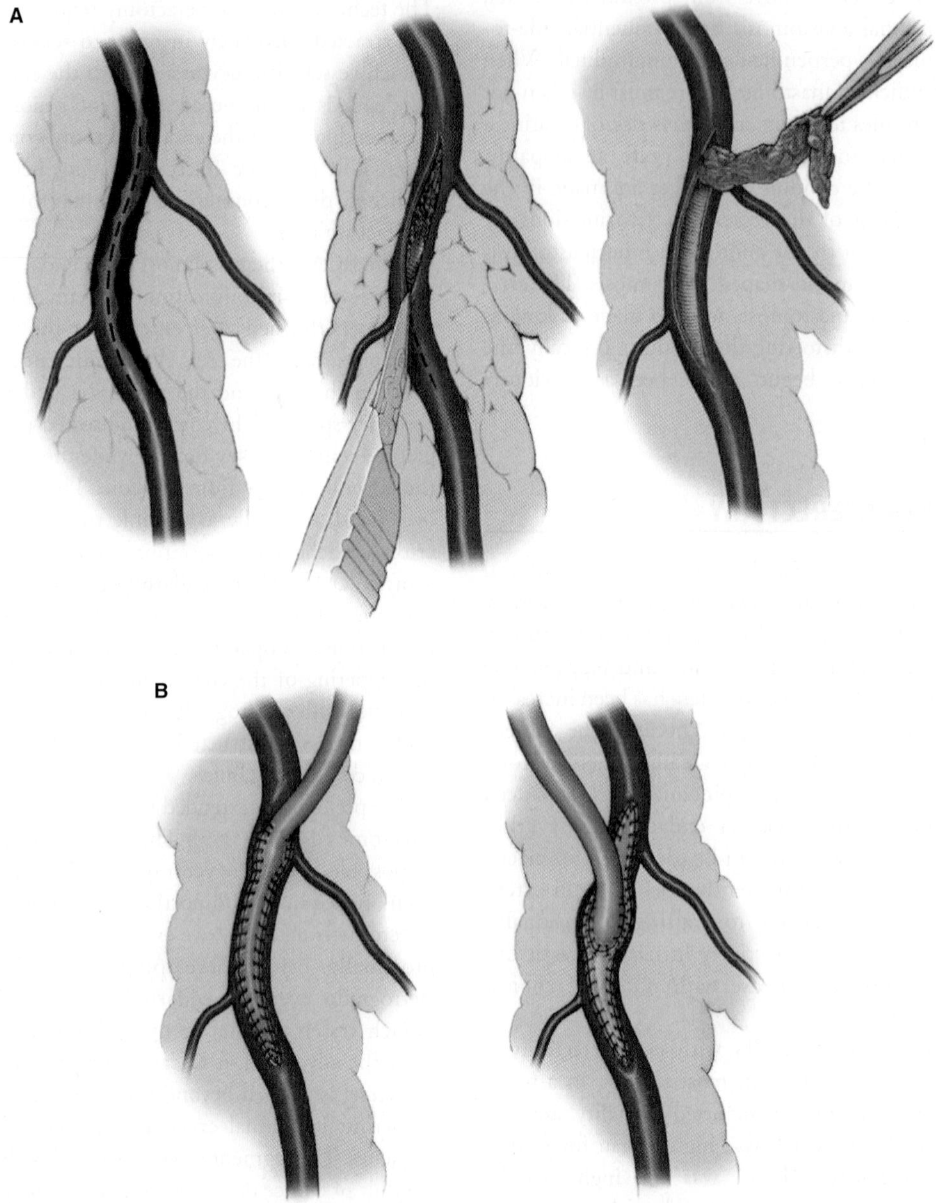

FIGURE 21-9 Coronary endarterectomy: Open extended technique. (A) The extent of disease is evaluated to plan the length of the arteriotomy and endarterectomy. The arteriotomy is performed and extended as proximal as needed before the circumferential plane of dissection between the core and the adventitia is developed with a fine coronary spatula. Once the core is separated from the adventitia, it is transected proximally at the heel and the vessel is opened beyond the takeoff of the major branches to permit individual eversion endarterectomy of each of the branches. (B) The segment is reconstructed with a long hood of the conduit of choice. The segment may be reconstructed with a vein patch into which the conduit is anastomosed. (*Copyrighted and used with permission of Mayo Foundation for Medical Education and Research, all rights reserved.*)

associated with a higher risk of neuropsychological deficits as compared with the single-clamp technique.[85]

Anastomotic Technique

Once an appropriate site for aortotomy is identified, the fatty tissue overlying the aorta is removed (Fig. 21-10). An arteriotomy is created with a no. 11 blade, and a 4.0-mm punch used to create a circular aortotomy. The size of the punch may vary depending on the size of the conduit graft. The graft is measured to length with the aorta, right heart, and pulmonary artery full of blood. The graft is cut and the proximal aspect of the conduit beveled and notched at the heel. A running 5-0 polypropylene suture is used for a venous graft and a 6-0 polypropylene suture for an arterial conduit. The long axis of the graft is aligned at an appropriate angle to the ascending aorta. The anastomosis can be completed with continuous stitches. Symmetry in the spacing of sutures is paramount to obtain a

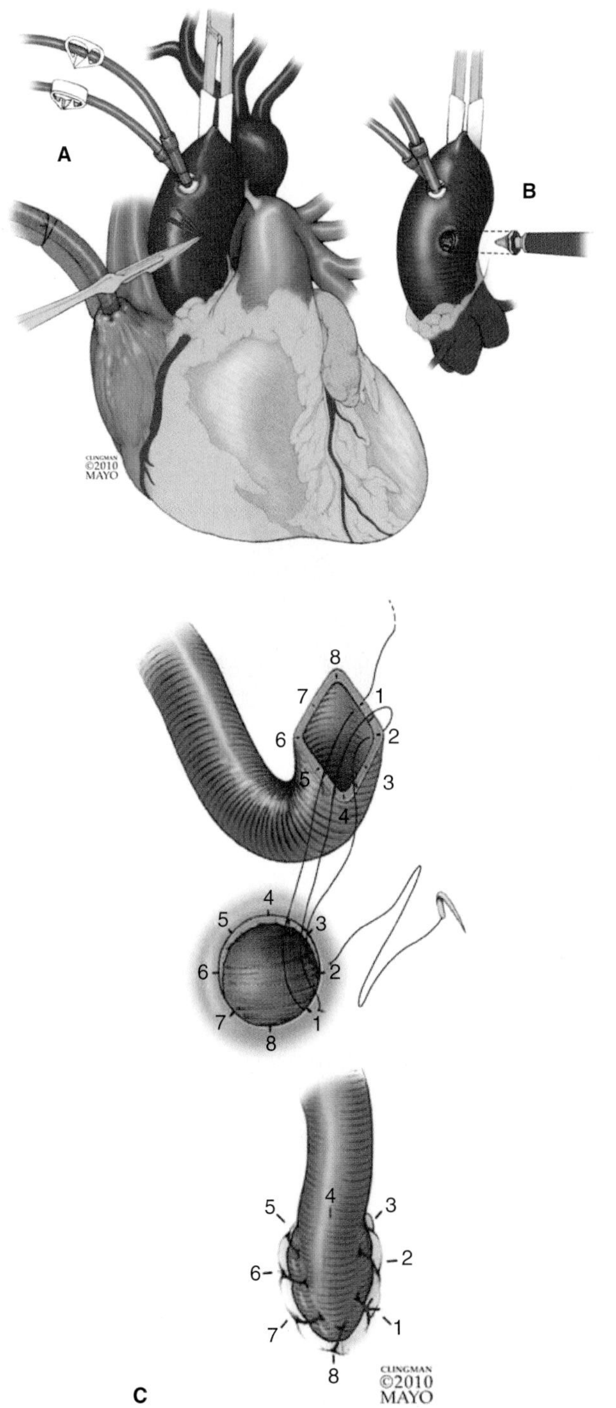

FIGURE 21-10 Proximal anastomosis. (A) The proximal anastomosis is performed using a single-clamp technique. The fatty tissue overlying the planned aortotomy site is removed. An arteriotomy is created with a no. 11 blade. (B) A 4- to 5-mm aortic punch is used to create a circular aortotomy. The size of the punch will vary depending on the size of the conduit graft. (C) The proximal aspect of the conduit is beveled and then notched at the heel. A running 5-0 or 6-0 polypropylene suture is used for a venous graft and a 6-0 or 7-0 polypropylene suture for an arterial conduit. The long axis of the graft is aligned at an appropriate angle to the ascending aorta. The anastomosis can be completed with eight stitches in most cases; symmetry in the spacing between stitches is of paramount importance to ensure hemostasis. *(Copyrighted and used with permission of Mayo Foundation for Medical Education and Research, all rights reserved.)*

hemostatic anastomosis. Free arterial grafts may also be sutured to the hood of a vein graft with continuous 7-0 Prolene suture.

Composite Grafts

As an alternative to proximal anastomosis to the aorta, a free graft can be anastomosed proximally to the pedicled ITA (Fig. 21-11). This technique has the theoretical advantage of providing a more physiologic arterial pressure waveform by attaching the conduit to a third-order vessel rather than to the aorta. Composite grafting is also a useful tool for the hostile, calcified ascending aorta or when there is a limited length of conduit available. It is also advantageous when there is a marked mismatch between aortic wall thickness and arterial conduit size.

A combination of composite and sequential grafting allows the opportunity to perform complete arterial revascularization with only ITA or with ITA and other arterial conduits (Fig. 21-12). Multiple configurations of Y- and T-grafts can be devised to best suit the anatomic characteristics of each patient. The LITA has been shown to have more than sufficient flow reserve to supply flow to the entire coronary circulation.[86] The free right ITA, the RA, or other arterial conduit can be based in this manner.

All-arterial Y-grafts are usually planned in advance and constructed before the initiation of cardiopulmonary bypass. Special care must be taken during construction of composite grafts to avoid tension, rotational torsion, or narrowing of the inflow anastomosis. Disadvantages include technical difficulty and reliance upon a single inflow source for two or more distal targets.

MANAGEMENT OF THE ATHEROSCLEROTIC ASCENDING AORTA

Ascending aortic atherosclerosis has been consistently identified as a very important risk factor for stroke in multiple series. Epiaortic ultrasound can be performed to define the extent of atherosclerosis of the ascending aorta and its likelihood of embolization. Patients with severe atherosclerosis of the ascending aorta may require alternative strategies to prevent embolization of aortic atheroma. If the ascending aorta is hostile, we favor cannulation of the right axillary artery. The axillary artery is a good option to achieve arterial inflow by using a chimney side graft. If needed, aortic clamping may be performed in areas free of atheroma, usually in the more proximal ascending aorta.

Coronary revascularization can be achieved with a variety of methods. Using a "no-touch" technique, revascularization can be done using only pedicled arterial conduits, and if proximal anastomoses are required they can be based off pedicled conduits or brachiocephalic vessels. Distal anastomoses can be performed under cold fibrillatory arrest without aortic cross-clamping, and they also can be accomplished using off-pump techniques. Proximal anastomoses can be performed under deep hypothermic circulatory arrest or after graft replacement of the ascending aorta if there are large mobile atheromas.[87]

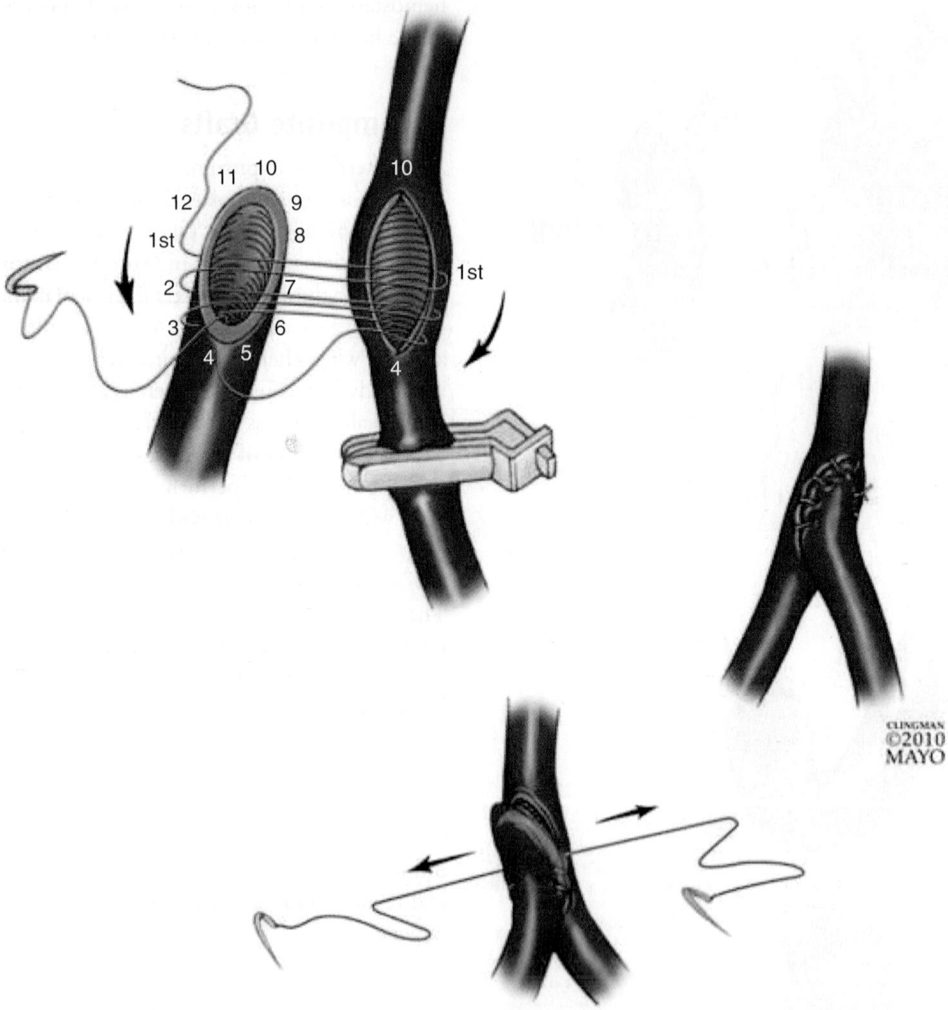

FIGURE 21-11 Composite Y-graft. Y-graft anastomotic technique: A coronary artery bypass graft (CABG) is used as a donor site for the proximal anastomosis of another conduit. An incision is created in the donor conduit. The proximal end of the recipient conduit is then anastomosed to the donor site in an end-to-side fashion as previously described for a distal anastomosis. The recipient conduit is then gently parachuted down onto the donor conduit. (*Copyrighted and used with permission of Mayo Foundation for Medical Education and Research, all rights reserved.*)

Weaning from Cardiopulmonary Bypass

On completion of all anastomoses, the aortic cross-clamp is removed and a stable heart rhythm established. Some advocate allowing the heart to recover on full bypass for 10 minutes for each 60 minutes of aortic cross-clamp time. During this time of recovery the patient is prepared for transition from supported circulation to native circulation. The aortic root vent and retrograde catheters are removed and the sites repaired with suture. The bypass grafts are checked for kinks, twists, or tension and for presence of hemostasis. The patient must be rewarmed to normothermia if cooled and the acid-base status and electrolyte abnormalities corrected. We place temporary atrial and ventricular pacing wires on all patients.

Weaning from cardiopulmonary bypass is otherwise the same as for other cardiac surgical cases. Issues particular to CABG include attention to avoid overdistention of the heart, which may place grafts on tension and disrupt anastomoses. If air has entered the heart, bubbles may pass into the aorta and down the bypass grafts causing arrhythmias and regional wall motion abnormalities. Treatment involves continued recovery on bypass and increasing the perfusion pressure as a means to drive the bubbles through the coronary circulation. Persistency of regional wall motion abnormalities may require bypass graft revision or placement of additional bypass grafts.

OUTCOMES

Operative Mortality

The risk profile of patients requiring isolated CABG in the United States has changed significantly in the past decade. Patients are older, with a greater number of comorbidities, decreased LVEF, and a higher burden of atherosclerotic disease; however, early outcomes after CABG continue to improve. The

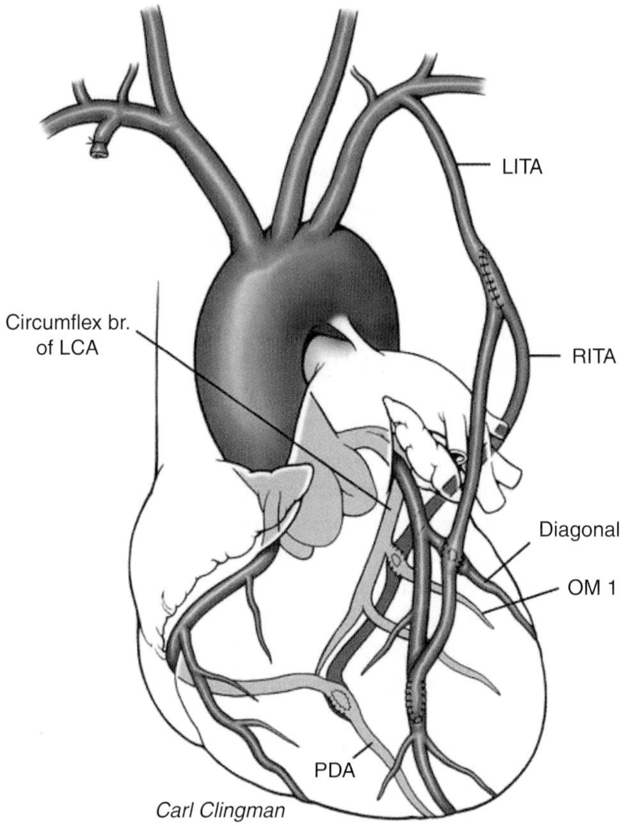

FIGURE 21-12 Total arterial revascularization: As shown, arterial revascularization can be performed using the right internal thoracic artery (RITA) off the left internal thoracic artery (LITA) as a Y-graft and liberal use of sequential grafting. (*Copyrighted and used with permission of Mayo Foundation for Medical Education and Research, all rights reserved.*)

STS database demonstrates that despite an increase in expected mortality from 2.6 to 3.4% (relative increase 30%) in the decade of the 1990s, the observed mortality has actually decreased from 3.9 to 3.0% (relative decrease 23%).[3]

Similar observations have been made using the Veterans Affairs mandatory national database, where the unadjusted mortality rate for isolated CABG fell from 4.3% in 1989 to 2.7% in the year 2000.[88] In the private sector similar trends have been observed. In an analysis of outcomes of patients undergoing isolated CABG in the HCA system, a nationwide for-profit health care system involving 200 hospitals in 23 states, Mack and associates reported an ongoing decrease in unadjusted operative mortality among 51,353 patients, 80% of whom received CABG with cardiopulmonary bypass. In this study the operative mortality decreased from 2.9% in 1999 to 2.2% in 2002.[89]

Causes of Death

In a multicenter prospective study performed by the Northern New England Cardiovascular Disease Study Group, 384 deaths among 8641 consecutive patients undergoing isolated CABG between 1990 and 1995 were analyzed with respect to the mode of death. The mode of death was defined as the seminal event that precipitated clinical deterioration and ultimately resulted in the patient's demise. Heart failure was judged to be the primary mode of death for 65% of the patients, followed in frequency by neurologic causes (7.3%), hemorrhage (7%), respiratory failure (5.5%), and dysrhythmia (5.5%). The greatest variability in mortality rates observed across surgeons in the study was attributable to differences in rates of heart failure.[90] Cardiac causes were also identified by Sergeant and colleagues as the most common causes of death in a series 5880 patients undergoing CABG between 1983 and 1988.[91]

Operative Morbidity

Myocardial Dysfunction

Postoperative myocardial dysfunction and cardiac failure after CABG may be related to preoperative ischemic injury, inadequate myocardial protection, incomplete revascularization, or postoperative graft failure. The spectrum of myocardial injury varies from subtle degrees of global myocardial ischemia to transmural infarction. The incidence of myocardial injury identified varies with the sensitivity of the method used for detection as well as the threshold set. Some studies have reported perioperative myocardial infarction rates as high as 10% of patients with associated worse clinical outcomes (death, MI, or revascularization).[92]

Some elevations of cardiac-specific enzymes are ubiquitous after CABG; however, most would agree that elevations in creatinine kinase-myocardial bound (CK-MB) greater than five times the upper limit of normal (ULN) value are considered significant. In a prospective study of 2918 patients undergoing CABG, 38% of patients had a CK-MB >5 ULN and 17% had a CK-MB >10 ULN with an incidence of new Q-wave MI of 4.7%.[93] Troponin may be a more sensitive marker than CK-MB, but its role in large populations of CABG patients is still to be defined.[94] Prominent elevations of CK-MB and troponin have been associated with global ischemia, MI, low cardiac output, and increased operative mortality, as well as increased midterm and long-term mortality.[93,94]

Transient myocardial dysfunction necessitating low-dose inotropic support for a short period of time is also common after CABG. Significant postoperative myocardial dysfunction manifest clinically as low cardiac output syndrome may be defined by the need for postoperative inotropic support or intra-aortic balloon pump support to maintain a systolic blood pressure >90 mm Hg or a cardiac index >2.2 L/min. The reported incidence of low output syndrome varies depending on the defining criteria and has a reported incidence of 4–9%.[95,96] Low output syndrome has been shown to be a marker for increased operative mortality by 10- to 15-fold.[97] Independent predictors of low output syndrome in order of importance include: LVEF <20%, reoperation, emergency operation, female gender, diabetes, age older than 70, left main disease, recent MI, and triple-vessel disease.[96]

Adverse Neurologic Outcome

Neurologic deficits after coronary surgery are divided into two types: type 1 deficits include major neurologic deficits, stupor, and coma; type 2 deficits are characterized by deterioration of intellectual function and memory. The incidence of type 1 deficits was reported to be 1.6% in a large review by the Northern New England Cardiovascular Disease Study Group with 1-, 5-, and 10-year survival rates significantly reduced in affected patients.[98] Perioperative mortality is similarly increased among those with type 1 injury at over 24%.[99] Type 2 deficits are more difficult to characterize and may be more related to the underlying atherosclerosis than to the bypass operation per se. In one nonrandomized study, there was no evidence that the cognitive test performance of coronary artery bypass grafting (CABG) patients differed from that of heart healthy control groups with coronary artery disease over a 1-year period.[100]

Predictors of neurologic deficits included advanced age (≥70 years of age), and history or presence of severe hypertension. Independent predictors of type 1 deficits included proximal aortic atherosclerosis, history of prior neurologic disease, need for IABP, diabetes, unstable angina, and perioperative hypotension. Predictors of type 2 deficits included history of alcohol consumption, dysrhythmias, prior CABG, peripheral vascular disease, congestive heart failure (CHF), and perioperative hypotension. Similar predictors of adverse neurologic outcomes have been observed in other studies.[101]

Deep Sternal Wound Infection

Deep sternal wound infection occurs in 1 to 4% of CABG patients and carries a mortality rate of 25%.[102] Proven methods to reduce postoperative wound complications include the use of preoperative showers with chlorhexidine gluconate on the evening and morning before the procedure, prophylactic intranasal application of mupirocin given on the evening and the morning before the procedure and twice daily for 5 days postoperatively, hair clipping the morning of surgery, and administration of intravenous prophylactic antibiotics before skin incision.[103–105] Application of a cyanoacrylate-based microbial skin sealant may further reduce surgical site infection.[106]

Obesity and diabetes are strong independent predictors of mediastinitis. Insulin-dependent diabetics are especially susceptible to deep sternal wound infection.[107–109] Recent data suggest that tight glycemic control in the postoperative period decreases the risk of mediastinitis in the diabetic population.[110,111] Other preoperative variables independently associated with an increased incidence of deep sternal wound infection include reoperation, longer operative times, reexploration for bleeding, and blood transfusions.[108,109,112]

The use of bilateral ITAs had been implicated as a risk factor for sternal would complications, especially in diabetics.[113] However, this risk appears to be mitigated in part by using a skeletonized ITA harvesting technique.[114] Bilateral ITA harvest should likely be avoided in obese diabetic women, in cases of repeat sternotomy, and in patients with severe COPD, because they exhibit a higher risk of deep sternal wound infection even with skeletonization of the ITA.[25,115]

Acute Renal Failure

Acute renal failure ensuing after CABG with cardiopulmonary bypass is an ominous event. In a prospective observational study conducted at 24 university centers in the United States, including data on 2222 CABG patients,[116] renal dysfunction not requiring dialysis occurred in 6.3%, and renal dysfunction requiring hemodialysis developed in 1.4%. Mortality was directly related to postoperative renal function. Patients with no renal dysfunction had 0.9% mortality.[116] Postoperative renal dysfunction increased mortality to 19% if no dialysis was needed and increased mortality to 63% if hemodialysis was required. Patients with large creatinine increases (≥ 50%) after CABG surgery also have higher 90-day mortality.[117]

Independent predictors of postoperative renal dysfunction included increasing age, CHF, reoperation, diabetes mellitus, chronic renal insufficiency, prolonged cardiopulmonary bypass time, and low cardiac output.[116] These findings were confirmed in another series of 42,733 patients with similar incidence and mortality associated with postoperative renal dysfunction.[118] One in four patients with preoperative chronic renal insufficiency (creatinine >1.6 mg/dL) will require renal replacement therapy post-CABG, and patients at highest risk are older than 70 years and have a baseline creatinine >2.5 mg/dL.[119]

Continuous infusion of low-dose recombinant human B-type natriuretic peptide (nesiritide) from the start of cardiopulmonary bypass has been evaluated as a method to effectively maintain postoperative renal function. In the prospective, randomized, NAPA Trial, 272 patients with ejection fraction ≤ 40% undergoing CABG who receive nesiritide experienced a significantly attenuated peak increase in serum creatinine and a greater urine output during the initial 24 hours after surgery. In addition, they had a shorter hospital stay and lower 180-day mortality.[120] Similar renal protective results were noted in a randomized trial using human atrial natriuretic peptide in 251 patients. The treated group had fewer postoperative complications, lower serum creatinine, and higher urinary creatinine and creatinine clearance. The maximum postoperative creatinine level and percent increase of creatinine were also significantly lower in the treatment group. No patient in the natriuretic group required hemodialysis.[121] We are awaiting further study before adopting natriuretic peptides in our routine CABG practice.

Long-Term Outcomes

Long-term outcomes of surgical myocardial revascularization depend on the complex interaction of patient-related and procedure-related factors. Important patient-related factors include anatomic distribution of the CAD, the extent and severity of coronary atherosclerosis, the physiologic impact of ischemia on ventricular function at the time of the original operation, age, gender, overall health status, severity of atherosclerotic burden throughout the body, the presence and severity of associated comorbidities, development of operative complications such as stroke, and need for permanent hemodialysis. The progression rate of native coronary atherosclerosis after surgery and the development of coronary bypass graft failure are of extreme importance in the development of post-CABG angina recurrence, MI, need for reintervention, and cardiac-related mortality. Procedure-related factors that influence long-term outcomes include completeness of revascularization, myocardial protection, and selection of bypass conduits.

Sergeant and colleagues at the Gasthuiberg University Hospital of the Katholieke Universiteit (KU) Leuven, Belgium have provided several reports detailing clinical outcomes after myocardial revascularization.[122–125] From 1971 to 1993, 9600 consecutive CABG patients were prospectively followed with special attention to clinical outcomes after surgical myocardial revascularization; the investigators achieved a 99.9% complete follow-up in this cohort. Clinical outcomes prospectively followed included mortality, return of angina, MI, and coronary reintervention.[122]

Defining the return of angina as the first occurrence of angina of any intensity or duration unless it was associated on the same day with MI or death, and recording the severity of this event, was also recorded. The overall non–risk-adjusted freedom from return of angina was 95% at 1 year, 82% at 5 years, 61% at 10 years, 38% at 15 years, and 21% at 20 years. The data suggest that if followed long enough after CABG, the return of angina is almost inevitable; by 12 years one-half of operated patients had return of angina. The initial episode of recurrent angina was rated as mild in 59% of patients.[123] In the Bypass Angioplasty Revascularization Investigation (BARI) trial of 914 patients with symptomatic multivessel disease randomly assigned to receive CABG, freedom from angina was 84% at 5 and 10 years.[126]

The overall non–risk-adjusted freedom from MI after CABG at the KU Leuven was 97% at 30 days, 94% at 5 years, 86% at 10 years, 73% at 15 years, and 56% at 20 years.[124] The overall non–risk-adjusted freedom from a coronary reintervention, either PCI or reoperative CABG, was 99.7% at 30 days, 97% at 5 years, 89% at 10 years, 72% at 15 years, and 48% at 20 years (125). In the BARI trial, freedom from subsequent coronary reintervention intervention at 10 years was 80%.[126]

Overall risk-unadjusted survival after CABG in the KU Leuven experience was 98% at 30 days, 92% at 5 years, 81% at 10 years, 66% at 15 years, and 51% at 20 years. Mortality after CABG was characterized by an initial period of high risk in the first month after surgery, then risk declined to its lowest at 1 year after the operation, and thereafter the mortality risk rose slowly and steadily for as long as the patient was followed. This slow and steady rise in the risk of death over time paralleled that of the general population when matched for sex, age, and ethnicity.[125] In the BARI trial, survival was 89% at 5 years and 74% at 10 years.[126]

The occurrence of ischemic clinical events after CABG negatively influences survival. In the KU Leuven study, overall survival was lessened by return of angina, with an observed survival of 83% at 5 years and 54% at 15 years; the more intense the severity of angina at its return, the greater its influence on survival.[123] The occurrence of MI after CABG has a greater negative effect on survival. Observed long-term survival after post-CABG infarction at the KU Leuven was 80% at 30 days, 65% at 5 years, 52% at 10 years, and 41% at 15 years.[124]

Progression of Disease in Native Coronary Arteries

Progression of atherosclerosis in the native coronary arteries continues after CABG. Bourassa and associates studied the progression of atherosclerosis in the native circulation 10 years after surgery and found that progression of CAD occurs in approximately 50% of nongrafted arteries.[127] The rate of progression of disease in nongrafted arteries was no different from that of grafted arteries with patent grafts; however, progression was more frequent in grafted arteries with occluded grafts. Progression of preexisting stenoses in native coronaries was more frequent than appearance of new stenoses, and it was related to the severity of the preexisting stenosis only in nongrafted arteries.

Progression of native CAD was associated with deterioration in left ventricular function. Native coronary atherosclerosis progressed at a similar rate to that of equally diseased arteries in nonoperated patients.[127] Low levels of high-density lipoprotein cholesterol and elevated levels of plasma low-density lipoprotein cholesterol correlated with native disease progression and development of new atherosclerotic lesions.[128,129] Diabetes has been related to accelerated atherosclerosis. The VICTORY trial will be the first cardiometabolic study to evaluate the antiatherosclerotic and metabolic effects of rosiglitazone is post-CABG patients with type 2 diabetes in patients 1 to 10 years after CABG.[130]

Vein Graft Failure

Although the use of the saphenous vein helped popularize coronary bypass grafting, the propensity of the saphenous vein graft to fail over time has been the limiting factor of the procedure. It has been reported that approximately 15% of vein grafts occlude in the first year after CABG, and by 6 and 10 years after surgery patency rates fall to approximately 75% and approximately 60%, respectively.18 Three entities are responsible for saphenous vein graft failure: thrombosis, intimal hyperplasia, and graft atherosclerosis

Thrombosis accounts for graft failure within the first month after CABG, and graft occlusion is found on angiography in 3 to 12% of all venous grafts. Even when performed under optimal conditions, the harvesting of venous conduits is associated with focal endothelial disruption. In particular, the high pressure distension used to overcome venospasm during harvesting causes prominent endothelial cell loss, medial damage, activation of local factors (ie, fibrinogen) influencing hemostasis. Additionally, the inherent antithrombotic properties of veins are comparatively weak. The propensity for early graft occlusion resulting from these prothrombotic effects may, on occasion, be amplified by technical factors that reduce graft flow, including intact venous valves, anastomotic stricture, or graft implantation proximal to an atheromatous segment.[18]

Intimal hyperplasia, defined as the accumulation of smooth muscle cells and extracellular matrix in the intimal compartment, is the major disease process in venous grafts between 1 month and 1 year after implantation. Nearly all veins implanted into the arterial circulation develop intimal thickening within 4 to 6 weeks, which may reduce the lumen by up to 25%. Intimal hyperplasia rarely produces significant stenosis per se; more importantly, however, is that it may provide the foundation for later development of graft atheroma.[131]

Progression of atherosclerosis in aortocoronary saphenous vein grafts is frequent and represents the predominant cause of late graft failure after CABG. Vein graft atherosclerosis may begin as early as the first year, but is fully developed only after about 5 years. Ten years after surgery, 50 to 60% of SVGs will be occluded and one-half of still patent grafts will show angiographic evidence of atherosclerosis; two-thirds of these lesions will have a luminal diameter reduction of 50% or greater. Vein graft atherosclerosis is the leading cause for reintervention following CABG, more so than progression of disease in native coronary arteries.[18]

Although the risk factors predisposing to vein graft atherosclerosis are broadly similar to those recognized for native coronary disease, the pathogenic effects of these risk factors are amplified by inherent deficiencies of the vein as a conduit when transposed into the coronary arterial circulation. A multifaceted strategy aimed at prevention of vein graft disease is emerging, elements of which include: continued improvements in surgical technique; more effective antiplatelet drugs; increasingly intensive risk factor modification, in particular early and aggressive lipid-lowering drug therapy; and a number of evolving therapies, such as gene transfer and nitric oxide donor administration, which target vein graft disease at an early and fundamental level. At present, a key measure is to circumvent the problem of vein graft disease by preferential selection of arterial conduits, in particular the internal mammary arteries, for coronary bypass surgery whenever possible.[18]

Extended Use of Arterial Grafting

Bilateral Internal Thoracic Artery Graft. In contrast to the easily demonstrated survival benefit conferred by an ITA graft to the LAD artery, it was more difficult to demonstrate a survival benefit to a second arterial graft. Buxton and colleagues studied 1243 patients undergoing primary CABG with bilateral ITA grafts compared with 1583 patients with single ITA grafts. This group demonstrated a 15% absolute improvement in actuarial survival rates 10 years after CABG with the use of bilateral ITA grafts, as compared with the use of a single ITA graft (10-year survival for bilateral ITA was 86 ± 3% versus 71 ± 5% for a single ITA).[131] Lytle and colleagues similarly demonstrated an improvement in survival at 12 years (79 versus 71%) as well as superior reoperation-free survival (77 versus 62%) among 2001 bilateral and 8123 single ITA graft patients.[132] The impact of selection bias in these studies is difficult to control, however, and although some surgeons have embraced bilateral ITA grafting, it still represents a small minority of cases reported to the STS database.

Complete Arterial Revascularization. The better long-term results achieved with the use of bilateral ITAs and the well-known time-related attrition in patency of venous conduits encouraged the exclusive use of arterial conduits for myocardial revascularization. Complete arterial revascularization can be achieved by a variety of strategies, including composite grafting using exclusively ITAs or secondary arterial conduits such as the RA and the GEA. The use of sequential anastomotic techniques maximizes the utilization of arterial conduits. Although technically demanding, sequential grafting can be performed safely and with excellent long-term results with reported 96% patency rates of 7.5 years of follow-up on 1150 sequential ITA anastomoses.[133]

Tector has championed complete arterial revascularization using bilateral ITAs in a T configuration with end-to-side anastomosis of one ITA as a free graft to the side of the second ITA, which is left as a pedicled graft, combined with liberal use of sequential anastomoses. In his series of 897 patients overall survival was 75%, and freedom from reintervention was 92% 8 years after revascularization.[134] Barner has reported similar encouraging results with composite grafting using one ITA and one RA.[135] Data from randomized studies are beginning to emerge supporting improvement in early outcomes with complete arterial revascularization compared with conventional CABG. Muneretto and associates randomized 200 patients to complete arterial revascularization (left ITA to the LAD artery and composite grafts with the right ITA, RA, or both) versus conventional CABG (left ITA to the LAD artery and SVGs). In midterm follow-up (20 months) superior event-free survival (freedom from non-fatal MI, angina recurrence, graft occlusion, need for percutaneous transluminal coronary angioplasty, and late death) was demonstrable in the complete arterial revascularization patients compared to conventional CABG.[136]

The same group conducted a second randomized trial comparing complete arterial revascularization to conventional CABG (ITA to LAD artery and SVG) in 160 patients older than 70 years of age undergoing first time nonemergent CABG. Early mortality was similar, but at 16 ± 3 months, there were significantly fewer graft occlusions and recurrences of angina among the complete arterial revascularization group. Independent predictors of graft occlusion and angina recurrence were use of SVGs, diabetes, and dyslipidemia.[137] The result of longer follow-up of these trials is still awaited.

CONCLUSION

Coronary artery bypass graft surgery with myocardial perfusion remains an excellent treatment strategy for myocardial ischemia. As the population grows older and acquires more relevant comorbidities, the risk of treatment will increase. New techniques and conduit choices, however, are proving effective as the associated morbidity and mortality of operation continue to decline. Alternative techniques such as off-pump CABG and PCI continue to be assessed against the current, best treatment option, CABG with cardiopulmonary bypass.

KEY POINTS

1. Coronary artery disease is the number one killer of Americans.
2. Coronary artery bypass is advantageous over medical therapy in patients with left main coronary artery stenosis, three-vessel disease with left ventricular dysfunction, two-vessel disease with proximal left anterior descending disease, and in patient with severe ischemia and multivessel disease.
3. The STS risk model for postoperative morbidity and mortality can be found on the STS web site (www.sts.org) and includes 30-day stroke and death rates of 1.6% and 3%, respectively.

4. The left internal mammary to left anterior descending coronary artery bypass graft confers a survival advantage to coronary artery bypass patients. In the BARI trial, patency rates at 1 and 4 years were 98% and 91%, respectively.
5. Skeletonization of the internal mammary artery is associated with reduced incidence of sternal wound complications.
6. Radial artery grafts have better 5 year patency (98% versus 86%) than saphenous vein grafts.
7. Cognitive test performance of patients after coronary artery bypass grafting is no different from that of heart healthy control groups over a 1-year period.
8. Freedom from angina after coronary artery bypass grafting in the BARI trial was 84% at 5 and 10 years.
9. Bilateral compared to single internal mammary artery bypass grafting is associated with improved survival, but the benefit is not noted until about 10 years after operation.

REFERENCES

1. American Heart Association Statistics Committee and Stroke Statistics Subcommittee. Heart disease and stroke statistics—2011 update: a report from the American Heart Association. *Circulation* 2011;123(4):e18-e209. Epub 2010; No abstract available. Erratum in: *Circulation* 2011; 123(6):e240.
2. U.S. Census Bureau: U.S. Interim Projections by Age, Sex, Race, and Hispanic Origin. http://www.census.gov/population/www/projections/usinterimproj/natprojtab02a.pdf. Accessed November 2009.
3. Ferguson TB Jr, Hammill BG, Peterson ED, et al: A decade of change—risk profiles and outcomes for isolated coronary artery bypass grafting procedures, 1990–1999: a report from the STS National Database Committee and the Duke Clinical Research Institute. Society of Thoracic Surgeons. *Ann Thorac Surg* 2002; 73:480.
4. Serruys PW, Morice MC, Kappetein AP, et al: Percutaneous coronary intervention versus coronary-artery bypass grafting for severe coronary artery disease. *NEJM* 2009; 360:961.
5. Shroyer AL, Grover FL, Hattler B, et al: On-pump versus off-pump coronary-artery bypass surgery. Veterans Affairs Randomized On/Off Bypass (ROOBY) Study Group. *NEJM* 2009; 361:1827.
6. Gibbon JH Jr: Application of a mechanical heart and lung apparatus to cardiac surgery. *Minn Med* 1954; 37:171.
7. Sones FM Jr, Shirey EK: Cine coronary arteriography. *Mod Concepts Cardiovasc Dis* 1962; 31:735.
8. Favaloro RG Effler DB, Groves LK, et al: Direct myocardial revascularization with saphenous vein autograft. Clinical experience in 100 cases. *Dis Chest* 1969; 56:279.
9. Johnson WD, Flemma RJ, Lepley D Jr, et al: Extended treatment of severe coronary artery disease: a total surgical approach. *Ann Surg* 1969; 170:460.
10. Eagle KA, Guyton RA, Davidoff R, et al: ACC/AHA 2004 guideline update for coronary artery bypass graft surgery. A report of the American College of Cardiology/American Heart Association Task Force on Practice Guidelines (Committee to Update the 1999 Guidelines for Coronary Artery Bypass Graft Surgery). *Circulation* 2004; 110:e340.
11. Anonymous: Long-term results of prospective randomized study of coronary artery bypass surgery in stable angina pectoris. European Coronary Surgery Study Group. *Lancet* 1982; 2:1173.
12. Anonymous: Coronary artery surgery study (CASS): a randomized trial of coronary artery bypass surgery. Survival data. *Circulation* 1983; 68:939.
13. Anonymous: Eleven-year survival in the Veterans Administration randomized trial of coronary bypass surgery for stable angina. The Veterans Administration Coronary Artery Bypass Surgery Cooperative Study Group. *NEJM* 1984; 311:1333.
14. Shroyer AL, Coombs LP, Peterson ED, et al: The Society of Thoracic Surgeons: 30-day operative mortality and morbidity risk models. *Ann Thorac Surg* 2003; 75:1856.
15. Berger JS, Frye CB, Harshaw Q, et al: Impact of clopidogrel in patients with acute coronary syndromes requiring coronary artery bypass surgery: a multicenter analysis. *J Am Coll Cardiol* 2008; 52:1693.
16. Lehmann KH, von Segesser L, Muller-Glauser W, et al: Internal-mammary coronary artery grafts: is their superiority also due to a basically intact endothelium? *Thorac Cardiovasc Surg* 1989; 37:187.
17. Cox JL, Chiasson DA, Gotlieb AI: Stranger in a strange land: the pathogenesis of saphenous vein graft stenosis with emphasis on structural and functional differences between veins and arteries. *Prog Cardiovasc Dis* 1991; 34:45.
18. Motwani JG, Topol EJ: Aortocoronary saphenous vein graft disease: pathogenesis, predisposition, and prevention. *Circulation* 1998; 97:916.
19. Gitter R, Anderson JM Jr, Jett GK: Influence of milrinone and norepinephrine on blood flow in canine internal mammary artery grafts. *Ann Thorac Surg* 1996; 61:1367.
20. Jett GK, Arcici JM Jr, Hatcher CR Jr, et al: Vasodilator drug effects on internal mammary artery and saphenous vein grafts. *J Am Coll Cardiol* 1988; 11:1317.
21. Gurne O, Chenu P, Buche M, et al: Adaptive mechanisms of arterial and venous coronary bypass grafts to an increase in flow demand. *Heart* 1999; 82:336.
22. Henriquez-Pino JA, Gomes WJ, Prates JC, et al: Surgical anatomy of the internal thoracic artery. *Ann Thorac Surg* 1997; 64:1041.
23. Cohen AJ, Lockman J, Lorberboym M, et al: Assessment of sternal vascularity with single photon emission computed tomography after harvesting of the internal thoracic artery. *J Thorac Cardiovasc Surg* 1999; 118:496.
24. Lorberboym M, Medalion B, Bder O, et al: 99mTc-MDP bone SPECT for the evaluation of sternal ischaemia following internal mammary artery dissection. *Nucl Med Commun* 2002; 23:47.
25. Matsa M, Paz Y, Gurevitch J, et al: Bilateral skeletonized internal thoracic artery grafts in patients with diabetes mellitus. *J Thorac Cardiovasc Surg* 2001; 121:668.
26. Calafiore AM, Vitolla G, Iaco AL, et al: Bilateral internal mammary artery grafting: midterm results of pedicled versus skeletonized conduits. *Ann Thorac Surg* 1999; 67:1637.
27. Noera G, Pensa P, Lodi R, et al: Influence of different harvesting techniques on the arterial wall of the internal mammary artery graft: microscopic analysis. *Thorac Cardiovasc Surg* 1993; 41:16.
28. Gaudino M, Trani C, Glieca F, et al: Early vasoreactive profile of skeletonized versus pedicled internal thoracic artery grafts. *J Thorac Cardiovasc Surg* 2003; 125:638.
29. Gaudino M, Toesca A, Nori SL, et al: Effect of skeletonization of the internal thoracic artery on vessel wall integrity. *Ann Thorac Surg* 1999; 68:1623.
30. Athanasiou T, Crossman MC, Asimakopoulos G, et al: Should the internal thoracic artery be skeletonized? *Ann Thorac Surg* 2004; 77:2238.
31. Raja SG, Dreyfus GD: Internal thoracic artery: to skeletonize or not to skeletonize? *Ann Thorac Surg* 2005; 79:1805.
32. Barner HB, Standeven JW, Reese J: Twelve-year experience with internal mammary artery for coronary artery bypass. *J Thorac Cardiovasc Surg* 1985; 90:668.
33. Loop FD, Lytle BE, Cosgrove DM, et al: Influence of the internal-mammary-artery graft on 10-year survival and other cardiac events. *NEJM* 1986; 314:1.
34. Whitlow PL, Dimas AP, Bashore TM, et al: Relationship of extent of revascularization with angina at one year in the Bypass Angioplasty Revascularization Investigation (BARI). *J Am Coll Cardiol* 1999; 34:1750.
35. Schwartz L, Kip KE, Frye RL, et al: Coronary bypass graft patency in patients with diabetes in the Bypass Angioplasty Revascularization Investigation (BARI). *Circulation* 2002; 106:2652.
36. Tatoulis J, Buxton BF, Fuller JA: Patencies of 2127 arterial to coronary conduits over 15 years. *Ann Thorac Surg* 2004; 77:93.
37. Carpenteier A: Selection of coronary bypass. Anatomic, physiological, and angiographic considerations of vein and mammary artery grafts. Discussion. *J Thorac Cardiovasc Surg* 1975; 70:414.
38. Acar C, Ramsheyi A, Pagny JY, et al: The radial artery for coronary artery bypass grafting: clinical and angiographic results at five years. *J Thorac Cardiovasc Surg* 1998; 116:981.
39. Tatoulis J, Royse AG, Buxton BF, et al: The radial artery in coronary surgery: a 5-year experience—clinical and angiographic results. *Ann Thorac Surg* 2002; 73:143.
40. Aca, C, Jebara VA, Portoghese M, et al: Comparative anatomy and histology of the radial artery and the internal thoracic artery. Implication for coronary artery bypass. *Surg Radiol Anat* 1991; 13:283.
41. Kaufer E, Factor SM, Frame R, Brodman RF: Pathology of the radial and internal thoracic arteries used as coronary artery bypass grafts. *Ann Thorac Surg* 1997; 63:1118.
42. Chardigny C, Jebara VA, Acar C, et al: Vasoreactivity of the radial artery. Comparison with the internal mammary and gastroepiploic arteries with implications for coronary artery surgery. *Circulation* 1993; 88(5 Pt 2):II115.
43. Cable DG, Caccitolo JA, Pearson PJ, et al: New approaches to prevention and treatment of radial artery graft vasospasm. *Circulation* 1998; 98(19 Suppl):10.

44. Shapira OM, Alkon JD, Macron DS, et al: Nitroglycerin is preferable to diltiazem for prevention of coronary bypass conduit spasm. *Ann Thorac Surg* 2000; 70:883.
45. Reyes AT, Frame R, Brodman RF: Technique for harvesting the radial artery as a coronary artery bypass graft. *Ann Thorac Surg* 1995; 59:118.
46. Shima H, Ohno K, Michi K, et al: An anatomical study on the forearm vascular system. *J Craniomaxillofac Surg* 1996; 24:293.
47. Agrifoglio M, Dainese L, Pasotti S, et al: Preoperative assessment of the radial artery for coronary artery bypass grafting: is the clinical Allen test adequate? *Ann Thorac Surg* 2005; 79:570.
48. Tatoulis J, Buxton BF, Fuller JA: Bilateral radial artery grafts in coronary reconstruction: technique and early results in 261 patients. *Ann Thorac Surg* 1998; 66:714.
49. Ronan JW, Perry LA, Barner HB, et al: Radial artery harvest: comparison of ultrasonic dissection with standard technique. *Ann Thorac Surg* 2000; 69:113.
50. Newman RV, Lammle WG: Radial artery harvest using endoscopic techniques. *Heart Surg Forum* 2003; 6:E194.
51. Mussa S, Choudhary BP, Taggart DP: Radial artery conduits for coronary artery bypass grafting: current perspective. *J Thorac Cardiovasc Surg* 2005; 129:250.
52. Denton TA, Trento L, Cohen M, et al: Radial artery harvesting for coronary bypass operations: neurologic complications and their potential mechanisms. *J Thorac Cardiovasc Surg* 2001; 121:951.
53. Moon MR, Barner HB, Bailey MS, et al: Long-term neurologic hand complications after radial artery harvesting using conventional cold and harmonic scalpel techniques. *Ann Thorac Surg* 2004; 78:535.
54. Meharwal ZS, Trehan N: Functional status of the hand after radial artery harvesting: results in 3,977 cases. *Ann Thorac Surg* 2001; 72:1557.
55. Acar C, Jebara VA, Portoghese M, et al: Revival of the radial artery for coronary artery bypass grafting. *Ann Thorac Surg* 1992; 54:652.
56. Desai ND, Cohen EA, Naylor CD, et al: A randomized comparison of radial-artery and saphenous-vein coronary bypass grafts. *NEJM* 2004; 351:2302.
57. Tatoulis J, Buxton BF, Fuller JA, et al: Long-term patency of 1108 radial arterial-coronary angiograms over 10 years. *Ann Thorac Surg* 2009: 88:23.
58. Hadinata IE, Hayward PA, Hare DL, et al: Choice of conduit for the right coronary system: 8-year analysis of Radial Artery Patency and Clinical Outcomes Trial. *Ann Thorac Surg* 2009; 88:1404.
59. Maniar HS, Barner HB, Bailey MS, et al: Radial artery patency: are aortocoronary conduits superior to composite grafting? *J Thorac Cardiovasc Surg* 2003; 76:1498.
60. Jung SH, Song H, Choo SJ, et al: Comparison of radial artery patency according to proximal anastomosis site: direct aorta to radial artery anastomosis is superior to radial artery composite grafting. *J Thorac Cardiovasc Surg* 2009; 138:76.
61. Collins P, Webb CM, Chong CF, et al: Radial artery versus saphenous vein patency randomized trail: five-year angiographic follow-up. *Circ* 2008; 117:2859.
62. Mangano DT and the Multicenter Study of Perioperative Ischemia Research Group: aspirin and mortality from coronary bypass surgery. *NEJM* 2002; 347:1309.
63. Anonymous: The effect of aggressive lowering of low-density lipoprotein cholesterol levels and low-dose anticoagulation on obstructive changes in saphenous-vein coronary-artery bypass grafts. The Post Coronary Artery Bypass Graft Trial Investigators. *NEJM* 1997; 336:153.
64. Hata M, Takayama T, Sezai A, et al: Efficacy of aggressive lipid controlling therapy for preventing saphenous vein graft disease. *Ann Thorac Surg* 2009; 88:1440.
65. Alexander JH, Hafley G, Harrington RA, et al: Efficacy and safety of edifoligide, an E2F transcription factor decoy, for prevention of vein graft failure following coronary artery bypass graft surgery: PREVENT IV: a randomized controlled trial. *JAMA* 2005; 294:2446.
66. Black EA, Guzik TJ, West NE, et al: Minimally invasive saphenous vein harvesting: effects on endothelial and smooth muscle function. *Ann Thorac Surg* 2001; 71:1503.
67. Yun KL, Wu Y, Aharonian V, et al: Randomized trial of endoscopic versus open vein harvest for coronary artery bypass grafting: six-month patency rates. *J Thorac Cardiovasc Surg* 2005; 129:496.
68. Lopes RD, Hafley GE, Allen KB, et al: Endoscopic versus open vein-graft harvesting in coronary-artery bypass surgery. *NEJM* 2009; 361:235.
69. Souza DS, Johansson B, Bojo L, et al. Harvesting the saphenous vein with surrounding tissue for CABG provides long-term graft patency comparable to the left internal thoracic artery: results of a randomized longitudinal trial. *J Thorac Cardiovasc Surg* 2006; 132:373.
70. Wijnberg DS, Boeve WJ, Ebels T, et al: Patency of arm vein grafts used in aorto-coronary bypass surgery. *Eur J Cardiothorac Surg* 1990; 4:510.
71. Christenson JT, Simonet F, Schmuziger M: Sequential vein bypass grafting: tactics and long-term results. *Cardiovasc Surg* 1998; 6:389.
72. Vural KM, Sener E, Tasdemir O: Long-term patency of sequential and individual saphenous vein coronary bypass grafts. *Eur J Cardiothorac Surg* 2001; 19:140.
73. McBride LR, Barner HB: The left internal mammary artery as a sequential graft to the left anterior descending system. *J Thorac Cardiovasc Surg* 1983; 86:703.
74. Bessone LN, Pupello DF, Hiro SP, et al: Sequential internal mammary artery grafting: a viable alternative in myocardial revascularization. *Cardiovasc Surg* 1995; 3:155.
75. Kootstra GJ, Pragliola C, Lanzillo G: Technique of sequential grafting the left internal mammary artery (LIMA) to the circumflex coronary system. *J Cardiovasc Surg* 1993; 34:523.
76. Ochi M, Bessho R, Saji Y, et al: Sequential grafting of the right gastroepiploic artery in coronary artery bypass surgery. *Ann Thorac Surg* 2001; 71:1205.
77. Shapira OM, Alkon JD, Aldea GS, et al: Clinical outcomes in patients undergoing coronary artery bypass grafting with preferred use of the radial artery. *J Card Surg* 1997; 12:381.
78. Hallen A, Bjork L, Bjork VO: Coronary thrombo-endarterectomy. *J Thorac Cardiovasc Surg* 1963; 45:216.
79. Sirivella S, Gielchinsky I, Parsonnet V: Results of coronary artery endarterectomy and coronary artery bypass grafting for diffuse coronary artery disease. *Ann Thorac Surg* 2005; 80:1738.
80. Brenowitz JB, Kayser KL, Johnson WD: Results of coronary artery endarterectomy and reconstruction. *J Thorac Cardiovasc Surg* 1988; 95:1.
81. Livesay JJ, Cooley DA, Hallman GL, et al: Early and late results of coronary endarterectomy. Analysis of 3,369 patients. *J Thorac Cardiovasc Surg* 1986; 92:649.
82. Beretta L, Lemma M, Vanelli P, et al: Coronary "open"endarterectomy and reconstruction: short- and long-term results of the revascularization with saphenous vein versus IMA-graft. *Eur J Cardiothorac Surg* 1992; 6:382.
83. Gill IS, Beanlands DS, Boyd WD, et al: Left anterior descending endartectomy and internal thoracic artery bypass for diffuse coronary disease. *Ann Thorac Surg* 1998; 65:659.
84. Sundt TM, 3rd, Camillo CJ, Mendeloff EN, et al: Reappraisal of coronary endarterectomy for the treatment of diffuse coronary artery disease. *Ann Thorac Surg* 1999; 68:1272.
85. Hammon JW, Stump DA, Butterworth JF, et al: Coronary artery bypass grafting with single cross-clamp results in fewer persistent neuropsychological deficits than multiple clamp or off-pump coronary artery bypass grafting. *Ann Thorac Surg* 2007; 84:1174.
86. Royse AG, Royse CF, Groves KL, et al: Blood flow in composite arterial grafts and effect of native coronary flow. *Ann Thorac Surg* 1999; 68:1619.
87. Rokkas CK and Kouchoukos NT: Surgical management of the severely atherosclerotic ascending aorta during cardiac operations. *Semin Thorac Cardiovasc Surg* 1998; 10:240.
88. Grover FL, Shroyer AL, Hammermeister K, et al: A decade's experience with quality improvement in cardiac surgery using the Veterans Affairs and Society of Thoracic Surgeons national databases. *Ann Surg* 2001; 234:464.
89. Mack MJ, Brown PP, Kugelmass AD, et al: Current status and outcomes of coronary revascularization 1999 to 2002: 148,396 surgical and percutaneous procedures. *Ann Thorac Surg* 2004; 77:761.
90. O'Connor GT, Birkmeyer JD, Dacey LJ, et al: Results of a regional study of modes of death associated with coronary artery bypass grafting. Northern New England Cardiovascular Disease Study Group. *Ann Thorac Surg* 1998; 66:1323.
91. Sergeant P, Lesaffre E, Flameng W, et al: Internal mammary artery: methods of use and their effect on survival after coronary bypass surgery. *Eur J Cardiothorac Surg* 1990; 4:72.
92. Yau JM, Alexander JH, Hafley G, et al: Impact of perioperative myocardial infarction on angiographic and clinical outcomes following coronary artery bypass grafting (from Project of Ex-vivo Vein graft Engineering via Transfection [PREVENT] IV). *Am J Cardiol* 2008; 102:546.
93. Klatte K, Chaitman BR, Theroux P, et al: Increased mortality after coronary artery bypass graft surgery is associated with increased levels of postoperative creatine kinase-myocardial band isoenzyme release: results from the GUARDIAN trial. *J Am Coll Cardiol* 2001; 38:1070.
94. Hashemzadeh K, Dehdilani M: Postoperative cardiac troponin I is an independent predictor of in-hospital death after coronary artery bypass grafting. *J Cardiovasc Surg (Torino)* 2009; 50:403.
95. Hogue CW Jr, Sundt T, 3rd, Barzilai B, et al: Cardiac and neurologic complications identify risks for mortality for both men and women undergoing coronary artery bypass graft surgery. *Anesthesiology* 2001; 95:1074.

96. Rao V, Ivanov J, Weisel RD, et al: Predictors of low cardiac output syndrome after coronary artery bypass. *J Thorac Cardiovasc Surg* 1996; 112:38.
97. Hausmann H, Potapov EV, Koster A, et al: Prognosis after the implantation of an intra-aortic balloon pump in cardiac surgery calculated with a new score. *Circulation* 2002; 106:I203
98. Roach GW, Kanchuger M, Mangano CM, et al: Adverse cerebral outcomes after coronary bypass surgery. Multicenter Study of Perioperative Ischemia Research Group and the Ischemia Research and Education Foundation Investigators. *NEJM* 1996; 335:1857.
99. Dacey LJ, Likosky DS, Leavitt BJ, et al: Perioperative stroke and long-term survival after coronary bypass graft surgery. *Ann Thorac Surg* 2005; 79:532.
100. McKhann GM, Grega MA, Borowicz LM Jr, et al: Is there cognitive decline 1 year after CABG? Comparison with surgical and nonsurgical controls. *Neurology* 2005; 65:991.
101. Frye RL, Kronmal R, Schaff HV, et al: Stroke in coronary artery bypass graft surgery: an analysis of the CASS experience. The participants in the Coronary Artery Surgery Study. *Int J Cardiol* 1992; 36:213.
102. Loop FD, Lytle BW, Cosgrove DM, et al: J. Maxwell Chamberlain memorial paper. Sternal wound complications after isolated coronary artery bypass grafting: early and late mortality, morbidity, and cost of care. *Ann Thorac Surg* 1990; 49:179.
103. Kaiser AB, Kernodle DS, Barg NL, et al: Influence of preoperative showers on staphylococcal skin colonization: a comparative trial of antiseptic skin cleansers. *Ann Thorac Surg* 1988; 45:35.
104. Cimochowski GE, Harostock MD, Brown R, et al: Intranasal mupirocin reduces sternal wound infection after open heart surgery in diabetics and nondiabetics. *Ann Thorac Surg* 2001; 71:1572.
105. Alexander JW, Fischer JE, Boyajian M, et al: The influence of hair-removal methods on wound infections. *Arch Surg* 1983; 118:347.
106. Dohmen PM, Gabbieri D, Weymann A, et al: Reduction in surgical site infection in patients treated with microbial sealant before coronary artery bypass graft surgery: a case-control study. *J Hosp Infect* 2009; 72:119.
107. Olsen MA, Lock-Buckley P, Hopkins D, et al: The risk factors for deep and superficial chest surgical-site infections after coronary artery bypass graft surgery are different. *J Thorac Cardiovasc Surg* 2002; 124:136.
108. Anonymous: Risk factors for deep sternal wound infection after sternotomy: a prospective multicenter study. The Parisian Mediastinitis Study Group. *J Thorac Cardiovasc Surg* 1996; 111:1200.
109. Milano CA, Kesler K, Archibald N, et al: Mediastinitis after coronary artery bypass graft surgery. Risk factors and long-term survival. *Circulation* 1995; 92:2245.
110. Zerr KJ, Furnary AP, Grunkemeier GL, et al: Glucose control lowers the risk of wound infection in diabetics after open heart operations. *Ann Thorac Surg* 1997; 63:356.
111. Furnary AP, Zerr KJ, Grunkemeier GL, et al: Continuous intravenous insulin infusion reduces the incidence of deep sternal wound infection in diabetic patients after cardiac surgical procedures. *Ann Thorac Surg* 1999; 67:352. [See comment in *Ann Thorac Surg* 2000; 69:668.]
112. Ottino G, De Paulis R, Pansini S, et al: Major sternal wound infection after open-heart surgery: a multivariate analysis of risk factors in 2,579 consecutive operative procedures. *Ann Thorac Surg* 1987; 44:173.
113. Gansera B, Schmidtler F, Gilrath G, et al: Does bilateral ITA grafting increase perioperative complications? Outcome of 4462 patients with bilateral versus 4204 patients with single ITA bypass. *Eur J Cardiothorac Surg* 2006; 30:318.
114. Toumpoulis IK, Theakos N, Dunning J: Does bilateral internal thoracic artery harvest increase the risk of mediastinitis? *Interact Cardiovasc Thorac Surg* 2007; 6:787.
115. Pevni D, Uretzky G, Mohr A, et al: Routine use of bilateral skeletonized internal thoracic artery grafting: long-term results. *Circulation* 2008; 118:705.
116. Mangano CM, Diamondstone LS, Ramsay JG, et al: Renal dysfunction after myocardial revascularization: risk factors, adverse outcomes, and hospital resource utilization. The Multicenter Study of Perioperative Ischemia Research Group. *Ann Intern Med* 1998; 128:194.
117. Brown JR, Cochran RP, Dacey LJ, et al: Perioperative increases in serum creatinine are predictive of increased 90-day mortality after coronary artery bypass graft surgery. *Circulation* 2006; 114:I409.
118. Chertow GM, Levy EM, Hammermeister KE, et al: Independent association between acute renal failure and mortality following cardiac surgery. *Am J Med* 1998; 104:343.
119. Samuels LE, Sharma S, Morris RJ, et al: Coronary artery bypass grafting in patients with chronic renal failure: A reappraisal. *J Card Surg* 1996; 11:128.
120. Mentzer RM Jr, Oz MC, Sladen RN, et al: Effects of perioperative nesiritide in patients with left ventricular dysfunction undergoing cardiac surgery: the NAPA trial. *J Am Coll Cardiol* 2007; 49:716.
121. Sezai A, Hata M, Niino T, et al: Influence of continuous infusion of low-dose human atrial natriuretic peptide on renal function during cardiac surgery: a randomized controlled study. *J Am Coll Cardiol* 2009; 54:1058.
122. Sergeant P, Blackstone E, Meyns B: Validation and interdependence with patient-variables of the influence of procedural variables on early and late survival after CABG. K. U. Leuven Coronary Surgery Program. *Eur J Cardiothorac Surg* 1997;12:1.
123. Sergeant P, Blackstone E, Meyns B: Is return of angina after coronary artery bypass grafting immutable, can it be delayed, and is it important? *J Thorac Cardiovasc Surg* 1998; 116:440.
124. Sergeant PT, Blackstone EG, Meyns BP: Does arterial revascularization decrease the risk of infarction after coronary artery bypass grafting? *Ann Thorac Surg* 1998; 66:1.
125. Sergeant P, Blackstone E, Meyns B, et al: First cardiological or cardiosurgical reintervention for ischemic heart disease after primary coronary artery bypass grafting. *Eur J Cardiothorac Surg* 1998; 14:480.
126. BARI investigators: The final 10-year follow-up results of the BARI randomized trial. *J Am Coll Cardiol* 2007; 49:1600.
127. Bourassa MG, Enjalbert M, Campeau L, et al: Progression of atherosclerosis in coronary arteries and bypass grafts: ten years later. *Am J Cardiol* 1984; 53:15.
128. Campeau L, Enjalbert M, Lesperance J, et al: Atherosclerosis and late closure of aortocoronary saphenous vein grafts: sequential angiographic studies at 2 weeks, 1 year, 5 to 7 years, and 10 to 12 years after surgery. *Circulation* 1983; 68(3 Pt 2):II1.
129. Campeau L, Enjalbert M, Lesperance J, et al: The relation of risk factors to the development of atherosclerosis in saphenous-vein bypass grafts and the progression of disease in the native circulation. A study 10 years after aortocoronary bypass surgery. *NEJM* 1984; 311:1329.
130. Bertrand OF, Poirier P, Rodes-Cabau J, et al: A multicentre, randomized, double-blind placebo-controlled trial evaluating rosiglitazone for the prevention of atherosclerosis progression after coronary artery bypass graft surgery in patients with type 2 diabetes. Design and rationale of the VeIn-Coronary aTherOsclerosis and Rosiglitazone after bypass surgery (VICTORY) trial. *Can J Cardiol* 2009; 25:509.
131. Buxton BF, Komeda M, Fuller JA, et al: Bilateral internal thoracic artery grafting may improve outcome of coronary artery surgery. Risk-adjusted survival. *Circulation* 1998; 98(19 Suppl):10.
132. Lytle BW, Blackstone EH, Loop FD, et al: Two internal thoracic artery grafts are better than one. *J Thorac Cardiovasc Surg* 1999; 117:855.
133. Dion R, Glineur D, Derouck D, et al: Long-term clinical and angiographic follow-up of sequential internal thoracic artery grafting. *Eur J Cardiothorac Surg* 2000; 17:407.
134. Tector AJ, McDonald ML, Kress DE, et al: Purely internal thoracic artery grafts: outcomes. *Ann Thorac Surg* 2001; 72:450.
135. Barner HB, Sundt TM, 3rd, Bailey M, et al: Midterm results of complete arterial revascularization in more than 1,000 patients using an internal thoracic artery/radial artery T graft. *Ann Thorac Surg* 2001; 234:447.
136. Muneretto C, Negri A, Manfredi J, et al: Safety and usefulness of composite grafts for total arterial myocardial revascularization: a prospective randomized evaluation. *J Thorac Cardiovasc Surg* 2003; 125:826.
137. Muneretto C, Bisleri G, Negri A, et al: Total arterial myocardial revascularization with composite grafts improves results of coronary surgery in elderly: a prospective randomized comparison with conventional coronary artery bypass. *Circulation* 2003; 108:9.

CHAPTER 22

Myocardial Revascularization without Cardiopulmonary Bypass

Michael E. Halkos
John D. Puskas

INTRODUCTION

Coronary artery bypass grafting (CABG) continues to be a valuable method of myocardial revascularization. Despite the increased prevalence of percutaneous coronary intervention to treat coronary disease, as well as improvements in medical therapy, surgical revascularization will continue to have a major role in patients with coronary disease. Currently, the majority of surgical revascularization is performed with the use of cardiopulmonary bypass, with most surgeons preferring to perform distal anastomoses on an arrested heart. Advocates of this approach cite low morbidity and mortality with outcomes that have continued to improve despite a surgical patient population with increasing comorbid conditions and more advanced and severe coronary disease. However, complications, albeit infrequent, continue to plague a small percentage of patients undergoing coronary artery bypass surgery. These include stroke, renal failure, and respiratory failure. These complications may occur not only because of the systemic inflammatory activation that occurs with extracorporeal circulation, but also because of the manipulation of the aorta required for cannulation, cardiopulmonary bypass, and aortic clamping. Off-pump coronary artery bypass grafting (OPCAB) has been increasingly used over the past decade for surgical coronary revascularization. The interest in off-pump techniques has largely been driven by the increased awareness of the deleterious effects of cardiopulmonary bypass and aortic manipulation. Although many centers have adopted this technique, OPCAB use appears to have reached a plateau in recent years and currently accounts for approximately 22% of coronary artery bypass cases (Data Analyses of the Society of Thoracic Surgeons National Adult Cardiac Database, 2008). For most surgeons, the lack of compelling evidence in randomized controlled trials supporting OPCAB over conventional on-pump coronary artery bypass (CCAB) has been an impediment to implementing this strategy in routine practice. Furthermore, many surgeons consider an off-pump approach more technically challenging, with new risks not familiar to on-pump surgery. It is important to note that the aforementioned randomized trials have enrolled predominantly low-risk patients and have sample sizes that are inadequate to demonstrate differences between groups for infrequently occurring events, such as death, stroke, and myocardial infarction. Nonetheless, randomized controlled trials have almost uniformly demonstrated reduced transfusion requirements, lower postoperative serum myocardial enzyme levels, and shorter length of stay. Moreover, there are many retrospective trials showing a survival benefit as well as reduced morbidity with OPCAB. These retrospective database studies have much larger sample size and include mixed-risk patients. However, inherent selection bias may limit the interpretation of these results, despite advanced statistical methodology. For many surgeons to consider implementing an off-pump approach, the following must be demonstrated: (1) equivalent short- and long-term patency rates; (2) complete revascularization; (3) reduced morbidity and even reduced mortality, especially in high-risk patients; and (4) cost efficiency both in the operating room and during the entire hospitalization. For certain high-risk subgroups, it would appear intuitive that avoiding the systemic effects of cardiopulmonary bypass as well as aortic manipulation would reduce the incidence of specific complications such as stroke and renal failure. However, until definitive studies yield superiority of one technique over the other, the preferred approach will ultimately be left to surgeon's discretion.

PREOPERATIVE CONSIDERATIONS

Surgeon Experience

The adoption of OPCAB into clinical practice requires a commitment to learning a unique skill set that has been associated with improved outcomes in certain patient subgroups. We consider that this is best achieved by routine adoption of OPCAB techniques such that the surgeon can employ this approach in patients likely to derive the most benefit. OPCAB surgery poses unique challenges to a surgeon who is accustomed to operating in a motionless and bloodless field. Furthermore, OPCAB requires an adept first and second assistant to provide exposure on a beating heart as well as excellent anesthesia management to maintain hemodynamics and alert the surgical team of potential hemodynamic problems. Thus, the commitment to OPCAB is usually tied to a belief that the technical challenges inherent in the procedure are worth overcoming so that the patient may benefit from the avoidance of cardiopulmonary bypass. Although the benefit may be small in low-risk patients, it is becoming apparent that certain high-risk subgroups may benefit from minimizing aortic manipulation as well as avoiding the systemic effects of cardiopulmonary bypass.

The inexperienced OPCAB surgeon embarking on the learning curve is best advised to choose his or her initial patients carefully and pay close attention to coronary anatomy as well as important patient variables. The surgeon must come to the operating room with an operative plan that is flexible enough to change as operative findings mandate. Unlike CCAB, in which graft sequence and hemodynamic management are relatively straightforward, OPCAB requires careful consideration of coronary anatomy, confounding patient variables, and attention to hemodynamic fluctuations. Early in a surgeon's experience, it is probably prudent to exclude patients with difficult lateral wall targets, especially multiple lateral wall targets, severe left ventricular dysfunction, left main disease, or other complex cases (Table 22-1). Ideal early candidates for OPCAB include those undergoing elective primary coronary revascularization with good target anatomy, preserved ventricular function, and one to three grafts with easily accessible or no lateral wall targets. When teaching OPCAB to residents, the left anterior descending coronary anastomosis is usually the easiest, given its anterior location. This is usually followed by easily accessible diagonal branches, then inferior wall vessels, and finally, lateral wall targets, which are the most difficult to expose and perform off-pump. As experience is gained in OPCAB, this technique can be safely and effectively applied to the vast majority of patients requiring coronary artery bypass surgery. Just as important, however, is the experience to know when it is better to use cardiopulmonary bypass in patients in which an off-pump approach will be exceedingly difficult, impractical, or poorly tolerated.

TABLE 22-1 Relative Exclusion Criteria during the Early Adoption of OPCAB

Recent myocardial infarction
More than three grafts required, especially multiple lateral wall targets
Left ventricular dysfunction
Intramyocardial coronary arteries
Small or diffusely diseased coronary arteries
Mild to moderate aortic or mitral regurgitation
Redosternotomy
Hemodynamically unstable
Pulmonary hypertension
Urgent/emergent cases
Difficult lateral wall targets
Left main coronary artery disease

Patient Variables

The preoperative evaluation of patients for OPCAB demands careful planning and consideration for certain risk factors. We routinely perform screening carotid duplex ultrasonography on all patients over the age of 65, smokers, those with a carotid bruit, history of transient ischemic attack or stroke, left main coronary disease, peripheral vascular disease, or history of prior carotid intervention. The remainder of the preoperative evaluation is similar to CCAB. In patients with a murmur, dyspnea, aortic or mitral regurgitation, or ventricular dysfunction on cardiac catheterization, preoperative echocardiography is also warranted. It is important to be aware of right ventricular dysfunction, valvular regurgitation, or pulmonary hypertension because positioning during OPCAB can result in dramatic changes in these parameters. Overall, the clinical condition of the patient, the urgency of the operation, and ventricular function need to be carefully assessed to determine whether an off-pump approach will be practical. Although patients operated on more acutely may benefit from an off-pump approach, it is important to have a backup plan explicitly prepared should an OPCAB approach be poorly tolerated. Patients with left ventricular dysfunction from a recent infarct pose a more difficult challenge than those with chronic ventricular dysfunction, with the former being much more sensitive to cardiac manipulation and displacement and more likely to develop intraoperative arrhythmias.

Anesthesia

As in other cardiac operations, all patients require invasive monitoring with a pulmonary artery catheter, arterial line, Foley catheter, and central venous line. We liberally use transesophageal echocardiography to provide valuable information about valvular regurgitation, regional myocardial function, and pulmonary hypertension. In our experience, a well-experienced anesthesia team is essential to maintaining stable hemodynamics and ensuring a smooth and uneventful operation. Unlike CCAB, which requires active coordination among surgeon, anesthesiologist, and perfusionist, the anesthesiologist and surgeon must work especially closely to maintain hemodynamic stability during OPCAB. Instead of relying on cardiopulmonary bypass to ensure adequate perfusion, other maneuvers are required to avoid dramatic fluctuations in hemodynamic status that can have detrimental consequences. Subtle changes in hemodynamic status, gradual elevation in pulmonary artery pressures, frequent boluses, or increased requirement of inotropes and vasopressors to maintain hemodynamic stability, and rhythm changes can herald cardiovascular collapse. Such an event can reliably be avoided if these changes are verbalized and discussed between anesthesiologist and surgeon preemptively. When manipulating the heart, it is important for the surgeon to communicate these abrupt maneuvers to the anesthesia team so that appropriate action can be taken and inappropriate reactions (bolusing vasopressors) avoided. Changes in table position (Trendelenburg) can provide dramatic volume changes that affect cardiac output and blood pressure. Indeed, autotransfusion of intravascular volume from the lower extremities by Trendelenburg positioning should be the first maneuver to maintain hemodynamic stability. Placing the patient in steep Trendelenburg can provide a rapid increase in preload and subsequent cardiac output and blood pressure, whereas reverse Trendelenburg can be helpful in lowering blood pressure if partial aortic clamping is required for proximal anastomoses. We prefer to avoid giving massive volumes of intravenous fluids which requires later postoperative diuresis. Instead, aggressive use of Trendelenburg positioning and judicious use of alpha-adrenergic agents provides stable hemodynamics in the large majority of patients undergoing OPCAB. This includes patients with pulmonary hypertension, mild or moderate ischemic mitral regurgitation, or left ventricular dysfunction in which cardiac manipulation and displacement as well as regional myocardial ischemia may be poorly tolerated without inotropic support. If preload conditions have been optimized, then vasopressor agents such as norepinephrine or Neo-Synephrine may be used to assist with maintaining adequate blood pressure during distal anastomoses. In our experience, effective communication with a well-experienced anesthesiologist is of paramount importance to ensure an uneventful off-pump operation.

Maintaining normothermia is critically important and requires more effort during OPCAB procedures, because the luxury of the cardiopulmonary bypass circuit for rewarming does not exist. This usually can be accomplished by infusing intravenous fluids through warmers, warming inhalational anesthetic agents, maintaining warm room temperatures before and during the procedure, and using convective forced-air warming systems. These can be placed around the patient before draping the patient to maintain normothermia, but sterile systems can also be placed on the lower body and extremities after graft harvesting (Bair Hugger; Arizant Healthcare, Eden Prairie, MN).

At our institution, anticoagulation regimens vary according to surgeon preference. For surgeons in their early experience, a full "pump" dose of heparin is reasonable in the event that conversion to cardiopulmonary bypass becomes necessary. Some of our surgeons continue to implement a full dose with 400 IU/kg to maintain an activated clotting time (ACT) of greater than 400 seconds; others use a half dose or 180 IU/kg, whereas others start with 10,000 U and administer additional doses (3000 IU every half-hour) to maintain an ACT of 275 to 300 seconds. Reversal of anticoagulation with varying doses of protamine is usually administered to facilitate hemostasis.

SURGICAL TECHNIQUE

Preparation

After the induction of anesthesia, patients are positioned, prepped, and draped in an identical fashion to an on-pump procedure. At our institution, patients receive an aspirin rectal suppository (1000 mg) after induction. Aspirin 81 mg and clopidogrel (150 mg postoperatively, then 75 mg/day) are routinely administered early in the postoperative period after mediastinal drainage decreases below 100 cc/h for 4 hours. This has not been associated with an increased risk of mediastinal reexploration.[1] Because of the absence of cardiopulmonary bypass–related coagulopathy, patients may have a relative hypercoagulable perioperative state, which theoretically may jeopardize early graft patency. Bednar and colleagues demonstrated a significantly higher expression of P-selectin, a marker of platelet activity, in the OPCAB patients compared with CCAB patients, suggesting a procoagulant state.[2] For this reason, we administer aspirin preoperatively, aspirin and clopidogrel early postoperatively, and then continue dual antiplatelet therapy in the postoperative period.

Although OPCAB allows for minimally invasive approaches, including small thoracotomy, endoscopic, and robotic-assisted coronary artery bypass, the most common approach is via median sternotomy. Endoscopic radial artery and saphenous vein conduits are harvested simultaneously during internal mammary artery harvest. It is our practice to administer 5000 U of heparin before endoscopic vein harvest to minimize thrombus formation within the conduit during the harvest. Concern over graft quality with endoscopic vein harvest has prompted increased vigilance in atraumatic harvest technique to ensure adequate conduits for bypass.[3] After single or bilateral internal mammary artery harvest, the full heparin dose is administered (see the preceding) and the arterial conduits divided distally. The pericardium is incised in an inverted T configuration, and then incised laterally along the diaphragm to facilitate with cardiac displacement. It is essential to free the left lateral pericardium from the diaphragm to allow the pericardium to be retracted to displace the heart and effectively expose the lateral wall of the left ventricle. Nonetheless, the phrenic nerves must be identified and preserved during pericardial mobilization. With left internal mammary artery harvest, we routinely dissect the vessel distally to the bifurcation to provide a long pedicle. Unlike CCAB, the heart is not decompressed and the extra length is often necessary to avoid tension on the anastomosis during rightward displacement for lateral or inferolateral wall grafting. Dividing or removing the endothoracic fascia, skeletonizing the internal mammary artery during harvest, and dividing the left pericardium vertically toward the left phrenic nerve at the level of the pulmonary artery all provide for extra length and less tension on the anastomosis.

Several pericardial traction sutures are placed to assist with exposure and lateral displacement of the heart. To avoid compression on the right heart during lateral displacement, the right pericardium can be dissected along the diaphragm or the right pleural space opened widely to allow the heart to fall into the right chest during lateral displacement. Additionally, one to two rolled towels placed along the inferior aspect of the right side of the retractor helps to elevate the right side of the sternum to allow the heart to be displaced toward or into the right chest. An important traction suture is the "deep stitch," which is placed approximately two-thirds of the way between the inferior vena cava and left pulmonary vein at the point where the pericardium reflects over the posterior left atrium (Fig. 22-1). Care should be taken with placement of this suture to avoid the underlying descending thoracic aorta, esophagus, left lung, and adjacent inferior pulmonary vein. This suture should be covered with a soft rubber catheter to prevent laceration of the epicardium during retraction. Furthermore, the manual elevation and compression of the heart required to take this stitch may be poorly tolerated in patients with marginal hemodynamics or significant left main coronary artery disease. In that case, grafting and reperfusion of the left anterior descending coronary artery should be accomplished before placing the deep pericardial traction suture.

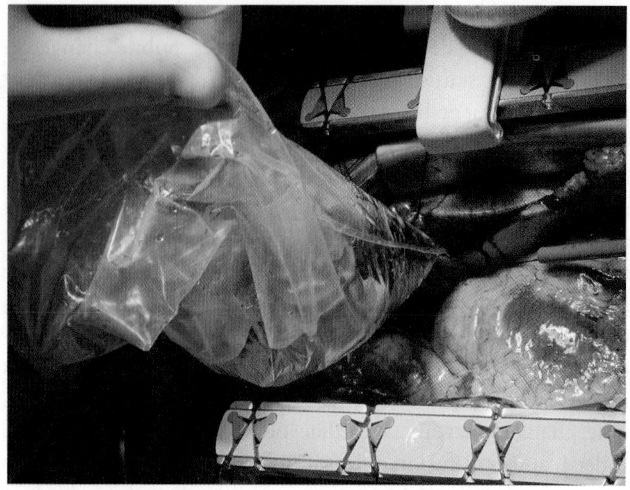

FIGURE 22-2 Epiaortic ultrasonography is performed in all patients prior to aortic manipulation. The 8.5-MHz linear array probe is placed inside a sterile sleeve filled with sterile saline to act as a medium between the probe and the surface of the aorta.

Epiaortic Ultrasound

Epiaortic ultrasonography is used in all of our patients undergoing cardiac surgery. It adds only 2 to 3 minutes to the procedure and provides both the surgeon and the anesthesiologist a simple noninvasive and inexpensive tool for assessing the extent of atheromatous disease in the ascending aorta in preparation for aortic clamping[4] or selection of an alternative clampless technique. Through the operative incision, the ascending aorta from the aortic root to the origin of the innominate artery is scanned directly by the surgeon using an ultrasound probe connected to an echocardiography ultrasound scanner. The 8.5-MHz linear array probe is placed inside a sterile sleeve filled with sterile saline to act as a medium between the probe and the surface of the aorta (Fig. 22-2). The information obtained often dictates changes in operative strategy depending on the grade of atherosclerosis. Similarly, it allows the surgeon to individualize placement of aortic clamps and proximal anastomotic devices to minimize the risk of atheroembolism. Few studies using epiaortic ultrasound for aortic screening have suggested improvements in outcome as a result of intraoperative modifications of the surgical plan.[5–7] Most of these studies have been inadequately powered, limiting the interpretation of their results. However, a study by Rosenberger and coworkers, which evaluated greater than 6000 patients with epiaortic ultrasound, suggested that the operative course was changed in 4% of patients because of the finding of aortic pathology, resulting in improved neurologic outcomes.[8] Smaller studies have shown that epiaortic ultrasonography changed the operative strategy in a larger percentage (10 to 12%) of patients.[5,9,10] Importantly, intraoperative epiaortic ultrasound has been shown to be superior to transesophageal echocardiography or palpation alone in identifying aortic atheromatous lesions, especially in the mid- to distal ascending aorta,[11–13] thus making it the modality of choice in identifying ascending aortic atheroma. Davila-Roman and coworkers also reported that there was greater than 1.5-fold increase in the incidence of both neurologic events and mortality as the severity of atherosclerosis increased from normal-mild to moderate, and a greater than threefold increase in the incidence of death and neurologic events as the severity of atherosclerosis increased from normal-mild to severe[14] (Table 22-2). Schachner et al. also found a higher rate of mortality in patients undergoing CABG that had ascending atheromatous disease.[15] Nonetheless, intraoperative epiaortic ultrasound scanning of the ascending aorta is performed in only a small minority of centers nationwide. More convincing data linking epiaortic ultrasonography to successful intraoperative decision making to reduce postoperative stoke are needed to drive

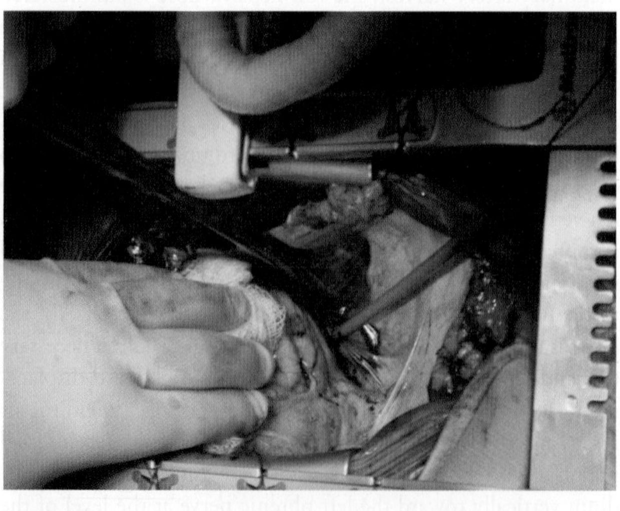

FIGURE 22-1 View from surgeon's side of the table. The heart is elevated toward the surgeon and superiorly for placement of the "deep stitch," which is placed two-thirds of the way between the inferior vena cava and inferior left pulmonary vein. With rightward retraction of the heart, the right-sided pericardial traction sutures should be relaxed to prevent compression of caval inflow.

TABLE 22-2 Epiaortic Ultrasound Grading System Used at Emory University

Epiaortic Ultrasound Grade of Ascending Aorta	Intimal Thickness/Severity of Disease
1	Normal (<2 mm)
2	Mild (2–3 mm)
3	Moderate (3–5 mm)
4	Severe (>5 mm)
5	Mobile plaque, irrespective of thickness

broader adoption and reimbursement of this promising diagnostic modality.

Exposure

Cardiac positioners and stabilizers have greatly increased the ability to manipulate the heart with minimal hemodynamic compromise. Two different systems are routinely used in our institution, the Medtronic Octopus Tissue Stabilizer and Starfish or Urchin Heart Positioner (Medtronic, Inc., Minneapolis, MN) and the Maquet ACROBAT stabilizer and XPOSE positioner (Maquet, GMBH & Co., Radstat, Germany). Cardiac positioning devices are frequently placed off of the apex, especially to the left of the apex, to expose the lateral wall and branches of the left circumflex coronary artery (Figs. 22-3 and 22-4). They are generally placed on the apex to expose the anterior wall (LAD territory) and inferior wall (posterior descending territory) of the heart and may be placed on the acute margin to expose the right coronary artery (Fig. 22-5). Because these suction-based

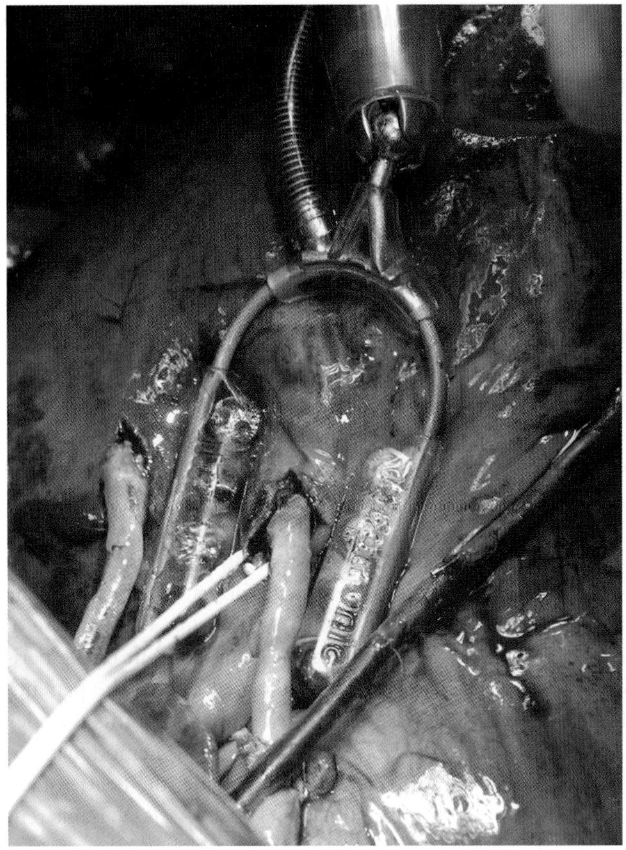

FIGURE 22-4 View from the head of table. An obtuse marginal artery is prepared for grafting. After positioning the coronary stabilizer, a Retract-o-tape is doubly looped around the proximal coronary artery to allow transient occlusion during the anastomosis.

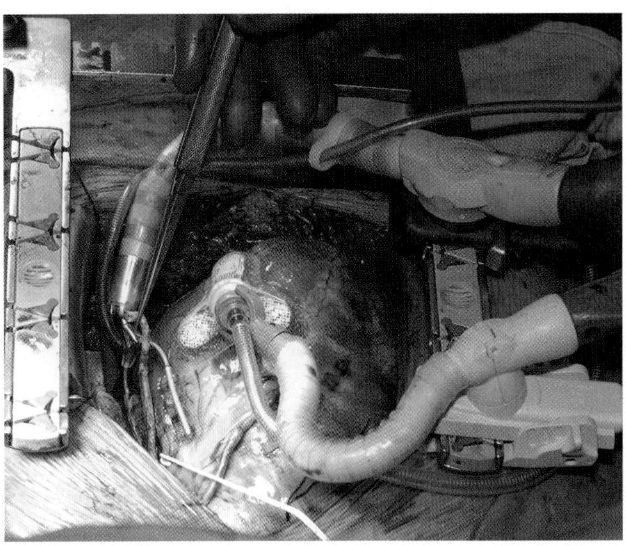

FIGURE 22-3 View from head of table. With the cardiac positioning device placed slightly off of the apex, the lateral wall can be exposed. The coronary stabilizers can then be placed to provide exposure of obtuse marginal vessels.

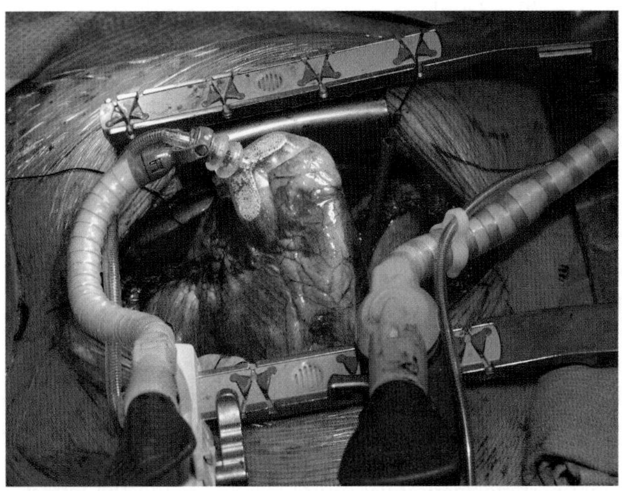

FIGURE 22-5 View from the surgeon's side of table. With cardiac positioner placed on the apex, the heart can be easily displaced to expose the inferior wall vessels. Because there is no compression used for displacement, this maneuver is usually accomplished with no hemodynamic sequelae. Note the positioning of the cardiac positioner and stabilizer on the surgeon's side of the retractor. Alternatively, the stabilizer can be placed on the assistant's side of the retractor. The right pericardial traction sutures are relaxed, and the "deep stitch" is retracted inferolaterally.

cardiac positioning devices pull the heart in the appropriate direction rather than pushing it, the heart is not compressed, functional geometry is maintained, and cardiac positioning is usually well tolerated. The coronary stabilizer devices can then be placed with minimal tension on the epicardium to allow for an area of mechanical stabilization. The anterior wall vessels often require only the coronary stabilizer for adequate exposure. The stabilizer is positioned along the caudal aspect of the retractor toward the left, with the retractor arm placed out of the way to prevent interference during the anastomosis. The location of these devices on the sternal retractor also requires consideration. For the lateral and inferior wall vessels, the cardiac positioner is usually placed on the surgeon's side at the most cephalad location of the retractor. The coronary stabilizers can then be placed on either side. A general rule is to put the stabilizer in the assistant's way instead of the surgeon's to prevent these devices from obstructing the surgeon's view or interfering with hand positioning during suture placement.

In addition to positioners and stabilizers, manipulating the traction sutures can greatly enhance exposure. The purpose of the "deep stitch" is to elevate the heart up and out of the pericardial well. When this suture is retracted toward the patient's feet, it elevates the heart toward the ceiling and points the apex vertically with remarkably little change in hemodynamics. When retracted toward the patient's left side, the heart rotates from left to right, exposing the lateral wall vessels. Variable tension on this stitch will enhance exposure to both the anterior and lateral wall. During positioning, the left-sided pericardial sutures should be pulled taut and the right-sided sutures completely relaxed to avoid compression on the right heart during cardiac displacement. Pericardial sutures on both the right and left sides are never under tension simultaneously when displacing the heart to expose coronary targets. Manipulation of the operating table can also facilitate exposure. Placing the patient in steep Trendelenburg exposes the inferior wall. Turning the table sharply toward the right will aid with exposure of the lateral wall targets. Usually, little manipulation is required for grafting the anterior wall vessels. The deep stitch can be pulled toward the patient's left side and clamped to the drapes or the retractor, and a coronary stabilizer can then be positioned to expose the target coronary artery (Fig. 22-6). Occasionally, a warm moist laparotomy pad can be placed between the heart and the "deep stitch" to assist with elevating the heart out of the pericardium.

In preparation for distal anastomosis, a soft silastic retractor tape mounted on a blunt needle (Retract-o-tape, Quest Medical, Inc., Allen, TX) is placed widely around the proximal vessel for transient occlusion. For inferior wall vessels, this suture can be displaced posteriorly and caudally by tying a more posterior pericardial suture loosely around the retractor tape (Fig. 22-7). The pericardial retraction suture serves as a "pulley" that not only enhances coronary exposure and the surgeon's view, but also keeps this retraction stitch from interfering with the sutures during the anastomosis. Similarly, this maneuver can be done for lateral wall targets. The field is kept free of blood with a humidified CO_2 blower (DLP, Medtronic, Inc.), which is managed by the scrub nurse or second assistant (Fig. 22-8). Occasionally an epicardial fat retractor can be used to expose the coronary target in patients with a large amount of epicardial fat.

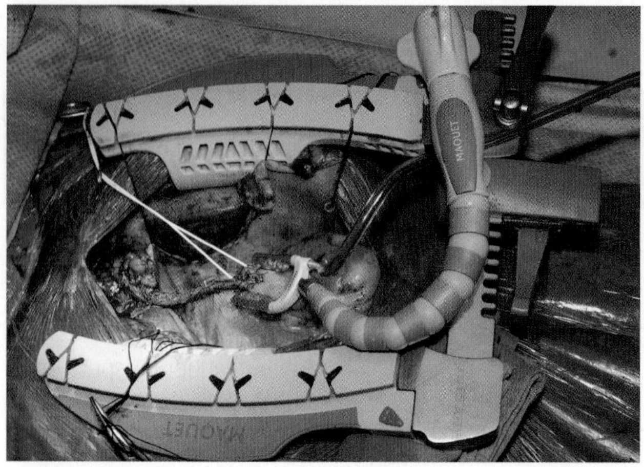

FIGURE 22-6 View from surgeon's side of table. With LAD grafting, excellent exposure can be obtained with lateral traction of the "deep stitch" and the coronary stabilizer. Note the right pericardial traction sutures are released from the retractor.

Although a well-trained first assistant is necessary for providing an effortless anastomosis, the second assistant, often the scrub nurse, also plays a major role in exposure. This assistant usually stands to the right of the surgeon, and controls the CO_2 blower and the Cell Saver (Haemonetics Corp, Braintree, MA). The blower is used to keep the field free of blood, but is also used to open the target vessel and graft during suture placement and can play a vital role in visualization during the anastomosis. During the inferior wall or lateral wall targets, the second assistant may occasionally provide better exposure by standing at the head of the bed, to the surgeon's left. In chronically occluded vessels that have collateral and/or retrograde flow, bleeding into the field can be controlled with another retractor tape distally,

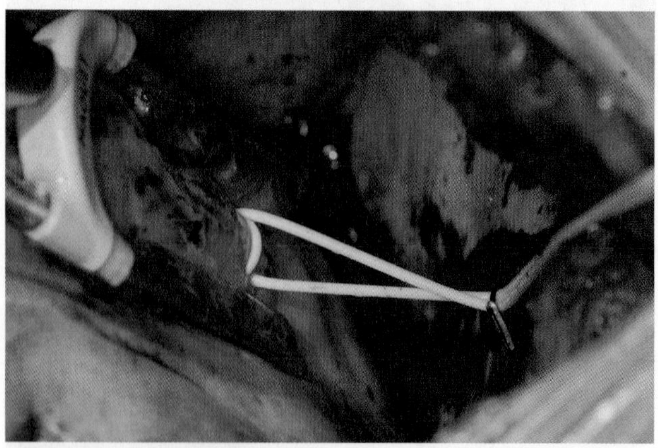

FIGURE 22-7 Close-up view from the surgeon's side of the table. For inferior vessel exposure (posterior descending or left ventricular branch) the Retract-o-tape is positioned as a "pulley" by placing a superficial pericardial traction suture posteriorly (below) to the placement around the coronary artery. A medium clip secures the suture and Retract-o-tape in place which can then be retracted to transiently occlude the artery.

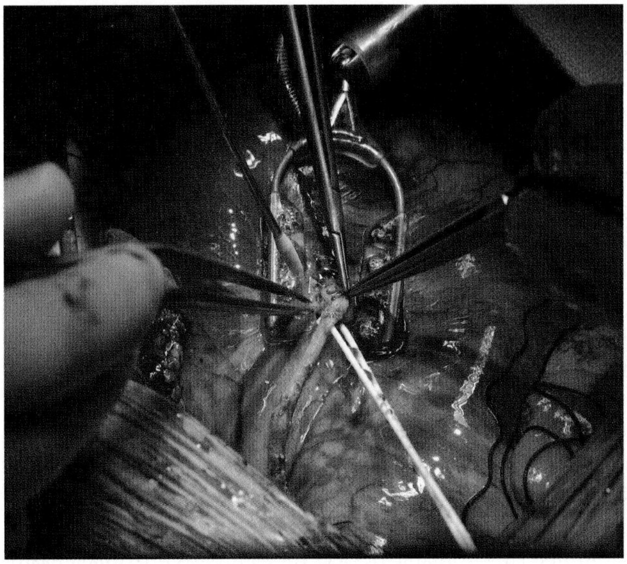

FIGURE 22-8 View from the head of the table. During the anastomosis, a humidified CO_2 blower managed by the second assistant or scrub nurse is used to expose the coronary artery (LAD in this figure).

a MyOcclude device (United States Surgical Corp., Norwalk, CT), or an intracoronary shunt.[16,17] A final preparatory measure is to place temporary atrial or ventricular pacing cables before positioning the heart. As the heart is rotated toward the right, visualization of the right atrium is more difficult, so it is often prudent to place and test these cables before positioning.

Coronary Grafting

The current generation of coronary stabilizers relies on epicardial suction rather than compression to maintain epicardial tissue capture and a motionless field in the region of grafting. A common mistake is to press down too hard on the epicardium, which will paradoxically cause increased movement in the target region. The malleable pods of the stabilizers can be bent or manipulated in any direction to stabilize the target vessel. Generally, gentle compression is applied to allow for epicardial capture. After positioning, the retractor tape can be placed and the coronary artery dissected. If there are concerns about hemodynamic stability during regional ischemia, the proximal vessel can be test occluded for 2 to 5 minutes. During this time the graft can be prepared. This gives the surgeon some assurance before committing to the anastomosis by creating an arteriotomy. After a brief period of reperfusion of 2 to 3 minutes, the vessel can be reoccluded and the artery prepared for anastomosis. The anastomosis is otherwise performed in a manner identical to on-pump grafting. It is essential to continue communication with the anesthesia team so that adequate steps can be promptly taken if hemodynamic conditions deteriorate. For example, if pulmonary artery pressures begin to rise and mean arterial pressures begin to fall during a lateral wall anastomosis, several steps can be taken to avoid cardiovascular collapse. Gently relaxing on the cardiac positioner or coronary stabilizer can often improve hemodynamics. Optimizing table positioning, fluid boluses, inotropes, vasopressors, or pacing may also help. However, if it appears that hemodynamic conditions are deteriorating, then the safe next step is to place an intracoronary shunt,[17] relax, and release both the stabilizer and positioner and allow the heart to recover. At this point a decision must be made to convert "electively" to an on-pump procedure or complete the procedure off-pump. With better preparation (eg, fluids, inotropes, vasopressors, pacing, shunt), the anastomosis can usually be completed off-pump. Another option that is frequently used in patients at high risk for complications of cardiopulmonary bypass is the use of intra-aortic balloon counterpulsation (IABP). An IABP can provide valuable mechanical support during cardiac displacement and positioning to enable safe and controlled completion of a distal anastomosis that would otherwise require cardiopulmonary bypass.

Sequence of Grafting

Careful assessment of the cardiac catheterization is imperative. During on-pump cases, the location and number of vessels requiring bypass usually suffice during evaluation of the catheterization films. However, when planning for OPCAB, particular attention needs to be paid to the collateralizing vessel, intramyocardial vessels, the size of the distal targets, the degree of stenosis, the complexity of coronary disease, and the number of lateral wall vessels requiring grafting. Careful attention must be paid to the sequence of grafting because regional myocardial perfusion is temporarily interrupted in the beating heart (Table 22-3). As

TABLE 22-3 Preferred Sequence of Grafting

Perform anastomosis to completely occluded or collateralized vessel first.
If LAD is not collateralizing vessel, perform LAD-LIMA anastomosis first to allow for anterior wall perfusion during lateral and inferior wall positioning.
Proximal anastomoses can be performed first to allow for perfusion of target vessels after each distal anastomosis. This can be helpful when cardiac positioning is not well tolerated.
Beware of large RCA with moderated proximal stenosis. Acute occlusion can cause bradycardia and hypotension. Be prepared for intracoronary shunt and epicardial pacing.
Patients with moderate MR may not tolerate prolonged cardiac displacement, which can exacerbate MR, and lead to elevated PA pressures and subsequent hemodynamic deterioration. Grafting the culprit causing papillary muscle dysfunction should be vessel performed early in the procedure.

a general rule, the collateralized vessel(s) is grafted first and the collateralizing vessel grafted last. For example, in patients with an occluded right coronary artery with a posterior descending artery supplied by collaterals from the left anterior descending artery, grafting the left anterior descending first would not only leave the anterior wall ischemic, but also disrupt flow to the septum, inferior wall, and right ventricle. Thus, a more reasonable approach would involve grafting the posterior descending artery first, then performing a proximal anastomosis to ensure adequate flow while the proximal left anterior descending is occluded during construction of the LAD anastomosis. Another scenario that may pose problems is a large moderately stenotic right coronary artery. Not uncommonly, temporary occlusion of this artery will result in profound bradycardia and hypotension. In these circumstances, the surgeon must be prepared to use an intracoronary shunt or provide temporary epicardial pacing. Additional options include a "proximals first" approach to allow adequate regional perfusion after completion of each distal anastomosis. Although concern for myocardial protection during OPCAB stems from the brief periods of coronary occlusion necessary to visualize distal target vessels, adequate perfusion can be achieved by maintaining adequate systemic perfusion pressure, selective use of coronary artery shunts, careful use of traction sutures and stabilizers, and proper sequencing of graft anastomoses. Careful placement of intracoronary shunts is important because at least one study demonstrated significant endothelial injury with the use of intracoronary shunts.[18]

Proximal Anastomosis

Traditionally, proximal anastomoses during OPCAB have been performed with the use of an aortic partial-occluding clamp. In preparation for an aortic clamp, the systolic blood pressure is lowered to less than 95 mm Hg. Once the clamp is applied, aortotomies can be made with a 4.0-mm aortic punch device. Proximal anastomoses are then performed using 5-0 or 6-0 polypropylene suture. Before tying down the most anterior proximal, the clamp is released and the aorta de-aired through the proximal anastomosis. After the suture is tied down, the vein grafts can be de-aired with a 25-gauge needle. Arterial grafts are not punctured but are allowed to bleed backward before clamp removal.

Unlike on-pump coronary artery bypass, OPCAB provides the opportunity to minimize or completely avoid manipulation of the aorta. Avoiding partial clamping during proximal anastomoses can be achieved by performing proximal anastomoses to in situ arterial grafts, or using proximal automated anastomotic connectors or facilitating devices.[19–22] This may be particularly relevant in patients with advanced aortic atheromatous disease detected by epiaortic ultrasound. Commercially available devices for clampless proximal anastomoses include the Heartstring III (Maquet Cardiovascular LLC, San Jose, CA) or PAS-Port Proximal Anastomosis System (Cardica Inc., Redwood City, CA). The Heartstring device creates a hemostatic seal with the inner surface of the ascending aorta that allows the creation of a hand-sewn anastomosis with a relatively bloodless field (Fig. 22-9). After completion of the anastomosis, the device is removed by unwinding the sealing cup from the aorta before tying down the suture. However, this device still requires a hand-sewn anastomosis to be performed between the graft and the aorta and can be associated with some blood loss. The PAS-Port Proximal Anastomosis System was specifically designed to create a consistent anastomosis between a saphenous vein graft and the aorta during either on- or off-pump coronary bypass surgery. It is a fully integrated, automated system that cuts the aortotomy and attaches the vein graft to the aorta in seconds, producing

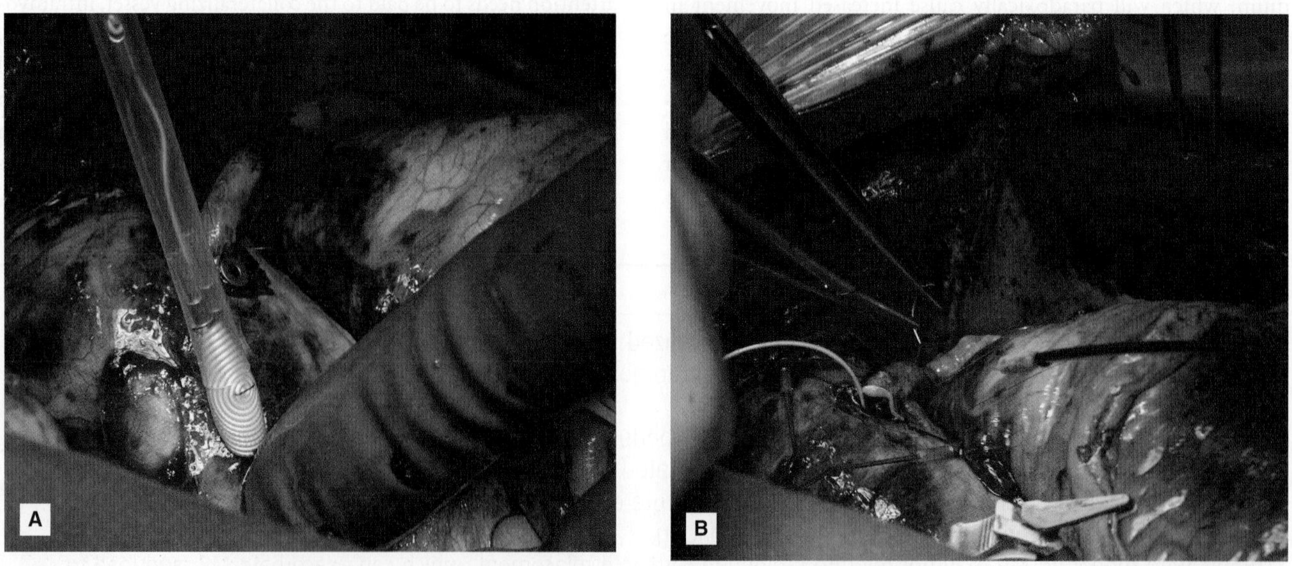

FIGURE 22-9 Proximal anastomoses can be performed without the use of an aortic clamp with either a Heartstring (in these figures) or PAS-Port device. The Heartstring device requires a hand-sewn anastomosis, whereas the PAS-Port device is an automated anastomosis.

consistent, reproducible anastomoses independent of surgical technique and skill.[22–24] Compared with earlier devices, the PAS-Port system allows the endothelium of the vein graft to be untouched during the loading and deployment process. Furthermore, there is no foreign material left within the graft lumen.[23,25–28]

On-Pump Beating Heart Coronary Artery Bypass

Performing coronary artery bypass with cardiopulmonary bypass support is especially useful in certain clinical scenarios such as acute coronary syndromes with cardiogenic shock or in patients with severe left ventricular dysfunction.[29,30] In many occasions, these patients already have tenuous hemodynamics and will not tolerate cardiac positioning and displacement during routine OPCAB maneuvers. One approach is to cannulate the ascending aorta and right atrium and complete the anastomoses on cardiopulmonary bypass with the heart beating but decompressed. This provides for hemodynamic support and also eliminates the global ischemic insult associated with cardioplegic arrest. Grafting can then be performed in a similar sequence as OPCAB. This approach has been supported in several recent studies,[31,32] specifically in the setting of acute coronary syndrome in an attempt to attenuate the ischemic insult associated with regional ischemia from acute coronary occlusion as well as global ischemia associated with cardioplegic arrest. Rastan and colleagues showed improved hospital outcomes in patients with acute coronary syndrome and cardiogenic shock who underwent revascularization with this strategy.[31] Miyahara and coworkers reported lower postoperative morbidity and mortality in patients undergoing emergency myocardial revascularization via an on-pump beating heart approach instead of conventional coronary artery bypass with cardioplegic arrest.[33]

OUTCOMES

Clinical outcomes between OPCAB and CCAB have been compared and reported for over a decade. Even with an abundance of literature, there is still no consensus for the optimal strategy, especially in low-risk patients. In higher-risk patients, it appears in recent studies that OPCAB may reduce both morbidity and mortality. These studies can generally be divided into smaller prospective randomized trials and larger observational or retrospective analyses. Prospective randomized trials provide the most accurate comparison between groups and avoid selection bias and confounding inherent to retrospective and observational analyses. However, these smaller studies are statistically underpowered to detect incremental improvements in morbidity or mortality rates that are already low with CCAB. This is especially true when predominantly low-risk patients are enrolled, which is the case for most of the randomized controlled trials. Furthermore, the cost associated with randomized trials usually prevents patients from being followed for extended periods of time after surgery. Retrospective and observational analyses provide much larger sample sizes with longer duration of follow-up but are limited by their retrospective nature and inherent selection bias despite the use of propensity matching or other advanced statistical methodologies designed to control for confounding variables. Because of their larger size, small differences in outcomes can often be detected. Taken together, both types of studies can provide valuable information to guide clinical practice. Because of the large number of patients required to adequately power important clinical outcomes such as death, stroke, and myocardial infarction, none of the randomized trials, even when analyzed by meta-analysis, are adequately powered to detect clinically or statistically significant differences. For these end points to be powered adequately to demonstrate a benefit in a randomized trial in the current clinical population would require approximately 85,000 patients to demonstrate a difference in death, 6000 patients to analyze any difference in stroke, and 12,000 patients to analyze any difference in myocardial infarction.[34] Most of the earlier trials focused on lower-risk patients. Recent trials, however, have focused on higher-risk cohorts such as elderly patients, those with renal dysfunction, or emergent patients in which a higher incidence of morbidity and mortality is expected.

Operative Mortality

Over the past decade, several randomized trials have documented the safety and efficacy of OPCAB.[28,35–47] However, none of these trials showed an in-hospital mortality advantage for OPCAB compared with CCAB. In a meta-analysis of 37 randomized trials (3369 predominantly low-risk patients), no significant differences were found for 30-day mortality (odds ratio [OR], 1.02; 95% confidence interval [CI] 0.58–1.80).[34] Only one randomized prospective study[48] has demonstrated a reduction in hospital mortality with OPCAB compared with CCAB, and this was in patients who underwent urgent/emergent surgery for ST-segment elevation myocardial infarction.

Several registry studies have been published that are adequately powered to detect differences in mortality outcomes. These retrospective studies, powered by their large sample size, are able to detect significant differences in adverse outcomes among a broad population of patients. In a study by Hannan et al.,[49] 49,830 patients from the New York State registry underwent risk-adjusted analysis (Cox proportional hazard models and propensity analysis) comparing outcomes after OPCAB versus CCAB. In this study, OPCAB patients had significantly lower 30-day mortality (adjusted OR 0.81, 95% CI 0.68 to 0.97, $p = .0022$). In a large registry study of California coronary artery bypass grafting outcomes, Li and colleagues also demonstrated a significant reduction in propensity-adjusted operative mortality with OPCAB compared with ONCAB (2.59% 95% CI 2.52 to 2.67% versus 3.22%, 95% CI 3.17 to 3.27%).[50] An intention-to-treat retrospective analysis of 42,477 patients from the Society of Thoracic Surgeons National Database showed a reduction in risk-adjusted operative mortality (adjusted OR 0.83, $p = .03$) as well as numerous morbidity outcomes favoring

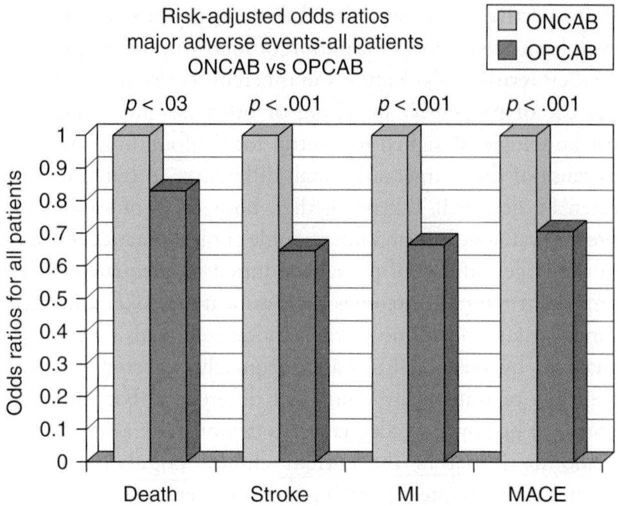

FIGURE 22-10 Risk-adjusted odds ratios for major adverse events in all patients undergoing on-pump coronary artery bypass (ONCAB, patterned bar) versus off-pump procedures (OPCAB, filled bar). MACE = Major adverse cardiac events; MI = myocardial infarction. (*Reproduced with permission from Puskas JD, Edwards FH, Pappas PA, et al: Off-pump techniques benefit men and women and narrow the disparity in mortality after coronary bypass grafting. Ann Thorac Surg 2007; 84(5):1447-1454; discussion 1454-1446.*)

patients undergoing OPCAB[51] (Fig. 22-10). These studies and others[52–56] have demonstrated that operative mortality may be reduced in patients undergoing OPCAB compared with CCAB (Fig. 22-11). Some other studies exist that challenge the aforementioned large registry and STS database conclusions. In a paper by Chu and associates that used an administrative database (Nationwide Inpatient Sample database) of 63,000 patients, there was no difference in hospital mortality between OPCAB and CCAB (3.0% versus 3.2%, $p = .14$).[57] Similarly, Williams and colleagues and Palmer and colleagues failed to show a difference in hospital mortality, although these studies had fewer than 6000 patients.[58,59]

Hospital Mortality in Patients Converted to On-Pump

A major complication of OPCAB is the occasional requirement of emergent conversion to cardiopulmonary support. In these circumstances, there is usually profound and acute hemodynamic compromise, either because of poorly tolerated regional ischemia, increased valvular regurgitation from positioning, bradycardia during right-sided or inferior wall grafting, hypotension during cardiac positioning and stabilization, or intractable ventricular tachycardia/fibrillation. It has become well recognized that an emergent conversion ("crash on pump") to CCAB is associated with significantly higher perioperative morbidity and mortality. There are five studies that quote mortality specifically for converted patients ranging from 6 to 15%.[60–64] Early skeptics of OPCAB appropriately criticized observational comparisons of outcomes after OPCAB versus CCAB because these observational studies were not analyzed on an intent-to-treat basis. Most publications now include patients who were converted urgently or emergently to on-pump in the OPCAB group. In more recent studies, Patel and colleagues reported an increased in-hospital mortality rate of 12% in those converted urgently to CCAB compared with 1.5% in those who did not require urgent conversion ($p = .001$).[65] Similarly, Jin and associates reported results from a large registry of greater than 70,000 patients. In this cohort, 5.8% of patients begun off-pump were converted to on-pump cases. In this group, hospital mortality was also significantly higher in converted patients compared with OPCAB patients or patients initially performed on-pump (9.9% versus 1.6% versus 3.0%, respectively).[66] Importantly, there does not appear to be an increased risk of complications in patients who are *electively* converted to CCAB. This usually occurs when the surgeon or anesthesiologist becomes aware of hemodynamic instability during a test period of regional ischemia or during initial cardiac positioning, displacement, or stabilization. In these circumstances, if these maneuvers are reversed, the hemodynamic status usually improves, and the decision can then be made to proceed with an on-pump approach under more controlled conditions.

Mid- and Long-Term Mortality

Because the previous edition of this textbook, mid- and long-term follow-up data has become available in patients undergoing OPCAB.[41,45,49,52,58,59,67] In all of these studies, which include data from two randomized prospective trials, mid- and long-term survival has been comparable among OPCAB and CCAB patients. In the observational study by Hannan et al., 3-year survival was equivalent in OPCAB versus CCAB patients (adjusted hazard ratio 1.01, 95% CI 0.92 to 1.10, $p = .89$; unadjusted 3-year survival 89.4% versus 90.1%, log-rank test, $p = .20$). Within our own institutional database, 10-year survival of over 12,000 patients was equivalent between OPCAB and CCAB groups.[52] In a long-term follow-up (6 to 8 years) study of two randomized trials, Angelini compared survival outcomes of OPCAB versus CCAB. In this study, there was no difference in long-term survival between the two groups (hazard ratio, 1.24; 95% CI 0.72 to 2.15, $p = .44$).[41] Based on these studies, it is reasonable to conclude that long-term survival after coronary artery bypass surgery is not affected by an on- or off-pump approach.

However, a recent randomized controlled trial (ROOBY) was published which reported a higher 1-year composite outcome of death, repeat revascularization, or nonfatal myocardial infarction for patients undergoing OPCAB compared with CCAB (9.9% versus 7.4%, $p = .04$),[47] although these individual end points were not statistically different. With sensitivity analysis, 1-year death from cardiac causes was slightly higher in the off-pump group compared with the on-pump group (2.7% versus 1.3%, $p = .03$). In this study, a minimum number of 20 cases performed off-pump for each study surgeon was required for study participation (median = 50 cases). The learning curve for OPCAB may extend well beyond this minimum number of cases, which may partly explain the difference in outcomes seen in this study.

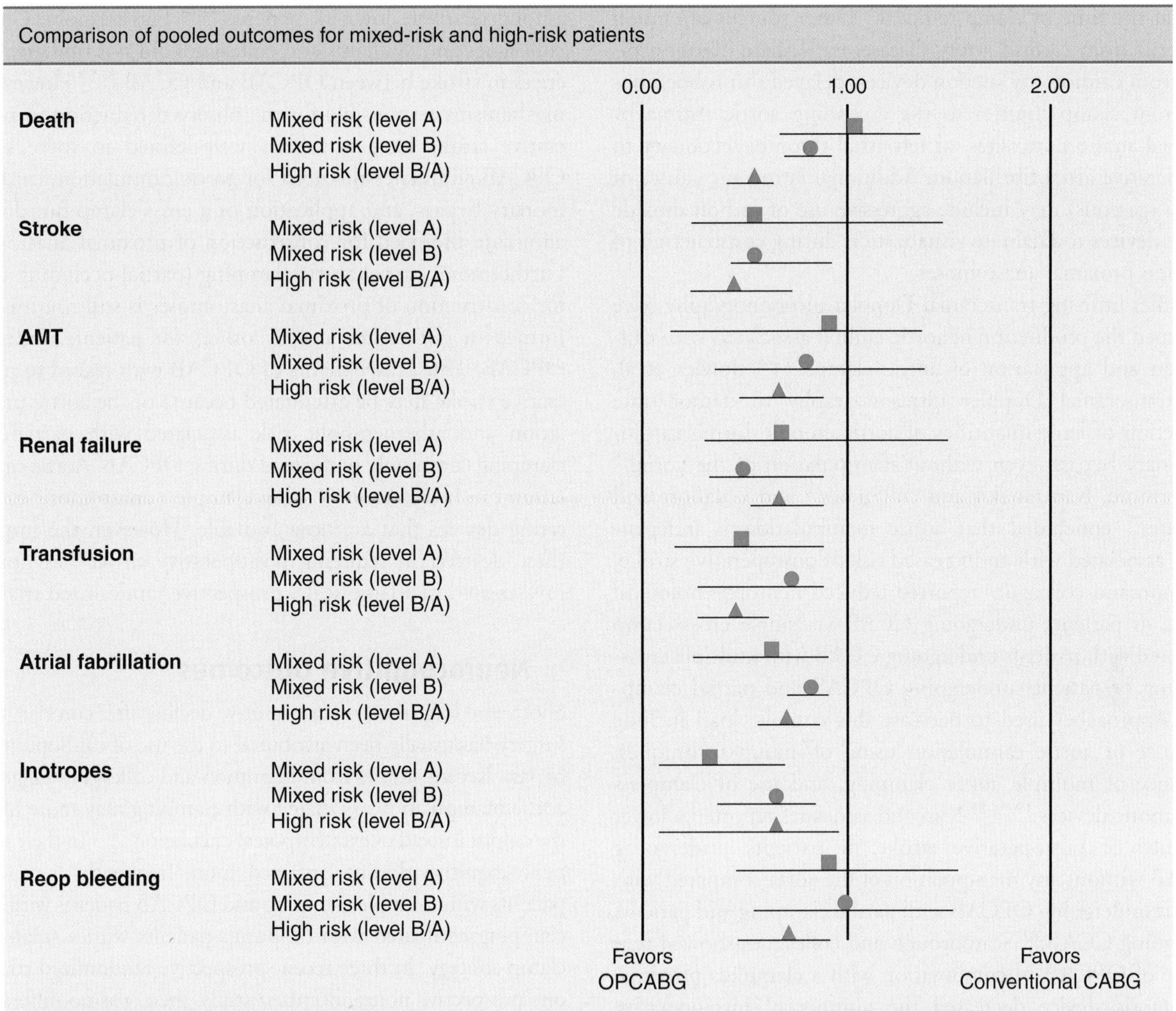

Note: **Mixed-risk patients (level A)** = Cheng 2004 (37 randomized trials; 3369 patients); **mixed-risk patients (level B)** = Beattie 2004 (13 nonrandomized trials; 198, 204 patients) or Reston 2003 (53 trials; 46,621 patients); **high-risk patients (level B/A)** = ISMICS Consensus Meta-analysis 2004 (42 nonrandomized trials and three randomized trials; 26,349 patients),
Used with permission from Puskas et al.

FIGURE 22-11 Comparison of pooled outcomes for mixed-risk and high-risk patients. Mixed-risk patients [Level A] = Cheng 2004 (37 randomized trials; 3369 patients). Mixed-risk patients [Level B] = Beattie 2004 (13 nonrandomized trials; 198,204 patients) or Reston 2003 (53 trials; 46,621 patients). High-risk patients [Level B/A] = ISMICS Consensus Meta-Analysis 2004 (42 nonrandomized trials and three randomized trials; 26,349 patients). (*Reproduced with permission from Puskas J, Cheng D, Knight J, et al: Off-pump versus conventional coronary artery bypass grafting: a meta-analysis and consensus statement from The 2004 ISMICS Consensus Conference. Innovations 2005; 1(1):3-27.*)

Perioperative Morbidity

In a meta-analysis of 37 randomized trials comparing OPCAB with CCAB, OPCAB was associated with a reduced incidence of atrial fibrillation (OR 0.58; 95% CI 0.44 to 0.77), transfusion requirements (OR, 0.43; 95% CI 0.29 to 0.65), inotrope requirements (OR, 0.48; 95% CI, 0.29 to 0.65), respiratory infections (OR, 0.41; 95% CI 0.23 to 0.74), ventilation time (weighted mean difference, –3.4 hours; 95% CI -5.1 to -1.7 hours), intensive care unit stay (OR weighted mean difference, -0.3 days; 95% CI -0.6 to -0.1 days), and hospital stay (weighted mean difference, -1.0 days; 95% CI -1.5 to -0.5 days).[34] However, at least one study has challenged these findings reporting equivalent morbidity outcomes between OPCAB and CCAB,[68] although this trial was relatively small with only 150 patients in each group.

Neurologic Outcomes

Stroke remains a significant cause of morbidity and mortality after coronary artery bypass grafting, occurring in approximately 1 to 14% of patients.[69,70] In addition, long-term survival of post-CABG stroke patients is negatively impacted with reductions in 1- and 5-year survival to 66 and 44% compared with 94 and 81% without stroke.[70] The incremental cost of a postoperative stroke has been reported to be an additional $19,000 to the health system when there are no other associated complications and greater than $58,000 when combined with two or more other complications.[71] As our understanding of the risk factors for stroke has increased, more attention is being focused on the observation that most strokes are embolic in nature. Most cerebral embolic events have been shown to occur at the time of clamp removal.[9] Other sources of emboli can occur from carotid artery disease, particulate matter aspirated from cardiotomy suction devices, delayed thromboembolism from clamp injuries to the ascending aortic intima or proximal anastomotic sites, or left atrial thrombi secondary to postoperative atrial fibrillation. Additional iatrogenic causes of emboli (gaseous) may include aggressive use of carbon dioxide blower devices to facilitate visualization during construction of clampless proximal anastomoses.

Studies utilizing transcranial Doppler ultrasonography have confirmed the production of aortic emboli associated with cannulation and application of aortic clamps.[72–74] Bowles et al. used transcranial Doppler ultrasonography to demonstrate production of large quantities of aortic emboli during cardiopulmonary bypass, even without manipulation of the aorta.[75] Furthermore, Kapetanakis and colleagues[76] and Calafiore and associates[77] concluded that aortic manipulation is independently associated with an increased risk of postoperative stroke. Hammon and colleagues reported reduced neuropsychological deficits in patients undergoing CCAB via single cross-clamp compared with patients undergoing CCAB with multiple cross-clamping or patients undergoing OPCAB and partial clamping.[78] Approaches used to decrease this embolic load include avoidance of aortic cannulation using off-pump techniques, avoidance of multiple aortic clamping, and use of clampless anastomotic devices.[19,79–81] Kim and associates reported a lower incidence of postoperative stroke in patients undergoing OPCAB without any manipulation of the aorta compared with patients undergoing OPCAB with partial clamping and patients undergoing CCAB.[82] Scarborough and colleagues showed that the use of OPCAB in combination with a clampless proximal anastomotic device decreased the number of intraoperative embolic events observed with transcranial Doppler monitoring in comparison with on-pump CABG with hand-sewn proximals.[80] Newer methods advocated to reduce the incidence of stroke include the use of proximal anastomotic devices that avoid the use of an aortic clamp and minimize aortic manipulation (eg, Heartstring or PAS-Port).

There are no prospective randomized trials or meta-analyses of randomized trials that have shown a reduction in stroke with OPCAB compared with CCAB. Large retrospective analyses[49,52,54,56,83,84] have shown that OPCAB may be associated with a reduced incidence of stroke compared with ONCAB. Hannan et al. reported a risk-adjusted decrease in postoperative stroke with OPCAB compared with CCAB (adjusted OR 0.70, 95% CI 0.57 to 0.86, $p = .0006$). Nishiyama and colleagues categorized postoperative strokes according to early (deficit upon awakening from anesthesia) or delayed (patient had a deficit after first awakening from anesthesia without a deficit).[85] In this study, OPCAB was associated with a significant reduction in early stroke compared with CCAB (0.1% versus 1.1%, $p = .0009$). Mishra and colleagues performed a propensity matched comparison of OPCAB versus ONCAB in 6991 patients with atheromatous aortic disease and found a significant decrease in hospital mortality and stroke incidence, with OPCAB being the only independent predictor of a decreased stroke rate.[86] On the contrary, postoperative stroke was not significantly reduced in two recent meta-analyses of off- versus on-pump CABG among relatively low-risk patients.[87,88] Furthermore, Chu and colleagues and Williams and colleagues did not find any differences in stroke between OPCAB and CCAB.[57,59] However, the mechanisms responsible for the observed reduction in postoperative stroke have not been well-defined in these studies. OPCAB eliminates the need for aortic cannulation, cardiopulmonary bypass, and application of a cross-clamp but does not eliminate the need for construction of proximal anastomoses. Furthermore, partial aortic clamping (partial-occluding clamp) for construction of proximal anastomoses is still routinely performed in our center and by others for patients undergoing OPCAB. Thus, the benefits of OPCAB with regard to postoperative stroke may be attenuated because of the aortic manipulation and atheroembolic risk associated with partial aortic clamping commonly performed during OPCAB. Aortic manipulation can be reduced by using clampless anastomotic or facilitating devices that are now available. However, the impact of these devices on reducing postoperative stroke has not been investigated in a large-scale, prospective randomized trial.

Neurocognitive Outcomes

Short- and long-term neurocognitive decline after coronary bypass surgery has usually been attributed to the use of cardiopulmonary bypass. Recent studies from Hammon and colleagues suggest that aortic manipulation associated with clamping may more likely be the culprit instead of extracorporeal circulation.[78,79] In their studies, neurocognitive decline occurred more frequently in on-pump patients with multiple clamping and OPCAB patients with partial clamping compared with on-pump patients with a single cross-clamp strategy. In three recent prospective randomized trials and one prospective nonrandomized study, there was no difference in short- or mid-term neurocognitive deficits between OPCAB and CCAB.[89–91] However, none of these trials differentiated the OPCAB cohort into those in which a partial occluding was used for proximals compared with the use of facilitating or anastomotic clampless devices or in patients in which no aorto-coronary proximal anastomoses were performed.

Renal Failure

Preoperative renal insufficiency is a significant predictor of postoperative renal failure and mortality in patients undergoing CABG.[92] In multiple studies, OPCAB has been shown to reduce morbidity and mortality in patients with normal renal function,[93,94] those with renal dysfunction not yet on hemodialysis[95] as well as those with end-stage renal failure on dialysis.[96] In a prospective randomized trial of 116 diabetic patients with preoperative non–dialysis-dependent renal insufficiency, Sajja et al.[95] demonstrated that the use of cardiopulmonary bypass was significantly associated with an adverse renal outcome. Two retrospective analyses, however, reported equivalent renal outcomes with either OPCAB or CCAB.[97,98] Therefore, the advantages of OPCAB to minimize or avoid renal dysfunction remain controversial.

High-Risk Patients

Several studies have documented improved outcomes in higher-risk patients undergoing OPCAB. Specifically, well-known higher-risk groups such as women, patients with left ventricular dysfunction, prior stroke, renal insufficiency, and previous sternotomy have been investigated retrospectively. Dewey et al. showed improved operative mortality in favor of OPCAB among patients with dialysis-dependent renal failure.[96] In patients with left ventricular dysfunction[99,100] previous sternotomy,[101] advanced age,[101–104] previous stroke,[84] and in female patients,[54] more favorable outcomes have been reported with OPCAB compared with CCAB. In a recent publication, Puskas and colleagues reported that patients in the highest-risk quartile had a significant reduction in hospital mortality with OPCAB compared with CCAB (3.2% versus 6.7%, $p < 0.0001$, OR 0.45 95% CI 0.33 to 0.63, $p < .0001$)[105] (Fig. 22-12).

The safety and feasibility of OPCAB in select emergency situations has been confirmed in several series.[106–109] In a randomized trial, Fattouch and colleagues reported that patients undergoing emergency off-pump revascularization for acute ST-elevation myocardial infarction had a significantly lower in-hospital mortality and lower incidence of low cardiac output syndrome.[106] Locker and colleagues[110] also reported a survival advantage for emergent patients undergoing revascularization without cardiopulmonary bypass. In their study there was a similar incidence of perioperative cardiogenic shock in both groups. In hemodynamically stable patients taken to the operating room during an evolving myocardial infarction, off-pump revascularization appears to be feasible and safe in our experience as well. However, this must be approached with caution for several reasons. Data on patients undergoing truly emergent revascularization off-pump are relatively sparse. In addition, unloading the ventricle with cardiopulmonary bypass lowers the workload and decreases oxygen demand of an ischemic heart and may be beneficial by that mechanism. Finally, those few published studies are limited by selection bias; the most unstable patients are likely to be revascularized using cardiopulmonary bypass, whereas hemodynamically stable patients may be done off-pump. As always, good surgical judgment based on individual patient risk factors and surgeon experience must guide decision making. "Beating heart" coronary bypass implies that the heart will continue to beat throughout the surgical procedure. Although we have performed many urgent and emergent coronary bypass operations off-pump, in our experience patients suffering ischemic arrhythmias are best revascularized on cardiopulmonary bypass. The onset of ischemic arrhythmias during either elective or urgent/emergent OPCAB mandates either immediate revascularization of the likely culprit lesion or prompt conversion to cardiopulmonary bypass in a controlled fashion.

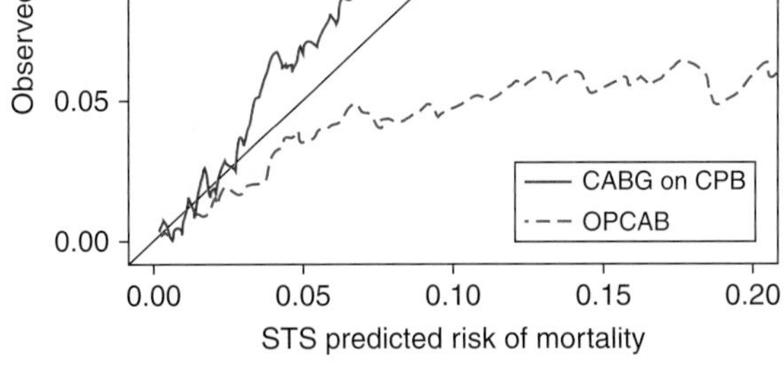

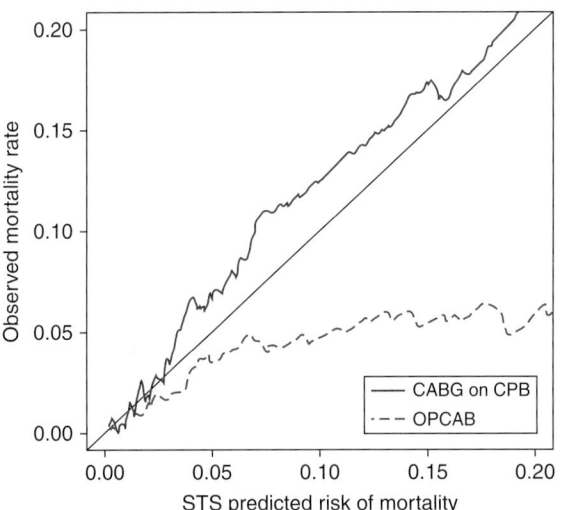

FIGURE 22-12 Regression curve comparison of observed mortality rates for off-pump coronary artery bypass grafting (OPCAB) and coronary artery bypass grafting (CABG) on cardiopulmonary bypass (CPB) across all levels of predicted risk. STS = The Society of Thoracic Surgeons. (*Reproduced with permission from Puskas JD, Thourani VH, Kilgo P, et al: Off-pump coronary artery bypass disproportionately benefits high-risk patients. Ann Thorac Surg 2009; 88(4):1142-1147.*)

Graft Patency, Completeness of Revascularization, and Need for Repeat Revascularization

Completeness of revascularization has been critical for the success and durable benefit of coronary artery bypass surger.[111,112] The detrimental effect of incomplete revascularization on long-term mortality was reported in a study by Synnergren and associates.[112] In this study, leaving two vascular segments without a bypass graft in three-vessel disease was associated with an increased hazard ratio for death (hazard ratio, 1.82; 95% CI, 1.15 to 2.85, $p = .01$). Although incomplete revascularization was more common in the off-pump group, there was no significant influence of the use of on/off-pump techniques after adjusting for incomplete revascularization.

Currently, the ability to provide complete revascularization with OPCAB techniques with equivalent graft patency has been challenged, although the majority of evidence from randomized trials suggests equivalent revascularization.[42,43,68,113,114] In a multicenter study from Veterans Affairs medical centers, Shroyer and colleagues found that fewer grafts completed than originally planned were higher in the OPCAB group (17.8% versus 11.1%). A study by Khan and colleagues found a higher rate of graft failure and incomplete revascularization in patients undergoing OPCAB compared with CCAB by surgeons with relatively little experience in off-pump techniques.[42] A meta-analysis of randomized trials has consistently shown a lower number of grafts per patient in off-pump versus on-pump CABG (2.6 versus 2.8, $p < .0001$).[55] Even analysis of later trials in which surgeon experience was greater still showed fewer grafts performed off-pump versus on-pump (2.7 versus 2.9 grafts).[54] Lattouf and colleagues revealed that patients requiring more than three grafts were more likely to have coronary bypass performed on-pump.[53] In this study, completeness of revascularization rather than number of grafts was associated with an improved long-term survival and that there was no difference in completeness of revascularization among groups. Therefore, completeness of revascularization and number of grafts should not be used synonymously. A common formula has been to divide the number of grafts performed by the number of grafts needed (number of graftable vessels with angiographically significant stenoses) by preoperative assessment of the cardiac catheterization. This value gives an index of complete revascularization. In a study of the Society of Thoracic Surgeons National Cardiac Database by Puskas and colleagues, OPCAB patients had a slightly lower index of complete revascularization than CCAB patients, although operative morbidity and mortality were significantly reduced in patients undergoing OPCAB.[51] In a recent study by Magee and coworkers, the number of grafts was fewer in the OPCAB group (2.75 ± 1.12) compared with the CCAB group (3.36 ± 1.01).[115] However, because the OPCAB group needed fewer grafts, the index of complete revascularization was comparable between OPCAB and CCAB (1.03 and 1.07, respectively). Thus, it appears that selection bias may be partly responsible for this observation, because surgeons may choose to use on-pump techniques on patients requiring more than three grafts. The issue of completeness of revascularization with OPCAB and its impact on long-term survival remains unsettled. Comparisons with older trials may not account for significant improvements in secondary medical prevention strategies or for advances in percutaneous coronary intervention. It is our policy that completeness of revascularization should not be compromised when deciding whether to use or avoid cardiopulmonary bypass unless the use of cardiopulmonary bypass poses obvious and significant risk for postoperative complications or mortality, which may be the case in patients with severe atherosclerotic disease of the ascending aorta. Because we perform the large majority of our coronary operations without cardiopulmonary bypass, complete revascularization, even in the more difficult lateral wall territory, is routinely accomplished.

Graft patency has been evaluated in five randomized trials from in-hospital to 1 year postoperatively. Puskas demonstrated no difference in graft patency at discharge and at 1 year,[114] whereas Khan showed a decreased graft patency in the off-pump group at 3 months.[42] Similarly, Widimsky and associates demonstrated equivalent arterial but reduced vein graft patency in OPCAB patients compared with CCAB patients.[28] Shroyer et al. found that the overall rate of graft patency (driven by vein graft patency) was lower in the OPCAB group compared with the CCAB group (82.6% versus 87.8%, $p < .001$).[47] Three other studies showed no difference in graft patency at 1 year.[26,43,116] Two meta-analyses reported no significant differences between off-pump and on-pump revascularization.[55,117] The largest study to challenge either completeness of revascularization or graft patency is the New York registry data from Hannan et al.[49] Although OPCAB was associated with lower in-hospital mortality and morbidity and equivalent long-term outcomes than CCAB, the need for repeat revascularization was greater in the OPCAB group (93.6% versus 89.9%). Because this was a retrospective analysis, this study was unable to differentiate whether this difference was a result of incomplete revascularization during OPCAB, reduced graft patency, or unrecognized confounding variables.

Minimally Invasive and Hybrid Approaches

Widespread familiarity with off-pump techniques has facilitated the development and application of minimally invasive revascularization procedures. Endoscopic atraumatic coronary artery bypass (EndoACAB) has been well described and involves a thoracoscopic or robotic-assisted left internal mammary artery dissection and harvest, followed by a direct off-pump anastomosis to the left anterior descending coronary artery via a left anterior minithoracotomy[118] (Fig. 22-13). So-called hybrid revascularization, which combines percutaneous intervention to non–left anterior descending targets with EndoACAB, has also been described[119] and is gaining in popularity, and early studies report acceptable outcomes.[120] Totally endoscopic coronary artery bypass, which is facilitated by off-pump and robotic techniques as well as anastomotic facilitating devices, has also been well described, and continued improvement in technology may make this approach more applicable.[121] The feasibility of these alternative minimally invasive approaches has been demonstrated and the use of minimally invasive techniques has generated much enthusiasm in the surgical and interventional communities. Nonetheless, these procedures remain technically challenging and have not become widespread to date.

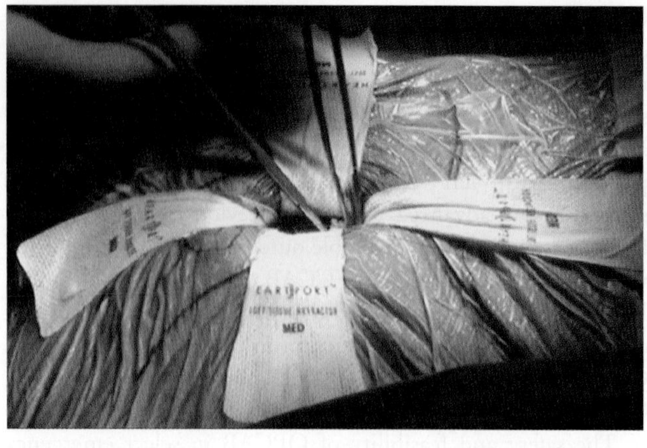

FIGURE 22-13 After endoscopic or robotic-assisted left internal mammary artery harvest, a direct hand-sewn anastomosis can be performed off-pump via a left anterolateral non-rib spreading minithoracotomy.

CONCLUSIONS

Despite the considerable amount of literature comparing OPCAB to CCAB, there is not widespread consensus about the relative advantages of these two techniques. Randomized controlled trials have reported equivalent short- and long-term mortality and major cardiovascular morbidity between groups. However, these trials are frequently underpowered to detect significant outcomes in relatively infrequent adverse events. Furthermore, most of these trials enrolled low-risk patients, thus further reducing their power. Randomized controlled trials have generally shown reduced incidence of myocardial enzyme release, fewer transfusions, shorter length of hospital stay, and reduced cost with OPCAB.[36]

Most retrospective and observational analyses have shown a benefit with regard to in-hospital mortality and both cardiovascular and noncardiac morbidity in favor of OPCAB. Such observational studies are usually larger, have more statistical power to identify significant differences, and include more high-risk patients. Although most evidence points to equivalent completeness of revascularization and short-term graft patency between OPCAB and CCAB, OPCAB patients tend to receive a lower number of grafts, which likely represents a selection bias. Some general conclusions can be made from the available data:

- Low-risk patients undergoing surgical revascularization can be safely revascularized with either off- or on-pump coronary artery bypass.
- With the appropriate use of modern stabilizers and heart positioning devices as well as adequate surgeon experience and careful patient selection, equivalent completeness of revascularization and graft patency can be achieved with OPCAB.
- Certain high-risk groups appear to have better in-hospital morbidity and mortality outcomes when revascularized without the use of cardiopulmonary bypass. This includes patients with advanced ascending aortic atherosclerosis, renal insufficiency, chronic obstructive pulmonary disease, females, and elderly patients. These benefits are likely caused not only by the avoidance of cardiopulmonary bypass, but also by minimizing aortic manipulation.
- Long-term survival outcomes are equivalent in patients undergoing on- or off-pump coronary artery bypass surgery
- There is an improvement in resource utilization with OPCAB, including reduced transfusion requirements, shorter length of stay, less intensive care and ventilator time, and reduced cost.
- The choice of OPCAB versus CCAB requires careful attention to preoperative and intraoperative patient variables that may influence operative circumstances as well as short- and long-term morbidity and mortality. There are certain circumstances in which advantages and disadvantages exist with either approach. Patients with ischemic arrhythmias or cardiogenic shock should be supported on cardiopulmonary bypass for surgical revascularization.
- Urgent or emergent conversion from OPCAB to CCAB is associated with higher in-hospital morbidity and mortality.
- The quality of the anastomosis and the completeness of revascularization should not be compromised when performing off-pump anastomoses. If complete revascularization cannot be performed or precise anastomoses are not possible with off-pump approaches, then an on-pump strategy is preferred, unless cardiopulmonary bypass poses excessive risk to the patient.

REFERENCES

1. Halkos ME, Cooper WA, Petersen R, et al: Early administration of clopidogrel is safe after off-pump coronary artery bypass surgery. *Ann Thorac Surg* 2006;81(3):815-819.
2. Bednar F, Osmancik P, Vanek T, et al: Platelet activity and aspirin efficacy after off-pump compared with on-pump coronary artery bypass surgery: results from the prospective randomized trial PRAGUE 11-Coronary Artery Bypass and REactivity of Thrombocytes (CABARET). *J Thorac Cardiovasc Surg* 2008; 136(4):1054-1060.
3. Lopes RD, Hafley GE, Allen KB, et al: Endoscopic versus open vein-graft harvesting in coronary-artery bypass surgery. *NEJM* 2009;361(3):235-244.
4. Whitley WS, Glas KE: An argument for routine ultrasound screening of the thoracic aorta in the cardiac surgery population. *Semin Cardiothorac Vasc Anesth* 2008; 12(4):290-297.
5. Wareing TH, Davila-Roman VG, Barzilai B, Murphy SF, Kouchoukos NT: Management of the severely atherosclerotic ascending aorta during cardiac operations. A strategy for detection and treatment. *J Thorac Cardiovasc Surg* 1992; 103(3):453-462.
6. Duda AM, Letwin LB, Sutter FP, Goldman SM: Does routine use of aortic ultrasonography decrease the stroke rate in coronary artery bypass surgery? *J Vasc Surg* 1995; 21(1):98-107; discussion 108-109.
7. Staples JR, Tanaka KA, Shanewise JS, et al: The use of the SonoSite ultrasound device for intraoperative evaluation of the aorta. *J Cardiothorac Vasc Anesth* 2004; 18(6):715-718.
8. Rosenberger P, Shernan SK, Loffler M, et al: The influence of epiaortic ultrasonography on intraoperative surgical management in 6051 cardiac surgical patients. *Ann Thorac Surg* 2008; 85(2):548-553.
9. Barbut D, Hinton RB, Szatrowski TP, et al: Cerebral emboli detected during bypass surgery are associated with clamp removal. *Stroke* 1994; 25(12):2398-2402.
10. Djaiani G, Ali M, Borger MA, et al: Epiaortic scanning modifies planned intraoperative surgical management but not cerebral embolic load during coronary artery bypass surgery. *Anesth Analg* 2008; 106(6):1611-1618.
11. Sylivris S, Calafiore P, Matalanis G, et al: The intraoperative assessment of ascending aortic atheroma: epiaortic imaging is superior to both transesophageal echocardiography and direct palpation. *J Cardiothorac Vasc Anesth* 1997; 11(6):704-707.
12. Bolotin G, Domany Y, de Perini L, et al: Use of intraoperative epiaortic ultrasonography to delineate aortic atheroma. *Chest* 2005; 127(1):60-65.
13. Suvarna S, Smith A, Stygall J, et al: An intraoperative assessment of the ascending aorta: a comparison of digital palpation, transesophageal echocardiography, and epiaortic ultrasonography. *J Cardiothorac Vasc Anesth* 2007; 21(6):805-809.
14. Davila-Roman VG, Murphy SF, Nickerson NJ, et al: Atherosclerosis of the ascending aorta is an independent predictor of long-term neurologic events and mortality. *J Am Coll Cardiol* 1999; 33(5):1308-1316.
15. Schachner T, Zimmer A, Nagele G, et al: The influence of ascending aortic atherosclerosis on the long-term survival after CABG. *Eur J Cardiothorac Surg* 2005; 28(4):558-562.
16. Collison SP, Agarwal A, Trehan N: Controversies in the use of intraluminal shunts during off-pump coronary artery bypass grafting surgery. *Ann Thorac Surg* 2006; 82(4):1559-1566.
17. Bergsland J, Lingaas PS, Skulstad H, et al: Intracoronary shunt prevents ischemia in off-pump coronary artery bypass surgery. *Ann Thorac Surg* 2009; 87(1):54-60.
18. Hangler H, Mueller L, Ruttmann E, Antretter H, Pfaller K: Shunt or snare: coronary endothelial damage due to hemostatic devices for beating heart coronary surgery. *Ann Thorac Surg* 2008; 86(6):1873-1877.
19. Guerrieri Wolf L, Abu-Omar Y, Choudhary BP, Pigott D, Taggart DP: Gaseous and solid cerebral microembolization during proximal aortic anastomoses in off-pump coronary surgery: the effect of an aortic side-biting clamp and two clampless devices. *J Thorac Cardiovasc Surg* 2007; 133(2):485-493.
20. Medalion B, Meirson D, Hauptman E, Sasson L, Schachner A: Initial experience with the Heartstring proximal anastomotic system. *J Thorac Cardiovasc Surg* 2004; 128(2):273-277.
21. Akpinar B, Guden M, Sagbas E, et al: Clinical experience with the Novare Enclose II manual proximal anastomotic device during off-pump coronary artery surgery. *Eur J Cardiothorac Surg* 2005; 27(6):1070-1073.
22. Puskas JD, Halkos ME, Balkhy H, et al: Evaluation of the PAS-Port Proximal Anastomosis System in coronary artery bypass surgery (the EPIC trial). *J Thorac Cardiovasc Surg* 2009; 138(1):125-132.
23. Kempfert J, Opfermann UT, Richter M, et al: Twelve-month patency with the PAS-port proximal connector device: a single center prospective randomized trial. *Ann Thorac Surg* 2008; 85(5):1579-1584.
24. Fujii T, Watanabe Y, Shiono N, et al: Study of coronary artery bypass using the PAS-Port device: assessment by multidetector computed tomography. *Gen Thorac Cardiovasc Surg* 2009; 57(2):79-86.
25. Alexander JH, Hafley G, Harrington RA, et al: Efficacy and safety of edifoligide, an E2F transcription factor decoy, for prevention of vein graft failure following coronary artery bypass graft surgery: PREVENT IV: a randomized controlled trial. *JAMA* 2005; 294(19):2446-2454.
26. Magee MJ, Alexander JH, Hafley G, et al: Coronary artery bypass graft failure after on-pump and off-pump coronary artery bypass: findings from PREVENT IV. *Ann Thorac Surg* 2008; 85(2):494-499; discussion 499-500.

27. Schwartz L, Kip KE, Frye RL, et al: Coronary bypass graft patency in patients with diabetes in the Bypass Angioplasty Revascularization Investigation (BARI). *Circulation* 2002; 106(21):2652-2658.
28. Widimsky P, Straka Z, Stros P, et al: One-year coronary bypass graft patency: a randomized comparison between off-pump and on-pump surgery angiographic results of the PRAGUE-4 trial. *Circulation* 2004; 110(22): 3418-3423.
29. Perrault LP, Menasche P, Peynet J, et al: On-pump, beating-heart coronary artery operations in high-risk patients: an acceptable trade-off? *Ann Thorac Surg* 1997; 64(5):1368-1373.
30. Izumi Y, Magishi K, Ishikawa N, Kimura F: On-pump beating-heart coronary artery bypass grafting for acute myocardial infarction. *Ann Thorac Surg* 2006; 81(2):573-576.
31. Rastan AJ, Eckenstein JI, Hentschel B, et al: Emergency coronary artery bypass graft surgery for acute coronary syndrome: beating heart versus conventional cardioplegic cardiac arrest strategies. *Circulation* 2006; 114(1 Suppl):I477-485.
32. Mizutani S, Matsuura A, Miyahara K, et al: On-pump beating-heart coronary artery bypass: a propensity matched analysis. *Ann Thorac Surg* 2007; 83(4):1368-1373.
33. Miyahara K, Matsuura A, Takemura H, et al: On-pump beating-heart coronary artery bypass grafting after acute myocardial infarction has lower mortality and morbidity. *J Thorac Cardiovasc Surg* 2008; 135(3):521-526.
34. Cheng DC, Bainbridge D, Martin JE, Novick RJ: Does off-pump coronary artery bypass reduce mortality, morbidity, and resource utilization when compared with conventional coronary artery bypass? A meta-analysis of randomized trials. *Anesthesiology* 2005; 102(1):188-203.
35. Gerola LR, Buffolo E, Jasbik W, et al: Off-pump versus on-pump myocardial revascularization in low-risk patients with one or two vessel disease: perioperative results in a multicenter randomized controlled trial. *Ann Thorac Surg* 2004; 77(2):569-573.
36. Puskas JD, Williams WH, Duke PG, et al: Off-pump coronary artery bypass grafting provides complete revascularization with reduced myocardial injury, transfusion requirements, and length of stay: a prospective randomized comparison of two hundred unselected patients undergoing off-pump versus conventional coronary artery bypass grafting. *J Thorac Cardiovasc Surg* 2003; 125(4):797-808.
37. Angelini GD, Taylor FC, Reeves BC, Ascione R: Early and midterm outcome after off-pump and on-pump surgery in Beating Heart Against Cardioplegic Arrest Studies (BHACAS 1 and 2): a pooled analysis of two randomised controlled trials. *Lancet* 2002; 359(9313):1194-1199.
38. Kobayashi J, Tashiro T, Ochi M, et al: Early outcome of a randomized comparison of off-pump and on-pump multiple arterial coronary revascularization. *Circulation* 2005; 112(9 Suppl):I338-343.
39. Muneretto C, Bisleri G, Negri A, et al: Off-pump coronary artery bypass surgery technique for total arterial myocardial revascularization: a prospective randomized study. *Ann Thorac Surg* 2003; 76(3):778-782; discussion 783.
40. van Dijk D, Nierich AP, Jansen EW, et al: Early outcome after off-pump versus on-pump coronary bypass surgery: results from a randomized study. *Circulation* 2001; 104(15):1761-1766.
41. Angelini GD, Culliford L, Smith DK, et al: Effects of on- and off-pump coronary artery surgery on graft patency, survival, and health-related quality of life: long-term follow-up of 2 randomized controlled trials. *J Thorac Cardiovasc Surg* 2009; 137(2):295-303.
42. Khan NE, De Souza A, Mister R, et al: A randomized comparison of off-pump and on-pump multivessel coronary-artery bypass surgery. *NEJM* 2004; 350(1):21-28.
43. Nathoe HM, van Dijk D, Jansen EW, et al: A comparison of on-pump and off-pump coronary bypass surgery in low-risk patients. *NEJM* 2003; 348(5):394-402.
44. Ascione R, Williams S, Lloyd CT, et al: Reduced postoperative blood loss and transfusion requirement after beating-heart coronary operations: a prospective randomized study. *J Thorac Cardiovasc Surg* 2001; 121(4): 689-696.
45. Karolak W, Hirsch G, Buth K, Legare JF: Medium-term outcomes of coronary artery bypass graft surgery on pump versus off pump: results from a randomized controlled trial. *Am Heart J* 2007; 153(4):689-695.
46. Fu SP, Zheng Z, Yuan X, et al: Impact of off-pump techniques on sex differences in early and late outcomes after isolated coronary artery bypass grafts. *Ann Thorac Surg* 2009; 87(4):1090-1096.
47. Shroyer AL, Grover FL, Hattler B, et al: On-pump versus off-pump coronary-artery bypass surgery. *NEJM* 2009; 361(19):1827-1837.
48. Fattouch K, Guccione F, Dioguardi P, et al: Off-pump versus on-pump myocardial revascularization in patients with ST-segment elevation myocardial infarction: a randomized trial. *J Thorac Cardiovasc Surg* 2009; 137(3):650-656; discussion 656-657.
49. Hannan EL, Wu C, Smith CR, et al: Off-pump versus on-pump coronary artery bypass graft surgery: differences in short-term outcomes and in long-term mortality and need for subsequent revascularization. *Circulation* 2007; 116(10):1145-1152.
50. Li Z, Yeo KK, Parker JP, et al: Off-pump coronary artery bypass graft surgery in California, 2003 to 2005. *Am Heart J* 2008; 156(6):1095-1102.
51. Puskas JD, Edwards FH, Pappas PA, et al: Off-pump techniques benefit men and women and narrow the disparity in mortality after coronary bypass grafting. *Ann Thorac Surg* 2007; 84(5):1447-1454; discussion 1454-1446.
52. Puskas JD, Kilgo PD, Lattouf OM, et al: Off-pump coronary bypass provides reduced mortality and morbidity and equivalent 10-year survival. *Ann Thorac Surg* 2008; 86(4):1139-1146; discussion 1146.
53. Lattouf OM, Thourani VH, Kilgo PD, et al: Influence of on-pump versus off-pump techniques and completeness of revascularization on long-term survival after coronary artery bypass. *Ann Thorac Surg* 2008; 86(3):797-805.
54. Puskas JD, Kilgo PD, Kutner M, et al: Off-pump techniques disproportionately benefit women and narrow the gender disparity in outcomes after coronary artery bypass surgery. *Circulation* 2007; 116(11 Suppl): I192-199.
55. Puskas J, Cheng D, Knight J, et al: Off-pump versus conventional coronary artery bypass grafting: a meta-analysis and consensus statement from The 2004 ISMICS Consensus Conference. *Innovations* 2005; 1(1):3-27.
56. Reston JT, Tregear SJ, Turkelson CM: Meta-analysis of short-term and mid-term outcomes following off-pump coronary artery bypass grafting. *Ann Thorac Surg* 2003; 76(5):1510-1515.
57. Chu D, Bakaeen FG, Dao TK, et al: On-pump versus off-pump coronary artery bypass grafting in a cohort of 63,000 patients. *Ann Thorac Surg* 2009; 87(6):1820-1826; discussion 1826-1827.
58. Palmer G, Herbert MA, Prince SL, et al: Coronary Artery Revascularization (CARE) registry: an observational study of on-pump and off-pump coronary artery revascularization. *Ann Thorac Surg* 2007; 83(3):986-991; discussion 991-982.
59. Williams ML, Muhlbaier LH, Schroder JN, et al: Risk-adjusted short- and long-term outcomes for on-pump versus off-pump coronary artery bypass surgery. *Circulation* 30 2005; 112(9 Suppl):I366-370.
60. Edgerton JR, Dewey TM, Magee MJ, et al: Conversion in off-pump coronary artery bypass grafting: an analysis of predictors and outcomes. *Ann Thorac Surg* 2003; 76(4):1138-1142; discussion 1142-1133.
61. Mathur AN, Pather R, Widjanarko J, Carrier RC, Garg R: Off-pump coronary artery bypass: the Sudbury experience. *Can J Cardiol* 2003; 19(11):1261-1269.
62. Soltoski P, Salerno T, Levinsky L, et al: Conversion to cardiopulmonary bypass in off-pump coronary artery bypass grafting: its effect on outcome. *J Card Surg* 1998; 13(5):328-334.
63. Iaco AL, Contini M, Teodori G, et al: Off or on bypass: what is the safety threshold? *Ann Thorac Surg* 1999; 68(4):1486-1489.
64. Mujanovic E, Kabil E, Hadziselimovic M, et al: Conversions in off-pump coronary surgery. *Heart Surg Forum* 2003; 6(3):135-137.
65. Patel NC, Patel NU, Loulmet DF, McCabe JC, Subramanian VA: Emergency conversion to cardiopulmonary bypass during attempted off-pump revascularization results in increased morbidity and mortality. *J Thorac Cardiovasc Surg* 2004; 128(5):655-661.
66. Jin R, Hiratzka LF, Grunkemeier GL, Krause A, Page US 3rd: Aborted off-pump coronary artery bypass patients have much worse outcomes than on-pump or successful off-pump patients. *Circulation* 2005; 112(9 Suppl): I332-337.
67. Motallebzadeh R, Bland JM, Markus HS, Kaski JC, Jahangiri M: Health-related quality of life outcome after on-pump versus off-pump coronary artery bypass graft surgery: a prospective randomized study. *Ann Thorac Surg* 2006; 82(2):615-619.
68. Legare JF, Buth KJ, King S, et al: Coronary bypass surgery performed off pump does not result in lower in-hospital morbidity than coronary artery bypass grafting performed on pump. *Circulation* 2004; 109(7): 887-892.
69. Filsoufi F, Rahmanian PB, Castillo JG, Bronster D, Adams DH: Incidence, topography, predictors and long-term survival after stroke in patients undergoing coronary artery bypass grafting. *Ann Thorac Surg* 2008; 85(3):862-870.
70. Puskas JD, Winston AD, Wright CE, et al: Stroke after coronary artery operation: incidence, correlates, outcome, and cost. *Ann Thorac Surg* 2000; 69(4):1053-1056.
71. Brown PP, Kugelmass AD, Cohen DJ, et al: The frequency and cost of complications associated with coronary artery bypass grafting surgery: results from the United States Medicare program. *Ann Thorac Surg* 2008; 85(6):1980-1986.

72. van der Linden J, Casimir-Ahn H: When do cerebral emboli appear during open heart operations? A transcranial Doppler study. *Ann Thorac Surg* 1991; 51(2):237-241.
73. Blauth CI: Macroemboli and microemboli during cardiopulmonary bypass. *Ann Thorac Surg* 1995; 59(5):1300-1303.
74. Barbut D, Yao FS, Lo YW, et al: Determination of size of aortic emboli and embolic load during coronary artery bypass grafting. *Ann Thorac Surg* 1997; 63(5):1262-1267.
75. Bowles BJ, Lee JD, Dang CR, et al: Coronary artery bypass performed without the use of cardiopulmonary bypass is associated with reduced cerebral microemboli and improved clinical results. *Chest* 2001; 119(1):25-30.
76. Kapetanakis EI, Stamou SC, Dullum MK, et al: The impact of aortic manipulation on neurologic outcomes after coronary artery bypass surgery: a risk-adjusted study. *Ann Thorac Surg* 2004; 78(5):1564-1571.
77. Calafiore AM, Di Mauro M, Teodori G, et al: Impact of aortic manipulation on incidence of cerebrovascular accidents after surgical myocardial revascularization. *Ann Thorac Surg* 2002; 73(5):1387-1393.
78. Hammon JW, Stump DA, Butterworth JF, et al: Coronary artery bypass grafting with single cross-clamp results in fewer persistent neuropsychological deficits than multiple clamp or off-pump coronary artery bypass grafting. *Ann Thorac Surg* 2007; 84(4):1174-1178; discussion 1178-1179.
79. Hammon JW, Stump DA, Butterworth JF, et al: Single crossclamp improves 6-month cognitive outcome in high-risk coronary bypass patients: the effect of reduced aortic manipulation. *J Thorac Cardiovasc Surg* 2006; 131(1):114-121.
80. Scarborough JE, White W, Derilus FE, et al: Combined use of off-pump techniques and a sutureless proximal aortic anastomotic device reduces cerebral microemboli generation during coronary artery bypass grafting. *J Thorac Cardiovasc Surg* 2003; 126(5):1561-1567.
81. Mark DB, Newman MF: Protecting the brain in coronary artery bypass graft surgery. *JAMA* 2002; 287(11):1448-1450.
82. Kim KB, Kang CH, Chang WI, et al: Off-pump coronary artery bypass with complete avoidance of aortic manipulation. *Ann Thorac Surg* 2002; 74(4):S1377-1382.
83. Sharony R, Grossi EA, Saunders PC, et al: Propensity case-matched analysis of off-pump coronary artery bypass grafting in patients with atheromatous aortic disease. *J Thorac Cardiovasc Surg* 2004; 127(2): 406-413.
84. Halkos ME, Puskas JD, Lattouf OM, et al: Impact of preoperative neurologic events on outcomes after coronary artery bypass grafting. *Ann Thorac Surg* 2008; 86(2):504-510; discussion 510.
85. Nishiyama K, Horiguchi M, Shizuta S, et al: Temporal pattern of strokes after on-pump and off-pump coronary artery bypass graft surgery. *Ann Thorac Surg* 2009; 87(6):1839-1844.
86. Mishra M, Malhotra R, Karlekar A, Mishra Y, Trehan N: Propensity case-matched analysis of off-pump versus on-pump coronary artery bypass grafting in patients with atheromatous aorta. *Ann Thorac Surg* 2006; 82(2):608-614.
87. Czerny M, Baumer H, Kilo J, et al: Complete revascularization in coronary artery bypass grafting with and without cardiopulmonary bypass. *Ann Thorac Surg* 2001; 71(1):165-169.
88. Alamanni F, Dainese L, Naliato M, et al: On- and off-pump coronary surgery and perioperative myocardial infarction: an issue between incomplete and extensive revascularization. *Eur J Cardiothorac Surg* 2008; 34(1):118-126.
89. van Dijk D, Spoor M, Hijman R, et al: Cognitive and cardiac outcomes 5 years after off-pump vs on-pump coronary artery bypass graft surgery. *JAMA* 2007; 297(7):701-708.
90. Hernandez F Jr, Brown JR, Likosky DS, et al: Neurocognitive outcomes of off-pump versus on-pump coronary artery bypass: a prospective randomized controlled trial. *Ann Thorac Surg* 2007; 84(6):1897-1903.
91. Jensen BO, Hughes P, Rasmussen LS, Pedersen PU, Steinbruchel DA: Cognitive outcomes in elderly high-risk patients after off-pump versus conventional coronary artery bypass grafting: a randomized trial. *Circulation* 2006; 113(24):2790-2795.
92. Cooper WA, O'Brien SM, Thourani VH, et al: Impact of renal dysfunction on outcomes of coronary artery bypass surgery: results from the Society of Thoracic Surgeons National Adult Cardiac Database. *Circulation* 2006; 113(8):1063-1070.
93. Massoudy P, Wagner S, Thielmann M, et al: Coronary artery bypass surgery and acute kidney injury—impact of the off-pump technique. *Nephrol Dial Transplant* 2008; 23(9):2853-2860.
94. Di Mauro M, Gagliardi M, Iaco AL, et al: Does off-pump coronary surgery reduce postoperative acute renal failure? The importance of preoperative renal function. *Ann Thorac Surg* 2007; 84(5):1496-1502.
95. Sajja LR, Mannam G, Chakravarthi RM, et al: Coronary artery bypass grafting with or without cardiopulmonary bypass in patients with preoperative non-dialysis dependent renal insufficiency: a randomized study. *J Thorac Cardiovasc Surg* 2007; 133(2):378-388.
96. Dewey TM, Herbert MA, Prince SL, et al: Does coronary artery bypass graft surgery improve survival among patients with end-stage renal disease? *Ann Thorac Surg* 2006; 81(2):591-598; discussion 598.
97. Schwann NM, Horrow JC, Strong MD 3rd, et al: Does off-pump coronary artery bypass reduce the incidence of clinically evident renal dysfunction after multivessel myocardial revascularization? *Anesth Analg* 2004; 99(4):959-964, table of contents.
98. Asimakopoulos G, Karagounis AP, Valencia O, et al: Renal function after cardiac surgery off- versus on-pump coronary artery bypass: analysis using the Cockroft-Gault formula for estimating creatinine clearance. *Ann Thorac Surg* 2005; 79(6):2024-2031.
99. Youn YN, Chang BC, Hong YS, Kwak YL, Yoo KJ: Early and mid-term impacts of cardiopulmonary bypass on coronary artery bypass grafting in patients with poor left ventricular dysfunction: a propensity score analysis. *Circ J* 2007; 71(9):1387-1394.
100. Darwazah AK, Abu Sham'a RA, Hussein E, Hawari MH, Ismail H: Myocardial revascularization in patients with low ejection fraction < or =35%: effect of pump technique on early morbidity and mortality. *J Card Surg* 2006; 21(1):22-27.
101. Mishra YK, Collison SP, Malhotra R, et al: Ten-year experience with single-vessel and multivessel reoperative off-pump coronary artery bypass grafting. *J Thorac Cardiovasc Surg* 2008; 135(3):527-532.
102. Panesar SS, Athanasiou T, Nair S, et al: Early outcomes in the elderly: a meta-analysis of 4921 patients undergoing coronary artery bypass grafting—comparison between off-pump and on-pump techniques. *Heart* 2006; 92(12):1808-1816.
103. Morris CD, Puskas JD, Pusca SV, et al: Outcomes after off-pump reoperative coronary artery bypass grafting. *Innovations* 2007; 2:29-32.
104. Vohra HA, Bahrami T, Farid S, et al: Propensity score analysis of early and late outcome after redo off-pump and on-pump coronary artery bypass grafting. *Eur J Cardiothorac Surg* 2008; 33(2):209-214.
105. Puskas JD, Thourani VH, Kilgo P, et al: Off-pump coronary artery bypass disproportionately benefits high-risk patients. *Ann Thorac Surg* 2009; 88(4):1142-1147.
106. Fattouch K, Bianco G, Sampognaro R, et al: Off-pump vs. on-pump CABG in patients with ST segment elevation myocardial infarction: a randomized, double-blind study. *American Association for Thoracic Surgery,* 2008; San Diego, CA.
107. Kerendi F, Puskas JD, Craver JM, et al: Emergency coronary artery bypass grafting can be performed safely without cardiopulmonary bypass in selected patients. *Ann Thorac Surg* 2005; 79(3):801-806.
108. Locker C, Mohr R, Paz Y, et al: Myocardial revascularization for acute myocardial infarction: benefits and drawbacks of avoiding cardiopulmonary bypass. *Ann Thorac Surg* 2003; 76(3):771-776; discussion 776-777.
109. Biancari F, Mahar MA, Mosorin M, et al: Immediate and intermediate outcome after off-pump and on-pump coronary artery bypass surgery in patients with unstable angina pectoris. *Ann Thorac Surg* 2008; 86(4): 1147-1152.
110. Locker C, Shapira I, Paz Y, et al: Emergency myocardial revascularization for acute myocardial infarction: survival benefits of avoiding cardiopulmonary bypass. *Eur J Cardiothorac Surg* 2000; 17(3):234-238.
111. Jones EL, Weintraub WS: The importance of completeness of revascularization during long-term follow-up after coronary artery operations. *J Thorac Cardiovasc Surg* 1996; 112(2):227-237.
112. Synnergren MJ, Ekroth R, Oden A, Rexius H, Wiklund L: Incomplete revascularization reduces survival benefit of coronary artery bypass grafting: role of off-pump surgery. *J Thorac Cardiovasc Surg* 2008; 136(1):29-36.
113. Covino E, Santise G, Di Lello F, et al: Surgical myocardial revascularization (CABG) in patients with pulmonary disease: beating heart versus cardiopulmonary bypass. *J Cardiovasc Surg (Torino)* 2001; 42(1):23-26.
114. Puskas JD, Williams WH, Mahoney EM, et al: Off-pump vs conventional coronary artery bypass grafting: early and 1-year graft patency, cost, and quality-of-life outcomes: a randomized trial. *JAMA* 2004; 291(15): 1841-1849.
115. Magee MJ, Hebert E, Herbert MA, et al: Fewer grafts performed in off-pump bypass surgery: patient selection or incomplete revascularization? *Ann Thorac Surg* 2009; 87(4):1113-1118; discussion 1118.
116. Lingaas PS, Hol PK, Lundblad R, et al: Clinical and radiologic outcome of off-pump coronary surgery at 12 months follow-up: a prospective randomized trial. *Ann Thorac Surg* 2006; 81(6):2089-2095.
117. Parolari A, Alamanni F, Polvani G, et al: Meta-analysis of randomized trials comparing off-pump with on-pump coronary artery bypass graft patency. *Ann Thorac Surg* 2005; 80(6):2121-2125.

118. Vassiliades TA, Jr., Reddy VS, Puskas JD, Guyton RA: Long-term results of the endoscopic atraumatic coronary artery bypass. *Ann Thorac Surg* 2007; 83(3):979-984; discussion 984-975.
119. Vassiliades TA Jr, Douglas JS, Morris DC, et al: Integrated coronary revascularization with drug-eluting stents: immediate and seven-month outcome. *J Thorac Cardiovasc Surg* 2006; 131(5):956-962.
120. Vassiliades TA, Kilgo PD, Douglas JS, et al: Clinical outcomes after hybrid coronary revascularization versus off-pump coronary artery bypass. *Innovations* 2009; 4:299-306.
121. Argenziano M, Katz M, Bonatti J, et al: Results of the prospective multicenter trial of robotically assisted totally endoscopic coronary artery bypass grafting. *Ann Thorac Surg* 2006; 81(5):1666-1674; discussion 1674-1665.

CHAPTER 23

Myocardial Revascularization with Carotid Artery Disease

Cary W. Akins
Richard P. Cambria

INTRODUCTION

Next to operative mortality, permanent stroke is the most dreaded complication of myocardial revascularization, not only because of the potential devastating consequences to the patient but also because of the increased cost of hospitalization and posthospital care. Perioperative stroke following coronary artery bypass grafting (CABG) is of increasing concern because as the average age of coronary bypass patients rises, so does the risk of stroke. This chapter investigates the relationship of carotid artery disease to neurologic complications following myocardial revascularization and evaluates treatment options for dealing with severe concomitant carotid and coronary artery disease (CAD).

PERIOPERATIVE STROKE

Incidence of Perioperative Stroke

The risk of stroke coincident with CABG is well defined. In 1986, Gardner and colleagues[1] found the risk of stroke to be a direct function of patient age. Patients younger than 45 years of age had a stroke rate of 0.2%, which rose to 3.0% for patients in their 60s and to 8.0% for patients older than age 75. Other risk factors associated with stroke were preexisting cerebrovascular disease, ascending aortic atherosclerosis, long cardiopulmonary bypass time, and perioperative hypotension.

Tuman and colleagues[2] in 1992 investigated the effect of age on cardiac performance and neurologic injury in coronary bypass patients. Whereas the rates of low cardiac output and myocardial infarction (MI) were constant as patient age increased, the incidence of neurologic damage rose exponentially after age 65. The stroke rate rose from 0.9% for patients younger than 65 years to 8.9% for patients older than age 75.

To place the problem of the increasing patient age into a more contemporary context, at our institution the mean age of coronary artery bypass (CABG) patients rose from 56 years in 1980 to older than 67 years in 2007. In 1980 only 6% of patients were age 70 or older, whereas by 2007 more than 41% were age 70 or older, and 10% were age 80 or older.

In 2000, John and colleagues[3] reported a stroke rate of 1.4% for 19,224 coronary bypass patients from the New York State Cardiac Surgical Database. Multivariable predictors of stroke included aortic calcification, renal failure, prior stroke, smoking, carotid artery disease, age, peripheral vascular disease, and diabetes. In their review of 10,860 patients having primary myocardial revascularization, Puskas and colleagues noted that stroke occurred in 2.2%.[4] Multivariable predictors of stroke were age, previous transient ischemic attack, and carotid bruits.

Cost of Perioperative Stroke

Puskas and colleagues also found that perioperative stroke was associated with significantly more in-hospital morbidity, longer length of stay, and almost twice the hospital cost.[4] Patients who suffered a perioperative stroke had a 23% hospital mortality rate. Roach and colleagues[5] noted a 21% mortality rate for patients suffering a perioperative stroke following coronary artery bypass grafting (CABG), with a mean hospital stay of 25 days among survivors.

Causes of Perioperative Stroke

Possible causes of perioperative neurologic injury are listed in Table 23-1. The most common cause of perioperative stroke is atherosclerotic or thrombotic emboli from the heart or major vessels. Intracardiac emboli can arise from mural thrombus secondary to MI, left atrial thrombus associated with valvular disease or atrial fibrillation, or suture lines in the aorta or left side of the heart. Catheters in the left side of the heart also can be a source of perioperative emboli. Less commonly, entrapped air may cause neurologic events, although rarely focal deficits.

The aorta is also a possible source of emboli. Cannulation of the ascending aorta for bypass, aortic occlusion clamps, and intra-aortic cardioplegia delivery devices may dislodge existing atherosclerotic material from the aorta. Wareing and colleagues[6] found aortic atherosclerosis to be a risk factor for perioperative stroke. Intraoperative echocardiography of the ascending aorta to identify atherosclerosis and the subsequent alteration of operative techniques to address identified problems improved the stroke risk in their patients. Studies that examine the anatomic distribution of perioperative strokes emphasize the importance of cardiac and aortic sources because diffuse anterior and posterior cerebral circulation beds are often affected.[7,8]

Embolism from atherosclerotic carotid bifurcation disease is a well-defined cause of perioperative neurologic injury. Carotid plaque morphology has an important impact on the stroke risk of patients with carotid stenosis. A companion study to the North American Symptomatic Carotid Endarterectomy Trial found that plaque ulceration was a significant incremental risk factor for stroke across all degrees of carotid stenosis.[9]

Many studies list flow-limiting carotid stenosis as a risk factor for perioperative stroke, but whether the carotid lesion is an etiologic factor or only a nonspecific marker of overall risk is unclear.[1,10–12] The Buffalo Cardiac Cerebral Study Group found that although carotid stenosis predicted increased risk of perioperative stroke and death, most strokes occurred more than 24 hours after the myocardial revascularization, and the anatomic distribution of the strokes did not correlate well with the site of the carotid lesion.[12,13]

TABLE 23-1 Potential Causes of Perioperative Neurologic Injury Associated with Coronary Artery Bypass Grafting

Vascular occlusion, usually embolic
Heart
Aorta
Innominate, carotid, or vertebral arteries
Low-flow phenomenon
Insufficient perfusion pressure on cardiopulmonary bypass
Bypass
Poor collateral circulation
Vascular spasm
Intracranial hemorrhage

Neurologic injury can result from inadequate blood flow on cardiopulmonary bypass. Schwartz and colleagues, found that cerebral blood flow depends on arterial perfusion pressures, not on cardiopulmonary bypass flow rates.[14] Low cerebral blood flow occurred with perfusion pressures of less than 60 mm Hg and was not influenced by the pump flow rate. Adequate perfusion pressure is very important in the presence of carotid stenosis, particularly with internal carotid occlusion.[10] Some investigators have shown a linear relationship between the degree of carotid stenosis and the risk of perioperative stroke; in such analyses patients with total ICA occlusion are typically the subgroup at highest risk for stroke.[7] Yet carotid revascularization is not possible in the circumstance of total ICA occlusion. When there is occlusion of carotid or intracerebral arteries, brain blood flow depends on collateral circulation, which, in turn, depends on perfusion pressure. Whether carotid or intracerebral vascular spasm can contribute to neurologic injury is unknown.

Finally, intracranial hemorrhage can lead to neurologic injury following cardiopulmonary bypass, but this is truly rare, despite the fact that patients are fully anticoagulated for cardiopulmonary bypass. We routinely use computed tomographic (CT) scanning to evaluate suspected perioperative stroke to guide anticoagulation, and the finding of primary intracerebral bleeding is extraordinarily uncommon. Indeed in a study of nearly 400 strokes after CABG, investigators of the Northern New England Cardiovascular Study Group identified hemorrhage as the cause of 1% of post-CABG strokes, and hypoperfusion as being responsible in about 10%.[8]

Of the potential causes of perioperative neurologic injury listed in Table 23-1, carotid stenosis is the one situation for which the surgeon can take action to remove the pathology. Because carotid stenosis is a significant risk factor for perioperative stroke, the need to define carotid disease before coronary artery grafting becomes obvious. The logical extension that surgical correction of carotid stenosis can decrease the risk of stroke has been the basis of our approach for many years. Although Level I evidence to support this approach does not exist, the safety of the combined operative approach, which is key to its continued application, has been verified, as will be discussed.

Relationship of Carotid Stenosis to Perioperative Stroke

Early studies relating the presence of carotid stenosis to perioperative stroke used auscultatory evidence of carotid disease as a surrogate for carotid stenosis. In 1988, Reed and colleagues from our institution documented a 3.9-fold increase in the risk for stroke after coronary artery bypass grafting in the presence of a preoperative carotid bruit.[15]

Yet carotid bruits are not reliable indicators of either the presence or degree of carotid stenosis. Sauve and colleagues[16] found poor correlation between carotid bruits and the degree of stenosis. Indeed, as carotid lesions progress to high degrees of stenosis, bruits may become inaudible. Despite these limitations, auscultation for carotid bruits is a common mode of detecting carotid stenosis, particularly in asymptomatic patients.

Currently, Doppler ultrasound–based noninvasive studies are the initially applied and often definitive (and sufficient) diagnostic testing modality for carotid stenosis. Although quality control is essential with noninvasive testing, verification of its accuracy has been demonstrated many times.[17,18]

Brener and colleagues[10] studied 4047 cardiac surgical patients and found a 9.2% rate of stroke or transient ischemic attack in patients with asymptomatic carotid stenosis, significantly greater than the 1.3% rate in patients with no carotid stenosis.

Faggioli and colleagues[19] in 1990 reported that routine carotid noninvasive testing in CABG patients with no ischemic neurologic symptoms yielded an odds ratio for stroke of 9.9 with greater than 75% carotid stenosis. In patients older than age 60 with greater than 75% carotid stenosis, the stroke rate was 15 versus 0.6% for patients of the same age with no carotid disease. Perioperative strokes occurred in 4 (14.3%) of 28 patients who had greater than 75% carotid stenosis who did not have concomitant carotid endarterectomy compared with no strokes in the 19 patients with greater than 75% carotid stenosis who had a prophylactic carotid endarterectomy with their CABG.

In 1992, Berens and colleagues,[20] using routine carotid duplex scanning for cardiac surgical patients 65 years of age or older, found that the risk of stroke was 2.5% for carotid stenoses greater than 50%, 7.6% for carotid stenoses greater than 50%, 10.9% for carotid stenoses greater than 80%, and 10.9% for unilateral carotid artery occlusion.

Thus, adequate evidence exists that significant carotid artery stenosis is an important incremental risk factor for the development of perioperative neurologic injury following CABG. In addition, the study by Faggioli and colleagues[19] suggested that carotid endarterectomy performed with CABG yielded a lower stroke rate.

Mechanism of Perioperative Stroke with Carotid Stenosis

How carotid stenoses cause perioperative strokes is not well understood, especially because patients are fully anticoagulated on cardiopulmonary bypass. Perioperative strokes may result from emboli from the carotid plaque, possibly caused by dynamic plaque events. Loss of pulsatile perfusion or inadequate perfusion pressure on bypass may lead to diminished flow distal to a significant stenosis, resulting in a watershed stroke. Indeed the belief that hypoperfusion is a mechanism whereby carotid lesions cause stroke is indirectly supported by several observations, including the high stroke risk in patients with total ICA occlusion. Hypoperfusion was identified as causing about 10% of strokes in one review of post-CABG stroke pathology.[8] However, Reed and colleagues[15] and Ricotta [12] found that more than one-half of strokes present after the immediate postoperative period. Such delayed strokes in patients with uncorrected carotid stenoses may be related to the prothrombotic milieu that occurs in the early days after cardiopulmonary bypass, potentially causing destabilization of a previously asymptomatic carotid lesion.

Relationship of Uncorrected Carotid Stenosis to Late Stroke

In 1985, Barnes [21] assessed the late risk of untreated asymptomatic carotid stenosis in 65 patients who had cardiovascular operations, of whom 40 had CABG. At mean follow-up of only 22 months, 10% of coronary bypass patients had died, and 17.5% had suffered a stroke. Noninvasive testing revealed progression of the carotid disease in one-half of the patients within 4 years. Ascher reported a 10% risk of stroke after CABG at a mean follow-up interval of 48 months when significant carotid disease was uncorrected, 10-fold higher than patients undergoing combined CABG and carotid endarterectomy.[22] Contemporary randomized trials of surgery versus medical therapy for significant carotid stenosis have defined the late risk of carotid-related stroke in medically treated patients. In the Asymptomatic Carotid Surgery Trial, actuarial risk of stroke at 5 years was 12% in medically treated patients with asymptomatic high-grade carotid stenosis.[23]

CAROTID STENOSIS IN CORONARY ARTERY BYPASS PATIENTS

Incidence of Carotid Stenosis in Coronary Artery Bypass Patients

In 1977, Mehigan and colleagues,[24] used noninvasive testing in 874 patients before coronary grafting and found a 6% incidence of significant extracranial cerebrovascular disease. Ivey and colleagues[25] reported that routine ultrasonic duplex scanning for a history of neurologic events or cervical bruits in 1035 patients having isolated CABG revealed significant carotid artery stenosis in 86 patients (8.3%). Faggioli evaluated 539 neurologically asymptomatic CABG patients and found 8.7% had a carotid stenosis greater than 75%.[19] The rate rose from 3.8% for patients less than age 60 to 11.3% for patients older than age 60. Berens and colleagues, using routine carotid artery scanning in 1087 cardiac surgery candidates 65 years of age or older (91% with coronary disease), found 186 (17.0%) had a greater than 50% carotid stenosis and 65 (5.9%) had a greater than 80% carotid stenosis.[20] Predictors of carotid artery disease were female gender, peripheral vascular disease, history of transient ischemic attacks (TIAs) or stroke, smoking history, and left main CAD. D'Agostino, using noninvasive testing in 1279 CABG candidates, found 262 (20.5%) had greater than 50% stenosis in at least one carotid artery and 23 (1.8%) had bilateral stenoses greater than 80%.[26] Significant multivariable predictors of carotid disease were age, diabetes, female sex, left main CAD, prior stroke, peripheral vascular disease, and smoking.

Virtually all studies have emphasized that patient age is the single highest risk variable. One report demonstrated a dramatic, statistically significant increase in patients older than 60 years of age. Diabetes, smoking, and hypertension were important associated risk factors, such that, with all three risk factors in patients older than age 60, the incidence of significant carotid stenosis nearly doubled from about 8% to 14%.[22]

Diagnosis of Carotid Artery Disease

Essentials of Noninvasive Testing

Ultrasound-based Doppler interrogation for carotid stenosis exploits the Doppler effect; namely, the reflected or altered frequency of an ultrasound wave is shifted in proportion to the velocities of the sampled, flowing blood, which are increased in regions of significant arterial stenosis.

Doppler interrogation produces two data sets—Doppler-shifted flow velocities in regions of interest, and spectral analysis of turbulent flow, which lends a qualitative determination of stenosis severity. Doppler samples must be obtained in the tightest portion of the stenosis for accuracy.

Derived Doppler velocities include peak systolic velocity (PSV), end-diastolic velocity (EDV), and the ratio between the PSV in the internal carotid artery and in the proximal common carotid artery (ICA/CCA ratio). The derived ratio corrects for baseline variations in hemodynamics, such as cardiac output and increased overall flows that might be noted in contralateral internal carotid occlusion. PSV is the single most important criterion, followed by the ICA/CCA ratio. EDV is helpful in discriminating severe versus "very severe" lesions. An ICA/CCA ratio of more than 4.0 equates to a greater than 70% diameter stenosis, the general threshold for a flow-reducing lesion at basal conditions according to the physics of critical arterial stenosis.

Some general comments about the efficacy of ultrasound-based carotid noninvasive tests are in order because many vascular surgeons proceed to carotid endarterectomy based solely on these preoperative studies.[15] Surgeons must be familiar with the specifics of noninvasive diagnostic criteria, and laboratories must have quality-control documentation of accuracy. Thorough knowledge of the translation of ultrasound-derived data to corresponding degrees of internal carotid artery stenosis is necessary.

Indications for Noninvasive Testing

Current indications for screening patients for carotid artery disease before surgical myocardial revascularization include:

1. An audible bruit in the neck
2. History of a prior stroke
3. History of transient ischemic attacks
4. Patients with severe peripheral vascular disease
5. Patients with a prior carotid endarterectomy
6. Elderly patients

All of these indications are self-explanatory except the last. Because the incidence of carotid stenosis rises dramatically in patients older than age 65, there must be an age above which it is cost-effective to screen all patients for carotid disease. However, that age has not yet been determined. One would have to demonstrate the cost advantage of routine carotid endarterectomy versus that of strokes related to uncorrected carotid stenoses.

Role of Carotid Imaging Modalities

Catheter-Based Carotid Angiography. Although catheter-based carotid angiography yields excellent detailed images of the carotid and intracranial vessels, angiography is expensive, requires potentially nephrotoxic contrast material, and is not without risks, including arterial dissection and stroke. Cholesterol embolization owing to catheter manipulation in a diseased aorta can cause emboli to other vascular distributions, especially renal and/or other visceral arteries. (Indeed, in the Asymptomatic Carotid Atherosclerosis Study, one-half of the 2.3% stroke risk with carotid endarterectomy was referable to mandated angiography.[27]) For these reasons, conventional carotid angiography had all but vanished from the practice of many vascular surgeons by the year 2000.[28] Ironically, current enthusiasm for carotid stenting has resurrected carotid angiography as a diagnostic and therapeutic tool.

Magnetic Resonance Angiography. Great enthusiasm in the 1990s arose for magnetic resonance angiography (MRA) to better define carotid lesions. Compared with catheter-based angiography, it was noninvasive, lacked nephrotoxicity, and when used with diffusion-weighted brain imaging, yielded an accurate map of the intracranial circulation. However, its limitations soon became obvious. Magnetic resonance vascular imaging relies on reflected magnetic pulses of flowing blood cells that vary as a function of flow turbulence. Because turbulent flow is characteristic of high-grade carotid stenoses, signal "dropout" in magnetic resonance imaging (MRI) is common. MRA suffers from low specificity with respect to detection of critical stenosis.[29] Indeed, MRA alone can overestimate carotid stenosis severity. Thus, in a reversal of prior algorithms, we insist that stenosis severity information from MRA be verified by a duplex study.

Computed Tomographic Angiography. Computed tomographic angiography (CTA) is the noninvasive test of choice when supplemental information is required after duplex scanning. Although CTA requires iodinated contrast material, it can provide excellent arterial mapping from the aortic arch to the intracranial vasculature, which can be important to both vascular and cardiac surgeons. Accurate assessment of residual lumen diameter within a carotid artery lesion is obtained from both axial and three-dimensional (3D) reconstructed images. Current processing capabilities and the generation of 3D models have improved CTA accuracy in highly calcified lesions.

EFFICACY OF CAROTID ENDARTERECTOMY AS A TREATMENT FOR CAROTID STENOSIS

C. Miller Fisher's original description of the relationship of ipsilateral hemispheric stroke to internal carotid artery occlusion in 1951[30] was followed by Eastcott's description of surgical therapy for symptomatic carotid artery atherosclerosis in 1953.[31] Thereafter, carotid endarterectomy became popular for stroke prevention until publication of the negative results in the multinational EC/IC bypass trial[32] in the mid-1980s. A vocal segment of the neurology community decried the apparent lack of evidence verifying the efficacy of carotid endarterectomy in stroke prevention, which led to a series of large-scale, prospective, randomized trials comparing carotid endarterectomy with medical therapy. In summary, there is now Level I evidence verifying the efficacy of carotid endarterectomy for stroke prevention in both symptomatic and asymptomatic patients.

Carotid Endarterectomy for Symptomatic Carotid Stenosis

In 1991, the results of the randomized North American Symptomatic Carotid Endarterectomy Trial (NASCET) of medical treatment or carotid endarterectomy were reported.[33] All patients had either hemispheric retinal TIAs or nondisabling strokes within 120 days of entry into the trial and 70 to 99% stenosis in the symptomatic carotid artery. The actuarial risk of any ipsilateral stroke at 2 years was significantly lower at 9% in the 328 surgical patients versus 26% in the 331 medical patients. The data-safety monitoring committee halted further randomization given the widely disparate 18-month follow-up data. For major or fatal ipsilateral strokes, the risk was 2.5% for surgical patients versus 13.1% for medical patients ($p < .001$). When all strokes and deaths were included, carotid endarterectomy still was better than medical treatment. Subsequent follow-up studies from this trial indicated that the benefit of carotid endarterectomy in symptomatic patients extended to those with even moderate (50 to 69%) carotid artery lesions.[34]

The Veterans Affairs Cooperative Study of symptomatic carotid stenosis reported in 1991 results of randomizing 189 men with stenoses greater than 50% to medical or surgical treatment.[35] After 1 year, there was a significant reduction in stroke or TIAs in the patients having carotid endarterectomy (7.7%) compared with medically treated patients (19.4%), with even more divergent results with carotid stenosis greater than 70%.

The European Carotid Surgery Trial randomized 2518 patients with nondisabling stroke, TIA, or retinal infarction in conjunction with ipsilateral carotid stenosis to medical or surgical treatment.[36] For the 778 patients with stenoses of 70 to 99%, the cumulative risk of stroke at carotid endarterectomy of 7.5%, plus an additional late stroke rate at 3 years of 2.8%, was less than the 16.8% rate for medically treated patients. At 3 years the cumulative risk of operative death, operative stroke, ipsilateral ischemic stroke, and any other stroke was 12.3% for the surgical cohort versus 21.9% for the medical group ($p < .01$). Finally, the risk of fatal or disabling ipsilateral stroke at 3 years was 6.0% for the carotid endarterectomy patients versus 11.0% for the medical control patients ($p < .05$).

Although the benefit of endarterectomy in these studies was due in part to the high risk of stroke in medically treated patients, the results were significant even in an era when the 30-day combined stroke and death risk of endarterectomy was about 7.5%. Although the combined stroke and death risk of carotid endarterectomy is higher in symptomatic versus asymptomatic patients,[37] the current combined risk is about 2 to 4%.[23,28,38–44]

Carotid Endarterectomy for Asymptomatic Carotid Stenosis

Early studies suggested a significant stroke risk reduction for carotid endarterectomy versus best medical therapy in asymptomatic patients.[40,41] Contemporary randomized studies subsequently verified this position.

The Veterans Affairs Cooperative Study of asymptomatic carotid stenosis, defined as greater than 50% diameter reduction by angiography, randomized 444 men to medical or surgical treatment.[42] At a mean follow-up of 4 years, the combined incidence of ipsilateral neurologic events was 8.0% for the surgical patients versus 20.6% for the medical patients ($p < .001$). The difference in stroke alone between the two groups (8 versus 20%) did not achieve statistical significance because of the study's sample size, nor was there a significant difference when all strokes and deaths were analyzed. Excessive late mortality (about 40% at 4 years in both groups) was caused largely by associated CAD. These mitigating factors limited definitive conclusions about the efficacy of carotid endarterectomy in asymptomatic patients in this trial.

In 1995, results of the Asymptomatic Carotid Atherosclerosis Study of 1662 patients randomized to surgical or medical treatment were published.[27] At mean follow-up of 2.7 years, aggregate risk for ipsilateral stroke and any perioperative stroke or death for the surgical group was 5.1%, significantly lower than the rate of ipsilateral stroke of 11.0% for the medical group, a benefit limited to male patients. Critics suggested that the low combined stroke and death rate (2.3%) in the surgical patients was not representative of results across a broader spectrum of hospitals. However, low morbidity for carotid endarterectomy in asymptomatic patients has been verified in multiple large studies.[43,44]

In 2004, the Asymptomatic Carotid Surgery Trial (ACST),[23] touted as the world's largest surgical trial from 126 hospitals in more than 30 countries, randomized over 3000 patients to carotid endarterectomy or medical therapy. Greater than 40% of patients had more than 3 years of follow-up. Risk of any stroke, any ipsilateral stroke, or any disabling stroke was halved in surgical patients, who had a combined stroke and death rate of about 3%. The time threshold to achieve statistical benefit, ie, cancel perioperative morbidity, by actuarial analysis was 2 years, suggesting that patients selected for endarterectomy should have a life expectancy of greater than 2 years. The only subgroup in which endarterectomy did not achieve statistical significance was in patients older than 75 years of age.

In summary, Level I evidence supports the advantage of carotid endarterectomy over medical management for patients with severe asymptomatic carotid artery stenoses. Of note, large contemporary studies verify the low perioperative morbidity with carotid endarterectomy, even across a spectrum of hospitals and surgeons. In a recent NSQIP study, whose methodology involved independent nurse reviewer adjudication of 30-day endpoints, some 4000 carotid endarterectomy procedures in both symptomatic and asymptomatic patients was accompanied by a 2.2% combined stroke and death risk.[43]

CAROTID STENTING

Following the success of percutaneous transluminal coronary angioplasty, particularly with adjunctive stenting, percutaneous interventionalists increasingly sought to treat carotid stenosis with angioplasty and stenting.[45–47] Technical aspects of the procedure to guard against procedure-related stroke are the dominant concern with this procedure. Emerging reports (mostly from industry-sponsored trials) indicate that carotid stenting can produce equivalent outcomes to carotid endarterectomy.[48–51] In one large series, the 30-day combined stroke and death rate was 7.4%, and most strokes were minor.[52] Results improved with experience, and late stroke-free survival was comparable with that for carotid endarterectomy.

In 2004, a randomized trial of carotid endarterectomy versus stenting with routine embolic protection, designed as a "noninferiority" trial, ie, insufficiently powered to detect superiority of one treatment, concluded that carotid stenting was not inferior to carotid endarterectomy in high-risk patients.[51] Study endpoints (composite death/stroke/MI at 30 days and 1 year), high 30-day combined stroke and death rate (5.7%) in asymptomatic patients, and small sample size limit the value of the data. Most large series and meta-analyses indicate a higher periprocedural complication rate for stenting versus endarterectomy.[53–57] In the French carotid endarterectomy versus stenting study in patients with symptomatic, severe carotid stenosis, stenting was associated with a 2.2-fold increased risk of stroke or death at 30 days compared with endarterectomy. The data-safety monitoring committee halted the trial after randomizing 527 patients.[58] The recently published International Carotid Stenting Study concluded that carotid endarterectomy, and not stenting, was the preferred treatment for symptomatic patients because of an unacceptable early stroke risk accompanying stenting.[59] A Society of Vascular Surgery registry study with risk adjustment methodology reported a nearly three-fold increased risk of 30-day stroke, death, and myocardial infarction with stenting as opposed to carotid endarterectomy.[54] Furthermore, published evidence documents an increased periprocedural risk of stroke after carotid stenting in elderly and symptomatic patients.[55,57,60,61]

Scant data are available about carotid stenting versus endarterectomy in patients requiring CABG. Investigators from the Cleveland Clinic compared patients treated with either carotid stenting before or carotid endarterectomy with open-heart surgery. After propensity scoring, the authors found no significant differences in combined stroke/death/MI in the two approaches.[62]

Given conflicting evidence to support combined carotid endarterectomy and CABG, not surprisingly many investigators have considered the strategy of antecedent carotid stenting, followed by interval CABG for combined disease. A logistic consideration in this strategy is the standard use of Clopidogrel with carotid stenting. One report from the Netherlands advocated such a strategy, but only if the CABG could be delayed for at least three weeks; overall death/stroke/myocardial infarction was still 8.7%.[63] Two collective reviews reflect the difficulty of improving upon reported results with combined carotid endarterectomy and CABG, and/or the conservative posture with respect to asymptomatic carotid stenosis in patients requiring CABG. Naylor collected 11 studies with 760 carotid stent procedures performed at variable intervals before CABG. The cumulative 30-day stroke/death risk was 9.1%, stated to be quite similar to the authors' prior review of concomitant carotid endarterectomy and CABG.[64,65] As in prior reports, that group supported a noninterventional approach in asymptomatic patients. Similarly, Guzman et al. reported a combined stroke/death rate of 12.3% for nearly 300 patients with carotid stenting followed by interval CABG performed at a mean of 32 days after the stenting. They concluded that the strategy of carotid stenting before CABG did not positively influence the stroke risk.[66]

MYOCARDIAL ISCHEMIC EVENTS IN PATIENTS AFTER CAROTID ENDARTERECTOMY

Although this chapter is focused primarily on managing CABG patients who have concomitant carotid artery disease, some comment on the impact of CAD on short- and long-term risks of carotid endarterectomy patients is appropriate.

Incidence of Coronary Artery Disease in Carotid Endarterectomy Patients

Mackey and colleagues[67] found that 53% of carotid endarterectomy patients had evidence of CAD by clinical history or electrocardiographic studies. Using thallium exercise testing in 106 carotid endarterectomy patients, Urbinati and colleagues[68] found that 27 (25%) had significant defects on myocardial scanning. In 1985, the Cleveland Clinic reported the results of routine preoperative coronary angiography in 506 carotid endarterectomy patients.[69] Only 7% of patients had normal coronary arteries, and 28% had mild to moderate CAD. However, 30% had advanced but compensated disease, 28% had severe, correctable disease, and 7% had severe, inoperable CAD.

Risk of Myocardial Ischemic Events

Short-Term Risks

The impact of CAD on short-term risks of carotid endarterectomy is well documented. In 1981, Hertzer and colleagues[70] reported hospital mortality in 335 carotid endarterectomy patients of 1.8%; 60% of deaths were caused by CAD. In the Mackey study cited earlier, carotid endarterectomy patients with clinical CAD had an operative mortality of 1.5% and an MI rate of 4.3% compared with no mortality and an MI rate of 0.5% for patients without CAD.[67] Although the frequent coexistence of CAD with carotid disease is often invoked as a principal cause of short- and long-term morbidity in carotid endarterectomy patients, the risk of perioperative MI vary with the risk profile of the cohort studied. For example, in the protected carotid artery stenting versus endarterectomy trial, 30-day non-Q wave MI occurred in 6.6%.[51] In our cohort of more than 2000 carotid endarterectomy patients, the perioperative MI rate was 1.2%.[28] A National Surgical Quality Improvement Program (NSQIP) database report of more than 13,000 endarterectomy procedures had a perioperative MI rate of 1.4%,[71] similar to results from the ACST trial.[23] In the Society for Vascular Surgery registry study myocardial infarction occurred in less than 1% of carotid endarterectomies.[54] Clearly, improved care, mostly in the form of adjunctive medical therapy with beta blockers, statins and aspirin, has substantially lowered the risk of coronary ischemic events complicating carotid endarterectomy.

Long-Term Risks

Mackey's study of carotid endarterectomy reported the 5- and 10-year survival rates of patients with CAD to be 68.6 and 44.9%, respectively, versus 86.4 and 72.3% for patients with no CAD.[67] Urbinati and colleagues reported the 7-year freedom from all cardiac events after carotid endarterectomy was 51% for patients with silent myocardial ischemia versus 98% for patients with normal thallium exercise testing.[68]

In the Hertzer study of 209 patients with clinically suspected CAD, 5-year mortality rate for hospital survivors was 27%, and 37% of late deaths were caused by MI.[70] Actuarial survival at 11 years was significantly better for the patients with CAD who had bypass grafting. A later study from the same group of 329 carotid endarterectomy patients followed to 10 years confirmed that MI caused more late deaths (37%) than did stroke (15%).[72] Again, 10-year survival was significantly better for patients having CABG.

In our Massachusetts General Hospital cohort of more than 2000 carotid endarterectomy patients treated between 1990 and 1999, 10-year actuarial survival was 45%. Among variables associated with increased late mortality, concomitant CAD [odds ratio (OR) 1.4; $p = .0002$] figured prominently.[28]

TIMING OF CAROTID AND CORONARY ARTERY SURGERY

If one accepts that (1) uncorrected carotid stenosis increases the risk of stroke for patients with severe carotid and CAD who have only isolated CABG, (2) carotid endarterectomy is the indicated treatment for severe symptomatic and asymptomatic carotid stenosis, (3) CAD increases the early and late risk of death for carotid endarterectomy patients, and (4) CABG is an indicated treatment for CAD, then the important question becomes not the indication for but the timing of the two operative procedures.

Staged Carotid and Coronary Artery Operations

One approach is to perform the carotid endarterectomy and CABG operations as staged procedures. By convention, doing the carotid endarterectomy before coronary bypass grafting is referred to as a *staged procedure,* whereas doing the CABG before the carotid artery operation is called a *reverse staged procedure.*

Most advocates of a sequential operative approach to patients with severe combined disease usually do the carotid endarterectomy first if the patient is hemodynamically stable and not ischemic. Improvements in patient management, especially use of regional anesthesia, may allow safe initial isolated carotid endarterectomy. Data from several studies powered to detect an impact of regional anesthesia have verified that composite outcomes of stroke/death/ MI after carotid endarterectomy are reduced significantly with use of regional anesthesia.[37,71] Alternatively, a large randomized study concluded that regional anesthesia for carotid endarterectomy had no significant impact on perioperative myocardial infarction when compared with general anesthesia.[73] Depending on the timing of the two procedures, practical considerations, such as imminent need for the large doses of heparin required for cardiopulmonary bypass, airway and/or neck swelling, and the risk of perioperative coronary ischemic events, remain real issues.

For unstable cardiac patients, particularly those with asymptomatic carotid stenosis, some cardiac surgeons opt to perform initial myocardial revascularization followed by an interval carotid endarterectomy. The principal risk with this approach is the potential for neurologic complications either during or shortly after the myocardial revascularization.

Currently, we advocate concomitant carotid and coronary artery operations for virtually all patients with severe combined disease. However, in patients with severe bilateral carotid stenosis, a staged approach may be appropriate, especially if the patient is cardiovascularly stable. We occasionally treat the more severe of the two carotid artery lesions with initial isolated endarterectomy, followed by combined CABG and endarterectomy of the other carotid artery within a few days. Use of a reversed staged approach, namely, doing one carotid endarterectomy with myocardial revascularization followed several days later by the other carotid endarterectomy, is rare because of an increased stroke risk with reversed staged procedures (to be discussed below).

Concomitant Carotid and Coronary Artery Operations

In 1972, Bernhard and colleagues[74] published the first report of successful combined carotid endarterectomy and CABG in 15 patients. The strategy of performing both operative procedures during one anesthetic is based on the premise that such an approach to severe combined disease ought to minimize cardiac events that frequently complicate isolated carotid endarterectomy and neurologic events that complicate isolated CABG.

Daily and colleagues[75] reported that doing both operative procedures together is more cost effective than a staged or reversed staged approach, which require two anesthetics and can incur the additional costs of two hospitalizations.

OPERATIVE TECHNIQUES FOR CONCOMITANT CAROTID AND CORONARY ARTERY OPERATIONS

Standard Approach

The usual operative technique for concomitant carotid endarterectomy and CABG has been to perform the carotid endarterectomy during harvesting of CAD conduits before cardiopulmonary bypass, the approach we use at our institution, where the carotid operation is performed by vascular surgeons as the cardiac surgical team harvests whatever saphenous vein or other conduits may be needed.

Technical aspects of carotid endarterectomy have evolved. Preoperative aspirin has been validated in large database studies.[76] We use routine electroencephalographic monitoring, selective shunting, and either eversion endarterectomy (presuming no need for a shunt) or patch closure. Simple primary closure is associated with a higher rate of restenosis.[77,78] After the carotid endarterectomy is completed, the neck incision is loosely approximated over a sponge. Final closure, usually over a plastic drain, is done after cardiopulmonary bypass is completed and heparinization is reversed.

Alternative Approaches

Minami and colleagues reported using some perceived advantages of cardiopulmonary bypass, namely, heparinization, hypothermia, and hemodynamic control, to perform carotid endarterectomy in 116 patients while on bypass for CABG.[79] Operative mortality was 1.7%, and total stroke risk was 4.3%. Weiss and colleagues perform the carotid endarterectomy on bypass with systemic hypothermia to 20° C with the heart protected with cardioplegia.[80] They had no neurologic events and one postoperative death in 23 patients. Theoretically, hypothermia on cardiopulmonary bypass provides an extra margin of ischemic protection for the brain during the carotid endarterectomy and avoids the need for intravascular shunting.

Whether performing the carotid and coronary artery operations on cardiopulmonary bypass saves total operative time is not proven, but it prolongs aortic occlusion and cardiopulmonary bypass times, something most cardiac surgeons would prefer to avoid. A deeper level of hypothermia is not favored by most cardiac surgeons, particularly as the trend toward using lesser degrees of hypothermia has become more popular.

HIGHLIGHTS OF POSTOPERATIVE MANAGEMENT

Our postoperative management of patients following concomitant carotid endarterectomy and CABG does not differ importantly from that of patients having isolated myocardial revascularization. We believe that maintenance of a good coronary perfusion pressure and, by extension, good cerebral perfusion pressure in the early postoperative hours is beneficial. Early clearing of perioperative edema with diuresis is efficacious.

The routine anticoagulation protocol for our myocardial revascularization patients, aspirin begun within 6 hours of completion of the operation, is also adequate for patients with concomitant carotid endarterectomy. Permanent aspirin therapy is indicated for both parts of the concomitant procedure.

If a surgeon decides not to treat a severe carotid stenosis either with a staged approach or concomitant operation, the increased incidence of stroke in the early days after isolated myocardial revascularization seen with the reversed staged approach suggests that heparinization is appropriate once the acute bleeding risk of the CAB operation is past.

RESULTS OF STAGED AND CONCOMITANT CAROTID AND CORONARY ARTERY OPERATIONS

Early Results

Staged Carotid and Coronary Artery Operations

Several studies report the results of staged operations for concomitant carotid and CAD, but only one study randomized patients to concomitant or reversed staged operation. Hertzer et al. randomized subgroup of patients with unstable coronary syndromes and incidental asymptomatic carotid stenosis.[81] Over 5 years they treated 275 patients with severe combined disease. Their criteria for carotid endarterectomy was symptomatic and/or severe (>70%) carotid artery disease. Only 24 (9%) of the patients had CAD that was stable enough to allow carotid endarterectomy before CABG. Of those 24 patients, 1 (4.2%) suffered a perioperative stroke after the carotid endarterectomy and died of an MI awaiting CABG. Symptomatic or severe bilateral carotid artery disease in 122 patients was treated with combined carotid and coronary artery operation with an operative mortality rate of 6.1% and a perioperative stroke rate of 7.1%.

The remaining 129 patients with unstable coronary symptoms and severe, unilateral, asymptomatic carotid stenoses were randomized to either a combined or a reversed staged operation. Patients having concomitant carotid and coronary operations had a mortality rate of 4.2% versus a combined rate of 5.3% for the two operations in the staged patients. Stroke rate in the concomitant operations was 2.8%, significantly lower than the 14% risk of the reversed staged operations (6.9% during the isolated CABG and 7.5% during the delayed isolated carotid endarterectomy). This randomized study emphasizes the advantage of concomitant operations over reversed staged procedures.

Several conclusions of this study were validated by a cumulative review from nearly 100 studies encompassing some 9000 patients. The authors noted that carotid endarterectomy very shortly after CABG was accompanied by an unacceptable stroke risk. They reported the stroke risk of the combined operation in their review was 4.6% and that of death/any stroke was 8.7%.[65] These data are similar to other large administrative database studies (stroke/death of 9.6% for combined operation), although such studies are inherently flawed because details for the procedures being staged or combined are often imprecise.[82]

In 1999, Borger and colleagues performed a meta-analysis of nonrandomized observational studies from centers reporting results with both staged and concomitant operations.[83] They identified a trend toward increased risk of stroke and death with combined operations. The results of this study need to be viewed with caution for several reasons. First, using meta-analysis to compare observational and nonrandomized studies limits its statistical power. Second, in most series, unstable patients had combined operations and stable patients had staged procedures. Third, the criterion for entry into these studies was operations completed, not intention to treat. Possibly some patients for whom a staged approach was planned were not studied because the second operation was never performed because of a poor result from the first procedure.

Concomitant Carotid and Coronary Artery Operations

Since the late 1970s, some surgeons in our group have taken an aggressive approach to patients with combined carotid and CAD, using concomitant operation as the standard approach. Staged operations were reserved for the patients with very stable CAD. Our first report in 1989 suggested that combined operation was safe (2% stroke or death risk). That study was among the first to document the disparate cardiac risk among patients having combined operations versus patients having isolated CABG.[84]

In 1995 we published our results of combined operations between 1979 and 1993 in the first 200 consecutive patients.[85] Hospital mortality was 3.5%, MI 2.5%, and perioperative stroke 4.0%.

More recently, we published results of concomitant operation between 1979 and 2001 in 500 patients.[86] Mean patient age was 69 years, about 6 years older than that for all CABG patients. Three-quarters of the patients had unstable angina pectoris, and 53% had prior MI. Although the distribution of single-, double-, and triple-vessel disease was as expected at 4%, 21%, and 75%, respectively, 42% of patients had significant left main CAD. Of the 500 patients, 329 (66%) were neurologically asymptomatic, 21% had transient ischemic attacks, and 13% had a prior stroke. Unilateral severe carotid stenosis was found in 336 patients (67%); 32% had disease in the contralateral carotid artery.

Urgent or emergency operations were required in 54% of patients; 3% were on the intra-aortic balloon preoperatively. The average number of grafts per patient was 3.7. Although only 50% of the first 200 patients received at least one mammary artery graft, 90% of the last 300 patients received a mammary artery graft.

Hospital mortality was 3.6%, MI was 2.0%, and stroke occurred in 4.6%. Of the 23 strokes, 12 were ipsilateral to the carotid endarterectomy and 11 contralateral or bilateral, suggesting that, in our experience, concomitant carotid endarterectomy and CABG have neutralized the impact of carotid stenosis as a risk factor for stroke during surgical myocardial revascularization.

Significant multivariate predictors of hospital death were preoperative TIAs, preoperative MI, and nonelective operation. Peripheral vascular disease predicted postoperative stroke. Significant predictors of prolonged postoperative hospital stay were failure to use a mammary artery graft, perioperative stroke, and advanced age.

Vermeulen and colleagues found that the only significant multivariate predictor of hospital death in 230 combined operations was left main CAD.[87] Postoperative neurologic events were predicted by severe left ventricular dysfunction and preoperative neurologic events, either stroke or TIAs.

Series of concomitant carotid endarterectomy and CABG published since 1985 are in Table 23-2. These results contrast to reports using administrative data. Brown reported a 17.7% stroke risk for combined operations in Medicare patients in Midwestern states.[88] In a Canadian study the combined risk of stroke and death for CABG alone was 4.9% versus 13% for combined carotid and coronary artery operations.[89] However, data from the New York State Registry indicate that such results can be explained largely by the disparate cardiac risk profiles of the two patient groups. Ricotta and colleagues used propensity scoring to match risk-factor profiling and found no difference

TABLE 23-2 Series of Combined Carotid and Coronary Operations with More than 100 Patients

Reference	Year	Patients (No.)	Mean Age (Y)	Deaths (%)	MI (%)	Stroke (%)
Dunn[92]	1986	130	60	6 (4.6)	—	13 (10.0)
Hertzer et al.[81]	1989	170	65	9 (5.3)	—	12 (7.1)
Vermeulen et al.[87]	1992	230	63	8 (3.5)	4 (1.8)	13 (5.6)
Rizzo et al.[91]	1992	127	65	7 (5.5)	6 (4.7)	8 (6.3)
Takach et al.[93]	1997	255	66	10 (3.9)	12 (4.7)	10 (3.9)
Darling et al.[94]	1998	420	69	10 (2.4)	1 (0.2)	13 (3.1)
Khaitan et al.[95]	2000	121	69	7 (5.8)	—	9 (7.4)
Minami et al.[96]	2000	340	65	9 (2.6)	2 (0.6)	16 (4.7)
Evagelopoulos et al.[97]	2000	313	66	28 (8.9)	10 (3.2)	7 (2.2)
Estes et al.[98]	2001	174	69	9 (5.2)	—	10 (5.7)
Zacharias et al.[99]	2002	189	69	5 (2.7)	2 (1.1)	5 (2.7)
Char et al.[100]	2002	154	68	6 (3.9)	—	6 (3.9)
Chiappini et al.[101]	2005	140	65	9 (6.4)	—	9 (6.4)
TOTAL		2763	65	123 (4.4)	37 (2.0)	131 (4.7)
Akins et al.[86]	2005	500	69	18 (3.6)	10 (2.0)	23 (4.6)

in combined stroke and death risk for the two operations after case-control matching.[11] Finally, Cywinski et al., using similar methodology for patient matching, reported in a Cleveland Clinic series of combined operations versus isolated CABG that overall morbidity was higher for the concomitant carotid and coronary operations. Of interest, their study endpoints, in which significant differences were noted between the two groups including overall morbidity and mortality, did not find a significant difference in the risk of stroke.[90]

Late Results

Follow-up in our series of combined operations revealed the following 10-year actuarial freedoms from late events: death, 43%; MI, 87%; percutaneous transluminal coronary angioplasty, 92%; reoperative myocardial revascularization, 96%; total stroke, 85%; and ipsilateral stroke, 90%.[86]

Vermeulen and colleagues found their 10-year actuarial freedom from cardiac events to be 50%, from neurologic events to be 81%, and from all events to be 41%.[87] The only significant multivariate predictors of late cardiac mortality were advanced age and severe left ventricular dysfunction.

In a study of 127 combined carotid and coronary operations, Rizzo et al. reported a 5-year survival rate of 70%, freedom from MI of 84%, and freedom from stroke of 88%.[91] Survival was worse for patients with low ejection fractions. Late strokes were fewer in patients who were neurologically asymptomatic preoperatively, more common in patients who were transiently symptomatic, and most frequent in patients with prior stroke.

CONCLUSION

The risk of perioperative stroke following myocardial revascularization rises with the increasing age of CABG patients, and increasing age is accompanied by an increased incidence of carotid artery disease. Several studies have defined severe, uncorrected carotid stenosis as a major risk factor for perioperative stroke. Patients with carotid bruits or a history of ischemic neurologic events, plus patients who are 65 years old or older ought to have noninvasive carotid artery evaluation before CABG. Randomized trials have established the safety and efficacy of carotid endarterectomy as the most appropriate treatment for both symptomatic and asymptomatic severe carotid stenosis. Another randomized study has demonstrated the advantage of concomitant carotid endarterectomy and CABG over reversed staged operations. Thus, we advocate combined carotid and coronary artery operations for virtually all patients with severe concomitant coronary and carotid artery disease, which on their own merits would require treatment.

REFERENCES

1. Gardner TJ, Horneffer PJ, Manolio TA, et al: Major stroke after coronary artery bypass surgery: changing magnitude of the problem. *J Vasc Surg* 1986; 3:684.
2. Tuman KJ, McCarthy RJ, Najafi H, Ivankovich AD: Differential effects of advanced age on neurologic and cardiac risks on coronary artery operations. *J Thorac Cardiovasc Surg* 1992; 104:1510.
3. John R, Choudhri AF, Weinberg AD, et al: Multicenter review of preoperative risk factors for stroke after coronary artery bypass grafting. *Ann Thorac Surg* 2000; 69:30.
4. Puskas JD, Winston D, Wright CE, et al: Stroke after coronary artery operation: Incidence, correlates, outcome, and cost. *Ann Thorac Surg* 2000; 69:1053.
5. Roach GW, Kanchuger M, Mangano CM, et al: Adverse cerebral outcomes after coronary bypass surgery. *NEJM* 1996; 335:1857.
6. Wareing TH, Davila-Roman VG, Barzilai B, et al: Management of the severely atherosclerotic ascending aorta during cardiac operations. *J Thorac Cardiovasc Surg* 1992; 103:453.
7. Li Y, Walicki D, Mathiesen C, et al: Strokes after cardiac surgery and relationship to carotid stenosis. *Arch Neurol* 2009; 66:1091.
8. Likosky DS, Marrin CAS, Caplan LR, et al. Determination of etiologic mechanisms of strokes secondary to coronary artery bypass graft surgery. *Stroke* 2003; 34:2830.
9. Eliasziw M, Streifler JY, Fox AJ, et al: Significance of plaque ulceration in symptomatic patients with high-grade carotid stenosis. *Stroke* 1994; 25:304.
10. Brener BJ, Brief DK, Alpert J, et al: The risk of stroke in patients with asymptomatic carotid stenosis undergoing cardiac surgery: a follow-up study. *J Vasc Surg* 1987; 5:269.
11. Ricotta JJ, Wall LP, Blackstone E: The influence of concurrent endarterectomy on coronary bypass: a case-controlled study. *J Vasc Surg* 2005; 41:397.
12. Ricotta JJ, Faggioli GL, Castilone A, Hassett JM: Risk factors for stroke after cardiac surgery: Buffalo Cardiac-Cerebral Study Group. *J Vasc Surg* 1995; 21:359.
13. Ricotta JJ, Char DJ, Cuadra SA, et al: Modeling stroke risk after coronary artery bypass and combined coronary artery bypass and carotid endarterectomy. *Stroke* 2003; 34:1212.
14. Schwartz AE, Sandhu AA, Kaplon RJ, et al: Cerebral blood flow is determined by arterial pressure and not cardiopulmonary bypass flow rate. *Ann Thorac Surg* 1995; 60:165.
15. Reed GL, Singer DE, Picard EH, DeSanctis RW: Stroke following coronary artery bypass surgery. *NEJM* 1988; 319:1246.
16. Sauve JS, Thorpe KE, Sackett DL, et al: Can bruits distinguish high-grade from moderate symptomatic carotid stenosis? *Ann Intern Med* 1994; 120:633.
17. Call GK, Abbott WM, Macdonald NR, et al: Correlation of continuous-wave Doppler special flow analysis with gross pathology in carotid stenosis. *Stroke* 1988; 19:584.
18. Gertler J, Cambria RP, Kistler JP, et al: Carotid surgery without angiography: non-invasive selection of patients. *Ann Vasc Surg* 1992; 5:253.
19. Faggioli GL, Curl GR, Ricotta JJ: The role of carotid screening before coronary artery bypass. *J Vasc Surg* 1990; 12:724.
20. Berens ES, Kouchoukos NT, Murphy SF, Wareing TH: Preoperative carotid artery screening in elderly patients undergoing cardiac surgery. *J Vasc Surg* 1992; 15:313.
21. Barnes RW, Nix ML, Sansonetti D, et al: Late outcome of untreated asymptomatic carotid disease following cardiovascular operations. *J Vasc Surg* 1985; 2:843.
22. Ascher E, Hingorani A, Yorkovich W, et al: Routine preoperative carotid duplex scanning in patients undergoing open heart surgery: Is it worthwhile? *Ann Vasc Surg* 2001; 15:669.
23. Halliday A, Mansfield A, Marro J, et al: Prevention of disabling and fatal strokes by successful carotid endarterectomy in patients without recent neurological symptoms: randomized, controlled trial. *Lancet* 2004; 363:1491.
24. Mehigan JT, Buch SW, Pipkin RD, et al: A planned approach to coexistent cerebrovascular disease in coronary artery bypass candidates. *Arch Surg* 1977; 112:1403.
25. Ivey TD, Strandness DE, Williams DB, et al: Management of patients with carotid bruit undergoing cardiopulmonary bypass. *J Thorac Cardiovasc Surg* 1984; 87:183.
26. D'Agostino RS, Svensson LG, Neumann DJ, et al: Screening carotid ultrasonography and risk factors for stroke in coronary artery surgery patients. *Ann Thorac Surg* 1996; 62:1714.
27. Executive Committee for the Asymptomatic Carotid Atherosclerosis Study: Endarterectomy for asymptomatic carotid artery stenosis. *JAMA* 1995; 273:1421.
28. LaMuraglia GM, Brewster DC, Moncure AC, et al: Carotid endarterectomy at the millenium: what interventional therapy must match. *Ann Surg* 2004; 240:535.
29. Jackson MR, Chang AS, Robles HA, et al. Determination of 60% or greater carotid stenosis: a prospective comparison of magnetic resonance angiography and duplex ultrasound with conventional angiography. *Ann Vasc Surg* 1998; 12:236.

30. Fisher CM: Occlusion of the internal carotid artery. *Arch Neurol Psychiatry* 1951; 65:346.
31. Eastcott HG, Pickering GW, Rob CG: Reconstruction of internal carotid artery in a patient with intermittent attacks of hemiplegia. *Lancet* 1954; 2:994.
32. EC/IC Bypass Study Group: Failure of extracranial-intracranial arterial bypass to reduce the risk of ischemic stroke: results of an international randomized trial. *NEJM* 1985; 313:1191.
33. North American Symptomatic Carotid Endarterectomy Trial Collaborators: Beneficial effect of carotid endarterectomy in symptomatic patients with high-grade carotid stenosis. *NEJM* 1991; 325:445.
34. Barnett H, Taylor DW, Eliaszew M, et al: Benefit of carotid endarterectomy in patients with symptomatic moderate or severe stenosis. *NEJM* 1998; 339:1415.
35. Mayberg MR, Wilson SE, Yatsu F, et al: Carotid endarterectomy and prevention of cerebral ischemia in symptomatic carotid stenosis. *JAMA* 1991; 266:3289.
36. European Carotid Surgery Trialists' Collaborative Group: MRC European Carotid Surgery Trial: Interim results for symptomatic patients with severe (70–99%) or with mild (0–29%) carotid stenosis. *Lancet* 1991; 337:1235.
37. Halm EA, Hannan EL, Rojas M, et al: Clinical and operative predictors of outcomes of carotid endarterectomy. *J Vasc Surg* 2005; 42:420.
38. Gaparis AP, Ricotta L, Cuadra SA, et al: High-risk carotid endarterectomy: fact or fiction? *J Vasc Surg* 2003; 37:40.
39. Reed AB, Graccione P, Belkin M, et al: Preoperative risk factors for carotid endarterectomy: defining the patient at high risk. *J Vasc Surg* 2003; 37:1191.
40. Hertzer NR, Flanagan RA, O'Hara PJ, Beven EG: Surgical versus nonoperative treatment of asymptomatic carotid stenosis. *Ann Surg* 1986; 204:163.
41. Moneta GL, Taylor DC, Nicholls SC, et al: Operative versus nonoperative management of asymptomatic high-grade internal carotid artery stenosis: improved results with endarterectomy. *Stroke* 1987; 18:1005.
42. Hobson RW, Weiss DG, Fields WS, et al: Efficacy of carotid endarterectomy for asymptomatic carotid stenosis. *NEJM* 1993; 328:221.
43. Kang JL, Chung TK, Lancaster RT, et al. Outcomes after carotid endarterectomy: Is there a high-risk population? A National Surgical Quality Improvement Program report. *J Vasc Surg* 2009; 49:331.
44. Matsen SL, Chang DC, Perler BA, et al. Trends in the in-hospital stroke rate following carotid endarterectomy in California and Maryland. *J Vasc Surg* 2006; 44:488.
45. Namaguchi Y, Puyau FA, Provenza LJ, Richardson DE: Percutaneous transluminal angioplasty of the carotid artery: its application to post surgical stenosis. *Neuroradiology* 1984; 26:527.
46. Roubin GS, Yadav S, Iyer SS, et al: Carotid stent-supported angioplasty: a neurovascular intervention to prevent stroke. *Am J Cardiol* 1996; 78:8.
47. Mathur A, Roubin GS, Piamsomboom C, et al: Predictors of stroke following carotid stenting: univariate and multivariate analysis. *Circulation* 1997; 96:A1710.
48. Eskandri MK, Longo GM, Matsumura JS, et al: Carotid stenting done exclusively by vascular surgeons: first 175 cases. *Ann Surg* 2005; 242:431.
49. CaRESS Steering Committee: Carotid Revascularization using Endarterectomy or Stenting Systems (CaRESS) phase I clinical trial: 1-year results. *J Vasc Surg* 2005; 42:213.
50. Bergeron P, Roux M, Khanovan P, et al: Long-term results of carotid stenting are competitive with surgery. *J Vasc Surg* 2005; 41:213.
51. Yadav JS, Wholey MH, Kuntz RE, et al: Protected carotid artery stenting versus endarterectomy in high-risk patients. *NEJM* 2004; 352:1493.
52. Roubin GS, New G, Iver SS, et al: Immediate and late clinical outcomes of carotid artery stenting in patients with symptomatic and asymptomatic carotid artery stenosis: a 5-year prospective analysis. *Circulation* 2001; 103:532.
53. Groenveld PW, Yang L, Greenhut A, Yang F. Comparative effectiveness of carotid arterial stenting versus endarterectomy. *J Vasc Surg* 2009; 50: 1040.
54. Sidawy AN, Zwolak RM, White RA, et al. Risk-adjusted 30-day outcomes of carotid stenting and endarterectomy: results from the SVS Vascular Registry. *J Vasc Surg* 2009; 49:71.
55. Murad MH, Flynn D, Elamin MB, et al. Endarterectomy vs stenting for carotid artery stenosis: a systematic review and meta-analysis. *J Vasc Surg* 2008; 48:497.
56. Brahmanandam S, Ding EL, Conte MS, et al. Clinical results of carotid artery stenting compared with carotid endarterectomy. *J Vasc Surg* 2008; 47:343.
57. Ringleb PA, Chatellier G, Hacke W, et al. Safety of endovascular treatment of carotid artery stenosis compared with surgical treatment: a meta-analysis. *J Vasc Surg* 2008; 47:350.
58. Mas J-L, Chatellier G, Beyssen B, et al: Endarterectomy versus stenting in patients with symptomatic severe carotid stenosis. *NEJM* 2006; 355:1660.
59. International Carotid Stenting Study investigators: Carotid artery stenting compared with endarterectomy in patients with symptomatic carotid stenosis (International Carotid Stenting Study): an interim analysis of a randomized controlled trial. *Lancet* 2010; 375:985.
60. Hobson RW, Howard VJ, Roubin GS: Carotid artery stenting is associated with increased complications in octogenarians: 30-day stroke and death rates in the CREST lead-in phase. *J Vasc Surg* 2004; 40:1106.
61. Stanziale SF, Marone LK, Boules TN, et al: Carotid artery stenting in octogenarians is associated with increased adverse outcomes. *J Vasc Surg* 2006; 43:297.
62. Ziada KM, Yadav JS, Mukherjee D, et al: Comparison of results of carotid stenting followed by open heart surgery versus combined carotid endarterectomy and open heart surgery (coronary bypass with or without another procedure). *Am J Cardiol* 2005; 96:519.
63. Van der Heyden J, Lans, HW, van Werkum JW. Will carotid angioplasty become the preferred alternative to staged or synchronous carotid endarterectomy in patients undergoing cardiac surgery? *Eur J Endovasc Surg* 2008; 36:379.
64. Naylor AR, Mehta Z, Rothwell PM. A systematic review and meta-analysis of 30-day outcomes following staged carotid artery stenting and coronary bypass. *Eur J Endovasc Surg* 2009; 37:379.
65. Naylor AR, Cuffe RL, Rothwell PM, et al. A systematic review of outcomes following staged and synchronous carotid endarterectomy and coronary artery bypass. *Eur J Endovasc Surg* 2003; 25:380.
66. Guzman LA, Costa MA, Angiolillo DM, et al. A systematic review of outcomes in patients with staged carotid artery stenting and coronary artery bypass graft surgery. *Stroke* 2008; 39:361.
67. Mackey WC, O'Donnell TF, Callow AD: Cardiac risk in patients undergoing carotid endarterectomy: impact on perioperative and long-term mortality. *J Vasc Surg* 1990; 11:226.
68. Urbinati S, DiPasquale G, Andreoli A, et al: Frequency and prognostic significance of silent coronary artery disease in patients with cerebral ischemia undergoing carotid endarterectomy. *Am J Cardiol* 1992; 69:1166.
69. Hertzer NR, Young JR, Beven EG, et al: Coronary angiography in 506 patients with extracranial cerebrovascular disease. *Arch Intern Med* 1985; 145:849.
70. Hertzer NR, Lees CD: Fatal myocardial infarction following carotid endarterectomy. *Ann Surg* 1981; 194:212.
71. Stoner MC, Abbott WM, Wong DR, et al: Defining the high-risk patients for carotid endarterectomy: an analysis of the prospective National Surgical Quality Improvement Program database. *J Vasc Surg* 2006; 43:285.
72. Hertzer NR, Arison R: Cumulative stroke and survival ten years after carotid endarterectomy. *J Vasc Surg* 1985; 2:661.
73. GALA Trial Collaborative Group, Lewis SC, Warlow CP, et al. General anaesthesia versus local anaesthesia for carotid surgery (GALA): a multicentre, randomized controlled trial. *Lancet* 2008; 372: 2132.
74. Bernhard VM, Johnson WD, Peterson JJ: Carotid artery stenosis: association with surgery for coronary artery disease. *Arch Surg* 1972; 105:837.
75. Daily PO, Freeman RK, Dembitsky WP, et al: Cost reduction by combined carotid endarterectomy and coronary artery bypass grafting. *J Thorac Cardiovasc Surg* 1996; 111:1185.
76. Kresowik TF, Brazlelr D, Karp HR, et al: Multistate utilization, processes, and outcomes of carotid endarterectomy. *J Vasc Surg* 2001; 33:227.
77. LaMuraglia GM, Stoner MC, Brewster DC, et al: Determinants of carotid endarterectomy anatomic durability: effects of serum lipids and lipid-lowering drugs. *J Vasc Surg* 2005; 41:762.
78. AbuRahma A. Processes of care for carotid endarterectomy: surgical and anesthesia considerations. *J Vasc Surg* 2009; 50:921.
79. Minami K, Gawaz M, Ohlmeier H, et al: Management of concomitant occlusive disease of coronary and carotid arteries using cardiopulmonary bypass for both procedures. *J Cardiovasc Surg* 1989; 30:723.
80. Weiss SJ, Sutter FP, Shannon TO, Goldman SM: Combined cardiac operation and carotid endarterectomy during aortic cross-clamping. *Ann Thorac Surg* 1992; 53:813.
81. Hertzer NR, Loop FD, Beven EG, et al: Surgical staging for simultaneous coronary and carotid disease: a study including prospective randomization. *J Vasc Surg* 1989; 9:455.
82. Dubinsky RM, Lai SM. Mortality from combined carotid endarterectomy and coronary artery bypass surgery in the US. *Neurology* 2007; 68:195.
83. Borger MA, Tremes SE, Weisel RD, et al: Coronary bypass and carotid endarterectomy: Does a combined approach increase risk? A meta-analysis. *Ann Thorac Surg* 1999; 68:14.

84. Cambria RP, Ivarsson BL, Akins CW, et al: Simultaneous carotid and coronary disease: safety of the combined approach. *J Vasc Surg* 1989; 9:56.
85. Akins CW, Moncure AC, Daggett WM, et al: Safety and efficacy of concomitant carotid and coronary artery operations. *Ann Thorac Surg* 1995; 60:311.
86. Akins CW, Hilgenberg AD, Vlahakes GJ, et al: Late results of combined carotid and coronary surgery using actual versus actuarial methodology. *Ann Thorac Surg* 2005; 80:2091.
87. Vermeulen FEE, Hamerlijnck RPHM, Defauw JJHM, Ernst SMPG: Synchronous operation for ischemic cardiac and cerebrovascular disease: early results and long-term follow-up. *Ann Thorac Surg* 1992; 53:381.
88. Brown KR, Kresowik TF, Chin MH, et al: Multistate population-based outcomes of combined carotid endarterectomy and coronary artery bypass. *J Vasc Surg* 2003; 37:32.
89. Hill MD, Shrive FM, Kennedy J, et al: Simultaneous carotid endarterectomy and coronary bypass surgery in Canada. *Neurology* 2005; 641:1435.
90. Cywinski JB, Koch CG, Krajewski LP, et al. Increased risk associated with combined carotid endarterectomy and coronary artery bypass graft surgery: a propensity-matched comparison with isolated coronary artery bypass graft surgery. *J Cardiothorac and Vasc Anesth* 2006; 20:796.
91. Rizzo RJ, Whittemore AD, Couper GS, et al: Combined carotid and coronary revascularization: the preferred approach to the severe vasculopath. *Ann Thorac Surg* 1992; 54:1099.
92. Dunn EJ: Concomitant cerebral and myocardial revascularization. *Surg Clin North Am* 1986; 66:385.
93. Takach TJ, Reul GJ, Cooley DA, et al: Is an integrated approach warranted for concomitant carotid and coronary artery disease? *Ann Thorac Surg* 1997; 64:16.
94. Darling RC, Dylewski M, Chang BB, et al: Combined carotid endarterectomy and coronary bypass grafting does not increase the risk of perioperative stroke. *Cardiovasc Surg* 1998; 6:448.
95. Khaitan L, Sutter FP, Goldman SM, et al: Simultaneous carotid endarterectomy and coronary revascularization. *Ann Thorac Surg* 2000; 69:421.
96. Minami K, Fukahara K, Boethig D, et al: Long-term results of simultaneous carotid endarterectomy and myocardial revascularization with cardiopulmonary bypass used for both procedures. *J Thorac Cardiovasc Surg* 2000; 119:764.
97. Evagelopoulos N, Trenz MT, Beckman A, Krian A: Simultaneous carotid endarterectomy and coronary artery bypass grafting in 313 patients. *Cardiovasc Surg* 2000; 8:31.
98. Estes JM, Khabbaz KR, Barnatan M, et al: Outcome after combined carotid endarterectomy and coronary artery bypass is related to patient selection. *J Vasc Surg* 2001; 33:1179.
99. Zacharias A, Schwann TA, Riordan CJ, et al: Operative and 5-year outcomes of combined carotid and coronary revascularization: review of a large contemporary experience. *Ann Thorac Surg* 2002; 73:491.
100. Char D, Chadra S, Ricotta JJ, et al: Combined coronary artery bypass and carotid endarterectomy: long-term results. *Cardiovasc Surg* 2002; 10:111.
101. Chiappini B, Dell'Amore A, DiMarco L, et al: Simultaneous carotid and coronary artery disease: staged or combined surgical approach? *J Card Surg* 2005; 23:234.

CHAPTER 24

Myocardial Revascularization after Acute Myocardial Infarction

Isaac George
Mathew Williams

INTRODUCTION

The ability of surgical interventions to minimize myocardial loss after myocardial infarction has advanced dramatically over the past two decades. Acute myocardial infarction still afflicts approximately 1.5 million individuals each year in the United States,[1] and 30% of these patients die before reaching the hospital, whereas 5% die during hospital admission.[1] Prompt medical attention, including transport to the hospital, diagnosis, and treatment of the myocardial infarction, is critical to patient survival. Since 1989, the death rate from acute myocardial infarctions has declined 24%, while the actual number of deaths declined only 7%.[2] Over the last 40 years, especially during the 1980s, new pharmacologic agents, interventional cardiology procedures, and coronary artery bypass surgical techniques have advanced and have led to a decrease in the overall morbidity and mortality associated with acute myocardial infarction. Despite this overall improvement, mechanical and electrical complications such as cardiogenic shock, rupture of the ventricular septum or free wall, acute mitral regurgitation, pericarditis, tamponade, and arrhythmias challenge the medical community caring for patients presenting with acute myocardial infarction on a daily basis.[3] Of these complications, cardiogenic shock complicating acute myocardial infarctions has the most significant impact on in-hospital mortality and long-term survival. The loss of more than 40% of functioning left ventricular mass and its accompanying systemic inflammatory response are major causes of cardiogenic shock and are determined by the degree of preinfarction ventricular dysfunction, the size of the infarcted vessel, and pathologic level of inflammatory mediators.[4,5] Restoration of blood flow to the threatened myocardium offers the best chance of survival following acute coronary occlusion, but the means and timing of revascularization continue to be a highly debated and studied topic. Thrombolytics, percutaneous transluminal coronary angioplasty (PTCA), intracoronary stenting, and coronary artery bypass (CABG) surgery have decreased the mortality associated with acute myocardial infarctions. Advances in myocardial preservation and mechanical support lead the surgical armamentarium in the treatment of acute myocardial infarctions.

PATHOGENESIS OF ACUTE OCCLUSION

Myocardial ischemia resulting from coronary occlusion for as little as 60 seconds causes ischemic zone changes from a state of active systolic shortening to one of passive systolic lengthening.[6] Occlusions for less than 20 minutes usually cause reversible cellular damage and depressed function with subsequent myocardial stunning. Furthermore, reperfusion of the infarct leads to variable amounts of salvageable myocardium. After 40 minutes of ischemia followed by reperfusion, 60 to 70% of the ultimate infarct is salvageable, but this decreases dramatically to 10% after 3 hours of ischemia.[7,8] Animal model evidence has also demonstrated that 6 hours of regional ischemia produces extensive transmural necrosis.[9] The exact timing in humans is even more difficult to analyze because of collateral flow, which is a major determinant of myocardial necrosis in the area at risk in humans.[8] The collateral blood supply is extremely variable, especially in patients with long-standing coronary disease. However, collateral flow is jeopardized with arrhythmias, hypotension, or the rise of left ventricular end-diastolic pressure above tissue capillary pressure.[7] Thus loss of collateral flow to the infarct area may lead to the cellular death of

TABLE 24-1 Factors That Influence the Evolution and Severity of Acute Myocardial Infarction

Anatomic
Site of lesion
Size of myocardium at risk
Collateral circulation
Physiologic
Arrhythmias
Coronary perfusion pressure
Myocardial oxygen consumption
Reperfusion injury
Stunned myocardium
Therapeutic options
Medical management
Revascularization
Thrombolysis
Percutaneous coronary angioplasty
Coronary artery surgery
Controlled reperfusion
Buckberg solution and technique
Mechanical circulatory support

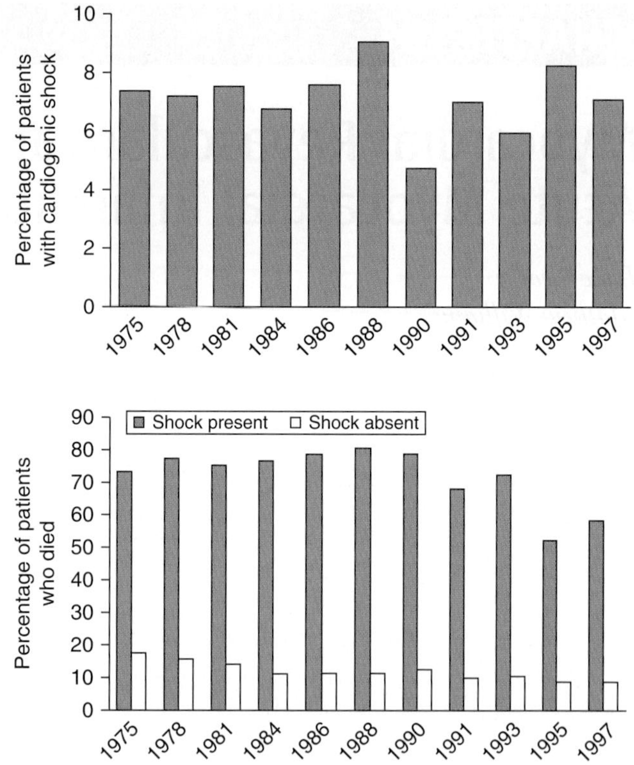

FIGURE 24-1 Trends in cardiogenic shock and survival based on presence or absence of shock. (*Reproduced with permission from Goldberg R, Samad N, Yarzebski J, et al: Temporal trends in cardiogenic shock complicating acute myocardial infarction. NEJM 1999; 340:1162.*)

salvageable myocardium. Control of blood pressure and prevention of arrhythmias are vital during this immediate time after infarction.

Table 24-1 outlines the effects of anatomic, physiologic, and therapeutic variables on the evolution of final infarct size.

CARDIOGENIC SHOCK

Definition

Cardiogenic shock is defined clinically as a systolic blood pressure below 80 mm Hg in the absence of hypovolemia, peripheral vasoconstriction with cold extremities, changes in mental status, and urine output of less than 20 mL/h. Hemodynamic parameters for cardiogenic shock include cardiac index less than 1.8 L/min/m^2, stroke volume index less than 20 mL/m^2, mean pulmonary capillary wedge pressure greater than 18 mm Hg, tachycardia, and a systemic vascular resistance of over 2400 dyn·sec/cm^5. These patients are defined as type IV by the Killip classification, a widely used system to classify myocardial infarctions.[10]

Prevalence

Shock is the most common cause of in-hospital mortality after myocardial infarction.[11] The in-hospital mortality associated with cardiogenic shock has remained unchanged at approximately 80% despite the development of new treatment modalities.[12] Cardiogenic shock occurs in 2.4 to 12.0% of patients with acute myocardial infarction.[13] Since 1975, the incidence of cardiogenic shock complicating acute myocardial infarctions has remained constant at 7.5%, ranging between 5 and 15% (Fig. 24-1).[11] The progressive reduction in time delay from symptom onset to treatment may account for these constant figures. Previously, patients with excessive time delays would have died before reaching the hospital or soon thereafter, as it is known that treatment delays increase 1-year mortality exponentially (Fig. 24-2).[14]

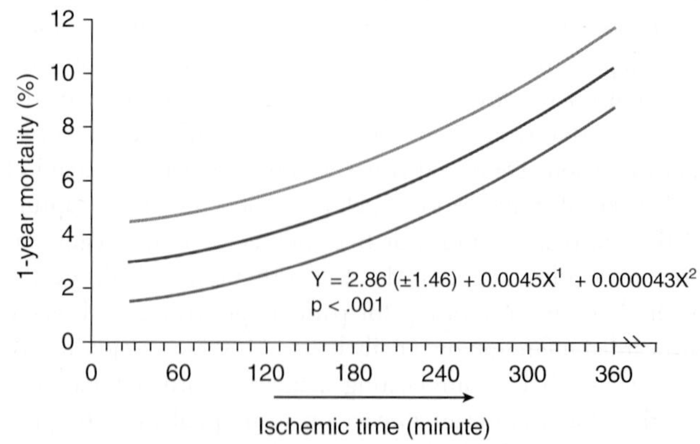

FIGURE 24-2 Relationship between time to treatment and 1-year mortality, as a continuous function, was assessed with a quadratic regression model. Dotted lines represent 95% confidence intervals of predicted mortality. (*Reproduced with permission from De Luca G, Suryapranata H, Ottervanger JP, et al: Time delay to treatment and mortality in primary angioplasty for acute myocardial infarction. Circulation 2004; 109:1223.*)

Pathophysiology and Infarct Size

Shock is directly related to the extent of the myocardium involved, and infarctions resulting in loss of at least 40% of the left ventricle have been found on autopsy in patients with cardiogenic shock.[4,15] Autopsy findings also revealed marginal extension of the recent infarct and focal areas of necrosis in patients with cardiogenic shock.[4] Extensive three-vessel disease is usually found in individuals with cardiogenic shock, and extension of the infarct is an important determinant in those individuals.[4,15] Limiting the size of the infarct and its extension is one of the key therapeutic interventions in patients with myocardial infarction.

MEDICAL MANAGEMENT OF MYOCARDIAL INFARCTION

The management of patients with acute myocardial infarctions demands expeditious treatment and decision making. With the ultimate goal of reperfusing the ischemic myocardium, treatment strategies should be directed toward reducing myocardial oxygen demand, maintaining circulatory support, and protecting the threatened myocardium before irreversible damage and expansion of the infarct occur.

Clinical assessment and risk stratification begins at triage during presentation, where electrocardiographic changes and cardiac biomarkers are used to identify patients suitable for revascularization versus medical management. At our center, clinical algorithms have been instituted to rapidly aid decision making.[16] Patients presenting with ongoing chest pain for more than 20 minutes and ST-segment elevation in two contiguous leads or new (or not known to be old) left bundle branch block *or* anterolateral ST depression are classified as having ST-segment Elevation Myocardial Infarction (STEMI). These patients are referred for primary percutaneous intervention in the cardiac catheterization suite 24 hours a day, 7 days a week, if no contraindications exist. The other group of patients, those with non–ST segment Elevation Myocardial Infarction (NSTEMI), present with chest pain at rest for 10 minutes or more and ST-segment depression greater than 0.5 mm or ST-segment elevation 0.6 to 1 mm or T-Wave inversions greater than 1 mm or positive troponin levels or a history of unstable angina in a patient with coronary artery disease risk factors. These patients are treated medically with a combination of antiplatelet therapy, intravenous heparin, and other traditional medications discussed in the following.

Both clinical and basic science research have demonstrated that reperfusion is the main treatment option for acute myocardial infarction. Unfortunately, the majority of patients with myocardial infarction receive only conservative medical management; only 40% of patients having an acute myocardial infarction receive thrombolytic therapy, the most common means of reperfusion.[17]

STATES OF IMPAIRED MYOCARDIUM

Coronary insufficiency can result in three states of impaired myocardium: infarcted, hibernating, and stunned. Each state requires separate clinical interventions and carries different prognostic implications. Infarcted myocardium is irreversible myocardial cell death owing to prolonged ischemia. Hibernating myocardium is a state of impaired myocardial and left ventricular function at rest resulting from reduced coronary blood flow and impaired coronary vasodilator reserve that can be restored to normal if a normal myocardial oxygen supply–demand relationship is reestablished.[18] Hibernating myocardium is defined as contractility-depressed myocardial function secondary to severe chronic ischemia that improves clinically immediately after myocardial revascularization. Stunned myocardium is left ventricular dysfunction without cell death that occurs after restoration of blood flow after an ischemic episode. If a patient survives the insult resulting from a temporary period of ischemia followed by reperfusion, the previously ischemic areas of cardiac muscle eventually demonstrate improved contractility (Table 24-2).

Hibernating Myocardium

Hibernation may be acute or chronic. Carlson and associates[31] showed that hibernating myocardium was present in up to 75% of patients with unstable angina and 28% with stable angina. The entity also occurs after myocardial infarction. Angina after myocardial infarction commonly occurs at a distance from the area of infarction.[19] In fact, mortality is significantly higher in patients with ischemia at a distance (72%) compared with ischemia adjacent to the infarct zone (33%).[19] It is the hibernating myocardium that may be in jeopardy and salvageable, although its presence is usually incidental to the occurrence of the acute infarction. By distinguishing between hibernating myocardium and irreversibly injured myocardium, a more aggressive approach to restoring or improving blood flow to the area at risk is reasonable. Function often improves immediately after revascularization of appropriately selected regions.

TABLE 24-2 States of Myocardial Cells after Periods of Ischemia

Condition	Viability of Cells	Cause of Injury	Return of Function
Infarcted	Nonviable	Prolonged ischemia	No recovery
Stunned viable	Limited ischemia	Delayed with reperfusion	Recovery
Hibernating	Viable	Ongoing ischemia	Prompt, sometimes unpredictable recovery

Stunned Myocardium

In the 1970s it was observed that after brief episodes of severe ischemia, prolonged dysfunction upon reperfusion with gradual return of contractile activity occurred. In 1982 Braunwald and Kloner[20] coined the phrase *stunned myocardium*. Stunning is a fully reversible process despite the severity and duration of the insult if the cells remain viable. However, myocardial dysfunction, biochemical alterations, and ultrastructural abnormalities continue to persist after return of blood flow. Within 60 seconds of coronary occlusion, the ischemic zone changes from a state of active shortening to one of passive shortening. Coronary occlusion lasting less than 20 minutes is the classic model reproducing the stunning phenomenon.[21] The most likely mechanisms of myocardial stunning are listed in Table 24-3.[21,22]

Stunned myocardium can occur adjacent to necrotic tissue after prolonged coronary occlusion and can be associated with demand-induced ischemia, coronary spasm, and cardioplegia-induced cardiac arrest during cardiopulmonary bypass. Clinically these regions are edematous, and even hemorrhagic, and can lead to both systolic and diastolic dysfunction.[23] They also have a propensity for arrhythmias, which can lead to more extensive ventricular stunning and hypotension with subsequent infarction of these regions.

Diagnosis of Viable Myocardium

Mechanisms to identify patients with myocardial stunning and hibernation include ECG findings, radionuclide imaging, positron emission tomography (PET), dobutamine echocardiography, and more recently magnetic resonance imaging (MRI). Thallium identifies perfusion-related defects of the myocardium and can distinguish between viable and scarred myocardium as well. However, early redistribution of thallium does not distinguish between hibernating and scarred myocardium because many segments with irreversible defects by thallium improve after reperfusion. Redistribution imaging and reinjection imaging improve the predictive value of thallium imaging in distinguishing hibernating myocardium.

PET measures the metabolic activity of myocardial cells. It has high positive and negative predictive values. It is now regarded as the best method to determine myocardial viability, particularly in patients with severe left ventricular dysfunction in whom other modalities are less accurate.[24]

Dobutamine echocardiography identifies hibernating and stunned myocardium by monitoring changes in segmental wall motion while the heart is stressed inotropically and chronotropically by dobutamine infusion. It has high specificity, sensitivity, and, more importantly, positive predictive value.[25]

MRI has also been established as an effective method to assess hibernating myocardium.[26] It has been proved to accurately diagnose the degree of both acute and chronic myocardial infarction and predict functional recovery.[27,28] A number of advantages exist with cardiac MRI, such as superior image resolution allowing accurate indentification of transmural infarction (Fig. 24-3). By providing morphologic, functional, and metabolic information, it may ultimately supplant other modalities for the diagnosis of cardiac injury and recovery.

Finally, multislice computed tomography has been used to measure hibernating myocardium, and early data suggest it may be a reliable and sensitive method compared with MRI, although its use in clinical practice is limited.[29]

TABLE 24-3 Mechanisms of Contractile Dysfunction after Myocardial Stunning

Generation of oxygen-derived free radicals*
Excitation-contraction uncoupling due to sarcoplasmic reticulum dysfunction
Calcium overload
Insufficient energy production by mitochondria
Impaired energy use by myofibrils
Impairment of sympathetic neural responsiveness
Impairment of myocardial perfusion
Damage of the extracellular collagen matrix
Decreased sensitivity of myofilaments to calcium

*Regarded as the primary mechanism of myocardial stunning.

Source: Modified with permission from Bolli R: Mechanism of myocardial stunning. Circulation 1990; 82:723.

RATIONALE FOR AGGRESSIVE MANAGEMENT OF MYOCARDIAL INFARCTION

Randomized trials have shown beneficial effects of early reperfusion within 12 hours and possibly up to 24 hours after acute myocardial infarction.[10,12,30,31] Early reperfusion clearly reduces infarct size in the major areas at risk. Controlled reperfusion may even be superior. The arguments are more difficult to make for patients outside the 24-hour window; however, patients with ongoing ischemia often have ischemic border regions that are prone to arrhythmias and necrosis. In addition, these patients are at risk for prolonged periods of hypotension with resulting end-organ injury and further left ventricular dysfunction. Even if revascularization does not appear critical, ventricular unloading with IABP or LVAD may provide the bridge to recovery needed in patients dying after myocardial infarction. The major limiting factors to aggressive surgical management are major comorbidities, which make continuation of life undesirable or unlikely, and an unclear neurologic status, especially after a period of cardiopulmonary arrest.

REPERFUSION

Although restoration of blood flow to ischemic regions is essential, the accompanying reperfusion injury initially can worsen rather than improve myocardial dysfunction. The area at risk is affected not only by reperfusion but also by the conditions of reperfusion and the composition of the reperfusate.[32] Thus controlling reperfusion itself may aid in reducing myocardial infarct size and ventricular injury.

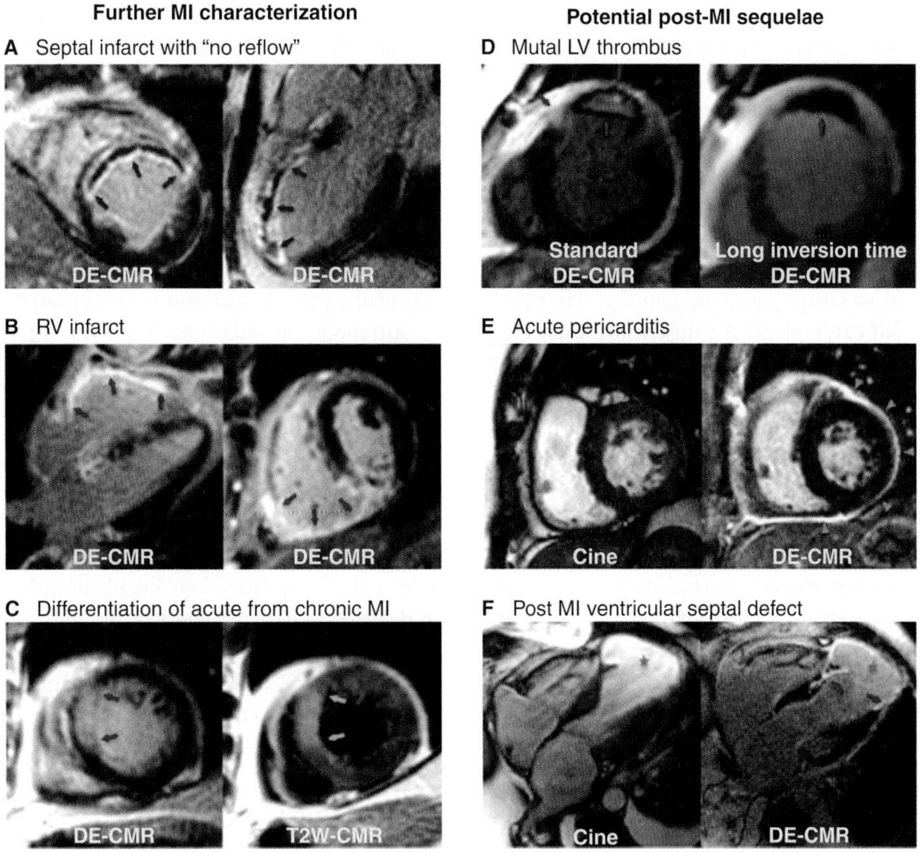

FIGURE 24-3 Cardiovascular MRI (CMR) characterization of myocardial infarction (MI) and post-myocardial infarction sequelae. Examples are shown of patients with myocardial infarction complicated by the presence of (A) microvascular damage (no reflow, *purple arrows*), and (B) right ventricular involvement (*red arrows*). (C) Acute infarcts (*red arrows*) can be differentiated from chronic infarcts by the use of T2-weighted imaging, which can show increased signal in areas of acute necrosis (*green arrows*). (D) Post-MI sequelae such as mural thrombus (*blue arrows*) can be identified by delayed-enhancement-CMR. Long-inversion-time imaging may improve detection because the image intensity of viable myocardium is gray rather than black. Thrombus is often immediately adjacent to infarcted myocardium (*red arrows*). (E) Acute pericarditis can be diagnosed by the presence of hyperenhanced pericardium (*orange arrowheads*). (F) CMR image may be used to define ventricular septal defect location (*orange stars*), extent of associated infarction (*red arrows*), and severity of shunting. (*Reproduced with permission from Kim HW, Farzaneh-Far A, Kim RJ: Cardiovascular magnetic resonance in patients with myocardial infarction. J Am Coll Cardiol 2010; 55:1-16.*)

At the cellular level, myocardial ischemia results in a change in energy production from aerobic to anaerobic metabolism. The consequences of ischemia vary from decreased adenosine triphosphate production and increased intracellular calcium to decreased amino acid precursors such as aspartate and glutamate. These changes can be reversed only by reperfusion.

However, as oxygen is reintroduced into a region, oxygen free radical generation ensues with resulting cellular damage. Cellular swelling and/or contracture leads to a "no-reflow phenomenon" that limits the recovery of some myocytes and possibly adds to irreversible injury of others. The production of oxygen free radicals during ischemia and at the time of reperfusion is the leading mechanism proposed to explain cellular injury. Four basic types of reperfusion injury have been described: lethal cell death, microvascular injury, stunned myocardium, and reperfusion arrhythmias (Table 24-4).

Buckberg and coworkers[33–38] conducted studies of controlled reperfusion after ischemia and produced a clinical application for controlled reperfusion. The surgical strategy of controlled

TABLE 24-4 Potential Types of Reperfusion Injury

Lethal	Cell death secondary to reperfusion
Vascular	Progressive damage causes an expanding zone of "no reflow" and deterioration of coronary flow reserve during the phase of reperfusion
Reperfusion arrhythmias	Arrhythmias, mainly ventricular, that occur shortly after reperfusion
Stunned myocardium	Postischemic ventricular dysfunction

Source: Modified with permission from Kloner RA: Does reperfusion injury exist in humans? J Am Coll Cardiol 1993; 21:537.

reperfusion, especially as espoused by Buckberg and associates, includes several elements. First, extracorporeal circulation is established as expeditiously as possible with venting of the left ventricle as required. Initially, antegrade cardioplegia is delivered using either a warm Buckberg solution to rebuild adenosine triphosphate stores or cold high-potassium cardioplegia to achieve rapid diastolic arrest. We routinely add retrograde cardioplegia to ensure global cooling, even in areas of active ischemia. The temperatures of the anterior and inferior walls of the ventricle are measured to ensure adequate cooling. After each distal anastomosis, cold cardioplegia is infused into each graft and the aorta at 200 mL/min over 1 minute. This is followed by retrograde infusion through the coronary sinus for 1 minute. After completion of the final distal anastomosis, warm substrate-enriched blood cardioplegia is given at 150 mL/min for 2 minutes into each anastomosis and the aorta. After removal of the aortic cross-clamp, regional blood cardioplegia is given at 50 mL/min into the graft supplying the region at risk for 18 minutes. This controlled rate of reperfusion minimizes cellular edema and myocyte damage. The proximal vein grafts are then completed, followed by reestablishment of normal blood flow. To decrease oxygen demand, the heart is allowed to beat in the empty state for 30 minutes. After this time, the patient is weaned off bypass.

Application of the Buckberg solution and technique has been shown to be effective in improving mortality rates and myocardial function after acute coronary occlusion. With ischemic times averaging 6 hours, a prevalence of multivessel disease, and cardiogenic shock, the overall mortality in patients with acute coronary arterial occlusions who underwent surgical revascularization applying this method of reperfusion was 3.9%. Postoperative ejection fractions averaged 50%.[39] Surgical revascularization in this series using controlled reperfusion compared favorably with PTCA in several large series. The superior results of this method for the treatment of cardiogenic shock, a 9% mortality, have brought this method to the forefront in the treatment of cardiogenic shock.

Methods of Reperfusion

Role of Thrombolytic Therapy

Because myocardial salvage depends on reperfusion of occluded coronary arteries, rapid dissolution of an occluding thrombus with thrombolytic therapy is an appealing intervention. Intracoronary streptokinase in patients with acute myocardial infarction demonstrates that thrombolytic therapy is a safe and efficient way to achieve the desired early reperfusion.[40] Following this study, a number of multi-institutional megatrials showed the effectiveness of thrombolytic therapy in treating acute myocardial infarctions.

The trial of the Italian Group for the Study of Streptokinase in Myocardial Infarction (Gruppo Italiano per lo Studio della Streptochinasi nell'Infarto Miocardio, [GISSI])[41] and the Second International Study of Infarct Survival [ISIS-2])[42] found a reduced hospital mortality in patients treated with streptokinase. The effectiveness of tissue-type t-PA also has been evaluated in randomized studies. The Thrombolysis in Myocardial Infarction (TIMI) study[43] and the European Cooperative Study Group (ECSG)[44] demonstrated the effectiveness of t-PA for the treatment of acute myocardial infarction.

When streptokinase and t-PA were compared, two studies failed to demonstrate any difference in mortality.[45,46] A third study, however, the Global Utilization of Streptokinase and Tissue Plasminogen Activator for Occluded Coronary Arteries (GUSTO) trial, supported the use of t-PA by demonstrating a more rapid and complete restoration of coronary flow that resulted in improved ventricular performance and reduced mortality.[47,48]

Although thrombolysis improves survival and ventricular function, the patency of infarct-related arteries is reported to be between 50 and 85%.[41–48] Normal flow should be achieved in 60% of patients by today's standards. Thrombolytic therapy works well but is not without complications, including bleeding and intracranial hemorrhage.[49] Bleeding is usually minor and occurs mostly at the sites of vascular puncture. Intracranial hemorrhage and stroke rates are around 1% and are an "acceptable" risk. The relative benefits of thrombolytic therapy appear to decrease as patient age increases, and a higher risk of intracranial hemorrhage in the elderly may partially account for these findings.[47,50,51] Careful selection of patients suitable for fibrinolytic therapy is warranted, especially in an increasingly older population.

Cardiogenic Shock

Thrombolytic therapy for patients presenting in cardiogenic shock or heart failure does not appear to improve survival in this population but may decrease the incidence of patients developing heart failure after myocardial infarction.[52]

Summary

Thrombolytic agents for the treatment of myocardial infarction have demonstrated several important points. Survival is improved by decreasing time to reperfusion. The GUSTO trial showed that patients treated within the first hour had the greatest improvement in survival, with a 1% reduction in mortality for each hour of time saved.[47,48] Thrombolytic therapy is easy to administer in the community by trained personnel, although a significant risk of bleeding exists in certain patients. Because the time to reperfusion is a critical element in preserving myocardium, thrombolytic therapy is ideal for most communities without percutaneous interventional capabilities. In this setting, thrombolytics may be used for treatment of patients with acute myocardial infarction.

Role of Percutaneous Transluminal Coronary Angioplasty

Since the first reported use of PTCA by Gruntzig and associates[74] in 1979, the efficacy of this procedure in the treatment of coronary artery disease has been well recognized. A number of studies have evaluated the efficacy of primary PTCA in the treatment of acute myocardial infarction. Overall, PTCA hospital mortality rates range from 6 to 9%.[53–56]

Several different strategies employing PTCA for acute myocardial infarction have been developed and examined through clinical trials. Primary, rescue, immediate, delayed, and elective PTCA are options for the treatment of acute myocardial infarction. Primary PTCA uses angioplasty as the method of reperfusion in patients presenting with acute myocardial infarction. Rescue, immediate, delayed, and elective PTCA all are done in conjunction with or following thrombolytic therapy. Rescue PTCA is done after recurrent angina or hemodynamic instability after thrombolytic therapy. Immediate PTCA is performed in conjunction with thrombolytic therapy, and delayed PTCA occurs during the intervening hospitalization. Finally, elective PTCA is done following thrombolytic therapy and medical management when a positive stress test is obtained during the same hospitalization or soon thereafter.

Primary PTCA functions in several roles for the treatment of acute myocardial infarctions. Because there are some absolute and relative contraindications to thrombolytics, PTCA is the one of best methods of reperfusion in patients with acute myocardial infarction, according to studies that evaluated PTCA as first-line therapy. Several studies evaluated the role of PTCA compared with thrombolytic therapy. The first study, the Primary Angioplasty in Myocardial Infarction Study Group trial in 1993, concluded that immediate PTCA without thrombolytics reduced occurrence of reinfarction and death and was associated with a lower rate of intracranial hemorrhage.[53] Since then, more than 20 studies have compared PTCA to thrombolysis. The results from these studies have consistently and conclusively demonstrated the superiority of PTCA to thrombolysis, regardless of the thrombolytic agent used. The findings include a lower short-term mortality rate, lower rates of reinfarction, reduced stroke and intracranial hemorrhage rates, and a decreased composite end point of death, reinfarction, and stroke.[57] These findings have been reconfirmed on long-term follow-up. A higher overall rate of bleeding was observed, likely because of vascular access complications. Myocardial salvage is similar for PTCA and thrombolytic therapy. However, primary PTCA may be slightly less costly than thrombolytic therapy.[54]

There are limits to the use of primary PTCA. Logistic and economic constraints apply to invasive modes of therapy. Catheterization laboratories and personnel must be ready at all times. This is not practical in most communities, and transportation to tertiary care centers raises costs considerably.

Intracoronary Stents

The use of intracoronary stents after myocardial infarction has expanded as PTCA has become more prevalent. Benefits of stenting include lowered rates of restenosis and abrupt closure, and a reduced need for target revascularization after PTCA. Although the STENT-PAMI trial in 1999 using first-generation stents showed lower restenosis rates compared with thrombolysis, a trend toward higher mortality was seen, and its effectiveness as first-line therapy was questioned.[58] Composite end points of death, reinfarction, and urgent target vessel revascularization at 30 days have now been shown to be lower in subsequent studies, such as the CADILLAC, ISAR-2, and ADMIRAL trials, which employed newer-generation stents.[59–61] In these trials, abciximab, a glycoprotein IIb/IIIa inhibitor, was added to primary stenting. A striking reduction in restenosis rates with stenting plus abciximab versus PTCA alone was evident at 12-month follow-up in the CADILLAC study (41 versus 22%).[59] Current data suggest that stenting combined with antiplatelet therapy provides superior benefit to PTCA alone. Drug-eluting stents offer the potential to lower restenosis even further through the use of anti-inflammatory medication delivered via the stent. Most recently, patients in the STRATEGY trial treated with drug-eluting stents after acute ST-elevation myocardial infarction (STEMI) had a significantly lower composite end point of death, reinfarction, stroke, and angiographic evidence of restenosis at 8-month follow-up compared with bare-metal stenting plus abciximab (50 versus 19%).[62] Using propensity score matching, retrospective analysis of patients post acute myocardial infarction in Massachusetts has shown a slight 2-year mortality benefit for drug-eluting stents when compared with bare-metal stents (10.7 versus 12.8%), as well as a lower need for repeat revascularization.[63] Further prospective studies are under way to determine if long-term data confirm these findings.

Antithrombotic agents continued for 12 to 18 hours after PTCA and stenting are an important adjunctive therapy to prevent further ischemic complications. Traditional agents, such as heparin, have been replaced by glycoprotein IIb/IIIa inhibitors, which may have survival benefit when used after PTCA.[64] Newer agents, such as direct thrombin inhibitors, have been introduced with the hope of reducing bleeding and/or heparin-associated complications. The Harmonizing Outcomes with Revascularization and Stents in Acute Myocardial Infarction (HORIZONS-AMI)[65,66] trial investigated bivalirudin, a direct thrombin inhibitor, versus heparin plus a glycoprotein IIb/IIIa inihibitor for use after primary PTCA with or without stenting. Both 30-day and 1-year outcomes revealed decreased hemorrhagic events, and 1-year cardiac mortality was lower in patients treated with bivalirudin, despite a higher 24-hour risk of stent thrombosis in the bivalirudin cohort. Concerns regarding increased thrombogenicity with drug-eluting stents persist; further research is warranted to ensure that late in-stent thrombosis does not preclude use in this setting. Intracoronary stenting with adjunctive antiplatlelet medications has been embraced by the medical community for off-label use after acute myocardial infarction since its recent introduction.

Cardiogenic Shock

Primary PTCA may play a greater role in patients presenting in cardiogenic shock, and percutaneous interventions have become more common over the past 10 years (Fig. 24-4). The GISSI-1 and GISSI-2 trials demonstrated no benefit from intravenous thrombolysis, with mortality rates of 70%.[41,45] In patients presenting in or developing cardiogenic shock after acute myocardial infarction, PTCA improved survival to 40 and 60%.[67] This improvement was even greater when angioplasty was successful; in-hospital survival rates increased to 70%. In most of these series an IABP was used in conjunction with PTCA. The SHOCK trial showed that revascularization by PTCA or CABG within 12 hours of the onset of cardiogenic shock results in improved 1- and 6-year survival rates versus medical stabilization followed by delayed revascularization (32.8 for PTCA/CABG versus 19.6% for initial medical stablization, 6-year follow-up)

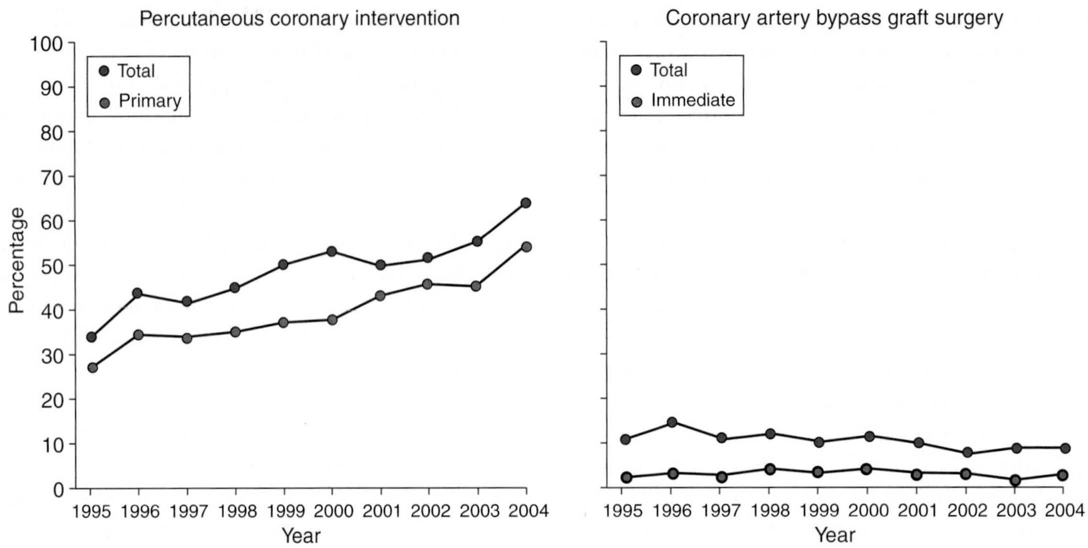

FIGURE 24-4 Survival estimates for early revascularization (n = 152) and initial medical stabilization (n = 150) groups in the SHOCK trial. Log-rank test, p = .03. ERV = early revascularization groups; IMS = initial medical stabilization group. (*Reproduced with permission from Hochman JS, Sleeper LA, White HD, et al: One-year survival following early revascularization for cardiogenic shock. JAMA 2001; 285:190.*)

in this high-risk group, particularly for those under the age of 75 years (Fig. 24-5).[12,30,31] Subgroup analysis in patients undergoing successful PTCA or with TIMI Grade 3 coronary flow after PTCA in the SHOCK trial revealed that 1-year survival was even higher, at 61%.[68] Independent predictors of mortality include age, hypotension, lower TIMI flow, and multivessel PTCA.

Summary

Primary PTCA or intracoronary stenting should be performed as first-line therapy in patients with acute myocardial infarction and those with contraindications to thrombolytic therapy. Patients with established or developing cardiogenic shock should be revascularized early by PTCA or stenting rather than initial medical stabilization by thrombolytic therapy. Specialized centers that have 24-hour catheterization facilities can provide primary PTCA or stenting as a first-line therapy. Rescue PTCA after failed thrombolytic therapy for patients with ongoing ischemia or clinical compromise is also recommended. Finally, elective PTCA should be performed on patients who have recurrent or provokable angina before hospital discharge.

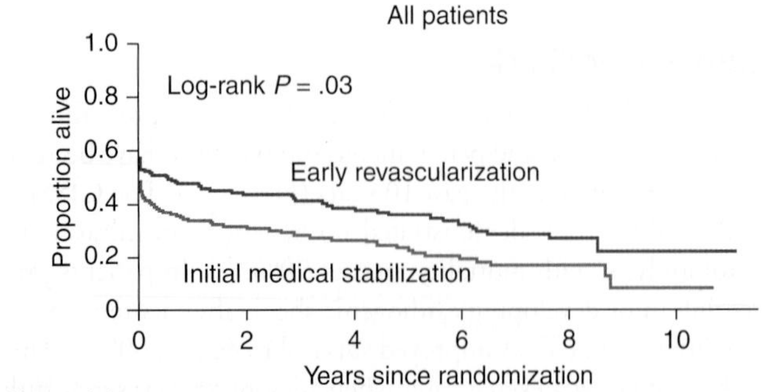

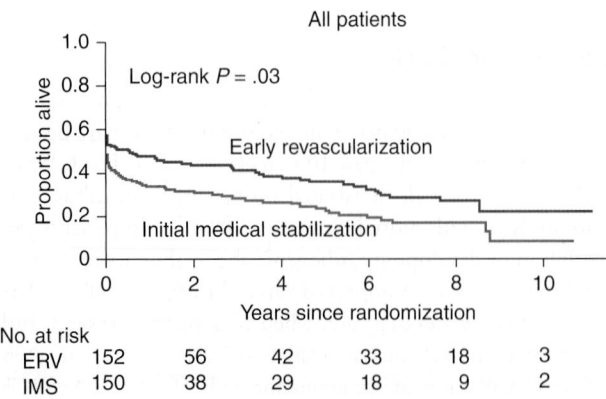

FIGURE 24-5 Revascularization rates in patients with cardiogenic shock at presentation (n = 7356). (*Reproduced with permission from Babaev A, Frederick PD, Pasta DJ, et al: Trends in management and outcomes of patients with acute myocardial infarction complicated by cardiogenic shock. JAMA 2005; 294:448.*)

Role of Coronary Artery Bypass Grafting

The role of surgical revascularization in the treatment of acute myocardial infarction has changed considerably over the past 30 years. Improvements in intraoperative management and myocardial preservation techniques have strengthened the surgeon's armamentarium. However, the development and use of thrombolytic therapy and PTCA offer effective alternatives to surgery.

During the 1980s, reports appeared recommending surgical revascularization in preference to medical therapy for acute myocardial infarction.[69,70] Mortality rates under 5% were reported. Critics argued that these studies lacked randomization or consecutive entry of patients, preoperative stratification was absent, and enzyme levels were not included. Inherent bias that favored surgery in low-risk patients was believed to be the reason for the excellent outcomes.[71]

At the time these reports surfaced, thrombolytic therapy and interventional cardiology were emerging as alternative options for acute infarction. With the availability of thrombolytics and PTCA, large multicenter trials began looking at the efficacy and usefulness of these two techniques. Randomized trials using CABG were not done, and thus this option was never established as an alternative for acute myocardial infarction.

However, several centers continued to use surgical revascularization to treat acute myocardial infarction. Excellent results were achieved by coordinated community and hospital systems. However, practical, logistic, and economic constraints relegate surgical revascularization to a third option behind thrombolytics and PTCA for the primary treatment of acute myocardial infarction.

There continue to be several scenarios that require emergent or urgent surgical revascularization. Failure of thrombolytics, PTCA, or intracoronary stenting with acute occlusion may require surgical intervention. Additionally, CABG for postinfarction angina has become a critical step in the pathway of treating acute myocardial infarction. Finally, surgical revascularization may be indicated in patients with multivessel disease or left main coronary artery disease developing cardiogenic shock after myocardial infarction.

Timing after Infarction

If surgical revascularization within 6 hours after the onset of symptoms is feasible, the mortality rate is improved over that of medically treated, nonrevascularized patients.[69,70] Although these early studies were not controlled and were criticized for selection bias, they did demonstrate that surgical revascularization may be performed with an acceptable mortality in the presence of acute myocardial infarction with improved myocardial protection, anesthesia, and surgical techniques. However, with the advent of thrombolytic therapy, PTCA, and an aging population, the surgical patient we encounter today bears little resemblance to the patient population represented in these early data.

Recent analyses of the New York State Cardiac Surgery Registry, which included every patient undergoing a cardiac operation in the last decade in the state of New York, resulted in valuable information regarding the optimal timing of CABG in acute myocardial infarction. In this large and contemporary patient population, there is a significant correlation between hospital mortality and time interval from acute myocardial infarction to time of operation, particularly if CABG was performed within 1 week of acute myocardial infarction. In addition, patients with transmural and nontransmural acute myocardial infarction have different trends in mortality when the time course is taken into consideration. Mortality for the nontransmural group peaked if the operation was performed within 6 hours of acute myocardial infarction, and then decreased precipitously (Table 24-5).[72] On the other hand, mortality for the transmural group remained high during the first 3 days before returning to baseline.[73] Multivariate analyses confirmed that CABG within 6 hours for the nontransmural group and 3 days for the transmural group were independently associated with in-hospital mortality.[72,73] Optimal timing of CABG in patients with acute myocardial infarction is a controversial subject. Early surgical intervention has the advantage of limiting the infarct expansion and ventricular remodeling that may result in possible ventricular aneurysm and rupture.[74] However, there is the theoretical risk of reperfusion injury, which may lead to hemorrhagic infarction resulting in extension of infarct size, poor infarct healing, and scar development.[75] The data from these studies caution against early revascularization, particularly among patients with transmural acute myocardial infarction within 3 days of onset.

TABLE 24-5 Comparison of Hospital Mortality with Respect to Time of Surgery—Transmural Versus Nontransmural Myocardial Infarction

	Mortality	
Time between CABG and MI	Transmural MI (%)	Nontransmural MI (%)
<6 h	14	13
6-23 h	14*	6*
1-7 d	5	4
>7 d	3	3

*p <.01 nontransmural versus transmural.
Source: Data compiled from the New York State Cardiac Surgery Registry, which included every patient undergoing a cardiac operation in the last decade in the state of New York.

Some have advocated the use of mechanical support to stabilize and allow elective rather than emergent surgery.[76,77] Using mechanical support "prophylactically" instead of CABG to improve outcome, however, would require placement of such support in many unnecessary cases. If revascularization cannot be delayed, aggressive mechanical support (such as an LVAD) must be available because mortality is most likely a result of pump failure. Furthermore, mechanical circulatory support has been shown to be efficacious as a bridge to ventricular recovery or transplantation for this patient cohort.[77] Although emergent cases such as structural complications and ongoing ischemia clearly cannot be delayed, nonemergent cases, particularly patients with transmural acute myocardial infarction, may benefit from delay of surgery. Early surgery after transmural acute myocardial infarction has a significantly higher risk and surgeons should be prepared to provide aggressive cardiac support including LVADs in this ailing population. Waiting in some cases may be warranted.

Risk Factors

In addition to timing of surgery as discussed in the preceding, risk factors include urgency of the operation, increasing patient age, renal insufficiency, number of previous myocardial infarctions, hypertension,[78] reoperation, cardiogenic shock, depressed left ventricular function, and the need for cardiopulmonary resuscitation, left main disease, female gender, left ventricular wall motion score, IABP, and transmural infarction.[79] Characteristics associated with better outcome early after myocardial infarction include preservation of left ventricular ejection fraction, male gender, younger patients, and subendocardial versus transmural myocardial infarction.

Cardiogenic Shock

Surgical revascularization in acute myocardial infarction complicated by cardiogenic shock has been shown to improve

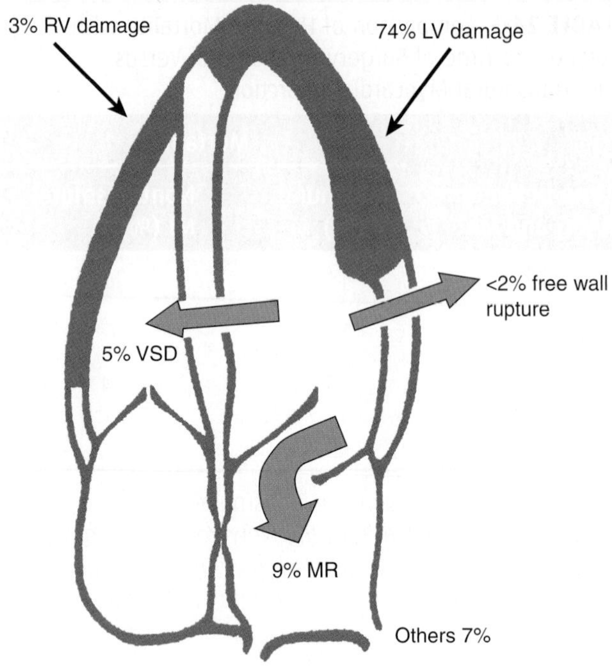

FIGURE 24-6 Mechanisms of cardiogenic shock. Apical four chamber echo view with relative incidence of the mechanisms responsible for cardiogenic shock in the SHOCK and MILIS 4 registries. LV = left ventricle; MR = mitral regurgitation; RV = right ventricle; VSD = ventricular septal defect. (*Reproduced with permission from Davies CH: Revascularization for cardiogenic shock. Q J Med 2001; 94:57.*)

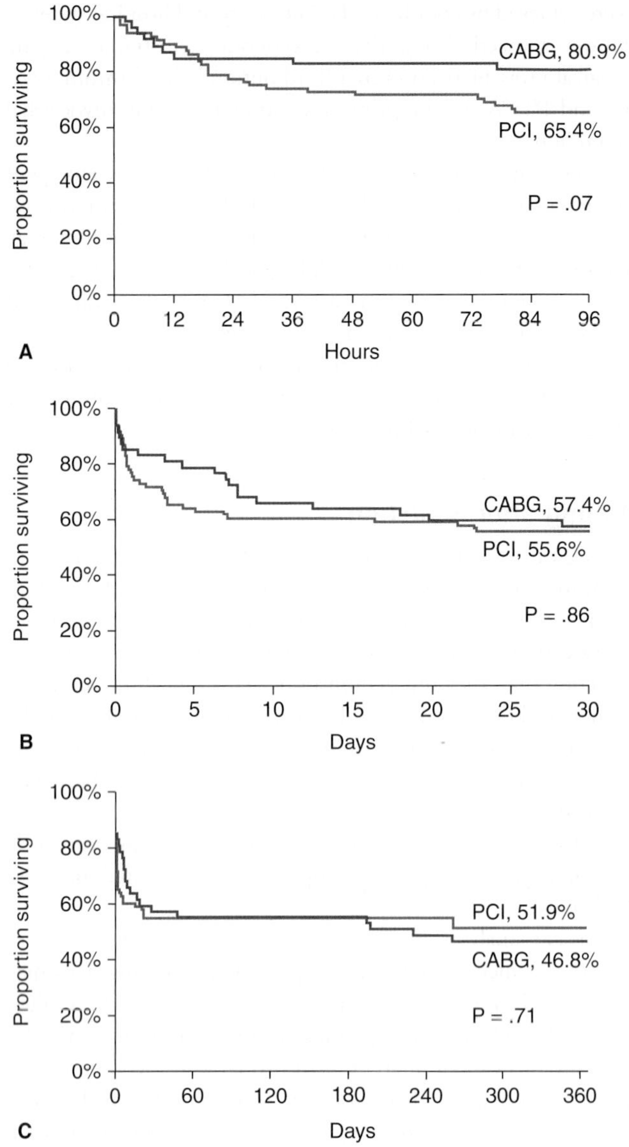

FIGURE 24-7 Kaplan-Meier survival estimates at 96 hours (**A**), 30 days (**B**), and 1 year (**C**) in patients treated with emergency percutaneous coronary intervention (PCI) versus emergency coronary artery bypass graft (CABG) in the SHOCK trial. (*Reproduced with permission from White HD, Assman SF, Sanborn TA, et al: Comparison of percutaneous coronary intervention and coronary artery bypass grafting after acute myocardial infarction complicated by cardiogenic shock. Circulation 2005; 112:1992.*)

survival. Cardiogenic shock, as discussed earlier, is accompanied by 80 to 90% mortality rates; various mechanisms of cardiogenic shock are shown in Fig. 24-6. DeWood and colleagues[80] were the first to demonstrate improved results with revascularization in patients with cardiogenic shock complicating acute myocardial infarction. Patients who were stabilized with an IABP and underwent emergent surgical revascularization had survival rates of 75%. Early surgical revascularization is associated with survival rates of 40 to 88% in patients in cardiogenic shock resulting from nonmechanical causes. Guyton and coworkers[81] reported an 88% in-hospital survival and a 3-year survival of 88%, with no late deaths reported. Furthermore, the SHOCK trial demonstrated survival benefit in early revascularization by CABG or PTCA within 12 hours of the diagnosis of cardiogenic shock for patients of all ages.[30,31] Patients comprising the CABG cohort in the SHOCK trial had more severe disease, with higher rates of three-vessel disease, left main coronary artery disease, diabetes, and elevated mean coronary jeopardy scores than the PTCA cohort.[82] Despite this, 87.2% of these patients achieved successful *and* complete revascularization with CABG, compared with successful revascularizaton in 77.2% with PTCA and only 23.1% with complete revascularization with PTCA. Overall, mortality was no different between groups at 1 year (Fig. 24-7). On subgroup analysis, patients older than age 75, with left main coronary disease or three-vessel disease, or with diabetes had trends toward better survival at 30 days and 1 year after CABG compared to PTCA. Thus, for patients in cardiogenic shock, surgical revascularization has become an established and viable option for select patient groups.

Advantages of Coronary Artery Bypass Grafting

Reported survival rates are similar for CABG and PTCA in the treatment of acute myocardial infarction. To date there have been no large randomized clinical trials comparing CABG with PTCA and thrombolytics after myocardial infarction. For patients with stable angina and elective revascularization for ischemic heart disease, a number of trials have been conducted comparing CABG with stenting.[83–86] In these studies, trends favoring CABG for multivessel disease were seen after 2 years in composite cardiac event end points, rate of reinfarction, and mortality; revascularization rates were five times higher in the stenting groups.[87] Most notably, survival after CABG for two or more diseased vessels was significantly higher than stenting with 2-year follow-up in a retrospective study of the New York State Cardiac Surgery Reporting System and Percutaneous Coronary Intervention Reporting System.[88] These results must be interpreted with caution, however, as patients with acute infarctions less than 24 hours pretreatment were excluded. Because of the lack of prospective, randomized trials, recommendations must be based on retrospective and observational studies. CABG offers several potential advantages. First, surgical revascularization is the most definitive form of treatment of the occlusion. CABG offers the longest patency of revascularized stenotic and occluded arteries in elective cases; 90% of internal mammary artery grafts are patent at 10 years. Second, CABG also offers more complete revascularization, because all vessel lesions are treated. This concept becomes especially important in patients with multivesssel disease or those in cardiogenic shock, in whom remote myocardium may continue to be comprised with only "culprit vessel" revascularization and inadequate restoration of collateral flow.[89] A complete revascularization returns global myocardial perfusion to normal levels and offers the best chance for myocardial salvage. Third, difficult distal obstructions can be reached. Fourth, there is controlled reperfusion to reverse ischemic injury and reduce reperfusion injury. Fifth, as with other forms of reperfusion, CABG interrupts the progression of ischemia and necrosis and limits infarct size.

Disadvantages of Coronary Artery Bypass Grafting

Disadvantages of immediate surgical revascularization include the high mortality associated with early CABG. Off-pump procedures may reduce perioperative complications in high-risk patients, but are not yet widely practiced and have limitations.[90] Rapid availability of catheterization and operating room personnel for emergency procedures imposes logistic and economic constraints. Thus, CABG is not readily applicable to the vast majority of patients in the community, and to provide this would strain health care resources. Second, it is difficult to analyze published results of CABG for acute myocardial infarction because randomized trials have not been done. Comparisons thus far have used medically treated patients as controls. Patients in the surgical group may be at lower risk; this might explain their progression to operation rather than continuing medical treatment. Crossover of patients from medical to surgical treatment also may have skewed the data.

Summary

Surgical revascularization following acute myocardial infarction can be performed with excellent results when the timing and patient cohort are appropriate. Most patients do not need such measures and would not benefit from this aggressive form of therapy. However, patients with mechanical complications, those in cardiogenic shock, and those with postinfarction angina are likely to benefit from early CABG.

USE OF THE INTRA-AORTIC BALLOON PUMP

The early use of aortic counterpulsation with an intra-aortic balloon pump (IABP) demonstrated the safety but not efficacy of this device for patients in cardiogenic shock following acute myocardial infarction.[91] Although survival was not improved, aortic counterpulsation did improve the myocardial oxygen requirements and myocardial energetics were reduced in patients in shock. The use of IABP is also effective for temporary hemodynamic stabilization in complications of acute myocardial infarction, such as ventricular septal rupture acute mitral valve insufficiency,[92] postinfarct angina,[93] ventricular arrythmias,[94] and acute heart failure following infarction.[95] As revascularization techniques for the repair of occluded coronary arteries of patients in cardiogenic shock have improved, use of aortic counterpulsation has found a role as an adjuvant to treatment protocols.

IABP counterpulsation in combination with early reperfusion is effective in the treatment of acute myocardial infarction complicated by cardiogenic shock.[80,96] Although the major improvement in survival is caused by early reperfusion, patients who had combined reperfusion and IABP additionally have improved long-term survival. IABP improves circulatory physiology and decreases end-organ damage in the early shock period before the myocardium is reperfused and recovers function.

Aortic counterpulsation decreases the reocclusion rate, recurrent ischemia, and need for emergency PTCA in patients who have coronary artery patency established by emergency cardiac catheterization after acute myocardial infarction.[97] Prophylactic counterpulsation for 48 hours sustains patency in coronary arteries after patency is reestablished after myocardial infarction. No increase in vascular or hemorrhagic complications is observed as compared with controls.[97]

Weaning from the IABP should take place only after there is clear evidence of myocardial and end-organ recovery. In general, inotropic requirements should be reduced first to minimize myocardial stress. The one exception is the development of limb ischemia resulting from the IABP catheter.

ROLE OF CIRCULATORY ASSIST

Circulatory support devices are reserved for patients who are hemodynamically unstable; however, intervention should not be delayed until after irreversible end-organ injury occurs. This group of shock patients has a mortality rate of 80%, and survival data with the use of assist devices reflect the critical condition of patients treated. Mortality rates have changed very little in the last 20 years despite improvements in medical and surgical therapy.

Patients in cardiogenic shock who are candidates for circulatory assist devices may be divided into two groups: individuals who have stunned myocardium and need a bridge to recovery, and those who have irreversible myocardial damage and need a bridge to cardiac transplantation. For example, if a patient with a previously normal ventricle develops a large myocardial infarction, we prefer short-term support, because enough recovery may occur to allow a fruitful existence with the native heart.

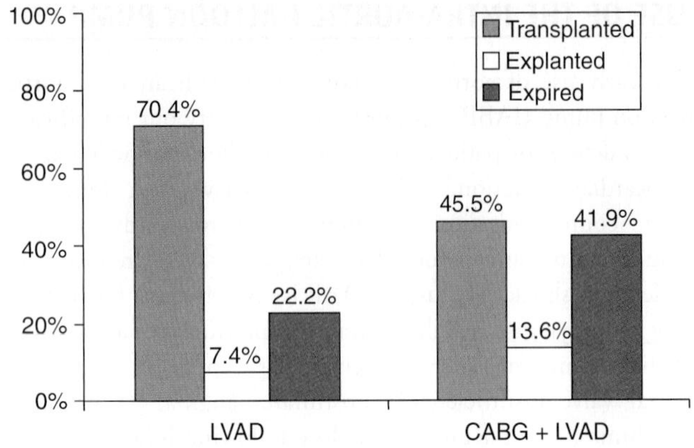

FIGURE 24-8 Outcomes of direct left ventricular assist device (LVAD) implantation versus coronary artery bypass graft (CABG) followed by LVAD implantation for cardiogenic shock. (*Reproduced with permission from Dang NC, Topkara VK, Leacche M, et al: Left ventricular assist device implantation after acute anterior wall myocardial infarction and cardiogenic shock: a two-center study. J Thorac Cardiovasc Surg 2005; 130:693.*)

However, if a patient with preexisting heart failure has another infarction, the need to definitively bridge the patient to transplant with a long-term implantable device is apparent. This approach is supported by results from a multicenter study, in which overall survival at 6 and 12 months was higher in patients who underwent direct LVAD implantation rather than revascularization followed by LVAD, in patients suffering cardiogenic shock (Fig. 24-8).[98] Difficulty arises in assessing the results of mechanical assistance for patients after acute myocardial infarction and cardiogenic shock because of these different objectives.

Mechanical assist devices augment systemic perfusion and prevent end-organ damage while resting the stunned ventricle with complete or partial pressure-volume unloading.[99] Early studies of implantable LVADs have shown that end-organ function is an early predictor of mortality. Treatment of patients before end-organ deterioration is essential to improving the odds for long-term survival. In addition to affecting end-organ function, assist devices promote "reverse remodeling" by improving myocardial contractility and calcium handling, altering the extracellular matrix, and decreasing myocardial fibrosis.[100,101] Recent studies have shown that circulatory support early after myocardial infarction improved survival and offered a feasible bridge to recovery or transplantation.[77,102]

Decisions regarding specific device use depend on the degree of circulatory support needed and many other factors. Selection criteria for device placement include:

1. Potential reversibility of cardiac dysfunction
2. Cause of the cardiac dysfunction
3. Degree of right and left ventricular dysfunction
4. Amount of circulatory support needed
5. Importance of the device for myocardial functional recovery
6. Patient size
7. Anatomical location of collapse or deterioration
8. Whether the patient is a candidate for cardiac transplantation
9. Whether the patient can be anticoagulated
10. Expected duration of support
11. The patient's age and severity of comorbid conditions

At the New York Presbyterian Hospital (Columbia Center), several circulatory assist devices are available to aid treatment of each group. Short-term devices that can be placed percutaneously include the IABP, extracorporeal membrane oxygenation, and percutaneous assist devices. Devices that require sternotomy and are beneficial for short-term use include both pulsatile and newer axial flow devices. These devices primarily treat stunned myocardium, but they are capable of bridging to transplant. These devices are easy to insert, do not require excision of ventricular muscle, and do not compromise ventricular function after device removal. These devices can be removed without the need to reinstitute cardiopulmonary bypass. These devices are effective in patients who require emergency support secondary to cardiogenic shock.

Percutaneous assist devices are an excellent option for patients in cardiogenic shock after catheter-based or surgical revascularization as a short-term bridge for recovery or transplant. Current devices include the Impella Recovery system (Impella Cardiosystems AG, Aachen, Germany) and the TandemHeart system (Cardiac Assist Inc., Pittsburgh, PA). These devices require vascular access, which can be obtained percutaneously, and angiography to guide placement. The TandemHeart provides up to 4 L/min of support producing a higher mean blood pressure and cardiac output, and lowering pulmonary capillary wedge pressure.[103] Clinical results of this device in a randomized trial in 42 patients suffering cardiogenic shock after acute myocardial infarction have shown an improvement in cardiac output, decreased pulmonary capillary wedge pressure, but no difference in 30-day overall mortality.[104] Likewise, the Impella device can provide either 2.5 L/min or 5 L/min depending on the model, and in small series, may offer superior hemodynamic support when compared with an IABP.[105]

Many of the implantable assist devices are suitable for bridging to transplantation. Initial reports of increased mortality in this high-risk patient population have been refuted by studies reporting higher than usual survival in acute myocardial infarction patients who received ventricular assist device support. At our facility, more than 80% of this patient cohort have survived until transplantation, a result threefold better than that seen in databases of extracorporeal systems.

Second-generation assist devices employ axial flow rotors that can generate up to 6 L of flow (partial unloading of the left ventricle). These devices are driven by an electromagnetically actuated impeller drive shaft, contain fewer moving parts, and are smaller than pulsatile devices, thus making them less prone to mechanical failure and driveline infections, at least in theory.[106] The major disadvantages to axial flow pumps are the need for systemic anticoagulation, the lack of pulsatile flow, and incomplete pressure-volume unloading of the left ventricle; these concerns have limited its use in the post-myocardial infarction setting and further research is needed to clarify its therapeutic potential for these patients.

A full discussion of short-term and long-term mechanical circulatory support is reported in Chapters 18 and 66.

SURGICAL MANAGEMENT

New York Presbyterian (Columbia Center) Approach

Patients who are potential transplant candidates and those who are dying of cardiogenic shock after myocardial infarction are all candidates for placement of a long-term implantable left ventricular assist device (LVAD) (Fig. 24-9). If at all possible, a coronary angiogram is obtained to allow revascularization with or without LVAD insertion. Surgery is delayed if the culprit vessel can be opened with angioplasty and the patient stabilized in the catheterization laboratory. If hemodynamics continue to deteriorate, the patient is taken directly to the operating suite, even if infarction occurred earlier than 6 hours before the planned procedure. Hemodynamic observations that favor early CABG are pulmonary artery pressures of less than 60/30 mm Hg and cardiac output of more than 3 L/min. If the hemodynamics are worse, early implantation of a long-term implantable LVAD may be needed, especially if the mixed venous oxygen saturation is less than or equal to 50%. The decision to place a long-term LVAD is influenced by the patient score on a screening scale designed for this purpose (Table 24-6). These scores were selected to identify end-organ dysfunction (lung, liver, or kidney) and operative constraints (right-sided heart failure and bleeding). We have nearly a 90% survival if the summed scores are less than 5 points, versus 30% survival with summed scores greater than 5 points.[107] For this reason, if the total score is greater than 5 points, an attempt is made to stabilize the patient before beginning long-term LVAD insertion. Patients with lower scores are offered temporary LVAD.

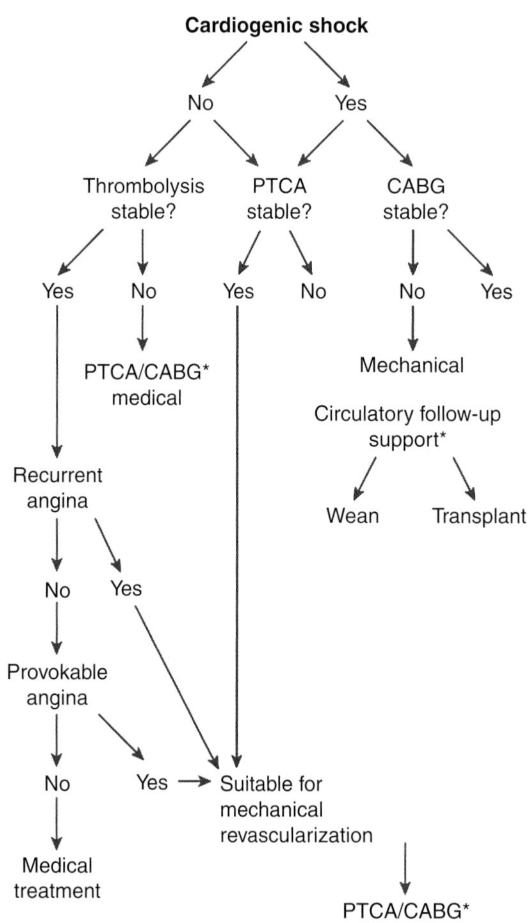

*PTCA = percutaneous transluminal coronary angioplasty; CABG = coronary artery bypass grafting. Choice of therapy is made based on the lesion(s) and comorbid factors.
†Choice of mechanical support is based on many factors (see text, along with other chapters).

FIGURE 24-9 Acute myocardial infarction algorithm.

TABLE 24-6 Preoperative Risk Scale for Left Ventricular Assist Device Placement*

Criteria	Points
Urine output <30 cc/h	3
Intubated	2
Prothrombin time >16 sec	2
Central venous pressure >16 mm Hg	2
Reoperation	1

*A combined score of >5 is associated with a 70% mortality risk.

If a patient is not a potential transplant candidate, our approach is more conservative, because we do not have a safety net if coronary revascularization fails and a temporary support device is inserted. An angiogram must be obtained; if hemodynamics are not favorable and no acute ischemia is present, we delay surgery until pulmonary arterial pressures fall. If the patient is ischemic, we proceed with CABG as described in the following. If the patient cannot be separated from bypass without high-dose inotropic support, including alpha agonists, if the cardiac index is less than 2 L/min/m^2, and if left-sided filling pressures remain high with mixed venous oxygen saturations of less than 50%, short-term LVAD support is instituted. IABP alone in this patient population often does not prevent death and almost always results in significant renal, hepatic, and pulmonary dysfunction that significantly complicates patient recovery even if adequate cardiac function returns. Most important, stressing the heart with high-dose inotropic agents and high filling pressures when it is weakest during the early reperfusion period after acute infarction may compromise border zone regions. This concern is especially true of patients with older infarctions (more than 6 hours). We err on the side of implanting this short-term device early, because the survival rate is only 7% if the device is inserted after a cardiac arrest in the recovery room.

Operative Techniques for Acute Myocardial Infarction

Anesthesia

Anesthesia is provided by a rapid narcotics-based regimen with perfusion and surgical teams prepared to respond to catastrophic hypotension or cardiac arrest. Transesophageal probes are always placed in these patients if possible. As the patient is prepped, a test dose followed by a loading dose of aprotinin is given.

Bleeding

Bleeding is a significant complication of emergency CABG and often results in further myocardial depression and pulmonary hypertension. Cytokine release induced by infusion of blood products and thromboxane A2 released by cardiopulmonary bypass stimulate pulmonary hypertension, which can be catastrophic in the setting of right ventricular ischemia. Use of aminocaproic acid for reoperative, emergency, or high-risk CABG is common in many institutions.

The use of clopidogrel deserves special mention, and its expanding administration can pose unique problems for the cardiac surgeon. Clopidogrel, an oral irreversible antagonist of the 5′-adenosine diphosphate that inhibits platelet activation and aggregation, is used extensively in patients with acute coronary syndromes and has been shown to lower cardiovascular risk by up to 20%, and reduce reinfarction and stroke rates;[108,109] in addition, it is commonly given before percutaneous interventions and after intracoronary stenting to prevent thrombosis. Higher loading doses have been used with increasing efficacy against ischemic complications, which will likely expand its use in the future.[110] However, patients frequently require surgical revascularization after medical therapy or cardiac catheterization while taking clopidogrel. The risk of bleeding after clopidogrel and cardiac surgery can be substantial. In multiple reports, the risk of reoperation for hemorrhage in patients receiving clopidogrel within 7 days of cardiac surgery is six times higher, and patients required more blood, platelet, and fresh-frozen plasma transfusions.[111,112] Because of these complication rates and the inability to reverse clopidogrel's effect on platelets, surgery is often delayed until platelet function is restored, which may take 7 to 10 days, or the life of the platelets. Emergent surgery while taking clopidogrel necessitates frequent blood product transfusions and confers significant morbidity, and possibly mortality. Further study is underway to determine if current dosing regimens after acute myocardial infarction can be reduced to lessen bleeding complications.

Choice of Conduits

For emergency cases, the choice of conduit should not differ from elective cases in most circumstances. The internal mammary artery is not associated with a higher number of complications compared with saphenous vein grafting in emergent situations and can be used in most circumstances.[113,114]

Intraoperative Considerations

Decompression of the ventricle during revascularization after acute coronary occlusion decreases muscle damage and improves functional outcome by decreasing wall tension and reducing oxygen consumption (Figs. 24-10 and 24-11).[38] Indeed, ventricular decompression reduces metabolic energy consumption by 60%. Diastolic basal arrest, by avoiding the energy of contraction, is the second most important means of minimizing oxygen consumption and further reduces metabolic energy consumption by 30%. Cooling of the patient and heart has an impact only on the final 10% of basal energy requirements.

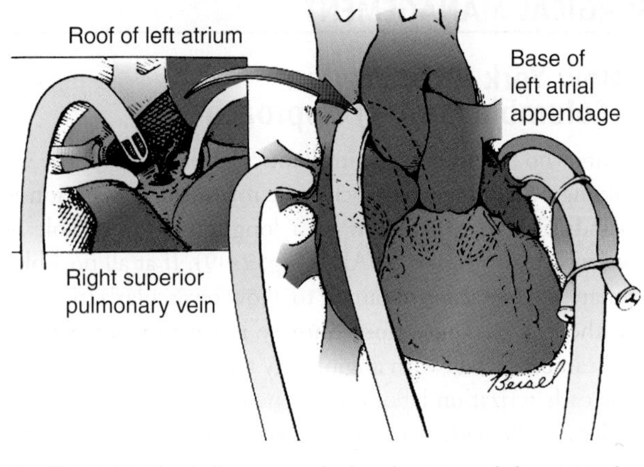

FIGURE 24-10 The inflow cannula for short-term left ventricular assist device support can be placed through the right superior pulmonary vein, the dome of the left atrium, or the left atrial appendage. Lighthouse tip cannulas allow improved venous return.

Reduction of myocardial energy consumption is best achieved by early institution of cardiopulmonary bypass to maintain a high perfusion pressure. If a coronary salvage catheter has been placed across a tight coronary lesion, the catheter is left in place until just before cross-clamping. Antegrade and retrograde catheters are placed before cross-clamping to allow quick instillation of retrograde cardioplegia and protection of the territory supplied by the occluded or compromised vessel. The standard Buckberg protocol is followed, including warm induction to allow regeneration of depleted adenosine triphosphate stores.

If the territory at risk is grafted by saphenous vein, this anastamosis is performed first to allow direct instillation of cardioplegia into the territory at risk. The proximal anastomoses should be performed before removal of the cross-clamp to allow complete perfusion of the entire heart upon removal of the cross-clamp. The role of off-pump CABG in this setting is appealing, but remains unproved.

Although large ventricular aneurysms are treated by resection and patch, debate surrounds smaller aneurysms. Our group does not resect small aneurysms, but some groups are more aggressive. If an aneurysm is resected, the defect is repaired with a patch of bovine pericardium sewn to the fibrotic rim of the endoaneurysm surface. The native left ventricular wall is closed over the patch.

Utilization of the Dor procedure (endoventricular circular patch plasty repair) in the post myocardial infarction setting is a controversial subject. Recent data have shown that surgical remodeling improves systolic function, ejection fraction, and intraventricular dyssynchrony, whereas other data suggest no added benefit when added to CABG.[115–118] Further investigation is needed to definitively answer this question.

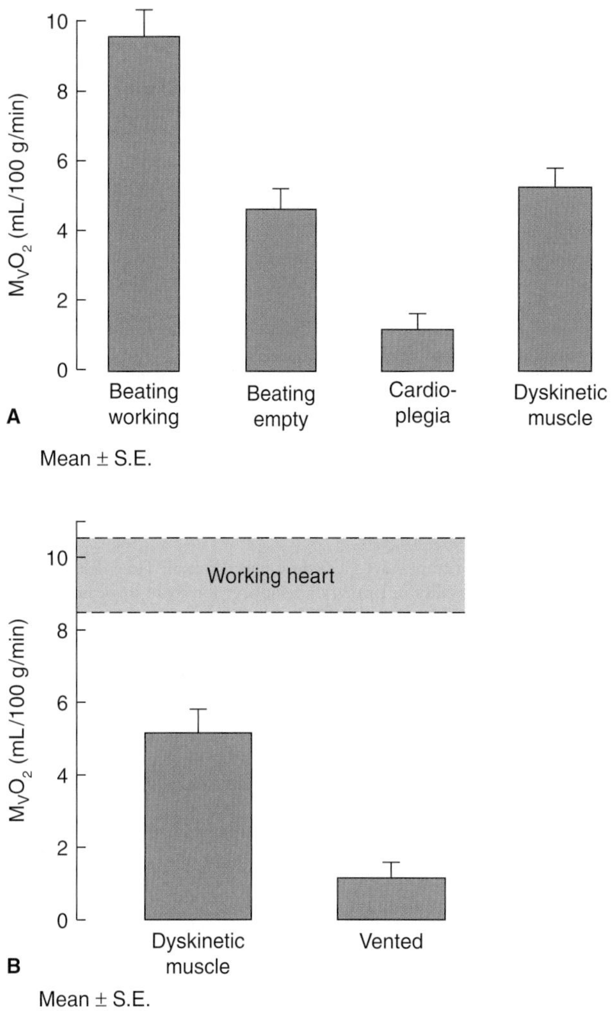

FIGURE 24-11 (A) Myocardial oxygen uptake (MvO_2), measured in milliliters per 100 grams per minute, in beating and working, beating and empty, and arrested hearts. Values after cardioplegia were determined both during cardiopulmonary bypass (cardioplegia) and during regional cardioplegic reperfusion in the working heart (dyskinetic muscle). Note (1) marked fall in MvO_2 with cardioplegia in the decompressed heart and (2) oxygen requirements of dyskinetic muscle increase fivefold over cardioplegia alone, and equal almost 55% of beating, working needs. (B) Regional oxygen uptake during selective cardioplegic reperfusion in dyskinetic and vented cardiac muscle. Stippled areas show requirements in working heart (8.5 to 10.5 mL/100 g/min). Note (1) high oxygen demands of dykinetic muscle and (2) marked reduction in demands when noncontracting muscle is decompressed by venting. *(Reproduced with permission from Allen BS, Rosenkranz ER, Buckberg GD, et al: Studies of controlled reperfusion after ischemia, VII: High oxygen requirements of dyskinetic cardiac muscle. J Thorac Cardiovasc Surg 1986; 92:543.)*

Postoperative Care

A higher incidence of complications in shock patients compared with nonshock emergencies has been reported. Guyton and associates[81] report a 47% complication rate associated with cardiogenic shock compared with 13% for patients with nonshock emergencies. This increase in complications probably reflects the preoperative condition of the patients rather than the treatment itself. Long-term follow-up in patients after emergency surgical revascularization shows that survival rates are closely correlated with postoperative ejection fraction and left ventricular size.[119,120]

FUTURE THERAPIES AND TRENDS

Improving outcomes in patients suffering acute myocardial infarction can occur through pharmacologic advances, optimization of existing practices, and application of new technology. Various medications have been described that reduce ischemic-reperfusion injury and limit infarct size in animal models, such as oxygen-derived free radical scavengers, folic acid, nitric oxide inhibitors, and others;[121] clinical study of these promising drugs will determine their efficacy. Sudden death after myocardial infarction may be reduced with administration of omega-3 fatty acids.[122] Reducing transport time to the hospital after the onset of symptoms and implementation of clinical guidelines have been initiatives of many hospitals and emergency services. The increased number of local hospitals able to perform primary percutaneous interventions has meant quicker revascularization, and thus improved outcomes.[14] This trend should continue in the future. Mechanical circulatory support has advanced greatly over the past 10 years, and pumps have become smaller, safer, less invasive, easier to use, and easier to implant. The indications for LVAD use are expanding in this population, and they may allow myocardial recovery to occur in select patients requiring hemodynamic support after acute infarction. The option of living long term with these devices has also become a reality. Finally, the rapidly emerging field of cellular therapy holds great promise for repair of damaged myocardium. A number of cell types, such as endothelial progenitor cells, mesenchymal stem cells, skeletal myoblasts, resident cardiac stem cells, and embryonic stem cells, are being investigated;[123] the optimal cell type, mode of delivery (intracoronary artery infusion, intravenous infusion, transendocardial injection, and transepicardial injection), and timing of administration have yet to be determined. Nevertheless, early clinical trials suggest that cellular therapy may offer benefits. One-year follow-up of 59 patients suffering acute myocardial infarction in the TOPCARE-AMI trial who received either circulating progenitor cells or bone marrow–derived progenitor cells demonstrated increased cardiac function and reduced ventricular dimensions, without adverse events.[124] Precultured mesenchymal cells also offer great promise by allowing cells from an unrelated donor to be administered without the complications of individual tissue harvest. The safety of these cells given intravenously after percutaneous revascularization in acute myocardial infarction was recently published, and efficacy studies are ongoing.[125] Numerous other clinical trials are underway to address questions regarding mechanisms of benefit, cell viability, and dosing. Future randomized clinical trials will be required to establish outcome benefit.

CONCLUSION

The treatment of acute myocardial infarction should be divided into two approaches. Uncomplicated acute myocardial infarction can be treated in most community hospitals. In most areas of the country, these patients are treated effectively with thrombolytic therapy and medical management. For communities and facilities that have catheterization laboratories, primary angioplasty may be more cost effective and produces improved results. At this time, emergency coronary artery bypass surgery is not the most cost-effective approach; randomized, controlled studies to demonstrate advantages of emergency CABG have not yet been performed.

The approach to acute myocardial infarctions complicated by cardiogenic shock presents a more difficult problem. Mortality rates are high with medical management. Reperfusion therapy is the only real hope for improved survival in this group of patients. Thrombolytic therapy is associated with poor outcomes. Early PTCA and CABG are the primary options in all patients, including those greater than age 75. Mechanical circulatory assistance has an important role for supporting patients until the myocardium recovers. Use of pharmacologic agents and means to control reperfusion are important areas of current research and development. Assist devices and artificial heart programs offer indispensable options and must be considered in this patient population, especially because all therapies offer suboptimal results.

KEY POINTS

1. Early reperfusion within 24 hours of acute myocardial infarction using thrombolysis, PTCA, intracoronary stenting, and CABG provides the best chance for myocardial salvage and long term survival.
2. Primary PTCA and intracoronary stenting are first-line therapies for patients suffering acute myocardial infarction, whereas thrombolysis is an acceptable alternative in select patient populations.
3. CABG after acute myocardial infarction may be appropriate for patients with ongoing angina or failure of percutaneous intervention, certain patients in cardiogenic shock, and those with structural complications of myocardial ischemia.
4. Circulatory assistance in the form of IABP and ventricular assist device insertion can provide temporary support until recovery or bridge to transplantation can occur in high-risk patients in cardiogenic shock.
5. Early institution of bypass, ventricular decompression, controlled reperfusion, and use of the Buckberg solution are important intraoperative techniques during CABG.

REFERENCES

1. Crossman AW, D'Agostino HJ, Geraci SA: Timing of coronary artery bypass graft surgery following acute myocardial infarction: a critical literature review. *Clin Cardiol* 2002; 25:406.
2. American Heart Association: Heart Disease and Stroke Statistics—2002 Update. Dallas, Tex, American Heart Association, 2002.
3. Goldberg RJ, Gore JM, Alpert JS, et al: Cardiogenic shock after acute myocardial infarction. *NEJM* 1991; 325:1117.
4. Page DL, Caulfield JB, Kastor JA, et al: Myocardial changes associated with cardiogenic shock. *NEJM* 1971; 285:133.
5. Hochman J: Cardiogenic shock complicating acute myocardial infarction: expanding the paradigm. *Circulation* 2003; 107:2998.
6. Tennant T, Wiggers CJ: Effect of coronary occlusion on myocardial contraction. *Am J Physiol* 1935; 112:351.
7. Jennings RB, Reimer KA: Factors involved in salvaging ischemic myocardium: effect of reperfusion of arterial blood. *Circulation* 1983; 68(Suppl I):I-25.
8. Schaper W: Experimental coronary artery occlusion, III: The determinants of collateral blood flow in acute coronary occlusion. *Basic Res Cardiol* 1978; 73:584.
9. Reimer KA, Jennings RB: The wavefront phenomenon of myocardial ischemic cell death, II: Transmural progression of necrosis within the framework of ischemic bed size (myocardium at risk) and collateral flow. *Lab Invest* 1979; 40:633.
10. Killip T 3rd, Kimball JT: Treatment of myocardial infarction in a coronary care unit: a two-year experience with 250 patients. *Am J Cardiol* 1972; 20:457.
11. Goldberg RJ, Gore JM, Alpert JS, et al: Cardiogenic shock after acute myocardial infarction. *NEJM* 1991; 325:1117.
12. Hochman JS, Sleeper LA, Webb JG, et al: Early revascularization in acute myocardial infarction complicated by cardiogenic shock. SHOCK Investigators. Should we emergently revascularize occluded coronaries for cardiogenic shock? *NEJM* 1999; 341:625.
13. Gacioch GM, Ellis SG, Lee L, et al: Cardiogenic shock complicating acute myocardial infarction: the use of coronary angioplasty and the integration of the new support devices into patient management. *J Am Coll Cardiol* 1992; 19:647.
14. De Luca G, Suryapranata H, Ottervanger JP, et al: Time delay to treatment and mortality in primary angioplasty for acute myocardial infarction. *Circulation* 2004; 109:1223.
15. Wackers FJ, Lie KI, Becker AE, et al: Coronary artery disease in patients dying from cardiogenic shock or congestive heart failure in the setting of acute myocardial infarction. *Br Heart J* 1976; 38:906.
16. Rabbani LE, Giglio J: Clinical pathways for acute coronary syndromes and chest pain. New York Hospital (Columbia Center) Guidelines, 2005.
17. Hennekens CH, O'Donnell CJ, Ridker PM, Marder VJ: Current issues concerning thrombolytic therapy for acute myocardial infarction. *J Am Coll Cardiol* 1995; 25(Suppl):18S.
18. Rahimtoola SH: The hibernating myocardium in ischemia and congestive heart failure. *Eur Heart J* 1993; 14 (Suppl A):22.
19. Schuster EH, Bulkley BH: Early post-infarction angina: ischemia at a distance and ischemia in the infarct zone. *NEJM* 1981; 305:1101.
20. Topol EJ, Ellis SH, Califf RM, et al: Combined tissue-type plasminogen activator and prostacyclin therapy for acute myocardial infarction. *J Am Coll Cardiol* 1989; 14:877.
21. Bolli R: Mechanism of myocardial stunning. *Circulation* 1990; 82:723.
22. Marban E: Myocardial stunning and hibernation: the physiology behind the colloquialisms. *Circulation* 1991; 83:681.
23. Bolli R: Basic and clinical aspects of myocardial stunning. *Prog Cardiovasc Dis* 1998; 40:477.
24. Underwood SR, Bax JJ, vom Dahl J, et al: Imaging techniques for the assessment of myocardial hibernation. *Eur Heart J* 2004; 25:815.
25. Charney R, Schwinger ME, Cohen MV, et al: Dobutamine echocardiography predicts recovery of hibernating myocardium following coronary revascularization. *J Am Coll Cardiol* 1992; 19:176A.
26. Klein C, Nekolla SG, Bengel FM, et al: Assessment of myocardial viability with contrast-enhanced magnetic resonance imaging: comparison with positron emission tomography. *Circulation* 2002; 105:162.
27. Kim HW, Farzaneh-Far A, Kim RJ: Cardiovascular magnetic resonance in patients with myocardial infarction. *J Am Coll Cardiol* 2010; 55:1-16.
28. Gerber BL, Garot J, Bluemke DA, et al: Accuracy of contrast enhanced magnetic resonance imaging in predicting improvement of regional myocardial function in patients after acute myocardial infarction. *Circulation* 2002; 106:1083.
29. Manhken AH, Koos R, Katoh M, et al: Assessment of myocardial viability in reperfused acute myocardial infarction using 16-slice computed tomography in comparison to magnetic resonance imaging. *J Am Coll Cardiol* 2005; 45:2042.
30. Hochman JS, Sleeper LA, White HD, et al: One-year survival following early revascularization for cardiogenic shock. *JAMA* 2001; 285:190.
31. Hochman JS, Sleeper LA, Webb JG, et al: Early revascularization and long-term survival in cardiogenic shock complicating acute myocardial infarction. *JAMA* 2006; 295:2511-2515.
32. Buckberg GD: Studies of controlled reperfusion after ischemia, I. When is cardiac muscle damaged irreversibly? *J Thorac Cardiovasc Surg* 1986; 92:483.
33. Vinten-Johansen J, Buckberg GD, Okamoto F, et al: Studies of controlled reperfusion after ischemia. V. Superiority of surgical versus medical reperfusion after regional ischemia. *J Thorac Cardiovasc Surg* 1986; 92:525.

34. Vinten-Johansen J, Rosenkranz ER, Buckberg GD, et al: Studies of controlled reperfusion after ischemia. VI. Metabolic and histochemical benefits of regional blood cardioplegic reperfusion without cardiopulmonary bypass. *J Thorac Cardiovasc Surg* 1986; 92:535.
35. Allen BS, Buckberg GD, Schwaiger M, et al: Studies of controlled reperfusion after ischemia. XVI. Early recovery of regional wall motion in patients following surgical revascularization after eight hours of acute coronary occlusion. *J Thorac Cardiovasc Surg* 1986; 92:636.
36. Allen BS, Okamoto F, Buckberg GD, et al: Studies of controlled reperfusion after ischemia, XIII: Reperfusion conditions—critical importance of total ventricular decompression during regional reperfusion. *J Thorac Cardiovasc Surg* 1986; 92:605.
37. Allen BS, Okamoto F, Buckberg GD, et al: Studies of controlled reperfusion after ischemia, XII: Effects of "duration" of reperfusate administration versus reperfusate "dose" on regional, functional, biochemical, and histological recovery. *J Thorac Cardiovasc Surg* 1986; 92:594.
38. Allen BS, Rosenkranz ER, Buckberg GD, et al: Studies of controlled reperfusion after ischemia. VII. High oxygen requirements of dyskinetic cardiac muscle. *J Thorac Cardiovasc Surg* 1986; 92:543.
39. Allen BS, Buckberg GD, Fontan FM, et al: Superiority of controlled surgical reperfusion versus percutaneous transluminal coronary angioplasty in acute coronary occlusion. *J Thorac Cardiovasc Surg* 1993; 105:864.
40. Rentrop P, Blanke H, Karsch KR, et al: Selective intracoronary thrombolysis in acute myocardial infarction and unstable angina pectoris. *Circulation* 1981; 63:307.
41. Gruppo Italiano per lo Studio della Streptokinasi: The effectiveness of intravenous thrombolytic treatment in acute myocardial infarction. *Lancet* 1986; 1:397.
42. ISSI-2 (Second International Study of Infarct Survival): Randomized trial of intravenous streptokinase, oral aspirin, both, or neither among 17187 cases of suspected acute myocardial infarction. *Lancet* 1988; 2:349.
43. The TIMI Study Group: Comparison of invasive and conservative strategies after treatment with intravenous tissue plasminogen activator in acute myocardial infarction. *NEJM* 1989; 320:618.
44. Simons ML, Betriu A, Col J, et al: Thrombolysis with tissue plasminogen activator in acute myocardial infarction: no additional benefit from immediate percutaneous coronary angioplasty. *Lancet* 1988; 1:197.
45. Gruppo Italiano per lo Studio della Streptokinasi: GISSI-2: A factorial randomized trial of alteplase versus streptokinase and heparin versus no heparin among 12,490 patients with acute myocardial infarction. *Lancet* 1990; 336:65.
46. ISIS-3 (Third International Study of Infarct Survival): ISIS-3: A randomized comparison of streptokinase vs. tissue plasminogen activator vs. anistreplase and of aspirin plus heparin vs. aspirin alone among 41,299 cases of suspected acute myocardial infarction. *Lancet* 1993; 339:753.
47. The GUSTO Angiographic Investigators: The effects of tissue plasminogen activator, streptokinase, or both on coronary patency, ventricular function, and survival after acute myocardial infarction. *NEJM* 1993; 329:1615.
48. The GUSTO Investigators: An international randomized trial comparing four thrombolytic strategies for acute myocardial infarction. *NEJM* 1993; 329:673.
49. Rentrop KP: Restoration of antegrade flow in acute myocardial infarction: The first 15 years. *J Am Coll Cardiol* 1995; 25(Suppl):1S.
50. Anonymous: Indications for fibrinolytic therapy in suspected acute myocardial infarction: collaborative overview of early mortality and major morbidity results from all randomized trials of more than 1000 patients. *Lancet* 1994; 343:311.
51. Angeja BG, Rundle AC, Gurwitz JH, et al: Death or nonfatal stroke in patients with acute myocardial infarction treated with tissue plasminogen activator. *Am J Cardiol* 2001; 87:627.
52. Bates ER, Topol EJ: Limitations of thrombolytic therapy for acute myocardial infarction complicated by congestive heart failure and cardiogenic shock. *J Am Coll Cardiol* 1991; 18:1077.
53. Grines CL, Browne KF, Marco J, et al: A comparison of immediate angioplasty with thrombolytic therapy in acute myocardial infarction. *NEJM* 1993; 328:673.
54. Goldman L: Cost and quality of life: thrombolysis and primary angioplasty. *J Am Coll Cardiol* 1995; 25(Suppl):38S.
55. Topol EJ, Califf RM, George BS, et al: A randomized trial of immediate versus delayed elective angioplasty after intravenous tissue plasminogen activator in acute myocardial infarction. *NEJM* 1987; 317:581.
56. Rogers WJ, Baim DS, Gore JM, et al: Comparison of immediate invasive, delayed invasive, and conservative strategies after tissue type plasminogen activator: results of the thrombolysis in myocardial infarction (TIMI) phase II-a trial. *Circulation* 1990; 81:1457.
57. Keeley EC, Boura JA, Grines CL: Primary angioplasty vs. intravenous thrombolytic therapy for acute myocardial infarction. *Lancet* 2003; 361:13.
58. Grines CL, Cox DA, Stone GW, et al: Coronary angioplasty with or without stent implantation for acute myocardial infarction. Stent Primary Angioplasty in Myocardial Infarction Study Group. *NEJM* 1999; 341:1949.
59. Stone GW, Grines CL, Cox DA, et al: Comparison of angioplasty with stenting, with or without abciximab, in acute myocardial infarction. *NEJM* 2002; 346:957.
60. Neumann FJ, Kastrati A, Schmitt C, et al: Effect of glycoprotein IIb/IIIa receptor blockade with abciximab on clinical and angiographic restenosis rate after the placement of coronary stents following acute myocardial infarction. *J Am Coll Cardiol* 2000; 35:915.
61. Montalescot G, Barragan P, Wittenberg O, et al: Platelet glycoprotein IIb/IIIa inhibition with coronary stenting for acute myocardial infarction. *NEJM* 2001; 344:1895.
62. Valgimigli M, Percoco G, Malagutti P, et al: STRATEGY Investigators: tirofiban and sirolimus-eluting stent vs. abciximab and bare-metal stent for acute myocardial infarction: a randomized trial. *JAMA* 2005; 293:2109.
63. Mauri L, Silbaugh TS, Garg P, et al: Drug-eluting or bare-metal stents for acute myocardial infarction. *NEJM* 2009; 359:1330-1342.
64. DeLuca G, Suryapranata H, Stone GW, et al: Abciximab as adjunctive therapy to reperfusion in acute ST-segment elevation myocardial infarction: a meta-analysis of randomized trials. *JAMA* 2005; 293:1759-1765.
65. Mehran R, Lansky AJ, Wiztenbichler W, et al: Bivalirudin in patients undergoing primary angioplasty for acute myocardial infarction (HORIZONS-AMI): 1-year results of a randomised controlled trial. *Lancet* 2009; 374:1149-1159.
66. Stone GW, Wiztenbichler B, Guagliumi G, et al: Bivalirudin during primary PCI in acute myocardial infarction. *NEJM* 2009; 358:2218-2230.
67. Lee L, Erbel R, Brown TM, et al: Multicenter registry of angioplasty therapy of cardiogenic shock: initial and long-term survival. *J Am Coll Cardiol* 1991; 17:599.
68. Webb JG, Lowe AM, Sanborn TA, et al: Percutaneous coronary intervention for cardiogenic shock in the SHOCK Trial. *J Am Coll Cardiol* 2003; 42:1380.
69. Berg R Jr, Selinger SL, Leonard JJ, et al: Immediate coronary artery bypass for acute evolving myocardial infarction. *J Thorac Cardiovasc Surg* 1981; 81:493.
70. DeWood MA, Spores J, Berg R Jr, et al: Acute myocardial infarction: a decade of experience with surgical reperfusion in 701 patients. *Circulation* 1983; 68(Suppl II):II-8.
71. Spencer FC: Emergency coronary bypass for acute infarction: an unproved clinical experiment. *Circulation* 1983; 68(Suppl II):II-17.
72. Lee DC, Oz MC, Weinberg AD, et al: Optimal timing of revascularization: transmural versus nontransmural acute myocardial infarction. *Ann Thorac Surg* 2001; 71:1198.
73. Lee DC, Oz MC, Weinberg AD, et al: Appropriate timing of surgical intervention after transmural acute myocardial infarction. *J Thorac Cardiovasc Surg* 2003; 125:115.
74. Weiss JL, Marino N, Shapiro EP: Myocardial infarct expansion: recognition, significance and pathology. *Am J Cardiol* 1991; 68:35.
75. Roberts CS, Schoen FJ, Kloner RA: Effects of coronary reperfusion on myocardial hemorrhage and infarct healing. *Am J Cardiol* 1983; 52:610.
76. Creswell LL, Rosenbloom M, Cox JL, et al: Intraaortic balloon counterpulsation: patterns of usage and outcome in cardiac surgical patients. *Ann Thorac Surg* 1992; 54:11.
77. Chen JM, DeRose JJ, Slater JP, et al: Improved survival rates support left ventricular assist device implantation early after myocardial infarction *J Am Coll Cardiol* 1999; 33:1903.
78. Creswell LR, Moulton MJ, Cox JL, Rosenbloom M: Revascularization after acute myocardial infarction. *Ann Thorac Surg* 1995; 60:19.
79. Stuart RS, Baumgartner WA, Soule L, et al: Predictors of perioperative mortality in patients with unstable postinfarction angina. *Circulation* 1988; 78(Suppl I):I-163.
80. DeWood MA, Notske RN, Hensley GR, et al: Intraaortic balloon counterpulsation with and without reperfusion for myocardial infarction shock. *Circulation* 1980; 61:1105.
81. Guyton RA, Arcidi JM, Langford DA, et al: Emergency coronary bypass for cardiogenic shock. *Circulation* 1987; 76(Suppl V):V-22.
82. White HD, Assman SF, Sanborn TA, et al: Comparison of percutaneous coronary intervention and coronary artery bypass grafting after acute myocardial infarction complicated by cardiogenic shock. *Circulation* 2005; 112:1992.
83. Serruys PW, Unger F, Sousa JE, et al (Group ARTS): Comparison of coronary-artery bypass surgery and stenting for the treatment of multivessel disease. *NEJM* 2001; 344:1117.
84. Rodriguez AE, Baldi J, Pereira CF, et al: Five-year follow-up of the Argentine randomized trial of coronary angioplasty with stenting versus coronary bypass surgery in patients with multiple vessel disease (ERACI II). *J Am Coll Cardiol* 2005; 46:582.

85. Eefting F, Nathoe H, van Dijk D, et al: Randomized comparison between stenting and off-pump bypass surgery in patients referred for angioplasty. *Circulation* 2003; 108:2870.
86. SoS Investigators: Coronary artery bypass surgery versus percutaneous coronary intervention with stent implantation in patients with multivessel coronary artery disease (the Stent or Surgery trial): a randomised controlled trial. *Lancet* 2002; 360:965.
87. Bakhai A, Hill RA, Dickson R, et al: Percutaneous transluminal coronary angioplasty with stents versus coronary artery bypass grafting for people with stable angina or acute coronary symptoms. *Cochrane Database Syst Rev* 2005; 4.
88. Hannan EL, Racz MJ, Walford G, et al: Long-term outcomes of coronary artery bypass grafting versus stent implantation. *NEJM* 2005; 352:2174.
89. Gersh BJ, Frye RL: Methods of coronary revascularization—things may not be as they seem. *NEJM* 2005; 352:2235.
90. Stamou SC, Jablonski KA, Hill PC, et al: Coronary revascularization without cardiopulmonary bypass versus the conventional approach in high-risk patients. *Ann Thorac Surg* 2005; 79:552.
91. Scheidt S, Wilner G, Mueller H, et al: Intra-aortic balloon counterpulsation in cardiogenic shock. *NEJM* 1973; 288:979.
92. Mueller HS: Role of intra-aortic counterpulsation in cardiogenic shock and acute myocardial infarction. *Cardiology* 1994; 84:168.
93. Gold HK Leinbach RC, Sanders CA, et al: Intra-aortic balloon pumping for control of recurrent myocardial ischemia. *Circulation* 1973; 47:1197.
94. Fotopoulos GD, Mason MJ, Walker S, et al: Stabilisation of medically refractory ventricular arrhythmias by intra-aortic balloon counterpulsation. *Heart* 1999; 82:96.
95. Stone GW, Ohman EM, Miller MF, et al: Contemporary utilization and outcomes of intra-aortic balloon counterpulsation in acute myocardial infarction. *J Am Coll Cardiol* 2003; 41:1940.
96. Waksman R, Weiss AT, Gotsman MS, Hasin Y: Intra-aortic balloon counterpulsation improves survival in cardiogenic shock complicating acute myocardial infarction. *Eur Heart J* 1993; 14:71.
97. Ohman EM, George BS, White CJ, et al: Use of aortic counterpulsation to improve sustained coronary artery patency during acute myocardial infarction. *Circulation* 1994; 90:792.
98. Dang NC, Topkara VK, Leacche M, et al: Left ventricular assist device implantation after acute anterior wall myocardial infarction and cardiogenic shock: a two-center study. *J Thorac Cardiovasc Surg* 2005; 130:693.
99. Ratcliffe MB, Bavaria JE, Wenger RK, et al: Left ventricular mechanics of ejecting postischemic hearts during left ventricular circulatory assistance. *J Thorac Cardiovasc Surg* 1991; 101:245.
100. Heerdt PM, Holmes JW, Cai B, et al: Chronic unloading by left ventricular assist device reverses contractile dysfunction and alters gene expression in end-stage heart failure. *Circulation* 2000; 102:2713.
101. Zafeiridis A, Jeevanandam V, Houser SR, et al: Regression of cellular hypertrophy after left ventricular assist device support. *Circulation* 1998; 98:656.
102. Mancini DM, Beniaminovitz A, Levin H, et al: Low incidence of myocardial recovery after left ventricular assist device implantation in patients with chronic heart failure. *Circulation* 1998; 98:2383.
103. Thiele H, Lauer B, Hambrecht R, et al: Reversal of cardiogenic shock by percutaneous left atrial-to-femoral artery bypass assisstance. *Circulation* 2001; 104:2917-2922.
104. Burkhoff D, Cohen H, Brunckhorst C, et al: A randomized multicenter clinical study to evaluate the safety and efficacy of the TandemHeart percutaneous ventricular assist device versus conventional therapy with intraaortic balloon pumping for treatment of cardiogenic shock. *Am Heart J* 2006; 152:469.e1-469.e8.
105. Seyfarth M, Sibbing D, Bauer I, et al: A randomized clinical trial to evaluate the safety and efficacy of a percutaneous left ventricular assist device versus intra-aortic balloon pumping for treatment of cardiogenic shock caused by myocardial infarction. *J Am Coll Cardiol* 2008; 52:1584-1588.
106. Lietz K, Miller L: Left ventricular assist devices: Evolving devices and indications for use in ischemic heart disease. *Curr Opin Cardiol* 2004; 7:174.
107. Oz MC, Pepino P, Goldstein DJ, et al: Selection scale predicts patients successfully receiving long-term, implantable left ventricular assist devices. *Circulation* 1994; 90:I-308.
108. CURE Study Investigators: The Clopidogrel in Unstable angina to prevent Recurrent Events (CURE) Trial Programme. *Eur Heart J* 2000; 21:2033.
109. Harker LA, Boisset JP, Pilgrim AJ, et al: Comparative safety and tolerability of clopidogrel and aspirin: results from CAPRIE. CAPRIE Steering Committee and Investigators. Clopidogrel vs. Aspirin in Patients at Risk of Ischaemic Events. *Drug Saf* 1999; 21:325.
110. Dangas G, Mehran R, Guagliumi G, et al: Role of clopidogrel loading dose in patients with st-segment elevation myocardial infarction undergoing primary angioplasty. *J Am Coll Cardiol* 2009: 54:1438-1446.
111. Hongo R, Ley J, Dick S, et al: The effect of clopidogrel in combination with aspirin when given before coronary artery bypass grafting. *J Am Coll Cardiol* 2002; 40:231.
112. Kapetanakis EI, Medlam DA, Boyce SW, et al: Clopidogrel administration prior to coronary artery bypass grafting surgery: The cardiologist's panacea or the surgeon's headache? *Eur Heart J* 2005; 26:576.
113. Caes FL, Van Nooten GJ: Use of internal mammary artery for emergency grafting after failed coronary angioplasty. *Ann Thorac Surg* 1994; 57:1295.
114. Zaplonski A, Rosenblum J, Myler RK, et al: Emergency coronary artery bypass surgery following failed balloon angioplasty: role of the internal mammary artery graft. *J Cardiac Surg* 1995; 10:32.
115. Di Donato M, Sabatier M, Dor V, et al: Effects of the Dor procedure on left ventricular dimension and shape and geometric correlates of mitral regurgitation one year after surgery. *J Thorac Cardiovasc Surg* 2001; 121:91.
116. Athanasuleas CL, Buckberg GD, Stanley AWH, et al: Surgical ventricular restoration in the treatment of congestive heart failure due to post-infarction ventricular dilation. *J Am Coll Cardiol* 2004; 44:1439.
117. DiDonato MD, Toso A, Dor V, et al: Surgical ventricular restoration improves mechanical intraventricular dyssynchrony in ischemic cardiomyopathy. *Circulation* 2004; 109:2536.
118. Jones RH, Velazquez EJ, Michler RE, et al: Coronary bypass surgery with or without surgical ventricular reconstruction. *NEJM* 2009; 309:1705-1717.
119. Applebaum R, House R, Rademaker A, et al: Coronary artery bypass grafting within thirty days of acute myocardial infarction. *J Thorac Cardiovasc Surg* 1991; 102:745.
120. Hochberg MS, Parsonnet V, Gielchinsky I, et al: Timing of coronary revascularization after acute myocardial infarction. *J Thorac Cardiovasc Surg* 1984; 88:914.
121. Moens AL, Claeys MJ, Timmermans JP, et al: Myocardial ischemia/reperfusion-injury, a clinical view on a complex pathophysiological process. *Int J Cardiol* 2005; 100:179.
122. Marchioli R, Barzi F, Bomba E, et al: Early protection against sudden death by n-3 polyunsaturated fatty acids after myocardial infarction: time course analysis of the results of the Gruppo Italiano per lo Studio della Sopravvivenza nell'Infarto Miocardico (GISSI)-Prevenzione. *Circulation* 2002; 105:1897.
123. Wollert KC, Drexler H: Clinical applications of stem cells for the heart. *Circ Res* 2005; 96:151.
124. Schachinger V, Assmus B, Britten MB, et al: Transplantation of progenitor cells and regeneration enhancement in acute myocardial infarction. Final one-year results of the TOPCARE-AMI Trial. *J Am Coll Cardiol* 2004; 44:1690.
125. Hare JM, Traverse JH, Henry TD, et al: A randomized, double-blind, placebo-controlled, dose-escalation study of intravenous adult human mesenchymal stem cell (prochymal) after acute myocardial infarction. *J Am Coll Cardiol* 2009; 54:2277-2286.

CHAPTER 25

Minimally Invasive Myocardial Revascularization

David M. Holzhey
Ardawan J. Rastan
Volkmar Falk
Friedrich W. Mohr

INTRODUCTION

The term *minimally invasive coronary artery bypass grafting* is not well defined. According to one definition, avoidance of cardiopulmonary bypass (CPB) is considered essential in decreasing the morbidity associated with conventional coronary artery bypass grafting (CABG).[1] Other authors consider the median sternotomy as a potential source for morbidity, referring to the risk of mediastinitis and the associated delayed return to daily life activities.[2] Accordingly, a number of surgical strategies have evolved to avoid the need for extracorporeal circulation and to minimize surgical access. Furthermore, operative strategies as avoidance of aortic manipulation or complete arterial revascularization focus on improved short- and long-term results. At the same time, it was widely recognized that open harvesting techniques for bypass grafts often are associated with wound-healing problems, especially in diabetic patients. As a consequence, endoscopic harvesting techniques for both venous and radial artery grafts have been developed.

OFF-PUMP CORONARY ARTERY BYPASS GRAFTING (OPCAB)

For decades, CABG was routinely performed with cardioplegic arrest and using CPB. An empty, nonbeating heart, a bloodless surgical field, and an easy exposure were regarded as essential for success of the procedure. Results were excellent, mortality declined constantly, and standard CABG became the "bread and butter" of our profession.[3] Anecdotal reports on the deleterious effects of CPB and systematic reports examining the pathophysiology of extracorporeal circulation started to question the dogma of "the pump is your friend." CPB is associated with (1) a systemic inflammatory response, (2) release of cytokines, (3) activation of the clotting cascade, (4) metabolic changes, (5) microembolization and numerous other adverse effects. Although tolerated in most cases, these effects alone or in combination may cause substantial morbidity and thus affect the results of the procedure. With an ever-aging population and increasing comorbidity, surgeons all over the world sought to further minimize the risk of CABG, and it seemed logical to question the role of CPB in CABG.

The evolution of *off-pump coronary artery bypass grafting* (OPCAB) is closely linked to the development of stabilizers that became available in the early 1990s. Initially, pure pressure stabilizers were engineered, but it soon became obvious that exposure of the back wall of the heart would require additional means of support. With the introduction of vacuum-assisted stabilizers by the Utrecht group, local myocardial immobilization was greatly facilitated and independent of the area of revascularization and OPCAB gained popularity. Despite better stabilizers, it was recognized that OPCAB requires a team approach and awareness of the sudden hemodynamic changes that may occur during the procedure.

Anesthesia Requirements

In most centers, general anesthesia is applied, and the patient is intubated. Incidental reports indicate that the operation is also possible on the awake, spontaneously breathing patient under high epidural anesthesia.[4] Standard monitoring is applied. In addition, some centers prefer online cardiac output measurement using the PICCO or similar methods.[5] A Swan-Ganz catheter is usually not helpful and can potentially cause arrhythmia when the heart is manipulated during the procedure. It is of utmost importance that the patient is kept warm at all times during the procedure. Temperature management includes placing the patient on a warming blanket, using warm infusions, and keeping the room temperature high. Volume management is essential because it is the preferred means for counterbalancing hemodynamic changes. Exposure of the back wall of the heart usually causes some degree of right ventricular outflow obstruction that can be treated adequately by increasing venous return by tilting the operating room table to the right with the head low. Because no CPB is used and filtering is not possible, intravenous volume overload must be avoided, especially in end-stage renal failure (ESRF) patients. The use of inotropes should be reserved for those with severe hemodynamic alterations only because they invariably increase the heart rate and thus complicate the procedure. In a review of human factors associated with manual control and tracking, it was pointed out that the human operator can at his or her best track a three-dimensional (3D) motion (such as the beating heart) only up to a frequency of 1 Hz, which happens to equal a heart rate of 60 beats per minute.[6] Higher frequencies cannot be tracked, thus the preferred heart rate should be kept in the range of 50 to 70 beats per minute to simplify suturing. In case of atrial fibrillation, pharmacologic slowing of the heart rate and temporary ventricular pacing using an epicardial pacing wire may facilitate the procedure. The use of a Cell Saver is recommended to minimize the risk for blood transfusion, which is rarely necessary. If less than 500 mL is collected, the blood usually is discarded.

Surgical Technique

After standard median sternotomy, single or bilateral internal thoracic artery (ITA) harvesting is performed. The patient is heparinized (150 to 200 units/kg, ie, about half of CPB dosage), keeping the activated clotting time (ACT) at a level above 300 seconds. In order to facilitate exposure of the heart, it is recommended to divide the pericardial and mediastinal attachments. Opening of the right pleura may become necessary in severely dilated hearts and some surgeons do it routinely to give the heart space during tilting, allowing easier access of the posterolateral wall. After the pericardium is opened, pericardial stay sutures are placed to aid in exposure of the heart. Numerous methods have been proposed for placing these sutures. Ideally, two or more sutures are placed beginning at the level of the right upper pulmonary vein all the way down distally to the lowest point of the epicardial sac (Fig. 25-1). To avoid damage to the myocardium, the sutures should be covered by plastic tubing; sponges may be used alternatively. Placement of the stay sutures should be done slowly because abrupt changes in positioning of the heart may cause undesired hemodynamic alterations or arrhythmia. The sequence for the grafts depends largely on the individual needs of the patient. In general, the left anterior descending (LAD) artery is the most important target vessel and the easiest to bypass. Therefore, revascularization should

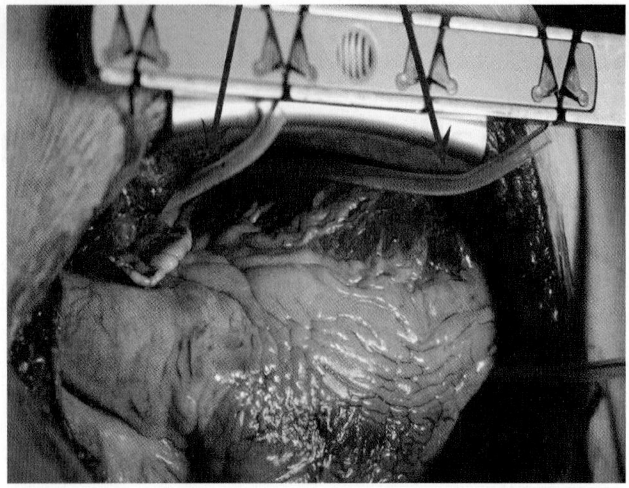

FIGURE 25-1 Setup for off-pump coronary artery bypass grafting. Placement of pericardial stay sutures.

start with an ITA graft to the LAD. By lifting the stay sutures, the LAD comes easily into view. The stabilizer is placed at the site of the anastomosis, and dissection of the surrounding tissue is begun. If the vessel is covered by excessive fat or muscle, low-energy cautery and clipping of epicardial veins may help to ensure minimal bleeding from the surrounding tissue. Once the site for the anastomosis is identified, the stabilizer is placed in a way to ensure enough space for suturing and equal distance to the stabilizer feet. Mechanical compromize of large diagonal branches should be avoided. Vacuum stabilizers should be locked only after vacuum is applied and the stabilizer sucks to the surface. Only a small amount of pressure will then be required to immobilize the heart. Excess pressure from the stabilizer will cause increasing wall motion as the heart works with more force against its compression. Temporary occlusion of the target vessel can be achieved in many ways. Surrounding 4-0 felt-pledgeted sutures or silastic tapes are used widely. The occlusion tapes ought to be placed at a distance of at least 5 to 10 mm from the anastomosis to avoid compression and distortion of the target vessel at the level of the anastomosis and thus allow for easy suturing. The suture needs to be placed deep enough in the tissue to avoid damage of the target vessel. The corresponding coronary vein should be respected to avoid disturbing side bleedings. Distal coronary artery occlusion should be avoided in general and is rarely necessary even in occluded vessels with strong backflow. Care must be taken to stay outside stented areas because the occlusion tapes may bend or kink an implanted stent. The incision usually is made before the occlusion suture is tightened to ensure complete filling of the vessel, which will minimize the risk of back wall injury. The suture then is tightened gently until bleeding stops. If there is only minimal coronary blood flow, eg, in chronic total vessel occusion, tightening may not at all be necessary. A CO_2 blower-mister is used to control residual bleeding from septal branches of the distal coronary at a rate not exceeding 5 L/min. Excessive blowing can cause dissection or injury to the intima of both the graft and the coronary artery or cause air embolism. The use of coronary artery shunts is controversial because they also may cause endothelial damage. If shunts are used, care must be taken to ensure atraumatic placement. A very new development is a transparent reverse thermosensitive gel (LeGoo, Pleuromed Inc., Woburn, MA) which can be injected after incision of the coronary vessel for temporary blockage of the blood flow allowing an almost bloodfree anastomotic site. The anstomosis can then be sutured without the need for a blower-mister, shunts, or occlusion snares. The gel completely dissolves with time (after approximately 15 minutes) or with the application of local cold.[7,8]

The circumflex artery and its branches are grafted next in a sequence that is dictated mainly by the individual coronary pathology and the preference of grafts. The distal circumflex artery is regarded as the most challenging vessel to graft during OPCAB because exposure may be difficult. In large hearts and more importantly in patients with right ventricular dysfunction, it may be necessary to open the right pleura and divide the right-sided pericardium low to the level of the phrenic nerve. This will allow displacement of the heart underneath the sternum into the right pleural cavity. This maneuver minimizes right outflow tract obstruction and exposes all posterior vessels. After the circumflex artery, the right coronary artery (RCA) and its branches are grafted. If the RCA is the dominant vessel and the stenosis is less than 80%, it may be necessary to use a shunt because ischemia of the atrioventricular (AV) nodal artery during occlusion of the RCA can cause acute total AV block. It is therefore advisable to place and connect a temporary pacing wire before occluding the vessel.

To maximize both the short- and long-term benefit of an OPCAB procedure, arterial grafting is preferred. This will obviate the need for aortic clamping, another source for emboli and independent predictor of stroke.[9] In fact, some authors see avoidance of aortic manipulation as the key factor to bring the stroke risk of CABG below the stroke risk of PCI (Table 25-1).

TABLE 25-1 Comparison of Stroke Rates Using Different Coronary Artery Bypass Techniques

	No. of patients	Strokes (%)
Vallely and colleagues[11]		
anaortic	1201	0.25
off-pump side clamp	557	1.08
on-pump	1599	1.81
Calafiore and colleagues[12]		
anaortic	1533	0.19
off-pump side clamp	460	1.09
on-pump	2830	1.44
Prapas and colleagues[13]		
anaortic	1359	0.22

Adapted from Brereton RJ, Misfeld M, Ross DE: Percutaneous coronary intervention versus coronary artery bypass grafting. NEJM 2009; 360(25):2673; author reply 2674-2675.

If vein grafts are used, the proximal or distal anastomosis can be performed first. It is of utmost importance to partially clamp the aorta under low pressure to minimize the risk of aortic embolie and to avoid aortic dissection. This can be achieved medically or by a brief period of inflow occlusion by manually compressing the inferior vena cava. This maneuver also should be repeated for declamping. Intraoperative graft patency control using transient-time Doppler or other means is recommended. If the operative field is dry, heparin usually is not completely antagonized. Postoperatively, aspirin is begun on the day of operation.

Special Situations

In patients with unstable angina, acute cardiogenic shock, or with ejection fraction (EF) below 20%, the preoperative implantation of an intra-aortic counterpulsation pump (IACP) may be useful. Alternatively these patients can be operated on-pump beating heart to combine the advantages of preserved native coronary blood flow, deloading the heart and adequate organ perfusion.[14,15] Patients with atrial fibrillation (AF) show an irregular contraction pattern that may distract during suturing (regular-motion patterns allow the development of coping strategies such as the "wait and see" strategy that are less effective when motion is unpredictable[5]). It therefore may be helpful to slow the heart rate pharmacologically and temporarily pace the patient in a VVI mode. If AF is paroxysmal, epicardial ablation for pulmonary vein isolation on the beating heart may be applied before bypass grafting.

Results

The number of OPCABs performed has reached 30% of all coronary revascularizations worldwide, in some countries especially with limited medical and financial resources exceeding today 80%. In some units, OPCAB is used almost exclusively with no patient selection.

When discussing outcomes, it is important to keep in mind that despite the fact that propensity scoring was applied for most analyses, some selection bias cannot be excluded. As pointed out by Sergeant and colleagues and also Puskas and coworkers, clinically relevant reductions of mortality, stroke, and renal failure with the OPCAB approach mandate large cohorts of patients to reach statistical significance in the presence of above-standard on-pump performance.[16,17]

When the first reports on OPCAB were published, concerns were raised regarding (1) incomplete revascularization[18–21] and (2) impaired graft patency owing to a more challenging technique.[22] These fears are fueled by some larger prospective studies. Khan and colleagues found a reduced graft patency in OPCAB patients after 3 months with no difference in all other outcome parameters.[22] In the ROOBY trial including more than a thousand patients in each group, the one-year outcome regarding cardiac death was inferior in the OPCAB group as well as the graft patency rate exept for the LIMA-LAD graft.[23] Other studies like the SMART and Prague IV study that provide angiographic data on graft patency reveal equal patency rates for on- and off-pump bypass surgery.[24–26]

Regarding operative and short-term mortality, most studies are in favor of OPCAB. In a retrospective analysis of the Society of Thoracic Surgeons database for the years 1999 and 2000, including 17,969 OPCAB patients (8.8% of total), a significant survival advantage with OPCAB compared with on-pump CABG was demonstrated by risk-adjusted multivariate logistic regression analysis (OR 0.76, 95% CI 0.68 to 0.84) and conditional logistic regression of propensity-matched groups (OR 0.83, 95% CI 0.73 to 0.96).[27] Similar results have been reported from another multicenter analysis consisting of some 7283 patients by Mack and colleagues. Following propensity score matching and multivariate regression analysis, the use of CPB was identified as an independent predictor of mortality (OR 2.08, 95% CI 1.52 to 2.83, $p < .001$).[28] Especially in high-risk populations (eg, the elderly, those with EFs below 30%, and obese patients), OPCAB seems to offer a survival benefit.[17,29–31] There are only sparse data on the midterm outcome. After 2 and 4 years, similar survival has been reported.[18,32]

There is growing evidence that neurocognitive outcome is better and stroke rate is reduced after OPCAB.[33–35] According to a number of studies, CPB is an independent predictor of adverse neurologic outcome.[36] The embolic burden measured by transit-time Doppler of the medial cerebral artery is reduced significantly during OPCAB.[37–39] The risk of acute renal failure is decreased in off-pump surgery,[40–42] especially in high-risk groups with preoperative renal insufficiency.[43,44]

The incidence of postoperative atrial fibrillation is reduced after OPCAB,[44,45] and biochemical markers for myocardial injury (eg, creatinine kinase and troponin) are reduced after OPCAB.[46–48] Blood loss is less, and transfusion rate is reduced.[17] Overall, OPCAB reduces hospital costs by 15 to 35%[31,49] possibly owing to decrease in length of stay and resource utilization.[31]

In a thorough meta-analysis, the International Society for Minimally Invasive Cardiac Surgery Consensus Group published the evidence for OPCAB.[17] Accordingly, OPCAB reduces mortality and length of stay and the incidence of postoperative myocardial infarction (MI), renal failure, AF, and transfusion rate in mixed-risk and high-risk patients (Fig. 25-2).

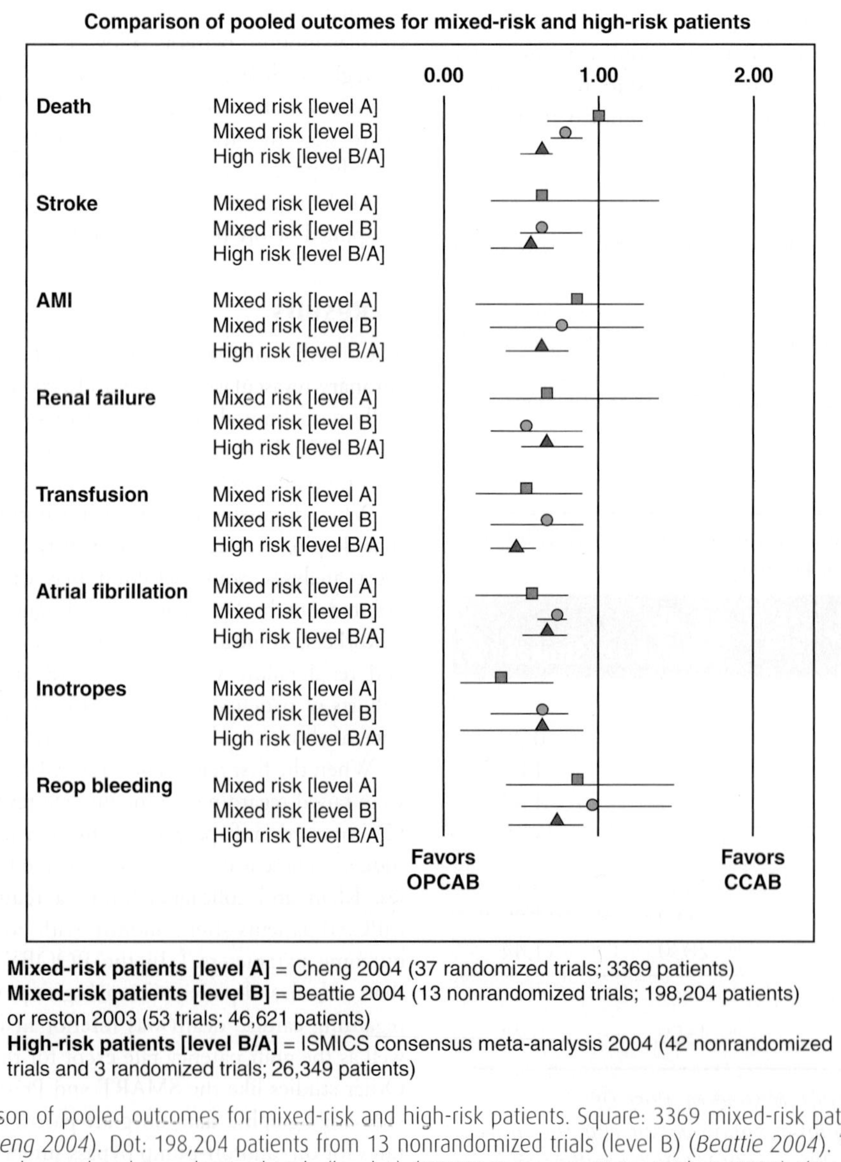

FIGURE 25-2 Comparison of pooled outcomes for mixed-risk and high-risk patients. Square: 3369 mixed-risk patients from 37 randomized trials (level A) (*Cheng 2004*). Dot: 198,204 patients from 13 nonrandomized trials (level B) (*Beattie 2004*). Triangle: 26,349 high-risk patients from 42 nonrandomized and 3 randomized trials (level A) (*ISMICS Consensus Meta-Analysis 2004*). *(Reprinted, with permission, from Puskas et al[20] with kind permission from Innovations)*

In conclusion, OPCAB is a highly demanding procedure with a prolonged learning curve compared with conventional byass graft surgery. Some surgeons perform OPCAB almost exclusively, whereas others never use it at all. Comparisons are therefore difficult and maybe OPCAB is not the best option for every patient or for all cardiac surgeons. It is, however, an important option and must be mastered with the same technical precision as conventional CABG.[50]

MINIMALLY INVASIVE DIRECT CORONARY ARTERY BYPASS (MIDCAB)

One goal of minimally invasive cardiac surgery has been to avoid sternotomy to reduce the amount of surgical trauma and avoid wound complications. Therefore, coronary artery bypass techniques on the beating heart without sternotomy were developed. The operation was termed *minimally invasive direct coronary artery bypass* (MIDCAB), and since its introduction in the mid-1990s,[51–55] it has found a widespread application. In some centers, MIDCAB is the preferred method of surgical revascularization for isolated coronary artery disease (CAD) of the LAD. In addition, MIDCAB is a valuable alternative to standard CABG or OPCAB in selected high-risk patients with multivessel disease and extensive comorbidity, who are at a prohibitively high risk for sternotomy.

Anesthesia

Standard monitoring is applied, and temperature management as for OPCAB is applied. Because single-lung ventilation is applied by using a double-lumen tube or bronchus blocker to provide selective right lung ventilation, short-acting anesthetics are used to allow for fast extubation.

Surgical Technique

Standard MIDCAB usually is performed through a left anterolateral minithoracotomy in a 10 to 20 degrees right lateral position. After making a 5- to 6-cm skin incision in the fifth intercostal space or the inframammary fold, the pectoralis muscle is displaced bluntly with minimal division following the muscle fiber orientation (muscle-sparing approach). This will decrease the likelihood of lung herniation that has been reported infrequently with this approach. The chest then usually is entered one intercostal space higher than the actual incision. Excessive rib spreading must be avoided at all times to prevent dislocation or fracture. Removal of a rib is almost never necessary. Take-down of the LITA usually is performed under direct vision, but endoscopic ITA takedown using a harmonic scalpel or telemanipulation systems has also been reported.[55–57]

The intrathoracic fascia is divided to facilitate take-down of the LITA, which usually is done in a pedicled manner. Takedown is performed from the fifth intercostal space to the origin of the subclavian artery. Using a sceletonized technique offers the advantage of gaining more graft length, but is, of course, more time consuming. Additional length can also be

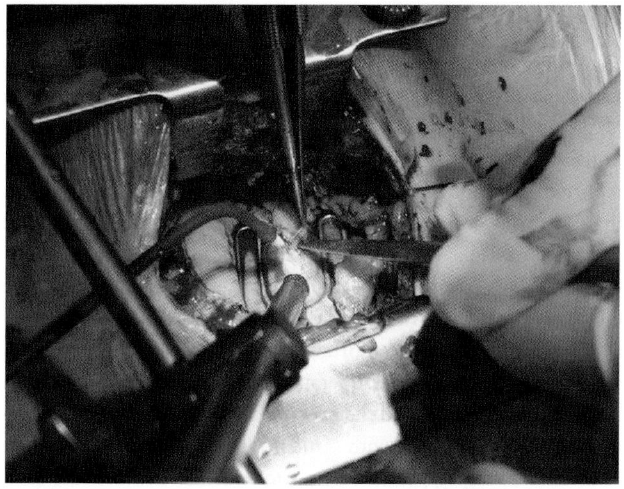

FIGURE 25-3 Minimally invasive direct coronary artery bypass. Through a muscle-sparing incision, the left anterior descending artery is easily exposed; standard pressure stabilizers are used.

gained by dividing the mammary vein at its junction with the subclavian vein. Side branches are clipped or cauterized based on the preference of the surgeon. Heparin is administered prior to distal transsection of the graft. As in sternotomy OPCAB the ACT is kept at a level above 300 seconds. The pericardium should be opened above the course of the LAD and extended to the groove between the aorta and the pulmonary artery. This will facilitate location of the target vessel if excess epicardial fat or an intramuscular course is present. After that the target vessel is identified. To enhance exposure, one or two pericardial stay sutures may be used to position the heart. It is of utmost importance to have the region of anastomosis in direct and comfortable view. Standard reusable pressure stabilizers are then used to immobilize the target region (Fig. 25-3). Vacuum stabilizers in general are too bulky and not required for a single anastomosis to the LAD. Proximal LAD occlusion is performed using a 4-0 felt-pledgeted suture or vessel loops. Ischemic preconditioning is not helpful, but some surgeons use it to feel more comfortable when knowing that ischemia is well tolterated. The use of shunts is rarely necessary, but they may be applied based on the preference of the surgeon and indicated when strong coronary backflow is evident. Distal occlusion should be avoided whenever possible (99% of patients). A blower-mister is used in all cases to achieve a bloodless field. The anastomosis then is performed in a standard fashion using a 7-0 or 8-0 polypropylene running suture. Finally the LITA can be fixed on the pericardial tissue. Graft patency assessment is performed routinely using transit-time Doppler. A single chest tube is inserted into the left pleural space, and intercostal nerve blockade is applied using local anesthetics. Before closing the chest with one or two strong rib sutures the single lung ventilation is stopped and the left lung is inflated under direct view to control tension free course of the LITA. This is facilitated by keeping the LITA aside to the mediastinum using the suction tip or long forceps. Extubation usually is performed on the table for a few hours postoperatively. Patients are routinely started on antiplatelet therapy on the day of operation.

Results

A number of papers have reported excellent results with this approach. Immediate angiographic patency rates are in the range of 94 to 98% and thus similar to those reported for conventional CABG.[54,58] At 6 months, patency rates of 94% have been reported.[59] Reported in-hospital mortality for MIDCAB is less than 1% and compares favorably with the off-pump single-bypass mortality of 1.4% and with the mortality of single bypass with CPB of 3.6% that was been reported in the registry of the German Society for Thoracic and Cardiovascular Surgery.[60] and is also lower than the 2.4% mortality that is reported from the STS database.[61] The rates of perioperative major complications such as myocardial infarction and the need for target-vessel reintervention are low and comparable with standard CABG. However, because of an aortic surgery perioperative stroke is rare and the rate considerably lower compared with conventional techniques.

In our own series of 1918 patients who underwent MIDCAB from 1996 to 2009, in-hospital mortality was 0.8% (predicted mortality by Euroscore 3.8%), and stroke rate was 0.3%. Conversion to sternotomy was necessary in 1.6%. A total of 745 patients received routine postoperative angiogram demonstrating a 96.3% early patency rate. At 6-month follow-up, graft patency was 95.2% ($n = 423$). Five-year survival is 91.5% (95% CI 89.51 to 93.5%). (Fig. 25-4A) The freedom from MACCE and angina after 5 and 7 years was 88.6% (95% CI 86.4 to 90.9%) (see Fig. 25-4B). These results are in accordance with the findings of other groups.[59,62,63]

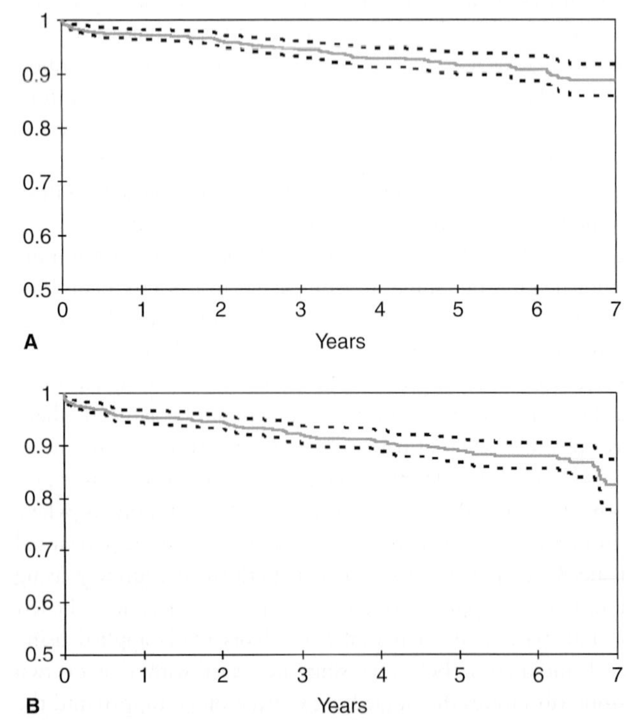

FIGURE 25-4 Kaplan-Meier (including 95% confidence interval) five-year survival curve (A) and event-free survival curve (freedom from death, myocardial infarction, stroke, freedom from angina, freedom from reintervention) (B) after minimally invasive direct coronary artery bypass. Data from 1483 patients undergoing MIDCAB at the Heartcenter Leipzig.

A few randomized trials comparing MIDCAB versus bare metal stenting in isolated proximal LAD lesions have demonstrated better early patency and superior freedom from target-vessel reintervention and angina for the MIDCAB group up to 5 years of follow-up.[64–69]

Some studies have pointed out that the lateral approach is associated with higher pain levels than sternotomy, mainly owing to the excessive rib spreading required for visualizing the LITA during takedown.[55] Rib dislocation or fracture has been reported infrequently with this approach. Direct harvesting of the LITA is regarded as technically challenging and has been one of the arguments for many surgeons to disregard MIDCAB as the primary operation for patients who require surgical revascularization of the LAD. Limited working space and incomplete vision are blamed for insufficient graft length, incomplete mobilization, and the occasional reports of LITA injury or injury of the subclavian vein.

MIDCAB is a highly demanding technical procedure that should be started by surgeons who have sufficient experience in conventional and off-pump surgery. It has been shown that the complication rate of MIDCAB (namely conversion to sternotomy, reexploration for bleeding, and reintervention on the target vessel) is significantly lowered after an experience of 100 to 150 MIDCAB procedures.[70] Therefore, it can be recommended to concentrate this operation on dedicated and experienced surgeons.

Even with improved outcomes of interventional procedures and less in-stent restenosis with the use of drug-eluting stents,[71] MIDCAB, based on its very good long-term results,[72] will remain an alternative revascularization strategy to PCI for patients with single-vessel disease, especially for complex ostial lesions, chronic occlusions, and in-stent restenosis.

TOTAL ENDOSCOPIC CORONARY ARTERY BYPASS GRAFTING (TECAB)

The possibly least invasive approach for surgical revascularization is *total endoscopic coronary artery bypass grafting* (TECAB) on the beating heart. Working through ports has long been known for limiting the available space to perform motions, for substantially decreasing the dexterity of the operator, and for altering the hand-eye coordination.[73] Active assistance, an indispensable component of open surgery, is difficult in thoracoscopic procedures. The transition from limited-access cardiac surgery to endoscopic cardiac surgery therefore complicates the procedure substantially and has rendered previous attempts at endoscopic CABG using conventional endoscopic instruments impossible. To overcome some of the instrument-related limitations, computer-enhanced instrumentation systems have been developed.

Principles of Telemanipulator-Assisted Cardiac Surgery

With the usage of telemanipulation devices the operator involved in the interaction is physically removed but not necessarily remote from the operation table. He instead operates at an *input manipulator* (surgical console, master console) from which he steers the *executing manipulator* (slave console) which is situated at the patient site. The slave console consists of all nessesary electromechanical equipment to operate two or three exchangable endoscopic instruments plus a high definition 3D endoscopic camera. Both haptic and visual information is fed back to the master console. This way a virtual 3D operative field is created wherein the surgeon can manipulate steering handles with a perfect hand-eye alignment. The introduction of telemanipulation technology to endoscopic surgery was able to address the key performance limitations of conventional endoscopic surgery, namely, reduced articulation, monocular vision, and loss of hand-eye coordination.

Surgical Technique

Standard monitoring for cardiac surgery is applied. Defibrillator pads are placed on the back and to the right side of the chest. Single-lung ventilation of the right lung is applied using a double-lumen endotracheal tube or a bronchus blocker. Temperature management follows the principles of OPCAB surgery. After draping the instrument arms and camera arm, camera and scope calibration are performed and the endostabilizer is prepared. A holding arm for the endostabilizer is mounted to the operating table rail on the patient's right side, and the operating table is rotated 10 to 15 degrees to raise the patient's left side.

After single right-lung ventilation is initiated, the camera port is placed in the fifth intercostal space 2 cm medial to the anterior axillary line. CO_2 insufflation is begun for adequate visualization and to create working space as tolerated hemodynamically (usually 10 to 12 mm Hg of insufflation pressure). A 30-degree scope angled up is used for takedown of the LITA. The right instrument port is placed in the third intercostal space medial to the anterior axillary line, and the left instrument port is placed in the seventh intercostal space medial to the anterior axillary line. The instrument arms are centered for optimal range of motion by adjusting the respective setup joints, and the instruments are inserted. LITA takedown starts by dividing the intrathoracic fascia covering the LITA with low-power monopolar cautery. The LITA is dissected bluntly off the chest wall moving from the lateral to the medial aspect as a pedicle, keeping the lateral veins. Side branches are cauterized or clipped. Dissection is performed from the first intercostal space to the level of the bifurcation. The pedicle is not detached from the chest wall until the anastomosis is finally performed to avoid torsion of the graft. The distal end of the graft is skeletonized to facilitate suturing of the anastomosis. Epicardial fat is removed, and the mediastinal and diaphragmatic attachments to the pericardium are dissected bluntly to widen the available space. The pericardiotomy is performed with a longitudinal incision in the pericardium over the suspected course of the LAD. The ideal site for the anastomosis is determined by the absence of visible atheromatous plaques and avoiding proximity to bifurcations. At this point, changing the angle of the endoscope from looking upward to looking downward may enhance visualization. After heparinization (an ACT of 300 seconds is recommended), a vascular clamp is placed approximately 2 cm proximal to the transsection site. The LITA is clipped distally, cut, and spatulated in preparation for the anastomosis in situ. Graft patency is confirmed by briefly releasing the vascular clamp.

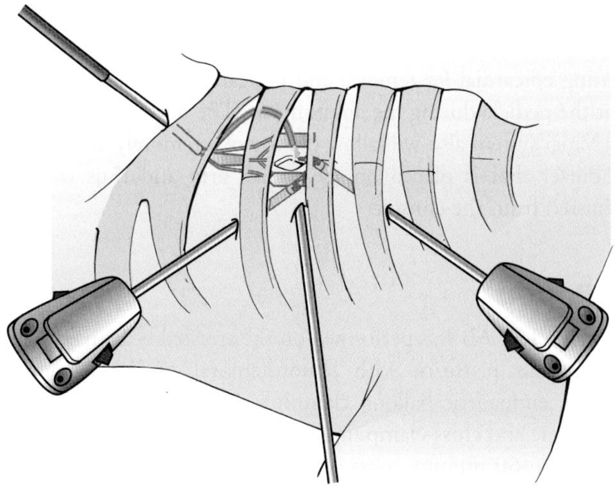

FIGURE 25-5 Setup for total endoscopic coronary artery bypass grafting. Two instrument ports, one central camera port, and a subxyphoidal port for the endostabilizer are required.

The LITA pedicle is still left attached to the chest wall in order to keep orientation of the graft until the anastomosis is performed. A 12-mm subxyphoid cannula is inserted under endoscopic vision. Before introduction of the endostabilizer, temporary silastic occlusion tapes and a 7-cm 7-0 double-armed Prolene suture are introduced through this port and stored in the mediastinum. Some surgeons prefer Gore-Tex sutures to avoid the memory effect. Alternatively, nitinol clips (U-clips) may be used. The endostabilizer then is introduced under endoscopic vision by the patient-side surgeon (Fig. 25-5). Vacuum lines and irrigating saline line are connected, and the multilink irrigator is advanced into the field of view. The console surgeon then positions the stabilizer feet parallel to the LAD target site. After suction is applied, the feet are locked into position. After blunt dissection of the anastomotic target site, the silastic tapes are placed proximal and distal to the anastomotic site, and temporary occlusion is applied. After a 5- to 6-mm arteriotomy is performed, transsection of the LITA is completed, and the graft is brought in close proximity of the target site. The anastomosis is best performed by beginning at the middle of the medial wall (12 o'clock position), suturing inside-out on the LITA and outside-in on the LAD toward and around the heel. Care has to be taken to tension the suture continuously. After the needles are broken off, an instrument knot is tied. The occlusion tapes and vascular clamp are released and evacuated through an instrument port. The pedicle may be fixed to the epicardium by stay sutures. For graft patency, control transient time Doppler flow measurements can be performed endoscopically if a probe without a handle is available. This probe can be advanced through the stabilizer port. Alternatively, intraoperative angiography has been performed using a mobile angiography unit or modern C-arm systems when TECAB operation is performed in a hybrid suite. After the pleural space is drained under vision, the stabilizer and instruments are withdrawn, and the left lung is ventilated. A chest tube is inserted through one of the port holes. In case a four-arm system is used, the fourth arm is introduced after harvesting of the LITA in the third intercostal space in the anterior axillary line. It may be used to provide countertraction during epicardial fat removal and pericardiotomy and to present the pedicle during the anastomosis. The new version of the da Vinci system also will allow the use of a remotely controlled stabilizer that is placed on the fourth arm and thus can be adjusted from the console.

Results

Initially, TECAB was performed on the arrested heart using the Port-Access platform with femorofemoral cardiopulmonary bypass, endoaortic balloon clamping, and cardioplegic arrest. CPB time and cross-clamp times were in the range of 80 to 120 and 40 to 60 minutes, respectively. The reported patency rate for the TECAB procedure on the arrested heart ranged from 95 to 100% prior to discharge and 96% at 3-month follow-up angiography.[74–77] A large single center study including 100 patients reported, besides good overall results and patency rates, anastomotic times of 10 to 30 minutes after a longer learning curve. Even more pronounced than in MIDCAB procedures (see previous) they also acknowledged that the learning curve continues beyond 100 operations.[78]

Endoscopic CABG on the beating heart is even more challenging.[74,79,80] Based on an intention to treat basis, the conversion rate (elective conversion to a MIDCAB procedure) in a five-center registry was 33% (37 of 117). Conversions were mostly because of calcified target vessels or the inability to locate or dissect the LAD and rarely because of other conditions such as arrhythmia or hemodynamic instability. The patency rates for completed beating-heart TECAB procedures are in the range of 92 to 94%.[61]

TECAB can be performed safely but is currently restricted to few indications (eg, single-vessel bypass grafting of the LAD and occasionally double-vessel grafting), but it has the potential for endoscopic multivessel procedures.[81,82] A more commonly applied technique is an endoscopic harvesting of both internal mammary arteries and direct coronary anastomosis via a minithoracotomy. This yields excellent results and very short recovery times for the patients.[82,83]

Despite the use of advanced telemanipulator technology, the TECAB procedure remains technically demanding and is performed infrequently worldwide. Long operation times, extensive use of material and operation room capacity combined with a stretched learning curve and well established minimally invasive alternatives have confined TECAB to few centers and single dedicated surgeons.

MULTIPLE BYPASS GRAFTING USING MINMALLY INVASIVE TECHNIQUES

Talking about minimally invasive surgical revascularization almost always means revascularization of the anterior wall with the left internal mammary artery. The classical MIDCAB operation is only rarely extended to bypass a diagonal or even intermediate branch as well, typically with a Y-graft using a vein or radial artery.

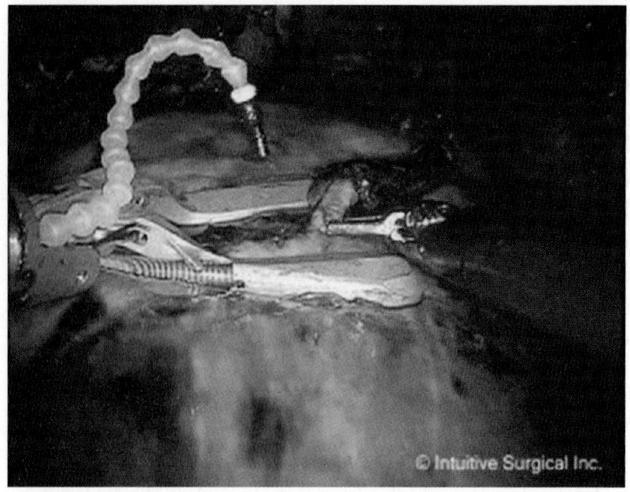

FIGURE 25-6 Endoscopic coronary artery bypass grafting. New endoscopic vacuum stabilizer including irrigating channel. The stabilizer is mounted to the fourth arm of the new da Vinci system and can be operated remotely by the surgeon at the console. (*Reproduced, with permission, from Intuitive Surgical, Inc, Sunnyvale, California.*)

Recent reports have proved the feasibility of complete revascularization for mutivessel disease. Through minimal incisions under direct vision or endoscopically with the help of a telemanipulator, harvesting of both mammary arteries is possible.[84] For proximal anastomoses the aorta can be mobilized and partially clamped or the mammary arteries serve as feeding grafts for a radial artery or saphenous vein.

Accessibility of all areas of the heart is made possible by special stabilizers and suction retractors that allow distal anastomoses even on the beating heart (Fig. 25-6). As an alterative, the Heartport system for endoaortic clamping and cardioplegia can be used.

These techniques have not yet found entry into the clinical routine. However, the published series of patients show excellent results often times superior to conventional CABG or OPCAB.[84] It can be assumed that all these operations were performed by dedicated, experienced surgeons on selected patients. Only a more widespread application of these procedures and the treatment of a broader variety of patients together with randomized studies would bring light to their significance in the future.

HYBRID REVASCULARISATION

The hybrid approach for patients with multivessel coronary artery disease seeks to combine the advantages of percutaneous coronary intervention (PCI) and minimally invasive CABG. The principle was first described by Angelini in 1996.[85] The goal is to minimize the surgical trauma but still gain complete revascularization. The rationale is that the excellent long-term results of LIMA to LAD grafting[72,86] cannot be transferred to other areas of revascularization. This is particularly true for the still widespread venous bypass grafting. Here PCI can potentially achieve similar long-term results, yet with a somewhat higher rate of reintervention. Although recent studies underline the superiority of complete surgical revascularization,[87] the avoidance of sternotomy seems to be very appealing to both patients and treating cardiologists.

However, combining the benefits of two different procedures also means adding the different risk inherent to each type of procedure. The risk of a surgical procedure, including the risk of general anesthesia and artificial ventilation, is combined with an increased risk of inferior PCI long-term outcome that includes the necessity of reinterventions and the possibility of eventual surgical multiple bypass grafting. Therefore the indication for hybrid revascularization should be discussed and agreed on by the treating cardiologist, cardiac surgeon, and, most important, the patient himself.

Indication for the Hybrid Approach

Current recommendations for coronary artery revascularization do not include hybrid procedures. This is because of limited availability of outcome data and a lack of randomized trials. Thus, choosing a hybrid approach is usually based on an individual decision. In all cases the patients with multivessel disease including the proximal LAD need to be informed that the best evidence-based treatment is a sternotomy CABG procedure. However, the different reasons for choosing a hybrid approach can be summarized as follows:

- *Multimorbid or high risk patients:* This is probably the best accepted indication and includes patients with a high risk for sternotomy associated problems such as mediastinitis or with reduced life expectancy. Patients with malignancies, redo patients with a history of deep sternal wound infections, patients dependent on crutches or a wheel chair or patients with additional risk factors such as diabetes, severe obesety, COPD, end stage peripheral occlusive disease, porcelain aorta, and history of stroke with paraplegia might also benefit from the hybrid aproach.
- *Rescue PCI of CX/RCA:* Patients with acute coronary syndromes presenting a culprit lesion in the circumflex or right coronary artery and additional stenosis of the LAD may undergo primary emergency PCI of the culprit lesion by the referring cardiologist. A MIDCAB procedure is usually scheduled 4 to 6 weeks later. A control angiogram confirming the patency of the stent should be done prior to surgery. In the presence of in-stent restenosis the patient can be scheduled for a standard bypass procedure.
- *Patient preference:* Some well informed patients want to avoid sternotomy and opt for a hybrid approach. Patients need to be informed that they might require future reinterventions including repeat target vessel revascularization or bypass surgery. Because the choice of the hybrid revascularization in these patients is not for medical reasons it deserves informed collaboration of patient, interventional cardiologist, and cardiac surgeon.

Timing of the Procedures

The optimal timing and order of revascularization is still discussed controversly.[88] All three possible scenarios have inherent benefits and drawbacks:

- *PCI before CABG:* Performing the percutaneous intervention first is usually associated with an increased bleeding risk for the subsequent surgery because of double antiplatelet therapy. This can be avoided in stable patients who received a bare metal stent by postponing the CABG procedure for more than 4 weeks. When the interval between the two procedures is even longer, a preoperative control angiogram is reasonable to exclude early in-stent restenosis.

  The PCI-first strategy is most commonly applied when a culprit lesion other than the LAD requires urgent therapy.[89]
- *CABG before PCI:* This is the most frequently applied order. The percutaneous intervention is done after the patient has recovered from surgery. After protection of the anterior wall, the percutaneous aproach to the other coronary vessels is safer, even for the left main.[90] A welcome side effect is the angiographic contoll of the minimally invasive bypass procedure.
- *Simultaneous revascularization:* The growing number of novel operating suites that provide true integration of surgical and fluoroscopic capabilities allows for complete hybrid revascularization in one session without moving the patient. After performing a standard MIDCAB/TECAB procedure the bypass quality is verified and the percutanous intervention is undertaken with the patient still under general anesthesia. In the rare case of a failed PCI easy conversion to conventional bypass surgery is possible. Patient acceptance for this approach is high yet it requires good collaboration and syncronizing of the schedules of the cardiologist and the cardiac surgeon.

Results

Although the concept of hybrid revascularization has been applied for almost 15 years the series of published results is not long and the reports oftentimes only involve some 20 to 50 patients. Additionally, the patients represent a very heterogeneous group with a wide range of risk profiles. The various means of revascularization both surgically (MIDCAB or TECAB) and interventionally (different types of bare metal stents and drug eluting stents) and their possible combinations further impair the comparibility. Randomized studies are not available.

There is a general consent that hybrid integrated revascularization is feasible and safe.[91–95] Friedrich and colleagues reviewed the published results of eighteen studies including 367 patients. At six months, the LIMA stenosis rate was 2% and in-stent restenosis was 12%.[91] A larger single center series was recently published by our group.[89] During the follow-up period (208 patient years) 8 patients died. Kaplan-Meier survival was 92.5% (95% CI 86.5% to 98.4%) at one year and 84.8% (95% CI 73.5% to 94.9%) at 5 years. Twenty-three patients had an angiogram for recurrent symptoms of angina. One patient showed an occluded LIMA bypass. Five patients showed significant in-stent restenosis with the need for reintervention. At one year freedom from MACCE and angina was 85.5% (95% CI 76.9% to 94.1%) and 75.5% (95% CI 62.7% to 87.3%), respectively. (Fig. 25-7)

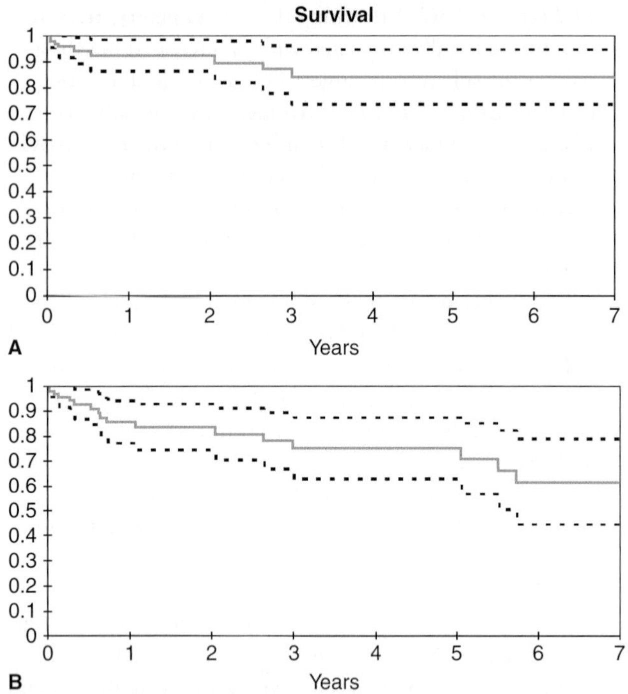

FIGURE 25-7 Kaplan-Meier (including 95% confidence interval) 5-year survival curve (**A**) and event-free survival curve (freedom from death, myocardial infarction, stroke, freedom from angina, freedom from reintervention) (**B**) after minimally invasive hybrid revascularization in 117 patients.

ENDOSCOPIC CONDUIT HARVEST

To minimize the overall trauma and wound healing problems of a bypass procedure, conduit harvest should be performed through limited incisions or endoscopically. There is a body of evidence indicating that although the quality of the conduit is not impaired by an endoscopic harvest, wound infections and other complications of the harvesting procedure are decreased substantially. The cosmetic advantage is obvious.

Endoscopic Saphenous Vein Harvesting

Despite the fact that arterial grafting yields better long-term results than venous grafting, and despite increased use of the IMA and other arterial grafts, the greater saphenous vein is still used frequently for CABG. The standard longitudinal open harvesting technique of the greater saphenous vein is associated with a 2 to 25% rate of wound complications (eg, dehiscence, delayed healing, infection, cellulitis, sepsis, and occasionally, limb amputation), complicating ambulation of the patient, prolonging hospitalization, and causing an economic burden.[96–99] In addition, open saphenous vein harvest is associated with postoperative pain, swelling, neuropathy, long-term pain, and scarring impairing patient satisfaction.

Various techniques for endoscopic vein harvest exist that require one or two 2-cm incisions. For a single-incision technique, the greater saphenous vein is identified through a 2-cm longitudinal incision at the crease of the knee posterior to the medial femoral condyle. A space anterior and posterior at the surface of the vein is dissected, and a subcutaneous retractor or dissection cannula is introduced. An endoscope is inserted into the subcutaneous tissue. Exposure can be enhanced by insufflating CO_2. The vein is mobilized circumferentially, and side branches are either clipped, coagulated using bipolar endoscopic cautery scissors, or vaporized using a harmonic scalpel. Whenever bipolar cautery is applied, a distance of at least 2 mm between the scissors and the vein should be kept in order to avoid thermal graft damage. Proximal and distal control of the greater saphenous vein is accomplished with endoscopic application of a Prolene suture, clips, or ligation loops. With this technique, the entire length of the vein can be harvested from the saphenous-femoral junction to the medial malleolus through a single incision. The wound is closed in a standard fashion, and the leg is wrapped circumferentially with bandages. In experienced hands, the procedure takes between 15 and 30 minutes.[100] As with all endoscopic techniques, a learning curve is associated with endoscopic vein harvesting, with training involving approximately 30 patients and a conversion rate ranging from 0 to 22%.

Results

The ISMICS Consensus Group reviewed the results of 1319 randomized and 8023 nonrandomized patients. In this meta-analysis, the risk of wound complications was reduced significantly by 69% with endoscopic vein harvesting compared with the open technique (OR 0.31, 95% CI 0.23 to 0.43; $p < .0001$).[101] The need for surgical intervention for wound infection also was reduced significantly (OR 0.29, 95% CI 0.12 to 0.70; $p = .007$). With regard to the incidence of moderate to severe postoperative pain, a reduction of 74% was found with endoscopic vein harvesting compared with the open technique (OR 0.26, 95% CI 0.12 to 0.55; $p < .0001$), and this reduction was 90% at 4 to 6-weeks follow-up (OR 0.10, 95% CI 0.03 to 0.37; $p < .0001$). The incidence of mobility disturbance at discharge was reduced by 69% (OR 0.31, 95% CI 0.15 to 0.65; $p = .002$).

One recent study reported worse angiographic and clinical outcome in patients after endoscopic vein harvest.[102] Most studies, however, found no difference for myocardial infarction, angina recurrence or reintervention, and death over the short and midterm.[101,103] However, the number of trials looking at cardiac outcomes and providing angiographic data on patency rates are too limited to allow any meaningful conclusion. The few trials that looked at vascular integrity and vessel wall trauma did not find a difference for the endoscopic versus open technique.[104,105]

Endoscopic Radial Artery Harvest

Use of the radial artery for CABG has regained popularity over the last decade. In conventional radial artery harvest, the incision runs from below the antecubital fossa to the wrist, along the medial border of the brachioradialis muscle. Although wound complications are reported infrequently, delayed healing of the forearm can cause severe discomfort.[106] Objective sensory loss in 10% of patients and forearm scar discomfort in 33% undergoing open radial artery harvest have been reported.[107,108] Endoscopic techniques for graft harvest have been developed subsequently.[109]

Surgical Technique

Collateral circulation from the ulnar artery to the palmar arch has to be verified pre- or intraoperatively using either the standard Allen test or modification of the test by applying Doppler or measuring oxygen saturation in patients in whom the signs of visual reperfusion are in doubt. In order to prevent brachial plexus injury, the arm should not be overextended above 90 degrees. One centimeter superior to the radial styloid prominence, a 2- to 3-cm incision is made, and the radial artery is identified and dissected. A subcutaneous retractor and a 5-mm, 30-degree endoscope are placed into the incision. By bluntly advancing the retractor through the subcutaneous tissue, the radial artery is visualized. Side branches and surrounding tissue are divided using an ultrasonic harmonic or thermowelding scalpel that is placed underneath the retractor. The fascia between the brachioradialis and flexor carpi radialis muscles is divided anterior to the radial artery with the scalpel to increase the space for insertion of the subcutaneous retractor.[110] After division of all side branches, a vessel retractor is advanced from the distal incision to verify complete isolation of the conduit. The proximal radial artery is occluded using an Endoloop or clipped distal to the origin of the ulnar artery branch and transsected with endoscopic scissors. The graft is recovered through the distal incision, and the distal end is ligated. The incision is closed in a standard fashion.

Results

The reported incidences of neurologic complications after standard open harvesting technique of the radial artery vary in the literature from 2.4 to 30% and can be related to injury of the superficial radial nerve or the lateral antebrachial cutaneous nerve. With endoscopic technique, the latter usually is not encountered, because the dissection is performed underneath the brachioradialis muscle. Superficial radial nerve injury, however, still may occur during distal dissection.[110] With regard to wound infections, endoscopic radial artery harvest is associated with a lower rate of infection (0 to 2.7%) compared with the open technique.[100,111]

Graft patency, clinical outcome, histological integrity, and in-vitro vasoreactivity are equal to open graft harvest.[112–114] Thus, endoscopic radial artery harvesting can be recommended for better patient satisfaction and fewer wound healing complications.[115]

CONCLUSION

In summary, minimally invasive bypass surgery continues to play an increasing role in surgical revascularization. There is growing evidence in favor of OPCAB, which is already the preferred method of bypass grafting in many centers. MIDCAB is still limited to patients with single-vessel disease, and excellent long-term data confirm the efficacy of this approach. Endoscopic bypass grafting using robotic assistance is still an evolving procedure that is applied only to selected patients, and its continued application will strongly depend on technological improvements. As for endoscopic vein graft harvesting, there is a body of evidence suggesting superior results compared with an open harvesting technique, which also may be true for the technique of endoscopic radial artery harvest in the future.

REFERENCES

1. Jansen EW, Borst C, Lahpor JR, Grundeman PF, Eefting FD, et al: Coronary artery bypass grafting without cardiopulmonary bypass using the octopus method: results in the first one hundred patients. *J Thorac Cardiovasc Surg* 1998; 116(1):60-67.
2. Vanermen H: What is minimally invasive cardiac surgery? *J Card Surg* 1998; 13(4):268-274.
3. Yusuf S, Zucker D, Peduzzi P, Fisher LD, Takaro T, et al: Effect of coronary artery bypass graft surgery on survival: overview of 10-year results from randomised trials by the Coronary Artery Bypass Graft Surgery Trialists Collaboration. *Lancet* 1994; 344(8922):563-570.
4. Aybek T, Kessler P, Khan MF, Dogan S, Neidhart G, et al: Operative techniques in awake coronary artery bypass grafting. *J Thorac Cardiovasc Surg* 2003; 125(6):1394-1400.
5. Leather HA, Vuylsteke A, Bert C, M'Fam W, Segers P, et al: Evaluation of a new continuous cardiac output monitor in off-pump coronary artery surgery. *Anaesthesia* 2004; 59(4):385-389.
6. Falk V: Manual control and tracking—a human factor analysis relevant for beating heart surgery. *Ann Thorac Surg* 2002; 74(2):624-628.
7. Bouchot O, Aubin MC, Carrier M, Cohn WE, Perrault LP: Temporary coronary artery occlusion during off-pump coronary artery bypass grafting with the new poloxamer P407 does not cause endothelial dysfunction in epicardial coronary arteries. *J Thorac Cardiovasc Surg* 2006; 132(5): 1144-1149.
8. Mommerot A, Aubin MC, Carrier M, Cohn W, Perrault LP: Use of the purified poloxamer 407 for temporary coronary occlusion in off-pump CABG does not cause myocardial injury. *Innovations* 2007; 2:201-204.
9. Lev-Ran O, Braunstein R, Sharony R, Kramer A, Paz Y, et al: No-touch aorta off-pump coronary surgery: the effect on stroke. *J Thorac Cardiovasc Surg* 2005; 129(2):307-313.
10. Brereton RJ, Misfeld M, Ross DE: Percutaneous coronary intervention versus coronary-artery bypass grafting. *NEJM* 2009; 360(25):2673; author reply 2674-2675.
11. Vallely MP, Potger K, McMillan D, Hemli JM, Brady PW, et al: Anaortic techniques reduce neurological morbidity after off-pump coronary artery bypass surgery. *Heart Lung Circ* 2008; 17(4):299-304.
12. Calafiore AM, Di Mauro M, Teodori G, Di Giammarco G, Cirmeni S, et al: Impact of aortic manipulation on incidence of cerebrovascular accidents after surgical myocardial revascularization. *Ann Thorac Surg* 2002; 73(5): 1387-1393.
13. Prapas SN, Panagiotopoulos IA, Hamed Abdelsalam A, Kotsis VN, Protogeros DA, et al: Predictors of prolonged mechanical ventilation following aorta no-touch off-pump coronary artery bypass surgery. *Eur J Cardiothorac Surg* 2007; 32(3):488-492.
14. Rastan AJ, Eckenstein JI, Hentschel B, Funkat AK, Gummert JF, et al: Emergency coronary artery bypass graft surgery for acute coronary syndrome: beating heart versus conventional cardioplegic cardiac arrest strategies. *Circulation* 2006; 114(1 Suppl):I477-485.
15. Edgerton JR, Herbert MA, Jones KK, Prince SL, Acuff T, et al: On-pump beating heart surgery offers an alternative for unstable patients undergoing coronary artery bypass grafting. *Heart Surg Forum* 2004; 7(1):8-15.
16. Sergeant P, Wouters P, Meyns B, Bert C, Van Hemelrijck J, et al: OPCAB versus early mortality and morbidity: an issue between clinical relevance and statistical significance. *Eur J Cardiothorac Surg* 2004; 25(5):779-785.
17. Puskas J, Cheng D, Knight J, Angelini G, DeCannier D, et al: Off-pump versus conventional coronary artery bypass grafting: a meta-analysis and consensus statement from The 2004 ISMICS Consensus Conference. *Innovations* 2005; 1(1):3-27.
18. Sabik JF, Blackstone EH, Lytle BW, Houghtaling PL, Gillinov AM, et al: Equivalent midterm outcomes after off-pump and on-pump coronary surgery. *J Thorac Cardiovasc Surg* 2004; 127(1):142-148.
19. Czerny M, Baumer H, Kilo J, Zuckermann A, Grubhofer G, et al: Complete revascularization in coronary artery bypass grafting with and without cardiopulmonary bypass. *Ann Thorac Surg* 2001; 71(1):165-169.
20. Calafiore AM, Di Mauro M, Canosa C, Di Giammarco G, Iaco AL, et al: Myocardial revascularization with and without cardiopulmonary bypass: advantages, disadvantages and similarities. *Eur J Cardiothorac Surg* 2003; 24(6):953-960.
21. van Dijk D, Nierich AP, Jansen EW, Nathoe HM, Suyker WJ, et al: Early outcome after off-pump versus on-pump coronary bypass surgery: results from a randomized study. *Circulation* 2001; 104(15):1761-1766.

22. Khan NE, De Souza A, Mister R, Flather M, Clague J, et al: A randomized comparison of off-pump and on-pump multivessel coronary-artery bypass surgery. *NEJM* 2004; 350(1):21-28.
23. Shroyer AL, Grover FL, Hattler B, Collins JF, McDonald GO, et al: On-pump versus off-pump coronary-artery bypass surgery. *NEJM* 2009; 361(19):1827-1837.
24. Puskas JD, Williams WH, Duke PG, Staples JR, Glas KE, et al: Off-pump coronary artery bypass grafting provides complete revascularization with reduced myocardial injury, transfusion requirements, and length of stay: a prospective randomized comparison of two hundred unselected patients undergoing off-pump versus conventional coronary artery bypass grafting. *J Thorac Cardiovasc Surg* 2003; 125(4):797-808.
25. Muneretto C, Bisleri G, Negri A, Manfredi J, Metra M, et al: Off-pump coronary artery bypass surgery technique for total arterial myocardial revascularization: a prospective randomized study. *Ann Thorac Surg* 2003; 76(3):778-782; discussion 783.
26. Widimsky P, Straka Z, Stros P, Jirasek K, Dvorak J, et al: One-year coronary bypass graft patency: a randomized comparison between off-pump and on-pump surgery angiographic results of the PRAGUE-4 trial. *Circulation* 2004; 110(22):3418-3423.
27. Magee MJ, Coombs LP, Peterson ED, Mack MJ: Patient selection and current practice strategy for off-pump coronary artery bypass surgery. *Circulation* 2003; 108 Suppl 1:II9-14.
28. Mack MJ, Pfister A, Bachand D, Emery R, Magee MJ, et al: Comparison of coronary bypass surgery with and without cardiopulmonary bypass in patients with multivessel disease. *J Thorac Cardiovasc Surg* 2004; 127(1): 167-173.
29. Stamou SC, Jablonski KA, Hill PC, Bafi AS, Boyce SW, Corso PJ: Coronary revascularization without cardiopulmonary bypass versus the conventional approach in high-risk patients. *Ann Thorac Surg* 2005; 79(2):552-557.
30. Ascione R, Reeves BC, Rees K, Angelini GD: Effectiveness of coronary artery bypass grafting with or without cardiopulmonary bypass in overweight patients. *Circulation* 2002; 106(14):1764-1770.
31. Cheng DC, Bainbridge D, Martin JE, Novick RJ: Does off-pump coronary artery bypass reduce mortality, morbidity, and resource utilization when compared with conventional coronary artery bypass? A meta-analysis of randomized trials. *Anesthesiology* 2005; 102(1):188-203.
32. Angelini GD, Taylor FC, Reeves BC, Ascione R: Early and midterm outcome after off-pump and on-pump surgery in Beating Heart Against Cardioplegic Arrest Studies (BHACAS 1 and 2): a pooled analysis of two randomised controlled trials. *Lancet* 2002; 359(9313):1194-1199.
33. Zamvar V, Williams D, Hall J, Payne N, Cann C, et al: Assessment of neurocognitive impairment after off-pump and on-pump techniques for coronary artery bypass graft surgery: prospective randomised controlled trial. *BMJ* 2002; 325(7375):1268.
34. Bucerius J, Gummert JF, Borger MA, Walther T, Doll N, et al: Predictors of delirium after cardiac surgery delirium: effect of beating-heart (off-pump) surgery. *J Thorac Cardiovasc Surg* 2004; 127(1):57-64.
35. Stamou SC, Jablonski KA, Pfister AJ, Hill PC, Dullum MK, et al: Stroke after conventional versus minimally invasive coronary artery bypass. *Ann Thorac Surg* 2002; 74(2):394-399.
36. Patel NC, Deodhar AP, Grayson AD, Pullan DM, Keenan DJ, et al: Neurological outcomes in coronary surgery: independent effect of avoiding cardiopulmonary bypass. *Ann Thorac Surg* 2002; 74(2):400-405; discussion 405-406.
37. Diegeler A, Hirsch R, Schneider F, Schilling LO, Falk V, et al: Neuromonitoring and neurocognitive outcome in off-pump versus conventional coronary bypass operation. *Ann Thorac Surg* 2000; 69(4):1162-1166.
38. Lee JD, Lee SJ, Tsushima WT, Yamauchi H, Lau WT, et al: Benefits of off-pump bypass on neurologic and clinical morbidity: a prospective randomized trial. *Ann Thorac Surg* 2003; 76(1):18-25; discussion 25-26.
39. Scarborough JE, White W, Derilus FE, Mathew JP, Newman MF, et al: Combined use of off-pump techniques and a sutureless proximal aortic anastomotic device reduces cerebral microemboli generation during coronary artery bypass grafting. *J Thorac Cardiovasc Surg* 2003; 126(5): 1561-1567.
40. Ascione R, Lloyd CT, Underwood MJ, Gomes WJ, Angelini GD: On-pump versus off-pump coronary revascularization: evaluation of renal function. *Ann Thorac Surg* 1999; 68(2):493-498.
41. Arom KV, Flavin TF, Emery RW, Kshettry VR, Janey PA, et al: Safety and efficacy of off-pump coronary artery bypass grafting. *Ann Thorac Surg* 2000; 69(3):704-710.
42. Bucerius J, Gummert JF, Walther T, Schmitt DV, Doll N, et al: On-pump versus off-pump coronary artery bypass grafting: impact on postoperative renal failure requiring renal replacement therapy. *Ann Thorac Surg* 2004; 77(4):1250-1256.
43. Ascione R, Nason G, Al-Ruzzeh S, Ko C, Ciulli F, et al: Coronary revascularization with or without cardiopulmonary bypass in patients with preoperative nondialysis-dependent renal insufficiency. *Ann Thorac Surg* 2001; 72(6):2020-2025.
44. Weerasinghe A, Athanasiou T, Al-Ruzzeh S, Casula R, Tekkis PP, et al: Functional renal outcome in on-pump and off-pump coronary revascularization: a propensity-based analysis. *Ann Thorac Surg* 2005; 79(5): 1577-1583.
45. Athanasiou T, Aziz O, Mangoush O, Al-Ruzzeh S, Nair S, et al: Does off-pump coronary artery bypass reduce the incidence of post-operative atrial fibrillation? A question revisited. *Eur J Cardiothorac Surg* 2004; 26(4):701-710.
46. Rastan AJ, Bittner HB, Gummert JF, Walther T, Schewick CV, et al: On-pump beating heart versus off-pump coronary artery bypass surgery-evidence of pump-induced myocardial injury. *Eur J Cardiothorac Surg* 2005; 27(6):1057-1064.
47. Dybdahl B, Wahba A, Haaverstad R, Kirkeby-Garstad I, Kierulf P, et al: On-pump versus off-pump coronary artery bypass grafting: more heat-shock protein 70 is released after on-pump surgery. *Eur J Cardiothorac Surg* 2004; 25(6):985-992.
48. Diegeler A, Doll N, Rauch T, Haberer D, Walther T, et al: Humoral immune response during coronary artery bypass grafting: a comparison of limited approach, "off-pump" technique, and conventional cardiopulmonary bypass. *Circulation* 2000; 102(19 Suppl 3):III95-100.
49. Nathoe HM, van Dijk D, Jansen EW, Suyker WJ, Diephuis JC, et al: A comparison of on-pump and off-pump coronary bypass surgery in low-risk patients. *NEJM* 2003; 348(5):394-402.
50. MacGillivray TE, Vlahakes GJ: Patency and the pump—the risks and benefits of off-pump CABG. *NEJM* 2004; 350(1):3-4.
51. Calafiore AM, Giammarco GD, Teodori G, Bosco G, D'Annunzio E, et al: Left anterior descending coronary artery grafting via left anterior small thoracotomy without cardiopulmonary bypass. *Ann Thorac Surg* 1996; 61(6):1658-1663; discussion 1664-1655.
52. Cremer J, Struber M, Wittwer T, Ruhparwar A, Harringer W, et al: Off-bypass coronary bypass grafting via minithoracotomy using mechanical epicardial stabilization. *Ann Thorac Surg* 1997; 63(6 Suppl):S79-83.
53. Subramanian VA, McCabe JC, Geller CM: Minimally invasive direct coronary artery bypass grafting: two-year clinical experience. *Ann Thorac Surg* 1997; 64(6):1648-1653; discussion 1654-1645.
54. Diegeler A, Matin M, Kayser S, Binner C, Autschbach R, et al: Angiographic results after minimally invasive coronary bypass grafting using the minimally invasive direct coronary bypass grafting (MIDCAB) approach. *Eur J Cardiothorac Surg* 1999; 15(5):680-684.
55. Bucerius J, Metz S, Walther T, Falk V, Doll N, et al: Endoscopic internal thoracic artery dissection leads to significant reduction of pain after minimally invasive direct coronary artery bypass graft surgery. *Ann Thorac Surg* 2002; 73(4):1180-1184.
56. Wolf RK, Ohtsuka T, Flege JB, Jr: Early results of thoracoscopic internal mammary artery harvest using an ultrasonic scalpel. *Eur J Cardiothorac Surg* 1998; 14 Suppl 1:S54-57.
57. Duhaylongsod FG, Mayfield WR, Wolf RK: Thoracoscopic harvest of the internal thoracic artery: a multicenter experience in 218 cases. *Ann Thorac Surg* 1998; 66(3):1012-1017.
58. Mack MJ, Magovern JA, Acuff TA, Landreneau RJ, Tennison DM, et al: Results of graft patency by immediate angiography in minimally invasive coronary artery surgery. *Ann Thorac Surg* 1999; 68(2):383-389; discussion 389-390.
59. Kettering K, Dapunt O, Baer FM: Minimally invasive direct coronary artery bypass grafting: a systematic review. *J Cardiovasc Surg* 2004; 45(3): 255-264.
60. Gummert JF, Funkat A, Krian A: Cardiac surgery in Germany during 2004: a report on behalf of the German Society for Thoracic and Cardiovascular Surgery. *Thorac Cardiovascular Surg* 2005; 53(6):391-399.
61. de Canniere D, Wimmer-Greinecker G, Cichon R, Gulielmos V, Van Praet F, et al: Feasibility, safety, and efficacy of totally endoscopic coronary artery bypass grafting: multicenter European experience. *J Thorac Cardiovasc Surg* 2007; 134(3):710-716.
62. Calafiore AM, Di Giammarco G, Teodori G, Gallina S, Maddestra N, et al: Midterm results after minimally invasive coronary surgery (LAST operation). *J Thorac Cardiovasc Surg* 1998; 115(4):763-771.
63. Mehran R, Dangas G, Stamou SC, Pfister AJ, Dullum MK, et al: One-year clinical outcome after minimally invasive direct coronary artery bypass. *Circulation* 2000; 102(23):2799-2802.
64. Mariani MA, Boonstra PW, Grandjean JG, Peels JO, Monnink SH, et al: Minimally invasive coronary artery bypass grafting versus coronary angioplasty for isolated type C stenosis of the left anterior descending artery. *J Thorac Cardiovasc Surg* 1997; 114(3):434-439.

65. Fraund S, Herrmann G, Witzke A, Hedderich J, Lutter G, et al: Midterm follow-up after minimally invasive direct coronary artery bypass grafting versus percutaneous coronary intervention techniques. *Ann Thorac Surg* 2005; 79(4):1225-1231.
66. Diegeler A, Thiele H, Falk V, Hambrecht R, Spyrantis N, et al: Comparison of stenting with minimally invasive bypass surgery for stenosis of the left anterior descending coronary artery. *NEJM* 2002; 347(8):561-566.
67. Shirai K, Lansky AJ, Mehran R, Dangas GD, Costantini CO, et al: Minimally invasive coronary artery bypass grafting versus stenting for patients with proximal left anterior descending coronary artery disease. *Am J Cardiol* 2004; 93(8):959-962.
68. Thiele H, Oettel S, Jacobs S, Hambrecht R, Sick P, et al: Comparison of bare-metal stenting with minimally invasive bypass surgery for stenosis of the left anterior descending coronary artery: a 5-year follow-up. *Circulation* 2005; 112(22):3445-3450.
69. Reeves BC, Angelini GD, Bryan AJ, Taylor FC, Cripps T, et al: A multicentre randomised controlled trial of minimally invasive direct coronary bypass grafting versus percutaneous transluminal coronary angioplasty with stenting for proximal stenosis of the left anterior descending coronary artery. *Health Technol Assess (Winchester, England)* 2004; 8(16):1-43.
70. Holzhey DM, Jacobs S, Walther T, Mochalski M, Mohr FW, et al: Cumulative sum failure analysis for eight surgeons performing minimally invasive direct coronary artery bypass. *J Thorac Cardiovasc Surg* 2007; 134(3):663-669.
71. Thiele H, Neumann-Schniedewind P, Jacobs S, Boudriot E, Walther T, et al: Randomized comparison of minimally invasive direct coronary artery bypass surgery versus sirolimus-eluting stenting in isolated proximal left anterior descending coronary artery stenosis. *J Am Coll Cardiol* 2009; 53(25):2324-2331.
72. Holzhey DM, Jacobs S, Mochalski M, Walther T, Thiele H, et al: Seven-year follow-up after minimally invasive direct coronary artery bypass: experience with more than 1300 patients. *Ann Thorac Surg* 2007; 83(1): 108-114.
73. Falk V, McLoughlin J, Guthart G, Salisbury JK, Walther T, et al: Dexterity enhancement in endoscopic surgery by a computer-controlled mechanical wrist. *Minim Invasive Ther Allied Technol* 1999; 8(4):235-242.
74. Falk V, Diegeler A, Walther T, Jacobs S, Raumans J, et al: Total endoscopic off-pump coronary artery bypass grafting. *Heart Surg Forum* 2000; 3(1):29-31.
75. Damiano RJ Jr, Ehrman WJ, Ducko CT, Tabaie HA, Stephenson ER Jr, et al: Initial United States clinical trial of robotically assisted endoscopic coronary artery bypass grafting. *J Thorac Cardiovasc Surg* 2000; 119(1):77-82.
76. Reichenspurner H, Damiano RJ, Mack M, Boehm DH, Gulbins H, et al: Use of the voice-controlled and computer-assisted surgical system ZEUS for endoscopic coronary artery bypass grafting. *J Thorac Cardiovasc Surg* 1999; 118(1):11-16.
77. Kappert U, Schneider J, Cichon R, Gulielmos V, Matschke K, et al: Wrist-enhanced instrumentation: moving toward totally endoscopic coronary artery bypass grafting. *Ann Thorac Surg* 2000; 70(3):1105-1108.
78. Bonatti J, Schachner T, Bonaros N, Oehlinger A, Wiedemann D, et al: Effectiveness and safety of total endoscopic left internal mammary artery bypass graft to the left anterior descending artery. *American J Cardiol* 2009; 104(12):1684-1688.
79. Falk V, Diegeler A, Walther T, Loscher N, Vogel B, et al: Endoscopic coronary artery bypass grafting on the beating heart using a computer enhanced telemanipulation system. *Heart Surg Forum* 1999; 2(3):199-205.
80. Falk V, Diegeler A, Walther T, Banusch J, Brucerius J, et al: Total endoscopic computer enhanced coronary artery bypass grafting. *Eur J Cardiothorac Surg* 2000; 17(1):38-45.
81. Kappert U, Cichon R, Schneider J, Gulielmos V, Ahmadzade T, et al: Technique of closed chest coronary artery surgery on the beating heart. *Eur J Cardiothorac Surg* 2001; 20(4):765-769.
82. Srivastava S, Gadasalli S, Agusala M, Kolluru R, Naidu J, et al: Use of bilateral internal thoracic arteries in CABG through lateral thoracotomy with robotic assistance in 150 patients. *Ann Thorac Surg* 2006; 81(3): 800-806; discussion 806.
83. Subramanian VA, Patel NU, Patel NC, Loulmet DF: Robotic assisted multivessel minimally invasive direct coronary artery bypass with port-access stabilization and cardiac positioning: paving the way for outpatient coronary surgery? *Ann Thorac Surg* 2005; 79(5):1590-1596; discussion 1590-1596.
84. McGinn JT Jr, Usman S, Lapierre H, Pothula VR, Mesana TG, et al: Minimally invasive coronary artery bypass grafting: dual-center experience in 450 consecutive patients. *Circulation* 2009; 120(11 Suppl):S78-84.
85. Angelini GD, Wilde P, Salerno TA, Bosco G, Calafiore AM: Integrated left small thoracotomy and angioplasty for multivessel coronary artery revascularisation. *Lancet* 1996; 347(9003):757-758.
86. Pick AW, Orszulak TA, Anderson BJ, Schaff HV: Single versus bilateral internal mammary artery grafts: 10-year outcome analysis. *Ann Thorac Surg* 1997; 64(3):599-605.
87. Serruys PW, Morice MC, Kappetein AP, Colombo A, Holmes DR, et al: Percutaneous coronary intervention versus coronary-artery bypass grafting for severe coronary artery disease. *NEJM* 2009; 360(10):961-972.
88. DeRose JJ: Current state of integrated "hybrid" coronary revascularization. *Semin Thorac Cardiovasc Surg* 2009; 21(3):229-236.
89. Holzhey DM, Jacobs S, Mochalski M, Merk D, Walther T, et al: Minimally invasive hybrid coronary artery revascularization. *Ann Thorac Surg* 2008; 86(6):1856-1860.
90. Mack MJ, Brown DL, Sankaran A: Minimally invasive coronary bypass for protected left main coronary stenosis angioplasty. *Ann Thorac Surg* 1997; 64(2):545-546.
91. Friedrich GJ, Bonatti J: Hybrid coronary artery revascularization—review and update 2007. *Heart Surg Forum* 2007; 10(4):E292-296.
92. Katz MR, Van Praet F, de Canniere D, Murphy D, Siwek L, et al: Integrated coronary revascularization: percutaneous coronary intervention plus robotic totally endoscopic coronary artery bypass. *Circulation* 2006; 114(1 Suppl):I473-476.
93. Bonatti J, Schachner T, Bonaros N, Jonetzko P, Ohlinger A, et al: Treatment of double vessel coronary artery disease by totally endoscopic bypass surgery and drug-eluting stent placement in one simultaneous hybrid session. *Heart Surg Forum* 2005; 8(4):E284-286.
94. Bonatti J, Schachner T, Bonaros N, Laufer G, Kolbitsch C, et al: Robotic totally endoscopic coronary artery bypass and catheter based coronary intervention in one operative session. *Ann Thorac Surg* 2005; 79(6):2138-2141.
95. Wittwer T, Haverich A, Cremer J, Boonstra P, Franke U, et al: Follow-up experience with coronary hybrid-revascularisation. *Thorac Cardiovasc Surg* 2000; 48(6):356-359.
96. Goldsborough MA, Miller MH, Gibson J, Creighton-Kelly S, Custer CA, et al: Prevalence of leg wound complications after coronary artery bypass grafting: determination of risk factors. *Am J Crit Care* 1999; 8(3):149-153.
97. Allen KB, Griffith GL, Heimansohn DA, Robison RJ, Matheny RG, et al: Endoscopic versus traditional saphenous vein harvesting: a prospective, randomized trial. *Ann Thorac Surg* 1998; 66(1):26-31; discussion 31-22.
98. Bonde P, Graham A, MacGowan S: Endoscopic vein harvest: early results of a prospective trial with open vein harvest. *Heart Surg Forum* 2002; 5 Suppl 4:S378-391.
99. Bonde P, Graham AN, MacGowan SW: Endoscopic vein harvest: advantages and limitations. *Ann Thorac Surg* 2004; 77(6):2076-2082.
100. Aziz O, Athanasiou T, Darzi A: Minimally invasive conduit harvesting: a systematic review. *Eur J Cardiothorac Surg* 2006; 29(3):324-333.
101. Cheng D, Allen K, Cohn W, Connolly M, Edgerton J, et al: Endoscopic vascular harvest in coronary artery bypass grafting surgery: a meta-analysis of randomized trials and controlled trials. *Innovations* 2005; 1(2):61-74.
102. Lopes RD, Hafley GE, Allen KB, Ferguson TB, Peterson ED, et al; Endoscopic versus open vein-graft harvesting in coronary-artery bypass surgery. *NEJM* 2009; 361(3):235-244.
103. Ouzounian M, Hassan A, Buth KJ, MacPherson C, Ali IM, et al: Impact of endoscopic versus open saphenous vein harvest techniques on outcomes after coronary artery bypass grafting. *Ann Thorac Surg* 2010; 89(2): 403-408.
104. Coppoolse R, Rees W, Krech R, Hufnagel M, Seufert K, et al: Routine minimal invasive vein harvesting reduces postoperative morbidity in cardiac bypass procedures. Clinical report of 1400 patients. *Eur J Cardiothorac Surg* 1999; 16 Suppl 2:S61-66.
105. Crouch JD, O'Hair DP, Keuler JP, Barragry TP, Werner PH, et al: Open versus endoscopic saphenous vein harvesting: wound complications and vein quality. *Ann Thorac Surg* 1999; 68(4):1513-1516.
106. Meharwal ZS, Trehan N: Functional status of the hand after radial artery harvesting: results in 3,977 cases. *Ann Thorac Surg* 2001; 72(5): 1557-1561.
107. Denton TA, Trento L, Cohen M, Kass RM, Blanche C, et al: Radial artery harvesting for coronary bypass operations: neurologic complications and their potential mechanisms. *J Thorac Cardiovasc Surg* 2001; 121(5):951-956.
108. Tatoulis J, Royse AG, Buxton BF, Fuller JA, Skillington PD, et al: The radial artery in coronary surgery: a 5-year experience—clinical and angiographic results. *Ann Thorac Surg* 2002; 73(1):143-147; discussion 147-148.
109. Connolly MW, Torrillo LD, Stauder MJ, Patel NU, McCabe JC, et al: Endoscopic radial artery harvesting: results of first 300 patients. *Ann Thorac Surg* 2002; 74(2):502-505; discussion 506.
110. Casselman FP, La Meir M, Cammu G, Wellens F, De Geest R, et al; Initial experience with an endoscopic radial artery harvesting technique. *J Thorac Cardiovasc Surg* 2004; 128(3):463-466.

111. Patel AN, Henry AC, Hunnicutt C, Cockerham CA, Willey B, et al: Endoscopic radial artery harvesting is better than the open technique. *Ann Thorac Surg* 2004; 78(1):149-153; discussion 149-153.
112. Medalion B, Tobar A, Yosibash Z, Stamler A, Sharoni E, et al: Vasoreactivity and histology of the radial artery: comparison of open versus endoscopic approaches. *Eur J Cardiothorac Surg* 2008; 34(4):845-849.
113. Ito N, Tashiro T, Morishige N, Iwahashi H, Nishimi M, et al: Endoscopic radial artery harvesting for coronary artery bypass grafting: the initial clinical experience and results of the first 50 patients. *Heart Surg Forum* 2009; 12(6):E310-315.
114. Bleiziffer S, Hettich I, Eisenhauer B, Ruzicka D, Wottke M, et al: Patency rates of endoscopically harvested radial arteries one year after coronary artery bypass grafting. *J Thorac Cardiovasc Surg* 2007; 134(3):649-656.
115. Nishida S, Kikuchi Y, Watanabe G, Takata M, Ito S, Kawachi K: Endoscopic radial artery harvesting: patient satisfaction and complications. *Asian Cardiovasc Thorac Ann* 2008; 16(1):43-46.

CHAPTER 26

Coronary Artery Reoperations

G. V. Gonzalez-Stawinski
Bruce W. Lytle

Coronary artery reoperations are more complicated than primary operations. Patients undergoing reoperations have distinct, more dangerous pathologies; reoperations are technically more difficult to perform; and the risks are greater.[1–12] Vein graft atherosclerosis, present in most reoperative candidates, is a unique and dangerous lesion. Reoperative candidates commonly have severe and diffuse native-vessel distal coronary artery disease (CAD), a problem that has had the time to develop only because these patients did not die from their original proximal coronary artery lesions. Aortic and noncardiac atherosclerosis are also often far advanced in many reoperative candidates. Some technical hazards, including the presence of patent arterial grafts and sternal reentry, are unique to reoperations, and others, such as lack of bypass conduits and difficult coronary artery exposure, are common.

INCIDENCE OF REOPERATION

After a primary bypass operation, the likelihood of a patient undergoing a reoperation depends on patient-related variables, primary operation-related variables, adherence to strict medical control of risk factors for disease progression after bypass surgery, the possibility of alternative treatments, physician opinion about the feasibility of reoperation, and time. Studies from our institution noted a cumulative incidence of reoperation of 3% by 5 years, 10% by 10 years, and 25% by 20 postoperative years[13] (Fig. 26-1). Factors associated statistically with an increased likelihood of reoperation have been variables predicting a favorable long-term survival (eg, young age, normal left ventricular function [LVF], and single- or double-vessel disease), variables designating an imperfect primary operation (eg, no internal thoracic artery [ITA] graft and incomplete revascularization), and symptom status (eg, class III or IV symptoms at primary operation). Young age at primary operation and incomplete revascularization are also markers of a severe atherogenic diathesis.

More recently, however, the proportion of isolated coronary artery operations that are reoperations has decreased. This decrease is related in part to the more aggressive use of coronary artery interventions for patients with previous bypass surgery and probably to more effective risk factor control. In 1990 about 37% of coronary artery revascularization operations were reoperative interventions, whereas in 2002 this figure decreased to 30%[14] (Fig. 26-2). Also, surgery has changed in directions that will decrease the rate of reoperation. Use of the left internal thoracic artery (LITA) to graft the left anterior descending (LAD) coronary artery decreases the risk of reoperation compared with the strategy of using only vein grafts, and the LITA-LAD graft has become a standard part of operations for coronary artery revascularization.[15] Furthermore, it now appears that use of bilateral ITA grafts decreases the likelihood of death and reoperation when compared with the single LITA-LAD strategy[16] (Fig. 26-3). The use of other arterial conduits such as the radial artery and the gastroepiploic artery in the context of total arterial revascularization may decrease the risk of reoperation further, but as yet the long-term data are insufficient to answer this question.

The patient population of reoperative candidates has evolved. Cleveland Clinic Foundation studies have shown that in the early years of bypass surgery (1967 to 1978), only 28% of patients underwent reoperation solely because of graft failure, and that graft failure often occurred early after the primary operation (mean postoperative interval of 28 months after primary operation). Reoperation because of the progression of atherosclerosis in nongrafted coronary arteries was common in

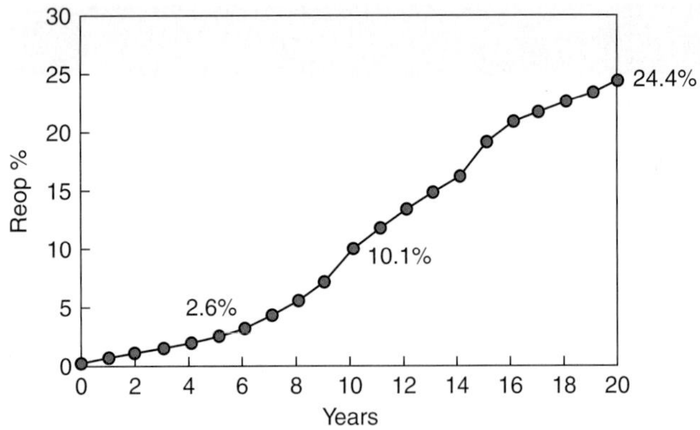

FIGURE 26-1 Study of 4000 patients who underwent bypass surgery from 1971 to 1974 showed that 25% of patients had undergone a reoperation within a period of 20 years after primary operation. (*Data from Cosgrove DM, Loop FD, Lytle BW, et al: Predictors of reoperation after myocardial revascularization. J Thorac Cardiovasc Surg 1986; 92:811.*)

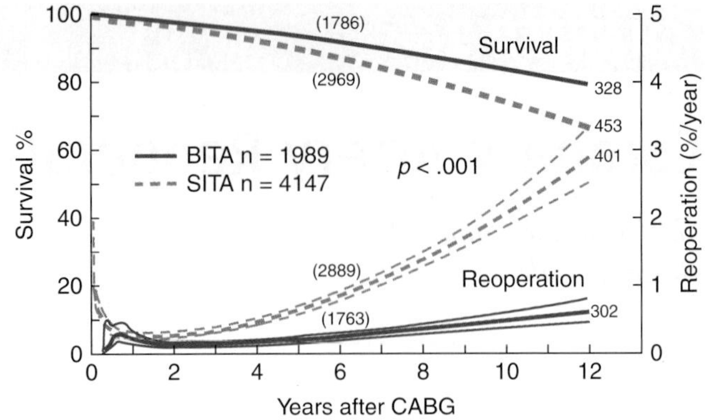

FIGURE 26-3 Comparison of survival and reoperation hazard function curves in the propensity-matched patients undergoing bilateral (BITA, *n* = 1989) or single ITA (SITA, *n* = 4147) CABG. (*Reproduced with permission from Lytle BW, Blackstone EH, Loop FD, et al: Two internal thoracic artery grafts are better than one. J Thorac Cardiovasc Surg 1999; 117:855.*)

the 1967 to 1978 time period (55% of patients).[1,2] Between 1988 and 1991, almost all patients had graft failure as at least part of the indication for reoperation (92%), but that graft failure occurred late after the primary operation at a mean interval of 116 months.[3] Today, patients undergoing reoperation usually had a successful primary operation at least 10 years previously for the treatment of multivessel CAD, and the angiographic indications for reoperation are progression of native-vessel distal CAD in combination with late graft failure caused by vein graft atherosclerosis.

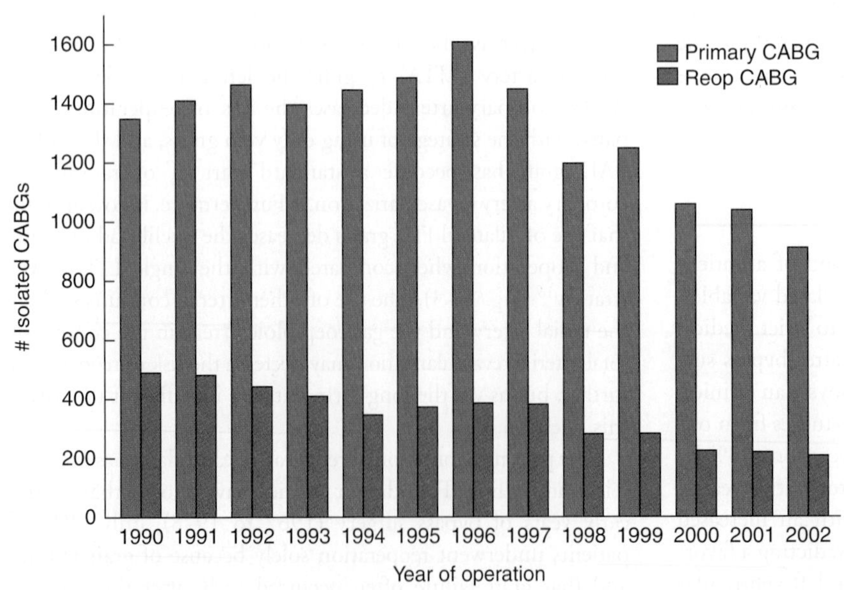

FIGURE 26-2 Study of 21,568 patients who underwent bypass surgery from 1990 to 2003 showed a steady decrease in the number of patients undergoing redo coronary artery operations. (*Data from Sabik JF, Blackstone EH, Houghtaling PL, et al: Is reoperation still a risk factor in coronary artery bypass surgery? Ann Thorac Surg 2005; 80:1719.*)

GRAFT FAILURE

An understanding of the pathology and causes of saphenous vein graft failure is important not only for an understanding of the causes of the need for reoperation, but also for understanding the dangers inherent in either the interventional or the conservative treatment of patients with previous bypass surgery. Saphenous vein to coronary artery grafts exhibit different pathologies at different intervals after operation.[17–20] Within a few months, they often have diffuse endothelial disruptions with associated mural thrombus. The mural thrombus usually is not obstructing, and when grafts do become occluded early after operation owing to thrombosis, it may not be a result of these intimal changes, but rather may be related to hemodynamic factors. Most saphenous vein grafts examined more than 2 to 3 months after operation have developed a proliferative intimal fibroplasia. This is a concentric cellular process, and it is diffuse, extending the entire length of the graft (Fig. 26-4). It evolves with time to a more fibrous lesion. It is not friable, and although intimal fibroplasia involves most vein grafts, it causes stenoses or occlusions of only a few.

Vein graft atherosclerosis is a distinct pathologic process that often is recognized as early as 3 to 4 years after operation and is characterized by lipid infiltration of areas of intimal fibroplasia (Fig. 26-5). The distribution of vein graft atherosclerosis mimics that of intimal fibroplasia in that it is concentric and diffuse, although as vein graft atherosclerosis progresses, stenotic lesions may become eccentric. In addition, vein graft atherosclerosis is a

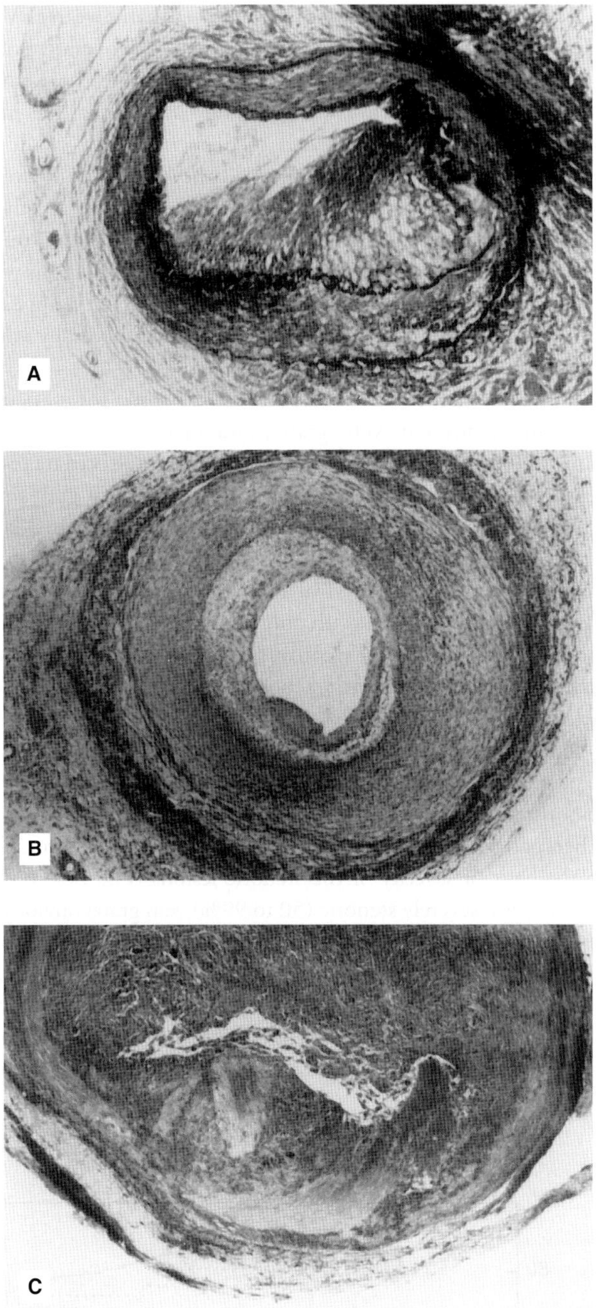

FIGURE 26-4 Pathology of (A) native coronary artery atherosclerosis, (B) vein graft intimal fibrosis, and (C) severe vein graft atherosclerosis. (*Reproduced with permission from Lytle BW, Cosgrove DM: Coronary artery bypass surgery, in Wells SA (ed): Current Problems in Surgery. Philadelphia, Saunders, 1992; p 733.*)

superficial lesion, it is very friable, and it is often associated with overlying mural thrombus. These characteristics make it different from native-vessel coronary atherosclerosis, a process that is segmental and proximal, eccentric, encapsulated, usually not friable, and usually not associated with overlying mural thrombus. Vein graft atherosclerosis is seen in a majority of grafts explanted more than 10 years after surgery whether or not those grafts are stenotic, and atherosclerotic lesions appear to account for almost all late saphenous vein graft (SVG)

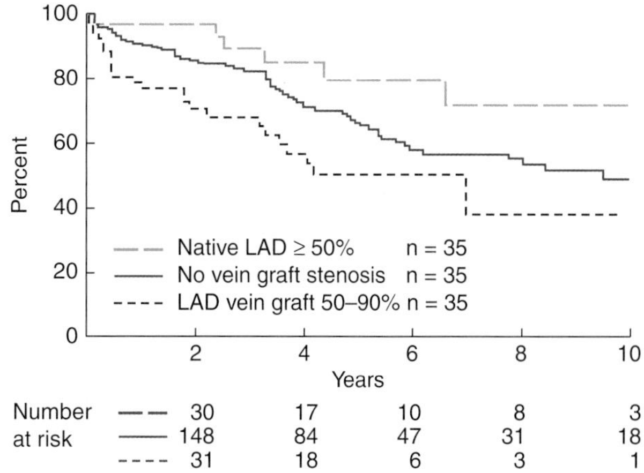

FIGURE 26-5 Patients with late stenoses in vein grafts to the LAD coronary artery had worse survival when compared with either patients with native coronary LAD stenoses or patients with no stenotic vein grafts. (*Reproduced with permission from Lytle BW, Loop FD, Taylor PC, et al: Vein graft disease: the clinical impact of stenoses in saphenous vein bypass grafts to coronary arteries. J Thorac Cardiovasc Surg 1992; 103:831.*)

stenoses. The extreme friability of vein graft atherosclerosis creates a substantial risk of distal coronary artery embolization during percutaneous interventions to treat stenotic lesions and during reoperations for patients with atherosclerotic vein grafts. It is also probable that spontaneous coronary artery embolization may occur from atherosclerotic grafts. In addition, atherosclerotic stenoses in vein grafts appear to predispose to graft thrombosis. Vein graft atherosclerosis appears to be an "active" event-producing lesion.

The exact incidence of late SVG stenoses and occlusions is difficult to determine even with prospective studies because death and reoperation are nonrandom events that remove patients from prospective populations available for late coronary artery angiography. However, it appears that by 10 years after operation, approximately 30% of vein grafts are totally occluded, and 30% of patent grafts exhibit some degree of stenosis or intimal irregularities characteristic of vein graft atherosclerosis.[21,22] Although vein graft atherosclerosis is not the only factor related to late SVG occlusion, it is an important one. Native-vessel stenoses distal to the insertion site of vein grafts may decrease SVG graft outflow and contribute to graft failure, but late graft occlusion usually occurs in the presence of vein graft atherosclerosis. Furthermore, when stenotic vein grafts are replaced at reoperation, the late patency rate of the new vein grafts is good.[2]

Progress has been made toward decreasing the rate of vein graft failure. The early patency rates of SVGs have been improved by the use of perioperative and long-term platelet inhibitors,[23–25] but the best data involving patients receiving platelet inhibitors indicate that the 10-year vein graft failure rate is approximately 35%. Some studies now indicate that lipid-lowering regimens decrease late vein graft disease and the risk of late cardiac events.[26,27] However, the overall level of improvement has been small.[26,27] So far, the only way known to avoid vein graft atherosclerosis is to avoid using vein grafts.

ITA grafts rarely develop late atherosclerosis, and the late attrition rate of patent ITA grafts is extremely low. Left ITA to LAD grafts have a very high late (20 years) patency rate, and for most patients, the LAD is a profoundly important coronary artery.[21,28] These factors account for the impact of the LITA-LAD graft not only in decreasing the rate of late death after primary bypass surgery, but also in decreasing the rate of reoperation.[15] Multiple ITA grafts provide incremental benefit in decreasing the risk of reoperation.[16] It is also important that ITA grafts do not develop graft atherosclerosis, and therefore do not create the risk of coronary artery embolization during reoperation. The presence of patent arterial grafts may create other technical problems during repeat surgery, but embolization is not among them.

INDICATIONS FOR REOPERATION

The randomized trials of bypass surgery versus medical management that were initiated in the 1970s provided a framework of information concerning the indications for bypass surgery, and subsequent observational studies have added substance to that framework. However, no randomized trials of medical versus surgical management pertain to patients with prior surgery. The coronary pathology of patients with previous bypass surgery is different from that of patients with only native-vessel stenoses, and we cannot assume that the natural history of, for example, triple-vessel disease based on atherosclerotic vein grafts, is equivalent to that of triple-native-vessel disease.

Two nonrandomized, retrospective studies of patients who had angiograms after bypass surgery addressed the issue of late survival.[29,30] One study showed that patients with early (fewer than 5 years after operation) stenoses in vein grafts and patients with no stenotic vein grafts had approximately the same outcomes and that these outcomes were relatively good.[29] *However, the presence of late (5 years or more after operation) stenoses in vein grafts predicted poor long-term outcomes, particularly if a stenotic vein graft supplied the LAD coronary artery. When late stenoses in LAD vein grafts were combined with other high-risk characteristics, the late survival rate was particularly dismal.* For example, patients with a 50 to 99% stenosis in an LAD vein graft combined with abnormal LVF and triple-vessel or left main stenoses had only a 46% 2-year survival without reoperation. Patients with late stenoses in an LAD vein graft had significantly worse long-term outcomes than did patients with the LAD jeopardized by a native lesion (see Fig. 26-5). This study showed that the difference in the pathology of early (intimal fibroplasia) and late (vein graft atherosclerosis) vein graft stenoses is associated with a difference in clinical outcome and that late stenoses in vein grafts are dangerous lesions.

A second study compared the outcomes of patients with stenotic vein grafts treated with reoperation (REOP group) versus those treated with medical treatment (MED group).[30] Again, this was a nonrandomized, retrospective study, and the patients in the REOP group were older and more symptomatic, had worse LVF, and had fewer patent grafts than the patients in the MED group.

The survival of patients with early (fewer than 5 years) SVG stenoses was not different in the two groups. The operative risk for the REOP group was low (no deaths among the 59 patients) and the long-term survival was good, but late survival was just as good for the patients treated medically (Fig. 26-6). It is important to note that the patients in the REOP group were more symptomatic to start with, and at late follow-up, they were less symptomatic than the patients in the MED group. Thus, reoperation for patients with early vein graft stenosis was an effective way of relieving symptoms of angina, but it appears that patients without symptoms can be treated medically with safety, at least over the short term.

However, the overall outcomes were worse for patients with late stenoses in vein grafts, and many subgroups had improved survival rates with reoperation. By multivariate testing (Table 26-1), a stenotic (20 to 99%) LAD vein graft predicted late death, and performing a reoperation increased late survival for these patients. Multivariate testing of smaller subgroups showed that the survival advantage for the REOP group was true even for patients with only class I or class II symptoms, and that reoperation still improved survival for the remaining patients when patients with stenoses in LAD vein grafts were excluded from the analysis.

Univariate comparisons for the REOP and MED subgroups of patients with stenotic LAD grafts are shown in Fig. 26-7, demonstrating the improved survival for the REOP group. When patients with stenotic LAD vein grafts were subgrouped on the basis of severity of the stenotic lesions (Fig. 26-8), the patients with severely stenotic (50 to 99%) vein grafts obviously benefited from surgery, exhibiting a decreased risk of death even early in the follow-up period. For patients with moderate stenoses (20 to 49%) in LAD vein grafts, the survivals of the MED and REOP groups were equivalent for about 2 years, but after that point survival of the patients in the MED group

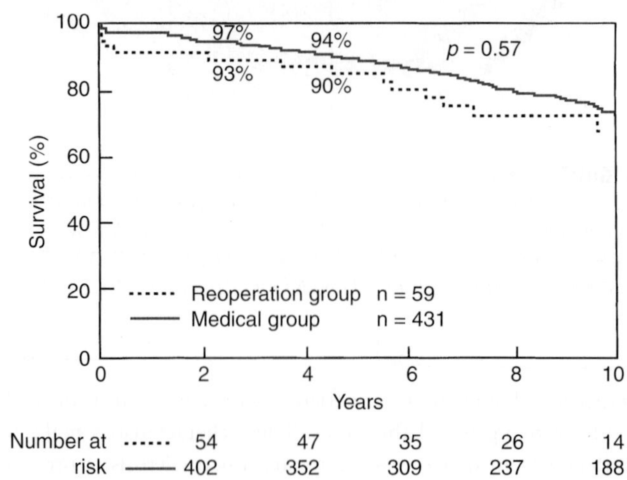

FIGURE 26-6 The survival of patients with early (<5 years after operation) stenoses in vein grafts was favorable with and without reoperation (p = NS). (*Reproduced with permission from Lytle BW, Loop FD, Taylor AC, et al: The effect of coronary reoperation on the survival of patients with stenoses in saphenous vein to coronary bypass grafts. J Thorac Cardiovasc Surg 1993; 105:605.*)

TABLE 26-1 Patients with Late Stenoses (≥5 y) in Saphenous Vein in Coronary Artery Bypass Grafts: Multivariate Model of Variables Influencing Late Survival

	p-Value	Relative Risk
Variables decreasing survival		
LVF moderate/severe	.0001	2.58
Age (at catheterization)	.0001	1.04*
3VD/LMT	.0011	2.87
LAD-SVG stenosis (20–99%)	.0019	1.90
Variable increasing survival	.0007	0.51
Reoperation		

LVF = left ventricular function: 3VD/LMT = triple-vessel disease and/or left main stenosis.
**Per year of age.*
Source: Reproduced with permission from Lytle BW, Loop FD, Taylor PC, et al: The effect of coronary reoperation on the survival of patients with stenoses in saphenous vein to coronary bypass grafts. J Thorac Cardiovasc Surg 1993; 105:605.

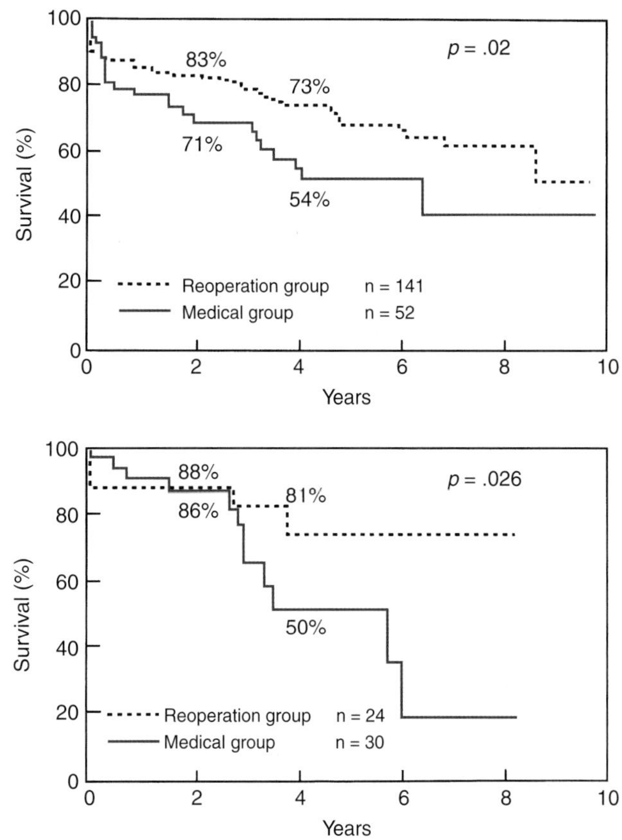

FIGURE 26-8 Patients with late stenoses in LAD vein grafts (*top*) had immediate improvement in their survival rate. Patients with moderate (20 to 49%) stenoses in LAD vein grafts had equivalent survival with or without reoperation for approximately 2 years, but after that point, the patients who did not have reoperation did poorly. (*Reproduced with permission from Lytle BW, Loop FD, Taylor PC, et al: The effect of coronary reoperation on the survival of patients with stenoses in saphenous vein to coronary bypass grafts. J Thorac Cardiovasc Surg 1993; 105:605.*)

became rapidly worse, so that by 3 to 4 years of follow-up, the survival benefit of reoperation became apparent. Although the patients in these studies did not have consistent functional testing, there is evidence that myocardial perfusion and functional studies can help to identify patients likely to benefit from reoperation.

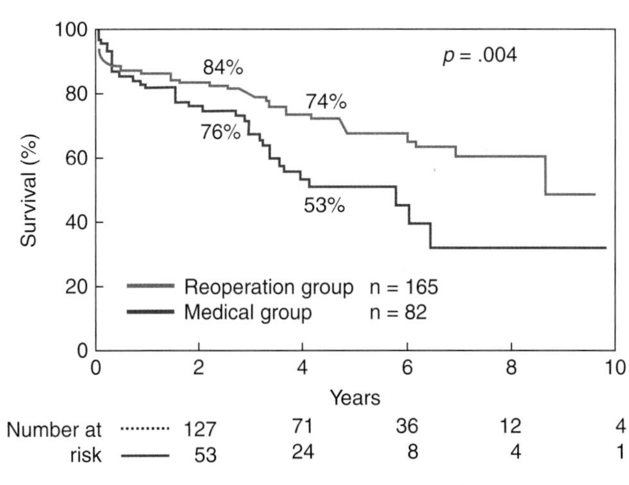

FIGURE 26-7 If patients had late (≥5 years after operation) stenoses in LAD vein grafts, they had a better survival rate (*p* = .004) with immediate reoperation than if they received initial nonoperative treatment. (*Reproduced with permission from Lytle BW, Loop FD, Taylor AC, et al: The effect of coronary reoperation on the survival of patients with stenoses in saphenous vein to coronary bypass grafts. J Thorac Cardiovasc Surg 1993; 105:605.*)

Lauer and colleagues studied 873 symptom-free postoperative patients with symptom-limited exercise thallium-201 studies and found that patients with reversible perfusion defects were more likely to die or experience major cardiac events during a 3-year follow-up.[31] Impaired exercise capacity also was strongly predictive of unfavorable outcomes.

Anatomical indications for reoperation to improve survival prognosis include: (1) atherosclerotic (late) stenoses in vein grafts that supply the LAD artery; (2) multiple stenotic vein grafts that supply large areas of myocardium; and (3) multivessel disease with a proximal LAD lesion and/or abnormal LVF based on either native-vessel lesions or stenotic vein grafts or a combination of the two pathologies. Reoperation is also effective in other anatomical situations in which severe symptoms are the indication for invasive treatment, including patients with a patent ITA to LAD graft combined with other ischemia-producing pathology and multiple early vein graft stenoses. The combination of the anatomical characteristics just noted and reversible ischemia and/or worsening LVF during stress constitutes a particularly strong indication for reoperation.

PERCUTANEOUS TREATMENT OF POSTOPERATIVE PATIENTS

Percutaneous treatments (PCTs) represent alternative anatomical treatments for postoperative patients and often are useful. The effectiveness of PCTs is related to the vascular pathology to be treated and the clinical implications of treatment failure. Today, native coronary artery stenoses often can be treated with a low restenosis rate as long as those vessels are large enough to allow intracoronary stenting. Unfortunately, many postoperative patients have very diffuse native coronary atherosclerosis that makes PCT difficult or ineffective. Also, PCT has not been as effective in the treatment of diabetic native CAD.

The rate of technologic change in interventional cardiology has been rapid, and multiple percutaneous technologies have been used to treat stenotic vein grafts. Balloon angioplasty, first-generation PCT, was relatively dangerous to perform and produced ineffective long-term revascularization, particularly when used to treat older (atherosclerotic) vein grafts.[32] Direct coronary atherectomy (DCA) increased the risk of coronary embolization at the time of the procedure without improving the restenosis rate.[33] It has been hoped that the use of intracoronary stents, particularly covered stents and drug-eluting stents (DESs), in stenotic vein grafts might provide better outcomes, and stenting does represent an improvement over balloon angioplasty.[32] The Randomized Evaluation of Polytetrafluoroethylene Covered Stent in Saphenous Vein Grafts (RECOVERS) trial, a randomized study designed to compare rates of SVG restenosis between CABG patients treated with covered stents and with bare stents, showed identical restenosis rates at 6 months of follow-up (24.2% versus 24.8%; $p = .24$).[34] In a nonrandomized retrospective study comparing the effects of DESs with those of bare metal stents in treating SVG stenosis, Ge and colleagues reported significant differences in in-stent stenosis between groups at 6 months of follow-up (10 versus 26%; $p = .03$).[35] However, other reports comparing DES with bare metal stents showed that the use of DES lowered the rate of restenosis but increased the risk of death.[36]

The kinetics of treatment failure after PCT for vein grafts are different from those for native coronary vessels. Restenosis and new stenotic lesions in vein grafts continue to appear with time, and the shoulder on the adverse outcome curve that appears at 6 months to 1 year after PCT for native vessels does not appear for vein grafts. Thus, there is still some uncertainty about the clinical impact of PCTs of stenotic vein grafts. Patients with previous bypass surgery are an extremely heterogeneous group; some subgroups are at low risk without any anatomical treatment at all, and some subgroups are at high risk without effective therapy. To date, the reported studies of PCT of SVG lesions have not included clinical risk stratifications that would allow comparison of patient survival rates.

Despite persistently high restenosis rates after percutaneous interventions, there are still many indications for their use in the treatment of patients with previous bypass surgery. Realistically, the ideal uses of PCTs are in situations in which failure of the anatomical treatment is not likely to be catastrophic as the impact of stenting on survival is unclear. These situations include symptomatic patients with: (1) early vein graft stenoses; (2) native coronary stenoses; or (3) focal late SVG stenoses in vein grafts not supplying the LAD artery. There are many patients with previous surgery who will fall into a middle ground where it is not clear whether percutaneous transluminal coronary angioplasty (PTCA) or reoperation is likely to yield the best outcome, and judgments must be made on the specific advantages and disadvantages of the treatments for those particular patients. Factors making PTCA more attractive than reoperation are listed in Table 26-2.

TABLE 26-2 Reoperation versus PTCA for Patients with Stenotic Vein Grafts

Factors Favoring Reoperation	Factors Favoring PTCA
Late (≥5 years) stenoses	Early (<5 years) stenoses
Multiple stenotic vein grafts	Single stenotic vein graft
Diffusely atherosclerotic vein grafts	Other patent vein grafts
Stenotic LAD vein graft	Focal graft lesions
No patent ITA graft	Patent ITA-LAD graft
Abnormal left ventricular function	Normal left ventricular function

There are patients with postsurgical repeat ischemic syndromes and very unfavorable coronary anatomy for whom good options for anatomical treatment do not exist. For reoperative coronary surgery to be of benefit there must be bypass conduits available to construct new grafts to graftable coronary arteries that subtend substantial areas of ischemic but viable myocardium. If these conditions do not exist, surgery may not be in the interest of even a symptomatic patient. Studies of diabetic patients undergoing postsurgical repeat revascularization with PCT or surgery have shown unfavorable 10-year survival rates.[37] Unless good coronary targets to receive bypass grafts are available, PCT may be the best choice for marginal candidates because of lower initial costs and, in some settings, lower initial mortality.

TECHNICAL ASPECTS OF CORONARY REOPERATIONS

Reoperations are more complicated than primary operations. The specific technical challenges that surgeons must recognize and solve that are unique to or more common during coronary reoperation are

1. Sternal reentry
2. Stenotic or patent vein or arterial bypass grafts
3. Aortic atherosclerosis
4. Diffuse native-vessel coronary artery disease
5. Coronary arteries located amid old grafts and epicardial scarring
6. Lack of bypass conduits

The overall problem of myocardial protection is more difficult during reoperations, with perioperative myocardial infarction still being the most common cause of in-hospital death.[3,6] The metabolic concepts of myocardial protection in use today are valid, but the reasons that myocardial protection sometimes fails during reoperation are related to anatomical causes of myocardial infarction. These anatomical causes of perioperative myocardial infarction include injury to bypass grafts, atherosclerotic embolization from vein grafts or the aorta to distal coronary arteries, myocardial devascularization secondary to graft removal, hypoperfusion through new grafts, failure to deliver cardioplegic solution, early vein graft thrombosis, incomplete revascularization, diffuse air embolization, and technical error.[3,38–42] To be consistently successful, coronary reoperations must be designed to avoid these causes of myocardial infarction.

Preoperative Assessment

A complete understanding of the patient's native coronary and bypass graft anatomy is essential. Achieving this goal is sometimes not as easy as it sounds, particularly if the patient has had multiple previous coronary operations. If bypass grafts, venous or arterial, are not demonstrated by a preoperative coronary angiogram, it usually means that they are occluded, but it is also possible that the angiogram simply has failed to demonstrate their location. Examination of old angiograms performed before previous operations and review of previous operative records often help to illustrate the patient's coronary anatomy.

It is also important to know that graftable stenotic coronary arteries supply viable myocardium. Myocardial scar and viability can be differentiated by thallium scanning, positron-emission tomography, and stress (exercise or dobutamine) echocardiography. The intricacies of establishing myocardial viability are beyond this discussion, but it is an important issue. Before embarking on a reoperation, it makes sense to be reasonably sure that there is a matchup between the patient's graftable arteries and some viable myocardium such that grafting those arteries will provide some long-term benefits.

It is also wise to have a preoperative plan for bypass conduit selection and to document that potential bypass conduits are available. ITA angiography often is helpful. Venous Doppler studies can be used to assess the presence of greater and lesser saphenous vein segments, and arterial Doppler studies can assess the radial and inferior epigastric arteries and establish the adequacy of flow to the digits during radial artery occlusion.

Median Sternotomy Incision, Conduit Preparation, and Cannulation

Most coronary reoperations are performed through a median sternotomy. Situations associated with increased risk during a repeat median sternotomy include right ventricular or aortic enlargement, a patent vein graft to the right coronary artery, an in situ right ITA graft patent to a left coronary artery branch, an in situ left ITA graft that curls under the sternum, multiple previous operations, and difficulty reopening the sternum during a previous reoperation. In such situations, vessels for arterial (via the femoral or axillary artery) and venous access for cardiopulmonary bypass are dissected out before sternal reentry. All bypass grafts except for the internal thoracic arteries may be prepared before sternal reentry. Preparation of radial artery and greater and lesser saphenous vein segments can be carried out simultaneously. The most common structure injured during reentry is a bypass graft.[4]

When reopening a median sternotomy, the incision is made to the level of the sternal wires; the wires are cut anteriorly and bent back but are not removed (Fig. 26-9). An oscillating saw is used to divide the anterior table of the sternum. When the anterior table has been divided, ventilation is stopped, and the assistants elevate each side of the sternum with rake retractors while the posterior table of the sternum is divided in a caudal-cranial direction. The sternal wires that have been left in place posterior to the sternum help to protect underlying structures. Once the posterior table of the sternum has been divided with the saw, the wires are removed, and sharp dissection with scissors is used to separate each side of the sternum from underlying structures. Once the sternum has been divided, it is important that the assistants retract in an upward direction, not laterally. The right ventricle is injured more often by lateral retraction while it is still adherent to the underside of the sternum than it is by a direct saw injury.

In high-risk situations, it can be helpful to perform a small anterolateral right thoracotomy (Fig. 26-10) before the repeat median sternotomy. Underlying structures, such as the aorta, patent bypass grafts, and the right atrium and ventricle, can be dissected away from the sternum via this approach, and thus, with the surgeon's hand placed behind the sternum, reentry is safe. This small additional incision contributes little morbidity.

Another technique for sternal reentry in high-risk patients is to heparinize, cannulate, and initiate cardiopulmonary bypass

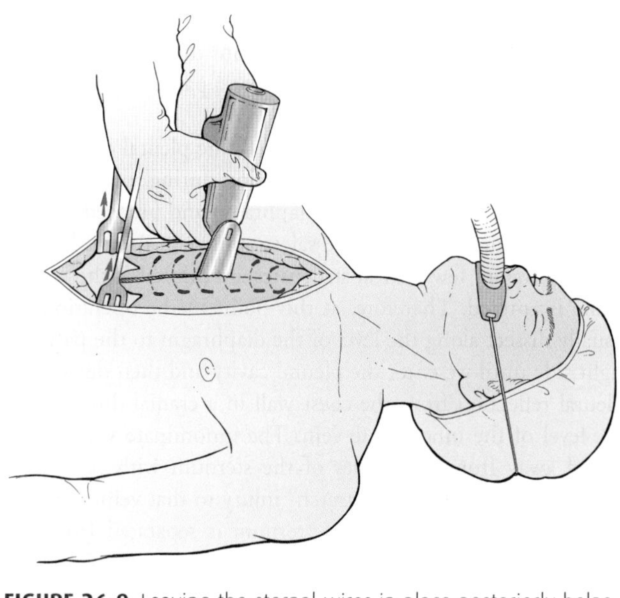

FIGURE 26-9 Leaving the sternal wires in place posteriorly helps to protect underlying structures while the posterior table of the sternum is divided with an oscillating saw. The direction of retraction with rake retractors should be anterior, not lateral.

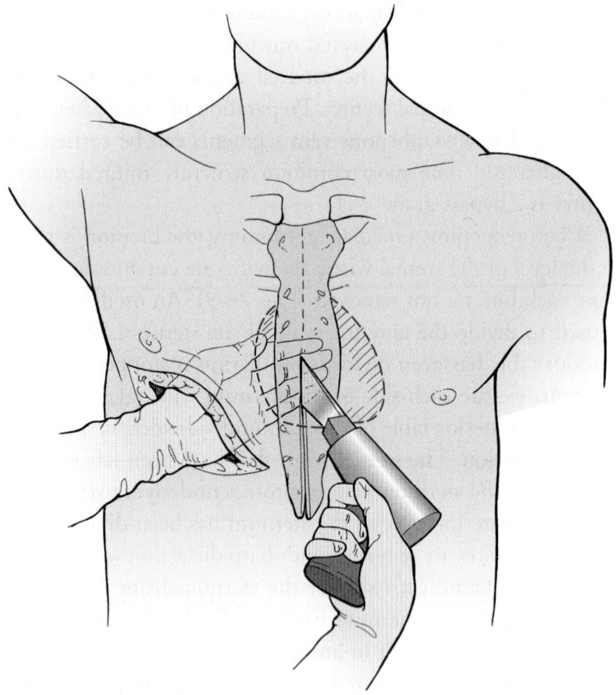

FIGURE 26-10 A small anterolateral right thoracotomy allows dissection of substernal structures such as patent grafts and the right ventricle or aorta away from the sternum under direct vision. While the sternum is being divided, the surgeon may place a hand behind the sternum for further safety.

before median sternotomy. The advantages of this strategy are that the heart can be emptied and allowed to fall away from the sternum, and cardiopulmonary bypass already has been initiated for protection if an injury does occur. The disadvantages of this approach are that extensive mediastinal dissection must be carried out in a heparinized patient, including dissection of the right internal thoracic artery if that is to be used. We rarely employ this approach except in situations in which adherence of an aortic aneurysm to the sternum or a patent right ITA-to-LAD graft creates a specific danger.

Once the sternum has been divided, the pleural cavities are entered. A general principle of dissection during reoperation is that starting at the level of the diaphragm and proceeding in a cranial direction is usually the safest approach. At the level of the diaphragm, few critical structures are injured if the wrong plane is entered. Therefore, at this point in the operation we usually dissect along the level of the diaphragm to the patient's right side until we enter the pleural cavity and then detach the pleural reflection from the chest wall in a cranial direction to the level of the innominate vein. The innominate vein is dissected away from both sides of the sternum with scissors, a maneuver that prevents a "stretch" injury to that vein.

Once the right side of the sternum is separated from the cardiac structures, it is usually possible to prepare a right ITA graft. Because of parietal pleural thickening, it is often more difficult to obtain length on ITA grafts during reoperation than it is during primary procedures, and the right ITA frequently is used as a "free" graft. Once the right ITA dissection is completed to the superior border of the first rib, an incision is made in the parietal pleura to separate the proximal ITA from the area of the phrenic nerve. Thus, if the right ITA needs to be converted to a "free" graft during aortic cross-clamping, it makes division at that point easier because the proximal ITA is clearly identifiable. Although intrapericardial dissection of the left side of the heart is left until later, freeing the left side of the anterior chest wall from the underlying structures (which may include a patent ITA graft) is undertaken now. This is difficult only if there is a patent ITA graft that is densely adherent to the chest wall. Again, it is best to enter the left pleural cavity at the level of the diaphragm and proceed in a cranial direction.

The most difficult point of dissection is usually at the level of the sternal angle, where a patent ITA graft may approach the midline and be adherent to the sternum or the aorta. There are no tricks for dissecting out a patent ITA graft except for being careful. The danger to a patent left ITA graft during sternal reentry and mediastinal dissection is entirely related to the location of the graft at the time of the primary operation. Ideally, the pericardium should be divided at a primary operation, and the left ITA graft should be allowed to run posterior to the lung through the incision in the pericardium and to the LAD or circumflex artery (Fig. 26-11). When this is done, the lung will lay anterior to the left ITA, and that graft will not become adherent to the aorta or to the chest wall.

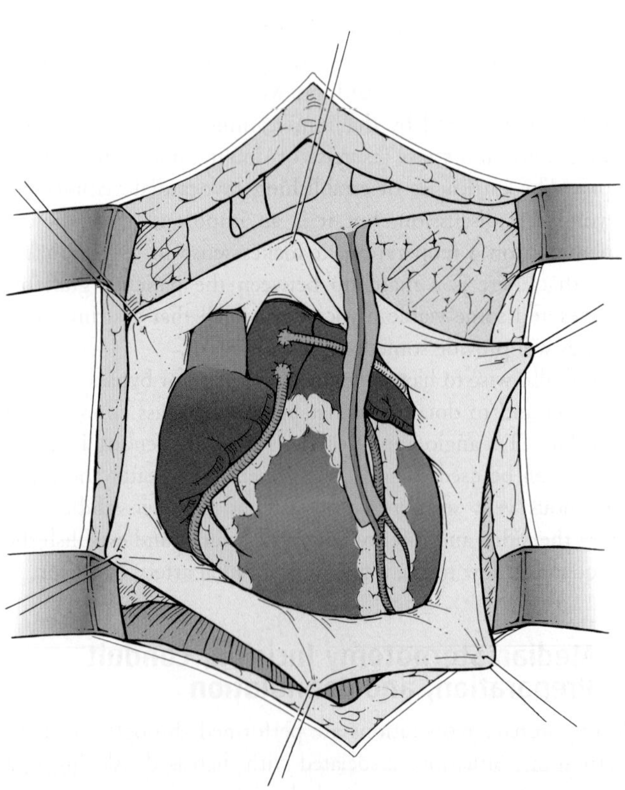

FIGURE 26-11 A patent left ITA-to-LAD graft should not pose a threat during reoperation. At a primary operation, the pericardium should be divided in a posterior direction, and the ITA graft should be placed in that incision. The ITA graft then will lie posterior to the lung and will not be pushed toward the midline by the lung or become adherent to the sternum.

Once the left side of the chest wall is free, the left IMA is prepared (if it has not been used at a previous operation), the sternal spreader is inserted, and the intrapericardial dissection of the aorta and right atrium is accomplished. Again, in most cases it is safest to find the correct dissection plane at the level of the diaphragm and then to continue around the right atrium to the aorta. The one situation in which this strategy may be dangerous is if an atherosclerotic vein graft to the right coronary artery lies over the right atrium. Manipulation of atherosclerotic vein grafts can cause embolization of atherosclerotic debris into coronary arteries, and it is best to employ a "no touch" technique with such grafts. If a vein graft to the right coronary artery lies in an awkward position over the right atrium, it is best to leave the right atrium alone and use the femoral vein and superior vena cava cannulation to establish venous drainage (Fig. 26-12). Once cardiopulmonary bypass has been established, the aorta has been cross-clamped, and cardioplegia has been given, the atherosclerotic vein graft then can be disconnected.

The goal of dissection of the ascending aorta is to obtain enough length for cannulation and cross-clamping and to avoid the most common error, aortic subadventitial dissection. The correct level of dissection on the aorta usually is found either by following the right atrium to the aorta in a caudal-to-cranial direction or by identifying the innominate vein and leaving all the tissue beneath the innominate vein on the aorta. At the level of the innominate vein, the pericardial reflection on each side of the aorta will be identifiable. Division of the pericardial reflection on the left side in a posterior direction will lead to the plane between the aorta and the pulmonary artery. Once the left side of the aorta is identified, the surgeon then may dissect posteriorly on the medial aspect of the left lung toward the hilum. The segment of tissue between these two dissection planes usually will include a patent left ITA graft, if present, and clamping that tissue will produce occlusion of the ITA graft.

When the aorta has been dissected out, heparin is given, and cannulation is undertaken. Cannulation of an atherosclerotic ascending aorta may cause atherosclerotic embolization leading to stroke, myocardial infarction, or multiorgan failure, so the ascending aorta should be studied with palpation and echocardiography to detect atherosclerosis before cannulation. Although the most widely used alternative arterial cannulation site is the femoral artery, arteriopathic patients often have severe femoral artery atherosclerosis. The axillary artery is an alternative arterial cannulation site that we have used with increasing frequency because atherosclerotic disease is usually not present in that vessel, and its cannulation allows antegrade perfusion[44] (Fig. 26-13). If atherosclerotic disease or calcification of the aorta makes any aortic occlusion hazardous, the options are off-pump bypass surgery (see Other Options) or replacement of the aorta with axillary artery cannulation, hypothermia, and circulatory arrest. Venous cannulation usually is accomplished with a single two-stage right atrial cannula. A transatrial coronary sinus cardioplegia cannula is inserted via a right atrial purse

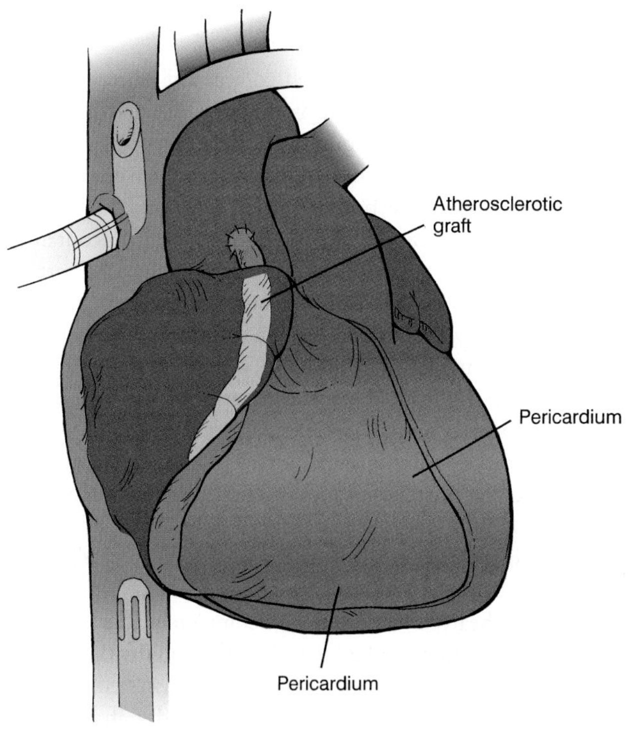

FIGURE 26-12 Manipulation of patent but atherosclerotic vein grafts should be avoided. If an atherosclerotic right coronary vein graft blocks access to the right atrium, femoral vein, and direct superior vena cava, cannulation is safer than mobilizing the vein graft so as to achieve right atrial cannulation.

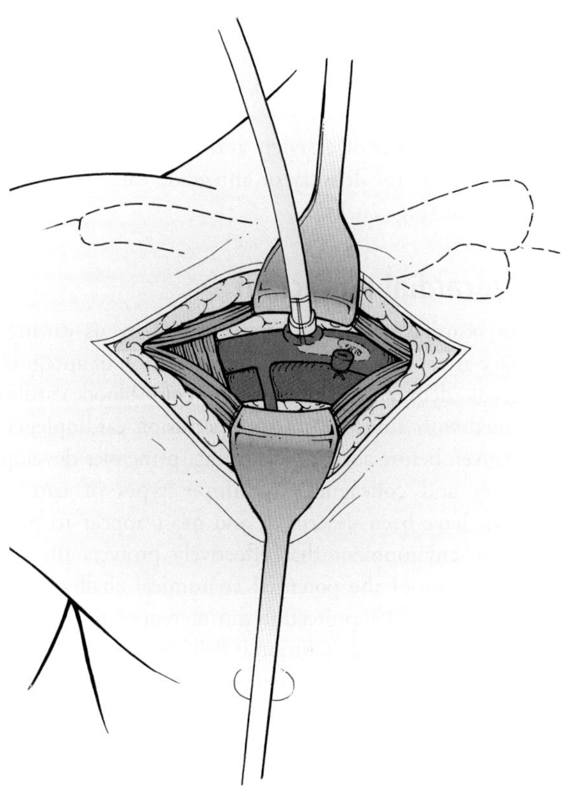

FIGURE 26-13 The axillary artery is an important alternative arterial cannulation site for patients with aortic and femoral artery atherosclerosis. A 21-gauge cannula will fit the axillary artery in most patients.

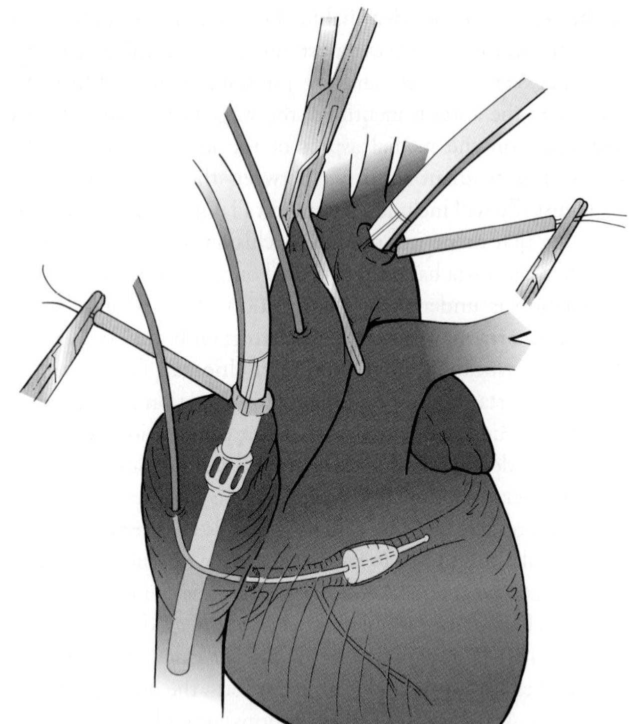

FIGURE 26-14 Standard cannulation for coronary artery reoperation includes aortic arterial cannulation, an aortic needle for antegrade delivery of cardioplegia and aortic root venting, a single two-stage venous cannula, and a transatrial coronary sinus catheter with a self-inflating balloon for delivery of retrograde cardioplegia. Cannulation is accomplished before dissection of the left ventricle.

string with the aid of a stylet, and a needle is placed in the ascending aorta for delivery of antegrade cardioplegia and for use as a vent (Fig. 26-14).

Myocardial Protection

The myocardial protection strategy used by us during most coronary artery reoperations is a combination of antegrade and retrograde delivery of intermittent cold blood cardioplegia combined with a dose of warm reperfusion cardioplegia ("hot shot") given before aortic unclamping, principles developed by Buckberg and colleagues.[45] Multiple types of cardioplegic solutions have been described, and most appear to provide a metabolic environment that effectively protects the myocardium. Because of the potential anatomical challenges to cardioplegic myocardial protection during reoperations, the details of how the cardioplegic solution is delivered are very important. In most primary bypass operations, antegrade cardioplegia works well by itself. During reoperations, however, antegrade cardioplegia may not be effective for areas of myocardium that are supplied by patent in situ arterial grafts and may be dangerous because of the risk of embolization of atherosclerotic debris into the coronary arteries from old vein grafts. The delivery of cardioplegia through the coronary sinus and through the cardiac venous system to the myocardium (retrograde cardioplegia) has been a step forward in myocardial protection during reoperations.[46,47] Retrograde cardioplegia delivery avoids atheroembolism from vein grafts, can be helpful in removing atherosclerotic debris and air from the coronary artery system, and can deliver cardioplegia to areas supplied by in situ arterial grafts. The biggest disadvantage of retrograde cardioplegia is that it is not always possible to place a catheter in the coronary sinuses that will deliver cardioplegia consistently. It is important to monitor the adequacy of cardioplegia delivery by measuring the pressure in the coronary sinus, noting the distention of cardiac veins with arterial blood, the cooling of the myocardium, and the return of desaturated blood from open coronary arteries.

Cardiopulmonary bypass is begun, the perfusionist empties the heart and produces mild systemic hypothermia (34°C), and the aorta is cross-clamped. We usually initiate cardioplegia induction with aortic root cardioplegia. To induce and maintain cardioplegic protection, it is helpful to be able to occlude patent arterial grafts. If it has not yet been possible to dissect out a patent arterial graft so that it can be clamped, the systemic perfusion temperature is decreased to 25°C until control of the graft is achieved. After antegrade cardioplegia has been given for 2 to 3 minutes, we shift to retrograde induction for another 2 to 3 minutes. Giving any antegrade cardioplegia does risk embolization from atherosclerotic vein grafts, but if these grafts have not yet been manipulated, that danger is relatively small. Once the adequacy of retrograde cardioplegia delivery has been established, it is often possible to use that route predominantly for maintenance doses.

Intrapericardial Dissection

When the heart has been arrested completely, intrapericardial dissection of the left ventricle is undertaken, starting at the diaphragm and extending out to the left of the apex of the heart. After the apex is identified, the surgeon divides the pericardium in a cranial direction on the left side of the LAD artery (Fig. 26-15). A patent LITA-to-LAD graft will be contained within the strip of pericardium that lies over the LAD artery. Dissection of this pedicle from the anterior aspect of the pulmonary artery will allow an atraumatic clamp to be placed across the patent ITA graft and also will allow the passage of new bypass grafts from the aorta underneath the patent ITA graft to left-sided coronary arteries. The advantages of waiting until after aortic clamping and arrest to dissect out the left ventricle are that dissection is more accurate, there is less damage to the epicardium and less bleeding, manipulation of atherosclerotic vein grafts is less likely to cause coronary embolization, and the dissection of patent ITA grafts is safer.

After the heart is dissected out completely, the coronary arteries to be grafted can be identified, the lengths that bypass conduits need to reach those vessels may be assessed, and the final operative plan can be established. The old grafts and epicardial scarring that are present during reoperations make the preoperative prediction of the lengths of conduits needed for bypass grafts quite difficult, particularly the lengths of arterial grafts, and it is wise to have some flexibility in the operative plan. Before the construction of the anastomoses, those patent

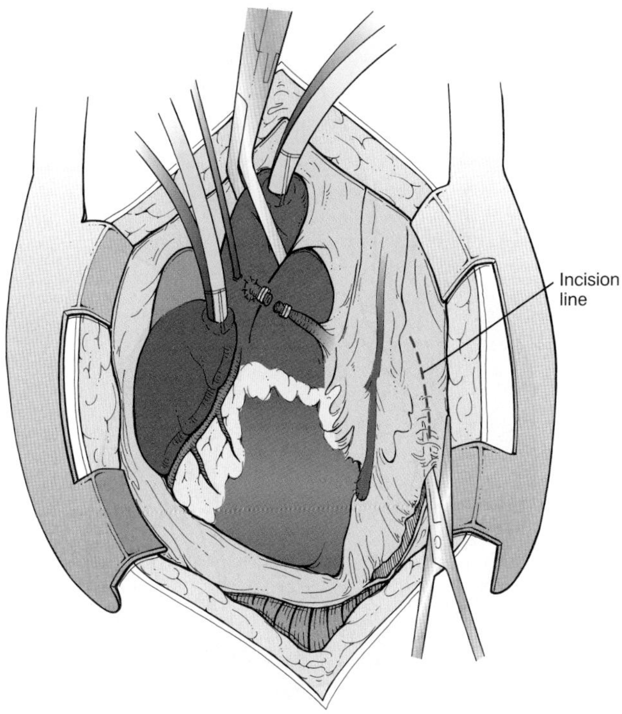

FIGURE 26-15 Division of the pericardium along the diaphragm allows the surgeon to reach a point to the left of the cardiac apex. From that point, the pericardium can be divided in a cranial direction to the left of the LAD artery, leaving a patent ITA graft in the strip of tissue overlying the LAD artery. Atherosclerotic vein grafts that are going to be replaced may be divided once a dose of antegrade cardioplegia is given.

but atherosclerotic vein grafts that are going to be disconnected are identified and are disconnected with a scalpel. The order of anastomosis construction that is used by the authors is: (1) distal vein graft anastomoses; (2) distal free arterial graft anastomoses; (3) distal in situ arterial graft anastomoses; and (4) proximal (aortic) anastomoses.

Stenotic Vein Grafts

When should patent or stenotic vein grafts be replaced, and with what should they be replaced? Atherosclerosis in vein grafts is common if those grafts are more than 5 years old, and leaving them in place risks embolization of atherosclerotic debris at the time of reoperation and subsequent development of premature graft stenoses or occlusions after reoperation. On the other hand, replacement of all vein grafts extends the operation and may use up available bypass conduits.

In the past, our general rule has been to replace all vein grafts that are more than 5 years old at the time of reoperation, even if those grafts are not diseased angiographically. However, this strategy assumes that conduits are available that can replace these old grafts. Today, many patients have very limited conduits at reoperation because of the large numbers of vein grafts used at primary surgery or because of multiple previous operations. Thus, graft replacement must be individualized. Inspection of vein grafts at reoperation occasionally will identify a graft that looks normal angiographically and does not appear to have any thickening or atherosclerosis on visual inspection. Often such vein grafts will be left alone.

Replacing old vein grafts with new vein grafts may often be accomplished by creating the new vein-to-coronary-artery anastomosis at the site of the previous distal anastomosis, leaving only 1 mm or so of the old vein in place (Fig. 26-16). If significant native-vessel stenoses have developed distal to the old vein graft, it is often best to place a new graft to the distal vessel in addition to replacing the vein graft. Many reoperative candidates have proximal occlusions of the native coronary artery system and multiple stenoses throughout the vessel, and if only new distal grafts are constructed, the proximal segments of coronary arteries and their branches that are supplied by atherosclerotic vein grafts may be jeopardized. More than one graft to a major coronary artery may be desirable during reoperation (Fig. 26-17).

Sequential vein grafts often are very helpful during reoperation because they allow more distal anastomoses and fewer proximal anastomoses. Sites for proximal anastomoses are often at a premium in the scarred reoperative aorta.

Artery-to-coronary-artery bypass grafts have many advantages during reoperations. First, they are often available. Second, the tendency of arteries to remain patent even when used as grafts to diffusely diseased coronary arteries makes them particularly applicable to reoperative candidates. Third, in situ arterial grafts do not require a proximal anastomosis. If the left ITA has not been used as a graft at a previous operation, a strong attempt should be made to use it as an in situ graft to the LAD artery. During primary operations, the right ITA usually can be crossed over as an in situ graft to left-sided vessels,

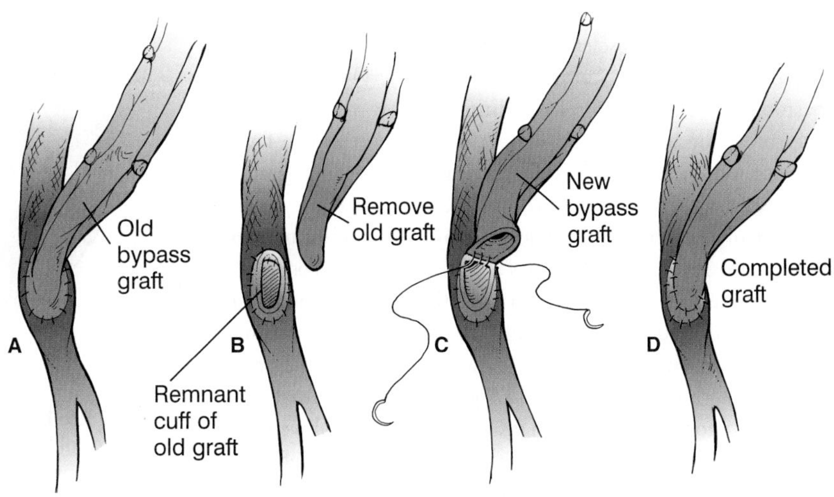

FIGURE 26-16 For patients with extensive native coronary atherosclerosis, the distal anastomotic site of an old vein graft is often the best spot for the distal anastomosis of a new graft. Only a small rim of the old graft should be left in place.

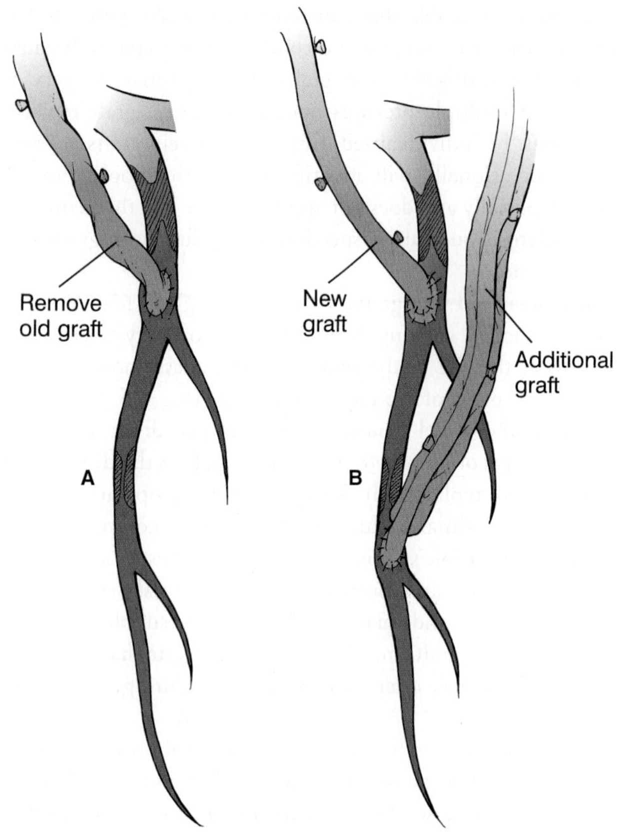

FIGURE 26-17 Extension of native-vessel coronary artery disease may indicate the placement of new distal grafts as well as replacement of diseased vein grafts supplying proximal coronary artery segments.

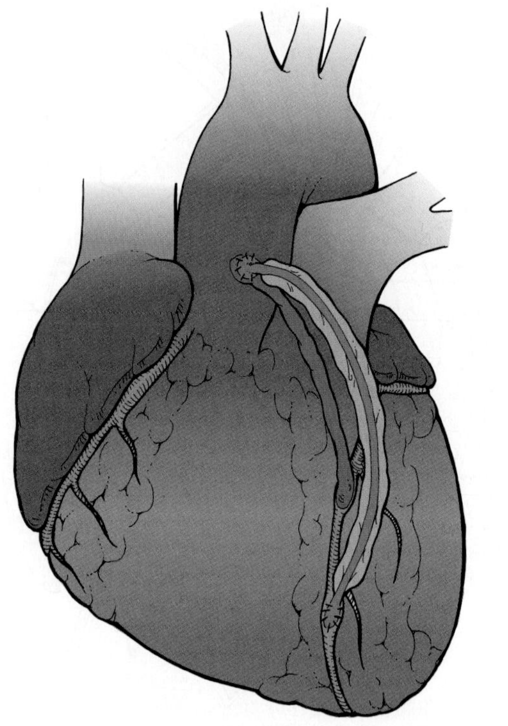

FIGURE 26-18 The hood of new or old vein grafts is often the best spot for the aortic anastomosis of free arterial grafts. Atherosclerosis rarely occurs in that "bubble" of vein.

but such a plan is more difficult during repeat surgery, so the right ITA is often used as a free graft.

Arterial graft proximal anastomoses are a problem at reoperation because the scarring and thickening of the reoperative aorta often make direct anastomoses of arterial grafts to the aorta unsatisfactory. However, when old vein grafts become occluded, there is usually a "bubble" of the hood of the old vein graft that is not atherosclerotic and that often is a good spot for construction of a free (aorta-to-coronary-artery) arterial graft anastomosis (Fig. 26-18). In addition, if new vein grafts are performed, the hood of that new vein graft represents a favorable location for an arterial graft anastomosis. Late angiographic data regarding this strategy are not available, but the relative freedom of the hood of vein grafts from the development of atherosclerosis means these grafts are likely to be successful.

Another effective strategy is to use either an old arterial graft or a newly constructed arterial graft for the proximal anastomosis of a free arterial graft (Fig. 26-19). Composite arterial grafts, usually using a new in situ left ITA graft at the proximal anastomotic site for a free right ITA graft, have been employed with increasing frequency, and early outcomes have been favorable.[48,49] This method is particularly useful during reoperations because it may avoid an aortic anastomosis, and less right ITA graft length is needed to reach distal circumflex arteries. Other advantages of using a previously performed patent ITA graft for

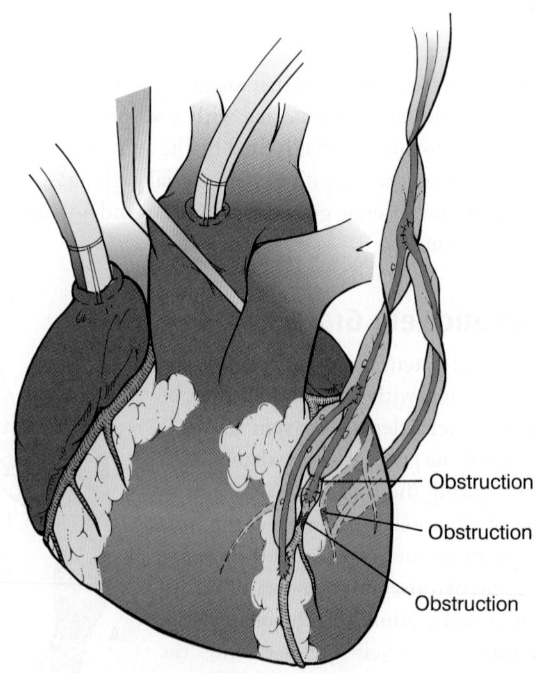

FIGURE 26-19 Composite arterial grafts can be constructed using a new or old left ITA graft as the inflow source. With its proximal anastomosis to the left ITA, a right ITA graft will easily reach the circumflex branches. Furthermore, a shorter segment of inferior epigastric artery or radial artery can be used to reach the distal LAD artery if intervening native LAD stenoses have limited the effectiveness of an old ITA graft.

the proximal anastomosis of a new arterial graft are that the old left ITA graft often has increased in size, and the preoperative angiogram has demonstrated its integrity. In situations in which the effectiveness of an LITA-to-LAD graft has been jeopardized by a distal LAD lesion, a short segment of a new arterial graft can be used to bridge that stenosis from the old arterial graft to the distal LAD artery (see Fig. 26-18).

Can an ITA graft be used to replace a vein graft during reoperation? When faced with replacing a stenotic or patent vein graft during reoperation, the surgeon has a number of options, all of which have some potential disadvantages:

1. The surgeon may leave the old vein graft in place and add an arterial graft to the same coronary vessel. The dangers of this approach are that atherosclerotic embolization from the old vein may occur during the reoperation, and competitive flow between the vein graft and the arterial graft may jeopardize the ITA graft after reoperation.
2. The surgeon may remove the old vein graft and replace it with an ITA graft. This decreases the likelihood of atherosclerotic embolization and competitive flow but risks hypoperfusion during reoperation if the arterial graft cannot supply all the flow that had been generated previously by the vein graft.
3. The surgeon may replace the old vein graft with a new vein graft. The disadvantage of this approach is a long-term one: The coronary vessel is left dependent on a vein graft.

When we examined these choices in a retrospective study of operations for patients with atherosclerotic vein grafts supplying the LAD artery, we found that the worst outcomes resulted from removing a patent (although stenotic) vein graft and replacing it with only an ITA graft.[39] This strategy was associated with a significant incidence of hypoperfusion and severe hemodynamic difficulties during reoperation that were treated effectively only by adding a vein graft to the same coronary artery. The incidence of myocardial infarction associated with leaving a stenotic vein graft in place was low. Thus, atherosclerotic embolization from an atherosclerotic vein graft is a danger, but it appears that with the use of retrograde cardioplegia, it is not commonly a major catastrophe.

Another potential disadvantage of the strategy of adding an ITA graft to a stenotic vein graft is that competition in flow from the stenotic vein graft may lead to failure of the new ITA graft. However, this is unlikely to occur as long as the stenosis in the SVG is severe.[50] Our usual approach, therefore, is to remove atherosclerotic vein grafts when replacing them with a new vein graft but leave stenotic vein grafts in place when grafting the same vessel with an arterial graft (Fig. 26-20).

Alternative arterial grafts often are very useful during reoperation. The radial artery has particular advantages during repeat surgery because it is larger and longer than other free arterial grafts. These qualities increase the range of coronary arteries that can be grafted. Early studies of radial artery grafts have shown favorable patency rates, but few long-term data currently exist. If the high patency rates that have been documented by early studies are confirmed by the tests of time, the radial artery will be used extensively during reoperations. The inferior epigastric artery often is too short to function as a

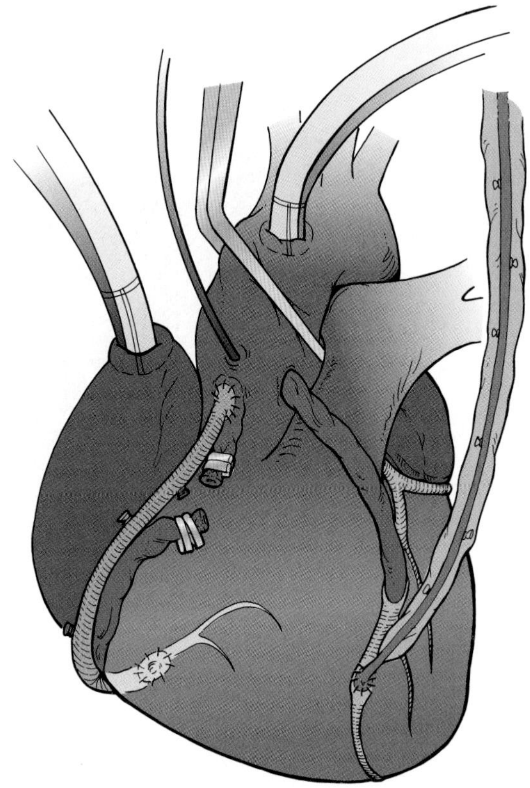

FIGURE 26-20 In this example, an atherosclerotic right coronary artery vein graft is disconnected and is replaced with a new vein graft. However, the stenotic vein graft to the LAD artery is left in place to avoid hypoperfusion, and a new ITA graft is added to the LAD artery.

separate aorta-to-coronary-artery graft during reoperation but can be extremely useful as a short composite arterial graft, as illustrated in Fig. 26-19.

The right gastroepiploic artery (RGEA) has established a good midterm graft patency rate record and often is useful during reoperation because it is an in situ graft.[51] Furthermore, it can be prepared before the median sternotomy. It is effective most often as an in situ graft to the posterior descending branch of the right coronary artery or the distal LAD artery (Fig. 26-21).

The aortic anastomoses of the vein and arterial grafts are performed last during the single period of aortic cross-clamping. Sites for aortic anastomoses are often at a premium owing to previous scarring, atherosclerotic disease, or the use of Teflon felt during the primary operation, and often the locations of the previous vein graft proximal anastomoses are the best locations for the new ones. The advantages of constructing aortic anastomoses during a single period of aortic cross-clamping are that it minimizes aortic trauma and allows excellent visualization of the proximal anastomoses. In addition, if patent or stenotic vein grafts have been removed and replaced, reperfusion is not accomplished by aortic declamping until the aortic anastomoses have been completed.

The disadvantage of this approach is that it prolongs the period of aortic cross-clamping. However, our strategies for reoperation are not based on trying to minimize myocardial

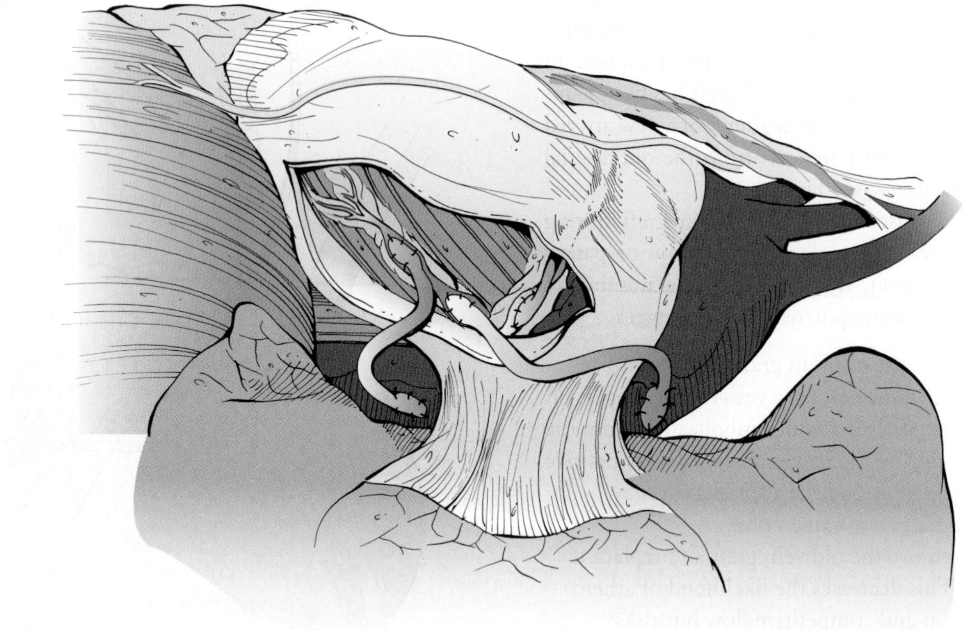

FIGURE 26-21 Circumflex vessels may be grafted through a left thoracotomy incision without cardiopulmonary bypass.

ischemic time. If cardioplegia can be delivered effectively, its metabolic concepts are valid, and myocardial protection is secure. Failure of myocardial protection usually is caused by anatomical events, not by metabolic failure. Once the proximal anastomosis has been constructed, a "hot shot" of substrate-enhanced blood cardioplegia is given, and the aortic cross-clamp is removed.

Other Options

Although most reoperations are performed through a median sternotomy with the use of cardiopulmonary bypass, the strategies of small-incision surgery and off-pump surgery that have been gaining increasing use for primary coronary artery operations also can be helpful during reoperations. Reoperations in situations in which a limited area of myocardium needs revascularization often can be accomplished through a limited incision and without the use of cardiopulmonary bypass (known as the *minimally invasive direct coronary artery bypass* [MIDCAB] *operation*). The distal LAD artery may be exposed with a small anterior thoracotomy, and the LAD or diagonal artery may be grafted with a left ITA graft. A stabilizing device usually is employed for anastomotic construction, although the intrapericardial adhesions provide some stability during reoperations. If the left ITA is not available, a segment of saphenous vein can be anastomosed to the subclavian artery and routed in a transthoracic path to the LAD artery. If the right ITA is to be used as an in situ graft to the LAD artery, a median sternotomy is indicated, but if this is the only graft, off-pump surgery usually is possible.

The lateral wall of the heart can be exposed through a left lateral thoracotomy (Fig. 26-22), and the circumflex and distal right coronary artery branches can be grafted with this approach. Often the LITA already has been used for a graft, but the descending thoracic aorta may be used as a site for the proximal anastomosis of a vein graft or a radial artery graft using a partial occluding clamp. The disadvantages of this

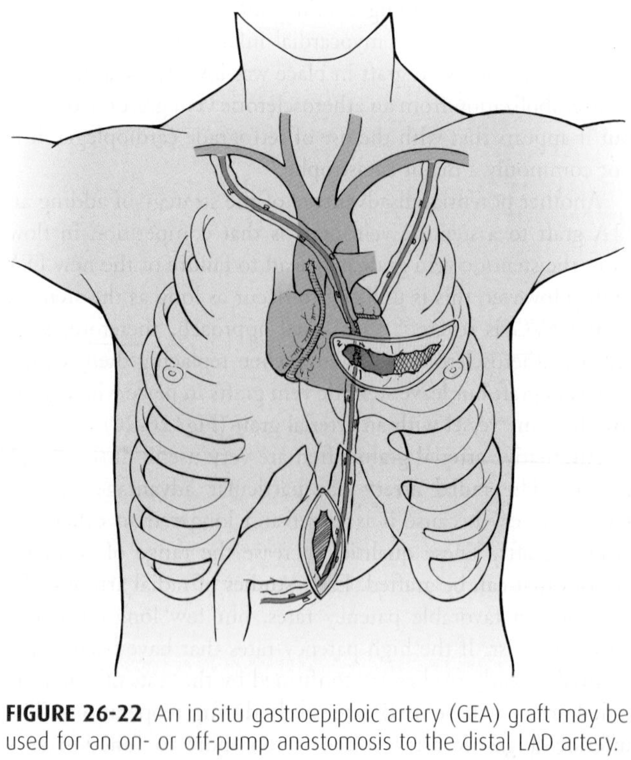

FIGURE 26-22 An in situ gastroepiploic artery (GEA) graft may be used for an on- or off-pump anastomosis to the distal LAD artery.

approach are that the right ITA is difficult to use as an in situ graft, and if the circumflex vessels are deeply intramyocardial, they may be difficult to expose and isolate with the off-pump strategy.

In addition to avoiding potential complications of cardiopulmonary bypass, the "limited-area, off-pump" approach also avoids extensive dissection of the heart and possible manipulation of atherosclerotic vein grafts. The disadvantage of this approach is that most patients who are candidates for reoperation need grafts to multiple vessels in multiple myocardial areas.

Use of a median sternotomy and the off-pump strategy to graft multiple myocardial areas is now a standard approach to primary coronary revascularization and also can be used during reoperation. However, because of the need to access all areas, extensive dissection sometimes is necessary for lysis of adhesions to be able to mobilize the heart. If patients have atherosclerotic vein grafts, dissection and manipulation create the dangers of embolization of atherosclerotic debris and myocardial infarction. This problem was encountered during the early years of bypass surgery when the risks of atherosclerotic embolization were less recognized. Another disadvantage of off-pump reoperative strategies is that reoperative candidates often have very distal and diffuse CAD, which leaves intramyocardial segments as the best areas for grafting. These characteristics stress off-pump isolation and immobilization techniques. In addition, the aortic anastomoses of vein or free arterial grafts may be difficult because of aortic atherosclerosis, adhesions, or previous aortic anastomoses that may limit the application of a partial occluding clamp. On the other hand, the use of off-pump techniques may minimize aortic trauma, particularly if in situ arterial grafts can be employed to provide inflow to new grafts.

In an individual case, the disadvantages of off-pump surgery may be important or irrelevant. Surgeons who perform reoperative coronary artery surgery in a wide spectrum of situations will find both on- and off-pump strategies helpful.

RESULTS OF CORONARY ARTERY REOPERATIONS

Coronary artery reoperations are riskier than primary operations. A study from the Society of Thoracic Surgeons (STS) database reported an in-hospital mortality rate of 6.95% associated with reoperations for the years 1991 to 1993, and in a multivariate analysis of all isolated coronary artery bypass surgery, "previous operation" was identified as a factor that increased the mortality rate.[12] At the Cleveland Clinic Foundation, the in-hospital mortality rate of a first reoperation ranged between 3 and 4% from 1967 through 1991, and the rate was 3.7% for 1663 patients having repeat surgery from 1988 through 1991.[1–3] Progress during the last decade has continued to lower this risk. In a recent report by Sabik and colleagues, the hospital mortality rate for patients undergoing reoperative CABG was reduced to 2.5% in 2002, and risk adjustment identified the comorbidity burden carried by reoperative patients as a factor that increased risk, not reoperative status itself.[14]

Recent mortality rates from other large series range from 4.2 to 11.4%, most being around 7%.[4–9,52] All these figures are two to five times higher than the rates we would expect for the risk of primary CABG.

Coronary artery reoperations have been associated with a higher in-hospital mortality mostly because of an increased risk of perioperative myocardial infarction. In the Cleveland Clinic Foundation series, the cause of perioperative death was cardiovascular in 85% of cases in the most recent cohort of patients undergoing reoperation, a figure that contrasts with recent studies of primary operations, in which noncardiac causes of death have been increasingly important.[3,15] Furthermore, in the reoperative series, in-hospital mortality was associated with new perioperative myocardial infarction in 67% of cases. Multiple causes of myocardial infarction have been identified, including incomplete revascularization owing to distal CAD, vein graft thrombosis, ITA graft failure, atherosclerotic embolization from vein grafts, injury to bypass grafts, hypoperfusion from arterial grafts, preoperative myocardial infarction, and complications of PTCA.

Sternal reentry still creates risk. In a study of 1847 patients undergoing reoperation, 7% were associated with an adverse event and only previous radiation and the number of previous operations could be identified as predictors of injury. Of the 127 patients sustaining an injury, 24 (19%) experienced a major adverse outcome (stroke, myocardial infarction, or death) compared with a risk of 6.2% for those without an injury.[43]

Multiple studies of patients undergoing reoperation have identified increased age, female gender, and emergency operation as clinical variables that have a high association with in-hospital mortality. Emergency operation is a particularly strong factor. Although there is not a standard definition of *emergency*, mortality rates after emergency reoperations that have been reported range from 13 to 40%.[3,5–8] Data from the STS for the year 1997 documented a risk of 5.2% for elective reoperations, 7.4% for urgent reoperations, 13.5% for emergency reoperations, and 40.7% for "salvage" reoperations. There is clearly a major increment in risk associated with emergency reoperations, a larger increment than has existed for patients undergoing primary surgery.

Advanced age, by itself, does not increase the risk of reoperation substantially but does so when combined with other variables. In a review of 739 patients aged 70 years or older undergoing reoperation, we noted an overall in-hospital mortality rate of 7.6% and identified emergency operation, female gender, left ventricular (LV) dysfunction, creatinine concentration greater than 1.6 μg/dL, and left main coronary artery stenosis as specific factors increasing risk. For patients with none of these characteristics, the in-hospital mortality rate was only 1.5%.[53]

Specific anatomical situations, in particular, the presence of patent ITA grafts and atherosclerotic vein grafts, can increase the risk of reoperation, but with experience, these technical factors largely have been neutralized. We have never documented an increased mortality rate for patients with patent ITA grafts but have noted that the risk of ITA damage has dropped from 8% in our early experience to 3.7% more recently, an improvement almost entirely related to increased surgical experience. With proper positioning of an ITA graft at primary operation, a patent LITA-to-LAD-artery or LITA-to-circumflex-artery graft should not represent an impediment to reoperation. Situations in which a patent in situ right ITA graft crosses the midline to supply the LAD or circumflex system are more difficult and require extreme care in reoperating using a median sternotomy incision. Although these situations are uncommon and provide difficult technical challenges, the risks for these patients have not been increased.

Studies from the past noted that the presence of atherosclerotic vein grafts did increase perioperative risk. Perrault and colleagues documented mortality rates of 7, 17, and 29% for patients with one, two, or three stenotic vein grafts, respectively, and in a previous study of patients with atherosclerotic vein grafts, we noted that the presence of an atherosclerotic vein graft to the LAD artery increased in-hospital risk.[30,36] However, in our more recent study we found that atherosclerotic vein grafts did not increase mortality, although there was a nonsignificant trend toward increased risk for patients with multiple stenotic grafts.[3] The favorable results for these patients have been based on a combination of improved technology, the use of retrograde cardioplegia delivery, and increased surgeon experience.

Although arterial grafts may offer advantages at reoperation, their use may prolong an already complex operation, and the influence of arterial grafting on perioperative risk has been a concern. However, we have specifically studied this issue and found that the use of single or double ITA grafts at reoperation does not increase perioperative risk, and in fact, not having an ITA graft at either the first or second operation appeared to be a factor associated with increased in-hospital mortality.[3] Graft selection in that study was not randomized, and it is certainly possible that the increased risk for patients receiving only vein grafts was related to patient-related variables rather than surgical strategy. It does appear, however, that the use of arterial grafts does not increase risk. Except for an increased incidence of perioperative myocardial infarction, in-hospital morbidity does not seem to be increased for patients undergoing reoperation. One important observation relates to wound complications. Multiple groups, including ours, have noted an increased risk of wound complications when diabetic patients have received bilateral (simultaneous) ITA grafts. However, there does not appear to be an increased risk of wound complications for diabetic patients who receive staged ITA grafts, one at the first and another at a second operation.

It is important to note that only the variables that can be identified and quantified are included in studies consistent enough to be identified as risk factors. For example, experience and logic dictate that severe atherosclerosis of the ascending aorta is a major risk factor, but this is rarely identified in large studies because patients do not routinely undergo echocardiography to identify the presence of aortic atherosclerosis.

Late Results

Patients who are undergoing reoperation are at a later stage in the progression of their native coronary atherosclerosis compared with the point when they underwent primary surgery, and the anatomical corrections achieved at reoperation are less perfect. Although the definition of *complete revascularization* varies widely, few reoperative candidates undergo an operation in which all diseased segments of all arteries receive bypass grafts. It is not surprising that the long-term results of reoperation have not been as favorable as the long-term results of primary operations.

The likelihood of recurrent angina after any bypass operation is related to time, but angina symptoms are more common after repeat surgery than they are after primary operation. Follow-up of our reoperative patients at a mean interval of 72 months after reoperation showed that 64% of patients were in New York Heart Association (NYHA) functional class I, although only 10% of patients had class III or class IV symptoms.[2] Weintraub and colleagues also noted at a 4-year follow-up that 41% of reoperative patients had experienced some angina.[6]

Late survival rates after reoperation are also inferior to those after primary surgery. Weintraub and colleagues noted 76% 5-year and 55% 10-year survival rates, and our most recent follow-up study found a 10-year survival rate of 69% for in-hospital survivors[2,6] (Fig. 26-23). The predictors of late survival have varied among studies, but LV dysfunction, advanced age, and diabetes consistently have been associated with a decreased late survival rate. The variables identified by multivariate testing as decreasing the late survival for 2429 hospital survivors of a first reoperation are listed in Table 26-3. The influence of ITA grafts on late survival has been difficult to determine for reoperations. We found a positive influence of a single ITA graft on late survival, as have others,[54] but the effect was not as dramatic as has been noted after primary operations. Weintraub and colleagues did not document an improved survival associated with ITA grafting.[6]

Multiple Coronary Artery Reoperations

Patients who have had more than one previous coronary artery operation are like patients undergoing first reoperations, only more so. Many patients undergoing multiple reoperations had their first procedure more than 15 years ago,

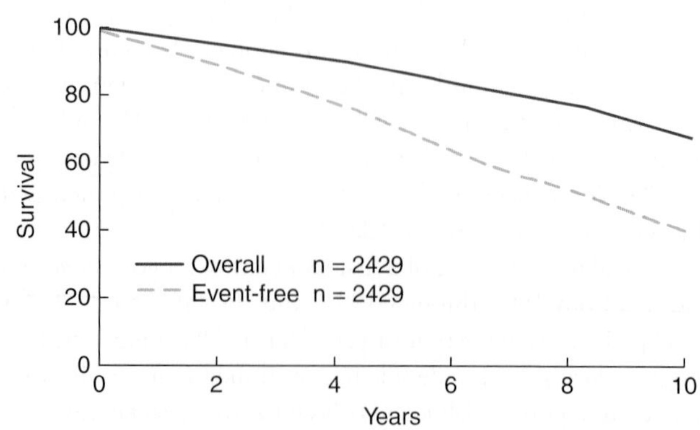

FIGURE 26-23 For 2429 hospital survivors who underwent reoperation between 1967 and 1987, the 10-year survival was 69%, and event-free survival was 41%. (*Reprinted with permission from Loop FD, Lytle BW, Cosgrove DM, et al: Reoperation for coronary atherosclerosis: changing practice in 2509 consecutive patients. Ann Surg 1990; 212:378.*)

TABLE 26-3 Factors Decreasing Late Survival after Reoperation: 1967 to 1987[2]

Factor	*p*-Value	Relative Risk
LV dysfunction	.0001	1.9
Age	.0001	1.04
Current cigarette smoking	.0001	1.6
Hypertension	.0002	1.4
Left main ≥50%	.0001	2.0
Triple-vessel disease	.0001	1.6
NYHA III/IV symptoms	.003	1.4
Peripheral vascular disease	.001	1.5
Interval >60 months	.006	1.003
No ITA at first operation	0.03	1.5

LV = left ventricular.
Source: Reproduced with permission from Loop FD, Lytle BW, Cosgrove DM, et al: Reoperation for coronary atherosclerosis: changing practice in 2509 consecutive patients. Ann Surg 1990; 212:378.

and severe native-vessel disease and lack of bypass conduits are a common combination of problems. Selection criteria vary widely among institutions, but in-hospital mortality rates are increased relative to first reoperations.[10,11] Through 1993, we reoperated on 392 patients who had more than one previous bypass operation, with an in-hospital mortality rate of 8%. Over the next 10 years, this mortality rate has decreased to 5.8%.[14] Follow-up of the in-hospital survivors in the former group found late survival rates of 84% at 5 and 66% at 10 postoperative years. Thus, although the in-hospital risks were increased for these patients, the long-term outcome has been relatively favorable. Age was a major determinant of outcome. Recently, in-hospital mortality for patients younger than 70 years of age has decreased to 1 to 2%, but for patients greater than age 70, it has remained higher than 10%. Furthermore, patients greater than age 70 who did survive operation in our series had only a 50% 5-year late survival.

CONCLUSION

Coronary artery reoperations continue to present adult cardiac surgeons with their most difficult challenges, in part because of the many technical pitfalls that exist, but also because significant comorbidity is common in reoperation candidates. The overall number of reoperations appears to be declining for multiple reasons, one important one being the increased use of arterial grafts at primary operations. However, when recurrent ischemia syndromes do occur reoperation will often be the best choice of therapy.

PEARLS

1. Make certain the end justifies the means before performing a coronary reoperation.
2. Avoid cardiac injury.
3. Do not replace a patent or stenotic vein graft with an ITA graft.
4. Dissect out the left side of the heart with the heart arrested.
5. Use the axillary artery as an alternative cannulation site.

REFERENCES

1. Lytle BW, Loop FD, Cosgrove DM, et al: Fifteen hundred coronary reoperations: results and determinants of early and late survival. *J Thorac Cardiovasc Surg* 1987; 93:847.
2. Loop FD, Lytle BW, Cosgrove DM, et al: Reoperation for coronary atherosclerosis: changing practice in 2509 consecutive patients. *Ann Surg* 1990; 212:378.
3. Lytle BW, McElroy D, McCarthy PM, et al: The influence of arterial coronary bypass grafts on the mortality of coronary reoperations. *J Thorac Cardiovasc Surg* 1994; 107:675.
4. Salomon NW, Page US, Bigelow JC, et al: Reoperative coronary surgery: comparative analysis of 6591 patients undergoing primary bypass and 508 patients undergoing reoperative coronary artery bypass. *J Thorac Cardiovasc Surg* 1990; 100:250.
5. Grinda JM, Zegdi R, Couetil JP, et al: Coronary reoperations: indications, techniques and operative results. Retrospective study of 240 coronary reoperations. *J Cardiol Surg* 2000; 41:703.
6. Weintraub WS, Jones EL, Craver JM, et al: In-hospital and long-term outcome after reoperative coronary artery bypass graft surgery. *Circulation* 1995; 92:II-50.
7. He GW, Acuff TE, Ryan WH, et al: Determinants of operative mortality in reoperative coronary artery bypass grafting. *J Thorac Cardiovasc Surg* 1995; 110:971.
8. Akins CW, Buckley MJ, Daggett WM, et al: Reoperative coronary grafting: changing patient profiles, operative indications, techniques, and results. *Ann Thorac Surg* 1994; 58:359.
9. Levy JH, Pifarre R, Schaff HV, et al: A multicenter double-blind placebo-controlled trial of aprotinin for reducing blood loss and the requirement for donor-blood transfusion in patients undergoing repeat coronary artery bypass grafting. *Circulation* 1995; 92:2236.
10. Lytle BW, Cosgrove DM, Taylor PC, et al: Multiple coronary reoperations: early and late results. *Circulation* 1989; 80:626.
11. Yau TM, Borger MA, Weisel RD, et al: The changing pattern of reoperative coronary surgery: trends in 1230 consecutive reoperations. *J Thorac Cardiovasc Surg* 2000; 120:156.
12. Edwards FH, Clark RE, Schwartz M: Coronary artery bypass grafting: The Society of Thoracic Surgeons National Database experience. *Ann Thorac Surg* 1994; 57:12.
13. Cosgrove DM, Loop FD, Lytle BW, et al: Predictors of reoperation after myocardial revascularization. *J Thorac Cardiovasc Surg* 1986; 92:811.
14. Sabik JF, Blackstone EH, Houghtaling PL, et al: Is reoperation still a risk factor in coronary artery bypass surgery? *Ann Thorac Surg* 2005; 80:1719.
15. Loop FD, Lytle BW, Cosgrove DM, et al: Influence of the internal mammary artery graft on 10-year survival and other cardiac events. *NEJM* 1986; 314:1.
16. Lytle BW, Blackstone EH, Loop FD, et al: Two internal thoracic artery grafts are better than one. *J Thorac Cardiovasc Surg* 1999; 117:855.
17. Neitzel GF, Barboriak JJ, Pintar K, et al: Atherosclerosis in aortocoronary bypass grafts: Morphologic study and risk factor analysis 6 to 12 years after surgery. *Arteriosclerosis* 1986; 6:594.
18. Ratliff NB, Myles JL: Rapidly progressive atherosclerosis in aortocoronary saphenous vein grafts: possible immune-mediated disease. *Arch Pathol Lab Med* 1989; 113:772.
19. Solymoss BC, Leung TK, Pelletier LC, et al: Pathologic changes in coronary artery saphenous vein grafts and related etiologic factors. *Cardiovasc Clin* 1991; 21:45.

20. Bourassa MG, Campeau L, Lesperance J: Changes in grafts and in coronary arteries after coronary bypass surgery. *Cardiovasc Clin* 1991; 21:83.
21. Lytle BW, Loop FD, Cosgrove DM, et al: Long-term (5 to 12 years) serial studies of internal mammary artery and saphenous vein coronary bypass grafts. *J Thorac Cardiovasc Surg* 1985; 89:248.
22. Fitzgibbon GM, Leach AJ, Kafka HP, et al: Coronary bypass graft fate: long-term angiographic study. *J Am Coll Cardiol* 1991; 17:1075.
23. Chesebro JH, Fuster V, Elveback LR, et al: Effect of dipyridamole and aspirin on late vein graft patency after coronary bypass operations. *NEJM* 1984; 310:209.
24. Goldman S, Copeland J, Moritz T, et al: Saphenous vein graft patency 1 year after coronary artery bypass surgery and effects of antiplatelet therapy. *Circulation* 1989; 80:1190.
25. Gavaghan TP, Gebski V, Baron DW: Immediate postoperative aspirin improves vein graft patency early and late after coronary artery bypass graft surgery: a placebo-controlled, randomized study. *Circulation* 1991; 83:1526.
26. Domanski M, Tian X, Fleg J, et al: Pleiotropic effect of Lovastatin, with and without Cholestyramine, in the Post Coronary Artery Bypass Graft (Post CABG) Trial. *Am J Cardiol* 2008;102:1023-1027.
27. Flaker GC, Warnica JW, Sacks EM, et al: Provastatin prevents clinical events in revascularized patients with average cholesterol concentrations: Cholesterol and Recurrent Events (CARE) investigators. *J Am Coll Cardiol* 1999;34:106.
28. Dion R, Verhelst R, Rousseau M, et al: Sequential mammary grafting: clinical, functional and angiographic assessment 6 months postoperatively in 231 consecutive patients. *J Thorac Cardiovasc Surg* 1989; 98:80.
29. Lytle BW, Loop FD, Taylor PC, et al: Vein graft disease: the clinical impact of stenoses in saphenous vein bypass grafts to coronary arteries. *J Thorac Cardiovasc Surg* 1992; 103:831.
30. Lytle BW, Loop FD, Taylor PC, et al: The effect of coronary reoperation on the survival of patients with stenoses in saphenous vein to coronary bypass grafts. *J Thorac Cardiovasc Surg* 1993; 105:605.
31. Lauer MS, Lytle B, Pashkow F, et al: Prediction of death and myocardial infarction by screening exercise-thallium testing after coronary-artery-bypass grafting. *Lancet* 1998; 351:615.
32. Brener SJ, Ellis SG, Apperson-Hansen C, et al: Comparison of stenting and balloon angioplasty for narrowings in aortocoronary saphenous vein conduits in place for more than five years. *Am J Cardiol* 1997; 79:13.
33. Holmes DR Jr., Topol EJ, Califf RM, et al: A multicenter, randomized trial of coronary angioplasty versus directional atherectomy for patients with saphenous vein bypass graft lesions. *Circulation* 1995; 91:1966.
34. Stankovic GA, Colombo A, Presbitero P, et al: Randomized evaluation of polytetrafluoroethylene-covered stent in saphenous vein grafts: the Randomized Evaluation of Polytetrafluoroethylene Covered Stent in Saphenous Vein Grafts (RECOVERS) trial. *Circulation* 2003; 108:37.
35. Ge L, Iakovou I, Sangiorgi GM, et al: Treatment of saphenous vein graft lesions with drug-eluting stents: Immediate and midterm outcome. *J Am Coll Cardiol* 2005; 45:989.
36. Vermeersch P, Agostoni P, Verheye S, et al: Increased late mortality after sirolimus-eluting stents versus bare-metal stents in diseased saphenous vein grafts. Results from the randomized DELAYED RRISC Trial. *J Am Coll Cardiol* 2007; 50:261-267.
37. Cole JH, Jones EL, Craver JM, et al: Outcomes of repeat revascularization in diabetic patients with prior coronary surgery. *J Am Coll Cardiol* 2002;40:1968-1975.
38. Perrault L, Carrier M, Cartier R, et al: Morbidity and mortality of reoperation for coronary artery bypass grafting: Significance of atheromatous vein grafts. *Can J Cardiol* 1991; 7:427.
39. Jain U, Sullivan HJ, Pifarre R, et al: Graft atheroembolism as the probable cause of failure to wean from cardiopulmonary bypass. *J Cardiothorac Anesth* 1990; 4:476.
40. Navia D, Cosgrove DM, Lytle BW, et al: Is the internal thoracic artery the conduit of choice to replace a stenotic vein graft? *Ann Thorac Surg* 1994; 57:40.
41. Keon WJ, Heggtveit HA, Leduc J: Perioperative myocardial infarction caused by atheroembolization. *J Thorac Cardiovasc Surg* 1982; 84:849.
42. Blauth CI, Cosgrove DM, Webb BW, et al: Atheroembolism from the ascending aorta: an emerging problem in cardiac surgery. *J Thorac Cardiovasc Surg* 1992; 103:1104.
43. Roselli EE, Pettersson GB, Blackstone EH, et al: Adverse events during reoperative cardiac surgery: frequency, characterization, and rescue. *J Thorac Cardiovasc Surg* 2008;135:316-323.
44. Sabik JF, Lytle BW, McCarthy PM, et al: Axillary artery: an alternative site of arterial cannulation for patients with extensive aortic and peripheral vascular disease. *J Thorac Cardiovasc Surg* 1995; 109:885.
45. Partington MT, Acar C, Buckberg GD, et al: Studies of retrograde cardioplegia: II. Advantages of antegrade/retrograde cardioplegia to optimize distribution in jeopardized myocardium. *J Thorac Cardiovasc Surg* 1989; 97:613.
46. Menasche P, Kural S, Fauchet M, et al: Retrograde coronary sinus perfusion: a safe alternative for ensuring cardioplegic delivery in aortic valve surgery. *Ann Thorac Surg* 1982; 34:647.
47. Gundry SR, Razzouk AJ, Vigesaa RE, et al: Optimal delivery of cardioplegic solution for "redo" operations. *J Thorac Cardiovasc Surg* 1992; 103:896.
48. Tector AJ, Amundsen S, Schmahl TM, et al: Total revascularization with T grafts. *Ann Thorac Surg* 1994; 57:33.
49. Calafiore AM, DiGiammarco G, Teodori G, Vitolla G: Myocardial revascularization with composite arterial grafts, in Possat GF, Suma H, Alessandria F (eds): *Proceedings of the Workshop on Arterial Conduits for Myocardial Revascularization.* Rome, 1995.
50. Turner FE, Lytle BW, Navia D, et al: Coronary reoperations: results of adding an internal mammary artery graft to a stenotic vein graft. *Ann Thorac Surg* 1994; 58:1353.
51. Suma H, Wanibuchi Y, Terada Y, et al: The right gastroepiploic artery graft: clinical and angiographic midterm results in 200 patients. *J Thorac Cardiovasc Surg* 1993; 105:615.
52. Di Mauro M, Iaco, AL, Contini M, et al: Reoperative coronary artery bypass grafting: analysis of early and late outcomes. *Ann Thorac Surg* 2005; 79:81.
53. Yamamuro M, Lytle BW, Sapp SK, et al: Risk factors and outcomes after coronary reoperation in 739 elderly patients. *Ann Thorac Surg* 2000; 69:464.
54. Dougenis D, Brown AH: Long-term results of reoperations for recurrent angina with internal mammary artery versus saphenous vein grafts. *Heart* 1998; 80:9.

CHAPTER 27

Transmyocardial Laser Revascularization and Extravascular Angiogenetic Techniques to Increase Myocardial Blood Flow

Keith A. Horvath
Yifu Zhou

TRANSMYOCARDIAL LASER REVASCULARIZATION (TMR) HISTORY

Despite the success of medical therapy, percutaneous coronary interventions (PCIs), and coronary artery bypass grafting (CABG) in the treatment of coronary artery disease (CAD), there are a significant number of patients with refractory angina owing to diffuse CAD that is not amenable to PCI or CABG. This severe CAD can lead to incomplete revascularization and is noted to occur in up to 25% of CABG surgery.[1] This incomplete revascularization is a powerful independent predictor of operative mortality and perioperative adverse events.[1,2] Additionally, the presence of diseased but nongrafted arteries carries a poor prognosis and poses a significant negative influence leading to an increased incidence of death, recurrent angina, myocardial infarction (MI), and the need for repeat CABG.[3,4]

Strategies to treat patients with end-stage coronary disease have sought to create or enhance myocardial angiogenesis. Such techniques include TMR as well as protein-, gene-, and cell-based therapies. TMR was founded, in part, on previous methods of providing direct perfusion to the myocardium. Prior attempts at direct perfusion were based on Wearn's description of sinusoids that allowed blood to flow directly from the ventricle into the myocardium.[5] These arterioluminal connections provide perfusion in more primitive vertebrate hearts and occur clinically in children with pulmonary atresia, an intact ventricular septum, and proximal obstruction of the coronary arteries. Sen and colleagues[6] used myocardial acupuncture to establish direct perfusion and theoretically to recreate a coronary microcirculation similar to that of the reptilian heart. Additional methods of attempting to improve myocardial blood flow include Beck's creation of a form of superficial angiogenesis as a response to epicardial and pericardial inflammation.[7] Combining the acupuncture, implantation, and inflammation techniques, Boffi[8] and Borst[9] used hollow tubes implanted in the myocardium to establish direct perfusion. Results from all these procedures yielded limited success. The angina relief obtained was not long lasting, was difficult to replicate, and most important, eventually was overshadowed by the ability to perform CABG. The mechanical trauma that resulted in poor long-term patency of myocardial acupuncture was overcome in theory by using a laser to create the channels. Although Mirhoseini and colleagues[10] and Okada and colleagues[11] pioneered the use of a laser to perform this type of revascularization in conjunction with CABG in the early 1980s, the use of a laser as sole therapy to establish its efficacy required advancements in the technology. The carbon dioxide (CO_2) laser used by Mirhoseini had a peak output of 80 W and, therefore, required a significant amount of time to complete a transmural channel. As a result, to perform TMR optimally, the heart had to be chilled and still. Increasing the output of the laser to 800 W allowed TMR to be performed on a beating heart. This breakthrough led to the widespread clinical application of TMR. Since then, more than 25,000 patients have been treated with TMR around the world, and results from individual institutions, multicenter studies, and prospective, randomized, controlled trials have been reported.[12–20]

CLINICAL TRIALS

The early nonrandomized trials demonstrated that sole-therapy TMR could be performed safely on patients with severe CAD who previously had no options. The significant angina relief seen in such patients led to prospective, randomized, controlled studies to further demonstrate the efficacy of TMR. In these pivotal trials, more than 1100 patients were enrolled and randomized to receive either TMR or medical management as treatment for their severe angina.[16–20] The trials employed a 1:1 randomization in which half the patients were treated with laser and those in the control group continued on maximal medical therapy. All patients were followed for 12 months.

TMR AS SOLE THERAPY

Patients

The entry criteria for these studies and for sole-therapy TMR in general are as follows. Patients had refractory angina that was not amenable to standard methods of revascularization, as verified by a recent angiogram; they had evidence of reversible ischemia based on myocardial perfusion scanning; and their left ventricular ejection fractions were greater than 25%.

The typical patient profiles of TMR patients in the randomized, controlled trials are listed in Table 27-1. Because the patients were equally randomized to the medical management group, there were no significant demographic differences between the TMR and control groups for any of these trials. Two different wavelengths of laser light were used. Two studies[16,17] employed a holmium:yttrium-aluminum-Garnett (Ho:YAG) laser, and three[18–20] used a CO_2 laser. The average patient age was 62 years, and most were male (86%). Although there were significant differences in the baseline distribution of patients according to Canadian Cardiovascular Society (CCS) angina class, the majority of the patients were in angina class IV (61%). The ejection fractions for all the patients were mildly diminished at 48 ± 10%. Many of the patients had suffered at least one previous MI, and most had some prior revascularization, CABG, and/or PCI. Two of the trials[16,18] permitted a crossover from the medical management group to laser treatment for the presence of unstable angina that necessitated intravenous antianginal therapy for which they were unweanable over a period of at least 48 hours. By definition, these crossover patients were less stable than and significantly different from those who had been randomized initially to TMR or medical management alone.

Operative Technique

For sole-therapy TMR, the patient is placed in a supine position with his or her left side slightly elevated. General anesthesia is established using a double-lumen endotracheal tube or a bronchial blocker to isolate the left lung. Although not mandatory,

TABLE 27-1 Patient Characteristics in RCTS of Sole-Therapy TMR

Characteristic	Allen	Frazier	Burkhoff	Schofield	Aaberge
Patients (*N*)	275	192	182	188	100
Age (years)	60	61	63	60	61
Male gender (%)	74	81	89	88	92
EF (%)	47	50	50	48	49
CCS class III/IV (%)	0/100	31/69	37/63	73/27	66/34
CHF (%)	17	34	NR	9	NR
Diabetes (%)	46	40	36	19	22
Hyperlipidemia (%)	79	57	77	NR	76
Hypertension (%)	70	65	74	NR	28
Prior MI (%)	64	82	70	73	70
Prior CABG (%)	86	92	90	95	80
Prior PCI (%)	48	47	53	29	38

Baseline patient demographics from prospective, randomized, controlled trials of TMR.
CABG = Coronary artery bypass grafting; CCS = Canadian Cardiovascular Society; CHF = congestive heart failure; EF = ejection fraction; MI = myocardial infarction; NR = not reported; PCI = percutaneous coronary intervention.

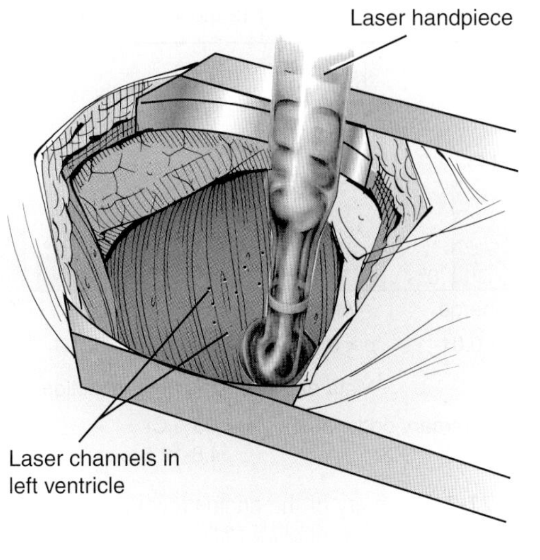

FIGURE 27-1 For TMR, channels of 1 mm diameter are created in a distribution of 1/cm^2 starting inferiorly and then working superiorly to the anterior surface of the heart. The number of channels created depends on the size of the heart and on the size of the ischemic area.

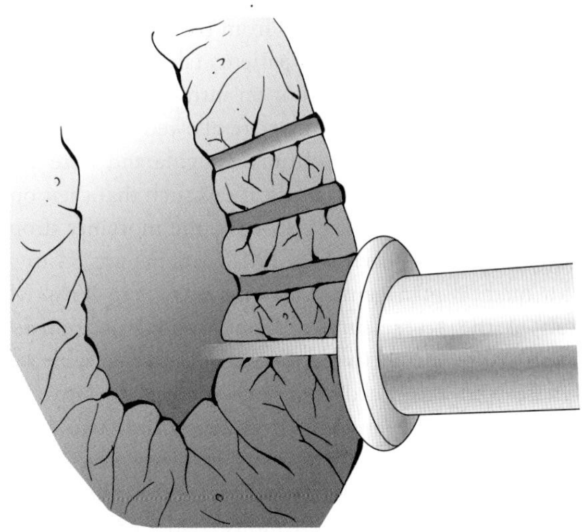

FIGURE 27-2 The CO_2 laser creates a transmural channel in a single 20-J pulse. Conceptually, direct perfusion may occur via the channel. Evidence indicates the laser stimulates angiogenesis in and around the channel that leads to improved perfusion.

this facilitates the operation, particularly because most of the patients have pleural and mediastinal adhesions from previous bypass surgery. Additionally, a thoracic epidural catheter can be employed to provide postoperative pain control.

A left anterior thoracotomy in the fifth intercostal space is the usual incision site. Once the ribs are spread by a retractor, the pericardium is opened to expose the epicardial surface of the heart (Fig. 27-1). Care must be taken to avoid previous bypass grafts. The left anterior descending (LAD) artery is identified and used as a landmark for the location of the septum. The inferior and posterolateral portions of the heart can be reached through this incision with a combination of manual traction, placement of packing behind the heart, and as illustrated, with the use of a right-angled laser handpiece. Channels are created starting near the base of the heart and then serially in a line approximately 1-cm apart toward the apex, starting inferiorly and working superiorly to the anterior surface of the heart. Because there is some bleeding from the channels, commencement of the TMR inferiorly keeps the anterior area clear and expedites the procedure. The number of channels created depends on the size of the heart and the size of the ischemic area. Myocardium that is thinned by scar, particularly when the scar is transmural, should be avoided because TMR will be of no benefit in these regions, and bleeding from channels in these areas may be problematic. The thoracotomy then is closed after placement of a chest tube, and in the majority of the cases the patient is extubated in the operating room.

The handpiece in Fig. 27-2 is from a CO_2 laser and illustrates one of the differences between the two lasers employed for TMR. The CO_2 laser energy is delivered via hollow tubes and is reflected by mirrors to reach the epicardial surface. One-millimeter channels are made with a 15- to 20-J pulse. Firing of the laser is synchronized to occur on the R wave of the electrocardiogram (ECG) to avoid arrhythmias. The transmural channel is created by a signal pulse in 40 milliseconds and can be confirmed by transesophageal echocardiography (TEE). The vaporization of blood by the laser energy as the laser beam enters the ventricle creates an obvious and characteristic acoustic effect on TEE. The Ho:YAG laser achieves a 1-mm channel by manually advancing a fiber bundle through the myocardium while the laser fires. Typical pulse energies are 2 J for this laser at a rate of five pulses per second; 10 to 20 pulses are required to traverse the myocardium. Detection of transmural penetration is done primarily by tactile and auditory feedback.

End Points

The principal subjective end point for all the trials was a change in angina symptoms. This was assessed by the investigator and/or a blinded independent observer. In addition to assigning an angina class, standardized questionnaires such as the Seattle Angina Questionnaire, the Short Form Questionnaire 36 (SF-36), and the Duke Activity Status Index were employed. These tests were used to detect changes in symptoms and quality of life. Objective measurements consisted of repeat exercise tolerance testing as well as repeat myocardial perfusion scans. Patients were reassessed at 3, 6, and 12 months after randomization.

RESULTS

Mortality

Before the randomized studies, mortality rates in the 10 to 20% range[12–15] were reported for TMR patients. In the randomized trials, lower perioperative mortality rates were reported ranging from 1 to 5%[16–20] One of the important lessons learned from these controlled trials that differs from the earlier studies was a decrease in the mortality when patients taken to the operating room were stable, specifically not on intravenous (IV) heparin or nitroglycerin. When patients were allowed to recover from their most recent episode of unstable angina and were able to be weaned from intravenous medications such that their operation could be performed 2 weeks later, the mortality dropped to 1%.[18] The 1-year survival for TMR patients was 84 to 95% and for medical management patients was 79 to 96%. Meta-analysis of the 1-year survival demonstrated no statistically significant difference between the patients treated with a laser and those who continued with their medical therapy. Long-term survival of the randomized patients from two of these studies has been reported. Four-year follow-up from Aaberge and colleagues, in which both the TMR and medical management groups were kept intact, demonstrated a 78% survival for TMR versus 76% for medical management (p = ns).[21] In a 5-year follow-up using an intent-to-treat analysis, Allen reported a survival for TMR patients at 65% versus 52% for medical management patients ($p = .05$).[22]

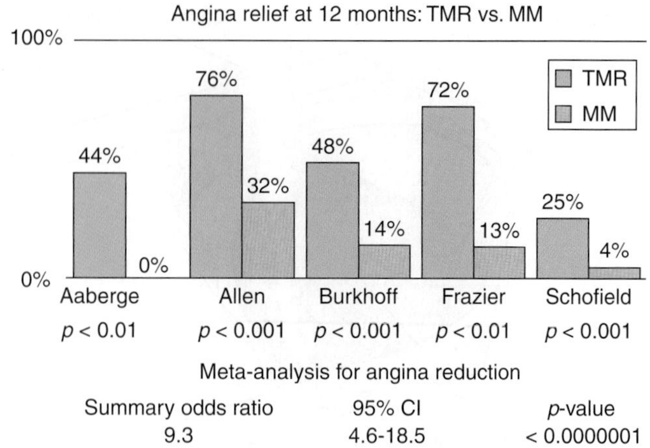

FIGURE 27-3 Summary of the angina relief results from five prospective, randomized, controlled trials comparing transmyocardial laser revascularization (TMR) and medical management (MM). Graph illustrates success rate for TMR or MM as measured by the percentage of patients that had a decrease of two or more angina classes. Meta-analysis of these results documents the significant advantage seen with TMR over MM.

Morbidity

Unlike mortality, the exact definition of various complications varied from one study protocol to the next, and therefore, morbidity data are difficult to pool. Nevertheless, the typical TMR patient's postoperative course had a lower incidence of MI, heart failure, and arrhythmias than what has been documented in a similar cohort of patients, those who have reoperative CABG.[16–20]

Angina Class

The principal reason for performing TMR is to reduce the patient's anginal symptoms. This can be quantified by assessing the angina class before and after the procedure. Angina class assessment was performed by a blinded independent observer in all studies. This was done as the only angina assessment or as comparison with the investigators' assessment. Significant symptomatic improvement was seen in all studies for patients treated with the laser. Using a definition of success as a decrease of two or more angina classes, all the studies demonstrated a significant success rate after TMR, with success rates ranging from 25 to 76% (Fig. 27-3). A meta-analysis of this angina reduction yielded a summary odds ratio of 9.3 (95% CI 4.6–18.5; $p < .000001$). Significantly fewer patients in the medical management group experienced symptomatic improvement, and the success rate for these patients ranged from 0 to 32%. The seemingly broad range of success is caused by differences among the baseline characteristics of the studies. It is more difficult to achieve a two-angina–class improvement if the baseline angina class is III. Studies that started with most of their patients in angina class III, not surprisingly, showed the lowest success rate. In contrast, the largest success rate for TMR was seen in the trial in which all the patients were in CCS class IV at enrollment. Of note, the medical management group in this study also showed the largest success rate.[16] This underscores some of the baseline differences among the studies.

Quality of Life and Myocardial Function

Quality-of-life indices as assessed by the Seattle Angina Questionnaire, the SF-36, and the Duke Activity Status Index demonstrated significant improvement for TMR-treated patients versus medical management in every study. Global assessment of myocardial function by ejection fraction using echocardiography or radionuclide multigated acquisition scans showed no significant change in overall ejection fraction for any of the patients regardless of group assignment or study.

Hospital Admission

Another indicator of the efficacy of TMR was demonstrated in a reduction in hospital admissions for unstable angina or cardiac-related events postprocedure. A meta-analysis of the data provided indicates that the 1-year hospitalization rate of patients in the laser-treated group was statistically significantly less than for those treated medically. Medical management patients were admitted four times more frequently than TMR patients over the year of follow-up.

Exercise Tolerance

Additional functional test assessment using exercise tolerance also was performed in three of the trials.[17,19,20] Although the method of treadmill testing differed among the trials, the results demonstrate an improvement in exercise tolerance for TMR-treated patients. Two studies showed an average of 65- to 70-second improvement in the TMR group at 12 months compared with their baseline, whereas the medical management group had either an average of 5-second improvement or a 46-second decrease in exercise time over the same interval.[19,20] One additional trial demonstrated that the time to chest pain during exercise increased significantly, and fewer patients were limited by chest pain in the TMR group, whereas the medical management group showed no improvement.[20]

Medical Treatment

All the studies employed protocols that continued all the patients on maximal medical therapy. For each study, the frequencies and dosages of antianginal and cardiovascular drugs were similar between the two groups at baseline. TMR patients, as a result of their symptomatic improvement, had a reduction in their medication use over the year of follow-up. Because many of these patients used a combination of short- and long-acting nitrates preoperatively, the trials demonstrated a significant decrease in the use of nitrates in TMR-treated patients, whereas the medical management patients showed a slight increase in their nitrate usage. At 1 year, the overall medication use decreased or remained unchanged in 83% of the TMR patients, and conversely, the use of medications increased or remained unchanged in 86% of the medical management patients.[18] The significant angina relief seen following TMR was not owing to medication changes or increases for the TMR-treated patients.

Myocardial Perfusion

As stated, myocardial perfusion scans were obtained preoperatively to verify the extent and severity of reversible ischemia. The four largest randomized trials included follow-up scans as part of the study.[16–19] These results reflect more than 800 of the patients randomized. The methodology of recording and analyzing these results differed in each study, so it is difficult to pool the data. Nevertheless, review of the results demonstrated an improvement in perfusion for CO_2 TMR-treated patients. Fixed (scar) and reversible (ischemic) defects were tallied for both the TMR-treated patients and the medical management groups. One study demonstrated a significant decrease in the number of reversible defects for both the TMR and the medical management patients.[19] This improvement in the reversible defects in the TMR group was seen without a significant increase in the fixed defects at the end of the study. However, the number of fixed defects in the medical management group had nearly doubled over the same 12-month interval. Similarly, there was a 20% improvement in the perfusion of previously ischemic areas in the CO_2 TMR group of another trial, and in that same trial there was a 27% worsening of the perfusion of the ischemic areas in the medical management group at 12 months.[18] There was no difference in the number of fixed defects among the groups at 12 months, nor was there a significant change in the number of fixed defects for each patient compared with his or her baseline scan. The remaining two Ho:YAG studies that obtained follow-up scans showed no significant difference between the TMR and medical management groups at 12 months and no significant improvement in perfusion in the TMR-treated patients over the same interval.[16,17]

Nonrandomized data previously had demonstrated an improvement in perfusion using dual isotope scanning at 1 and 2 years after CO_2 TMR.[12] Additionally, using N-13 ammonia position-emission tomographic (PET) assessment, subendocardial perfusion improved significantly compared with subepicardial perfusion after CO_2 TMR treatment.[23]

Long-Term Results

Two reports of long-term follow-up of prospectively randomized patients are available. Similar to the 1-year results, intention-to-treat analyses determined that significantly more TMR than medical management patients continued to experience at least two-class angina improvement from baseline (88% versus 44%; $p < .001$) or were free from angina symptoms altogether (33% versus 11%; $p = .02$) at a mean of 5 years.[22] In long-term follow-up of the randomized trial that kept both the TMR and medical management groups intact (ie, no crossover), it was shown that angina symptoms still were improved significantly (24% versus 3%, TMR versus medical management; $p = .001$), and unstable angina hospitalizations were reduced significantly ($p < .05$) at a mean follow-up of 43 months.[21] Follow-up of a series of nonrandomized patients who received TMR and survived long term support these findings.[24] At a mean of 5 years and up to 7 years postprocedure, 81% of these patients improved to class II or better, 68% were found to have improved at least two angina classes from baseline, 17% were angina-free, and quality of life remained significantly improved. These last two reports reflect the sustained angina relief seen with CO_2 TMR because these patients had no additional procedures to account for their symptom improvement over the long term.

Based on an assessment of the cumulative results from these multiple randomized trials, the recently updated American College of Cardiology/American Heart Association (ACC/AHA) practice guidelines[25] and the Society of Thoracic Surgeons (STS) practice guidelines[26] have determined that the weight of the evidence favors the use of TMR in the treatment of stable, medically refractory angina patients.

TMR AS AN ADJUNCT TO CABG

Clinical Trials

Owing to its success as sole therapy, TMR has been evaluated in conjunction with CABG in patients with diffuse CAD who would be incompletely revascularized by CABG alone. The safety and effectiveness of adjunctive TMR have been somewhat difficult to assess owing to the influence of coronary bypass grafts and the lack of randomized control arms in some studies.[27–29]

Two prospective, randomized, controlled multicentered trials have been performed using TMR adjunctively with CABG in patients. In these studies, patients with one or more viable myocardial target areas served by coronary vessels that were not amenable to bypass grafting received either CABG plus TMR or CABG alone.[30,31] Baseline and operative characteristics were similar between groups, including the location and number of bypass grafts placed (3.1 ± 1.2, CABG + TMR; 3.4 ± 1.2, CABG alone; $p = .07$). Patients were blinded to their treatment group through 1-year follow-up.

RESULTS

Mortality

Improved outcomes following TMR + CABG versus CABG alone in terms of a reduced operative mortality rate (1.5% versus 7.6%; $p = .02$), reduced postoperative inotropic support requirements (30% versus 55%; $p = .001$), increased 30-day freedom from major adverse cardiac events (97% versus 91%; $p = .04$), and improved 1-year Kaplan-Meier survival (95% versus 89%; $p = .05$) have been reported.[30] Multivariable predictors of operative mortality were CABG alone (OR 5.3; $p = 0.04$) and increased age (OR 1.1; $p = .03$).[30] A similar trend in operative mortality following TMR + CABG versus CABG alone (9% versus 33%; $p = .09$) was reported in a study of high-risk patients.[31]

Efficacy

The use of TMR adjunctively with CABG has been shown to decrease intensive care unit (ICU) times and length of hospitalization stay.[29] In a long-term follow-up of the randomized, controlled trial, the effectiveness of TMR + CABG versus CABG alone has been reported.[32] At a mean of 5 years, both groups experienced significant angina improvement from baseline; however, the TMR + CABG group had a lower mean number of angina-free patients (78% versus 63%; $p = .08$) compared with the CABG-alone group. Long-term survival was similar between randomized groups.

Observational data on the practice of TMR + CABG have been collected in the STS National Cardiac Database.[33] From 1998 to 2003, 5618 patients underwent TMR + CABG. These were compared with 932,715 patients who underwent CABG-only operations. The TMR + CABG patients therefore account for 0.6% of the surgical revascularization practice in the database. Table 27-2 outlines the significant baseline differences between the CABG-only patients and the TMR + CABG patients. The TMR + CABG patients have an increased incidence of every surrogate marker of diffuse arterial disease, and therefore, it is not surprising that their observed mortality was higher at 3.8% (versus 2.7% for CABG-only patients; $p < .001$). When unstable angina patients were removed, the observed mortality for TMR + CABG was decreased to 2.7%, and the observed:expected (*O*/*E*) ratio was 0.87. Comparison of use and outcomes from sites that have a TMR laser versus those that showed no evidence of overuse of TMR or difference in outcomes.[33]

TABLE 27-2 Comparison of CABG Only versus TMR + CABG Patients, STS Adult Cardiac Database 1998–2003

Characteristic	CABG Only	TMR + CABG	*p*-Value
N	932,715	5,618	
Body surface area, m² (SD)	1.96 (0.24)	1.99 (0.23)	<.001
Diabetes (all types)	34%	50%	<.001
Insulin-dependent diabetes	10%	19%	<.001
Renal failure	5%	7%	<.001
Dialysis	1%	2%	<.001
CVA	7%	9%	<.001
Chronic lung disease	14%	17%	<.001
Peripheral vascular disease	16%	20%	<.001
Cerebral vascular disease	12%	17%	<.001
MI	46%	49%	<.001
Reoperation	9%	26%	<.001
Three-vessel CAD	71%	80%	<.001
Hypercholesterolemia	62%	73%	<.001
Hypertension	72%	80%	<.001

Baseline demographics of TMR combined with CABG patients enrolled in the Society of Thoracic Surgeons (STS) National Adult Cardiac Database.
CAD = coronary artery disease; CVA = cerebral vascular accident; MI = myocardial infarction.

MECHANISMS

Laser–Tissue Interactions

Understanding the mechanism of TMR starts with understanding the laser-tissue interaction. While numerous devices,[34] including ultrasound,[35] cryogenic ablation,[36] radiofrequency revascularization,[37,38] heated needles,[39,40] and the aforementioned hollow and solid needles have been used; none has engendered the same response that is seen with a laser. Additionally, numerous wavelengths of laser light also have been employed. These include xenon chloride (XCl),[41] neodymium:YAG (Nd:YAG),[42] erbium:YAG (Er:YAG),[43] and thulium-holmium-chromium:YAG lasers (THC:YAG).[44] All these devices have been explored experimentally but have not been pursued on a significant scale clinically. Only CO_2 and Ho:YAG lasers are used for TMR. The result of any laser–tissue interaction depends on both laser and tissue variables.[43–45] A CO_2 laser has a wavelength of 10,600 nanometers, whereas a Ho:YAG laser has a wavelength of 2120 nanometers. These infrared wavelengths are absorbed primarily in water and therefore rely on thermal energy to ablate tissue. One significant difference, however, is that the Ho:YAG laser is pulsed, and the arrival of two successive pulses must be separated by time to allow for thermal dissipation. Otherwise, the accumulated heat will cause the tissue to explode under pressure. Such explosions create acoustic waves that travel along the planes of lower resistance between muscle fibers and cause structural trauma as well as thermocoagulation.[45] The standard operating parameters for the Ho:YAG laser are pulse energies of 1 to 2 J and 6 to 8 W/pulse. The energy is delivered at a rate of five pulses per second through a flexible 1 mm optical fiber bundle. Despite the low energy level and short pulse duration, very high levels of peak power are delivered to the tissue so that with each pulse there is an explosion (Fig. 27-4). Additionally, the fiber is advanced manually through the myocardium, and it is therefore impossible to know whether the channel is being created by the kinetic energy delivered via the mechanical effects of the fiber or there has been enough time for thermal dissipation before the next pulse.

In contrast, the CO_2 laser was used at an energy level of 15 to 20 J/pulse with a pulse duration of 25 to 40 milliseconds. At this level, the laser photons do not cause explosive ablation, and the extent of structural damage is limited. Additionally, a transmural channel can be created with a single pulse (see Fig. 27-4). Confirmation of this transmurality is obtained by observing the vaporization of blood within the ventricle using TEE.

Finally, the CO_2 laser is synchronized to fire on the R wave, and with its short pulse duration, arrhythmic complications are minimized. The Ho:YAG device is unsynchronized and, owing to the motion of the fiber through the myocardium over several cardiac cycles, is more prone to produce ventricular arrhythmias.

Patent Channels

As noted, the original concept of TMR was to create perfusion via channels connecting the ventricle with the myocardium. Clinical work has demonstrated some evidence of long term patency.[46] Additional experimental work showed some evidence of patency as well.[47–49] There are also significant reports from autopsy series and laboratories that indicate that the channels do not remain patent.[50–52] The consensus is that while channels occasionally may remain patent, this is not the principal mechanism of TMR.

Denervation

In contrast to the open-channel mechanism, damage to the sympathetic nerve fibers may explain the angina relief noted in clinical trials. The nervous system of the heart can function independent of inputs from extracardiac neurons to regulate regional cardiac function by reflex action. This intrinsic system contains afferent neurons, sympathetic efferent postganglionic neurons, and parasympathetic efferent postganglionic neurons. Because of this complex system, it is difficult to demonstrate true denervation. However, several experimental studies have demonstrated that denervation indeed may play a role in Ho:YAG TMR.[53,54] Experimental evidence to the contrary was performed in a nonischemic animal model.[55] Although the studies were carried out carefully, it is difficult to isolate the sympathetic afferent nerve fibers, and the experiments were in the acute setting and only address short-term effects. Regardless of the methodology employed in the laboratory, there is significant evidence of sympathetic denervation following PET scanning of Ho:YAG TMR–treated patients.[56]

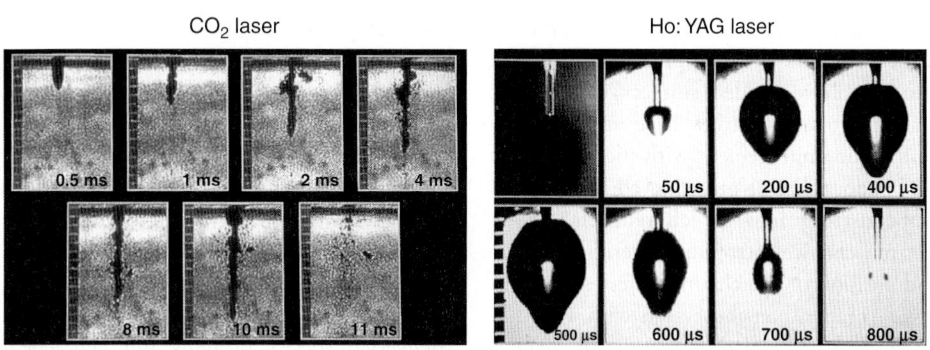

FIGURE 27-4 Sequential photography of the firing of a single pulse from a CO_2 laser and a Ho: YAG laser into water. The pulse duration and energy levels are the same as those employed clinically.

Angiogenesis

The likely underlying mechanism for the clinical efficacy of TMR is the stimulation of angiogenesis. This mechanism fits the clinical picture of significant improvement in symptoms over time, as well as a concomitant improvement in perfusion, as seen with the CO_2 laser. Numerous reports have demonstrated a histologic increase in neovascularization as a result of TMR channels.[51,57–61] More molecular evidence of this angiogenic phenomenon was derived from work that demonstrated an upregulation of vascular endothelial growth factor (VEGF) messenger RNA, expression of fibroblast growth factor 2 (FGF2), and matrix metalloproteinases following TMR.[62–64] Histologically, similar degrees of neovascularization have been noted after mechanical injury of various types. Needle injury has been demonstrated by immunohistochemistry to also stimulate growth factor expression and angiogenesis. The conclusion is that TMR-induced angiogenesis is a nonspecific response to injury.[65,66] Investigation of this using hot and cold needles, radiofrequency energy, and laser energy to perform TMR clearly demonstrates a spectrum of tissue response to the injury.[39] The results in a model of chronic myocardial ischemia to mimic the clinical scenario indicate that indeed neovascularization can occur after mechanical TMR, but if these new blood vessels grow in the midst of a scar, there will be little functional contribution from blood flow through these new vessels. The recovery of function with laser TMR was to the result of a minimization of scar formation and maximization of angiogenesis.

This then becomes a critical question: If TMR induces angiogenesis, is there an ensuing improvement in function? Clinically, this has been demonstrated subjectively with quality-of-life assessments, but more important, it has been demonstrated objectively with multiple techniques, including dobutamine stress echocardiography,[67] PET scanning,[23] and cardiac magnetic resonance imaging (MRI).[68,69] As further evidence of the angiogenic response, experimental data have mirrored the clinical perfusion results noted, with improvements in perfusion in porcine models of chronic ischemia where the ischemic zone was treated with CO_2 TMR.[70–73] This improved perfusion did lead to an improvement in myocardial function as well.

PERCUTANEOUS MYOCARDIAL LASER REVASCULARIZATION

Myocardial laser revascularization has been performed percutaneously,[74] thoracoscopically,[75] via thoracotomy,[16–20] and via sternotomy.[27–30] Aside from the PMR approach, any of the other surgical approaches have yielded similar symptomatic improvement. Several percutaneous trials have attempted to demonstrate a symptomatic improvement with the creation of 2- to 3-mm deep subendocardial divots achieved with a laser fiber fed via a peripheral artery into the left ventricle.[74] Even with the use of electromechanical mapping to verify the position of the fiber and creation of the channel, the results from PMR have been less favorable than those seen with TMR. A double-blinded, randomized, controlled trial showed no benefit to the laser-treated patients compared with the untreated control group.[74] Because the patients were blinded to their treatment, the possibility of a significant placebo effect for PMR has been raised. Of note, the morbidity and mortality of PMR reportedly are similar to those seen with TMR. As a result, the U.S. Food and Drug Administration (FDA) rendered PMR unapprovable.

The failure of PMR to achieve the same clinical results that have been seen with TMR may result from several significant limitations, the first of which is the partial-thickness treatment of the left ventricle. Even at the maximal estimated depth of 6 mm that has been reported with PMR, this is significantly less than the full-thickness treatment of the myocardium that is achieved with an open TMR approach. Furthermore, typically fewer of these partial-thickness channels are created with PMR. The exact location of the channel and the establishment of a wide distribution of the channels from inside a moving ventricle are also problematic. Finally, the limitations of Ho:YAG TMR are also applicable to PMR because that is the wavelength of light that has been employed.

FUTURE USES OF TMR

Other potential applications include the use of TMR in the treatment of cardiac transplant graft atherosclerosis. Although the procedure has been performed on a small number of patients, the results have indicated a benefit.[76] Finally, the combination of TMR plus other methods of angiogenesis may provide an even more robust response. Experimental work investigating these combinations has verified a synergistic effect with regard to histologic evidence of significant angiogenesis and, perhaps more important, an improvement in myocardial function with a combination of TMR and gene therapy versus either therapy alone.[77–79]

Cardiothoracic surgeons increasingly are faced with a more complex patient who has developed a pattern of diffuse CAD and has exhausted nonsurgical options. Results replicated in multiple randomized, controlled trials augmented by recently available long-term results have validated the safety, effectiveness, and substantially improved health outcomes achieved through application of TMR for the treatment of selected patients with severe angina owing to diffuse disease when used alone and as adjunctive therapy to achieve a more complete revascularization.

EXTRAVASCULAR ANGIOGENETIC TECHNIQUES

Before TMR, investigators have been trying different mechanical strategies to increase blood flow in ischemic hearts since the 1930s by obliterating the pericardial sac with mechanical abrasion and the addition of asbestos powder, tacking omentum to ischemic hearts, removing the epicardium, or combining several of these with the addition of implanting the internal mammary artery into the myocardium. Subsequently, pharmacologic strategies were employed in both experimental and clinical studies to ischemic hearts by using heparin and growth factors such as VEGF and fibroblast growth factors (FGF1 and FGF2). The angiogenic growth factors were first applied via direct delivery of specific proteins, and then gene delivery techniques, in both experimental and clinical studies. In the late 1990s, cell-based therapy was introduced in therapeutic angiogenesis for ischemic heart diseases and has been the most rapidly progressing and hot research field over the past 12 years. This section discusses the topic of protein-, gene-, and cell-based therapeutic angiogenesis for the treatment of ischemic cardiovascular diseases.

Proteins

Experimental Studies

In early in vitro studies, VEGF, FGF1, and FGF2 proteins showed angiogenic potential.[80,81] These studies were followed by in vivo work showing that these factors actually do stimulate the growth of new vessels.[82] The more recent genetic studies of vasculogenesis in mouse embryogenesis documented the critical importance of synergetic effects of multiple molecules, such as VEGF and angiopoietin-1, to the development of mature, branching blood vessels.[83]

Basic FGF and VEGF proteins stimulate the development of collaterals to tissues supplied by an obstructed artery and augment tissue blood flow were first demonstrated in the early 1990s. In experiments on myocardial ischemia, a portion of the left ventricle of dogs was made ischemic by gradual occlusion of the circumflex coronary artery. The intracoronary or left atrial administration of bFGF or intracoronary administration of VEGF proteins daily for 28 days significantly increased collateral flow.[84] Likewise, studies in the rabbit ischemic hind limb model demonstrated that intramuscular administration of bFGF protein daily for 2 weeks improved limb perfusion significantly.[85]

However, when the effect of VEGF protein studied in the canine myocardial ischemia model using two different methods, controversial results were observed: While 28 days of administering boluses of VEGF into the left atrium improved collateral flow, 7 days of administration did not,[86] and although 7 and as few as 2 days of intracoronary administration of bFGF improved collateral flow, a single bolus injection did not.[87] These results demonstrated, at least in this model of myocardial ischemia, that the duration of exposure of the vessels supplying the ischemic tissue to angiogenesis factors is critical for a therapeutically relevant effect.

Additional studies employing[125] I-labeled bFGF demonstrated that route of administration is another critical factor in determining local tissue uptake and, potentially, therapeutic response.[88] The results showed that whereas 3 to 5% of an intracoronary dose of bFGF was recovered in the myocardium, only 0.5% of an intravenous dose was. The most plausible explanation of these findings derives from the fact that myocardial uptake depends on peak serum concentration; because bFGF has a heparin-binding domain, considerable first-pass uptake in the lungs will occur after intravenous administration (the lungs contain large amounts of heparin sulfates), resulting in a blunted peak serum concentration presented to the myocardium when compared with the very high concentrations presented to the myocardium with bolus injection directly into the coronary artery.

The biologic consequences of these differences were demonstrated in angiogenesis studies of the same canine ischemia model. Collateral flow improved with intracoronary administration of bFGF but did not increase when the drug was given intravenously, despite its being given for 1 week.[87] Although similar uptake studies have not been performed with VEGF, its 165 isoform ($VEGF_{165}$) also has a heparin-binding domain (whereas $VEGF_{121}$ does not), suggesting that similar results would be seen.

Animal studies that appear to be at variance with these results also have been reported. Thus, Lopez and colleagues[89] delivered $VEGF_{165}$ to a porcine model of myocardial ischemia (ameroid occlusion of the circumflex coronary artery) by three different local intracoronary delivery systems (via an InfusaSleeve catheter, intracoronary bolus infusion, and epicardial implantation of an osmotic delivery system). VEGF was administered 3 weeks after ameroid placement, and indices of collateral function were assessed at that time (baseline) and 3 weeks later. Whereas there was no significant improvement in circumflex territory perfusion in control pigs, improved circumflex perfusion was demonstrable within each VEGF-treated group using paired *t*-tests to compare pretreatment and posttreatment perfusion values. Although these data are suggestive of a VEGF treatment effect, they are not convincing. First, ongoing collateral development has been observed in pigs throughout the 6-week period after circumflex ameroid placement.[90] In the Lopez study, however, the control group did not exhibit the expected increase in circumflex territory perfusion during that interval. Second, direct comparisons between individual VEGF treatment groups and the control group were not statistically significant. Only when all three VEGF treatment groups were combined in a post hoc analysis was a statistically significant difference demonstrable between VEGF groups and the control group. Third, there were three deaths in VEGF-treated animals during the investigation. Elimination of three animals in a small study such as this could have an important effect on the results through selection bias. Thus, while suggestive, the data from this experiment do not demonstrate unequivocally that a *single* bolus intracoronary injection of VEGF is capable of increasing collateral flow to a greater extent than that which occurs in the absence of therapy.

Hariawala and colleagues[91] also reported improved flow in a similar model. However, this study is flawed by the fact that intracoronary bolus administration of VEGF (2 mg) caused severe hypotension that led to the acute death of four of eight animals in the treated group; hence the surviving animals, which were found to have greater collateral flow than the untreated controls, may have survived only *because* they had greater intrinsic collateral flow. These investigators also demonstrated in the rabbit hind limb model of ischemia that a single dose of intrafemoral bFGF or $VEGF_{165}$ improves collateral flow and, surprisingly, that a single intravenous dose of $VEGF_{165}$ also improves flow.[92] The conflicting results are reported in the literature relating to whether a *single* intra-arterial bolus injection of VEGF or bFGF protein improves collateral flow and whether improvement occurs following intravenous administration, at least for heparin-binding agents.

Clinical Trials

The clinical trials of protein-based angiogenesis have been reported by using growth factors like FGF and VEGF families.

The effect of FGF-1 on the ischemic myocardium was first performed by Schumacher and colleagues[93] in a series of 20 patients. In the study, 0.01 mg/kg of FGF-1 protein was injected directly into the ischemic myocardium along LAD while patients were undergoing bypass surgery. Three months later, neoangiogenesis, together with the development of a normal vascular appearance, was demonstrated angiographically. The first randomized, double-blind, placebo-controlled clinical trial for basic FGF was reported by the Simons' group.[94] Twenty-four patients undergoing CABG were randomized to three groups, receiving either 10 μg or 100 μg of bFGF, or placebo through delivery of microcapsules capable of sustained-release which were implanted in ischemic myocardium. During 16 months of follow-up, all patients in the 100 μg bFGF remained angina-free and a stress nuclear perfusion imaging test at baseline and 3 months showed significant improvement. The efficacy of single intracoronary infusion of FGF-2 (0, 0.3, 3, or 30 μg/kg; $n = 337$ patients) was tested by a multicenter FIRST trial.[95] At 90 days, in all FGF-2 treated groups angina symptoms were significantly reduced compared with placebo, but not in 180 days because of the continued improvement in the placebo. The effect of intracoronary injection of recombinant human VEGF on myocardial perfusion was first performed on 14 severe CAD patients,[96] and followed by a multicenter VIVA trial on a total of 178 patients.[97] In the small patients group study, seven patients who received high-dose VEGF (0.05–0.167 μg/kg) showed improvement in resting myocardial perfusion and collateral count density at 60 days follow-up.[96] In the VIVA trial, patients were randomized to receive a 20-minute intracoronary infusion of placebo, low-dose (17 ng/kg/min) or high-dose (50 ng/kg/min) rhVEGF and followed by 4-hour intravenous infusion on days 3, 6, and 9. However, the study showed no significant differences in primary end point of the trial and ETT time compared with placebo at 60 days follow-up. At day 120, high-dose patients showed improvement in angina class and favorable trends in exercise treadmill test time and quality of life.[97]

Genes

Experimental Studies

Gene therapy presents one of the solutions to the possible dosing conundrum because gene therapy can be considered a sophisticated form of a sustained delivery system. Once transfected, the target cell expresses gene product for days, weeks, or longer depending on the specific tissue transfected and the specific vector used.

Proof of concept that gene therapy can improve collateral function was demonstrated by Giordano and colleagues.[98] They found in a porcine model of myocardial ischemia (ameroid occlusion of the circumflex coronary artery) that a single-dose intracoronary administration of an adenoviral vector carrying the FGF5 transgene into the nonoccluded right coronary artery increased myocardial flow and function. Surprisingly, they found that about 95% first-pass myocardial uptake was achieved with intracoronary administration. Hammond and colleagues have since demonstrated that FGF4 produces similar effects in restoring myocardial flow and function.[99] Improvement of myocardial contractility in a porcine model of chronic ischemia has been reported recently by using a combined TMR and FGF-2 gene therapy approach.[100] In this study, adenoviral vector encoded FGF-2 was formulated in a collagen-based matrix and directly injected into ischemic myocardium. Other investigators also have performed studies employing the rabbit hind limb model of ischemia and have reported that injection into the femoral artery of the $VEGF_{165}$ transgene carried in a plasmid vector improves collateral flow.[101]

Direct Intramyocardial Injection

No matter how efficient first-pass uptake is, a considerable proportion of an angiogenesis factor *injected into an artery* supplying the target tissue will enter the systemic circulation and thereby expose nontarget tissues to its biologic effects.[102] Although there is no definitive evidence yet that such systemic spillover will produce serious side effects, there is always that possibility (see the following). Therefore, it appears that if *direct intramuscular injection* of the angiogenesis factor, either by the transepicardial or transendocardial route, does result in enhanced collateral flow, such an approach might be preferable.

A protein injected once intramuscularly would be unlikely to persist in the tissue long enough to exert an important biologic effect.[102] Although multiple injections of protein might well improve collateral flow,[85] such a strategy has practical limitations. Therefore, once it was demonstrated that an adenoviral vector carrying a reporter transgene efficiently expresses its gene product after intramyocardial injection,[103] this approach to gene delivery was explored as an approach for gene therapy.

Proof of concept that intramyocardial injection could enhance collateral flow and improve impaired myocardial function was demonstrated in a porcine model of myocardial ischemia. This was achieved by the transepicardial injection of an adenoviral vector carrying the $VEGF_{121}$ transgene performed after thoracotomy.[104] The feasibility of catheter-based transendocardial delivery of angiogenesis genes has been shown recently,[105] demonstrating that the direct injection of angiogenesis factors into the myocardium can be accomplished without the need for thoracotomy.

However, because VEGF induces marked increases in vascular permeability and tissue edema, excessive VEGF administration could develop deleterious effects. Recent reports showed that in a chronic ischemic rabbit ear model, both adenoviral encoded VEGF and Angiopoietin-1 (Ang-1) increased flow at one week after injection. However, Ang-1-induced flow was localized to larger vessels, with no visible inflammatory response, but VEGF produced a diffuse increase in flow that was associated with pronounced swelling, vessel leakage, and inflammatory cell infiltration. At 4 weeks, the flow in the VEGF treated group decreased from pretreatment values. In contrast, the Ang-1–induced improvement was maintained.[106] Similar deleterious effects of VEGF were also reported by Masaki et al in their mouse hind limb ischemia model.[107]

Clinical Trials

The first clinical trial on gene-based therapy using adenoviral vector was reported by Rosengart and colleagues.[108] In this phase I trial, 15 patients received adenoVEGF121 by direct intramyocardial injection as an adjunct to conventional CABG and six patients received gene-therapy only. Thirty days after the treatment, all patients showed improvement of wall motion in the area of vector administration by coronary angiography and stress ^{99m}Tc-sestamibi perfusion scan, as well as improvement in angina class after therapy. There was no evidence of systemic or cardiac-related adverse events related to vector administration. The effect of plasmid encoded VEGF2 on chronic myocardial ischemia was studied in 19 patients using catheter-based delivery.[109] In this small phase 1/2 study, Losordo and colleagues used an injecting catheter device guided by NOGA mapping technique and administered 200 to 800 μg of phVEGF2 plasmid directly into the endomyocardium. The end point analysis at 3 months disclosed improvement in angina class and strong trends favoring efficacy of phVEGF2 versus placebo in exercise duration, functional improvement, and Seattle Angina Questionnaire data. The adenoviral encoded FGF4 was studied by AGENT trial by Grines et al. in a group of 79 patients with chronic stable angina pectoris.[110] In this trial, patients received one time intracoronary injection of five different doses of adenoviral encoded FGF4 (from 3.3×10^8 to 10^{11} viral particles in half-log increments). In this first report of a randomized, double-blind and placebo-controlled trial, ad5-FGF4 showed a trend to have greater improvements in exercise time versus placebo at 4 weeks' follow-up. The same group also reported an AGENT-2 study of 52 patients with chronic stable angina using a single dose of 10^{10} viral particle of ad5FGF4 intracoronary infusion. At 8 weeks after treatment, ischemic defect size was significantly decreased in ad5-FGF4–injected patients compared with placebo-treated patients and the viral vector was well tolerated and did not result in any permanent adverse sequelae.[111] Hedman et al. conducted a phase II Kuopio Angiogenesis Trial (KAT) to study the effects of VEGF on restenosis and chronic myocardial ischemia by intracoronary injection of either adenoviral or plasmid encoded VEGF165 on 103 patients who underwent PTCA and stenting.[112] At 6 months' follow-up, no difference was found in restenosis rate or minimal lumen diameter between all study groups. However, myocardial perfusion showed a significant improvement in the adenoVEGF treated group. Recently, the Euroinject One Trial was reported by Kastrup and colleagues[113] on direct intramyocardial plasmid VEGF-A_{165} gene therapy in patients with stable severe angina pectoris. In this study, 80 "no option" patients with severe stable ischemic heart disease were randomly assigned to receive either 0.5 mg of phVEGFA_{165} or placebo plasmid in the myocardial region showing stress-induced perfusion defects under the guidance of the NOGA-MyoStar system. At 3 months' follow-up, the VEGF gene transfer did not significantly improve stress-induced myocardial perfusion defect compared with placebo. However, improved regional wall motion indicated a favorable anti-ischemic effect.

In summary, single protein or gene-based therapy so far has not achieved significant convincing beneficial results in improving myocardial perfusion both experimentally and clinically. More clinical studies are needed to determine how to achieve optimal myocardial angiogenesis. Many aspects of gene transfer, including the appropriate vector dose, formulation, and administration route, are still to be tested.

Cell-Based Therapy

Two classical concepts have been challenged in recent years by cell-based therapy using either embryonic or adult stem cells. First, vasculogenesis, which previously referred to a process that occurred only in the embryo, in which the vascular system develops from mesodermal precursor cells called *angioblasts* that invade the different embryonic organs and assemble in situ to form the primary capillary plexus. However, many investigators now believe that in adults, bone marrow–derived stem cells or endothelial progenitor cells can be recruited to and incorporated into tissues undergoing neovascularization. Second, cardiac myocytes originally were considered to be terminally differentiated cells that cannot be regenerated in adulthood. However, recent studies have shown that a limited number of cardiomyocytes may be regenerated by locally sited or recruited circulating stem cells. Therefore, stem cells, which include hematopoietic stem cells (HSCs), endothelial progenitor cells (EPCs), mesenchymal stem cells/stromal stem cells (MSCs), myoblasts, and undifferentiated side population cells, have been used as an alternative therapeutic strategy for ischemic cardiovascular diseases that cannot be treated by routine interventional approaches. Theoretically, embryonic stem cells have more potential to differentiate into cardiomyocytes; however, clinical trials are now only limited to adult stem cells owing to the fact that they are relatively easier to handle, and autologous transplantation can be performed in clinical patients. Several centers around the world, including the United States, had reported an improved functional status in experimental animals and clinical patients after such therapy; however, it is still unclear how bone marrow–derived stem/progenitor cells are mobilized and recruited into ischemic tissues, if the injected cells in clinical trial patients differentiated into functional cardiomyocytes, and what particular cell type is better to use compared with others. This section focuses on the progress status of clinical trials, mechanisms of involving functional improvements by stem cell therapy, limitations for applications, and potential risks.

Clinical Trials

Intracoronary Infusion of Autologous Bone Marrow–Derived Cells.

TOPCARE-AMI. Assmus and colleagues first reported cell-based therapy for 20 acute myocardial infarction (AMI) patients in 2002.[114] In this study, the authors performed intracoronary infusion of autologous bone marrow–derived mononuclear cells (n = 9) or circulating blood-derived progenitor cells (n = 11) 4 to 5 days after AMI. The circulating blood-derived progenitor cells were expanded ex vivo for 3 days before injection. The bone marrow–derived cells were extracted on the same day as injection without expansion. At 4 months after cell injection, patients' cardiac function was improved compared with 11 matched controls. The authors also reported postinfarction remodeling outcome using serial contrast-enhanced MRI.[115] A total of 28 patients with reperfused AMI who received bone marrow–derived cells or circulating blood progenitor cells were analyzed. They found that intracoronary infusion of adult progenitor cells in patients with AMI beneficially affects postinfarction remodeling processes. The migratory capacity of the infused cells is a major determinant of infarct remodeling, suggesting a causal effect of progenitor cell therapy on regeneration enhancement.[115] In 2004, the same group reported final 1-year results of 59 patients that showed similar functional improvements.[116]

TOPCARE-CHD. Assmus and colleagues also performed a clinical study of using functional competent BMCs in chronic postinfarction heart failure patients. In this study, 121 patients treated with BMCs showed statistically significant improvement in the serum level of natriuretic peptide and favorable clinical outcomes.[117]

Strauer and colleagues conducted a study to test the effect of autologous bone marrow–derived mononuclear cells (BMCs) on myocardial repair or regeneration. The authors first reported the data with 10 AMI patients who received BMCs by intracoronary injection and compared with 10 compatible patients treated with standard therapy alone. At 3 months after cell therapy, they found that the infarct region had decreased significantly and wall motion also significantly improved.[118] More recently, the same group reported another study using same cell therapy technique on 18 patients with chronic MI (5 months to 8.5 years old) for their effects on myocardial regeneration.[119] At 3 months, the patients with cell therapy showed that the infarct size was reduced by 30% and global left ventricular ejection fraction and infarction wall movement velocity increased significantly, whereas in the control group no significant changes were observed. The authors also found that following BMC transplantation there were improvements in maximum oxygen uptake and regional ^{18}F-fluor-desoxyglucose uptake into infarct tissue suggesting a regeneration of myocardium after infarction.

BOOST Trial. The initial BOne marrOw transfer to enhance ST-elevation infarct regeneration (BOOST) trial was reported by Meyer GP and colleagues,[120] which showed significant improvements in global and regional left ventricular systolic function. However, the 5-year follow-up from this trial proved that a single intracoronary infusion of BMCs did not promote a sustained improvement of LVEF in ST-elevation myocardial infarction patients.[121]

Catheter-Based Transendocardial Cell Injection. Perin and colleagues[122] reported their results using a NOGA catheter technique to transendocardialy inject autologous bone marrow stem cells for severe chronic ischemic heart failure patients. Fourteen patients who received cell injection showed significant functional improvement compared with seven controls. Similar methods also were reported by Fuchs and colleagues in Washington Hospital Center in 10 no-option patients with advanced CAD. The authors first initiated a porcine ischemic model to test the effect of freshly extracted autologous bone marrow on myocardial blood perfusion. Improved collateral flow and contractility in a treated group of animals was found.[123] Subsequently, in a pilot clinical study, the 10 no-option patients with advanced CAD autologous bone marrow direct myocardial injection induced a significant improved Canadian Cardiovascular Society angina score and stress-induced ischemia occurring within the injected territories.[124]

Intracoronary Injection of Extra Vivo Expanded BMCs. Chen and colleagues[125] were the first group to use autologous ex vivo expanded bone marrow–derived mesenchymal stem cells in patients with AMI. In their study, a total of 69 patients who received PCI 12 hours after AMI were chosen randomly for either cell injection ($n = 34$) or control ($n = 35$). The bone marrow–derived mononuclear cells were cultured in vitro for 10 days, and then patients underwent intracoronary injection of the fibroblast-like mesenchymal stem cells. Patients who received mononuclear stem cell injection showed significant improvement in left ventricular (LV) function at 3 to 6 months of follow-up.

Mobilized Peripheral Blood Mononuclear Cell Studies. Kang and colleagues[126] reported a mobilized peripheral blood mononuclear cell study for AMI patients after coronary stenting. A total of 27 patients with AMI who underwent PCI 48 hours later were studied. Ten patients received intracoronary injection of mobilized (granulocyte colony-stimulation factor [G-CSF] 10 μg/kg for 4 days) PBMC, and 10 patients received injection of G-CSF alone, seven as control. At 6 months, the cell infusion group showed improvement in LV function compared with the other two groups.

However, from later randomized placebo-controlled trials (REVIVAL-2) reported by Zohlnhofer and colleagues[127] showed that stem cells mobilized by G-CSF therapy did not improve the infarct size, left ventricular function, or coronary restenosis in patients with acute myocardial infarction who had successful mechanical reperfusion.

Autologous Myoclast Studies. Taylor and colleagues[128] first reported to use autologously transplanted skeletal myoblasts to improve ventricular function in animal models of heart failure. This has been a hot topic in the field of cell-based therapy for the last 10 years. However, recently reported first randomized placebo-controlled clinical study of autologous myoblast transplantation showed no evidence of functional improvement of the left ventricle, but did show an increased number of early postoperative arrhythmic events.[129]

Direct Epimyocardial Cell Transplantation. Patel and colleagues[130] recently reported direct myocardial injection of autologous bone marrow–derived stem cells in 10 patients who underwent bypass surgery. Six months later, the cell injection patients showed improvement in LV function compared with 10 patients who received bypass surgery alone. No side effects were found with this direct stem cell injection.

Allogenic Human Mesenchymal Stem Cell Therapy

Most recently, Osiris Therapeutics Inc. completed its first allogenic hMSCs clinical trial reported by Hare and colleagues.[131] In this study, hMSCs, developed by Osiris Therapeutics Inc. more than 10 years ago, were administered intravenously to patients with acute myocardial infarction at a dose range of 0.5, 1.6, and 5 million cells/kg. They found that the allogenic stem cell therapy was safe, and the arrhythmia events were significantly reduced, global symptom score and LV ejection fraction in a subset of anterior MI patients was significantly better in hMSCs treated compared with placebo patients. The study suggested the potential usage of allogenic cell therapy in the future.

Safety and Efficacy

Potential for Deleterious Effects

For most potent therapeutic interventions, therapeutic efficacy is rarely free of the potential for harmful effects to occur. The biologic activities of most of the angiogenesis agents currently being tested clinically are very potent, and it is likely that the same activities that lead to a therapeutic effect also could cause unwanted side effects. It is therefore probable that some side effects consequent to the cellular effects of these agents inevitably will occur. If this concept is true, then the critical question we will have to address in large clinical trials is whether the incidence of these risks is sufficiently low that they will be outweighed by the therapeutic benefits.

Among the side effects that might occur as a result of the biologic effects of these agents is the development of new blood vessels in nontargeted tissues, a complication that would be particularly devastating if it were to occur, for example, in the retina. It is possible that this particular complication may not develop unless a tissue is "primed" to respond with an angiogenesis response. That is, quiescent cells have low constitutive expression of receptors for the VEGF and FGF family of agents—thus, unless the tissue is exposed to very high doses of the ligands for prolonged periods, it is possible that normal tissue is resistant to the neovascularization effects of angiogenesis factors, a result suggested by the study by Banai and colleagues.[132]

Other VEGF-specific complications could develop as a result of the potent activity of VEGF as an inducer of vascular permeability.[133] Although angiogenesis and vascular permeability might be considered two separate biologic activities, it is also possible that the vascular permeability properties of VEGF are essential for angiogenesis to occur.

Whatever the interrelation between these two actions, if vascular permeability increases in tissues other than the tissue targeted for angiogenesis, serious consequences could accrue. That this could occur was demonstrated in a recent study in which the effects of overexpression of VEGF (achieved by injecting an adenovirus carrying the VEGF transgene) in adult mice was investigated.[133] The mice, as expected, developed elevated circulating levels of VEGF following injection of the adenoviral vector. However, a high percentage died within days, developing increased vascular permeability and severe multiple-organ edema.

Other potential complications based on biologic activities are the expansion and induction of instability of atherogenic plaque and the growth of tumors. For example, Flugelman and colleagues demonstrated an association between unstable angina and the intraplaque presence of aFGF and bFGF.[134] They suggested that these agents might play a role in plaque instability. In addition, the broad range of cells on which the FGF family of agents exerts mitogenic effects could result in the growth of cells resident within plaques or of malignant cells.

Although the direct mitogenic effects of VEGF are limited largely to endothelial cells, it is of note that VEGF and its receptors, VEGFR1 and VEGFR2 (flt-1 and Flk-1), are overexpressed in atherosclerotic lesions.[135] Moreover, a number of nonendothelial tumor cells have been found to possess low levels of functional VEGFR1 and VEGFR2.[136] Also of possible relevance is the fact that the uterus possesses functional VEGF receptor tyrosine kinases[137] and VEGF is mitogenic for uterine smooth muscle. These observations raise the possibility that the atherosclerotic lesion, certain tumors, and the common leiomyoma (fibroid) could at least theoretically respond to direct exogenous stimulation by VEGF.

There is also increasing evidence suggesting that growth of microvessels into plaque or tumors, through angiogenesis processes, is critical to growth of both tumor and plaque.[138,139] Thus, microvascular angiogenesis per se, an activity inherent in most angiogenesis factors, could predispose to plaque or tumor growth. In addition, the potent vascular permeability effect of VEGF could result in exposing a plaque or tumor to many cytokines and growth factors that normally are confined to the plasma and through this indirect mechanism stimulate their growth.

It must be emphasized that there have been *no* conclusive reports in clinical studies demonstrating that angiogenesis agents actually induce new tumor development, increase growth of in situ tumors, or increase plaque size. However, several experimental studies have demonstrated that prolonged exposure of skeletal muscle or myocardium to high local levels of VEGF or FGF family peptides can cause hemangioma-like tumors and vascular malformations[140] and can increase neointimal development.[141]

A phase I randomized, dose-escalation trial also demonstrated that high doses of bFGF can lead to the development of thrombocytopenia and renal toxicity.[142] In addition, the immune surveillance system is not normally exposed to large amounts of these proteins. Therefore, it is possible that antibodies can develop to these cytokines and these could either impair the efficacy of repeated administration of the agents or even possibly lead to immunopathogenic processes. It also should be noted that one of the clinical trials in progress employs FGF2 of porcine origin[94,95]; although the high homology between the FGFs in different species makes it unlikely that recognition of nonself protein will occur, this certainly is not beyond the realm of possibility.

FGF and VEGF proteins, administered acutely, can produce hypotension through, at least in part, a nitric oxide–mediated pathway[143] and, in the case of FGF2, a potassium channel–mediated mechanism.[144] The hypotensive effect has resulted in the death of pigs that had chronic myocardial ischemia and were treated with the intracoronary injection of $VEGF_{165}$ protein[91] and in a prolonged hypotensive episode of a patient entered into a phase I study testing the safety of intracoronary administration of bFGF.[142] This complication appears to occur only when high systemic levels of bFGF and VEGF develop rapidly. Thus, it would appear to be of little or no concern if bFGF and VEGF proteins are not administered rapidly and of no concern when the factors are given as genes—which express the proteins they encode slowly.

We also need to consider, in the case of gene therapy employing viral vectors, the potential for the vectors themselves to cause deleterious effects. The administration of large amounts of virus can lead to massive immune responses that could cause serious, even fatal immunopathology. Such responses are unlikely given the amount of adenovirus administered in current clinical cardiovascular protocols. However, the foreign proteins presented by the virus, even when administered in relatively small amounts, probably will induce immune responses that conceivably could decrease subsequent sensitivity to the beneficial effects of the transgene delivered by the virus if administered repeatedly or could possibly lead to immune-mediated tissue damage.

In cell-based therapy, most of the clinical trials so far are using non ex vivo expanded or short term expanded (4 to 5 days) cells. In animal studies, stem cells potentially can transform via in vitro expansion. These transformed cells can create tumors in nude mice.[145] Similar incidents have occurred occasionally in adult human bone marrow–derived mesenchymal stem cells as well. It is still not clear which cell type is best for myocardial ischemia patients; however, if it is decided to use ex vivo expanded cells, one has to be sure that they are not tumorigenic. It is absolutely necessary to test these cells for tumorigenic potential in nude mice and to perform a karyotyping test before injecting the cells into patients.

REFERENCES

1. Weintraub WS, Jone EL, Craver JM, et al: Frequency of repeat coronary bypass or coronary angioplasty after coronary artery bypass surgery using saphenous venous grafts. *Am J Cardiol* 1994; 73:103.
2. Osswald B, Blackstone E, Tochtermann U, et al: Does the completeness of revascularization affect early survival after coronary artery bypass grafting in elderly patients? *Eur J Cardiothorac Surg* 2001; 20:120.
3. Lawrie GM, Morris GC, Silvers A, et al: The influence of residual disease after coronary bypass on the 5-year survival rate of 1274 men with coronary artery disease. *Circulation* 1982; 66:717.
4. Schaff H, Gersh B, Pluth J, et al: Survival and functional status after coronary artery bypass grafting: results 10 to 12 years after surgery in 500 patients. *Circulation* 1983; 68:200.
5. Wearn J, Mettier S, Klumpp T, et al: The nature of the vascular communications between the coronary arteries and the chambers of the heart. *Am Heart J* 1933; 9:143.
6. Sen P, Udwadia T, Kinare S, et al: Transmyocardial revascularization: a new approach to myocardial revascularization. *J Thorac Cardiovasc Surg* 1965; 50:181.
7. Beck CS: The development of a new blood supply to the heart by operation. *Ann Surg* 1935; 102:801.
8. Massimo C, Boffi L: Myocardial revascularization by a new method of carrying blood directly from the left ventricular cavity into the coronary circulation. *J Thorac Surg* 1957; 34:257.
9. Walter P, Hundeshagen H, Borst HG: Treatment of acute myocardial infarction by transmural blood supply from the ventricular cavity. *Eur Surg Res* 1971; 3:130.
10. Mirhoseini M, Muckerheide M, Cayton MM: Transventricular revascularization by laser. *Lasers Surg Med* 1982; 2:187.
11. Okada M, Ikuta H, Shimizu OK, et al: Alternative method of myocardial revascularization by laser: experimental and clinical study. *Kobe J Med Sci* 1986; 32:151.
12. Horvath KA, Mannting F, Cummings N, et al: Transmyocardial laser revascularization: operative techniques and clinical results at two years. *J Thorac Cardiovasc Surg* 1996; 111:1047.
13. Cooley DA, Frazier OH, Kadipasaoglu KA, et al: Transmyocardial laser revascularization: clinical experience with 12-month follow-up. *J Thorac Cardiovasc Surg* 1996; 111:791.
14. Horvath KA, Cohn LC, Cooley DA, et al: Transmyocardial laser revascularization: results of a multicenter trial using TLR as sole therapy for end-stage coronary artery disease. *J Thorac Cardiovasc Surg* 1997; 113:645.
15. Milano A, Pratali S, Tartarini G, et al: Early results of transmyocardial revascularization with a holmium laser. *Ann Thorac Surg* 1998; 65:700.
16. Allen KB, Dowling RD, Fudge TL, et al: Comparison of transmyocardial revascularization with medical therapy in patients with refractory angina. *NEJM* 1999; 341:1029.
17. Burkhoff D, Schmidt S, Schulman SP, et al: Transmyocardial laser revascularization compared with continued medical therapy for treatment of refractory angina pectoris: a prospective, randomized trial. *Lancet* 1999; 354:885.
18. Frazier OH, March RJ, Horvath KA: Transmyocardial revascularization with a carbon dioxide laser in patients with end-stage coronary artery disease. *NEJM* 1999; 341:1021.
19. Schofield PM, Sharples LD, Caine N, et al: Transmyocardial laser revascularization in patients with refractory angina: a randomized, controlled trial. *Lancet* 1999; 353:519.
20. Aaberge L, Nordstrand K, Dragsund M, et al: Transmyocardial revascularization with CO_2 laser in patients with refractory angina pectoris: clinical results from the Norwegian randomized trial. *J Am Coll Cardiol* 2000; 35:1170.
21. Aaberge L, Rootwelt K, Blomhoff S, et al: Continued symptomatic improvement three to five years after transmyocardial revascularization with CO_2 laser: a late clinical follow-up of the Norwegian randomized trial with transmyocardial revascularization. *J Am Coll Cardiol* 2002; 39:1588.
22. Allen KB, Dowling RD, Angell W, et al: Transmyocardial revascularization: five-year follow-up of a prospective, randomized, multicenter trial. *Ann Thorac Surg* 2004; 77:1228.
23. Frazier OH, Cooley DA, Kadipasaoglu KA, et al: Myocardial revascularization with laser: preliminary findings. *Circulation* 1995; 92:58.
24. Horvath KA, Aranki SF, Cohn LH, et al: Sustained angina relief 5 years after transmyocardial laser revascularization with a CO_2 laser. *Circulation* 2001; 104:I-181.
25. Gibbons R, Abrams J, Chatterjee K, et al: ACC/AHA 2002 guideline update for the management of patients with chronic stable angina-summary article: a report of the American College of Cardiology/American Heart Association Task Force on Practice Guidelines (Committee on the Management of Patients with Chronic Stable Angina). *Circulation* 2003; 107:149.
26. Bridges CR, Horvath KA, Nugent B, et al: Society of Thoracic Surgeons practice guideline: transmyocardial laser revascularization. *Ann Thorac Surg* 2004; 77:1484.
27. Trehan J, Mishra M, Bapna R, et al: Transmyocardial laser revascularization combined with coronary artery bypass grafting without cardiopulmonary bypass. *Eur J Cardiothorac Surg* 1997; 12:276.
28. Stamou SC, Boyce SW, Cooke RH, et al: One-year outcome after combined coronary artery bypass grafting and transmyocardial laser revascularization for refractory angina pectoris. *J Am Coll Cardiol* 2002; 89:1365.
29. Wehberg KE, Julian JS, Todd JC, et al: Improved patient outcomes when transmyocardial revascularization is used as adjunctive revascularization. *Heart Surg Forum* 2003; 6:1.
30. Allen KB, Dowling R, DelRossi A, et al: Transmyocardial revascularization combined with coronary artery bypass grafting: a multicenter, blinded, prospective, randomized, controlled trial. *J Thorac Cardiovasc Surg* 2000; 119:540.
31. Frazier OH, Boyce SW, Griffith BP, et al: Transmyocardial revascularization using a synchronized CO_2 laser as adjunct to coronary artery bypass grafting: results of a prospective, randomized multi-center trial with 12-month follow-up. *Circulation* 1999; 100:I-1248.
32. Allen KB, Dowling RD, Schuch D, et al: Adjunctive transmyocardial revascularization: 5-year follow-up of a prospective, randomized, trial. *Ann Thorac Surg* 2004; 78:458.
33. Horvath KA, Ferguson TB, Guyton RA, et al: The impact of unstable angina on outcomes of transmyocardial laser revascularization combined with coronary artery bypass grafting. *Ann Thorac Surg* 2005; 80:2082.
34. Malekah R, Reynolds C, Narula N, et al: Angiogenesis in transmyocardial laser revascularization: a nonspecific response to injury. *Circulation* 1998; 9:II-62.
35. Smith NB, Hynynen K: The feasibility of using focused ultrasound for transmyocardial revascularization. *Ultrasound Med Biol* 1998; 24:1045.
36. Khairy P, Dubuc M, Gallo R: Cryoapplication induces neovascularization: a novel approach to percutaneous myocardial revascularization. *J Am Coll Cardiol* 2000; 35:5A.
37. Yamamoto N, Gu AG, Derosa CM, et al: Radiofrequency transmyocardial revascularization enhances angiogenesis and causes myocardial denervation in a canine model. *Lasers Surg Med* 2000; 27:18.
38. Dietz U, Darius H, Eick O, et al: Transmyocardial revascularization using temperature-controlled HF energy creates reproducible intramyocardial channels. *Circulation* 1998; 98:3770
39. Horvath KA, Belkind N, Wu I, et al: Functional comparison of transmyocardial revascularization by mechanical and laser means. *Ann Thorac Surg* 2001; 72:1997.

40. Whittaker P, Rakusan K, Kloner RA: Transmural channels can protect ischemic tissue: assessment of long-term myocardial response to laser- and needle-made channels. *Circulation* 1996; 93:143.
41. Hughes GC, Kypson AP, Annex BH, et al: Induction of angiogenesis after TMR: a comparison of holmium:YAG, CO_2, and excimer lasers. *Ann Thorac Surg* 2000; 70:504.
42. Whittaker P, Spariosu K, Ho ZZ: Success of transmyocardial laser revascularization is determined by the amount and organization of scar tissue produced in response to initial injury: results of ultraviolet laser treatment. *Lasers Surg Med* 1999; 24:253.
43. Genyk IA, Frenz M, Ott B, et al: Acute and chronic effects of transmyocardial laser revascularization in the nonischemic pig myocardium by using three laser systems. *Lasers Surg Med* 2000; 27:438.
44. Jeevanandam V, Auteri JS, Oz MC, et al: Myocardial revascularization by laser-induced channels. *Surg Forum* 1990; 41:225.
45. Kadipasaoglu KA, Sartori M, Masai T, et al: Intraoperative arrhythmias and tissue damage during transmyocardial laser revascularization. *Ann Thorac Surg* 1999; 67:423.
46. Cooley DA, Frazier OH, Kadipasaoglu KA, et al: Transmyocardial laser revascularization: anatomic evidence of long-term channel patency. *Texas Heart Inst J* 1994; 21:220.
47. Horvath KA, Smith WJ, Laurence RG, et al: Recovery and viability of an acute myocardial infarct after transmyocardial laser revascularization. *J Am Coll Cardiol* 1995; 25:258.
48. Krabatsch T, Schaper F, Leder C, et al: Histologic findings after transmyocardial laser revascularization. *J Card Surg* 1996; 11:326.
49. Lutter G, Martin J, Ameer K, et al: Microperfusion enhancement after TMLR in chronically ischemic porcine hearts. *Cardiovasc Surg* 2001; 9:281.
50. Gassler N, Wintzer HO, Stubbe HM, et al: Transmyocardial laser revascularization: histological features in human nonresponder myocardium. *Circulation* 1997; 95:371.
51. Burkhoff D, Fisher PE, Apfelbaum M, et al: Histologic appearance of transmyocardial laser channels after 41/2 weeks. *Ann Thorac Surg* 1996; 61:1532.
52. Sigel JE, Abramovitch CM, Lytle BW, et al: Transmyocardial laser revascularization: three sequential autopsy cases. *J Thorac Cardiovasc Surg* 1998; 115:1381.
53. Kwong KF, Kanellopoulos GK, Nikols JC, et al: Transmyocardial laser treatment denervates canine myocardium. *J Thorac Cardiovasc Surg* 1997; 114:883.
54. Hirsch GM, Thompson GW, Arora RC, et al: Transmyocardial laser revascularization does not denervate the canine heart. *Ann Thorac Surg* 1999; 68:460.
55. Minisi AJ, Topaz O, Quinn MS, et al: Cardiac nociceptive reflexes after tansmyocardial laser revascularization: implications for the neural hypothesis of angina relief. *J Thorac Cardiovasc Surg* 2001; 122:712.
56. Al-Sheikh T, Allen KB, Straka SP, et al: Cardiac sympathetic denervation after transmyocardial laser revascularization. *Circulation* 1999; 100:135.
57. Fisher PE, Khomoto T, DeRosa CM, et al: Histologic analysis of transmyocardial channels: comparison of CO_2 and holmium:YAG lasers. *Ann Thorac Surg* 1997; 64:466.
58. Zlotnick AY, Ahmad RM, Reul RM: Neovascularization occurs at the site of closed laser channels after transmyocardial laser revascularization. *Surg Forum* 1996; 48:286.
59. Kohmoto T, Fisher PE, DeRosa, C, et al: Evidence of angiogenesis in regions treated with transmyocardial laser revascularization. *Circulation* 1996; 94:1294.
60. Spanier T, Smith CR, Burkhoff D: Angiogenesis: a possible mechanism underlying the clinical benefits of transmyocardial laser revascularization. *J Clin Laser Med Surg* 1997; 15:269.
61. Hughes GC, Lowe JE, Kypson AP, et al: Neovascularization after transmyocardial laser revascularization in a model of chronic ischemia. *Ann Thorac Surg* 1998; 66:2029.
62. Horvath KA, Chiu E, Maun DC, et al: Up-regulation of VEGF mRNA and angiogenesis after transmyocardial laser revascularization. *Ann Thorac Surg* 1999; 68:825.
63. Li W, Chiba Y, Kimura T, et al: Transmyocardial laser revascularization induced angiogenesis correlated with the expression of matrix metalloproteinase and platelet-derived endothelial cell growth factor. *Eur J Cardiothorac Surg* 2001; 19:156.
64. Pelletier MP, Giaid A, Sivaraman S, et al: Angiogenesis and growth factor expression in a model of transmyocardial revascularization. *Ann Thorac Surg* 1998; 66:12.
65. Chu VF, Giaid A, Kuagn JQ, et al: Angiogenesis in transmyocardial revascularization: comparison of laser versus mechanical punctures. *Ann Thorac Surg* 1999; 68:301.
66. Malekan R, Reynolds C, Narula N, et al: Angiogenesis in transmyocardial laser revascularization: a nonspecific response to injury. *Circulation* 1998; 98:II-62.
67. Donovan CL, Landolfo KP, Lowe JE, et al: Improvement in inducible ischemic during dobutamine stress echocardiography after transmyocardial laser revascularization in patients with refractory angina pectoris. *J Am Coll Cardiol* 1997; 30:607.
68. Laham RJ, Simons M, Pearlman JD, et al: Magnetic resonance imaging demonstrates improved regional systolic wall motion and thickening and myocardial perfusion of myocardial territories treated by laser myocardial revascularization. *J Am Coll Cardiol* 2002; 39:1.
69. Horvath KA, Kim RJ, Judd RM, et al: Contrast enhanced MRI assessment of microinfarction after transmyocardial laser revascularization. *Circulation* 2000; 102:II-765.
70. Horvath KA, Greene R, Belkind N, et al: Left ventricular functional improvement after transmyocardial laser revascularization. *Ann Thorac Surg* 1998; 66:721.
71. Hughes GC, Kypson AP, St Louis JD, et al: Improved perfusion and contractile reserve after transmyocardial laser revascularization in a model of hibernating myocardium. *Ann Thorac Surg* 1999; 67:1714.
72. Krabatsch T, Modersohn D, Konertz W, et al: Acute changes in functional and metabolic parameters following transmyocardial laser revascularization: an experimental study. *Ann Thorac Cardiovasc Surg* 2000; 6:383.
73. Lutter G, Martin J, von Samson P, et al: Microperfusion enhancement after TMLR in chronically ischemic porcine hearts. *Cardiovasc Surg* 2001; 9:281.
74. Stone GW, Teirstein PS, Rubenstein R, et al: A prospective, multi-center, randomized trial of percutaneous transmyocardial laser revascularization in patients with nonrecanalizable chronic total occlusions. *J Am Coll Cardiol* 2002; 39:1581.
75. Horvath KA: Thoracoscopic transmyocardial laser revascularization. *Ann Thorac Surg* 1998; 65:1439.
76. Frazier OH, Kadipasaoglu KA, Radovancevic B, et al: Transmyocardial laser revascularization in allograft coronary artery disease. *Ann Thorac Surg* 1998; 65:1138.
77. Sayeed-Shah U, Mann MJ, Martin J, et al: Complete reversal of ischemic wall motion abnormalities by combined use of gene therapy with transmyocardial laser revascularization. *J Thorac Cardiovasc Surg* 1998; 116:763.
78. Doukas J, Ma CL, Craig D, et al: Therapeutic angiogenesis induced by *FGF-2* gene delivery combined with laser transmyocardial revascularization. *Circulation* 2000; 102:1214.
79. Lutter G, Dern P, Attmann T, et al: Combined use of transmyocardial laser revascularization with basic fibroblastic growth factor in chronically ischemic porcine hearts. *Circulation* 2000; 102:3693.
80. Esch F, Baird A, Ling N, et al: Primary structure of bovine pituitary basic fibroblast growth factor (FGF) and comparison with the amino-terminal sequence of bovine brain acidic FGF. *Proc Natl Acad Sci USA* 1985; 82:6507.
81. Connolly DT, Heuvelman DM, Nelson R, et al: Tumor vascular permeability factor stimulates endothelial cell growth and angiogenesis. *J Clin Invest* 1989; 84:1470.
82. Wilting J, Christ B, Weich HA: The effects of growth factors on the day 13 chorioallantoic membrane (CAM): a study of $VEGF_{165}$ and PDGF-BB. *Anat Embryol* 1992; 186:251.
83. Yancopoulos GD, Davis S, Gale NW, et al: Vascular-specific growth factors and blood vessel formation. *Nature* 2000; 407:242.
84. Unger EF, Banai S, Shou M, et al: Basic fibroblast growth factor enhances myocardial collateral flow in a canine model. *Am J Physiol* 1994; 266: H1588.
85. Baffour R, Berman J, Garb JL, et al: Enhanced angiogenesis and growth of collaterals by in vivo administration of recombinant basic fibroblast growth factor in a rabbit model of acute lower limb ischemia: dose-response effect of basic fibroblast growth factor. *J Vasc Surg* 1992; 16:181.
86. Lazarous DF, Shou M, Scheinowitz M, et al: Comparative effects of basic fibroblast growth factor and vascular endothelial growth factor on coronary collateral development and the arterial response to injury. *Circulation* 1996; 94:1074.
87. Rajanayagam MA, Shou M, Thirumurti V, et al: Intracoronary basic fibroblast growth factor enhances myocardial collateral per-fusion in dogs. *J Am Coll Cardiol* 2000; 35:519.
88. Lazarous DF, Shou M, Stiber JA, et al: Pharmacodynamics of basic fibroblast growth factor: route of administration determines myocardial and systemic distribution. *Cardiovasc Res* 1997; 36:78.
89. Lopez JJ, Laham RJ, Stamler A, et al: VEGF administration in chronic myocardial ischemia in pigs. *Cardiovasc Res* 1998; 40:272.

90. Roth D, Maruoka Y, Rogers J, et al: Development of coronary collateral circulation in left circumflex ameroid-occluded swine myocardium. *Am J Physiol* 1987; 253:H1279.
91. Hariawala MD, Horowitz JR, Esakof D, et al: VEGF improves myocardial blood flow but produces EDRF-mediated hypotension in porcine hearts. *J Surg Res* 1996; 63:77.
92. Bauters C, Asahara T, Zheng LP, et al: Site-specific therapeutic angiogenesis after systemic administration of vascular endothelial growth factor. *J Vasc Surg* 1995; 21:314.
93. Schumacher B, Pecher P, von Specht BU, et al: Induction of neoangiogenesis in ischemic myocardium by human growth factors: first clinical results of a new treatment of coronary heart disease. *Circulation* 1998; 97:645.
94. Simons M, Annex BH, Laham RJ, et al: Pharmacological treatment of coronary artery disease with recombinant fibroblast growth factor-2. Double-blind, randomized, controlled clinical trial. *Circulation* 2002; 105:788.
95. Laham RJ, Sellke FW, Edelman ER, et al: Local perivascular delivery of basic fibroblast growth factor in patients undergoing coronary bypass surgery: results of a Phase I randomized, double-blind, placebo-controlled trial. *Circulation* 1999; 100:1865
96. Hendel RC, Henry TD, Rocha-Singh K, et al: Effect of intracoronary recombinant human vascular endothelial growth factor on myocardial perfusion: evidence for a dose-dependent effect. *Circulation* 2000; 101:118.
97. Henry TD, Annex BH, McKendall GR, et al: The VIVA trial. Vascular endothelial growth factor in ischemia for vascular angiogenesis. *Circulation* 2003; 107:1359.
98. Giordano FJ, Ping P, Mckirnan D, et al: Intracoronary gene transfer of fibroblast growth factor-5 increases blood flow and contractile function in an ischemic region of the heart. *Nature Med* 1996; 2:534.
99. Gao MH, Lai NC, Mckirnan MD, et al: Increased regional function and perfusion after intracoronary delivery of adenovirus encoding fibroblast growth factor 4: report of preclinical data. *Hum Gene Ther* 2004; 15:574.
100. Horvath KA, Lu CYJ, Robert E, et al: Improvement of myocardial contractility in a porcine model of chronic ischemia using a combined transmyocardial revascularization and gene therapy approach. *J Thorac Cardiovasc Surg* 2005; 129:1071.
101. Witzenbichler B, Asahara T, Murohara T, et al: Vascular endothelial growth factor-C (VEGF-C/VEGF-2) promotes angiogenesis in the setting of tissue ischemia. *Am J Pathol* 1998; 153:381.
102. Laham RJ, Rezaee M, Post M, et al: Intrapericardial administration of basic fibroblast growth factor: myocardial and tissue distribution and comparison with intracoronary and intravenous administration. *Catheter Cardiovasc Interv* 2003; 58:375.
103. Guzman RJ, Lemarchand P, Crystal RG, et al: Efficient gene transfer into myocardium by direct injection of adenovirus vectors. *Circ Res* 1993; 73:1202.
104. Mack CA, Patel SR, Schwartz EA, et al: Biologic bypass with the use of adenovirus-mediated gene transfer of the complementary deoxyribonucleic acid for VEGF-12, improves myocardial perfusion and function in the ischemic porcine heart. *J Thorac Cardiovasc Surg* 1998; 115:168.
105. Vale PR, Losordo DW, Tkebuchava T, et al: Catheter-based myocardial gene transfer utilizing nonfluoroscopic electromechanical left ventricular mapping. *J Am Coll Cardiol* 1999; 34:246.
106. Zhou YF, Stabile E, Walker J, et al: Effects of gene delivery on collateral development in chronic hypoperfusion: diverse effects of angiopoietin-1 versus vascular endothelial growth factor. *J Am Coll Cardiol* 2004; 44:897.
107. Masaki I, Yonemitsu Y, Yamashita A, et al: Angiogenic gene therapy for experimental critical limb ischemia. Acceration of limb loss by overexpression of vascular endothelial growth factor 165 but not fibrobast growth factor-2. *Circ Res* 2002; 90:966.
108. Rosengart TK, Lee LY, Patel SR, et al: Angiogenesis gene therapy: phase I assessment of direct intramyocardial administration of an adenovirus vector expressing VEGF121 cDNA to individuals with clinically significant severe coronary artery disease. *Circulation* 1999; 100:468.
109. Losordo DW, Vale PR, Hendel RC, et al: Phase 1/2 placebo-controlled, double-blind, dose-escalating trial of myocardial vascular endothelial growth factor2 gene transfer by catheter delivery in patients with chronic myocardial ischemia. *Circulation* 2002; 105:2012.
110. Grines CL, Watkins MW, Helmer G, et al: Angiogenic gene therapy (AGENT) trial patients with stable angina pectoris. *Circulation* 2002; 105:1291.
111. Grines CL, Watkins MW, Mahamarian JJ, et al: A randomized, double blind, placebo-controlled trial of Ad5FGF-4 gene therapy and its effect on myocardial perfusion in patients with stable angina. *J Am Coll Cardiol* 2003; 42:1339.
112. Hedman M, Hartikainen J, Syvänne M, et al: Safety and feasibility of catheter-based local intracoronary vascular endothelial growth factor gene transfer in the prevention of postangioplasty and instent restenosis and in the treatment of chronic myocardial ischemia. Phase II results of the Kuopio Angiogenesis Trial (KAT). *Circulation* 2003; 107:2677.
113. Kastrup J, Jørgensen E, Rück A, et al: Direct intramyocardial plasmid vascular endothelial growth factor-A_{165} gene therapy in patients with stable severe angina pectoris. A randomized double-blind placebo-controlled study: the Euroinject One Trial. *J Am Coll Cardiol* 2005; 45:982.
114. Assmus B, Schächinger V, Teupe C, et al: Transplantation of progenitor cells and regeneration enhancement in acute myocardial infarction (TOPCARE-AMI). *Circulation* 2002; 106:3009.
115. Britten MB, Abolmaali ND, Assmus B, et al: Infarct remodeling after intracoronary progenitor cell treatment in patients with acute myocardial infarction (TOPCARE-AMI)-mechanistic insights from serial contrast-enhanced magnetic resonance imaging. *Circulation* 2003; 108:2212.
116. Schächinger V, Assmus B, Britten MB, et al: Transplantation of progenitor cells and regeneration enhancement in acute myocardial infarction—final one-year results of the TOPCARE-AMI trial. *J Am Coll Cardiol* 2004; 44:1690.
117. Assmus B, Ulrich FR, Honold J, et al: Transcoronary transplantation of functionally competent BMCs is associated with a decrease in natriuretic peptide serum levels and improved survival of patients with chronic postinfarction heart failure-results of the TOPCARE-CHD registry. Circ Res. 2007; 100;1234-1241.
118. Strauer BE, Brehm M, Zeus T, et al: Repair of infarcted myocardium by autologous intracoronary mononuclear bone marrow cell transplantation in humans. *Circulation* 2002; 106:1913.
119. Strauer BE, Brehm M, Zeus T, et al: Regeneration of human infarcted heart muscle by intracoronary autologous bone marrow cell transplantation in chronic coronary artery disease the IACT study. *J Am Coll Cardiol* 2005; 46:1651.
120. Wollert KC, Meyer GP, Lotz J, et al: Intracoronary autologous bone-marrow cell transfer after myocardial infarction: the BOOST randomized controlled clinical trial. Lancet 2004; 364:141-148.
121. Meyer GP, Wollert KC, Lotz J, et al: Intracoronary autologous bone-marrow cell transfer after myocardial infarction: 5-year follow-up from randomized-controlled BOOST trial. *Eur Heart J* 2009; 30: 2978-2984.
122. Perin EC, Dohmann HFR, Borojevic R, et al: Transendocardial, autologous bone marrow cell transplantation for severe, chronic ischemic heart failure. *Circulation* 2003; 107:2294.
123. Fuchs S, Baffour R, Zhou YF, et al: Transendocardial delivery of autologous bone marrow enhances collateral perfusion and regional function in pigs with chronic experimental myocardial ischemia. *J Am Coll Cardiol* 2001; 37:1726.
124. Fuchs S, Satler LF, Kornowski R, et al: Catheter-based autologous bone marrow myocardial injection in no-option patients with advanced coronary artery disease. *J Am Coll Cardiol* 2003; 41:1721.
125. Chen SL, Fang WW, Ye F, et al: Effect on left ventricular function of intracoronary transplantation of autologous bone marrow mesenchymal stem cell in patients with acute myocardial infarction. *Am J Cardiol* 2004; 94:92.
126. Kang HJ, Kim HS, Zhang SY, et al: Effects of intracoronary infusion of peripheral blood stem cells mobilized with granulocyte colony stimulating factor on left ventricular systolic function and restenosis after coronary stenting in myocardial infarction: the MAGIC cell randomized clinical trial. *Lancet* 2004; 363:751.
127. Zohlnhofer D, Ott I, Mehilli J, et al: Stem cell mobilization by granulocyte colony-stimulating factor in patients with acute myocardial infarction-a randomized controlled trial. *JAMA* 2006; 295:1003-1010.
128. Taylor DA, Atkins BZ, Hungspreugs P, et al: Regenerating functional myocardium: improved performance after skeletal myoblast transplantation. *Nat Med* 1998; 4:929-933.
129. Menasché P, Alfieri O, Janssens S, et al: The myoblast autologous grafting in ischemic cardiomyopathy (MAGIC) trial-first randomized placebo-controlled study of myoblast transplantation. *Circulation* 2008; 117:1189-1200.
130. Patel AN, Geffner L, Vina RF, et al: Congestive heart hailure with autologous adult stem cell transplantation: a prospective randomized study. *J Thorac Cardiovasc Surg* 2005; 130:1631.
131. Hare JM, Traverse JH, Henry TD, et al: A randomized, double-blind, placebo-controlled, dose-escalation study of intravenous adult human mesenchymal stem cells (Prochymal) after acute myocardial infarction. *J Am Coll Cardiol* 2009; 54:2277-2286.
132. Banai S, Jaklitsch MT, Casscells W, et al: Effects of acidic fibroblast growth factor on normal and ischemic myocardium. *Circ Res* 1991; 69:76.

133. Thurston G, Rudge JS, Ioffe E, et al: Angiopoietin-1 protects the adult vasculature against plasma leakage. *Nat Med* 2000; 6:460.
134. Flugelman MY, Virmani R, Correa R, et al: Smooth muscle cell abundance and fibroblast growth factors in coronary lesions of patients with nonfatal unstable angina: a clue to the mechanism of transformation from the stable to the unstable clinical state. *Circulation* 1993; 88:2493.
135. Inoue M, Itoh H, Ueda M, et al: Vascular endothelial growth factor (VEGF) expression in human coronary atherosclerotic lesions: possible pathophysiological significance of VEGF in progression of atherosclerosis. *Circulation* 1998; 98:2108.
136. Herold-Mende C, Steiner HH, Andl T, et al: Expression and functional significance of vascular endothelial growth factor receptors in human tumor cells. *Lab Invest* 1999; 79:1573.
137. Brown LF, Detmar M, Tognazzi K, et al: Uterine smooth muscle cells express functional receptors (flt-1 and KDR) for vascular permeability factor/vascular endothelial growth factor. *Lab Invest* 1997; 76:245.
138. Hanahan D, Folkman J: Patterns and emerging mechanisms of the angiogenic switch during tumorigenesis. *Cell* 1996; 86:353.
139. O'Brien ER, Garvin MR, Dev R, et al: Angiogenesis in human coronary atherosclerotic plaques. *Am J Pathol* 1994; 145:883.
140. Schwarz ER, Speakman MT, Patterson M, et al: Evaluation of the effects of intramyocardial injection of DNA expressing vascular endothelial growth factor (VEGF) in a myocardial infarction model in the rat: angiogenesis and angioma formation. *J Am Coll Cardiol* 2000; 35:1323.
141. Nabel EG, Yang ZY, Plautz G, et al: Recombinant fibroblast growth factor-1 promotes intimal hyperplasia and angiogenesis in arteries in vivo. *Nature* 1993; 362:844.
142. Unger EF, Goncalves L, Epstein SE, et al: Effects of a single intra-coronary injection of basic fibroblast growth factor in stable angina pectoris. *Am J Cardiol* 2000; 85:1414.
143. Horowitz JR, Rivard A, van der Zee R, et al: Vascular endothelial growth factor/vascular permeability factor produces nitric oxide-dependent hypotension: evidence for a maintenance role in quiescent adult endothelium. *Arterioscler Thromb Vasc Biol* 1997; 17:2793.
144. Cuevas P, Carceller F, Ortega S, et al: Hypotensive activity of fibroblast growth factor. *Science* 1991; 254:1208.
145. Zhou YF, Bosch-Marce M, Okuyama H, et al: Spontaneous transformation of cultured mouse bone marrow–derived stromal cells. *Cancer Res* 2006; 66:10849.

CHAPTER 28

Surgical Treatment of Complications of Acute Myocardial Infarction: Postinfarction Ventricular Septal Defect and Free Wall Rupture

Arvind K. Agnihotri
Joren C. Madsen
Willard M. Daggett, Jr.

INTRODUCTION

Rupture of the ventricular chamber (septum or free wall) after myocardial infarction is a relatively infrequent condition with high mortality. An *acute* postinfarction VSD is a perforation of the muscular ventricular septum occurring in an area of acutely infarcted myocardium. A ventricular septal rupture may be termed *chronic* when it has been present for more than 4 to 6 weeks. A *postinfarction ventricular rupture* is a perforation of the ventricular free wall occurring in an area of acutely infarcted myocardium. These conditions, resulting from transmural infarction, may cause rapid hemodynamic compromise and early death precluding surgical repair. Free wall rupture can result in tamponade and sudden cardiovascular collapse. In ventricular septal rupture, there is a variable amount of left-to-right shunting, but such defects typically lead to symptoms of heart failure. The clinical presentation ranges from an asymptomatic murmur to cardiogenic shock and sudden death.

The early evolution of successful surgical repair of an acute postinfarction ventricular septal rupture involved differentiating the surgical treatment of these acquired lesions from surgical approaches used to repair congenital ventricular septal defects (VSDs), which are for the most part not applicable. Initial success was achieved with methods involving infarctectomy and patching. Specific methods were developed for differing anatomical locations of postinfarction VSDs, including location of the cardiotomy and patch methodology. With experience, there was gradual appreciation of different clinical courses pursued by patients after postinfarction ventricular septal rupture, both in terms of location of the defect and the degree of right ventricular functional impairment, led to an increased urgency relative to the timing of surgical repair. An important paradigm shift had resulted from improved results utsing a technique of endocardial patching with infarct exclusion. Surgical management requires an understanding of the various approaches. The incorporation of specific anatomic concepts of surgical repair and a better understanding of the physiologic basis of the disease has led to an integrated approach to the patient that has improved salvage of patients suffering this catastrophic complication of acute myocardial infarction (AMI).

History

In 1845 Latham[1] described a postinfarction ventricular septal rupture at autopsy, but it was not until 1923 that Brunn[2] first made the diagnosis antemortem. Sager[3] in 1934 added the 18th case to the world literature and established specific clinical criteria for diagnosis, stressing the association of postinfarction septal rupture with coronary artery disease (CAD).

The treatment of this entity was medical and strictly palliative until 1956, when Cooley and associates[4] performed the first successful surgical repair in a patient 9 weeks after the diagnosis of septal rupture. These first patients who underwent similar repairs in the early 1960s usually presented with congestive heart failure (CHF), having survived for more than a month after acute septal perforation.[5,6] The success of operation in these patients and the precipitous, acute course of other patients with this complication gave rise to the belief that operative repair should be limited to patients surviving for 1 month or longer.[6,7] This purportedly allowed for scarring at the edges of the defect, which was thought to be crucial to the secure and long-lasting closure of the septal rupture.[8,9]

In the late 1960s, more rapid recognition of septal rupture after infarction led to the recommendation that operation be attempted earlier in patients who were hemodynamically deteriorating. Notable among these was a superb early study by Heimbecker and associates of infarctectomy and its clinical application to patients with postinfarction VSDs. The surgical management of these patients was further refined by the inclusion of infarctectomy and aneurysmectomy and the development of techniques to repair perforations in different areas of the septum.[10–12] Improved surgical techniques, newer prosthetic materials, enhanced myocardial protection, and improved perioperative mechanical and pharmacologic support have led to more favorable results in the surgical management of patients with postinfarction septal rupture.

Incidence

Postinfarction ventricular septal defects complicate approximately 1 to 2% of cases of AMIs and account for about 5% of early deaths after MI.[13,14] The average time from infarction to rupture has been reported to be between 2 and 4 days, but it may be as short as a few hours or as long as 2 weeks.[15,16] These observations correlate well with the pathologic findings, which demonstrate that necrotic tissue is most abundant and ingrowth of blood vessels and connective tissue is only beginning 4 to 21 days after an MI.[17] Postinfarction ventricular septal defects occur in men more often than women (3:2), but more women experience rupture than what would be expected from the incidence of CAD in women. The average age of patients with this complication is 62.5 years, although there is some evidence that more elderly patients are being seen in the recent era. The vast majority of patients who experience ventricular septal rupture do so after their initial infarction.[18] The overall incidence of postinfarction ventricular septal rupture may have decreased slightly during the past decade as a result of aggressive pharmacologic treatment of ischemia and thrombolytic and interventional therapy in patients with evolving MI, as well as the prompt control of hypertension in these patients. The effect of widespread use of percutaneous angioplasty and stenting on the appearance of this complication of MI is not well documented, but several large centers, including ours, have had a decreased number of post-MI VSD patients in the past 10 years.

Angiographic evaluation of patients with postinfarction ventricular rupture indicates that septal rupture is usually associated with complete occlusion rather than severe stenosis of a coronary artery.[19] On average, these patients have slightly less extensive CAD, as well as less developed septal collaterals than do other patients with CAD.[20] The lack of collateral flow noted acutely may be secondary to anatomical configuration, edema, or associated arterial disease. Hill and associates,[21] in reviewing 19 cases of postinfarction ventricular septal rupture, found single-vessel disease in 64%, double-vessel disease in 7%, and triple-vessel disease in 29%. However, the frequency of single-, double-, and triple-vessel CAD is more evenly distributed in other series.[16,22]

Postinfarction ventricular septal defects are most commonly located in the anteroapical septum as the result of a full-thickness anterior infarction (in approximately 60% of cases). These anterior septal ruptures are caused by anteroseptal MI after occlusion of the left anterior descending (LAD) artery. In about 40% of patients, the rupture occurs in the posterior septum after an inferoseptal infarction, which is usually owing to occlusion of a dominant right coronary artery, or less frequently, a dominant circumflex artery. Thus, ventricular septal perforations occur most frequently in 65-year-old men with single-vessel coronary disease and poor collateral flow who present 2 to 4 days after their first anterior MI.

Pathogenesis

The infarct associated with septal rupture is transmural and generally quite extensive, involving, on average, 26% of the left ventricular wall in hearts with septal rupture, compared with only 15% in other acute infarctions.[14] In an autopsy study, Cummings and colleagues[23] found that in patients with acute anterior or inferior infarctions, the amount of right ventricular infarction was much greater in the hearts with septal ruptures as compared with those without septal defects. Likewise, hearts with posterior septal rupture had more extensive left ventricular necrosis than did hearts with inferior infarctions and no septal defects.

Why certain hearts rupture and others do not is not fully understood. Slippage of myocytes during infarct expansion may allow blood to dissect through the necrotic myocardium and enter either the right ventricle or pericardial space. Hyaline degeneration of cardiomyocytes with subsequent fragmentation and enzymatic digestion may allow fissures to form, predisposing to rupture.[24–26]

There are two types of rupture: simple, consisting of a direct through-and-through defect usually located anteriorly; and complex, consisting of a serpiginous dissection tract remote from the primary septal defect, which is usually located inferiorly. Multiple defects, which may develop within several days of each other, occur in 5 to 11% of cases and are probably caused by infarct extension. Because a successful surgical outcome is related to adequacy of closure of septal defects, multiple defects must be sought preoperatively if possible, and certainly at the time of operative repair.

Of the small number of patients who survive the early period of ventricular septal rupture, 35 to 68% go on to develop ventricular aneurysms through the process of ventricular remodeling.[27] This compares with an approximately 12% incidence of aneurysm formation in patients suffering an infarction but no septal rupture,[28] and probably relates to the size and transmural nature of the infarction associated with septal rupture. Postinfarction septal rupture, especially in the posterior septum, may be accompanied by mitral valve regurgitation resulting from papillary muscle infarction or dysfunction. In approximately one-third of cases of septal rupture, there is a degree of mitral insufficiency, usually functional in nature, secondary to left ventricular (LV) dysfunction with mitral annular dilation, which usually resolves with repair of the defect.[20]

Pathophysiology

The most important determinant of early outcome after postinfarction ventricular septal rupture is the development of heart failure (left, right, or both). The associated cardiogenic shock leads to end-organ malperfusion, which may be irreversible.

The degree to which heart failure develops depends on the size of the ventricular infarction and the magnitude of the left-to-right shunt. Left ventricular dysfunction resulting from extensive necrosis of the left ventricle is the primary determinant of CHF and cardiogenic shock in patients with anterior septal rupture, whereas right ventricular dysfunction secondary to extensive infarction of the right ventricle is the principal determinant of heart failure and cardiogenic shock in patients with posterior septal rupture. However, the development of CHF and cardiogenic shock in a patient with postinfarction VSDs is not explained solely by the degree of damage sustained by the ventricle.

The magnitude of the left-to-right shunt is the other key variable in the development of hemodynamic compromise. With the opening of a VSD, the heart is challenged by an increase in pulmonary blood flow, and a decrease in systemic blood flow, as a portion of each stroke volume is diverted to the pulmonary circuit. As a consequence of the sudden increase in hemodynamic load imposed on a heart already compromised by acute infarction, and possibly by a ventricular aneurysm, mitral valve dysfunction, or a combination of these problems, a severe low cardiac output state results. The normally compliant right ventricle is especially susceptible to failure in this circumstance.[29,30] Patients with posterior ventricular septal rupture and right ventricular dysfunction may display shunt reversal during diastole because the end-diastolic pressure in the right ventricle can be higher than in the left. Ultimately, persistence of a low cardiac output state results in peripheral organ failure.

Diagnosis

The typical presentation of a ventricular septal rupture is that of a patient who has suffered an AMI, and who after convalescing for a few days develops a new systolic murmur, recurrent chest pain, and an abrupt deterioration in hemodynamics. The development of a loud systolic murmur, usually within the first week after an AMI, is the most consistent physical finding of postinfarction ventricular septal rupture (present in greater than 90% of patients). The murmur is usually harsh, pansystolic, and best heard at the left lower sternal border. The murmur is often associated with a palpable thrill. Depending on the location of the septal defect, the murmur may radiate to the left axilla, thereby mimicking mitral regurgitation. Up to one-half of these patients experience postinfarction chest pain in association with the appearance of the murmur.[14] Coincident with the onset of the murmur, there is usually an abrupt decline in the patient's clinical course, with the onset of congestive failure and often cardiogenic shock. The findings of cardiac failure that occur acutely in these patients are primarily the result of right-sided heart failure, with pulmonary edema being less prominent than that occurring in patients with acute mitral regurgitation caused by a ruptured papillary muscle.[32]

The electrocardiographic (ECG) findings in patients with acute septal rupture relate to the changes associated with antecedent anterior, inferior, posterior, or septal infarction. The localization of infarction by ECG correlates highly with the location of the associated septal perforation. In our review[18] of 55 patients with postinfarction septal rupture, the location of the defect corresponded to the territory of transmural infarction as determined by ECG in all but three patients. Up to one-third of patients develop some degree of atrioventricular conduction block (usually transient) that may precede rupture,[33] but there is no pathognomonic prognostic indicator of impending perforation. The chest radiograph usually shows increased pulmonary vascularity consistent with pulmonary venous hypertension.

It is important to realize that the sudden appearance of a systolic murmur and hemodynamic deterioration after infarction may also result from acute mitral regurgitation caused by a ruptured papillary muscle. Distinguishing these two lesions clinically is difficult, and an urgent echocardiogram should be obtained. A number of points may help with the initial evaluation. First, the systolic murmur associated with a septal rupture is more prominent at the left sternal border, whereas the murmur resulting from a ruptured papillary muscle is best heard at the apex. Second, the murmur associated with septal perforation is loud and associated with a thrill (in greater than 50% of patients), whereas the murmur of acute mitral regurgitation is softer and has no associated thrill. Third, septal rupture is often associated with anterior infarctions and conduction abnormalities, whereas papillary muscle rupture is commonly associated with an inferior infarction and no conduction defects. Finally, it should be noted that septal rupture and papillary muscle rupture may coexist after infarction.[34,35]

Historically, the mainstay of differentiating septal rupture from mitral valve dysfunction has been right heart catheterization using the Swan-Ganz catheter.[36] With septal rupture, there is an oxygen saturation step-up between the right atrium and pulmonary artery. Step-up in oxygen saturation greater than 9% between the right atrium and pulmonary artery confirms the presence of a shunt. The pulmonary-to-systemic flow ratios (Qp:Qs) obtained from oxygen saturation samples range from 1.4:1 to greater than 8:1 and roughly correlate with the size of the defect. In contrast, with acute mitral regurgitation secondary to papillary muscle rupture, there are classic giant V waves in the pulmonary artery wedge pressure trace. It should be noted, however, that up to one-third of patients with septal rupture also have mild mitral regurgitation secondary to LV dysfunction.[37]

Advances in transthoracic and transesophageal echocardiography, especially color flow Doppler mapping, have revolutionized the diagnosis of both the presence and site of septal rupture. Echocardiography can detect the defect, localize its site and size, determine right and left ventricular function, assess pulmonary artery and right ventricular pressures, and exclude coexisting mitral regurgitation or free wall rupture. Twenty years ago, Smyllie and associates[38] reported 100% specificity and 100% sensitivity when color flow Doppler mapping was used to differentiate ventricular septal rupture from acute severe mitral regurgitation following AMI. It also correctly demonstrated the site of septal rupture in 41 of 42 patients. Widespread use of this technology has made this imaging the primary method of diagnosis. Indeed, the trend in the past two decades toward early surgical referral and prompt operative repair is at least partially explained by the routine use of color Doppler echocardiography for diagnosis in peripheral centers.

The necessity of preoperative left heart catheterization with coronary angiography has been a matter of debate. On one hand, left heart catheterization provides important information concerning associated CAD, left ventricular wall motion, and specifics of valvular dysfunction, which are all important in planning operative correction of postinfarction septal rupture. In most series, greater than 60% of patients with septal rupture have significant involvement of at least one vessel other than the one supplying the infarcted area. Arguably, bypassing associated CAD may increase long-term survival when compared with patients with unbypassed CAD.[39] However, left heart catheterization has disadvantages—it is time consuming, requires use of nephrotoxic dye, and may contribute to both the mortality and morbidity of these already compromised patients. Thus, some centers do not carry out preoperative left heart catheterization. Others use it selectively, avoiding invasive studies in patients with septal rupture caused by anterior wall infarction, which is associated with a much lower incidence of multiple-vessel disease than septal defects resulting from posterior infarctions. The issue of concomitant coronary bypassing is discussed in greater detail below.

Natural History

Reviews by Oyamada and Queen,[40] and Kirklin and coworkers[41] reveal that nearly 25% of patients with postinfarction septal rupture and no surgical intervention died within the first 24 hours, 50% died within 1 week, 65% within 2 weeks, and 80% within 4 weeks; only 7% lived longer than 1 year. Lemery and associates[42] reported that of 25 patients with postinfarction VSDs treated medically, 19 died within 1 month. Thus, the risk of death after postinfarction VSD is highest immediately after infarction and septal rupture, and then gradually declines. Interestingly, there are reports of spontaneous closure of small defects, although this is so rare that it would be unreasonable to manage a patient with the expectation of closure.

Despite the many advances in the nonoperative treatment of CHF and cardiogenic shock, including the intra-aortic balloon pump and a multitude of new inotropic agents and vasodilators, these do not supplant the need for operative intervention in these critically ill patients.

Management

It has become clear that the early practice of waiting for several weeks after ventricular septal rupture before proceeding with intervention only selects out the small minority of patients in whom the hemodynamic insult is less severe and is better tolerated.[22,24] Likewise, it has also become clear that to manage most patients supportively, in hopes of deferring intervention, is to deprive the great majority of those with postinfarction ventricular septal rupture of the benefits of definitive surgery before irreversible damage resulting from peripheral organ ischemia has occurred.[43]

In addition to definitive surgical closure, early intervention can include mechanical support and device closure. The routine use of the intra-aortic balloon pump (IABP), whenever technically feasible, frequently results in *transient* reversal of the hemodynamic deterioration. This period of stability often makes it possible to complete left heart catheterization before proceeding to operation, but should not significantly delay definitive surgical treatment. In general, an IABP should be placed once the diagnosis is made, unless more aggressive mechanical support is immediately planned. In patients who are deemed to be at unacceptable risk for definitive surgery, there may be a role for left or biventricular support to bridge the patient to surgery (see the following). The high-risk patient may also represent a category in whom catheter-based device placement may greatly improve hemodynamic function and lead to stabilization, with a planned operation after recovery from the acute illness (see the following).

Although we as well as others have advocated early intervention since the middle of the 1970s, some continue to prefer to defer operation in patients who are easily supported and exhibit no further hemodynamic deterioration. Persistence of CHF or marginal stabilization with rising blood urea nitrogen and borderline urine output necessitate aggressive therapy and prompt operation. Patients with septal rupture rarely die of cardiac failure per se, but rather of end-organ failure as a consequence of shock.

Our experience and the experience of others suggest that patients in cardiogenic shock represent a true surgical emergency requiring immediate intervention, which may include surgery, mechanical support, or catheter options. Because deaths in these patients result from multisystem failure secondary to organ hypoperfusion, delay in operative repair (or mechanical support) for patients in cardiogenic shock represents a failed therapeutic strategy. Those few patients who are completely stable, with no clinical deterioration, and who require no hemodynamic support, can undergo operative repair when convenient during that hospitalization. The large group of patients who are in an intermediate position between those with shock and those in stable condition should have intervention early (usually within 12 to 24 hours) after appropriate preoperative evaluation. Because the group of patients in stable condition constitutes 5% or less of the total population of patients with postinfarction ventricular septal rupture, the overwhelming majority of patients require prompt treatment.

Rarely, because of a delayed referral, a patient will be seen for surgical therapy who is already in a state of multisystem failure or has developed septic complications. Such a patient is unlikely to survive an emergency operation and thus may benefit from prolonged support with an IABP before an attempted operative repair. We have found it necessary to treat a small number of patients (3 of 92) in this fashion. Baillot and colleagues[44] have reported individual successes with such an approach, which we consider the exception rather than the rule.

Preoperative Management

Preoperative management is directed toward stabilization of the hemodynamic condition so that peripheral organ perfusion can be best maintained while any further diagnostic studies are obtained and while deciding on the optimal time for surgical intervention. Although the early clinical course of patients with postinfarction ventricular septal rupture can be quite variable, 50 to 60% present with severe CHF and a low cardiac output state requiring intensive therapy.[45,74]

The goals of preoperative management are to: (1) reduce the systemic vascular resistance, and thus the left-to-right shunt; (2) maintain cardiac output and arterial pressure to ensure peripheral organ perfusion; and (3) maintain or improve coronary artery blood flow. This is best accomplished by the IABP. Counterpulsation reduces left ventricular afterload, thereby increasing cardiac output and decreasing the left-to-right shunt, as reported by Gold and associates in 1973.[46] In addition, IABP support is associated with decreased myocardial oxygen consumption, as well as improved myocardial and peripheral organ perfusion. Although counterpulsation produces an overall improvement in the patient's condition, a complete correction of the hemodynamic picture cannot be obtained.[47] Peak improvement occurs within 24 hours and no further benefit has been observed with prolonged balloon pumping.[48]

Pharmacologic therapy with inotropic agents and diuretics should be instituted promptly. The addition of vasodilators (ie, sodium nitroprusside or intravenous nitroglycerine) makes good theoretical sense, because it can decrease the left-to-right shunting associated with the mechanical defect, and thus increase cardiac output. However, these effects are often associated with a marked fall in mean arterial blood pressure and reduced coronary perfusion, both poorly tolerated in these critically ill patients. It must be stressed that pharmacologic therapy is intended primarily to support the patient in preparation for operation and should not in any way delay urgent operation in the critically ill patient. We now admit patients with postinfarction septal rupture directly to the surgical intensive care unit rather than to the coronary care or medical intensive care unit.

Other techniques that have been tried in an effort to improve the hemodynamics of patients with interventricular septal rupture include left ventricular mechanical support, venoarterial extracorporeal membrane oxygenation, and inflation of a balloon in the right ventricular outflow tract to decrease the left-to-right shunt. At the present, we believe these techniques should be reserved for patients with severe end-organ malperfusion deemed unlikely to survive surgery. To avoid shunting across the lesion (right to left at the ventricular level), atrial cannulation is necessary. Use of a catheter-mounted axial flow pump (Hemopump, Impella) in stabilizing these patients is controversial because of the risk of acute pump failure resulting from catheter blockage from pieces of necrotic tissue.[49]

Operative Techniques

Historical Development

The first repair by Cooley and colleagues of an acquired VSD was accomplished using an approach through the right ventricle with incision of the right ventricular outflow tract.[4] This approach, which was adapted from surgical techniques for closure of congenital VSDs, proved to be disadvantageous for many reasons. Exposure of the defect was frequently less than optimal, particularly for defects located in the apical septum. It involved unnecessary injury to normal right ventricular muscle and interruption of collaterals from the right coronary artery. Finally, it failed to eliminate the paradoxic bulging segment of infarcted left ventricular wall. Subsequently, Heimbecker and associates[9] introduced a left-sided approach (left ventriculotomy) with incision through the area of infarction. Such an approach frequently incorporates infarctectomy and aneurysmectomy, together with repair of septal rupture.[50]

Overview

For the purpose of planning an operative repair, there are three locations of defects: apical, anterior, and posterior/inferior. The apical defect can be considered as a subset of the anterior location, and provides the surgeon the possibility of a straightforward repair, similar to an aneurysmectomy. There are two very different surgical paradigms for repair, one using infarctectomy, and the other infarct exclusion. Posterior lesions are the most challenging with the infarctectomy technique, and there is now a general trend to approach those lesions with exclusion methods. As described in the following, the surgical approach to lesion in various locations requires specific considerations, but certain general principles apply (Tables 28-1A and 28-1B).

Anesthesia and Perfusion

Patients are anesthetized using a fentanyl-based regimen. Pancuronium is selected as the muscle relaxant so as to prevent bradycardia. Pulmonary bed vasodilators such as dobutamine are avoided to minimize the left-to-right shunt fraction. Preoperative

TABLE 28-1A Principles of Infarctectomy Repair of Postinfarction VSD

Transinfarct approach to ventricular septal defect

1. Thorough trimming of the left ventricular margins of the infarct back to viable muscle to prevent delayed rupture of the closure
2. Conservative trimming of the right ventricular muscle as required for complete visualization of the margins of the defect
3. Inspection of the left ventricular papillary muscles and concomitant replacement of the mitral valve only if there is frank papillary muscular rupture
4. Closure of the septal defect without tension, which in most instances will require the use of prosthetic material
5. Closure of the infarctectomy without tension with generous use of prosthetic material as indicated, and epicardial placement of the patch to the free wall to avoid strain on the friable endocardial tissue
6. Buttressing of the suture lines with pledgets or strips of Teflon felt or similar material to prevent sutures from cutting through friable muscle

Source: Heitmiller R, Jacobs ML, Daggett WM: Surgical management of postinfarction ventricular septal rupture. Ann Thorac Surg 1986; 41:683.

TABLE 28-1B Principles of Exclusion Repair of Postinfarction VSD

Transinfarct approach to ventricular septal defect

1. No infarctectomy unless necrotic muscle along ventriculotomy is sloughing during closure
2. Bovine pericardial patch in either an oval (anterior defect) or triangular (posterior defect) shape is sutured securely with continuous Prolene around the defect to exclude it from the LV cavity
3. Where necessary, full-thickness bites are taken to the epicardial surface and anchored by strips of pericardium or Teflon (see text for details)
4. An anterior patch is anchored to noninfarcted septum below the defect, then the noninfarcted endocardium of the anterolateral ventricular wall. If the infarct involves the base of the anterior muscle, full thickness anchoring bites are used.
5. A posterior patch is anchored to the mitral annulus, noninfarcted septum, and through the infarcted posterior wall along a line corresponding to the medial margin of the posteromedial papillary muscle (with full thickness anchoring).
6. Closure of the infarctectomy using strips of pericardium or Teflon
7. When possible, infarcted right ventricular free wall is left undisturbed during closure

Source: David TE, Dale L, Sun Z: Postinfarction ventricular septal rupture: repair by endocardial patch with infarct exclusion. J Thorac Cardiovasc Surg 1995; 110:1315.

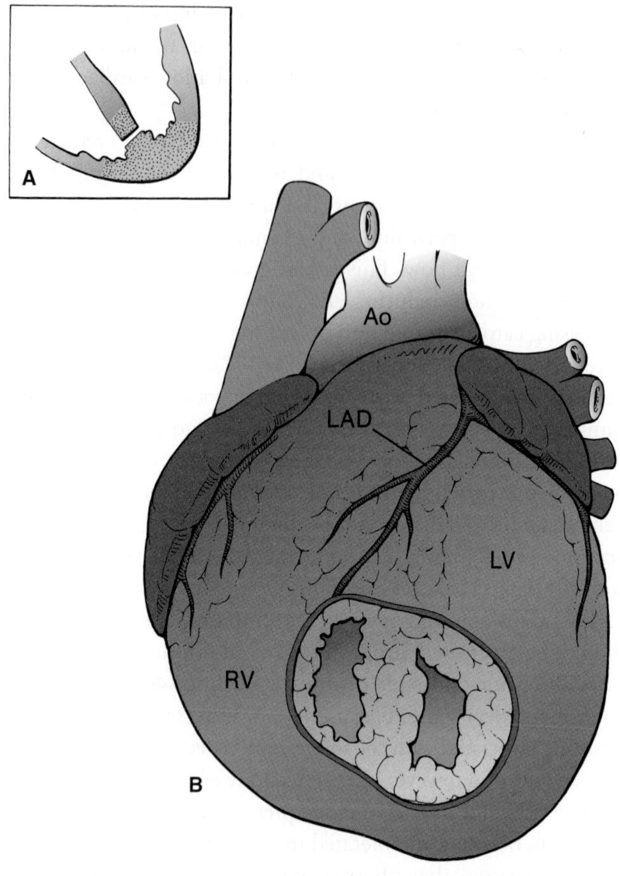

FIGURE 28-1 (A) Apical postinfarction ventricular septal defect. (B) View of the apical septal rupture, which is exposed by amputating the apex of the left and right ventricles. Ao = aorta; LAD = left anterior descending coronary artery; LV = left ventricle; RV = right ventricle; stippled region = infarcted myocardium.

antibiotics include both cefazolin and vancomycin, given the fact that prosthetic material may be left in the patient.

Cardiopulmonary bypass is accomplished with bicaval venous drainage. Standard techniques of myocardial protection for injured hearts are employed. Systemic cooling is begun to 25 to 30°C. Although a number of myocardial protection strategies are currently available, including warm continuous blood, we continue to use cold oxygenated, dilute blood cardioplegia to protect the heart during surgical correction of a VSD.[51] A total of 1200 to 2000 mL of cardioplegia solution is delivered, depending on the size of the heart and the degree of hypertrophy. Although we have not employed warm cardioplegic induction, we do administer warm reperfusion cardioplegia just before removing the aortic cross-clamp.[52] Patients with multivessel coronary disease and critical coronary stenoses are revascularized before opening the heart to optimize myocardial protection. In most of these patients, the saphenous vein rather than the left internal mammary artery is used.

Repair of Apical Septal Rupture

The technique of apical amputation was described by Daggett and colleagues in 1970.[11] An incision is made through the infarcted apex of the left ventricle. Excision of the necrotic myocardium back to healthy muscle results in amputation of the apical portion of the left ventricle, right ventricle, and septum (Figs. 28-1 A and B). The remaining apical portions of the left and right ventricle free walls are then approximated to the apical septum. This is accomplished by means of a row of interrupted mattress sutures of 1-0 Tevdek that are passed sequentially through a buttressing strip of Teflon felt, the left ventricular wall, a second strip of felt, the interventricular septum, a third strip of felt, the right ventricular wall, and a fourth strip of felt (Figs. 28-2 A and B). After all sutures have been tied, the closure is reinforced with an additional over-and-over suture, as in ventricular aneurysm repair, to ensure hemostasis of the ventriculotomy closure.

Anterior Repair with Infarctectomy

The approach to these defects is by a left ventricular transinfarct incision with infarctectomy (Fig. 28-3). Small defects beneath anterior infarcts can be closed by the technique of plication as suggested by Shumacker.[53] This involves approximation of the free anterior edge of the septum to the right ventricular free wall using mattress sutures of 1-0 Tevdek over strips of felt (Fig. 28-4A). The transinfarct incision is then closed with a second row of mattress sutures buttressed with strips of Teflon

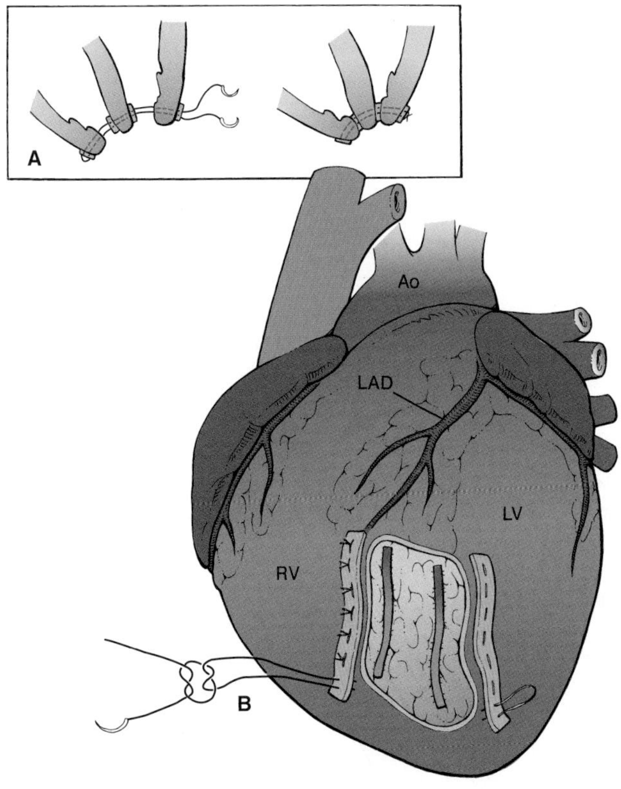

FIGURE 28-2 (A) The necrotic infarct and the apical septum have been débrided back to healthy muscle. Repair is made by approximating the left ventricle, apical septum, and right ventricle using interrupted mattress sutures of 1-0 Tevdek with but tressing strips of Teflon felt. Felt strips are used within the interior of the left and right ventricles as well as on the epicardial surface of each ventricle. (B) All sutures are placed before any are tied. A second running over-and-over suture (not shown) is used, as in left ventricular aneurysm repair, to ensure a secure hemostatic ventriculotomy closure. Ao = aorta; LAD = left anterior descending coronary artery; LV = left ventricle; RV = right ventricle. (*Adapted with permission from Daggett et al. 16*)

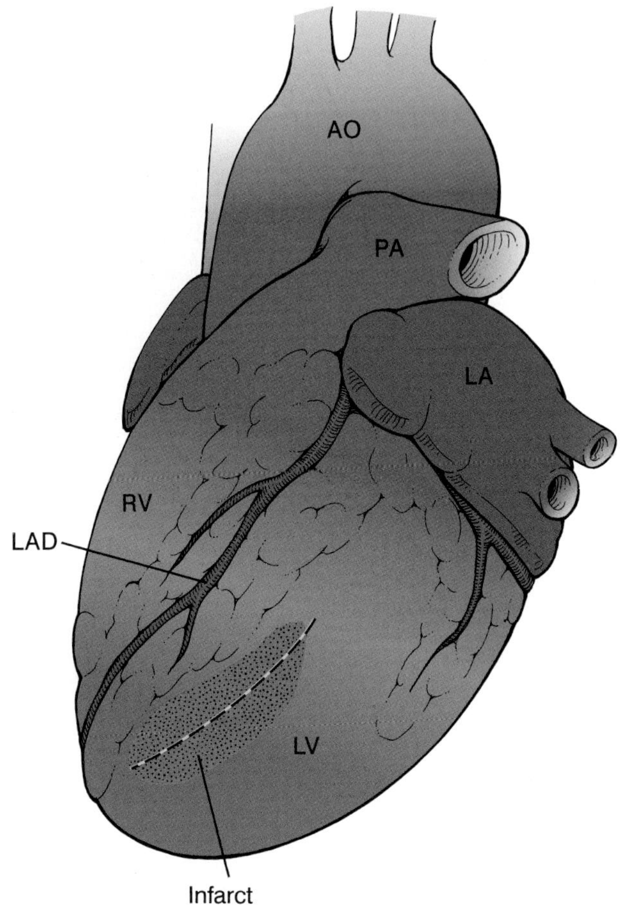

FIGURE 28-3 Transinfarct left ventricular incision to expose an anterior septal rupture. An incision (dashed line) is made parallel to the anterior descending branch of the left coronary artery (LAD) through the center of the infarct (stippled area) in the anterior left ventricle (LV). Ao = aorta; LA = left atrium; PA = pulmonary artery; RV = right ventricle.

felt (see Figs. 28-4 B–D). An over-and-over running suture completes the ventriculotomy closure.

Most anterior defects require closure with a prosthetic patch (DeBakey Elastic Dacron fabric, USCI Division of C.R. Bard, Inc., Billerica, MA) or pericardium to avoid tension that could lead to disruption of the repair (Fig. 28-5). After debridement of necrotic septum and left ventricular muscle, a series of pledgeted interrupted mattress sutures are placed around the perimeter of the defect (see Fig. 28-5A). Along the posterior aspect of the defect, sutures are passed through the septum from right to left. Along the anterior edge of the defect, sutures are passed from the epicardial surface of the right ventricle to the endocardial surface. All sutures are placed before the patch is inserted, and then passed through the edge of a synthetic patch, which is seated on the left side of the septum (see Fig. 28-5B). Each suture is then passed through an additional pledget and all are tied. We use additional pledgets on the left ventricular side overlying the patch (see Fig. 28-5C) to cushion each suture as it is tied down to prevent cutting through the friable muscle. The edges of the ventriculotomy are then approximated by a two-layer closure consisting of interrupted mattress sutures passed through buttressing strips of Teflon felt (or glutaraldehyde-preserved bovine pericardium) and a final over-and-over running suture.

Posterior/Inferior Repair with Infarctectomy

Closure of inferoposterior septal defects, which result from transmural infarction in the distribution of the posterior descending artery, has posed the greatest technical challenge.[54,55] Because of the difficulty in surgical management of these defects by the method of infarctectomy, many surgeons now feel that these defects may be better suited to repair using exclusion techniques, which are described in detail in the next section.

Early attempts at primary closure of these posterior/inferior defects by simple plication techniques similar to those used in the repair of anterior defects were frequently unsuccessful because of the sutures tearing out of soft, friable myocardium that had been closed under tension. This resulted in either reopening of the defect or catastrophic disruption of the infarctectomy closure. It was, in large part, the analysis of such early

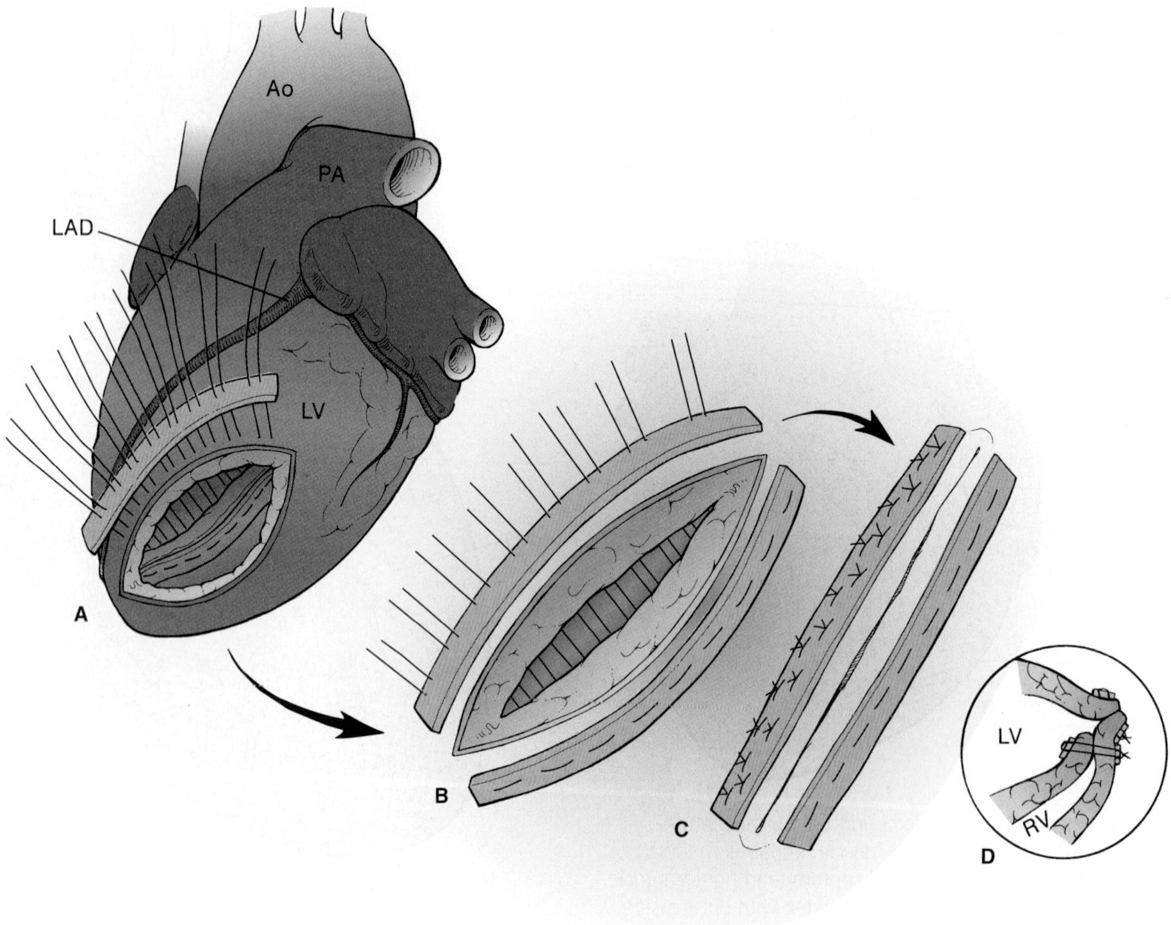

FIGURE 28-4 (A) Repair of an anterior septal rupture by plicating the free anterior edge of the septum to the right ventricular free wall with interrupted 1-0 Tevdek mattress sutures buttressed with strips of Teflon felt. (B, C, and D) The left ventriculotomy is then closed as a separate suture line, again with interrupted mattress sutures of 1-0 Tevdek buttressed with felt strips. A second running suture (not shown) is used to ensure a secure left ventriculotomy closure. Ao = aorta; LAD = left anterior descending coronary artery; LV = left ventricle; PA = pulmonary artery; RV = right ventricle. *(Adapted with permission from Guyton SW, Daggett WM: Surgical repair of post-infarction ventricular septal rupture, in Cohn LH (ed): Modern Techniques in Surgery: Cardiac/Thoracic Surgery. Mt.Kisco, NY, Futura, 1983; installment 9, p 61-1.)*

results that led to the evolution of the operative principles enumerated in Table 28-1A.

Use of the following techniques has been associated with an improved operative survival. After the establishment of bypass with bicaval cannulation, the left side of the heart is vented via the right superior pulmonary vein. The heart is retracted out of the pericardial well as for bypass to the posterior descending coronary artery. The margins of the defect may involve the inferior aspects of both ventricles, or of the left ventricle only (Fig. 28-6A). A transinfarct incision is made in the left ventricle, and the left ventricular portion of the infarct is excised (see Fig. 28-6B), exposing the septal defect. The left ventricular papillary muscles are inspected. Only if there is frank papillary muscle rupture is mitral valve replacement performed. When it is indicated, we prefer to perform mitral valve replacement through a separate conventional left atrial incision, to avoid trauma to the friable ventricular muscle. After all infarcted left ventricular muscle has been excised, a less aggressive debridement of the right ventricle is accomplished, with the goal of resecting only as much muscle as is necessary to afford complete visualization of the defect(s). Using this technique, delayed rupture of the right ventricle has not been a problem. If the posterior septum has cracked or split from the adjacent ventricular free wall without loss of a great deal of septal tissue, then the septal rim of the posterior defect may be approximated to the edge of the diaphragmatic right ventricular free wall using mattress sutures buttressed with strips of Teflon felt or bovine pericardium (see Figs. 28-6 C and D).

Larger posterior defects require patch closure (Fig. 28-7). Pledgeted mattress sutures are placed from the right side of the septum and from the epicardial side of the right ventricular free wall (see Fig. 28-7B). All sutures are passed through the perimeter of the patch and then through additional pledgets, and are then tied (see Fig. 28-7C). Thus, as in closure of large anterior defects, the patch is secured on the left ventricular side of the septum. Direct closure of the remaining infarctectomy is rarely possible because of tension required to pull together the edges of the gaping defect. A prosthetic patch is generally required.

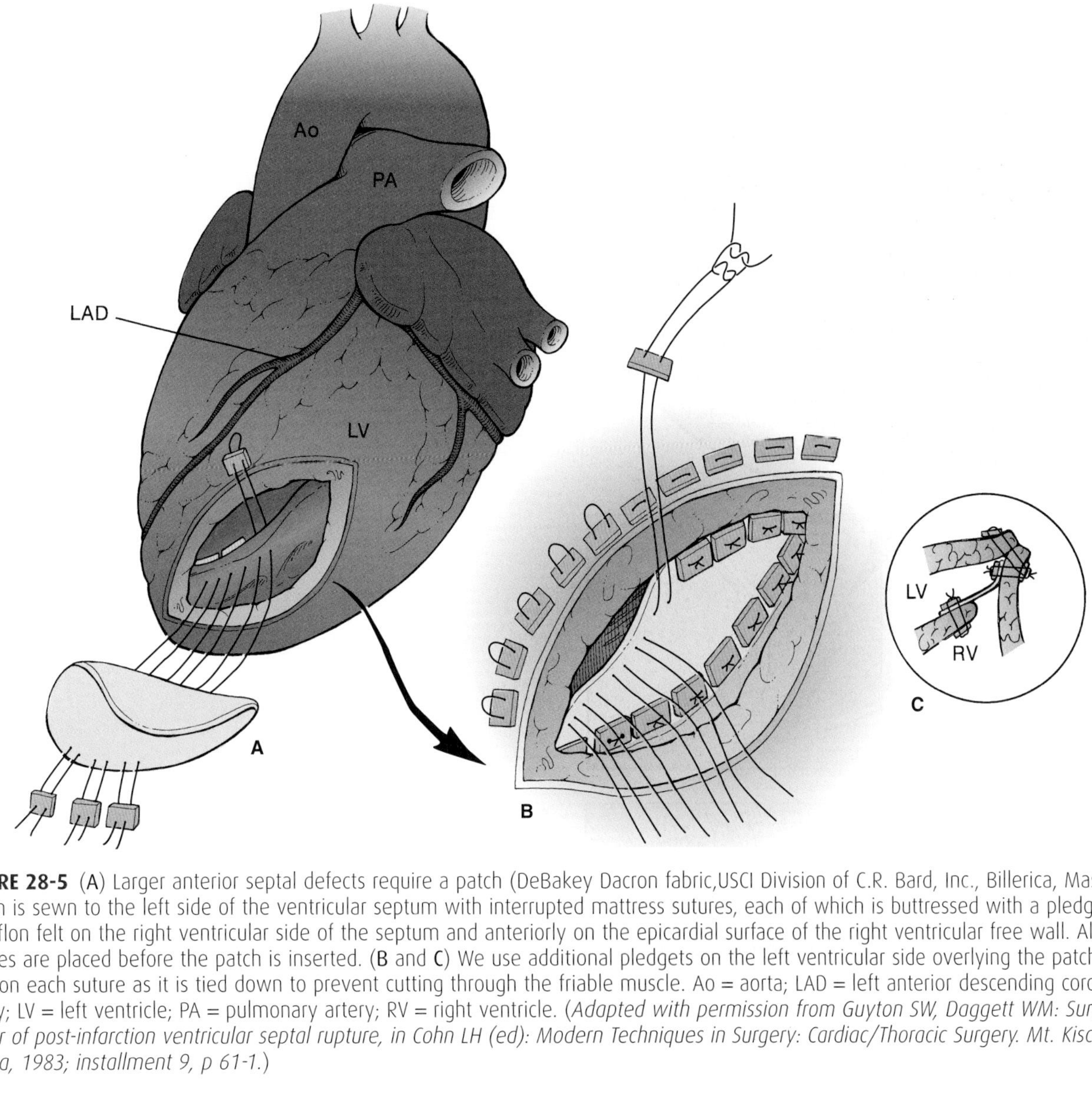

FIGURE 28-5 (A) Larger anterior septal defects require a patch (DeBakey Dacron fabric,USCI Division of C.R. Bard, Inc., Billerica, Mass), which is sewn to the left side of the ventricular septum with interrupted mattress sutures, each of which is buttressed with a pledget of Teflon felt on the right ventricular side of the septum and anteriorly on the epicardial surface of the right ventricular free wall. All sutures are placed before the patch is inserted. (B and C) We use additional pledgets on the left ventricular side overlying the patch to cushion each suture as it is tied down to prevent cutting through the friable muscle. Ao = aorta; LAD = left anterior descending coronary artery; LV = left ventricle; PA = pulmonary artery; RV = right ventricle. (*Adapted with permission from Guyton SW, Daggett WM: Surgical repair of post-infarction ventricular septal rupture, in Cohn LH (ed): Modern Techniques in Surgery: Cardiac/Thoracic Surgery. Mt. Kisco, NY, Futura, 1983; installment 9, p 61-1.*)

Originally, we cut an oval patch from a Cooley low-porosity woven Dacron tube graft (Meadox Medicals, Inc., Oakland, NJ). Currently, we cut this patch from a Hemashield woven double velour Dacron collagen impregnated graft (Meadox Medicals). Pledgeted mattress sutures are passed out through the margin of the infarctectomy (endocardium to epicardium) and then through the patch (see Fig. 28-7D), which is seated on the epicardial surface of the heart. After each suture is passed through an additional pledget, all sutures are tied (see Fig. 28-7E). The cross-sectional view of the completed repair (Fig. 28-8) illustrates the restoration of relatively normal ventricular geometry, which is accomplished by the use of appropriately sized prosthetic patches.

Repair of Anterior and Posterior Defects by Infarct Exclusion

The concept that the preservation of left ventricular geometry plays a crucial role in the preservation of left ventricular function has laid the groundwork for evolution in the surgical approach to postinfarction VSDs—the technique of endocardial patch repair of postinfarction VSDs described by David,[50] Cooley,[56] and then by Ross[57] in the early 1990s. This operative technique, which is an application to ventricular septal rupture repair of Dor's technique of ventricular endoaneurysmorrhaphy,[58] involves intracavitary placement of an endocardial patch to exclude infarcted myocardium while maintaining ventricular geometry. Thus, instead of closing the septal defect, it is simply *excluded* from the high-pressure zone of the left ventricle. Some institutions have reported impressive results using infarct exclusion, but results in for other centers have been mixed. We currently consider this a particular helpful technique in selected patients with posterior/inferior defects, given the complexity of a infarctectomy repair in this location. The description that follows is based in large part on the work of David.[46]

In patients with anterior septal rupture, the interventricular septum is exposed via a left ventriculotomy, which is made through the infarcted anterolateral wall starting at the apex and

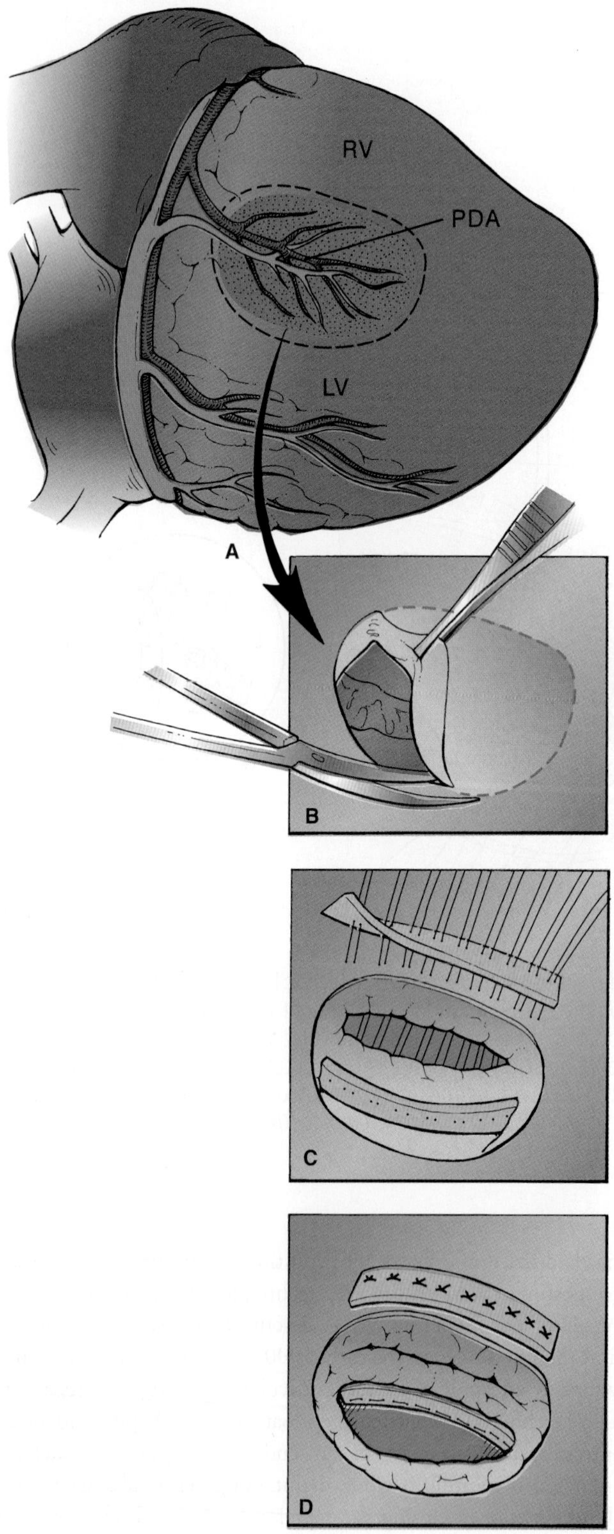

FIGURE 28-6 (A) View of an inferior infarct (stippled area) associated with posterior septal rupture. The apex of the heart is to the right. Exposure at operation is achieved by dislocating the heart up and out of the pericardial sac, and then retracting its cephalad, as in the performance of distal vein bypass and anastomosis to the posterior descending artery. (B) The inferoposterior infarct is excised to expose the posterior septal defect. Complete excision of the left ventricular portion of the infarct is important to prevent delayed rupture of the ventriculotomy repair. The free edge of the right ventricle is progressively shaved back to expose the margins of the defect clearly. (C and D) Repair of the posterior septal rupture is accomplished by approximating the edge of the posterior septum to the free wall of the diaphragmatic right ventricle with felt-buttressed mattress sutures. The repair is possible when the septum has cracked or split off from the posterior ventricular wall without necrosis of a great deal of septal muscle. The surgeon can perform repair of posterior septal rupture to best advantage by standing at the left side of the supine patient. The left ventriculotomy is then closed as a separate suture line, again with interrupted mattress sutures of 1-0 Tevdek buttressed with felt strips. A second running suture is used to ensure a secure left ventriculotomy closure (not shown). LV = posterior left ventricle; PDA = posterior descending artery; RV = diaphragmatic surface of the right ventricle. (*Adapted with permission from Daggett. 21*)

extending proximally parallel to, but 1 to 2 cm away from, the anterior descending artery (Fig. 28-9A). Stay sutures are passed through the margins of the ventriculotomy to aid in the exposure of the infarcted septum. The septal defect is located and the margins of the infarcted muscle identified. A glutaraldehyde-fixed bovine pericardial patch is tailored to the shape of the left ventricular infarction as seen from the endocardium but 1 to 2 cm larger. The patch is usually oval and measures approximately 4 × 6 cm in most patients. The pericardial patch is then sutured to healthy endocardium all around the infarct (see Fig. 28-9B). Suturing begins in the lowest and most proximal part of the noninfarcted endocardium of the septum with a continuous 3-0 polypropylene suture. Interrupted mattress sutures with felt pledgets may be used to reinforce the repair.[57] The

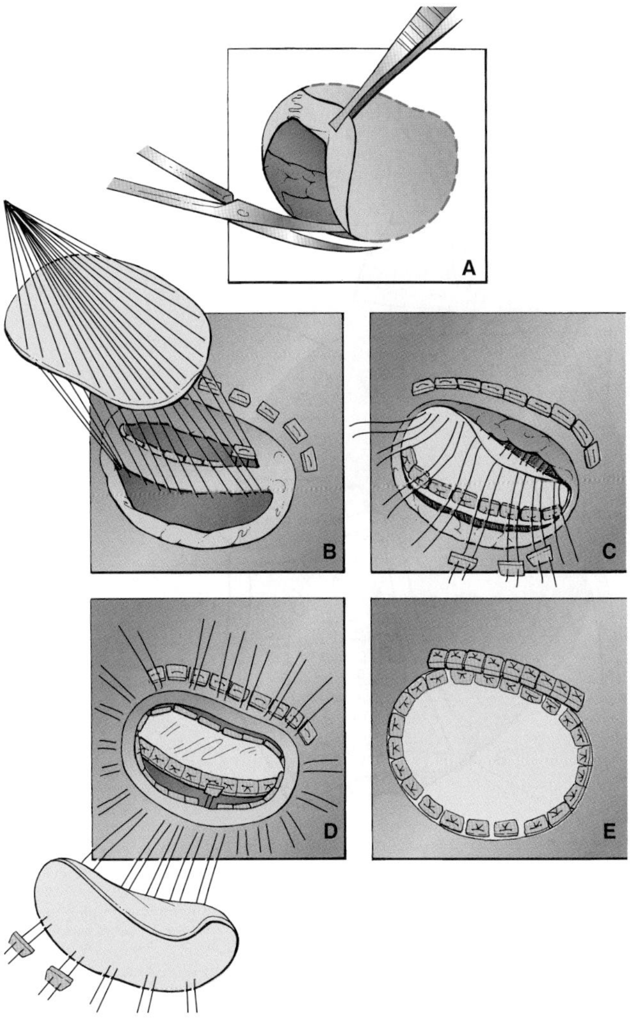

FIGURE 28-7 (A) Repair of posterior septal rupture when necrosis of a substantial portion of the posterior septum requires the use of patches. (B) Interrupted mattress sutures of 2-0 Tevdek are placed circumferentially around the defect. These sutures are buttressed with felt pledgets on the right ventricular side of the septum and on the epicardial surface of the diaphragmatic right ventricle. (C) All sutures are placed and then the patch (DeBakey elastic Dacron fabric) is slid into place on the left ventricular side of the septum. The patch sutures are tied down with an additional felt pledget placed on top of the patch (left ventricular side) as each suture is tied, to cushion the tie and prevent cutting through the friable muscle. These maneuvers are viewed by the authors as essential to the success of early repair of the posterior septal rupture. (D) Remaining to be repaired is the posterior left ventricular free wall defect created by infarctectomy. Mattress sutures of 2-0 Tevdek are placed circumferentially around the margins of the posterior left ventricular free wall defect. Each suture is buttressed with a Teflon felt pledget on the endocardial side of the left ventricle. With all sutures in place, a circular patch, fashioned from a Hemashield woven double velour Dacron collagen-impregnated graft (Meadox Medicals Inc., Oakland, NJ), is slid down onto the epicardial surface of the left ventricle. An additional pledget of Teflon felt is placed under each suture (on top of the patch) as it is tied to cushion the tie and prevent cutting through the friable underlying muscle. This onlay technique of patch placement prevents the cracking of friable left ventricular muscle that occurred with the eversion technique of patch insertion. (E) Completed repair. *(Adapted with permission from Daggett. 21)*

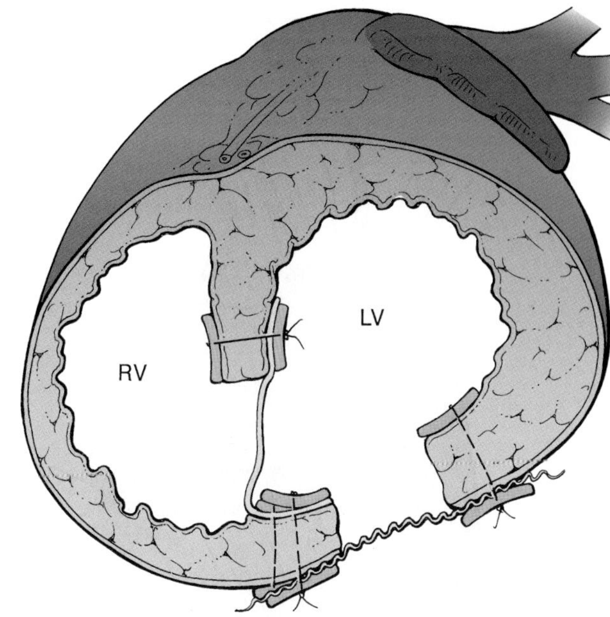

FIGURE 28-8 Cross-sectional view of the completed repair of posterior septal rupture with prosthetic patch placement of the posterior left ventricular free wall defect created by infarctectomy. LV = left ventricular cavity; RV = right vent ricular cavity. *(Adapted with permission from Daggett. 21)*

patch is also sutured to the noninfarcted endocardium of the anterolateral ventricular wall. The stitches should be inserted 5 to 7 mm deep in the muscle and 4 to 5 mm apart. The stitches in the patch should be at least 5 to 7 mm from its free margin so as to allow the patch to cover the area between the entrance and exit of the suture in the myocardium. This technique minimizes the risk of tearing muscle as the suture is pulled taut. If the infarct involves the base of the anterior papillary muscle, the suture is brought outside of the heart and buttressed on a strip of bovine pericardium or Teflon felt applied to the epicardial surface of the left ventricle. Once the patch is completely secured to the endocardium of the left ventricle, the left ventricular cavity becomes largely excluded from the infarcted myocardium. The ventriculotomy is closed in two layers over two strips of bovine pericardium or Teflon felt using 2-0 or 3-0 polypropylene sutures, as illustrated in Fig. 28-9C. No infarctectomy is performed unless the necrotic muscle along the ventriculotomy is sloughing at the time of its closure, and even then it is minimized, because infarcted muscle will not be exposed to left ventricular pressures when the heart begins to work (see Fig. 28-9D). Alternatively, sutures can be passed through the ventricular free wall and through a tailored external patch of Teflon or pericardium (Fig. 28-10).

In patients with posterior septal defects, an incision is made in the inferior wall of the left ventricle 1 or 2 mm from the posterior descending artery (Fig. 28-11A). This incision is started at the midportion of the inferior wall and extended proximally toward the mitral annulus and distally toward the apex of the ventricle. Care is taken to avoid damage to the posterolateral papillary muscle. Stay sutures are passed through the fat pad of the apex of the ventricle and margins of the ventriculotomy to

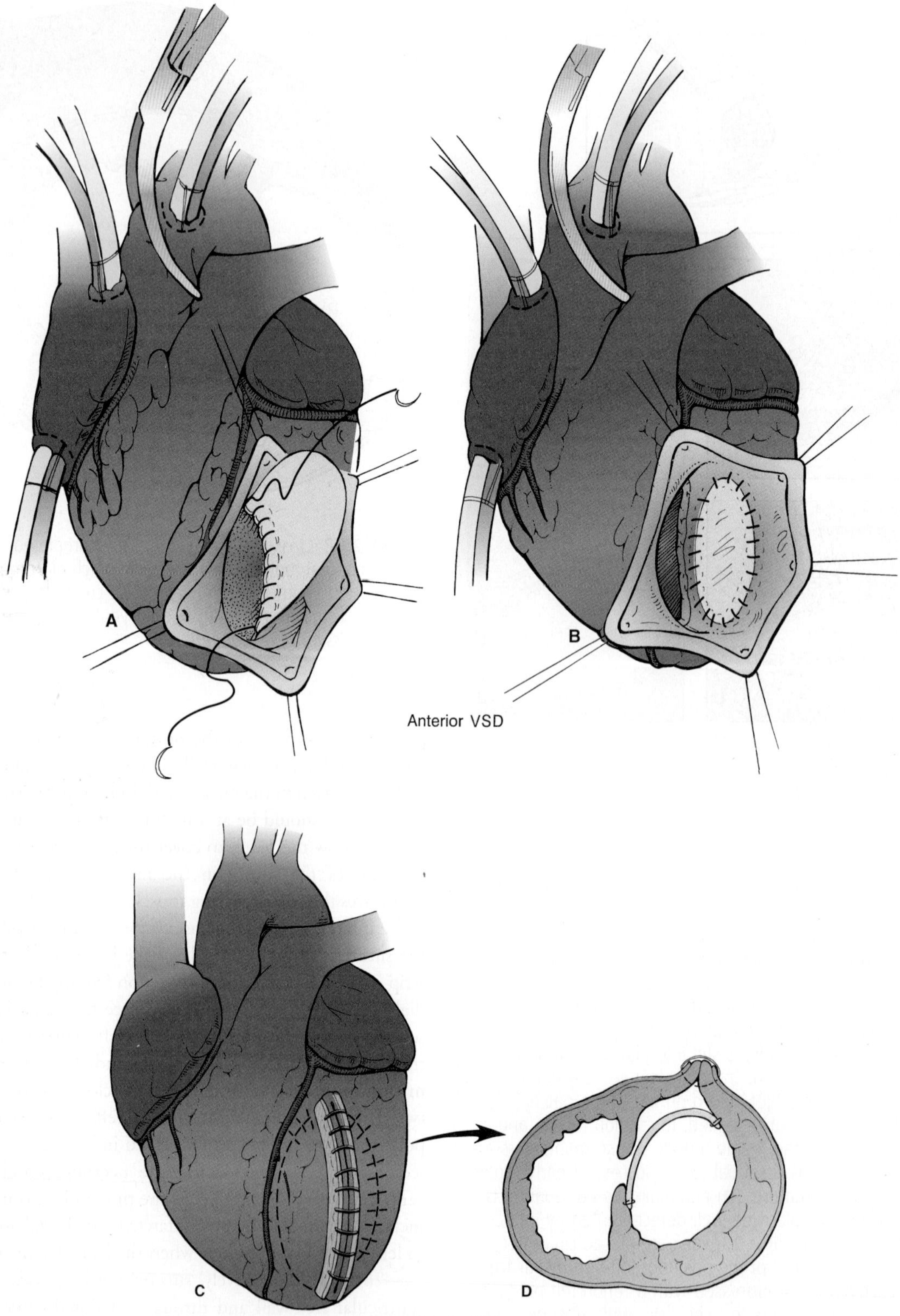

FIGURE 28-9 Repair of an anterior postinfarction ventricular septal rupture using the technique of infarct exclusion. (A) The standard ventriculotomy is made in the infarcted area of left ventricular free wall. An interior patch of Dacron (Meadox Medicals Inc., Oakland, NJ), polytetrafluoroethylene, or glutaraldehyde-fixed pericardium is fashioned to replace and/or cover the diseased areas (ventricular septal defect [VSD], septal infarction, or free wall infarction). (B) The internal patch is secured to normal endocardium with a continuous monofilament suture, which may be reinforced with pledgeted mattress sutures. There is little, if any, resection of myocardium and no attempt is made to close the septal defect. Repair of an anterior postinfarction ventricular septal rupture using the technique of infarct exclusion. (C) The ventriculotomy, which is outside the pressure zone of the left ventricle, may be repaired with a continuous suture. (D) On transverse section, one can see that the endocardial patch is secured at three levels: above and below the septal rupture and beyond the ventriculotomy. (*Adapted with permission from David et al. 46*)

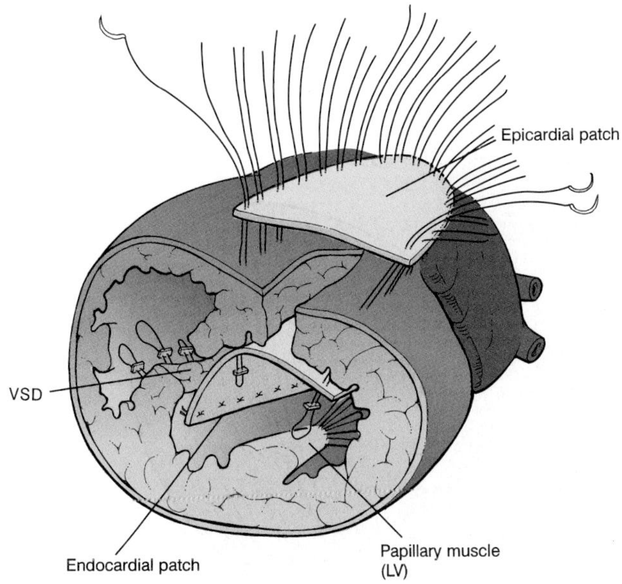

FIGURE 28-10 Repair of an anterior postinfarction ventricular septal rupture using the technique of infarct exclusion with external patching of the ventricular free wall with tailored Teflon or pericardium. LV = left ventricle; VSD = ventricular septal defect. *(Adapted with permission from Cooley. 93)*

facilitate exposure of the ventricular cavity. In most cases, the rupture is found in the proximal half of the posterior septum and the posteromedial papillary muscle is involved by the infarction. A bovine pericardial patch is tailored in a triangular shape of approximately 4 × 7 cm in most patients. The base of the triangular-shaped patch is sutured to the fibrous annulus of the mitral valve with a continuous 3-0 polypropylene suture starting at a point corresponding to the level of the posteromedial papillary muscle and moving medially toward the septum until the noninfarcted endocardium is reached (see Fig. 28-11B). At that level, the suture is interrupted and any excess patch material trimmed. The medial margin of the triangular-shaped patch is sewn to healthy septal endocardium with a continuous 3-0 or 4-0 polypropylene suture taking bites the same size as those described for anterior defects. In this area of the septum, reinforcing pledgeted sutures may be required. The lateral side of the patch is sutured to the posterior wall of the left ventricle along a line corresponding to the medial margin of the base of the posteromedial papillary muscle. Because the posterior wall of the left ventricle is infarcted, it is usually necessary to use full-thickness bites and anchor the sutures on a strip of pericardium or Teflon felt applied on the epicardial surface of the posterior wall of the left ventricle right at the level of the posteromedial papillary muscle insertion, as shown in Fig. 28-11B. Once the patch is completely sutured to the mitral valve annulus, the endocardium of the interventricular septum, and the full thickness of the posterior wall (see Fig. 28-11C), the ventriculotomy is closed in two layers of full-thickness sutures buttressed on strips of pericardium or Teflon felt (see Fig. 28-11D). The infarcted right ventricular wall is left undisturbed. If the posteromedial papillary muscle is ruptured, mitral valve replacement is necessary.

There are several theoretical advantages in the technique of infarct exclusion: (1) It does not require resection of myocardium; excessive resection results in depression of ventricular function and insufficient resection predisposes to recurrence of septal rupture; (2) it maintains ventricular geometry, which enhances ventricular function; and (3) it avoids tension on friable muscle, which may diminish postoperative bleeding.

Other Techniques

Most other operative techniques that have resulted in successful management of postinfarction of ventricular septal rupture have adhered to the same general principles described in the preceding. For example, Tashiro and colleagues[59] described an extended endocardial repair in which a *saccular* patch of glutaraldehyde-fixed equine pericardium was used to exclude an anterior septal rupture. Usui and coworkers[60] reported the successful repair of a posterior septal rupture using two sheets of equine pericardium to sandwich the infarcted myocardium, including the septal defect and ventriculotomy. Others have modified the exclusion technique by using multiple patches or use of tissue sealants to aid in the septal closure.[61,62]

Percutaneous Closure

Successful transcatheter closure of postinfarction ventricular septal rupture has been reported using several types of catheter-deployed devices. Early experience was with the CardioSEAL device, a nitinol double-umbrella prosthesis. The device consists of two attached and opposing umbrellas formed by hinged steel arms covered in a Dacron meshwork that theoretically promotes endothelialization. The arms are manually everted to allow the device to be passed through a narrow percutaneous deployment system. When extruded from the guiding catheter, the arms spring backward, resembling a clamshell. The device approaches the septum via the systemic veins and through the atrial septum (or alternatively via the arterial system through the aortic valve). As reported by Landzberg and Lock,[63] the experience at Boston Children's Hospital and Brigham and Women's Hospital indicates that although the device can be routinely deployed in the setting of an acute infarction, the continued necrosis of septal tissue led to decompensation and death in four of seven patients. In contrast, they reported success in six of six patients treated for residual or recurrent septal defects discovered after primary operative repair. Other catheter devices have also been attempted, including the Amplatzer septal occluder and the Rashkind double umbrella.[64]

The recently developed Amplatzer VSD device allows closure of muscular and membranous VSDs, and it can be used for larger postinfarction defects, with the septal Amplatzer device favored for smaller lesions.[65] The device features a longer waist (10 mm) connecting the two umbrella ends, which corresponds more closely to the thickness expected for the adult ventricular septum

Results with device closure have been mixed. In a recent report involving use of these devices as a primary treatment strategy, "procedural success" was reported as 86%, but 41% of patients had important complications that included left ventricular rupture, device embolization, and major residual shunting.[66]

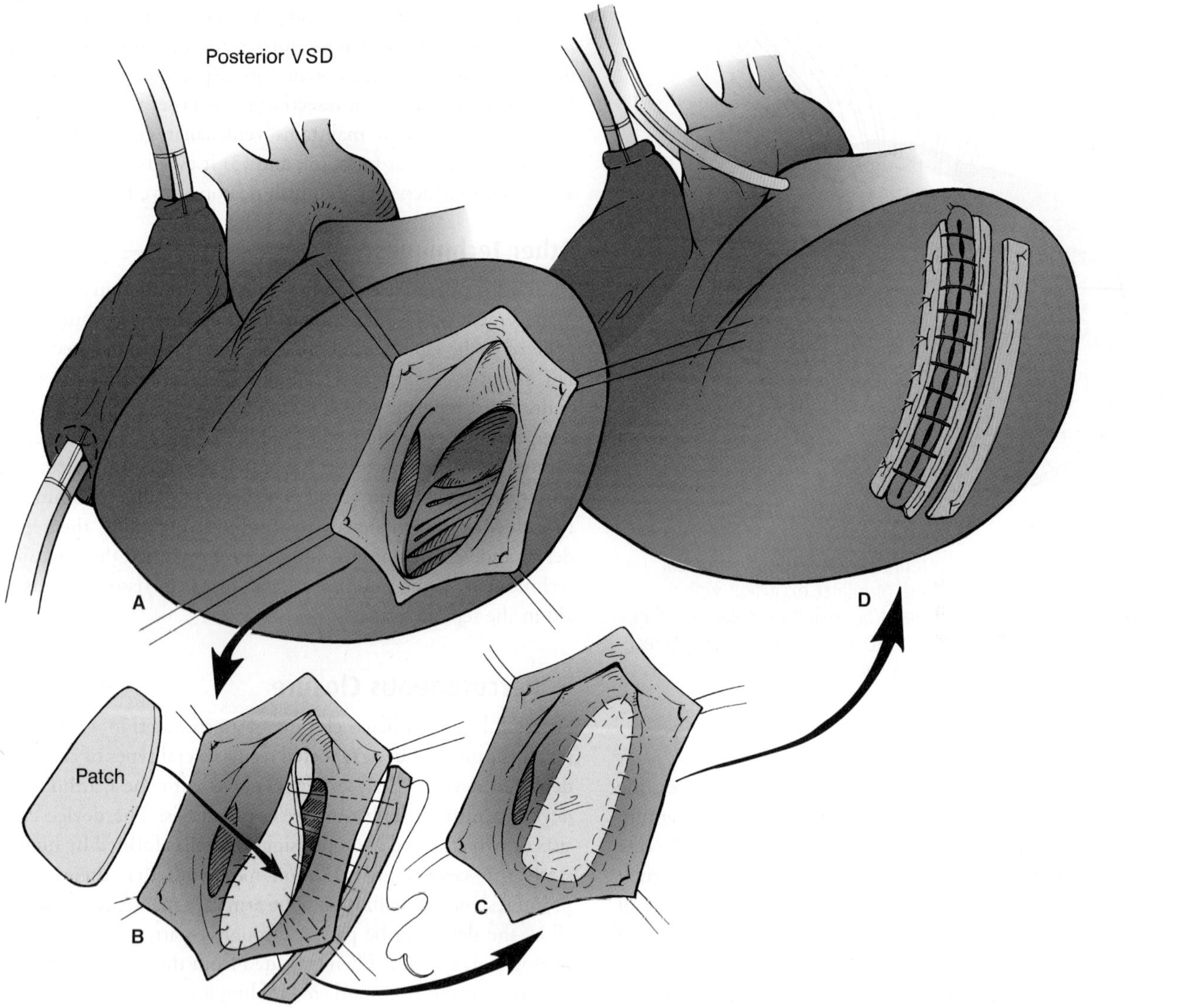

FIGURE 28-11 Endocardial repair of a posterior postinfarction ventricular septal rupture using the technique of infarct exclusion. (A) An incision is made in the inferior wall of the left ventricle 1 or 2 mm from the posterior descending artery starting at the midportion of the inferior wall and extended proximally toward the mitral annulus and distally toward the apex of the ventricle. Care is taken to avoid damage to the posterolateral papillary muscle. (B) A bovine pericardial patch is tailored in a triangular shape.The base of the triangular-shaped patch is sutured to the fibrous annulus of the mitral valve with a continuous 3-0 polypropylene suture starting at a point corresponding to the level of the posteromedial papillary muscle and moving medially toward the septum until the noninfarcted endocardium is reached. (C) The medial margin of the triangular-shaped patch is sewn to healthy septal endocardium with a continuous 3-0 or 4-0 polypropylene suture.The lateral side of the patch is sutured to the posterior wall of the left ventricle along a line corresponding to the medial margin of the base of the posteromedial papillary muscle. At this point, it is usually necessary to use full-thickness bites and anchor the sutures on a strip of pericardium or Teflon felt applied on the epicardial surface of the posterior wall of the left ventricle. (D) Once the patch is completely sutured to the mitral valve annulus, the endocardium of the interventricular septum, and the full thickness of the posterior wall, the ventriculotomy is closed in two layers of full-thickness sutures buttressed on strips of pericardium or Teflon felt. The infarcted right ventricular wall is left undisturbed. (*Adapted with permission from David et al. 46*)

The 30-day survival rate was only 35%. Others have also reported that residual shunts are the norm, although often greatly improved by the procedure. Several series noted a poor outcome when this approach was attempted early after infarction, when the defect margins are fragile, but after about 2 weeks the results were considered acceptable.[67–69] Of course, surgical results after a delay are also considerably better, but many patients would die in the first 2 weeks without intervention.

The best use of such devices in an overall treatment strategy is unclear. As a primary treatment, data suggest that the devices have a high early failure rate, but their potential role in improving the risk of an unstable surgical patient is not yet well characterized. Currently, catheter approaches appear to be most effective in treatment of recurrent or residual defects,[70] and we preferentially employ them for these conditions. Device development is an ongoing process, and the future undoubtedly will see use of new devices, especially in the high-risk patient with multisystem failure. An additional area of use for catheter devices is to reduce shunt fraction in an attempt to stabilize a patient for a planned delayed operation. We are employing this technique when we deem early surgery to be at extreme risk, with a planned operation either immediately if device closure is unsuccessful, or at approximately 6 to 8 weeks if stabilization is obtained.

Of interest, two centers have reported using a standard Swan-Ganz balloon catheter from the groin to abolish the shunt in unstable patients with postinfarction septal rupture.[71,72] Hemodynamic improvement was immediate in both patients, who underwent subsequent surgical repair of the defect.

Role of Ventricular Assist Devices

In patients who present for operation with evidence of potentially reversible multiorgan dysfunction, or in patients who have intractable failure after repair, there may be a role for temporary mechanical heart support. There have been multiple anecdotal cases of unstable patients being successfully managed by mechanical support followed by definitive operation.

The theoretical advantages that make mechanical support attractive as an initial therapy in very sick patients with postinfarction VSD include: (1) the potential to reverse end-organ dysfunction; (2) maturation of the infarct leading to firmer tissue, making the closure less prone to technical failure; and (3) recovery of the stunned and energy-depleted myocardium. However, there are potential hazards with mechanical support that are specific to the patient with postinfarction VSD. High right-to-left shunting across the ventricular septum has been reported to cause hypoxic brain injury in a postinfarction VSD patient placed on a Heart-Mate left ventricular support device.[107] This observation suggests that either partial left heart support or preferably biventricular support should be considered when using mechanical assistance in these patients. In a report using the Hemopump axial flow device, two of two patients supported experienced lethal pump failure. Examination of the device at autopsy disclosed necrotic material clogging the catheter system.[73a]

Simultaneous Myocardial Revascularization

There has been controversy in the literature concerning the advantages and disadvantages of concurrent coronary artery grafting in patients undergoing emergent repair of postinfarction ventricular septal rupture. The potential benefit of revascularization in a patient with significant lesions to living muscle is obvious: improved myocardial distribution, protection from postoperative ischemic, and reduced late ischemic events. However, in patients with postinfarction VSDs, there is already a completed myocardial injury and the involved territory is unlikely to benefit. For this reason, some have argued that revascularization provides no survival benefit and subjects patients to preoperative left heart catheterization, a time-consuming and potentially dangerous diagnostic procedure. Loisance and associates[73b] base their policy of not revascularizing patients with postinfarction septal ruptures on the fact that none of their 20 long-term survivors (five of whom were bypassed) had incapacitating angina or recurrent myocardial infarction.

Some groups use left heart catheterization and coronary bypassing selectively. Davies and colleagues[74] found that of 60 long-term survivors (median 70 months; range 1 to 174 months), only five patients developed exertional angina during follow-up and none required revascularization. Their current policy is to avoid left heart catheterization of patients in whom an acquired septal defect is suspected to be a consequence of their first anterior infarction, provided that the patient has no history of angina or electrocardiographic evidence of previous infarction in another territory.

Weaning from Cardiopulmonary Bypass

The two most common problems encountered in separating from bypass after repair of a postinfarction VSD are low cardiac output and bleeding. Although the treatment of low cardiac output after cardiac surgery is beyond the scope of this chapter, a few agents and principles are worth mentioning. First, most of these patients will have had an IABP inserted before surgery. If not, one should be inserted in the operating room, especially if the low-output state is secondary to LV dysfunction. Also, an IABP may benefit patients with right ventricular failure by improving right coronary artery blood flow resulting from diastolic augmentation. We have found intravenous milrinone, a phosphodiesterase inhibitor, to be very effective in reversing low-output states secondary to LV dysfunction. Milrinone possesses a balance of inotropic and vasodilatory properties that together produce an increase in cardiac output and reduction in right and left filling pressures and systemic vascular resistance. It is less arrhythmogenic than dobutamine, causes less hypotension than amrinone, and is not associated with thrombocytopenia.

Posterior defects are commonly associated with mitral regurgitation and right heart dysfunction secondary to extensive right ventricular infarction. Management of right heart failure is aimed at reducing right ventricular afterload while maintaining systemic pressure. Initial steps to manage right ventricular dysfunction include volume loading, inotropic support, and correction of acidosis, hypoxemia, and hypercarbia. If patients remain unresponsive to these measures, we have successfully treated right ventricular failure with a prostaglandin E_1 infusion (0.5 to 2.0 μg/min) into the right heart, counterbalanced with a norepinephrine infusion titrated into the left atrium.[75] Inhaled nitric oxide (20 to 80 ppm), which selectively dilates the pulmonary circuit, has also proved efficacious in the treatment of right heart failure.[76]

If a patient cannot be weaned from bypass using conventional therapy, we consider using a ventricular assist device. Indications for a left ventricular assist device are a cardiac index less than 1.8 L/min/m^2, a left atrial pressure above 18 to 25 mm Hg, a right atrial pressure below 15 mm Hg, and an aortic pressure below 90 mm Hg peak systolic. Indications for a right ventricular assist device are a cardiac index less than 1.8 L/min/m^2, an aortic pressure below 90 mm Hg peak systolic, and a left atrial pressure less than 15 mm Hg despite volume loading to a right atrial pressure of 25 mm Hg with a competent tricuspid valve. Important points to remember when instituting ventricular assistance are:

1. Right ventricular failure may not become evident until left ventricular assistance is instituted.
2. Once refractory ventricular failure has been identified, delay in initiating support is associated with increased morbidity and mortality.

3. Closure of a patent foramen ovale is mandatory before left ventricular support.
4. Postoperative hemorrhage should be treated aggressively and completely controlled.
5. Residual septal defects may result in right-to-left shunting and severe hypoxia when only left heart support is used.

Hemostatic Measures

To prevent postpump coagulopathy, we begin antifibrinolytic with ε-aminocaproic acid (Amicar) before commencing cardiopulmonary bypass. Amicar is administered by loading patients with 10 g before commencing bypass and then adding another 10 g to the pump prime. During the procedure Amicar is continuously infused at 1 g/h for the duration of surgery. Aprotinin was previously used routinely for this condition, but concerns regarding early and late complication led this drug to be withdrawn from the US market.

Postpump suture line bleeding may be reduced by application of a fibrin sealant to the ventricular septum around the septal defect *before* formal repair.[77] Biological glue may be effective in controlling bleeding suture lines after repair. As a last resort, Baldwin and Cooley[78] have suggested insertion of a left ventricular assist device solely as an adjunct to the repair of friable or damaged myocardium to reduce left ventricular distention and thus control bleeding. Finally, for intractable bleeding, there may be role for Factor VII concentrate, although results and risks of administration in cardiac surgery are limited.

Highlights of Postoperative Care

Early postoperative diuresis and positive end-expiratory pressure ventilation are used to decrease the alveolar-arterial gradient induced by the increased extravascular pulmonary water associated with cardiopulmonary bypass. Once the patient has warmed, we commonly use an intravenous infusion of furosemide combined with mannitol or, if needed, continuous venovenous hemofiltration is employed postoperatively.

Intractable postoperative ventricular arrhythmias secondary to reperfusion injury are sometimes difficult to control using standard therapy. We have been impressed with the efficacy of intravenous amiodarone in these situations (10 to 20 mg/kg over 24 hours).

Operative Mortality and Risk Factors for Death

Table 28-2 summarizes recently reported experience from several centers. Operative mortality, defined as death before discharge *or* within 30 days of operation, ranged from 30 to 50%. In the Massachusetts General Hospital experience of 114 patients, operative mortality was 37% (Fig. 28-12A). The risk for death

TABLE 28-2 Selected Recent Clinical Experience with Surgical Repair of Postinfarction Ventricular Septal Defect

Institution	City	Year	No.	Hospital Mortality	5-Year Survival	Reference
Johann-Wolfgang-Goethe	Frankfurt	2009	32	31.2%	41%	79
Sweden (multi-institutional)	Sweden	2005	189	41% (30-day)	38%	80
Ospedale di Circolo-Fondazione Macchi	Varese, Italy	2005	50	36%	47%	81
Northwest England (multi-institutional)	England	2003	65	23% (30-day)	—	82
Hospital Haut-Lévêque	Bordeaux	2002	85	42%	33%	83
Massachusetts General Hospital	Boston	2002	114	37%	45%	84
University Hospital	Zurich	2000	54	26%	52%*	85
Glenfield General Hospital	Leicester	2000	117	37% (30-day)	46%	86
Texas Heart Institute	Houston	1998	126	46%	—	87
The Toronto Hospital	Toronto	1998	52	19%	65%*	88
Southampton General	Southampton	1998	179	27%	49%	89
Cedars-Sinai	Los Angeles	1998	31	32%	—	90
Mid America Heart Institute	Kansas City	1997	76	41%	41%	91
St. Anthonius Hospital	Nieuwegein	1996	109	28% (30-day)	—	92
Green Lane Hospital	Auckland	1995	35	31% (30-day)	60%*	93
Hospital Cardiologique du Haut-Lévèque	Bordeaux	1991	62	38%	44%	22
CHU Henri Mondor	Créteil	1991	66	45%	44%	94

*Value estimated from published graphical or tabular data.
Note: Series with fewer than 30 patients were excluded from the table.

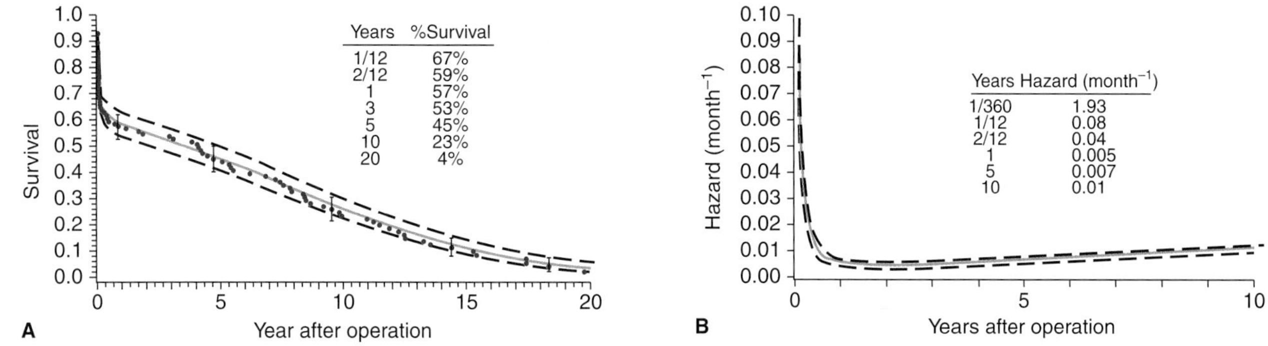

FIGURE 28-12 (A) Time-related survival after repair of postinfarction ventricular septal defect at the Massachusetts General Hospital (n = 114). Note that the horizontal axis extends to 20 years. Circles represent each death, positioned on the horizontal axis at the interval from operation to death, and actuarially (Kaplan-Meier method) along the vertical axis. The vertical bars represent 70% confidence limits (± 1 SD). The solid line represents the parametrically estimated freedom from death, and the dashed lines enclose the 70% confidence limits of that estimate. The table shows the nonparametric estimates at specified intervals. (B) Hazard function for death after repair of postinfarction ventricular septal defect (n = 114). The horizontal axis is expanded for better visualization of early risk. The hazard function has two phases, consisting of an early, rapidly declining phase, which gives way to a slowly rising phase at about 6 months.The estimate is shown with 70% confidence limits.

was found to be very high initially, but dropped rapidly (see Fig. 28-12B). We identified independent risk factors for early and late death using multivariate methods (Table 28-3). The most important predictor of operative mortality in our study, and in other reports, was preoperative hemodynamic instability. Patients in this group are usually in cardiogenic shock, are emergency cases, are on inotropic support, and usually have intra-aortic balloon pumps. Several variables are highly correlated with hemodynamic instability, and different multivariate models may use one or more of these indicators of severe hemodynamic failure in their final model.

Additional risk factors for early and late death include the presence of left main CAD, previous MI, renal dysfunction, and right heart failure (Fig. 28-13). Other factors have been found to increase the risk of early death. Posterior location of the septal rupture has been associated with an increased operative mortality.[22,23,29,31] This has been attributed to a more technically difficult repair, the increased risk of associated mitral regurgitation, and associated right ventricular dysfunction that is an independent predictor of early mortality after posterior infarction. A short time interval between infarction and operation selects for sicker patients unable to be managed medically. Older patient age has also been associated with an increased early mortality, but in our analysis, we found that the impact of age was more pronounced in the high-risk patient. Thus, age alone should not be used as a reason for denying surgery in an otherwise low-risk candidate (Fig. 28-14).

Our review of the Massachusetts General Hospital experience underscored the large variability of risk to which

TABLE 28-3 Incremental Risk Factors for Death after Repair of Postinfarct VSD

Risk Factor	Hazard Phase	
	Early	Late
Demographic		
Age (older)	•	•
Clinical history		
Previous MI		•
Clinical status		
BUN (higher)	•	
Creatinine (higher)		•
"Emergency"	•	
Right atrial P (higher)	•	•
Catecholamines	•	
Coronary/VSD anatomy		
Left main Dz		•

MGH; n = 114; 95 events.

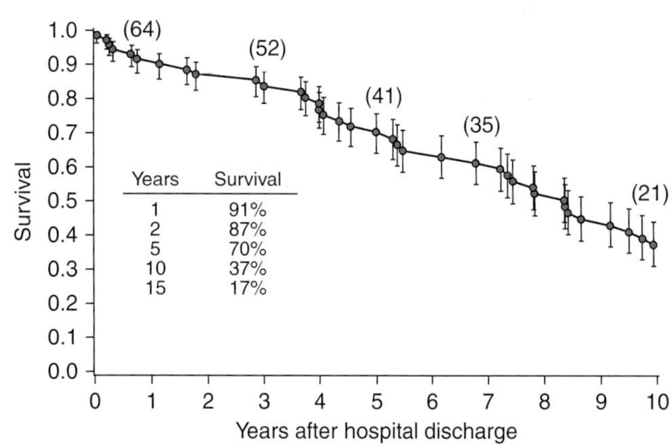

FIGURE 28-13 Survival in patients who were discharged after repair of postinfarction ventricular septal defect (Massachusetts General Hospital, n = 72). The horizontal axis is expanded and represents the time from hospital discharge to death. The depiction is otherwise similar to that seen in Fig. 28-12A.

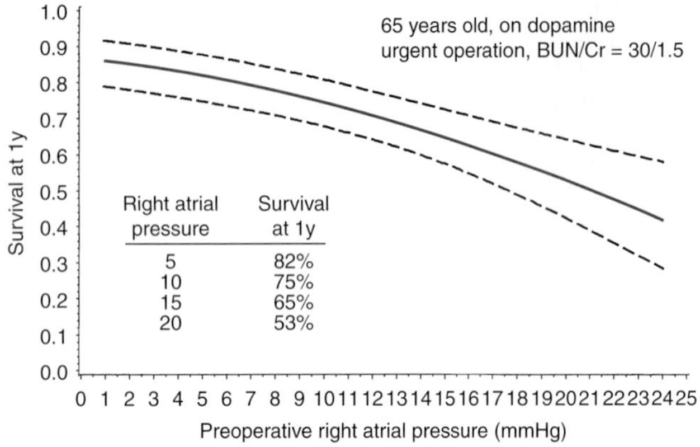

FIGURE 28-14 Survival at 1 year vs. preoperative right atrial pressure (Massachusetts General Hospital; n = 114). The depiction is a solution of the multivariate equation for a 65-year-old with a blood urea nitrogen of 30 mg/dL, a creatinine of 1.5 mg/dL, not on catecholamines, not an "emergency" case, and without a history of myocardial infarction or left main coronary artery disease.

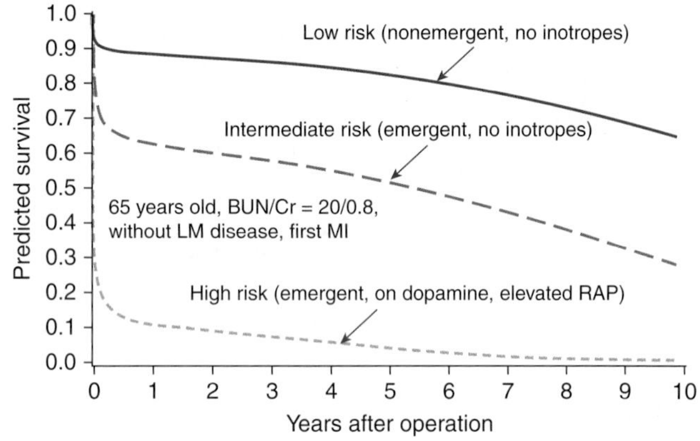

FIGURE 28-16 Nomograms (specific solutions of the multivariate equation) depicting the predicted survival in three hypothetical 65-year-old patients who present with ventricular septal defect. Each solution is for a patient who has no history of myocardial infarction and without left main coronary artery disease,blood urea nitrogen of 20 mg/dL, and creatinine of 0.8 mg/dL. The "low-risk" patient is nonemergent and not on inotropes with right atrial pressure (RAP) of 8 mm Hg. The "intermediaterisk" patient is emergent and not on inotropes with RAP of 12 mm Hg. The "high-risk"patient is emergent and on inotropes with RAP of 20 mm Hg. Confidence limits have been eliminated to improve clarity.

patients could be segregated using a few clinical variables (Figs. 28-15 and 28-16), most notably indicators of hemodynamic instability (emergency surgery and use of inotropes). The result was that a small group of high-risk patients dramatically affected the overall mortality rate. We believe that this phenomenon makes it very difficult to compare mortality among institutions. A slight difference in practice patterns, such as a tendency of a surgeon or referring cardiologist to deny operation, could substantially affect results. Additionally, any difference in transport dynamics to certain centers could lead to loss of unstable patients, which could create another type of selection bias. In our opinion, these issues are by far the most important source of mortality differences in modern series.

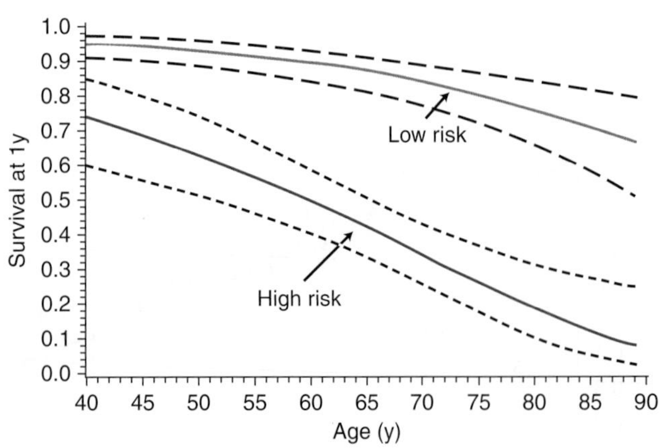

FIGURE 28-15 Nomograms (specific solutions to the multivariate equation) depicting the effect of age on risk in two different hypothetical patients. In both curves the patient was considered to have no left main disease, a blood urea nitrogen of 30 mg/dL, creatinine of 1.5 mg/dL, and no history of previous myocardial infarction. The curve for "low-risk" was solved for a patient who was not emergent and not on catecholamines.The curve for "high-risk"was for an emergent patient on inotropes. The vertical axis represents the calculated survival at 1 year.

Several centers have reported improved early results with an "exclusion" repair.[87,95] Our group has not been able to replicate these results, with a 60% mortality in 10 patients (higher than the rate achieved historically with traditional techniques). This is likely to the result of our tendency to use this technique on the most challenging type of defects in whom we anticipate a long and complex repair, and continued use of infarctectomy in the lower risk patients with anterior or apical defects.

Regardless of the technique, the most common cause of death after repair of acute postinfarction VSD was low cardiac output syndrome (52%). Technical failures, most commonly recurrent or residual VSD, but including bleeding, were the second most common (23%). Other causes of death include sepsis (17%), recurrent infarction (9%), cerebrovascular complications (4%), and intractable ventricular arrhythmias.

Long-Term Results

Long-term results have been favorable with regard to both mortality risk and functional rehabilitation. Actuarial survival at 5 years for most recent series generally ranges between 40 and 60% (see Table 28-2). Because of the overall high risk of the operation, it is rewarding to note that hospital survivors enjoy excellent longevity, with 1-, 5-, and 10-year survival of 91, 70, and 37%, respectively. They also are quite functional—among 15 of our patients contacted during follow-up of long-term survivors, 75% were in New York Heart Association functional class I, and 12.5% were class II.[18]

Recurrent Ventricular Septal Defects

Recurrent or residual septal defects have been diagnosed by Doppler color flow mapping early or late postoperatively in 10 to 25% of patients.[96] They may be caused by reopening of a closed defect, to the presence of an overlooked defect, or to the development of a new septal rupture during the early postoperative period. These recurrent defects should be closed when they cause symptoms or signs of heart failure or when the calculated shunt fraction (pulmonary-to-systemic flow ratio) is large (Qp:Qs >2.0). When they are small (Qp:Qs <2.0) and either asymptomatic or controlled with minimal diuretic therapy, a conservative approach is reasonable and late spontaneous closure can occur. Intervention in the catheterization laboratory may be useful in closing symptomatic residual or recurrent defects postoperatively.

Chronic Ventricular Septal Defects

In 1987 Rousou and associates reported successful closure of an acquired posterior VSD by means of a right transatrial approach.[97] Filgueira and colleagues have used the transatrial approach for *delayed* repair of chronic acquired posterior septal defects.[98] Approaching a postinfarction VSD through the tricuspid valve should not be used in acute cases because of the friability of the necrotic septum, poor exposure, and because this technique does not involve infarctectomy, and thus cannot achieve the hemodynamic advantages of elimination of a paradoxically bulging segment of ventricular wall. However, the right heart approach can be used in chronic postinfarction VSD when the septum is well scarred and the patch can be safely sutured to it from the right atrium. We emphasize that although the transatrial approach may be used selectively for the closure of chronic defects, it is unlikely to be an appropriate choice for the closure of acute defects, except perhaps in the rare circumstance when an infarct is localized to the septum with no evidence of necrosis of the free wall of the left ventricle.[25]

POSTINFARCTION VENTRICULAR FREE WALL RUPTURE

History

William Harvey first described rupture of the free wall of the heart after AMI in 1647.[99] In 1765, Morgagni reported 11 cases of myocardial rupture found postmortem.[100] Ironically, Morgagni later died of myocardial rupture.[101] Hatcher and colleagues from Emory University reported the first successful operation for free wall rupture of the right ventricle in 1970.[101] FitzGibbon and associates[102] in 1971 and Montegut[103] in 1972 reported the first successful repairs of left ventricular ruptures associated with ischemic heart disease.

Incidence

Autopsy studies reveal that ventricular free wall rupture occurs about 10 times more frequently than postinfarction ventricular septal rupture, occurring in about 11% of patients after AMI.[104] The incidence has been found to be as high as 31% in autopsy studies of anterior MI.[105] Ventricular rupture and cardiogenic shock are now the leading causes of death after AMI, and together account for greater than two-thirds of early deaths in patients suffering their first acute infarction. Postinfarction ventricular ruptures are more common in elderly women (mean age of 63 years) suffering their first infarction.[106] In the prethrombolytic era, 90% of ruptures occurred within 2 weeks after infarction with the peak incidence at 5 days.[107] In contrast, the time to cardiac rupture (not frequency of rupture) seems to be accelerated by thrombolysis and coronary reperfusion, sometimes occurring within hours from the onset of symptoms.[108]

Opinions differ as to the most common site of left ventricular rupture. The older literature suggests that the anterior wall is the most frequent site; however, more recent series have observed a preponderance of lateral and posterior wall ruptures.[104,105] Lateral wall infarction may be more likely to rupture than an anterior or inferior injury, but because anterior infarctions are much more frequent than lateral infarctions, overall the most common site of rupture is the anterior wall. Like postinfarction ventricular septal rupture, free wall ruptures may be simple or complex. A simple rupture results from a straight through-and-through tear that is perpendicular to the endothelial and epicardial surfaces, whereas a complex rupture results from a more serpiginous tear, often oblique to the endocardial and epicardial surfaces. Batts and coworkers[107] reported 100 consecutive cases of left ventricular free wall rupture and found that half were simple ruptures and the rest were complex.

Pathogenesis and Pathophysiology

Left ventricular free wall rupture can be divided into three clinicopathologic categories: acute, subacute, and chronic. An *acute* or "blow-out" rupture is characterized by sudden recurrent chest pain, electrical mechanical dissociation, profound shock, and death within a few minutes because of massive hemorrhage into the pericardial cavity. This type of rupture is probably not amenable to current management. A *subacute* rupture is characterized by a smaller tear, which may be temporarily sealed by clot or fibrinous pericardial adhesions. These usually present with the signs and symptoms of cardiac tamponade, and eventually cardiogenic shock. Subacute rupture may mimic other complications of AMI, such as infarct extension and right ventricular failure, and may be compatible with life for several hours or days or even longer.[109] A *chronic* rupture with *false aneurysm* formation occurs when the leakage of blood is slow and when surrounding pressure on the epicardium temporarily controls the hemorrhage. Adhesions form between the epicardium and pericardium, which reinforce and contain the rupture. The most common clinical presentation of patients with false aneurysms of the left ventricle is CHF.[110] A false aneurysm may also be an echocardiographic finding in an otherwise asymptomatic patient recovering from AMI. Angina, syncope, arrhythmias, and thromboembolic complications occur in a small percentage of patients. There are four major differences between a true and false aneurysm of the left ventricle:

1. The wall of a false aneurysm contains no myocardial cells.
2. False aneurysms are more likely to form posteriorly.
3. False aneurysms usually have a narrow neck.
4. False aneurysms have a great propensity for rupture.

Rupture of the free wall of the left ventricle may occur in isolation or with rupture of other ventricular structures such as the interventricular septum, papillary muscles, or right ventricle.[110,111]

The pathogenesis of cardiac rupture remains poorly understood. However, cardiac rupture occurs only with transmural MIs and infarction expansion appears to play an important role in its pathogenesis.[24,27,112] Infarct expansion is an acute regional thinning and dilatation of the infarct zone, seen as early as 24 hours after acute transmural MI and not related to additional myocardial necrosis.[113] This regional thinning and dilatation of the infarct zone is a consequence of slippage between muscle bundles, resulting in a reduction in the number of myocytes across the infarcted area. Infarct expansion increases the size of the ventricular cavity, with a consequent increase in wall tension (Laplace effect) that subjects the infarct zone to more tension and predisposes to endocardial tearing.[109] Systemic hypertension aggravates the problem of thinning and dilatation of the infarct wall and increases the probability of rupture.[114] Lack of collateral flow may also promote ventricular rupture.[115]

Because myocardial rupture occurs in regions of complete transmural myocardial necrosis, usually after extensive hemorrhagic transformation of the acute infarct, and because thrombolytic therapy is associated with the conversion of a bland infarct into a hemorrhagic infarct, there has been an ongoing concern that thrombolysis might increase the likelihood of ventricular rupture.[117] Honan and associates[116] performed a meta-analysis of four large clinical trials (1638 patients) in which streptokinase was used to treat AMIs and concluded that the risk of cardiac rupture was directly related to the timing of thrombolytic therapy. Early treatment (within 7 hours from the onset of symptoms) decreased the risk of cardiac rupture, whereas late treatment (after 17 hours) increased the risk of this complication even though, surprisingly, the overall mortality rate was diminished when streptokinase was given late after acute infarction. In a prospective ancillary study of 5711 patients, Late Assessment of Thrombolytic Efficacy, Becker and colleagues[108] were unable to show an increased risk of cardiac rupture in patients treated with recombinant tissue plasminogen activator 6 to 24 hours after the onset of symptoms. Thus, there is general agreement that early successful thrombolysis decreases the overall risk of cardiac rupture, probably by limiting the extent of necrosis, resulting in a nontransmural instead of transmural infarct, but the impact of late thrombolytic therapy on cardiac rupture remains unclear.

Diagnosis

The clinical picture of a subacute ventricular rupture is primarily that of pericardial tamponade, with pulsus paradoxus, distended neck veins, and cardiogenic shock. Although 5 to 37% of patients with AMI but no rupture may develop a pericardial effusion, echocardiographic signs that increase the sensitivity and specificity for cardiac rupture include effusion thickness greater than 10 mm, echodense masses in the effusion, ventricular wall defects, and signs of tamponade (eg, right atrial and right ventricular early diastolic collapse and increased respiratory variation in transvalvular blood flow velocities).[118,119] Pericardiocentesis and aspiration of uncoagulated blood have historically been considered the most reliable criteria of subacute ventricular rupture; however, false-positive and -negative diagnoses have been reported. The demonstration of a clear pericardial fluid on pericardiocentesis definitively excludes cardiac rupture.[118] Pericardiocentesis is of therapeutic value in some patients, often providing short-term circulatory improvement.

In an attempt to define symptomatic, electrocardiographic, and hemodynamic markers that may permit the prospective identification of patients prone to rupture of the heart after AMI, Oliva and colleagues[104] retrospectively studied 70 consecutive patients with rupture and 100 comparison patients with AMI but without rupture. They found a number of markers that were associated with a significant increase in the risk of rupture (Table 28-4). The presence of a lateral infarction,

TABLE 28-4 Sensitivity, Specificity and Predictive Value of Symptoms and Electrocardiographic Criteria for Cardiac Rupture

	Sensitivity (%)	Specificity (%)	Predictive value (%)
Pericarditis	86	72	68
Repetitive emesis	64	95	90
Restlessness, agitation	55	95	86
Two or more symptoms	84	97	95
ST segment deviations	61	72	58
T wave deviations	94	66	66
ST-T wave deviations	61	68	64

From Oliva PB, Hammill SC, Edwards WD: Cardiac rupture, a clinically predictable complication of acute myocardial infarction: report of 70 cases with clinicopathologic correlations. J Am Coll Cardiol 1993; 22:720.

especially with associated inferior or posterior infarction, identified a subset of patients at increased risk for rupture. Persistent, progressive, or recurrent ST-segment elevation, and especially persistent T-wave changes after 48 to 72 hours, or the gradual reversal of initially inverted T waves, are associated with an increased risk of rupture. Finally, the development of pericarditis, repetitive emesis, or restlessness and agitation, particularly two or three of these symptoms, conveyed predictive value.[105]

Natural History

Acute rupture of the free wall of the left ventricle is invariably fatal, with death usually occurring within minutes of the onset of recurrent chest pain.[107,109] In most of these cases, the sequence of events leading to death is so rapid that there is not enough time for surgical intervention. In contrast, patients with a subacute rupture usually survive hours or days, rarely weeks, following the myocardial tear. Pollack and colleagues[119] found that in 24 patients with postinfarction subacute rupture, survival time (ie, time from critical event to death) varied between 45 minutes and 6.5 weeks, with a median survival of 8 hours. Núñez and coworkers[120] found that in 29 patients with subacute rupture, 20 (69%) died within minutes of the onset of symptoms, and 9 (31%) lived several hours, allowing time for treatment. Subacute ventricular ruptures are generally considered to be less common than acute free wall ruptures. In recent studies, with high autopsy rates, 21 to 42% of all postinfarction free wall ruptures followed a subacute course.[119,121,122]

Because of its rarity, the natural history of false aneurysm of the left ventricle has not been well established. It is believed to have a poor prognosis because of its high probability of rupture;[122,123] however, there are patients in whom the diagnosis was made many years after MI.[124,125] The increasingly wide application of echocardiography after AMI gives promise of altering clinical outcome for many patients with the various forms of ventricular wall rupture.

Preoperative Management

Usually the sequence of events leading to death is so rapid in patients with acute rupture of the free wall of the left ventricle that there is not enough time for surgical intervention. These patients typically die within minutes of the onset of recurrent chest pain.[120] However, a high index of suspicion, emergent surgery, perhaps combined with a novel technique of percutaneous intrapericardial infusion of fibrin glue immediately after pericardiocentesis,[126] may afford at least a chance of survival in this surgically untreatable subgroup of patients.

In contrast, patients with subacute left ventricular rupture can be saved with surgery. Once the diagnosis of rupture of the free wall is established, the patient should be immediately transferred to the operating room. No time should be wasted attempting to perform coronary angiography.[108,110,125] Inotropic agents and fluids should be started while preparing for surgery. Pericardiocentesis often improves hemodynamics temporarily, and insertion of an intra-aortic balloon pump may be beneficial, even though the principal problem is cardiac tamponade.

The timing of surgery after the diagnosis of false aneurysm of the left ventricle is dependent upon the age of the MI. When a false aneurysm is discovered within the first 2 to 3 months after coronary infarction, surgery is urgently recommended after coronary angiography and ventriculography because of the unpredictability of rupture.[111,127] However, when the diagnosis is made several months or years after MI, the urgency of the operation is not determined so much by the risk of rupture, but rather by symptoms and the severity of the CAD.[109,124]

Operative Techniques

Subacute Rupture of the Free Wall

As soon as the diagnosis of rupture of the free wall of the left ventricle is confirmed by echocardiography, the patient should be transferred to the operating room. In patients with tamponade, severe hypotension may result during the induction of anesthesia. Therefore, we usually complete the sterile preparation and draping of the patient before inducing anesthesia, with preparations for rapid cannulation of the groin if needed. A median sternotomy is performed and upon decompressing the pericardium, the blood pressure commonly rises quickly. This should be anticipated and controlled because hypertension can cause ventricular bleeding to start again, or may even increase the size of the ventricular rent. In most cases, however, the ventricular tear is sealed off by clot, and there is no active bleeding.

Traditionally postinfarction rupture of the free wall of the left heart has been repaired on cardiopulmonary bypass; however, some surgeons have suggested that cardiopulmonary bypass is not necessary except perhaps in patients with posterior wall rupture, severe mitral regurgitation, ventricular septal rupture, or graftable CAD.[109,127] Although the ventricular tear can be repaired without aortic cross-clamping, cardiac standstill and left ventricular decompression make the procedure easier when the rupture is in the posterior wall of the left ventricle.[109]

The term *ventricular double rupture* has been applied when there is rupture of two of the following three structures: the ventricular septum, ventricular free wall, and papillary muscle.

Four surgical techniques have been used to control ventricular rupture. The first technique involves closing the rent with large horizontal mattress sutures buttressed with two strips of Teflon felt.[101] This method is not recommended because the sutures are placed into necrotic, friable myocardium that can easily tear. The second method combines infarct excision and closure of the defect with interrupted, pledgeted sutures[102,128] or a Dacron patch.[129] This method usually requires aortic cross-clamping and is probably best reserved for those patients who have an associated VSD. The third technique, described by Núñez and colleagues,[120] involves closing the defect with horizontal mattress sutures buttressed with two strips of Teflon felt, and then covering the closed ventricular tear and surrounding infarcted myocardium with a Teflon patch sutured to healthy epicardium with a continuous polypropylene suture (Fig. 28-17). Good control of active ventricular hemorrhage has been achieved with this method. The fourth method consists of simply gluing a patch of either Teflon[127] or autologous glutaraldehyde-preserved bovine pericardium to the ventricular tear and infarcted area

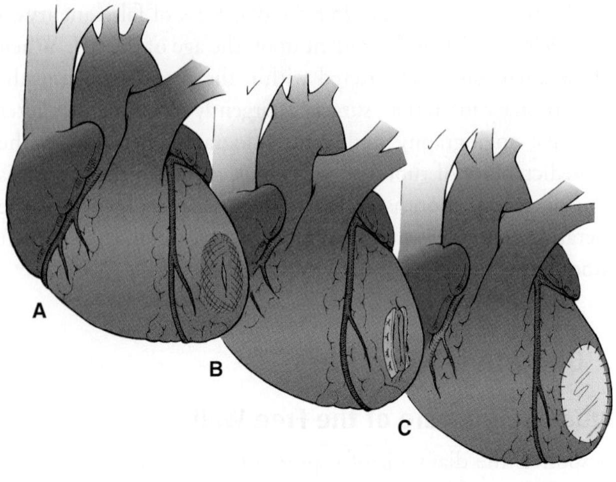

FIGURE 28-17 Technique to repair rupture of the free wall of the left ventricle. (A) Left ventricular free wall rupture. (B) A limited infarctectomy is closed with horizontal mattress sutures buttressed with two strips of Teflon felt. (C) Then the whole area is covered with a Teflon patch sutured to healthy epicardium with a continuous polypropylene suture. Alternatively, the Teflon patch can be glued to the ventricular tear and the infarcted area using a biocompatible glue. (*Adapted with permission from David.*[138])

using a biocompatible glue of either fibrin (Tissucol, Immuno AG, Vienna, Austria), butyl-2-cyanoacrylate monomer (Histoacryl Blue, B. Braun, Melsungen AG, Germany), or gelatin-resorcin-formaldehyde (Pharmacie Centrale, C.H.V. Henry Mondor, Créteil, France). This technique does not necessarily require institution of cardiopulmonary bypass and, because of its simplicity, may be the repair of choice when the ventricle is not actively bleeding.

False Aneurysm of the Left Ventricle

Acute false aneurysms are probably best repaired with an endocardial patch using the same methods as those used in repairing true ventricular aneurysms.[109] Chronic anterior false aneurysms can usually be closed primarily if the neck is fibrotic. However, primary closure of the neck of a posterior false aneurysm may exacerbate mitral regurgitation, and it therefore probably should be reconstructed with a patch of Dacron graft or glutaraldehyde-fixed bovine pericardium.[110,111]

Results

Subacute Rupture of the Free Wall

The surgical experience with this entity is largely anecdotal. The single largest experience with surgical repair of postinfarction left ventricular free wall rupture was reported by Padró and colleagues.[127] They treated 13 patients using a Teflon patch glued onto the ventricular tear and surrounding infarcted muscle, and used cardiopulmonary bypass in only one patient who presented with a posterior defect. All of their patients survived and were alive after a mean follow-up of 26 months. Eleven of them were asymptomatic and two had exertional angina. Núñez and associates[120] operated on seven patients, four of whom survived. Recently the use of unsupported felt secured with cyanoacrylate glue has been described by several authors with encouraging results.[130,131]

In ventricular double rupture involving the free wall and the septum, a recent series achieved an operative survival of 60% in five patients.[132] Four of the patients initially had only septal rupture but progressed to include free wall rupture, making this diagnosis a consideration in acute deterioration of medically managed patients with postinfarct VSD.

Although operative risk cannot be determined from these small numbers, it is likely that without surgery all these patients would have died, and patients who survive surgery tend to do well afterward.[109]

False Aneurysm of the Left Ventricle

Komeda and David[110] treated 12 patients with postinfarction left ventricular false aneurysms; four of them also had mitral valve replacements, one had repair of a fistula between the false aneurysm and the right ventricle, and nine had coronary artery bypass surgery. There were three operative deaths, all in patients who needed mitral valve replacements. Of the eight patients who underwent isolated repair of false aneurysms, all were alive after a mean follow-up of 62 months. Seven patients were asymptomatic and one had angina pectoris. Overall, the literature suggests that patients who have isolated repair of false aneurysms of the left ventricle have low operative mortality.

REFERENCES

1. Latham PM: *Lectures on Subjects Connected with Clinical Medicine Comprising Diseases of the Heart.* London, Longman Rees, 1845.
2. Brunn F: Diagnostik der erworbenen ruptur der kammerscheidewand des herzens. *Wien Arch Inn Med* 1923; 6:533.
3. Sager R: Coronary thrombosis: perforation of the infarcted interventricular septum. *Arch Intern Med* 1934; 53:140.
4. Cooley DA, Belmonte BA, Zeis LB, Schnur S: Surgical repair of ruptured interventricular septum following acute myocardial infarction. *Surgery* 1957; 41:930.
5. Effler DB, Tapia FA, McCormack LJ: Rupture of the ventricular myocardium and perforation of the interventricular septum complicating acute myocardial infarction. *Circulation* 1959; 20:128.
6. Payne WS, Hunt JC, Kirklin JW: Surgical repair of ventricular septal defect due to myocardial infarction: report of a case. *JAMA* 1963; 183:603.
7. Lee WY, Cardon L, Slodki SV: Perforation of infarcted interventricular septum. *Arch Intern Med* 1962; 109:135.
8. Dobell ARC, Scott HJ, Cronin RFP, Reid EAS: Surgical closure of interventricular septal perforation complicating myocardial infarction. *J Thorac Cardiovasc Surg* 1962; 43:802.
9. Heimbecker RO, Lemire G, Chen C: Surgery for massive myocardial infarction. *Circulation* 1968; 11(Suppl 2):37.
10. Lojos TZ, Greene DG, Bunnell IL, et al: Surgery for acute myocardial infarction. *Ann Thorac Surg* 1969; 8:452.
11. Daggett WM, Burwell LR, Lawson DW, Austen WG: Resection of acute ventricular aneurysm and ruptured interventricular septum after myocardial infarction. *NEJM* 1970; 283:1507.
12. Stinson EB, Becker J, Shumway NE: Successful repair of postinfarction ventricular septal defect and biventricular aneurysm. *J Thorac Cardiovasc Surg* 1969; 58:20.
13. Lundberg S, Sodestrom J: Perforation of the interventricular septum in myocardial infarction: a study based on autopsy material. *Acta Med Scand* 1962; 172:413.
14. Hutchins GM: Rupture of the interventricular septum complicating myocardial infarction: pathological analysis of 10 patients with clinically diagnosed perforation. *Am Heart J* 1979; 97:165.
15. Selzer A, Gerbode F, Keith WJ: Clinical, hemodynamic and surgical considerations of rupture of the ventricular septum after myocardial infarction. *Am Heart J* 1969; 78:598.

16. Mann JM, Robert WC: Acquired ventricular septal defect during acute myocardial infarction: analysis of 38 unoperated necropsy patients and comparison with 50 unoperated necropsy patients without rupture. *Am J Cardiol* 1988; 62:8.
17. Silver MD, Butany J, Chiasson DA: The pathology of myocardial infarction and its mechanical complications, in David TE (ed): *Mechanical Complications of Myocardial Infarction.* Austin, TX, RG Landes, 1993; p 4.
18. Daggett WM, Buckley MJ, Akins CW, et al: Improved results of surgical management of postinfarction ventricular septal rupture. *Ann Surg* 1982; 196:269.
19. Skehan JD, Carey C, Norrell MS, et al: Patterns of coronary artery disease in post-infarction ventricular septal rupture. *Br Heart J* 1989; 62:268.
20. Miller S, Dinsmore RE, Grenne RE, Daggett WM: Coronary, ventricular, and pulmonary abnormalities associated with rupture of the interventricular septum complicating myocardial infarction. *Am J Radiol* 1978; 131:571.
21. Hill JD, Lary D, Keith WJ, Gerbode F: Acquired ventricular septal defects: evolution of an operation, surgical technique and results. *J Thorac Cardiovasc Surg* 1975; 70:440.
22. Deville C, Fontan F, Chevalier JM, et al: Surgery of post-infarction ventricular defect: risk factors for hospital death and long-term results. *Eur J Cardiothorac Surg* 1991; 5:167.
23. Cummings RG, Reimer KA, Catliff R, et al: Quantitative analysis of right and left ventricular infarction in the presence of postinfarction ventricular septal defect. *Circulation* 1988; 77:33.
24. Weisman HF, Healy B: Myocardial infarct expansion, infarct extension, and reinfarction: pathophysiologic concepts. *Prog Cardiovasc Dis* 1987; 30:73.
25. David TE: Surgery for postinfarction ventricular septal defects, in David TE (ed): *Mechanical Complications of Myocardial Infarction.* Austin, TX, RG Landes, 1993; p 175.
26. Beranek JT: Hyaline degeneration. Present in heart infarction and implicated in pathogenesis of heart rupture. *Chest* 1994; 106:981.
27. Pfeffer MA, Braunwald E: Ventricular remodeling after myocardial infarction: clinical observations and clinical implications. *Circulation* 1990; 81:1161.
28. Abrams D, Edilist A, Luria M, Miller A: Ventricular aneurysms. *Circulation* 1963; 27:164.
29. Moore CA, Nygaard TW, Kaiser DL, et al: Postinfarction ventricular septal rupture: the importance of location of infarction and right ventricular function in determining survival. *Circulation* 1986; 74:45.
30. Zehender M, Kasper W, Kauder E: Right ventricular infarction as an independent predictor of prognosis after acute inferior myocardial infarction. *NEJM* 1993; 328:981.
31. Anderson DR, Adams S, Bhat A, Pepper JR: Postinfarction ventricular septal defect: the importance of site of infarction and cardiogenic shock on outcome. *Eur J Cardiothorac Surg* 1989; 3:554.
32. Campion BL, Harrison CE, Guiliani ER, et al: Ventricular septal defect after myocardial infarction. *Ann Intern Med* 1969; 70:251.
33. Vlodaver Z, Edwards JE: Rupture of ventricular septum or papillary muscle complicating myocardial infarction. *Circulation* 1977; 55:815.
34. Rawlins MO, Mendel D, Braimbridge MV: Ventricular septal defect and mitral regurgitation secondary to myocardial infarction. *Br Heart J* 1972; 34:323.
35. Taylor FH, Citron DS, Robicsek F, Sanger PW: Simultaneous repair of ventricular septal defect and left ventricular aneurysm following myocardial infarction. *Ann Thorac Surg* 1965; 1:72.
36. Meister SG, Helfant RH: Rapid differentiation of ruptured interventricular septum from acute mitral insufficiency. *NEJM* 1972; 287:1024.
37. Buckley MJ, Mundth ED, Daggett WM, et al: Surgical therapy for early complications of myocardial infarction. *Surgery* 1971; 70:814.
38. Smyllie JH, Sutherland GR, Geuskens R, et al: Doppler color flow mapping in the diagnosis of ventricular septal rupture and acute mitral regurgitation after myocardial infarction. *J Am Coll Cardiol* 1990; 15:1455.
39. Blanche C, Khan SS, Matloff JM, et al: Results of early repair of ventricular septal defect after an acute myocardial infarction. *J Thorac Cardiovasc Surg* 1992; 104:961.
40. Oyamada A, Queen FB: Spontaneous rupture of the interventricular septum following acute myocardial infarction with some clinico-pathologic observations on survival in five cases unpublished, 1961.
41. Berger TJ, Blackstone EH, Kirklin JW: Postinfarction ventricular septal defect, in Kirklin JW, Barratt-Boyes BG (eds): *Cardiac Surgery.* New York, Churchill Livingstone, 1993; p 403.
42. Lemery R, Smith HC, Giuliani ER, Gersh BJ: Prognosis in rupture of the ventricular septum after acute myocardial infarction and role of early surgical intervention. *Am J Cardiol* 1992; 70:147.
43. Heitmiller R, Jacobs ML, Daggett WM: Surgical management of postinfarction ventricular septal rupture. *Ann Thorac Surg* 1986; 41:683.
44. Baillot R, Pelletier C, Trivino-Marin J, Castonguay Y: Postinfarction ventricular septal defect: delayed closure with prolonged mechanical circulatory support. *Ann Thorac Surg* 1983; 35:138.
45. Gaudiani VA, Miller DC, Oyer PE, et al: Post-infarction ventricular septal defect: an argument for early operation. *Surgery* 1981; 89:48.
46. Gold HK, Leinbach RC, Sanders CA, et al: Intra-aortic balloon pumping for ventricular septal defect or mitral regurgitation complicating acute myocardial infarction. *Circulation* 1973; 47:1191.
47. Montoya A: Ventricular septal rupture secondary to acute myocardial infarction, in Pifarre R (ed): *Cardiac Surgery: Acute Myocardial Infarction and Its Complications.* Philadelphia, Hanley & Belfus, 1992; p 159.
48. Scanlon PJ, Monatoya A, Johnson SA: Urgent surgery for ventricular septal rupture complicating myocardial infarction. *Circulation* 1985; 72(Suppl 2):185.
49. Samuels L, Entwistle J, Holmes E, et al: Mechanical support of the unrepaired postinfarction ventricular septal defect with the Abiomed BVS 5000 ventricular assist device. *J Thorac Cardiovasc Surg* 2003; 126:2100.
50. David H, Hunter JA, Najafi H, et al: Left ventricular approach for the repair of ventricular septal perforation and infarctectomy. *J Thorac Cardiovasc Surg* 1972; 63:14.
51. Daggett WM, Randolph JD, Jacobs ML, et al: The superiority of cold oxygenated dilute blood cardioplegia. *Ann Thorac Surg* 1987; 43:397.
52. Teoh KH, Christakis GT, Weisel RD, et al: Accelerated myocardial metabolic recovery with terminal warm blood cardioplegia. *J Thorac Cardiovasc Surg* 1986; 91:888.
53. Shumacker H: Suggestions concerning operative management of postinfarction ventricular septal defects. *J Thorac Cardiovasc Surg* 1972; 64:452.
54. Daggett WM, Mundth ED, Gold HK, et al: Early repair of ventricular septal defects complicating inferior myocardial infarction. *Circulation* 1974; 50(Suppl 3):112.
55. Daggett WM: Surgical technique for early repair of posterior ventricular septal rupture. *J Thorac Cardiovasc Surg* 1982; 84:306.
56. Cooley DA: Repair of the difficult ventriculotomy. *Ann Thorac Surg* 1990; 49:150.
57. Cooley DA: Repair of postinfarction ventricular septal defect. *J Card Surg* 1994; 9:427.
58. Dor V, Saab M, Coste P, et al: Left ventricular aneurysm: a new surgical approach. *Thorac Cardiovasc Surg* 1989; 37:11.
59. Tashiro T, Todo K, Haruta Y, et al: Extended endocardial repair of postinfarction ventricular septal rupture: new operative technique modification of the Komeda-David operation. *J Card Surg* 1994; 9:97.
60. Usui A, Murase M, Maeda M, et al: Sandwich repair with two sheets of equine pericardial patch for acute posterior post-infarction ventricular septal defect. *Eur J Cardiothorac Surg* 1993; 7:47.
61. Imagawa H, Takano S, Shiozaki T, et al: Two-patch technique for postinfarction inferoposterior ventricular septal defect. *Ann Thorac Surg* 2009; 88:692-694.
62. Fujimoto K, Kawahito K, Yamaguchi A, et al: Percutaneous extracorporeal life support for treatment of fatal mechanical complications associated with acute myocardial infarction. *Artif Organs* 2001; 25:1000.
63. Landzberg MJ, Lock JE: Transcatheter management of ventricular septal rupture after myocardial infarction. *Semin Thorac Cardiovasc Surg* 1998; 10:128.
64. Lock JE, Block PC, McKay RG, et al: Transcatheter closure of ventricular septal defects. *Circulation* 1988; 78:361.
65. Michel-Behnke I, Le Trong-Phi, Waldecker B, et al: Percutaneous closure of congenital and acquired ventricular septal defects—considerations on selection of the occlusion device. *J Interventr Cardiol* 2005; 18:89.
66. Thiele H, Kaulfersch C, Daehnert I, et al: Immediate primary transcatheter closure of postinfarction ventricular septal defects. *Eur Heart J* 2009; 30:81-89.
67. Szkutnik M, Bialkowski J, Kusa J, et al: Postinfarction ventricular septal defect closure with Amplatzer occluders. *Eur J Cardiothorac Surg* 2003; 23:323.
68. Papadopoulos N, Moritz A, Dzemali O, et al: Long-term results of postinfarction ventricular septal rupture by infarct exclusion technique. Ann Thorac Surg 2009; 87:1421-1425.
69. Thiele H, Kaulfersch C, Daehnert I, et al: Immediate primary transcatheter closure of postinfarction ventricular septal defects. *Eur Heart J* 2009; 30(1):81-88.
70. Maree A, Jneid H, Palacios I: Percutaneous closure of a postinfarction ventricular septal defect that recurred after surgical repair. *Eur Heart J* 2006; 27:1626.
71. Hachida M, Nakano H, Hirai M, Shi CY: Percutaneous transaortic closure of postinfarction ventricular septal rupture. *Ann Thorac Surg* 1991; 51:655.

72. Abhyankar A, Jagtap P: Post-infarction ventricular septal defect: percutaneous transvenous closure using a Swan-Ganz catheter. *Catheter Cardiovasc Interv* 1999; 47:208.
73a. Meyns B, Vanermen H, Vanhaecke J, et al: Hemopump fails as bridge to transplantation in postinfarction ventricular septal defect. *J Heart Lung Transplant* 1994; 13:1133.
73b. Loisance DP, Lordez JM, Deleuze PH, et al: Acute postinfarction septal rupture: long-term results. *Ann Thorac Surg* 1991; 52:474.
74. Davies RH, Dawkins KD, Skillington PD, et al: Late functional results after surgical closure of acquired ventricular septal defect. *J Thorac Cardiovasc Surg* 1992; 106:592.
75. D'Ambra MN, LaRaia PJ, Philbin DM, et al: Prostaglandin E_1: a new therapy for refractory right heart failure and pulmonary hypertension after mitral valve replacement. *J Thorac Cardiovasc Surg* 1985; 89:567.
76. Rich GF, Murphy GD Jr, Roos CM, Johns RA: Inhaled nitric oxide: selective pulmonary vasodilatation in cardiac surgical patients. *Anesthesiology* 1993; 78:1028.
77. Seguin JR, Frapier JM, Colson P, Chaptal PA: Fibrin sealant for early repair of acquired ventricular septal defect. *J Thorac Cardiovasc Surg* 1992; 104:748.
78. Baldwin RT, Cooley DA: Mechanical support for intraventricular decompression in repair of left ventricular disruption. *Ann Thorac Surg* 1992; 54:176.
79. Papadopoulos N, Moritz A, Dzemali O, et al: Long-term results of postinfarction ventricular septal rupture by infarct exclusion technique. *Ann Thorac Surg* 2009; 87:1421-1425.
80. Jeppsson A, Liden H, Johnson P, et al: Surgical repair of post infarction ventricular septal defects: a national experience. *Eur J Cardiothorac Surg* 2005; 27:216.
81. Mantovani V, Mariscalco G, Leva C, et al: Surgical repair of postinfarction ventricular septal defect: 19 years of experience. *Int J Cardiol* 2005; 108:202.
82. Barker TA, Ramnarine IR, Woo EB, et al: Repair of post-infarct ventricular septal defect with or without coronary artery bypass grafting in the northwest of England: a 5-year multi-institutional experience. *Eur J Cardiothorac Surg* 2003; 24:940.
83. Labrousse L, Choukroun E, Chevalier JM, et al: Surgery for post infarction ventricular septal defect (VSD): risk factors for hospital death and long term results. *Eur J Cardiothorac Surg* 2002; 21:725.
84. Agnihotri AK, Madsen J, Daggett WM: Unpublished data from Massachusetts General Hospital experience, complied 2006.
85. Pretre R, Ye Q, Grúnefelfder J, et al: Role of myocardial revascularization in postinfarction ventricular septal rupture. *Ann Thorac Surg* 2000; 69:51.
86. Deja MA, Szostek J, Widenka K, et al: Post infarction ventricular septal defect—can we do better? *Eur J Cardiothorac Surg* 2000; 18:194.
87. Cooley DA: Postinfarction ventricular septal rupture. *Semin Thorac Cardiovasc Surg* 1998; 10:100.
88. David TE, Armstrong S: Surgical repair of postinfarction ventricular septal defect by infarct exclusion. *Semin Thorac Cardiovasc Surg* 1998; 10:105.
89. Dalrymple-Hay MJR, Monro JL, Livesey SA, Lamb RK: Postinfarction ventricular septal rupture: the Wessex experience. *Semin Thorac Cardiovasc Surg* 1998; 10:111.
90. Chaux A, Blanch C, Matloff JM, et al: Postinfarction ventricular septal defect. *Semin Thorac Cardiovasc Surg* 1998; 10:93.
91. Killen DA, Piehler JM, Borkon AM, et al: Early repair of postinfarction ventricular septal rupture. *Ann Thorac Surg* 1997; 63:138.
92. Cox FF, Morshuis WJ, Plokker T, et al: Early mortality after repair of postinfarction ventricular septal rupture: importance of rupture location. *Ann Thorac Surg* 1996; 61:1752.
93. Ellis CJ, Parkinson GF, Jaffe WM, et al: Good long-term outcome following surgical repair of post-infarction ventricular septal defect. *Aust NZ J Med* 1995; 25:330.
94. Loisance DY, Lordex JM, Deluze PH, et al: Acute postinfarction septal rupture: long-term results. *Ann Thorac Surg* 1991; 52:474.
95. David TE, Dale L, Sun Z: Postinfarction ventricular septal rupture: repair by endocardial patch with infarct exclusion. *J Thorac Cardiovasc Surg* 1995; 110:1315.
96. Skillington PD, Davies RH, Luff AJ, et al: Surgical treatment for infarct-related ventricular septal defects. *J Thorac Cardiovasc Surg* 1990; 99:798.
97. Rousou JA, Engelman RM, Breyer RH, et al: Transatrial repair of postinfarction posterior ventricular septal defect. *Ann Thorac Surg* 1987; 43:665.
98. Filgueira JL, Battistessa SA, Estable H, et al: Delayed repair of an acquired posterior septal defect through a right atrial approach. *Ann Thorac Surg* 1986; 42:208.
99. Willius FA, Dry TJ: *A History of the Heart and Circulation*. Philadelphia, WB Saunders, 1948.
100. Morgagni JB: *The Seat and Causes of Disease Investigated by Anatomy*. London, A. Millau & T. Cadell, 1769; p 811.
101. Hatcher CR Jr, Mansour K, Logan WD Jr, et al: Surgical complications of myocardial infarction. *Am Surg* 1970; 36:163.
102. FitzGibbon GM, Hooper GD, Heggtveit HA: Successful surgical treatment of postinfarction external cardiac rupture. *J Thorac Cardiovasc Surg* 1972; 63:622.
103. Montegut FJ Jr: Left ventricular rupture secondary to myocardial infarction. *Ann Thorac Surg* 1972; 14:75.
104. Oliva PB, Hammill SC, Edwards WD: Cardiac rupture, a clinically predictable complication of acute myocardial infarction: report of 70 cases with clinicopathologic correlations. *J Am Coll Cardiol* 1993; 22:720.
105. Hutchins KD, Skurnick J, Lavendar M, et al: Cardiac rupture in acute myocardial infarction: a reassessment. *Am J Forensic Med Pathol* 2002; 23:78.
106. Herlitz J, Samuelsson SO, Richter A, Hjalmarson Å: Prediction of rupture in acute myocardial infarction. *Clin Cardiol* 1988; 11:63.
107. Batts KP, Ackermann DM, Edwards WD: Post-infarction rupture of the left ventricular free wall: clinicopathologic correlates in 100 consecutive autopsy cases. *Hum Pathol* 1990; 21:530.
108. Becker RC, Charlesworth A, Wilcox RG, et al: Cardiac rupture associated with thrombolytic therapy: impact of time to treatment in the Late Assessment of Thrombolytic Efficacy (LATE) study. *J Am Coll Cardiol* 1995; 25:1063.
109. David TE: Surgery for postinfarction rupture of the free wall of the ventricle, in David TE (ed): *Mechanical Complications of Myocardial Infarction*. Austin, TX, RG Landes, 1993; p 142.
110. Komeda M, David TE: Surgical treatment of postinfarction false aneurysm of the left ventricle. *J Thorac Cardiovasc Surg* 1993; 106:1189.
111. Mascarenhas DAN, Benotti JR, Daggett WM, et al: Postinfarction septal aneurysm with delayed formation of left-to-right shunt. *Am Heart J* 1991; 122:226.
112. Schuster EH, Bulkley BH: Expansion of transmural myocardial infarction: a pathophysiologic factor in cardiac rupture. *Circulation* 1979; 60:1532.
113. Hutchins GM, Bulkley BH: Infarct expansion versus extension: two different complications of acute myocardial infarction. *Am J Cardiol* 1978; 41:1127.
114. Christensen DJ, Ford M, Reading J, Castle CH: Effects of hypertension in myocardial rupture after acute myocardial infarction. *Chest* 1977; 72:618.
115. Pohjola-Sintonen S, Muller JE, Stone PH, et al: Ventricular septal and free wall rupture complicating acute myocardial infarction: experience in the multicenter investigation of limitation of infarct size. *Am Heart J* 1989; 117:809.
116. Honan MB, Harrell FE, Reimer KA, et al: Cardiac rupture, mortality and timing of thrombolytic therapy: a meta-analysis. *J Am Coll Cardiol* 1990; 16:359.
117. Westaby S, Parry A, Ormerod O, et al: Thrombolysis and postinfarction ventricular septal rupture. *J Thorac Cardiovasc Surg* 1992; 104:1506.
118. López-Sendón J, González A, López De Sá E, et al: Diagnosis of subacute ventricular wall rupture after acute myocardial infarction: sensitivity and specificity of clinical, hemodynamic and echocardiographic criteria. *J Am Coll Cardiol* 1992; 19:1145.
119. Pollack H, Diez W, Spiel R, et al: Early diagnosis of subacute free wall rupture complicating acute myocardial infarction. *Eur Heart J* 1993; 14:640.
120. Núñez L, de la Llana R, López Sendón J, et al: Diagnosis and treatment of subacute free wall ventricular rupture after infarction. *Ann Thorac Surg* 1982; 35:525.
121. Feneley MP, Chang VP, O'Rourke MF: Myocardial rupture after acute myocardial infarction: ten year review. *Br Heart J* 1983; 49:550.
122. Dellborg M, Held P, Swedberg K, Vedin A: Rupture of the myocardium: occurrence and risk factors. *Br Heart J* 1985; 54:11.
123. Epstein JI, Hutchins GM: Subepicardial aneurysms: a rare complication of myocardial infarction. *Am J Cardiol* 1983; 75:639.
124. Harper RW, Sloman G, Westlake G: Successful surgical resection of a chronic false aneurysm of the left ventricle. *Chest* 1975; 67:359.
125. Shabbo FP, Dymond DS, Rees GM, Hill IM: Surgical treatment of false aneurysm of the left ventricle after myocardial infarction. *Thorax* 1983; 38:25.
126. Kyo S, Ogiwara M, Miyamoto N, et al: Percutaneous intrapericardial fibrin-glue infusion therapy for rupture of the left ventricle free wall following acute myocardial infarction. *J Am Coll Cardiol* 1996; 27:327A.
127. Padró JM, Mesa J, Silvestre J, et al: Subacute cardiac rupture: repair with a sutureless technique. *Ann Thorac Surg* 1993; 55:20.
128. Eisenmann B, Bareiss P, Pacifico AD, et al: Anatomic, clinical, and therapeutic features of acute cardiac rupture. *J Thorac Cardiovasc Surg* 1978; 76:78.

129. Levett JM, Southgate TJ, Jose AB, et al: Technique for repair of left ventricular free wall rupture. *Ann Thorac Surg* 1988; 46:248.
130. Pappas PJ, Cernaianu AC, Baldino WA, et al: Ventricular free-wall rupture after myocardial infarction: treatment and outcome. *Chest* 1991; 4:892.
131. Lachapelle K, deVarennes B, Ergina PL: Sutureless patch technique for postinfarction left ventricular rupture. *Ann Thorac Surg* 2002; 74:96.
132. Tanaka K, Sato N, Yasutake M, et al: Clinicopathological characteristics of 10 patients with rupture of both the ventricular free wall and septum (double rupture) after acute myocardial infarction. *J Nippon Med Sch* 2003; 70:21.

CHAPTER 29

Ischemic Mitral Regurgitation

Pavan Atluri
Robert C. Gorman
Joseph H. Gorman III
Michael A. Acker

INTRODUCTION

Ischemic mitral regurgitation (IMR), often termed *functional* mitral regurgitation, is mitral insufficiency as a result of myocardial ischemia or infarction. By definition, the mitral valve leaflets are structurally normal in IMR. The malcoaptation of the leaflets and resultant regurgitation of the mitral valve in IMR is a result of either acute papillary muscle dysfunction or rupture, or chronic changes with left ventricular remodeling and subsequent changes in geometry.

Ischemic mitral regurgitation (IMR) is associated with decreased quality of life and long-term survival. Although extensive mechanistic research has been conducted, the optimal management of IMR remains elusive. Clinical studies in the past often included MR of multiple etiologies, including degenerative or nonischemic origin and IMR grouped into the same category, leading to confusion and incorrect conclusions regarding the natural history and true long-term impact of IMR. It is important to distinguish IMR from mitral regurgitation resulting from nonischemic etiologies. Mitral regurgitation is often associated with coronary artery disease without a direct cause-and-effect relationship. Given the prevalence of coronary artery disease, the association of myocardial infarction and nonischemic mitral regurgitation is a common clinical association. IMR must be distinguished from mitral insufficiency caused by degenerative, rheumatic, congenital, and infectious etiologies, as well as that arising from idiopathic dilated cardiomyopathy. Our recognition of IMR as a distinct clinical entity has improved the understanding of the pathophysiology and natural history of this distinct disease process.

IMR can produce a variety of very variable clinical presentations depending on infarct characteristics and subsequent postinfarction ventricular remodeling. The size, location, and transmurality of the myocardial infarction (MI) sets in motion varying degrees of left ventricular remodeling that subsequently determine the severity, time course, and clinical manifestations of IMR. The presentation may be either acute and immediately life threatening, or develop insidiously over time in association with congestive heart failure (CHF).

PREVALENCE

The advancement in catheter-based intervention for coronary artery disease and medical therapy has resulted in dramatically improved survival from ischemic heart disease and acute myocardial infarctions (AMI). Although survival following an AMI has improved, there has been a subsequent increase in the incidence of congestive heart failure. The American Heart Association estimates that 5.7 million Americans were in various stages of congestive heart failure in 2006.[1] An increasing number of ischemic cardiomyopathy patients will develop left ventricular dysfunction and IMR as a result of annular dilatation and/or papillary muscle displacement.

Early after an acute myocardial infarction (AMI), between 11 and 55% of patients develop clinical (mitral systolic murmur), echocardiographic, or angiographic evidence of IMR. A recent echocardiographic study investigating the incidence of mechanical complications after acute myocardial infarction found a significantly reduced incidence of mitral regurgitation in the percutaneous coronary intervention (PCI) era, but still noted a very large incidence of post-MI acute ischemic MR, 28 versus 53%.[2] Many of the murmurs early after acute myocardial infarction are transient and disappear by the time of discharge without further intervention, implying a correction of acute MR without intervention.

In one study, 19% of 11,748 patients who had elective cardiac catheterization for symptomatic coronary artery disease (CAD) had ventriculographic evidence of mitral regurgitation (MR).[3] In most of these patients the degree of mitral insufficiency was mild, but in 7.2% the degree of regurgitation was 2+ or greater, and in 3.4% MR was severe with evidence of heart failure.[3] In another study of consecutive cardiac catheterizations, 10.9% of 1739 patients with CAD had MR.[4]

Collectively, these data indicate that IMR is frequent early after AMI, but in many patients it is mild or disappears completely. The relatively high incidence of IMR in catheterized patients with symptomatic CAD suggests that chronic IMR persists in many patients after acute infarction and/or may subsequently develop in others. Approximately 16.8 million Americans have CAD, 7.9 million have had at least one myocardial infarction, 9.8 million suffer from angina, and millions more have asymptomatic coronary atherosclerosis that remains to be diagnosed.[1] Using these figures, the incidence of IMR in the United States is estimated to be 1.2 to 2.1 million patients, with approximately 425,000 patients having moderate or severe IMR with heart failure.[3,5]

CLASSIFICATION

IMR has traditionally been classified based on the time course of clinical presentation. Acute IMR occurs in the immediate postinfarction period, and the patients are often in hemodynamic distress. Fortunately, this population of patients represents a minority of the IMR cohort. Chronic IMR represents the clinical presentation for the majority of patients with IMR. The chronic presentation is one of progressive and insidious nature and is often associated with decremental decrease in left ventricular function.

In his landmark American Association for Thoracic Surgery–invited distiguinshed lecture and corresponding 1983 paper, *Cardiac Valve Surgery: The French Correction,* Dr. Carpentier provided an insightful way to mechanistically approach MR, including IMR. This classification scheme categorizes the improper leaflet coaptation of mitral regurgitation into three subsets based on leaflet and chordal pathology. In type I dysfuction, leaflet motion is normal and mitral regurgitation results from mitral annular dilatation. Type II is mitral regurgitation as a result of leaflet prolapse or excessive motion. In type III dysfunction, there is leaflet restriction or tethering, and is further subclassified into "a" (tethering during diastole) and "b" (tethering during systole and diastole).

IMR can result from type I, II, or IIIb dysfunction. Acute postinfarct mitral regurgitation can be a result of type II dysfunction, in which there is papillary muscle rupture. However, acute IMR is more often associated with much more subtle changes in the mitral valve apparatus. Chronic IMR classically presents as either type I or IIIb dysfunction. Pure annular dilatation with normal leaflets (type I) results from left ventricular remodeling and its geometric sequalae on the mitral valve apparatus. Type IIIb is the more common dysfunction associated with chronic IMR, and is the result of papillary muscle displacement and subsequent tethering of leaflets that results from ventricular dilatation and remodeling that occurs with ischemic cardiomyopathy. Often, a combination of type I and IIIb dysfunctions are seen in patients with chronic IMR and cardiomyopathy.

PATHOPHYSIOLOGY

Normal Valve Function

The mitral valve has six anatomical components: leaflets, chordae tendineae, annulus, papillary muscles, left ventricle (LV), and left atrium. The mitral annulus is saddle-shaped (hyperbolic paraboloid with two-directional curvature) with cephalad promontories near the mid portions of the anterior and posterior leaflets and caudad depressions at the commissures (Fig. 29-1).[6] This unique shape, which is present in all mammalian mitral valves, has been shown, using finite element analysis, to reduce leaflet, annular, and chordal stress.[7] Function of the normal mitral valve is complex and involves precisely timed interactions among the six components. These interactions are most easily described by relating the changes in each of the six components during a cardiac cycle. For this description the cardiac cycle is divided into four periods: systole, diastole, isovolumetric relaxation (IVR), and isovolumetric contraction (IVC), as defined in the following.

End systole (ES) is defined as the maximum negative left ventricular dP/dt and end diastole (ED) is defined as the peak of the QRS complex. End isovolumetric contraction (EIVC) is defined as the first time point at which the aortic root dP/dt is greater than zero. End isovolumetric relaxation (EIVR) is defined as the time at which the LVP is 10% of LVP_{max} and the left ventricular dP/dt less than 0.

During isovolumetric contraction (IVC), left atrial filling begins immediately after the mitral valve closes and before the

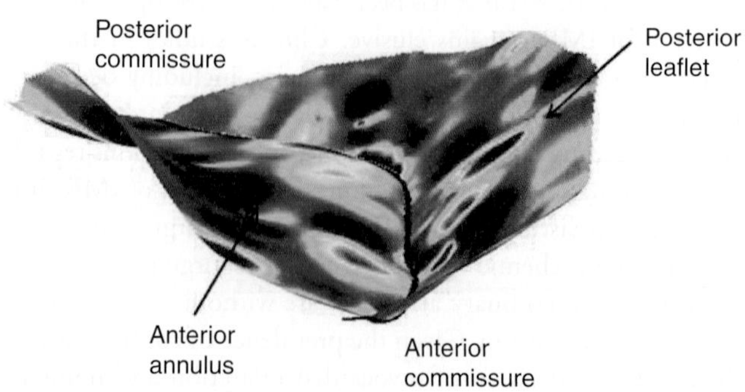

FIGURE 29-1 A rendering of a normal human mitral valve using an image analysis algorithm recently developed at the University of Pennsylvania. The technique uses real-time 3D echocardiography to assess mitral annular geometry and leaflet curvature. The pseudocolor map in the figure depicts regional Gaussian curvature in the anterior and posterior mitral leaflets. Deeper blue colors represent more negative Gaussian curvature, which is indicative of a hyperbolic (saddle-shaped) curvature and reduced leaflet stress.

aortic valve opens. Flow through the mitral valve briefly reverses as the leaflets coapt and bulge toward the atrium.

During systole the left atrium rapidly fills and reaches maximum volume near ES. The position of the annulus ascends (away from the apex) slightly during atrial contraction, which occurs during late diastole, does not change during IVC, and descends progressively 1 to 1.5 cm toward the apex throughout systole. The annulus asymmetrically contracts during atrial and ventricular systole and in humans reaches a minimal area (mean reduction of 27%) in mid systole.[8–10] Immediately after atrial contraction, the mitral leaflets approach each other and close within 20 to 60 milliseconds after pressure crossover when LV pressure exceeds LA pressure. Because the total area of leaflet tissue is approximately twice the total area of the annulus, the apposition point of the two leaflets at the time of pressure crossover is very near the plane of the annulus. At closure, approximately 30% of the anterior cusp and 50% of the longer posterior cusp are in apposition. Chordae tendineae attached to the free edges and body of the leaflets restrict the upward movement of the slightly compliant leaflets and produce a tight seal along the line of apposition. Chordal tension peaks in early systole and begins to fall slowly in late systole and rapidly during IVR. Papillary muscles begin to shorten during late IVC and throughout systole in synchrony with shortening of the adjacent ventricular wall. The actual distance the papillary muscles shorten is small and ranges between 2 and 4 mm.[11,12] During systole, the directions and timing of left ventricular contraction are not necessarily uniform throughout because of the complex anatomical arrangement of muscle bundles and the timing produced by the impulse conduction pattern.[13] LV shortening is greater in both equatorial axes than in the long axis.[13] LV wall thickness increases during IVC and decreases rapidly during IVR.[14] Peak wall thickness occurs near ES, but timing of the exact peak varies slightly between ventricular wall segments. During systole the ventricle progressively twists counterclockwise (as viewed from the apex) along its longitudinal axis to reach a maximum at ES.[15]

During IVR the left atrium begins to empty when left atrial pressure crosses over and exceeds LV pressure. The atrium empties rapidly in early diastole and further diminishes with atrial contraction in late diastole just before IVC. The LV may actually generate negative pressure in early diastole if left atrial pressures are low. During IVR, the mitral annulus to LV apex distance lengthens as the mitral annulus ascends in early diastole, descends slightly, and ascends again with atrial contraction. The area of the mitral orifice increases slightly during IVR and continues to increase during diastole until it reaches a maximum just before the left atrium contracts. In humans, the annular area index reaches a maximum of 3.9 ± 0.7 cm^2/m^2.[10] As the annular area increases, its shape changes asymmetrically; most of the area increase is caused by lengthening in the posterior and lateral parts of the annulus (away from the fibrous trigone).[8] During IVR the mitral leaflets separate approximately 30 milliseconds before left atrial pressure exceeds LV pressure.[16] Peak blood flow through the valve occurs early in diastole, but the mitral leaflets reach their maximal open position before peak flow occurs and begin closing while flow is still accelerating.

The papillary muscles may shorten very slightly during early IVR, but do not begin to lengthen until the beginning of diastole. Papillary muscles reach maximum length shortly after ED during IVC. Chordal tension decreases rapidly during IVR and remains near zero until late diastole, when a small increase occurs. The left ventricle relaxes and dilates after ES and reverses the complex deformations of LV shape produced by systole. During early diastole, and the period of rapid filling, the ventricle dilates primarily along both equatorial axes and much less along the longitudinal, base-to-apex axis. Only a little shape change occurs in mid diastole and after atrial contraction. Ventricular wall thickness decreases primarily during IVR. Last, the ventricle rapidly untwists (rotating clockwise) during early diastole and more gradually during mid and late diastole.

Mechanism of Ischemic Mitral Regurgitation

Acute Ischemic Mitral Regurgitation

Papillary muscle rupture is a rare, often fatal complication, occuring in 1 to 5% of patients who die after myocardial infarction, as determined by autopsy studies.[17] The rupture involves the posteromedial papillary muscle in approximately two-thirds of acute, severe IMR. The vascular supply to the posteromedial papillary muscle is dependent on a single coronary artery (the right coronary artery, or the circumflex coronary artery in a left-dominant system), whereas the anterolateral papillary muscle receives dual supply from the left anterior descending and circumflex coronary arteries. Papillary muscle rupture results in prolapse of the mitral leaflets, often causing severe acute IMR, hemodynamic instability, and acute pulmonary edema. Acute mitral regurgitation in this setting carries a poor prognosis with a high mortality rate.

More often, acute IMR occurs with subtle changes in the mitral valve apparatus in the absence of leaflet prolapse. Annular dilatation has traditionally been regarded as the mechanism of acute IMR. Laboratory work involving an ovine model from the Stanford group has demonstrated the importance of the septolateral (SL) dimension of the mitral annulus in the pathophysiology of IMR.[18–20] The SL dimension, the vertical distance of the mitral annulus from the middle of the anterior annulus to the middle of the posterior annulus, is clinically referred as the *anteroposterior* (AP) dimension. Timek and coworkers demonstrated that correcting SL distance alone may abolish acute IMR.[19]

However, other experimental studies have demonstrated subvalvular geometric changes as important contributors to the pathophysiology of acute IMR. With ischemia or infarction, the posterior papillary muscle elongates 2 to 4 mm in the sheep and dog[12,21]; the tip moves 1.5 to 3.0 mm closer to the annulus.[12,22] In the sheep model of acute IMR, the uninfarcted, preserved anterior papillary muscle contracts earlier and more vigorously than before infarction. This moves the tip 4 to 5 mm further away from the annular plane at mid systole than before infarction.[23] The Stanford group has meticulously characterized this discoordination of normal synchronous papillary muscle contraction and its complex effect on leaflet coaptation.[24,25] Tibayan and coworkers demonstrated that by using mitral suture

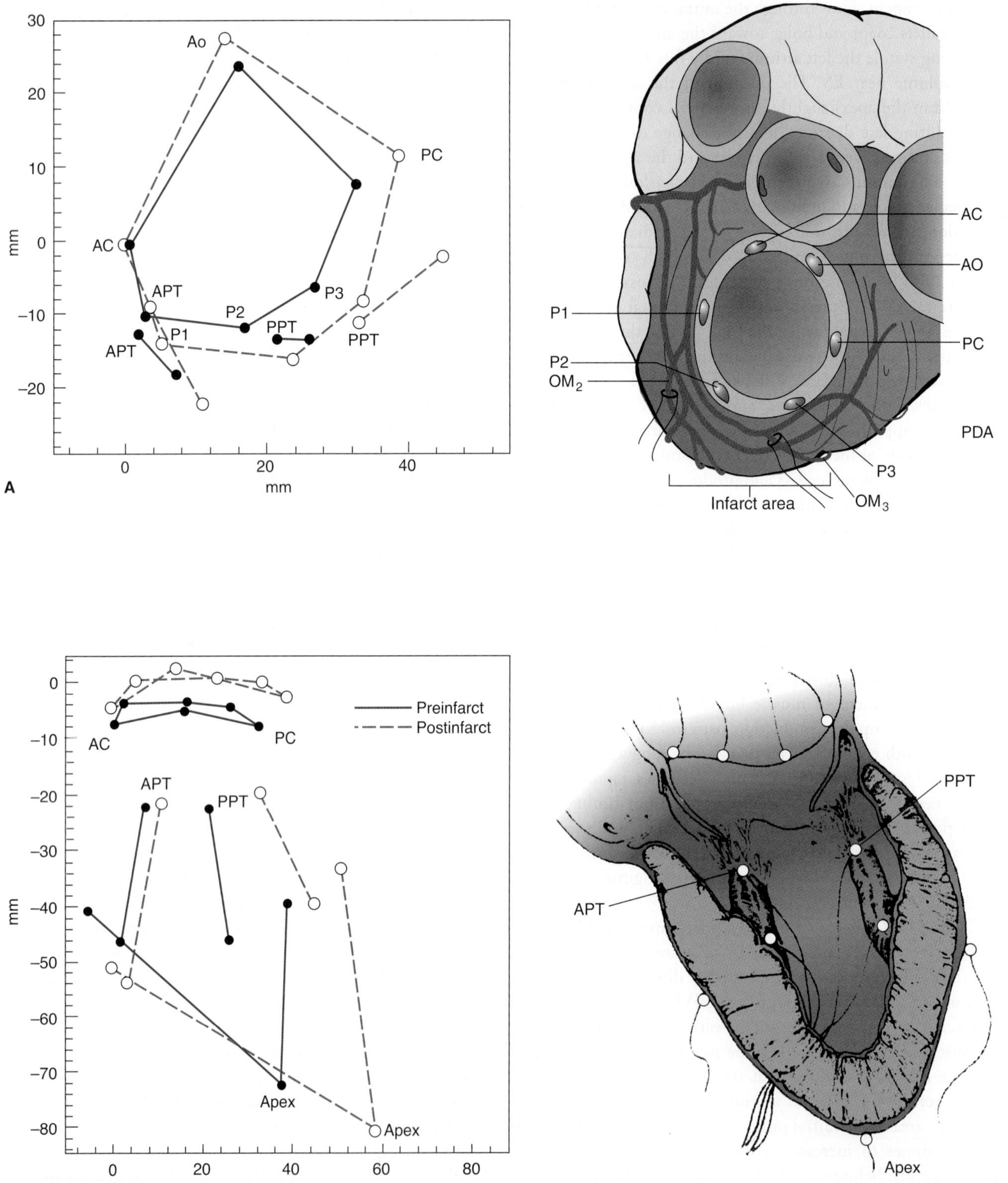

FIGURE 29-2 (A) *Left:* Two-dimensional axial view of the mitral valve annulus and papillary muscle transducers before (*solid line*) and 8 weeks after infarction (*dashed line*). *Right*: An artist's drawing of how the transducers are placed in relation to the mitral annulus and the location of the infarct. Note the stretching of both the posterior part of the aortic portion of the annulus (Ao to PC) and the anterior part of the mural portion of the annulus (Ao to P1 to P2). Also, note how the portion of the annulus between P2 and PC along with the posterior papillary muscle tip (PPT) pulls away from the relatively fixed anterior commissure. (B) *Left*: Two-dimensional sagital view of the sheep mitral annulus and its relationship to the LV and papillary muscles before and 8 weeks after infarction. *Right*: An artist's drawing is provided for orientation of the sonomicrometry transducers. Note how the PPT and the posterior annulus are retracted away form the anterior commissure. The heart shown in this figure is the same one shown in Figure 28-2. (*Reproduced with permission from Gorman JH III, Gorman RC, Jackson BM, et al: Annuloplasty ring selection for chronic ischemic mitral regurgitation: lessons from the ovine model. Ann Thorac Surg 2003; 76:1556-1563.*)

annuloplasty (Paneth-type), altered annular and subvalvular geometry can be corrected, and acute IMR is abolished.[26] Neilsen and coworkers in a pig model of acute IMR demonstrated that imbalanced chordal force distribution is directly related to the development of acute IMR.[27] The authors showed a decrease in tension of the primary chorda from the ischemic posterior left ventricular wall to the anterior leaflet, whereas the tension of the chorda from the nonischemic anterior left ventricluar wall to the anterior leaflet increased.

These data suggest that acute IMR is a result of complex interaction of small changes in the mitral valvular complex, and not merely simple annular dilatation, as previously believed.[23,28,29] These small changes are difficult to demonstrate by standard imaging techniques, making repair challenging in this acute setting. In addition, finite element analysis of the mitral annulus has suggested an association between the normal annular saddle shape of the mitral valve and its competency.[30]

Chronic Ischemic Mitral Regurgitation

In chronic IMR, mitral valve prolapse has been described in occasional patients, but the vast majority have incomplete mitral valve closure owing to left ventricular remodeling and papillary muscle displacement. Remodeling often manifests as annular dilatation with papillary muscle and chordal restriction of leaflet motion. Pathologic studies consistently show fibrosis and atrophy of infarcted papillary muscles, and none demonstrate papillary muscle or chordal elongation.[31–34] Nevertheless, surgeons describe elongated chordae in some patients with myocardial infarction and mitral regurgitation. Elongated chordae and mitral valve prolapse without mitral regurgitation probably antedate the infarction in these patients.[35] In a patient with preexisting mitral valve prolapse, ventricular infarction may cause the previously competent valve to leak. This hypothesis explains sporadic observations of mitral valve prolapse in patients with chronic IMR, but requires preinfarction echocardiograms for confirmation.

Ovine experiments using sonomicrometry array localization to study postinfarction MR that evolves during the first 8 weeks after infarction have added insight relevant to the pathogenesis of chronic IMR. As a result of ischemic left ventricular remodeling, a combination of asymmetric annular dilatation and leaflet tethering by *both* papillary muscles occurs to alter the normal saddle shape of the annulus and produce chronic IMR.[36] Previously thought to be fixed, the anterior portion of the annulus does dilate.[37] The intertrigonal distance has been shown to increase, in addition to the increase in the SL dimension.[38] The annular area dilates by at least 60% at all time points during systolic ejection, but the dilatation involves all of the muscular annulus. The posterior or mural portion of the annulus directly adjacent to the infarct moves away from the relatively fixed anterior commissure (at the anterior fibrous trigone) and stretches the anterior portion of the mural annulus and the posterior portion of the aortic-based annulus, which are remote from the infarct. This finding illustrates how a moderately sized (21% of the LV mass) localized infarct remodels and distorts remote, uninfarcted myocardium including the mitral valve annulus (Fig. 29-2A).[39]

Lateral displacement of the posterior papillary muscle appears to play a major role in the development of chronic IMR.[38] Interestingly, the posterior papillary muscle tip to posterior commissure relationship does not change significantly. Both these points are displaced together, away from the relatively fixed anterior commissure as a result of the remodeling process (Fig. 29-2B). This indicates that the posterior papillary muscle tethering is more pronounced at its most anterior connection with both leaflets near the center of the coaptation line and not at the commissure. The anterior papillary muscle tip is displaced significantly from both commissures but further from the posterior commissure. This indicates that the tethering effect of the anterior papillary muscle is greatest along both leaflets from the anterior commissure to the middle of the coaptation line. Together, these findings suggest that in this model, the postinfarction ventricular remodeling process tethers the anterior portion of both leaflets.

The concept of leaflet tethering as a contributing factor in the pathogenesis of chronic IMR is not new. Two echocardiographic reports, one studying the same sheep model presented here and one human study, demonstrated findings consistent with the experimental results cited in the preceding. Otsuji and coworkers applied a very effective three-dimensional echocardiographic technique to quantify leaflet tethering in the same ovine model.[40] These authors also reported mid-systolic distortions between both papillary muscle tips and the anterior commissure, but did not observe changes between papillary muscle tips and the posterior commissure or annular dilatation. Yiu and coworkers used quantitative two-dimensional echocardiography to corroborate these findings clinically by comparing normal controls with a cohort of patients with varying degrees of chronic IMR.[41] They found that ventricular distortions, which most closely correlated with the degree of mitral regurgitation, occurred between the posterior papillary muscle tip and anterior commissure and posterior displacement of the anterior papillary muscle tip.

To summarize, the geometric changes that lead to acute IMR are multiple but extremely subtle (<5 mm) and are not reliably imaged by currently available clinical modalities. Chronic IMR involves larger changes (1 to 2 cm) that cause moderate annular dilatation and complex leaflet tethering along the anterior and mid leaflet coaptation line. It is a process resulting from complex geometrical alteration of the mitral valve apparatus as a result of ischemic left ventricular remodeling (Fig. 29-3).

CLINICAL PRESENTATION AND MANAGEMENT

Acute Ischemic Mitral Regurgitation

Clinical Presentation

Clinically, acute IMR usually presents abruptly with chest pain and/or shortness of breath. The presentation is that of an acute myocardial infarction and occasionally may be silent. These patients are often hemodynamically unstable, in cardiogenic shock. They often present in extremis with symptoms of congestive heart failure, including pulmonary edema, systemic

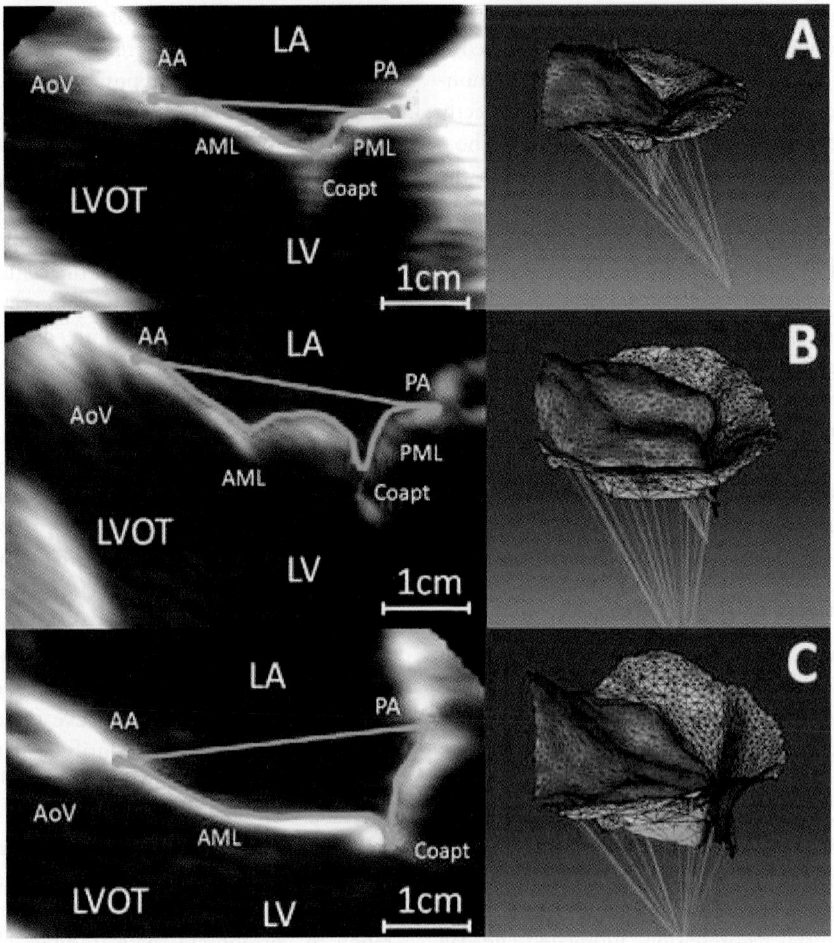

FIGURE 29-3 Three-dimensional rendering to compare normal mitral valve with ischemic mitral valve with either severe or minimal leaflet tethering. (**A**) A normal valve. (**B**) Ischemic mitral valve (3+ MR) with mild leaflet tethering. (**C**) An ischemic mitral valve (4+ MR) with severe bileaflet tethering. The left picture in each panel demonstrates the leaflet tracing technique used in serial 2D slices through the valve. The right picture in each panel demonstrates the completely traced valve rendered three-dimensionally from 1-mm slices through the valve. (Chordal structures have been added to help orient the viewer.)

hypotension, oliguria, acidosis, and poor periperhal perfusion. On physical examination, in the setting of profound MR, most patients have a loud apical, holosystolic murmur that radiates to the left axilla; but with lesser degrees of MR, a murmur is inconsistently detected.

Nearly all electrocardiograms are abnormal,[17,42,43] but only slightly more than half are diagnostic of AMI. Some of the nondiagnostic changes include right or left bundle branch block and nonspecific ST- and T-wave changes in the anteroseptal, lateral, or inferior leads.[17,42,44] Most patients are in sinus rhythm. In autopsy series, the incidence of subendocardial infarctions is approximately equal to the incidence of transmural infarctions.[17,43] Frequently patients with papillary muscle rupture have electrocardiographic evidence of an inferior MI. When the ECG is diagnostic, inferior wall infarctions are much more common than anterior and lateral wall infarctions. Conduction abnormalities are relatively uncommon and are more often found in patients with postinfarction ventricular septal defects. Chest x-rays nearly always show signs of pulmonary congestion, interstitial pulmonary edema, and pulmonary venous engorgement.[42] Cardiomegaly is usually not present, and there is usually no sign of left atrial enlargement in acute MR.[17]

The differential diagnosis for acute IMR includes postinfarction ventricular septal defect, massive AMI without significant MR, and ruptured chordae tendineae without AMI. Right heart catheterization usually shows elevated pulmonary arterial pressures with prominent V waves reaching 40 mm Hg or higher.[42,45] Mean pulmonary artery wedge pressures are greater than 20 mm Hg unless cardiac output is very low. Mixed venous oxygen saturations are often well below 50% and reflect low cardiac output with indices that range from 1.0 to 2.9 L/m^2/min.[45] In the presence of a loud systolic murmur, absence of an oxygen step-up in the pulmonary artery is strong evidence against the diagnosis of postinfarction ventricular septal defect. Electrocardiographic evidence of AMI distinguishes acute IMR from acute chordal rupture, but the lack of EKG changes does not differentiate the two diseases.[42]

Transthoracic echocardiography (TTE) assesses the degree of MR, confirms wall motion abnormalities, and may demonstrate flail mitral leaflets. However, transesophageal (TEE) echocardiography is the diagnostic imaging tool of choice. This modality definitively documents the degree and characteristics of the MR jet of IMR, associated wall motion abnormalities, and the status of the posterior papillary muscle. In the modern era, the information provided by TEE is vital in making an accurate decision to repair versus replace the mitral valve. Typically the left atrium is not enlarged, but the left ventricle shows signs of volume overload and segmental wall motion abnormalities. Color flow Doppler velocity mapping documents the presence of MR after myocardial infarction and semiquantitates its severity. Ejection fractions vary widely, but do not reflect the extent of the LV infarction.

Despite hemodynamic instability, most patients have a diagnostic cardiac catheterization primarily for definition of coronary arterial anatomy. However, the wisdom of prescribing cardiac catheterization for patients in cardiogenic shock is highly questionable in that revascularization of obstructed, remote coronary vessels is not likely to improve a patient's chances for immediate survival. Approximately half of catheterized patients have single-vessel disease, most often of the right coronary artery.[42,45] Most of the remainder have three-vessel disease.[17,42–44] Ventriculography shows increased LV volume at both end diastole and end systole, severe MR, segmental wall motion abnormalities, and a wide range of ejection fractions, which are generally over 40% and frequently over 60%.[44,45] LV end-diastolic pressures are usually elevated, with prominent left atrial V waves and moderate pulmonary hypertension. Occasionally patients may have mild or moderate tricuspid regurgitation. Cardiac output is usually very low in this disease process.

Indication for Surgery

Immediate surgery is the best chance for survival for most patients with acute, severe postinfarction MR. The goal of medical therapy is to stabilize the patient and optimize hemodynamcs in preparation for surgical intervention. A few, highly selected patients without papillary muscle rupture early in their presentation have been treated by emergency PCI and/or thrombolytic therapy in an attempt to reduce the size of the infarct and thereby reduce mitral regurgitation.[46–49] PCI or thrombolysis carried out within 4 hours of the onset of AMI may on occasion produce spectacular reversal of both the infarction and mitral regurgitation.[47–49] However, less rapid PCI may not succeed in preempting the infarct and aborting mitral regurgitation.[49] PCI and thrombolysis in catheterized patients are potentially worth trying if patients reach medical attention soon after the onset of symptoms, are sufficiently stable, and can be followed by echocardiography. However, in many patients PCI and thrombolysis do not provide a favorable outcome.[46] In one study, 17% of patients with acute IMR and successful thrombolysis died in the hospital; in those with successful PCI, 50% died shortly afterward, and 77% were dead in 1 year.[46] Of the survivors, the majority continue to have 3+ or 4+ MR.[46]

For patients who have acute postinfarction angina with 1+ or 2+ MR, urgent myocardial revascularization is indicated to relieve angina and prevent extension of the infarction. It is important to prevent progression of MR and the development of congestive heart failure or cardiogenic shock. This is usually accomplished by thrombolysis or PCI. If these measures are unsuccessful, operation is rarely completed in time to reverse the infarction, but early operation may reduce the size of the ultimate infarct.[50–52] The presence of mild to moderate IMR does not increase operative mortality, but the presence of congestive heart failure is a risk factor.[53] In these patients, the mitral valve is generally not addressed unless intraoperative transesophageal echocardiography indicates 3+ or 4+ MR.

Indications for emergency surgery for acute, severe postinfarction MR vary among institutions and probably explain wide discrepancies in reports of hospital mortality.[54,55] In this group of patients, medical therapy does not produce survivors and patients denied operation are not reported.[42,44] Aged patients are less likely to survive operation, and there are only anecdotal reports of successful operation in octogenarians.[47,54,56] Other risk factors for hospital death are severe congestive heart failure, the number and severity of comorbid diseases such as renal or pulmonary problems, presence of an intra-aortic balloon pump, reduced ejection fraction, and greater number of diseased coronary arteries.[57]

Surgical intervention for acute, severe postinfarction MR consists of mitral valve repair or replacement with or without myocardial revascularization. Nearly all surgeons recommend revascularization of all significantly obstructed coronary vessels away from the site of the infarction.[55] Improved methods of cardioplegia support this recommendation even in patients with preoperative cardiogenic shock who have had cardiac catheterization. The wisdom of blind revascularization of remote coronary vessels in patients who have not had preoperative cardiac catheterization and revascularization of the infarct artery more than 4 to 6 hours after onset of pain is less clear.[58] On a statistical basis, only half of patients with acute IMR have multivessel coronary artery disease.[17,42,45] Revascularization of completed infarctions favorably influences subsequent ventricular remodeling.[51,52,59]

With echocardiographic findings amenable to repair, a simple, central regurgitant jet, minimally tethered leaflets, and no papillary muscle pathlogy such as rupture, a simple repair with an annuloplasty ring can be enterained. However, replacement of the diseased valve should be considered if the effectiveness and durability of the repair are at all in question. These patients are often critically ill, and will not tolerate the increased cardiopulmonary bypass time associated with mitral valve replacement after failed mitral repair. When performing mitral valve replacement, it is important to preserve the chordal attachments to the annulus to limit adverse ventricular remodeling (Fig. 29-4). Bioprosthetic valves are a reasonable choice since anticoagulation is not benign and durability is a relatively minor concern in these patients with poor long-term prognosis.[60,61]

Results

Published results of mitral valve replacement for acute IMR are poor. Hospital mortality ranges from 31 to 69% and probably reflects the selection process more than quality of care. Variables that increase early mortality include patient age, cardiogenic shock, comorbid conditions, the amount of infarcted myocardium, and delay in operation.[42,44,45,54] More recent experience

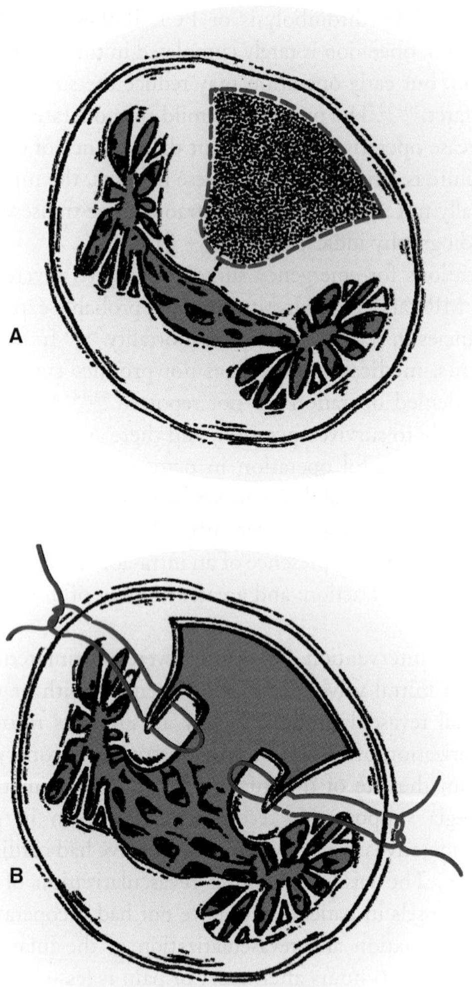

FIGURE 29-4 Okita's method for retaining chordal attachment to the mitral annulus during replacement of the mitral valve. (A) Diagram showing the mitral valve from the left atrium. The center of the anterior leaflet is excised (*shaded area*) and the leaflet is divided retaining the chordae from each papillary muscle attached to the residual anterior leaflet tissue. The posterior leaflet may be divided at its midpoint if necessary. (B) Remnants of the anterior leaflets are sutured to the annulus using a single stitch as shown. This tissue is later included in sutures used in sewing the valve to the annulus. (*Modified slightly with permission from Okita Y, Miki S, Kusuhara K, et al: Analysis of left ventricular motion after mitral valve replacement with a technique of preservation of all chordae tendineae. J Thorac Cardiovasc Surg 1992; 104:786.*)

may be better because of prompt diagnosis, early surgery, complete revascularization, and application of chordal preservation techniques that better preserve left ventricular function.[60–67] Several techniques are available for preserving chordae (see Fig. 29-4).[62,68,69]

Controversy exists over whether the mitral valve should be repaired or replaced in the setting of acute IMR. Repair of the valve in acute IMR potentially enhances the complexity of the operation as well as the cardiopulmonary bypass time as compared with mitral valve replacement. As demonstrated, the anatomical derangements in the acute IMR setting may be very subtle, resulting in annular dilatation and malcoaptation of the leaflets, in which case an undersized ring annuloplasty is a reasonable option. Long-term (5-year) survival in patients who survive the perioperative period is poor and even in modern reports hovers around 50%.[60,61] Even with poor prognosis, we believe mitral valve annuloplasty ring is a reasonable option for pathology amenable to repair.

Papillary muscle rupture is less common as the etiology for acute ischemic mitral regurgitation, and this subset of patients is usually much less ill. A recent retrospective analysis of post-MI papillary muscle rupture patients noted a marked improvement in postoperative survival when either valve repair (reimplantation of the papillary muscle and annuloplasty) or replacement was performed in combination with concomitant revascularization. It is encouraging that the authors noted normalization in 5-year survival (79%) and freedom from congestive heart failure to that of matched MI controls without papillary mucle rupture (28 ± 8% versus 36 ± 6%) was noted, predicting an optimistic outcome for this patient population in the modern surgical era.[70]

Chronic Ischemic Mitral Regurgitation

Clinical Presentation

Chronic IMR represents the majority of patients with IMR. Between 10.9 and 19.0% of patients with symptomatic coronary artery disease who have cardiac catheterization[3,4] and 3.5 to 7.0% of patients who have myocardial revascularization have IMR.[71–74] The majority of these patients have 1+ to 2+ mitral regurgitation, without evidence of heart failure.[3,4,71–73] In patients with chronic IMR, three major variables interrelate to produce the clinical spectrum of patients with varying combinations of symptomatic ischemia and heart failure. As with acute IMR, the three major variables are: (1) the presence and severity of ischemia, (2) the severity of mitral regurgitation, and (3) the magnitude of left ventricular dysfunction. First, patients with obstructive coronary artery disease may be asymptomatic or have stable, progressive, unstable, or postinfarction angina or its equivalent. Because of disabling symptoms, threat to left ventricular mass or statistically shortened survival, ischemia is a compelling problem that must be addressed therapeutically. The approach and methods do not differ from similar patients who do not have IMR.

The second variable is the severity of mitral regurgitation. At present, 1+ or 2+ mitral regurgitation in patients without symptoms of heart failure does not compel invasive therapy for mitral regurgitation. Severe mitral regurgitation and/or symptoms of heart failure require evaluation for possible operation irrespective of the therapy needed for ischemia. The third variable is the degree of left ventricular dysfunction. LV dysfunction is the most difficult to assess in the presence of mitral regurgitation. Symptoms of heart failure may be caused by left ventricular dysfunction secondary to ischemia, mitral regurgitation, or both.

The primary purpose of diagnostic studies is to determine the severity of coronary artery disease and its anatomy, the severity and mechanism of mitral regurgitation, and the degree of left ventricular dysfunction. In chronic IMR, the ventricular geometry and function reflect remodeling owing to both the mitral regurgitation and infarction; therefore, these patients may require diagnostic studies and perhaps operative procedures that are different from patients with CAD associated with mitral regurgitation. It is also important to define comorbidity of other organ systems by appropriate diagnostic studies dictated by the patient's history, physical examination, and screening laboratory findings.

In patients with IMR, the ECG usually shows evidence of a prior myocardial infarction. The incidence of arrhythmias varies but atrial fibrillation as noted earlier is quite common. In patients without failure and mild mitral regurgitation, heart size by chest x-ray is normal or slightly enlarged; the left atrium is seldom enlarged. In those with moderate or severe mitral regurgitation and/or severe left ventricular dysfunction, the heart is enlarged and usually the left atrium is also enlarged.

Transthoracic echocardiography and TEE are useful in determining the etiology of mitral regurgitation. Two-dimensional echocardiography reliably detects ruptured chordae, annular calcification, and myxomatous degeneration, which are not features of chronic IMR, and differentiates rheumatic valve disease, endocarditis, and degenerative valve disease. Echocardiography also effectively assesses regional wall motion abnormalities and global left ventricular function. The degree of mitral regurgitation is also well quantified by color flow Doppler measurements. Characteristics of the mitral regurgitation demonstrated by TEE will also aid in the decision to repair or replace the mitral valve. Extremely dilated annulus with severe bileaflet tethering (Carpentier Type IIIB) and eccentric or complex regurgitation jet are echocardiographic findings that repair may not be effective or durable.

Cardiac catheterization provides information regarding the coronary arterial anatomy and pathology. Ventriculograms add little to the data provided by TTE or TEE and should be avoided, especially in patients with impaired renal function. Measurements of chamber pressures and estimates of cardiac output contribute to the overall evaluation of left ventricular function. Pulmonary hypertension, when present, is typically moderate and correlates with the degree of left ventricular dysfunction and/or severity of mitral regurgitation.

Indications for Surgery

The decision to intervene surgically in IMR can be a challenging process. Chronic IMR represents a set of patients with symptoms of insidious onset and often of chronic duration. Patients may primarily present with symptoms of ischemic coronary artery disease, and on preoperative workup are found to have significant concomitant mitral regurgitation. Although this group of patients may have preserved left ventricular function, compromised ventricular function is not uncommon. The surgical indication in this group of patients is coronary artery disease requiring CABG with coexistent significant mitral regurgitation. Important factors to consider in the decision to intervene on mitral regurgitation include the following: the impact of coronary artery bypass grafting (CABG) alone on the progression of IMR; the impact of CABG with or without MVR on survival; the additional risk of MVR at the time of CABG; and the choice of valve repair and replacement.

Other patients may primarily present with symptoms of congestive heart failure and signs of significant mitral regurgitation. Preoperative catheterization subsequently may reveal significant CAD. These patients tend to have more compromised left ventricular function compared with the first group. The indication for surgery is congestive heart failure. In reality, most patients present in a clinical spectrum somewhere along the two clinical scenerios. In this section, however, the indications for surgery of each scenerio are discussed separately.

Ischemic Mitral Regurgitation and Coronary Artery Disease

The optimal management of concomitant IMR at the time of CABG remains to be determined. Most surgeons agree that concomitant severe (4+) mitral regurgitation should be addressed at the time of CABG and that revascularization alone will not ameliorate severe mitral regurgitation. Similarly, most surgeons agree that trace to mild (1+) mitral regurgitation should be left alone because it will not adversly affect long-term symptomatology or prognosis. Yet, the optimal management of mild to moderate (2+) mitral regurgitation remains controversial.

Multiple factors must be addressed in deciding on the management of IMR at the time of CABG. First, IMR has been demonstrated to have a negative impact on long-term survival. Numerous studies have documented the negative impact of IMR on long-term survival after an acute MI.[75–78] Similarly, in patients undergoing PCI for acute coronary syndromes, IMR has been demonstrated to have a negative impact on survival. Three-year survival in this group ranges from 46 to 76%, based on the severity of mitral regurgitation.[79] Moreover, in the setting of CABG, myocardial revascularization alone in patients with chronic IMR has a higher hospital mortality than in patients without IMR.[74] Mild (1+) IMR increases operative mortality from 3.4 to 4.5%[72–74,80] and moderate (2+) IMR raises operative mortality from 6 to 11%.[72–74,81] Two-year survival for revascularization alone in patients with 1+ and 2+ mitral regurgitation is 78 and 88%, respectively.[82] Five-year survival rates for patients with mild mitral regurgitation range between 70 and 80%.[3,72,83,84] For moderate mitral regurgitation, 5-year survival ranges between 60 and 70%.[85,86] Many surgeons argue that these data suggest that concomitant IMR should be addressed during CABG to affect survival.

Those who advocate the conservative approach of revascularization alone, without treatment of the IMR, argue that revascularization will improve regional wall motion abnormalities, papillary muscle function, and potentially correct IMR.[71,87,88] Moreover, there are data that suggest that survival and long-term functional status are not improved with concomitant MVR,[89,90] thus bringing into question the benefit of the higher operative risk associated with simultaneous MVR. Surgeons who advocate mitral valve repair/replacement for moderate IMR during CABG cite studies that suggest revascularization does not correct IMR,[91] and that uncorrected IMR may result in late symptoms and decreased long-term survival.[76,82]

Furthermore, mitral valve repair with annuloplasty ring is nearly always technically feasible, obviating the need for valve replacement and the associated anticoagulation of mechanical valves or subsequent valve replacement required of bioprosthetic valves. Operative risk with combined CABG/MV repair today is much better than the older series, with operative mortality in the 3 to 4% range.[92–94] Kron and collegues have concluded that the addition of MVR does not increase the operative risk of CABG in ischemic cardiomyopathy.[95] Considering the increased complexity associated with redo sternotomy with patent grafts for MVR for recurrent or progressive IMR, some feel aggressive management of IMR is justified on initial sternotomy and revascularization, given simplicity of repair when compared with subsequent redo-operation.

The impact of isolated CABG without MVR on the progression of moderate IMR has been examined. Previous studies suggest that CABG alone improves IMR grade and functional status.[71,87,88] However, in contrast recent reports have suggested that CABG alone is not the optimal therapy for moderate IMR.[91,96,97] A study from the Cleveland Clinic Foundation reported that moderate (2+) IMR does not resolve with CABG alone, and furthermore, is associated with reduced survival.[98] Between 1980 to 2000, 467 patients with moderate IMR underwent CABG alone. Longitudinal analysis of 267 follow-up echocardiograms from 156 patients demonstrated that early postoperative improvements in IMR did not persist. IMR of moderate or greater severity was present in 60% of patients by postoperative week 6. Interestingly, postoperative IMR severity was not predicted by cardiac function or extent of CAD. Furthermore, early survival of patients with unrepaired moderate IMR was reduced compared with similar patients without IMR. Based on their results, the authors concluded that a mitral valve procedure is warranted for such patients at the time of CABG. A retrospective registry review of the progression of mitral regurgitation following isolated coronary artery bypass surgery, examined 438 patients with preoperative mitral regurgitation of less than or equal to 2+ requiring CABG.[99] New 3+ to 4+ mitral regurgitation developed in 10% of patients with no prior mitral regurgitation, 12% with pre-CABG 1+ mitral regurgitation, and 25% with pre-CABG 2+ mitral regurgitation, thereby implying significant progression of IMR without treatment. Preoperative left ventricular dysfunction and large left ventricular size were identified as predictors of mitral regurgitation progression post-CABG. Although no correlation was identified between the extent of CAD or the number of grafts performed, incomplete revascularization in the PDA territory was identified as a significant predictor of mitral regurgitation progression, suggesting a role for incomplete revascularization and left ventricular remodeling in the progression of IMR.

To directly address the impact of MVR for moderate IMR, studies have compared the results of CABG alone versus CABG with concomitant MVR in the setting of IMR.[100–105] The results do suggest that post-operative mitral regurgitation is improved with CABG with concomitant MVR. However, whether there exists an improvement in long-term survival remains unclear. Several studies suggest no improvement in survival following CABG with concomitant MVR.[102,104–107] In contrast, two studies[100,101] comparing CABG versus CABG/MVR in patients with CAD and IMR have found a significant improvement in survival. Both studies involved patients with 2+ to 3+ IMR with depressed LVEF. A recent study[103] examining 111 patients with moderate to severe IMR and multivessel CAD undergoing either medical therapy, isolated CABG, or CABG/MVR found a greater than 50% reduction in mortality in the CABG and CABG/MVR groups when compared with medical therapy. However, only CABG/MVR independently predicted survival. Moreover, a history of CHF was an independent predictor of cardiac death. Five-year survival has been found to be influenced by the severity of left ventricular dysfunction at the time of operation, age, and comorbid disease.[57] Collectively, these studies suggested that concomitant MVR with CABG may improve late survival, especially in the setting of LV dysfunction and CHF, but the definitive answer remains elusive. To clarify the appropriate management of moderate IMR during CABG, a multi-institutional randomized, prospective NIH NHLBI–sponsored clinical trial has begun. In this study, patients with moderate IMR at the time of CABG are randomized to either repair of the MR or isolated CABG alone.

The final factor to address when dealing with IMR is the decision to repair or replace the valve. Gillinov demonstrated the short-term efficacy of mitral valve repair in 97% of patients undergoing elective surgery for 3+ to 4+ chronic IMR.[60] Ring annuloplasty was employed in 98% of these repairs and was the sole surgical maneuver on the valve in greater than 80%. There was a distinct inclination in this study to undersize the annuloplasty ring; 79% of the rings were 30 mm or less. Iatrogenic mitral stenosis was not seen even in patients who received 26-mm annuloplasty devices. However, there was no benefit to repair versus replacement in high-risk patients, including older age, higher NYHA functional class, significant wall motion abnormalities, and renal dysfunction. In contrast, Calafiore and colleagues have found no difference in either short- or long-term mortality between MV repair and replacement for patients with 2+ to 4+ IMR.[92] Similarly, a recent study found no difference in either operative or 6-year mortality following MV repair as compared with replacement. A prospective, randomized multi-institutional NIH NHLBI–sponsored study is presently underway to definitively determine if there is a difference between MV repair and replacement in the setting of severe ischemic mitral regurgitation.

In summary, patients with CAD with concomitant moderate to severe (3+ to 4+) IMR should undergo CABG/MVR. In patients with moderate (2+) IMR, recent studies may suggest that CABG/MVR may be justified, given the lower rate of morbidity and mortality in the modern surgical era, but this remains to be determined. Left ventricular dysfunction and increased left ventricular dimension along with incomplete revascularization may predict a higher rate of progression of IMR, suggesting CABG/MVR should be performed in this particular group of patients. Patients with symptoms of CHF appear to benefit most from CABG/MVR. Mild (1+) IMR should be left alone, unless: (1) preoperative signs and symptoms are suggestive of periods of more severe mitral regurgitation; and (2) intraoperative TEE demonstrate anatomical findings requiring MVR (ie, significant annular dilatation, leaflet tenting). Most patients with IMR benefit from mitral valve repair. In the most complex, high-risk settings, replacement may be preferable, with no demonstrable difference in survival between repair and replacement.

Ischemic Mitral Regurgitation and Congestive Heart Failure

The ischemic cardiomyopathy patient subset is a complex population to manage. In the current era of aggressive medical management and revascularization, there has been a dramatic decrease in the incidence of acute myocardial infarction and death. However, there is a significant increase in the number of patients suffering from ischemic cardiomyopathy. This disease is often coincident with ischemic mitral regurgitation. As described in previous sections, postinfarction LV remodeling is characterized by progressive LV dilatation with a change to a spherical shape with resultant functional MR secondary to annular dilatation, papillary muscle displacement, and chordal tethering. With functional MR there is increased ventricular volume overload (preload), myocardial wall tension, and LV workload; all of which further contribute to a deleterious cycle of progressive heart failure.

In the past, operative repair of mitral regurgitation was associated with a prohibitively high perioperative mortality, making surgeons cautious about MVR and MVR/CABG in the setting of left ventricular dysfunction. The traditional teaching incorporated the "popoff" valve hypothesis, which believed that the mitral valve functioned as a low-pressure runoff to decompress the failing ventricle. It was believed that surgical correction of mitral regurgitation in the failing ventricle would further contribute to ventricular overload and further contribute to myocardial failure.

However, this hypothesis has been challenged and disproved by Bolling who believes that there is an "annular solution for the ventricular problem."[108–111] It is believed that correction of mitral regurgitation alleviates excessive ventricular workload, improves ventricular geometry, and enhances ventricular function; a process referred to as reverse remodeling. The Stanford group has reported in an ovine model of ischemic mitral regurgitation, that reduction of the annulus by an undersized ring reduces the radius of curvature of the left ventricle at the base, equiatorial, and apical levels.[112] This decrease in the radius of curvature supports the concept that a small ring can restore a more elliptical shape. Reduction of left ventricular dimensions to a more elliptical shape, reverse remodeling, after annuloplasty have also been demonstrated by clinical studies.[113–115]

The previously published high operative mortality associated with mitral valve replacement was most likely the result of loss of the subvalvular apparatus, thus indicating the importance of maintaining the integrity of the annular and subvalvular continuity during mitral valve surgery. More recent series have indeed demonstrated much lower perioperative morbidity and mortality (1.6 to 5%), demonstrating safety in carefully selected patients.[60,61,116,117]

Data from most recently published series have demonstrated improvements in left ventricular ejection fraction, mitral regurgitation, clinical symptoms (NYHA classification), and left ventricular reverse remodeling with surgical intervention.[89,100,107–109,118–121] However, questions remain regarding improvements in long-term survival and its overall effect on the natural history of IMR. Some have recently raised questions, despite previous data, about the potential improvement in long-term survival in patients with IMR in the setting of depressed LVEF. In perhaps the largest experience of MVR in patients with severe left ventricular dysfunction, Wu and coworkers examined the impact of mitral valve annuloplasty on mortality risk in patients with mitral regurgitation and left ventricular dysfunction.[122] Reviewing their echocardiographic database ($n = 682$), the authors identified 419 patients who met the criteria for surgical intervention. One hundred twenty-six patients underwent MVR, whereas 263 continued conservative medical therapy. It should be noted that the etiology of mitral regurgitation included both ischemic and nonischemic subtypes. Their analysis demonstrated no improvements in long-term survival in the MVR group versus medical therapy. Talkwalkar and coworkers[89] reported a series of 338 patients who underwent MVR. Compared with the control group, patients with depressed left ventricular ejection fraction were more likely to be associated with IMR, concomitant CABG, and NYHA class IV symptoms. Five-year survival was 54%, and when associated with prior CABG, prior myocardial infarction, or concomitant CABG, it was 0, 37, and 63%, respectively.

In agreement with previous reports, these recent studies confirmed the poor prognosis associated with IMR in the presence of LV dysfunction. In Wu's series,[122] 5-year survival in the setting of IMR and left ventricular dysfunction is less than 50%, regardless of surgical versus medical therapy. A randomized study comparing surgical versus medical therapy for IMR is needed to clarify the benefit of mitral valve surgery in this population of patients.

Patients who present primarily with symptoms of congestive heart failure and IMR provide surgeons with a fairly straightforward indication for intervention. Although it remains unclear if there is a survival benefit with repair, it is clear that there are improvements in symptoms, exercise tolerance, and ventricular remodeling. Given the low operative mortality associated with modern surgical techniques it is reasonable to correct severe IMR in the setting of heart failure. The operative indications for this group of patients are similar to mitral regurgitation of nonischemic origin. Symptoms of CHF and depressed left ventricular function are indications for surgical mitral repair or replacement. The current ACC/AHA valve disease guidelines include a cautious recommendation for consideration of MV surgery in patients with advanced heart failure, but only if MV repair or replacement with chordal sparing are options. Most surgeons agree that concomitant CABG is indicated in the presence of significant CAD.

Results

An undersized annuloplasty ring is effective in the acute correction or reduction of IMR in the majority of patients. However, recurrent mitral regurgitation after annuloplasty has been reported to be present in 30 to 40% of patients. Although these studies are criticized for not addressing the appropriate annuloplasty ring selection and adequately downsizing the ring, both of which have been demonstrated to be vital in adequate long-term correction of IMR. These studies have often used flexible bands or partial rings, which fail to address the dilatation that occurs along the anterior annulus and fail to adequately fix the septal-lateral dimension of the valve.

The Cleveland Clinic reported its series of 585 patients who underwent annuloplasty alone for IMR between 1985 and 2002 in which 678 postoperative echocardiograms were evaulated in 422 patients. The majority of recurrent IMR occurred within the first 6 months. Overall, 28% of patients 6 months after surgery demonstrated 3+ to 4+ mitral regurgitation.[123] These results stand in contrast to the findings by Spoor and Bolling, in which minimal recurrent MR was seen up to 4 years after mitral repair with rigid annuloplasty using a ring that was downsized by two sizes.[121] It has been found that there is an almost fourfold increase in recurrence rate of IMR with the use of a flexible ring as compared with a nonflexible ring in patients with a preoperative ejection fraction less than 30%.[124]

Evidence of left ventricular reverse remodeling after annuloplasty ring has been demonstrated in small clinical studies, with excellent results and freedom from recurrent IMR for up to 2 years.[113-115] Braun and coworkers reported a series of 87 patients with IMR and depressed left ventricular function (mean LVEF 32%) who underwent undersized mitral annuloplasty and coronary revascularization. Mitral regurgitation grade decreased significantly from a mean of 3.1 to 0.6 at 18 months. Both left ventricular end-systolic and end-diastolic dimensions decreased significantly when compared with preoperative echocardiograms. Interestingly, the left ventricular end-diastolic dimension was found to be the best predictor of reverse remodeling. Left ventricular end-diastolic dimension exceeding 65 mm was associated with a lower probability of reverse remodeling, suggesting a relationship between recurrent IMR and ventricular geometric dimension. Further studies would be useful to identify preoperative echocardiographic parameters predictive of durable mitral valve repair.

Operative results for mitral valve surgery with or without concomitant CABG have improved, with recent series reporting operative mortality of 3-4%.[60,61,116,117] However, 5-year survival remains very low, with reported values as low as 30 to 40%, depending on the series (Fig. 29-5).[3,72,73,83,125] More recently, Gillinov and coworkers reported 5-year survival in the propensity-matched best risk group of 58% for valve repair and 36% for replacement. This group had significantly fewer NYHA class IV patients and less severe mitral regurgitation preoperatively. In the propensity-matched poorer risk groups (more severe CHF, mitral regurgitation, and emergency surgery) and for the group as a whole, there was no difference between repair and replacement and 5-year survival was uniformly less than 50%.[60]

There has been no randomized study demonstrating a survival benefit with mitral valve repair/replacement in IMR. In a restrospective analysis of cardiomyopathy including both ischemic and nonischemic etiology, Wu and coworkers reported in their series 5-year survival of less than 50%, regardless of surgical versus medical therapy in patients with mitral regurgitation and left ventricular dysfunction.[122] Other series have also demonstrated no survival benefit with mitral valve surgery in patients with IMR.[104-106] The similarity of results between surgical and medical therapy points out a need for better understanding of the pathophysiology of IMR and left ventricular remodeling. A randomized study examining the clinical outcome and survival benefit of mitral valve surgery for IMR is warranted.

OPERATIVE TECHNIQUE

Given the unstable presentation of patients with acute, severe postinfarction mitral regurgitation, operative intervention is often emergent. A very large percentage of these patients require

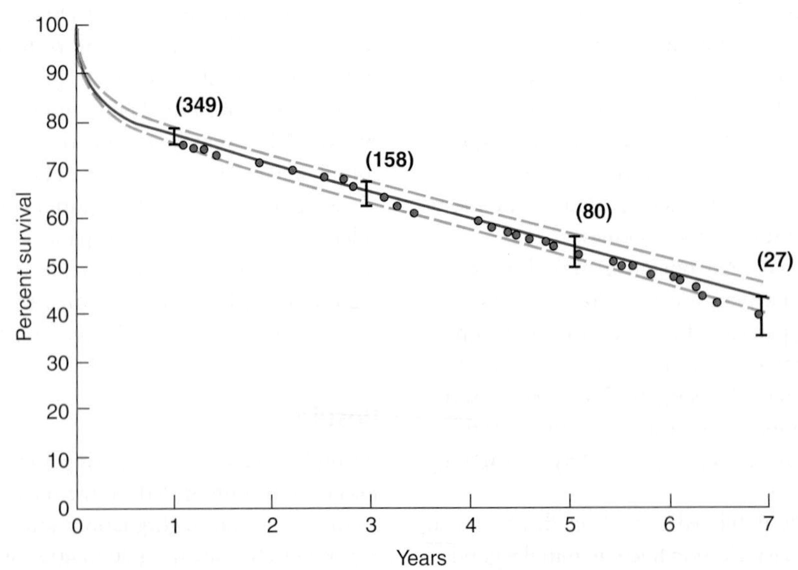

FIGURE 29-5 Survival after mitral valve surgery for all patients with ischemic mitral regurgitation. Each symbol represents a death according to Kaplan-Meier estimator. *Vertical bars* enclose asymmetric 68% confidence limits. *Solid lines* represent parametric survival estimates; these are enclosed between *dashed* 68% confidence limits. *Numbers in parentheses* are numbers of patients traced beyond that point. (*Reproduced with permission from Gillinov AM, Wierup PN, Blackstone EH, et al: Is repair preferable to replacement for ischemic mitral regurgitation? J Thorac Cardiovasc Surg 2001; 122[6]:1125-1141.*)

high-dose pharmacologic support or intra-aortic balloon pump counterpulsation for hemodynamic stablization in the immediate preoperative period.[45,58] Although intraoperative monitoring is very institution dependent, typical monitors include electrocardiogram, arterial blood pressure, pulmonary artery catheter with mixed venous oxygen electrode, nasopharyngeal and core body temperatures, and a urinary catheter for urine output. Additionally, a large proportion of centers use intraoperative TEE for optimal management of valvular repair and myocardial optimization.

Chronic IMR is most often performed in an elective manner, except in patients with uncontrolled symptoms of coronary ischemia who may require emergency or urgent operation to prevent myocardial infarction. Preoperative preparation and intraoperative monitors are similar to other cardiac operations. Transesophageal echocardiography and color flow Doppler velocity mapping are considered the standard of care in most centers that perform large volume valve repairs/replacements. After induction of anesthesia, TEE is used to assess: (1) anatomy of the valve; (2) degree of mitral regurgitation, include characteristics of the regurgitant jet; and (3) dimensions and segmental wall motion of the left ventricle. General anesthesia reduces systemic vascular resistance and afterload, thereby masking the degree of mitral regurgitation; therefore, assessment of the valve after administration of vasopressors to enhance afterload may unmask more severe mitral regurgitation. If the amount of mitral regurgitation remains in question or is only mild to moderate, then transfusion after aortic cannulation to increase preload to 1.5 to 2.0 times resting pulmonary capillary wedge pressure may further unmask more severe mitral regurgitation and prompt a decision to expose and repair the valve at the time of other cardiac interventions (ie, CABG). If there is a significant discrepancy between the intraoperative degree of mitral regurgitation and that diagnosed by preoperative TEE, it is probably best to treat according to the preoperative value because this is likely what the patient experiences under normal loading conditions. In patients with marginal left ventricular function, a pulmonary artery catheter with continuous cardiac output and mixed venous oxygen sensing capabilities along with a femoral arterial catheter for rapid intra-aortic balloon insertion, if needed to wean from cardiopulmonary bypass, are recommended.

The most common exposure to the mitral valve is via a median sternotomy, although over the past decade port-access and robotic platforms have afforded many surgeons expertise in exposure to the valve via the right pleural space. If revascularization is required, arterial and venous conduits are harvested before cannulation and initation of cardiopulmonary bypass. Bicaval cannulation is preferred for exposure of the mitral valve. Both antegrade and retrograde cardioplegia are recommended to minimize myocardial stunning and post-bypass ventricular dysfunction. After initiation of cardipulmonary bypass, the aorta is cross-clamped and cardioplegia is given in a standard fashion. If revascularization is needed, the distal coronary anastomoses are performed first to reduce manipulation of the heart and prevent potential atrioventricular disruption after mitral valve repair or replacement.

In patients with a history of CABG, right thoracotomy is an option to avoid injury to previous bypass grafts during a redo sternotomy. Patent grafts, especially the left internal mammary (LIMA) graft to the left anterior descending artery, may be immediately under the sternal table from previous surgery. Because of the inability to isolate and control the LIMA graft from a right thoracotomy, fibrillatory arrest is needed.

Once exposed, the left atrium is opened after developing the interatrial groove, Sondegaard's groove, extending the incision behind the inferior vena cava to the oblique sinus. In cases of redo sternotomy or acute IMR (in which case the left atrium may be small), exposure to the mitral valve can be diffcult and a transeptal approach via the right atrium may be required. Improved exposure may also be obtained by extending the atrial incision superiorly behind the superior caval–right atrial junction. Using a specialized mitral retractor (Cosgrove retractor), the left atrium is lifted and the mitral valve should be exposed for inspection. If further exposure is required the superior vena cava can be transected and the left atriotomy further extended. This is later reanastomosed much like is performed in a bicaval orthotopic heart transplant.

The first and most important step in mitral valve surgery is valve analysis. Inspection will reveal the degree of annular dilatation and leaflet and chordal pathology, and may indicate segments of the mural annulus that appear disproportionately elongated. Traction sutures in the annulus at each commissure elevate the valve and facilitate exposure of the leaflets, chordae, and papillary muscles. Careful inspection should include searching for ruptured, elongated, or sclerosed chordae; fibrotic, atrophied papillary muscle, and redundant or defective leaflet tissue. Most often the entire valve appears normal; sometimes the posterior papillary muscle seems slightly more yellowish brown than the rest of the ventricle and the posterior part of the mural annulus seems slightly elongated.

Echocardiographic evaluation of the valve is important in the decision to repair or replace the valve. A central regurgitant jet with a dilated annulus is suggestive of a successful simple repair with an annuloplasty ring. In contrast, eccentric, complex regurgitant jets with severe bileaflet tethering and papillary muscle pathology such as elongation or rupture suggest that mitral replacement may be the best durable option. In this scenario mitral valve repair may not be a long-term solution. Magne and coworkers have found that preoperative echocardiographic assessment of posterior-leaflet angle greater than 45 degrees to the annulus determines a higher rate of failure of mitral repair using an annuloplasty ring (Fig. 29-6).[126]

For mitral valves amenable to annuloplasty repair, 2-0 braided suture is routinely used. Often, exposure to posterior and medial portions of the mitral annulus is easiest to achieve. These sutures should be placed first and used to place tension on the mitral annulus to faciliate exposure of the lateral and anterior portions of the annulus. It is essential that the full curve of the needle be used to ensure optimal placement of the sutures in the mitral annulus. Significant tension can develop when the dilated annulus is downsized, so sutures should be placed close together and overlap may be warranted. It is vital that the sutures are placed in the annulus and not in the atrial tissue to avoid subsequent annuloplasty ring dehiscence.

Sizing of the annuloplasty ring can be performed before or after placement of the annuloplasty sutures, depending on the

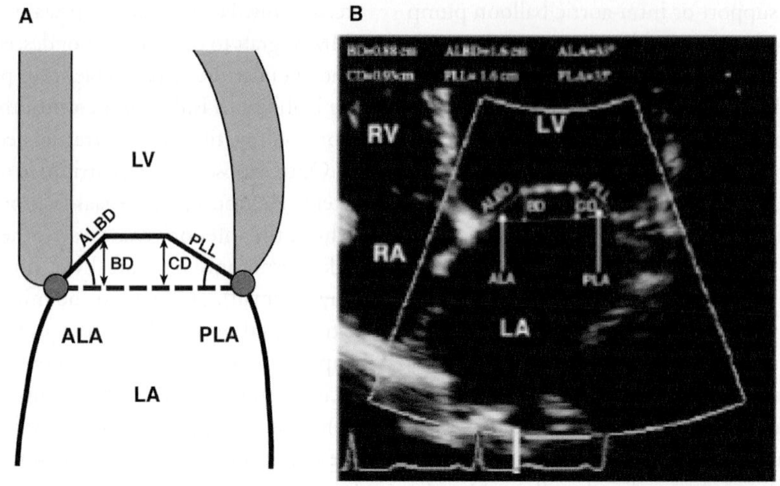

FIGURE 29-6 Method of mitral leaflet angle quantification. (A) Schema of transthoracic echocardiographic four-chamber view in mid-systole. (B) Echocardiographic image demonstrating technique of measurements of anterior leaflet angle (ALA) and posterior leaflet angle (PLA) using coaptation distance (CD), bending distance (BD), anterior leaflet bending distance (ALBD), and posterior leaflet length (PLL). RA = right atrial; RV = right ventricle. (*Reproduced with permission from Magne J, Pibarot P, Dagenais F, et al: Preoperative posterior leaflet angle accurately predicts outcome after restrictive mitral valve annuloplasty for ischemic mitral regurgitation. Circulation 2007; 115:782-791.*)

size of the left atrium and adequate exposure. Introduced by Bolling, the concept of reducing annular dilatation with aggressive annuloplasty downsizing aims to optimize leaflet coaptation. When choosing an annuloplasty ring, the intertrigonal distance and/or the surface area of the anterior leaflet are measured. Aggressive downsizing of the annulus (two sizes smaller than predicted by measuring the fibrous intertrigonal annulus) can be achieved with minimal risk of the development of systolic anterior motion, because the posterior leaflet in IMR is often tethered and restricted. Gorman and colleagues have demonstrated that use of a saddle-shaped annuloplasty ring restores normal annular geometry, decreases leaflet strain, and may increase repair durability.[127,128] Therefore, it may be prudent to choose a saddle-shaped annuloplasty ring as compared with a flat ring (Fig. 29-7). After the size of the ring is chosen, the annuloplasty sutures are placed in accordance with the geometry of the mitral annulus. Once all sutures are placed, the annuloplasty ring is slid down onto the mitral valve annulus and sutures tied to secure the ring. At this point, a saline test is usually employed to interrogate the competency of the mitral valve repair. If satisfied with the repair, the left atrium is then closed.

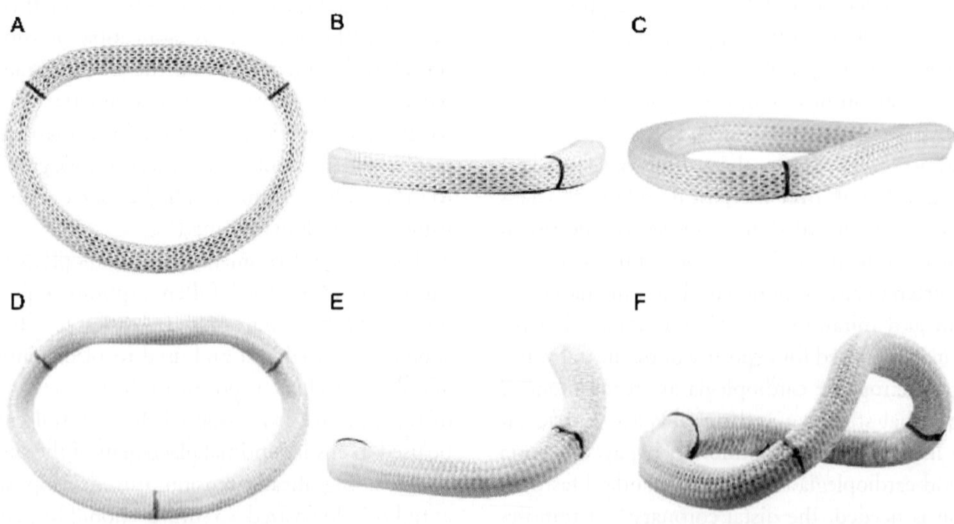

FIGURE 29-7 Images of the (A–C) Physio and (D–F) saddle ring as viewed from several orientations are provided. Subtle differences in the shape of the flow orifice (although the mitral annular areas are quite similar) can be appreciated in the short-axis views (A and D), whereas dramatic differences in annular height and nonplanarity are evident in the intercommissural (B and E) and oblique (C and F) views. (*Reproduced with permission from Ryan LP, Jackson BM, Hamamoto H, et al: The influence of annuloplasty ring geometry on mitral leaflet curvature. Ann Thorac Surg 2008; 86[3]:749-760.*)

If on inspection the valve is not amenable to annuloplasty repair, mitral valve replacement should be performed. Chordal sparing techniques[62–64,68,69,129] should be used if the valve is replaced. These methods have significantly reduced postoperative ventricular dysfunction observed after valve excision and have been found to produce no more left ventricular dysfunction than reparative operations.[69] Aged patients in sinus rhythm and patients with a life expectancy of less than 10 years who otherwise do not need anticoagulation are candidates for bioprosthetic valves; mechanical valves are recommended for others. The valve is inserted after excising a portion of anterior leaflet[63,69] and transposing[68] the remaining leaflet tissue to the commissures (see Fig. 29-4). Pledgeted everting sutures (atrial to ventricular, intra-annular placement) are used for intra-annular placement if downsizing and/or low profile valve (ie, mechanical valve) is desired. Noneverting, pledgeted sutures (ventricular to atrial, supra-annular placement) may be used for high-profile bioprosthetic valves or when a friable annulus is encountered. The mural leaflet is plicated into the valve insertion suture line and the struts of the prosthetic valve are placed along the commissural plane to prevent interference with the valve mechanism and left ventricular outflow tract obstruction.

The atriotomy is closed using running sutures, and any proximal coronary anastomoses are completed. Before removing the aortic clamp, all air is evacuated from the ventricle and the mitral valve is kept incompetent using a transvalvular catheter with ventricular and atrial holes. Absence of air and assessment of ventricular wall motion is made by transesophageal echocardiography. Anticipated pharmacologic support is started and satisfactory left ventricular contractility is established before loading the heart. After weaning, cardiopulmonary bypass is restarted. If the left ventricle begins to dilate and wall motion deteriorates, every effort is made to prevent any distention of the ventricle that might reduce myocardial contractile force. This may require placement of a pulmonary artery vent. Decisions for using intra-aortic balloon pump counterpulsation or even temporary left ventricular mechanical assistance are better made early than after multiple attempts to wean from cardiopulmonary bypass have failed.

FUTURE DIRECTIONS

There have been significant preliminary advances in novel approaches to treating mitral regurgitation, this has included subvalvar approaches, external fixation, and percutaneous repair strategies. Chordal cutting of two critical basal chordae of the anterior leaflet first described by Messas[130,131] has been shown to be effective in treating IMR. By relieving leaflet restriction and eliminating the angulation of the anterior leaflet, chordal cutting improves leaflet coaptation while the intact marginal chordae continue to prevent prolapse. Conflicting data from the Stanford group[132,133] demonstrate that cutting of second-order chords neither prevented nor decreased the severity of IMR in a sheep. Further investigation is required before this treatment modality is brought into mainstream management of IMR.

Kron and coworkers have reported a successful subvavular repair as an adjunct to standard annuloplasty.[134] Direct reposition of the displaced posterior papillary muscle toward the right fibrous trigone appear to ameliorate IMR. In a sheep model, Langer and coworkers confirmed Kron's findings.[135] Anchoring a suture at the right fibrous trigone and passing it through the posterior papillary muscle tip and left ventricular wall, the investigators demonstrated reduction of IMR by tightening the suture. Other groups have demonstrated that reapproximation of both papillary muscles may be beneficial in reducing leaflet tethering and IMR.[136–138]

Recent evidence argues that the development of IMR is a complex, multifactorial process resulting from left ventricular remodeling involving the entire mitral apparatus. Many investigators postulate that adjunctive surgical therapy directed at the remodeled ventricle may prove to be potential therapeutic strategies at treating IMR. Many have stated that IMR is not a valvular process, but a ventricular disease process. In a sheep model, Moaine and coworkers demonstrated that external restraint of the infarct zone attenuated remodeling and reduced chronic IMR.[139] Furthermore, external infarct restraint with mesh before infarction prevented left ventricular remodeling compared with the annuloplasty group. The data suggested that left ventricular remodeling associated with infarct expansion may serve as an important therapeutic target. The Acorn cardiac restrain device (CorCap) is a mesh device that is implanted around the heart to reduce wall stress and address left ventricular remodeling. Clinical trials with the Acorn device have shown that it is safe and effective in patients with advanced heart failure and remodeled ventricles, of mostly dilated etiology.[140–142] Further investigation is needed before definitive conclusions can be made.

Percutaneous therapies for MR have been attempted in multiple derivations. Rigid coronary sinus–based mitral annuloplasty devices deployed percutaneously have been demonstrated to reduce IMR in animal model.[143–145] Subseqent clinical trials have demonstrated clinical feasiblity.[146] A percutaneous approach to a modified Alfieri repair utilizing a clip to approximate the anterior and posterior mitral leaflets while creating a double outlet mitral valve has also been clinically tested. Initial results suggest feasibility and an acute reduction in MR.[147] Finally, the advent of percutaneous valve replacement technology has expanded to include transcatheter mitral valve prosthesis. Animal studies have been formulated and feasibility remains to be determined. The long-term results of these novel therapies remain to be elucidated. Further work is needed to explore the potential effectiveness and clinical applicability of these new technologies.

REFERENCES

1. Lloyd-Jones D, Adams R, Carnethon M, et al: Heart disease and stroke statistics—2009 update: a report from the American Heart Association Statistics Committee and Stroke Statistics Subcommittee. *Circulation* 2009; 119(3):480-486.
2. Gueret P, Khalife K, Jobic Y, et al: Echocardiographic assessment of the incidence of mechanical complications during the early phase of myocardial infarction in the reperfusion era: a French multicentre prospective registry. *Arch Cardiovasc Dis* 2008; 101(1):41-47.
3. Hickey MS, Smith LR, Muhlbaier LH, et al: Current prognosis of ischemic mitral regurgitation. Implications for future management. *Circulation* 1988; 78(3 Pt 2):I51-59.

4. Frantz E, Weininger F, Oswald H, Fleck E: Predictors for mitral regurgitation in coronary artery disease, in Vetter HO, Hetzer R, Schmutzler H (eds): *Ischemic Mitral Incompetence.* New York, Springer-Verlag, 1991; p 57.
5. *Heart and Stroke Facts: 1995 Statistical Supplement.* Dallas, American Heart Association, 1996.
6. Levine RA, Handschumacher MD, Sanfilippo AJ, et al: Three-dimensional echocardiographic reconstruction of the mitral valve, with implications for the diagnosis of mitral valve prolapse. *Circulation* 1989; 80(3):589-598.
7. Salgo IS, Gorman JH III, Gorman RC, et al: Effect of annular shape on leaflet curvature in reducing mitral leaflet stress. *Circulation* 2002; 106(6):711-717.
8. Tsakiris AG, Von Bernuth G, Rastelli GC, et al: Size and motion of the mitral valve annulus in anesthetized intact dogs. *J Appl Physiol* 1971; 30(5): 611-618.
9. Tsakiris AG, Sturm RE, Wood EH: Experimental studies on the mechanisms of closure of cardiac valves with use of roentgen videodensitometry. *Am J Cardiol* 1973; 32(2):136-143.
10. Ormiston JA, Shah PM, Tei C, Wong M: Size and motion of the mitral valve annulus in man. II. Abnormalities in mitral valve prolapse. *Circulation* 1982; 65(4):713-719.
11. Boltwood CM, Tei C, Wong M, Shah PM: Quantitative echocardiography of the mitral complex in dilated cardiomyopathy: the mechanism of functional mitral regurgitation. *Circulation* 1983; 68(3):498-508.
12. Gorman RC, McCaughan JS, Ratcliffe MB, et al: A three-dimensional analysis of papillary muscle spatial relationships in acute postinfarction mitral insufficiency. *Surg Forum* 1994; 45:330.
13. Walley KR, Grover M, Raff GL, et al: Left ventricular dynamic geometry in the intact and open chest dog. *Circ Res* 1982; 50(4):573-589.
14. Pandian NG, Kerber RE: Two-dimensional echocardiography in experimental coronary stenosis. I. Sensitivity and specificity in detecting transient myocardial dyskinesis: comparison with sonomicrometers. *Circulation* 1982; 66(3):597-602.
15. Moon MR, Ingels NB Jr, Daughters GT II, et al: Alterations in left ventricular twist mechanics with inotropic stimulation and volume loading in human subjects. *Circulation* 1994; 89(1):142-150.
16. Tsakiris AG, Gordon DA, Padiyar R, Frechette D: Relation of mitral valve opening and closure to left atrial and ventricular pressures in the intact dog. *Am J Physiol* 1978; 234(2):H146-151.
17. Wei JY, Hutchins GM, Bulkley BH: Papillary muscle rupture in fatal acute myocardial infarction: a potentially treatable form of cardiogenic shock. *Ann Intern Med* 1979; 90(2):149-152.
18. Tibayan FA, Rodriguez F, Langer F, et al: Does septal-lateral annular cinching work for chronic ischemic mitral regurgitation? *J Thorac Cardiovasc Surg* 2004; 127(3):654-663.
19. Timek TA, Lai DT, Tibayan F, et al: Septal-lateral annular cinching abolishes acute ischemic mitral regurgitation. *J Thorac Cardiovasc Surg* 2002; 123(5):881-888.
20. Timek TA, Lai DT, Liang D, et al: Effects of paracommissural septal-lateral annular cinching on acute ischemic mitral regurgitation. *Circulation* 2004; 110(11 Suppl 1):II79-184.
21. Hirakawa S, Sasayama S, Tomoike H, et al: In situ measurement of papillary muscle dynamics in the dog left ventricle. *Am J Physiol* 1977; 233(3): H384-91.
22. Tei C, Sakamaki T, Shah PM, et al: Mitral valve prolapse in short-term experimental coronary occlusion: a possible mechanism of ischemic mitral regurgitation. *Circulation* 1983; 68(1):183-189.
23. Gorman JH III, Jackson BM, Gorman RC, et al: Papillary muscle discoordination rather than increased annular area facilitates mitral regurgitation after acute posterior myocardial infarction. *Circulation* 1997; 96(9 Suppl): II-124-127.
24. Glasson JR, Komeda M, Daughters GT, et al: Early systolic mitral leaflet "loitering" during acute ischemic mitral regurgitation. *J Thorac Cardiovasc Surg* 1998; 116(2):193-205.
25. Komeda M, Glasson JR, Bolger AF, et al: Geometric determinants of ischemic mitral regurgitation. *Circulation* 1997; 96(9 Suppl):II-128-133.
26. Tibayan FA, Rodriguez F, Langer F, et al: Mitral suture annuloplasty corrects both annular and subvalvular geometry in acute ischemic mitral regurgitation. *J Heart Valve Dis* 2004; 13(3):414-420.
27. Nielsen SL, Timek TA, Green GR, et al: Influence of anterior mitral leaflet second-order chordae tendineae on left ventricular systolic function. *Circulation* 2003; 108(4):486-491.
28. Gorman RC, McCaughan JS, Ratcliffe MB, et al: Pathogenesis of acute ischemic mitral regurgitation in three dimensions. *J Thorac Cardiovasc Surg* 1995; 109(4):684-693.
29. Gorman JH III, Gorman RC, Jackson BM, et al: Distortions of the mitral valve in acute ischemic mitral regurgitation. *Ann Thorac Surg* 1997; 64(4): 1026-1031.
30. Gorman JH III, Jackson BM, Enomoto Y, Gorman RC: The effect of regional ischemia on mitral valve annular saddle shape. *Ann Thorac Surg* 2004; 77(2):544-548.
31. Sharma SK, Seckler J, Israel DH, Borrico S, Ambrose JA: Clinical, angiographic and anatomic findings in acute severe ischemic mitral regurgitation. *Am J Cardiol* 1992; 70(3):277-280.
32. Heikkila J: Mitral incompetence as a complication of acute myocardial infarction. *Acta Med Scand* 1967; 475:1-149.
33. Roberts WC, Cohen LS: Left ventricular papillary muscles. Description of the normal and a survey of conditions causing them to be abnormal. *Circulation* 1972; 46(1):138-154.
34. Llaneras MR, Nance ML, Streicher JT, et al: Large animal model of ischemic mitral regurgitation. *Ann Thorac Surg* 1994; 57(2):432-439.
35. Braunwald E: Valvular heart disease, in Braunwald E (ed): *Heart Disease,* 4th ed. Philadelphia, Saunders, 1992; p 1007.
36. Gorman JH 3rd, Gorman RC, Jackson BM, et al: Annuloplasty ring selection for chronic ischemic mitral regurgitation: lessons from the ovine model. *Ann Thorac Surg* 2003; 76(5):1556-1563.
37. Parish LM, Jackson BM, Enomoto Y, Gorman RC, Gorman JH III: The dynamic anterior mitral annulus. *Ann Thorac Surg* 2004; 78(4):1248-1255.
38. Tibayan FA, Rodriguez F, Zasio MK, et al: Geometric distortions of the mitral valvular-ventricular complex in chronic ischemic mitral regurgitation. *Circulation* 2003; 108(Suppl 1):II116-121.
39. Jackson BM, Gorman JH, Moainie SL, et al: Extension of borderzone myocardium in postinfarction dilated cardiomyopathy. *J Am Coll Cardiol* 2002; 40(6):1160-1167; discussion 68-71.
40. Otsuji Y, Handschumacher MD, Schwammenthal E, et al: Insights from three-dimensional echocardiography into the mechanism of functional mitral regurgitation: direct in vivo demonstration of altered leaflet tethering geometry. *Circulation* 1997; 96(6):1999-2008.
41. Yiu SF, Enriquez-Sarano M, Tribouilloy C, Seward JB, Tajik AJ: Determinants of the degree of functional mitral regurgitation in patients with systolic left ventricular dysfunction: a quantitative clinical study. *Circulation* 2000; 102(12):1400-1406.
42. Loisance DY, Deleuze P, Hillion ML, Cachera JP: Are there indications for reconstructive surgery in severe mitral regurgitation after acute myocardial infarction? *Eur J Cardiothorac Surg* 1990; 4(7):394-397.
43. Barbour DJ, Roberts WC: Rupture of a left ventricular papillary muscle during acute myocardial infarction: analysis of 22 necropsy patients. *J Am Coll Cardiol* 1986; 8(3):558-565.
44. Nishimura RA, Schaff HV, Shub C, et al: Papillary muscle rupture complicating acute myocardial infarction: analysis of 17 patients. *Am J Cardiol* 1983; 51(3):373-377.
45. Tepe NA, Edmunds LH Jr: Operation for acute postinfarction mitral insufficiency and cardiogenic shock. *J Thorac Cardiovasc Surg* 1985; 89(4): 525-530.
46. Tcheng JE, Jackman JD Jr, Nelson CL, et al: Outcome of patients sustaining acute ischemic mitral regurgitation during myocardial infarction. *Ann Intern Med* 1992; 117(1):18-24.
47. Le Feuvre C, Metzger JP, Lachurie ML, et al: Treatment of severe mitral regurgitation caused by ischemic papillary muscle dysfunction: indications for coronary angioplasty. *Am Heart J* 1992; 123(4 Pt 1):860-865.
48. Heuser RR, Maddoux GL, Goss JE, et al: Coronary angioplasty for acute mitral regurgitation due to myocardial infarction. A nonsurgical treatment preserving mitral valve integrity. *Ann Intern Med* 1987; 107(6):852-855.
49. Shawl FA, Forman MB, Punja S, Goldbaum TS: Emergent coronary angioplasty in the treatment of acute ischemic mitral regurgitation: long-term results in five cases. *J Am Coll Cardiol* 1989; 14(4):986-991.
50. Bates ER, Califf RM, Stack RS, et al: Thrombolysis and Angioplasty in Myocardial Infarction (TAMI-1) trial: influence of infarct location on arterial patency, left ventricular function and mortality. *J Am Coll Cardiol* 1989; 13(1):12-18.
51. Pfeffer MA, Braunwald E: Ventricular remodeling after myocardial infarction. Experimental observations and clinical implications. *Circulation* 1990; 81(4):1161-1172.
52. Marino P, Zanolla L, Zardini P: Effect of streptokinase on left ventricular modeling and function after myocardial infarction: the GISSI (Gruppo Italiano per lo Studio della Streptochinasi nell'Infarto Miocardico) Trial. *J Am Coll Cardiol* 1989; 14(5):1149-1158.
53. Kennedy JW, Ivey TD, Misbach G, et al: Coronary artery bypass graft surgery early after acute myocardial infarction. *Circulation* 1989; 79(6 Pt 2): I73-78.
54. Rankin JS, Hickey MS, Smith LR, et al: Ischemic mitral regurgitation. *Circulation* 1989; 79(6 Pt 2):I116-121.
55. Replogle RL, Campbell CD: Surgery for mitral regurgitation associated with ischemic heart disease. Results and strategies. *Circulation* 1989; 79(6 Pt 2): I122-125.

56. Gorman JH III, Jackson BM, Kolansky DM, Gorman RC: Emergency mitral valve replacement in the octogenarian. *Ann Thorac Surg* 2003; 76(1): 269-271.
57. Kono T, Sabbah HN, Stein PD, Brymer JF, Khaja F: Left ventricular shape as a determinant of functional mitral regurgitation in patients with severe heart failure secondary to either coronary artery disease or idiopathic dilated cardiomyopathy. *Am J Cardiol* 1991; 68(4):355-359.
58. Piwnica A, Menasche PH, Kucharski C, et al: Surgery for acute ischemic mitral incompentence, in Vetter HO, Hetzer H, Schmutzler H (eds): *Ischemic Mitral Incompetence.* New York, Springer-Verlag, 1991; p 193.
59. Hochman JS, Choo H: Limitation of myocardial infarct expansion by reperfusion independent of myocardial salvage. *Circulation* 1987; 75(1): 299-306.
60. Gillinov AM, Wierup PN, Blackstone EH, et al: Is repair preferable to replacement for ischemic mitral regurgitation? *J Thorac Cardiovasc Surg* 2001; 122(6):1125-1141.
61. Grossi EA, Goldberg JD, LaPietra A, et al: Ischemic mitral valve reconstruction and replacement: comparison of long-term survival and complications. *J Thorac Cardiovasc Surg* 2001; 122(6):1107-1124.
62. Lillehei CW, Levy MJ, Bonnabeau RC Jr: Mitral valve replacement with preservation of papillary muscles and chordae tendineae. *J Thorac Cardiovasc Surg* 1964; 47:532-543.
63. David TE, Uden DE, Strauss HD: The importance of the mitral apparatus in left ventricular function after correction of mitral regurgitation. *Circulation* 1983; 68(3 Pt 2):II76-82.
64. Sarris GE, Fann JI, Niczyporuk MA, et al: Global and regional left ventricular systolic performance in the in situ ejecting canine heart. Importance of the mitral apparatus. *Circulation* 1989; 80(3 Pt 1):I24-42.
65. Yun KL, Niczyporuk MA, Sarris GE, Fann JI, Miller DC: Importance of mitral subvalvular apparatus in terms of cardiac energetics and systolic mechanics in the ejecting canine heart. *J Clin Invest* 1991; 87(1):247-254.
66. Yun KL, Rayhill SC, Niczyporuk MA, et al: Mitral valve replacement in dilated canine hearts with chronic mitral regurgitation. Importance of the mitral subvalvular apparatus. *Circulation* 1991; 84(5 Suppl):III112-124.
67. David TE: Techniques and results of mitral valve repair for ischemic mitral regurgitation. *J Card Surg* 1994; 9(2 Suppl):274-277.
68. Oury JH, Cleveland JC, Duran CG, Angell WW: Ischemic mitral valve disease: classification and systemic approach to management. *J Card Surg* 1994; 9(2 Suppl):262-273.
69. Okita Y, Miki S, Kusuhara K, et al: Analysis of left ventricular motion after mitral valve replacement with a technique of preservation of all chordae tendineae. Comparison with conventional mitral valve replacement or mitral valve repair. *J Thorac Cardiovasc Surg* 1992; 104(3):786-795.
70. Russo A, Suri RM, Grigioni F, et al: Clinical outcome after surgical correction of mitral regurgitation due to papillary muscle rupture. *Circulation* 2008; 118(15):1528-1534.
71. Balu V, Hershowitz S, Zaki Masud AR, Bhayana JN, Dean DC: Mitral regurgitation in coronary artery disease. *Chest* 1982; 81(5):550-555.
72. Pinson CW, Cobanoglu A, Metzdorff MT, et al: Late surgical results for ischemic mitral regurgitation. Role of wall motion score and severity of regurgitation. *J Thorac Cardiovasc Surg* 1984; 88(5 Pt 1):663-672.
73. Connolly MW, Gelbfish JS, Jacobowitz IJ, et al: Surgical results for mitral regurgitation from coronary artery disease. *J Thorac Cardiovasc Surg* 1986; 91(3):379-388.
74. Karp RB, Mills N, Edmunds LH Jr: Coronary artery bypass grafting in the presence of valvular disease. *Circulation* 1989; 79(6 Pt 2):I182-184.
75. Bursi F, Enriquez-Sarano M, Nkomo VT, et al: Heart failure and death after myocardial infarction in the community: the emerging role of mitral regurgitation. *Circulation* 2005; 111(3):295-301.
76. Calafiore AM, Mazzei V, Iaco AL, et al: Impact of ischemic mitral regurgitation on long-term outcome of patients with ejection fraction above 0.30 undergoing first isolated myocardial revascularization. *Ann Thorac Surg* 2008; 86(2):458-464; discussion 64-65.
77. Kumanohoso T, Otsuji Y, Yoshifuku S, et al: Mechanism of higher incidence of ischemic mitral regurgitation in patients with inferior myocardial infarction: quantitative analysis of left ventricular and mitral valve geometry in 103 patients with prior myocardial infarction. *J Thorac Cardiovasc Surg* 2003; 125(1):135-143.
78. Aronson D, Goldsher N, Zukermann R, et al: Ischemic mitral regurgitation and risk of heart failure after myocardial infarction. *Arch Intern Med* 2006; 166(21):2362-2368.
79. Ellis SG, Whitlow PL, Raymond RE, Schneider JP: Impact of mitral regurgitation on long-term survival after percutaneous coronary intervention. *Am J Cardiol* 2002; 89(3):315-318.
80. Waibel AW, Hausdorf G, Vetter HO, et al: Results of surgical therapy in ischemic mitral regurgitation, in Vetter HO, Hetzer H, Schmutzler H (eds): *Ischemic Mitral Incompetence.* New York, Springer-Verlag, 1991; p 149.
81. Downing SW, Savage EB, Streicher JS, et al: The stretched ventricle. Myocardial creep and contractile dysfunction after acute nonischemic ventricular distention. *J Thorac Cardiovasc Surg* 1992; 104(4):996-1005.
82. Adler DS, Goldman L, O'Neil A, et al: Long-term survival of more than 2,000 patients after coronary artery bypass grafting. *Am J Cardiol* 1986; 58(3):195-202.
83. Arcidi JM Jr, Hebeler RF, Craver JM, et al: Treatment of moderate mitral regurgitation and coronary disease by coronary bypass alone. *J Thorac Cardiovasc Surg* 1988; 95(6):951-959.
84. Dion R: Ischemic mitral regurgitation: when and how should it be corrected? *J Heart Valve Dis* 1993; 2(5):536-543.
85. Tamaki N, Kawamoto M, Tadamura E, et al: Prediction of reversible ischemia after revascularization. Perfusion and metabolic studies with positron emission tomography. *Circulation* 1995; 91(6):1697-1705.
86. Schelbert HR: Different roads to the assessment of myocardial viability. Lessons from PET for SPECT. *Circulation* 1995; 91(6):1894-1895.
87. Christenson JT, Simonet F, Bloch A, et al: Should a mild to moderate ischemic mitral valve regurgitation in patients with poor left ventricular function be repaired or not? *J Heart Valve Dis* 1995; 4(5):484-488; discussion 8-9.
88. Tolis GA Jr, Korkolis DP, Kopf GS, Elefteriades JA: Revascularization alone (without mitral valve repair) suffices in patients with advanced ischemic cardiomyopathy and mild-to-moderate mitral regurgitation. *Ann Thorac Surg* 2002; 74(5):1476-1480; discussion 80-81.
89. Talwalkar NG, Earle NR, Earle EA, Lawrie GM: Mitral valve repair in patients with low left ventricular ejection fractions: early and late results. *Chest* 2004; 126(3):709-715.
90. Mihaljevic T, Lam BK, Rajeswaran J, et al: Impact of mitral valve annuloplasty combined with revascularization in patients with functional ischemic mitral regurgitation. *J Am Coll Cardiol* 2007; 49(22):2191-2201.
91. Aklog L, Filsoufi F, Flores KQ, et al: Does coronary artery bypass grafting alone correct moderate ischemic mitral regurgitation? *Circulation* 2001; 104(12 Suppl 1):I68-75.
92. Calafiore AM, Di Mauro M, Gallina S, et al: Mitral valve surgery for chronic ischemic mitral regurgitation. *Ann Thorac Surg* 2004; 77(6):1989-1997.
93. Bolling SF, Deeb GM, Bach DS: Mitral valve reconstruction in elderly, ischemic patients. *Chest* 1996; 109(1):35-40.
94. Gangemi JJ, Tribble CG, Ross SD, et al: Does the additive risk of mitral valve repair in patients with ischemic cardiomyopathy prohibit surgical intervention? *Ann Surg* 2000; 231(5):710-714.
95. Fedoruk LM, Tribble CG, Kern JA, Peeler BB, Kron IL: Predicting operative mortality after surgery for ischemic cardiomyopathy. *Ann Thorac Surg* 2007; 83(6):2029-2035; discussion 35.
96. Czer LS, Maurer G, Bolger AF, DeRobertis M, Chaux A, Matloff JM: Revascularization alone or combined with suture annuloplasty for ischemic mitral regurgitation. Evaluation by color Doppler echocardiography. *Tex Heart Inst J* 1996; 23(4):270-278.
97. Fukushima S, Kobayashi J, Bando K, et al: Late outcomes after isolated coronary artery bypass grafting for ischemic mitral regurgitation. *Jpn J Thorac Cardiovasc Surg* 2005; 53(7):354-360.
98. Lam BK, Gillinov AM, Blackstone EH, et al: Importance of moderate ischemic mitral regurgitation. *Ann Thorac Surg* 2005; 79(2):462-470; discussion 70.
99. Campwala SZ, Bansal RC, Wang N, Razzouk A, Pai RG: Mitral regurgitation progression following isolated coronary artery bypass surgery: frequency, risk factors, and potential prevention strategies. *Eur J Cardiothorac Surg* 2006; 29(3):348-353.
100. Prifti E, Bonacchi M, Frati G, et al: Ischemic mitral valve regurgitation grade II-III: correction in patients with impaired left ventricular function undergoing simultaneous coronary revascularization. *J Heart Valve Dis* 2001; 10(6):754-762.
101. Harris KM, Sundt TM III, Aeppli D, Sharma R, Barzilai B: Can late survival of patients with moderate ischemic mitral regurgitation be impacted by intervention on the valve? *Ann Thorac Surg* 2002; 74(5):1468-1475.
102. Wong DR, Agnihotri AK, Hung JW, et al: Long-term survival after surgical revascularization for moderate ischemic mitral regurgitation. *Ann Thorac Surg* 2005; 80(2):570-577.
103. Buja P, Tarantini G, Del Bianco F, et al: Moderate-to-severe ischemic mitral regurgitation and multivessel coronary artery disease: Impact of different treatment on survival and rehospitalization. *Int J Cardiol* 2006; 111(1):26-33. Epub 2005.
104. Kim YH, Czer LS, Soukiasian HJ, et al: Ischemic mitral regurgitation: revascularization alone versus revascularization and mitral valve repair. *Ann Thorac Surg* 2005; 79(6):1895-1901.
105. Diodato MD, Moon MR, Pasque MK, et al: Repair of ischemic mitral regurgitation does not increase mortality or improve long-term survival in patients undergoing coronary artery revascularization: a propensity analysis. *Ann Thorac Surg* 2004; 78(3):794-799; discussion 9.

106. Trichon BH, Glower DD, Shaw LK, et al: Survival after coronary revascularization, with and without mitral valve surgery, in patients with ischemic mitral regurgitation. *Circulation* 2003; 108(Suppl 1):II103-110.
107. Fattouch K, Guccione F, Sampognaro R, et al: POINT: Efficacy of adding mitral valve restrictive annuloplasty to coronary artery bypass grafting in patients with moderate ischemic mitral valve regurgitation: a randomized trial. *J Thorac Cardiovasc Surg* 2009; 138(2):278-285.
108. Bolling SF, Pagani FD, Deeb GM, Bach DS: Intermediate-term outcome of mitral reconstruction in cardiomyopathy. *J Thorac Cardiovasc Surg* 1998; 115(2):381-386; discussion 7-8.
109. Bach DS, Bolling SF: Improvement following correction of secondary mitral regurgitation in end-stage cardiomyopathy with mitral annuloplasty. *Am J Cardiol* 1996; 78(8):966-969.
110. Badhwar V, Bolling SF: Mitral valve surgery in the patient with left ventricular dysfunction. *Semin Thorac Cardiovasc Surg* 2002; 14(2):133-136.
111. Romano MA, Bolling SF: Update on mitral repair in dilated cardiomyopathy. *J Card Surg* 2004; 19(5):396-400.
112. Tibayan FA, Rodriguez F, Langer F, et al: Undersized mitral annuloplasty alters left ventricular shape during acute ischemic mitral regurgitation. *Circulation* 2004; 110(11 Suppl 1):II98-102.
113. Bax JJ, Braun J, Somer ST, et al: Restrictive annuloplasty and coronary revascularization in ischemic mitral regurgitation results in reverse left ventricular remodeling. *Circulation* 2004; 110(11 Suppl 1):II103-108.
114. Braun J, Bax JJ, Versteegh MI, et al: Preoperative left ventricular dimensions predict reverse remodeling following restrictive mitral annuloplasty in ischemic mitral regurgitation. *Eur J Cardiothorac Surg* 2005; 27(5):847-853.
115. Geidel S, Lass M, Schneider C, et al: Downsizing of the mitral valve and coronary revascularization in severe ischemic mitral regurgitation results in reverse left ventricular and left atrial remodeling. *Eur J Cardiothorac Surg* 2005; 27(6):1011-1016.
116. Filsoufi F, Salzberg SP, Adams DH: Current management of ischemic mitral regurgitation. *Mt Sinai J Med* 2005; 72(2):105-115.
117. Adams DH, Filsoufi F, Aklog L: Surgical treatment of the ischemic mitral valve. *J Heart Valve Dis* 2002; 11(Suppl 1):S21-25.
118. Szalay ZA, Civelek A, Hohe S, et al: Mitral annuloplasty in patients with ischemic versus dilated cardiomyopathy. *Eur J Cardiothorac Surg* 2003; 23(4):567-572.
119. Rothenburger M, Rukosujew A, Hammel D, et al: Mitral valve surgery in patients with poor left ventricular function. *Thorac Cardiovasc Surg* 2002; 50(6):351-354.
120. Gummert JF, Rahmel A, Bucerius J, et al: Mitral valve repair in patients with end stage cardiomyopathy: who benefits? *Eur J Cardiothorac Surg* 2003; 23(6):1017-1022; discussion 22.
121. Braun J, van de Veire NR, Klautz RJ, et al: Restrictive mitral annuloplasty cures ischemic mitral regurgitation and heart failure. *Ann Thorac Surg* 2008; 85(2):430-436; discussion 6-7.
122. Wu AH, Aaronson KD, Bolling SF, et al: Impact of mitral valve annuloplasty on mortality risk in patients with mitral regurgitation and left ventricular systolic dysfunction. *J Am Coll Cardiol* 2005; 45(3):381-387.
123. McGee EC, Gillinov AM, Blackstone EH, et al: Recurrent mitral regurgitation after annuloplasty for functional ischemic mitral regurgitation. *J Thorac Cardiovasc Surg* 2004; 128(6):916-924.
124. Spoor MT, Geltz A, Bolling SF: Flexible versus nonflexible mitral valve rings for congestive heart failure: differential durability of repair. *Circulation* 2006; 114(1 Suppl):I67-71.
125. Hendren WG, Nemec JJ, Lytle BW, et al: Mitral valve repair for ischemic mitral insufficiency. *Ann Thorac Surg* 1991; 52(6):1246-1251; discussion 51-52.
126. Magne J, Pibarot P, Dagenais F, et al: Preoperative posterior leaflet angle accurately predicts outcome after restrictive mitral valve annuloplasty for ischemic mitral regurgitation. *Circulation* 2007; 115(6):782-791.
127. Jimenez JH, Liou SW, Padala M, et al: A saddle-shaped annulus reduces systolic strain on the central region of the mitral valve anterior leaflet. *J Thorac Cardiovasc Surg* 2007; 134(6):1562-1568.
128. Ryan LP, Jackson BM, Hamamoto H, et al: The influence of annuloplasty ring geometry on mitral leaflet curvature. *Ann Thorac Surg* 2008; 86(3): 749-760; discussion 60.
129. Cooley DA, Ingram MT: Intravalvular implantation of mitral valve prostheses. *Tex Heart Inst J* 1987; 14(2):188-193.
130. Messas E, Guerrero JL, Handschumacher MD, et al: Chordal cutting: a new therapeutic approach for ischemic mitral regurgitation. *Circulation* 2001; 104(16):1958-1963.
131. Messas E, Pouzet B, Touchot B, et al: Efficacy of chordal cutting to relieve chronic persistent ischemic mitral regurgitation. *Circulation* 2003; 108(Suppl 1):II111-115.
132. Rodriguez F, Langer F, Harrington KB, et al: Cutting second-order chords does not prevent acute ischemic mitral regurgitation. *Circulation* 2004; 110(11 Suppl 1):II91-97.
133. Rodriguez F, Langer F, Harrington KB, et al: Importance of mitral valve second-order chordae for left ventricular geometry, wall thickening mechanics, and global systolic function. *Circulation* 2004; 110(11 Suppl 1): II115-122.
134. Kron IL, Green GR, Cope JT: Surgical relocation of the posterior papillary muscle in chronic ischemic mitral regurgitation. *Ann Thorac Surg* 2002; 74(2):600-601.
135. Langer F, Rodriguez F, Ortiz S, et al: Subvalvular repair: the key to repairing ischemic mitral regurgitation? *Circulation* 2005; 112(9 Suppl):I383-389.
136. Matsui Y, Suto Y, Shimura S, et al: Impact of papillary muscles approximation on the adequacy of mitral coaptation in functional mitral regurgitation due to dilated cardiomyopathy. *Ann Thorac Cardiovasc Surg* 2005; 11(3):164-171.
137. Nair RU, Williams SG, Nwafor KU, Hall AS, Tan LB: Left ventricular volume reduction without ventriculectomy. *Ann Thorac Surg* 2001; 71(6): 2046-2049.
138. Menicanti L, Di Donato M, Frigiola A, et al: Ischemic mitral regurgitation: intraventricular papillary muscle imbrication without mitral ring during left ventricular restoration. *J Thorac Cardiovasc Surg* 2002; 123(6): 1041-1050.
139. Moainie SL, Guy TS, Gorman JH III, et al: Infarct restraint attenuates remodeling and reduces chronic ischemic mitral regurgitation after posterolateral infarction. *Ann Thorac Surg* 2002; 74(2):444-449; discussion 9.
140. Acker MA, Bolling S, Shemin R, et al: Mitral valve surgery in heart failure: insights from the Acorn Clinical Trial. *J Thorac Cardiovasc Surg* 2006; 132(3): 568-577, 77 e1-4.
141. Acker MA: Clinical results with the Acorn cardiac restraint device with and without mitral valve surgery. *Semin Thorac Cardiovasc Surg* 2005; 17(4):361-363.
142. Oz MC, Konertz WF, Kleber FX, et al: Global surgical experience with the Acorn cardiac support device. *J Thorac Cardiovasc Surg* 2003; 126(4): 983-991.
143. Daimon M, Shiota T, Gillinov AM, et al: Percutaneous mitral valve repair for chronic ischemic mitral regurgitation: a real-time three-dimensional echocardiographic study in an ovine model. *Circulation* 2005; 111(17): 2183-2189.
144. Kaye DM, Byrne M, Alferness C, Power J: Feasibility and short-term efficacy of percutaneous mitral annular reduction for the therapy of heart failure-induced mitral regurgitation. *Circulation* 2003; 108(15):1795-1797.
145. Liddicoat JR, Mac Neill BD, Gillinov AM, et al: Percutaneous mitral valve repair: a feasibility study in an ovine model of acute ischemic mitral regurgitation. *Catheter Cardiovasc Interv* 2003; 60(3):410-416.
146. Schofer J, Siminiak T, Haude M, et al: Percutaneous mitral annuloplasty for functional mitral regurgitation: results of the CARILLON Mitral Annuloplasty Device European Union Study. *Circulation* 2009; 120(4):326-333.
147. Feldman T, Kar S, Rinaldi M, et al: Percutaneous mitral repair with the MitraClip system: safety and midterm durability in the initial EVEREST (Endovascular Valve Edge-to-Edge REpair Study) cohort. *J Am Coll Cardiol* 2009; 54(8):686-694.

CHAPTER 30

Left Ventricular Aneurysm

Donald D. Glower
James E. Lowe

DEFINITION

Left ventricular aneurysm has been strictly defined as a distinct area of abnormal left ventricular diastolic contour with systolic dyskinesia or paradoxical bulging (Fig. 30-1).[1,2] Yet, a growing number of authors favor defining left ventricular aneurysm more loosely as any large area of left ventricular akinesia or dyskinesia that reduces left ventricular ejection fraction.[3–5] This broader definition has been justified by data suggesting that the pathophysiology and treatment may be the same for ventricular akinesia and for ventricular dyskinesia.[4,6] However, recent studies suggest that the optimal treatment and outcomes of patients with akinetic segments versus dyskinetic segments might be different.[7,8] Intraoperatively, a left ventricular aneurysm may also be identified as an area that collapses upon left ventricular decompression.[3,6,9] True left ventricular aneurysms involve bulging of the full thickness of the left ventricular wall, whereas a false aneurysm of the left ventricle is, in fact, a rupture of the left ventricular wall contained by surrounding pericardium.

HISTORY

Left ventricular aneurysms have long been described at autopsy, but left ventricular aneurysm was not recognized to be a consequence of coronary artery disease until 1881.[10] The angiographic diagnosis of left ventricular aneurysm was first made in 1951.[10] A congenital left ventricular aneurysm was first treated surgically by Weitland in 1912 using aneurysm ligation. In 1944, Beck[11] described fasciae latae plication to treat left ventricular aneurysms. Likoff and Bailey[12] successfully resected a left ventricular aneurysm through a thoracotomy in 1955 using a special clamp without cardiopulmonary bypass. The modern treatment era began in 1958 when Cooley et al.[13] successfully performed a linear repair of a left ventricular aneurysm using cardiopulmonary bypass. More geometric ventricular reconstruction or restoration techniques were subsequently devised by Stoney et al.,[14] Daggett et al.,[15] Dor et al.,[16] Jatene,[17] and Cooley et al.[18,19]

INCIDENCE

The incidence of left ventricular aneurysm in patients suffering from myocardial infarction has varied between 10 and 35% depending on the definition and the methods used. Of patients undergoing cardiac catheterization in the CASS study, 7.6% had angiographic evidence of left ventricular aneurysms.[20] The absolute incidence of left ventricular aneurysms may be declining because of the increased use of thrombolytics and revascularization after myocardial infarction.[21,22]

ETIOLOGY

More than 95% of true left ventricular aneurysms reported in the English literature result from coronary artery disease and myocardial infarction. True left ventricular aneurysms also may result from trauma,[23] Chagas' disease,[24] or sarcoidosis.[25] A very small number of congenital left ventricular aneurysms also have been reported and have been termed *diverticula* of the left ventricle.[26]

False aneurysms of the left ventricle result most commonly from contained rupture of the ventricle 5 to 10 days after myocardial infarction and often occur after circumflex coronary arterial occlusion. False aneurysm of the left ventricle also may result from submitral rupture of the ventricular wall, a dramatic event that generally occurs after mitral valve replacement with resection of the mitral valve apparatus.[27] Left ventricular pseudoaneurysm may also result from septic pericarditis[28] or any prior operation on the left ventricle, aortic annulus, or mitral annulus.

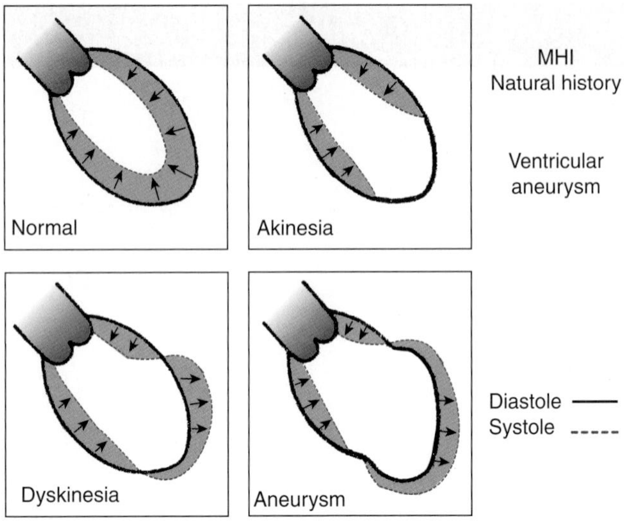

FIGURE 30-1 Diagrammatic distinction between aneurysm and other states of the left ventricle. (*Reproduced with permission from Grondin P, Kretz JG, Bical O, et al: Natural history of saccular aneurysm of the left ventricle. J Thorac Cardiovasc Surg 1979; 77:57.*)

PATHOPHYSIOLOGY

The development of a true left ventricular aneurysm involves two principal phases: early expansion and late remodeling.

Early Expansion Phase

The early expansion phase begins with the onset of myocardial infarction. Ventriculography can demonstrate left ventricular aneurysm formation within 48 hours of infarction in 50% of patients who develop ventricular aneurysms. The remaining patients have evidence of aneurysm formation by 2 weeks after infarction.[29]

True aneurysm of the left ventricle generally follows transmural myocardial infarction because of acute occlusion of the left anterior descending or dominant right coronary artery.

Lack of angiographic collaterals is strongly associated with aneurysm formation in patients with acute myocardial infarction and left anterior descending artery occlusion,[30] and absence of re-formed collateral circulation is probably a prerequisite for formation of a dyskinetic left ventricular aneurysm (Table 30-1).

TABLE 30-1 Factors Contributing to Left Ventricular Aneurysm Formation

Preserved contractility of surrounding myocardium
Transmural infarction
Lack of collateral circulation
Lack of reperfusion
Preserved contractility of surrounding myocardium
Elevated wall stress
Hypertension
Ventricular dilation
Wall thinning

At least 88% of dyskinetic ventricular aneurysms result from anterior infarction, and the remainder follow inferior infarction.[10] Posterior infarctions that produce a distinct dyskinetic left ventricular aneurysm are relatively unusual.

In experimental transmural infarction without collateral circulation, myocyte death begins 19 minutes after coronary occlusion. Infarctions that result in dyskinetic aneurysm formation are almost always transmural and may show gross thinning of the infarct zone within hours of infarction. Within a few days, the endocardial surface of the developing aneurysm becomes smooth with loss of trabeculae and deposition of fibrin and thrombus on the endocardial surface in at least 50% of patients. Because most myocytes within the infarct are necrotic, viable myocytes often remain within the infarct zone. In a minority of patients, extravascular hemorrhage occurs in the infarcted tissue and may further depress systolic and diastolic function of involved myocardium. Inflammatory cells migrate into the infarct zone by 2 to 3 days after infarction and contribute to lysis of necrotic myocytes by 5 to 10 days after infarction. Electron microscopy demonstrates disruption of the native collagen network several days after infarction. Collagen disruption and myocyte necrosis produce a nadir of myocardial tensile strength between 5 and 10 days after infarction, when rupture of the myocardial wall is most common. Left ventricular rupture is relatively rare after the ventricular aneurysmal wall becomes replaced with fibrous tissue.

Loss of systolic contraction in the large infarcted zone and preserved contraction of surrounding myocardium cause systolic bulging and thinning of the infarct. By Laplace's law ($T = Pr/2h$), at a constant ventricular pressure, P, increased radius of curvature, r, and decreased wall thickness, h, in the infarcted zone both contribute to increased muscle fiber tension, T, and further stretch the infarcted ventricular wall.

Relative to normal myocardium, ischemically injured or infarcted myocardium displays greater *plasticity* or *creep,* defined as deformation or stretch over time under a constant load.[31] Thus increased systolic and diastolic wall stress in the infarcted zone tends to produce progressive stretch of the infarcted myocardium (termed *infarct expansion*)[32] until healing reduces the plasticity of infarcted myocardium.

Transmural infarction without significant hibernating myocardium within the infarct region is necessary for subsequent development of a true left ventricular aneurysm. Angiographic ventricular aneurysms with evidence of hibernating myocardium (lack of Q waves or presence of uptake on technetium scan; Takotsubo cardiomyopathy, for example) may resolve over days to weeks and thus do not represent true left ventricular aneurysms by strict criteria.[33,34]

Because of increased diastolic stretch or preload and elevated catecholamines, remaining noninfarcted myocardium may demonstrate increased fiber shortening and, ultimately, myocardial hypertrophy in the presence of a left ventricular aneurysm.[35] This increased shortening and increased wall stress increase oxygen demand for noninfarcted myocardium and for the left ventricle as a whole.

In addition to increased regional wall stresses, left ventricular aneurysm can increase ventricular oxygen demand and decrease net forward cardiac output by producing a ventricular volume load because a portion of the stroke volume goes into the aneurysm instead of out the aortic valve. Net mechanical efficiency of the left ventricle (external stroke work minus myocardial oxygen consumption) is decreased by reducing external stroke work (volume times pressure) and increasing myocardial oxygen consumption.

Left ventricular aneurysms can produce both systolic and diastolic ventricular dysfunction. Diastolic dysfunction results from increased stiffness of the distended and fibrotic aneurysmal wall, which impairs diastolic filling and increases left ventricular end-diastolic pressure.

Late Remodeling Phase

The remodeling phase of ventricular aneurysm formation begins 2 to 4 weeks after infarction when highly vascularized granulation tissue appears. This granulation tissue is subsequently replaced by fibrous tissue 6 to 8 weeks after infarction. As myocytes are lost, ventricular wall thickness decreases as the myocardium becomes largely replaced by fibrous tissue. In larger infarcts, the thin scar is often lined with mural thrombus.[36]

After acute myocardial infarction, animal studies show that ventricular load reduction with 8 weeks of nitrate therapy may reduce expected infarct thinning, decrease infarct stretch, and lessen hypertrophy of noninfarcted myocardium.[37] Interestingly, nitrate therapy for only 2 weeks after infarction does not prevent aneurysm formation. This observation emphasizes the importance of late remodeling from 2 to 8 weeks after infarction. Angiotensin converting-enzyme (ACE) inhibitors also reduce infarct expansion and subsequent development of ventricular aneurysm.[38] Because animal studies show that ACE inhibitors nonspecifically suppress ventricular hypertrophy, it is not clear whether suppression of the compensatory hypertrophy of surrounding myocardium is ultimately beneficial or harmful. Intravenous administration of atrial natriuretic factor for 4 weeks has improved ventricular function, dimensions, and fibrosis in rats.[39]

Lack of coronary reperfusion is probably prerequisite for development of left ventricular aneurysm. In humans, reperfusion of the infarct vessel either spontaneously,[33] by thrombolysis,[40] or by angioplasty[41] has been associated with a lower incidence of aneurysm formation. It is speculated that coronary reperfusion as late as 2 weeks after infarction prevents aneurysm formation by improving blood flow and fibroblast migration into the infarcted myocardium. The role of delayed infarct healing in aneurysm development is supported by observations that steroids after myocardial infarction may increase the likelihood of aneurysm formation.[42]

Arrhythmias such as ventricular tachycardia may occur at any time during the development of ventricular aneurysm, and all these patients have the substrate for reentrant conduction pathways within the heterogeneous ventricular myocardium. These pathways tend to involve border zones surrounding the ventricular aneurysm (see Chapter 57).

NATURAL HISTORY

The excellent prognosis of asymptomatic patients with dyskinetic ventricular aneurysms who were treated medically was demonstrated in a series of 40 patients followed for a mean of 5 years.[2] Of 18 initially asymptomatic patients, 6 developed class II symptoms and 12 remained asymptomatic. Ten-year survival was 90% for these patients but was only 46% at 10 years in patients who presented with symptoms (Fig. 30-2).

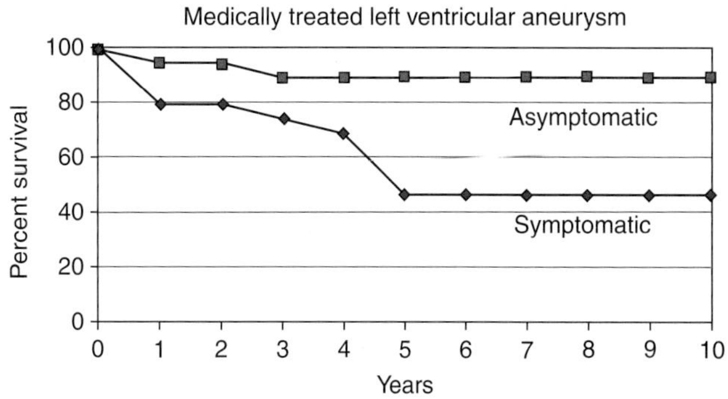

FIGURE 30-2 Survival in medically treated patients with left ventricular aneurysm based on presence (group B) or absence (group A) of symptoms. (*Based on Grondin P, Kretz JG, Bical O, et al: Natural history of saccular aneurysm of the left ventricle. J Thorac Cardiovasc Surg 1979; 77:57.*)

Although earlier autopsy series reported relatively poor survival in patients with medically managed left ventricular dyskinetic aneurysms (12% at 5 years), most recent studies report 5-year survival from 47 to 70%.[2,20,43–45] Causes of death include arrhythmia in 44%, heart failure in 33%, recurrent myocardial infarction in 11%, and noncardiac causes in 22%.[2] The natural history of patients with akinetic rather than dyskinetic left ventricular aneurysms is less well documented.[7]

Factors that influence survival with medically managed left ventricular dyskinetic aneurysm include age, heart failure score, extent of coronary disease, duration of angina, prior infarction, mitral regurgitation, ventricular arrhythmias, aneurysm size, function of residual ventricle, and left ventricular end-diastolic pressure.[2,45] Early development of aneurysm within 48 hours after infarction also diminishes survival.[29]

In general, the risk of thromboembolism is low for patients with aneurysms (0.35% per patient-year),[43] and long-term anticoagulation is not usually recommended. However, in the 50% of patients with mural thrombus visible by echocardiography after myocardial infarction, 19% develop thromboembolism over a mean follow-up of 24 months.[46] In these patients, anticoagulation and close echocardiographic follow-up may be indicated. Atrial fibrillation and large aneurysmal size are additional risk factors for thromboembolism.

The natural history of left ventricular pseudoaneurysm is not well documented. Frank rupture of chronic left ventricular pseudoaneurysms is less common than one might expect.[47] Rupture of left ventricular pseudoaneurysms may be most likely in the acute phase or in large sized pseudoaneurymsms.[48] Left ventricular pseudoaneurysms tend to behave similarly to true aneurysms in that they may present a volume load to the left ventricle or may be a source of embolization or endocarditis. Left ventricular pseudoaneurysms after prior cardiac surgery have also been reported to compress adjacent structures such as the pulmonary artery or esophagus.

CLINICAL PRESENTATION

Angina is the most frequent symptom in most series of operated patients with left ventricular aneurysm. Given that three-vessel coronary disease is present in 60% or more of these patients, the frequency of angina is not surprising.[49]

Dyspnea is the second most common symptom of ventricular aneurysm and often develops when 20% or more of the ventricular wall is infarcted. Dyspnea may occur from a combination of decreased systolic function and diastolic dysfunction.

Either atrial or ventricular arrhythmias may produce palpitations, syncope, or sudden death, or aggravate angina and dyspnea in up to one-third of patients.[49] Thromboembolism is unusual but may produce symptoms of stroke, myocardial infarction, or limb or visceral ischemia.

DIAGNOSIS

The electrocardiogram frequently demonstrates Q waves in the anterior leads along with persistent anterior ST-segment elevation (Fig. 30-3). The chest radiograph may show left ventricular enlargement and cardiomegaly (Fig. 30-4), but the chest radiograph is not usually specific for left ventricular aneurysm.

Left ventriculography is the gold standard for diagnosis of left ventricular aneurysm. The diagnosis is made by demonstrating a large, discrete area of dyskinesia (or akinesia), generally in the anteroseptal-apical walls. Occasionally, left ventriculography also may demonstrate mural thrombus. Quantitative definition of left ventricular aneurysms has been accomplished using a centerline analysis of left ventricular wall motion on left ventriculography in the 30 degree right anterior oblique view.[5] Hypocontractile segments contracting more than two standard deviations out of normal range have also been defined as aneurysmal (Fig. 30-5).[50] Outward motion is termed *dyskinetic*, and remaining aneurysmal segments are termed *akinetic*. The fraction of total left ventricular circumference that is aneurysmal can thus be computed as the value %A.[5]

Two-dimensional echocardiography is also a sensitive and specific means of diagnosing left ventricular aneurysm (Fig. 30-6). Echocardiography can detect mural thrombus or mitral valve regurgitation, and echocardiography can often distinguish false aneurysm from true aneurysm by demonstrating a defect in the true ventricular wall.

Magnetic resonance imaging (MRI) is the most reliable means of assessing left ventricular volume in the presence of left ventricular aneurysm.[51] Magnetic resonance imaging (MRI) can accurately define left ventricular aneurysms and can detect mural thrombus.[51] Yet, distinguishing true aneurysms from pseudoaneurysms remains difficult, even with magnetic resonance imaging.[52] Gated radionuclide angiography reliably detects left ventricular aneurysms, and thallium scanning or positron emission tomography (PET) can be helpful early after infarction to differentiate true aneurysm from hibernating myocardium with reversible dysfunction.

INDICATIONS FOR OPERATION

Because of the relatively good prognosis for asymptomatic left ventricular aneurysm,[2] no indications for repairing chronic, asymptomatic aneurysms are established. Yet, in low-risk patients during operation for associated coronary disease, investigators report repairing large, minimally symptomatic aneurysms.[10,53]

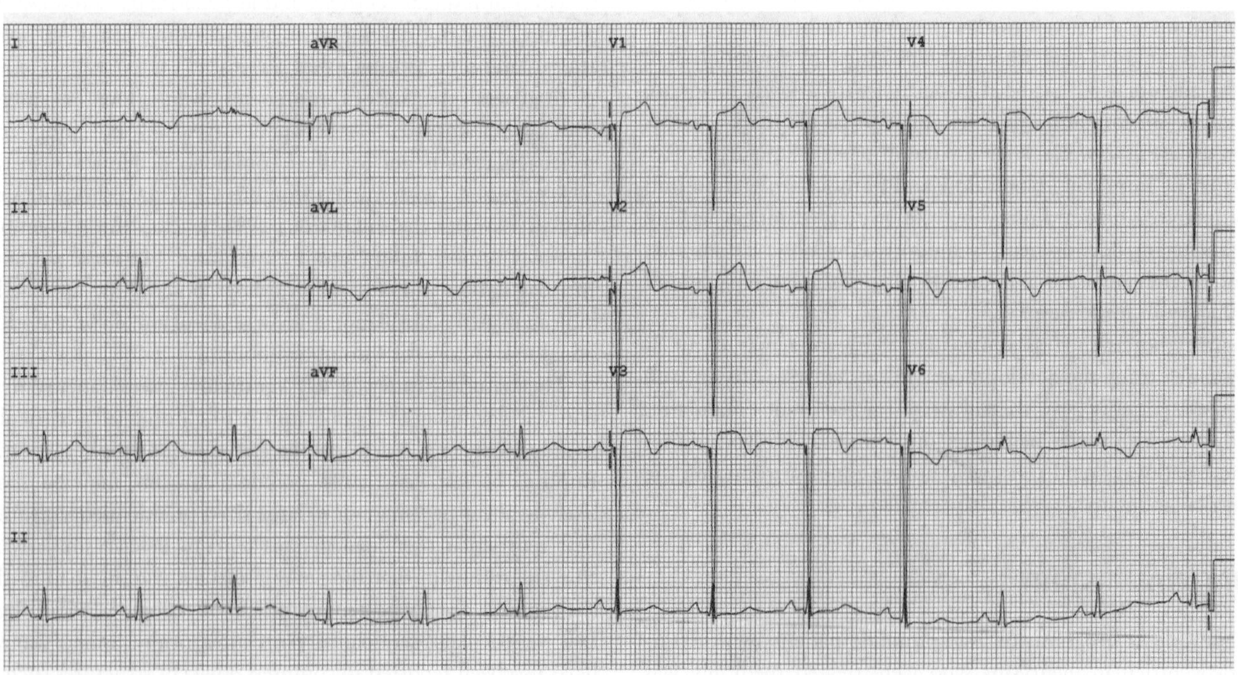

FIGURE 30-3 Electrocardiogram showing persistent ST-segment elevation with pathologic Q waves in a 72-year-old man with left ventricular aneurysm.

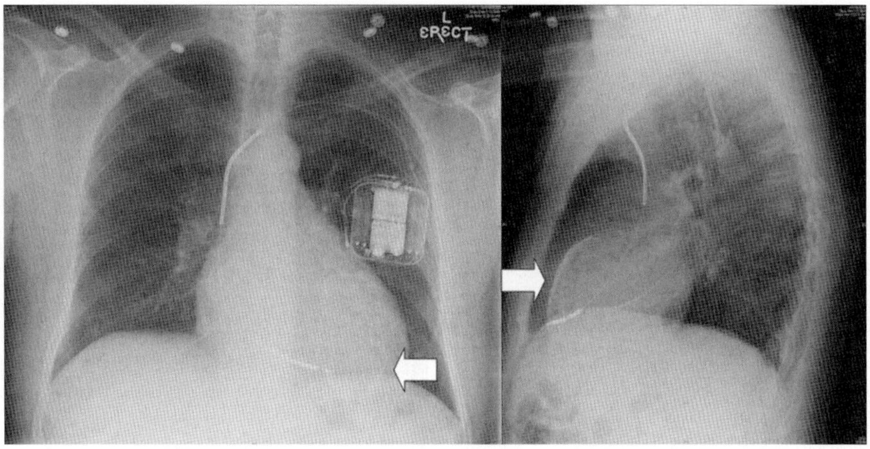

FIGURE 30-4 Posteroanterior and lateral chest radiograph in a patient with an anteroapical left ventricular aneurysm with calcification (*arrows*).

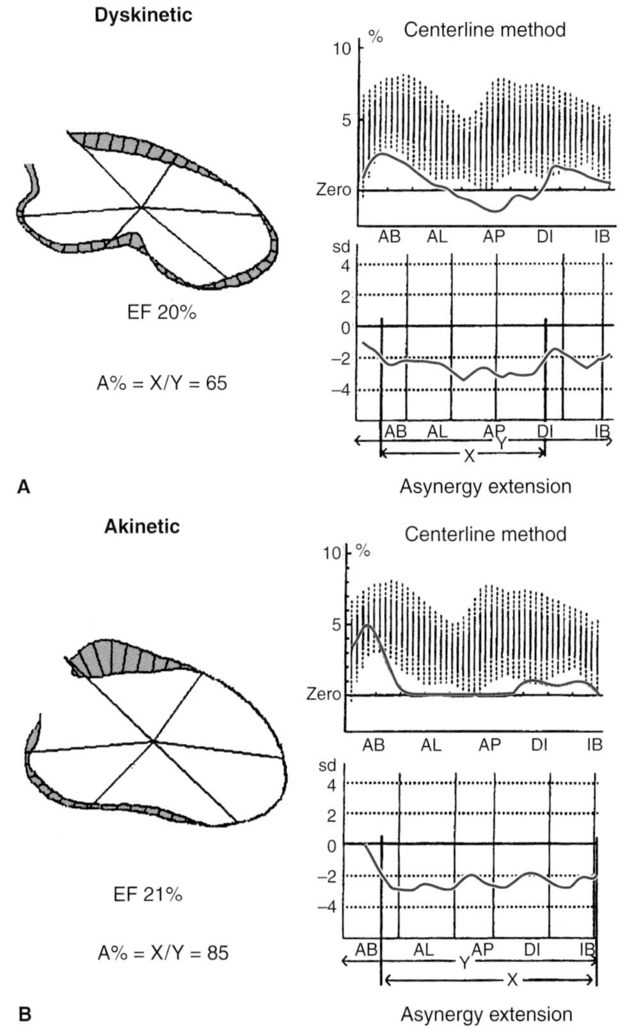

FIGURE 30-5 Examples of preoperative centerline analysis in dyskinetic (A) and akinetic (B) LV aneurysms. Vertical lines indicate the extent of asynergy. AB = anterobasal; AL = anterolateral; AP = apical; DI = diaphragmatic; EF = ejection fraction; IB = inferobasal. (*Reproduced with permission from Dor V, Sabatier M, DiDonato M: Efficacy of endoventricular patch plasty in large postinfarction akinetic scar and severe left ventricular dysfunction: comparison with a series of large dyskinetic scars. J Thorac Cardiovasc Surg 1998; 116:50.*)

On the other hand, operation is indicated for symptoms of angina, congestive heart failure, or selected ventricular arrhythmias (see Chapter 57) (Table 30-2). For these symptomatic patients, operation offers better outcome than medical therapy.

To be worthy of operation, a dyskinetic or akinetic left ventricular aneurysm should significantly enlarge left ventricular end-systolic volume index (>80 mL/m^2) and end-diastolic volume (>120 mL/m^2). These volume criteria are, however, poorly defined and limited by technical difficulty measuring left ventricular volume in aneurysmal left ventricles. Because of data suggesting that akinetic versus dyskinetic aneurysms have similar results, Dor and others feel that dyskinesia is not a prerequisite for aneurysm repair.[4,5] Nonetheless, the only randomized trial (the STICH trial) has suggested that little benefit is obtained in terms of survival or symptoms in patients who on average have smaller, akinetic aneurysmal segments (end-systolic volume index 82 mL/m^2 and 50 to 56% of anterior wall involved).[7]

Operation is indicated in viable patients with contained cardiac rupture, with or without development of a false aneurysm. Because left ventricular pseudoaneurysms may have a tendency to rupture when acute or of larger size (either with or without symptoms), operation is indicated.[47,48,54] Similarly, congenital aneurysms have a presumed risk of rupture and should undergo repair independently of symptoms. Rarely, embolism is an indication for operation in medically treated patients at high risk for repeated thromboembolism. The role of operation in asymptomatic patients with very large aneurysms or documented expansion of aneurysms is uncertain.

Relative contraindications to operation for left ventricular aneurysm include excessive anesthetic risk, impaired function of residual myocardium outside the aneurysm, resting cardiac index less than 2.0 L/min/m^2, significant mitral regurgitation, evidence of nontransmural infarction (hibernating myocardium), and lack of a discrete, thin-walled aneurysm with distinct margins. Global ejection fraction may be less useful than ejection fraction of the basal, contractile portion of the heart in determining operability.[55]

Angioplasty has an uncertain role in the treatment of left ventricular aneurysms but may be indicated in patients with

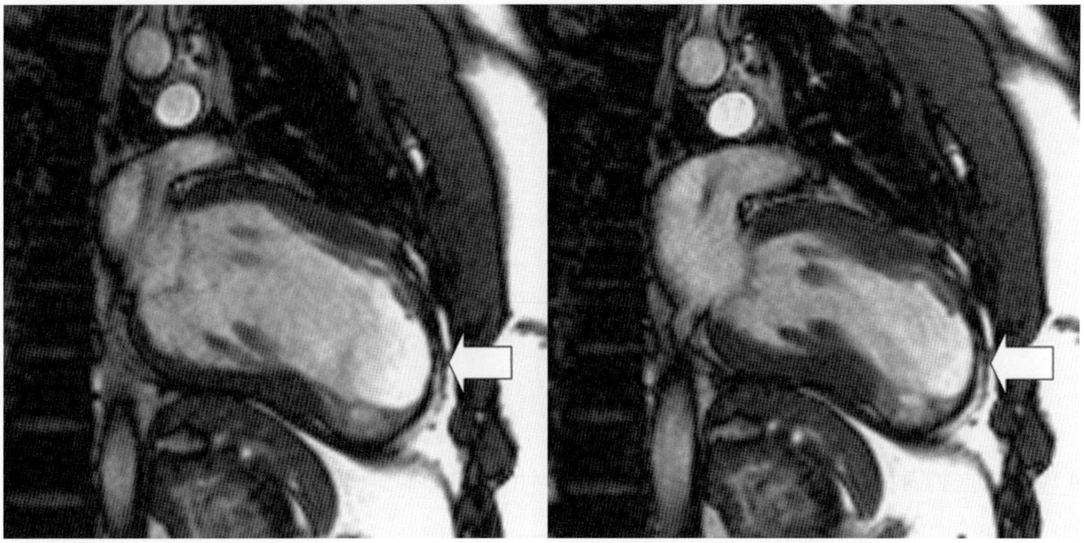

FIGURE 30-6 Magnetic resonance images of an apical left ventricular aneurysm during diastole (*left panel*) and systole (*right panel*).

suitable coronary anatomy, one- or two-vessel disease, a contraindication for operation, or asymptomatic status with inducible ischemia.

PREPARATION FOR OPERATION

All patients being considered for operation should undergo right- and left-sided heart catheterization with coronary arteriography and left ventriculography. Patients with at least 2+ mitral regurgitation at cardiac catheterization should have echocardiography to assess the mitral valve and to look for intrinsic mitral valve disease not amenable to annuloplasty. Magnetic resonance imaging can be helpful to assess left ventricular volumes and aid in planning the size and extent of left ventricular reconstruction.[51]

Preoperative electrophysiologic study is clearly indicated in any patient with preoperative ventricular tachycardia or ventricular fibrillation. The decision to perform an electrophysiologic study in patients without preoperative ventricular arrhythmias is controversial, because the incidence of postoperative ventricular arrhythmias is low and not changed by endocardial resection at the time of operation.[10] Electrophysiologic study is frequently not helpful in patients with polymorphic ventricular tachycardia occurring within 6 weeks of myocardial infarction.[10]

TABLE 30-2 Relative Indications for Ventricular Aneurysm Operation

Documented expansion/large size
Angina
Congestive heart failure
Arrhythmia
Rupture
Pseudoaneurysm
Congenital aneurysm
Embolism
Documented expansion/large size

OPERATIVE TECHNIQUES

General Operation

Operation for left ventricular aneurysm (aneurysmectomy, aneurysmorrhaphy, ventricular restoration) requires cardiopulmonary bypass and a balanced anesthetic technique, as generally used for coronary bypass grafting. After induction of anesthesia and endotracheal intubation, an electrocardiogram monitor, a Foley catheter, a radial arterial line, and a Swan-Ganz catheter are placed. A median sternotomy is performed, and the patient is given heparin. Saphenous vein or arterial conduits are prepared.

Cardiopulmonary bypass is begun after cannulating the ascending aorta. A single, two-stage cannula is generally adequate to cannulate the right atrium, but dual venous cannulation should be considered if the right ventricle is to be opened. Epicardial mapping is performed if necessary. The left ventricle is inspected to identify an appropriate area of thinned ventricular wall. A linear vertical ventriculotomy, generally on the anterior wall 3 to 4 cm from the left anterior descending coronary artery, is made (Fig. 30-7). The left ventricle is opened (Fig. 30-8), all mural thrombus is carefully removed, and endocardial mapping is performed if necessary. A left ventricular vent is now placed through the right superior pulmonary vein–left atrial junction after mural thrombus is removed. Coronary arteries to be grafted are identified. Endocardial scar, if present, is resected, and afterwards, endocardial mapping is repeated. Body temperature is maintained at 37°C until intraoperative mapping is completed; thereafter, temperature is decreased to 28 to 32°C.

The ascending aorta is clamped, and the heart is arrested with cold anterograde and/or retrograde cardioplegic solution.

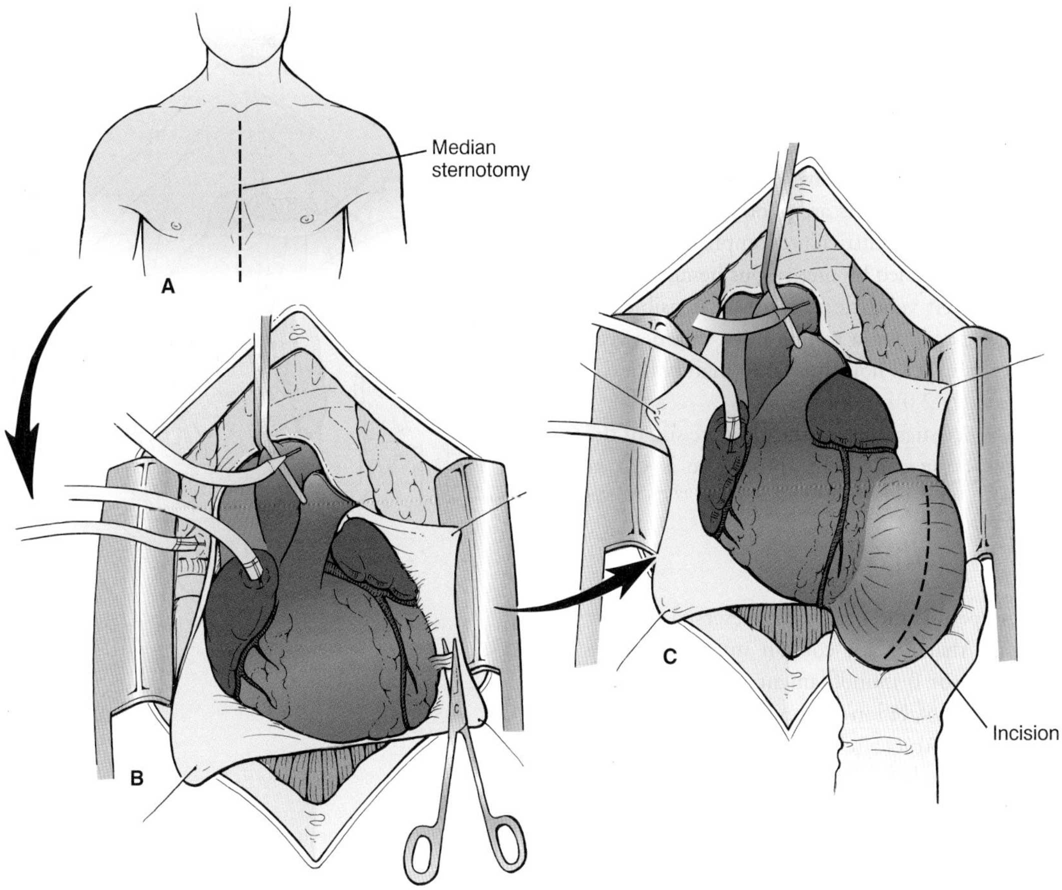

FIGURE 30-7 Technique of exposure for left ventricular aneurysm repair through a median sternotomy. The ascending aorta and right atrium are cannulated. A left ventricular vent is placed through the right superior pulmonary vein. Pericardial adhesions are divided, and the aneurysm is opened.

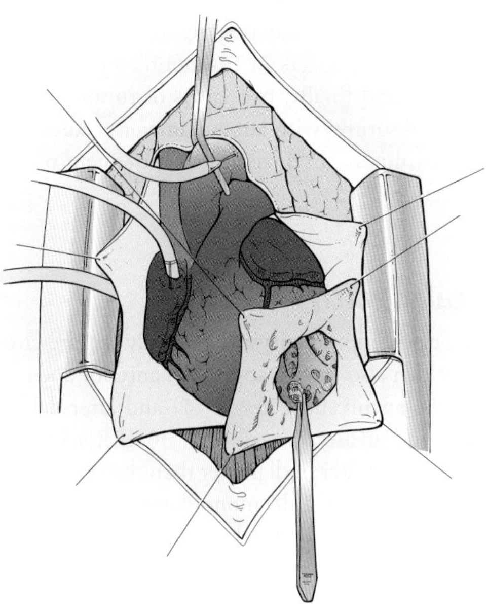

FIGURE 30-8 With the aneurysm wall opened, thrombus is removed, without injury to the papillary muscles.

Alternatively, the aorta is not clamped and the entire procedure is done during hypothermic fibrillation. The left ventricular aneurysm is repaired using one of the techniques described below. The distal coronary anastomoses are performed, followed by releasing the aortic clamp.[56] Air is removed by venting the ascending aorta and left ventricle while filling the heart and ventilating the lungs with the patient in the Trendelenberg position. The patient is rewarmed, and proximal coronary anastomoses are performed. Once normothermia is achieved, an electrophysiologic study may be repeated if indicated. Temporary pacing wires are placed on the right atrium and right ventricle, cardiopulmonary bypass is discontinued, and heparin is reversed. The heart is decannulated, and the median sternotomy is closed with mediastinal drains after hemostasis is achieved.

Weaning from cardiopulmonary bypass frequently requires some degree of inotropic support. Typically 5 μg/kg/min of dopamine, nitroglycerin to prevent coronary spasm, and nitroprusside for afterload reduction are used. An intraaortic balloon pump may be needed in patients with borderline ventricular function. Transesophageal echocardiography is useful for assessing left ventricular function and to detect residual intracardiac air.

Additional inotropic support may not increase cardiac output significantly because of abnormal ventricular compliance and may produce arrhythmias and poorly tolerated tachycardia. Hypokalemia and hypomagnesemia are corrected immediately to minimize arrhythmias. Intraoperative and postoperative ventricular ectopy is treated aggressively with intravenous lidocaine. Intravascular volume shifts are poorly tolerated in these patients because of poor ventricular compliance; therefore, rapid transfusions are avoided by meticulous hemostasis before closing. Because the left ventricle is poorly distensible, stroke volume is relatively fixed, and a resting heart rate between 90 and 115 beats per minute is not unusual to maintain a cardiac index of approximately 2.0 L/min/m^2.

Growing experience suggests that the ultimate size of the left ventricular cavity at the end of the procedure is critical to patient outcome.

Plication

Plication without opening the aneurysm is reserved for only the smallest aneurysms that do not contain mural thrombus. A two-layer suture line of 0 monofilament is placed across the aneurysm using a strip of Teflon felt on either side. The suture line is oriented to reconstruct a relatively normal left ventricular contour and does not exclude all aneurysmal tissue.

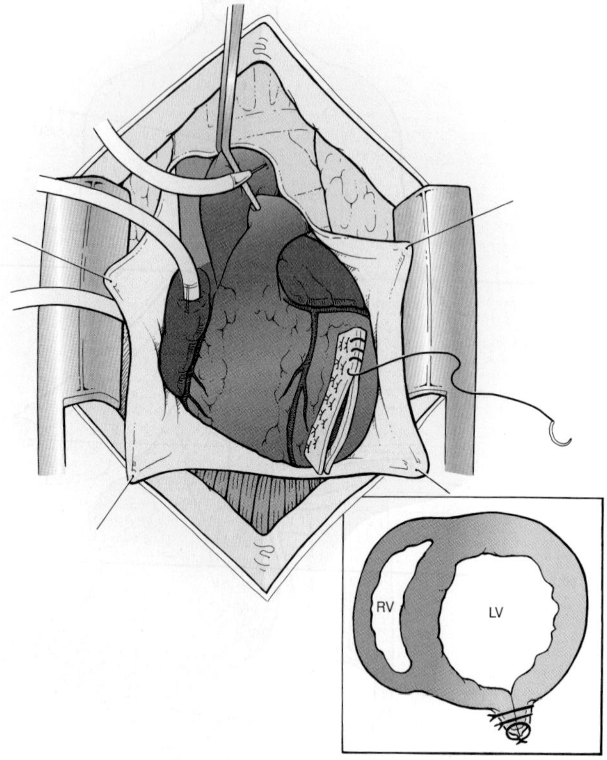

FIGURE 30-10 Linear repair. The aneurysm walls are closed in a vertical line between two layers of Teflon felt. Two layers of 0 monofilament interrupted horizontal mattress sutures are reinforced with two layers of running 2-0 monofilament sutures.

Linear Closure

After removing all mural thrombus, the aneurysmal wall is trimmed, leaving a 3-cm rim of scar to allow reconstruction of the normal left ventricular contour (Fig. 30-9). Care is taken not to resect too much aneurysmal wall and overly reduce ventricular cavity size. A monofilament 2-0 suture may be used to reduce the neck of the aneurysm to the proper size before closure of the ventricular wall.[17] Anterior aneurysm defects are closed vertically between two external 1.5-cm strips of Teflon felt, two layers of 0 monofilament horizontal mattress sutures, and finally, two layers of running 2-0 monofilament vertical sutures with large-diameter needles (Fig. 30-10). Similar techniques can be used in less frequent posterior aneurysm resections.[57]

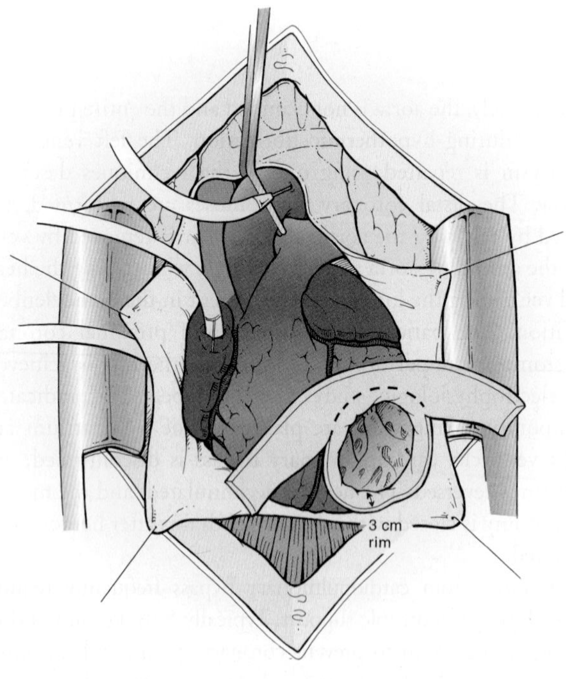

FIGURE 30-9 Linear repair. The fibrous aneurysm wall is excised, leaving a 3-cm rim of fibrous aneurysm wall attached to healthy muscle.

Circular Patch

Inferior or posterior aneurysms generally require circular patch closure, which also can be applied to anterior aneurysms. After opening the aneurysm (Fig. 30-11) and after debridement of thrombus and aneurysm wall (Fig. 30-12), a Dacron patch is cut to be 2 cm greater in diameter than the ventricular opening. Interrupted, pledgeted 0 monofilament horizontal mattress sutures are placed through the ventriculotomy rim and then through the patch, leaving the pledgets outside the ventricular cavity (Fig. 30-13). Sutures are tied, and additional interrupted sutures or a second layer of running 2-0 monofilament is placed for hemostasis.

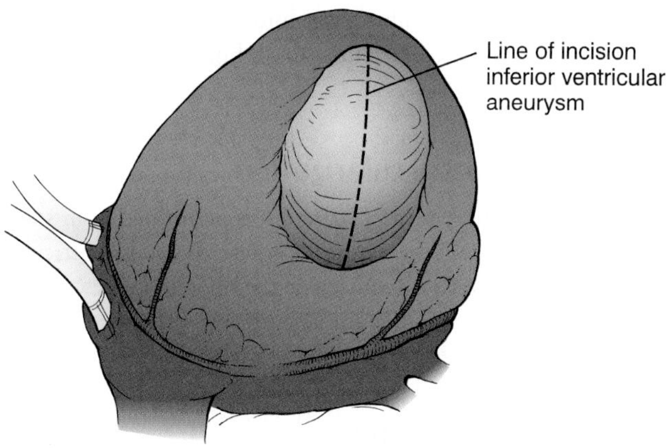

FIGURE 30-11 Circular patch repair. The aneurysm wall is incised. An inferior aneurysm is shown.

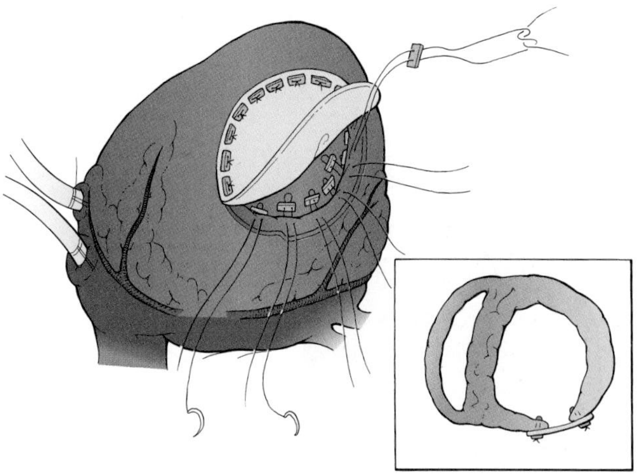

FIGURE 30-13 Circular patch repair. The aneurysmal defect is closed with a Dacron patch using interrupted 2-0 monofilament horizontal mattress sutures with reinforcing pledgets.

Endoventricular Patch

The endoventricular patch technique is suitable for anterior aneurysms but is less suited for inferior or posterior aneurysms, for which the standard (circular) patch technique is used. After debridement of thrombus, a running 2-0 polypropylene suture may be placed at the aneurysm rim to optimize left ventricular size.[4,17,50,55] Optimizing patch size and residual left ventricular cavity size can be facilitated with plastic or balloon forms (Chase Medical, Richardson, Texas) chosen to leave a left ventricular end-diastolic volume index of 50 to 60 mL/m^2.[58] If the remaining ventricular defect is small (<3 cm), then the ventricular wall may be closed linearly.[17] More commonly, a patch (bovine pericardium, Dacron cloth, or polytetrafluoroethylene) is cut to size sufficient to restore normal ventricular size and geometry when secured to the aneurysmal rim (Fig. 30-14). The patch is sutured to normal muscle at the aneurysmal circumference using a running 3-0 polypropylene suture that is secured with single sutures at three or four places around the patch circumference. The patch may extend onto the interventricular septum,[4,50,55] or aneurysmal septum may be plicated.[17] Interrupted 3-0 sutures are placed as needed to ensure good fit. Care is taken not to distort the papillary muscles. The aneurysmal rim is trimmed to allow primary closure of the native

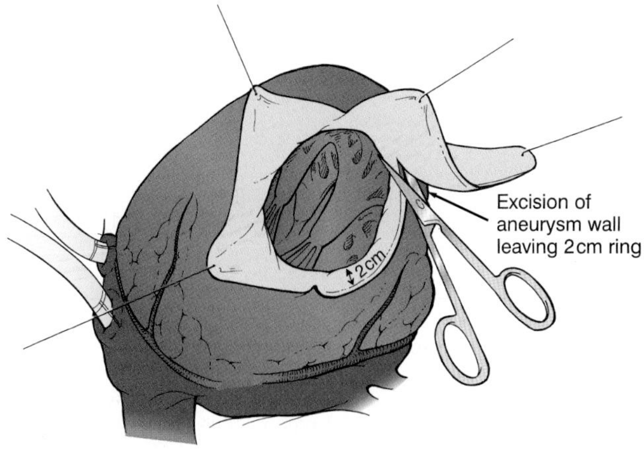

FIGURE 30-12 Circular patch repair. The aneurysmal wall is excised, leaving a 2-cm rim of fibrous aneurysmal wall attached to healthy muscle.

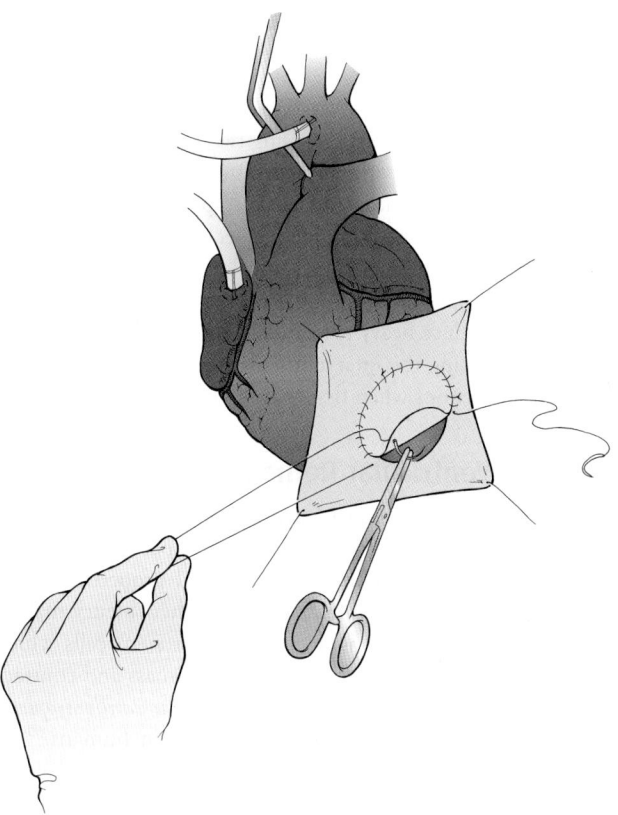

FIGURE 30-14 Endocardial patch. Without excising the aneurysm wall, the ventricular defect is closed with a Teflon felt patch using 3-0 polypropylene suture secured at three or four points along the suture line. Additional 3-0 pledgeted horizontal mattress sutures may be used to achieve hemostasis.

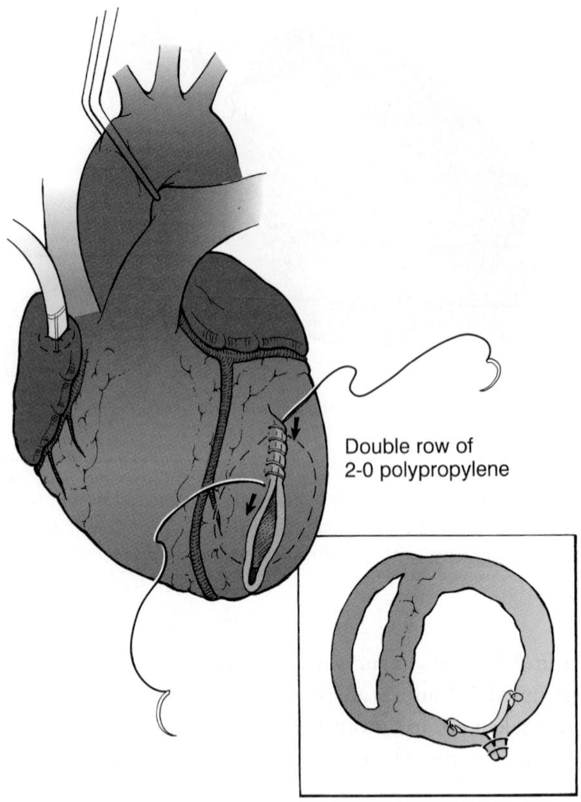

FIGURE 30-15 Endocardial patch. The aneurysm wall is closed over a Teflon patch after resecting excess aneurysm tissue. A double row of running vertical 2-0 polypropylene suture is used.

aneurysmal wall over the patch using two layers of running 2-0 monofilament suture without pledgets (Fig. 30-15).

Compared with linear and circular patch techniques, the endoventricular patch technique has technical advantages. An endoventricular patch preserves the left anterior descending artery for possible grafting and leaves no external prosthetic material to produce heavy pericardial adhesions. The technique facilitates patching the interventricular septum, and is suitable for acute infarctions when tissues are friable.[10,19,58,59]

Other Ventricular Remodeling Techniques

In addition to the techniques listed above where left ventricular infarct tissue is excised and/or replaced with patch material, an alternative would be to alter the biological properties of the infarct scar. Remaining infarct scar (whether aneurysmal or not) can then be seeded with myoblasts or stem cells which offer the potential to restore cardiac muscle mass and contraction. This technique has been termed *cellular cardiomyoplasty* and has been done only on a limited basis in humans.[60] In animals, cellular cardiomyoplasty has successfully improved global left ventricular performance and geometry using either myoblasts, stem cells that differentiate into myocytes, fibrocytes, or cells seeded onto a graft matrix.[61–63] Cellular cardiomyoplasty could be done by direct injection of cells at the time of coronary revascularization, or even by transcoronary or intramyocardial injection in the cardiac catheterization laboratory. Percutaneous insertion of a parachute-like device into the left ventricular apex has had some early success in humans in Europe (Cardiokinetix, Redwood City, CA).

Coronary Revascularization

Concurrent coronary revascularization is performed as in standard coronary bypass procedures. Because the endoventricular patch technique does not encroach on the left anterior descending coronary, the left internal mammary artery may be used to graft the left anterior descending coronary artery.

Mitral Regurgitation

The severity of mitral regurgitation should be evaluated before cardiopulmonary bypass by intraoperative transesophageal echocardiography. The need for concurrent mitral valve operation increases as the preoperative ejection fraction decreases (Fig 30-16).[64] The mitral valve is also inspected from below after opening the aneurysm and beginning repair of the aneurysm. Transventricular mitral valve repair may be done by placing pledgeted polypropylene sutures at both mitral commissures to reduce the circumference of the annulus.[57] This technique produces satisfactory short-term results, but long-term results are not known. Usually the mitral valve is repaired via left atriotomy after completion of the distal coronary anastomoses and before releasing the aortic cross-clamp. If mitral regurgitation results from annular dilatation and systolic restriction of leaflet motion (Carpentier type IIIB), an undersized, complete, rigid mitral annuloplasty is generally done.[65]

Cardiac Transplantation

In symptomatic patients with sufficient depression of global left ventricular function to preclude aneurysm repair, transplantation is a reasonable alternative and may have survival and

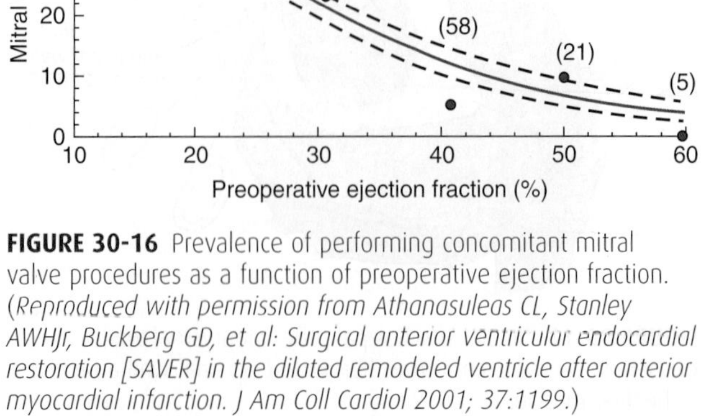

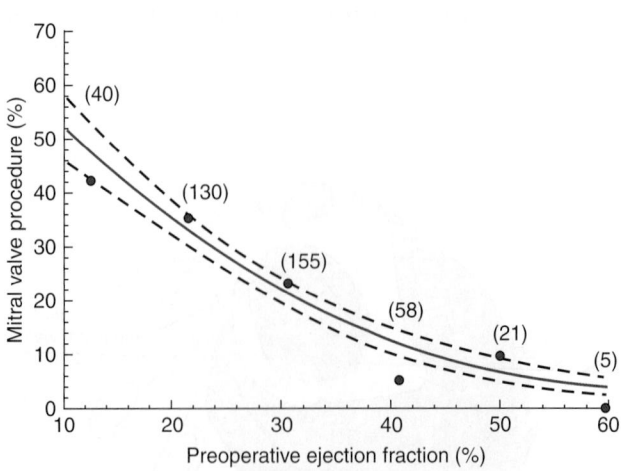

FIGURE 30-16 Prevalence of performing concomitant mitral valve procedures as a function of preoperative ejection fraction. (*Reproduced with permission from Athanasuleas CL, Stanley AWHJr, Buckberg GD, et al: Surgical anterior ventricular endocardial restoration [SAVER] in the dilated remodeled ventricle after anterior myocardial infarction. J Am Coll Cardiol 2001; 37:1199.*)

symptomatic benefit similar to ventricular aneurysm repair at a higher dollar cost.[66]

Ventricular False Aneurysm

Ventricular false aneurysms are repaired with the same techniques used for true ventricular aneurysms based according to the location and size of the aneurysm. The circular patch technique is particularly useful in that inferior false aneurysms are common and typically have narrow necks. Usually the wall of the false aneurysm is inadequate to close over the defect.

Ventricular Rupture

Any of the techniques described above may be used to manage a contained ventricular rupture. Because infarcted tissue is particularly friable 5 to 10 days after rupture, closure may be difficult. The endoventricular technique is particularly well suited for this uncommon operation because the patch can be sewn to the margins of healthy endocardium, which may be at some distance from the site of rupture. Patient survival also has been reported by gluing a biologic patch to the ventricular epicardium over the site of the rupture.

EARLY RESULTS

Hospital Mortality

In a compilation of 3439 operations for left ventricular aneurysm between 1972 and 1987[21] and in a series of 731 ventricular restoration patients from 2002 to 2004,[67] hospital mortality was 9.9 and 9.3% respectively and ranged from 2 to 19%. More recent reports suggest that hospital mortality can be as low as 3 to 7% using either patch[10,19,64,68,69] or linear closures.[22,53,69] The most common cause of hospital mortality is left ventricular failure, which occurs in 64% of deaths.[53]

Risk factors for hospital mortality include increased age,[21,53,64,67,69] incomplete revascularization,[53] increased heart failure class,[21,67,69–71] female gender,[21,67] emergent operation,[21] ejection fraction less than 20 to 30%,[64,69,70] concurrent mitral valve replacement,[10,21,64,67] preoperative cardiac index < 2.1 L/min/m^2,[5,67] mean pulmonary artery pressure >33 mmHg,[5] serum creatinine >1.8 mg/dl,[5] and failure to use the internal mammary artery.[71]

In-Hospital Complications

The most common in-hospital complications are shown in Table 30-3 and include low cardiac output, ventricular arrhythmias, and respiratory failure.[21,22,68,67,69,72] Low cardiac output may be more common in patients undergoing intraoperative mapping because of perioperative cardiac injury.[73]

Left Ventricular Function

The preponderance of data from the last two decades have shown that left ventricular function improves in most patients undergoing operation for left ventricular aneurysm. Operation improves ejection fraction whether linear repair[6,11,74–76] or

TABLE 30-3 In-Hospital Complications of Ventricular Aneurysm Repair

Low cardiac output 22–39%
Ventricular arrhythmias 9–19%
Respiratory failure 4–21%
Bleeding 4–7%
Dialysis-dependent renal failure 4%
Stroke 3–4%

patch repair[16,19,64,77–80] is used (Fig. 30-17). Both techniques decrease end-diastolic and end-systolic volumes[64,75,78,80] and improve exercise response[19,76] (Fig. 30-18). Aneurysmal repair in general may improve diastolic filling, left ventricular diastolic compliance, left ventricular contractility, effective arterial elastance (Ea), and left ventricular efficiency.[35,79–82] However, recent studies have suggested little improvement or even worsening of left ventricular diastolic compliance, particularly in patients with large resections or small ventricular size or without large dyskinetic aneurysms preoperatively.[83]

Controversy remains strong regarding whether patch techniques provide results superior to those achieved with linear closures. Stoney et al.[14,84] noted lower left ventricular end-diastolic pressure when more geometric reconstructions were performed. Hutchins and Brawley[85] first noted at autopsy that some patients had severe reduction and distortion of ventricular volume after linear repair. The authors proposed that a more geometric repair might avert these problems. Although no prospective studies compare results from the two procedures, several very experienced groups attribute improved symptoms, less low cardiac output, and greater improvement in ejection fraction to a switch to patch techniques.[10,19,86] In other retrospective

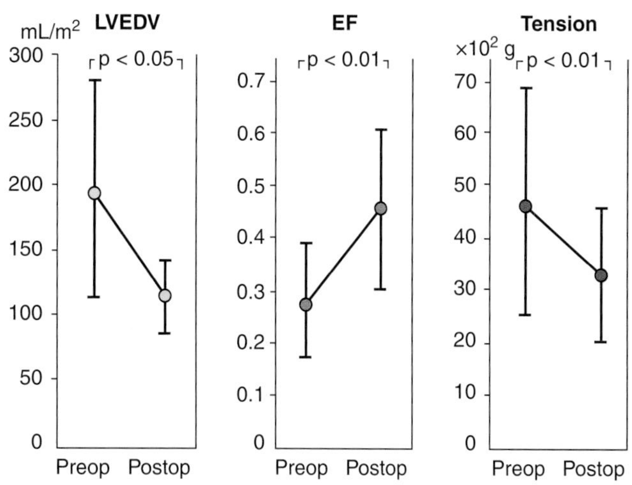

FIGURE 30-17 Effects of linear aneurysmectomy on left ventricular end-diastolic volume (LVEDV), ejection fraction (EF), and wall tension. *(Reproduced with permission from Kawachi K, Kitamura S, Kawata T, et al: Hemodynamic assessment during exercise after left ventricular aneurysmectomy. J Thorac Cardiovasc Surg 1994; 107:178.)*

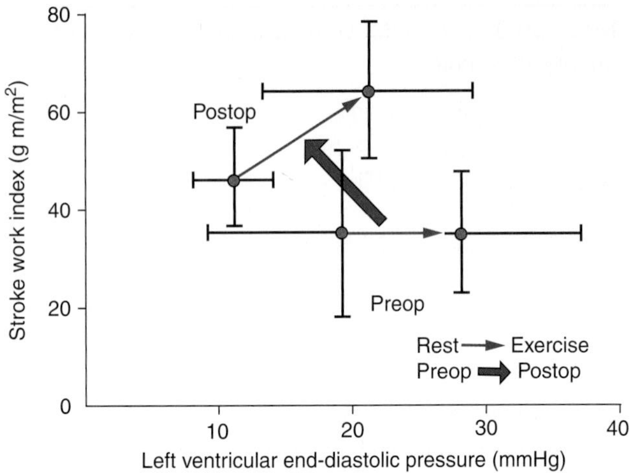

FIGURE 30-18 Relationship between stroke work index and left ventricular end-diastolic pressure. Data are shown at rest and during exercise before (preop) and after (postop) linear aneurysmectomy. Stroke work index increased only with exercise postoperatively. (*Reproduced with permission from Kawachi K, Kitamura S, Kawata T, et al: Hemodynamic assessment during exercise after left ventricular aneurysmectomy. J Thorac Cardiovasc Surg 1994; 107:178.*)

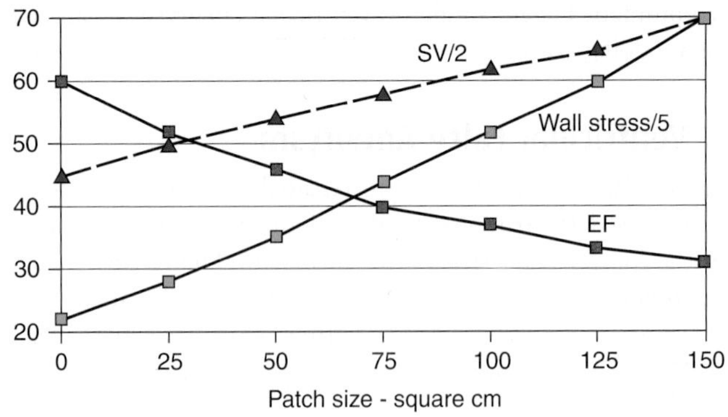

FIGURE 30-19 Computer prediction of the effects of patch size on stroke volume (SV), ejection fraction (EF), and wall stress (afterload) at a chamber pressure of 100 mm Hg. Predictions are based on data from an animal model of simulated aneurysm repair, neglecting the effects of afterload on stroke volume. Because increasing afterload in reality decreases muscle shortening, patch reconstruction can increase stroke volume only if contractile reserve is sufficient to overcome the afterload from increased ventricular size. (*Based on Nicolosi AC, Weng ZC, Detwiler PW, et al: Simulated left ventricular aneurysm and aneurysm repair in swine. J Thorac Cardiovasc Surg 1990; 100:745.*)

comparisons, no differences were seen in postoperative symptoms, ejection fraction, echocardiographic ventricular dimensions, or late survival between linear and patch repairs.[75,86–89] In an animal model of simulated aneurysm repair, Nicolosi et al.[83] found no difference in left ventricular systolic or diastolic function between linear and patch techniques. Two groups reported that switch to patch techniques was associated with increased operative mortality, perhaps because of excessive volume reduction, [90,91] whereas other groups found improved survival when switching from linear to patch techniques.[92] One meta-analysis has suggested that the better results with patch techniques are the result of more experience in more recent series.[86]

The durability of functional benefit from aneurysm repair remains poorly documented. In animals and humans, there is a tendency for the initial improvement in ejection fraction, ventricular volume, and filling pressures to diminish over the next 6 weeks to 12 months,[93,94] especially in patients with residual mitral regurgitation.

Although technical differences exist between patch and linear repairs, good functional results are possible with either technique. Suboptimal outcomes result from either technique when left ventricular cavitary volume is overly reduced with resultant decreased stroke volume and impaired diastolic filling.[85,94] Excessively small patches reduce stroke volume and impair diastolic filling, but excessively large patches reduce ejection fraction and increase wall stress (Fig. 30-19).

LATE RESULTS

Survival

Survival after operation for left ventricular aneurysm is variable, largely because of differences between patient populations. Five-year survival in recent series varies between 58 and 80%,[6,70] 10-year overall survival is 34%,[70] and 10-year cardiac survival is 57%[53] (Fig. 30-20). Cardiac causes are responsible for 57% of late deaths,[73] and most cardiac deaths result from new myocardial infarctions. In aneurysm patients randomized to medical or surgical therapy in the CASS study (most of the patients had minimal symptoms), survival was not different between medical or surgical therapy, except for patients with three-vessel disease.[45] These patients had better survival with surgery (Fig. 30-21).

Preoperative risk factors for late death include age, heart failure score, ejection fraction less than 35%, cardiomegaly on chest radiograph, left ventricular end-diastolic pressure greater than 20 mm Hg, and mitral regurgitation[45,53,73] (Fig. 30-22, Fig. 30-23).

The prospective, randomized STICH trial of 1000 patients with ejection fraction of 35% or less and anatomy amenable to ventricular restoration showed that, on average, left ventricular restoration techniques did not affect survival relative to coronary bypass grafting alone (see Fig 30-20).[7] The failure to see benefit in the STICH trial probably resulted from inclusion of relatively few patients with large, classical, dyskinetic aneurysms (mean reduction of end-systolic volume index of 16 mL/m^2 versus 48 mL/m^2 seen in classical aneurysms).[7,8] Although unproven, the net sum of evidence suggests that patients with large, classical, dyskinetic aneurysms probably obtain more benefit from aneurysm repair than do patients with diffuse ventricular dysfunction or small akinetic segments.[8]

SYMPTOMATIC IMPROVEMENT

Studies consistently demonstrate improvement in symptoms after operation relative to preoperative symptoms[6,74] (Fig. 30-24). In the study of Elefteriades et al.,[74] using a linear repair, mean angina class improved from 3.5 to 1.2 and mean CHF class

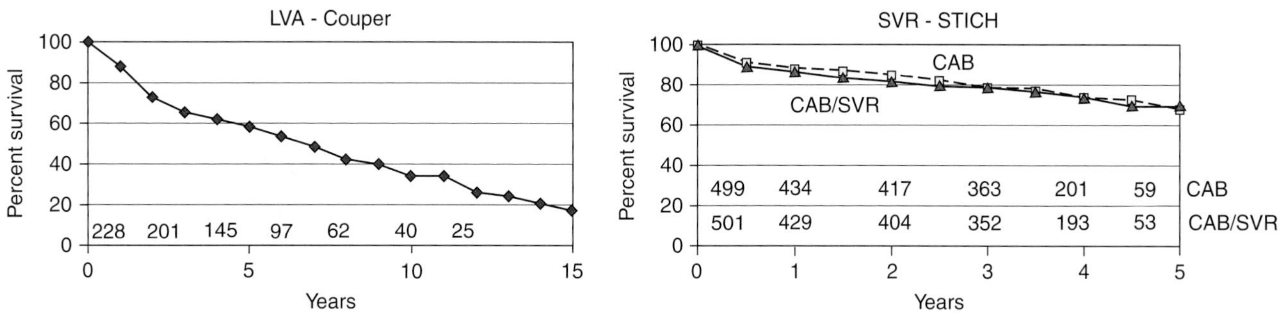

FIGURE 30-20 Survival in 303 patients undergoing left ventricular aneurysmectomy (LVA)(left panel). (*Based on Couper GS, Bunton RW, Birjiniuk V, et al: Relative risks of left ventricular aneurysmectomy in patients with akinetic scars versus true dyskinetic aneurysms. Circulation 1990; 82[Suppl IV]:248.*). Survival in 1000 patients randomized to coronary bypass (CAB) or CAB and ventricular restoration (SVR)(*right panel*). (*Based on Jones RH, Velazquez EJ, Michler RE, et al: Coronary bypass surgery with or without surgical ventricular restoration. NEJM 2009; 360:1705*).

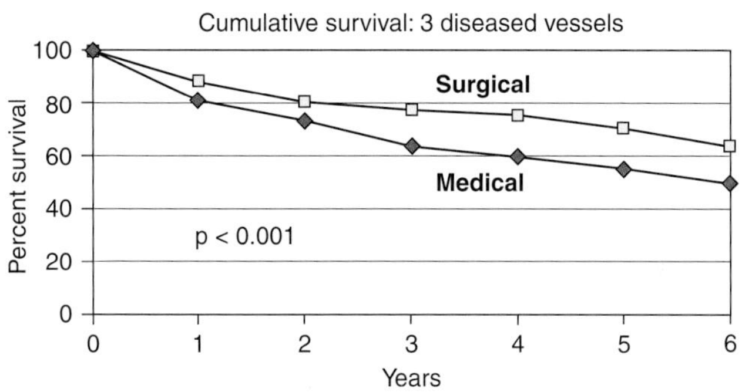

FIGURE 30-21 Survival in patients with left ventricular aneurysm and three-vessel coronary disease treated with medical or surgical therapy. (*Based on Faxon DP, Myers WO, McCabe CH: The influence of surgery on the natural history of angiographically documented left ventricular aneurysm: the Coronary Artery Surgery Study. Circulation 1986; 74:110.*)

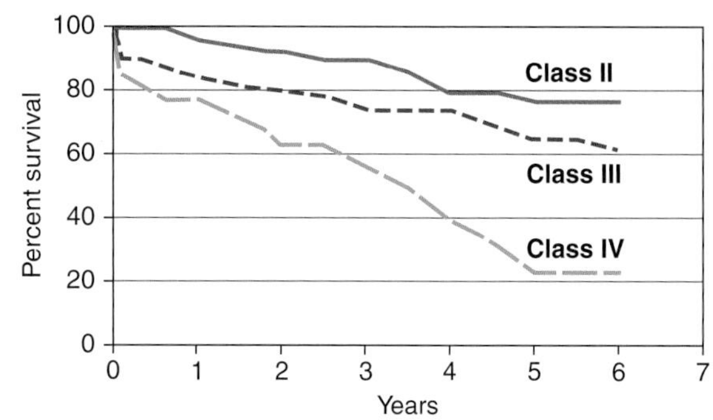

FIGURE 30-22 Effects of preoperative NYHA functional class on survival after ventricular aneurysm repair and myocardial revascularization. (*Based on Vauthy JN, Berry DW, Snyder DW, et al: Left ventricular aneurysm repair with myocardial revascularization: an analysis of 246 consecutive patients over 15 years. Ann Thorac Surg 1988; 46:29.*)

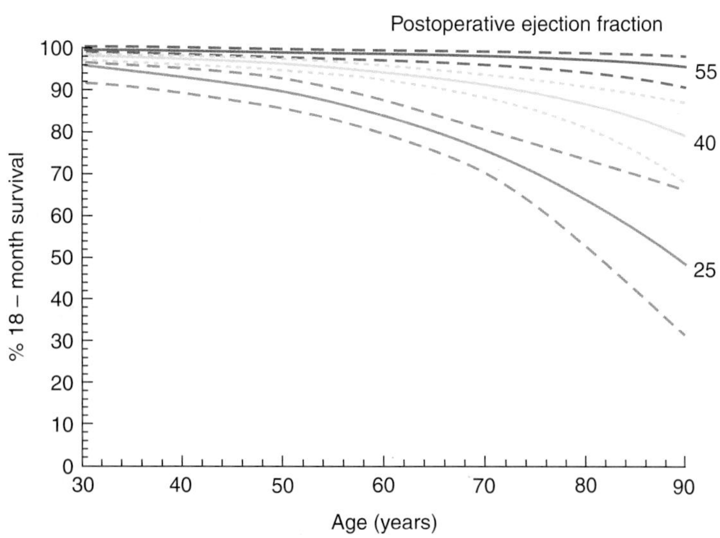

FIGURE 30-23 Nomogram of 18-month survival after ventricular restoration as a function of patient age and postoperative ejection fraction. (*Reproduced with permission from Athanasuleas CL, Stanley AWH Jr, Buckberg GD, et al: Surgical anterior ventricular endocardial restoration [SAVER] in the dilated remodeled ventricle after anterior myocardial infarction. J Am Coll Cardiol 2001; 37:1199.*)

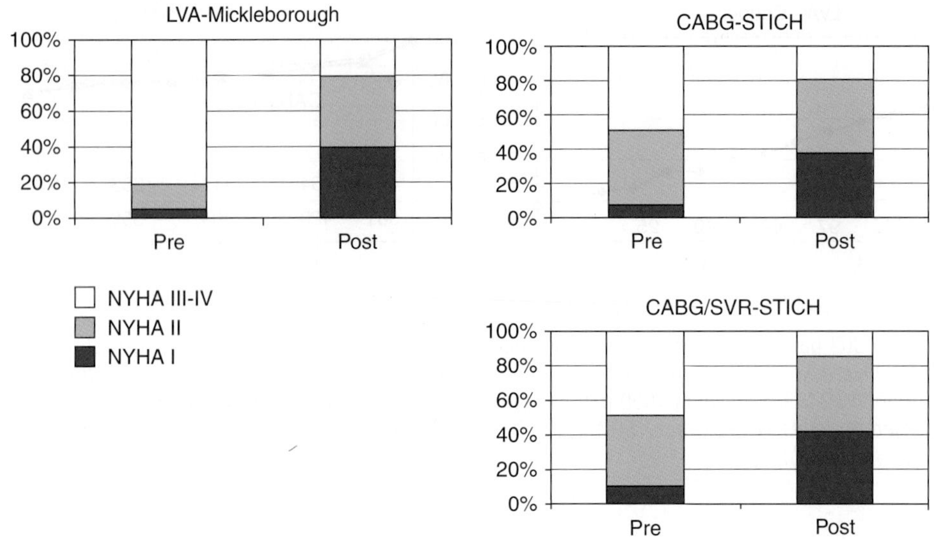

FIGURE 30-24 Preoperative (PRE) and latest follow-up (POST) symptoms of congestive heart failure (NYHA class) in patients undergoing coronary bypass alone (CABG) or CABG plus ventricular restoration (CABG/SVR) in the randomized STICH trial ($p = 0.7$ CABG versus CABG/SVR) (*Based on Jones RH, Velazquez EJ, Michler RE, et al: Coronary bypass surgery with or without surgical ventricular restoration. NEJM 2009; 360:1705.*)

improved from 3.0 to 1.7. In the randomized CASS study, the subset of patients with left ventricular aneurysm achieved a better heart failure class with surgical therapy than with medicine, and rehospitalization for heart failure was less common for the surgical therapy group than for the medicine group.[45] At 18 months, 85% of patients are free of rehospitalization for congestive heart failure, with rehospitalization peaking at 2 to 4 months.[64] Prucz found in a small, nonrandomized case-control study that ventricular restoration reduced hospitalization rate relative to coronary bypass alone.[95] However, the STICH trial found no benefit on average in symptoms or quality of life relative to coronary bypass alone.[7,96] (Fig 30-24) The STICH trial found that ventricular restoration significantly increased hospital cost by $14,500 or 26%.[96]

REFERENCES

1. Rutherford JD, Braunwald E, Cohn PE: Chronic ischemic heart disease, in Braunwald E (ed): *Heart Disease: A Textbook of Cardiovascular Medicine.* Philadelphia, Saunders, 1988; p 1364.
2. Grondin P, Kretz JG, Bical O, et al: Natural history of saccular aneurysm of the left ventricle. *J Thorac Cardiovasc Surg* 1979; 77:57.
3. Buckberg GD: Defining the relationship between akinesia and dyskinesia and the cause of left ventricular failure after anterior infarction and reversal of remodeling to restoration. *J Thorac Cardiovasc Surg* 1998; 116:47.
4. Dor V, Sabatier M, DiDonato M: Efficacy of endoventricular patch plasty in large postinfarction akinetic scar and severe left ventricular dysfunction: comparison with a series of large dyskinetic scars. *J Thorac Cardiovasc Surg* 1998; 116:50.
5. DiDonato M, Sabatier M, Dor V, et al: Akinetic versus dyskinetic postinfarction scar: relation to surgical outcome in patients undergoing endoventricular circular patch plasty repair. *J Am Coll Cardiol* 1997; 29:1569.
6. Mickleborough LL, Carson S, Ivanov J: Repair of dyskinetic or akinetic left ventricular aneurysm: results obtained with a modified linear closure. *J Thorac Cardiovasc Surg* 2001; 121:675.
7. Jones RH, Velazquez EJ, Michler RE, et al: Coronary bypass surgery with or without surgical ventricular restoration. *NEJM* 2009; 360:1705.
8. DiDonato M, Castelvecchio S, Kukulski T, et al: Surgical ventricular restoration: left ventricular shape influence on cardiac function, clinical status, and survival. *Ann Thorac Surg* 2009; 87:455.
9. Cox JL: Left ventricular aneurysms: pathophysiologic observations and standard resection. *Sem Thorac Cardiovasc Surg* 1997; 9:113.
10. Mills NL, Everson CT, Hockmuth DR: Technical advances in the treatment of left ventricular aneurysm. *Ann Thorac Surg* 1993; 55:792.
11. Beck CS: Operation for aneurysm of the heart. *Ann Surg* 1944; 120:34.
12. Likoff W, Bailey CP: Ventriculoplasty: excision of myocardial aneurysm. *JAMA* 1955; 158:915.
13. Cooley DA, Collins HA, Morris GC, et al: Ventricular aneurysm after myocardial infarction: surgical excision with use of temporary cardiopulmonary bypass. *JAMA* 1958; 167:557.
14. Stoney WS, Alford WC Jr, Burrus GR, et al: Repair of anteroseptal ventricular aneurysm. *Ann Thorac Surg* 1973; 15:394.
15. Daggett WM, Guyton RA, Mundth ED: Surgery for post-myocardial infarct ventricular septal defect. *Ann Surg* 1977; 86:260.
16. Dor V, Saab M, Coste P, et al: Left ventricular aneurysm: a new surgical approach. *Thorac Cardiovasc Surg* 1989; 37:11.
17. Jatene AD: Left ventricular aneurysmectomy: resection of reconstruction. *J Thorac Cardiovasc Surg* 1985; 89:321.
18. Cooley DA: Ventricular endoaneurysmorrhaphy: a simplified repair for extensive postinfarction aneurysm. *J Cardiac Surg* 1989; 4:200.
19. Cooley DA, Frazier OH, Duncan JM, et al: Intracavitary repair of ventricular aneurysm and regional dyskinesia. *Ann Surg* 1992; 215:417.
20. Faxon DP, Ryan TJ, David KB: Prognostic significance of angiographically documented left ventricular aneurysm from the Coronary Artery Surgery Study (CASS). *Am J Cardiol* 1982; 50:157.
21. Cosgrove DM, Lytle BW, Taylor PC, et al: Ventricular aneurysm resection: trends in surgical risk. *Circulation* 1989; 79(Suppl I):97.
22. Coltharp WH, Hoff SJ, Stoney WS, et al: Ventricular aneurysmectomy: a 25-year experience. *Ann Surg* 1994; 219:707.
23. Grieco JG, Montoya A, Sullivan HJ, et al: Ventricular aneurysm due to blunt chest injury. *Ann Thorac Surg* 1989; 47:322.
24. de Oliveira JA: Heart aneurysm in Chagas' disease. *Revista Instit Medic Trop Sao Paulo* 1998; 40:301.
25. Silverman KJ, Hutchins GM, Bulkley BH: Cardiac sarcoid: a clinicopathological study of 84 unselected patients with systemic sarcoidosis. *Circulation* 1978; 58:1204.
26. Davila JC, Enriquez F, Bergoglio S, et al: Congenital aneurysm of the left ventricle. *Ann Thorac Surg* 1965; 1:697.
27. Antunes MJ: Submitral left ventricular aneurysms. *J Thorac Cardiovasc Surg* 1987; 94:241.

28. de Boer HD, Elzenga NJ, de Boer WJ, et al: Pseudoaneurysm of the left ventricle after isolated pericarditis and Staphylococcus aureus septicemia. *Eur J Cardio-Thorac Surg* 1999; 15:97.
29. Meizlish JL, Berger MJ, Plaukey M, et al: Functional left ventricular aneurysm formation after acute anterior transmural myocardial infarction: incidence, natural history, and prognostic implications. *NEJM* 1984; 311:1001.
30. Forman MB, Collins HW, Kopelman HA, et al: Determinants of left ventricular aneurysm formation after anterior myocardial infarction: a clinical and angiographic study. *J Am Coll Cardiol* 1986; 8:1256.
31. Glower DD, Schaper J, Kabas JS, et al: Relation between reversal of diastolic creep and recovery of systolic function after ischemic myocardial injury in conscious dogs. *Circ Res* 1987; 60:850.
32. Eaton LW, Weiss JL, Bulkley BH, et al: Regional cardiac dilation after acute myocardial infarction: recognition by two-dimensional echocardiography. *NEJM* 1979; 300:57.
33. Iwasaki K, Kita T, Taniguichi G, Kusachi S: Improvement of left ventricular aneurysm after myocardial infarction: report of three cases. *Clin Cardiol* 1991; 14:355.
34. Leurent G, Larralde A, Boulmier D, et al: Cardiac MRI studies of transient left ventricular apical ballooning syndrome (Takotsubo cardiomyopathy): a systematic review. *Int J Cardiol* 2009; 135:146.
35. Sakaguchi G, Young RL, Komeda M, et al: Left ventricular aneurysm repair in rats: structural, functional, and molecular consequences. *J Thorac Cardiovasc Surg* 2001; 121:750.
36. Markowitz LJ, Savage EB, Ratcliffe MB, et al: Large animal model of left ventricular aneurysm. *Ann Thorac Surg* 1989; 48:838.
37. Jugdutt BI, Khan MI: Effect of prolonged nitrate therapy on left ventricular modeling after canine acute myocardial infarction. *Circulation* 1994; 89:2297.
38. Nomoto T, Nishina T, Tsuneyoshi H, et al: Effects of two inhibitors of renin-angiotensin system on attenuation of postoperative remodeling after left ventricular aneurysm repair in rats. *J Card Surg* 2003; 18:S61.
39. Tsuneyoshi H, Nishina T, Nomoto T, et al: Atrial natriuretic peptide helps prevent late remodeling after left ventricular aneurysm repair. *Circulation* 2004; 110:II174.
40. Kayden DS, Wackers FJ, Zaret BL: Left ventricular aneurysm formation after thrombolytic therapy for anterior infarction. TIMI phase I and open label 1985–1986. *Circulation* 1987; 76(Suppl IV):97.
41. Chen JS, Hwang CL, Lee DY, et al: Regression of left ventricular aneurysm after delayed percutaneous transluminal coronary angioplasty (PTCA) in patients with acute myocardial infarction. *Int J Cardiol* 1995; 48:39.
42. Bulkley BH, Roberts WC: Steroid therapy during acute myocardial infarction: a cause of delayed healing and of ventricular aneurysm. *Am J Med* 1974; 58:244.
43. Lapeyre AC III, Steele PM, Kazimer FJ, et al: Systemic embolism in chronic left ventricular aneurysm: incidence and the role of anticoagulation. *Am J Cardiol* 1985; 6:534.
44. Benediktsson R, Eyjolfsson O, Thorgeirsson G: Natural history of chronic left ventricular aneurysm: a population based cohort study. *J Clin Epidemiol* 1991; 44:1131.
45. Faxon DP, Myers WO, McCabe CH: The influence of surgery on the natural history of angiographically documented left ventricular aneurysm: the Coronary Artery Surgery Study. *Circulation* 1986; 74:110.
46. Keren A, Goldberg S, Gottlieb S, et al: Natural history of left ventricular thrombi: their appearance and resolution in the posthospitalization period of acute myocardial infarction. *J Am Coll Cardiol* 1990; 15:790.
47. Yeo TC, Malouf JF, Reeder GS, et al: Clinical characteristics and outcome in postinfarction pseudoaneurysm. *Am J Cardiol* 1999; 84:592.
48. Pretre R, Linka A, Jenni R, et al: Surgical treatment of acquired left ventricular pseudoaneurysms. *Ann Thorac Surg* 2000; 70:553.
49. Ba'albaki HA, Clements SD Jr: Left ventricular aneurysm: a review. *Clin Cardiol* 1989; 12:5.
50. Dor V: Reconstructive left ventricular surgery for post-ischemic akinetic dilatation. *Sem Thorac Cardiovasc Surg* 1997; 9:139.
51. Lloyd SG, Buckberg GD, RESTORE Group: Use of cardiac magnetic resonance imaging in surgical ventriclar restoration. *Eur J Cardio-Thorac Surg* 2006; 295:S216.
52. Konen E, Merchant N, Gutierrez C, et al: True versus false left ventricular aneurysm: differentiation with MR imaging–initial experience. *Radiology* 2005; 236:65.
53. Baciewicz PA, Weintraub WS, Jones EL, et al: Late follow-up after repair of left ventricular aneurysm and (usually) associated coronary bypass grafting. *Am J Cardiol* 1991; 68:193.
54. Vlodaver Z, Coe JE, Edwards JE: True and false left ventricular aneurysm: propensity for the latter to rupture. *Circulation* 1975; 51:567.
55. Dor V, Saab M, Coste P, Sabatier M, Montiglio F: Endoventricular patch plasties with septal exclusion for repair of ischemic left ventricle: technique, results and indications from a series of 781 cases. *Jap J Thorac Cardiovasc Surg* 1998; 46:389.
56. Akins CW: Resection of left ventricular aneurysm during hypothermic fibrillatory arrest without aortic occlusion. *J Thorac Cardiovasc Surg* 1986; 91:610.
57. Rankin JS, Hickey MSJ, Smith LR, et al: Current management of mitral valve incompetence associated with coronary artery disease. *J Cardiac Surg* 1989; 4:25.
58. Menicanti L, DiDonato M, Castelvecchio V, et al: Functional ischemic mitral regurgitation in anterior ventricular remodeling: results of surgical ventricular restoration with and without mitral repair. *Heart Failure Rev* 2004; 9:317.
59. Cox JL: Surgical management of left ventricular aneurysms: a clarification of the similarities and differences between the Jatene and Dor techniques. *Sem Thorac Cardiovasc Surg* 1997; 9:131.
60. Menasche P, Hagege A, Scorsin M, et al: Autologous skeletal myoblast transplantation for cardiac insufficiency. First clinical case. *Arch Maladies Coeur Vaisseaux* 2001; 94:180.
61. Taylor DA, Atkins BZ, Hungspreugs P, et al: Regenerating functional myocardium: improved performance after skeletal myoblast transplantation. *Nat Med* 1998; 4:929.
62. Matsubayashi K, Fedak PW, Mickle DA, et al: Improved left ventricular aneurysm repair with bioengineered vascular smooth muscle grafts. *Circulation* 2003; 108:II219.
63. Sakakibara Y, Tambara K, Lu F, et al: Combined procedure of surgical repair and cell transplantation for left ventricular aneurysm: an experimental study. *Circulation* 2002; 106:I193.
64. Athanasuleas CL, Stanley AWH Jr, Buckberg GD, et al: Surgical anterior ventricular endocardial restoration (SAVER) in the dilated remodeled ventricle after anterior myocardial infarction. *J Am Coll Cardiol* 2001; 37:1199.
65. Wellens F, Degreick Y, Deferm H, et al: Surgical treatment of left ventricular aneurysm and ischemic mitral incompetence. *Acta Chir Belg* 1991; 91:44.
66. Williams JA, Weiss ES, Patel ND, et al: Surgical ventricular restoration versus cardiac transplantation: a comparison of cost, outcomes, and survival. *J Card Fail* 14; 547:2008.
67. Hernandez AF, Velazquez EJ, Dullum MKC, et al: Contemporary performance of surgical ventricular restoration procedures: data from the Society of Thoracic Surgeons' national cardiac database. Am Heart J 2006; 152:494.
68. Dor V: Left ventricular aneurysms: the endoventricular circular patch plasty. *Sem Thorac Cardiovasc Surg* 1997; 9:123.
69. Komeda M, David TE, Malik A, et al: Operative risks and long-term results of operation for left ventricular aneurysm. *Ann Thorac Surg* 1992; 53:22.
70. Couper GS, Bunton RW, Birjiniuk V, et al: Relative risks of left ventricular aneurysmectomy in patients with akinetic scars versus true dyskinetic aneurysms. *Circulation* 1990; 82(Suppl IV):248.
71. Stahle E, Bergstrom R, Nystrom SO, et al: Surgical treatment of left ventricular aneurysm assessment of risk factors for early and late mortality. *Eur J Cardio-Thorac Surg* 1994; 8:67.
72. Silveira WL, Leite AF, Soares EC, et al: Short-term follow-up of patients after aneurysmectomy of the left ventricle. *Arquivos Bras Cardiol* 2000; 75:401.
73. Vauthy JN, Berry DW, Snyder DW, et al: Left ventricular aneurysm repair with myocardial revascularization: an analysis of 246 consecutive patients over 15 years. *Ann Thorac Surg* 1988; 46:29.
74. Elefteriades JA, Solomon LW, Salazar AM, et al: Linear left ventricular aneurysmectomy: modern imaging studies reveal improved morphology and function. *Ann Thorac Surg* 1993; 56:242.
75. Kesler KA, Fiore AC, Naunheim KS, et al: Anterior wall left ventricular aneurysm repair: a comparison of linear versus circular closure. *J Thorac Cardiovasc Surg* 1992; 103:841.
76. Kawachi K, Kitamura S, Kawata T, et al: Hemodynamic assessment during exercise after left ventricular aneurysmectomy. *J Thorac Cardiovasc Surg* 1994; 107:178.
77. David TE: Surgical treatment of mechanical complications of myocardial infarction, in Spence PA, Chitwood RA (eds): *Cardiac Surgery: State of the Art Reviews,* Vol 5. Philadelphia, Hanley and Belfus, 1991; p 423.
78. DiDonato M, Barletta G, Maioli M, et al: Early hemodynamic results of left ventricular reconstructive surgery for anterior wall left ventricular aneurysm. *Am J Cardiol* 1992; 69:886.
79. Kawata T, Kitamura S, Kawachi K, et al: Systolic and diastolic function after patch reconstruction of left ventricular aneurysms. *Ann Thorac Surg* 1995; 59:403.

80. Tanoue Y, Ando H, Fukamura F, et al: Ventricular energetics in endoventricular circular patch plasty for dyskinetic anterior left ventricular aneurysm. *Ann Thorac Surg* 2003; 75:1205.
81. Schreuder JJ, Castiglioni A, Maisano F, et al: Acute decrease of left ventricular mechanical dyssynchrony and improvement of contractile state and energy efficiency after left ventricular restoration. *J Thorac Cardiovasc Surg* 2005; 129:138.
82. Fantini F, Barletta G, Toso A, et al: Effects of reconstructive surgery for left ventricular anterior aneurysm on ventriculoarterial coupling. *Heart* 1999; 81:171.
83. Nicolosi AC, Weng ZC, Detwiler PW, et al: Simulated left ventricular aneurysm and aneurysm repair in swine. *J Thorac Cardiovasc Surg* 1990; 100:745.
84. Walker WE, Stoney WS, Alford WC, et al: Results of surgical management of acute left ventricular aneurysm. *Circulation* 1978; 62(Suppl II):75.
85. Hutchins GM, Brawley RK: The influence of cardiac geometry on the results of ventricular aneurysm repair. *Am J Pathol* 1980; 99:221.
86. Parolari A, Naliato M, Loardi C, et al. Surgery of left ventricular aneurysm: a meta-analysis of early outcomes following different reconstruction techniques. *Ann Thorac Surg* 2007; 83:2009.
87. Doss M, Martens S, Sayour S, et al: Long term follow up of left ventricular function after repair of left ventricular aneurysm. A comparison of linear closure versus patch plasty. *Eur J Cardio-Thorac Surg* 2001; 20:783.
88. Antunes PE, Silva R, Ferrao de Oliveira J, Antunes MJ: Left ventricular aneurysms: early and long-term results of two types of repair. *Eur J Cardio-Thorac Surg* 2005; 27:210.
89. Marchenko AV, Cherniavsky AM, Volokitina TL, Alsov SA, Karaskov AM: Left ventricular dimension and shape after postinfarction aneurysm repair. *Eur J Cardio-Thorac Surg* 2005; 27:475.
90. Vicol C, Rupp G, Fischer S, et al: Linear repair versus ventricular reconstruction for treatment of left ventricular aneurysm: a 10-year experience. *J Cardiovasc Surg* 1998; 39:461.
91. Salati M, Paje A, Di Biasi P, et al: Severe diastolic dysfunction after endoventriculoplasty. *J Thorac Cardiovasc Surg* 1995; 109:694.
92. Lundblad R, Abdelnoor M, Svennevig JL: Surgery for left ventricular aneurysm: early and late survival after simple linear repair and endoventricular patch plasty. *J Thorac Cardiovasc Surg* 2004; 128:449.
93. Ratcliffe MB, Wallace AW, Salahieh A, et al: Ventricular volume, chamber stiffness, and function after anteroapical aneurysm plication in the sheep. *J Thorac Cardiovasc Surg* 2000; 119:115.
94. Di Mattia DG, Di Biasi P, Salati M, et al: Surgical treatment of left ventricular post-infarction aneurysm with endoventriculoplasty: late clinical and functional results. *Eur J Cardio-Thorac Surg* 1999; 15:413.
95. Prucz RB, Weiss ES, Patel ND, et al: Coronary artery bypass grafting with or without surgical ventricular restoration: a comparison. *Ann Thorac Surg* 2008; 86:806.
96. Mark DB, Knight JD, Velazquez EJ, et al: Quality of life and economic outcomes with surgical ventricular reconstruction in ischemic heart failure: results from the Surgical Treatment for Ischemic Heart Failure Trial. *Am Heart J* 2009; 157:837.

PART 4A

VALVULAR HEART DISEASE (AORTIC)

CHAPTER 31

Pathophysiology of Aortic Valve Disease

Craig M. Jarrett
Samuel Edwards
A. Marc Gillinov
Tomislav Mihaljevic

INTRODUCTION

The aortic valve (AV) is a semilunar valve positioned at the end of the left ventricular outflow tract (LVOT) between the left ventricle and aorta. Proper functioning of this valve is critical in maintaining efficient cardiac function. This chapter explores the anatomical and physiologic properties of the AV.

EMBRYOLOGIC DEVELOPMENT

Embryologic development of the AV is closely associated with development of the LVOT. In the primary heart tube, blood travels from the primitive ventricle into the bulbous cordis and out the aortic roots. The midportion of the bulbous cordis, the conus cordis, develops into the outflow tracts of the ventricles. The distal portion of the bulbous cordis, the truncus arteriosus (TA), develops into the proximal portion of the aorta and pulmonary arteries. During the fifth week of development, pairs of opposing swellings appear in the conus cordis and TA (Fig. 31-1). These conotruncal, or bulbar, ridges grow toward each other and fuse to form the aorticopulmonary (AP) septum. The AP septum divides the conus cordis into the left and right ventricular outflow tracts and the TA into the ascending aorta and pulmonary trunk.

When partitioning of the TA is nearly completed, the AV begins to develop from three swellings of subendocardial tissue (see Fig. 31-1). Two swellings arising from the fused truncal ridges develop into the right and left AV leaflets. A third dorsal swelling develops into the posterior leaflet. These swellings are reshaped and hollowed out to form the three thin-walled cusps of the fully developed AV. The pulmonary valve develops in a similar manner.

ANATOMY

The AV separates the terminal portion of the LVOT from the aorta. The normal AV consists of three semilunar leaflets or cusps projecting outward and upward into the lumen of the ascending aorta (Fig. 31-2). The space between the free edge of each leaflet and the points of attachment to the aorta comprise the sinuses of Valsalva. Because the coronary arteries arise from two of the three sinuses, the sinuses and the respective leaflets are named the right coronary, left coronary, and posterior (noncoronary) sinuses and leaflets. The ostia of coronary arteries arise from the upper part of the sinuses, with the ostium of the left coronary artery positioned slightly higher than the ostium of the right. The leaflets are separated from one another at the aorta by the right-left, right-posterior, and left-posterior commissures (Fig. 31-3). The area adjacent to the left-posterior commissure is the fibrous continuity, which interconnects the aorta and the mitral valve annulus. The area beneath this commissure is the aortomitral curtain, which is an important anatomical landmark for root enlargement procedures. The posterior leaflet attaches above the posterior diverticulum of the LVOT and opposes the right atrial wall. The right-posterior commissure is positioned directly above the penetrating atrioventricular bundle and membranous septum. The right-left commissure opposes the posterior commissure of the pulmonary valve and the two associated aortic cusps oppose the right ventricular infundibulum. The lateral part of the left coronary sinus is the only part of the AV that is not closely related to another cardiac chamber and is in direct relationship with the free pericardial space.

The AV leaflets meet centrally along a line of coaptation, at the center of which are the thickened nodules of Arantius.

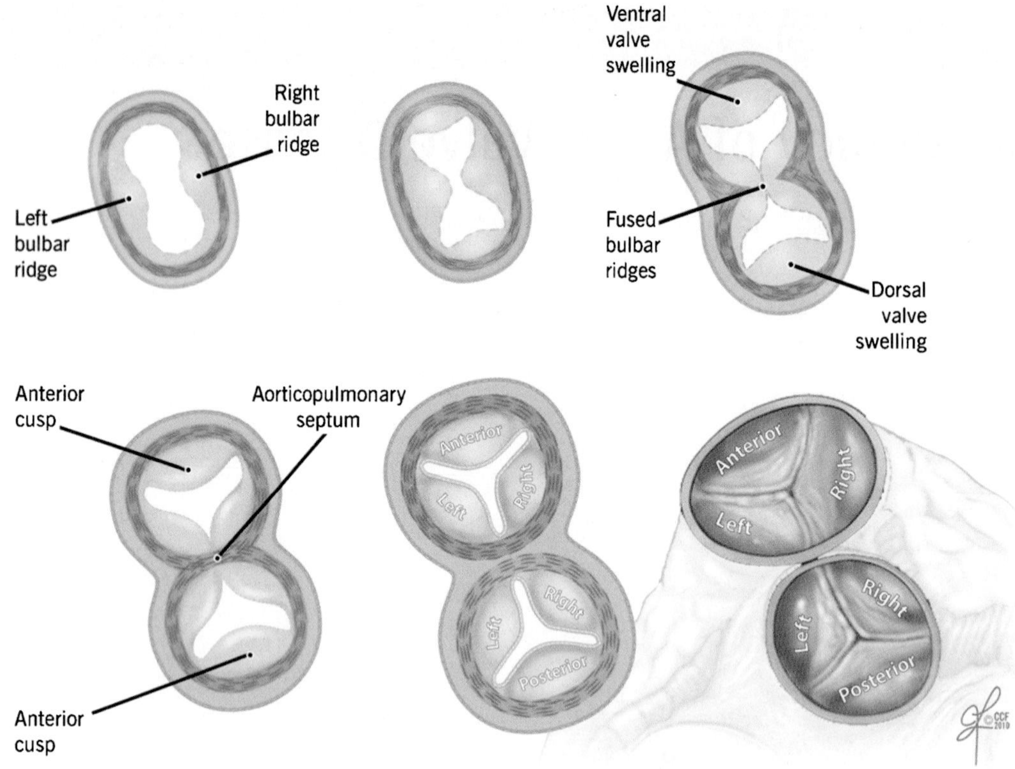

FIGURE 31-1 Schematic representation of development of the left and right ventricular outflow tracts and aortic and pulmonary valves. (*Top left*) Cross-section through the cordis showing the conotruncal ridges beginning to develop. (*Top right*) Aorticopulmonary septum forming from fusion of the conotruncal ridges and subendocardial swellings beginning to develop into the aortic and pulmonary valve leaflets. (*Bottom left*) Left and right ventricular outflow tracts separated by the aorticopulmonary septum and further development of the subendocardial swellings. (*Bottom right*) Aortic and pulmonary valves in the adult. (*Reproduced with permission of the Cleveland Clinic, Cleveland, OH.*)

Because of the semilunar shape of the leaflets, the AV does not have a true annulus in the traditional sense of a ringlike attachment. Instead, the leaflets have semilunar attachments along a hollow cylinder or cuff of tissue interconnecting the left ventricular (LV) chamber and the proximal aorta (Fig. 31-4).[1] The distal border of the cuff is the sinotubular junction, which is defined by imaginary lines connecting the commissures. The proximal border is the ventriculoarterial (VA) junction, which has both hemodynamic and anatomic parts. The hemodynamic VA junction is marked by the semilunar attachments of the leaflets, whereas, the anatomic VA junction is marked by the circular attachment of the proximal aorta and the muscular and membranous ventricular septums.

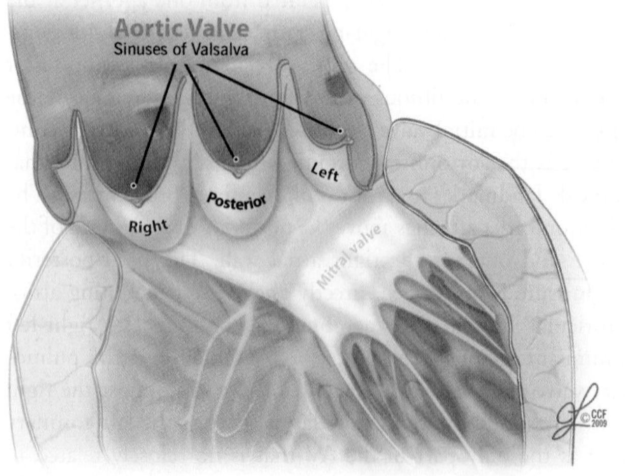

FIGURE 31-2 Anatomical relationship between the aortic valve leaflets and surrounding structures. (*Reproduced with permission of the Cleveland Clinic, Cleveland, OH.*)

The valve leaflets consist of three layers of endothelially invested connective tissue of distinctly different density and composition. There is no demarcation between the outer layers of the aortic and ventricular sides of the leaflets and outer layers of the corresponding aortic and ventricular walls; that is, leaflet endothelial cells form a continuum with aortic and ventricular endothelial cells (Fig. 31-5).[2,3] Endothelial cells of both the aortic and ventricular surfaces of the AV are arranged circumferentially. Beneath the endothelium, there are extensions of the aortic intima and ventricular endocardium, termed the *arterialis* and *ventricularis,* respectively. The next layer is the lamina fibrosa, which is composed of dense collagen mostly in a circumferential pattern. Because of the thickness and density of this layer, it is the strongest layer and important for bearing the stress of diastolic pressure. The middle layer, referred to as the *spongiosa,* forms the core of the leaflets at

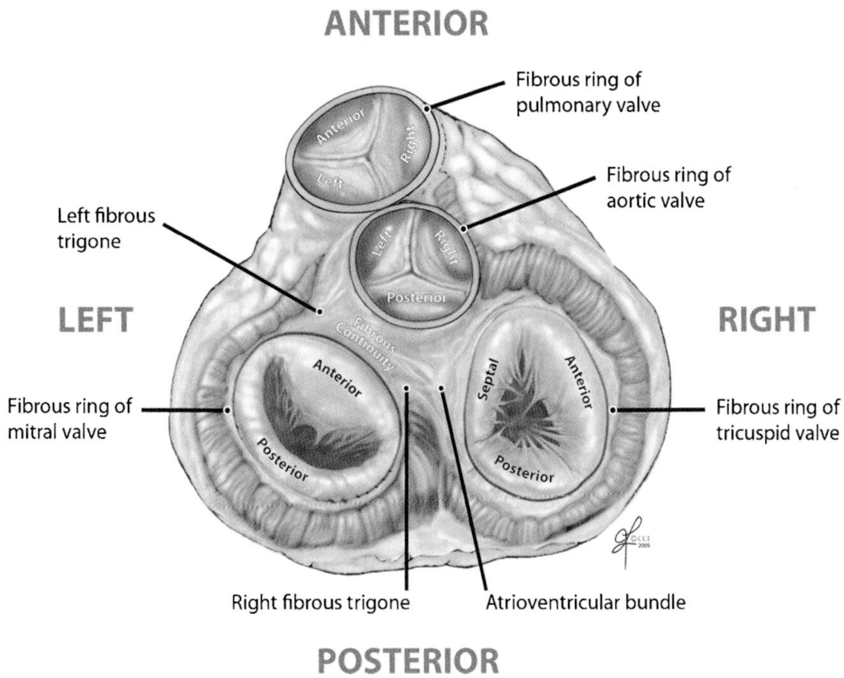

FIGURE 31-3 Anatomical relationship between the aortic valve and surrounding structures. (*Reproduced with permission of the Cleveland Clinic, Cleveland, OH.*)

their bases. It is made of loose connective tissue consisting of water and glycosaminoglycans with sparse fibers and cellularity. The semifluid nature of this layer gives the leaflet considerable plasticity.

MECHANICS OF MOVEMENT

The AV passively opens and closes in response to pressure differences between the left ventricle and aorta during the cardiac cycle. Pressure generated from ventricular contraction leads to valve opening, and the subsequent relatively higher pressure of the aorta leads to valve closure. The mechanical properties of the AV allow it to open with minimal transvalvular gradient and close completely with minimal flow reversal.

Opening

Pressure differences between the aorta and the ventricle coupled with compliance of the aortic root cause aortic root dilation and constriction during the cardiac cycle. This dynamic

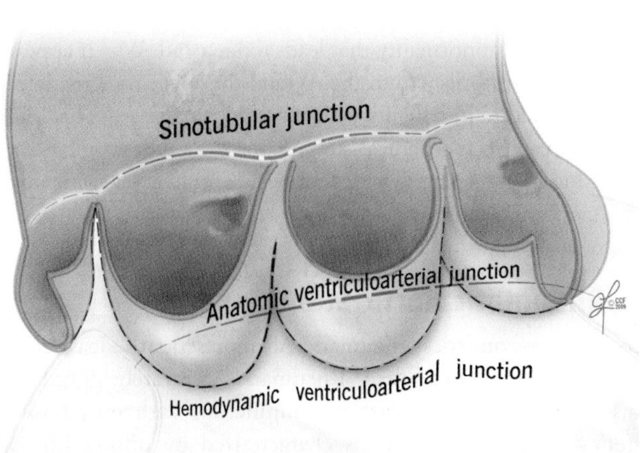

FIGURE 31-4 Schematic representation of the aortic valve cuff. The sinotubular junction marks the distal border. The ventriculoarterial junction, which has both hemodynamic and anatomic parts, marks the proximal border. (*Reproduced with permission of the Cleveland Clinic, Cleveland, OH.*)

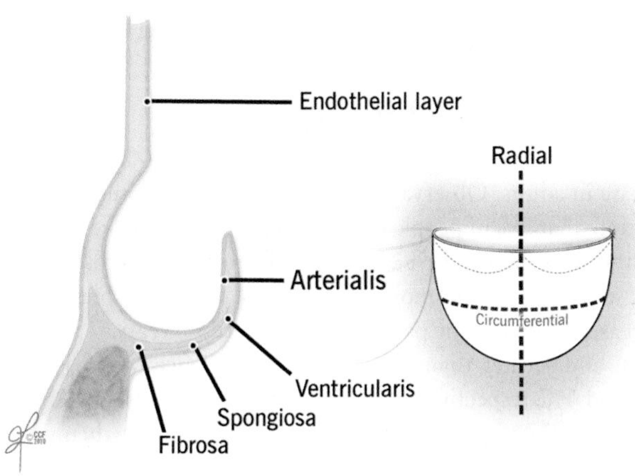

FIGURE 31-5 Schematic representation of a cross-section through the aortic valve leaflet showing the continuity of endocardial and endothelial components with the aortic valve. Inset illustrates the radial and circumferential axes of the valve leaflet. *(Reproduced with permission of the Cleveland Clinic, Cleveland, OH.)*

motion of the root plays an important role in opening and closure of the AV. During late diastole, as blood fills the ventricle, a 12% expansion of the aortic root occurs 20 to 40 msec before AV opening.[4,5] The leaflets begin to open as a result of root dilation even before any generation of positive pressure from ventricular contraction. Root dilation alone opens the leaflets about 20%.[6] As pressure rises in the LVOT, tension across the leaflets produced from root dilation lessens. As pressure continues to rise, the pressure difference across the leaflets is minimal, and no tension is present within the leaflet.[4] This loss of tension allows the aortic root to further dilate and allows the valve to open rapidly at the beginning of ejection. Under normal circumstances, the AV presents little or no obstruction to flow because the specific gravity of the leaflets is equal to that of blood.[7] These mechanisms permit rapid opening of the valve and minimal resistance to ejection.[8]

Closure

Closure of the AV is an elegant mechanism, which has interested investigators since the time of Leonardo da Vinci.[9] A principal theory involved in closure is vortex theory, which recognizes the importance of the sinuses of Valsalva in valve closure.[10] As ejection occurs, blood creates small eddy currents or vortices along the aortic wall. At the end of ejection and before valve closure, these vortices fill the sinuses and balloon the leaflets away from the aortic wall toward the aortic axis. After the pressure difference across the open AV equalizes, a small flow reversal forces the leaflets completely closed. Apposition of the valve leaflets occurs briskly and the ensuing second heart sound occurs after complete closure of the AV. Upon closing, the elastic leaflets stretch and recoil to generate compression and expansion of blood. The subsequent pressure changes produce the second heart sound; the sound is not produced by physical apposition of the valve leaflets.[11]

AORTIC STENOSIS

Aortic stenosis (AS) is incomplete opening of the AV, which restricts blood flow out of the left ventricle during systole.

Prevalence and Etiology

In developed countries, AS is the most prevalent valvular heart disease in adults. Observational echocardiography studies demonstrate that 2% of people 65 years of age or older have isolated calcific AS, whereas 29% exhibit age-related AV sclerosis without stenosis.[12] AS is more common in men and prevalence increases with age. In patients aged 65 to 75 years, 75 to 85 years, and greater than 85 years, the prevalence of AS is 1.3, 2.4, and 4%, respectively.[13] The most common causes of AS are acquired degenerative disease, bicuspid AV, and rheumatic heart disease.

Acquired Aortic Stenosis

The most common cause of AS is degenerative calcification of the AV, which typically occurs in septuagenarians and octogenarians. Progressive calcification, initially along the flexion lines at the leaflet bases, leads to immobilization of the cusps. The characteristic pathologic findings are discrete, focal lesions on the aortic side of the leaflets that can extend deep into the aortic annulus. The deposits may involve the sinuses of Valsalva and the ascending aorta. Although long considered to be the result of years of mechanical stress on an otherwise normal valve, it is now understood that the mechanical stress leads to proliferative and inflammatory changes, with lipid accumulation, upregulation of angiotensin-converting enzyme (ACE) activity, and infiltration of macrophages and T lymphocytes in a process similar to atherosclerosis.[13–18] The risk factors for the development of calcific AS are also similar to those for atherosclerosis and include elevated serum levels of low-density lipoprotein (LDL) cholesterol, diabetes, smoking, and hypertension.[13] Therefore, coronary artery disease is commonly present in patients with AS. Age-related AV sclerosis is associated with an increased risk of cardiovascular death and myocardial infarction (MI).

Calcific AS is also observed in a number of other conditions, including Paget's disease of bone and end-stage renal disease.[19] Ochronosis with alkaptonuria is another rare cause of AS, which also can cause a rare greenish discoloration of the AV.[20]

Bicuspid Aortic Stenosis

A calcified bicuspid AV represents the most common form of congenital AS. Bicuspid AVs are present in approximately 2% of the general population. Gradual calcification of the bicuspid AV results in significant stenosis most often in the fifth and sixth decades of life, earlier in unicommissural than in bicuspid valves and earlier in men than women. The abnormal architecture of the unicommissural or bicuspid AV induces turbulent flow, which injures the leaflets and leads to fibrosis, increased rigidity, leaflet calcification, and narrowing of the AV orifice.[21] Bicuspid valves are often associated with dilatation of the ascending aorta related to accelerated degeneration of the aortic media that in some cases may progress to aneurysm formation. Recent work suggests that a DNA transcriptional error in the gene encoding endothelial nitric oxide synthetase may be implicated in the genetic abnormality that leads to bicuspid AV.[22] It appears that the microfibrils within the AV and the aortic root are defective in structure in patients with bicuspid AV disease. This leads to a decrease in mechanical support for the valve, thereby contributing to accelerated "wear and tear," and hence degenerative changes in the valve matrix.

Rheumatic Aortic Stenosis

In Western countries, rheumatic AS represents the least common form of AS in adults.[23] Rheumatic AS is rarely an isolated disease and usually occurs in conjunction with mitral valve stenosis.[24] Rheumatic AS is characterized by diffuse fibrous leaflet thickening with fusion, to a variable extent, of one or more commissures. The early stage of rheumatic AS is characterized by edema, lymphocytic infiltration, and revascularization of the leaflets, whereas the later stages are characterized by thickening, commissural fusion, and scarred leaflet edges.[25]

Pathophysiology

In adults with calcific disease, the AV slowly thickens over time. Early, it causes little hemodynamic disturbance as the valve area is reduced from the normal 3 to 4 cm^2 to 1.5 to 2 cm^2.[13] Past this point, hemodynamically significant obstruction of LV outflow develops with a concomitant increase in LV pressure and lengthening of the LV ejection time. The elevated LV pressure increases wall stress. Wall stress is normalized by increased wall thickness and LV hypertrophy (LVH). As it hypertrophies, the left ventricle becomes less compliant and LV end-diastolic pressure (LVEDP) increases without chamber dilatation. This reflects diastolic dysfunction and the ventricle becomes increasingly dependent on atrial systole for filling.[26] Hence, if a patient develops an atrial arrhythmia, he or she can rapidly decompensate.

Although adaptive, the concentric hypertrophy that develops has adverse consequences. LVH, increased systolic pressure, and prolonged ejection time all contribute to an increase in myocardial oxygen consumption. Increased diastolic pressure increases endocardial compression of the coronary arteries, reducing coronary flow reserve (or maximal coronary flow).[27] Prolonged ejection also results in decreased time in diastole and therefore reduced myocardial perfusion time. The increased demand of the hypertrophied ventricle and decreased delivery capacity can yield subendocardial ischemia with activity. This can result in angina and LV dysfunction. LVH also makes the heart more susceptible to ischemic injury. Severe LVH is only partly reversed by AV replacement (AVR) and is associated with decreased long-term survival even after initially successful surgery.[28]

In late stages of severe AS, the left ventricle decompensates with resulting dilated cardiomyopathy and heart failure. Cardiac output (CO) declines and the pulmonary artery pressure rises, leading to pulmonary hypertension.

Myocardial hypertrophy in patients with AS is characterized by increased gene expression for collagen I and II, and fibronectin that is associated with activation of the renin-angiotensin system.[22] Reduction in renin-angiotensin parallels regression of hypertrophy after AVR.[29] Experimental studies have indicated a role of apoptotic mechanisms in the progression to LVH and heart failure in patients with AS.[30] For 50% of patients who present with symptoms of congestive heart failure (CHF), mean survival is less than 1 year.[31]

Hemodynamics

The severity of AS can be assessed by measuring the AV orifice area (AVA), mean pressure gradient, and peak jet velocity. AVA is calculated by using CO, heart rate (HR), systolic ejection period (SEP), and mean pressure gradient in the Gorlin formula, which describes the fundamental relationships linking the area of an orifice to the flow and pressure drop across the orifice. The Gorlin formula is:

$$\text{AVA} = \frac{\text{CO}\left(\frac{\text{mL}}{\text{min}}\right)}{44.3 \times \text{HR}\left(\frac{\text{beats}}{\text{min}}\right) \times \text{SEP(sec)} \times \sqrt{\text{mean pressure gradient (mmHg)}}}$$

CO can be measured using the Fick or thermodilution technique. SEP is the time from AV opening to closure. The normal AVA is 2.6 to 3.5 cm^2 in adults. Valve areas of less than 1.0 cm^2 represent severe AS. In low-output states, the Gorlin formula may systematically predict smaller valve areas than are actually present. Several reports also indicate that the AVA from the Gorlin formula increases with increases in CO.[32]

In patients with AS, the transvalvular pressure gradient can be measured by simultaneous catheter pressure measurements in the left ventricle and proximal aorta. The peak-to-peak gradient, measured as the difference between peak LV pressure and peak aortic pressure, is used commonly to quantify the valve gradient.

Invasive measurements of AS severity have been largely replaced by echocardiographic measurements, which are currently the clinical standard. The Doppler acquired jet velocity is converted to a gradient using the Bernoulli equation, which is:

$$\text{Gradient} = 4 \times (\text{velocity})^2$$

Transesophageal echocardiography (TEE) is an alternative method for assessment of AVA that uses planimetry of the systolic short-axis view of the AV (Fig. 31-6).[33] Planimetry of the valve area is challenging because the valve orifice is a complex, three-dimensional shape, and area measurements assume the valve orifice lies entirely within the image plane.

Clinical Presentation

Symptoms

The cardinal symptoms of AS are angina pectoris, syncope, and symptoms of CHF (dyspnea, orthopnea, and paroxysmal nocturnal dyspnea).[34] Although the mechanisms of angina and heart failure are well understood, the mechanism of syncope is less clear. A common theory is that the augmented stroke volume that usually accompanies exercise is limited by the narrowed outflow orifice. With exercise-induced reduction in peripheral

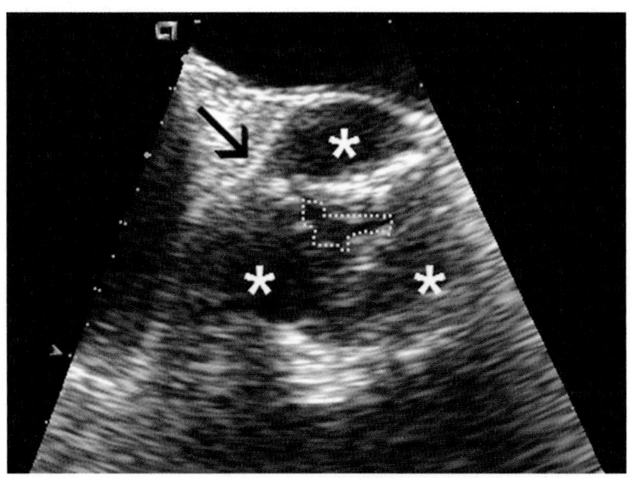

FIGURE 31-6 Transesophageal echocardiographic image of aortic stenosis resulting from severe degenerative calcification. Transverse section of the aortic root at the level of the aortic valve orifice showing the aortic ring (*arrow*), the sinuses of Valsalva (*asterisks*), and a significantly reduced aortic valve orifice area of 0.44 cm^2 (*dotted line*).

arterial resistance, blood pressure drops, leading to cerebral hypoperfusion and syncope.[35] Syncope also may be the result of dysfunction of baroreceptor mechanisms and a vasodepressor response to the increased LV systolic pressure during exercise. Besides these cardinal symptoms, patients also commonly present with more subtle symptoms, such as fatigue, decreased exercise tolerance, and dyspnea on exertion.[36]

Another rare presentation of AS is gastrointestinal bleeding secondary to angiodysplasia occurring predominantly in the right colon as well as the small bowel or stomach. This complication arises from shear-stress–induced platelet aggregation with reduction in high-molecular-weight multimers of von Willebrand factor and increases in proteolytic subunit fragments. These abnormalities correlate with the severity of AS and are correctable by AVR.[37] Other late manifestations of severe AS include atrial fibrillation and pulmonary hypertension. Infective endocarditis can occur in younger patients with AS; it is less common in elderly patients with a severely calcified valve.

Patients who develop severe AS have a long period of asymptomatic progression in which morbidity and mortality is relatively low (Fig. 31-7). Sudden death from AS before the onset of symptoms is estimated to be approximately 1% per year.[38] With the onset of symptoms, survival is dramatically reduced without surgical intervention. Of the 35% of patients who present with angina, 50% survive for 5 years. Of the 15% who present with syncope, 50% survive for 3 years, and mean survival for those who present with CHF is 2 years.[34]

Signs

AS is frequently first diagnosed before symptom onset by auscultation of a murmur on physical exam. Classically, AS causes a systolic crescendo-decrescendo murmur, heard loudest at the right upper sternal border. Another sign of AS is a delayed second heart sound (S_2) because of prolongation of the systolic ejection time. S_2 also may be single when the aortic component is absent, and if the aortic component is audible, this may give rise to a paradoxical splitting of S_2.

The classic pulsus parvus (small pulse) is a sign of severe AS or decompensated AS and occurs when stroke volume and systolic and pulse pressures fall. A wide pulse pressure is also characteristic of AS. Prolongation of the ejection phase with slow rise in the arterial pressure also gives rise to the pulsus tardus (late pulse). Pulsus parvus et tardus is diagnosed by palpation.

LVH is evident as a sustained apical thrust or heave. This sign is present only when failure occurs because until failure occurs, the hypertrophy is not accompanied by dilatation, and the apical impulse is not displaced. Conversely, absence of an apical thrust (except in muscular patients, or those with emphysema or adiposity) suggests mild or moderate AS. Other physical findings of significant AS include a prominent atrial kick and prominence of the jugular venous *a* wave secondary to decreased right ventricular compliance caused by right ventricular hypertrophy.[39]

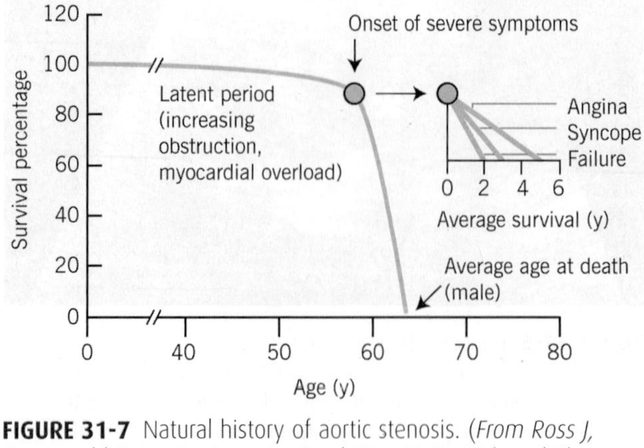

FIGURE 31-7 Natural history of aortic stenosis. *(From Ross J, Braunwald E. Aortic stenosis. Circulation 1968; 38(suppl 5): 61-67.)*

Electrocardiogram

Most patients with severe AS present with QRS complex or ST-T interval abnormalities reflecting LVH. Patients with a higher gradient are more likely to show a "strain" or "systolic overload" pattern. The conduction abnormalities may result from septal trauma secondary to high intramyocardial tension from hypoxic damage to the conducting fibers or from extension of valvular calcifications into the fibrous septum.

Roentgenogram

The roentgenographic characteristics of compensated AS include concentric hypertrophy of the left ventricle without cardiomegaly, poststenotic dilatation of the aorta, and calcification of the valve cusps. With decompensation, there is cardiomegaly in the posteroanterior projection and pulmonary venous congestion. It is important to recognize that a routine chest x-ray may be within normal limits in patients with hemodynamically compensated AS. The rounding of the lower-left heart border may be subtle, the poststenotic aortic dilatation may be equivocal, and the valvular calcification may be invisible on the posteroanterior view. Of equal importance, the presence of cardiomegaly in a normotensive patient with isolated AS indicates decompensated AS.

Echocardiography

Echocardiography is the diagnostic tool of choice for confirming the diagnosis of AS and quantification of disease severity. Echocardiography is used to define: (1) the severity and etiology of AS; (2) coexisting valvular abnormalities; and (3) cardiac chamber size and function.

The development of diastolic dysfunction in patients with AS can lead to symptom development, and may increase late mortality after AVR.[28,40] Hence, the quantification of diastolic dysfunction is important in the assessment of AS. LV filling pressures can be assessed by combining transmitral flow velocity and annular velocity obtained at the level of the mitral annulus with tissue Doppler (E/E').[41] In patients with normal LV function (LVF), stress echocardiography is used to determine if symptom development during exercise is due to diastolic dysfunction.[42] Diastolic dysfunction in patients with normal LVF may cause exercise intolerance for several reasons: (1) elevated LV diastolic and pulmonary venous pressures increase the work of breathing and cause dyspnea; (2) patients with LVH exhibit a limited ability to use the Frank-Starling mechanism during exercise, resulting in a decrease in CO during exercise; and (3) elevated LV diastolic and pulmonary venous pressures result in abnormalities in the diastolic properties of the ventricle.

When AS is suspected, an initial Doppler echocardiogram can confirm the diagnosis and assess the severity. Periodic reexamination, every 5 years for mild AS, every 2 years for moderate AS, and annually for severe AS, is recommended to identify worsening stenosis, LV dysfunction, LVH, and mitral regurgitation.[43] Although AS is best understood as a disease continuum, severity can be graded by echocardiographic evaluation of hemodynamics. The current guidelines use definitions based on the AVA, mean pressure gradient, and peak jet velocity (Table 31-1).

Exercise Testing

Traditionally, severe AS has been regarded as a relative contraindication to exercise testing. Exercise testing should be avoided in symptomatic patients with AS as well. Recent studies have indicated that quantitative exercise Doppler echocardiography can be performed safely in asymptomatic patients and may be useful for identifying patients who at higher risk of becoming symptomatic and/or requiring AVR. Several studies have shown that asymptomatic patients with severe AS who become symptomatic on exercise stress testing, have a higher rate of cardiac death or progression to AVR.[44,45] Dobutamine stress echocardiography is occasionally used in severe AS, specifically to assess contractile reserve in patients with moderate to severe AS with a low AV gradient and depressed LVF.[46,47]

TABLE 31-1 Classification of Aortic Stenosis Severity

Indicator	Mild	Moderate	Severe
Aortic valve area (cm^2)	>1.5	1.0–1.5	<1.0
Aortic valve area index (cm^2 per m^2)			<0.6
Mean pressure gradient (mm Hg)	<25	25–40	>40
Peak jet velocity (m/sec)	<3.0	3.0–4.0	>4.0

Adapted from Bonow RO, Carabello BA, Chatterjee K, de Leon AC Jr, Faxon DP, et al: 2008 focused update incorporated into the ACC/AHA 2006 guidelines for the management of patients with valvular heart disease: a report of the American College of Cardiology/American Heart Association Task Force on Practice Guidelines (Writing Committee to revise the 1998 guidelines for the management of patients with valvular heart disease). Endorsed by the Society of Cardiovascular Anesthesiologists, Society for Cardiovascular Angiography and Interventions, and Society of Thoracic Surgeons. J Am Coll Cardiol 2008; 52(13):e1-142.

Cardiac Catheterization

Although Doppler echocardiography is well validated, cardiac catheterization remains the gold standard for measuring the transvalvular gradient. Because coronary artery disease is common in patients with AS, coronary angiography is usually performed in patients with severe AS to assess coronary anatomy and evaluate the need for combined AVR and myocardial revascularization. Right-sided heart catheterization is also used to calculate the AVA based on the Gorlin equation, as described earlier. Cardiac catheterization can also provide an assessment of ejection fraction (EF) through ventriculography and also may provide information about the presence or absence of other valve lesions.

Computed Tomography

Computed tomography (CT) can be used to assess progression of AS. Electrocardiographically gated multidetector row CT has shown high accuracy and reproducibility in quantifying AV calcification and its progression[48] and estimating AVA by planimetry.[49] The quantification of calcification may develop into clinical applications with respect to the prognostic relevance of AV sclerosis, as well as the problem of calcification of bioprostheses after surgery.

Magnetic Resonance Imaging

Cardiac magnetic resonance imaging (MRI) has emerged as an alternative noninvasive imaging modality for AS.[50] Similar to echocardiography, cardiac MRI records images throughout the cardiac cycle. Cardiac MRI uses a range of pulse sequences to assess structural heart disease. The steady-state free precession (SSFP) cine pulse sequence is commonly used in cardiac MRI and provides detailed images of AV leaflet number, leaflet thickening, valve calcification, and commissural fusion. This sequence is also useful for assessing the effects of AS, including LVH and LVF.[51] MRI is useful when acoustic windows in the echocardiogram are poor or there are discordant imaging and catheterization results.[52,53] MRI has also been used to demonstrate improvement in LVF, myocardial metabolism, and diastolic function, as well as reduced hypertrophy after AVR for AS.[54]

Management

Symptomatic Patients

There is no effective medical therapy for AS. Given the biologic similarity of the calcific lesions of AS to atherosclerosis, there has been substantial effort to investigate the role of lipid-lowering agents in slowing the progression of AS, but to date prospective randomized trials have not found any benefit.[55,56] Prophylactic antibiotics are recommended before any dental or surgical procedures as a prevention strategy for endocarditis.[43] Management of CHF from AS has traditionally consisted of diuretics and ionotropes. Beta-blockers are avoided as reduced inotropy may lead to decreased CO in an overloaded ventricle. Classically, vasodilators are avoided in AS because their administration can lead to hypotension, syncope, and reduced coronary perfusion.

Percutaneous balloon valvuloplasty (valvotomy) is effective in congenital AS, but in adults the valve tends to re-stenose, and the procedure has no effect on long-term mortality.[17] Currently, valvuloplasty is recommended only as a possible bridge to surgical intervention or a palliative measure.[43] AV repair for AS has yielded poor results compared with AVR.[57]

The definitive treatment for severe AS is AVR, and onset of symptoms is the primary indication for AVR. As the risk of asymptomatic severe AS is perceived to be low, symptom onset remains the primary indication. Survival after successful AVR is reduced in younger patients but mimics that of the normal population in older patients.[28,58,59]

Percutaneous AVR represents a novel, less invasive approach to the treatment of AS. This approach has been applied successfully in high-risk patients with severe symptomatic AS who were not deemed candidates for conventional surgery.[60]

Asymptomatic Patients

AVR in asymptomatic patients is currently controversial. Current guidelines recommend AVR for patients with symptomatic AS, for patients with asymptomatic moderate or severe AS who also require coronary revascularization or surgery of the aorta, and for patients with severe AS and reduced EF.[43] As AVR has become a safer procedure and technology for assessing disease severity has improved, it is likely that an identifiable high-risk subset of asymptomatic patients with severe AS could benefit from AVR. Studies show that asymptomatic patients with an aortic jet velocity greater than 4 m/sec,[36] patients with high rates of aortic jet velocity progression and valve calcification,[61] and those with small AVAs and LVH[38] progress to symptom development quickly and will soon require AVR. Exercise stress testing, as described earlier, is also useful to stratify high-risk patients.

A number of recent studies have explored the potential benefit of AVR in asymptomatic patients. In studies of propensity matched cohorts of asymptomatic patients with severe AS, those who had AVR had significantly improved survival.[62,63] It has also been shown that, among patients undergoing AVR for severe AS, LVH is only partly reversed and is associated with decreased long-term survival even after initially successful surgery. This suggests that intervening before development of LVH may improve outcomes.[28] In summary, there is increasing evidence that AVR can be beneficial in a subset of asymptomatic patients with severe AS.

AORTIC REGURGITATION

Aortic regurgitation (AR) is the diastolic reflux of blood from the aorta into the left ventricle due to failure of coaptation of the valve leaflets at the onset of diastole.

Prevalence and Etiology

AR has numerous causes, which can be grouped according to the structural components of the valve apparatus affected. AR may be caused by primary disease of the aortic leaflets and/or disease of the aortic root.

Aortic leaflet calcific degeneration, myxomatous degeneration, infective endocarditis, rheumatic disease, a bicuspid AV, and anorectic medications, such as fenfluramine and phentermine, all lead to distortion of the valve leaflets and prevent proper coaptation.[64–67] Aortic root dilatation caused by aortic dissection; trauma; chronic systemic hypertension; aortitis from syphilis, viral syndromes, or other systemic arteritides (eg, giant cell and Takayasu); and connective tissue disorders, such as Marfan's syndrome, Reiter's disease, Ehlers-Danlos syndrome, osteogenesis imperfecta, and rheumatoid arthritis, leads to improper leaflet coaptation and consequent AR.[68–73] AR is seen most commonly in combination with AS due to calcific or rheumatic disease in which some degree (usually mild) of AR is present in the vast majority of patients. However, AR secondary to aortic dilation is now more common than primary valve disease in patients undergoing AVR for pure AR.[74]

Pathophysiology

The pathophysiology of AR varies according to the onset and duration of the disease process.

Acute Aortic Regurgitation

AR that presents in the acute setting is typically caused by aortic dissection, endocarditis, or trauma. By definition, acute AR is a significant aortic incompetence of sudden onset across a previously competent AV. The blood returned to the left ventricle in diastole causes a sudden increase in LV end-diastolic volume (LVEDV) and reduces the effective or forward stroke volume. LVEDV only increases mildly (20 to 30%) because the ability of the left ventricle to dilate acutely is limited. This leads to a rapid increase in LVEDP. This increase is greatest in the less compliant, concentrically thickened, hypertrophic myocardium seen in those with AS or chronic systemic hypertension. Increased LVEDP results in increased mean LA and pulmonary venous pressures and produces varying degrees of pulmonary edema.[75] The rapid rise in LVEDP also blunts or abolishes the normally widened pulse pressure seen in chronic AR.[76] In the acute setting, two compensatory mechanisms attempt to maintain an effective CO: an increase in contractility attributable to the Frank-Starling mechanism and an increase in HR. The maintenance of an appropriate effective CO depends on the adequacy of these mechanisms, especially systolic pump function.

Chronic Aortic Regurgitation

In contrast, chronic AR is a slow, insidious process, which sets in motion numerous compensatory mechanisms. The diastolic regurgitant flow in AR increases LVEDV, LVEDP, and wall stress. Adaptive signals lead to an increase in myocyte length and addition of sarcomeres in series in a pattern of remodeling known as *eccentric hypertrophy.* Typically there is a modest increase in LV wall thickness such that the ratio of wall thickness to radius is close to normal. Chamber enlargement in the setting of normal systolic function increases total stroke volume and maintains forward stroke volume (total stroke volume minus regurgitant volume).[77] The increased total stroke volume coupled with a normal to slightly elevated LVEDP is responsible for the wide pulse pressure seen in chronic AR. Forward stroke volume in AR is increased by any physiologic change that decreases afterload or increases HR. Increasing HR increases forward stroke volume by itself, but it also decreases diastolic filling time and hence regurgitant flow time and volume. The peripheral vasodilatation and increased HR that accompany exercise increase forward stroke volume in this manner.[78] This also illustrates the physiologic basis for vasodilator therapy in the treatment of AR, and explains why bradycardia and use of negative chronotropic agents should be avoided.

As AR progresses, the hypertrophic response becomes inadequate,[79] and/or the preload reserve is eventually exhausted.[80] Thereafter, any further increase in afterload creates afterload mismatch and results in a reduction in EF. Although the hypertrophied myocardium may provide adequate compensation for many years, eventually maladaptive signals, which lead to decreased myocyte survival and fibrosis, predominate. The myocardium becomes incapable of sustaining the increased work load imposed upon it and heart failure ensues.

Myocardial ischemia in AR, which can result from both decreased coronary artery perfusion and increased myocardial oxygen demand, may lead to further impairment of LVF. The decrease in diastolic coronary perfusion that occurs with a severe reduction in aortic diastolic pressure is only partially compensated by increased coronary arterial flow during systole. In severe AR, there may even be reversal of coronary arterial flow. Superimposed CAD only exacerbates the effect of decreased diastolic coronary perfusion pressure. On the other hand, increased LV muscle mass, wall tension, and systolic ventricular pressure all contribute to increased myocardial oxygen demand. The subsequent ischemia caused by decreased perfusion and increased oxygen demand can lead to cell death and fibrosis, and chronically, can contribute to systolic dysfunction.

Clinical Presentation

Symptoms

The presentation varies depending on the acuity of onset, severity of regurgitation, compliance of the ventricle and aorta, and hemodynamic conditions present at the time. Acute AR can be debilitating and life threatening if not treated emergently, whereas chronic AR is usually well tolerated for years. Severe acute AR commonly presents catastrophically with sudden cardiovascular collapse. Patients also often present with ischemic chest pain caused by decreased coronary blood flow coupled with rapidly increased myocardial oxygen consumption.

Patients with chronic, compensated AR remain asymptomatic for prolonged periods of time while the left ventricle gradually enlarges. Symptoms of heart failure, such as exertional dyspnea, orthopnea, and paroxysmal nocturnal dyspnea, usually develop gradually only after considerable ventricular hypertrophy and decompensation. Patients with severe AR may experience palpitations during emotional stress or exertion; an uncomfortable awareness of each heartbeat, especially at the ventricular apex; angina pectoris; nocturnal angina; or atypical chest pain syndromes, such as thoracic pain owing to pounding of the heart against the chest wall.[81]

Signs

Physical examination findings of AR vary with the chronicity of the disease process. Many of the classic findings of chronic AR are a result of the widened pulse pressure. They include a "water-hammer pulse" (Corrigan pulse), head bobbing with each heartbeat (De Musset sign), capillary pulsations in the lips and fingers (Quincke pulses), pulsus bisferiens, "pistol shot sounds" on auscultation of the femoral artery (Traube sign), pulsations of the uvula (Müller sign). Although interesting, these signs are not necessarily clinically useful. The classic auscultatory finding of AR is an immediate to early diastolic, blowing, decrescendo murmur. It is best heard with the diaphragm at the left sternal border while the patient is sitting, leaning forward, and holding respiration in deep exhalation. The murmur is often better heard along the right sternal border when AR is caused primarily by root disease.[82] When it is soft, isometric exercise, such as handgrip, can increase its intensity by increasing aortic diastolic pressure. In severe AR, the murmur may be holodiastolic. S_1 is usually soft because the mitral leaflets are close to each other at the onset of systole. S_2 is usually single because the AV does not close properly, or because LV ejection time is prolonged and P_2 is obscured by the early diastolic murmur. Other findings, if present, are associated with CHF, for example, rales, S3, etc.[81] As discussed, the pulse pressure in acute AR is not widened, hence many of the classic signs of chronic AR are not seen in the acute setting. Instead, signs of CHF predominate.

Electrocardiogram

The increased LV mass in chronic AR leads to left axis deviation and increased QRS complex amplitude. A strain pattern and reduction in the total QRS complex amplitude in patients with chronic severe AR is highly predictive of severe depression of EF resulting from inadequate hypertrophy.[83] Q waves in leads I, V1, and V3 through V6 are indicative of diastolic volume overload.[84] LV conduction defects occur late in the course and are usually associated with LV dysfunction. Overall, ECG is an inaccurate predictor of AR severity.

Roentgenogram

The chest radiograph typically shows a "normal"-sized heart with pulmonary edema, although there may be some enlargement of all cardiac chambers and the main pulmonary artery. The aorta may be dilated if aortic root disease is the cause of AR. There may be signs of pulmonary emboli in AR caused by endocarditis when there is concomitant tricuspid valve endocarditis.

Echocardiography

Echocardiography is the most useful diagnostic modality in both the initial diagnosis and continued monitoring of patients with AR. Transthoracic echocardiography (TTE) is the most commonly used imaging tool. TTE provides noninvasive assessment of the AV and aortic anatomy; the presence, severity, and etiology of regurgitation; and the size and function of the left ventricle. TEE is used when the patient's body habitus does not allow for adequate assessment with TTE and to evaluate the

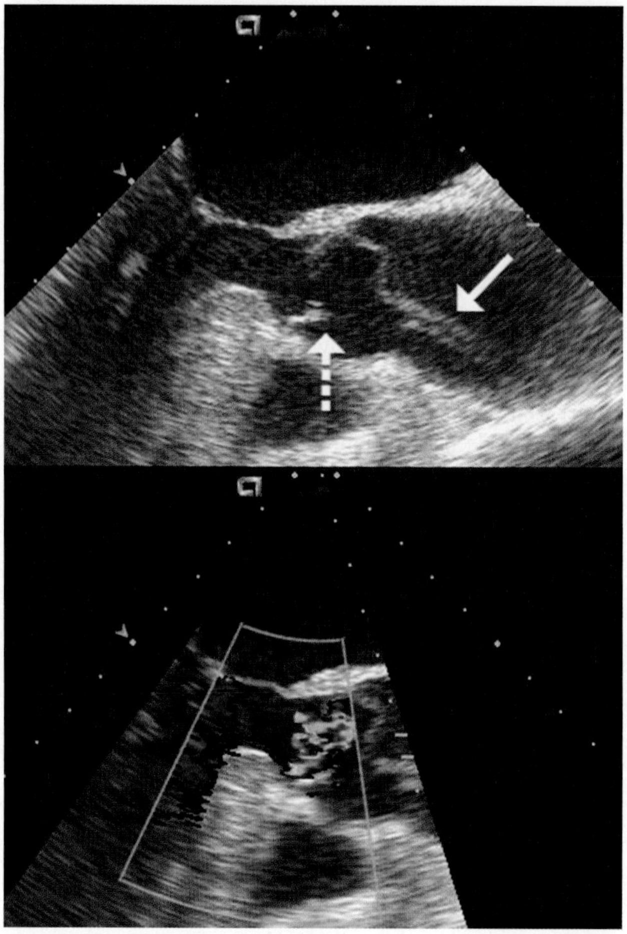

FIGURE 31-8 Transesophageal echocardiographic images of aortic regurgitation due to acute aortic dissection. (*Top*) Showing dilated annulus, prolapse of aortic valve leaflet (*dotted arrow*), and intimal flap (*solid arrow*). (*Bottom*) Color Doppler showing regurgitant flow.

AV and ascending aorta in patients with suspected aortic dissection (Fig. 31-8).

Two-dimensional (2D) echocardiography with Doppler color-flow mapping has been used routinely to assess the severity of AR.[85–87] The color-flow jets are typically composed of three components: (1) a proximal flow convergence zone (area of acceleration into the orifice); (2) the vena contracta (the narrowest and highest-velocity region of the jet); and (3) the distal jet itself in the LV cavity. Assessment of the severity of AR is determined qualitatively by jet width and vena contracta width, and quantitatively by regurgitant volume, regurgitant fraction, and regurgitant orifice area (Table 31-2). The regurgitant orifice area is calculated by dividing the regurgitant volume by the velocity time integral of the AR jet calculated by continuous wave Doppler.[88] Measurement of LV dimensions, such as end-systolic and end-diastolic volumes and wall thickness, are useful for determining LV changes and function. Additional echocardiographic findings in AR include premature closure of the mitral valve, diastolic fluttering of the anterior mitral leaflet from regurgitant flow, and less commonly, diastolic fluttering of the posterior mitral leaflet.[89]

TABLE 31-2 Classification of Aortic Regurgitation Severity

Indicator	Mild	Moderate	Severe
Angiographic grade	1+	2+	3-4+
Jet width	<25% LVOT	25–65% LVOT	>65% LVOT
Vena contracta width (cm)	<0.3	0.3–0.6	>0.6
Regurgitant volume (mL per beat)	<30	30–59	≥60
Regurgitant fraction (%)	<30	30–49	≥50
Regurgitant orifice area (cm²)	<0.10	0.10–0.29	≥0.30

Exercise Stress Testing

Exercise stress testing can provide valuable information in patients with AR, especially in those whose symptoms are equivocal or difficult to assess. In the management of AR, the presence of symptoms with exercise testing is equivalent to symptoms at rest because both circumstances warrant AVR.

Cardiac Catheterization

Cardiac catheterization is less frequently used to assess the severity of AR. It is most commonly used during preoperative assessment of coronary anatomy in patients requiring AV repair or replacement. The amount of regurgitant flow can be determined by calculating the angiographic stroke volume minus a measured fixed stroke volume. The difference between these two measured volumes divided by the angiographic stroke volume determines the regurgitant fraction. LVEDP is measured directly and EF is estimated roughly.

Computed Tomography

CT can be used to assess the severity of AR by measurement of the regurgitant orifice area, but currently the results are inferior to echocardiography.[90] Several studies have demonstrated the utility of CT to detect moderate and severe AR, but inaccuracies are seen with lesser degrees of AR.[91–93]

Magnetic Resonance Imaging

With the recent advancements in MRI technology, MRI cineangiography is able to provide some of the same information provided by TTE and TEE. MRI in some aspects provides superior resolution of the valves and better quantification of regurgitant flow and LVF. The regurgitant volume can be calculated by quantitative assessment, wherein aortic flow is subtracted from the ventricular stroke volume measured by the volumetric technique. It also can be assessed using flow mapping downstream from the AV by measuring the retrograde volume flow after valve closure. This method is more reproducible and is used more frequently for follow-up studies. However, MRI is costly, and expertise is not available in most centers. Future improvements in technology may reduce costs and increase its availability, thereby making it a standard imaging modality along with or in substitution for echocardiography.[94–96]

Management

Acute AR is treated by early AV repair or replacement, depending on the etiology. With inadequate time for the left ventricle to compensate by eccentric hypertrophy, progressive CHF, tachycardia, and diminished CO occur rapidly. Vasodilators and inotropic agents, which augment forward flow and reduce LVEDP, may be helpful to manage the patient temporarily before surgery.

Compensated chronic AR is well tolerated by most patients.[97–99] Current recommendations for the management of chronic AR depend on the presence of symptoms, LVF, and LV dimensions. Patients with symptoms or EFs less than or equal to 50% should undergo AV repair or replacement.[100] Surgery is currently not recommended for patients who are asymptomatic, even with severe chronic AR. However, these patients must have normal LVF and LV dimensions. In asymptomatic patients with normal LVF, it is reasonable to perform surgery with an LV end-diastolic dimension (LVEDD) approaching 75 mm or an LV end-systolic dimension (LVESD) approaching 55 mm.[100]

After surgery, LVEDV and LVEDP decrease significantly and with the decrease in preload, EF also decreases.[101] LV size and function eventually return to normal if the operation is timed correctly.[102–113] The best postoperative predictor of recovery in systolic function is reduction in LVEDD because the magnitude of reduction correlates well with the magnitude of increase in EF.[102] Importantly, 80% of the total reduction in LVEDD after AVR occurs within 10 to 14 days after surgery.[102,107,114] Additional changes postoperatively include regression of myocardial hypertrophy, normalization of mass-to-volume ratio, increase in diastolic coronary perfusion, and decrease in peak systolic wall stress.[102,114,115]

Despite surgery, LV dilation and/or impaired LVF may continue in some patients. The best predictors of persistent LV dilation are greater preoperative LVESD and end-diastolic radius to wall thickness ratio.[116,117] In addition to these measures, greater preoperative LVEDD and duration of LV dysfunction, and reduced EF and fractional shortening predict persistent LV dysfunction.[102,106,118–121]

Medical management with chronic vasodilator therapy is indicated in patients with severe AR who have symptoms or LV dysfunction, and are poor candidates for surgery. Vasodilator therapy may be beneficial in asymptomatic patients with severe AR, normal LVF, and LV dilation. Other than these instances, chronic therapy with vasodilators is not indicated in patients with AR.

In asymptomatic patients with normal LVF, the overall rate of progression to symptoms or LV dysfunction averages 4.5% per year and the mortality rate is 0.2% per year.[100] Predictors for the development of future symptoms, LV dysfunction, or death include age, LVESV, LVEDV, and EF during exercise.[97,122–125] Currently, there is insufficient evidence to determine if EF during exercise is a reliable predictor because exercise EF is dependent on too many factors, such as myocardial contractility,[126] severity of volume overload,[97,126–128] and exercise-induced changes in preload and PVR.[128]

REFERENCES

1. Anderson RH, Devine WA, Ho SY, Smith A, McKay R: The myth of the aortic annulus: the anatomy of the subaortic outflow tract. *Ann Thorac Surg* 1991; 52(3):640-646.
2. Broom ND: The Third George Swanson Christie memorial lecture. Connective tissue function and malfunction: a biomechanical perspective. *Pathology* 1988; 20(2):93-104.
3. Deck JD: Endothelial cell orientation on aortic valve leaflets. *Cardiovasc Res* 1986; 20(10):760-767.
4. Deck JD, Thubrikar MJ, Schneider PJ, Nolan SP: Structure, stress, and tissue repair in aortic valve leaflets. *Cardiovasc Res* 1988; 22(1):7-16.
5. Thubrikar M, Harry R, Nolan SP: Normal aortic valve function in dogs. *Am J Cardiol* 1977; 40(4):563-568.
6. Gnyaneshwar R, Kumar RK, Balakrishnan KR: Dynamic analysis of the aortic valve using a finite element model. *Ann Thorac Surg* 2002; 73(4): 1122-1129.
7. Zimmerman J: The functional and surgical anatomy of the aortic valve. *Isr J Med Sci* 1969; 5(4):862-866.
8. Mercer JL: The movements of the dog's aortic valve studied by high speed cineangiography. *Br J Radiol* 1973; 46(545):344-349.
9. Robicsek F: Leonardo da Vinci and the sinuses of Valsalva. *Ann Thorac Surg* 1991; 52(2):328-335.
10. Bellhouse BJ, Reid KG: Fluid mechanics of the aortic valve. *Br Heart J* 1969; 31(3):391.
11. Sabbah HN, Stein PD: Investigation of the theory and mechanism of the origin of the second heart sound. *Circ Res* 1976; 39(6):874-882.
12. Nkomo VT, Gardin JM, Skelton TN, Gottdiener JS, Scott CG, et al: Burden of valvular heart diseases: a population-based study. *Lancet* 2006; 368(9540):1005-1011.
13. Otto CM, Lind BK, Kitzman DW, Gersh BJ, Siscovick DS: Association of aortic-valve sclerosis with cardiovascular mortality and morbidity in the elderly. *NEJM* 1999; 341(3):142-147.
14. Ghaisas NK, Foley JB, O'Briain DS, Crean P, Kelleher D, et al: Adhesion molecules in nonrheumatic aortic valve disease: endothelial expression, serum levels and effects of valve replacement. *J Am Coll Cardiol* 2000; 36(7):2257-2262.
15. O'Brien KD, Shavelle DM, Caulfield MT, McDonald TO, Olin-Lewis K, et al: Association of angiotensin-converting enzyme with low-density lipoprotein in aortic valvular lesions and in human plasma. *Circulation* 2002; 106(17):2224-2230.
16. Olsson M, Thyberg J, Nilsson J: Presence of oxidized low density lipoprotein in nonrheumatic stenotic aortic valves. *Arterioscleros Thromb Vasc Biol* 1999; 19(5):1218-1222.
17. Otto CM, Kuusisto J, Reichenbach DD, Gown AM, O'Brien KD: Characterization of the early lesion of 'degenerative' valvular aortic stenosis. Histological and immunohistochemical studies. *Circulation* 1994; 90(2): 844-853.
18. Rajamannan NM, Gersh B, Bonow RO: Calcific aortic stenosis: from bench to the bedside—emerging clinical and cellular concepts. *Heart Br Card Soc* 2003; 89(7):801-805.
19. Hultgren HN: Osteitis deformans (Paget's disease) and calcific disease of the heart valves. *Am J Cardiol* 1998; 81(12):1461-1464.
20. Hangaishi M, Taguchi J, Ikari Y, Ohno M, Kurokawa K, et al: Aortic valve stenosis in alkaptonuria. Images in cardiovascular medicine. *Circulation* 1998; 98(11):1148-1149.
21. Fedak PW, Verma S, David TE, Leask RL, Weisel RD, et al: Clinical and pathophysiological implications of a bicuspid aortic valve. *Circulation* 2002; 106(8):900-904.
22. Fielitz J, Hein S, Mitrovic V, Pregla R, Zurbrugg HR, et al: Activation of the cardiac renin-angiotensin system and increased myocardial collagen expression in human aortic valve disease. *J Am Coll Cardiol* 2001; 37(5):1443-1449.
23. Roberts WC: Anatomically isolated aortic valvular disease. The case against its being of rheumatic etiology. *Am J Med* 1970; 49(2):151-159.
24. Passik CS, Ackermann DM, Pluth JR, Edwards WD: Temporal changes in the causes of aortic stenosis: a surgical pathologic study of 646 cases. *Mayo Clin Proc* 1987; 62(2):119-123.
25. Roberts WC, Ko JM: Frequency by decades of unicuspid, bicuspid, and tricuspid aortic valves in adults having isolated aortic valve replacement for aortic stenosis, with or without associated aortic regurgitation. *Circulation* 2005; 111(7):920-925.

26. Hess OM, Ritter M, Schneider J, Grimm J, Turina M, et al: Diastolic stiffness and myocardial structure in aortic valve disease before and after valve replacement. *Circulation* 1984; 69(5):855-865.
27. Marcus ML, Doty DB, Hiratzka LF, Wright CB, Eastham CL: Decreased coronary reserve: a mechanism for angina pectoris in patients with aortic stenosis and normal coronary arteries. *NEJM* 1982; 307(22):1362-1366.
28. Mihaljevic T, Nowicki ER, Rajeswaran J, Blackstone EH, Lagazzi L, et al: Survival after valve replacement for aortic stenosis: implications for decision making. *J Thorac Cardiovasc Surg* 2008; 135(6):1270-1278; discussion 1278-1279.
29. Walther T, Schubert A, Falk V, Binner C, Walther C, et al: Left ventricular reverse remodeling after surgical therapy for aortic stenosis: correlation to Renin-Angiotensin system gene expression. *Circulation* 2002; 106(12 Suppl 1): I23-26.
30. Yussman MG, Toyokawa T, Odley A, Lynch RA, Wu G, et al: Mitochondrial death protein Nix is induced in cardiac hypertrophy and triggers apoptotic cardiomyopathy. *Nat med* 2002; 8(7):725-730.
31. Pellikka PA, Nishimura RA, Bailey KR, Tajik AJ: The natural history of adults with asymptomatic, hemodynamically significant aortic stenosis. *J Am Coll Cardiol* 1990; 15(5):1012-1017.
32. Tardif JC, Rodrigues AG, Hardy JF, Leclerc Y, Petitclerc R, et al: Simultaneous determination of aortic valve area by the Gorlin formula and by transesophageal echocardiography under different transvalvular flow conditions. Evidence that anatomic aortic valve area does not change with variations in flow in aortic stenosis. *J Am Coll Cardiol* 1997; 29(6): 1296-1302.
33. Blumberg FC, Pfeifer M, Holmer SR, Kromer EP, Riegger GA, et al: Transgastric Doppler echocardiographic assessment of the severity of aortic stenosis using multiplane transesophageal echocardiography. *Am J Cardiol* 1997; 79(9):1273-1275.
34. Ross J Jr, Braunwald E: Aortic stenosis. *Circulation* 1968; 38(1 Suppl): 61-67.
35. Schwartz LS, Goldfischer J, Sprague GJ, Schwartz SP: Syncope and sudden death in aortic stenosis. *Am J Cardiol* 1969; 23(5):647-658.
36. Otto CM, Burwash IG, Legget ME, Munt BI, Fujioka M, et al: Prospective study of asymptomatic valvular aortic stenosis. Clinical, echocardiographic, and exercise predictors of outcome. *Circulation* 1997; 95(9):2262-2270.
37. Vincentelli A, Susen S, Le Tourneau T, Six I, Fabre O, et al: Acquired von Willebrand syndrome in aortic stenosis. *NEJM* 2003; 349(4):343-349.
38. Pellikka PA, Sarano ME, Nishimura RA, Malouf JF, Bailey KR, et al: Outcome of 622 adults with asymptomatic, hemodynamically significant aortic stenosis during prolonged follow-up. *Circulation* 2005; 111(24): 3290-3295.
39. Selzer A: Changing aspects of the natural history of valvular aortic stenosis. *NEJM* 1987; 317(2):91-98.
40. Gjertsson P, Caidahl K, Farasati M, Oden A, Bech-Hanssen O: Preoperative moderate to severe diastolic dysfunction: a novel Doppler echocardiographic long-term prognostic factor in patients with severe aortic stenosis. *J Thorac Cardiovasc Surg* 2005; 129(4):890-896.
41. Maurer MS, Spevack D, Burkhoff D, Kronzon I: Diastolic dysfunction: can it be diagnosed by Doppler echocardiography? *J Am Coll Cardiol* 2004; 44(8):1543-1549.
42. Agricola E, Oppizzi M, Pisani M, Margonato A: Stress echocardiography in heart failure. *Cardiovasc Ultrasound* 2004; 2:11.
43. Bonow RO, Carabello BA, Chatterjee K, de Leon AC Jr, Faxon DP, et al: 2008 focused update incorporated into the ACC/AHA 2006 guidelines for the management of patients with valvular heart disease: a report of the American College of Cardiology/American Heart Association Task Force on Practice Guidelines (Writing Committee to revise the 1998 guidelines for the management of patients with valvular heart disease). Endorsed by the Society of Cardiovascular Anesthesiologists, Society for Cardiovascular Angiography and Interventions, and Society of Thoracic Surgeons. *J Am Coll Cardiol* 2008; 52(13):e1-142.
44. Amato MC, Moffa PJ, Werner KE, Ramires JA: Treatment decision in asymptomatic aortic valve stenosis: role of exercise testing. *Heart Br Card Soc* 2001; 86(4):381-386.
45. Das P, Rimington H, Chambers J: Exercise testing to stratify risk in aortic stenosis. *Eur Heart J* 2005; 26(13):1309-1313.
46. deFilippi CR, Willett DL, Brickner ME, Appleton CP, Yancy CW, et al: Usefulness of dobutamine echocardiography in distinguishing severe from nonsevere valvular aortic stenosis in patients with depressed left ventricular function and low transvalvular gradients. *Am J Cardiol* 1995; 75(2):191-194.
47. Monin JL, Quere JP, Monchi M, Petit H, Baleynaud S, et al: Low-gradient aortic stenosis: operative risk stratification and predictors for long-term outcome: a multicenter study using dobutamine stress hemodynamics. *Circulation* 2003; 108(3):319-324.
48. Melina G, Scott MJ, Cunanan CM, Rubens MB, Yacoub MH: In-vitro verification of the electron beam tomography method for measurement of heart valve calcification. *J Heart Valve Dis* 2002; 11(3):402-407; discussion 408.
49. Alkadhi H, Wildermuth S, Plass A, Bettex D, Baumert B, et al: Aortic stenosis: comparative evaluation of 16-detector row CT and echocardiography. *Radiology* 2006; 240(1):47-55.
50. Cawley PJ, Maki JH, Otto CM: Cardiovascular magnetic resonance imaging for valvular heart disease: technique and validation. *Circulation* 2009; 119(3):468-478.
51. Cranney GB, Lotan CS, Dean L, Baxley W, Bouchard A, et al: Left ventricular volume measurement using cardiac axis nuclear magnetic resonance imaging. Validation by calibrated ventricular angiography. *Circulation* 1990; 82(1):154-163.
52. Caruthers SD, Lin SJ, Brown P, Watkins MP, Williams TA, et al: Practical value of cardiac magnetic resonance imaging for clinical quantification of aortic valve stenosis: comparison with echocardiography. *Circulation* 2003; 108(18):2236-2243.
53. John AS, Dill T, Brandt RR, Rau M, Ricken W, et al: Magnetic resonance to assess the aortic valve area in aortic stenosis: how does it compare to current diagnostic standards? *J Am Coll Cardiol* 2003; 42(3):519-526.
54. Beyerbacht HP, Lamb HJ, van Der Laarse A, Vliegen HW, Leujes F, et al: Aortic valve replacement in patients with aortic valve stenosis improves myocardial metabolism and diastolic function. *Radiology* 2001; 219(3): 637-643.
55. Cowell SJ, Newby DE, Prescott RJ, Bloomfield P, Reid J, et al: A randomized trial of intensive lipid-lowering therapy in calcific aortic stenosis. *NEJM* 2005; 352(23):2389-2397.
56. Rossebo AB, Pedersen TR, Boman K, Brudi P, Chambers JB, et al: Intensive lipid lowering with simvastatin and ezetimibe in aortic stenosis. *NEJM* 2008; 359(13):1343-1356.
57. Craver JM: Aortic valve debridement by ultrasonic surgical aspirator: a word of caution. *Ann Thorac Surg* 1990; 49(5):746-752; discussion 752-743.
58. Lindblom D, Lindblom U, Qvist J, Lundstrom H: Long-term relative survival rates after heart valve replacement. *J Am Coll Cardiol* 1990; 15(3): 566-573.
59. Gillinov AM, Lytle BW, Hoang V, Cosgrove DM, Banbury MK, et al: The atherosclerotic aorta at aortic valve replacement: surgical strategies and results. *J Thorac Cardiovasc Surg* 2000; 120(5):957-963.
60. Kapadia SR, Goel SS, Svensson L, Roselli E, Savage RM, et al: Characterization and outcome of patients with severe symptomatic aortic stenosis referred for percutaneous aortic valve replacement. *J Thorac Cardiovasc Surg* 2009; 137(6):1430-1435.
61. Rosenhek R, Binder T, Porenta G, Lang I, Christ G, et al: Predictors of outcome in severe, asymptomatic aortic stenosis. *NEJM* 2000; 343(9):611-617.
62. Pai RG, Kapoor N, Bansal RC, Varadarajan P: Malignant natural history of asymptomatic severe aortic stenosis: benefit of aortic valve replacement. *Ann Thorac Surg* 2006; 82(6):2116-2122.
63. Varadarajan P, Kapoor N, Bansal RC, Pai RG: Survival in elderly patients with severe aortic stenosis is dramatically improved by aortic valve replacement: results from a cohort of 277 patients aged > or = 80 years. *Eur J Cardiothoracic Surg* 2006; 30(5):722-727.
64. Carabello BA: Progress in mitral and aortic regurgitation. *Prog Cardiovasc Dis* 2001; 43(6):457-475.
65. Fedak PW, Verma S, David TE, Leask RL, Weisel RD, et al: Clinical and pathophysiological implications of a bicuspid aortic valve. *Circulation* 2002; 106(8):900-904.
66. Maurer G: Aortic regurgitation. *Heart* 2006; 92(7):994-1000.
67. Tonnemacher D, Reid C, Kawanishi D, Cummings T, Chandrasoma P, et al: Frequency of myxomatous degeneration of the aortic valve as a cause of isolated aortic regurgitation severe enough to warrant aortic valve replacement. *Am J Cardiol* 1987; 60(14):1194-1196.
68. Carter JB, Sethi S, Lee GB, Edwards JE: Prolapse of semilunar cusps as causes of aortic insufficiency. *Circulation* 1971; 43(6):922-932.
69. Emanuel R, Ng RA, Marcomichelakis J, Moores EC, Jefferson KE, et al: Formes frustes of Marfan's syndrome presenting with severe aortic regurgitation. Clinicogenetic study of 18 families. *Br Heart J* 1977; 39(2):190-197.
70. Heppner RL, Babitt HI, Bianchine JW, Warbasse JR: Aortic regurgitation and aneurysm of sinus of Valsalva associated with osteogenesis imperfecta. *Am J Cardiol* 1973; 31(5):654-657.
71. Roberts WC: Aortic dissection: anatomy, consequences, and causes. *Am Heart J* 1981; 101(2):195-214.
72. Roldan CA: Valvular disease associated with systemic illness. *Cardiol Clin* 1998; 16(3):531-550.
73. Roldan CA, Chavez J, Wiest PW, Qualls CR, Crawford MH: Aortic root disease and valve disease associated with ankylosing spondylitis. *J Am Coll Cardiol* 1998; 32(5):1397-1404.

74. Roberts WC, Ko JM, Moore TR, Jones WH 3rd: Causes of pure aortic regurgitation in patients having isolated aortic valve replacement at a single US tertiary hospital (1993 to 2005). *Circulation* 2006; 114(5):422-429.
75. Rahimtoola SH: Recognition and management of acute aortic regurgitation. *Heart Dis Stroke* 1993; 2(3):217-221.
76. Reimold SC, Maier SE, Fleischmann KE, Khatri M, Piwnica-Worms D, et al: Dynamic nature of the aortic regurgitant orifice area during diastole in patients with chronic aortic regurgitation. *Circulation* 1994; 89(5): 2085-2092.
77. Grossman W, Jones D, McLaurin LP: Wall stress and patterns of hypertrophy in the human left ventricle. *J Clin Invest* 1975; 56(1):56-64.
78. Slordahl SA, Piene H: Haemodynamic effects of arterial compliance, total peripheral resistance, and glyceryl trinitrate on regurgitant volume in aortic regurgitation. *Cardiovasc Res* 1991; 25(10):869-874.
79. Gaasch WH: Left ventricular radius to wall thickness ratio. *Am J Cardiol* 1979; 43(6):1189-1194.
80. Ross J Jr: Afterload mismatch in aortic and mitral valve disease: implications for surgical therapy. *J Am Coll Cardiol* 1985; 5(4):811-826.
81. DeGowin RL, DeGowin EL, Brown DD, Christensen J: *DeGowin & DeGowin's Diagnostic Examination*. New York: McGraw-Hill; 1994.
82. Bonow RO. *Valvular Heart Disease*, 3rd ed. Philadelphia: Lippincott Williams & Wilkins; 2000.
83. Scognamiglio R, Fasoli G, Bruni A, Dalla-Volta S: Observations on the capability of the electrocardiogram to detect left ventricular function in chronic severe aortic regurgitation. *Eur Heart J* 1988; 9(1):54-60.
84. Schamroth L, Schamroth CL, Sareli P, Hummel D: Electrocardiographic differentiation of the causes of left ventricular diastolic overload. *Chest* 1986; 89(1):95-99.
85. Aurigemma G, Whitfield S, Sweeney A, Fox M, Weiner B: Color Doppler mapping of aortic regurgitation in aortic stenosis: comparison with angiography. *Cardiology* 1992; 81(4-5):251-257.
86. Bouchard A, Yock P, Schiller NB, Blumlein S, Botvinick EH, et al: Value of color Doppler estimation of regurgitant volume in patients with chronic aortic insufficiency. *Am Heart J* 1989; 117(5):1099-1105.
87. Enriquez-Sarano M, Bailey KR, Seward JB, Tajik AJ, Krohn MJ, et al: Quantitative Doppler assessment of valvular regurgitation. *Circulation* 1993; 87(3):841-848.
88. Perry GJ, Helmcke F, Nanda NC, Byard C, Soto B: Evaluation of aortic insufficiency by Doppler color flow mapping. *J Am Coll Cardiol* 1987; 9(4):952-959.
89. Chia BL: Mitral valve fluttering in aortic insufficiency. *J Clin Ultrasound* 1981; 9(4):198-200.
90. LaBounty TM, Glasofer S, Devereux RB, Lin FY, Weinsaft JW, et al: Comparison of cardiac computed tomographic angiography to transesophageal echocardiography for evaluation of patients with native valvular heart disease. *Am J Cardiol* 2009; 104(10):1421-1428.
91. Feuchtner GM, Dichtl W, Muller S, Jodocy D, Schachner T, et al: 64-MDCT for diagnosis of aortic regurgitation in patients referred to CT coronary angiography. *Am J Roentgenol* 2008; 191(1):W1-7.
92. Feuchtner GM, Dichtl W, Schachner T, Muller S, Mallouhi A, et al: Diagnostic performance of MDCT for detecting aortic valve regurgitation. *Am J Roentgenol* 2006; 186(6):1676-1681.
93. Jassal DS, Shapiro MD, Neilan TG, Chaithiraphan V, Ferencik M, et al: 64-slice multidetector computed tomography (MDCT) for detection of aortic regurgitation and quantification of severity. *Invest Radiol* 2007; 42(7):507-512.
94. Benjelloun H, Cranney GB, Kirk KA, Blackwell GG, Lotan CS, et al: Interstudy reproducibility of biplane cine nuclear magnetic resonance measurements of left ventricular function. *Am J Cardiol* 1991; 67(16): 1413-1420.
95. Cranney GB, Lotan CS, Dean L, Baxley W, Bouchard A, et al: Left ventricular volume measurement using cardiac axis nuclear magnetic resonance imaging. Validation by calibrated ventricular angiography. *Circulation* 1990; 82(1):154-163.
96. Dulce MC, Mostbeck GH, O'Sullivan M, Cheitlin M, Caputo GR, et al: Severity of aortic regurgitation: interstudy reproducibility of measurements with velocity-encoded cine MR imaging. *Radiology* 1992; 185(1):235-240.
97. Bonow RO, Lakatos E, Maron BJ, Epstein SE: Serial long-term assessment of the natural history of asymptomatic patients with chronic aortic regurgitation and normal left ventricular systolic function. *Circulation* 1991; 84(4):1625-1635.
98. Ishii K, Hirota Y, Suwa M, Kita Y, Onaka H, et al: Natural history and left ventricular response in chronic aortic regurgitation. *Am J Cardiol* 1996; 78(3):357-361.
99. Tornos MP, Olona M, Permanyer-Miralda G, Herrejon MP, Camprecios M, et al: Clinical outcome of severe asymptomatic chronic aortic regurgitation: a long-term prospective follow-up study. *Am Heart J* 1995; 130(2):333-339.
100. Bonow RO, Carabello BA, Chatterjee K, de Leon AC Jr, Faxon DP, et al: 2008 Focused update incorporated into the ACC/AHA 2006 guidelines for the management of patients with valvular heart disease: a report of the American College of Cardiology/American Heart Association Task Force on Practice Guidelines (Writing Committee to Revise the 1998 Guidelines for the Management of Patients With Valvular Heart Disease): endorsed by the Society of Cardiovascular Anesthesiologists, Society for Cardiovascular Angiography and Interventions, and Society of Thoracic Surgeons. *Circulation* 2008; 118(15):e523-661.
101. Boucher CA, Bingham JB, Osbakken MD, Okada RD, Strauss HW, et al: Early changes in left ventricular size and function after correction of left ventricular volume overload. *Am J Cardiol* 1981; 47(5):991-1004.
102. Bonow RO, Dodd JT, Maron BJ, O'Gara PT, White GG, et al: Long-term serial changes in left ventricular function and reversal of ventricular dilatation after valve replacement for chronic aortic regurgitation. *Circulation* 1988; 78(5 Pt 1):1108-1120.
103. Bonow RO, Rosing DR, Maron BJ, McIntosh CL, Jones M, et al: Reversal of left ventricular dysfunction after aortic valve replacement for chronic aortic regurgitation: influence of duration of preoperative left ventricular dysfunction. *Circulation* 1984; 70(4):570-579.
104. Borer JS, Herrold EM, Hochreiter C, Roman M, Supino P, et al: Natural history of left ventricular performance at rest and during exercise after aortic valve replacement for aortic regurgitation. *Circulation* 1991; 84(5 Suppl): III133-139.
105. Borer JS, Rosing DR, Kent KM, Bacharach SL, Green MV, et al: Left ventricular function at rest and during exercise after aortic valve replacement in patients with aortic regurgitation. *Am J Cardiol* 1979; 44(7):1297-1305.
106. Carabello BA, Usher BW, Hendrix GH, Assey ME, Crawford FA, et al: Predictors of outcome for aortic valve replacement in patients with aortic regurgitation and left ventricular dysfunction: a change in the measuring stick. *J Am Coll Cardiol* 1987; 10(5):991-997.
107. Carroll JD, Gaasch WH, Zile MR, Levine HJ: Serial changes in left ventricular function after correction of chronic aortic regurgitation. Dependence on early changes in preload and subsequent regression of hypertrophy. *Am J Cardiol* 1983; 51(3):476-482.
108. Clark DG, McAnulty JH, Rahimtoola SH: Valve replacement in aortic insufficiency with left ventricular dysfunction. *Circulation* 1980; 61(2): 411-421.
109. Fioretti P, Roelandt J, Sclavo M, Domenicucci S, Haalebos M, et al: Postoperative regression of left ventricular dimensions in aortic insufficiency: a long-term echocardiographic study. *J Am Coll Cardiol* 1985; 5(4):856-861.
110. Gaasch WH, Andrias CW, Levine HJ: Chronic aortic regurgitation: the effect of aortic valve replacement on left ventricular volume, mass and function. *Circulation* 1978; 58(5):825-836.
111. Schwarz F, Flameng W, Langebartels F, Sesto M, Walter P, et al: Impaired left ventricular function in chronic aortic valve disease: survival and function after replacement by Bjork-Shiley prosthesis. *Circulation* 1979; 60(1):48-58.
112. Taniguchi K, Nakano S, Hirose H, Matsuda H, Shirakura R, et al: Preoperative left ventricular function: minimal requirement for successful late results of valve replacement for aortic regurgitation. *J Am Coll Cardiol* 1987; 10(3):510-518.
113. Toussaint C, Cribier A, Cazor JL, Soyer R, Letac B: Hemodynamic and angiographic evaluation of aortic regurgitation 8 and 27 months after aortic valve replacement. *Circulation* 1981; 64(3):456-463.
114. Schuler G, Peterson KL, Johnson AD, Francis G, Ashburn W, et al: Serial noninvasive assessment of left ventricular hypertrophy and function after surgical correction of aortic regurgitation. *Am J Cardiol* 1979; 44(4):585-594.
115. Fujiwara T, Nogami A, Masaki H, Yamane H, Kanazawa S, et al: Coronary flow characteristics of left coronary artery in aortic regurgitation before and after aortic valve replacement. *Ann Thorac Surg* 1988; 46(1):79-84.
116. Gaasch WH, Carroll JD, Levine HJ, Criscitiello MG: Chronic aortic regurgitation: prognostic value of left ventricular end-systolic dimension and end-diastolic radius/thickness ratio. *J Am Coll Cardiol* 1983; 1(3): 775-782.
117. Kumpuris AG, Quinones MA, Waggoner AD, Kanon DJ, Nelson JG, et al: Importance of preoperative hypertrophy, wall stress and end-systolic dimension as echocardiographic predictors of normalization of left ventricular dilatation after valve replacement in chronic aortic insufficiency. *Am J Cardiol* 1982; 49(5):1091-1100.
118. Bonow RO, Picone AL, McIntosh CL, Jones M, Rosing DR, et al: Survival and functional results after valve replacement for aortic regurgitation from 1976 to 1983: impact of preoperative left ventricular function. *Circulation* 1985; 72(6):1244-1256.

119. Fioretti P, Roelandt J, Bos RJ, Meltzer RS, van Hoogenhuijze D, et al: Echocardiography in chronic aortic insufficiency. Is valve replacement too late when left ventricular end-systolic dimension reaches 55 mm? *Circulation* 1983; 67(1):216-221.
120. Michel PL, Iung B, Abou Jaoude S, Cormier B, Porte JM, et al: The effect of left ventricular systolic function on long term survival in mitral and aortic regurgitation. *J Heart Valve Dis* 1995; 4(Suppl 2):S160-168; discussion S168-169.
121. Stone PH, Clark RD, Goldschlager N, Selzer A, Cohn K: Determinants of prognosis of patients with aortic regurgitation who undergo aortic valve replacement. *J Am Coll Cardiol* 1984; 3(5):1118-1126.
122. Borer JS, Hochreiter C, Herrold EM, Supino P, Aschermann M, et al: Prediction of indications for valve replacement among asymptomatic or minimally symptomatic patients with chronic aortic regurgitation and normal left ventricular performance. *Circulation* 1998; 97(6):525-534.
123. Scognamiglio R, Rahimtoola SH, Fasoli G, Nistri S, Dalla Volta S: Nifedipine in asymptomatic patients with severe aortic regurgitation and normal left ventricular function. *NEJM* 1994; 331(11):689-694.
124. Siemienczuk D, Greenberg B, Morris C, Massie B, Wilson RA, et al: Chronic aortic insufficiency: factors associated with progression to aortic valve replacement. *Ann Intern Med* 1989; 110(8):587-592.
125. Tarasoutchi F, Grinberg M, Spina GS, Sampaio RO, Cardoso LF, et al: Ten-year clinical laboratory follow-up after application of a symptom-based therapeutic strategy to patients with severe chronic aortic regurgitation of predominant rheumatic etiology. *J Am Coll Cardiol* 2003; 41(8): 1316-1324.
126. Shen WF, Roubin GS, Choong CY, Hutton BF, Harris PJ, et al: Evaluation of relationship between myocardial contractile state and left ventricular function in patients with aortic regurgitation. *Circulation* 1985; 71(1):31-38.
127. Greenberg B, Massie B, Bristow JD, Cheitlin M, Siemienczuk D, et al: Long-term vasodilator therapy of chronic aortic insufficiency. A randomized double-blinded, placebo-controlled clinical trial. *Circulation* 1988; 78(1):92-103.
128. Kawanishi DT, McKay CR, Chandraratna PA, Nanna M, Reid CL, et al: Cardiovascular response to dynamic exercise in patients with chronic symptomatic mild-to-moderate and severe aortic regurgitation. *Circulation* 1986; 73(1):62-72.

CHAPTER 32

Aortic Valve Replacement with a Mechanical Cardiac Valve Prosthesis

Robert W. Emery
Ann M. Emery
Jan Hommerding
Goya V. Raikar

INTRODUCTION

In 1931, Paul Dudley White stated, "There is no treatment for aortic stenosis." Even today the medical therapy of aortic stenosis has not significantly advanced (Fig. 32-1).[1] Conversely, patients may tolerate aortic insufficiency for many years, but as the ventricle starts to dilate, a progressive downhill course begins and early operation is warranted.[2] Definitive therapy for aortic valve disease was unavailable until the advent of cardiopulmonary bypass. Innovative cardiovascular surgeons then began to develop cardiac valve prostheses. Over the subsequent 50 years[3] the variety of prostheses that have become available for use have expanded greatly. Available aortic valve substitutes include mechanical valve prostheses, stented biologic valve prostheses, stentless biologic valve prostheses, human homograft tissue (both as isolated valve replacement and aortic root replacement), percutaneous or transapical biologic valves and a combination of a biologic valve using a pulmonary autograft, and pulmonary outflow tract replacement with heterograft prostheses (Ross procedure). This chapter focuses on the use of mechanical valve replacement in the aortic position.

HISTORY

In 1952, Hufnagel used an aortic valve ball and cage prosthesis heterotopically in the descending thoracic aorta to treat aortic insufficiency.[4] After the advent of cardiopulmonary bypass, initial attempts at aortic valve replacement (AVR) consisted of replacement of the individual aortic cusps with Ivalon gussets sewn to the annulus. When successful, these prostheses often calcified and results were short lived. Shortly thereafter, surgical pioneers Starr, Braunwald, and Harkin began replacement of the aortic valve in the orthotopic position. First-generation aortic valve prostheses, the ball and cage, became the standard for AVR for more than a decade (Fig. 32-2). Many of these prostheses have remained durable for up to 40 years.[5,6] Multiple modifications ensued, including changing the material of the ball from silastic to stellite, changes in the shape of the cage, depression of the ball occluder, the addition of cloth coating to the sewing ring and the cage, and changes in the sewing ring itself. These valves, however, required intense anticoagulation.[7] Hemodynamic performance was compromised because there were three areas of potential outflow obstruction: (1) the annular size of the sewing ring (the effective orifice area of the valve); (2) the distance between the cage and the walls of the ascending aorta (particularly in the small aortic root); and (3) obstruction to outflow by the ball itself distal to the tissue annulus. Flow patterns were also abnormal (Fig. 32-3). These problems led to the development of the next generation of aortic valve prostheses—the tilting disc valve. Innovators such as Björk, Hall, Kaster, and Lillehei developed three models of tilting disc prostheses that became the second generation of commonly implanted aortic valve replacement devices between 1968 and 1980. The low-profile configuration simplified surgical implantation (Fig. 32-4). Problems with the tilting disc valve included stasis and eddy current formation at the minor flow orifice (see Fig. 32-3), and sticking or embolization of the leaflet, the latter leading to discontinuation of the Björk prosthesis in spite of otherwise good

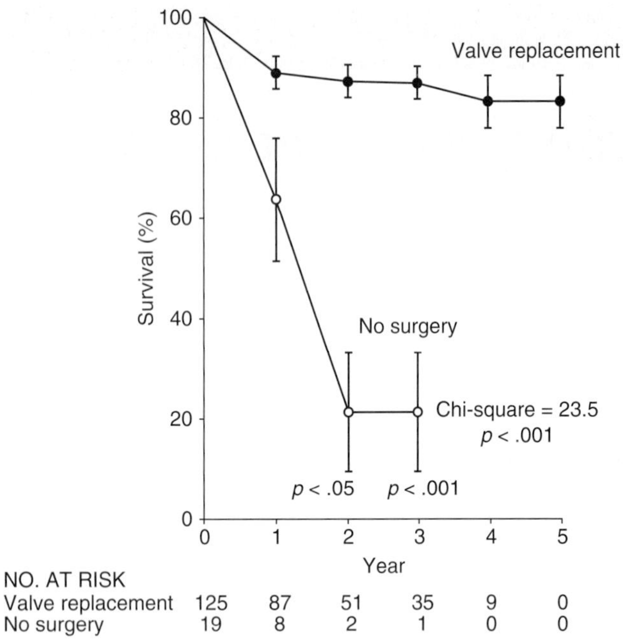

FIGURE 32-1 Survival of patients having aortic valve replacement compared to those not having valve replacement. (*Reproduced with permission from Carabello BA: Clinical practice. Aortic stenosis. NEJM 2002; 346:677.*)

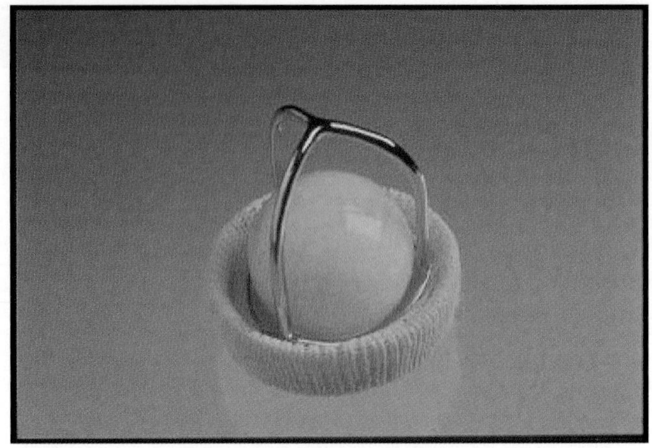

FIGURE 32-2 Prototype model of a ball and cage valve, an early Starr-Edwards model.

long-term results.[8] The Lillehei-Kaster prosthesis has evolved into the Omniscience valve. The Medtronic Hall valve, the third tilting disc prosthesis, now discontinued (Fig. 32-5).

Kalke and Lillehei developed the first rigid bileaflet valve, but it had very limited clinical use. In 1977, the St. Jude Medical (SJM) prosthesis was developed and implanted by Nicoloff and associates (Fig. 32-6).[3,9] Over the following

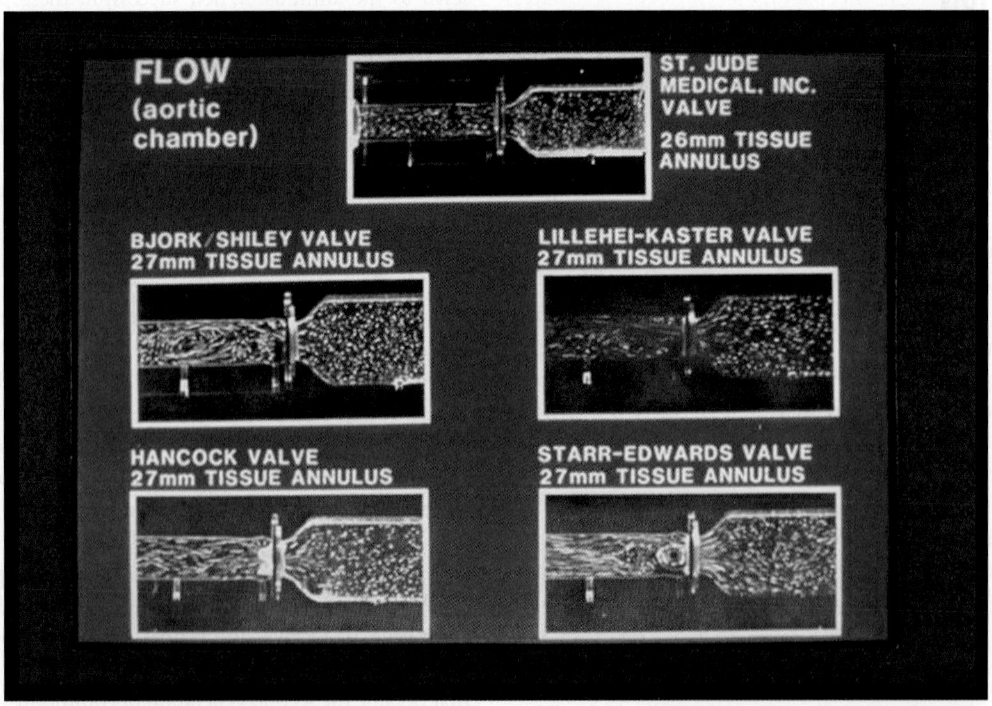

FIGURE 32-3 Prosthetic valve flow patterns using the Weiting CBA-77-03 pulse duplicator with high-speed photography and resin particles. Note the laminar flow with the bileaflet aortic valve as opposed to other clinically available prostheses and the flow similarity between the bileaflet valve and the tissue valve in the lower left corner. Tilting disk valves show directional flow, stasis at the minor flow orifice, and eddy current formation distally. The ball valve demonstrates stasis beyond the ball and eddy current formation around the ball itself. Note that the ball is obstructive to outflow, as is the proximity of the ball cage to the walls of the outflow chamber. (*Reproduced with permission from Emery RW, Nicoloff DM: The St. Jude Medical cardiac valve prosthesis: in vitro studies. J Thorac Cardiovasc Surg 1979; 78:269.*)

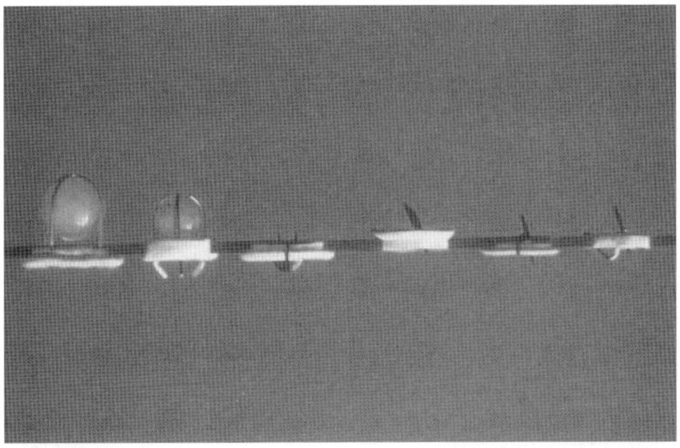

FIGURE 32-4 Low-profile prostheses simplify the surgical implant. The lowest profile is that of the bileaflet valve, and orientation of the leaflets is most commonly not necessary, as compared with tilting disc prostheses, for which the major flow orifice should be directed along the greater curvature of the aorta.

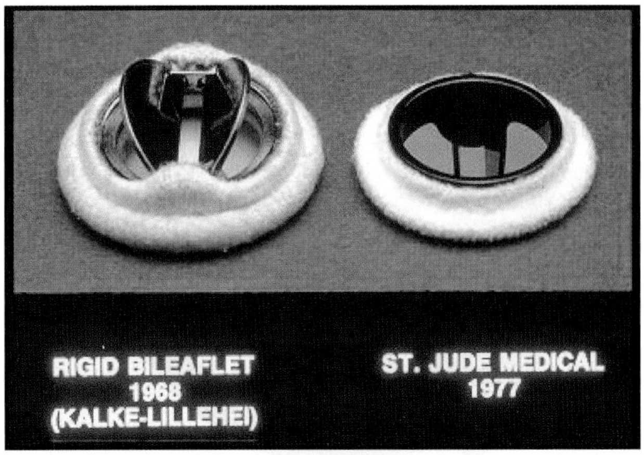

FIGURE 32-6 The original Kalke-Lillehei bileaflet valve as compared to the St. Jude Medical valve introduced nearly a decade later.

decades, the dramatic step of a bileaflet prosthesis nearly obviated the use of all other kinds of mechanical prosthetic valves in the United States and to a large extent elsewhere. The SJM valve demonstrated low aortic gradients, minimal aortic insufficiency, and low rates of thromboembolism (TE) (Fig. 32-7).[9–11] Anticoagulation continued to be necessary, but to a lesser extent than with previous design models.[12] Because of the low-profile design and lesser need for orientation, surgical implant was further simplified. After the introduction of the SJM valve, several other third-generation models of bileaflet prostheses were introduced, including the Sulzer Carbomedics valve (Sorin S.p.A., Milan, Italy) (Fig. 32-8), the ATS Medical prosthesis

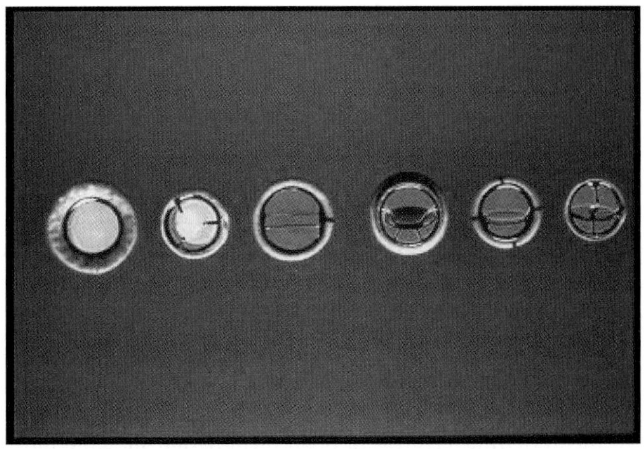

FIGURE 32-7 The increased flow orifice of the bileaflet valve is clearly shown as compared with ball valves and tilting disc valves available at the time of introduction of the bileaflet bioprosthesis.

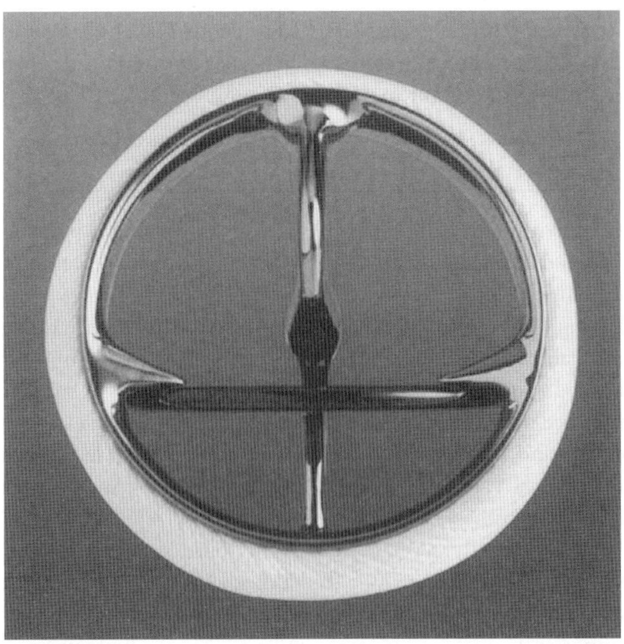

FIGURE 32-5 The Medtronic Hall valve.

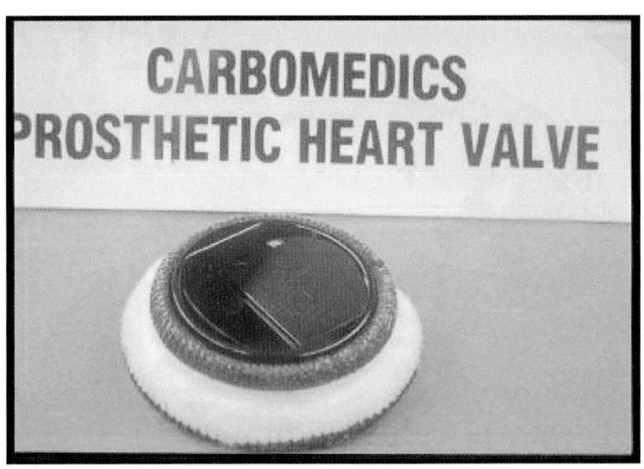

FIGURE 32-8 Carbomedics Top Hat valve.

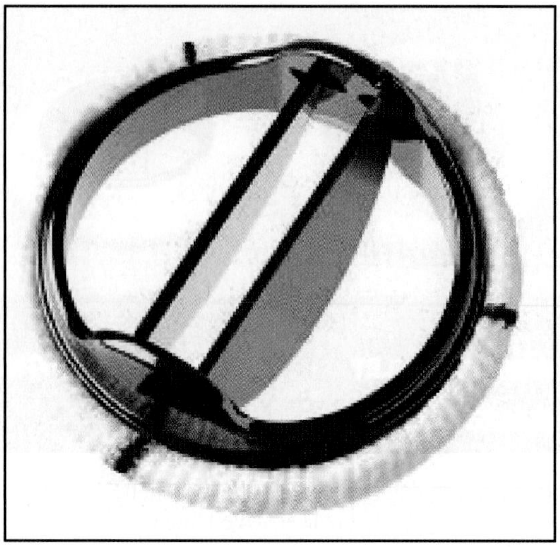

FIGURE 32-9 ATS Medical valve. Note the open pivot design maintaining leaflet insertion.

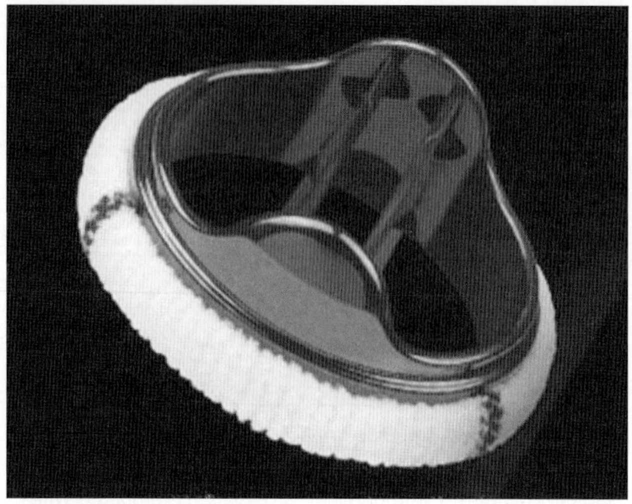

FIGURE 32-11 St. Jude Medical Regent valve.

(Medtronic, Minneapolis, MN) (Fig. 32-9), and the On-X prosthesis (On-X Life Technologies, Inc., Austen, TX) (Fig. 32-10). Since the introduction of the bileaflet valve, more than 2 million implants on a global basis have been accomplished and extensive literature has developed. Surgeons have become more confident in earlier aortic valve replacement, and guidelines for anticoagulation necessary for all mechanical valves have been developed for each generation of prosthesis at progressively decreasing target levels.[12]

Over the past 25 years, design and configurational changes have been made in bileaflet prostheses. The ATS Medical valve changed the "rabbit ears" pivot style of other bileaflet prostheses, incorporating a convex or open-pivot design allowing more complete washing of the moving parts of the valve and possibly a quieter valve closing.[13,14] The sewing ring of the SJM valve has changed (SJM HP) to allow a larger valve size implantation for any given tissue annulus, as has ATS Medical with its AP design. The sewing ring of the Sulzer Carbomedics valve has been modified such that this valve is implanted in a supravalvular position (top hat model). The On-X valve incorporates advanced pyrolytic carbon technology using a purer, more flexible coating to allow flanging of the inflow portion of the valve housing, mimicking the normal flow pattern.

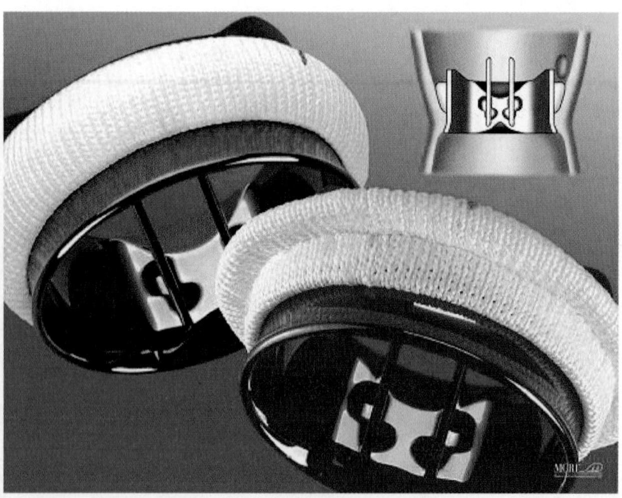

FIGURE 32-10 On-X valve. Note the flange of the inflow portion of the valve housing, which seats in the left ventricular outflow tract.

The most recent development in bileaflet valve design was the introduction of the SJM Regent valve (Fig. 32-11). This valve model not only modified the sewing ring, but also redefined the external profile in a nonintrinsic structural portion of the valve, increasing the effective flow orifice area. Thus, a larger prosthesis could be implanted for any given tissue annulus diameter. This was the first mechanical prosthesis to demonstrate left ventricular mass regression across all valve sizes.[15,16] The Regent valve is seated supra-annular with only the pivot guards protruding into the aortic annulus.[17]

PATIENT SELECTION

As with any medical therapy, AVR with a mechanical prosthesis is not indicated for all patients. Several prospective randomized studies have shown no difference in survival in patients having biologic or mechanical valve prostheses or among mechanical prostheses per se.[18–22] However, follow-up was limited. Conversely, in other nonrandomized studies of patients followed over longer time frames, freedom from all valve-related events and from reoperation were improved in patients with mechanical valve prostheses as compared with patients with biologic prostheses.[8,23]

Most recently several publications have shown improved survival in patients having bileaflet mechanical valve prosthesis, most likely related to improved and longer patient follow-up.[24,25] Importantly quality of life was similar to that of a biologic prosthesis; even in elderly patients.[25]

Although the advantages of large effective flow orifice and durability with a mechanical valve are paramount, the confounding effects resulting from the necessity for anticoagulation continue. Patients who are transient, noncompliant, or incapable of managing medications are not good candidates for long-term chronic anticoagulation, nor are those with dangerous lifestyles or hobbies.[26] Patients with higher levels of education, and those from geographic areas with a sophisticated medical infrastructure and a static population have better compliance with necessary medication, anticoagulant monitoring, and fewer risk factors for TE are good candidate for AVR with a mechanical valve prothesis.[27]

A mechanical valve prosthesis is recommended to patients having second valve reoperations regardless of the nature of the first procedure, as re-reoperative risks are substantial.[28,29] Some studies report low mortality for reoperation of patients with failed biologic valves, but failures can occur abruptly, creating more risk.[30] Reoperative risk is also higher in those patients having combined procedures[28,31] or after prior coronary bypass.

Many surgeons have opted for an age of greater than 70 years as the indication for bioprosthetic AVR, based on data by Akins and associates.[28] In patients younger than 60 years of age, most would opt for a mechanical prosthesis based on prosthesis durability.[32] In the decade between 60 and 70 years of age, other factors have to be taken into account.[33,34]

SURGICAL TECHNIQUES

Implantation of mechanical valve prostheses has been previously described and is straightforward.[11] Historically, high-profile aortic valve prostheses could be difficult to implant, particularly in small aortic roots. In such cases, a hockey-stick aortotomy is used to "unroll" the aorta and expose the annulus. Although the implantation of low-profile bileaflet prostheses is simpler, problems can still arise in the small aortic root. If a tilting disc prosthesis is used, orienting the major flow orifice toward the greater curve of the aorta is necessary. Because bileaflet prostheses are the most commonly used, the surgical technique for implantation of these devices is described: A midline incision and sternotomy is made and a pericardial well created. Alternatively, a right anterior thoracotomy approach with femoral cannulation has been reported. A partial sternotomy is also an alternative in thin patients, creating a sternal T at the fourth inter-space.[35] These alternative techniques are particularly amenable to the implantation of low-profile aortic valve prostheses. The patient is cannulated via the aorta and a single atrial venous cannula. Most commonly, retrograde cardioplegic solution is used and a left ventricular vent is placed via the right superior pulmonary vein to maintain a dry operative field. After cross-clamping of the aorta, a transverse aortotomy is made approximately 1 cm above the takeoff of the right coronary artery, slightly above the level of the sinotubular ridge (Fig. 32-12). The incision is extended three-quarters of the way around the aorta, leaving the posterior one-quarter of the aorta intact, and allowing excellent visualization of the native aortic valve and annulus. The leaflets of the aortic valve are excised to the level of the annulus and the annulus is thoroughly debrided of any calcium. Extensive decalcification will minimize the risk of paravalvular leak, particularly in newer-generation prostheses with thinner sewing rings, and allows for better seating of the valve prosthesis. Braided 2-0 sutures with pledgets are used. Beginning at the noncoronary commissure, the annulus is encircled with interrupted mattress sutures (Fig. 32-13) extending from the aortic to the ventricular surface (everting). Alternatively, multiple single interrupted sutures may be placed. After placement, the suture bundles are divided into two equal portions and two individual sutures placed into the sewing ring at the level of the pivot guards, orienting the pivot guard toward the ostia of the

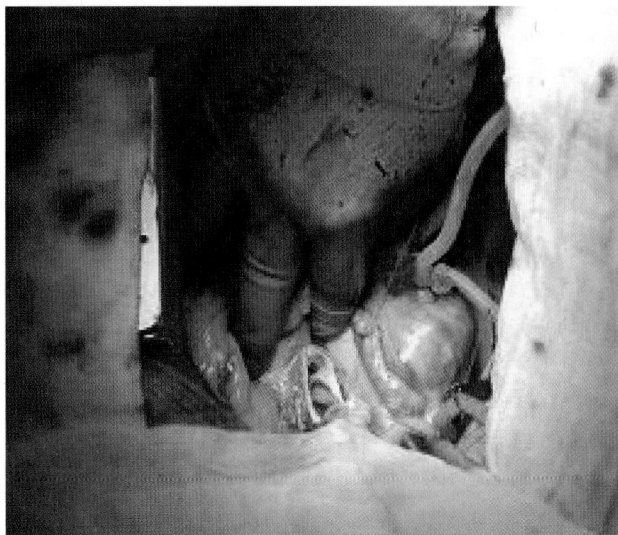

FIGURE 32-12 A transverse aortotomy has been made above the level of the sinotubular ridge. The diseased valve can be visualized readily and excised in toto.

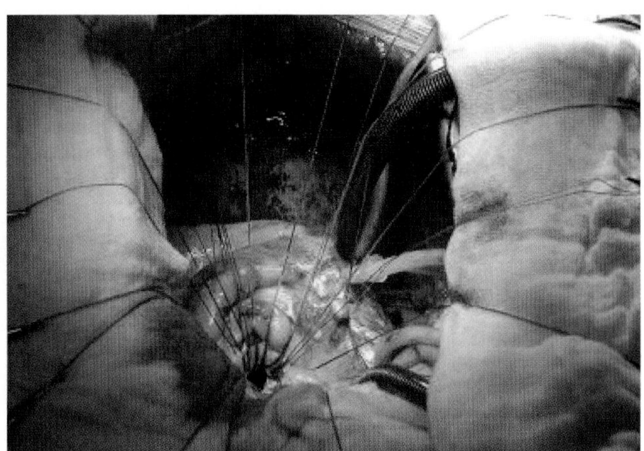

FIGURE 32-13 The annulus has been encircled with multiple interrupted pledgeted mattress sutures of 2-0 braided suture. The annulus can be readily visualized and all calcification has been extensively debrided.

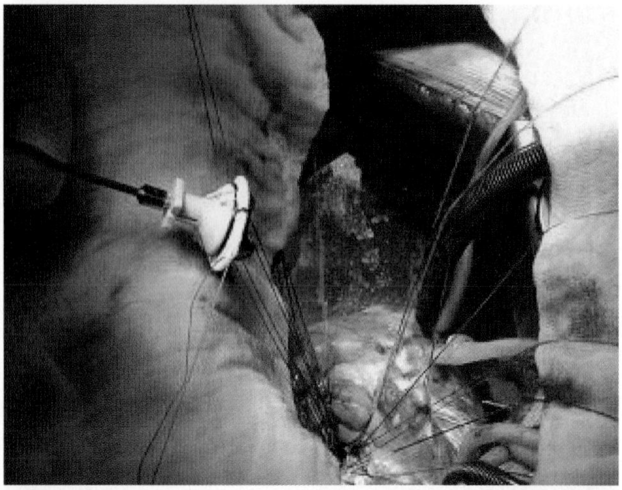

FIGURE 32-14 The pivot guard sutures have been placed aligning the pivot guards with the right and the left coronary arteries.

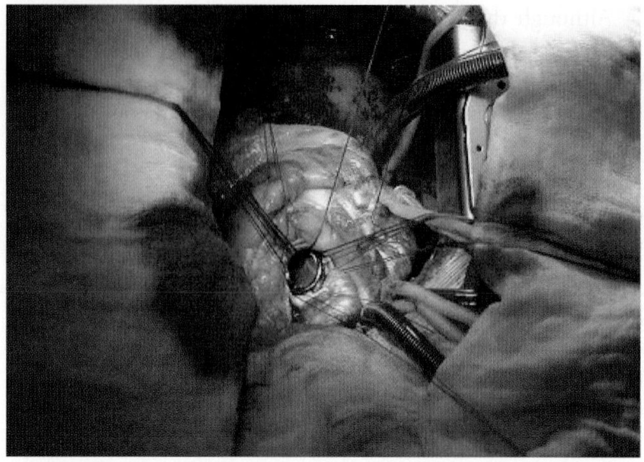

FIGURE 32-16 All sutures have been passed through the sewing ring and the valve is lowered to the aortic annulus and seated appropriately by placing gentle leverage on the valve sewing ring and traction on the suture bundles.

left and right coronary artery (Fig. 32-14). Next, each half of the suture bundles are implanted in the sewing ring and the prosthesis seated (Figs. 32-15 and 32-16).

The pivot guard sutures are tied first followed by the sutures beginning at the left coronary cusp extending to the mid-portion of the right coronary cusp. The sutures of the noncoronary cusp are secured last, seating the valve appropriately. In a small aortic root, if a valve is not able to be seated, a paravalvular leak can be prevented if the unseated area of the valve is in the noncoronary cusp. External aortic sutures can be placed from outside the aorta to the valve sewing ring, securing the prosthesis and preventing regurgitation. Because of the low-profile nature of the leaflets, opening and closing can still occur unimpeded. Leaflet motion should always be checked, and the surgeon must be assured that the coronary arteries are not obstructed. The aortotomy is closed with a double layer of polypropylene suture consisting of an underlying mattress suture and a more superficial over-and-over suture. The patient is placed in the Trendelenburg position and the heart filled with blood and cardioplegic solution, vented, and the cross-clamp removed. After resuscitation and de-airing of the heart, the procedure is completed and the patient transferred to the intensive care unit. On the first postoperative day the chest tubes are removed if output is less than 125 mL in the previous 8 hours. After the removal of the chest tube, the patient is begun on subcutaneous heparin (5000 U every 8 hours) or low molecular weight heparin (1 mg/kg twice a day), and warfarin therapy started. Valve implantation usually can be accomplished in less than 40 minutes of aortic cross-clamping and with cardiopulmonary bypass times of approximately 1 hour, allowing limited coagulopathic and homeopathic alterations.

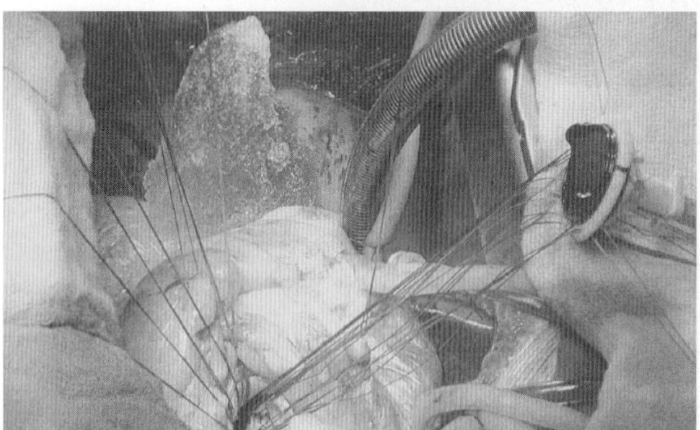

FIGURE 32-15 The first half of the remaining suture bundles has been passed through the sewing ring of the valve. The valve has been moved to the opposite side of the patient and the remaining suture bundle is to be placed.

When coronary bypass grafting is indicated, the order of the operation changes. The diseased valve is excised, distal vein or free arterial grafts constructed, the valve is replaced, and the aortotomy closed. Proximal anastomoses are then completed, with one left untied for de-airing. The distal anastomoses of pedicled grafts (internal mammary artery, IMA) are then completed. De-airing is accomplished through the untied proximal anastomosis.

ANTICOAGULATION

The durability and function of mechanical valve prostheses, particularly those of the modern generation, is unquestioned.[23,32,36–39] It is the process of anticoagulation that is key and drives long-term success. The international normalized ratio (INR) is the standard to which anticoagulation levels should be targeted.[26,40] Anticoagulation is begun slowly after removal of the chest tubes, as the danger of overshooting target INR to dangerous levels is common.[41] Current data on anticoagulant regimens indicate that a one-size-fits-all recipe is inadequate to obtain excellent long-term results.[12,27] Horstkotte and associates noted that complications occur during fluctuations in the INR, and less often during steady-state levels, whether high or low.[42] When levels

TABLE 32-1 Traditional Risk Factors for Thromboembolism

Atrial fibrillation
Increased left ventricular cavity size
Regional wall motion abnormality
Depressed ejection fraction
Hypercoagulability
Increased age

of INR increase, bleeding episodes become more common, and when levels of INR decrease, thromboembolic episodes become more common, both on the slope of the change. These events are opposite ends of the continuum of anticoagulation-related complications. The presence of a mechanical valve prosthesis is also not the only risk factor for TE.[27,43] Traditional risk factors for TE listed in Table 32-1 predispose patients to thromboembolic episodes, and as such higher therapeutic INRs are warranted. Similarly, as shown in Table 32-2, nontraditional risk factors for thromboembolism will also predispose patients to embolic events.[27,43] Butchart has noted that the more of these risk factors patients have, the greater the incidence of events and the greater the need for a higher target INR (Fig. 32-17).[27] Thus, it is imperative in the modern era that patient risk factors be taken into account and the INR individualized for a given patient.[12] Recommendations for INR target levels in our practice are shown in Table 32-3. These levels are more liberal than those offered by the American College of Cardiology/American Heart Association (ACC/AHA) and the American College of Chest Physicians (ACCP) guidelines, but more conservative than those recommended by the European self-anticoagulation

TABLE 32-2 Nontraditional Risk Factors for Thromboembolism

Cancer
Systemic infection
Diabetes
Prior event
IgA against *Chlamydia pneumoniae* (CP)
Eosinophilia
Hypertension

Reproduced with permission from Butchart EG, Ionescu A, Payne N, et al: A new scoring system to determine thromboembolic risk after heart valve replacement. Circulation 2003; 108(Suppl II):II-68.

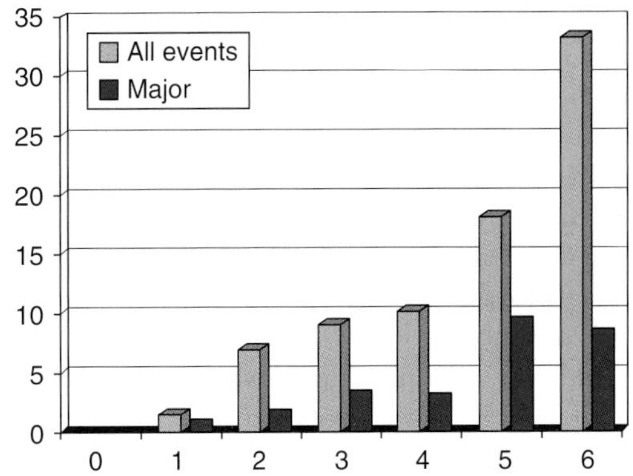

FIGURE 32-17 The correlation of number of risk factors to thromboembolic events. (*Reproduced with permission from Butchart EG, Ionescu A, Payne N, et al: A new scoring system to determine thromboembolic risk after heart valve replacement. Circulation 2003; 108[Suppl II]:II-68.*)

trials.[44–46] These later reports are especially relevant, because they demonstrate that a lower INR is consistent with a lower incidence of TE if patients are maintained in the therapeutic target range.[44,47] Patients with home testing were maintained in the therapeutic range a substantially greater percentage of the time than those whose status was monitored at anticoagulation clinics.[44,47] Starting self-management early after mechanical valve replacement further reduced valve-related events.[41] In the United States, home testing has not become commonplace or popular. However, home testing could certainly be expected to lower the incidence of valve-related thromboembolic and bleeding events. It has recently been approved for reimbursement for weekly testing in patients with a mechanical valve prosthesis or atrial fibrillation, but only after a 3-month waiting period. Obtaining appropriate funding for access in the immediate postoperative period would be an important initiative that could acutely reduce the incidence of valve-related events.

A recent report of patients followed over 25 years noted that approximately 40% of the bleeding episodes occurred in the first year after surgery. It is thus important during this initial postoperative time frame when the patient's anticoagulant levels are more likely to fluctuate, that INR be measured more frequently.[32] In the early postoperative period, INR can occasionally jump to

TABLE 32-3 Target INR Recommendations

Normal ejection fraction and cavity size, NSR: INR 1.82.0, ASA
Any single factor: INR 2.0–2.5, ASA
Multiple factors or atrial fibrillation: INR 2.5–3.5
? Antiplatelet only

ASA = aspirin; INR = international normalized ratio; NSR = normal sinus rhythm.

supratherapeutic levels and result in significant bleeding events. This is an independent risk factor for mortality at 60 days.[48] Furthermore, the most important independent predictor of reduced survival is anticoagulant variability.[26] We and others therefore recommend in the early postoperative period that one proceed slowly to bring the INR to target levels while the patient is under the protection of subcutaneous enoxaparin (100 IU/kg twice a day) or heparin (5000 U every 8 hours) until the INR is therapeutic.[12,32,49,50]

The addition of aspirin to a warfarin regimen can be expected to result in a lower incidence of TE at any given therapeutic INR with a low probability for bleeding events and so is recommended.[51,52]

An educational program to teach patients how to manage their anticoagulation is an important part of the overall operative process. Patients should be instructed on the influence of alcohol and diet on anticoagulant levels, the need for regular dosing, and the potential impact of travel and gastrointestinal illnesses on fluctuations in anticoagulant levels. Warfarin is well known to be high-risk, as is insulin, yet both drugs can be managed with proper compliance and education so that the impact on lifestyle and quality of life is minimal.[7,25,53] Patient age does not appear to be a risk factor for anticoagulation[53–56] as long as there are no specific contraindications to anticoagulation. The presence of a mechanical valve is not a risk factor for long-term neurocognitive dysfunction.[57] The importance of regular testing cannot be overstated.

Newer antithrombin agents may obviate several of the issues discussed in the preceding. These agents are showing promise in the treatment of atrial fibrillation, with a lower incidence of embolism and bleeding complications. The drugs are expensive, require multiple administrations per day, and may cause hepatic dysfunction, yet they do not require blood testing or physician visits to maintain the therapeutic effect.[58] Their application to mechanical valve prostheses is as yet unknown.

Of importance platelet activation may be more important in the long-term therapy of an aortic prosthesis than mitral, where areas of stasis predominate.[10] This is likely the reason there is no difference in the freedom from embolic events in mechanical versus biologic prosthesis over the long term.[23] Thus aortic valve prostheses could in theory be managed with newer strong antiplatelet therapy. Garcia-Renaldi has tested this theory in 178 patients followed out to 7.8 years treated only with clopidogrel. Results were excellent, with few bleeding episodes and minimal thromboembolic events.[59] Importantly, this group found the majority of patients having thromboembolic events when tested were resistant to the drug or had been removed from the drug by themselves or a physician. The authors stressed the importance of measurement of platelet responsiveness if only antiplatelet therapy is used.[59] A prospective randomized trial is warranted to confirm those results.

RESULTS

Outcomes from aortic valve replacement with mechanical valve prostheses vary among reports depending on the patient population. Patients with higher-risk factors for TE and those with risk factors for anticoagulation will have a higher incidence of valve-related events, making meta-analyses less meaningful.[60] Older patients are at higher risk for valve-related events, particularly thromboembolic episodes, because of the greater number of risk factors that accumulate with aging.[27] The incidence of valve-related events is also determined by the intensity with which the investigators follow their patients. A higher incidence of early hemorrhagic events may also be diluted over the longer periods of follow-up.[61] Compliance is vital to good long-term outcomes. Traditional and nontraditional risk factors for embolism and risk factors for anticoagulation and valve-related events must be considered.[27,43] Several trials have indicated no significant differences in events among various mechanical prostheses, but follow-up was short.[19,21,62] There are, however, certain standards within which one should expect a mechanical valve to perform, and within which the medical decisions for anticoagulation must be made. The majority of valve-related morbidity is related to TE and anticoagulation-related hemorrhage.[26,29,39] The sections that follow deal with specific valve-related complications and acceptable current incidence.

Valve Type

Freedom from all valve-related events over the long term is shown in Fig. 32-18. In the early follow-up period, anticoagulation-related hemorrhage is the most common untoward event for mechanical valve prostheses. Thus, over the first 10 years of follow-up there is a higher incidence of valve-related events in patients with mechanical prostheses as opposed to those with biologic valves.[23] However, over the subsequent period of 10 to 20 years, the incidence of biologic valve failure changes this ratio such that the valve-related complications of biologic prostheses become more common than those with mechanical valve

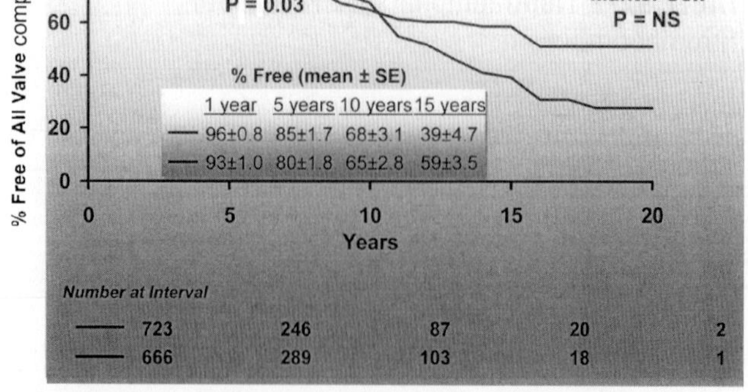

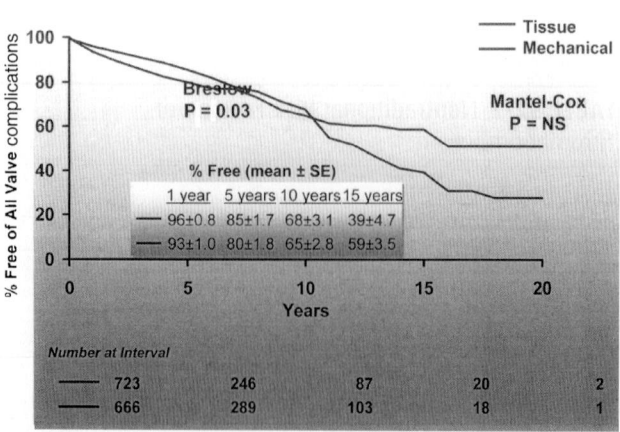

FIGURE 32-18 Freedom from all valve-related complications over 20 years. Note that in the first 10-year period of follow-up, complications related to mechanical valves exceeded those of tissue valves. The lines cross at approximately 10 years, and over the following period, complications from tissue valves were more frequent than those from mechanical valves. (*Reproduced with permission from Khan SS, Trento A, DeRobertis M, et al: Twenty-year comparison of tissue and mechanical valve replacement. J Thorac Cardiovasc Surg 2001; 122:257.*)

prostheses. In a series of aortic reoperations, Potter has noted that the time to biologic valve failure was only 7.6 years and Maganti 11 years.[30,63] This failure rate will increase over time.[23,64] Overall, freedom from valve-related events is more strongly influenced by preexisting comorbidities than the presence of a mechanical prosthesis per se.[23,27,32,36]

Anticoagulant-Related Hemorrhage

Anticoagulation-related hemorrhage (ARH) is the most common valve-related event. The more intense the anticoagulation regimen, the higher the incidence of valve-related hemorrhage. Most commonly ARH occurs during fluctuations in INR values commonly related to changes in warfarin dosing or medical or drug interactions.[42] The most common site for ARH is the gastrointestinal tract, and the second is the central nervous system.[32] ARH also accounts for the highest incidence of patient mortality for valve-related events. Acceptable ARH rates range from 1.0 to 2.5% per patient-year in long-term reports.[8,23,32,36–39] These long-term reports dilute the short-term impact, because ARH risks are higher early after valve replacement.[32,39,61] With individualized and home-monitored anticoagulant regimens, both related events, TE and ARH, are diminished.[44] Freedom from anticoagulation at 10 and 20 years are 75 to 80% and 65 to 70%, respectively. Importantly, one long-term study noted that nearly 40% of all ARH that occurred over a 25-year follow-up period occurred during the first year of anticoagulation (Fig. 32-19), indicating that a slow increase to therapeutic levels, coupled with close follow-up during this early period is warranted.[12,32,48,49] Results of the European self-anticoagulation study indicate that a lower INR target is appropriate if home testing is initiated, because greater time is spent in the therapeutic range.[44] Mortality more commonly occurs in relation to bleeding events than to thromboembolic events.[12,32]

Thromboembolism

Thromboembolic episodes are the second most common valve-related event and are the major reason that chronic anticoagulation is warranted. Khan and associates reported in a large series of patients that the incidence of thromboembolic events between bioprostheses and mechanical prostheses are the same (Fig. 32-20), but the mechanical valve patients are on warfarin.[23] Acceptable thromboembolic rates range between 0.8 and 2.3% per patient-year.[8,23,32,36–39,65] Approximately one-half of these events are neurologic, 40% are transient, and 10% peripheral.[32] Freedom from thromboembolic events at 10 and 20 years is approximately 80 to 85% and 65 to 70%, respectively.

Thromboembolism is a continuous risk factor that is present throughout the life of the mechanical valve prosthesis. As patients age, risk factors for TE increase, so one must be on guard to maintain therapeutic anticoagulant levels. Changes in the target INR may be necessary as individual risks increase.

Interestingly, not all neurologic events classified historically as embolic are indeed embolic. Piper and coworkers report a study of patients prospectively admitted to a single institution with a neurologic event postmechanical valve replacement and intensively worked up. More than 75% were found to have

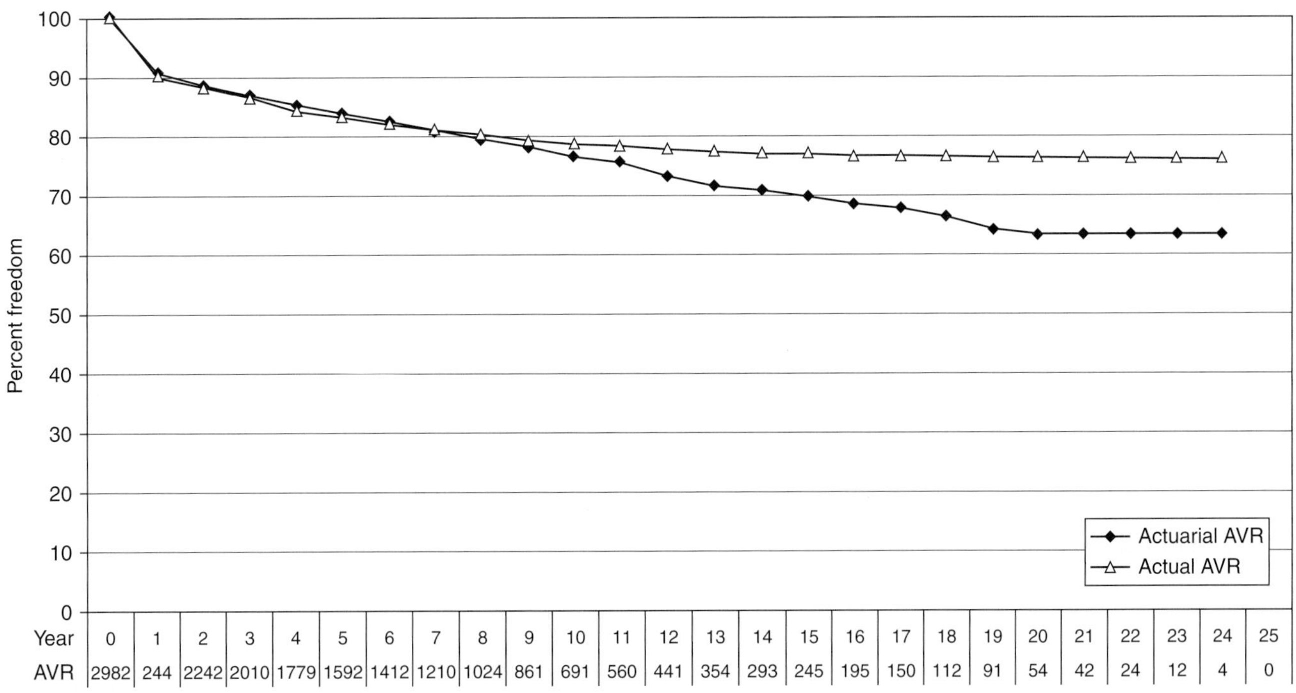

Year	0	1	2	3	4	5	6	7	8	9	10	11	12	13	14	15	16	17	18	19	20	21	22	23	24	25
AVR	2982	244	2242	2010	1779	1592	1412	1210	1024	861	691	560	441	354	293	245	195	150	112	91	54	42	24	12	4	0

FIGURE 32-19 Kaplan-Meier curve of freedom from anticoagulation-related hemorrhage for patients having aortic valve replacement. *(Reproduced with permission from Emery RW, Krogh CC, Arom DV, et al: The St. Jude Medical cardiac valve prosthesis: a 25-year experience with single valve replacement. Ann Thorac Surg 2005; 79:776.)*

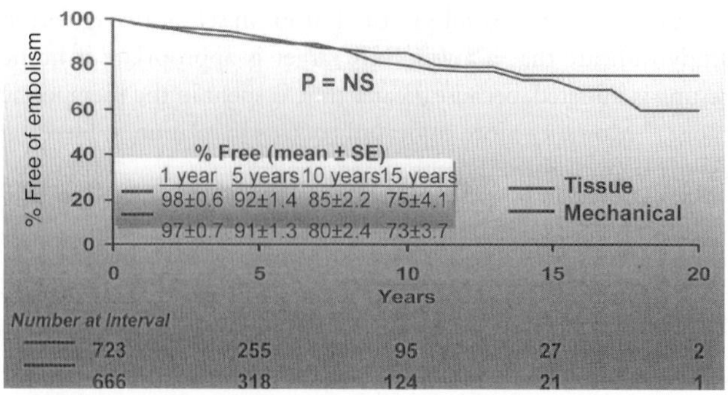

FIGURE 32-20 Freedom from thromboembolism in patients followed for 20 years. Note that there is no difference in the incidence of thromboembolic events between mechanical and tissue valves. (*Reproduced with permission from Khan SS, Trento A, DeRobertis M, et al: Twenty-year comparison of tissue and mechanical valve replacement. J Thorac Cardiovasc Surg 2001; 122:257.*)

intracerebral hemorrhage as the etiology of the event as opposed to embolic. This would indicate that target anticoagulant levels may be artificially high, and that not all neurologic events that appear to be embolic in fact are so.[66]

Valve Thrombosis

Valve thrombosis in the aortic position is an unusual event that occurs late after valve replacement and is most commonly a result of inadequate anticoagulation or noncompliance.[67,68] In bileaflet valves, thrombus formation impinging valve function occurs at the pivot guards and in the crevices of the valve. Only one bileaflet design does not have convexities into which the leaflets fit.[69] In tilting disc valves, thrombus is most common at the minor flow orifice. The incidence of thrombosis is approximately less than 0.3% per patient-year, and freedom from valve thrombosis at 20 years is greater than 97%.[8,23,32,36–39]

Prosthetic Valve Endocarditis

Prosthetic valve endocarditis is also a rare event in the modern era with prophylactic antibiotics. Approximately 60% of events occur early and are associated with staphylococci. The mortality for this event is high. The remainder appear late (>60 days). Prosthetic valve endocarditis is also a continuous variable, and patients must be cautioned to take prophylactic antibiotics for any invasive procedure. Freedom from endocarditis with mechanical valve prostheses is 97 to 98% at 20 to 25 years.[32,39]

Paravalvular Leak

Paravalvular leak is an operative complication and is most commonly related to operative technique but occasionally to endocarditis. With annular decalcification and closely placed sutures, these events can be minimized. The Silzone experience showed an increased incidence of paravalvular leak wherein the silver impregnated in the sewing ring not only impeded bacterial growth, but also healing of the annular ring, doubling the accepted rate of this complication.[70] The Silzone-coated sewing ring was removed from the market. There may be an anatomical predisposition to paravalvular leak in the area of the annulus extending from the right and noncoronary commissure, one-third the distance along the right coronary cusp, and two-thirds the distance to the noncoronary cusp, owing to intrinsic weakness in this area of the annulus.[71] The acceptable range of paravalvular leak is approximately less than .01% per patient-year, with early postoperative occurrence predominating.[29,32]

Structural Failure

Structural failure of bileaflet aortic prostheses resulting from wear has not been observed or reported in long-term studies totaling more than 50,000 patient-years of follow-up. This indicates the high structural integrity of these modern aortic devices.[23,32,39] In a single study totaling 21,742 patient-years with 94% complete follow-up, there was no structural failure.[49]

Freedom from Reoperation

The long-term durability of modern mechanical valve prostheses is excellent, and a valve replacement rate of less than 2% over 25 years (Fig. 32-21) can be expected, and re-reoperation after AVR replacement is even more rare.[29] Subvalvular pannus formation is also rare with aortic bileaflet valves.[32,39] The most common reasons for prosthetic valve reimplantation are preoperative and postoperative endocarditis, paravalvular leak, and valve thrombosis.

SPECIAL CIRCUMSTANCES

Technical Considerations

Although the technique of implanting a mechanical valve prosthesis is very straightforward, special circumstances arise. Because of the large size of the valve housing of the St. Jude Medical Regent valve compared to the tissue annulus, entry into the aorta can sometimes be difficult. Occasionally, patients have the smallest diameter of their aortic root at the sinotubular ridge. Although the sizer will pass readily through the aortic annulus, seating the Regent valve itself into the annulus can sometimes be difficult and frustrating. It is important to gently rock the valve back and forth through the sinotubular ridge, tilting the valve circumferentially through the narrowest part. Once the valve is below the level of the sinotubular ridge, it will seat readily in the annulus if sizing has been correct. When tying the valve into the annulus, sutures in the pivot guards and the left and right coronary cusps should be completed first. The last sutures ligated are those of the noncoronary cusp for two reasons. It may seem like the Regent valve will not seat because of the large-sized valve housing; however, with gentle persistence seating can be completed as long as sizing has been correct. The Regent valve sits supra-annular and only the pivot guards lie inside the annulus (Fig. 32-22). Therefore one should leave the last sutures to be tied in the mid-part of the noncoronary cusp with the valve oriented so the leaflets are parallel to the ventricular septum.[72] With proper annular decalcification and

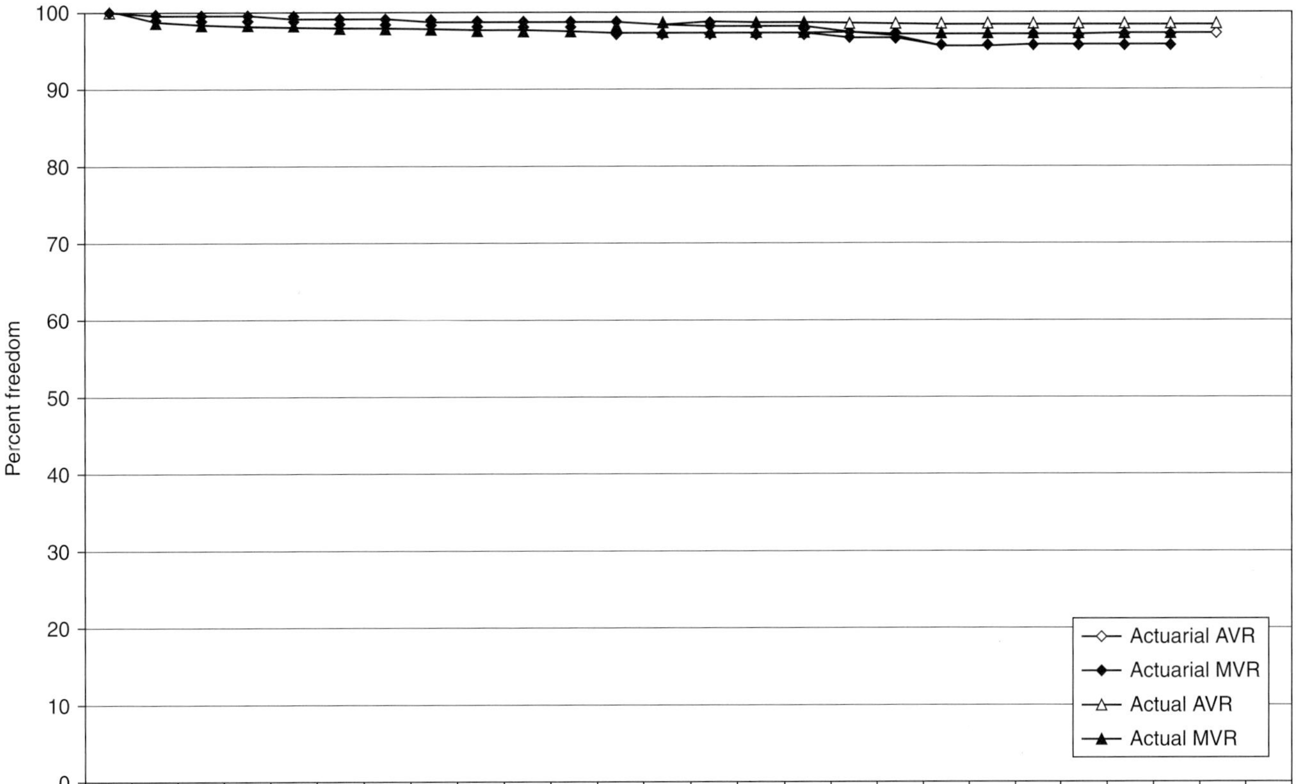

Year	0	1	2	3	4	5	6	7	8	9	10	11	12	13	14	15	16	17	18	19	20	21	22	23	24	25
AVR	2982	2652	2472	2240	2004	1814	1619	1404	1194	1010	811	668	542	452	373	309	246	193	142	118	71	52	33	14	6	0
MVR	1498	1231	1145	1047	932	822	729	631	541	476	405	345	291	237	201	160	136	94	75	57	40	23	15	1	0	0

FIGURE 32-21 Freedom from reoperations in patients having mechanical valve replacement followed over 25 years. Note that the rate of reoperation in patients with aortic valve replacement is less than 2% in over 21,000 patient-years of follow-up. (*Reproduced with permission from Emery RW, Krogh CC, Arom DV, et al: The St. Jude Medical cardiac valve prosthesis: a 25-year experience with single valve replacement. Ann Thorac Surg 2005; 79:776.*)

flexibility of the annulus, we have not seen a Regent valve that has not been able to be seated properly.

Similarly, when using the On-X valve one has to be sure that the flare of the valve inflow is seated properly in the left ventricular outflow tract. Gentle manipulation and patience may be necessary. Walther and colleagues note that exact sizing requires some experience.[20]

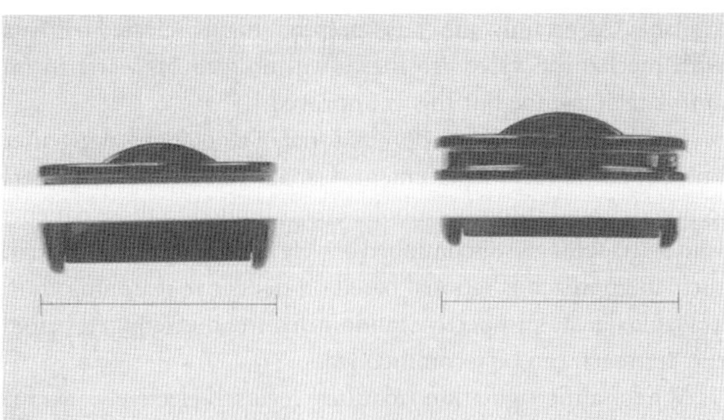

FIGURE 32-22 The St. Jude Medical Regent valve on the right, compared with the St. Jude Medical HP valve on the left. With the Regent valve only the pivot guards insert into the annulus, allowing a larger valve housing for any given tissue annulus diameter. (*Reproduced with permission from Emery RW, Krogh CC, Arom KV, et al: The St. Jude Medical cardiac valve prosthesis: a 25-year experience with single valve replacement. Ann Thorac Surg 2005; 79:776.*)

If an oversized bileaflet valve has been implanted purposefully in a small aortic root, the valve can be tilted and will still function without coronary obstruction as long as the highest portion of the valve is in the noncoronary cusp. Pledgeted sutures placed from outside the aorta through the sewing ring of the valve can prevent paravalvular leak, and opening and closing can still occur because of the low-profile nature of the prosthetic valve. In our review of nearly 3000 bileaflet aortic valve replacements, no annular enlarging procedures were completed.[49]

Patient-Prosthesis Mismatch

Patient-prosthesis mismatch (PPM) is a concept first described by Rahimtoola and popularized by Pibarot and Dumesnil.[73,74] Unfortunately, views are varied on the importance of PPM.[75–78] This is because virtually all contributions to the literature study mixtures of mechanical and biologic prostheses and varying types of each. In a 25-year follow-up of patients with a single model mechanical valve prosthesis, no difference was found in overall valve-related mortality for patients who had severe PPM, moderate PPM, or insignificant PPM according to the criteria described by Blais and associates.[77] This similarity in long-term

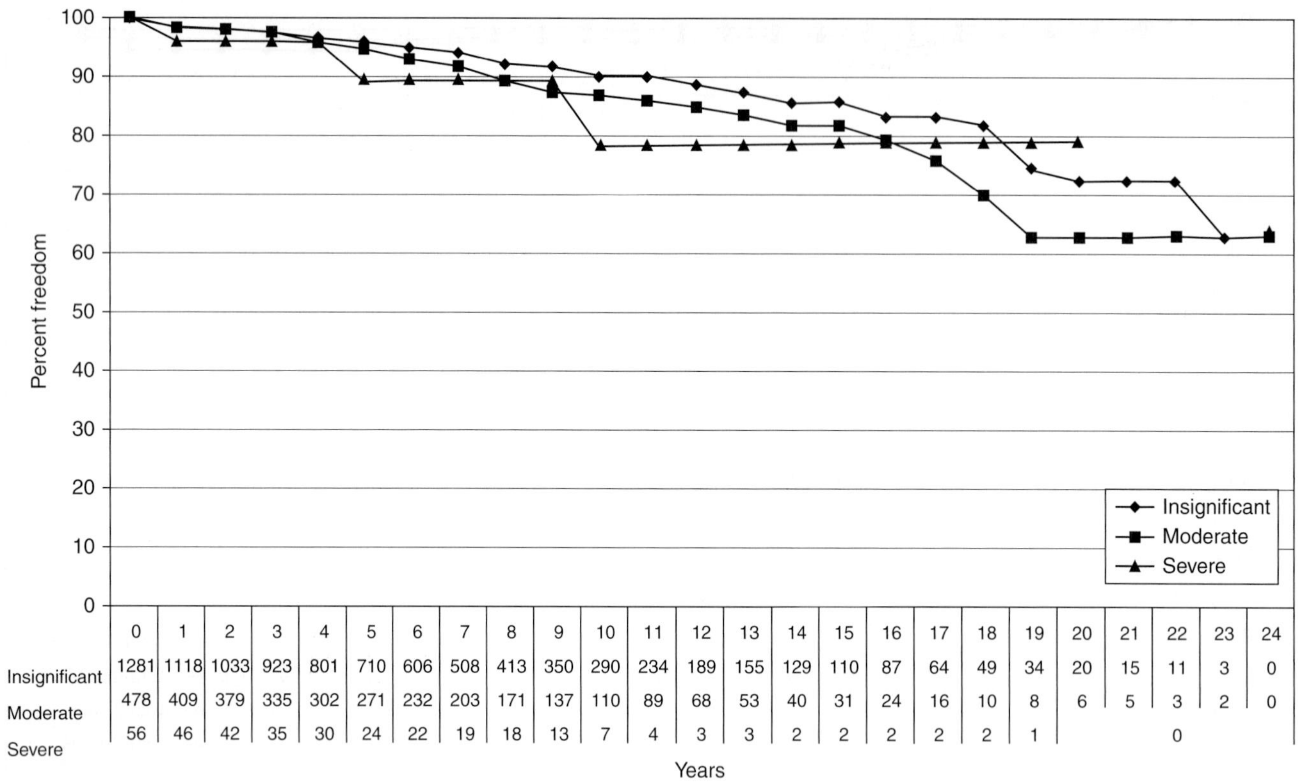

FIGURE 32-23 Kaplan-Meier determination of valve-related late mortality in patients having insignificant, moderate, or severe patient-prosthesis mismatch according to the criteria of Pibarot and colleagues. After implant of a bileaflet prosthesis, in vitro determination is calculated from the geometric flow orifice by the manufacturer. Note there is no difference in these three curves. Numbers at the bottom of the figure represent patients available for follow-up.

survival was sustained whether the effective area was measured by in vitro (internal geometric valve area) or in vivo criteria (echo-calculated valve area) as shown in Figs. 32-23 and 32-24. This study also found no difference in valve-related events, including operative mortality, long-term cumulative mortality, anticoagulant-related hemorrhage, TE, valve thrombosis, paravalvular leak, or diagnosis of congestive heart failure. Follow-up in this study was 94% complete and extended over 13,000 patient-years.[79] Therefore, with bileaflet mechanical valve prostheses, PPM does not appear to be an issue. This study was limited in that it did not address patient age (ie, younger versus older), patient activity, or ventricular function. Thus, it is likely that PPM is important in patients with small biologic prostheses, because as the valve leaflets stiffen, clinical aortic stenosis becomes prominent early in the postoperative follow-up period, affecting symptoms and survival in younger and more active patients and those with depressed ventricular function. However, if one is concerned about PPM, the indexed effective orifice area can be calculated for any given prosthetic valve and a determination made whether an annular enlarging procedure or a different model prosthesis with a larger effective orifice area is warranted.[80] PPM has been minimized by the new-generation Regent valve and is very rare with this prosthesis.[16,49]

Off Anticoagulation

Anticoagulation is recommended in all patients with mechanical valve prostheses. Limited trials have been undertaken with low-risk patients, but only after a several-month course of systemic anticoagulation. An increased incidence of valve thrombosis but with little increase in the incidence of TE has been reported in patients not taking chronic anticoagulation if antiplatelet agents are used.[67,81,82] One study found no significant differences in valve-related events in patients on warfarin as compared with antiplatelet therapy alone, but follow-up was limited.[83] One prospective study is currently ongoing, consisting of a randomized trial of antiplatelet therapy versus warfarin after 3 months of formal anticoagulation, but the results are not yet available.[84] Certainly one can expect that highly selected patients with mechanical valve prostheses will do well off warfarin on antiplatelet agents, but this is unproved.[17,85]

In a prospective nonrandomized trial of clopidogrel along after bileaflet aortic valve replacement, Garcia-Rinaldi and coworkers as noted, found thromboembolic events limited to those patients who had clopidogrel discontinued or were nonresponders. Although such an approach is rational based on deductive reasoning from available data, a prospective randomized trend is required before this approach can be recommended.

When anticoagulation requires reversal electively, as for scheduled surgery, the INR is allowed to slowly drift toward normal over 5 days and the patient is admitted for intravenous heparin therapy 24 hours before the procedure. Anticoagulation is restarted after the procedure with antiplatelet therapy, and subcutaneous heparin with warfarin restarted on postoperative day one. Abrupt reversal of INR in patients who have bleeding episodes may be warranted, but carries increased risk of TE. Fresh-frozen plasma will gently reverse INR when necessary,

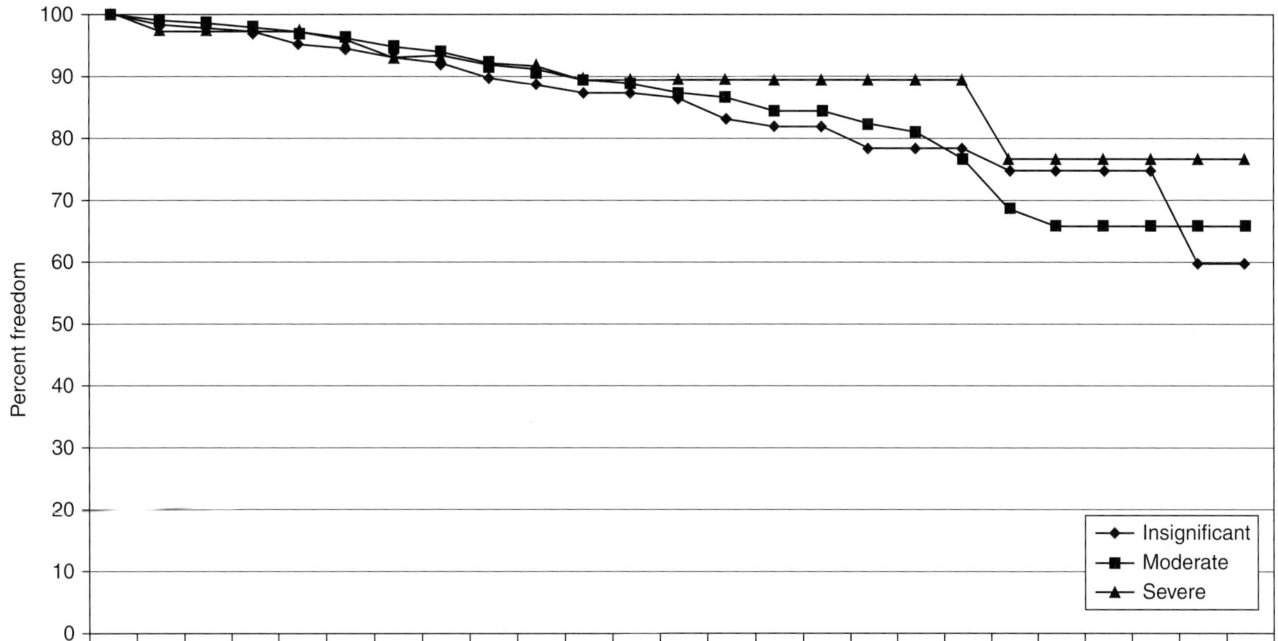

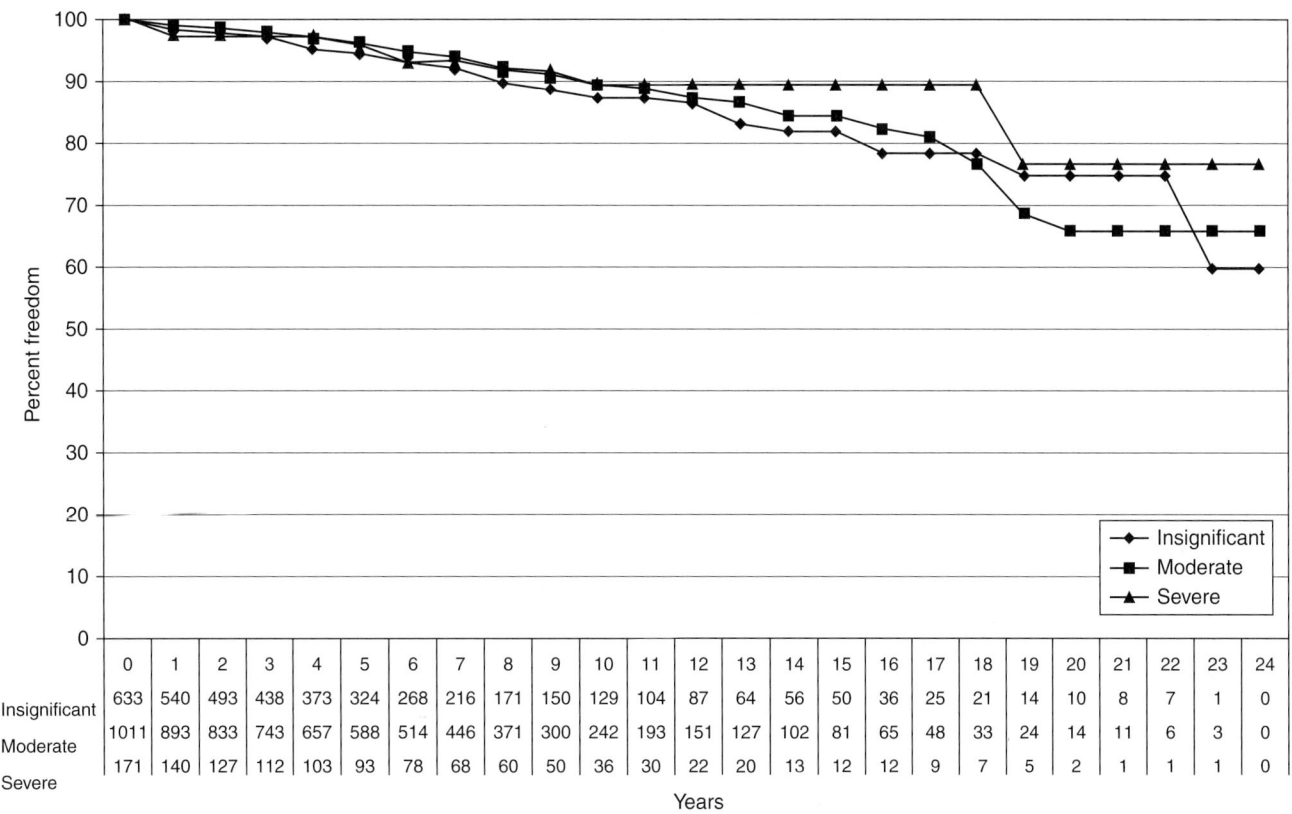

Years	0	1	2	3	4	5	6	7	8	9	10	11	12	13	14	15	16	17	18	19	20	21	22	23	24
Insignificant	633	540	493	438	373	324	268	216	171	150	129	104	87	64	56	50	36	25	21	14	10	8	7	1	0
Moderate	1011	893	833	743	657	588	514	446	371	300	242	193	151	127	102	81	65	48	33	24	14	11	6	3	0
Severe	171	140	127	112	103	93	78	68	60	50	36	30	22	20	13	12	12	9	7	5	2	1	1	1	0

FIGURE 32-24 Kaplan-Meier determination of valve-related late mortality in patients having insignificant, moderate, or severe patient-prosthesis mismatch by the in vivo criteria according to Blais and associates determined echocardiographically. There is no difference in the survival curves after implant of a bileaflet prosthesis. The numbers at the bottom of the graph represent patients available for follow-up.

but it is best to avoid the use of vitamin K. Frequent INR checks are warranted.

After ARH episodes, when feasible, because of the high incidence of recurrent bleeding, anticoagulant therapy is withheld up to 2 weeks or until the source of the bleeding has been identified and definitively treated, using antiplatelet agents only.[82] For those patients in whom anticoagulant therapy cannot be restarted, antiplatelet therapy is warranted, but the patient should be informed of an increased incidence of thromboembolism to approximately 4% per patient-year and that of valve thrombosis to 2% per patient-year with bileaflet valves.[67,81,82,86]

Mechanical Valve Replacement in the Younger Patient

A major deterrent to mechanical valve replacement in the younger patient is the impact of long-term anticoagulation. Mechanical valves are, however, more ideal for younger patients because of their excellent durability characteristics. Most importantly, younger patients (i.e., patients less than age 50) are a low-risk subset for valve-related events. These individuals have very few risk factors for TE, and thus anticoagulation can be run at the lower end of the therapeutic target range, decreasing the incidence of anticoagulant-related hemorrhage without altering the incidence of TE. In fact, many infants and children have been managed with only aspirin with quite good long-term results.[87] Although this is not recommended in patients older than infants, it is a feasible alternative. A recent study in patients under 50 years of age followed 254 patients for up to 20 years and found an exceedingly low rate of valve-related events (Table 32-4), an exceptional long-term overall survival of nearly 88%, and event-free survival probability of 92% at 19 years.[88]

TABLE 32-4 Valve-Related Events with the St. Jude Medical Prosthetic Valve

Event	No. of Events	Percent Per Patient-Year	No. of Deaths
Endocarditis	3	0.15	0
Paravalvular leak	6	0.30	2
Embolism	6	0.30	0
Valve thrombosis	2	0.10	0
Bleeding	6	0.10	2
Structural failure	0	0	0

Source: Data from Emery RW, Erickson CA, Arom KV, et al: Replacement of the aortic valve in patients under 50 years old with the St Jude Medical Prosthesis. Ann Thorac Surg 2003; 75:1815.

TABLE 32-5 Indications for Mechanical Valve Replacement

High probability for anticoagulant use
Need for chronic anticoagulation (any age)
Preferences of patient
Surgical risk for reoperation
Age <60 years
Age 60–70 years with patient discussion
Reoperations
Good medical infrastructure

The longest surviving patient in a series of bileaflet valve replacement patients is currently more than 30 years from his procedure, which was completed in his early forties and has been without complication.[30] The low incidence of valve-related complications in younger patients should drive a discussion of the alternative prostheses available for such individuals, especially with new aggressive antiplatelet drugs. Operative mortality increases with each succeeding procedure; therefore, discussion of durability with patients becomes mandatory.[28–30]

Follow-up

With the use of any valve prosthesis, long-term follow-up is a vital factor. Ten years is certainly not long enough to ascertain the true durability of a prosthesis. Grunkemeier reviewed several types of biologic prostheses and found that the 10-year durability was excellent, but between 12 and 18 years durability fell off and prosthetic replacement was necessary.[64] These data were echoed by Khan and colleagues.[23] Valve-related failure of all biologic alternatives, including stented prosthetic replacements, stentless prostheses, and homograft and autograft replacements have all shown long-term durability to be less than that of modern mechanical valve prostheses.

Even with some mechanical valve prostheses, durability after 10 years has not been adequate. In recommending mechanical valve replacement, one should be assured to have clinically available data on the prostheses that extend beyond 15 years.

In conclusion, with proper selection of patients for mechanical valve replacement, one can expect excellent long-term results, long-term survival, and a low incidence of valve-related complications. Current indications for recommending aortic valve replacement with mechanical prostheses are shown in Table 32-5.

REFERENCES

1. Carabello BA: Clinical practice. Aortic stenosis. *NEJM* 2002; 346:677.
2. Tornos P, Sambola A, Permanyer Miralda G, et al: Long-term outcome of surgically treated aortic regurgitation: influence of guideline adherence toward early surgery. *J Am Coll Cardiol* 2006; 47:1012.
3. Gott VL, Alejo DE, Cameron DE: Mechanical heart valves: 50 years of evolution. *Ann Thorac Surg* 2003; 76:S2230.
4. Hufnagel CA, Harvey WP: The surgical correction of aortic regurgitation preliminary report. *Bull Georgetown Univ Med Cent* 1953; 6:60.
5. Shiono M, Sezai Y, Sezai A, et al: Long-term results of the cloth-covered Starr-Edwards ball valve. *Ann Thorac Surg* 2005; 80:204.
6. Gao G, Wu Y, Grunkemeier GL, et al: Forty-year survival with the Starr-Edwards heart valve prosthesis. *J Heart Valve Dis* 2004; 13:91.
7. Ezekowitz MD: Anticoagulation management of valve replacement patients. *J Heart Valve Dis* 2002; 11(Suppl 1):S56.
8. Oxenham H, Bloomfield P, Wheatley DJ, et al: Twenty-year comparison of a Bjork-Shiley mechanical heart valve with porcine bioprostheses. *Heart* 2003; 89:697.
9. Emery RW, Anderson RW, Lindsay WG, et al: Clinical and hemodynamic results with the St. Jude Medical aortic valve prosthesis. *Surg Forum* 1979; 30:235.
10. Emery RW, Nicoloff DM: The St. Jude Medical cardiac valve prosthesis: in vitro studies. *J Thorac Cardiovasc Surg* 1979; 78:269.
11. Nicoloff DM, Emery RW, Arom KV, et al: Clinical and hemodynamic results with the St. Jude Medical cardiac valve prosthesis. *J Thorac Cardiovasc Surg* 1982; 82:674.
12. Emery RW, Emery AM, Raikar GV, et al: Anticoagulation for mechanical heart valves: a role for patient based therapy. *J Thrombosis Thrombolysis* 2008;25:18-25.
13. Sezai A, Shiono M, Orime Y, et al: Evaluation of valve sound and its effects on ATS prosthetic valves in patients' quality of life. *Ann Thorac Surg* 2000; 69:507.
14. Emery RW, Krogh CC, Jones DJ, et al: Five-year follow up of the ATS mechanical heart valve. *J Heart Valve Dis* 2004; 13:231.
15. Bach DS, Sakwa MP, Goldbach M, et al: Hemodynamics and early clinical performance of the St. Jude Medical Regent mechanical aortic valve. *Ann Thorac Surg* 2002; 74:2003.
16. Gelsomino S, Morocutti G, Da Col P, et al: Preliminary experience with the St. Jude Medical Regent mechanical heart valve in the aortic position: early in vivo hemodynamic results. *Ann Thorac Surg* 2002; 73:1830.
17. Emery RW, Emery AM: Letter to the editor. *J Thorac Cardiovasc Surg* 2006; 131:760.
18. Hammermeister KE, Sethi GK, Henderson WG, et al: A comparison of outcomes in men 11 years after heart valve replacement with a mechanical valve or bioprosthesis. *NEJM* 1993; 328:1289.
19. Autschbach R, Walther T, Falk V: Prospectively randomized comparison of different mechanical aortic valves. *Circulation* 2000; 102:III-1.
20. Walther T, Falk V, Tigges R, et al: Comparison of On-X and SJM HP bileaflet aortic valves. *J Heart Valve Dis* 2000; 9:403.
21. Masters RG, Helou J, Pipe AL, Keon WJ: Comparative clinical outcomes with St. Jude Medical, Medtronic Hall and Carbomedics mechanical heart valves. *J Heart Valve Dis* 2001; 10:403.
22. Chambers J, Roxburgh J, Blauth C, et al: A randomized comparison of the MCRI On-X and Carbomedics Top Hat bileaflet mechanical replacement aortic valves: early postoperative hemodynamic function and clinical events. *J Thorac Cardiovasc Surg* 2005; 130:759.
23. Khan SS, Trento A, DeRobertis M, et al: Twenty-year comparison of tissue and mechanical valve replacement. *J Thorac Cardiovasc Surg* 2001; 122:257.
24. Brown ML, Schare HV, Lahr BD, et al: Aortic valve replacement in patients aged 50 to 70 years: Improved outcome with mechanical versus biologic prosthesis. *J Thorac Cardiovasc Surg* 2008;135:878.
25. deVincentiis C, Kunkl AB, Trimarchi S, et al. Aortic valve replacement in octogenarians: is biologic valve the unique solution? *Ann Thorac Surg* 2008; 85:1296-1301
26. Butchart EG, Payne N, Li H, et al: Better anticoagulation control improves survival after valve replacement. *J Thorac Cardiovasc Surg* 2002; 123:715.
27. Butchart EG, Ionescu A, Payne N, et al: A new scoring system to determine thromboembolic risk after heart valve replacement. *Circulation* 2003; 108(Suppl II):II-68.
28. Akins CW, Buckley MJ, Daggett WM, et al: Risk of reoperative valve replacement for failed mitral and aortic bioprostheses. *Ann Thorac Surg* 1998; 65:1545.
29. Emery RW, Arom KV, Krogh CC, et al: Reoperative valve replacement with the St. Jude Medical valve prosthesis: long-term follow up. *J Am Coll Cardiol* 2004; 435:438A.
30. Potter DD, Sundt TM 3rd, Zehr KJ, et al: Operative risk of reoperative aortic valve replacement. *J Thorac Cardiovasc Surg* 2005; 129:94.
31. Harrington JT: My three valves. *NEJM* 1993; 328:1345.
32. Emery RW, Krogh CC, Arom DV, et al: The St. Jude Medical cardiac valve prosthesis: a 25-year experience with single valve replacement. *Ann Thorac Surg* 2005; 79:776.
33. Emery RW, Arom KV, Nicoloff DM: Utilization of the St. Jude Medical prosthesis in the aortic position. *Semin Thorac Cardiovasc Surg* 1996; 8:231.

34. Emery RW, Arom KV, Kshettry VR, et al: Decision making in the choice of heart valve for replacement in patients aged 60–70 years: twenty-year follow up of the St. Jude Medical aortic valve prostheses. *J Heart Valve Dis* 2002; 11(Suppl 1):S37.
35. Bakir MD, Casselman FP, Wellens F, et al: Minimally invasive versus standard approach aortic valve replacement: a study in 506 patients. *Ann Thorac Surg* 2006;81:1599-1604
36. Lund O, Nielsen SL, Arildsen H, et al: Standard aortic St. Jude valve at 18 years: performance, profile and determinants of outcome. *Ann Thorac Surg* 2000; 69:1459.
37. Aagaard J, Tingleff J, Hansen CN, et al: Twelve years' clinical experience with the Carbomedics prosthetic heart valve. *J Heart Valve Dis* 2001; 10:177.
38. Butchart EG, Li H, Payne N, et al: Twenty years' experience with the Medtronic Hall valve. *J Thorac Cardiovasc Surg* 2001; 121:1090.
39. Ikonomidis JS, Kratz JM, Crumbley AJ, et al: Twenty-year experience with the St. Jude Medical mechanical valve prosthesis. *J Thorac Cardiovasc Surg* 2003; 126:20022.
40. Koertke H, Korfer R: International normalized ratio self-management after mechanical heart valve replacement: is an early start advantageous? *Ann Thorac Surg* 2001; 72:44.
41. Montalescot G, Polle V, Collet JP, et al: Low molecular weight heparin after mechanical heart valve replacement. *Circulation* 2000; 101:1083.
42. Horstkotte D, Schulte H, Bircks W, Strauer B: Unexpected findings concerning thromboembolic complications and anticoagulation after complete 10-year follow-up of patients with St. Jude Medical prostheses. *J Heart Valve Dis* 1993; 2:291.
43. Butchart EG, Lewis PA, Bethel JA, Breckenridge IM: Adjusting anticoagulation to prosthesis thrombogenicity and patient risk factors. *Circulation* 1991; 84(Suppl III):III-61.
44. Koertke H, Minami K, Boethig D, et al: INR self-management permits lower anticoagulation levels after mechanical heart valve replacement. *Circulation* 2003; 108(Suppl II):II-75.
45. Bonow RO, Carabello BA, Chatterjee BA, et al: ACC/AHA 2006 guidelines for the management of patients with valvular heart disease. *J Am Coll Cardiol* 2008;52;e1-142
46. American College of Chest Physicians: Sixth (2000) ACCP guidelines for antithrombotic therapy for prevention and treatment of thrombosis. *Chest* 2001; 119(1 Suppl):1S.
47. Horstkotte D, Piper C, Wiener X, et al: Improvement of prognosis by home control in patients with lifelong anticoagulant therapy. *Ann Hematol* 1996; 72(suppl D):AE3.
48. Koo S, Kucher N, Nguyen PL, et al: The effect of excessive anticoagulation on mortality and morbidity in hospitalized patients with anticoagulant-related major hemorrhage. *Arch Intern Med* 2004; 164:1557.
49. Emery RW, Arom KV, Krogh CC, Joyce LD: Long-term results with the St. Jude Medical aortic valve: a 25-year experience. *J Am Coll Cardiol* 2004; 435:429A.
50. Horstkotte D, Schulte HD, Bircks W, Strauer BE: Lower intensity anticoagulation therapy results in lower complication rates with the St. Jude Medical prosthesis. *J Thorac Cardiovasc Surg* 1994; 107:1136.
51. Turpie A, Gent M, Laupacis A, et al: A comparison of aspirin with placebo in patients treated with warfarin after heart valve replacement. *NEJM* 1993; 329:524.
52. Massel D, Little SH: Risk and benefits of adding antiplatelet therapy to warfarin among patients with prosthetic heart valves: a meta-analysis. *J Am Coll Cardiol* 2001; 37:569.
53. Accola KD, Scott ML, Spector SD, et al: Is the St. Jude Medical mechanical valve an appropriate choice for elderly patients? A long-term retrospective study measuring quality of life. *J Heart Valve Dis* 2006; 15:57.
54. Arom KV, Emery RW, Nicoloff DM, Petersen RJ: Anticoagulant related complications in elderly patients with St. Jude mechanical valve prostheses. *J Heart Valve Dis* 1996; 5:505.
55. Masters RG, Semelhago LC, Pipe AL, Keon WJ: Are older patients with mechanical heart valves at increased risk? *Ann Thorac Surg* 1999; 68:2169.
56. Davis EA, Greene PS, Cameron DE, et al: Bioprosthetic versus mechanical prostheses for aortic valve replacement in the elderly. *Circulation* 1996; 94(9 Suppl):II121.
57. Zimpfer D, Czerny M, Schuch P, et al: Long-term neurocognitive function after mechanical aortic valve replacement. *Ann Thorac Surg* 2006; 81:29.
58. Lip GY, Hart RG, Conway DS: Antithrombotic therapy for atrial fibrillation. *BMJ* 2002; 325:1022.
59. Garcia-Rinaldi R, Carro-Pagan C, Schaer HV, et al: Initial experience with dual antiplatelet thrombo prophylaxis with clopidogrel and aspirin in patients with mechanical aortic prosthesis. *J Heart Valve Dis* 2009;18:617
60. Horstkotte D: Letter to the editor. *Ann Thorac Surg* 1996; 62:1566.
61. Akins CW: Results with mechanical cardiac valvular prostheses. *Ann Thorac Surg* 1995; 60:1836.
62. David TE, Gott VL, Harker LA, et al: Mechanical valves. *Ann Thorac Surg* 1996; 62:1567.
63. Maganti M, Rao V, Armstrong S, et al: Redo valvular surgery in elderly patients. *Ann Thorac Surg* 2009;87:521-525
64. Grunkemeier GL, Li HH, Naftel DC, et al: Long-term performance of heart valve prostheses. *Curr Probl Cardiol* 2000; 25:73.
65. Sawant D, Singh AK, Feng WC, et al: St. Jude Medical cardiac valves in small aortic roots: follow-up to sixteen. *J Thorac Cardiovasc Surg* 1997; 113:499.
66. Piper C, Hering D, Langer C, Horstkotte D: Etiology of stroke after mechanical heart valve replacement: results from a ten-year prospective study. *J Heart Valve Dis* 2008; 17:413-417.
67. Czer LS, Matloff JM, Chaux A, et al: The St. Jude valve: analysis of thromboembolism, warfarin-related hemorrhage, and survival. *Am Heart J* 1987; 114:389.
68. Durrleman N, Pellerin M, Bouchard D, et al: Prosthetic valve thrombosis: twenty-year experience at the Montreal Heart Institute. *J Thorac Cardiovasc Surg* 2004; 127:1388.
69. Van Nooten GJ, Van Belleghem Y, Caes F, et al: Lower-intensity anticoagulation for mechanical heart valves: a new concept with the ATS bileaflet aortic valve. *J Heart Valve Dis* 2003; 12:495.
70. Schaff HV, Carrel TP, Jamieson WRE, et al: Paravalvular leak and other events in silzone-coated mechanical heart valves: a report from AVERT. *Ann Thorac Surg* 2002; 73:785.
71. De Cicco G, Lorusso R, Colli A, et al: Aortic valve periprosthetic leakage, anatomic observations and surgical results. *Ann Thorac Surg* 2005; 79:1480.
72. Baudet EM, Oca CC, Roques XF, et al: A 5½ year experience with the St. Jude Medical cardiac valve prosthesis. Early and late results of 737 valve replacements in 671 patients. *J Thorac Cardiovasc Surg* 1985; 90:137.
73. Rahimtoola SH: The problem of valve prosthesis patient mismatch. *Circulation* 1978; 58:20.
74. Pibarot P, Dumesnil JG: Hemodynamic and clinical impact of prosthesis-patient mismatch in the aortic valve position and its prevention. *J Am Coll Cardiol* 2000; 36:1131.
75. Hanayama N, Christakis GT, Mallidi HR, et al: Patient prosthesis mismatch is rare after aortic valve replacement: valve size may be irrelevant. *Ann Thorac Surg* 2002; 73:1822.
76. Blackstone EH, Cosgrove DM, Jamieson WRE, et al: Prosthesis size and long-term survival after aortic valve replacement. *J Thorac Cardiovasc Surg* 2003; 126:783.
77. Blais C, Dumesnil JG, Baillot R, et al: Impact of valve prosthesis patient mismatch on short-term mortality after aortic valve replacement. *Circulation* 2003; 108:983.
78. Moon MR, Pasque MK, Munfakh NA, et al: Prosthesis-patient mismatch after aortic valve replacement: impact of age and body size on late survival. *Ann Thorac Surg* 2006; 81:481.
79. Emery RW, Krogh CC, Arom KV, et al: Patient-prosthesis mismatch: Impact on patient survival and valve related events: a 25-year experience with the St. Jude Medical valve prosthesis. Presented at the Society of Thoracic Surgeons at the 41st Annual Meeting, San Antonio, TX. January 2005.
80. Pibarot P, Dumesnil JG: Patient-prosthesis mismatch and the predictive use of indexed effective orifice area: is it relevant? *Cardiac Surg Today* 2003; 1:43.
81. Riberiro PA, Al Zaibag M, Idris M, et al: Antiplatelet drugs and the incidence of thromboembolic complications of the St. Jude Medical aortic prosthesis in patients with rheumatic heart disease. *J Thoracic Cardiovasc Surg* 1986; 91:92.
82. Ananthasubramaniam K, Beattie JN, Rosman HS, et al: How safely and for how long can warfarin therapy be withheld in prosthetic heart valve patients hospitalized with a major hemorrhage? *Chest* 2001; 119:478.
83. Hartz RS, LoCicero J 3rd, Kucich V, et al: Comparative study of warfarin versus antiplatelet therapy in patients with a St. Jude Medical valve in the aortic position. *J Thorac Cardiovasc Surg* 1986; 92:684.
84. Garcia-Rinaldi R: Letter to the editor. *Ann Thorac Surg* 2006; 81:787.
85. Emery RW, Emery AM: Letter to the editor: reply to Garcia-Rinaldi. *Ann Thorac Surg* 2006; 81:788.
86. Cannegieter SC, Rosendaal FR, Briet E: Thromboembolic and bleeding complications in patients with mechanical heart valve prostheses. *Circulation* 1994; 89:635.
87. Cabalka AK, Emery RW, Petersen RJ: Long-term follow-up of the St. Jude Medical prosthesis in pediatric patients. *Ann Thorac Surg* 1995; 60:S618.
88. Emery RW, Erickson CA, Arom KV, et al: Replacement of the aortic valve in patients under 50 years old with the St. Jude Medical prosthesis. *Ann Thorac Surg* 2003; 75:1815.

CHAPTER 33

Bioprosthetic Aortic Valve Replacement: Stented Pericardial and Porcine Valves

Bobby Yanagawa
George T. Christakis

INTRODUCTION

This chapter provides an overview of aortic valve replacement (AVR) with stented bioprostheses. The *indications for aortic valve surgery* are reviewed, with an emphasis on current evidence-based guidelines, and currently available stented aortic bioprostheses are described. Clinical and physiologic outcomes of aortic valve surgery are critically evaluated to create a rational basis for prosthesis selection.

NATURAL HISTORY AND INDICATIONS FOR OPERATION

Aortic Stenosis

Natural History

Aortic stenosis (AS) may be caused by: (1) degenerative calcification; (2) congenital malformations, most commonly bicuspid aortic valve; or (3) rheumatic fever. It is uncommonly associated with systemic diseases such as Paget's disease of bone and end-stage renal disease. Degenerative calcification is common in the elderly population and moderate to severe calcific AS is the most common pathology among patients undergoing AVR. The incidence of calcific AS is expected to rise with the increase in age of population in developed countries.

Valvular degenerative calcification is characterized as a progressive reduction of orifice cross-sectional area caused by calcification of the cusps. The pathogenesis of inflammation and lipid accumulation is reminiscent of atherosclerosis.[1] The normal human aortic valve area (AVA) is between 3.0 and 4.0 cm^2 with minimal to no gradient. Aortic stenosis is defined as mild, moderate, and severe AS, and the corresponding AVA, mean gradients, and peak jet velocities are shown in Table 33-1. In the presence of normal cardiac output, transvalvular gradient is usually greater than 50 mm Hg when the AVA is less than 1.0 cm^2.[2] A rapid increase in transvalvular gradient is seen when AVA is less than 0.8 to 1.0 cm^2.

Obstruction to flow created by the reduced orifice area of the aortic valve elevates intracavitary pressures, and resultant wall stress leads to compensatory concentric hypertrophy to maintain normal cardiac output.[3] With progressive hypertrophy, ventricular compliance progressively decreases and end-diastolic pressure rises.[4] In this situation, the contribution of atrial contraction to preload becomes more significant and loss of sinus rhythm may lead to rapid progression of symptoms.

Symptomatic Patients

As AS progresses to become hemodynamically significant, initial compensation occurs by left ventricular hypertrophy (LVH). The average AVA is 0.6 to 0.8 cm^2 at the onset of symptoms.[3] Gradual progression of outflow obstruction and ventricular hypertrophy lead to the cardinal symptoms of AS, which are: (1) angina, (2) syncope, and (3) dyspnea or congestive heart failure (CHF). Classic natural history studies have demonstrated that average life expectancy in patients with hemodynamically significant AS is 4 years with angina, 3 years with syncope, and 2 years with CHF.[5] Symptom development in the context of AS is an absolute indication for surgical intervention.[6] Excessive delay of AVR in symptomatic patients is associated with rate of sudden death of greater than 10% per year. Once a patient is symptomatic, average survival is less than 3 years typically from ventricular arrhythmia or CHF.[7]

TABLE 33-1 Classification of Aortic Stenosis (AS)

	Mild	Moderate	Severe
AVA (cm^2)	>1.5	1.5–1.0	<1.0
Mean gradient (mm Hg)	<25	25–40	>40
Peak jet velocity (m/s)	<3.0	3.0–4.0	>4.0

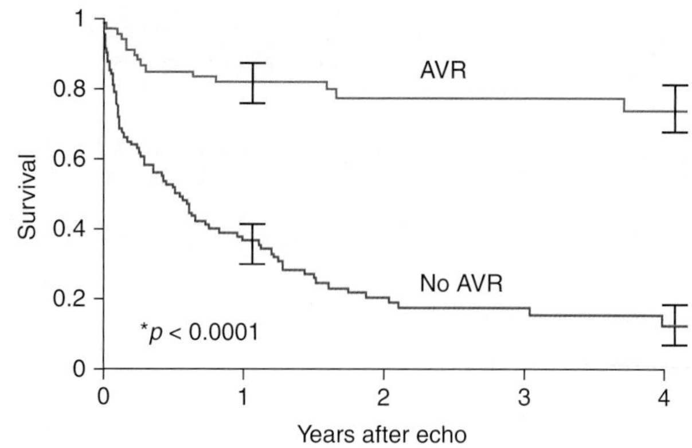

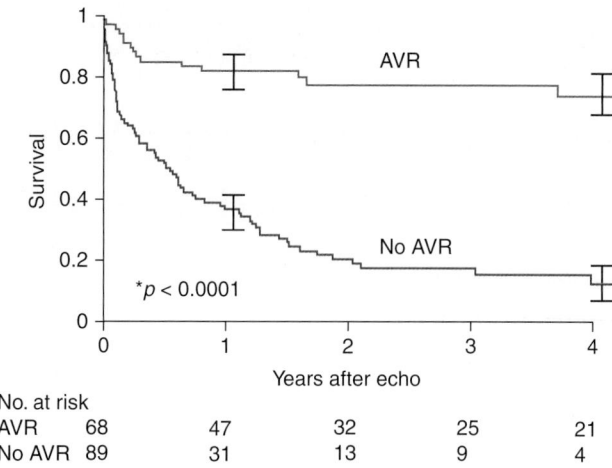

FIGURE 33-1 Impact of aortic valve replacement on survival in patients with low-gradient aortic stenosis. Survival by Kaplan-Meier analysis among all propensity-matched patients in the aortic valve replacement (AVR) and control (No AVR) groups ($p < .0001$). The number of patients at risk during follow-up is shown on the x-axis. *(Reproduced with permission from Pereira JJ, Lauer MS, Bashir M, et al: Survival after aortic valve replacement for severe aortic stenosis with low transvalvular gradients and severe left ventricular dysfunction. J Am Coll Cardiol 2002; 39:1356.)*

ASYMPTOMATIC PATIENTS

Managing asymptomatic patients with hemodynamically significant AS remains controversial. The average decrease in AVA is 0.12 cm^2 per year, whereas the average increase in transvalvular pressure is often 10 to 15 mm Hg per year.[8] However, considerable variation does exist in the rate of disease progression and many patients do not experience any change in gradient for several years. As such, there may exist a prolonged and stochastic latent periods before symptoms emerge. During this period, concentric LVH progresses as ventricle adapts to elevated chamber pressures.

Sudden death is rather uncommon in the asymptomatic patient unless the degree of AS is severe, in which case the rate is approximately 1% per year. However, the vast majority of patients who experience sudden death will become symptomatic in the months immediately before the fatal event.[9]

When considering AVR, the risk of sudden death should be weighed against the contemporary STS database surgical mortality of 3.5%. Although it is difficult to predict who will need surgical intervention, asymptomatic patients with increases in peak velocity jet greater than 0.45 m/s per year are substantially more likely to need an operation.[9] Overall, up to 7% of asymptomatic patients with AS experience death or aortic valve surgery 1 year after diagnosis.[10] After 5 years, the incidence of death or aortic valve surgery surges to 38%. Of note, early and late outcomes were similar among patients with severe AS who underwent surgery with or without symptoms.[11]

Low-Gradient Severe Aortic Stenosis

The significance of AS is often unclear in patients with very poor ventricular function (ejection fraction <20%) who have severely stenotic valves but small (<30 mm Hg) transvalvular gradients. Compromised left ventricular function (LVF) in these patients may be caused by afterload mismatch created by the stenotic valve or by intrinsic cardiomyopathy, particularly in the setting of chronic ischemia from diffuse coronary disease. In these patients, measurement of transvalvular gradient and valve area at rest and with positive inotropy (eg, dobutamine infusion) may distinguish cardiomyopathy versus true valvular stenosis as the most responsible diagnosis. Most patients with poor LVF and severe AS experience a significant survival benefit from valve replacement[12] (Fig. 33-1). However, a subset of patients with a preponderance of cardiomyopathy do not experience significant benefit.[13] A multivariate analysis to determine factors that predict poor LVF after AVR for AS identified poor preoperative LVF as the most significant predictor, indicating suboptimal outcome in the low-gradient group of patients.[14]

Medical Therapy

No known medical therapy has been shown to alter the natural history of AS. Although several small nonrandomized studies have shown a reduction in disease progression with antilipid therapy,[15] a recent prospective randomized clinical trial of aggressive antilipid therapy with atorvastatin did not demonstrate decreased rates of disease progression[16] (Fig. 33-2).

Indications for Operation

In 1998, a joint task force of the American College of Cardiology (ACC) and the American Heart Association (AHA) developed evidence-based consensus guidelines for management of valvular heart disease.[17] These were subsequently updated in 2006.[18] Their recommendations for AVR in the setting of AS are summarized in Table 33-2.

Aortic valve replacement is indicated in all symptomatic patients with severe AS or those with severe asymptomatic AS who require concomitant coronary bypass, aortic surgery, or other valve replacement. At Sunnybrook Health Sciences Center, it is our practice to perform AVR on patients with moderate AS requiring concomitant cardiac surgery. We do not routinely perform AVR on patients with mild AS undergoing concomitant cardiac surgery unless the aortic valve is heavily calcified and the stenosis likely to progress rapidly. Aortic valve replacement is commonly performed in otherwise asymptomatic patients with severe AS and severe left ventricular dysfunction (LVD), exercise-induced symptoms, significant hypertrophy, or ventricular arrhythmia. Asymptomatic patients with very high transvalvular gradients (>60 mm Hg) or highly stenotic valves (valve

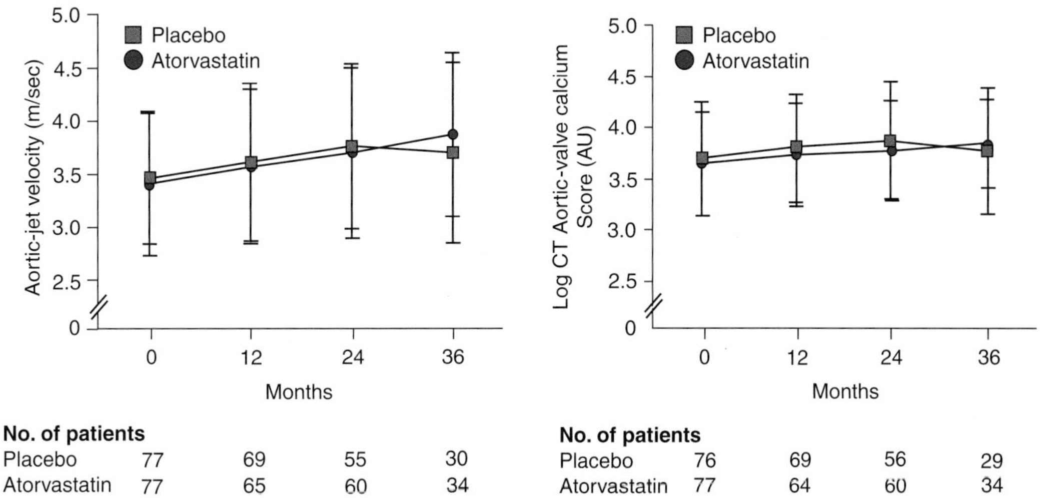

FIGURE 33-2 Progression of aortic valve jet velocity and calcification in patients treated with intensive atorvastatin therapy or matched placebo. *(Reproduced with permission from Cowell SJ, Newby DE, Prescott RJ, et al: A randomized trial of intensive lipid-lowering therapy in calcific aortic stenosis. NEJM 2005; 352:2389.)*

area <0.6 cm^2) are at higher risk for progression to symptoms and should have valve replacement before significant ventricular decompensation or sudden death.

Aortic Regurgitation

Acute Aortic Regurgitation

Acute aortic regurgitation (AR) is caused by: (1) acute dilatation of the aortic annulus preventing adequate cusp coaptation; or (2) disruption of the valve cusps themselves. The specific causes of AR include aortic dissection, infective endocarditis, trauma, aortic cusp prolapse secondary to VSD, aortitis (syphilitic or giant cell, and iatrogenic, such as postaortic balloon valvotomy).

The heart is rather intolerant of acute AR. Because the left ventricle is unable to compensate for the sudden increase in end-diastolic volume caused by a large regurgitant volume load, a dramatic reduction in forward stroke volume ensues.[19] In the context of a hypertrophic and poorly compliant LV, hemodynamic decompensation is significantly more dramatic.

TABLE 33-2 ACC/AHA Guidelines for Aortic Valve Replacement in Patients with Aortic Stenosis (AS)

Indication	Class
1. Symptomatic patients with severe AS	I
2. Patients with severe AS undergoing coronary bypass surgery	I
3. Patients with severe AS undergoing surgery on the aorta or other heart valves	I
4. Patients with severe AS and left ventricular systolic dysfunction (ejection fraction <50%)	I
5. Patients with moderate AS undergoing coronary artery bypass or other aortic or valvular surgery	IIA
6. Asymptomatic patients with severe AS and:	
a. Abnormal response to exercise (hypotension)	IIB
b. Likelihood of rapid progression (age, calcification, or coronary artery disease)	IIB
c. Ventricular tachycardia	IIB
d. Valve area <0.6 cm^2, mean gradient >60 mm Hg, jet velocity >5.0 m/s	IIB
7. Patients with mild AS and moderate to severe valve calcification undergoing coronary bypass surgery	IIB
8. Prevention of sudden death in an asymptomatic patient with none of the findings in 5–7	III

Source: Adapted with permission from Bonow RO, Carabello BA, Chatterjee K, et al: ACC/AHA 2006 guidelines for the management of patients with valvular heart disease: a report of the American College of Cardiology/American Heart Association Task Force on Practice Guidelines (Writing Committee to Develop Guidelines for the Management of Patients with Valvular Heart Disease). Available at: http://www.americanheart.org.

Tachycardia is the initial compensatory response to acute decline in forward stroke volume. Volume overload causes the left ventricular end-diastolic pressure to acutely rise above left atrial pressure, resulting in early closure of the mitral valve.[20] Although this protects the pulmonary venous circulation from excessively high end-diastolic pressures, rapid progression of pulmonary edema and cardiogenic shock are unavoidable. Death secondary to progressive cardiogenic shock and malignant ventricular arrhythmias is the common endpoint of acute AR regardless of etiology. Thus urgent surgical treatment is warranted for all causes of hemodynamically significant acute AR.

Chronic Aortic Regurgitation

Chronic AR is caused by either slow enlargement of the aortic root or dysfunction of the valve cusps. Common causes of chronic AR include congenital abnormalities (eg, bicuspid, unicuspid, quadricuspid aortic valve), calcific cusp degeneration, rheumatic fever, endocarditis, Marfan's syndrome, Ehlers-Danlos syndrome, myxomatous proliferation, osteogenesis imperfecta, and ankylosing spondylitis.

Chronic AR causes a persistent volume overload of the left ventricle. This volume burden leads to progressive chamber enlargement without increasing end-diastolic pressure during the asymptomatic phase of the disease. Chamber enlargement is accompanied by adaptive eccentric hypertrophy, associated at the cellular level with sarcomere replication and elongation of myocytes. The combination of chamber dilatation and hypertrophy leads to a massive increase in left ventricular mass. Initially, the ratio of wall thickness to chamber diameter, ejection fraction (EF), and fractional shortening are maintained.[21] However, a vicious cycle of chamber enlargement, continually increasing wall stress, and maladaptive ventricular hypertrophy ensues. Development of interstitial fibrosis is an important pathogenic mechanism that limits further ventricular dilitation, elevating end-diastolic pressure and leading to left ventricular systolic dysfunction, and CHF.[22] Vasodilator therapy may delay progression of ventricular dysfunction by decreasing afterload thus reducing regurgitant flow. Vasodilator therapy is currently indicated in asymptomatic patients with hypertension; asymptomatic patients with severe AR, ventricular dilatation, and preserved systolic function; and for short-term hemodynamic tailoring before operation. This therapy is not recommended in patients with severe AR and LVD, as it does not improve survival but may be used if such patients are considered inoperable.

The time course from diagnosis of AR to the development of symptoms is highly variable. Natural history studies of AR show that symptoms, LVD, or both develop in less than 6% of patients per year.[23] Progression to LVD without symptoms occurs in less than 4% of patients per year, and sudden death occurs in less than 0.2% per year.[24] Independent predictors of progression to symptoms, LVD, or death in asymptomatic patients include age, left ventricular end-systolic dimension, rate of change in end-systolic dimension, and resting EF LVD develops, the onset of symptoms occur at a rate exceeding 25% per year.[26] Because symptoms such as angina and dyspnea develop only after significant ventricular decompensation has occurred, surgery is advocated before the symptomatic phase of the disease. Symptomatic patients experience greater than 10% mortality per year; thus surgery is absolutely indicated.[27]

Indications for Operation

Surgical intervention for asymptomatic patients is based on the identification of subtle but measurable changes in myocardial function before they become irreversible and negatively affect the patient's long-term prognosis. Unfortunately, such deleterious changes are often missed by current imaging modalities. Patients with more severe LVD have decreased perioperative and late survival because of irreversible ventricular remodeling, including hypertrophy and interstitial fibrosis.[26,28] The decision to operate on this patient population is indeed challenging because the outcomes are poor with surgery or medical therapy.[4] A summary of the revised ACC/AHA Task Force guidelines for AVR for chronic AR is presented in Table 33-3.[18]

CORONARY ANGIOGRAPHY AND AORTIC VALVE REPLACEMENT

Many patients requiring AVR have coexistent coronary artery disease (CAD). In North America, more than one-third of AVR procedures are accompanied with coronary bypass graft surgery. This proportion will indeed increase as the surgical population continues to age. Risk assessment for ischemic heart disease is complicated in patients with aortic valve disease because angina may be related to true ischemia from hemodynamically significant coronary lesions, or other causes such as left ventricular wall stress with subendocardial ischemia or chamber enlargement in the setting of reduced coronary flow reserve. Because traditional coronary risk stratification is unreliable in aortic valve patients, at Sunnybrook Health Sciences Center, it is our practice to routinely perform diagnostic coronary angiography on all patients greater than age 35.

Technique of Operation

Myocardial Protection and Cardiopulmonary Bypass

Isolated AVR is performed using a single, two-stage right atrial venous cannula and an arterial cannula into the ascending aorta for systemic perfusion of oxygenated blood. A retrograde cardioplegia cannula may be placed into the coronary sinus via the right atrium. A left ventricular vent cannula is placed in the right superior pulmonary vein and advanced into the left ventricle to ensure a bloodless field and prevent ventricular distention with aortic insufficiency. Once cardiopulmonary bypass (CPB) is initiated, aorta and pulmonary artery are dissected to expose the anterior aortic root to the left coronary artery. Careful dissection of the pulmonary artery from the aorta ensures that the cross-clamp will be fully occlusive on the aorta and prevents inadvertent opening of the pulmonary artery with the aortotomy incision. Care is needed to present pulmonary artery injury, as this tissue is substantially more friable than the aorta.

After the cross-clamp is applied, myocardial protection is initially delivered as a single dose of high potassium blood through the ascending aorta. This will trigger prompt diastolic

TABLE 33-3 ACC/AHA Recommendations for Aortic Valve Replacement (AVR) in Chronic Severe Aortic Regurgitation (AR)

Indication	Class
1. AVR is indicated for symptomatic patients with severe AR irrespective of left ventricular systolic function	I
2. AVR is indicated for asymptomatic patients with chronic severe AR and left ventricular systolic dysfunction (ejection fraction ≤0.50) at rest	I
3. AVR is indicated for patients with chronic severe AR while undergoing coronary artery bypass graft or surgery on the aorta or other heart valves	I
4. AVR is reasonable for asymptomatic patients with severe AR with normal left ventricular systolic function (ejection fraction >0.50) but with severe left ventricular dilatation (end-diastolic dimension >75 mm or end-systolic dimension >55 mm)*	IIA
5. AVR may be considered in patients with moderate AR while undergoing surgery on the ascending aorta	IIB
6. AVR may be considered in patients with moderate AR while undergoing coronary artery bypass graft surgery	IIB
7. AVR may be considered for asymptomatic patients with severe AR and normal left ventricular systolic function at rest (ejection fraction >0.50) when the degree of left ventricular dilatation exceeds an end-diastolic dimension of 70 mm or end-systolic dimension of 50 mm, when there is evidence of progressive left ventricular dilatation, declining exercise tolerance, or abnormal hemodynamic responses to exercise*	IIB
8. AVR is not indicated for asymptomatic patients with mild, moderate, or severe AR and normal left ventricular systolic function at rest (ejection fraction >0.50) when the degree of dilatation is not moderate or severe (end-diastolic dimension <70 mm, and those with end-diastolic dimension >70 mm should have aortic valve replacement if there is evidence of serial deterioration of ventricular function or exercise intolerance)*	III

**Consider lower threshold values for patients of small stature of either gender.*
Source: Adapted with permission from Bonow RO, Carabello BA, Chatterjee K, et al: ACC/AHA 2006 guidelines for the management of patients with valvular heart disease: a report of the American College of Cardiology/American Heart Association Task Force on Practice Guidelines (Writing Committee to Develop Guidelines for the Management of Patients with Valvular Heart Disease). Available at: http://www.americanheart.org.

arrest unless there is moderate to severe AR. Myocardial protection is maintained by continuous infusion of cold or tepid oxygenated blood cardioplegia delivered via direct cannulation of both coronary ostia after the aorta has been opened. In the case of the short left main coronary artery, antegrade cannulation may preferentially perfuse either the LAD or circumflex system. In the presence of severe coronary artery disease, antegrade cardioplegia may not perfuse myocardial segments distal to significant coronary obstruction. Furthermore, direct cannulation of left main coronary artery risks endothelial injury and potential dissection or promotion of atherosclerosis development.

An alternative method of cardioprotection in aortic valve cases is retrograde cardioplegia, in either intermittent or continuous forms, and used in isolation or in combination with antegrade cardioplegia. This is helpful in patients with significant AR or severe concomitant coronary disease. However, there are some questions regarding the quality of RV perfusion using retrograde alone. If retrograde cannula cannot be guided into the coronary sinus, conversion to bicaval cannulation will allow opening the right atrium and direct placement of the cannula into the coronary sinus. Do not place the retrograde cannula beyond the origin of the right coronary vein ostium in the coronary sinus to ensure adequate right ventricular myocardial protection.

Aortotomy, Valve Excision, and Debridement

Once the cross-clamp has been applied and cardioplegic arrest has been achieved, the aorta is opened either with a transverse or oblique aortotomy. The low transverse aortotomy is a common approach to the aortic valve when using stented bioprostheses or mechanical valves. The aortotomy is started approximately 10 to 15 mm above the origin of the right coronary artery (RCA) and extended anteriorly and posteriorly. The initial transverse incision over the RCA may also be extended obliquely in the posterior direction into the noncoronary sinus or the commissure between the left and noncoronary cusps (Fig. 33-3). The oblique incision is often used in patients with small aortic roots, in whom root enlargement procedures may be required

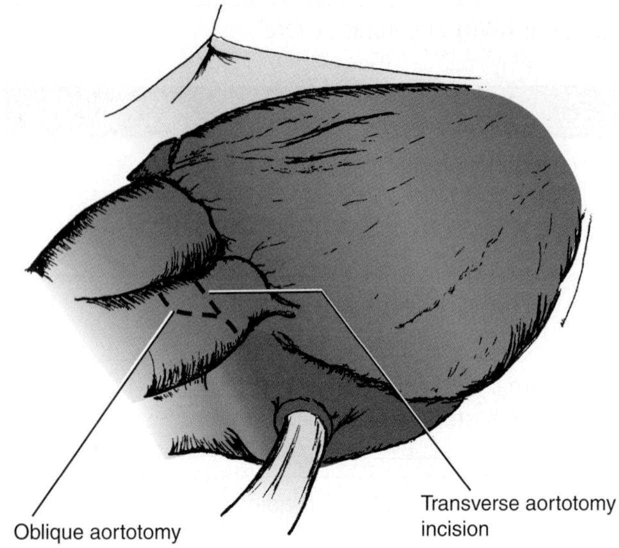

FIGURE 33-3 Exposure and aortotomy incision. A two-stage venous cannula is in place in the right atrial appendage. The aortotomy (*dashed line*) may be made in the transverse or oblique direction.

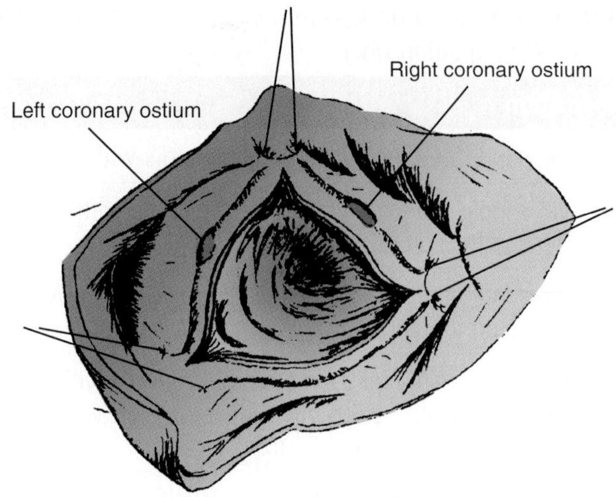

FIGURE 33-5 The aortic valve after leaflet excision.

(see the following) and may also be used to tailor a larger ascending aorta.

Morphology of the valve is then inspected (Fig. 33-4). The valve cusps are incised with scissors at the right cusp between the right coronary ostium and the commissure between the right and noncoronary cusps (Fig. 33-5). Mayo scissors or special right-angled valve scissors are usually used at this stage and the calcific deposits are removed from the aortic wall. One to two millimeters of tissue are left behind to support a sewing surface. Right cusp excision is carried first toward the left coronary cusp and then toward the noncoronary cusp and the cusp is removed as a single piece if possible. Excision is then carried toward the left and noncoronary commissure along the noncoronary cusp and then the left coronary cusp. A moistened radiopaque sponge is placed into the outflow area to catch calcific debris, which must be removed before placing the valve sutures. Thorough decalcification is then performed with a scalpel or rongeur. Debridement of all calcium deposits back to soft tissue improves seating of the prosthesis and decreases the incidence of paravalvular leak and dehiscence.

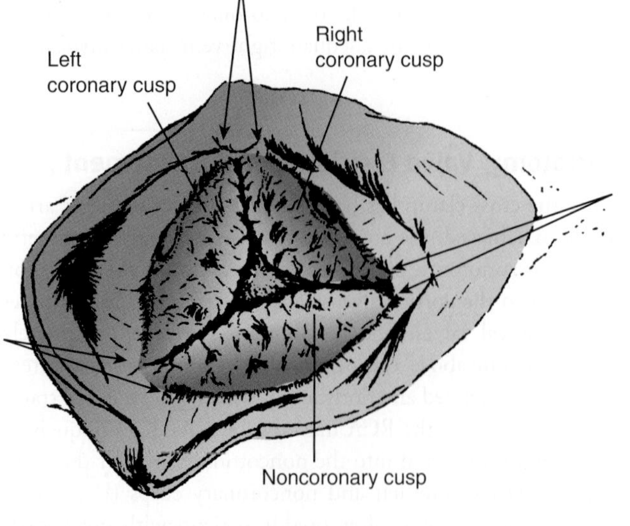

FIGURE 33-4 The exposed aortic valve.

Care must be taken to prevent aortic perforation while calcific deposits are debrided from the aortic wall, particularly at the commissure between the left and noncoronary cusps, where perforation is most likely. Several anatomic relationships must be respected during valve excision (Fig. 33-6). The bundle of His (conduction system) is located below the junction of the right and noncoronary cusps in the membranous septum. Deep debridement in this area can result in permanent heart block. The anterior leaflet of the mitral valve is in direct continuity with the left aortic valve cusp. If it is damaged during decalcification, an autologous pericardial patch is used to repair the defect.

Once debridement is completed, the aortic root is copiously flushed with saline while the left ventricular vent is stopped. To prevent pushing debris into the left ventricle, saline in a bulb syringe is flushed through the left ventricular vent and out the aortic valve in an antegrade manner instead of retrograde through the valve. The irrigation solution is suctioned with the external wall suction and not into the cardiotomy suction.

Valve Implantation

After the native valve has been excised, the annulus is sized with a valve-sizer designed for the selected prosthetic device. The valve is secured to the annulus using 12 to 16 double-needled interrupted 2-0 synthetic braided pledgeted sutures that are alternating in color. The pledgets can be left on the inflow/ventricular side or the outflow/aortic side of the aortic annulus (Figs. 33-7 and 33-8). Placing the pledgets on the inside of the annulus allows supra-annular placement of the valve and generally

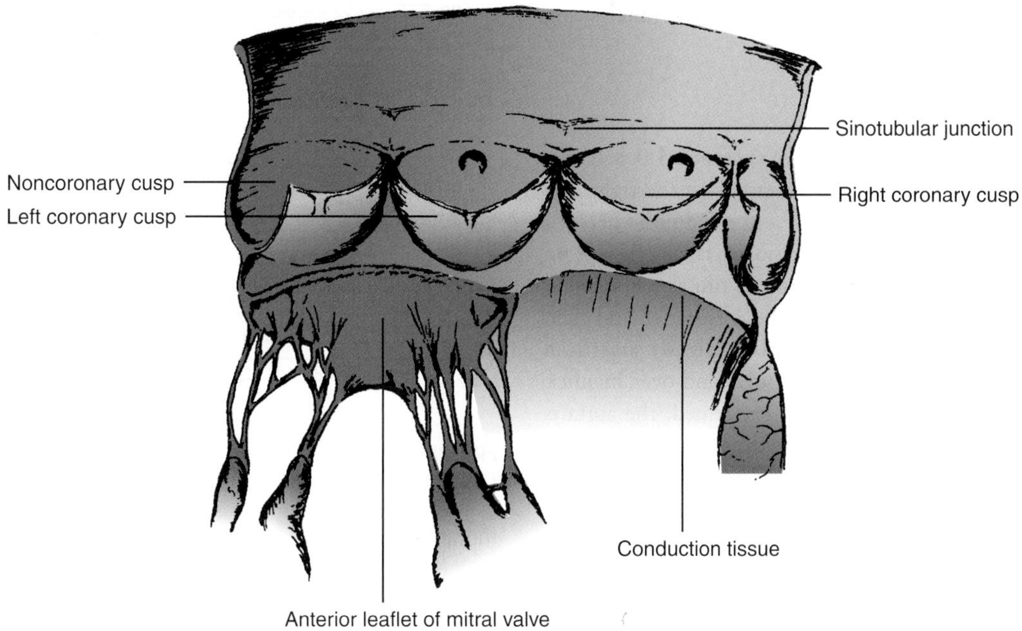

FIGURE 33-6 Anatomical relationships of the aortic valve.

will allow implantation of a slightly larger prosthesis. In cases in which the coronary ostia are close to the annulus, supra-annular placement may only be possible along the noncoronary cusp. Mattress sutures are first placed in the three commissures and retracted to assist visualization. Some surgeons will place the commissural suture between the right and noncoronary cusps from the outside of the aorta (ie, the pledget is left on the outside of the aorta) to prevent injury to the conduction system. Pledgeted mattress sutures are then placed in a clockwise fashion typically starting in the noncoronary cusp. Sutures may be placed into the sewing ring of the prosthetic valve with each annular suture or after all annular sutures are placed. The sutures for each of the three cusps are held separately with three hemostats and retracted while the prosthesis is slid into the annulus.

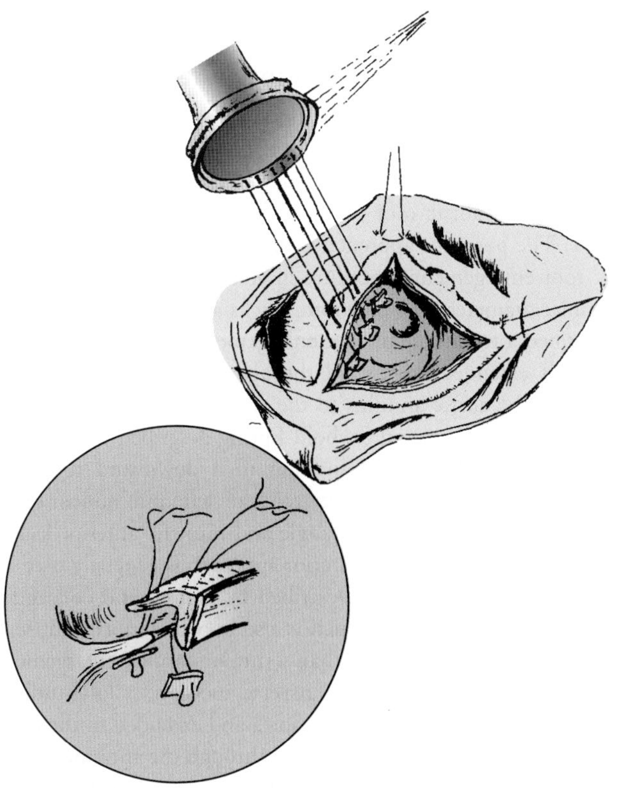

FIGURE 33-7 Placement of sutures with pledgets below the annulus.

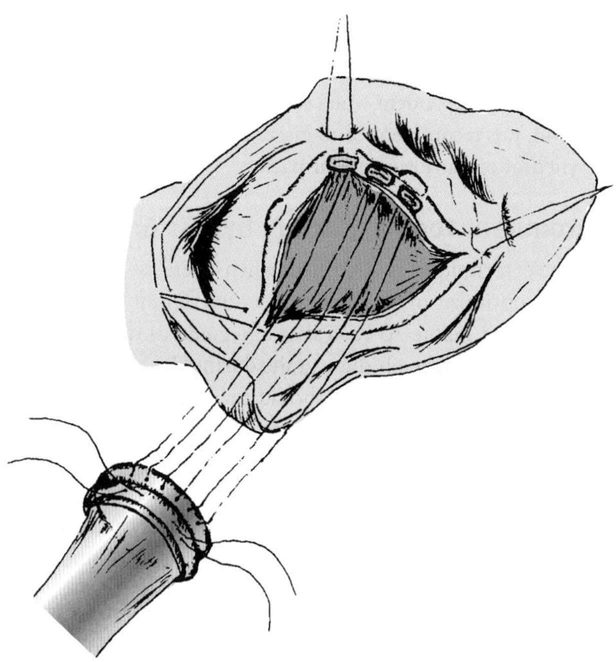

FIGURE 33-8 Placement of sutures with pledgets above the annulus.

Sutures are then tied down in a balanced fashion alternating among the three cusps.

Aortic Closure and De-airing

The aorta is closed with a double row of synthetic 4-0 polypropylene sutures. The first suture line is started on the right side at the posterior end of the aortotomy, and the double-needled suture is secured slightly beyond the incision to ensure there is no leak in this region. One end of the suture is run as a horizontal mattress anteriorly to the midpoint of the aortotomy, and then the second end of the suture is run anteriorly, slightly superficial to the horizontal mattress suture, in an over-and-over manner. On the left side, a similar technique is performed, the aorta is de-aired (described in the following), and the two sutures are tied to themselves and to each other at the aortotomy midpoint.

During AVR, air is entrained into the left atrium and ventricle, and aorta. This must be removed to prevent catastrophic air embolization. Immediately before tying the suture of the aortotomy, the heart is allowed to fill, the vent in the superior pulmonary vein is stopped, the lungs are inflated, and the cross-clamp is briefly partially opened. The influx of blood should expel most air from these cavities out of the partially open aortotomy. Closure of the aortotomy is then completed and the cross-clamp is fully removed. The cardioplegia cannula in the ascending aorta and the left ventricular vent are then placed on suction to remove any residual air as the heart begins electrical activity. A small needle (21-gauge) is used to aspirate the apex of the left ventricle and the dome of the left atrium. To prevent air entrainment, the left ventricular vent must be removed while the pericardium is filled with saline irrigation. De-airing maneuvers are verified with visualization using transesophageal echocardiography to verify that all air has been removed from the left side of the heart. Vigorous shaking and careful manual compression of the heart while suctioning through the aortic vent (ie, cardioplegia tack) is helpful to remove air trapped within trabeculations. Once de-airing is complete, the aortic vent is removed. The patient is then weaned from CPB and decannulated in the standard fashion. If patients are pacemaker-dependent when weaned from CPB in the operating room, it is recommended to insert atrial pacing wires to allow for synchronous atrioventricular pacing.

Concomitant Coronary Artery Bypass Grafting

Operative technique is modified when there is concomitant CAD to optimize myocardial protection. Distal anastomoses are performed before AVR so that antegrade cardioplegia may be administered through these grafts during the operation. The left internal mammary artery should be used for revascularization of the left anterior descending artery, because this may improve long-term survival in aortic valve patients.[29] This anastomosis is performed after the aortotomy is closed to ensure that the coronary circulation is not exposed to systemic circulation during cardioplegic arrest and to prevent trauma to the anastomosis during manipulation of the heart.

Concomitant Ascending Aortic Replacement

In general, the ascending aorta is replaced electively when maximal diameter exceeds 5.5 to 6.0 cm; however, with Marfan's syndrome or equivalent connective tissue disorder the cutoff is 4.5 to 5.0 cm. In the setting of concomitant AVR, aortic replacement is advised if the ascending aortic diameter is greater than 5.0 cm. Patients with bicuspid aortic valves have an underlying aortopathy that leads to significant risk of late ascending aortic complications, and these patients should have replacement of their ascending aorta if its diameter exceeds 4.5 cm at the time of AVR[30] (Fig. 33-9).

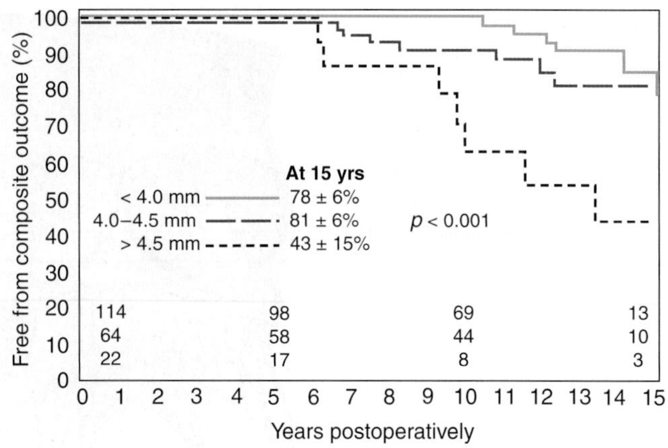

FIGURE 33-9 Freedom from ascending aortic complications for patients with a bicuspid aortic valve with an ascending aortic diameter of less than 4 cm, 4.0 to 4.5 cm, and 4.5 to 4.9 cm at the time of aortic valve replacement. (*Reproduced with permission from Borger MA, et al: Should the ascending aorta be replaced more frequently in patients with bicuspid aortic valve disease? J Thorac Cardiovasc Surg 2004; 128:677.*)

Aortic Root Enlargement Procedures

Detailed descriptions of aortic root enlargement procedures are presented in a later chapter. Briefly, either an anterior or posterior annular enlargement procedure may be performed in a patient with a small aortic root to allow for implantation of a larger valve. The posterior approach is the most commonly used aortic root enlargement procedure in adults and can increase the annular diameter by 2 to 4 mm. Nicks and colleagues in 1970 described a technique of root enlargement in which the aortotomy is extended downward through the noncoronary cusp, through the aortic annulus to the anterior mitral leaftlet.[31] In 1979, Manouguian and Seybold-Epting described a procedure extending the aortotomy incision in a downward direction through the commissure between the left and noncoronary cusps into the interleaflet triangle and into the anterior leaflet of the mitral valve.[32] The anterior approach is generally used in the pediatric population. Described by Konno and colleagues in 1975, this technique, which is also known as aortoventriculoplasty, is used when more than 4 mm of annular enlargement is required.[33] Instead of a transverse incision, a longitudinal incision is made in the anterior aorta and extended to the right coronary sinus of Valsalva and then through the anterior wall of the right ventricle to open the right ventricular outflow tract. The ventricular septum is incised, allowing significant expansion of the aortic annulus and left ventricular outflow tract.

Reoperative Aortic Valve Surgery

Repeat sternotomy after AVR may be performed for valve-related complications, progressive ascending aortic disease, or CAD. Valve-related causes include structural valve deterioration, prosthetic endocarditis, prosthesis thrombosis, or paravalvular leak. Chest re-entry is the most hazardous portion of any repeat cardiac procedure. At Sunnybrook Health Sciences Center, our routine practice is to obtain an adequate lateral chest x-ray and computed tomography scan to determine the proximity of cardiac structures to the posterior sternum. Cardiopulmonary bypass is instituted through the femoral vessels for any concerns about chest re-entry. An oscillating saw is used to open the sternum and the dissection is kept as limited as possible. Extreme caution must be employed during dissection when there are patent bypass grafts.

Once cardioplegic arrest is established, the old prosthesis is excised with sharp dissection. Care must be taken to remove all sutures and pledgets from the annulus. Annular injuries caused while excising the prosthesis are repaired with pledgeted interrupted sutures. Removal of stentless prostheses may be particularly difficult in this regard. In the setting of endocarditis, aggressive debridement of infected tissue must be performed with appropriate annular reconstruction with pericardium when root abscesses are present.[34] All foreign graft material, including Dacron aortic grafts, must be excised in the presence of active endocarditis.

In the presence of a Dacron prosthesis in the ascending aorta, chest re-entry may be extremely hazardous because exsanguination will occur if the graft is inadvertently opened during dissection. To limit the systemic consequences of exsanguination at normothermia, the patient should be placed on femoro-femoral CPB and cooled to 20°C before chest reentry. If the Dacron graft is accidentally opened, local control of the bleeding is established and CPB is stopped. Under circulatory arrest, atrial venous cannulation is instituted and the graft is controlled distal to the tear. Cardiopulmonary bypass may then be restarted. In all repeat aortic procedures, rigorous myocardial protection must be applied because these procedures often have very long ischemic times. Antegrade cold blood cardioplegia is usually employed in a continuous fashion throughout the case by selective cannulation of the coronary ostia. Retrograde cardioplegia may have benefit in the setting of patent old saphenous vein grafts.[35]

POSTOPERATIVE MANAGEMENT

Special consideration must be given to the underlying pathologic changes to the ventricle during the immediate postoperative period. The severely hypertrophied, noncompliant LV resulting from AS is highly dependent on sufficient preload for adequate filling. Filling pressures should be carefully titrated between 15 and 18 mm Hg with intravenous volume infusion. In such cases, subvalvular left ventricular outflow obstruction with systolic anterior wall motion of the mitral valve may occur. Intravenous beta-adrenergic blockage may relieve this obstruction by decreasing inotropy. In extreme cases, reoperation and surgical myectomy may be required.

Maintenance of sinus rhythm is also essential because up to one-third of cardiac output is derived from atrial contraction in a noncompliant ventricle. Up to 10% of patients will experience low cardiac output syndrome in the immediate postoperative period. If pacing is required postoperatively, synchronous atrioventricular pacing is beneficial in preventing low cardiac output syndrome.

Complete heart block occurs in 3 to 5% of AVR patients. This complication may be caused by suture placement or injury from debridement near the conduction system. Transient complete heart block caused by perioperative edema usually resolves in 4 to 6 days. After this time, insertion of a permanent pacemaker is recommended if there is no resolution.

Profound peripheral vasodilation, often seen in patients with aortic insufficiency, is treated with vasoconstrictors, including alpha-adrenergic agonists or vasopressin. Adequate filling of the dilated left ventricle may also require volume infusion.

STENTED BIOPROSTHETIC AORTIC VALVE REPLACEMENT DEVICES

Stented biologic prostheses may be constructed of porcine aortic valves or bovine pericardium. Over the past 40 years, advances in tissue fixation methodology and chemical treatments have been developed to prevent extracellular matrix and calcium deposition. All heterograft valves are preserved with glutaraldehyde, which acts by cross-linking collagen fibers to reduce tissue antigenicity. Glutaraldehyde also ameliorates in vivo enzymatic degradation and causes the loss of cell viability, thereby preventing extracellular matrix turnover.[36] Glutaraldehyde fixation of porcine valves can be performed at high pressure (60 to 80 mm Hg), low pressure (0.1 to 2 mm Hg), or zero pressure (0 mm Hg). Pericardial prostheses are fixed in low- or zero-pressure conditions. Porcine prostheses fixed at zero pressure retain the collagen architecture of the relaxed aortic valve cusp.[37] When comparing various bioprostheses, it is important to be aware of lack of standardization in methodologies for labeling valve sizes by the different manufacturers. In general, label sizes refer to either the internal or external diameter of the stent, not the external diameter of the sewing cuff or the maximal opening diameter of the valve leaflets. Thus, the same aortic annulus will likely fit different-sized valves from different manufacturers, depending on the convention they use and the size of their sewing cuff. Figure 33-10 compares internal and external sizes for a variety of prostheses.

First-Generation Prostheses

First-generation bioprostheses were preserved with high-pressure fixation and were placed in the annular position. They include the Medtronic Hancock Standard and Modified Orifice (Medtronic, Minneapolis, MN), and Carpentier-Edwards Standard porcine prostheses (Edwards Life Sciences, Irvine, CA).

Second-Generation Prostheses

Second-generation prostheses are treated with low- or zero-pressure fixation. Several second-generation prostheses may also be placed

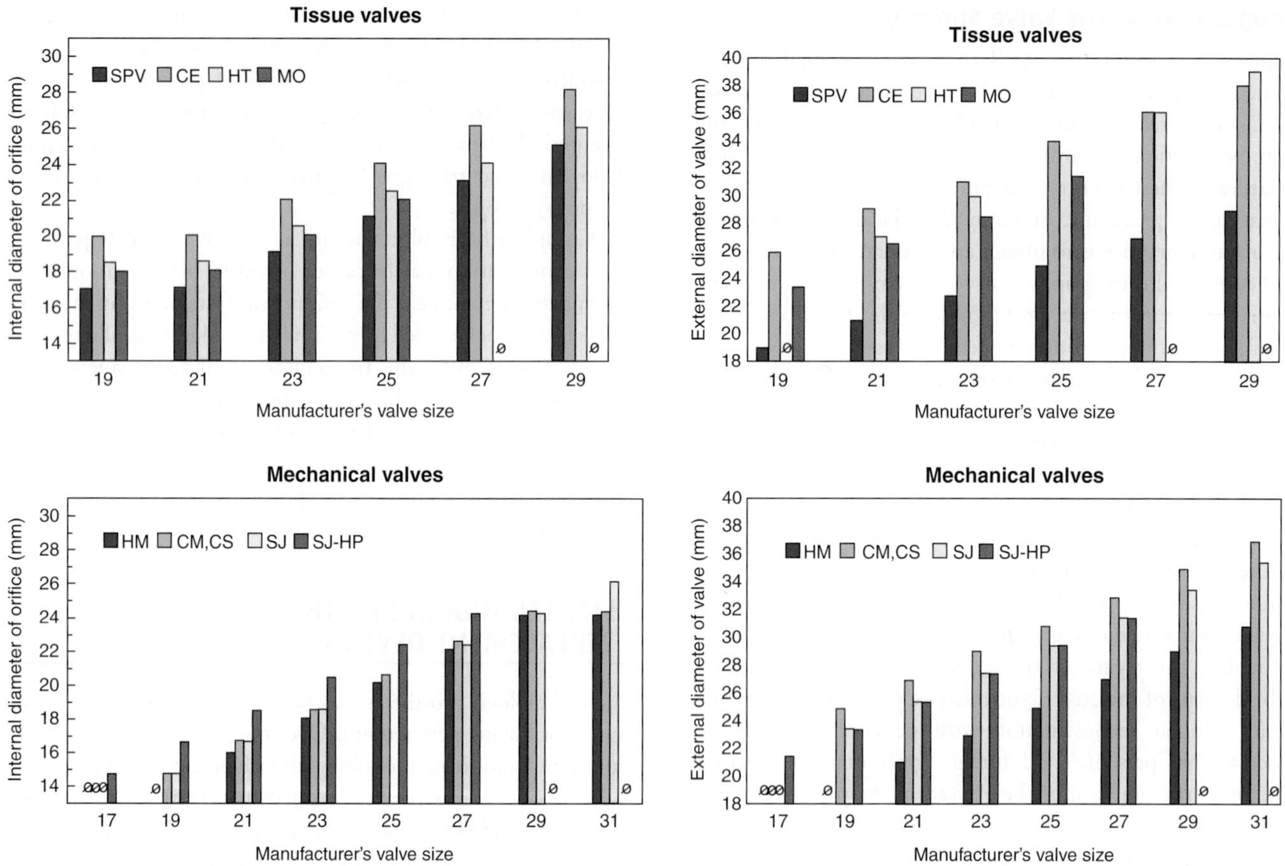

FIGURE 33-10 Comparison of the internal and external diameter of prosthetic aortic valves to the manufacturer's labeled size of each valve. No two manufacturers' valves have the same internal diameter for a given labeled size. CE = Carpentier-Edwards Pericardial valve; CM = Carbomedics Standard valve; CS = Carbomedics Supra-annular valve; HM = Medtronic Hall valve; HT = Hancock II Bioprosthesis; MO = Hancock Modified Orifice Bioprosthesis; SJ = St. Jude Standard valve; SJ-HP = St. Jude Hemodynamic Plus valve; SPV = stentless porcine valve. (*Reproduced with permission from Christakis GT, et al: Inaccurate and misleading valve sizing: a proposed standard for valve size nomenclature. Ann Thorac Surg 1998; 66:1198.*)

in the supra-annular position, which allows placement of a slightly larger prosthesis. Porcine second-generation prostheses include the Medtronic Hancock II valve (Medtronic), the Medtronic Intact porcine valve (Medtronic), and the Carpentier-Edwards Supraannular valve (SAV) (Edwards Life Sciences). Second-generation pericardial prostheses include the Carpentier-Edwards Perimount (Edwards Life Sciences), and the Pericarbon (Sorin Biomedica, Saluggia, Italy) prostheses.

Third-Generation Prostheses

Newer-generation prostheses incorporate zero- or low-pressure fixation with antimineralization processes that are designed to reduce material fatigue and calcification. Stents have become progressively thinner, have a lower profile, are more flexible, and sewing rings have become scalloped for supra-annular placement. The Medtronic Mosaic porcine valve (Medtronic) is fixed in a "physiologic" environment with equal pressure (40 mm Hg) applied to the ventricular and aortic sides of the leaflets, resulting in net zero pressure on the leaflets themselves (Figs. 33-11 and 33-12). The St. Jude Medical Epic valve (St. Jude Medical, Inc.) is a porcine valve with a very low stent post and base profile to minimize protrusion into the aortic wall and facilitate coronary clearance (Fig. 33-13). The Carpentier-Edwards Perimount Magna valve (Edwards Life Sciences) is the evolution of the Perimount pericardial valve, with a narrower sewing cuff and scalloped design for supra-annular placement (Fig. 33-14). The Mitroflow Pericardial aortic prosthesis (Carbomedics) is a pericardial valve that is unique in that the pericardium is placed around the exterior of the stent, presumably allowing for a larger opening diameter (Fig. 33-15).

OUTCOMES OF AORTIC VALVE REPLACEMENT

Operative Mortality

Operative mortality is defined as all-cause mortality within 30 days of operation or during the same hospital admission.[38] Contemporary series describe a very low operative mortality for isolated AVR between 1 and 8%, depending on the patient population, the presence of coronary disease, and the era of study.[39–43] In 1999, the Society of Thoracic Surgeons' (STS) database reviewed the results of 86,580 valve procedures to find an overall mortality of 4.3% for isolated AVR, and 8.0% for AVR

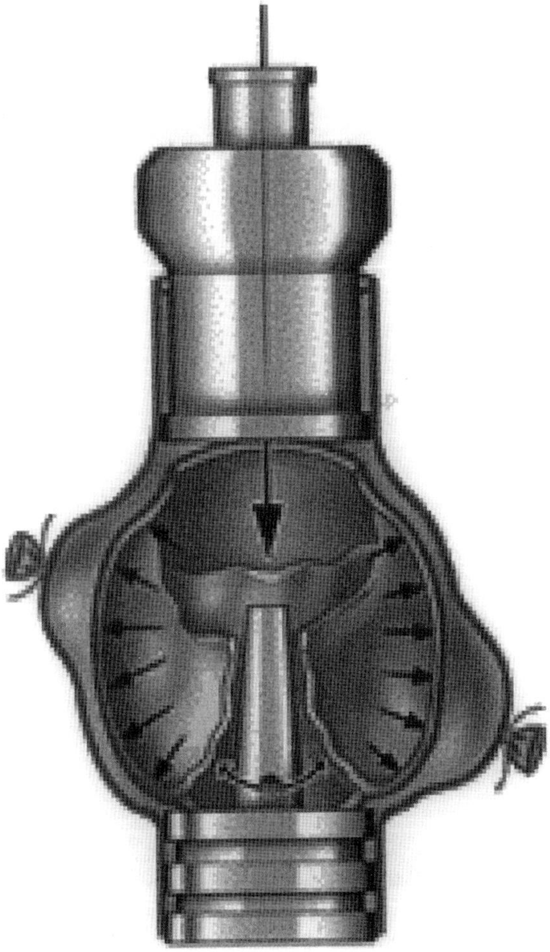

FIGURE 33-11 "Physiologic" fixation process. Simultaneous application of pressure to the inflow and outflow portions of a porcine bioprosthesis place zero net pressure on leaflets within a pressurized root. (*Figure courtesy of Medtronic Inc., Minneapolis, MN.*)

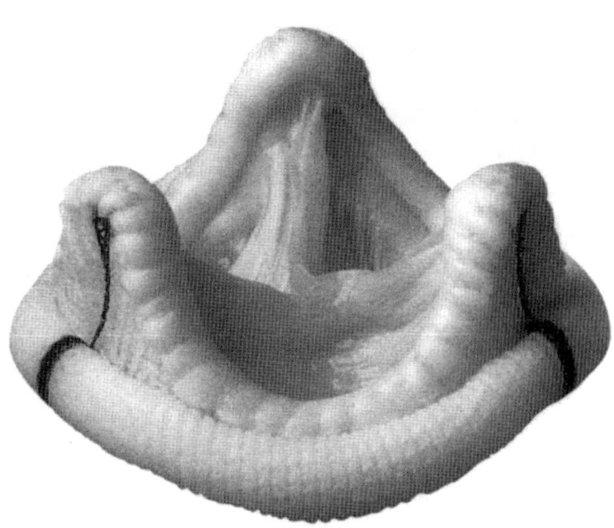

FIGURE 33-13 The St. Jude Epic porcine aortic prosthesis. (*Figure courtesy of St. Jude Medical Inc., Minneapolis, MN.*)

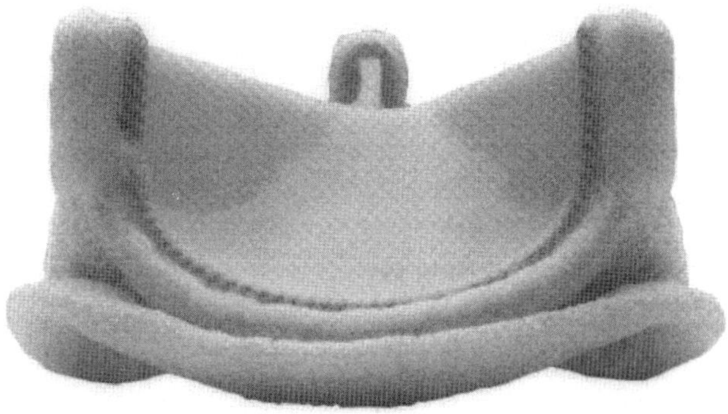

FIGURE 33-14 The Carpentier-Edwards Magna pericardial pros-thesis. (*Figure courtesy of Edwards Life Sciences Inc., Irvine, CA.*)

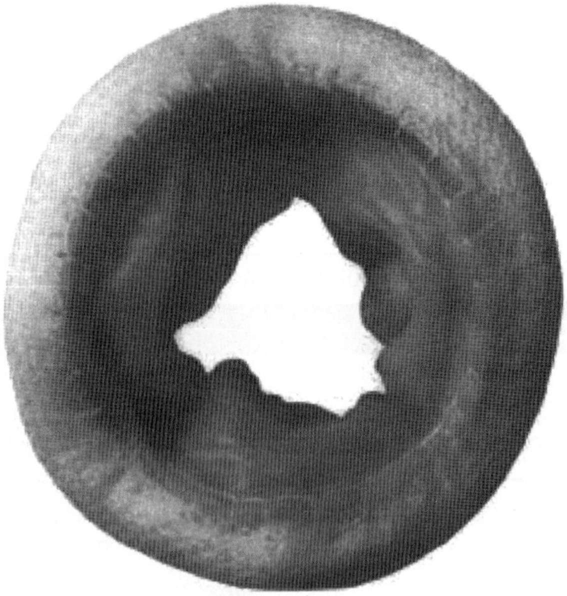

FIGURE 33-12 The Medtronic Mosaic porcine aortic prosthesis. (*Figure courtesy of Medtronic Inc., Minneapolis, MN.*)

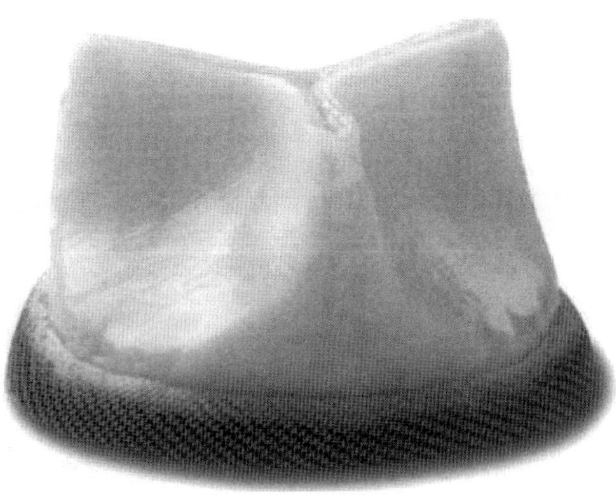

FIGURE 33-15 The Mitroflow Pericardial aortic prosthesis. (*Figure courtesy of Carbomedics Inc., Austin, TX.*)

TABLE 33-4 Operative Mortality Rates for Aortic Valve Replacement (AVR) Procedures from the Society of Thoracic Surgeons' Database

Operative Category	Number	Operative Mortality (%)
AVR (isolated)	26,317	4.3
Multiple valve replacement	3840	9.6
AVR + coronary artery bypass	22,713	8.0
Multiple valve replacement + coronary artery bypass	1424	18.8
AVR + any valve repair	938	7.4
Aortic valve repair	597	5.9
AVR + aortic aneurysm repair	1723	9.7
AVR + other*	356	8.4

*Other includes left ventricular aneurysm, ventricular septal defect, atrial septal defect, congenital defect, cardiac trauma, cardiac transplant, permanent pacemaker, automatic implanted cardioverter-defibrillator, aortic aneurysm, or carotid endarterectomy. Isolated aortic valve replacement and aortic aneurysm are not included in aortic valve replacement + other.

Source: Adapted from Jamieson WR, Edwards FH, Schwartz M, et al: Risk stratification for cardiac valve replacement. National Cardiac Surgery Database. Database Committee of the Society of Thoracic Surgeons. Ann Thorac Surg 1999; 67:943.

with CABG.[44] Aortic valve replacement with ascending aortic aneurysm repair was shown to have an increased operative mortality of 9.7%. The results of this study are summarized in Table 33-4. Then in 2009, they reviewed 67,292 cases of AVR and found 3.2% mortality rate (Table 33-5).[45] It is important to note that information in this database is voluntarily submitted and includes both low- and high-volume centers.

The preoperative risk factors of operative mortality for AVR derived from the STS database are presented in Table 33-6.[43,46–48] Most early deaths are attributable to renal failure, emergency status, and reoperations. In Table 33-7, mortality data for AVR-related procedures from an update of the STS database are presented describing the operative risk of isolated and combined valve procedures.[49]

Long-Term Survival

Longitudinal analysis demonstrates no difference in survival between patients receiving mechanical and bioprosthetic valves when they are implanted in similar age cohorts over 10 years of follow-up.[50] However, at 15 years' follow-up, structural valve deterioration in bioprosthetic valves leads to a survival benefit for patients with mechanical valves. In a prospective trial, 15-year mortality was 79 and 66% for bioprosthetic and mechanical

TABLE 33-5 Frequency of Endpoints for AVR in Overall Study of Population from 2002 to 2006

	Mort	CVA	RF	Vent	DSWI	Reop	Comp	PLOS	SLOS
N	67,292	67,292	65,828	67,292	67,292	67,292	67,292	67,292	67,292
Events	2157	1007	2774	7323	197	5369	11,706	5308	26,144
%	3.2	1.5	4.1	10.9	0.3	8	17.4	7.9	38.9

AVR = aortic valve replacement; Comp = composite adverse event (any); CVA = cerebrovascular accident (stroke); DSWI = deep sternal wound infection; Mort = mortality; PLOS = prolonged length of stay; Reop = reoperation; RF = renal failure; SLOS = short length of stay; Vent = prolonged ventilation.

Source: Adapted from O'Brien SM, Shahian DM, Filardo G, et al: The Society of Thoracic Surgeons 2008 cardiac surgery risk models: part 2—isolated valve surgery. Ann Thorac Surg 2009; 88:S23.

TABLE 33-6 Independent Risk Factors for Operative Mortality (Odds Ratios) for Isolated Aortic Valve Replacement and Aortic Valve Replacement Plus Coronary Artery Bypass from the Society of Thoracic Surgeons' Database

Aortic Valve Replacement			Aortic Valve Replacement Plus Coronary Artery Bypass		
Risk Factor	**Odds Ratio**	**CI**	**Risk Factor**	**Odds Ratio**	**CI**
Salvage status	7.12	4.69-10.68	Salvage status	7.00	4.74-10.33
DDRF	4.32	2.83-6.43	DDRF	4.60	3.10-6.70
ES	3.46	2.62-4.52	Reoperation	2.40	2.11-2.73
Multiple reoperations	2.27	1.57-3.21	NDRF	2.11	1.77-2.51
NDRF	2.20	1.76-2.73	ES	1.89	1.50-2.36
Resuscitation	1.77	1.05-2.91	Preoperative IABP	1.82	1.43-2.30
First reoperation	1.70	1.44-1.99	Female gender	1.61	1.45-1.80
CS	1.67	1.14-2.40	CS	1.57	1.14-2.13
NYHA IV	1.56	1.35-1.81	NYHA IV	1.36	1.21-1.52
Inotropic agent used	1.47	1.10-1.95	TVD	1.31	1.18-1.45
CVA	1.44	1.14-1.80	CVA	1.24	1.03-1.48
MI	1.36	1.12-1.65	Diabetes	1.23	1.10-1.38
Female gender	1.25	1.10-1.42	Obesity	1.23	1.04-1.44
US	1.25	1.05-1.48	COPD	1.21	1.06-1.37
Diabetes	1.23	1.04-1.44	LMD	1.20	1.04-1.38
CHF	1.22	1.07-1.40	PVD	1.17	1.00-1.36
Arr	1.16	1.01-1.31	Diuretics	1.16	1.05-1.29
Age (mean = 68.7)	1.03	1.03-1.04	MI	1.16	1.03-1.29
EF (mean = 49.9%)	0.99	0.99-1.00	Arr	1.14	1.01-1.29
			Age	1.04	1.03-1.05
			EF	1.00	0.99-1.00

Arr = arrhythmia; CHF = congestive heart failure; CI = 95% confidence interval; COPD = chronic obstructive pulmonary disease; CS = cardiogenic shock; CVA = cerebrovascular accident; DDRF = dialysis-dependent renal failure; EF = ejection fraction; ES = emergency status; IABP = intra-aortic balloon pump; LMD = left main disease; MI = myocardial infarction; NDRF = nondialysis-dependent renal failure; NYHA IV = New York Heart Association class IV; PVD = peripheral vascular disease; TVD = triple vessel disease; US = urgent status.
Source: Adapted from Jamieson WR, Edwards FH, Schwartz M, et al: Risk stratification for cardiac valve replacement. National Cardiac Surgery Database. Database Committee of the Society of Thoracic Surgeons. Ann Thorac Surg 1999; 67:943.

valves, respectively.[51] Substantially more bleeding events were found in patients with mechanical valves. It is important to note that increased bioprosthetic structural deterioration was likely influenced by the use of a first-generation prosthesis more prone to structural failure than newer devices.

In most published series, the expected survival after AVR is approximately 80 to 85% at 5 years, 65 to 75% at 10 years, and 45 to 55% at 15 years.[52–54] The outcomes of AVR are highly dependent on the functional status, comorbidities, and age of each individual patient.[55] The effect of age at the time of

TABLE 33-7 Distribution of Operative Mortality in AVR Alone and in Conjunction with Other Valve Replacement from the Society of Thoracic Surgeons' Database

	No.	% Concomitant		Unadjusted Mortality
		CAB	"Other"	
Single valve				
A	216,245	50.00%	11.70%	5.70%
Double valve				
A, M	24,608	38.30%	13.00%	11.50%
A, T	1183	29.60%	24.80%	14.00%
A, P	2574	10.20%	25.00%	3.10%
Triple valve				
A, M, T	3121	27.10%	20.50%	15.30%
A, M, P	92	20.70%	18.50%	5.40%
A, T, P	23	17.40%	26.10%	4.40%
Quadruple valve				
A, M, T, P	47	61.70%	27.70%	8.50%

A = aortic valve; CAB = coronary artery bypass; M = mitral valve; P = pulmonic valve; R = aortic root reconstruction; T = tricuspid valve.
Source: Adapted from Rankin JS, Hammill BG, Ferguson TB Jr, et al: Determinants of operative mortality in valvular heart surgery. J Thorac Cardiovasc Surg 2006; 131:547.

surgery on late mortality for a variety of prostheses is depicted in Fig. 33-16. The comorbidities of age, concomitant CAD, LVD, and poor functional status on middle to late survival after bioprosthetic AVR are additive (Table 33-8).[56] Other risk factors for late mortality include concomitant renal disease, female gender, concomitant cardiac or vascular procedure, and atrial fibrillation.[57,58] Studies of mechanical valves often show superior long-term survival but patients are significantly younger at the time of operation. No prospective series of comparable patients has shown any survival benefit comparing pericardial with porcine valves in similar eras.

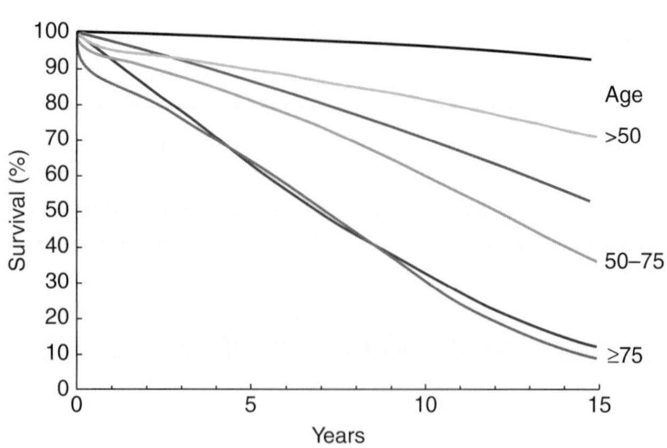

FIGURE 33-16 Projected long-term survival after aortic valve replacement stratified by age at time of surgery. For each age group the age-, race-, and ethnicity-matched population life table curve is shown as a dot-dashed line. Note that younger patients show more marked departure from normal life expectancy. (*Reproduced with permission from Blackstone EH, Kirklin JW: Death and other time-related events after valve replacement. Circulation 1985; 72:753.*)

Valve-Related Mortality

Long-term survival data distinguishes between valve-related mortality, non–valve-related cardiac mortality, and mortality from other causes. A revised consensus document from the STS and the American Association of Thoracic Surgeons (AATS) outlines a standardized method to report valve-related complications in prosthetic and repaired heart valves.[59] This panel defined valve-related mortality as all deaths caused by structural valve deterioration, nonstructural valve dysfunction, valve thrombosis, embolism, bleeding event, operated valvular endocarditis, or death related to reoperation of an operated valve. Sudden, unexplained, unexpected deaths of patients with an operated valve are included as valve-related mortality. Deaths caused by progressive heart failure in patients with satisfactorily functioning cardiac valves are not included. In the Hammermeister series, valve-related deaths accounted for 37% of all deaths in patients with mechanical valves and 41% of all deaths in patients with bioprostheses at 15 years.[51] Nonvalvular cardiac deaths accounted for 17 and 21% of deaths at 15 years in patients with mechanical and bioprostheses, respectively.[38] There are no well-designed prospective randomized series comparing the long-term outcomes of specific pericardial or porcine prostheses to each other.

TABLE 33-8 Survival Probability Calculated from an Accelerated Time Failure Model for Combinations of Risk Factors*

CAD	Age >65	NYHA Class IV	LV Grade III or IV	Predicted 5-year Survival (%)	Predicted 10-year Survival (%)
				89.1 (73,100)	83.9 (73, 95)
X				83.4 (70, 97)	76.2 (67, 85)
	X			84.5 (71, 98)	77.7 (69, 86)
		X		83.6 (70, 97)	76.6 (68, 85)
			X	82.3 (69, 96)	74.8 (66, 84)
X	X			77.1 (66, 88)	68.2 (61, 75)
X		X		75.9 (65, 87)	66.8 (60, 74)
X			X	74.1 (63, 85)	64.6 (58, 72)
	X	X		77.4 (66, 88)	68.6 (62, 76)
	X		X	75.7 (65, 86)	66.5 (59, 74)
		X	X	74.5 (64, 85)	65.1 (58, 72)
X	X	X		67.8 (59, 77)	57.4 (52, 63)
X	X		X	65.7 (57, 75)	55.0 (49, 61)
	X	X	X	66.2 (57, 75)	55.5 (50, 61)
X	X	X	X	54.6 (47, 62)	43.5 (39, 48)

*Each of these four risk factors was entered into the model as a dichotomous variable (ie, NYHA IV versus NYHA I, II, or III; left ventricular grades 3 or 4 versus left ventricular grades 1 or 2). The X indicates that the risk factor is present. These four risk factors are not present for the first row of estimates. The upper and lower 95% confidence interval for the predicted survival probabilities are given in parentheses.

CAD = coronary artery disease; NYHA = New York Heart Association.

Source: Reproduced with permission from Cohen G, David TE, Ivanov J, et al: The impact of age, coronary artery disease, and cardiac comorbidity on late survival after bio-prosthetic aortic valve replacement. J Thorac Cardiovasc Surg 1999; 117:273.

Nonfatal Valve Events

The joint STS/AATS panel defined specific guidelines for reporting outcomes on structural and nonstructural valve deterioration, valve thrombosis, embolic events, bleeding events, and prosthetic endocarditis.[60] *Structural valve deterioration* refers to any change in function of an operated valve resulting from an intrinsic abnormality of the valve that causes stenosis or regurgitation (eg, leaflet tears, suture line disruption). *Nonstructural dysfunction* is any abnormality of an operated valve resulting in stenosis or regurgitation that is caused by factors not intrinsic to the valve itself (eg, pannus overgrowth, inappropriate sizing, or paravalvular leak). *Valve thrombosis* is any thrombus that interferes with valve function in the absence of infection. *Embolism* is any embolic event that occurs after the immediate postoperative period when perioperative anesthesia has been completely reversed. *Cerebral embolic events* are subclassified into: *transient ischemic attacks,* which are fully reversible neurologic events lasting less than 24 hours; *reversible ischemic neurologic deficits,* which are fully reversible neurologic events lasting between 24 hours and 3 weeks; and *strokes,* which are permanent neurologic deficits lasting longer than 3 weeks or causing death. A *bleeding event* is any episode of major internal or external bleeding that causes death, hospitalization, or permanent injury, or requires transfusion, regardless of the patient's anticoagulation status. This does not include embolic stroke followed by hemorrhagic transformation and intracranial bleed. Finally, *operated valvular endocarditis* is any infection involving an operated valve; or any structural or nonstructural valvular dysfunction, thrombosis, or embolic event associated with operated valvular endocarditis.

TABLE 33–9 Structural Deterioration of Stented Bioprosthetic Valves in the Aortic Position: Long-term Follow-up Over 12–15 years

Study	Prosthesis	No. of Patients	Mean Age (years)	Mean Follow-Up (months)	Time of SVD Estimate (years)	Actuarial Freedom from SVD	Actuarial Freedom from Reoperation
David et al	Hancock II Porcine	723	65 ± 12	68 ± 40	12	94 ± 2	89 ± 5
Dellgren et al	CE Pericardial	254	71 ± 9	60 ± 31	12	86 ± 9	83 ± 9
Poirier et al	CE Pericardial	598	65 ± 8	57.7	12	93 ± 2	91 ± 2
					14	80 ± 5	72 ± 6
Corbineau et al	Medtronic Intact	188	72 ± 8	86.4 ± 50.4	13	91 ± 3.3	
Jamieson et al	CE SA Porcine	1657	65.5 ± 11.9	70.8 ± 58.8	12	83.4 ± 2.1	
					14	57.4 ± 9.2	52.9 ± 2.8
Burdon et al	Hancock I and MO	857	59 ± 11	87.6	15	63 ± 3	57 ± 3

CE = Carpentier-Edwards; MO = modified orifice; SA = supra-annular; SVD = structural valve deterioration

Structural Valve Deterioration

Stented Bioprostheses

Several large series describe long-term follow-up of first- and second-generation stented bioprostheses. These series are not directly comparable because they took place in different patient populations or different eras. Structural valve deterioration is the most common nonfatal valve-related complication in bioprosthetic aortic valve (Table 33-9). Long-term follow-up of currently available second-generation stented bioprostheses, including the Medtronic Hancock II porcine and Carpentier-Edwards pericardial valves, show freedom from structural valve deterioration less than 90% at 12-year follow-up.[52,61,62] However, beyond 15-year follow-up, freedom from SVD falls rapidly.[63] No good evidence exists to suggest that comparable, well-established second-generation pericardial or porcine prostheses differ in longevity; thus decisions regarding specific prosthesis should be made based on surgeon comfort and familiarity with the prosthesis and its sizing. Although newer third-generation prostheses with advanced tissue treatments eventually may be shown to have superior longevity, data about these prostheses are currently limited to 5- to 6-year outcomes, which appear comparable with those of the second-generation prostheses.[64]

Importantly, younger patients are predisposed to premature bioprosthetic SVD, particularly those less than the age of 40 years (Table 33-10).[65,66] Structural valve deterioration may be less common in elderly patients because of the decreased hemodynamic stress placed on the valve. The freedom from SVD may be underestimated in the literature because most series report SVD by the actuarial method instead of the actual or cumulative incidence method.[67] Actuarial statistical analysis overestimates SVD in older patients because it assumes that patients who have died of other causes will continue to be at risk for SVD.

Bioprostheses have a higher rate of reoperation then mechanical valves owing to structural valve dysfunction. In large series, freedom from reoperation is greater than 95% at 5 years, greater than 90% at 10 years, but less than 70% at 15 years.[52,68–73] The long-term freedom from reoperation for several commonly available valves is presented in Table 33-10.

Optimal Antithrombotic Therapy

Bioprosthetic Valves

Bioprosthetic valves thus do not require long-term anticoagulation with warfarin unless the patient is at high risk for

TABLE 33–10 Bioprosthetic Valve Failure 10 years After Valve Replacement According to the Patient's Age at the Time of Implantation

Patient's Age (y)	Valve Failure After 10 Years (%)
<40	42
40–49	30
50–59	21
60–69	15
>70	10

Source: Based on data adapted from Vongpatanasin et al[65] and from Grunkemeier et al.[66]

thromboembolism or has had a thromboembolic event with his or her prosthesis. Stented bioprostheses have a linearized risk for thromboembolism between 0.5 and 1% per year. This risk appears to be lower in patients with stentless heterograft, allograft, or autograft valves.[74–76] An increased hazard function exists for thromboembolism before the exposed surfaces of stented bioprostheses endothelialize.[77] The current ACC/AHA guidelines recommend anticoagulation with warfarin to an INR between 2.0 and 3.0 for the first 3 months for bioprosthetic valves as a class IIB recommendation.[18] This is discontinued at the end of the third month unless the patient is at high risk for thromboembolism. Low-dose aspirin is continued as monotherapy in low-risk patients. Aspirin significantly decreases the risk of thromboembolism in low-risk patients with bioprostheses versus no antiplatelet therapy.[78,79] High-risk patients require lifetime aspirin and warfarin treatment, which has a survival benefit over warfarin alone.[78] If a patient has identified high-risk factors for thrombosis preoperatively, a mechanical prosthesis should be implanted unless the risk factor is amenable to correction because formal anticoagulation with warfarin will still be necessary. With aspirin, bioprosthetic valves have approximately the same risk of thromboembolism as fully anticoagulated mechanical valves, with fewer bleeding complications.

Prosthesis Thrombosis

Prosthesis thrombosis is a rare but potentially devastating outcome after AVR. The incidence of prosthesis thrombosis is less than 0.2% per year and occurs more often in mechanical prostheses.[80] Thrombolytic therapy may be used in some patients but it is often ineffective. Thrombolysis is recommended in patients with left-sided thrombosis who are experiencing significant heart failure (NYHA class III or IV) and are considered too high risk for surgery.[81,82] Cerebral or peripheral thromboembolism occurs in 12% of patients after thrombolytic therapy.[81] Surgical treatment includes replacement of the valve or open thrombectomy, and mortality from either procedure is similar at approximately 10 to 15%.[81] Recurrent thrombosis after de-clotting occurs in up to 40% of patients and we recommend valve replacement in virtually all patients who are managed operatively.

Prosthetic Valve Endocarditis

Prosthetic valve endocarditis (PVE) is separated into two time frames: early (<60 days postimplantation) and late (>60 days postimplantation). Early PVE is usually a sequela of perioperative bacterial seeding of the valve, either during implantation or postoperatively from wound or intravascular catheter infections. *Staphylococcus aureus, S. epidermidis,* gram-negative bacteria, and fungal infections are common in this period.[52,72,83–86] Although most cases of late PVE are caused by septicemia from noncardiac sources, a small proportion of late cases in the first year are attributable to less virulent organisms introduced in the perioperative period, particularly *S. epidermidis.* Organisms responsible for late PVE include *Streptococcus* and *Staphylococcus* species and other organisms commonly found in native valve infectious endocarditis. All unexplained fevers should be meticulously investigated for PVE with serial blood cultures and TEE and/or TTE. Transesophageal echocardiography provides more detailed anatomical information such as the presence of vegetations, abscesses, and fistulas. Transthoracic views may provide better views of the anterior portion of the valve. The annual risk of PVE in the aortic position is 0.6 to 0.9% per patient year.[85–87] The 5-year freedom from PVE reported in many major series is greater than 97%.[52,85] Mechanical valves may have a slightly higher early hazard for PVE than stented bioprostheses.[86] However, no difference exists in risk between patients with mechanical and stented bioprosthetic prostheses after the early phase. Stentless porcine heterografts and allografts are less likely to develop PVE because they have less prosthetic material that may serve as a nidus of infection.[87] These valves may be particularly helpful in valve re-replacement for PVE.

Outcome for patients with PVE is very poor. Invasive paravalvular infection occurs in up to 40% of cases of PVE.[84] Early PVE is associated with 30 to 80% mortality, whereas late PVE is associated with 20 to 40% mortality.[52] Surgical indications for PVE include early PVE; concomitant heart failure and valvular dysfunction; paravalvular leak or partial dehiscence; presence of a new conduction defect, abscess, aneurysm, or fistula; persistent bacteremia despite a maximum of 5 days of appropriate antibiotic therapy and no other source of infection; vegetations (>10 mm); and multiple systemic emboli. Notably, all fungal and most virulent strains of *Staphylococcus aureus, Serratia marcescens,* and *Pseudomonas aeruginosa* require operation, as these organisms are highly invasive and antibiotic therapy is generally ineffective.

Paravalvular Leak and Hemolysis

Paravalvular leak is uncommon when pledgeted sutures are routinely used outside of the setting of infective endocarditis. Technical errors may result in inappropriately large gaps between sutures, leaving a small portion of the prosthesis unattached to the annulus. If paravalvular leak is sufficient to cause significant hemolysis, surgical correction may be performed with a few interrupted pledgeted sutures. Pannus overgrowth and prosthetic structural degeneration interfering with normal valve opening and closure may cause hemolysis severe enough to warrant reoperation. Milder cases of hemolysis may be managed conservatively by dietary supplementation with iron and folic acid, and routine measurement of hemoglobin, serum haptoglobin, and lactate dehydrogenase.

HEMODYNAMIC PERFORMANCE AND VENTRICULAR REMODELING

Left Ventricular Mass Regression

Pressure and volume overload caused by aortic valve disease leads to increased intracavitary left ventricular pressures and compensatory LVH. In severe AS, concentric ventricular hypertrophy occurs without increasing end-diastolic dimension until late in the disease process, thus maintaining the ventricular wall thickness:cavity radius ratio. On the other hand, severe AR causes volume overload with an increase in left ventricular end-diastolic volume and eccentric hypertrophy, but may not change the ratio of ventricular wall thickness to cavity radius. Both pathologies result in an increase in LV mass (LVM), which has a strong negative prognostic effect.[88,89] The overall goal of AVR is to alleviate the pressure and volume overload on the left ventricle, allowing myocardial remodeling and regression of left ventricular mass.

The clinical impact of LVM regression is not as well understood, despite its widespread acceptance as a measure of outcome after aortic valve surgery. In hypertensive patients undergoing medical treatment, reduction of LVM was associated with fewer cardiac events than those whose left ventricular mass did not change or increased.[135] In patients after AVR for isolated AS, LVM generally regresses significantly over the first 18 months and returns to normal limits.[90,91] Ventricular mass regression may continue for up to 5 years after valve replacement.[92] However, some patients do not experience adequate ventricular mass regression. The prognostic implications of LVM regression after aortic valve surgery have not been rigorously studied but it is reasonable to suppose that lack of LVM regression is associated with poor clinical outcome. Several authors have identified a situation, referred to as patient-prosthesis mismatch (PPM), in which poor hemodynamic performance of a prosthesis results in poor regression of LVH and poor patient outcome.

Prosthesis-Patient Mismatch

Definitions

The term PPM has been applied to several different clinical situations. It has been used to describe absolute small valve size (ie, <21 mm), small valve size in a patient with a large body surface area, excessive transvalvular gradient postimplantation, increased transvalvular gradient with exercise, indexed effective orifice area, and various combinations of these variables. Rahimtoola defined PPM as a condition that occurs when the valve area of a prosthetic valve is less than the area of that patient's normal valve.[93] He further described a clinical condition in which the patient experienced either no relief or worsening of symptoms owing to the obstructive nature of the prosthesis, which creates a residual stenosis resulting in an elevated transvalvular gradient. To varying degrees, all valve prostheses are inherently stenotic.[94] The presence of rigid sewing rings, and in the case of stented bioprostheses, struts to hold the valve commissures, cause obstruction to outflow and will therefore cause a residual gradient despite normal prosthesis function. The EOA of commonly-available bioprosthetic valves are shown in Table 33-11. PPM is further exacerbated by annular fibrosis, annular calcification, and LVH, as seen in AS, that cause contraction of the native annulus, leading to the implantation of a smaller prosthesis. Two distinct terms are commonly used to describe the size of prosthetic valves: *effective orifice area* and *geometric orifice area.*

Effective Orifice Area

The most commonly cited definition of PPM is a low indexed effective orifice area (IEOA). The IEOA is calculated by dividing the echocardiographically determined effective orifice area (EOA) by the body surface area. Effective orifice area is calculated by a reconfiguration of the continuity equation:

$$EOA = (CSA_{LVOT} \times TVI_{LVOT})/TVI_{AO}$$

where EOA is effective orifice area (cm^2), CSA_{LVOT} is cross-sectional area of the LV outflow tract (LVOT; cm^2), TVI_{LVOT} is velocity time integral of forward blood flow (cm) as derived from pulse-wave Doppler in the LVOT, and TVI_{AO} is velocity

TABLE 33-11 The Effective Orifice Area (EOA) and Mean Systolic Gradient (MSG) of Commonly Available Bioprostheses

	19 mm		21 mm		23 mm		25 mm		27 mm	
Prosthesis and References	EOA (cm^2)	MSG (mm Hg)	EOA (cm^2)	MSG (mm Hg)	EOA (cm^2)	MSG (mm Hg)	EOA (cm^2)	MSG (mm Hg)	EOA (cm^2)	MSG (mm Hg)
Hancock II			1.2		1.3		1.5		1.6	
Medtronic Mosaic	1.2	16	1.3	14–15	1.5	12–13	1.8	11–12	2	9–10
CE Pericardial	0.95	18–19	1.1	13–14	1.5	11–14	1.4	10–11	1.6	10
Mitroflow Pericardial	1.3		1.4		1.7					
Medtronic Freestyle	1.0–1.4	18–22	1.3–1.4	7–13	1.4–1.5	7–14	1.7–2.0	5–9	2.0-2.3	5–7

CE = Carpentier-Edwards.

time integral of forward blood flow (cm) as derived from software integration of transvalvular continuous wave Doppler.

The EOA and mean systolic gradient of several commonly available bioprostheses are shown in Table 33-11.

Several authors suggest that PPM occurs at an IEOA of less than 0.85 cm^2/m^2.[95,96] Dumesnil and Pibarot have redefined PPM as a condition "when the EOA of the prosthesis is too small in relation to the patient's body size, resulting in abnormally high postoperative gradients."[96] This definition is based on the assumption that transvalvular gradients begin to rise substantially at IEOAs below this value, and that these elevated gradients result in increased left ventricular work preventing regression of LVH.[97]

The EOA is a functional estimate of the minimal cross-sectional area of the transvalvular flow jet downstream of a valve and dependent on the: (1) geometric area of the prosthesis, (2) shape and size of the LVOT and ascending aorta, (3) blood pressure, and (4) cardiac output (Fig. 33-17). Doppler-derived EOA correlates best with catheter-derived EOA (as determined by the Gorlin formula) when the ascending aortic diameter is 4 cm, but tends to underestimate EOA in patients with smaller aortic diameters.[98] The EOA cannot be known for a specific valve in a specific patient until the valve has actually been implanted. Studies examining the effect of low IEOA on clinical outcomes have typically used published tables of EOA derived from historical controls instead of actually measuring true in vivo postoperative EOA. Moreover, these tables have been derived from relatively small numbers of valves in each size for each manufacturer with wide variability between studies. EOA correlates with postoperative valve gradients, which is not surprising considering that they are mathematically related. Echocardiographic mean and peak gradients are calculated according to the Bernoulli equation:

$$\text{Peak gradient (mm Hg)} = 4 \times (V_{AVmax}{}^2 - V_{LVOTmax}{}^2)$$
$$\text{Mean gradient (mm Hg)} = 4 \times (V_{AVmean}{}^2 - V_{LVOTmean}{}^2)$$

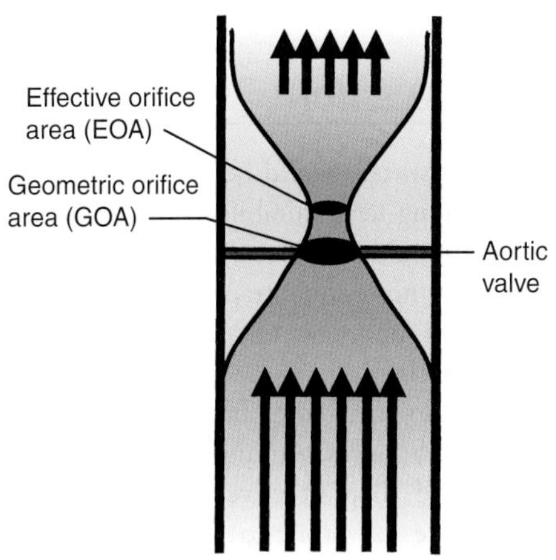

FIGURE 33-17 Diagrammatic representation of effective orifice area and geometric orifice area in relation to the left ventricular outflow tract and aortic root.

Geometric Orifice Area

Alternatively the geometric orifice area (GOA; also known as the internal geometric area) of the valve is the maximal cross-sectional area of the valve opening that does not vary significantly between same-sized valves from the same manufacturer. It is a static measure that is known preoperatively for any given prosthesis based on manufacturer specifications or by measurement with calipers. As seen in Fig. 33-17, the GOA is always larger than the EOA for any given prosthesis.

Clinical Significance

The significance of PPM is still controversial. Several studies have found that that lower IEOA is associated with diminished short- and long-term clinical results. Pibarot and Dumesnil[97] studied PPM in 1266 patients undergoing AVR and found moderate (IEOA <0.85 cm^2/m^2) or severe (IEOA <0.65 cm^2/m^2) PPM to be present in 38% of patients. Multivariate analysis showed that moderate and severe PPM are associated with a twofold and 11-fold increase of perioperative mortality, respectively. Retrospective analysis of PPM in 2154 patients undergoing AVR at two large centers showed similar overall mortality with and without PPM, but higher valve-related mortality with PPM at 10 years. A single-center analysis of 1563 mechanical and tissue aortic prostheses found that IEOA less than 0.8 cm^2/m^2 was associated with increased prevalence of heart failure symptoms at a mean follow-up time of 4.3 years but not with mortality.[99] Ruel and colleagues showed that overall survival and LVM regression was poorer in patients with PPM and LVD than those who had LVD without PPM.[100] In a series of 1400 patients, PPM affected long-term survival in patients less than 60 years old but not in older patients.[101]

On the other hand, several studies have also shown that PPM does not influence clinical outcomes. Medalion and colleagues studied 892 AVRs and demonstrated no differences in 15-year survival between patients with or without PPM, despite 25% of patients with an indexed internal orifice area less than two standard below predicted.[102] Hanayama and colleagues reported in 1129 patients with PPM post-AVR, no differences in LVM index or survival at midterm follow-up between patients with normal and abnormal gradients over a 10-year period.[103] They defined PPM as: (1) IEOA less than the 90th percentile in the study population (0.6 cm^2/m^2); and (2) valve gradient in the highest 90th percentile of the study population (peak gradient and mean gradient were 38 and 21 mm Hg), which would be considered severe by most groups. Fig. 33-18 shows no differences in LVM index or survival at midterm follow-up between patients with or without PPM. The average labeled size of valve in the low-IEOA and high-gradient groups were 22.4 and 23 mm, respectively. The only multivariate predictor of elevated postoperative gradient was valve size.

Blackstone and colleagues have compiled the largest and most statistically sound examination of the role of PPM in short- and long-term outcomes.[104] In a multi-institutional study of over 13,000 aortic prostheses, presence of an indexed GOA in the lowest 10th percentile was associated with a 1 to 2% increase in perioperative (30-day) mortality and had no effect

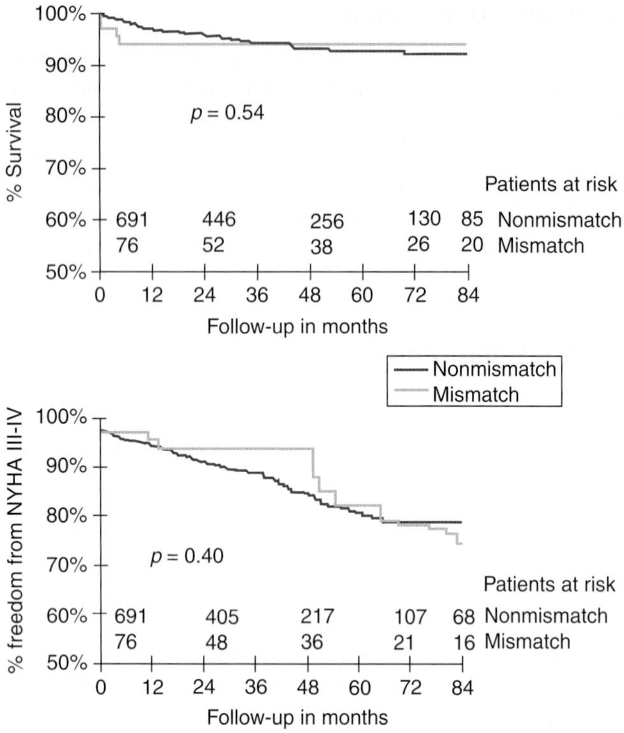

FIGURE 33-18 Actuarial survival and freedom from NYHA class III or IV in patients with and without prosthesis-patient mismatch. There were no significant differences in the two groups. (*Reproduced with permission from Hanayama N, Christakis GT, Mallidi HR, et al: Patient prosthesis mismatch is rare after aortic valve replacement: valve size may be irrelevant. Ann Thorac Surg 2002; 73:1822.*)

on medium- or long-term survival (Fig. 33-19). An important finding in this study was that virtually no stented bioprostheses were in the group of patients in the lowest 10th percentile of indexed GOA, who predominantly received mechanical prostheses. In a subsequent study from the same group, there was no relationship between indexed GOA and Duke Activity Status Index in 1108 patients undergoing AVR at a mean follow-up of 8.3 months. Predictors of postoperative functional status are presented in Table 33-12.

Small Aortic Root

Many surgeons express concern regarding postoperative outcomes in patients with small aortic roots in whom only very small (19 mm or smaller) valves can be implanted. However, several studies have shown no difference in LVM regression, NYHA functional class, CHF or survival with small diameter AVRs. [105–107] Khan and colleagues studied 19 mm to 23 mm Carpentier-Edwards pericardial valves and found that significant LVM regression occurred with each valve size, including 19 mm valves.[108] Studies by DePaulis and colleagues show no difference in LVM regression between patients receiving 19 and 21 mm mechanical valves versus those with 23 or 25 mm valves.[106] Kratz and associates also reported that small valve size was not predictive of CHF or late death.[107]

Data Synthesis

Although the literature regarding the clinical significance of PPM remains divided, proponents of the concept advocate use of mechanical prostheses. The presumption is less obstructive than stented bioprostheses, aortic root enlargement, and stentless valves when used in the subcoronary position and as full root replacement. However, whether mechanical prostheses alleviate PPM versus the current generation of tissue valves is an open question and indeed, they may even result in greater PPM.[109] Aortic root enlargement procedures require significant experience operating on the aortic root and may carry excessive mortality and wide variability in surgical outcomes even among highly experienced centers.

Alternatively, a stentless prosthesis in the subcoronary position may be a lower profile alternative but requires additional technical skill and cross-clamp time. Rao and colleagues compared hemodynamic data between stented Carpentier-Edwards pericardial valves and Toronto stentless porcine valves of equivalent diameter and found no hemodynamic differences in peak or mean gradient.[110]

Aortic root replacement in patients without ascending aortic pathology, solely to diminish the potential long-term effects of PPM, is a potentially high-risk strategy and is discouraged.

When faced with potential PPM in the operating room, the decision to perform a more complex, higher-risk procedure must be balanced carefully with the potential benefits of implanting a larger prosthesis. Some reports have shown that transvalvular gradients in patients with lower IEOA often rise substantially with exercise.[97,111] Although the majority of patients undergoing AVR are elderly and unlikely to experience functional limitations from this situation, in younger, highly active patients either root enlargement or stentless prostheses may provide better functional outcome with lower transvalvular gradients. In the rare circumstance of anticipated extreme mismatch (ie, IEOA <0.6 cm^2/m^2), root enlargement is an acceptable approach in the hands of an experienced surgeon. Except in these circumstances, given the paucity of long-term data to support more complex procedures and well-documented increased risk, routine AVR with modern standard prostheses is acceptable and preferable.

PROSTHESIS SELECTION

An ideal aortic prosthesis would be simple to implant, widely available, possess long-term durability, would have no intrinsic thrombogenicity, would not have a predilection for endocarditis, and would have no residual transvalvular pressure gradient. Such a valve does not currently exist. Currently available options include mechanical valves, stented biologic heterograft valves, stentless biologic heterograft valves, allograft valves, and pulmonary autograft valves. Among these options pulmonary autograft valves and allograft valves are the most physiologic prostheses. They are less prone to thrombosis or endocarditis and have excellent hemodynamic characteristics.[112,113] The longevity of such valves is dependent on patient factors, the preparation of the valve, and the technical skill of the operating surgeon. Despite their potential benefits, these prostheses are

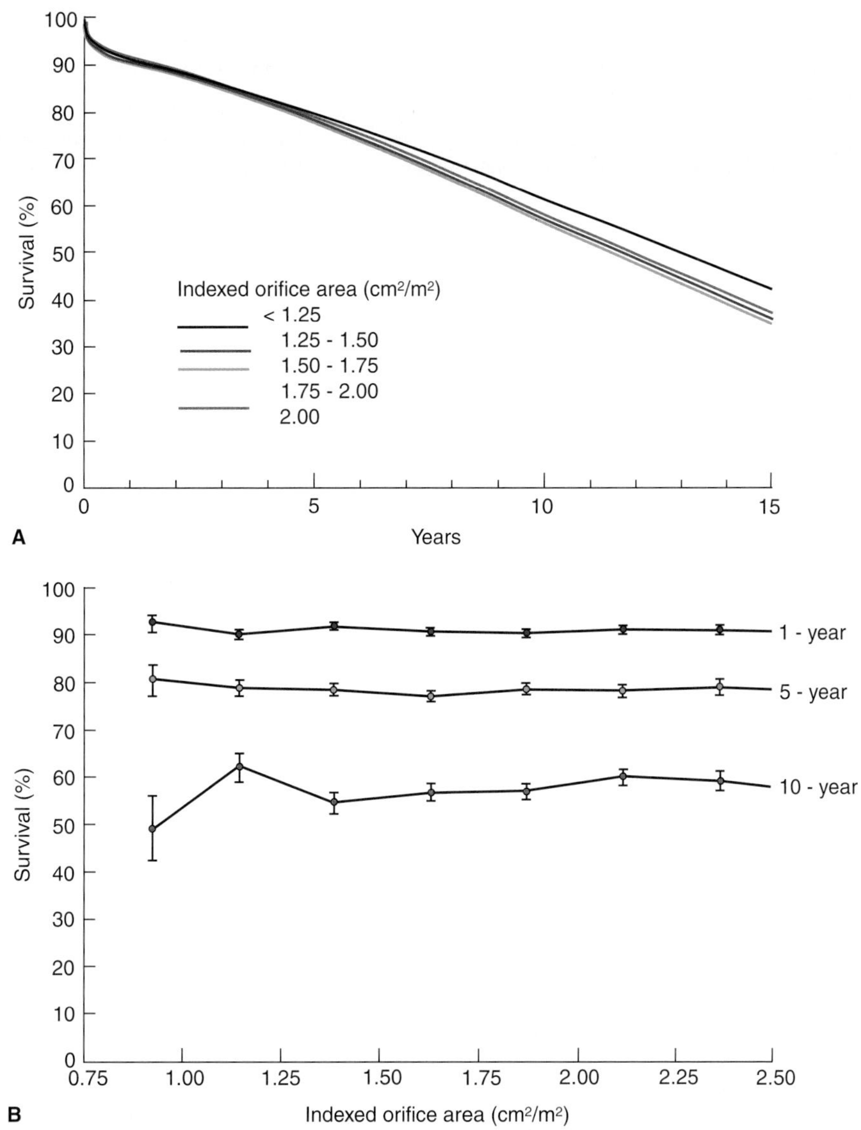

FIGURE 33-19 (A) Effect of indexed orifice area on non–risk-adjusted survival. (B) Time-related survival stratified by indexed orifice area. These are Kaplan-Meier estimates of 1-, 5-, and 10-year survivals in finely grouped strata of indexed orifice area. (*Reproduced with permission from Blackstone EH, Cosgrove DM, Jamieson WR, et al: Prosthesis size and long-term survival after aortic valve replacement. J Thorac Cardiovasc Surg 2003; 126:783.*)

not readily available and can be very technically demanding to implant compared with standard mechanical or stented bioprostheses. They are most beneficial in children and younger adults. Allograft valves may also improve the results of AVR in active endocarditis.[114] A further discussion of these valves is presented in subsequent chapters. As their use has remained confined to a few centers that perform such operations regularly, the remainder of this discussion focuses on issues regarding selection of mechanical or bioprosthetic valves.

Mechanical versus Biologic Valves

When selecting between mechanical and biologic heart valves, the surgeon and patient together must balance the risks and benefits of each choice. Mechanical valves are much less likely to undergo structural deterioration necessitating reoperation. Mechanical valves are more thrombogenic than bioprosthetic valves and require formal anticoagulation with oral warfarin, which carries a significantly increased risk of bleeding complications. Patients with mechanical valves and adequate anticoagulation do not have a greater risk of thromboembolic events than do those with bioprosthetic valves.[115] There is no difference in actuarial freedom from bacterial endocarditis between mechanical and bioprosthetic valves. Regarding overall survival, two randomized comparisons of mechanical and bioprosthetic aortic valves performed in the 1970s demonstrated equivalent survival between valve types at 12 years of follow-up.[116,117] Long-term survival beyond 15 years was superior in the mechanical valve groups as the risks of reoperation and structural failures of bioprostheses became more common.[118] However, the rate of structural valve deterioration was higher with first-generation prostheses than with newer-generation models.

TABLE 33-12 Multivariate Predictors of Functional Recovery after Aortic Valve Replacement

Follow-Up DASI	Factor	Estimate ± Standard Error	Estimated Odds Ratio (95% Upper and Lower Confidence Intervals)	*p*	Reliability (%)
	Standardized orifice	0.0040 ± 0.074	1.00 (0.87, 1.16)	0.96	1
	Balancing score	0.11 ± 0.11	1.11 (0.90, 1.37)	0.3	
Worse	Female sex	−0.50 ± 0.14	0.61 (0.46, 0.80)	<0.001	79
Worse	Age*	−0.39 ± 0.075	0.68 (0.58, 0.78)	<0.001	81
Better	Preoperative DASI	0.018 ± 0.0041	1.02 (1.01, 1.03)	<0.001	94
Worse	Preoperative creatinine (mg/dL)	−0.37 ± 0.094	0.69 (0.58, 0.83)	<0.001	41
Worse	Central venous pressure in the intensive care unit (mm Hg)	−0.037 ± 0.014	0.96 (0.94, 0.99)	0.01	46
Worse	Red blood cells transfused (units)	−0.45 ± 0.14	0.64 (0.49, 0.83)	0.001	82

*Age was transformed as exponent of age in years/50.
DASI = Duke Activity Status Index.
Source: Adapted with permission from Koch CG, Khandwala F, Estafanous FG, Loop FD, et al: Impact of prosthesis-patient size on functional recovery after aortic valve replacement. Circulation 2005; 111:3221.

Special Patient Groups

Patients with an absolute requirement for long-term anticoagulation such as atrial fibrillation, previous thromboembolic events, hypercoagulable state, severe LVD, another mechanical heart valve in place, or intracardiac thrombus, should receive a mechanical valve regardless of age.

Patients in whom anticoagulation with warfarin is contraindicated, such as women of child-bearing age wishing to become pregnant, patients with other bleeding disorders, or those who refuse anticoagulation should receive a bioprosthesis. Alternatively, implantation of mechanical prostheses in such women combined with anticoagulation using subcutaneous low-molecular weight heparin injections during the pregnancy is a possibility.

Patients with end-stage renal failure were previously believed to have significantly elevated risk for early bioprosthetic structural valve deterioration. However, increased anticoagulation-related complications are also more likely in this group, and the current ACC/AHA guidelines do not recommend routine use of mechanical prostheses in these patients.

Further considerations that may affect future patient decisions include testing for genetic variants of the *CYP2C9* and *VKORC1* genes, which influence warfarin response, use of devices to facilitate home INR monitoring, and use of novel nonwarfarin oral anticoagulants. A detailed and comprehensive discussion of these risks and benefits of prosthesis selection should occur with all patients and their families before entering the operating room.

Age Considerations

Currently available bioprostheses, such as the Medtronic Hancock II porcine and Carpentier-Edwards pericardial valve, have greater than 90% freedom from structural valve dysfunction and greater than 90% freedom from reoperation at 12-year follow-up.[52,60,61] The rate of structural deterioration is lower in patients over 65 to 70 years. Hence, patients greater than 65 years at the time of surgery should receive a biologic valve. Patients less than age 60 should have a mechanical prosthesis to minimize the risk of structural failure requiring repeat AVR as an octogenarian. Patients between 60 and 65 represent the group in whom there is still considerable debate regarding prosthesis selection. Those patients who have comorbidities such as severe CAD may be less likely to outlive their prosthesis and should receive a biologic valve. Prompted by improvements in durability of bioprostheses and lower reoperation risks, a recent retrospective study of patients 50 to 70 with AVR demonstrated worse 10-year unadjusted survival (50 versus 65%) and freedom from reoperation (91 versus 98%) with tissue compared with mechanical AVR.[11] On the other hand, Ruel et al.[119] found no difference in overall survival for patients less than 60 years old with tissue AVR versus those with mechanical AVR over a 20-year follow-up. Although age alone usually does not preclude one from surgery, advanced age and associated comorbidities may make someone a poor candidate for a classic valve replacement. In such patients, transcatheter aortic valve replacement (TAVR), discussed later, may be an alternative to medical management or balloon aortic valvuloplasty.

Stented versus Stentless Biologic Valves

Stentless porcine valves have gained popularity in cardiac surgery owing to the pioneering work done by Tirone David at the

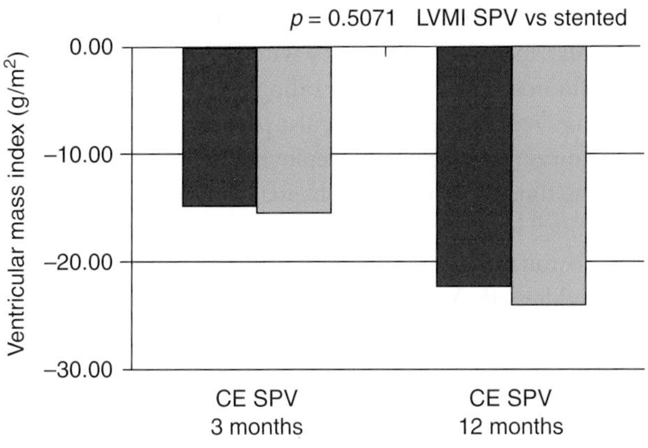

FIGURE 33-20 Indexed ventricular mass regression in stentless and stented valve patients over time. There were no significant differences in the two groups. CE = Carpentier-Edwards stented valve; LVMI = left ventricular mass index; SPV = Toronto stentless porcine valve. (*Reproduced with permission from Cohen G, Christakis GT, Joyner CD, et al: Are stentless valves hemodynamically superior to stented valves? A prospective randomized trial. Ann Thorac Surg 2002; 73:767.*)

Toronto General Hospital in 1988.[120] Stentless valves lack obstructive stents and strut posts, thus have residual gradients that are similar to those of freehand allografts. However, their use involves a more complex operation as they are more difficult to implant and require a longer cross-clamp time. Cohen and colleagues found no differences in aortic root size, IEOA, or LVM regression (Fig. 33-20) or functional outcome at 1 year between patients randomized to receive Carpentier-Edwards pericardial valves and Toronto stentless porcine valves (Fig. 33-21).[121] These findings challenge the notion that stentless porcine valves provide increased IEOA or hemodynamic or clinically

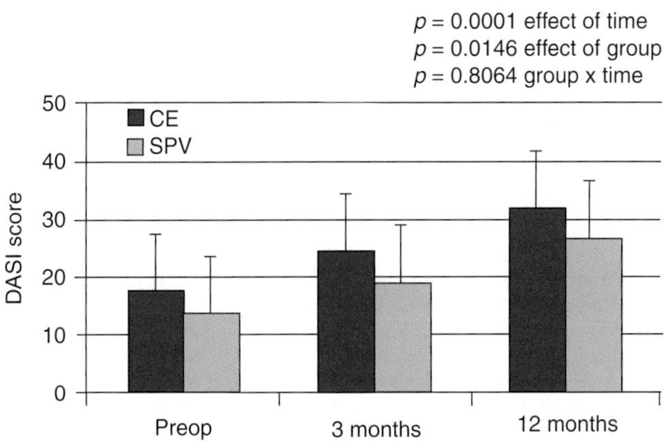

FIGURE 33-21 Change in Duke Activity Status Index (DASI) scores in stentless and stented valve patients over time. There were no significant differences in the two groups. CE = Carpentier-Edwards stented valve; SPV = Toronto stentless porcine valve; Preop = preoperative. (*Reproduced with permission from Cohen G, Christakis GT, Joyner CD, et al: Are stentless valves hemodynamically superior to stented valves? A prospective randomized trial. Ann Thorac Surg 2002; 73:767.*)

significant benefit. In a randomized trial comparing St. Jude Toronto stentless porcine valves with Carpentier-Edwards pericardial valves, Chambers and colleagues found no difference in IEOA, LVM regression, or mortality between groups. Arenaza and colleagues also performed a multicenter randomized trial comparing the Medtronic Freestyle valve with the Medtonic Mosaic valve and found increased IEOA in the stentless group, but no differences in LVM regression or clinical outcomes at 1 year.

However, Walther and colleagues performed a small randomized trial comparing the ability of stented porcine and stentless porcine valves which cause regression of LVH.[122] They showed that patients in the stentless valve group received larger valves for a given annular size and had a slightly higher degree of LVM regression. Borger and colleagues showed modestly lower mean gradients in stentless prostheses versus stented prostheses (9 versus 15 mm Hg) and LVMI (100 versus 107 g/m^2) but no difference in survival.[123]

Hence, conflicting evidence exists regarding benefit of stentless valves in LVM regression or clinical outcomes over stented bioprostheses. There is also little evidence that incremental improvements in LVM provide additional clinical benefit. Thus, the routine use of stentless bioprostheses cannot be recommended for most patients with small aortic roots based on currently available data. At this time, stentless porcine valves are most useful in a relatively younger patient with a small aortic root who is active and likely to be limited by the elevated residual gradient a small stented bioprosthesis may create.

PERCUTANEOUS VALVULAR INTERVENTIONS

Percutaneous Aortic Balloon Valvotomy

As an alternative to surgical management for AS, aortic balloon valvotomy has been performed percutaneously via a femoral artery puncture to treat AS.[124] Inflation of the balloon within the valve orifice can stretch the annular tissue and fracture calcified areas or open fused commissures. There is no role for valvotomy in the patient with significant AR, as this will become significantly worse after the procedure.[125,126] Balloon valvotomy is rarely successful if significant calcification is present and carries a prohibitive risk of stroke from calcific emboli.[127] The long-term outcomes of this procedure in adult patients are dismal, with restenosis usually occurring within 1 year.[126,127] Patients with severe symptomatic AS who are too hemodynamically unstable to tolerate operation or have comorbid illnesses, such as advanced malignancy, which contraindicate operation, may benefit from palliative balloon valvotomy.[128,129] More recently, techniques have developed to implant prosthetic valves using transfemoral and transapical catheter-based approaches.

Transcatheter Aortic Valve Replacement

Although surgical aortic valve replacement is the definitive treatment for aortic valve stenosis, up to one-third of patients are not candidates due to increasing age, heart failure, or other comorbidities.[130] The first clinical description of human transcatheter valve implantation took place in 2002.[131] Transcatheter

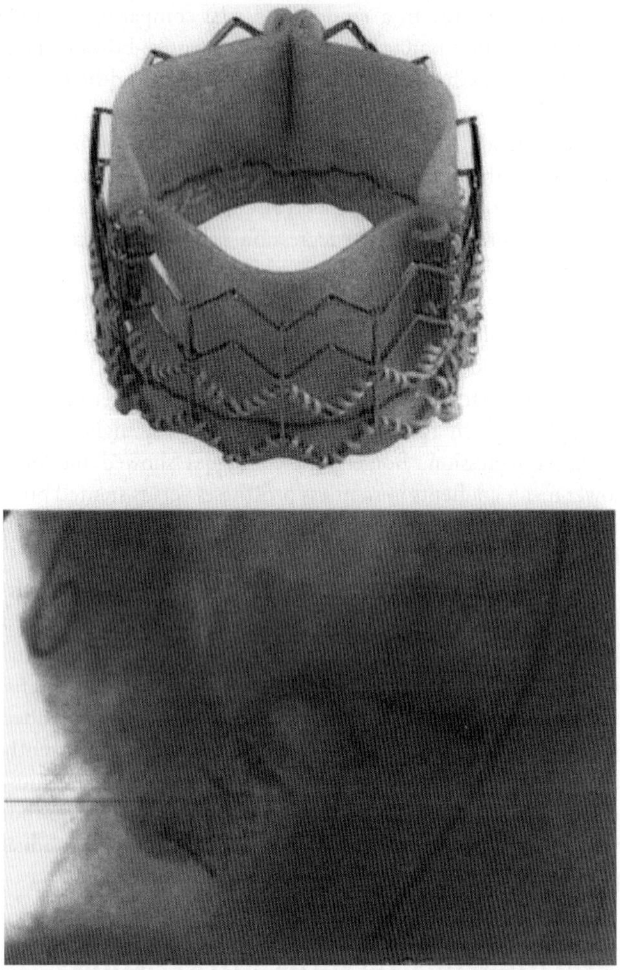

FIGURE 33-22 The Edwards Sapien aortic percutaneous heart valve (*upper panel*) and fluoroscopic view of this prosthesis deployed in the aortic root (*lower panel*). (*Figure courtesy of Edwards Life Sciences Inc., Irvine, CA.*)

heart valve technologies are now a clinical reality and have been shown to offer symptom relief and survival benefit to high-risk, elderly, and nonoperative patients.[132] Early experience from Webb and coworkers demonstrate overall mortality of 14.3% in the initial half to 8.3% in the second half of the study, and 74% 1-year survival with both percutaneous and transapical procedures.[133]

Currently, the two most extensively studied valve systems include the Edwards Sapien Valve and the CoreValve, although various other valves exist in different stages of development and evaluation (Fig. 33-22). Each valve system includes: (1) the valve prosthesis, (2) the stent or frame, (3) the loading system, and (4) the delivery system. The Edwards Lifesciences SAPIEN THV valve (Edwards Lifesciences Inc., Irvine, CA) is composed of a bovine pericardial valve on a balloon-expandable stent, whereas the CoreValve (Medtronic) is a porcine pericardial valve on a self-expanding nitonol frame.

The approach is accomplished via a retrograde transarterial or transapical manner. The percutaneous retrograde femoral approach involves femoral artery access, retrograde cannulation of the aortic valve, balloon dilatation, and device delivery. Alternatively, transapical transcatheter valve delivery involves creating a small thoracotomy, direct cannulation of the left ventricular apex, and passing of a wire and stent-mounted valve under fluoroscopic and echocardiographic guidance.[134] Both techniques require rapid ventricular pacing to ensure there is no cardiac output during device deployment.

At the time of writing this chapter, clinical trials are in progress in which issues regarding prosthesis durability, periprocedural stroke, coronary artery injury, and hemodynamic performance will be addressed. At present, these techniques are enabling very high-risk patients to experience some relief of their symptoms without undergoing a complex operation. Given the excellent current results of open operative AVR, the use of these procedures in lower-risk patients is not currently warranted.

REFERENCES

1. Selzer A: Changing aspects of the natural history of valvular aortic stenosis. *NEJM* 1987; 317:91.
2. Rahimtoola SH: Valvular heart disease: a perspective. *J Am Coll Cardiol* 1983; 1:199.
3. Braunwald E: Valvular heart disease, in Braunwald E (ed): *Braunwald: Heart Disease: A Textbook of Cardiovascular Medicine*, 6th ed. New York, WB Saunders, 2001; p 1643.
4. Hess OM, Ritter M, Schneider J, et al: Diastolic stiffness and myocardial structure in aortic valve disease before and after valve replacement. *Circulation* 1984; 69:855.
5. Horstkotte D, Loogen F: The natural history of aortic valve stenosis. *Eur Heart J* 1988; 9(Suppl E):57.
6. Lund O, Nielsen TT, Emmertsen K, et al: Mortality and worsening of prognostic profile during waiting time for valve replacement in aortic stenosis. *Thorac Cardiovasc Surg* 1996; 44:289.
7. Schwarz F, Baumann P, Manthey J, et al: The effect of aortic valve replacement on survival. *Circulation* 1982; 66:1105.
8. Otto CM, Burwash IG, Legget ME, et al: Prospective study of asymptomatic valvular aortic stenosis. Clinical, echocardiographic, and exercise predictors of outcome. *Circulation* 1997; 95:2262.
9. Rosenhek R, Binder T, Porenta G, et al: Predictors of outcome in severe, asymptomatic aortic stenosis. *NEJM* 2000; 343:611.
10. Otto CM, Burwash IG, Legget ME, et al: Prospective study of asymptomatic valvular aortic stenosis. Clinical, echocardiographic, and exercise predictors of outcome. *Circulation* 1997; 95:2262.
11. Brown ML, Pellikka PA, Schaff HV, et al: The benefits of early valve replacement in asymptomatic patients with severe aortic stenosis. *J Thorac Cardiovasc Surg* 2008; 135:308.
12. deFilippi CR, Willett DL, Brickner ME, et al: Usefulness of dobuta-mine echocardiography in distinguishing severe from nonsevere valvular aortic stenosis in patients with depressed left ventricular function and low transvalvular gradients. *Am J Cardiol* 1995; 75:191.
13. Pereira JJ, Lauer MS, Bashir M, et al: Survival after aortic valve replacement for severe aortic stenosis with low transvalvular gradients and severe left ventricular dysfunction. *J Am Coll Cardiol* 2002; 39:1356.
14. Hwang MH, Hammermeister KE, Oprian C, et al: Preoperative identification of patients likely to have left ventricular dysfunction after aortic valve replacement. Participants in the Veterans Administration Cooperative Study on Valvular Heart Disease. *Circulation* 1989; 80(3 Pt 1):I65.
15. Rosenhek R: Statins for aortic stenosis. *NEJM* 2005; 352:2441.
16. Cowell SJ, Newby DE, Prescott RJ, et al: A randomized trial of intensive lipid-lowering therapy in calcific aortic stenosis. *NEJM* 2005; 352:2389.
17. American College of Cardiology/American Heart Association: ACC/AHA guidelines for the management of patients with valvular heart disease. A report of the American College of Cardiology/American Heart Association. Task Force on Practice Guidelines (Committee on Management of Patients with Valvular Heart Disease). *J Am Coll Cardiol* 1998; 32:1486.
18. Bonow RO, Carabello BA, Chatterjee K, et al: ACC/AHA 2006 guidelines for the management of patients with valvular heart disease: a report of the American College of Cardiology/American Heart Association Task Force on Practice Guidelines (Writing Committee to Revise the 1998 Guidelines for the Management of Patients with Valvular Heart Disease) developed in collaboration with the Society of Cardiovascular Anesthesiologists endorsed by the Society for Cardiovascular Angiography and Interventions and the Society of Thoracic Surgeons. *J Am Coll Cardiol* 2006; 48:e1.

19. Braunwald E: Aortic valve replacement: an update at the turn of the millennium. *Eur Heart J* 2000; 21:1032.
20. Downes TR, Nomeir AM, Hackshaw BT, et al: Diastolic mitral regurgitation in acute but not chronic aortic regurgitation: implications regarding the mechanism of mitral closure. *Am Heart J* 1989; 117:1106.
21. Grossman W, Jones D, McLaurin LP: Wall stress and patterns of hypertrophy in the human left ventricle. *J Clin Invest* 1975; 56:56.
22. Starling MR, Kirsh MM, Montgomery DG, Gross MD: Mechanisms for left ventricular systolic dysfunction in aortic regurgitation: importance for predicting the functional response to aortic valve replacement. *J Am Coll Cardiol* 1991; 17:887.
23. Bonow RO: Asymptomatic aortic regurgitation: indications for operation. *J Cardiol Surg* 1994; 9(2 Suppl):170.
24. Bonow RO, Rosing DR, McIntosh CL, et al: The natural history of asymptomatic patients with aortic regurgitation and normal left ventricular function. *Circulation* 1983; 68:509.
25. Bonow RO, Lakatos E, Maron BJ, Epstein SE: Serial long-term assessment of the natural history of asymptomatic patients with chronic aortic regurgitation and normal left ventricular systolic function. *Circulation* 1991; 84:1625.
26. Tornos MP, Olona M, Permanyer-Miralda G, et al: Clinical outcome of severe asymptomatic chronic aortic regurgitation: a long-term prospective follow-up study. *Am Heart J* 1995; 130:333.
27. Rapaport E: Natural history of aortic and mitral valve disease. *Am J Cardiol* 1975; 35:221.
28. Bonow RO, Nikas D, Elefteriades JA: Valve replacement for regurgitant lesions of the aortic or mitral valve in advanced left ventricular dysfunction. *Cardiol Clin* 1995; 13:73,85.
29. Gall S Jr, Lowe JE, Wolfe WG, et al: Efficacy of the internal mammary artery in combined aortic valve replacement-coronary artery bypass grafting. *Ann Thorac Surg* 2000; 69:524.
30. Borger MA, David TE: Management of the valve and ascending aorta in adults with bicuspid aortic valve disease. *Semin Thorac Cardiovasc Surg* 2005; 17:143.
31. Nicks R, Cartmill T, Bernstein L: Hypoplasia of the aortic root. The problem of aortic valve replacement. *Thorax* 1970; 25:339.
32. Manouguian S, Seybold-Epting W: Patch enlargement of the aortic valve ring by extending the aortic incision into the anterior mitral leaflet. New operative technique. *J Thorac Cardiovasc Surg* 1979; 78:402.
33. Konno S, Imai Y, Iida Y, et al: A new method for prosthetic valve replacement in congenital aortic stenosis associated with hypoplasia of the aortic valve ring. *J Thorac Cardiovasc Surg* 1975; 70:909.
34. David TE: Surgical management of aortic root abscess. *J Cardiol Surg* 1997; 12(2 Suppl):262.
35. Borger MA, Rao V, Weisel RD, et al: Reoperative coronary bypass surgery: effect of patent grafts and retrograde cardioplegia. *J Thorac Cardiovasc Surg* 2001; 121:83.
36. Hilbert SL, Ferrans VJ: Porcine aortic valve bioprostheses: morphologic and functional considerations. *J Long Term Eff Med Implants* 1992; 2:99.
37. Flomenbaum MA, Schoen FJ: Effects of fixation back pressure and antimineralization treatment on the morphology of porcine aortic bioprosthetic valves. *J Thorac Cardiovasc Surg* 1993; 105:154.
38. Edmunds LH Jr, Clark RE, Cohn LH, et al: Guidelines for reporting morbidity and mortality after cardiac valvular operations. Ad Hoc Liaison Committee for Standardizing Definitions of Prosthetic Heart Valve Morbidity of The American Association for Thoracic Surgery and The Society of Thoracic Surgeons. *J Thorac Cardiovasc Surg* 1996; 112:708.
39. Bloodwell RD, Okies JE, Hallman GL, Cooley DA: Aortic valve replacement. Long-term results. *J Thorac Cardiovasc Surg* 1969; 58:457.
40. Christakis GT, Weisel RD, David TE, et al: Predictors of operative survival after valve replacement. *Circulation* 1988; 78(3 Pt 2):I25.
41. Craver JM, Weintraub WS, Jones EL, et al: Predictors of mortality, complications, and length of stay in aortic valve replacement for aortic stenosis. *Circulation* 1988; 78(3 Pt 2):I85.
42. Edwards FH, Peterson ED, Coombs LP, et al: Prediction of operative mortality after valve replacement surgery. *J Am Coll Cardiol* 2001; 37:885.
43. Scott WC, Miller DC, Haverich A, et al: Determinants of operative mortality for patients undergoing aortic valve replacement. Discriminant analysis of 1,479 operations. *J Thorac Cardiovasc Surg* 1985; 89:400.
44. Edwards FH, Peterson ED, Coombs LP, et al: Prediction of operative mortality after valve replacement surgery. *J Am Coll Cardiol* 2001; 37:885.
45. O'Brien SM, Shahian DM, Filardo G, et al: The Society of Thoracic Surgeons 2008 cardiac surgery risk models: part 2—isolated valve surgery. *Ann Thorac Surg* 2009; 88:S23.
46. Rao V, Christakis GT, Weisel RD, et al: Changing pattern of valve surgery. *Circulation* 1996; 94(9 Suppl):II113.
47. He GW, Acuff TE, Ryan WH, et al: Aortic valve replacement: determinants of operative mortality. *Ann Thorac Surg* 1994; 57:1140.
48. Lytle BW, Cosgrove DM, Loop FD, et al: Replacement of aortic valve combined with myocardial revascularization: determinants of early and late risk for 500 patients, 1967-1981. *Circulation* 1983; 68:1149.
49. Rankin JS, Hammill BG, Ferguson TB Jr, et al: Determinants of operative mortality in valvular heart surgery. *J Thorac Cardiovasc Surg* 2006; 131:547.
50. Hammermeister KE, Sethi GK, Henderson WG, et al: A comparison of outcomes in men 11 years after heart-valve replacement with a mechanical valve or bioprosthesis. Veterans Affairs Cooperative Study on Valvular Heart Disease. *NEJM* 1993; 328:1289.
51. Hammermeister K, Sethi GK, Henderson WG, et al: Outcomes 15 years after valve replacement with a mechanical versus a bioprosthetic valve: final report of the Veterans Affairs randomized trial. *J Am Coll Cardiol* 2000; 36:1152.
52. David TE, Ivanov J, Armstrong S, et al: Late results of heart valve replacement with the Hancock II bioprosthesis. *J Thorac Cardiovasc Surg* 2001; 121:268.
53. Dellgren G, David TE, Raanani E, et al: Late hemodynamic and clinical outcomes of aortic valve replacement with the Carpentier-Edwards Perimount pericardial bioprosthesis. *J Thorac Cardiovasc Surg* 2002; 124:146.
54. Stahle E, Kvidal P, Nystrom SO, Bergstrom R: Long-term relative survival after primary heart valve replacement. *Eur J Cardiothorac Surg* 1997; 11(81):146.
55. Cohen G, David TE, Ivanov J, et al: The impact of age, coronary artery disease, and cardiac comorbidity on late survival after bio-prosthetic aortic valve replacement. *J Thorac Cardiovasc Surg* 1999; 117:273.
56. Verheul HA, van den Brink RB, Bouma BJ, et al: Analysis of risk factors for excess mortality after aortic valve replacement. *J Am Coll Cardiol* 1995; 26:1280.
57. Lytle BW, Cosgrove DM, Taylor PC, et al: Primary isolated aortic valve replacement. Early and late results. *J Thorac Cardiovasc Surg* 1989; 97:675.
58. Aranki SF, Rizzo RJ, Couper GS, et al: Aortic valve replacement in the elderly. Effect of gender and coronary artery disease on operative mortality. *Circulation* 1993; 88(5 Pt 2):II17.
59. Edmunds LH Jr, Clark RE, Cohn LH, et al: Guidelines for reporting morbidity and mortality after cardiac valvular operations. *Eur J Cardiothorac Surg* 1996; 10:812.
60. Poirer NC, Pelletier LC, Pellerin M, Carrier M: 15-Year experience with the Carpentier-Edwards pericardial bioprosthesis. *Ann Thorac Surg* 1998; 66(6 Suppl):S57.
61. Dellgren G, David TE, Raanani E, et al: Late hemodynamic and clinical outcomes of aortic valve replacement with the Carpentier-Edwards Perimount pericardial bioprosthesis. *J Thorac Cardiovasc Surg* 2002; 124:146.
62. Rizzoli G, Mirone S, Ius P, et al: Fifteen-year results with the Hancock II valve: a multicenter experience. *J Thorac Cardiovasc Surg* 2006; 132:602,609.
63. Jamieson WR, Fradet GJ, MacNab JS, et al: Medtronic mosaic porcine bioprosthesis: investigational center experience to six years. *J Heart Valve Dis* 2005; 14:54.
64. Grunkemeier GL, Jamieson WR, Miller DC, Starr A: Actuarial versus actual risk of porcine structural valve deterioration. *J Thorac Cardiovasc Surg* 1994; 108:709.
65. Vongpatanasin W, Hillis LD, Lange RA: Prosthetic heart valves. *NEJM* 1996; 335:407.
66. Grunkemeier GL, Wu Y: Actual versus actuarial event-free percentages. *Ann Thorac Surg* 2001; 72:677.
67. Mahoney CB, Miller DC, Khan SS, et al: Twenty-year, three-institution evaluation of the Hancock Modified Orifice aortic valve durability. Comparison of actual and actuarial estimates. *Circulation* 1998; 98(19 Suppl):II88.
68. Akins CW, Carroll DL, Buckley MJ, et al: Late results with Carpentier-Edwards porcine bioprosthesis. *Circulation* 1990; 82(5 Suppl):IV65.
69. Glower DD, White WD, Hatton AC, et al: Determinants of reoperation after 960 valve replacements with Carpentier-Edwards pros-theses. *J Thorac Cardiovasc Surg* 1994; 107:381.
70. Jamieson WR, Ling H, Burr LH, et al: Carpentier-Edwards supraannular porcine bioprosthesis evaluation over 15 years. *Ann Thorac Surg* 1998; 66(6 Suppl):S49.
71. Corbineau H, De La TB, Verhoye JP, et al: Carpentier-Edwards supraannular porcine bioprosthesis in aortic position: 16-year experience. *Ann Thorac Surg* 2001; 71(5 Suppl):S228.
72. David TE, Armstrong S, Sun Z: The Hancock II bioprosthesis at 12 years. *Ann Thorac Surg* 1998; 66(6 Suppl):S95.
73. Burdon TA, Miller DC, Oyer PE, et al: Durability of porcine valves at fifteen years in a representative North American patient population. *J Thorac Cardiovasc Surg* 1992; 103:238.

74. O'Brien MF, Stafford EG, Gardner MA, et al: Allograft aortic valve replacement: long-term follow-up. *Ann Thorac Surg* 1995; 60 (2 Suppl):S65.
75. Bodnar E, Wain WH, Martelli V, Ross DN: Long term performance of 580 homograft and autograft valves used for aortic valve replacement. *Thorac Cardiovasc Surg* 1979; 27:31.
76. Gross C, Harringer W, Beran H, et al: Aortic valve replacement: is the stentless xenograft an alternative to the homograft? Midterm results. *Ann Thorac Surg* 1999; 68:919.
77. Heras M, Chesebro JH, Fuster V, et al: High risk of thromboemboli early after bioprosthetic cardiac valve replacement. *J Am Coll Cardiol* 1995; 25:1111.
78. David TE, Ho WI, Christakis GT: Thromboembolism in patients with aortic porcine bioprostheses. *Ann Thorac Surg* 1985; 40:229.
79. Goldsmith I, Lip GY, Mukundan S, Rosin MD: Experience with low-dose aspirin as thromboprophylaxis for the Tissuemed porcine aortic bioprosthesis: a survey of five years' experience. *J Heart Valve Dis* 1998; 7:574.
80. Lengyel M, Vandor L: The role of thrombolysis in the management of left-sided prosthetic valve thrombosis: a study of 85 cases diagnosed by transesophageal echocardiography. *J Heart Valve Dis* 2001; 10:636.
81. Bonow RO, Carabello B, de Leon AC, et al: ACC/AHA Guidelines for the Management of Patients With Valvular Heart Disease. Executive Summary. A report of the American College of Cardiology/American Heart Association Task Force on Practice Guidelines (Committee on Management of Patients With Valvular Heart Disease). *J Heart Valve Dis* 1998; 7:672.
82. Lengyel M, Fuster V, Keltai M, et al: Guidelines for management of left-sided prosthetic valve thrombosis: a role for thrombolytic therapy. Consensus Conference on Prosthetic Valve Thrombosis. *J Am Coll Cardiol* 1997; 30:1521.
83. Calderwood SB, Swinski LA, Waternaux CM, et al: Risk factors for the development of prosthetic valve endocarditis. *Circulation* 1985; 72:31.
84. Vongpatanasin W, Hillis LD, Lange RA: Prosthetic heart valves. *NEJM* 1996; 335:407.
85. Blackstone EH, Kirklin JW: Death and other time-related events after valve replacement. *Circulation* 1985; 72:753.
86. Ivert TS, Dismukes WE, Cobbs CG, et al: Prosthetic valve endocarditis. *Circulation* 1984; 69:223.
87. Haydock D, Barratt-Boyes B, Macedo T, et al: Aortic valve replacement for active infectious endocarditis in 108 patients. A comparison of free-hand allograft valves with mechanical prostheses and bioprostheses. *J Thorac Cardiovasc Surg* 1992; 103:130.
88. Levy D, Garrison RJ, Savage DD, et al: Prognostic implications of echocardiographically determined left ventricular mass in the Framingham Heart Study. *NEJM* 1990; 322:1561.
89. Haider AW, Larson MG, Benjamin EJ, Levy D: Increased left ventricular mass and hypertrophy are associated with increased risk for sudden death. *J Am Coll Cardiol* 1998; 32:1454.
90. Christakis GT, Joyner CD, Morgan CD, et al: Left ventricular mass regression early after aortic valve replacement. *Ann Thorac Surg* 1996; 62:1084.
91. Kuhl HP, Franke A, Puschmann D, et al: Regression of left ventricular mass one year after aortic valve replacement for pure severe aortic stenosis. *Am J Cardiol* 2002; 89:408.
92. Kennedy JW, Doces J, Stewart DK: Left ventricular function before and following aortic valve replacement. *Circulation* 1977; 56:944.
93. Rahimtoola SH: The problem of valve prosthesis-patient mismatch. *Circulation* 1978; 58:20.
94. Hanayama N, Christakis GT, Mallidi HR, et al: Patient prosthesis mismatch is rare after aortic valve replacement: valve size may be irrelevant. *Ann Thorac Surg* 2002; 73:1822.
95. Yun KL, Jamieson WR, Khonsari S, et al: Prosthesis-patient mismatch: hemodynamic comparison of stented and stentless aortic valves. *Semin Thorac Cardiovasc Surg* 1999; 11(4 Suppl 1):98.
96. Dumesnil JG, Pibarot P: Prosthesis-patient mismatch and clinical outcomes: the evidence continues to accumulate. *J Thorac Cardiovasc Surg* 2006; 131:952.
97. Pibarot P, Dumesnil JG: Hemodynamic and clinical impact of prosthesis-patient mismatch in the aortic valve position and its prevention. *J Am Coll Cardiol* 2000; 36:1131.
98. Garcia D, Dumesnil JG, Durand LG, et al: Discrepancies between catheter and Doppler estimates of valve effective orifice area can be predicted from the pressure recovery phenomenon: practical implications with regard to quantification of aortic stenosis severity. *J Am Coll Cardiol* 2003; 41:435.
99. Rao V, Jamieson WR, Ivanov J, et al: Prosthesis-patient mismatch affects survival after aortic valve replacement. *Circulation* 2002; 102 (19 Suppl 3):III5.
100. Ruel M, Al-Faleh H, Kulik A, et al: Prosthesis-patient mismatch after aortic valve replacement predominantly affects patients with preexisting left ventricular dysfunction: effect on survival, freedom from heart failure, and left ventricular mass regression. *J Thorac Cardiovasc Surg* 2006; 131:1036.
101. Moon MR, Pasque MK, Munfakh NA, et al: Prosthesis-patient mismatch after aortic valve replacement: impact of age and body size on late survival. *Ann Thorac Surg* 2006; 81:481.
102. Medalion B, Blackstone EH, Lytle BW, et al: Aortic valve replacement: is valve size important? *J Thorac Cardiovasc Surg* 2000; 119:963.
103. Hanayama N, Christakis GT, Mallidi HR, et al: Patient prosthesis mismatch is rare after aortic valve replacement: valve size may be irrelevant. *Ann Thorac Surg* 2002; 73:1822.
104. Blackstone EH, Cosgrove DM, Jamieson WR, et al: Prosthesis size and long-term survival after aortic valve replacement. *J Thorac Cardiovasc Surg* 2003; 126:783.
105. Sawant D, Singh AK, Feng WC, et al: St. Jude Medical cardiac valves in small aortic roots: follow-up to sixteen years. *J Thorac Cardiovasc Surg* 1997; 113:499.
106. De Paulis R, Sommariva L, Colagrande L, et al: Regression of left ventricular hypertrophy after aortic valve replacement for aortic stenosis with different valve substitutes. *J Thorac Cardiovasc Surg* 1998; 116:590.
107. Kratz JM, Sade RM, Crawford FA Jr, et al: The risk of small St. Jude aortic valve prostheses. *Ann Thorac Surg* 1994; 57:1114.
108. Khan SS, Siegel RJ, DeRobertis MA, et al: Regression of hypertrophy after Carpentier-Edwards pericardial aortic valve replacement. *Ann Thorac Surg* 2000; 69:531.
109. Blackstone EH, Cosgrove DM, Jamieson WR, et al: Prosthesis size and long-term survival after aortic valve replacement. *J Thorac Cardiovasc Surg* 2003; 126:783.
110. Rao V, Christakis GT, Sever J, et al: A novel comparison of stentless versus stented valves in the small aortic root. *J Thorac Cardiovasc Surg* 1999; 117:431.
111. Pibarot P, Dumesnil JG: Effect of exercise on bioprosthetic valve hemodynamics. *Am J Cardiol* 1999; 83:1593.
112. Lund O, Chandrasekaran V, Grocott-Mason R, et al: Primary aortic valve replacement with allografts over twenty-five years: valve-related and procedure-related determinants of outcome. *J Thorac Cardiovasc Surg* 1999; 117:77.
113. O'Brien MF, Stafford EG, Gardner MA, et al: Allograft aortic valve replacement: long-term follow-up. *Ann Thorac Surg* 1995; 60(2 Suppl):S65.
114. Lupinetti FM, Lemmer JH Jr: Comparison of allografts and prosthetic valves when used for emergency aortic valve replacement for active infective endocarditis. *Am J Cardiol* 1991; 68:637.
115. Hammermeister K, Sethi GK, Henderson WG, et al: Outcomes 15 years after valve replacement with a mechanical versus a bioprosthetic valve: final report of the Veterans Affairs randomized trial. *J Am Coll Cardiol* 2000; 36:1152.
116. Hammermeister KE, Henderson WG, Burchfiel CM, et al: Comparison of outcome after valve replacement with a bioprosthesis versus a mechanical prosthesis: initial 5 year results of a randomized trial. *J Am Coll Cardiol* 1987; 10:719.
117. Bloomfield P, Kitchin AH, Wheatley DJ, et al: A prospective evaluation of the Bjork-Shiley, Hancock, and Carpentier-Edwards heart valve prostheses. *Circulation* 1986; 73:1213.
118. Oxenham H, Bloomfield P, Wheatley DJ, et al: Twenty year comparison of a Bjork-Shiley mechanical heart valve with porcine bioprostheses. *Heart* 2003; 89:715.
119. Ruel M, Chan V, Bédard P, et al: Very long-term survival implications of heart valve replacement with tissue versus mechanical prostheses in adults <60 years of age. *Circulation* 2007; 116:294.
120. David TE, Ropchan GC, Butany JW: Aortic valve replacement with stentless porcine bioprostheses. *J Cardiol Surg* 1988; 3:501.
121. Cohen G, Christakis GT, Joyner CD, et al: Are stentless valves hemodynamically superior to stented valves? A prospective randomized trial. *Ann Thorac Surg* 2002; 73:767.
122. Walther T, Falk V, Langebartels G, et al: Prospectively randomized evaluation of stentless versus conventional biological aortic valves: impact on early regression of left ventricular hypertrophy. *Circulation* 1999; 100 (19 Suppl):II6.
123. Borger MA, Carson SM, Ivanov J, et al: Stentless aortic valves are hemodynamically superior to stented valves during mid-term follow-up: a large retrospective study. *Ann Thorac Surg* 2005; 80:2180.
124. Safian RD, Berman AD, Diver DJ, et al: Balloon aortic valvuloplasty in 170 consecutive patients. *NEJM* 1988; 319:125.

125. Kuntz RE, Tosteson AN, Berman AD, et al: Predictors of event-free survival after balloon aortic valvuloplasty. *NEJM* 1991; 325:17.
126. Percutaneous balloon aortic valvuloplasty. Acute and 30-day follow-up results in 674 patients from the NHLBI Balloon Valvuloplasty Registry. *Circulation* 1991; 84:2383.
127. Bernard Y, Etievent J, Mourand JL, et al: Long-term results of percutaneous aortic valvuloplasty compared with aortic valve replacement in patients more than 75 years old. *J Am Coll Cardiol* 1992; 20:796.
128. Smedira NG, Ports TA, Merrick SH, Rankin JS: Balloon aortic valvuloplasty as a bridge to aortic valve replacement in critically ill patients. *Ann Thorac Surg* 1993; 55:914.
129. Cormier B, Vahanian A: Indications and outcome of valvuloplasty. *Curr Opin Cardiol* 1992; 7:222.
130. Zajarias A, Cribier AG: Outcomes and safety of percutaneous aortic valve replacement. *J Am Coll Cardiol* 2009; 53:1829.
131. Cribier A, Eltchaninoff H, Bash A, et al: Percutaneous transcatheter implantation of an aortic valve prosthesis for calcific aortic stenosis: first human case description. *Circulation* 2002; 106:3006.
132. Webb JG, Pasupati S, Humphries K, et al: Percutaneous transarterial aortic valve replacement in selected high-risk patients with aortic stenosis. *Circulation* 2007; 116:755.
133. Webb JG, Altwegg L, Boone RH, et al: Transcatheter aortic valve implantation: impact on clinical and valve-related outcomes. *Circulation* 2009; 119:3009.
134. Ye J, Cheung A, Lichtenstein SV, et al: Transapical transcatheter aortic valve implantation: 1-year outcome in 26 patients. *J Thorac Cardiovasc Surg* 2009; 137:167.

CHAPTER 34

Stentless Aortic Valve Replacement: Autograft/Homograft

Paul Stelzer
Robin Varghese

INTRODUCTION

Unique among the many options now available for aortic valve surgery are the very old, but still useful "human" valve options, including the aortic homograft and the pulmonary autograft (Ross procedure) alternatives. Having reviewed the subject more than 20 years ago,[1] it is interesting to note how some things have changed but much has remained the same. Table 34-1 summarizes advantages and disadvantages of current replacement options.

HISTORICAL PERSPECTIVE

The first choice for aortic valve replacement was the homograft aortic valve. Gordon Murray created an animal model to implant an aortic homograft valve in the descending aorta[2] and was the first to apply the concept in the human demonstrating function for up to 4 years.[3]

Duran and Gunning at Oxford described a method for orthotopic (subcoronary) implantation of an aortic homograft valve in 1962,[4] and in 1962 both Donald Ross in London[5] and Sir Brian Barratt-Boyes in Auckland[6] did this successfully in humans.

Initially, homograft aortic valves were implanted shortly after collection.[7] This impractical method was rapidly supplanted by techniques to sterilize and preserve the valve for later use. Early methods employed beta-propiolactone[6,8] or 0.02% chlorhexidine,[9] followed by ethylene oxide[9] or radiation exposure.[10] Some were preserved by freeze-drying.[6,11] Recognizing that the incidence of valve rupture was high in chemically treated valves, Barratt-Boyes introduced antibiotic sterilization of homografts in 1968.[12] Cryopreservation of homografts was introduced in 1975 by O'Brien and continues to be the predominant method.[13,15] Experimental use of autologous valve transplantation began in 1961 when Lower and colleagues at Stanford transposed the autologous pulmonic valve to the mitral position in dogs[14] and shortly thereafter to the aortic position.[15] Donald Ross applied this to humans, reporting in 1967 clinical experience replacing either the aortic or mitral valve with a pulmonary autograft.[16] Nearly 20 years later the autograft was finally done in America by Elkins and Stelzer.[17] The operation came to be known as the Ross procedure. After an initial surge of interest in the 1990s (more than 240 surgeons worldwide reported their experience to the Ross Procedure International Registry[18]), its use diminished in the next decade.

HOMOGRAFTS

Procurement and Preservation

Homograft valves can be obtained from donors whose beating hearts are not suitable for transplantation but the larger source is tissue from nonbeating heart donors. This has been poorly understood and underappreciated by both medical professionals and the lay public.[19] Regional transplant organizations now participate in procurement of both solid organs and tissues. Specialized homograft processing centers receive hearts in sterile, refrigerated containers. Donor history is reviewed and serology tested for transmissible disease. The great vessels with their valves are separated from the heart under sterile conditions, carefully inspected for defects, measured, cultured, and immersed in antibiotic solution before being sealed in multiple-layer packaging containing dimethylsulfoxide, which prevents

TABLE 34-1 Comparison of Mechanical and Tissue Alternatives for Aortic Valve Replacement

	Mechanical	Stented Bioprosthetic	Stentless Bioprosthetic	Homograft	Autograft
Advantages	Long durability Easy implantation Good EOAI	Easy implantation No anticoagulation	Larger EOAI than stented valve Root replacement is available option	Excellent EOAI All biologic material good for use in endocarditis	Excellent EOAI Living valve Long durability possible
Disadvantages	Anticoagulation Emboli/bleeding Noise	Durability limited Poor EOAI in small valve sizes	Durability limited More complex operative technique Harder reoperation	Complex technique Availability limited Durability limited	Complex operation Double valve or root replacement with potential late failure of either or both

EOAI = effective orifice area index.

cellular rupture during the carefully controlled freezing process.[20] The homografts are then placed in vapor phase liquid nitrogen storage (about −195°C) until used.

Cellular and Immunologic Aspects of Homografts

The normal living valve contains multiple viable cell types, including endothelial cells, fibroblasts, and smooth muscle cells incorporated in a complex extracellular matrix. The cells and matrix elements are in a constant state of remodeling under the influence of regulatory systems that optimize the structure and function of the valve mechanism. It is understandable, therefore, that efforts to preserve homograft structure and function were translated into efforts to maintain homograft cellular viability. Radiation and chemical treatment led to very early failure and were quickly abandoned.[6,8,10,12,21] Antibiotic sterilization of homografts and storage at 4°C does not maintain cellular viability beyond a few days.[22,23] Cryopreservation became the gold standard when donor fibroblast viability was shown after implantation.[13] Although antigenicity of the fibroblast is low and other cell types do not survive the freezing process, panel reactive antibody (PRA) and donor-specific HLA I and II antibody testing is positive in 60 to 80% of homograft recipients.[24–26] The potential advantages of viability may be defeated by the detrimental effects of this on immune system reponse.[26] Animal studies have confirmed an immune mechanism by demonstrating that deterioration in homograft valve function is prevented by immunosuppression[27] and does not occur in T-cell–deficient rats.[28] Clinical use of immunosuppression, however, could not be justified for homograft patients.

Tissue engineering concepts led to decellularization, which lyses cells and "rinses" out antigenic proteins, leaving an inert matrix and intact structural framework. Preserved mechanical properties and structural integrity were demonstrated in a sheep model of such a scaffold. In addition, the empty matrix seemed to attract circulating recipient stem cells, which repopulated the framework and differentiated into appropriate cell lines capable of maintaining the matrix.[29] Initial use of the decellularized aortic homograft in humans demonstrated that structural integrity could be maintained with low, stable gradients and minimal regurgitation similar to standard cryopreserved homografts.[30] The same concept has been applied to the pulmonary homograft used in the Ross operation.[31,32] A decellularized xenograft valved conduit has also been used successfully for the right ventricular outflow (RVOT) reconstruction with the Ross.[33] Long-term studies are needed to determine if native cell ingrowth occurs reliably.

In summary, despite intensive investigation over decades, the relative contribution of the immune response, preservation techniques, and warm ischemia time to ultimate valve degeneration is not clear. More importantly, after consideration of the structural benefits and the immune-reaction risks, the net advantage of maintaining cellular (particularly fibroblast) viability in the homograft is not well defined.[34]

Indications for Aortic Homografts

Aortic valve replacement (AVR) with an aortic homograft has a number of advantages, including excellent hemodynamic profile with low transvalvular gradients and possibly enhanced regression of left ventricular mass,[35] low risk of thromboembolism without the need for systemic anticoagulation, and low risk of prosthetic valve infection. However, homografts are subject to structural deterioration which is inversely related to recipient age. Older donor age may also increase rates of degeneration. Furthermore, the availability of homografts is still limited, especially the larger sizes.

The strongest indication for a homograft is for treatment of active aortic valve endocarditis, particularly in patients with root abscess, fistula formation, or prosthetic valve infection.[36] The pliable handling characteristics, ease of coronary reimplantation, the potential for using the attached donor mitral anterior leaflet, and the ability to reconstruct the debrided root with all biological material to minimize risk of persistent infection, all make the homograft exceptionally well suited to this challenging task. The homograft's very low early hazard rate for endocarditis sets it apart from other valve alternatives.[37]

Aortic homograft is also a reasonable option in the older patient (>60) with a small aortic root. The hemodynamic advantages of the homograft translate into better relief of outflow obstruction and improved exercise tolerance. Given its resistance to thromboembolic complications the aortic homograft can also be considered for younger patients requiring composite aortic valve or root replacement who cannot be anticoagulated. However, recent data from a prospective randomized trial would argue that most of the advantages of the homograft can be duplicated by the stentless porcine root replacement which has a significantly lower rate of calcification and valve dysfunction in this study.[38]

Preoperative Evaluation

Preoperative transthoracic echocardiography (TTE) is an invaluable diagnostic tool for evaluation of the AV and associated anatomic structures. Echo measurement of the left ventricular outflow tract (LVOT) can accurately predict aortic annulus diameter and thus the size of the homograft required.[39–41]

Computed tomographic angiography (CTA) or cardiac magnetic resonance (CMR) imaging can also be very useful in the evaluation of potential homograft patients, particularly those with aortic root abscess (Fig. 34-1). Coronary angiography should be employed with the standard indications but may be hazardous in patients with mobile vegetations on the aortic leaflets. Standard chest computed tomography with and without contrast should be considered in any reoperative setting to assess proximity of vital structures to the sternum and extent of ascending aortic or arch calcification or aneurysm. Heavy calcification around the coronary ostia may preclude safe reimplantation of coronary "buttons" or even a distal subcoronary suture line.

Transesophageal echocardiography (TEE) is often necessary to establish the presence of a root abscess, but its major role is for intraoperative confirmation of the anatomy and assessment of both valve and ventricular function.

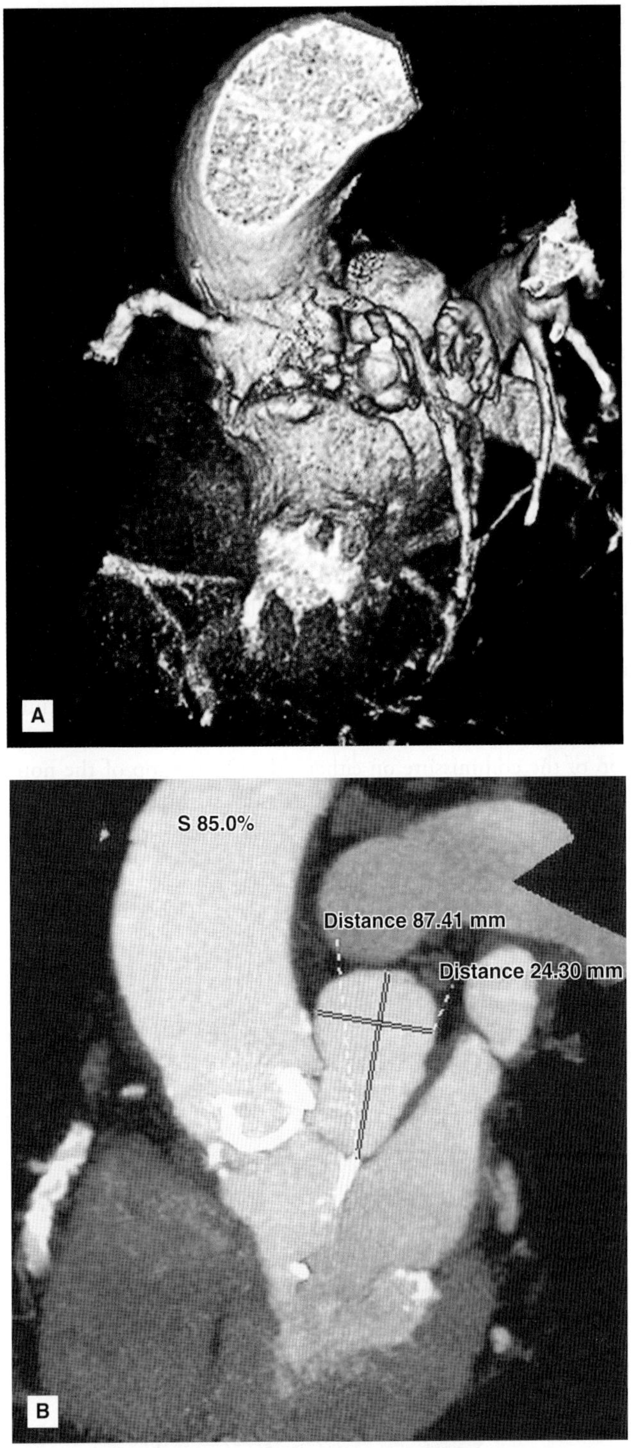

FIGURE 34-1 CTA of root abscess in setting of prosthetic aortic valve endocarditis. The abscess projects from under the valve sewing ring near the left main coronary extending over the left atrial roof under the right pulmonary artery. (A) 3D reconstruction. (B) Standard CT showing prosthetic valve outline.

Operative Technique

General Preparation

Routine cardiac surgical monitoring including TEE is considered the standard of care. An antifibrinolytic agent such as epsilon-aminocaproic acid is helpful. A standard midline sternotomy incision provides full exposure of the heart, ease in cannulation, and access for optimal myocardial protection. Routine distal aortic cannulation and a dual-stage venous cannula usually can be employed.

Unless circulatory arrest is needed, minimal systemic cooling (32°C) is adequate if the heart is maintained at 10 to 15°C using a standard insulating pad and directly monitoring the myocardial septal temperature. A combination of antegrade and retrograde cold blood cardioplegia can be used with the bulk of the protection coming from the retrograde. The open aortic root reveals coronary return from both ostia to confirm effective retrograde.

A transverse aortotomy high above (1.5 to 2 cm) the commissures is usually best. The diseased aortic valve is excised and the annulus is measured with cylindrical sizers. The sinotubular junction should also be evaluated for the subcoronary technique. The homograft is trimmed appropriately. In general, 2 to 3 mm of tissue, proximal to the nadir of each cusp, is advised for security in suture placement, leaving even more for full root replacements.

Techniques of Homograft Placement

Subcoronary Implant Technique

The subcoronary method involves two suture lines within the native root. The homograft is usually oriented anatomically to properly align the commissures and the coronaries. The proximal end of the homograft is sewn to the native annulus in a circular plane at the level of the nadir of each sinus curving upward slightly in the membranous septum to avoid injury to the conduction system. This anastomosis can be done with either interrupted or continuous sutures (Fig. 34-2).

The top of each commissure is tacked to the aortic wall. The right and left sinus walls are then scalloped out to a point 3 to 5 mm from the leaflets. The noncoronary sinus can also be removed but is usually left intact. A 4-0 or 5-0 polypropylene suture is started at the lowest point under each coronary ostium and a continuous suture line constructed from there up to the top of the commissure on either side. On the top of the noncoronary sinus, excess homograft tissue is trimmed down and tacked to the top of the aortotomy. The aortotomy is then closed with continuous 4-0 polypropylene suture incorporating the top of the homograft noncoronary sinus with the native aortic wall (Fig. 34-3). The ascending aorta is vented as the aortic clamp is removed. TEE can quickly assess any regurgitation at this point. Distention of the ventricle should be avoided by prompt defibrillation (if necessary) and pacing if required.

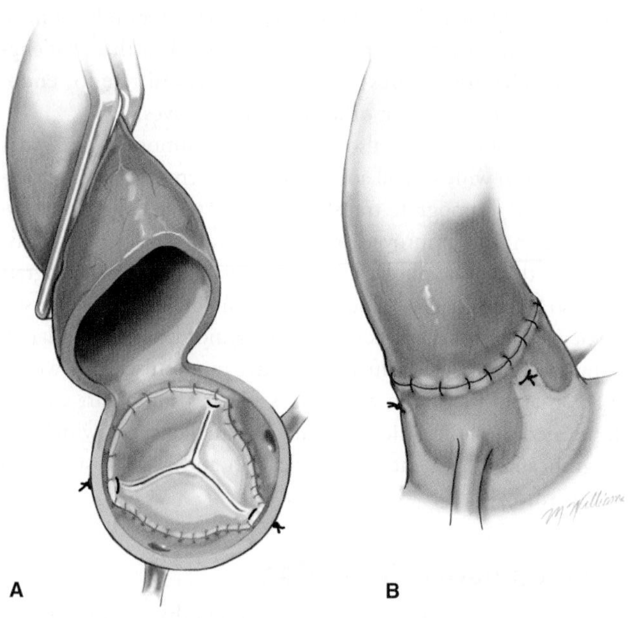

FIGURE 34-3 Distal homograft suture line. (A) The subcoronary implant is completed by tacking the aortic wall of the homograft to the recipient aortic wall with continuous fine polypropylene suture after trimming out the tissue in the coronary sinuses to allow blood flow to the native coronaries. The noncoronary sinus is usually left intact. (B) The aortotomy is closed in standard fashion incorporating the top of the homograft in the process.

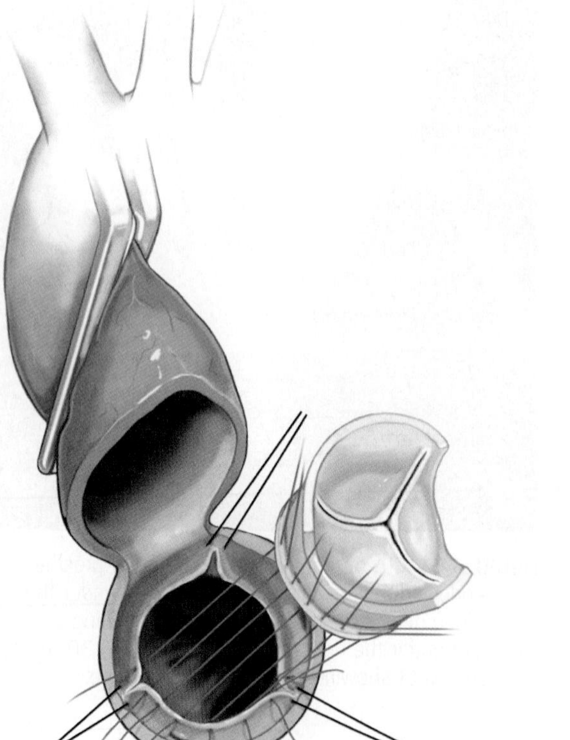

FIGURE 34-2 Subcoronary homograft implantation. The homograft is oriented anatomically and the proximal end attached in a circular plane at the level of the nadir of the recipient sinuses using either interrupted or continuous sutures.

Because even slight malalignment of the commissures can result in regurgitation, the subcoronary implant technique is considered more demanding than the other homograft techniques and may have poorer long-term results than the other methods.[42–46] It is a good technique for patients with small, symmetric aortic roots and sinotubular junctions, whereas it is a poor choice for those with dilated, asymmetric, or severely diseased roots.

Homograft Cylinder–Inclusion Root Technique

The cylinder modification of the subcoronary technique was developed in an attempt to preserve the native geometry of the homograft inside the recipient aortic root. The proximal suture line is identical to the subcoronary method but the sinuses are not scalloped out. Instead, a buttonhole is made in the right and left sinuses in such a way as to allow the homograft wall to be sewn to the native sinus wall around the coronary ostia. After the coronaries are secure, the distal end of the homograft is attached at the commissures and then incorporated circumferentially into the aortotomy closure. This method is the most difficult technically and is seldom used.

Homograft Root Replacement

The root replacement technique can be used in any root and is particularly useful in small roots or those destroyed by endocarditis. The root replacement allows size flexibility, which allows thawing an appropriate homograft without wasting clamp time. Very large roots may require commissural plication as described by Northrup.[47]

The aorta is opened transversely well above the commissures of the valve. The diseased valve is excised and annulus debrided. The aorta is transected and the coronary ostial buttons are mobilized in standard fashion. Antegrade cardioplegia should be avoided after this point to avoid injury to the mobilized ostia.

The homograft root is usually oriented anatomically, which makes matching the two roots easiest. The proximal suture line can be constructed with either continuous or interrupted technique. Interrupted is best in difficult reoperations, especially for prosthetic valve endocarditis because it allows for very accurate, deep placement of individual stitches. A strip of autologous (or bovine) pericardium is used to reinforce this crucial anastomosis. Polypropylene sutures of 3-0 or 4-0 are used and organization scrupulously maintained on suture guides. The homograft parachutes down as the sutures are carefully tightened (Fig. 34-4).

Routine cases can be expedited with a continuous suture technique with 4-0 polypropylene begun at the right-left commissure. The fibrous trigones and commissures of the native and homograft roots serve as anatomical landmarks and should match up as one proceeds around. The initially loose suture line is tightened carefully with nerve hooks and tied securely.

The coronary buttons are attached with continuous 5-0 or 6-0 polypropylene after excising the homograft coronary stumps. The distal end of the homograft and the native aorta are trimmed and sewn together with continuous 4-0 polypropylene incorporating another strip of pericardium for support. The native aorta is vented anteriorly and systemic flow rate lowered as the cross-clamp is removed.

Care is taken to avoid systemic hypertension or vigorous traction on the reconstructed root to avoid bleeding. Topical hemostatic agents and biological glues can be used, but they should not be routinely necessary. Blood and blood products are not routinely required unless the patient is coagulopathic.

Postreplacement Assessment

Ventricular function, regional wall motion abnormalities, and valve function may all be accurately determined with TEE. With appropriate loading conditions, moderate to severe AR warrants inspection and revision of the homograft. Mild AR is usually tolerated well and does not warrant reexploration.

Postoperative Management

Even mild hypertension should be avoided to prevent disruption of crucial aortic suture lines. Coagulopathic bleeding is best addressed with products targeted to specific abnormalities defined by laboratory studies.

Adequate volume replacement is required to keep the stiff ventricle of aortic stenosis filled and alpha adrenergic support is often required for the patient who is vasodilated. Atrial rhythm

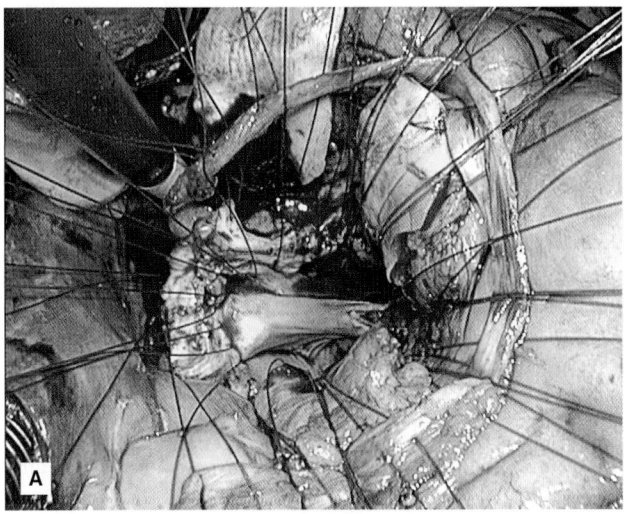

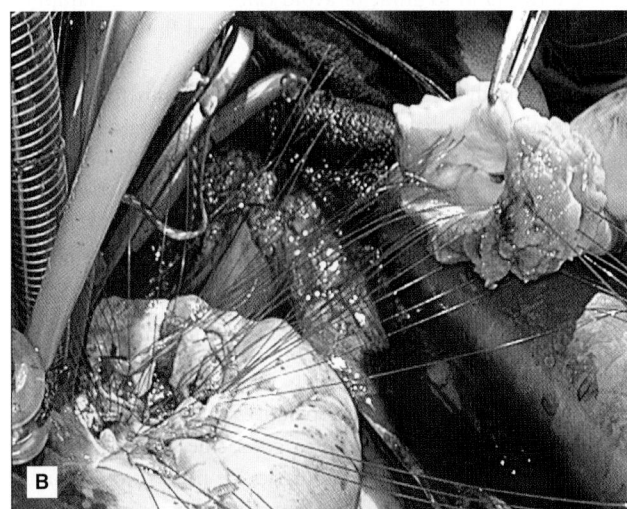

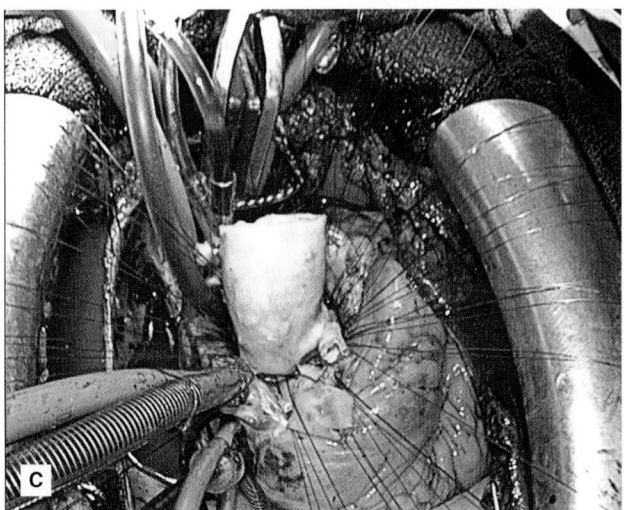

FIGURE 34-4 Homograft root replacement. (A) Interrupted 3-0 or 4-0 polypropylene sutures are placed deep in solid tissue, then passed through a pericardial strip and organization is scrupulously maintained on suture guides. (B) Sutures are then passed through the homograft from inside out. (C) The homograft parachutes down as the sutures are carefully tightened maintaining organization until each suture is tied precisely.

disturbances should be treated aggressively. Elderly patients, particularly females, with aortic stenosis and diastolic dysfunction are at increased risk of morbidity and even mortality from postoperative atrial fibrillation. The increased volume loading needed to overcome the loss of atrial transport often leads to pulmonary congestion requiring reintubation and prolonged support. Forward cardiac output is impaired and renal function deteriorates. Cardioversion should be considered early in these patients and loading with intravenous amiodarone is usually indicated. Preoperatively loading with amiodarone may minimize the incidence and consequences of this arrhythmia.[48]

Temporary pacing, preferably atrial as well as ventricular, should be enabled. Permanent pacing is indicated if epicardial wires become unreliable, heart block was present preoperatively, or the underlying rhythm fails to return within a week after surgery.

Stroke risk can be minimized by careful intraoperative epiaortic ultrasound to guide or avoid cannulation and clamping. TEE-guided evacuation of air is essential and flooding the field with carbon dioxide may be helpful.

Myocardial dysfunction is best prevented by careful temperature-monitored myocardial protection but long operations may still require temporary inotropic support. Caution must be used in the hyperdynamic ventricle with diastolic dysfunction. The combination of a hyperdynamic left ventricle and a dysfunctional right heart is very challenging. These patients may benefit from atrial pacing (if pacing is required), phosphodiesterase inhibitors, adequate volume replacement, and alpha agonists.

Renal insufficiency is a risk minimized by maintenance of adequate flows and pressure during bypass and generous volume administration in the early postoperative period. A thirsty patient with dry mucous membranes is a good clue that intravascular volume is still depleted. Later, diuretics are needed to encourage mobilization and excretion of this extra fluid. Hypotension should be avoided but vasopressors can have direct negative effects on renal blood flow.

Low-dose aspirin is often recommended for homograft patients, but is not necessary and formal anticoagulation with warfarin is not required at all unless dictated by other conditions. A routine predischarge echo should be done to confirm valve function, ventricular function, and freedom from pericardial effusion.

Results

Perioperative Complications

In patients without active endocarditis at the time of surgery, operative mortality in the current era is 1 to 5%.[44,49,50] The risk in experienced hands is comparable to using a stented bioprosthetic or mechanical valve. Ischemic time for a root replacement with either stentless porcine or aortic homograft is approximately 90 minutes.[51] A contemporary series of 100 consecutive aortic homografts (virtually all root replacements including 13 reoperations) demonstrated no hospital mortality with 100% survival at 1 year and 98% at 5 years.[52]

In contrast, patients with active endocarditis have a higher early mortality ranging from 8 to 16%.[44,53–56] Prosthetic valve endocarditis (17.9 to 18.8%) is worse than native (2.6 to 10%).[53,57]

Hemorrhage, heart block, stroke, myocardial infarction, and wound complications occur with similar frequency to those of other AVRs, but early risk of endocarditis is lower with homografts than any other replacement valve.[37]

Hemodynamics and Exercise Capacity

Hemodynamic characteristics of homografts are excellent at short- and medium-term follow-up, both at rest and during exercise.[58,59] A study of 31 patients demonstrated increases in peak and mean gradients of 6.6 and 3.0 mm Hg, respectively, without a significant change in effective orifice area (EOA).[58] Importantly, the EOA of even the 17- to 19-mm homografts was 1.7 cm^2 and larger valves approximated the normal aortic valve areas as high as 2.7 cm^2 for 24- to 27-mm homografts.

The typical subcoronary homograft implant demonstrates a 1- to 2-mm Hg drop in mean transvalvular gradient over the first 6 months but with full root replacement, the hemodynamic benefit is fully realized immediately. In the randomized trial of homograft versus stentless porcine root replacement the mean gradients were only 6 ± 1 mm Hg in the stentless and 5 ± 2 mm Hg in the homografts. Only one patient in each group had mild regurgitation after 5 years.[51] These authors concluded that stentless and homograft root replacements are hemodynamically equivalent in the mid-term.

Long-Term Outcomes

Long-term outcome has been shown to be technique dependent in a meta-analysis of more than 3000 patients (37% full root, 63% subcoronary) from 18 studies with a mean follow-up of 12.5 years. Reoperation was significantly lower in the root replacement group.[60] There may have been some bias against reoperation in failing roots, in which failing subcoronary implants were more readily subjected to reoperation.

The pioneering work of Mark O'Brien in Brisbane, Australia, produced a huge series of homograft patients over nearly three decades with 99.3% follow-up.[50] This series demonstrated that rates of reoperation were lower in the full root patients ($n = 3$, 0.85%) than the subcoronary ($n = 18$, 3.3%). Of note, operative mortality was only 1.13% in 352 root patients.

Long-term durability was compromised by young age of recipient to the point that those less than 20 years of age had a 47% rate of reoperation for structural valve degeneration at 10 years. Conversely, those more than 60 had a 94% freedom from reoperation at 15 years, and those between 21 and 60 had 81 to 85% freedom at 15 years. This series confirmed the very low incidence of thromboembolic phenomena (without anticoagulation) and a low but not insignificant rate of endocarditis.

Lund reported crude survival at 10 and 20 years to be 67 and 35%, respectively,[44] whereas Langley and O'Brien reported actuarial survival at 10, 20, and 25 years to be 81,[49] 58,[49] and 19%, respectively.[50]

Structural valve failure of homografts increases with time, and approximates 19 to 38% at 10 years and 69 to 82% at 20 years.[44,49] Freedom from repeat AVR, for any reason, parallels structural valve failure and is 86.5 and 38.8% at 10 and 20 years, respectively.[49] As heterograft tissue technology has progressed, the difference between homograft and heterograft durability has narrowed to the point of near equivalency, with both showing a dramatic age-dependent relationship with youngest patients failing most rapidly.[61]

Freedom from endocarditis at 10 years is 93 to 98%,[49,50] and at 20 years 89 to 95%.[44,49,50] Freedom from thromboembolism at 15 and 20 years is 92 and 83%, respectively.[50] Thrombosis of a homograft has been reported, but in the setting of lupus anticardiolipin antibody syndrome.[62]

In patients with active endocarditis requiring AVR, results may be poorer, with survival ranging from 58% at 5 years[53] to 91% at 10 years,[56] and is significantly lower in patients with prosthetic valve endocarditis (PVE).[54] Of note, however, the risk of recurrent endocarditis is less than 4% up to 4 years postoperatively.[43,53,54,56] These results still compare favorably with alternatives; therefore, aortic homograft is considered by many to be the valve of choice for aortic valve or root replacement in patients with active endocarditis.

Homograft Reoperation

Because of extensive calcification after many years the risk at reoperation after homograft replacement can be as high as 20%.[63] The subcoronary implants may be easier in this regard because the native aortic root is preserved. The full root replacement is more of a problem. Up to about 10 years, calcification is limited and it is theoretically possible to place a new valve inside the homograft annulus after removing the leaflets.[64] Ultimately, however, the conduit becomes so rigid as to preclude such an alternative and complete re-replacement of the root is required (Fig. 34-5). The most hazardous part of this operation is related to the coronary ostial buttons, which must be protected and available for use again.

Reoperation can be made easier by anticipating the need for this at the original operation. Keeping the coronary buttons large at the initial operation is one way to avoid problems with dissecting them again. The homograft root should be kept as short as possible to minimize the extent of ultimately calcified wall and maximize the amount of normal aorta available for subsequent cannulation and clamping. Closing the pericardium or using a pericardial substitute can make sternal re-entry safer. Careful assessment of the aorta and mediastinum on CT preoperatively can alert one to the need for early peripheral cannulation and even sternotomy under circulatory arrest.

Clamping the aorta distal to the main pulmonary artery is very useful in these cases and avoids the hazards of entering a great vessel while dissecting between them before the clamp is on. Complete excision of the calcified wall is often the best policy, but leaving a little margin around each coronary ostium may make reconstruction easier. Another homograft is often an excellent solution because it is easier to reimplant the coronary ostia, but even a Ross operation can be done in this setting, as was done for the 40-year-old man shown in Fig. 34-5.

An increasingly attractive option in the future for older patients is transcatheter valve replacement, which should be well-suited to the calcified homograft root as reported from Milan[65] (Fig. 34-6).

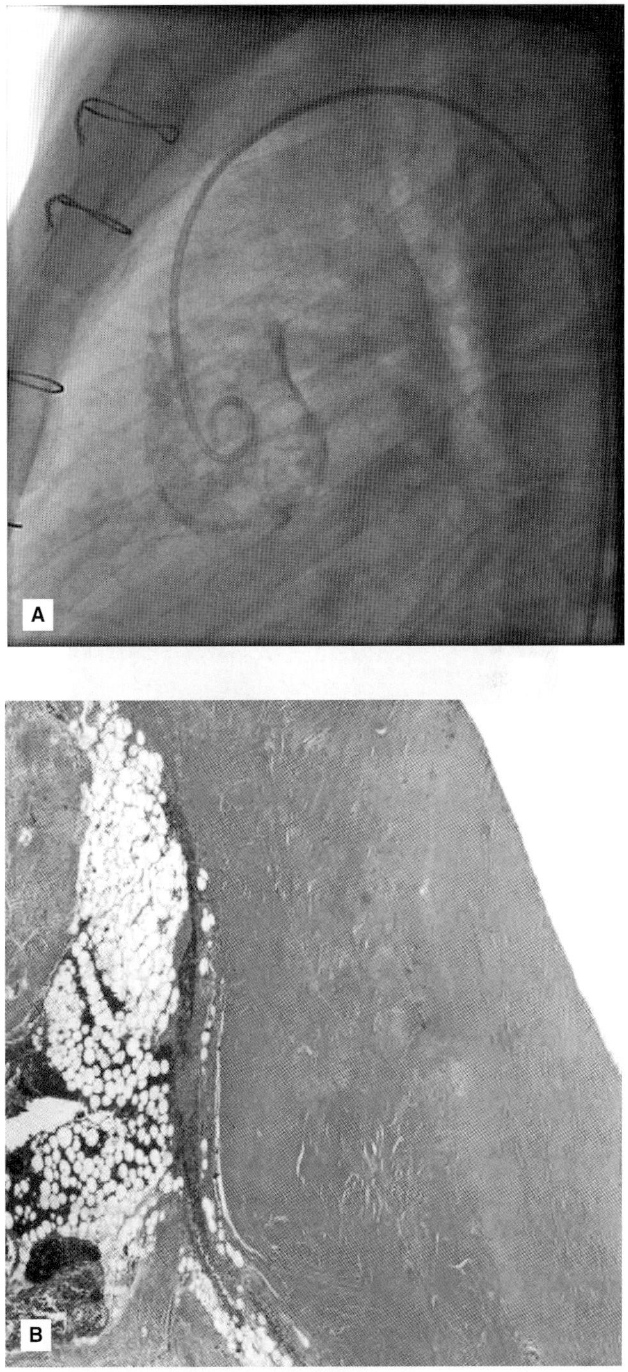

FIGURE 34-5 Calcified aortic homograft. (A) Lateral view of calcified homograft at catheterization 23 years after implantation. (B) Microscopic appearance of this homograft showing fibrosis with essentially acellular mass of collagen fibers.

Conclusions

Between the lack of availability of homografts and the improvements in readily available alternatives such as stentless porcine devices, homograft replacement of the aortic valve is less common than it was 20 years ago. However, it remains a versatile, highly effective tool with potential advantages in small aortic roots greater than age 60 and in settings of severe aortic root endocarditis. The homograft can be placed with a low operative

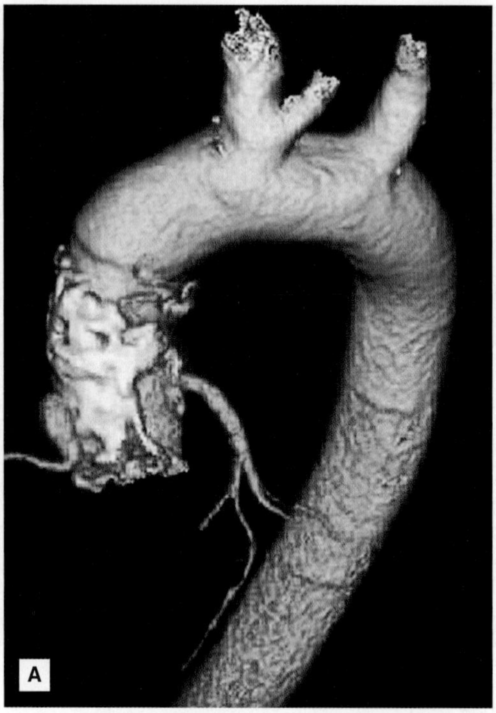

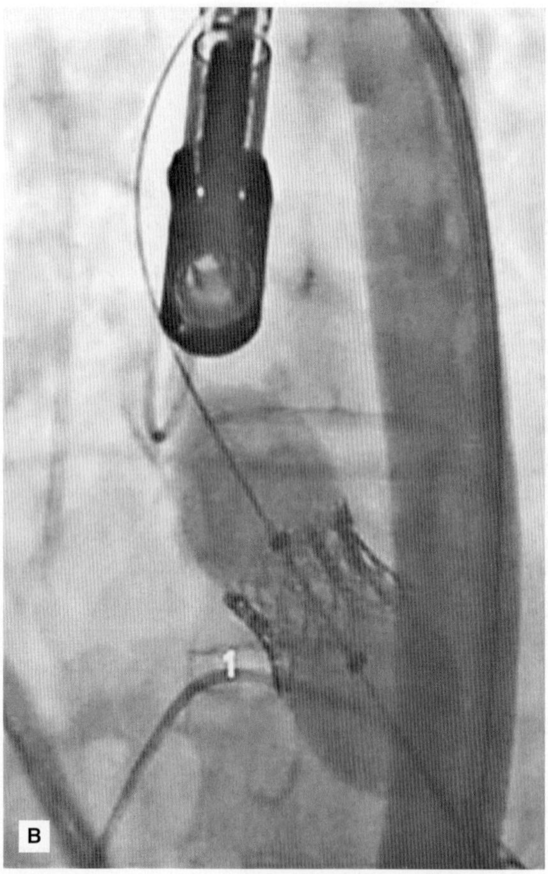

FIGURE 34-6 Percutaneous valve placement in calcified homograft root. (A) CTA appearance of heavily calcified homograft root. (B) Percutaneous valve being deployed in this root. (*Adapted from Dainese L, Fusari M, Trabattoni P, Biglioli P: Redo in aortic homograft replacement: Transcatheter aortic valve as a valid alternative to surgical replacement. J Thorac Cardiovasc Surg 2009; 2[2]:e6-7.*)

mortality risk and provide excellent hemodynamic function immediately without the need for any anticoagulation. Its major downside is the inexorable deterioration of its structure over time, which makes it a poor choice in very young patients. Those patients may well be best served by the autograft operation.

PULMONARY AUTOGRAFT: ROSS PROCEDURE

Theoretical Considerations

The pulmonary autograft shares the hemodynamic advantages and anti-thrombotic features of the homograft but is the only valve which has the benefit of being a fully viable autologous tissue. Pulmonary leaflets have been found to have equivalent breaking strain compared to aortic leaflets and even higher tensile strength.[66] The living pulmonary valve demonstrates the adaptability of human biology to change in response to changing physiologic conditions. The histologic features of this adaptation have been elegantly described and illustrated.[67] The initial response is to lay down a collagen-rich support on the ventricular aspect of the leaflets. This thins out later but remains slightly thicker than normal aortic leaflets. All three layers of the leaflets, fibrosa, spongiosa, and ventricularis contain viable cells which maintain a rich extracellular matrix to support the leaflet function. Endothelial cells are transformed to become capable of smooth muscle actin production becoming more like the aortic than the pulmonary phenotype. The autograft (pulmonary artery) walls are a different story. There is rapid loss of elastin with fragmentation and loss of cellularity and increasing collagen deposition. This may reflect the need to sacrifice elasticity for strength to withstand systemic pressure.

Patient Selection

The cardinal principle in selecting patients for the Ross procedure is that they must have a life expectancy of at least 20 to 25 years. Other simpler alternatives can be expected to give 10 to 15 years, even in young patients, although durability of tissue valves in patients less than 35 years of age can be very limited. Active lifestyle, potential for childbearing, and contraindications to anticoagulation favor the Ross procedure. Many young people seek out this option specifically to avoid the issues of anticoagulation and even to allow extreme athletic activity, such as mountain biking and triathlons. Practically speaking, the ideal patient is under 50 years of age but special circumstances can extend this to 65 or even slightly higher.

The generally accepted contraindications are significant pulmonary valve disease, congenitally abnormal pulmonary valves (eg, bicuspid or quadricuspid), Marfan's syndrome, other connective tissue disorders, complex coronary anomalies, and probably severe coexisting autoimmune disease, particularly if it is the cause of the aortic valve disease. Active rheumatic disease is a relative contraindication because the autograft can be attacked early by the acute rheumatic process and lead to early failure.[68] Bacterial endocarditis is not a contraindication for the Ross procedure, although it is best used when only leaflet destruction is present or root involvement can be reconstructed without distortion.[69]

Comorbid conditions should also be considered before offering this operation to any given patient. These conditions often limit life expectancy and also influence the ability of the patient to withstand this longer procedure. Poor left ventricular function, multivessel coronary disease, and need for complex mitral repair are examples. Ascending aortic dilatation or aneurysm have been considered contraindications by some, but these can be and should be easily addressed. Previous AVR or other open cardiac operations are not a contraindication to the Ross procedure, but all the standard considerations of reoperative surgery apply including appropriate imaging to allow safe sternal re-entry.

Bicuspid aortic valves (BAV) are the most common etiology of severe aortic stenosis or regurgitation in patients less than 65 years of age. Some have felt this group should not undergo the Ross procedure because of potential complications of intrinsic aortopathy, which is common in BAV patients.[70] Because this is the largest group of patients potentially to benefit from the operation, it has been the quest of Ross surgeons to find ways to make the operation safe and durable in this situation. Controversy still exists as to whether primary aortic regurgitation (AR) is less favorable than primary aortic stenosis.[71,72] The patient with aortic stenosis (AS) is more likely to have a smaller annulus, which is resistant to dilatation, as opposed to the AR patient, whose annulus is often dilated and continues to dilate if not supported. There is also more of a tendency to distal aortic dilatation in the setting of AR as opposed to AS. These issues are addressable by technical modifications, which is discussed later in detail.

Preoperative Evaluation

Because most candidates for the Ross procedure are less than 50 years of age, it is not usually necessary to subject them to cardiac catheterization. CTA is an excellent tool to evaluate the entire ascending aorta and arch as well as the proximal coronary arteries. Cardiac magnetic resonance (CMR) can be used as well but does not give as much resolution as CTA for the coronaries. Both give excellent imaging of the entire aorta (Fig. 34-7). Transthoracic echocardiography gives excellent assessment of the aortic valve, ventricular function, and aortic root. Approximately 1% of patients are found to have a bicuspid pulmonary valve at surgery. Unfortunately, echo, CTA, and CMR have all been limited in their ability to define the morphology of the pulmonary valve. With proper gating, timing of contrast, and attention to the pulmonary trunk, however, this can be determined fairly reliably (Fig. 34-8).

Technique

The original description by Donald Ross involved a fully scalloped subcoronary implant of the pulmonary autograft using essentially the same technique he had used for a subcoronary homograft implant. Modifications were adopted to decrease the immediate incidence of regurgitation by maintaining the cylindrical geometry of the autograft either within the aortic root or as a complete replacement thereof. The root replacement has become the most commonly employed technique.

Full median sternotomy is usually the best incision. Aortic cannulation should be kept high and bicaval cannulation is preferable because the open RVOT is a constant source of air. Initial antegrade and then generous retrograde cold blood cardioplegia is employed insulating the heart from surrounding structures and monitoring the effectiveness of myocardial

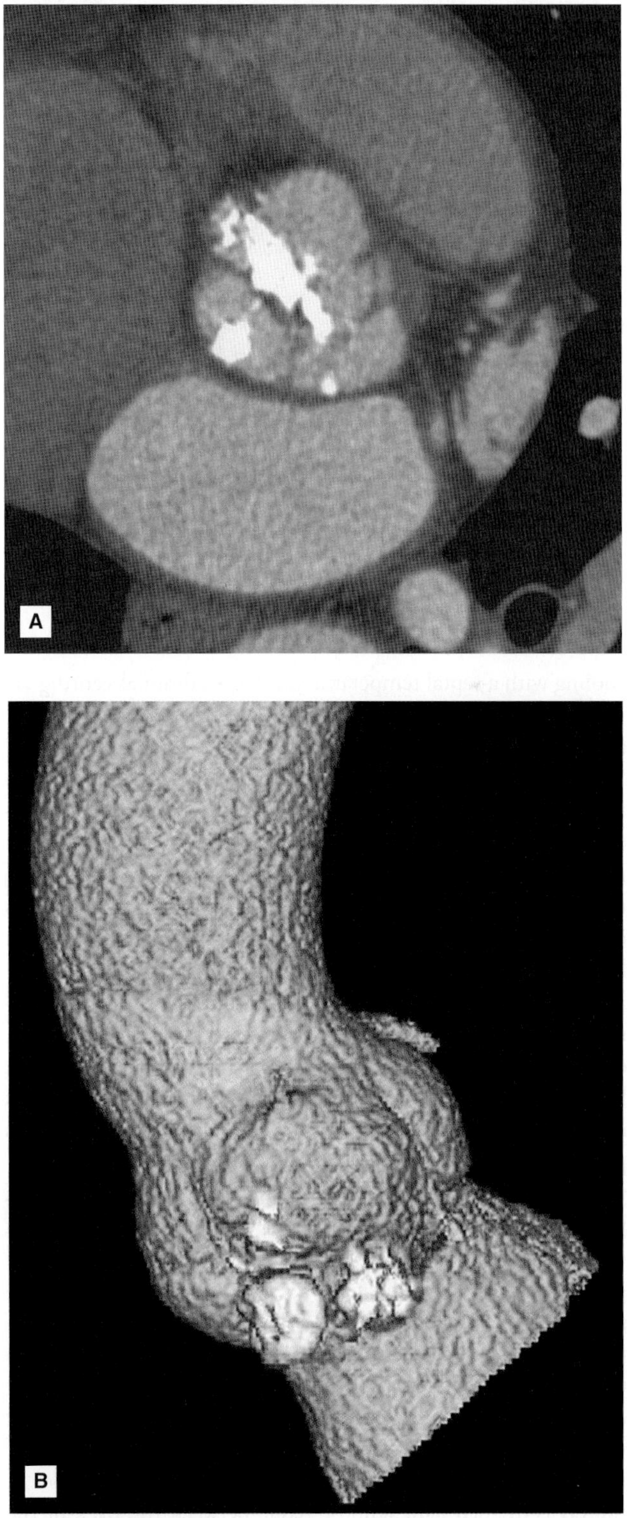

FIGURE 34-7 Preoperative imaging of the aorta. (A, B) Computed tomographic angiography. (C) Cardiac magnetic resonance.

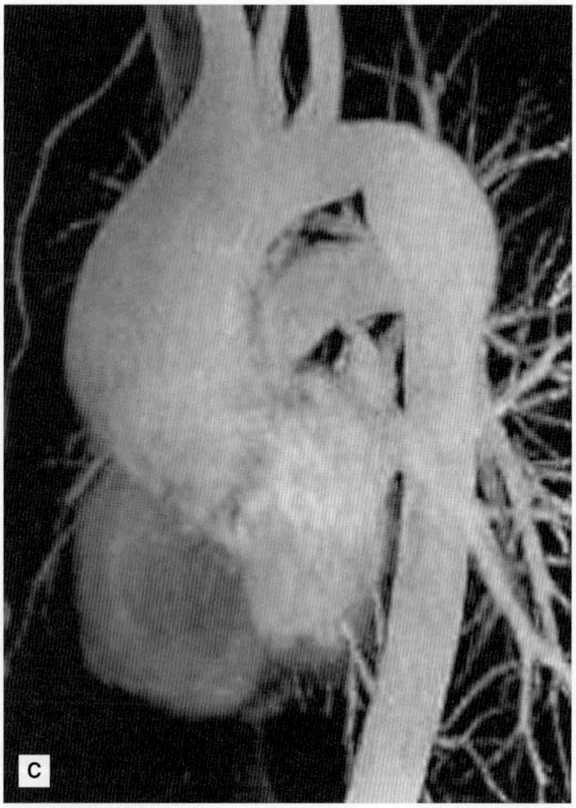

FIGURE 34-7 *(Continued)*

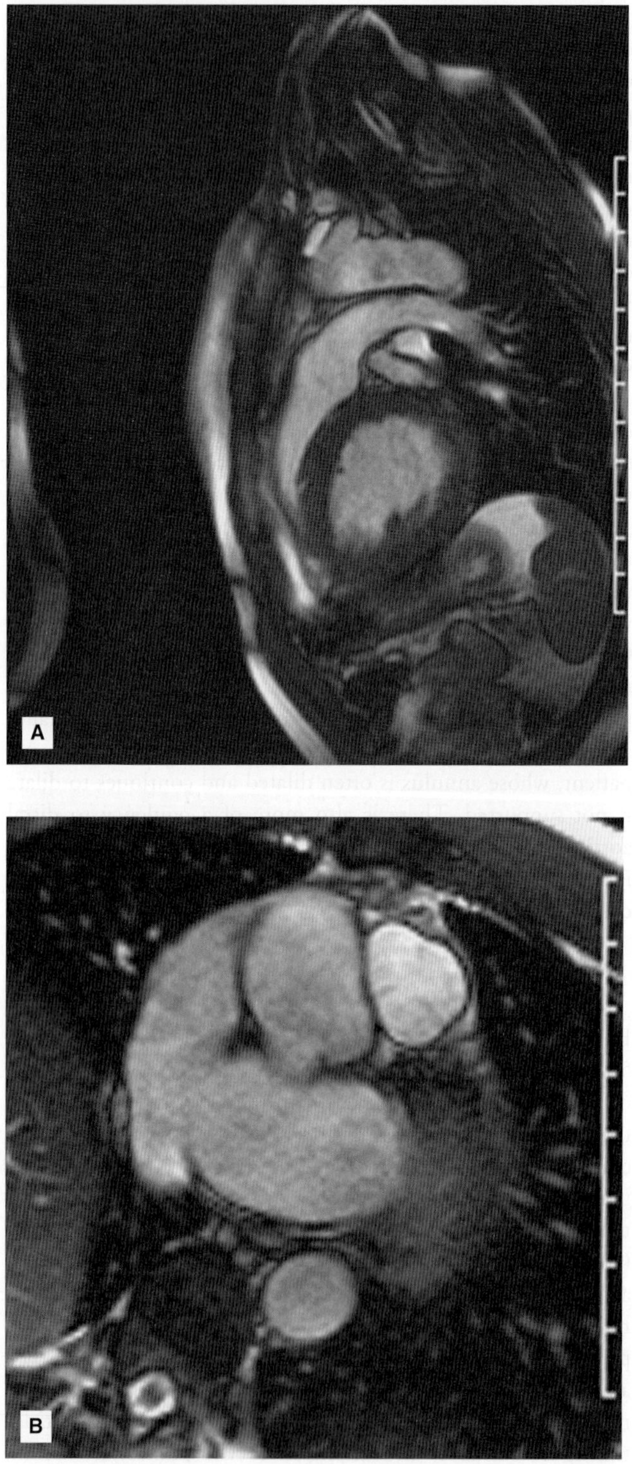

FIGURE 34-8 Evaluation of pulmonic valve by CMR. (A) Longitudinal view. (B) Cross-sectional view showing three distinct leaflets and sinuses.

cooling with a septal temperature probe. Traditional venting via the right superior pulmonary vein is not necessary because the open pulmonary artery serves that purpose.

Extensive dissection between the great vessels allows retraction of the aorta with an umbilical tape and keeps the cross-clamp off the right pulmonary artery. After clamping the aorta, the space between the aortic and pulmonary roots is dissected until the roots are completely separated. Final separation is often safest after the aorta is opened and coronary locations can be readily identified.

A rather high transverse aortotomy incision keeps all technique options open, but if a subcoronary implant is planned, extending an oblique incision into the noncoronary sinus can be employed. The aortic valve pathology is inspected as well as coronary ostial positions. A stenotic valve can be excised at this point and the annulus debrided and measured.

Common to any of the techniques is the need to harvest the pulmonary autograft from the right ventricular outflow tract (RVOT). The close proximity of the left coronary system and general constraints of this maneuver are obvious from the elegant anatomical casts published by Muresian.[73] The main pulmonary artery is incised transversely just distal to the valve and the opening extended to either side taking care to avoid the left coronary. A flexible sucker can be placed in the distal PA as a vent. The pulmonic valve is inspected to make sure it is a healthy, three-leaflet valve with minimal fenestrations. The remainder of the PA is divided. The adipose tissue between the back of the PA and the left main is gently dissected down to the muscle in the back of the RVOT with the cautery.

The RVOT is opened with a no. 15 blade well below the anterior commissure as determined by palpation or by passing a suture or clamp through the muscle about 5- to 6-mm below the valve from inside out (Fig. 34-9). The initial incision is cautiously extended until the leaflet can be clearly seen. The dissection then continues around each side leaving 3 to 4 mm of

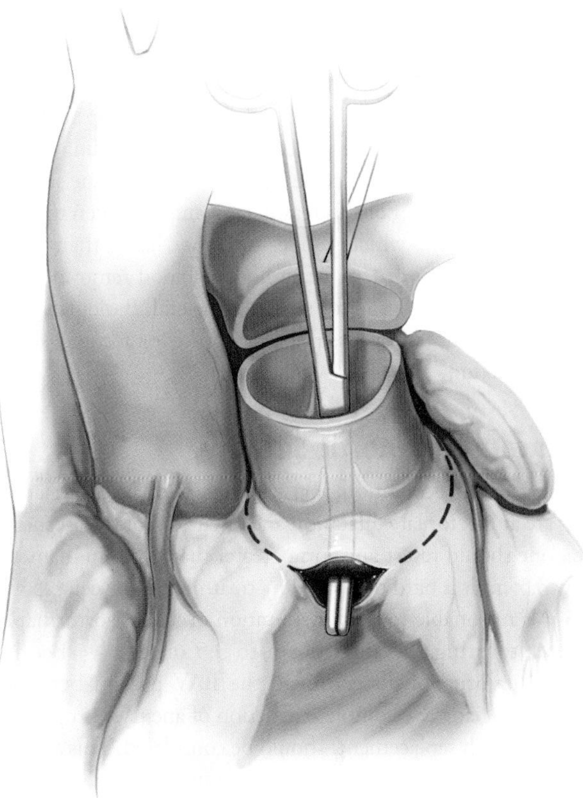

FIGURE 34-9 Pulmonary autograft harvest. A right-angle clamp can be passed through the right ventricular outflow tract muscle below the anterior commissure to assure safe beginning of the harvest incision.

muscle cuff. Posteriorly, a natural plane can be appreciated between the right and left ventricular septal components. The septal perforators are always in the left side and can be avoided by taking only the right ventricular part of the septum. Most often they are not seen. Small branches of the coronary sinus posteriorly can be the source of annoying venous bleeding at the end, so gentle administration of retrograde can identify these and allow control at this point.

The autograft is trimmed by following the curvilinear course of the leaflets on the inflow end leaving a smooth 3- to 4-mm cuff of muscle. The inflow end is measured by gently inserting cylindrical sizers. The RVOT opening can also be measured at this time. An appropriate pulmonary homograft can then be thawed.

Subcoronary Technique

If the subcoronary or inclusion cylinder technique is chosen, the operation proceeds similarly to subcoronary homograft replacement. Proximal and distal suture lines are constructed as described. Of note, the aortic root must match the autograft at both the annulus and the sinotubular junction. Accordingly, tailoring of the root with annuloplasty and/or downsizing the sinotubular junction may be required.[74] The potential advantage of this technique is to preserve the native root support around the autograft, which may prevent autograft dilatation and insufficiency. However, if the native aorta dilates, the autograft will do so as well.

Root Replacement Technique

In preparation for full root replacement the aortic transection is completed and the coronary ostial buttons are dissected out and mobilized appropriately. The native noncoronary sinus and the "pillar" of tissue between the right and the left buttons are preserved for later "re-inclusion" around the autograft root. The best orientation for the autograft is determined by placing it in the aortic root. Usually the bare area from the back of the PA is positioned in the left coronary sinus.

A strip of Teflon felt about 5- to 7-mm wide is cut to length around a size 2 mm larger than the inflow size of the autograft. The proximal autograft suture line is constructed incorporating the felt strip. This can be done with interrupted 3-0 or 4-0 simple sutures best organized on suture guides. Continuous 4-0 polypropylene can also be used beginning under the right-left commissure and working down the left sinus. The noncoronary and right sinuses follow. The sutures are left loose and slightly remote to facilitate visibility (Fig. 34-10). When completed, the suture line is carefully tightened with nerve hooks and tied securely.

The coronary buttons are then reimplanted with continuous 6-0 Prolene. The position of the right coronary is always higher than anticipated, usually just at the sinotubular junction of the autograft.

Excess pulmonary artery wall is trimmed from the autograft down to just above the commissures and very close to the tops

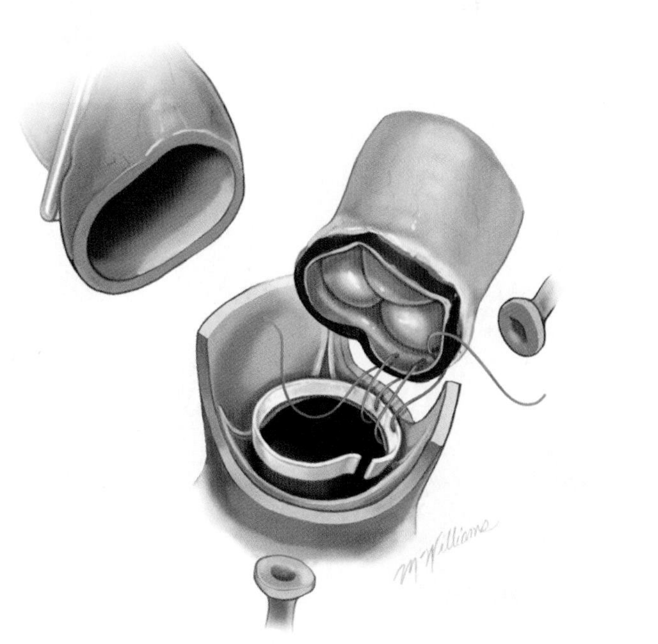

FIGURE 34-10 Proximal autograft suture line. The continuous suture technique is facilitated by leaving the sutures loose enough to easily see the leaflets to optimize depth and spacing and minimize tearing of this delicate muscle cuff. A measured strip of felt is incorporated in this suture line. Note that the noncoronary sinus tissue and the "pillar" of tissue between the coronary buttons has been preserved for later inclusion around the autograft root.

of the coronary buttons. The native aortic wall elements that were preserved earlier are now brought up beside the autograft and shortened if necessary. If the native root was dilated or frankly aneurismal, artificial support can be employed using felt patches or vascular graft material.

The distal autograft is attached to the ascending aorta with continuous 4-0 polypropylene incorporating the natural and/or fabric support elements along with another strip of felt placing the sutures right at the tops of the commissures to establish a new sinotubular junction (Fig. 34-11). With the aorta closed, antegrade cardioplegia can be administered to give a test of valve competence and integrity of the coronary and distal suture lines.

The pulmonary homograft is now attached to the RVOT with continuous 4-0 polypropylene. Care is taken to take long and superficial bites posteriorly over the area of the septal perforator. The distal suture line is completed with continuous 4-0 or 5-0 polypropylene.

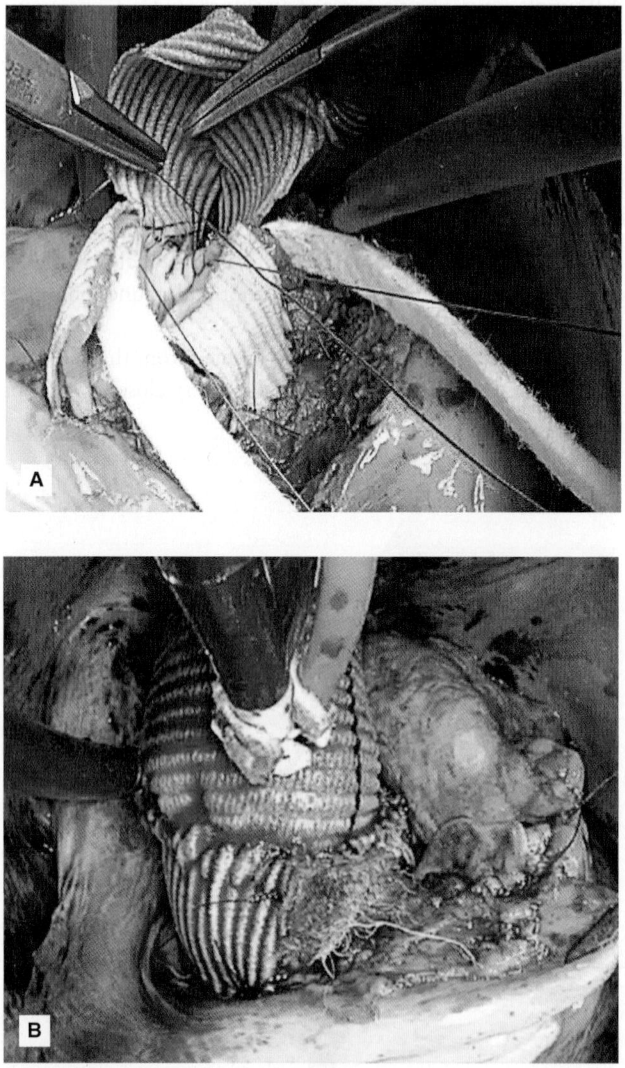

FIGURE 34-11 Fabric support of autograft wall. (A) The arterial wall of the autograft is supported by segments of vascular graft material especially when native aortic wall is intrinsically poor. The entire autograft is enclosed with a combination of native aortic wall and vascular graft material and attached to the ascending aortic graft incorporating another strip of felt. (B) Completed Ross with external fabric support and ascending aortic replacement as well.

The ascending aorta is vented and the cross-clamp removed. Generous reperfusion time is recommended. Bleeding is certainly a risk with so many needle holes in delicate tissue submitted to aortic pressure. For this reason care must be taken to avoid vigorous retraction, which can cause more harm than good. Amicar is recommended, as is autologous blood removal at the beginning of the operation for return at the end. Biological glues can be helpful but their use is not a substitute for accurate suture line construction.

Concomitant Aortic Surgery

Because of the recognition that patients with bicuspid aortic valves are at risk for late dilatation and aneurysm of the ascending aorta, one should resect any aorta greater than 5 cm in diameter. Below 3.5 cm it is hard to justify any treatment. Between 3.5 and 5 cm it is reasonable to employ plication or lateral aortorrhaphy concepts to bring the aorta down to 3.5 or less.[75,76] Because the vast majority of dissection in the BAV patient begins in the ascending aorta,[77] complete resection of aneurysms up to the arch (hemi-arch replacement) should be considered. This actually adds very little time to the operation if planned appropriately. The proximal end of the aortic graft is attached to the (usually reinforced) autograft root to restore aortic continuity.

Operative Risk

According to the International Ross Registry, overall perioperative mortality (i.e., <30 days) was 4.1% (129 deaths in 3922 patients).[18] Given the 1% risk of alternative operations, this may be unacceptably high. Like so many highly technical procedures, experience makes a big difference. The author's own experience demonstrated a "learning curve" with three deaths in the first 30, three more in the next 178 and no deaths in the next 260. Clearly the complexities of reoperative status, need for circulatory arrest, replacement of ascending aneurysm, and concomitant mitral repair should encourage referral to an experienced surgeon if a Ross procedure is to be considered. Individualized discussion with each patient should examine the options and consider the potential risks and benefits of each. Because a volume–outcome relationship may be apparent, the option of referral to regional "centers of excellence" should be included in this discussion.

Results

Pioneer Series Results

No discussion of the Ross operation could be complete without a careful look back at the pioneer series of patients treated by Donald Ross.[78] The 1997 paper from this seminal source analyzed 131 hospital survivors followed for 9 to 26 years with a mean of 20 years. The technical problems that led to early reoperation with the subcoronary technique were recognized in that series and the cylinder modification adopted. Even the full root replacement method was employed as an alternative by

Ross in 20 patients beginning as early as 1974.[79] Survival at 10 and 20 years was a remarkable 85 and 61%, respectively. Freedom from autograft replacement was 88 and 75%, where freedom from homograft replacement was 89 and 80% each at 10 and 20 years. Of 53 late deaths, 46 were cardiac. Importantly, of the 30 autografts that were explanted, only three had evidence of degenerative change, which was patchy and did not involve all leaflets. The remainder had completely viable structure as long as 24 years after implantation. Clearly, the transplanted pulmonary autograft is and remains a fully living valve. Homograft stenosis accounted for all but 1 of 20 late reoperations on the right side. Thromboembolic phenomena were documented in 20 patients, but only one did not have another systemic risk factor for a source.

Exercise Hemodynamics of the Ross Operation

Multiple studies demonstrate the excellent hemodynamic profile offered by the autograft in the Ross operation. A comparison with normal age- and gender-matched controls showed peak gradients going from only 2 to 4 mm Hg in both groups with exercise.[80] Effective orifice areas of 3.5 cm^2 (EOAI 1.9 cm^2/m^2) did not change with exercise in either group. Full root Ross patients had better hemodynamics than subcoronary Ross patients, but the difference (1.98 ± 0.57 versus 1.64 ± 0.43 cm^2/m^2) was more important statistically than it was clinically.[81] This study also documented the superiority of the Ross hemodynamics over stented and stentless valves and even over aortic homografts.

It is important to remember that the Ross operation includes RVOT reconstruction, and the hemodynamics of that structure can adversely affect exercise capacity. One study documented an average resting gradient of 14 ± 10 mm Hg rising to 25 ± 22 mm Hg for the pulmonary homografts of Ross patients compared with only 3 ± 1 mm Hg at rest and 5 ± 4 mm Hg with exercise in the normal native RVOT of aortic homograft recipients.[82] The higher gradients in the RVOT may contribute to slightly lower maximal oxygen consumption compared with normal controls, even though Ross patients easily exceeded 100% of predicted consumption.

Contemporary Results

With operative mortality now approaching that of alternative valve replacements, the long-term results are the vital point in considering the Ross operation for any given patient. The comparative incidence of reoperation for structural valve deterioration with present-generation tissue valves and the continuing risks of thromboembolism and anticoagulant-related hemorrhage with modern mechanical devices must be fairly presented to patients along with the data for the Ross.

A thorough review of available series confirms that survival is extremely good after the Ross operation and approximates that of the normal age-matched population.[83] Combined with its low incidence of thromboembolic complications and endocarditis as well as avoidance of anticoagulation with its risks of bleeding, the Ross is a very attractive option for young people. Some of these patients will undoubtedly require further surgery, but the outcomes of subsequent surgery have also been extremely good, which contributes to the long-term survival.

Elkins reported results in 487 patients operated on between 1986 and 2002.[84] Hospital mortality was 19 to 3.9%. Of 15 late deaths, none were owing to reoperation but only 7 were not cardiac related. Actuarial freedom from all cause mortality was $92 \pm 2\%$ at 10 years and $82\% \pm 6\%$ at 16 years. There was only one documented thromboembolic event. Actuarial freedom from endocarditis was $95 \pm 6\%$ at 16 years. Of 38 patients who needed further surgery, autograft reoperation was more common than homograft reoperation. Importantly, the vast majority of these patients had bicuspid or even unicuspid morphology, but their risk of reoperation was actually lower than the 9/78 three-leaflet valve patients. Patients with primary aortic regurgitation fared significantly worse until 1996 when the institution of routine annular reduction and fixation was initiated. Subsequent results in AR were then only slightly inferior to those in AS in whom the 15-year freedom from autograft valve failure was $82 \pm 6\%$. Technique seemed important as only 21/389 full roots required reoperation where 17/79 intra-aortic implants did.

Pulmonary Autograft Dysfunction

Pulmonary autograft stenosis has never been reported but the incidence of regurgitation increases with time and seems to be due to autograft or native aortic dilatation or both. The recognition of early AR due to technical problems with intra-aortic implants led to widespread acceptance of the root replacement method when we reported this in 1989.[85] Unfortunately, the totally unsupported autograft as a freestanding aortic root replacement proved to have potential for dilatation with root aneurysm and AR as a result. Annular dilatation was appreciated early and addressed with annuloplasty and external fixation with fixed pericardium or prosthetic material. Dilatation at the sinus and sinotubular junction levels was not appreciated and addressed until about a decade later. Incidence of this problem has been difficult to define and risk factors have been controversial. Autograft function can often remain excellent even with significant root dilatation (Fig. 34-12).

Brown found that preoperative ascending aortic dilatation, male gender, and postoperative systemic hypertension were significant in a Cox proportional hazard analysis for the development of moderate neo-aortic regurgitation.[86] Hypertension, particularly early postoperatively, can cause acute dilatation and damage to the delicate autograft leaflets before they have time to adapt to the systemic pressure environment. The unsupported root technique having failed in 22 of 142 patients in Rotterdam over a 17-year period, the adult Ross procedure was abandoned at Erasmus.[87] David expressed concern about the potential for dilatation at multiple levels particularly in bicuspid valve patients because of a higher incidence of aortic wall pathology.[88]

Multiple approaches have been developed to solve the dilatation problem. Sievers has demonstrated that a rigorously selected population of patients with frequent "tailoring" of the native aortic root can be treated with a subcoronary Ross implant with excellent results up to at least 10 years.[74] Others including this

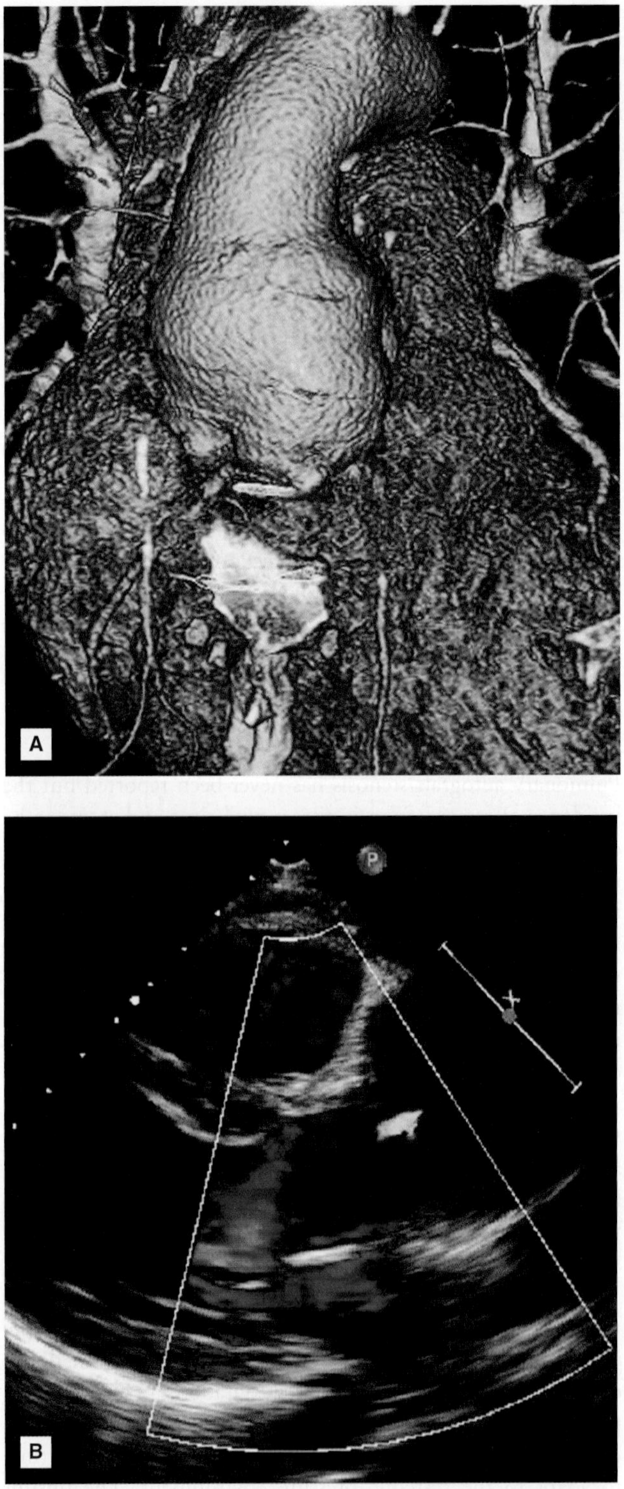

FIGURE 34-12 Dilated Ross procedure at 10 years. (A) CTA appearance. (B) Echocardiogram showing minimal central AR.

author[89] and Oswalt [90] stressed the need for multilevel fixation to support the autograft. Still others have suggested use of absorbable mesh,[91] pericardial,[92] or fabric[93] wrapping to completely enclose the autograft. The restrictive nature of this approach may produce other problems by compressing the pliable, dynamic autograft into a rigid cylinder with decrease in potential for vascular ingrowth. Clearly the patient with root and ascending aneurysm cannot be treated by a simple inclusion cylinder implant, but the patient with normal root anatomy and good size match can be served quite well by this alternative. Individualization is required to make sure that the autograft whether inside the intact or "tailored" aortic root or implanted as a full root has appropriate supporting autologous tissue and/or prosthetic material of appropriate dimensions to allow normal valve function and prevent late dilatation. With this approach it is not unreasonable to anticipate autograft failure rates of less than or equal to 10% at ten years and less than or equal to 20% at twenty years.

Pulmonary Homograft Dysfunction

As part of the Ross operation, the single aortic valve operation becomes a double valve operation also leaving the RVOT substitute at risk for future problems. The pioneer series clearly demonstrated the homograft to be superior to other alternatives of that day, but controversy remains particularly over the advantages and disadvantages of homograft viability on the right side. Although the initial hemodynamics of the cryopreserved pulmonary homografts are excellent, consistent increase in transvalvular gradients occurs within 6 to 12 months. This early increase in gradient usually stabilizes by 2 years, but can be progressive in 1 to 2% of patients. An immune system response has been implicated, but the mechanisms are poorly understood.[94]

The pulmonary homograft can develop extensive calcification of the inflow end indicative of an intense scar response to the homograft muscle cuff (Fig. 34-13). Schmidtke and associates tried to minimize this with a unique trimming of the muscle and replacing it with a cuff of pericardium.[95] This proved effective over the first two years but failed to make a long-term difference. An intense adventitial inflammatory reaction with diffuse thickening along the entire homograft was described with elegant MRI flow studies by Carr-White.[96] This caused extrinsic compression of the conduit portion of the homograft.

The incidence of homograft stenosis is probably 5 to 10% at 10 years. Risk factors proposed include younger donor age, shorter time of cryopreservation, and homograft size.[97] Because small size is the most consistent risk factor, oversizing helps reduce the effect of shrinkage.

Most patients tolerate peak gradients up to 50 mm Hg without symptoms so the clinical significance is less than the incidence of stenosis. In the Oklahoma series, homograft failure (reoperation or percutaneous intervention) occurred in 33 of 487 patients giving actuarial freedom from failure of 90 ± 2% at 10 years and 82 ± 4% at 16 years.[84] The advent of catheter-based valve replacement has made it possible to treat some of these patients percutaneously.[98]

Moderate or even severe homograft regurgitation may also be detected by echocardiography in as much as 10% of patients by 10 years but this lesion is well tolerated by the right ventricle in the absence of pulmonary hypertension. It is probable that most pulmonary homografts will ultimately suffer this mode of failure but the majority will last 20 to 25 years before they reach this point.

After four decades of use and research, the cryopreserved pulmonary homograft is the best RVOT substitute documented for use in the Ross procedure. Rarely, a stentless porcine

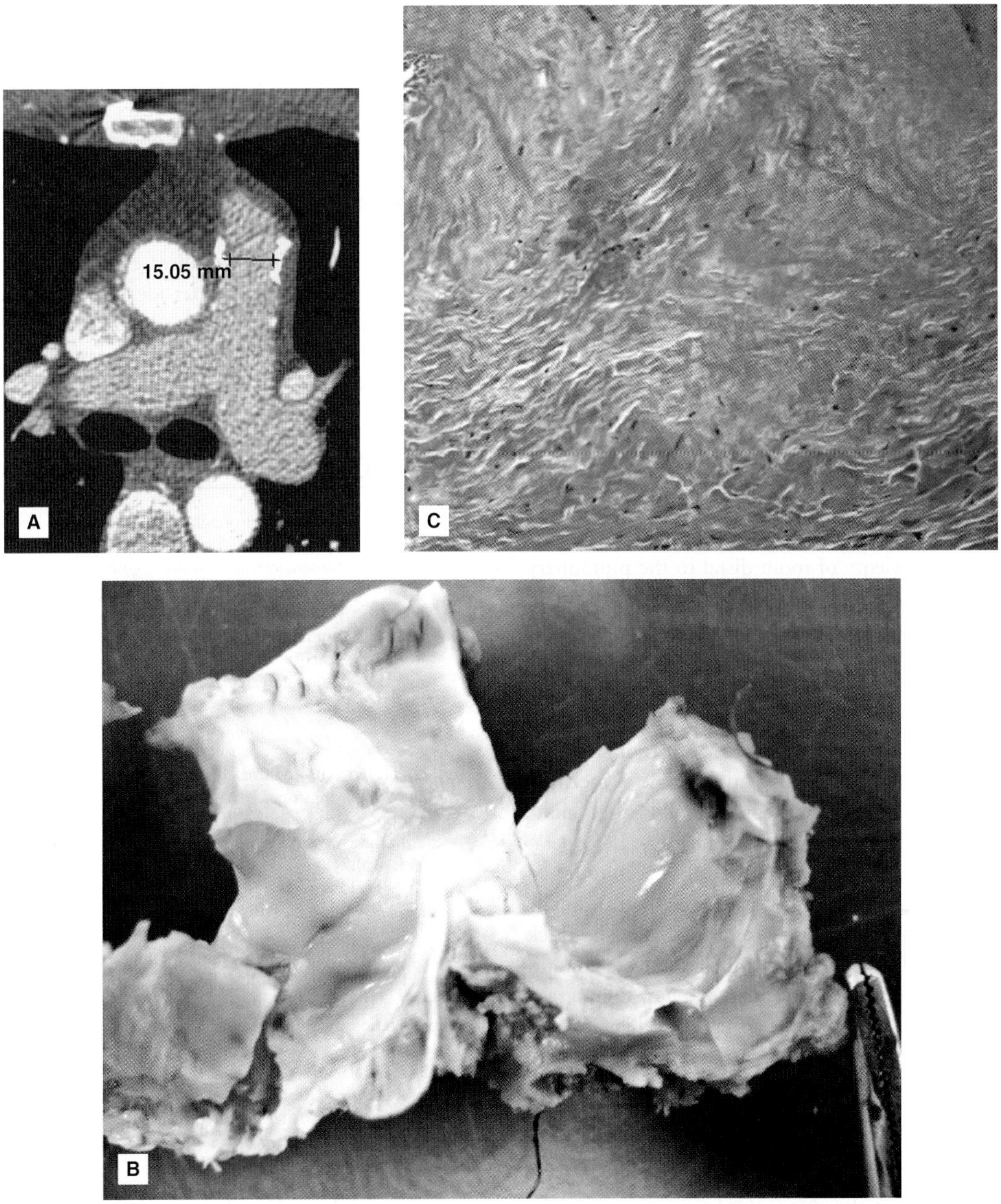

FIGURE 34-13 Calcified pulmonary homograft. The inflow anastomosis of this pulmonary homograft is markedly narrowed and calcified 16 years after a Ross procedure. Gradient was only 28 at rest but 75 mm Hg with exercise. (A) Appearance on CT scan. (B) Gross specimen at explant. (C) Microscopic showing acellular scar.

bioprosthesis has been used. Tissue engineering concepts seem ideally suited to this low pressure area where a decellularized homograft or even heterograft matrix can perform nicely while providing an environment suitable for maturation of new cellular elements derived from circulating stem cells, adjacent ingrowth, or preoperative seeding. Initial clinical studies with both show promise but await long term follow up.[33,99]

REOPERATION POST-ROSS PROCEDURE

The prospect of reoperation after a Ross procedure has been regarded as a complex and hazardous undertaking.[87] Concern about dissection and rupture is largely unsupported. Rupture of the autograft has never been reported. Localized dissection of the autograft does occur but does not extend across circumferential suture lines that protect the distal aorta and the coronary ostia. The wall of the autograft, although thinner than native aorta, is encased in scar tissue from the original surgery, making leakage into a free pericardial space extremely unlikely.

If moderate autograft regurgitation has developed with root dilatation, a policy of waiting for symptoms or ventricular dysfunction/dilatation typically indicative for surgical intervention should be considered appropriate, not just treating a sinus dimension. If distal native aorta dilates to 5.0 cm or greater, it may be reasonable to intervene before it gets to 5.5 cm in the setting of original bicuspid aortic valve disease. If other valve disease or coronary disease dictates operative intervention, the dilated autograft should not be ignored. If the autograft has been supported at the inflow end with felt, the Yacoub valve–sparing approach may be appropriate because the annulus is already supported. If there is strictly a leaflet problem, such as prolapse or perforation, repair might be considered, but only if a durable repair can be anticipated. Complete redo root replacement should be considered if both the leaflets and the sinuses are problematic. The living, pliable autograft makes this much easier than a redo after a standard Bentall.

Safe reoperation begins with appropriate planning at the original operation where closure of the pericardium or coverage of the heart with pericardial substitute will allow safe sternal re-entry. Central cannulation is almost always possible, but peripheral cannulation should be considered in multiple reoperative settings or when preoperative imaging suggests perilous re-entry. Crucial to safe conduct of these operations is avoidance of the plane between the pulmonary homograft and the aorta. There is usually plenty of room distal to the pulmonary artery to clamp the aorta before this plane needs to be addressed. Coronary buttons are often very close to the distal autograft anastomosis, so aortotomy at reoperation should never be proximal to this suture line. The complete spectrum of replacement options is open at reoperation, including simple mechanical or stented tissue valves, subcoronary or full root stentless, aortic homograft, or Bentall operation with biologic or mechanical valved conduit. The RVOT homograft should be left alone unless grossly abnormal by preoperative evaluation. If reoperation is required for RVOT obstruction, this can be accomplished on the beating heart. The old conduit is opened longitudinally from normal right ventricular muscle to normal PA. The thick proximal scar is resected carefully and as much of the old conduit is removed as necessary to allow placement of a new homograft. The posterior wall and that facing the aorta can be left intact to avoid injury to the autograft and coronary tree.

SUMMARY

Of all the substitutes for the diseased aortic valve, only the pulmonary autograft has all the biologic advantages of a truly living structure. It is delicate and demands precise implantation technique for immediate and long-term success. Appropriate aortic tailoring or support is needed in the majority of patients to prevent late autograft dilatation and dysfunction. Approximately 20% of patients will probably require additional surgery for either the neo-aortic or the neo-pulmonary aspects of this operation by 20 years, but they will not require anticoagulation and will not be limited in activity or lifestyle during that time. In appropriate hands, this operation can be done very safely and is a durable and excellent choice for young active people with aortic valve disease. Compared with the virtually 100% reoperation rate at 20 years for animal tissue valves, unavoidable and ongoing risks of thromboembolic and hemorrhagic complications with mechanical valves, and proven advantage of the Ross procedure over aortic homograft in randomized prospective trial,[100] the Ross procedure is a very viable option. Long-term survival may actually be superior to any other aortic valve operation.

Appropriate imaging of patients after these patients is essential and should include a thorough echo evaluation at least every 2 years. CT or MRI evaluation of the aorta should probably be done at least every 10 years and more frequently if progressive aortic dilatation is observed. Reoperation when required can be done safely in experienced centers with preservation of the autograft possible in some cases. The Ross operation should be offered as an option for any patient under the age of 50 with aortic valve disease and a life expectancy in excess of 20 to 25 years. Under ideal circumstances, it can be considered in the 50- to 65-year-old population where the Ross procedure has the possibility of lasting to the end of a normal life span.

REFERENCES

1. Stelzer P, Elkins RC: Homograft valves and conduits: applications in cardiac surgery. *Curr Probl Surg* 1989; 26(6):381-452.
2. Murray G: Homologous aortic-valve-segment transplants as surgical treatment for aortic and mitral insufficiency. *Angiology* 1956; 7(5):466-471.
3. Murray G: Aortic valve transplants. *Angiology* 1960; 11:99-102.
4. Duran C, Gunning AJ: A method for placing a total homologous aortic valve in the subcoronary position. *Lancet* 1962; 2(7254):488-489.
5. Ross DN: Homograft replacement of the aortic valve. *Lancet* 1962; 2(7254):487.
6. Barratt-Boyes BG: Homograft aortic valve replacement in aortic incompetence and stenosis. *Thorax* 1964; 19:131-150.
7. Kirklin JK, Barratt-Boyes BG, eds. *Cardiac Surgery,* 2nd ed. London, Churchill Livingstone, 1993.
8. Logrippo GA, Overhulse PR, Szilagyi DE, Hartman FW: Procedure for sterilization of arterial homografts with beta-propiolactone. *Lab Invest* 1955; 4(3):217-231.
9. Davies H, Lessof MH, Roberts CI, Ross DN: Homograft replacement of the aortic valve: follow-up studies in twelve patients. *Lancet* 1965; 1(7392): 926-929.
10. Pacifico AD, Karp RB, Kirklin JW: Homografts for replacement of the aortic valve. *Circulation* 1972; 45(1 Suppl):I36-43.
11. Sands MP, Nelson RJ, Mohri H, Merendino KA: The procurement and preparation of aortic valve homografts. *Surgery* 62(5):839-842.
12. Barratt-Boyes B: Long-term follow-up of aortic valvar grafts. *Br Heart J* 1971; 33:60-65.
13. O'Brien MF, Stafford EG, Gardner MA, Pohlner PG, McGiffin DC: A comparison of aortic valve replacement with viable cryopreserved and fresh allograft valves, with a note on chromosomal studies. *J Thorac Cardiovasc Surg* 1987; 94(6):812-823.
14. Lower RR, Stofer RC, Shumway NE: Total excision of the mitral valve and replacement with the autologous pulmonic valve. *J Thorac Cardiovasc Surg* 1961; 42:696-702.
15. Pillsbury RC, Shumway NE: Replacement of the aortic valve with the autologous pulmonic valve. *Surg Forum* 1966; 17:176-177.
16. Ross DN: Replacement of aortic and mitral valves with a pulmonary autograft. *Lancet* 1967; 2(7523):956-958.
17. Stelzer P, Elkins RC: Pulmonary autograft: an American experience. *J Card Surg* 1987; 2(4):429-433.
18. Oury JH, Hiro SP, Maxwell JM, Lamberti JJ, Duran CM: The Ross Procedure: current registry results. *Ann Thorac Surg* 1998; 66(6 Suppl): S162-165.
19. Jones DJ, Hance ML, Stelzer P, Elkins RC: Procurement of hearts for valve homografts: one year's experience. *J Okla State Med Assoc* 1988; 81(8): 510-512.
20. Bank HL, Brockbank KG: Basic principles of cryobiology. *J Card Surg* 1987; 2(1 Suppl):137-143.
21. Smith JC: The pathology of human aortic valve homografts. *Thorax* 1967; 22(2):114-138.
22. Armiger LC: Viability studies of human valves prepared for use as allografts. *Ann Thorac Surg* 1995; 60:S118; discussion S120.
23. O'Brien MF, Stafford G, Gardner M, et al: The viable cryopreserved allograft aortic valve. *J Card Surg* 1987; 2(1 Suppl):153-167.
24. Hoekstra F, Witvliet M, Knoop C, et al: Donor-specific anti-human leukocyte antigen class I antibodies after implantation of cardiac valve allografts. *J Heart Lung Transplant* 1997; 16(5):570-572.

25. Shaddy RE, Hunter DD, Osborn KA, et al: Prospective analysis of HLA immunogenicity of cryopreserved valved allografts used in pediatric heart surgery. *Circulation* 1996; 94(5):1063-1067.
26. Smith JD, Ogino H, Hunt D, et al: Humoral immune response to human aortic valve homografts. *Ann Thorac Surg* 1995; 60(2 Suppl):S127-130.
27. Green MK, Walsh MD, Dare A, et al: Histologic and immunohistochemical responses after aortic valve allografts in the rat. *Ann Thorac Surg* 1998; 66(6 Suppl):S216-220.
28. Legare JF, Lee TD, Ross DB: Cryopreservation of rat aortic valves results in increased structural failure. *Circulation* 2000; 102(19 Suppl 3): III75-78.
29. Baraki H, Tudorache I, Braun M, et al: Orthotopic replacement of the aortic valve with decellularized allograft in a sheep model. *Biomaterials* 2009; 30(31):6240-6246.
30. Zehr KJ, Yagubyan M, Connolly HM, Nelson SM, Schaff HV: Aortic root replacement with a novel decellularized cryopreserved aortic homograft: postoperative immunoreactivity and early results. *J Thorac Cardiovasc Surg* 2005; 130(4):1010-1015.
31. Brown JW, Ruzmetov M, Rodefeld MD, Turrentine MW: Right ventricular outflow tract reconstruction in Ross patients: does the homograft fare better? *Ann Thorac Surg* 2008; 86(5):1607-1612.
32. Elkins RC, Dawson PE, Goldstein S, Walsh SP, Black KS: Decellularized human valve allografts. *Ann Thorac Surg* 2001; 71(5 Suppl):S428-432.
33. Konertz W, Dohmen PM, Liu J, et al: Hemodynamic characteristics of the Matrix P decellularized xenograft for pulmonary valve replacement during the Ross operation. *J Heart Valve Dis* 2005; 14(1):78-81.
34. Armiger LC: Postimplantation leaflet cellularity of valve allografts: are donor cells beneficial or detrimental? *Ann Thorac Surg* 1998; 66(6 Suppl): S233-235.
35. Maselli D, Pizio R, Bruno LP, Di Bella I, De Gasperis C: Left ventricular mass reduction after aortic valve replacement: homografts, stentless and stented valves. *Ann Thorac Surg* 1999; 67(4):966-971.
36. Foghsgaard S, Bruun N, Kjaergard H: Outcome of aortic homograft implantation in 24 cases of severe infective endocarditis. *Scand J Infect Dis* 2008; 40(3):216-220.
37. McGiffin DC, Kirklin JK: The impact of aortic valve homografts on the treatment of aortic prosthetic valve endocarditis. *Semin Thorac Cardiovasc Surg* 1995; 7(1):25-31.
38. El-Hamamsy I, Clark L, Stevens LM, et al: Late outcomes following freestyle versus homograft aortic root replacement results from a prospective randomized trial. *J Am Coll Cardiol* 2010; 55(4):368-376.
39. Greaves SC, Reimold SC, Lee RT, Cooke KA, Aranki SF: Preoperative prediction of prosthetic aortic valve annulus diameter by two-dimensional echocardiography. *J Heart Valve Dis* 1995; 4(1):14-17.
40. Moscucci M, Weinert L, Karp RB, Neumann A: Prediction of aortic annulus diameter by two-dimensional echocardiography. Application in the preoperative selection and preparation of homograft aortic valves. *Circulation* 1991; 84(5 Suppl):III76-80.
41. Weinert L, Karp R, Vignon P, Bales A, Lang RM: Feasibility of aortic diameter measurement by multiplane transesophageal echocardiography for preoperative selection and preparation of homograft aortic valves. *J Thorac Cardiovasc Surg* 1996; 112(4):954-961.
42. Daicoff GR, Botero LM, Quintessenza JA: Allograft replacement of the aortic valve versus the miniroot and valve. *Ann Thorac Surg* 1993; 55(4): 855-858; discussion 859.
43. Dearani JA, Orszulak TA, Daly RC, et al: Comparison of techniques for implantation of aortic valve allografts. *Ann Thorac Surg* 1996; 62(4): 1069-1075.
44. Lund O, Chandrasekaran V, Grocott-Mason R, et al: Primary aortic valve replacement with allografts over twenty-five years: valve-related and procedure-related determinants of outcome. *J Thorac Cardiovasc Surg* 1999; 117(1):77-90; discussion 90-71.
45. McGiffin DC, O'Brien MF: A technique for aortic root replacement by an aortic allograft. *Ann Thorac Surg* 1989; 47(4):625-627.
46. Rubay JE, Raphael D, Sluysmans T, et al: Aortic valve replacement with allograft/autograft: subcoronary versus intraluminal cylinder or root. *Ann Thorac Surg* 1995; 60(2 Suppl):S78-82.
47. Northrup WF 3rd, Kshettry VR: Implantation technique of aortic homograft root: emphasis on matching the host root to the graft. *Ann Thorac Surg* 1998; 66(1):280-284.
48. Mitchell LB, Exner DV, Wyse DG, et al: Prophylactic oral amiodarone for the prevention of arrhythmias that begin early after revascularization, valve replacement, or repair: PAPABEAR: a randomized controlled trial. *JAMA* 2005; 294(24):3093-3100.
49. Langley SM, McGuirk SP, Chaudhry MA, et al: Twenty-year follow-up of aortic valve replacement with antibiotic sterilized homografts in 200 patients. *Semin Thorac Cardiovasc Surg* 1999; 11(4 Suppl 1):28-34.
50. O'Brien MF, Harrocks S, Stafford EG, et al: The homograft aortic valve: a 29-year, 99.3% follow up of 1,022 valve replacements. *J Heart Valve Dis* 2001; 10(3):334-344; discussion 335.
51. Melina G, De Robertis F, Gaer JA, et al: Mid-term pattern of survival, hemodynamic performance and rate of complications after medtronic freestyle versus homograft full aortic root replacement: results from a prospective randomized trial. *J Heart Valve Dis* 2004; 13(6):972-975; discussion 975-976.
52. Byrne JG, Karavas AN, Mihaljevic T, et al: Role of the cryopreserved homograft in isolated elective aortic valve replacement. *J Am Coll Cardiol* 2003; 91(5):616-619.
53. Dearani JA, Orszulak TA, Schaff HV, et al: Results of allograft aortic valve replacement for complex endocarditis. *J Thorac Cardiovasc Surg* 1997; 113(2):285-291.
54. Niwaya K, Knott-Craig CJ, Santangelo K, et al: Advantage of autograft and homograft valve replacement for complex aortic valve endocarditis. *Ann Thorac Surg* 1999; 67(6):1603-1608.
55. Yacoub M, Rasmi NR, Sundt TM, et al: Fourteen-year experience with homovital homografts for aortic valve replacement. *J Thorac Cardiovasc Surg* 1995; 110(1):186-193; discussion 193-194.
56. Yankah AC, Klose H, Petzina R, et al: Surgical management of acute aortic root endocarditis with viable homograft: 13-year experience. *Eur J Cardiothorac Surg* 2002; 21(2):260-267.
57. Grinda JM, Mainardi JL, D'Attellis N, et al: Cryopreserved aortic viable homograft for active aortic endocarditis. *Ann Thorac Surg* 2005; 79(3): 767-771.
58. Eriksson MJ, Kallner G, Rosfors S, Ivert T, Brodin LA: Hemodynamic performance of cryopreserved aortic homograft valves during midterm follow-up. *J Am Coll Cardiol* 1998; 32(4):1002-1008.
59. Hasegawa J, Kitamura S, Taniguchi S, et al: Comparative rest and exercise hemodynamics of allograft and prosthetic valves in the aortic position. *Ann Thorac Surg* 1997; 64(6):1753-1756.
60. Athanasiou T, Jones C, Jin R, Grunkemeier GL, Ross DN: Homograft implantation techniques in the aortic position: to preserve or replace the aortic root? *Ann Thorac Surg* 2006; 81(5):1578-1585.
61. Smedira NG, Blackstone EH, Roselli EE, Laffey CC, Cosgrove DM: Are allografts the biologic valve of choice for aortic valve replacement in nonelderly patients? Comparison of explantation for structural valve deterioration of allograft and pericardial prostheses. *J Thorac Cardiovasc Surg* 2006; 131(3):558-564; e554.
62. Unger P, Plein D, Pradier O, LeClerc JL: Thrombosis of aortic valve homograft associated with lupus anticoagulant antibodies. *Ann Thorac Surg* 2004; 77(1):312-314.
63. Sadowski J, Kapelak B, Bartus K, et al: Reoperation after fresh homograft replacement: 23 years' experience with 655 patients. *Eur J Cardiothorac Surg* 2003; 23(6):996-1000; discussion 1000-1001.
64. Joudinaud TM, Baron F, Raffoul R, et al: Redo aortic root surgery for failure of an aortic homograft is a major technical challenge. *Eur J Cardiothorac Surg* 2008; 33(6):989-994.
65. Dainese L, Fusari M, Trabattoni P, Biglioli P: Redo in aortic homograft replacement: Transcatheter aortic valve as a valid alternative to surgical replacement. *J Thorac Cardiovasc Surg* 2009; 2(2):e6-7.
66. Gorczynski A, Trenkner M, Anisimowicz L, et al: Biomechanics of the pulmonary autograft valve in the aortic position. *Thorax* 1982; 37(7):535-539.
67. Rabkin-Aikawa E, Aikawa M, Farber M, et al: Clinical pulmonary autograft valves: pathologic evidence of adaptive remodeling in the aortic site. *J Thorac Cardiovasc Surg* 2004; 128(4):552-561.
68. Pieters FA, Al-Halees Z, Hatle L, Shahid MS, Al-Amri M: Results of the Ross operation in rheumatic versus non-rheumatic aortic valve disease. *J Heart Valve Dis* 2000; 9(1):38-44.
69. Oswalt JD, Dewan SJ: Aortic infective endocarditis managed by the Ross procedure. *J Heart Valve Dis* 1993; 2(4):380-384.
70. de Sa M, Moshkovitz Y, Butany J, David TE: Histologic abnormalities of the ascending aorta and pulmonary trunk in patients with bicuspid aortic valve disease: clinical relevance to the Ross procedure. *J Thorac Cardiovasc Surg* 1999; 118(4):588-594.
71. Elkins RC: The Ross operation: a 12-year experience. *Ann Thorac Surg* 1999; 68(3 Suppl):S14-18.
72. Stelzer P: Technique and results of the modified Ross procedure in aortic regurgitation versus aortic stenosis. *Adv Cardiol* 2002; 39:93-99.
73. Muresian H: The Ross procedure: new insights into the surgical anatomy. *Ann Thorac Surg* 2006; 81(2):495-501.
74. Sievers H, Dahmen G, Graf B, et al: Midterm results of the Ross procedure preserving the patient's aortic root. *Circulation* 2003; 108(Suppl 1):II55-60.
75. Polvani G, Barili F, Dainese L, et al: Reduction ascending aortoplasty: midterm follow-up and predictors of redilatation. *Ann Thorac Surg* 2006; 82(2):586-591.

76. Bauer M, Pasic M, Schaffarzyk R, et al: Reduction aortoplasty for dilatation of the ascending aorta in patients with bicuspid aortic valve. *Ann Thorac Surg* 2002; 73(3):720-723; discussion 724.
77. Roberts CS, Roberts WC: Dissection of the aorta associated with congenital malformation of the aortic valve. *J Am Coll Cardiol* 1991; 17(3): 712-716.
78. Chambers JC, Somerville J, Stone S, Ross DN: Pulmonary autograft procedure for aortic valve disease: long-term results of the pioneer series. *Circulation* 1997; 96(7):2206-2214.
79. Gerosa G, McKay R, Ross DN: Replacement of the aortic valve or root with a pulmonary autograft in children. *Ann Thorac Surg* 1991; 51(3): 424-429.
80. Pibarot P, Dumesnil JG, Briand M, Laforest I, Cartier P: Hemodynamic performance during maximum exercise in adult patients with the Ross operation and comparison with normal controls and patients with aortic bioprostheses. *J Am Coll Cardiol* 2000; 86(9):982-988.
81. Bohm JO, Botha CA, Hemmer W, et al: Hemodynamic performance following the Ross operation: comparison of two different techniques. *J Heart Valve Dis* 2004; 13(2):174-180; discussion 180-181.
82. Wang A, Jaggers J, Ungerleider RM, Lim CS, Ryan T: Exercise echocardiographic comparison of pulmonary autograft and aortic homograft replacements for aortic valve disease in adults. *J Heart Valve Dis* 2003; 12(2):202-208.
83. Takkenberg JJ, Klieverik LM, Schoof PH, et al: The Ross procedure: a systematic review and meta-analysis. *Circulation* 2009; 119(2):222-228.
84. Elkins RC, Thompson DM, Lane MM, Elkins CC, Peyton MD: Ross operation: 16-year experience. *J Thorac Cardiovasc Surg* 2008; 136(3):623-630, 630; e621-625.
85. Stelzer P, Jones DJ, Elkins RC: Aortic root replacement with pulmonary autograft. *Circulation* Nov 1989; 80(5 Pt 2):III209-213.
86. Brown JW, Ruzmetov M, Rodefeld MD, Mahomed Y, Turrentine MW: Incidence of and risk factors for pulmonary autograft dilation after Ross aortic valve replacement. *Ann Thorac Surg* 2007; 83(5):1781-1787; discussion 1787-1789.
87. Klieverik LM, Takkenberg JJ, Bekkers JA, et al: The Ross operation: a Trojan horse? *Eur Heart J* 2007; 28(16):1993-2000.
88. David TE, Omran A, Ivanov J, et al: Dilation of the pulmonary autograft after the Ross procedure. *J Thorac Cardiovasc Surg* 2000; 119(2):210-220.
89. Stelzer P: Reoperation for dilatation of the pulmonary autograft after the Ross procedure. *J Thorac Cardiovasc Surg* 2002; 124(2):417-418; author reply 418.
90. Oswalt JD, Dewan SJ, Mueller MC, Nelson S: Highlights of a ten-year experience with the Ross procedure. *Ann Thorac Surg* 2001; 71(5 Suppl): S332-335.
91. Mortiz A, Domanig E, Marx M, Moidl R, et al: Pulmonary autograft valve replacement in the dilated and asymmetric aortic root. *Eur J Cardiothorac Surg* 1993; 7(8):405-408.
92. Pacifico AD, Kirklin JK, McGiffin DC, et al: The Ross operation—early echocardiographic comparison of different operative techniques. *J Heart Valve Dis* 1994; 3(4):365-370.
93. Slater M, Shen I, Welke K, Komanapalli C, Ungerleider R: Modification to the Ross procedure to prevent autograft dilatation. *Semin Thorac Cardiovasc Surg Pediatr Card Surg Annu* 2005:181-184.
94. Lang SJ, Giordano MS, Cardon-Cardo C, et al: Biochemical and cellular characterization of cardiac valve tissue after cryopreservation or antibiotic preservation. *J Thorac Cardiovasc Surg* 1994; 108(1):63-67.
95. Schmidtke C, Dahmen G, Graf B, Sievers HH: Pulmonary homograft muscle reduction to reduce the risk of homograft stenosis in the Ross procedure. *J Thorac Cardiovasc Surg* 2007; 133(1):190-195.
96. Carr-White GS, Glennan S, Edwards S, et al: Pulmonary autograft versus aortic homograft for rereplacement of the aortic valve: results from a subset of a prospective randomized trial. *Circulation* 1999; 100(19 Suppl): II103-106.
97. Raanani E, Yau TM, David TE, et al: Risk factors for late pulmonary homograft stenosis after the Ross procedure. *Ann Thorac Surg* 2000; 70(6):1953-1957.
98. Boudjemline Y, Khambadkone S, Bonnet D, et al: Images in cardiovascular medicine. Percutaneous replacement of the pulmonary valve in a 12-year-old child. *Circulation* 2004; 110(22):e516.
99. Konuma T, Devaney EJ, Bove EL, et al: Performance of CryoValve SG decellularized pulmonary allografts compared with standard cryopreserved allografts. *Ann Thorac Surg* 2009; 88(3):849-854; discussion 854-845.
100. Aklog L, Carr-White GS, Birks EJ, Yacoub MH: Pulmonary autograft versus aortic homograft for aortic valve replacement: interim results from a prospective randomized trial. *J Heart Valve Dis* 2000; 9(2):176-188; discussion 188-179.

CHAPTER 35

Aortic Valve Replacement with a Stentless Bioprosthetic Valve: Porcine or Pericardial

Edward H. Kincaid
Neal D. Kon

INTRODUCTION

The history of stentless xenograft aortic valves follows in the footsteps of the aortic homograft, which was considered historically as the best biologic prosthesis for management of root pathology and for optimizing hemodynamics in the absence of root pathology. The original concept behind creating a stentless xenograft valve was to maintain the excellent hemodynamics of the homograft, while improving on the availability, durability, technical complexity, and costs associated with homografts.

Stentless, or "natural valve" substitutes closely mimic the native aortic root anatomy and are implanted without a stent, large sewing ring, or other supporting apparatus that can lead to persistent LV obstruction sometimes observed with stented bioprostheses or mechanical valves. In general, use of stentless valves also allows for implantation of larger prostheses with resultant larger effective orifice area for any given LV outflow tract diameter. Comparing homografts, autografts and xenografts, stentless porcine constructs have the most opportunity for wide-spread application because of their ready shelf availability and ease of implantation. Compared with traditional stented bioprostheses, touted advantages of stentless valves include better hemodynamics,[1-3] improved regression of left ventricular mass,[3-5] less risk of patient-prosthesis mismatch (ppm) in the small aortic root,[6] and possibly improved long-term survival.[7,8] Because of these advantages, over the past 15 years, aortic valve replacement (AVR) with stentless porcine bioprostheses has become an accepted technique for routine treatment of aortic valve and root diseases. Some of these advantages appear to be maximized with implantation using a total root replacement technique, which also is associated with less risk of late valve failure.[9] However, the potential benefits of stentless valves implanted as total roots may come at the cost of increased operative risks, including a potential for higher operative mortality compared with subcoronary stentless or stented AVR.[9] Although other large series have reported low operative mortality with stentless root replacement,[10-12] a learning curve of over 20 cases has been described.[13] Besides a learning curve for this more complex procedure, other factors that could potentially contribute to excess mortality include longer perfusion and myocardial ischemic times, and more suture lines exposed to the pericardial space. Thus, the use of stentless aortic bioprostheses has become a controversial topic within the cardiothoracic surgical community.

AVAILABLE PROSTHESES

Many stentless xenograft valves have come and gone in the marketplace over the past decade. Currently, the only two stentless prostheses available are the Medtronic Freestyle bioprosthesis and the ATS 3F valve, which has only recently been introduced to the North American market.

Medtronic Freestyle

The Medtronic Freestyle valve followed closely behind the development of the St Jude Toronto SPV, which is now out of production. From its beginning, the Freestyle valve had several options of implantation techniques, similar to the homograft, including full root, root inclusion, and subcoronary positions. The Freestyle valve began clinical application in the early 1990s, thus making some long-term outcome data available. The Freestyle is a complete porcine root with minimal polyester fabric covering all exposed porcine myocardium (Figs. 35-1, 35-2). This

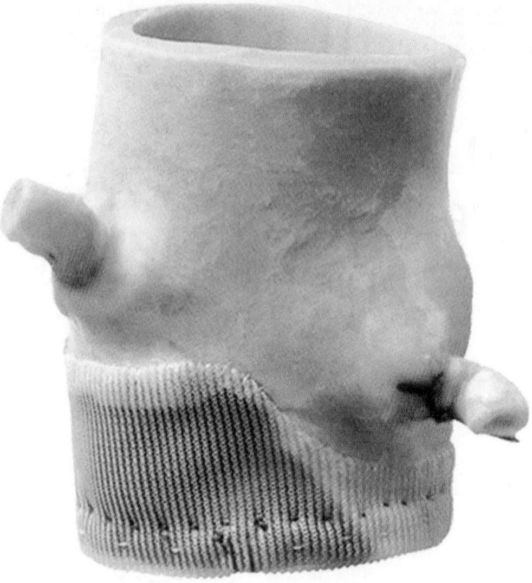

FIGURE 35-1 The Medtronic Freestyle Aortic Root Bioprosthesis. The longitudinal view shows the fabric covering of the porcine septal muscle and the associated higher position of the right coronary stump. (*Reproduced with permission from Medtronic, Inc., Minneapolis, MN.*)

serves to strengthen the proximal (inflow) suture line and reduce antigenicity. There is a green demarcation line around the inner circumference of the polyester fabric covering indicating the suturing area. There are also markers for each commissure to aid in suture placement. The Freestyle tissue is crosslinked in a dilute glutaraldehyde solution using a tissue fixation method that allows valves to maintain natural leaflet structure and natural root geometry by simultaneously applying 40 mm Hg (diastolic pressure of the pig) to the inflow and outflow portions of the bioprosthesis, allowing the leaflets to relax at net zero pressure differential with a pressurized root.[14] This results in leaflets fixed under no load but in an anatomically distended root. Potential advantages of this process include maintenance of radial leaflet distensibility (corrugations), circumferential leaflet stability (crimp), maintenance of strength with elasticity, and mitigation of kinking. Using a combination of accelerated wear testing in a pulse duplicator and biaxial mechanical testing of the tissue, Christie and colleagues demonstrated better preservation of both circumferential and radial stretch in the Freestyle leaflets compared with leaflets fixed even at low pressure, which flattens the native collagen crimp.[15] The Freestyle bioprosthesis is treated with an alpha-amino oleic acid (AOA), a compound derived from oleic acid, designed to mitigate both leaflet and wall calcification. Various anticalcification treatments are now commonly used by all manufacturers with data based on animal and some short-term human efficacy studies. Minimal long-term human data exists on the effectiveness of any of these proprietary anticalcification treatments, although the group at Harefield recently reported lower calcium scores in Freestyle valves compared with homografts at 8 years.[16]

ATS 3F Valve

The ATS Aortic Bioprosthesis, Model 1000 is a stentless pericardial aortic heart valve replacement designed as a tubular structure and constructed from three equal sections of equine pericardium, with each section cut roughly in the shape of a square (Fig. 35-3). This unique construction design was based on the development of the embryonic tubular aortic valve subjected to computer modeling. The choice of equine pericardium is reportedly based on its strength in the areas of the leaflets where stress was found to be greatest. For the 3F valve,

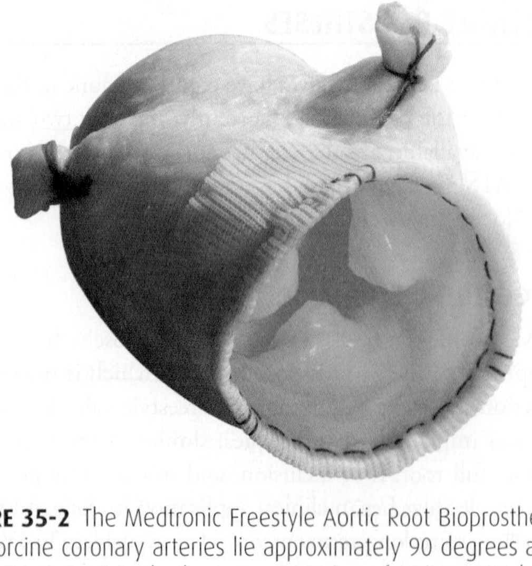

FIGURE 35-2 The Medtronic Freestyle Aortic Root Bioprosthesis. The porcine coronary arteries lie approximately 90 degrees apart. This is in contrast to the human orientation of 140 to 160 degrees apart.

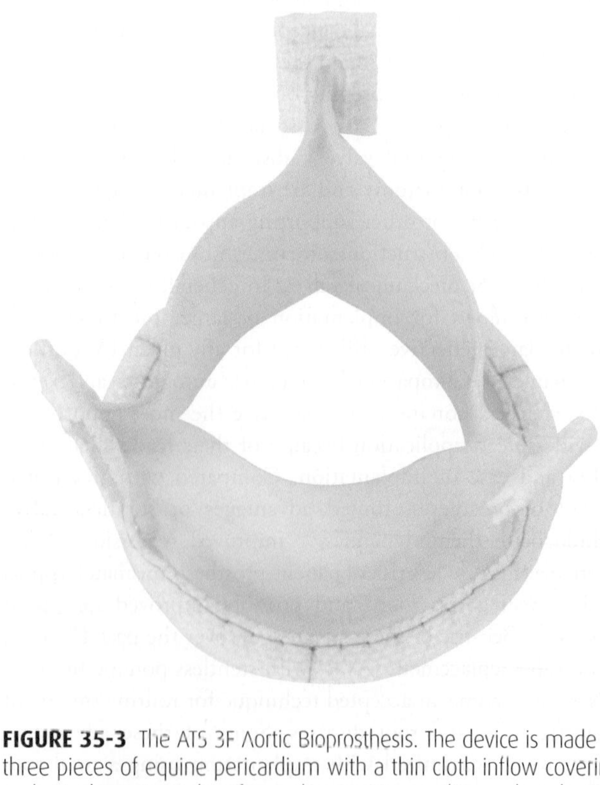

FIGURE 35-3 The ATS 3F Aortic Bioprosthesis. The device is made of three pieces of equine pericardium with a thin cloth inflow covering and attachment patches for each commissure. (*Reproduced with permission from ATS Medical, Minneapolis, MN.*)

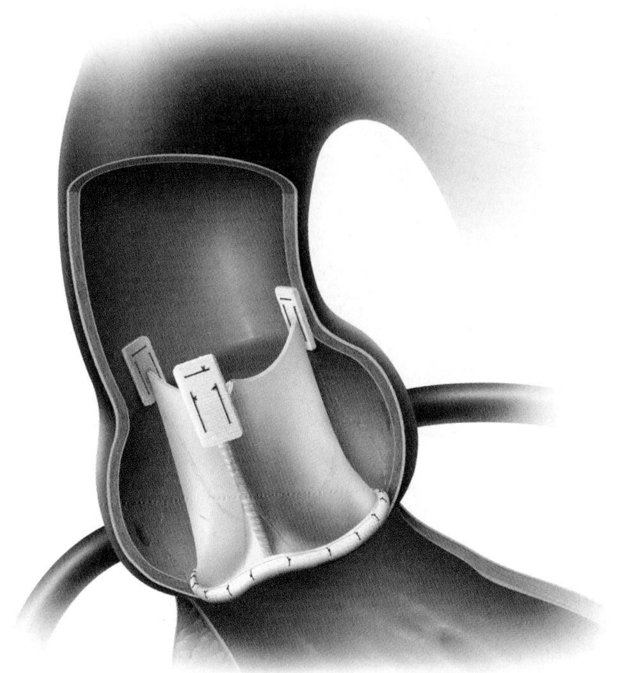

FIGURE 35-4 The ATS 3F Aortic Bioprosthesis. The tubular design allows the omission of the full subcoronary suture line. Instead, the three commissures are attached to the aorta at 120-degree spacing at appropriate height from the annulus. (*Reproduced with permission from ATS Medical, Minneapolis, MN.*)

this highest stress area is the midportion or "belly" of the leaflet. Equine pericardium is also reportedly thinner and more consistent in thickness compared with bovine pericardium. The equine pericardium is fixed with 0.25% buffered glutaraldehyde to preserve its collagen matrix and reduce its immunogenic and thrombogenic potentials while preserving its strength and flexibility. Anticalcification agents are not used. The proximal orifice of the valve has an attached thin polyester sewing ring used to attach the bioprosthesis to the aortic root orifice after resection of the diseased aortic valve. The distal portion of the valve has three commissural tabs, formed from contiguous sections of each of the leaflets and reinforcing polyester material that are used to attach the commissures to the native aortic wall. Similar to traditional subcoronary stentless valves, the 3F relies on normal root/annular ratios and geometry during implantation. The tubular design of the valve, however, allows the omission of the full subcoronary (outflow) suture line. Instead, the three commissures are attached to the aorta at 120-degree spacing at appropriate height from the annulus (Fig. 35-4).

Currently little data exist on the performance of the 3F valve, although at one year in a study of 35 implants, mean gradients ranged from 9 to13 mm Hg and there was minimal AI and no structural deterioration.[17]

INDICATIONS FOR STENTLESS AORTIC VALVES

Stentless aortic valves placed as a subcoronary or full root implant are indicated for the small aortic root, and root replacement provides better hemodynamic function than traditional root enlarging procedures. Stentless aortic valves placed as a total root are also useful in the following situations:

1. Aortic root disease when bioprosthesis is desired
2. Elderly patients with poor tissues. It is simpler to replace fragile disease tissues with synthetic material, thereby eliminating working with poor tissues and tension on critical suture lines.
3. Aortic dissection, when valve needs replacement. Extensive dissection in the sinuses of Valsalva is easily handled with a stentless root bioprosthesis.
4. Endocarditis. Similar to the homograft, the stentless root bioprosthesis allows maximal debridement prior to reconstruction, but has the advantage of immediate availability in all sizes.

IMPLANTATION METHODS

Subcoronary and Modified Subcoronary

Function of the subcoronary stentless valve relies on the intact native sinus geometry. For this reason, an oblique aortotomy should not be used to approach the aortic valve, and instead, a transverse aortotomy or complete aortic transsection should be used. At least 1 to 1.5 cm of clearance is needed to place the stentless device within the root and still close it above the tips of the commissures of the new valve. Complete transsection of the aorta is often helpful in gaining full exposure for implantation. For traditional subcoronary technique, all three sinuses of the prosthesis are scalloped out. For modified subcoronary implantation, the noncoronary sinus is left intact. The advantages are higher suture line, and two posts are fixed. The proximal suture line is usually done with simple interrupted technique using 2-0 to 4-0 braided sutures. Approximately 20 to 30 sutures are used depending on the size of the annulus (Fig. 35-5). Suture guides are very helpful in keeping these many sutures organized. The device is parachuted down into the root and the sutures tied and cut. The right and left sinuses are scalloped out either before or after this step (Fig. 35-6). A distal suture line of continuous small (4-0) caliber polypropylene suture is then constructed coursing below the coronary ostia, taking care not to buckle the stentless tissue or distort the positions of the commissural posts. Stay sutures can be placed at the top of each commissure to help maintain orientation. One suture is begun at the bottom of the left and another at the bottom of the right sinus and run up to the top of each commissure (Fig. 35-7). The porcine tissue and especially the cloth-covered portion of some devices must not encroach on the ostium of either coronary, because obstructive granulation tissue may form in this location. The top of the device is trimmed down to the level of the native aorta, taking care to stay above the top of each commissure. If the noncoronary sinus of the stentless valve is kept intact, the distal suture line can be completed by running along the top to join the two sutures. The aortotomy is closed with continuous suture incorporating the tops of the commissures and the retained noncoronary sinus edge. The completed concept of the complete and modified subcoronary implant technique is shown in Figs. 35-8 and 35-9.

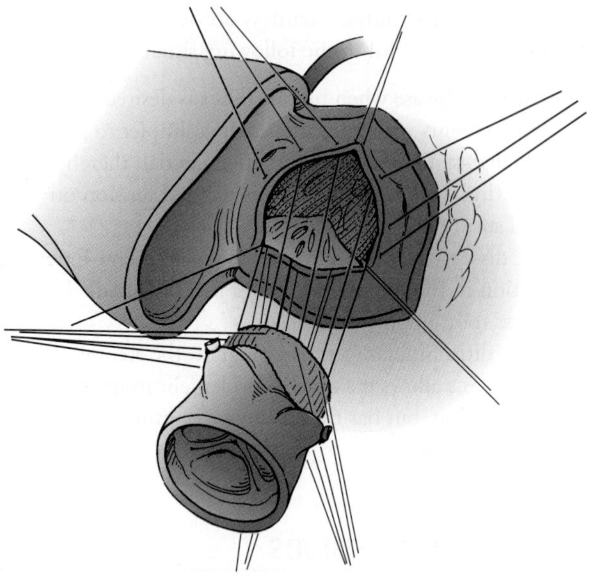

FIGURE 35-5 Modified subcoronary technique—proximal suture line. Interrupted sutures are placed in a circular plane coursing through the annulus itself at the lowest point of each sinus, but well below the commissures except anteriorly where the conduction system must be avoided. These are best organized on suture guides using alternating colors, then divided in thirds and passed through the inflow end of the stentless valve. (*Modified and reproduced, with permission, from Kon ND, Westaby S, Amarasena N, et al: Comparison of implantation techniques using Freestyle stentless porcine aortic valve. Ann Thorac Surg 1995; 59:857.*)

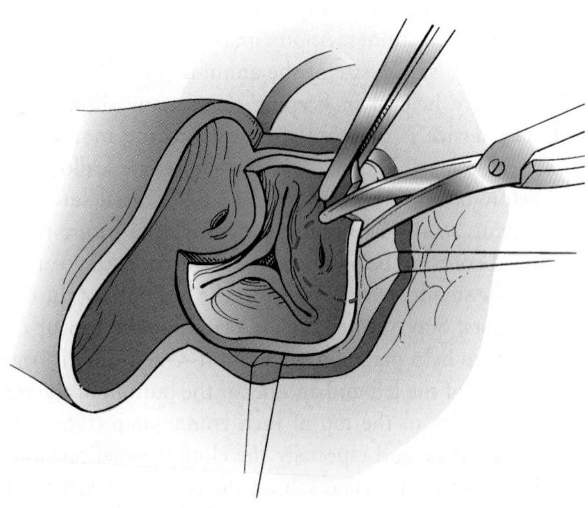

FIGURE 35-6 Modified subcoronary technique—preparing the sinuses. Either before or after the device is slid down and the proximal sutures tied, the sinuses facing the native left and right coronary ostia are scalloped out below the level of those recipient coronaries. Care is taken to avoid cutting into any cloth covering or getting too close to the leaflets of the new valve. (*Modified and reproduced, with permission, from Kon ND, Westaby S, Amarasena N, et al: Comparison of implantation techniques using Freestyle stentless porcine aortic valve. Ann Thorac Surg 1995; 59:857.*)

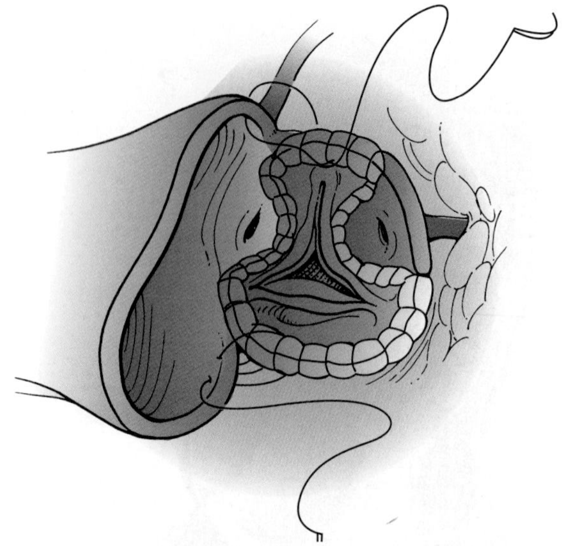

FIGURE 35-7 Modified subcoronary technique—distal suture line. A continuous 4-0 polypropylene suture is begun at the bottom of each sinus below the coronary ostium. This is brought around and up to the top of the adjacent commissures, where the top of the device is trimmed down to the level of the native aorta to allow completion of the suture line. This demonstrates the completed distal suture line and beginning of the aortic closure, which incorporates the tops of the commissures again as well as the top of the retained noncoronary sinus. (*Modified and reproduced, with permission, from Kon ND, Westaby S, Amarasena N, et al: Comparison of implantation techniques using Freestyle stentless porcine aortic valve. Ann Thorac Surg 1995; 59:857.*)

An expanding hematoma in the space between the native and the porcine noncoronary sinus walls is undesirable, but a small, fixed collection in this area usually resorbs over time. One technique to minimize this problem is to rotate the Freestyle root 120 degrees to put the porcine right coronary stump in the patient's noncoronary sinus. A small cut in the sinus allows the porcine stump to be extruded to the outside of the native

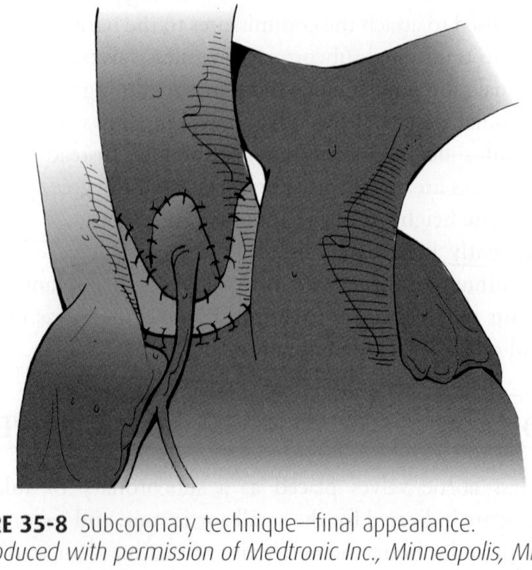

FIGURE 35-8 Subcoronary technique—final appearance. (*Reproduced with permission of Medtronic Inc., Minneapolis, MN.*)

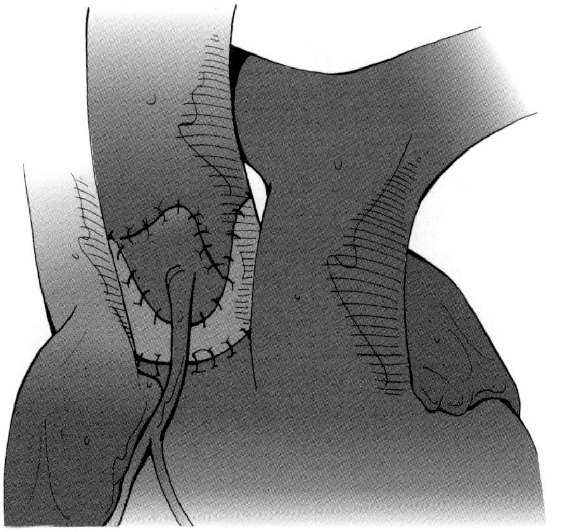

FIGURE 35-9 Modified subcoronary technique—final appearance. (*Reproduced with permission of Medtronic Inc., Minneapolis, MN.*)

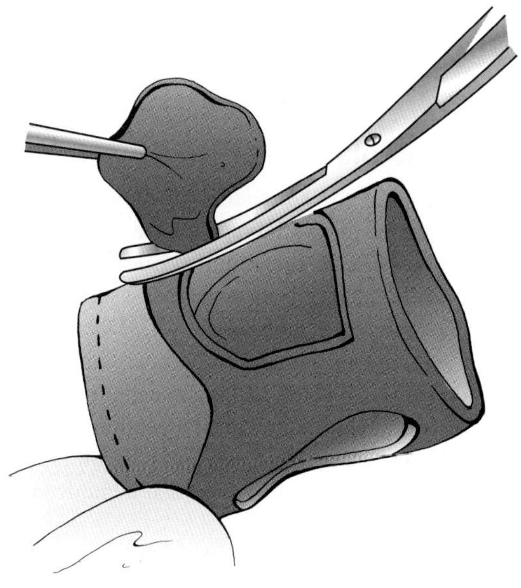

FIGURE 35-10 Root inclusion technique—trimming out sinuses. Very generous openings are made in the two appropriate sinuses facing the native coronaries without violating the sinotubular junction of the stentless valve. (*Modified and reproduced, with permission from Krause AH: Technique for complete subcoronary implantation of the Medtronic Freestyle porcine bioprosthesis. Ann Thorac Surg 1997; 64:1495.*)

sinus where it is secured with a pledgeted mattress suture of 4-0 polypropylene.

The subcoronary method has been preferred by most early adopters of the stentless valve because the first available, the Toronto SPV, was a completely scalloped device that required this method of implantation. In general, sizing and implantation of the subcoronary stentless valve is more prone to error compared with stented and full-root replacement operations. To assure valve competency, the recipient must have a normal ratio between annulus and ST junction diameter (<3 mm difference). Because relative dilatation of the ST junction can create valvular insufficiency, many surgeons choose a valve size based on this diameter, not the annular diameter. Sinus dilation can also cause insufficiency, but this would be unusual without concomitant ST junction effacement.

Oversizing of the stentless valve leads to higher transvalvular gradients. This is because of the compressible nature of the valve such that when placed in a fixed space such as the aortic root, excess tissue can lead to obstruction. Inflow buckling of the prosthesis may also lead to insufficiency and excessive turbulence. Undersizing leads to insufficiency by stretching of the prosthetic tissue with resultant loss of coaptation.

Root Inclusion

In an effort to completely preserve the three-dimensional geometry of the bioprosthetic root devices without completely replacing the native root, a minority of users have chosen to employ the root inclusion method. This involves a proximal suture line (continuous or interrupted) like the subcoronary technique in a circular plane coursing below the commissures. Generous openings are made by excising the sinuses facing the right and left main coronary ostia (Fig. 35-10). These are then tacked around the ostia much as a root inclusion Bentall procedure with continuous 4-0 polypropylene suture. The aortotomy is then closed in standard fashion after trimming the device top down as necessary to incorporate in the closure, making sure that the complete circle of the sinotubular junction is left intact. The only difference between the root inclusion method and the subcoronary technique is that the complete sinotubular ring of the stentless device is preserved, thus preventing any chance of dilatation at that level in the future. The top of the device is incorporated in the closure of the aortotomy (Fig. 35-11). Practically, this method is the most difficult and should not be used unless the root is large enough to place a 23-mm or larger device. It may, however, be the most desirable in a younger patient with a larger aortic root. The bioprosthetic sinotubular junction will not dilate over time, and at a subsequent

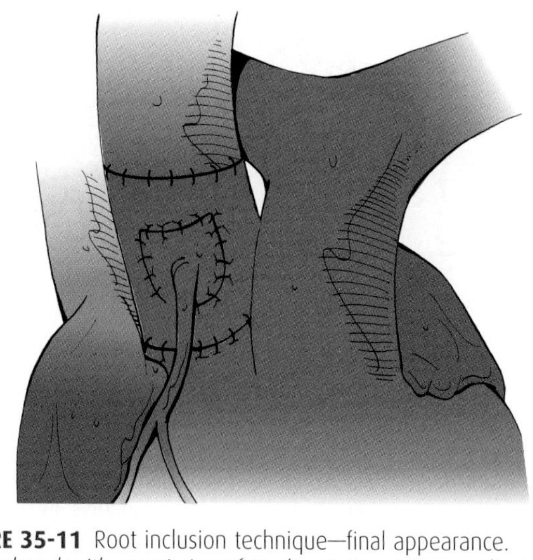

FIGURE 35-11 Root inclusion technique—final appearance. (*Reproduced with permission of Medtronic Inc., Minneapolis, MN.*)

operation, after gently removing this device, the entire native aortic root will be available for a complete range of replacement choices.

Full Root Replacement

Total replacement of the aortic root in most respects is the easiest and most reliable technique for stentless aortic valve replacement. Exposure of the annulus, calcified leaflets, and LV outflow tract is enhanced when the root is removed and the coronary ostia are mobilized out of the way. Decalcification of the annulus and aortomitral curtain becomes straightforward. Each suture is simple to place, making malalignment and poor bites of tissue less likely. Treatment of ascending aorta pathology with a Dacron tube graft extension becomes easy and logical. Perhaps most importantly, optimal hemodynamics are obtained.

The procedure begins with transection of the aorta just above the sinotubular junction (Fig. 35-12). Both coronary ostia are mobilized on generous buttons of aortic wall (Fig. 35-13). The remaining tissue of each sinus of Valsalva and the diseased aortic valve are excised. The valve is sized by identifying the largest sizer that will pass into the left ventricular cavity, then choosing one size larger valve so that the internal orifice of the prosthesis will match the left ventricular outflow tract diameter (Fig. 35-14). The proximal or inflow anastomosis is accomplished using 28 to 35 simple interrupted sutures of 3-0 braided Dacron tied around a 3-mm strip of Teflon felt (Fig. 35-15). The sutures are placed in a single plane in the left ventricular outflow tract to conform to the round inflow of the prosthesis. The coronary arteries on their buttons of aortic wall are sewn end-to-side to the corresponding sinus of Valsalva of the bioprosthesis with a continuous 5-0 polypropylene suture (Fig. 35-16). The distal end of the bioprosthesis is sewn end-to-end to the aorta with a continuous 5-0 polypropylene suture to complete the root replacement (Fig. 35-17).

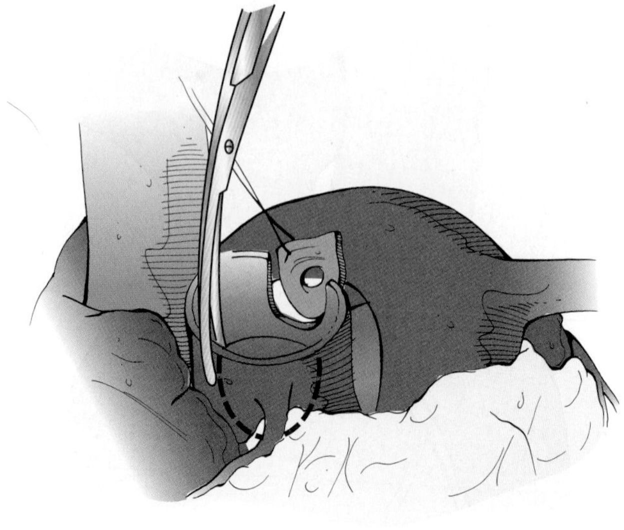

FIGURE 35-13 The coronary arteries are mobilized on generous buttons of aorta. A traction suture at the top of the button helps to maintain orientation.

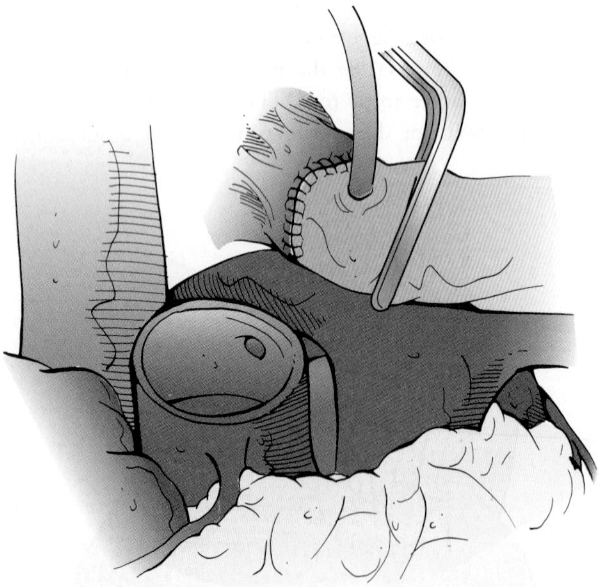

FIGURE 35-12 Placement of the stentless valve as a total root replacement begins with complete transaction of the aorta approximately 3-mm above the sinotubular junction. In this drawing, the ascending aorta has been replaced with a prosthetic graft.

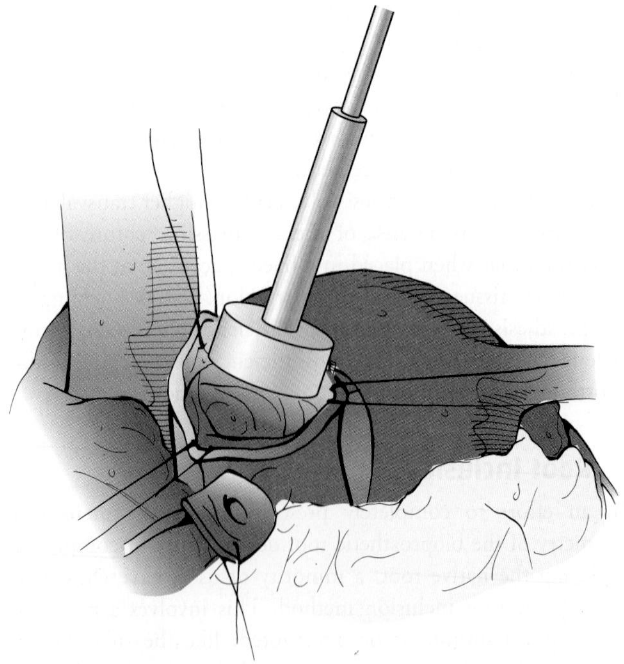

FIGURE 35-14 After excising the remaining tissue of each sinus of Valsalva and the diseased aortic valve, the valve is sized. After identifying the largest size that will pass into the left ventricular cavity, the valve chosen should be one size larger valve so that the internal orifice of the prosthesis will match the left ventricular outflow tract diameter. This will allow the entire orifice of the prosthesis to be exposed to the left ventricular outflow tract.

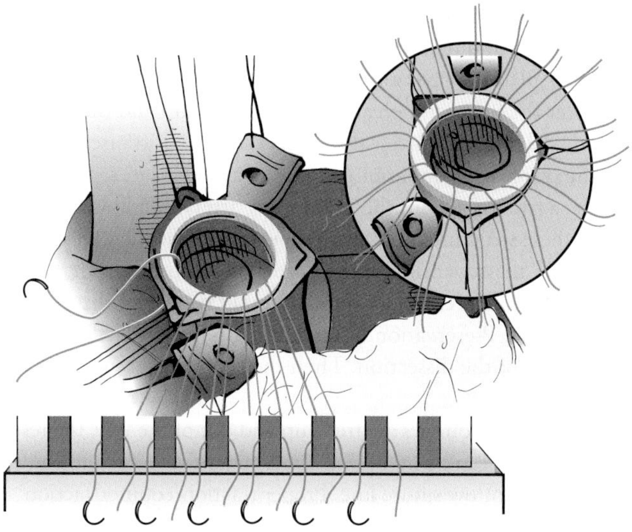

FIGURE 35-15 Valve sutures of 3-0 braided polyester are then placed in simple fashion through the LV outflow tract and around a narrow (approximately 3 mm) felt strip, which helps with hemostasis. The typical number of valve sutures used usually varies between 28 and 32. Use of suture guides simplifies placement and organization.

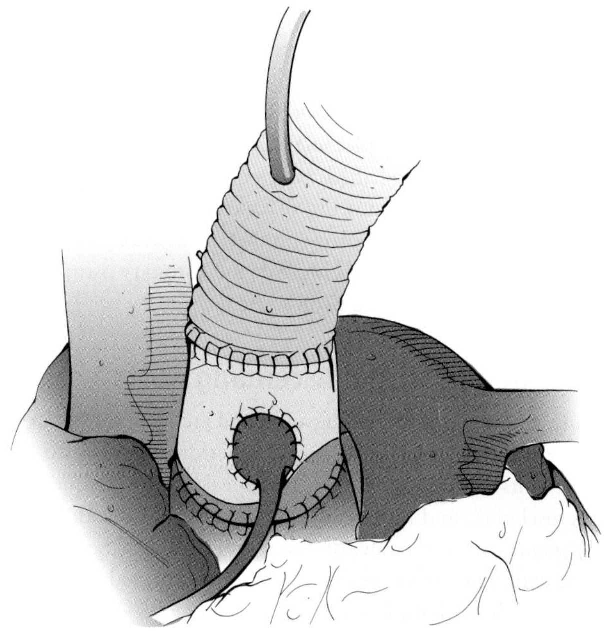

FIGURE 35-17 The native ascending aorta or vascular graft is then trimmed to appropriate level, and an end-to-end anastomosis is constructed using running monofilament suture.

TIPS AND PITFALLS FOR STENTLESS AORTIC ROOT REPLACEMENT

Coronary Alignment

To correctly align the coronary buttons on the porcine full root prosthesis, the similarities and differences between human and porcine aortic root anatomy must be appreciated. The anatomy between the two roots is similar in that the left main arises from the middle of the left sinus of Valsalva with similar heights from the annulus in both human and pig. Also similar to both roots, the right coronary artery is situated slightly higher (more distal) above the annulus. The right coronary artery arises closer to the left coronary in the pig compared with the human. Specifically, porcine coronary arteries are oriented approximately 90 to 110 degrees apart compared with human coronaries, which normally lie 140 to 160 degrees apart, but up to 180 degrees apart in patients with truly bicuspid valves. Practically, this means that the porcine root will need to be rotated 120 degrees during implantation in most situations, so that the porcine noncoronary sinus will be used for reimplantation of either the right or left coronary artery. Flexibility is crucial during coronary alignment, given the inherent anatomic differences seen between patients and prostheses. Native orientation and height must be maintained to prevent coronary insufficiency, an unusual event that most commonly involves the right coronary artery.[18] Signs of right coronary insufficiency include right ventricular dilatation, EKG changes, and otherwise unexplained arrhythmias. Frequently, these findings are only present upon ventricular filling, which may exacerbate a kinked or malaligned proximal right coronary artery. Saphenous vein grafting without repeat cross clamping should be liberally performed if there is any unexplained ventricular abnormality that prevents easy wean from cardiopulmonary bypass.

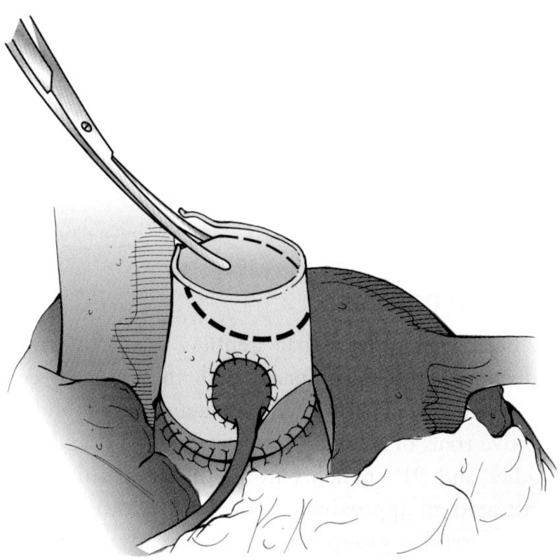

FIGURE 35-16 The coronary buttons are then sewn to the bioprosthesis using running 5-0 monofilament suture, taking care to maintain proper orientation. Excess tissue from the distal end of the bioprosthesis is removed, with more taken from the lesser curve of the ascending aorta to help reproduce its natural contour.

Calcified Coronary Buttons

Severe calcification of the sinuses of Valsalva is often cited as a contraindication to total root replacement. Typically, this calcification will not be isolated to the sinuses, and traditional stented or mechanical valves are often difficult to place as well, with higher risks of paravalvular leak, bleeding from anastomoses, and coronary dissection. With appropriate recognition and button management, severe root calcification is often best managed with total root replacement, which allows for the most effective removal of calcified and poor quality tissue. Tailoring button size to avoid suturing of calcified sinus tissue is one option to facilitate reimplantation, as is ligation and bypass grafting. Usually, endarterectomy of the coronary ostium must be performed to achieve a hemostatic ligation.

Pathology of the Ascending Aorta

Replacement of the ascending aorta and arch is a natural extension of full root replacement and is performed in up to 55% of patients in large series.[10,19] This speaks to the frequency of atherosclerotic and aneurysmal changes of the ascending aorta in patients with aortic valve disease. Replacement of the ascending aorta with a prosthetic graft, even when performed with a brief period of hypothermic circulatory arrest, adds no additional morbidity or mortality.[20]

Bleeding

Increased risk of bleeding complications is often cited as a reason to avoid total root replacement. Bleeding can occur from any of the four suture lines, but is uncommon when adequate resection of calcified tissue is performed. We have found that placement of an interrupted proximal suture line as described along with careful inspection of the coronary button anastomoses has made bleeding complications less frequent than might be expected. Bleeding from the proximal suture line is usually not manifest until the left ventricle is ejecting, and usually requires reclamping of the aorta, especially early in a surgeon's experience. Coronary buttons may need to be removed to access proximal suture lines in these locations. Other potential areas of bleeding include the right ventricle underneath the right coronary button, and small venous or arterial branches on the adventitia of the mobilized left coronary artery or medial aspect of the main or right pulmonary artery.

Reoperation

Reoperation for a failed stentless bioprosthesis can be challenging. We believe that a full root replacement for the reoperation is preferable if the root or sinuses are extensively calcified. If the reoperation is performed early, ie, for a paravalvular leak with a subcoronary implant, a prosthesis can be inserted inside the previously placed valve after leaflet removal. However, most patients with degenerated calcified aortic root prostheses will be best served with redo total root replacement.

Technical Tips to Facilitate Redo Total Root Replacement

1. Preoperative cardiac CT scan. This tells you the location within the mediastinum of any previous coronary bypass grafts. Knowledge of how close vascular structures reside to the underside of the sternum simplifies the process of reopening the sternum. The presence or absence of coronary anomalies or atherosclerotic vascular disease also helps plan the operation.
2. After the heart and great vessels are freed up and the aorta is cross clamped to arrest the heart, the aorta is transected at the prior distal anastomosis. Next one begins to separate the aortic root from the pulmonary artery. If adherence of these structures is excessive, one can develop a safer plane within the adventitia of the degenerated porcine root.
3. The left main coronary button should be re-mobilized at this time. Preservation of the left main button facilitates the rest of the dissection. Then the right main button is mobilized.
4. Once the coronaries are freed up and out of the way, the rest of the root can be mobilized circumferentially down to the previous inflow suture line. Proper traction/countertraction simplifies this dissection.
5. At this point one can simply cut the rest of the old aortic root out at its junction with the left ventricular outflow tract out.

The surgical field is now ready for the new total root replacement.

RESULTS OF STENTLESS AORTIC VALVE REPLACEMENT

Evaluating the short and long term outcomes of stentless valves in the literature is difficult for several reasons: many manufactured valves are no longer in clinical use; long-term data is scarce; there exists little randomized prospective data comparing stentless versus stented valves; studies generally mix various AVR indications together (patients with root pathology differ from those with a small annulus undergoing stentless valves for avoidance of patient-prosthesis mismatch); and most importantly, the majority of studies on stentless valves include both subcoronary and full root implants together in the "stentless" arm. This results in a heterogeneous population undergoing surgery for differing indications, by surgeons with bias towards one technique over another, and using techniques that can result in vastly different hemodynamic and potentially long-term results.

Hemodynamics

It has been well proven that stentless valves offer superior hemodynamic profiles compared with their stented counterparts. Kunadian et al performed a meta-analysis of randomized, prospective trials of stentless versus stented AVR and included 10 studies and 919 patients from European centers.[21] They demonstrated an approximately 6-mm Hg lower peak gradient for the stentless group, but no survival advantage at 1 year. Importantly, the vast majority of the stentless valves were implanted by subcoronary technique. As a full root replacement, stentless valve hemodynamics compare favorably to homografts, with nonsignificant differences in mean gradients reported between the two prostheses.[22] Freedom from aortic insufficiency and degenerative changes also favors the Freestyle root over the homograft.[23] Compared with subcoronary implantation, stentless full root replacement achieves lower gradients, larger effective orifice area, and greater freedom from at least moderate aortic insufficiency after 10 years of follow up.[9] Studies on the subcoronary implant technique have consistently shown a decrease in gradient and increase in EOA over time. Early and late gradients are both low for total root replacement and generally do not change over time. This discrepancy is most likely related to absorption of hematoma in the potential space between the porcine and native aortic walls, which occurs when performing a subcoronary implant.

Reverse Remodeling and Survival

Regardless of valve substitute, AVR in patients with severe, symptomatic AS consistently results in improvements in both structural and clinical outcome compared with medical treatment. However, long-term survival after AVR remains lower than age-matched populations, for known and unknown reasons.[24-26] Known factors related to higher death rates include bleeding with anticoagulation required for mechanical valves, thrombotic complications, endocarditis, and structural valve degeneration. Additionally, in patients with advanced myocardial damage and fibrosis, AVR would not be expected to allow for complete reverse remodeling, and lower long-term survival in this condition is intuitive. Indeed, low preoperative ejection fraction is perhaps the strongest predictor of long-term outcome.[27,28] In patients with less advanced structural disease, however, incomplete reverse remodeling of the pressure overload state is an unknown prognostic variable. Even seven years after AVR with stented or mechanical valves, increased muscle fiber diameter and percent interstitial fibrosis compared with normal is observed,[29] possibly because of persistent prosthetic LV obstruction and residual gradient.

To overcome the problem of residual gradient after AVR, stentless valves have been proposed as ideal for allowing reverse remodeling to occur. Using LV mass as the predominant surrogate marker, multiple small randomized and nonrandomized studies have attempted to assess for differences in reverse remodeling after AVR with different valve substitutes. Although demonstrating conflicting results, regression of LV mass does appear to be associated with achieving valvular competence and a low transvalvular gradient, regardless of prosthetic choice, and with treatment of postoperative hypertension.[30] The ASSERT trial[31] is one of the few randomized studies comparing the effects of stented versus stentless AVR on LV mass. In this study performed in Europe, 190 patients with aortic annulus size ≤25 mm were randomized to receive a Medtronic stented Mosaic porcine prosthesis or Medtronic stentless Freestyle prosthesis, implanted using a subcoronary technique. After one year, both groups demonstrated similar reductions in LV mass despite significant differences in effective orifice areas and flow velocities in favor of the stentless valves. Operative and postoperative clinical outcomes were also similar. A significant weaknesses of the study, however, was the use of the subcoronary technique for implantation of the stentless valve, which leads to higher gradients, more aortic insufficiency, and higher rates of late valve failure compared with the total root technique.[9,32] Additionally, one year follow-up may be an inadequate time to detect for differences in LV hypertrophy, because changes in LV geometry occur over many years after AVR.[33,34] This concept is supported by a small, randomized study of stented versus stentless valves that found no difference in LV mass regression at 6 months but a significant difference in favor of the stentless valve at 32 months.[35] The most recent large randomized study compared Edwards Lifesciences stented and nonstented subcoronary prostheses in 161 patients and again demonstrated similar reductions in LV mass at 1 year. However, in patients with LV ejection fraction less than 60%, subsequent improvement in ejection fraction was greater in the stentless group.[36] Because of these conflicting data, some have questioned the overall clinical importance of LV mass regression after AVR. Despite the known adverse prognostic implication of LV hypertrophy in the population as a whole, and importance of regression with treatment of hypertension, it has not been conclusively determined that regression after AVR correlates with survival.[37]

Gender issues are important to the topic of remodeling in aortic stenosis. For example, left ventricular adaptation to severe aortic stenosis is gender specific, with less compensatory increase in LV mass and wall tension in females compared with males.[38,39] Perhaps a better indicator of hypertrophy is the LV mass/volume ratio, a parameter that is increased in women with aortic stenosis compared with men.[39,40] Consequently, women with aortic stenosis tend to have worse diastolic function and exercise capacity compared with men.[41] Patient-prosthesis mismatch (PPM) is also more common in women and refers to implantation of a valve too small for a patient's size. Although PPM is generally defined as an in vivo effective orifice area indexed to body surface area (EOAI) of ≤ 0.75 to 0.85 cm^2/m^2,[42] EOAI may be preferentially evaluated on a continuum, similar to native aortic valve stenosis. Depending on definition, PPM is present in 20 to 60% of patients after AVR.[43-45] EOAI incorporates both size and functional considerations because postoperative gradients (ie, persistent LV pressure-overload state) are related to the area available for blood to leave the LV and to flow, or cardiac output in this instance, which correlates well with body size. Although controversial,[46-48] the preponderance of data, all retrospective, suggests that the presence of PPM is associated with reduced mid- and long-term survival.[45,49-54] Techniques to prevent PPM include annular enlargement procedures and implantation of stentless valves.

Durability

History teaches a good lesson in the story of the Toronto SPV stentless valve. Pioneered by David, this was the first prosthesis widely available for use. The Toronto SPV was designed to be implanted only by subcoronary technique. Numerous reports identified the hemodynamic advantages over stented valves, and remarkably, David reported improved survival over stented valves in midterm follow-up.[55] At 9 years, durability and hemodynamics were found to be excellent, with 90% freedom from structural failure.[56] At 12 years, however, freedom from structural valve degeneration was only 69%, and only 52% for patients under 65 years of age at time of implant.[57] Freedom from moderate or severe aortic insufficiency was only 48% for the group as a whole. The mechanism for this finding was postulated to be dilatation of the sinotubular junction, and such a mechanism could theoretically affect late results of any subcoronary stentless valve. In a group of mostly subcoronary Freestyle implants, however, Bach et al reported 92% freedom from structural degeneration at 12 years with equivalent rates in patients less than 60 years of age at the time of implant.[58] One possible explanation, although not proven, for the discrepancy between SPV and Freestyle longevity is that most Freestyles have been implanted with the modified subcoronary technique compared with complete subcoronary for the Toronto SPV. The preservation of two commissural posts may create more sinotubular junction stability over time. In general, though, the lessons to be learned from the SPV data are that all valves are not created equal, even when implanted in similar manners, and that long-term and ongoing follow up is required to assess for durability because all bioprosthetic valves will eventually fail.

Operative Risk

Contemporary series of patients implanted with stentless valves do not support a higher operative risk, even with total root replacement. It is clear that the procedure requires slightly longer aortic cross-clamp and CPB times,[21] but this has not translated into higher mortality. Florath et al examined factors related to operative mortality in 1400 patients undergoing AVR, and neither stentless nor stented valve use was found to be predictive.[12]

CONCLUSIONS

As newer valve designs continue to be introduced to the market, ease and safety of implantation will continue to dominate as factors important for patients and surgeons. Closely followed in importance will be hemodynamic performance and durability. With the advent of transcatheter aortic valves, the bar will be set high for both implantation ease and hemodynamics. Already, effective orifice areas for first generation transcatheter valves exceeds those for 3rd generation stented bioprostheses,[59] albeit at the expense of trace-to-moderate aortic regurgitation. This issue will continue to drive the debate over the importance of patient-prosthesis mismatch. In the coming years, these issues may also highlight the hemodynamic advantages of stentless valves over stented and may also define the importance of different valves as platforms for performing transcatheter valve-in-valve implantation. Stentless total roots may have an advantage over other aortic valve prostheses in this setting given the larger orifices and root anatomy that is equivalent to the anatomy used during transcatheter valve development.

In summary, the stentless aortic valve, when implanted as a total root replacement, is an undeniably important tool for management of aortic root pathology. The debate continues, however, over the use of stentless valves in the absence of root pathology. Given that survival and functional outcomes often remain impaired after AVR for aortic stenosis, and that this suboptimal outcome appears to coincide with incomplete reverse remodeling of the left ventricle, surgeons should continue to seek the best option for long-term quantity and quality of life. Placement of larger valve substitutes intuitively will result in lower residual transvalvular gradients and may allow for better myocardial structural and functional outcomes. Use of stentless valves optimally achieves these surgical goals and may be appropriate for broader applications.

KEY POINTS

- The indication for subcoronary or modified subcoronary stentless AVR is for prevention of patient-prosthesis mismatch and can be considered an alternative to annular enlargement procedures.
- Stentless valves placed as full roots maximize the hemodynamic advantages of stentless technology and can be placed without excess mortality.
- Stentless valves placed as full roots are an excellent alternative to homografts when a bioprosthesis is desired for treatment of aortic root pathology.
- Long-term data on currently available stentless valves reveals acceptable rates of structural degeneration.
- Tips for successful stentless root replacement include paying close attention to coronary alignment, interrupted proximal suture line, complete resection of calcified or poor quality tissue, and close inspection of coronary button suture lines.
- All stentless valves are not the same. Various techniques are utilized for implantation resulting in heterogeneous populations for different indications with different valves by surgeons with bias towards one technique over another. The result is vastly different hemodynamic profiles and long term outcomes.

REFERENCES

1. Sensky PR, Loubani M, Keal RP, Samani NJ, Sosnowski AW, et al: Does the type of prosthesis influence early left ventricular mass regression after aortic valve replacement? Assessment with magnetic resonance imaging. *Am Heart J* 2003; 146:e13.
2. Maselli D, Pizio R, Bruno LP, Di Bella I, De Gasperix C: Left ventricular mass reduction after aortic valve replacement: homografts, stentless and stented valves. *Ann Thorac Surg* 1999; 67:966-971.
3. Walther T, Falk V, Langebartels G, Kruger M, Bernhardt U, et al: Prospectively randomized evaluation of stentless versus conventional biological aortic valves: impact on early regression of left ventricular hypertrophy. *Circulation* 1999; 100:II6-10.
4. Jin XY, Zhang ZM, Gibson DG, Yacoub MH, Pepper JR: Effects of valve substitute on changes in left ventricular function and hypertrophy after aortic valve replacement. *Ann Thorac Surg* 1996; 62:683-690.
5. Thomson HL, O'Brien MF, Almeida AA, Tesar PJ, Davison MB, et al: Haemodynamics and left ventricular mass regression: a comparison of the stentless, stented and mechanical aortic valve replacement. *Eur J Cardiothorac Surg* 1998; 13:572-575.
6. Yun KL, Jamieson WR, Khonsari S, Burr LH, Munro AI, et al: Prosthesis-patient mismatch: hemodynamic comparison of stented and stentless aortic valves. *Semin Thorac Cardiovasc Surg* 1999; 11:98-102.
7. Luciani GB, Casali G, Auriemma S, Santini F, Mazzucco A: Survival after stentless and stented xenograft aortic valve replacement: a concurrent, controlled trial. *Ann Thorac Surg* 2002; 74:1443-1449.
8. Casali G, Auriemma S, Santini F, Mazzucco A, Luciani GB: Survival after stentless and stented xenograft aortic valve replacement: a concurrent, case-match trial. *Ital Heart J* 2004; 5:282-289.
9. Bach DS, Kon ND, Dumesnil JG, Sintek CF, Doty DB: Ten-year outcome after aortic valve replacement with the freestyle stentless bioprosthesis. *Ann Thorac Surg* 2005; 80:480-486.

10. Kon ND, Riley RD, Adair SM, Kitzman DW, Cordell AR: Eight-year results of aortic root replacement with the freestyle stentless porcine aortic root bioprosthesis. *Ann Thorac Surg* 2002; 73:1817-1821.
11. Westaby S, Katsumata T, Vaccari G: Aortic root replacement with coronary button re-implantation: low risk and predictable outcome. *Eur J Cardiothorac Surg* 2000; 17:259-565.
12. Florath I, Rosendahl UP, Mortasawi A, Bauer SF, Dalladaku F, et al: Current determinants of operative mortality in 1400 patients requiring aortic valve replacement. *Ann Thorac Surg* 2003; 76:75-83.
13. Sonnad SS, Bach DS, Bolling SF, Armstrong WF, Pagani FD, et al: The impact of new technology on a clinical practice. *Semin Thorac Cardiovasc Surg* 1999; 11:79-82.
14. Vesely I: Effects of "zero- pressure" fixation. Analysis of the Medtronic Intact bioprosthetic valve. *J Thorac Cardiovasc Surg* 1991; 101:90-99.
15. Christie GW, Gross JF, Eberhardt CE: Fatigue-induced changes to the biaxial mechanical properties of glutaraldehyde-fixed porcine aortic valve leaflets. *Semin Thorac Cardiovasc Surg* 1999; 11(4 Suppl 1):201-205.
16. El-Hamamsy I, Zaki M, Stevens LM, Clark LA, Rubens M, et al: Rate of progression and functional significance of aortic root calcification after homograft versus freestyle aortic root replacement. *Circulation* 2009; 120(11 Suppl):S269-275.
17. Linneweber J, Kossagk C, Rogge ML, Dushe S, Dohmen P, et al: Clinical experience with the 3F stentless aortic bioprosthesis: one-year follow up. *J Heart Valve Dis* 2006; 15(4):545-548.
18. Kincaid EH, Cordell, AR, Hammon JW, Adair SM, Kon ND: Coronary insufficiency after stentless aortic root replacement: risk factors and solutions. *Ann Thorac Surg* 2007; 83:964-968.
19. Gleason TG, David TE, Coselli JS, Hammon JW Jr, Bavaria JE: St. Jude Medical Toronto biologic aortic root prosthesis: early FDA phase II IDE study results. *Ann Thorac Surg* 2004; 78:786-793.
20. Reece TB, Singh RR, Stiles BM, Peeler BB, Kern JA, et al: Replacement of the proximal aorta adds no further risk to aortic valve procedures. *Ann Thorac Surg* 2007; 84(2):473-478.
21. Kunadian B, Vijayalakshmi K, Thornley AR, et al: Meta-analysis of valve hemodynamics and left ventricular mass regression for stentless versus stented aortic valves. *Ann Thorac Surg* 2007; 84:73-79.
22. Melina G, De Robertis F, Gaer JA, Amrani M, Khaghani A, et al: Mid-term pattern of survival, hemodynamic performance and rate of complications after medtronic freestyle versus homograft full aortic root replacement: results from a prospective randomized trial. *J Heart Valve Dis* 2004; 13(6): 972-975.
23. El-Hamamsy I, Clark L, Stevens LM, Sarang Z, Melina G, et al: Late outcomes following freestyle versus homograft aortic root replacement results from a prospective randomized trial. *J Am Coll Cardiol* 2010; 55(4): 368-376.
24. Ruel M, Kulik A, Lam BK, Rubens FD, Hendry PJ, et al: Long-term outcomes of valve replacement with modern prostheses in young adults. *Eur J Cardiothorac Surg* 2005; 27:425-433.
25. Blackstone EH, Kirklin JW: Death and other time-related events after valve replacement. *Circulation* 1985; 72:753-767.
26. McGiffin DC, O'Brien MF, Galbraith AJ, McLachlan GJ, Stafford EG, et al: An analysis of risk factors for death and mode-specific death after aortic valve replacement with allograft, xenograft and mechanical valves. *J Thorac Cardiovasc Surg* 1993; 106:895-911.
27. Lund O, Flo C, Jensen FT, et al: Left ventricular systolic and diastolic function in aortic stenosis. Prognostic value after valve replacement and underlying mechanisms. *Eur Heart J* 1997; 18:1977-1987.
28. Connolly HM, Oh JK, Orszulak TA, et al: Aortic valve replacement for aortic stenosis with severe left ventricular dysfunction. Prognostic indicators. *Circulation* 1997; 95:2395-2400.
29. Krayenbuehl HP, Hess OM, Monrad ES, Schneider J, Mall G, et al: Left ventricular myocardial structure in aortic valve disease before, intermediate, and late after aortic valve replacement. *Circulation* 1989; 79:744-755.
30. Imanaka K, Kohmoto O, Nishimura S, Yokote Y, Kyo S: Impact of post-operative blood pressure control on regression of left ventricular mass following valve replacement for aortic stenosis. *Eur J Cardiothorac Surg* 2005; 27:994-999.
31. Perez de Arenaza D, Lees B, Flather M, et al: Randomized comparison of stentless versus stented valves for aortic stenosis: effects on left ventricular mass. *Circulation* 2005; 112:2696-2702.
32. Bach DS et al: Freestyle Valve Study Group: Impact of implant technique following freestyle stentless aortic valve replacement. *Ann Thorac Surg* 2002; 74:1107-1113.
33. Lund O, Erlandsen M, Dorup I, Emmertsen K, Flo C, et al:. Predictable changes in left ventricular mass and function during ten years after valve replacement for aortic stenosis. *J Heart Valve Dis* 2004; 13:357-368.
34. Pela G, La Canna G, Metra M, Ceconi C, Berra Centurini P, et al: Long-term changes in left ventricular mass, chamber size and function after valve replacement in patients with severe aortic stenosis and depressed ejection fraction. *Cardiology* 1997; 88:315-322.
35. Williams RJ, Muir DF, Pathi V, MacArthur K, Berg GA: Randomized controlled trial of stented and stentless aortic bioprostheses: hemodynamic performance at 3 years. *Semin Thorac Cardiovasc Surg* 1999; 11:93-97.
36. Ali A, Halstead JC, Cafferty F, et al: Are stentless valves superior to modern stented valves? A prospective randomized trial. *Circulation* 2006; 114: I535-I540.
37. Gaudino M, Alessandrini F, Glieca F, et al: Survival after aortic valve replacement for aortic stenosis: does left ventricular mass regression have a clinical correlate? *Eur Heart J* 2005; 26:51-57.
38. Favero L, Giordan M, Tarantini G, Ramondo AB, Cardaioli P, et al: Gender differences in left ventricular function in patients with isolated aortic stenosis. *J Heart Valve Dis* 2003; 12:313-318.
39. Bech-Hanssen O, Wallentin I, Houltz E, Beckman Suurkula M, Larsson S, et al: Gender differences in patients with severe aortic stenosis: impact on preoperative left ventricular geometry and function, as well as early postoperative morbidity and mortality. *Eur J Cardiothorac Surg* 1999; 15: 24-30.
40. Rohde LE, Zhi G, Aranki SF, Beckel NE, Lee RT, et al: Gender-associated differences in left ventricular geometry in patients with aortic valve disease and effect of distinct overload subsets. *Am J Cardiol* 1997; 80:475-480.
41. Legget ME, Kuusisto J, Healy NL, Fujioka M, Schwaegler RG, et al: Gender differences in left ventricular function at rest and with exercise in asymptomatic aortic stenosis. *Am Heart J* 1996; 131:94-100.
42. Dumesnil JG, Pibarot P: Prosthesis-patient mismatch and clinical outcomes: the evidence continues to accumulate. *J Thorac Cardiovasc Surg* 2006; 131: 952-955.
43. Pibarot P, Dumesnil JG: Hemodynamic and clinical impact of prosthesis-patient mismatch in the aortic valve position and its prevention. *J Am Coll Cardiol* 2000; 36:1131-1141.
44. Ruel M, Al-Faleh H, Kulik A, Chan K, Mesana T, et al: Prosthesis–patient mismatch after aortic valve replacement predominantly affects patients with preexisting left ventricular dysfunction: effect on survival, freedom from heart failure, and left ventricular mass regression. *J Thorac Cardiovasc Surg* 2006; 131:1036-1044.
45. Blais C, Dumesnil JG, Baillot R, Simard S, Doyle D, et al: Impact of prosthesis-patient mismatch on short-term mortality after aortic valve replacement. *Circulation* 2003; 108:983-988.
46. Medalion B, Blackstone EH, Lytle BW, White J, Arnold JH, et al: Aortic valve replacement: is valve size important? *J Thorac Cardiovasc Surg* 2000; 119:963-974.
47. Howell NJ, Keogh BE, Barnet V, Bonser RS, Graham TR, et al: Patient-prosthesis mismatch does not affect survival following aortic valve replacement. *Eur J Cardiothorac Surg* 2006; 30:10-14.
48. Blackstone EH, Cosgrove DM, Jamieson WR, et al: Prosthesis size and long-term survival after aortic valve replacement. *J Thorac Cardiovasc Surg* 2003; 126:783-796.
49. Tasca G, Mhagna Z, Perotti S, et al: Impact of prosthesis-patient mismatch on cardiac events and midterm mortality after aortic valve replacement in patients with pure aortic stenosis. *Circulation* 2006; 113:570-576.
50. Rao V, Jamieson WRE, Ivanov J, Armstrong S, David TE: Prosthesis-patient mismatch affects survival following aortic valve replacement. *Circulation* 2000; 102:III5-III9.
51. Ruel M, Rubens FD, Masters RG, et al: Late incidence and predictors of persistent or recurrent heart failure in patients with aortic prosthetic valves. *J Thorac Cardiovas Surg* 2004; 127:149-159.
52. Walther T, Rastan A, Falk V, Lehmann S, Garbade J, et al: Patient prosthesis mismatch affects short- and long-term outcomes after aortic valve replacement. *Eur J Cardiothorac Surg* 2006; 30:15-19.
53. Mohty-Euhahidi D, Girard SE, Malouf JF, et al: Impact of prosthesis-patient mismatch on long-term survival in patients with small St Jude mechanical prosthesis in the aortic position. *Circulation* 2006; 113: 420-426.
54. Botzenhardt F, Eichinger WB, Bleiziffer S, Guenzinger R, Wagner IM, et al: Hemodynamic comparison of bioprostheses for complete supra-annular position in patients with small aortic annulus. *J Am Coll Cardiol* 2005; 45:2054-2060.
55. David TE, Puschmann R, Ivanov J, Bos J, Armstrong S, et al: Aortic valve replacement with stentless and stented porcine valves: a case-match study. *J Thorac Cardiovasc Surg* 1998; 116:236-241.
56. Bach DS, Goldman B, Verrier E, Petracek M, Wood J, et al: Durability and prevalence of aortic regurgitation nine years after aortic valve replacement with the Toronto SPV stentless bioprosthesis. *J Heart Valve Dis* 2004; 13(1):64-72.

57. David TE, Feindel CM, Bos J, Ivanov J, Armstrong S: Aortic valve replacement with Toronto SPV bioprosthesis: optimal patient survival but suboptimal valve durability. *J Thorac Cardiovasc Surg* 2008; 135(1): 19-24.
58. Bach DS, Metras J, Doty JR, Yun KL, Dumesnil JG, et al: Freedom from structural valve deterioration among patients aged < or = 60 years undergoing Freestyle stentless aortic valve replacement. *J Heart Valve Dis* 2007; 16: 649-655.
59. Clavel MA, Webb JG, Pibarot P, Altwegg L, Dumont E, et al: Comparison of the hemodynamic performance of percutaneous and surgical bioprostheses for the treatment of severe aortic stenosis. *J Am Coll Cardiol* 2009; 53(20):1883-1891.

CHAPTER 36

Aortic Valve Repair and Aortic Valve-Sparing Operations

Tirone E. David

FUNCTIONAL ANATOMY OF THE AORTIC VALVE

The aortic valve is a complex structure that is best described as a functional and anatomic unit, the aortic root. The aortic root has four components: aorto-ventricular junction or aortic annulus, aortic cusps, aortic sinuses, and sinotubular junction. In addition, the triangles beneath the commissures of the aortic valve, although part of the left ventricular outflow tract, are also important for valve function.

The aortic annulus unites the aortic cusps and aortic sinuses to the left ventricle. It is attached to ventricular myocardium (interventricular septum) in approximately 45% of its circumference and to fibrous structures (anterior leaflet of the mitral valve and membranous septum) in the remaining 55% (Fig. 36-1). The aortic annulus has a scalloped shape. Histologic examination of the aortic annulus reveals that it is a fibrous structure with strands attaching itself to the muscular interventricular septum and has a fibrous continuity with the mitral valve and membranous septum. The fibrous structure that separates the aortic annulus from the anterior leaflet of the mitral valve is the intervalvular fibrous body. An important structure immediately below the membranous septum is the bundle of His. The atrioventricular node lies in the floor of the right atrium between the annulus of the septal leaflet of the tricuspid valve and the coronary sinus. This node gives origin to the bundle of His, which travels through the right fibrous trigone along the posterior edge of the membranous septum to the muscular interventricular septum. At this point, the bundle of His divides into left and right bundle branches that extend subendocardially along both sides of the muscular interventricular septum.

The aortic cusps are attached to the aortic annulus in a scalloped fashion (see Fig. 36-1). The aortic cusps have a semilunar shape whereby the length of the base is approximately 1.5 times longer than the length of the free margin, as illustrated in Fig. 36-2. There are three cusps and three aortic sinuses: left, right, and noncoronary. The aortic sinuses are also referred to as sinuses of Valsalva. The left coronary artery arises from the left aortic sinus and the right coronary artery arises from the right aortic sinus. The left coronary artery orifice is closer to the aortic annulus than is the right coronary artery orifice. The highest point where two cusps meet is called the commissure, and it is located immediately below the sinotubular junction. The scalloped shape of the aortic annulus creates three triangular spaces underneath the commissures. The two triangles beneath the commissures of the noncoronary cusp are fibrous structures, whereas the triangular space beneath the commissure between the left and right cusps is mostly muscular. These three triangles are seen in Fig. 36-1. The aortic annulus evolves along three horizontal planes within a cylindrical structure. Thus, the annulus of each cusp inserts itself in the aortic root along a single horizontal plane. The sinotubular junction represents the end of the aortic root. It is an important component of the aortic root because the commissures of the aortic valve are immediately below it and changes in the diameter of the sinotubular junction affect the function of the aortic cusps.

The geometry of the aortic root and its anatomic components varies among individuals, but the geometry of these components is somewhat interrelated. For instance, the larger the aortic cusps, the larger are the diameters of the aortic annulus and sinotubular junction. The aortic cusps are semilunar (crescent shape) and their bases are attached to the annulus; the free margins extend from commissure to commissure, and the cusps coapt centrally during diastole. The size of the aortic cusps varies among individuals and within the same person, but as a rule the noncoronary cusp is slightly larger than the right and left. The left is usually the smallest of the three. Because of the crescent

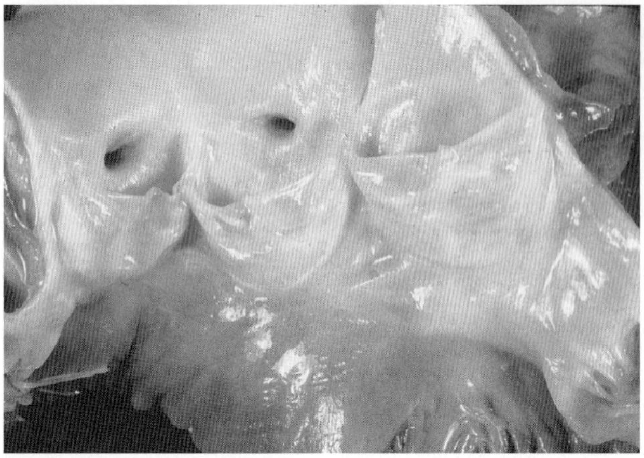

FIGURE 36-1 A photograph of a human left ventricular outflow tract and aortic root.

shape of the aortic cusps and the fact that their free margins extend from commissure to commissure, the diameter of the aortic valve orifice must be smaller than the length of the free margins. Indeed, anatomic studies of fresh human aortic roots demonstrated that the average length of the free margins of the aortic cusps was one-third longer than the diameter of the aortic orifice. The diameter of the aortic annulus is 15 to 20% larger than the diameter of the sinotubular junction in children, but this relationship changes with age and the diameter of the aortic annulus is often smaller than the diameter of aortic annulus in older persons (see Fig. 36-2).

The aortic annulus, the aortic cusps, and the sinotubular junction play an important role in maintaining valve competence. On the other hand, the aortic sinuses play no role in valve competence, but they are believed to be important in minimizing mechanical stress on the aortic cusps during the cardiac cycle by creating eddies currents between the cusps and the aortic sinuses.

All components of the aortic root are very elastic and compliant in children but compliance decreases with aging as elastic fibers are replaced by fibrous tissue. Expansion and contraction of the aortic annulus during the cardiac cycle are heterogeneous

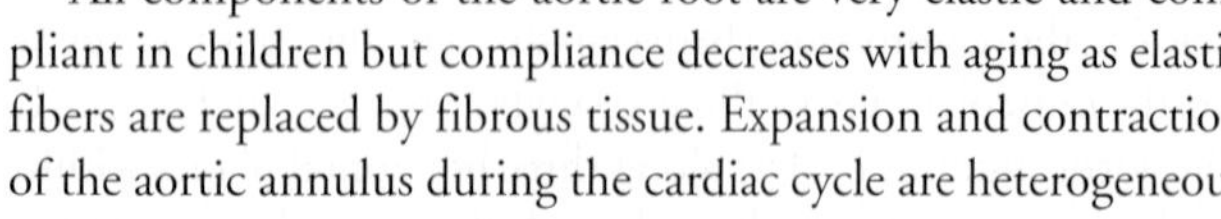

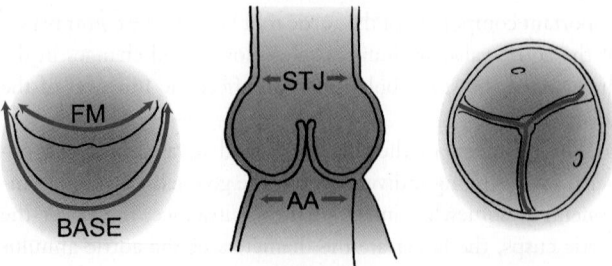

FIGURE 36-2 Geometric relationships of various components of the aortic root. The base of the aortic cusp is 1.5 times longer than its free margin. The diameter of the aortic annulus is 10 to 15% larger than the diameter of the sinotubular junction in children and young adults but it tends to become equal with aging. Three semilunar cusps seal the aortic orifice. The height of the cusps must be longer than the radius of the aortic annulus.

probably because of its attachments to contractile myocardium as well as to fibrous structures such as the membranous septum and intervalvular fibrous body. On the other hand, the expansion and contraction of the sinotubular junction are more uniform. The aortic root also displays some degree of torsion during isovolumic contraction and ejection of the left ventricle. The movements of the aortic annulus, cusps, sinuses, and sinotubular junction also change with aging as elastic fibers are replaced by fibrous tissue.

AORTIC VALVE PATHOLOGY

Anatomically normal aortic cusps may become calcified late in life and cause aortic stenosis. This type of lesion is called dystrophic calcification, senile calcification, or degenerative calcification. The range of histopathologic lesions includes calcification, chondroid and osseous metaplasia, neorevascularization, inflammation, and lipid deposition.

Bicuspid aortic valve is believed to occur in 1 to 2% of the population. Movahed and colleagues[1] recently reviewed the echocardiograms of 24,265 patients who had the study for various clinical reasons and 1742 teenage athletes in Southern California, and found a prevalence of bicuspid aortic valve of 0.6% in the large cohort and 0.5% in the smaller one. Males are affected more than females at a ratio of 4:1. There is a relatively high incidence of familial clustering, which suggests an autosomal dominant inheritance with reduced penetrance.[2] Extensive research in the genetics of bicuspid aortic valve is being presently conducted and this disorder is likely heritable. Most patients with bicuspid aortic valve have three aortic sinuses and two cusps of different sizes. The larger cusp often contains a raphe instead of a commissure. The raphe extends from the mid portion of the cusp to the aortic annulus, and its insertion in the aortic root is at a lower level than the other two commissures. Bicuspid aortic valves with two aortic sinuses and no raphe are least common and called "type 0"; the most common is with one raphe and is called "type 1"; and finally with two raphes is "type 2."[3] Types 1 and 2 can be subclassified according to the fused cusps: L-R is the most common form (a raphe in between the left and right cusps). Most patients with bicuspid aortic valves have a dominant circumflex artery and a small right coronary artery. Bicuspid aortic valve may function satisfactorily until late in life when it may become calcified and stenotic.[4] It may also become incompetent, particularly in younger patients and is often associated with dilated aortic annulus and cusp prolapsed.

Other congenital anomalies of the aortic valve are the unicusp and quadricuspid valves. Subaortic membranous ventricular septal defect can cause aortic insufficiency because of distortion of the aortic annulus and prolapse of the right cusp.

Numerous connective tissue disorders (ankylosing spondylitis, osteogenesis imperfecta, rheumatoid arthritis, Reiter's syndrome, lupus, etc.) can cause aortic insufficiency. The anorexigenic drugs phentermine and fenfluramine can also cause aortic insufficiency. Rheumatic aortic valve disease is still prevalent in developing countries and can cause aortic stenosis and/or insufficiency by causing fusion, fibrosis, and contraction of the cusps.

AORTIC ROOT AND ASCENDING AORTA PATHOLOGY

Degenerative diseases of the media with aneurysm formation are the most common disorders of the aortic root and ascending aorta. A broad spectrum of pathologic and clinical entities is grouped under degenerative disorders, and it ranges from severe degeneration of the media, which can become clinically important early in life in cases such as Loyes-Dietz syndrome, to cases of the not so important mild dilation of the ascending aorta in elderly patients. Bicuspid and unicusp aortic valve disease often display premature degeneration of the media with dilation of the aorta. Atherosclerosis, infectious and noninfectious aortitis are other pathologic entities.

Aneurysms of the ascending aorta are often caused by cystic medial degeneration (cystic medial necrosis). Histologically, necrosis and disappearance of muscle cells in the elastic lamina, and cystic spaces filled with mucoid material are often observed. Although these changes occur more often in the ascending aorta, they may affect any portion or the entire aorta. These changes weaken the arterial wall, which dilates and forms a fusiform aneurysm. The aortic root may be involved in this pathologic process, and in patients with Marfan syndrome, the aneurysm usually begins in the aortic sinuses. A large proportion of patients with aortic root aneurysms do not fulfill the criteria of diagnosis of Marfan syndrome, but the gross appearance of the aneurysm and the histology of the arterial wall may be indistinguishable from that of Marfan syndrome. These cases are referred to as *forma frusta* of Marfan syndrome.

Patients with aortic root aneurysms are usually in their second or third decade of life when the diagnosis is made. These patients develop aortic insufficiency because of dilation of the sinotubular junction and/or aortic annulus (Fig. 36-3). Annuloaortic ectasia is a term used to describe dilation of the aortic annulus.

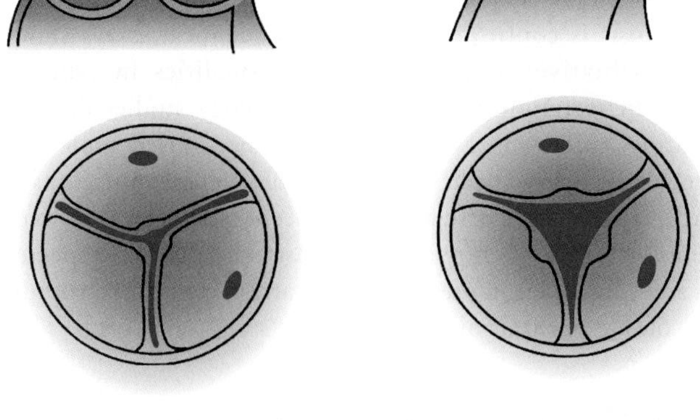

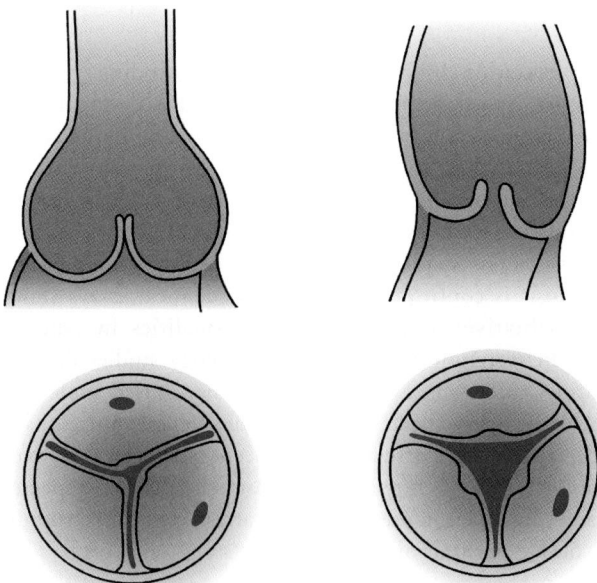

FIGURE 36-3 Dilation of the sinotubular junction causes aortic insufficiency because it displaces the commissures outward and prevents the cusps to coapt centrally.

Other patients have relatively normal aortic roots but develop ascending aortic aneurysms. These patients are usually in their fifth or sixth decade of life. Finally, certain patients have extensive degenerative disease of the entire aorta and develop the so-called mega-aorta syndrome with dilation of the entire thoracic and abdominal aorta. Ascending aortic aneurysm may cause dilation of the sinotubular junction with consequent aortic insufficiency (Fig. 36-3).

Marfan Syndrome

Marfan syndrome is an autosomal dominant variably penetrant inherited disorder of the connective tissue in which cardiovascular, skeletal, ocular, and other abnormalities may be present to a variable degree. The prevalence is estimated to be around 1 in 5000 individuals. It is caused by mutations in the gene that encodes fibrillin-1 (FBN1) on chromosome 15. This is a large gene (approximately 10,000 nucleotides in the mRNA), and identification of the mutation is a complex task. More than 1000 mutations in FBN1 have been identified. The phenotype presents a highly variable degree because of varying genotype expression.

The clinical features of Marfan syndrome were thought to be a result of weaker connective tissues caused by defects in fibrillin-1, a glycoprotein, and principal component of the extracellular matrix microfibril. This concept was inadequate to explain the overgrowth of long bones, osteopenia, reduced muscular mass, and adiposity and craniofacial abnormalities often seen in Marfan syndrome.[5] Dietz and colleagues[5,6] showed in an experimental mouse with Marfan syndrome that many findings are the result of abnormal levels of activation of tranforming growth factor beta (TGF-β), a potent stimulator of inflammation, fibrosis, and activation of certain matrix metalloproteinases, especially matrix metalloproteinases 2 and 9. Excess TGF-β activation in tissues correlates with failure of lung septation, development of a myxomatous mitral valve, and aortic root dilation in mice. This combination of structural microfibril matrix abnormality, dysregulation of matrix homestasis mediated by excess TGF-β, and abnormal cell-matrix interactions is responsible for the phenotype features of the Marfan syndrome. Ongoing destruction of the elastic and collagen lamelae and medial degeneration result in progressive dilation of the aortic root, as well as a predisposition to aortic dissection from the loss of appropriate medial layer support. Loss of elasticity in the media causes increased aortic stiffness and decreased distensibility.

The diagnosis of Marfan syndrome is made on clinical grounds, and it is not always simple because of the variability in clinical expression. A multidisciplinary approach is needed to diagnose and manage patients afflicted with this syndrome. Table 36-1 shows the criteria for the diagnosis of Marfan syndrome. The presence of major criteria in two separate systems and involvement of a third (minor or major) are needed to establish the diagnosis.[7]

The most common cardiovascular features are aortic root aneurysm and mitral valve prolapse. These anatomical abnormalities may cause aortic rupture, aortic dissection, aortic insufficiency, and mitral insufficiency.

TABLE 36-1 Diagnosis Criteria for Marfan Syndrome

Criteria	Major	Minor
Family history	Independent diagnosis in parent, child, sibling	None
Genetics	Mutation FBN1	None
Cardiovascular	Aortic root dilation Dissection of ascending aorta	Mitral valve prolapse Calcification of the mitral valve (<40 years) Dilation of the pulmonary artery Dilation or dissection of the descending aorta
Ocular	Ectopia lentis	(Two needed:) Flat cornea Myopia Elongated globe
Skeletal	(Four needed:) Pectus excavatum needing surgery Pectus carinatum Pes planus Wrist and thumb sign Scoliosis >20 degrees or spondylolisthesis Arm span–height ratio >1.05 Protrusio acetabulae (x-ray, MRI) Diminished extension elbows (<170 degrees)	(Two major or one major and two minor signs) Moderate pectus excavatum High narrowly arched palate Typical facies Joint hypermobility
Pulmonary		Spontaneous pneumothorax Apical bulla
Skin		Unexplained stretch marks (striae) Recurrent or incisional herniae
Central nervous system	Lumbosacral dural ectasia (CT or MRI)	

LOEYS-DIETZ SYNDROME

Mutations in the genes encoding TGF-ß receptors 1 and 2 have been found in association with a continuum of clinical features. On the mild end, the mutation have been found in association with presentation similar to that of the Marfan syndrome or with familial thoracic aneurysm and dissection, and on the severe end, they are associated with a complex phenotype in which aortic dissection or rupture commonly occurs in childhood.[8] This complex phenotype is characterized by the triad of hypertelorism, bifid uvula or cleft palate, and generalized arterial tortuosity with widespread vascular aneurysm and dissection. This phenotype has been classified as Loeys-Dietz syndrome. Affected patients have a high risk of aortic dissection or rupture at an early age and at relatively small diameters. CT angiograms should be obtained from head to pelvis.

Ehlers–Danlos Syndrome

Vascular Ehlers–Danlos syndrome is a rare autosomal dominant inherited disorder of the connective tissue resulting from mutation of the COL3A1 gene encoding type III collagen. Spontaneous rupture without dissection of large and medium-caliber arteries such as the abdominal aorta and its branches, the branches of the aortic arch, and the large arteries of the limbs accounts for most deaths. Aortic root dilation was present in 28% in a series of 71 patients with Ehlers–Danlos syndrome.[9] Aortic dissection is uncommon. Diagnosis is confirmed either by biochemical assays showing qualitative or quantitative abnormalities in type III collagen secretion or by molecular biology studies demonstrating mutation of the COL3A1 gene. Varied molecular mechanisms have been observed with different mutations in each family. No correlation has been established between genotype and phenotype. Diagnosis should be suspected in any young person presenting with arterial or visceral rupture or colonic perforation.

Other Pathologies

Atherosclerotic aneurysms of the ascending aorta are uncommon. They are more common in the abdominal aorta and to a lesser degree in the descending thoracic aorta. Atherosclerosis often causes irregular and saccular aneurysms of the ascending aorta rather than a more fusiform shape as those caused by degenerative disease of the media.

Infectious aneurysms of the ascending aorta are rare. Syphilis was a common cause of aneurysm of the ascending aorta but it is seldom seen. The spirochetal infection destroys the muscular and elastic fibers of the media, which are replaced by fibrous and other inflammatory tissues. The ascending aorta is the most common site of involvement and the aneurysm is usually saccular. The wall of the ascending aorta is frequently calcified. Syphilitic aortitis also causes coronary ostial stenosis and aortic valve insufficiency. Other bacteria can also cause aneurysm of the ascending aorta.

Various types of aortitis may involve the ascending aorta. Giant cell arteritis is among the more common and it involves medium-sized arteries, but the aorta and its branches are involved in approximately 15% of the cases. The etiology is unknown. The characteristic lesion is a granulomatous inflammation of the media of large and medium-caliber arteries such as the temporal artery. Occasionally the inflammatory process weakens the aorta leading to aneurysm formation, aortoannular ectasia, and aortic insufficiency.

Ankylosinsg spondylitis, Reiter's syndrome, psoriatic arthritis, and polyarteritis nodosa can cause aortic insufficiency because of annuloaortic ectasia. Behçet's disease can cause aneurysm of the ascending aorta.

NATURAL HISTORY OF AORTIC VALVE DISEASE

Aortic Stenosis

Asymptomatic patients with aortic stenosis have a good prognosis.[10] Sudden death in asymptomatic patients is uncommon. However, when symptoms develop, the prognosis becomes poor and the average survival is 2 to 3 years for patients with symptoms of angina and syncope, and 1 to 2 years for those with congestive heart failure.[11]

Aortic Insufficiency

The prognosis of symptomatic patients with aortic insufficiency is poor with death occurring within 4 years after development of angina and within 2 years after the onset of congestive heart failure.[12]

Bicuspid Aortic Valve Disease

A prospective follow-up on 642 adult patients (mean age 35±9 years) with bicuspid aortic valve during a mean 9±5 years in our institution revealed a late survival similar to that of the general population in spite the fact that 161 patients had an adverse event (cardiac death, aortic valve/ascending aorta surgery, dissection or congestive heart failure).[13] Age greater than 30 years, and moderate or severe aortic stenosis or insufficiency were independent predictors of adverse event.[13] In a study from the Mayo Clinic on 212 patients (mean age 32±20 years) with normal or minimally dysfunctional bicuspid aortic valve who lived in Olmsted County and followed for a mean of 15±6 years revealed a 20-year survival similar to that of the general population but the incidence of surgery on the aortic valve and/or ascending aorta was 27±4% and the total adverse cardiovascular events was 42±5%.[4]

Aortic Root and Ascending Aortic Aneurysms

Aortic root/ascending aortic aneurysm can cause aortic insufficiency, aortic dissection or rupture. The transverse diameter of the aneurysm is the most important predictor of rupture or dissection. In a study by Coady and associates[14] on 370 patients with thoracic aneurysms (201 ascending aortic aneurysms), during a mean follow-up of 29.4 months the incidence of acute dissection or rupture was 8.8% for aneurysms less than 4 cm, 9.5% for aneurysms of 4 to 4.9 cm, 17.8% for 5 to 5.9 cm, and 27.9% for those greater than 6 cm. The median size of the ascending aortic aneurysm at the time of rupture or dissection was 5.9 cm. The growth rates of thoracic aneurysms are exponential.[14] In Coady's study, the growth rate ranged from 0.08 cm/year for small (<4 cm) aneurysms to 0.16 cm/year for large (8 cm) aneurysms.[14] The growth rates for chronic dissecting aneurysms were much higher than for chronic nondissecting aneurysms.

The growth rates for aortic root aneurysms may be higher than in ascending aortic aneurysms, particularly in patients with Marfan syndrome. Aortic dissection is rare in aortic root aneurysm of less than 50 mm, unless the patients have family history of aortic dissection. Without surgery most patients with Marfan syndrome die in the third decade of their lives from complications of aortic root aneurysm such as rupture, aortic dissection, or aortic insufficiency.[15] Pregnancy in women with Marfan syndrome has two potential problems: the risk of having a child who will inherit the disorder and the risk of acute aortic dissection during the third trimester, parturition, or the first month postpartum. The offspring has a 50% risk of inheriting the syndrome.

Patients affected with Loeys-Dietz syndrome have a high risk of aortic dissection or rupture at an early age and at relatively small aortic root diameters. Surgery is recommended in adults when the aortic root exceeds 4 cm.

Patients with bicuspid aortic valve had larger aortas than patients with tricuspid aortic valve and the rate of dilation of the ascending aorta was higher (0.19 cm versus 0.13 cm per year respectively) in a study by Davies et al.[16] Among patients with bicuspid aortic valve, those with aortic stensois had a higher risk of rupture, dissection, or death.

DIAGNOSIS OF AORTIC VALVE/ROOT DISEASE

Patients with aortic stenosis remain asymptomatic for many years. Symptoms usually appear late in the course of the disease. The symptoms are: angina pectoris, syncope, congestive heart failure, and syncope. The clinical presentation of patients with aortic insufficiency is dependent on the rapidity with which aortic insufficiency develops. Patients with chronic aortic insufficiency remain asymptomatic for many years while the heart slowly enlarges. Palpitations and head pounding may occur during exertion. Angina pectoris may occur, but it is not as common as with aortic stenosis. Syncope is rare. Symptoms of congestive heart failure are usually an indication of left ventricular dysfunction. Acute aortic insufficiency is frequently associated with cardiovascular collapse, with extreme fatigue, dyspnea, and hypotension resulting from reduced stroke volume and elevated left atrial pressure. Echocardiography confirms the diagnosis of aortic valve dysfunction and provides information regarding its mechanism. Radionuclide imaging is useful in assessing the left ventricular function at rest and during exercise, valuable information in asymptomatic patients.

Most patients with aortic root aneurysm are asymptomatic and have no physical signs if the aortic valve is competent. Some patients may complain of vague chest pain. Severe chest pain is suggestive of rapid expansion or intimal tear with dissection. Echocardiography establishes the diagnosis and provides information regarding the aortic cusps. CT scan and MRI of the chest are also diagnostic and it is useful to provide information regarding the thoracic aorta.

INDICATIONS FOR SURGERY

Surgeons must be familiar with the guidelines for heart valve surgery established by a joint committee of the ACC and AHA.[17]

SELECTION OF PATIENTS FOR AORTIC VALVE REPAIR

Most candidates for aortic valve repair have aortic insufficiency or normally functioning aortic valve with aortic root aneurysm. Transesophageal echocardiography is the best diagnostic tool to study the aortic valve and the mechanism of aortic insufficiency. Each component of the aortic root must be carefully interrogated, and in particular the aortic cusps. The number of cusps, their thickness, the appearance of their free margins, and the excursion of each cusp during the cardiac cycle must be examined in multiple views. The lines of coaptation of the aortic cusps should be interrogated by color Doppler imaging. The direction and size of the regurgitant jets recorded in many views. Information regarding the morphologic features of the aortic annulus, aortic sinuses, sinotubular junction, and ascending aorta should be obtained.

Obviously, the aortic cusps are the most important determinant of aortic valve repair. If the cusps are thin, mobile, and smooth free margins, the feasibility of aortic valve repair is very high, including bicuspid aortic valve. Calcified or scarred and fibrotic aortic cusps preclude aortic valve repair unless autologous or xenograft glutaraldehyde fixed pericardium is used for cusp augmentation.

Patients with aortic root aneurysm often have normal or minimally stretched aortic cusps and reconstruction of the aortic root with preservation of the native aortic cusps is feasible. Grossly dilated aortic annulus and/or sinotubular junction are likely to have overstretched, thinned out aortic cusps with stress fenestrations along the commissural areas and may not be suitable for repair.

TECHNIQUES OF AORTIC VALVE REPAIR

Cusp Perforation

Occasionally a cups perforation is the sole reason for aortic insufficiency. The perforation may be iatrogenic, a sequelae of healed endocarditis, or the result of resection of a papillary fibroelastoma. A simple patch of fresh or glutaraldehyde fixed autologous pericardium is adequate to correct the problem. Fresh autologous pericardium can also be used to repair small holes (<5 mm) but the patch should be larger than the defect because it retracts during healing. We use a continuous 7-0 polypropylene to suture the patch around the defect on the aortic side of the cusp.

Cusp Extension

Cusp augmentation has been used to repair incompetent aortic valves due rheumatic and congenital disease. Glutaraldehyde-fixed bovine or autologous pericardium has been used for this purpose.

Cusp Prolapse

Cusp prolapse is caused by elongation of the free margin. This is corrected by plication along the nodule of Arantius as illustrated in Fig. 36-4. The degree of shortening is determined by examining the other cusps and their level of coaptation.

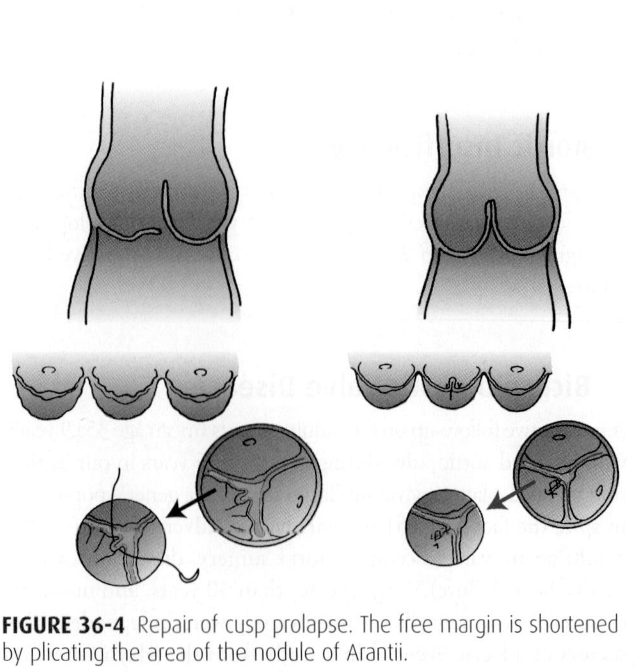

FIGURE 36-4 Repair of cusp prolapse. The free margin is shortened by plicating the area of the nodule of Arantii.

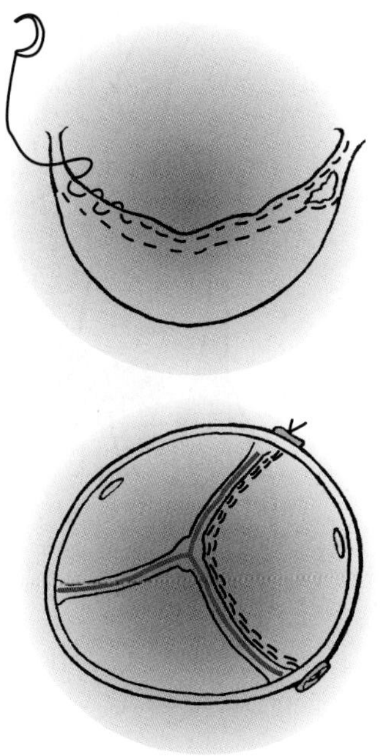

FIGURE 36-5 Reinforcement of the free margin with a double layer of 6-0 expanded polytetrafluoroethylene suture. This is often done in patients with stress fenestration.

Cusp with Stress Fenestration

Dilation of the sinotubular junction increases the mechanical stress along the free margin of the cusp near the commissures and may cause a stress fenestration with thinning and sometimes even detachment from the commissure. This type of lesion has been successfully corrected by weaving a double layer of 6-0 expanded polytetrafluoroethylene suture along the free margin of the cusp as illustrated in Fig. 36-5.

Bicuspid Aortic Valve

The most commonly performed aortic valve repair in adults is for bicuspid aortic valve with prolapse of one cusp. Although the anatomic arrangement of the bicuspid aortic valve varies, most patients have an anterior cusp attached to the interventricular septum and a posterior cusp attached to the fibrous components of the left ventricular outflow tract. The anterior cusp often contains a raphe at approximately where the commissure between the right and left cusps would be (Type 1, L-R). This cusp is usually the one that is elongated and prolapsed. As long as the posterior cusp is normal, repair is feasible and relatively simple. The raphe is excised and the free margin of the anterior cusp is shortened with plicating sutures as illustrated in Fig. 36-6. The lengths of the free margins of both cusps should be similar and should coapt at the same level. Suspending the arterial walls immediately above the commissures and observing the level of coaptation of each cusp gives an estimate of the level of coaptation of the cusps.

Because most patients with incompetent bicuspid aortic valves have dilated aortic annulus, aortic valve sparing operation may be more appropriate procedure than simple cusp repair. However, if the aortic sinuses are not aneurismal and the annulus is only mildly dilated, a reduction annuloplasty to increase the coaptation area of the cusps can be done. This is accomplished by plicating the subcommissural triangles using horizontal mattress sutures of 4-0 polypropylene with Teflon felt pledgets on the outside of the aortic root (Fig. 36-7). The suture is first passed from the outside to the inside of the aorta through the aortic annulus of both cusps 2 mm below their commissure. The same suture is passed again through the annulus and subcommissural triangle 4 or 5 mm below the first one and the ends are tied together over Teflon felt pledgets on the outside of the aorta.

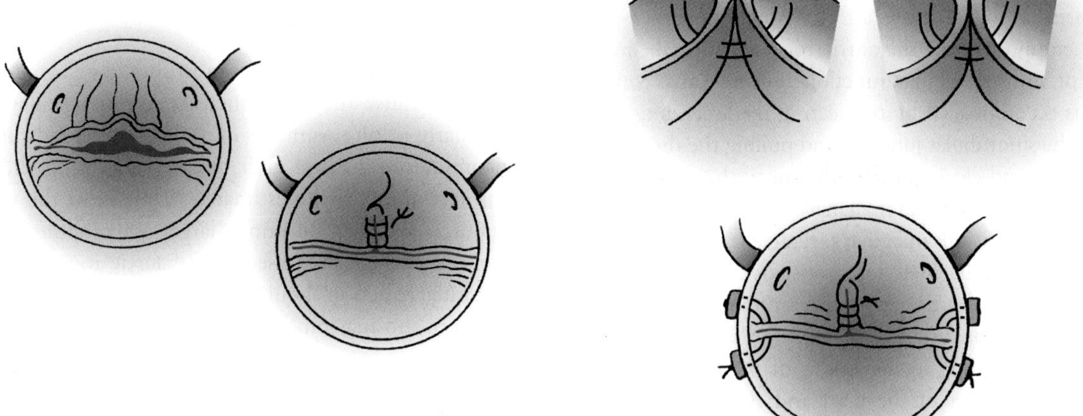

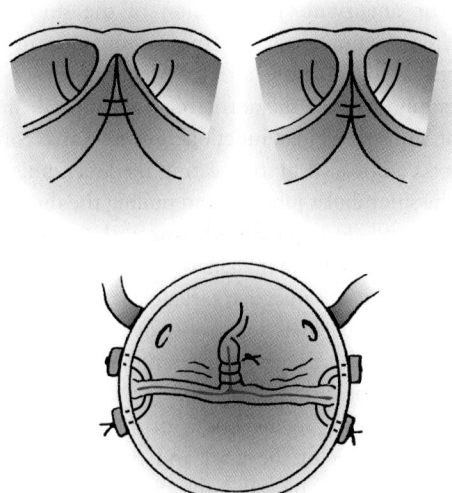

FIGURE 36-6 Repair of incompetent bicuspid aortic valve. The elongated cusp is shortened and the sub-commissural triangles narrowed with sutures.

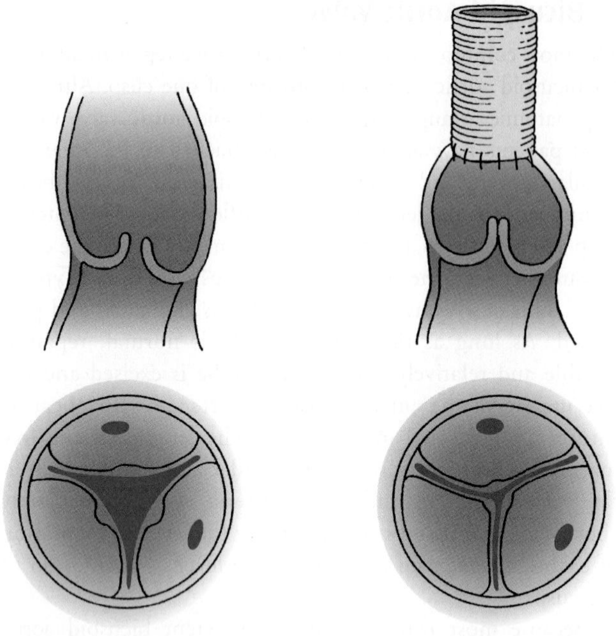

FIGURE 36-7 Dilation of the sinotubular junction causes aortic insufficiency. Correction of the dilation with a tubular Dacron graft of appropriate diameter corrects aortic insufficiency.

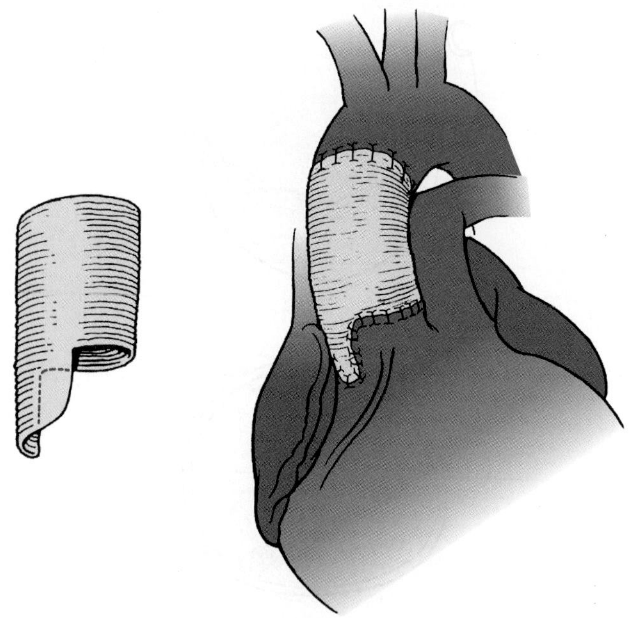

FIGURE 36-8 Correction of the sinotubular junction and replacement of the noncoronary aortic sinus.

AORTIC VALVE SPARING OPERATIONS

Aortic valve sparing operations include various procedures used to preserve the aortic cusps in patients with aortic root aneurysm or ascending aortic aneurysm with aortic insufficiency.[18,19]

Ascending Aortic Aneurysm with Aortic Insufficiency

Dilation of the sinotubular junction displaces the commissures of the aortic valve outward and prevents the cusps from coapting during diastole (see Fig. 36-3). These patients are often on the sixth, seventh, or eighth decade of their lives and have ascending aortic aneurysm. The dilation of the sinotubular junction is often asymmetrical, and the commissures of noncoronary aortic cusp are more affected than the other two. If the other components of the aortic root are normal, simple adjustment of the sinotubular junction restores valve competence. This is accomplished by transecting the ascending aorta 5 mm above the sinotubular junction and pulling the three commissures upward and close to each other until the cusps coapt. The three commissures form an imaginary triangle. The diameter of a circle that contains this imaginary triangle is the diameter of the graft that should be used to reconstruct the sinotubular junction. Because the aortic cusps and sinuses have different sizes, this triangle is not always equilateral and the commissures must be spaced according to the length of the free margin of each cusp. The diameter of the graft and the space between commissures are facilitated by sizing the diameter of the circle that contains all three commissures with a transparent valve sizer, such as the one used to size the aortic annulus for a stentless porcine aortic valve. Those valve sizers have three equidistant marks, and one can determine the space between the commissures by comparing to the distance between marks. The tubular Dacron graft is sutured right at the level of the sinotubular junction with a continuous 4-0 polypropylene suture (see Fig. 36-7). If after adjusting the sinotubular junction, the cusps do not coapt at the same level, one or more cusps may be elongated and the free margin has to be shortened as illustrated in Fig. 36-4. Aortic valve competence can be tested at this time by injecting cardioplegia into the graft under pressure and observing the left ventricle for distension.

If the noncoronary aortic sinus is dilated or altered by aortic dissection, a neosinus can be created by tailoring the graft with tongue of tissue that is sutured directly to the aortic annulus as illustrated in Fig. 36-8. The height of the neosinus of Dacron should be 3 or 4 mm more than the diameter of the graft, and the width should be 3 or 4 mm more than the estimated intercommissural distance to allow the graft to bulge and create a neoaortic sinus.

Small diameter grafts (<24 mm) should be avoided in adult patients because they may increase left ventricular afterload, particularly if long segments of aorta are replaced such as with concomitant transverse arch replacement using the elephant trunk technique. If the estimated diameter of the sinotubular junction is less than 24 mm, a larger graft should be used and the end that is anastomosed to the aortic root to recreate the sinotubular junction should be reduced by plicating the graft in the area of the anastomosis.

Aortic Root Aneurysm

A large proportion of patients with aortic root aneurysm have normal or minimally stretched aortic cusps and an aortic valve sparing operation is feasible. There are basically two types of

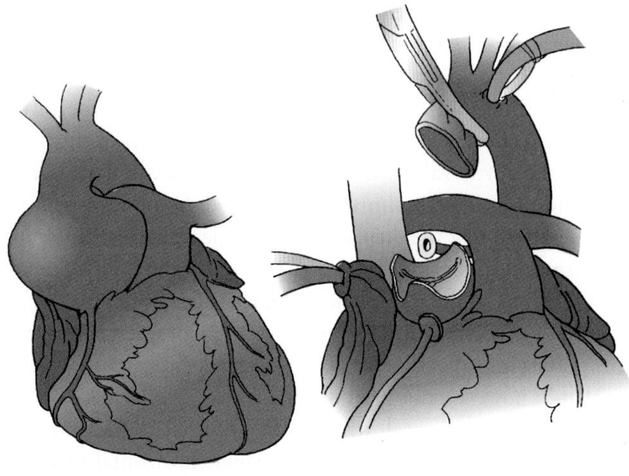

FIGURE 36-9 Remodeling of the aortic root. The aortic sinuses are excised leaving 4 to 6 mm of arterial wall attached to the aortic annulus and around the coronary arteries.

aortic valve-sparing operations for patients with aortic root aneurysm: remodeling of the aortic root and reimplantation of the aortic valve.[18,19]

Remodeling of the Aortic Root

The ascending aorta is transected and the aortic root is dissected circumferentially down to the level of the aortic annulus. All three aortic sinuses are excised, leaving approximately 4 to 6 mm of arterial wall attached to the aortic annulus and around the coronary artery orifices as illustrated in Fig. 36-9. The three commissures are gently pulled vertically and approximated until the cusps coapt. The three commissures form a triangle and the diameter of the circle that contains that triangle is the diameter of the graft to be used for remodeling. In our experience, most grafts are 24, 26, or 28 mm in diameter. Here again the stentless valve sizers are very useful to determine the diameter of the graft and also the distance between commissures because they may not be equidistant. The spaces in between the commissures are marked in one of the ends of the graft, and the graft is tailored to create three neo-aortic sinuses (Fig. 36-10). The heights of these neosinuses should be approximately equal to the diameter of the graft. The three commissures are suspended in the graft (Fig. 36-11), which is then sutured to the remnants of the aortic wall as close as possible to aortic annulus with continuous 4-0 polypropylene sutures. The coronary arteries are reimplanted into their respective neosinuses. The aortic cusps are inspected to make sure that all three coapt at the same level and well above the nadir of the aortic annulus. If one or more cusp is prolapsing, the free margin is shortened as described previously. If one or two cusps have stress fenestrations, the free margin should be reinforced with a fine expanded polytetrafluoroethylene suture. Aortic valve competence can be assessed by injecting cardioplegia under pressure into the reconstructed aortic root and observing the left ventricle for distension or by turning the echocardiography machine on. The graft is then anastomosed to the distal ascending aorta or transverse aortic arch graft depending on the extent of the aneurysm (Fig. 36-11).

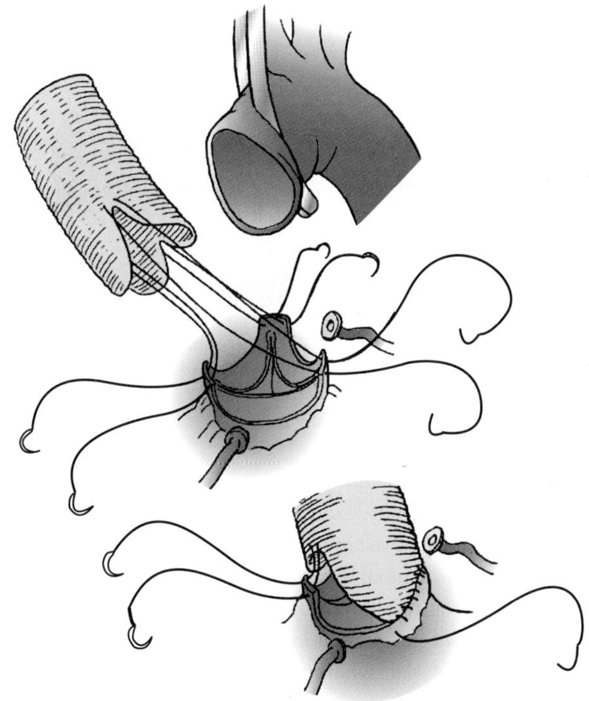

FIGURE 36-10 A graft of diameter equal to the diameter of the sinotubular junction is tailored to recreate three aortic sinuses. The three commissures are suspended into the tailored graft and the neoaortic sinuses are sutured to the aortic annulus and remnants of arterial wall.

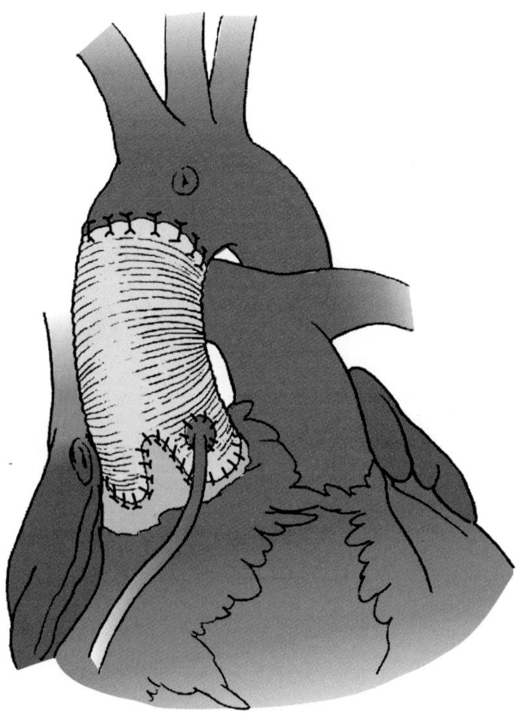

FIGURE 36-11 Remodeling of the aortic root. The coronary arteries are reimplanted into their respective neo-aortic sinuses and the graft anastomosed to the distal aorta.

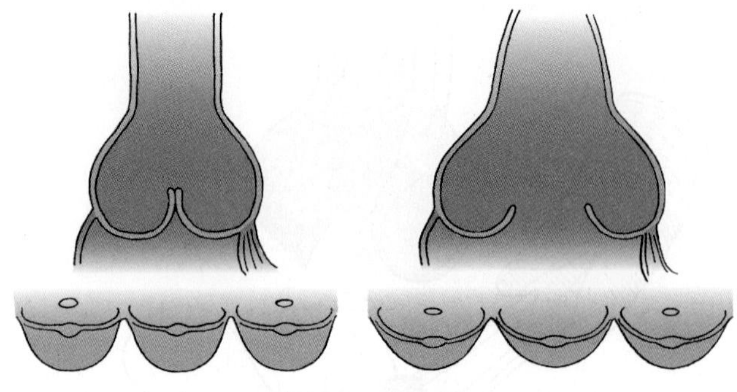

FIGURE 36-12 Annuloaortic ectasia. The subcommissural triangles of the noncoronary aortic cusps are flattened by dilation of the fibrous tissue.

Remodeling of the aortic root may be inappropriate for patients with Marfan syndrome or annuloaortic ectasia because the annulus may continue to dilate and cause aortic insufficiency. An aortic annuloplasty along the fibrous component of the left ventricular outflow tract[18] did not prevent late dilation of the aortic annulus in patients with Marfan syndrome in our experience. Thus, reimplantation of the aortic valve may be a better operative procedure for patients with annuloaortic ectasia (Fig. 36-12) because this operative procedure corrects and prevents annular dilation whereas remodeling of the aortic root may be more suitable for patients with normal aortic annulus.

Reimplantation of the Aortic Valve

This procedure can be performed in all patients with aortic root aneurysm, but it is particularly valuable in patients with annuloaortic ectasia and in those with acute type A aortic dissection. It is technically more demanding than remodeling of the aortic root because it requires greater knowledge of the functional anatomy of the aortic root. This is because the aortic annulus, the aortic sinuses, the sinotubular junction, and even the aortic cusps are reconstructed. In the original description of this procedure, the aortic valve was reimplanted into a tubular Dacron graft and no neoaortic sinuses were created. Some investigators have suggested that the presence of the aortic sinuses is important for normal cusp motion, and potentially, cusp durability. Several modifications to the reimplantation procedure were introduced to create neoaortic sinuses. There is now a commercially available graft with sinuses of Valsalva (Vascutek Ltd. Renfrewshire, Scotland); however, this graft distorts the aortic annulus because its sinuses are spherical whereas the normal aortic annulus develops along a crescent shape on a single horizontal plane. A cylindrical graft with neoaortic aortic sinuses that permits reimplantation of the aortic annulus along single horizontal planes has also been developed in Germany.[20]

Following is a description of this procedure as we have been performing it during the past decade, with excellent functional results. The three aortic sinuses are excised as described for the remodeling procedure (see Fig. 36-9). Multiple horizontal mattress sutures of 2-0 or 3-0 polyester are passed from the inside to the outside of the left ventricular outflow tract, immediately below the nadir of the aortic annulus, through a single horizontal plane along the fibrous portion of the outflow tract and along its scalloped shape in the interventricular septum as illustrated in Fig. 36-13. If the fibrous portion is thin, sutures with Teflon felt pledgets should be used. A tubular Dacron graft of diameter equal to double the average height of the cusps is selected and three equidistant marks placed in one of its ends. A small triangular segment is cut off along the mark that

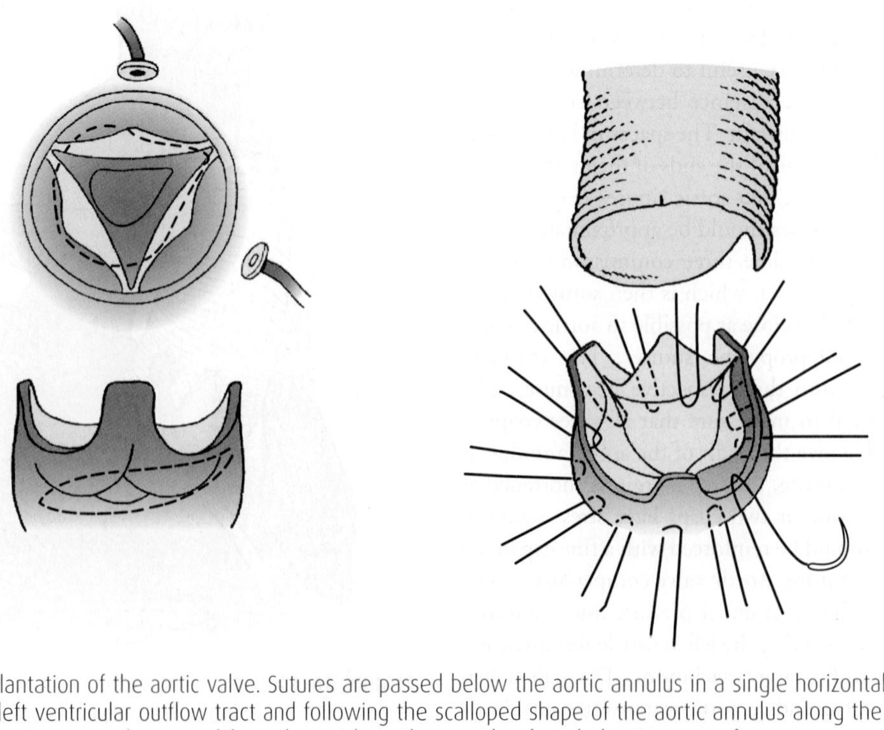

FIGURE 36-13 Reimplantation of the aortic valve. Sutures are passed below the aortic annulus in a single horizontal plane along the fibrous portion of the left ventricular outflow tract and following the scalloped shape of the aortic annulus along the muscular interventricular septum. These sutures are also passed from the inside to the outside of a tubular Dacron graft.

corresponds to the subcommissural triangle of the left and right cusps. If the diameter of the aortic annulus is smaller than the diameter of the graft by 10 mm or more, the diameter of the graft is reduced by plicating it in the areas corresponding to the nadir of the aortic annulus. The sutures previously placed in the left ventricular outflow tract are now passed through the graft. The sutures should be spaced symmetrically if the aortic annulus is not dilated. If there is obvious dilation of the aortic annulus, the sutures should be spaced symmetrically along the muscular interventricular septum and around the nadirs of the aortic annulus but closer together beneath the subcommissural triangles of the noncoronary cusp because that is where dilation occurs in patients with connective disorders. The sutures are then tied on the outside of the graft. Care must be exercised not to purse-string this suture line. The graft is then cut in a length of approximately 5 cm and pulled gently, and the three commissures are also pulled vertically and temporarily secured to the graft with transfixing 4-0 polypropylene sutures buttressed on small Teflon felt pledgets, but these sutures are not tied. Once all three commissures are suspended inside the graft, the commissures and the cusps are inspected to make sure they are all correctly aligned. The subcommissural triangles should also be inspected to make sure they are as narrow as the diameter of the graft allows, i.e., the triangles should have a narrower base than before surgery. Next, the sutures are tied on the outside of the graft and used to secure the aortic annulus into the graft. This is accomplished by passing the suture sequentially from the inside to the outside right at the level of the annulus and from the outside to the inside at the level of the remnants of the arterial wall. We start at the level of the commissure and stop at the nadir of the aortic annulus where the sutures are tied together. The coronary arteries are reimplanted into their respective sinuses (Fig. 36-14). The coaptation of the aortic cusps is inspected and prolapse is corrected if necessary. It is important that the coaptation level is well above the aortic annulus. Neoaortic sinuses are created by plicating the graft at the level of the commissure as illustrated in Fig. 36-15. Valve competence can be assessed by occluding the distal graft and injecting cardioplegia under pressure. If the ventricle does not distend, no more than trace aortic insufficiency is present. The aortic valve can also be examined by echocardiography during injection of cardioplegia. The distal anastomosis is performed either to the distal ascending aorta or transverse aortic arch depending on the pathology. The graft sizes in our patients ranged from 26 to 34 mm, mean of 31 mm.

RESULTS OF AORTIC VALVE REPAIR

One of the earliest series of aortic valve repair for aortic insufficiency caused by prolapse of bicuspid aortic valve came from the Cleveland Clinic.[21] In a series of 94 patients with a mean age of 38 years, the freedom from reoperation was 84% at 7 years.[21] The only factor predictive of reoperation was residual aortic insufficiency at the time of repair.[21]

The appropriateness of aortic valve repair in patients with incompetent bicuspid aortic valve remains unclear. Competent bicuspid aortic valves appear to be durable because a large proportion of patients who require aortic valve replacement for aortic stenosis in their fifth, sixth, or seventh decades of life are found to have bicuspid aortic valve. Thus, aortic valve repair for incompetent bicuspid aortic valves is a reasonable surgical approach in young adults but the best type of repair remains to be determined. Incompetent bicuspid aortic valves are often

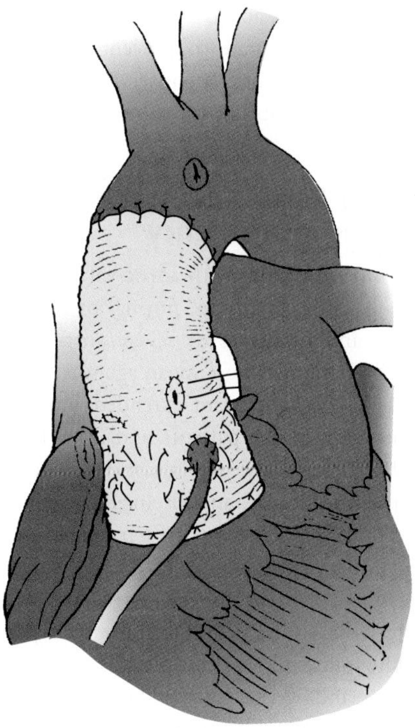

FIGURE 36-14 Reimplantation of the aortic valve. The commissures and the aortic annulus are sutured inside the graft and the coronary arteries reimplanted.

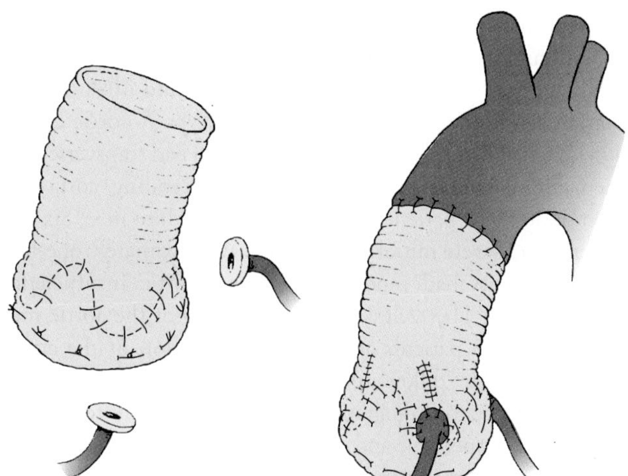

FIGURE 36-15 Reimplantation of the aortic valve. Neoaortic sinuses can be created by plicating the graft in the spaces in between the commissures at the level of the sinotubular junction.

associated with dilated aortic annulus and subcommissural plication may be inadequate to prevent future dilation and recurrent aortic insufficiency. A conservative aortic root procedure may be more appropriate for some of these patients.

Ascending Aortic Aneurysm with Aortic Insufficiency

We reported our experience with aortic valve repair in patients with ascending aortic aneurysm, normal or minimally dilated aortic sinuses, and moderate or severe aortic insufficiency.[22] There were 103 patients whose mean age was 65±12 years and 53% were men. The aneurysm extended into the transverse aortic arch in 60% of the patients and 20% had mega-aorta syndrome. The aortic valve repair consisted in adjusting the diameter of the sinotubular junction in all patients. In addition, repair of cusp prolapse was needed in 36 patients, and replacement of the noncoronary aortic sinus in 8. Associated procedures were: replacement of the transverse aortic arch in 62 patients, coronary artery bypass in 28, and mitral valve repair or replacement in 7. The follow-up was complete at 5.8±2.3 years. There were 2 operative and 30 late deaths. The survival at 10 years was 54±7%. Independent predictors of late death were transverse arch aneurysm, the use of elephant trunk technique to replace the arch and mega-aorta syndrome. Only 2 patients required aortic valve replacement: one for endocarditis and one for severe aortic insufficiency. The freedom from aortic valve replacement at 10 years was 98%. Only one patient developed severe and six developed moderate aortic insufficiency during the follow-up. The freedom from severe or moderate aortic insufficiency at 10 years was 80±7%. These findings suggest that aortic valve repair in these patients is an excellent alternative to valve replacement and the repair remains stable in most patients during the follow-up. Late survival was suboptimal because of the extensiveness of the vascular disease.

Aortic Root Aneurysm

We reported our current experience with aortic valve sparing operations for aortic root aneurysm in 220 patients.[23] Their mean age was 46±15 years, 78% were men and 40% had the Marfan syndrome. In addition, 17% had type A aortic dissection, 7% had bicuspid aortic valve, and 22% had transverse arch aneurysm. Previous replacement of the ascending aorta had been done in 10 patients and the Ross procedure in 2. Sixteen patients had severe mitral insufficiency. Approximately one-half of the patients had moderate or severe aortic insufficiency before surgery. The technique of remodeling of the aortic root was used in 53 patients and the reimplantation of the aortic valve in 167. The follow-up was complete at 5.2±3.7 years. All patients had echocardiographic studies during the follow-up. There were 3 operative and 13 late deaths. Patients' survival at 10 years was 88±3% and was similar to that of the general population of Ontario. Age greater than 65 years, advanced functional class, and ejection fraction less than 40% were independent predictors of death. Seven patients developed moderate and 5 developed severe aortic insufficiency. Overall freedom from moderate or severe aortic insufficiency at 10 years was 85±5%, but it was 94±4% after reimplantation of the aortic valve and 75 ±10% remodeling of the aortic root ($p = 0.04$). Five patients required aortic valve replacement; the freedom at 10 years was 95±3%. One patient developed endocarditis 11 years postoperatively, and 8 suffered thromboembolic events. At the latest follow-up 88% of the patients were in functional class I, and 10% were in class II. These findings suggested that reimplantation of the aortic valve provides more stable aortic valve function than remodeling of the aortic root.

Yacoub et al.[24] who used exclusively the remodeling of the aortic root to treat 158 patients with aortic root and ascending aortic aneurysms, reported a freedom from aortic valve replacement of 89% at 10 years, and moderate aortic insufficiency in one-third of the patients.

Aicher et al.[25] who also used the remodeling of the aortic root in 274 patients (mean age 59±15 years, 193 tricuspid and 81 bicuspid valves) reported a freedom from aortic insufficiency grade II or greater of 91% for bicuspid and 87% for tricuspid at 10 years, and a freedom from aortic valve replacement of 98% at 5 and at 10 years.

We recently reported the long-term results with aortic valve sparing operations in patients with Marfan syndrome.[26] A cohort of 103 consecutive patients with Marfan syndrome with a mean age of 37±12 years underwent either remodeling of the aortic root (26 patients) or reimplantation of the aortic valve (77 patients) and were prospectively followed for a mean of 7.3±4.2 years with annual echocardiography. The survival at 15 years was 87.2%, somewhat lower than the 95.6% for the general population largely because of complications of aortic dissection. The freedom from aortic insufficiency greater than mild was 79.2%. Only 3 patients required aortic valve replacement, two for aortic insufficiency and one for endocarditis.

There are several reports on early clinical and hemodynamic outcomes on these two types of aortic valve sparing procedures.[27-30] Most comparative studies suggest that the reimplantation of the aortic valve provides a more stable aortic valve function than the remodeling of the aortic root, particularly in patients with dilated aortic annulus, Marfan syndrome, and acute type A aortic dissection. Hemodynamic studies suggest that cusp motion and flow patterns across the reconstructed aortic root are more physiologic after remodeling of the aortic root than reimplantation of the aortic valve.[29] In patients who had the reimplantation procedure, flow patterns and cusp motion are better with neoaortic sinuses than without.[30] However, in our series of reimplantations of the aortic valve, there was no difference in aortic valve function after 10 years in patients with a straight tube or with neoaortic sinuses. Aortic sinuses seem to decrease the mechanical stress on the aortic cusps but it is not clinically apparent during the first decade of follow-up as far as durability of the procedure.

Aortic valve sparing operations may be inappropriate for young children because of future mismatch between the size of the graft and somatic growth.

Another important question regarding aortic valve sparing operations is whether they are better than the Bentall procedure with mechanical valves. There has been no randomized clinical trial comparing these two procedures for the treatment of aortic root aneurysms or ascending aortic aneurysm but retrospective studies in patients with Marfan syndrome suggest that the outcomes may be similar.

We believe that aortic valve sparing operations offer an ideal method for treating patients with aortic root aneurysm and normal or minimally diseased aortic cusps. When correctly performed, they provide excellent results and are associated with very low rates of valve-related complications. However, because they are technically demanding operations, only surgeons with extensive experience in aortic surgery should perform them. The surgeon must have a sound knowledge of anatomy and pathology of the aortic valve and be able to apply the concepts of functional anatomy to create an anatomically and functionally satisfactory new aortic root.

REFERENCES

1. Movahed MR, Hepner AD, Ahmadi-Kashani M: Echocardiographic prevalence of bicuspid aortic valve in the population. *Heart Lung Circ* 2006; 15:297.
2. Huntington K, Hunter AG, Char KL: A prospective study to assess the frequency of familial clustering of congenital bicuspid aortic valve. *J Am Coll Cardiol* 1997; 30:1809.
3. Sievers HH, Schmidtke C: A classification system for the bicuspid aortic valve from 304 surgical specimens. *J Thorac Cardiovasc Surg* 2007; 133: 1226-1233.
4. Michelena HI, Desjardins V, Avierinos JF, et al: Natural history of asymptomatic patients with normally functioning or minimally dysfunctional bicuspid aortic valve in the community. *Circulation* 2008; 117:2776.
5. Dietz HC, Loeys BL, Carta L, Ramirez F: Recent progress towards a molecular understanding of Marfan syndrome. *Am J Med Genet* 2005; 139C:4.
6. Bee KJ, Wilkes D, Devereux RB, et al: Structural and functional genetic disorders of the great vessels and outflow tracts. *Ann N Y Acad Sci* 2006; 1085:256.
7. De Paepe A, Devereux RB, Dietz HC, et al: Revised diagnostic criteria for the Marfan syndrome. *Am J Med Genet* 1996; 62:417.
8. Loeys BL, Chen J, Neptune ER, et al: A syndrome of altered cardiovascular, craniofacial, neurocognitive and skeletal development caused by mutations in TGFBR1 or TGFBR2. *Nat Genet* 2005; 37:275.
9. Wenstrup RJ, Meyer RA, Lyle JS, et al: Prevalence of aortic root dilation in the Ehlers-Danlos syndrome. *Genet Med* 2002; 4:112.
10. Pellika PA, Nishimura RA, Bailey KR, et al: The natural history of adults with asymptomatic hemodynamically significant aortic stenosis. *J Am Coll Cardiol* 1990; 15:1018.
11. Frank S, Johnson A, Ross J Jr: Natural history of valvular aortic stenosis. *Br Heart J* 1997; 35:41.
12. Goldschlager N, Pfeifer J, Cohn K, et al: Natural history of aortic regurgitation: a clinical and hemodynamic study. *Am J Med* 1973; 54:577.
13. Tzemos N, Terrien J, Yip J, et al: Outcomes in adults with bicuspid aortic valves. *JAMA* 2008; 300:1317.
14. Coady MA, Rizzo JA, Hammond GL, et al: Surgical intervention criteria for thoracic aortic aneurysms: a study of growth rates and complications. *Ann Thorac Surg* 1999; 67:1922.
15. Silverman DI, Burton KJ, Gray J: Life expectancy in the Marfan syndrome. *Am J Cardiol* 1995; 75:157.
16. Davies RR, Kaple RK, Mandapati D, et al: Natural history of ascending aortic aneurysms in the setting of an unreplaced bicuspid aortic valve. *Ann Thorac Surg* 2007; 83:1338-1344.
17. Bonow RO, Carabello BA, Kanu C, et al: ACC/AHA 2006 guidelines for the management of patients with valvular heart disease: a report of the American College of Cardiology/American Heart Association Task Force on Practice Guidelines. *Circulation* 2006; 114:84.
18. David TE: Remodeling of the aortic root and preservation of the native aortic valve. *Op Tech Cardiac Thorac Surg* 1996; 1:44-56.
19. Sarsam MA, Yacoub M: Remodeling of the aortic valve anulus. *J Thorac Cardiovasc Surg* 1993; 105:435-438.
20. Richardt D, Karluß A, Sievers HH, Scharfschwerdt M: A new sinus prosthesis for aortic valve sparing surgery maintaining the shape of the root at systemic pressure. *Ann Thorac Surg* 2010; 89:943-946.
21. Casselman FP, Gillinov AM, Akhrass R, et al: Intermediate-term durability of bicuspid aortic valve repair for prolapsing leaflet. *Eur J Cardiothorac Surg* 1999; 15:302.
22. David TE, Feindel CM, Armstrong S, Maganti M: Replacement of the ascending aorta with reduction of the diameter of the sinotubular junction to treat aortic insufficiency in patients with ascending aortic aneurysm. *J Thorac Cardiovasc Surg* 2007; 133:414-418.
23. David TE, Armstrong S, Maganti M, Colman J, Bradley TJ: Long-term results of aortic valve-sparing operations in patients with Marfan syndrome. *J Thorac Cardiovasc Surg* 2009; 138:859-864.
24. Yacoub MH, Gehle P, Chandrasekaran V, et al: Late results of a valve-preserving operation in patients with aneurysm of the ascending aorta and root. *J Thorac Cardiovasc Surg* 1998; 115:1080.
25. Aicher D, Langer F, Lausberg H, Bierbach B, Schäfers HJ: Aortic root remodeling: ten-year experience with 274 patients. *J Thorac Cardiovasc Surg* 2007; 134:909-915.
26. David T, Armstrong S, Maganti M, Colman J, Bradley TJ: Long-term results of aortic valve–sparing operations in patients with Marfan syndrome. *J Thorac Cardiovasc Surg* 2009; 138:859-856.
27. Hanke T, Charitos EI, Stierle U, et al: Factors associated with the development of aortic valve regurgitation over time after two different techniques of valve-sparing aortic root surgery. *J Thorac Cardiovasc Surg* 2009; 137: 314-319.
28. Kvitting JP, Ebbers T, Wigstrom L, et al: Flow patterns in the aortic root and the aorta studied with time-resolved, 3-dimensional, phase contrast magnetic resonance imaging: implications for aortic valve-sparing surgery. *J Thorac Cardiovasc Surg* 2004; 127:1602.
29. Leyh RG, Schmidtke C, Sievers HH, et al: Opening and closing characteristics of the aortic valve after different types of valve-preserving surgery. *Circulation* 1999; 100:2153.
30. De Paulis R, De Matteis GM, Nardi P, et al: Opening and closing characteristics of the aortic valve after valve-sparing procedures using a new aortic root conduit. *Ann Thorac Surg* 2001; 72:487.

CHAPTER 37

Surgical Treatment of Aortic Valve Endocarditis

Tirone E. David

INTRODUCTION

Infective endocarditis is a disease in which a microorganism colonizes a focus in the heart, producing fever, heart murmur, splenomegaly, embolic manifestations, and bacteremia or fungemia. Early diagnosis of this condition is extremely important because it almost invariably leads to devastating complications and death if not treated with antibiotics, combined or not with surgery. Infective endocarditis is defined as community-acquired or health care–associated infection. The latter can be nosocomial or non–nosocomial health care associated.

EPIDEMIOLOGY

Predisposing factors for infective endocarditis are cardiac abnormalities that disrupt the endocardium by means of a jet injury, as well as the presence of blood-borne microorganisms that colonize these abnormal surfaces. Among patients with aortic valve endocarditis, congenitally bicuspid aortic valve is the most common predisposing lesion.[1] Other congenital abnormalities of the aortic valve, degenerative calcific aortic stenosis, aortic insufficiency secondary to connective tissue disorders, and rheumatic aortic valve disease, are also predisposing lesions for infection. Depending on the virulence of the offending microorganism, normal aortic valves can also be affected. Patients with prosthetic heart valves have a constant risk of developing infective endocarditis.

It is difficult to determine the incidence and prevalence of native aortic valve endocarditis in the general population because this disease is continuously changing.[2] The annual incidence of infective endocarditis is estimated to range from 1.7 to 7.0 episodes per 100,000 person-years in North America.[3–5]

Patients with prosthetic aortic valves are reported to have an incidence of infective endocarditis of 0.2 to 1.4 episodes per 100 patient-years, which varies with the type of aortic valve.[6–12] Approximately 1.4% of patients undergoing aortic valve replacement develop prosthetic valve endocarditis during the first postoperative year.[13]

The incidence of nosocomial endocarditis is increasing because more patients undergo invasive procedures. Infective endocarditis in hemodialysis patients is relatively infrequent, but it is associated with high mortality.[14] Dental extractions have been demonstrated to produce bacteremia. Dental flossing can produce bacteremia in periodontally healthy and periodontally diseased individuals at a rate comparable with that caused by some dental treatments, for which antibiotic prophylaxis is usually given to prevent endocarditis.[15] Endoscopic procedures may also produce bacteremia. Intravenous drug users are particularly susceptible to infective endocarditis, which often occurs in structurally normal heart valves. (Please see prophylaxis of infective endocarditis elsewhere in this chapter.)

PATHOGENESIS AND PATHOLOGY

In 1928, Grant and colleagues[16] theorized that platelet-fibrin thrombi on the heart valve served as a nidus for bacteria adherence. In 1963, Angrist and Oka[17] introduced the term *nonbacterial thrombotic endocarditis* to describe sterile vegetations on a heart valve and provided experimental animal evidence supporting the role of these vegetations in the pathogenesis of endocarditis. Experimental inoculation in animals with preexisting nonbacterial thrombotic endocarditis produced by mechanical abrasion of the endothelial covering of heart valves causes a prompt leukocytic infiltration of the thrombi.[18] As the microorganism multiplies, more leukocytes and thrombotic material accumulate in the area and a verrucous vegetation begins to form.

Depending on the virulence of the microorganism and the resistance of the host, the aortic valve can be destroyed and the infection may spread into the annulus and surrounding structures with abscess formation. The abscess may rupture into the pericardial or a cardiac cavity.

Infective endocarditis of the aortic valve not only causes destruction of the aortic cusps, paravalvular abscess, and cardiac fistulas but also can cause coronary and systemic embolization of vegetations.[19] Cerebral infarction, either ischemic because of arterial occlusion, or hemorrhagic, because of rupture of the mycotic aneurysm, is common in these patients.[20,21] Mycotic aneurysms, infarcts, and abscesses of other organs such as spleen, liver, kidneys, and limbs are also common.[18] Aortic valve endocarditis with a large vegetation that prolapses into the left ventricle and comes in contact with the anterior leaflet of the mitral valve can cause secondary involvement of this valve.[22,23]

Infection of a mechanical heart valve is usually located in its sewing ring.[24,25] Infection of a porcine or pericardial valve may involve the cusps, the sewing ring, or both.[26,27] Infection in aortic valve homografts and pulmonary autografts resembles that of the native aortic valve: It begins in the aortic cusps and destroys them, causing aortic insufficiency, but it may also extend into surrounding structures.[28] Endocarditis after aortic root replacement with mechanical valves frequently causes dehiscence of the valve from the aortic annulus with consequent false aneurysm.[29]

MICROBIOLOGY

The microbiology of infective endocarditis of the aortic valve depends on whether the valve is native or prosthetic, and whether the infection is hospital or community acquired. *Staphylococcus aureus* and *Streptococcus viridans* are the most common microorganisms responsible for native aortic valve endocarditis.[30,31] *Staphylococcus aureus* is extremely virulent and able to cause infection in patients with normal aortic valves. *Streptococcus viridans* is not as virulent and causes infection that often follows a protracted course. *Staphylococcus epidermidis* and various other streptococci can also cause endocarditis. Coagulase-negative staphylococci have emerged as an important cause of native valve endocarditis in both community and health care settings.[32]

Endocarditis caused by gram-negative bacteria is uncommon, but it is often resistant to antibiotic therapy and may cause serious complications. *Haemophilus, Actinobacillus, Cardiobacterium, Eikenella,* and *Kingella* (the HACEK group) are gram-negative bacilli grouped together because of their characteristic fastidiousness requiring a prolonged incubation period before growth. Endocarditis resulting from the HACEK group is also uncommon. Fungal endocarditis is rare but extremely serious. *Candida albicans* and *Aspergillus fumigatus* are the usual agents.

The microbiology of prosthetic aortic valve endocarditis is somewhat different from that of the native valve.[25,33] Prosthetic valve endocarditis has been arbitrarily classified as *early* when it occurs within the first 2 months after surgery and *late* when it occurs after 2 months.[34] However, it is possible that many cases of prosthetic valve endocarditis that occur during the first year after surgery are acquired at the time of implantation of the artificial heart valve.[35,36] This may be particularly true when the infection is caused by coagulase-negative staphylococci and the HACEK group of bacteria. Early prosthetic valve endocarditis is caused by contamination of the valve at the time of implantation by perioperative bacteremia.[13] *Staphylococcus epidermidis, S. aureus,* and *Enterococcus faecalis* are among the more common microorganisms responsible for early prosthetic valve endocarditis.[13,33,36] The sources of late prosthetic valve endocarditis are more difficult to determine. Bacteremia is probably the principal cause of late endocarditis. Although streptococci and staphylococci are commonly encountered in these patients, a myriad of microorganisms can cause late prosthetic valve endocarditis.[33,36]

Nosocomial infections are often caused by *S. aureus* or other staphylococci.

In a small proportion of cases of aortic valve endocarditis, no microorganism can be cultured from either the blood or surgical specimens.[33,36] This is called "culture-negative endocarditis," but it is important to rule out fastidious microorganisms and every effort should be made to identify them.

CLINICAL PRESENTATION AND DIAGNOSIS

It is helpful to classify infective endocarditis as acute and subacute because there are major differences between these two clinical presentations. Subacute endocarditis is often caused by less virulent microorganisms such as *S. viridans.* When this organism affects a diseased aortic valve, the clinical course is protracted and antibiotics alone cure most cases. On the other hand, acute endocarditis is frequently caused by a virulent microorganism such as *S. aureus* and may affect a normal aortic valve. The clinical course is acute, and antibiotics alone often fail to cure the infection.

The onset of subacute endocarditis in most cases is subtle, with low-grade fever and malaise. Patients think they have the "flu" and are often treated with oral antibiotics for a week to 10 days with improvement of symptoms. However, in most cases the symptoms recur a few days after stopping antibiotics. In the majority of cases no predisposing factor is identified. An aortic valve murmur is present in nearly all patients because they have preexisting aortic valve disease. Splenomegaly is common. Clubbing of the fingers and toes may develop in long-standing cases. Skin and mucous membrane signs occur late in this form of endocarditis. Petechiae appear on any part of the body. Small areas of hemorrhage may be seen in the ocular fundi. Hemorrhages in the nail beds usually have a linear distribution near the distal end, hence the name splinter hemorrhages. Osler nodes are acute, tender, barely palpable nodular lesions in the pulp of the fingers and toes. Bacteria have been cultured from these lesions. Embolization of large vegetation fragments may cause dramatic clinical events such as acute myocardial infarction (AMI), stroke, or splenic or hepatic infarcts. Any other organ also may be involved. Destruction of the aortic cusps causes aortic insufficiency and heart failure. The blood pathology is not distinctive in subacute endocarditis. Anemia without reticulocytosis develops in patients untreated for more than a few weeks. The leukocyte count is moderately elevated. Blood cultures frequently identify the offending microorganism.

The clinical course of acute endocarditis is often fulminating. A preexisting source of bacteremia may be identified. This form of endocarditis can present with all the symptoms and signs described under subacute endocarditis, but they are more acute and patients are often sicker with overwhelming signs of sepsis. Early metastatic infections are common. Two physical signs are seen only in acute endocarditis: the Janeway lesion (a painless red-blue hemorrhagic lesion a few millimeters in diameter found in the palms of the hands and the soles of the feet) and the Roth spot (an oval pale area surrounded by hemorrhage near the optic disc). Acute endocarditis is common in patients with no preexisting aortic valve disease. Early cardiac decompensation caused by aortic insufficiency is common. Paravalvular abscess is also common, and depending on the location of the abscess, the electrocardiogram may show an increased PR interval or heart block. The blood picture is one of acute sepsis. Blood culture often isolates the infecting agent.

Prosthetic valve endocarditis may present as acute or subacute endocarditis.

Doppler echocardiography is very useful in the diagnosis and management of infective endocarditis.[37–40] Transesophageal echocardiography is usually better than transthoracic echocardiography and multiplane is better than monoplane for the diagnosis of endocarditis. Echocardiography can detect vegetations as small as 1 or 2 mm in size, but it is more reliable in native than prosthetic valve endocarditis. It is more useful for tissue than for mechanical valves because of the acoustic shadowing of ball, disc, or leaflet motion of mechanical heart valves. Echocardiography is also highly sensitive for detecting paravalvular abscess and cardiac fistulas.[40,41]

Clinical investigators from Duke University proposed certain criteria for confirming or rejecting the diagnosis of infective endocarditis.[42] These criteria have been confirmed by other investigators and their limitations addressed by others.[43–45] A modified version of the Duke criteria has been proposed[45] and it is shown in Table 37-1.

Heart catheterization and coronary angiography increase the risk of embolization in patients with aortic valve vegetations and should be avoided. Newer computed tomography (CT) imaging techniques to diagnose coronary artery disease are useful in these patients.

The investigators of the International Collaboration on Endocarditis–Prospective Cohort Study (ICE-PCS), an international and multicenter database on patients with confirmed endocarditis maintained at the Duke Clinical Research Institute recently reported on the clinical presentation, etiology, and outcome of infective endocarditis with definite diagnosis according to Duke criteria (see Table 37-1).[31] The ICE-PCS report included a cohort of 2781 patients whose median age was 57.9 years. The endocarditis was native in 72%, prosthetic in 21% and pacemaker/ICD related in 7%. Approximately one-fourth of the patients had history of recent health care exposure. The mitral valve was infected in 41.1% of the patients and the aortic valve in 37.6%. *Staphylococcus aureus* was the offending microorganism in 31.2% of all cases. The diagnosis of stroke was made in 16.9% and other emboli were diagnosed in 22.6%. Congestive heart failure (CHF) developed 32.2%. Paravalvular abscess occurred in 14% of the patients. Surgical treatment was common for the entire cohort (48.2%), and overall in-hospital mortality was 17.7%.

TREATMENT

An appropriate antibiotic is the most important aspect of the management of patients with infective endocarditis.[30,31,36] Antibiotic therapy should be started soon after obtaining several blood cultures. The initial choice of antibiotics is based on clinical circumstances and the suspected source of infection. Patients who had recent dental work should receive antibiotics to counteract bacteria from the oral cavity; those who had recent urinary or colonic procedures should be treated with antibiotics that are effective against gram-negative bacteria.

Intravenous drug users are usually infected with *S. aureus* or coagulase-negative *staphylococci*, and antibiotics should be chosen accordingly. Once the microorganism is identified by blood cultures and its sensitivity to specific antibiotics is known, antibiotic therapy is adjusted accordingly. A combination of two or three antibiotics that potentiate each other is often needed in the treatment of endocarditis caused by virulent microorganisms. Intravenous antibiotic therapy is continued for 6 weeks.

It is difficult to eradicate infection caused by virulent microorganisms with antibiotics alone because these microorganisms often destroy the native aortic valve very rapidly and cause aortic insufficiency and CHF. These infections are usually caused by *S. aureus, Pseudomonas aeruginosa, Serratia marcescens,* or fungi.

Surveillance blood cultures are performed in 48 hours to monitor the efficacy of antibiotic therapy. The patient must be watched closely for signs of CHF, coronary and systemic embolization, and persistent infection. Daily electrocardiograms and frequent echocardiograms are performed during the first 2 weeks of treatment. With any evidence of increasing aortic insufficiency, enlarging vegetations, recurrent embolism, paravalvular abscess, or persistent infection, surgery should be immediately performed. It is important to operate on patients before they develop intractable heart failure, cardiogenic or septic shock, or extensive aortic root abscesses. Patients with vegetations larger than 10 mm present a clinical problem because they are more likely to develop serious complications and early surgery is justifiable.[37–39]

Anticoagulation is not effective in preventing embolization of vegetations in native and biologic valves and is associated with an increased risk of neurologic complications.[46,47]

Surgical treatment should be considered in patients with signs of CHF, acute valve dysfunction, paravalvular abscess or cardiac fistulas, recurrent systemic embolization when aortic valve vegetations are present, and persistent sepsis despite adequate antibiotic therapy for more than 4 to 5 days.

Patients with neurologic deficits should have CT or magnetic resonance imaging performed to determine if the cerebrovascular accident is ischemic or hemorrhagic. Ischemic damage

TABLE 37-1 Modified Duke Criteria for the Diagnosis of Infective Endocarditis

Major Criteria

- Blood culture positive for infective endocarditis
  - Typical microorganisms consistent with infective endocarditis from two separate blood cultures: *Streptococcus viridans, S. bovis* HACEK group, *S. aureus,* or community-acquired enterococci, in the absence of a primary focus, or Microorganisms consistent with infective endocarditis from a persistently positive blood culture, defined as follows:
    - At least two positive cultures of blood drawn >12 hours apart, or
    - All of three or a majority of >four separate cultures of blood (with the first and last samples drawn at least 1 hour apart)
    - Single positive blood culture for *Coxiella burnetii* or phase I IgG antibody titer to *C. burnetii*> 1:800
- Evidence of endocardial involvement:
- Echocardiogram positive for infective endocarditis: TEE recommended in patients with prosthetic valves, rated at least as "possible endocarditis" by clinical criteria, or complicated endocarditis, such as endocarditis with paravalvular abscess; TTE as the first test in other patients as follows:
  - Oscillating intracardiac mass on valve or supporting structures, in the path of regurgitant jets, or on implanted material in the absence of an alternative anatomic explanation;
  - Abscess:
  - New partial dehiscence of prosthetic valve
- New valvular regurgitation (worsening or changing of preexisting murmur not sufficient)

Minor Criteria

- Predisposition, predisposing heart condition, or injection drug use
- Fever
- Vascular phenomena: major arterial emboli, septic pulmonary infarcts, mycotic aneurysm, intracranial hemorrhage, conjunctival hemorrhages, and Janeway lesions
- Immunologic phenomena: glomerulonephritis, Osler nodes, Roth spots, and rheumatoid factor
- Microbiologic evidence: positive blood culture but does not meet a major criterion as noted above, or serologic evidence of active infection with an organism consistent with infective endocarditis
- Echocardiographic minor criteria eliminated

Definite endocarditis = two major criteria, or one major + three minor criteria, or five minor criteria
Possible endocarditis = one major + one minor, or three minor criteria
HACEK group = Haemophilus, Actinobacillus, Cardiobacterium, Eikenella, and Kingella; IE = infective endocarditis; TEE = transesophageal echocardiography; TTE = transthoracic echocardiography
Source: Used with permission from Li JS, Sexton DJ, Mick N, et al: Proposed modifications to the Duke Criteria for the diagnosis of infective endocarditis. Clin Infect Dis 2000; 30:633.

is far more common than hemorrhagic damage, but both are associated with increased mortality and morbidity.[46–49] Mycotic aneurysms should be treated before valve surgery. Aortic valve replacement should be postponed for 2 weeks after an ischemic stroke and 4 weeks after a hemorrhagic stroke if possible.[49]

SURGICAL TREATMENT

Patients who need surgery are often very sick and may be in CHF. For this reason and because they often require complex and long surgical procedures, myocardial protection is of utmost importance. Another important aspect of surgery for endocarditis is avoidance of contamination of the surgical field, instruments, drapes, and gloves with vegetations and pus. Instruments used to extirpate contaminated areas in the heart should be discarded before reconstruction of the ventricle and aortic root begins. In addition, local drapes, suction equipment, and surgical gloves should all be changed.

When the infection is limited to the cusps of the native aortic valve or a bioprosthetic valve, complete removal of the valve and implantation of a biologic or mechanical valve usually resolves the problem. There is no evidence that bioprostheses are better than mechanical valves in patients with active infective endocarditis.[50] Some investigators believe that aortic valve homograft is ideal for patients with active endocarditis,[51–53] but the fact is that it can become infected like other valves and there is no evidence that the risk of persistent or recurrent infection is different from other valves.[54,55] Some surgeons favor the pulmonary autograft, particularly in young patients.[56]

If the aortic annulus is involved in the infective process, resection of the necrotic or inflamed area is needed before a prosthetic valve can be implanted. The defect created by the resection should be patched before a prosthetic valve is implanted. We prefer to use fresh autologous pericardium to patch small defects (1 or 2 cm wide) in the aortic root and left ventricular outflow tract (LVOT), and glutaraldehyde-fixed bovine pericardium for larger defects.[57,58] Some surgeons also use Dacron fabric to reconstruct the aortic root.[59,60] Here again, aortic valve homograft is believed to be ideal for reconstruction of the aortic root and LVOT.[52,61–63] The mitral valve of the aortic valve homograft can be used to patch defects in the LVOT by correctly orienting the homograft. However, an aortic valve homograft is by no means a substitute for radical resection of all infected tissues, because persistent infection can occur with this biologic valve.[64,65] The pulmonary autograft has also been used in cases of extensive destruction of the aortic root,[66] but again, this valve is no substitute for radical resection of all infected tissues.

Surgery for aortic root abscess and/or cardiac fistulas is challenging. The most important aspect in the surgical treatment of these patients is radical resection of all infected tissues.[25,55,57,58] We believe that the type of valve implanted is less important than complete extirpation of all infected and edematous tissues.[58] These patients frequently require replacement of the entire aortic root and reconstruction of the surrounding structures that are also involved by the abscess. These operations must be individualized because the pathology of aortic root abscess is variable. Extensive resection and reconstruction may be needed.[58,67–69] Thus, patching of the interventricular septum, dome of the left atrium, intervalvular fibrous body, right atrium, and pulmonary artery may be necessary, as well as repair of the left and/or right coronary arteries. The aortic root is often replaced with a valved conduit.

Aortic root abscess extending into the intervalvular fibrous body or into a prosthetic mitral valve is particularly difficult to treat.[67–69] In these cases, the resection and reconstruction can be performed through the aortic root and dome of the atrium.[67–69] When an aortic valve homograft is used for this type of reconstruction, the anterior leaflet of the mitral valve of the homograft can be used as patch material for the new fibrous body between the aortic and mitral valves. Actually, aortic and mitral valve homografts in a single bloc of tissue have been used to treat this condition.[70]

Postoperative complications are common after surgery for active infective endocarditis. Septic patients may have severe coagulopathy and may bleed excessively after cardiopulmonary bypass. Antifibrinolytic agents such as tranexaminic acid or aminocaproic acid should be used in addition to platelets, cryoprecipitate, and fresh-frozen plasma in patients with coagulopathy. The administration of recombinant Factor VII may also be necessary after correction of thrombocytopenia, fibrinogen level, and thromboplastin and prothrombin times. Radical resection of aortic root abscess may cause heart block, for which a permanent pacemaker will be needed postoperatively. Depending on the patient's clinical condition before surgery, multiorgan failure may develop postoperatively. Neurologic deterioration may occur in patients with preexisting cerebral emboli. Pulmonary, splenic, hepatic, and other metastatic abscesses seldom require surgical treatment. Large metastatic abscesses may have to be drained, and in the case of the spleen, splenectomy should be performed because of the risk of rupture.[71]

Clinical Results

The prognosis of aortic valve endocarditis depends largely on when the disease is diagnosed, on the offending microorganism, and how promptly it is treated.[30,31,72] Patients with prosthetic aortic valve endocarditis have a more serious prognosis than patients with native aortic valve endocarditis,[31,36] and nosocomial infections are associated with higher mortality than community-acquired infections.[73,74] The results of surgery for infective endocarditis have improved significantly since the introduction of antibiotics and surgery, but in-hospital mortality remains high at approximately 18%.[31] Prosthetic valve endocarditis, increasing age, pulmonary edema, *S. aureus* infection, coagulase-negative staphylococcal infection, mitral valve vegetation, and paravalvular abscess were associated with an increased risk of in-hospital mortality at the ICE-PCS report on 2781 patients.[31] Approximately one-half of those patients required surgery as part of their treatment.[31]

The operative mortality for patients with infection limited to the cusps of the aortic valve is largely dependent on the patients' clinical presentation at the time of surgery, age, and comorbidities. Most reports indicate that the operative mortality is under 10%.[36,55,75] The operative mortality is higher for prosthetic valve endocarditis and ranges from 20 to 30%.[25,26,31,76] Similarly, surgery for aortic root abscess is associated with higher operative mortality.[58–63]

We reviewed our 25-year experience with surgery for infective endocarditis in 383 consecutive patients.[36] There were 226 patients with native and 117 with prosthetic valve endocarditis. The overall operative mortality was 12%. Preoperative shock, prosthetic valve endocarditis, paravalvular abscess and *S. aureus* were independent predictors of operative mortality. The 15-year survival for patients with native valve endocarditis was 59% and for patients with prosthetic valve endocarditis was 25% ($p < .01$). The freedom from recurrent infective endocarditis at 15 years was 86%, and similar for patients with native and prosthetic valve endocarditis. In most of these patients, a different microorganism caused the second episode of endocarditis.

PROPHYLAXIS OF INFECTIVE ENDOCARDITIS

The American Heart Association guidelines for prophylaxis of infective endocarditis were updated in 2007.[77]

The major changes in the updated recommendations include the following: (1) The Committee concluded that only an extremely small number of cases of infective endocarditis might be prevented by antibiotic prophylaxis for dental procedures even if such prophylactic therapy were 100% effective. (2) Infective endocarditis prophylaxis for dental procedures is reasonable only for patients with underlying cardiac conditions associated with the highest risk of adverse outcome from infective endocarditis. (3) For patients with these underlying cardiac conditions, prophylaxis is reasonable for all dental procedures that involve manipulation of gingival tissue or the periapical region of teeth or perforation of the oral mucosa. (4) Prophylaxis is not recommended based solely on an increased lifetime risk of acquisition of infective endocarditis. (5) Administration of antibiotics solely to prevent endocarditis is not recommended for patients who undergo a genitourinary or gastrointestinal tract procedure. These changes are intended to define more clearly when infective endocarditis prophylaxis is or is not recommended and provide more uniform and consistent global recommendations.

These new recommendations represent a dramatic shift with regard to which patients should receive antibiotic prophylaxis for prevention of infective endocarditis. However, they are "guidelines" and physicians caring for patients with organic heart valve disease should advise them according to the perceived risk of endocarditis and potential benefit of antibiotic prophylaxis.

REFERENCES

1. Lamas CC, Eykyn SJ: Bicuspid aortic valve—a silent danger: analysis of 50 cases of infective endocarditis. *Clin Infect Dis* 2000; 30:336.
2. Dyson C, Barnes RA, Harrison GA: Infective endocarditis: an epidemiological review of 128 episodes. *J Infect* 2000; 40:99.
3. King JW, Nguyen VQ, Conrad SA: Results of a prospective statewide reporting system for infective endocarditis. *Am J Med Sci* 1988; 295:517.
4. Berlin JA, Abrutyn E, Strom BL, et al: Incidence of infective endocarditis in the Delaware Valley, 1988–1990. *Am J Cardiol* 1995; 76:933.
5. Tleyjeh IM, Steckelber JM, Murad HS, et al: Temporal trends in infective endocarditis: a population-based study in Olmsted County, Minnesota. *JAMA* 2005; 293:3022.
6. Cabell CH, Fowler VG Jr, Chamber JC, Sommerville J, Stone S, et al: Pulmonary autograft procedure for aortic valve disease: long-term results of a pioneer series. *Circulation* 1997; 96:2206.
7. Lund O, Chandrasekaran V, Grocott-Mason R, et al: Primary aortic valve replacement with allografts over twenty-five years: valve-related and procedure-related determinants of outcomes. *J Thorac Cardiovasc Surg* 1999; 117:77.
8. David TE, Ivanov J, Armstrong S, et al: Late results of heart valve replacement with the Hancock II bioprosthesis. *J Thorac Cardiovasc Surg* 2001; 121:268.
9. Jamieson WRE, Janusz MT, Burr LH, et al: Carpentier-Edwards supra-annular porcine bioprosthesis: second generation prosthesis in aortic valve replacement. *Ann Thorac Surg* 2001; 71:S224.
10. Poirier NC, Pelletier LC, Pellerin M, et al: 15-Year experience with the Carpentier-Edwards pericardial bioprosthesis. *Ann Thorac Surg* 1998; 66:S57.
11. Emery RW, Krogh CC, Arom KV, et al: The St. Jude Medical valve: a 25-year experience with single valve replacement. *Ann Thorac Surg* 2005; 79:776.
12. Hammermeister KE, Sethi GK, Henderson WG, et al: Outcomes 15 years after valve replacement with a mechanical versus a bioprosthetic valve: final report of the Veterans Affairs randomized trial. *J Am Coll Cardiol* 2000; 36:1152.
13. Gordon SM, Serkey JM, Longworth DL, et al: Early onset prosthetic valve endocarditis: the Cleveland Clinic experience 1992–1997. *Ann Thorac Surg* 2000; 69:1388.
14. McCarthy JT, Steckelberg JM: Infective endocarditis in patients receiving long-term hemodialysis. *Mayo Clin Proc* 2000; 75:1008.
15. Crasta K, Daly CG, Mitchell D, et al: Bacteraemia due to dental flossing. *J Clin Periodontol* 2009;36:323-32.
16. Grant RT, Wood JR Jr, Jones TS: Heart valve irregularities in relation to subacute bacterial endocarditis. *Heart* 1928; 14:247.
17. Angrist AA, Oka M: Pathogenesis of bacterial endocarditis. *JAMA* 1963; 181:249.
18. Durack DT, Beeson PB, Petersdorf RG: Experimental bacterial endocarditis, III: production and progress of the disease in rabbits. *Br J Exp Pathol* 1973; 54:142.
19. Mylonakis E, Calderwood SB: Infective endocarditis in adults. *NEJM* 2001; 345:1318.
20. Salgado AV, Furlan AJ, Keys TF, et al: Neurologic complications of endocarditis: a 12-year experience. *Neurology* 1989; 39:173.
21. Kanter MC, Hart RG: Neurologic complications of infective endocarditis. *Neurology* 1991; 41:1015.
22. Piper C, Hetzer R, Korfer R, et al: The importance of secondary mitral valve involvement in primary aortic valve endocarditis: the mitral kissing vegetation. *Heart* 2002; 23:79.
23. Gillinov AM, Diaz R, Blackstone EH, et al: Double valve endocarditis. *Ann Thorac Surg* 2001; 71:1874.
24. Arnett EN, Roberts WC: Prosthetic valve endocarditis: clinicopathologic analysis of 22 necropsy patients with active infective endocarditis involving natural left-sided cardiac valves. *Am J Cardiol* 1976; 38:282.
25. David TE: The surgical treatment of patients with prosthetic valve endocarditis. *Semin Thorac Cardiovasc Surg* 1995; 7:47.
26. Sett SS, Hudon MPJ, Jamieson WRE, et al: Prosthetic valve endocarditis: experience with porcine bioprostheses. *J Thorac Cardiovasc Surg* 1993; 105:428.
27. Fernicola DJ, Roberts WC: Frequency of ring abscess and cuspal infection in active infective endocarditis involving bioprosthetic valves. *Am J Cardiol* 1993; 72:314.
28. Clarkson PM, Barratt-Boyes BG: Bacterial endocarditis following homograft replacement of the aortic valve. *Circulation* 1970; 42:987.
29. Ralph-Edwards A, David TE, Bos J: Infective endocarditis in patients who had replacement of the aortic root. *Ann Thorac Surg* 1994; 35:429.
30. Watanakunakorn C, Burket T: Infective endocarditis at a large community teaching hospital, 1980–1990: a review of 210 episodes. *Medicine* 1993; 72:90.
31. Murdoch DR, Corey GR, Hoen B, et al: Clinical presentation, etiology, and outcome of infective endocarditis in the 21st century: the International Collaboration on Endocarditis-Prospective Cohort Study. *Arch Intern Med* 2009; 169:463.
32. Chu VH, Woods CW, Miro JM, et al: Emergence of coagulase-negative staphylococci as a cause of native valve endocarditis. *Clin Infect Dis* 2008; 46:232.
33. Fang G, Keys TF, Gentry LO, et al: Prosthetic valve endocarditis resulting from nosocomial bacteremia: a prospective, multicenter study. *Ann Intern Med* 1993; 119:560.
34. Calderwood SB, Swinsk LA, Waternaux CM, et al: Risk factors for development of prosthetic valve endocarditis. *Circulation* 1985; 72:31.
35. Chu VH, Miro JM, Hoen B, et al. Coagulase-negative staphylococcal prosthetic valve endocarditis—a contemporary update based on the International Collaboration on Endocarditis: prospective cohort study. *Heart* 2009; 95:570.
36. David TE, Gavra G, Feindel CM, et al: Surgical treatment of active infective endocarditis: a continued challenge. *J Thorac Cardiovasc Surg* 2007; 133:144.
37. Buda AJ, Zotx RJ, Lemire MS, Back DS: Prognostic significance of vegetations detected by two-dimensional echocardiography in infective endocarditis. *Am Heart J* 1986; 112:1291.
38. Lowry RW, Zoghbi WA, Baker WB, et al: Clinical impact of transesophageal echocardiography in the diagnosis and management of infective endocarditis. *Am J Cardiol* 1994; 73:1089.
39. DiSalvo G, Habib G, Pergola V, et al: Echocardiography predicts embolic events in infective endocarditis. *J Am Coll Cardiol* 2001; 15:1069.
40. Daniel WG, Mugge A, Martin RP, et al: Improvement in the diagnosis of abscesses associated with endocarditis by transesophageal echocardiography. *NEJM* 1991; 324:795.
41. Anguera I, Quaglio G, Miro JM, et al: Aortocardiac fistulas complicating infective endocarditis. *Am J Cardiol* 2001; 87:652.
42. Durack DT, Lukes AS, Bright DK: New criteria for diagnosis of infective endocarditis: utilization of specific echocardiographic findings. *Am J Cardiol* 1994; 96:200.
43. Sekeres MA, Abrutyn E, Berlin JA, et al: An assessment of the usefulness of the Duke criteria for diagnosing active infective endocarditis. *Clin Infect Dis* 1997; 24:1185.
44. Habib G, Derumeaux G, Avierinos JF, et al: Value and limitations of the Duke criteria for the diagnosis of infective endocarditis. *J Am Coll Cardiol* 1999; 33:2023.
45. Li JS, Sexton DJ, Mick N, et al: Proposed modifications to the Duke Criteria for the diagnosis of infective endocarditis. *Clin Infect Dis* 2000; 30:633.
46. Davenport J, Hart RG: Prosthetic valve endocarditis 1976–1987: antibiotics, anticoagulation, and stroke. *Stroke* 1990; 21:993.
47. Ting W, Silverman N, Levistky S: Valve replacement in patients with endocarditis and cerebral septic emboli. *Ann Thorac Surg* 1991; 51:18.
48. Matsushita K, Kuriyama Y, Sawada T, et al: Hemorrhagic and ischemic cerebrovascular complications of active infective endocarditis of native valve. *Eur Neurol* 1993; 33:267.
49. Gillinov AM, Shah RV, Curtis WE, et al: Valve replacement in patients with endocarditis and acute neurologic deficit. *Ann Thorac Surg* 1996; 61:1125.
50. Moon MR, Miller DC, Moore KA, et al: Treatment of endocarditis with valve replacement: the question of tissue versus mechanical prosthesis. *Ann Thorac Surg* 2001; 71:1164.
51. Haydock D, Barratt-Boyes B, Macedo T, et al: Aortic valve replacement for active infective endocarditis in 108 patients: a comparison of free-hand allograft valves with mechanical prostheses and bioprostheses. *J Thorac Cardiovasc Surg* 1992; 103:130.

52. Yankah AC, Pasic M, Klose H, et al: Homograft reconstruction of the aortic root for endocarditis with periannular abscess: a 17-year study. *Eur J Cardiothorac Surg* 2005; 28:69.
53. Grinda JM, Mainardi JL, D'Attellis N, et al: Cryopreserved aortic viable homograft for active aortic endocarditis. *Ann Thorac Surg* 2005; 79:767.
54. Kilian E, Oberhoffer M, Gulbins H, et al: Ten years' experience in aortic valve replacement with homografts in 389 cases. *J Heart Valve Dis* 2004; 13:554.
55. Klieverik LM, Yacoub MH, Edwards S, et al: Surgical treatment of active native aortic valve endocarditis with allografts and mechanical prostheses. *Ann Thorac Surg* 2009; 88:1814.
56. Oswalt JD, Dewan SJ, Mueller MC, et al: Highlights of a ten-year experience with the Ross procedure. *Ann Thorac Surg* 2001; 71:S332.
57. David TE, Komeda M, Brofman PR: Surgical treatment of aortic root abscess. *Circulation* 1989; 80(Suppl 1):26.
58. David TE, Regesta T, Gavra G, Armstrong S, Maganti MD: Surgical treatment of paravalvular abscess: long-term results. *Eur J Cardiothorac Surg* 2007; 31:43.
59. Jault F, Gandjbakhch I, Chastre JC, et al: Prosthetic valve endocarditis with ring abscesses: surgical management and long-term results. *J Thorac Cardiovasc Surg* 1993; 105:1106.
60. Fiore AC, Ivey TD, McKeown PP, et al: Patch closure of aortic annulus mycotic aneurysm. *Ann Thorac Surg* 1986; 42:372.
61. Glazier JJ, Verwilghen J, Donaldson RM, et al: Treatment of complicated prosthetic aortic valve endocarditis with annular abscess formation by homograft root replacement. *J Am Coll Cardiol* 1991; 17:1177.
62. Dossche KM, Defauw JJ, Ernst SM, et al: Allograft aortic root replacement in prosthetic aortic valve endocarditis: a review of 32 patients. *Ann Thorac Surg* 1997; 63:1644.
63. Knosalla C, Weng Y, Yankah AC, et al: Surgical treatment of active infective aortic valve endocarditis with associated periannular abscess—11 year results. *Eur Heart J* 2000; 21:421.
64. Ritter M, von Segesser L, Lenni R: Persistent root abscess after emergency repair with an aortic homograft. *Br Heart J* 1994; 72:495.
65. Joyce FS, McCarthy PM, Stewart WJ, et al: Left ventricle to right atrial fistula after aortic homograft replacement for endocarditis. *Eur J Cardiothorac Surg* 1994; 8:100.
66. Pettersson G, Tingleff J, Joyce FS: Treatment of aortic valve endocarditis with the Ross procedure. *Eur J Cardiothorac Surg* 1998; 13:678.
67. David TE, Feindel CM, Armstrong S, et al: Reconstruction of the mitral annulus: a ten-year experience. *J Thorac Cardiovasc Surg* 1995; 110:1323.
68. David TE, Kuo J, Armstrong S: Aortic and mitral valve replacement with reconstruction of the intervalvular fibrous body. *J Thorac Cardiovasc Surg* 1997; 114:766.
69. Krasopoulos G, David TE, Armstrong S: Custom-tailored valved conduit for complex aortic root disease. *J Thorac Cardiovasc Surg* 2008; 135:3.
70. Obadia JF, Raisky O, Sebbag L, et al: Monobloc aorto-mitral homo-graft as a treatment of complex cases of endocarditis. *J Thorac Cardiovasc Surg* 2001; 121:584.
71. Ting W, Silverman NA, Levitsky S: Splenic septic emboli in endocarditis. *Circulation* 1990; 82(Suppl V):105.
72. Miro JM, Anguera I, Cabell CH, et al: *Staphylococcus aureus* native valve endocarditis: report of 566 episodes from the International Collaboration on Endocarditis Merged Database. *Clin Infect Dis* 2005; 41:507.
73. Hoen B, Alla F, Selton-Suty C, et al: Changing profile of infective endocarditis—Results of a 1-year survey in France. *JAMA* 2002; 288:75.
74. Chu VH, Cabell CH, Benjamin DK, et al: Early predictors of inhospital death in infective endocarditis. *Circulation* 2004; 109:1745.
75. Alexiou C, Langley SM, Stafford H, et al: Surgery for active culture-positive endocarditis: determinants of early and late outcome. *Ann Thorac Surg* 2000; 69:1448.
76. Alonso-Valle H, Fariñas-Álvarez C, García-Palomo JD. Clinical course and predictors of death in prosthetic valve endocarditis over a 20-year period. *J Thorac Cardiovasc Surg* 2009.
77. Wilson W, Taubert KA, Gewitz M, et al: Prevention of infective endocarditis: guidelines from the American Heart Association: a guideline from the American Heart Association Rheumatic Fever, Endocarditis, and Kawasaki Disease Committee, Council on Cardiovascular Disease in the Young, and the Council on Clinical Cardiology, Council on Cardiovascular Surgery and Anesthesia, and the Quality of Care and Outcomes Research Interdisciplinary Working Group. *Circulation* 2007; 116:1736.

CHAPTER 38

Minimally Invasive Aortic Valve Surgery

Prem S. Shekar
Lawrence H. Cohn

INTRODUCTION

Aortic valve surgery started with the implantation of the Hufnagel valve in the descending thoracic aorta in 1956. Its evolution over time has culminated with the advent of percutaneous catheter based aortic valve replacement techniques. There is a flurry of recent activity in the world literature about this new approach. As a new paradigm in aortic valve replacement is ushered, there will be new challenges for the cardiac surgeons to not only maintain the efficacy and outcomes of conventional valve replacement but to provide it in a less invasive approach. Modern techniques will be measured against conventional procedures, especially in the older patients with multiple comorbidities. Minimally invasive aortic valve surgery holds promise as an effective operation with reduced pain, improved respiratory function, early recovery and an overall reduction in trauma.

ESSENTIALS OF MINIMAL ACCESS AORTIC VALVE SURGERY

Reoperative minimal access aortic valve surgery is discussed in detail at the end of this chapter. We will first outline the known benefits and salient principles of and the essential ingredients for the conduct of primary minimal access aortic valve surgery.

There are many benefits of minimal access aortic valve surgery.

1. It provides a cosmetically superior incision.
2. There is reduced postoperative pain.
3. There is faster postoperative recovery.
4. There is improved postoperative respiratory function from preservation of a part of the sternum and the integrity of the costal margin.
5. It can be performed with the same degree of ease and speed as a conventional operation with no difference in mortality.
6. It provides access to the relevant parts of the heart and reduces dissection of other areas.
7. It greatly facilitates a reoperation at a later date as the lower part of the pericardium remains closed.

There are some salient inviolate principles of minimal access aortic valve surgery:

1. Ability to safely apply a stable aortic cross-clamp
2. Ability to visualize the aortic valve completely and perform a successful replacement with the standard techniques
3. Ability to achieve the same degree of myocardial protection as through a midline sternotomy approach
4. Ability to deal with issues of the aortic root, ascending and arch of the aorta with relative ease and without the need for conversion
5. Ability to quickly convert to a standard midline sternotomy if compromising situations arise

The safety and reproducibility of minimal access aortic valve surgery depend on:

1. Availability of experienced cardiac anesthesiologists
2. Availability of transesophageal echocardiography (TEE) in every case and an experienced echocardiographer to interpret findings
3. Ability to place pulmonary artery catheters with pacing capabilities and transjugular coronary sinus catheters, if and when necessary
4. Ability to place percutaneous arterial and venous cardiopulmonary bypass canulae
5. Ability to use vacuum-assisted venous drainage on cardiopulmonary bypass
6. Availability of minimal access retractors and other relevant instruments that facilitate this operation

7. Ability to remotely monitor myocardial protection and distention by TEE
8. Availability of surgeons experienced with conventional aortic valve surgery and minimal access surgery

Whatever the surgical approach, today aortic valve replacement is done with the use of cardiopulmonary bypass and diastolic arrest of the heart. There are at least four different minimal access surgical approaches to the aortic valve:

1. Upper hemisternotomy
2. Right parasternal approach
3. Right anterior thoracotomy
4. Transverse sternotomy

THE UPPER HEMISTERNOTOMY APPROACH

This is undoubtedly the most popular of all minimal access approaches to the aortic valve. This has been popularized by the surgeons of the Cleveland Clinic and Brigham and Women's Hospital.[1,2]

This is performed through a 6- to 8-cm vertical midline incision over the upper part of the sternum, starting at or just above the level of the manubrio-sternal angle. The sternotomy is performed with the standard saw starting at the level of the sternal notch up to the level of the third or fourth intercostal space (Fig. 38-1). The sternotomy is then T'd off into the right or left third or fourth intercostal space using a narrow blade oscillating saw, taking care not to dive too deeply with it for risk of injuring mediastinal or pericardial structures. The decision to T into the third or fourth space can be made preoperatively with the chest x-ray being a guide to the amount of exposure that will be needed. We favor the fourth interspace because this almost always produces the ideal exposure. It is very important to ensure that the sternotomy is absolutely midline and that the midline sternotomy is not carried beyond the level of the transverse T. Failure to adhere to these principles will result in either a lateral fracture with resultant three sternal fragments or a continued lower extension of midline fracture which with retraction could result in a slow ongoing intraoperative or postoperative blood loss and also difficulty in closure. There is no need to prophylactically divide the right or left internal mammary arteries with this incision. If care is taken not to damage them, they will usually gently retract away.

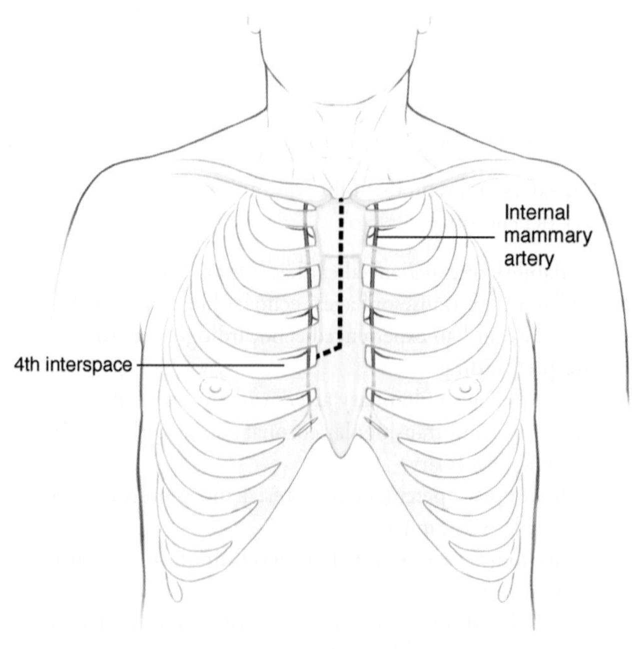

FIGURE 38-1 Upper hemisternotomy incision.

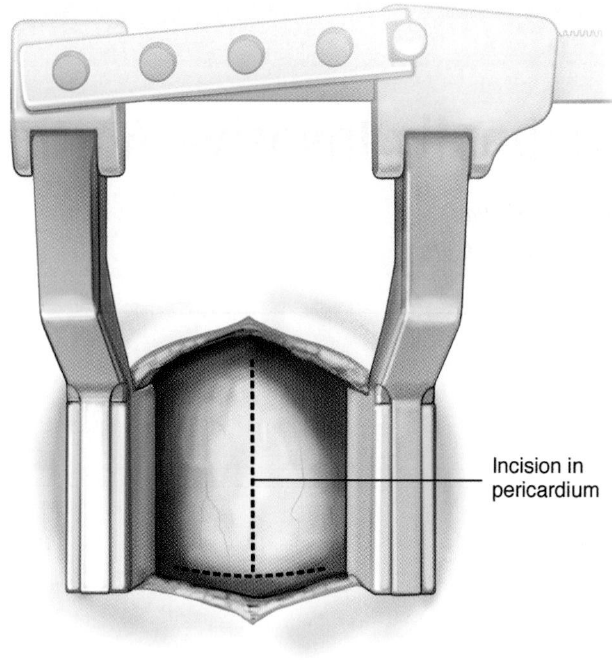

FIGURE 38-2 Midline incision in the pericardium.

We use a Kuros-Baxter® retractor to retract the sternal edges. The pericardium is opened in the midline (Fig. 38-2), T'd inferiorly, and at least three pericardial stay sutures are applied to either side and the needles are left on. The retractor is removed and the pericardium is tacked to the dermis of the skin and tied down. This facilitates exposure by elevating the pericardial contents forward into the operating field. The Kuros-Baxter® retractor is then replaced. Care must be taken during reopening the retractor because sudden retraction with elevated cardiac structures could impede venous return, causing a sudden drop in cardiac output, and leading to acute refractory decompensation in patients with severe aortic stenosis.

We perform an epiaortic ultrasound to exclude atheromatous disease in the ascending aorta before proceeding to systemic heparinization and ascending aortic cannulation in the standard fashion. Right atrial venous cannulation is accomplished directly through the appendage (when easily accessible) (Fig. 38-3) or with a percutaneous venous canula inserted via the right or left femoral vein. There are a variety of custom long venous canulae that are available for the same (usually 20- or 22-French), and they are inserted using the Seldinger technique. The canula is positioned within the right atrium with the tip in the superior venacava using transesophageal echocardiographic guidance. The patient is then placed on cardiopulmonary

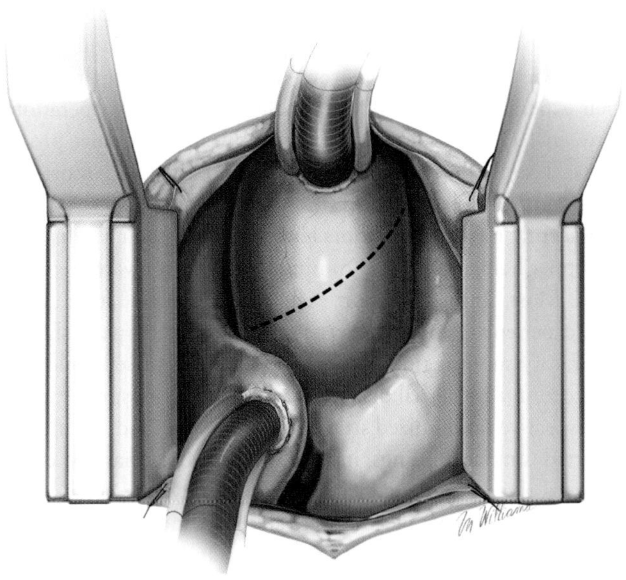

FIGURE 38-3 The pericardium has been tacked up and the patient has been canulated in the standard fashion. Oblique aortotomy has been marked.

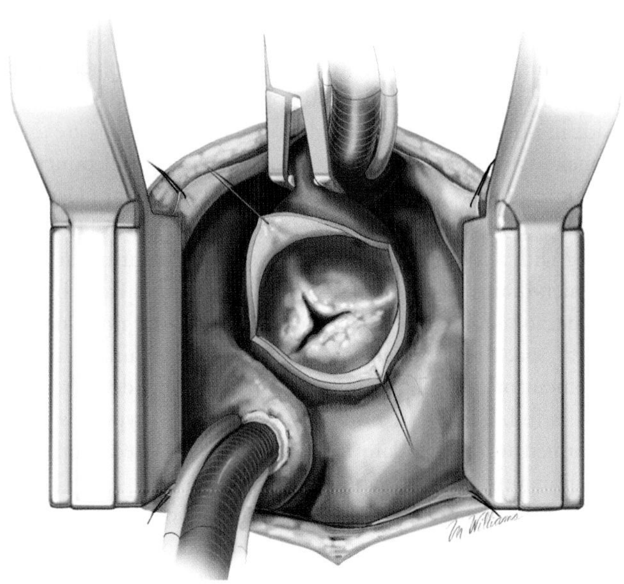

FIGURE 38-4 The aorta was opened after cross-clamping, exposing a calcified trileaflet aortic valve.

bypass. We use tepid bypass with core cooling to 34 to 35°C. The need for vacuum-assisted venous drainage to facilitate this operation cannot be overemphasized.

A retrograde cardioplegia catheter can be placed in the coronary sinus via the right atrial appendage. This may require a minor adjustment to reduce the angulation of the catheter and its insertion can be facilitated by the use of transesophageal echocardiography. Alternatively, this catheter can be placed by the anesthesiologists before surgical incision via the transjugular route. Although we routinely use a transaortic left ventricular vent, a right superior pulmonary vein or a left atrial dome vent can also be easily placed via this incision.

The operation then proceeds as usual. The aorta is cross-clamped and we use 1 L of 8:1 cold blood antegrade cardioplegia. TEE is used to monitor left ventricular distention in patients who may have aortic insufficiency. Retrograde cardioplegia and additional doses of cardioplegia are administered as necessary. Standard aortic valve replacement is then carried through an oblique aortotomy (Fig. 38-4). Upon completion of the procedure, the patient is rewarmed and the aortotomy is closed. A de-airing needle is placed in the ascending aorta before removal of the aortic cross-clamp.

Almost always the heart recovers spontaneous sinus rhythm. When the heart recovers into ventricular fibrillation, it will need to be defibrillated using the external defibrillator pads placed before commencement of the operation. Defibrillation can be facilitated by turning the cardiopulmonary bypass flows down to decompress the heart and other appropriate pharmacologic maneuvers. It is usually quite difficult to introduce internal defibrillator blades through this incision, although pediatric blades can be placed successfully on occasion. Appropriate preoperative placement of external defibrillator pads are of paramount importance. The heart is de-aired using TEE guidance. In the absence of the ability to reach in and agitate the heart, a combination of ventricular filling, table positioning, and external compression is used to successfully de-air the left heart. Although this can always be successfully completed, patience may be an important tool to facilitate this. It is important remember that successful and complete de-airing does not occur until the blood has begun to circulate through the pulmonary and systemic circuits and the heart has started to eject normally.

Before emergence from bypass, pacing wires and drainage tubes will have to be placed (Fig. 38-5). It is very important to perform these placements with the heart decompressed on bypass so as to prevent injury. Invariably, there is an adequate

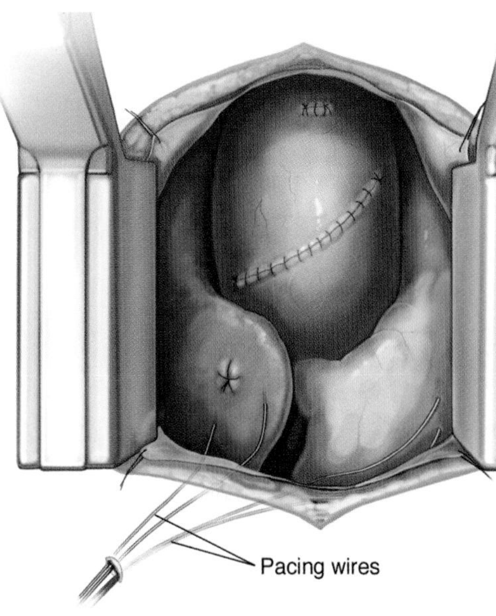

FIGURE 38-5 The aortotomy was closed after valve replacement, and epicardial pacing wires were placed.

amount of atrial and ventricular myocardium exposed to place pacing wires. We usually bring these wires out in the right inframammary area through the right-sided T. We place fluted silastic drains from a subxiphoid approach. Small incisions are made in the subxiphoid area and long grabbing forceps are used to make two retrosternal tunnels, one of which will puncture the pericardium to facilitate placement of a pericardial drain and the other will remain in the retrosternal plane. These are placed with a combination of tactile and visual control. In cases in which drains were not placed before separation from bypass and decannulation, we recommend opening the right or left pleural space and placement of transpleural drainage tubes. Placement of subxiphoid drains is not recommended after the heart is full. The wean from cardiopulmonary bypass is then performed in the standard fashion followed by decannulation and protamine administration.

The pericardium is left open. While policing the area for bleeding, some of the important sites are the coronary sinus from the placement of the retrograde catheter (which will need full sternotomy conversion for control), areas of pacing wire placement and drainage tube entry (which may or may not require conversion to full sternotomy and/or institution of bypass for visualization and control), sites of left ventricular vents, the lower edge of the sternotomy/pericardiotomy, and the internal mammary vessels on the side of the T. The sternum is closed using three or four horizontal sternal wires and an oblique wire placed between the lower intact segment of the sternum and the T'd off segment (Fig. 38-6).

Minimally invasive aortic valve replacement via the upper hemisternotomy approach was originally developed by Cosgrove and colleagues at the Cleveland Clinic[1] and soon after by Cohn and colleagues at the Brigham and Women's Hospital in Boston.[2] Gillinov and colleagues reported their excellent results in 365 cases

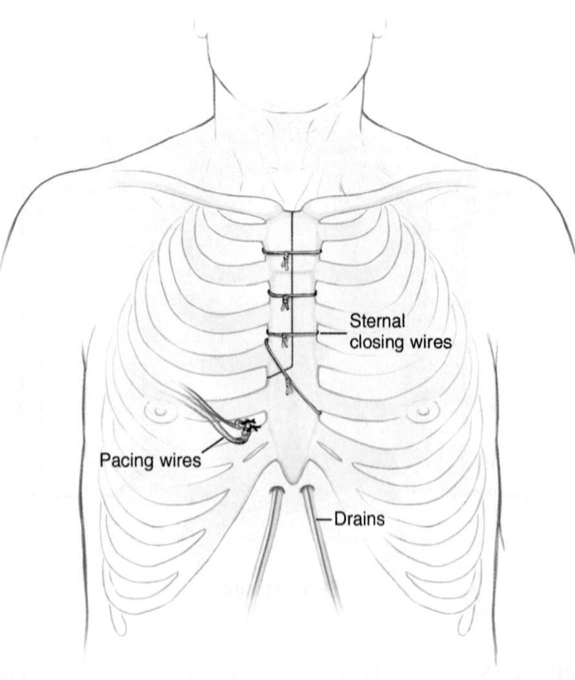

FIGURE 38-6 Final closure of the hemisternotomy incision.

by 2000,[3] and today upper hemisternotomy is the approach of choice for isolated aortic valve surgery at the Cleveland Clinic. Mihaljevic[4] and colleagues from the Brigham group reported their experience with 1000 minimally invasive valve operations between 1996 and 2003, of which 526 were aortic valve procedures. They reported low levels of morbidity and mortality equal to or better than conventional techniques.

Recently numerous authors have published their results with the upper hemisternotomy minimal access aortic valve replacement. Most, if not all, report excellent outcomes. Liu et al,[5] in their experience, reported easier surgical access, less pain, shorter respiratory support time, lower blood loss, decreased incidence of infection and sternal dehiscence, and shorter hospital stay. In a prospective randomized study, Bonacchi et al[6] and Bakir et al[7] reported similar findings in 2002 and 2006. Sharony et al[8] reported their experience with minimally invasive aortic valve surgery in elderly people and were able to demonstrate its safety in this fragile population with morbidity and mortality comparable to standard techniques.

Foghsgaard et al[9] demonstrated a lower incidence of left lower lobe atelectasis in the cardiac intensive care unit than patients who had AVR through a full sternotomy.

The surgeons from the Brigham and Women's Hospital continue to report excellent results from this approach. Tabata et al[10] demonstrated in 2007 that a minimal access AVR can be safely performed in patients with left ventricular dysfunction with mortality and morbidity outcomes similar to a full sternotomy approach. Tabata et al[11] reported excellent early and late results with this technique for their first 1000 patients.

THE RIGHT PARASTERNAL APPROACH

The first foray into the world of minimal access aortic valve surgery was with use of this approach. This approach seemed to be the most logical and elegant at a time when the focus was on the morbidity of the sternotomy and surgeons were compelled to come up with this alternative.

This was performed via a vertical upper right parasternal incision. The second, third, and fourth costal cartilages were removed and the right internal mammary vessels were usually ligated and divided. It provided a similar approach to the aortic valve as an upper hemisternotomy incision described before and techniques of cannulation, cardiopulmonary bypass, myocardial protection, and valve replacement were the same. It soon gave way to the more elegant and simple upper hemisternotomy approach. One particular problem associated with the right parasternal approach was the incidence of lung herniation, which was physiologically disturbing aside from being a cosmetic disaster and often required a second operation and mesh closure of the defect.

Cohn[12] and Minale et al[13] described their experiences with the right parasternal incision for aortic valve replacement in 1998. They reported fairly low mortality and morbidity rates and had, at that time, recommended the approach for minimal access aortic valve surgery, but soon moved to a hemisternotomy approach because of occasional right lung herniation.

THE RIGHT ANTERIOR THORACOTOMY APPROACH

This is another method to perform minimal access primary aortic valve replacement in adults.

This is usually performed via the second right intercostal space. Owing to the relatively high nature of the thoracotomy, it never reaches around to become a true anterolateral thoracotomy. One can visualize why this would be unappealing for a female patient because the incision would traverse horizontally across the upper part of the right breast, which could lead to scarring and disfigurement. This incision is carried to the right sternal edge and through this incision the right side of the aorta is easily visualized; and with appropriate strategically placed pericardial retraction sutures the area of interest could easily be moved into the operative field. Aortic and venous cannulation could be performed centrally or peripherally. The rest of the operation is fairly routine for any minimal access aortic valve surgery. Special cross-clamps may be required to facilitate this procedure.

This operation has some relevance and indication for patients requiring isolated aortic valve surgery in whom sternotomy needs to be avoided at all costs. A unique subset of such patients is those who are disabled and routinely ambulate with the use of shoulder crutches. These patients could be made to ambulate early with the use of their crutches without the risk of sternal dehiscence by the use of this approach. Another possible subset of patients includes those with heavily irradiated or damaged sternum.

The exposure via this incision could be optimized in cases with poor exposure by extending it across the sternum with a transverse sternotomy through the manubrio-sternal angle. Reoperative aortic valve replacement is particularly difficult via this incision and the authors sincerely discourage the approach for a reoperation.

Yakub et al[14] and Benetti et al[15] reported their results with the minimally invasive aortic valve replacement via the right anterior thoracotomy approach. Their small series report excellent operative exposure and low mortality and morbidity. Minale et al[16] reported a small series of submammary right thoracotomy approach to aortic valve replacement in women with excellent results, especially cosmesis.

More recently, in 2009, Plass et al[17] reported their series of 160 patients who underwent minimal access aortic valve replacement through a right minithoracotomy. They emphasize the need for careful evaluation of the preoperative multislice computed tomography for surgical planning. They had excellent results and reduced complication rates.

THE TRANSVERSE STERNOTOMY APPROACH

There are anecdotal reports of this incision for minimal access aortic valve surgery.

Typically an 8- to 10-cm transverse incision is made over the manubrio-sternal angle extending onto either side. Bilateral second costal cartilages have to be excised and both internal mammary pedicles have to be ligated and divided. A transverse sternotomy is performed across the sternal angle. The retractor is placed and the sternal edges are retracted in a craniocaudal plane. Adequate exposure is obtained through this incision to permit central aortic cannulation and a routine aortic valve replacement; however, venous cannulation, retrograde coronary sinus catheter placement and vent placement (except transaortic) may have to be performed percutaneously.

For reasons that the mammary arteries are sacrificed, this incision never gained much popularity.

Lee et al,[18] De Amicis et al,[19] and Aris et al[20] reported their small experiences with the transverse sternotomy approach and good results. However, Bridgewater et al[21] reported an unacceptably high incidence of morbidity (re-exploration for bleeding, paravalvular leaks, and longer hospital stay) and mortality with this approach.

Karimov et al,[22] from Italy, reported a series of 85 patients who underwent an upper V-type ministernotomy in the second intercostal space with excellent results.

REOPERATIVE MINIMAL ACCESS AORTIC VALVE SURGERY

The Brigham and Women's Hospital has pioneered minimal access reoperative aortic valve replacement in patients who previously have undergone coronary artery bypass grafting or other cardiac surgery. We popularized and published our data and have since had more experience with the technique.

According to the STS database, patients requiring a reoperative aortic valve replacement after previous coronary artery bypass grafting have a mortality risk of about 8 to 12% from the procedure. The risks are associated with the performance of a reoperation in an older patient with more comorbidities and patent/diseased bypass grafts.

The Need for This Operation

1. There is a definite subgroup of patients who have undergone coronary bypass surgery who had mild or no aortic stenosis at the time of their original operation who will eventually progress to have severe aortic stenosis over time. This has sparked off a whole discussion on the management of moderate aortic stenosis with coronary artery disease.[23]
2. These patients are older, sicker and have many comorbid conditions.
3. They need a simple, safe, and effective operation.
4. The areas of interest are the ascending aorta and aortic root.
5. Dissection of the rest of the heart and bypass grafts provide no additional benefit and are potentially harmful.
6. Clipping the left internal mammary artery is not mandatory with alternative protection strategies.

Operative Strategy

Preoperatively, a computed tomogram of the chest with angiography and three-dimensional reconstruction is performed to ascertain the exact location of the old bypass grafts and their relative location to the sternum (especially the left internal mammary artery).[24] Coronary angiography and percutaneous coronary and graft intervention with drug-eluting stents are done as appropriate to optimize the revascularization as far as possible. Heart failure is controlled medically.

All patients need intraoperative transesophageal echocardiography and a pulmonary artery catheter with atrial and ventricular pacing wire placement capabilities, which should ideally be placed before incision. Accurate placement of external defibrillator pads is emphasized because internal paddles cannot be introduced in these patients.

All patients need peripheral cannulation for cardiopulmonary bypass. We prefer right axillary and percutaneous femoral venous cannulation. Appropriate arterial line placement is needed to facilitate need for circulatory arrest and antegrade cerebral perfusion if required.[25] A standard upper hemisternotomy incision is made with a T into the right fourth intercostal space (Figs. 38-7 and 38-8). The anterior table split is performed with the use of an oscillating saw, whereas the posterior table split is performed on cardiopulmonary bypass using straight Mayo scissors starting from the top down (preferably from the assistant's side of the table). When the left internal mammary artery graft is close to the left side or the middle of the sternum, a preplanned one-third to two-thirds sternotomy to the right is performed. The right pleural space is widely opened. Only 5 to 10 mm dissection is performed underneath the left sternal edge, enough to facilitate the placement of the Kuros-Baxter® retractor. The rest of the mediastinal and aortic dissection is performed on cardiopulmonary bypass. Care is taken not to injure previous saphenous vein or radial arterial bypasses. It is not necessary to visualize the left internal mammary artery graft.

We start core cooling to 25°C only after there is an ability to place an aortic cross-clamp. Moderate to deep hypothermia facilitates low flow states and reduces myocardial oxygen demand, which is important because the left internal mammary artery will continue to perfuse the heart for the duration of the operation. A retrograde coronary sinus catheter is placed through the right atrial appendage using TEE guidance. Usually, enough right atrial appendage is seen to place this catheter. Alternatively, a transjugular catheter can be placed before incision. After cross-clamping the aorta, 1 L antegrade cold blood cardioplegia is delivered through the aortic root. Thereafter, 500 cc of cold retrograde blood cardioplegia is used. Simultaneously, systemic hyperkalemia is achieved by instilling 40 mEq of potassium into the cardiopulmonary bypass. Systemic hyperkalemia will achieve diastolic arrest in the left anterior descending artery territory that is perfused by the left internal mammary artery distal to the aortic cross-clamp. All through the operation, frequent doses of antegrade (through the coronaries and grafts using perfusion canulae) and retrograde cardioplegia are delivered. Systemic hyperkalemia is maintained at a level of 6 to 7 mEq/L. This keeps the myocardium fairly quiescent during the procedure. Needless to say, heavy doses of potassium may leave the patient with severe hyperkalemia that may not be cleared in the setting of renal dysfunction. In addition to being judicious in such cases, it is imperative that the perfusion technologists be able to provide ultrafiltration as well.

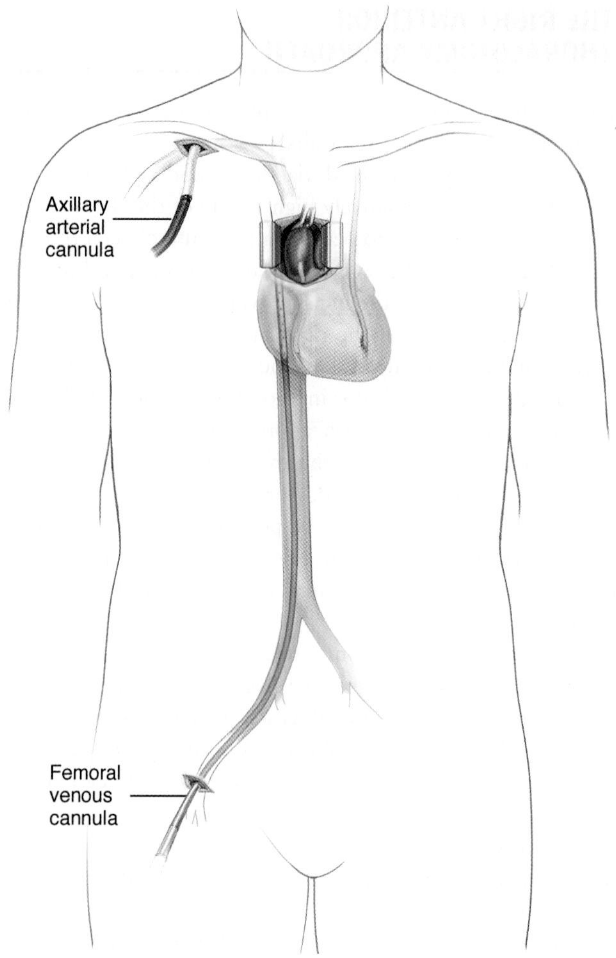

FIGURE 38-8 Peripheral cannulation for cardiopulmonary bypass.

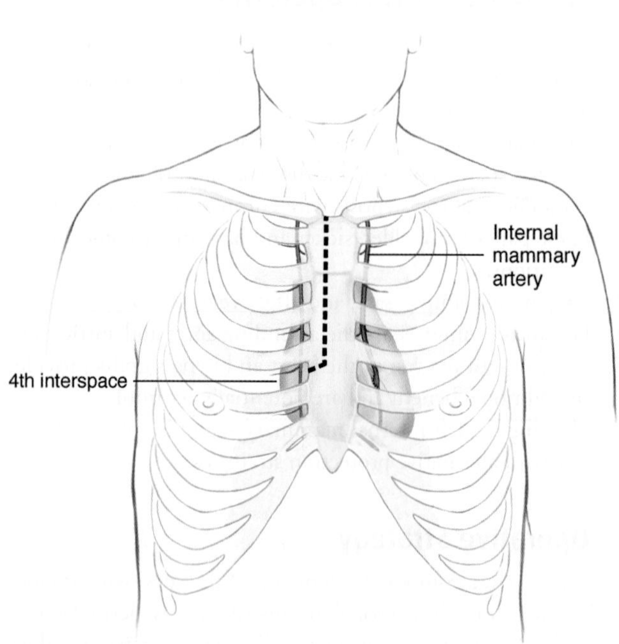

FIGURE 38-7 The upper hemisternotomy incision has been marked.

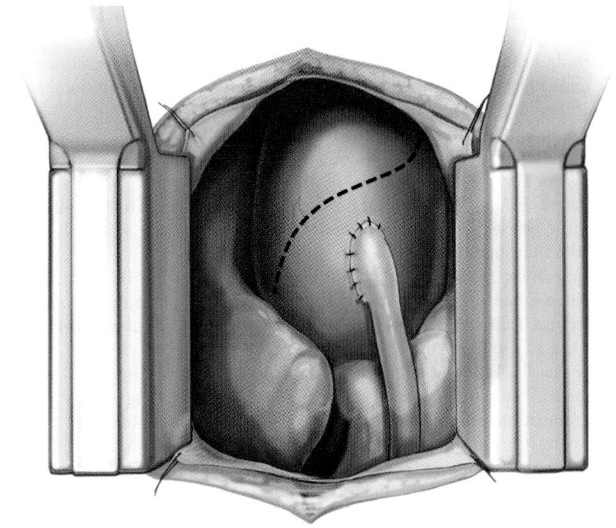

FIGURE 38-9 This is a lazy S oblique aortotomy keeping the grafts to the left.

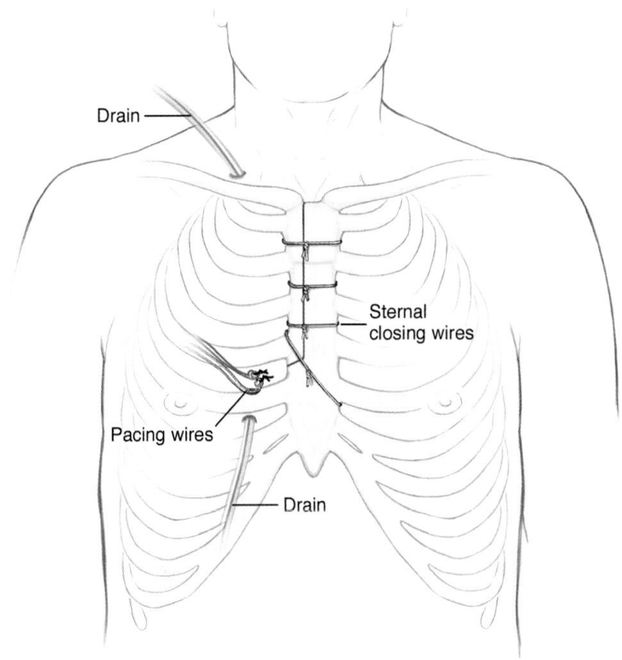

FIGURE 38-10 Final closure, also showing an occasional drainage tube in the supraclavicular space.

The aortotomy is dictated by the location of previous bypass grafts. Although in some cases a standard oblique aortotomy can be made, most cases require a modified aortotomy such as a lazy S or a lateral vertical aortotomy (Fig. 38-9). The exposure should be adequate and an expeditious valve replacement is the key to success. We aim to keep the cross-clamp time under 60 minutes. In most cases, there will be continuous back-bleeding through the left main orifice from the open left internal mammary artery graft. During debridement and suture placement in the left coronary area, the bypass flows can be reduced or briefly turned off to facilitate exposure. Rewarming is started after the valve is seated. The aortotomy is closed in the standard fashion and a de-airing needle is placed before removal of the aortic cross-clamp. The heart often recovers spontaneous sinus rhythm. Defibrillation is achieved via the external pads if required. The de-airing and wean from cardiopulmonary bypass is as described before.

Drainage tubes are always placed through the right pleural space. Subxiphoid placement is not possible and strongly discouraged. Rarely, when the right pleural space is completely fused, the silastic drain could be brought out in the supraclavicular area. It may be possible to place atrial pacing wires, but placement of ventricular wires is almost always quite difficult. We have routinely switched to the use of pulmonary artery catheter based pacing leads with good success. Closure is fairly standard, as described before, and care must be taken during the placement of wires on the left side of the sternum and the oblique lower wire (Fig. 38-10).

Our Experience with This Technique

Byrne et al[26–28] first published the Brigham experience with reoperative minimal access aortic valve replacement in patients who had previously undergone coronary artery bypass grafting or other cardiac surgery and compared it with conventional surgery through a full sternotomy approach. Patients having a conventional full sternotomy redo AVR had more blood loss, more transfusions, and longer operations.

Our positive experience has encouraged others to pursue this technique. Dell'Amore et al[29] report the suitability of this technique in their modest report of 10 patients, and Bakir et al[30] report similarly.

As of 2008, the Brigham experience has grown to 146 patients, reported by Tabata et al[31] The median times for cardiopulmonary bypass and aortic cross-clamp were 150 and 80 minutes, respectively, which are quite acceptable. The operative mortality was 4.1%.

This technique is clearly advantageous but has a fairly steep learning curve. When perfected, it can accomplish a successful operation, with lower mortality and morbidity in an older patient with multiple comorbidities who needs a redo AVR.

REFERENCES

1. Cosgrove DM 3rd, Sabik JF: Minimally invasive approach for aortic valve operations. *Ann Thorac Surg* 1996; 62(2):596-597.
2. Cohn LH, Adams DH, Couper GS, Bichell DP, Rosborough DM, et al: Minimally invasive cardiac valve surgery improves patient satisfaction while reducing costs of cardiac valve replacement and repair. *Ann Surg* 1997; 226(4):421-426; discussion 427-428.
3. Gillinov AM, Banbury MK, Cosgrove DM: Hemisternotomy approach for aortic and mitral valve surgery. *J Card Surg* 2000; 15(1):15-20.
4. Mihaljevic T, Cohn LH, Unic D, Aranki SF, Couper GS, et al: One thousand minimally invasive valve operations: early and late results. *Ann Surg* 2004; 240(3):529-534; discussion 534.
5. Liu J, Sidiropoulos A, Konertz W: Minimally invasive aortic valve replacement (AVR) compared to standard AVR. *Eur J Cardiothorac Surg* 1999; 16(Suppl 2):S80-83.
6. Bonacchi M, Prifti E, Giunti G, Frati G, Sani G: Does ministernotomy improve postoperative outcome in aortic valve operation? A prospective randomized study. *Ann Thorac Surg* 2002; 73(2):460-465; discussion 465-466.

7. Bakir I, Casselman FP, Wellens F, Jeanmart H, De Geest R, et al: Minimally invasive versus standard approach aortic valve replacement: a study in 506 patients. *Ann Thorac Surg* 2006; 81(5):1599-1604.
8. Sharony R, Grossi EA, Saunders PC, Schwartz CF, Ribakove GH, et al: Minimally invasive aortic valve surgery in the elderly: a case-control study. *Circulation* 2003; 108(Suppl 1):II43-47.
9. Foghsgaard S, Gazi D, Bach K, Hansen H, Schmidt TA, et al: Minimally invasive aortic valve replacement reduces atelectasis in cardiac intensive care. *Acute Card Care* 2009; 24:1-4.
10. Tabata M, Aranki SF, Fox JA, Couper GS, Cohn LH, et al: Minimally invasive aortic valve replacement in left ventricular dysfunction. *Asian Cardiovasc Thorac Ann* 2007; 15(3):225-228.
11. Tabata M, Umakanthan R, Cohn LH, Bolman RM 3rd, Shekar PS, et al: Early and late outcomes of 1000 minimally invasive aortic valve operations. *Eur J Cardiothorac Surg* 2008; 33(4):537-541.
12. Cohn LH: Minimally invasive aortic valve surgery: technical considerations and results with the parasternal approach. *J Card Surg* 1998; 13(4):302-305.
13. Minale C, Reifschneider HJ, Schmitz E, Uckmann FP: Minimally invasive aortic valve replacement without sternotomy. Experience with the first 50 cases. *Eur J Cardiothorac Surg* 1998; 14(Suppl 1):S126-129.
14. Yakub MA, Pau KK, Awang Y: Minimally invasive "pocket incision" aortic valve surgery. *Ann Thorac Cardiovasc Surg* 1999; 5(1):36-39.
15. Benetti F, Rizzardi JL, Concetti C, Bergese M, Zappetti A: Minimally aortic valve surgery avoiding sternotomy. *Eur J Cardiothorac Surg* 1999; 16(Suppl 2): S84-85.
16. Minale C, Tomasco B, Di Natale M: A cosmetic access for minimally invasive aortic valve replacement without sternotomy in women. *Ital Heart J* 2002; 3(8):473-475.
17. Plass A, Scheffel H, Alkadhi H, Kaufmann P, Genoni M, et al: Aortic valve replacement through a minimally invasive approach: preoperative planning, surgical technique and outcome. *Ann Thorac Surg* 2009; 88(6):1851-1856.
18. Lee JW, Lee SK, Choo SJ, Song H, Song MG: Routine minimally invasive aortic valve procedures. *Cardiovasc Surg* 2000; 8(6):484-490.
19. De Amicis V, Ascione R, Iannelli G, Di Tommaso L, Monaco M, et al: Aortic valve replacement through a minimally invasive approach. *Tex Heart Inst J* 1997; 24(4):353-355.
20. Aris A, Padro JM, Camara ML: Minimally invasive aortic valve replacement. *Rev Esp Cardiol* 1997; 50(11):778-781.
21. Bridgewater B, Steyn RS, Ray S, Hooper T: Minimally invasive aortic valve replacement through a transverse sternotomy: a word of caution. *Heart* 1998; 79(6):605-607.
22. Karimov JH, Santarelli F, Murzi M, Glauber M: A technique of an upper V-type ministernotomy in the second intercostal space. *Interact Cardiovasc Thorac Surg* 2009; 9(6):1021-1022.
23. Filsoufi F, Aklog L, Adams DH, Byrne JG: Management of mild to moderate aortic stenosis at the time of coronary artery bypass grafting. *J Heart Valve Dis* 2002; 11(Suppl 1):S45-49.
24. Gasparovic H, Rybicki FJ, Millstine J, Unic D, Byrne JG, et al: Three dimensional computed tomographic imaging in planning the surgical approach for redo cardiac surgery after coronary revascularization. *Eur J Cardiothorac Surg* 2005; 28(2):244-249.
25. Shekar PS, Ehsan A, Gilfeather MS, Lekowski RW Jr, Couper GS: Arterial pressure monitoring during cardiopulmonary bypass using axillary arterial cannulation. *J Cardiothorac Vasc Anesth* 2005; 19(5):665-666.
26. Byrne JG, Karavas AN, Adams DH, Aklog L, Aranki SF, et al: Partial upper re-sternotomy for aortic valve replacement or re-replacement after previous cardiac surgery. *Eur J Cardiothorac Surg* 2000; 18(3):282-286.
27. Byrne JG, Karavas AN, Filsoufi F, Mihaljevic T, Aklog L, et al: Aortic valve surgery after previous coronary artery bypass grafting with functioning internal mammary artery grafts. *Ann Thorac Surg* 2002; 73(3):779-784.
28. Byrne JG, Aranki SF, Couper GS, Adams DH, Allred EN, et al: Reoperative aortic valve replacement: partial hemisternotomy versus conventional full sternotomy. *J Thorac Cardiovasc Surg* 1999; 118(6):991-997.
29. Dell'Amore A, Del Giglio M, Calvi S, Pagliaro M, Fedeli C, et al: Mini re-sternotomy for aortic valve replacement in patients with patent coronary bypass grafts. *Interact Cardiovasc Thorac Surg* 2009; 9(1):94-97.
30. Bakir I, Casselman FP, De Geest R, Wellens F, Degrieck I, et al: Should minimally invasive aortic valve replacement be restricted to primary interventions. *Thorac Cardiovasc Surg* 2007; 55(5):304-309.
31. Tabata M, Khalpey Z, Shekar PS, Cohn LH: Reoperative minimal access aortic valve surgery: minimal mediastinal dissection and minimal injury risk. *J Thorac Cardiovasc Surg* 2008; 136(6):1564-1568.

CHAPTER 39

Percutaneous Treatment of Aortic Valve Disease

Lars G. Svensson

INTRODUCTION

Over the last few years, data have accumulated that untreated aortic valve disease, particularly in elderly people, is a problem despite the success of surgery and newer methods of treatment.[1–32]

The history of percutaneous treatment of aortic valve disease with various types of device goes back to the work of Danish researcher, H.R. Andersen, who in the late 1980s experimented in an animal lab with a balloon-expandable stented valve.[15] The technology was later acquired by PVT Company and further developed and later sold to Edwards. The early work was done by Alain Cribier[21,22] and subsequently the expandable stented valve was adopted in the United States and further modified. The initial approach taken by Cribier was to insert the valve via the femoral vein and then using a transeptal technique to snake the catheter through the mitral valve and left ventricle to access the aortic annulus. This turned out to be a fairly cumbersome and difficult operation to do with a fairly high mortality rate and an 8.1% stroke rate. At the same time, animal experiments were carried out by Michael Mack, Todd Dewey, and Lars Svensson,[17,25] to use a transapical approach to insert the aortic valve. During this time period, John Webb and colleagues[18,19] were also developing a transapical aortic valve method, and subsequently they introduced the retrograde transfemoral artery approach. This latter technique became feasible once Edwards developed a catheter that could be flexed to get around the aortic arch to access the aortic valve.

The Revival Trial was started in the United States in 55 patients using the retrograde transarterial transfemoral approach (Transapical aortic valve insert, TFAVI; Figs. 39-1 to 39-3).[24] A separate Revival trial also included a transapical approach in 40 patients.[25] In the United States, the three centers involved in these studies were Cleveland Clinic in Ohio, Columbia in New York, and Medical City in Dallas. In the first transfemoral Revival series of patients, the mortality rate was 7% and the stroke rate 9.2%. The transapical (TA-AVI) (Figs. 39-4 to 39-6) had a higher mortality rate of 17% in the first 40 patients with no immediate strokes after successful insertion, although two patients did develop strokes, one after an open replacement for aortic valve disease in a very heavily calcified ascending aorta and the other in a patient who developed atrial fibrillation a few days after surgery. Based on the feasibility studies, the FDA then approved a prospective randomized trial to further evaluate the device technology.

At the same time as the Edwards balloon-expandable valve was being developed, Core-valve introduced a nitinol-based percutaneous valve system that was also inserted transfemorally but did not require balloon expansion, but rather expanded over time as the nitinol stretched the aortic valve and seated in the aortic valve annulus.

DESIGN

The Edwards balloon-expandable valve has evolved over time with two principal changes, which include the stent steel cage having a higher skirt sewn to the base of it and switching from equine to bovine biological leaflets. Furthermore, the bovine leaflets are manufactured to the same thickness as those found in regular pericardial valves. In the pulse duplicators the valve was tested to exceed the equivalent of some 10.4 years of implantation. To try and reduce the bulk of the stainless steel cage, newer modifications are going to become available that

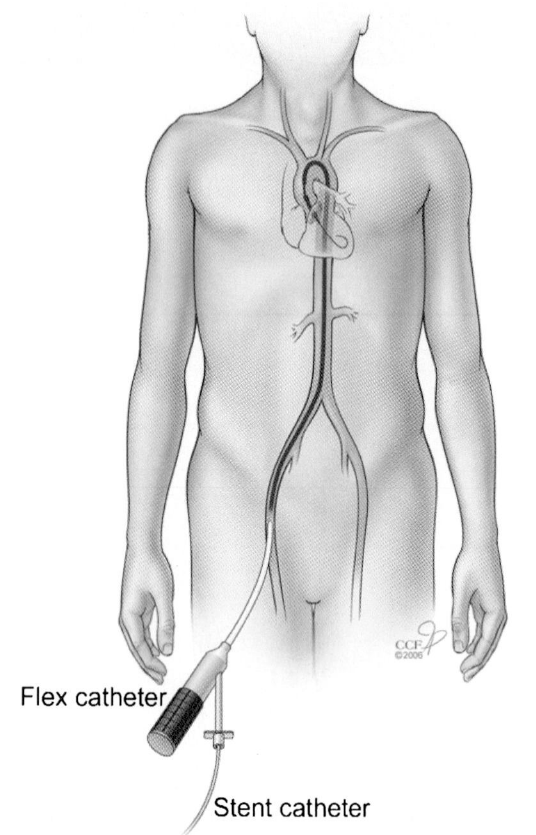

FIGURE 39-1 Transfemoral artery catheter insertion. (*Reproduced with permission of the Cleveland Clinic, Cleveland, OH.*)

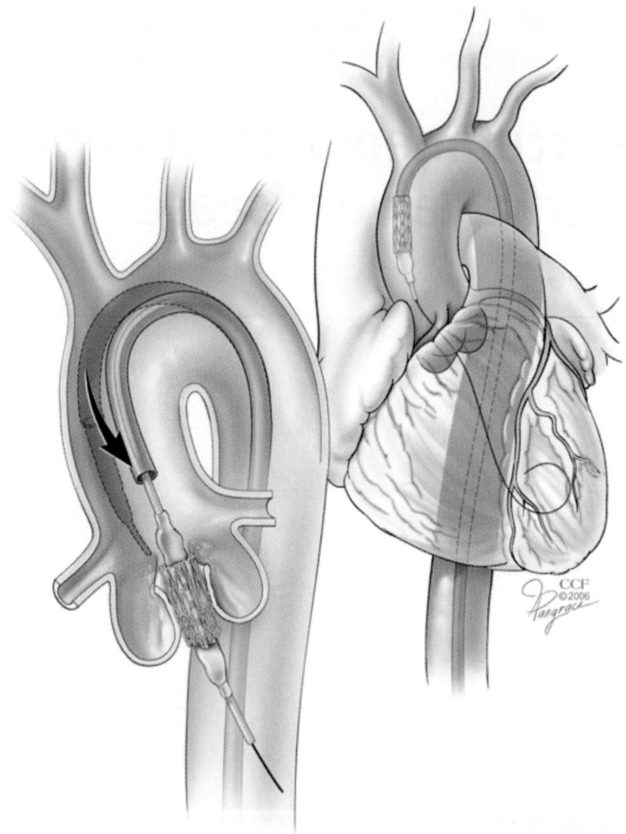

FIGURE 39-2 Catheter for delivery across the arch. (*Reproduced with permission of the Cleveland Clinic, Cleveland, OH.*)

involve the use of a different metal, altering the existing mounting system for the valve on the catheter for balloon expansion. Thus, the intent is that the valve will be able to be inserted in an "18-sheath system." The long-term durability of the bovine valve leaflets appears to be excellent with few reported failure of the devices at this time on long-term follow-up of the patients with the important caveat that the valve is both full and symmetrically expanded. Clearly, endocarditis is still a risk factor over time and has occurred occasionally, but leaflet calcification or tearing, at least in the first few years, has not been a problem. It is likely that further development of the valve skirt will reduce the incidence and the degree of perivalvular leak by changes in the cuff and height of the cuff of the balloon-expandable valve.

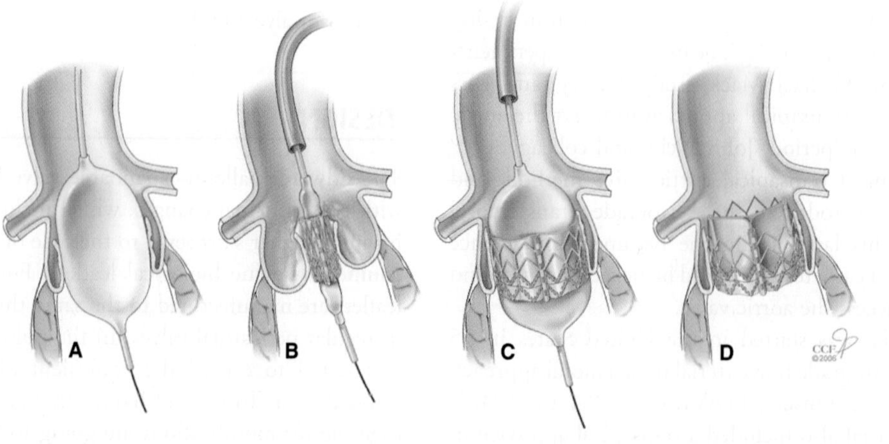

FIGURE 39-3 Positioning and deployment of the valve. (*Reproduced with permission of the Cleveland Clinic, Cleveland, OH.*)

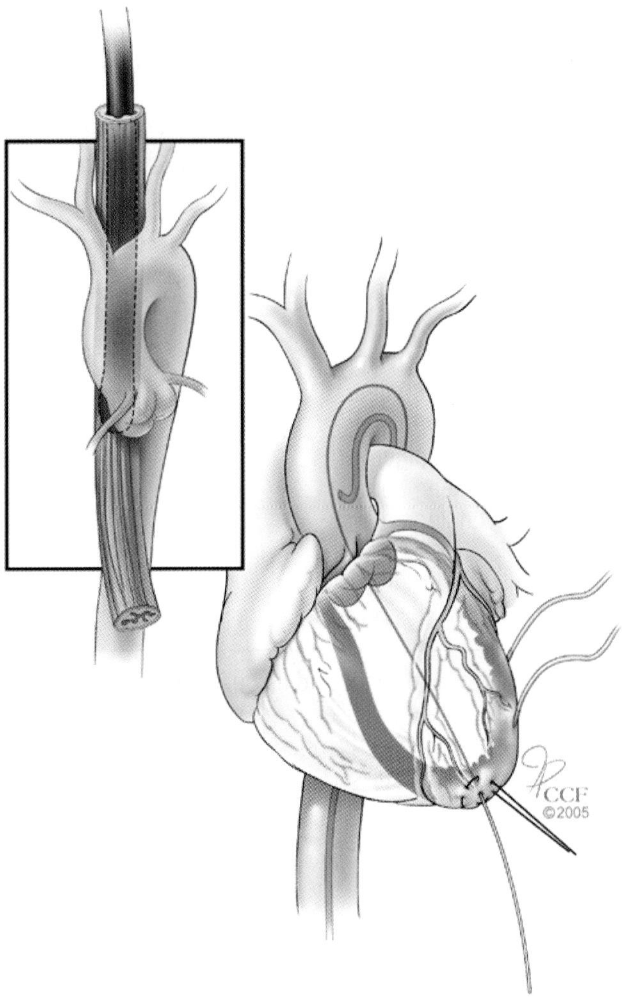

FIGURE 39-4 Transapical purse string and wire. (*Reproduced with permission of the Cleveland Clinic, Cleveland, OH.*)

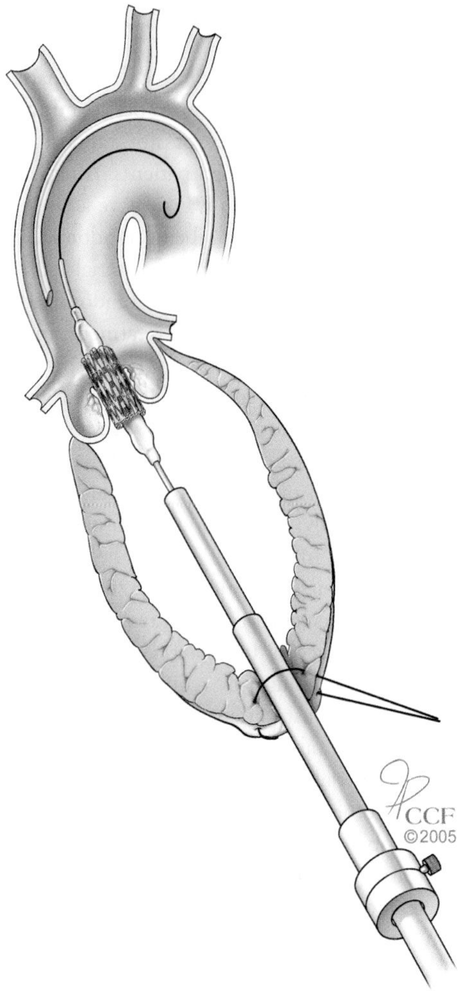

FIGURE 39-5 Sheath and valve insertion. (*Reproduced with permission of the Cleveland Clinic, Cleveland, OH.*)

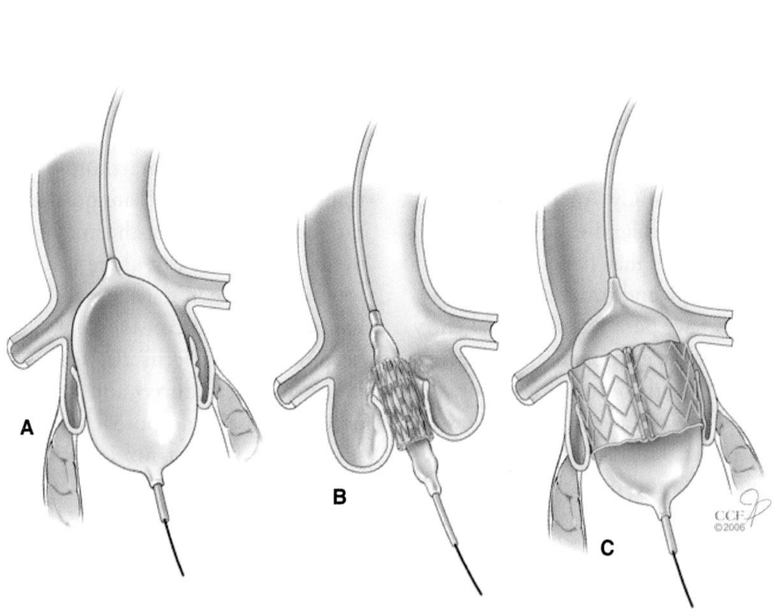

FIGURE 39-6 Valve deployment sequence. (*Reproduced with permission of the Cleveland Clinic, Cleveland, OH.*)

PROSPECTIVE RANDOMIZED TRIAL

The PARTNER Prospective Randomized Trial consisted of two arms. There was much debate as how to best conduct the study as far as methods, and whether or not randomization was needed and which groups to assign patients. After negotiations with the FDA, the final decision was to have a Group A and a Group B, with Group A patients being randomized either to regular open surgery, or transfemoral arterial or transapical valve insertion. Group B patients were randomized to either transfemoral insertion or best medical treatment, including the use of balloon valvuloplasty. The Group A patients in the treatment arm were to be compared with the open surgical patients on the basis of noninferiority, and in Group B the treated patients were to be compared with the best medical treatment control arm on the basis of superiority. A total of 1040 patients were placed in the study, with 450 in the Group B arm, which was completed in the first half of 2009. The Group A part of the study was completed on August 28, 2009, and thereafter patients will still be screened and will require approval by the panel for continued access in either Group B or Group A. Randomization will no longer be required.

Entry criteria for most patients in Group A was having an STS score above 10, a valve area of less than 0.8, and, thereafter, depending on arterial access of the groins, patients were assigned either to the transapical arm or the transfemoral arm. Patients in the open surgical arm were not allowed to undergo any coronary artery bypass surgery or any other valvular procedure but were allowed to have the ascending aorta replaced for calcification using deep hypothermia and circulatory arrest. Group B patients require a combined risk of serious morbidity or mortality exceeding at least 50% and two surgeons agreeing the patient was inoperable. Exclusions included bicuspid valve pathology, left ventricular outflow tract smaller than 1.8 cm or larger than 2.4 cm, creatinine above 2.5 or dialysis, infection within 6 months, and a PCI procedure within 30 days.

There are important caveats to bear in mind when considering the trial. In our experience at the Cleveland Clinic (Table 39-1) it is only patients greater than age 80 undergoing reoperation in whom the risk of aortic valve replacement and the risk of death exceeds 5%. Hence, most patients in the trial are elderly with severe comorbid disease and usually undergoing a reoperation. Indeed, a 90-year-old patient with no comorbid disease requiring a reoperation may not qualify for the study. Another important caveat is the influence of peripheral vascular disease on outcome. We showed in a study of our patients that peripheral vascular disease increased the risk of both death and stroke after surgery.[30] Hence, because TA-AVI patients have poor access by trial entry criteria, they are also at greater risk of death or complications.

The Group B patient data will clearly be available before the Group A randomized patients and in both categories, the follow-up required will be 30 days plus 1 year. The data will then be presented to the FDA and panel evaluation. In both groups, mortality at 1 year is the most important variable, although there are also the composite end points of outcomes for analysis. (See "PARTNER Results Update" at the end of this chapter.)

While the PARTNER Trial data is being evaluated, ongoing studies are being continued in Europe in which patients have not been randomized but are being followed. The method of insertion has varied somewhat from site to site, with some sites, for example the group in Leipzig, prefer a transapical approach, whereas those in other centers prefer a transfemoral approach. In the centers in which the transapical approach has been used almost exclusively in patients, the reported results have so far been equivalent to those for the transfemoral approach. We note that the perceived advantages for the transapical approach are a quicker time for insertion, less contrast, and less risk of stroke. On the other hand, patients with severe lung disease and oxygen dependency do not tolerate this procedure well because it requires a minithoracotomy. The obvious benefits for the transfemoral approach are quicker recovery and earlier mobilization of patients, but this may be burdened with a higher risk of stroke and, clearly, there is a risk of vascular injury, which was 17% in the initial series in the Revival trial. This, however, has been reduced considerably and with the 18-French device becoming available in 2010, it is likely that both the rate of injury will be reduced and also the number of patients who need a transapical approach. The other option is to use the subclavian artery or mini aortic approach for insertion of the device.

Core valve has been inserted in 79 patients in Europe via the left subclavian artery, with a 9% risk of death, but what has been more daunting has been the 38% risk of requirement for pacemaker insertion after the procedure. This may be related to the proximal stent sitting a little bit lower in the left ventricular

TABLE 39-1 Death Rates for Aortic Valve Procedures, Including Complex Aortic Procedures, at Cleveland Clinic: 2001 to December 2007

Group	N	Death Rate
Primary AVR <70 years	720	0.28%*
Primary AVR >70 years	426	1.6%*
Primary AVR >80 years	139	1.4%*
Primary AVR >90 years	3	0%*
Reoperative AVR <70 years	217	2.3%*
Reoperative AVR >70 years	238	2.9%*
Reoperative AVR >80 years	89	5.6%
Reoperative AVR >90 years	3	0
Valve-sparing technique	418	1.4%†
Repair of ascending aorta	2812	4.2%‡
Repair of ascending aorta and aortic arch	985	4.6%‡
Use of "elephant trunk" technique	275	7.3%‡

*Including those with endocarditis but excluding those with coronary artery disease.
†Including those with aortic dissection.
‡Including those with dissection and endocarditis involving the aorta.
AVR = aortic valve replacement.

on-flow tract, leading to continued expansion of pressure on the bundle of His, and thus resulting in the need for pacemaker insertion.

INSERTION OF THE VALVES: TRANSFEMORAL APPROACH

In our most recent patients at the Cleveland Clinic, the modified approach we have used for insertion of the transfemoral approach is to introduce the femoral, arterial, and venous lines percutaneously using a closure device at the end of the procedure. Thus, a venous pacing wire is inserted into the right ventricle and then two arterial wires are inserted into the groin, one for the pigtail catheter and the other for the insertion of the device. Typically, the patient is heparinized so the ACT is between 250 and 350 seconds. The sequence of insertion is the introduction of a straight wire via the straight catheter through the aortic valve and into the left ventricle. This is then exchanged with an extra stiff or Lunderquist wire, which is placed in the left ventricle after sliding the sheath across the aortic valve. A 3- or 5-cm balloon is then threaded over the guidewire and positioned across the aortic valve using fluoroscopy and then during rapid pacing, and breath holding, expanded to crack the calcium. If the balloon does not move, then the balloon is removed and the femoral 14-French sheath exchanged for progressive-sized Cook dilators and finally the largest-sized Edwards dilators are inserted into the femoral artery and into the distal abdominal aorta. The size is dependent on the valve selection, namely, a size 23 or 26 valve. The large sheath is then inserted. The size 23-mm valve is used for patients with left ventricular outflow tracts of 1.8 to approximately 2.1 to 2.2 cm, and the larger 26-mm valve is used for left ventricular outflow tract sizes from 2.2 to 2.4 cm. Generally, patients with left ventricular outflow tracts of 2.5 cm or larger are excluded from the study until the new 29-mm valve becomes available.

As a rule, patients who need the smaller-sized valve should have a femoral artery of at least 7 mm and for the size 26 valve a 7.5- to 8-mm external iliac artery, depending on the tortuosity of the vessel and degree of calcification. If there is more than 90-degree angulation of the iliac arteries, then generally it would be difficult to insert the large sheath unless the vessel straightens very easily with a Lunderquist wire. In measuring for the 22-mm-French sheath (internal diameter) the size varies from 7.45 to 7.72 mm for the internal diameter and external measurements vary from 8.21 to 8.50 mm. The 22-French sheath is used for the size 23-mm valve. In other words, the true internal size is 23-mm French and 25.5 French external diameter using a conversion factor of 0.333. For the 26-mm valve, a size 24-French sheath is used, which has an internal size measurement between 8.20 and 8.40 mm and an external size of 8.94 to 9.90 mm. By converting this to French sizes this would be equivalent to a 25.3 internal and 27.3 external French size. The 28 dilator sheath diameter is 9.24 mm, which is used before introducing the big 24-French sheath.

Once the sheath is inserted and the valve mounted on the balloon, it is checked to be correctly loaded, and is then threaded over the stiff wire and the loader pushed into the sheath to the black mark but not beyond it. Note that with the new sheath this requirement is not as critical. The valve is then pushed and threaded across the aortic arch with the steerable catheter being flexed to get around the aortic arch and then fed down to the aortic valve. With the flex-three system, the insertion and retraction of the dilators are much easier. Essentially, the valve with the leading little cone is fed across the valve to cross the valve and then the cone is pushed further into the ventricle so that the stent valve is free. Once the balloon is inflated, it can be expanded without limitation from the cone. We consider it very important to carefully check on the positioning of the valve across the hinged point of the native valve using both echocardiography and fluoroscopy and root injections with contrast via the pigtail catheter. With the flex-three system the valve is positioned at the valve hinged points, approximately 50/50 aortic/ventricular. Once everybody agrees that the position is correct, the patient's breath is held, the patient is paced at approximately 180 beats per minute, the balloon is inflated in position and then deflated, the pacer is switched off, and the patient is put back on the ventilator. There is virtually always some perivalvular regurgitation in the region of the noncoronary–left main leaflet commissure, probably because this is an area of less flexibility and a lot of calcium. Echocardiography is then used to inspect the function of the valve. Thereafter, cone is first withdrawn from the left ventricle followed by removal of the catheter and sheath, and lastly the previous closure device is tied down at the insertion sites.

TRANSAPICAL INSERTION

In the United States, the transapical approach is reserved for those patients who do not have access and, as such, they generally have more comorbidity than transfemoral patients based on comparative studies.

The way we prefer to do it at the Cleveland Clinic is to have the patient lie flat on his or her back on pillows rather than at a traditional left thoracotomy position, because this interferes with the positioning of the C-arms. All patients before surgery undergo an aortic root injection from which the ideal planes are calculated for positioning the valve with the nadir of each cusp being in the same plane. This is also obtained with the computer tomographic scans, which are done preoperatively to check for potential calcium obstruction of the native coronary arteries.

Once the patient is positioned, he or she is prepped in the usual manner with exposure of the groin and left chest. The femoral artery and vein are exposed on the right side and the left femoral venous pacing wires inserted. The femoral artery exposure is performed in case the patient has to be placed on a pump.

We continue to have all of our patients undergo general anesthesia but, more recently, we have not used a double-lumen tube for the transapical valves. Before opening the chest, an echo probe is placed on the chest to try to better define where the left ventricular apex is, and CAT scan images are also inspected to find the ideal place to open the left chest. Typically, the fifth intercostal space is entered and the apex of the left ventricle palpated. Once the apex of the left ventricle has been palpated, a short piece of rib is removed to expose the apex. Originally we did not do this and rather spread the ribs, but we found that some patients had severe pain as with the mid-cab experience. We therefore opted to resect a short piece of rib to obtain both a better exposure and less pain after surgery, particularly because many of these patients have severe lung disease. The pericardium is then opened and stay sutures placed and then two pursestring sutures with Teflon felt pledgets are placed around the left ventricular apex. The site is selected by tapping on the left ventricular apex and then looking at the echo to make sure that the left ventricular apex is correctly identified. This is important because the heart can be anywhere from the fourth intercostal space to the seventh or eighth intercostal space. In addition, a horizontal mattress suture is also placed in the apex. A needle is then inserted followed by a guidewire into the left ventricle; then we insert a Berman catheter into the left ventricle, through the aortic valve, and across the aortic arch down to the renal arteries. An extra stiff wire is also fed down at the same time. The Berman catheter is then removed and the 14-gauge sheath exchanged for the large-bore introduction sheath. Balloon valvuloplasty is performed through this in the same sequence with rapid pacing as for the transfemoral approach. The valve is then loaded onto the sheath and pushed into position and the pusher retracted into the sheath. With the valve situated approximately 60% aortic and with rapid pacing the balloon is then inflated at this point. The balloon is then withdrawn into the left ventricle before stopping pacing. If all appears well, the sheath and wire are then removed and the pursestring sutures are tied down.

PARTNER RESULTS UPDATE

PARTNER B showed that TFAVI significantly improved 1 year survival despite a 30-day death rate of 6.4% and stroke/TIA rate of 5.5%. PARTNER A showed transcatheter aortic valve replacement (TAVR) was noninferior to open surgery for both 30-day and 1-year mortalities; however, the rate of stroke/TIA was higher for TAVR.

CONCLUSION

Percutaneous aortic valve procedures continue to improve and, despite our early skepticism with the approach based on early animal work that showed a high embolization rate in the animal valves, the procedure has established itself as a very effective way of treating high-risk patients with severe aortic valve stenosis. Undoubtedly with new iterations the procedure will become safer and even better, likely with retrievable devices and easier positioning of the devices.

REFERENCES

1. Varadarajan P, Kapoor N, Bansal RC, Pai RG: Clinical profile and natural history of 453 nonsurgically managed patients with severe aortic stenosis. *Ann Thorac Surg* 2006; 82(6):2111-2115.
2. Pai RG, Kapoor N, Bansal RC, Varadarajan P: Malignant natural history of asymptomatic severe aortic stenosis: benefit of aortic valve replacement. *Ann Thorac Surg* 2006; 82(6):2116-2122.
3. Soler-Soler J, Galve E: Worldwide perspective of valve disease. *Heart* 2000; 83(6):721-725.
4. Stuge O, Liddicoat J: Emerging opportunities for cardiac surgeons within structural heart disease. *J Thorac Cardiovasc Surg* 2006; 132(6): 1258-1261.
5. Lung B, Baron G, Butchart EG, Delahaye F, Gohlke-ärwolf C, et al: A prospective survey of patients with valvular heart disease in Europe: The Euro Heart Survey on Valvular Heart Disease. *Eur Heart J* 2003; 24(13): 1231-1243.
6. Lindroos M, Kupari M, Heikkilä J, Tilvis R: Prevalence of aortic valve abnormalities in the elderly: an echocardiographic study of a random population sample. *J Am Coll Cardiol* 1993; 21(5):1220-1225.
7. Pellikka PA, Sarano ME, Nishimura RA, Malouf JF, Bailey KR, et al: Outcome of 622 adults with asymptomatic, hemodynamically significant aortic stenosis during prolonged follow-up. *Circulation* 2005; 111(24): 3290-3295.
8. Bonow RO, Carabello B, de Leon AC, Edmunds LH Jr, Fedderly BJ, et al: ACC/AHA Guidelines for the Management of Patients With Valvular Heart Disease. Executive Summary.
9. Banbury MK, Cosgrove DM 3rd, Thomas JD, Blackstone EH, Rajeswaran J, et al: Hemodynamic stability during 17 years of the Carpentier-Edwards aortic pericardial bioprosthesis. *Ann Thorac Surg* 2002; 73(5):1460-1465.
10. Blackstone EH, Cosgrove DM, Jamieson WR, Birkmeyer NJ, Lemmer JH Jr, et al: Prosthesis size and long-term survival after aortic valve replacement. *J Thorac Cardiovasc Surg* 2003; 126(3):783-796.
11. Svensson LG, Blackstone EH, Cosgrove DM 3rd: Surgical options in young adults with aortic valve disease. *Curr Probl Cardiol* 2003; 28(7): 417-480.
12. Schwarz F, Baumann P, Manthey J, Hoffmann M, Schuler G, et al: The effect of aortic valve replacement on survival. *Circulation* 1982; 66(5): 1105-1110.
13. Smith N, McAnulty JH, Rahimtoola SH: Severe aortic stenosis with impaired left ventricular function and clinical heart failure: results of valve replacement. *Circulation* 1978; 58(2):255-264.
14. Otto CM, Mickel MC, Kennedy JW, Alderman EL, Bashore TM, et al: Three-year outcome after balloon aortic valvuloplasty. Insights into prognosis of valvular aortic stenosis. *Circulation* 1994; 89(2):642-650.
15. Andersen HR, Knudsen LL, Hasenkam JM: Transluminal implantation of artificial heart valves. Description of a new expandable aortic valve and initial results with implantation by catheter technique in closed chest pigs. *Eur Heart J* 1992; 13(5):704-708.
16. Walther T, Simon P, Dewey T, Wimmer-Greinecker G, Falk V, et al: Transapical minimally invasive aortic valve implantation: multicenter experience. *Circulation* 2007; 116(11 Suppl):I240-245.
17. Dewey TM, Walther T, Doss M, Brown D, Ryan WH, et al: Transapical aortic valve implantation: an animal feasibility study. *Ann Thorac Surg* 2006; 82(1):110-116.
18. Lichtenstein SV, Cheung A, Ye J, Thompson CR, Carere RG, et al: Transapical transcatheter aortic valve implantation in humans: initial clinical experience. *Circulation* 2006; 114(6):591-596.
19. Webb JG, Pasupati S, Humphries K, Thompson C, Altwegg L, et al: Percutaneous transarterial aortic valve replacement in selected high-risk patients with aortic stenosis. *Circulation* 2007; 116(7):755-763.
20. Webb JG, Chandavimol M, Thompson CR, Ricci DR, Carere RG, et al: Percutaneous aortic valve implantation retrograde from the femoral artery. *Circulation* 2006; 113(6):842-850.
21. Cribier A, Eltchaninoff H, Bash A, Borenstein N, Tron C, et al: Percutaneous transcatheter implantation of an aortic valve prosthesis for calcific aortic stenosis: first human case description. *Circulation* 2002; 106(24): 3006-3008.
22. Cribier A, Eltchaninoff H, Tron C, Bauer F, Agatiello C, et al: Early experience with percutaneous transcatheter implantation of heart valve prosthesis for the treatment of end-stage inoperable patients with calcific aortic stenosis. *J Am Coll Cardiol* 2004; 43(4):698-703.
23. Grube E, Laborde JC, Gerckens U, Felderhoff T, Sauren B, et al: Percutaneous implantation of the CoreValve self-expanding valve prosthesis in high-risk patients with aortic valve disease: the Siegburg first-in-man study. *Circulation* 2006; 114(15):1616-1624.
24. Leon MB, Kodali S, Williams M, Oz M, Smith C, et al: Transcatheter aortic valve replacement in patients with critical aortic stenosis: rationale, device descriptions, early clinical experiences, and perspectives. *Semin Thorac Cardiovasc Surg* 2006; 18(2):165-174.
25. Svensson LG, Dewey T, Kapadia S, Roselli EE, Stewart A, et al: United States feasibility study of transcatheter insertion of a stented aortic valve by the left ventricular apex. *Ann Thorac Surg* 2008; 86(1):46-54.
26. Webb JG, Altwegg L, Boone RH, Cheung A, Ye J, et al: Transcatheter aortic valve implantation: impact on clinical and valve-related outcomes. *Circulation* 2009; 119(23):3009-3016.

27. Schoenhagen P, Tuzcu EM, Kapadia SR, Desai MY, Svensson LG: Three-dimensional imaging of the aortic valve and aortic root with computed tomography: new standards in an era of transcatheter valve repair/implantation. *Eur Heart J* 2009; 30(17):2079-2086.
28. Kurra V, Schoenhagen P, Roselli EE, Kapadia SR, Tuzcu EM, et al: Prevalence of significant peripheral artery disease in patients evaluated for percutaneous aortic valve insertion: preprocedural assessment with multidetector computed tomography. *J Thorac Cardiovasc Surg* 2009; 137(5):1258-1264.
29. Akhtar M, Tuzcu EM, Kapadia SR, Svensson LG, Greenberg RK, et al: Aortic root morphology in patients undergoing percutaneous aortic valve replacement: evidence of aortic root remodeling. *J Thorac Cardiovasc Surg* 2009; 137(4):950-956.
30. Svensson LG: Evolution and results of aortic valve surgery, and a 'disruptive' technology. *Cleveland Clin J Med* 2008; 75(11):802, 804.
31. Svensson LG: Aortic valve stenosis and regurgitation: an overview of management. *J Cardiovasc Surg (Torino)* 2008; 49(2):297-303.
32. Svensson LG: Minimally invasive surgery with a partial sternotomy "J" approach. *Semin Thorac Cardiovasc Surg* 2007; 19(4):299-303.

PART 4B

VALVULAR HEART DISEASE (MITRAL)

CHAPTER 40

Pathophysiology of Mitral Valve Disease

James I. Fann
Neil B. Ingels, Jr.
D. Craig Miller

THE NORMAL MITRAL VALVE

Anatomy

The mitral annulus is a pliable junctional zone of discontinuous fibrous and muscular tissue that joins the left atrium and left ventricle and anchors the hinge portions of the anterior and posterior mitral leaflets.[1–8] The annulus has two major collagenous structures: (1) the right fibrous trigone, which is part of the central fibrous body and is located at the intersection of the membranous septum, the tricuspid annulus, and the aortic annulus; and (2) the left fibrous trigone, which is located near the aortic annulus under the left aortic cusp (Fig. 40-1). The anterior mitral leaflet spans the distance between the commissures (including the trigones) and is in direct fibrous continuity with the aortic annulus under the left and noncoronary aortic valve cusps, including the fibrous triangle between the left and noncoronary aortic valve cusps. The posterior half to two-thirds of the annulus, which subtends the posterior leaflet, is primarily muscular with little or no fibrous tissue.[4]

The mitral valve has two major leaflets, the larger anterior (or aortic or septal) leaflet and the smaller posterior (or mural) leaflet; the latter usually contains three or more scallops separated by fetal clefts or *subcommissures,* which are developed to variable degrees in different individuals.[9] The three posterior leaflet scallops are anatomically termed anterolateral (P1), middle (P2), and posteromedial (P3) scallops (Fig. 40-2). The portions of the leaflets near the free margin on the atrial surface are called the *rough zone,* with the remainder of the leaflet surface closer to the annulus being termed the *smooth* (or *bare* or *membranous*) *zone.* The ratio of the height of the rough zone to the height of the clear zone is 0.6 for the anterior leaflet and 1.4 for the posterior leaflet because the clear zone on the posterior scallops occupies only about 2 mm.[9] The two leaflets are separated by the posteromedial and anterolateral commissures, which usually are distinctly developed but occasionally are incomplete.

The histologic structure of the leaflets includes three layers: (1) the fibrosa, the solid collagenous core that is continuous with the chordae tendineae; (2) the spongiosa, which is on the atrial surface and forms the leaflet leading edge (it consists of few collagen fibers but has abundant proteoglycans, elastin, and mixed connective tissue cells); and (3) a thin fibroelastic covering of most of the leaflets.[4] On the atrial aspect of both leaflets, this surface (the atrialis) is rich in elastin. The ventricular side of the fibroelastic cover (the ventricularis) is much thicker, confined mostly to the anterior leaflet, and densely packed with elastin. The fibroelastic layers become thickened with advancing age as a result of elaboration of more elastin and more collagen formation; accelerated similar changes also accompany the progression of myxomatous (degenerative or "floppy") mitral valvular disease in young patients with the Barlow syndrome. In addition to these complex connective tissue structures, the mitral leaflets contain myocardium, smooth muscle, contractile valvular interstitial cells, and blood vessels, as well as both adrenergic and cholinergic afferent and efferent nerves.[10–24] Leaflet contractile tissue is neurally controlled and plays a role in mitral valve function.[8,11–14,25–32] The atrial surface of the anterior leaflet exhibits a depolarizing electrocardiogram spike shortly before the onset of the QRS complex, and the resulting contraction of leaflet muscle (which can be abolished by beta-blockade), along with contraction of smooth muscle and valvular interstitial cells, possibly aids leaflet coaptation before the onset of systole, as well as stiffens the leaflet in response to rising left ventricular (LV) pressure.[11–14,29,31,33,34–38] Mitral leaflet stretch of 10% or

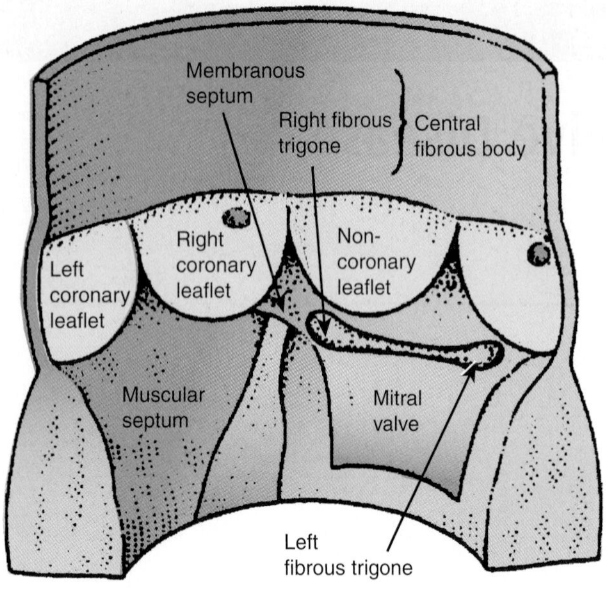

FIGURE 40-1 Diagram from a pathologic perspective with division of the septum illustrating the fibrous continuity between the mitral and aortic valves. (*Reproduced with permission from Anderson RH, Wilcox BR: The anatomy of the mitral valve, in Wells FC, Shapiro LM [eds]: Mitral Valve Disease. Oxford, England, Butterworth-Heinemann, 1996; p 4.*)

more also leads to an action potential that initiates leaflet muscle contraction.[34,39]

Annular Size, Shape, and Dynamics

The average mitral annular cross-sectional area ranges from 5.0 to 11.4 cm^2 in normal human hearts (average is 7.6 cm^2).[40] The annular perimeter of the posterior leaflet is longer than that subtending the anterior leaflet by a ratio of 2:1; ie, the posterior annulus circumscribes approximately two-thirds of the mitral annulus.[12] Annular area varies during the cardiac cycle and is influenced directly by both left atrial (LA) and LV contraction, size, and pressure.[41,42] The mitral annular area changes by 20 to 40% during the cardiac cycle.[6,41–47] Annular size increases beginning in late systole and continues through isovolumic relaxation and into diastole; maximal annular area occurs in late diastole around the time of the P wave on the electrocardiogram.[6,41,43,46,48] Importantly, half to two-thirds of the total decrease in annular area occurs during atrial contraction (or *presystolic*); this component of annular area change is smaller when the PR interval is short and is abolished completely when atrial fibrillation or ventricular pacing is present. Annular area decreases further (if LV end-diastolic volume is not abnormally elevated) to a minimum in early to midsystole.[5,6,41–43]

The normal human mitral annulus is roughly elliptical (or kidney-shaped), with greater eccentricity (ie, being less circular) in systole than in diastole.[3,6,40–42,45,47,49] In its most elliptical configuration, the ratio of minor to major diameters is approximately 0.75. In three-dimensional space, the annulus is saddle shaped (or more precisely, a hyperbolic paraboloid), with the highest point (farthest from the LV apex) located anteriorly in the middle of the anterior leaflet; this point is termed the *fibrosa* in the echocardiography literature and the *saddle horn* by surgeons, and is readily identified in echocardiographic images owing to the common junction with the aortic valve. The low points are located posteromedially and anterolaterally in the commissures, and another less prominent high point is located directly posterior.[41,50,51] During the cardiac cycle, annular regions adjacent to the posterior leaflet (where the leaflet attaches directly to the atrial and ventricular endocardium) move toward (during systole) and away (during diastole) from the relatively immobile anterior annulus.[41,47]

The mitral annulus moves upward into the left atrium in diastole and toward the LV apex during systole; the duration, average rate, and magnitude of annular displacement correlate with (and perhaps influence) the rate of LA filling and emptying.[6,41,43,46,52,53] The annulus moves slightly during late diastole (2 to 4 mm toward the left atrium during atrial systole). This movement does not occur in the presence of atrial fibrillation and may be an atriogenic contractile property. The annulus moves a greater distance (3 to 16 mm toward the

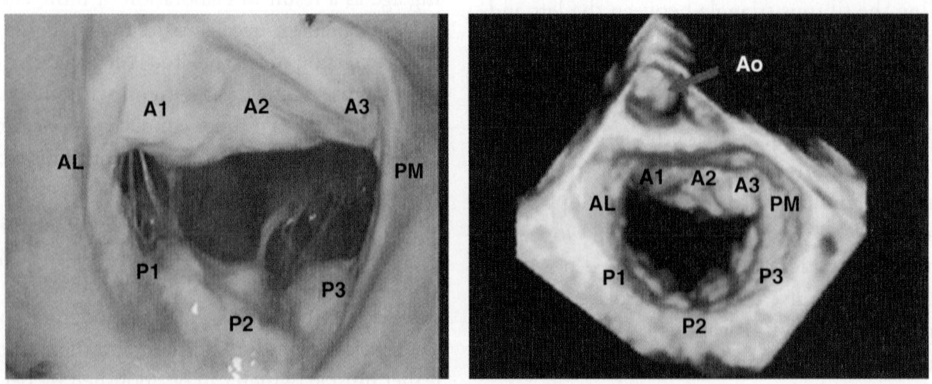

FIGURE 40-2 The operative view of the mitral valve is shown (*left*), and the corresponding "surgical view" obtained with real-time three-dimensional transesophageal echocardiography volume rendering (*right*). Images are from patient with type IIIb dysfunction (*see text*). A1, A2, A3 = anterior mitral valve scallops; AL = anterolateral; P1, P2, P3 = posterior mitral valve scallops; PM = posteromedial. (*Reproduced with permission from O'Gara P, Sugeng L, Lang R, et al: The role of imaging in chronic degenerative mitral regurgitation. J Am Coll Cardiol Img 2008; 1:221.*)

LV apex) during isovolumic contraction and ventricular ejection. This systolic motion, which aids subsequent LA filling, occurs in the presence or absence of atrial fibrillation and is related to the extent of ventricular emptying; thus, it is likely driven by LV contraction.[6,41,45,46,52–55] Subsequently, the annulus moves very little during isovolumic relaxation but then exhibits rapid recoil toward the left atrium in early diastole. This recoiling increases the net velocity of mitral inflow by as much as 20%.[46,56] Annular motion can be responsible for up to 20% of LV filling and ejection.[57]

Dynamic Leaflet Motion

The posterior mitral leaflet is attached to thinner chordae tendineae than the anterior leaflet, and its motion is restrained by chordae during both systole and diastole.[9,52] Regions of both leaflets are concave toward the left ventricle during systole,[58–60] but leaflet shape is complex, and anterior leaflet curvature near the annulus is convex to the left ventricle during systole, thus resulting in a sigmoid shape.[48,50,51,61] Leaflet opening does not start with the free margin but rather in the center of the leaflet; leaflet curvature flattens initially and then becomes reversed (making the leaflet convex toward the left ventricle) while the edges are still approximated.[48,59,60] The leading edge then moves into the left ventricle (like a traveling wave), and the leaflet straightens. The leaflet edges in the middle of the valve appear to separate before those portions closer to the commissures, and posterior leaflet opening occurs approximately 8 to 40 ms later.[60–63] Early leaflet opening (*e* wave) is very rapid; once reaching maximum opening, the edges exhibit a slow to-and-fro movement (like a flag flapping in a breeze) until another less forceful opening impulse occurs, associated with the *a* wave. During late diastole, the leaflets move gradually away from the LV wall.

Valve closure starts with the leaflet bulging toward the atrium at its attachment point to the annulus. The closure rate of the anterior leaflet is almost twice that of the posterior leaflet, thereby ensuring arrival of both cusps at their closed positions simultaneously (because the anterior leaflet is opened more widely than the posterior leaflet at the onset of ventricular systole).[63] The anterior leaflet actually arrives at the plane of the annulus in a bulged shape (concave to the ventricle), but as the closing movement proceeds and the leaflet ascends toward the atrium, this curvature appears to run through the whole leaflet, from the annulus toward the edge, in a rolling manner. The leaflet edge is the last part of the leaflet to approach the annular plane. Leaflet curvature is more pronounced with the onset of systolic ejection.[59,60]

Chordae Tendineae and Papillary Muscles

Epicardial fibers in the left ventricle descend from the base of the heart and proceed inward at the apex to form the two papillary muscles, which are characterized by vertically oriented myocardial fibers.[64,65] The anterolateral papillary muscle usually has one major head and is a more prominent structure; the posteromedial papillary muscle can have two or more subheads and is flatter.[9] A loop from the papillary muscles to the mitral annulus is completed by the chordae tendineae continuing into the mitral leaflets, which then are attached to the annulus. The posteromedial papillary muscle usually is supplied by the right coronary artery (or a dominant left circumflex artery in 10% of patients); the anterolateral papillary muscle is supplied by blood flow from both the left anterior descending and circumflex coronary arteries.[7,64,66,67]

The posteromedial and anterolateral papillary muscles give rise to chordae tendineae going to both leaflets[9] (Fig. 40-3). Classically, the chordae are divided functionally into three groups.[64,68] First-order chordae originate near the papillary muscle tips, divide progressively, and insert on the leading edge of the leaflets; these primary chordae prevent valve-edge prolapse during systole. The second-order chordae (including two or more larger and less branched "strut" chordae) originate from the same location and tend to be thicker and fewer in number;[9,68] they insert on the ventricular surface of the leaflets at the junction of the rough and clear zones, which is demarcated by a subtle ridge on the leaflet corresponding to the line of leaflet coaptation. The second-order chordae (including the strut chordae) serve to anchor the valve, are more prominent on the anterior leaflet, and are important for optimal ventricular systolic function. Second-order chordae also may arborize from large chordae that also give rise to first-order chordae. The third-order chordae, also called *tertiary* or *basal chordae,* originate directly from the trabeculae carneae of the ventricular wall, attach to the posterior leaflet near the annulus, and can be identified by their fan-shaped patterns.[68] Additionally, distinct commissural chordae and cleft chordae exist in the commissures. In total, about 25 major chordal trunks (range 15 to 32) arise from the papillary muscles in humans, equally divided between those going to the anterior and posterior leaflets; on the other end, greater than 100 smaller individual chordae attach to the leaflets.[68] Studies of porcine mitral valves demonstrate that the chordae have different microstructures based on chordal type.[69] The presence of blood vessels characterizes the chordae as complex living components that work in coordination with the other elements of the valvular and subvalvular apparatus.

During diastole, the papillary muscles form an inflow tract. During systole, they create an outflow tract that later becomes obliterated owing to systolic thickening of the papillary muscles, thereby augmenting LV ejection by volume displacement.[65] The contribution of the papillary muscles to LV chamber volume is 5 to 8% during diastole but 15 to 30% during systole.[65,70] The anterolateral and posteromedial papillary muscles contract simultaneously and are innervated by both sympathetic and parasympathetic (vagal) nerves.[71,72]

Studies of papillary muscle function during the cardiac cycle have yielded discordant results.[71,73–76] Although the papillary muscles shorten at some point during systole (by more than one-fourth their maximum length), this contraction may be isometric or substantially less than that of the LV free wall fibers.[73–75,77–80] In addition, there is no consensus as to the exact timing of papillary muscle contraction and elongation during the cardiac cycle.[71–73,75,76,78,79] Some studies suggest that the papillary muscles contract before the LV free wall so that the

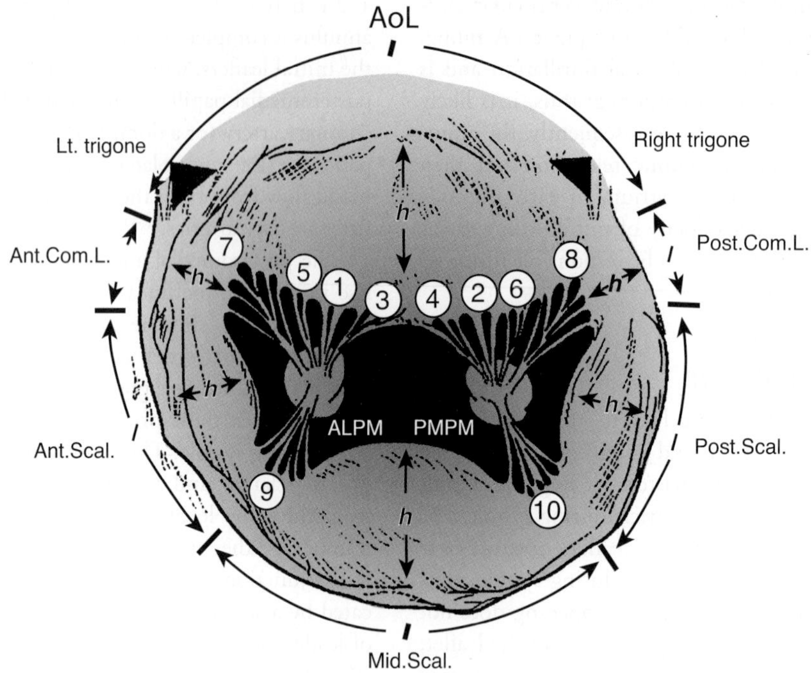

FIGURE 40-3 Mitral valve and subvalvular apparatus. ALPM = anterolateral papillary muscle; Ant.Com.L. = anterior commissural leaflet; Ant.Scal. = anterior scallop; AoL = aortic leaflet; h = height of leaflet; l = length of attachment of leaflet; Lt.Trigone = left fibrous trigone; Mid.Scal. = middle scallop; PMPM = posteromedial papillary muscle; Post.Com.L. = posterior commissural leaflet; Post.Scal. = posterior scallop; Rt.Trigone = right fibrous trigone; 1 = anterior main chorda; 2 = posterior main chorda; 3 = anterior paramedial chorda; 4 = posterior paramedial chorda; 5 = anterior paracommissural chorda; 6 = posterior paracommissural chorda; 7 = anterior commissural chorda; 8 = posterior commissural chorda; 9 = anterior cleft chorda; 10 = posterior cleft chorda. (*Reproduced with permission from Sakai T, Okita Y, Ueda Y, et al: Distance between mitral annulus and papillary muscles: anatomic study in normal human hearts. J Thorac Cardiovasc Surg 1999; 118:636.*)

mitral valve leaflets are supported during early LV ejection;[76] others, however, show that papillary muscles lengthen during isovolumic contraction and shorten during ejection, as well as during isovolumic relaxation.[72,75] From the standpoint of electromechanics, although papillary muscle excitation occurs simultaneously with the rest of the endocardial surface of the ventricle, the papillary muscles may contract just after the onset of LV contraction.[71,78] Papillary muscle shortening throughout isovolumic relaxation may play a role in opening the mitral valve, and elongation in late diastole may be necessary to permit proper valve closure.[78]

Experimentally, both papillary muscles closely mimic general LV dynamics; ie, the papillary muscles shorten during ejection, lengthen during diastole, and change length minimally during the isovolumic periods[73] (Fig. 40-4). These findings suggest that earlier studies suggesting that papillary muscle lengthens during isovolumic contraction and shortens during isovolumic relaxation may have been confounded by some form of myocardial injury or surgical trauma during instrumentation.[73]

MITRAL STENOSIS

Etiology

Mitral stenosis generally is the result of rheumatic heart disease.[81–88] Nonrheumatic causes of mitral stenosis or LV inflow obstruction include severe mitral annular and/or leaflet calcification in elderly people, congenital mitral valve deformities, malignant carcinoid syndrome, neoplasm, LA thrombus, endocarditic vegetations, certain inherited metabolic diseases, and those cases related to previous commissurotomy or an

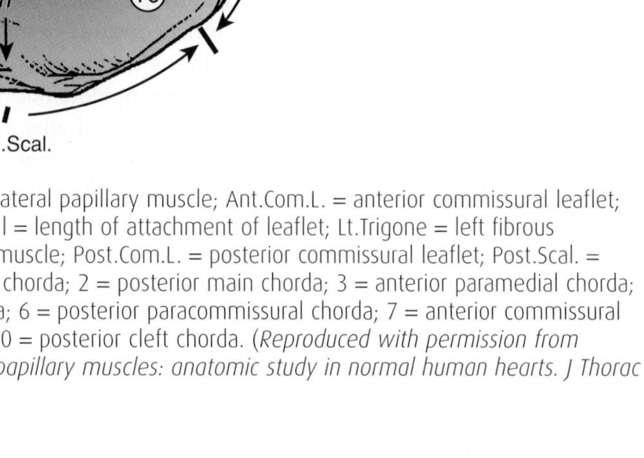

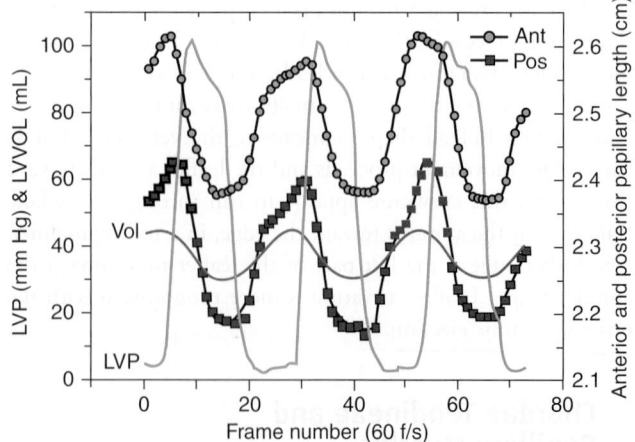

FIGURE 40-4 Graph showing typical dynamics of the left ventricle and papillary muscles. The papillary muscle lengths are temporally related closely to changes in LV volume (LV VOL). ANT = anterior papillary muscle; POST = posterior papillary muscle. (*Modified with permission from Rayhill SC, Daughters GT, Castro LJ, et al: Dynamics of normal and ischemic canine papillary muscles. Circ Res 1994; 74:1179.*)

implanted prosthesis.[84–90] A definite history of rheumatic fever can be obtained in only about 50 to 60% of patients; women are affected more often than men by a 2:1 to 3:1 ratio. Nearly always acquired before age 20, rheumatic valvular disease becomes clinically evident one to three decades later.

Approximately 20 million cases of rheumatic fever occur in developing countries annually.[91] In the United States, Western Europe, and other developed countries, the prevalence of mitral stenosis has decreased markedly. The etiologic agent for acute rheumatic fever is group A beta-hemolytic streptococcus, but the specific immunologic and inflammatory mechanisms leading to the valvulitis are less clear.[91–94] Streptococcal antigens cross-react with human tissues, known as *molecular mimicry*, and may stimulate immunologic responses. Components implicated in the organism's virulence include the hyaluronic acid capsule and the antigenic streptococcal M protein and its peptides.[91–93] Mimicry between streptococcal antigens and heart tissue proteins, combined with high inflammatory cytokine and low interleukin-4 production, leads to the development of autoimmune reactions and cardiac tissue damage.[92,93]

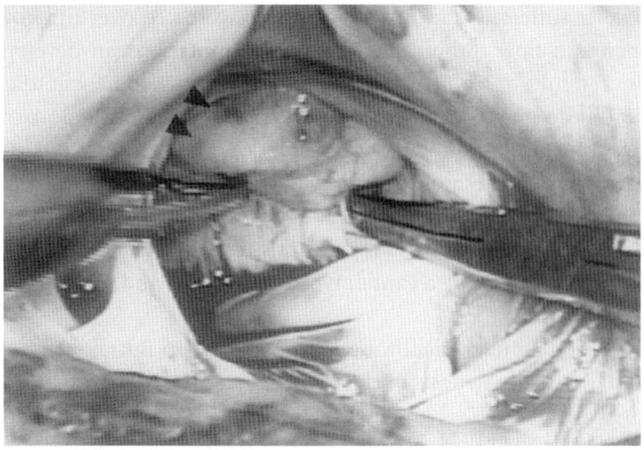

FIGURE 40-5 Intraoperative photograph of mitral stenosis as a result of rheumatic heart disease. The mitral leaflets are markedly restricted. The arrowheads point to the anterior leaflet near the anterolateral commissure.

In addition to affecting the cardiac valves, rheumatic heart disease is a pancarditis affecting to various degrees the endocardium, myocardium, and pericardium[81–83,87] (Fig. 40-5). In rheumatic valvulitis, mitral valve involvement is the most common (isolated mitral stenosis is found in 40% of patients), followed by combined aortic and mitral valve disease, and least frequently, isolated aortic valve disease, with or without tricuspid involvement. Pathoanatomical characteristics of mitral valvulitis include commissural fusion, leaflet fibrosis with stiffening and retraction, and chordal fusion and shortening (Fig. 40-6).[82,88]

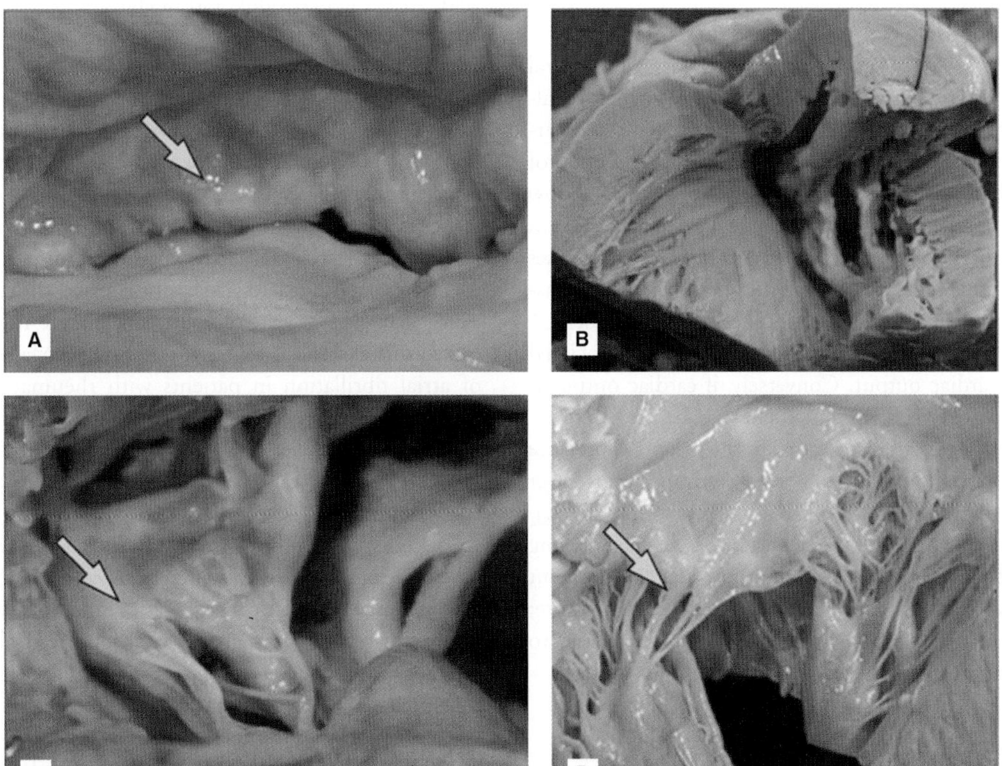

FIGURE 40-6 Pathology of the mitral valve in mitral stenosis. Thickened, rigid nodular appearance of the mitral valve leaflets viewed from the atria (A) and ventricle (B). Calcium is present in the commissure and the commissures are fused, resulting in a valve shaped like a fish mouth. Subvalvular apparatus is thick, fused, and shortened (B, C). Healthy mitral valve leaflets (D). (*Reproduced with permission from Chandrashekhar Y, Westaby S, Narula J. Mitral stenosis. Lancet 2009; 374:1271.*)

Leaflet stiffening and fibrosis can be exacerbated over time by increased flow turbulence. Valvular regurgitation can develop as a result of chordal fusion and shortening. The chordae tendineae may become so retracted that the leaflets appear to insert directly into the papillary muscles. The degree of calcification varies. It is more common and of greater severity in men, older patients, and those with a higher transvalvular gradient.[83] In some cases, rheumatic myocarditis results in left ventricular dilatation caused by a cardiomyopathic process and progressive heart failure.

Mitral annular calcification may progress to mitral sclerosis and eventually stenosis in elderly people or those who are dialysis dependent.[88,90] The anterior leaflet can become thick and immobile; LV inflow obstruction also results from calcification of the posterior mitral valve leaflet. Calcific protrusions into the ventricle and extension of the calcium into the leaflets further narrow the valve orifice, resulting in mitral stenosis.[88,90] In these cases, the left ventricle typically is small, hypertrophied, and noncompliant.

Hemodynamics

In patients with mitral stenosis, an early, middle, and late diastolic transvalvular gradient is present between the left atrium and ventricle; as the degree of mitral stenosis worsens, a progressively higher gradient occurs, especially late in diastole.[84,95–97] The average left atrial pressure in patients with severe mitral stenosis may be in the range of 15 to 20 mm Hg at rest, with a mean transvalvular gradient of 10 to 15 mm Hg.[95,97] With exercise, the LA pressure and gradient rise substantially.

Another physiologic measurement in patients with mitral stenosis is the (derived) cross-sectional valve area, which is calculated from the mean transvalvular pressure gradient and cardiac output. The transvalvular pressure gradient is a function of the square of the transvalvular flow rate; eg, doubling the flow quadruples the gradient. Mitral transvalvular flow depends on cardiac output and heart rate. An increase in heart rate decreases the duration of transvalvular LV filling during diastole; the transvalvular mean gradient increases, and consequently, so does LA pressure.[96,98] A high transvalvular gradient may be associated with a normal cardiac output. Conversely, if cardiac output is low, only a modest transvalvular gradient may be present.

Because of effective atrial contraction, the mean LA pressure in patients with mitral stenosis and normal sinus rhythm is lower than that in patients with atrial fibrillation.[99,100] Sinus rhythm further augments flow through the stenotic valve, thereby helping to maintain adequate forward cardiac output. The development of atrial fibrillation decreases cardiac output by 20% or more; atrial fibrillation with a rapid ventricular response can lead to acute dyspnea and pulmonary edema.[81,99]

Ventricular Adaptation

In patients with isolated mitral stenosis and restricted LV inflow, LV chamber size (end-diastolic volume) is normal or smaller than normal, and the end-diastolic pressure typically is low.[84,101,102] The peak filling rate is reduced, as is stroke volume. Cardiac output thus is diminished as a result of inflow obstruction leading to underfilling of the ventricle rather than LV pump failure.[103] During exercise, the LV ejection fraction may increase slightly; however, LV filling is compromised by the shorter diastolic filling periods at higher heart rates, resulting in a smaller end-diastolic volume (or LV preload). Therefore, stroke volume and a blunted increase (or even decrease) in cardiac output can occur.[102]

Approximately 25 to 50% of patients with severe mitral stenosis have LV systolic dysfunction as a consequence of associated problems (eg, mitral regurgitation, aortic valve disease, ischemic heart disease, rheumatic myocarditis or pancarditis, and myocardial fibrosis) or internal constraint of a rigid mitral valve, reduced preload, and reflex increase in afterload.[83,88,97,102] In these patients, LV end-systolic and -diastolic volumes may be larger than normal. Diastolic dysfunction and abnormal chamber compliance are sometimes evident.[88] Also, because right ventricular afterload increases as pulmonary hypertension develops in these patients, right ventricular systolic performance deteriorates.[84,104]

Atrial Adaptation

In patients with mitral stenosis who are in normal sinus rhythm, the LA pressure tracing is characterized by an elevated mean LA pressure with a prominent *a* wave, which is followed by a gradual pressure decline.[81,100] Because of the stenotic valve, coordinated LA contraction is important in maintaining adequate transvalvular flow.[100] The high LA pressure gradually leads to LA hypertrophy and dilatation, atrial fibrillation, and atrial thrombus formation.[83,102,105] The degree of LA enlargement and fibrosis does not correlate with the severity of the valvular stenosis partly because of the marked variation in duration of the stenotic lesion and atrial involvement by the underlying rheumatic inflammatory process.[102] Disorganization of atrial muscle fibers is associated with abnormal conduction velocities and inhomogeneous refractory periods. Premature atrial activation owing to increased automaticity or reentry eventually may lead to atrial fibrillation, which is present in more than half of patients with either pure mitral stenosis or mixed mitral stenosis and regurgitation.[105] Major determinants of atrial fibrillation in patients with rheumatic heart disease include older age and larger LA diameter.[105]

Pulmonary Changes

In patients with mild to moderate mitral stenosis, pulmonary vascular resistance is not increased, and pulmonary arterial pressure may remain normal at rest, rising only with exertion or increased heart rate.[95] In severe chronic mitral stenosis with elevated pulmonary vascular resistance, pulmonary arterial pressure is elevated at rest and can approach systemic pressure with exercise. A pulmonary arterial systolic pressure greater than 60 mm Hg significantly increases impedance to right ventricular emptying and produces high right ventricular end-diastolic and right atrial pressures.

LA hypertension produces pulmonary vasoconstriction, which exacerbates the elevated pulmonary vascular resistance.[83,104] As the mean LA pressure exceeds 30 mm Hg above oncotic pressure, transudation of fluid into the pulmonary interstitium occurs, leading to reduced lung compliance. Pulmonary hypertension develops as a result of passive transmission of high LA pressure, pulmonary venous hypertension, pulmonary arteriolar constriction, and eventually, pulmonary vascular obliterative changes. Early changes in the pulmonary vascular bed may be considered protective in that the elevated pulmonary vascular resistance protects the pulmonary capillary bed from excessively high pressures. However, the pulmonary hypertension worsens progressively, leading to right-sided heart failure, tricuspid insufficiency, and occasionally, pulmonic valve insufficiency.[84,104]

Clinical Evaluation

Because of the gradual development of mitral stenosis, patients may remain asymptomatic for many years.[81,88,95] Characteristic symptoms of mitral stenosis eventually develop and are associated primarily with pulmonary venous congestion or low cardiac output, eg, dyspnea on exertion, orthopnea, or paroxysmal nocturnal dyspnea and fatigue. With progressive stenosis (valve area between 1 and 2 cm^2), patients become symptomatic with less effort. When mitral valve area decreases to about 1 cm^2, symptoms become more pronounced. As pulmonary hypertension and right-sided heart failure subsequently develop, signs of tricuspid regurgitation, hepatomegaly, peripheral edema, and ascites can be found.

As a result of high LA pressure and increased pulmonary blood volume, hemoptysis may develop secondary to rupture of dilated bronchial veins (or submucosal varices).[81,88,104] Over time, pulmonary vascular resistance becomes higher, and the likelihood of hemoptysis decreases. Hemoptysis also may result from pulmonary infarction, which is a late complication of chronic heart failure. Acute pulmonary edema with pink frothy sputum can occur as a result of alveolar capillary rupture.

Systemic thromboembolism, occurring in approximately 20% of patients, may be the first symptom of mitral stenosis; recurrent embolization occurs in 25% of patients.[81,106] The incidence of thromboembolic events is higher in patients with mitral stenosis or mixed mitral stenosis–mitral regurgitation than in those with pure mitral regurgitation. At least 40% of all clinically important embolic events involve the cerebral circulation, approximately 15% involve the visceral vessels, and 15% affect the lower extremities.[81,107] Embolization to coronary arteries may lead to angina, arrhythmias, or myocardial infarction; renal embolization can result in hypertension.[81] Factors that increase the risk of thromboembolic events include low cardiac output, LA dilatation, atrial fibrillation, left atrial thrombus, absence of tricuspid or aortic regurgitation, and the presence of echocardiographic "smoke" in the atrium, an indicator of stagnant flow. Patients with these risk factors should be anticoagulated.[81,106,107] If an episode of systemic embolization occurs in patients in sinus rhythm, infective endocarditis, which is more common in mild than in severe mitral stenosis, should be considered.

Patients with chronic mitral stenosis are often thin and frail (cardiac cachexia), indicative of longstanding low cardiac output, congestive heart failure, and inanition.[81] The peripheral arterial pulse generally is normal, except in patients with a decreased LV stroke volume, in which case the pulse amplitude is diminished. Heart size usually is normal, with a normal apical impulse on chest palpation. An apical diastolic thrill may be present. In patients with pulmonary hypertension, a right ventricular lift can be felt in the left parasternal region. Auscultatory findings include a presystolic murmur, a loud S_1, an opening snap, and an apical diastolic rumble.[81,88,108–110] The presystolic murmur, which occurs because of closing of the anterior mitral leaflet, is a consistent finding and begins earlier in those in sinus rhythm than in those in atrial fibrillation.[110] S_1 is accentuated in mitral stenosis when the leaflets are pliable but diminished in later phases of the disease when the leaflets are thickened or calcified. As pulmonary artery pressure becomes elevated, S_2 becomes prominent.[111] With progressive pulmonary hypertension, the normal splitting of S_2 narrows because of reduced pulmonary vascular compliance. Other signs of pulmonary hypertension include a murmur of tricuspid and/or pulmonic regurgitation and an S_4 originating from the right ventricle. Best heard at the apex, the early diastolic mitral opening snap is caused by sudden tensing of the pliable leaflets during valve opening and is absent when the leaflets are rigid or immobile.[81,108,109] In mild mitral stenosis, the diastolic rumble is soft and of short duration; a long or holodiastolic murmur indicates severe mitral stenosis. The intensity of the murmur does not necessarily correlate with the severity of the stenosis; indeed, no diastolic murmur may be detectable in patients with severe stenosis, calcified leaflets, or low cardiac output.[110] Coagulation abnormalities common in mitral stenosis include changes in platelet and fibrinolytic activity and increased concentration of fibrinopeptide A, thrombin-antithrombin III complex, and d-dimer.[88]

On chest radiography, LA enlargement is the earliest change found in patients with mitral stenosis; it is suggested by posterior bulging of the left atrium seen on the lateral view, a double contour of the right heart border seen on the posteroanterior film, and elevation of the left main stem bronchus.[95] The overall cardiac size often is normal. Prominence of the pulmonary arteries coupled with LA enlargement may obliterate the normal concavity between the aorta and left ventricle to produce a straight left heart border. In the lung fields, pulmonary congestion may be recognized as distention of the pulmonary arteries and veins in the upper lung fields and pleural effusions. If mitral stenosis is severe, engorged pulmonary lymphatics are seen as distinct horizontal linear opacities in the lower lung fields (Kerley B lines).

The electrocardiogram is not accurate in assessing the severity of mitral stenosis and in many cases may be completely normal. In patients with severe mitral stenosis and normal sinus rhythm, LA enlargement is the earliest change (a wide notched P wave in lead II and a biphasic P wave in lead V1).[88,95,112] Atrial arrhythmias are common in patients with advanced degrees of mitral stenosis. In those with pulmonary hypertension, right ventricular hypertrophy may develop and is associated with right-axis deviation, a tall R wave in V_1, and secondary ST-T-wave changes; however, the electrocardiogram is not a sensitive indicator of right ventricular hypertrophy or the degree of pulmonary hypertension.[112] Because multivalvular disease may be present in patients with rheumatic heart disease, signs of left and right ventricular hypertrophy can be identified on the electrocardiogram in cases of combined mitral and aortic stenosis. Right atrial enlargement and right ventricular dilatation and hypertrophy, however, also can mask the changes indicative of LV hypertrophy on the electrocardiographic tracing in patients with multivalvular disease.[112]

Echocardiography has become the primary diagnostic method for assessing mitral valve pathology and pathophysiology.[7,88,113–116] Cross-sectional valve area and LA and LV dimensions can be quantified using two-dimensional transthoracic echocardiography (TTE). Best appreciated in the parasternal long-axis view, features of rheumatic mitral stenosis include reduced diastolic excursion of the leaflets (Carpentier type IIIa leaflet motion) and thickening or calcification of the valvular and subvalvular apparatus (Fig. 40-7). M-mode findings include thickening, reduced motion, and parallel movement of the anterior and posterior leaflets during diastole. The mitral valve area can be planimetered directly in the short-axis view, but this measurement has limited clinical value. Doppler echocardiography accurately determines peak and mean transvalvular mitral pressure gradients that correlate closely with cardiac catheterization measurements.[81,113] To estimate mitral valve area, the pressure half-time (time required for the initial diastolic gradient to decline by 50%) has been employed; the more prolonged the half-time, the more severe is the reduction in orifice area.[113] Using the pressure half-time determination, mitral valve area is equal to 220 (an empirical value) divided by the pressure half-time. Deriving mitral valve area using the pressure half-time method, however, generally has fallen out of favor. The mean mitral gradient at rest and with bicycle or supine exercise measured using Doppler echocardiography is more useful clinically than estimating mitral valve area; the simultaneous increase in right ventricular systolic pressure (estimated from continuous-wave or pulse-wave Doppler envelopes of the tricuspid regurgitation signal) during exercise is also revealing. The mitral separation index, which is the average of the maximum separation of the mitral leaflet tips in diastole in parasternal and apical four-chamber views, shows good correlation with mitral valve area measured by planimetry and pressure half-time and may be able to discriminate between hemodynamically significant and insignificant mitral stenosis.[117] TEE can provide more information in the evaluation of mitral stenosis; although rarely needed, it is better than the transthoracic approach for visualizing details of valvular pathology, such as valve mobility and thickness, subvalvular apparatus involvement, and extent of leaflet or commissural calcification.[88,113,114]

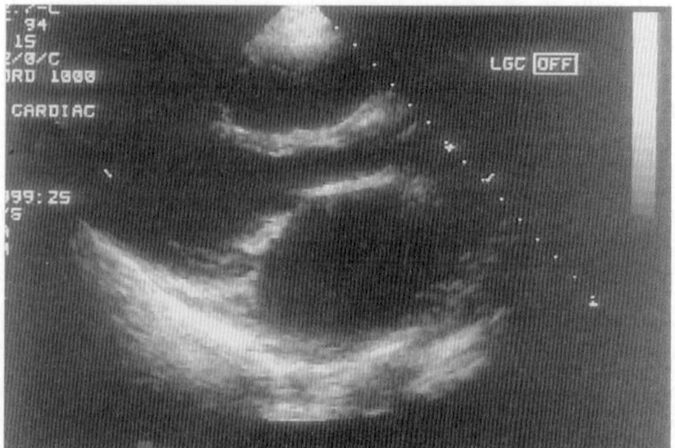

FIGURE 40-7 Echocardiogram (long axis) of a patient with severe mitral stenosis caused by rheumatic heart disease. A thickened, stenotic valve separates an enlarged left atrium (*right*) and the left ventricle (*left*) and outflow tract (*above*).

Three-dimensional (3D) echocardiography facilitates spatial recognition of intracardiac structures and can evaluate cardiac valvular and congenital heart disease using both real-time three-dimensional TTE and TEE images.[116,118,119] The addition of color-flow Doppler to 3D echocardiography provides better visualization of regurgitant lesions and promises to improve quantitative assessment of such lesions. Measurements of LV volume using 3D echocardiography correlate tightly with measurements obtained using both contrast ventriculography and magnetic resonance imaging (MRI). Cardiac MRI technology continues to be refined but remains inferior to echocardiography for depiction of valvular morphology and motion.[120,121] Multidetector computed tomography (CT) may emerge as a technique that can evaluate both cardiac structure and function. Experience with gated multidetector CT has yielded good visualization of valve leaflet hinges, commissures, and the mitral annulus.[122] Main limitations of this technology include image noise, the time required for postprocessing, and the radiation dose.

Cardiac catheterization is not necessary to establish the diagnosis of mitral stenosis; however, it provides information regarding coronary artery status.[123] Historically, left ventriculography permits assessment of the mitral valve and LV contractility and calculation of ejection fraction, but its role has been totally replaced by echocardiography. Left-sided heart catheterization allows determination of LV end-diastolic pressure; right-sided heart catheterization is performed to measure cardiac index and the degree of pulmonary hypertension. Rarely, cardiac catheterization is used to evaluate the reversibility of severe pulmonary hypertension using pharmacologic interventions, including inhaled nitric oxide when indicated.

Postprocedure Outcome

Whereas LV systolic function is used to predict the natural history and postprocedure prognosis of patients with other valvular lesions, there are few data linking LV function to outcome in patients with mitral stenosis. Not surprisingly, the best indicator is related to the degree of clinical impairment. Untreated mitral stenosis is associated with a poor prognosis once severe symptoms occur.[88] Percutaneous balloon valvuloplasty is the mainstay of treatment of mitral stenosis provided the anatomy is favorable (Fig. 40-8).[88] Generally, the technique immediately doubles mitral valve area and decreases the gradient substantially in properly selected patients with rheumatic mitral stenosis. Approximately 90% of patients improve clinically if a valve area greater than 1.5 cm^2 without significant regurgitation can be achieved.[124] Surgical intervention (eg, open mitral commissurotomy or mitral valve replacement) substantially improves functional capacity and long-term survival of patients with mitral stenosis; 67 to 90% of patients are alive at 10 years.[112,125–127]

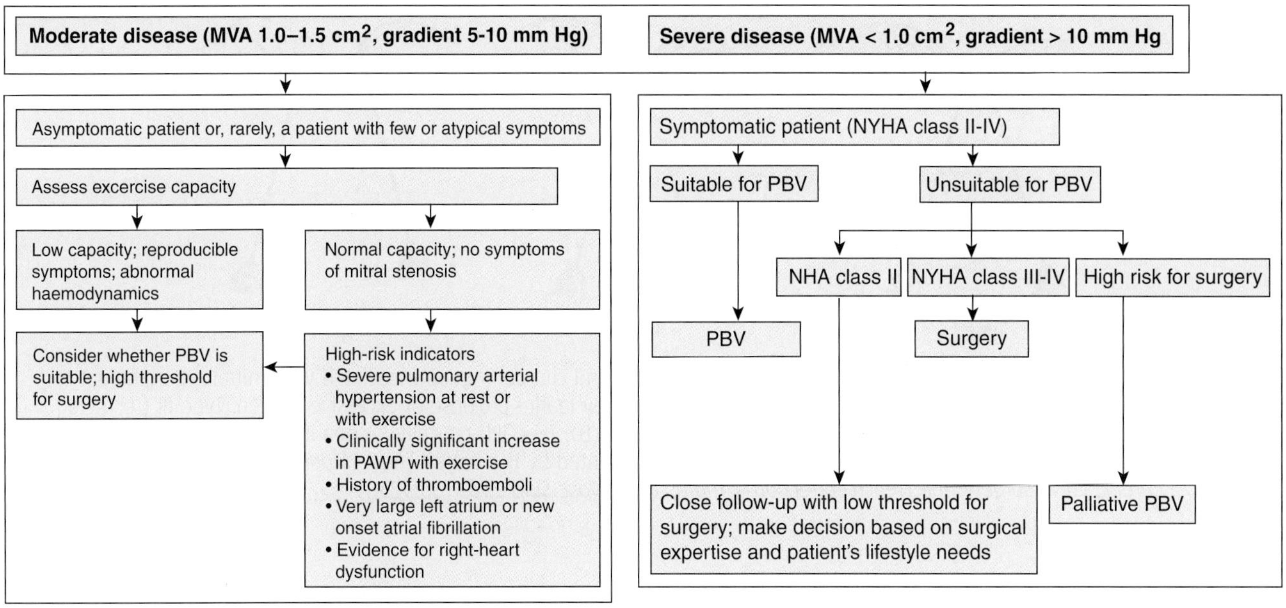

FIGURE 40-8 Treatment strategies for mitral stenosis. MVA = mitral valve area; NYHA = New York Heart Association functional class; PAWP = pulmonary artery wedge pressure; PBV = percutaneous balloon valvuloplasty. Severe mitral stenosis is rarely asymptomatic and, for such patients, we suggest use of the algorithm for assessment of patients with moderate disease. (*Reproduced with permission from Chandrashekhar Y, Westaby S, Narula J. Mitral stenosis. Lancet 2009; 374:1271.*)

Despite a higher operative risk for patients with severe pulmonary hypertension and right-sided heart failure, these individuals usually improve postoperatively with a reduction in pulmonary vascular pressures.[84,128] If there is not excessive scarring of the subvalvular mitral apparatus, mitral valve replacement using chordal-sparing techniques can be performed in patients with rheumatic mitral valve disease, particularly those with mixed stenotic and regurgitant lesions; this results in a reduction in LV end-systolic and end-diastolic volumes and preservation of LV systolic pump performance.[129,130] Alternatively, the valve and the entire subvalvular apparatus have to be resected during mitral valve replacement when the disease process is very advanced and all structures are densely calcified and extremely scarred, which frequently is the case in older patients.

Summary

Mitral stenosis generally is caused by rheumatic heart disease. With worsening mitral stenosis, a progressively higher transvalvular pressure gradient develops. Mitral transvalvular flow depends on cardiac output and heart rate; an increase in heart rate decreases the duration of transvalvular filling during diastole and reduces forward cardiac output, causing symptoms. In mild to moderate mitral stenosis, pulmonary vascular resistance may not be elevated; pulmonary arterial pressure may be normal at rest and rise only with exercise or increased heart rate. In patients with severe mitral stenosis with elevated pulmonary vascular resistance, the pulmonary arterial pressure usually is high at rest. Characteristic symptoms of mitral stenosis are associated with pulmonary venous congestion and/or low cardiac output. Echocardiography remains the best technique for assessing mitral valve pathology. Percutaneous or surgical intervention can improve functional capacity and long-term survival of patients with mitral stenosis.

MITRAL REGURGITATION

Etiology

The functional competence of the mitral valve relies on proper, coordinated interaction of the mitral annulus and leaflets, chordae tendineae, papillary muscles, left atrium, and left ventricle, what we refer to as the *valvular-ventricular complex*.[64,66,131–134] Normal LV geometry and alignment of the papillary muscles and chordae tendineae permit leaflet coaptation and prevent prolapse during ventricular systole. Dysfunction of any one or more of the components of this valvular–ventricular complex can lead to mitral regurgitation. Regurgitation also can occur in diastole (*presystolic mitral regurgitation*) as a result of delayed ventricular contraction or permanent ventricular pacing, but this phenomenon appears to have few clinical implications.[135]

Important causes of systolic mitral regurgitation include ischemic heart disease with ischemic mitral regurgitation (IMR), dilated cardiomyopathy [for which the general term *functional mitral regurgitation* (FMR) is used], myxomatous degeneration, rheumatic valve disease, mitral annular calcification, infective endocarditis, congenital anomalies, endocardial fibrosis, myocarditis and collagen-vascular disorders.[83,86,87,136–138] IMR is considered a specific subset of FMR. Acute mitral regurgitation also may be the result of ventricular dysfunction from rapidly developing cardiomyopathy, such as Takotsubo cardiomyopathy, in which the mitral regurgitation is caused by left ventricular outflow tract obstruction and systolic anterior motion of the mitral valve from apical ballooning.[139]

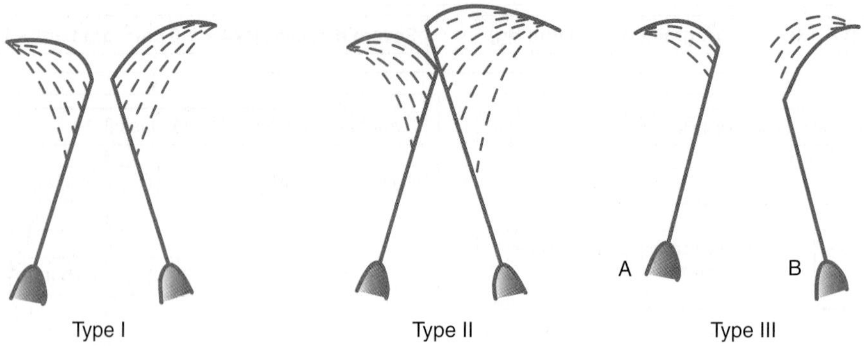

FIGURE 40-9 Carpentier's functional classification of the types of leaflet and chordal motion associated with mitral regurgitation. In type I, the leaflet motion is normal. Type II mitral regurgitation is caused by leaflet prolapse or excessive motion. Type III (restricted leaflet motion) is subdivided into restriction during diastole (A) or systole (B). Type IIIb typically is seen in patients with ischemic mitral regurgitation. The course of the leaflets during the cardiac cycle is represented by the dotted lines. (*Modified with permission from Carpentier A: Cardiac valve surgery: the French correction. J Thorac Cardiovasc Surg 1983; 86:323.*)

In general, four types of structural changes of the mitral valve apparatus may produce regurgitation: Leaflet retraction from fibrosis and calcification, annular dilatation, chordal abnormalities (including rupture, elongation, or shortening), and LV dysfunction with or without papillary muscle involvement.[64,66,140–146] Carpentier classified mitral regurgitation into three main pathoanatomic types based on leaflet motion: normal leaflet motion (type I), leaflet prolapse or excessive motion (type II), and restricted leaflet motion (type III).[140,141] Type III is further subdivided into types IIIa and IIIb based on leaflet restriction during diastole (type IIIa), as seen in rheumatic disease, or during systole (type IIIb), which is typically seen in IMR (Fig. 40-9). Mitral regurgitation with normal leaflet motion can be the result of annular dilatation, which is often secondary to LV dilatation, eg, patients with dilated cardiomyopathy or ischemic cardiomyopathy. Normal leaflet motion also includes patients with leaflet perforation secondary to endocarditis. Leaflet prolapse typically results from a floppy mitral valve with chordal elongation and/or rupture, but rarely also can be seen in patients with coronary artery disease who have papillary muscle elongation or rupture. Mitral regurgitation caused by restricted leaflet motion is associated with rheumatic valve disease (types IIIa and IIIb), ischemic heart disease (IMR with type IIIb restricted systolic leaflet motion secondary to apical tethering or tenting), and dilated cardiomyopathy (type IIIb).[141,142]

Functional and Ischemic Mitral Regurgitation

Functional mitral regurgitation (FMR) is the result of incomplete mitral leaflet coaptation in the setting of LV dysfunction and dilatation with or without annular dilatation (eg, dilated cardiomyopathy or ischemic cardiomyopathy).[143–146] LV systolic dysfunction and dilatation also may be associated with longstanding mitral regurgitation caused by severe chronic LV volume overload. Most commonly, the etiology of nonischemic cardiomyopathy is unknown or idiopathic; the second most common cause is advanced valvular disease. FMR occurs in 40% of patients with heart failure caused by dilated cardiomyopathy.[146] In the past, the leaflet morphology in patients with FMR was considered normal, but further analyses have shown the leaflets to be biochemically different, with extracellular matrix changes associated with altered cardiac dimensions.[147,148] In recipient hearts obtained at time of transplantation, mitral leaflets have up to 78% more deoxyribonucleic acid, 59% more glycosaminoglycans, 15% more collagen, but 7% less water than autopsy control leaflets.[147,148] Radially and circumferentially oriented anterior mitral leaflet strips from failing hearts are 50 to 61% stiffer and less viscous.[148] Experimentally, in tachycardia-induced cardiomyopathy, there is significant heterogeneous remodeling with increased collagen and elastic fiber turnover and myofibroblast phenotype of the mitral valve leaflet.[149] Thus, the mitral leaflets in heart failure have altered intrinsic structural properties, suggesting that the permanently distended and fibrotic tissue is unable to stretch sufficiently to cover the valve orifice and that mitral regurgitation in these patients is not purely functional.[147–149]

IMR, a subset of FMR, is becoming more widely appreciated as the population ages and more patients survive acute myocardial infarction. In those with acute infarction, IMR occurs in approximately 15% of patients with anterior wall involvement and up to 40% of patients with an inferior infarct.[85,86,150] Generally, the severity of mitral regurgitation is related to the size of the area of LV akinesia or dyskinesia. The pathophysiology of IMR can be attributed to changes in global and regional LV function or geometry, alterations in mitral annular geometry, abnormal leaflet motion and malcoaptation, increased interpapillary distance, and papillary muscle malalignment leading to apical tethering of the leaflets with restricted systolic leaflet motion (type IIIb) (Fig. 40-10).[140,143,144,150–163] Because of the interdependence of the elements constituting the valvular–ventricular complex in IMR, perturbation of any component, such as LV systolic function and geometry, annular geometry, leaflet motion and morphology, and papillary and chordal relationship, may result in mitral regurgitation.

Left Ventricular Systolic Function and Geometry. Although LV dilatation and dysfunction are less pronounced in the setting of inferior myocardial infarction than that affecting the anterior wall, the incidence and severity of mitral regurgitation

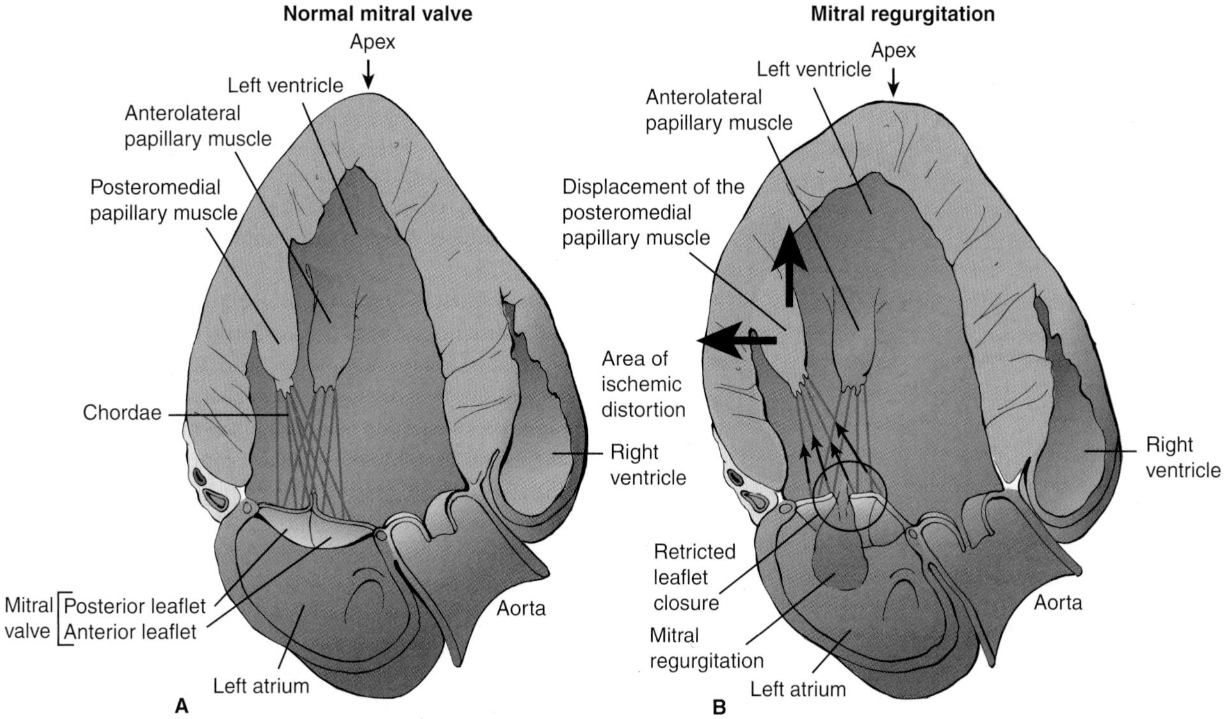

FIGURE 40-10 Mechanism of mitral regurgitation. A normal mitral valve is shown in (A). Ischemic mitral regurgitation, in which the leaflets cannot close effectively, is shown in (B). The orientation of the figure is typical of ultrasound imaging.

are greater in patients with inferior infarctions.[85,86,150,152,155] Over time, as the left ventricle dilates and changes shape after the ischemic event (postinfarction remodeling), the degree of IMR progresses.[145,155,164] Geometric changes associated with ventricular remodeling, such as posteromedial papillary muscle dislocation in the lateral axis, may lead to leaflet tenting, as reflected by a larger distance from the middle of the anterior annulus (saddle horn on echocardiography) to the posteromedial papillary muscle tip, and increased annular diameter.[145,156,157,164] At the ventricular level, myocardial infarction associated with chronic IMR is associated with greater adverse perturbations in LV systolic torsion and diastolic recoil than myocardial infarction without chronic IMR.[165] These abnormalities may be linked to more LV dilatation, which possibly reduces the effectiveness of fiber shortening on torsion generation. Altered LV torsion and recoil may contribute to the "ventricular disease" component of chronic IMR, with increased gradients of myocardial oxygen consumption adversely affecting cardiac efficiency and impaired early diastolic filling.[165] Additionally, in a subacute model of IMR (less than 7 weeks), there is an equivalent increase in LV end-diastolic volume in those with mild mitral regurgitation compared to those with more severe mitral regurgitation, coupled with unchanged end-diastolic and -systolic remodeling strains, including systolic circumferential, longitudinal, and radial strains; these findings in aggregate argue against an intracellular (cardiomyocyte) mechanism for the LV dysfunction.[166] Instead, differences in subepicardial shear strains suggest a causal role of altered interfiber interactions, and the mechanical impairment may be in extracellular matrix between the fibers and the microtubules in the cytoskeleton that couple cardiomyocyte shortening to LV wall thickening.[166]

Annular Geometry. In IMR, there may be increased mitral annular area, annular stretching (involving both anterior and posterior components of the annulus), increased septal-lateral annular dimension (also termed the *anteroposterior axis*), which is perpendicular to the line of leaflet coaptation), lateral displacement of posteromedial papillary muscle, and apically tethered posterior leaflet with restricted closing motion, all of which contribute to leaflet malcoaptation[152,153,156,157] (Fig. 40-11). The septal-lateral annular dilatation and diminished LV systolic function determine mitral systolic tenting area, which in turn is predictive of the severity of the IMR.[152] LV dilatation and larger annular dimensions after inferior myocardial infarction require the mitral leaflets to cover more area during closing, exceeding their normal redundancy or "reserve," which is exacerbated by restricted leaflet closure (type IIIb motion) owing to apical leaflet tenting. Additionally, the distinctive saddle shape of the normal annulus, which becomes accentuated during systole, is eliminated, suggesting an association between maintaining the saddle shape and valvular competence.[152,167–169] Furthermore, in patients with IMR, the anterior and posterior annular perimeters and annular orifice area (9.1 cm^2 compared with 5.7 cm^2 normally) are increased accompanied by an increase in the intertrigonal (anterior) annular distance and restriction of annular motion.[157]

Leaflet Motion and Morphology. Acute IMR from proximal left circumflex artery occlusion experimentally results in

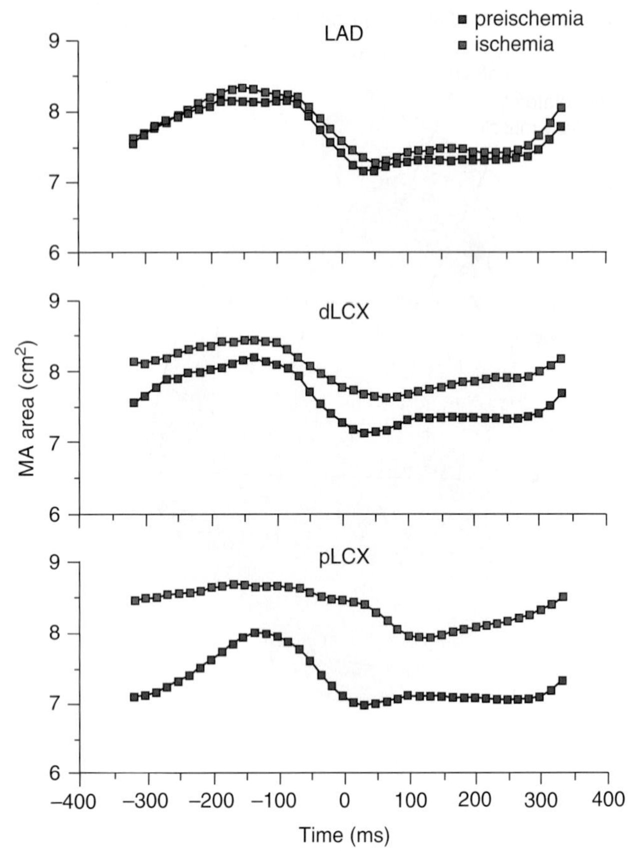

FIGURE 40-11 Average mitral annular area (in cm^2) before (*solid squares*) and during (*open circles*) acute LV ischemia induced by balloon occlusion of either the LAD artery (*top*), the dLCx coronary artery (*middle*), or the pLCx coronary artery (*bottom*). A 650-ms time interval centered at end-diastole (t = 0) is shown. dLCx = Distal to second obtuse marginal artery; LAD = proximal left anterior descending artery; MA = mitral annular; pLCx proximal to second obtuse marginal artery. (*Reproduced with permission from Timek TA et al: Ischemia in three left ventricular regions: insights into the pathogenesis of acute ischemic mitral regurgitation. J Thorac Cardiovasc Surg 2003; 125:559.*)

delayed valve closure in early systole (termed *leaflet loitering*) and increased leaflet edge separation throughout ejection in three leaflet coaptation sites across the valve, specifically near the anterior commissure, the valve center, and near the posterior commissure.[151,153] In addition, there is lateral displacement of the central scallop of the posterior leaflet, suggesting that interscallop malcoaptation, which is mechanistically owing to septal-lateral annular dilatation, can contribute to IMR in certain circumstances.[163] Clinically, chronic IMR is associated with apical systolic restriction of the posterior leaflet, thereby effectively preventing competent valve closure. Chronic IMR is also associated with posterior leaflet displacement in the posterior direction and lateral displacement of both leaflets. When the position of each leaflet edge is assessed independently, the anterior leaflet is not displaced apically after inferior infarction, although with more time and further remodeling, apical restriction of this leaflet may occur.[156] A strong echocardiographic determinant of leaflet tenting height is the distance from the tips of the papillary muscles to the saddle horn of the anterior annulus; LV end-diastolic volume is only weakly correlated with tenting height.[170] Recent startling human observations have revealed that in some patients with IMR/FMR, there is growth or elongation of the leaflets associated with leaflet thickening that compensates for the larger orifice area and minimizes the amount of mitral regurgitation. In others, however, the leaflets do not become larger and cannot coapt normally across the large orifice, which causes more leaks.[171]

Papillary Muscle and Chordal Relationships. The papillary-annular distances in the LV long axis remain relatively constant in normal hearts throughout the cardiac cycle.[144] During acute ischemia, however, these distances change, which reflects repositioning or dislocation of the papillary muscle tips with respect to the mitral annulus. This can also contribute to apical tenting of the leaflets during systole.[140,144,156,159] With proximal circumflex artery occlusion and resulting IMR in an ovine model, the interpapillary distance and LV end-diastolic volume both increase. There is also increased mitral annular area and displacement of both (but predominantly the posteromedial) papillary muscle tips away from the septal annulus throughout ejection and at end-systole.[156,159] Posteromedial papillary muscle tip displacement probably results from failure of the ischemic papillary muscle to shorten during systole, lengthening of the ischemic papillary muscle over time, and dyskinesia of the ischemic LV wall subtending the papillary muscle. Since posterior papillary muscle displacement in the apical and posterior directions also occurs in sheep that did not develop substantial degrees of IMR, the additional posteromedial papillary muscle displacement in the lateral direction is a dominant factor in the development of IMR.[156] In the setting of posterolateral ischemia, a larger distance from the papillary muscle tips to the midseptal annulus is an important determinant of mitral regurgitant jet area and volume.[150,156] The nonischemic anterolateral papillary muscle also may play a role in apical leaflet restriction because this papillary muscle is displaced apically at end-systole relative to baseline. In sheep with mitral regurgitation, posteromedial papillary muscle tethering distance, papillary muscle depth, and papillary muscle angle are unchanged, and the anterolateral papillary muscle depth and papillary muscle angle decrease with decreasing ejection fraction.[159] Reduced systolic shortening of either papillary muscle in isolation, on the other hand, does not result in mitral regurgitation; thus, the previous notion that papillary muscle dysfunction by itself is responsible for IMR is not correct. In fact, papillary muscle dysfunction paradoxically can decrease mitral regurgitation resulting from inferobasal ischemia by reducing leaflet tethering, which improves leaflet coaptation.[172] Further insult to the LV wall underlying the papillary muscles is likely needed before valvular incompetence occurs. Finally, acute IMR from experimental posterior LV ischemia is associated with chordal and leaflet tethering at the nonischemic commissural portion of the mitral valve and a paradoxical decrease of the chordal forces and relative prolapse at the ischemic commissural site.[160] Thus a combination of systolic annular dilatation and shape change and altered posteromedial (and possibly anterolateral) papillary muscle position and motion contributes to incomplete leaflet coaptation and IMR during acute inferior or posterolateral ischemia.

Papillary Muscle Ischemia. Papillary muscle dysfunction in patients with ischemic heart disease has been thought to contribute to mitral regurgitation, although the significance of its role in IMR remains in question.[64,66,67,85,86,144,156,159,172] The papillary muscles are particularly susceptible to ischemia, more so the posteromedial papillary muscle (supplied only by the posterior descending artery in 63% of cases) than the anterolateral papillary muscle (supplied by both the left anterior descending and the circumflex arteries in 71% of cases).[64,66,67] Hence, myocardial infarction leading to papillary muscle dysfunction occurs more frequently with the posteromedial papillary muscle after an inferior myocardial infarction. Although papillary muscle necrosis can complicate myocardial infarction, frank rupture of a papillary muscle is rare. Total papillary muscle rupture usually is fatal as a result of severe mitral regurgitation and LV pump failure; survival long enough to reach the operating room in reasonable condition is possible with rupture of one or two of the subheads of a papillary muscle, which is associated with a lesser degree of acute mitral regurgitation. Papillary muscle rupture usually occurs 2 to 7 days after myocardial infarction; without urgent surgery, approximately 50 to 75% of such patients may die within 24 hours.[173,174]

Myxomatous Degeneration

Myxomatous degeneration of the mitral valve, also known as *floppy mitral valve* or *mitral valve prolapse,* is the most common cause of mitral regurgitation in patients undergoing surgical evaluation in the United States.[64,175–178] The etiology of mitral valve prolapse is both acquired (*fibroelastic deficiency* in older patients) and congenital or heritable, with excess spongy, weak fibroelastic connective tissue constituting the leaflets and chordae tendineae (*Barlow's valve* in younger patients)[83,179–182] (Fig. 40-12). Frequently associated with connective tissue disorders, such as Marfan syndrome, Ehlers-Danlos and osteogenesis imperfecta, mitral valve prolapse at a young age can be sporadic or familial with autosomal dominant and X-linked inheritance.[182,183] Although three different loci on chromosomes 16, 11, and 13 (autosomal dominant) are linked to mitral valve prolapse, no specific gene has yet been incriminated.[182,183] Also, a locus on chromosome X cosegregates with a rare form of mitral valve prolapse called *X-linked myxomatous mitral valve dystrophy.*[183] Some degree of mitral valve prolapse is seen echocardiographically in 5 to 6% of the female population.[179,184] The risk of endocarditis is increased only if valvular regurgitation is present and accompanied by a murmur. Mitral valve prolapse appears to be more widespread in women, but severe mitral regurgitation resulting from mitral valve prolapse is more common in men. Subtle signs of heart failure, usually manifest as declining stamina and fatigue, may be the presenting complaint in 25 to 40% of symptomatic patients with mitral valve prolapse. As strictly defined originally by John Barlow, Barlow's syndrome includes prolapse of the posterior leaflet and chest pain, and occasionally palpitations, syncope, and dyspnea; in younger patients, the initial clinical sign is a midsystolic nonejection click, which later evolves into a click followed by a late systolic murmur.[179] This latter scenario is seen typically in young patients with Barlow's valves, in which large amounts of excessive leaflet tissue and marked annular dilatation are coupled with extensive hooding and billowing of both leaflets.

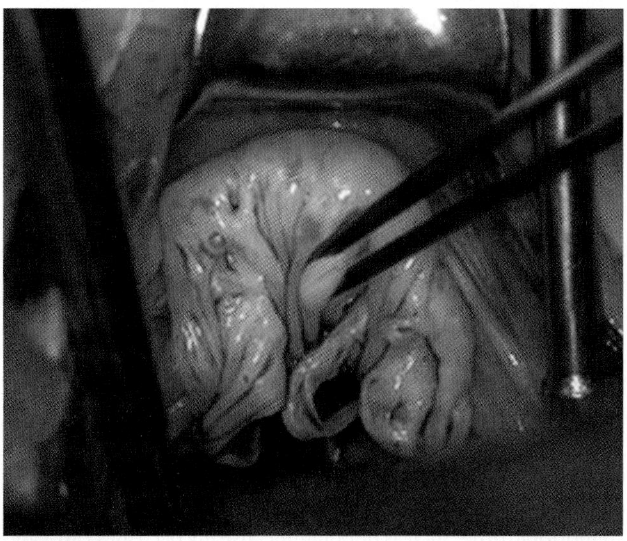

FIGURE 40-12 Intraoperative photograph of mitral regurgitation caused by a floppy mitral valve (Barlow's valve).

Pathologically, the atrial aspect of the prolapsing mitral leaflet often is thickened focally, whereas the changes on the ventricular surface of the leaflet consist of connective tissue thickening primarily on the interchordal segments with fibrous proliferation into adjacent chordae and onto the ventricular endocardium.[83,179,181] Histologically, elastic fiber and collagen fragmentation and disorganization are present, and acid mucopolysaccharide material accumulates in the leaflets. Myxomatous degeneration commonly involves the annulus, resulting in annular thickening and dilatation. All these changes are pronounced in young patients with Barlow's valves but can be minimal in older subjects with fibroelastic deficiency, in whom the noninvolved posterior leaflet scallops and anterior leaflet are normal and thin (termed *pellucid* by Carpentier). It is important to recognize that these two distinct varieties of mitral valve prolapse exist and can be segregated on clinical grounds, even if pathologists have difficulty discriminating between the two, because the repair techniques differ in major ways. The main visual and pathologic difference is the extent and degree of degenerative changes. Many centers like the Mayo Clinic encounter mainly elderly patients with coronary artery disease and fibroelastic deficiency (78% of their surgical "flail" leaflet surgical population were greater than 60 years old and/or required concomitant coronary artery bypass grafting), in whom the valvular pathology is limited, and simple repair techniques, such as the small McGoon triangular excision of the middle scallop of the posterior leaflet, are applicable and work well.[185] In contrast, other institutions attract younger patients who have Barlow's valves or severely myxomatous mitral valves, circumstances that demand much more extensive repair techniques and different expertise.

Only 5 to 10% of patients with mitral valve prolapse progress to develop severe mitral regurgitation, and they can surprisingly remain relatively asymptomatic until very late.[179,180] Mechanisms accounting for severe mitral regurgitation in those with mitral valve prolapse include annular dilatation and rupture or elongation of the first-order chordae (58%), annular dilatation without chordal rupture (19%), and chordal rupture without annular dilatation (19%).[181] Chordal rupture, probably related to defective collagen, underlying papillary muscle fibrosis or dysfunction, or bacterial endocarditis, typically is the culprit when mitral regurgitation develops acutely in patients without any previous symptoms of heart disease or suddenly becomes worse in those with known mitral valve prolapse.[64,66,83,85,86,137,186] Chordal rupture is typically found in older patients with prolapse owing to fibroelastic degeneration without much accompanying leaflet pathology. Chordal rupture is evident in 14 to 23% of surgically excised purely regurgitant valve specimens; in 73 to 93% of these patients, the underlying pathology is degenerative or floppy mitral valves.[85,86,137] Posterior chordal rupture, usually subtending just the middle scallop, is the most frequent finding, followed by anterior chordal rupture and then combined anterior and posterior chordal rupture.[85,86,137]

Rheumatic Disease

With decreasing incidence in the United States, rheumatic fever remains a common cause of mitral regurgitation in developing countries.[64,85–87,136–138,187] It is unknown why rheumatic fever leads to valvular stenosis in some patients and pure regurgitation in others. The pathoanatomical changes of the purely regurgitant rheumatic valve differ from those in a stenotic valve. In chronic rheumatic mitral regurgitation, the valves have diffuse fibrous thickening of the leaflets with minimal calcific deposits and relatively nonfused commissures; chordae tendineae usually are not extremely thickened or fused.[85–87] There also may be shortening of the chordae tendineae, fibrous infiltration of the papillary muscle, and asymmetric annular dilatation primarily in the posteromedial portion. During the first episodes of rheumatic fever (average age is 9 years), patients may develop acute mitral regurgitation, which is more frequently related to annular dilatation and prolapse of the anterior or posterior mitral valve leaflet.[87,187] Those with anterior leaflet prolapse tend to improve with medical management; however, those with prolapse of the posterior leaflet have a less favorable outcome and often require early surgical repair.[187]

Mitral Annular Calcification

Mitral annular calcification is a degenerative disorder that usually is confined to elderly individuals; most patients are older than 60 years of age, and women are affected more often than men.[64,90] The pathogenesis of mitral annular calcification is not known, but it appears to be a stress-induced phenomenon; annular calcification also can be associated with systemic hypertension, hypertrophic cardiomyopathy, aortic stenosis, and occasionally, advanced Barlow's disease. Other predisposing conditions include chronic renal failure and diabetes mellitus. Aortic valve calcification is an associated finding in 50% of patients with severe mitral annular calcification.

The gross appearance of mitral annular calcification may vary from small, localized calcified spicules to massive, rigid bars up to 2 cm in thickness in the annulus and leaflets.[90] Initially, calcification begins at the midportion of the posterior annulus; as the process progresses, the leaflets become upwardly deformed, stretching the chordae tendineae, and a rigid curved bar of calcium surrounding the entire posterior annulus in a horseshoe shape or even a complete ring of calcium may encircle the entire mitral orifice. The calcific deposit spurs extend into the LV myocardium and the conduction system, which can result in atrioventricular and/or intraventricular conduction defects. Annular calcification causes mitral regurgitation by displacing and immobilizing the mitral leaflets (thereby preventing their normal systolic coaptation) or impairing the presystolic sphincteric action of the annulus.[90] As the degree of mitral regurgitation worsens over time, LV volume overload can lead to heart failure. Systemic embolization can occur if the annular calcific debris is extensive and friable.

Hemodynamics

The pathophysiology of acute mitral regurgitation differs from that of chronic mitral regurgitation. Acute regurgitation may result from spontaneous chordal rupture, myocardial ischemia or infarction, infective endocarditis, or chest trauma.[64,66,173,174,186] The clinical impact of acute mitral incompetence is modulated largely by the compliance of the left atrium and the pulmonary vasculature. In a normal left atrium with a relatively low compliance, acute mitral regurgitation results in high LA pressure, which can lead rapidly to pulmonary edema. Such is not the situation in patients with chronic mitral regurgitation, in whom compensatory changes over time increase LA and pulmonary bed venous compliance so that symptoms of pulmonary congestion may not occur for many years.

With mitral regurgitation, the impedance to LV emptying is lowered because the mitral orifice is in parallel with the LV outflow tract.[64,97,188] The volume of mitral regurgitation depends on the square root of the systolic pressure gradient between the left ventricle and the atrium, the time duration of regurgitation, and the effective regurgitant orifice (ERO).[64,170,189,190] The ERO is determined echocardiographically using two-dimensional color Doppler imaging to measure the cross-sectional area of the vena contracta (narrowest width of the regurgitant jet) and the proximal isovelocity surface area (PISA), or continuous-wave Doppler measuring the ratio of regurgitant volume to regurgitant time-velocity integral.[170,191] Regurgitation into the left atrium increases LA pressure and reduces forward cardiac output. LA pressure even may remain elevated at end-diastole (transient 5- to 10-mm Hg transvalvular gradient), representing a functional gradient associated with the increased diastolic LV filling rate.

If the mitral annulus is not rigid, various diagnostic and therapeutic interventions can alter ERO. Altered loading conditions (elevated preload and afterload) and decreased contractility result in progressive LV dilatation and a larger ERO.[192] When LV size is reduced by medical management (eg, digoxin, diuretics, and most importantly, arteriolar vasodilators), ERO, and regurgitant volume fall.[193,194] Stress echocardiography using an inotropic drug, such as dobutamine, usually decreases ERO and the degree of mitral regurgitation in patients with FMR and IMR because the LV chamber is smaller at the beginning of systole (end-diastole) and throughout systole secondary to enhanced LV contractility.[195]

Ventricular Adaptation

The loading conditions induced by mitral regurgitation promote more LV ejection because ventricular preload is increased and afterload is normal or decreased secondary to backward flow across the mitral valve. In terms of cardiac energetics, reduced LV impedance in patients with mitral regurgitation allows a greater proportion of contractile energy to be expended in myocardial fiber shortening than in tension development.[64,188] Because increased fiber shortening is less of a determinant of myocardial oxygen consumption than other components, such as tension (or pressure) development and heart rate, mitral regurgitation causes only small increases in myocardial oxygen consumption.[188] Reduction in developed tension as a result of lower LV systolic wall stress (LV afterload) permits the ventricle to adapt to the substantial regurgitant volume by increasing LV end-diastolic volume to maintain adequate forward output. Along with lower afterload, this increase in preload (LV end-diastolic volume or, more precisely, LV end-diastolic wall stress) allows the heart to compensate for chronic mitral regurgitation for a long time before symptoms occur.[64,196,197] A fundamental response to increased preload is augmented stroke volume and stroke work, although effective forward stroke volume may be normal or subnormal. High LV preload eventually leads to LV dilatation and shape change, ie, more spherical remodeling, owing to replication of sarcomeres in series as a consequence of chronic elevation of LV end-diastolic wall stress.[196,197] This process is in contrast to LV hypertrophy secondary to chronic pressure overload (elevated systolic wall stress), which leads to sarcomere replication in parallel. In chronic mitral regurgitation, LV mass also increases; however, the degree of hypertrophy correlates with the amount of chamber dilatation so that the ratio of LV mass to end-diastolic volume remains in the normal range (unlike the situation in patients with LV pressure overload).[198–200] The contractile dysfunction that evolves due to chronic LV volume overload is accompanied by increased myocyte length as well as reduced myofibril content.[197,198] The basic changes thus are a combination of myofibrillar loss and the absence of significant hypertrophy in response to the progressive decrease in left ventricular pump function. The defect is intrinsic to the myocyte per se, but changes in the extracellular matrix also play a role.[166,201] Conversely, in acute mitral regurgitation, the ratio of LV mass to end-diastolic volume is reduced because chamber dilatation occurs suddenly, and the LV wall becomes acutely thinned; this increase in LV end-diastolic volume is associated with sarcomere lengthening along the length-tension curve.[197]

After the initial compensatory phase, LV systolic contractility becomes progressively impaired as mitral regurgitation progresses chronically.[199–202] Because of the low impedance during systole, however, ejection-phase indexes of LV systolic function, such as ejection fraction, stroke volume, and fractional circumferential fiber shortening (%FSc), still can be normal even if the contractility is severely depressed.[201,203,204] An ejection fraction of less than 55 to 60% or %FSc less than 28% in the presence of severe mitral regurgitation indicates an advanced degree of myocardial dysfunction. The ejection-phase indexes commonly used clinically to estimate LV pump performance, eg, ejection fraction, %FSc, cardiac output, stroke volume, stroke work, etc. are all affected by changes in LV preload and afterload.

Because of abnormal LV loading conditions in the setting of mitral regurgitation, load-independent indexes of LV contractility (eg, end-systolic elastance derived from the end-systolic pressure–volume relationship [ESPVR]) or preload recruitable stroke work (PRSW, also termed *linearized Frank-Starling relationship*) are preferred to measure LV systolic function and mechanics.[199,200,202,205,206] In hypertrophied and dilated hearts, as seen in chronic mitral regurgitation, however, the utility of end-systolic elastance may be limited because of LV chamber shape and size changes. It is necessary to use the end-systolic stress-volume relationship in these circumstances. One other problem inherent in the use of end-systolic elastance or stress-volume data is that end-systole and -ejection are dissociated in patients with mitral regurgitation. End-ejection is defined as minimum LV volume and end-systole as the instant when LV elastance reaches its maximal value. Because of this temporal dissociation of end-systole from minimal ventricular volume, end-ejection pressure–volume relations do not correlate with maximal elastance values derived using isochronal methods.[205] End-systolic dimension or LV end-systolic volume (LVESV) is less dependent on LV loading conditions than is ejection fraction, and therefore is a better measure of LV systolic contractile function. LVESV varies directly and linearly with afterload, and inversely with contractile state.[202,207–209] The larger the LVESV becomes, the worse LV contractility. Correcting LVESV for chamber geometry, wall thickness and afterload [ie, end-systolic wall stress (ESS)], and body size (LV end-systolic volume index [LVESVI]) provides good indexes of LV systolic function that are less influenced by loading conditions and variation in patient size.[207,208] Thus, preoperative LVESV or LVESVI is a better predictor of outcome in terms of postoperative LV systolic performance and cardiac death than is ejection fraction, end-diastolic volume, or end-diastolic pressure.[209]

Based on load-independent indexes of LV contractility in experimental mitral regurgitation, the normalized end-systolic pressure–volume and end-systolic stress-volume relationships decline after 3 months of mitral regurgitation.[199] PRSW (the relation of stroke work to LV end-diastolic volume) and preload-recruitable pressure–volume area (the relation of stroke work to LV pressure–volume area) also fall, along with a decrease in efficiency of energy transfer from pressure–volume area to external pressure–volume work at matched LV end-diastolic volume. Furthermore, there is deterioration in ventriculoarterial coupling over time; ie, a mismatch develops between the ventricle and the total (forward and regurgitant) vascular load.[199] Although the overall (systemic plus LA) effective arterial elastance is decreased, there is a proportionally greater reduction in LV end-systolic elastance. Thus, LV systolic mechanics become impaired along with deterioration in global LV energetics and efficiency, and a mismatch develops in coupling between the left ventricle and the arterial bed.[199] Additionally, progression from acute to chronic mitral regurgitation (at 3 months) is associated with a decrease in maximum

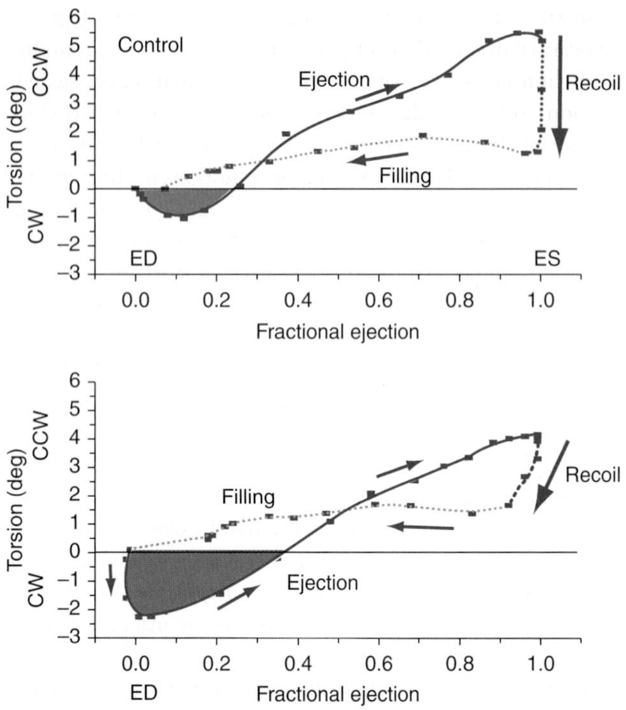

FIGURE 40-13 Torsional deformation versus fractional ejection with acute (*top*) and chronic (*bottom*) mitral regurgitation in a representative animal. With acute mitral regurgitation, systole (*solid line*) is characterized by a slight clockwise rotation followed by counterclockwise torsion that peaks at end-ejection. Early diastole (*dashed line*) shows steeper torsional recoil than middle to late diastole (*dotted line*). With chronic mitral regurgitation, the initial clockwise torsion is larger, the maximum positive torsion is decreased, and less recoil occurs during early diastole. (*Reproduced with permission from Tibayan FA, Yun KL, Fann JI, et al: Torsional dynamics in the evolution from acute to chronic mitral regurgitation. J Heart Valve Dis 2002; 11:39.*)

LV systolic torsional deformation from 6.3 to 4.7 degrees and a decrease in early diastolic LV recoil from +3.8 to −1.5 degrees[210] (Fig. 40-13). Because torsion is a mechanism by which the left ventricle equalizes transmural gradients of fiber strain and oxygen demand, a decrease in systolic torsion in chronic mitral regurgitation may play a role in the inexorable and progressive decline of LV performance.[210] The left ventricle responds to decreased forward cardiac output resulting from mitral regurgitation by dilating; such dilatation equalizes the lengths of the endocardial and epicardial radii and thereby decreases systolic LV torsion. In assessing transmural 3D myocardial deformations in an ovine model of isolated mitral regurgitation, early changes in LV function at 12 weeks was evidenced by alterations in transmural strain (which may be detected before the onset of global LV dysfunction), but not by changes in B-type natriuretic peptide or PRSW.[211] The associated increase in transmural gradient of fiber strain and oxygen supply–demand imbalance results in a further decrease in forward cardiac output, leading to more LV dilatation and continuing the vicious cycle.

Diastolic inflow into the ventricle must increase as total stroke volume increases during the evolution of mitral regurgitation and ventricular dilatation.[212–215] Acute mitral regurgitation enhances LV diastolic function by increasing the early diastolic filling rate and decreasing chamber stiffness. Flow across the mitral valve during early diastole is determined by the LA-LV pressure gradient, even though other factors, such as diastolic restoring forces and LV diastolic recoil (creating LV suction) during isovolumic relaxation also influence early LV filling.[212] In middle and late diastole, the lower LV chamber stiffness in patients with acute mitral regurgitation (evidenced by a shift of the LV diastolic pressure dimension or pressure–volume relationship to the right) allows the LV mean and LV end-diastolic pressures (and stresses) to remain in the normal range. In patients with chronic mitral regurgitation and preserved ejection fraction, LV chamber stiffness is also lower, similar to that during acute mitral regurgitation. Conversely, in those with impaired LV systolic function, chamber stiffness usually is normal.[214] In general, chronic mitral regurgitation causes a decrease in LV systolic contractile function but an increase in early diastolic function (as evidenced by an increase in early diastolic filling rate and a decrease in chamber stiffness).[215,216] The reduced chamber stiffness may be the result of altered ventricular geometry (more spherical or less eccentric shape); this shape change can exacerbate the degree of mitral regurgitation by distorting annular dimensions and dislocating the papillary muscles.[214,217] Although the LV chamber stiffness is less owing to the change in geometry, the LV myocardium may be stiffer as a result of myocyte hypertrophy and interstitial fibrosis.[214,215]

Regarding the impact of mitral regurgitation on right ventricular contractility, reduction in right ventricular systolic function is associated with a worse prognosis, emphasizing the adverse impact of pulmonary hypertension in this disease.[218] Patients with a right ventricular ejection fraction of less than 30% are at risk for a suboptimal outcome.

Atrial Adaptation

Regurgitant flow into the left atrium leads to progressive atrial enlargement, the degree of which does not correspond directly with the severity of mitral regurgitation.[101,188] Also, the LA *v* wave in mitral regurgitation does not correlate with LA volume. Compared with patients with mitral stenosis, LA size can be larger in patients with longstanding mitral regurgitation, but thrombus formation and systemic thromboembolization occur less frequently because of the absence of atrial stasis.[101,104] Atrial fibrillation occurs less often in those with mitral regurgitation than in individuals with mitral stenosis.[104]

LA compliance is an important component of the patient's overall hemodynamic status if mitral regurgitation is present.[64,186,188,219] With sudden development of mitral regurgitation from chordal rupture, papillary muscle infarction, or leaflet perforation, LA compliance is normal or reduced. The left atrium is not enlarged, but the mean LA pressure and *v* wave are high. Gradually, the left atrial myocardium becomes hypertrophied, proliferative changes develop in the pulmonary vasculature, and pulmonary vascular resistance rises. As the mitral regurgitation becomes chronic and more severe, the left atrium becomes markedly enlarged, atrial compliance is increased, the atrial wall is fibrotic, but LA pressure remains normal or only slightly elevated.[219] In this situation, pulmonary artery pressure and pulmonary vascular resistance usually are still in the normal range or are elevated only modestly.

Pulmonary Changes

Because chronic mitral regurgitation is associated with LA enlargement and only mild elevations in LA pressure, pronounced increases in pulmonary vascular resistance usually do not develop. In patients with acute mitral regurgitation with normal or reduced LA compliance, a sudden increase in LA pressure initially elevates pulmonary vascular resistance, and occasionally acute right-sided heart failure occurs.[64,186] Pulmonary edema is seen less frequently in patients with chronic mitral regurgitation than in those with mitral stenosis because elevated LA pressure is uncommon. In patients with IMR and heart failure, however, acute pulmonary edema is associated with the dynamic changes in IMR and the resulting increase in pulmonary vascular pressure.[220] Exercise-induced changes in ERO, tricuspid regurgitant pressure gradient (estimate of systolic pulmonary artery pressure), and LV ejection fraction are independently associated with the development of pulmonary edema.[220] From the standpoint of pulmonary parenchymal function and respiratory mechanics in patients with chronic mitral regurgitation, there is a decline in vital capacity, total lung capacity, forced expiratory volume, and maximal expiratory flow at 50% vital capacity.[74] These patients also may have a positive response to methacholine challenge; this bronchial hyperresponsiveness may result from increased vagal tone owing to longstanding pulmonary congestion.

Clinical Evaluation

Patients with mild to moderate mitral regurgitation may remain asymptomatic for many years as the left ventricle adapts to the increased workload and maintains normal forward cardiac output. Gradually, symptoms reflecting decreased cardiac output with physical activity and/or pulmonary congestion develop insidiously, such as weakness, fatigue, palpitations, and dyspnea on exertion. If right-sided heart failure appears late in the course of the disease, hepatomegaly, peripheral edema, and ascites occur and can be associated with rapid clinical deterioration.[106,221] Conversely, acute mitral regurgitation usually is associated with marked sudden pulmonary congestion and pulmonary edema. Patients with coronary artery disease can present with myocardial ischemia or infarction and associated mitral regurgitation. Acute papillary muscle rupture may clinically mimic the presentation of a patient with a postinfarction ventricular septal defect.[222]

On physical examination, the cardiac impulse in patients with mitral regurgitation is hyperdynamic and displaced laterally; the forcefulness of the apical impulse is indicative of the degree of LV enlargement. In patients with chronic mitral regurgitation, S_1 usually is diminished. S_2 may be single, closely split, normally split, or even widely split as a consequence of the reduced resistance to LV ejection; a common finding is a widely split S_2 that results from shortening of LV systole and early closure of the aortic valve.[223] An S_3 gallop may be appreciated from the increased transmitral diastolic flow rate during the rapid filling phase. The apical systolic murmur of mitral regurgitation can be blowing, moderately harsh, or even soft and usually radiates to the axilla and left or right sternal border and occasionally to the neck or the vertebral column.[223] The murmur is best appreciated in early systole in patients with FMR or IMR. With rupture of the posterior leaflet first-order chordae, the mitral regurgitation jet is directed superiorly and impinges on the atrial septum near the base of the aorta, which can produce a murmur heard best along the right sternal border and radiating to the neck.[223,224] In cases of ruptured anterior leaflet first-order chordae, the leakage is aimed laterally and toward the posterior LA wall; the murmur may be transmitted posteriorly. Although there is no correlation between the intensity of the systolic murmur and the hemodynamic severity of the mitral regurgitation, a holosystolic murmur is characteristic of more regurgitant flow.[223] In younger patients with Barlow's valves (severe bileaflet mitral billowing with prolapse), early in the disease process, a characteristic midsystolic click is heard, followed by a late systolic murmur; as the annulus and left ventricle dilate, the murmur over time becomes holosystolic, and the midsystolic click may become inaudible.

On chest radiography, cardiomegaly indicative of LV and LA enlargement is found commonly in patients with longstanding moderate to severe mitral regurgitation.[123] Acute mitral regurgitation often is not associated with an enlarged heart shadow. Chest x-ray findings of congested lung fields are less prominent in patients with mitral regurgitation than in those with mitral stenosis, but interstitial edema is seen frequently in individuals with acute mitral regurgitation and those with progressive LV failure secondary to chronic mitral regurgitation.

Changes on the electrocardiogram are not particularly useful and depend on the etiology, severity, and duration of the mitral regurgitation.[112,223] Atrial fibrillation can occur late in the natural history of the disease and usually causes sudden exacerbation of symptoms. In cases of chronic mitral regurgitation, LV volume overload leads to LA and LV dilatation, and eventually to LV hypertrophy. Electrocardiographic evidence of LV enlargement or hypertrophy occurs in half of patients, 15% have right ventricular hypertrophy owing to increased pulmonary vascular resistance, and 5% have combined left and right ventricular hypertrophy.[112] Ventricular arrhythmias may be noted on ambulatory ECG recording or event monitors, especially in patients with LV systolic dysfunction. In those with acute mitral regurgitation, LA and/or LV dilatation may not be evident, and the electrocardiogram may be normal or show only nonspecific findings, including sinus tachycardia or ST-T-wave alterations.[112] Findings of myocardial ischemia or infarction, more commonly noted in the inferior leads, may be present when acute mitral regurgitation is related to acute inferior myocardial infarction or myocardial ischemia; in these cases, first-degree AV block is a common coexisting finding.

In the majority of individuals with mitral valve prolapse, particularly those who are asymptomatic, the resting electrocardiogram is normal.[112,184] In symptomatic patients, a variety of ST-T-wave changes, including T-wave inversion and sometimes ST-segment depression, particularly in the inferior leads, can be found.[179,184] QTc prolongation also may be seen. Arrhythmias may be observed on ambulatory electrocardiograms, including premature atrial contractions, supraventricular tachycardia, AV block, bradyarrhythmias, and premature ventricular contractions.[184] Atrial arrhythmias may be present in upward of 14% of patients, and ventricular arrhythmias are present in 30% of patients.[112,184]

Transthoracic echocardiography (TTE) is the diagnostic mainstay in patients with valvular heart disease. In those with chronic mitral regurgitation, this modality is used to follow the progression of LA and LV dilatation and changes in the amount of mitral regurgitation and leaflet morphology.[7,64,116,191,225–227] Echocardiography identifies abnormalities in leaflet and chordal morphology and function, including myxomatous degeneration with or without leaflet prolapse, restricted systolic leaflet motion (as in IMR) or diastolic opening motion (as in rheumatic valve disease), lack of adequate coaptation due to annular dilatation or rheumatic valvulitis (fused subvalvular apparatus), and leaflet destruction by endocarditis[7,64,113,116,191,227] (Fig. 40-14). The degree of mitral regurgitation is assessed using 2D color Doppler echocardiography, which permits visualization of the origin, extent, direction, duration, and velocity of disturbed backward flow of the regurgitant leak.[113,191,227] Chordal rupture or elongation causing a flail leaflet is characterized by excessive motion of the leaflet tip backward into the left atrium beyond the normal leaflet coaptation zone. Papillary muscle rupture after myocardial infarction and annular dilatation can be visualized (Fig. 40-15). In patients with IMR or FMR, apical systolic tethering of the leaflets, tenting area and height, and leaflet opening angles can be quantitated using echocardiography, including important pathoanatomic differences between ischemic cardiomyopathy and idiopathic dilated cardiomyopathy[170,189,191,228] (Fig. 40-16). When the regurgitant leak is caused in part or totally by annular dilatation, usually in the septal-lateral dimension, the coaptation height of the anterior and posterior leaflets can be measured.

In mitral regurgitation, ERO and regurgitant volume can be estimated quantitatively in many but not all patients using 2D color Doppler echocardiography.[170,190,191] ERO was an important predictor of outcome in a sample of Mayo Clinic patients with mitral regurgitation and has been proposed as an indicator of when to proceed with mitral repair in asymptomatic patients with prolapse.[190] However, accurate quantification of the degree of mitral regurgitation using ERO and regurgitant volume is demanding, time consuming, and may not be available at all institutions. The hemodynamic magnitude or severity of the mitral regurgitation also can be estimated semiquantitatively by calculating mitral and aortic stroke volumes, with regurgitant volume being the difference between these two stroke volumes. Cardiac MRI is an accurate method to measure regurgitant volume and regurgitant fraction by comparing right- with left-sided flow.[121,229,230]

Interest in the timing of the regurgitant leak has helped clinicians discern subtle details about the mechanism(s) responsible for the mitral regurgitation, infer information about the overall hemodynamic burden imposed by the LV volume overload, and predict the likelihood of successful and durable mitral repair.[170,189–191,228] IMR is primarily an early-systolic leak, FMR occurs during early and middle systole (can be a biphasic pattern), and prolapse is associated with late-systolic leaks. Although detected by pulse- and continuous-wave Doppler

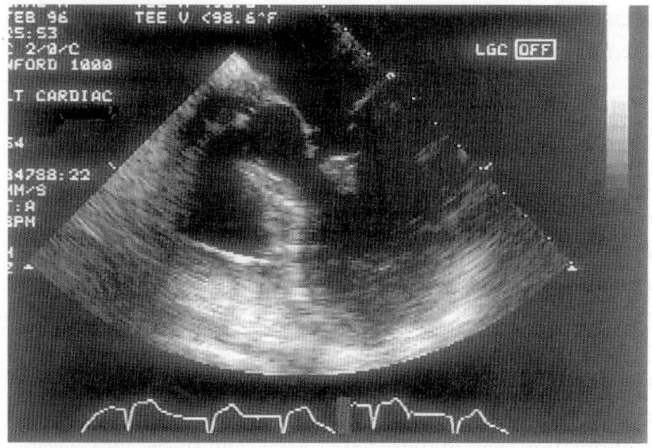

FIGURE 40-15 Echocardiogram (two-chamber view) of a patient with mitral regurgitation from ruptured papillary muscle.

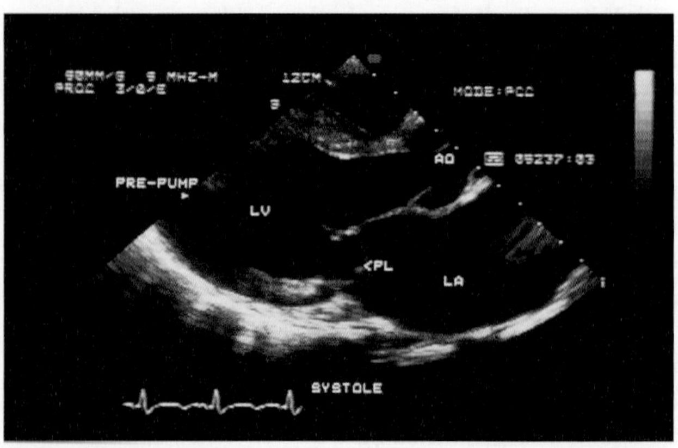

FIGURE 40-14 Echocardiogram (long-axis) of a patient with mitral regurgitation resulting from floppy mitral valve. The leaflets billow back into the left atrium during systole.

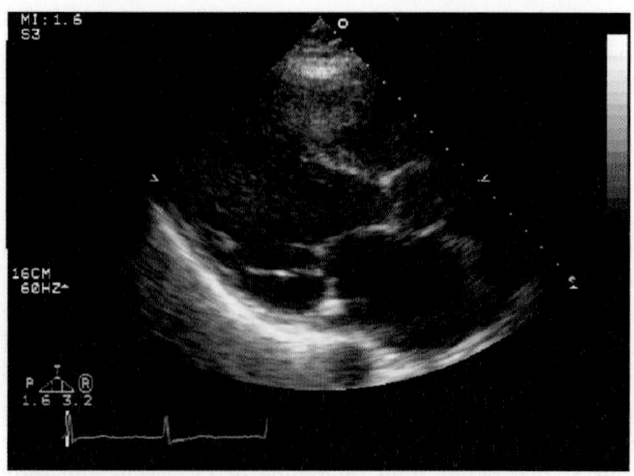

FIGURE 40-16 Echocardiogram of a patient with ischemic mitral regurgitation and apical systolic leaflet tenting.

echocardiography for years, the timing of the mitral regurgitation has become more widely appreciated as a result of a resurgence of interest in color Doppler M-mode echocardiography, which has a much faster temporal resolution (sampling frequency) than does 2D color Doppler echocardiography. Cardiac surgeons should study these color Doppler M-mode images carefully because the timing of the regurgitant leak yields important information about the mechanisms responsible for the MR.

TTE is usually adequate to learn all that is necessary, but if high-quality TTE images cannot be obtained because of the patient's habitus or advanced emphysema, transesophageal echocardiography (TEE) provides superior image quality and can reveal additional anatomical and pathophysiologic information, including details of the valvular pathoanatomy and the mechanism, origin, direction, timing, and severity of the regurgitant leak.[7,64,116,191,226,227,231] TEE can detect small mitral vegetations, ruptured chordae, leaflet perforations or clefts, calcification, and other inflammatory changes and can be useful in patients with annular or leaflet calcification. TEE also is useful in patients with a previously implanted aortic valve prosthesis that can interfere with TTE assessment of mitral regurgitation owing to acoustic shadowing. Although intraoperative TEE during mitral valve repair is essential, a major limitation must always be remembered. The vascular unloading effects (vasodilatation) of general anesthesia downgrade the severity of mitral regurgitation.[232,233] The judgment about how much mitral regurgitation is present must be made on the basis of an awake TTE study when the patient has a normal ambulatory blood pressure. This concept is imperative in assessing the degree of mitral regurgitation in patients with IMR when deciding whether to add a mitral valve procedure at the time of coronary artery bypass grafting. For patients in whom the degree of mitral regurgitation has been minimized by the effects of anesthesia, intraoperative TEE provocative testing using vasoconstrictor drugs with or without volume infusion is mandatory to guide surgical decision making. Testing consists of reproducing the patient's normal awake or active ambulatory hemodynamic condition with preload challenge and afterload augmentation.[232,233] Preload challenge is performed after aortic cannulation for cardiopulmonary bypass by rapidly infusing volume from the pump until the pulmonary capillary wedge pressure reaches 15 to 18 mm Hg. If severe mitral regurgitation is not produced, LV afterload is increased by intravenous boluses of phenylephrine until the arterial systolic pressure climbs to the 130- to 150-mm Hg range. In patients undergoing coronary artery bypass grafting, if both tests are negative, or regurgitation is induced but associated with new regional LV systolic wall motion abnormalities (ie, the regurgitation is caused by acute ischemia of viable myocardium), the valve may not require visual inspection because coronary revascularization usually is all that is necessary if the inferior wall myocardium is viable. If these tests confirm the presence of moderate to severe mitral regurgitation, the valve is inspected and usually is repaired at the time of coronary revascularization.

Real-time 3D echocardiography is helpful in the visual assessment of congenital and acquired valvular disease[7,116,118,228,234,235] (Fig. 40-17). In patients with mitral regurgitation, this modality is fairly accurate in elucidating the dynamic mechanisms of the regurgitant leak(s). The addition of color-flow Doppler to 3D imaging provides improved visualization and may offer improved quantitative assessment of regurgitant valvular lesions.[7,116,118] Additionally, 3D echocardiography may provide more insight into the geometric deformities of the mitral leaflets and annulus, maximum tenting site of the mitral leaflet, and quantitative measurements of mitral valve tenting and annular deformity in patients with IMR.[7,116,118,228,235] Real-time 3D color Doppler echocardiographic imaging provides direct measurement of vena contracta area.[7,234] The quantification of mitral regurgitant flow directly at the lesion using color Doppler echocardiography, however, has been prevented because of multiple aliasing from high flow velocities. De-aliasing of color Doppler flow at the vena contracta is feasible and appears promising for measuring severity of mitral regurgitation. This novel approach can be readily implemented in current systems to provide regurgitant flow volume and regurgitant fraction.[7,234]

Cardiac catheterization and coronary angiography are rarely needed in patients with mitral regurgitation when it is prudent to determine coronary artery anatomy in older patients with prolapse before repair and those with IMR.[64,111,196] Other techniques, such as calculating mitral regurgitant fraction (regurgitant volume determined as the difference between total LV angiographic stroke volume and the effective forward stroke volume measured by the Fick method), are limited. By measuring rest and exercise (supine bicycle) pulmonary artery pressures and cardiac output, right-sided heart catheterization can be useful occasionally to identify patients with primary myocardial disease who present with LV dilatation and relatively mild degrees of mitral regurgitation (who may not have a high likelihood of benefiting from mitral valve surgery) and those with severe mitral regurgitation who deny symptoms to see if they develop pulmonary hypertension with exercise.

Cardiac MRI can be employed to assess the cardiovascular system, including cardiac structure and function.[120,121,229,236,230] Specialized MRI techniques, such as moving-slice velocity mapping, the control-volume method, planimetry, or real-time color-flow MRI have been used to evaluate and quantify the degree of mitral regurgitation. The presence of valvular regurgitation can be determined, LV volumes and mitral regurgitant fraction estimated, and information obtained concerning mitral and coronary anatomy. Direct measurement by MRI is a promising method for assessment of the severity of mitral regurgitation; MRI planimetry of the anatomical mitral regurgitant lesion permits quantification of regurgitation with good agreement with cardiac catheterization and echocardiography.[230] Constraints of MRI, such as pacemakers or implanted defibrillators, morbid obesity, and claustrophobia, hamper the wider use of cardiac MRI. Multidetector CT has emerged as an imaging technique that can fully evaluate both cardiac structure and function, including coronary artery anatomy; this technology has yielded good visualization of valve leaflets, commissures, and mitral annulus.[122] Limitations still include image noise, requirement for a regular rhythm and a slow heart rate during imaging, time required for postprocessing data analysis, and radiation dose.

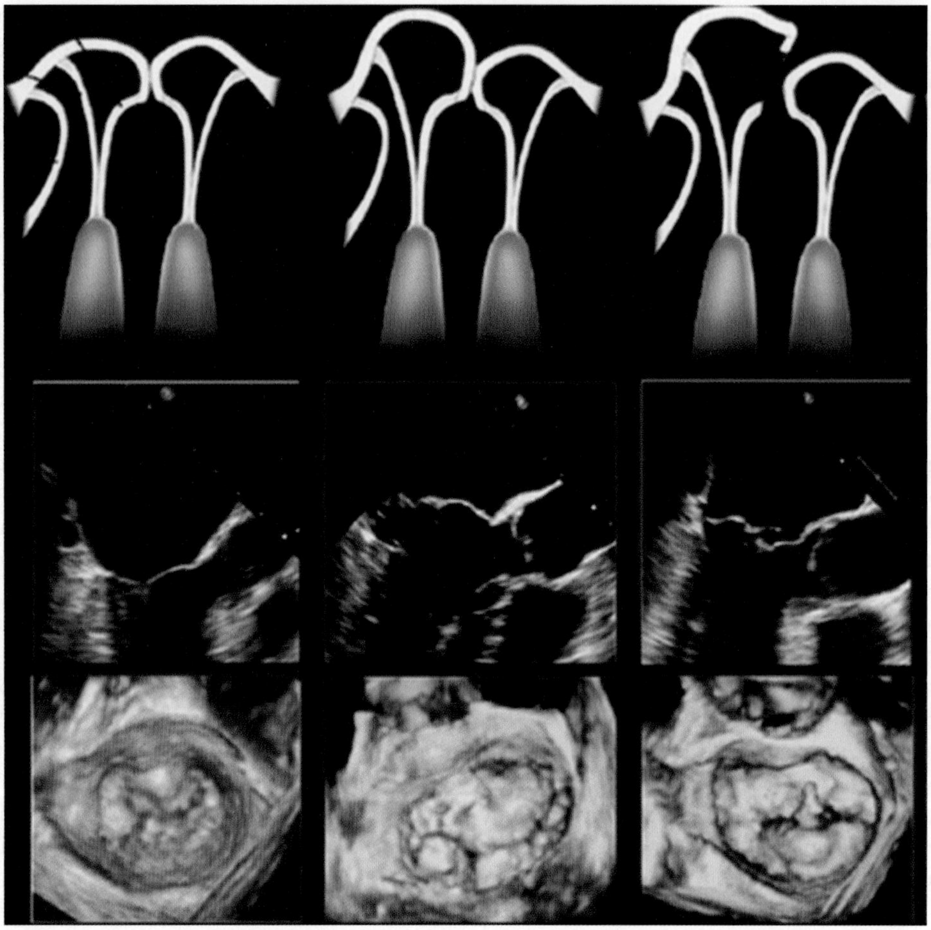

FIGURE 40-17 Intraoperative two-dimensional and three-dimensional transesophageal echocardiographic depiction of mitral valve prolapse and leaflet flail. Schematic (*upper row*) and two-dimensional and three-dimensional echocardiographic images of a patient with normal mitral valve (*left panels*), mitral valve prolapse (P1, *middle panels*), and a flail mitral valve (P2, *right panels*) as visualized with two-dimensional transesophageal echocardiography: long-axis mid-esophageal views (*middle row*) and real-time three-dimensional transesophageal echocardiographic volume rendering from the left atrial perspective (*bottom row*). (*Reproduced with permission from O'Gara P, Sugeng L, Lang R, et al: The role of imaging in chronic degenerative mitral regurgitation. J Am Coll Cardiol Img 2008; 1:221.*)

Postoperative LV Function and Surgical Outcomes

General

Successful mitral valve repair or replacement usually is associated with clinical improvement, augmented forward stroke volume with lower total stroke volume, smaller LV end-diastolic volume, and regression of LV hypertrophy.[177,127,238–243] Correction of mitral regurgitation can preserve LV contractility, particularly in patients with a normal preoperative ejection fraction who have minimal ventricular dilatation and those without significant coronary artery disease. On the other hand, in patients with LV dysfunction preoperatively, improvement in LV systolic function may not necessarily occur after operation.[209,237] An LVESVI exceeding 30 mL/m^2 is associated with decreased postoperative LV function.[209,237] Thus, patients with chronic mitral regurgitation should be referred for mitral valve surgery before LVESVI exceeds 40 to 50 mL/m^2 or when LV end-systolic dimension reaches 4 cm, consistent with the 2006 American College of Cardiology/American Heart Association (ACC/AHA) practice guidelines (Fig. 40-18).[209,238] LVESVI corrected for LV wall stress, a single-point ratio of end-systolic wall stress to end-systolic volume index (or ESS:LVESVI) is a good index of LV systolic function and accurately predicts surgical outcome in patients with mitral regurgitation.[207,208] Specifically, an ESS:LVESVI ratio of less than 2.6 portends a poor medium-term prognosis, whereas a normal or high ESS:LVESVI ratio is associated with a favorable outcome.[208] Significant determinants of increased operative risk also include older age, higher New York Heart Association (NYHA) functional class, associated coronary artery disease, increased LV end-diastolic pressure, elevated LV end-diastolic volume index, elevated LV end-systolic dimension, reduced LV ESS index, depressed resting ejection fraction, decreased fractional shortening, reduced cardiac index, elevated capillary wedge or right ventricular end-diastolic pressure, concomitant operative procedures, and previous cardiac surgery.[209,237,238,244–247] The abnormal LV diastolic properties (including early diastolic filling rate, myocardial relaxation,

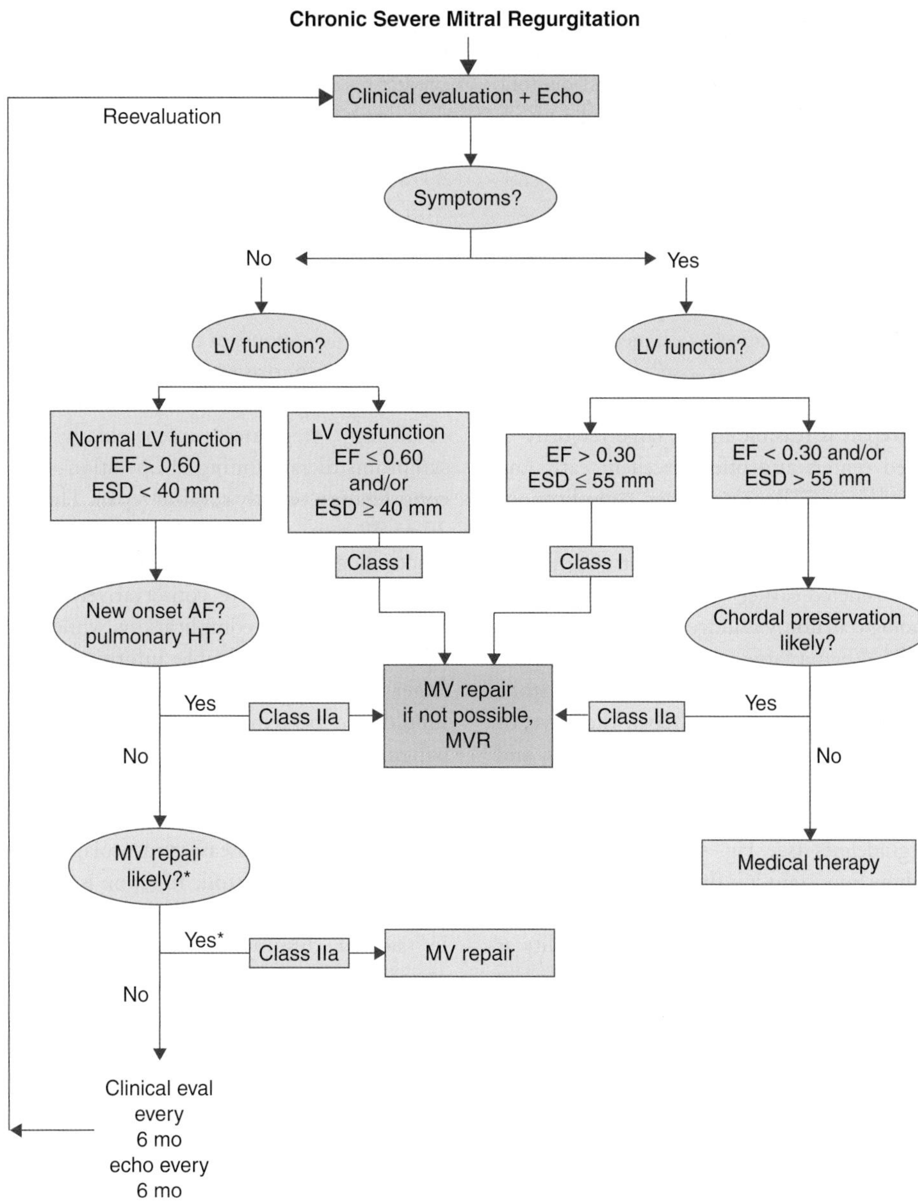

FIGURE 40-18 Management strategy for patients with chronic severe mitral regurgitation. *Mitral valve repair may be performed in asymptomatic patients with normal left ventricular function if performed by an experienced surgical team and if the likelihood of successful repair is greater than 90%. AF = atrial fibrillation; EF = ejection fraction; ESD = end-systolic dimension; eval = evaluation; HT = hypertension; LV = left ventricular; MV = mitral valve; MVR = mitral valve replacement. (*Reproduced with permission from Bonow RO et al: ACC/AHA 2006 guidelines for the management of patients with valvular heart disease. J Am Coll Cardiol 2006; 48:e1.*)

chamber stiffness, myocardial stiffness, and end-diastolic pressure) also may be reversible after mitral valve surgery.[215] If surgical correction of mitral regurgitation is carried out before the volume-overload cardiomyopathy reaches an irreversible stage, LV diastolic filling characteristics and systolic contractile function return toward normal values. Furthermore, LV volume and the LV volume:mass ratio (or dimension:thickness ratio) usually normalize postoperatively, but mild LV hypertrophy may persist.[215]

The decline in ejection fraction after mitral valve replacement for chronic mitral regurgitation historically was thought to result from an increase in LV afterload as a result of closure of the low-resistance early-systolic "pop-off" into the left atrium and the surgical excision of the subvalvular apparatus. A spherical mathematical model defining the relations among LV end-diastolic dimension, systolic wall stress, and ejection fraction, demonstrated that postoperative changes in systolic stress are related directly to changes in chamber size, and LV afterload may *decrease* postoperatively if chordal-preservation valve replacement techniques are used.[248] In terms of exercise performance after surgery for nonischemic mitral regurgitation, although patients generally report symptomatic improvement, cardiopulmonary exercise testing at 7 months is not better than preoperatively, and abnormal neurohumoral activation persists, probably reflective of incomplete recovery of LV contractility.[249] Regarding long-term clinical outcome, risk factors portending postoperative cardiac deterioration include larger LV end-diastolic dimension, increased LV end-systolic dimension, increased LVESV, diminished fractional shortening, reduced LV ESS index, large LA size, decreased LV wall thickness/cavity dimension at end-systole, and associated coronary artery disease.[209,246,250–252]

Patients with mitral regurgitation from a flail leaflet usually are asymptomatic, yet this entity is associated with a risk of progressive LV dysfunction and a suboptimal prognosis if not treated surgically. If managed conservatively with medical therapy, mitral regurgitation from a flail leaflet is associated with high annual mortality risk (6.3%) and morbidity rates.[178,253] In these patients, mitral valve repair is feasible in the large majority of patients in experienced centers and offers excellent early and late functional results.[177,254,255] Because fewer complications and lower operative mortality risk are associated with valve repair compared with valve replacement in this patient population, operation should be considered earlier in the natural history of the disease if the pathologic anatomy is judged favorable for valve repair.[141,177,178,250,253,254] When a large preoperative LVESVI or end-systolic dimension indicates the presence of LV systolic dysfunction, every effort should be made to repair the valve, or at least preserve all chordae tendineae (to both the anterior and posterior leaflets) if valve replacement is necessary.[238] Importantly, these surgical technical details have been emphasized in the 2006 ACC/AHA practice guidelines (see Fig. 40-16). Furthermore, these guidelines state how important it is that patients be referred to surgical centers that have demonstrated track records of excellence for mitral repair, including long-term repair durability as assessed by serial echocardiography.[238]

In a Mayo Clinic study focusing on the management of asymptomatic patients with organic mitral regurgitation, 456 asymptomatic patients with at least mild holosystolic mitral regurgitation defined echocardiographically were enrolled prospectively from 1991 to 2000.[190] At entry, baseline ejection fraction was 70%, LV end-systolic dimension was 3.4 ± 6 cm, LV end-diastolic dimension was 5.6 ± 8 cm, LVESVI was 33 ± 130 mL/m^2, and regurgitant volume was 66 ± 40 mL/beat. Management was at the discretion of the primary physician, including when to proceed to surgical intervention. At 5 years, 54% of patients had been operated on after an average of 1.2 ± 2 years of medical treatment when symptoms occurred or when worrisome echocardiographic findings were detected (based on the older 1998 ACC/AHA practice guidelines). Among the 230 patients who underwent a mitral valve procedure, 91% received a valve repair; the operative mortality rate was low at 1%. The patients were stratified by degree of regurgitation; mild, moderate, and severe were defined as regurgitant volumes of less than 30, 30 to 59, and 60 or more mL/beat, and ERO was defined as less than 20, 20 to 39, and 40 or greater mm^2, respectively. For the medically treated patients, 5-year survival compared with U.S. Census life tables was significantly inferior for those with moderate regurgitation (ERO of 20 to 39 mm^2, 66% versus 84%) and severe regurgitation (ERO of 40 mm^2 or more, 58% versus 78%).[190] Independent risk factors for death in the medically treated patients were advancing age, diabetes mellitus, and larger ERO. Even when adjusted for age, gender, diabetes, atrial fibrillation, and ejection fraction, ERO still predicted survival. The influence of ERO also held true for predicting cardiac deaths and all cardiac events. The 5-year cardiac death rate was 36% for patients with an ERO of 40 mm^2 or greater compared with 20% for those with an ERO of 20 to 39 mm^2 and only 3% for those with an ERO of less than 20 mm^2. Mitral valve operation was an independent determinant of fewer deaths, cardiac deaths, and cardiac events, especially in those with a larger ERO.[190] This important study, which focuses on the predictive effects of the severity of the regurgitation instead of the response of the ventricle, has prompted a rethinking in the approach to asymptomatic patients with mitral regurgitation owing to prolapse. All asymptomatic patients with an ERO of 40 mm^2 or greater—except elderly people, in whom only symptoms dictate timing of operation—should be referred for consideration of early surgical repair. Those with an ERO in the 20 to 39 mm^2 range should be monitored closely using serial echocardiography. Finally, those with the smallest ERO (<20 mm^2) can be followed more conservatively and are at low risk of developing cardiac complications while being managed medically. Despite the valuable information in this study, future larger prospective trials are necessary to validate these results; it should also be remembered that most of these Mayo Clinic patients were older and their prolapse was caused by fibroelastic degeneration, not younger individuals with Barlow's valves. Further, the critical ERO threshold for mitral regurgitation from degenerative disease and prolapse (40 mm^2) in patients with preserved LV systolic function is twice the 20 mm^2 critical value of ERO that predicts an adverse outcome in patients with LV systolic dysfunction and IMR or FMR.[170,189] In other words, it only takes a regurgitant orifice one-half as large to portend an unfavorable outcome if one has impaired LV systolic function owing to ischemic or idiopathic cardiomyopathy.

Because many patients with substantial mitral regurgitation report no symptoms, and symptoms have been the mainstay of when to consider surgical repair, cardiopulmonary exercise testing has been used to evaluate asymptomatic patients with organic mitral regurgitation (owing to prolapse in 93% of cases).[256] Of 134 asymptomatic patients with an average ejection fraction of 73%, 57% had severe mitral regurgitation with a regurgitant volume of 68 ± 24 mL/beat (range of 30 to 146 mL/beat) and an ERO of 35 ± 14 mm^2 (range 14 to 83 mm^2). Surprisingly, functional capacity was markedly reduced (defined as 84% or less than expected) in 19% of these "asymptomatic" patients. Those with impaired functional capacity were roughly equally distributed according to regurgitant volume of less than or greater than 60 mL/beat and ERO of less than or greater than 40 mm^2. When patients with extraneous reasons for impaired functional capacity were excluded, 14% had a reduced functional capacity, and their regurgitant volume and ERO were larger than those with a normal functional capacity. Determinants of reduced functional capacity were impaired LV diastolic function, lower forward stroke volume, and atrial fibrillation; ERO had no significant influence on functional capacity.[257] Thus, it was the consequences of chronic mitral regurgitation and not the magnitude of the leak that predicted impaired functional capacity. Follow-up at over 2 years revealed that 66% of patients with impaired functional capacity sustained some adverse event or required mitral surgery (versus 29% of those with normal functional capacity) after adjusting for age, ERO, gender, and ejection fraction. Thus, the evidence supports that asymptomatic patients with substantial mitral regurgitation should undergo periodic cardiopulmonary exercise testing to detect subclinical impairment in functional capacity, and that mitral valve repair should be recommended to those with impaired capacity.

Even after mitral valve surgery for chronic mitral regurgitation, some patients continue to be limited by heart failure symptoms and have suboptimal long-term postoperative outcomes. The incidence of congestive heart failure in patients who survive surgery (combined series of valve repair and valve replacement) for pure mitral regurgitation has been 23%, 33%, and 37% at 5, 10, and 14 years.[258] Valve repair is not a predictor of decreased incidence of congestive heart failure; however, using a combined end point of congestive heart failure and death, valve repair compared with valve replacement in patients with mitral regurgitation appears to confer a survival advantage. Patient survival after the first episode of congestive heart failure is dismal, being only 44% at 5 years. Causes of congestive heart failure include LV dysfunction in two-thirds of patients and valvular problems in the remaining one-third. Predictors of postoperative heart failure are lower preoperative ejection fraction, coronary artery disease, and higher NYHA functional class.[258] Importantly, preoperative functional class III/IV symptoms are associated with markedly decreased postoperative medium- and long-term survival independent of all other baseline characteristics.[259]

Ischemic Mitral Regurgitation

To risk stratify patients after myocardial infarction, detecting and quantifying IMR are essential.[189,260–262] In a report from the Mayo Clinic, medically managed patients who developed IMR late after myocardial infarction had a very high mortality rate (62% at 5 years) compared with those with an infarction who did not develop IMR (39% at 5 years).[189] Medium-term survival for patients with IMR and LV systolic dysfunction was inversely related to the ERO and regurgitant volume. After 5 years, the survival rate was 47% for patients with an ERO of less than 20 mm^2 and 29% for those with an ERO of 20 mm^2 or greater. Survival at 5 years was 35% when the regurgitant volume was 30 mL/beat or greater compared with 44% for those with a regurgitant volume of less than 30 mL/beat. The relative risk ratio for cardiac death for patients with IMR was 1.56 for patients with an ERO of less than 20 mm^2 versus 2.38 for those with an ERO of greater than 20 mm^2. It must be remembered this ERO threshold was twice as large (40 mm^2 or greater) in patients with prolapse or flail leaflets.[190] An ERO of more than 40 mm^2 was considered to reflect severe regurgitation in either disease, but the compound injury of coexisting LV dysfunction made the prognostic impact of even a "mild" leak (ERO of about 20 mm^2) very strong in patients with IMR.[262] In patients with myocardial infarction, the incidences of congestive heart failure or cardiac death were high even in patients with no or minimal symptoms at baseline and even higher in patients with IMR.[261] Determinants of congestive heart failure were ejection fraction, sodium plasma level, and presence and degree of IMR. At 5 years, the rate of congestive heart failure was 18% without IMR compared with 53% if IMR was present. If the ERO was less than 20 mm^2, the incidence of congestive heart failure was 46% compared with 68% when the ERO was 20 mm^2 or greater. The relative risk of congestive heart failure was 3.65 if IMR was present but 4.42 if ERO was 20 mm^2 or greater. At 5 years, the rate of congestive heart failure or cardiac death was 52%; the relative risk of congestive heart failure or cardiac death was 2.97 if IMR was present and 4.4 if ERO was 20 mm^2 or greater[261] (Fig. 40-19). Moderate or severe IMR was associated with a relative risk of 3.44 for congestive heart failure and 1.55 for death among 30-day survivors independent of age, gender, ejection fraction, and Killip class.[260]

Mitral repair or replacement for patients with IMR has been associated with higher operative risk (4 to 30%) than for patients with nonischemic chronic mitral regurgitation, which reflects the concomitant adverse consequences of previous myocardial infarction and ischemia.[241,242,263–268] Most investigators believe that coronary revascularization alone in the setting of moderate or severe IMR leaves many patients (up to 40%) with significant residual mitral regurgitation and heart failure symptoms.[143,269–271] Immediately postoperatively, IMR is absent or mild in 73% and severe in 6%; on the other hand, by 6 weeks, only 40% of patients have absent or mild mitral regurgitation, and 22% have severe mitral regurgitation[270] (Fig. 40-20). Postoperative residual or recurrent IMR is not associated with the preoperative extent of coronary artery disease or LV dysfunction. The 5-year survival rate of patients without IMR undergoing isolated coronary artery bypass grafting is 85% compared with 73% for patients with moderate IMR.[270] Because moderate IMR does not reliably resolve with bypass grafting alone, valve repair (or even chordal-sparing valve replacement) should

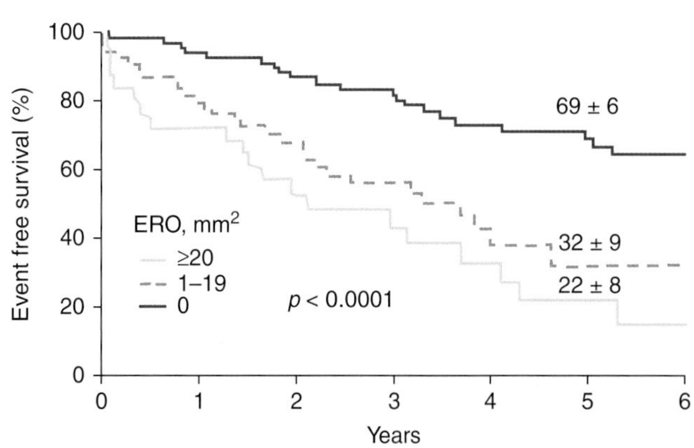

FIGURE 40-19 Survival free of congestive heart failure or cardiac death (event-free survival) in asymptomatic patients after myocardial infarction according to degree of ischemic mitral regurgitation measured by effective regurgitant orifice (ERO) of 20 mm^2 or more (*green line*), 1 to 19 mm^2 (*dashed red line*), and no mitral regurgitation (ERO = 0) (*blue line*) at diagnosis. The events at 5 years are indicated ± standard error. (*Reproduced with permission from Grigioni F et al: Contribution of ischemic mitral regurgitation to congestive heart failure after myocardial infarction. J Am Coll Cardiol 2005; 45:260.*)

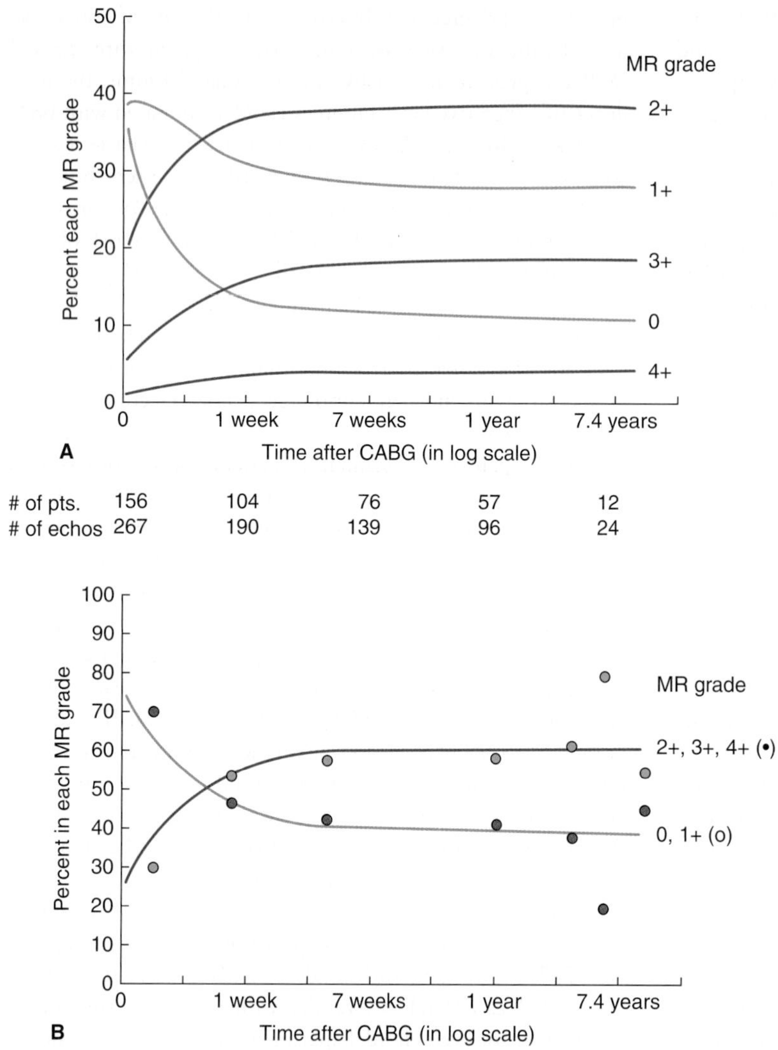

FIGURE 40-20 Course of mitral regurgitation after isolated coronary revascularization. Horizontal axis is time after coronary artery bypass grafting on a logarithmic scale. 1+ is mild regurgitation, 2+ moderate, 3+ moderately severe, and 4+ severe. (A) All grades of mitral regurgitation. (B) Mitral regurgitation grades 0 or 1+ compared with 2+, 3+, or 4+. Symbols (*open circles, solid circles*) represent aggregated raw echocardiographic values for mitral regurgitation grade. CABG = Coronary artery bypass grafting; MR = mitral regurgitation. (*Reproduced with permission from Lam BK et al: Importance of moderate ischemic mitral regurgitation. Ann Thorac Surg 2005; 79:462.*)

be considered in these patients because it potentially can reduce cardiac morbidity and may improve long-term survival.[143,269–270] Others argue that patients with moderate IMR undergoing coronary revascularization and concomitant mitral annuloplasty have less postoperative IMR but no improvement in long-term survival.[155,264,266,272,273] The Yale group postulated that isolated coronary grafting without valve repair is adequate in most patients with ischemic cardiomyopathy and mild to moderate mitral regurgitation, yielding survival rates of 88% at 1 year and 50% at 5 years; however, this study was small, and only a few patients had clinically important degrees of IMR.[274] Others have shown that for patients with moderate or moderately severe IMR, isolated coronary surgery and coronary revascularization combined with mitral annuloplasty provide similar long-term outcome with survival rates of 82 to 92% at 1 year, 40 to 75% at 5 years, and 37 to 47% at 10 years[264–266,273–275] (Fig. 40-21). Predictors of long-term mortality are older age, prior myocardial infarction, unstable angina, chronic renal failure, atrial fibrillation, absence of an internal mammary artery graft, lack of beta blocker use, lower ejection fraction, smaller left atrial size, global LV wall motion abnormalities, severe lateral wall motion abnormalities, ST segment elevation in the lateral leads, higher voltage sum, mitral leaflet restriction, and fewer bypass grafts.[264,266,273] Combined mitral valve repair and coronary revascularization does not emerge as a predictor of long-term survival in these series. In order to elucidate preoperatively those that would more likely benefit from isolated coronary artery bypass grafting, the Prague group evaluated 135 patients with ischemic heart disease and moderate IMR undergoing isolated coronary artery bypass surgery; of these, 42% of the patients had no or mild mitral regurgitation postoperatively, whereas 47% failed to improve.[276] Before surgery, the improvement group had significantly more viable myocardium and less dyssynchrony between papillary muscles than the failure group. Thus, reliable improvement in moderate IMR by isolated coronary artery bypass graft surgery is likely only in patients with concomitant presence of viable myocardium and absence of dyssynchrony between papillary muscles.[276] In a pilot study of cardiac MRI in patients with ischemic mitral regurgitation and ischemic cardiomyopathy, extensive scarring and severe wall motion abnormalities in the region of posterior papillary muscle correlated with recurrent mitral regurgitation after coronary artery bypass grafting and mitral annuloplasty.[277] Routinely assessing scar burden may identify patients for whom annuloplasty alone is insufficient to eliminate mitral regurgitation. Therefore, although some investigators report that annuloplasty can be added to coronary grafting in high-risk patients without increasing early mortality, the potential benefit with respect to late survival and functional status is not proved and may be limited because of the underlying ischemic cardiomyopathy.[264–266,272]

In the Brigham and Women's Hospital experience, patients with IMR and annular dilatation or type IIIb restricted systolic leaflet motion (not chordal or papillary muscle rupture) who underwent valve repair and coronary revascularization had a worse long-term outcome than those who underwent valve replacement and coronary revascularization.[263] Notably, the pathophysiology or cause of the IMR was a stronger determinant of long-term survival than was the type of valve procedure. Conversely, the New York University group reported a higher complication-free survival rate (64% at 5 years) for patients undergoing mitral valve repair compared with 47% at 5 years for those in whom

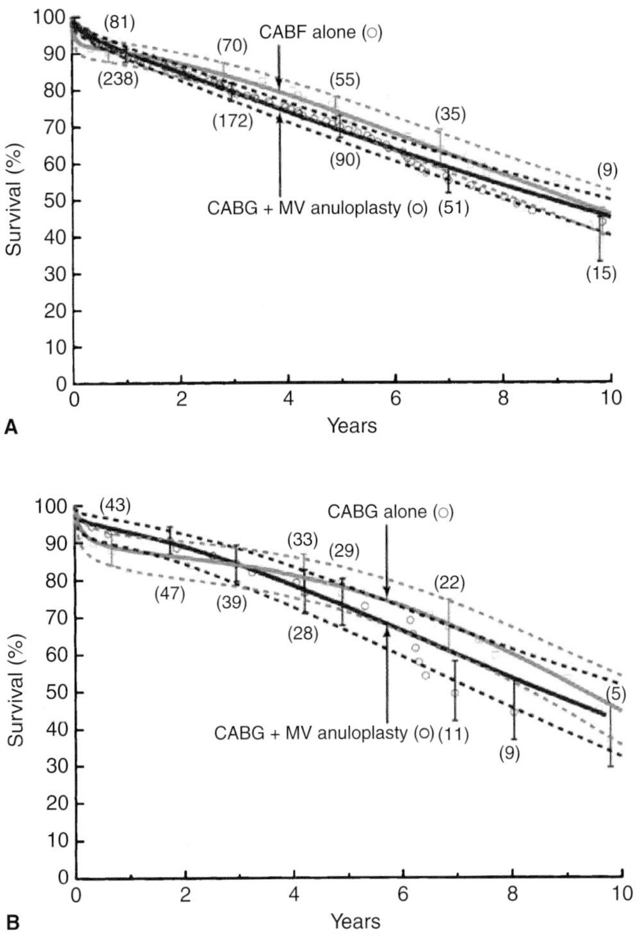

FIGURE 40-21 Survival after coronary artery bypass grafting (CABG) alone or with concomitant mitral valve (MV) annuloplasty for ischemic mitral regurgitation. Vertical bars are 68% confidence limits. Numbers in parentheses are patients alive and remaining at risk. Solid lines are parametric estimates enclosed within 68% confidence limits. (A) Unadjusted survival, based on 37 deaths after CABG alone and 92 after CABG + MV annuloplasty. (B) Propensity-matched survival, based on 19 deaths after CABG alone and 19 after CABG + MV annuloplasty. (*Reproduced with permission from Mihaljevic T, Lam BK, Rajeswaran J, Takagaki M, Lauer MS, et al: Impact of mitral valve annuloplasty combined with revascularization in patients with functional ischemic mitral regurgitation. J Am Coll Cardiol 2007; 49:2191.*)

the valve had to be replaced.[278] The analysis of the early mortality risk for patients with IMR undergoing mitral valve repair versus valve replacement was confounded by many other factors, including functional disability and degree of angina. Excluding these two variables, further analysis showed that the early mortality rate was lower for patients undergoing valve repair than for those undergoing valve replacement.[278] Based on propensity-score analysis, the Cleveland Clinic group found that in the lower-risk quintiles of patients with IMR, valve repair conferred a survival advantage (58% at 5 years) over those who underwent valve replacement (36% at 5 years); however, in the highest-risk patients, late survival after valve repair and valve replacement was similarly poor, and valve replacement actually conferred a small survival advantage.[279] In their experience, when patients with severe IMR underwent mitral valve surgery, undersized annuloplasty resulted in a durable repair in 70 to 85% of cases.[280] Although mitral valve repair is the procedure of choice in the majority of patients having surgery for IMR, in the most severely ill patients and those with certain echocardiographic characteristics (eg, severe bileaflet tethering), complete chordal-sparing mitral valve replacement may be preferable to repair.[280] At the Laval University in Quebec, 370 patients with IMR underwent mitral valve repair or mitral valve replacement.[281] The operative mortality was lower in the repair group (10%) compared with the replacement group (17%), but 6-year survival estimates were similar at 73% and 67%, respectively (Fig. 40-22). The type of valve procedure did not emerge as a risk factor for a poor outcome. Therefore, in patients with

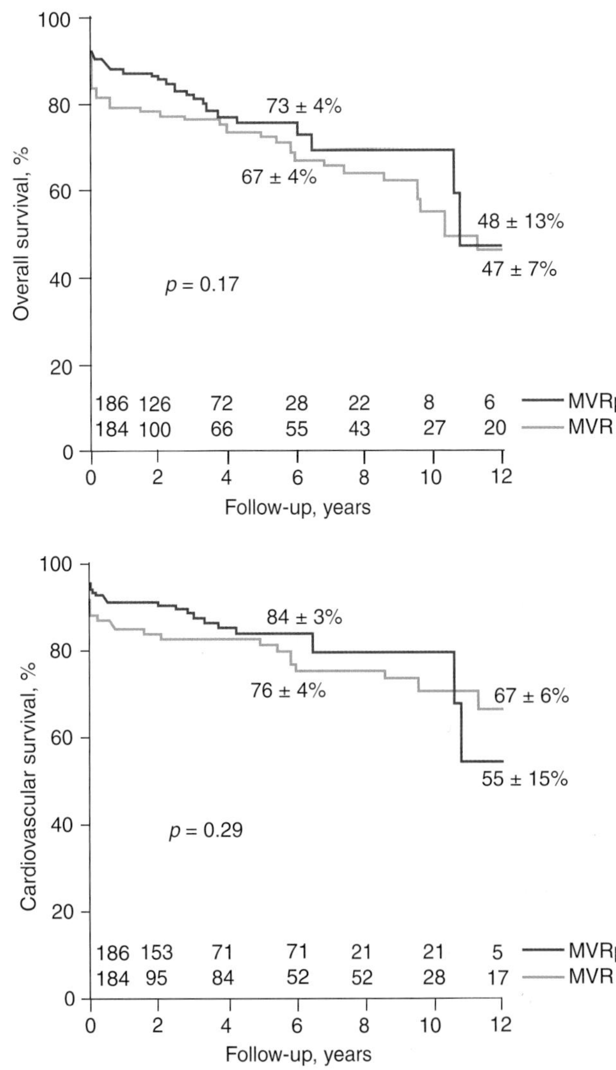

FIGURE 40-22 Comparison of mitral valve repair (MVRp) versus mitral valve replacement (MVR) with respect to overall (A) and cardiovascular (B) survival. (*Reproduced with permission from Magne J, Girerd N, Senechal M, et al. Mitral repair versus replacement for ischemic mitral regurgitation: comparison of short-term and long-term survival. Circulation 2009; 120[Suppl 1]:S-104.*)

IMR, mitral valve repair is not necessarily superior to replacement in terms of overall survival.[281]

Analysis of the etiology of the mitral regurgitation (degenerative versus ischemic) in patients with coronary artery disease after combined mitral valve repair and coronary revascularization showed that those with IMR had more extensive coronary disease, worse ventricular function, more comorbidities, and more preoperative symptoms.[282] Unadjusted 5-year survival estimates were 64 and 82% for patients with IMR and degenerative mitral regurgitation, respectively; however, matched pairs had equivalent but poor 5-year survival rates (66 and 65%, respectively). Long-term survival varied widely among patients with degenerative mitral regurgitation and coronary artery disease, depending largely on ischemic burden and extent of LV dysfunction.[282] Similarly, in the Duke experience, the survival discrepancy between patients with IMR and those with degenerative mitral regurgitation combined with coronary artery disease was attributed to patient-related differences.[268] In 535 patients (26% with IMR, 74% with nonischemic etiology) undergoing mitral valve repair with or without coronary artery bypass grafting, the 30-day mortality was 4.3% for those with IMR and 1.3% for nonischemic group; the 5 year survival was 56% for IMR and 84% for those with nonischemic mitral regurgitation.[268] Only the number of preoperative comorbidities and advanced age emerged as predictors of survival, whereas ischemic etiology, gender, ejection fraction, NYHA functional class, coronary artery disease, reoperation, and year of operation did not achieve statistical significance. Because survival was not different between patients with IMR and those with nonischemic mitral regurgitation after routine use of a rigid-ring annuloplasty during coronary artery grafting, long-term patient survival was more influenced by baseline patient characteristics and comorbidity than by the etiology of the mitral regurgitation per se[268] (Fig. 40-23). Additionally, investigators at the Mayo Clinic concluded that the decision as to whether to repair or replace the valve should be based on patient condition and not on whether the mitral regurgitation results from ischemia.[267] Older age, ejection fraction of 35% or less, three-vessel coronary disease, mitral valve replacement, and residual mitral regurgitation at discharge were risk factors for death. The cause of the mitral regurgitation, ischemic versus degenerative, was not a predictor of long-term survival, class III or IV congestive heart failure, or recurrent regurgitation.[267] Thus, survival after mitral valve surgery and coronary artery bypass grafting was determined more by the extent of coronary disease and LV systolic dysfunction and the success of the valve procedure.[267,268] These reports highlight the poor prognosis of patients with IMR and how the patient's clinical condition and LV functional status are more powerful determinants of outcome than type of operative procedure performed. The University of Virginia group proposed that despite the multiple comorbidities in patients with IMR, mitral valve repair for IMR and degenerative mitral regurgitation produced comparable and satisfactory outcomes.[283] The operative mortality rate for the IMR group was impressively low at 1.9% (compared with 1.2% in the degenerative group). The 5-year survival rate for those undergoing mitral valve repair was higher than expected at 84%, but significantly less that the 94% survival rate for patients with the

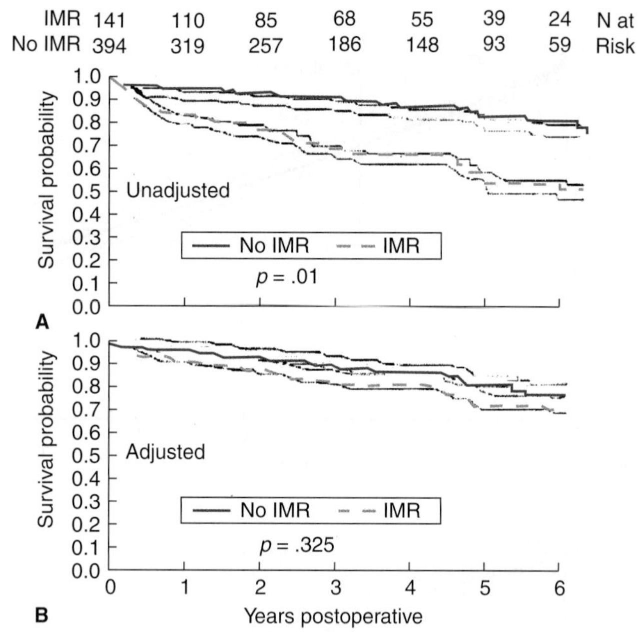

FIGURE 40-23 Survival of patients undergoing mitral valve repair with ischemic mitral regurgitation versus nonischemic mitral regurgitation before (**A**) and after (**B**) adjustment for differences in baseline patient characteristics. IMR = ischemic mitral regurgitation; NMR = nonischemic mitral regurgitation. (*Reproduced with permission from Glower DD et al: Patient survival characteristics after routine mitral valve repair for ischemic mitral regurgitation. J Thoracic Cardiovasc Surg 2005; 129:860.*)

degenerative MR. At longer follow-up, however, the survival trend for the IMR group diminished rapidly consistent with previous reported data (Fig. 40-24).[268,283] Recurrent mitral regurgitation and the 5-year rates of freedom from reoperation were similar between the IMR and degenerative groups in the Virginia experience.[283] Thus, an aggressive approach to repair patients with IMR, including treatment of leaflet tethering, may lead to acceptable results.

A compelling explanation for the generally poor long-term outcome of patients who undergo mitral valve repair for IMR is the presence of residual and/or recurrent mitral regurgitation postoperatively.[284–286] Persistence of IMR after mitral annuloplasty is due predominantly to augmented posterior leaflet apical tethering with no improvement in anterior leaflet tethering and no increase in coaptation length.[286] In a Cleveland Clinic report of annuloplasty (95% with concomitant coronary artery bypass grafting) for IMR, the proportion of patients with 0 or 1+ mitral regurgitation decreased from 71% preoperatively to 41% postoperatively, but the proportion with 3+ or 4+ residual or recurrent IMR increased from 13 to 28% during the first 6 months after repair[284] (Fig. 40-25). The temporal pattern of development of severe regurgitation was similar for those who received a Cosgrove partial, flexible band or a semirigid, complete Carpentier Edwards ring (25%), but it was substantially worse for those who received a strip of glutaraldehyde-preserved xenograft pericardium for annuloplasty (66%).[284] Smaller annuloplasty ring size apparently did not influence postoperative mitral regurgitation. At the Montreal Heart Institute, 78 patients

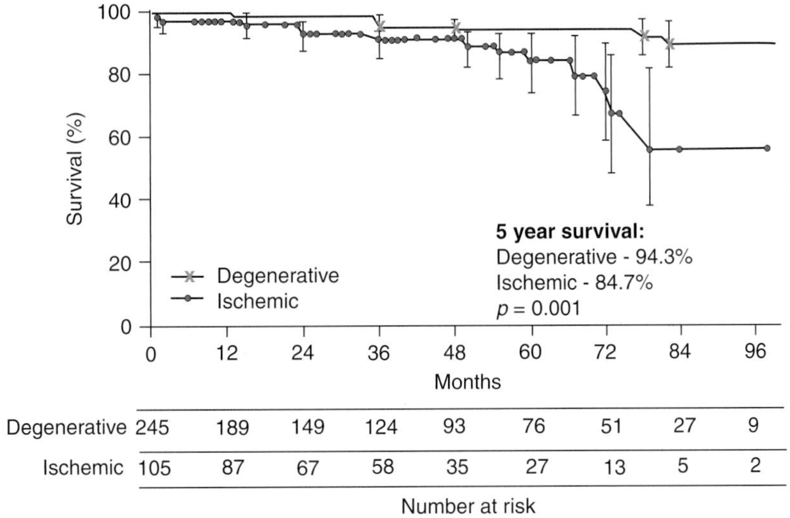

FIGURE 40-24 Kaplan-Meier survival estimates for patients with degenerative (x) versus ischemic (o) mitral regurgitation. (*Reproduced with permission from Gazoni LM, Kern JA, Swenson BR, Dent JM, Smith PW, et al: A change in perspective: results for ischemic mitral valve repair are similar to mitral valve repair for degenerative disease. Ann Thorac Surg 2007; 84:750.*)

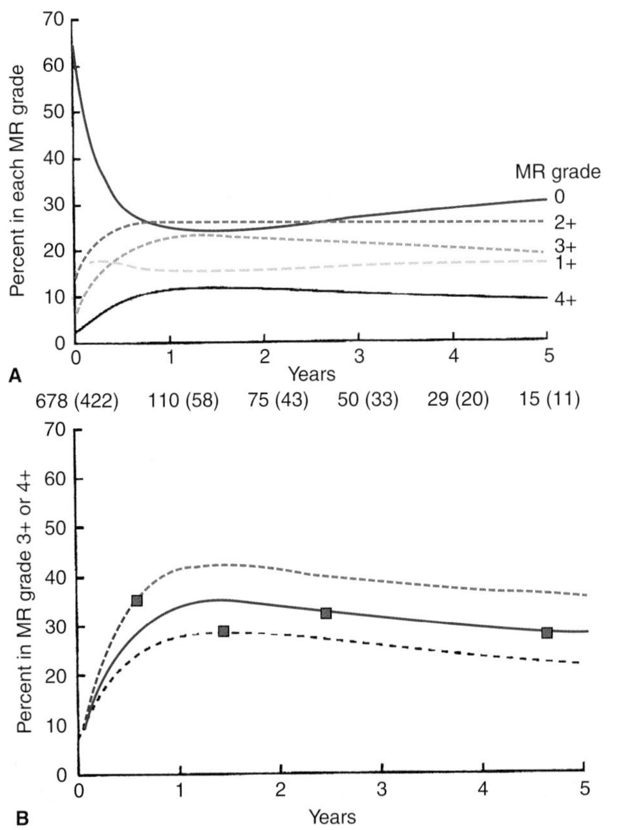

FIGURE 40-25 Progression of mitral regurgitation after surgical annuloplasty overall. (A) All grades of mitral regurgitation. Curves for each regurgitation grade represent average temporal prevalence, and they sum up to 100% at each point in time. Numbers below the horizontal axis represent echocardiograms available at various time points, with the number of patients in parentheses. (B) Prevalence of regurgitation grades 3+ or 4+. Dashed lines are 68% confidence limits of average prevalence. MR = Mitral regurgitation. (*Reproduced with permission from McGee EC Jr et al: Recurrent mitral regurgitation after annuloplasty for functional ischemic mitral regurgitation. J Thorac Cardiovasc Surg 2004; 128:916.*)

underwent mitral valve repair for IMR.[287] The operative mortality was 12.3% and the 5-year survival was 68%.[287] Recurrent moderate mitral regurgitation was 37% and severe regurgitation was present in 20% at mean follow-up of 28 months. Only age and less marked preoperative posterior tethering were predictive of recurrent mitral regurgitation. Patients with preoperative NYHA class greater than II and recurrent MR greater than 2+ had lower survival rates (Fig. 40-26). This finding again highlights the need for improved repair techniques, better patient selection, or possibly chordal-sparing mitral valve replacement in certain patients.[283,284,287]

Mitral Subvalvular Apparatus and LV Systolic Function

Originally proposed by Lillehei and colleagues in 1964, the mitral subvalvular apparatus (or valvular–ventricular complex), including chordal and papillary muscle function, is important for optimal postoperative LV geometry and systolic pump function.[131–134,199,200,288–292] After mitral valve replacement with total chordal excision, LV performance declines along with depression of regional and global LV elastance, dyssynergy of contraction, and dyskinesia at the papillary muscle insertion sites. Conversely, valve replacement with total or partial chordal preservation maintains LV contractile function.[131–133,216,292] Experimentally, severing either the anterior or the posterior leaflet chordae impairs global LV systolic function, as evidenced by reduced maximal elastance, but this is reversible if chordal reattachment is carried out.[132] In a canine model of chronic mitral regurgitation, mitral valve replacement with chordal preservation (compared with chordal severing) optimized postoperative LV energetics and ventriculovascular coupling in addition to enhancing systolic performance.[200] Chordal interruption decreased global LV end-systolic elastance and depressed the end-systolic stress–volume relationship. In terms of myocardial energetics, the slopes of the LV stroke work–end-diastolic

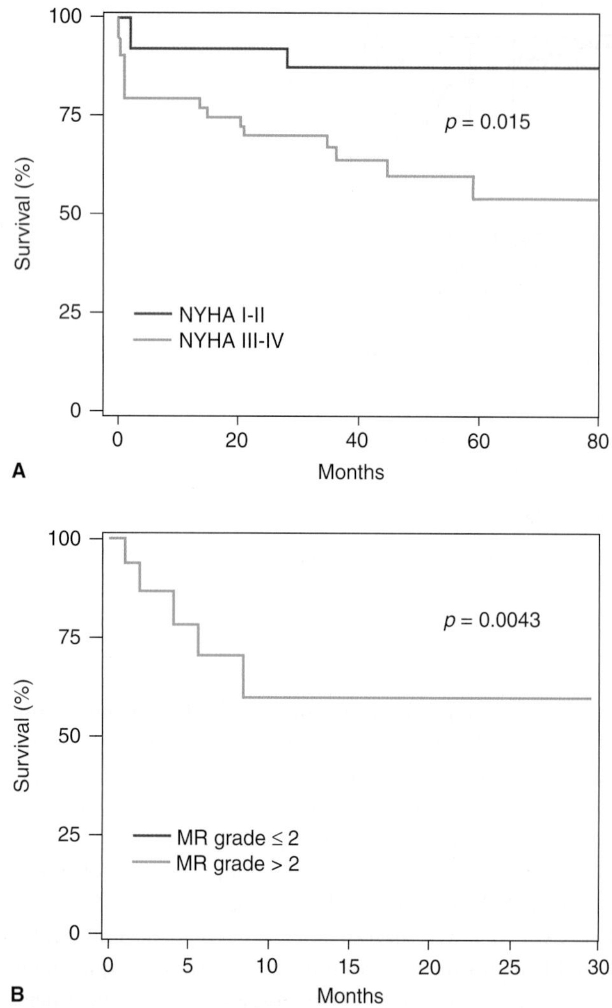

FIGURE 40-26 Kaplan-Meier survival curves according to preoperative NYHA class (A) and postoperative mitral regurgitation (MR) grade (B). (A) $n = 73$ patients. Time "0" represents date of surgery. (B) $n = 60$ Patients having survived to echocardiography. Time "0" represents date of latest available echocardiogram. *(Reproduced with permission from Serri K, Bouchard D, Demers P, Coutu M, Pellerin M, et al: Is a good perioperative echocardiographic result predictive of durability in ischemic mitral valve repair? J Thorac Cardiovasc Surg 2006; 131:565.)*

volume (preload recruitable stroke work, or PRSW) and pressure–volume area–end-diastolic volume relations also declined, indicating a reduction in external stroke work and mechanical energy generated at any given level of preload.

Clinically, mitral valve replacement with chordal division is associated with reduced rest and exercise LV ejection fraction owing in part to an increase in LV end-systolic stress (ESS).[291] Mitral valve repair does not perturb rest and exercise ejection indexes of LV function primarily as a consequence of reducing ESS and maintaining a more ellipsoidal chamber geometry. Mitral valve replacement with complete chordal transection results in no postoperative change in LV end-diastolic volume, an increase in LVESV, an increase in ESS, and a decrease in ejection fraction.[290] Patients who undergo chordal-sparing valve replacement, on the other hand, have a smaller LV end-diastolic volume and LVESV, decreased ESS, and unchanged ejection fraction. These findings suggest that smaller chamber size, reduced systolic afterload, and preservation of ventricular contractile function act in concert to maintain ejection performance after chordal-sparing mitral valve replacement. In contrast, increased LV chamber size, increased systolic afterload, and probable reduction in LV contractile function leading to reduced ejection performance occur in patients who undergo valve replacement with chordal transaction.[290] Indeed, the 2006 ACC/AHA valve practice guidelines stipulate that the subvalvular apparatus be preserved whenever possible when the mitral valve must be replaced in patients with MR, including chordae to both mitral leaflets.[238]

The loss of ventricular function after mitral valve replacement with chordal division may be caused by heterogeneity of regional LV wall stress and not local depression of regional contractile function.[293] After valve replacement with chordal transection in an experimental model, outward displacement of the ventricular wall and transverse shearing deformation occurred in the LV region papillary muscle insertion during isovolumic contraction.[293] Circumferential and radial strains during ejection were maintained at the basal LV site and enhanced in the apical LV site. Chordal transection augmented regional myocardial loading at the papillary muscle insertion site; the resulting heterogeneity of regional systolic function might be the mechanism for reduced global LV function and slowed ventricular relaxation. Anterior chordal transection with mitral valve replacement caused impaired regional LV function and also impaired regional right ventricular function,[294] whereas radionuclide angiography before and after mitral valve repair showed that LV ejection fraction did not change and right ventricular ejection fraction improved. In the region of the anterolateral papillary muscle insertion, local LV contractile function deteriorated after valve replacement with chordal transection, and right ventricular apicoseptal region was similarly impaired.[294]

In patients with chronic IMR, surgical division of the second-order chordae subtending the infarcted wall (usually those originating from the posteromedial papillary muscle) has been proposed to treat IMR.[295,296] It is postulated that if the apical systolic tethering is eliminated, the normal redundancy of the mitral leaflet area creates better coaptation with the intact first-order or marginal chordae preventing leaflet prolapse. Clinically, the Toronto group compared the outcomes of patients who underwent chordal-cutting mitral valve repair (n = 43) and those undergoing conventional mitral valve repair (n = 49) for ischemic mitral regurgitation.[196] The reduction in tenting height before-to-after repair was similar in the two groups of patients, but those undergoing chordal cutting had a greater reduction in tenting area. The chordal-cutting group also had greater mobility of the anterior leaflet, as measured by a reduction in the distance between the free edge of the anterior mitral valve leaflet and the posterior left ventricular wall. Additionally, those undergoing conventional mitral valve repair had a higher incidence of recurrent mitral regurgitation during 2 years of follow-up.[296] Chordal cutting did not adversely affect postoperative left ventricular ejection fraction (10% relative increase in EF compared with 11% in the control group). The authors proposed that chordal cutting improves mitral valve leaflet mobility and reduces mitral regurgitation recurrence in patients with ischemic mitral regurgitation, without any obvious deleterious effects on left ventricular function.[296] It is known, however, that division of the chordae, especially the second-order or "strut" chordae, impairs LV systolic function.[154,297,298] Dividing the second-order chordae in an acute ovine preparation is associated with regional LV systolic dysfunction near the chordal insertion sites and neither prevents nor decreases the severity of acute IMR, septal-lateral annular dilatation, leaflet tenting area, or leaflet tenting volume.[154,297] Cutting the anterior mitral leaflet second-order chordae alters LV chamber long-axis and subvalvular geometry, remodels end-diastolic transmural myocardial architecture in the equatorial lateral LV region, perturbs systolic transmural LV wall-thickening mechanics (thereby decreasing subendocardial "microtorsion") and wall thickening, changes systolic temporal dynamics with delayed ejection, and impairs global LV systolic function (decreased end-systolic elastance and PRSW).[298] Because of the importance of the chordae for LV structure and function, we believe that caution is necessary when considering procedures that cut second-order chordae to treat patients with IMR because of the resulting compromise in LV systolic function in ventricles that are already impaired.[154,297,298]

Summary

The functional competence of the mitral valve relies on the interaction of the mitral annulus and leaflets, chordae tendineae, papillary muscles, left atrium, and left ventricle. Dysfunction of any one or more components of this valvuloventricular complex can lead to mitral regurgitation. Important causes of mitral regurgitation include ischemic heart disease with IMR, dilated cardiomyopathy leading to FMR, myxomatous degeneration and prolapse, rheumatic valve disease, mitral annular calcification, and infective endocarditis. Four structural changes of the mitral valve apparatus may produce regurgitation: leaflet retraction from fibrosis and calcification, annular dilatation, chordal abnormalities, and LV systolic dysfunction with or without papillary muscle involvement. In IMR, changes in global and regional LV function and geometry, alterations in mitral annular geometry, abnormal leaflet (type IIIb) motion, leaflet malcoaptation, increased interpapillary distance, and papillary muscle lateral displacement and malalignment all may result in apical tenting of the leaflets and mitral incompetence.

With mitral regurgitation, the impedance to LV emptying is lower because the mitral orifice is parallel with the LV outflow tract. Reduced LV impedance allows a greater proportion of contractile energy to be expended in myocardial fiber shortening than in tension development. After the initial compensatory phase, LV contractility becomes progressively more impaired with chronic mitral regurgitation and chronic LV volume overload. Importantly, because of the low impedance during systole, clinical indexes of systolic function, such as ejection fraction, can be normal even if depressed LV contractility is already present. LVESV is less dependent on preload than is ejection fraction and is a better measure of LV contractile reserve. Preoperative LVESV is a good predictor of postoperative outcome. Surgical mitral valve repair (or, if repair is judged not to be durable, mitral valve replacement with total chordal preservation) for chronic mitral regurgitation can preserve LV contractility, particularly in patients with a normal preoperative ejection fraction who have minimal ventricular dilatation and those without major coronary disease. In patients with impaired preoperative LV contractility, LV systolic function may not necessarily improve after ring annuloplasty and definitely will not improve if the subvalvular apparatus and chordae are divided during mitral valve replacement.

IMR is generally associated with a higher operative risk than is nonischemic chronic mitral regurgitation. In patients with ischemic cardiomyopathy and mild mitral regurgitation, isolated coronary artery bypass grafting may suffice if most of the ventricle is still viable. Other workers argue that coronary revascularization alone in the setting of moderate IMR leaves many patients with substantial residual mitral regurgitation, heart failure symptoms, and a grave prognosis. Because moderate IMR does not resolve reliably with coronary revascularization alone, valve repair (undersized mitral annuloplasty with or without other adjunctive techniques) should be considered because it can reduce complications and possibly may improve long-term survival. Survival after mitral valve surgery and coronary artery bypass grafting may be more determined by the extent of coronary artery disease and LV dysfunction than by the etiology of mitral regurgitation. IMR may be a manifestation rather than an important impetus for postinfarct LV remodeling.

The mitral subvalvular apparatus is a key component of LV ejection performance; an intact mitral subvalvular apparatus, including second-order chordae tendineae to both leaflets, is necessary to maintain optimal postoperative LV geometry and maximize postoperative systolic pump function. After mitral valve replacement with chordal transection, LV systolic performance declines (depressed regional and global LV elastance, dyssynergy of contraction, and dyskinesia at the papillary muscle insertion sites). Experimental and clinical findings suggests that reduced LV chamber size, reduced LV systolic afterload, and preservation of ventricular contractile function act in concert to maintain ejection performance after mitral valve repair or total chordal-sparing valve replacement.

REFERENCES

1. van Gils FA: The fibrous skeleton in the human heart: embryological and pathogenetic considerations. *Virchows Arch A Pathol Anat Histol* 1981; 393:61.
2. Davila JC, Palmer TE: The mitral valve: anatomy and pathology for the surgeon. *Arch Surg* 1962; 84:174.
3. Silverman ME, Hurst JW: The mitral complex: Interaction of the anatomy, physiology, and pathology of the mitral annulus, mitral valve leaflets, chordae tendineae, and papillary muscles. *Am Heart J* 1968; 76:399.
4. Anderson RH, Wilcox BR: The anatomy of the mitral valve, in Wells FC, Shapiro LM (eds): *Mitral Valve Disease.* Oxford, England, Butterworth-Heinemann, 1996; p 4.
5. Walmsley R: Anatomy of human mitral valve in adult cadaver and comparative anatomy of the valve. *Br Heart J* 1978; 40:351.
6. Ormiston JA, Shah PM, Tei C, et al: Size and motion of the mitral valve annulus in man: I. A two-dimensional echocardiographic method and findings in normal subjects. *Circulation* 1981; 64:113.
7. O'Gara P, Sugeng L, Lang R, et al: The role of imaging in chronic degenerative mitral regurgitation. *J Am Coll Cardiol Img* 2008; 1:221.
8. Fenoglio J Jr, Tuan DP, Wit AL, et al: Canine mitral complex: ultrastructure and electromechanical properties. *Circ Res* 1972; 31:417.
9. Ranganathan N, Lam JH, Wigle ED, et al: Morphology of the human mitral valve: II. The valve leaflets. *Circulation* 1970; 41:459.

10. Wit AL, Fenoglio J Jr, Hordof AJ, Reemtsma K: Ultrastructure and transmembrane potentials of cardiac muscle in the human anterior mitral valve leaflet. *Circulation* 1979; 59:1284.
11. Curtis MB, Priola DV: Mechanical properties of the canine mitral valve: effects of autonomic stimulation. *Am J Physiol* 1992; 262:H56.
12. Marron K, Yacoub MH, Polak JM, et al: Innervation of human atrioventricular and arterial valves. *Circulation* 1996; 94:368.
13. Ahmed A, Johansson O, Folan-Curran J: Distribution of PGP 9.5, TH, NPY, SP and CGRP immunoreactive nerves in the rat and guinea pig atrioventricular valves and chordae tendinae. *J Anat* 1997; 191:547.
14. Filip DA, Radu A, Simionescu M: Interstitial cells of the heart valves possess characteristics similar to smooth muscle cells. *Circ Res* 1986; 59:310.
15. De Biasi S, Vitellaro-Zuccarello L, Blum I: Histochemical and ultrastructural study on the innervation of human and porcine atrio-ventricular valves. *Anat Embryol (Berl)* 1984; 169:159.
16. Boucek RJ, Bouckova B, Levy S: Anatomical arrangement of muscle tissue in the anterior mitral leaflet in man. *Cardiovasc Res* 1978; 12:675.
17. Williams TH: Fast-conducting fibres in the mitral valve. *Br Heart J* 1964; 26:554.
18. Smith RB: Intrinsic innervation of the atrioventricular and semi-lunar valves in various mammals. *J Anat* 1971; 108:115.
19. Hibbs RG, Ellison JP: The atrioventricular valves of the guinea pig: II. An ultrastructural study. *Am J Anat* 1973; 138:347.
20. Williams TH, Folan JC, Jew JY, et al: Variations in atrioventricular valve innervation in four species of mammals. *Am J Anat* 1990; 187:193.
21. Jew JY, Fink CA, Williams TH: Tyrosine hydroxylase-and nitric oxide synthase–immunoreactive nerve fibers in mitral valve of young adult and aged Fischer 344 rats. *J Auton Nerv Syst* 1996; 58:35.
22. Mulholland DL, Gotlieb AI: Cell biology of valvular interstitial cells. *Can J Cardiol* 1996; 12:231.
23. Williams TH: Mitral and tricuspid valve innervation. *Br Heart J* 1964; 26:105.
24. Swanson JC, Davis LR, Arata K, et al: Characterization of mitral valve anterior leaflet perfusion patterns. *J Heart Valve Dis* 2009; 18:488-495.
25. Erlanger J: A note on the contractility of the musculature of the auriculo-ventricular valves. *Am J Physiol* 1916; 40:150.
26. Dean AL Jr: The movements of the mitral cusps in relation to the cardiac cycle. *Am J Physiol* 1916; 40:206.
27. Sarnoff SJ, Gilmore JP, Mitchell JH: Influence of atrial contraction and relaxation on closure of mitral valve. *Circ Res* 1962; 11:26.
28. Sonnenblick EH, Napolitano LM, Daggett WM, Cooper T: An intrinsic neuromuscular basis for mitral valve motion in the dog. *Circ Res* 1967; 21:9.
29. Cooper T, Sonnenblick EH, Priola DV, et al: An intrinsic neuromuscular basis for mitral valve motion, in Brewer LA (ed): *Prosthetic Heart Valves.* Springfield, IL, Charles C Thomas, 1969; Chap 2.
30. Anderson RH: The disposition and innervation of atrioventricular ring specialized tissue in rats and rabbits. *J Anat* 1972; 113:197.
31. Kawano H, Kawai S, Shirai T, et al: Morphological study on vagal innervation in human atrioventricular valves using histochemical method. *Jpn Circ J* 1993; 57:753.
32. Timek TA, Lai DTM, Dagum P, et al: Ablation of mitral annular and leaflet muscle: effects on annular and leaflet dynamics. *Am J Physiol Heart Circ Physiol* 2003; 285:H1668-H1674.
33. Priola DV, Fellows C, Moorehouse J, Sanchez R: Mechanical activity of canine mitral valve in situ. *Am J Physiol* 1970; 219:1647.
34. Wit AL, Fenoglio J Jr, Wagner BM, Bassett AL: Electrophysiological properties of cardiac muscle in the anterior mitral valve leaflet and the adjacent atrium in the dog: possible implications for the genesis of atrial dysrhythmias. *Circ Res* 1973; 32:731.
35. Rozanski GJ: Electrophysiological properties of automatic fibers in rabbit atrioventricular valves. *Am J Physiol* 1987; 253:H720.
36. Williams TH, Jew JY: Is the mitral valve passive flap theory overstated? An active valve is hypothesized. *Med Hypoth* 2004; 62:605.
37. Krishnamurthy G, Itoh A, Swanson JC, et al: Regional stiffening of the mitral valve anterior leaflet in the beating ovine heart. *J Biomechanics* 2009, 42:2697.
38. Itoh A, Krishnamurthy G, Swanson JC, et al: Active stiffening of mitral valve leaflets in the beating heart. *Am J Physiol Heart Circ Physiol* 2009; 296:H1766-H1773.
39. Rozanski GJ, Jalife J: Automaticity in atrioventricular valve leaflets of rabbit heart. *Am J Physiol* 1986; 250:H397.
40. Police C, Piton M, Filly K, et al: Mitral and aortic valve orifice area in normal subjects and in patients with congestive cardiomyopathy: determination by two-dimensional echocardiography. *Am J Cardiol* 1982; 49:1191.
41. Tsakiris AG, Von Bernuth G, Rastelli GC, et al: Size and motion of the mitral valve annulus in anesthetized intact dogs. *J Appl Physiol* 1971; 30:611.
42. Tsakiris AG, Strum RE, Wood EH: Experimental studies on the mechanisms of closure of cardiac valves with use of roentgen videodensitometry. *Am J Cardiol* 1973; 32:136.
43. Davis PKB, Kinmonth JB: The movements of the annulus of the mitral valve. *J Cardiovasc Surg* 1963; 4:427.
44. Padula RT, Cowan G Jr, Camishion RC: Photographic analysis of the active and passive components of cardiac valvular action. *J Thorac Cardiovasc Surg* 1968; 56:790.
45. Ormiston JA, Shah PM, Tei C, Wong M: Size and motion of the mitral valve annulus in man: II. Abnormalities in mitral valve prolapse. *Circulation* 1982; 65:713.
46. Keren G, Sonnenblick EH, LeJemtel TH: Mitral annulus motion: Relation to pulmonary venous and transmitral flows in normal subjects and in patients with dilated cardiomyopathy. *Circulation* 1988; 78:621.
47. van Rijk-Zwikker GL, Mast F, Schipperheyn JJ, et al: Comparison of rigid and flexible rings for annuloplasty of the porcine mitral valve. *Circulation* 1990; 82:V-58.
48. Karlsson MO, Glasson JR, Bolger AF, et al: Mitral valve opening in the ovine heart. *Am J Physiol* 1998; 274:H552.
49. Roberts WC, Perloff JK: Mitral valvular disease: A clinicopatho-logic survey of the conditions causing the mitral valve to function abnormally. *Ann Intern Med* 1972; 77:939.
50. Levine RA, Triulzi MO, Harrigan P, Weyman AE: The relationship of mitral annular shape to the diagnosis of mitral valve prolapse. *Circulation* 1987; 75:756.
51. Levine RA, Handschumacher MD, Sanfilippo AJ, et al: Three-dimensional echocardiographic reconstruction of the mitral valve, with implications for the diagnosis of mitral valve prolapse. *Circulation* 1989; 80:589.
52. Rushmer R, Finlayson B, Nash A: Movements of the mitral valve. *Circ Res* 1956; 4:337.
53. Tsakiris AG, Gordon DA, Padiyar R, et al: The role of displacement of the mitral annulus in left atrial filling and emptying in the intact dog. *Can J Physiol Pharmacol* 1978; 56:447.
54. Rushmer RF: Initial phase of ventricular systole: asynchronous contraction. *Am J Physiol* 1956; 184:188.
55. Popp RL, Harrison DC: Ultrasonic cardiac echography for determining stroke volume and valvular regurgitation. *Circulation* 1970; 41:493.
56. Toumanidis ST, Sideris DA, Papamichael CM, et al: The role of mitral annulus motion in left ventricular function. *Acta Cardiol* 1992; 47:331.
57. Carlhall C, Kindberg K, Wigstrom L, et al: Contribution of mitral annular dynamics to LV diastolic filling with alteration in preload and inotropic state. *Am J Physio Heart Circ Physiol* 2007; 293:H1473-H1479.
58. Chiechi MA, Lees M, Thompson R: Functional anatomy of the normal mitral valve. *J Thorac Cardiovasc Surg* 1956; 32:378.
59. Sovak M, Lynch PR, Stewart GH: Movement of the mitral valve and its correlation with the first heart sound: selective valvular visualization and high-speed cineradiography in intact dogs. *Invest Radiol* 1973; 8:150.
60. Pohost GM, Dinsmore RE, Rubenstein JJ, et al: The echocardiogram of the anterior leaflet of the mitral valve: correlation with hemodynamic and cineroentgenographic studies in dogs. *Circulation* 1975; 51:88.
61. Rodriguez F, Langer F, Harrington KB, et al: Effect of cutting second-order chordae on in-vivo anterial mitral leaflet compound curvature. *J Heart Valve Dis* 2005; 14:592.
62. Edler I, Gustafson A, Karlefors T, et al: Mitral and aortic valve movements recorded by an ultra-sonic echo method: an experimental study in ultrasound cardiology. *Acta Med Scand* 1961; 370:68.
63. Tsakiris AG, Gordon DA, Mathieu Y, et al: Motion of both mitral valve leaflets: a cineroentgenographic study in intact dogs. *J Appl Physiol* 1975; 39:359.
64. Fenster MS, Feldman MD: Mitral regurgitation: an overview. *Curr Probl Cardiol* 1995; 20:193.
65. Armour JA, Randall WC: Structural basis for cardiac function. *Am J Physiol* 1970; 218:1517.
66. Luther RR, Meyers SN: Acute mitral insufficiency secondary to ruptured chordae tendineae. *Arch Intern Med* 1974; 134:568.
67. Voci P, Bilotta F, Caretta Q, et al: Papillary muscle perfusion pattern: a hypothesis for ischemic papillary muscle dysfunction. *Circulation* 1995; 91:1714.
68. Lam JHC, Ranganathan N, Wigle ED, et al: Morphology of the human mitral valve: I. Chordae tendineae: a new classification. *Circulation* 1970; 41:449.
69. Ritchie J, Warnock JN, Yoganathan AP: Structural characterization of the chordae tendineae in native porcine mitral valves. *Ann Thorac Surg* 2005; 80:189.

70. Ross J Jr, Sonnenblick EH, Covell JW, et al: The architecture of the heart in systole and diastole. *Circ Res* 1967; 21:409.
71. Armour JA, Randall WC: Electrical and mechanical activity of papillary muscle. *Am J Physiol* 1978; 218:1710.
72. Cronin R, Armour JA, Randall WC: Function of the in-situ papillary muscle in the canine left ventricle. *Circ Res* 1969; 25:67.
73. Rayhill SC, Daughters GT, Castro LJ, et al: Dynamics of normal and ischemic canine papillary muscles. *Circ Res* 1994; 74:1179.
74. Karas S, Elkins RC: Mechanism of function of the mitral valve leaflets, chordae tendineae and left ventricular papillary muscles in dogs. *Circ Res* 1970; 26:689.
75. Semafuko WEB, Bowie WC: Papillary muscle dynamics: In situ function and responses of the papillary muscle. *Am J Physiol* 1975; 228:1800.
76. Burch GE, DePasquale NP: Time course of tension in papillary muscle of the heart. *JAMA* 1965; 192:701.
77. Grimm AF, Lendrum BL, Lin HL: Papillary muscle shortening in the intact dog. *Circ Res* 1975; 36:49.
78. Marzilli M, Sabbah HN, Lee T, et al: Role of the papillary muscle in opening and closure of the mitral valve. *Am J Physiol* 1980; 238:H348.
79. Marzilli M, Sabbah HN, Goldstein S, et al: Assessment of papillary muscle function in the intact heart. *Circulation* 1985; 71:1017.
80. Hirakawa S, Sasayama S, Tomoike H, et al: In situ measurement of papillary muscle dynamics in the dog left ventricle. *Am J Physiol* 1977; 233:H384.
81. Wood P: An appreciation of mitral stenosis. *BMJ* 1954; 1:1051.
82. Spencer FC: A plea for early, open mitral commissurotomy. *Am Heart J* 1978; 95:668.
83. Roberts WC: Morphologic aspects of cardiac valve dysfunction. *Am Heart J* 1992; 123:1610.
84. Carabello BA: Timing of surgery in mitral and aortic stenosis. *Cardiol Clin* 1991; 9:229.
85. Waller BF, Howard J, Fess S: Pathology of mitral valve stenosis and pure mitral regurgitation, part I. *Clin Cardiol* 1994; 17:330.
86. Waller BF, Howard J, Fess S: Pathology of mitral valve stenosis and pure mitral regurgitation, part II. *Clin Cardiol* 1994; 17:395.
87. Essop MR, Nkomo VT: Rheumatic and nonrheumatic valvular heart disease: epidemiology, management, and prevention in Africa. *Circulation* 2005; 112:3584.
88. Chandrashekhar Y, Westaby S, Narula J: Mitral stenosis. *Lancet* 2009; 374:1271-1283.
89. Khalil KG, Shapiro I, Kilman JW: Congenital mitral stenosis. *J Thorac Cardiovasc Surg* 1975; 70:40.
90. Korn D, DeSanctis RW, Sell S: Massive calcification of the mitral annulus. *NEJM* 1962; 267:900.
91. Burge DJ, DeHoratious RJ: Acute rheumatic fever. *Cardiovasc Clin* 1993; 23:3.
92. Fae KC, Oshiro SE, Toubert A, et al: How an autoimmune reaction triggered by molecular mimicry between streptococcal M protein and cardiac tissue proteins leads to heart lesions in rheumatic heart disease. *J Autoimmun* 2005; 24:101.
93. Guilherme L, Cury P, Demarchi LM, et al: Rheumatic heart disease: proinflammatory cytokines play a role in the progression and maintenance of valvular lesions. *Am J Pathol* 2004; 165:1583.
94. Davutoglu V, Celik A, Aksoy M: Contribution of selected serum inflammatory mediators to the progression of chronic rheumatic valve disease, subsequent valve calcification and NYHA functional class. *J Heart Valve Dis* 2005; 14:151.
95. Hygenholtz PG, Ryan TJ, Stein SW, et al: The spectrum of pure mitral stenosis. *Am J Cardiol* 1962; 10:773.
96. Arani DT, Carleton RA: The deleterious role of tachycardia in mitral stenosis. *Circulation* 1967; 36:511.
97. Schofield PM: Invasive investigation of the mitral valve, in Wells FC, Shapiro LM (eds): *Mitral Valve Disease.* Oxford, England, Butterworth-Heinemann, 1996; p 84.
98. Braunwald E, Turi ZG: Pathophysiology of mitral valve disease, in Wells FC, Shapiro LM (eds): *Mitral Valve Disease.* Oxford, England, Butterworth-Heinemann, 1996; p 28.
99. Thompson ME, Shaver JA, Leon DF: Effect of tachycardia on atrial transport in mitral stenosis. *Am Heart J* 1977; 94:297.
100. Stott DK, Marpole DGF, Bristow JD, et al: The role of left atrial transport in aortic and mitral stenosis. *Circulation* 1970; 41:1031.
101. Kennedy JW, Yarnall SR, Murray JA, et al: Quantitative angiocardiography: relationships of left atrial and ventricular pressure and volume in mitral valve disease. *Circulation* 1970; 41:817.
102. Choi BW, Bacharach SL, Barcour DJ, et al: Left ventricular systolic dysfunction: diastolic filling characteristics and exercise cardiac reserve in mitral stenosis. *Am J Cardiol* 1995; 75:526.
103. Bolen JL, Lopes MG, Harrison DC, et al: Analysis of left ventricular function in response to afterload changes in patients with mitral stenosis. *Circulation* 1975; 52:894.
104. Schwartz R, Myerson RM, Lawrence LT, et al: Mitral stenosis, massive pulmonary hemorrhage, and emergency valve replacement. *NEJM* 1966; 275:755.
105. Diker E, Aydogdu S, Ozdemir M, et al: Prevalence and predictors of atrial fibrillation in rheumatic valvular heart disease. *Am J Cardiol* 1996; 77:96.
106. Chiang CW, Lo SK, Kuo CT, et al: Noninvasive predictors of systemic embolism in mitral stenosis. *Chest* 1994; 106:396.
107. Daley R, Mattingly TW, Holt CL, et al: Systemic arterial embolism in rheumatic heart disease. *Am Heart J* 1951; 42:566.
108. McCall BW, Price JL: Movement of mitral valve cusps in relation to first heart sound and opening snap in patients with mitral stenosis. *Br Heart J* 1967; 29:417.
109. Kalmanson D, Veyrat C, Bernier A, et al: Opening snap and isovolumic relaxation period in relation to mitral valve flow in patients with mitral stenosis. *Br Heart J* 1976; 38:135.
110. Toutouzas P, Koidakis A, Velimezis A, et al: Mechanism of diastolic rumble and presystolic murmur in mitral stenosis. *Br Heart J* 1974; 36:1096.
111. Perloff JK: Auscultatory and phonocardiographic manifestations of pulmonary hypertension. *Prog Cardiovasc Dis* 1967; 9:303.
112. Goldstein MA, Michelson EL, Dreifus LS: The electrocardiogram in valvular heart disease. *Cardiovasc Clin* 1993; 23:55.
113. Kotler MN, Jacobs LE, Podolsky LA, et al: Echo-Doppler in valvular heart disease. *Cardiovasc Clin* 1993; 23:77.
114. Stoddard MF, Prince CR, Ammash NM, et al: Two-dimensional transesophageal echocardiographic of mitral valve area in adults with mitral stenosis. *Am Heart J* 1994; 127:1348.
115. Wu WC, Aziz GF, Sadaniantz A: The use of stress echocardiography in the assessment of mitral valvular disease. *Echocardiography* 2004; 21:451.
116. Hung J, Lang R, Flachskampf F, et al. 3D echocardiography: a review of the current status and future directions. *J Am Soc Echocardiogr* 2007; 20: 213-233.
117. Seow SC, Koh LP, Yeo TC: Hemodynamic significance of mitral stenosis: use of a simple, novel index by two-dimensional echocardiography. *J Am Soc Echocardiogr* 2006; 19:102.
118. Lange A, Palka P, Burstow DJ, et al: Three-dimensional echocardiography: Historical development and current applications. *J Am Soc Echocardiogr* 2001; 14:403.
119. Fabricius AM, Walther T, Falk V, et al: Three-dimensional echocardiography for planning of mitral valve surgery: current applicability? *Ann Thorac Surg* 2004; 78:575.
120. Nayak KS, Pauly JM, Kerr AB, et al: Real-time color flow MRI. *J Magn Reson Med* 2000; 43:251.
121. Han Y, Peters DC, Salton CJ, et al. Cardiovascular magnetic resonance: characterization of mitral valve prolapse. *J Am Coll Cardiol Img* 2008; 1:294-303.
122. Alkadhi H, Bettex D, Wildermuth S, et al: Dynamic cine imaging of the mitral valve with 16-MDCT: a feasibility study. *AJR* 2005; 185:636.
123. Amplatz K: The roentgenographic diagnosis of mitral and aortic valvular disease. *Am Heart J* 1962; 64:556.
124. Iung B, Nicoud-Houel A, Fondard O, et al. Temporal trends in percutaneous mitral commissurotomy over a 15-year period. *Eur Heart J* 2004; 25:701-707.
125. Cohn LH, Allred EN, Cohn LA, et al: Long-term results of open mitral valve reconstruction for mitral stenosis. *Am J Cardiol* 1985; 55:731.
126. Detter C, Fischlein T, Feldmeier C, et al: Mitral commissurotomy, a technique outdated? Long-term follow-up over a period of 35 years. *Ann Thorac Surg* 1999; 68:2112.
127. Glower DD, Landolfo KP, Davis RD, et al: Comparison of open mitral commissurotomy with mitral valve replacement with or without chordal preservation in patients with mitral stenosis. *Circulation* 1998; 98:II-120.
128. Zener JC, Hancock EW, Shumway NE, et al: Regression of extreme pulmonary hypertension after mitral valve surgery. *Am J Cardiol* 1972; 30:820.
129. Chowdhury UK, Kumar AS, Mittal AB, et al: Mitral valve replacement with and without chordal preservation in a rheumatic population: serial echocardiographic assessment of left ventricular size and function. *Ann Thorac Surg* 2005; 79:1926.
130. Sugita T, Matsumoto M, Nishizawa J, et al: Long-term outcome after mitral valve replacement with preservation of continuity between the mitral annulus and the papillary muscle in patients with mitral stenosis. *J Heart Valve Dis* 2004; 13:931.
131. Hansen DE, Sarris GE, Niczyporuk MA, et al: Physiologic role of the mitral apparatus in left ventricular regional mechanics, contraction synergy, and global systolic performance. *J Thorac Cardiovasc Surg* 1989; 97:521.

132. Sarris GE, Cahill PD, Hansen DE, et al: Restoration of left ventricular systolic performance after reattachment of the mitral chordae tendineae. *J Thorac Cardiovasc Surg* 1988; 95:969.
133. Yun KL, Fann JI, Rayhill SC, et al: Importance of the mitral subvalvular apparatus for left ventricular segmental systolic mechanics. *Circulation* 1990; 82:IV-89.
134. Yun KL, Niczyporuk MA, Sarris GE, et al: Importance of mitral subvalvular apparatus in terms of cardiac energetics and systolic mechanics in the ejecting canine heart. *J Clin Invest* 1991; 87:247.
135. Covalesky VA, Ross J, Chandrasekaran, et al: Detection of diastolic atrioventricular valvular regurgitation by M-mode color Doppler echocardiography. *Am J Cardiol* 1989; 64:809.
136. Hanson TP, Edwards BS, Edwards JE: Pathology of surgically excised mitral valves: one hundred consecutive cases. *Arch Pathol Lab Med* 1985; 109:823.
137. Olson LJ, Subramanian R, Ackermann DM, et al: Surgical pathology of the mitral valve: a study of 812 cases spanning 21 years. *Mayo Clin Proc* 1987; 62:22.
138. Waller BF, Morrow AG, Maron BJ, et al: Etiology of clinically isolated, severe, chronic, pure, mitral regurgitation: analysis of 97 patients over 30 years of age having mitral valve replacement. *Am Heart J* 1982; 104:188.
139. Brunetti ND, Ieva R, Rossi G, et al: Ventricular outflow tract obstruction, systolic anterior motion and acute mitral regurgitation in Tako-Tsubo syndrome. *Int J Cardiol* 2008; 127:e152-e157.
140. Carpentier A: Cardiac valve surgery: the French correction. *J Thorac Cardiovasc Surg* 1983; 86:323.
141. Carpentier A, Chauvaud S, Fabiani J, et al: Reconstructive surgery of mitral valve incompetence: ten-year appraisal. *J Thorac Cardiovasc Surg* 1980; 79:338.
142. Wells FC: Conservation and surgical repair of the mitral valve, in Wells FC, Shapiro LM (eds): *Mitral Valve Disease.* Oxford, England, Butterworth-Heinemann, 1996; p 114.
143. Miller DC: Ischemic mitral regurgitation redux: to repair or to replace? *J Thorac Cardiovasc Surg* 2001; 122:1059.
144. Dagum P, Timek TA, Green GR, et al: Coordinate-free analysis of mitral valve dynamics in normal and ischemic hearts. *Circulation* 2000; 102:III-62.
145. Otsuji Y, Handschumacher MD, Liel-Cohen N, et al: Mechanism of ischemic mitral regurgitation with segmental left ventricular dysfunction: three-dimensional echocardiographic studies in models of acute and chronic progressive regurgitation. *J Am Coll Cardiol* 2001; 37:641.
146. Ngaage DL, Schaff HV: Mitral valve surgery in non-ischemic cardiomyopathy. *J Cardiovasc Surg* 2004; 45:477.
147. Grande-Allen KJ, Borowski AG, Troughton RW, et al: Apparently normal mitral valves in patients with heart failure demonstrate biochemical and structural derangements. *J Am Coll Cardiol* 2005; 45:54.
148. Grande-Allen KJ, Barber JE, Klatka KM, et al: Mitral valve stiffening in end-stage heart failure: evidence of an organic contribution to functional mitral regurgitation. *J Thorac Cardiovasc Surg* 2005; 130:783.
149. Stephens EH, Timek TA, Daughters GT, et al. Significant changes in mitral valve leaflet matrix composition and turnover with tachycardia-induced cardiomyopathy. *Circulation* 2009; 120(Suppl 1):S-112-S-119.
150. Kumanohoso T, Otsuji Y, Yoshifuku S, et al: Mechanism of higher incidence of ischemic mitral regurgitation in patients with inferior myocardial infarction: quantitative analysis of left ventricular and mitral valve geometry in 103 patients with prior myocardial infarction. *J Thorac Cardiovasc Surg* 2003; 125:135.
151. Glasson J, Komeda M, Daughters GT, et al: Early systolic mitral leaflet "loitering" during acute ischemic mitral regurgitation. *J Thorac Cardiovasc Surg* 1998; 116:193.
152. Srichai MB, Grimm RA, Stillman AE, et al: Ischemic mitral regurgitation: Impact of the left ventricle and mitral valve in patients with left ventricular systolic dysfunction. *Ann Thorac Surg* 2005; 80:170.
153. Timek TA, Lai DT, Tibayan F, et al: Ischemia in three left ventricular regions: insights into the pathogenesis of acute ischemic mitral regurgitation. *J Thorac Cardiovasc Surg* 2003; 125:559.
154. Rodriguez F, Langer F, Harrington KB, et al: Cutting second-order chords does not prevent acute ischemic mitral regurgitation. *Circulation* 2004; 110:II-91.
155. Enomoto Y, Gorman JH III, Moainie SL, et al: Surgical treatment of ischemic mitral regurgitation might not influence ventricular remodeling. *J Thorac Cardiovasc Surg* 2005; 129:504.
156. Tibayan FA, Rodriguez F, Zasio MK, et al: Geometric distortions of the mitral valvular-ventricular complex in chronic ischemic mitral regurgitation. *Circulation* 2003; 108:II-116.
157. Ahmad RM, Gillinov AM, McCarthy PM, et al: Annular geometry and motion in human ischemic mitral regurgitation: novel assessment with three-dimensional echocardiography and computer reconstruction. *Ann Thorac Surg* 2004; 78:2063.
158. Popovic ZB, Martin M, Fukamachi K, et al: Mitral annulus size links ventricular dilatation to functional mitral regurgitation. *J Am Soc Echocardiogr* 2005; 18:959.
159. Matsunaga A, Tahta SA, Duran CMG: Failure of reduction annuloplasty for functional ischemic mitral regurgitation. *J Heart Valve Dis* 2004; 13:390.
160. Nielsen SL, Hansen SB, Nielsen KO, et al: Imbalanced chordal force distribution causes acute ischemic mitral regurgitation: mechanistic insights from chordae tendineae force measurements in pigs. *J Thorac Cardiovasc Surg* 2005; 129:525.
161. Levine RA: Dynamic mitral regurgitation: more than meets the eye. *NEJM* 2004; 351:16.
162. Lai DT, Timek TA, Tibayan FA, et al: The effects of mitral annuloplasty rings on mitral valve complex 3D geometry during left ventricular ischemia. *Eur J Cardiothorac Surg* 2002; 22:808.
163. Lai DT, Tibayan FA, Myrmel T, et al: Mechanistic insights into posterior mitral leaflet interscallop malcoaptation during acute ischemic mitral regurgitation. *Circulation* 2002; 106:I-40.
164. Liel-Cohen N, Guerrero JL, Otsuji Y, et al: Design of a new surgical approach for ventricular remodeling to relieve ischemic mitral regurgitation. *Circulation* 2000; 101:2756.
165. Tibayan FA, Rodriguez F, Langer F, et al: Alterations in left ventricular torsion and diastolic recoil after myocardial infarction with and without chronic ischemic mitral regurgitation. *Circulation* 2004; 110:II-109.
166. Nguyen TC, Cheng A, Langer F, et al: Altered myocardial shear strains are associated with chronic mitral regurgitation. *Ann Thorac Surg* 2007; 83:47.
167. Gorman JH III, Jackson BM, Enomoto Y, et al: The effect of regional ischemia on mitral valve annular saddle shape. *Ann Thorac Surg* 2004; 77:544.
168. Watanabe N, Ogasawara Y, Yamaura Y, et al: Geometric deformity of the mitral annulus in patients with ischemic mitral regurgitation: a real-time three-dimensional echocardiographic study. *J Heart Valve Dis* 2005; 14:447.
169. Watanabe N, Ogasawara Y, Yamaura Y, et al: Mitral annulus flat-tens in ischemic mitral regurgitation: geometric differences between inferior and anterior myocardial infarction. *Circulation* 2005; 112:I-458.
170. Yiu SF, Enriquez-Sarano M, Tribouilloy C, et al: Determinants of the degree of functional mitral regurgitation in patients with systolic left ventricular dysfunction. *Circulation* 2000; 102:1400.
171. Chaput M, Handschumacher MD, Guerrero JL, et al. Mitral leaflet adaptation to ventricular remodeling: prospective changes in a model of ischemic mitral regurgitation. *Circulation* 2009; 120(Suppl 1):S-99-S-103.
172. Messas E, Guerrero JL, Handschumacher MD, et al: Paradoxic decrease in ischemic mitral regurgitation with papillary muscle dysfunction. *Circulation* 2001; 104:1952.
173. Kishon Y, Oh JK, Schaff HV, et al: Mitral valve operation in postinfarction rupture of a papillary muscle: immediate results and long-term follow-up in 22 patients. *Mayo Clin Proc* 1992; 67:1023.
174. LeFeuvre C, Metzger JP, Lachurie ML, et al: Treatment of severe mitral regurgitation caused by ischemic papillary muscle dysfunction: indications for coronary angioplasty. *Am Heart J* 1992; 123:860.
175. Olsen LJ, Subramanian R, Ackerman DM, et al: Surgical pathology of the mitral valve: a study of 712 cases spanning 21 years. *Mayo Clin Proc* 1987; 62:22.
176. Hayek E, Gring CN, Griffin BP: Mitral valve prolapse. *Lancet* 2005; 365:507.
177. David TE, Ivanov J, Armstrong S, et al: Late outcomes of mitral valve repair for floppy valves: implications for asymptomatic patients. *J Thorac Cardiovasc Surg* 2003; 125:1143.
178. Ling LH, Enriquez-Sarano M, Seward JB, et al: Early surgery in patients with mitral regurgitation due to flail leaflets. *Circulation* 1997; 96:1819.
179. Barlow JB, Pocock WA: Mitral valve prolapse, the specific billowing mitral leaflet syndrome, or an insignificant non-ejection systolic click. *Am Heart J* 1979; 97:277.
180. Abrams J: Mitral valve prolapse: a plea for unanimity. *Am Heart J* 1976; 92:413.
181. Roberts WC, McIntosh CL, Wallace RB: Mechanisms of severe mitral regurgitation in mitral valve prolapse determined from analysis of operatively excised valves. *Am Heart J* 1987; 113:1316.
182. Nesta F, Leyne M, Yosefy C, et al: New locus for autosomal dominant mitral valve prolapse on chromosome 13: clinical insights from genetic studies. *Circulation* 2005; 112:2022.
183. Grau JB, Pirelli L, Yu PJ, et al: The genetics of mitral valve prolapse. *Clin Genet* 2007; 72:288.

184. Procacci PM, Savran SV, Schreiter SL, et al: Prevalence of clinical mitral-valve prolapse in 1169 young women. *NEJM* 1976; 294:1086.
185. Enriquez-Sarano M, Schaff HV, Frye RL: Mitral regurgitation: what causes the leakage is fundamental to the outcome of valve repair. *Circulation* 2003; 108:253.
186. Roberts WC, Braunwald E, Morrow AG: Acute severe mitral regurgitation secondary to ruptured chordae tendineae. *Circulation* 1966; 33:58.
187. Kamblock J, N'Guyen L, Pagis B, et al: Acute severe mitral regurgitation during first attacks of rheumatic fever: clinical spectrum, mechanisms and prognostic factors. *J Heart Valve Dis* 2005; 14:440.
188. Braunwald E: Mitral regurgitation: physiologic, clinical and surgical considerations. *NEJM* 1969; 281:425.
189. Grigioni F, Enriquez-Sarano M, Zehr KJ, et al: Ischemic mitral regurgitation: long-term outcome and prognostic implications with quantitative Doppler assessment. *Circulation* 2001; 103:1759.
190. Enriquez-Sarano M, Avierinos JF, Messika-Zeitoun D, et al: Quantitative determinants of the outcome of asymptomatic mitral regurgitation. *NEJM* 2005; 352:875.
191. Zoghbi WA, Enriquez-Sarano M, Foster E, et al: Recommendations for evaluation of the severity of native valve regurgitation with two-dimensional and Doppler echocardiography. *J Am Soc Echocardiogr* 2003; 16:777.
192. Yoran C, Yellin EL, Becker RM, et al: Dynamic aspects of acute mitral regurgitation: effects of ventricular volume, pressure and contractility on the effective regurgitant orifice area. *Circulation* 1979; 60:170.
193. Keren G, Laniado S, Sonnenblick EH, et al: Dynamics of functional mitral regurgitation during dobutamine therapy in patients with severe congestive heart failure: a Doppler echocardiographic study. *Am Heart J* 1989; 118:748.
194. Keren G, Katz S, Strom J, et al: Dynamic mitral regurgitation: an important determinant of the hemodynamic response to load alterations and inotropic therapy in severe heart failure. *Circulation* 1989; 80:306.
195. Abe Y, Imai T, Ohue K, et al: Relation between reduction in ischaemic mitral regurgitation and improvement in regional left ventricular contractility during low dose dobutamine stress echocardiography. *Heart* 2005; 91:1092.
196. Grossman W: Profiles in valvular heart disease, in Baim DS, Grossman W (eds.): *Cardiac Catheterization, Angiography and Intervention,* 5th ed. Baltimore, Williams & Wilkins, 1996; p 735.
197. Ross J Jr: Adaptations of the left ventricle to chronic volume overload. *Circ Res* 1974; 34-35:II-64.
198. Spinale FG, Ishihra K, Zile M, et al: Structural basis for changes in left ventricular function and geometry because of chronic mitral regurgitation and after correction of volume overload. *J Thorac Cardiovasc Surg* 1993; 106:1147.
199. Yun KL, Rayhill SC, Niczyporuk MA, et al: Left ventricular mechanics and energetics in the dilated canine heart: acute versus chronic mitral regurgitation. *J Thorac Cardiovasc Surg* 1992; 104:26.
200. Yun KL, Rayhill SC, Niczyporuk MA, et al: Mitral valve replacement in dilated canine hearts with chronic mitral regurgitation. *Circulation* 1991; 84:III-112.
201. Urabe Y, Mann DL, Kent RL, et al: Cellular and ventricular contractile dysfunction in experimental canine mitral regurgitation. *Circ Res* 1992; 70:131.
202. Carabello BA, Crawford FA Jr: Valvular heart disease. *NEJM* 1997; 337:32.
203. Starling MR, Kirsh MM, Montgomery DG, et al: Impaired left ventricular contractile function in patients with long-term mitral regurgitation and normal ejection fraction. *J Am Coll Cardiol* 1993; 22:239.
204. Nakano K, Swindle MM, Spinale F, et al: Depressed contractile function due to canine mitral regurgitation improves after correction of the volume overload. *J Clin Invest* 1991; 87:2077.
205. Brickner ME, Starling MR: Dissociation of end systole from end ejection in patients with long-term mitral regurgitation. *Circulation* 1990; 81:1277.
206. Glower DD, Spratt JA, Snow ND, et al: Linearity of the Frank-Starling relationship in the intact heart: the concept of preload recruitable stroke work. *Circulation* 1985; 71:994.
207. Carabello BA, Nolan SP, McGuire LB: Assessment of preoperative left ventricular function in patients with mitral regurgitation: value of the end-systolic wall stress–end-systolic volume ratio. *Circulation* 1981; 64:1212.
208. Carabello BA, Williams H, Gash AK, et al: Hemodynamic predictors of outcome in patients undergoing valve replacement. *Circulation* 1986; 74:1309.
209. Borow KM, Green LH, Mann T, et al: End-systolic volume as a predictor of postoperative left ventricular performance in volume overload from valvular regurgitation. *Am J Med* 1980; 68:655.
210. Tibayan FA, Yun KL, Fann JI, et al: Torsion dynamics in the evolution from acute to chronic mitral regurgitation. *J Heart Valve Dis* 2002; 11:39.
211. Carlhall CJ, Nguyen TC, Itoh A, et al: Alterations in transmural myocardial strain: an early marker of left ventricular dysfunction in mitral regurgitation? *Circulation* 2008; 118(Suppl 1):S-256.
212. Yellin EL, Nikolic S, Frater RWM: Left ventricular filling dynamics and diastolic function. *Prog Cardiovasc Dis* 1990; 32:333.
213. Zile MR, Tomita M, Nakano K, et al: Effects of left ventricular volume overload produced by mitral regurgitation on diastolic function. *Am J Physiol* 1991; 261:H471.
214. Corin WJ, Murakami T, Monrad ES, et al: Left ventricular passive diastolic properties in chronic mitral regurgitation. *Circulation* 1991; 83:797.
215. Zile MR, Tomita M, Ishihara K, et al: Changes in diastolic function during development and correction of chronic left ventricular volume overload produced by mitral regurgitation. *Circulation* 1993; 87:1378.
216. Corin WJ, Sutsch G, Murakami T, et al: Left ventricular function in chronic mitral regurgitation: preoperative and postoperative comparison. *J Am Coll Cardiol* 1995; 25:113.
217. Sabbah HN, Kono T, Rosman H, et al: Left ventricular shape: a factor in the etiology of functional mitral regurgitation in heart failure. *Am Heart J* 1992; 123:961.
218. Borer JS, Hochreiter C, Rosen S: Right ventricular function in severe non-ischemic mitral insufficiency. *Eur Heart J* 1991; 12:22.
219. Braunwald E, Awe WC: The syndrome of severe mitral regurgitation with normal left atrial pressure. *Circulation* 1963; 27:29.
220. Pierard LA, Lancellotti P: The role of ischemic mitral regurgitation in the pathogenesis of acute pulmonary edema. *NEJM* 2004; 351:1627.
221. Gray RJ, Helfant RH: Timing of surgery in valvular heart disease. *Cardiovasc Clin* 1993; 23:209.
222. Harrison MR, MacPhail B, Gurley JC, et al: Usefulness of color Doppler flow imaging to distinguish ventricular septal defect from acute mitral regurgitation complicating acute myocardial infarction. *Am J Cardiol* 1989; 64:697.
223. Perloff JK, Harvey WP: Auscultatory and phonocardiographic manifestations of pure mitral regurgitation. *Prog Cardiovasc Dis* 1962; 5:172.
224. Antman EM, Angoff GH, Sloss LJ: Demonstration of the mechanism by which mitral regurgitation mimics aortic stenosis. *Am J Cardiol* 1978; 42:1044.
225. Wann LS, Weyman AE, Feigenbaum H, et al: Determination of mitral valve area by cross-sectional echocardiography. *Ann Intern Med* 1978; 88:337.
226. Karalis DG, Ross JJ, Brown BM, et al: Transesophageal echocardiography in valvular heart disease. *Cardiovasc Clin* 1993; 23:105.
227. Smith MD, Cassidy JM, Gurley JC, et al: Echo Doppler evaluation of patients with acute mitral regurgitation: superiority of transesophageal echocardiography with color flow imaging. *Am Heart J* 1995; 129:967.
228. Kwan J, Shiota T, Agler DA, et al: Geometric differences of the mitral apparatus between ischemic and dilated cardiomyopathy with significant mitral regurgitation: real-time three-dimensional echocardiography study. *Circulation* 2003; 107:1135.
229. Kozerke S, Schwitter J, Pedersen EM, et al: Aortic and mitral regurgitation: quantification using moving slice velocity mapping. *J Magn Reson Imag* 2001; 14:106.
230. Buchner S, Debl K, Poschenrieder F, et al: Cardiovascular magnetic resonance for direct assessment of anatomic regurgitant orifice in mitral regurgitation. *Circ Cardiovasc Imaging.* 2008; 1:148.
231. Pieper EPG, Hellemans IM, Hamer HPM, et al: Additional value of biplane transesophageal echocardiography in assessing the genesis of mitral regurgitation and the feasibility of valve repair. *Am J Cardiol* 1995; 75:489.
232. Grewal KS, Malkowsi MJ, Piracha AR, et al: Effect of general anesthesia on the severity of mitral regurgitation by transesophageal echocardiography. *Am J Cardiol* 2000; 85:199.
233. Byrne JG, Aklog L, Adams DH: Assessment and management of functional or ischemic mitral regurgitation. *Lancet* 2000; 355:1743.
234. Plicht B, Kahlert P, Goldwasser R, et al: Direct quantification of mitral regurgitant flow volume by real-time three-dimensional echocardiography using dealiasing of color Doppler flow at the vena contracta. *J Am Soc Echocardiogr* 2008; 21:1337.
235. Ryan LP, Salgo IS, Gorman RC, Gorman JH III: The emerging role of three-dimensional echocardiography in mitral valve repair. *Semin Thorac Cardiovasc Surg* 2006; 18:126-134.
236. Hundley WG, Li HF, Willard JE, et al: Magnetic resonance imaging assessment of the severity of mitral regurgitation. *Circulation* 1995; 92:1151.
237. Starling MR: Effects of valve surgery on left ventricular contractile function in patients with long-term mitral regurgitation. *Circulation* 1995; 92:811.

238. Bonow RO, Carabello BA, Chatterjee K, et al: ACC/AHA 2006 guidelines for the management of patients with valvular heart disease. *J Am Coll Cardiol* 2006; 48:598.
239. Suri RM, Schaff HV, Dearani JA, et al: Survival advantage and improved durability of mitral repair for leaflet prolapse subsets in the current era. *Ann Thorac Surg* 2006; 82:819.
240. DeBonis M, Lapenna E, Verzini A, et al: Recurrence of mitral regurgitation parallels the absence of left ventricular reverse remodeling after mitral repair in advanced dilated cardiomyopathy. *Ann Thorac Surg* 2008; 85:932.
241. Braun J, Bax JJ, Versteegh MIM, et al: Preoperative left ventricular dimensions predict reverse remodeling following restrictive mitral annuloplasty in ischemic mitral regurgitation. *Eur J Cardiothorac Surg* 2005; 27:847.
242. Bax JJ, Braun J, Somer ST, et al: Restrictive annuloplasty and coronary revascularization in ischemic mitral regurgitation results in reverse left ventricular remodeling. *Circulation* 2004; 110:II-103.
243. Onorati F, Santarpino G, Marturano D, et al: Successful surgical treatment of chronic ischemic mitral regurgitation achieves left ventricular reverse remodeling but does not affect right ventricular function. *J Thorac Cardiovasc Surg* 2009; 138:341.
244. Wisenbaugh T, Skudicky D, Sarelli P: Prediction of outcome after valve replacement for rheumatic mitral regurgitation in the era of chordal preservation. *Circulation* 1994; 89:191.
245. Crawford MH, Souchek J, Oprian CA, et al: Determinants of survival and left ventricular performance after mitral valve replacement. *Circulation* 1990; 81:1173.
246. Levine HJ: Is valve surgery indicated in patients with severe mitral regurgitation even if they are asymptomatic? *Cardiovasc Clin* 1990; 21:161.
247. Davis EA, Gardner TJ, Gillinov AM, et al: Valvular disease in the elderly: influence on surgical results. *Ann Thorac Surg* 1993; 55:333.
248. Goldfine H, Aurigemma GP, Zile MR, et al: Left ventricular length-force-shortening relations before and after surgical correction of chronic mitral regurgitation. *J Am Coll Cardiol* 1998; 31:180.
249. LeTourneau T, deGroote P, Millaire A, et al: Effect of mitral valve surgery on exercise capacity, ventricular ejection fraction and neurohumoral activation in patients with severe mitral regurgitation. *J Am Coll Cardiol* 2000; 36:2263.
250. Salomon NW, Stinson EB, Griepp RB, et al: Patient-related risk factors as predictors of results following isolated mitral valve replacement. *Ann Thorac Surg* 1977; 24:520.
251. Michel PL, Iung B, Blanchard B, et al: Long-term results of mitral valve repair for non-ischemic mitral regurgitation. *Eur Heart J* 1991; 12:39.
252. Reed D, Abbott R, Smucker M, et al: Prediction of outcome after mitral valve replacement in patients with symptomatic chronic mitral regurgitation: the importance of left atrial size. *Circulation* 1991; 84:23.
253. Ling LH, Enriquez-Sarano M, Seward JB, et al: Clinical outcome of mitral regurgitation due to flail leaflet. *NEJM* 1996; 335:1417.
254. Cohn LH, Couper GS, Aranki SF, et al: Long-term results of mitral valve reconstruction for regurgitation of the myxomatous mitral valve. *J Thorac Cardiovasc Surg* 1994; 107:143.
255. Deloche A, Jebara V, Relland J, et al: Valve repair with Carpentier techniques: the second decade. *J Thorac Cardiovasc Surg* 1990; 99:990.
256. Kim HJ, Ahn SJ, Park SW, et al. Cardiopulmonary exercise testing before and one year after mitral valve repair for severe mitral regurgitation. *Am J Cardiol* 2004; 93:1187.
257. Messika-Zeitoun D, Johnson BD, Nkomo V, et al: Cardiopulmonary exercise testing determination of functional capacity in mitral regurgitation physiologic and outcome implications. *J Am Coll Cardiol* 2006; 47:2521.
258. Enriquez-Sarano M, Schaff HV, Orszulak TA, et al: Congestive heart failure after surgical correction of mitral regurgitation. *Circulation* 1995; 92:2496.
259. Tribouilloy CM, Enriquez-Sarano M, Schaff HV, et al: Impact of preoperative symptoms on survival after surgical correction of organic mitral regurgitation. *Circulation* 1999; 99:400.
260. Bursi F, Enriquez-Sarano M, Nkomo VT, et al: Heart failure and death after myocardial infarction in the community. *Circulation* 2005; 111:295.
261. Grigioni F, Detaint D, Avierinos JF, et al: Contribution of ischemic mitral regurgitation to congestive heart failure after myocardial infarction. *J Am Coll Cardiol* 2005; 45:260.
262. Dujardin KS, Enriquez-Sarano M, Bailey KR, et al: Grading of mitral regurgitation by quantitative Doppler echocardiography: calibration by left ventricular angiography in routine clinical practice. *Circulation* 1997; 96:3409.
263. Cohn LH, Rizzo RJ, Adams DH, et al: The effect of pathophysiology on the surgical treatment of ischemic mitral regurgitation: operative and late risks of repair versus replacement. *Eur J Cardiothorac Surg* 1995; 9:568.
264. Diodato MD, Moon MR, Pasque MK, et al: Repair of ischemic mitral regurgitation does not increase mortality or improve long-term survival in patients undergoing coronary artery revascularization: a propensity analysis. *Ann Thorac Surg* 2004; 78:794.
265. Kim YH, Czer LSC, Soukiasian HJ, et al: Ischemic mitral regurgitation: Revascularization alone versus revascularization and mitral valve repair. *Ann Thorac Surg* 2005; 79:1895.
266. Wong DR, Agnihotri AK, Hung JW, et al: Long-term survival after surgical revascularization for moderate ischemic mitral regurgitation. *Ann Thorac Surg* 2005; 80:570.
267. Dahlberg PS, Orszulak TA, Mullany CJ, et al: Late outcome of mitral valve surgery for patients with coronary artery disease. *Ann Thorac Surg* 2003; 76:1539.
268. Glower DD, Tuttle RH, Shaw LK, et al: Patient survival characteristics after routine mitral valve repair in ischemic mitral regurgitation. *J Thorac Cardiovasc Surg* 2005; 129:860.
269. Aklog L, Filshoufi F, Flores KQ, et al: Does coronary artery bypass grafting alone correct moderate ischemic mitral regurgitation? *Circulation* 2001; 104:I-68.
270. Lam BK, Gillinov AM, Blackstone EH, et al: Importance of moderate ischemic mitral regurgitation. *Ann Thorac Surg* 2005; 79:462.
271. Grossi EA, Crooke GA, DiGiorgi PL, et al: Impact of moderate functional mitral insufficiency in patients undergoing surgical revascularization. *Circulation* 2006; 114(suppl I):I-573.
272. Trichon BH, Glower DD, Shaw LK, et al: Survival after coronary revascularization, with and without mitral valve surgery, in patients with ischemic mitral regurgitation. *Circulation* 2003; 108:II-103.
273. Mihaljevic T, Lam BK, Rajeswaran J, et al: Impact of mitral valve annuloplasty combined with revascularization in patients with functional ischemic mitral regurgitation. *J Am Coll Cardiol* 2007; 49:2191.
274. Tolis GA Jr., Korkolis DP, Kopf GS, et al: Revascularization alone (without mitral valve repair) suffices in patients with advanced ischemic cardiomyopathy and mild-to-moderate mitral regurgitation. *Ann Thorac Surg* 2003; 74:1476.
275. Harris KM, Sundt TM III, Aeppli D, et al: Can late survival of patients with moderate ischemic mitral regurgitation be impacted by intervention on the valve? *Ann Thorac Surg* 2002; 74:1468.
276. Penicka M, Linkova H, Lang O, et al: Predictors of improvement of unrepaired moderate ischemic mitral regurgitation in patients undergoing elective isolated coronary artery bypass graft surgery. *Circulation* 2009; 120:1474.
277. Flynn M, Curtin R, Nowicki ER, et al: Regional wall motion abnormalities and scarring in severe functional ischemic mitral regurgitation: a pilot cardiovascular magnetic resonance imaging study. *J Thorac Cardiovasc Surg* 2009; 137:1063.
278. Grossi EA, Goldberg JD, LaPietra A, et al: Ischemic mitral valve reconstruction and replacement: comparison of long-term survival and complications. *J Thorac Cardiovasc Surg* 2001; 122:1107.
279. Gillinov AM, Wieryp PN, Blackstone EH, et al: Is repair preferable to replacement for ischemic mitral regurgitation? *J Thorac Cardiovasc Surg* 2001; 122:1125.
280. Gillinov AM: Is ischemic mitral regurgitation an indication for surgical repair or replacement? *Heart Fail Rev* 2006; 11:231-239.
281. Magne J, Girerd N, Senechal M, et al: Mitral repair versus replacement for ischemic mitral regurgitation: comparison of short-term and long-term survival. *Circulation* 2009; 120(Suppl 1):S-104-S-111.
282. Gillinov AM, Blackstone EH, Rajeswaran J, et al: Ischemic versus degenerative mitral regurgitation: does etiology affect survival? *Ann Thorac Surg* 2005; 80:811.
283. Gazoni LM, Kern JA, Swenson BR, et al: A change in perspective: Results for ischemic mitral valve repair are similar to mitral valve repair for degenerative disease. *Ann Thorac Surg* 2007; 84:750.
284. McGee EC, Gillinov AM, Blackstone EH, et al: Recurrent mitral regurgitation after annuloplasty for functional ischemic mitral regurgitation. *J Thorac Cardiovasc Surg* 2004; 128:916.
285. Tahta SA, Oury JH, Maxwell JM, et al: Outcome after mitral valve repair for functional ischemic mitral regurgitation. *J Heart Valve Dis* 2002; 11:11.
286. Zhu F, Otsuji Y, Yotsumoto G, et al: Mechanism of persistent ischemic mitral regurgitation after annuloplasty. *Circulation* 2005; 112:I-396.
287. Serri K, Bouchard D, Demers P, et al: Is a good perioperative echocardiographic result predictive of durability in ischemic mitral valve repair? *J Thorac Cardiovasc Surg* 2006; 131:565.
288. Lillehei CW, Levy MJ, Bonnabeau RC: Mitral valve replacement with preservation of papillary muscles and chordae tendineae. *J Thorac Cardiovasc Surg* 1964; 47:532.
289. David TE, Burns RJ, Bacchus CM, et al: Mitral valve replacement for mitral regurgitation with and without preservation of chordae tendineae. *J Thorac Cardiovasc Surg* 1984; 88:718.

290. Rozich JD, Carabello BA, Usher BW, et al: Mitral valve replacement with and without chordal preservation in chronic mitral regurgitation. *Circulation* 1992; 86:1718.
291. Tischler MD, Cooper KA, Rowen M, et al: Mitral valve replacement versus mitral valve repair: a Doppler and quantitative stress echocardiographic study. *Circulation* 1994; 89:132.
292. Pitarys CJ, Forman MB, Panayiotou H, et al: Long-term effects of excision of the mitral apparatus on global and regional ventricular function in humans. *J Am Coll Cardiol* 1990; 15:557.
293. Takayama Y, Holmes JW, LeGrice I, et al: Enhanced regional deformation at the anterior papillary muscle insertion site after chordal transection. *Circulation* 1996; 93:585.
294. Le Tourneau T, Grandmougin D, Foucher C, et al: Anterior chordal transection impairs not only regional left ventricular function but also regional right ventricular function in mitral regurgitation. *Circulation* 2001; 104:I-41.
295. Messas E, Pouzet B, Touchot B, et al: Efficacy of chordal cutting to relieve chronic persistent ischemic mitral regurgitation. *Circulation* 2003; 108:II-111.
296. Borger MA, Murphy PM, et al: Initial results of the chordal-cutting operation for ischemic mitral regurgitation. *J Thorac Cardiovasc Surg* 2007; 133:1483.
297. Nielsen SL, Timek TA, Green GR, et al: Influence of anterior mitral leaflet second-order chordae tendineae on left ventricular systolic function. *Circulation* 2003; 103:486.
298. Rodriguez F, Langer F, Harrington KB, et al: Importance of mitral valve second-order chordae for left ventricular geometry, wall thickening mechanics, and global systolic function. *Circulation* 2004; 110:II-115.

CHAPTER 41

Mitral Valve Repair

Frederick Y. Chen
Lawrence H. Cohn

INTRODUCTION

Sir Thomas Lauder Brunton, a Scottish physician, first introduced the concept of surgical repair of the mitral valve in 1902.[1] Twenty-one years later, Elliot Cutler, the future Moseley Professor of Surgery at the Peter Bent Brigham Hospital in Boston, performed the world's first successful mitral valve operation in 1923 by carrying out a transventricular commissurotomy with a neurosurgical tenotomy knife. A new era in surgery was introduced as well as the reality of mitral valve repair.[2] Cutler had worked assiduously on this problem in the Surgical Research Laboratories of Harvard Medical School before turning his attention to a critically ill, bed-bound 12-year-old girl, performing mitral valvulotomy on May 20, 1923. With that seminal operation, the idea of surgically restoring normal anatomy to the pathologic mitral valve came to fruition. Subsequent attempts at transventricular valvulotomy with a cardiovalvutome to produce graded mitral regurgitation resulted in several deaths and Cutler eventually abandoned the procedure.[3] Of Cutler's contemporaries, Henry Souttar of England performed a single successful transatrial finger commissurotomy in 1925, but received no further referrals.[4] After Souttar there remained little activity in mitral valve repair until Dwight Harken, then the Chief of Cardiothoracic Surgery at the Peter Bent Brigham Hospital, published his groundbreaking series of valvuloplasty patients for mitral stenosis[5] concomitantly with Charles Bailey in Philadelphia.[6]

That early era focused on mitral stenosis created by rheumatic heart disease, which was extremely common at the time. Surgical treatment of mitral regurgitation for prolapse was first introduced in the 1950s[7–9] but with limited success. Later, in the '60s, '70s, and '80s, the visionary concepts and ideas disseminated by Carpentier,[10] McGoon,[11] and Duran,[12] and later promulgated by others,[13–15] stimulated the field. Initially, those ideas, like any other groundbreaking idea, were met with resistance that has gradually dissipated as long term results by these surgeons have been validated. In particular, the idea that repair of mitral regurgitation might damage a weakened left ventricle by eliminating the left atrium as a low-resistance "pop-off" valve[16] proved a significant barrier to referral that only in the past decade has been overcome. What has now become firmly established is the significant contribution to overall left ventricular function of the papillary muscle–annular interaction.[17] As a result of these contributions, mitral valve repair, if technically possible, has now become recognized as the procedure of choice for mitral valve pathology of virtually all etiologies, to the extent that mitral valve repair is always considered first in virtually any clinical situation in which the mitral valve is regurgitant.

This chapter will focus on repair of the myxomatous, degenerated valve with some consideration of the repair of the rheumatic mitral valve. Repair of ischemic or infected mitral valves is presented in detail in Chapters 29 and 43, respectively. Detailed pathophysiology of the mitral valve is presented in Chapter 40 and detailed echo findings are shown in Chapter 11 by Sarano.

ANATOMY OF THE MITRAL VALVE

A surgical dictum is that form follows function and this is particularly apropos for the mitral valve. The bicuspid mitral valve is one of the most complex structures of the human heart; its complexity lies in its multifaceted anatomy. Because each part of the anatomy is intimately related to function, there are a variety of pathways whereby regurgitation may be created. If one part of the valvular apparatus fails, regurgitation results. There are five discrete components to the mitral valve complex: the annulus, the two leaflets (anterior and posterior), the chordae, the papillary muscles, and the left ventricle (Fig. 41-1A.)

As part of the fibrous skeleton of the heart, the annulus is the myocardial connective tissue area where the mitral valve leaflets attach to the intersection of the left atrium and left ventricle. It is surrounded by vitally important structures that the cardiac surgeon must avoid for safe surgery: the circumflex coronary artery laterally, the coronary sinus medially, the aortic root superiorly, and the atrioventricular node superior-medially. In myxomatous disease it is the posterior annulus that usually dilates.[18] Previous dictum held that the anterior annulus does not dilate, but recent data suggest that it may dilate a limited amount.[19] Of critical importance to the surgeon are the right and left fibrous trigones. These are intimately related to the anterior annulus and are contiguous with the aortic valve curtain and must be identified during surgery. The trigones, as part of the essential structural framework of the heart, form the anchoring points for ring annuloplasty.

The anterior leaflet of the mitral valve (AML) is in continuity with the left and noncoronary cusps of the aortic valve and is located directly beneath the left ventricular outflow tract (LVOT).

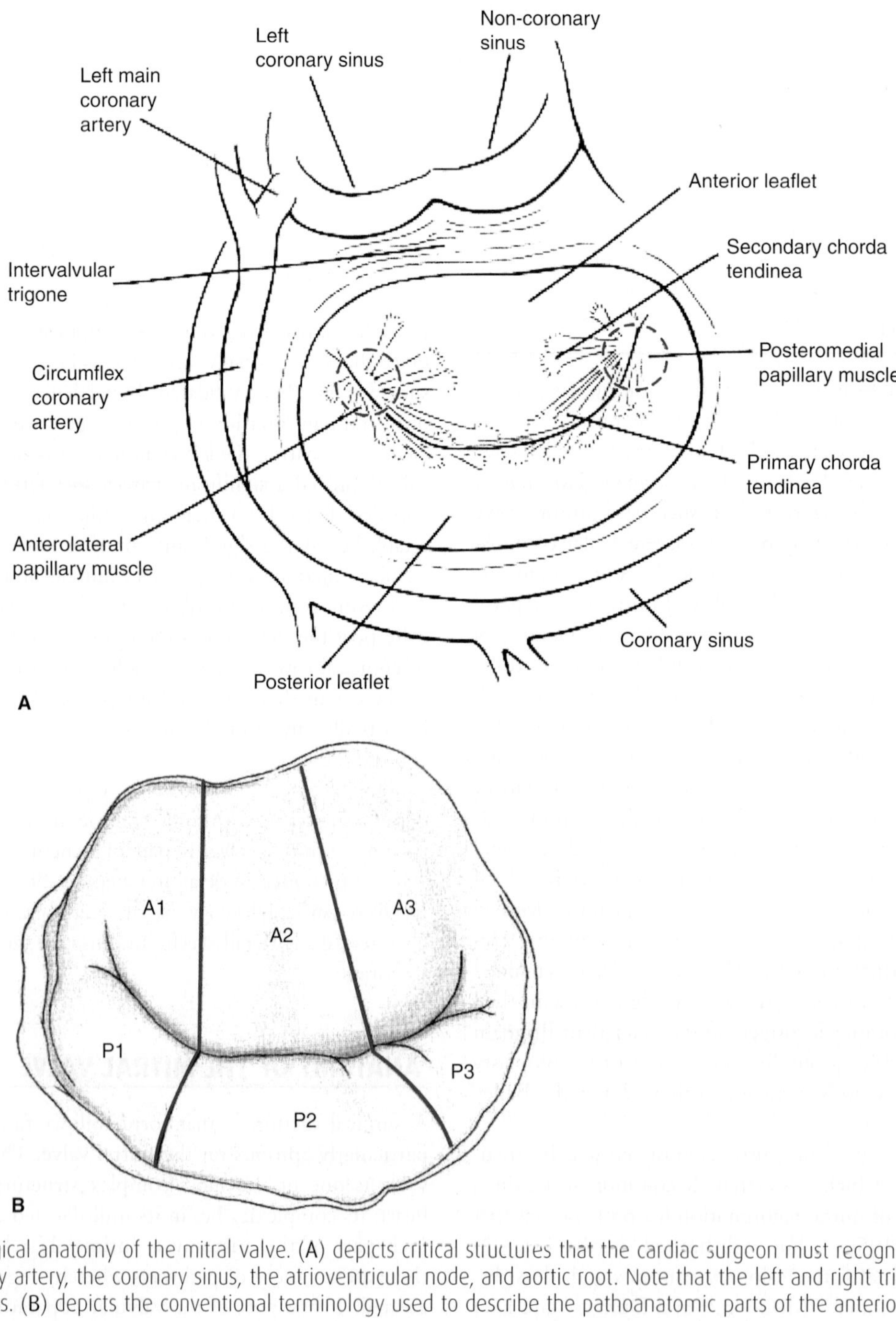

FIGURE 41-1 Surgical anatomy of the mitral valve. (A) depicts critical structures that the cardiac surgeon must recognize, including the circumflex coronary artery, the coronary sinus, the atrioventricular node, and aortic root. Note that the left and right trigones are superior to the commissures. (B) depicts the conventional terminology used to describe the pathoanatomic parts of the anterior and posterior leaflets.

It typically accounts for approximately 40% of the circumference of the annulus, with the posterior leaflet accounting for the rest.[20] The posterior mitral valve leaflet (PML) is crescent-shaped and dilates more commonly in degenerative disease. For surgical decision making and analysis, both the anterior and posterior leaflet are divided into three parts, corresponding to the three scalloped areas of each leaflet (A1, A2, A3 for the anterior leaflet; P1, P2, and P3 for the posterior leaflet; 1 refers to the leftmost, or lateral scallop; 2 the middle scallop; and 3 the rightmost, or medial scallop; Fig. 41-1B).

There are two papillary muscles, the anterolateral and the posteromedial. Each muscle is attached to the leaflets by the chordae tendinae, chords of stringlike fibrous connective tissue. Primary chords are those that attach to the edge of the leaflet. Secondary chords are those that attach to the underside of the leaflet. Tertiary chords (only the posterior leaflet has tertiary chords) are those that attach to the undersurface of the leaflet directly from the ventricular wall instead of from the papillary muscle. The papillary muscles each give off chordae to both leaflets and correspond to the anterolateral and posteromedial commissures of the mitral valve. The anterolateral papillary muscle receives blood from both the left anterior descending artery as well as the circumflex artery; the posteromedial one receives blood usually from only the posterior descending artery or a branch of the circumflex artery. Because of its single coronary blood supply, the posteromedial papillary muscle is more susceptible to infarction and rupture than the anterolateral one.

The left ventricle acts in concert with the papillary muscles via the chordae to pull in the leaflet edges during systole, thereby maintaining the line of coaptation and therefore valve competency. If the left ventricle dilates from any etiology, failure of central leaflet coaptation may occur and regurgitation created. Such regurgitation in a valve with *normal leaflets but dilated annulus* is termed *functional* MR.

MYXOMATOUS MITRAL VALVE DISEASE

Etiology and Pathophysiology

The underlying etiology of myxomatous disease is a defect in the fibroelastic connective tissue of the valvular leaflets, chordae, and annulus.[21] The myxomatous defect leads to an abnormal elongation and redundancy of valve tissue and chordae. Each particular anatomic redundancy creates mitral regurgitation in its own particular manner. Annular dilatation (Fig. 41-2) obliterates the normal coaptation line between the anterior and posterior leaflet, causing regurgitation. If primarily posterior annular dilatation occurs, there is a separation in the middle of the valve between the two leaflets and blood leaks through during ventricular contraction. Leaflet redundancy results in a movement of the redundant leaflet into the left atrium during diastole. If severe enough, that movement leads to a compromised coaptation line and mitral regurgitation (MR) then occurs. Elongation of the chordae also causes leaflet tissue to move into the atrium during diastole, also resulting in compromised coaptation. Ruptured or flail leaflets are often the result

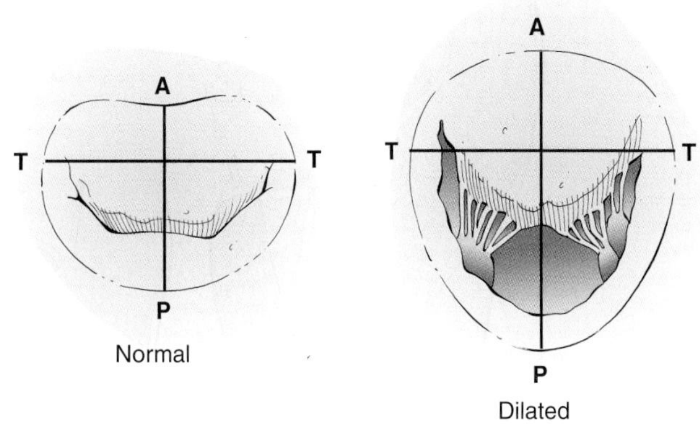

FIGURE 41-2 Annular dilatation. A = anterior; P = posterior; T = trigone.

of systolic stresses fracturing weakened chordae, causing severe regurgitation.

Mitral regurgitation represents pure volume overload for the left ventricle.[22] In myxomatous disease, MR is typically of the chronic compensated variety.[23] A vicious circle is perpetuated whereby the excess volume load over time results in ventricular failure. Ventricular failure itself implies ventricular dilatation, which results in a greater degree of MR. Thus, MR begets more MR, so a vicious downward spiral is created.[17] MR created by left ventricular failure occurs primarily by ventricular dilatation. Successful repair will result in left ventricular mass reduction.[24] By dint of the papillary muscles, ventricular dilatation "pulls" or "tethers" the leaflets open, thereby impinging on coaptation. In degenerative disease of the mitral valve, however, the left ventricle itself per se does not primarily cause MR in the early course of the disease.

Carpentier[10] has developed a mitral valve analysis protocol and surgical philosophy for repair of all types of valves (Fig. 41-3). Myxomatous disease has become the pathology responsible for the vast majority of patients with mitral regurgitation in the United States.[25] Currently, mitral valve prolapse, as a part of the spectrum of degenerative disease, is present in about 5% of the general population,[26] with about 10% of these patients exhibiting severe MR requiring surgery.[27] Whatever the ultimate pathologic pathway creating regurgitation, more than 90% of all degenerative disease should be amenable to successful repair.

Diagnostic Work-Up and Indications for Operation

Patient presentation is typically quite varied depending on the degree of MR as well as the chronicity of the disease. Patients may be floridly symptomatic or completely asymptomatic. Symptomatology is usually of two varieties. Heart failure symptoms are secondary to pulmonary venous hypertension as well as fluid retention. This may include shortness of breath, limited exertional capacity, fluid overload, and in the late stage of the disease, frank heart failure. Embolization sequelae and arrhythmias form a second set of symptoms and include atrial fibrillation and increased stroke risk;[28] regurgitation predisposes the

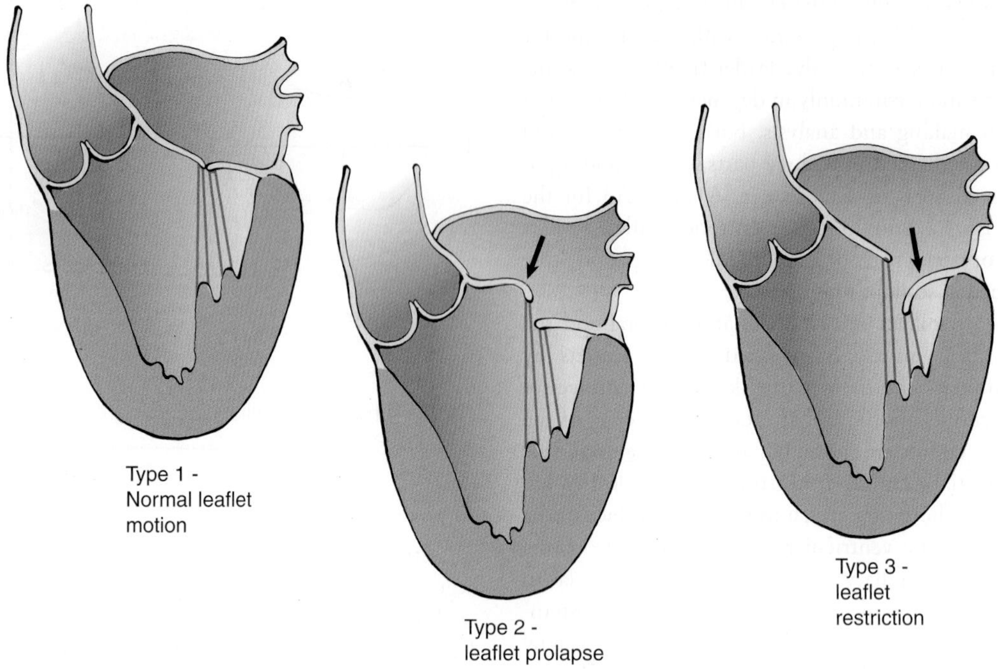

FIGURE 41-3 Carpentier classic mitral valve classification.

valve to infectious endocarditis.[29] Abnormal hemodynamics create pathologic shear stresses and turbulence that generates vulnerability to infection in the valve.

The critical question for any valvular pathology is the timing of surgery. The first consideration is the MR itself. The key information obtained from echocardiography is the degree of MR, its associated pathophysiology, cardiac chamber dimensions, and left ventricular functional analysis. Transthoracic echocardiography is usually the first modality employed. However, if images from transthoracic echocardiography are of insufficient quality, then transesophageal echocardiography (TEE) is required. Mitral regurgitation is graded on a scale from mild to severe with severe typically referring to a reversal of pulmonary venous blood flow in the left atrium.[30] Methods used to determine the degree of regurgitation commonly include regurgitant volume, regurgitant fraction, and orifice area.[30] Echocardiographic analysis of the MR (eg, flail leaflet, ruptured chordae, or anterior or posterior prolapse) is extremely helpful in planning the operative intervention. Other crucial information obtained by the preoperative echo includes left atrial size, ventricular function, ventricular dilatation, aortic valve function, and tricuspid valve function. A large left atrium implies chronic MR. A small LA and hyperdynamic LV implies acute MR. Ventricular function is a key component in assessing operative candidacy; a left ventricular ejection fraction below the norm of 60% indicates some degree of myocardial decompensation secondary to volume overload. Indeed, in the presence of severe MR, the ejection fraction will often decline postoperatively even if the preop ejection fraction is normal. A corollary of this fact is a normal preoperative ejection fraction does not necessarily mean normal ventricular function.

What, precisely, are the indications for operation? In general, as surgical results improve, the indications for surgery are broadening. Patients who would never have been considered for surgery previously are now routinely being offered repair surgery at much earlier stages of their disease. The indications for mitral valve repair have widened as the success of repair has so dramatically improved over the last several years. Better myocardial protection and cardiopulmonary bypass technology, minimally invasive incisions, increased incidence of repair, and better intensive care unit support have all contributed to the phenomenon.[31] The biggest change has been an overall broadening of the indications for mitral valve repair and lowering of the threshold for operation because of these factors,[32] even in the elderly.[33] Increasingly, asymptomatic mitral regurgitation, even without symptoms, is becoming accepted as a reasonable strategy.[34]

Repair itself, as opposed to replacement, is now accepted as the superior treatment for myxomatous mitral regurgitation. Out of a long laboratory and clinical experience has come the conclusions that repair is associated with better survival, enhanced preservation of ventricular function (by preserving the chordae and papillary muscles), and decreased late thromboembolic complications.[35–42]

Whether or not a patient is offered valve repair depends on the degree of regurgitation, the pathophysiology of the regurgitation, ventricular function, and surgeons' consistent ability to perform mitral valve repair. At Brigham and Women's Hospital, virtually any patient with severe myxomatous MR is offered mitral valve repair, regardless of symptoms and ventricular function, unless other comorbidities make repair problematic. Asymptomatic patients are offered valve repair if evidence exists of myocardial decompensation by echocardiography, such as cardiac chamber enlargement or pulmonary hypertension. Such patients will usually demonstrate left ventricular or left atrial dilatation or both. Atrial fibrillation, either paroxysmal or chronic, is also a relative indication for surgery.

For all patients with moderate to severe MR and moderately decreased ventricular function (left ventricular ejection fraction <60%) valve repair is offered, because the ventricle has exhibited signs of decompensation even with a lesser degree of MR; repair in this setting is much more urgent, because severe decompensation can occur in a matter of months as left ventricular function begins to deteriorate.

The standard of care for patients with severe cardiomyopathy and severe MR is unclear presently and is one of the most controversial topics in cardiac surgery. This situation typically does not occur with myxomatous disease but rather ischemia or idiopathic cardiomyopathy and such regurgitation is functional in nature. In longstanding myxomatous disease, however, LV dysfunction may be present.

The intermediate situation of moderate mitral regurgitation and preserved ventricular function is the one in which the most judgment must be exercised. Consider the situation of a structurally normal mitral valve with moderate functional MR, but with concomitant critical aortic stenosis. The patient is to undergo an aortic valve replacement. Should the mitral valve be repaired? Perhaps not, as the moderate MR here is typically exacerbated by the patient's aortic stenosis and volume overload, and correction of the aortic stenosis and euvoluemia would likely reduce or eliminate the MR in this structurally normal valve.[39,40] However, should repair be undertaken, ring annuloplasty would be needed to correct the posterior annular dilatation. If the same situation exists, however, with a structurally abnormal valve, such as a prolapsed P2 or markedly dilated mitral annulus in a myxomatous valve, then mitral repair should always be undertaken, because there is a structural abnormality that aortic valve replacement will not correct. What of moderate MR secondary to myxomatous disease (and not ischemia) in a patient who is to undergo coronary bypass grafting? That patient would likely be offered concomitant valve repair, because bypass grafting would not impact on the pathophysiology of the MR in this case. What of the situation of moderate to severe, isolated MR secondary to myxomatous disease and borderline normal ventricular function? Even without symptoms of heart failure, this patient should have repair performed on an elective basis. Once left ventricular function begins to deteriorate from the normal 60 to 70% left ventricular ejection fraction, decline may be unpredictably rapid and hence intervention warranted. Increasingly, moderate ischemic, as well as degenerative, MR is thought to be detrimental for long-term survival.[41,42]

In general, no matter what the chronological age is, adequate functional status before valve repair is preferred. If symptoms of heart failure exist before surgery, optimal diuresis should be undertaken before operation. If the procedure involves coronary artery bypass grafting, the conduit status should be determined. Dental clearance on all patients should be obtained before any valvular procedure. If neurologic symptoms exist or if the patient has a history of a previous cerebrovascular disease, then preoperative carotid noninvasive studies are warranted to assess carotid arterial stenosis. All patients older than 40 years should undergo coronary angiography. Since the late 1990s patients with MR without coronary artery disease have been offered minimally invasive valve repair as the standard procedure at Brigham and Women's Hospital.[43,45]

Whatever the scenario, the decision to operate and repair the valve is a decision made preoperatively as opposed to intraoperatively. Once the patient is under anesthesia, loading conditions are not physiologic and the mitral regurgitation assessed then is inevitably underestimated. Maneuvers used to "bring out the MR," such as increasing afterload with vasoactive drugs, do not reflect true physiology, but should be used in surgical decision making and may be helpful in some situations. Recent discussions of earlier referral for the treatment of MR clearly depend on a high rate of valve repair in any center.[46,47]

Operative Philosophy

Despite the success of mitral valve repair in specialized centers, there still persists a general reluctance to perform repair, particularly in severe degenerative disease. In 2003, for example, the Society of Thoracic Surgeons database indicated that only 36% of valves that could be repaired actually were repaired,[48] although this percentage has recently improved. Recent studies indicate that this percentage may now be as high as 69%.[49]

Beginning in the 1980s, we have developed what we think is a simple, reproducible algorithm that can be used to repair the degenerative mitral valve in most patients. Overriding this philosophy is the belief that mitral valve repair is not an esoteric "art form" that is difficult to explain, perform, or learn. Rather, we think it is a procedure like any other that should and can be simplified, disseminated, and reproduced with success. In keeping with this philosophy, we have reduced complicated bileaflet prolapse to a competent valve with simplified and straightforward maneuvers that we have found effective with good long-term results. Our overall philosophy and technique is as follows:

1. Expose the valve well through the complete development of Sondergaard's groove, division of pericardial attachments of the superior and inferior venae cavae, release of the left pericardial retraction stitches.
2. Assess the valve through saline injection and corroborate the intraoperative findings with transesophageal echocardiography.
3. Perform basic, obvious leaflet repair procedures first (eg, quadrangular resections to the posterior leaflet).
4. Implant the annuloplasty ring sized by the height of the anterior leaflet (not the trigones or commissures).
5. Test the repair.
6. Perform additional reparative procedures as needed, ie, cleft closure.

With the above maneuvers, we estimate that approximately 95% of all degenerative valves can be repaired.

Collaborative involvement with cardiac anesthesia colleagues is essential in utilizing the invaluable tool of transesophageal echocardiogram monitoring for pre and postrepair assessment. In our clinic, standard TEE monitoring (either two-dimensional or three-dimensional) is now utilized for every patient undergoing mitral valve repair. In addition to documenting the efficacy of repair, TEE is essential in preventing and assessing the potential or persistence of systolic anterior motion of the anterior valve.

Operative Exposure

Because the mitral valve is such a complex anatomic structure and the maneuvers involved in correcting a regurgitant valve may vary from the simple to the very complex, adequate exposure is an absolute requirement in every operative plan. This becomes more important if minimally invasive techniques are employed. Mitral valve exposure is more challenging than exposure of the aortic or tricuspid valve. Why? From the surgeon's side, the mitral valve is furthest away from the operating surgeon than any other valve. In addition, the valve in its native position naturally faces above and/or towards the surgeon's left shoulder at an oblique angle such that the surgeon does not see the valve en face.

The first critical aspect to the standard valve repair is the complete and thorough development of the Sondergaard plane reflecting the right atrium off the left atrium to the atrial septum, as depicted in Fig. 41-4. This was first described in the 1950s by the Danish surgeon Sondergaard,[50] to expose the atrial septum for noncardiopulmonary bypass treatment of atrial septal defects. In 1990 we stressed the importance of this particular technique for exposure in mitral valve surgery.[51] Regardless of even previous procedures, it should always be possible to dissect out the groove without significant difficulty. The complete and full development of the groove is a most important aspect to obtain adequate exposure of the mitral valve. With this technique, via blunt and sharp dissection we typically have not needed any other incision for mitral valve repair or replacement, whether for primary surgery or reoperation. This incision usually brings the surgeon very close to the mitral valve. Once the right atrium is dissected off the left atrium, a generous incision in the left atrium is made, avoiding the atrial septum.

The second aspect of exposure is to bring the valve as close to an en face position to the operating surgeon as possible. Pericardial stay sutures are released on the left side. The operating table is maneuvered head up and to the left. If necessary, the left pericardium is opened and the apex of the heart moved laterally to the left pleural space. Exposure of the left trigone can be particularly challenging for stitch placement. This can be facilitated with local epicardial displacement of the midlateral LV wall medially with a spongestick.

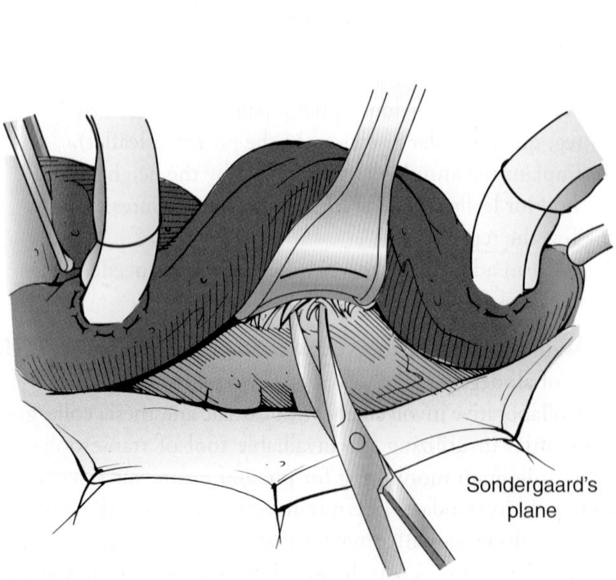

FIGURE 41-4 Dissection of Sondergaard's plane. Sondergaard's plane should be dissected at least 2 to 4 cm from the right superior pulmonary vein for adequate exposure of the mitral valve.

Minimally Invasive Techniques

With the development of minimally invasive incisions for adult cardiac surgery this past decade, mitral valve surgery has undergone an evolution. Isolated minimally invasive mitral valve repair has been offered at Brigham and Women's Hospital since 1996 as a lower hemisternotomy via a 6- to 8-cm skin incision[43,44,71] (Fig. 41-5A). Cannulation is typically performed with a percutaneous venous cannula via the femoral vein and vacuum-assisted drainage is employed (Fig. 41-5B). The vacuum applied never exceeds 80 mm Hg of suction. TEE guidance is used to place the venous cannula into the superior vena cava through the right atrium. The aorta is cannulated directly with a flexible 20F aortic perfusor. If venous drainage is inadequate even with vacuum assist, we cannulate the superior vena cava with an additional cannula. Other minimally invasive techniques are detailed in Chapter 44.

In obese patients, or those with large anterior posterior dimensions, minimally invasive techniques may not be feasible. In these situations, a full sternotomy should be performed. Furthermore, a transseptal incision may be more optimal than Sondergard's groove for these patients.

Cardiopulmonary Bypass

For cardiopulmonary bypass, we use a 22F percutaneous femoral vein venous catheter placed into the right atrium via the right femoral vein with TEE control. The cannula can even be advanced into the superior vena cava if desired. Because the cannula has multiple holes, is flexible and thus can still drain the inferior vena cava, this one cannula is sometimes all that is needed for drainage of both the superior and inferior vena cava. If performing a concomitant bypass procedure requiring a full sternotomy, then venous cannulation should be bicaval via the atria. One venous cannula should be placed in the superior vena cava above the right atrial/superior vena caval junction and the other through the lowest part of the right atrium into the mouth of the inferior vena cava. The arterial cannula should be placed directly into the distal ascending aorta.

Once on cardiopulmonary bypass, systemic temperature is allowed to drift to 34°, the ascending aorta is cross-clamped, and the heart arrested by cold blood cardioplegia. For isolated valve repair, some debate still exists regarding the use of retrograde or antegrade blood cardioplegia after cross-clamping. If there is concomitant coronary artery disease, myocardial protection in this circumstance should be antegrade and retrograde, because the coronary artery bypass graft/mitral operation presents one of the highest-risk operative settings in cardiac surgery.[36]

After the heart is arrested, the left atrium is opened well above the right superior pulmonary vein near the septum inferiorly. Retractors are placed (Fig. 41-6). The patient's bed is

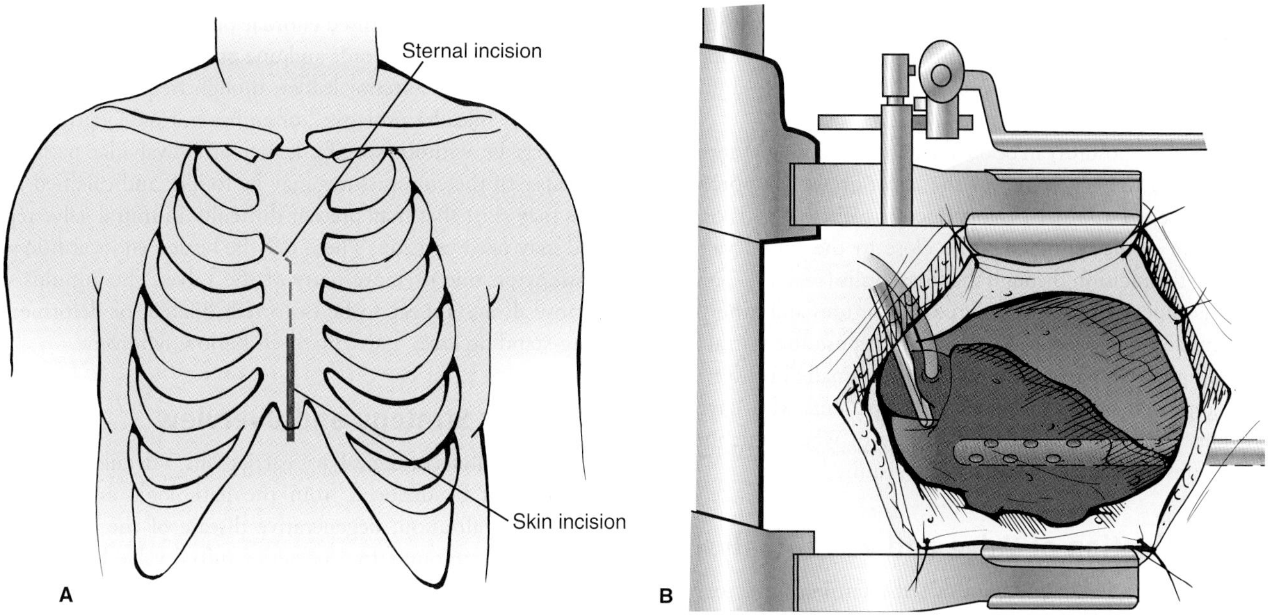

FIGURE 41-5 Minimally invasive mitral valve repair. (A) Via a 6- to 8-cm skin incision, a lower hemisternotomy through the right second interspace is performed. (B) Venous cannulation is percutaneous with vacuum assist. Aortic cannulation, cross-clamping, and cardioplegia administration are performed in the standard manner.

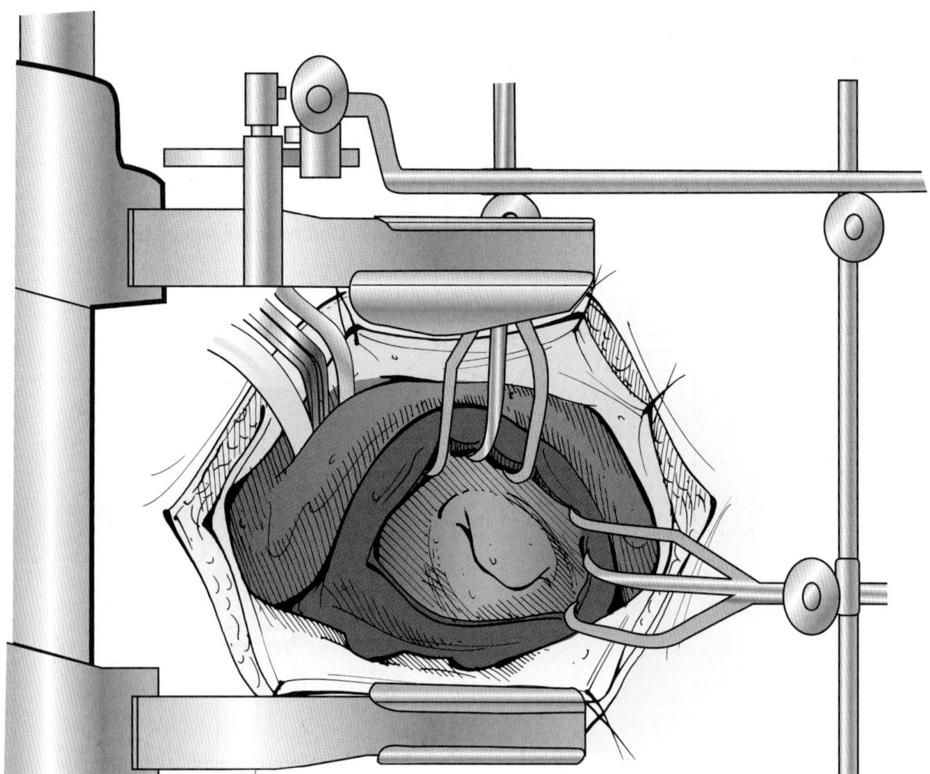

FIGURE 41-6 Minimally invasive operative exposure. After the retractors are placed, the patient is positioned with head up and the operative bed tilted to the left. Exposure is excellent.

placed head up with a tilt to the left. A wire-reinforced suction catheter is placed in the left inferior pulmonary vein (the most dependent portion of the left atrium in this position) for drainage of collateral blood flow. Carbon dioxide is infused to minimize intracardiac air.

Alternate exposures can be obtained by the transseptal approach through the right atrium[52] or the superior septal approach.[53] The transseptal approach is a perfectly acceptable incision that allows the cardiac surgeon to be close to the mitral valve by carrying the incision through the fossa ovalis (Fig. 41-7) and up into the superior vena cava. Retraction sutures and other types of retraction devices can be utilized to expose the mitral valve exceedingly well, particularly in these minimally invasive cases. This approach may also be helpful in patients who have had previous operations on the mitral valve or when concomitant procedures on the tricuspid valve are required.

Examination of Valve and Valve Analysis

Once exposure is obtained and a self-retaining retractor is in place, inspection of the valve is carried out. Valve analysis takes a few minutes utilizing nerve hooks, forceps, and insufflation of the ventricle with saline to determine and corroborate the pathology already diagnosed by intraoperative TEE. Valve analysis may reveal ruptured chordae or simply a prolapse of the valve with elongated chords and one or more prolapsed sections of the valve. The anterior leaflet, though frequently advertised as part of "bileaflet prolapse," often has normal length chordae and may be without specific leaflet or subvalvular pathology. Prolapse of the commissures may be found, and calcified nodules may exist that may present difficulty in mitral valve repair and may need excision. There may be healed endocarditic vegetations on one or more parts of the valve. The annulus will almost always appear to be distorted, dilated, or deformed in long-standing cases, particularly in Barlow syndrome.

Repair Strategy and Overview

After the analysis of the valve is carried out, a detailed reparative strategy can be deduced from the pathologic analysis. In a broad generalization, degenerative disease of the mitral valve creates what amounts to a posterior mitral valve leaflet that is too large, with or without flail segments, in an annulus that is functionally too small for the anterior leaflet. In degenerative disease, the posterior leaflet is typically pathologic whereas the anterior leaflet usually is not.

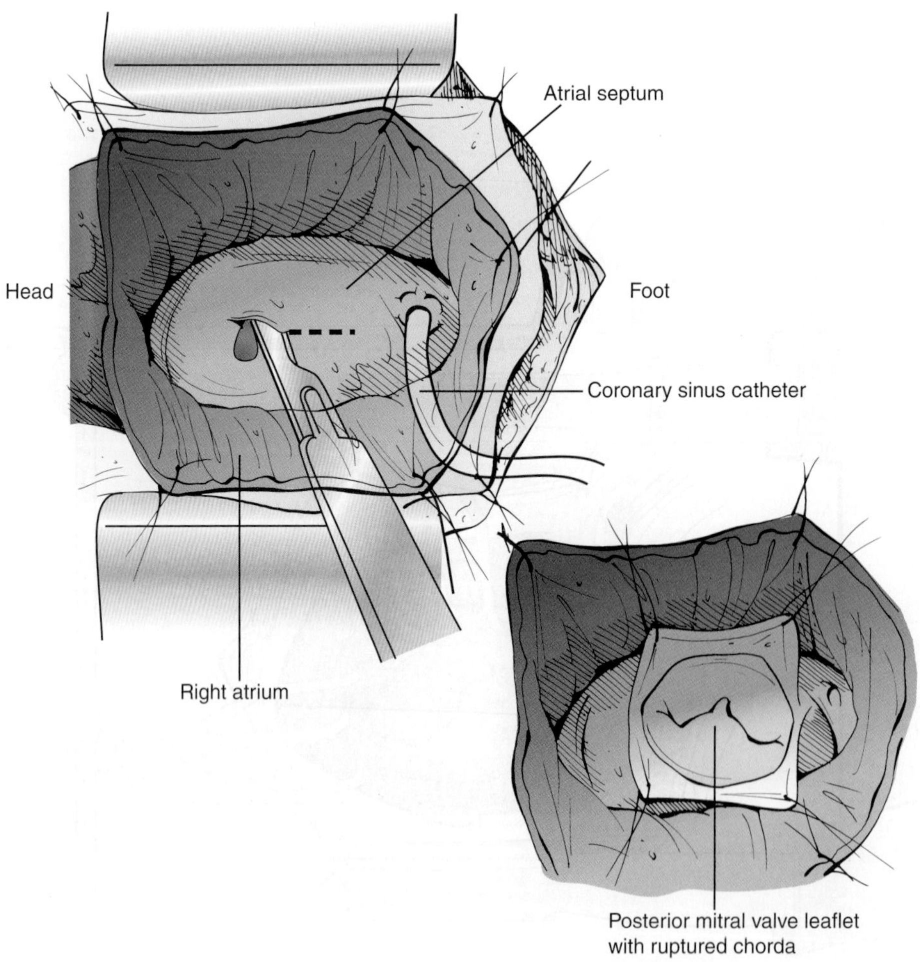

FIGURE 41-7 Transseptal exposure of the mitral valve. After the right atrium is incised, the septum is divided across the fossa ovalis, and stay sutures are placed. This incision allows very good access to the mitral valve and is an alternative to the Sondergaard plane.

The first principle of the repair is to reduce or obliterate the enlarged segments and to reduce the overall height of the abnormally large posterior leaflet. This reduction reconstructs the correct coaptation line with the anterior leaflet, and, just as importantly, prevents systolic anterior motion (SAM) of the anterior leaflet. If the height of the posterior leaflet is too high, it will push the anterior leaflet into the LVOT and create SAM. In general, the height of the posterior leaflet should be no more than 1 to 1.5 cm in average-sized patients once the repair is complete. The normal sections of the posterior leaflet should be used as a marker to guide the reduction of the redundant parts. Ultimately, the reconstructed posterior leaflet should appear like a "smile." Once the posterior leaflet reduction is performed, one must ensure that the anterior leaflet coapts with the subsequently reduced posterior leaflet within the correct plane using the saline test. The resulting repair should result in a coaptation line at the level of the annulus during systole. Specific methods to lower the height of the posterior leaflet and anterior leaflet will be addressed below.

The second principle is that a remodeling annuloplasty ring is essential for all repairs. This is a fundamental concept of Carpentier[18] and Duran,[54] both of whom developed mitral valve annuloplasty rings early in the history of mitral valve regurgitation surgery and advocated remodeling of the distorted annulus as a key principle of mitral valve repair. The annulus, after many years of regurgitation, is often deformed and in myxomatous disease, it is floppy and dilated. The best approach to conceptualize the floppy and dilated annulus in myxomatous disease is to consider it functionally too small for the anterior leaflet. Why too small if it is floppy and dilated? If floppy with redundant tissue, the annulus will not provide the relatively stable skeleton necessary for the anterior leaflet to spread out completely and thus coapt at the correct line and in the correct plane with the posterior leaflet. Rather, the floppy annulus will buckle and have an effectively smaller radius, and cause the anterior leaflet to appear as though it is "prolapsing" because the leaflet cannot spread out correctly. In reality the pathology is within the annulus. That is why we believe that oversizing the ring in degenerative disease is important. The ring then recreates the relatively rigid, broad annulus that allows the anterior leaflet to spread out and coapt in the correct plane, at the correct coaptation line, without "prolapsing." A structurally sound annulus is necessary for the correct physiologic function of the anterior leaflet. Hence, our protocol is to place the annuloplasty ring after posterior leaflet repair and then reassess for any anterior or complex leaflet pathology afterward. Our belief is that annular pathology often falsely gives the appearance of leaflet pathology, and by following the steps outlined above, many unnecessary procedures are prevented.

By utilizing the two principles outlined above, we believe that the proper and necessary attention is given to the correct physiologic functioning of the valve in a manner that is surgically relevant. The height of the posterior leaflet is reduced to prevent SAM as well as to allow the correct coaptation plane. The two leaflets are made to coapt at the correct line by reinforcing the annulus with a remodeling ring. As outlined above, in our experience at the Brigham and that of others,[55] many times the so-called bileaflet prolapse is completely eliminated by adequate posterior leaflet resection and a large remodeling annuloplasty ring without any further anterior leaflet intervention.

There is clear evidence supporting the integral and essential necessity of the ring for a lasting repair. In an early paper on mitral valve repair, we compared a repair group that had no annuloplasty ring to another group in whom a ring was implanted at the time of valve repair.[56] All valves were competent at the time of surgery, but after several years of follow-up, the rate of mitral regurgitation in the no-ring group was five times that of the ring group. Recent studies have supported the importance of ring annuloplasty.[57] Thus, a remodeling ring is critical to a long-lasting physiologic mitral valve repair.

SPECIFIC SURGICAL TECHNIQUES

Posterior Leaflet Quadrangular Resection

The most common mitral valve pathologies (approximately 80%) encountered in the myxomatous, degenerated valve are ruptured and elongated chords from the middle section of the posterior leaflet (Fig. 41-8A). In one approach limited resection of this diseased section of leaflet is shown in Fig. 41-8B. To fill the gap produced by removing the pathologic section, leaflet advancement of the remaining leaflet sections is carried out (Fig. 41-8C and D) and the cut edges of the valve are reapproximated with running monofilament suture (Fig. 41-8E, F, and G). An annuloplasty ring is then implanted (Fig. 41-8H, I, and J). This scenario is the most common pathophysiology encountered and operative strategy employed. Interestingly, recent results by Perier[58] and Lawrie[59] have reported successful results with use of only artificial polytetrafluoroethylene (PTFE) chords to preserve the posterior leaflet instead of resecting it, a technique that has traditionally been applied only to the anterior leaflet.

For cardiac surgeons who perform a modest number of valve repairs, incising the posterior leaflet off the annulus may be somewhat daunting. In our own experience, a prolapsed leaflet without ruptured chordae at P2 may simply be obliterated by a few sutures to bring the leading edge of the prolapsed leaflet to the underside of the annular connection, thus reducing the height, preserving all the chords, and accomplishing what might be done with a resection.[61]

If the repair includes a resection of a flail segment, then some form of the leaflet advancement technique popularized by Carpentier should be employed.[60] In this technique the two remaining sections are advanced upon each other to close the gap produced by the resected area. This includes separating each remaining segment off the annulus for a short segment. Of all the traditional techniques, this is the one that has produced some concern for surgeons who perform only moderate numbers of valve repairs because of the necessity of incising the posterior leaflet off the annulus and then reanastomosing the leaflet to the annulus.

We have evolved a simplified technique for limited PML resections in which leaflet advancement may be more easily performed, and yet still accomplish the exact same result in much less time. We have named this the "fold-over leaflet advancement." In this technique the remaining enlarged segments of P2, on either side of the elongated resected leaflet with supporting

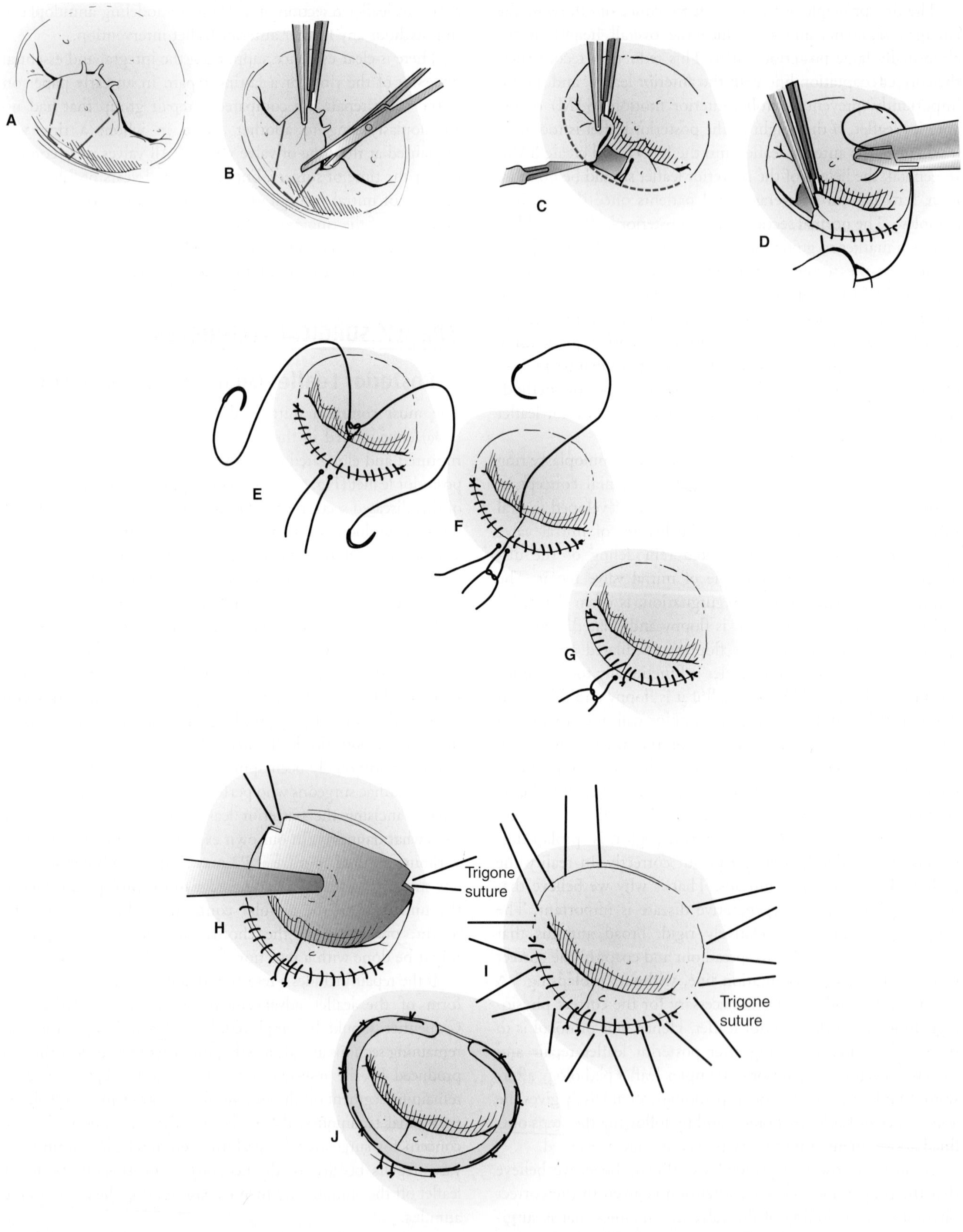

FIGURE 41-8 Repair of P2 with flail segment with ruptured chordae. (A) demonstrates the classic flail P2 segment. (B) demonstrates resection of this flail segment. (C) and (D) demonstrates the classic sliding valvuloplasty and advancement, in which each segment of the valve adjacent to the resected P2 segment is separated from the annulus. The valve is then reattached with the gap eliminated. At the same time, the height of the posterior leaflet is reduced. (E), (F), and (G) demonstrates completion of the classic sliding valvuloplasty. (H), (I), and (J) illustrates placement of the annuloplasty stitches and ring placement. Sizing of the ring is done by the size of the anterior leaflet.

chordae, are simply folded over by a continuous polypropylene suture to the annular gap produced by the limited posterior leaflet resection, without any further incision (Fig. 41-9). The fold-over advancement accomplishes the same goals as the traditional leaflet advancement. The small gap distance, created by the small area of resected flail segment, is eliminated and the height of the posterior leaflet is reduced. We have found the fold-over advancement to be extremely effective for small resections of the posterior leaflet in any position without the necessity of incising the leaflet off the annulus.

That being stated, many situations exist with true Barlow syndrome with elongation and elevation of almost the entire posterior leaflet. In essence, the whole posterior leaflet is elongated. In these particular pathologic situations, the classic techniques are mandatory. The entire posterior leaflet on both sides of the resected area, including P1 and P3, must be incised off the annulus and a careful and detailed valve advancement carried out, beginning at each commissure, with running 4-0 polypropylene (see Fig. 41-8C and D). The height of the leaflet is lowered to avoid creation of SAM and provide a good coaptation point for the anterior leaflet. Because some of these leaflets may be as high as 3 to 4 cm, if the height of the leaflet is not shortened significantly, SAM is highly likely. While performing the leaflet advancement, imbrication of PML segment areas may also be effective if there is focal enlargement at a particular area of the leaflet. This simplifies the surgical technique, reduces operative time, and achieves the same result. Multiple interrupted mattress sutures may be used.

Commissural Prolapse

As the most straightforward example of pathologic valve prolapse, chordal rupture or elongation at the anteriorlateral or posteriormedial commissure provides the surgeon with the most obvious strategy of repair. Many surgeons still recommend resection of this area, but commissuroplasty is by far the most simple, direct, and efficient way to handle this particular problem. The prolapsed area is obliterated by one to

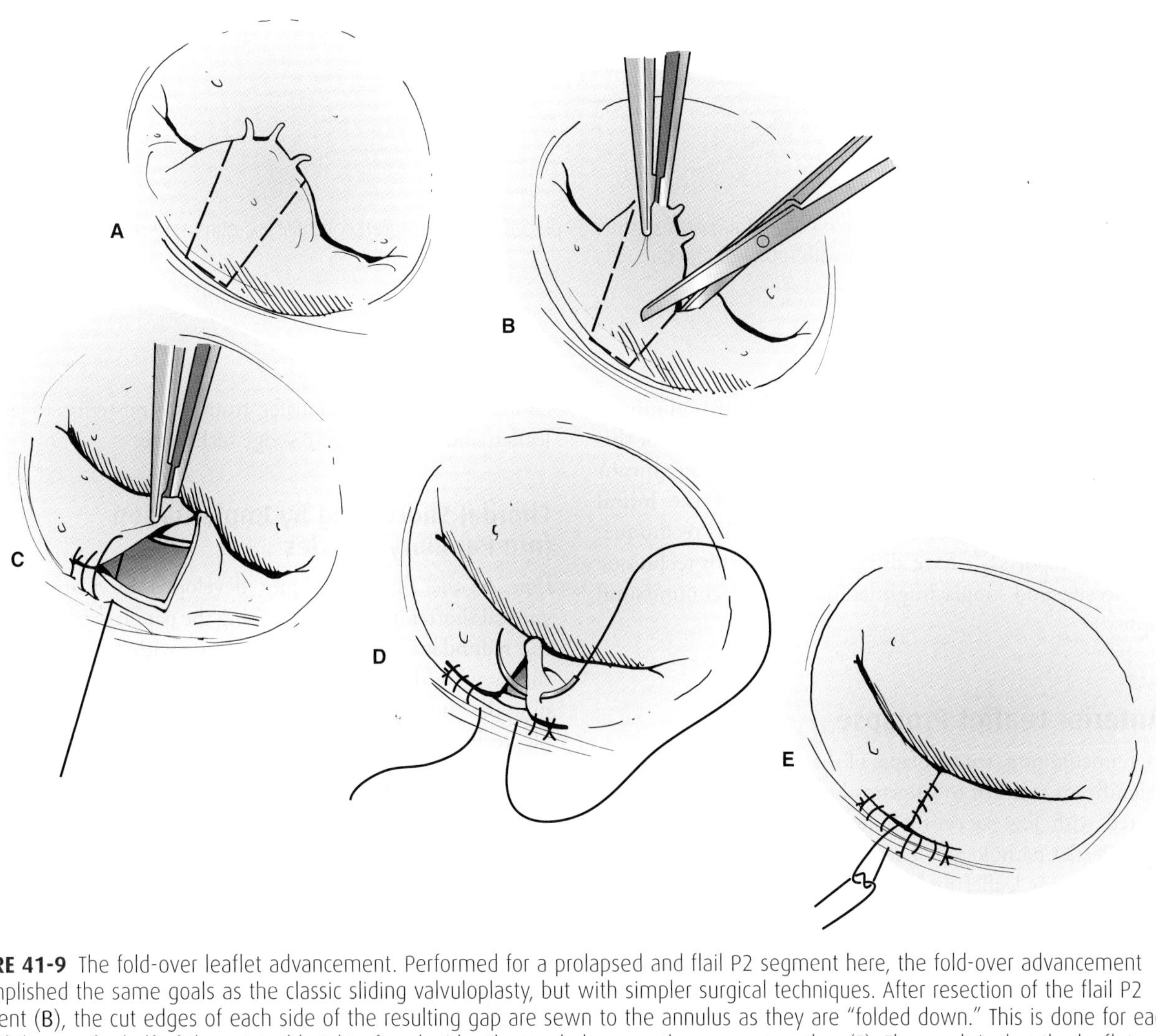

FIGURE 41-9 The fold-over leaflet advancement. Performed for a prolapsed and flail P2 segment here, the fold-over advancement accomplished the same goals as the classic sliding valvuloplasty, but with simpler surgical techniques. After resection of the flail P2 segment (B), the cut edges of each side of the resulting gap are sewn to the annulus as they are "folded down." This is done for each side of the gap for half of the original height of each side. The top halves are then sewn together (E). The result is that the leaflet gap is eliminated and the height of the leaflet reduced.

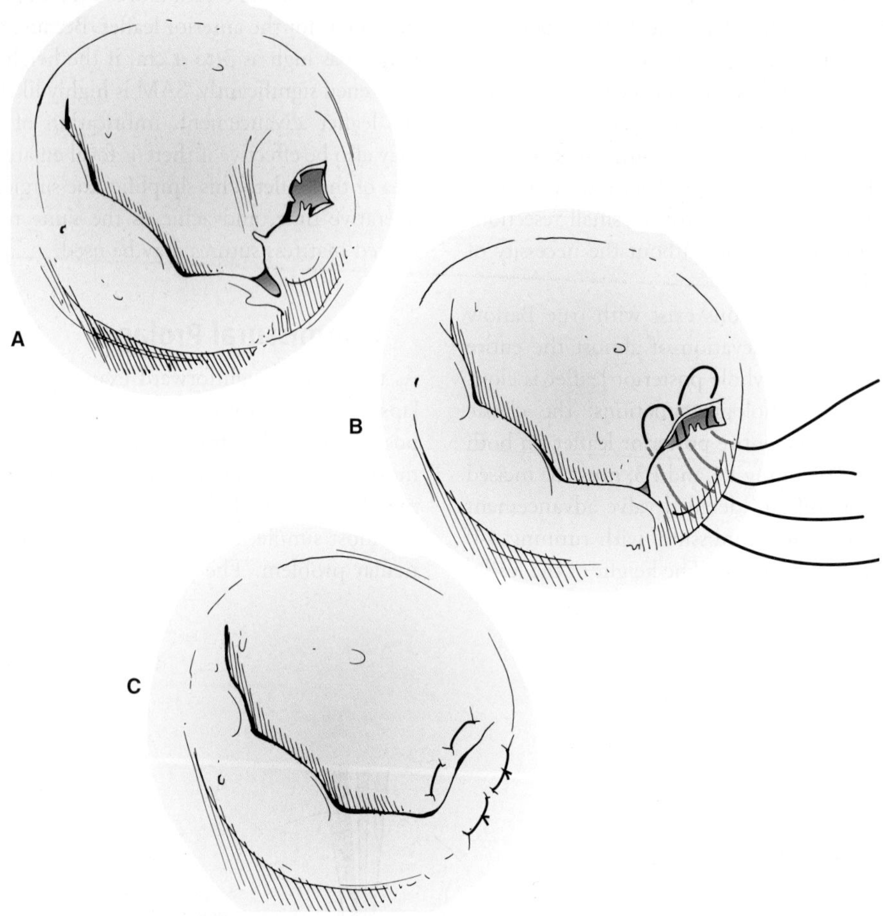

FIGURE 41-10 Commissuroplasty. Simple horizontal mattress stitches placed in the ruptured commissure eliminate regurgitation without need for further leaflet resection, even with ruptured chordae.

three polypropylene mattress stitches (Fig. 41-10), eliminating the regurgitation at that point. A small obliteration of this area at A1 and P1 or A3 and P3 will not make any significant difference in the overall cross-sectional area of the mitral valve, so mitral stenosis is of no concern with this technique. Several other reports[62,63] have also documented this technique as an effective and longlasting method to treat commissural prolapse.

Anterior Leaflet Prolapse

Though uncommon, true prolapse of the anterior leaflet engenders significant concern to surgeons because such pathology is associated with less successful long term repair results than posterior leaflet pathology.[64] The height of the chordae underlying the anterior leaflet must be assessed and chords may be grossly elongated or ruptured and make the AML flail. This problem may be addressed by a variety of techniques and the long-term follow-up on many of these techniques has been quite promising. There are four basic techniques to repair true prolapse of the anterior leaflet. They are: (1) reduction of the chordal height by implantation techniques; (2) artificial PTFE chordae; (3) chordal transfer from the posterior to anterior leaflet; and (4) the edge-to-edge technique.

Chordal Shortening by Implantation into Papillary Muscles

One of the first techniques developed by Carpentier[10] of chordal shortening involves incising the papillary muscle, placing the redundant anterior leaflet chords within the muscle, and then sewing the papillary muscle over the chord, thus entrapping the chordae and shortening it (Fig. 41-11). This is a simple technique, but it has gone out of favor, as reports by Cosgrove and coworkers[65] have demonstrated that additional chordal ruptures may occur after use of this technique. They postulate that the potential sawing action of the papillary muscle on the buried chord is the cause. Other techniques of this type include papillary muscle repositioning[66] and chordal plication and free edge (AML) remodeling.[67]

Artificial Chordae

Artificial chordae with PTFE is the technique that is perhaps the most popular current technique for AML pathology.

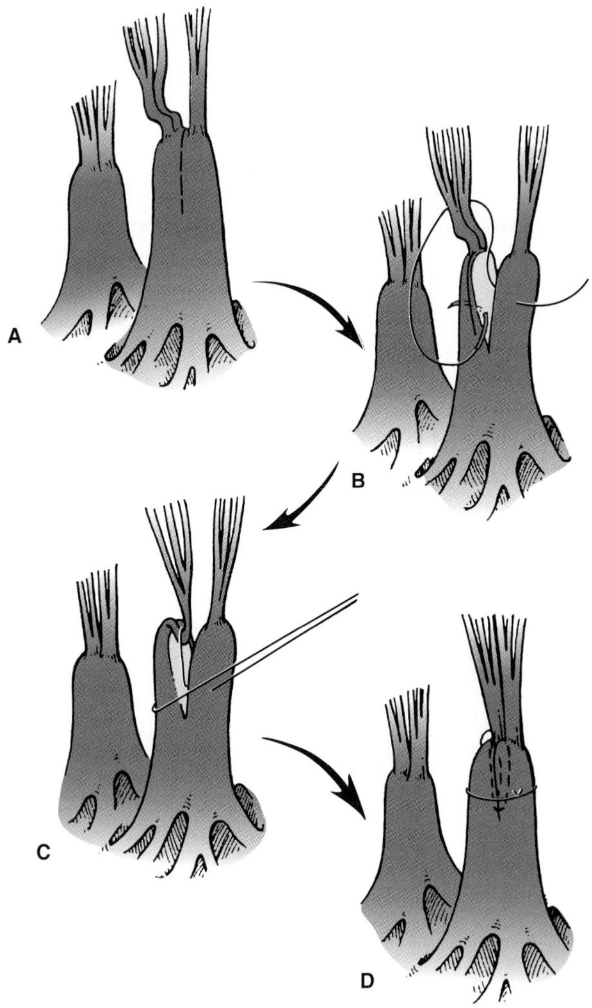

FIGURE 41-11 Anterior leaflet chordal shortening. The papillary muscle is incised and the redundant chord folded into it. The excess chord is held in place with pledgeted sutures.

Originally described by Frater and Zussa,[68,69] this technique has grown in popularity over the past several years.[64,70] Lawrie[59] has also recently reported excellent results in applying PTFE neochords for the anterior and posterior leaflet repair. Duran has devised a method for more precise measurement of the correct height for these new chordal structures.[70] This technique (Fig. 41-12) involves placing a mattress suture with a pledget on the papillary muscle to which the redundant or ruptured chord has been attached. The two ends of the double-armed PTFE are then brought up through the edge of the leaflet that needs to be lowered. The critical part of this technique is determining the degree to which the leaflet is lowered and hence how tightly the stitch is tied down. This is determined by ascertaining the optimal position of the two leaflets in systole. Both the anterior and posterior leaflets should be in apposition at this point, and thus the leaflet's height in systole should be the level to which the chords are adjusted. We have used tenting of the posterior leaflet as our guide while carefully tying down the chord (Fig. 41-12B). Whatever the technique employed, the end result should be that the anterior leaflet now coapts at the same level as the posterior leaflet with left ventricular contraction. Some surgeons advocate neo chordae, as opposed to leaflet resection, as the repair technique of choice for leaflet prolapse.[61]

Chordal Transfer

The third technique for true anterior prolapse is chordal transfer from the posterior leaflet to the anterior leaflet. This was originally described by Carpentier[10] and has been popularized by the Cleveland Clinic[65] and Duran and coworkers.[72] Figure 41-13 illustrates the operative steps. A resection of the flail chordae of the anterior leaflet is carried out, and an adjacent segment of the posterior leaflet is then resected from the posterior leaflet and then transferred to the gap produced by the anterior leaflet resection. This technique has had reportedly good long-term results, but may involve both leaflets when only single leaflet pathology exists.[73]

Edge-to-Edge Technique

The edge-to-edge repair is a technique in which the anterior leaflet and posterior leaflet are sewn together at the coaptation line, producing a double-orifice mitral valve.[74] This has gained considerable popularity and even percutaneous interventional attempts to emulate this surgical maneuver are being pursued.[75] Developed by Alfieri and coworkers,[76] their theory is that with Barlow syndrome or truly redundant anterior leaflets, apposition of the midportion of the anterior leaflet to the midportion of the posterior leaflet will prevent the elevation of the anterior leaflet above the level of the posterior leaflet, thus eliminating mitral regurgitation. This technique greatly simplifies the repair of the true bileaflet prolapse and has been adopted as standard therapy for AML pathology by several groups, especially in those patients with a high probability of postrepair SAM. In particular, with anterior leaflet chordal rupture or marked elongation of the chordae to the anterior leaflet, repair consists of a single stitch carefully placed.

Figure 41-14 illustrates our technique. A figure-of-eight braided polyester suture is placed at the apposition points of the anterior and the posterior leaflet. We use this stronger suture, because there have been reports of the more commonly used polypropylene sutures rupturing. An important point of the surgical technique is our strong belief that the stitch should be placed only with myxomatous valves, so as to avoid producing mitral stenosis as has been the case with ischemic MR.[77] To ensure the adequacy of each orifice created by the edge-to-edge technique, we also measure the diameter of each orifice and confirm that it is at least 2 cm in diameter. If the orifices are less than 2 cm in diameter, the technique is abandoned. This technique is a very valuable adjunct in patients who have the potential for systolic anterior motion of the mitral valve.[78,79] In fact, prevention of SAM may be the best utilization of this technique at present. In our small series of 20 patients with SAM potential, all were treated and SAM was prevented in all patients. A competent mitral valve was maintained in all at 8 years postoperatively.[78]

Medium-term results of this surgical maneuver are satisfactory and compatible with all other commonly used repair techniques, according to studies by Alfieri and coworkers,[76,80] but there have been no comparative, prospective, randomized studies comparing the classic repair techniques to this approach in the long term.

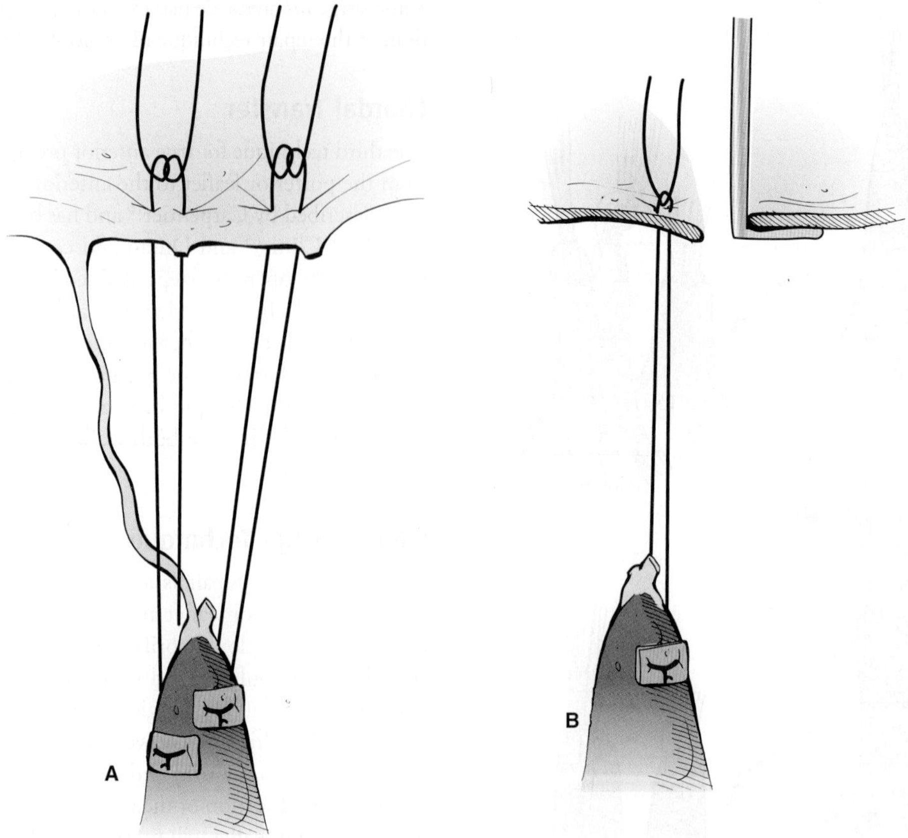

FIGURE 41-12 Artificial PTFE chords for the anterior leaflet. (A) Pledgeted PTFE stitches are placed through a papillary muscle and brought through the leading edge of the anterior leaflet. Using the tented-up posterior leaflet (B), the correct length of artificial chord is created.

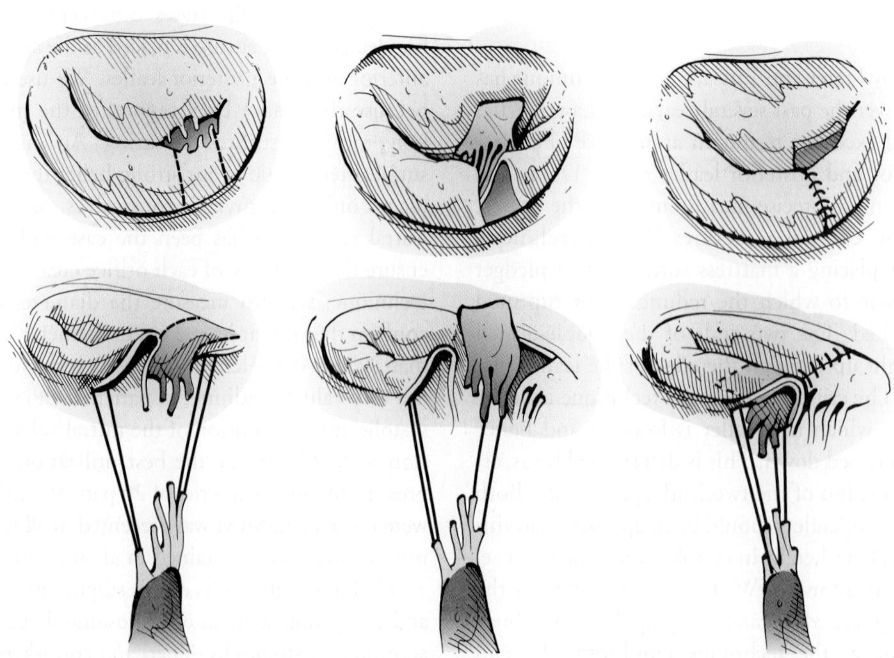

FIGURE 41-13 Chordal transfer. For an isolated flail anterior leaflet segment, first the prolapsed section of anterior leaflet is resected. An adjoining section of posterior leaflet is then resected and transposed over to the gap created by the anterior resection.

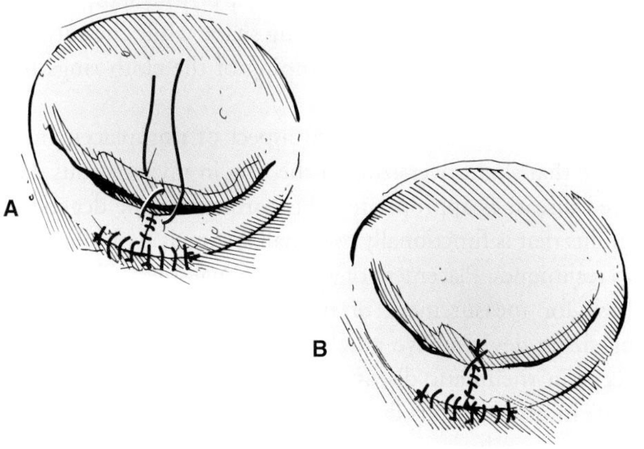

FIGURE 41-14 Edge-to-edge technique. The technique involves a braided polyester figure-of-eight stitch at apposition of A2 and P2.

Resection of the Anterior Leaflet

It has been well established that the body of the anterior leaflet should be treated with great respect, and preservation of AML tissue is important. Resections can be carried out, but only as a small triangular resection for ruptured chords to reduce the bulk of a large anterior leaflet.[81] For anterior mitral valve prolapse associated with idiopathic hypertrophic subaortic stenosis, or as an alternative technique for reduction of the AML height, creation of a longitudinal periannular anterior leaflet resection with reconstruction of the leaflet has also been advocated to reduce the height of the anterior leaflet with some success.[82,83]

SPECIAL PROBLEMS AND CONSIDERATIONS

The Calcified Annulus

Calcification, particularly of the posterior annulus, is a complicating aspect of mitral valve repair. Calcification makes repair more difficult, as stitches are more difficult to place and the risk of paravalvular leak is increased. Severe annular calcification, however, does not necessarily rule out an effective mitral valve repair. Partial or total removal of the calcified bar may be done safely. Carpentier has promulgated removal of the entire calcified bar in radical fashion, which in essence partially detaches the left ventricle from the left atrium.[84] Partial and selective calcification removal may also be quite effective and potentially safer.[85] Partial removal of calcium with leaflet advancement can be performed without the need for a radical debridement in many patients. Only the amount of calcium should be removed that allows adequate stitch placement and leaflet and annular flexibility. Obviously, calcification of the chordae or a substantial part of the leaflet tissue is a poor prognostic factor for long term freedom from valve repair, and an extensively calcified valve usually indicates valve replacement.

Systolic Anterior Motion of the Mitral Valve

As mentioned above, persistent systolic anterior motion of the anterior leaflet is an adverse outcome after valve repair. In this condition, the anterior leaflet obstructs the LVOT. Clearly, increased redundancy of leaflet tissue is a risk factor with a small annuloplasty ring. After repair, if the line of leaflet coaptation is displaced anteriorly, then the anterior leaflet will be displaced into the LVOT and cause LVOT obstruction.[86,87] The etiology is usually inadequate reduction of the height of the posterior leaflet, which then pushes the anterior leaflet into the LVOT. SAM is particularly prevalent in patients with bileaflet prolapse or those with extremely enlarged anterior leaflets. Thus, the PML height reduction has to be meticulously carried out, and in myxomatous valve disease, an upsizing rather than a downsizing of the mitral valve annuloplasty ring should be done. As indicated above, if the anterior leaflet is supported by a relatively small annulus, the anterior leaflet will not spread out and instead will appear to have redundant tissue above the correct plane of coaptation, predisposing to SAM.[78]

Several investigators have looked at the potential echocardiographic risk factors for systolic anterior motion. Echocardiographic details that are associated with a high risk of systolic anterior motion include proximity of the mitral valve coaptation point to the interventricular septum, as well as asymmetry between the anterior and posterior leaflets. If the posterior leaflet is relatively large with respect to the anterior leaflet, then SAM is potentiated. If the medial portion of A2 is larger than the medial portion of A2, then SAM is also potentiated. We look for this information before surgery and take such data into account as the repair strategy is finalized in the operating room.[78,79]

If the probability is high that SAM will occur, our practice is to use the Alfieri edge-to-edge technique to reduce such a risk after lowering the height of the posterior leaflet.[78] By forcing the coaptation line to be correct with a single stitch in the situation of high SAM probability, the probability of SAM is reduced. Another strategy to consider in this circumstance is implantation of PTFE anterior chordae to lower the AML. That will reduce the height of the anterior leaflet, and thus further reduce the potential of SAM. In our own experience long-term competency is maintained in this group.

If SAM appears by TEE following what appears to be an excellent repair, filling the left ventricle with fluid volume post-cardiopulmonary bypass will relieve systolic anterior motion in approximately 90% of patients. In rare circumstances, if an adequate reduction of the posterior leaflet has not been carried out, more posterior leaflet may have to be resected or the ring size increased. The most common alternative in our clinic is the edge-to-edge technique, as mentioned above, for situations where postrepair SAM still exists despite all techniques to reduce it.[78]

Remodeling Ring Annuloplasty

Remodeling the annulus by ring annuloplasty after mitral valve repair is essential to a complete and long lasting repair. The remodeling concept, promulgated by Carpentier[18] and Duran[54] is that the distorted mitral annulus requires restorative structural support. There is debate on which type of ring should be used for remodeling: rigid or soft, complete or partial? Our thought is that it is probably not critical which type of ring is used for myxomatous valve degeneration as long as there is a relative upsizing of the ring and a secure attachment to the trigone area of the anterior mitral leaflet. There is some evidence to suggest that flexible rings may incur less possibility of SAM and that partial rings are safer with respect to SAM.[88] As none of this has been studied in a prospective randomized fashion, these opinions will continue to exist. Though we prefer the Cosgrove ring for mitral valve prolapse, our belief based on over 2000 mitral valve repairs is that the existing evidence is not compelling for any particular ring, and that the type of ring implanted is far less important than a correctly performed operation and appropriate sizing of the ring.

The technical aspects of ring implantation are important to avoid circumflex artery compromise, atrioventricular dissociation, or dehiscence of the ring. Implantation of currently available annuloplasty rings requires the placement of mattress sutures, parallel to the annulus, at the conjunction of the posterior leaflet and the annulus. Radially oriented bites are to be avoided because by definition they exert radial stresses and thus will pull to some extent on the circumflex artery. Bites should be deep with the needle entering the annulus, then into the left ventricular cavity, and then coming out on the atrial side again. Of paramount importance is the requirement that the plane of the needle bite should be orthogonal to the annular plane. If this is done, it is impossible for the stitch to impinge or distort the circumflex artery. That is why such bites may be made deep. Wide bites are taken such that there is not an excess number of sutures. A partial mitral ring should require approximately 9 to 12 sutures depending on the size of the annulus. The sutures are not pledgeted unless there is extreme fragility of the annular structures. Annular integrity will of course depend on the pathology. Sutures are then passed through the fabric part of the ring. The central stabilizer frame is kept in place to maintain the ring shape while the sutures are tied down, thus preventing crimping of the cloth rings in the nonrigid or semi-rigid rings.

Sizing is the most important aspect of ring placement. We believe that slight oversizing of the ring in myxomatous degenerated disease is appropriate. This corrects for the degenerative annulus that is functionally too small. Sizing is typically done by two techniques. Placement of aortic trigonal stitches (Fig. 41-15) allows for measurement of the intertrigonal distance. Many ring-sizing devices have notches on the rings to facilitate this. Except in rheumatic disease, we do not rely on this measurement. In myxomatous disease, the height of the anterior leaflet from the annulus to the highest point on the leaflet when it is stretched is the most important criterion for sizing, a concept originally espoused by Carpentier.[10] This height of the leaflet is the critical dimension that must be carefully measured so that during systole there is minimal redundancy that may lead to SAM. Using trigonal sizing may, in fact, downsize the ring and cause either systolic anterior motion or ring dehiscence because of the huge disparity between ring size and annulus size. In our re-repair series, either improved sizing or placing the ring below the commissures were the most common remedies.[89] Therefore, using the sizer to evaluate anterior leaflet size is the most critical maneuver. Echocardiographic dimensions of the anterior leaflet correlate well with in vivo sizing, and calculating the anterior leaflet size by standard echocardiogram techniques is performed in every case. Deployment of a ring matching the anterior leaflet size in our experience has been most efficacious and has rarely led to systolic anterior motion.[78]

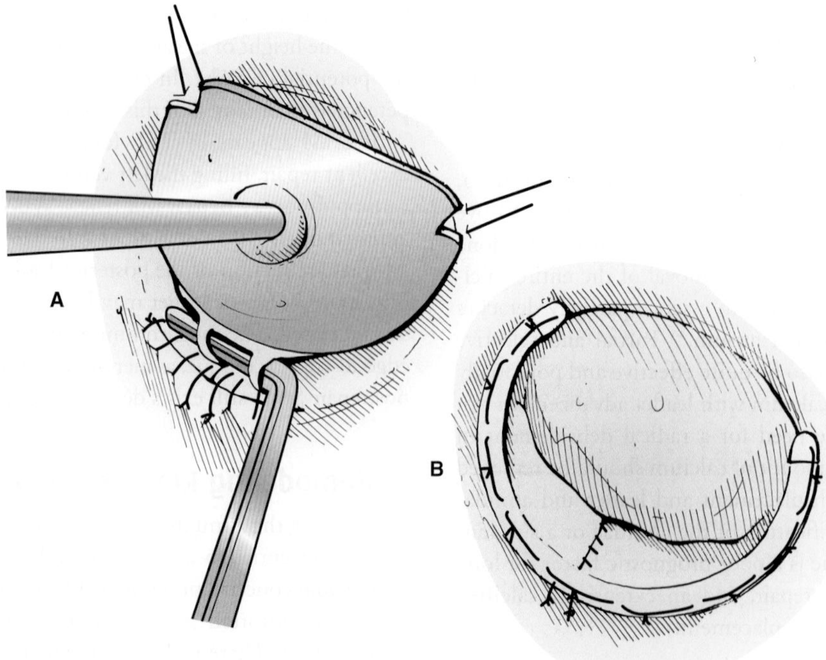

FIGURE 41-15 Ring annuloplasty sizing and insertion. The ring for degenerative disease should be slightly oversized. Sizing should be done to match the height of the anterior leaflet, not the distance between the trigones or commissures. Nine to eleven mattress sutures are usually needed.

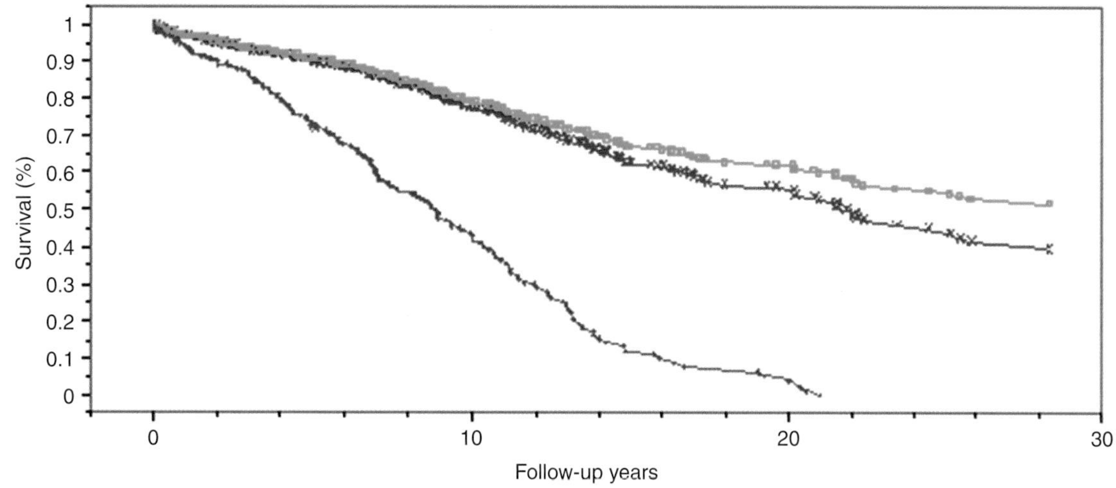

Number at risk:							
Myxomatous	1002	521	230	79	19	2	1
Rheumatic	183	146	110	87	62	34	14
FMR	230	64	25	9	5	1	

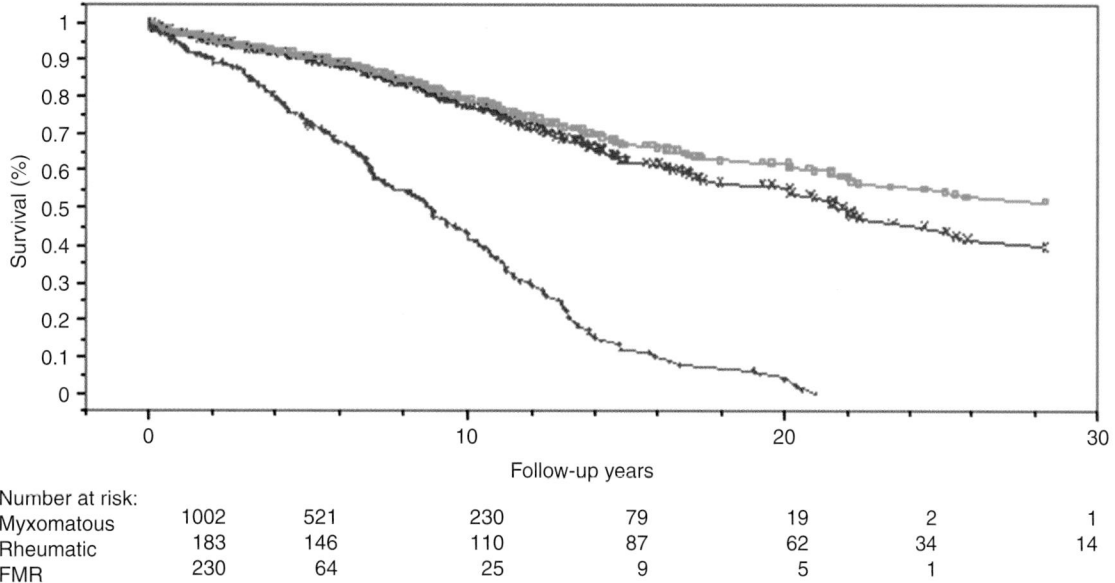

FIGURE 41-16 Etiology of mitral regurgitation determines longevity. (*Reproduced, with permission, from Dibardino DJ, Elbardissi AW, McClure RS, Razo-Vasquez OA, Kelly NE, Cohn LH: Four decades of experience with mitral valve repair: analysis of differential indications, technical evolution, and long-term outcome. J Thoracic Cardiovasc Surg 2010; 139:76-84.*)

Results

Based on long-term studies, the probability of a durable mitral valve repair at 10 years is greater than 90%.[42,53,56,64,90] Thromboembolic incidence is also exceedingly low; longterm anticoagulation is not required unless patients are in atrial fibrillation. Recently, we reviewed our personal operative experiencc (LHC) over four decades of mitral valve surgery.[91] This study has confirmed many commonly believed relationships between the etiology of MR and the durability of mitral valve repair. Etiology of regurgitation was noted to be the primary determinant of repair longevity and freedom from reoperation. Although repair of rheumatic disease was noted to ultimately require reoperation, myxomatous repair resulted in outstanding long-term freedom from recurrent MR and reoperation (Figure 41-16).

RHEUMATIC MITRAL VALVE DISEASE

The incidence of rheumatic fever and its valvular sequelae have dropped precipitously in North America and Europe during the last few decades. This has resulted in far fewer rheumatic valves requiring surgery. The disease is still seen, however, in individuals from undeveloped countries where rheumatic valve disease is still quite prevalent.[92] The primary lesion of rheumatic mitral valve disease is mitral stenosis caused by a fibrotic restriction at both commissures of the mitral valve. Open commissurotomy evolved from the early efforts in the 1940s and 1950s with closed mitral valvotomy and commissurotomy (Harken)[93,94] and was carried out successfully with a very low rate of recurrence and with a high probability of symptom relief.

Over the last several years, balloon mitral valvuloplasty has been the treatment of choice for noncalcified rheumatic mitral stenosis.[95] This technique has been widely used and has proved to be extremely efficacious in the noncalcified, nonregurgitant mitral valve. Nonetheless, there are still a number of patients with rheumatic valve disease who present primarily with severe mitral regurgitation secondary to varying degrees of restricted leaflet motion, thickening of the subvalvular apparatus, and commissural fusion. In most instances, if the valve is severely calcified and there is obliteration of the subvalvular chordal structure by fibrosis, repair will be fruitless and replacement carried out. In younger patients, with preservation of the chordal apparatus and minimal calcification, a satisfactory repair for mitral regurgitation can be carried out. Thickening of the valve may require, however, some thinning of the valve by removal of some of the rheumatic scarification process.

Techniques of rheumatic repair should always employ commissural incisions of the stenosis leaving a 2- to 3-mm edge to the annulus. Debridement of calcium and scar and incising the papillary muscles and chordae may improve mobility. Several European surgeons, particularly Duran and colleagues,[96] have devised techniques that include lengthening the anterior leaflet of the mitral valve, and even in some instances the use of PTFE chords to improve the flexibility of the posterior leaflet and retraction caused by the chordal scarring and fibrosis.

Particularly in patients with severe mitral regurgitation related to rheumatic mitral disease, a remodeling annuloplasty ring will be necessary. Repair is possible with combined mitral stenosis and regurgitation because alleviation of stenosis may improve the mobility of the anterior leaflet, which then allows for a corrective operation rather than replacement. Finally, the absence or presence of fibrosis of the subannular chordal structure may often determine mitral valve replacement versus mitral valve repair. In young patients, however, every effort should be made to repair these valves by the techniques outlined above, because repair results are better in the long term than valve replacement.[97]

However, given the near certainty of reoperation, every measure should be taken during the first procedure to ease any future reoperation, ie, Gore-Tex for reapproximating the pericardium.

SUMMARY

Mitral valve repair for degenerative disease has undergone a virtual revolution in the previous 30 years. What was once viewed skeptically is now well accepted as the ideal treatment for mitral regurgitation based on improved physiology and lower valve-related morbidity than valve replacement. In major valve referral centers, repair is commonplace and routine. However, for many cardiac surgeons mitral valve repair is still surrounded by mystical references to such surgery as "a special art," one that is difficult to understand and requires special esoteric skills to master. Repair should be part of every cardiac surgeon's standard toolbox and should be considered as simply another procedure to be mastered.

REFERENCES

1. Brunton L, Edin MD: Preliminary note on the possibility of treating mitral stenosis by surgical methods. *Lancet* 1902; 1:352.
2. Cutler EC, Levine SA: Cardiotomy and valvulotomy for mitral stenosis: experimental observations and clinical notes concerning an operated case with recovery. *Boston Med Surg J* 1923; 188:1023.
3. Cutler EC, Beck CS: The present status of surgical procedures in chronic valvular disease of the heart: final report of all surgical cases. *Arch Surg* 1929; 18:403.
4. Souttar HS: Surgical treatment of mitral stenosis. *BMJ* 1925; 2:603.
5. Harken DE, Ellis LB, Ware PF, et al: The surgical treatment of mitral stenosis. I. Valvuloplasty. *NEJM* 1948; 239:801.
6. Bailey CP: The surgical treatment of mitral stenosis (mitral commissurotomy). *Dis Chest* 1949; 15:377.
7. Davila JC, Glover RP: Circumferential suture of the mitral valve for the correction of regurgitation. *Am J Cardiol* 1958; 2:267.
8. Nichols HT: Mitral insufficiency: treatment by polar cross fusion of the mitral annulus fibrosis. *J Thorac Cardiovasc Surg* 1957; 33:102.
9. Kay EB, Mendelsohn D, Zimmerman HA: Evaluation of the surgical correction of mitral regurgitation. *Circulation* 1961; 23:813.
10. Carpentier A: Cardiac valve surgery: the "French correction." *J Thorac Cardiovasc Surg* 1983; 86:323.
11. McGoon DC: Repair of mitral insufficiency due to ruptured chordae tendineae. *J Thorac Cardiovasc Surg* 1960; 39:357.
12. Duran CG, Pomar JL, Revuelta JM, et al: Conservative operation for mitral insufficiency. Critical analysis supported by postoperative hemodynamic studies of 72 patients. *J Thorac Cardiovasc Surg* 1980; 79:326.
13. Orszulak TA, Schaff HV, Danielson GK, et al: Mitral regurgitation due to ruptured chordae tendinae. Early and late results of mitral valve repair. *J Thorac Cardiovasc Surg* 1985; 89:491.
14. Cohn LH, Couper GS, Kinchla NM, et al: Decreased operative risk of surgical treatment of mitral regurgitation with or without coronary artery disease. *J Am Coll Cardiol* 1990; 16:1575.
15. Cosgrove DM, Chavez AM, Lytle BW, et al: Results of mitral valve reconstruction. *Circulation* 1986; 74:I82.
16. Kirklin JW: Replacement of the mitral valve for mitral incompetence. *Surgery* 1972; 72:827.
17. Sarris GE, Cahill PD, Hansen DE, et al: Restoration of left ventricular systolic performance after reattachment of the mitral chordae tendineae: the importance of valvular-ventricular interaction. *J Thorac Cardiovasc Surg* 1988; 95:969.
18. Carpentier A, Deloche A, Dauptain J, et al: A new reconstructive operation for correction of mitral and tricuspid insufficiency. *J Thorac Cardiovasc Surg* 1971; 61:1.
19. McCarthy PM: Does the intertrigonal distance dilate? Never say never. *J Thorac Cardiovasc Surg* 2002; 124:1078.
20. Du Plessis LA, Marchano P: The anatomy of the mitral valve and its associated structures. *Thorax* 1964; 19:221.
21. Roberts WC: Morphologic aspects of cardiac valve dysfunction. *Am Heart J* 1992; 123:1610.
22. Wisenbaugh T, Spann JF, Carabello BA: Differences in myocardial performance and load between patients with similar amounts of chronic aortic versus chronic mitral regurgitation. *J Am Coll Cardiol* 1984; 3:916.
23. Carabello BA: Indications for mitral valve surgery. *J Cardiovasc Surg* 2004; 45:407.
24. Shyu KG, Chin JJ, Lin FY, et al: Regression of left ventricular mass after mitral valve repair of pure mitral regurgitation. *Ann Thorac Surg* 1994; 58:1670.
25. Deloche A, Jebara VA, Relland FYM, et al: Valve repair with Carpentier techniques: The second decade. *J Thorac Cardiovasc Surg* 1990; 99:990.
26. Freed LA, Levy D, Levine RA, et al: Prevalence and clinical outcome of mitral-valve prolapse. *NEJM* 1999; 341:1.
27. Mills P, Rose J, Hollingsworth J, et al: Long-term prognosis of mitral-valve prolapse. *NEJM* 1977; 297:13.
28. Marks AR, Choong CY, Sanfilippo AJ, et al: Identification of high-risk and low-risk subgroups of patients with mitral valve prolapse. *NEJM* 1989; 320:1031.
29. Danchin N, Voiriot P, Briancon S, et al: Mitral valve prolapse as a risk factor for infective endocarditis. *Lancet* 1989; 1:743.
30. Enriquez-Sarano M, Dujardin KS, Tribouilloy CM, et al: Determinants of pulmonary venous flow reversal in mitral regurgitation and its usefulness in determining the severity of regurgitation. *Am J Cardiol* 1999; 83:535.
31. Chen FY, Cohn LH: Valvular surgery in cardiomyopathy, in Baughman KL, Baumgartner WA (eds): *Treatment of Advanced Heart Disease.* New York, Taylor and Francis, 2006; .
32. Stewart WJ: Choosing the "golden moment" for mitral valve repair. *J Am Coll Cardiol* 1994; 24:1544.
33. Gogbashian A, Sepic J, Soltesz EG, et al: Operative and long-term survival of elderly is significantly improved by mitral valve repair. *Am Heart J* 2006; 151:1325.
34. Kang DH, Kim JH, Rim JH, et al: Comparison of early surgery versus conventional treatment in asymptomatic severe mitral regurgitation. *Circulation* 2009; 119:797.
35. Cosgrove DM, Stewart WJ: Mitral valvuloplasty. *Curr Probl Cardiol* 1989; 14:359.
36. Sand ME, Naftel DC, Blackstone EH, et al: A comparison of repair and replacement for mitral valve incompetence. *J Thorac Cardiovasc Surg* 1987; 94:208.
37. Lawrie GM: Mitral valve repair vs. replacement: current recommendations and long-term results. *Cardiol Clin* 1998; 16:437.
38. Gillinov AM, Cosgrove DM, Blackston EH, et al: Durability of mitral valve repair for degernerative disease. *J Thorac Cardiovasc Surg* 1998; 116:734.
39. Vanden Eynden F, Bouchard D, El-Hamamsy I, Butnaru A, et al: Effect of aortic valve replacement for aortic stenosis on severity of mitral regurgitation. *Ann Thorac Surg* 2007; 83:1279.
40. Wan CK, Suri RM, Li Z, et al: Management of moderate functional mitral regurgitation at the time of aortic valve replacement: is concomitant valve repair necessary? *J Thorac Cardiovasc Surg* 2009; 137:635.
41. Enriquez-Sarano M, Avierinos JF, Messika-Zeitoun D, et al: Quantitative determinants of the outcome of asymptomatic mitral regurgitation. *NEJM* 2005; 352:875.
42. Ling LH, Enriquez-Sarano M, Seward JB, et al: Clinical outcome of mitral regurgitation due to flail leaflet. *NEJM* 1996; 335:1417.
43. Greelish JP, Cohn LH, Leacche M, et al: Minimally invasive mitral valve repair suggests earlier operations for mitral valve disease. *J Thorac Cardiovasc Surg* 2003; 126:365.
44. McClure RS, Cohn LH, Wiegerinck E, et al: Early and late outcomes in minimally invasive mitral valve repair: an eleven-year experience in 707. *J Thorac Cardiovasc Surg* 2009; 137:70.
45. Mihaljevic T, Cohn LH, Unic D, et al: One thousand minimally invasive valve operations: early and late results. *Ann Surg* 2004; 240:529.
46. Spencer FC, Galloway AC, Grossi EA, et al: Recent developments and evolving techniques of mitral valve reconstruction. *Ann Thorac Surg* 1998; 65:307.
47. Mohty D, Orszulak TA, Schaff HV, et al: Very long-term survival and durability of mitral valve repair for mitral valve prolapse. *Circulation* 2001; 104(Suppl I):I-1.
48. Savage EB, Ferguson TB Jr., DiSesa VJ: Use of mitral valve repair: analysis of contemporary United States experience reported to the Society of Thoracic Surgeons National Cardiac Database. *Ann Thorac Surg* 2003; 75:820.
49. Gammie JS, Sheng S, Griffith BP, et al: Trends in mitral valve surgery in the United States: results from the Society of Thoracic Surgeons Adult Cardiac Surgery Database. *Ann Thorac Surg* 2009; 87:1431.
50. Sondergaard T, Gotzsche M, Ottosen P, et al: Surgical closure of interatrial septal defects by circumclusion. *Acta Chir Scand* 1955; 109:188.

51. Larbalestier RI, Chard RB, Cohn LH: Optimal approach to the mitral valve: dissection of the interatrial groove. *Ann Thorac Surg* 1992; 54:1186.
52. Cohn LH: Mitral valve repair. *Op Techniques Thorac Cardiovasc Surg* 1998; 3:109.
53. Khonsari S, Sintek CF: Transatrial approach revisited. *Ann Thorac Surg* 1990; 50:1002.
54. Duran CG, Ubago JLM: Clinical and hemodynamic performance of a totally flexible prosthetic ring for atrioventricular valve reconstruction. *Ann Thorac Surg* 1976; 22:458.
55. Gillinov AM, Cosgrove DM 3rd, Wahi S, et al: Is anterior leaflet repair always necessary in repair of bileaflet mitral valve prolapse? *Ann Thorac Surg* 1999; 68:820.
56. Cohn LH, Couper GS, Aranki SF, et al: Long-term results of mitral valve reconstruction for regurgitation of the myxomatous mitral valve. *J Thorac Cardiovasc Surg* 1994; 107:143.
57. Gillinov AM, Tantiwongkosri K, Blackstone EH, et al: Is prosthetic annuloplasty necessary for durable mitral valve repair? *Ann Thorac Surg* 2009; 88:76.
58. Perier P: A new paradigm for the repair of posterior leaflet prolapse: respect rather than resect. *Op Techniques Thorac Cardiovasc Surg* 2005; 10:180.
59. Lawrie GM, Earle EA, Earle NR: Feasibility and intermediate term outcome of repair of prolapsing anterior mitral leaflets with artificial chordal replacement in 152 patients. *Ann Thorac Surg* 2006; 81:849.
60. Perier P, Clausnizer B, Mistraz K: Carpentier "sliding leaflet" technique for repair of the mitral valve: Early results. *Ann Thorac Surg* 1994; 57:383.
61. Tabata M, Ghanta RK, Shekar PS, Cohn LH: Early and midterm outcomes of folding valvuloplasty without leaflet resection for myxomatous mitral valve disease. *Ann Thorac Surg* 2008; 86:1288.
62. Gillinov AM, Shortt KG, Cosgrove DM 3rd: Commissural closure for repair of mitral commissural prolapse. *Ann Thorac Surg* 2005; 80:1135.
63. Aubert S, Barreda T, Acar C, et al: Mitral valve repair for commissural prolapse: surgical techniques and long term results. *Eur J Cardiothorac Surg* 2005; 28:443.
64. David TE, Ivanov J, Armstrong S, et al: A comparison of outcomes of mitral valve repair for degenerative disease with posterior, anterior, and bileaflet prolapse. *J Thorac Cardiovasc Surg* 2005; 130:1242.
65. Smedira NG, Selman R, Cosgrove DM, et al: Repair of anterior leaflet prolapse: chordal transfer is superior to chordal shortening. *J Thorac Cardiovasc Surg* 1996; 112:287.
66. Dreyfus GD, Bahrami T, Alayle N, et al: Repair of anterior leaflet prolapse by papillary muscle repositioning: a new surgical option. *Ann Thorac Surg* 2001; 71:1464.
67. Pino F, Moneta A, Villa E, et al: Chordal plication and free edge remodeling for mitral anterior leaflet prolapse repair: 8-year follow-up. *Ann Thorac Surg* 2001; 72:1515.
68. Frater RW, Vetter HO, Zussa C, et al: Chordal replacement in mitral valve repair. *Circulation* 1990; 82(5 Suppl):IV125.
69. Zussa C, Polesel E, Da Col U, et al: Seven-year experience with chordal replacement with expanded polytetrafluoroethylene in floppy mitral valve. *J Thorac Cardiovasc Surg* 1991; 108:37.
70. Duran CM, Pekar F: Techniques for ensuring the correct length of new chords. *J Heart Valve Dis* 2003; 12:156.
71. Falk V, Seeburger J, Czesla M, et al: How does the use of polytetrafluoroethylene neochordae for posterior mitral valve prolapse (loop technique) compare with leaflet resection? A prospective randomized trial. *J Thorac Cardiovasc Surg* 2008; 136:1205
72. Duran CM: Surgical techniques for the repair of anterior mitral leaflet prolapse. *J Card Surg* 1999; 14:471.
73. Uva MS, Grare P, Jebara V, et al: Transposition of chordae in mitral valve repair: mid-term results. *Circulation* 1993; 88:35.
74. Maisano F, Torracca L, Oppizzi M, et al: The edge-to-edge technique: a simplified method to correct mitral insufficiency. *Eur J Cardiothorac Surg* 1998; 13:240.
75. Condado JA, Acquatella H, Rodriguez L, et al: Percutaneous edge-to-edge mitral valve repair: 2-year follow-up in the first human case. *Catheter Cardiovasc Intervent* 2006; 67:323.
76. Alfieri O, Maisano F, De Bonis M, et al: The double-orifice technique in mitral valve repair: A simple solution for complex problems. *J Thorac Cardiovasc Surg* 2001; 122:674.
77. Bhudia SK, McCarthy PM, Smedira NG: Edge-to-edge (Alfieri) mitral repair: results in diverse clinical settings. *Ann Thorac Surg* 2004; 77:1598.
78. Brinster DR, Unic D, D'Ambra MN, et al: Mid term results of the edge to edge technique for complex mitral repair. *Ann Thorac Surg* 2006; 81:1612.
79. Maslow AD, Regan MM, Haering JM, et al: Echocardiographic predictors of left ventricular outflow tract obstruction and systolic anterior motion of the mitral valve after mitral valve reconstruction for myxomatous valve disease. *J Am Coll Cardiol* 1999; 34:2096.
80. De Bonis M, Lorusso R, Lapenna E, et al: Similar long-term results of mitral valve repair for anterior compared with posterior leaflet prolapse. *J Thorac Cardiovasc Surg* 2006; 131:364.
81. Suri RM, Orszulak TA: Triangular resection for repair of mitral regurgitation due to degenerative disease. *Op Techniques Thorac Cardiovasc Surg* 2005; 10:194.
82. Duran CMG: Surgical techniques for the repair of anterior mitral leaflet prolapse. *J Card Surg* 1999; 14:471.
83. Chauvaud S, Jebara V, Chachques JC, et al: Valve extension with glutaraldehyde-preserved autologous pericardium. Results in mitral valve repair. *J Thorac Cardiovasc Surg* 1991; 102:171.
84. el Asmar B, Acker M, Couetil JP, et al: Mitral valve repair in the extensively calcified mitral valve annulus. *Ann Thorac Surg* 1991; 52:66.
85. Bichell DP, Adams DH, Aranki SF, et al: Repair of mitral regurgitation from myxomatous degeneration in the patient with a severely calcified posterior annulus. *J Card Surg* 1995; 10(4 Pt 1):281.
86. Lee KS, Stewart WJ, Lever HM, et al: Mechanism of outflow tract obstruction causing failed valve repair: anterior displacement of leaflet coaptation. *Circulation* 1993; 88(5 Pt 2):II24.
87. Mihaileanu S, Marino JP, Chauvaud S, et al: Left ventricular outflow obstruction after mitral repair (Carpentier's technique): proposed mechanism of disease. *Circulation* 1988; 78(3 Pt 2):78.
88. Gillinov AM, Cosgrove DM, Shiota T, et al: Cosgrove-Edwards annuloplasty system: Midterm results. *Ann Thorac Surg* 2000; 69:717.
89. Shekar PS, Couper GS, Cohn LH: Mitral valve re-repair. *J Heart Valve Dis* 2005; 14:583.
90. Braunberger E, Deloche A, Berrebi A: Very long-term results (more than 20 years) of valve repair with Carpentier's techniques in nonrheumatic mitral valve insufficiency. *Circulation* 2001;104:I-8.
91. Dibardino DJ, Elbardissi AW, McClure RS, et al: Four decades of experience with mitral valve repair: analysis of differential indications, technical evolution, and long-term outcome. *J Thoracic Cardiovasc Surg* 2010; 139:76.
92. Bitar FF, Hayek P, Obeid M: Rheumatic fever in children: a 15-year experience in a developing country. *Pediatr Cardiol* 2000; 21:119.
93. Hickey MSJ, Blackstone EH, Kirklin JW, et al: Outcome probabilities and life history after surgical mitral commissurotomy. *J Am Coll Cardiol* 1991; 17:29.
94. Cohn LH, Allred EN, Cohn LA, et al: Long-term results of open mitral valve reconstruction for mitral stenosis. *Am J Cardiol* 1985; 55:731.
95. Palacios IF, Block PC, Wilins GT, et al: Follow up of patients undergoing percutaneous mitral balloon valvuloplasty: analysis of factors determining restenosis. *Circulation* 1989; 79:573.
96. Duran CMG, Gometza B, Saad E: Valve repair in rheumatic mitral disease: an unsolved problem. *J Card Surg* 1994; 9(2 Suppl):282.
97. Yau TM, El-Ghoneimi YA, Armstong S, et al: Mitral valve repair and replacement for rheumatic disease. *J Thorac Cardiovasc Surg* 2000; 119:53.

CHAPTER 42

Mitral Valve Replacement

Robert P. Gallegos
Tomas Gudbjartsson
Sary Aranki

INTRODUCTION

This chapter discusses the surgical indications, operative techniques, and early and late follow-up after implantation of mechanical and bioprosthetic mitral valve devices. The valves that are discussed are those that are currently (2010) approved by the FDA. Figure 42-1 shows the current FDA-approved prosthetic mitral valve devices, including the Starr-Edwards ball-and-cage valve (historical relevance only), the Omnicarbon tilting-disk valve, the Medtronic Hall tilting-disk valve, the St. Jude Medical bileaflet valve, the Carbomedics bileaflet valve, the ATS bileaflet valve, and the On-X bileaflet valve. The FDA-approved bioprosthetic valve devices are shown in Fig. 42-2 and include the Hancock II porcine valve, the Carpentier-Edwards porcine valve, the Carpentier-Edwards pericardial valve, the Mosaic porcine valve, and the Biocor porcine valve.

Heart valve prostheses are continually undergoing iterative advancement by the manufacturers, and the future device of choice has yet to be developed. This ideal replacement valve prosthetic would have longevity of a mechanical prosthetic combined with the superior hemodynamic function of the native biologic tissue valve. As a result this hypostatic ideal replacement device would not require anticoagulation and carrying no risk of either thromboembolic events or valve thrombosis. To achieve this goal will require major advancement away from current design.

INDICATIONS FOR MITRAL VALVE REPLACEMENT

The indications for mitral valve replacement are variable and undergoing evolution. Because of increasing use of reparative techniques, particularly for mitral regurgitation, replacement or repair of a mitral valve often depends on the experience of the operating surgeon. Current indications for valve replacement pertain to those types of valve problems that are unlikely to be repaired by most surgeons or which have been shown to have poor long-term success after reconstruction. Indications are discussed according to: (1) pathophysiologic states; and (2) type of valve required (ie, mechanical or bioprosthetic).

MITRAL STENOSIS

Mitral stenosis is almost exclusively caused by rheumatic fever, even though a definite clinical history can be obtained in only about 50% of patients. The incidence of mitral stenosis has decreased substantially in the United States in the last several decades because of effective prophylaxis of rheumatic fever, nevertheless in certain developing countries mitral stenosis is still very common. Two-thirds of patients with rheumatic mitral stenosis are female.

The pathologic changes associated with rheumatic valvulitis are mainly fusion of the valve leaflets at the commissures, shortening and fusion of the cordae tendineae, and thickening of the leaflets owing to fibrosis with subsequent stiffening, contraction, and calcification. Approximately 25% of patients have pure mitral stenosis, but an additional 40% have combined mitral stenosis and mitral regurgitation.[1]

Stenosis usually develops one or two decades after the acute illness of rheumatic fever with no or slow onset of symptoms until the stenosis becomes more severe. Limitation of exercise tolerance usually is the first symptom, followed by dyspnea that can progress to pulmonary edema. New-onset atrial fibrillation and the risk for thromboembolism, hemoptysis, and pulmonary hypertension are other common symptoms in patients with mitral stenosis.

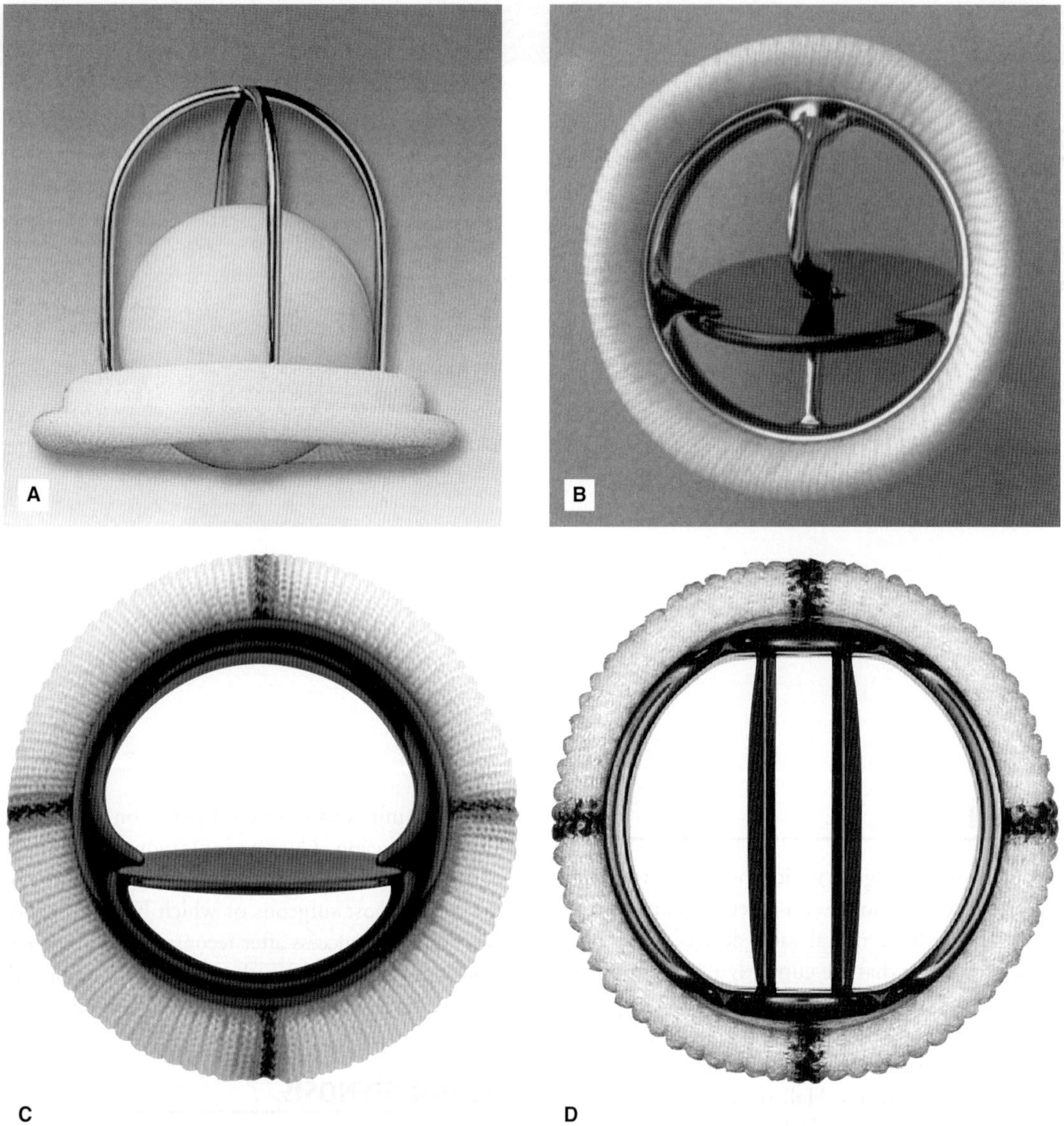

FIGURE 42-1 FDA-approved mechanical mitral valves. (**A**) Starr-Edwards ball-and-cage. (**B**) Medtronic Hall tilting-disk. (**C**) Omnicarbon tilting-disk. (**D**) St. Jude Medical bifleaflet. (**E**) Carbomedics bileaflet. (**F**) ATS bileaflet. (**G**) On-X bileaflet.

The diagnostic workup of the symptomatic patient with mitral stenosis should include a complete cardiac catheterization, including coronary angiography in any patient greater than age of 40. Under age 40, echocardiographic findings of the mitral valve suffice in most symptomatic patients for the definition of mitral valve pathology unless there is a history of chest pain or coronary artery disease. Cardiac catheterization establishes the extent of mitral valve stenosis by determining valve gradients and valve area. Pulmonary artery pressure, which may be extremely high in longstanding cases of mitral stenosis, is also documented. In general, operation is prescribed when the mean valve area is 1.0 cm^2 or less[2] (normal mitral valve area is 4 to 6 cm^2); however, with a "mixed" lesion of mitral stenosis and mitral regurgitation, the valve area in symptomatic patients occasionally may be as large as 1.5 cm^2. Asymptomatic patients generally are not considered for surgery,[1] but some authors recommend operation in asymptomatic patients with significant hemodynamic mitral stensosis.[2] The degree of pulmonary artery pressure elevation secondary to mitral stenosis continues to be an area of concern for the mitral valve surgeon. There is still no definitive answer to this question, but most surgeons operate on patients with severe pulmonary hypertension (suprasystemic patients) with the knowledge that intensive postoperative respiratory and diuretic therapy is necessary to maintain relatively dry lungs and reduce the risk of severe right ventricular failure. It has been known for more than 40 years that after mitral valve replacement for mitral stenosis, pulmonary artery pressure decreases within hours in most patients and decreases more gradually over weeks to months in others.[4–6]

Success with closed commissurotomy after World War II and the development of the Starr-Edwards valve in the early

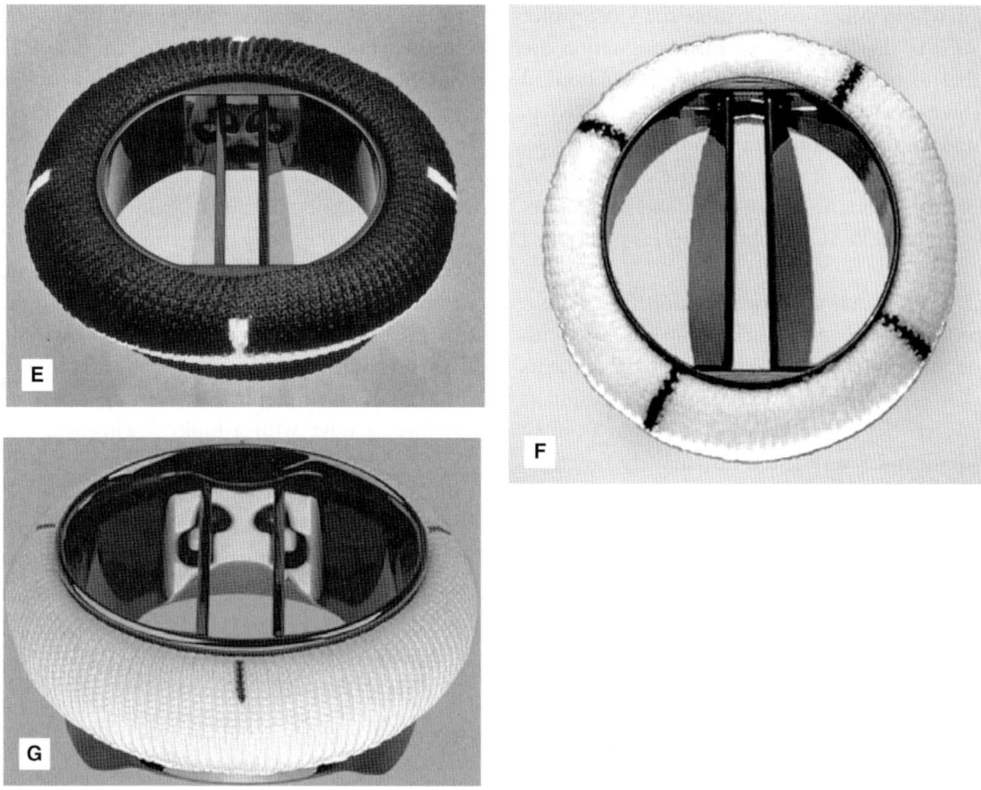

FIGURE 42-1 *(Continued)*

1960s led to an enormous increase in operations for rheumatic mitral valve disease. In the 1990s, balloon dilation of fibrotic, stenotic mitral valves became increasingly common.[6,7] At the present time, percutaneous mitral balloon valve dilation is used in most cases of symptomatic noncalcified, fibrotic mitral stenosis. But even though this technique has been shown to be equivalent in the short run to closed mitral commissurotomy, especially in young patients, it is only indicated in a minority of patients, that is, those with optimal valvular characteristiscs.[1,8] Open mitral commissurotomy and valvuloplasty for such patients can be a successful operation,[9,10] but other studies have shown better long-term results with mitral valve replacement using a mechanical valve.[11] Many patients with chronic mitral stenosis now require valve replacement because the valve has developed significant dystrophic changes, including marked thickening and shortening of all chordae, obliteration of the subvalvular space, agglutination of the papillary muscles, and calcification in both annular and leaflet tissue. Aggressive decalcification and heroic reconstructive techniques for these extremely advanced pathologic valves generally have produced poor long-term results; nevertheless, some surgeons still advocate aggressive repairs in this subset of patients.[12]

MITRAL REGURGITATION

The etiology of mitral regurgitation is very diverse, and the decision to recommend operation for patients with mitral regurgitation is more complex than for patients with mitral stenosis, except in patients with acute ischemic mitral regurgitation

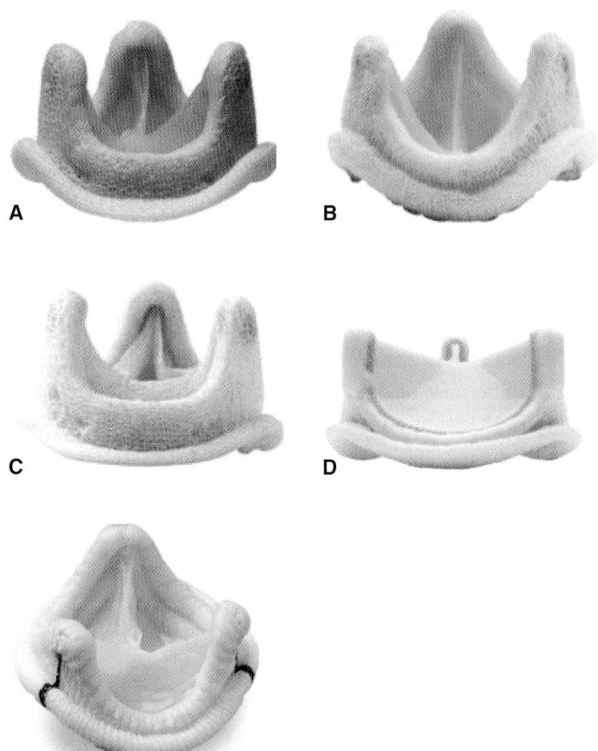

FIGURE 42-2 FDA-approved bioprosthetic mitral valves. (A) Hancock II porcine heterograft. (B) Carpentier-Edwards standard porcine heterograft. (C) Mosaic porcine heterograft. (D) Carpentier-Edwards pericardial bovine heterograft. (E) St. Jude Biocor porcine heterograft.

and endocarditis, in whom indications are more straightforward. The pathologic subsets that produce mitral regurgitation are related to a number of metabolic, functional, and anatomical abnormalities.[1] These can be categorized into degenerative (eg, mitral prolapse and ruptured/elongated chordae), rheumatic, infectious, and ischemic diseases of the mitral valve. Most of these entities are now amenable to mitral valve repair and reconstruction with or without the use of annuloplasty rings, as mentioned in Chapter 41.

It is important to stress that depressed ejection fraction is a poor indicator of left ventricular function in patients with mitral regurgitation. Ejection fraction can be preserved in patients with irreversible left ventricular failure because of regurgitant flow through the valve.[20,21] Depressed cardiac output (<40%) therefore usually indicates severe left ventricular dysfunction, and results of surgery are not as favorable in these patients as they are in those with normal ventricles.[22,23] Compared with ejection fraction, measurements of end-systolic volume and diameter are more reliable noninvasive parameters to evaluate the status of the left ventricle and determine the optimal time for operation[24,25]

Once the valve is exposed, indications for mitral valve replacement in patients with mitral regurgitation depend on the extent of the pathology in each patient and the reparative experience of the operating surgeon. Thus, in regurgitation from degenerative prolapsing myxomatous valves that have a high probability of reconstruction, mitral valve repair is indicated if the prolapse is generalized and local findings that decrease the probability of a successful repair are absent.[26–30] Similarly, if rheumatic mitral regurgitation, calcific deposits throughout the leaflet substance, and shortened chordae and papillary muscles are encountered, mitral valve replacement is often the most prudent operation because the probability of successful repair is low.[31] However, good results with reconstructive surgery in this patient group have been reported.[32] In ischemic mitral regurgitation, pathology that precludes satisfactory repair includes restrictive valve motion from shortened, scarred papillary muscles, an acutely infarcted papillary muscle, and rupture of chordae associated with extensive calcification of valve leaflets.[33–35] In endocarditis, mitral valve replacement may be required because of destruction of the valve leaflets and subvalvular mechanisms and annular abscess formation. Although repair of the valve and avoidance of prosthetic material are very desirable in septic situations, the extent of the destruction may preclude repair. Therefore, mitral valve replacement is required after careful debridement of the infectious tissue and reconstruction of the valve annulus.[36–38]

CHOICE OF VALVE TYPE

Indications for Mechanical Valve Replacement

Currently available prosthetic valves in the United States are the bileaflet and the tilting disk designs. For young patients, patients in chronic atrial fibrillation who require long-term anticoagulation, and any patient who wants to minimize the chance of reoperation, a prosthetic valve should be chosen if valve replacement is required. The St. Jude Medical bileaflet valve is the most widely used prosthetic mitral valve at present because it has good hemodynamic characteristics and is easy to insert. Recent interest in the On-X mechanical valve relates primarily to the possibility for limited anticoagulation, although this remains to be borne out from current clinical trial.[39] Indications to choose one prosthetic or another vary primarily by surgeon preference and occasionally depending on the state of the annulus and whether or not there have been multiple previous operations. For example, infrequently, the mitral annulus provides poor anchorage with subsequent perivalvular leak with the bileaflet or tilting-disk valve, which requires an everting-suture technique. In this instance, a valve with a bulky sewing ring may be chosen to reduce the probability of subsequent perivalvular leak. A low-profile mechanical valve is preferable in a patient with a small left ventricular cavity to prevent obstruction of left ventricular outflow and impingement of the myocardium.

Indications for Bioprosthetic Valve Replacement

Patients in any age group in sinus rhythm who wish to avoid anticoagulation may prefer a bioprosthetic valve. This is especially true for patients in whom anticoagulation is contraindicated; for example, patients with a history of gastrointestinal bleeding or those who have a high-risk occupation or lifestyle.[1] A bioprosthetic valve is preferred in patients greater than age 65 and in sinus rhythm because these valves deteriorate more slowly in older patients.[40]In addition, some 60-year-old patients may not outlive their prosthetic valves because of comorbid disease.[41,42] Specifically, patients who require combined mitral valve replacement and coronary bypass grafting for ischemic mitral regurgitation and coronary artery disease have significantly reduced long-term survival as compared with patients who do not have concomitant coronary artery disease.[43–48] These individuals may avoid anticoagulation with little risk of reoperation.

As 20-year results have become available for various bioprostheses, it is clear that structural valve degeneration (SVD) is the most prominent complication of these valves.[49–54] The durability of porcine mitral valves is less than with aortic bioprostheses. The more rapid deterioration of mitral bioprostheses may be caused by higher ventricular systolic pressures against the mitral cusps compared with the diastolic pressures resisted by aortic bioprosthetic leaflets. Durability of bioprosthetic valves is directly proportional to age[50]; deterioration occurs within months or years in children and young adults and only gradually over years in septuagenarians and octogenarians.[49,55] Essentially all valves implanted into patients younger than 60 years of age have to be replaced ultimately, and valve failure is prohibitively rapid in children and adults younger than 35 to 40 years of age; therefore, bioprostheses are not advisable in these age groups.[56] Nevertheless, there are still indications for mitral porcine bioprosthetic valves in young patients. In a woman who desires to become pregnant, a bioprosthesis may be used to avoid warfarin anticoagulation and fetal damage during pregnancy.[57–60]

In patients with chronic renal failure and hypercalcemia related to hyperparathyroidism, bioprostheses have extremely limited durability and therefore should be avoided.

Over the last decade several reports, mainly from European centers, on the use of unstented cryopreserved homografts[61–64] and stentless heterografts[65–68] for mitral valve replacements, particularly in patients with endocarditis. The prosthetic valve is transplanted, donor papillary muscles are reattached to recipient papillary muscles, and the annulus is sutured circumferentially. This technique has been shown to be safe and reproducible, but it does not always provide durable results and therefore should not be used in young patients.[65] Other reports suggest that these operations may be a feasible alternative to stented valve replacement in patients with endocarditis. Pulmonary autografts also have been used for replacing the mitral valve (Ross II procedure), but these series are small, and follow-up is relatively short.[69–71]

TRENDS IN MITRAL VALVE SURGERY

Mitral valve surgery has been in a state of constant evolution since its inception. Data regarding all cardiac surgical procedures reported to the Society of Thoracic Surgeons Adult Cardiac Surgery Database (STS ACSD) demonstrate this dynamic state as more surgeons begin to repair rather than replace mitral valves. Gammie et al. recently evaluated trends in mitral valve surgery in the United States using the STS ACSD evaluating the years between 2000 and 2007.[192] In this time period, 210,529 mitral valve procedures were performed in all settings. From the study population 58,370 patients undergoing primary mitral valve operations were identified. Over this 7-year study time line, a 50% increase in repair rates was documented. When considering the valve procedures involving replacement, a 100% increase in use of bioprosthetic devices coincided with a concomitant reduction in use of mechanical valves.

Gammie and coworkers identified clear trends with respect to patient selection as well.[192] Compared with patients undergoing mitral valve repair, those undergoing mitral replacement tended to be older, female, more likely to have multiple comorbidities (eg, diabetes mellitus, hypertension, chronic lung disease, stroke), concomitant tricuspid valve disease, and mitral stenosis, and were less likely to be asymptomatic. With respect to survival, overall risk adjusted mortality was lower for mitral valve repair versus replacement (OR 0.52, 95% CI: 0.45 to 0.59, $p < .0001$). The outcome with respect to choice of valve type and survival was not addressed but was felt to be confounded by patient factors that led to the initial device selection.

Needless to say, the role for mitral valve replacement as a whole is being diminished by improvements in mitral repair technique. Most importantly, these technical advancements have simplified repair procedures such that more surgeons can perform the procedure while not compromising on repair results. Each individual surgeon must assess their own outcomes to judge whether their ability to repair the valve can offer the same if not superior results when compared with replacement in their hands.

HEMODYNAMIC OF MITRAL VALVES DEVICES

Mechanical Prosthesis

The designs of mechanical and bioprosthetic heart valves have evolved over the last five decades in an effort to develop the ideal replacement for the pathologic mitral valve. Biochemical and engineering advances have produced hemodynamic improvements and reduced morbidity from valve-related complications. The ideal valve, however, is not available, and the positive and negative characteristics of current valves must be considered when choosing the most appropriate valve for an individual patient. The optimal heart valve exerts minimal resistance to forward blood flow and allows only trivial regurgitant backflow as the occluder closes. The design must cause minimal turbulence and stasis in vivo during physiologic flow conditions. The valve must be durable enough to last a lifetime and must be constructed of biomaterials that are nonantigenic, nontoxic, nonimmunogenic, nondegradable, and noncarcinogenic. The valve also must have a low incidence of thromboembolism.

The opening resistance to blood flow is determined by the orifice diameter; the size, shape, and weight of the occluder; the opening angle; and the orientation of leaflet or disk occluders with respect to the plane of the mitral annular orifice for any given annular size. Least resistance to transvalvular blood flow during diastole for valves in the mitral position is provided by a large ratio of orifice to total annular area. A wide opening angle also improves the effective orifice area and results in decreased diastolic pressure gradients. With an increasing orifice diameter, however, more energy is lost across the valve as more backflow passes through the valve at end diastole and early systole. Table 42-1 shows hemodynamic assessments of each of the FDA-approved mitral valve prostheses for the most commonly used mitral valve sizes.[72–75] The results of in vivo assessments at rest by invasive (catheterization) or noninvasive (Doppler echocardiography) techniques are tabulated.

Blood turbulence flowing across mitral valve devices results from impedance to forward or reverse flow. This impedance can be minimized by occluder design and orientation, central flow through the orifice, and limited struts or pivots extending into flow areas (Fig. 42-3). Hemolysis is the product of red blood cell destruction that is caused by cavitation and shearing stresses of turbulence, high-velocity flow, regurgitation, and mechanical damage during valve closure.[76] Areas of perivalvular blood stagnation and turbulence increase platelet aggregation, activation of the coagulation proteins, and thrombus formation.

Dynamic regurgitation is a feature of all prosthetic valves and is the sum of the closing volume during occluder closure and the leakage volume that passes through the valve while it is closed. The closing volume is a function of the effective orifice area and the time needed for closure. Closure time is influenced by the difference between the opening and closing angles of the occluder and valve ring. Leakage volume is inherent to the design of the valve and depends on the amount of time the valve remains in the closed position.[77] A small amount of regurgitant volume can be beneficial by minimizing stasis and reducing platelet aggregation; this decreases the incidence of valve thrombosis and valve-related thromboembolism.

TABLE 42-1 Hemodynamics of Mitral Valve Prostheses

Valve	Reference (Year)						EOA (cm^2)				
		25 mm	27 mm	29 mm	31 mm	33 mm	25 mm	27 mm	29 mm	31 mm	33 mm
Starr-Edwards	Pyle (1978)		1.4	1.4	1.9			8.0	10.0	5.0	
	Sala (1982)							7.9	6.7	5.0	
	Horskotte (1987)		1.8					6.3			
Omniscience/Omnicarbon	Mikhail (1989)							6.1		5.4	
	Messner-Pellenc (1993)		1.9	2.2	2.0	2.0	4.3	3.6	3.5	2.0	
	Fehsk (1994)						6	6	5	6	4
	di Summa (2002)	1.7	1.9	1.6	1.9		9	4.1	5.1	5.6	
Medtronic Hall	Hall (1985)							3.0	2.7	2.0	
	Fiore (1998)						4.0	4.3	3.1	2.9	2.7
St. Jude	Chaux (1981)			2.1	2.8	3.1			1.9	1.8	1.6
	Horskotte (1987)			3.1					2.3		
	Fiore (1998)						3.0	3.3	3.8	1.5	2.5
	Hasegawa (2000)	2.6	2.5	2.4							
Carbomedics	Johnston (1992)			3.3					3.8		
	Chambers (1993)		2.1	2.1	1.8			3.9	3.3	3.3	
	Carbomedics (1993)		2.9	3.0	3.0			3.9	4.6	4.6	
	Carrier (2006)						5.3	4.9	4.6	4.4	4.9
ATS	Westaby (1996)		3	2	2	2					
	Shiono (1996)						5	6	4.5		
	Hasegawa (2000)	2.3	2.6	2.7							
	Emery (2001)						7.8	5	6	4	3
Hancock standard	Johnson (1975)		1.0	2.5	1.8			12.0	5.0	5.0	
	Ubago (1982)		1.3	1.0	1.0			7.0	7.6	7.4	
	Khuri (1988)		1.5	2.0	1.8			7.0	7.0	7.0	

Carpentier-Edwards porcine	Chaitman (1979)		1.7	2.2	2.8			7.0	6.7	5.0	
	Levine (1981)			3.0	3.2				2.0	2.6	
	Pelletier (1982)		1.7	2.4	2.5			6.5	7.4	5.3	
Carpentier-Edwards pericardial	Aupart (1997)	2.6	2.7	2.6	3.1		4.1	3.0	3.0	3.0	3.1
Mosaic	Thomson (2001)			1.7 (all sizes)							
	Eichinger (2002)	2.6	1.5	1.8	2.1		4.6	3.8	4.4	2.7	
	Fradet (2004)	1.1	0.9	1.0	0.9		4.2	5.8	4.8	4.0	
Biocor	Rizzoli (2005)			3.1	3.3	3.6			6.7	6.2	5.4
Normal				4.6					0		
Severe stenosis				>1.0					>12		
Desired postoperative				>1.5					>10		

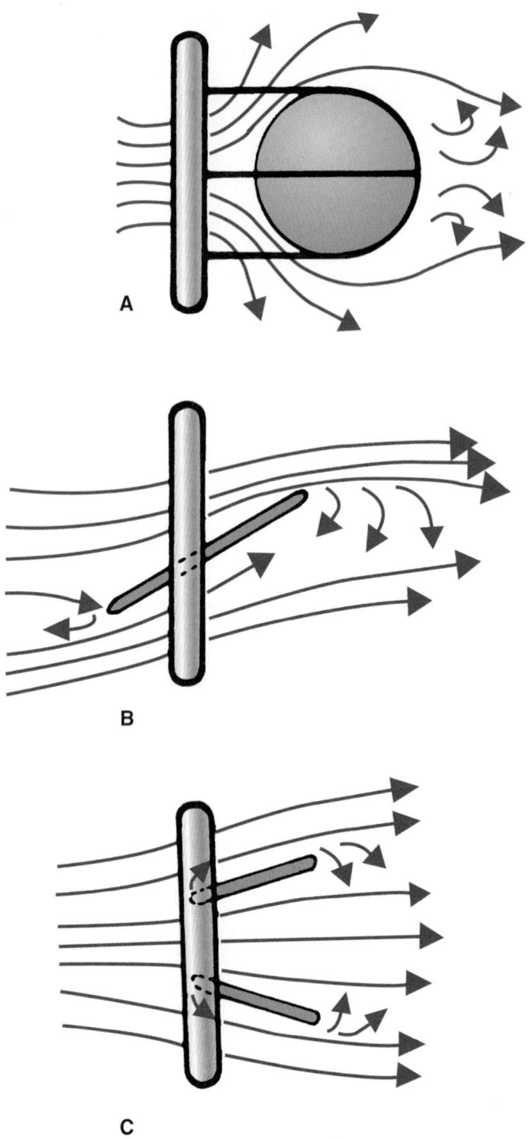

FIGURE 42-3 Flow characteristics of different mechanical valve designs. (A) Ball-and-cage. (B) Tilting-disk. (C) Bileaflet.

The Starr-Edwards Model 6120 is the only ball-and-cage mitral valve prosthesis currently approved for use in the United States by the FDA. It was introduced with its current design in 1965 after undergoing several engineering modifications and has been in use longer than any other type of mechanical valve (see Fig. 42-1A). The occluder is a barium-impregnated Silastic ball in a Stellite alloy cage that projects into the left ventricle. This valve has a large Teflon/polypropylene sewing ring that produces a relatively smaller effective orifice and larger diastolic pressure gradients than other prosthetic valves of similar annular sizes. Leakage volumes are not inherent in the ball-and-cage design, and in contrast with other mechanical valves, the presence of regurgitation may indicate a pathologic process. The central ball occluder causes lateralization of forward flow and results in turbulence and cavitation that increase the risk of hemolysis and thromboembolic complications (see Fig. 42-3A). The incidence of thromboembolism has been shown to be higher with the Starr-Edwards valve than with bileaflet valves in most studies[78,79] but not all.[80] Because the cage projects into the left ventricle, it is unwise to implant this valve in small left ventricles, where the cage may contact the ventricular wall or cause ventricular outflow obstruction.

Tilting-disk mitral valve prostheses have better hemodynamic characteristics than ball-and-cage valves (see Fig.42-3B). The Medtronic Hall central pivoting-disk valve was introduced in 1977 and is based on engineering design modifications of the earlier Hall-Kaster valve[81] (see Fig. 42-1B). The axis of the tilting disk was moved more centrally to allow greater blood flow through the minor orifice and to reduce stagnation in areas of low flow. The opening angle originally was increased to 78 degrees to decrease resistance to forward flow and later narrowed to 70 degrees when in vitro studies revealed an unacceptable regurgitant volume. The opening angle of 70 degrees produced regurgitation volumes of less than 5% of left ventricular stroke volume without significantly compromising forward flow. The disk occluder was allowed to slide out of the housing at the end of the closing cycle to provide a gap through which blood could flow to minimize stasis at the contact surfaces.[110] The large opening angle and slim disk occluder, along with a thinner sewing ring, provide improved hemodynamics with comparably larger effective orifice areas and lower mean diastolic pressure gradients for each valve size. During implantation, the larger orifice should be oriented posteriorly when using the larger valve sizes to minimize the potential for disk impingement. Smaller valves (27 mm or less) should be oriented with the larger orifice anteriorly to optimize in vivo hemodynamics.[73,82]

The Omniscience tilting-disk valve is a second-generation device derived from improvements to the design of the Lillehei-Kaster pivoting-disk valve.[83] This low-profile device has a pyrolytic disk located eccentrically in a one-piece titanium housing attached to a seamless Teflon sewing ring. Introduced in 1978, the Omniscience prosthesis includes several engineering modifications from prior devices in an effort to improve its hemodynamic function. The orifice-to-annular-area ratio was increased to minimize resistance to forward flow. The opening angle of 80 degrees is relatively large to allow flow reserve in patients with high cardiac outputs and during exercise. Resulting increases in regurgitant volumes are minimized by the disk design. Turbulence is reduced by the curvature of the disk, and areas of stasis and shear stress are reduced by the eccentric location of the pivot axis in an effort to decrease the risk of thrombosis, thromboembolism, and hemolysis. Retaining prongs are not used, and the lower profile reduces the risk of impingement. A potential hemodynamic disadvantage that has been the subject of debate is the possibility of incomplete disk opening in vivo. Clinical studies report postoperative mean opening angles of between 44.8[73] and 75.9 degrees.[84] Implicated factors causing this variation include valve sizing, orientation during implantation, and anticoagulation status.[84,85] A subsequent generation of the Omniscience valve is the all-carbon Omnicarbon monoleaflet valve that was released in 2001 in the United States but has been in clinical use in Europe since 1984 (see Fig. 42-1C). The housing material is made of pyrolytic carbon instead of titanium. As a result of this change, the incidence of thromboembolism, valvular thrombosis, and reoperations was decreased significantly compared with the Omniscience valve protheses.[86] For all the tilting-disk valves, meticulous surgical technique is important because retained leaflets or chordae can cause subvalvular interference and leakage.

The unique design of the bileaflet St. Jude Medical valve was introduced in 1977, and it is currently the prosthesis used most commonly worldwide (see Fig. 42-1D). Two separate pyrolytic carbon semidisks in a pyrolytic carbon housing are attached to a Dacron sewing ring. The housing has two pivot guards that project into the left atrium. The bileaflet design produces three different flow areas through the valve orifice that provide overall a more uniform, central, and laminar flow than in the caged-ball and monoleaflet tilting-disk designs. The improved flow results in less turbulence and decreased transmitral diastolic pressure gradients[77,87] (see Fig. 42-3C) at any annulus diameter size and cardiac output compared with the caged-ball and single-leaflet tilting valves.[88] The favorable hemodynamics in smaller sizes makes it especially useful in children. The central opening angle is 85 degrees, with a closing angle of 30 to 35 degrees, which along with a thin sewing ring, provides a large effective orifice area for each valve size at the expense of greater regurgitant volumes, especially at low heart rates. Asynchronous closure of the valve leaflets in vivo also contributes to the regurgitant volume.[89] The design of this prosthesis provides excellent hemodynamic function even in small sizes in any rotational plane.[90] The antianatomical plane, however, with the central slit between the leaflets oriented perpendicular to the opening axis of the native valve leaflets decreases the potential risk of leaflet impingement by the posterior left ventricular wall.[91]

The Carbomedics bileaflet valve was approved by the FDA in 1986 (see Fig. 42-1E). This low-profile device is constructed of pyrolytic carbon and has no pivot guards, struts, or orifice projections to decrease blood flow impedance and turbulence through the valve.[77] It has a rotatable sewing cuff design and is available with a more generous and flexible sewing cuff (the OptiForm variant) that confirms more easily to different patient anatomies and allows sub-, intra-, or supra-annular suture placement. The leaflet opening angle is 78 degrees, which with the bileaflet design provides a relatively large effective orifice area and transvalvular diastolic pressure differences only slightly greater than the St. Jude Medical bileaflet valve. Rapid synchronous leaflet closure reduces closing regurgitant volumes to less than that of the Björk-Shiley pivoting-disk prosthesis, which has an opening angle of 60 degrees. Leakage volume, however, is greater with Carbomedics valves because of backflow through gaps around pivots. Because of its narrow closing angle and large leakage volume, the Carbomedics valve does not reduce the relatively large regurgitant volume associated with the bileaflet design. Although this valve has good hemodynamic function overall, in the mitral position, the 25-mm Carbomedics valve has a relatively high diastolic pressure gradient and large regurgitant energy loss across the valve, especially at high flows. Hemodynamic studies suggest that the Carbomedics valve should be avoided in patients with a small mitral valve orifice.[77]

The ATS (Advancing The Standard) mechanical prosthesis has been in clinical use in the United States since 2000. Similar to the Carbomedics valve, the ATS valve is a low-profile bileaflet prosthesis with a pyrolytic housing and pyrolytic carbon leaflets containing graphite substrate (see Fig. 42-1F). The pivot areas are located entirely within the orifice ring, and the valve leaflets hinge on convex pivot guides on the carbon orifice ring. This design minimizes the overall height of the valve and provides a wider orifice area, and the absence of cavities in the valve ring theoretically reduces stasis or eddy currents that may develop. Valve noise, a bothersome problem for some patients, also is reduced by this design.[91] The opening angle is up to 85 degrees, and the sewing cuff is constructed of double velour polyester fabric that is mounted to a titanium stiffening ring, which enables the surgeon to rotate the valve orifice during and after implantation.

The On-X prosthesis was approved by the FDA in 2002. It has a bileaflet design similar to the St. Jude Medical, Carbomedics, and ATS prostheses with comparable hemodynamic performance, ie, a relatively large orifice diameter and a wide opening angle (90 degrees) (see Fig. 42-1G). Instead of silicon-alloyed pyrolytic carbon, as used in the other mechanical prostheses, the On-X valve is made of pure pyrolytic carbon. This material is stronger and tougher than silicon-alloyed carbon and allows incorporation of hydrodynamically efficient features into the valve orifice, such as increased orifice length and a flared inlet that reduces transvalvular gradient. Early clinical results are promising and the valve produces very little hemolysis with postoperative levels of serum lactate dehydrogenase in the normal range.[95,96]

Bioprostheses

Porcine Valves

The porcine bioprosthetic mitral valves are designed to mimic the flow characteristics of the in situ aortic valve. The Hancock I mitral valve bioprosthesis was introduced in 1970. It has three glutaraldehyde-preserved porcine aortic valve leaflets on a polypropylene stent attached to a Dacron-covered silicone sewing ring. The design allows for central laminar flow through the valve, which tends to decrease diastolic pressure gradients and minimize turbulence.[87] The stent, however, impedes forward flow and results in relatively large diastolic pressure gradients across the bioprosthesis. The stent and the large sewing ring contribute to effective orifice areas that are smaller than those of size-matched mechanical valves (see Table 42-1).

The Hancock II porcine bioprosthesis (see Fig. 42-2A) is the more modern version of the Hancock I prosthesis. The stent is made of Delrin with a scalloped sewing ring and reduced stent profile. The leaflets are fixed in glutaraldehyde at low pressure and subsequently for a prolonged period at high pressure. To retard calcification, the leaflets are treated with sodium dodecyl sulfate.

The Carpentier-Edwards porcine valve uses a flexible stent to decrease the stress of leaflet flexion while maintaining its overall configuration (see Fig. 42-2B). The effective orifice-to-total-annulus-area ratio for the Carpentier-Edwards valve is relatively small, but exercise studies show that the effective orifice area increases significantly with increased blood flow across the valve; diastolic gradients also increase, although to a lesser degree.[74,75,97,] Porcine bioprostheses in the mitral position should be avoided in patients with small left ventricles because of the possibility of ventricular rupture or left ventricular outflow obstruction caused by the large struts.[97]

The Mosaic porcine bioprosthesis is a third-generation bioprosthesis using the Hancock II stent (see Fig. 42-2C). It was introduced in the United States in 2000 and has a Delrin stent, scalloped sewing ring, and reduced stent profile. The valve tissue is pressure-free fixed with glutaraldehyde, and the prosthesis is treated with alpha-oleic acid (AOA) to retard calcification.

In 2005, the FDA approved the Biocor porcine bioprosthesis (St. Jude Medical); however, it has been used and investigated for almost two decades in Europe. It belongs to the third generation of bioprostheses, and the valve tissue is pretreated in glutaraldehyde at very low pressure (<1 mm Hg), making the valve cusps less stiff with less tendency to tissue fatigue.

Pericardial Valves

Previous studies indicated poor durability of pericardial valves, namely, the Ionescu-Shiley valve, caused by leaflet tearing. This led to significant changes in design, including mounting of the pericardium completely within the stent, causing less leaflet abrasion and increased durability. The Carpentier-Edwards pericardial valve uses bovine pericardium as material to fabricate a trileaflet valve that is cut, fitted, and sewn onto a flexible Elgiloy wire frame for stress reduction (see Fig. 42-2D). The tissue is preserved with glutaraldehyde with no applied pressure, and the leaflets are treated with the calcium mitigation agent XenoLogiX. Compared with the Carpentier-Edwards porcine bioprosthesis, the stent profile is reduced. Long-term durability for the Carpentier-Edwards pericardial valve is strong, and compared with third-generation porcine valves, valve-related complications are similar (see discussion later in this chapter).

Hemodynamically, pericardial valves provide the best solution to flow problems. The design maximizes use of the flow area, which results in minimal flow resistance. Figure 42-4A shows how the cone shape of the open valve and circular valve orifice minimizes flow disturbance compared with the more irregular cone shape of the porcine valves that allow for central unimpeded flow (see Fig. 42-4B).

Structural valve deterioration is seen after long-term follow-up of patients with both porcine and pericardial bioprostheses and results in mitral stenosis or regurgitation or both. Hemodynamic studies early after operation and at 5 years reveal higher average diastolic pressure gradients and smaller effective orifice areas when compared in the same patients at the follow-up study. In some patients, these changes are sufficiently severe to require reoperation as soon as 4 to 5 years postoperatively, and by 10 years the rate of primary tissue failure averages 30%. It then accelerates, and by 15 years postoperatively, the actuarial freedom from bioprosthetic primary tissue failure has ranged from 35 to 71%[49,51,53,54,72] (Table 42-2). Most of these patients show hemodynamic evidence of valvular deterioration before any clinical signs or symptoms.[75] Bioprosthetic valves have the advantage of low thrombogenicity, which must be weighed against poor long-term durability and subsequent hemodynamic deterioration and the risk of reoperation.

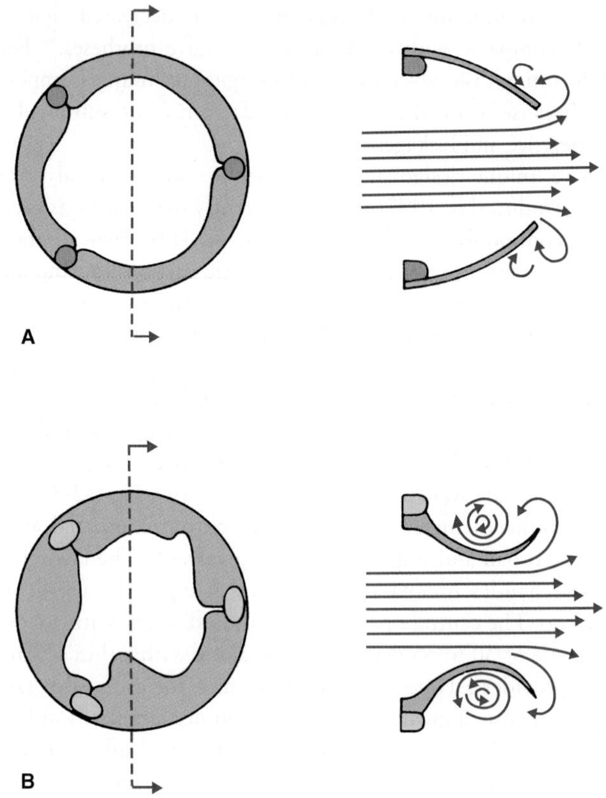

FIGURE 42-4 Flow patterns for bioprosthetic valves. (A) Pericardial bioprosthesis. (B) Porcine bioprosthesis.

OPERATIVE TECHNIQUES

Preoperative Management and Anesthetic Preparation

Congestive heart failure secondary to mitral stenosis usually can be treated with aggressive diuretic therapy and sodium restriction preoperatively. If the patient is in rapid atrial fibrillation, digoxin, beta blockers, and calcium channel antagonists can be used to slow down the ventricular rate. Patients with acute mitral regurgitation often are in cardiogenic shock, and they can be stabilized preoperatively with inotropes and arterial vasodilators to reduce systemic afterload. Intra-aortic balloon counterpulsation also can be used for this purpose. Symptoms of congestive heart failure in patients with chronic mitral regurgitation are treated with diuretics and oral vasodilators. The vasodilators lower the peripheral vascular resistance, and forward cardiac output is increased by reducing the regurgitant volume into the left atrium.

Preferred anesthesia for mitral valve replacement typically involves a combination of narcotic and inhalational agents. Ultimately, anesthetic management is dictated by the wide range of functional disabilities and hemodynamic abnormalities of patients who present for mitral valve replacement. For example, a cachectic patient with functional class IV mitral stenosis and severe pulmonary hypertension may require postoperative positive-pressure mechanical ventilation for 1 or 2 days to remove excess pulmonary fluid by diuresis, facilitate bronchial toileting, and provide optimal conditions for adequate gas exchange.

TABLE 42-2 Freedom (Actuarial) from Structural Valve Deterioration after Mitral Valve Replacement with Bioprotheses

Valve	Reference (year)	5 y	10 y	15 y	20 y
Hancock Standard	Cohn (1989)	98%	75%	45%	
	Burdon (1992)	98%	80%	44%	
	Bortolotti (1995)	94%	73%	35%	
	Khan (1998)				65%
Hancock II	Legarra (1999)		65%		33% (18 y)
	David (2001)	100%	86%	66%	
	Rizzoli (2003)	99%	86%	60%	
	Masters (2004)		98% (8 y)		
Carpentier-Edwards porcine	Perier (1989)	89%	65%		
	Sarris (1993)	97%	60%		
	Jamieson (1995)	98%	72%	49%	
	Van Doorn (1995)	97%	71%		
	Corbineau (2001)	98%	83%	48%	
Carpentier-Edwards pericardial	Pelletier (1995)	100%	79% (8 y)		
	Takahara (1995)		84% (9 y)		
	Aupart (1997)	100%	76%		
	Marchand (1998)	98%	85% (11 y)		
	Neville (1998)	100%	78% (12 y)		
	Poirer (1998)	100%	81%		
Mosaic	Jasinski (2000)	100% (2 y)			
	Thomson (2001)	100% (4 y)			
	Eichinger (2002)	100%			
	Fradet (2004)	100% (7 y)			
	Jamieson (2005)	98% (6 y)			
Biocor	Myken (2000)		100% (8 y)	92%	
	Rizzoli (2005)				

Alternatively, young patients who require mitral valve surgery and present with less preoperative comorbidity may benefit from a short-acting, balanced anesthetic that can facilitate extubation within 6 hours of surgery.[98]

Monitoring should include arterial and venous lines, a urinary catheter, and a pulmonary artery catheter placed before bypass to measure pulmonary pressures and cardiac output. After valve replacement, occasionally a left atrial catheter directly inserted through the left atrial incision can be helpful to allow measurement of pulmonary vascular resistance, but we do not use it routinely. Preoperative intravenous prophylactic antibiotics are administered to all patients and are continued for 2 postoperative days until lines are removed. Temporary ventricular pacing wires are placed, and in many instances temporary atrial pacing wires are placed for possible pacing or diagnosis of various atrial arrhythmias.

Cardiopulmonary Bypass for Mitral Valve Replacement

Cardiopulmonary bypass is instituted by placing two right-angle cannulas into the superior and inferior venae cavae. We place a small (22 French) plastic or metal cannula directly into the superior vena cava, above the sinoatrial node. The inferior caval cannula is placed at the entrance of the inferior vena cava, low in the right atrium. These insertion sites keep the caval catheters out of the operative field and yet maintain excellent bicaval drainage. An arterial cannula is placed in the distal ascending aorta. Bypass flows are approximately 1.5 L/m^2 per minute, and moderate hypothermia 28 to 32°C is used with vacuum-assisted suction. Myocardial protection includes antegrade and retrograde blood cardioplegia and profound myocardial hypothermia.[99] Retrograde cardioplegia is useful for all valve surgery to protect the ischemic left ventricle and help remove ascending aorta bubbles. Antegrade cardioplegia, used as an initial loading dose, is augmented by intermittent retrograde cardioplegia every 20 minutes. This provides safer delivery of cardioplegia because when the atrium is retracted during valve replacement, the aortic valve is distorted, and antegrade cardioplegia tends to fill the ventricle.

Exposure of the Mitral Valve

Evolution of meticulous and complicated methods of mitral valve repair and reconstruction has required optimal exposure

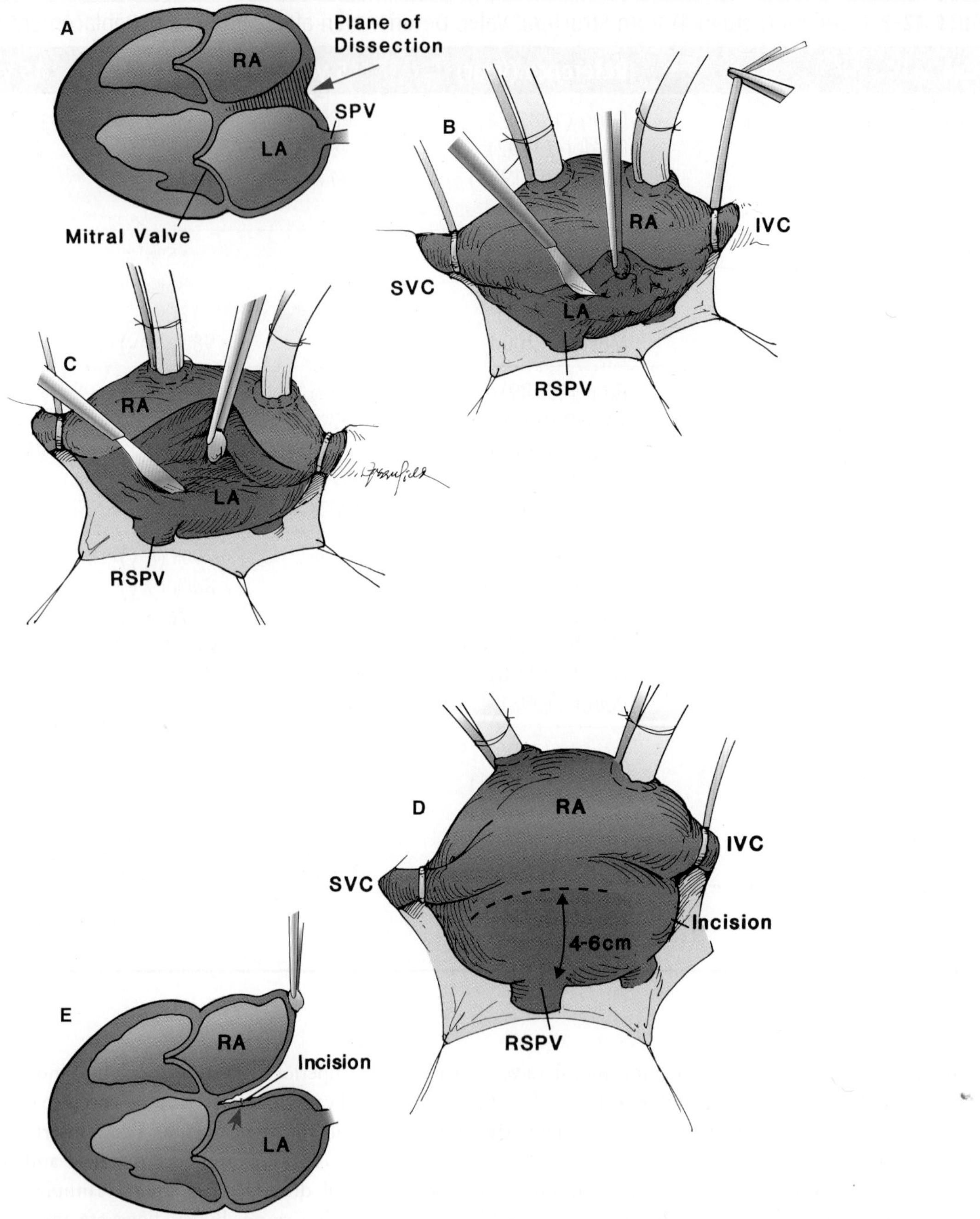

FIGURE 42-5 Exposure of the mitral valve. (**A**) Location of Sondergaard's plane. (**B**,**C**) Development of the interatrial plane. (**D**) Location of the left atrial incision. (**E**) Cross-sectional view.

of the mitral valve. In primary operations, median sternotomy, development of Sondergaard's plane, and incision of the left atrium close to the atrial septum provide excellent exposure[100,101] (Fig. 42-5). This incision is a ubiquitous one, and we have rarely seen indications for use of other incisions, such as the superior approach through the dome of the left atrium,[102,103] the so-called biatrial incision popularized by Guiraudon and colleagues,[105] division of the superior vena cava,[106,107] and the less common but occasionally useful trans–right atrial septal incision.[108] The trans–right atrial incision has in some studies been related to higher incidence of junctional and nonsinus rhythm postoperatively,[109] although this has not been confirmed by other studies.[110]

Minimally Invasive Mitral Valve Replacement

After advances in videoscopic and other minimally invasive techniques in many areas of surgery in the 1990s, similar techniques are now being used increasingly in cardiac surgery, especially in mitral valve surgery. In 1996, we began minimally invasive valve surgery for patients who have isolated valvular pathology without concomitant coronary artery disease. Our experience at Brigham and Women's Hospital now totals over 1000 patients, including mitral valve repairs and aortic and mitral valve replacements.[110] The minimally invasive approach for mitral valve surgery is well described in Chapter 44.

Safety and efficacy of minimally invasive mitral valve surgery have been confirmed in several reports.[31,109–111] Trauma seems to be less with the minimally invasive incisions, which is beneficial in regard to infections (including mediastinitis) and bleeding from the incision and the operative field, leading to lesser usage of homologous blood.[111] There is also improved cosmesis with these incisions, and postoperative pain seems to be considerably less than in patients with the median sternotomy. This can result in fewer requirements for pain medication and faster return to normal activity with less dependence on after-hospital stay and after-hospital care without compromising results.

Intracardiac Technique

Operation entails secure fixation of a valve prosthesis to the annulus by reliable suture techniques without damage to adjacent structures or myocardium and without tissue interference with valve function. Implantation should prevent injury to anatomical structures surrounding the mitral valve annulus. Figure 42-6 shows the proximity of important cardiac structures near the mitral valve annulus. These include the circumflex coronary artery within the atrioventricular (AV) groove, the left atrial appendage, the aortic valve in continuity with the anterior mitral curtain, and the AV node.

An accumulation of laboratory and clinical evidence indicates that preservation of papillary muscle–chordal attachments to the annulus is important for maintenance of left ventricular function. In patients with mitral stenosis with agglutinated, fibrotic chordae and papillary muscles, preservation of these structures probably has little effect on left ventricular dysfunction but does protect the AV groove from rupture by preserving the posterior leaflet. However, preservation of the posterior mitral leaflet may preclude use of an adequately sized prosthesis. If fibrotic, agglutinated chordae and the posterior leaflet are excised, placement of artificial Gore-Tex chordae to reattach the papillary muscles to the annulus may improve early and late preservation of cardiac output.[112] In patients with mitral regurgitation, however, it is important to preserve as much of the papillary muscle and annular interaction as possible. This can be achieved by a variety of techniques, as shown in Fig. 42-7. The anterior leaflet may be partially excised and brought to the posterior leaflet[113] (see Fig. 42-7A) or can be partially excised and "furled" to the anterior annulus by a running Prolene suture[114,115] (see Fig. 42-7B).

Experimental and clinical evidence suggest that preservation of the conical shape of the ventricle is important to maintain

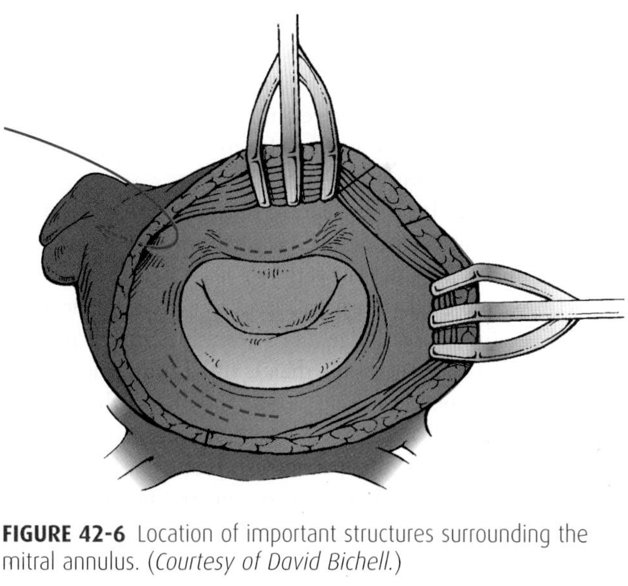

FIGURE 42-6 Location of important structures surrounding the mitral annulus. (*Courtesy of David Bichell.*)

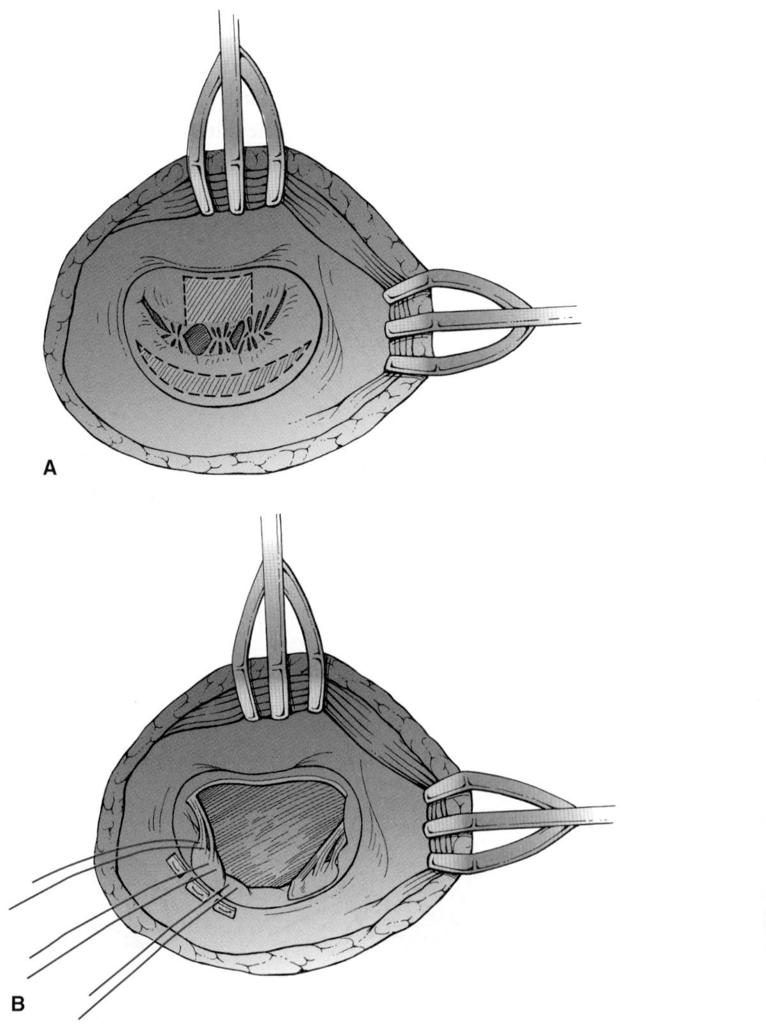

FIGURE 42-7 Techniques to maintain annular–papillary muscle continuity. (A) An ellipse is removed from the posterior leaflet, and a flap is cut from the central portion of the anterior leaflet. The anterior flap is flipped to the posterior annulus and tacked to the caudad edge of the posterior leaflet and the posterior annulus. Sutures anchoring the prosthesis include the annulus and anterior and posterior leaflet remnants to which chordae are attached. (B) The anterior leaflet is partially excised, and remnants are "furled" to the annulus by sutures used to insert the prosthesis.

normal cardiac output[116–119] and that assumption of a globular shape from cutting papillary muscles is deleterious to left ventricular function. Furthermore, preservation of the posterior leaflet and chordae has reduced the incidence of perforation of the left ventricle and atrioventricular separation dramatically during mitral valve replacement.[10,120,121]

Suturing techniques vary according to the type of valve that is implanted. The bioprosthetic valve is inserted preferentially with the sutures placed from ventricle to atrium (noneverting or subannular). This has been shown to be the strongest type of suturing technique to the mitral annulus and is used with this valve and with the central-flow Starr-Edwards ball-and-cage valve (Fig. 42-8A).

To ensure adequate function of bileaflet or tilting-disk valves, everting sutures (atrium to ventricle to sewing ring) should be used (see Fig. 42-8B). This technique pushes the prosthetic valve out into the center of the orifice and minimizes any tissue interference of the prosthetic valve leaflets. This is particularly important if annular-chordal attachments are preserved. Teflon-pledgeted sutures, particularly with the thin sewing rings of the currently available bileaflet and tilting-disk valves, should be used. If a bioprosthetic valve is inserted, a dental mirror is used to ensure that no annular suture is wrapped around a stent strut. A running Prolene suture for implantation of mitral valves has been advocated by some surgeons.[123,124] This technique makes a very clean suture line with minimal knots but runs the risk of valve dehiscence if an infection occurs.[125]

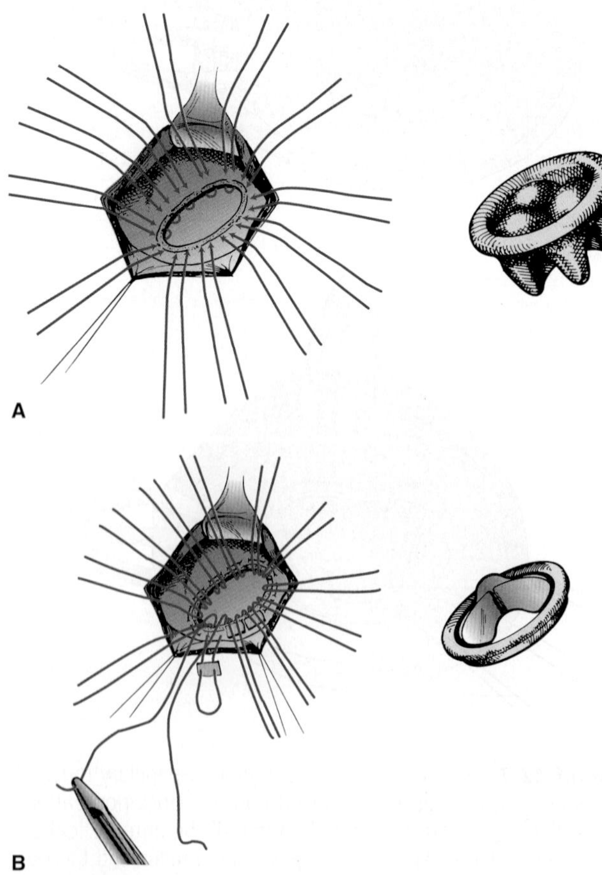

A

B

FIGURE 42-8 Suturing techniques for prosthetic mitral valve implantation. (A) Noneverting (subannular) sutures placed from ventricle to atrium for bioprosthetic or Starr-Edwards valves. (B) Everting (supra-annular) sutures placed from atrium to ventricle for bileaflet or tilting-disk valves.

Before closure, the left atrial appendage is ligated by suture or stapled to prevent clot formation in patients with chronic atrial fibrillation, enlarged left atrium, or left atrial thrombus.[126] The atrium is closed by a running Prolene suture, making sure that endocardial surfaces are approximated. If needed, a left atrial catheter can be inserted through the suture line.

ASSOCIATED OPERATIONS/PROCEDURES

Coronary bypass is the most common procedure performed with mitral valve replacement and should be performed first. This reduces lifting of the heart after the rigid mitral valve prosthesis is in place, which can cause rupture of the myocardium or the atrioventricular groove. This also allows cardioplegia to be delivered through the bypass grafts.

Tricuspid valve repair or replacements usually are performed after replacing the mitral valve. In these cases, the mitral valve often is approached through the right atrium and a transseptal incision. After the mitral valve prosthesis is in place, the septum is closed, and the aortic cross-clamp is removed before proceeding with the tricuspid valve procedure.[127]

When both the aortic and mitral valves are replaced at the same operation, most surgeons begin with excising the aortic valve before proceeding with the mitral valve procedure. When excising the anterior mitral valve leaflet, care must be taken not to injure the aortic annulus and the intra-annular region. The aortic valve then is sewn in after the mitral valve is in place.

Weaning Off Cardiopulmonary Bypass

We use transesophageal echocardiography for every valve operation and particularly for mitral valves, where excellent images can be obtained. If transesophageal echocardiography is contraindicated (eg, because of esophageal disease), direct epicardial echocardiography can be used. The echocardiograms provide information about valve and left ventricular function, possible retained material in the left atrium including thrombus, and removal of intracardiac air.

A careful de-airing at the end of the operation is essential. The heart is vented through the left atrium and the ascending aorta and sometimes the left ventricle. Before the aortic cross-clamp is removed, the patient's head is lowered and the lungs inflated carefully to dislodge any air bubbles in the pulmonary vein. The operating table then is tilted from side to side, the left atrial appendage is inverted, and the cardiac chambers are aspirated if necessary. Once de-airing maneuvers are completed, and after the patient is completely rewarmed, venous return is partially occluded, and the heart is gradually volume loaded. Pulmonary artery pressures are monitored carefully. Pharmacologic agents, such as amrinone or dobutamine, particularly for right ventricular overload, are used frequently.

De-airing the heart after a minimally invasive approach is more complex because the heart is only partially visible through the 5- to 7-cm sternal incision, and the apex of the heart is not accessible. Flooding the operative field with continuous CO_2 can be beneficial in reducing intracardial air.[128] In addition, by filling the left ventricle with cardioplegia through the left atriotomy suture line, and manipulating the volume of the heart on bypass and alternating the position of the patient, air can be evacuated effectively.

POSTOPERATIVE CARE

Postoperative care is directed toward the resumption of normal cardiac output, respiratory function, temperature control, electrolyte management, adequate renal flow, and prophylaxis against bleeding. Patients with low cardiac output are managed with a variety of pharmacologic agents after providing adequate volume loading. Left atrial and especially pulmonary arterial catheters are particularly helpful in determining optimal balancing of volume loading and myocardial function in the first hours after operation.

Reduction in pulmonary interstitial fluid is pursued aggressively by diuresis in the intensive care unit in patients with severe pulmonary hypertension. Most patients with severe pulmonary hypertension can be extubated within 48 hours of surgery. Nutritional, respiratory, and general metabolic support is provided. Many patients with severe, longstanding mitral valve disease are cachectic and, despite preoperative nutritional support, are severely catabolic at the time of operation. These patients generally require longer periods of ventilatory support owing to lack of respiratory muscle strength. They need aggressive nutritional support with nasogastric hyperalimentation to increase respiratory muscle strength. In patients with severe pulmonary hypertension and cardiac cachexia who require prolonged intubation, tracheostomy may be necessary to reduce ventilatory dead space and facilitate faster weaning and better pulmonary toilet. Tracheostomy usually is performed by the end of the first postoperative week.

Postoperative atrial arrhythmias are so common that their absence is unusual. Arrhythmias vary from rapid supraventricular tachycardias, usually atrial fibrillation, to junctional rhythm and heart block. These arrhythmias are treated by pharmacologic agents, pacemakers, or both. If rapid atrial fibrillation cannot be controlled pharmacologically and is destabilizing hemodynamically, emergency cardioversion is done to improve cardiac output. Pharmacologic management of supraventricular tachycardia usually is required but may precipitate the need for a prophylactic transvenous pacemaker if severe slowing of the heart rate occurs.

Anticoagulation is prescribed for all patients undergoing mitral valve replacement with either a mechanical or bioprosthetic valve. In the first 6 weeks after operation, the incidence of atrial and other arrhythmias is high; thus, these fluctuating rhythms mandate anticoagulation even if the basic rhythm is sinus. In addition to rhythm concerns, the left atrial incisions and the possibility of stasis in the left atrial appendage justify full anticoagulation with warfarin for all patients. Some surgeons advocate immediate intravenous heparin until therapeutic warfarin doses can be reached.[129,130] Low molecular weight heparin (LMWH) also can be used.[131,132]

The therapeutic international normalized ratio (INR) after mitral valve replacement is 2.5 to 3.5 depending on the type of valve, cardiac rhythm, and presence or absence of the aforementioned intraoperative risk factors for thromboembolism.[2,126,130,131] Anticoagulation levels are in the low range for patients in sinus rhythm who received tissue valves. Patients who have mechanical valves need lifelong anticoagulation. Patients who have bioprosthetic valves are evaluated at 6 to 12 weeks for cardiac rhythm abnormalities. If they are in predominantly sinus rhythm, warfarin is stopped, and one aspirin tablet is given daily indefinitely. If the patient has continuous atrial fibrillation or fluctuating rhythms, anticoagulation with warfarin is continued. This is also true for patients with a history of previous embolism or in whom thrombus is found in the left atrium at operation.

Warfarin usually is started on the second postoperative day. Addition of aspirin, 80 to 150 mg daily, to the warfarin may reduce the risk of thromboembolism[133,134] and may have a role in patients with prosthetic valves.[135]

RESULTS

Early Results

The hospital mortality for mitral valve replacement with and without coronary bypass grafting has decreased significantly since the inception of mitral valve surgery. The current risk (2006) of elective primary mitral valve replacement with and without coronary bypass grafting is 5 to 9% in most studies (range 3.3 to 13.1%).[72] Operative (30-day) mortality is related to myocardial failure, multisystem organ failure, bleeding, respiratory failure in the chronically ill, debilitated individual, diabetes, infection, stroke, and, very rarely, technical problems.[27,45] Mortality is correlated with preoperative functional class, age, and preexisting coronary artery disease.[138]

Published results on mitral valve surgery have improved in recent years,[139] probably because of preservation of papillary muscles, preventing midventricular rupture,[120,121] and preservation of the normal geometry of the left ventricle, which aids in the maintenance of early postoperative cardiac output.[116,117,140] Mitral valve replacement and coronary artery bypass surgery 20 to 25 years ago had an associated mortality of about 10 to 20%.[44,141] This mortality risk also has decreased as myocardial protection has improved with the use of blood cardioplegia and retrograde methods of administration.[99,142] Some studies have indicated that the risk of combined mitral valve replacement–coronary artery bypass grafting is now no greater than that of mitral valve repair with an annuloplasty ring or mitral valve replacement without coronary artery bypass grafting.[116,143] Other studies have shown significantly increased morbidity and mortality with the addition of coronary artery bypass grafting.[48,144] Figures from the database of the Society of Thoracic Surgeons indicate that both reoperation and emergency operation increase operative mortality[145] (Fig. 42-9).

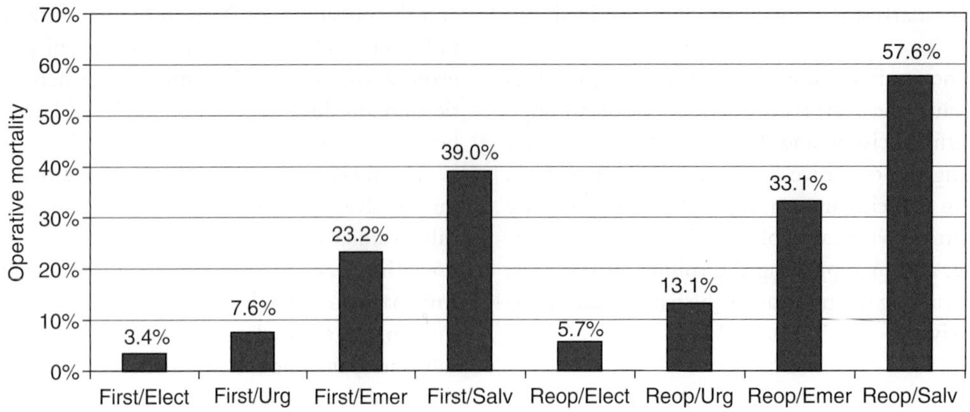

FIGURE 42-9 Operative mortality for elective, urgent, emergency, and salvage procedures for primary operations and reoperations for mitral valvular replacements. (*Data used with permission from Society of Thoracic Surgeons.*)

Late Results

Functional Improvement

In more than 90% of patients after mitral valve replacement, functional class improves to at least class II. A small group of patients remains in class III or IV depending on left ventricular function before surgery or other coexisting morbidity.

Survival

The causes of late death in patients after mitral valve replacement are primarily chronic myocardial dysfunction, thromboemboli and stroke, endocarditis, anticoagulant-related hemorrhage, and coronary artery disease. The extent of left ventricular dysfunction and patient age, particularly if myocardial and coronary diseases are combined, also correlate with late mortality. The probability of survival after mitral valve replacement at 10 years is usually around 50 to 60% (range 42 to 81%)[72] (Table 42-3). Long-term patient survival seems to be similar for patients with biologic and mechanical mitral valves.[147–149] Unlike patients with severe aortic regurgitation or aortic stenosis, arrhythmias seldom cause sudden death in patients after mitral valve replacement; however, a few patients die from thromboembolic stroke owing to chronic atrial fibrillation. The fact that more than 50% of patients after mitral valve replacement are in chronic atrial fibrillation increases the propensity for thromboembolic stroke despite anticoagulation and for mechanical valve thrombosis if the anticoagulation protocol is altered. In addition, patients with older types of prosthetic valves who receive higher-intensity anticoagulation may develop severe anticoagulant hemorrhage.[150]

In patients with bioprosthetic valves, one of the important determinants of mortality is reoperation secondary to structural valve degeneration[53,54,72] (Table 42-4). Reoperative mitral valve replacement mortality has decreased significantly in the last 15 years to under 10%, even in patients who have required multiple mitral valve reoperations.[142] At the Brigham and Women's Hospital, operative mortality was less than 6% for reoperative mitral valve operations from 1990 to 1995.[142] Improved myocardial protection, earlier selection of patients for reoperation, and better perfusion techniques, including frequent femorofemoral bypass to protect the right ventricle during incision and dissection of the heart, are factors contributing to decreased mortality.[116,142,152–154]

Late Morbidity

The major morbidity in patients after mitral valve replacement is structural valve deterioration of a bioprosthetic valve and thromboembolism and anticoagulant hemorrhage with a mechanical prosthesis. Both valve types develop perivalvular leak and infection.

Thromboembolism. Thromboembolism is perhaps the most common complication of both biologic and mechanical mitral prostheses but is more frequent in patients with mechanical valves. Chronic atrial fibrillation and local atrial factors, discussed earlier, increase the risk of thromboembolism in patients with mitral prostheses.[203,236] A number of recent studies have summarized the thromboembolic potential of various valves (Table 42-5), and it appears that the better the valve hemodynamics, the lower is the probability of thromboemboli. The incidence of thromboemboli in currently available bileaflet and tilting-disk valves is similar to that in bioprosthetic valves—about 1.5 to 2.0% per patient-year. Thromboembolism in patients with mitral valve replacement is lower in those with a small left atrium, sinus rhythm, and normal cardiac output. It is much higher in patients with a large left atrium, chronic atrial fibrillation, and the presence of intra-atrial clot.[126,169] Thrombosis of a mechanical valve, once a feared complication of tilting-disk valves,[170,171] is now relatively rare unless anticoagulation is stopped for any period of time. Valve thrombosis can be treated with thrombolytic agents if the patient is not in cardiogenic shock but requires surgery if the circulation is inadequate.[172,173]

Anticoagulant Hemorrhage. Bleeding related to anticoagulation is seen most commonly in the gastrointestinal, urogenital, and central nervous systems and usually is proportionate to the INR. The incidence of anticoagulant-related hemorrhage has decreased markedly with hemodynamic improvements in

TABLE 42-3 Actuarial Survival after Mitral Valve Replacement

		Actuarial Survival				
Valve	**Reference (year)**	**5 y**	**10 y**	**15 y**	**20 y**	**30 y**
Starr-Edwards	Teply (1981)	78%	56%			
	Sala (1982)	78%	72%			
	Miller (1983)	71%	47%			
	Godje (1997)	85%	75%	56%	37%	23%
	Murday (2003)		57% (8 y)			
	Gao (2004)		51%		23%	8%
Omniscience/Omnicarbon	Damle (1987)	91% (4 y)				
	Peter (1993)	77% (4 y)				
	Otaki (1993)	82% (6 y)				
	Misawa (1993)	94% (3 y)				
	Thevenet (1995)		88% (9 y)			
	Iguro (1999)	88%				
	Torregrosa (1999)		81%			
	di Summa (2002)		61%			
Medtronic Hall	Vallejo (1990)	79%				
	Masters (1995)	70%	67%			
	Fiore (1998)	70%	58%			
	Butchart (2001)		58%	36%		
	Masters (2001)	75%	63%			
St. Jude	DiSesa (1989)	65% (4 y)				
	Kratz (1993)	80%	63%			
	Aoyagi (1994)	88%	81%			
	Fiore (1998)	65%	53%			
	Camilleri (2001)	89% (4 y)				
	Remadi (2001)	88%	76%	61%		
	Masters (2001)	75%	52%			
	Lim (2003)	72%				
	Murday (2003)		44% (8 y)			
Carbomedics	Bortolotti (1991)	90%				
	Rabelo (1991)	75% (4 y)				
	De Luca (1993)	93% (3 y)				
	Copeland (1995)	81%				
	Nistal (1996)	83%				
	Yamauchi (1996)	92%				
	Masters (2001)	76%				
	Santini (2002)	86%	86%			
	Lim (2002)	72%				
	Soga (2002)	88%				
	Ikonamidis (2003)		61%		39%	
	Tominaga (2005)	95%	94%			
	Kang (2005)		89%			
	Carrier (2006)	76%	59%	40%		
	Wu (2006)	74%	54%			
On-X	Williams (2006)	87% (4 y)				
Hancock standard	Cohn (1989)	82%	60%			
	Burdon (1992)	74%	55%			
	Sarris (1993)	79%	58%			
	Khan (1998)		50%	29%	14%	

(Continued)

TABLE 42-3 Actuarial Survival after Mitral Valve Replacement (*Continued*)

			Actuarial Survival			
Valve	**Reference (year)**	**5 y**	**10 y**	**15 y**	**20 y**	**30 y**
Hancock II	Legarra (1999)		65%		33% (18 y)	
	Rizzoli (2003)	72%	49%	37%		
	Masters (2004)		57% (8 y)			
	Borger (2006)		50%		6%	
Carpentier-Edwards standard	Akins (1990)	53%	45%			
	Louagie (1992)	61%	46%			
	Bernal (1995)	89%	80%			
	Pelletier (1995)	83%	62% (8 y)			
	van Doorn (1995)	75%	53%			
	Murakami (1996)		75%			
	Marchand (1998)		53% (11 y)			
Carpentier-Edwards pericardial	Takahara (1995)		59% (9 y)			
	Aupart (1997)	78%	71%			
	Marchand (1998)		53% (11 y)			
	Neville (1998)		54% (12 y)			
	Porier (1998)	84%	58%			
Mosaic	Jasinski (2000)	100% (3 y)				
	Thomson (2001)	79% (4 y)				
	Fradet (2004)	83 (7 y)				
	Jamieson (2005)	74% (6 y)				
Biocor	Myken (2000)		55%	25%		
	Rizzoli (2005)	55%	51%			

mitral valve prostheses. New valves do not require the intensity of anticoagulation of older prostheses. For example, the distinctive Starr-Edwards ball-and-cage valve requires an INR of 3.5 to 4.5.[150] Patients with streamlined bileaflet or tilting-disk valves require an INR of between 2.5 and 3.5; thus, the incidence of anticoagulant hemorrhage is reduced significantly in the newer, hemodynamically improved prostheses.[174] Table 42-5 lists the incidence of anticoagulant hemorrhage with various bioprostheses and mechanical valves.

Structural Valve Degeneration

Structural valve degeneration (SVD) is the most important complication of the bioprosthetic valve. The probability of structural failure with currently available porcine valves (Hancock or Carpentier-Edwards) begins to increase 8 years after operation and reaches more than 60% at 15 years.[51,53] This finite durability is a major impediment to long-term success of these biologic prostheses, even though the failure rate in a patient 70 years of age or older is significantly less than in younger age groups (Table 42-6). Structural valve degeneration presents as mitral regurgitation from leaflet tear, calcific mitral stenosis owing to calcification of valve leaflets, or both. The appearance of a new murmur with new congestive symptoms should prompt a noninvasive investigation of the prosthesis and elective re-replacement if dysfunction is documented. Structural valve degeneration leading to reoperation is the cause for at least two-thirds of the reoperations in patients with bioprostheses.[152,153] The probabilities of structural valve degeneration at 5, 10, and 15 years of the six most commonly used biologic prostheses are shown in Table 42-2. With current quality controls, the incidence of structural valve degeneration is virtually zero for bileaflet, tilting-disk, and ball-and-cage valves.

Perivalvular Leak

Perivalvular leak is an uncommon complication that usually depends on technical factors. Patient-related factors such as endocarditis and calcifications involving the annulus are also important. Perivalvular leak usually causes refractory hemolytic anemia in contrast with the milder chronic hemolysis seen after implantation of some of the mechanical valves, especially the tilting-disk valves.[175]

Because of improved surgical techniques and the use of Teflon pledgets, the incidence of perivalvular leak has fallen and is about 0 to 1.5% per patient-year for both mechanical and biologic valves.[158,168,176] Perivalvular leak is slightly more common with the bileaflet valve than with the porcine valve because

TABLE 42-4 Freedom from Reoperation

		Actuarial Freedom from Reoperation		
Valve	Reference (year)	5 y	10 y	15 y
Hancock	Cohn (1989)	96%	79%	41%
	Perier (1989)	88%	59%	
	Bernal (1991)	92%	69%	25%
	Sarris (1993)	93%	69%	
	Khan (1998)		44%	
Hancock II	Legarra (1999)		77%	37% (18 y)
	David (2001)	98%	85%	69%
	Rizzoli (2003)	97%	88%	70%
	Borger (2006)		88%	44 (20 y)
Carpentier-Edwards standard	Perier (1989)	91%	64%	
	Jamieson (1991)	94%	64%	39%
	Sarris (1993)	91%	57% (8 y)	
	Van Doorn (1995)	95%	69%	
	Glower (1998)	94%	65%	30%
Carpentier-Edwards pericardial	Pelletier (1995)	98%	67% (8 y)	
	Murakami (1996)	100%	77%	
	Aupart (1997)		90%	
	Marchand (1998)		83% (11 y)	
	Neville (1998)		76% (12 y)	
	Poirer (1998)	99%	76%	
Mosaic	Jasinski (2000)	100% (3 y)		
	Eichinger (2002)	95%		
	Fradet (2004)	97% (7 y)		
Biocor	Myken (1995)			79%
	Rizzoli (2005)	95%	91%	

of the need for the everting suture technique and less bulky sewing ring.[177,178] Surgery should be offered to all symptomatic patients and even patients with mild symptoms who require blood transfusions.[176]

Endocarditis

Mitral valve endocarditis is considerably less common than aortic prosthetic valve endocarditis,[179] but when it does appear, it may present as septicemia, malignant burrowing infections, abscess formation, and septic emboli. This often results in difficult management problems related to timing of operation, type of operation, ability to fix the prosthesis securely, and operative and late survival. With better antibiotic prophylaxis at the time of mitral surgery and improved prophylaxis for all patients having dental or other surgical procedures, the incidence of endocarditis has been reduced substantially.

The incidence of prosthetic endocarditis is highest during the initial 6 months after surgery and thereafter declines to a lower but persistent risk.[1] The probability of freedom from this morbid event is shown in Table 42-7 for both mechanical and bioprosthetic valves. Biologic and mechanical valves have a similar incidence of endocarditis, except for the initial months after valve implantation, when mechanical prostheses carry a greater risk of infection.[184]

The diagnosis of prosthetic endocarditis is made by the presence of symptoms, appearance of a new murmur, a septic embolus, or large vegetation on echocardiogram. Blood cultures usually are positive, although a small percentage of patients have culture-negative endocarditis. Echocardiograms may show a rocking motion of the prosthesis and the presence of vegetations. The most frequent organisms are still *Streptococcus* and *Staphylococcus;* the latter is usually hospital acquired. Antibiotic therapy depends on the sensitivity of the organisms, but immediate high-dose intravenous therapy must begin as soon as possible. Experience indicates that a number of patients with bioprosthetic valvular endocarditis can be "cured" of low-potency organisms such as *Streptococcus.* However, it is unlikely that antibiotics alone can sterilize more virulent mitral valve infections, particularly *Staphylococcus.* These infections usually require urgent and sometimes emergent surgery because of invasion of the cardiac exoskeleton.

TABLE 42-5 Incidence of Thromboembolism and Anticoagulant-Related Hemorrhage

Valve	Reference (year)	Incidence of Thromboembolism (%/pt-y)	Incidence of Anticoagulant-Related Bleeding (%/pt-y)
Starr-Edwards	Miller (1983)	5.7	3.7
	Akins (1987)	3.9	2.4
	Agathos (1993)	6.6	2.2
	Godje (1997)	1.3	0.6
Omniscience/Omnicarbon	Cortina (1986)		2.7
	Damle (1987)	2.5	
	Akalin (1992)	1.0	2.7
	Peter (1993)	1.7	0.9
	Otaki (1993)	0.7	0.0
	Misawa (1993)	1.8	0.0
	Ohta (1995)	1.1	0.8
	Thevenet (1995)	0.9	1.1
	Iguro (1999)	1.0	0.6
	Torregrosa (1999)	0.6	0.8
	di Summa (2002)	0.4	0.2
Medtronic Hall	Antunes (1988)	4.2	1.5
	Beaudet (1988)	2.1	3.2
	Akins (1991)	1.8	3.2
	Butchar (2001)	4.0	1.4
St. Jude	Czer (1990)	1.9	2.1
	Kratz (1993)	2.9	2.2
	Jegaden (1994)	1.5	0.9
	Aoyagi (1994)	1.1	0.3
	Nistal (1996)	3.7	2.8
	Camilleri (2001)	1.9	1.5
	Khan (2001)	3.0	1.9
	Ramadi (2001)	0.7	0.9
	Emery (2005)	2.8	2.7
Carbomedics	De Luca (1993)	0.8	0.0
	Copeland (1995)	0.6	1.5
	Nistal (1996)	0.9	2.8
	Yamauchi (1996)	1.6	1.5
	Jamieson (2000)	4.6	2.7
	Soga (2002)	0.8	1.3
	Santini (2002)	2.2	
	Tominaga (2005)	1.8	0.9
	Carrier (2006)	0.7	0.7
	Wu (2006)	0.5	0.4
ATS	Shiono (1996)		0.0
	Westaby (1996)	0.0	
	Emery (2004)	3.0	2.3
	Stefanitis (2005)	0.5	0.0
On-X	Laczkovics (2001)	1.8	0.0
	Moidl (2002)	1.7	1.4
	McNicholas (2006)	1.6	3.1
	Williams (2006)	1.5	1.0

(*Continued*)

TABLE 42-5 Incidence of Thromboembolism and Anticoagulant-Related Hemorrhage (*Continued*)

Valve	Reference (year)	Incidence of Thromboembolism (%/pt-y)	Incidence of Anticoagulant-Related Bleeding (%/pt-y)
Hancock standard	Cohn (1989)	2.4	0.4
	Perier (1989)	1.1	1.0
	Bortolotti (1995)	1.4	0.7
Hancock II	Rizzoli (2003)	1.7	1.1
	Borger (2006)		
Carpentier-Edwards Porcine	Perier (1989)	0.8	1.0
	Akins (1990)	1.4	1.2
	Jamieson(1987)	2.4	0.7
	van Doorn (1995)	1.9	
	Glower (1998)	1.7	0.7
Carpentier-Edwards Pericardial	Pelletier (1995)	1.5	0.3
	Murakami (1996)	0.6	0.0
	Aupart (1997)	0.7	1.2
	Marchand (1998)	1.2	1.0
	Neville (1998)	0.6	1.1
	Poirer (1998)	1.7	0.3
Mosaic	Fradet (2001)	1.4	1.1
	Thomson (2001)	0.2	0.9
	Eichinger (2002)	0.8	2.0
Biocor	Myken (2000)	2.1	1.1
	Rizzoli (2005)	2.0	1.1

The indications for surgical intervention in mitral valve prosthetic endocarditis are persistent sepsis, organism, congestive failure, perivalvular leak, large vegetations, or systemic infected emboli.[37,38,185] Operative technique is similar to other mitral procedures with respect to anesthesia, monitoring, cardioplegia, left atrial incision, and exposure of the valve. Critical to successful resolution is the complete excision of the prosthetic device and débridement of all infected tissues. Surgical technique is described in Chapter 43. Postoperative care should include at least 6 weeks of appropriate intravenous antibiotics. Hospital mortality is related primarily to ongoing sepsis, multisystem organ failure, or failure to eradicate the local infection and subsequent recurrent perivalvular leak.[187,188] Recurrence of infection depends on the type of organism and the surgeon's ability to remove all areas of infection completely. Recurrence of infection is the single most important long-term complication.

Patient–Prosthesis Mismatch

The concept of patient–prosthesis mismatch is not new, but was first described in relationship to aortic valve replacement by Rahimtoola in 1978.[189] Since his introduction, the deleterious effects of patient–prosthesis mismatch in LV remodeling, function, and early and late survival with aortic valve replacement have been well documented. The notion of mitral valve patient prosthesis mismatch (MVPPM) in the adult was first proposed in a case report in 1981 again by Rahimtoola.[190] Most MVPPM was described in relation to pediatric mitral valve surgery, resulting in re-replacement rates approaching 30%, largely the result of somatic growth versus fixed prosthesis size. Recently, the possibility of such patient prosthesis mismatch in the mitral position has become an area of increased interest among adult cardiac surgeons. At this time, MCPPM has been studied through in vitro pulse generator analysis demonstrating that an index geometric orifice area (IGOA) less than 1.3 to 1.5 cm^2/m^2 could potentially result any patient having a high postoperative transprosthetic gradient. Similar studies performed in the clinical arena suggest that an index effective orifice area (IEOA) less than 1.3 to 1.5 cm^2/m^2 as measured by the continuity equation may increase the risk for MVPPM. Using this criterion, Lam and coworkers demonstrated a potential for MVPPM of roughly 32% in a recent series of 884 patients. In this population, patients at elevated risk for MVPPM measured at IEOA 1.0 to 1.25 cm^2/m^2 were at a significantly higher risk for development of postoperative congestive heart failure than those with IEOA greater than 1.25 cm^2/m^2. Although a weak association with CHF and pulmonary hypertension was noted, no direct correlation

TABLE 42-6 Freedom (Actuarial) from SVD by Age

			Freedom from SVD		
Valve	**Reference (year)**	**Age**	**5 y**	**10 y**	**15 y**
Hancock	Cohn (1989)	≤40		68%	
		41–69		84%	
		≥70		84%	
Hancock II	David (2001)	<65			76%
		≥65			89%
	Rizzoli (2003)	<65			82%
		≥65			92%
	Borger (2006)	<65			27% (20 y)
		≥65			59% (20 y)
Carpentier-Edwards standard	Akins (1990)	≤40		7%	
		41–50		82%	
		51–60		65%	
		61–70		79%	
		≤70		98%	
	Jamieson (1995)	≤35	79%	51%	
		36–40	99%	68%	48%
		51–64	98%	72%	42%
		65–69	98%	74%	64%
		≥70	100%	9%	90%
	Corbineau (2001)	≤35			0% (14 y)
		36–50			22% (14 y)
		51–60			34% (14 y)
		61–65			50% (14 y)
		66–70			93% (14 y)
		≥70			96% (14 y)
Carpentier-Edwards pericardial	Aupart (1997)	<60	47%		
		≥60	100%		
	Pelletier (1995)	≤59	100%	64% (8 y)	
		60–69	100%	91% (8 y)	
		≥70	100%	100% (8 y)	
	Marchand (1998)	≤60		78% (11 y)	
		61–70		89% (11 y)	
		>70		100% (11 y)	
	Neville (1998)	<60		70%	
		≥60		100%	
	Poirer (1998)	<60	100%	78%	
		60–6	100%	78%	
		≥70	100%	100%	
Biocor	Myken(2000)	<50			71%
		51–60			90%
		>61			100%

was found between MVPPM and the development of postoperative pulmonary hypertension.

Jamieson and coworkers recently evaluated the potential impact of MVPPM and long-term survival.[191] In contrast to prior reports, this study of nearly 2500 patients refuted the notion that MVPPM had any relation to mortality. Instead predictors of overall mortality included age, New York Heart Association III or IV, competent coronary artery disease, ventricular dysfunction, prosthesis type, BMI, and pre-existing pulmonary hypertension.

Certainly some degree of patient prosthesis mismatch may occur as a result of mitral valve replacement. The surgeon

TABLE 42-7 Prosthetic Valve Endocarditis

Valve	Reference (year)	PVE Rate (%/pt-y)	Freedom from PVE at 5 y
Starr-Edwards	Miller (1983)	0.5	97%
	Akins (1987)	0.4	95%
	Agathos 1993)	0.6	
	Godje (1997)		99% (10 y)
Omniscience/Omnicarbon	Carrier (1987)	0.8	98%
	Damle (1987)	0.8	98%
	Peter (1993)	0.0	100%
	Otaki (1993)	1.5	
	Misawa (1993)	0.0	100% (3 y)
	Ohta (1995)	0.5	
	Thenevet (1995)	0.2	
	Torregrosa (1999)	0.2	99% (10 y)
	di Summa (2002)	0.0	100% (10 y)
Medtronic Hall	Keenan (1990)	0.5	98%
	Akins (1991)	0.1	100%
	Fiore (1998)		94% (10 y)
	Masters (1995)	0.1	
	Butchart (2001)	0.4	94% (10 y)
	Masters (2001)	0.6	
St. Jude	Antunes (1988)	0.5	97%
	Kratz (1993)	0.4	
	Aoyagi (1994)	0.1	100%
	Fiore (1998)		100% (10 y)
	Camilleri (2001)	0.8	
	Masters (2001)	0.4	
	Khan (2001)	0.3	
	Ikonamidis (2003)		98% (10 y)
	Emery (2005)	0.3	
Carbomedics	De Luca (1993)	0.0	100%
	Copeland (1995)	0.3	96%
	Nistal (1996)	0.0	100%
	Yamauchi (1996)	0.0	100%
	Jamieson (2000)	0.4	
	Masters (2001)	0.6	
	Santini (2002)		100%
	Soga (2002)	0.0	100%
	Tominaga (2005)	0.3	97% (10 y)
	Carrier (2006)	0.3	97% (15 y)
	Wu (2006)	0.4	98% (10 y)
ATS	Emery (2004)	0.4	
	Stefanitis (2005)	0.0	100%
On-X	Laczkovics (2001)	0.5	
	Moidl (2002)	0.7	99% (2 y)
	Williams (2006)		95% (4 y)
	McNicholas (2006)	0.0	100%
Hancock standard	Cohn (1989)		93%
	Bernal (1991)	0.3	
	Sarris (1993)		93%
	Bortolotti (1995)	0.3	

(Continued)

TABLE 42-7 Prosthetic Valve Endocarditis (*Continued*)

Valve	Reference (year)	PVE Rate (%/pt-y)	Freedom from PVE at 5 y	
Hancock II	Legarra (1999)		97% (15 y)	
	David (2001)		91% (15 y)	
	Rizzoli (2003)	0.4	96% (15 y)	
	Masters (2004)		99% (8 y)	
	Borger (2006)		85% (20 y)	
Carpentier-Edwards porcine	Pelletier (1989)	0.4		
	Akins (1990)	1.0		
	Louagie (1992)	0.0	100%	
	Sarris (1993)		91%	
	van Doorn (1995)		97%	92% (10 y)
	Glower (1998)	0.3	97%	96% (10 y)
Carpentier-Edwards pericardial	Pelletier (1995)	0.3%	93% (10 y)	
	Murakami (1996)	0.86	94% (10 y)	
	Aupart (1997)	0.4%	97% (10 y)	
	Marchand (1998)	0.1%		
	Neville (1998)	0.6%	94% (12 y)	
	Poirer (1998)	0.3%	95% (10 y)	
Mosaic	Jasinski (2000)		100% (3 y)	
	Fradet (2004)	0.8	98% (7 y)	
	Thomson (2001)	0.8		
	Eichinger (2002)	0.8	94%	
Biocor	Myken (2000)	0.7	93% (15 y)	
	Rizzoli1 (2005)		94% (8 y)	

should be aware of the potential for MVPPM, particularly in the setting of particularly small annulus size in patients resulting in the need for implantation of a small prosthetic device resulting in a high transprosthetic gradient. As such, foreknowledge of the devices specific IGOA may assist allowing the surgeon to choose a device that might minimize MVPPM. Unfortunately, unlike the aortic position, in which aortic root enlargement will allow for valve upsizing, the mitral position cannot be corrected as simply. As a result, in patients with particularly small mitral valve area, some degree of patient prosthesis mismatch may be unavoidable. This phenomenon remains an area of active clinical investigation. Its resolution will require larger meta-analysis.

CONCLUSIONS

Mitral valve replacement by mechanical or bioprosthetic valves revolutionized the care of patients with severe mitral valve disease. Reconstructive operations of the mitral valve now have assumed an equally important role for mitral regurgitation. A number of advanced lesions of the mitral valve still require mitral valve replacement with reliable devices. The bileaflet, tilting-disk, and ball-and-cage prosthetic valves are extremely reliable in terms of durability but require long-term anticoagulation and have a high risk of thromboembolism or thrombosis without anticoagulation. Bioprosthetic porcine valves, conversely, in patients in sinus rhythm do not need long-term anticoagulation and are used mainly in elderly patients who are not likely to outlive the valve and in women who plan to become pregnant and do not wish to accept the risks of warfarin or heparin. The long-term durability of these valves is limited, and the probability of valve failure at 15 years is at least 40%. Improvements in mechanical valve design and biologic valve preservation of collagen structure and resistance to calcification are ongoing and are the hope for the future. In addition, there is renewed interest in homograft mitral valves, which may offer better long-term durability, as has been observed with cryopreserved homograft aortic valves. Improved valve design and development of better biomaterials eventually will improve clinical results; however, current FDA restrictions on the development and evaluation of new prosthetic valves have an important impact on this process.

REFERENCES

1. Zipes DP, Braunwald E: *A Textbook of Cardiovascular Medicine.* Philadelphia, Saunders, 2004.
2. Bonow RO, Carabello B, de Leon AC Jr, et al: Guidelines for the management of patients with valvular heart disease: executive summary. A report of the American College of Cardiology/American Heart Association Task Force on Practice Guidelines (Committee on Management of Patients with Valvular Heart Disease). *Circulation* 1998; 98:1949.

3. Spencer FC: A plea for early, open mitral commissurotomy. *Am Heart J* 1978; 95:668.
4. Vincens JJ, Temizer D, Post JR, et al: Long-term outcome of cardiac surgery in patients with mitral stenosis and severe pulmonary hypertension. *Circulation* 1995; 92:II137.
5. Li M, Dumesnil JG, Mathieu P, Pibarot P: Impact of valve prosthesis-patient mismatch on pulmonary arterial pressure after mitral valve replacement. *J Am Coll Cardiol* 2005; 45:1034.
6. Palacios IF, Tuzcu ME, Weyman AE, et al: Clinical follow-up of patients undergoing percutaneous mitral balloon valvotomy. *Circulation* 1995; 91:671.
7. Reyes VP, Raju BS, Wynne J, et al: Percutaneous balloon valvuloplasty compared with open surgical commissurotomy for mitral stenosis. *NEJM* 1994; 331:961.
8. National Heart, Lung, and Blood Institute Balloon Valvuloplasty Registry: Complications and mortality of percutaneous balloon commissurotomy. *Circulation* 1992; 85:2014.
9. Cohn LH, Allred EN, Cohn LA, et al: Long-term results of open mitral valve reconstruction for mitral stenosis. *Am J Cardiol* 1985; 55:731.
10. Glower DD, Landolfo KP, Davis RD, et al: Comparison of open mitral commissurotomy with mitral valve replacement with or without chordal preservation in patients with mitral stenosis. *Circulation* 1998; 98:II-120.
11. el Asmar B, Acker M, Couetil JP, et al: Mitral valve repair in the extensively calcified mitral valve annulus. *Ann Thorac Surg* 1991; 52:66.
12. Enriquez-Sarano M, Tajik AJ, Schaff HV, et al: Echocardiographic prediction of survival after surgical correction of organic mitral regurgitation. *Circulation* 1994; 90:830.
13. Hellgren L, Kvidal P, Horte LG, et al: Survival after mitral valve replacement: rationale for surgery before occurrence of severe symptoms. *Ann Thorac Surg* 2004; 78:1241.
14. Ling LH, Enriquez-Sarano M, Seward JB, et al: Clinical outcome of mitral regurgitation due to flail leaflet. *NEJM* 1996; 335:1417.
15. Stewart WJ: Choosing the "golden moment" for mitral valve repair. *J Am Coll Cardiol* 1994; 24:1544.
16. Tavel ME, Carabello BA: Chronic mitral regurgitation: when and how to operate. *Chest* 1998; 113:1399.
17. Tribouilloy CM, Enriquez-Sarano M, Schaff HV, et al: Impact of preoperative symptoms on survival after surgical correction of organic mitral regurgitation: rationale for optimizing surgical indications. *Circulation* 1999; 99:400.
18. Kizilbash AM, Hundley WG, Willett DL, et al: Comparison of quantitative Doppler with magnetic resonance imaging for assessment of the severity of mitral regurgitation. *Am J Cardiol* 1998; 81:792.
19. Malm S, Frigstad S, Sagberg E, et al: Accurate and reproducible measurement of left ventricular volume and ejection fraction by contrast echocardiography: a comparison with magnetic resonance imaging. *J Am Coll Cardiol* 2004; 44:1030.
20. Enriquez-Sarano M, Tajik AJ, Schaff HV, et al: Echocardiographic prediction of left ventricular function after correction of mitral regurgitation: results and clinical implications. *J Am Coll Cardiol* 1994; 24:1536.
21. Timmis SB, Kirsh MM, Montgomery DG, Starling MR: Evaluation of left ventricular ejection fraction as a measure of pump performance in patients with chronic mitral regurgitation. *Cathet Cardiovasc Intervent* 2000; 49:290.
22. Kontos GJ Jr, Schaff HV, Gersh BJ, Bove AA: Left ventricular function in subacute and chronic mitral regurgitation: effect on function early postoperatively. *J Thorac Cardiovasc Surg* 1989; 98:163.
23. Nakano S, Sakai K, Taniguchi K, et al: Relation of impaired left ventricular function in mitral regurgitation to left ventricular contractile state after mitral valve replacement. *Am J Cardiol* 1994; 73:70.
24. Matsumura T, Ohtaki E, Tanaka K, et al: Echocardiographic prediction of left ventricular dysfunction after mitral valve repair for mitral regurgitation as an indicator to decide the optimal timing of repair. *J Am Coll Cardiol* 2003; 42:458.
25. Wisenbaugh TSD, Sareli P: Prediction of outcome after valve replacement for rheumatic mitral regurgitation in the era of chordal preservation. *Circulation* 1994; 89:191.
26. Braunberger E, Deloche A, Berrebi A, et al: Very long-term results (more than 20 years) of valve repair with Carpentier's techniques in nonrheumatic mitral valve insufficiency. *Circulation* 2001; 104:I-8.
27. Cohn LH, Allred EN, Cohn LA, et al: Early and late risk of mitral valve replacement. A 12-year concomitant comparison of the porcine bioprosthetic and prosthetic disc mitral valves. *J Thorac Cardiovasc Surg* 1985; 90:872.
28. Cohn LH, Couper GS, Aranki SF, et al: The long-term results of mitral valve reconstruction for the "floppy" valve. *J Card Surg* 1994; 9:278.
29. Cosgrove DM, Chavez AM, Lytle BW, et al: Results of mitral valve reconstruction. *Circulation* 1986; 74:I-82.
30. Greelish JP, Cohn LH, Leacche M, et al: Minimally invasive mitral valve repair suggests earlier operations for mitral valve disease. *J Thorac Cardiovasc Surg* 2003; 126:365; discussion 371.
31. Asmar BE, Perrier P, Couetil J, Carpentier A: Failures in reconstructive mitral valve surgery. *J Med Liban* 1991; 39:7.
32. Chauvaud S, Fuzellier JF, Berrebi A, et al: Long-term (29 years) results of reconstructive surgery in rheumatic mitral valve insufficiency. *Circulation* 2001; 104:I-12.
33. Byrne JG, Aranki SF, Cohn LH: Repair versus replacement of mitral valve for treating severe ischemic mitral regurgitation. *Coron Artery Dis* 2000; 11:31.
34. Cohn LH, Rizzo RJ, Adams DH, et al: The effect of pathophysiology on the surgical treatment of ischemic mitral regurgitation: operative and late risks of repair versus replacement. *Eur J Cardiothorac Surg* 1995; 9:568.
35. Grossi EA, Goldberg JD, LaPietra A, et al: Ischemic mitral valve reconstruction and replacement: comparison of long-term survival and complications. *J Thorac Cardiovasc Surg* 2001; 122:1107.
36. Alexiou C, Langley SM, Stafford H, et al: Surgical treatment of infective mitral valve endocarditis: predictors of early and late outcome. *J Heart Valve Dis* 2000; 9:327.
37. Aranki SF, Adams DH, Rizzo RJ, et al: Determinants of early mortality and late survival in mitral valve endocarditis. *Circulation* 1995; 92:II-143.
38. Mihaljevic T, Paul S, Leacche M, et al: Tailored surgical therapy for acute native mitral valve endocarditis. *J Heart Valve Dis* 2004; 13:210.
39. Williams MA, van Riet S: The On-X heart valve: mid-term results in a poorly anticoagulated population. *J Heart Valve Dis* 2006; 15(1):80-86.
40. Jamieson WR, von Lipinski O, Miyagishima RT, et al: Performance of bioprostheses and mechanical prostheses assessed by composites of valve-related complications to 15 years after mitral valve replacement. *J Thorac Cardiovasc Surg* 2005; 129:1301.
41. Grunkemeier GL, Jamieson WR, Miller DC, Starr A: Actuarial versus actual risk of porcine structural valve deterioration. *J Thorac Cardiovasc Surg* 1994; 108:709.
42. Peterseim DS, Cen YY, Cheruvu S, et al: Long-term outcome after biologic versus mechanical aortic valve replacement in 841 patients. *J Thorac Cardiovasc Surg* 1999; 117:890.
43. Angell WW, Pupello DF, Bessone LN, et al: Influence of coronary artery disease on structural deterioration of porcine bioprostheses. *Ann Thorac Surg* 1995; 60:S276.
44. DiSesa VJ, Cohn LH, Collins JJ Jr, et al: Determinants of operative survival following combined mitral valve replacement and coronary revascularization. *Ann Thorac Surg* 1982; 34:482.
45. Edwards FH, Peterson ED, Coombs LP, et al: Prediction of operative mortality after valve replacement surgery. *J Am Coll Cardiol* 2001; 37:885.
46. Jones EL, Weintraub WS, Craver JM, et al: Interaction of age and coronary disease after valve replacement: implications for valve selection. *Ann Thorac Surg* 1994; 58:378; discussion 384.
47. Schoen FJ, Collins JJ Jr, Cohn LH: Long-term failure rate and morphologic correlations in porcine bioprosthetic heart valves. *Am J Cardiol* 1983; 51:957.
48. Thourani VH, Weintraub WS, Craver JM, et al: Influence of concomitant CABG and urgent/emergent status on mitral valve replacement surgery. *Ann Thorac Surg* 2000; 70:778; discussion 783.
49. Burdon TA, Miller DC, Oyer PE, et al: Durability of porcine valves at fifteen years in a representative North American patient population. *J Thorac Cardiovasc Surg* 1992; 103:238; discussion 251.
50. Cohn LH, Collins JJ Jr, Rizzo RJ, et al: Twenty-year follow-up of the Hancock modified orifice porcine aortic valve. *Ann Thorac Surg* 1998; 66:S30.
51. Corbineau H, Du Haut Cilly FB, Langanay T, et al: Structural durability in Carpentier Edwards standard bioprosthesis in the mitral position: a 20-year experience. *J Heart Valve Dis* 2001; 10:443.
52. Jamieson WR, Burr LH, Munro AI, Miyagishima RT: Carpentier-Edwards standard porcine bioprosthesis: a 21-year experience. *Ann Thorac Surg* 1998; 66:S40.
53. Khan SS, Chaux A, Blanche C, et al: A 20-year experience with the Hancock porcine xenograft in the elderly. *Ann Thorac Surg* 1998; 66:S35.
54. van Doorn CA, Stoodley KD, Saunders NR, et al: Mitral valve replacement with the Carpentier-Edwards standard bioprosthesis: performance into the second decade. *Eur J Cardiothorac Surg* 1995; 9:253.
55. Pupello DF, Bessone LN, Hiro SP, et al: Bioprosthetic valve longevity in the elderly: an 18-year longitudinal study. *Ann Thorac Surg* 1995; 60:S270; discussion S275.
56. Jamieson WR, Tyers GF, Janusz MT, et al: Age as a determinant for selection of porcine bioprostheses for cardiac valve replacement: experience with Carpentier-Edwards standard bioprosthesis. *Can J Cardiol* 1991; 7:181.

57. Badduke BR, Jamieson WR, Miyagishima RT, et al: Pregnancy and childbearing in a population with biologic valvular prostheses. *J Thorac Cardiovasc Surg* 1991; 102:179.
58. Jamieson WR, Miller DC, Akins CW, et al: Pregnancy and bioprostheses: influence on structural valve deterioration. *Ann Thorac Surg* 1995; 60:S282; discussion S287.
59. Mihaljevic T, Paul S, Leacche M, et al: Valve replacement in women of childbearing age: influences on mother, fetus and neonate. *J Heart Valve Dis* 2005; 14:151.
60. Sareli P, England MJ, Berk MR, et al: Maternal and fetal sequelae of anticoagulation during pregnancy in patients with mechanical heart valve prostheses. *Am J Cardiol* 1989; 63:1462.
61. Ali M, Iung B, Lansac E, et al: Homograft replacement of the mitral valve: eight-year results. *J Thorac Cardiovasc Surg* 2004; 128:529.
62. Deac RF, Simionescu D, Deac D: New evolution in mitral physiology and surgery: mitral stentless pericardial valve. *Ann Thorac Surg* 1995; 60:S433.
63. Gulbins H, Kreuzer E, Uhlig A, Reichart B: Mitral valve surgery utilizing homografts: early results. *J Heart Valve Dis* 2000; 9:222.
64. Kumar AS, Choudhary SK, Mathur A, et al: Homograft mitral valve replacement: five years' results. *J Thorac Cardiovasc Surg* 2000; 120:450.
65. Chauvaud S, Waldmann T, d'Attellis N, et al: Homograft replacement of the mitral valve in young recipients: midterm results. *Eur J Cardiothorac Surg* 2003; 23:560.
66. Hofmann B, Cichon R, Knaut M, et al: Early experience with a quadrileaflet stentless mitral valve. *Ann Thorac Surg* 2001; 71:S323.
67. Lehmann S, Walther T, Kempfert J, et al: Stentless mitral valve implantation in comparison to conventional mitral valve repair or replacement at five years. *Thorac Cardiovasc Surg* 2006; 54:10.
68. Vrandecic MO, Fantini FA, Gontijo BF, et al: Surgical technique of implanting the stentless porcine mitral valve. *Ann Thorac Surg* 1995; 60:S439.
69. Athanasiou T, Cherian A, Ross D: The Ross II procedure: pulmonary autograft in the mitral position. *Ann Thorac Surg* 2004; 78:1489.
70. Brown JW, Ruzmetov M, Turrentine MW, Rodefeld MD: Mitral valve replacement with the pulmonary autograft: Ross II procedure with Kabanni modification. *Semin Thorac Cardiovasc Surg Pediatr Card Surg Annu* 2004; 7:107.
71. Kabbani SS, Jamil H, Hammoud A, et al: The mitral pulmonary autograft: assessment at midterm. *Ann Thorac Surg* 2004; 78:60; discussion 65.
72. Cohn LH: *Cardiac Surgery in the Adult.* New York, McGraw Hill, 2008.
73. Cordoba M, Almeida P, Martinez P, et al: *Invasive Assessment of Mitral Valve Prostheses.* New York, Futura, 1987; p 369.
74. Khuri SF, Folland ED, Sethi GK, et al: Six month postoperative hemodynamics of the Hancock heterograft and the Bjork-Shiley prosthesis: results of a Veterans Administration cooperative prospective, randomized trial. *J Am Coll Cardiol* 1988; 12:8.
75. Pelletier C, Chaitman B, Bonan R, Dyrda I: *Hemodynamic Evaluation of the Carpentier-Edwards Standard and Improved Annulus Bioprostheses.* New York, Yorke Medical Books, 1982; p 96.
76. Horskotte D, Loogen F, Birckson B: *Is the Late Outcome of Heart Valve Replacement Influenced by the Hemodynamics of the Heart Valve Substitute?* New York, Springer-Verlag, 1986; p 55.
77. Butterfield M, Fisher J, Davies GA, Spyt TJ: Comparative study of the hydrodynamic function of the CarboMedics valve. *Ann Thorac Surg* 1991; 52:815.
78. Agathos EA, Starr A: Mitral valve replacement. *Curr Probl Surg* 1993; 30:481.
79. Miller DC, Oyer PE, Stinson EB, et al: Ten to fifteen year reassessment of the performance characteristics of the Starr-Edwards Model 6120 mitral valve prosthesis. *J Thorac Cardiovasc Surg* 1983; 85:1.
80. Murday AJ, Hochstitzky A, Mansfield J, et al: A prospective, controlled trial of St Jude versus Starr-Edwards aortic and mitral valve prostheses. *Ann Thorac Surg* 2003; 76:66; discussion 73.
81. Hall KV: The Medtronic-Hall valve: a design in 1977 to improve the results of valve replacement. *Eur J Cardiothorac Surg* 1992; 6:S64.
82. Butchart E: Early clinical and hemodynamic results with Hall-Kaster valve, in *Medtronic International Valve Symposium.* Lisbon, Portugal, Congress Books, 1981; p 159.
83. Grunkemeier GL, Starr A, Rahimtoola SH: Prosthetic heart valve performance: long-term follow-up. *Curr Probl Cardiol* 1992; 17:329.
84. Akalin H, Corapcioglu ET, Ozyurda U, et al: Clinical evaluation of the Omniscience cardiac valve prosthesis: follow-up of up to 6 years. *J Thorac Cardiovasc Surg* 1992; 103:259.
85. DeWall R, Pelletier LC, Panebianco A, et al: Five-year clinical experience with the Omniscience cardiac valve. *Ann Thorac Surg* 1984; 38:275.
86. Watanabe N, Abe T, Yamada O, et al: Comparative analysis of Omniscience and Omnicarbon prosthesis after aortic valve replacement. *Jpn J Artif Organs* 1989; 18:773.
87. Emery RW, Nicoloff DM: St Jude Medical cardiac valve prosthesis: in vitro studies. *J Thorac Cardiovasc Surg* 1979; 78:269.
88. Nair CK, Mohiuddin SM, Hilleman DE, et al: Ten-year results with the St Jude Medical prosthesis. *Am J Cardiol* 1990; 65:217.
89. Champsaur G, Gressier M, Niret J, et al: *When Are Hemodynamics Important for the Selection of a Prosthetic Heart Valve?* New York, Springer-Verlag, 1986; p 71.
90. D'Alessandro L, Narducci C, Pucci A, et al: *The Use of Mechanical Valves in the Treatment of Valvular Heart Disease.* New York, Springer-Verlag, 1986; p 31.
91. Laub GW, Muralidharan S, Pollock SB, et al: The experimental relationship between leaflet clearance and orientation of the St Jude Medical valve in the mitral position. *J Thorac Cardiovasc Surg* 1992; 103:638.
92. Sezai A, Shiono M, Orime Y, et al: Evaluation of valve sound and its effects on ATS prosthetic valves in patients' quality of life. *Ann Thorac Surg* 2000; 69:507.
93. Ely JL, Emken MR, Accuntius JA, et al: Pure pyrolytic carbon: preparation and properties of a new material, On-X carbon for mechanical heart valve prostheses. *J Heart Valve Dis* 1998; 7:626.
94. Laczkovics A, Heidt M, Oelert H, et al: Early clinical experience with the On-X prosthetic heart valve. *J Heart Valve Dis* 2001; 10:94.
95. Birnbaum D, Laczkovics A, Heidt M, et al: Examination of hemolytic potential with the On-X(R) prosthetic heart valve. *J Heart Valve Dis* 2000;
96. McNicholas KW, Ivey TD, Metras J, et al: North American multicenter experience with the On-X prosthetic heart valve. *J Heart Valve Dis* 2006; 15:73.
97. Gallucci V, Valfre C, Mazzucco A, et al: *Heart Valve Replacement with the Hancock Bioprosthesis: A 5- to 11-Year Follow-up.* New York, Yorke Medical Books, 1982; p 96.
98. D'Attellis N, Nicolas-Robin A, Delayance S, et al: Early extubation after mitral valve surgery: a target-controlled infusion of propofol and low-dose sufentanil. *J Cardiothorac Vasc Anesth* 1997; 11:467.
99. Buckberg GD: Development of blood cardioplegia and retrograde techniques: the experimenter/observer complex. *J Card Surg* 1998; 13:163.
100. Larbalestier RI, Chard RB, Cohn LH: Optimal approach to the mitral valve: dissection of the interatrial groove. *Ann Thorac Surg* 1992; 54:1186.
101. Sondergaard T, Gotzsche M, Ottosen P, Schultz J: Surgical closure of interatrial septal defects by circumclusion. *Acta Chir Scand* 1955; 109:188.
102. Hirt SW, Frimpong-Boateng K, Borst HG: The superior approach to the mitral valve: is it worthwhile? *Eur J Cardiothorac Surg* 1988; 2:372.
103. Utley JR, Leyland SA, Nguyenduy T: Comparison of outcomes with three atrial incisions for mitral valve operations: right lateral, superior septal, and transseptal. *J Thorac Cardiovasc Surg* 1995; 109:582.
104. Guiraudon GM, Ofiesh JG, Kaushik R: Extended vertical transatrial septal approach to the mitral valve. *Ann Thorac Surg* 1991; 52:1058; discussion 1060.
105. Barner HB: Combined superior and right lateral left atriotomy with division of the superior vena cava for exposure of the mitral valve. *Ann Thorac Surg* 1985; 40:365.
106. Selle JG: Temporary division of the superior vena cava for exceptional mitral valve exposure. *J Thorac Cardiovasc Surg* 1984; 88:302.
107. Kon ND, Tucker WY, Mills SA, et al: Mitral valve operation via an extended transseptal approach. *Ann Thorac Surg* 1993; 55:1413; discussion 1416.
108. Kumar N, Saad E, Prabhakar G, et al: Extended transseptal versus conventional left atriotomy: early postoperative study. *Ann Thorac Surg* 1995; 60:426.
109. Cosgrove DM 3d, Sabik JF, Navia JL: Minimally invasive valve operations. *Ann Thorac Surg* 1998; 65:1535; discussion 1538.
110. Mihaljevic T, Cohn LH, Unic D, et al: One thousand minimally invasive valve operations: early and late results. *Ann Surg* 2004; 240:529; discussion 534.
111. Cohn LH, Adams DH, Couper GS, et al: Minimally invasive cardiac valve surgery improves patient satisfaction while reducing costs of cardiac valve replacement and repair. *Ann Surg* 1997; 226:421; discussion 427.
112. Cohn LH, Couper GS, Aranki SF, et al: The long-term results of mitral valve reconstruction for the "floppy" valve. *J Card Surg* 1994; 9:278.
113. Douglas JJ: *Mitral Valve Replacement.* Philadelphia, Saunders, 1995; p 393.
114. David TE, Armstrong S, Sun Z: Left ventricular function after mitral valve surgery. *J Heart Valve Dis* 1995; 4:S175.
115. Lillehei C, Levy M, Bonnabeau R: Mitral valve replacement with preservation of papillary muscles and chordae tendinae. *J Thorac Cardiovasc Surg* 1964; 47:532.
116. Cohn LH, Couper GS, Kinchla NM, Collins JJ Jr: Decreased operative risk of surgical treatment of mitral regurgitation with or without coronary artery disease. *J Am Coll Cardiol* 1990; 16:1575.

117. Horskotte D, Schulte HD, Bircks W, Strauer BE: The effect of chordal preservation on late outcome after mitral valve replacement: a randomized study. *J Heart Valve Dis* 1993; 2:150.
118. Okita Y, Miki S, Ueda Y, et al: Midterm results of mitral valve replacement combined with chordae tendineae replacement in patients with mitral stenosis. *J Heart Valve Dis* 1997; 6:37.
119. Sugita T, Matsumoto M, Nishizawa J, et al: Long-term outcome after mitral valve replacement with preservation of continuity between the mitral annulus and the papillary muscle in patients with mitral stenosis. *J Heart Valve Dis* 2004; 13:931.
120. Karlson KJ, Ashraf MM, Berger RL: Rupture of left ventricle following mitral valve replacement. *Ann Thorac Surg* 1988; 46:590.
121. Spencer FC, Galloway AC, Colvin SB: A clinical evaluation of the hypothesis that rupture of the left ventricle following mitral valve replacement can be prevented by preservation of the chordae of the mural leaflet. *Ann Surg* 1985; 202:673.
122. Chambers EP Jr, Heath BJ: Comparison of supra-annular and subannular pledgeted sutures in mitral valve replacement. *Ann Thorac Surg* 1991; 51:60; discussion 63.
123. Antunes MJ: Technique of implantation of the Medtronic-Hall valve and other modern tilting-disc prostheses. *J Card Surg* 1990; 5:86.
124. Cooley DA: Simplified techniques of valve replacement. *J Card Surg* 1992; 7:357.
125. Dhasmana JP, Blackstone EH, Kirklin JW, Kouchoukos NT: Factors associated with periprosthetic leakage following primary mitral valve replacement: with special consideration of the suture technique. *Ann Thorac Surg* 1983; 35:170.
126. DiSesa VJ, Tam S, Cohn LH: Ligation of the left atrial appendage using an automatic surgical stapler. *Ann Thorac Surg* 1988; 46:652.
127. Cohn LH: Tricuspid regurgitation secondary to mitral valve disease: when and how to repair. *J Card Surg* 1994; 9:237.
128. Svenarud P, Persson M, van der Linden J: Effect of CO_2 insufflation on the number and behavior of air microemboli in open-heart surgery: a randomized clinical trial. *Circulation* 2004; 109:1127.
129. Heras M, Chesebro JH, Fuster V, et al: High risk of thromboemboli early after bioprosthetic cardiac valve replacement. *J Am Coll Cardiol* 1995; 25:1111.
130. Jegaden O, Eker A, Delahaye F, et al: Thromboembolic risk and late survival after mitral valve replacement with the St Jude Medical valve. *Ann Thorac Surg* 1994; 58:1721; discussion 1727.
131. Ezekowitz MD: Anticoagulation management of valve replacement patients. *J Heart Valve Dis* 2002; 11:S56.
132. Meurin P, Tabet JY, Weber H, et al: Low-molecular-weight heparin as a bridging anticoagulant early after mechanical heart valve replacement. *Circulation* 2006; 113:564.
133. Laffort P, Roudaut R, Roques X, et al: Early and long-term (one-year) effects of the association of aspirin and oral anticoagulant on thrombi and morbidity after replacement of the mitral valve with the St Jude Medical prosthesis: a clinical and transesophageal echocardiographic study. *J Am Coll Cardiol* 2000; 35:739.
134. Yamak B, Iscan Z, Mavitas B, et al: Low-dose oral anticoagulation and antiplatelet therapy with St Jude Medical heart valve prosthesis. *J Heart Valve Dis* 1999; 8:665.
135. Braunwald E: *Valvular Heart Diseases.* Philadelphia, Saunders, 2001; p 1699.
136. Aoyagi S, Oryoji A, Nishi Y, et al: Long-term results of valve replacement with the St Jude Medical valve. *J Thorac Cardiovasc Surg* 1994; 108:1021.
137. Emery RW, Krogh CC, Arom KV, et al: The St Jude Medical cardiac valve prosthesis: a 25-year experience with single valve replacement. *Ann Thorac Surg* 2005; 79:776; discussion 782.
138. Remadi JP, Bizouarn P, Baron O, et al: Mitral valve replacement with the St Jude Medical prosthesis: a 15-year follow-up. *Ann Thorac Surg* 1998; 66:762.
139. Birkmeyer NJ, Marrin CA, Morton JR, et al: Decreasing mortality for aortic and mitral valve surgery in northern New England. Northern New England Cardiovascular Disease Study Group. *Ann Thorac Surg* 2000; 70:432.
140. Okita Y, Miki S, Ueda Y, et al: Left ventricular function after mitral valve replacement with or without chordal preservation. *J Heart Valve Dis* 1995; 4:S181; discussion S192.
141. Arom KV, Nicoloff DM, Kersten TE, et al: Six years of experience with the St Jude Medical valvular prosthesis. *Circulation* 1985; 72:II-153.
142. Cohn LH, Aranki SF, Rizzo RJ, et al: Decrease in operative risk of reoperative valve surgery. *Ann Thorac Surg* 1993; 56:15; discussion 20.
143. Oury JH, Cleveland JC, Duran CG, Angell WW: Ischemic mitral valve disease: classification and systemic approach to management. *J Card Surg* 1994; 9:262.
144. Thourani VH, Weintraub WS, Guyton RA, et al: Outcomes and long-term survival for patients undergoing mitral valve repair versus replacement: effect of age and concomitant coronary artery bypass grafting. *Circulation* 2003; 108:298.
145. Society of Thoracic Surgeons: *Data Analysis of the Society of Thoracic Surgeons National Cardiac Surgery Database: The Fifth Year—January 1996.* Minneapolis: Summit Medical Systems, 1996.
146. Bortolotti U, Milano A, Testolin L, et al: The Carbomedics bileaflet prothesis: initial experience at the University of Padova. *Clin Rep* 1991; 4.
147. Grossi EA, Galloway AC, Miller JS, et al: Valve repair versus replacement for mitral insufficiency: when is a mechanical valve still indicated? *J Thorac Cardiovasc Surg* 1998; 115:389; discussion 394.
148. Hammermeister K, Sethi GK, Henderson WG, et al: Outcomes 15 years after valve replacement with a mechanical versus a bioprosthetic valve: final report of the Veterans Affairs randomized trial. *J Am Coll Cardiol* 2000; 36:1152.
149. Sidhu P, O'Kane H, Ali N, et al: Mechanical or bioprosthetic valves in the elderly: a 20-year comparison. *Ann Thorac Surg* 2001; 71:S257.
150. Starr A: The Starr-Edwards valve. *J Am Coll Cardiol* 1985; 6:899.
151. Bernal JM, Rabasa JM, Cagigas JC, et al: Valve-related complications with the Hancock I porcine bioprosthesis: a twelve- to fourteen-year follow-up study. *J Thorac Cardiovasc Surg* 1991; 101:871.
152. Cohn LH, Peigh PS, Sell J, DiSesa VJ: Right thoracotomy, femoro-femoral bypass, and deep hypothermia for re-replacement of the mitral valve. *Ann Thorac Surg* 1989; 48:69.
153. Perier P, Swanson J, Takriti A, et al: *Decreasing Operative Risk in Isolated Valve Re-replacement.* New York, Yorke Medical Books, 1986; p 333.
154. Wideman FE, Blackstone EH, Kirklin JW, et al: Hospital mortality of re-replacement of the aortic valve: incremental risk factors. *J Thorac Cardiovasc Surg* 1981; 82:692.
155. Myken PS, Caidahl K, Larsson P, et al: Mechanical versus biological valve prosthesis: a ten-year comparison regarding function and quality of life. *Ann Thorac Surg* 1995; 60:S447.
156. Akins C, Buckley M, Daggett W, et al: *Ten-Year Follow-up of the Starr-Edwards Prosthesis.* New York: Futura, 1987.
157. Akins CW: Mechanical cardiac valvular prostheses. *Ann Thorac Surg* 1991; 52:161.
158. Antunes MJ, Wessels A, Sadowski RG, et al: Medtronic Hall valve replacement in a third-world population group: a review of the performance of 1000 prostheses. *J Thorac Cardiovasc Surg* 1988; 95:980.
159. Beaudet RL, Nakhle G, Beaulieu CR, et al: Medtronic-Hall prosthesis: valve-related deaths and complications. *Can J Cardiol* 1988; 4:376.
160. Cortina JM, Martinell J, Artiz V, et al: Comparative clinical results with Omniscience (STM1), Medtronic-Hall, and Bjork-Shiley convexo-concave (70 degrees) prostheses in mitral valve replacement. *J Thorac Cardiovasc Surg* 1986; 91:174.
161. Emery RW, Krogh CC, Jones DJ, et al: Five-year follow up of the ATS mechanical heart valve. *J Heart Valve Dis* 2004; 13:231.
162. Jamieson WR, Fradet GJ, Miyagishima RT, et al: CarboMedics mechanical prosthesis: performance at eight years. *J Heart Valve Dis* 2000; 9:678.
163. Khan SS, Trento A, DeRobertis M, et al: Twenty-year comparison of tissue and mechanical valve replacement. *J Thorac Cardiovasc Surg* 2001; 122:257.
164. Moidl R, Simon P, Wolner E: The On-X prosthetic heart valve at five years. *Ann Thorac Surg* 2002; 74:S1312.
165. Ohta S, Ohuchi M, Katsumoto K, et al: Comparison of long-term clinical results of the three models of the Bjork-Shiley valve prosthesis and the Omnicarbon valve prosthesis. *Nippon Kyobu Geka Gakkai Zasshi* 1995; 43:1569.
166. Stefanidis C, Nana AM, De Canniere D, et al: 10-year experience with the ATS mechanical valve in the mitral position. *Ann Thorac Surg* 2005; 79:1934.
167. Fradet GJ, Bleese N, Burgess J, Cartier PC: Mosaic valve international clinical trial: early performance results. *Ann Thorac Surg* 2001; 71:S273.
168. Jamieson W, Burr L, Allen P, et al: *Quality of Life Afforded by Porcine Bioprostheses Illustrated by the New-Generation Carpentier-Edwards Porcine Bioprothesis.* New York, Futura, 1987.
169. Cohn LH, Sanders JH, Collins JJ Jr: Actuarial comparison of Hancock porcine and prosthetic disc valves for isolated mitral valve replacement. *Circulation* 1976; 54:III-60.
170. Edmunds L: Thrombotic complications with the Omniscience valve. *J Thorac Cardiovasc Surg* 1989; 98:300.
171. Levantino M, Tartarini G, Barzaghi C, et al: Survival despite almost complete occlusion by chronic thrombosis of a Bjork-Shiley mitral prosthesis. *J Heart Valve Dis* 1995; 4:103.
172. Manteiga R, Carlos Souto J, Altes A, et al: Short-course thrombolysis as the first line of therapy for cardiac valve thrombosis. *J Thorac Cardiovasc Surg* 1998; 115:780.

173. Silber H, Khan SS, Matloff JM, et al: The St Jude valve: thrombolysis as the first line of therapy for cardiac valve thrombosis. *Circulation* 1993; 87:30.
174. Hering D, Piper C, Bergemann R, et al: Thromboembolic and bleeding complications following St Jude Medical valve replacement: results of the German Experience with Low-Intensity Anticoagulation Study. *Chest* 2005; 127:53.
175. Ahmad R, Manohitharajah SM, Deverall PB, Watson DA: Chronic hemolysis following mitral valve replacement: a comparative study of the Bjork-Shiley, composite-seat Starr-Edwards, and frame-mounted aortic homograft valves. *J Thorac Cardiovasc Surg* 1976; 71:212.
176. Genoni M, Franzen D, Vogt P, et al: Paravalvular leakage after mitral valve replacement: improved long-term survival with aggressive surgery? *Eur J Cardiothorac Surg* 2000; 17:14.
177. Burckhardt D, Striebel D, Vogt S, et al: Heart valve replacement with St Jude Medical valve prosthesis: long-term experience in 743 patients in Switzerland. *Circulation* 1988; 78:I-18.
178. Gallucci V, Mazzucco A, Bortolotti U, et al: The standard Hancock porcine bioprosthesis: overall experience at the University of Padova. *J Card Surg* 1988; 3:337.
179. Baumgartner WA, Miller DC, Reitz BA, et al: Surgical treatment of prosthetic valve endocarditis. *Ann Thorac Surg* 1983; 35:87.
180. Carrier M, Martineau JP, Bonan R, Pelletier LC: Clinical and hemodynamic assessment of the Omniscience prosthetic heart valve. *J Thorac Cardiovasc Surg* 1987; 93:300.
181. Copeland JG 3d, Sethi GK: Four-year experience with the CarboMedics valve: the North American experience. North American team of clinical investigators for the CarboMedics prosthetic heart valve. *Ann Thorac Surg* 1994; 58:630; discussion 637.
182. Keenan RJ, Armitage JM, Trento A, et al: Clinical experience with the Medtronic-Hall valve prosthesis. *Ann Thorac Surg* 1990; 50:748.
183. Pelletier LC, Carrier M, Leclerc Y, et al: Porcine versus pericardial bioprostheses: a comparison of late results in 1593 patients. *Ann Thorac Surg* 1989; 47:352.
184. Calderwood SB, Swinski LA, Waternaux CM, et al: Risk factors for the development of prosthetic valve endocarditis. *Circulation* 1985; 72:31.
185. Verheul HA, van den Brink RB, van Vreeland T, et al: Effects of changes in management of active infective endocarditis on outcome in a 25-year period. *Am J Cardiol* 1993; 72:682.
186. Cachera JP, Loisance D, Mourtada A, et al: Surgical techniques for treatment of bacterial endocarditis of the mitral valve. *J Card Surg* 1987; 2:265.
187. Edwards MB, Ratnatunga CP, Dore CJ, Taylor KM: Thirty-day mortality and long-term survival following surgery for prosthetic endocarditis: a study from the UK heart valve registry. *Eur J Cardiothorac Surg* 1998; 14:156.
188. Jault F, Gandjbakhch I, Rama A, et al: Active native valve endocarditis: determinants of operative death and late mortality. *Ann Thorac Surg* 1997; 63:1737.
189. Rahimtoola SH: The problem of valve prosthesis-patient mismatch. *Circulation* 1978; 58:20-24.
190. Rahimtoola SH, Murphy E: Valve prosthesis-patient mismatch. A long-term sequela. *Br Heart J* 1981; 45:331-335.
191. Jamieson WRE, Germann E, Ye J, et al: Effect of prosthesis-patient mismatch on long-term survival with mitral valve replacement: assessment to 15 years. *Ann Thorac Surg* 2009; 87:1135-1142.
192. Gammie JS, Sheng S, Griffith BP, et al: Trends in mitral valve surgery in the United States: results from the Society of Thoracic Surgeons Adult Cardiac Surgery Database. *Ann Thorac Surg* 2009; 87(5):1431-1437; discussion 1437-1439. PMID: 19379881.

CHAPTER 43

Surgical Treatment of Mitral Valve Endocarditis

Gosta B. Pettersson
A. Marc Gillinov
Sotiris C. Stamou

INTRODUCTION

Mitral valve infective endocarditis is one of the more devastating complications of heart valve disease, and, if left untreated, is universally fatal. Although the distribution of causes of mitral valve dysfunction has changed in recent years, the incidence of infective endocarditis has remained constant over the past several decades.[1] Underlying rheumatic valvular disease, which was a frequent predisposing factor to infective endocarditis in the 1980s, is now rare in industrialized nations.[2] Other predisposing factors more frequently encountered today include intravenous drug abuse, immunosuppression, degenerative valvular disease, intravascular prostheses and devices, hemodialysis catheters, and nosocomial infections. Several of these predisposing factors are consequences of advances that characterize modern medicine.[3]

Today, more effective antimicrobial agents have improved early and long-term outcomes of patients treated for endocarditis. However, endocarditis is still associated with high rates of morbidity and mortality and frequently requires operation for cure.[4] Increased experience and improvements in surgical technique have improved success rates with these challenging operations.

PATHOLOGY

Native Mitral Valve Endocarditis

Native valve endocarditis (NVE) refers to infectious endocarditis involving a patient's own (native) heart valve. Crude incidence of NVE is 6.2 per 100,000 people per year, and is highest in older age groups.[5] The pathogenesis of NVE begins with endocardial trauma resulting in alteration of the valvular endocardial surface; this allows deposition of fibrin and platelets with subsequent attachment of bacteria. Endocardial injury may be secondary to rheumatic valvulitis or other leaflet disease, or valvular or annular calcification.[5] Common reasons for bacteremia or fungemia predisposing to NVE include use of long-term indwelling catheters, intravenous drug abuse, and fungemia associated with prolonged antibiotic therapy.[6,7] Although vegetations may be seen anywhere on the leaflets or the chordae, the usual site at which infective NVE of the mitral valve causes valvular destruction and invasion is at the base of the atrial aspect of the mitral valve leaflets. Annular or subannular invasion may cause separation at the atrioventricular (AV) junction. Fortunately, mitral annular invasion is shallow in most cases. Invasion into the AV groove fat with abscess formation is more serious and necessitates radical debridement. Destruction of the fibrous trigones and intervalvular fibrosa between the anterior mitral valve leaflet and the aorta is usually a consequence of aortic valve endocarditis with secondary mitral involvement. Occasionally "drop lesions" from an infected aortic valve seed the anterior mitral leaflet or the tensor apparatus of the mitral valve, resulting in double-valve endocarditis; the mechanism may be a large vegetation directly infecting the mitral leaflet or a jet lesion that becomes infected.

Prosthetic Mitral Valve Endocarditis

Prosthetic valve endocarditis (PVE) or replacement device endocarditis is infectious endocarditis involving a surgically implanted heart valve. The number of cases of PVE is on the rise as the number of patients with prosthetic heart valves continues to increase. In contradistinction to NVE, wherein the mitral valve is more likely to be infected,[8] PVE is more common in the aortic than in the mitral position.[9] The risk of PVE appears to be greatest approximately 5 weeks after valve implantation and thereafter declines.[10–13]

PVE identified within the first postoperative year is considered early endocarditis, and those cases appearing more than 1 year after operation are termed late.[13,14] The incidence of early PVE is 1%.[14] Once past the early phase, the incidence of late PVE is 0.5 to 1% per year.[15–18] The type of prosthesis (mechanical versus bioprosthetic) does not influence the risk of PVE.

Early PVE is usually the result of intraoperative infection.[19] Common portals of entry for bacteria that cause PVE are intravascular catheters and skin infection.[20,21] Nosocomial infections contribute to late PVE, particularly in patients with medical comorbidities that require frequent hospital admission or instrumentation (eg, hemodialysis patients) or immunosuppression (eg, organ transplantation).[19]

Early PVE usually affects the sewing ring or the interface of the prosthetic valve and the annulus (often a site of clot formation), resulting in periprosthetic leak. Involvement of the sewing ring starts locally but eventually becomes circumferential. Enzymatic degradation of the tissue holding the sutures results in dehiscence of the prosthesis and periprosthetic leak. Progression of the infection and invasion may lead to abscess formation. Mitral PVE may extend anteriorly to the fibrous trigone or posteriorly, causing AV separation. PVE may be classified into different subgroups based on the anatomic distribution of the infection. According to this classification, PVE cases are classified as those involving the prosthesis alone, those involving the prosthesis–native annular junction (annular infection), and those extending beyond the annulus (extensive infection).[13,19] Another useful classification that applies to both NVE and PVE involves the distinction between *active* and *healed* endocarditis. The latter includes cases in which organisms cannot be demonstrated but remote infection is still presumed.[13,22]

MICROBIOLOGY

Endocarditis of native valves is most often caused by *Streptococcus viridans, Staphylococcus aureus* or *epidermidis,* or *Enterococci.* The distribution of microorganisms responsible for early PVE includes coagulase-negative staphylococci (52%), *S. aureus* (10%), *Enterococci* (8%), *S. viridans* (5%), and gram-negative organisms (6%).[19] Fungi account for 10% of cases of early PVE (*Candida albicans* in 8 of 10). Although gram-positive cocci are dominant in both early and late PVE, in early PVE staphylococci predominate whereas in late PVE streptococci are the most common organisms isolated.[9] *Haemophilus* spp., *Actinobacillus actinomycetemcomitans, Cardiobacterium hominis, Eikenella corrodens,* and *Kingella kingae* are collectively termed the HACEK group and account for 3% of culture-negative late PVE.[23] Patients with PVE and negative cultures may be infected by fastidious organisms. In general, late PVE is more amenable to successful antibiotic therapy than is early PVE; however, once the sewing ring is involved, cure is unlikely. PVE always warrants surgical consideration.

DIAGNOSIS

Clinical Presentation

The most common clinical finding is fever;[9] however, it is nonspecific. Other findings include a new murmur or a change in an existing murmur. Embolic phenomena may cause petechiae, Roth spots, Osler nodes, and Janeway lesions. Splenomegaly may be present in both NVE and PVE.

Laboratory findings include a white blood cell count >12,000/mm^3, anemia (hematocrit <34%), and hematuria.[9] Blood cultures from separate sites are usually positive in patients with bacterial endocarditis; two of three positive cultures is considered diagnostic. However, cultures in patients with fastidious organisms or fungi may take more than 3 weeks to become positive. Blood cultures should be drawn before antibiotics are started.

Electrocardiographic Findings

Conduction abnormalities are present in up to 23% of patients with NVE and 47% of patients with PVE. This usually indicates extension of the infection and formation of a paravalvular abscess.[24]

Echocardiographic Findings

The present gold standard diagnostic modality for documenting infective endocarditis is transesophageal echocardiography. Specificity for transesophageal echocardiography is approximately 90% and sensitivity is 95%.[26,27] In contrast, transthoracic echocardiography is more operator dependent and its images may be compromised by surrounding structures; it is only 50% sensitive and 90% specific for infective endocarditis.[25] Echocardiographic findings of endocarditis include vegetations, periprosthetic leak in patients with PVE, intracardiac fistulae, and abscesses. The echocardiographic examination is very good at evaluating valve function but less reliable for assessing the severity and invasiveness of the infection. A negative echocardiogram does not exclude the diagnosis of endocarditis. In situations with strong suspicion of endocarditis, the diagnosis may be pursued by magnetic resonance imaging (MRI). In the majority of patients with endocarditis, MRI will demonstrate abnormal consistency of tissue in the annulus. Metastatic infection is a possibility and patients with infective endocarditis and abdominal symptoms should be investigated with computed tomography (CT) scanning to rule out splenic or hepatic abscesses. Metastatic infection of viscera is typically caused by staphylococcal organisms.[5] The brain is the most frequent site for emboli.[28,29] Any neurologic deficit or abnormality should trigger investigation with CT or MRI of the brain, funduscopic examination, and occasionally cerebrospinal fluid examination. CT or MRI of the brain is also justified in the absence of symptoms if there are stigmata of other embolic events. Preoperative coronary angiography is indicated in patients with coronary artery disease or history of previous revascularization procedures and in patients in whom coronary embolization is suspected.

Duke Criteria

The Duke University criteria were developed to improve the specificity and sensitivity of the diagnosis of infective endocarditis. These criteria include echocardiographic results along with clinical, microbiologic, and pathologic findings.[30] Most authorities accept a modification of these criteria for PVE that includes progressive heart failure in the presence of positive blood cultures and new conduction disturbances (Table 43-1). The Duke criteria are classified as "major criteria" (typical positive blood culture and positive echocardiogram) and "minor" criteria (predisposition, fever, vascular phenomena, immunologic phenomena, suggestive echocardiogram, suggestive microbiologic findings, and new-onset heart failure or conduction disturbances). There are three diagnostic categories: (1) patients with a *low clinical likelihood of infective endocarditis* are those with resolution of manifestations of endocarditis with antibiotic therapy for 4 days or less, or no pathologic evidence of infective endocarditis at surgery or autopsy after antibiotic therapy for 4 days or less; (2) patients with *possible endocarditis* have one or two minor clinical criteria of the Duke classification system; and (3) patients with a *definite* diagnosis of infective endocarditis are those (a) in whom pathologic specimens from surgery or autopsy reveal positive histology and/or culture, (b) who have two major criteria, (c) who have one major and three minor criteria, or (d) who have five minor criteria.[30] Understandably, the Duke criteria are not particularly relevant in patients who have had surgical treatment, those in whom the

TABLE 43-1 Duke Criteria for Native Valve Endocarditis and Prosthetic Valve Endocarditis

Major Criteria
Positive Blood Cultures for Infective Endocarditis
Typical microorganism for infective endocarditis from two separate blood cultures: *Streptococcus viridans, S. bovis*, and HACEK group or community-acquired *Staphylococcus aureus* or *enterococci* in the absence of a primary focus, or
Persistently positive blood cultures, defined as recovery of a microorganism consistent with infective endocarditis from:
Blood cultures drawn >12 hours apart or
All of three or most of four or more separate blood cultures, with the first and last drawn at least 1 hour apart
Evidence of Endocardial Involvement
Positive echocardiogram for infective endocarditis
Oscillating intracardiac mass on valve or supporting structures or in the path of regurgitant jets or on implanted material in the absence of an alternative anatomic explanation, abscess, new partial dehiscence of prosthetic valve, or new valvular regurgitation (increase or change in preexisting murmur not sufficient)
Minor Criteria
Predisposition: predisposing heart condition or intravenous drug use
Fever: temperature ≥38°C (100.4°F)
Vascular phenomena: major arterial emboli, septic pulmonary infarcts, mycotic aneurysm, intracranial hemorrhage, conjunctival hemorrhage, and Janeway lesions
Immunologic phenomena: glomerulonephritis, Osler nodes, Roth spots, rheumatoid factor
Microbiologic evidence: positive blood culture but not meeting major criterion as noted previously or serologic evidence of active infection with organisms consistent with infective endocarditis
Echocardiogram: consistent with infective endocarditis but not meeting major criterion as noted previously
New-onset heart failure
New conduction disturbances

HACEK group = Haemophilus spp., Actinobacillus actinomycetemcomitans, Cardiobacterium hominis, Eikenella corrodens, and Kingella kingae
Source: Modified with permission from Perez-Vasquez et al.[55] *(permission from Muehrcke et al.*[43]*)*

diagnosis is based on surgical findings, and those with analysis of surgical specimens by microscopy, culture, and polymerase chain reaction.

INDICATIONS FOR SURGERY

Surgery plays a pivotal role in the management of native mitral valve endocarditis. Indications for surgical intervention in patients with NVE and PVE are presented in Table 43-2. Congestive heart failure is the most common indication for surgery.

The majority of patients with PVE require surgery.[31,32] Indications for surgical intervention in patients with PVE include heart failure, new heart block (possibly secondary to a myocardial abscess), ongoing sepsis, valve dehiscence, recurrent systemic embolism, relapse of infection, and fungal infection. Operation for large mobile vegetations to prevent embolization in both NVE and PVE remains a controversial indication in the absence of hemodynamic compromise or other surgical indications. Fungal PVE is uncommon but is more difficult to cure than is PVE caused by other organisms. The operative strategy should include perioperative intravenous amphotericin B, radical debridement of infected tissue, reconstruction using biologic tissue whenever possible, and lifelong oral suppressive antifungal therapy after completion of intravenous therapy.[33]

TIMING OF SURGERY

Many patients with NVE and the majority of patients with PVE require surgical intervention, and the challenge for the surgeon is to determine the appropriate timing of surgery.[31] In most cases, the operation should not be delayed once surgical indications are present. Patients with PVE caused by *S. aureus,* even without periannular abscess formation, should have early operation to prevent an aggressive infection with rapid progression and invasion. The same principle applies to fungal infective endocarditis, because a mortality rate as high as 93% has been reported.[9]

However, delaying repair is usually advised in the presence of central nervous system complications.[28] Before undergoing valve surgery, patients with endocarditis should have careful neurologic evaluation and significant findings should be evaluated by head CT or MRI. Occasionally, angiography is required to exclude a mycotic aneurysm. Patients with hemorrhagic strokes should have surgery delayed for 4 weeks to reduce the risk of further intracranial bleeding during heart surgery. Intracranial hemorrhage in the setting of PVE has been associated with mortality as high as 28 to 69%.[35] The main concern with nonhemorrhagic embolic stroke is transformation of an ischemic infarct into a hemorrhagic infarct as a complication of the anticoagulation required during cardiopulmonary bypass.[34] Patients who suffered recent ischemic stroke should have their operation delayed for 2 to 4 weeks, particularly if the stroke is large.[36,37] The risk of worsening neurologic symptoms as a consequence of operation is time-related, decreasing with increasing interval from the initial neurologic event. This risk must be weighed against the indications for surgery and the risk of additional emboli during the waiting period.

OPERATIVE TECHNIQUES

General Principles

Operations for endocarditis are guided by some basic principles: optimal timing of surgery as discussed above, good exposure of the valve, radical debridement, optimal choice for reconstruction of the heart and repair or replacement of the valve, and adequate postoperative antibiotic treatment. Radical debridement with removal of all infected and necrotic tissue and foreign material is more difficult to accomplish in mitral cases with AV groove invasion and abscess formation, particularly when compared with aortic root infections. In addition, reconstruction after invasion of the AV groove and AV separation entails closing off the infected space, leaving it without drainage.

TABLE 43-2 Surgical Indications for Native Valve Endocarditis and Prosthetic Valve Endocarditis

1. Severe mitral regurgitation, with or without symptoms of congestive heart failure
2. Uncontrolled sepsis despite proper antibiotic therapy
3. Presence of an antibiotic-resistant organism
4. Fungal endocarditis or endocarditis caused by *Staphylococcus aureus* or gram-negative bacteria
5. Presence of mitral annular abscess, extension of infection to intervalvular fibrous body, or formation of intracardiac fistulas
6. Onset of a new conduction disturbance
7. Large vegetations (>1 cm), particularly those that are mobile and located on the anterior leaflet, and thus at high risk for embolic complications
8. Multiple emboli despite appropriate antibiotic therapy

Native Mitral Valve Endocarditis

Intraoperative transesophageal echocardiography should be performed in all cases to evaluate the valve before commencing the procedure. Surgical treatment options for NVE affecting the mitral valve include valve replacement and valve repair. Although there is some experience with the mitral valve allograft for treatment of mitral valve endocarditis, there are too few data available to support this strategy.[38]

Most operations for NVE are best conducted through a full median sternotomy. Cannulation for cardiopulmonary bypass involves arterial return via the ascending aorta and bicaval cannulation for venous return. In case of large mobile vegetations, it is advisable to arrest the heart before placing a transatrial retrograde cardioplegia catheter. Protection is achieved using antegrade and retrograde substrate-enhanced cardioplegia.[39]

The mitral valve is exposed via a left atriotomy through the interatrial groove or transseptally. If the left atrium is small, an extended transseptal approach is employed. Once exposure of the mitral valve is accomplished, the valve is evaluated to assess for presence of paravalvular abscesses, intracardiac fistulae, or intervalvular fibrous body/ventricular involvement. Radical resection of all necrotic tissue is performed with a margin of normal tissue. All grossly infected tissue is removed without concern for the possibility of repair. Specimens are sent for microbiologic analysis and culture.

For NVE, our approach is to attempt repair if feasible. Mitral valve repair can be performed safely provided there is sufficient remaining tissue to allow valvular reconstruction without tension.[40–44] In the event of extensive destruction of the subvalvular apparatus, prosthetic valve replacement is performed. Regardless of the mitral procedure performed, all patients with active infection receive 6 weeks of postoperative antibiotic therapy.

Anterior Leaflet Repair

"Drop lesions" of the anterior leaflet encountered in association with aortic endocarditis can be repaired with autologous or glutaraldehyde-preserved pericardium.[38] A patch of pericardium is fixed to the remaining tissue of the anterior leaflet with running polypropylene suture (Fig. 43-1). The smooth surface of the patch should face the atrium to decrease the risk of thromboembolic complications.[37] More extensive destruction involving both the aortic valve and the anterior leaflet of the mitral valve can be repaired using a free-standing aortic root homograft with the anterior leaflet of the mitral valve still attached. The homograft's attached aortomitral curtain can be used to reconstruct the base of the native anterior mitral leaflet.[37,45]

Involvement of the free margin of the anterior leaflet can be managed with triangular resection and closure with interrupted fine sutures. Anterior leaflet chordal rupture can be repaired with chordal transposition from the posterior leaflet or with secondary chordal transfer to the free margin of the anterior leaflet. Artificial chordae may also be used to replace ruptured anterior leaflet chordae.

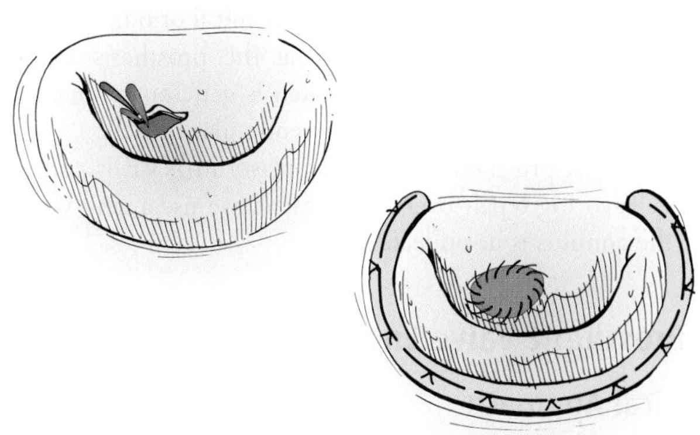

FIGURE 43-1 Repair of anterior leaflet perforation by patch with autologous pericardium followed by annuloplasty.

Posterior Leaflet Repair

The middle scallop (P_2 segment) of the posterior segment is frequently affected by the infectious process. Repair can be performed with quadrangular resection of the middle scallop, and a sliding repair is frequently required to close the gap between the remaining two scallops (Fig. 43-2). Extensive destruction of the posterior annulus requires removal of all devitalized tissue and annular reconstruction with autologous pericardium. Occasionally, repair of the annulus and the posterior leaflet can be accomplished with the same patch if chordal support to the leaflet is good. A running polypropylene suture is used on the ventricular, atrial, and valvular aspects of the

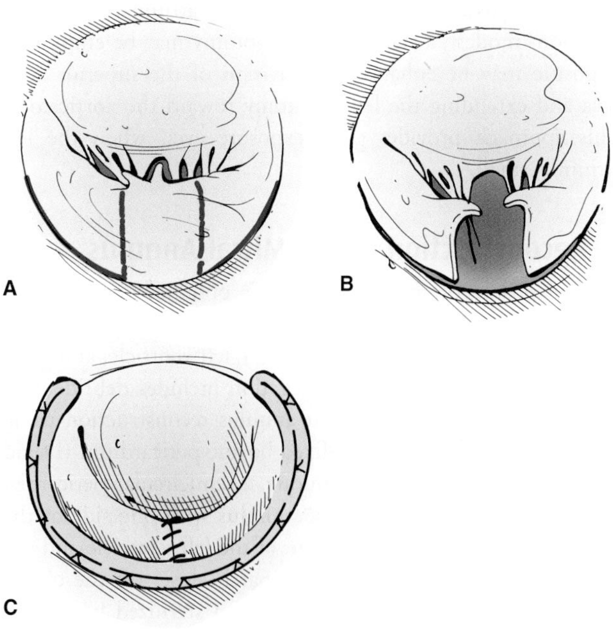

FIGURE 43-2 Quadrangular resection and sliding repair for posterior leaflet vegetation with ruptured chordae. (A,B) Segment of posterior leaflet is resected and a portion of leaflet detached from the annulus. (C) Leaflet remnants are sutured to the annulus, taking deep bites to reduce leaflet height. Leaflet edges are reapproximated in the center. Annuloplasty completes the repair.

patch. If replacement is required, a mechanical or bioprosthetic valve may then be inserted, affixing the prosthesis to the patch.[45] It is important that the patch is generous enough to minimize tension on the sutures in ventricular muscle.

The use of prosthetic ring annuloplasty in NVE is controversial. Favoring repair over replacement, we use a ring whenever the annulus is not infected.

Prosthetic Valve Endocarditis

Surgical Approach

Operations for PVE are reoperations, usually performed via a median sternotomy. An alternative approach is right anterolateral thoracotomy in the fourth intercostal space; this is particularly useful in patients with multiple previous sternotomies, bypass grafts near the sternum, or a history of mediastinal radiation and/or mediastinitis.[46,47] However, a right thoracotomy for mitral reoperations allows limited access, sometimes denies aortic cross-clamping, and may be associated with a risk of stroke.

Myocardial Protection

Cardiopulmonary bypass is instituted using the ascending aorta and bicaval cannulation. A transatrial retrograde cardioplegia cannula is used and myocardial protection is achieved using antegrade and retrograde cardioplegia.

Mitral Valve Exposure

The main issues in achieving mitral valve exposure are related to obtaining mobility of the right atrium and vena cavae.[19] Our usual approach to obtain mitral valve exposure is to use an extended transseptal approach. If the left atrium is large and adhesions modest, a standard left atriotomy may be employed. Exposure may be enhanced by division of the superior vena cava and extending the left atriotomy toward the aortic root. This approach provides good exposure even when the left atrium is small.

Reconstruction of the Mitral Annulus

Once exposure of the mitral valve is obtained, the infected prosthesis is removed. Mitral valve PVE may produce an abscess cavity separating the left atrium, left ventricle, and prosthesis. In these situations the operation includes debridement of the annulus with subsequent annulus reconstruction using autologous or glutaraldehyde-fixed bovine pericardium (David technique).[48,49] With this technique, a semicircular pericardial patch is used to reconstruct the annulus with one side of the patch sutured to the endocardium of the left ventricle and the other side to the left atrium. This patch closes off the cavity, which must be thoroughly debrided and sterilized before the patch is affixed. The new valve prosthesis is affixed to this reconstructed annulus (Fig. 43-3). The patch should be large in order to minimize tension on suture lines. In most situations with annular reconstruction we employ a bioprosthesis because of the larger and softer sewing ring and to avoid anticoagulation in the postoperative period.

An alternative technique for mitral annular reconstruction is the technique described by Carpentier and colleagues.[50] This technique involves using figure-of-eight atrial and ventricular sutures to reconstruct the AV junction. Exerting traction on

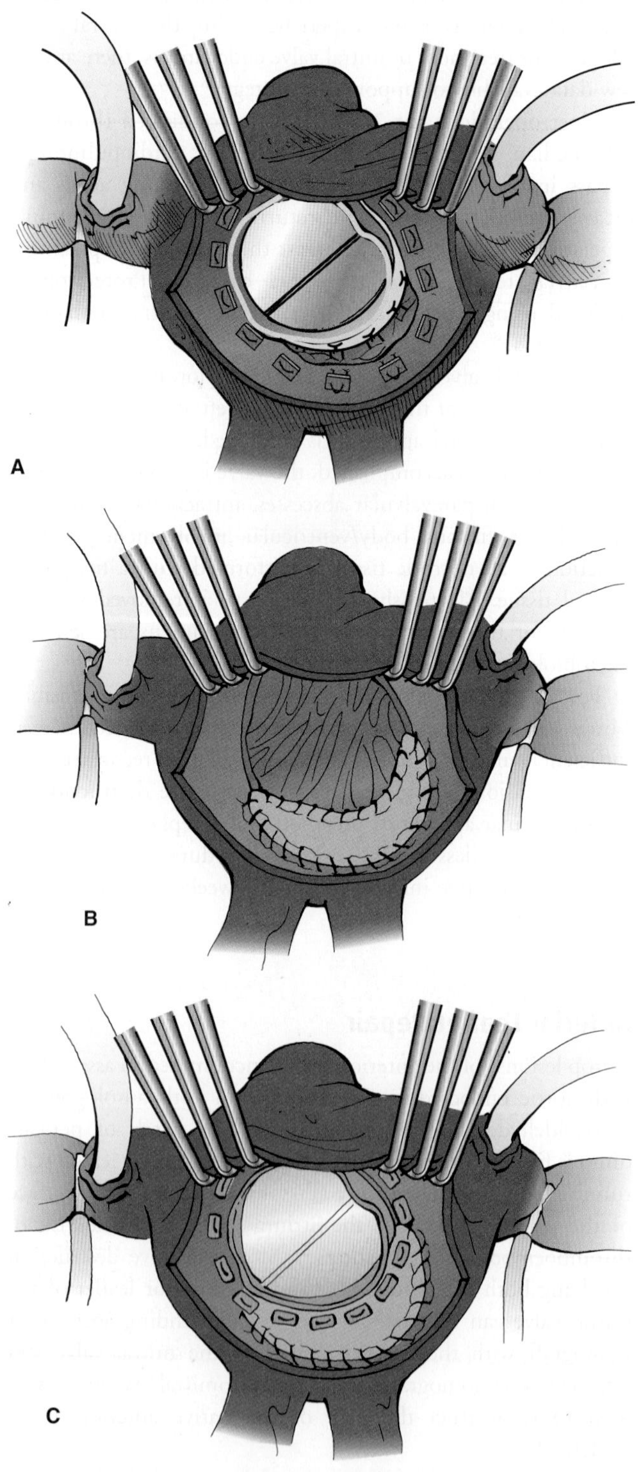

FIGURE 43-3 (A) Prosthetic valve endocarditis with posterior perivalvular abscess. (B) The valve is removed and the abscess debrided. A pericardial patch sewn to the ventricle and atrium excludes the abscess cavity and reconstructs the annulus. (C) A new prosthesis is affixed to the pericardial patch and annulus. (*Reproduced with permission from the Cleveland Clinic Foundation.*)

these sutures reduces the size of the annulus and closes the AV groove without injury to the circumflex vessels. The main potential disadvantage of this technique is that sutures may pull through stiff and noncompliant ventricular tissue.[19] We have observed pseudoaneurysm formation after application of this technique.

Reconstruction of the Fibrous Trigones

Extension of PVE into the intervalular fibrosa/fibrous trigones may necessitate replacement of both mitral and aortic valves. This usually occurs in the setting of PVE affecting both the aortic and the mitral valves and seldom with isolated mitral valve endocarditis. Reconstruction of the intervalvular fibrosa as well as replacement of both the aortic and mitral valve are required (Fig. 43-4). In such circumstances the fibrous trigones may be reconstructed with autologous or bovine pericardium that is used to secure the new prosthesis.[13,19] Perfect exposure is mandatory whether it is provided by the extended transseptal approach or by dividing the superior vena cava and extending the left atriotomy from anterior to the right superior pulmonary vein toward the dome of the left atrium. This approach

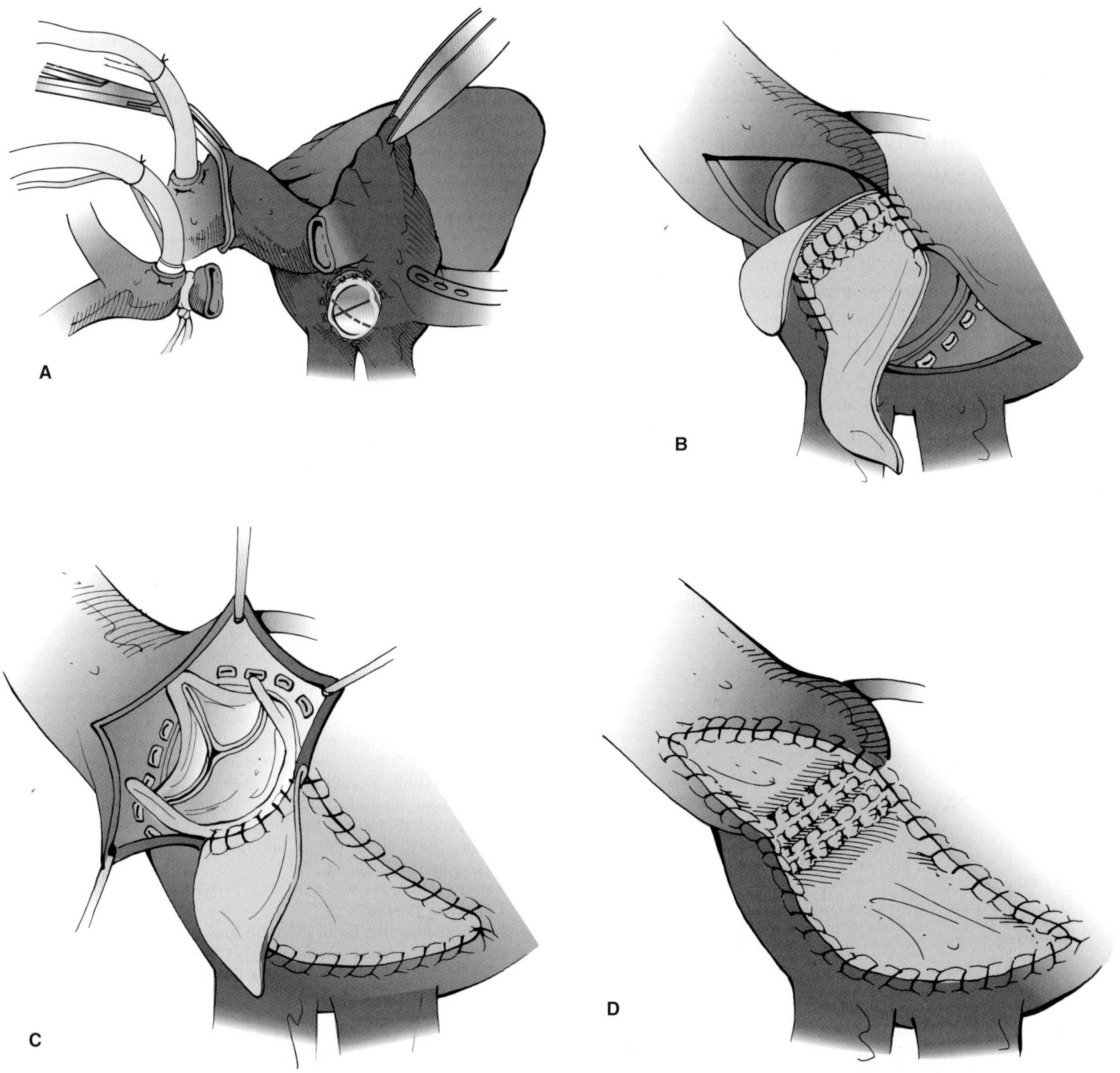

FIGURE 43-4 Reconstruction of the fibrous trigones. (A) Infection involves the mitral and aortic valves. Division of the superior vena cava facilitates exposure of the aortic valve, mitral valve, and fibrous trigones. (B) The new prosthetic mitral valve is sewn to the annulus posteriorly, medially, and laterally, but the superior portion of the mitral valve annulus is reconstructed by a pericardial patch that recreates the fibrous trigone. The valve is then sewn to this patch with horizontal mattress sutures. (C) Once the mitral valve prosthesis is in place, the aortic valve prosthesis is secured throughout most of the annulus. The pericardial patch reconstructs the medial part of the aortic valve annulus and the aortic valve is then sewn to the patch. (D) After the valve replacements are complete, the pericardial patch is extended to finish the closure of the aorta and the left atrium. (*Reproduced with permission from the Cleveland Clinic Foundation.*)

allows debridement of the aortic and mitral valves, as well as the fibrous trigones. The prosthetic mitral valve is then sewn to the annulus posteriorly, medially, and laterally, and the superior portion of the mitral valve annulus is reconstructed with a pericardial patch that replaces the fibrous trigones. The valve is then sewn to the patch with horizontal mattress sutures. Once the mitral valve is secured in place, the aortic valve prosthesis is affixed to the aortic annulus. The pericardial patch is used to reconstruct the medial part of the aortic valve annulus. The aortic valve is then sewn to that patch.[13,19] An alternative option is aortic valve and root allograft replacement in an anatomic position and orientation, suturing the intervalvular fibrosa/mitral valve of the allograft to the mitral valve prosthesis.

RESULTS

Native Mitral Valve Endocarditis

In patients with NVE, mitral valve repair is preferable to mitral valve replacement, because repair has been associated with lower hospital mortality and improved long-term survival (Fig. 43-5).[43,51] In our series of 146 patients having surgery for NVE, patients undergoing repair had a lower hospital mortality ($p = 0.008$) and improved long-term survival ($p = 0.05$) compared with those having replacement.[43] Several recent series have reported excellent results with valve repair in the setting of mitral valve endocarditis, with mortality rates ranging between 0 and 9%.[40–43,52] The infection-free survival is also better for mitral valve repair compared with replacement with a less than 1% per year reinfection rate.[43] The likely explanations for these excellent outcomes are the avoidance of prosthetic material in the infected field and the preservation of left ventricular function associated with repairing mitral valves.[43] Second, the replacement group contains the sickest patients with the most advanced and destructive disease.

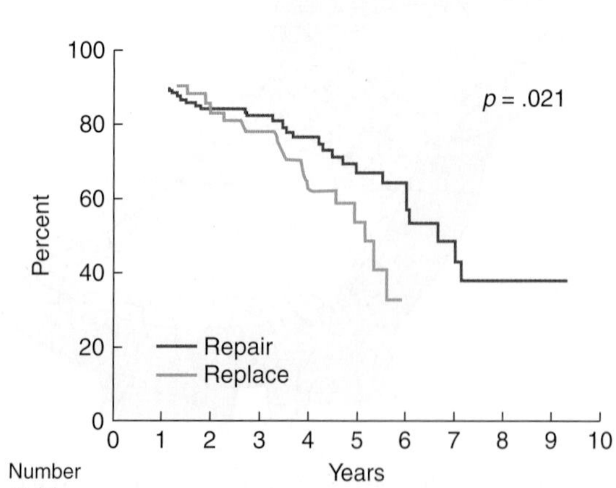

Number at risk											
Repair	99	87	74	54	40	26	18	10	5	3	2
Replace	36	32	28	26	16	9	2	0	0	0	0

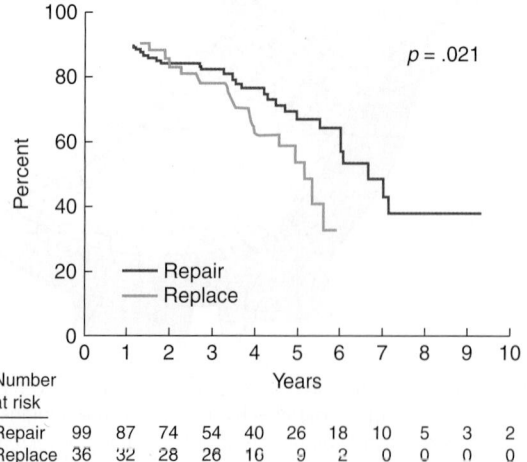

FIGURE 43-5 Event-free survival for all patients undergoing mitral valve repair or replacement. (*Reproduced with permission from Muehrcke et al.*[43])

Prosthetic Valve Endocarditis

PVE is associated with a much higher operative mortality than is native valve endocarditis.[24,49,53,54] Despite improved antimicrobial regimens, outcomes of medical therapy without reoperation are poor in PVE, particularly for patients with annular involvement or early endocarditis after valve surgery.[13] The success of allografts in the aortic position has led to attempts to use mitral valve allografts to treat mitral valve PVE. That strategy seems to offer no advantage over standard prostheses and remains experimental.

For all patients with mitral valve PVE, prolonged postoperative treatment with intravenous antibiotics is required. Most patients with active endocarditis are treated for at least 6 weeks after surgery and are followed with transesophageal echo studies. In comparison with aortic valve endocarditis, radical debridement and drainage of posterior mitral annulus abscesses is far more difficult. Patients with fungal endocarditis require 2 months of intravenous antifungal therapy followed by indefinite oral antifungal therapy.[33]

REFERENCES

1. Moreillon P, Que YA: Infective endocarditis. *Lancet* 2004; 363:144.
2. Hoen B, Alla F, Selton-Suty C, et al: Changing profile of infective endocarditis: results of a 1-year survey in France. *JAMA* 2002; 288:75.
3. Bouza E, Menasalvas A, Munoz P, et al: Infective endocarditis—A prospective study at the end of the twentieth century: new predisposing conditions, new etiologic agents, and still a high mortality. *Medicine (Baltimore)* 2001; 80:298.
4. Fullerton D, Frederick LG: Prosthetic valve endocarditis, in Sellke FW, Del Nido P, Swanson SJ (eds): *Sabiston & Spencer Surgery of the Chest*, 6th ed. Duke University, Durham, NC, WB Saunders, 2004; p 1355.
5. Kouchoukos N, Blackstone E, Doty D, et al: Infective endocarditis. In Kouchoukos N, Blackstone E, Doty D, et al. (eds): *Cardiac Surgery*, 3rd ed. Missouri Baptist Medical Center, St. Louis, Churchill Livingstone, 2003: p 689.
6. McKinsey DS, Ratts TE, Bisno AL: Underlying cardiac lesions in adults with infective endocarditis. The changing spectrum. *Am J Med* 1987; 82:681.
7. Weinstein L, Schlesinger JJ: Pathoanatomic, pathophysiologic and clinical correlations in endocarditis (second of two parts). *NEJM* 1974; 291:1122.
8. Raanani E, David TE, Dellgren G, et al: Redo aortic root replacement: experience with 31 patients. *Ann Thorac Surg* 2001; 71:1460.
9. Cowgill LD, Addonizio VP, Hopeman AR, Harken AH: A practical approach to prosthetic valve endocarditis. *Ann Thorac Surg* 1987; 43:450.
10. Calderwood SB, Swinski LA, Waternaux CM, et al: Risk factors for the development of prosthetic valve endocarditis. *Circulation* 1985; 72:31.
11. Calderwood SB, Swinski LA, Karchmer AW, et al: Prosthetic valve endocarditis. Analysis of factors affecting outcome of therapy. *J Thorac Cardiovasc Surg* 1986; 92:776.
12. Ivert TS, Dismukes WE, Cobbs CG, et al: Prosthetic valve endocarditis. *Circulation* 1984; 69:223.
13. Lytle BW, Priest BP, Taylor PC, et al: Surgical treatment of prosthetic valve endocarditis. *J Thorac Cardiovasc Surg* 1996; 111:198.
14. Gordon SM, Serkey JM, Longworth DL, et al: Early onset prosthetic valve endocarditis: The Cleveland Clinic experience 1992-1997. *Ann Thorac Surg* 2000; 69:1388.
15. Agnihotri AK, McGiffin DC, Galbraith AJ, O'Brien MF: The prevalence of infective endocarditis after aortic valve replacement. *J Thorac Cardiovasc Surg* 1995; 110:1708.
16. Grover FL, Cohen DJ, Oprian C, et al: Determinants of the occurrence of and survival from prosthetic valve endocarditis. Experience of the Veterans Affairs Cooperative Study on Valvular Heart Disease. *J Thorac Cardiovasc Surg* 1994; 108:207.
17. Hammermeister KE, Sethi GK, Henderson WG, et al: A comparison of outcomes in men 11 years after heart-valve replacement with a mechanical valve or bioprosthesis. Veterans Affairs Cooperative Study on Valvular Heart Disease. *NEJM* 1993; 328:1289.

18. Lytle BW, Cosgrove DM, Taylor PC, et al: Primary isolated aortic valve replacement. Early and late results. *J Thorac Cardiovasc Surg* 1989; 97:675.
19. Lytle BW: Prosthetic valve endocarditis, in Vlessis AA, Bolling SF (eds): *Endocarditis: a Multidisciplinary Approach to Modern Treatment.* Armonk, NY, Futura Publishing, 1999; p 344.
20. Keys TF: Do patients with total joint replacements need antibiotics before dental work? *Cleve Clin J Med* 2003; 70:351.
21. Fang G, Keys TF, Gentry LO, et al: Prosthetic valve endocarditis resulting from nosocomial bacteremia. A prospective, multicenter study. *Ann Intern Med* 1993; 119:560.
22. Sabik JF, Lytle BW, Blackstone EH, et al: Aortic root replacement with cryopreserved allograft for prosthetic valve endocarditis. *Ann Thorac Surg* 2002; 74:650.
23. Berbari EF, Cockerill FR 3rd, Steckelberg JM: Infective endocarditis due to unusual or fastidious microorganisms. *Mayo Clin Proc* 1997; 72:532.
24. Miller DC: Predictors of outcome in patients with prosthetic valve endocarditis (PVE) and potential advantages of homograft aortic root replacement for prosthetic ascending aortic valve-graft infections. *J Card Surg* 1990; 5:53.
25. Birmingham GD, Rahko PS, Ballantyne F 3rd: Improved detection of infective endocarditis with transesophageal echocardiography. *Am Heart J* 1992; 123:774.
26. Daniel WG, Mugge A, Grote J, et al: Comparison of transthoracic and transesophageal echocardiography for detection of abnormalities of prosthetic and bioprosthetic valves in the mitral and aortic positions. *Am J Cardiol* 1993; 71:210.
27. Stein PD, Harken DE, Dexter L: The nature and prevention of prosthetic valve endocarditis. *Am Heart J* 1966; 71:393.
28. Gillinov AM, Shah RV, Curtis WE, et al: Valve replacement in patients with endocarditis and acute neurologic deficit. *Ann Thorac Surg* 1996; 61:1125.
29. Sandre RM, Shafran SD: Infective endocarditis: review of 135 cases over 9 years. *Clin Infect Dis* 1996; 22:276.
30. Durack DT, Lukes AS, Bright DK: New criteria for diagnosis of infective endocarditis: utilization of specific echocardiographic findings. Duke Endocarditis Service. *Am J Med* 1994; 96:200.
31. Okita Y, Franciosi G, Matsuki O, et al: Early and late results of aortic root replacement with antibiotic-sterilized aortic homograft. *J Thorac Cardiovasc Surg* 1988; 95:696.
32. Olaison L, Pettersson G: Current best practices and guidelines: indications for surgical intervention in infective endocarditis. *Infect Dis Clin North Am* 2002; 16:453.
33. Muehrcke DD, Lytle BW, Cosgrove DM 3rd: Surgical and long-term antifungal therapy for fungal prosthetic valve endocarditis. *Ann Thorac Surg* 1995; 60:538.
34. Ting W, Silverman N, Levitsky S: Valve replacement in patients with endocarditis and cerebral septic emboli. *Ann Thorac Surg* 1991; 51:18.
35. Davenport J, Hart RG: Prosthetic valve endocarditis 1976–1987. Antibiotics, anticoagulation, and stroke. *Stroke* 1990; 21:993.
36. Eishi K, Kawazoe K, Kuriyama Y, et al: Surgical management of infective endocarditis associated with cerebral complications. Multi-center retrospective study in Japan. *J Thorac Cardiovasc Surg* 1995; 110:1745.
37. Filsoufi F, Adams D: Surgical treatment of mitral valve endocarditis, in Edmunds LH, Cohn LH (eds): *Cardiac Surgery in the Adult*, 2nd ed. New York, McGraw-Hill Professional, 2003; p 987.
38. Gillinov AM, Diaz R, Blackstone EH, et al: Double valve endocarditis. *Ann Thorac Surg* 2001; 71:1874.
39. Buckberg GD: When is cardiac muscle damaged irreversibly? *J Thorac Cardiovasc Surg* 1986; 92:483.
40. Dreyfus G, Serraf A, Jebara VA, et al: Valve repair in acute endocarditis. *Ann Thorac Surg* 1990; 49:706.
41. Hendren WG, Morris AS, Rosenkranz ER, et al: Mitral valve repair for bacterial endocarditis. *J Thorac Cardiovasc Surg* 1992; 103:124.
42. Pagani FD, Monaghan HL, Deeb GM, Bolling SF: Mitral valve reconstruction for active and healed endocarditis. *Circulation* 1996; 94(9 Suppl): II133.
43. Muehrcke DD, Cosgrove DM 3rd, Lytle BW, et al: Is there an advantage to repairing infected mitral valves? *Ann Thorac Surg* 1997; 63:1718.
44. Sternik L, Zehr KJ, Orszulak TA, et al: The advantage of repair of mitral valve in acute endocarditis. *J Heart Valve Dis* 2002; 11:91.
45. Gardner TJ, Spray TL: *Operative Cardiac Surgery*, 5th ed. London, Arnold Publishers, 2004.
46. Byrne JG, Karavas AN, Adams DH, et al: The preferred approach for mitral valve surgery after CABG: right thoracotomy, hypothermia and avoidance of LIMA-LAD graft. *J Heart Valve Dis* 2001; 10:584.
47. Adams DH, Filsoufi F, Byrne JG, et al: Mitral valve repair in redo cardiac surgery. *J Card Surg* 2002; 17:40.
48. David TE, Feindel CM: Reconstruction of the mitral annulus. A ten-year experience. *J Thorac Cardiovasc Surg* 1995; 110:1323.
49. David TE; The surgical treatment of patients with prosthetic valve endocarditis. *Semin Thorac Cardiovasc Surg* 1995; 7:47.
50. Carpentier AF, Pellerin M, Fuzellier JF, Relland JY: Extensive calcification of the mitral valve annulus: pathology and surgical management. *J Thorac Cardiovasc Surg* 1996; 111:718.
51. Ruttmann E, Legit C, Poelzl G, et al: Mitral valve repair provides improved outcome over replacement in active infective endocarditis. *J Thorac Cardiovasc Surg* 2005; 130:765.
52. Zegdi R, Debieche M, Latremouille C, et al: Long-term results of mitral valve repair in active endocarditis. *Circulation* 2005; 111:2532.
53. Aranki SF, Adams DH, Rizzo RJ, et al: Determinants of early mortality and late survival in mitral valve endocarditis. *Circulation* 1995; 92(9 Suppl): II143.
54. Moon MR, Miller DC, Moore KA, et al: Treatment of endocarditis with valve replacement: the question of tissue versus mechanical prosthesis. *Ann Thorac Surg* 2001; 71:1164.
55. Perez-Vasquez A, Farinas MC, Garcia-Palomo JD, et al: Evaluation of the Duke criteria in 93 episodes of prosthetic valve endocarditis. *Arch Intern Med* 2000; 160:1185.

CHAPTER 44

Minimally Invasive and Robotic Mitral Valve Surgery

Eric J. Lehr
Evelio Rodriguez
W. Randolph Chitwood, Jr.

INTRODUCTION

Minimally invasive mitral valve surgery (MIMVS) does not refer to a single approach, but rather to a collection of new techniques and operation-specific technologies. These include enhanced visualization and instrumentation systems as well as modified perfusion methods, all directed toward minimizing surgical trauma by reducing the incision size. Cohn and Cosgrove, along with several European surgeons, first modified cardiopulmonary bypass techniques and reduced incision sizes to enable safe, effective, minimally invasive aortic and mitral valve surgery.[1–3] Concurrently, port-access methods using endoaortic balloon occluders were developed.[4] Despite expanding enthusiasm for minimally invasive valve surgery, many surgeons remained skeptical and became critical of complex operations done through small incisions, owing to possibilities of unsafe operations, unknown operative complexities, and inferior results.[5,6]

Despite circumspect reticence, significant advances were made and various institutions have published favorable results as single-center observational and comparative studies. Most surgeons who performed MIMVS in this era selected either a variation of a sternal incision or a minithoracotomy, and used direct vision with longer instruments. Simultaneous advances in cardiopulmonary perfusion, intracardiac visualization, instrumentation, and robotic telemanipulation hastened a technologic shift, with more surgeons adopting minimally invasive valve surgery in their practice. Less surgical trauma, blood loss, transfusions, and pain, translating into shorter hospital stays, faster return to normal activities, less use of rehabilitation resources, and overall healthcare savings, has driven further development in this field. Today, replacing and repairing cardiac valves through small incisions have become standard practices for many surgeons as patients become more aware of its increasing availability. Changes in surgical indications, largely because of a better understanding of the natural history of organic mitral regurgitation and improved repair techniques, have increased the number of less symptomatic patients with degenerative disease being referred for an elective repair.[7,8] For MIMVS to become widely accepted, equivalent, if not better, short- and long-term outcomes have to be demonstrated compared with sternotomy operations.

EVOLUTION OF MINIMALLY INVASIVE MITRAL VALVE SURGERY

To perform the ideal cardiac valve operation (Table 44-1) surgeons need to operate in restricted spaces through tiny incisions, which necessitate assisted vision and advanced instrumentation. Although the ultimate goal of a completely endoscopic mitral valve repair has not been widely achieved, MIMVS has continued to evolve, with many surgeons performing procedures along the minimally invasive continuum, utilizing a variety of techniques including either limited incisions, video-assistance, video-directed operations, or robotic techniques. Heretofore, completely endoscopic mitral valve repair was difficult but telemanipulators now offer ideal endoscopic techniques to mitral valve surgeons and their patients. However, the steep learning curve still can be an impediment to more widespread adoption. Video-assisted and direct vision techniques have placed MIMVS within the reach of most cardiac surgeons.

TABLE 44-1 The Ideal Cardiac Valve Operation

Single small endoscopic port
Central antegrade perfusion
Tactile feedback
Clear visualization
Facile, secure valve attachment
Wide Intracardiac access
No instrument conflicts
Minimal requirements for
Cardiopulmonary perfusion
Blood product usage
Ventilation and ICU care
Extended hospitalization
Same or better quality as open procedures
Valve repairs in greater than 80%
Few reoperations (<2%)
Low mortality (<1.5%)
Computerized surgical pathway memory
Instrument navigation systems

Minimally invasive cardiac surgery has not enjoyed a standardized nomenclature. The terms *minimally invasive* or *limited access* cardiac surgery have suggested reduced size of the incision, the avoidance of a sternotomy, the use of a partial sternotomy or mini-thoracotomy, or lack of need for cardiopulmonary bypass. The development of less invasive heart surgery may be considered analogous to the ascent of Mount Everest. Embarking from a conventional median sternotomy-based operation or "base camp," surgeons advance progressively toward less invasiveness through experience and methodological acclimatization. Nomenclature paralleling this "mountaineering" analogy is shown in Table 44-2. In this schema entry levels of technical complexity are mastered before advancing past small-incision, direct-vision approaches (Level 1), toward more complex video-assisted procedures (Level 2 or 3), and finally to completely endoscopic robotic valve operations (Level 4). With the constant evolution of new technology and surgical expertise, many established surgeons have already attained "comfort zones" along this trek. Advancements in robotic surgery have allowed more and more surgeons to flatten this curve, favoring robotic mitral repairs.

TABLE 44-2 Levels of Ascent in Minimally Invasive Cardiac Surgery

Level 1
Direct vision: Limited (10- to 12-cm) incisions
Level 2
Direct vision/video assisted: Mini (4- to 6-cm) incisions
Level 3
Video-directed and robot-assisted: Micro (1.2- to 4-cm) incisions
Level 4
Robotic (computer telemanipulation): Port (<1.2cm) incisions

Level 1: Direct Vision

The first steps toward MIMVS were to establish the safety and efficacy of less invasive cardiac operations. Early minimally invasive valve operations were based solely on modifications of previous incisions, and nearly all operations were done under direct vision. In 1996 the first truly minimally invasive aortic valve operations were reported.[3,9] At that time surgeons found that minimal access incisions provided adequate exposure of the mitral valve.[10–12] Using either a ministernal or parasternal incision, Arom, Cohn, Cosgrove, and Gundry showed encouraging results with low surgical mortality (1 to 3%) and morbidity.[1,2,13,14] In Cosgrove's first 50 minimally invasive aortic operations, perfusion and cardioplegia times approximated those of conventional operations and his operative mortality was 2%. Over half the patients were discharged by postoperative day 5.[2] In early 1997 Cohn described 41 minimally invasive aortic operations and first defined the economic benefits of these operations.[1]

In early 1996, the Stanford group performed the first MIMVS using intra-aortic balloon occlusion (port-access) and cardioplegia.[11,14–16] Subsequently, surgeons at the University of Leipzig reported 24 mitral valve repairs done through a minithoracotomy using port-access techniques.[4] This group later reported a high incidence of retrograde aortic dissections and neurologic complications with their initial cases, seemingly related to new catheter technology and limited surgeon experience.[17] By early 1997 Colvin and Galloway had performed 27 direct-vision, port-access mitral repairs or replacements with a single death. None of their patients experienced an aortic dissection, and 63% of patients had mitral valve repairs with no reoperations for leakage.[18] By December 1998, Cosgrove had performed 250 minimally invasive mitral valve operations through either a ministernotomy or parasternal incision with no mortality.[3] The successes of these early MIMVS procedures became the springboard to the current direct-vision techniques described herein.

Level 2: Direct Vision/Video Assisted

Radical endoscopic surgical techniques of the 1980s became routine general, urologic, orthopedic, and gynecologic operations in the 1990s. This advancement was related primarily to successes with extirpative or ablative endoscopic operations. In contrast, fine vascular anastomotic and complex reparative procedures are the centerpieces of cardiac surgery. Limited video technology and instrumentation with only four degrees of freedom hindered the fine dexterity required for these operations, and cardiac surgeons were reluctant to explore the benefits of operative video assistance.

In early 1996, Carpentier performed the first video-assisted mitral valve repair through a minithoracotomy using hypothermic ventricular fibrillation.[19] Shortly thereafter, we reported the first video-assisted mitral valve replacement, completed through a mini-thoracotomy, using a percutaneous transthoracic aortic clamp and antegrade cardioplegia.[20,21] This clamping and visualization technique was simple, cost-effective, and has remained the mainstay of isolated mitral valve operations at several centers.[17,22] In 1997, Mohr reported 51 minimally invasive mitral valve operations, performed with port-access cardioplegia techniques, a 4-cm incision, and for the first time three-dimensional (3D) videoscopy.[23] In this series 3D assistance aided mitral replacement; however, these surgeons found that even simple reconstructions were significantly more difficult than those done through a sternotomy. At about the same time Loulmet and Carpentier deployed an intracardiac "mini-camera" for lighting and subvalvular visualization; however, they also concluded that two-dimensional (2D) visualization was inadequate for detailed repairs.[24] Concurrently, our group reported 31 successful mitral valve operations done using 2D video-assistance.[25] Complex repairs were possible, and these included quadrangular resections, sliding valvuloplasties, chordal transfers, and synthetic chordal replacements. Our initial results were encouraging.

Level 3: Video-Directed

In 1997, Mohr first used the Aesop 3000 voice-activated camera robot (Intuitive Surgical, Inc., Mountainview, CA) in minimally invasive videoscopic mitral valve surgery.[23] Six months later we began using the Aesop 3000 routinely to perform both video-assisted and video-directed minimally invasive mitral valve repairs.[26] We continued to use this device during most isolated mitral valve operations, including reoperations. This device provided surgeons camera-site voice activation, precluding translation errors inherent with verbal transmission to an assistant. Camera motion was shown to be much smoother, more predictable, and requiring less lens cleaning than during manual direction. At one point along our progression, we completed over 90% of mitral repairs under video direction with the Aesop 3000. This device, however, is no longer in production and other camera scope holders have been found to be equally effective. Mohr first termed this method "solo mitral surgery" and reported 8 patients undergoing successful mitral repairs using this semirobotic technique.[23] Vanermen perfected his method to perform repairs completely endoscopically with excellent results. In nearly 1000 mitral valve operations, he and his colleagues have shown that after a significant learning curve totally video-directed repairs could be done with excellent results using long-shafted instruments.[27,28]

Level 4: Robotic (Computer Telemanipulation)

In June 1998, Carpentier and Mohr completed the first true robotic mitral valve operations using the da Vinci surgical system.[29,30] In May 2000, the East Carolina University group performed the first da Vinci mitral valve repair in the United States.[31] This computer-driven system provides both tele- and micromanipulation of tissues in small spaces. The surgeon operates from a console through end-effecter, microwrist instruments, which are mounted on robotic arms that are inserted through the chest wall (Fig. 44-1). These devices emulate human X-Y-Z axis' wrist motion throughout seven degrees of manipulative excursion. Movement occurs through two joints that together control pitch, yaw, and rotation. Additionally, arm insertion and rotation, as well as variable grip strength, give additional freedom to the operating "wrist."[30,32] Grossi and associates performed a partial mitral valve repair but had limited ergonomic freedom using the Zeus system.[33] Lange and associates in Munich were the first to perform a totally robotic mitral valve repair using only 1-cm ports and the da Vinci device.[34] To date, Chitwood, Murphy, and Smith have the largest experiences with robotic mitral valve repairs, and have independently shown da Vinci to be very effective, even for performing complex bileaflet repairs.[32,35] Together, they have successfully completed well over 1000 mitral valve repairs and now routinely perform these procedures using only ports and a 2- to 4-cm mini-incision. Still further technological development will eventually lead to better improved learning curves. To this end, we are on the cusp of developing a closed-chest operation that can be done by many surgeons.

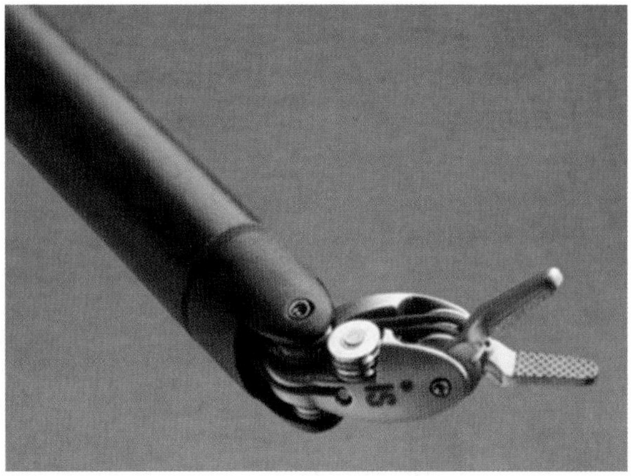

FIGURE 44-1 The da Vinci MicroWrist needle-holder instrument. This instrument is inserted into the robotic arm and controlled from the surgeon's console.

INCISIONS

The type and size of the musculoskeletal incision remains central to discussions around minimally invasive cardiac surgery. A myriad of modified small sternal, para-sternal, and minithoracotomy incisions are used to access the cardiac valves. In the largest patient series modified sternal incisions have been used.[36–38] Although many surgeons prefer the hemisternotomy approach, a right minithoracotomy yields excellent exposure for both direct-vision and videoscopic mitral valve access (Fig. 44-2A and B). To access the left atrium for direct vision, using a limited access mini-thoracotomy, a 4- to 6-cm submammary incision is placed along the anterior axillary line. The small sections of the pectoralis and intercostal muscles fibers are divided, and the thorax is entered through the fourth intercostal space with minimal rib distraction and no rib cutting. The New York University group has been quite successful in combining this incision with port-access methods and direct vision for both mitral and tricuspid repairs/replacements.[39,40] A smaller 3- to 5-cm incision with

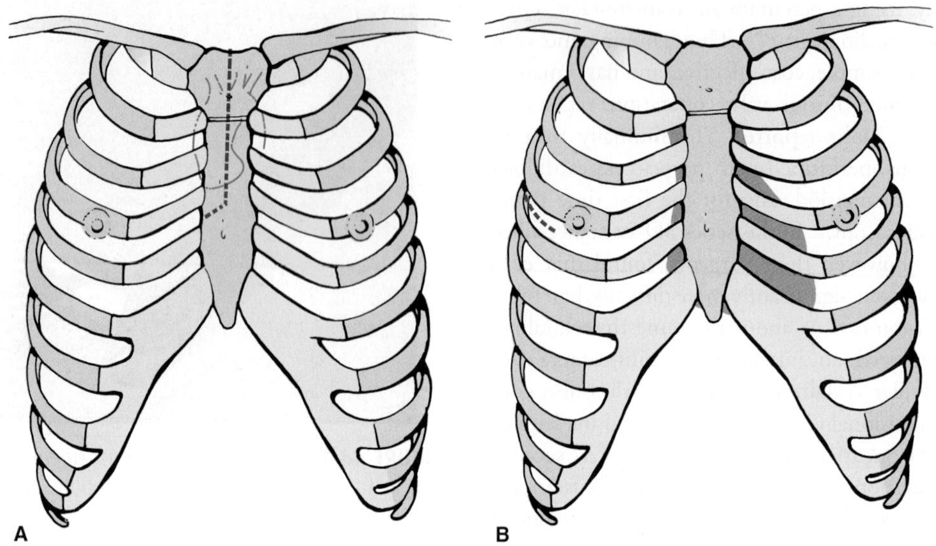

FIGURE 44-2 (A) The hemisternotomy, used for minimally invasive mitral and aortic valve surgery. (B) The minithoracotomy, used for minimally invasive mitral valve surgery.

minimal rib retraction can be used in video-assisted cases and is large enough for prosthesis passage (Fig. 44-3). Vanermen and Mohr perform video-assisted mitral operations routinely through 4-cm, nonretracted thoracic incisions with excellent results.[41–43] Minimal rib spreading to prevent intercostal nerve injury and use of intraoperative local anesthetics are the keys to minimize postoperative discomfort. We generally use a soft tissue retractor to enhance visualization without the need for rib spreading. Tricuspid operations can be performed through this incision when combined with bicaval cannulation and drainage isolation. Murphy and colleagues prefer a more lateral approach for access in robotic mitral valve surgery.[44]

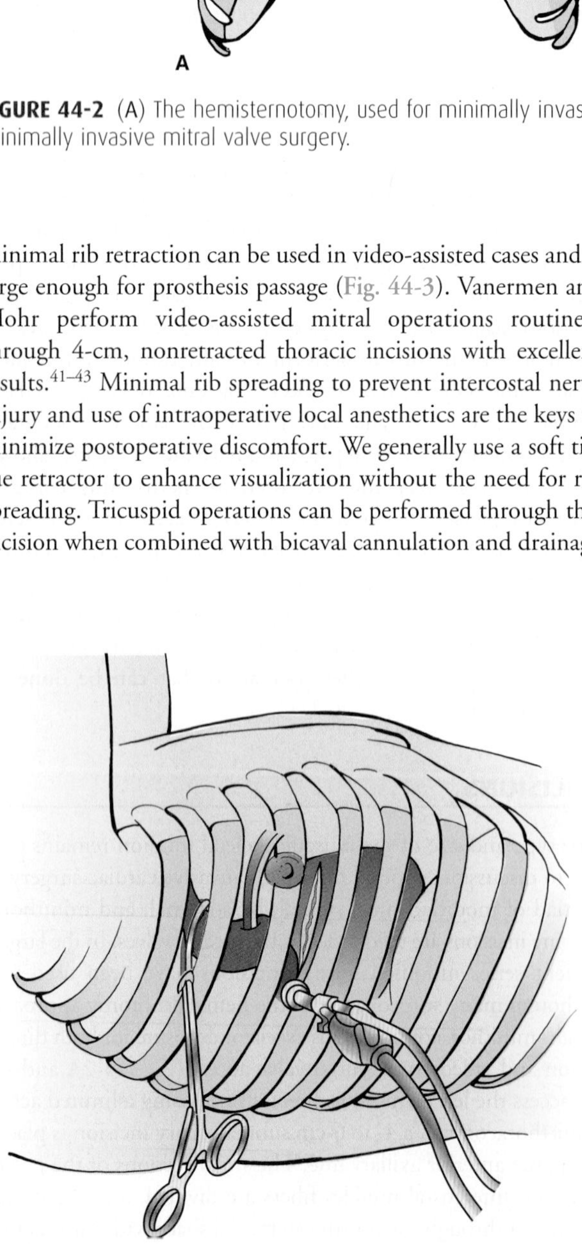

FIGURE 44-3 Right minithoracotomy and video access. The right minithoracotomy allows aortic access for the transthoracic clamp shown here as well as the video camera. With this arrangement minimal rib spreading is needed to perform mitral surgery.

We consider the term *minimally invasive* to include the size of the actual cardiac incision. Most superior and transseptal mitral valve approaches, through a hemisternotomy, require a larger cardiac incision. For aortic, mitral, and tricuspid valve operations, surgeons at the Cleveland Clinic use a hemisternotomy, extended to the fourth interspace, with direct aortic arch and right atrial cannulation.[3,9] To access the mitral valve, they extend the atriotomy from the right atrium, across the left atrial roof, and continuing caudally to divide the interatrial septum (Fig. 44-4A and B). This incision provides excellent exposure for aortic, mitral, and tricuspid valve replacements as well as repairs. Although the septal artery is divided, the incidence of atrial arrhythmias seems to parallel traditional interatrial groove atriotomies. For mitral and aortic surgery, Gundry suggested a similar hemisternotomy with single right atrial cannulation. This incision provides similar exposure to that described by opening the atrial roof, between the superior vena cava and aorta, without entering the right atrium.[14] Cohn now prefers a lower hemisternotomy for mitral surgery and uses a transseptal approach for valve exposure.[45] Loulmet and Carpentier reported using a midsternal, C-shaped, partial sternotomy for exposing mitral valves through the interatrial septum.[24] All of these incisions provide generous direct-vision exposure, if combined with pericardial retraction.

PERFUSION AND MYOCARDIAL PROTECTION

Cannulation for cardiopulmonary perfusion can be accomplished through a number of approaches for MIMVS. By combining modified traditional perfusion methods and new technology, surgeons have been able to speed the development of less invasive mitral operations. Thin-walled arterial and venous cannulas, transthoracic aortic cannulas, endoaortic balloon

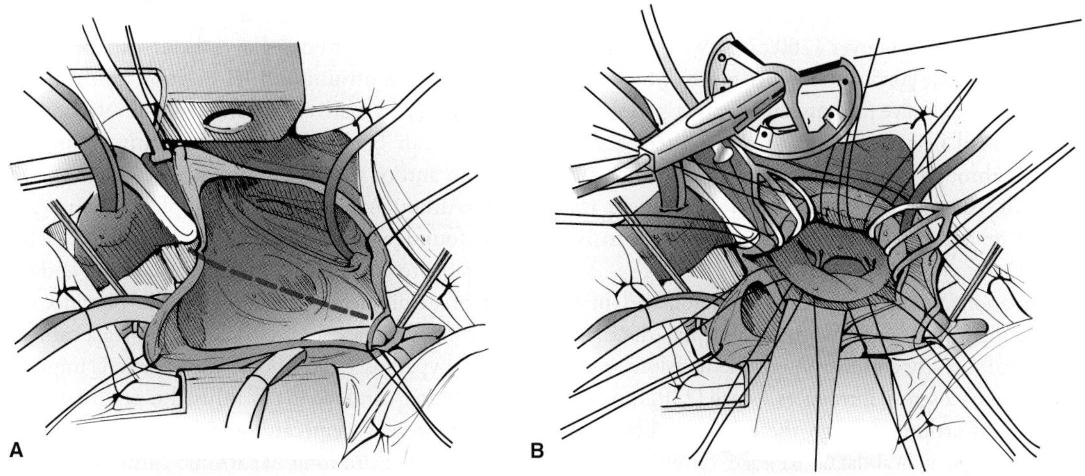

FIGURE 44-4 (A) Hemisternotomy with an extended atrial incision. Popularized by Dr. Cosgrove, the incision begins along the ventral right atrium and extends over the dome of the left atrium and through the left atrial wall and interatrial septum. (B) Mitral valve exposure is excellent through this hemisternotomy with an extended atrial incision, and complex repairs are similar in difficulty to full sternotomy operations. (*Courtesy of Dr. D.M. Cosgrove.*)

occluders, modified aortic clamping devices, longer direct aortic antegrade cardioplegia catheters, percutaneous retrograde coronary sinus cardioplegia catheters, and assisted venous drainage all have assisted the evolution of these operations.

We prefer to establish arterial access via femoral cannulation, employing a small wire-wound Bio-Medicus (Medtronic, Inc., Minneapolis, MN) arterial cannula (17 to 21F) inserted over a guidewire (Fig. 44-5). Exposure of the femoral artery is through a 1.5-cm transverse incision placed in the right groin crease. We ask our referring cardiologists to perform cardiac catheterizations via the left groin to avoid hematoma and scar formation. However, if the right groin vessels were used at catheterization, we still use the right femoral vessels for cannulation, because the trajectory is better when introducing the cannula into the femoral-iliac venous system. Minimal dissection of the femoral vessels is performed without encircling the vessels. Less dissection has reduced seroma formation, which is now rare. For both venous and arterial cannulation, we believe that transesophageal echocardiographic guidance is mandatory to ensure proper guidewire insertion before passing dilators and the cannulae.

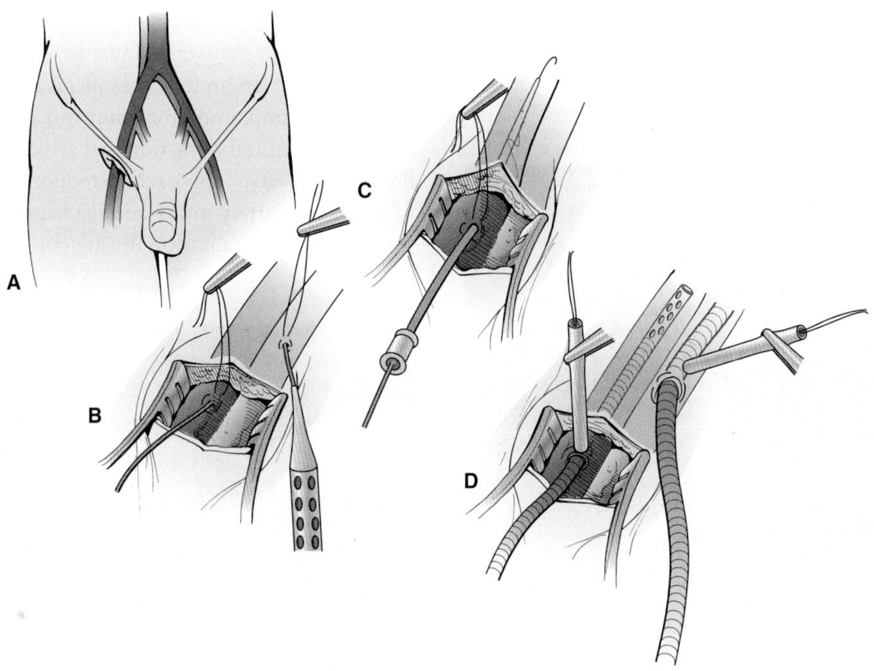

FIGURE 44-5 Thin-walled (A) arterial perfusion cannula from Bio-Medicus (Medtronic Inc., Minneapolis, MN) and (B) percutaneous Carpentier dual-stage venous drainage cannula (Medtronic Inc., Minneapolis, MN). (C, D) These cannulas are inserted from the femoral approach using the Seldinger guidewire method.

Using this method excellent flow rates have been attained with acceptable perfusion pressures in over 1200 cases. We have experienced only two retrograde aortic dissections, one of which was in a reoperative case. Mitral valve patients having either peripheral atherosclerosis or small iliac vessels may require direct aortic cannulation either through the incision or via a transthoracic Seldinger approach. Alternatively, cannulation of the right (as in aortic surgery) or left axillary artery also has proved to be very effective.[46]

Venous cannulation and drainage can be established in a variety of ways. At the Brigham and Women's Hospital, the right atrium is cannulated directly either through the incision or via a separate skin incision. Cosgrove introduces a small (23F) cannula directly into the right atrium through the mini-sternotomy.[40] Gundry and Konertz insert an oval-flat or "pancake" cannula directly into the right atrium to maximize hemisternotomy exposure.[9,14] Assisted venous drainage has been a major advancement by enhancing the efficiency of smaller cannulas. At our institution we use the Bio-Medicus centrifugal vortex pump to create variable negative pressures for venous drainage. Similarly, by combining wall suction (<40-cm H_2O pressure) and a closed-bag or hard-shell cardiotomy reservoir, a safe, simple, and economical assisted venous drainage system can be developed. For superior caval drainage a 15 to 17F Biomedicus cannula is placed by the anesthesia team via the right internal jugular vein using the Seldinger technique, positioning the tip at the pericardial-caval junction (Fig. 44-6). In addition, a 22 or 25F Cardiovations (Johnson & Johnson, Inc., Sommerville, NJ) or a 21 or 23F Biomedicus cannula is inserted via the right femoral vein and advanced over a guidewire into the right atrium. Again, it is important to use transesophageal echocardiographic guidance for proper cannula placement and safety.

Myocardial preservation techniques used with MIMVS are similar to those used in sternotomy-based operations. We cool systemically to 28°C, because the ambient cardiac temperature generally is warmer than during conventional valve operations.

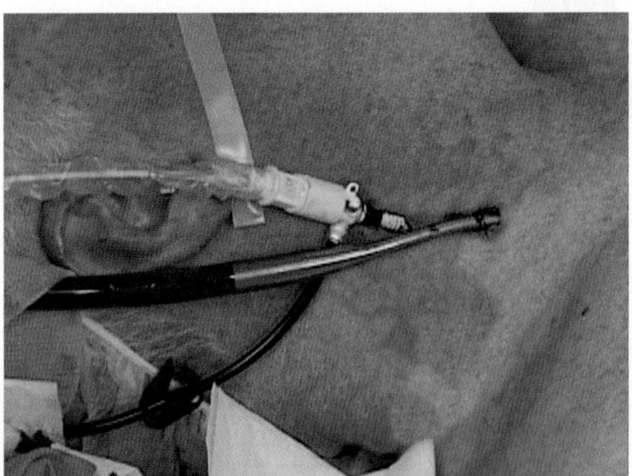

FIGURE 44-6 A right internal jugular venous catheter (15 or 17F) is combined with femoro-atrial active venous drainage for full bicaval access. This is important during atrial retraction in a near closed chest where the cavae can be kinked with distraction.

With either a ministernotomy or minithoracotomy, a retrograde coronary sinus cardioplegia catheter can be inserted directly into the right atrium and its position confirmed by echocardiography. Alternatively, a percutaneous retrograde cardioplegia catheter can be introduced preoperatively using echocardiographic and/or fluoroscopic guidance via the internal jugular vein. Although retrograde cardioplegia seems preferable, we have found antegrade cold blood cardioplegia efficient and preferable to ensure uniform cardiac cooling and even distribution of cardioplegia solutions. In the presence of significant aortic insufficiency, a retrograde cardioplegia catheter is inserted before bypass is established. After aortic clamping, cold antegrade blood cardioplegia is infused every 15 minutes into the aortic root via a vent/cardioplegia cannula passed through the incision. An extra long Medtronic cardioplegia catheter facilitates its positioning in the aortic root. During both videoscopic and robotic mitral surgery, we place a flexible sucker via the left atriotomy directly into the left superior pulmonary vein to clear residual blood from the surgical field.

For partial sternotomy based mitral valve surgery, aortic occlusion can be achieved using a standard cross-clamp applied through the incision. Cosgrove developed a flexible-handle aortic clamp to increase exposure through the hemisternotomy while minimizing inadvertent dislodgment (Fig. 44-7). For minithoracotomy mitral operations we use a percutaneous transthoracic aortic cross-clamp (Scanlan International, Minneapolis, MN), which is inserted through a 4-mm incision placed in the lateral right third intercostal space toward the axilla. The posterior immobile "tine" of the clamp is positioned through the transverse sinus dorsal to the aorta (see Figs. 44-3, and 44-8A and B).[47] During placement, attention is necessary to prevent injury to the left atrial appendage and right pulmonary artery behind the aorta. This clamp has provided very secure occlusion without any aortic injuries. Occasionally we will apply this clamp in the "verso" direction with the mobile tine posterior to the aorta in the transverse sinus. In a short aorta this approach provides more length for cardioplegia needle insertion, and also arches the clamp away from the atriocaval junction, improving atrial septal ventral retraction and avoiding left robotic arm collisions. The "verso" approach introduces a somewhat greater risk of pulmonary artery injury and inadequate aortic occlusion, and thus excellent visualization during deployment is essential.

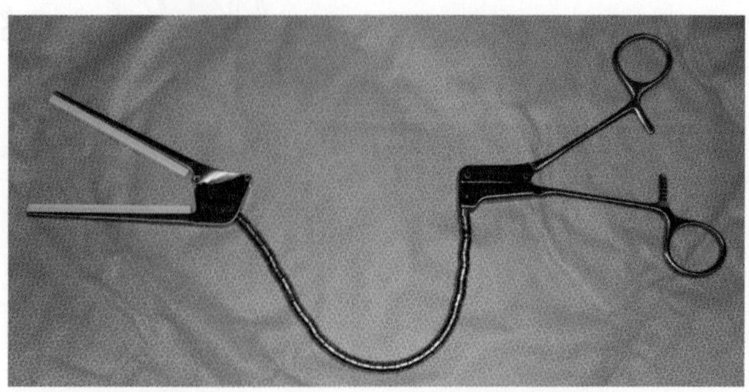

FIGURE 44-7 Flexible arm Cosgrove Aortic Clamp (V Muller Inc.). This mobile arm clamp allows complete aortic occlusion through limited access incisions, such as the ministernotomy. We have also used it for transthoracic aortic occlusion in mitral valve surgery.

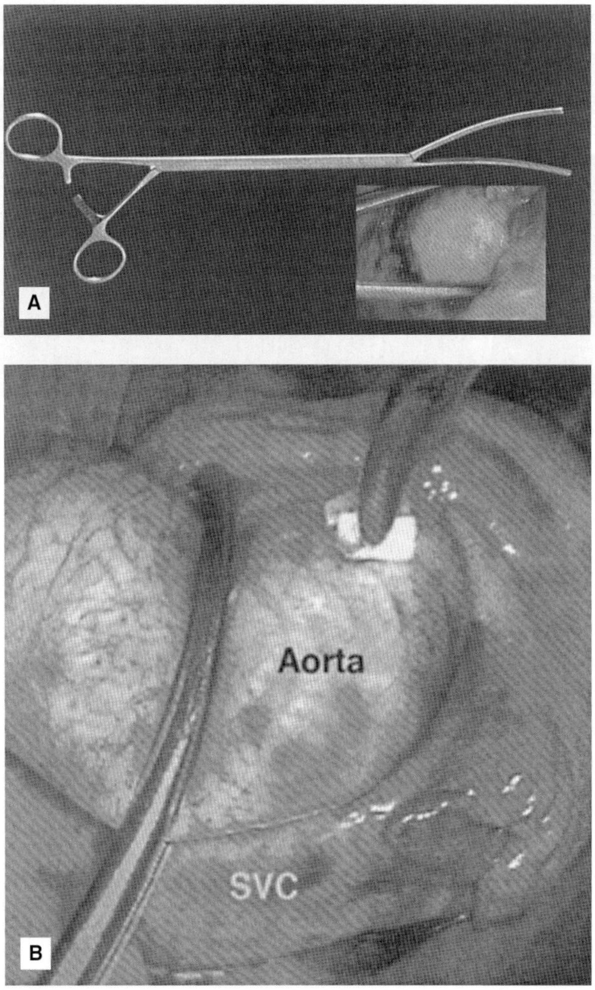

FIGURE 44-8 (A) The Chitwood transthoracic aortic cross-clamp (Scanlan International Inc., Minneapolis, MN). The shaft is 4 mm in diameter and is passed through the third intercostal space (*inset*). The posterior or fixed prong of the clamp is passed through the transverse sinus under direct or video visualization to avoid injury to the right pulmonary artery, left atrial appendage, or left main coronary artery. The mobile prong is passed ventral to the aorta as far as the main pulmonary artery. (B) A videoscopic view of the deployed transthoracic aortic clamp. The aorta is fully compressed and an antegrade cardioplegia needle is shown in position just distal to the right coronary artery origin.

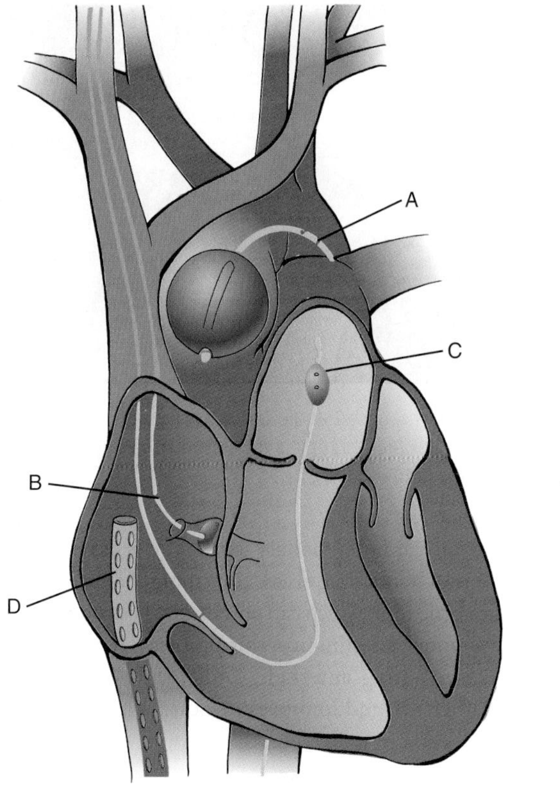

FIGURE 44-9 Port-access system with transfemoral artery endoaortic balloon occluder (*A*), percutaneous internal jugular retrograde coronary sinus cardioplegia catheter (*B*), pulmonary artery vent (*C*), and femoral venous drainage catheter (*D*). (*Courtesy Cardiovations, Ethicon, Inc., Norwalk, CN.*)

Vanermen, Murphy, Colvin, and Hargrove continue to be strong advocates for intra-aortic balloon occlusion for minimally invasive and robotic mitral surgery.[27,28,44,48] Most commonly these devices are introduced retrograde through the femoral artery. The occlusive balloon should be positioned, under echocardiographic control, just above the sinotubular junction in the ascending aorta (Fig. 44-9).[4,49] Balloon pressures often reach 400 torr during complete occlusion. Antegrade cardioplegia is delivered via the central lumen of the catheter. Balloon dislodgment can cause innominate artery occlusion, potentially causing neurologic injury, or prolapse into the left ventricle with inferior myocardial preservation. Thus, continuous echocardiographic monitoring and the comparison of right and left radial artery pressures are essential to detect balloon migration. Balloon occlusion may be advantageous compared with the transthoracic clamp method when there is limited access to the aorta. Aortic dissection is a feared complication of using the endoballoon, but experience with the technique dramatically reduces the risk of this adverse event. Regardless, Reichenspurner and colleagues demonstrated increased morbidity, cost, and operative/cross-clamp times when the endoballoon technique was used for mitral valve surgery.[22]

Meticulous intracardiac air removal is most important in these operations, because difficulty exists in manipulating and deairing the left ventricular apex. Also, in the right anterolateral minithoracotomy, air tends to be retained along the more dorsal ventricular septum and in the right pulmonary veins. Continuous carbon dioxide (CO_2) insufflation has been helpful in minimizing intracardiac air and should begin before opening any cardiac chamber. CO_2 displaces air efficiently and is much more soluble than air in blood. We continuously infuse CO_2 (4 to 5 L/min) into the thorax via a 14-gauge angiocatheter throughout the case. Before releasing the cross-clamp, both lungs are ventilated vigorously to deair the pulmonary veins. After atriotomy closure and following cross-clamp release, suction is applied to the aortic root vent, and the right coronary artery origin is compressed during early ejection. As the heart beats, nonatherosclerotic aortas can be partially reclamped to expel residual air into the vent suction. Constant transesophageal echocardiographic monitoring is essential to ensure adequate air removal before

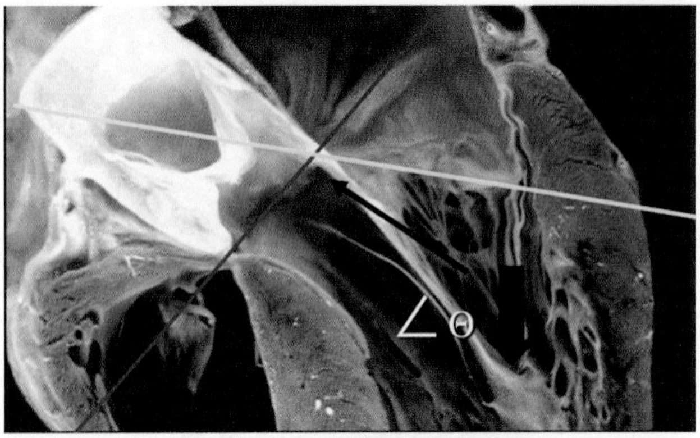

FIGURE 44-10 A reduced angle between the mitral valve and the aortic annular plane predicts increased risk of systolic motion of the anterior mitral leaflet.

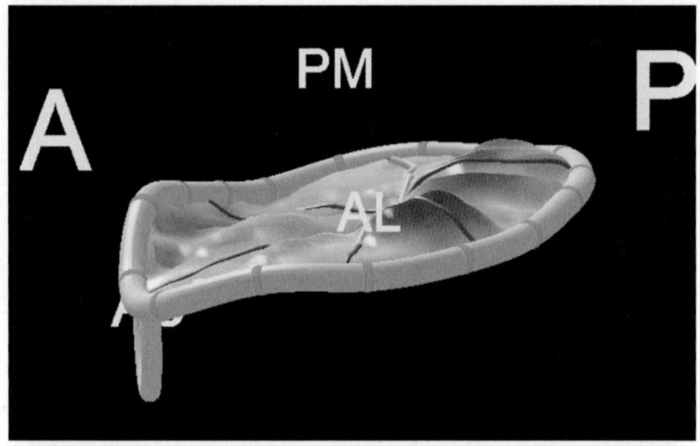

FIGURE 44-11 A topographic map is constructed using intraoperative three dimensional TEE. Each valve segment is measured and the C-septal distance (distance between the septum at the hinge point of the aortic valve cusp and the coaptation point of the mitral valve leaflets) and thickness of interventricular septum are measured.

weaning from cardiopulmonary bypass. We have found that during ventral retraction fixed transthoracic atrial retractors distort the aortic root, which can entrain air. The robotic retractor can be positioned to minimize this problem. Moreover, reducing retraction during antegrade cardioplegia delivery reduces aortic insufficiency and improves myocardial protection.

Preoperative Mitral Valve Repair Plan

Successful mitral valve repair begins with a comprehensive assessment and understanding of the mitral valve pathology by the surgeon in conjunction with the cardiologists and/or anesthesiologists. High quality intraoperative 3D transesophageal echocardiography (TEE) has become a critical aspect of planning mitral valve repair and is more accurate than 2D TEE in mapping mitral valve prolapse[50]; we now rely almost exclusively on TEE imaging to plan the repair. Each valve segment is measured using TEE. We pay particular attention to the angle between the mitral valve and the aortic annular plane (Fig. 44-10), the C-septal distance (distance between the septum at the hinge point of the aortic valve cusp and the coaptation point of the mitral valve leaflets), and the thickness of the interventricular septum, to minimize the potential for systolic anterior motion (SAM) of the anterior leaflet. We rely solely on measurements acquired by TEE to construct a topographic model, size the annuloplasty band, and plan the operation (Fig. 44-11). A saline test is performed intraoperatively to confirm the echocardiographic findings, but occasionally we still measure the valve segments directly (Fig. 44-12).

Mitral Valve Exposure

Using a hemisternotomy, exposure of the mitral valve is best accomplished through either an extended right to left atrial incision

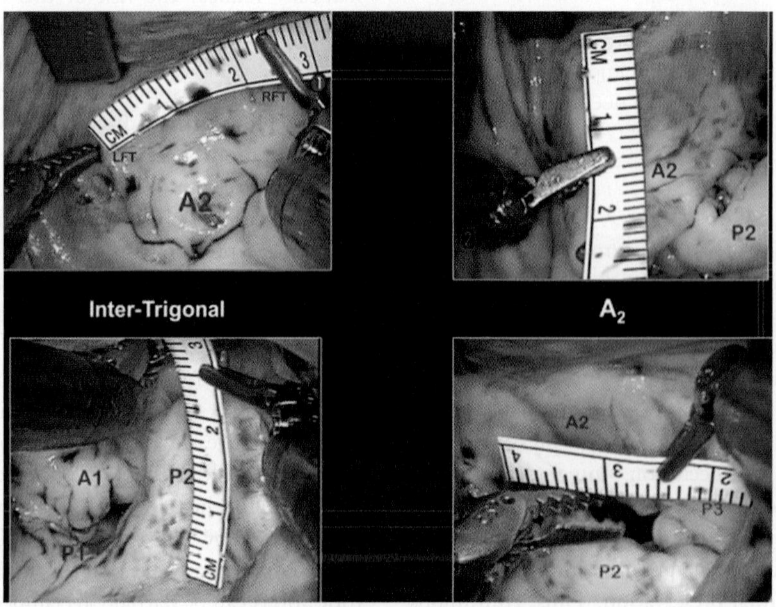

FIGURE 44-12 A saline test is performed intraoperatively to confirm the echocardiographic findings, but occasionally, we still measure the valve segments directly.

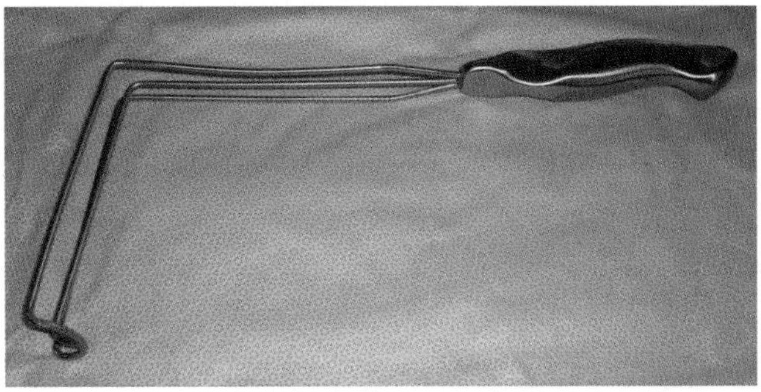

FIGURE 44-13 Chitwood hand-held left atrial retractor.

or the transseptal approach championed by Cosgrove and Cohn, respectively (see Figs. 44-2A and 44-4A and B). A hand-held retractor placed through the incision facilitates valvular exposure using these incisions. For endoscopic and robotic mitral repairs most of us have favored a fixed-blade transthoracic retractor immobilized by a table-mounted clamp. Blades of various sizes are available; however, after fixed-retractor deployment, movement to provide additional exposure becomes limited. For reoperative mitral surgery through a minithoracotomy, we prefer to use the hand-held retractor shown in Fig. 44-13. It allows variable access to all parts of the left atrium and subvalvular structures; moreover, it can provide access in very deep chests. The second and subsequent generations of the da Vinci system includes a fourth robotic arm that can be used to dynamically manipulate a left atrial retractor (Fig. 44-14) that is activated alternately through the left instrument arm control. This retractor provides variable exposure of the mitral valve by altering blade positions, length, rotation, and flexion. The retractor arm is inserted via a third interspace port in men and a fourth interspace port in women, medial to the anterior thoracotomy in both cases.

Robotic Mitral Valve Surgery

For both video-assisted and robotic mitral surgery we position the patient as shown in Fig. 44-15 with the right arm at the side

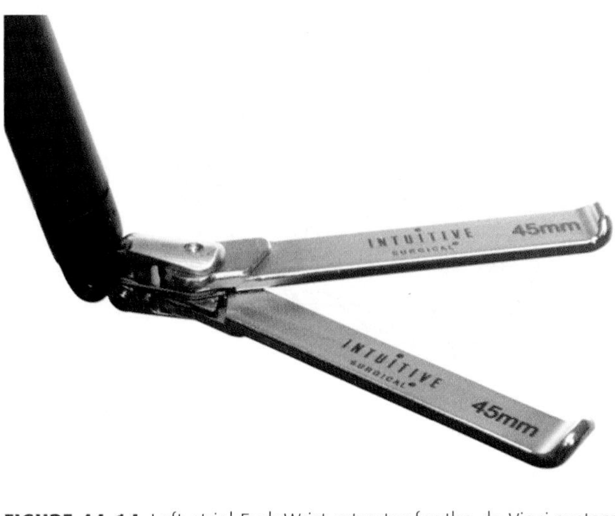

FIGURE 44-14 Left atrial EndoWrist retractor for the da Vinci system.

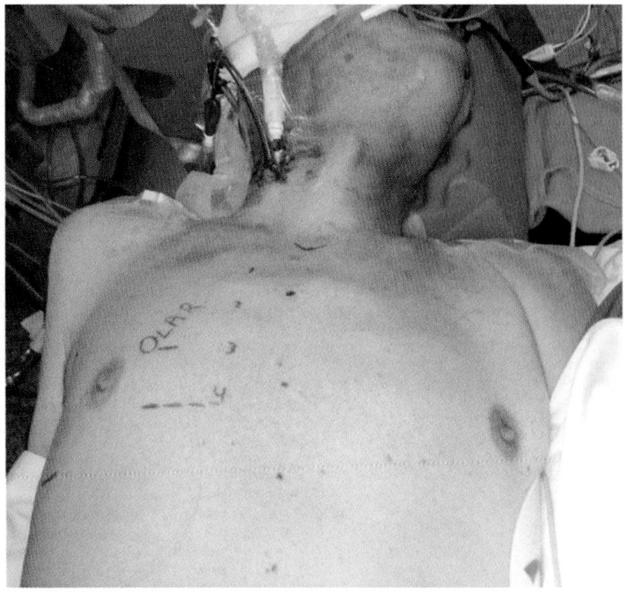

FIGURE 44-15 The patient is positioned in the semi–left lateral decubitus position. In most patients the arm is best left on the side, obviating the need for an arm rest, which allows more room for positioning the da Vinci robotic arms. The sternum and intercostal spaces are marked.

facilitating application of the cross-clamp through the midaxilla. A simple Olympus endoscope holder attached to the operating table now is used for our minimally invasive video-assisted approach. Using video-assistance, surgeons operate with long instruments in a 2D operative field (Fig. 44-16). Knots are tied and sutures cut using specialized hand-held long-shafted instruments (Figs. 44-17A and B and 44-18).

The da Vinci surgical system is comprised of three components: a surgeon console, an instrument cart, and a visioning platform (Fig. 44-19A and B).[51] This system provides intracardiac telepresence and facile tissue micromanipulation. The operative console is removed physically from the patient and allows the surgeon to sit comfortably, resting the arms ergonomically with his or her head positioned in a 3D vision array. The da Vinci Si Surgical System released in April 2009 provides dual-console capability, extending the potential for either two surgeons to work together, or to enhance training with a "student-driver" model. Instruments are positioned through 8-mm ports around the operative sites in the thorax, and the camera is passed either through the working port used for suture and prosthesis passage (Fig. 44-20A) or a separate port incision. The surgeon's finger and wrist movements are registered by sensors in the masters, transformed by a computer and then transferred to the instrument cart, which operates end-effecter instruments. Wristlike instrument articulation emulates precisely the surgeon's actions at the tissue level, and dexterity becomes enhanced through combined tremor suppression and motion scaling. These features allow increased precision and dexterity with the surgeon becoming truly "ambidextrous." A clutching mechanism enables readjustment of hand positions to maintain an optimal ergonomic attitude with respect to the visual field. The clutch acts very much like a computer mouse, which can be

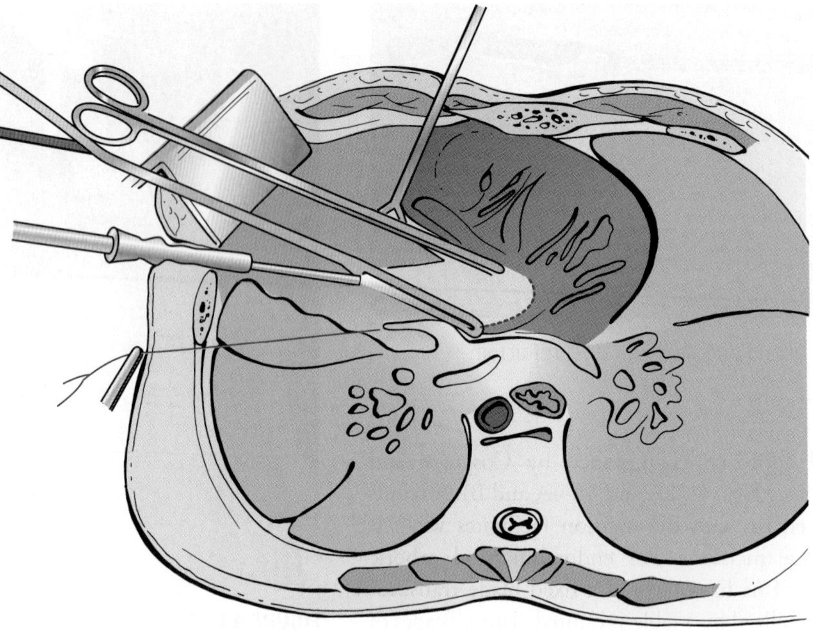

FIGURE 44-16 Mini right thoracotomy approach for mitral surgery. Long instruments are required to operate in a two-dimensional operative field.

reoriented by lifting and repositioning it to reestablish unrestrained freedom of computer activation. The SI system provides the surgeon with depth perception as a 3D image of the surgical field in full high definition (1080i) with up to 10× magnification. The operator becomes ensconced in the 3D operative topography and can perform extremely precise surgical manipulations, devoid of traditional distractions. Both 0-degree and 30-degree endoscopes can be manipulated electronically to look either "up" or "down" within the heart. Access to and visualization of the internal thoracic artery, coronary arteries, and mitral apparatus have been shown to be excellent. Figure 44-20B shows the surgeon's operative field during a da Vinci mitral repair. Perfusion technology is the same as described above for video-assisted operations and a larger mini-thoracotomy.

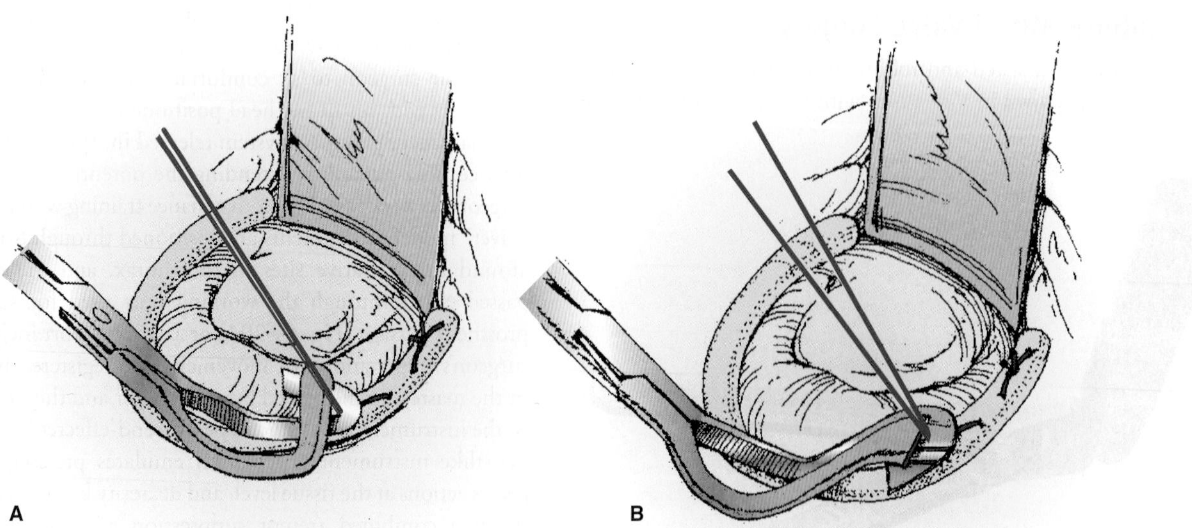

FIGURE 44-17 Knot pusher (A) and cutter (B).

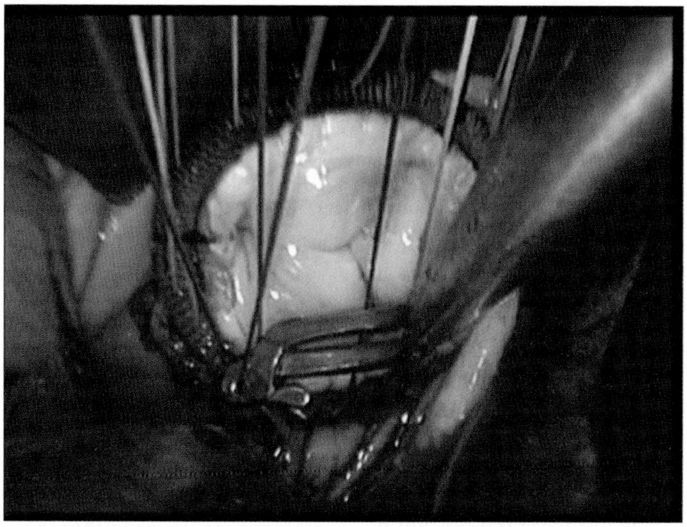

FIGURE 44-18 Knot pusher used to secure knots during annuloplasty band and valve placement.

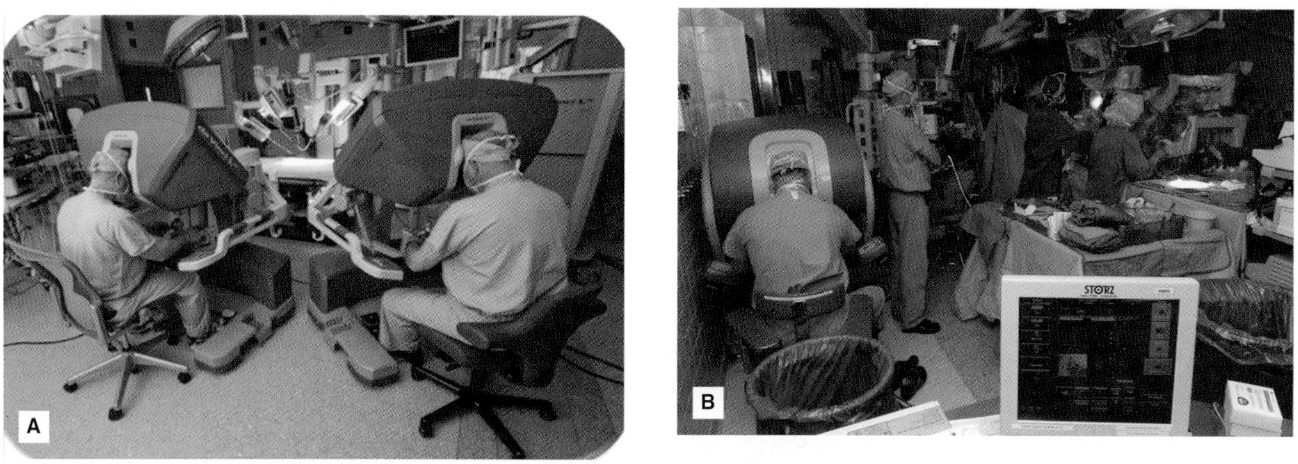

FIGURE 44-19 (A) The da Vinci Robotic Telemanipulation System. The operative console is in the foreground; the instrument cart is at the table. Both the operating surgeon and patient-side assistant are shown. (B) da Vinci robotic mitral valve repair. The surgeon is positioned approximately 10 feet from the patient. The instrument cart is placed on the left side of the tilted patient with arms entering the right thorax.

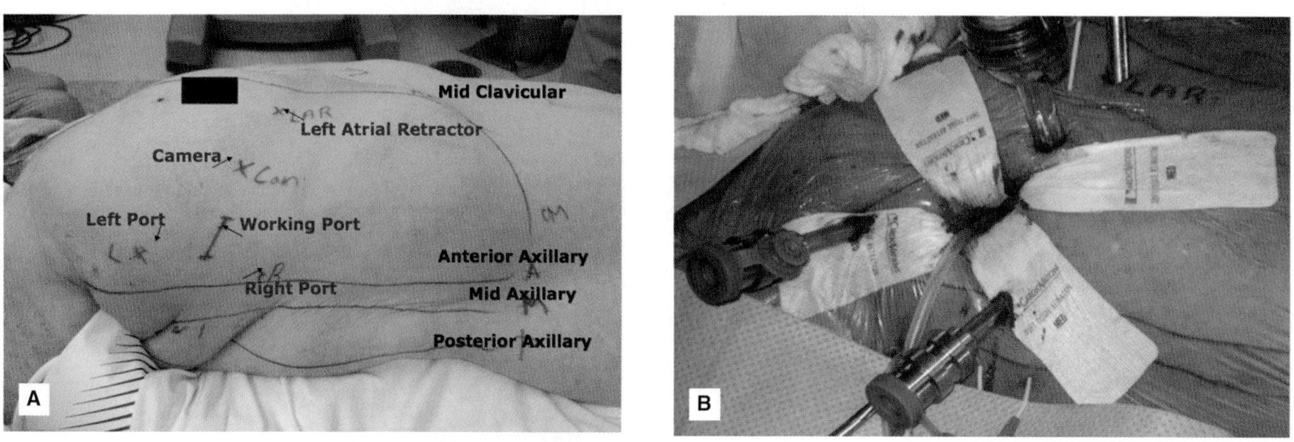

FIGURE 44-20 da Vinci bedside setup for mitral valve surgery. (A and B) A 3- to 4-cm incision is made in the inframammary fold. The chest is entered via the fourth intercostal space. Ports are positioned around the incision for the left and right robot arms, the left atrial retractor and the camera. A cardioplegia line is inserted either through the incision or above the camera port. Carbon dioxide floods the field through an angiocatheter posterior to the right arm port and a flexible sucker placed through the incision returns blood to the bypass machine.

COMPLEX MITRAL VALVE REPAIRS WITH THE DA VINCI SYSTEM

Heretofore, many surgeons avoided repairing valves with large bileaflet defects. However, we have found that repairs of these maladies are particularly amenable to robotic telemanipulation because of high-definition 3D magnified vision and the ability to translocate multiple individual chordae tendineae to new leaflet sites. After the first 50 mitral repairs our group began to repair more complex valves as well as develop and use new adjunctive technology during robotic surgery. Figures 44-21 through 44-28 illustrate the variety of methods we use routinely for both simple and complex repairs. The mainstay of our repair techniques for posterior leaflet prolapse secondary to ruptured or redundant chordae has been a modification of the classic quadrangular resection. As seen in Fig. 44-21, a trapezoidal or triangular resection is made in the central portion of redundant posterior leaflet segment. By conserving the annular distance that must be closed, tension along the posterior annulus is limited, especially when one of the scallops is much larger than the others as is often the case in P2 prolapse, where P1 and P3 may be diminutive. The minor base of the trapezoid is closed with a figure-of-eight braided suture (2-0 Cardioflon [Peters, Inc., Paris, France]). Often we conserve leaflet tissue by decreasing the size of P2. When the leading edges are approximated, chordae are effectively shortened as they assume a new angle with the leaflet insertions which brings the line of coaptation below the annular plane. When there is an isolated anterior leaflet prolapse, chordae can either be transferred from the posterior leaflet (Fig. 44-22A and B) or the redundancy reduced using PTFE neochords (Fig. 44-23A and B). When any posterior leaflet scallop is radially higher than 2 cm or the anterior leaflet is longer than 3 cm, there is increased risk of systolic anterior motion of the anterior leaflet. This is especially true when the aortic outflow is narrowed by a thickened interventricular septum or a relatively acute angle exists (>120 degrees) between the aortic and mitral valve annular planes (see Fig. 44-10). Generally, systolic anterior motion can be avoided by reducing the posterior leaflet height with a sliding-plasty after prolapsing segments are resected (Fig. 44-24A through C).

Traditional repair techniques employing resection become complicated in the presence of a large P2 scallop with multiple ruptured or redundant chords and either significant annular calcification, thin leaflets, or deficient P1 or P3 scallops that are too small to slide successfully. In addition, standard repair techniques usually render the posterior leaflet immobile, leaving the

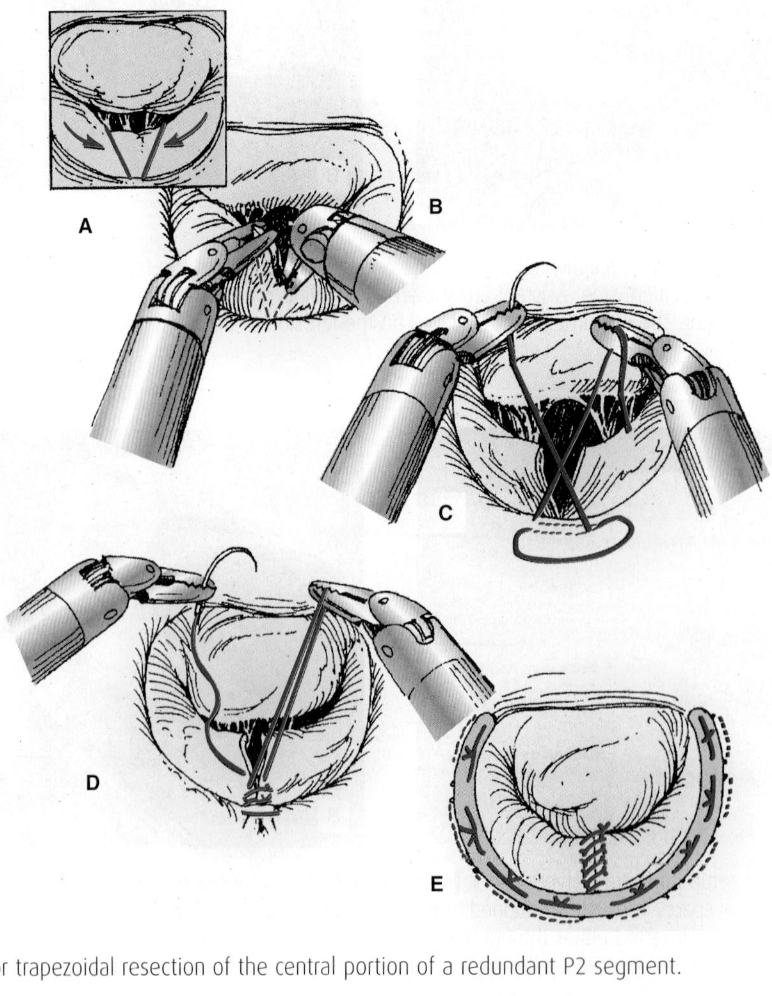

FIGURE 44-21 Triangular or trapezoidal resection of the central portion of a redundant P2 segment.

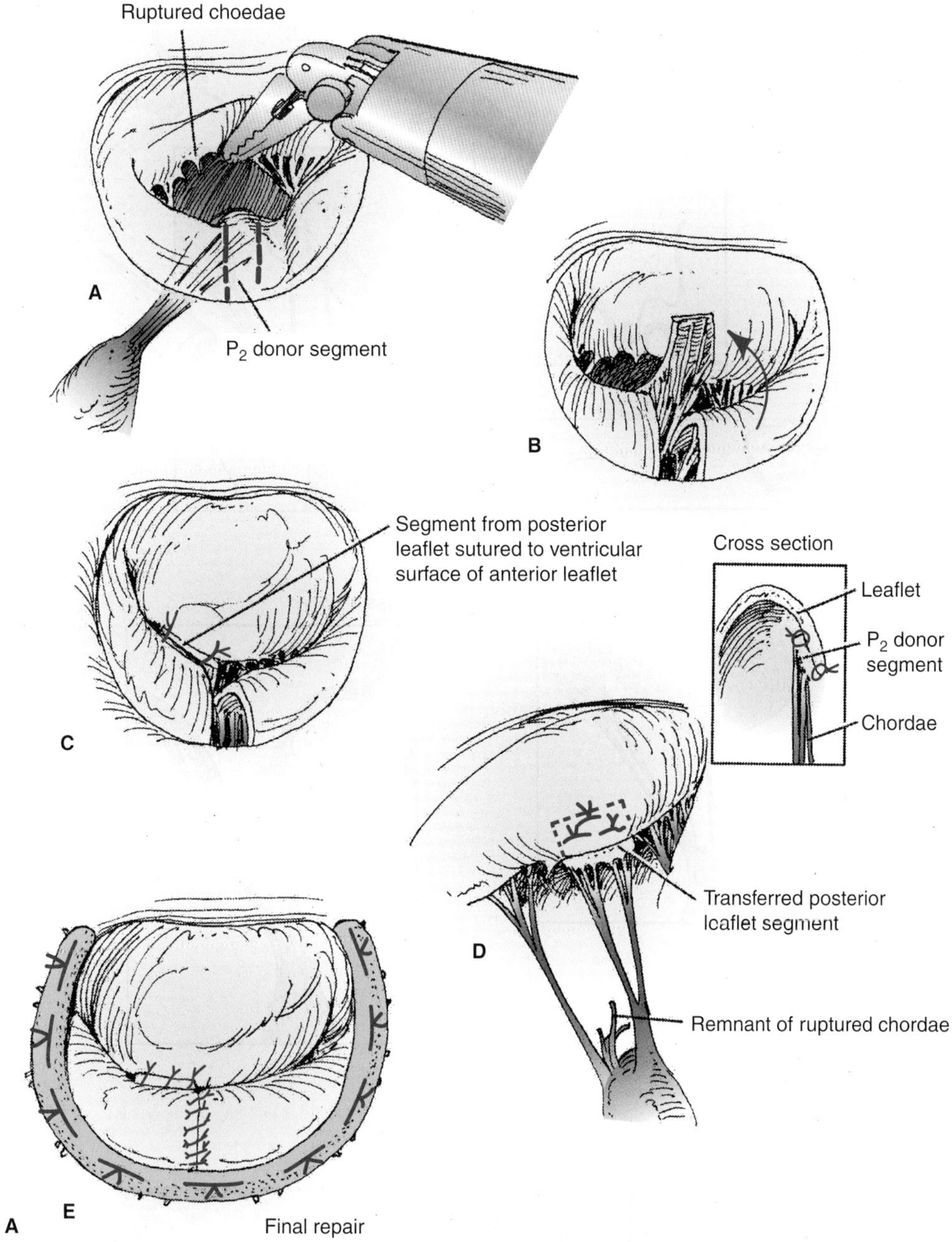

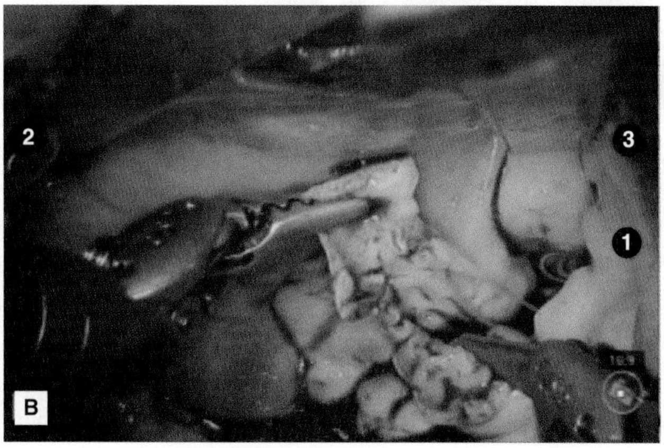

FIGURE 44-22 (A,B) Chordal transfer from posterior leaflet for the treatment of isolated anterior leaflet prolapse.

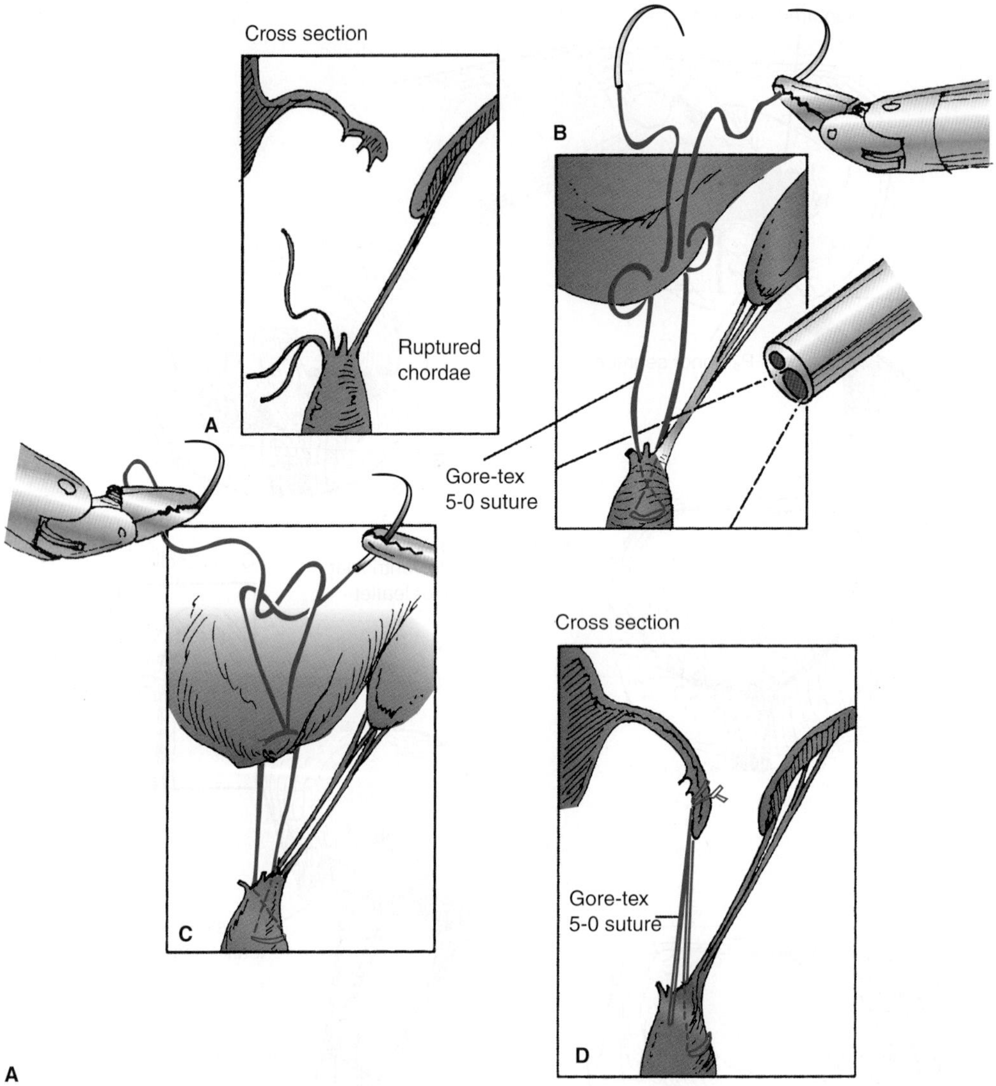

A

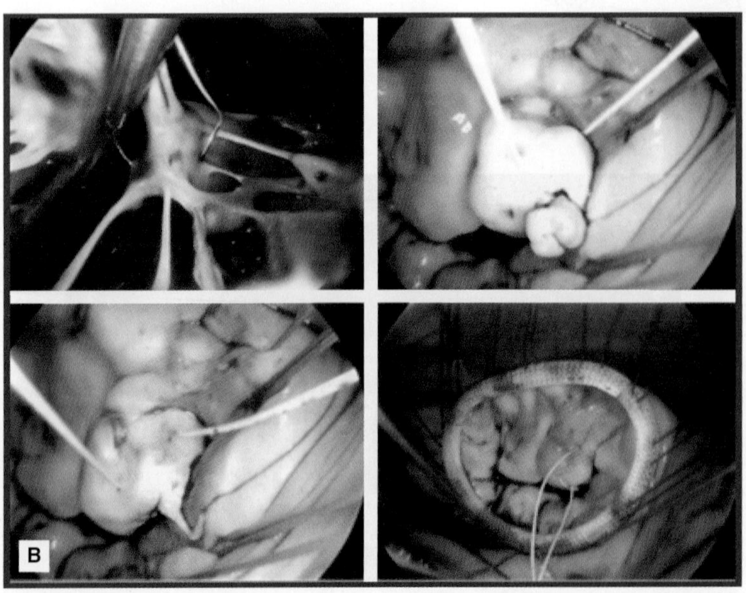

FIGURE 44-23 (A,B) Gore-Tex neochords are used for treating leaflet prolapse and/or for the replacement of ruptured chords.

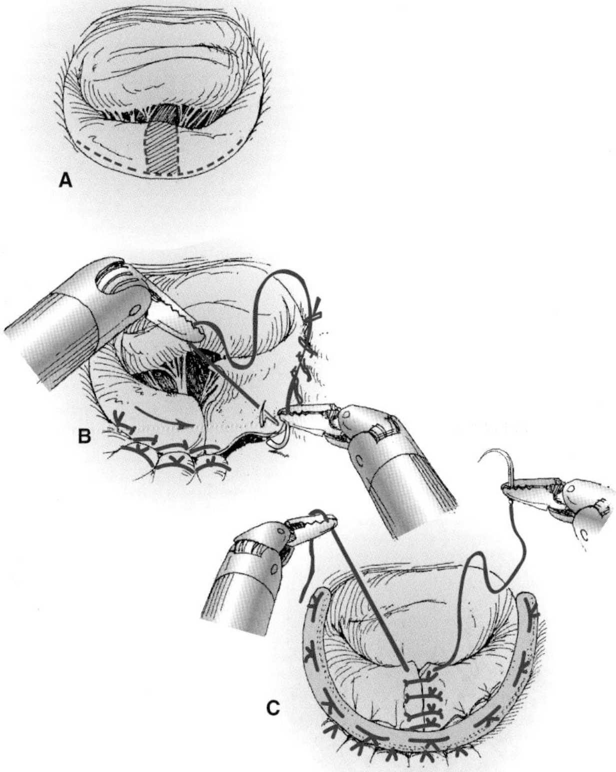

FIGURE 44-24 A da Vinci mitral valve repair. (**A**) The P2 segment of the posterior leaflet is being resected by robotic microscissors. (**B**) The annulus is reduced, the sliding-plasty is completed (**C**), and both P1 and P3 are approximated.

MV with one functional leaflet. Advances in robotic technology, including three-dimensional visualization and improved dexterity with enhanced operative precision, have facilitated the development of new repair techniques for MR. In 2006 we introduced the "Haircut" repair technique. The limits of the prolapsing P2 segment with associated ruptured or redundant chords are identified (Fig. 44-25A) and the height (annulus to tip) of each scallop is measured. Lateral P2 scallop edges are imbricated concomitantly with P1-P2 and P2-P3 cleft closure (4-0 Cardionyl; Péters, Surgical, Bobigny, France). Incomplete natural clefts can be closed during imbrication. Completion of this part of the repair generally reduces the P2 segment prolapse substantially. Thereafter, excess P2 tissue is resected to the measured height of adjacent P1 and P3 scallops (Fig. 44-25B), with the goal of achieving a posterior leaflet height less than 15 mm. With this resection ruptured chords and excess P2 lengths get a "haircut." Redundant chords are preserved along with a tiny piece of leaflet-anchoring tissue and are reattached to the free edge of the P2 chord, restoring the line of coaptation (Fig. 44-25C). If all P2 chords require resection, adjacent secondary chords can be transferred from either the posterior or anterior leaflet. Alternately, polytetrafluoroethylene neochords can be substituted. The repair is completed with an annuloplasty band (Cosgrove-Edwards; Edwards Lifesciences, Irvine, CA) (Fig. 44-25D). We implant the band using 2-0 Cardioflon sutures (Péters Surgical, Paris, France), which have excellent handling characteristics and require only four knots, facilitating a more expeditious repair. A photograph of the completed repair is shown in Fig. 25E.[52]

In patients with bileaflet prolapse, or Barlow's disease, part of the resected segments from the posterior leaflet are transposed to the redundant anterior leaflet segments and attached with 4-0 monofilament sutures. Again, "swinging" a chord-bearing piece of posterior leaflet to the undersurface of the anterior leaflet generally reduces the prolapse of the latter (Figs. 44-26A through E).

To date, all of our nearly 600 robotic repairs have been supported either by an annuloplasty using a Cosgrove-Edwards (Edwards Lifesciences, Inc., Irvine, CA) or an ATS annuloplasty band. We use either single-arm 2-0 braided sutures as shown in Fig. 44-27A or nitinol U-clips (Medtronic, Inc., Minneapolis, MN) as shown in Figs. 44-27B and C and 44-28 to secure the band. For insertion of a band alone or with limited resection, we prefer to use U-clips, which enable faster deployment. However, when greater tension is required, as in larger resections and sliding-plasties, the compressive force of sutures provides seemingly better reinforcement of the repair.

CURRENT STATUS OF MINIMALLY INVASIVE MITRAL VALVE SURGERY

Cosgrove and Gundry have consistently promoted the hemisternotomy for mitral valve surgery. They have considered this technique to be the most reproducible for surgeons with variable experiences and abilities, as well as small clinical volumes. Complex replacements and repairs have been performed through this incision and to date few repair failures have resulted from this exposure method. Between 1995 and early 2004, Cosgrove and his Cleveland Clinic group performed 2124 minimally invasive mitral operations, using direct vision through either a right paramedian incision or partial sternotomy using modified perfusion methods, compared with 1047 standard sternotomy procedures during the same time period. As noted earlier, the extended atriotomy, first proposed by Guiardon and used continually by the Cleveland Clinic group, apparently has caused excessive atrial arrhythmias, which have been lessened by modifying the atriotomy.[53] Of the patients undergoing a minimally invasive approach, 85% had degenerative and 9% had rheumatic disease and 90% were repaired using standard techniques. In a propensity-matched subset of 590 patient pairs, perfusion and aortic occlusion times averaged 85 and 65 minutes, respectively, and were only slightly longer compared with a full sternotomy. For propensity-matched patients, mortality was less than 1% for both groups with no differences in stroke, renal failure, myocardial infarction, or infection. However, patients undergoing minimally invasive procedures experienced less mediastinal drainage and received fewer blood transfusions. In addition, more patients in the minimally invasive group were extubated in the operating room and had higher postoperative forced expiratory volume in 1-second and lower pain scores. Their conversion rate to full sternotomy was 1.9%.[54]

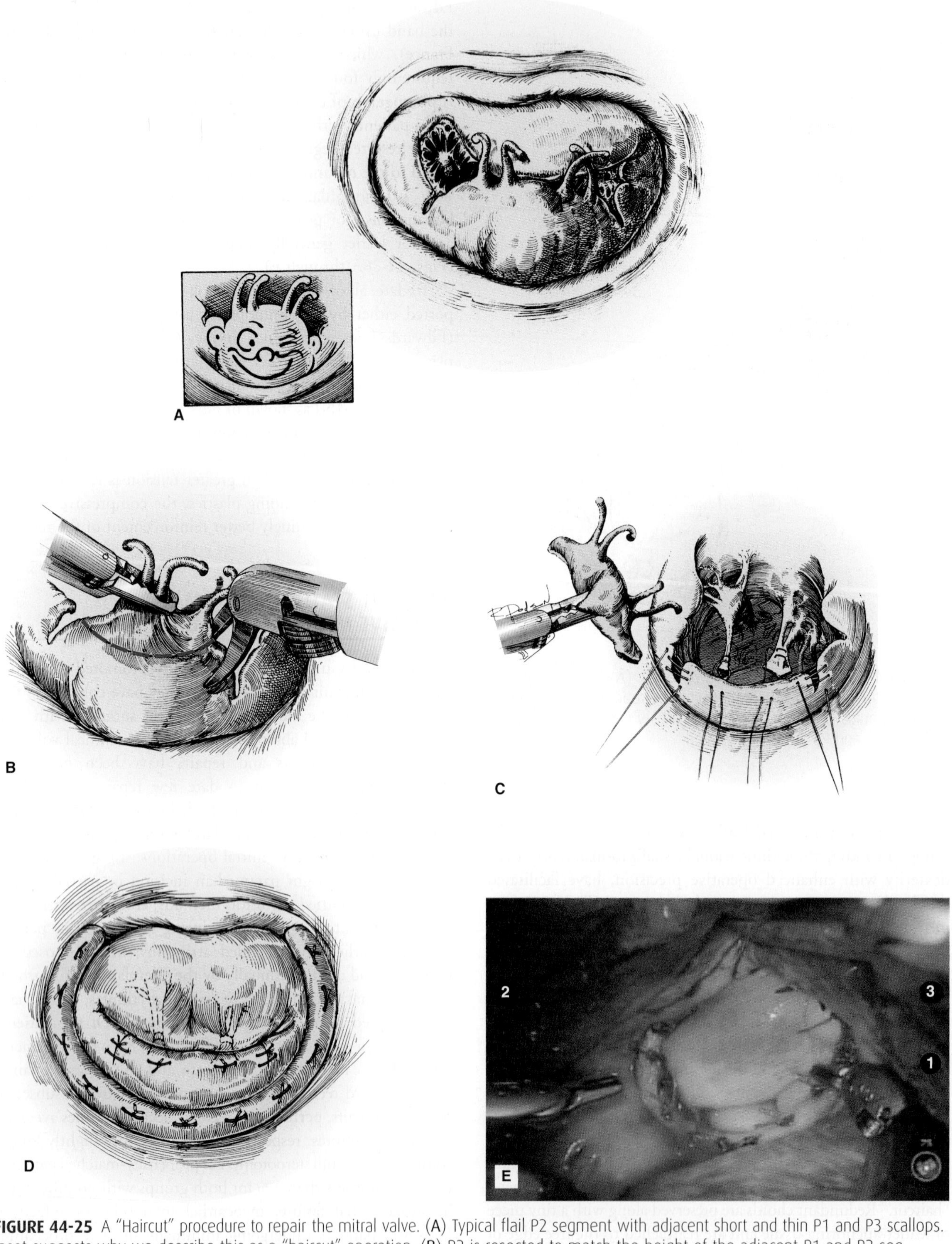

FIGURE 44-25 A "Haircut" procedure to repair the mitral valve. (A) Typical flail P2 segment with adjacent short and thin P1 and P3 scallops. Inset suggests why we describe this as a "haircut" operation. (B) P2 is resected to match the height of the adjacent P1 and P2 segments. (C) Preserved posterior leaflet chords can be reattached to free edge of P2 segment to pull the leaflet edge down into the ventricle and provide leaflet support. If adequate chords cannot be saved, secondary chords can be transferred from either the posterior or anterior leaflet. Posterior leaflet clefts are plicated. (D) Repair is completed with band annuloplasty. (E) Completed repair. *(Adapted with permission from Chu MWA, Gersch KA, Rodriguez E, et al: Robotic "haircut" mitral valve repair: posterior leaflet-plasty. Ann Thorac Surg 2008;85:1461.)*

After initially using a right parasternal incision Cohn and associates now prefer a lower hemisternotomy with direct aortic arterial cannulation and vacuum-assisted percutaneous femoral venous drainage, accessing the mitral valve via a standard left atriotomy. Of the 707 mitral patients operated between 1996 and 2007, the most common mitral valve pathology was myxomatous degeneration (88%) including 184 patients with anterior or bileaflet prolapse, rheumatic disease (3.5%), and endocarditis (3.1%). Their thirty-day mortality was 0.4%. Bleeding requiring reoperation occurred in 2% of patients. Strokes occurred in 1.7% of patients, myocardial infarctions in 0.7% and vascular complications in 4.4%. Patients were hospitalized for a mean of 5 days and 6.9% required additional rehabilitation before discharge. Survival at 11.2 years was 83%

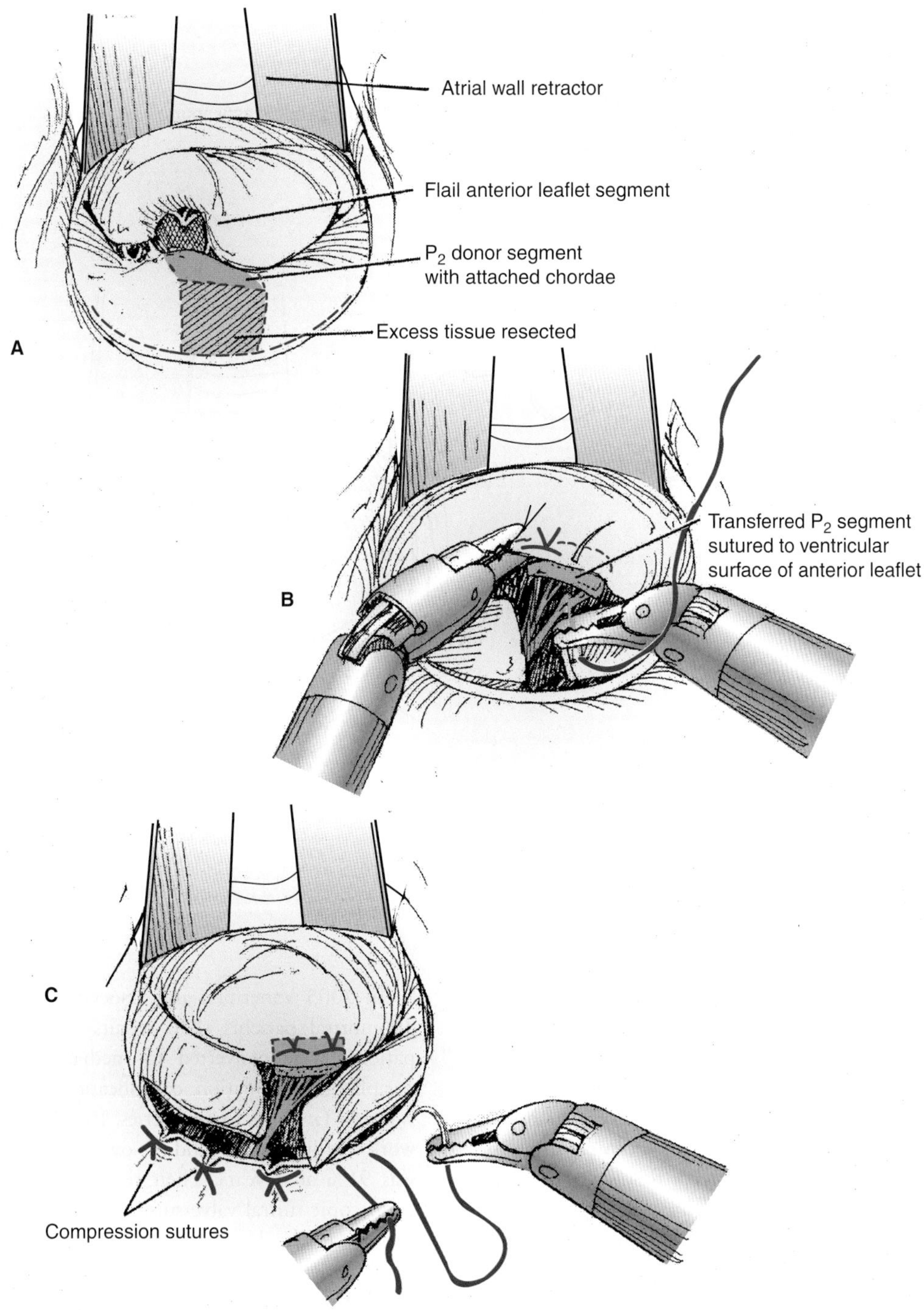

FIGURE 44-26 Repair of Barlow's or bileaflet disease. Resection of P2 maintaining the chordal apparatus intact is performed (A) followed by transfer of this segment to the anterior leaflet (B). The posterior annulus is then reduced (C). The sliding-plasty is then completed (D) followed by approximation of P1 and P3 (E).

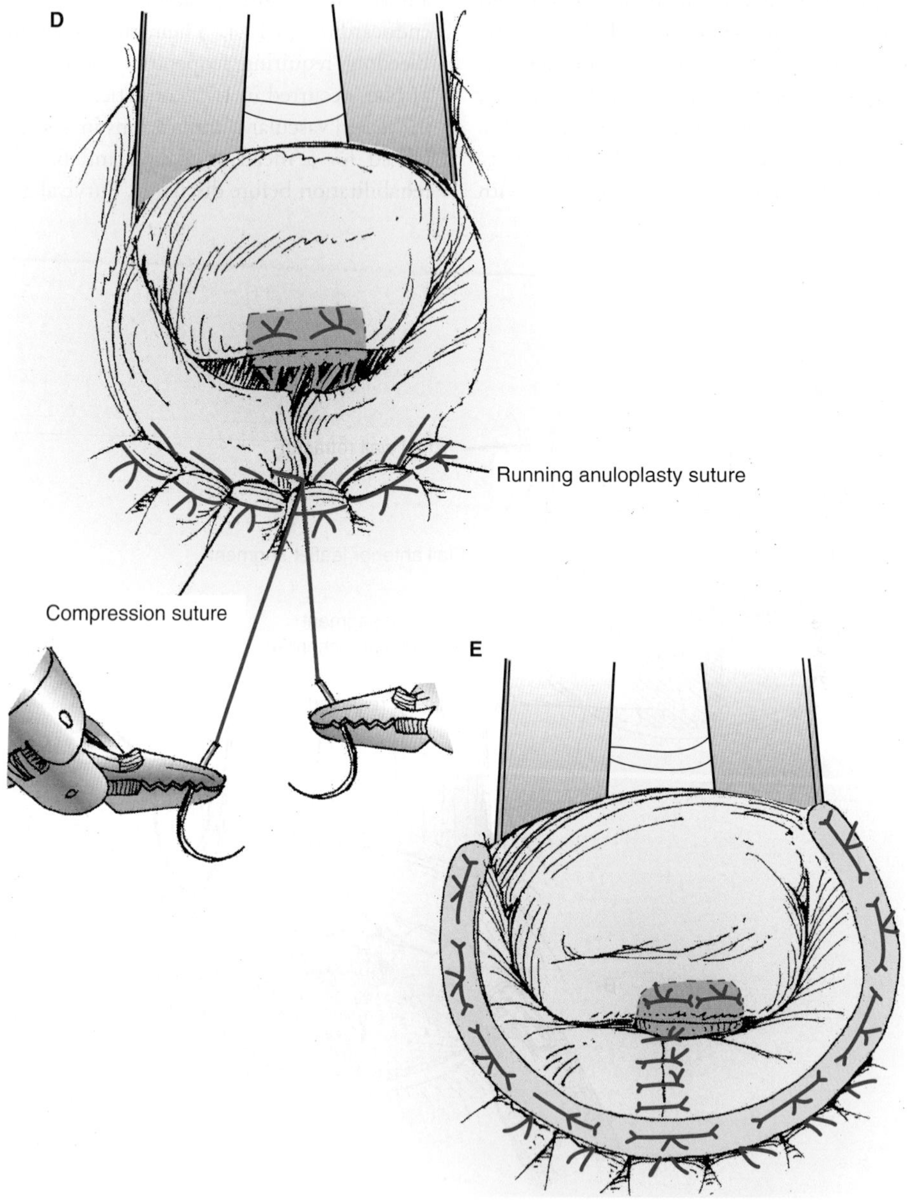

FIGURE 44-26 *(Continued)*

and freedom from reoperation was 92%. Late mitral regurgitation occurred in 12%. Anterior leaflet prolapse and lack of an annuloplasty ring were involved in 65% of failed repairs.[55]

In early 2002, Vanermen described 187 patients undergoing totally video-directed repairs using the port-access method and no rib spreading. He used a 2D endoscopic camera to perform complex repairs with excellent results at follow-up 19 months later.[41] The hospital mortality was 0.5%, and there were only two conversions to a sternotomy for bleeding. Freedom from reoperation was 95% at 4 years. Over 90% of patients had minimal postoperative pain. Although this and other series had not been randomized, these series strongly suggest that mitral valve surgery has entered a new era, and that minimally invasive and video techniques can facilitate these operations.

In 2003 Vanermen and associates updated their results in 306 mitral patients (226 repairs and 80 replacements). Six patients were converted to median sternotomy because of peripheral cannulation complications, and 30-day mortality was 1% (n = 3). In this series 46% of patients were back to work within 4 weeks, and the overall freedom from reoperation was 91% at 4 years. Their results continued to suggest that endoscopic mitral valve surgery is safe with excellent results.[56] Mohr and the University of Leipzig group recently reported 1536 patients undergoing video-assisted mitral valve surgery for mitral regurgitation using peripheral perfusion and Bretschneider cardioplegia administered at intervals of 90 to 120 minutes. The repair rate was 87.2% and the conversion rate was only 0.3%. Thirty-day mortality was 2.4% and 5 year

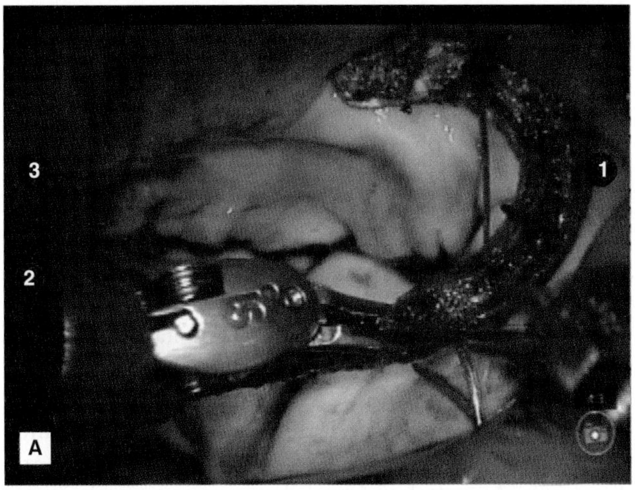

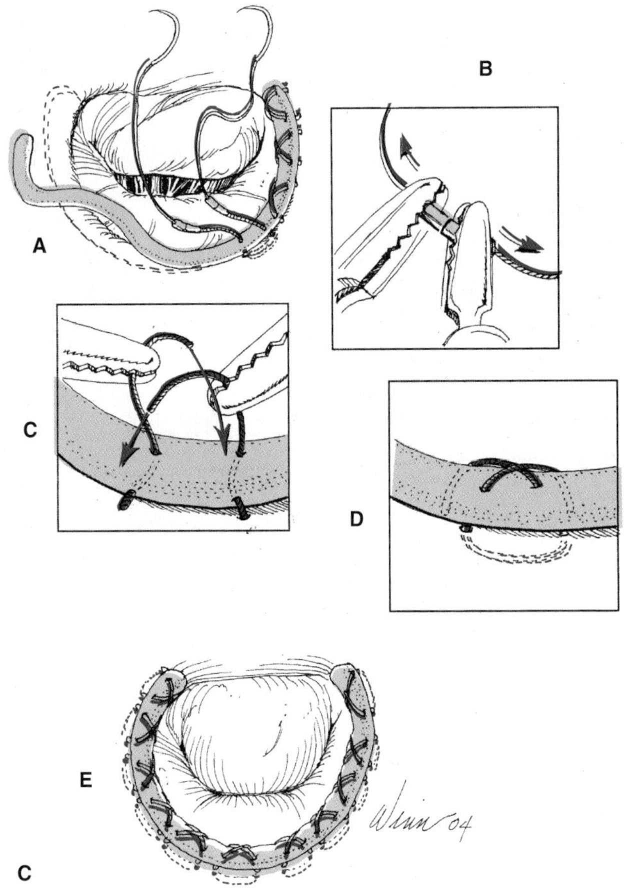

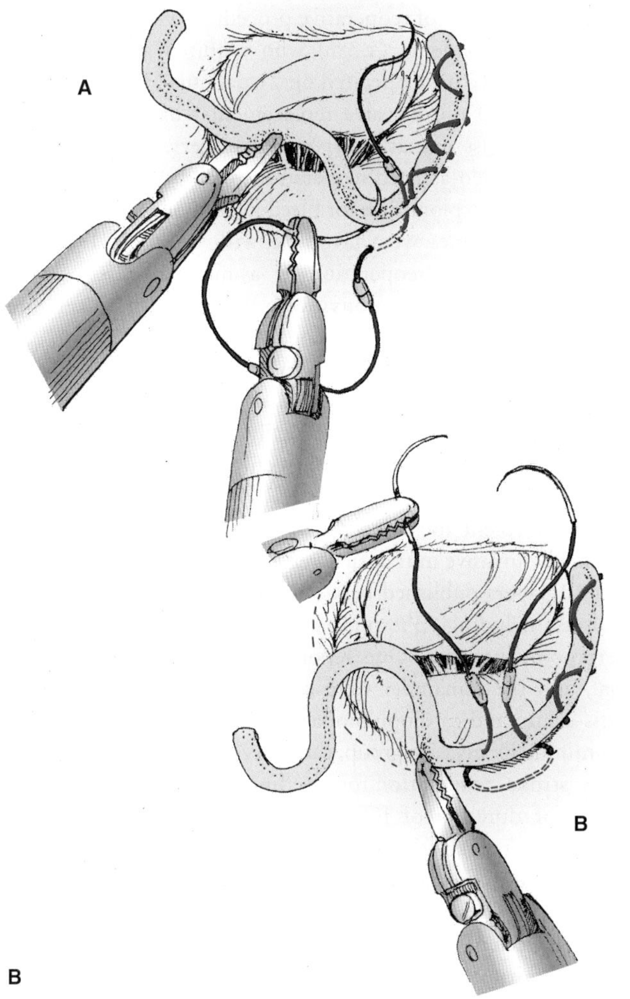

FIGURE 44-27 Annuloplasty bands are secured with single-arm 2-0 braided suture (A) or with nitinol U-clips (B,C) using the da Vinci system.

Kaplan-Meier survival was 82.6%. Their freedom from reoperation was 96.3% at 5 years.[57] Subsequently, this group compared results from a subset of patients undergoing complex mitral valve repair with patients undergoing simple posterior leaflet repairs. They determined that long-term results and reoperation rates for anterior mitral valve leaflet repair and bileaflet repair were similar to posterior leaflet repairs.[58]

The East Carolina University group reported a combined series with Hargrove consisting of 1178 successful video-assisted mitral valve operations between 1996 and 2008.[59]

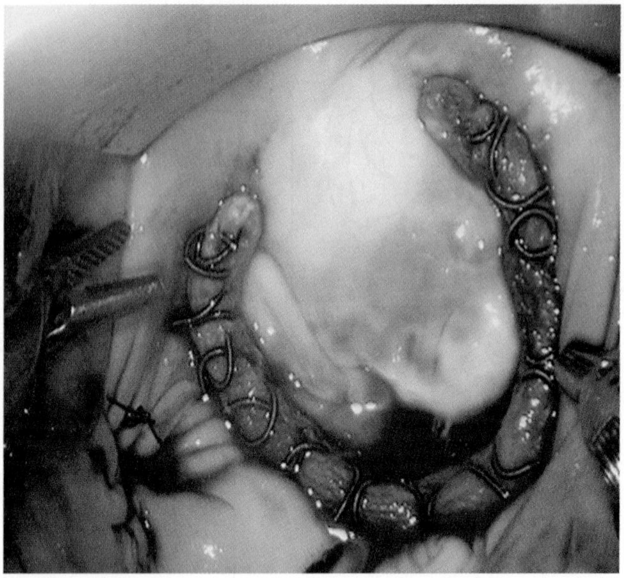

FIGURE 44-28 Completed repair using nitinol U-clips to secure the annuloplasty band.

At first, patients with anterior leaflet pathology and annular calcification were avoided. However, these patients are now operated on using video-assisted techniques. Table 44-3 details our current criteria for patient selection. The majority of patients had degenerative disease and 79.9% of the total group underwent a repair. In this series repairs included ring annuloplasties with quadrangular resections, sliding plasties, chordal transfers and PTFE neochordae placement procedures. The operative mortality for mitral valve repair and replacement for this two center series was 2.1% and 4.6%, respectively, but only 0.2% for isolated primary mitral valve repair. Cross-clamp (100 minutes) and perfusion (142 minutes) times still remained longer than those of conventional operations. Currently, at our institution cardiac arrest and perfusion times for video-assisted mitral operations have fallen to 70 and 100 minutes, respectively, Myocardial protection strategies included transthoracic clamping (48.7%), endoaortic balloon occlusion (40.7%), and hypothermic fibrillation (10.1%). A trend for increased stroke and aortic dissection was found, especially when using the endoballoon. Interestingly, we have seen no difference in bleeding and transfusion requirements between our conventional and minimally invasive cases. However, hospital length of stay averaged 6 days compared with 8 days for conventional operations. Of these 1178 patients there were 19 (1.6%) conversions to a sternotomy, 23 (2.0%) had strokes, 63 (5.4%) required re-exploration for bleeding, and 9 (0.8%) sustained aortic dissections. A total of 45.5% of the patients received a blood product transfusion. Postoperative repair transesophageal echocardiograms showed no more than trivial insufficiency in 97.1% of patients having mitral valve repair. We previously reported our series of reoperative procedures via this approach including 14 patients (4.3%) who required a mitral valve reoperation. We have operated on 71 patients (31 mitral valve repairs and 40 mitral valve replacements) having had prior coronary bypass operation or mitral surgery. These patients underwent video-assisted reoperations with 9.8% mortality as well as four re-explorations for bleeding and one stroke (1.4%) Midterm outcomes were favorable with only 22 (1.9%) of patients requiring reoperation at a mean of 732 days.[60] Hargrove has become convinced that small-incision and videoscopic mitral surgery is safe, effective, economical, and better accepted by patients than conventional sternotomy operations. The long-term results of all of the above series continue to confirm that minimally invasive mitral operations have already taken a prominent position in the evolution of cardiac surgery.

TABLE 44-3 Current Patient Selection: Videoscopic or Video-Assisted Mitral Valve Surgery

Unsuitable candidates
Highly calcified mitral annulus
Severe pulmonary hypertension, especially with a small right coronary artery
Significant untreated coronary disease
Severe peripheral atherosclerosis
Prior right chest surgery
Concomitant aortic or aortic valve pathology requiring surgical interventions
Suitable candidates
Patients with primary mitral valve disease
Reoperative mitral valve patients
Bileaflet and/or anterior leaflet disease
Combined tricuspid and mitral operations
Mild annular calcification
Obese or large patients
Elderly patients

In our recent meta-analysis of 43 manuscripts comparing minimally invasive mitral valve repair to sternotomy, we identified 10 papers published between 1998 and 2005 suitable for analysis, including 1358 minimally invasive patients and 1469 sternotomy patients. One report was a randomized control trial, and the remainder were case-control studies. Although cross-clamp and cardiopulmonary bypass times were longer in the minimally invasive group, there were no differences in mortality, stroke, reoperation for bleeding, new onset atrial fibrillation, or duration of ICU or hospital stay. Freedom from reoperation ranged from 91 to 99%.[61]

Grossi and associates at New York University have reported the longest outcomes for minimally invasive mitral surgery to date. Between 1996 and 2008 they performed 1071 minimally invasive mitral valve repairs and compared their results with a cohort of 1601 conventional procedures. This group uses a 6- to 8-cm minithoracotomy and operates under direct vision. They now prefer to use direct aortic cannulation with an external aortic clamp. Venous drainage is via a femoral cannula and cardioplegia is administered by a coronary sinus catheter inserted through the right atrium. Approximately one third of the minimally invasive repairs included an anterior leaflet procedure and all patients received an annuloplasty device. They reported a perioperative mortality of 1.3% in both groups with isolated mitral valve repair and no differences in major adverse events. Long-term results were equivalent to sternotomy techniques. In isolated mitral valve repair, eight-year freedom from reoperation or severe recurrent insufficiency was 93% and freedom from all valve-related complications was 90%. Their results suggest that minimally invasive mitral operations can be done safely using limited incisions and direct aortic clamping methods with similar results as conventional operations and with no added mortality or morbidity. At the same time they had fewer transfusions, shorter lengths of hospital stay, and fewer septic complications.[62]

The right chest minithoracotomy provides significant benefits in re-operative settings by avoiding sternal re-entry and limited dissection of adhesions, avoiding the risk of injury to cardiac structures or patent grafts, and limiting the amount of postoperative bleeding. Vanermen reported 80 adults undergoing endoscopic mitral valve and tricuspid valve re-operative surgery with an operative mortality of 3.8%. There were three perioperative strokes, and survival at 1 and 4 years was 93.6 and 85.6%, respectively.[63] A recent case control study, comparing re-sternotomy to the right minithoracotomy for redo mitral valve surgery, noted no difference in mortality or perfusion times but significantly reduced intubation times, blood transfusions, and hospital stays with the minimally invasive approach.[60]

Robotic Mitral Valve Surgery

The East Carolina University group performed the first da Vinci system robotic mitral valve repair in North America in May 2000. Since then, we have performed nearly 600 robotic mitral valve repairs. The first Food and Drug Administration (FDA) safety and efficacy trial was conducted at our institution in 2000 and included 20 patients.[32] Leaflet resections, sliding-plasties, chordal transfers, neochord insertions, and annuloplasties were all performed successfully. This initial study demonstrated that although operative times were longer, when compared with conventional mitral valve sternotomy operations, the results were comparable. There were no device-related complications. Postoperative hospital stays averaged 4 days, and all patients returned to normal activity by 1 month following surgery. Early postoperative echocardiograms at 3 months demonstrated that none of the patients had more than trace mitral regurgitation.

These initial results were encouraging and prompted a phase II multicenter FDA trial, which was completed in 2002.[35] A total of 112 patients were enrolled at 10 different institutions and all types of repairs were performed. Following surgery, nine patients (8%) had grade 2 or higher mitral regurgitation, and six patients (5%) required a reoperation. Although the reoperative number was high for the number of patients, failures were distributed evenly among centers, with some centers having performed fewer than 10 procedures and were still early in their learning curve phase. There were no deaths, strokes, or device-related complications. These results prompted FDA approval (2002) of the da Vinci system for mitral valve surgery.

Other early robotic assisted mitral valve surgery reports included:

1. Tatooles et al. reported their experience with 25 patients and demonstrated excellent results with no mortality, device-related complications, strokes or reoperations for bleeding. One patient had a transient ischemic attack 7 days after surgery. The CPB and XC times were 126.6±25.7 minutes and 87.7±20.9 minutes, respectively. Eighty-four percent were extubated in the operating room, 8 were discharged home within 24 hours, and the mean hospital stay was 2.7 days. However, there was a 28% rate of readmission using this aggressive discharge policy and two patients required interval mitral valve replacement.[64]
2. Jones et al. reported a series of 32 robotic mitral repair patient from a community hospital. They performed concomitant procedures in five patients (tricuspid valve repair $n = 3$ and MAZE procedure $n = 2$). There were two deaths in this series where neither was reported as a device-related complication. Complications included reoperations for repair failure ($n = 3$), stroke ($n = 1$), groin lymphocele ($n = 1$) and pulmonary embolism ($n = 1$).[65]
3. In a nonrandomized single surgeon experience from the University of Pennsylvania, Woo et al. demonstrated that robotic surgery patients had a significant reduction in blood transfusions and length of stay compared with sternotomy patients.[66]
4. Folliguet et al. compared patients undergoing robotically-assisted mitral valve repair with a matched cohort undergoing a sternotomy ($n = 25$ each). The robotic group had a shorter hospital stay (7 days versus 9 days, $p = 0.05$) but besides this there were no differences between the 2 groups.[67]

More recent and larger series include:

1. Murphy et al. reported their experience in 127 patients undergoing robotic mitral surgery of which five were converted to a median sternotomy and one to a thoracotomy; seven patients had a valve replacement and 114 had a repair. There was a single in-hospital death, one late death, two strokes and 22 patients developed new onset of atrial fibrillation. Blood product transfusion was required in 31% of patients and two (1.7%) patients required a reoperation. Postdischarge echocardiograms were available in 98 patients at a mean follow-up of 8.4 months with no more than 1+ residual MR in 96.2%.[44]
2. Our report from the East Carolina University included the first 300 patients undergoing robotic mitral valve repair between May 2000 and November 2006. Mean patient age was 57 years and 36% were female. Cardiopulmonary bypass times were 159 minutes, and cross-clamp times were 122 minutes. Repairs included quadrangular resections, sliding-plasties, chordal transfers, chordal shortening, neochord insertion, edge-to-edge repairs, and annuloplasties. Echocardiographic and survival follow-up was complete in 93% and 100% of patients, respectively.[68]

There were 2 (0.7%) 30-day mortalities and 6 (2.0%) late mortalities. No conversions to sternotomy or mitral valve replacements were required. Immediate postrepair echocardiograms showed the following degrees of mitral regurgitation: none/trivial, 294 (98%); mild, 3 (1.0%); moderate, 3 (1.0%); and severe, 0 (0.0%). Complications included two (0.7%) strokes, two (0.7%) transient ischemic attacks, three (1.0%) myocardial infarctions, and seven (2.3%) reoperations for bleeding. The mean hospital stay was 5.2 ±4.2 (standard deviation) days. Sixteen (5.3%) patients required a reoperation. Echocardiographic follow-up demonstrated the following degrees of mitral regurgitation: none/trivial, 192 (68.8%); mild, 66 (23.6%); moderate, 15 (5.4%); and severe, 6 (2.2%). Within this series, 66 patients underwent complex repairs for anterior leaflet or bileaflet prolapse. In this subgroup, 90% of patients had moderate or less mitral regurgitation postoperatively, and the 5-year freedom from reoperation was approximately 90%.[69]

We have also used the da Vinci system to perform mitral valve replacements as well as combined mitral valve repairs with atrial fibrillation ablation.[70] As we continue to perform further robotic mitral operations, the operative times have continued to decrease. In addition, we are able to repair more complex valves because of the enhanced visualization and fine dexterity offered by the evolved da Vinci system.

MINIMALLY INVASIVE HEART VALVE SURGERY: CONCLUSIONS

Over the last decade there has been a transformation in the way cardiac surgeons, cardiologists and patients approach cardiac therapies. Indeed, current STS data shows that 11.3% of isolated mitral valve repairs are performed with robotic assistance. Up to 20% of surgeons are using some minimally invasive method for their repairs. Nevertheless, fewer than 60% of repairable mitral valves are currently being repaired, no matter the approach. Less invasive mitral valve repair procedures are more demanding, but proven safety, efficacy, and durability are still demanded with new techniques. Evidence presented herein demonstrates that minimally invasive mitral valve surgery is associated with equal mortality and neurological events to sternotomy methods, despite longer cardiopulmonary bypass and aortic cross-clamp times. However, there is less morbidity in terms of reduced need for reoperation for bleeding, a trend towards shorter hospital stays, less pain, and faster return to preoperative function levels than conventional sternotomy-based surgery. It is expected that these results will translate into improved utilization of limited healthcare resources. With follow-up now of almost 7 years it is clear that long-term outcomes are equivalent to those of conventional surgery. Data for minimally invasive mitral valve surgery after previous cardiac surgery is limited but consistently demonstrates reduced blood loss, fewer transfusions and faster recovery compared with reoperative sternotomy. Almost all patients who undergo a minimally invasive mitral valve operation as their second procedure feel their recovery is more rapid and less painful than their original sternotomy.

As for the future, minimally invasive cardiac surgery is likely to become more widely adopted and less of a niche market. Although operative philosophies, patient populations, and surgeon abilities differ among centers, the compendium of recent results remains very encouraging. The ultimate goal is to perform safe completely endoscopic surgery. To successfully perform these operations, surgeons and engineers will need to continue to improve methods by which instruments are directed by computers. Recent successes with direct-vision, videoscopic, and robotic minimally invasive surgery all have reaffirmed that this evolution can be extremely fast, albeit through various pathways.

Patient requirements, technology developments, and surgeon capabilities all must become aligned to drive these needed changes. In addition, we must work closer with our cardiology colleagues in these developments. This is an evolutionary process, and even the greatest skeptics must concede that progress has been made. However, curmudgeons and surgical scientists alike must continue to interject their concerns. Caution cannot be overemphasized. Traditional valve operations enjoy proven long-term success with ever-decreasing morbidity and mortality, and remain the gold standard. Less invasive approaches to treating valve disease cannot capitulate to poorer operative quality or unsatisfactory valve and/or patient longevity. Nevertheless, patients are opting for less invasive operations.

REFERENCES

1. Cohn LH, Adams DH, Couper GS, Bichell DP: Minimally invasive aortic valve replacement. *Semin Thorac Cardiovasc Surg* 1997; 9:331-336.
2. Cosgrove DM, III, Sabik JF: Minimally invasive approach for aortic valve operations. *Ann Thorac Surg* 1996; 62:596-597.
3. Cosgrove DM, III, Sabik JF, Navia JL: Minimally invasive valve operations. *Ann Thorac Surg* 1998; 65:1535-1538.
4. Falk V, Walther T, Diegeler A, Wendler R, Autschbach R, et al: Echocardiographic monitoring of minimally invasive mitral valve surgery using an endoaortic clamp. *J Heart Valve Dis* 1996; 5:630-637.
5. Baldwin JC: Editorial (con) re minimally invasive port-access mitral valve surgery. *J Thorac Cardiovasc Surg* 1998; 115:563-564.
6. Cooley DA: Antagonist's view of minimally invasive heart valve surgery. *J Card Surg* 2000; 15:3-5.
7. Enriquez-Sarano M, Avierinos JF, Messika-Zeitoun D, Detaint D: Quantitative determinants of the outcome of asymptomatic mitral regurgitation. *NEJM* 2005; 352:875-883.
8. Tribouilloy CM, Enriquez-Sarano M, Schaff HV, Orszulak TA, Bailey KR, et al: Impact of preoperative symptoms on survival after surgical correction of organic mitral regurgitation: rationale for optimizing surgical indications. *Circulation* 1999; 99:400-405.
9. Konertz W, Waldenberger F, Schmutzler M, Ritter J, Liu J: Minimal access valve surgery through superior partial sternotomy: a preliminary study. *J Heart Valve Dis* 1996; 5:638-640.
10. Arom KV, Emery RW, Kshettry VR, Janey PA: Comparison between port-access and less invasive valve surgery. *Ann Thorac Surg* 1999; 68:1525-1528.
11. Cohn LH, Adams DH, Couper GS, Bichell DP, Rosborough DM, et al: Minimally invasive cardiac valve surgery improves patient satisfaction while reducing costs of cardiac valve replacement and repair. *Ann Surg* 1997; 226:421-426.
12. Navia JL, Cosgrove DM, III: Minimally invasive mitral valve operations. *Ann Thorac Surg* 1996; 62:1542-1544.
13. Arom KV, Emery RW: Minimally invasive mitral operations. *Ann Thorac Surg* 1997; 63:1219-1220.
14. Gundry SR, Shattuck OH, Razzouk AJ, del Rio MJ, Sardari FF, et al: Facile minimally invasive cardiac surgery via ministernotomy. *Ann Thorac Surg* 1998; 65:1100-1104.
15. Fann JI, Pompili MF, Burdon TA, Stevens JH, St Goar FG, et al:. Minimally invasive mitral valve surgery. *Semin Thorac Cardiovasc Surg* 1997; 9:320-330.
16. Fann JI, Pompili MF, Stevens JH, Siegel LC, St Goar FG, et al: Port-access cardiac operations with cardioplegic arrest. *Ann Thorac Surg* 1997; 63:S35-S39.

17. Mohr FW, Falk V, Diegeler A, Walther T, van Son JA, Autschbach R: Minimally invasive port-access mitral valve surgery. *J Thorac Cardiovasc Surg* 1998; 115:567-574.
18. Spencer FC, Galloway AC, Grossi EA, Ribakove GH, Delianides J, et al: Recent developments and evolving techniques of mitral valve reconstruction. *Ann Thorac Surg* 1998; 65:307-313.
19. Carpentier A, Loulmet D, Carpentier A, Le Bret E, Haugades B, et al: Open heart operation under video surgery and minithoracotomy. First case (mitral valvuloplasty) operated with success. *C R Acad Sci III* 1996; 319: 219-223.
20. Chitwood WR, Jr., Elbeery JR, Chapman WH, Moran JM, Lust RL, et al: Video-assisted minimally invasive mitral valve surgery: the "micro-mitral" operation. *J Thorac Cardiovasc Surg* 1997; 113:413-414.
21. Chitwood WR, Jr., Elbeery JR, Moran JF: Minimally invasive mitral valve repair using transthoracic aortic occlusion. *Ann Thorac Surg* 1997; 63: 1477-1479.
22. Reichenspurner H, Detter C, Deuse T, Boehm DH, Treede H: Video and robotic-assisted minimally invasive mitral valve surgery: a comparison of the Port-Access and transthoracic clamp techniques. *Ann Thorac Surg* 2005; 79:485-490.
23. Falk V, Walther T, Autschbach R, Diegeler A, Battellini R: Robot-assisted minimally invasive solo mitral valve operation. *J Thorac Cardiovasc Surg* 1998; 115:470-471.
24. Loulmet DF, Carpentier A, Cho PW, Berrebi A, d'Attellis N, et al: Less invasive techniques for mitral valve surgery. *J Thorac Cardiovasc Surg* 1998; 115:772-779.
25. Chitwood WR, Jr., Wixon CL, Elbeery JR, Moran JF, Chapman WH, et al: Video-assisted minimally invasive mitral valve surgery. *J Thorac Cardiovasc Surg* 1997; 114:773-780.
26. Felger JE, Chitwood WR, Jr., Nifong LW, Holbert D: Evolution of mitral valve surgery: toward a totally endoscopic approach. *Ann Thorac Surg* 2001; 72:1203-1208.
27. Vanermen H, Farhat F, Wellens F, De Geest R, Degrieck I, et al: Minimally invasive video-assisted mitral valve surgery: from Port-Access towards a totally endoscopic procedure. *J Card Surg* 2000; 15:51-60.
28. Vanermen H, Wellens F, De Geest R, Degrieck I, Van Praet F: Video-assisted Port-Access mitral valve surgery: from debut to routine surgery. Will Trocar-Port-Access cardiac surgery ultimately lead to robotic cardiac surgery? *Semin Thorac Cardiovasc Surg* 1999; 11:223-234.
29. Carpentier A, Loulmet D, Aupecle B, Kieffer JP, Tournay D, et al: Computer assisted open heart surgery. First case operated on with success. *C R Acad Sci III* 1998; 321:437-442.
30. Mohr FW, Falk V, Diegeler A, Autschback R: Computer-enhanced coronary artery bypass surgery. *J Thorac Cardiovasc Surg* 1999; 117:1212-1214.
31. Chitwood WR, Jr., Nifong LW, Elbeery JE, Chapman WH, Albrecht R, et al: Robotic mitral valve repair: trapezoidal resection and prosthetic annuloplasty with the da Vinci surgical system. *J Thorac Cardiovasc Surg* 2000; 120:1171-1172.
32. Nifong LW, Chu VF, Bailey BM, Maziarz DM, Sorrell VL, et al: Robotic mitral valve repair: experience with the da Vinci system. *Ann Thorac Surg* 2003; 75:438-442.
33. Grossi EA, Lapietra A, Applebaum RM, Ribakove GH, Galloway AC, et al: Case report of robotic instrument-enhanced mitral valve surgery. *J Thorac Cardiovasc Surg* 2000; 120:1169-1171.
34. Mehmanesh H, Henze R, Lange R: Totally endoscopic mitral valve repair. *J Thorac Cardiovasc Surg* 2002; 123:96-97.
35. Nifong LW, Chitwood WR, Pappas PS, Smith CR, Argenziano M, et al: Robotic mitral valve surgery: a United States multicenter trial. *J Thorac Cardiovasc Surg* 2005; 129:1395-1404.
36. Gillinov AM, Banbury MK, Cosgrove DM: Hemisternotomy approach for aortic and mitral valve surgery. *J Card Surg* 2000; 15:15-20.
37. Gillinov AM, Cosgrove DM: Minimally invasive mitral valve surgery: mini-sternotomy with extended transseptal approach. *Semin Thorac Cardiovasc Surg* 1999; 11:206-211.
38. Byrne JG, Hsin MK, Adams DH, Aklog L, Aranki SF, et al: Minimally invasive direct access heart valve surgery. *J Card Surg* 2000; 15:21-34.
39. Grossi EA, Lapietra A, Ribakove GH, Delianides J, Esposito R, et al: Minimally invasive versus sternotomy approaches for mitral reconstruction: comparison of intermediate-term results. *J Thorac Cardiovasc Surg* 2001; 121:708-713.
40. Cosgrove DM, Gillinov AM: Partial sternotomy for mitral valve operations. In Cox JL, Sundt TM (eds): *Operative Techniques in Cardiac and Thoracic Surgery; a comparative Atlas.* Philadelphia, W.B. Saunders Co, 1998; p 62.
41. Casselman FP, Van Slycke S, Dom H, Lambrechts DL, Vermeulen Y, et al: Endoscopic mitral valve repair: feasible, reproducible, and durable. *J Thorac Cardiovasc Surg* 2003; 125:273-282.
42. Schroeyers P, Wellens F, De Geest R, Degrieck I, Van Praet F, et al: Minimally invasive video-assisted mitral valve surgery: our lessons after a 4-year experience. *Ann Thorac Surg* 2001; 72:S1050-S1054.
43. Mohr FW, Onnasch JF, Falk V, Walther T, Diegeler A, et al: The evolution of minimally invasive valve surgery---2 year experience. *Eur J Cardiothorac Surg* 1999; 15:233-238.
44. Murphy DA, Miller JS, Langford DA, Snyder AB: Endoscopic robotic mitral valve surgery. *J Thorac Cardiovasc Surg* 2006; 132:776-781.
45. Cohn LH: Minimally invasive valve surgery. *J Card Surg* 2001; 16: 260-265.
46. Bonatti J, Garcia J, Rehman A, Odonkor P, Haque R, et al: On-pump beating-heart with axillary artery perfusion: a solution for robotic totally endoscopic coronary artery bypass grafting? *Heart Surg Forum* 2009; 12: E131-E133.
47. Chitwood WR: Minimally invasive video-assisted mitral valve surgery using the Chitwood clamp. In: Cox JL, Sundt TM (eds): *Operative Techniques in Cardiac and Thoracic Surgery; a comparative Atlas.* Philadelphia, W.B. Saunders Co, 1998; p 1.
48. Colvin SB, Galloway AC, Ribakove G, Grossi EA, Zakow P, et al: Port-Access mitral valve surgery: summary of results. *J Card Surg* 1998; 13:286-289.
49. Grossi EA, Ribakove G, Schwartz DS, et al: Port-access approach for minimally invasive mitral valve surgery. In, Cox JL, Sundt TM (eds): *Operative Techniques in Cardiac and Thoracic Surgery: a comparative Atlas.* Philadelphia, W.B. Saunders Co, 1998; p 32.
50. La Canna G, Arendar I, Maisano F, Monaco F, Collu E, et al: Real-time three-dimensional transesophageal echocardiography for assessment of mitral valve functional anatomy in patients with prolapse-related regurgitation. *The American Journal of Cardiology* 2011 May; 107:1365-1374.
51. Chitwood WR, Nifong LW: Robotic assistance in cardiac surgery. In, Talamini MA (ed): *Problems in General Surgery.* Philadelphia, Lippincott Williams & Wilkins, 2001; p 9.
52. Chu MW, Gersch KA, Rodriguez E, Nifong LW, Chitwood WR, Jr: Robotic "haircut" mitral valve repair: posterior leaflet-plasty. *Ann Thorac Surg* 2008; 85:1460-1462.
53. Svensson LG: Minimally invasive surgery with a partial sternotomy "J" approach. *Semin Thorac Cardiovasc Surg* 2007; 19:299-303.
54. Svensson LG, Atik FA, Cosgrove DM, Blackstone EH, Rajeswaran J, et al: Minimally invasive versus conventional mitral valve surgery: a propensity-matched comparison. *J Thorac Cardiovasc Surg* 2009; 139:926-932.
55. McClure RS, Cohn LH, Wiegerinck E, Couper GS, Aranki SF, et al: Early and late outcomes in minimally invasive mitral valve repair: an eleven-year experience in 707 patients. *J Thorac Cardiovasc Surg* 2009; 137:70-75.
56. Casselman FP, Van Slycke S, Wellens F, De Geest R, Degrieck I, et al: Mitral valve surgery can now routinely be performed endoscopically. *Circulation* 2003; 108 Suppl 1:II48-II54.
57. Seeburger J, Borger MA, Falk V, Kuntze T, Czesla M, et al: Minimal invasive mitral valve repair for mitral regurgitation: results of 1339 consecutive patients. *Eur J Cardiothorac Surg* 2008; 34:760-765.
58. Seeburger J, Borger MA, Doll N, Walther T, Passage J, et al: Comparison of outcomes of minimally invasive mitral valve surgery for posterior, anterior and bileaflet prolapse. *Eur J Cardiothorac Surg* 2009; 36:532-538.
59. Modi P, Rodriguez E, Hargrove WC, III, Hassan A, Szeto WY, et al: Minimally invasive video-assisted mitral valve surgery: a 12-year, 2-center experience in 1178 patients. *J Thorac Cardiovasc Surg* 2009; 137:1481-1487.
60. Bolotin G, Kypson AP, Reade CC, Chu VF, Freund WL, Jr., et al: Should a video-assisted mini-thoracotomy be the approach of choice for reoperative mitral valve surgery? *J Heart Valve Dis* 2004; 13:155-158.
61. Modi P, Hassan A, Chitwood WR, Jr: Minimally invasive mitral valve surgery: a systematic review and meta-analysis. *Eur J Cardiothorac Surg* 2008; 34:943-952.
62. Galloway AC, Schwartz CF, Ribakove GH, Crooke GA, Gogoladze G, et al: A decade of minimally invasive mitral repair: long-term outcomes. *Ann Thorac Surg* 2009; 88:1180-1184.
63. Casselman FP, La Meir M, Jeanmart H, Mazzarro E, Coddens J, et al: Endoscopic mitral and tricuspid valve surgery after previous cardiac surgery. *Circulation* 2007; 116:I270-I275.
64. Tatooles AJ, Pappas PS, Gordon PJ, Slaughter MS: Minimally invasive mitral valve repair using the da Vinci robotic system. *Ann Thorac Surg* 2004; 77:1978-1982.
65. Jones BA, Krueger S, Howell D, Meinecke B, Dunn S: Robotic mitral valve repair: a community hospital experience. *Tex Heart Inst J* 2005; 32: 143-146.
66. Woo YJ, Nacke EA: Robotic minimally invasive mitral valve reconstruction yields less blood product transfusion and shorter length of stay. *Surgery* 2006; 140:263-267.

67. Folliguet T, Vanhuyse F, Constantino X, Realli M, Laborde F: Mitral valve repair robotic versus sternotomy. *Eur J Cardiothorac Surg* 2006; 29:362-366.
68. Chitwood WR, Jr., Rodriguez E, Chu MW, Hassan A, Ferguson TB, et al: Robotic mitral valve repairs in 300 patients: a single-center experience. *J Thorac Cardiovasc Surg* 2008; 136:436-441
69. Rodriguez E, Nifong LW, Chu MW, Wood W, Vos PW, et al: Robotic mitral valve repair for anterior leaflet and bileaflet prolapse. *Ann Thorac Surg* 2008; 85:438-444.
70. Reade CC, Johnson JO, Bolotin G, Freund WL, Jr., Jenkins NL, et al: Combining robotic mitral valve repair and microwave atrial fibrillation ablation: techniques and initial results. *Ann Thorac Surg* 2005; 79:480-484.

CHAPTER 45

Percutaneous Catheter-Based Mitral Valve Repair

Michael J. Mack

PERCUTANEOUS MITRAL VALVE REPAIR

There has been intense interest over the past decade in developing percutaneous catheter-based techniques to manage valvular heart disease.[1–4] Although the success has been rapid to the point of being disruptive in catheter treatment of aortic stenosis, progress has been much more modest in correcting mitral regurgitation (MR) percutaneously.[5] The success of catheter-based treatment of aortic stenosis can be attributed to a singular pathophysiology of the disease and the successful development of delivery systems and techniques to treat this disorder using conventional imaging techniques. The field of percutaneous mitral valve repair, however, has not progressed nearly as rapidly for a host of reasons. These include the complex pathophysiology of MR with diverse causes as well as challenging imaging and complex delivery issues. These obstacles have led to slower than anticipated clinical adoption of catheter-based approaches for the treatment of MR. To understand the potential for successful therapy, it is first instructive to examine the pathophysiology of the various mechanisms of the disease.

Pathophysiology of Mitral Regurgitation

The mitral valve is a complex structure composed of two leaflets, a fibrous annulus with varying degrees of continuity and integrity, and a subvalvular apparatus consisting of chordae tendinea and papillary muscles attached to the wall of the left ventricle (LV). The causes of mitral regurgitation range from intrinsic disease of the leaflets mainly owing to degenerative disease or fibroelastic deficiency in patients with mitral valve prolapse, although connective tissue diseases, including Barlow's syndrome, also occur, to functional mitral regurgitation (FMR) in which the valve is anatomically normal but stretched because of tethering and annular dilatation.[6] Although the mitral regurgitation in intrinsic disease occurs initially as leaflet disease, secondary annular dilatation occurs in the large majority of patients by the time they present for treatment. The larger proportion of patients with mitral regurgitation, however, are those without intrinsic disease of the leaflets, or FMR. FMR is not a primary valvular pathology but a secondary one caused by ventricular dilation, which leads to apical and lateral distraction of the papillary muscles tethering the mitral leaflets causing central regurgitation owing to failure of coaptation during systole of the anatomically normal leaflets[7] (Fig. 45-1). The causes and prognosis are inherently different from intrinsic disease. Although annular dilatation also occurs in this disease, it also is a secondary phenomenon. Surgical correction of FMR is based upon overcorrection of the annular dilatation component by performing an undersized annuloplasty to restore leaflet coaptation.

Transcatheter Approaches to the Treatment of Mitral Regurgitation

There is a wide spectrum of ingenious devices and creative approaches to manage MR from a percutaneous or transcatheter approach[8] (Table 45-1). Most of these are based on techniques that have been developed and proved to be effective in open surgical mitral valve surgery. Examples include the edge-to-edge techniques, annular remodeling, and placement of artificial chords. However, the challenges in adapting these techniques to catheter-based treatment are significant and center mainly on device delivery and imaging. In addition, totally new concepts have also been developed, including a "mitral spacer" to augment leaflet coaptation and use of

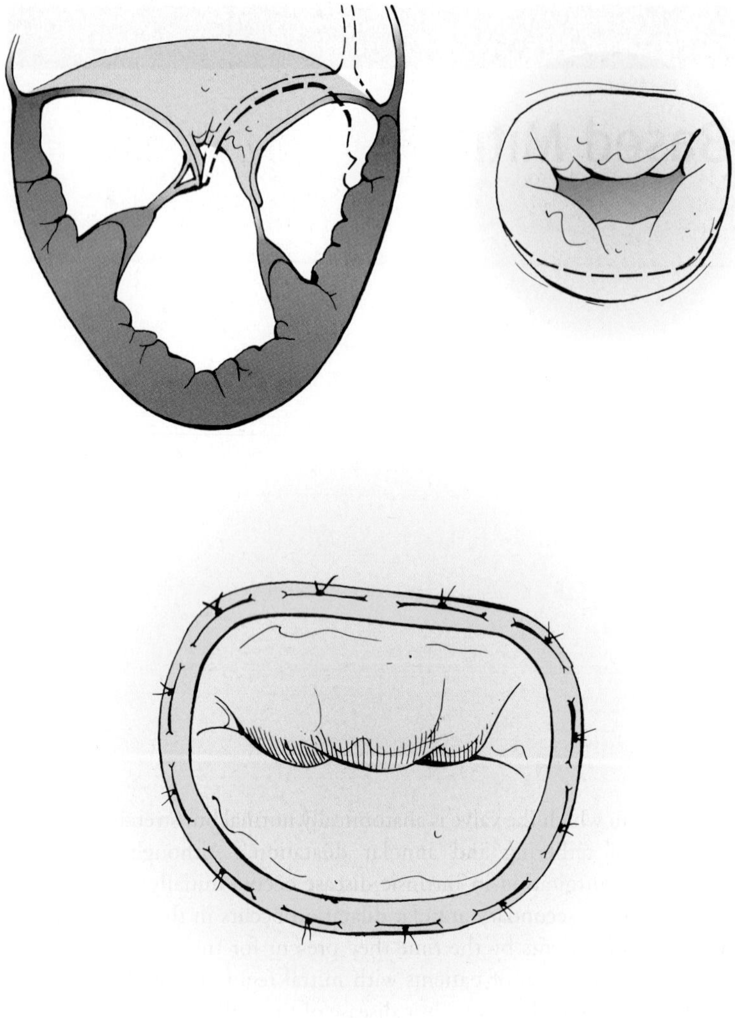

FIGURE 45-1 Pathophysiology of functional mitral regurgitation with concept of correction of leaflet malcoaptation by a complete and undersized ring annuloplasty.

external devices and energy sources to remodel the mitral annulus. Although some devices such as the Evalve MitraClip (Abbott Vascular, Irvine, CA) have been employed to treat both intrinsic disease as well as FMR, most of the devices have been designed to treat only one, with the majority devoted to FMR because of the larger clinical unmet need as well as the existence of excellent surgical repair techniques for intrinsic disease. This chapter reviews the procedures and devices for the management of degenerative mitral disease.

TABLE 45-1 Concepts of Transcatheter Techniques for the Management of Mitral Regurgitation

Degenerative Disease
Edge-to-edge repair
Artificial chord placement
Functional
Edge-to-edge repair
Coronary sinus annuloplasty
Direct annuloplasty
Indirect annuloplasty
Extracardiac annuloplasty
Mitral "spacer"
Mitral valve replacement

Percutaneous Techniques for Degenerative Disease of the Mitral Leaflets

Percutaneous Edge-to-Edge Repair

Two devices have been developed based on the surgical edge-to-edge repair technique of Alfieri (Fig. 45-2).[9] The Evalve MitraClip and the Mobius Mitral leaflet repair system (Edwards Lifesciences, Irvine, CA) both simulate the Alfieri surgical edge-to-edge repair technique; the former by placement of a clip between the free edges of the anterior and posterior leaflets, and the latter by employing a suture-based system.[10,11] The Mobius device underwent an early clinical feasibility trial in 15 patients, and because of disappointing results and arduous delivery and placement, further development of this device was abandoned. Modification of this device to create artificial chords attached to the free edge of the leaflet is now being developed.

The Evalve MitraClip system is a catheter-based device designed to perform endovascular reconstruction of the regurgitant mitral valve while the heart is beating. It includes a clip device (MitraClip) and a delivery system that is a steerable guide catheter that enables placement of the clip on the free edges of the mitral valve leaflets, resulting in permanent leaflet approximate approximation and a double orifice mitral valve (Fig. 45-3). The procedure is

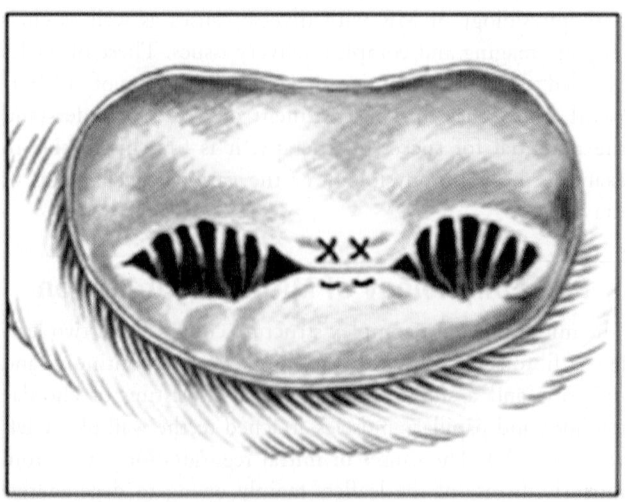

FIGURE 45-2 Concept of correction of mitral regurgitation by attaching the free edges if the mitral leaflets, creating a double orifice valve.

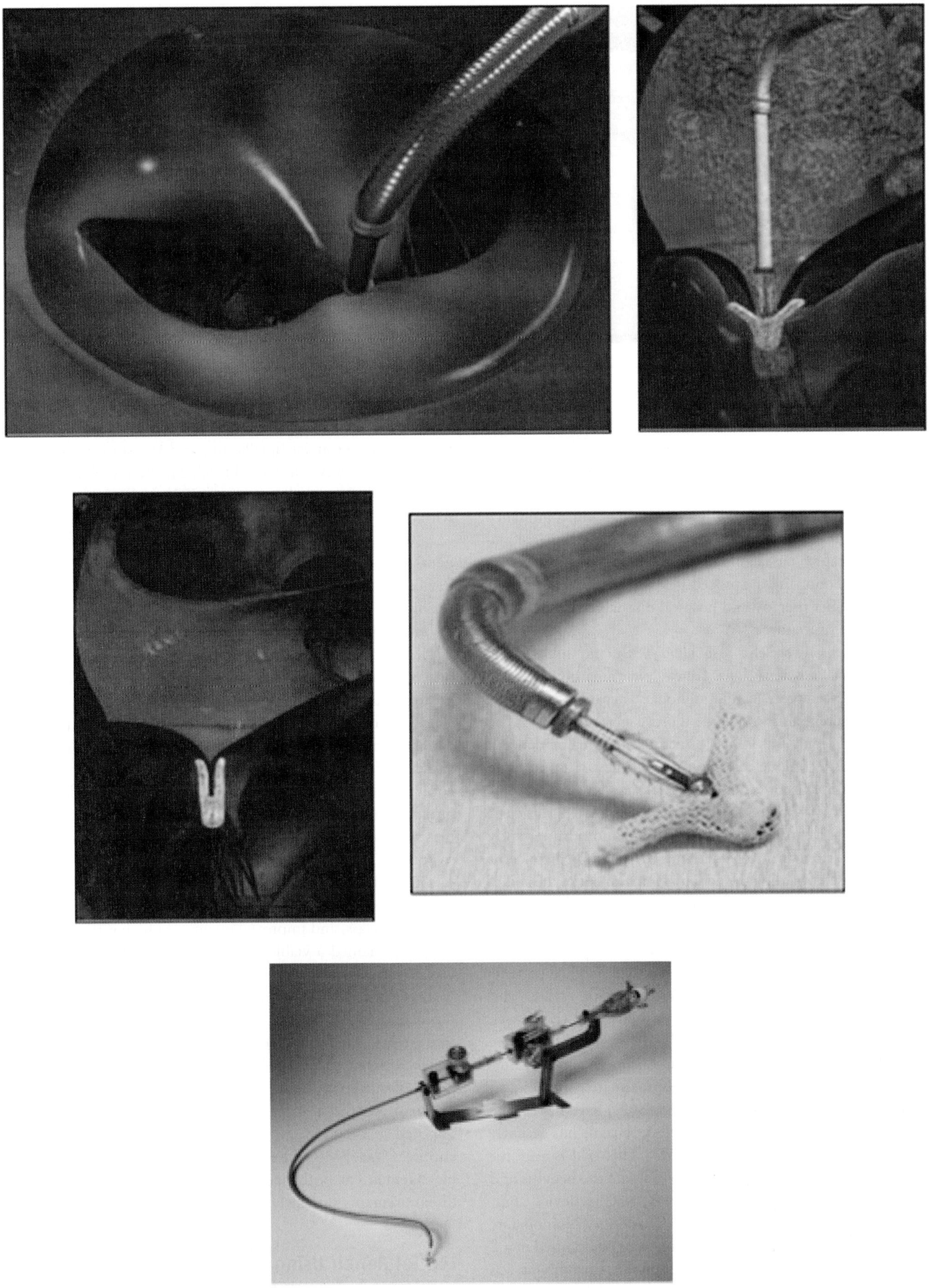

FIGURE 45-3 The Evalve MitraClip with delivery system. (*Reproduced with permission from Abbott Laboratories, Abbott Park, IL.*)

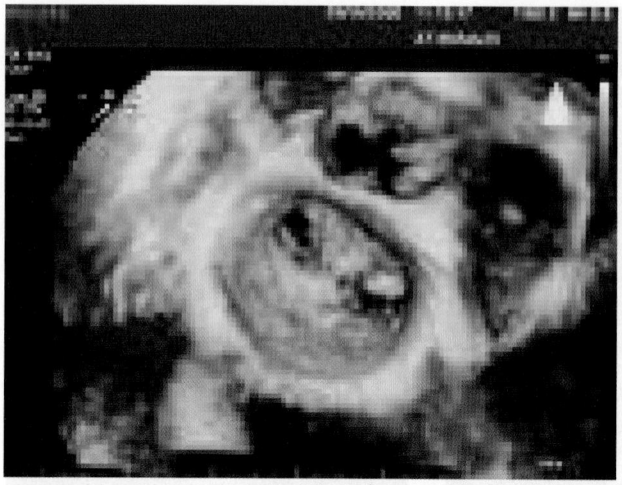

FIGURE 45-4 Three-dimensional echocardiogram demonstrating the MitraClip in position. (*Reproduced with permission from Abbott Laboratories, Abbott Park, IL.*)

performed percutaneously via the femoral vein in a cardiac catheterization laboratory with echocardiographic guidance under general anesthesia. The addition of three-dimensional echocardiography has significantly facilitated the procedure (Fig. 45-4). Following the procedure, patients are treated with dual antiplatelet therapy and hospital discharge is usually the day after the procedure.

The potential benefit associated with the use of the MitraClip includes repairing MR while eliminating the need for open chest surgery, cardiopulmonary bypass, and cardiac arrest. The potential risks include those associated with cardiac catheterization and transseptal puncture. The major concern regarding this technique centers on the efficacy of a procedure with a less complete correction of the MR than is usually accomplished surgically. Whether partial reduction of MR is sufficient to translate to ventricular remodeling and more importantly clinical benefit remains to be determined. Additional concerns have been raised regarding the potential impairment of the ability to perform a subsequent surgical valve repair should that prove necessary.[12]

Evalve MitraClip has undergone significant clinical testing over the past 7 years. As of early 2010 a total of 1316 patients had been entered into the various clinical trials and registries.[13–15] In the initial clinical feasibility trial (Everest I), 55 patients were enrolled with safety and efficacy of the device demonstrated. Subsequent high-risk, European, and continued access registries have enrolled approximately 1000 additional patients, the majority of whom (~80%) have FMR. The pivotal trial of this system, the Everest II trial, has recently been completed and results presented.[16] This trial is a multicenter randomized controlled trial to evaluate the benefits and risks of mitral valve repair using the MitraClip device compared with open mitral valve surgery in patients with moderate or severe mitral regurgitation. Patients were randomized in a 2 to 1 ratio of device versus mitral valve surgery. Enrollment was 279 patients at 37 sites with 184 patients receiving the device and 95 patients receiving surgical repair or replacement. There were very specific anatomical criteria, including moderate or severe MR defined as 3 to 4+, with the primary regurgitant jet originating from between the A2 and P2 scallops. Important exclusion criteria included ejection fraction less than 25% and left ventricular and systolic dimension greater than 55 mm. The width of the flail segment could not be greater than 15 mm nor was the flail gap greater than 10 mm. If leaflet tethering was present, a coaptation depth of greater than 11 mm or a vertical co-optation length less than 2 mm would be excluded. Severe mitral annular calcification, calcification of the leaflets, a significant cleft in the A2 or P2 scallops, and bileaflet flail or severe bileaflet prolapse were also excluded.

There were both safety and efficacy primary end points in the randomized trial. The primary safety end point was major adverse event rate at 30 days on a per-protocol analysis based upon a superiority hypothesis. Predefined major adverse events included death, major stroke, reoperation of the mitral valve, urgent or emergent cardiovascular surgery, myocardial infarction, renal failure, wound infection, prolonged ventilation, new onset atrial fibrillation, and transfusion of greater than or equal to two units of blood. The major adverse events in the surgical control arm were 657% at 30 days compared with 9.6% in the device arm for an observed absolute difference of 47.4%. Although transfusion was the major component of the composite safety end point in the surgical arm, the device still met noninferiority hypothesis criteria even if transfusion was eliminated.

The primary effectiveness end point was based on the clinical success rate defined as freedom from the combined outcome of death, mitral valve surgery or reoperation, or greater than 2+ mitral regurgitation at 12 months. It also was a per-protocol analysis, but on a noninferiority hypothesis. The trial also met the noninferiority hypothesis of clinical success rate at 12 months. The clinical success rate in the control group was 87.8% compared with 72.4% in the device group. The absolute observed difference of 15.4% met the prespecified margin of 31%, satisfying the noninferiority hypothesis.

Patient benefit was also demonstrated in the trial as defined by improved left ventricular ejection function, improved NYHA functional class, and improved quality of life. For the most part surgery remained a viable option after a MitraClip procedure was performed.

Experience with this device is ongoing in a continued access protocol, which will allow enrollment until the results of this trial are presented to the Food and Drug Administration expert panel expected to be late 2010. Approximately 70% of the patients currently being enrolled in the continued access protocol are those with functional mitral regurgitation, as opposed to the randomized trial, in which only 20% of the enrollees had FMR. The ultimate role of this device in the management of both patients with intrinsic and functional disease remains presently unclear.[17]

Leaflet Repair Using Artificial Chords

Another unique concept for repair of the prolapsing or flail mitral leaflet percutaneously is placement of artificial chords by

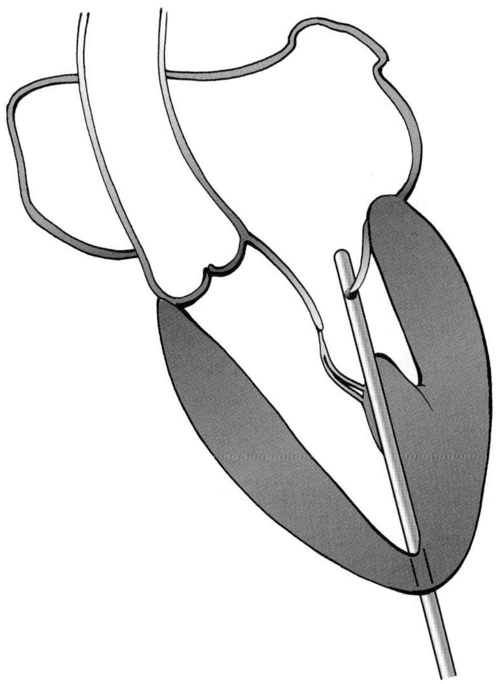

FIGURE 45-5 Placement of artificial chords from the left ventricular apex under echocardiographic guidance.

a transapical approach. The access for this procedure is a left minithoracotomy through which a pursestring is placed at the apex of the heart. A delivery device that contains an infrared sensor grasps the edge of the prolapsing leaflet. Using the device a suture is passed through the grasped free edge. The two ends of the suture that are passed through the edge of the leaflet are then brought through the apex of the heart and tied on the epicardial surface (Fig. 45-5). Proper chordal length is determined by adjustment under echocardiographic guidance. The chords can be either lengthened or shortened based on the color jet seen on echo. Early clinical feasibility testing with this device is currently under way in Europe with eight patients enrolled in a 30-patient feasibility trial.

Functional Mitral Regurgitation

Functional mitral regurgitation when treated surgically is most commonly managed by reduction in the septal lateral diameter of the dilated mitral annulus by an undersized, complete, and rigid annuloplasty ring. Although there is dilatation of the whole mitral annulus in patients with FMR, the greatest degree of dilation is in the posterior annulus and the greatest increase in dimension is in the septal lateral (or anterior posterior) diameter.[18,19] A key element of this surgical repair includes anchoring a complete ring to the central fibrous skeleton of the heart at the fibrous trigones. Anchoring the ring away from the mitral annulus in the atrial wall or in the leaflet tissue leads to less effective reduction in annular dimensions. Similarly, it has been well proved in the surgical arena that a partial posterior annuloplasty is less effective in annular reduction and treating mitral regurgitation.[20–22] Correction of the septal lateral diameter by as little as 5 to 8 mm has been demonstrated to reconstitute leaflet coaptation and improve MR. Transcatheter approaches to FMR are based on this concept of remodeling the mitral annulus with the goal of decreasing the septal lateral diameter. There is no shortage of ingenious strategies to accomplish this goal[23–28] (see Table 45-1). Some devices take advantage of the anatomical relationship between the coronary sinus and posterior mitral annulus. Other devices take a direct approach to plicating the posterior annulus; still others rely on distraction of the left ventricle or left atrial walls to decrease the septal lateral diameter.

Coronary Sinus Annuloplasty

The close proximity of the coronary sinus to the posterior mitral annulus has served as an attractive entrée for placement of devices to remodel the mitral valve[29–33] (Fig. 45-6). The easy access by a transvenous route led to great early optimism. However, the variability in the relationship of the coronary sinus to the mitral annulus has been problematic in obtaining consistent decrease in annular dimensions. Although most commonly the coronary sinus is located adjacent to the posterior annulus, it is frequently located along the free wall of the left atrium and superior to the mitral annulus.[34,35] The smallest separation between the coronary sinus in the mitral annulus is usually at the entry to the sinus. Separation of the coronary sinus from the mitral annulus is maximal at the posterolateral commissure, as demonstrated in an anatomical study by Miselli of coronary sinus anatomy in 61 human cadaver hearts.[36] The distances between the inferior border of the coronary sinus and the mitral annulus at the P2 and P3 mitral segments averaged 9.7 mm. It is important to note that in patients with severe MR, the distance between the coronary sinus and the mitral annulus is usually much greater compared with patients without severe regurgitation. In addition, the relationship between

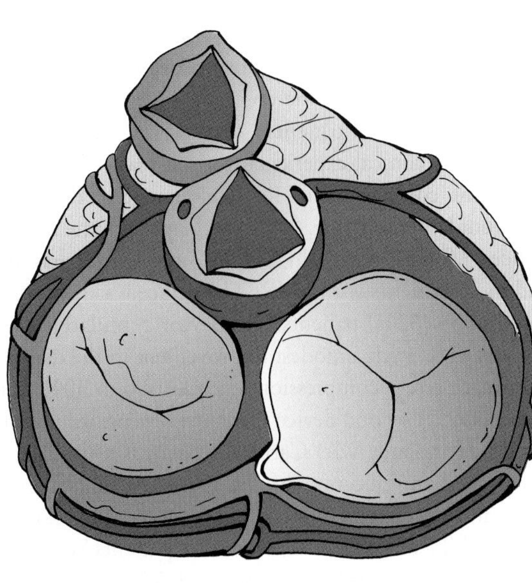

FIGURE 45-6 Concept of a posterior mitral annulus plication performed by a device placed through the coronary sinus.

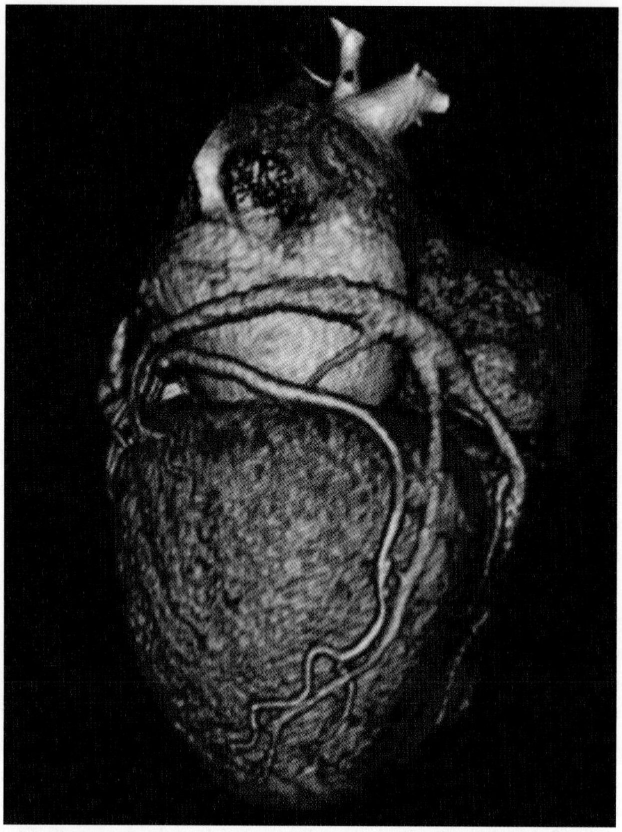

FIGURE 45-7 Example demonstrating by computerized tomography the relationships between the coronary sinus and the mitral annulus. Note the intervening circumflex coronary artery. (*Reproduced with permission from Choure AJ, Garcia MJ, Hesse B, et al: In vivo analysis of the anatomical relationship of coronary sinus to mitral annulus and left circumflex coronary artery using cardiac multidetector computed tomography: implications for percutaneous coronary sinus mitral annuloplasty. J Am Coll Cardiol 2006; 48:1938-1945.*)

the circumflex coronary artery or its branches intervening between the coronary sinus and mitral annulus is of significant concern. The left circumflex artery or major branches has been reported to course between the coronary sinus and the mitral annulus in up to 80% of patients[37] (Fig. 45-7).

There now is clinical experience with at least three devices that access the coronary sinus for deployment of devices for posterior annular remodeling.[38–42] Experience with the Edwards Lifesciences Monarc device in the Evolution Trial has been reported in 72 patients with FMR. The device was successfully implanted in 59 (82%) patients. The 1-year cumulative event-free rate was 81%, with a modest improvement in the degree of MR. Coronary artery compression has occurred in 30% of the implanted cases. A second device Cardiac Dimensions (Cardiac Dimensions, Kirkland, WA) Carillon System is a fixed-length device designed for plication of the coronary sinus between deployable anchors placed via internal jugular access. In two trials, Amadeus and Titan trials, a total of 113 patients with FMR have been attempted. Implant success rate is 58% (66/113).[39,40] The primary end point was 30-day major adverse events, and secondary end points included decrease MR severity. At 30 days the major adverse event rate was 13% and there was reduction in only two of the four parameters used to measure degree of MR. There was a modest improvement on patients' 6-minute walk tests. Coronary artery compression occurred in 12% of cases. Although the study was declared successful by the investigators, the accompanying editorial expressed a much more modest interpretation of the results.[39,40]

The third device is the Viacor (Viacor, Inc., Wilmington, MA) PTMA system, in which a distributed anatomical bending with variable diameter nitinol rods are delivered through subclavian access.[41,42] This has been tested in 27 patients with FMR in the Ptolemy Trial. The device was successfully implanted in 13 (48%) patients attempted.

Direct Mitral Annular Remodeling

There are a number of devices designed to remodel the mitral annulus by direct plication The Mitralign system (Mitralign, Inc., Tewksbury, MA), which is placed retrograde through the aortic valve on the ventricular side of the mitral annulus performs suture-based placation of the posterior annulus. Two sutures are placed in two locations placating P1-P2 and P2-P3 (Fig. 45-8). The GDS Accucinch (Guided Delivery Systems, Santa Clara, CA) selectively places a tensioning wire directly into the posterior mitral annulus. Another device, the Valtech Cardioband (Valtech, Inc., Tel Aviv, Israel) places a tensioning member anchored by screws placed into the mitral annulus. The tensioning band is then adjusted under echocardiographic guidance until the regurgitant jet disappears. Other systems include the Mitral Solutions (Fort Lauderdale, FL) Cordis DPA, and MiCardia for direct annular plication.

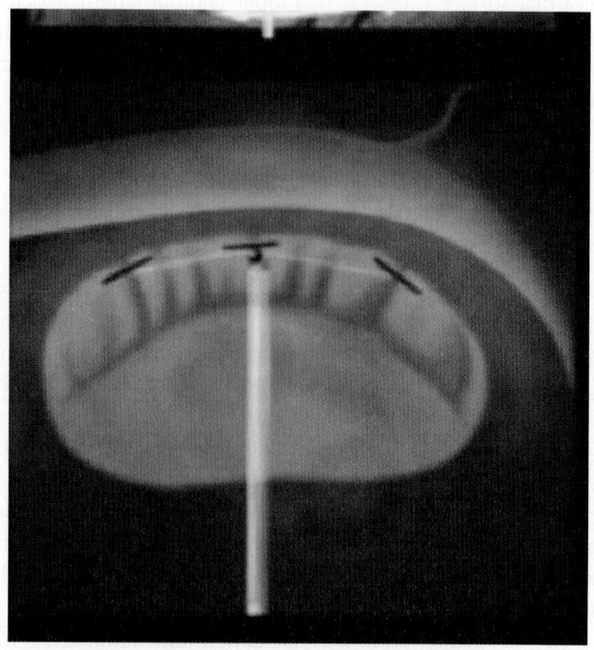

FIGURE 45-8 Plication of the posterior mitral annulus by a percutaneous transventricular approach. (*Reproduced with permission from Mitralign, Inc., Tewksbury, MA.*)

Another interesting concept that is still in the preclinical proof of concept stage is the QuantumCor (QuantumCor, Inc., Lake Forest, CA) device. This concept is designed to remodel the posterior mitral annulus by delivery of radiofrequency energy directly to the posterior annulus causing shrinkage. A similar concept uses radiofrequency energy to shrink the mitral leaflet and/or chords.[43]

Indirect Mitral Annuloplasty

Another concept is that of indirect annuloplasty. This conception relies on compression of either the left ventricle or the left atrium to distract the mitral annulus and decrease the septal lateral diameter and thus the degree of mitral regurgitation.[44–50] Both of the devices pursuing this concept, i-Coapsys for the ventricle and Ample Medical for the atrium, have been shelved after early human feasibility studies.

Other Concepts

Other intriguing concepts include cinching devices placed in an extracardiac location to compress the anteroposterior diameter of the mitral annulus. The devices are placed by a thoracoscopic transpericardial approach and placed on the atrioventricular groove causing compression of the annulus. These C-shaped devices have undergone animal proof of concept testing and early human trials in open surgical settings during concomitant CABG.

Another unique concept is the placement of a prosthetic "spacer" into the mitral valve orifice (Fig. 45-9). With this concept, a prosthetic device anchored in the apex of the left ventricle fills the regurgitant space in the mitral valve orifice. Rather than repairing the mitral regurgitation by leaflet-to-leaflet coaptation, leaflet-to-device-to-leaflet coaptation is the mechanism of intended correction.

Percutaneous Mitral Valve Replacement

The last and perhaps most intriguing concept for the percutaneous treatment of functional mitral regurgitation is mitral valve replacement (Fig. 45-10). One of the issues with surgical annuloplasty for the treatment of FMR is the subsequent recurrence of regurgitation as the left ventricle continues to dilate. Although the annuloplasty performed by either a surgical or percutaneous approach completely corrected the regurgitation at the time of the index procedure, the ongoing ventricular disease process causes further dilation, causing further tethering of the papillary muscles and free edges of the leaflets, causing a recurrence of the regurgitation. The concept of mitral valve replacement rather than repair would theoretically prevent recurrence of mitral regurgitation if further left ventricular dilation occurs. This concept of surgical mitral valve replacement with preservation of the mitral leaflets and subvalvular apparatus compared with ring annuloplasty is the current subject of a National Institutes of Health Cardiothoracic Surgery Network randomized trial.

Two devices, Endovalve (Endovalve, Inc., Princeton, NJ) and CardiAQ (CardiAQ, Inc., Irvine, CA) have been developed to perform percutaneous valve sparing mitral valve replacement. In both of these concepts a delivery system placed from the femoral vein across the interatrial septum under fluoroscopic and echocardiographic guidance positions a valve in the mitral annulus. A nitinol-based anchoring system is deployed to keep the valve in place. Both of these devices have undergone proof of concept animal testing. Numerous issues exist, including the complexity of the delivery system, mechanisms of anchoring, and then translation of these concepts into the clinical arena.

In summary, there are a host of unique and intriguing concepts for the transcatheter treatment of mitral regurgitation. Although progress in the transcatheter treatment of aortic stenosis has rapid and promising, progress with mitral regurgitation has been much slower. There are a host of reasons for this, including complex valvular anatomy, variable pathology,

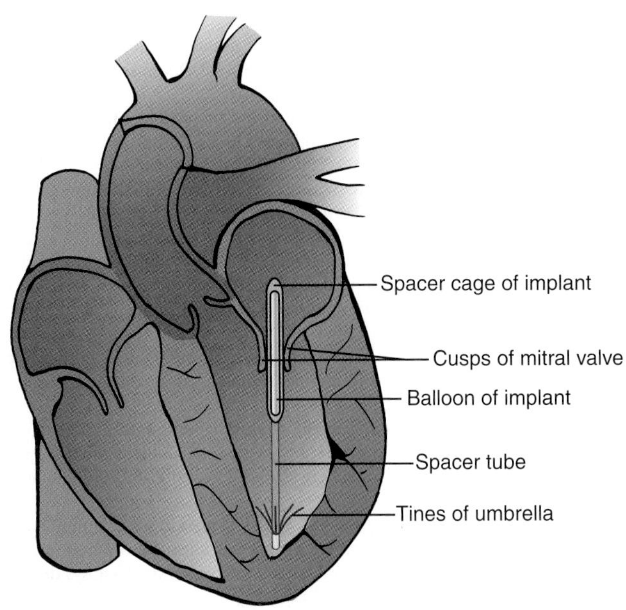

FIGURE 45-9 Placement of a "spacer" anchored in the left ventricular apex to fill the gap between the noncoapting leaflets.

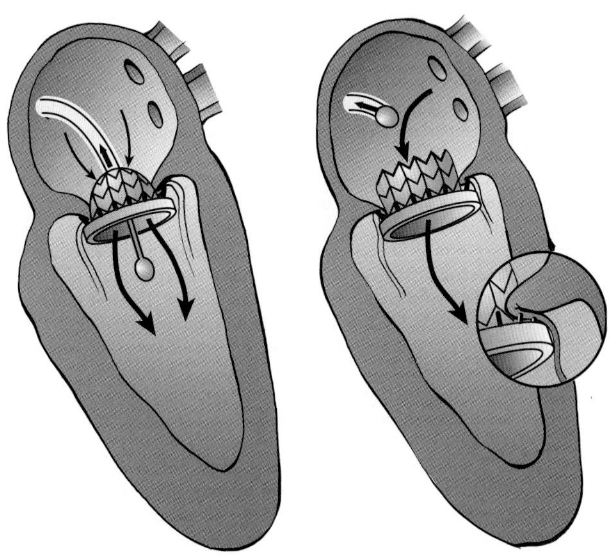

FIGURE 45-10 Concept of percutaneous mitral valve replacement.

the necessity for complex delivery systems, limited early success in clinical trials, and the existence of effective established therapy. In addition, trial design has proved problematic, with the ability to demonstrate clinical benefit a significant challenge. However, the clinical unmet need is huge and with a host of unique concepts significant progress can be expected. However, the timeline will be a long one and none of these devices will have a significant clinical impact on the management of patients with mitral regurgitation in the near future.

REFERENCES

1. Feldman T: Percutaneous mitral valve repair. *J Interv Cardiol* 2007; 20:488- 494.
2. Carabello BA: The current therapy for mitral regurgitation. *J Am Coll Cardiol* 2008; 52:319-326.
3. Mack M: Fool me once, shame on you; fool me twice, shame on me! A perspective on the emerging world of percutaneous heart valve therapy. *J Thorac Cardiovasc Surg* 2008; 136:816-819.
4. Masson JB, Webb JD: Percutaneous treatment of mitral regurgitation. *Circ Cardiovasc Interv* 2009; 2:140-146.
5. Mack M: Percutaneous treatment of mitral regurgitation: so near, yet so far! *J Thorac Cardiovasc Surg* 2008; 135:237-239.
6. Carpentier A: Cardiac valve surgery—the "French correction." *J Thorac Cardiovasc Surg*1983; 86(3):323-337.
7. Bach DS, Bolling SF: Improvement following correction of secondary mitral regurgitation in end-stage cardiomyopathy with mitral annuloplasty. *Am J Cardiol* 1996; 78(8):966-969.
8. Fedak PW, McCarthy PM, Bonow RO: Evolving concepts and technologies in mitral valve repair. *Circulation* 2008; 117:963-974.
9. Alfieri O, Elefteriades JA, Chapolini RJ, et al: Novel suture device for beating heart mitral leaflet approximation. *Ann Thorac Surg* 2002; 74(5):14.
10. Feldman T, Wasserman HS, Herrmann HC, et al: Percutaneous mitral valve repair using the edge-to-edge technique: six-month results of the EVEREST Phase I Clinical Trial. *J Am Coll Cardiol* 2005; 46(11):2134-2140.
11. Herrmann HC, Rohatgi S, Wasserman HS, et al: Mitral valve hemodynamic effects of percutaneous edge-to-edge repair with the MitraClip device for mitral regurgitation. *Catheter Cardiovasc Interv* 2006; 68:821-828.
12. Dang NC, Aboodi MS, Sakaguchi T, et al: Surgical revision after percutaneous mitral valve repair with a clip: initial multicenter experience. *Ann Thorac Surg* 2005; 80(6):233.
13. Feldman T, Glower D: Patient selection for percutaneous mitral valve repair: insight from early clinical trial applications. *Nat Clin Pract Cardiovasc Med* 2008; 5:84-90.
14. Condado JA, Acquatella H, Rodriguez L, et al: Percutaneous edge-to-edge mitral valve repair: 2-year follow-up in the first human case. *Catheter Cardiovasc Interv* 2006; 67:323-325.
15. Tamburino C, Ussia GP: Percutaneous mitral valve repair with the MitraClip system: acute results from a real world setting. *Eur Heart J* 2010; 31(11):1382-1389.
16. Feldman T: Endovascular Valve Edge-to-Edge REpair Study (EVEREST II) randomized clinical trial: primary safety and efficacy endpoints. Presented at American College of Cardiology Annual Meeting, Atlanta, GA, March, 2010.
17. Vahanian A, Iung B: Edge to edge percutaneous mitral valve repair in mitral regurgitation: it can be done but should it be done? *Eur Heart J* 2010; 31(11):1301-1304.
18. Wu AH, Aaronson KD, Bolling SF, et al: Impact of mitral valve annuloplasty on mortality risk in patients with mitral regurgitation and left ventricular systolic dysfunction. *J Am Coll Cardiol* 2005; 45(3):381-387.
19. Acker MA, Bolling S, Shemin R, et al: Mitral valve surgery in heart failure: insights from the Acorn Clinical Trial. *J Thorac Cardiovasc Surg* 2006; 132(3):568-577, 577.e1-4.
20. Nguyen TC, Cheng A, Tibayan FA, et al: Septal-lateral annular cinching perturbs basal left ventricular transmural strains. *Eur J Cardiothorac Surg* 2007; 31(3):423-429.
21. Mihaljevic T, Lam BK, Rajeswaran J, et al: Impact of mitral valve annuloplasty combined with revascularization in patients with functional ischemic mitral regurgitation. *J Am Coll Cardiol* 2007; 49(22):2191-2201.
22. Ruiz CE, Kronzon I: The wishful thinking of indirect mitral annuloplasty: will it ever become a reality? *Circ Cardiovasc Intervent* 2009; 2:271-272.
23. Duffy SJ, Federman J, Farrington C, et al: Feasibility and short-term efficacy of percutaneous mitral annular reduction for the therapy of functional mitral regurgitation in patients with heart failure. *Catheter Cardiovasc Interv* 2006; 68:205-210.
24. Dubreuil O, Basmadjian A, Ducharme A, et al: Percutaneous mitral valve annuloplasty for ischemic mitral regurgitation: first in man experience with a temporary implant. *Catheter Cardiovasc Interv* 2007; 69(7):1053-1061.
25. Duffy SJ, Federman J, Farrington C, et al: Feasibility and short-term efficacy of percutaneous mitral annular reduction for the therapy of functional mitral regurgitation in patients with heart failure. *Catheter Cardiovasc Interv* 2006; 68:205-210.
26. Fukamachi K: Percutaneous and off-pump treatments for functional mitral regurgitation. *J Artif Organs* 2008; 11:12-18.
27. Kaye DM, Byrne M, Alferness C, Power J: Feasibility and short-term efficacy of percutaneous mitral annular reduction for the therapy of heart failure-induced mitral regurgitation. *Circulation* 2003; 108:1795-1797.
28. Mack MJ: Coronary sinus in the management of functional mitral regurgitation: the mother lode or fool's gold? *Circulation* 2006; 114:363-364.
29. Sorajja P, Nishimura RA, Thompson J, Zehr K: A novel method of percutaneous mitral valve repair for ischaemic mitral regurgitation. *J Am Coll Cardiol Intv* 2008; 1:663-672.
30. Tops LF, Kapadia SR, Tuzcu EM, et al: Percutaneous valve procedure: an update. *Curr Probl Cardiol* 2008; 33:409-458.
31. Sack S, Kahlert P, et al: Percutaneous transvenous mitral annuloplasty: initial human experience with a novel coronary sinus implant device. *Circ Cardiovasc Interv* 2009; 2:277-284.
32. Webb JG, Harnek J, Munt BI, et al: Percutaneous transvenous mitral annuloplasty: initial human experience with device implantation in the coronary sinus. *Circulation* 2006; 113(6):851-855.
33. Piazza N, Bonan R: Transcatheter mitral valve repair for functional mitral regurgitation: coronary sinus approach. *J Interv Cardiol* 2007; 20:495-508.
34. Tops LF, Van de Veire NR, Schuijf JD, et al: Noninvasive evaluation of coronary sinus anatomy and its relation to the mitral valve annulus: implications for percutaneous mitral annuloplasty. *Circulation* 2007; 115(11): 1426-1432.
35. Lansac E, Di Centa I, Al Attar N, et al: Percutaneous mitral annuloplasty through the coronary sinus: an anatomic point of view. *J Thorac Cardiovasc Surg* 2008; 135:376-381.
36. Maselli D, Guarracino F, Chiaramonti F, et al: Percutaneous mitral annuloplasty: an anatomic study of human coronary sinus and its relation with mitral valve annulus and coronary arteries. *Circulation* 2006; 114(5):377-380.
37. Choure AJ, Garcia MJ, Hesse B, et al: In vivo analysis of the anatomical relationship of coronary sinus to mitral annulus and left circumflex coronary artery using cardiac multidetector computed tomography: implications for percutaneous coronary sinus mitral annuloplasty. *J Am Coll Cardiol* 2006; 48:1938-1945.
38. Siminiak T, Firek L, Jerzykowska O, et al: Percutaneous valve repair for mitral regurgitation using the Carillon Mitral Contour System. Description of the method and case report. *Kardiol Pol* 2007; 65(3):272-278 [discussion: 279].
39. Schofer J, Siminiak T, et al: Percutaneous mitral annuloplasty for functional mitral regurgitation: results of the CARILLON mitral annuloplasty device. *EU Study Circ* 2009; 120:326-333.
40. Bach DS: Functional mitral regurgitation and transcatheter mitral annuloplasty: The Carillon Mitral Annuloplasty Device European Union Study in perspective. *Circulation* 2009; 120:272-274.
41. Sack S, Kahlert P, et al: Percutaneous transvenous mitral annuloplasty: initial human experience with a novel coronary sinus implant device. *Circ Cardiovasc Intervent* 2009; 2:277-284.
42. Dubreuil O, Basmadjian A, Ducharme A, et al: Percutaneous mitral valve annuloplasty for ischemic mitral regurgitation: first in man experience with a temporary implant. *Catheter Cardiovasc Interv* 2007; 69(7): 1053-1061.
43. Williams JL, Toyoda Y, Ota T, et al: Feasibility of myxomatous mitral valve repair using direct leaflet and chordal radiofrequency ablation. *J Interv Cardiol* 2008; 21(6):547-554.
44. Fukamachi K, Inoue M, Popovic ZB, et al: Off-pump mitral valve repair using the Coapsys device: a pilot study in a pacing-induced mitral regurgitation model. *Ann Thorac Surg* 2004; 77(2):688-692 [discussion: 692-693].
45. Fukamachi K, Popovic ZB, Inoue M, et al: Changes in mitral annular and left ventricular dimensions and left ventricular pressure-volume relations after off pump treatment of mitral regurgitation with the Coapsys device. *Eur J Cardiothorac Surg* 2004; 25(3):352-357.
46. Fukamachi K: Percutaneous and off-pump treatments for functional mitral regurgitation. *J Artif Organs* 2008; 11:12-18.

47. Fukamachi K, Inoue M, Popovic ZB, et al: Off-pump mitral valve repair using the Coapsys device: a pilot study in a pacing-induced mitral regurgitation model. *Ann Thorac Surg* 2004; 77(2):688-692 [discussion: 692-693].
48. Inoue M, McCarthy PM, Popovic ZB, et al: The Coapsys device to treat functional mitral regurgitation: in vivo long-term canine study. *J Thorac Cardiovasc Surg* 2004; 127(4):1068-1076 [discussion: 1076-1077].
49. Grossi EA, Woo YJ, Schwartz CF, et al: Comparison of Coapsys annuloplasty and internal reduction mitral annuloplasty in the randomized treatment of functional ischemic mitral regurgitation: impact on the left ventricle. *J Thorac Cardiovasc Surg* 2006; 131:1095-1098.
50. Grossi EA, Saunders PC, Woo YJ, et al: Intraoperative effects of the Coapsys annuloplasty system in a randomized evaluation (RESTOR-MV) of functional ischemic mitral regurgitation. *Ann Thorac Surg* 2005; 80:1706-1711.

PART 4C

VALVULAR HEART DISEASE (OTHER)

CHAPTER 46

Tricuspid Valve Disease

Richard J. Shemin

INTRODUCTION

The tricuspid valve consists of three leaflets (anterior, posterior, and septal), the chordae tendinea, two discrete papillary muscles, the fibrous tricuspid annulus, and the right atrial and right ventricular myocardium (Fig. 46-1A). Valve function depends on coordination of all these components. The anterior leaflet is the largest. The septal leaflet is the smallest and arises medially directly from the tricuspid annulus above the interventricular septum. Because the small septal wall leaflet is fixed and is relatively spared from annular dilation, tricuspid annular sizing has been based on the dimension of the base of the septal leaflet.[1,2] The posterior leaflet often has multiple scallops. The anterior papillary muscle provides chordae to the anterior and posterior leaflets, and the medial papillary muscle provides chordae to the posterior and septal leaflets. The septal wall gives chordae to the anterior and septal leaflets. There may be accessory chordal attachments to the right ventricular free wall and the moderator band.

Right ventricular dysfunction and dilation lead to chordal tethering contributing to loss of leaflet apposition.[2] In addition, dilation of the free wall of the right ventricle results in tricuspid annular enlargement, primarily in its anterior/posterior (mural) aspect, resulting in significant functional TR (fTR) as a result of leaflet malcoaptation[3] (Fig. 46-1B).

The tricuspid annulus has a complex three-dimensional structure, which differs from the more symmetric "saddle-shaped" mitral annulus. The tricuspid annulus is dynamic and can change markedly with loading conditions. During the cardiac cycle, there is a ~20% reduction in annular circumference (~30% reduction in annular area) with atrial systole.[4,5] This distinct shape has implications for the design and application of currently available annuloplasty rings in the tricuspid position. Most commercially available rings or bands are essentially planar except for the Edwards MC^3 annuloplasty system.

Fukuda et al.[4] studied the shape and movement of the healthy and diseased tricuspid annulus performing a real-time three-dimensional transthoracic echocardiographic study. Healthy subjects had a nonplanar, elliptical-shaped tricuspid annulus, with the posteroseptal portion being "lowest" (toward the right ventricular apex) and the anteroseptal portion the "highest" (Fig. 46-2). Patients with functional TR generally had a more planar annulus, which was dilated primarily in the septal-lateral direction, resulting in a more circular shape as compared with the elliptical shape in healthy subjects.

CLINICAL PRESENTATION

The most common presentation of TR is secondary to cardiac valvular pathology (mostly mitral valve disease) on the left side of the heart. As pulmonary hypertension develops, leading to right ventricular dilatation, the tricuspid valve annulus will dilate. The circumference of the annulus lengthens primarily along the attachments of the anterior and posterior leaflets. The septal leaflet is fixed between the fibrous trigones, preventing lengthening (Fig. 46-1B). With progressive annular and ventricular dilatation, the chordal papillary muscle complex becomes functionally shortened, causing leaflet tethering. This combination prevents leaflet apposition, resulting in valvular incompetence.[6–9]

Eisenmenger syndrome and primary pulmonary hypertension lead to the same pathophysiology of progressive right ventricular dilatation, tricuspid annular enlargement, and valvular incompetence. A right ventricular infarction produces either disruption of the papillary muscle or a severe regional wall motion abnormality. This prevents normal leaflet apposition by a tethering effect on the leaflets. Marfan's syndrome and other variations of myxomatous disease affecting the mitral and tricuspid valves can lead to prolapsing leaflets, elongation of chordae, or chordal rupture, producing valvular incompetence.

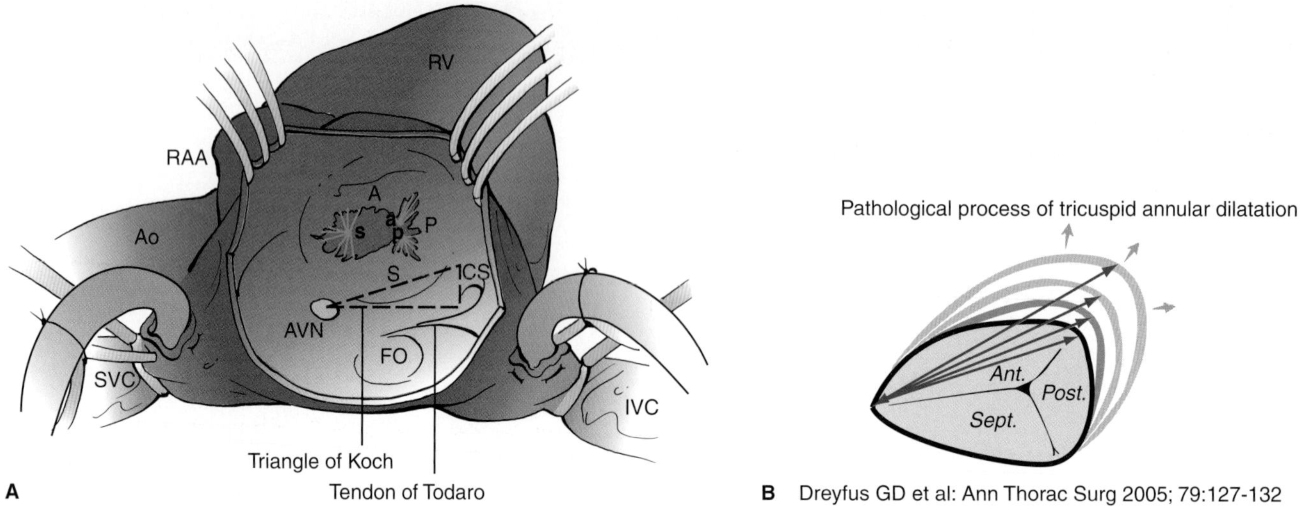

FIGURE 46-1 (A) Surgical view of the tricuspid valve complex. The tricuspid valve consists of three leaflets: anterior (A), posterior (P), and septal (S). There are two main papillary muscles, anterior (a) and posterior (p). The septal papillary muscle (s) is rudimentary, and chordae tendinea arise directly from the ventricular septum. Adjacent structures include the atrioventricular node (AVN), coronary sinus ostium (CS), and the tendon of Todaro, forming the triangle of Koch. *Ao = Aorta; FO = foramen ovale; IVC = inferior vena cava; RAA = right atrial appendage; RV = right ventricle; SVC = superior vena cava.* (B) *Direction of progressive tricuspid valve annular dilatation.* (*B reproduced, with permission, from Dreyfus GD et al: Ann Thorac Surg 2005; 79:127-132.*)

Blunt or penetrating chest trauma may disrupt the structural components of the tricuspid valve. Dilated cardiomyopathy in the late stages of biventricular failure and pulmonary hypertension produces TR.[10–13] Infectious endocarditis can destroy leaflet tissue, mostly in drug addicts with staphylococcal infection.[14–16]

The carcinoid syndrome leads to either focal or diffuse deposits of fibrous tissue on the endocardium of valve cusps, cardiac chambers, intima of the great vessels, and coronary sinus. The white fibrous carcinoid plaques, if present on the ventricular side of the tricuspid valve cusps, adhere the leaflet tissue to the right ventricular wall, preventing leaflet coaptation.[17–19] Rheumatic disease of the tricuspid valve is always associated with mitral valve involvement, and the deformity of the tricuspid tissue results in a tricuspid valve stenosis as well as regurgitation[20] (Table 46-1).

A unique cause of TR is the result of pacemaker or defibrillator leads, which cross from the right atrium into the right ventricle and may directly interfere with leaflet coaptation. This

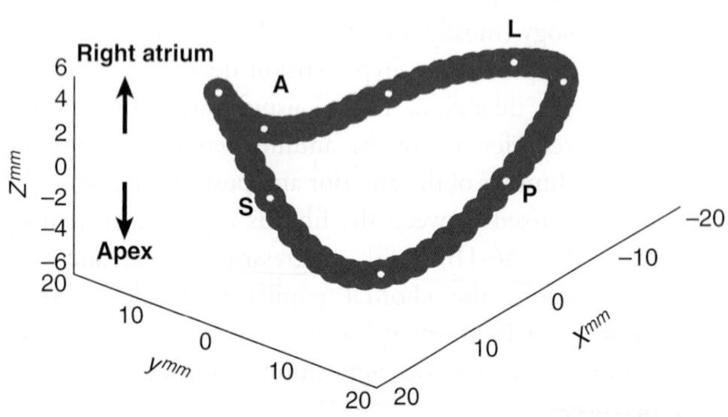

FIGURE 46-2 Three-dimensional shape of the tricuspid annulus based on a three-dimensional transthoracic echocardiographic study in healthy subjects. Note that the annulus is not planar and an optimally shaped annuloplasty ring may need to mimic this configuration. A indicates anterior; L, lateral; P, posterior; S, septal. (*Copyright 2006, the American Heart Association. Reproduced with permission from Fukuda S, Saracino G, Matsumura Y, et al: Three-dimensional geometry of the tricuspid annulus in healthy subjects and in patients with functional tricuspid regurgitation: a real-time, 3-dimensional echocardiographic study. Circulation 2006; 114[Suppl]:I-492-I-498.*)

TABLE 46-1 Causes of Tricuspid Regurgitation

Primary causes (25%)
Rheumatic
myxomatous
Ebstein anomaly
Endomyocardial fibrosis
Endocarditis
Carcinoid disease
Traumatic (blunt chest injury, laceration)
Latrogenic (pacemaker/defibrillator lead, RV biopsy)
Secondary causes (75%)
Left heart disease (LV dysfunction or value disease) resulting in pulmonary hypertension
Any cause of pulmonary hypertension (chronic lung disease, pulmonary thromboembolism, left to right shunt)
Any cause of RV dysfunction (myocardial disease, RV ischemia/infarction)

RV indicates right ventricular, LV, left ventricular.

entity has been reported in case reports and small series but is likely more significant and prevalent than currently perceived. In a recent report by Kim et al., the effect of transtricuspid permanent pacemaker or implantable cardiac defibrillator leads on 248 subjects with echocardiograms before and after device placement was studied TR worsened by one grade or more after implant in 24.2% of subjects and that TR worsening was more common with implantable cardiac defibrillators than permanent pacemakers.[21,22]

The current guidelines do not recommend lead extraction for patients with existing TR and transtricuspid pacing leads, because the risks of lead extraction are significant and there is potential for injury to the tricuspid valve if the lead is adherent to the valve apparatus.[23]

It has also been shown at 5 years after successful tricuspid valve repair, 42% of patients with a pacemaker had severe TR, almost double the incidence of those without pacemaker implantation.[24] This suggests removing a transtricuspid lead and replacing it with an epicardial lead at the time of tricuspid valve surgery may reduce late repair failure.

Tricuspid Regurgitation

Patients with TR have the presenting symptoms of fatigue and weakness related to a reduction in cardiac output. Atrial fibrillation is common. Jugular vein distention is found, especially during inspiration, when a physiologic increase in venous return is accentuated. Right-sided heart failure leads to ascites, congestive hepatosplenomegaly, pulsatile liver, pleural effusions, and peripheral edema. In the late stages, these patients are wasted with cachexia, cyanosis, and jaundice. Hepatic cardiac cirrhosis can develop in neglected cases.

Echocardiography is routinely used to assess the severity of TR in clinical practice. The exam is performed in an integrative manner using color Doppler flow mapping of the direction and size of the TR jet. In addition, the morphology of continuous wave Doppler recordings across the valve and pulsed wave Doppler of the hepatic veins can be used.[25]

Serial assessments of TR must be interpreted within the clinical context, because functional mitral regurgitation severity can be affected by multiple factors, such as volume status (preload) and afterload. Right ventricular shape is complex as compared with the left ventricle, appearing crescent shaped in cross-section and triangular when viewed en face.[26] Right ventricular function can be assessed quantitatively in the four-chamber view by measuring the end-diastolic and end-systolic area to calculate the fractional area change of the right ventricle.[27] Although right ventricular chamber dimensions may be obtained during echocardiography, magnetic resonance imaging is emerging as an improved technique for assessing right ventricular diastolic and systolic volumes.[28]

Other echocardiographic findings include a shift in the atrial septum to the left and paradoxical septal motion, consistent with right ventricular diastolic overload. Pulsed Doppler and color-flow studies help to identify systolic right ventricular to right atrial flow with inferior vena cava and hepatic vein flow reversal. Contrast-enhanced echocardiography can be useful, with a rapid saline bolus injection producing microcavities that are visible on echo, demonstrating to-and-fro motion across the valve orifice and reversal into the inferior vena cava and hepatic veins. Possible ASD or patent foramen ovale should be sought. Endocarditis vegetations are clearly visible on echocardiography. The valve may be destroyed, and septic pulmonary emboli are a common feature. The tricuspid valve in carcinoid syndrome is thickened with retracted leaflets fixed in a semi-open position throughout the cardiac cycle.[29–34]

Tricuspid Stenosis

Tricuspid stenosis (TS) is most commonly rheumatic. It is extremely rare to have isolated tricuspid stenosis because some degree of TR will be present.[35–37] Mitral valve disease coexists with occasional involvement of the aortic valve. The third still have a significant prevalence of rheumatic mitral and tricuspid valvular disease. The anatomical features are similar to those of mitral stenosis, with fusion and shortening of the chordae and leaflet thickening. Fusion along the free edges and calcific deposits on the valve are found late in the disease. The preponderance of cases are in young women.

The diastolic gradient between the right atrium and right ventricle is significantly elevated even at 2 to 5 mm Hg mean pressure. As the right atrial pressure increases, venous congestion leads to distention of the jugular veins, ascites, pleural effusion, and peripheral edema. The right atrial wall thickens, and the atrial chamber dilates.

Clinical features are consistent with reduced cardiac output producing the symptoms of fatigue and malaise. Significant liver engorgement produces right upper quadrant tenderness with a palpable liver with a presystolic pulse. Ascites produces increased abdominal girth. Significant peripheral edema or anasarca can develop. Severe TS may mask or reduce the pulmonary congestion of mitral stenosis owing to reduced blood flow to the left side of the heart. The low output state of the patient is prominent.

Echocardiography reveals the diagnostic features of diastolic doming of the thickened tricuspid valve leaflets, reduced leaflet mobility, and a reduced orifice of flow. The Doppler flow pattern across the tricuspid valve has a prolonged slope of antegrade flow.

Functional Tricuspid Regurgitation (fTR)

Without treatment, fTR may become worse over time, leading to severe symptoms, biventricular heart failure, and death.[24] In a large retrospective echocardiographic analysis of 5223 Veterans Administration patients by Nath et al.[38] showed that independent of echo-derived pulmonary artery systolic pressure, left ventricular ejection fraction, inferior vena cava size, and right ventricular size and function, survival is worse for patients with moderate and severe TR than for those with no TR.

Pulmonary artery hypertension from any cause is known to be associated with the development of secondary tricuspid regurgitation. However, not all patients with pulmonary hypertension develop significant tricuspid regurgitation, and the mechanisms of secondary TR are multifactorial.

Mutlak et al.[39] studied 2139 subjects with mild (<50), moderate (50 to 69), or severe (≥70) elevations in pulmonary artery systolic pressure. In their analysis, increasing PASP was independently associated with greater degrees of TR (odds ratio, 2.26 per 10 mm Hg increase). However, many patients with high PASP had only mild TR (mild TR in 65.4% of patients with PASP 50 to 69 mm Hg and in 45.6% of patients with PASP ≥70 mm Hg). Other factors, such as atrial fibrillation, pacemaker leads, and right heart enlargement, were also importantly associated with TR severity. The authors concluded that the cause of TR in patients with pulmonary hypertension is only partially related to an increase in transtricuspid pressure gradient. It remains unproved if surgical annuloplasty, in the setting of pulmonary hypertension, alters the natural course of right ventricular dilation and recurrent TR.

Thus, functional tricuspid incompetence is progressive. Surgical treatment of left-sided valvular lesions are not always adequate to resolve or prevent progressive TR. This is particularly true when pulmonary hypertension persists.

SURGICAL DECISIONS

The cardiologist and the cardiac surgeon face the decision as to when to intervene and when to surgically repair or replace the tricuspid valve. The choice of reparative technique to use for a durable result must be evaluated, as well as which type of valve, mechanical or bioprosthesis, to employ to maximize durability and minimize complications (ie, thrombosis and thromboembolism). The surgical literature can be misleading because of case selection bias and the various time frames of retrospective reviews. This is particularly true during the era that cage-ball and single-disk mechanical valves were in use.

SURGICAL EXPOSURE

Tricuspid valve annuloplasty performed with either mitral and/or aortic valve operations is accomplished either through a full or partial lower sternotomy approach or less invasive right minithoracotomy exposure with mitral valve procedures. Bicaval venous cannulation with caval snares is essential to isolate the right atrium. The cannula can be placed conventionally via the right atrium or less invasively via the femoral vein. A superior vena cava cannula can be inserted via the internal jugular vein.

Left-sided valve repair or replacement (mitral and/or aortic) is performed under blood cardioplegia arrest with antegrade and/or retrograde administration, moderate systemic hypothermia, and optional surface cooling. The mitral valve can be exposed through a left atrial incision posterior to the intra-atrial septum or through a transseptal incision (Fig. 46-3). The transseptal incision is particularly useful when there is an aortic valve prosthesis or in a reoperation.

After completing the mitral valve procedure and the de-airing maneuvers, the aorta is unclamped and caval snares are tightened around the venous drainage cannula. Attention can be turned to the tricuspid valve while rewarming and return of a cardiac rhythm. During tricuspid valve suturing, misplacement of a suture adversely affecting the cardiac conduction system can be assessed immediately and corrected.

In a reoperative setting, approaching the tricuspid valve through a right mini-thoracotomy has the advantage of avoiding adhesions and possible injury to the right ventricle during repeat sternotomy. Femoral vein and internal jugular vein cannula are positioned outside the right atrium and confirmed by echo. Caval snares below the cannula tips ensure venous drainage. Coronary sinus return is controlled by a sucker in the coronary sinus.

If the operation will include the mitral valve, exposure can be simplified by using a right atrial incision and transseptal approach. If atrial fibrillation is present, a Maze procedure can be added to the technical maneuvers.

ANNULOPLASTY TECHNIQUES

Techniques to deal with a dilated tricuspid valve annulus with normal leaflets and chordal structures include plication of the posterior leaflet's annulus (bicuspidization), partial purse-string reduction of the anterior and posterior leaflet annulus (DeVega-style techniques), and rigid or flexible rings or bands placed to reduce the annular size and achieve leaflet coaptation (Fig. 46-4). Preoperative and intraoperative echocardiograms are valuable assessment tools to help the surgeon understand the structure and function of the valve.[30–34]

The degree of pulmonary hypertension, right ventricular dilatation, and systolic function, coupled with the size of the right atrium, must be factored into the surgical decision making. The classical technique of inserting a finger via a pursestring suture, into the right atrium to palpate the tricuspid valve and withdrawing the fingertip 2 to 3 cm from the valve orifice, so as to access the force of the regurgitant jet is of historical importance in the current era of cardiac surgery. The intraoperative transesophageal echocardiogram (TEE) allows the surgeon to access the degree of tricuspid regurgitation and look for reversal of flow in the inferior cava. The TEE assessment after the repair and under the appropriate loading conditions ensures leaving the operating room with confidence that the repair is functioning satisfactorily.

Classic surgical teaching has been that patients with minimal right atrial enlargement and +1 to +2 regurgitation do well and resolve the TR after successful surgery on left-sided valve lesions, especially if the pulmonary hypertension resolves. Recent literature has documented the variability in the resolution of TR after dealing effectively with the left-sided valvular lesions.

The pathologic process of functional TR (fTR) requires an understanding that the tricuspid annulus is a component of both the tricuspid valve and the right ventricular myocardium. For the tricuspid valve to leak, the tricuspid annulus; therefore, the right ventricle have to be dilated. If the tricuspid annulus and the right ventricle are not dilated, there is a very low probability that TR can occur.

Dilation of the tricuspid annulus occurs in the anterior and posterior directions (see Fig. 46-1B) corresponding to the free wall of the right ventricle. In addition to tricuspid dilatation, the degree of TR is also directly related to three important factors: the preload, afterload, and right ventricular function. Thus, TR is difficult to assess accurately because these factors can interfere with the observed severity of TR under different conditions. Significant TR may not be detected echocardiographically despite considerable annular dilatation in the tricuspid valve annulus.

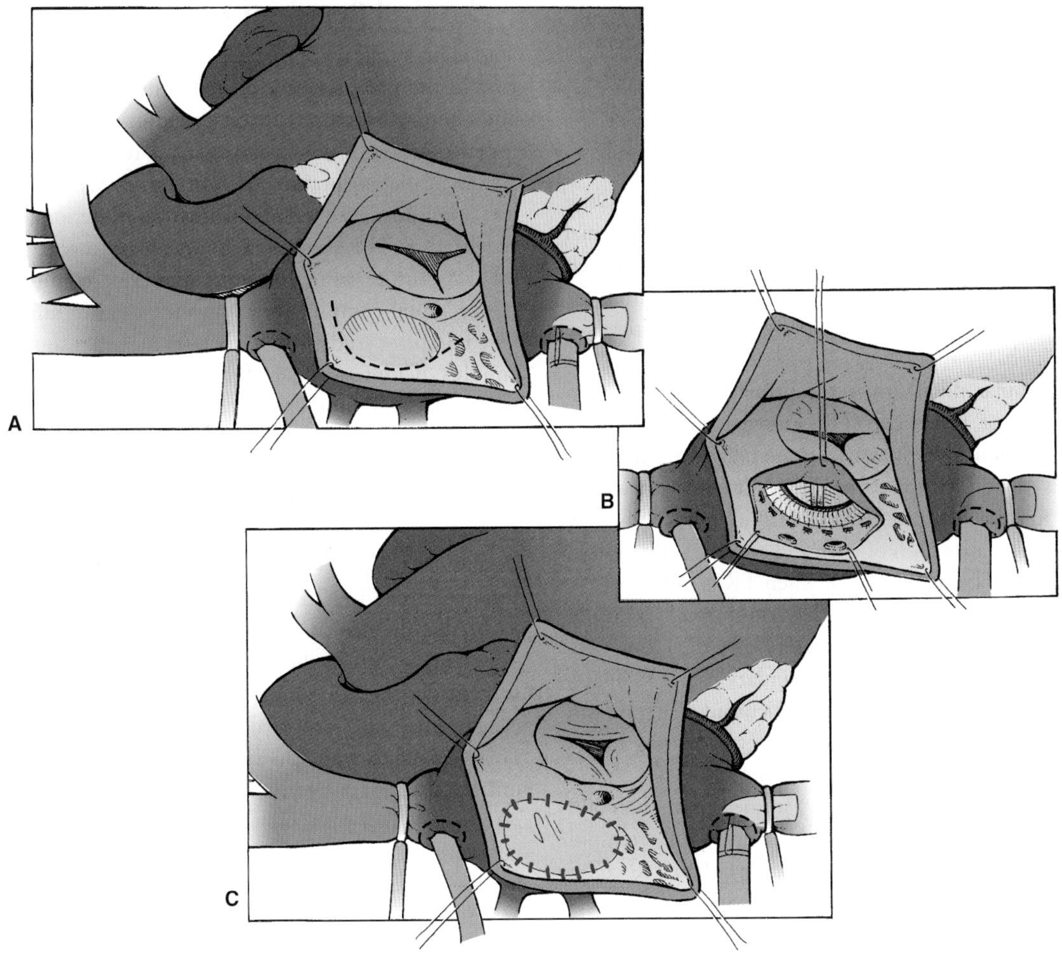

FIGURE 46-3 (A) The superior and inferior venae cavae are cannulated, an oblique atriotomy incision is made, and stay sutures are placed on the right atrial wall to aid exposure. For transatrial exposure of the mitral valve, an incision is placed in the fossa ovale and extended superiorly through the interatrial septum. The superior aspect of the septal incision is extended, if necessary, into the dome of the left atrium behind the aorta. (B) Stay sutures in the interatrial septum are used for retraction. Use of retractors is avoided to prevent injury to the AV node. The mitral prosthesis is implanted in an anti anatomic orientation. (C) The interatrial septum is closed primarily or by using a pericardial patch with a continuous 4-0 Prolene suture.

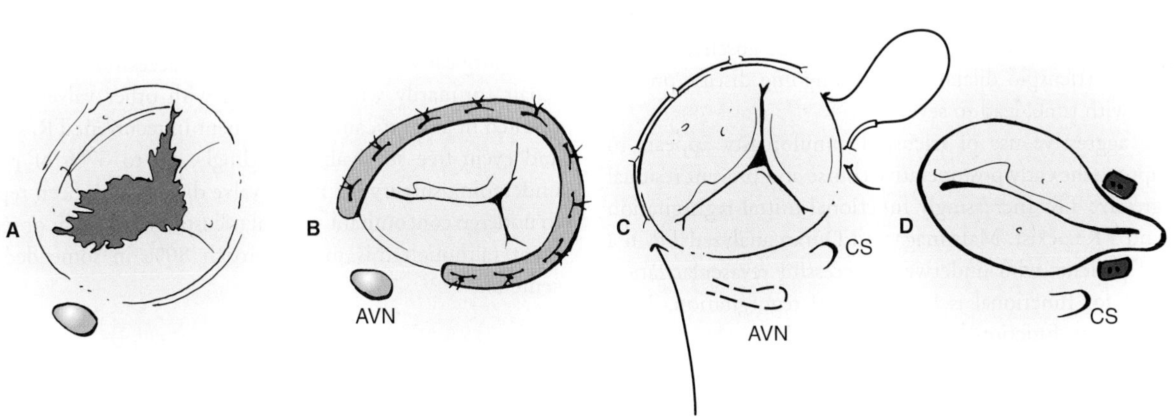

FIGURE 46-4 Predominant surgical repair techniques for functional tricuspid regurgitation (TR) in the presence of a dilated annulus. (A) Dilated tricuspid annulus with abnormal circular shape, failure of leaflet coaptation, and resultant TR. (B) Rigid or flexible annuloplasty bands are used to restore a more normal annular size and shape (ovoid), thereby reducing or eliminating TR. The open rings spares the atrioventricular node (AVN), reducing the incidence of heart block. (C) DeVega suture annuloplasty partially plicate the annulus reducing annular circumference and diameter. (D) Suture bicuspidalization is performed by placement of a mattress suture from the anteroposterior to the posteroseptal commissure along the posterior annulus. *CS = Coronary sinus.*

An understanding of these important fundamental concepts seem to contradict current practice regarding the management of secondary TR, which focuses on assessment of the severity of TR and advocates treatment of the primary lesion alone (ie, mitral valve disease). Treatment of the mitral valve lesion alone only decreases the afterload. It does not correct tricuspid dilatation, nor does it affect preload or right ventricular function. Once the tricuspid annulus is dilated, its size cannot return to normal spontaneously, and it may in fact continue to dilate further. This explains why some patients require a second operation for TR years after the initial mitral valve surgery. The reoperative risks are very high.

Tricuspid annular dilatation is the primary mechanism in the development of functional TR. Dreyfus and colleagues postulated that annular size may be a more reliable indicator of late outcomes than the degree of TR. Moreover, successful treatment of functional (secondary) tricuspid valve pathology may necessitate the correction of tricuspid annular dilatation in addition to mitral valve surgery even when TR is mild.

Over a 12-year period, these authors performed tricuspid valve repair (TVR) for secondary tricuspid valve dilatation irrespective of the severity of TR because secondary tricuspid dilatation may or not be accompanied by TR. Tricuspid dilatation can be measured objectively, whereas TR can vary according to the preload, afterload, and right ventricular function.

Dreyfus and colleagues prospectively studied more than 300 patients to determine whether surgical repair of the tricuspid valve, based on tricuspid dilatation alone rather than TR, could lead to potential benefits. Tricuspid annuloplasty was performed only if the tricuspid annular diameter was greater than twice the normal size (≥70 mm) regardless of the grade of regurgitation. Patients in group 1 (163 patients, 52.4%) received mitral valve repair (MVR) alone. Patients in group 2 (148 patients, 47.6%) received MVR plus tricuspid annuloplasty. Tricuspid regurgitation increased by more than two grades in 48% of the patients in group 1 and in only 2% of the patients in group 2 ($p < .001$).

The authors concluded that remodeling annuloplasty of the tricuspid valve based on tricuspid dilatation improved functional status irrespective of the grade of regurgitation. Considerable tricuspid dilatation can be present even in the absence of substantial TR. Tricuspid dilatation is an ongoing disease process that will, with time, lead to severe TR.[40]

More aggressive use of tricuspid annuloplasty appears to help improve the early postoperative course and prevent residual or progressive TR. Increasingly functional mitral regurgitation (MR) and TR coexist. Matsunaga and Duran analyzed TR in a group of patients who underwent successful revascularization and MVR for functional ischemic mitral regurgitation. They concluded that functional TR is frequently associated with functional ischemic MR. After MVR, close to 50% of patients have residual TR that increases over time. The annular size may become the objective criteria, regardless of the degree of TR, to determine the need for a tricuspid annuloplasty.[41]

Special note should be taken in assessing the foramen ovale for patency. If patent the foramen should always be sutured closed, reducing the possibility of arterial desaturation from right-to-left shunting or paradoxic embolization.

Surgical Repair of the TV

The main surgical approaches to rectify functional TR (occurring in the presence of a dilated annulus with normal leaflets and chordal structures) involve rigid or flexible annular bands (open or closed), which are used to reduce annular size and achieve leaflet coaptation, as with mitral valve disease. Another less commonly used technique involves posterior annular bicuspidalization. This surgical technique places a pledget-supported mattress suture from the anteroposterior commissure to the posteroseptal commissure along the posterior annulus. This is based on prior studies by Deloche et al.[42] that showed posterior annulus dilation occurs in functional TR and that a focal posterior tricuspid annuloplasty can be effective in selected cases. Other approaches include edge-to-edge (Alfieri-type) repairs as described by Castedo et al.[43,44] and partial purse-string suture techniques to reduce the anterior and posterior portions of the annulus (DeVega-style techniques; see Fig. 46-4). DeVega and flexible annuloplasty bands appear to have a lower freedom from recurrent TR than rigid annuloplasty rings.[24,45–47]

In the absence of simultaneous tricuspid valve repair, the prevalence of TR in the postoperative period after mitral valve surgery depends to some degree on the mechanism of MR. Matsuyama et al.[48] reported in a study of 174 patients that only 16% of patients who underwent nonischemic (ie, degenerative) mitral valve surgery without tricuspid valve surgery developed 3 to 4+ TR at 8-year follow-up. Conversely, TR appears to be far more prevalent in patients undergoing mitral valve repair for functional ischemic mitral regurgitation. In the series by Matsunaga et al.[49] of 70 patients undergoing mitral valve repair for functional ischemic mitral regurgitation, 30% of patients (21/70) had at least moderate TR before surgery. In the postoperative period, the prevalence of at least moderate TR increased over time, from 25% at less than 1 year, 53% at 1 to 3 years, and 74% at greater than 3 years of follow-up.

Significant residual tricuspid valve insufficiency contributes to a poor postoperative result, even after successful mitral valve repair. King et al.[50] studied patients requiring subsequent tricuspid valve surgery after mitral valve surgery. They had high early and late mortality. The authors encouraged a policy of liberal use of tricuspid annuloplasty at initial mitral valve surgery. Surgical series have shown that successful tricuspid valve repair (primarily when combined with other valve surgeries) resulted in a significant improvement in recurrent TR, survival, and event-free survival. Accordingly, 50 to 67% of patients undergoing surgery for mitral valve disease have been reported to undergo concomitant surgical tricuspid valve repair or replacement (although this may approach 80% in some dedicated centers).[45,51,52]

Specific Techniques

Bicuspidization

After the caval snares are tightened, the right atrium is opened via an oblique incision. Exposure and assessment of all aspects of the tricuspid valve structure should be performed before choosing the technique of annuloplasty. Suture plication to deal with mild dilatation of the annulus is accomplished by placing

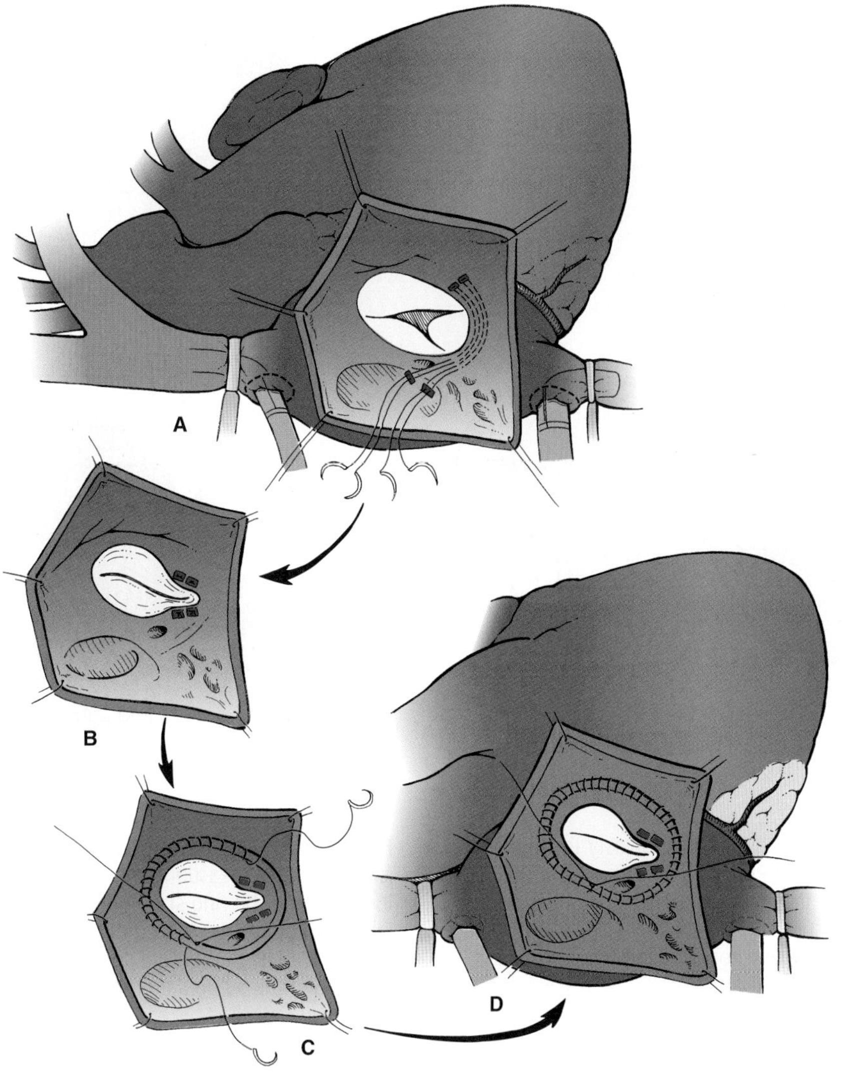

FIGURE 46-5 (A) Tricuspid valve bicuspidization is accomplished by plicating the annulus along the posterior leaflet. Two concentric, pledgeted 2-0 Ethibond sutures are used. (B) The sutures are tied, obliterating the posterior leaflet, effectively creating a bicuspid AV valve. Saline is injected into the right ventricle to test the competency of the repair. (C) As an option to support the bicuspidization repair, a flexible ring may be placed. Prior to ring implantation, measuring the intertrigonal distance determines the annular size. As an option, the ring can be inserted using a continuous 4-0 Prolene suture. Care is taken to avoid the AV node. As another option, the ring can be implanted above the coronary sinus.

pledgeted mattress sutures from the center of the posterior leaflet to the commissure between the septal and posterior leaflets. A second suture often is necessary to further reduce the annulus, ensuring proper leaflet coaptation while providing an adequate orifice for flow. An annuloplasty ring can be inserted to further support the annular reduction (Fig. 46-5).

DeVega Technique

The DeVega technique also can be employed for mild to moderate annular dilatation.[53] The technique employs a 2-0 Prolene or Dacron polyester suture placed at the junction of the annulus and right ventricular free wall, running from the anteroseptal commissure to the posteroseptal commissure. The second limb of the suture is placed through a pledget and run parallel and close to the first suture line in the same clockwise direction, placing it through a second pledget at the posteroseptal commissure. The suture is tightened, producing a pursestring effect and reducing the length of the anterior and posterior annulus to provide adequate leaflet coaptation and orifice of flow (Fig. 46-6).

The judgment regarding the degree of annular reduction has varied from the guideline of being able to insert two and one-half to three fingerbreadths snugly through the valve orifice to using the ring annuloplasty sizers designed for the tricuspid valve. An annuloplasty sizer, chosen by measuring the intertrigonal distance, can be used as a template while tying the pursestring suture to achieve the proper degree of reduction. The DeVega and suture plication techniques should be reserved for mild annular reductions and situations in which the structural integrity of the annulus is not absolutely necessary for long-term success (ie, functional TR expected to resolve over time). In these situations, the annuloplasty provides a competent tricuspid valve

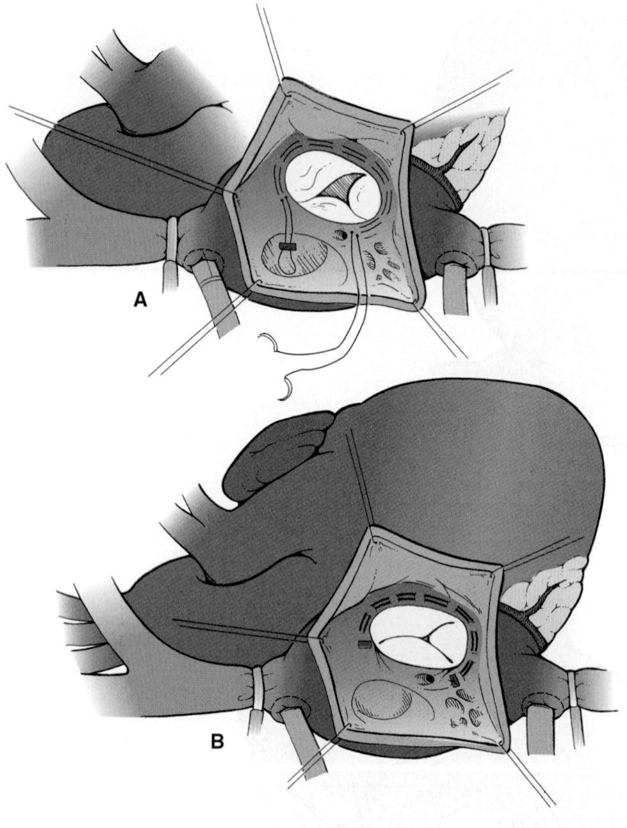

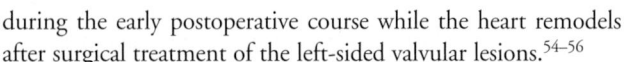

FIGURE 46-6 (A) A modified DeVega annuloplasty technique is shown. A single pledgeted 2-0 Prolene suture is placed. Care is taken to avoid the area of the AV node. (B) The suture is tied, completing the annuloplasty. Injecting saline into the right ventricle using a bulb syringe and compressing the pulmonary artery tests the valve for competency.

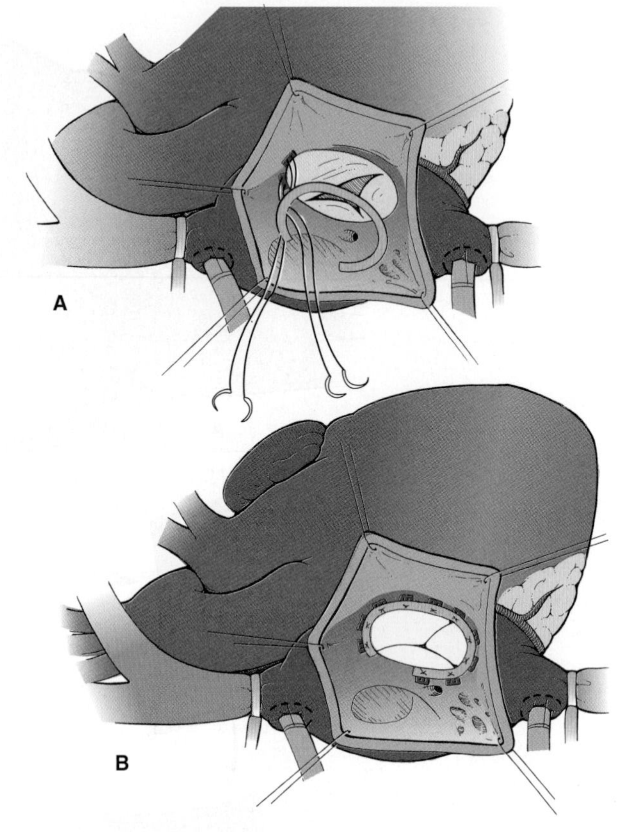

FIGURE 46-7 (A) The Carpentier-Edwards ring annuloplasty is shown. A sizer measuring the intertrigonal distance was used to determine the ring size. Multiple interrupted, pledgeted 2-0 Ethibond sutures are placed at the atrioannular junction. All sutures are inserted before seating the ring. (B) The valve is seated and the sutures are tied.

during the early postoperative course while the heart remodels after surgical treatment of the left-sided valvular lesions.[54–56]

Rings and Bands

Significant degrees of annular reduction requiring durability are best accomplished with rigid rings (eg, Carpentier-Edwards and MC3), flexible rings (eg, Duran), or flexible bands (eg, Cosgrove annuloplasty system). The length of the base of the septal leaflet (ie, the intertrigonal distance) determines the size of the ring or band. These devices avoid suture placement in the region of the atrioventricular (AV) node (apex of the triangle of Koch) to avoid postoperative conduction problems. The mattress sutures are placed circumferentially, with wider bites on the annulus and smaller corresponding bites through the fabric of the ring or band, producing the annular plication mostly along the length of the posterior leaflet. The result allows the tricuspid valve orifice to be occluded primarily by the leaflet tissue of the anterior and septal leaflets. Overly aggressive annular reduction can lead to ring dehiscence owing to excessive tension on the tenuous tricuspid valve annular tissue[57,58] (Fig. 46-7).

A recent review of a 790-patient series for the durability and risk factors for failure of a repair was reported by McCarthy and colleagues. The authors reported that TR 1 week after annuloplasty was 3+ or 4+ in 14% of patients. Regurgitation severity remained stable over time with the Carpentier-Edwards ring (p = .7), increased slowly with the Cosgrove-Edwards band (p = .05), and rose more rapidly with the DeVega (p = .002) and Peri-Guard (p = .0009) procedures. Risk factors for worsening regurgitation included higher preoperative regurgitation grade, poor left ventricular function, permanent pacemaker, and repair type other than ring annuloplasty. Right ventricular systolic pressure, ring size, preoperative New York Heart Association (NYHA) functional class, and concomitant surgery were not risk factors. Tricuspid reoperation was rare (3% at 8 years), and hospital mortality after reoperation was 37%. The authors concluded that tricuspid valve annuloplasty did not consistently eliminate functional regurgitation, and over time, regurgitation increased importantly after Peri-Guard and DeVega annuloplasty. Therefore, these repair techniques should be abandoned, and transtricuspid pacing leads should be replaced with epicardial leads.[59]

INTRAOPERATIVE ASSESSMENT OF THE REPAIR

Assessment of tricuspid valve competence after the annuloplasty requires filling the right ventricle with saline and observing leaflet coaptation. This assessment is best performed with the heart beating and the pulmonary artery occluded to allow right ventricular volume to generate enough intracavitary pressure to close the tricuspid valve tightly. If the result appears inadequate, downsizing the ring or ring replacement should be performed. Final assessment is by TEE examination after completely weaning from cardiopulmonary bypass with appropriate volume and afterload adjustment.

TRICUSPID VALVE REPLACEMENT

The technique for secure fixation of a tricuspid valve is with pledgeted mattress sutures using an everting suture technique for mechanical valves and either a supra-annular or an intra-annular technique for a bioprosthesis. The tricuspid valve leaflets are left in place, preserving the subvalvular structures and helping to avoid injury to the conduction system (Fig. 46-8). If there is concern that the anterior leaflet could billow and obstruct the right ventricular outflow tract, the central portion of the leaflet can be excised and still preserve the chordal attachments.

Tricuspid valve replacement with a homograft is more complicated. The homograft tissue is a mitral valve.[60–62] Sizing is performed by measuring the intratrigonal distances. Fixation of the papillary muscles is either intracavity (right ventricle) or through the wall of the right ventricle. This requires judgment

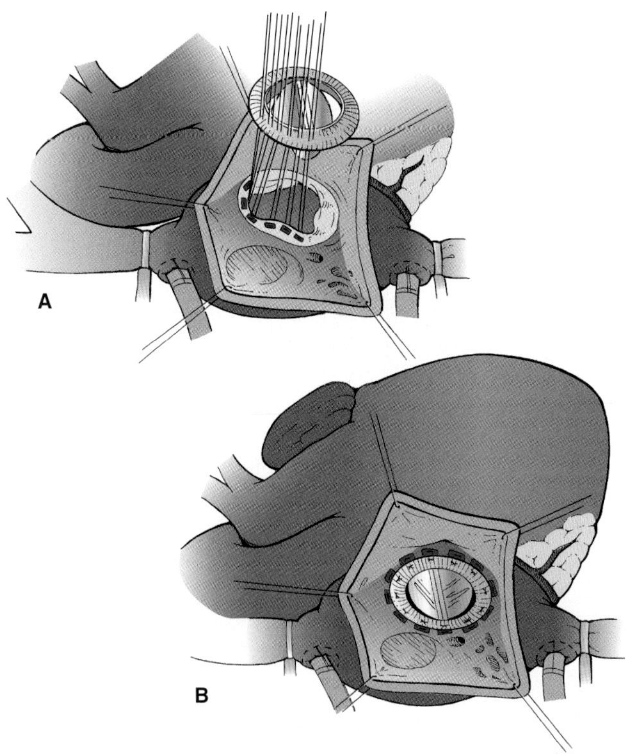

FIGURE 46-8 (A) Tricuspid valve replacement is performed with a St. Jude Medical valve. The native leaflets are left in situ, and the pledgeted 2-0 Ethibond sutures are passed through the annulus and the edges of the leaflets. (B) The valve is seated, and the sutures are tied. The subvalvular apparatus is visualized to ensure that there is no impingement of the prosthetic valve leaflets. The valve can be rotated if necessary to prevent leaflet contact with tissue.

and experience to gauge proper chordal length. The annulus is run with a monofilament suture line. An annuloplasty ring is inserted to prevent dilatation and ensure adequate leaflet coaptation. Special care is necessary in suture placement to avoid conduction disturbances. Suture placement and tying with the heart beating provide immediate detection of rhythm disturbances. Similar to mitral valve replacement, leaflet and chordal preservation should be performed, or Gore-Tex suture should used as artificial chordae to maintain annular papillary muscle continuity.

A recent report documented the use of a stentless porcine valve in endocarditis in which the commissural posts were anchored to the right ventricular septal, anterior, and posterior walls. Orientation is critical to be sure that the right ventricular outflow tract is straddled by two of the commissural posts.[63] Low profile AV bioprosthesis should be chosen.

Carpentier techniques for MVR can be applied to the tricuspid valve. Traumatic disruptions, occasionally endocarditis with healed lesions and perforations, or the rare myxomatous valve can be repaired. Pericardial patching of perforations, partial leaflet resections of the anterior (limited) or posterior (extensive) leaflets, chordal transfer, artificial Gore-Tex chordae, Alfieri suture and ring annuloplasty are standard techniques used to produce competent valves and avoid replacement.[64–66]

ENDOCARDITIS

Tricuspid valve excision is possible if pulmonary pressures and the pulmonary vascular resistance are not elevated and the degree of infection is extensive.[66–68] Blood flows passively through the right side of the heart to the lungs. After eradication of the infection, a second-stage procedure with valve replacement can be performed months to years later.

In patients with tricuspid valve endocarditis owing to drug addiction, the second-stage valve insertion should be performed preferably after controlling the drug dependence or hopefully curing the accompanying addiction. Late survival and reinfection are correlated directly with continued drug use. Patients with less severe endocarditis can have one-stage procedures with prosthetic replacement or localized leaflet excision and repair.[69,70] Homograft tissue often is versatile for partial or total tricuspid valve repair or replacement but has the limitations of availability, technical difficulty, and limited follow-up. The stentless aortic porcine valve is a novel option.[63,64]

PROSTHETIC VALVE CHOICE

The choice of prosthesis follows an algorithm similar to that used for valve replacement in other cardiac valve positions. The patient's age, anticoagulation considerations, whether the patient is a young woman during her childbearing years, and social issues must be considered. The previously reported poor results with mechanical valves in the tricuspid position were caused by valve thrombosis. Most of these reports were during the era of cage-ball and tilting-disk prostheses.[71] Reports with the St. Jude bileaflet valve have provided encouraging data, allowing the surgeon to recommend a mechanical valve with

TABLE 46-2 Reports of Bioprosthetic and Mechanical Valves in the Tricuspid Position

			Operative Mortality						Actuarial Freedom From								
						Death			Structural Degeneration			Nonstructural Degeneration			Tricuspid Reoperation		
Reference	Series Dates	Patients (no.)	Bioprosthesis (B)	Mechanical (M)	Overall (A)	B	M	A	B	M	A	B	M	A	B	M	A
Nakano[74]	1979–1992	39		8%			55% @14 y;		100%			72%				100% @14 y	
Nakano[79]	1978–1995	98	15%			77% @5 y; 69% @10 y; and 18 y			98% @5 y; 96% @18 y			99% @5 y; 82% @10 y; 77% @18 y*			97% @5 y; 76% @10 y; 63% @18 y		
Ratnatunga[77]	1966–1997	425	19%	16%	17%	71% @1 y; 62% @5 y; 48% @10 y	74% 58% 34%	72% 60% 43%							99% @1 y; 98% @10 y;	98% 97%	
Glower[70]	1972–1993	129			27% (14% 1st Operation)	56% @5 y; 48% @10 y; 31% @14 y									96% @5 y; 93% @10 y; 49% @14 y		
Ohata[81]	1984–1998	88	7%			88% @5 y; 81% @10 y; 69% 14 y			100% @14 y			†			88% @14 y		
Van Nooton[69]	1967–1987	146			16%			74% @5 y; 23% @10y									

Singh[72]	1981–1984	14		8%			50% @10 y					
Munro[75]	1975–1992	94	15%	14%	14%				97% @5, 7 y, and 10 y	100%	97%	87%
Kaplan[70]	1980–2000	122			25%	55% @20 y	68% @20 y	65% @20y	90% @20 y	97%‡ @20y		
Scully[71]	1975–1993	60			27%		50% @15 y					

*Thick fibrous pannus in 35% of survivors; freedom from nonstructural valve dysfunction at 18 y = 24%.
†Thick pannus noted in reoperative case.
‡Freedom from deterioration, endocarditis, leakage, and thromboembolism 93% @20 y.

confidence to younger patients who do not have a contraindication to anticoagulation.[72–78]

This strategy will avoid the not uncommon situation in the past in which patients received a bioprosthetic on the right side and a mechanical prosthesis on the left. Bioprostheses, both porcine and of pericardial tissue, have functioned well in the tricuspid position.[79–82] The data demonstrate a longer duration of freedom from structural valve dysfunction or re-replacement for a bioprosthetic valve in the tricuspid compared with the mitral valve position.[83]

Table 46-2 summarizes multiple reports from the literature. The reports either compare bioprosthetic and mechanical valves in the tricuspid position or present follow-up of bioprosthetic valves alone. The bioprosthesis, either porcine or pericardial valves, have excellent freedom from degeneration and re-replacement for structural valve degeneration. In 1984, Cohen and colleagues reported on six simultaneously implanted and then explanted valves from the mitral and tricuspid positions. Degenerative changes were less extensive for the bioprosthetic valves in the tricuspid position than in the mitral position. However, thrombus and pannus formation (interpreted as organized thrombotic material) were observed more frequently in the tricuspid position.[83]

Nakano's review of the Carpentier-Edwards bovine pericardial valve reported a freedom from structural degeneration of 100% at 9 years, but nonstructural dysfunction was 72.8%. The cause of nonstructural dysfunction was pannus formation on the ventricular side of the cusps. This finding is often subclinical. Echocardiographic follow-up revealed a 35% incidence of this anatomical finding in patients with at least 5 years of follow-up.[81]

Guerra reported similar changes in simultaneously explanted porcine valves. The tricuspid position had less structural tissue degeneration and calcification than the mitral position. The report described the presence of pannus formation on the ventricular side of the cusps in tricuspid porcine valves. The pannus interfered with cuspal pliability and function.[84]

Nakano's 2001 report of bioprosthetic tricuspid valves reported an 18-year freedom from reoperation of 63%.[80] The freedom from structural deterioration was 96%, and nonstructural dysfunction was 77%. Reoperation replacing previously placed bioprosthetic valves occurred in 12 of 58 survivors. In 6 of the 12 patients, the primary indication for reoperation was tricuspid dysfunction, and 7 of the 12 had pannus formation on the ventricular side of the cusps (Fig. 46-9). This rate of degeneration and the subclinically high incidence of pannus formation, often eventually leading to reoperation, are major concerns. Tricuspid bioprosthetic valves require echocardiographic follow-up. Possible anticoagulation of bioprosthetic valves in the tricuspid position can reduce the incidence of pannus formation. The reported data in the literature categorize this pannus formation as nonstructural degeneration; therefore, clinical surgeons should be aware of future reports following this potentially serious clinical problem.

In the tricuspid position it is always possible to place large bioprosthetic or mechanical valves. Prostheses with more than a 27-mm internal diameter do not have clinically significant gradients. Therefore, hemodynamic performance is rarely an issue for tricuspid valve replacement. The data demonstrate excellent results with modern bileaflet mechanical valves. Series comparing bioprosthetic and mechanical valves have been consistent in demonstrating equality during the period of follow-up. The development of thrombus on a bileaflet valve can be treated successfully with thrombolysis.

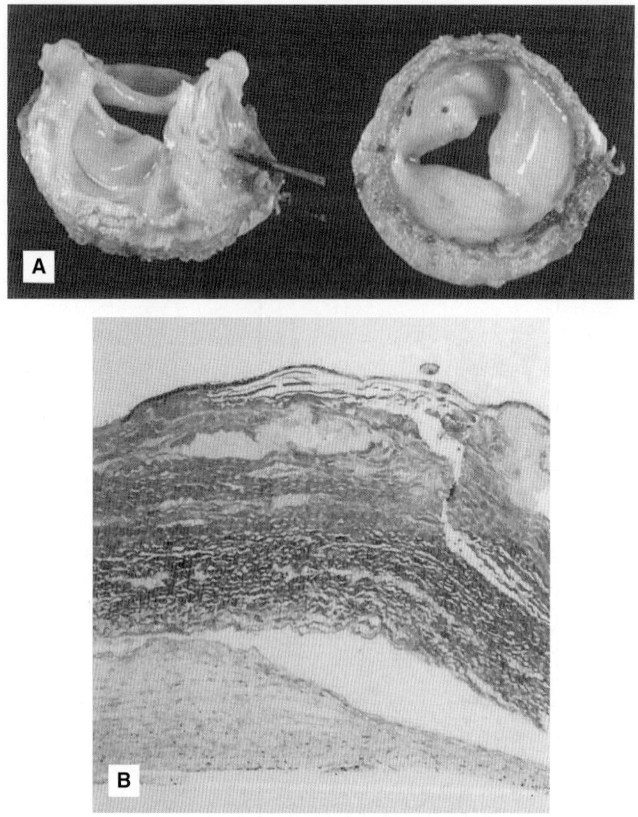

FIGURE 46-9 (A) Fibrous pannus observed 8 years after implantation of a Carpentier-Edwards pericardial valve. (B) Photomicrograph of a pericardial leaflet. The bottom of the leaflet has pannus, a dense fibrous tissue on the ventricular side. (*Reprinted with permission from the Society of Thoracic Surgeons and Nakano K, Ishibashi-Ueda H, Kobayashi J, et al: Tricuspid valve replacement with bioprostheses: Long-term results and causes of valve dysfunction. Ann Thorac Surg 2001; 71:105.*)

A recent review by Filsoufi and a meta-analysis of biologic or mechanical prostheses in the tricuspid position both conclude that there is no survival benefit of a bioprosthesis over a mechanical valve[85–87] (Fig. 46-10). Some patients with mitral valve disease and TR undergoing surgery do not require surgical treatment of the tricuspid valve. Guidelines to identify these patients are poorly developed. Experience has shown that careful observation of the patient preoperatively is quite valuable. Absence of tricuspid valve regurgitation during periods of good medical control, absence of TR by transesophageal echocardiography (TEE) at the time of operation, minimal elevation of pulmonary vascular resistance, and absence of right atrial enlargement are helpful findings that permit the surgeon to replace the mitral valve confidently without performing an annuloplasty or replacement of the tricuspid valve. If unrepaired, reassessment of the tricuspid valve by TEE after weaning from cardiopulmonary bypass is essential.

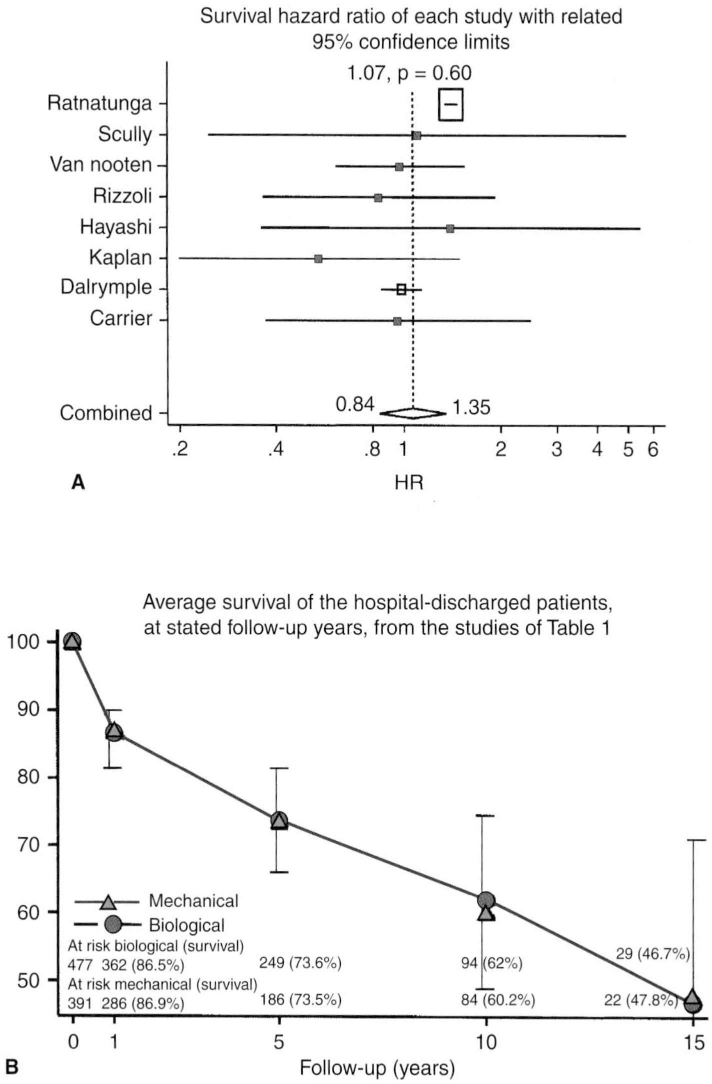

FIGURE 46-10 Meta-analysis of bioprosthetic vs mechanical valves replacing the tricuspid valve. (A) Survival hazard. (B) Survival curve of hospital survivors.

If TR persists and elevated right atrial pressures greater than left atrial pressures are encountered with an underfilled, well-contracting left ventricle, tricuspid repair should be performed. A patent foramen ovale with interatrial shunting must be identified and closed surgically. Hemodynamically, when right atrial pressure is greater than left atrial pressure, the foramen may open, leading to systemic desaturation from a right-to-left shunt.

Temporary right ventricular dysfunction caused by RCA air embolism often requires a brief return to cardiopulmonary bypass, repeat of air maneuvers, elevation of the blood pressure, TEE evaluation for residual intracavity air, and a search for the characteristic echogenic brightness in the myocardial distribution of the RCA confirming the suspicion of air embolism. Treatment should include 10 to 15 minutes of cardiopulmonary bypass support and reweaning from cardiopulmonary bypass, with inotropic support for right ventricular dysfunction, elevated blood pressure, and reassessment of the TR and cardiac function.

CONCLUSION

Historical clinical experience has demonstrated that up to 20% of patients undergoing mitral valve replacement receive a tricuspid annuloplasty, but less than 2% require replacement. The surgeon's clinical judgment and experience have guided the approach to tricuspid valve surgery, ultimately leading to variability in reported clinical data. The accuracy of these judgments can have been guided by assessment of the risk factors for persistent or progressive tricuspid valve regurgitation. Recent studies have taught us that our ability to make these judgments is flawed and unpredictable. We have learned about the dilated tricuspid valve annulus, the progression of TR in spite of successful left-sided surgery, and the unpredictable resolution of pulmonary hypertension. Failure to improve can have adverse impacts on late morbidity, mortality, and residual or progressive TR. Therefore, the current recommendation is to aggressively pursue tricuspid annuloplasty with remodeling rings or bands.

Older studies showed patients undergoing a tricuspid valve annuloplasty during a mitral valve replacement have more advanced disease than those having mitral valve replacement alone. This is evidenced by the elevation in operative mortality (approximately 12 versus 3%) and the progressive increased hazard of late death (5-year survival of 80 versus 70%) despite good valve function. However, these patients achieved good functional results (NYHA Class 1–2). It is unknown what the survival and functional result would have been if tricuspid repair had not been performed in these patients, but one presumes that it would have been worse. In the current era adding an annuloplasty can have minimal adverse impact in the perioperative period and seems to confer long-term benefit.

The durability of simple annuloplasty techniques such as bicuspidization and the DeVega technique has been satisfactory when employed only for mild to moderate degrees of functional TR with successful resolution of pulmonary hypertension after the mitral valve operation. Extensive experience with the tricuspid annuloplasty using the Duran, Carpentier-Edwards, and MC^3 rings or bands have resulted in an 85% freedom from moderate to severe TR at 6 years. The subsequent requirement for tricuspid reoperation is very low. Inadequate resolution of the mitral disease and persistent pulmonary hypertension with right ventricular dilatation and dysfunction are the major predictors of poor late results.

The American College of Cardiology/American Heart Association 2006 Practice Guidelines for the surgical management of patients with TR (Table 46-3)[88] are driven by the individual patient's clinical status and the cause of their tricuspid valve abnormality. The guidelines state that the timing of surgical intervention for TR remains controversial, as do the surgical techniques. At present, surgery on the tricuspid valve for significant TR should occur at the time of mitral valve surgery, as TR does not reliably resolve after mitral valve surgery. TR associated with dilatation of the tricuspid annulus should be repaired, to prevent tricuspid annular dilation progressing and producing severe TR.[89–96]

TABLE 46-3 2006 ACC/AHA Guidelines Pertaining to the Surgical Management of Tricuspid Value Disease/Regurgitation

Class I

Tricuspid value repair is beneficial for severe TR in patients MV disease requiring MV surgery. *(Level of Evidence: B)*

Class IIa

1. Tricuspid value replacement or annuloplasty is reasonable for severe primary TR when symptomatic. *(Level of Evidence: C)*
2. Tricuspid value replacement is reasonable for severe TR secondary to disease/abnormal tricuspid value leaflets not amenable to annuloplasty or repair. *(Level of Evidence: C)*

Class IIb

Tricuspid annuloplasty may be considered for less than severe TR in patients undergoing MV surgery when there is pulmonary hypertension or tricuspid annular dilatation. *(Level of Evidence: C)*

Class III

1. Tricuspid value replacement or annuloplasty is not indicated in asymptomatic patients with TR whose pulmonay artery systolic pressure is less than 60 mm Hg in the pressure of a normal MV. *(Level of Evidence: C)*
2. Tricuspid value replacement or annuloplasty is not indicated in patients with mild primary TR. *(Level of Evidence: C)*

ACC indicates Amercian College of Cardiology; AHA, Amercian Heart Association; TR, tricuspid regurgitation; and MV, mitral value.

Patients requiring tricuspid and mitral valve replacement have operative mortalities from 5 to 10% by current standards. Actuarial survival rates are 55% at 10 years (Fig. 46-10 A,B). Advanced right ventricular failure or arrhythmia causes late death. Patients who need valve replacement for endocarditis comprise a unique subgroup with the additional risk for death owing to sepsis, reinfection, and the complications related to drug addiction.

Complete heart block can occur immediately postoperatively owing to damage to the conduction system during mitral and tricuspid valve surgery. This complication can be minimized intraoperatively by performing the tricuspid valve procedure on the perfused beating heart, as described earlier. Late heart block remains a persistent risk with a 25% actuarial incidence at 10 years for patients with mitral and tricuspid prostheses. The presence of two rigid prosthetic sewing rings can produce ongoing trauma and lead to AV node dysfunction over time. Late development of heart block rarely occurs after mitral valve replacement and tricuspid annuloplasty.

The surgical treatment of tricuspid valve disease presents the surgeon with challenges requiring clinical and intraoperative judgment. Following the principles presented in this chapter, appropriate decisions should lead to optimal clinical outcomes. The data support the safe use of mechanical bileaflet prostheses in select patients. A lingering concern is the pannus formation on the ventricular side of bioprosthetic cusps. This observation should be followed closely as future clinical series are reported.

REFERENCES

1. Yiwu L, Yingchun C, Jianqun Z, Bin Y, Ping B: Exact quantitative selective annuloplasty of the tricuspid valve. *J Thorac Cardiovasc Surg,* 2001; 122: 611-614.
2. Cohn LH: Tricuspid regurgitation secondary to mitral valve disease: when and how to repair. *J Card Surg* 199; 9:237-241.
3. Ewy G: Tricuspid valve disease, in Alpert JS, Dalen JE, Rahimtoola SH (eds): *Valvular Heart Disease,* 3rd ed. Philadelphia, Lippincott Williams & Wilkins, 2000; pp 377-392.
4. Fukuda S, Saracino G, Matsumura Y, et al: Three-dimensional geometry of the tricuspid annulus in healthy subjects and in patients with functional tricuspid regurgitation: a real-time, 3-dimensional echocardiographic study. *Circulation* 2006; 114(Suppl):I-492-I-498.
5. Tei C, Pilgrim JP, Shah PM, Ormiston JA, Wong M: The tricuspid valve annulus: study of size and motion in normal subjects and in patients with tricuspid regurgitation. *Circulation* 1982; 66:665-671.

6. Cohen ST, Sell JE, McIntosh CL, et al: Tricuspid regurgitation in patients with acquired, chronic, pure mitral regurgitation: I. Prevalence, diagnosis, and comparison of preoperative clinical and hemodynamic features in patients with and without tricuspid regurgitation. *J Thorac Cardiovasc Surg* 1987; 94:481.
7. Cohen SR, Sell JE, McIntosh CL, et al: Tricuspid regurgitation in patients with acquired, chronic, pure mitral regurgitation: II. Nonoperative management, tricuspid valve annuloplasty, and tricuspid valve replacement. *J Thorac Cardiovasc Surg* 1987; 94:488.
8. Tei C, Pilgrim JP, Shah PM, et al: The tricuspid valve annulus: study of size and motion in normal subjects and in patients with tricuspid regurgitation. *Circulation* 1982; 66:665.
9. Ubago JL, Figueroa A, Ochotcco A, et al: Analysis of the amount of tricuspid valve annular dilation required to produce functional tricuspid regurgitation. *Am J Cardiol* 1983; 52:155.
10. Come PC, Riley MF: Tricuspid annular dilatation and failure of tricuspid leaflet coaptation in tricuspid regurgitation. *Am J Cardiol* 1985; 55:599.
11. Waller BF, Moriarty AT, Able JN, et al: Etiology of pure tricuspid regurgitation based on annular circumference and leaflet area: analysis of 45 necropsy patients with clinical and morphologic evidence of pure tricuspid regurgitation. *J Am Coll Cardiol* 1986; 7:1063.
12. Miller MJ, McKay RG, Ferguson JJ, et al: Right atrial pressure-volume relationships in tricuspid regurgitation. *Circulation* 1986; 73:799.
13. Morrison DA, Ovit T, Hammermeister KE, et al: Functional tricuspid regurgitation and right ventricular dysfunction in pulmonary hypertension. *Am J Cardiol* 1988; 62:108.
14. Atbulu A, Holmes RJ, Asfaw I: Surgical treatment of intractable right-sided infective endocarditis in drug addicts: 25 years' experience. *J Heart Valve Dis* 1993; 2:129.
15. Bayer AS, Blomquist IK, Bello E, et al: Tricuspid valve endocarditis due to *Staphylococcus aureus*. *Chest* 1988; 93:247.
16. Tanaka M, Abe T, Hosokawa ST, et al: Tricuspid valve *Candida* endocarditis cured by valve-sparing debridement. *Ann Thorac Surg* 1989; 48:857.
17. Robiolio PA, Rigolin VH, Harrison JK, et al: Predictors of outcome of tricuspid valve replacement in carcinoid heart disease. *Am J Cardiol* 1995, 75:485.
18. Ohri SK, Schofield JB, Hodgson H, et al: Carcinoid heart disease: early failure of an allograft valve replacement. *Ann Thorac Surg* 1994; 58:1161.
19. Lundin I, Norheim I, Landelius J, et al: Carcinoid heart disease: relationship of circulating vasoactive substances to ultrasound-detectable cardiac abnormalities. *Circulation* 1988; 77:264.
20. Fujii S, Funaki K, Denzunn N: Isolated rheumatic tricuspid regurgitation and stenosis. *Clin Cardiol* 1966; 9:353.
21. Kim JB, Spevack DM, Tunick PA, et al: The effect of transvenous pacemaker and implantable cardioverter defibrillator lead placement on tricuspid valve function: an observational study. *J Am Soc Echocardiogr.* 2008; 21:284-287.
22. Taira K, Suzuki A, Fujino A, et al: Tricuspid valve stenosis related to subvalvular adhesion of pacemaker lead: a case report. *J Cardiol* 2006; 47: 301-306.
23. Love CJ, Wilkoff BL, Byrd CL, et al: Recommendations for extraction of chronically implanted transvenous pacing and defibrillator leads: indications, facilities, training: North American Society of Pacing and Electrophysiology Lead Extraction Conference Faculty. *Pacing Clin Electrophysiol* 2000; 23: 544-551.
24. McCarthy PM, Bhudia SK, Rajeswaran J, et al: Tricuspid valve repair: durability and risk factors for failure. *J Thorac Cardiovasc Surg* 2004; 127: 674-685.
25. Zoghbi WA, Enriquez-Sarano M, Foster E, et al: Recommendations for evaluation of the severity of native valvular regurgitation with two-dimensional and Doppler echocardiography. *J Am Soc Echocardiogr* 2003; 16: 777-802.
26. Lorenz CH, Walker ES, Morgan VL, Klein SS, Graham TP Jr: Normal human right and left ventricular mass, systolic function, and gender differences by cine magnetic resonance imaging. *J Cardiovasc Magn Reson* 1999; 1:7-21.
27. Zornoff LA, Skali H, Pfeffer MA, et al: Right ventricular dysfunction and risk of heart failure and mortality after myocardial infarction. *J Am Coll Cardiol* 2002; 39:1450-1455.
28. Nesser HJ, Tkalec W, Patel AR, et al: Quantitation of right ventricular volumes and ejection fraction by three-dimensional echocardiography in patients: comparison with magnetic resonance imaging and radionuclide ventriculography. *Echocardiography* 2006; 23:666-680.
29. Brown AK, Anderson V: The value of contrast cross-sectional echocardiography in the diagnosis of tricuspid regurgitation. *Eur Heart J* 1984; 5:62.
30. Child JS: Improved guides to tricuspid valve repair: two-dimensional echocardiographic analysis of tricuspid annulus function and color flow imaging of severity of tricuspid regurgitation. *J Am Coll Cardiol* 1989; 14:1275.
31. Wong M, Matsumura M, Kutsuzawa S, et al: The value of Doppler echocardiography in the treatment of tricuspid regurgitation in patients with mitral valve replacement. *J Thorac Cardiovasc Surg* 1990; 99:1003.
32. Czer LSC, Maurer G, Bolger A, et al: Tricuspid valve repair, operative and follow-up evaluation by Doppler color flow mapping. *J Thorac Cardiovasc Surg* 1989; 98:101.
33. DeSimone R, Lange R, Saggau W, et al: Intraoperative transesophageal echocardiography for the evaluation of mutual, aortic and tricuspid valve repair. *Eur J Cardiothorac Surg* 1992; 6:665.
34. Maurer G, Siegel RJ, Czer LSC: The use of color-flow mapping for intraoperative assessment of valve repair. *Circulation* 1991; 84:I-250.
35. Gibson R, Wood P: The diagnosis of tricuspid stenosis. *Br Heart J* 1955; 17:552.
36. Keefe JF, Wolk MJ, Levine HJ: Isolated tricuspid valvular stenosis. *Am J Cardiol* 1970; 25(2):252-257.
37. Roberts WC, Sullivan MF: Combined mitral valve stenosis and tricuspid valve stenosis: morphologic observations after mitral and tricuspid valve replacements or mitral replacement and tricuspid valve commissurotomy. *Am J Cardiol* 1986; 58:850.
38. Nath J, Foster E, Heidenreich PA: Impact of tricuspid regurgitation on long-term survival. *J Am Coll Cardiol* 2004; 43:405-409.
39. Mutlak D, Aronson D, Lessick J, et al: Functional tricuspid regurgitation in patients with pulmonary hypertension: is pulmonary artery pressure the only determinant of regurgitation severity? *Chest* 2009; 135:115-121.
40. Dreyfus GD, Corbi PJ, Chan KMJ, Toufan Bahrami T: Secondary tricuspid regurgitation or dilatation: which should be the criterion for surgical repair? *Ann Thorac Surg* 2005; 79:127.
42. Matsunaga A, Duran CM: Progression of tricuspid regurgitation after repaired functional ischemic mitral regurgitation. *Circulation* 2005; 112: I-453.
43. Deloche A, Guerinon J, Fabiani JN, et al: Anatomical study of rheumatic tricuspid valve diseases: application to the various valvuloplasties [in French]. *Ann Chir Thorac Cardiovasc.* 1973; 12:343-349.
44. Castedo E, Canas A, Cabo RA, Burgos R, Ugarte J: Edge-to-edge tricuspid repair for redeveloped valve incompetence after DeVega's annuloplasty. *Ann Thorac Surg* 2003; 75:605-606.
44. Castedo E, Monguio E, Cabo RA, Ugarte J: Edge-to-edge technique for correction of tricuspid valve regurgitation due to complex lesions. *Eur J Cardiothorac Surg* 2005; 27:933-934.
45. Tang GH, David TE, Singh SK, et al: Tricuspid valve repair with an annuloplasty ring results in improved long-term outcomes. *Circulation* 2006; 114 (suppl): I-577-I-581.
46. DeVega NG: La anuloplastia selective, reguable y permanente. *Rev Esp Cardiol* 1972; 25:6-9.
47. Ghanta RK, Chen R, Narayanasamy N, et al: Suture bicuspidization of the tricuspid valve versus ring annuloplasty for repair of functional tricuspid regurgitation: midterm results of 237 consecutive patients. *J Thorac Cardiovasc Surg* 2007; 133:117-126.
48. Matsuyama K, Matsumoto M, Sugita T, et al: Predictors of residual tricuspid regurgitation after mitral valve surgery. *Ann Thorac Surg* 2003; 75:1826-1828.
49. Matsunaga A, Duran CM: Progression of tricuspid regurgitation after repaired functional ischemic mitral regurgitation. *Circulation* 2005; 112(Suppl): I-453-I-457.
50. King RM, Schaff HV, Danielson GK, et al: Surgery for tricuspid regurgitation late after mitral valve replacement. *Circulation* 1984; 70(Suppl): I-193-I-197.
51. Singh SK, Tang GH, Maganti MD, et al: Midterm outcomes of tricuspid valve repair versus replacement for organic tricuspid disease. *Ann Thorac Surg* 2006; 82:1735-1741.
52. Silver MD, Lam JH, Ranganathan N, Wigle ED: Morphology of the human tricuspid valve. *Circulation* 1971; 43:333-348.
53. Cohn L: Tricuspid regurgitation secondary to mitral valve disease: when and how to repair. *J Card Surg* 1994; 9(Suppl):237.
54. Duran CM, Kumar N, Prabhakar G, et al: Vanishing DeVega annuloplasty for functional tricuspid regurgitation. *J Thorac Cardiovasc Surg* 1993; 106:609.
55. Chidambaram M, Abdulali SA, Baliga BG, et al: Long-term results of DeVega tricuspid annuloplasty. *Ann Thorac Surg* 1987; 43:185.
56. Carpentier A, Deloche A, Dauptain J, et al: A new reconstructive operation for correction of mitral and tricuspid insufficiency. *J Thorac Cardiovasc Surg* 1971; 61:1.
57. Brugger JJ, Egloff L, Rothlin M, et al: Tricuspid annuloplasty: results and complications. *Thorac Cardiovasc Surg* 1982; 30:284.
58. Gatti G, Maffei G, Lusa A, et al: Tricuspid valve repair with Cosgrove-Edwards annuloplasty system: early clinical and echocardiographic results. *Ann Thorac Surg* 2001; 72:764.
59. McCarthy PM, Bhudia SK, Rajeswaran J, et al: Tricuspid valve repair: durability and risk factors for failure. *J Thorac Cardiovasc Surg* 2004; 127:67

60. Pomar JI, Mestres CA, Pate JC, et al: Management of persistent tricuspid endocarditis with transplantation of cryopreserved mitral homografts. *J Thorac Cardiovasc Surg* 1994; 107:1460.
61. Hvass U, Baron F, Fourchy D, et al: Mitral homografts for total tricuspid valve replacement: comparison of two techniques. *J Thorac Cardiovasc Surg* 2001; 3:592.
62. Katz NM, Pallas RS: Traumatic rupture of the tricuspid valve: repair by chordal replacements and annuloplasty. *J Thorac Cardiovasc Surg* 1986; 91:310.
63. Cardarelli MG, Gammie JS, Brown JM, et al: A novel approach to tricuspid valve replacement: the upside down stentless aortic bioprosthesis. *Ann Thorac Surg* 2005; 80:507.
64. Sutlic Z, Schmid C, Borst HG: Repair of flail anterior leaflets of tricuspid and mitral valves by cusp remodeling. *Ann Thorac Cardiovasc Surg* 1990; 50:927.
65. Doty JR, Cameron DE, Elmaci T, et al: Penetrating trauma to the tricuspid valve and ventricular septum: delayed repair. *Ann Thorac Surg* 1999; 67:252.
66. Arbulu A, Asfaw I: Tricuspid valvulectomy without prosthetic replacement. *J Thorac Cardiovasc Surg* 1981; 82:684.
67. Arbulu A, Thoms NW, Wilson RI: Valvulectomy without prosthetic replacement: a lifesaving operation for tricuspid Pseudomonas endocarditis. *J Cardiovasc Surg (Torino)* 1972; 74:103.
67. Walther T, Falk V, Schneider J, et al: Stentless tricuspid valve replacement. *Ann Thorac Surg* 1999; 68:1858.
68. Arbulu A, Holmes RJ, Asfaw I: Tricuspid valvulectomy without replacement: twenty years' experience. *J Thorac Cardiovasc Surg* 1991; 102:917.
69. Turley K: Surgery of right-sided endocarditis: valve preservation versus replacement. *J Card Surg* 1989; 4:317.
70. Van Nooten G, Caes F, Tacymans Y, et al: Tricuspid valve replacement: postoperative and long-term results. *J Thorac Cardiovasc Surg* 1995; 110:672.
71. Kaplan M, Kut MS, Demirtas MM, et al: Prosthetic replacement of tricuspid valve: bioprosthetic or mechanical. *Ann Thorac Surg* 2002; 73:467.
72. Scully HE, Armstrong CS: Tricuspid valve replacement: fifteen years of experience with mechanical prostheses and bioprostheses. *J Thorac Cardiovasc Surg* 1995; 109:1035.
73. Singh AK, Feng WC, Sanofsky SJ: Long-term results of St Jude Medical valve in the tricuspid position. *Ann Thorac Surg* 1992; 54:538.
74. Kaplan M, Kut MS, Demirtas MM, et al: Prosthetic replacement of tricuspid valve: bioprosthetic or mechanical. *Ann Thorac Surg* 2002; 73:467.
75. Nakano K, Koyanagi H, Hashimoto A, et al: Tricuspid valve replacement with the bileaflet St Jude Medical valve prosthesis. *J Thorac Cardiovasc Surg* 1994; 108:888.
76. Munro AI, Jamieson WRE, Tyers FO, et al: Tricuspid valve replacement: porcine bioprostheses and mechanical prostheses. *Ann Thorac Surg* 1995; 59:S470.
77. Ohata T, Kigawa I, Tohda E, et al: Comparison of durability of bioprostheses in tricuspid and mitral positions. *Ann Thorac Surg* 2001; 71:S240.
78. Ratnatunga C, Edwards M-B, Dore C, et al: Tricuspid valve replacement: UK heart valve registry midterm results comparing mechanical and biological prostheses. *Ann Thorac Surg* 1998; 66:1940.
79. Glower DD, White WD, Smith LR, et al: In-hospital and long-term outcome after porcine tricuspid valve replacement. *J Thorac Cardiovasc Surg* 1995; 109:877.
80. Nakano K, Ishibashi-Ueda H, Kobayashi J, et al: Tricuspid valve replacement with bioprostheses: long-term results and causes of valve dysfunction. *Ann Thorac Surg* 2001; 71:105.
81. Nakano K, Eishi K, Kosakai Y, et al: Ten-year experience with the Carpentier-Edwards pericardial xenograft in the tricuspid position. *J Thorac Cardiovasc Surg* 1996; 111:605.
82. Ohata T, Kigawa I, Yamashita Y, et al: Surgical strategy for severe tricuspid valve regurgitation complicated by advanced mitral valve disease: long-term outcome of tricuspid valve supra-annular implantation in eighty-eight cases. *J Thorac Cardiovasc Surg* 2000; 120:280.
83. Cohen SR, Silver MA, McIntosh CL, Roberts WC: Comparison of late (62 to 104 months) degenerative changes in simultaneously implanted and explanted porcine (Hancock) bioprosthesis in the tricuspid and mitral positions in six patients. *Am J Cardiol* 1984; 53:1599.
84. Guerra F, Bortolotti U, Thiene G, et al: Long-term performance of the Hancock porcine bioprosthesis in the tricuspid position: a review of 45 patients with 14 visit follow-up. *J Thorac Cardiovasc Surg* 1990; 99:838.
85. Filsoufi F, Anyanwu AC, Salzberg SP, et al: Long-term outcomes of tricuspid valve replacement in the current era. *Ann Thorac Surg* 2005; 80:845.
86. Solomon NAG, Lim CH, Nand P, Graham KJ: Tricuspid valve replacement: bioprosthetic or mechanical valve? *Asian Cardiovasc Thorac Ann* 2004; 12:143.
87. Rizzoli G, Vendramin I, Nesseris G, et al: Biological or mechanical prostheses in tricuspid position? A meta-analysis of intrainstitutional results. *Ann Thorac Surg* 2004; 77:1607.
88. Bonow RO, Carabello BA, Kanu C, et al: ACC/AHA 2006 guidelines for the management of patients with valvular heart disease: a report of the American College of Cardiology/American Heart Association Task Force on Practice Guidelines (writing committee to revise the 1998 Guidelines for the Management of Patients With Valvular Heart Disease): developed in collaboration with the Society of Cardiovascular Anesthesiologists: endorsed by the Society for Cardiovascular Angiography and Interventions and the Society of Thoracic Surgeons. *Circulation* 2006; 114:e84-e231.
89. Aoyagi S, Tanaka K, Hara H, et al: Modified De Vega's annuloplasty for functional tricuspid regurgitation: early and late results. *The Kurume Med J* 1992; 39:23-32.
90. Fukuda S, Song JM, Gillinov AM, et al: Tricuspid valve tethering predicts residual tricuspid regurgitation after tricuspid annuloplasty. *Circulation* 2005; 111:975-979.
91. Holper K, Haehnel JC, Augustin N, Sebening F: Surgery for tricuspid insufficiency: long-term follow-up after De Vega annuloplasty. *Thorac Cardiovasc Surg* 1993; 41:1-8.
92. Minale C, Lambertz H, Nikol S, Gerich N, Messmer BJ: Selective annuloplasty of the tricuspid valve: two-year experience. *J Thorac Cardiovasc Surg* 1990; 99:846-851.
93. Paulis RD, Bobbio M, Ottino G, DeVega N: The De Vega tricuspid annuloplasty: perioperative mortality and long term follow-up. *J Cardiovasc Surg (Torino)* 1990; 31:512-517.
94. Peltola T, Lepojarvi M, Ikaheimo M, Karkola P: De Vega's annuloplasty for tricuspid regurgitation. *Ann Chir Gynaecol* 1996; 85:40-43.
95. Kirklin JW, Barratt-Boyes BG (eds): *Cardiac Surgery,* vol. 1, 2nd ed. New York, Churchill-Livingstone, 1992; p 598.
96. Rogers JH, Bolling SF: The tricuspid valve: current perspective and evolving management of tricuspid regurgitation. *Circulation* 2009; 119:2718-2725.

CHAPTER 47

Multiple Valve Disease

Hartzell V. Schaff
Rakesh M. Suri

INTRODUCTION

Pathologic changes in the cardiac valves requiring surgical correction of more than one valve can result from rheumatic heart disease, degenerative valve diseases, infective endocarditis, and a number of miscellaneous causes. Further, valve dysfunction may be primary; that is, a direct result of a disease process, or secondary; that is, caused by cardiac enlargement and/or pulmonary hypertension. Surgical management is influenced both by the underlying cause of valve dysfunction and, when valves are involved secondarily, by the anticipated response to replacement or repair of the primary valve lesion. In addition, the consequences of various combinations of diseased valves on left and right ventricular geometry and function frequently are different from the remodeling as a result of single-valve disease. This chapter addresses pathophysiologic considerations in multivalvular heart disease, surgical techniques, and management of commonly encountered etiologies.

Repair of multiple lesions was necessary even in the early development of operative management of valvular heart disease (Table 47-1). The first triple-valve replacement during a single operation was reported in 1960, and simultaneous replacement of all four valves was reported in 1992.[1]

Experience from clinical practice indicates that multiple valve disease requiring surgical correction occurs in a few common combinations. As seen in Table 47-2, multiple procedures account for approximately 15% of all operations on cardiac valves; 80% of these operations involve the aortic and mitral positions. Replacement of the mitral and tricuspid valves (with or without aortic replacement) accounts for 20% of operations. Only rarely is the combination of aortic and tricuspid disease encountered.

PATHOPHYSIOLOGY OF MULTIPLE VALVE DISEASE

Valvular regurgitation may result from the pathologic process affecting the valve directly or may be secondary to alterations in ventricular morphology caused by other valve lesions; this secondary or functional regurgitation affects the atrioventricular valves. In some patients, secondary valvular regurgitation may be expected to improve with repair or replacement of the primarily diseased valve. In other patients, the secondary disease process may have advanced to the stage that valve function will not improve following correction of the primary lesion, and thus simultaneous surgical correction should be considered.

Primary Aortic Valve Disease with Secondary Mitral Regurgitation

Isolated aortic valve lesions can cause secondary regurgitation of the mitral valve and rarely, the tricuspid valve. Severe aortic valve stenosis with or without left ventricular dilatation frequently is associated with some degree of mitral valve regurgitation. In one series, 67% of patients with severe aortic valve stenosis had associated mitral valve leakage.[2]

When the mitral valve is structurally normal, its regurgitation would be expected to improve with relief of left ventricular outflow obstruction[3]; mild mitral valve regurgitation would be expected to resolve almost completely after aortic valve replacement. Improvement in mitral valve regurgitation results from both decreased intraventricular pressure and ventricular remodeling.[4] If mitral valve regurgitation is severe, some degree of persistent regurgitation is expected after aortic valve replacement, and mitral valve annuloplasty may be required. In contrast,

TABLE 47-1 History of Multiple Valve Operations

Event	Year	Institution
Staged mitral then tricuspid commissurotomy	1952	Doctor's Hospital, Philadelphia, PA[164]
Simultaneous mitral and tricuspid commissurotomy	1953	Cleveland, OH[165]
Simultaneous mitral commissurotomy and aortic valvuloplasty using cardiopulmonary bypass	1956	University of Minnesota, Minneapolis, MN[166]
Simultaneous mitral and aortic valve replacement	1961	St. Francis General Hospital, Pittsburgh, PA[123]
Simultaneous triple-valve replacement	1963	University of Oregon, Portland, OR
Simultaneous quadruple valve replacement	1992	Mayo Clinic, Rochester, MN[120]

Source: Modified with permission from Acker M, Hargrove WC, Stephenson LW: Multiple valve replacement. Cardiol Clin 1985; 3:425.

with aortic valve stenosis and mitral valve regurgitation associated with a structurally abnormal mitral valve, repair or replacement of the mitral valve usually is necessary. A recent report alleges that moderate mitral regurgitation has an adverse impact on survival in elderly patients undergoing aortic valve replacement and suggests that those with intrinsic mitral valve disease should be considered for concurrent correction.[5]

Thus determination of the morphology and pathophysiologic severity of each valve lesion is critically important in planning surgical management, and preoperative and intraoperative echocardiographic studies are necessary in all patients suspected of having multiple valve disease. Often, transthoracic echocardiography can define the etiology of mitral and tricuspid valvular regurgitation. When valve regurgitation is entirely secondary, the mitral valve leaflets will appear thin and freely mobile, without prolapsing segments. Mitral (and tricuspid) valve regurgitation secondary to rheumatic disease is readily identified when leaflets are thickened and chordae are shortened; fibrosis

TABLE 47-2 Prevalence of Multiple Cardiac Valve Replacement According to Institution

	University of Alabama	Mayo Clinic	Texas Heart Institute	University of Oregon	Percentage of all Valve Surgery (11,026 cases)	Percentage of Multiple Valve Surgery (1662 cases)
Years involved	1967–1976	1963–1972	1962–1974	1960–1980		
Total number of all valve operations	2555	2166	4170	2135		
All multiple valve procedures	383 (15%)	437 (20%)	541 (13%)	301 (14%)	15 (1662)	100
M-A	298 (11.6%)	320 (14.7%)	459 (11%)	253 (11.8%)	12 (1330)	80
M-A-T	40 (1.6%)	55 (2.5%)	55 (2.5%)	48 (2.2%)	2 (198)	12
M-T	41 (1.6%)	58 (2.5%)	26 (0.6%)	—	1.5 (125)	8
A-T	4 (0.1%)	4 (0.2%)	1 (0.02%)	—	0.1 (9)	5

M = mitral valve; A = aortic valve; T = tricuspid valve.
Source: Modified with permission from Acker M, Hargrove WC, Stephenson LW: Multiple valve replacement. Cardiol Clin 1985; 3:425.

of these structures restricts leaflet mobility. Leaflet prolapse with or without ruptured chordae tendineae also may cause atrioventricular valve regurgitation.

Transesophageal echocardiography images the heart from a retrocardiac position, which avoids interference from interposed ribs, lungs, and subcutaneous tissue. A high-frequency (5-MHz) transducer is employed, which yields better resolution than that of images obtained with routine transthoracic imaging with 2.25- to 3.5-MHz transducers.[6] Thus transesophageal echocardiography provides the best image of the mitral and tricuspid valves and may be obtained preoperatively. Intraoperative transesophageal Doppler echocardiography should be employed in all patients having valve repair or replacement, and the technique is especially important for assessment of response of mitral regurgitation to relief of left ventricular outflow obstruction.[7] In some cases, preoperative left ventriculography may help to quantify left atrioventricular valve leakage. Right ventricular angiocardiography also can be useful in determining the degree of tricuspid valve dysfunction, but it is rarely employed in current practice.[8]

Tricuspid Valve Regurgitation Secondary to Other Valvular Disease

Secondary tricuspid valve regurgitation commonly is associated with rheumatic mitral valve stenosis, and the exact cause is unknown.[9,10] Some authors believe that secondary tricuspid valve regurgitation is a result of pulmonary artery hypertension and right ventricular dilatation.[11] As with the mitral valve, tricuspid valve annular dilatation in those with severe TR is asymmetric. Most enlargement occurs in the annulus subtended by the free wall of the right ventricle, and there is little dilation of the annulus adjacent to the septal leaflet of the tricuspid valve.[12,13] Although pulmonary artery hypertension with secondary enlargement of the right ventricle and tricuspid valve annulus may be an important contributing factor in secondary tricuspid regurgitation, it is not the sole mechanism. For example, congenital heart lesions such as tetralogy of Fallot produce systemic pressure in the right ventricle, yet severe tricuspid valve regurgitation rarely is seen in these patients. Similarly, important tricuspid valve regurgitation is uncommon in children with ventricular septal defects who have enlargement of the right ventricle associated with variable degrees of pulmonary hypertension.

Furthermore, clinical experience suggests that other mechanisms must play a role in development of secondary tricuspid valve regurgitation. Patients who have had mitral valve replacement for rheumatic mitral valve stenosis may develop regurgitation of their native tricuspid valve years after initial operation, and many patients have only modest elevation of pulmonary artery pressure.[14,15] Recent evidence points to a progressive immunologic process in rheumatic valve disease, which can lead to severe TR many years after successful percutaneous or surgical management of the mitral valve.[16]

It is useful to classify secondary mitral and tricuspid valve regurgitation as mild, moderate, and severe.[13] Usually, patients with mild tricuspid valve regurgitation do not have clinical signs and symptoms of right-sided heart failure. Also, mild tricuspid regurgitation demonstrated by preoperative echocardiography may appear even less severe in the operating room under general anesthesia. In most instances, mild secondary tricuspid regurgitation does not require intervention.

Patients with echocardiographic evidence of significant regurgitation who do not have symptoms or have their symptoms controlled by medical treatment can be classified as having moderate tricuspid regurgitation. These patients usually are managed with a DeVega suture annuloplasty or a partial-ring annuloplasty.[17] Patients with severe secondary tricuspid regurgitation and clinical evidence of right-sided heart failure (eg, pulsatile liver, distended neck veins, and peripheral edema with or without ascites) are most frequently managed by concomitant ring annuloplasty or tricuspid valve replacement.

The degree of pulmonary hypertension may influence surgical management of secondary tricuspid valve regurgitation. Kaul and colleagues[18] grouped 86 patients with functional tricuspid regurgitation in association with rheumatic mitral valve disease according to the degree of pulmonary hypertension. One group had severe pulmonary hypertension (mean pulmonary pressure 78 mm Hg), and a second group had moderate pulmonary hypertension (mean pulmonary artery pressure 41 mm Hg). Patients with moderate pulmonary hypertension preoperatively had more advanced right-sided heart failure and right ventricular dilatation, and many of these patients continued to have tricuspid valve regurgitation following mitral valve surgery without tricuspid valve surgery. The patients with severe pulmonary hypertension all showed regression of tricuspid regurgitation, and 28% had complete resolution following mitral valve surgery without operation on the tricuspid valve.

Excluding hospital mortality, about 40% of patients undergoing tricuspid valve surgery have premature death.[8] It is also important to understand that mild to moderate (2+) regurgitation is a risk factor for late failure of tricuspid valve repair, and severe (4+) regurgitation preoperatively is a predictor of early residual regurgitation.[19] Finally, there is recent evidence to suggest that remodeling annuloplasty in the setting of tricuspid annular dilatation (≥70 mm) at the time of mitral repair significantly decreases the risk of subsequent functional deterioration as compared with those not having annular correction.[20]

The difficulty with interpretation and generalization of current literature guiding management of secondary functional TR is the significant heterogeneity in both patient disease substrate and surgical procedure performed. The incidence of severe late TR has been reported to be approximately 68% up to 30 years following mitral replacement for rheumatic disease.[21] The risk of significant late secondary TR is as high as 74% 3 years following repair of ischemic MR.[22] The most frequently identified risk factors for TR progression from these series include older age, female gender, rheumatic etiology, atrial fibrillation, the absence of a Maze operation.[21–24] Therefore, most would agree that correction of moderate or greater TR at the time of surgery for rheumatic mitral disease is indicated to prevent the development of symptoms associated with TR progression.[25] Less clear however is whether long-term survival is improved by such intervention.[24] Furthermore, reliance on tricuspid annular dilation alone as suggested by Dreyfus and coworkers[20] has recently been challenged.[26]

In contrast, although mitral valve prolapse is the most frequent cause of mitral regurgitation in the developed world, there are few reports addressing the incidence and fate of functional TR following successful mitral valve repair. Recent data suggest that moderate or less functional TR does not progress as aggressively following repair of leaflet prolapse as in rheumatic or ischemic mitral disease subsets.[27] Outcomes following isolated mitral valve repair for degenerative MR with less than severe coexistent functional TR at Mayo Clinic support this assertion; with only one patient out of 699 requiring tricuspid valve reoperation during long-term follow up.

VALVE SELECTION FOR MULTIPLE VALVE REPLACEMENT

When multiple valve replacement is confined to the left ventricle, replacement valves should be chosen from the same class with respect to the need for anticoagulation and projected longevity. There are no theoretical or practical advantages to use of a tissue valve and a mechanical valve for mitral and aortic valve replacement, and studies show no reduction in the risk of thromboembolism, valve-related morbidity, or late death.[29,30] In addition, a lower reoperation rate is reported for patients with two mechanical valves in the left ventricle compared with patients with one mechanical and one tissue valve.[29]

For tricuspid valve replacement, alone or in conjunction with other valve procedures, use of a bioprosthesis may have advantages in regard to minimizing risk of valve thrombosis.[31,32] Furthermore, there are few hemodynamic considerations in selecting a tricuspid prosthesis; the greater hemodynamic efficiency of mechanical valves compared with bioprostheses rarely is an issue in atrioventricular valve replacement, especially the tricuspid valve, in which the annulus diameter in adults is often 33 mm or more. In vitro studies demonstrate only minimal hemodynamic improvement with atrioventricular valves larger than 25 mm.[33]

SURGICAL METHODS

Aortic and Mitral Valve Replacement

Cannulation

Arterial inflow is established by cannulation of the distal ascending aorta near the pericardial reflection just to the left of the origin of the innominate artery (Fig. 47-1A). Venous cannulation is simplified by using a two-stage cannula in the right atrium for venous return. Individual cannulation of the superior and inferior venae cavae is reserved for operations that require right atrial or ventricular incisions (Fig. 47-2A). Provisions for intraoperative autotransfusion are used routinely, and antifibrinolytic drugs such as aprotinin or epsilon-aminocaproic acid (Amicar) may be useful, especially in reoperations, in which pericardial adhesions may worsen bleeding.[34]

Cardioplegia

If the aortic valve is competent, myocardial protection during aortic cross-clamping is achieved by initial infusion of cold (4 to 8°C) blood cardioplegia through a tack vent placed in the aorta proximal to the clamp. The volume of cardioplegia needed to achieve diastolic arrest and uniform hypothermia depends on the heart size and the presence of aortic valve regurgitation. Generally, the initial volume of cardioplegia required for hearts with multiple valve disease is higher than that required for coronary revascularization because of myocardial hypertrophy. For patients without cardiac enlargement, we infuse approximately 10 mL/kg of body weight, whereas 15 mL/kg of body weight is used for patients with significant degrees of myocardial hypertrophy. Repeat infusions of 400 mL of cardioplegia are given directly into the coronary ostia at 20-minute intervals during aortic occlusion. We use custom-designed, soft-tipped coronary perfusion catheters to minimize the potential for trauma to the coronary ostia during intubation and infusion.[35]

If aortic valve regurgitation is moderate or severe, cardioplegia is infused directly into the coronary ostia. Initial aortotomy is facilitated by emptying the heart using suction on an aortic tack vent and temporarily reducing the cardiopulmonary bypass flow rate to maximize venous return. Some surgeons prefer retrograde infusion of cardioplegia,[36] and if this method is used, even larger volumes are necessary because of nonnutritive flow through the coronary venous system and variation in coronary venous anatomy.[37,38]

Procedure

After cardioplegia, the aortic valve is inspected through an oblique aortotomy extended into the noncoronary aortic sinus (see Fig. 47-1B). Aortic valve regurgitation caused by cuspal perforation or prolapse of a congenitally bicuspid valve often can be repaired,[39] but the decision for or against aortic valve repair should take into consideration whether or not a mitral valve prosthesis will be needed. For example, even though aortic valve repair might seem technically possible, prosthetic replacement may be the best option for a patient who requires mitral valve replacement and will be maintained on warfarin for long-term anticoagulation.

Severe calcification of the valve, whether it is bicuspid or tricuspid, necessitates replacement;[40] therefore, the cusps are excised and annular calcium debrided carefully. The aortic annulus then is calibrated; experience has shown that subsequent replacement of the mitral valve usually reduces the aortic annular diameter by shortening the circumference that is in continuity with the attachment of the anterior mitral valve leaflet. Therefore, we routinely identify (but do not break the sterile packaging of) two aortic prostheses: One corresponds to the calibrated dimension, and the other is the next size smaller. Final selection of the aortic prosthesis is made after mitral valve replacement or repair.

Although exposed first, the aortic valve usually is replaced after mitral valve repair or insertion of the mitral valve prosthesis. Sutures placed in the portion of the aortic valve annulus that is continuous with the anterior leaflet of the mitral valve pull the anterior leaflet superiorly toward the left ventricular outflow area and thus hinder exposure of this area as viewed through the left atriotomy.

If the aortic annulus is small, it can be enlarged with a patch of pericardium.[41] This technique increases annular diameter by

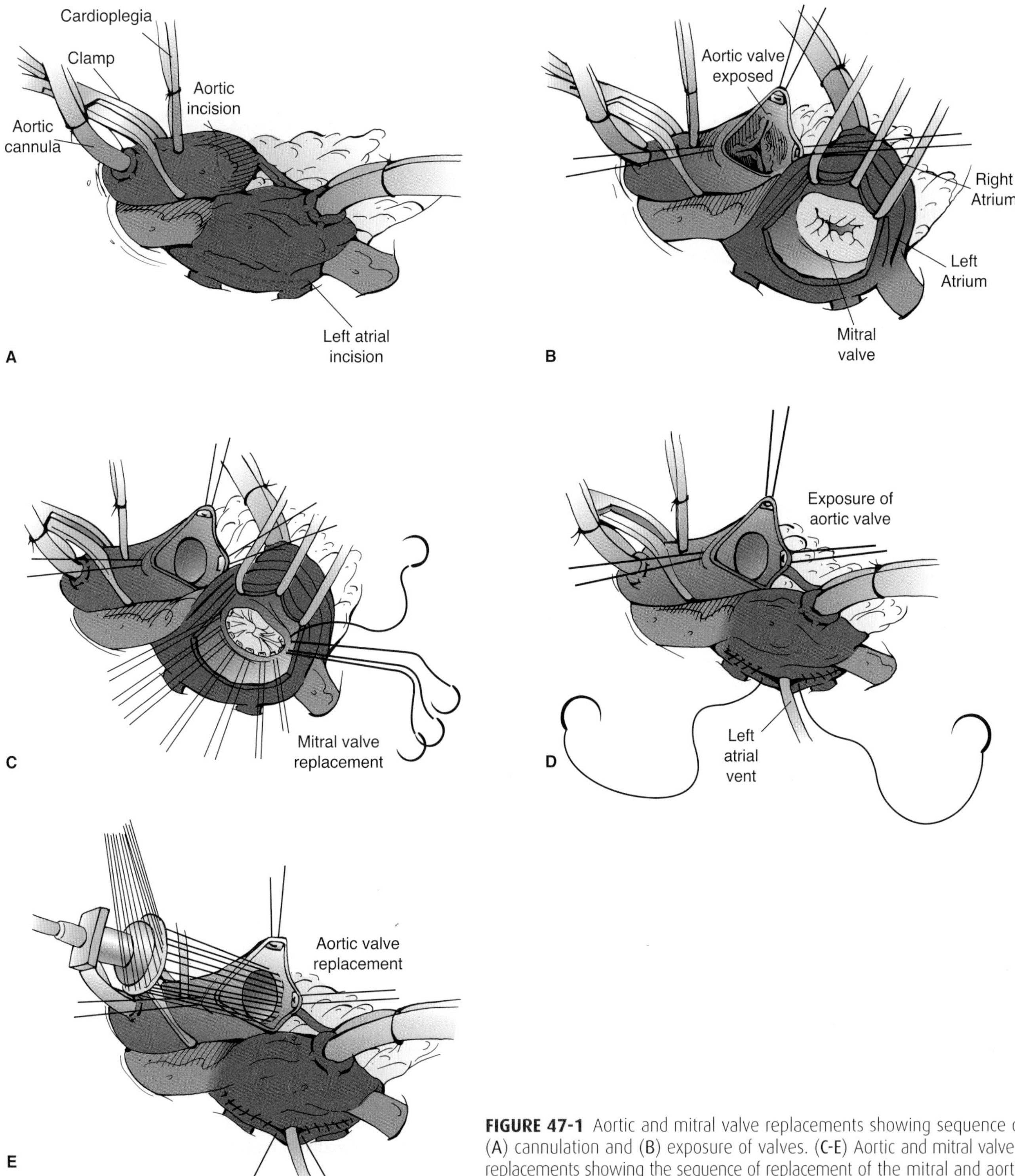

FIGURE 47-1 Aortic and mitral valve replacements showing sequence of (A) cannulation and (B) exposure of valves. (C-E) Aortic and mitral valve replacements showing the sequence of replacement of the mitral and aortic valves.

2 to 4 mm or more, and only rarely are more radical techniques necessary.[42–44] Another maneuver to accommodate as large a prosthesis as possible is to place the necessary sutures for the mitral valve repair or replacement but not secure the mitral prosthesis until the aortic valve is implanted. This eliminates downsizing of the aortic prosthesis but does not compromise insertion of sutures in the superior portion of the mitral valve annulus.

After removal of the aortic valve, the right atrial cannula is repositioned, and the mitral valve is exposed through an incision posterior to the interatrial groove (see Fig. 47-1B). The presence or absence of thrombi in the left atrium is noted, and the mitral valve is inspected. When there is rheumatic disease of the aortic valve, the mitral valve almost always will be involved to some extent. If aortic valve replacement is necessary, the surgeon should have a low threshold for replacing a diseased mitral

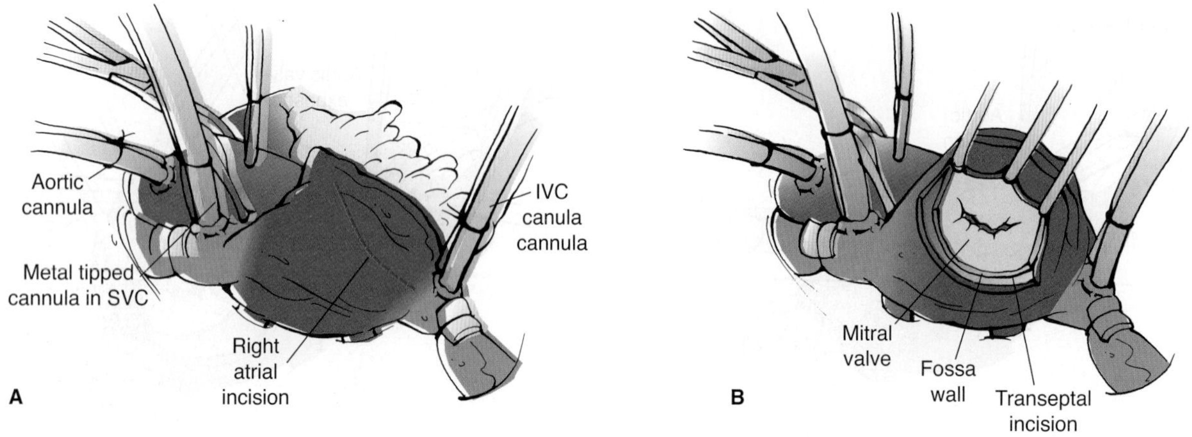

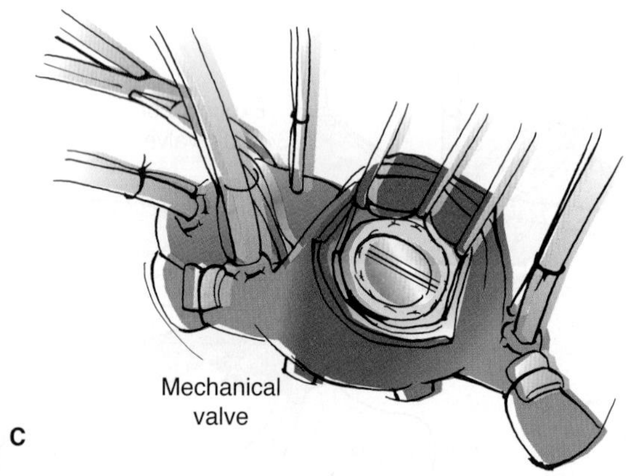

FIGURE 47-2 Combined mitral valve and tricuspid valve operation. The panels illustrate (A) cannulation (B) and transseptal incision. (C) Combined mital valve and tricuspid valve operation: mitral replacement. (Superior vena cava snare not shown.)

valve because scarring and fibrosis of the rheumatic process are progressive, and mitral valve repair (commissurotomy for stenosis or leaflet repair and annuloplasty for regurgitation) is less durable than repair for degenerative disease.[45–47] In contrast, when aortic valve replacement is necessary because of calcification of a bicuspid valve or senescent calcification, repair of mitral valve regurgitation owing to degenerative causes can be expected to give predictably good long-term results. Repair of the mitral valve is described in Chapter 41.

In preparation for replacement, the anterior leaflet of the mitral valve is excised, and when possible, a portion of the posterior leaflet with its chordal attachments is preserved to maintain left ventricular papillary muscle–annular continuity.[48–50] Some surgeons make a special effort to preserve the anterior leaflet and its chordal attachments, believing that this has a further beneficial effect on ventricular performance.[51] The mitral prosthesis is implanted using interrupted mattress sutures of 2-0 braided polyester reinforced with felt pledgets, which can be situated on the atrial or ventricular side of the valve annulus (see Fig. 47-1C). The leaflets of mechanical valves should be tested for free mobility following valve seating.

When atrial fibrillation is present preoperatively, we obliterate the left atrial appendage by oversewing its orifice from within the left atrium or ligating it externally. The left atriotomy is closed from each end with running polypropylene sutures. Vent tubing is inserted through the partially closed left atriotomy and left in place while the aortic valve is being replaced (see Fig. 47-1D).

After appropriate exposure, the aortic prosthesis is sewn in place with interrupted 2-0 polyester mattress sutures backed with felt pledgets, and the aortotomy is closed, usually with two layers of 4-0 polypropylene. Any remaining air is evacuated from the heart with the usual maneuvers, and a tack vent in the ascending aorta is placed on suction as the aortic clamp is removed. The vent is removed from the left atrium, and closure of the left atriotomy is secured.

In patients with annuloaortic ectasia, the mitral valve sometimes can be visualized and replaced through the enlarged aortic annulus.[52]

Aortic Valve Replacement and Mitral Valve Repair

Intraoperative transesophageal echocardiography is useful in assessing the degree of mitral regurgitation and, importantly, in identifying the cause of valve leakage. When mitral valve regurgitation is only moderate and leaflet morphology is normal, we expect mitral valve function to improve following relief of severe aortic stenosis. In all other instances, the valve should be inspected directly to determine the need for repair or replacement.

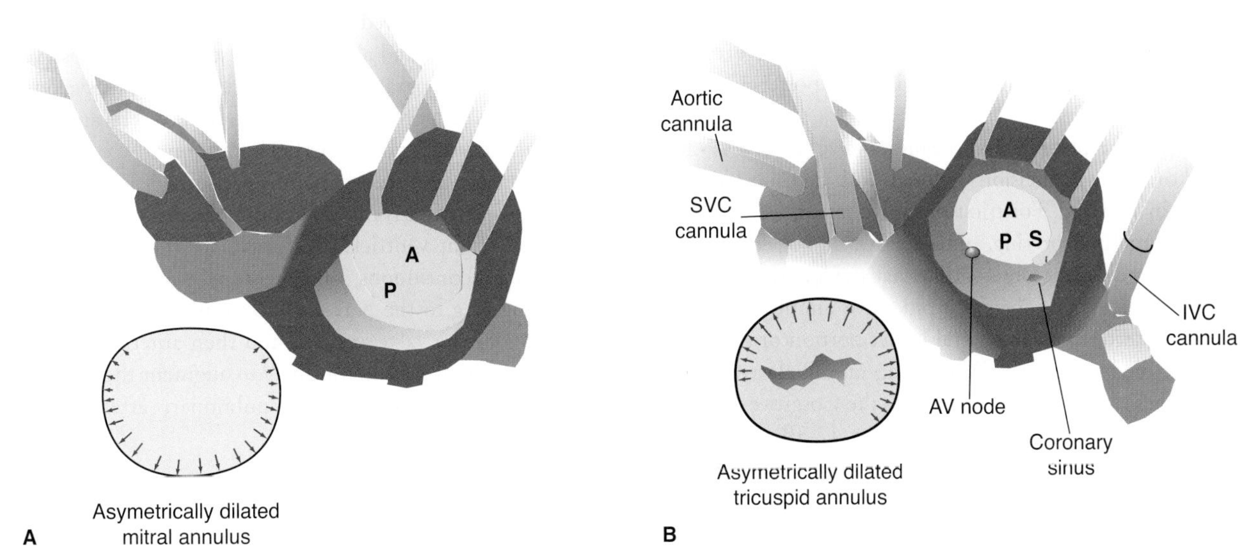

FIGURE 47-3 (A) Mitral valve repair and (B) tricuspid valve repair using a partial-ring annuloplasty. (Superior and inferior venae cavae snares not shown.)

Sternotomy, cannulation, and assessment of the aortic valve proceed as described previously. When there is no indication of tricuspid valve disease and no other right atrial procedures are planned, venous return is obtained through a single two-staged cannula (Fig. 47-3A). Specific techniques of mitral valve repair depend on operative findings.[53] Localized prolapse of a portion of the posterior leaflet with or without ruptured chordae usually is managed by triangular excision of that segment and repair with continuous 4-0 polypropylene suture.[54] Ruptured chordae to the anterior leaflet are replaced with 4-0 or 5-0 polytetrafluoroethylene (PTFE) sutures inserted into papillary muscle and through the free edge of the prolapsing leaflet.[55]

Almost all leaflet repairs are supplemented with a posterior annuloplasty. Interrupted 2-0 braided polyester mattress sutures are placed along the posterior circumference of the annulus ending at the right and left fibrous trigones (see Fig. 47-3A). Sutures then are spaced evenly through a flexible 6.0- to 6.5-cm–long partial ring; this standard length can be obtained by using a flexible 63-mm posterior annuloplasty band.[47,56] Following annuloplasty, competence of the mitral valve is tested by filling the ventricle with saline or blood; the atrium then is closed, and the aortic valve prosthesis is sewn into place.

Mitral Valve Replacement and Tricuspid Valve Replacement or Repair

In most instances, tricuspid valve regurgitation is caused by annular dilatation.[57] The severity of tricuspid valve leakage can be determined by transesophageal echocardiography before bypass and by digital exploration of the right atrium just before venous cannulation. Under general anesthesia, changes in blood volume and cardiac output can cause significant fluctuation in the amount of regurgitation, and most often the severity of tricuspid valve leakage is lessened in the immediate prebypass period.

The patient's clinical condition must be correlated with echocardiographic findings and intraoperative assessment of the tricuspid valve. Patients with an enlarged, pulsatile liver, peripheral edema, and jugular venous distention are likely to require tricuspid valvuloplasty following mitral valve replacement or repair. Patients without the stigmata of right-sided heart failure usually have less severe valve leakage, and tricuspid valve function may improve without direct repair or replacement after left-sided valvular lesions are corrected.

The decision for repair or replacement of functional tricuspid valve regurgitation at the time of mitral valve replacement is important because the risk of subsequent reoperation is high. In our earlier experience, operative mortality was 25% in patients who required later reoperation for tricuspid valve regurgitation. Further, tricuspid regurgitation progresses in 10 to 15% of patients after replacement of rheumatic mitral valves.[58] Therefore, we maintain a liberal policy for annuloplasty or prosthetic replacement at initial operation.[59]

Procedure

For operations on the tricuspid valve, insertion of a Swan-Ganz catheter is optional; if one is used, the catheter is withdrawn from the right heart chambers during inspection and assessment of the tricuspid valve. We prefer direct cannulation of the inferior and superior venae cavae.[60] After commencement of cardiopulmonary bypass and cardioplegia, the cavae are snared around the venous cannulae, and the interatrial septum and tricuspid valve are exposed through a right atriotomy (see Fig. 47-2A). A decision for repair or replacement of the tricuspid valve is made, and the necessary prosthesis is identified.

When the tricuspid valve is also addressed, we tend to expose the mitral valve through an incision in the interatrial septum, which crosses the fossa ovalis and can be extended superiorly (see Fig. 47-2B). Care should be taken during retraction to avoid tearing the septum inferiorly toward the coronary sinus and triangle of Koch. Alternatively, the mitral valve can be exposed through a standard left atriotomy posterior to the interatrial groove.

After repair or replacement of the mitral valve (see Fig. 47-2C), the septal or left atrial incision is closed, and the tricuspid valve is repaired or replaced. For tricuspid valve repair, we use either the DeVega method or ring annuloplasty.[11,17,61,62] Both techniques are based on the observation that the anterior and posterior valve portions of the tricuspid valve annulus are more prone to dilatation than the septal leaflet portion of the annulus, as described previously. When ring annuloplasty is indicated, we prefer a flexible device such as the Cosgrove-Edwards prosthesis[63] or a partial Duran ring (see Fig. 47-3B). The use of a partial ring avoids placement of sutures in the annulus near the penetrating bundle of His and reduces risk of injury to conduction tissue. There have been conflicting reports regarding the superiority of DeVega procedure versus prosthetic annuloplasty in improving freedom from recurrent TR.[64–66]

Minimally Invasive Approaches

Although addressed elsewhere in this textbook, minimally invasive approaches to primary and reoperative left and right-sided valvular heart disease have been proposed. Various cannulation and cardioplegia techniques have been described as determined by the pattern of valve disease and patient anatomy.[67]

Tricuspid Valve Replacement and Pulmonary Valve Replacement for Carcinoid Heart Disease

If there is no involvement of the mitral and aortic valves,[57,68] tricuspid and pulmonary valve replacement usually can be performed without the need for aortic occlusion and cardioplegic arrest. It is important to exclude the presence of a patent foramen ovale to eliminate the risk of air entering the left atrium, and if a defect in the atrial septum is identified, it is closed using a brief period of aortic occlusion. In the past, our strategy for patients with carcinoid heart disease was to replace the tricuspid valve and excise the diseased pulmonary valve.

Subsequent experience has suggested that right ventricular function is better preserved with a competent pulmonary valve, so we now favor pulmonary valve replacement rather than valvectomy.[69] Tricuspid valve replacement always is indicated, and it is usually necessary only to remove the anterior leaflet. A recent review of 200 patients with carcinoid heart disease at our institution demonstrated that prognosis has improved in the current era and that valve replacement surgery was independently associated with prolonged survival.[70]

Carcinoid disease produces fibrosis and retraction of the leaflets, so anchoring sutures (interrupted mattress sutures of 2-0 braided polyester backed with felt pledgets) can be inserted into the remaining septal and posterior leaflets. We prefer to position the pledgets on the ventricular side of the valve annulus. If exposure is difficult, a brief period of aortic clamping and cardioplegic arrest is used during placement of sutures in the posterior and septal leaflets; the aortic cross-clamp is removed, and the heart is allowed to beat rhythmically. The remaining sutures are placed, and all sutures are secured with observation of the electrocardiogram. If atrioventricular block develops, the sutures in the area of the penetrating bundle of His are removed and reinserted in a more superficial location.

Pulmonary valve replacement is performed through a longitudinal incision across the valve annulus onto the outflow portion of the right ventricle. We prefer to insert the prosthetic valve using a continuous 3-0 polypropylene suture, anchoring the sewing ring to the native valve annulus for approximately two-thirds of the valve annulus and then anteriorly to a pericardial patch that is used routinely to augment the valve annulus and facilitate closure of the pulmonary artery and right ventricle.

Triple-Valve Replacement

Operative preparation is similar to that described previously. Usually left-sided valvular lesions are corrected before tricuspid valve procedures. Again, if there is aortic valve regurgitation, the aortotomy is performed first, and cardioplegia is administered; simultaneously, we snare the cavae and open the right atrium. After excision of the aortic valve and calibration of the annulus, the interatrial septum is incised, and the mitral valve is repaired or replaced. Next, the aortic valve is implanted, and after closure of the aortotomy and septotomy, the tricuspid valvuloplasty or prosthetic replacement can be performed without aortic cross-clamping.[71]

RHEUMATIC HEART DISEASE AFFECTING MULTIPLE VALVES

As shown in Table 47-3, rheumatic valvulitis is a common cause of multiple valve disease. Autopsy studies show that almost all patients with rheumatic heart disease have some involvement of the mitral valve, although it is not always evident clinically.[72] The percentages of multiple valve involvement in two autopsy studies of patients with rheumatic heart disease are shown in Table 47-4.

Forty-seven percent of those studied had involvement of more than one valve. Mitral and aortic valve disease was the most common combination and was present in 34% of patients; the second most common combination was mitral, aortic, and tricuspid valve disease (9%). A recent report has suggested that all four valves might be involved with the rheumatic process.[73]

Long-term follow-up of children with rheumatic heart disease suggests that approximately 50% of patients have multivalvular involvement.[74,75] In a study of patients undergoing mitral valvotomy for rheumatic mitral stenosis (Table 47-5), 13% had clinical evidence of other rheumatic valve stenosis or regurgitation. Most of these patients had associated rheumatic aortic disease.[76]

Rheumatic heart disease can cause valve stenosis, regurgitation, or a combination of lesions. The percentages of 290 patients with specific valvular lesions from four studies of multiple valve disease are shown in Table 47-6. Mixed lesions producing stenosis and regurgitation were encountered most commonly in both aortic and mitral valves.

TABLE 47-3 Reports of Operations for Multiple Valve Disease, Showing the High Incidence of Rheumatic Heart Disease

Study	Patients (no.)	Patients with Rheumatic Heart Disease, % (no.)
Combined mitral and aortic replacement[155]	86	100 (86)
Combined mitral and aortic replacement[130]	92	100 (92)
Combined mitral and aortic replacement with tricuspid repair[60]	109	98 (107)
Triple valve replacement[160]	48	100 (48)
Combined mitral and aortic replacement[100]	54	85 (46)
Multiple valve procedures[135]	50	86 (43)
Triple valve replacement[31]	91	100 (91)
Combined mitral and aortic replacement[134]	65	80 (52)
Mitral replacement and tricuspid surgery[14]	32	81 (26)
Combined mitral and aortic replacement[169]	166	64 (106)
Mitral and aortic procedures[78]	124	100 (124)
Multiple valve procedures[170]	102	100 (102)
Combined mitral and aortic replacement[171]	33	82 (27)
Mitral and aortic regurgitation[93]	39	67 (26)
Mitral and aortic stenosis[86]	32	100 (32)
Mitral and aortic stenosis[84]	141	100 (141)

TABLE 47-4 Results of Autopsy Series (1910–1937) Showing Multiple Valve Involvement in 996 Patients with Rheumatic Heart Disease

Valve Lesion at Autopsy	Clawson[172]	Cooke and White[173]	Percentage of 996 Patients Studied
All combinations	321	147	47
M-A	221	100	32
M-A-T	52	35	9
M-T	31	7	4
M-A-T-P	14	5	2
A-T	2	0	0.2
A-M-P	1	0	0.1

A = aortic valve; M = mitral valve; T = tricuspid valve; P = pulmonary valve.
Source: Modified with permission from Acker M, Hargrove WC, Stephenson LW: Multiple valve replacement. Cardiol Clin 1985; 3:425.

TABLE 47-5 Patients with Rheumatic Mitral Stenosis Undergoing Valvotomy with Clinical Evidence of Multiple Valve Disease

Valve Lesion at Surgery	No.	Percentage of 1000 Patients with Rheumatic Mitral Stenosis
All combinations	127	12.7
M-A	121	12.1
M-T	6	0.6

A = aortic valve; M = mitral valve; T = tricuspid valve. Does not include patients with tricuspid regurgitation. Source: Modified with permission from Ellis LB, Harken DE, Black H: A clinical study of 1000 consecutive cases of mitral stenosis two to nine years after mitral valvuloplasty. Circulation 1959; 19:803.

TABLE 47-7 Characteristics of Patients with Combined Mitral Stenosis and Aortic Regurgitation

Mitral Stenosis and Aortic Regurgitation	Terzaki[78]
Number of patients	26
Symptom of dyspnea	100% (26)
Electrocardiographic evidence of LVH	62% (16)
Roentgenographic evidence of LVH	54% (14)
Symptom of angina	23% (6)
Aortic diastolic pressure >70 mm Hg	46% (12)
Elevated LVEDP	38% (10)

LVEDP = left ventricular end-diastolic pressure; LVH = left ventricular hypertrophy.

Rheumatic Mitral Stenosis with Rheumatic Aortic Regurgitation

Approximately 10% of patients with rheumatic mitral valve stenosis also have rheumatic aortic regurgitation.[77,78] Clinical and laboratory characteristics of patients with mitral stenosis and aortic regurgitation are summarized in Table 47-7.

Pathophysiology

In patients with mitral valve stenosis and aortic valve regurgitation, decreased cardiac output minimizes the classic signs of aortic regurgitation (eg, waterhammer pulse, head bobbing, visibly pulsating capillaries). Also, concomitant mitral stenosis reduces left ventricular volume overload, which is a characteristic of isolated aortic regurgitation.[79] The underfilling of the left ventricle characteristic of mitral stenosis is offset by overfilling secondary to aortic valve regurgitation. Pulmonary artery hypertension characteristic of mitral stenosis usually is present.

Operative Decision Making

Patients with rheumatic mitral stenosis and rheumatic aortic regurgitation of more than a mild degree usually require replacement of both valves. Aortic valve repair is possible using techniques such as cuspal extension with glutaraldehyde-treated bovine or autologous pericardium[80] or the Trussler technique.[81]

TABLE 47-6 Hemodynamic Classification in Patients Undergoing Multiple Valve Surgery for Rheumatic Valvular Disease

	Combined Mitral and Aortic Surgery[78]	Triple-Valve Replacement[160]	Combined Mitral and Aortic Replacement[171]	Triple-Valve Replacement[31]	Totals
Number in study	124	48	27	91	290
MS	53% (66)	19% (9)	30% (8)	22% (20)	35.5% (103/290)
MR	47% (58)	10% (5)	52% (14)	12% (11)	30.3% (88/290)
MS/MR	—	71% (34)	19% (5)	66% (169)	34.1% (99/290)
AS	53% (66)	10% (5)	44% (12)	10% (9)	31.7% (92/290)
AR	47% (58)	35% (17)	41% (11)	33% (30)	40% (116/290)
AS/AR	—	54% (26)	15% (4)	57% (52)	28.3% (82/290)

AR = aortic regurgitation; AS = aortic stenosis; MR = mitral regurgitation; MS = mitral stenosis.

Although early results with cuspal extension have been good, inexorable progression of valve fibrosis may necessitate later prosthetic replacement for many patients.[82]

Preoperative transthoracic and intraoperative transesophageal echocardiography aids in assessing function of the aortic valve in patients requiring surgery for mitral stenosis. At operation, the degree of ventricular filling and amount of aortic root distention with infusion of cardioplegia are clues to important aortic valve regurgitation. As stated previously, if mitral valve replacement is necessary, serious consideration should be given to replacement of the aortic valve when there is moderate or worse leakage owing to rheumatic valvulitis.

Great care should be exercised to avoid ventricular distention if ventricular fibrillation occurs before aortic clamping. If ventricular fibrillation develops, distention of the heart can be prevented by inserting a left ventricular vent and compressing the heart manually. Also, even mild or moderate degrees of aortic regurgitation can complicate cardioplegia delivery through the proximal aorta.

Rheumatic Mitral Stenosis with Rheumatic Aortic Stenosis

Pathophysiology

In contrast to isolated mitral stenosis, in which ventricular function frequently is preserved, the combination of mitral and aortic stenosis is associated with ventricular hypertrophy and diastolic dysfunction. The pressure load from the aortic stenosis causes a concentric hypertrophy with a small, noncompliant ventricular cavity.[78] Mitral stenosis compromises the ventricle's ability to maintain cardiac output (in contrast to isolated aortic stenosis, in which cardiac output is maintained).[83,84] The decrease in cardiac output minimizes the signs and symptoms of aortic stenosis and may make the diagnosis of aortic stenosis difficult.[85] Other hemodynamic parameters are similar to those of isolated mitral stenosis, eg, elevation of left atrial and pulmonary arterial pressures.[84,86]

Operative Decision Making

Although mitral valve stenosis sometimes can be treated effectively with valvuloplasty, commissurotomy for rheumatic aortic stenosis is indicated rarely. Thus, for patients with both aortic and mitral valve stenoses caused by rheumatic heart disease, we favor prosthetic replacement with mechanical prostheses if patients can manage long-term anticoagulation. If aortic valve stenosis is only mild and the decision is made not to replace the aortic valve at the time of mitral valve replacement, then the patient should be followed carefully, because more than 50% will develop moderate to severe disease by 15 years postoperatively.[87] The combination of aortic stenosis and mitral stenosis may present unique problems for the surgeon. First, concentric hypertrophy of the left ventricle may displace the mitral valve orifice anteriorly, producing poor exposure through a standard atriotomy; several maneuvers and alternative incisions are described for patients in whom mitral valve exposure is difficult.[85,88–92] Also, the small left ventricular cavity may impinge on struts of a stent-mounted bioprosthesis. There is also the potential for left ventricular outflow obstruction from high-profile prostheses in the mitral position in patients with aortic and mitral valve stenoses and small left ventricular cavity size.

Rheumatic Mitral Regurgitation with Rheumatic Aortic Regurgitation

Pathophysiology

The combination of mitral and aortic valve regurgitation produces severe volume overload of the left ventricle. The reduction of impedance to ejection allows the ventricle to empty further, reducing ventricular wall tension with a resulting increase in the velocity of shortening.[94] Chronic volume overload increases stroke volume and distention of the left ventricle so that a larger stroke volume can be achieved with less myocardial fiber shortening than in normal hearts.[78] Patients who respond to increased volume load by left ventricular dilatation appear to tolerate surgical correction better than patients with left ventricular hypertrophy owing to an increased pressure load.[78] Patients with aortic valve regurgitation have augmented stroke volume to maintain an adequate cardiac output, but when mitral regurgitation coexists, part of the augmented stroke regurgitates into the left atrium and pulmonary veins. For this reason, when aortic regurgitation is severe, concomitant mitral regurgitation greatly reduces systemic cardiac output and can produce severe pulmonary congestion.[95]

Operative Decision Making

As stated previously, aortic valves involved with rheumatic disease usually require replacement. When the mitral valve also has rheumatic involvement, we replace the mitral valve at the time of aortic valve operation. After the aortic valve is excised, the mitral valve is inspected visually if it is suspected of being diseased or the degree of regurgitation is severe.

MYXOMATOUS AND PROLAPSING VALVE DISEASE AFFECTING MULTIPLE VALVES

Myxomatous degeneration is the most common etiology of mitral regurgitation requiring surgical correction in North America, and myxomatous aortic valve disease with annular dilatation is perhaps the most common cause of aortic regurgitation.[96–98] Most cases of isolated mitral or aortic valve prolapse are not associated with known connective tissue disorders. However, the coexistence of both mitral and aortic valvular prolapse together frequently can be seen in patients with connective tissue diseases such as Marfan's syndrome, Ehlers-Danlos syndrome, osteogenesis imperfecta, and others.[95]

Aortic valve regurgitation in patients with Marfan's syndrome is caused by progressive enlargement of the sinus portion of the aorta and the aortic valve annulus, ie, annuloaortic ectasia.[99,100] The principal causes of mitral regurgitation in patients with Marfan's syndrome are mitral annular dilatation, floppy or prolapsing leaflets, and mitral annular calcification.[100] The pathologic lesion in Marfan's syndrome is cystic medial necrosis, which is characterized by degeneration of elastic fibers and infrequent cysts.[100] Alterations in the synthesis and cellular secretion of

TABLE 47-8 Incidence of Echocardiographic Evidence of Aortic Valve Prolapse in Patients with Mitral Valve Prolapse

	Ogawa[103]	Rippe[102]	Mardelli[174]	Total
Number of patients with MVP	50	400	75	525
Aortic valve prolapse	24% (12)	3% (11)	20% (15)	7% (38/525)
Aortic regurgitation	16% (8)	1% (4)	—	3% (12/450)
Aortic and mitral valve replacement	2% (1)	—	—	2% (1/50)

MVP = mitral valve prolapse.
Number of patients in parentheses.

fibrillin are responsible for the phenotypic characteristics of many patients with Marfan's syndrome.[101] Some patients have myxomatous cardiovascular lesions and annuloaortic ectasia without the other clinical characteristics of Marfan's syndrome.

Two-dimensional echocardiographic studies show that the frequency of aortic valve prolapse in patients with mitral valve prolapse varies between 3% and 24%[102,103] (Table 47-8). In one necropsy study, the frequency of mitral regurgitation in Marfan patients with aortic aneurysms (most with aortic regurgitation) was 54% (7 of 13).[100] About 17% of patients who undergo surgery for myxomatous aortic valve require surgical correction of mitral regurgitation (Table 47-9).

Although multiple valve involvement with myxomatous degeneration usually manifests as mitral regurgitation in combination with aortic regurgitation, in some cases, all four valves may be involved.[105] It is not clear whether the underlying pathology of isolated mitral valve prolapse is the same as the cardiovascular lesions that occur in Marfan's syndrome and other multiple-floppy-valve syndromes.[106,107]

Diagnosis, Signs, and Symptoms

Signs and symptoms of aortic and mitral valve regurgitation are reviewed in the section on rheumatic valvular disease. In addition to complete evaluation of the aortic and mitral valves and proximal aorta, patients with Marfan's syndrome should have assessment of the descending aorta for aneurysm or chronic dissection.

Operative Decision Making

If annuloaortic ectasia is not present, patients with mitral and aortic valve regurgitation caused by myxomatous degeneration are candidates for repair of both valves. The aortic valve is inspected initially, and the decision for repair or prosthetic replacement is made depending on cuspal morphology. If tissue is sturdy and there is little prolapse or prolapse is limited to one cusp, repair can be undertaken with commissural narrowing and cusp resuspension. Often, aortic valve regurgitation is central, and simply narrowing the annulus by commissural plication restores valvular competence. Outcome of repair of both mitral and aortic valves has been good in terms of patient survival and freedom from valve-related complications, but reoperation is necessary in 35% of patients 10 years after the initial procedure; patients with most severe aortic valve regurgitation have an increased risk of late reoperation.[108] If tissue is attenuated, or if multiple cusps have severe prolapse, the valve is replaced.

In most instances, patients with Marfan's syndrome and aortic regurgitation require composite replacement of the aortic valve and ascending aorta.[109] Occasionally, moderate aortic regurgitation can be repaired at the time of aortic replacement by suspending the aortic valve inside a tube graft or remodeling the sinus portion of the aorta.[110] Even if the aortic valve is replaced with a composite graft and mechanical valve, the surgeon should favor repair of associated mitral regurgitation.[111] Gillinov and colleagues reported that valvuloplasty is possible in approximately 80% of patients with mitral regurgitation and Marfan's syndrome and that 5 years postoperatively 88% of patients are free of significant mitral valve insufficiency.[112]

Myxomatous Mitral Regurgitation with Tricuspid Regurgitation

Myxomatous degeneration also may involve the tricuspid valve, and presentation of mitral and tricuspid valve regurgitation

TABLE 47-9 Frequency of Mitral Valve Procedures in Patients Undergoing Aortic Valve Repair or Replacement for Myxomatous Degeneration, Prolapse, or Root Dilation

	David[175]	Gott[176]	Shigenobu[96]	Agozzino[99]	Bellitti[98]	Total
All aortic surgery	18	270	13	69	25	395
Number requiring concomitant mitral surgery	3 (17%)	36 (13%)	5 (38%)	16 (23%)	3 (12%)	73 (16%)

owing to degenerative disease is not uncommon. In one study, 54% of patients with mitral valve prolapse also had tricuspid valve prolapse; however, most of these patients did not have significant regurgitation.[95] As with tricuspid regurgitation associated with rheumatic mitral disease, preoperative and intraoperative echocardiography is important in evaluating tricuspid disease in patients with myxomatous mitral regurgitation. In contrast with rheumatic disease, myxomatous mitral and tricuspid regurgitation almost always lends itself to valve repair.

TABLE 47-10 Comparison of Early Outcome Between Patients Having Multiple Valve Surgery for Infective Endocarditis and Patients Having Multiple Valve Surgery for other Reasons[8,106]

	Class II	Class III	Class IV
Multiple valve procedures for infective endocarditis	20% (15)	33% (3)	20% (5)
Multiple valve procedures for other causes	16% (25)	12% (25)	36% (25)

Operative mortality is expressed as percentage, and numbers of patients are in parentheses.

SENILE CALCIFIC AORTIC VALVE DISEASE WITH MULTIPLE VALVE INVOLVEMENT

Unlike aortic stenosis caused by rheumatic disease, in which associated mitral valve disease is common, senile calcific aortic stenosis usually presents as an isolated lesion. Although the combination of mitral valve disease and senile calcific aortic stenosis is uncommon, senile aortic calcification is a frequent cause of aortic valve stenosis.[97] The incidence of senile calcific aortic disease has increased steadily in the last 20 years. Therefore, although mitral valve disease associated with calcific aortic stenosis is less common than that seen with rheumatic disease of the aortic valve, as the incidence of calcific aortic stenosis increases, so does the likelihood of encountering patients with disease of both valves.

Patterns of Multiple Valve Involvement with Calcific Aortic Stenosis

Calcific Aortic Stenosis with Infective Endocarditis of the Mitral Valve

Stenotic aortic valves frequently are sites of infective endocarditis. As discussed in the section on endocarditis, the mitral valve may become involved with infective endocarditis by common abscess, by verrucous extension, or from a jet lesion, and infection may cause mitral valve aneurysm, perforation, and/or chordae disruption.[113] Management of these patients usually requires aortic valve replacement and assessment of the mitral valve at the time of operation. Vegetations of the mitral valve sometimes can be removed and perforations patched if the remaining tissue is sturdy and appears healthy.

Calcific Aortic Stenosis with Functional Mitral Valve Disease

Senile calcification of the aortic valve may lead to mixed stenosis and regurgitation,[97] and the volume load from regurgitation may lead to left ventricular dilatation and secondary mitral regurgitation of an otherwise normal mitral valve.[97] Mitral regurgitation secondary to aortic valvular disease is discussed in the section on pathophysiology of multiple valve disease.

Calcific Aortic Stenosis with Calcification of the Mitral Valve

Degenerative calcification is an age-related process usually affecting the aortic and mitral valves. In a study of patients older than 75 years of age, one-third had degenerative aortic or mitral calcification.[95] About 25 to 50% of patients with calcific aortic stenosis have calcification of the mitral valve annulus. Generally, patients with associated mitral annular calcification are older, have more severe aortic stenosis, and are more often female when compared with patients with aortic stenosis without mitral annular calcification.[104] Mills reported 17 patients undergoing mitral valve replacement for valvular disease related to severe annular calcification. Four of these patients also had concomitant aortic valve replacement.[114] Mitral annular calcification may exist in the setting of rheumatic or myxomatous disease.[115] These patients may have increased incidence of conduction defects,[116] aortic outflow murmurs, coronary artery disease,[117] and stroke.[118] Mitral repair or replacement is facilitated in some circumstances by removal of the annular calcium bar and pericardial reconstruction.[119]

Table 47-10 compares New York Heart Association (NYHA) class-matched groups that had multiple valve procedures for infective endocarditis and for other reasons.

CARCINOID HEART DISEASE AFFECTING MULTIPLE VALVES

Valvular heart disease develops in about 50% of patients with carcinoid tumors; patients with primary carcinoid tumor in the small intestine are more likely to have carcinoid heart disease than those with carcinoid tumors in other locations.[1] In most cases, the tricuspid and pulmonary valves are involved. We have offered valvular surgery to patients with severe symptoms of right-sided heart failure caused by carcinoid heart disease whose systemic carcinoid symptoms are controlled by octreotide and/or hepatic dearterialization.[123] Patients who are being considered for complete resection of hepatic metastases after control of the primary tumor are also candidates for extirpation of cardiac disease and valve replacement. A recent review of 200 patients with carcinoid heart disease from our institution revealed that survival has improved over the past decade. Multivariate analysis indicated that valve replacement surgery was associated with a risk reduction of 0.48.[68]

Diagnosis, Signs, and Symptoms

Jugular venous distention with v waves (from tricuspid regurgitation) and a waves (from tricuspid stenosis) can be evident. Right ventricular enlargement can produce a pericardial lift. Most patients have murmurs from the tricuspid and pulmonary valves.[123] Patients often demonstrate ascites and liver enlargement as a result of either right-sided heart failure or hepatic metastases or both. Therefore, these findings are not necessarily indicative of severe tricuspid valve regurgitation.

The electrocardiogram of patients with carcinoid heart disease often shows low voltage (85%), right bundle-branch block (42%), and evidence of right atrial enlargement (35%).[1,123] The chest x-ray characteristically shows cardiomegaly (69%), pleural effusions (58%), and pleural thickening (35%).[123]

Echocardiography

Echocardiographic findings of carcinoid heart disease include thickening and reduced motion of the tricuspid valve leaflets; the pulmonic valve cusps may be thickened and retracted. Fusion of the pulmonary valve commissures results in a stiff fibrotic ring that may cause a stricture in the entire pulmonary orifice. Pulmonary regurgitation and stenosis both may be present.[124]

Invasive Studies

Cardiac catheterization is not necessary unless ischemic symptoms or a history of myocardial infarction suggests coronary artery disease.

Pathophysiology

Carcinoid heart disease results from deposition of plaques on the endocardium of the valves and atria; this usually occurs on the right side of the heart. However, plaques can develop on the mitral and aortic valves when there is carcinoid tumor in the lungs or in the presence of intracardiac shunting that bypasses the lungs. Valves are damaged by exposure to circulating substances released from carcinoid tumors such as serotonin and bradykinin. Both these components are inactivated by the lungs and the liver; the relationship between tumor location and the location of cardiac lesions is summarized in Table 47-11.[125] The plaques usually deposit on the downstream side of the cardiac valves, causing adherence of the leaflet to the underlying structures and producing functional regurgitation. Carcinoid plaque deposition also may constrict the valve annulus and produce stenosis.[1]

The dominant functional lesion of carcinoid heart disease is tricuspid valve regurgitation; the valve is fixed in a semiopen position so that some degree of stenosis is present. Fibrosis and plaque deposition also affect the pulmonary valve, causing mixed stenosis and regurgitation, which increases the degree of tricuspid regurgitation.[1]

TABLE 47-11 A Comparison of Venous Drainage, Presence of Liver Metastases, and Carcinoid Plaque Location in Relation to Location of Primary Carcinoid Tumor[121]

Tumor Location	Venous Drainage	Liver Metastases	Plaque Location
Gut	Portal	Yes	Right-sided
Ovary	Systemic	No	Right-sided
Bronchial	Pulmonary	No	Left-sided

Operative Decision Making

Timing of Operation

The primary indications for surgery are increasing symptoms of congestive failure with objective evidence of valvular disease.[122] Again, it should be noted that some of the signs of right-sided heart failure, such as peripheral edema, ascites, and hepatomegaly, can be caused by the primary disease. Another indication for operation may be progressive right ventricular enlargement in the absence of symptoms. In a small series of carcinoid patients, right ventricular size and function did not correlate with operative or late mortality.[123] Currently, we employ exercise testing to provide an objective assessment of the functional status and a guideline to the timing of cardiac surgery. If the primary cause for debilitation is right-sided heart failure, it is reasonable to offer valve replacement even though the prognosis may be guarded.[126]

Tricuspid Valve Operation

The tricuspid valve always requires replacement, and in our earlier experience, we used mechanical prostheses because of the possibility of carcinoid plaque formation on a bioprosthesis. However, review of our patients and those reported previously shows little difference in patient survival with mechanical or tissue valves. Bioprostheses are selected for patients who have liver dysfunction that would complicate anticoagulation with Coumadin and those who will undergo subsequent hepatic resection or hepatic artery embolization.

Pulmonary Valve Options

As stated previously, we now advise valve replacement rather than excision when the pulmonary valve is involved.

Management of the carcinoid syndrome during and early after operation is critically important, and this has been simplified greatly by treatment with long-acting octreotide; this is supplemented intraoperatively with intravenous administration of short-acting octreotide when there is evidence of flushing and vasodilatation.[127] Preoperative steroids and antihistamines also can be used to prevent adverse effects from tumor-released mediators.[127,128] We usually give octreotide, 500 μg intravenously, before induction of anesthesia, with additional intravenous doses given as needed at the onset and termination of cardiopulmonary bypass. Postoperatively, octreotide is continued, and the dose is adjusted according to the severity of the flushing and vasodilatation. Aprotinin, a kallikrein inhibitor, may mitigate the effects of substances released by carcinoid tumors during anesthesia and reduce intraoperative and postoperative bleeding.[127]

RARE CAUSES OF MULTIPLE VALVE DISEASE

Table 47-12 lists some rare causes of multiple heart valve disease that require surgical correction.

RESULTS OF MULTIPLE VALVE SURGERY

Long- and Short-Term Mortality

Survival following multiple valve surgery has improved along with refinements in myocardial protection; for example, mortality for multiple valve operations performed using normothermic ischemic arrest was approximately 40%[129]; the use of cardioplegic arrest reduced operative risk by three-fourths.[78,129,130] In recent reports,[131] operative mortality (30-day mortality or hospital mortality) ranges from about 6 to 17% (Table 47-13, part A). The 5-year actuarial survival is 60 to 88% (see Table 47-13, part B), and the 10-year actuarial survival is 43 to 81% (see Table 47-13, part C). Risk factors identified for morbidity and mortality following multiple valve surgery include advanced NYHA class,[132–134] advanced age,[132–136] current or prior myocardial revascularization,[135] ejection fraction,[132] presence of coronary artery disease,[132,133] aortic stenosis,[137] elevated pulmonary artery pressure,[135] tricuspid regurgitation,[137] and diabetes mellitus.[135]

Clearly, operative mortality is influenced by patient selection,[134] and comparisons among studies are of limited value.[134] Causes of death after multiple valve surgery are low cardiac output,[134,137–140] myocardial infarction,[135] technical failure,[140] multiple-organ failure,[32] ventricular rupture,[100,135,138] and mechanical obstruction of the prosthetic leaflet.[100,139] Comparisons of late survival between patients having multiple valve versus single-valve replacement are inconsistent. Some studies show poorer survival[133] after multiple valve replacement, and others report no significant difference in survival.[32,126,129,136–141] The discrepancy in these results may be because the majority of deaths in many reports are secondary to progression of coronary artery disease and noncardiac causes rather than valve-related issues.[130,132] The presence of coronary artery disease and concomitant coronary artery surgery increases mortality following multiple valve surgery.[135,146,147]

Some causes of early death following multiple valve surgery are perhaps less common today owing to changes in practice. In a necropsy study from 1963 to 1985 of patients who died early following double-valve replacement, prosthetic valve dysfunction secondary to mechanical interference was evident in almost 50%, and ventricular rupture had occurred in 15% of patients.[100] Most of these patients received Starr-Edwards caged-ball prosthetic valves. Mechanical failure of low-profile tilting-disk prostheses that are in current use is rare, and early valve-related death with this type of prosthesis is very unusual.[32,133,134,148] The current practice of preserving the posterior leaflet and chordal attachments of the mitral valve during prosthetic replacement may decrease the chance of ventricular disruption.[149]

TABLE 47-12 Rare Causes of Multiple Valve Disease Requiring Surgery

Disease	Valves Replaced or Repaired
Methysergide/ergotamine toxicity[95]	Aortic and mitral
Fenfluramine–phentermine[156]	Left and right heart valves
Ergot-derived dopamine agonists[157]	Left and right heart valves
3,4 methylenedioxymethamphetamine (Ecstasy)[158]	Mitral and tricuspid
Radiation injury[121,177]	Mitral and tricuspid
Q-fever endocarditis[178]	Aortic and mitral
Ectodermal anhydrotic dysplasia[179]	Aortic and mitral
Maroteaux-Lamy syndrome (mucopoly-saccharidosis type VI)[180]	Aortic and mitral
Werner syndrome (adult progeria)[181]	Aortic and mitral
Blunt trauma[182]	Mitral and tricuspid
Lymphoma[183]	Aortic and mitral
Relapsing polychondritis[184]	Aortic and mitral
Systemic lupus erythematosus[185]	Mitral and tricuspid
Secondary hyperparathyroidism[186]	Aortic and mitral
Urticarial vasculitis syndrome (HUVS) with Jaccoud hands deformity[187]	Aortic and mitral

Thromboembolism

Thromboembolic rates following multiple valve replacement are shown in Table 47-13, part D, and range from 1 to 7% per patient-year for double-valve replacement. Ten years postoperatively, freedom from thromboembolic events ranges from 77 to 89% (see Table 47-13, part E). Although the data presented in Table 47-13, part D, along with other sources,[150] do not indicate significant differences between single and multiple valve replacement, some reports suggest that both mechanical[151] and bioprosthetic[152] valves have an increased risk of thromboembolism in the mitral position. This risk is present early (90 days after operation) in patients undergoing multiple valve replacement that includes a bioprosthetic mitral valve.[152]

Anticoagulation-Related Hemorrhage

Rates of anticoagulant-related hemorrhage following multiple valve replacement, as with single-valve surgery, depend on

TABLE 47-13 Summary of Morbidity and Mortality Following Multiple Valve Surgery

	DVR	MVR	AVR	*p*-Value	Valve Type	Reference
A. Operative mortality (percent)	5.6				Various*	Teoh[133]
	5.9	4.3	2	—	SJM	Horstkotte[149]
	6.3	5.2	3.1	—	SJM	Smith[143]
	6.5				SJM	Armenti[130]
	7.2	4.7	3.9	—	SJM	Aoyagi[120]
	8.0	—	—	—	SJM	Emery[188]
	8.2	4.3	2.4	—	SJM	Ibrahim[189]
	10				Hancock II	David[190]
	10.5				C-E	Jamieson[191]
	10.8	11.3	7.8	—	Sorin Disc	Milano[192]
	10.8				Various*	Galloway[131]
	11.6	7.5	5.1	—	C-E	Bernal[140]
	15.5	—	—	—	Various	Leavitt[193]
	17.5				Various*	Mattila[135]
B. 5-Year actuarial survival (percent)	88	88	91	N.S.	SJM	Aoyagi[120]
	86	86	94	MVR or DVR < AVR $p < .05$	<SJM	Smith[143]
	78				Various*	Galloway[131]
	75				C-E	Bernal[140]
	73				Hancock II	David[190]
	70				C-E	Jamieson[191]
	62				MIPB	Lemieux[194]
	61	65	75	DVR < MVR or AVR $p < .01$	SJM	Khan[129]
	60				SJM	Armenti[130]
	****	****	****	DVR < AVR or MVR $p < .006$	B-S	Alvarez[137]
C. 10-Year actuarial survival (percent)	81	80	81	N.S.	SJM	Aoyagi[120]
	72	78	85	—	SJM	Horstkotte[149]
	60	59	71	N.S.	SJM	Ibrahim[189]
	55	63	65	—	B-S	Orszulak[195]
D. Thromboembolism (percent per patient-year)	0.3	0.3	0.6	—	SJM	Smith[143]
	0.79	1.6	1.3	—	SJM	Nakano[196]
	1.3	1.1	1.0	N.S.	SJM	Aoyagi[120]
	2.1				Various*	Mattila[135]
	2.1	1.2	1.3	N.S.	Sorin Disc	Milano[192]
	4.5				Various*	Mullany[60]
	4.6				SJM	Armenti[130]
	4.6	4.3	2.1	—	B-S	Orszulak[195]
	5.0	4.4	2.4	—	SJM	Ibrahim[189]
	6.6	5.1	3.7	—	SJM	Horstkotte[149]
E. 10-Year freedom from thromboembolism (percent)	89	92	91	—	C-E pericardial	Pelletier[197]
	89	89	94	N.S.	SJM	Aoyagi[120]
	89	83	—	—	C-E	van Doorn[198]
	86	88	80	—	Hancock II	David[190]
	77	79	87	—	B-S	Orszulak[195]
	ξ	ξ	ξ	N.S.	B-S	Alvarez[137]
F. Anticoagulation-related hemorrhage (percent per patient-year)	0.1	0.2	0.1	—	SJM	Nakano[196]
	0.5	0.3	0.4	—	SJM	Aoyagi[120]
	0.9	0.9	0.9	N.S.	Sorin Disc	Milano[192]
	1.2				SJM	Armenti[130]
	1.2	0.7	0.2	—	SJM†	Horstkotte[149]
	4.5	2.1	1.2	—	SJM‡	Horstkotte[149]
	ξ	ξ	ξ	DVR > AVR or MVR $p < .05$	B-S	Alvarez[137]

TABLE 47-13 Summary of Morbidity and Mortality Following Multiple Valve Surgery (*Continued*)

	DVR	MVR	AVR	*p*-Value	Valve Type	Reference
G. Endocarditis (percent per patient-year)	0.2	0.06	0.21	—	St. Jude	Nakano[196]
	0.3	0.03	0.4	—	St. Jude	Aoyagi[120]
	2.1				Various*	Mattila[135]
	2.5				SJM	Armenti[130]
	ξ	ξ	ξ	DVR > AVR or MVR $p < .05$	B-S	Alvarez[137]
H. 8-, 10-, and 15-year freedom from structural deterioration for bioprostheses (percent)	77	79	87	—	C-E pericardial	Pelletier[197]
	59.6	70.8		—	C-E	van Doorn[198]
	44	33	62	$p < .03$	C-E	Bernal[150]
	38	58	80	DVR < MVR, AVR $p < .05$	MP	Pomar[146]

*Includes some patients with concomitant tricuspid procedures.
†dR INR 1.75 2.75.
‡INR 4 = 6.
ξResults reported graphically.
Comparisons to isolated aortic and mitral valve procedures from the same series are included when available. If statistical analysis between the results of multiple and single valve procedures was reported, the p values are included. If a series was limited to a single valve type, it is listed.
AVR = isolated aortic valve replacement; B-S = Björk-Shiley; C-E = Carpentier-Edwards; DVR = double valve replacement; MIPB = medtronic intact porcine bioprosthesis; MP = mitroflow pericardial; MVR = isolated mitral valve replacement; N.S. = not statistically significant; SJM = St. Jude Medical.

target international normalization ratio (INR).[153] Risks of hemorrhage are reported to be 0.1 to 4.5% per patient-year following multiple valve surgery (see Table 47-13, part F). Alvarez reported a significantly higher rate of anticoagulant-related hemorrhage following multiple valve replacement than following single-valve replacement.[137]

Prosthetic Valve Infective Endocarditis

Rates of infective endocarditis following multiple valve surgery range from 0.2 to 2.5% per patient-year, as shown in Table 47-13, part G. In comparison with isolated valve surgery, Alvarez reports that prosthesis infection is more frequent following double valve replacement than following either isolated aortic ($p < .05$) or mitral valve replacement ($p < .001$).[137]

Valve Performance

Rates of bioprosthetic structural deterioration relate to valve position; tissue valves appear to fail earlier in the mitral position than in the aortic position. When multiple valve replacements include the mitral valve, the rates of deterioration are similar[154] or even worse than[150] isolated mitral valve replacement (see Table 47-13, part H).

COMPARISON OF BIOPROSTHETIC VALVES TO MECHANICAL VALVES

Comparisons of outcomes of patients with two or more mechanical prostheses with those of patients with two or more bioprostheses show similar rates of thromboembolism,[27,153] but freedom from operation favors those with multiple mechanical valves.[29,155,159] As might be expected, anticoagulation-related hemorrhage is less in patients with two bioprosthetic valves,[155,160] but there is no clear advantage of one prosthesis over the other in terms of early and late mortality.[29,155,160]

Results of Tricuspid Valve Procedures with Other Valve Procedures

Results of Mitral and Tricuspid Valve Surgeries

Reported operative mortality following mitral valve replacement and tricuspid valve repair or replacement is approximately 12 to 15%,[161] and 65 to 75% of patients are alive 5 years postoperatively.[135,161] Outlook for patients with lesser degrees of tricuspid regurgitation at the time of mitral valve replacement is good; 5-year actuarial survival for patients with tricuspid regurgitation who do not have tricuspid valve repair or replacement is 80 to 84%, and 10-year survival is 62 to 77%.[162]

Triple-Valve Replacement

The operative mortality following triple-valve replacement is higher than that for double-valve replacement and ranges from 5 to 25%.[31,135] As with double-valve replacement, advanced age and higher NYHA class are associated risk factors for early mortality.[31,163] Causes of perioperative death are similar to those following double-valve replacement and include low cardiac output, multiorgan failure, hemorrhage, and dysrhythmia.[31]

Five-year actuarial survival after triple-valve replacement is 53 to 78%, and 10- and 15-year survivals are 40% and 25%, respectively (Table 47-14).

TABLE 47-14 Results of Triple Valve Surgery by Author

	Han[199]	Gersh[31]	Galloway[131]	Brown[151]	Mullany[60]	Kara[159]
Years studied	1985–2005	1962–1984	1976–1985		1965–1984	1972–1983
Number of patients	871	91	61	40	109	107
Type of procedure	Triple valve procedure	Triple valve replacement	Triple valve procedure	Triple valve replacement	Double valve replacement with tricuspid repair	Triple valve procedure
Valve type		Various (mostly S-E)	Various	Various	Various (60% S-E)	S-E, Björk, or St. Jude
Operative mortality	8%	24%	23%		21%	20%
Actuarial 5-year survival	75%	55%	62%	78%	70%	53%
Thromboembolism rate	0.98% pt-y	12.3% pt-y		32% at 5 years combined with hemorrhage	4.5% pt-y	
Prosthetic infective endocarditis rate	0.6% pt-y	6%			3%	
Hemorrhage rate	1.6% pt-y	22%		17%		
Significant risk factors	Age, NYHA Class IV, lower LV EF	Age, NYHA Class IV			Age, NYHA Class IV	Higher NYHA class, emergent operation, tricuspid replacement

LVEF = left ventricular ejection fraction; NYHA = New York Heart Association functional class; S-E = Starr-Edwards.

Considering only perioperative survivors of triple-valve replacement, late survival is comparable with that of patients undergoing isolated valve replacement.[31,164] Reports of thromboembolic rates following triple-valve replacement range from 5 to 12% per patient-year (see Table 47-14).

Double-Valve Replacement and Tricuspid Annuloplasty

Operative mortality for patients undergoing double-valve replacement with tricuspid valve repair is about 25%,[60] and the 10- and 15-year survival rates are 35% and 27%, generally comparable with those of patients having triple-valve replacement.[60] Rates of thromboembolism in this group are reported to be 5% per patient-year.[60]

Other Results

The operative mortality for double re-replacement is about 10 to 20%.[133,165] Incidence of postoperative ventricular arrhythmias is higher in patients having combined valve surgery than in those having single-valve surgery.[166] Hemolysis may be more common with multiple valve disease or following multiple valve replacement.[167,168]

The incidence of perivalvular leak following multiple valve surgery is about 4% per patient-year and may be more frequent following multiple valve surgery than following single-valve surgery.[139,141]

When multiple valve surgery is combined with myocardial revascularization, the morbidity and mortality are 12 to 24%.[146,169] Early death in this group of patients is associated with prolonged perfusion time, the need for postoperative inotropic support, and high blood loss.[165]

CONCLUSION

The challenges of multiple valve replacement and repair include not only the technical maneuvers of operation but also the identification of associated valve lesions and correct judgment in surgical management. Echocardiography is the essential tool in preoperative diagnosis, and surgeons should become as familiar and facile with interpretation of ultrasound assessment of cardiac valves as with analysis of coronary angiograms. Finally, the various etiologies of multiple valve disease occur in certain combinations, and understanding the pathophysiology and pathologic anatomy is necessary to select the best procedure and to optimize early and late operative results.

REFERENCES

1. Knott-Craig CJ, Schaff HV, Mullany CJ, et al: Carcinoid disease of the heart: surgical management of 10 patients. *J Thorac Cardiovasc Surg* 1992; 104:475.
2. Schulman DS, Remetz MS, Elefteriades J, et al: Mild mitral insufficiency is a marker of impaired left ventricular performance in aortic stenosis. *J Am Coll Cardiol* 1989; 13:796.
3. Christenson JT, Jordan B, Bloch A, et al: Should a regurgitant mitral valve be replaced simultaneously with a stenotic aortic valve? *Texas Heart Inst J* 2000; 27:350.
4. Harris KM, Malenka DJ, Haney MF, et al: Improvement in mitral regurgitation after aortic valve replacement. *Am J Cardiol* 1997; 80:741.
5. Barreiro CJ, Patel ND, Fitton TP, et al: Aortic valve replacement and concomitant mitral valve regurgitation in the elderly: impact on survival and functional outcome. *Circulation* 2005; 112:I-443.
6. Freeman WK, Seward JB, Khandheria BK, et al: *Transesophageal Echocardiography.* Boston, Little, Brown, 1994.
7. Nowrangi SK, Connolly HM, Freeman WK, et al: Impact of intra-operative transesophageal echocardiography among patients undergoing aortic valve replacement for aortic stenosis. *J Am Soc Echocardiogr* 2001; 14:863.
8. McGrath L, Gonzalez-Lavin L, Bailey B, et al: Tricuspid valve operations in 530 patients: twenty-five-year assessment of early and late phase events. *J Thorac Cardiovasc Surg* 1990; 99:124.
9. Farid L, Dayem MK, Guindy R, et al: The importance of tricuspid valve structure and function in the surgical treatment of rheumatic mitral and aortic disease. *Eur Heart J* 1992; 13:366.
10. Pellegrini A, Colombo T, Donatelli F, et al: Evaluation and treatment of secondary tricuspid insufficiency. *Eur J Cardiothorac Surg* 1992; 6:288.
11. Carpentier A, Deloche A, Hannia G, et al: Surgical management of acquired tricuspid valve disease. *J Thorac Cardiovasc Surg* 1974; 67:53.
12. Wilson WR, Danielson GK, Giuliani ER, et al: Cardiac valve replacement in congestive heart failure due to infective endocarditis. *Mayo Clin Proc* 1979; 54:223.
13. Cohn LH: Tricuspid regurgitation secondary to mitral valve disease: when and how to repair. *J Cardiol Surg* 1994; 9:237.
14. King RM, Schaff HV, Danielson GK, et al: Surgery for tricuspid regurgitation, late after mitral valve replacement. *Circulation* 1984; 70:193.
15. Izumi C, Iga K, Konishi T: Progression of isolated tricuspid regurgitation late after mitral valve surgery for rheumatic mitral valve disease. *J Heart Valve Dis* 2002; 11:353.
16. Henein MY, O'Sullivan CA, Li W, et al: Evidence for rheumatic valve disease in patients with severe tricuspid regurgitation long after mitral valve surgery: the role of 3D echo reconstruction. *J Heart Valve Dis* 2003; 12(5):566-572.
17. DeVega NG: La anuloplastia selectiva reguable y permanente. *Rev Esp Cardiol* 1972; 25:6.
18. Kaul TK, Ramsdale DR, Mercer JL: Functional tricuspid regurgitation following replacement of the mitral valve. *Int J Cardiol* 1991; 33:305.
19. Kuwaki K, Morishita K, Tsukamoto M, et al: Tricuspid valve surgery for functional tricuspid valve regurgitation associated with left-sided valvular disease. *Eur J Cardiothorac Surg* 2001; 20:577.
20. Dreyfus GD, Corbi PJ, Chan KM, Bahrami T: Secondary tricuspid regurgitation or dilatation: which should be the criterion for surgical repair? *Ann Thorac Surg* 2005; 79:127.
21. Porter A, Shapira Y, Wurzel M, et al: Tricuspid regurgitation late after mitral valve replacement: clinical and echocardiographic evaluation. *J Heart Valve Dis* 1999; 8(1):57-62.
22. Matsunaga A, Duran CM: Progression of tricuspid regurgitation after repaired functional ischemic mitral regurgitation. *Circulation* 2005; 112(9 Suppl):I453-457.
23. Kim HK, Kim YJ, Kim KI, et al: Impact of the maze operation combined with left-sided valve surgery on the change in tricuspid regurgitation over time. *Circulation* 2005; 112(9 Suppl):I14-19.
24. Je HG, Song H, Jung SH, et al: Impact of the Maze operation on the progression of mild functional tricuspid regurgitation. *J Thorac Cardiovasc Surg* 2008; 136(5):1187-1192.
25. Kwak JJ, Kim YG, Kim MK, et al: Development of tricuspid regurgitation late after left-sided valve surgery: a single-center experience with long-term echocardiographic examinations. *Am Heart J* 2008; 155(4): 732-737.
26. Chan V, Burwash IG, Lam BK, et al: Clinical and echocardiographic impact of functional tricuspid regurgitation repair at the time of mitral valve replacement. *Ann Thorac Surg* 2009; 88(4):1209-1215.
27. Calafiore AM, Gallina S, Iaco AL, et al: Mitral valve surgery for functional mitral regurgitation: should moderate-or-more tricuspid regurgitation be treated? A propensity score analysis. *Ann Thorac Surg* 2009; 87(3): 698-703.
28. Shiran A, Sagie A: Tricuspid regurgitation in mitral valve disease incidence, prognostic implications, mechanism, and management. *J Am Coll Cardiol* 2009; 53(5):401-408.
29. Bortolotti U, Milano A, Testolin L, et al: Influence of type of prosthesis on late results after combined mitral-aortic valve replacement. *Ann Thorac Surg* 1991; 52:84.
30. Brown PJ, Roberts CS, McIntosh CL, et al: Relation between choice of prostheses and late outcome in double-valve replacement. *Ann Thorac Surg* 1993; 55:631.
31. Gersh BJ, Schaff HV, Vatterott PJ, et al: Results of triple valve replacement in 91 patients: perioperative mortality and long-term follow-up. *Circulation* 1985; 72:130.
32. Kawano H, Oda T, Fukunaga S, et al: Tricuspid valve replacement with the St Jude Medical valve: 19 years of experience. *Eur J Cardiothorac Surg* 2000; 18:565.
33. Struber M, Campbell A, Richard G, et al: Hydrodynamic performance of Carbomedics valves in double valve replacement. *J Heart Valve Dis* 1994; 3:667.
34. Levi M, Cromheecke ME, de Jonge E, et al: Pharmacological strategies to decrease excessive blood loss in cardiac surgery: a meta-analysis of clinically relevant endpoints. *Lancet* 1999; 354:1940.
35. Tyner JJ, Hunter JA, Najafi H: Postperfusion coronary stenosis. *Ann Thorac Surg* 1987; 44:418.
36. Talwalkar NG, Lawrie GM, Earle N: Can retrograde cardioplegia alone provide adequate protection for cardiac valve surgery? *Chest* 1999; 115:1359.
37. Villanueva FS, Spotnitz WD, Glasheen WP, et al: New insights into the physiology of retrograde cardioplegia delivery. *Am J Physiol* 1995; 268:H1555.
38. Ruengsakulrach P, Buxton BF: Anatomic and hemodynamic considerations influencing the efficiency of retrograde cardioplegia. *Ann Thorac Surg* 2001; 71:1389.
39. Fraser CD Jr, Wang N, Mee RB, et al: Repair of insufficient bicuspid aortic valves. *Ann Thorac Surg* 1994; 58:386.
40. Cosgrove DM, Ratliff NB, Schaff HV, Eards WD: Aortic valve decalcification: history repeated with a new result. *Ann Thorac Surg* 1994; 49:689.
41. Piehler JM, Danielson GK, Pluth JR, et al: Enlargement of the aortic root or annulus with autogenous pericardial patch during aortic valve replacement: long-term follow-up. *J Thorac Cardiovasc Surg* 1983; 86:350.
42. Ross DB, Trusler GA, Coles JG, et al: Successful reconstruction of aorto-left atrial fistula following aortic valve replacement and root enlargement by the Manouguian procedure. *J Cardiol Surg* 1994; 9:392.
43. de Vivie ER, Borowski A, Mehlhorn U: Reduction of the left-ventricular outflow-tract obstruction by aortoventriculoplasty: long-term results of 96 patients. *Thorac Cardiovasc Surg* 1993; 41:216.
44. Manouguian S: [A new method for patch enlargement of hypoplastic aortic annulus: an experimental study (author's translation).] *Thoraxchir Vaskulare Chir* 1976; 24:418.
45. Skoularigis J, Sinovich V, Joubert G, Sareli P: Evaluation of the long-term results of mitral valve repair in 254 young patients with rheumatic mitral regurgitation. *Circulation* 1994; 90:II-167.
46. Enriquez-Sarano M, Tajik AJ, Schaff HV, et al: Echocardiographic prediction of survival after surgical correction of organic mitral regurgitation. *Circulation* 1994; 90:830.
47. Enriquez-Sarano M, Schaff HV, Orszulak TA, et al: Valve repair improves the outcome of surgery for mitral regurgitation: a multivariate analysis. *Circulation* 1995; 91:1022.
48. Liao K, Wu JJ, Frater RW: Comparative evaluation of left ventricular performance after mitral valve repair or valve replacement with or without chordal preservation. *J Heart Valve Dis* 1993; 2:159.
49. David TE: Papillary muscle-annular continuity: is it important? *J Cardiol Surg* 1994; 9:252.
50. Suzuki N, Takanashi Y, Tokuhiro K, et al: Mitral valve replacement with and without chordal preservation in patients with chronic mitral regurgitation: Mechanisms for differences. *Circulation* 1992; 86:1718.

51. Wasir H, Choudhary SK, Airan B, et al: Mitral valve replacement with chordal preservation in a rheumatic population. *J Heart Valve Dis* 2001; 10:84.
52. Crawford ES, Coselli JS: Marfan's syndrome: combined composite valve graft replacement of the aortic root and transaortic mitral valve replacement. *Ann Thorac Surg* 1988; 45:296.
53. Seccombe JF, Schaff HV: Mitral valve repair: current techniques and indications, in Franco L, Verrier ED (eds): *Advanced Therapy in Cardiac Surgery.* Hanover, PA, Sheridan Press, 1999; p 220.
54. Suri R, Orszulak T: Triangular resection for repair of mitral regurgitation due to degenerative disease. *Op Tech Thorac Cardiovasc Surg* 2005; 10:194.
55. Phillips MR, Daly RC, Schaff HV, et al: Repair of anterior leaflet mitral valve prolapse: chordal replacement versus chordal shortening. *Ann Thorac Surg* 2000; 69:25.
56. Odell JA, Schaff HV, Orszulak TA: Early results of a simplified method of mitral valve annuloplasty. *Circulation* 1995; 92:150.
57. Acar C, Perier P, Fontaliran F, et al: Anatomical study of the tricuspid valve and its variations. *Surg Radiol Anat* 1990; 12:229.
58. Izumi C, Iga K, Konishi T: Progression of isolated tricuspid regurgitation late after mitral valve surgery for rheumatic mitral valve disease. *J Heart Valve Dis* 2002; 11:353.
59. King RM, Schaff HV, Danielson GK, et al: Surgical treatment of tricuspid insufficiency late after mitral valve replacement. *Circulation* 1983; 68:III.
60. Mullany CJ, Gersh BJ, Orszulak TA, et al: Repair of tricuspid valve insufficiency in patients undergoing double (aortic and mitral) valve replacement: perioperative mortality and long-term (1 to 20 years) follow-up in 109 patients. *J Thorac Cardiovasc Surg* 1987; 94:740.
61. Duran CG, Ubago JL: Clinical and hemodynamic performance of a totally flexible prosthetic ring for atrioventricular valve reconstruction. *Ann Thorac Surg* 1976; 22:458.
62. Kay JH, Maselli-Capagna G, Tsuji HK: Surgical treatment of tricuspid insufficiency. *Ann Surg* 1965; 162:53.
63. McCarthy JF, Cosgrove DM: Tricuspid valve repair with the Cosgrove-Edwards annuloplasty system. *Ann Thorac Surg* 1997; 64:267.
64. McCarthy PM, Bhudia SK, Rajeswaran J, et al: Tricuspid valve repair: durability and risk factors for failure. *J Thorac Cardiovasc Surg* 2004; 127(3):674-685.
65. Morishita A, Kitamura M, Noji S, et al: Long-term results after De Vega's tricuspid annuloplasty. *J Cardiovasc Surg (Torino)* 2002; 43(6):773-777.
66. Tang GH, David TE, Singh SK, et al: Tricuspid valve repair with an annuloplasty ring results in improved long-term outcomes. *Circulation* 2006; 114(1 Suppl):I577-581.
67. Karimov JH, Bevilacqua S, Solinas M, Glauber M: Triple heart valve surgery through a right antero-lateral minithoracotomy. *Int Cardiovasc Thorac Surg* 2009; 9(2):360-362; Meyer SR, Szeto WY, Augoustides JG, et al: Reoperative mitral valve surgery by the port access minithoracotomy approach is safe and effective. *Ann Thorac Surg* 2009; 87(5):1426-1430.
68. Connolly HM, Schaff HV, Mullany CJ, et al: Surgical management of left-sided carcinoid heart disease. *Circulation* 2001; 104:I-36.
69. Connolly HM, Schaff HV, Larson RA, et al: Carcinoid heart disease: impact of pulmonary valve replacement on right ventricular function and remodeling. *Circulation* 2001; 104:II-685.
70. Moller JE, Pellikka PA, Bernheim AM, et al: Prognosis of carcinoid heart disease: analysis of 200 cases over two decades. *Circulation* 2005; 112:3320.
71. Kirklin J, Barratt-Boyes B: Combined aortic and mitral valve disease with and without tricuspid valve disease, in Kirklin JW, Barratt-Boyes B (eds): *Cardiac Surgery.* New York, Wiley, 1993; p 431.
72. Roberts WC, Virmani R: Aschoff bodies at necropsy in valvular heart disease. *Circulation* 1978; 57:803.
73. Jai Shankar K, Jaiswal PK, Cherian KM: Rheumatic involvement of all four cardiac valves. *Heart* 2005; 91:e50.
74. Bland EF, Jones TD: Rheumatic fever and rheumatic heart disease: a 20-year report on 1000 patients followed since childhood. *Circulation* 1951; 4:836.
75. Wilson MG, Lubschez R: Longevity in rheumatic fever. *JAMA* 1948; 121:1.
76. Ellis LB, Harken DE, Black H: A clinical study of 1000 consecutive cases of mitral stenosis two to nine years after mitral valvuloplasty. *Circulation* 1959; 19:803.
77. Kern MJ, Aguirre F, Donohue T, et al: Interpretation of cardiac pathophysiology from pressure waveform analysis: multivalvular regurgitant lesions. *Cath Cardiovasc Diag* 1993; 28:167.
78. Terzaki AK, Cokkinos DV, Leachman RD, et al: Combined mitral and aortic valve disease. *Am J Cardiol* 1970; 25:588.
79. Gash AK, Carabello BA, Kent RL, et al: Left ventricular performance in patients with coexistent mitral stenosis and aortic insufficiency. *J Am Coll Cardiol* 1984; 67:148.
80. Grinda JM, Latremouille C, Berrebi AJ, et al: Aortic cusp extension valvuloplasty for rheumatic aortic valve disease: midterm results. *Ann Thorac Surg* 2002; 74:438.
81. Liuzzo JP, Shin YT, Lucariello R, et al: Triple valve repair for rheumatic heart disease. *J Cardiol Surg* 2005; 20:358.
82. Prabhakar G, Kumar N, Gometza B, et al: Triple-valve operation in the young rheumatic patient. *Ann Thorac Surg* 1993; 55:1492.
83. Katznelson G, Jreissaty RM, Levinson GE, et al: Combined aortic and mitral stenosis: a clinical and physiological study. *Am J Med* 1960; 29:242.
84. Uricchio JF, Sinha KP, Bentivoglio L, et al: A study of combined mitral and aortic stenosis. *Ann Intern Med* 1959; 51:668.
85. Kumar N, Saad E, Prabhakar G, et al: Extended transseptal versus conventional left atriotomy: early postoperative study. *Ann Thorac Surg* 1995; 60:426.
86. Honey M: Clinical and haemodynamic observations on combined mitral and aortic stenoses. *Br Heart J* 1961; 23:545.
87. Choudhary SK, Talwar S, Juneja R, et al: Fate of mild aortic valve disease after mitral valve intervention. *J Thorac Cardiovasc Surg* 2001; 122:583.
88. Larbalestier RI, Chard RB, Cohn LH: Optimal approach to the mitral valve: dissection of the interatrial groove. *Ann Thorac Surg* 1992; 54:1186.
89. Barner HB: Combined superior and right lateral left atriotomy with division of the superior vena cava for exposure of the mitral valve. *Ann Thorac Surg* 1992; 54:594.
90. Smith CR: Septal-superior exposure of the mitral valve: the transplant approach. *J Thorac Cardiovasc Surg* 1992; 103:623.
91. Couetil JP, Ramsheyi A, Tolan MJ, et al: Biatrial inferior transseptal approach to the mitral valve. *Ann Thorac Surg* 1995; 60:1432.
92. Brawley RK: Improved exposure of the mitral valve in patients with a small left atrium. *Ann Thorac Surg* 1980; 29:179.
93. Shine KI, DeSanctis RW, Sanders CA, et al: Combined aortic and mitral incompetence: clinical features and surgical. *Am Heart J* 1968; 76:728.
94. Urschel CW, Covell JW, Sonnenblick EH, et al: Myocardial mechanics in aortic and mitral valvular regurgitation: the concept of instantaneous impedance as a determinant of the performance of the intact heart. *J Clin Invest* 1968; 47:867.
95. Boucher C: Multivalvular heart disease, in Eagle K, Haber E, DeSanctis R, et al (eds): *The Practice of Cardiology,* 2nd ed. Boston, Little, Brown, 1989; p 765.
96. Shigenobu M, Senoo Y, Teramoto S: Results of surgery for aortic regurgitation due to aortic valve prolapse. *Acta Med Okayama* 1988; 42:343.
97. Dare AJ, Veinot JP, Edwards WD, et al: New observations on the etiology of aortic valve disease: a surgical pathologic study of 236 cases from 1990. *Hum Pathol* 1993; 24:1330.
98. Bellitti R, Caruso A, Festa M, et al: Prolapse of the floppy aortic valve as a cause of aortic regurgitation: a clinicomorphologic study. *Int J Cardiol* 1985; 9:399.
99. Agozzino L, de Vivo F, Falco A, et al: Non-inflammatory aortic root disease and floppy aortic valve as cause of isolated regurgitation: a clinicomorphologic study. *Int J Cardiol* 1994; 45:129.
100. Roberts WC, Sullivan MF: Clinical and necropsy observations early after simultaneous replacement of the mitral and aortic valves. *Am J Cardiol* 1986; 58:1067.
101. Milewicz DM, Pyeritz RE, Crawford ES, et al: Marfan syndrome: defective synthesis, secretion, and extracellular matrix formation of fibrillin by cultured dermal fibroblasts. *J Clin Invest* 1992; 89:79.
102. Rippe LM, Angoff G, Sloss LJ: Multiple floppy valves: an echocardiographic syndrome. *Am J Med* 1979; 66:817.
103. Ogawa S, Hayashi J, Sasaki H, et al: Evaluation of combined valvular prolapse syndrome by two-dimensional echocardiography. *Circulation* 1982; 65:174.
104. Lakier JB, Copans H, Rosman HS, et al: Idiopathic degeneration of the aortic valve: a common cause of isolated aortic regurgitation. *J Am Coll Cardiol* 1985; 5:347.
105. Tomaru T, Uchida Y, Mohri N, et al: Postinflammatory mitral and aortic valve prolapse: a clinical and pathological study. *Circulation* 1987; 76:68.
106. Gillinov AM, Blackstone EH, White J, et al: Durability of combined aortic and mitral valve repair. *Ann Thorac Surg* 2001; 72:20.
107. Gott VL, Cameron DE, Alejo DE, et al: Aortic root replacement in 271 Marfan patients: a 24-year experience. *Ann Thorac Surg* 2002; 73:438.
108. David TE: Aortic valve-sparing operations for aortic root aneurysm. *Semin Thorac Cardiovasc Surg* 2001; 13:291.
109. Bozbuga N, Erentug V, Kirali K, et al: Surgical management of mitral regurgitation in patients with Marfan syndrome. *J Heart Valve Dis* 2003; 12:717.
110. Gillinov AM, Hulyalkar A, Cameron DE, et al: Mitral valve operation in patients with the Marfan syndrome. *J Thorac Cardiovasc Surg* 1994; 107:724.

111. Fernicola DJ, Roberts WC: Pure mitral regurgitation associated with a malfunctioning congenitally bicuspid aortic valve necessitating combined mitral and aortic valve replacement. *Am J Cardiol* 1994; 74:619.
112. Mills NL, McIntosh CL, Mills LJ: Techniques for management of the calcified mitral annulus. *J Cardiol Surg* 1986; 1:347.
113. Utley JR, Mills J, Hutchinson JC, et al: Valve replacement for bacterial and fungal endocarditis: a comparative study. *Circulation* 1973; 3:42.
114. Nair CK, Aronow WS, Sketch MH, et al: Clinical and echocardiography characteristics of patients with mitral annular calcification: comparison with age- and sex-matched control subjects. *Am J Cardiol* 1983; 51:992.
115. Kim HK, Park SJ, Suh JW, et al: Association between cardiac valvular calcification and coronary artery disease in a low-risk population. *Coronary Artery Dis* 2004; 15:1.
116. Kizer JR, Wiebers DO, Whisnant JP, et al: Mitral annular calcification, aortic valve sclerosis, and incident stroke in adults free of clinical cardiovascular disease: The Strong Heart Study. *Stroke* 2005; 36:2533.
117. Feindel CM, Tufail Z, David TE, et al: Mitral valve surgery in patients with extensive calcification of the mitral annulus. *J Thorac Cardiovasc Surg* 2003; 126:777.
118. Buchbinder NA, Roberts WC: Left-sided valvular active infective endocarditis: a study of forty-five necropsy patients. *Am J Med* 1972; 53:20.
119. Mathew J, Addai T, Anand A, et al: Clinical features, site of involvement, bacteriologic findings, and outcome of infective endocarditis in intravenous drug users. *Arch Intern Med* 1995; 155:1641.
120. Aoyagi S, Oryoji A, Nishi Y, et al: Long-term results of valve replacement with the St Jude Medical valve. *J Thorac Cardiovasc Surg* 1994; 108:1021.
121. Schoen FJ, Berger BM, Guerina NG: Cardiac effects of noncardiac neoplasms (review). *Cardiol Clin* 1984; 2:657.
122. Connolly HM: Carcinoid heart disease: medical and surgical considerations. *Cancer Control* 2001; 8:454.
123. Propst JW, Siegel LC, Stover EP: Anesthetic considerations for valve replacement surgery in a patient with carcinoid syndrome. *J Cardiothorac Vasc Anesth* 1994; 8:209.
124. Neustein SM, Cohen E, Reich D, et al: Transoesophageal echocardiography and the intraoperative diagnosis of left atrial invasion by carcinoid tumour. *Can J Anaesth* 1993; 40:664.
125. Cartwright RS, Giacobine JW, Ratan RS, et al: Combined aortic and mitral valve replacement. *J Thorac Cardiovasc Surg* 1963; 45:35.
126. Stephenson LW, Edie RN, Harken AH, et al: Combined aortic and mitral valve replacement: changes in practice and prognosis. *Circulation* 1984; 69:640.
127. Sakamoto Y, Hashimoto K, Okuyama H, et al: Long-term results of triple-valve procedure. *Asian Cardiovasc Thorac Ann* 2006; 14:47.
128. LaSalle CW, Csicsko JF, Mirro MJ: Double cardiac valve replacement: a community hospital experience. *Ind Med* 1993; 86:422.
129. Khan S, Chaux A, Matloff J, et al: The St Jude medical valve: experience with 1000 cases. *J Thorac Cardiovasc Surg* 1994; 108:1010.
130. Armenti F, Stephenson LW, Edmunds LH Jr.: Simultaneous implantation of St Jude Medical aortic and mitral prostheses. *J Thorac Cardiovasc Surg* 1987; 94:733.
131. Galloway A, Grossi E, Bauman F, et al: Multiple valve operation for advanced valvular heart disease: results and risk factors in 513 patients. *J Am Coll Cardiol* 1992; 19:725.
132. Fiore AC, Swartz MT, Sharp TG, et al: Double-valve replacement with Medtronic-Hall or St Jude valve. *Ann Thorac Surg* 1995; 59:1113.
133. Teoh KH, Christakis GT, Weisel RD, et al: The determinants of mortality and morbidity after multiple-valve operations. *Ann Thorac Surg* 1987; 43:353.
134. Donahoo JS, Lechman MJ, MacVaugh H 3d: Combined aortic and mitral valve replacement: a 6-year experience. *Cardiol Clin* 1985; 3:417.
135. Mattila S, Harjula A, Kupari M, et al: Combined multiple-valve procedures: factors influencing the early and late results. Sc and *J Thorac Cardiovasc Surg* 1985; 19:33.
136. He G, Acuff T, Ryan W, et al: Aortic valve replacement: determinants of operative mortality. *Ann Thorac Surg* 1994; 57:1140.
137. Alvarez L, Escudero C, Figuera D, et al: The Bjork-Shiley valve prosthesis: analysis of long-term evolution. *J Thorac Cardiovasc Surg* 1992; 104:1249.
138. Jegaden O, Eker A, Delahaye F, et al: Thromboembolic risk and late survival after mitral valve replacement with the St Jude medical valve. *Ann Thorac Surg* 1994; 58:1721.
139. Copeland J 3d: An international experience with the Carbo-Medics prosthetic heart valve. *J Heart Valve Dis* 1995; 4:56.
140. Bernal JM, Rabasa JM, Cagigas JC, et al: Valve-related complications with the Hancock I porcine bioprosthesis: a twelve- to fourteen-year follow-up study. *J Thorac Cardiovasc Surg* 1991; 101:871.
141. Loisance DY, Mazzucotelli JP, Bertrand PC, et al: Mitroflow pericardial valve: long-term durability (see comments). *Ann Thorac Surg* 1993; 56:131.
142. Akins CW, Buckley MJ, Daggett WM, et al: Myocardial revascularization with combined aortic and mitral valve replacements. *J Thorac Cardiovasc Surg* 1985; 90:272.
143. Smith JA, Westlake GW, Mullerworth MH, et al: Excellent long-term results of cardiac valve replacement with the St Jude Medical valve prosthesis. *Circulation* 1993; 88:II-49.
144. Sante P, Renzulli A, Festa M, et al: Acute postoperative block of mechanical prostheses: incidence and treatment. *Cardiovasc Surg* 1994; 2:403.
145. Craver JM, Jones EL, Guyton RA, et al: Avoidance of transverse midventricular disruption following mitral valve replacement. *Ann Thorac Surg* 1985; 40:163.
146. Pomar JL, Jamieson WR, Pelletier LC, et al: Mitroflow pericardial bioprosthesis: clinical performance to ten years. *Ann Thorac Surg* 1995; 60:S305.
147. Cannegieter SC, Rosendaal FR, Briet E: Thromboembolic and bleeding complications in patients with mechanical heart valve prostheses (review). *Circulation* 1994; 89:635.
148. Heras M, Chesebro JH, Fuster V, et al: High risk of thromboembolism early after bioprosthetic cardiac valve replacement. *J Am Coll Cardiol* 1995; 25:1111.
149. Horstkotte D, Schulte HD, Bircks W, et al: Lower intensity anticoagulation therapy results in lower complication rates with the St Jude medical prosthesis. *J Thorac Cardiovasc Surg* 1994; 107:1136.
150. Bernal JM, Rabasa JM, Lopez R, et al: Durability of the Carpen-tier-Edwards porcine bioprosthesis: role of age and valve position. *Ann Thorac Surg* 1995; 60:S248.
151. Brown PJ, Roberts CS, McIntosh CL, et al: Late results after triple-valve replacement with various substitute valves. *Ann Thorac Surg* 1993; 55:502.
152. Hamamoto M, Bando K, Kobayashi J, et al: Durability and outcome of aortic valve replacement with mitral valve repair versus double valve replacement. *Ann Thorac Surg* 2003; 75:28.
153. Munro AI, Jamieson WR, Burr LH, et al: Comparison of porcine bioprostheses and mechanical prostheses in multiple valve replacement operations. *Ann Thorac Surg* 1995; 60:S459.
154. Pellegrini A, Colombo T, Donatelli F, et al: Evaluation and treatment of secondary tricuspid insufficiency. *Eur J Cardiothorac Surg* 1992; 6:288.
155. Kaul TK, Ramsdale DR, Mercer JL: Functional tricuspid regurgitation following replacement of the mitral valve. *Int J Cardiol* 1991; 33:305.
156. Connolly HM, Crary JL, McGoon MD, et al: Left and right heart valves: valvular heart disease associated with fenfluramine-phentermine. *NEJM* 1997; 337:581-588.
157. Pritchett AM, Morrison JF, Edwards WD, et al: Left and right heart valves: valvular heart disease in patients taking pergolide. *Mayo Clin Proc* 2002; 77:1280-1286.
158. Droogmans S, Cosyns B, D'Haenen H, et al: Mitral and tricuspid: possible association between 3,4-methylenedioxymethamphetamine abuse and valvular heart disease. *Am J Cardiol* 2007; 100:1442-1525.
159. Kara M, Langlet MF, Blin D, et al: Triple valve procedures: an analysis of early and late results. *Thorac Cardiovasc Surg* 1986; 34:17.
160. Macmanus Q, Grunkemeier G, Starr A: Late results of triple valve replacement: a 14-year review. *Ann Thorac Surg* 1978; 25:402.
161. Cohn L, Aranki S, Rizzo R, et al: Decrease in operative risk of reoperative valve surgery. *Ann Thorac Surg* 1993; 56:15.
162. Konishi Y, Matsuda K, Nishiwaki N, et al: Ventricular arrhythmias late after aortic and/or mitral valve replacement. *Jpn Circ J* 1985; 49:576.
163. Konstantopoulos K, Kasparian T, Sideris J, et al: Mechanical hemolysis associated with a bioprosthetic mitral valve combined with a calcified aortic valve stenosis. *Acta Haematol* 1994; 91:164.
164. Skoularigis J, Essop M, Skudicky D, et al: Valvular heart disease: frequency and severity of intravascular hemolysis after left-sided cardiac valve replacement with Medtronic Hall and St Jude medical prostheses, and influence of prosthetic type, position, size and number. *Am J Cardiol* 1993; 71:587.
165. Page RD, Jeffrey RR, Fabri BM, et al: Combined multiple valve procedures and myocardial revascularisation. *Thorac Cardiovasc Surg* 1990; 38:308.
166. Trace HD, Bailey CP, Wendkos MH: Tricuspid valve commissurotomy with one-year follow-up. *Am Heart J* 1954; 47:613.
167. Brofman BL: Right auriculoventricular pressure gradient with special reference to tricuspid stenosis. *J Lab Clin Med* 1953; 42:789.
168. Lillehei CW, Gott VL, DeWall RA, et al: The surgical treatment of stenotic and regurgitant lesions of the mitral and aortic valves by direct utilization of a pump oxygenator. *J Thorac Surg* 1958; 35:154.
169. Aberg B: Surgical treatment of combined aortic and mitral valvular disease. *Scand J Thorac Cardiovasc Surg* 1980; 25:1.

170. West PN, Ferguson TB, Clark RE, et al: Multiple valve replacement: changing status. *Ann Thorac Surg* 1978; 26:32.
171. Lemole GM, Cuasay R: Improved technique of double valve replacement. *J Thorac Cardiovasc Surg* 1976; 71:759.
172. Clawson BJ: Rheumatic heart disease: an analysis of 796 cases. *Am Heart J* 1940; 20:454.
173. Cooke WT, White PD: Tricuspid stenosis with particular reference to diagnosis and prognosis. *Br Heart J* 1941; 3:141.
174. Mardelli TJ, Morganroth J, Naito M, et al: Cross-sectional echocardiographic identification of aortic valve prolapse (abstract). *Circulation* 1979; 60:II-204.
175. David TE: Aortic valve repair in patients with Marfan syndrome and ascending aorta aneurysms due to degenerative disease. *J Cardiol Surg* 1994; 9:182.
176. Gott VL, Gillinov AM, Pyeritz RE, et al: Aortic root replacement: risk factor analysis of a seventeen-year experience with 270 patients. *J Thorac Cardiovasc Surg* 1995; 109:536.
177. Raviprasad GS, Salem BI, Gowda S, et al: Radiation-induced mitral and tricuspid regurgitation with severe ostial coronary artery disease: a case report with successful surgical treatment [review]. *Cathet Cardiovasc Diag* 1995; 35:146.
178. Blanche C, Freimark D, Valenza M, et al: Heart transplantation for Q fever endocarditis. *Ann Thorac Surg* 1994; 58:1768.
179. Rozycka CB, Hryniewiecki T, Solik TA, et al: Mitral and aortic valve replacement in a patient with ectodermal anhydrotic dysplasia: a case report. *J Heart Valve Dis* 1994; 3:224.
180. Tan C, Schaff H, Miller F, et al: Clinical investigation: valvular heart disease in four patients with Maroteaux-Lamy syndrome. *Circulation* 1992; 85:188.
181. Carrel T, Pasic M, Tkebuchava T, et al: Aortic homograft and mitral valve repair in a patient with Werner's syndrome. *Ann Thorac Surg* 1994; 57:1319.
182. Pellegrini RV, Copeland CE, DiMarco RF, et al: Blunt rupture of both atrioventricular valves. *Ann Thorac Surg* 1986; 42:471.
183. Gabarre J, Gessain A, Raphael M, et al: Adult T-cell leukemia/ lymphoma revealed by a surgically cured cardiac valve lymphomatous involvement in an Iranian woman: clinical, immunopathological and viromolecular studies. *Leukemia* 1993; 7:1904.
184. Lang LL, Hvass U, Paillole C, et al: Cardiac valve replacement in relapsing polychondritis: a review. *J Heart Valve Dis* 1995; 4:227.
185. Ames DE, Asherson RA, Coltart JD, et al: Systemic lupus erythematosus complicated by tricuspid stenosis and regurgitation: successful treatment by valve transplantation. *Ann Rheum Dis* 1992; 51:120.
186. Fujise K, Amerling R, Sherman W: Rapid progression of mitral and aortic stenosis in a patient with secondary hyperparathyroidism. *Br Heart J* 1993; 70:282.
187. Palazzo E, Bourgeois P, Meyer O, et al: Hypocomplementemic urticarial vasculitis syndrome, Jaccoud's syndrome, valvulopathy: a new syndromic combination. *J Rheumatol* 1993; 20:1236.
188. Emery RW, Emery AM, Krogh C, et al: The St. Jude Medical cardiac valve prosthesis: long-term follow up of patients having double valve replacement. *J Heart Valve Dis* 2007; 16(6):634-640.
189. Ibrahim M, O'Kane H, Cleland J, et al: The St Jude Medical pros-thesis: a thirteen-year experience. *J Thorac Cardiovasc Surg* 1994; 108:221.
190. David TE, Armstrong S, Sun Z: The Hancock II bioprosthesis at ten years. *Ann Thorac Surg* 1995; 60:S229.
191. Jamieson WR, Burr LH, Tyers GF, et al: Carpentier-Edwards supraannular porcine bioprosthesis: clinical performance to twelve years. *Ann Thorac Surg* 1995; 60:S235.
192. Milano A, Bortolotti U, Mazzucco A, et al: Heart valve replacement with the Sorin tilting-disk prosthesis: a 10-year experience. *J Thorac Cardiovasc Surg* 1992; 103:267.
193. Leavitt BJ, Baribeau YR, DiScipio AW, Northern New England Cardiovascular Disease Study Group, et al: Outcomes of patients undergoing concomitant aortic and mitral valve surgery in northern New England. *Circulation* 2009; 120(11 Suppl):S155-162.
194. Lemieux MD, Jamieson WR, Landymore RW, et al: Medtronic intact porcine bioprosthesis: clinical performance to seven years. *Ann Thorac Surg* 1995; 60:S258.
195. Orszulak TA, Schaff HV, DeSmet JM, et al: Late results of valve replacement with the Bjork-Shiley valve (1973 to 1982) (see comments). *J Thorac Cardiovasc Surg* 1993; 105:302.
196. Nakano K, Koyanagi H, Hashimoto A, et al: Twelve years' experience with the St Jude Medical valve prosthesis. *Ann Thorac Surg* 1994; 57:697.
197. Pelletier LC, Carrier M, Leclerc Y, et al: The Carpentier-Edwards pericardial bioprosthesis: clinical experience with 600 patients. *Ann Thorac Surg* 1995; 60:S297.
198. van Doorn C, Stoodley K, Saunders N, et al: Mitral valve replacement with the Carpentier-Edwards standard bioprosthesis: performance into the second decade. *Eur J Cardiothoracic Surg* 1995; 9:253.
199. Han QQ, Xu ZY, Zhang BR, et al: Primary triple valve surgery for advanced rheumatic heart disease in Mainland China: a single-center experience with 871 clinical cases. *Eur J Cardiothorac Surg* 2007; 31(5): 845-850.

CHAPTER 48

Valvular and Ischemic Heart Disease

Verdi J. DiSesa

INTRODUCTION

In recent years, there has been a great deal of progress in coronary artery surgery, nonsurgical treatment of coronary artery disease, and the surgical treatment of valvular heart disease. As thoroughly described in previous chapters, surgery on the beating heart has become commonplace. Interventional therapies for coronary artery obstruction have extended to multivessel disease and continue to change the number and the nature of patients referred for bypass surgery. The options for treatment of valvular disease have continued to expand with advances in techniques for repair of aortic and mitral valves, as well as increases in the choices of valve type for replacement. Techniques for aortic valve replacement on the beating heart via a retrograde transvascular or transapical approach are now under investigation. Other areas of rapidly growing interest are surgical treatment of atrial arrhythmias and the surgical approach to the failing ventricle in dilated ischemic cardiomyopathy. Some of these topics are discussed in other chapters. All are issues that the surgeon must consider when planning a strategy for the treatment of the patient with combined valvular and coronary artery disease. More patients are now presenting with increasingly complex pathology. It is less often that the surgeon sees a patient with simple aortic stenosis and proximal coronary artery disease. Rather, that patient now may have been managed with more aggressive medical therapy or even catheter interventions, and is referred at an older age and is sicker, with more diffuse disease, arrhythmias, and worsening ventricular function. As a result those patients who present for surgery have a higher-risk profile than was previously the case, and may require a more flexible and thoughtful approach.

The interaction between the pathophysiologies of valvular heart disease and coronary artery disease is complex. Valvular heart disease alters ventricular function. Coronary artery disease may have an additional impact because of its potential to affect ventricular morphology and physiology. In addition to decreases in contractile strength, regional myocardial infarction may lead to distortion of ventricular shape with resulting effects not only on ventricular function, but also on mitral valve performance. In patients with valvular heart disease, coronary obstructions may be symptomatic or asymptomatic, but the decision to intervene surgically is often made regardless of the presence of symptoms and in order to have a positive effect on the pathophysiology of both diseases.

Under most circumstances, surgeons attempt to treat both valvular and coronary artery diseases simultaneously. At the least, this makes for a longer and more complicated operation with longer myocardial ischemia times. Because of this, combined coronary artery and valve operations usually have a higher risk for early and late mortality than operations for isolated valvular heart disease (Fig. 48-1). This complexity increases the need for careful preoperative assessment of myocardial function and an understanding of the impact on ventricular function of the changing afterload and preload associated with valve surgery. Therefore, in adult patients with combined valvular and ischemic heart disease, the assessment of intrinsic left ventricular function assumes paramount importance. Clinical signs and symptoms of left ventricular failure should be sought. In addition to history, physical examination, and routine laboratory tests, preoperative echocardiography is mandatory. Transesophageal echocardiography often is the diagnostic technique of choice for accurate planning when operative repair of the mitral valve is considered. It is also important to distinguish heart failure resulting from valvular disease from reversible or irreversible myocardial dysfunction owing to coronary ischemia. Dobutamine stress echocardiography may be useful in eliciting ventricular size and shape changes that occur under stress and that may exacerbate underlying pathology, especially of the mitral valve. At cardiac catheterization, left ventricular end-diastolic pressure and pulmonary

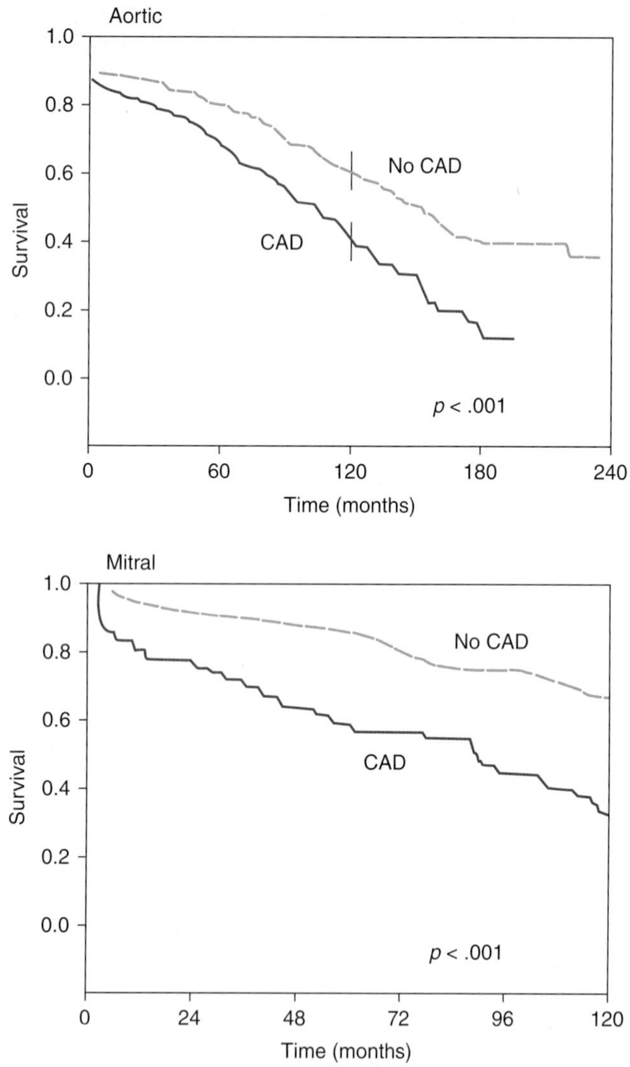

FIGURE 48-1 Survival after aortic or mitral valve replacement in patients with and without coronary artery disease (CAD). In both cases, long-term survival is significantly worse in patients with coronary disease. *(Adapted with permission from Jones EL, Weintraub WS, Craver JM, et al: Interaction of age and coronary disease after valve replacement: implications for valve selection. Ann Thorac Surg 1994; 58:378.)*

pressures give additional information about left and right ventricular function and supplement noninvasive evaluation of valve function and coronary anatomy. In centers where it is available, positron emission tomography (PET) scans can help distinguish areas of viable myocardium with reversible ischemia and ischemic dysfunction from irreversibly scarred muscle. These assessments are important before embarking on combined valve and coronary artery surgery, for they are crucial in estimating operative risk and planning the operative approach.

The assessment of valve pathology is covered in detail in previous chapters on isolated valvular heart disease. As has been noted, coronary angiography is not necessarily required in all patients with valvular pathology who are about to undergo valve surgery. However, given the prevalence of coronary artery disease in aging Western populations, coronary angiography is usually performed in all patients greater than 40 years of age, and select younger patients with suggestive symptoms or significant risk factors.

With present technology and techniques, myocardial revascularization can be added to any valve procedure. What is needed are a rational approach, more time, and good myocardial protection. Because of the wide pathophysiologic spectrum of valvular and coronary artery diseases, several frequently encountered valve and coronary artery combinations are considered in this chapter, including: (1) aortic stenosis with coronary artery disease (CAD), (2) aortic regurgitation plus CAD, (3) mitral regurgitation plus CAD, (4) mitral stenosis plus CAD, (5) aortic stenosis and mitral regurgitation plus CAD, and (6) aortic regurgitation and mitral regurgitation plus CAD.

Of course, patients may have combined lesions of stenosis and insufficiency, but to avoid unproductive complexity, and because one lesion usually dominates, the somewhat arbitrary categorization noted above will be maintained during the ensuing discussion. For each entity, the clinical presentation, the pathophysiology of the disease state and its correction, the operative and management approach, and short- and long-term results are discussed. The surgeon also must acknowledge and understand the potential and evolving roles of new techniques, such as coronary artery stenting, beating heart revascularization, and percutaneous aortic valve replacement in the management of patients with combined valve and coronary artery disease.[3–7] At this time, none of these techniques represents the standard of care for patients who are candidates for a major cardiovascular surgical procedure.

AORTIC STENOSIS AND CORONARY ARTERY DISEASE

Aortic stenosis is one of the more frequently encountered valvular lesions in adult populations. Because degenerative calcific aortic stenosis is most common in patients in their sixties, seventies, and eighties[1,2] and because congenitally bicuspid valves that become stenotic are more frequent in men who are susceptible to CAD at an earlier age than are women,[8] it is not surprising that the combination of aortic stenosis and CAD is encountered frequently. This disease combination is usually gratifying to treat because the response to surgical relief of aortic stenosis and coronary artery obstructions is significant, immediate, and relatively durable.

Clinical Presentation

Patients with aortic stenosis are asymptomatic initially, but eventually present with angina pectoris, congestive heart failure, syncope, or some combination of these. When significant coronary artery obstructions are present in addition to valvular obstruction, angina pectoris is almost always present. However, angina pectoris can occur in the absence of significant coronary artery obstructions. It is relatively easy to identify symptoms of myocardial ischemia or congestive heart failure in these patients. Neurologic symptoms may be more difficult to elicit, and careful questioning regarding transient symptomatology is required. Symptoms suggestive of carotid artery obstruction should be sought. Specific studies of the carotid arteries may be necessary, especially because the murmur of aortic stenosis may radiate into the carotids and obscure the detection of bruits.

Prominent findings on physical examination include the typical crescendo/decrescendo systolic murmur heard in the aortic area. Signs of congestive heart failure with rales and edema may be present. The electrocardiogram may show left ventricular strain. If the patient suffered recent or old myocardial infarction, electrocardiographic abnormalities typical of infarction also may be present. The echocardiogram usually shows calcified and immobile aortic valve leaflets producing a constricted aortic orifice with the resultant hypertrophied left ventricle. All patients with angina pectoris and all patients with aortic valve disease who are greater than 40 years of age should have coronary angiography to define coronary anatomy. Right- and left-sided heart catheterization should be performed simultaneously so that complete evaluation of myocardial performance, including measurement of left ventricular end-diastolic pressure and the pulmonary artery pressure, can be obtained. The transaortic valvular gradient also can be determined at catheterization.

The preoperative evaluation of patients with aortic stenosis, coronary artery disease, and poor ventricular function is complicated. Patients with poor ventricular function often generate relatively low transaortic valve gradients. This renders the calculation of valve area and the assessment of critical aortic stenosis less accurate. The morphology of the valve with immobile leaflets and heavy calcification as seen on echocardiography is often an important confirmatory sign that critical aortic stenosis is present. Even in the presence of a small gradient, if echocardiographic signs of significant valve stenosis are present, and if left ventricular intracavitary pressure exceeds 120 mm Hg in systole, mortality rates are acceptable, and response to valve replacement surgery is usually good. A poorly contractile, thinned-out ventricle with low transvalvular gradient and low intracavitary systolic pressure usually suggests that the operation is of high risk and may be of limited or no benefit. A poorly contractile ventricle with normal or increased wall thickness may recover contractile force if a substantial amount of reversibly ischemic myocardium is present and if the degree of aortic stenosis is significant. In addition to ventricular function, other important determinants of the risks and advisability of surgery include patient age, presence of previous cardiac operations, and overall organ function, especially renal function.

The optimal management of a patient with coronary artery disease and mild or moderate aortic stenosis presently remains a matter of some controversy. The dilemma is whether to subject a patient to the lifelong limitations of a valve replacement procedure that may not be necessary, or the prospect of a repeat cardiac operation, perhaps in only a few years, should the aortic stenosis progress. There is now evidence that favors valve replacement in patients with moderate aortic stenosis who are referred for surgical myocardial revascularization.[9–12] In one study,[9] survival rates at both 1 year and 8 years were superior for patients who underwent valve replacement for moderate aortic stenosis (gradient >30 mm Hg or gradient <40 mm Hg with valve area between 1.0 and 1.5 cm^2). One-year survival was 90% in those having valve replacement compared to 85% in patients having coronary artery bypass graft (CABG) alone. Similarly, 8-year survival (55% versus 39%) was statistically significantly better ($p < .001$).

The rate of progression of aortic stenosis may also provide an indication for valve replacement even without hemodynamically critical disease.[11] For slow progression (<3 mm Hg per year), isolated CABG is preferred for patients with valve gradients less than 50 mm Hg. In contrast, rapid progression (>10 mm Hg per year) favors valve replacement at the time of CABG surgery. One possible exception is in octogenarians with valve gradients less than 25 mm Hg. Of course, other individual patient characteristics (life expectancy and other significant comorbidity) may influence the decision to replace the aortic valve at the time of revascularization surgery.

Pathophysiology

Aortic stenosis produces obstruction to left ventricular emptying during systole, which ultimately is the source of all the symptoms and signs of aortic stenosis. Most patients with aortic stenosis have hypertrophied and thick-walled left ventricles. Contractile function is initially good, and ejection fraction may be maintained. In later stages of the disease, the ventricle begins to fail with enlargement and global diminution of contractile function. At any stage of the disease, the presence of critical coronary artery obstruction can cause regional wall motion abnormalities. Significant three-vessel CAD may itself lead to global ventricular dysfunction, which may be reversible with revascularization.

In patients with critical aortic stenosis and good ventricular function, valve replacement immediately reduces left ventricular afterload. Because most patients with aortic stenosis have hypertrophied and thick-walled ventricles, intraoperative subendocardial ischemia may be more difficult to avoid during aortic cross-clamping. Although revascularization should not decrease left ventricular contractility and may increase it, some myocardial stunning with a temporary decrease in global and regional left ventricular contractility inevitably results from the surgical procedure.[13–16] This, of course, assumes more important pathophysiologic significance in patients with poor ventricular function preoperatively. Diastolic dysfunction may also occur, causing a less compliant left ventricle. The most extreme example of this was the so-called "stone heart" that plagued surgical pioneers who attempted aortic valve replacement surgery. Modern techniques of myocardial preservation have eliminated this feared complication.

Postoperatively, patients may have dramatic improvement in symptoms. Relief of left ventricular outflow obstruction immediately leads to enhanced cardiac output and perfusion of vital organs. In addition, left ventricular function improves both immediately and over time after relief of outflow obstruction and as remodeling ensues. Correction of myocardial ischemia can lead to recruitment of formerly hibernating myocardium[10] with further enhancement of ventricular function.[8]

Operative Management

Monitoring for surgery of the aortic valve and coronary arteries includes catheters and measurements that have become standard for most cardiac surgical operations. These include an arterial line (usually in the radial artery for blood pressure and blood gases) and a pulmonary artery catheter for measurement of pulmonary artery pressures, and cardiac output by thermodilution, with optical sensors for continuous estimation of mixed venous oxygen saturation. While the pulmonary artery catheter has a balloon at its tip, occlusion wedge pressure is rarely measured in the perioperative period because of the danger of pulmonary artery rupture. Particularly useful information is provided by continuous measurement of mixed venous oxygen saturation.

The perfusion setup is standard and similar to that for isolated coronary artery bypass (Fig. 48-2). A single aortic cannula is ordinarily placed in the distal ascending aorta. A single two-stage venous cannula is placed via the right atrial appendage with its tip positioned in the inferior vena cava. After establishment of cardiopulmonary bypass, the patient is usually cooled to 32 to 34°C, during which time a left ventricular vent is positioned via the right superior pulmonary vein. With the heart well emptied, the aortic cross-clamp is applied during a temporary reduction in pump flow. Thereafter, the heart is arrested with cold (4°C) potassium blood cardioplegia and topical irrigation is applied with iced saline solution. After the aorta is opened, the endocardium is intermittently irrigated with iced saline solution to enhance myocardial cooling.

A combination of antegrade and retrograde cardioplegia is optimal. The initial dose of cardioplegia usually is given both ways.

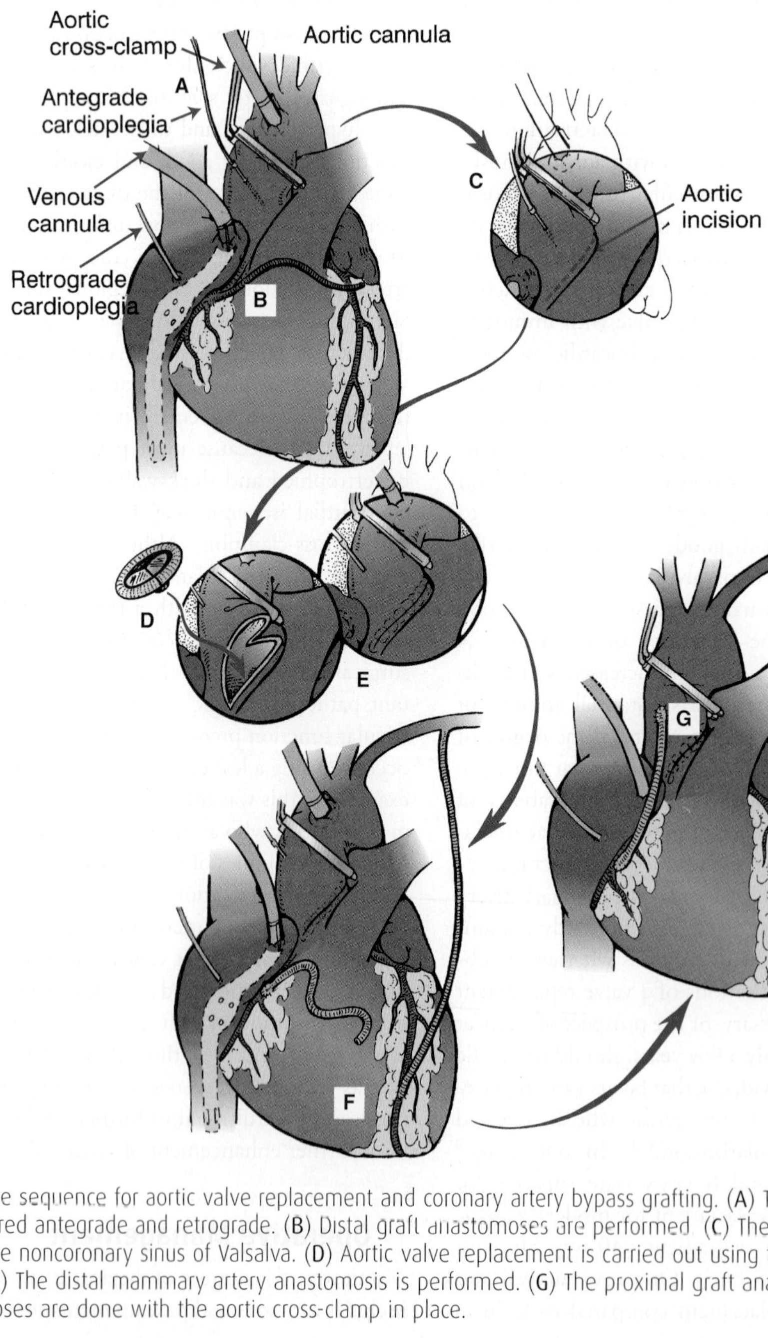

FIGURE 48-2 Operative sequence for aortic valve replacement and coronary artery bypass grafting. (A) The aorta is cross-clamped and cardioplegia administered antegrade and retrograde. (B) Distal graft anastomoses are performed. (C) The aortotomy is made with an oblique incision into the noncoronary sinus of Valsalva. (D) Aortic valve replacement is carried out using the prosthesis of choice. (E) The aortotomy is closed. (F) The distal mammary artery anastomosis is performed. (G) The proximal graft anastomoses are done. In this case, the proximal anastomoses are done with the aortic cross-clamp in place.

Approximately 15 mL/kg is given as the initial dose. Subsequent doses of cardioplegia are given retrograde throughout the operation. This is particularly convenient because retrograde cardioplegia can be given even after the aortic root is opened without significantly disrupting the flow of the operation. Cardioplegia may also be given antegrade via radial artery and vein saphenous bypass grafts after distal anastomoses are completed. This is especially important if a graft has been placed in the right coronary system, as retrograde cardioplegia is not well delivered to the right ventricle and may not protect it well.

The left internal mammary artery is almost always used to graft the left anterior descending artery when it has a significant obstruction. In general, reversed greater saphenous veins and radial arteries are used for other bypass grafts. The reasoning behind the choice of valve prosthesis is nearly identical to that used in the treatment of isolated valvular heart disease. Any type of prosthesis may be used, but several issues must be considered. The indications for all types of tissue valves are stronger, as these patients' life expectancies are often shorter. However, these sicker patients may not tolerate well the longer clamp times necessary for the more complex implantation of nonstented tissue valves.

The multiple steps in the combined operation follow a logical sequence. After establishment of cardiopulmonary bypass and insertion of the left ventricular vent, the aorta is clamped and the heart arrested as described. The first step in the operation is performance of the distal radial artery and/or saphenous vein bypass grafts. When these are complete, the ventricles may be wrapped in a cooling pad, after which the aorta is opened and aortic valve replacement is carried out using the prosthesis of choice. The aorta is closed completely at this point. The distal anastomosis of the internal mammary artery graft is then made. Following completion of this, air is evacuated from the heart and the aortic cross-clamp is released. A partially occluding clamp is applied to the aorta, and proximal anastomoses are performed when necessary. Alternatively, the proximal anastomoses can be performed with the aortic cross-clamp still in place. Although this prolongs the ischemia time, it avoids application of a second clamp to the aorta with the potential for disruption of atheromatous debris or injury to the aortic suture line. This consideration is particularly important in patients undergoing reoperations, because the presence of previous bypass grafts can make application of a partially occluding clamp on the aorta difficult. Coordinated sinus rhythm is established after temporary atrial and ventricular pacing wires are positioned. After the heart is resuscitated and de-airing is confirmed by transesophageal echocardiography, the left ventricular vent is removed. Of note, atrial-ventricular sequential activation is particularly important to optimize hemodynamic performance in patients with aortic stenosis. This is because as much as 30% of the cardiac output may be derived from atrial contraction as the hypertrophied and noncompliant ventricle that is typical of the patient with aortic stenosis does not fill completely during the earlier phases of diastole.

Weaning from cardiopulmonary bypass is performed gradually with stepwise diminution of pump flow and increased left ventricular filling. Simultaneous monitoring of the appearance of the heart, pulmonary artery and systemic blood pressures, and mixed venous oxygen saturation is done during weaning. In patients with hypertrophied ventricles, it may be important to pay particular attention to keeping the poorly compliant left ventricle filled to ensure adequate preload and cardiac output.

In patients with particularly severe ventricular dysfunction who do not wean from bypass, the intra-aortic balloon pump may be used. Two to three attempts to wean from cardiopulmonary bypass using inotropic drugs should be made over a period of 20 to 30 minutes. If weaning from cardiopulmonary bypass is not successful at this point, an intra-aortic balloon pump should be inserted. In some patients, a ventricular assist device is required. Persistent attempts to wean from bypass without mechanical support may be counterproductive because complications from prolonged cardiopulmonary bypass may ensue beyond 30 minutes of elapsed time. As the hypertrophied heart recovers after the ischemic insult, inotropic and mechanical support often can be weaned rapidly. In patients with more impaired ventricular function, weaning, of necessity, occurs more gradually and may take days.

Results

Early hospital mortality after aortic valve replacement and CABG ranges from approximately 2 to 10%.[8,17] Higher mortality is observed in patients with more severe symptoms of heart failure and impaired ventricular function preoperatively. The most frequent causes of operative death are low-output cardiac failure, myocardial infarction, and arrhythmia. Incremental risk factors for hospital death include patient age, functional class, and several measures of ventricular function. In a number of studies, late survival has ranged from 60 to 80% at 5 years and 50 to 75% at 8 years postoperatively (Fig. 48-3).[18–23] By multivariate analysis, risk factors for reduced late survival include older age, cardiac enlargement, and more severe preoperative clinical symptoms. The use of a mechanical prosthesis at valve replacement has been associated with lower long-term survival and

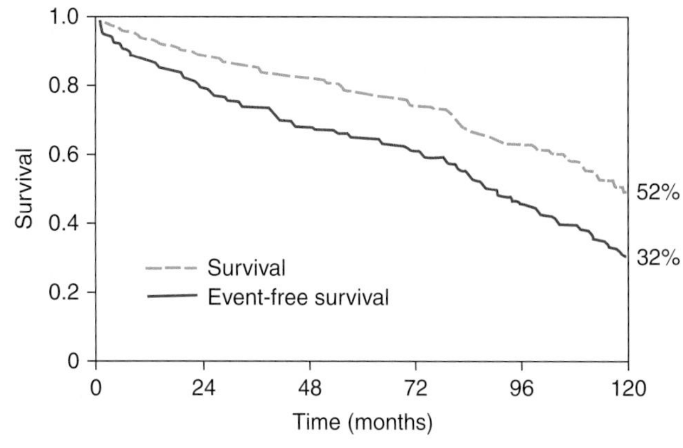

FIGURE 48-3 Long-term survival and event-free survival after aortic valve replacement and coronary artery bypass grafting in 471 patients. (*Adapted with permission from Lytle BW, Cosgrove DM, Gill CC, et al: Aortic valve replacement combined with myocardial revascularization. J Thorac Cardiovasc Surg 1988; 95:402.*)

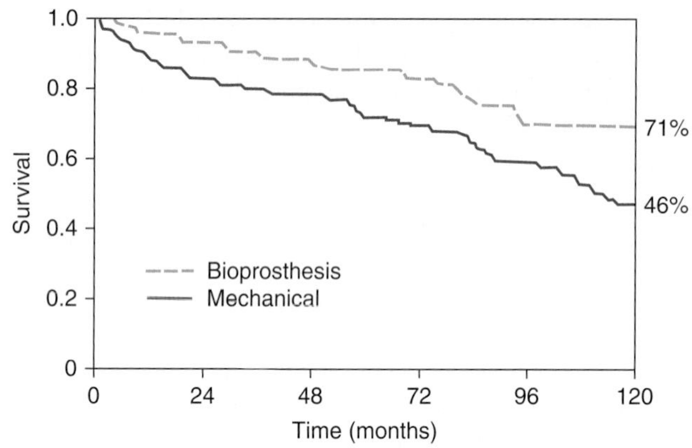

FIGURE 48-4 Long-term survival advantage for patients undergoing aortic valve replacement and coronary artery bypass grafting using a bioprosthesis (n = 218) versus a mechanical valve (n = 253). *(Adapted with permission from Lytle BW, Cosgrove DM, Gill CC, et al: Aortic valve replacement combined with myocardial revascularization. J Thorac Cardiovasc Surg 1988; 95:402.)*

lower long-term event-free survival (Fig. 48-4). Nonetheless, elderly patients have acceptable results following relief of aortic stenosis, even with redo valve surgery combined with coronary revascularization.[24,25] As discussed, choice of valve type is a complex issue in combined valve–coronary artery surgery. This is a decision that cannot be made without consultation with the patient. A frank discussion of the advantages and drawbacks of each approach continues to be an important component of the preoperative evaluation and planning for this type of surgery. Similar consideration should apply to consideration of "hybrid" procedures such as coronary artery stenting followed by valve replacement.[3,6] This approach has at least the one clear advantage of permitting aortic valve replacement through a smaller incision (partial sternotomy, anterior thoracotomy).

AORTIC REGURGITATION AND CORONARY ARTERY DISEASE

Significant aortic regurgitation occurs less often in older populations, and is also less often encountered with CAD. Most series of patients undergoing aortic valve replacement and CABG include a relatively small number (10 to 25%) of patients with aortic insufficiency.[8,17–20] Although the operative management of patients with aortic regurgitation and CAD is similar to that previously described, aortic insufficiency produces different pathophysiology that has implications for perioperative management, and the presence of an incompetent aortic valve introduces nuances to the intraoperative management of these patients.

Clinical Presentation

Patients with aortic regurgitation and coronary artery disease usually present in one of three ways. The aortic regurgitation may be asymptomatic and detected incidentally during evaluation for symptomatic coronary disease. Second, the patient may be asymptomatic, yet a routine physical examination reveals a murmur of aortic insufficiency that leads to cardiac evaluation and detection of coronary disease. Finally, patients may present relatively late in the course of valvular heart disease with congestive heart failure caused by decompensation of the volume-overloaded left ventricle or ischemic damage or both. Patients therefore may present with no symptoms and essentially normal physiology, a classic ischemic syndrome, or congestive heart failure. The physical signs also depend on the nature of the presentation. In general, all patients with aortic insufficiency have an audible early diastolic blowing murmur. In late stages of the disease, signs of congestive heart failure, including rales and peripheral edema, may be present.

The preoperative evaluation of a patient with aortic insufficiency and CAD is no different from that previously described for patients with aortic stenosis and ischemic heart disease. Echocardiography is particularly useful in detecting aortic regurgitation because the murmur is sometimes difficult to detect. In addition, echocardiography gives important information regarding both ventricular contractile function and ventricular size. Because many patients with aortic regurgitation are asymptomatic, careful evaluation for changes in ventricular size or function is important, as the presence of these changes may constitute an indication to proceed with surgical intervention in the absence of symptoms.

Pathophysiology

Aortic regurgitation increases left ventricular preload and causes left ventricular dilatation. Dilatation does not occur acutely, and patients with acute aortic insufficiency are often severely symptomatic owing to a sudden increase in left ventricular end-diastolic pressure and decrease in net forward cardiac output. Global left ventricular dysfunction caused by CAD also can produce left ventricular dilatation. Valve replacement relieves some of the preload but does not immediately result in improved left ventricular contractility. Revascularization may produce improved contractility by recruitment of hibernating myocardium.[13,16] This operation does not increase left ventricular afterload.

The indications for surgery in aortic regurgitation continue to be somewhat controversial, and are reviewed in depth in the section on aortic valve disease. The evaluation of valvular pathology proceeds along similar lines to those described above, with emphasis on echocardiographic results. However, this evaluation is somewhat more difficult when CAD is also present, because the presence of coronary disease might have an impact on ventricular function that revascularization may or may not improve. Nevertheless, except in advanced stages of diffuse three-vessel coronary artery disease, myocardial abnormalities caused by coronary artery obstructions are usually regional and can be distinguished from global dysfunction caused by volume overload from the insufficient valve. Making this distinction is of paramount importance in the preoperative assessment and risk stratification of these patients because regional abnormalities are likely to improve after myocardial revascularization. In difficult cases an evaluation of myocardial viability (with thallium or PET scanning) may be helpful in evaluating candidates for surgery. Decisions about timing of aortic valve surgery in the presence of CAD are different from those in cases of isolated valvular disease, with the usual result that the valve is replaced earlier in the course of the disease.

Operative Management

The operation is conducted in a fashion similar to that described for aortic stenosis and CAD. However, in the presence of aortic insufficiency, antegrade cardioplegia in the aortic root cannot be given because the cardioplegia solution leaks into the left ventricle. In general, retrograde cardioplegia is used under these circumstances, with doses of antegrade cardioplegia given into the coronary ostia, especially on the right, with hand-held catheters after the aorta has been opened.

Considerations in weaning from cardiopulmonary bypass are somewhat different from those described for aortic stenosis. Patients with aortic regurgitation are more likely to have dilated ventricles that tolerate increases in afterload poorly. Therefore, successful perioperative management of these patients requires careful attention to adjustments in preload and afterload. In patients with volume-overloaded ventricles caused by aortic insufficiency, vasodilators may be an important component of postoperative management. Drugs such as milrinone and dobutamine have a role because they provide both inotropic support and ventricular unloading. The mechanical ventricular unloading device—the intra-aortic balloon pump—also may be used. It is rare that mechanical circulatory assistance with a ventricular assist device is required. Its use should be reserved for younger patients without comorbid conditions in whom prompt improvement in ventricular function is anticipated.

Results

Early results after operation for aortic regurgitation and CAD include an expected hospital mortality rate of less than 10%.[8,17] Incremental risk factors for hospital death are similar to those described previously, with advanced age and poor ventricular function having the greatest impact. Late survival after this operation is similar to that for aortic stenosis and CAD (see Fig. 48-3).[18–23] Despite the impression that patients with aortic insufficiency and CAD do not do as well as those with aortic stenosis, aortic insufficiency has not been an independent risk factor for early or late mortality.[8] Interestingly, recovery of ventricular ejection fraction does have a favorable impact on late mortality. When ventricular dilatation and diminution in ventricular systolic function occur in the setting of aortic regurgitation, these often are irreversible changes. Although some improvement of function can occur with elimination of the volume overload and revascularization in patients with combined valvular and coronary artery diseases, there may be less recovery of ejection fraction in patients with aortic insufficiency compared with aortic stenosis. This observation is the primary reason that valve replacement is recommended before changes in ventricular morphology and function have occurred. Failure of recovery of ventricular function in this setting may have an impact on long-term survival, but not one so great as to render aortic insufficiency an independent risk factor for late death.

MITRAL REGURGITATION AND CORONARY ARTERY DISEASE

Successful management of patients with mitral regurgitation and CAD remains one of the greater challenges in adult cardiac surgery. This group of patients tends to be sicker, and their surgical care is accomplished at higher risk.[1,26–30] This is almost certainly because of the complex interaction between the function of the left ventricle and that of the mitral valve. Normal valve function depends on normal function of the entire mitral apparatus, which includes the ventricular wall and the papillary muscles. Similarly, normal ventricular function depends on competence of the mitral valve. Therefore, there is unique potential for CAD and mitral valve disease to interact, making the patient sicker, the pathophysiology more complicated, and the surgical management more difficult.

In patients with preserved ventricular function, the pathophysiology and management strategies are not significantly different from those for treatment of isolated mitral regurgitation or CAD. Of course, the operation is more complex and longer, and therefore, as has been described previously, a carefully conceived operative plan with special attention to myocardial preservation is important. However, the more interesting problems are in those patients with mitral insufficiency and CAD who do not have normal hearts, and in fact, most patients with this disease combination do not have normal ventricular function.

Clinical Presentation

The spectrum of clinical presentation ranges from patients who are asymptomatic to those who are moribund in cardiogenic shock. The patient may have no signs or symptoms of heart disease, or may have predominant symptoms of failure, ischemia, or both. Finally, patients may present with acute syndromes often related to myocardial infarction and the sudden development of mitral insufficiency. These patients are extremely ill when they present in congestive heart failure and cardiogenic shock. Management of these patients is the most difficult.

Findings on physical examination obviously relate to the nature of the presentation, and can range from signs of mild mitral insufficiency to severe congestive failure or cardiogenic shock. An electrocardiogram may show evidence of ischemic heart disease. All patients should undergo echocardiography. The echocardiogram is particularly useful because it gives information both about the valve and about ventricular geometry and function. Transesophageal echocardiography is especially useful in the evaluation of mitral anatomy and function. Assessments of mitral valve leaflet structure and function, chordal anatomy, and functioning of the papillary muscles and adjacent ventricular wall via transesophageal echocardiography are invaluable. All these data are important in planning the operative approach to the mitral valve and assessing the risk of surgery. Cardiac catheterization is performed in these patients for the same reasons outlined for patients with aortic valve disease. Any patient with angina pectoris or a positive stress test and any patient greater than the age of 40 with mitral insufficiency should have coronary angiography before surgery. As noted, cardiac catheterization also provides information about hemodynamics that is important in planning the operation and estimating the risk.

Pathophysiology

Mitral regurgitation increases left ventricular preload and decreases afterload at the expense of cardiac output. Ischemic damage causes ventricular dilatation with decreased contractility and an increase in left ventricular filling pressures. These lesions combined cause synergistic decompensation and can produce pulmonary hypertension and secondary tricuspid regurgitation. Cardiac output may be very low, especially in patients with acute mitral insufficiency. Mitral insufficiency may occur in association with CAD, but often the CAD is the cause of mitral insufficiency. The pathophysiology of primary mitral insufficiency can be caused by involvement of the valve leaflets, the annulus, the subvalvular apparatus, or some combination of all of these. A detailed understanding of the pathophysiology of primary mitral insufficiency is important for planning the operative approach.

When CAD is the cause of mitral insufficiency by its effect on regional and global ventricular function, the pathophysiology is more complicated. Global ventricular dysfunction from CAD can produce ventricular dilatation with mitral annular dilatation and subsequent mitral insufficiency. The jet of mitral regurgitation is usually central and often can be managed with annuloplasty. Alternatively, regional wall motion abnormalities involving the papillary muscle and adjacent ventricular wall can produce dynamic changes that produce insufficiency of the mitral valve. These abnormalities are now becoming better understood and are discussed more completely in Chapter 40.

Correction of mitral insufficiency either by valve repair or valve replacement produces an instantaneous increase in left ventricular afterload. The ventricle no longer has the low-impedance left atrial chamber into which to eject blood and must overcome systemic afterload in systole. Even when myocardial ischemia is reversible, recruitment of hibernating myocardium may take time. These factors in combination with the sudden increase in left ventricular afterload contribute to the difficulty and increased risk of managing this entity. Secondary right ventricular failure may be present or ensue because pulmonary hypertension does not decrease immediately after mitral valve repair or replacement, and CAD also may affect right ventricular function.

Symptomatic mitral insufficiency and symptomatic CAD are the usual indicators for combined surgery. As noted, patients with acute illnesses may be in extremis. Ventricular dysfunction is not per se a contraindication to surgery, especially if it is caused by reversible ischemia. Patients with global irreversible cardiomyopathy and mitral insufficiency should not be operated on because the ventricle tolerates the increase in afterload poorly and results are unsatisfactory. Estimation of the viability of the myocardium and demonstration of reversible ischemia using thallium or PET scanning therefore are important. With the left atrial enlargement that is common, patients often present with chronic or recent-onset atrial fibrillation. This condition often contributes to the reduction in cardiac output and ablation of the arrhythmia at the time of surgery may confer additional benefit. Finally a hybrid approach with catheter-based treatment of coronary disease followed by mitral surgery through a less invasive approach may be an attractive option.[3,6]

Operative Management

One important preoperative decision in patients with mitral regurgitation and CAD is whether there is, in fact, any need for valve surgery. Because mitral regurgitation in the presence of CAD may be functional and caused by reversible myocardial ischemia, revascularization alone may improve mitral regurgitation. It is important, therefore, to distinguish organic from functional mitral insufficiency. Intraoperative transesophageal echocardiography is an essential tool for assessment of mitral valve function in this setting.[31] Patients with no preoperative congestive heart failure, absent or only transient murmurs of mitral insufficiency, normal pulmonary pressures in the operating room, and trace to mild mitral insufficiency by transesophageal echocardiography after induction of anesthesia probably do not need mitral valve surgery at all.[32] Many of these patients will appear to have more mitral regurgitation and higher pulmonary pressures at catheterization or when they are ischemic than when they are under anesthesia. On the other hand, many, if not all, patients with moderate to severe insufficiency will need to have the valve regurgitation addressed.[5,33] If the patient has no symptoms of mitral valve disease and the morphology of the valve is normal, it is often unclear whether a valve repair operation is necessary. Myocardial revascularization itself, by its effect on ventricular function, may be associated with or is likely often the cause in improvement of mitral valve function even in the absence of a procedure on the valve itself. This may be a situation in which a staged hybrid procedure is particularly useful. For example, percutaneous coronary artery stenting, perhaps of multiple vessels, can be performed in association with expectant treatment of the moderate mitral valve insufficiency. If revascularization also contributes to amelioration of valve function, the patient may avoid an intracardiac procedure without sacrificing long-term benefit.[34]

Several recent studies suggest that the quality of modern surgical results justifies a more aggressive approach to valve repair in patients with moderate mitral insufficiency and CAD.[35–39] Some patients with ventricular enlargement and annular dilation secondary to CAD and/or mitral insufficiency may be managed with annuloplasty alone. Patients with organic mitral valve disease such as leaflet prolapse, chordal rupture, or chordal elongation need primary repair. Restricted leaflet motion is frequently a complication of ischemic changes in ventricular shape. In other cases, standard leaflet resection techniques for posterior flail segments may be indicated. In sicker patients, and those with restricted leaflet motion or more complex lesions (severe myxomatous degeneration), an edge-to-edge leaflet approximation (the "Alfieri stitch") may be appropriate.[40] This is especially true in patients with extensive calcification of the posterior annulus or severely restricted posterior leaflet motion.[41] As noted elsewhere, results of mitral repair and CABG are superior to those of mitral valve replacement, which should be avoided except in the setting of acute, severe mitral insufficiency caused by papillary muscle rupture.[42]

Anesthetic considerations are similar to those described previously, although it must be recognized that these patients are in general sicker than patients with aortic valve disease and in some cases are among the sickest patients treated. Monitoring includes a radial artery line and a pulmonary artery catheter. As suggested earlier, intraoperative transesophageal echocardiography is particularly important in this group of patients for operative planning, intraoperative monitoring, and post-repair assessment of valve function. Setup for cardiopulmonary bypass is similar to that described earlier. However, both venae cavae are cannulated for venous return (Fig. 48-5). This is usually accomplished by introducing the cannulas through pursestrings in the superior vena cava and low in the right atrium. Vena caval tourniquets may be used to establish total cardiopulmonary bypass and facilitate visualization of the mitral valve and subvalvar apparatus. After clamping the aorta, cardioplegia is administered antegrade and then retrograde. Subsequent doses of cardioplegia are given retrograde. As with aortic disease, special attention must be paid to protecting the right ventricle during periods of prolonged retrograde cardioplegia.

The most common incision providing access to the mitral valve is in the wall of the left atrium anterior to the right pulmonary veins. Preparative dissection of the interatrial groove facilitates exposure using this incision. Another choice for exposure of the mitral valve is the transseptal approach with the primary incision in the right atrium. This allows for direct visual insertion of the retrograde cardioplegia catheter through a pursestring, and affords an excellent view of the mitral valve, especially if the left atrium is not enlarged, without excessive stretching of the right atrium or the cavae. If necessary, the incision can be carried up into the dome of the left atrium for even greater exposure. This approach is particularly useful when a procedure on the tricuspid valve is indicated as well. Other incisions are discussed in the section on mitral valve disease.

The first choice in surgery for mitral insufficiency is valve repair. When valve repair is impossible, valve replacement follows the same guidelines set forth in Chapter 42. However, in patients with the combination of coronary artery and mitral valve disease and an abbreviated life expectancy, a stronger rationale for use of a tissue prosthesis may exist.[43] Regardless of

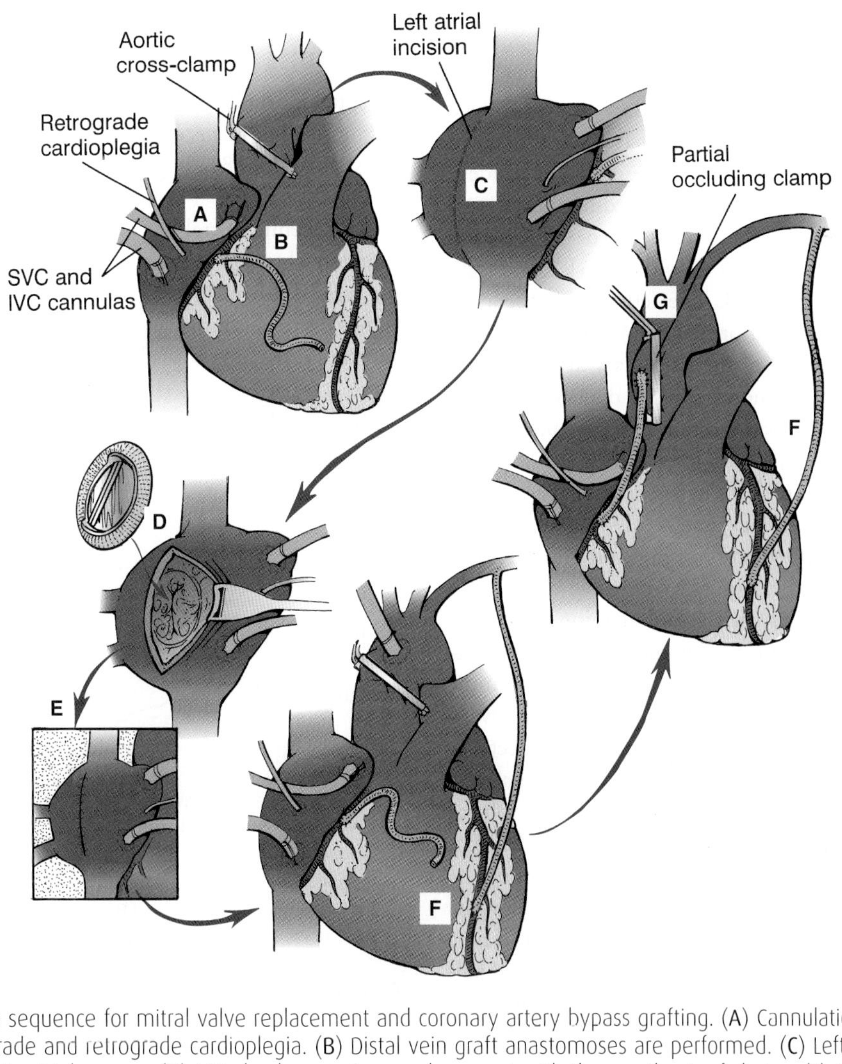

FIGURE 48-5 Operative sequence for mitral valve replacement and coronary artery bypass grafting. (A) Cannulation and cross-clamping of the aorta with antegrade and retrograde cardioplegia. (B) Distal vein graft anastomoses are performed. (C) Left atriotomy is performed after dissection in the interatrial groove. (D) Mitral valve repair or replacement with the prosthesis of choice. (E) Closure of left atriotomy. (F) Distal anastomosis using the mammary artery is performed. (G) Proximal graft anastomosis is done. In this case, the cross-clamp has been removed and a partially occluding aortic clamp used.

the type of prosthesis, an effort should be made to retain continuity between the papillary muscles and the mitral annulus. The attachments to the posterior leaflet usually can be retained in their entirety without interfering with prosthesis function. The anterior leaflet must be resected either in whole or in part to avoid left ventricular outflow tract obstruction or interference with mechanical valve function. However, major chordal attachments may still be preserved and incorporated into the annular suture line. Regardless, standard practice is to retain continuity between the mitral annulus and the subvalvular apparatus whenever the mitral valve is replaced. Short- and long-term ventricular function has been demonstrated to be superior when this is done. Obviously, in this clinical setting, in which ventricular function has a significant impact on short- and long-term results, all steps should be taken to ensure optimal myocardial performance postoperatively.

Patients with papillary muscle rupture caused by infarction are usually extremely sick. Valve replacement is almost always required. Some surgeons have reported success with reimplantation of the papillary muscle. This strategy is risky in these sick patients because the operation must be both expeditious and effective. Multiple attempts to achieve mitral valve competence are tolerated poorly. A reimplanted, infarcted papillary muscle does not necessarily restore mitral valve competence and also may be subject to early or late breakdown.

As in combined aortic valve and coronary artery surgery, distal graft anastomoses are performed first (see Fig. 48-5). At this point, after the atrium has been opened, it may be prudent to undertake an arrhythmia ablation procedure in selected patients with atrial fibrillation. Radiofrequency or cryoablation probes can be used to create a lesion set within the left and right atria, as described in Chapter 58. The left atrial appendage should be oversewn. Valve repair or replacement is then carried out, followed by performance of the mammary artery anastomosis. Proximal graft anastomoses can be done either after release of the cross-clamp and application of a partially occluding clamp or with the cross-clamp in place.

Weaning from cardiopulmonary bypass is similar to that in patients with aortic insufficiency and CAD. Again, in this group of patients, afterload reduction using drugs or the intra-aortic balloon pump may be required. Inotropic drugs with afterload-reducing capabilities such as dobutamine and milrinone may be indicated. The surgeon should have a low threshold for adding a drug such as milrinone to catecholamine agents because this combination has some theoretical advantages as a result of positive inotropic and unloading effects, as well as a reduction in pulmonary artery pressures. Alternatively dobutamine, which has both central inotropic and peripheral afterload-reducing effects, may be a first-choice drug. Because some of these patients are particularly sick, little time should be wasted in futile attempts to wean from cardiopulmonary bypass on medications and without the intra-aortic balloon. There should be a low threshold for insertion of the intra-aortic balloon in patients whose hemodynamics may be quite tenuous for hours to days after surgery, especially when the operation is an emergency.

Another consideration for a select subset of patients with this disease is the incorporation of ventricular remodeling into the operation. There now is evidence that patients with anterior infarctions and dilated cardiomyopathy, mitral insufficiency, and CAD will benefit from exclusion of the infarcted area and remodeling of the left ventricle so as to restore an elliptical shape.[44] This can be performed safely, along with mitral repair and coronary revascularization, in carefully selected patients. The result can be an increase in ejection fraction with improved postoperative function.

Strict attention must be paid to right ventricular function and therefore to right ventricular myocardial protection in this group of patients, although right ventricular failure is more common in the setting of mitral stenosis. Right ventricular failure must be anticipated and correctly diagnosed and managed. The presence of a falling systemic blood pressure and cardiac output with falling pulmonary artery pressure and/or pulmonary capillary wedge pressure should prompt a search for right ventricular failure, which is manifested by a rising central venous pressure. Failure to recognize this and inappropriate administration of fluid can lead to irreversible right ventricular failure. As noted, less invasive approaches to mitral valve repair and coronary revascularization may become increasingly useful in these patients.[45]

Results

Hospital mortality for this group of patients is higher than that for most other forms of acquired heart disease. Early mortality rates range from 3% in good-risk patients to 60% in the sickest patients.[21–23,26–29,46] The higher mortality is seen in patients with acute ischemic mitral valve disease and severe ventricular dysfunction who require emergency surgery. Incremental risk factors for early death include age, functional class, ventricular function, elevated pulmonary pressures, and cardiogenic shock. Late survival in patients with this entity is 55 to 85% at 5 years and 30 to 45% at 10 years (Fig. 48-6).[21–23,26–29,47–50]

In general, patients who survive surgery have good relief of symptoms, although recurrent mitral insufficiency remains an

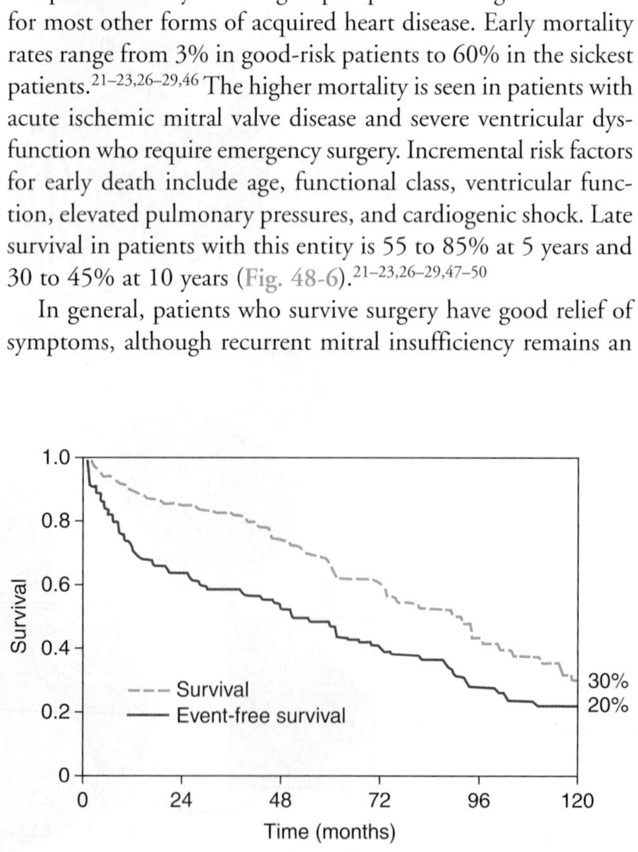

FIGURE 48-6 Survival and event-free survival after mitral valve replacement combined with coronary artery bypass grafting in 278 patients. (*Adapted with permission from Lytle BW, Cosgrove DM, Gill CC, et al: Mitral valve replacement combined with myocardial revascularization: early and late results for 300 patients, 1970 to 1983. Circulation 1985; 71:1179.*)

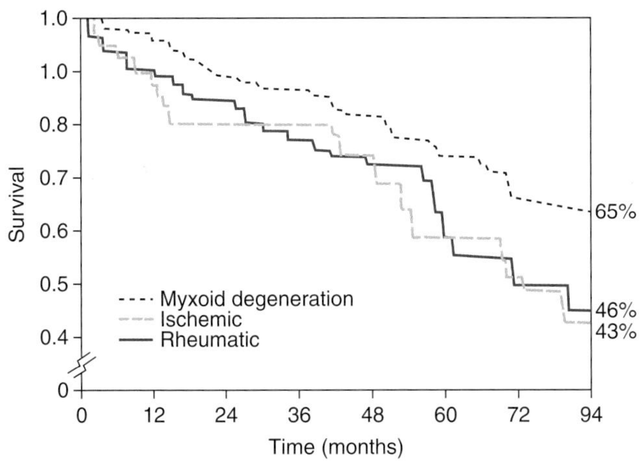

FIGURE 48-7 Survival after mitral valve replacement and coronary artery bypass grafting based on the etiology of mitral valve disease. A survival advantage for patients with myxoid degeneration of the mitral valve is demonstrated. (*Adapted with permission from Lytle BW, Cosgrove DM, Gill CC, et al: Mitral valve replacement combined with myocardial revascularization: early and late results for 300 patients, 1970 to 1983. Circulation 1985; 71:1179.*)

issue for some patients who have undergone restrictive annuloplasty.[51] The risk factors for this complication remain incompletely identified, although abnormal ventricular morphology and regional function appear to play a role. Significant risk factors for late death include preoperative functional class, left ventricular function, and an ischemic as opposed to a degenerative etiology for mitral insufficiency (Fig. 48-7).

MITRAL STENOSIS AND CORONARY ARTERY DISEASE

Patients with mitral stenosis and CAD usually have good left ventricular function and often are a relatively easy group of patients to take care of because the mitral stenosis does not subject the left ventricle to abnormal hemodynamic loads. CAD may cause left ventricular dysfunction, but this is unusual. A more usual concern is right ventricular dysfunction postoperatively, because pulmonary hypertension, with its potential to produce right ventricular failure and tricuspid insufficiency, is often encountered in patients with mitral stenosis.

Clinical Presentation

As implied earlier, mitral stenosis is usually the dominant lesion in patients with mitral stenosis and CAD; therefore, symptoms are typically caused by the valvular lesion. Patients may have congestive heart failure with shortness of breath, orthopnea, and fatigue. Atrial fibrillation is a common presenting symptom with mitral stenosis. Patients with mitral stenosis and CAD infrequently have angina as a presenting symptom. The electrocardiogram may show evidence of right ventricular strain and hypertrophy. Transesophageal echocardiography confirms the diagnosis of mitral stenosis and usually shows a small left ventricle with preserved contractile function. The right ventricle may be enlarged and hypertrophied. Cardiac catheterization further confirms the diagnosis by showing a gradient across the mitral valve. Other important information gleaned from invasive catheterization includes a measurement of the pulmonary artery pressures and central venous pressure. The degree of pulmonary hypertension is a marker of the severity and duration of mitral stenosis and alerts the surgeon to the potential for right ventricular failure postoperatively. An elevated central venous pressure is a potential sign that right ventricular decompensation has already occurred. Coronary angiography should be done in all patients with angina pectoris, and as noted before, in any patient greater than age 40 in whom mitral valve surgery is anticipated.

Pathophysiology

Unlike the other entities described, mitral stenosis and CAD do not have significantly synergistic pathologic effects on the heart. CAD usually has more profound effects on the left ventricle, which remains protected in patients with mitral stenosis until late in the disease. The right ventricle is the chamber most vulnerable to the effects of long-standing mitral stenosis, as noted. However, even with right ventricular hypertension, the potential impact of CAD on right ventricular function in adults is usually not significant. In the rare patient with diffuse CAD and ischemic cardiomyopathy, the risk of surgery is enhanced because of global ventricular dysfunction.

The indications for surgery, not surprisingly, are usually determined by the severity of the mitral stenosis. Patients with significant heart failure and low cardiac output from mitral stenosis whose calculated valve area is less than 1 cm^2 should have a mitral valve operation and associated bypass grafting if significant CAD is present. A rare patient may have significant CAD and mild mitral stenosis detected incidentally. These patients may be managed with CABG and mitral commissurotomy if this is technically feasible. Another alternative in the modern era is the combination of percutaneous revascularization with stents and balloon mitral valvuloplasty. The number of patients suitable for the latter procedure is relatively small and thus far there are no definitive data supporting this kind of hybrid transcatheter approach to these lesions.

Operative Management

Monitoring, perfusion setup, and operative sequence are identical to those described for treatment of mitral regurgitation and CAD. Transesophageal echocardiography is useful to assess both the feasibility of mitral commissurotomy (or more extensive mitral repair) and the results of valvuloplasty. In most patients with mitral stenosis, valve replacement is required because irreversible damage to the leaflets and subvalvular apparatus is usually extensive. A mechanical prosthesis is used most often because the majority of patients have chronic atrial fibrillation from left atrial enlargement, and long-term anticoagulation is indicated. However, the potential benefits of an ablation procedure (as discussed) within the left and right atria also may have an impact on prosthetic choice. Particular attention must be directed to preservation of the right ventricle. In practice, this means that initial and subsequent doses of cardioplegia should be given antegrade as well as retrograde because the latter approach usually offers relatively poor distribution of cardioplegia to the right ventricle.

Transesophageal echocardiography is often important in monitoring both right and left ventricular function postoperatively. The early differentiation between left and right ventricular failure is facilitated by the use of this modality during weaning from cardiopulmonary bypass. If inotropic drugs are required, their selection should be based in part on the consideration that pulmonary hypertension and right ventricular failure might be important components of the clinical syndrome. Drugs such as isoproterenol, dobutamine, and especially milrinone (the latter often in combination with norepinephrine or other catecholamine) may be indicated for their combined beneficial effects on right ventricular contractility and pulmonary vascular resistance. Judicious use of inotropic drugs and careful administration of fluid usually are sufficient to restore cardiac output. The intra-aortic balloon is almost never useful in these patients because right ventricular problems predominate, and the intra-aortic balloon has little direct effect on right ventricular function. Temporary support with a right ventricular assist device may be employed because once the acute phase is past, mitral valve replacement can lead to dramatic decreases in pulmonary artery pressures and subsequent recovery of right ventricular function.

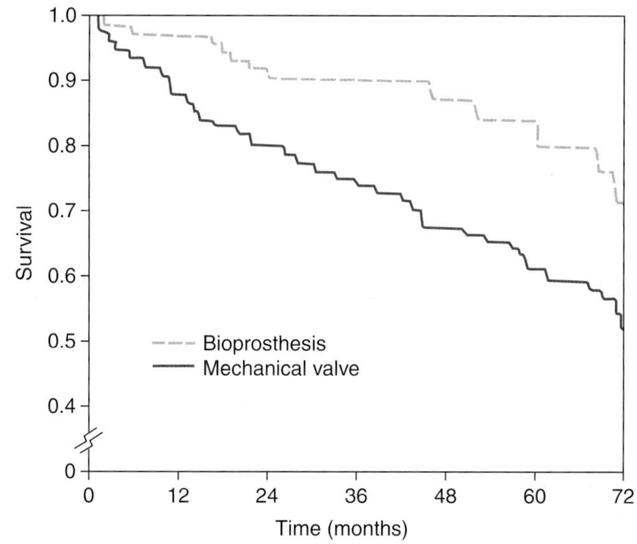

FIGURE 48-8 Comparative survival after mitral valve replacement and coronary artery bypass grafting for patients having mitral valve replacement with a bioprosthesis (n = 82) or mechanical valve (n = 100). (*Adapted with permission from Lytle BW, Cosgrove DM, Gill CC, et al: Mitral valve replacement combined with myocardial revascularization: early and late results for 300 patients, 1970 to 1983. Circulation 1985; 71:1179.*)

Results

Early mortality after combined surgery for mitral stenosis and CAD is approximately 8%.[18–21,26,37] This is not significantly different from results of surgery in lower-risk patients with mitral regurgitation and CAD. Long-term probability of survival is approximately 50% at 7 years and in one series was not significantly different from that for patients with ischemic mitral insufficiency.[21–23,27–29,47] Interestingly, long-term survival of patients with myxoid degeneration of the mitral valve and CAD (65%) was significantly better than survival of the patients with rheumatic or ischemic mitral valve disease and CAD in at least one series (see Fig. 48-7).[27] As implied, rheumatic valve pathology is a risk factor for late death, as is poor preoperative left ventricular function and the presence of ventricular arrhythmias. Interestingly, the use of a bioprosthesis without anticoagulants confers both a survival advantage and an event-free survival advantage in these patients (Fig. 48-8). These data lend support to the hypothesis that biologic valves may be appropriate for mitral replacement in older patients and those with CAD, whose expected life span may be shorter than the anticipated durability of the replacement device.[43]

AORTIC STENOSIS, MITRAL REGURGITATION, AND CORONARY ARTERY DISEASE

Patients with aortic stenosis, mitral regurgitation, and CAD often present with aortic stenosis as the predominant lesion. It is important to note that functional mitral regurgitation may improve after relief of aortic stenosis with concomitant reduction in left ventricular systolic pressure. If the mitral valve is not intrinsically diseased, it may not require surgery.

Clinical Presentation

Patients with these diseases often present identically with patients with aortic stenosis and CAD, but may do so earlier because of the combined valvular lesions. Angina, congestive heart failure, and syncope may be presenting symptoms alone or together. It is relatively uncommon for symptoms resulting from mitral insufficiency to be predominant. Echocardiography is an extremely important tool in this disease combination. Careful evaluation of the mitral valve, often using transesophageal echocardiography, is necessary to determine the degree of intrinsic mitral valve disease, because improvement in mitral insufficiency is expected after aortic valve replacement and relief of left ventricular outflow obstruction.[52] It is critical to determine whether or not the mitral valve has anatomical abnormalities that might not reverse with aortic surgery alone.[53] Of course, cardiac catheterization is required, as it is for the other disease entities described.

Pathophysiology

Aortic stenosis increases left ventricular afterload and therefore can contribute to increasing the amount of mitral regurgitation. Because the combined lesions may cause patients to present earlier in the course of the disease, the left ventricle may be better preserved in this setting than in patients with isolated mitral insufficiency and CAD. Also as noted, the mitral valve may not be structurally diseased. Because of earlier presentation, pulmonary hypertension and subsequent right ventricular failure and tricuspid valve incompetence are usually not prominent features. Because relief of outflow obstruction helps left ventricular function immediately, these patients often do quite well.

The indications for surgery are usually the same as for aortic stenosis and CAD. Critical aortic stenosis, when documented, requires valve replacement; if significant CAD is present, coronary artery bypass grafts are also done. Mitral valve repair is almost always necessary and possible when mitral insufficiency is moderate to severe and/or anatomical abnormalities of the valve are detected. End-stage ventricular dysfunction with ventricular dilatation and myocardial thinning are the primary cardiac contraindications to surgery.

Operative Management

Anesthesia and perfusion setup are identical to those described for mitral valve and coronary artery surgery. In this entity, intraoperative transesophageal echocardiographic monitoring plays an important role because the intraoperative assessment of mitral valve structure and function before and after bypass is critical. The choice of valve for aortic replacement is the same as described previously. In most situations, however, bioprosthetic valves should be considered, especially if the mitral valve is to be repaired.

Under almost all circumstances in which anatomical abnormalities of the mitral valve are detected or in which mitral insufficiency is severe, mitral valve repair should be considered. Annuloplasty may be all that is required if the mitral insufficiency results from annular dilatation and the insufficiency is symmetric and central. More complex disease may require more extensive repair or even replacement of the mitral valve. When the decision is made not to operate on the mitral valve, transesophageal echocardiography is done to assess residual mitral valve dysfunction following aortic valve replacement and coronary artery bypass surgery. If moderate or severe mitral regurgitation remains, the valve should be repaired or replaced. This is technically more difficult after the aortic valve has been replaced, because the prosthesis in the aortic position hinders exposure of the mitral valve. Therefore, every effort must be made to assess mitral valvular morphology and function before starting cardiopulmonary bypass.

As in the other entities described, distal graft anastomoses are performed first (Fig. 48-9). After these grafts are completed, the aorta is opened and the aortic valve is resected. Replacement of the aortic valve, however, is deferred until after the mitral valve operation. However, it is important to resect the aortic valve before replacing the mitral valve to improve exposure of the latter. In addition, because of the fibrous continuity between the aortic and mitral valves, sutures used for mitral valve repair or replacement, if placed first, may become disrupted during resection or debridement of the aortic valve and annulus. After resection of the aortic valve, the atrium is opened and the mitral operation is performed. The atrium is closed with a vent across the mitral valve. The aortic valve is then replaced and the aorta is closed. The internal mammary artery graft is done last. Proximal graft anastomoses can be done with the aortic cross-clamp in place or after removal of the cross-clamp and placement of a partially occluding clamp, as described previously. It is conceivable that at some point in the future patients with this combination of lesions may undergo catheter-based coronary revascularization, catheter-based aortic valve replacement, and catheter-based mitral valve repair.[54,55] That day, however, has not arrived yet.

As noted, this group of patients may have preserved ventricular function, and weaning from cardiopulmonary bypass may be relatively easy. Inotropic drugs and the intra-aortic balloon can be used as indicated.

Results

Early hospital mortality is 12 to 16%.[56,57] Not surprisingly, predictors of early death include severe mitral regurgitation, lower ejection fraction with more severe symptoms of heart failure, and the presence of triple-vessel CAD. Late survival is approximately 60% at 72 months (Fig. 48-10). Multivariate predictors of late mortality include advanced symptoms of heart failure and increased severity of mitral insufficiency.

AORTIC AND MITRAL REGURGITATION AND CORONARY ARTERY DISEASE

Relatively few patients have insufficiency of both the aortic and mitral valves combined with CAD. Those patients who do usually have rheumatic heart disease and present early in the course of the valvular heart disease. Aortic regurgitation may be the predominant valve pathology in a patient with simultaneous significant CAD. The mitral valve problem may be secondary to left ventricular dilatation from the aortic lesion and/or from ischemia resulting from the coronary obstructions. Morphologic mitral valve disease may not be present. Because of the interaction of the valve and coronary pathologies, assessment of left ventricular contractility may be difficult for the reason that both preload and afterload are altered. In addition, the presence of reversible ischemia may obscure accurate measurement of ventricular function and reserve. Therefore, assessment of myocardial viability in these patients is often important.

Clinical Presentation

Most patients with this combination of cardiac lesions present with congestive heart failure. It is unusual to see a patient who has significant insufficiency of both the aortic and mitral valves present with angina as the primary symptom. Typical murmurs of aortic and mitral insufficiency are present, and the patient may have other signs of chronic congestive heart failure, including rales and peripheral edema. If myocardial infarction is a significant component of the pathophysiology and presentation of the disease, evidence of it may be seen on electrocardiogram and echocardiogram. On echocardiography, patients may have regional wall motion abnormalities if infarction has occurred, as well as global ventricular dilatation and dysfunction from the combined valvular lesions and/or diffuse CAD. Cardiac catheterization defines the coronary anatomy and helps to assess the severity of the valvular insufficiency and ventricular dysfunction. Accurate assessment of true left ventricular function is difficult in this entity. Mitral insufficiency may abnormally inflate visual measurements of ejection fraction because the ventricle can eject into the low-pressure pulmonary venous circuit. The misleading ejection fraction combined with the

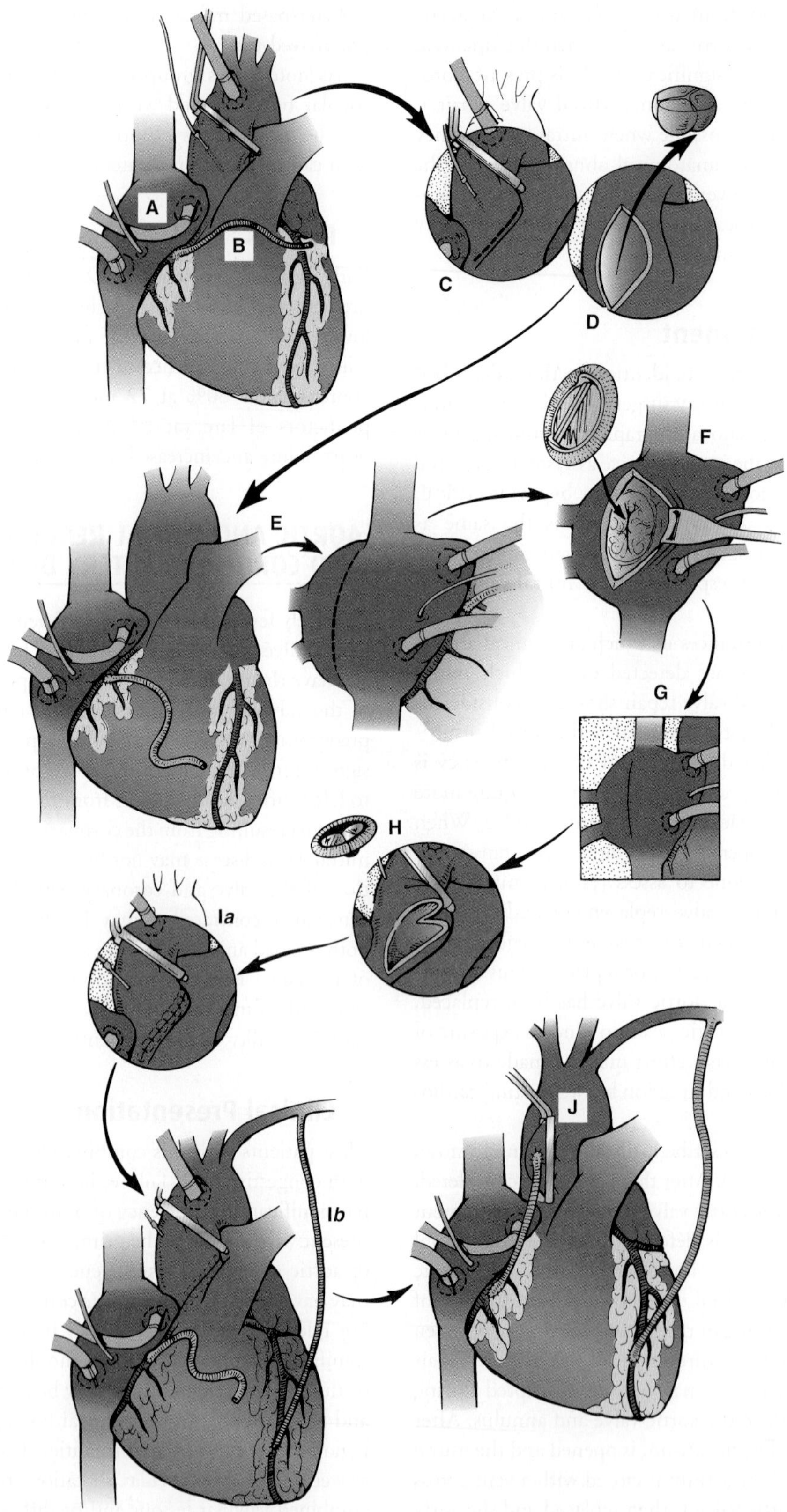

FIGURE 48-9 Operative sequence for aortic valve replacement, mitral valve replacement, and coronary artery bypass grafting. (A) Cannulation with cross-clamping of the aorta and administration of antegrade and retrograde cardioplegia. (B) Distal graft anastomoses are performed. (C) Aortotomy with standard oblique incision. (D) The aortic valve is resected but not replaced. (E) Standard left atriotomy after dissection in the interatrial groove. (F) Mitral valve repair or replacement with the prosthesis of choice. (G) Closure of the left atriotomy. (H) Aortic valve replacement with prosthesis of choice. (I*a* and *b*) Closure of aortotomy and performance of distal anastomosis with the internal mammary artery. (J) Proximal graft anastomoses are performed. In this illustration, a partially occluding clamp has been applied to the aorta.

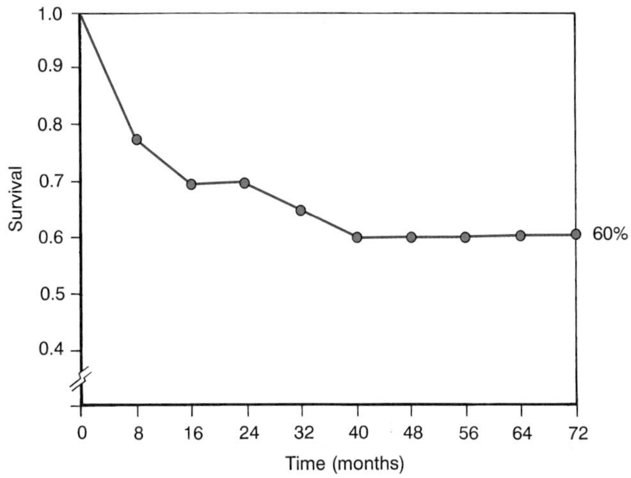

FIGURE 48-10 Long-term survival after combined aortic and mitral valve replacement and coronary artery bypass grafting. *(Adapted with permission from Akins CW, Buckley MJ, Daggett WM, et al: Myocardial revascularization with combined aortic and mitral valve replacements. J Thorac Cardiovasc Surg 1985; 90:272.)*

multiple volume overloads of insufficient aortic and mitral valves and the potential contribution of dysfunctional myocardium from ischemia make it very difficult to get an accurate estimation of preoperative left ventricular function. Thallium or PET scans may be useful to assess which areas of dysfunctional myocardium may be viable and potentially recruitable after revascularization.

Pathophysiology

Symptoms and signs of left ventricular failure develop as the left ventricle dilates. In patients with rheumatic disease with both valves intrinsically damaged, ischemic disease may be minimal. In the more common setting of patients with aortic regurgitation and significant ischemia, mitral regurgitation is more likely to be secondary to both of these processes, and valve repair should be possible. Correction of aortic regurgitation reduces preload, whereas correction of mitral insufficiency increases afterload. The dilated myopathic ventricle may not have sufficient reserves to maintain adequate output under these circumstances. Higher postoperative preload may need to be maintained while afterload is reduced. Any additional contractility as a result of revascularization should improve output further. Hence, forward flow will improve if ventricular contractility is maintained or increased. However, because of the multiple, uncontrollable variables that inhibit preoperative assessment of ventricular function, prediction of expected improvement after this operation is difficult.

This consideration is extremely important. Patients with severe and irreversible ischemic myocardial disease and poor ventricular function will not do well with operative treatment of this entity. Therefore, preoperative assessments of myocardial viability and reversible ischemia are important. It is also important to assess whether organic mitral valve disease is present. The best results in these patients are in those in whom no mitral operation, or at most annuloplasty, is required.

Operative Management

Details of the operative technique are similar to those described previously. Because of the presence of aortic insufficiency, retrograde cardioplegia must be used in conjunction with handheld ostial cannulas to deliver cardioplegia antegrade. For the reasons enunciated, excellent myocardial protection is important in these patients. Transesophageal echocardiography is required in the operating room for the assessment of mitral valve function. Residual 1+ to 2+ mitral regurgitation may be acceptable in certain patients because relief of aortic regurgitation can be expected to reduce ventricular size, which may lead to improvement of mitral regurgitation as the ventricle remodels with time. Similarly, myocardial revascularization also may lead to ultimate improvement in ventricular and mitral valve function.

In weaning from cardiopulmonary bypass, afterload reduction is extremely important because of the large preoperative volume overload of the heart. Drugs that reduce ventricular afterload, including vasodilators and inotropic drugs such as milrinone, may be particularly appropriate. The intra-aortic balloon pump may be needed.

Results

Early hospital mortality in this group of patients may be high, and if myocardial failure is severe, overall mortality rates exceed the range already noted for double-valve and coronary artery surgery.[56,57] Important determinants of risk in these patients are the familiar ones. In several series, predictors of hospital death and late events included severe mitral regurgitation, lower ejection fraction, more severe symptoms of congestive heart failure, and severe triple-vessel CAD.

SUMMARY

This chapter has reviewed the surgical management of patients with valvular and ischemic heart disease. The discussion has focused on management of disease of the aortic and mitral valves, because these are the valves most frequently affected in adults who present with these combined diseases.

Rather than concentrating on the details of the technical aspects of valve implantation or coronary artery grafting, the discussion has focused on the particular problems for surgical management that the combined pathophysiology of valvular and ischemic heart disease produces. As has been noted often during the discussion, there is usually an interaction among valve function, myocardial perfusion, and ventricular performance. Dysfunction of the aortic and mitral valves has secondary effects on ventricular function, and the addition of CAD can make this interaction more complex. Therefore, the pathophysiology of these disease states can be complicated. To manage these entities successfully, this pathophysiology must be understood so that accurate estimates of risk and reasonable expectations for results can be achieved.

In almost every case, ventricular function and severity of mitral incompetence are important short- and long-term risk factors. Also, functional mitral insufficiency in the absence of anatomical abnormalities of the mitral valve may resolve after aortic and/or coronary artery surgery, and therefore an operation on the mitral valve may not be required. Data from several sources suggest that patients with both coronary artery and valvular heart disease should be considered for a tissue prosthesis because of reduced life expectancy and the benefits of avoiding long-term anticoagulation. The ultimate role of catheter-based therapies for valvular and coronary artery disease in these patients remains to be defined. It is a certainty, however, that as these techniques are perfected, they will be applied to more patients, some of whom may have been considered at too high a risk for direct surgical therapy.

Finally, the complex interaction among ventricular function, valvular function, and coronary ischemia requires that the operation be well planned with attention paid to expeditious surgery, short myocardial ischemia times, and good myocardial preservation. Much of the discussion in this chapter, therefore, has focused on the operative plan and the development of a rational approach to intraoperative and postoperative management of these patients.

REFERENCES

1. Davis EA, Gardner TJ, Gillinov AM, et al: Valvular disease in the elderly: influence on surgical results. *Ann Thorac Surg* 1993; 55:333.
2. Freeman WK, Schaff HV, O'Brien PC, et al: Cardiac surgery in the octogenarian: perioperative outcome and clinical follow-up. *J Am Coll Cardiol* 1991; 18:29.
3. Byrne JG, Leacche M, Vaughan DE, Zhao DX: Hybrid cardiovascular procedures. *JACC Cardiovasc Interv* 2008; 1:459.
4. Piazza N, Serruys PW, de Jaegere P: Feasibility of complex coronary intervention in combination with percutaneous aortic valve implantation in patients with aortic stenosis suing percutaneous left ventricular assist device (TandemHeart). *Catheter Cardiovasc Interv* 2009; 73:161.
5. Harris KM, Pastorius CA, Duval S, et al: Practice variation among cardiovascular physicians in management of patients with mitral regurgitation. *Am J Cardiol* 2009; 103:255.
6. Peels JO, Jessurun GA, Boonstra PW, et al: Hybrid approach for complex coronary artery and valve disease: a clinical follow-up study. *Neth Heart J* 2007; 15:327.
7. Lu JC, Shaw M, Grayson AD, et al: Do beating heart techniques applied to combined valve and graft operations reduce myocardial damage? *Interact Cardiovasc Thorac Surg* 2008; 7:111.
8. Morris JJ, Schaff HV, Mullany CJ, et al: Determinants of survival and recovery of left ventricular function after aortic valve replacement. *Ann Thorac Surg* 1993; 56:22.
9. Pereira JJ, Balaban K, Lauer MS, et al: Aortic valve replacement in patients with mild or moderate aortic stenosis and coronary bypass surgery. *Am J Med* 2005; 118:735.
10. Gillinov AM, Garcia MJ: When is concomitant aortic valve replacement indicated in patients with mild to moderate stenosis undergoing coronary revascularization? *Curr Cardiol Rep* 2005; 7:101.
11. Smith WT IV, Ferguson TB Jr, Ryan T, et al: Should coronary artery bypass graft surgery patients with mild or moderate aortic stenosis undergo concomitant aortic valve replacement? A decision analysis approach to the surgical dilemma. *J Am Coll Cardiol* 2004; 15:1241.
12. Boning A, Burger S, Fraaund S, et al: Should the aortic valve be replaced in patients with mild aortic stenosis admitted for coronary surgery? *Thorac Cardiovasc Surg* 2008; 56:467.
13. Ren JF, Panidis IP, Kotler MN, et al: Effect of coronary bypass surgery and valve replacement on left ventricular function: assessment by intraoperative two-dimensional echocardiography. *Am Heart J* 1985; 103:281.
14. Braunwald E, Kloner RA: The stunned myocardium: prolonged postischemic ventricular dysfunction. *Circulation* 1982; 66:1146.
15. Braunwald E: The stunned myocardium: newer insights into mechanisms and clinical applications. *J Thorac Cardiovasc Surg* 1990; 100:310.
16. Marban E: Myocardial stunning and hibernation: the physiology behind the colloquialisms. *Circulation* 1991; 83:681.
17. Shahle E, Bergstrom R, Nystrom SO, Hansson HE: Early results of aortic valve replacement with or without concomitant coronary artery bypass grafting. *Scand J Thorac Cardiovasc Surg* 1991; 25:29.
18. Lytle BW, Cosgrove DM, Gill CC, et al: Aortic valve replacement combined with myocardial revascularization. *J Thorac Cardiovasc Surg* 1988; 95:402.
19. Kay PH, Nunley D, Grunkemeier GL, et al: Ten-year survival following aortic valve bypass as a risk factor: a multivariate analysis of coronary replacement. *J Cardiovasc Surg* 1986; 27:494.
20. Mullany CJ, Elveback LR, Frye FL, et al: Coronary artery disease and its management: influence on survival in patients undergoing aortic valve replacement. *J Am Coll Cardiol* 1987; 10:66.
21. Kirklin JK, Nartel DC, Blackstone EH, et al: Risk factors for mortality after primary combined valvular and coronary artery surgery. *Circulation* 1989; 79(Suppl I):I-180.
22. Karp RB, Mills N, Edmunds LH Jr: Coronary artery bypass grafting in the presence of valvular disease. *Circulation* 1989; 79(Suppl I):I-182.
23. Tsai TP, Matloff JM, Chaux A, et al: Combined valve and coronary artery bypass procedures in septuagenarians and octogenarians: results in 120 patients. *Ann Thorac Surg* 1986; 42:681.
24. Maganti M, Rao V, Armstrong S, et al: Redo valvular surgery in elderly patients. *Ann Thorac Surg* 2009; 87:521.
25. Pedersen WR, Klaassen PJ, Pedersen CW, et al: Comparison of outcomes in high-risk patients >70 years of age with aortic valvuloplasty and percutaneous coronary intervention versus aortic valvuloplasty alone. *Am J Cardiol* 2008; 101:1309.
26. Andrade IG, Cartier R, Panisi P, et al: Factors influencing early and late survival in patients with combined mitral valve replacement and myocardial revascularization and in those with isolated replacement. *Ann Thorac Surg* 1987; 44:607.
27. Lytle BW, Cosgrove DM, Gill CC, et al: Mitral valve replacement combined with myocardial revascularization: early and late results for 300 patients, 1970 to 1983. *Circulation* 1985; 71:1179.
28. Ashraf SS, Shaukat N, Odom N, et al: Early and late results following combined coronary bypass surgery and mitral valve replacement. *Eur J Cardiothorac Surg* 1994; 8:57.
29. Szecsi J, Herrijgers P, Sergeant P, et al: Mitral valve surgery combined with coronary bypass grafting: multivariate analysis of factors predicting early and late results. *J Heart Valve Dis* 1994; 3:236.
30. Crabtree TD, Bailey MS, Moon MR, et al: Recurrent mitral regurgitation and risk factors for early and late mortality after mitral valve repair for functional ischemic mitral regurgitation. *Ann Thorac Surg* 2008; 85:1537.
31. Sheikh KH, Bengtson JR, Rankin JS, et al: Intraoperative transesophageal Doppler color flow imaging used to guide patient selection and operative treatment of ischemic mitral regurgitation. *Circulation* 1991; 84:594.
32. Dion R: Ischemic mitral regurgitation: when and how should it be corrected? *J Heart Valve Dis* 1993; 2:536.
33. Aklog L, Filsoufi F, Flores KQ, et al: Does coronary artery bypass grafting alone correct moderate ischemic mitral regurgitation? *Circulation* 2001; 75:I-68.
34. Ho PC, Nguyen ME: Multivessel coronary drug-eluting stenting alone in patients with significant ischemic mitral regurgitation: a 4-year follow up. *J Invasive Cardiol* 2008; 20:41.
35. Lam BK, Gillinov AM, Blackstone EH, et al: Importance of moderate ischemic mitral regurgitation. *Ann Thorac Surg* 2005; 79:462.
36. Filsoufi F, Aklog L, Byrne JG, et al: Current results of combined coronary artery bypass grafting and mitral annuloplasty in patients with moderate ischemic mitral regurgitation. *J Heart Valve Dis* 2004; 13:747.
37. Bax JJ, Braun J, Somer ST, et al: Restrictive annuloplasty and coronary revascularization in ischemic mitral regurgitation results in reverse left ventricular remodeling. *Circulation* 2004; 110:II103.
38. Diodato MD, Moon MR, Pasque MK, et al: Repair of ischemic mitral regurgitation does not increase mortality or improve long-term survival in patients undergoing coronary artery revascularization: a propensity analysis. *Ann Thorac Surg* 2004; 78:794.
39. Geidel S, Lass M, Osstermeyer J: Restrictive mitral valve annuloplasty for chronic ischemic mitral regurgitation: a 5-year clinical experience with the physio ring. *Heart Surg Forum* 2008; 11:E225.
40. Maisano F, Schreuder JJ, Oppizzi M, et al: The double-orifice technique as a standardized approach to treat mitral regurgitation due to severe myxomatous disease: surgical technique. *Eur J Cardiothorac Surg* 2000; 17:201.
41. Alfieri O, Maisano F, DeBonis M, et al: The double-orifice technique in mitral valve repair: a simple solution for complex problems. *J Thorac Cardiovasc Surg* 2001; 122:674.

42. Cohn LH, Kowalker W, Bhatia S, et al: Comparative morbidity of mitral valve repair versus replacement for mitral regurgitation with and without coronary artery disease. *Ann Thorac Surg* 1988; 45:284.
43. Jones EL, Weintraub WS, Craver JM, et al: Interaction of age and coronary disease after valve replacement: implications for valve selection. *Ann Thorac Surg* 1994; 58:378.
44. Cox JL, Buckberg GD: Ventricular shape and function in health and disease. *Semin Thorac Cardiovasc Surg* 2001; 13:298.
45. Guy TS, Brzezinski M, Stechert MM, Tseng E: Robotic mammary artery harvest and anastomotic device allows minimally invasive mitral valve repair and coronary bypass. *J Card Surg* 2009; 24:170.
46. Cohn LH, Couper GS, Kinchla NM, Collins JJ Jr: Decreased operative risk of surgical treatment of mitral regurgitation with or without coronary artery disease. *J Am Coll Cardiol* 1990; 16:1575.
47. Kay PH, Nunley DL, Grunkemeier GL, et al: Late results of combined mitral valve replacement and coronary bypass surgery. *J Am Coll Cardiol* 1985; 5:29.
48. Chiappini B, Minuti U, Gregorini R, et al: Early and long-term outcome of mitral valve repair with a Cosgrove band combined with coronary revascularization in patients with ischemic cardiomyopathy and moderate-severe mitral regurgitation. *J Heart Valve Dis 2008*; 17:396.
49. Milano CA, Daneshmand MA, Rankin JS, et al: Survival prognosis and surgical management of ischemic mitral regurgitation. *Ann Thor Surg* 2008; 86:735.
50. Sirivella S, Gielchinsky I: Results of coronary bypass and valve operations for valve regurgitation. *Asian Cardiovasc Thorac Ann* 2007; 5:396.
51. Gelsomino S, Lorusso R, De Cicco G, et al: Five-year echocardiographic results of combined undersized mitral ring annuloplasty and coronary artery bypass grafting for chronic ischaemic mitral regurgitation. *Eur Heart J 2008*; 29:231.
52. Waisbren EC, Stevens LM, Avery EG, et al: Changes in mitral regurgitation after replacement of the stenotic aortic valve. *Ann Thorac Surg* 2008; 86:56.
53. Wan CK, Suri RM, Li Z, Orszulak TA et al: Management of moderate functional mitral regurgitation at the time of aortic valve replacement: is concomitant mitral valve repair necessary? *J Thorac Cardiovasc Surg* 2009; 137:635.
54. Masson JB, Webb JG: Percutaneous mitral annuloplasty. *Coron Artery Dis* 2009; 20:183.
55. Davidson MJ, Cohn LG: Surgeons' perspective on percutaneous valve repair. *Coron Artery Dis* 2009; 20:192.
56. Akins CW, Buckley MJ, Daggett WM, et al: Myocardial revascularization with combined aortic and mitral valve replacements. *J Thorac Cardiovasc Surg* 1985; 90:272.
57. Johnson WD, Kayser KL, Pedraza PM, Brenowitz JB: Combined valve replacement and coronary bypass surgery: results in 127 operations stratified by surgical risk factors. *Chest* 1986; 90:338.

CHAPTER 49

Reoperative Valve Surgery

James P. Greelish
John G. Byrne

INTRODUCTION

The number of patients undergoing reoperation for valvular heart disease is increasing and will continue to increase as the general population ages.[1] These reoperations most commonly involve structural deterioration of a bioprosthesis or progression of native-valve disease after nonvalve surgery. In fact, structural failure of a biologic valve should be considered part of the natural evolution of tissue valves and should be fully appreciated by both the surgeon and the patient prior to implantation.[2] Reoperations are technically more difficult than primary operations because of adhesions around the heart with an associated risk of reentry, the presence of more advanced cardiac pathology, and the existence of more frequent comorbidities such as pulmonary hypertension. Perhaps most important, reoperative replacement operations often are performed in functionally compromised patients who tolerate complications poorly or who have little reserve.[3] As a consequence of these and other factors, reoperative valve surgery historically has been associated with a considerably higher operative mortality than primary valve surgery, particularly in patients who have had multiple prior replacements.[4] In the modern era, however, with the use of alternative surgical approaches and advanced perioperative care, there has been significant improvement in outcomes.[5–9]

Reductions in operative risk and postoperative morbidity after reoperative valve surgery have been made in the past few years through advances in myocardial protection, as well as alternative perfusion strategies such as the proper use of deep hypothermic cardiac arrest.[10] In addition, use of peripheral cannulation techniques to institute cardiopulmonary bypass has become a relatively standard practice in reoperative cases.[11–13] Early institution of cardiopulmonary bypass prior to reentry is known to prevent injury to the distended right ventricle or patent coronary artery bypass grafts during reoperative sternotomy. In addition, this technique reduces myocardial oxygen consumption by decreasing myocardial distension.[4]

Successful replacement of the degenerate cardiac valve usually results in gratifying symptomatic and hemodynamic improvement. Maintenance of this improved state, however, depends on persistence of prosthetic valve function. In this regard, improvements in valve design have mitigated but not eliminated primary bioprosthetic failure.[14–16] As such, the risk of re-replacement for bioprosthetic failure remains a significant factor to be considered in the selection of valve type for implantation.[17]

MECHANICAL VERSUS BIOLOGIC VALVES

The most appropriate valve substitute for an individual patient remains a source of much controversy. This choice should be adapted to each individual patient depending on age, life expectancy, valve size, and cardiac as well as noncardiac comorbidities.[18] Some studies comparing the long-term outcomes between biologic and mechanical aortic valve prostheses have yielded similar results with regard to overall valve-related complications.[19–22] However, most recent large studies have documented that anticoagulant-related bleeding with mechanical valves must be balanced against life expectation and the risk of biologic valve re-replacement.[23–25] Bioprosthetic valves are known to undergo a time-dependent process of structural deterioration that results in a freedom of reoperation of 80% at 15 years.[20] Consequently, structural degeneration of a bioprosthesis is the most frequent indication for reoperation in patients with tissue valves.[19,26]

Despite this, recently improved durability of tissue valves, as well as the availability of stentless valves and homografts, has led to surgeons placing bioprostheses in progressively younger age groups.[18,27–30] Contributing to this trend, many patients do not accept the risk of anticoagulant-related hemorrhage associated with mechanical valves: major events 0.5% per patient-year and minor events 2 to 4% per patient-year.[31]

Mechanical prostheses usually are selected for younger recipients because of their proven durability over time. However, the risk of anticoagulant-related bleeding, as well as thromboembolic events (TEs), in these valves is not trivial and depends on valve design, structural materials, and host-related interactions.[31] In a 12-year comparison of Bjork-Shiley versus porcine valves, Bloomfield and colleagues documented severe bleeding complications in 18.6% versus 7.1%, respectively.[32] Moreover, although endocarditis, dehiscence, perivalvular leak, and pannus formation are associated with both biologic and mechanical valves, acute prosthetic thrombosis is exclusively a complication of mechanical valves.[33,34] In considering mechanical valve durability, these associated risks cannot be ignored and must be weighed against the anticipated rate of tissue-valve failure and the need for reoperation.

RISK FACTORS IN REOPERATIVE VALVE SURGERY (TABLE 49-1)

In evaluating patients for reoperative valve surgery, certain factors are associated with added risk. For example, Husebye and colleagues, in a review of their 20-year experience[17] with reoperative valve surgery, found specific issues to carry higher risk. Overall operative mortality was 7% for the second and 14% for the third reoperation. Operative mortality for the first reoperation (n = 530 patients) was 5.9% in the aortic position and 19.6% in the mitral position. In the aortic position, operative mortality was 2.4% for New York Heart Association (NYHA) class I, 1.6% for NYHA class II, 6.3% for NYHA class III, and 20.8% for NYHA class IV, emphasizing the significance of early referral. Regarding the urgency of surgery, the mortality for elective mitral valve reoperations was 1.4%; for urgent procedures, 8%; and for emergency procedures, 37.5%. Based on these findings, the authors have recommended that referral for reoperation be made when valve dysfunction is first noted, ie, before a significant decrement in myocardial function.[17] Similarly, Jones and colleagues reviewed their experience with first heart valve reoperations in 671 patients between 1969 and 1998.[6] Their overall operative mortality for first-time heart valve reoperation was 8.6%, similar to the results published by Lytle[35] (10.9%), Cohn[4] (10.1%), Akins[36] (7.3%), Pansini[2] (9.6%), and Tyers[37] (11.0%). In the Jones and colleagues series, mortality increased from 3.0% for reoperation on a new valve site to 10.6% for prosthetic valve dysfunction or periprosthetic leak; mortality was highest (29.4%) for associated endocarditis or valve thrombosis. Concomitant coronary artery bypass grafting carried a higher associated mortality (15.4%) than when it was not required (8.2%). Among the 336 patients requiring re-replacement of prosthetic valves, mortality was 26.1% for re-replacement of a mechanical valve compared with 8.6% for re-replacement of a tissue valve. The authors concluded through multivariable analysis that significant predictors of mortality were year of reoperation, patient age, indication, concomitant coronary artery bypass grafting, and the replacement of a mechanical valve rather than a tissue valve.[6]

TABLE 49-1 Risk Factors for Reoperative Valve Surgery

Advanced age
Impaired ejection fraction (EF), congestive heart failure (CHF), or advanced preoperative functional class (NYHA)
Urgency of operation or unstable status preoperatively
Preoperative shock
Concomitant coronary artery bypass graft (CABG) or the presence of previous bypass grafts
Prosthetic valve endocarditis
Surgery for perivalvular leaks, valve thrombosis, or prosthetic dysfunction
Renal dysfunction
Chronic obstructive pulmonary disease (COPD)

REOPERATIVE AORTIC VALVE SURGERY

Historical Points

Historically, aortic valve surgery typically involved the placement of a mechanical valve. In the past, there were only a few generally accepted indications to use a bioprosthesis for primary, isolated aortic valve replacement: (1) the presence of well-established contraindications to continuous anticoagulation, (2) the inability to monitor prothrombin levels adequately, and (3) patients whose survival was limited and more dependent on non-valve–related issues.[18,26] In recent years, however, the use of biologic valves in the aortic position has become more common.[24,38]

As mentioned, reoperations are technically demanding, and many patients present in a poor functional state that further increases their mortality, in some series up to 19%.[32,39,40] Generally, optimal planning for reoperation prior to deterioration to NYHA class III to IV levels and before unfavorable comorbid conditions have arisen is imperative to ensure good outcomes.[9] Following these guidelines in the modern era, elective re-replacement of malfunctioning aortic bioprostheses can be performed with results similar to those of the primary operation.[18,23,41] The Mayo Clinic, for example, recently reviewed its experience with 162 reoperative aortic valve replacements (AVRs). Early mortality for reoperative AVR was not statistically different from that for primary AVR.[42] In light of recent lower operative mortality in reoperative valve surgery, a more conservative approach toward issues such as "prophylactic" AVR in patients with asymptomatic mild to moderate aortic stenosis at the time of coronary artery bypass grafting (CABG) also may be more appropriate.[43]

In evaluating the reoperative patient, the presence of concomitant coronary artery disease and pulmonary hypertension has been shown consistently to be independent risk factors.[18]

Patients with these risk factors therefore need careful surveillance once the probability of bioprosthetic dysfunction begins increasing (ie, 6 to 10 years after implantation).[16] Regarding valve surveillance and timing of reoperation, the following variables are relevant to the clinical management of patients with an aortic bioprosthesis: a history of endocarditis before the first operation, perioperative infectious complications, coronary artery disease acquired after the first operation, an increase in pulmonary artery pressure, and a decrease in left ventricular function during the interoperative interval.[18] Proper timing of the reoperation therefore is paramount because duration of clinical signs with a dysfunctional aortic bioprosthesis may be misleading. This is further supported by the fact that the need for emergency reoperation is the most ominous risk factor and consistently yields a high early mortality rate of 25 to 44%.[44]

Approaches and Techniques

Conventional Resternotomy

The evolution of cardiac surgery through the last few decades has led to the popularization of various surgical approaches. Thoracotomy, for example, once was used extensively to gain access to mediastinal structures. Then median sternotomy became the standard approach. In reoperative cases, however, repeating the sternotomy carries definite surgical risks. Before proceeding with a resternotomy, the relationship between certain anterior mediastinal structures (eg, the right ventricle and the aorta) and the posterior aspect of the sternum must be assessed carefully.[45] This generally can be visualized on chest radiograph or more accurately with a chest computed tomographic (CT) scan. Recently, it has been shown that multidetector computed tomographic (MDCT) scanning, in combination with retrospective electrocardiographic gating, can be used as a noninvasive way to assess not only the heart's location in relation to the sternum, but also graft location and patency.[46–48]

Exposure of the femoral vessels and preparation for emergency femoral-femoral cardiopulmonary bypass should be considered before resternotomy. In cases of heightened concern for right ventricle–graft injury or in cases in which a left internal mammary artery (LIMA) graft is patent, the surgeon should consider the use of cardiopulmonary bypass before chest reentry. Sternal wires from the previous operation should be undone carefully but left in place as a posterior safeguard during initial sternal division. An oscillating (not reciprocating) bone saw can be used to divide the anterior sternal table. An Army-Navy retractor, placed inferiorly in-line with the sternotomy can be used to stent open the wound during opening of the posterior table. Most authors recommend dividing the posterior table using a combination of scissors and anterolateral rake retraction.[45,48,49] Following this, bilateral pleural spaces should be entered inferiorly, followed by careful dissection of other mediastinal structures. The pericardial dissection plane can be developed by starting at the cardiophrenic angle and advancing slowly cephalad and laterally on the surface of the right side of the heart. Cephalad dissection should start with freeing the innominate vein before spreading the retractor to avoid its injury. Further dissection then is carried down to the superior vena cava, being careful to note the location of the right phrenic nerve. An area of consistently dense adhesions is the right atrial appendage, and caution should be used here. In addition, great care should be taken to avoid "deadventializing" the aorta. The area where the aorta apposes the pulmonary artery is another site of potential injury.

Repairing small ventricular or atrial lacerations should not be attempted before releasing the tension of the surrounding adhesions. Repair of great vessel injuries or severe right ventricle injuries is best done under cardiopulmonary bypass.[45] Severe active hemorrhage during a second sternotomy usually is caused by adherence of the heart or great vessels to the posterior sternum. Prevention of this ominous complication by interposition of pericardium or other mediastinal tissue at the time of the first operation has been suggested but has debatable relevance.[48] The incidence of resternotomy hemorrhage is between 2 and 6% per patient reoperation.[50–52] In a report of 552 patients who had undergone reoperative prosthetic valve surgery, 23 patients (4%) had complications related directly to sternal opening.[17] Of these, five patients had entry into the right atrium, seven patients had lacerated right ventricles, nine patients had injuries to the aorta, and two patients had a previously placed coronary artery graft divided. Nineteen of the 23 complications occurred during a first reoperation. Overall, there were two operative deaths related to resternotomy. The first death involved division of a previously placed coronary artery graft during reentry. The second death was caused by laceration of the aorta with subsequent exsanguination.[17] Of note, prior use of a right internal mammary artery (RIMA) graft can be particularly challenging because it frequently crosses the midline, and extreme caution must be used in first dissecting out this vessel.

Macanus and colleagues reviewed their experience with 100 patients undergoing repeat median sternotomy.[51] Eighty-one patients had one repeat sternotomy, whereas the others had undergone multiple sternotomies. All had had a previous valve procedure and were reoperated on for progressive rheumatic valvular disease or for complications related to the prosthesis. Complications included operative hemorrhage in eight patients, postoperative hemorrhage in two, seroma in four, and dehiscence, wound infection, and hematoma in one patient each. There was one operative death directly related to resternotomy hemorrhage.[51] When major hemorrhage does occur on sternal reentry, attempts at resternotomy should be abandoned, and the chest should be reapproximated by pushing toward the midline. The patient should be heparinized immediately while obtaining femoral arterial and venous cannulation. Blood loss from the resternotomy should be aspirated with cardiotomy suction and returned to the pump. Once bypass has been established, core cooling should be commenced with anticipation of the need for circulatory arrest. Once cool, flow rates can be reduced, and the remaining sternal division can be completed, followed by direct repair of the underlying injury.[48] Anticipating the possibility of this scenario, we frequently expose peripheral cannulation sites prior to beginning a resternotomy. In cases of heightened concern for right ventricle or graft injury, or in patients with a patent LIMA to left anterior descending (LAD) artery graft, cardiopulmonary bypass and cardiac decompression may be initiated *before* sternal reentry. After safe sternal entry, the patient may be weaned from bypass for further dissection of adhesions to avoid prolonged pump times.

Minimally Invasive Reoperative AVR

Reoperative procedures are challenging owing to diffuse mediastinal and pericardial adhesions. A large incision that increases the operative exposure also has been associated with a higher risk of injury to cardiac structures and coronary artery bypass grafts and results in greater bleeding with its associated transfusion requirements.[53–56] A smaller incision with a limited sternotomy, on the other hand, reduces the area of pericardiolysis, thus mitigating these effects. The intact lower sternum that remains also preserves the integrity of the caudal chest wall, thereby enhancing sternal stability and promoting earlier extubation.[57,58] *Minimally invasive* valve procedures gradually have become more accepted as new technologies and instrumentation have been developed.[57] Reoperative procedures in which there is risk for graft injury are an area where minimally invasive strategies may be of direct benefit.[59,60] Our surgical approach in reoperative AVR is shown in Fig. 49-1.[57] In our series of patients, peripheral cannulation sites were exposed or cannulated before beginning the partial upper resternotomy. An external defibrillator was placed on the patient before draping for anticipated defibrillation as necessary. Transesophageal echocardiography (TEE) was used in every patient. A partial upper resternotomy was carried out to the third or fourth intercostal space depending on the estimated position of the aortic valve as documented by chest x-ray (CXR)/TEE and then was "T'd to the right."[61] The oscillating saw was used to divide the anterior sternal table, whereas the straight Mayo scissors, under direct visualization, was used to divide the posterior sternal table. In the setting of a patent LIMA-LAD graft or other anterior coronary artery bypass grafts, patients were placed on cardiopulmonary bypass before partial resternotomy. Mediastinal dissection was limited to only the ascending aorta as was necessary for clamping and aortotomy. The right atrium was dissected only if it was cannulated. Although intrathoracic cannulation was preferred, we frequently used peripheral cannulation to avoid clutter in the chest. Retrograde cardioplegia, if necessary, was delivered via a transjugular coronary sinus catheter or with right atrial placement under TEE guidance. Vacuum assistance of venous drainage was used in the majority of patients. Once on cardiopulmonary bypass, all patients were systemically cooled to 20 to 25°C. Patients with patent LIMA-LAD grafts were cooled routinely to 20°C for additional myocardial protection and in so doing avoided the need and potential hazard of dissecting out the LIMA for clamping in an attempt to avoid cardioplegia washout. If flow from the patent LIMA-LAD graft led to significant blood flow out of the coronary ostium and obscured the operative field, pump flows were turned down temporarily to allow visualization. Venting was accomplished by placing a pediatric vent through the aortic annulus. The aortic valve surgery then was performed based on patient indications. While closing the aortotomy, intracardiac air was removed by insufflating the lungs and decreasing flows on cardiopulmonary bypass. Carbon dioxide was used and flooded the operative field. Patients also were tilted from side to side to

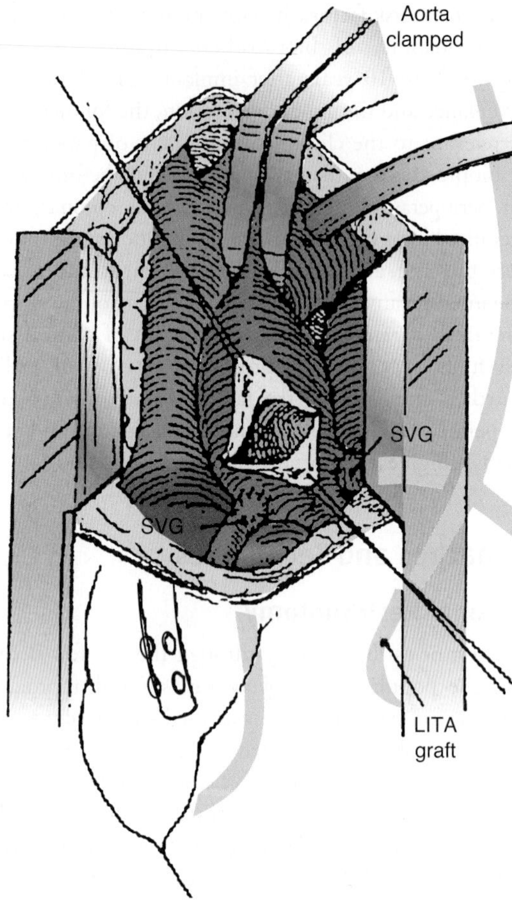

FIGURE 49-1 Partial upper resternotomy for reoperative AVR. The previous sternotomy incision is exposed to the third or fourth intercostal space depending on the position of the aortic valve, as documented by TEE. After dissection of the ascending aorta, paying particular attention to the position of coronary artery bypass grafts and their proximal anastomoses, cannulation is carried out. In this figure, the ascending aorta and innominate vein are cannulated. Frequently, however, other cannulation sites are required owing to space limitations in the chest. The ascending aorta is cross-clamped, and the aortic valve re-replacement is conducted in a standard fashion. (*Used with permission from Byrne JG, Karavas AN, Adams DH, et al: Partial upper re-sternotomy for aortic valve replacement or re-replacement after previous cardiac surgery. Eur J Cardiothorac Surg 2000; 18[3]:282.*)

help with deairing, and the ascending aortic vent was left open until separation from cardiopulmonary bypass. Temporary epicardial pacing wires were placed on the anterior surface of the right ventricle while the heart was decompressed and before the aortic cross-clamp was removed. Two 32 French right-angled submammary chest tubes then were placed through the right pleural space, one angled medially into the mediastinum and one angled posterior into the pleural space. Decannulation and closure then were performed in the standard manner.

With our increasing experience in minimally invasive reoperative AVR, we have refined our technique as an alternative to conventional full resternotomy.[57] In so doing, we have ascertained the technical details of the partial upper resternotomy

TABLE 49-2 Thirteen Technical Details for Successful Aortic Valve Replacement After Previous Cardiac Surgery by Use of Partial Upper Resternotomy

1. Routine exposure of peripheral cannulation sites prior to partial upper resternotomy
2. Placement of Zoll (Zoll, Inc., Burlington, MA) defibrillator pads before prepping
3. Use of intraoperative transesophageal echocardiography for air removal and inspection of valve
4. In patients with patent left internal mammary artery to left anterior descending coronary artery (LIMA-LAD) graft, peripheral cannulation, and cardiopulmonary bypass (CPB) established before partial upper resternotomy
5. Mediastinal dissection limited to ascending aorta for clamping and aortotomy and atrium (RA), only if RA is cannulated
6. Use of peripheral cannulation to avoid clutter in the chest
7. Use of vacuum assistance on CPB
8. Use of retrograde cardioplegia (CP) delivered by transjugular retrograde CP catheter in addition to antegrade CP
9. Use of aprotinin unless absolute contraindication
10. Cooling to at least 25°C in all patients primarily for myocardial protection; if a patent LIMA-LAD graft is present, cooling to 20°C without isolation and clamping LIMA graft
11. If visualization is poor because of LIMA-LAD collaterals flowing from coronary ostia, temporary low flows on CPB to improve visualization
12. Venting with a pediatric vent placed through the aortic annulus
13. Placement of temporary pacing wires on the right ventricular free wall before aortic clamp removal

Source: Reproduced with permission from Byrne J, Karavas A, Adams D, et al: Partial upper re-sternotomy for aortic valve replacement or re-replacement after previous cardiac surgery. Eur J Cardiothorac Surg 2000; 18:282.

approach (Table 49-2). By following these guidelines, we have yet to convert any patient to a full resternotomy. Lateral CXR and/or TEE is helpful in locating the level of the aortic valve and determining the proximity of the aorta to the posterior aspect of the sternum.[61] If necessary, additional information can be obtained with CT scanning or magnetic resonance imaging (MRI) preoperatively. Also, extension of the sternal incision laterally on both sides through the intercostal spaces helps to later reapproximate the sternum. We have tried to limit mediastinal and pericardial dissection primarily to the aorta, believing that this is the principal reason for decreased bleeding and transfusion requirements postoperatively.[57,60,62,63] The right ventricle, which often is attached to the sternum, does not need to be dissected. Also, injuries to patent but atherosclerotic vein grafts can be reduced with this "no touch" technique.[64]

Arterial and venous cannulation sites can vary considerably, reflecting the individual choice of the operating surgeon and the sufficiency of intrathoracic space. Possible cannulation sites, other than standard ones, include the axillary artery, innominate vein, and percutaneous femoral vein.[13,65] Innominate vein or percutaneous femoral vein cannulation, as well as the use of TEE to place the retrograde cardioplegia catheter, has been extremely helpful in minimizing dissection of the right atrium. At present, we consider this approach to be useful for isolated, elective reoperative aortic valve surgery.[57]

Reoperative AVR after Homograft/Root/Allograft

AVR with homografts and autografts was performed increasingly because of excellent freedom from thromboembolism, resistance to infection, and reasonable hemodynamic performance.[27] Although improved durability of current tissue valves has slowed this trend, autografts and, to a lesser degree, homografts remain popular in younger patients owing to durability and, in the case of autografts, the potential for growth.[30,66] Consequently, many patients will require aortic valve re-replacement for structural degeneration of their homograft or autograft valve.[67] It is expected that about one third of patients younger than 40 years of age will require aortic valve re-replacement within 12 years of homograft placement. This is owing primarily to calcification and structural valve degeneration. As such, the issue of homograft or autograft durability is particularly pertinent in this subgroup of younger patients who are expected to live beyond 15 years from time of operation.[66]

The incidence of patients with homografts or autografts in need of a second valve operation is expected to increase owing to the aforementioned recent popularity and availability of these conduits. Also, there is varied opinion as to the optimal surgical method of primary homograft AVR, with increased rates of aortic insufficiency in patients with the subcoronary implantation technique. Importantly, the selected technique of primary homograft operation may have relevance at reoperation because calcification or aneurysmal dilatation of the homograft may pose surgical challenges at reoperation. Despite these challenges, Sundt and others[29,68,69] have documented the feasibility of aortic valve re-replacement after full-root replacement with a homograft. In our own series of 18 patients, full-root, mini-root, and subcoronary techniques all were amenable to valve re-replacement.[27]

How to best approach the reoperative root scenario and which valve to reimplant, however, have been debated. At one extreme, Hasnet and colleagues documented the results of 144 patients who underwent a *second* aortic homograft replacement with a hospital mortality rate of only 3.5%.[67] Although Kumar and colleagues, in a multivariate analysis of reoperative aortic valve surgery, did not show that a previous homograft added significant risk,[70] the technical aspects of reoperative AVR in this patient population consistently have been found to be challenging owing to the heavy calcific degeneration that invariably occurs. With this in mind, and owing to the typical absence of the need for a second root operation, we and others[71] believe that a more simplified approach to reoperative aortic valve surgery in patients with previously placed homografts may be optimal. Our approach has been to perform aortic valve re-replacement using a mechanical valve or, less commonly, a stented xenograft while reserving a second homograft and root operation for specific indications such as endocarditis, associated root pathology, or a very young patient with contraindications to a mechanical valve.

Homograft re-replacement nonetheless is performed but it is much less common, and hospital mortality varies widely across many centers, ranging between 2.5 and 50%.[29,68,69] David and colleagues, for example, recently reviewed their experience with root operations in 165 patients who previously had undergone cardiac surgery. Of these, 28 had a previous root operation. Overall, 12 operative (7%) and 20 late deaths (12%) occurred.[72] Variations in sample size, valve selection, surgical techniques, and patient factors, as well as the experience of the surgeons, may account for these wide differences.

AORTIC VALVE BYPASS SURGERY

Aortic valve bypass surgery (AVB), also known as apical aortic conduit surgery, is an alternative for high-risk and "inoperable" reoperative patients with aortic stenosis. It has been used in cases with reduced LV function,[73] porcelain aorta,[74] severe patient prosthetic mismatch,[75] excessive comorbidities, and vulnerable functional grafts[76] leading to prohibitive risk for conventional reoperative aortic valve replacement. AVB surgery works by shunting blood from the apex of the left ventricle to the descending aorta through a surgically placed valve conduit (Fig. 49-2). This approach avoids cross-clamping, cardioplegic arrest, potentially cardiopulmonary bypass,[77] debridement of the native valve, and injury to patent grafts because the procedure is performed through the left chest. Patient-prosthesis mismatch is also unlikely as the indexed effective orifice area (EOAi) is the sum of the valves in both the native position and conduit.

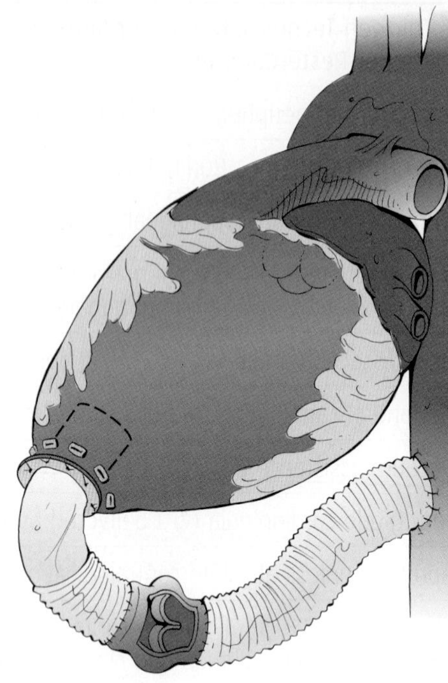

FIGURE 49-2 Apical aortic conduit. Aortic valve bypass surgery performed via left thoracotomy avoids sternotomy in difficult reoperative cases. (*With permission from Gammie JS, Krowsoski LS, Brown JM, et al: Aortic valve bypass surgery: midterm clinical outcomes in a high-risk aortic stenosis population. Circulation 2008; 118[14]:1460-1466.*)

Contraindications to this procedure include moderate aortic insufficiency. Relative contraindications include a heavily diseased descending aorta or significant mitral valve regurgitation. However, Gammie et al. showed that the degree of mitral regurgitation is reduced after placement of the conduit and moderate MR patients are still considered.

The procedure[78,79] is performed using a left ventricular apical connector with a silicon sewing ring and a heart valve (typically a stentless porcine valve with the coronaries over sewn) sewn to a Dacron graft at the beginning of the procedure. An 8-mm side branch off the Dacron graft may be used for direct inflow from the cardiopulmonary bypass machine if performed on pump. The patient is positioned in the right lateral decubitus position with a double lumen endotracheal tube. TEE is used to exclude apical thrombus, calcification of the descending aorta and ensure proper conduit positioning. If going on bypass an arterial and venous cannula are place in groin. A fifth- to sixth-intercostal space thoracotomy is performed and the apex of the heart and descending thoracic aorta exposed. The valve conduit with apical connector is then oriented with connector aimed at the apex of the heart. After heparinization the distal anastomosis is performed after placement of a partial occluding clamp on the descending thoracic aorta. The clamp is removed and hemostasis achieved. Stentless valve competency will prevent blood flow out of the apical connector. The pericardium is then opened and tacked up and a mark is made 1 to 2 cm lateral to the true apex of the left ventricle: 2-0 monofilament pledgeted sutures are used in an interrupted fashion around this marked area with deep bites of nearly full thickness. These are then taken through the sewing ring of the apical connector. If cardiopulmonary bypass is to be initiated, it is done at this time. The patient is placed in steep Trendelenburg position and the ventricle is then paced at 200 beats/min to reduce ventricular ejection. A hole is made in the marked apical area and a 14 French Foley catheter is placed into the left ventricle. Tension is placed on the Foley catheter and a coring knife is used to remove a plug of apical myocardium. A coring knife 85% of the diameter of the apical connector is selected to ensure a proper fit and optimize hemostasis. The Foley catheter is then removed and the apical connector is placed in the left ventricle. The sutures are tied down. The graft is de-aired and the chest is closed. When complete blood flow from the left ventricle travels out of the native valve and the conduit where it will primarily travel distally in the aorta with some flow in the retrograde direction. Studies have shown that approximately one third of the flow travels out the native valve, whereas two thirds travel out the conduit.[76] The procedure has been shown to be highly efficacious, dropping the mean aortic valve gradients in one study from 43 to 10 mm.[76] The durability of the apical aortic conduit procedure is also apparent, with some patients now more than 25 years out from their operations.

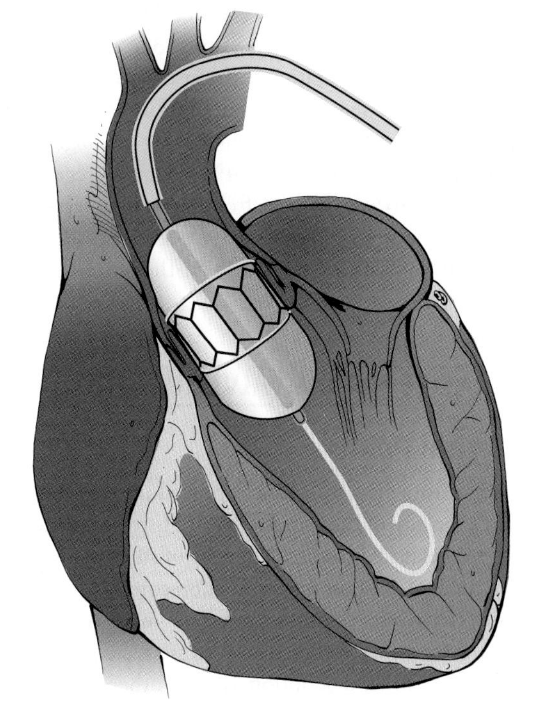

FIGURE 49-3 Transcatheter aortic valve replacement. Retrograde transcatheter approach for aortic valve replacement via femoral artery avoids sternotomy in reoperative cases. (*With permission from Brinkman WT, Mack MJ: Transcatheter cardiac valve interventions. Surg Clin North Am 2009; 89[4]:951-966.*)

TRANSCATHETER AORTIC VALVES

Percutaneous aortic valves are currently not available in the United States except for investigational use. However, their promising results indicate that they are sure to impact the approach to the high-risk reoperative patient in the future. Currently, two valves have received clinical approval in Europe: the Edwards Lifesciences, Inc. (Irvine, CA) SAPIEN THV device and the Medtronic (Minneapolis, MN) CoreValve, Inc. (Irvine, CA) Revalving device. The Edwards SAPIEN THV device is currently undergoing evaluation against medical management and traditional AVR in the PARTNERS trial in the United States, with commercial approval expected around 2011. The CoreValve randomized clinical trial is also planned. The SAPIEN THV is a trileaflet bovine pericardium valve mounted within a balloon expandable stainless steel stent with a fabric sealing cuff. Two sizes are being investigated (23 and 26 mm and require a 22 French (8-mm OD) and a 24 French (9-mm OD) sheath, respectively, for the percutaneous placement, and 26 French sheath for transapical approach).

The Medtronic CoreValve device is a trileaflet porcine pericardial valve prosthesis built in a self-expanding nitinol frame with a narrowing waist at its mid-section to allow coronary perfusion. It is currently available in 26- and 29-mm sizes. The first generation device used bovine pericardial tissue and a 25 French delivery system, whereas the second-generation valve was built using porcine tissue with a 21 French catheter. A third-generation device with an 18 French catheter delivery system is now available.

Two surgical approaches are used for placement of percutaneous valves; the transapical antegrade and transfemoral retrograde approaches. The retrograde approach uses femoral artery access with positioning of the valve in a retrograde fashion through the aortic arch and into the subcoronary position (Fig. 49-3). As such, this approach has advantages in the context of reoperative valve placement. The transapical approach requires a minimally invasive thoracotomy over the left ventricular apex. The apex is exposed and entered and the valve positioned in an antegrade fashion. Rapid ventricular pacing is used at the time of valve positioning and expansion to reduce the aortic outflow. Challenges to delivery of these transcatheter valve systems include the relatively large catheters needed for placement, valve positioning to avoid coronary obstruction, valve migration or embolization, and proper valve sizing to avoid perivalvular leak or coronary obstruction.[80] Buchbinder at the 2008 EuroPCR meeting reported the results of the CoreValve percutaneous aortic valve replacement in registry data. Five hundred thirty-six procedures were performed in high-risk patients, of which one fifth were reoperative patients with prior CABG. Procedural success was achieved in 97% of cases, with 94% of patients discharged from the hospital. Mean procedural time was 128 min (±47 min). AVA (cm^2) increased from 0.64 ± 0.20 [0.2 – 1.7] to 1.90 ± 0.40 [1.3 – 2.6], with mean aortic valve pressure gradient (mm Hg) decreasing from 49.7 ± 17.63 [12 – 114] to 2.71 ± 4.73 [0 – 27]. The percentage of patients in NYHA Class III/IV decreased from 86 to 8% at 30 days. Procedural failures occurred in only 3% of patients and included device malplacement, aortic root perforation, aortic dissection, access vessel bleeding, LV perforation, RV perforation, and conversion to surgery. Complications included less than

1% MI, less than 1% aortic dissection, 0% coronary impairment, 1% acute vascular complications, 3% stroke/TIA, 9% pacemaker, and 1% reoperation for nonstructural dysfunction. Clinically acceptable regurgitation defined as less than 3 to 4+ occurred in all patients, with 30% having no regurgitation, 56% having 1+ regurgitation and 14% having 2+ regurgitation. Thirty-day mortality was 8%, 4% from procedural related death, and 4% from nonprocedural/non-valve–related deaths. No structural deterioration or migration of the valve occurred in any patient.

REOPERATIVE MITRAL VALVE SURGERY

Historical Points

Fundamental to a flawless surgical procedure is excellent and consistent exposure of the mitral valve.[81] Historically, the mitral valve has been exposed through a variety of surgical approaches, including median sternotomy, right thoracotomy, left thoracotomy, and transverse sternotomy.[82] The median sternotomy and right thoracotomy will be discussed in detail in the following; however, a brief description of the other approaches is warranted.

The *left* thoracotomy has been used in recent years to gain access to the mitral valve in situations in which a right thoracotomy is precluded (eg, mastectomy/radiation or pleurodesis). This incision is made through the fourth intercostal space, and the left pleural cavity is entered in the standard fashion.[82] Surgery is performed under fibrillatory arrest or with the beating-heart technique. Of importance, the mitral valve orientation is noted to be upside down with this approach, with the posterior annulus found anteriorly.[83] Thompson and colleagues recently reported their experience with the beating-heart left thoracotomy approach for reoperative mitral valve surgery. Of the 125 patients undergoing this technique, 86% were in NYHA class III or IV, and 28% had undergone two or more sternotomies. Thirty-day mortality was 6.4% with low complication rates.[84] Although occasionally useful, this approach provides limited access to the other cardiac chambers as well as poor visibility. This left-sided approach is rarely needed and typically reserved for patients in whom reoperative sternotomy or right thoracotomy is considered unacceptable. A bilateral anterior thoracotomy (ie, transverse sternotomy) carried out through the fourth intercostal space also has been described.[83,85] Rarely used today, this incision transects the sternum transversely, requiring ligation of both internal mammary arteries.

Regardless of the actual approach, once cardiopulmonary bypass has been established and the heart exposed, there are several incisions that can be employed to view the underlying mitral valve. The standard left atriotomy begins with blunt dissection of the interatrial groove (ie, Waterston's groove), allowing the right atrium to be retracted medially and anteriorly (see Fig. 49-4). The right superior pulmonary vein at its junction with the left atrium then is exposed, and the left atrium is opened at the midpoint between the right superior pulmonary vein insertion and the interatrial groove. This incision is extended longitudinally both superiorly and inferiorly to give enough exposure of the mitral valve. Care must be taken to avoid inadvertent injury to the posterior wall of the left atrium, and when closing, one must avoid including the posterior wall of the right pulmonary vein. The right atrial transeptal approach has become popular in recent years, especially in reoperative valve surgery. After opening the right atrium, the interatrial septum is incised starting at the fossa ovalis and moving vertically upward for a few centimeters (Figs. 49-5 and 49-6). This technique is especially helpful in reoperative surgery because it minimizes the amount of dissection required. Superior biatrial atriotomy, left ventriculotomy, and aortotomy all have been well described[15,56,81,82,86,87] as approaches to the mitral valve; each one has varying advantages and disadvantages.

Approaches and Techniques

Resternotomy

Resternotomy is still a common approach in reoperative mitral valve surgery. In many cases, this incision provides full and adequate exposure. This is especially true when concomitant procedures are necessary. However, reoperative median sternotomy has known risks, including injury to or embolism from prior grafts, sternal dehiscence, excessive hemorrhage, and inadvertent cardiac injury.[88] Patients with valvular heart disease may be especially prone to these complications because atrial dilatation can result in significant cardiomegaly, atrial thinning, and adherence of the heart to the posterior sternum. As discussed, patients undergoing prosthetic valve reoperation have a 4% incidence of complications directly related to sternal reentry that can result directly in intraoperative death.[17,35] Resternotomy also has been noted to be particularly hazardous in the presence of patent internal mammary grafts. Injury to a patent LIMA graft has an associated mortality rate approaching 50%.[48,61] Furthermore, manipulation of patent but diseased saphenous vein grafts can result in embolization into the native coronary circulation with resulting morbidity and mortality.[88,89] Patients with previous aortic valve replacements can have difficult exposure of the mitral valve owing to anterior fixation and probably are best served by an anterolateral thoracotomy approach. In general, in the setting of reoperative surgery, the resternotomy is likely to be the most dangerous part of the operation.[90] In this situation, we also have employed techniques that avoid resternotomy, such as right thoracotomy.

Right Thoracotomy

The right anterolateral thoracotomy approach was one of the first surgical approaches to the mitral valve, and it has become a safe alternative to resternotomy for mitral valve replacement[10,48,91,92] (see Fig. 49-5). This approach provides excellent exposure of the valves (mitral and tricuspid) with minimal need for dissection within the pericardium. In our recent experience with this approach,[90,93–96] all patients had double-lumen endotracheal tubes placed, and operations were performed in the right lateral thoracotomy position. We routinely prepared and draped the right groin to allow femoral cannulation, if necessary. Preoperative and intraoperative Doppler TEE was performed in all patients, as well as standard intraoperative cardiac monitoring and

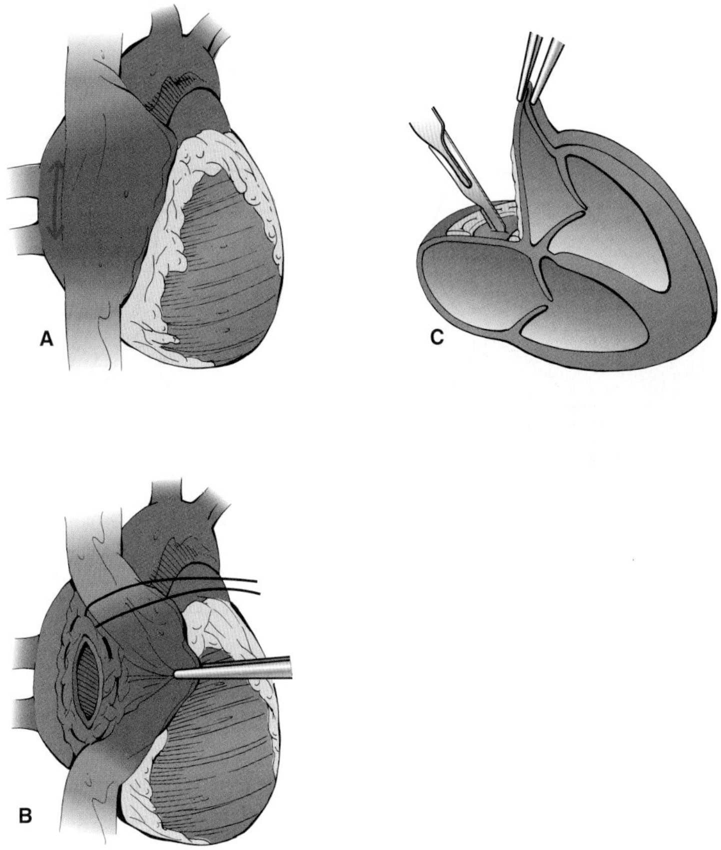

FIGURE 49-4 Sondergaard's groove approach. The left atrium enlarges to the right, increasing visualization from the right thoracotomy approach. The interatrial groove (Sondergaard's groove) is dissected approximately 1-cm deep, down to the left atrial wall. The purse-string suture is placed in the nondissected area. This prevents tearing of the dissected left atrial wall when the suture is tied down. Sagittal view shows location of the mitral valve in relation to the atriotomy. (*Used with permission from De DH, Pessella AT: Closed mitral commissurotomy utilizing right thoracotomy approach. Asian Cardiovasc Thorac Ann 2000; 8:192.*)

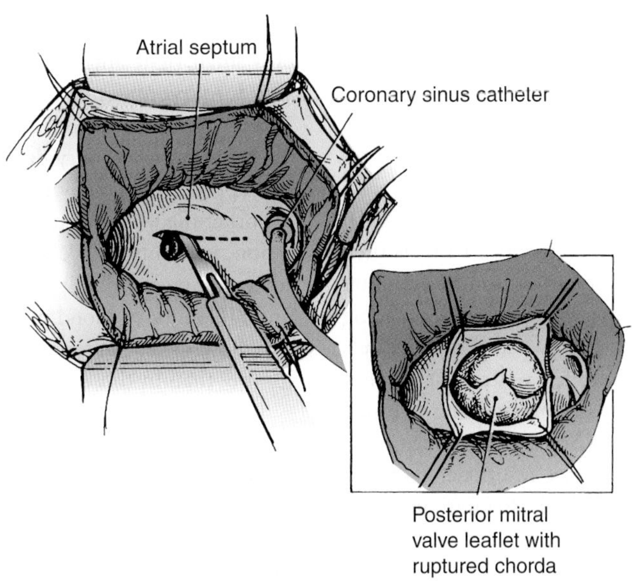

FIGURE 49-5 Atrial incision through the fossa ovalis. When the right atrium is incised, an incision is made in the atrial septum through the fossa ovalis. Retraction sutures on both the right atrium and the atrial septum of 2-0 silk then are used to elevate the septum and to keep the left atrium open. The mitral valve then will be exposed (*inset*). (*Used with permission from Byrne JG, Mitchell ME, Adams DH, et al: Minimally invasive direct access mitral valve surgery. Semin Thorac Cardiovasc Surg 1999; 11[3]:212.*)

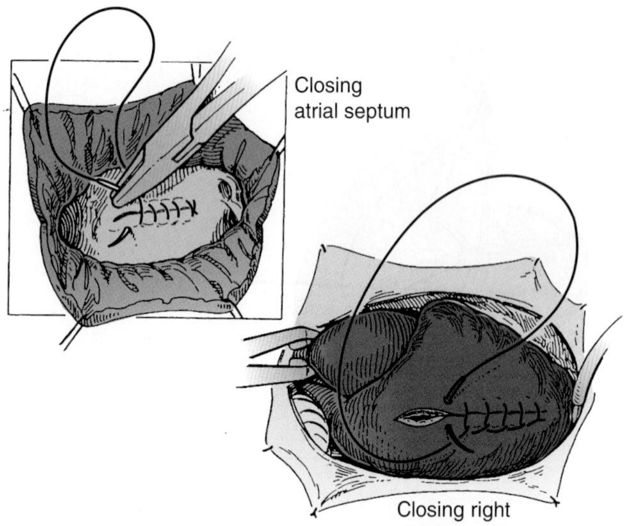

FIGURE 49-6 Closure. In the transeptal approach, the atrial septum is approximated with running 4-0 Prolene sutures and is left open until the aortic cross-clamp is removed and the air is evacuated. The left ventricle should be filled with fluid before removal of the cross-clamp to help dislodgment of intraventricular air. Once the cross-clamp has been removed, air is evacuated vigorously from the left atrium through the septum or the left atrium itself, and the sutures are tied. The right atrium is then closed with running 4-0 Prolene sutures in two layers. TEE has been very important in helping to monitor the clearing of air from the intracardiac structures. We consider it mandatory in the minimally invasive technique, in which access to the entire cardiac structure is limited. (*Used with permission from Byrne JG, Mitchell ME, Adams DH, et al: Minimally invasive direct access mitral valve surgery. Semin Thorac Cardiovasc Surg 1999; 11[3]:212.*)

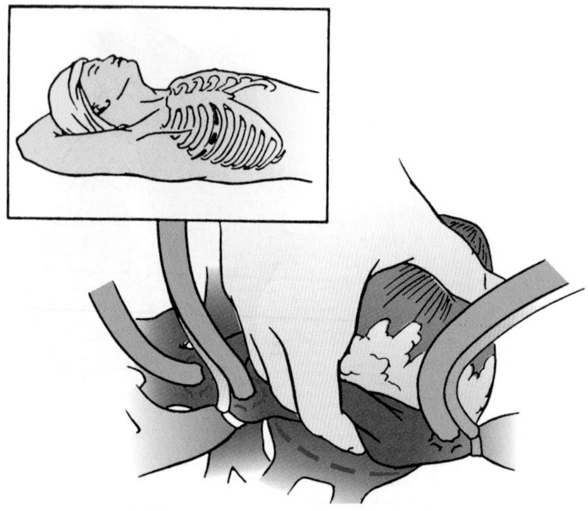

FIGURE 49-7 Right anterolateral thoracotomy through the fourth intercostal space and standard left atriotomy. (*Used with permission from Balasundaram SG, Duran C: Surgical approaches to the mitral valve. J Card Surg 1990; 5(3):163.*)

thermodilution Swan-Ganz catheterization. A right thoracotomy was made, and the chest was entered through the bed of the fourth or fifth rib. Adhesions of the right lung to the chest wall or pericardium were divided by electrocautery. The pericardium was entered anterior to the phrenic nerve. Arterial cannulation was performed via the ascending aorta with the use of a flexible aortic cannula or, alternatively, through the groin. Bicaval venous cannulation was carried out with a 28 French (DLP) cannula in the superior vena cava and a 32 French (USCI) flexible cannula in the inferior vena cava. Patients then were cooled to 20 to 25°C. Fibrillatory arrest occurred spontaneously in the majority of patients. Alternatively, a pacing Swan-Ganz catheter can be used to rapidly paced the ventricle into fibrillation. If care is used to avoid left ventricular ejection by keeping the left ventricle empty (ie, maintaining laminar, nonpulsatile arterial line tracing), a beating-heart technique also may be used. In the absence of aortic insufficiency, aortic cross-clamping usually was not required. Regurgitant flow through the aortic valve occasionally required temporary low pump flow at appropriate temperatures to avoid cerebral injury. The mitral valve then was approached through the left atrium directly by dissection of the intra-atrial (Sundergaard's) groove (see Fig. 49-4) or through the right atrium via the atrial septum (see Fig. 49-6). As the valve procedure was completed, rewarming was initiated (Fig. 49-7). Carbon dioxide (CO_2) can flood into the field and be infused directly into the left atrium and left ventricle to reduce the time spent de-airing. In addition, perfusing blood via a cannula (eg, the left ventricular vent) positioned across the mitral valve and into the left ventricle will serve to displace residual air. An aortic root vent kept on suction in the ascending aorta is used to remove any ejected air. Patients then were placed in the Trendelenburg position and de-airing ascertained under 2D TEE guidance. When core temperatures reached 37°C, the patient was weaned from cardiopulmonary bypass. Temporary atrial and ventricular pacing wires were placed and exteriorized through the chest wall. Closure then was routine. At the conclusion of the procedure, patients were returned to the supine position and reintubated with a single-lumen endotracheal tube for postoperative ventilation. The use of a small right anterior thoracotomy, femorofemoral bypass, and deep hypothermia has increased since our initial report in 1989.[97] Reduced blood use and decreased risk of LIMA or cardiac structural injury during sternal reentry make it a desirable approach for many complicated mitral reoperations. Deep hypothermia (~20°C) and low-flow femorofemoral bypass perfusion, without the necessity of aortic cross-clamping, provide adequate myocardial protection.[98] Cardiopulmonary bypass times, blood loss, blood product usage, and LIMA injury rates have been lower in reoperative patients undergoing right thoracotomy than in those with resternotomy.[35,84,87,96,98–100]

Certain issues must be considered before the right thoracotomy approach is entertained. Patients who require simultaneous coronary artery bypass grafting generally will require a median sternotomy, although isolated right-sided grafting may be performed with a thoracotomy. Simultaneous replacement of the aortic valve is difficult from a thoracotomy approach and generally should be performed through a resternotomy. Significant aortic insufficiency can make effective perfusion on cardiopulmonary bypass difficult because, after opening the left atrium, blood will be returned to the pump via the cardiotomy suction.

Unless the ascending aorta is clamped, effective end-organ perfusion will not be achieved. Also, in the setting of aortic insufficiency (AI), exposure of the mitral valve may be difficult owing to this regurgitant flow into the surgical field. Left ventricular distension and myocardial stretch injury also can occur with fibrillatory arrest in patients with and occasionally without AI. Patients with greater than minimal aortic insufficiency therefore should either be excluded from a right thoracotomy approach or expected to require aortic cross-clamping either with traditional clamping or rarely with balloon occlusion. Significant right pleural disease, especially scarring in the right hemithorax, previously has been a relative contraindication to a right thoracotomy, although our series includes two patients with a previous right thoracotomy who did not represent an overwhelming challenge.[101]

Holman and colleagues[98] reported their experience in 84 patients undergoing reoperative mitral valve surgery via right thoracotomy. Myocardial management included ventricular fibrillation in 10 patients, a beating-heart procedure in 58 patients, and hypothermic blood cardioplegia in 16 patients. The mean duration of cardiopulmonary bypass was 63 ± 56 minutes. There were no perioperative strokes, and the operative risk for patients who received cardioplegic arrest was significantly greater than in the other two groups ($p = .007$). The authors concluded that procedures on the beating or fibrillating heart were feasible in most patients and are at least as safe as surgery using cardioplegic arrest.[98]

Minimally Invasive/Port Access Right-Sided Techniques

An alternative approach to reoperative mitral valve is with minimally invasive or port access techniques. From January 2000 to July 2005, 517 patients underwent a simplified port access mitral valve procedure performed at St. Thomas Hospital in Nashville, TN. Of these 517 patients, 110 (21%) had a previous sternotomy, with 58 (11%) having a previous mitral valve procedure. All 110 operations were done with a 5-cm anterolateral thoracotomy incision through the fourth or fifth interspace under hypothermic fibrillatory arrest. Standard single-lumen endotracheal intubation was used. Cardiopulmonary bypass was instituted via femoral cannulation and vacuum-assisted venous return. Twenty-three patients (21%) had an ejection fraction of less than 30%, and 7 (6%) had an ejection fraction of less than 20%. There were no operative deaths. Skin-to-skin operative times averaged 3 hours and 18 minutes. Thirty-two percent of the patients were discharged in 5 days or less and 68% in 7 days or less (Michael R. Petracek, personal series, unpublished data). By not cross-clamping, the need for cardioplegia is eliminated, and there is minimal myocardial ischemia. The only dissection is at Waterston's groove; therefore, bleeding is decreased.

Some authors have noted that the distance to the mitral valve with the right thoracotomy approach at times can be limiting. Chitwood and colleagues recently reported use of a minithoracotomy aided by the voice-activated robotic camera AESOP.[102] Vleissus also reported 22 patients who underwent a "minimally invasive" right thoracotomy approach to the atrioventricular valves.[103] The procedures performed included mitral valve repair ($n = 12$), mitral valve replacement ($n = 5$), prosthetic mitral valve re-replacement ($n = 4$), repair of a perivalvular leak ($n = 3$), tricuspid valve repair ($n = 5$), and closure of an atrial septal defect ($n = 7$). Mean bypass time was 109 minutes with a mean fibrillatory time of 62 minutes. Operative mortality in this group was 0%, and none of the patients experienced a wound complication. At follow-up, all reoperative patients thought that their recovery from this approach was more rapid and less painful than their original sternotomy.[103] Burfeind and colleagues recently reviewed Duke University's experience with the port access technique.[104] In their series of 60 patients, a 6-cm right anterolateral thoracotomy was used with standard port access technique. Forty-five percent of patients underwent cardiac arrest with the EndoClamp technique, whereas ventricular fibrillation was used in 55% of patients. Femoral cannulation was used in all patients. When compared with concurrent cohorts of patients undergoing reoperative sternotomy or right anterolateral thoracotomy, patients undergoing the port access technique had lower mortality and decreased transfusion requirements but significantly longer cardiopulmonary bypass times. Although similar results have been found by other groups, one should be mindful of the potential hazards of the port access technique, namely, EndoClamp migration.[105–108]

Additional Techniques of Reoperative Mitral Surgery

A less common indication for reoperative mitral valve surgery but one that can be challenging is periprosthetic leak. The incidence of perivalvular leak for both mechanical and biologic valves is about 0 to 1.5% per patient-year. Of note, perivalvular leak is slightly more common with mechanical than with tissue valves, possibly owing to differences in suture technique for each and sewing ring characteristics. The regurgitant flow across the perivalvular area frequently leads to hemolysis and, through denuding of the endocardium, endocarditis. The antibacteriocidic Silzone coating on St. Jude prostheses has been shown recently to have a particular predilection for this complication.[109]

In evaluating patients with a periprosthetic leak, an assessment of valve function is important. If the valve itself is competent, direct repair of the leak avoids the hazards of valve replacement. Although pledgeted suturing may be attempted for smaller leaks, fibrotic tethering of surrounding tissue and the size of the defect may require a bovine or autologous pericardial patch. In cases of significant dehiscence or associated valvular dysfunction, removal of the valve is necessary. Replacement in this situation, however, is prone to leak recurrence because the annulus is partially intact, often calcified, and otherwise less than ideal for suture placement. In these cases, a bovine pericardial skirt can be fashioned and sewn to the sewing ring of the valve. Annular sutures then are placed in a typical fashion through the sewing ring, and the valve is seated. A running suture then can be used to sew this skirt to the left atrium (Fig. 49-8).

An additional risk of reoperative mitral valve replacement is atrioventricular disruption. Care must be used in removing the original valve sewing ring because it is frequently "socked in," and inadvertent removal of excessive annular tissue may occur.

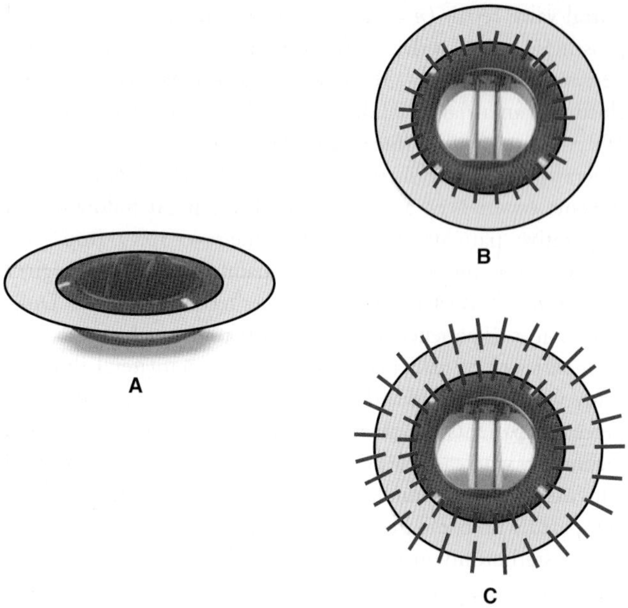

FIGURE 49-8 Pericardial skirt. Bovine pericardium can be fashioned as a skirt (**A**) and sewn to the sewing ring of the mitral prosthesis (**B**). Standard annular valve sutures are then taken through the sewing ring, the valve is seated, and the skirt is sewn to the left atrium with running technique (**C**). (Carbomedics mechanical valve shown.)

Any evidence of disruption of the posterior annulus necessitates patch repair with pericardium (autologous or bovine) before placement of annular sutures.[110] When faced with less than ideal annular tissue, and in an attempt to ensure stability, bites must not be overly aggressive in depth. Left circumflex injury can occur and will lead to significant morbidity and mortality (Fig. 49-9). When removal of the old sewing ring will result in severe annular disruption, the ring may be left in place and used as a "neoannulus" for suturing.

The benefits of preservation of the subvalvular apparatus have been clearly demonstrated during first-time mitral valve replacement.[111] Aside from improved contractile function, disruption of the posterior mitral annulus is avoided. David and colleagues found that preservation of the subvalvular apparatus is also important in reoperative patients.[112] Of 513 reoperative mitral valve replacements, preservation of the posterior subvalvular apparatus was accomplished in 103 (21%) patients, with anterior and posterior preservation occurring in 31 patients (6%). Gore-Tex neochordal construction was performed in 135 reoperative mitral valve replacement patients (26%). Perioperative mortality occurred in 3.6% of redo patients with a preserved subvalvular apparatus (native tissue and/or Gore-Tex reconstruction) versus 13.3% of redo patients without preservation ($p < .001$). Attempts at preservation of the subvalvular apparatus in reoperative patients therefore should be made.

REOPERATIVE TRICUSPID VALVE SURGERY

The need for reoperative tricuspid valve surgery most frequently occurs in high-risk patients. In a recent series of tricuspid valve replacements (TVR) by Filsoufi and colleagues,[113] 72% ($n = 58$) were reoperations. The overall operative mortality in this group was 22% ($n = 18$). Risk factors for mortality included urgent/emergent status, age greater than 50 years, functional etiology, and elevated pulmonary artery pressure. Of the 60 survivors, 26 (43%) died during follow-up. The authors concluded that patients requiring TVR are at high risk, frequently at end-stage functional class. As such, serious consideration of the risks should occur before embarking on such procedures.

Tricuspid valve endocarditis is most commonly the result of seeding of the tricuspid valve leaflets during sustained bacteremia.[114] Continued sepsis despite antibiotic therapy, heart failure owing to tricuspid insufficiency, and recurrent multiple pulmonary emboli are indications to intervene surgically in tricuspid valve endocarditis. Complete excision of the tricuspid valve (without subsequent replacement) was first advocated by Arbulu and colleagues.[114] From an infectious disease standpoint, this surgical approach has the obvious advantage of complete extirpation of the infected tissue and avoids placement of any prosthetic material. Although it is tolerated initially, the extirpation procedure inevitably leads to late-onset right-sided failure in the majority of patients.[114–116] In a 20-year follow-up of the originally reported series of 55 patients with intractable

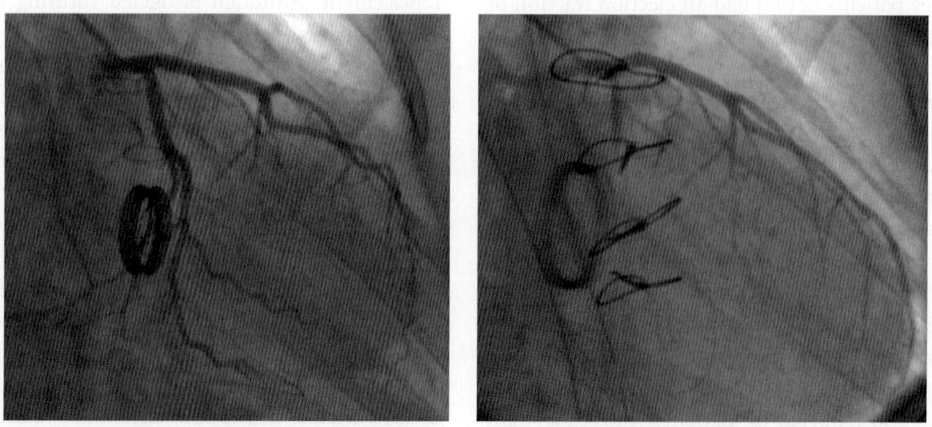

FIGURE 49-9 Left circumflex artery injury. Preoperative (*left*) and postoperative (*right*) angiograms demonstrating excessive depth of annular sutures leading to left circumflex occlusion.

right-sided endocarditis who underwent tricuspid valvectomy without replacement, two patients (4%) died in the postoperative period owing to right-sided failure. Six patients (11%) required prosthetic valve insertion 2 days to 13 years later for medically refractory right-sided heart failure. Of those who underwent reoperation (n = 6), four (66%) died. As such, severe hepatic congestion and the need for reoperative valve replacement have made this approach (without replacement) untenable to some practitioners. An alternative treatment option is to perform valvectomy followed by delayed valve replacement 3 to 9 months later.[117]

THE HYBRID APPROACH

Recently, hybrid approaches that combine percutaneous intervention (PCI) and valve surgery have been advocated for high-risk reoperative patients. In Byrne's[118] series of 26 patients undergoing initial PCI of culprit lesions followed by valve surgery (*staged hybrid* approach), almost half (46%) the patients underwent reoperation. In this way, surgical time and complexity were minimized. As a consequence, a marked reduction in mortality was observed (3.8%) compared with the predicted mortality calculated by STS algorithms (22%, range 3.5 to 63.5%). These results and those of other similar reports have led to popularization of the hybrid approach to reoperative valve surgery, as well as prompting the creation of hybrid operating rooms (combined catheter laboratory and operating room) throughout the United States.

CONCLUSION

The most common indication for valve re-replacement is structural valve degeneration of a bioprosthesis.[4] After 8 to 10 years of follow-up, biologic valves begin to deteriorate structurally, especially in young patients and in the mitral position, which exposes the valve to higher pressure gradients than seen by the aortic valve. Therefore, close follow-up should be encouraged in these patients to avoid missing early degeneration. When patients have been allowed to degenerate into higher NYHA classes, the mortality of reoperative surgery is affected directly (see Table 49-3).

KEY POINTS

1. Reoperative valve surgery most commonly involves structural deterioration of a bioprosthesis or progression of native valve disease after nonvalve surgery.
2. Bioprosthetic valves are known to undergo a time-dependent process of structural deterioration that results in a freedom of reoperation of 80% at 15 years.
3. Major risk factors in reoperative valve surgery include advanced age, impaired ejection fraction, congestive heart failure, urgency of operation, preoperative shock, concomitant coronary artery bypass surgery or presence of previous bypass grafts, prosthetic valve endocarditis, surgery for perivalvular leaks, valve thrombosis, or prosthetic dysfunction, renal dysfunction, chronic obstructive pulmonary disease, and pulmonary hypertension.

TABLE 49-3 Technical Considerations for Reoperative Valve Surgery

Consider reoperation before decline in functional status (NYHA class). Assess RV/aortic proximity to sternum preoperatively with CXR or CT scan.
Consider alternate approaches (especially with patent bypass grafts) Right thoracotomy for reoperative MVR Mini-sternotomy for reoperative AVR
Consider alternate cannulation techniques to gain safe entry, eg, groin, axillary
Address the LIMA-LAD graft if present Dissect it out and clamp it, or Cool and ignore it
Consider ease of implantation in valve choice, eg, mechanical in homograft
Use "no-touch" technique of bypass grafts
Use a conservative myocardial protection strategy Antegrade and retrograde Systemic cooling Glutamate-aspartate Warm induction/final dose ("hot shot")
If using hypothermic fibrillatory arrest, beware of AI leading to LV distension and/or obscuring operative field
Place external defibrillator pads
Consider the use of antifibrinolytic agents, eg, aprotinin, Amicar

4. The technical details listed in Table 49-2 lead to a successful aortic valve replacement after previous cardiac surgery.
5. Reoperative aortic valve surgery after homograft or root replacement can be difficult and should be simplified by replacement with a mechanical valve when possible. Reoperative root operations should be avoided if not indicated.
6. Aortic valve bypass surgery is an alternative for reoperative AVR in extremely difficult reoperative cases.
7. Transcatheter valves are likely to play a significant role in reoperative AVR in the future.
8. The right thoracotomy approach to reoperative mitral and tricuspid valves provides excellent exposure with minimal need for dissection while also avoiding prior bypass grafts. Significant aortic insufficiency and the need for bypass grafting preclude this approach.
9. Most commonly, periprosthetic leaks should be patched, rather than treated with valve replacement if the valve is functioning normally.
10. Reoperative tricuspid valve surgery occurs in high-risk patients with pulmonary hypertension with variable degrees of right heart failure. As such, this operation should be carefully considered.

REFERENCES

1. Fremes SE, Goldman BS, Ivanov J, et al: Valvular surgery in the elderly. *Circulation* 1989; 80(3 Pt 1):I77-90.
2. Pansini S, Ottino G, Forsennati PG, et al: Reoperations on heart valve prostheses: an analysis of operative risks and late results. *Ann Thorac Surg* 1990; 50(4):590-596.
3. Kirsch M, Nakashima K, Kubota S, et al: The risk of reoperative heart valve procedures in Octogenarian patients. *J Heart Valve Dis* 2004; 13(6): 991-996; discussion 6.
4. Cohn LH, Aranki SF, Rizzo RJ, et al: Decrease in operative risk of reoperative valve surgery. *Ann Thorac Surg* 1993; 56(1):15-20; discussion -1.
5. Weerasinghe A, Edwards MB, Taylor KM: First redo heart valve replacement: a 10-year analysis. *Circulation* 1999; 99(5):655-658.
6. Jones JM, O'Kane H, Gladstone DJ, et al: Repeat heart valve surgery: risk factors for operative mortality. *J Thorac Cardiovasc Surg* 2001; 122(5): 913-918.
7. Cohn LH: Evolution of redo cardiac surgery: review of personal experience. *J Cardiac Surg* 2004; 19(4):320-324.
8. Wauthy P, Goldstein JP, Demanet H, Deuvaert FE: Redo valve surgery nowadays: what have we learned? *Acta Chirurg Belgica* 2003; 103(5): 475-480.
9. O'Brien MF, Harrocks S, Clarke A, Garlick B, Barnett AG: Experiences with redo aortic valve surgery. *J Cardiac Surg* 2002; 17(1):35-39.
10. Cohn LH, Peigh PS, Sell J, DiSesa VJ: Right thoracotomy, femorofemoral bypass, and deep hypothermia for re-replacement of the mitral valve. *Ann Thorac Surg* 1989; 48(1):69-71.
11. Jones RE, Fitzgerald D, Cohn LH: Reoperative cardiac surgery using a new femoral venous right atrial cannula. *J Cardiac Surg* 1990; 5(3):170-173.
12. Aranki SF, Adams DH, Rizzo RJ, et al: Femoral veno-arterial extracorporeal life support with minimal or no heparin. *Ann Thorac Surg* 1993; 56(1):149-155.
13. Bichell DP, Balaguer JM, Aranki SF, et al: Axilloaxillary cardiopulmonary bypass: a practical alternative to femorofemoral bypass. *Ann Thorac Surg* 1997; 64(3):702-705.
14. Cohn LH, Koster JK Jr, VandeVanter S, Collins JJ Jr: The in-hospital risk of rereplacement of dysfunctional mitral and aortic valves. *Circulation* 1982; 66(2 Pt 2):I153-156.
15. Antunes MJ: Reoperations on cardiac valves. *J Heart Valve Dis* 1992; 1(1): 15-28.
16. Turina J, Hess OM, Turina M, Krayenbuehl HP: Cardiac bioprostheses in the 1990s. *Circulation* 1993; 88(2):775-781.
17. Husebye DG, Pluth JR, Piehler JM, et al: Reoperation on prosthetic heart valves. An analysis of risk factors in 552 patients. *J Thorac Cardiovasc Surg* 1983; 86(4):543-552.
18. Vogt PR, Brunner-LaRocca H, Sidler P, et al: Reoperative surgery for degenerated aortic bioprostheses: predictors for emergency surgery and reoperative mortality. *Eur J Cardiothorac Surg* 2000; 17(2):134-139.
19. Cohn LH, Couper GS, Aranki SF, Kinchla NM, Collins JJ Jr: The long-term follow-up of the Hancock Modified Orifice porcine bioprosthetic valve. *J Cardiac Surg* 1991; 6(4 Suppl):557-561.
20. Starr A, Grunkemeier GL: The expected lifetime of porcine valves. *Ann Thorac Surg* 1989; 48(3):317-318.
21. Myken PS, Caidahl K, Larsson P, et al: Mechanical versus biological valve prosthesis: a ten-year comparison regarding function and quality of life. *Ann Thorac Surg* 1995; 60(2 Suppl):S447-452.
22. Milano A, Guglielmi C, De Carlo M, et al: Valve-related complications in elderly patients with biological and mechanical aortic valves. *Ann Thorac Surg* 1998; 66(6 Suppl):S82-87.
23. Barwinsky J, Cohen M, Bhattacharya S, Kim S, Teskey J: Bjork-Shiley cardiac valves long term results: Winnipeg experience. *Can J Cardiol* 1988; 4(7):366-371.
24. Birkmeyer NJ, Marrin CA, Morton JR, et al: Decreasing mortality for aortic and mitral valve surgery in Northern New England. Northern New England Cardiovascular Disease Study Group. *Ann Thorac Surg* 2000; 70(2):432-437.
25. Peterseim DS, Cen YY, Cheruvu S, et al: Long-term outcome after biologic versus mechanical aortic valve replacement in 841 patients. *J Thorac Cardiovasc Surg* 1999; 117(5):890-897.
26. Borkon AM, Soule LM, Baughman KL, et al: Aortic valve selection in the elderly patient. *Ann Thorac Surg* 1988; 46(3):270-277.
27. Byrne JG, Karavas AN, Aklog L, et al: Aortic valve reoperation after homograft or autograft replacement. *J Heart Valve Dis* 2001; 10(4): 451-457.
28. Kouchoukos NT: Aortic allografts and pulmonary autografts for replacement of the aortic valve and aortic root. *Ann Thorac Surg* 1999; 67(6): 1846-1848; discussion 53-56.
29. Albertucci M, Wong K, Petrou M, et al: The use of unstented homograft valves for aortic valve reoperations. Review of a twenty-three-year experience. *J Thorac Cardiovasc Surg* 1994; 107(1):152-161.
30. O'Brien MF, McGiffin DC, Stafford EG, et al: Allograft aortic valve replacement: long-term comparative clinical analysis of the viable cryopreserved and antibiotic 4 degrees C stored valves. *J Cardiac Surg* 1991; 6(4 Suppl):534-543.
31. Edmunds LH Jr: Thrombotic and bleeding complications of prosthetic heart valves. *Ann Thorac Surg* 1987; 44(4):430-445.
32. Bloomfield P, Wheatley DJ, Prescott RJ, Miller HC: Twelve-year comparison of a Bjork-Shiley mechanical heart valve with porcine bioprostheses. *NEJM* 1991; 324(9):573-579.
33. Rizzoli G, Guglielmi C, Toscano G, et al: Reoperations for acute prosthetic thrombosis and pannus: an assessment of rates, relationship and risk. *Eur J Cardiothorac Surg* 1999; 16(1):74-80.
34. Deviri E, Sareli P, Wisenbaugh T, Cronje SL: Obstruction of mechanical heart valve prostheses: clinical aspects and surgical management. *J Am Coll Cardiol* 1991; 17(3):646-650.
35. Lytle BW, Cosgrove DM, Taylor PC, et al: Reoperations for valve surgery: perioperative mortality and determinants of risk for 1,000 patients, 1958-1984. *Ann Thorac Surg* 1986; 42(6):632-643.
36. Akins CW, Buckley MJ, Daggett WM, et al: Risk of reoperative valve replacement for failed mitral and aortic bioprostheses. *Ann Thorac Surg* 1998; 65(6):1545-1551; discussion 51-52.
37. Tyers GF, Jamieson WR, Munro AI, et al: Reoperation in biological and mechanical valve populations: fate of the reoperative patient. *Ann Thorac Surg* 1995; 60(2 Suppl):S464-468; discussion S8-9.
38. Birkmeyer NJ, Birkmeyer JD, Tosteson AN, et al: Prosthetic valve type for patients undergoing aortic valve replacement: a decision analysis. *Ann Thorac Surg* 2000; 70(6):1946-1952.
39. Cohn LH, Collins JJ Jr, DiSesa VJ, et al: Fifteen-year experience with 1678 Hancock porcine bioprosthetic heart valve replacements. *Ann Surg* 1989; 210(4):435-442; discussion 42-43.
40. Jamieson WR, Munro AI, Miyagishima RT, et al: Carpentier-Edwards standard porcine bioprosthesis: clinical performance to seventeen years. *Ann Thorac Surg* 1995; 60(4):999-1006; discussion 7.
41. Gaudiani VA, Grunkemeier GL, Castro LJ, Fisher AL, Wu Y: The risks and benefits of reoperative aortic valve replacement. *Heart Surg Forum* 2004; 7(2):E170-173.
42. Potter DD, Sundt TM 3rd, Zehr KJ, et al: Operative risk of reoperative aortic valve replacement. *J Thorac Cardiovasc Surg* 2005; 129(1): 94-103.

43. Phillips BJ, Karavas AN, Aranki SF, et al: Management of mild aortic stenosis during coronary artery bypass surgery: an update, 1992-2001. *J Cardiac Surg* 2003; 18(6):507-511.
44. Bortolotti U, Guerra F, Magni A, et al: Emergency reoperation for primary tissue failure of porcine bioprostheses. *Am J Cardiol* 1987; 60(10): 920-921.
45. Ban T, Soga Y: [Re-sternotomy]. *Nippon Geka Gakkai zasshi* 1998; 99(2): 63-67.
46. Aviram G, Sharony R, Kramer A, et al: Modification of surgical planning based on cardiac multidetector computed tomography in reoperative heart surgery. *Ann Thorac Surg* 2005; 79(2):589-595.
47. Gilkeson RC, Markowitz AH, Ciancibello L: Multisection CT evaluation of the reoperative cardiac surgery patient. *Radiographics* 2003; 23 Spec No:S3-17.
48. Dobell AR, Jain AK: Catastrophic hemorrhage during redo sternotomy. *Ann Thorac Surg* 1984; 37(4):273-278.
49. Elami A, Laks H, Merin G: Technique for reoperative median sternotomy in the presence of a patent left internal mammary artery graft. *J Cardiac Surg* 1994; 9(2):123-127.
50. English TA, Milstein BB: Repeat open intracardiac operation. Analysis of fifty operations. *J Thorac Cardiovasc Surg* 1978; 76(1):56-60.
51. Macmanus Q, Okies JE, Phillips SJ, Starr A: Surgical considerations in patients undergoing repeat median sternotomy. *J Thorac Cardiovasc Surg* 1975; 69(1):138-143.
52. Wideman FE, Blackstone EH, Kirklin JW, et al:Hospital mortality of re-replacement of the aortic valve. Incremental risk factors. *J Thorac Cardiovasc Surg* 1981; 82(5):692-698.
53. Cosgrove DM 3rd, Sabik JF, Navia JL: Minimally invasive valve operations. *Ann Thorac Surg* 1998; 65(6):1535-1538; discussion 8-9.
54. Cosgrove DM 3rd, Sabik JF: Minimally invasive approach for aortic valve operations. *Ann Thorac Surg* 1996; 62(2):596-597.
55. Hearn CJ, Kraenzler EJ, Wallace LK, et al: Minimally invasive aortic valve surgery: anesthetic considerations. *Anesthes Analges* 1996; 83(6):1342-1344.
56. Aklog L, Adams DH, Couper GS, et al: Techniques and results of direct-access minimally invasive mitral valve surgery: a paradigm for the future. *J Thorac Cardiovasc Surg* 1998; 116(5):705-715.
57. Byrne JG, Karavas AN, Adams DH, et al: Partial upper re-sternotomy for aortic valve replacement or re-replacement after previous cardiac surgery. *Eur J Cardiothorac Surg* 2000; 18(3):282-286.
58. Machler HE, Bergmann P, Anelli-Monti M, et al: Minimally invasive versus conventional aortic valve operations: a prospective study in 120 patients. *Ann Thorac Surg* 1999; 67(4):1001-1005.
59. Tam RK, Garlick RB, Almeida AA: Minimally invasive redo aortic valve replacement. *J Thorac Cardiovasc Surg* 1997; 114(4):682-683.
60. Byrne JG, Aranki SF, Couper GS, et al: Reoperative aortic valve replacement: partial upper hemisternotomy versus conventional full sternotomy. *J Thorac Cardiovasc Surg* 1999; 118(6):991-997.
61. Gundry SR, Shattuck OH, Razzouk AJ, et al: Facile minimally invasive cardiac surgery via ministernotomy. *Ann Thorac Surg* 1998; 65(4): 1100-1104.
62. Luciani GB, Casali G, Santini F, Mazzucco A: Aortic root replacement in adolescents and young adults: composite graft versus homograft or autograft. *Ann Thorac Surg* 1998; 66(6 Suppl):S189-193.
63. Byrne JG, Karavas AN, Cohn LH, Adams DH: Minimal access aortic root, valve, and complex ascending aortic surgery. *Curr Cardiol Repts* 2000; 2(6):549-557.
64. Byrne JG, Aranki SF, Cohn LH: Aortic valve operations under deep hypothermic circulatory arrest for the porcelain aorta: "no-touch" technique. *Ann Thorac Surg* 1998; 65(5):1313-1315.
65. Zlotnick AY, Gilfeather MS, Adams DH, Cohn LH, Couper GS: Innominate vein cannulation for venous drainage in minimally invasive aortic valve replacement. *Ann Thorac Surg* 1999; 67(3):864-865.
66. McGiffin DC, Galbraith AJ, O'Brien MF, et al: An analysis of valve re-replacement after aortic valve replacement with biologic devices. *J Thorac Cardiovasc Surg* 1997; 113(2):311-318.
67. Hasnat K, Birks EJ, Liddicoat J, et al: Patient outcome and valve performance following a second aortic valve homograft replacement. *Circulation* 1999; 100(19 Suppl):II42-47.
68. Sundt TM 3rd, Rasmi N, Wong K, et al: Reoperative aortic valve operation after homograft root replacement: surgical options and results. *Ann Thorac Surg* 1995; 60(2 Suppl):S95-99; discussion S100.
69. Yacoub M, Rasmi NR, Sundt TM, et al: Fourteen-year experience with homovital homografts for aortic valve replacement. *J Thorac Cardiovasc Surg* 1995; 110(1):186-193; discussion 93-94.
70. Kumar P, Athanasiou T, Ali A, et al: Re-do aortic valve replacement: does a previous homograft influence the operative outcome? *J Heart Valve Dis* 2004; 13(6):904-912; discussion 12-13.
71. Sadowski J, Kapelak B, Bartus K, et al: Reoperation after fresh homograft replacement: 23 years' experience with 655 patients. *Eur J Cardiothorac Surg* 2003; 23(6):996-1000; discussion 1.
72. David TE, Feindel CM, Ivanov J, Armstrong S: Aortic root replacement in patients with previous heart surgery. *J Cardiac Surg* 2004; 19(4): 325-328.
73. Matsushita T, Kawase T, Tsuda E, Kawazoe K: Apicoaortic conduit for the dilated phase of hypertrophic obstructive cardiomyopathy as an alternative to heart transplantation. *Int Cardiovasc Thorac Surg* 2009; 8(2):232-234.
74. Hirota M, Oi M, Omoto T, Tedoriya T: Apico-aortic conduit for aortic stenosis with a porcelain aorta; technical modification for apical outflow. *Int Cardiovasc Thorac Surg* 2009; 9(4):703-705.
75. Chahine JH, El-Rassi I, Jebara V: Apico-aortic valved conduit as an alternative for aortic valve re-replacement in severe prosthesis-patient mismatch. *Int Cardiovasc Thorac Surg* 2009; 9(4):680-682.
76. Gammie JS, Krowsoski LS, Brown JM, et al: Aortic valve bypass surgery: midterm clinical outcomes in a high-risk aortic stenosis population. *Circulation* 2008; 118(14):1460-1466.
77. Vassiliades TA Jr: Off-pump apicoaortic conduit insertion for high-risk patients with aortic stenosis. *Eur J Cardiothorac Surg* 2003; 23(2): 156-158.
78. Left ventricular apico-aortic conduit. CTSNet.org, 2008. (Accessed 2008, at http://www.ctsnet.org/sections/clinicalresources/videos/vg2008_luckraz_left_ventric.html.)
79. Aortic Valve Bypass Surgery: Beating Heart Therapy for Aortic Stenosis. STSA Surgical Motion Picture 2008 Annual Meeting. CTSNet.org, 2008. (Accessed 2008, at http://www.ctsnet.org/sections/clinicalresources/videos/vg2008_gammie_AorticValveBypass.html.)
80. Brinkman WT, Mack MJ: Transcatheter cardiac valve interventions. *Surg Clin North Am* 2009; 89(4):951-966.
81. McCarthy JF, Cosgrove DM 3rd: Optimizing mitral valve exposure with conventional left atriotomy. *Ann Thorac Surg* 1998; 65(4):1161-1162.
82. Balasundaram SG, Duran C: Surgical approaches to the mitral valve. *J Cardiac Surg* 1990; 5(3):163-169.
83. Saunders PC, Grossi EA, Sharony R, et al: Minimally invasive technology for mitral valve surgery via left thoracotomy: experience with forty cases. *J Thorac Cardiovasc Surg* 2004; 127(4):1026-1031; discussion 31-32.
84. Thompson MJ, Behranwala A, Campanella C, Walker WS, Cameron EW: Immediate and long-term results of mitral prosthetic replacement using a right thoracotomy beating heart technique. *Eur J Cardiothorac Surg* 2003; 24(1):47-51.
85. Brawley RK: Improved exposure of the mitral valve in patients with a small left atrium. *Ann Thorac Surg* 1980; 29(2):179-181.
86. Praeger PI, Pooley RW, Moggio RA, et al: Simplified method for reoperation on the mitral valve. *Ann Thorac Surg* 1989; 48(6):835-837.
87. Bonchek LI: Mitral valve reoperation. *Ann Thorac Surg* 1991; 51(1):160.
88. Keon WJ, Heggtveit HA, Leduc J: Perioperative myocardial infarction caused by atheroembolism. *J Thorac Cardiovasc Surg* 1982; 84(6): 849-855.
89. Grondin CM, Pomar JL, Hebert Y, et al: Reoperation in patients with patent atherosclerotic coronary vein grafts. A different approach to a different disease. *J Thorac Cardiovasc Surg* 1984; 87(3):379-385.
90. Byrne JG, Aranki SF, Adams DH, et al: Mitral valve surgery after previous CABG with functioning IMA grafts. *Ann Thorac Surg* 1999; 68(6): 2243-2247.
91. Tribble CG, Killinger WA Jr, Harman PK, et al: Anterolateral thoracotomy as an alternative to repeat median sternotomy for replacement of the mitral valve. *Ann Thorac Surg* 1987; 43(4):380-382.
92. Londe S, Sugg WL: The challenge of reoperation in cardiac surgery. *Ann Thorac Surg* 1974; 17(2):157-162.
93. Byrne JG, Hsin MK, Adams DH, et al: Minimally invasive direct access heart valve surgery. *J Cardiac Surg* 2000; 15(1):21-34.
94. Byrne JG, Mitchell ME, Adams DH, et al: Minimally invasive direct access mitral valve surgery. *Semin Thorac Cardiovasc Surg* 1999; 11(3):212-222.
95. Adams DH, Filsoufi F, Byrne JG, Karavas AN, Aklog L: Mitral valve repair in redo cardiac surgery. *J Cardiac Surg* 2002; 17(1):40-45.
96. Byrne JG, Karavas AN, Adams DH, et al: The preferred approach for mitral valve surgery after CABG: right thoracotomy, hypothermia and avoidance of LIMA-LAD graft. *J Heart Valve Dis* 2001; 10(5): 584-590.
97. Cohn LH: As originally published in 1989: Right thoracotomy, femorofemoral bypass, and deep hypothermia for re-replacement of the mitral valve. Updated in 1997. *Ann Thorac Surg* 1997; 64(2):578-579.
98. Holman WL, Goldberg SP, Early LJ, et al: Right thoracotomy for mitral reoperation: analysis of technique and outcome. *Ann Thorac Surg* 2000; 70(6):1970-1973.

99. Berreklouw E, Alfieri O: Revival of right thoracotomy to approach atrio-ventricular valves in reoperations. *Thorac Cardiovasc Surg* 1984; 32(5):331-333.
100. Braxton JH, Higgins RS, Schwann TA, et al: Reoperative mitral valve surgery via right thoracotomy: decreased blood loss and improved hemodynamics. *J Heart Valve Dis* 1996; 5(2):169-173.
101. Steimle CN, Bolling SF: Outcome of reoperative valve surgery via right thoracotomy. *Circulation* 1996; 94(9 Suppl):II126-28.
102. Bolotin G, Kypson AP, Reade CC, et al: Should a video-assisted minithoracotomy be the approach of choice for reoperative mitral valve surgery? *J Heart Valve Dis* 2004; 13(2):155-158; discussion 8.
103. Vleissis AA, Bolling SF: Mini-reoperative mitral valve surgery. *J Cardiac Surg* 1998; 13(6):468-470.
104. Burfeind WR, Glower DD, Davis RD, et al:Mitral surgery after prior cardiac operation: port-access versus sternotomy or thoracotomy. *Ann Thorac Surg* 2002; 74(4):S1323-1325.
105. Trehan N, Mishra YK, Mathew SG, et al: Redo mitral valve surgery using the port-access system. *Asian Cardiovasc Thorac Ann* 2002; 10(3): 215-218.
106. Greco E, Barriuso C, Castro MA, Fita G, Pomar JL: Port-Access cardiac surgery: from a learning process to the standard. *Heart Surg Forum* 2002; 5(2):145-149.
107. Schneider F, Falk V, Walther T, Mohr FW: Control of endoaortic clamp position during Port-Access mitral valve operations using transcranial Doppler echography. *Ann Thorac Surg* 1998; 65(5):1481-1482.
108. Onnasch JF, Schneider F, Falk V, et al: Minimally invasive approach for redo mitral valve surgery: a true benefit for the patient. *J Cardiac Surg* 2002; 17(1):14-19.
109. Schaff H, Carrel T, Steckelberg JM, et al: Artificial Valve Endocarditis Reduction Trial (AVERT): protocol of a multicenter randomized trial. *J Heart Valve Dis* 1999; 8(2):131-139.
110. Yoshikai M, Ito T, Murayama J, Kamohara K: Mitral annular reconstruction. *Asian Cardiovasc Thorac Ann* 2002; 10(4):344-345.
111. Hansen DE, Cahill PD, DeCampli WM, et al: Valvular-ventricular interaction: importance of the mitral apparatus in canine left ventricular systolic performance. *Circulation* 1986; 73(6):1310-1320.
112. Borger MA, Yau TM, Rao V, Scully HE, David TE: Reoperative mitral valve replacement: importance of preservation of the subvalvular apparatus. *Ann Thorac Surg* 2002; 74(5):1482-1487.
113. Filsoufi F, Anyanwu AC, Salzberg SP, et al: Long-term outcomes of tricuspid valve replacement in the current era. *Ann Thorac Surg* 2005; 80(3): 845-850.
114. Arbulu A, Holmes RJ, Asfaw I: Surgical treatment of intractable right-sided infective endocarditis in drug addicts: 25 years experience. *J Heart Valve Dis* 1993; 2(2):129-137; discussion 38-39.
115. Khonsari S, Sintek C, Ardehali A. *Cardiac Surgery: Safeguards and Pitfalls in Operative Technique*, 4th ed. Philadelphia, Lippincott Williams & Wilkins; 2008.
116. Yee ES, Ullyot DJ: Reparative approach for right-sided endocarditis. Operative considerations and results of valvuloplasty. *J Thorac Cardiovasc Surg* 1988; 96(1):133-140.
117. Greelish JP, Cohn LH, Leacche M, et al: Minimally invasive mitral valve repair suggests earlier operations for mitral valve disease. *J Thorac Cardiovasc Surg* 2003; 126(2):365-371; discussion 71-73.
118. Byrne JG, Leacche M, Unic D, et al: Staged initial percutaneous coronary intervention followed by valve surgery ("hybrid approach") for patients with complex coronary and valve disease. *J Am Coll Cardiol* 2005; 45(1):14-18.

PART 5

DISEASES OF THE GREAT VESSELS

CHAPTER 50

Aortic Dissection

Carlos M. Mery
T. Brett Reece
Irving L. Kron

INTRODUCTION

Thoracic aortic dissection occurs when an intimal tear allows redirection of blood flow from the aorta (true lumen) through the intimal defect into the media of the aortic wall (false lumen). A dissection plane that separates the intima from the overlying adventitia forms within the media. The acute form of aortic dissection is often rapidly lethal, whereas those surviving the initial event go on to develop a chronic dissection with more protean manifestations. The purpose of this chapter is to review the etiology and pathogenesis of aortic dissection, examine current diagnostic algorithms, and provide detailed descriptions of contemporary surgical techniques for treatment. Additional information regarding follow-up and the subsequent management of these patients is presented to provide a comprehensive understanding of a clinical entity that has challenged physicians and surgeons for centuries.

HISTORY

Sennertus is credited with the first description of the dissection process, but the earliest detailed descriptions of the clinical entity appeared in the seventeenth and eighteenth centuries, during which time Maunoir named the process aortic "dissection." Laennec defined the propensity of the chronically dissected aorta to become aneurysmal. Aortic dissection was exclusively a postmortem diagnosis until the first part of the twentieth century, but in 1935 Gurin attempted surgical intervention with the first aortic fenestration procedure to treat malperfusion syndrome.[1] In 1949, Abbott and Paulin advanced surgical treatment by theoretically preventing aortic rupture by wrapping the aorta with cellophane. Other attempts at surgical treatment over the years met with limited clinical success, although certain concepts regarding surgical management are still in use today.[2] With the advent of cardiopulmonary bypass, DeBakey and Cooley forever altered the natural history of aortic dissection by successfully performing primary surgical repair using techniques not remarkably different from contemporary procedures.[3] Investigators such as Wheat made substantial contributions by defining physiologically based medical management algorithms to complement surgical correction.[4] There is still considerable controversy regarding surgical versus medical treatment of certain forms of acute thoracic aortic dissection.

CLASSIFICATION

The classification systems used for aortic dissection are based on the location and extent of dissection. The particular type is then subclassified based on the timing of dissection. Acute dissection has traditionally been used to describe presentation within the first 2 weeks, whereas the term *chronic* is reserved for those patients presenting at more than 2 months after the initial event. The more recently added subacute designation is sometimes used to describe the period between 2 weeks and 2 months.

Two classification systems are most frequently used in clinical practice: the DeBakey and the Stanford systems (Fig. 50-1). The DeBakey system differentiates patients based on the location and extent of aortic dissection.[5] The advantage of this system is that four different groups of patients with different forms of aortic dissection emerge. This structure provides the greatest opportunity for subsequent comparative research. In contrast, the Stanford system proposed by Daily et al. is a functional classification system.[6] All dissections that involve the

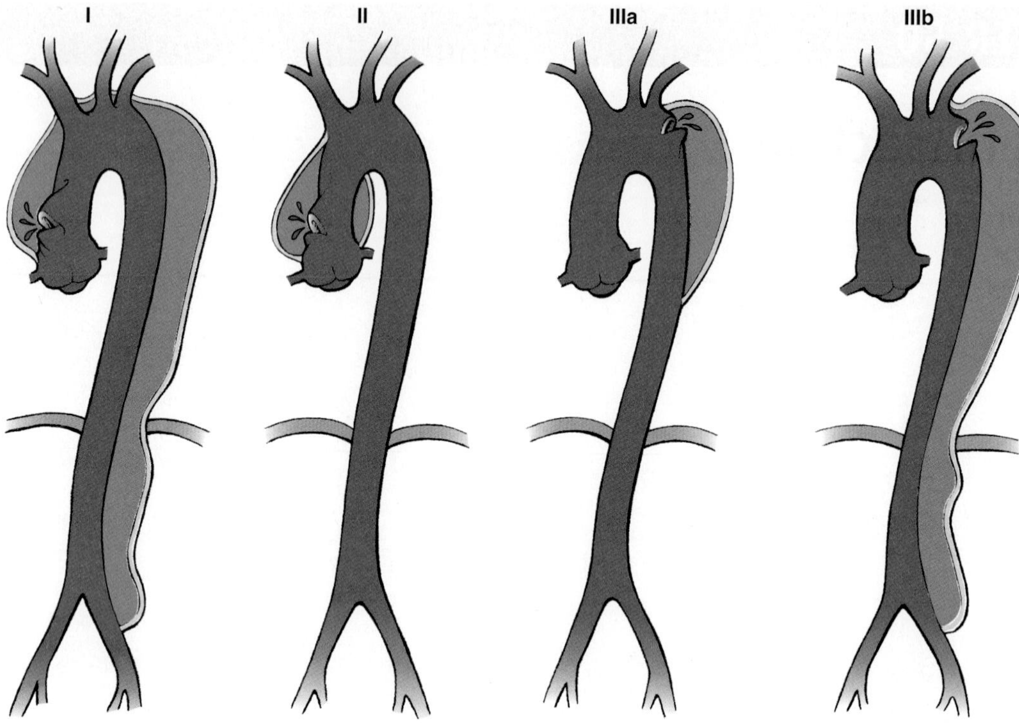

FIGURE 50-1 Classification of aortic dissection. DeBakey type I and Stanford type A include dissections that involve the proximal aorta, arch, and descending thoracic aorta. DeBakey type II only involves the ascending aorta; this dissection is included in the Stanford type A. DeBakey type III and Stanford type B include dissections that originate in the descending thoracic and thoracoabdominal aorta regardless of any retrograde involvement of the arch. These are subdivided into subtypes a and b, depending on abdominal aortic involvement.

ascending aorta are grouped together as type A, regardless of the position of the primary tear or the distal extent of the dissection. Proponents of the simpler Stanford system contend that the clinical behavior of patients with aortic dissection is essentially determined by involvement of the ascending aorta. Critics, however, suggest that individual patients in the type A classification may be quite different from one another depending on the distal extent. Drawing clinical conclusions from such a potentially heterogeneous patient population has inherent limitations. However, because of its simplicity, practicality, and widespread use, the Stanford system is used throughout this chapter.

INCIDENCE

Aortic dissection is the most frequently diagnosed lethal condition of the aorta. Dissection occurs nearly three times as frequently as rupture of abdominal aortic aneurysm in the United States.[7] There is an estimated worldwide prevalence of 0.5 to 2.95 per 100,000 per year; the prevalence ranges from 0.2 to 0.8 per 100,000 per year in the United States, resulting in roughly 2000 new cases per year.[8] These figures are only an estimate. In one autopsy series, the antemortem diagnosis was made in only 15% of patients, revealing that many immediately fatal events go undiagnosed.[9] Clinically, type A dissections occur with an overall greater frequency (Table 50-1).

ETIOLOGY AND PATHOGENESIS

Several hypotheses exist regarding the etiology of the intimal disruption (primary tear) that permits aortic blood flow to create a cleavage plane within the media of the aortic wall. This was originally viewed as a consequence of a biochemical abnormality within the media on which normal mechanical forces in the aorta acted to create an intimal tear. The link between the abnormal media, termed *cystic medial necrosis* or *degeneration*, and the primary tear has not been scientifically established. In fact, medial degeneration is found in only a minority of patients with acute aortic dissection, and most are children.[10] This theory has lost support over the years.

Alternatively, there are data supporting a relationship between aortic dissections and intramural hematoma. Advocates of this theory suggest that bleeding from vasa vasorum into the media creates a mass that results in localized areas of increased stress in the intima during diastole. These areas then permit intimal disruption. In fact, between 10 and 20% of patients thought to have acute aortic dissection are found to have intramural hematoma, suggesting that it may be a precursor to dissection.[11] Penetrating atherosclerotic ulcers have been implicated as the source of intimal disruption in some cases; thus many centers treat penetrating ulcers of the ascending aorta similarly to true dissections.[12] Although it may apply to certain patients, enthusiasm for the penetrating ulcer mechanism causing all dissections has waned. The pattern of atherosclerotic

TABLE 50-1 Clinical Characteristics of Patients Presenting with Acute Type A and B Thoracic Aortic Dissections

	Type A	Type B
Frequency	60–75%	25–40%
Sex (M:F)	1.7–2.6:1	2.3–3:1
Age (y)	50–56	60–70
Hypertension	++	+++
Connective tissue disorder	++	+
Pain		
Retrosternal	+++	+, −
Interscapular	+, −	+++
Syncope	++	+−
Cerebrovascular accident	+	−
Congestive heart failure	+	−
Aortic valve regurgitation	++	+, −
Myocardial infarction	+	−
Pericardial effusion	+, −	+++
Pleural effusion	+, −	+, −
Abdominal pain	+, −	+, −
Peripheral pulse deficit	Upper and lower extremities	Lower extremities

TABLE 50-2 Risk Factors for Type A and B Thoracic Aortic Dissection

Hypertension
Connective tissue disorders Ehlers-Danlos syndrome Marfan's disease Turner's syndrome
Cystic medial disease of aorta
Aortitis
Iatrogenic
Atherosclerosis
Thoracic aortic aneurysm
Bicuspid aortic valve
Trauma
Pharmacologic
Coarctation of the aorta
Hypervolemia (pregnancy)
Congenital aortic stenosis
Polycystic kidney disease
Pheochromocytoma
Sheehan's syndrome
Cushing's syndrome

involvement of the thoracic aorta resulting in penetrating ulcer and the frequency of dissection throughout the aorta do not support this theory.

Although no single disorder is responsible for aortic dissection, several risk factors have been identified that can damage the aortic wall and lead to dissection (Table 50-2). These include direct mechanical forces on the aortic wall (ie, hypertension, hypervolemia, derangements of aortic flow) and forces that affect the composition of the aortic wall (ie, connective tissue disorders or direct chemical destruction). Hypertension is the mechanical force most often associated with dissection and is found in greater than 75% of cases.[8] Although the role of increased strain on the aortic wall is intuitive, the mechanism by which hypertension actually leads to dissection is unclear. Similarly, hypervolemia, high cardiac output, and an abnormal hormonal milieu certainly contribute to the increased incidence of dissection in pregnancy, but the mechanism is unclear. Atherosclerosis is not a risk factor for aortic dissection except in preexisting aneurysms or in the case of atherosclerotic ulceration.

Iatrogenic trauma to the aortic intima may result in dissection. Catheterization procedures, aortic root and femoral artery cannulation for cardiopulmonary bypass, aortic cross-clamping, surgical procedures performed on the aorta (aortic valve replacement and aorto-coronary bypass grafting), and placement of intra-aortic balloon pumps have all been reported to result in dissection. Aortic transection as a result of trauma rarely results in excessive dissection and deserves differentiation from the process of aortic dissection. This process is usually limited to the aortic isthmus and in addition to the risk of rupture may present as a circular prolapse of the intima and media producing aortic obstruction referred to as "pseudo-coarctation" (Fig. 50-2).

Once a cleavage plane exists in the media, the aortic wall floating within the lumen is termed the *dissection flap* and is composed of the aortic intima and partial-thickness media. The primary tear is usually greater than 50% of the circumference of the aorta. Full aortic circumference is rarely involved, but may carry a worse prognosis. The primary tear in type A dissection is usually located on the right anterior aspect of the ascending aorta and follows a somewhat predictable course, spiraling around the arch and into the descending thoracic and abdominal aorta on the left and posteriorly. The dissection may propagate in

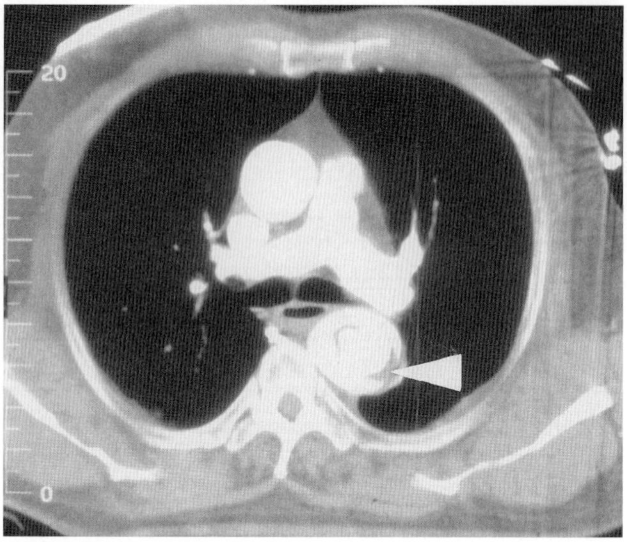

FIGURE 50-2 Axial image of CT arteriogram showing a nearly circumferential dissection flap (*arrowhead*) as a result of acute traumatic aortic dissection.

a retrograde fashion for a variable distance as well to involve the coronary ostia; this occurs in roughly 11% of all dissections.[11] Myocardial ischemia or aortic rupture into the pericardium are the causes of death in as many as 80% of mortalities from acute dissection. Often the distal false lumen communicates with the true lumen through one or more fenestrations within the dissection flap. The false lumen may also end blindly in as many as 4 to 12% of patients, in which case blood in the false lumen frequently thromboses. The false lumen may also penetrate the adventitia, causing rupture and death. Regardless of whether the true and false lumens communicate, perfusion of aortic side branches may be compromised by the dissection, resulting in end-organ ischemia (Fig. 50-3). If these acute complications are avoided, the weakened outer aortic wall, composed of partial media and the adventitia, may dilate over time, resulting in aneurysm formation. This evolving dilatation is the reason for operation in the majority of chronic dissections regardless of type.

The remaining adventitia provides most of the tensile strength of the aortic wall with minimal contribution from the media. The media is composed of concentrically arranged smooth muscle interposed with connective tissue proteins such as collagen, elastin, and fibrillin within the ground substance. Abnormal constituents of the media, as in certain connective tissue disorders such as Marfan's disease and Ehlers-Danlos syndrome, are associated with aortic dissection. Marfan's syndrome is an autosomal dominant inherited disorder in which a point mutation in the fibrillin-1 gene (FBN1) located on the long arm of chromosome 15 results in an abnormal media. The incidence of Marfan's syndrome is approximately 1 per 5000 live births.[13] There are, however, many incomplete forms of the disease, and as many as 25% may be sporadic in which no known fibrillin abnormalities are observed. Type IV Ehlers-Danlos syndrome is a connective tissue disorder of the proα1(III) chain of type III collagen with an incidence of 1 in 5000.[14] The structurally abnormal media is susceptible to dissection. Of note, there are also familial aggregations of dissection without discernable biochemical or genetic abnormalities.[7]

CLINICAL PRESENTATION

Signs and Symptoms

As many as 40% of patients suffering from acute aortic dissection die immediately. Those surviving the initial event may be stabilized with medical management, and it is these patients in whom subsequent therapeutic intervention on aortic dissection has altered the natural history of the disease. The clinical outcome is eventually determined by dissection type and timing of presentation, patient-related factors, and the quality and experience of the individuals and institution providing care.

The initial evaluation of a stable patient with suspected aortic dissection includes a detailed history and physical

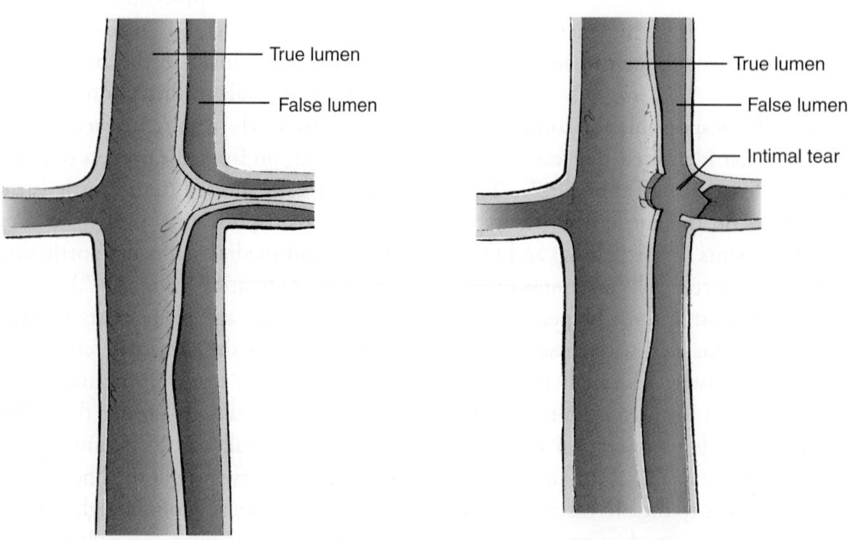

FIGURE 50-3 Diagram of aortic dissection. (A) An intact dissection membrane compresses the true lumen and causes malperfusion of a branch artery. (B) Rupture of the dissection membrane that may or may not restore blood flow to the branch.

examination focusing on those elements likely to rule in the diagnosis. Most importantly, the diagnosis of aortic dissection requires a high level of suspicion. Up to 30% of patients ultimately diagnosed with acute dissection are first thought to have another diagnosis. Aortic dissection should always be considered in the setting of severe, unrelenting chest pain, which is present in most patients. Patients usually have no previous episodes of similar pain, which often causes anxiety. Pain is usually located in the midsternum for ascending aortic dissection, while in the interscapular region for descending thoracic aortic dissection (see Table 50-1). The location of maximum pain tends to change as the dissection extends in an antegrade or retrograde direction. Such "migratory pain" should arouse clinical suspicion. The character of the pain is often described as "ripping" or "tearing." The pain is constant with greatest intensity at the onset. Although painless dissection has been described, it usually occurs in the setting of an existing aneurysm in which the pain of a new dissection may not be differentiated from chronic aneurysm pain. Patients may also present with signs or symptoms related to malperfusion of the brain, limbs, or visceral organs. These findings confuse the true diagnosis, as the obvious signs of ischemia distract the historian from a less apparent initial episode of pain.

Elements of the past medical history such as primary hypertension, presence of aneurysmal disease of the aorta, or familial connective tissue disorders are useful as risk factors to help establish the diagnosis. Illicit drug use is an increasingly important predisposition to ascertain during the initial evaluation. The differential diagnosis of chest pain as a result of aortic dissection includes diagnoses such as myocardial ischemia, aortic aneurysm, acute aortic regurgitation, pericarditis, musculoskeletal pain, and pulmonary embolus. It is essential to consider aortic dissection in each case, as specific therapy (eg, thrombolytic therapy for acute myocardial infarction) may impact the survivability of acute dissection.

Patients suffering acute dissection appear ill. Tachycardia is usually accompanied by hypertension in the setting of baseline essential hypertension and increased catecholamine levels from pain and anxiety. Hypotension and tachycardia may result from aortic rupture, pericardial tamponade, acute aortic valve regurgitation, or even acute myocardial ischemia with involvement of the coronary ostia. An abnormal peripheral vascular examination is present in a minority of patients with acute aortic dissection, but when present an abnormal pulse exam may indicate the type of dissection. Absence of pulses in the upper extremity suggests ascending aortic involvement, whereas pulse deficits in the lower extremities speak to involvement of the distal aorta. These findings are subject to change as the dissection progresses or reentry into the true lumen occurs. Auscultation of the heart may reveal a diastolic murmur consistent with acute aortic regurgitation or an S3, indicating left heart volume overload. Physical exam findings such as jugular venous distention and a pulsus paradoxus are signs of pericardial tamponade that should be identified in any unstable patient to initiate the correct diagnostic and treatment algorithms. Unilateral loss of breath sounds, usually the left, may indicate hemothorax as a result of aortic leak or rupture with hemothorax. Alternatively, a pleural effusion may exist secondary to pleural inflammation related to the dissection. This finding requires additional evaluation before treatment.

A complete central and peripheral neurologic exam is critical in that abnormalities are present in up to 40% of acute type A dissections. Involvement of the brachiocephalic vessels with loss of brain perfusion may result in transient syncope or stroke. Syncope may also result from rupture into the pericardium and is an ominous sign. Stroke rarely improves with restoration of blood flow and may even cause hemorrhage and brain death, yet surgery is indicated in such patients. Fortunately, stroke is a presenting feature in fewer than 5% of patients with acute type A dissection. Loss of perfusion to intercostals or lumbar arteries may result in spinal cord ischemia and paraplegia. Peripheral nerve ischemia as a result of malperfusion may yield findings similar to spinal cord malperfusion and should be discerned as these patients often improve with restoration of blood flow. Acute aortic dissection may also cause superior vena cava syndrome, vocal cord paralysis, hematemesis, Horner's syndrome, hemoptysis, and airway compression as a result of local compression and mass effect.

Malperfusion of aortic branch vessels may occur from the coronary ostia to the aortic bifurcation and may dominate the presentation of certain patients. Although autopsy series yield a greater percentage of patients with evidence of malperfusion, clinical series reveal that dissection is not infrequently complicated by malperfusion of at least one organ system (Table 50-3).[15] Compression of the true lumen by the false lumen is the mechanism by which aortic branch vessel occlusion occurs in the majority of cases. Branch vessels may also be completely sheared off the true lumen and perfused to various degrees by the false lumen.

Chronic aortic dissection is usually asymptomatic. It may be incidentally discovered following an asymptomatic acute dissection, most often in patients with a preexisting aortic aneurysm. Some patients eventually require surgical treatment for chronic dissection and most do so as a result of aneurysmal dilatation of a chronically dissected aortic segment. Presenting complaints often include intermittent, dull chest pain, or even severe skeletal pain from erosion into the bony thorax with large or rapidly expanding aneurysms. Aortic insufficiency may develop with chronic type A dissection and present with typical

TABLE 50-3 Frequency and Location of Malperfusion in Acute Type A and B Thoracic Aortic Dissection

Vascular System	Frequency
Renal	23–75%
Extremities (upper and lower)	25–60%
Mesenteric	10–20%
Coronary	5–11%
Cerebral	3–13%
Spinal	2–9%

features of congestive failure, including fatigue, dyspnea, and mild, dull chest pain. Infrequently, chronic dissection may result in paralysis/paraplegia from loss of vital intercostal arteries or even distal embolization of thrombus or atheroma from the false lumen. Malperfusion syndrome is an uncommon presentation for patients with chronic dissection given the likelihood that the true and false lumens communicate.

Diagnostic Studies

Routine diagnostic studies including blood tests, chest x-ray, and electrocardiogram (ECG) should be obtained, but are often not sufficient to establish the diagnosis of acute aortic dissection. ECG often reveals no ischemic changes. Obvious ischemic changes are present in up to 20% of acute type A dissections, whereas only nonspecific repolarization abnormalities are present in nearly one third of patients with coronary ostial involvement. The ECG may also reveal left ventricular hypertrophy in those patients with long-standing hypertension. The chest x-ray is abnormal in 60% to 90% of patients with acute dissection (Fig. 50-4). Although most patients have at least one, if not several abnormal findings, a normal chest x-ray does not rule out the diagnosis. Blood should be drawn and sent for complete blood count, serum and electrolytes, creatine kinase with myocardial isoenzymes, troponin, and blood type and screen. These tests obtained at the time of initial observation are usually unremarkable. There is frequently a mild to moderate leukocytosis. Anemia may result from sequestration of blood or hemolysis. Liver function tests, serum creatinine, myoglobin, and lactic acid may all be abnormal in the setting of certain malperfusion syndromes.

Diagnostic Imaging

Diagnostic imaging is essential to clarify the anatomy of an acute aortic dissection, regardless of clinical certainty of diagnosis or the acuity of the patient. The diagnosis should be made rapidly with minimal distress for the patient. Two imaging modalities currently meet these criteria and are used to diagnose acute aortic dissection: computed tomography (CT) and echocardiography. Magnetic resonance imaging (MRI) and aortography, with or without intravascular ultrasound (IVUS), are used to diagnose acute aortic dissection but are second-line modalities for various reasons. The benefits, disadvantages, and diagnostic accuracy of each are useful when choosing the most appropriate study for a particular clinical situation (Table 50-4). Each test provides disruption, reentry points, whether there is flow or thrombus in the false lumen, status of the aortic valve, presence and nature of myocardial ischemia, and brachiocephalic and aortic branch vessel involvement. Specific data may be necessary for operative planning and subsequent management to define the imaging study most appropriate for a particular patient.

TABLE 50-4 Sensitivity and Specificity of Various Imaging Modalities Useful for the Diagnosis of Thoracic Aortic Dissection

Imaging Study	Sensitivity	Specificity
Aortography	80–90%	88–93%
Computed tomography	90–100%	90–100%
Intravascular ultrasound	94–100%	97–100%
Echocardiography		
Transthoracic	60–80%	80–96%
Transesophageal	90–99%	85–98%
Magnetic resonance imaging	98–100%	98–100%

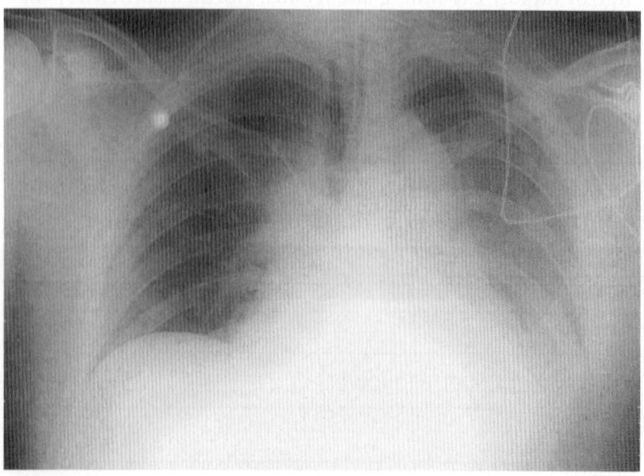

FIGURE 50-4 Plain chest x-ray exhibiting many features of acute type A dissection, such as a widened mediastinum, rightward tracheal displacement, irregular aortic contour with loss of the aortic knob, an indistinct aortopulmonary window, and a left pleural effusion.

Helical CT scanning is widely available and is now the most frequently used test to diagnose acute aortic dissection. It requires intravenous contrast medium that may limit its use in certain clinical situations but generates images familiar to most practitioners and has a high sensitivity and specificity. This technique can be performed quickly, fulfilling the requirements for use in the early management of acute dissection. Additional structures such as the pleural and pericardial spaces are imaged. When performed and formatted as an arteriogram, aortic branch vessels may also be evaluated: Involvement of the brachiocephalic vessels is identified with nearly 96% accuracy. The diagnosis of dissection requires two or more channels separated by a dissection flap (Fig. 50-5). Transaxial two-dimensional images can be reconstructed to display three-dimensional images of the aorta that not only aid in diagnosis but also are useful for operative planning.

Transesophageal echocardiography (TEE) is currently the second most frequently used study for making the diagnosis of acute aortic dissection. It is widely available, requires no intravenous contrast or radiation, and generates dynamic images of the aorta from which the diagnosis can be made (Fig. 50-6). It requires operator expertise both to acquire the necessary images and to conduct the examination safely. Although the safest

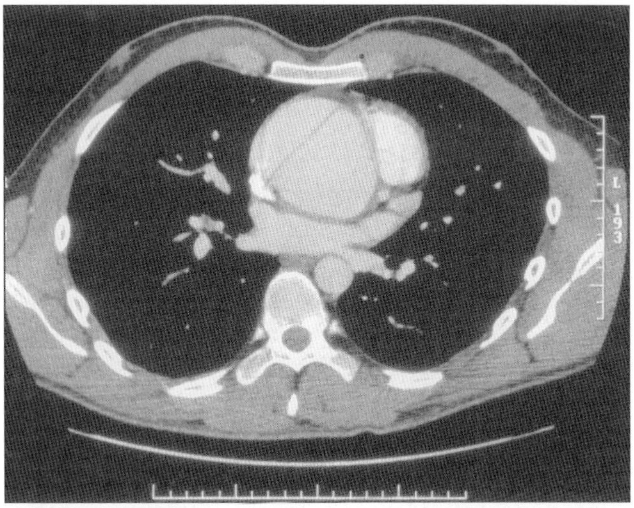

FIGURE 50-5 Axial image of CT arteriogram of acute type A dissection showing a dissection flap in the mid-ascending aorta.

setting in which to perform TEE is the operating room under general anesthesia, it can be performed in a monitored setting using topical anesthesia and light sedation. Patient comfort is paramount in this situation as rupture has been reported during difficult studies and a complete examination of the entire aorta is necessary to exclude the diagnosis of acute dissection. Absolute contraindications to TEE include esophageal abnormalities such as varices, stricture, or tumor. A full stomach or recent meal are relative contraindications, but recognition of these conditions permits safe examination with few complications in the vast majority of patients. Criteria for making the diagnosis of acute aortic dissection include visualization of an echogenic surface separating two distinct lumens, repeatedly, in more than one view, and that can be differentiated from normal surrounding cardiac structures. The true lumen is identified by expansion during systole and collapse during diastole. Communication of the false lumen is found by identifying distal tears in the flap and flow in the false lumen with the addition of color Doppler. Similarly, the absence of flow indicates false lumen thrombosis. TEE additionally may provide high-quality images of the aortic valve and pericardial space. The coronary ostia are directly evaluated and regional left ventricular function may be assessed to identify myocardial ischemia indirectly. Color flow Doppler reliably quantifies aortic regurgitation and may be used to assess for additional valvular abnormalities. The pericardium and pleural space are also visualized and therefore effusions may be identified.

Transthoracic echocardiography (TTE) provides images of the ascending aorta and sections of the aortic arch that may yield the diagnosis but with much less sensitivity than transesophageal imaging. As such, transthoracic imaging may prove useful but is generally insufficient to reliably establish the diagnosis. Transthoracic evaluation is additionally limited by patient-related factors including body habitus, emphysema, and mechanical ventilation. A negative transthoracic study should be complemented by a transesophageal study, which provides greater detail of the entire aorta.

Aortography was the first study used to diagnose acute dissection in 1939 and until recently was considered the gold standard for diagnosis. It is an invasive test requiring nephrotoxic contrast media in which the aorta is visualized in multiple two-dimensional projections. The diagnosis of dissection depends on visualization of the intimal flap, two distinct lumens, or compression of the true lumen by flow through an adjacent false lumen (Fig. 50-7). Indirect signs of dissection include the presence of branch vessel abnormalities and abnormal intimal contour on injection of the false lumen. The status of the aortic valve may be evaluated and coronary angiography in the setting of type A dissections is possible only with this diagnostic test. However, coronary angiography is not recommended given that the coronary ostia are involved in 10 to 20% of acute type A dissections and are easily evaluated at the time of surgery. Coronary atherosclerosis is present in 25% of all patients with acute aortic dissection, but even in those patients repair of the dissection should take precedence. Aortography is sometimes useful in acute type B dissections with evidence of mesenteric ischemia or oliguria and in type A dissections with signs of malperfusion because catheter-based intervention may be possible. Aortography can have a high false-negative rate

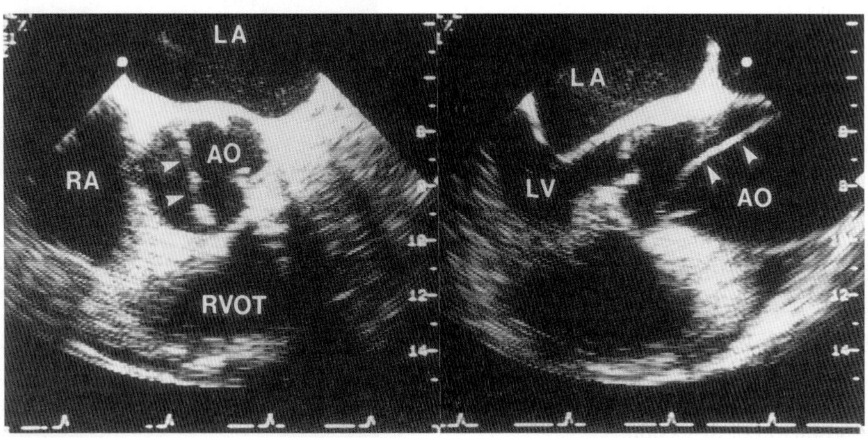

FIGURE 50-6 Transesophageal echocardiogram showing the dissection membrane (*arrows*) in the short (*left panel*) and long (*right panel*) views of a type A dissection.

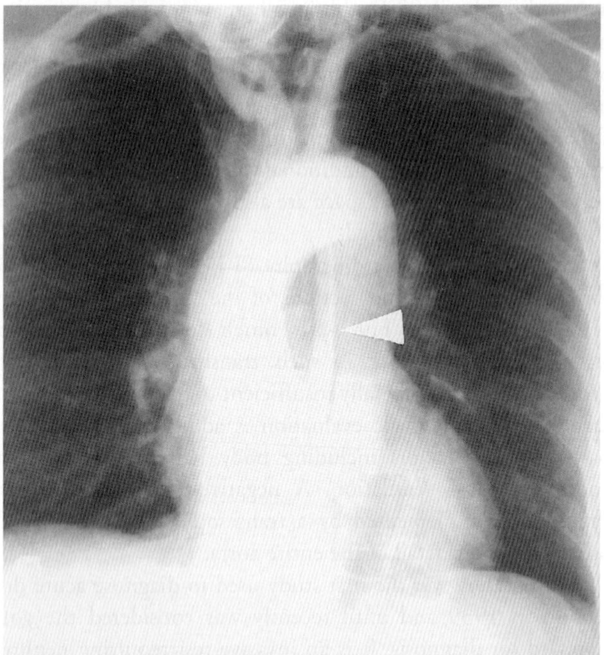

FIGURE 50-7 Aortogram of acute type B dissection illustrating differential contrast enhancement of the true and false lumens in the descending thoracic aorta. The intimal flap (*arrowhead*) can be seen separating the two lumens.

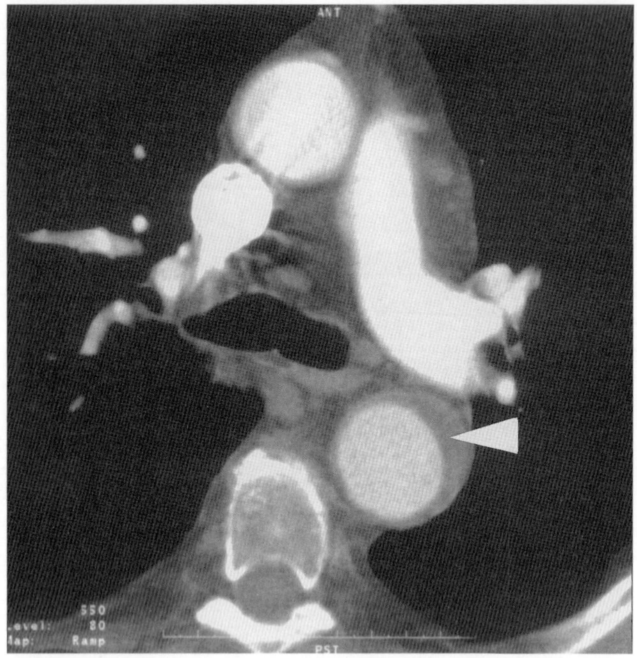

FIGURE 50-8 Axial image from a CT arteriogram showing an intramural hematoma of the descending thoracic aorta (*arrowhead*).

secondary to thrombosis of one lumen or when contrast equally opacifies each lumen, impairing distinction of a separate true and false lumen.[9] The diagnosis of intramural hematoma may also be difficult given the absence of intimal disruption, whereas penetrating atherosclerotic ulcer is usually easily visualized. Visualization of the dissection variants is best accomplished with either CT scanning or MRI (Figs. 50-8 and 50-9). One major limitation to the use of aortography in the acute setting is the need for skilled personnel. The time required to assemble this team varies with each institution, rendering aortography less useful when compared with other immediately available diagnostic tests. Aortography also requires arterial access, which can be painful and precipitate rupture or dissection extension.

IVUS is a catheter-based imaging tool that provides dynamic imaging of the aortic wall and an intimal flap in patients with aortic dissection. It is particularly useful in delineating the proximal and distal extent of dissection and for identifying the true and false lumens in questionable cases during aortography. High-resolution images of the normal three-layered aortic wall are differentiated to identify the abnormally thin wall adjacent to the false lumen. Because the aortic wall itself is imaged, intramural hematoma and penetrating atherosclerotic ulcers may also be identified. Currently, as an isolated imaging study, it is time consuming and requires skilled personnel, as with aortography, and generally is not useful as an initial study in the acute setting. It may be most useful in combination with aortography when the initial imaging studies are negative, yet there remains a high clinical suspicion of dissection.

MRI and the newer contrast-enhanced magnetic resonance angiography (MRA) generate superior images reliably demonstrating aortic dissection (Fig. 50-10). In fact, some consider this the gold standard imaging study given the published diagnostic accuracy. Dissection is identified as an intraluminal membrane separating two or more channels (Fig. 50-11). MRI provides detailed images of the entire aorta, the pericardium,

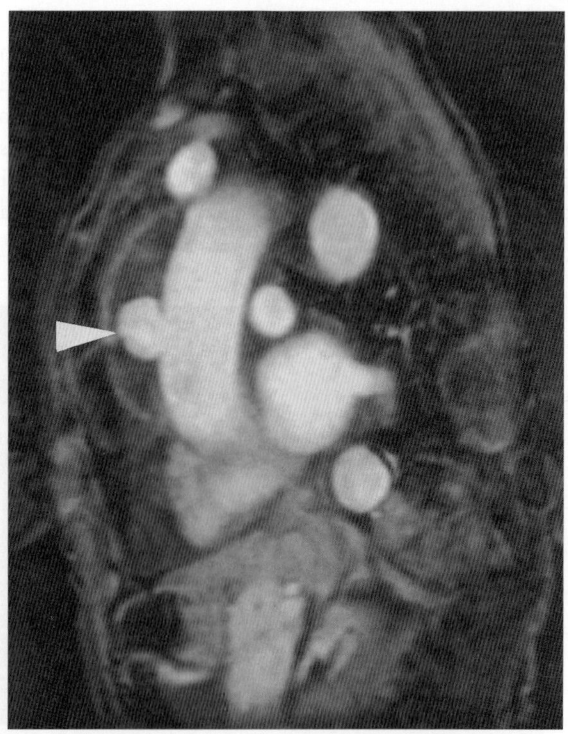

FIGURE 50-9 Sagittal contrast-enhanced MRI of penetrating atherosclerotic ulcer of the ascending aorta (*arrowhead*).

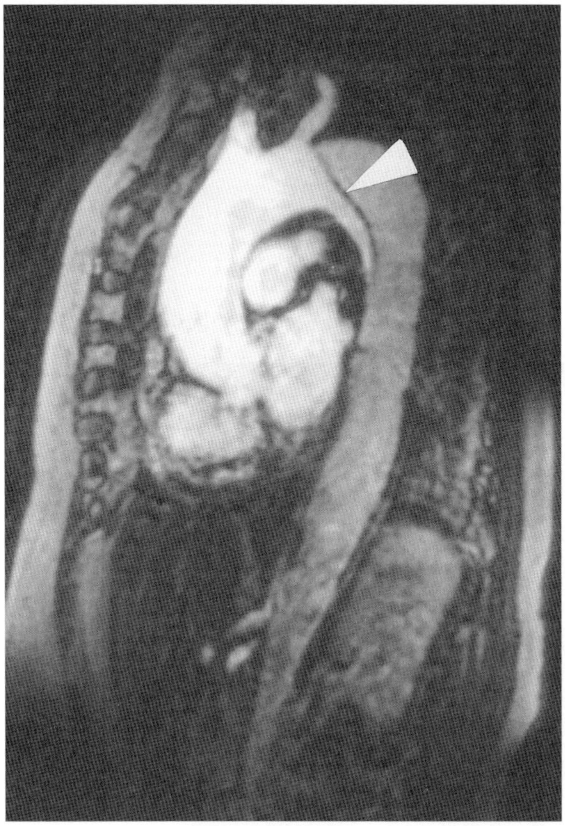

FIGURE 50-10 Sagittal contrast-enhanced MRI of a chronic type B dissection. The dissection flap (*arrowhead*) is clearly identified and the false lumen appears to extend the entire length of the thoracic and abdominal aorta (*darker posterior lumen*).

and pleural spaces similar to those obtained with CT. Cine imaging may also be used to evaluate left ventricular function, the status of the aortic valve, and flow in aortic branch vessels as well as flow in the false lumen. It is, however, not widely available and the presence of ferromagnetic metal contraindicates its use. Another disadvantage of MRI is that artifact is identified in up to 64% of studies, which underscores the need for expert radiologic interpretation of the images. These factors account for its infrequent use in the acute setting.

Diagnostic Strategy

The evaluation of suspected acute aortic dissection begins with a determination of the clinical likelihood that the diagnosis is correct and an evaluation of the hemodynamic stability of the patient. The unstable patient should undergo ECG to rule out acute coronary syndrome and be transferred immediately to the operating room. Medical management may be initiated as soon as the diagnosis is suspected. It is our practice to intubate and mechanically ventilate such patients while essential monitoring lines are placed. A TEE is then performed. If TEE fails to reveal acute aortic dissection, a hemodynamically unstable patient will then have a protected airway and invasive monitoring lines for subsequent evaluation of alternative diagnoses and continued resuscitation. If acute dissection is suspected despite a negative TEE, CT arteriogram (CTA) or aortography (potentially with IVUS) is the next study of choice.

Clinically and hemodynamically stable patients permit a more detailed history and physical examination with imaging decisions tailored to specific aspects of the presentation. At the University of Virginia, such patients are first evaluated with a CTA. A CT scanner is located in the emergency room and these data may be obtained in less than 15 minutes. If that study is negative yet the diagnosis still entertained, TEE is performed. In a recent review, an average of 1.8 imaging studies was used to correctly diagnose acute aortic dissection.[9] Although TTE is a relatively insensitive study (especially in the descending thoracic aorta), patients with suspected acute type A dissection may first undergo that study. If positive, subsequent confirmation using TEE may be performed in the operating room to expedite surgical management; if negative, either CT scanning or TEE performed in the ICU is appropriate.

Diagnostic imaging of chronic aortic dissection is usually performed for surveillance, but may also be necessary in patients with symptoms attributable to dissection and for operative planning. Routine follow-up for acute dissection occurs on a scheduled basis and is usually done with either CT or MRI. We prefer CT scanning for patients with normal renal function and no contrast allergy because CT is usually the original imaging study obtained during the acute dissection. The improved accuracy that comes with comparing similar studies combined with the availability, cost, and patient satisfaction make CT favorable for this purpose. MRI is used mostly as a follow-up study for patients with renal insufficiency, but is the study of choice to provide precise anatomical detail for operative planning. TTE is useful to follow chronic type A dissection when there is aortic insufficiency. It can provide cross-sectional images of the ascending aorta, but generating images useful for comparison to previous studies is highly dependent on the skill of the operator. For that reason, we use echocardiography to follow patients with aortic insufficiency but also obtain a CT scan to assess ascending aortic diameter. Aortography is used primarily for operative planning. Patients older than 50 years and those with risk factors for coronary artery disease routinely undergo coronary arteriography before operation, and images of the aorta are obtained at that time. Aortography is especially useful to determine the origin of aortic branch vessels for operative planning when noninvasive imaging is inadequate (Fig. 50-12).

MANAGEMENT OF ACUTE TYPE A AORTIC DISSECTION

Natural History

Acute type A aortic dissection is impressively morbid. Fifty percent of patients suffering acute type A aortic dissection are dead within 48 hours if untreated.[16] Data such as these suggests that acute type A dissection carries a "1% per hour" mortality for missed diagnoses. More contemporary data reveal a different prognosis such that medical management may be considered in certain high-risk groups. In one such study in

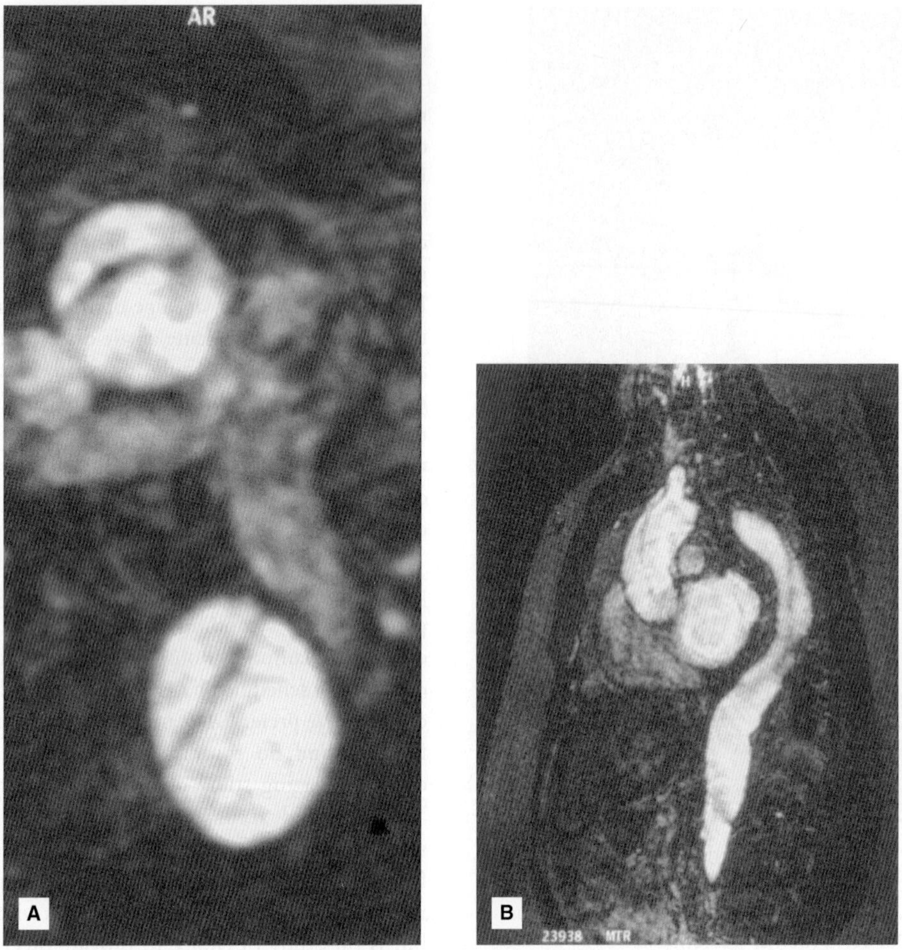

FIGURE 50-11 Axial (A) and sagittal (B) contrast-enhanced MRI of a chronic type A dissection.

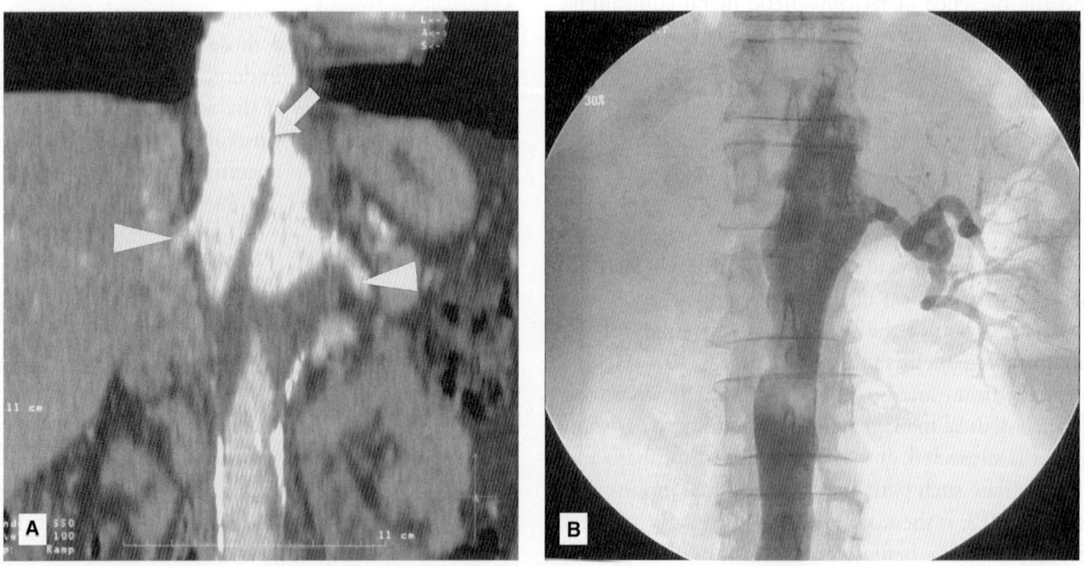

FIGURE 50-12 Coronal view of contrast-enhanced MRI (A) demonstrating chronic type B dissection with renal arteries (*arrowheads*) separated by the dissection flap (*arrow*). Aortogram (B) of the same patient revealing that each renal artery is perfused exclusively by either the true or false lumen. Such tests are often complementary and may influence surgical strategy.

octogenarians, type A dissection was managed medically in 28% of patients for various reasons with a 58% in-hospital mortality.[8] Regardless, because of the extreme mortality with medical management, patients surviving acute type A aortic dissections must be aggressively diagnosed and treated with surgical intervention.

Initial Medical Management

The high morbidity of acute type A aortic dissection dictates that management should precede confirmation of diagnosis in highly suspicious cases. The initial patient encounter centers on making the diagnosis while identifying factors that require immediate treatment. The site of this initial evaluation and resuscitation is determined primarily by the hemodynamic stability of the patient. The unstable patient belongs in the operating room, whereas a more detailed diagnostic approach and subsequent management can be undertaken in stable patients. Therefore, the hypotensive patient, whether from hemorrhagic shock or tamponade, requires the aforementioned evaluation and resuscitation on transfer to the operating room. It is preferable to avoid procedures such as TEE or central line placement on an awake patient outside the operating room because hypertension resulting from patient discomfort may precipitate aortic rupture or propagation of dissection. However, as in any patient with potential aortic rupture, anesthetic induction remains dangerous in patients compensating for impaired preload, whether from pericardial fluid or hypovolemia. The operating room must be prepared for prompt decompressive pericardiotomy and/or initiation of cardiopulmonary bypass.

In the hemodynamically stable patient, blood pressure is measured in both arms and both legs. These dissections can propagate in either direction, but proximal propagation can quickly destabilize the situation. In general, the goals of hypertension management in acute aortic dissection, regardless of anatomy, are twofold.[4] First, transmural aortic wall stress is diminished by decreasing the systolic blood pressure, which reduces the possibility of rupture. Second, shear stress on the aorta is decreased by minimizing the rate of rise of aortic pressure to decrease the likelihood of dissection propagation, so-called anti-impulse therapy. Specifically, the immediate goal for this situation remains to achieve a target systolic blood pressure between 90 and 110 mm Hg with a target heart rate of less than 60 beats per minute.

Pain control is important to reduce catecholamine release and decrease the risk of rupture. Therefore, therapy begins with pain control using narcotic analgesics. The drugs most commonly used for anti-impulse therapy are beta-blockers and peripheral vasodilators. In most cases, beta-blockers such as esmolol should be used first because adequate heart rate control may be difficult if the blood pressure is controlled by peripheral vasodilators first and because vasodilators may increase ventricular ejection and aortic shear stress if used unopposed. Short-acting beta-blockers should be titrated to a heart rate less than 60 beats per minute. After beta-blocker treatment has been initiated, vasodilators such as sodium nitroprusside are used for further blood pressure control. Sodium nitroprusside is a direct arterial vasodilator with a short onset and duration of action, which makes it ideal to rapidly achieve the target systolic blood pressure. Loading doses for esmolol and sodium nitroprusside should be avoided to prevent hypotension. Alternative beta-1 blocking drugs such as propranolol or metoprolol, and the combined alpha- and beta-blocker labetalol are appropriate in the subacute phase. Calcium channel blockers may be necessary to reduce systolic blood pressure in those patients with a contraindication to beta-blocker use. A commonly used alternative to nitroprusside is nicardipine. This is also a calcium channel-blocker devoid of any cardiac effects which is easily titrated to a goal blood pressure.

Operative Indications

The goals of surgery in acute type A dissection are to prevent or treat an aortic catastrophe while restoring blood flow to the true lumen of the aorta. Aortic catastrophe includes aortic rupture into the pericardium or pleural space, dissection and occlusion of the coronary ostia, and progression to aortic valvular incompetence. The presence of ascending aortic involvement is therefore an indication for operative management in all but the highest-risk patients (Table 50-5). The difficulty arises in determining which patients are high risk and which additional factors should affect the management algorithm. Patient age, for example, is not regarded as an absolute contraindication to surgery. However, this factor should be considered given the relative worse outcomes of operative treatment for acute type A dissection for patients greater than 80 years of age. Neurologic

TABLE 50-5 Operative Indications for Acute and Chronic Type A and B Thoracic Aortic Dissection

Dissection Type	Operative Indication
Acute	
Type A	Presence
Type B	Failure of medical management (persistent or recurrent pain, medically uncontrolled hypertension) Expanding aortic diameter Progressive dissection Impending or actual rupture Malperfusion
Chronic	Impending or actual rupture Symptoms related to dissection (congestive heart failure, angina, aortic regurgitation, stroke, pain) Malperfusion Aneurysm ≥5.5 cm (type A), ≥6.5 cm (type B) Aortic expansion >1 cm/yr

status at the time of presentation can also affect the decision to operate. Although most agree that obtunded or comatose patients are unlikely to improve with surgical repair, complications such as stroke or paraplegia at the time of presentation are not contraindications to surgical correction. It must be acknowledged that dissection repair will most likely not improve neurologic condition, and may even make it worse. Neither the distal extent nor the thrombosis of the false lumen obviates the need for surgical repair because the risk of developing an aortic catastrophe remains. Similarly, patients with subacute type A dissection who present or are referred after 2 weeks of dissection onset require operation. Scholl et al demonstrated that these patients have avoided the early complications of dissection and may safely undergo elective operation rather than emergency repair.[17]

Surgical Therapy

Anesthesia and Monitoring

Anesthesia used during the repair of aortic dissections is often narcotic based with inhalational agents for maintenance. Single-lumen endotracheal tubes are used for procedures performed through a median sternotomy, whereas double-lumen endotracheal tubes are useful but not mandatory for procedures performed through a left thoracotomy. Monitoring lines often include central venous access with a pulmonary artery catheter and one or more arterial pressure monitoring lines specific to the operation performed. Preparation must be made for all possibilities in these cases, most importantly for the possible need for hypothermic circulatory arrest. Arterial monitoring should be tailored to both the anatomy of the dissection and the method of cannulation. One or two radial arterial lines and at least one femoral line may be required to ensure adequate perfusion of the upper and lower body. All patients require a TEE probe. Core body temperature is monitored in the bladder using a Foley catheter and in the esophagus using a nasopharyngeal probe. A wide skin preparation to include the axillary and femoral arteries is essential to provide all possible cannulation options.

Neurologic monitoring is available, but its utility remains controversial even in elective cases. Advocates of both cerebral and spinal cord monitoring argue that these monitors are able to detect injury to neurons before irreversible cellular injury.[18] Thus, this warning allows for detection of imminent injury and subsequent evasion of injury. Opponents argue that there is a significant learning curve and that the injury has already occurred once these monitors can identify ischemic neurologic changes. The optimal type of monitoring depends on the location of the dissection and the resultant details of required vascular control. Manipulation of the ascending aorta and arch can affect cerebral perfusion. In these cases, transcranial Doppler (TCD) or near-infrared spectroscopy (NIRS) have been used. Intraoperative TCD monitoring is used to identify malpositioned cannulas or document the need for adjustment of retrograde perfusion.[19] Opponents of TCD argue difficulty with low baseline flow and poor signal in patients with thick temporal bones, which confuses interpretation of the results and the response to them. Continuous noninvasive NIRS can be used to monitor cerebral oxygenation, marker of cerebral blood flow. Although the role of NIRS in aortic dissection has not been elucidated, advocates extrapolate use from studies on carotid endarterectomy and coronary bypass. NIRS can be used for identification of regional oxygenation changes during the case, which may be particularly useful during normothermic periods of these cases.[18] Somatosensory evoked potentials (SSEP) is argued to be useful in identifying neurologic injury ranging anywhere from the peripheral nerve to the brain. These studies may even identify ischemic cerebral injury during hypothermic circulatory arrest earlier than electroencephalography (EEG).[20] SSEP can also be useful in the detection of spinal cord ischemia to identify crucial spinal cord vasculature requiring reimplantation. The use of SSEP at some centers has led to reduced intraoperative and postoperative paraplegia in retrospective studies.[21] Neurologic monitoring remains a relatively new technology that is operator dependent, but probably is useful in experienced hands.

Hemostasis

Open aortic dissection repair is commonly associated with significant blood loss caused by weak tissues and coagulopathy from bleeding or hypothermia. Strict blood conservation is an important aspect of the operation. At least one cell-saver device should be available. Packed red blood cells, platelets, and fresh-frozen plasma should be in the operating room at the start of the operation. Coagulopathy as a result of the preoperative status of the patient, cardiopulmonary bypass, and deep hypothermic circulatory arrest contribute to excessive blood loss. Antifibrinolytic drugs can be useful hemostatic adjuncts. Patients will often require transfusion of fresh-frozen plasma, platelets, and possibly cryoprecipitate. Fibrin glues and hemostatic materials such as Surgicel and Gelfoam are useful as systemic coagulopathy is corrected.

Cardiopulmonary Bypass

Cannulation for type A dissection repair requires thoughtful evaluation of the dissection anatomy while taking into consideration the extent of the repair to be undertaken. The crucial point is to provide arterial flow into the true lumen of the aorta with proof of sufficient end-organ perfusion, in particular as dynamic flaps may alter perfusion. Some flexibility regarding arterial access should be exercised. In certain situations, a patient may require multiple cannulation sites to adequately perfuse the entire body. Various options for cannulation exist, but the optimal choice of cannulation in aortic dissection requires tailoring to the combination of surgeon preference with dissection anatomy.

Venous cannulation remains relatively straightforward. Venous cannulation is obtained commonly through the right atrium using a two-stage venous cannula, whereas bicaval cannulation is used for certain cases in which retrograde cerebral perfusion is used during hypothermic circulatory arrest. A left ventricular vent is necessary in the setting of aortic valve incompetence and is easily placed through the right superior pulmonary vein or rarely through the left ventricular apex wall.

Cardioplegia is administered in a retrograde fashion through a coronary sinus catheter with additional protection via direct cannulation of the undissected coronary ostia.

Arterial cannulation requires a much more thoughtful process. Historically, femoral cannulation was the site of choice for arterial cannulation for type A dissection. However, the optimal site of cannulation should be tailored based on the combined goals of surgery and the specific anatomy of the patient, with contingency plans for evidence of malperfusion.

The goals of surgery, in terms of distal extent of the repair, depend to a certain extent on surgeon's preference. Many surgeons feel that optimal repair should be limited to the ascending aorta. This scenario can be accomplished by cannulation at most sites with flow directed into the true lumen of the aorta. Femoral cannulation has been a traditional mainstay in dissection repair. The most favorable side of femoral cannulation has been debated in the past, but as long as there is perfusion into the true lumen, the side most likely does not matter. Reports from the University of Virginia, among others, have also shown that the dissection itself can be cannulated safely with echocardiographic guidance.[22] This technique involves confirming access to the true lumen of the aorta with echocardiography of the descending aorta. Then, using the Seldinger technique, a percutaneous cannula can be properly positioned. Direct cannulation should be avoided through areas with evidence of hematoma. Proper perfusion of the true lumen must be confirmed with ultrasound or echocardiography. A potential salvage maneuver involves cannulation of the ventricular apex with advancement of the cannula though the aortic valve and into the true lumen of the aorta. This technique also requires confirmation of true lumen perfusion. Aortic cannulation of either the dissection area or the apex mandates cannulation of the graft after repair in most cases.

Other surgeons believe that resection of the maximal amount of abnormal aorta possible is ideal. Because this resection commonly involves the aortic arch, many choose to cannulate in a way that allows for antegrade cerebral perfusion. Although cannulation of the innominate and the left common carotid artery have been described, the most common cannulation site for arch cases has become right axillary cannulation.[23] The right axillary artery provides direct access to the right carotid artery for selective antegrade perfusion. This can be done by sewing a graft to the artery or directly cannulating it. However, direct axillary cannulation appears to cause more morbidity than graft cannulation, including further dissection, brachial plexus injury, and limb ischemia. Axillary cannulation may be suboptimal in cases in which the axillary, right common carotid, or innominate artery are dissected. Similar techniques have been described in cannulation approaches to the innominate and left carotid arteries. Finally, the open aorta allows direct access to the lumen of the innominate and the left common carotid, which can be cannulated during hypothermic circulatory arrest for selective antegrade perfusion. No matter the preferred site of arterial cannulation, the surgeon must be cognizant of whole body perfusion. Patients that are not cooling properly or show other signs of malperfusion may require more than one arterial cannulation sites for cardiopulmonary bypass. Routine confirmation of blood flow in the carotids as well as the descending aorta can be critical to avoid malperfusion.

Cerebral Protection

Type A dissection repair involving the arch disrupts blood flow to the brachiocephalic arteries during a period of circulatory arrest. Cerebral protection during that period is critical to neurologic outcome. Cerebral protection is optimized through deep hypothermia with or without potential neuroprotective adjuncts. Straight hypothermia during circulatory arrest was the first method used to perform operations on the aortic arch and remains an effective method for shorter procedures. Two alternative primary end points for cooling are employed: goal temperature or EEG silence.

The published temperature goals vary widely, namely anywhere from 14 to 32°C. The ischemic tolerance of the brain improves with colder temperatures. However, cooling to a temperature below 14°C can result in a form of nonischemic brain injury and is therefore not recommended. The neurologic protection from straight hypothermic circulatory arrest can be very good, especially for short ischemic times. Most data suggest that straight hypothermic circulatory arrest up to 20 minutes is safe. However, increased ischemic time is directly related to increased incidence of neurologic deficits.[24] Proponents of straight hypothermic circulatory arrest have suggested in elective patients that longer times can be used safely without significant adverse cognitive outcomes but circulatory arrest should be limited to as short a time as possible.[25]

For these cases, temperature is being used as a proxy for metabolic function. Unfortunately, nasopharyngeal and tympanic temperature may be imperfect estimates of brain temperature. Moreover, temperature does not directly relate to neurologic activity. For these reasons, some groups use EEG silence to determine the appropriate point at which to discontinue cooling and perfusion. The patients are cooled until EEG silence is obtained. After 5 minutes at this temperature, the circulatory arrest period can be initiated, usually at a temperature between 15 and 22°C. Using this technique, the group from the University of Pennsylvania achieved EEG silence in 90% of patients after 45 minutes of cooling and had a postoperative stroke rate of less than 5%.[26] As a result, in the absence of EEG monitoring, they cool for at least 45 minutes in almost all cases to optimize brain protection. Although EEG is attractive in theory, it is not always available when patients with dissections are taken to the operating room.

Continued cerebral perfusion during the period of circulatory arrest is an alternative technique for cerebral protection, especially for circulatory arrest times greater than 20 minutes. Cerebral blood flow may be delivered in either a retrograde or antegrade fashion. The technique for retrograde cerebral perfusion depends on the venous cannulation strategy. If bicaval cannulation is used, reversing flow through the superior vena caval cannula with a proximally placed tourniquet is simple and effective. Use of retrograde flow with dual-stage venous cannulation requires placement of a retrograde "coronary sinus" catheter into the superior vena cava through a pursestring suture. The superior vena cava is then occluded with an umbilical tape to direct flow toward the head. Retrograde cerebral perfusion has the added benefit of flushing atherosclerotic material and air from the brachiocephalic vessels. A flow rate necessary to produce a superior vena caval pressure of 15 to 25 mm Hg is considered optimal.

Selective antegrade cerebral perfusion has recently gained popularity. Once the aortic arch is open, the innominate artery and the left common carotid artery are encircled with vessel occluders and each lumen cannulated with a retrograde "coronary sinus" cannula. With the left subclavian artery occluded, flow rates are slowly increased to achieve perfusion pressures of 50 to 70 mm Hg at the desired circulatory arrest temperature. These cannulae are then removed just before completing the anastomosis of the brachiocephalic vessels to the vascular graft, at which time cardiopulmonary bypass may be reinstituted.

A few basic principles apply to all approaches. During cooling on cardiopulmonary bypass, a maximum temperature gradient between perfusate and patient of less than 10°C is ideal. The head is then packed in ice to maintain a low brain temperature. To ensure maximal protection, the goal temperature should be maintained for 5 minutes before initiation of hypothermic circulatory arrest. Similarly, the body should be reperfused for 5 minutes at the colder temperature before beginning the rewarming process. Rewarming too early can exacerbate neurologic injury. Rewarming proceeds without exceeding a 10°C perfusate-patient temperature gradient to at least 37°C as core body temperature often falls briefly after cessation of active warming and separation from cardiopulmonary bypass.

Pharmacologic adjuncts are believed by some to decrease metabolic rate with hopes of reducing injury. Although methylprednisolone continues to be used in these cases by many, barbiturate administration during cooling has fallen mostly out of favor. If used, methylprednisolone should be given early as the steroid effects require incorporation into the cell nucleus. Others give lidocaine and magnesium before the arrest period to stabilize the neuronal cell membrane. Furosemide and mannitol can be administered to initiate diuresis and promote free radical scavenging after circulatory arrest. The results of all these techniques are not fully substantiated yet.

Operative Technique

The exposure for procedures performed on the ascending aorta and proximal arch is through a median sternotomy. This can be modified with supraclavicular, cervical, or trapdoor incisions to gain exposure to the brachiocephalic vessels or descending thoracic aorta. When dissecting the distal arch, it is important to identify and protect both the left vagus nerve with its recurrent branch and the left phrenic nerve. Replacement of the ascending aorta in type A dissections is best performed by an open distal anastomosis technique if the arch is involved (30%) or if arch involvement is unknown. The open distal anastomotic technique requires clamping the mid ascending aorta and producing cardiac arrest via administration of antegrade and/or retrograde cardioplegic solution. The dissected ascending aorta proximal to the clamp is then opened. Evaluation and surgical correction of the aortic valve is ideally performed at this time while systemic cooling continues. If the dissection does not involve the aortic root, the aorta is transected 5 to 10 mm distal to the sinotubular ridge. When the dissection involves the sinotubular ridge, the proximal aorta is reconstructed by reuniting the dissected aortic layers between one or two strips of Teflon felt using either 3-0 or 4-0 Prolene suture. Safi et al use a technique of interrupted pledgeted horizontal mattress sutures as compared with the felt sandwich technique.[27] In their experience, this provides superior stabilization and decreases the potential for subsequent aortic stenosis. The University of Pennsylvania has described aortic reconstruction using felt as a neomedia giving a stable platform to sew the graft to otherwise friable tissue.[26]

Once the temperature reaches 18 to 20°C, perfusion is discontinued during a brief period of circulatory arrest. When using antegrade or retrograde cerebral perfusion, the selected perfusion is initiated at this time. The aortic clamp is released and the intima of the aortic arch is inspected and repaired accordingly (Fig. 50-13). If the intima is intact, the distal anastomosis is performed and the graft is cannulated, deaired, and clamped for resumption of cardiopulmonary bypass with systemic warming. If the intima of the arch is violated, then a hemiarch reconstruction is performed (Fig. 50-14). We have only rarely found it necessary to perform a complete arch resection for an acute dissection. If a complex aortic root procedure is required, it is often useful to repair the aortic root with one vascular graft and use a separate graft to create the distal aortic anastomosis. The two grafts are then measured, cut, and anastomosed to provide the correct length and orientation for aortic replacement.

If the ascending aorta cannot be cross-clamped, the patient is cooled to 20°C with subsequent circulatory arrest. The distal aortic reconstruction is performed first in this circumstance, at which time the graft is cannulated and proximally clamped with resumption of cardiopulmonary bypass and systemic rewarming.

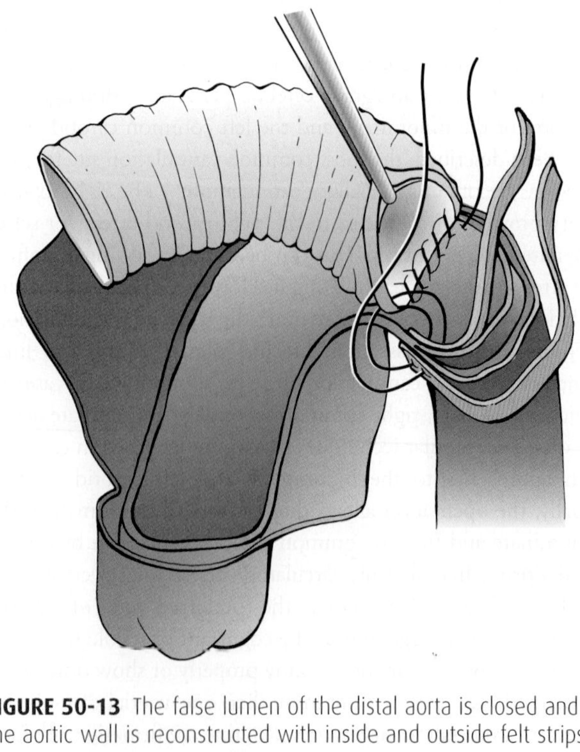

FIGURE 50-13 The false lumen of the distal aorta is closed and the aortic wall is reconstructed with inside and outside felt strips.

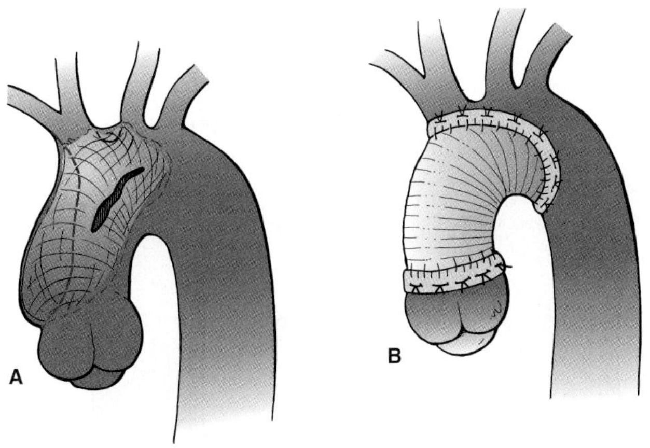

FIGURE 50-14 (A) The type A dissection extends into the proximal aortic arch. (B) The distal dissected aortic wall is reconstructed with inside and outside felt strips to replace part of the arch and ascending aorta.

Cannulation of the graft for antegrade systemic perfusion and rewarming is associated with improved neurologic outcomes compared with retrograde perfusion and should be performed whenever possible. Because a cross-clamp is not applied, the left ventricle must be decompressed once fibrillation starts during systemic cooling (approximately 20°C) to prevent distention and irreversible myocardial injury. Proximal ascending aortic repair is completed during the period of rewarming.

An alternative to the open distal technique is possible when the dissection is limited to the ascending aorta or the proximal arch away from the origin of the brachiocephalic vessels. Antegrade arterial perfusion is achieved through distal arch or right subclavian artery cannulation; retrograde perfusion via cannulation of a femoral artery has traditionally provided acceptable results. An aortic cross-clamp is applied tangentially just proximal to the innominate artery. The ascending aorta is resected to include the inferior aspect of the arch. The layers of the dissected aorta proximal to the clamp are then reunited if necessary and the ascending aorta replaced with an appropriately sized, beveled vascular graft. The proximal reconstruction and anastomosis may then be created and the entire procedure performed without requiring deep hypothermia and circulatory arrest.

Isolated dissection of the aortic arch is rare. Classified as a type A dissection, it requires resection of the arch at the site of intimal disruption and aortic replacement. Surgical management of the brachiocephalic vessels is determined by the integrity of the adjacent intima. If intact, the brachiocephalic vessels are reimplanted as a Carrel patch into a vascular graft after repair (Fig. 50-15). If the dissection involves individual vessels, each may require repair and reimplantation individually into the graft used for arch replacement (Fig. 50-16).

Aortic root dissection often fails to violate the intima of the coronary ostia. Repair of the ascending aorta at the sinotubular junction is therefore sufficient to reunite the aortic root layers and provide uninterrupted coronary blood flow. Minimal disruption of the coronary ostial intima should be repaired primarily with 5-0 or 6-0 Prolene suture. If, however, the ostium is circumferentially dissected and an aortic root replacement is necessary, an aortic button should be excised and the layers reunited with running 5-0 Prolene suture, glue, or both. Coronary buttons are then reimplanted into the vascular graft or to a separate 8-mm vascular graft as part of a Cabrol repair

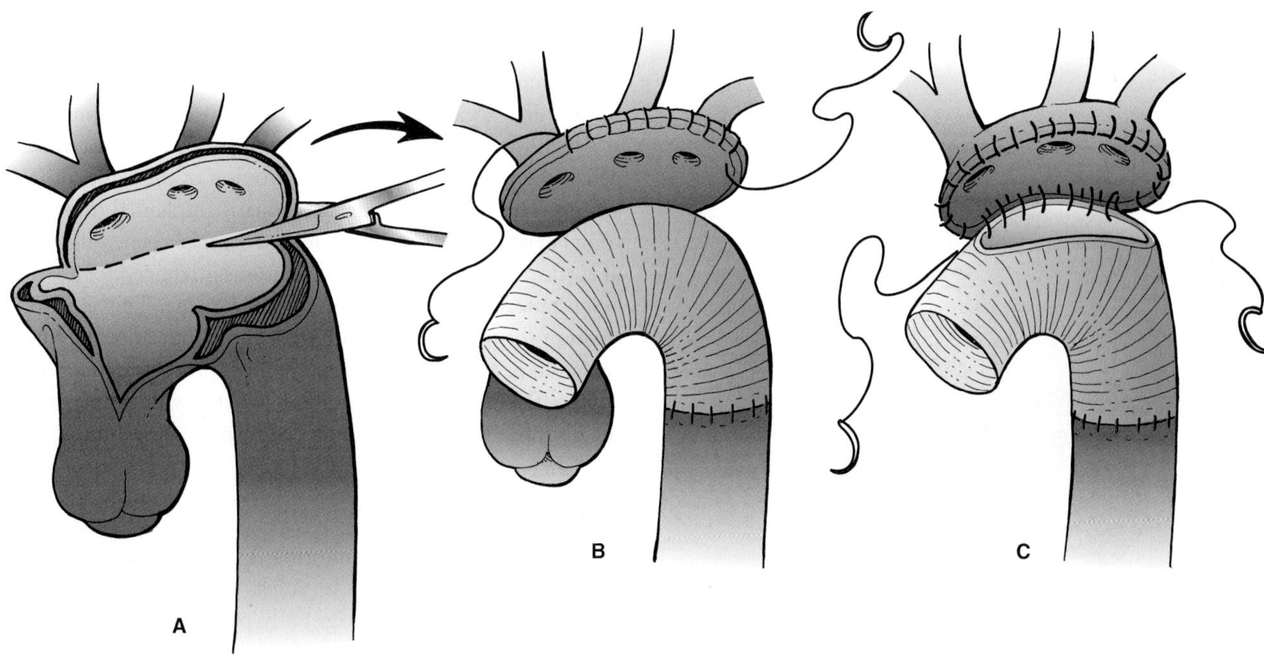

FIGURE 50-15 Brachiocephalic vessels can be reattached to an arch graft as a unit if the inner cylinder of origin of each vessel remains intact. (A) The arch vessels are excised as a unit from the superior surface of the dissected aortic arch. (B) The separated layers of the brachiocephalic patch are reunited using inner and outer felt strips and continuous suture. (C) A corresponding hole is cut in the aortic graft and the continuous brachiocephalic unit is sutured into place.

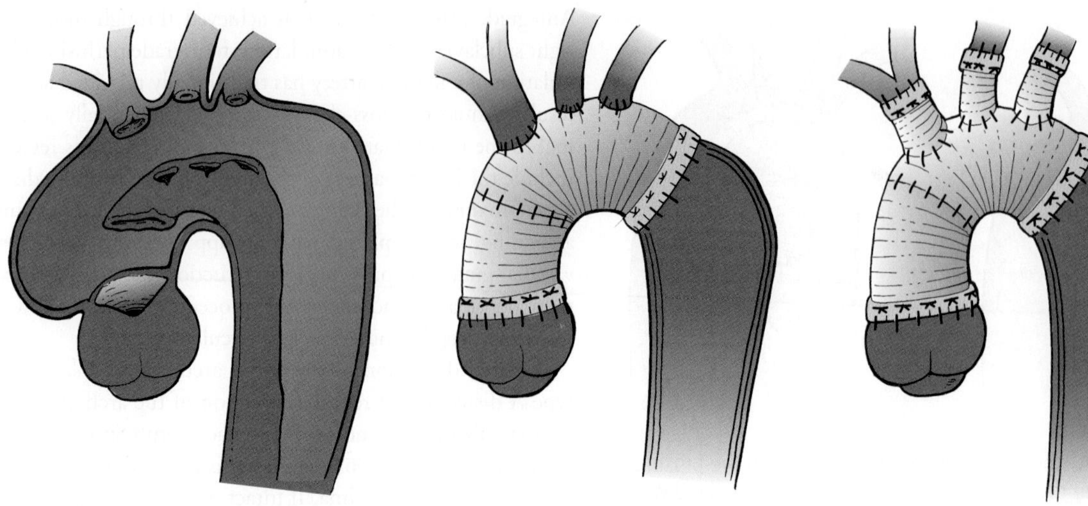

FIGURE 50-16 The brachiocephalic vessels are separated from the true lumen by the dissected false lumen (*left panel*). If individual brachiocephalic vessels are also damaged beyond repair, short interposition grafts are added to reconnect each artery to the aortic graft (*right panel*).

(Fig. 50-17). Aortocoronary bypass grafting is performed only when the coronary ostium is not reconstructable and as a last resort.

Acute type A dissection is complicated by aortic valve insufficiency in up to 75% of patients. Fortunately, preservation of the native valve is successful nearly 85% of the time. The mechanism of aortic insufficiency in most cases is the loss of commissural support of the valve leaflets. This is repaired using pledgeted 4-0 Prolene sutures to reposition each of the commissures at the sinotubular ridge (Fig. 50-18). The dissected aortic root layers are then reunited using 3-0 Prolene suture and either one or two strips of Teflon felt to recreate the sinotubular junction and reform the sinuses of Valsalva. Aortic valve preservation must

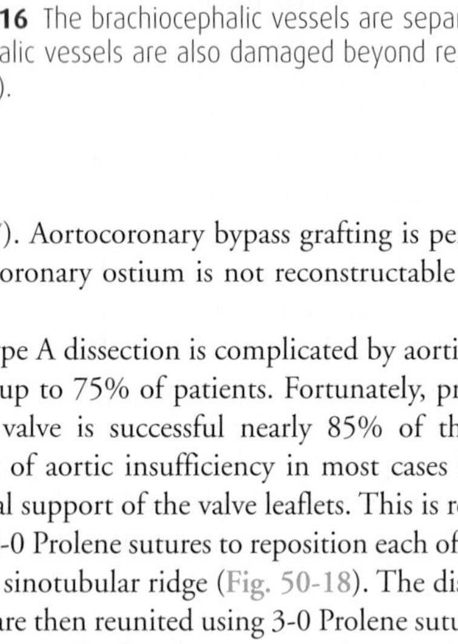

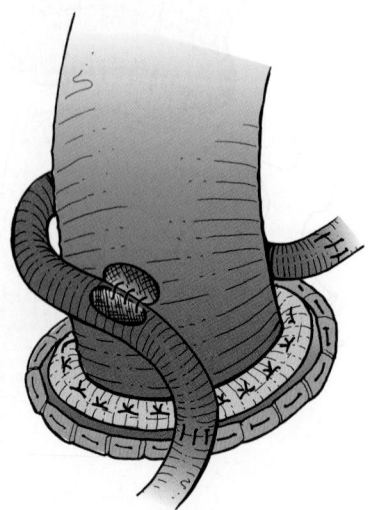

FIGURE 50-17 Illustration showing the attachment of the coronary ostia to the graft using the Cabrol technique. The ends of a 60-mm Dacron graft are sewn end to end to each coronary ostium. A side-to-side anastomosis is made between the intercoronary tube graft and the aortic graft.

always be performed using intraoperative TEE to assess the valve postoperatively. No more than mild aortic insufficiency should be present. In addition to commissural resuspension, techniques exist to spare the aortic valve and replace the aortic root in acute type A dissection, but the experience is early and the number of patients few. This topic is covered in greater detail in the section on surgical techniques for chronic type A dissection.

If the aortic valve cannot be spared, replacement of the ascending aorta and valve should be performed using a composite valve graft or homograft. The composite valve graft is implanted using horizontal mattress 2-0 Tycron sutures to encircle the annulus and to seat the valved conduit (Fig. 50-19). The previously excised and reconstituted coronary buttons are reimplanted into the vascular graft with running 5-0 Prolene suture (Fig. 50-20). The left coronary button is implanted first, at which time the graft is clamped and placed under pressure to define the proper orientation and position of the right coronary button. The aortic homograft is similarly implanted using horizontal mattress 2-0 Tycron sutures, except that a generous margin of aortic root below the coronary buttons is retained for a second hemostatic suture line of running 4-0 Prolene. This is an ideal solution for individuals who have a contraindication to anticoagulation or for young females. The Ross procedure (pulmonary autograft) is not applicable in those patients with connective tissue disorders and not recommended in acute dissection.

Postoperative Management

Invasive hemodynamic monitoring is used to ensure adequate end-organ perfusion with a target systolic blood pressure between 90 and 110 mm Hg. Early postoperative blood pressure control begins with adequate analgesia and sedation using narcotics and sedative/hypnotic agents. The patient should, however, be allowed to emerge from general anesthesia briefly for a gross neurologic examination. The patient is then sedated for a period to ensure continued hemodynamic stability and

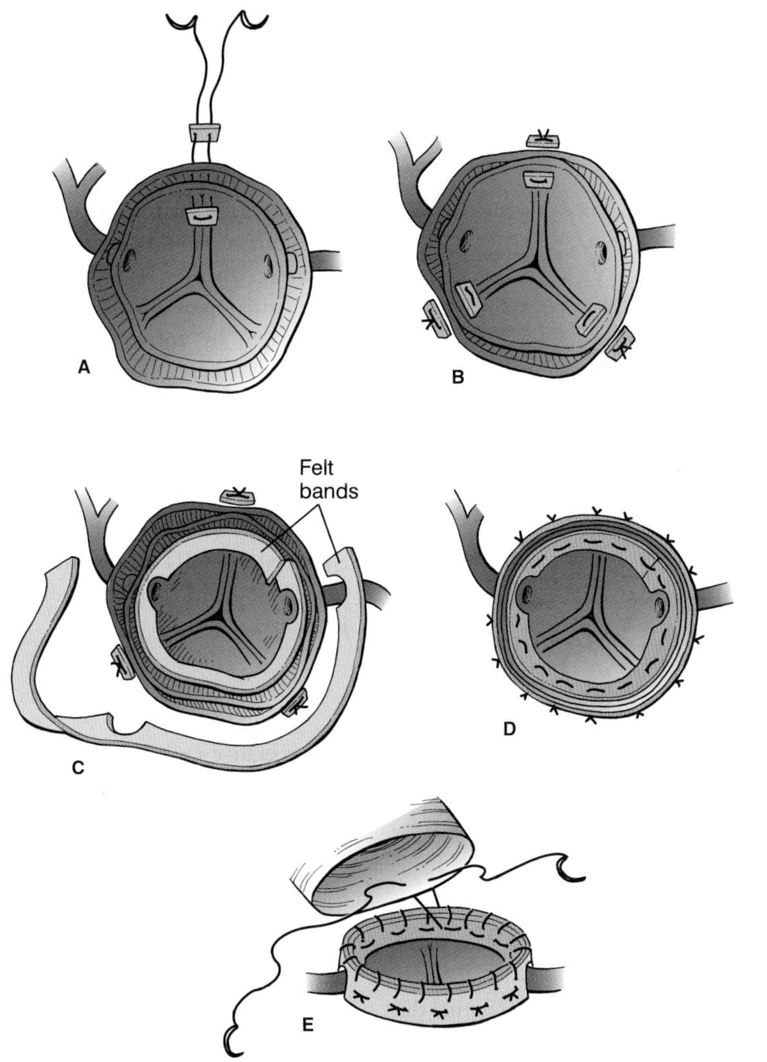

FIGURE 50-18 Resuspension and preservation of the native aortic valve in a type A dissection. (A) The dissected layers are approximated at each commissure with double-pledgeted mattress sutures. (B) The aortic valve commissures are completely resuspended. (C) Thin felt strips (8- to 10-mm wide) are placed inside and outside from the circumference of the aorta. The coronary ostia are not compromised. (D) The aortic walls are sandwiched between the felt strips with a horizontal mattress. (E) A vascular graft is sutured to the reconstructed proximal aorta.

facilitate hemostasis. Coagulopathy is aggressively treated with blood products and antifibrinolytic agents as necessary, and by warming the patient. Hematocrit, platelet count, coagulation studies, and serum electrolytes are obtained and corrected as necessary. An ECG and chest radiograph are used to assess for abnormalities and to serve as baseline studies. A full physical exam, including complete peripheral vascular exam, is performed on arrival. Despite adequate repair of the dissection, perfusion of the false lumen may persist; therefore, malperfusion syndrome remains possible. If an abdominal malperfusion syndrome is suspected postoperatively, this should be aggressively evaluated with ultrasound and subsequent angiography if positive. A strong clinical suspicion is enough to warrant this evaluation given the consequences of failed recognition. The patient can be extubated once extubation criteria are met if the patient has been hemodynamically stable without excessive bleeding and the results of a neurologic exam are normal. Management is routine from that point forward.

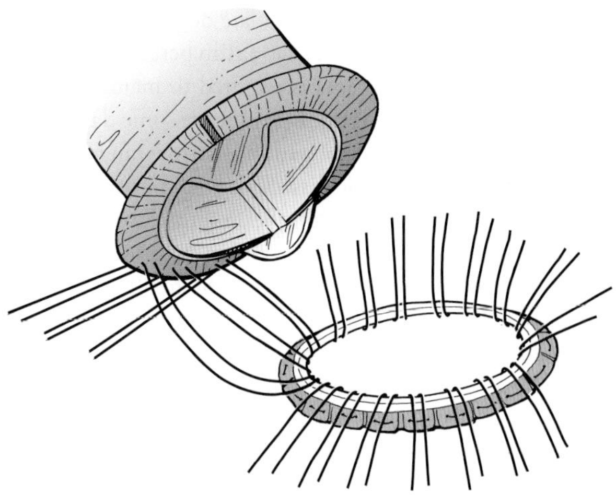

FIGURE 50-19 Everting 2-0 pledgeted mattress sutures are placed shoulder to shoulder around the aortic annulus to anchor a composite graft containing a St. Jude prosthesis.

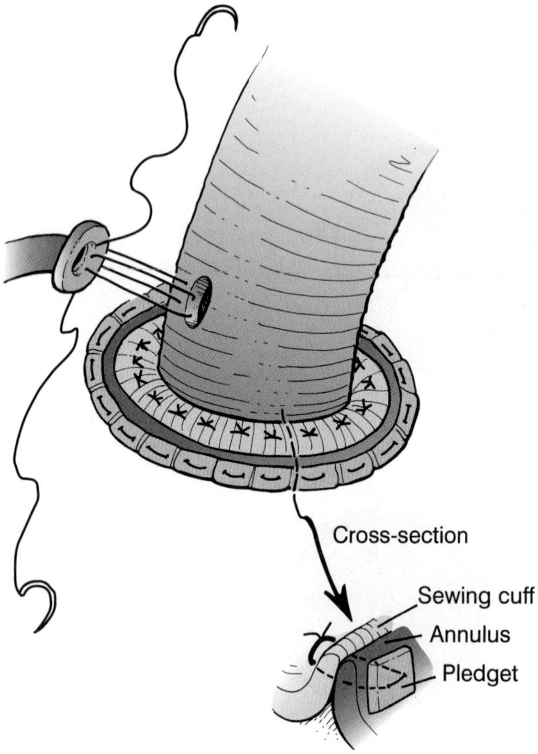

FIGURE 50-20 The coronary ostia are attached to the graft by the button technique using continuous 5-0 polypropylene suture.

Long-Term Management

Surviving the operation for acute dissection represents the beginning of a lifelong requirement for meticulous medical management and continued close observation. It has been estimated that replacement of the ascending aorta for type A dissection obliterates flow in the distal false lumen in fewer than 10% of patients. As a result, the natural history of repaired dissection may involve dilatation and potential rupture of the chronically dissected distal aorta. This was the reason for the late death in nearly 30% of DeBakey's original series in 1982 and is currently the leading cause of late death following surgical repair.[28] Often a multidrug antihypertensive regimen including beta-blocking agents is required to maintain systolic blood pressure below 120 mm Hg. There are some data indicating that blood pressure control within a narrow range may alter the natural history of chronic dissection by diminishing the rate of aneurysmal dilatation. The long-term durability of the aortic valve after supracoronary reconstruction is quite good with freedom from aortic valve replacement of 80 to 90% at 10 years. Progressive aortic insufficiency of the native valve is possible and should be followed with TEE in some patients.

Follow-up diagnostic imaging is required to monitor aortic diameter in patients after repair. Spiral CT arteriogram and MRI are the imaging studies of choice. MRI and ultrasound are useful in patients with renal insufficiency and those requiring only imaging of the abdominal aorta. Echocardiography is useful for imaging the ascending aorta and provides additional information regarding the aortic valve. It is important to recognize the resolution limitations of each imaging modality and inherent imprecision of comparing different imaging modalities to evaluate changes. In general, measurements should be made at the same anatomical level with respect to reproducible anatomical structures (ie, the sinotubular ridge, proximal to the innominate or left subclavian arteries or at the diaphragmatic hiatus). It is important to recognize that the false lumen should be included in measurements of aortic diameter whether it is perfused or not. Three-dimensional reconstruction of spiral CT and MRI scans minimizes the error introduced by aortic eccentricity when comparing imaging studies and has simplified following this patient population. The current recommendations are to obtain a baseline study before hospital discharge and at 6-month intervals during the first year. If the aortic diameter remains unchanged at 1 year, studies are obtained yearly. Aortic enlargement of more than 0.5 cm within a 6-month period and greater eccentricity on comparison of 3D reconstruction images are high-risk changes for which the interval is decreased to 3 months if surgery is not indicated.

Results

The operative mortality for repair of acute type A aortic dissection has fallen since DeBakey's original 40% mortality was reported in 1965. Improved ICU and floor care of these patients, earlier recognition of dissection through improved imaging modalities, development of hemostatic vascular graft material, more effective hemostatic agents, and improvements in the safety of cardiopulmonary bypass are likely responsible. In the last two decades, most centers consistently report an operative mortality for acute type A dissection of between 10 and 30%. The high early mortality in acute dissection parallels the number of patients who present profoundly hypotensive and in shock. The mode of death is stroke, myocardial ischemia/heart failure, aortic rupture, or malperfusion in most cases.

The International Registry of Acute Aortic Dissections (IRAD) recently reported on the results of 526 patients with acute type A aortic dissection who underwent surgical treatment in 18 large tertiary centers.[29] Surgery in these patients included replacement of the ascending aorta in 92%, aortic root in 32%, partial arch in 23%, complete arch in 12%, and descending aorta in 4%. Overall in-hospital mortality was 25%; 31% for hemodynamically unstable patients and 17% for stable patients. Causes of death were aortic rupture (33%), neurologic complications (14%), visceral ischemia (12%), tamponade (3%), or nonspecified (42%).

Age is not an absolute contraindication to surgical treatment of type A aortic dissections. However, operative mortality increases with age. Retrospective series show that operative mortality increases from 20 to 30% for patients younger than 75 years of age to greater than 45 to 50% for those 80 years or older.[30]

The published results for long-term survival following surgically treated acute type A aortic dissection over the last decade is roughly 71 to 89% at 5 years and between 54 and 66% at 10 years.[31–33] Survival for patients who are discharged alive from the hospital after surgical repair of type A aortic dissection carries a survival rate of 96% at 1 year and 91% at 3 years.[34]

MANAGEMENT OF ACUTE TYPE B AORTIC DISSECTION

Natural History

Type B aortic dissections account for approximately 40% of all acute aortic dissections.[8] Their natural course is more benign than that of acute type A dissections.

Most patients with acute type B aortic dissections survive the acute and subacute phases with medical management alone. Approximately 20 to 30% of patients present with complicated type B dissection, which require urgent operative (surgical or endovascular) intervention. Complicated dissection can be defined as imminent or actual aortic rupture, aortic expansion, hemodynamic instability, persistent pain despite medical management, drug-resistant hypertension, and malperfusion syndrome.[8,35] The most frequent causes of death in acute type B dissection are aortic rupture and visceral malperfusion.

The relative success with medical management has relegated surgical treatment for acute type B dissections to patients with complicated dissections or those with progression of the disease (see Table 50-5). Medical therapy of uncomplicated type B aortic dissection confers a relatively good short-term prognosis with in-hospital survival of approximately 90%.[35] Medical management in these patients has survival rates of approximately 85% at 1 year and 71% at 5 years.[36]

On the contrary, patients with complicated dissections that require open surgical intervention have a 30-day mortality of approximately 30%.[8] More recently though, endovascular techniques have been used in these complicated dissections with reduced perioperative mortality and morbidity. Endovascular treatment of acute type B dissections was first described in 1999 by Dake et al.[37] and Nienaber et al.[38] As endovascular treatment of complicated dissections has expanded, the results have improved, with studies now reporting a mortality of around 5%.[39]

Medical Management

Historically, the mortality of open surgical approaches for type B aortic dissections exceeded 50%, whereas medical management carried a mortality risk of 30% or less. Therefore, medical management has played a pivotal role in the management of these patients. Medical management is identical to that described in the initial management of the acute type A aortic dissection. The goals are control of the heart rate and blood pressure to decrease the shear stress on the aorta and limit expansion of the false lumen and propagation of the dissection.

Medical management initially requires an adequate airway and intravenous access. Patients with suspected or confirmed type B aortic dissection should be admitted to the intensive care unit for close monitoring. Pain control is important to reduce catecholamine release and is best achieved with narcotic medications, in particular morphine sulfate. Management is initiated with beta-blockers such as esmolol or propranolol.[9] These medications should be titrated to achieve optimal blood pressure (ie, systolic pressure of 100 to 120 mm Hg) and heart rate while allowing for adequate renal, gut, and brain perfusion. Heart rate control to a goal of less than 60 bpm has been shown to decrease the risk of secondary adverse events such as aortic expansion, recurrent dissection, and aortic rupture.[40]

Vasodilators such as sodium nitroprusside can be used as an adjunct to beta-blockers if blood pressure is still not adequately controlled. Vasodilators can increase the force of ventricular ejection and aortic shear stress and should therefore be only used concurrently with beta-blockade. Calcium channel blockers can also be used to control blood pressure, especially in patients intolerant to beta-blockers. However, their use has not been appropriately studied in patients with aortic dissection. Patients with normal or decreased low blood pressure at presentation, without evidence of cardiac tamponade or heart failure, may benefit from judicious intravenous volume administration.

Once the patient with uncomplicated type B aortic dissection has been stabilized, blood pressure medications should be transitioned to an oral regimen. The patient can then be discharged home with close follow-up, including imaging and clinical assessment in 3 months and every 6 months thereafter.

Operative Indications

Operative management of acute type B aortic dissection, either by endovascular or open surgical techniques, is currently limited to the prevention or relief of life-threatening complications.[9,41] Operative treatment is indicated for patients with persistent or recurrent pain, medically uncontrolled hypertension, rapidly expanding aortic diameter, progression of dissection despite maximal medical management, signs of impending or actual aortic rupture (ie, periaortic or mediastinal hematoma), or malperfusion to limbs, kidneys, or gut (see Table 50-5).

Endovascular Therapy

General Considerations

Given the poor outcomes of open surgical approaches, endovascular therapy has transitioned to the frontline of therapy for complicated type B dissections. Endovascular treatments can include placement of thoracic endovascular graft prostheses, endovascular creation of flap fenestrations, and/or placement of uncovered stents in affected branch vessels to treat malperfusion. Because of the relative simplicity and recent improvements in outcomes, endovascular grafts have become the preferred endovascular technique for treatment of aortic dissections.

The goals of endovascular graft therapy in complicated acute aortic dissection are to restore flow to the true lumen and perfusion to the distal aorta and branch vessels. Coverage of the primary tear is frequently necessary to achieve these goals, especially if the tear is in the proximal descending aorta. Obliteration of the false lumen is desirable as well because it improves the prognosis, but it is not always possible. Endoluminal treatment of these cases usually requires coverage of the entire descending thoracic aorta because of the presence of multiple tears in the intima. The optimal outcome occurs when the prosthesis covers the primary tear, reapposes the dissected layers of the aorta, and prevents blood flow into the false lumen, therefore leading to

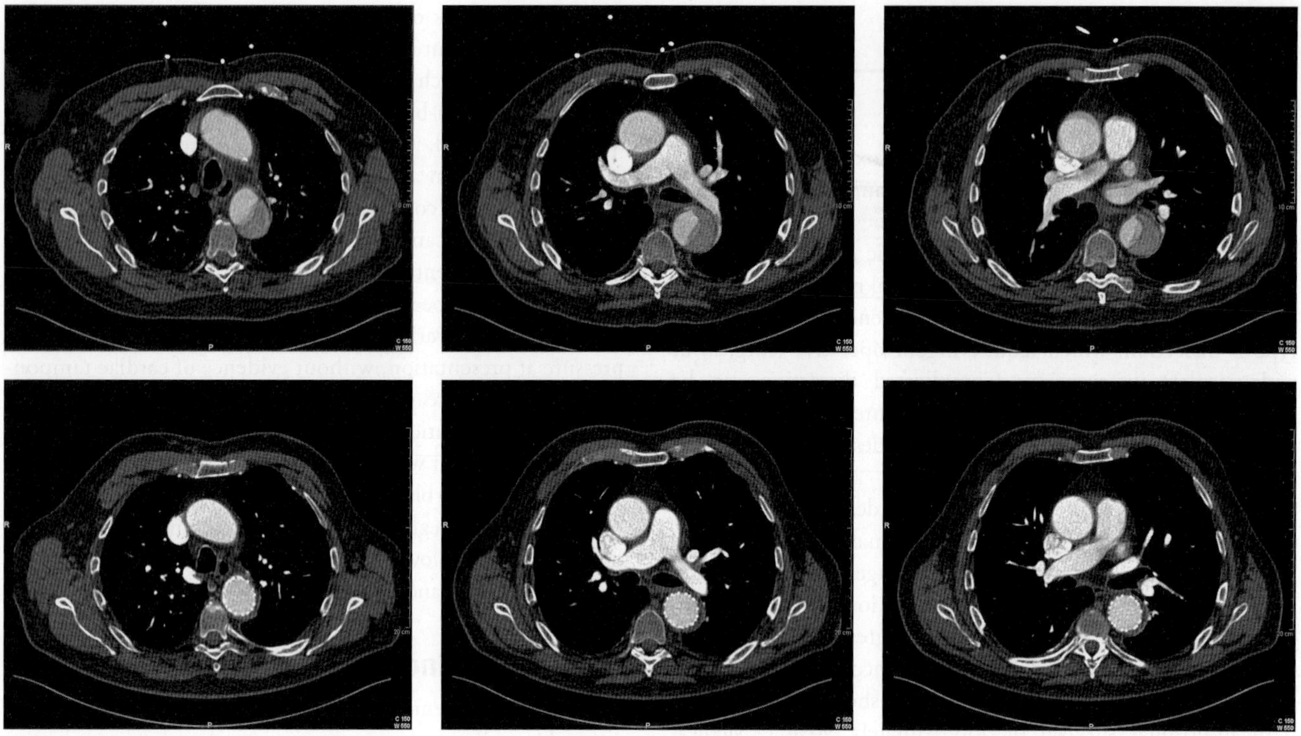

FIGURE 50-21 Endovascular stent grafting in a 77-year-old male with an acute type B aortic dissection. *Upper panel:* CTA at initial presentation showing a long dissection flap involving the descending thoracic aorta. *Lower panel:* CTA on the same patient one year after placement of an endovascular stent graft showing aortic remodeling with obliteration of the false lumen. (*Images courtesy of John Kern.*)

thrombosis of the false lumen, expansion of the true lumen, and restoration of branch vessel patency (Fig. 50-21).

An alternative technique used to treat branch malperfusion from aortic dissection is percutaneous fenestration with or without stenting of the malperfused branch vessels. According to this technique, a communication is created between the true and the false aortic lumens so as to provide flow to both of them. Percutaneous fenestration is performed by pulling an inflated balloon or a fenestration knife through the dissection flap to create communication between both lumens. An uncovered stent can then be placed in the true lumen at the region of the affected branch vessel or vessels to alleviate dynamic obstruction (occlusion of the branch by prolapse of the dissection flap into the branch vessel).[42] If static obstruction (extension of the dissection into the branch vessel with reduction of the true lumen) is also present, a stent is deployed directly into the branch vessel (Fig. 50-22). The major limitation of percutaneous fenestration for treatment of aortic dissection when compared with endovascular grafting, is that it does not induce thrombosis of the false lumen. False lumen thrombosis has been shown to induce aortic remodeling and decrease the long-term risk of aortic dilatation and rupture.[43]

Percutaneous fenestration and stenting can also be used as an adjunct to endovascular grafting when closure of the primary tear fails to improve distal malperfusion. Another technique that can be used to improve malperfusion after endovascular grafting is the PETTICOAT (provisional extension to induce complete attachment) technique.[44] According to this technique, a bare metal stent is placed as a distal extension of the previously implanted stent graft in order to expand the true lumen.

Preoperative Planning

The endovascular treatment of aortic dissections requires meticulous preoperative planning. The anatomy of the aorta and the actual dissection should be studied in detail with the use of imaging technology.

Preoperative imaging for endovascular repair of aortic dissections is accomplished with either computed tomographic angiography (CTA) or magnetic resonance angiography (MRA). Three-dimensional sagittal and coronal reconstructions are useful to assess details of the anatomy of the aorta. Preoperative imaging allows the surgeon to size the aorta for selection of the device, ascertain the presence of adequate proximal and distal landing zones for adequate apposition of the graft, and assess the femoral and iliac vessels to plan the delivery of the device.

The left subclavian artery may be occluded in certain situations without the need for revascularization. Exclusion of the left subclavian artery without concomitant revascularization should be avoided in patients with a patent left internal mammary artery coronary bypass, those with an incomplete posterior cerebral circulation, a dominant left vertebral vessel, or a stenosed or occluded right vertebral artery.[45] Left subclavian revascularization should also be considered in those patients in whom a long segment of the aorta is being covered or those with a history of prior

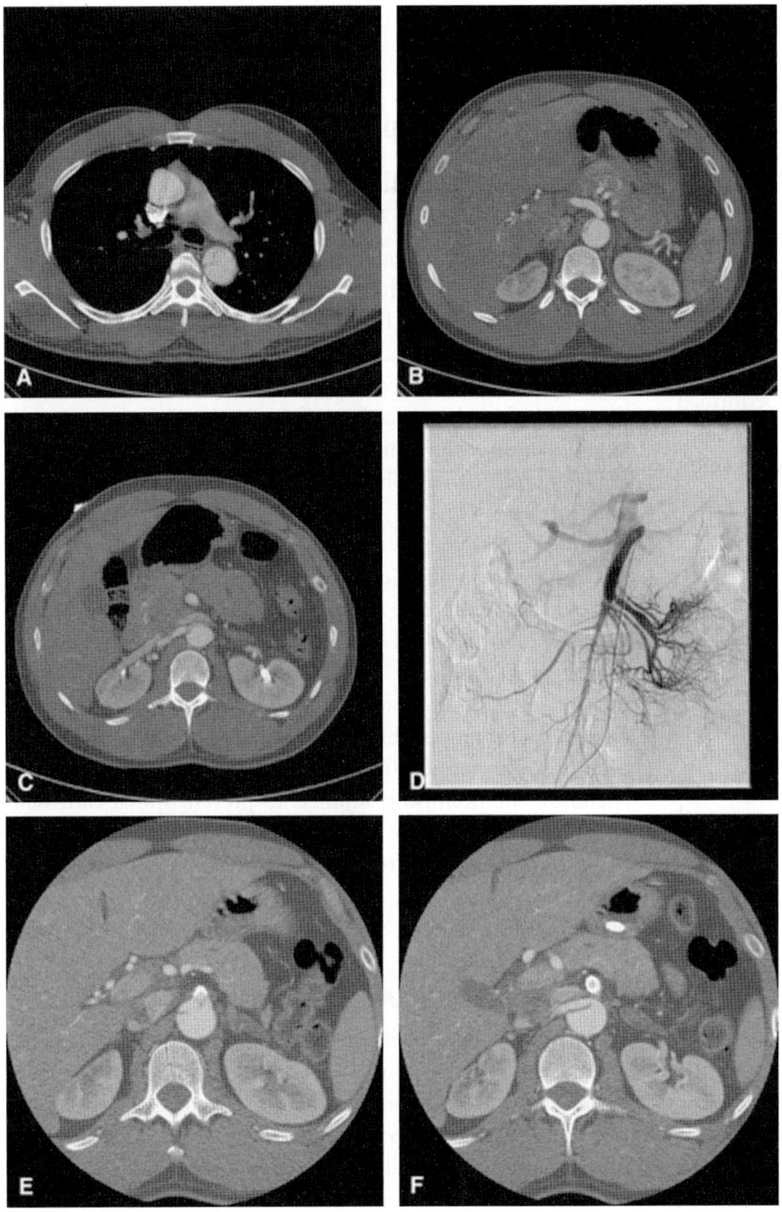

FIGURE 50-22 Endovascular treatment of visceral ischemia with fenestration and stenting of the aortic true lumen and the superior mesenteric artery (SMA) on a 40-year-old man with type B aortic dissection. (**A**) Near-total aortic true lumen collapse of the proximal descending aorta. (**B**) Dynamic compromise of the celiac artery origin. (**C**) Collapsed true lumen and dissection flap within the SMA suggesting both dynamic and static obstructions of this vessel. (**D**) Angiogram showing the dissection flap extending into the SMA. (**E, F**) Follow-up imaging at 1 month after percutaneous fenestration, true lumen stenting of the aorta at the level of the celiac artery, and placement of a stent into the SMA shows a patent fenestration tear in the dissection flap and a patent vessel. *(Reprinted from Patel HJ, Williams DM, Meerkov M, et al: Long-term results of percutaneous management of malperfusion in acute type B aortic dissection: implications for thoracic aortic endovascular repair. J Thorac Cardiovasc Surg 2009; 138:300-308, with permission from Elsevier.)*

aortic surgeries because of the increased risk of spinal ischemia. Left subclavian revascularization is usually accomplished with the creation of a left carotid to subclavian bypass, or less commonly, left subclavian artery transposition. To assess the cerebral circulation, a head and neck CTA should be performed preoperatively in every patient in whom left subclavian exclusion is a possibility. In our experience, the left subclavian artery is covered in approximately 50% of the cases, with 25% of these patients requiring revascularization because of concerns of cerebral circulation or arm claudication.[46]

Adequate vascular access for delivery of the device is an important requirement for endovascular therapy of the aorta. Both iliofemoral systems are evaluated preoperatively with CTA or MRA with particular attention to size, tortuosity, and presence of calcification that may preclude safe delivery of the device. The minimum size required for the access vessels is determined by the outer diameter of the introducer sheath. Current devices require insertion through a vessel of at least 6 to 8 mm in diameter (equivalent to ~20 French delivery device). When the femoral vessels have an adequate caliber, no tortuosity, and minimal calcification, total percutaneous access is possible, using automated percutaneous closure devices to seal the entry point. Alternatively, an open approach to control the common femoral arteries may be used. If the caliber of the femoral vessels is not appropriate for insertion of the device, retroperitoneal exposure of the iliac artery with placement of a 10-mm tube graft may be necessary as a surgical conduit for insertion of the device.

Endovascular stenting of the aorta is associated with a risk of paraplegia in recent series of 0 to 3.4%.[35,47] Preoperative insertion of a lumbar catheter for drainage of cerebrospinal fluid (CSF) may decrease the risk of permanent paraplegia. In our institutions, we perform selective preoperative placement of lumbar catheters at the discretion of the surgeon, taking into account the region and length of planned aortic exclusion, and previous history of aortic surgery.[45] If there is no evidence of paraplegia postoperatively, these drains are usually discontinued 48 to 72 hours after surgery.

Operative Technique

The endovascular stenting procedure can be performed either in the angiography suite or an operating room with advanced imaging capabilities. At our institutions, the procedure is performed in the angiography suite by a team of cardiovascular surgeons and interventional radiologists. The procedure is usually performed under general anesthesia, although local or epidural anesthesia can also be used, depending on the comorbidities and clinical status of the patient. Monitoring lines are placed, including a radial arterial line in the right upper extremity. A lumbar drain for CSF drainage is placed preoperatively at the discretion of the surgeon, as stated. Antibiotic prophylaxis is administered.

In most cases, bilateral iliofemoral arterial access is used for the procedure. The larger side with less calcification and tortuosity is chosen for the delivery of the device. The other side is used for percutaneous insertion of a 5 French pigtail catheter for diagnostic contrast injection. If only one side is appropriate for use, the diagnostic pigtail catheter may be inserted through one of the brachial arteries.

If there is significant calcification of the vessel or the surgeon does not feel comfortable with the use of a percutaneous vascular closure device, the femoral artery is surgically exposed and controlled. In our experience, approximately 20% of patients have femoral vessels of an inadequate caliber to accommodate the delivery device. In these patients, a flank incision is performed and the retroperitoneal common iliac artery is exposed. A 10-mm polyester surgical conduit is then anastomosed to the common iliac artery and used as access for delivery of the device.

The pigtail catheter is inserted percutaneously and advanced to the arch of the aorta. Aortography or IVUS is then used to confirm the location of the catheter within the true lumen, define the anatomy, localize the entry tear, and create a roadmap for the procedure. The confirmation of the device being in the true lumen cannot be overemphasized. Many centers use only IVUS for these procedures. From these images, the decision is made regarding the site of deployment. The left subclavian artery may need to be covered to ensure an adequate proximal landing zone and completely exclude the primary tear. The proximal landing zone is usually visualized best at a fluoroscopic angle of approximately 45 to 75 degrees left anterior oblique (LAO).

A super-stiff wire is then inserted through a sheath placed into the iliofemoral vessel previously chosen for device delivery, and advanced into the aortic arch. The patient is heparinized to an ACT of greater than or equal to 200 seconds. The appropriate sheath is advanced into the abdominal aorta under direct fluoroscopic visualization. The device is then advanced to the selected point of delivery. Placement of the sheath and the device into the aorta are probably the most dangerous parts of this procedure. Before the deployment of the device, blood pressure and heart rate should be pharmacologically controlled so as to avoid undue strain on the heart and migration of the endograft on deployment. The device is then deployed. The optimal placement of the prosthesis is confirmed by angiography or IVUS. Although the device may need to be ballooned for full opening and apposition to the aortic wall, this maneuver has inherent risks given the weakness of the aortic wall and the pressure required to expand the stent grafts.

It is important to confirm the correct placement of the device, the absence of endoleaks, and the resolution of malperfusion to branch vessels at the end of the procedure. For this purpose, an angiogram is performed through the diagnostic pigtail catheter. If there is evidence of persistent malperfusion, adjunctive therapies should be considered such as percutaneous fenestration or deployment of additional bare-metal stents on the distal aspect of the prosthesis to expand the true lumen (PETTICOAT technique). Branch vessel stenting may also be necessary to relieve static obstruction.[42] In case of a ruptured dissection, the endovascular prosthesis should cover both the site of the primary tear and the site of rupture. Furthermore, in patients with significant hemothorax the dissection should be treated before draining the chest, as this may be tamponading the rupture.

Surgical Therapy

General Considerations

Open surgical intervention for type B aortic dissections is performed under general anesthesia with narcotic and inhalational agents. Double-lumen endotracheal intubation allows for lung isolation, which is critical in exposure of the thoracic aorta. Central venous access, right radial and femoral arterial lines, and in selected cases a pulmonary artery catheter, are inserted before the procedure. Core body temperature is usually measured with the use of a temperature probe in the Foley catheter and/or an esophageal probe. Antibiotic prophylaxis is administered.

Spinal cord ischemia resulting in paraplegia or paraparesis is a recognized complication of acute dissection repair that may be partially preventable and even reversible. The incidence of spinal cord ischemia is between 19 and 36% after repair of acute type B dissection.[48,49] Whereas various strategies exist to prevent spinal cord ischemia during repair of a chronic dissection, very few are feasible in the acute setting. Pharmacologic agents such as steroids, free radical scavengers, vasodilators, and adenosine are promising adjuncts to prevent spinal cord ischemia but presently have little to no proven clinical utility. We presently use left atrial to femoral artery bypass and reimplant key intercostals arteries and selectively use cerebrospinal fluid drainage as outlined by Safi et al.[50]

Operative Technique

The patient is positioned in right lateral decubitus. The pelvis is canted posteriorly to allow access to both femoral vessels. A posterolateral thoracotomy in the fourth intercostal space provides sufficient access to the aorta; notching the fifth and sixth ribs posteriorly can facilitate wider exposure of the thorax. A thoracoabdominal incision may be required to access the abdominal aorta in the case of visceral malperfusion. This may be performed through either a transperitoneal or a retroperitoneal approach. The left hemidiaphragm is divided in a radial fashion while marking adjacent sites on each side of the division with metal clips for later reapproximation.

The ideal open acute type B aortic dissection repair involves replacement of as little of the descending thoracic aorta as necessary. The extent of replacement rarely exceeds the proximal third, which includes the primary tear in most cases. Such a strategy optimizes perfusion of the spinal cord by preserving more intercostals arteries.[48] This point is controversial, however, and some groups advocate replacement of the entire thoracic aorta. Any less extensive aortic replacement leaves dissected aorta with the potential for late aneurysmal dilation when there is perfusion of the false lumen. The ideal strategy to minimize spinal cord malperfusion yet resect all involved aorta has not been proved.

Once the thoracic aorta has been exposed, the operation continues with division of the mediastinal pleura between the left subclavian and the left common carotid arteries. It is essential that the left vagus and recurrent laryngeal nerves are identified and preserved during the course of the dissection. The left subclavian artery is encircled with an umbilical tape and Rummel tourniquet. Ultimately, the entire distal arch must be free enough to place an aortic clamp between the left common carotid and left subclavian arteries. Next, the proximal descending thoracic aorta is circumferentially mobilized, dividing intercostal arteries in the segment to be excised.

The formerly popular "clamp and sew" technique used for repair of acute type B dissection has largely been replaced by the use of partial left heart bypass. To institute left heart bypass, the left inferior pulmonary vein is dissected and a 4-0 Prolene pursestring suture placed posteriorly for cannulation. Arterial cannulation sites for this technique include the distal thoracic aorta for limited dissections of the proximal descending thoracic aorta or the femoral artery for those extending into the abdomen. It is important to assure that distal perfusion during cannulation is directed into the true lumen. Following the administration of 100 U/kg of intravenous heparin, 14 French cannulae are inserted into the left inferior pulmonary vein and either a normal-appearing area of descending thoracic aorta or percutaneously into either femoral artery. Bypass is then initiated with flow rates between 1 and 2 L/min.

The left subclavian artery is controlled and vascular clamps are placed on the aorta proximal to the left subclavian artery and distally on the mid-thoracic aorta. Right radial artery pressure is measured to maintain proximal aortic systolic pressure between 100 and 140 mm Hg and mean femoral artery pressure greater than 60 mm Hg.[49] The aorta is then opened longitudinally and bleeding from intercostals arteries is controlled by suture ligation. Transection of the aorta distal to the origin of the left subclavian artery provides a site for the proximal anastomosis. This is performed using 3-0 Prolene suture and may require external reinforcement with Teflon felt strips.

The graft inclusion technique is another procedure in which the posterior aspect of the proximal aorta is not fully transected. The proximal anastomosis is then created to the intact posterior aspect of the aorta. We do not recommend this technique because one cannot be certain of including all layers of the aorta in the anastomosis.

The size of the vascular graft is based on the diameter of the distal aorta and beveled to match the aorta proximally. This anastomosis may include the origin of the left subclavian to treat dissection in this vessel. A separate 6- to 8-mm Dacron graft can be used if there is intimal disruption involving the proximal segment of the left subclavian artery. Once the proximal anastomosis is completed, the proximal clamp is released and repositioned on the vascular graft to inspect the anastomosis. The distal anastomosis is then completed, the clamps are released, and partial left heart bypass is terminated. Percutaneously placed femoral artery cannulae 14 French or smaller may be removed without direct repair of the vessel. When cannulae 15 French or larger are required, open surgical repair of the femoral arteriotomy is indicated.

Rupture of the thoracic aorta before or during repair is a catastrophic event often leading to operative death. Successful management requires immediate cannulation of the femoral artery and vein for cardiopulmonary bypass and eventual deep hypothermic circulatory arrest. Assisted venous drainage through the femoral vein is often adequate, but direct cannulation of the right ventricle through the pulmonary artery may also be performed. A left atrial vent is placed through the left inferior pulmonary vein once the heart begins to fibrillate; the left ventricle may be vented as well directly through the apex. Once the nasopharyngeal temperature reaches 15°C, the vent is occluded and cardiopulmonary bypass is stopped. The head is placed down and the aorta opened for repair under circulatory arrest. The distal aorta should be clamped to minimize blood loss. Once the proximal anastomosis is performed, the proximal clamp is moved onto the graft and the graft cannulated to resume cardiopulmonary bypass.

Malperfusion of intra-abdominal viscera or lower extremities may be apparent at the time of presentation or may follow surgical repair of aortic dissections. Proximal repair of the dissection is standard treatment and may be sufficient to treat the malperfusion syndrome. However, if malperfusion presents or persists after surgical repair, percutaneous or surgical fenestration may be necessary. As specified, percutaneous fenestration is accomplished by using a balloon or a percutaneous knife to create a communication between the false and the true lumens. Surgical fenestration is performed through a midline laparotomy or left flank incision to provide exposure of the infrarenal aorta (Fig. 50-23). Occasionally, fenestration of intra-abdominal aortic branch vessels may be required if

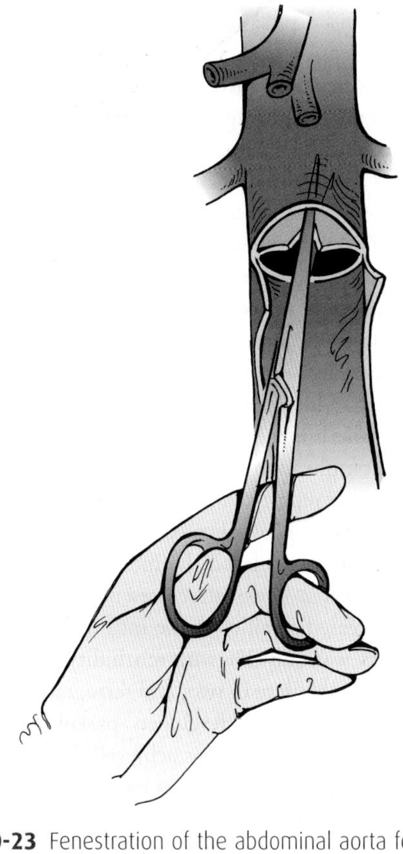

FIGURE 50-23 Fenestration of the abdominal aorta for visceral malperfusion. A transverse incision is made into the aorta, preferably into a nondissected aorta. The proximal dissection membrane is incised and then excised to decompress the false lumen as far proximally as possible. The dissected layers are reconstructed with Teflon felt or glue and the aortotomy is closed directly.

the intima is violated beyond the ostia. If the dissection flap cannot be completely excised, the distal vessel layers must be reunited. Consideration should be given to patch angioplasty to prevent narrowing when closing smaller vessels. In the event that perfusion is not reestablished, extra-anatomic bypass may be required.

Obstruction of the terminal aorta or malperfusion of the lower extremities following operative repair is best treated with percutaneous fenestration. Surgical fenestration remains an option if percutaneous techniques fail to reestablish blood flow. In the event that surgical fenestration fails, the best solution is femoral-femoral bypass grafting in the setting of unilateral malperfusion or axilla-femoral and femoral-femoral bypass if bilateral lower extremity malperfusion exists.

Results

Medical management remains the mainstay of treatment for acute uncomplicated type B aortic dissections. Early medical management alone is an adequate treatment in approximately 68 to 85% of patients presenting with acute type B dissection and leads to a 30-day survival rate of 89 to 93%.[35,51] The long-term outcomes of medical management are not as favorable. In the IRAD series, only 78% of 189 patients discharged alive from the hospital after medical management of type B dissections were alive at 3 years.[34] Predictors of follow-up mortality were female gender, history of prior aneurysm, history of atherosclerosis, in-hospital renal failure, pleural effusion, and in-hospital hypotension or shock. In a separate series of patients, 87% of patients managed medically were alive at 5 years, with 25% of patients requiring aortic-related interventions.[52] Similarly, in a series of 122 patients with type B aortic dissections managed medically over 36 years, Umaña et al reported survival rates of 85% at 1 year and 71% at 5 years, with reoperation rates of 14% at 5 years.[36]

These outcomes have prompted some authors to consider operative treatment of uncomplicated dissections in an attempt to prevent long-term aortic-related complications. The rationale for this consideration also comes from the fact that endovascular stenting induces thrombosis of the false lumen in 75% of cases[39] and false lumen patency is associated with long-term aortic-related complications and mortality.[53]

Xu et al recently reported a series of 63 patients with type B aortic dissections (59 uncomplicated) treated with endovascular grafting.[54] The authors delayed the intervention in uncomplicated patients until 2 weeks after presentation so as to allow fibrosis and increased stability of the intimal flap. The perioperative mortality was only 3% with morbidity including stroke in one patient, renal failure in two, and retrograde aortic dissection in two. No patients developed paraplegia. Complete thrombosis of the false lumen was achieved in 98% of patients at 1 year, and the 4-year survival was nearly 90%.

Two European randomized clinical trials have been designed to answer the question of whether uncomplicated type B dissections should be treated with endovascular grafting or with medical management alone. The results of the first trial, the INSTEAD (INvestigation of STEnt Grafts in Aortic Dissection) trial, have been recently published.[55] This trial randomized 140 patients with subacute or chronic type B aortic dissection (>14 days but <1 year) to either elective stent graft placement or optimal medical management alone. Survival was not significantly different between both groups with 2-year survival rates of 96 and 89% after optimal medical therapy and endovascular stenting, respectively. There were also no differences in the rates of a combined end point, including aortic-related deaths or reinterventions. Complete thrombosis of the false lumen was more common among patients with endovascular stenting (91% with stenting versus 19% with medical management). Aortic expansion to greater than 6 cm was also more common in the group with medical management, requiring crossover to stent grafting in 16% of cases and conversion to open surgery in 4%. All crossover patients had uneventful outcomes and no deaths. Therefore, the trial supported the use of optimal medical management for treatment of uncomplicated type B aortic dissections and reserving endovascular interventions for those patients that develop complications or other indications for intervention. The second trial, the ADSORB (Acute Uncomplicated Aortic Dissection Type B) trial has been designed to study patients with acute uncomplicated dissection (<14 days) by randomizing them to optimal medical management or endovascular stenting.[56] The trial started enrollment in 2007 and is underway. No results are currently available.

Based on these results, medical management remains the standard of care for *uncomplicated* type B aortic dissection.

Approximately 20% of patients with acute type B aortic dissection present with complications requiring operative intervention.[35] In the past, surgical intervention was the only therapy available for these patients. The development of endovascular techniques has provided an additional treatment option that is now preferred in the majority of cases.

Surgical treatment of aortic dissection was traditionally poised with dismal outcomes. Even though morbidity and mortality remain high, outcomes from surgical management have improved over the last few decades, from as high as 50% in the 1960s to as low as 13% in more recent times.[57] In a series of 76 patients treated emergently with surgery for acute complicated type B aortic dissection including 22% patients with aortic rupture, Bozinovski et al reported an in-hospital mortality of 22% with a risk of stroke of 7%, paraplegia of 7%, and renal failure of 20%.[58] Similarly, as part of the IRAD series, 82 patients surgically treated for acute type B aortic dissection had an in-hospital mortality of 29% with a risk of stroke of 9%, paraplegia of 5%, and acute renal failure of 8%.[59]

Because of the unfavorable outcomes of open surgical therapy for acute complicated type B aortic dissection, endovascular therapies have been increasingly used in this patient population. Table 50-6 summarizes the current experience with endovascular therapy for treatment of type B aortic dissections.[35,37,38,42,46,47,54,60–68]

A recent meta-analysis of 39 studies involving 609 patients using endovascular repair of aortic dissections between 1999 and 2004 showed a procedural success of 98% with emergency surgical conversion of 1%. In-hospital complications occurred in 14% of patients including neurological complications in 3%, retrograde dissection in 2%, and a perioperative mortality

TABLE 50-6 Selected Retrospective Series with Endovascular Treatment of Type B Aortic Dissection

Study	N	Type of Dissection	Technique	Technical Success	Perioperative Mortality	Morbidity	Permanent Paraplegia	Endoleak	Median Follow Up (mo)	Long-Term Survival	False Lumen Thrombosis
Böckler, 2009[47]	54	Acute and chronic	Stent graft	93%	11%	19%	0%		32	66%	60% complete, 13% partial
Dake, 1999[37]	19	Acute	Stent graft	100%	16%	21%	0%	15%	13	79%	79% complete, 21% partial
Dialetto, 2005[68]	28	Acute	Stent graft	100%	11%		0%		18	86%	
Duebener, 2004[67]	10	Acute	Stent graft	90%	20%	50%	10%		25	80%	
Fattori, 2008[35]	66	Acute	65% stent graft, 35% fenestration	94% stent graft, 50% fenestration	10.6%	20.8%	3.4%				
Hutschala, 2002[66]	9	Acute	Stent graft	100%	0%	11%	0%		3		22% complete, 78% partial
Khoynezhad, 2009[65]	28	Acute	Stent graft	90%	11%		0%	28%	36	78%	88% complete, 12% partial
Kische, 2009[64]	171	Acute and chronic	Stent graft	98%	5%	17%	1.7%	29%	22	81%	
Nathanson, 2005[63]	40	Acute and chronic	Stent graft	95%	2.5%	38%	2.5%	2.5%	20	85%	79%
Nienaber, 1999[38]	12	Chronic	Stent graft	100%	0%	0%	0%		12	100%	100%
Nienaber, 2002[62]	127	Acute	Stent graft	100%	1.6%	3%	0.8%		28	97%	
Palma, 2002[61]	70	Acute	Stent graft	93%	5.7%	31.4%	0%		29	91%	
Patel, 2009[42]	69	Acute	Fenestration and/or branch stenting	96%	17.4%	21.7%	2.9%*		42	64%	—
Pitton, 2008[60]	13	Acute	Stent graft	100%	15%	31%	7.7%*		13	66%	
Siefert, 2008[46]	34	Acute and chronic	Stent graft	100%	0%	11.7%	0%	38%		86%	
Xu, 2006[54]	63	Acute and chronic	Stent graft	95%	3.2%	19%	0%		12	90%	98%

*Patients presented preoperatively with paraplegia.

of 5%.[39] Survival rates at 2 years were 89% with a risk of aortic rupture at follow-up of 2%.

Most of these studies have used endografts, rather than percutaneous fenestrations, as the endovascular treatment of choice. In one of the largest series of percutaneous fenestration for treatment of type B aortic dissection, Patel et al reports the experience from the University of Michigan from 1997 to 2008.[42] During this period, 69 patients with type B aortic dissection and malperfusion by angiography were treated with endovascular flap fenestration and/or branch vessel stenting. Overall technical success for flow restoration was 96% with an early mortality of 17%. Complications included stroke in 4%, acute renal failure requiring dialysis in 14%, and permanent spinal cord ischemia in two patients that presented initially with paraplegia from their dissection. However, despite these encouraging outcomes all-cause mortality at follow-up was as high as 36% with 7% risk of aortic rupture, likely related to the obligate persistence of the false lumen as part of the fenestration procedure.

Despite the multiple isolated series reporting outcomes after different treatment strategies for acute type B aortic dissection, there are currently no randomized controlled trials addressing this issue. The most recent retrospective report by IRAD comparing the different strategies included 571 patients with acute complicated or uncomplicated type B aortic dissection between 1996 and 2005. Of these, 390 patients (68%) were treated medically and 125 required intervention for complicated dissection; 59 (10%) underwent open surgical procedures and 66 (11%) had endovascular treatment with either stent grafts or percutaneous fenestration. In-hospital mortality was significantly higher for patients that underwent surgery (34%) when compared to those that had endovascular procedures (11%) (Fig. 50-24). In-hospital complications occurred in 40% of

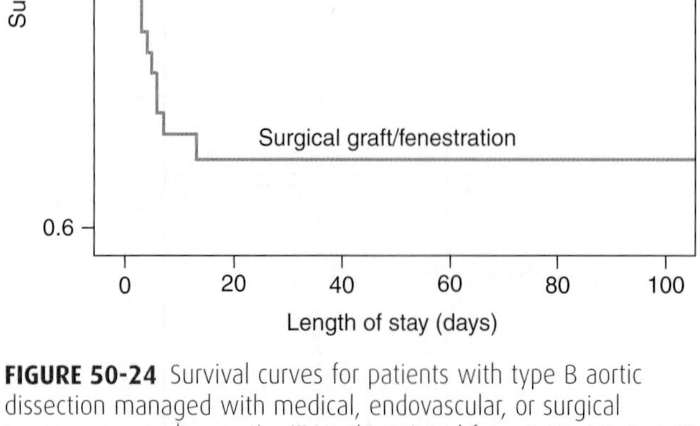

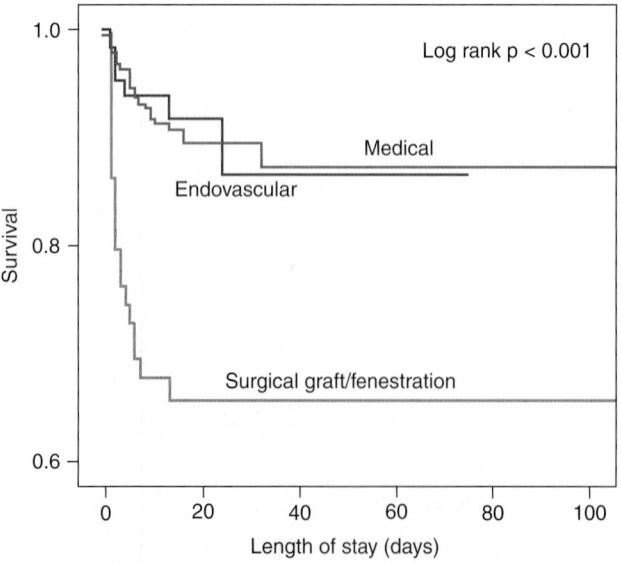

FIGURE 50-24 Survival curves for patients with type B aortic dissection managed with medical, endovascular, or surgical treatment according to the IRAD. (*Reprinted from Fattori R, Tsai TT, Myrmel T, et al: Complicated acute type B dissection: is surgery still the best option? A report from the International Registry of Acute Aortic Dissection. JACC Cardiovasc Intervent 2008; 1:395-402, with permission from Elsevier.*)

patients undergoing surgical treatment and in 21% of those undergoing endovascular therapy. These findings remained true even after comparing patients with similar comorbidities. Interestingly, in-hospital mortality was similar for those patients that underwent endovascular therapy and those that were treated medically, and significantly better than in those that underwent surgery. The low mortality risk of patients treated medically is obviously related to the fact that most of these patients presented with uncomplicated disease and were deemed eligible for medical management. However, the data suggest that endovascular therapies may improve outcomes of patients with *complicated* type B aortic dissection to the rate of those with uncomplicated dissections managed medically. The data have to be interpreted with caution though, because part of these findings may be associated to selection bias in treatment modality based on patient characteristics not accounted for, or in differing treatment strategies in different institutions.

MANAGEMENT OF CHRONIC AORTIC DISSECTION

Natural History

Chronic type A dissection develops in patients who fail to undergo immediate surgical treatment of the acute dissection. Patients with chronic type B aortic dissection include those that have been successfully managed medically after an acute dissection and those with repaired type A aortic dissections that have retained segments of dissected descending thoracic aorta.

Patients with a history of acute aortic dissection, especially those with retained dissected segments, require close surveillance indefinitely. Our preference for follow-up imaging in patients with normal renal function and no contrast allergy is CTA. CTA provides good imaging, is cost effective, and is usually the technique used for the original acute dissection, making it ideal for longitudinal comparison of studies. MRA is utilized mostly as a follow-up study for patients with renal insufficiency but is the study of choice to provide precise anatomical detail for operative planning.

Many patients treated for aortic dissection, especially those with persistent communication between true and false lumens, can progress to develop aneurysmal dilatation of the aorta. They carry similar risk for aortic rupture that that of atherosclerotic aneurysms. Chronic dissections have an annual rate of expansion of 0.9 to 7.2 mm per year.[69–71] Despite appropriate medical management and close follow-up, approximately 20 to 40% of patients have aortic enlargement during follow up.[69,72] This number is probably even higher in those patients with connective tissue disorders. In one study of 50 patients over a period of 40 months, 18% had fatal rupture and another 20% underwent surgical repair because of symptoms or aneurysm enlargement, emphasizing the need for diligent follow-up care.[69] Risk factors for rupture of chronic type B dissection include older age, COPD, and hypertension. Chronic beta-blocker treatment reduces the rate of aortic dilatation as well as the incidence of dissection-related hospital admissions and procedures.[72]

The presence of a patent false lumen is a significant predictor of aortic enlargement and is associated with a higher incidence of aortic-related complications and death.[53,70] In a study of 101 patients followed after medical management for type B uncomplicated dissections, the most important risk factors for aortic enlargement were a maximum aortic diameter of 4 cm or more and a patent false lumen.[73]

Operative Indications

The operative indications for chronic type A and B dissection are shown in Table 50-5. Chronic type A dissection is rarely symptomatic yet a minority of patients will present with chest pain as a result of aneurysm expansion or heart failure related to aortic regurgitation. Chronic type B dissection may present with intermittent dull chest or back pain, or infrequently, with malperfusion syndrome. Although each of these findings is an indication for intervention, the most common indications for operative management are aneurysmal dilatation of the aorta, rapid expansion, or aortic rupture. The size criteria for intervention in aortic dissection are controversial, but the one generally used is similar to that for general thoracic aortic aneurysms. Based on these criteria, aortic intervention is indicated at a size of 5.5 cm for type A dissections and 6.5 cm for type B dissections, or slightly less if there is a family history or physical stigmata of a connective tissue disorder.[74] Similarly, aortic expansion greater than 1 cm per year should be considered an indication for repair.

Recent retrospective studies from Japan have shown that patients with aortic diameters greater than or equal to 4 cm and a patent false lumen have a high likelihood of aortic-related complications (up to 50% in 6 months).[73,75] Based on these findings, it has been suggested that these patients should be considered for early repair depending on their operative risk. This issue is controversial and further studies are required before making more definitive recommendations.

Techniques for Chronic Type A Aortic Dissection

Chronic type A dissection, with or without aneurysmal enlargement, is treated using similar operative techniques described for acute dissection. The particular operation performed depends on the specific pathology involving the aortic root, status of the aortic valve, distal extent of dissection, and brachiocephalic vessel involvement. The pathology of each of these components can be very different in a chronic dissection as compared with the acute process. These differences underlie the need for surgical techniques appropriate to each unique abnormality. In general, the ascending aorta is replaced using a vascular graft to include the entire diseased segment as in acute dissection, but surgical treatment of the aortic valve and creation of the distal anastomosis differ.

Whereas the aortic valve can be repaired in most cases of acute type A dissection by simple commissural resuspension, the rate of aortic valve replacement is much higher in patients with chronic dissection. Preservation of the aortic valve is complicated by morphologic changes in the valvular apparatus such as leaflet elongation and annuloaortic ectasia, which render the valve irreparable in as many as 50% of cases. More severe grades of preoperative aortic regurgitation portend a lower probability of valve preservation. In cases in which the aortic valve cannot be preserved with simple commissural reattachment, three options exist to treat aortic insufficiency: composite root replacement, aortic valve replacement with separate ascending aortic replacement, and finally, valve-sparing aortic root repair. The technical aspects of composite valve-graft repair were covered under the surgical management of acute type A dissection. Separate aortic valve and ascending aortic replacement are appropriate when there is an operative indication to repair the ascending aorta in the setting of a normal aortic root and structural aortic valve disease. Note that this operation is not appropriate for patients with connective tissue disease. In this situation, aortic root replacement is required.

Several methods for aortic valve preservation have been described for cases affecting the aortic root. One such technique is performed by reimplanting the valve commissures into an appropriately sized vascular graft, which is secured to the left ventricular outflow tract using multiple horizontal mattress sutures.[76] Another elegant yet time-consuming technique requires resection of the sinuses of Valsalva leaving a 5-mm rim of aorta circumferentially around the leaflets.[77] Scallops are then created in the vascular graft to resuspend the commissures and remodel the aortic root. David et al advocate Teflon felt reinforcement of the aortic annulus to prevent late annular dilatation and recurrent aortic insufficiency for the remodeling technique.[78] The mid-term outcome of such operations revealed a freedom from reoperation rate of 97 to 99% at 5 years and a 5-year survival for the aortic dissection subgroup of 84%. Cochran et al devised a similar technique to recreate the sinuses of Valsalva, which may be more important than previously recognized and contribute to improved long-term valve durability.[79] Such data in patients with chronic dissection are lacking. These techniques appear appropriate for patients with Marfan disease and in those with congenitally bicuspid aortic valves.

Treatment of the distal aorta in chronic type A dissection is somewhat controversial. Some advocate obliteration of flow in the false lumen with distal aortic repair, whereas others purposely maintain flow into both the true and false lumen using distal resection of the intimal flap. Those who reunite the chronically dissected aortic layers to perfuse only the true lumen maintain that false lumen perfusion continues through distal reentry tears in greater than 50% of cases. There is a theoretical concern that important side branches arise exclusively from the false lumen and perfusion may be interrupted with this technique. Our practice at the University of Virginia is to resect the distal chronic dissection flap as far as possible to obviate such concerns. The distal anastomosis is therefore made to the outer wall of the aorta, which has been strengthened over time. Malperfusion of the brachiocephalic vessels as a result of chronic type A dissection is treated with resection of the dissection flap from the arch. Infrequently, the chronic dissection flap extends into more distal branch vessels and may present as transient ischemic attacks or stroke. In such cases it is often necessary to resect the dissection flap into the branch vessel or reunite the layers distally before reimplantation.

Infrequently, chronic type A dissection results in extensive aneurysmal dilatation of the aorta extending from the ascending aorta through the arch and into the descending thoracic aorta. Surgical treatment of such extensive disease has traditionally been performed as a staged procedure in which the ascending aorta and arch are replaced first through a sternotomy. The second stage of the so-called elephant trunk procedure is performed 6 weeks later through a left thoracotomy for replacement of the descending aorta using a second vascular graft. Originally described by Borst et al, this technique has been used extensively with good results.[80] In some cases, the aorta distal to the left subclavian artery may be so large as to preclude the use of a two-stage repair. Kouchoukos et al. have described a single-stage repair performed through a bilateral anterior thoracotomy in which the arch is repaired first during a brief period of circulatory arrest. Right subclavian and femoral artery cannulation for cardiopulmonary bypass provide proximal and distal perfusion during the subsequent ascending and descending aortic replacement. The hospital mortality was 6.2% and there were no adverse neurologic outcomes in the small series.[81] Postoperative and long-term management of these cases are identical to the acute repairs, but with an emphasis on monitoring for evidence of malperfusion.

Techniques for Chronic Type B Aortic Dissection

Endovascular Therapy

Endovascular therapy has been recently used for management of chronic type B aortic dissections[38,46,47,54,63,64] (see Table 50-6). The goal of endovascular therapy is to seal any dissection entry points, promote thrombosis of the false lumen, induce aortic remodeling, and prevent further aneurysmal dilatation, rupture, or malperfusion.

The general considerations, preoperative assessment, and operative technique for endovascular therapies in chronic dissection are similar to the ones described for acute type B dissection. Although percutaneous fenestrations may be used in cases of malperfusion, most chronic dissections require treatment for aneurysmal dilatation and aortic expansion because of the persistence of a false lumen, an obligate consequence of fenestrations. Therefore, the endovascular treatment of choice for most chronic dissections is endovascular grafting. Because of the increased risk of spinal malperfusion, lumbar drainage for spinal protection is used liberally in chronic dissections.

Preoperative planning with CTA or MRA is important to define the anatomy and plan the deployment of the endovascular graft. Multiple connections between the true and the false lumen may be identified in chronic dissections. It is important to seal all entry points with the endovascular graft to depressurize the false lumen. Follow-up imaging and close surveillance after the endovascular procedure are necessary.

Surgical Therapy

The purpose of surgical intervention in chronic aortic dissection is to replace all segments of dissected aorta at risk for rupture and prevent the possibility of subsequent malperfusion syndrome. The conduct of the operation including surgical approach, monitoring lines required, anesthetic technique, and cardiopulmonary bypass is similar to that described for acute dissections. Greater emphasis is placed on methods of spinal cord protection.

The incidence of paraplegia after repair of thoracoabdominal aneurysms resulting from aortic dissection is reportedly as high as 25%.[82] Both mechanical and pharmacologic interventions have been advocated over the last decade to reduce this risk. Partial left heart bypass alone for replacement of the thoracic aorta above the level of T9 can reduce paraplegia rate to between 5 and 8%.[83] We routinely use a lumbar drain for aneurysms extending below T9.[50] Reimplanting intercostals and lumbar arteries between T9 and L1 can be an important adjunct.[84] The aortic cross-clamp is sequentially moved distally to perfuse branches as they are reimplanted. The combination of distal perfusion, cerebrospinal fluid drainage, and reimplanting large intercostal and lumbar arteries has significantly reduced the incidence of paraplegia at our institutions. Additional techniques used for spinal cord protection include measurement of sensory and motor evoked potentials, regional epidural cooling, and the use of a variety of pharmacologic agents for cellular protection.

The techniques used for replacement of the descending thoracic aorta are identical to those described for treatment of acute type B dissection. The extent of resection, however, for chronic type B dissection is usually greater with the goal to remove all dissected aorta at risk for rupture or symptoms. Usually these operations can be performed through the left chest, but more extensive aneurysms or cases of visceral malperfusion require a thoracoabdominal incision or a staged repair. The proximal anastomosis is ideally made to undissected normal aorta but infrequently the distal arch is involved, which requires alteration in surgical strategy.

As mentioned, we prefer the combination of partial left heart bypass and cerebrospinal fluid drainage for spinal cord protection. Sites for cannulation are the left inferior pulmonary vein and the left femoral artery or descending thoracic aorta. Depending on location and extent of aneurysm, the distal arch is mobilized first. The area between the left common carotid and left subclavian artery is circumferentially dissected, and the left subclavian artery is independently controlled. Partial left heart bypass is then initiated. Ideally, clamps are placed between the left subclavian and left common carotid arteries and on the aorta distal to the involved segment. If the entire descending thoracic aorta is diseased, the clamp is placed on the mid-thoracic aorta to perform the proximal anastomosis first. The aorta is opened and small intercostal arteries are oversewn. The proximal anastomosis is made to normal aorta whenever possible with running 3-0 Prolene; 4-0 Prolene is used if the tissue is fragile. The clamp is moved distally onto the graft to inspect the proximal anastomosis and achieve hemostasis. Several centimeters of the dissection flap is then resected from the lumen of the distal aorta and the distal anastomosis created to the adventitia of the chronic dissection. In more extensive thoracoabdominal disease, the clamp is progressively moved distal as intercostal arteries below T7 to L2 and visceral vessels are reimplanted (Fig. 50-25). Bypass is terminated and the operation completed.

Full cardiopulmonary bypass with deep hypothermic circulatory arrest may be necessary in cases in which the proximal

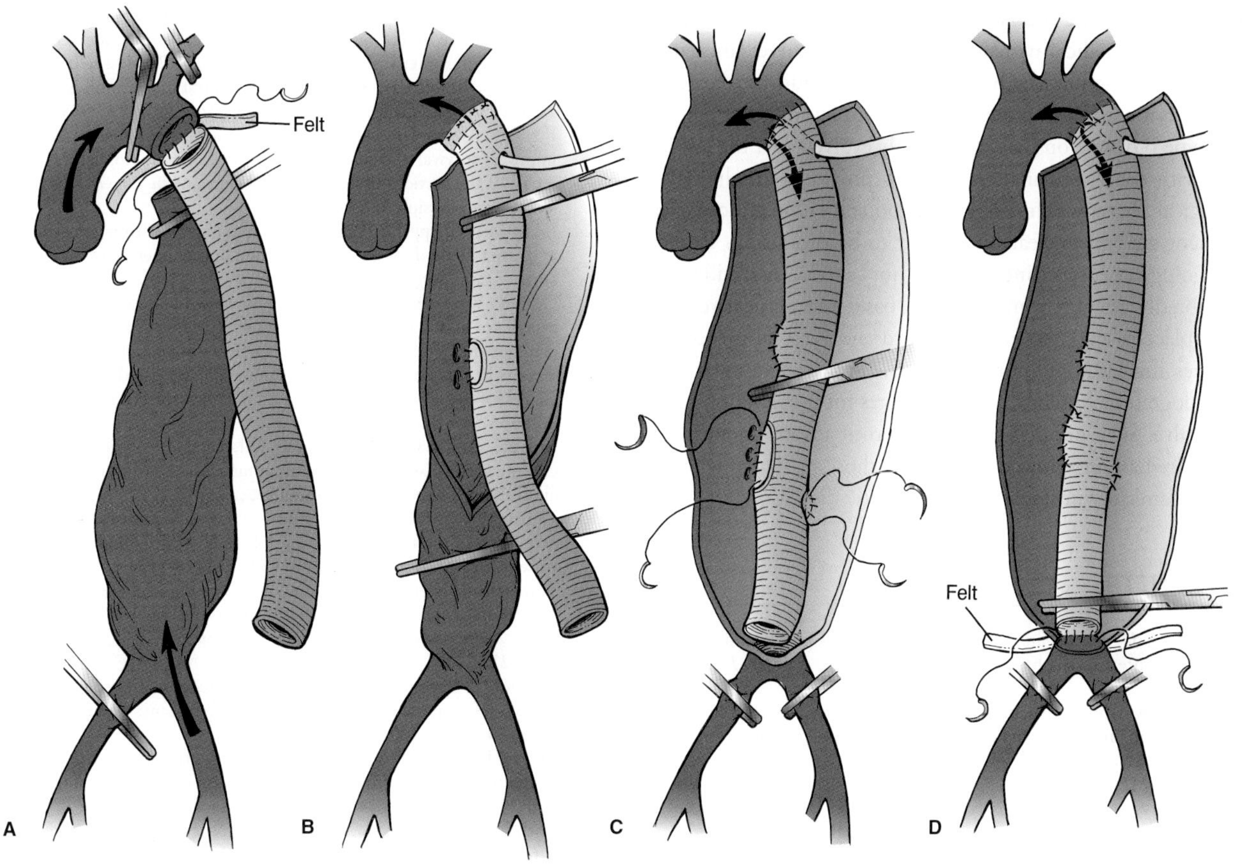

FIGURE 50-25 Replacement of the thoracoabdominal aorta. (A) A left femoral cannula perfuses the lower body and viscera while the heart continues to eject. The arch is transected near or at the left subclavian and any dissection involving the proximal cuff is repaired. (B) The clamp is moved down and a second arterial cannula is inserted into the proximal graft to perfuse the upper body and heart. The anterior wall of the dissection is incised longitudinally and bleeding intercostals of the upper six pairs are oversewn. A group of lower intercostal arteries above the celiac axis is sutured to the graft. (C) The clamp is moved down and the distal aortic clamp is moved to the left common iliac artery. A patch of aorta containing the celiac, superior mesenteric, and right renal artery is sewn into the graft. The left renal artery is sutured separately to the graft. (D) The proximal clamp is moved below the visceral anastomoses and the distal aortic anastomosis is made to the aortic bifurcation.

anastomosis cannot be safely or adequately performed with a clamp in the usual position.

Results

The operative mortality for chronic type A dissections is between 4 and 17%.[84,85] The stroke rate after repair is 4%, with early neurologic complications occurring in 9%.[27] Regular follow-up of the aortic valve is necessary when the native valve is preserved at the initial operation. This is best performed using TTE on a yearly basis. Early reports indicated that nearly 20% of patients require reoperation secondary to progressive aortic regurgitation. The most recent data from David et al., however, reveal a 90 ± 4% 5-year freedom from severe or moderate aortic insufficiency in patients with aortic root aneurysm and 98 ± 2% in patients with ascending aortic aneurysm following valve-sparing operation.[78]

The perioperative mortality after surgical treatment of chronic type B dissections has been reported to be as low as 10% with a rate of permanent paraplegia of 9%.[27] Long-term survival for type A and B chronic dissections is similar with rates at 1, 5, 10, and 15 years after surgery of 78, 60, 45, and 27%, respectively.[86] Approximately one third of deaths are cardiac-related, and at least 15% of deaths are related to complications or extension of the aortic dissection.

Recently, endovascular therapies have been used for management of chronic type B aortic dissections. The outcomes cited on Table 50-6 are similar to the outcomes after endovascular treatment of acute dissections. Although the results of these studies look promising, this topic needs to be studied further before recommendations or indications of endovascular repair in chronic type B dissections are elucidated.

CONCLUSION

Considerable improvement in the treatment of patients with acute and chronic aortic dissection has occurred over the last 50 years. The management of aortic dissections will continue to evolve as improved medical, endovascular, and surgical techniques are refined. At the present time, surgical therapy remains the standard of care for acute type A aortic dissections.

Uncomplicated type B dissections should continue to be treated with optimal medical management and close surveillance until further studies define whether "prophylactic" endovascular repair will play a role in these patients. The treatment of acute complicated type B dissections has significantly evolved over the last few years, with endovascular therapies now providing an alternative to surgical therapy. The long-term outcomes of endovascular treatment are still unclear but appear to be promising. Patients undergoing operative intervention for aortic dissection will undoubtedly benefit from the novel basic and clinical research taking place in the areas of spinal cord and cerebral protection, strategies for cardiopulmonary bypass, improved vascular graft and endograft technology, and procedures for preservation of the aortic valve. Such progress may even permit advancement in our greatest remaining clinical challenge, those patients who are hemodynamically unstable following aortic dissection.

REFERENCES

1. Gurin D: Dissecting aneurysms of the aorta: diagnosis and operative relief of acute arterial obstruction due to this cause. *NY State J Med* 1935; 35:1.
2. Abbott OA: Clinical experiences with the application of polythene cellophane upon the aneurysms of the thoracic vessels. *J Thorac Surg* 1949; 18:435-461.
3. DeBakey ME, Cooley DA, Creech JO: Surgical considerations of dissecting aneurysm of the aorta. *Ann Surg* 1955; 14:24.
4. Wheat MW Jr, Palmer RF, Bartley TD, Seelman RC: Treatment of dissecting aneurysms of the aorta without surgery. *J Thorac Cardiovasc Surg* 1965; 50:364-373.
5. Beall AC Jr, Lewis JM, Weibel J, Crawford ES, DeBakey ME: Angiographic evaluation of the vascular surgery patient. *Surg Clin North Am* 1966; 46:843-862.
6. Daily PO, Trueblood HW, Stinson EB, et al: Management of acute aortic dissections. *Ann Thorac Surg* 1970; 10.
7. Coady MA, Rizzo JA, Goldstein LJ, Elefteriades JA: Natural history, pathogenesis, and etiology of thoracic aortic aneurysms and dissections. *Cardiol Clin* 1999; 17:615-635; vii.
8. Hagan PG, Nienaber CA, Isselbacher EM, et al: The International Registry of Acute Aortic Dissection (IRAD): new insights into an old disease. *JAMA* 2000; 283:897-903.
9. Erbel R, Alfonso F, Boileau C, et al: Diagnosis and management of aortic dissection. *Eur Heart J* 2001; 22:1642-1681.
10. Larson EW, Edwards WD: Risk factors for aortic dissection: a necropsy study of 161 cases. *Am J Cardiol* 1984; 53:849-855.
11. Coady MA, Rizzo JA, Elefteriades JA: Pathologic variants of thoracic aortic dissections. Penetrating atherosclerotic ulcers and intramural hematomas. *Cardiol Clin* 1999; 17:637-657.
12. Sundt TM: Intramural hematoma and penetrating atherosclerotic ulcer of the aorta. *Ann Thorac Surg* 2007; 83:S835-841; discussion S846-850.
13 Robinson PN, Booms P: The molecular pathogenesis of the Marfan syndrome. *Cell Mol Life Sci* 2001; 58:1698-1707.
14. Callewaert B, Malfait F, Loeys B, De Paepe A: Ehlers-Danlos syndromes and Marfan syndrome. *Best Pract Res Clin Rheumatol* 2008; 22:165-189.
15. Cambria RP, Brewster DC, Gertler J, et al: Vascular complications associated with spontaneous aortic dissection. *J Vasc Surg* 1988; 7:199-209.
16. Anagnostopoulos CE, Prabhakar MJ, Kittle CF: Aortic dissections and dissecting aneurysms. *Am J Cardiol* 1972; 30:263-273.
17. Scholl FG, Coady MA, Davies R, et al: Interval or permanent nonoperative management of acute type A aortic dissection. *Arch Surg* 1999; 134:402-405; discussion 405-406.
18. Kohl BA, McGarvey ML. Anesthesia and neurocerebral monitoring for aortic dissection. *Semin Thorac Cardiovasc Surg* 2005; 17:236-246.
19. Estrera AL, Garami Z, Miller CC 3rd, et al: Cerebral monitoring with transcranial Doppler ultrasonography improves neurologic outcome during repairs of acute type A aortic dissection. *J Thorac Cardiovasc Surg* 2005, 129:277-285.
20. Stecker MM, Cheung AT, Pochettino A, et al: Deep hypothermic circulatory arrest: II. Changes in electroencephalogram and evoked potentials during rewarming. *Ann Thorac Surg* 2001; 71:22-28.
21. Schepens M, Dossche K, Morshuis W, et al: Introduction of adjuncts and their influence on changing results in 402 consecutive thoracoabdominal aortic aneurysm repairs. *Eur J Cardiothorac Surg* 2004; 25:701-707.
22. Reece TB, Tribble CG, Smith RL, et al: Central cannulation is safe in acute aortic dissection repair. *J Thorac Cardiovasc Surg* 2007; 133:428-434.
23. Etz CD, Plestis KA, Kari FA, et al: Axillary cannulation significantly improves survival and neurologic outcome after atherosclerotic aneurysm repair of the aortic root and ascending aorta. *Ann Thorac Surg* 2008; 86: 441-446; discussion 446-447.
24. Ergin MA, Griepp EB, Lansman SL, et al: Hypothermic circulatory arrest and other methods of cerebral protection during operations on the thoracic aorta. *J Card Surg* 1994; 9:525-537
25. Gega A, Rizzo JA, Johnson MH, et al: Straight deep hypothermic arrest: experience in 394 patients supports its effectiveness as a sole means of brain preservation. *Ann Thorac Surg* 2007; 84:759-766; discussion 766-757.
26. Bavaria JE, Pochettino A, Brinster DR, et al: New paradigms and improved results for the surgical treatment of acute type A dissection. *Ann Surg* 2001; 234:336-342; discussion 342-333.
27. Safi HJ, Miller CC 3rd, Reardon MJ, et al: Operation for acute and chronic aortic dissection: recent outcome with regard to neurologic deficit and early death. *Ann Thorac Surg* 1998; 66:402-411.
28. DeBakey ME, McCollum CH, Crawford ES, et al: Dissection and dissecting aneurysms of the aorta: twenty-year follow-up of five hundred twenty-seven patients treated surgically. *Surgery* 1982; 92:1118-1134.
29. Trimarchi S, Nienaber CA, Rampoldi V, et al: Contemporary results of surgery in acute type A aortic dissection: The International Registry of Acute Aortic Dissection experience. *J Thorac Cardiovasc Surg* 2005; 129: 112-122.
30. Piccardo A, Regesta T, Zannis K, et al: Outcomes after surgical treatment for type A acute aortic dissection in octogenarians: a multicenter study. *Ann Thorac Surg* 2009; 88:491-497.
31. Driever R, Botsios S, Schmitz E, et al: Long-term effectiveness of operative procedures for Stanford type a aortic dissections. *J Card Surg* 2004; 19: 240-245
32. Ehrlich MP, Ergin MA, McCullough JN, et al: Results of immediate surgical treatment of all acute type A dissections. *Circulation* 2000; 102:III248-252.
33. Kallenbach K, Oelze T, Salcher R, et al: Evolving strategies for treatment of acute aortic dissection type A. *Circulation* 2004; 110:II243-249.
34. Tsai TT, Evangelista A, Nienaber CA, et al: Long-term survival in patients presenting with type A acute aortic dissection: insights from the International Registry of Acute Aortic Dissection (IRAD). *Circulation* 2006; 114:I350-356.
35. Fattori R, Tsai TT, Myrmel T, et al: Complicated acute type B dissection: is surgery still the best option? A report from the International Registry of Acute Aortic Dissection. *JACC Cardiovasc Interv* 2008; 1:395-402.
36. Umana JP, Lai DT, Mitchell RS, et al: Is medical therapy still the optimal treatment strategy for patients with acute type B aortic dissections? *J Thorac Cardiovasc Surg* 2002; 124:896-910.
37. Dake MD, Kato N, Mitchell RS, et al: Endovascular stent-graft placement for the treatment of acute aortic dissection. *NEJM* 1999; 340:1546-1552.
38. Nienaber CA, Fattori R, Lund G, et al: Nonsurgical reconstruction of thoracic aortic dissection by stent-graft placement. *NEJM* 1999; 340: 1539-1545.
39. Eggebrecht H, Nienaber CA, Neuhauser M, et al: Endovascular stent-graft placement in aortic dissection: a meta-analysis. *Eur Heart J* 2006; 27:489-498.
40. Kodama K, Nishigami K, Sakamoto T, et al: Tight heart rate control reduces secondary adverse events in patients with type B acute aortic dissection. *Circulation* 2008; 118:S167-170.
41. Tsai TT, Nienaber CA, Eagle KA: Acute aortic syndromes. *Circulation* 2005; 112:3802-3813.
42. Patel HJ, Williams DM, Meerkov M, et al: Long-term results of percutaneous management of malperfusion in acute type B aortic dissection: implications for thoracic aortic endovascular repair. *J Thorac Cardiovasc Surg* 2009; 138: 300-308.
43. Rodriguez JA, Olsen DM, Lucas L, et al: Aortic remodeling after endografting of thoracoabdominal aortic dissection. *J Vasc Surg* 2008; 47:1188-1194.
44. Nienaber CA, Kische S, Zeller T, et al: Provisional extension to induce complete attachment after stent-graft placement in type B aortic dissection: the PETTICOAT concept. *J Endovasc Ther* 2006; 13:738-746.
45. Adams JD, Garcia LM, Kern JA: Endovascular repair of the thoracic aorta. *Surg Clin North Am* 2009; 89:895-912, ix.
46. Siefert SA, Ailawadi G, Thompson RB, et al: Is limited stent grafting a viable treatment option in type B aortic dissections? 55th Annual Meeting, Southern Thoracic Surgical Association. Austin, TX; 174.

47. Bockler D, Hyhlik-Durr A, Hakimi M, Weber TF, Geisbusch P: Type B aortic dissections: treating the many to benefit the few? *J Endovasc Ther* 2009; 16(Suppl 1):I80-90.
48. Coselli JS, LeMaire SA, de Figueiredo LP, Kirby RP: Paraplegia after thoracoabdominal aortic aneurysm repair: is dissection a risk factor? *Ann Thorac Surg* 1997; 63:28-35; discussion 35-26.
49. Cunningham JN Jr, Laschinger JC, Spencer FC: Monitoring of somatosensory evoked potentials during surgical procedures on the thoracoabdominal aorta. IV. Clinical observations and results. *J Thorac Cardiovasc Surg* 1987; 94:275-285.
50. Safi HJ, Hess KR, Randel M, et al: Cerebrospinal fluid drainage and distal aortic perfusion: reducing neurologic complications in repair of thoracoabdominal aortic aneurysm types I and II. *J Vasc Surg* 1996; 23:223-228; discussion 229.
51. Estrera AL, Miller CC, Goodrick J, et al: Update on outcomes of acute type B aortic dissection. *Ann Thorac Surg* 2007; 83:S842-845; discussion S846-850.
52. Schor JS, Yerlioglu ME, Galla JD, et al: Selective management of acute type B aortic dissection: long-term follow-up. *Ann Thorac Surg* 1996; 61:1339-1341.
53. Bernard Y, Zimmermann H, Chocron S, et al: False lumen patency as a predictor of late outcome in aortic dissection. *Am J Cardiol* 2001; 87:1378-1382.
54. Xu SD, Huang FJ, Yang JF, et al: Endovascular repair of acute type B aortic dissection: early and mid-term results. *J Vasc Surg* 2006; 43:1090-1095.
55. Nienaber CA, Rousseau H, Eggebrecht H, et al: Randomized comparison of strategies for type B aortic dissection: the INvestigation of STEnt Grafts in Aortic Dissection (INSTEAD) trial. *Circulation* 2009; 120: 2519-2528.
56. Tang DG, Dake MD: TEVAR for acute uncomplicated aortic dissection: immediate repair versus medical therapy. *Semin Vasc Surg* 2009; 22:145-151.
57. Miller DC, Mitchell RS, Oyer PE, et al: Independent determinants of operative mortality for patients with aortic dissections. *Circulation* 1984; 70:I153-164.
58. Bozinovski J, Coselli JS: Outcomes and survival in surgical treatment of descending thoracic aorta with acute dissection. *Ann Thorac Surg* 2008; 85:965-970; discussion 970-961
59. Trimarchi S, Nienaber CA, Rampoldi V, et al: Role and results of surgery in acute type B aortic dissection: insights from the International Registry of Acute Aortic Dissection (IRAD). *Circulation* 2006; 114:I357-364.
60. Pitton MB, Herber S, Schmiedt W, et al: Long-term follow-up after endovascular treatment of acute aortic emergencies. *Cardiovasc Intervent Radiol* 2008; 31:23-35.
61. Palma JH, de Souza JA, Rodrigues Alves CM, et al: Self-expandable aortic stent-grafts for treatment of descending aortic dissections. *Ann Thorac Surg* 2002; 73:1138-1141; discussion 1141-1132.
62. Nienaber CA, Ince H, Petzsch M, et al: Endovascular treatment of thoracic aortic dissection and its variants. *Acta Chir Belg* 2002; 102:292-298.
63. Nathanson DR, Rodriguez-Lopez JA, Ramaiah VG, et al: Endoluminal stent-graft stabilization for thoracic aortic dissection. *J Endovasc Ther* 2005; 12:354-359.
64. Kische S, Ehrlich MP, Nienaber CA, et al: Endovascular treatment of acute and chronic aortic dissection: midterm results from the Talent Thoracic Retrospective Registry. *J Thorac Cardiovasc Surg* 2009; 138:115-124.
65. Khoynezhad A, Donayre CE, Omari BO, et al: Midterm results of endovascular treatment of complicated acute type B aortic dissection. *J Thorac Cardiovasc Surg* 2009; 138:625-631.
66. Hutschala D, Fleck T, Czerny M, et al: Endoluminal stent-graft placement in patients with acute aortic dissection type B. *Eur J Cardiothorac Surg* 2002; 21:964-969.
67. Duebener LF, Lorenzen P, Richardt G, et al: Emergency endovascular stent-grafting for life-threatening acute type B aortic dissections. *Ann Thorac Surg* 2004; 78:1261-1266; discussion 1266-1267.
68. Dialetto G, Covino FE, Scognamiglio G, et al: Treatment of type B aortic dissection: endoluminal repair or conventional medical therapy? *Eur J Cardiothorac Surg* 2005; 27:826-830.
69. Juvonen T, Ergin MA, Galla JD, et al: Risk factors for rupture of chronic type B dissections. *J Thorac Cardiovasc Surg* 1999; 117:776-786.
70. Sueyoshi E, Sakamoto I, Hayashi K, Yamaguchi T, Imada T: Growth rate of aortic diameter in patients with type B aortic dissection during the chronic phase. *Circulation* 2004; 110:II256-261.
71. Hata M, Shiono M, Inoue T, et al: Optimal treatment of type B acute aortic dissection: long-term medical follow-up results. *Ann Thorac Surg* 2003; 75:1781-1784.
72. Genoni M, Paul M, Jenni R, et al: Chronic beta-blocker therapy improves outcome and reduces treatment costs in chronic type B aortic dissection. *Eur J Cardiothorac Surg* 2001; 19:606-610.
73. Marui A, Mochizuki T, Mitsui N, et al: Toward the best treatment for uncomplicated patients with type B acute aortic dissection: a consideration for sound surgical indication. *Circulation* 1999; 100:II275-280.
74. Coady MA, Rizzo JA, Hammond GL, et al: What is the appropriate size criterion for resection of thoracic aortic aneurysms? *J Thorac Cardiovasc Surg* 1997; 113:476-491; discussion 489-491.
75. Kato M, Bai H, Sato K, et al: Determining surgical indications for acute type B dissection based on enlargement of aortic diameter during the chronic phase. *Circulation* 1995; 92:II107-112.
76. David TE, Feindel CM: An aortic valve-sparing operation for patients with aortic incompetence and aneurysm of the ascending aorta. *J Thorac Cardiovasc Surg* 1992; 103:617-621; discussion 622.
77. Yacoub MH, Gehle P, Chandrasekaran V, et al: Late results of a valve-preserving operation in patients with aneurysms of the ascending aorta and root. *J Thorac Cardiovasc Surg* 1998; 115:1080-1090.
78. David TE, Armstrong S, Ivanov J, et al: Results of aortic valve-sparing operations. *J Thorac Cardiovasc Surg* 2001; 122:39-46.
79. Cochran RP, Kunzelman KS: Methods of pseudosinus creation in an aortic valve-sparing operation for aneurysmal disease. *J Card Surg* 2000; 15:428-433.
80. Borst HG, Walterbusch G, Schaps D: Extensive aortic replacement using "elephant trunk" prosthesis. *Thorac Cardiovasc Surg* 1983; 31:37-40.
81. Kouchoukos NT, Masetti P, Rokkas CK, Murphy SF, Blackstone EH: Safety and efficacy of hypothermic cardiopulmonary bypass and circulatory arrest for operations on the descending thoracic and thoracoabdominal aorta. *Ann Thorac Surg* 2001; 72:699-707; discussion 707-698.
82. Panneton JM, Hollier LH: Dissecting descending thoracic and thoracoabdominal aortic aneurysms: Part II. *Ann Vasc Surg* 1995; 9:596-605.
83. Coselli JS, LeMaire SA: Left heart bypass reduces paraplegia rates after thoracoabdominal aortic aneurysm repair. *Ann Thorac Surg* 1999; 67:1931-1934; discussion 1953-1938.
84. Safi HJ, Miller CC 3rd, Carr C, et al: Importance of intercostal artery reattachment during thoracoabdominal aortic aneurysm repair. *J Vasc Surg* 1998; 27:58-66; discussion 66-58.
85. Sabik JF, Lytle BW, Blackstone EH, et al: Long-term effectiveness of operations for ascending aortic dissections. *J Thorac Cardiovasc Surg* 2000; 119:946-962.
86. Fann JI, Smith JA, Miller DC, et al: Surgical management of aortic dissection during a 30-year period. *Circulation* 1995; 92:II113-121.

CHAPTER 51

Ascending Aortic Aneurysms

Nimesh D. Desai
Joseph E. Bavaria

INTRODUCTION

The Greek physician Galen first described superficial false aneurysms arising from venisection in the antecubital fossa and in gladiators injured during battle in the second century AD.[1] Antyllos, during the same time period, distinguished between true and false aneurysms and attempted surgical treatment with proximal and distal ligation, opening of the aneurysmal sac, and removal of its contents.[2]

In 1542, the French physician Jean Francois Fernel described aneurysms, "in the chest, or about the spleen and mesentery where a violent throbbing is frequently observable."[3] In 1543, Andeas Versalius described a thoracic aortic aneurysm. In the late 1500s, Ambroise Paré described a death by a ruptured thoracic aortic aneurysm, and either Fernel or Paré proposed that syphilis played a causative role in some aortic aneurysms.[1] In 1760, Morgagni reported the first cases of aortic dissection, and in 1773, Alexander Monro described three coats of the arterial wall and the destruction of the wall in the formation of true and false aneurysms.[1]

Peripheral arterial ligation was developed in the 1800s by John Hunter, who demonstrated safe and reproducible means of ligating certain peripheral arteries.[4] Innovative measures used to cause thrombosis of aneurysms included the insertion of long segments of wire[5] with the application of an electric current,[6] and wrapping of aneurysms with cellophane or other irritating materials.[7,8]

In 1888, Rudolph Matas introduced obliterative endoaneurysmorrhaphy, in which stitches placed from within the aneurysm sac obliterated the arterial openings.[9] This allowed closure of large aneurysms that would have been difficult to ligate externally. Recognizing the importance of maintaining arterial continuity for certain aneurysms, he subsequently devised techniques of restorative or reconstructive endoaneurysmorrhaphy, in which diseased segments of the aneurysm wall were resected and the remaining vessel wall was reconstructed to reestablish flow.[10] The number of aneurysms to which these techniques could be applied, however, was very limited. The broad application of surgical treatment for major arterial aneurysms would have to await the development of satisfactory conduits and the techniques to insert them.

The first report of a descending aortic repair was described by Cooley and DeBakey in 1952. The technique involved lateral resection and aortorrhaphy performed on a saccular aneurysm without cardiopulmonary bypass.[11] In 1956, Cooley and DeBakey performed replacement of the ascending aorta with a segment of homograft with cardiopulmonary bypass.[12] Polyester cloth grafts were introduced by DeBakey, who discovered it in a Houston department store, and it soon became the artificial conduit of choice for aortic replacement.[13] Technical improvements in graft replacements included the impregnation of polyester grafts with albumin, collagen, or gelatin, which has greatly reduced the blood loss through the grafts.[14]

Wheat and colleagues, in 1964, resected the ascending aorta and entire aortic root except for the aortic tissue surrounding the coronary arteries.[15] They then performed a mechanical valve insertion and fashioned the proximal tube graft to accommodate the coronary arteries, which were left in situ. The first composite aortic root replacement was performed by Bentall and De Bono in 1963 to treat an ascending aortic aneurysm in a patient with Marfan's syndrome who had severe thinning of the aortic wall in the sinus segment.[16] The original technique involved hand sewing a Starr no. 13 mechanical prosthesis to a preclotted graft (Fig. 51-1). An inclusion-type technique with aortic wrap in which the coronary buttons were left in situ and anastomosed to holes made in the graft was performed. Because of concerns about coronary malposition, in 1981 Cabrol and colleagues described the use of an 8- to 10-mm Dacron graft to

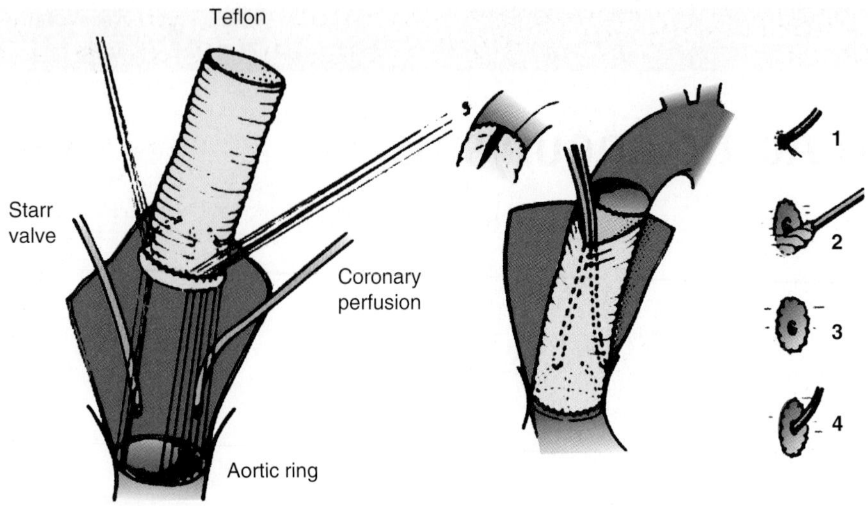

FIGURE 51-1 The original root replacement operation as described by Bentall and De Bono. (*Reproduced with permission from Bentall H, De Bono A: A technique for complete replacement of the ascending aorta. Thorax 1968; 23:338.*)

attach to independently mobilized coronary artery buttons.[17] Techniques eventually evolved to the current method of individual coronary button reimplantation as described by Kouchoukas and Karp with end-to-end anastomoses as opposed to the inclusion technique, which tended to be prone to pseudoaneurysm formation.[18]

SURGICAL ANATOMY

The aortic root is an extension of the left ventricular outflow tract and that provides the scaffolding for the elements of the aortic valve and connects to the descending aorta. Its components include the aortic valve cusps, the sinuses of Valsalva, the aortic annulus and subcommissural triangles, and the sinotubular junction (Fig. 51-2).[19] The aortic valve cusps attach to the aortic annulus at hinge point following a semilunar contour being a three pointed crown-type arrangement not a circular or oval ring. The annular tissue itself is typically 50 to 60% fibrous tissue along the hinge point between the aortic and mitral valves as well as the membranous portion of the septum, and the remainder is muscular. Small projections of collagen anchor the aortic root to the ventricular muscle.[20] The apices of the attachments of the cusps to the aortic annulus are known as *commissures,* and the most superior aspect of the commissures interrelates with the sinotubular junction. The sinotubular junction is a ridge that marks the beginning of the ascending aorta. The sinotubular junction diameter is typically 15 to 20% smaller than annular diameter in younger patients.[21] With aging the sinotubular junction diameter becomes larger. When the sinotubular junction is more than 10% larger than the annular diameter, there is frequently resultant aortic insufficiency

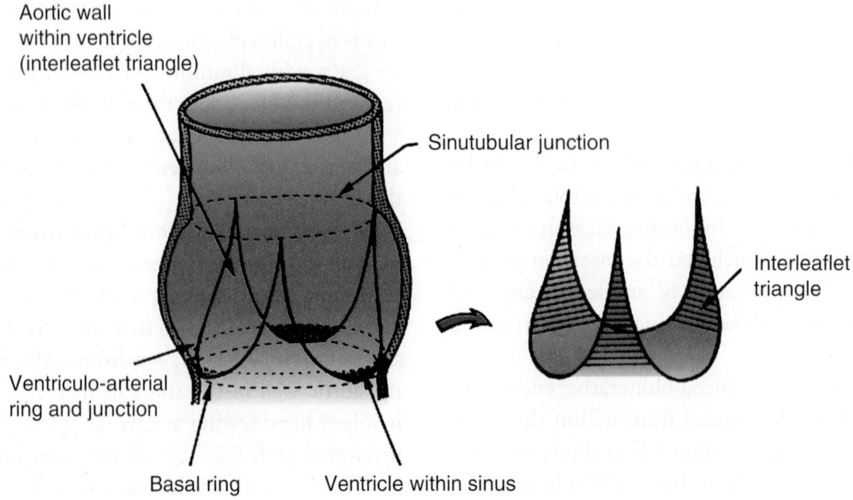

FIGURE 51-2 Aortic root geometry. (*Reproduced with permission from Sutton JP 3rd, Ho SY, Anderson RH: The forgotten interleaflet triangles: a review of the surgical anatomy of the aortic valve. Ann Thorac Surg 1995; 59[2]:419-427.*)

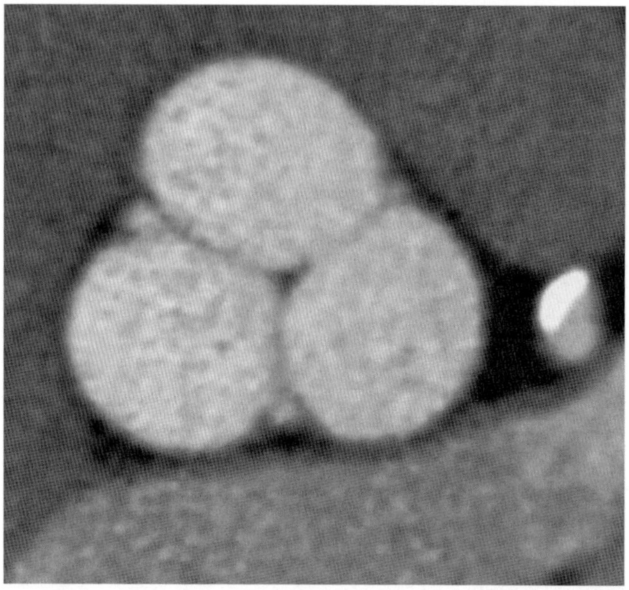

FIGURE 51-3 Anatomy of the aortic root from a cardiac gated CT angiogram. Note the "cloverleaf" orientation of the sinuses.

because the leaflets were no longer coapt owing to displacement of the commissures.

Between the sinotubular junction and the aortic annulus are expanded segments of the aorta referred to as the sinuses of Valsalva. The sinuses form a cloverleaf rather than circular alignment when viewed in cross-section (Fig. 51-3).[22] Dilatation of the aortic sinuses and annulus are referred to as *aortoannular ectasia*. Each sinus is named for its corresponding coronary artery right, left, and noncoronary.

The noncoronary sinus is anatomically related to the left and right atria as well as the transverse sinus. The left coronary sinus anatomically relates to the left atrium, and the right coronary sinus is related to the right atrium and right ventricle. The subcommissural triangle between the right and noncoronary arteries is anatomically related to the conduction system within the membranous septum as well as the septal leaflet of the tricuspid valve. The left and noncoronary subcommissural triangle are related to the anterior leaflet of the mitral valve. The ascending aorta starts at the level the sinotubular junction and ascends to the level of the takeoff of the innominate artery.

PATHOPHYSIOLOGY

The ascending aorta histologically contains a high proportion of compliant elastic tissue allowing it to serve as a reservoir and that stores kinetic energy from the systolic pulse wave as it expands and uses it to maintain flow during diastole via elastic recoil. The ascending aorta is a three-layered structure composed of a smooth intimal layer composed of a single layer of endothelial cells adhered to a basal lamina; a medial layer composed of layers of elastin sheets, collagen, smooth muscle cells, and extracellular matrix; and an outer layer of adventitial tissue, which includes the vaso-vasorum and nerves.[23] The elastin content of the aorta decreases distally and in the abdominal aorta is less than half of that in the ascending aorta.[24] The principal biologic causes of aneurysm formation in the ascending aorta are related to degenerative processes in the elastic media, as compared with primarily atherosclerotic changes in the descending and abdominal aortas.[25]

Ascending aortic aneurysm formation is the result of several biologic and mechanical mechanisms. Disruption of the balance between homeostatic mechanisms within the aortic wall, including elastic and collagen elements, proteoglycans, proteolytic enzymes and their inhibitors, and inflammatory mediators, causes a spectrum of aortic pathology that manifests in the final pathway as aortic enlargement, eventually leading to rupture or dissection. Fragmentation of the extracellular matrix of the aortic media occurs because of matrix-degrading enzymes such as matrix metalloproteinases and cathepsin groups.[26–30] Matrix metalloproteinases comprise a family of proteases that are capable of degrading virtually all components of the extracellular milieu and perform a variety of tasks necessary for normal homeostasis, including maintenance of the dynamic integrity of the extracellular structure within arteries.[26–28] Aneurysms form as elastic layers fragment, smooth muscle cells become dysfunctional and eventually elastic, and smooth muscle components are replaced with a cystic appearing mucoid material (Fig. 51-4).[31]

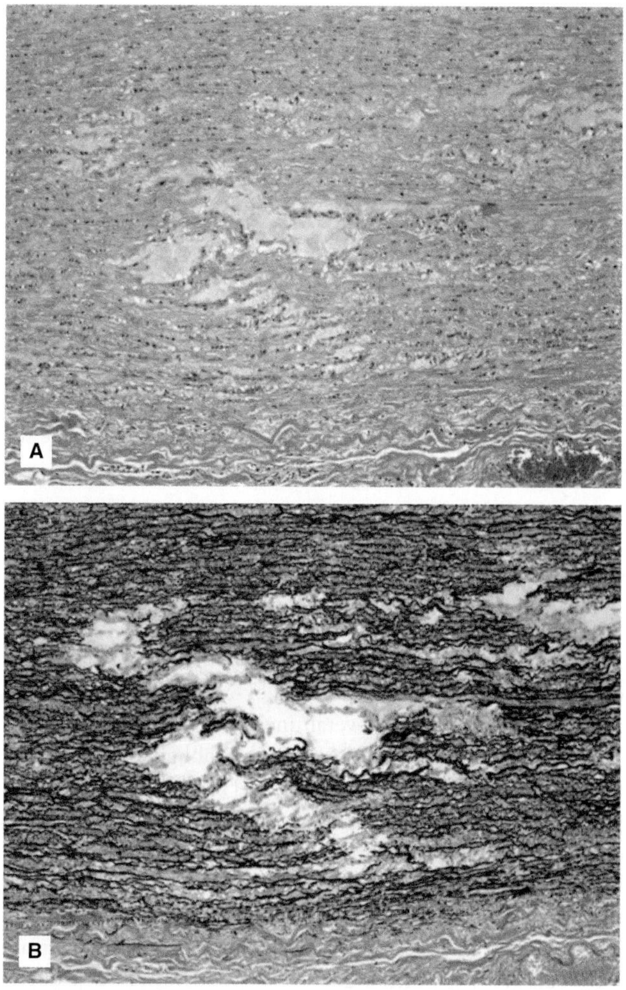

FIGURE 51-4 Cystic medial degeneration with (A) pools of glycosaminoglycans with 25% transmural extent, and (B) associated loss of elastic fibers.

This process is referred to as *cystic medial degeneration.* The term *cystic medial necrosis* has also been applied to this condition, but has been largely abandoned because there is no true necrotic process involved. To a lesser extent, mild degeneration of the aortic wall is common with advanced age and is responsible for the slow dilation of the ascending aorta with age. Smoking tends to exacerbate this degeneration.[32]

Mechanical changes to aortic wall characteristics such as alterations in cross-sectional symmetry, compliance, and stress–strain relationships likely predate dilatation. The Young–Laplace relationship describes the association between aortic diameter and wall tension, in which increases in aortic wall diameter lead to increases in wall stress at similar pressures (tension = pressure × radius). Changes in aortic wall compliance, broadly defined as the change in volume of the vessel with a change in pressure, lead to increased stress applied to the aortic wall during the systolic impulse and further exacerbate the biologic derangements leading to aneurysm formation.[33] The coupling between mechanical forces on the arterial wall and the biochemical changes leading to aneurysm formation (mechano-transduction) are not yet clearly elucidated.

Degenerative aortic aneurysms cause asymmetric enlargement of the ascending aorta because the segment of aorta along the inner curvature is adherent to the pulmonary artery[34]; hence, there is significant rightward and anterior displacement of the aortic wall. This causes a relative elongation of the ascending aorta in an asymmetric fashion, which tends to push the heart into a horizontal arrangement. This also causes a significant change in the orientation of the aortic valve annulus to a more oblique arrangement.[34] Aneurysmal widening will typically involve the aorta to the level of the sinotubular junction and frequently involves the noncoronary sinus to a lesser extent.[35] This widening at the level of the sinotubular junction is responsible for aortic insufficiency in these cases, and frequent placement of tube graft to the sinotubular junction will resolve significant central aortic insufficiency. The left and noncoronary sinuses are fairly normal in these cases. The noncoronary aortic valve cusp may be elongated along its free margin to compensate for the asymmetric enlargement of the noncoronary sinus.

SPECIFIC ETIOLOGIES

Marfan's Syndrome

Marfan's syndrome is an autosomal dominant syndrome with complete penetrance. Up to 25% of Marfan cases are from sporadic dictation in the overall incidence is one per 3000 to 10,000 live births.[36] Traditionally, it is thought to have been caused by alterations in the gene (FBM1) coding the aortic wall protein fibrillin-1, leading to elastin derangement, medial degeneration, and aneurysm formation.[37,38] More recently, homology between fibrillin-1 molecules and latent TGF beta-binding proteins has led investigators to infer that altered sequestration of the latent form of TGF beta in the extracellular matrix may increase TGF beta activity, which negatively affect smooth muscle development and the extracellular matrix.[39] Approximately 80% of patients with Marfan's syndrome develop aortic root aneurysms and nearly half develop mitral regurgitation.[40] The clinical

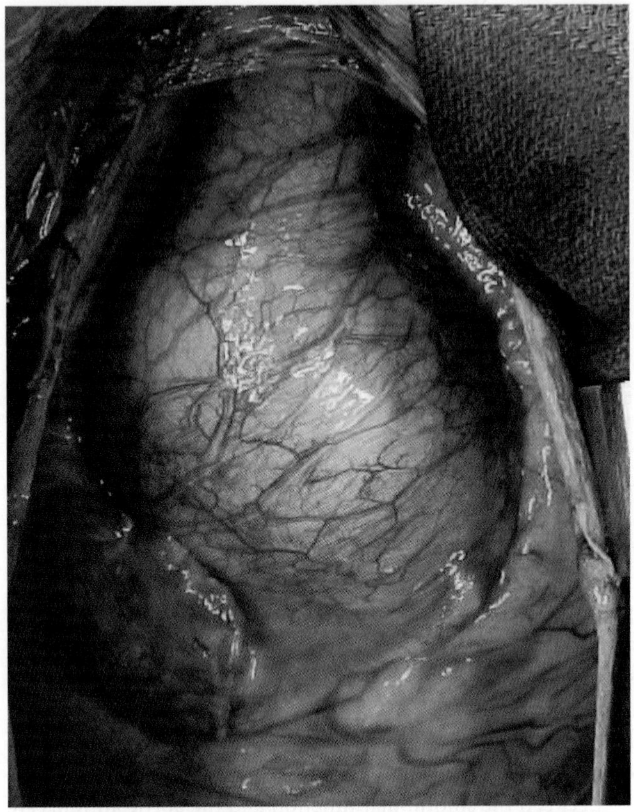

FIGURE 51-5 Massively dilated aortic root in a Marfan's syndrome patient. Note the severe dilation of the aortic annulus and relative sparing of the proximal arch.

manifestations of Marfan's syndrome involve multiple organ systems because it is a systemic disease. Diagnosis has traditionally been made using the Ghent criteria, although it is now made definitively using genotyping.[41] Anatomically, Marfan's syndrome results in severe aortoannular ectasia and massively dilated sinuses and aortic annulus (Fig. 51-5).

More recently, reports have shown that the use of angiotensin-converting enzyme inhibitors can prolong the life expectancy of smooth muscle cells in the aortic tissue of Marfan patients via an angiotensin-2 type II receptor blockade mechanism, which may antagonize TGF beta.[42] This has led to the clinical application of the angiotensin receptor blocker losartan as a prophylactic therapy to diminish aortic degeneration and aneurysm formation, which has been shown in animal models to be effective when given in the early stages of the disease.[43] A small clinical study of 18 pediatric patients also showed decreased aortic growth rate with treatment of losartan.[44]

Loeys-Deitz Syndrome

Loeys-Deitz syndrome is a more recently described autosomal-dominant syndrome.[45] Rather than a fibrillin-1 defect, however, there is a mutation in transforming growth factor (TGF) beta receptor 1 and 2. Characteristics of Loeys-Deitz syndrome include cleft palate, bifid uvula, scoliosis, orbital hypertelorism, pectus deformities, developmental abnormalities, and congenital heart defects, including persistent patent ductus arteriosus and atrial septal defects.[45] Patients may phenotypically have characteristics that overlapped between Loeys-Deitz syndrome and Marfan's syndrome.[46] Histologically, it is associated with increased medial collagen and a subtle but diffuse form of elastic fiber fragmentation and extracellular matrix deposition.[47] Loeys-Deitz syndrome has a more rapid clinical course than Marfan's syndrome and prophylactic aortic root replacement or reimplantation is often recommended at younger ages and with smaller aortic dimensions.

Ehlers-Danlos Syndrome

Ehlers-Danlos syndrome is caused by either sporadic mutation or inherited autosomal dominant trait, resulting in a connective tissue disorder derived from defective type III collagen synthesis. The type IV variant of the Ehlers-Danlos syndrome is associated with spontaneous arterial rupture. Most commonly this occurs in the mesenteric or carotid arteries. However, spontaneous rupture of the descending aorta and aortic arch has been described.[48] The arterial wall of these patients is extremely thin and friable. Ascending aortic involvement may occur as a consequence of retrograde extension of a primary brachiocephalic branch pathology.

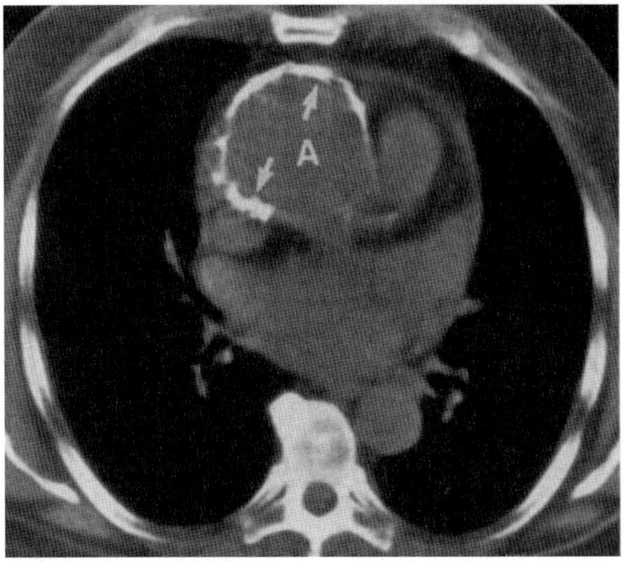

FIGURE 51-6 Syphilitic aortic aneurysm. (*A*) Extensive calcified plaques are noted in cross-section. (*Reproduced permission from Kuniyoshi Y, Koja K, Miyagi K, et al: A ruptured syphilitic descending thoracic aortic aneurysm. The characteristic findings on computed tomography for the etiological diagnosis of aneurysm. Ann Thorac Cardiovasc Surg 1998; 4[2]:99-102.*)

INFECTIOUS AND INFLAMMATORY ETIOLOGIES

Infections and systemic inflammatory disorders can occasionally cause damage to the wall of the ascending aorta, leading to aneurysm formation. Frequently, despite high-quality preoperative imaging and even with intraoperative tissue pathology, is not possible to definitively distinguish between the different possible etiologies.

Ascending aortic aneurysms caused by infection are extremely uncommon. Such mycotic ascending aortic aneurysms are frequently related to concomitant left-sided valvular endocarditis. Most common organisms include, in order of decreasing frequency, *Staphylococcus aureus, Staphylococcus epidermidis, Salmonella,* and *Streptococcus.*[49] In cases of atherosclerotic aneurysm, if there is intraluminal clot in the ascending aorta, transient bacteremia may lead to infected clot leading to a mycotic aneurysm.[50]

Syphilis, caused by the spirochete *Treponema pallidum,* was the predominant cause of ascending aortic aneurysms in the preantibiotic era and accounted for 5 to 10% of all cardiovascular deaths.[51] Typically syphilitic aortitis involves the thoracic aorta with a particular predilection for the ascending aorta, likely owing to its rich vascular and lymphatic supply. The pathologic process involves a multifocal lymphoplasmacytic infiltrate of the vasa vasorum leading to degeneration of the medial elastic fibers. The intima develops wrinkles ridges and plaques described as a "tree bark appearance" (Fig. 51-6).[52] Inflammation around the coronary artery ostia may lead to high-grade proximal occlusions. The inflammatory process may either be patchy or diffusely involve a large section of aorta. Once established, treatment of syphilis with antibiotics does not reverse the vascular lesions.

Other systemic arteritis conditions may also produce ascending aortic aneurysms. Takayasu's arteritis is associated with inflammation of the vasa vasorum and medial necrosis, and may also have intimal changes similar to syphilis. It is typically seen in women between 15 and 30 years of age and frequently involves occlusive lesions to major branch vessels of the arch.[53] Although syphilis aortitis often in leads to rapid aneurysmal degeneration, this is much less common in Takayasu's aortitis, occurring only 15% of cases.[54] Giant cell arteritis is a systemic arteritis that occurs in elderly patients, most commonly affecting the temporal artery. It is also more common in females and is also associated with polymyalgia rheumatica. Giant cell arteritis is an inflammatory process with inflammatory infiltration with lymphocytes, plasma cells, and histiocytes. There is a variable presence of giant cells.[55] Aortitis leading to aortic aneurysm may also be associated rarely with Behçet's disease, rheumatoid arthritis, sarcoidosis, ankylosing spondylitis, lupus erythematosus, and Wegener's granulomatosis.

Bicuspid Aortopathy

Bicuspid aortic valve is a complex familial syndrome, with a male predominance of 3 to 1.[56] It is also associated with Turner's syndrome. There is a 9% prevalence of bicuspid aortic valve disease in first-degree relatives of patients with bicuspid aortic valve disease.[57] More than half of patients with aortic coarctation have an associated bicuspid aortic valve.[58] Several genetic defects have been implicated in the formation of bicuspid aortic valve disease; however, no single genetic etiology has been derived. Aortic dilatation is frequently associated with bicuspid aortic valve disease; however, the mechanism for this is not well delineated. Originally thought to be a sequela of poststenotic dilatation, aortic aneurysm formation in patients with bicuspid aortic valve may occur without any significant aortic stenosis, although there is clearly flow perturbation in the proximal sinuses of Valsalva and descending aorta in patients with bicuspid aortic valve.[59] Recent investigation has shown that embryologically, the aortic valve and ascending aorta arise from the neural crest cells, implicating a potential common mechanism for the development of a bicuspid aortic valve and subsequent aneurysm formation.[60] The aortic wall in bicuspid aortic valve disease patients shows increased elastic fragmentation, fibrillin-1 deficiency, matrix disruption, increased levels of matrix metallic proteinases, and smooth muscle cell apoptosis.[60–65]

Fazel and colleagues using a cluster-type analysis identified four distinct patterns of aortic dilatation including: aortic root alone (13%), ascending aorta alone (10%), ascending aorta and proximal transverse arch (28%), and aortic root, ascending aorta, and proximal transverse arch (45%) (Fig. 51-7).[66] This study suggests that for younger patients, definitive treatment of bicuspid aortic valve disease with aortic dilatation requires strategies that address the aortic root, ascending aorta, and proximal transverse hemiarch. It is advisable to perform an aggressive hemiarch, resecting all aortic tissue along the lesser curve to the level of the subclavian artery takeoff in younger bicuspid aortic valve patients to eliminate as much of the diseased aorta as possible. However, total arch replacement with brachiocephalic branch reimplantation is rarely necessary because the aneurysmal component rarely involves the distal aspect of the transverse arch.

Isolated Sinus of Valsalva Aneurysm

Aneurysms of the sinuses of Valsalva that occur as isolated lesions are rare abnormalities caused by either a congenital defect in the continuity between the medial layer of the affected sinus and the aortic valve annulus or, less commonly, acquired causes such as endocarditis, syphilis, tuberculosis, focal dissection, or iatrogenic causes.[67] They are more common in males and may be associated with subaortic stenosis, ventricular septal defects, and aortic insufficiency. In greater than 90% of cases, they involve the right coronary sinus (Fig. 51-8).[68,69] The noncoronary sinus of the second most common location and these aneurysms are extremely uncommon in a left coronary sinus. They are generally asymptomatic until they rupture, when they usually cause intracardiac shunts. Right sinus of Valsalva aneurysms typically ruptures into the right ventricle, effectively causing a hemodynamic defect similar to a ventricular septal defect. Aneurysms of the noncoronary sinus typically rupture into the right atrium and the left coronary sinus ruptures into the pulmonary artery or left ventricle. Occasionally an unruptured left coronary sinus of Valsalva aneurysm may compress the left main coronary artery.[69]

Other Familial Aneurysms

Specific families often exhibit strong tendencies for thoracic aortic aneurysm formation without any clearly definable connective tissue disorder such as Marfan's syndrome. There is no defect in fibrillin-1 expression in these patients. It is postulated that aneurysms in these patients are inherited in an autosomal-dominant manner with no gender bias, incomplete penetrance, variable expression, and variable age of aneurysm onset.[70] A wide variety of potential genes have been implicated and relate to processes involving collagen formation, extracellular matrix hemostasis, and smooth muscle proteins.[71–74]

CLINICAL PRESENTATION

Symptoms

Most ascending aortic aneurysms are asymptomatic when diagnosed, being incidentally noted on chest x-ray or echocardiogram. Anterior chest pain is the most frequent symptom. The pain may be acute in onset signifying impending rupture, or a chronic gnawing pain from compression of the overlying sternum. Occasionally signs of superior vena cava or airway compression are present. Hoarseness resulting from stretch injury of the left recurrent laryngeal nerve suggests involvement of the distal aortic arch or proximal descending thoracic aorta. Less commonly, aneurysms of the ascending aorta or aortic root can rupture into the right atrium or the superior vena cava, presenting with high-output cardiac failure, or bleed into the lungs with ensuing hemoptysis. Acute dissection of the ascending aorta presents with severe tearing pain in greater than 75% of patients.[75]

Physical Examination

Physical examination is often unremarkable. If there is related aortic insufficiency, a widened pulse pressure or diastolic murmur may be present. If dilation is isolated to the ascending aorta, however, the aneurysm can reach large dimensions without producing physical findings. A thorough vascular examination should be carried out to look for any concomitant peripheral vascular disease, carotid disease, or abdominal aortic aneurysm. Abdominal aortic aneurysms may be present in 10 to 20% of patients with atherosclerotic involvement of an ascending aortic aneurysm.[76]

DIAGNOSTIC STUDIES

Electrocardiogram

With significant aortic insufficiency, left ventricular hypertrophy or strain is evident. Patients with generalized atherosclerosis may show evidence of concomitant coronary artery disease or previous myocardial injury.

Chest Radiography

Many asymptomatic ascending aortic aneurysms are first detected on chest x-ray. The enlarged ascending aorta produces a convex contour of the right superior mediastinum (Fig. 51-9A). In the lateral view, there is loss of the retrosternal air space (Fig. 51-9B). Aneurysms confined to the aortic root can be obscured by the cardiac silhouette and may not be evident on chest radiograph.[77]

Echocardiography

Transesophageal echocardiography (TEE) is a portable diagnostic tool that accurately detects and differentiates among

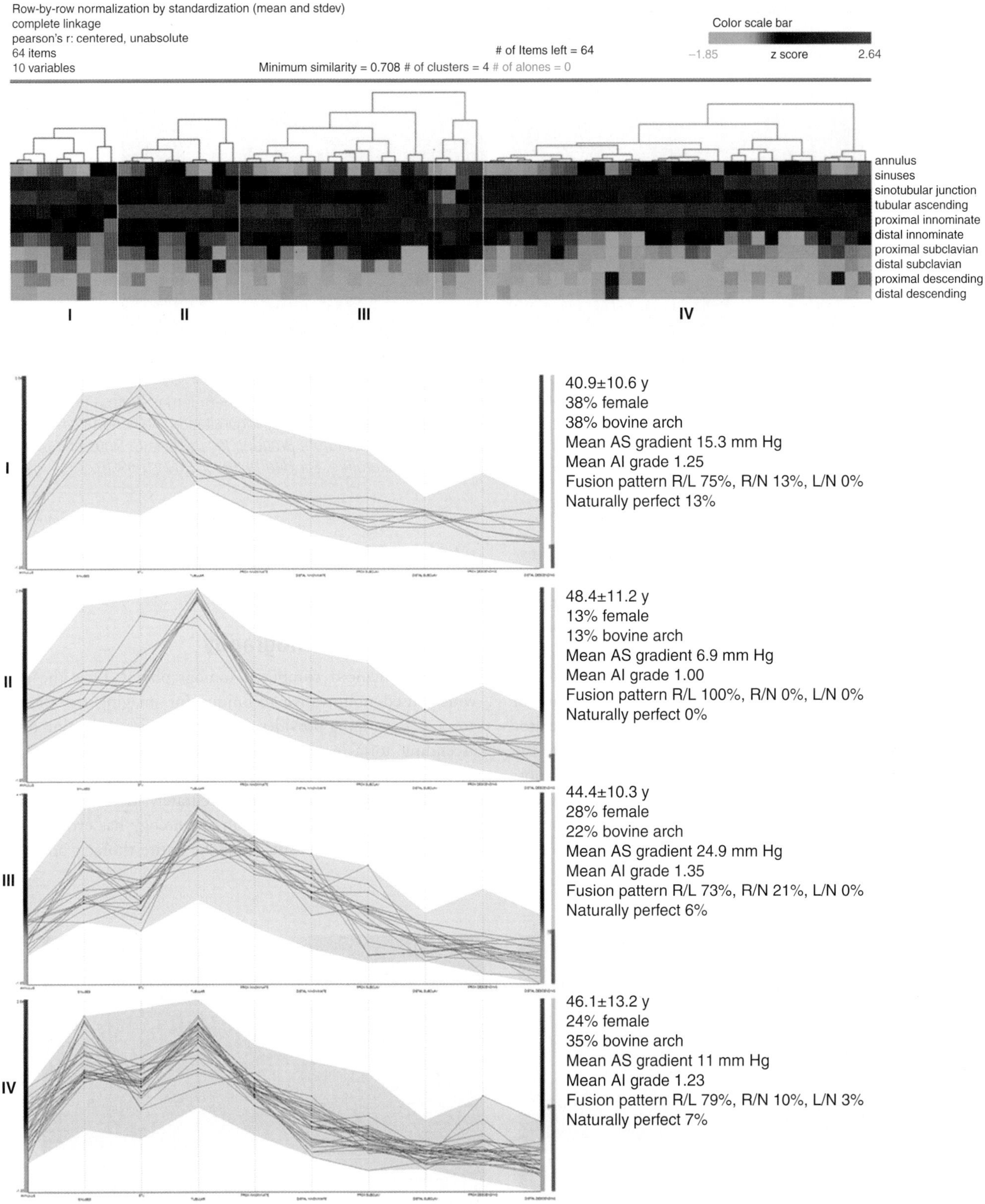

FIGURE 51-7 Patterns of aortic pathology in bicuspid aortopathy patients using hierarchal clustering methodology. The top panel shows a "heat map" in which each column represents a patient and each row represents aortic diameters that have been color coded according to the calculated within-patient *z* scores on a continuous scale shown on the top right corner of the panel. Cluster I patients had predominant involvement of the aortic root (n = 8). Cluster II patients had predominant involvement of the tubular portion of the ascending aorta (n = 9). Cluster III patients had involvement of the tubular portion of the ascending aorta and the transverse arch (n = 18). Cluster IV patients had diffuse involvement of the thoracic aorta with dilation extending from the aortic root to the midtransverse arch (n = 29). The four clusters are shown again in the bottom four panels, which depict the metric aortic diameters across the thoracic aorta for each individual patient. The clinical data for each cluster are summarized to the right of each cluster panel. AI = aortic insufficiency; AS = aortic stenosis. (*Reproduced with permission from Fazel SS, Mallidi HR, Lee RS, et al: The aortopathy of bicuspid aortic valve disease has distinctive patterns and usually involves the transverse aortic arch. J Thorac Cardiovasc Surg 2008; 135[4]:901-907.*)

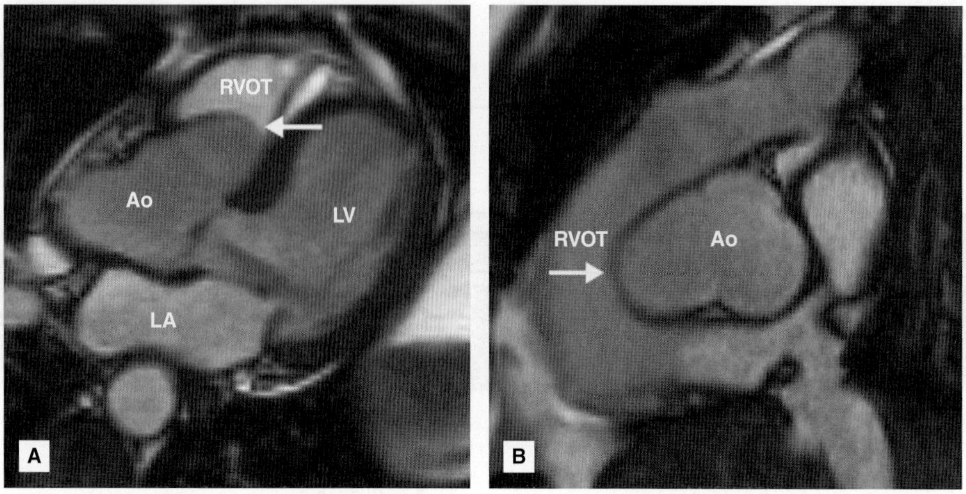

FIGURE 51-8 Contrast MR showing three-chamber view (*left panel*) and the aortic valve plane (*right panel*) demonstrate a right SVA protruding into the right ventricular outflow tract (*arrows*). There is an associated turbulent jet of aortic regurgitation. Ao = Aorta; LA = left atrium; LV = left ventricle; RVOT = right ventricular outflow tract. (*Reproduced with permission from Brandt J, Jögi P, Lührs C: Sinus of Valsalva aneurysm obstructing coronary arterial flow: case report and collective review of the literature. Eur Heart J 1985; 6[12]:1069-1073.*)

ascending aortic aneurysms, dissections, and intramural hematoma (Fig. 51-10).[78–80] TEE is an invasive imaging modality and carries a small risk of esophageal perforation, respiratory compromise, and hemodynamic instability. Imaging of the distal ascending aorta is obscured on TEE by air in the tracheobronchial tree, with up to 40% of its distal extent not well visualized, although this is somewhat mitigated with the use of modern multiplanar probes.[81] Although somewhat operator dependent, TEE provides a reliable technique to measure the annular, sinus, sinotubular junction, and ascending dimensions. It is uniquely well suited to examine the most proximal aspects of the aortic root, which are often blurred by motion artifact on computed tomography scans. Transthoracic echocardiography is far less reliable but may be useful for assessing the severity of aortic regurgitation.

Computed Tomography

Contrast-enhanced computed tomography (CT) is the most widely used noninvasive technique for imaging the thoracic aorta. CT scanning provides rapid and precise evaluation of the ascending aorta in regard to size, extent, and location of the disease process (Fig. 51-11). CT scanning detects areas of calcification, and modern scanner accurately identify dissections and mural thrombus.[82] CT scan technology has evolved with multidetector scanners such that the entire thoracic aorta can

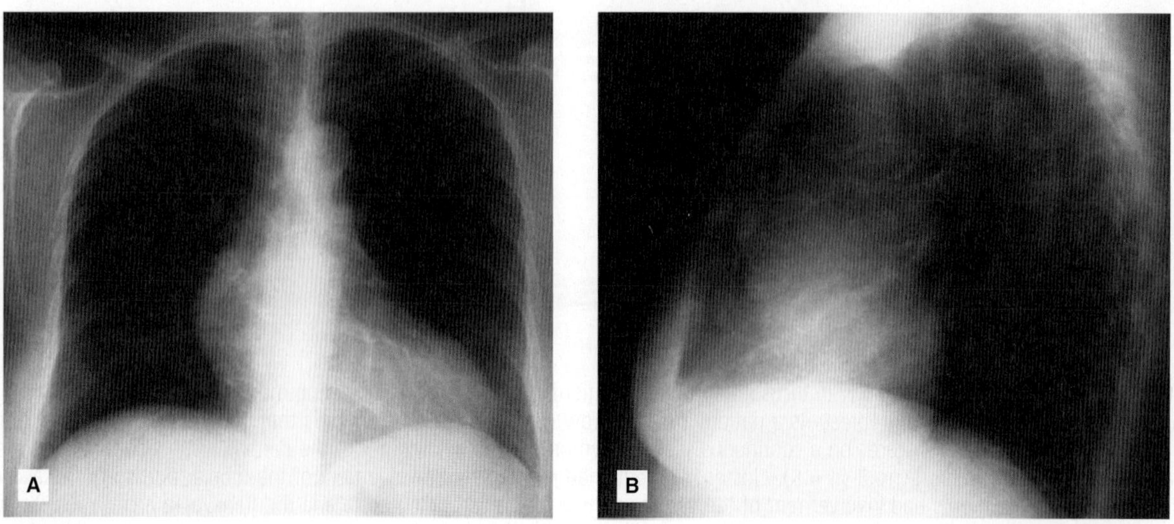

FIGURE 51-9 Posteroanterior and lateral chest radiograph of a patient with an ascending aortic aneurysm. (A) The posteroanterior view shows convexity of the right mediastinum; and (B) the lateral view shows loss of the normal retrosternal air space. *(Reproduced with permission from Downing SW, Kouchokos NT: Ascending aortic aneurysm, in Edmunds LH Jr [ed]: Cardiac Surgery in the Adult. New York, McGraw-Hill, 1997; p 1163.)*

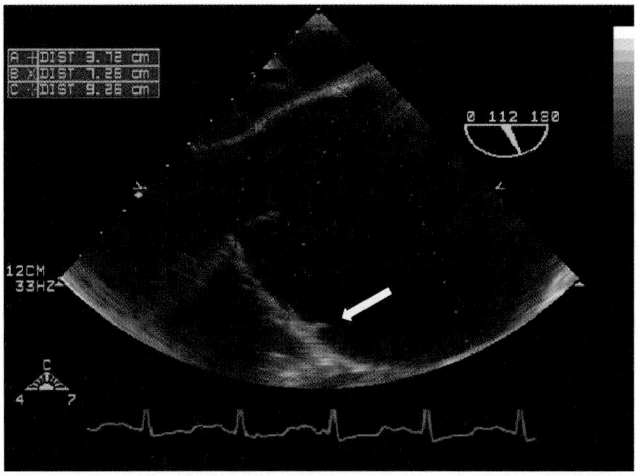

FIGURE 51-10 Transesophageal echocardiogram of a massive aortic root aneurysm with dissection (*arrow*).

be evaluated on one breath-hold and the distance between axial slices can be as small as 0.5 mm. Three-dimensional volume rendering is a highly useful tool for determining true in-plane aortic diameters and the proximal and distal extent of aortic disease relative to the arch vessels, which can aid the surgeon in operative planning (Fig. 51-12). Ideally, the entire thoracic and abdominal aorta should be examined for evidence of concomitant aneurysm disease in the arterial tree. Gating to the electrocardiogram during image acquisition eliminates the motion artifact that may be seen in the most proximal aspects of the aortic root and can also allow for assessment of the coronary arteries.[83] The main disadvantage of CT scans is the need for contrast solution for optimal resolution, which may be contraindicated in those patients with renal insufficiency or a history of a dye allergy. Noncontrast CT scans allow for assessment of aortic diameters but cannot identify dissection flaps or other acute pathologies.

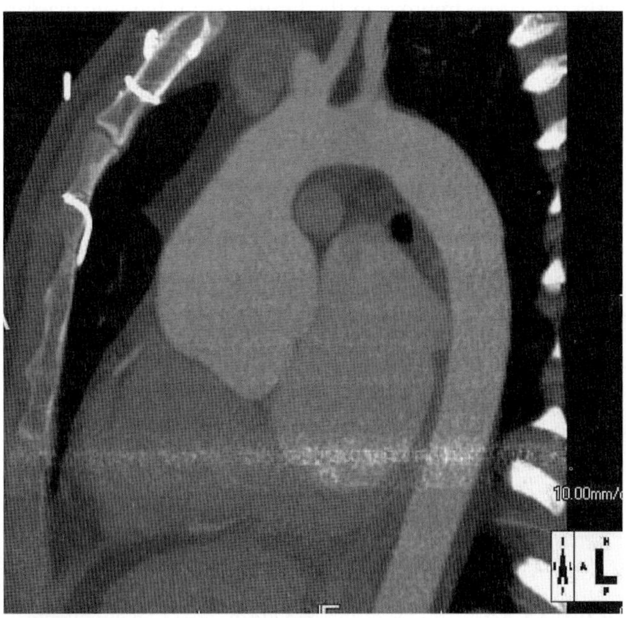

FIGURE 51-11 CT angiogram of an enlarged aortic root in a Marfan patient.

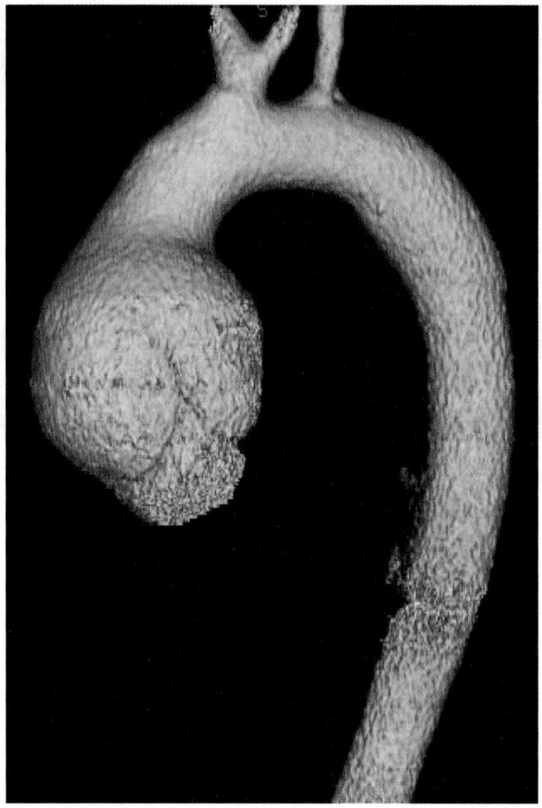

FIGURE 51-12 Three-dimensional reconstruction of an aortic root aneurysm in a Marfan patient.

Magnetic Resonance Imaging

Magnetic resonance imaging (MRI) can provide axial and three-dimensional reconstruction of the ascending aorta with the avoidance of iodinated contrast agents and radiation exposure. Contrast-enhanced MR angiography with gadolinium allows more precise measurements of the aorta and its major branches with images comparable with conventional angiography.[84] MRI scanners are relatively unsuitable for those patients connected to mechanical ventilators or hemodynamic monitoring equipment. MRI is more expensive, less readily available, and requires significantly more acquisition time than CT scanning and is used less frequently.

NATURAL HISTORY

Elective aortic replacement is used as a means to prophylactically prevent aortic catastrophe such as dissection and rupture, which carry high mortality. Recent data from the International Registry of Acute Aortic Dissections (IRAD) shows an operative mortality for emergent type A aortic dissection repair of 26%, although this is generally lower in more experienced centers.[85] Bickerstaff and colleagues examined the natural history of 72 patients who were diagnosed with aortic aneurysms and did

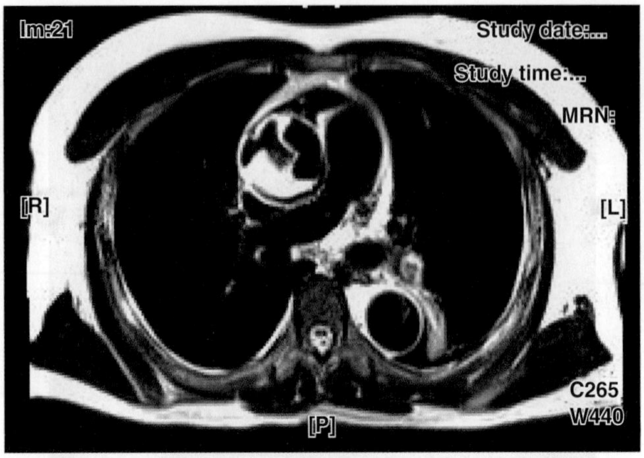

FIGURE 51-13 MR angiogram (without contrast) depicting an acute type A dissection. The partially thrombosed false lumen is denoted by the arrow.

not undergo surgery.[86] Over a 5-year follow-up period, 74% of patients experienced aortic rupture or dissection (Fig. 51-14). Of these, 94% died. The overall 5-year survival was only 13% in untreated aneurysm patients, compared with 75% in control patients without aortic aneurysms.

Traditionally, the most important criterion for ascending aortic replacement on an elective basis is maximal aortic diameter. In natural history studies by Coady and colleagues, patients with 3.5- to 3.9-cm aortic aneurysms were very unlikely to rupture within 3 to 4 years, and each incremental 1-cm increase from this point increased rupture risk (Fig. 51-15).[87] Patients with aneurysms greater than 5 cm showed substantially higher dissection and rupture risk within the first year. Using a logistic regression model, they found that the aneurysm with maximal diameter of 6.0 to 6.9 cm had a 4.3 times greater increased risk of rupture or dissection than an aneurysm that is 4.0 to 4.9 cm in diameter. Growth rates for aortic aneurysms less than 4 cm are about 0.1 cm per year, and this increases gradually as aortic size increases up to 0.4 cm per year.[88,89] Uncontrolled hypertension, smoking, and presence of connective tissue disorders are associated with more rapid aortic growth.[88] Patients with Marfan's syndrome are at particularly high risk for rupture or dissection of smaller sizes, and dissection is frequently seen with a maximal ascending aortic dimension of less than 5 to 6 cm

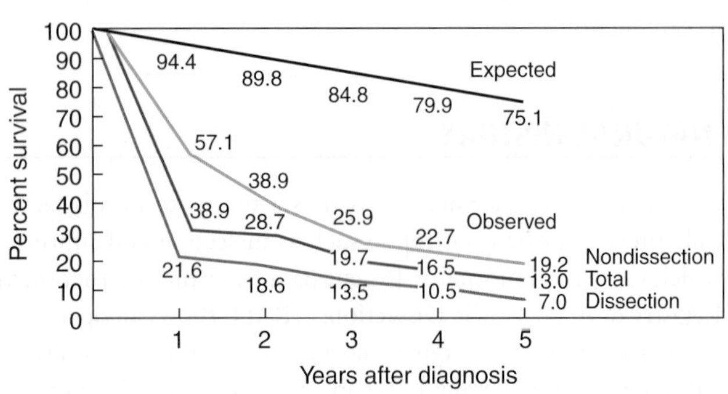

FIGURE 51-14 Actuarial survival estimates of 72 patients followed nonoperatively with thoracic aneurysms and dissections.

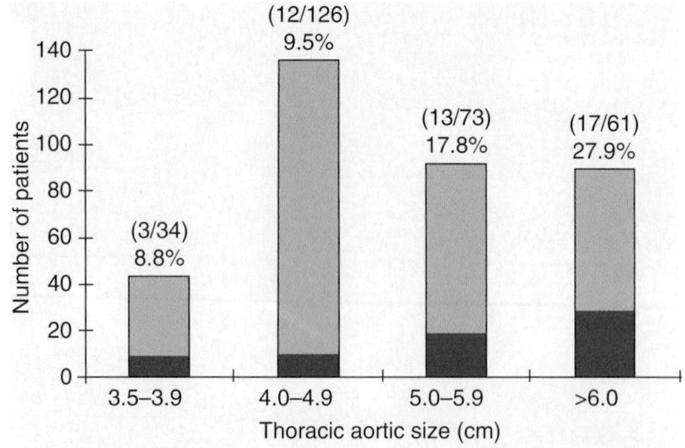

FIGURE 51-15 The incidence of acute dissection or rupture of thoracic aneurysms according to size. The height of the column corresponds to the total number of patients and the black area to the proportion of patients who suffered complications of dissection or rupture. (*Reproduced with permission from Coady MA, Rizzo JA, Hammond GL, et al: What is the appropriate size criterion for resection of thoracic aortic aneurysms? J Thorac Cardiovasc Surg 1997; 113:476.*)

(Fig. 51-16).[90] Strikingly, the average age of death for untreated patients with Marfan's syndrome is 32 years, with complications of the aortic root being responsible for 60 to 80% of these deaths.[91] Marfan's patients with a family history of early dissection or rupture are at the highest risk for aortic catastrophe occurring at smaller dimensions.[92]

Although size clearly correlates with rupture risk, it is important to note that many aortic dissections occur in ascending aortas that are less than 5.5 cm in diameter. In the IRAD registry, more than 59% of 591 enrolled patients with acute type A aortic dissections had maximum aortic dimensions less than 5.5 cm and 40% were less than 5.0 cm (Fig. 51-17).[93] As the understanding of the biologic mechanisms behind aortic aneurysm formation improve in the future, serum biologic markers and sensitive imaging techniques that can detect subtle changes in aortic strain characteristics or compliance may provide more accurate identification of the high-risk aorta.

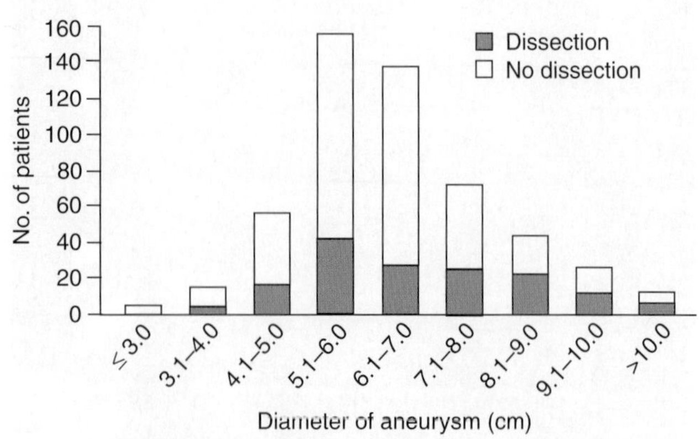

FIGURE 51-16 Diameter of the aneurysm in 524 adult patients with Marfan's syndrome, according to the presence of aortic dissection.

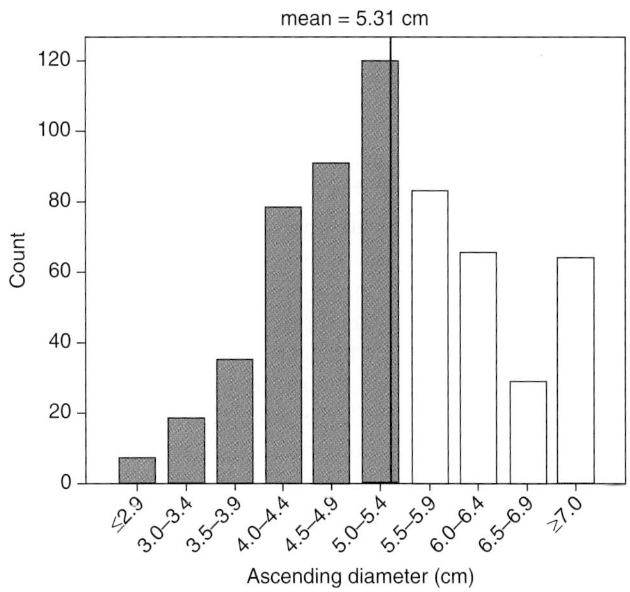

FIGURE 51-17 Distribution of aortic size at time of presentation with acute type A aortic dissection (cm). (*Reproduced with permission from Pape LA, Tsai TT, Isselbacher EM, et al: Aortic diameter > or = 5.5 cm is not a good predictor of type A aortic dissection: observations from the International Registry of Acute Aortic Dissection [IRAD]. Circulation 2007; 116[10]:1120-1127.*)

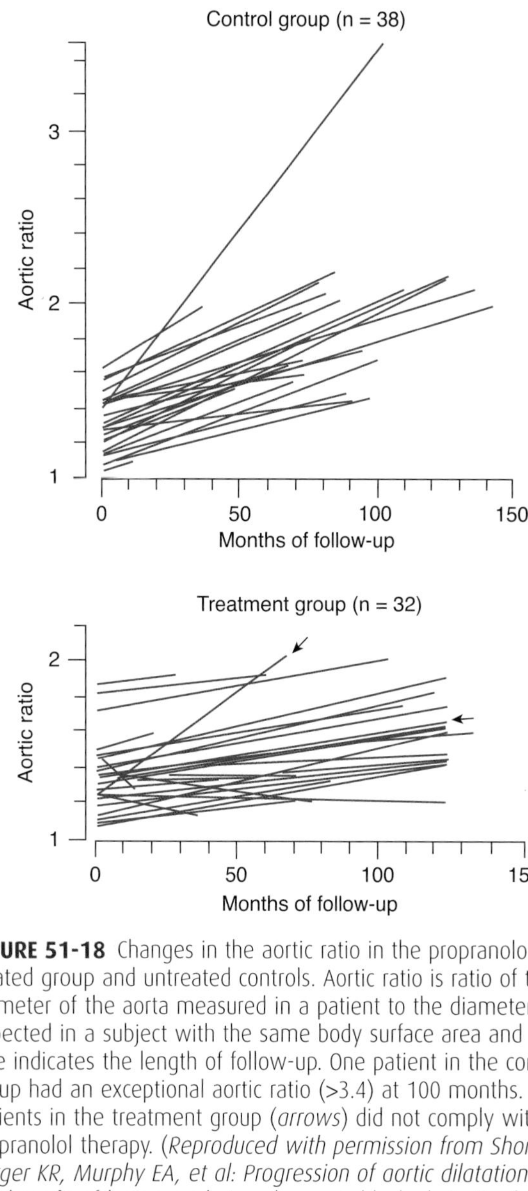

FIGURE 51-18 Changes in the aortic ratio in the propranolol-treated group and untreated controls. Aortic ratio is ratio of the diameter of the aorta measured in a patient to the diameter expected in a subject with the same body surface area and age. Line indicates the length of follow-up. One patient in the control group had an exceptional aortic ratio (>3.4) at 100 months. Two patients in the treatment group (*arrows*) did not comply with propranolol therapy. (*Reproduced with permission from Shores J, Berger KR, Murphy EA, et al: Progression of aortic dilatation and the benefit of long-term beta-adrenergic blockade in Marfan's syndrome. NEJM 1994; 330[19]:1335-1341.*)

MEDICAL TREATMENT OF ASCENDING AORTIC ANEURYSMS

Therapies designed to limit the growth of aortic aneurysms are targeted at mechanisms to diminish stress on the aortic wall and prevent deleterious degenerative biochemical changes. In general, patients with aortic aneurysms should avoid high-intensity isometric exercise, such as weightlifting, because aortic pressures may increase rapidly and exert significant stress on the aortic wall. Weight lifting restriction should be less than one-third to one-half of the patient's body weight. Additionally, exercises with rapid bursts of acceleration and deceleration, such as basketball, may place excessive stress on the aortic wall.

Anti-impulse therapies are the mainstay treatment for thoracic aortic aneurysms. Because of their negative chronotropic and inotropic effects, beta-blockers are typically used as a first-line treatment.[94] The primary goals of beta-blocker therapy are to decrease overall blood pressure and decrease the change in aortic pressure over time (dP/dT), to diminish the stress applied to the aorta in systole and thereby limit damage to the media layer. The rationale for using beta-blockers was initially established with an ex vivo plastic model of aortic dissection by Wheat and colleagues in which a tear created in an artificial intimal layer of rubber cement in the plastic tubing propagated less when the pulse pressure was artificially flattened, whereas variation of mean blood pressure and flow rates had no effect.[95] Studies performed on turkeys, which are uniquely prone to aortic dissection, showed the combination of sodium nitroprusside and propranolol were effective at preventing rupture, whereas lowering blood pressure with nitroprusside alone was ineffective and may have actually increased dP/dT owing to reflex sympathetic stimulation, causing increased chronotropy and inotropy.[96] In a landmark study by Shores and colleagues, young patients with Marfan's syndrome randomized to a regimen of beta-blocker therapy had significantly less aortic dilatation over a 10-year follow-up period (Fig. 51-18), and also had a lower incidence of a composite end point of death, congestive heart failure, aortic dissection, severe regurgitation, or aortic root surgery versus controls.[97] These results have been extrapolated to a wider variety of patients with ascending aortic aneurysms in whom beta-blockade is used extensively.

INDICATIONS FOR SURGERY

Nonelective Indications

Any new onset acute dissection, rupture or intramural hematoma generally warrants immediate surgery. The presence of symptoms of chest pain in patients with ascending aortic aneurysms greater than 4.5 to 5 cm is a sign of impending rupture and should also be managed operatively with expediency. Acute severe congestive heart failure secondary to root dilatation and loss of sinotubular junction definition either from rapid aneurysm expansion or chronic dissection also warrants early operative management, although aggressive diuresis and cardiac optimization for one to two days before surgery is frequently helpful.

Elective Indications

Despite the limitations of size criteria, decisions to intervene are still largely decided based on maximal aortic diameter and growth rate. For degenerative aneurysms in the absence of connective tissue disorders or other cardiac pathology, elective repair is reasonable at an absolute maximal diameter of 5.5 cm.[98] A growth rate of greater than 1 cm per year is generally accepted as a strong indication to proceed with surgery for degenerative aneurysms regardless of diameter.[99] Some groups have also advocated the use of normalized aortic dimensions to body size to provide a more accurate reflection of the aneurysm dimension for an individual patient.[100]

The aortic ratio is calculated as measured diameter divided by predicted diameter for a given age body surface area. Using this method, elective replacement is warranted at an aortic ratio of 1.5 in an asymptomatic patient without a connective tissue disorder or other complicating factor.[101] This leads to intervention at a size of only 4.8 to 5.0 cm in an adult less than 40 years of age with a body surface area of 2 m^2.[101] Because the ascending aorta normally increases in size with age, the diameter for intervention is higher in a patient more than 40 years old.

Special Considerations

Patients with Marfan's syndrome are at higher risk for rupture, and the ascending aorta should be replaced prophylactically at a diameter of 4.5 cm or an aortic ratio of 1.3 to 1.4.[101,102] Among patients with bicuspid aortic valves, current consensus is that aortas greater than 4.5 cm or aortic ratio of 1.3 to 1.4 should be replaced at the time of aortic valve replacement.[101,103] In the context of a well-functioning bicuspid aortic valve, the ascending aorta should be replaced at a maximal dimension of 5.0 cm.[104] In chronic aortic dissections, in which the external aortic wall is supported only by the residual outer third of the medial and adventitial layers, replacement should be performed when aortic diameters reach 4.5 cm or ratio of 1.3 to 1.4 because of the intrinsic weakness of the aortic wall.[101] In the setting of connective tissue disorders, bicuspid aortic valve, or chronic dissection, a growth rate of greater than 0.5 cm per year should warrant repair. Pseudoaneurysms, which are frequently from previous aortic suture lines, should be repaired on diagnosis because of high rupture risk related to their extremely thin walls.

In younger patients, in whom aortic root reimplantation is preferred to avoid lifelong anticoagulation, earlier repair may prevent the development of aortic valve cusp pathology and improve the chances of successful repair. Among patients undergoing aortic valve replacement who have ascending aortic aneurysms, Prenger and colleagues reported a 27% incidence of aortic dissection if the aorta was greater than 5 cm versus 0.6% incidence if aortic size was normal.[105] In general, in the setting of other cardiac surgery, ascending aortas with a maximal dimension of 5.0 cm or a ratio of 1.5 should be replaced.[101,105]

PREOPERATIVE PREPARATION

Nearly one-third of patients undergoing surgery for thoracic aortic disease have chronic obstructive pulmonary disease.[106] Patients with suspect pulmonary function should have spirometry and room air arterial blood gases. Smoking cessation, antibiotic treatment of chronic bronchitis, and chest physiotherapy may prove beneficial in elective situations. Normal renal function should be ensured with the appropriate blood work, and abnormal results should prompt further investigation. Because unaddressed severe carotid disease is a risk factor for stroke during ascending aortic operations, patients greater than age 65 should have duplex imaging of their carotids.[107] Younger patients with peripheral vascular disease, extensive coronary artery disease, carotid bruits, or a history suspicious for cerebral ischemia should be investigated as well. CT or MRI of the thoracic and abdominal aorta is usually indicated. Coronary angiography should be performed in all patients to evaluate for significant coronary atherosclerosis, and lesions with greater than 50 to 60% stenosis should be bypassed. Coronary angiography also helps define the coronary anatomy to identify anomalous or intramural coronary arteries, which may complicate root replacement.[108]

AN ALGORITHMIC APPROACH TO DECISION MAKING IN THE ASCENDING AORTA

Choice of procedure when managing ascending aortic aneurysms is predicated on a detailed understanding of individual patient anatomy and pathophysiology. The potential operative decisions include whether to replace the aortic valve, aortic sinuses, ascending aorta, or aortic arch. Any combination of these procedures is theoretically possible. A systematic approach to evaluate the aorta and aortic root begins with determining if there is a suspicion for connective tissue disorder. Patients with Marfan's syndrome, Ehler's Danlos, Loeys-Dietz, bicuspid valve–related aortopathy, or strong family history of aortic dissection or rupture should generally be treated more aggressively by replacing the sinus segment, ascending aorta, and proximal arch, because late reintervention is more likely in this group.[109] Proximal reconstruction in these patients may be accomplished by either root replacement or a valve-sparing root reimplantation procedure.[110]

The next step is to determine the pathology of the aortic valve. Moderate or worse aortic stenosis with or without insufficiency generally requires replacement, whereas the management of pure aortic insufficiency is more complex. Aortic insufficiency caused solely by dilatation of the sinotubular junction, typically from an atherosclerotic aneurysm in an elderly patient, may be fully addressed with tube graft replacement of the ascending aorta alone with anastomosis to the sinotubular junction (Fig. 51-19). Care must be taken in this instance to appropriately size the graft to within 10% of the annular dimension to allow full coaptation of the aortic valve leaflets.[111] The sinus segment must also be closely interrogated. If it is particularly

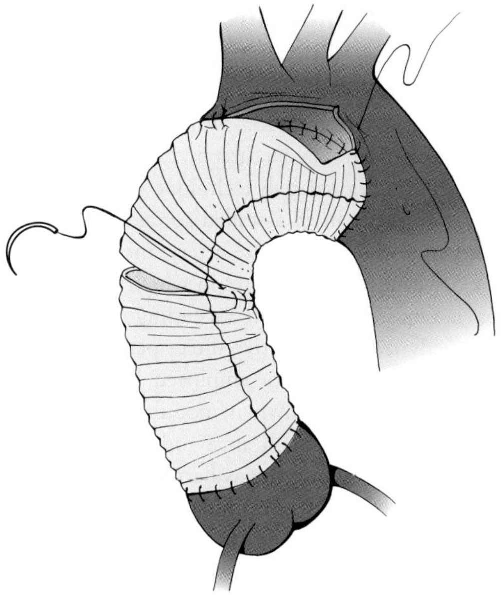

FIGURE 51-19 Replacement of the ascending aorta and transverse arch with an aggressive hemiarch anastomosis.

thin or aneurysmal, it should be replaced. Normal dimensions of the sinus of Valsalva are typically 30 to 32 mm when the aortic annulus measures 23 to 24 mm and the sinotubular junction measures 24 to 25 mm.[112] If there are aneurysmal sinuses and annular dilatation (aortoannular ectasia), but the leaflets appear fairly normal, then a valve-sparing aortic valve reimplantation is often feasible (Fig. 51-20). Technical details of this procedure are discussed in a previous chapter. If the annulus or sinuses are dilated and the leaflets are abnormal and not repairable, root replacement is performed. Prosthesis options include

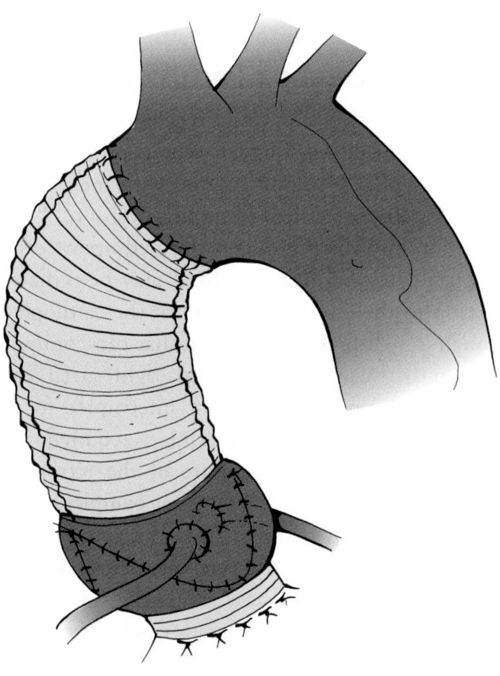

FIGURE 51-20 Valve-sparing aortic root reimplantation using a Dacron graft with a premade sinus of Valsalva segment.

prefashioned composite mechanical root prostheses, sewing a stented tissue valve to a conduit, or using a porcine bioroot. Prosthesis selection is based on several competing factors, including the elevated hazard for structural deterioration of biologic prostheses in younger patients, anticoagulant-related complications with mechanical prostheses, complexity and difficulty of performing future redo root replacements for bioprosthetic failure, and the growing trend toward the avoidance of warfarin in younger patients. The innovation of transcatheter valves, which have the potential to extend the life of a biologic root prosthesis without repeat sternotomy, has generated interest in using these prostheses in younger patients.[113] Pulmonary autografts may also be used as root replacements, but their practicality in aneurysm patients is somewhat limited because degenerative aneurysms tend to occur in older patients who would not benefit from the durability of the pulmonary autograft. Younger aneurysm patients, who could potentially benefit, frequently have bicuspid pathology or connective tissue disorders that may lead to early valve failure. Bicuspid patients have been shown to have significant histologic arterial wall derangements, including the cystic medial necrosis, elastic fragmentation, and changes in the smooth muscle cell orientation in the autograft root.[114]

In patients in whom there is an isolated dilatation of the noncoronary sinus in degenerative aneurysms with preserved sinus dimensions in the coronary sinuses, In the noncoronary sinus may be individually excised and a "tongue" of the ascending aortic graft may be used to reconstruct this sinus with the rest of the graft anastomosed above the native annulus; that is, a Yacoub-type remodeling procedure isolated to the noncoronary sinus.[115] Such a procedure carries the risk of late dilatation or suture-line disruption because the remaining aortic tissue is often thin and weak. It is also possible to perform an isolated noncoronary sinus reimplantation as described by David and Feindel.[116] Unless operative risk is prohibitive, it is preferential to perform a full root replacement or reimplantation in such patients rather than treat only one sinus.

In patients in whom the aortic valve needs to be replaced because of leaflet pathology, the sinus segment is not aneurysmal, and there is an ascending aneurysm, a modified Wheat procedure with replacement of the aortic valve and placement of a tube graft to the sinotubular junction is used (Fig. 51-21).[15] This approach is especially useful in elderly patients who have mild to moderate sinus segment dilatation, but a root replacement carries significant extra perioperative risk and the likelihood of future proximal reoperation is negligible.

Distal repair may be done as either a total arch, hemiarch, open distal, or clamped distal anastomosis. Total arch replacement with or without elephant trunk extension is typically reserved for patients with full arch aneurysms extending into the thoracic aorta or mega-aorta syndrome. Aneurysmal extension into the proximal aortic arch is a common variant and is well treated with an aggressive hemiarch. Resection of the ascending aorta to the innominate artery on the greater curve and to the level of the subclavian takeoff on the lesser curve provides excellent protection from future aneurysmal degeneration of the arch (see Fig. 51-21). Although clamped techniques for the distal anastomosis are suitable for isolated root pathologies such

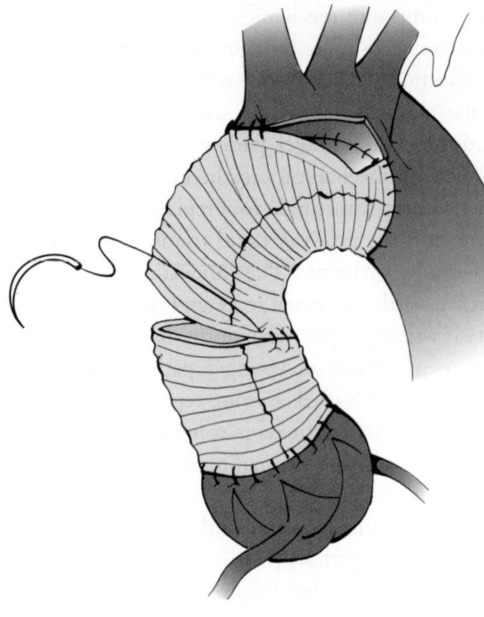

FIGURE 51-21 Separate ascending aortic replacement and aortic valve replacement with retention of the native sinus segment.

as complex endocarditis repair, in aneurysm cases it is preferable to excise the cross-clamped portion of aorta and perform an open distal anastomosis.

OPERATIVE MANAGEMENT

Monitoring and Anesthesia

All procedures are performed using central venous access and a pulmonary artery catheter. Location of arterial line for blood pressure monitoring should be discussed with the anesthesia team preoperatively, although generally right radial is preferred. Nasopharyngeal and bladder temperature monitors are used. Bilateral near-infrared spectroscopy (NIRS) is employed to provide real-time estimation of cerebral saturation throughout the bypass run.[117] Precipitous drops in cerebral saturations are managed with increasing perfusion pressure and hematocrit to the cerebral circulation. In circulatory arrest cases, EEG monitoring is also employed to ensure EEG silence during interruption of cerebral circulation.

Transesophageal echocardiography plays a critical role in diagnosis, particularly of degree of aortic insufficiency and sinus segment and sinotubular junction anatomy that is not well assessed by CT angiography. It is also critical for hemodynamic management separating from cardiopulmonary bypass.

Anesthesia management includes fentanyl, 25 to 50 μg/kg; midazolam, 0.1 to 0.2 mg/kg; isoflurane, 0.5 to 1.5%, end-tidal concentration, in oxygen and pancuronium, 0.1 to 0.2 mg/kg. Aminocaproic acid is dosed initially as an intravenous bolus of 5 g, followed by a maintenance intravenous infusion of 1 g/h and stopped within 2 hours of patient admission to the intensive care unit. Pharmacologic adjuncts in circulatory arrest cases include 1 g of methylprednisolone, 1 g of magnesium sulfate, 2.5 mg/kg of lidocaine, and 12.5 g of mannitol.[118]

Circulation Management

Cannulation strategies vary significantly with individual pathology and the modern cardiovascular surgeon must be proficient in several different techniques. With experience, ascending aortas as large as 7 cm may be directly cannulated. This can be done with the traditional stab technique or using a Seldinger technique over a wire in thin-walled aortas. In aneurysms that terminate before the innominate artery, the transverse arch is easily directly cannulated. In cases in which antegrade cerebral perfusion is required, either the ascending aorta may be cannulated directly if using selective direct perfusion cannulas or the right axillary artery may be employed. Right axillary artery cannulation, which has grown in popularity in recent years, should be performed through an 8- or 10-mm Dacron graft anastomosed end-to-side to the axillary artery, because there is risk of dissection from direct cannulation of this friable artery. In some instances, femoral artery cannulation can be employed, but should be avoided in patients with atheroma in the thoracic aorta by CT scan or TEE.

A standard two-stage venous cannula is used unless performing concomitant mitral or tricuspid surgery. For retrograde cerebral perfusion, a 24-French wire reinforced cannula is placed cephalad to the azygous vein in the superior vena cava and secured with a caval tape. Cooling is performed maintaining less than a 2 to 3°C gradient between arterial inflow temperature and venous return temperature to ensure even cooling. Rather than arbitrarily choosing a particular time or temperature threshold, cooling to EEG silence provides maximal potential brain protection. Data from Cheung and colleagues has shown that only 60% of subjects undergoing hypothermic circulatory arrest achieve EEG silence at a core temperature of 18°C or a cooling time of 30 minutes.[119] In cases in which EEG monitor is not available, a safer technique is to cool for a minimum of 50 minutes, at which point 100% of patients have EEG silence.

Retrograde Cerebral Perfusion

Retrograde cerebral perfusion with oxygenated blood is adjusted to maintain a right internal jugular venous pressure of 25 mm Hg, a flow rate of 200 to 300 cc/min, with the patient in an approximately 10-degree Trendelenburg position.[120] Minimal exsanguination into the pump is performed upon cessation of bypass to facilitate later deairing. RCP may be initiated via a Y-connection to the arterial line or from the cardioplegia system through a high-pressure stopcock that can connect to the Y-connection between the SVC and right atrial cannulas. Retrograde cerebral perfusion may be interrupted for variable periods of time during deep hypothermia as required by various surgical maneuvers. The temperature of the retrograde perfusate is maintained at 12 to 18°C. After completion of aortic arch anastomoses, air is removed from the aorta and graft by allowing it to fill by retrograde cerebral perfusion. After arch deairing, a cross-clamp is placed across the ascending aortic graft, and standard CPB with antegrade cerebral perfusion, that is, antegrade graft perfusion, is reinstituted for the final repair and rewarming. Our practice is to always reestablish antegrade flow via direct cannulation of the ascending graft using either a prefabricated 8- or 10-mm side-arm or by placing a pursestring suture in the graft and directly cannulating it.

Antegrade Cerebral Perfusion

Used routinely by many centers, antegrade cerebral perfusion is primarily beneficial over RCP in situations in which the expected circulatory arrest time is greater than 35 to 45 minutes. Common strategies include direct cannulation of the head vessels with balloon-tip catheters as described by Kazui or by right axillary cannulation.[121] When performing direct arch vessel cannulation, it is advisable to use balloon tip catheters that have individual pressure-monitoring lines so the true perfusion pressures can be monitored to avoid cerebral hypertension. Right radial artery monitoring may also be helpful. Perfusion is typically performed at 10 cc/kg/min and mean pressures are maintained at 40 to 70 mm Hg. Perfusate temperature should approximate the core temperature. Optimal protection is gained by direct perfusion of all three arch branches, not just the left common carotid and innominate arteries.

Axillary cannulation is performed via cutdown to the right axillary artery with an 8- to 10-mm Dacron graft sewn in an end-to-side fashion (Fig. 51-22). The graft is ligated at the end of the procedure. Given the fragility of the axillary artery, few surgeons cannulate it directly. As with direct cerebral vessel perfusion, perfusion pressure is maintained at 10 cc/kg/min and mean pressures are 40 to 70 mm Hg. The innominate artery is either snared or clamped at its origin. Although antegrade cerebral perfusion via this method is rapid and effective, it only provides unilateral perfusion; contralateral ischemia may still occur. To maintain adequate cerebral perfusion pressure and eliminate the effect of arterial–arterial collaterals stealing flow, ideally the left common carotid and subclavian artery origins are controlled as well.[122]

Myocardial Protection

Typically, 1 L of cold blood hyperkalemic cardioplegia (4°C) is given antegrade into the aortic root. A left ventricular vent is employed to prevent distention. In cases of severe aortic insufficiency, the aorta is opened and the coronary ostia are cannulated directly with handheld cannula. A temperature probe is placed through the anterior myocardium into the septum and a myocardial temperature of 6 to 8°C is achieved. Retrograde cardioplegia is administered at least every 20 minutes and continuously when possible. It is important to give cardioplegia immediately before commencing circulatory arrest and at its conclusion.

SPECIFIC OPERATIVE TECHNIQUES

Ascending Aortic Replacement

After the aortic cross-clamp is applied and cardioplegic arrest is achieved as described in the preceding, the ascending aorta is transected about 1 cm below the clamp and resected to the level of the sinotubular junction. The aorta is carefully freed from the pulmonary artery using low-energy electrocautery. Using a metric sizer, the diameter of the sinotubular junction that provides adequate leaflet coaptation is determined; this should be within 10% of the annular diameter. The aortic valve is inspected to ensure that it is trileaflet and free from significant calcification or leaflet pathology. If the aortic valve is to be replaced, this is performed at this point using standard techniques. An appropriate-size graft is then anastomosed to the sinotubular junction using a running 4-0 polypropylene. The external aspect may be reinforced with Teflon felt if the aorta appears especially thin and a root replacement is not feasible. In cases of acute dissection, individual pledgeted sutures are placed at upper aspects of the commissures to resuspend the aortic valve and Teflon felt is placed inside between the dissected layers to form a robust neomedia that can hold sutures.

Composite Root Replacement

Aortic root replacement involves excision of the entire ascending aorta to the native valve annulus with mobilization of coronary buttons and placement of a composite valve and polyester

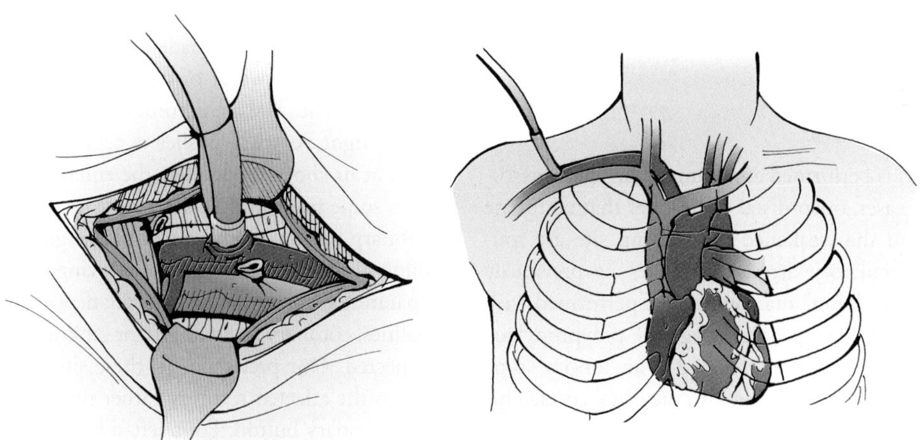

A B

FIGURE 51-22 (A) Direct cannulation of axillary artery with right-angle arterial cannula (note division of crossing vein). (B) Cannulation of axillary artery with a side graft. A straight arterial cannula is inserted into graft.

graft conduit into the annulus. After cross-clamping and administration of cardioplegia, the ascending aorta is resected to the level of the sinotubular junction. The sinuses are mobilized off of the pulmonary arteries and right ventricle and the coronary buttons are mobilized as described in the following. Unless a root reimplantation procedure is being performed, excessive proximal mobilization of the root is unnecessary.

The aortic valve leaflets are excised. The annular dimension is sized and an appropriately sized prosthesis is selected. Mechanical composite prostheses come prefabricated with either a polyester straight tube graft or artificial neosinuses created by changing the orientation of the polyester in the sinus segment. If a tissue valve is desired, a polyester graft that is either straight or has neo-sinuses is anastomosed with a running 3-0 or 4-0 polypropylene suture to an appropriately sized stented tissue valve. If using a Dacron graft with neo-sinuses, this should be sewn 3 to 4 mm below the start of the neo-sinus segment. The valve sutures must pass through both the valve sewing ring and the Dacron graft to ensure hemostasis.

The composite prosthesis may be placed with either pledgeted everting; that is, "intra-annular," mattress sutures with pledgets on the outside of the annulus or in a "supra-annular" configuration with pledgets on the ventricular side of the annulus. Typically, the everting technique is used because it is hemostatic and strong. Implanting the root with pledgets on the ventricular side requires less mobilization of the sinuses, which may be advantageous in certain situations and may allow for a slightly larger prosthesis. When implanting a mechanical prosthesis, the everting technique is preferred because it is less prone to pannus formation, which may interfere with valve function. Care must be taken with either technique not to shorten the mitral valve anterior leaflet with excessively large bites with the annular sutures along the left and noncoronary sinuses. Polyester, braided 2-0 sutures with a larger needle than used for aortic valve replacement is employed.

Once the valve-conduit is tied down, the coronary buttons are anastomosed using 5-0 Prolene sutures as described in the following (Fig. 51-23). Pressurization of the new root by inserting a catheter into the proximal graft, running cardioplegia and clamping the graft distally after de-airing the neoroot allows assessment of all suture lines.

Implantation of stentless bioroots, homograft roots, pulmonary autografts, and valve-sparing procedures is discussed in previous chapters.

Distal Anastomosis

Distal reconstruction is performed as a clamped or open anastomosis. In aneurysm cases, open distal techniques that eliminate all diseased aorta and the weakened cross-clamp site are routinely employed. Circulatory arrest techniques as previously described are employed. Distal anastomoses are performed with a beveled polyester graft using a running 4-0 polypropylene suture. The distal anastomosis is performed as an "on-lay" type anastomosis with the graft invaginated into the distal aorta. This pushes the graft material into the native aorta when the aorta is pressurized and prevents leaks. In cases of extremely friable aorta, Teflon felt placed along the outer aspect may also be beneficial but does not substitute for a proper "on-lay" technique.

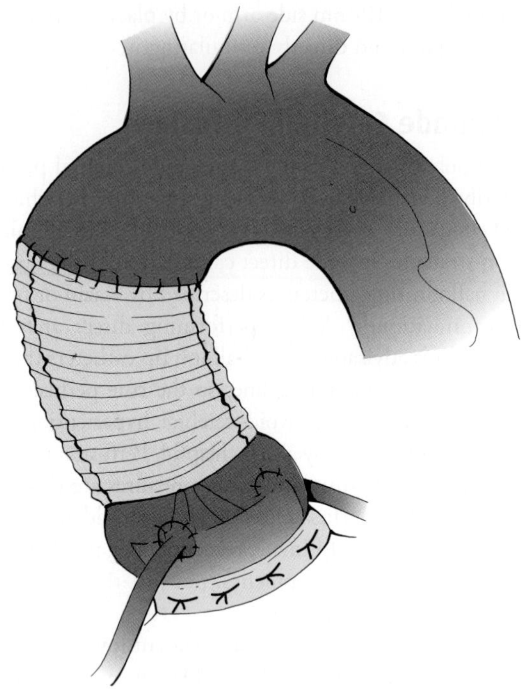

FIGURE 51-23 Composite root replacement with a mechanical prosthesis.

Management of Coronary Arteries

Mobilization of the coronary artery buttons in root operations remains the most technically demanding and least forgiving aspect of root operations. The left main button is mobilized after the aorta has been fully dissected from the pulmonary artery. It is frequently useful to work from the inside of the aorta outward, gently scoring the dissection plane with low-intensity electrocautery. Generally, 1 to 2 cm of freedom of motion in all directions is required for adequate mobilization. Care must be taken mobilizing the right coronary artery to ensure the right ventricle is not inadvertently entered. Application of retrograde and direct antegrade cardioplegia into the coronaries after mobilization will identify any small branch disruptions or major injuries while they are still repairable.

When anastomosing the left coronary button to the aortic graft, if a graft with premade sinuses of Valsalva is used, the button is typically sewn at or below the level of the equator of the sinus segment. The right coronary, which is more likely to kink as the right ventricle pushes it cephalad once the heart fills, is sewn at or above the level of the equator. When using a straight graft, some surgeons will determine the final position of the right coronary button after completing the graft-to-graft anastomosis, filling the heart and briefly removing the cross-clamp. When separating from bypass, if there are new gross wall motion abnormalities, coronary artery injury or kinking should be immediately suspected. Our preference in these situations is to immediately bypass the affected territory rather than attempt to salvage a friable coronary button. For a left-sided problem, a LIMA to LAD bypass will typically resolve the difficulty expediently.

In complex endocarditis, dissection, severe calcification, or reoperative cases, coronary artery buttons may be too damaged

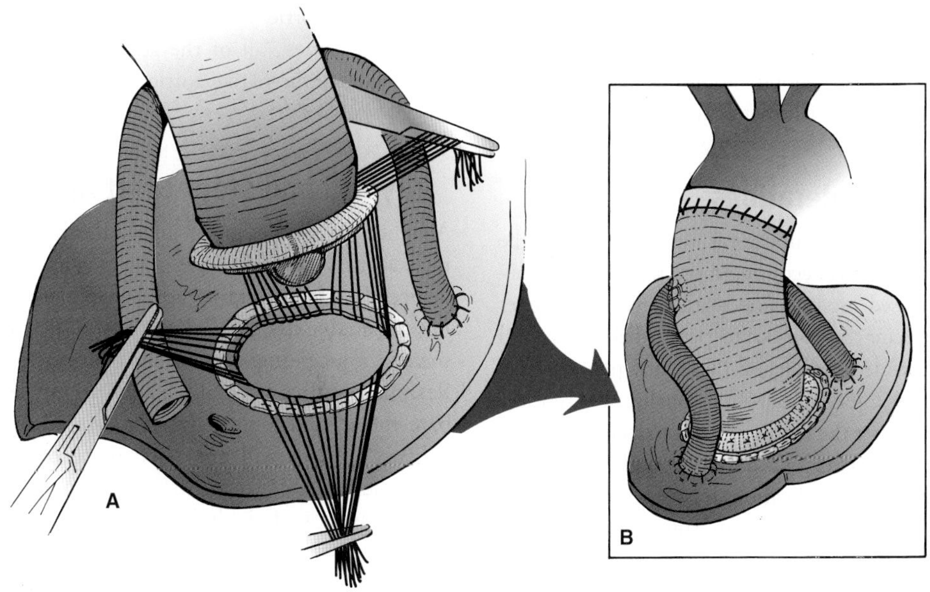

FIGURE 51-24 Classic Cabrol technique for coronary reimplantation. (A) An 8- to 10-mm Dacron tube graft is anastomosed end-to-end to the aortic tissue surrounding the left and right coronary ostia. (B) An opening is made in the midportion of the coronary graft and in an appropriate position in the aortic graft and an anastomosis is formed. The modified Cabrol technique involves the formation of individual coronary buttons allowing the small-caliber Dacron graft to be sewn to the full thickness of the aortic tissue surrounding the coronary ostia.

or immobile to directly attach to the graft. In such situations, a Cabrol-type coronary anastomosis, where the coronary os are anastomosed to an 8- to 10-mm Dacron grafts in a "moustache" configuration, may be employed (Fig. 51-24). Alternatively, segments of reversed saphenous vein can be used as interposition grafts. Typically these grafts are 3 to 5 cm in length, are anastomosed fairly high on the aortic graft, and follow a gentle S-shaped curve to prevent kinking. In cases of right coronary button problems, proximal ligation and bypass to the main right coronary artery is another alternative.

Aortic Wrapping and Reduction Aortoplasty

Reduction ascending aortoplasty and aortic wrapping are less common techniques to address ascending aortic aneurysms typically reserved for patients undergoing concomitant aortic valve replacement but who are deemed too high risk for either composite root or ascending aortic replacement or who have ascending aortic dimensions less than the recommendations for replacement as a prophylactic measure to prevent aneurysm formation. Reduction aortoplasty involves excision of a segment of the ascending aorta to achieve a normal radial maximal dimension. It may be performed either with a side-biting aortic clamp, cross-clamped or with open technique depending on the length of aortoplasty and technique used.[123–125] The excised segment may be taken in the long axis of the aorta down to the sinotubular junction (true reduction annuloplasty), or lesser plication techniques may be employed. External reinforcement can also be performed in conjunction with reduction aortoplasty. Concerns regarding this technique include dehiscence or aortic rupture at the suture line, which is constantly under tension from the radial force on the aortic wall during systole.

Aortic wrapping of girdling is either performed by itself or in conjunction with reduction aortoplasty. Wrapping has been performed with cellophane, polyester grafts and meshes, PTFE, and other materials. Neri and colleagues described two patients required reoperation because of development of false aneurysms after aortic valve replacement with aortoplasty and wrapping.[126] The unwrapped parts of the ascending aorta in both patients appeared normal; conversely, the aortic wall underlying the wrap was severely atrophic, a phenomenon previously reported with abdominal aneurysms that were wrapped without aortoplasty. In a larger series by Cohen and colleagues, among 102 patients who underwent aortic wrapping with a polyester mesh followed for a median of 4.7 years, there were no instances of major aortic complications and an average aneurysm growth of 2.6 mm over the follow-up period.[127]

Concomitant Mitral Surgery

Mitral valve disease is frequently encountered in patients with aortic aneurysms. This is particularly true for patients with Marfan's syndrome, in whom the incidence approaches 30%.[128] Patients who have evidence of moderate to severe mitral regurgitation should undergo mitral valve repair at the time of aortic replacement. Gillinov and colleagues reported results of mitral valve repair in patients with Marfan's syndrome, many of whom also had simultaneous replacement of the aortic root.[129] They observed an 88% actuarial rate of freedom from significant mitral regurgitation at 5 years. A fairly liberal approach to mitral valve intervention is warranted in aortic root replacement patients as reoperation for late mitral regurgitation may be particularly technically difficult. Additionally, care must be taken when taking the annular stitches along the aorto-mitral continuity to avoid shortening the anterior leaflet of the mitral valve.

Reoperative Considerations

Reoperative surgery on the ascending aorta and aortic root can be particularly challenging but is becoming more frequent in experienced centers. Increased use of tissue aortic valves in younger patients, biologic porcine or composite pericardial roots, and homografts in past few decades suggest that many patients may require reoperative root intervention. Additionally, root replacement may be required after the development of ascending aortic aneurysms in bicuspid patients who have previously undergone aortic valve replacement only. Indications for reoperation include aortic insufficiency, development of aneurysms or dissections in remaining segments of the thoracic aorta, false aneurysms, prosthetic valve dysfunction, infection or thrombosis, or degeneration of biologic prostheses.

Re-entry is usually accomplished with a repeat sternotomy incision, although for complex arch operations involving the proximal descending aorta, a thoracosternotomy approach may be required.[130] In cases of massive ascending aortic aneurysm, adhesion of the aorta to the posterior table of the sternum or contained ruptures, exposure of alternative cannulation site such as the right axillary artery or femoral artery is necessary. Massive aortic hemorrhage upon sternal entry should by locally controlled by forcibly reapproximating the sternum, heparinizing the patient, instituting peripheral cardiopulmonary bypass, and cooling to deep hypothermia such that the sternal reentry can be completed under lower flow conditions with active pump-suction in the operative field. If entering the aorta on re-entry is felt to be inevitable, staring cardiopulmonary bypass and cooling before sternotomy may be a superior strategy. In cases of moderate to severe aortic insufficiency, venting of the left ventricle prior to cardiac fibrillation is mandatory and can be accomplished by a small left anterior thoracotomy incision and direct venting of the apex.

Cross-clamping in the reoperative scenario may also be hazardous as previous graft material may cause severe adhesions to the pulmonary artery making the dissection of a clamping site difficult. Previous use of a porcine root prosthesis or left-sided bypass grafts makes this dissection particularly difficult. If the pulmonary artery is inadvertently entered, patching with a pericardial substitute is usually necessary.

Mobilization of the coronary arteries is frequently difficult and creation of a Cabrol-type anastomosis, interposition grafts, or bypass grafts are frequently necessary. Previous coronary bypass grafts should be reimplanted, and frequently, interposition vein grafts are required to accomplish this. Direct cardioplegia administration down bypass grafts is preferred but avoided when there is diffuse vein graft disease.[131] Retrograde cardioplegia is extremely helpful in this circumstance.

In cases of reoperation for failed porcine bioroots, root replacement is preferable to simple aortic valve implantation within the porcine root because there is a higher likelihood for valve dehiscence owing to the degenerative nature of the root tissue.[132] If aortic valve implantation into a porcine root is being performed, all of the aortic valve implantation sutures must traverse the native aortic root tissue, not just the porcine tissue.

Hybrid and Stent Graft Approaches

Advances in the design of highly flexible and low-profile thoracic aortic stent grafts have generated an interest in using these devices for the ascending aorta in patients who are otherwise not reasonable risk surgical candidates. Essential design requirements for ascending aortic stent grafts include a high degree of flexibility and conformability, short graft lengths, no exposed bare metal, and long delivery systems, because most TEVAR delivery systems will not reach the proximal ascending aorta from the femoral artery. Alternative approaches for access sites for the stent graft include axillary artery, carotid artery, and perhaps most promising, transapical artery. Graft lengths are more critical in the ascending aorta than in the thoracic aorta as the distance between sinotubular junction and/or coronary ostia and the takeoff of the innominate artery is typically shorter than 10 cm, and is therefore shorter than most thoracic devices. The antegrade transapical technique may also offer potential advantage by limiting the distance between the sheath and the device, thereby minimizing the potential for device migration during deployment, as is seen in transapical deployment of transcatheter aortic valves. Stent graft placement has been described to treat focal ascending aneurysms in nonoperative candidates (Fig. 51-25).[133]

EARLY COMPLICATIONS

Bleeding

Woven Dacron grafts impregnated with collagen or gelatin are relatively impervious to blood and have reduced blood loss following replacement of the ascending aorta compared with knitted grafts. Precise suturing with careful attention to avoid torque on the suture needles while constructing anastomoses is critical to avoid the inevitable needle-hole bleeding at the end of the surgery. Tension must be avoided at the sites of coronary reimplantation, because this is a frequent site of bleeding. The modified Cabrol method or an interposition graft should be used when any tension is present. The inclusion technique of graft insertion is associated with an increased incidence of bleeding and pseudoaneurysm formation and has largely been abandoned. In very friable aortas, Teflon felt may be used to reinforce the suture line on the outside of the anastomosis in which a thin strip of felt is slipped into the suture line as it is tightened. Alternatively, it may be sewn to the inside, outside or both sides of the native aorta with a running polypropylene stitch before sewing the graft.

In cases of refractory coagulopathy, the anastomosis can be wrapped tightly with a small segment of polyester graft or Teflon felt to reduce tension on the suture line and reduce needle hole bleeding (Fig. 51-26). Blood transfusion can be avoided in a significant number of patients with the use of blood conservation techniques such as Cell Savers, autologous blood donation,

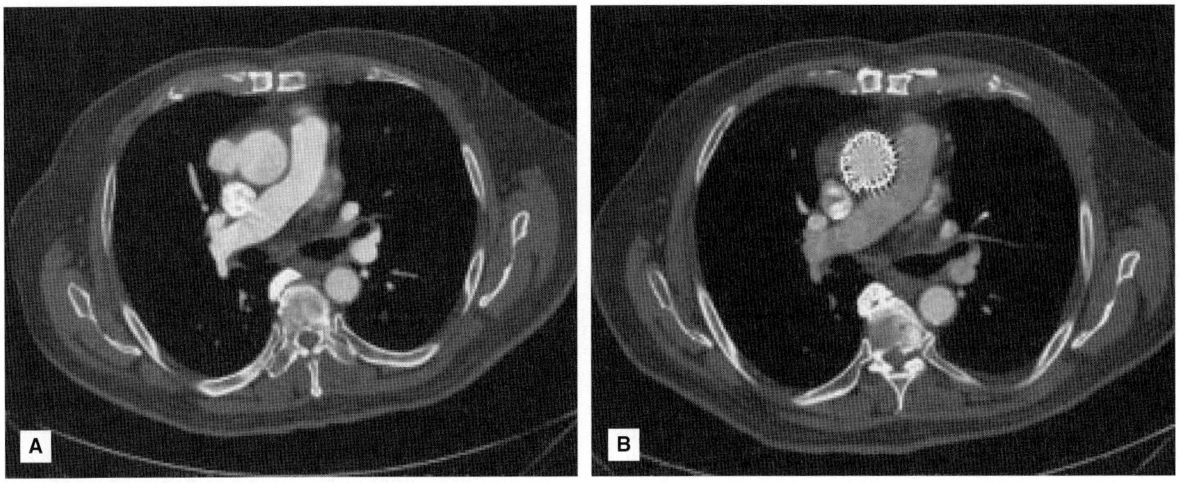

FIGURE 51-25 Placement of a covered stent graft in the ascending aorta to treat a pseudoaneurysm after previous cardiac surgery. (A) Preoperative CT angiogram demonstrates a saccular pseudoaneurysm in the ascending aorta after previous coronary artery bypass graft. (B) Postoperative CT angiogram demonstrates exclusion of pseudoaneurysm with no evidence of endoleak. (*Reproduced with permission from Szeto WY, Moser WG, Desai ND, et al: Transapical deployment of endovascular thoracic aortic stent graft for an ascending aortic pseudoaneurysm. Ann Thorac Surg 2010; 89[2]:616-618.*)

plateletpheresis, the reinfusion of chest tube drainage, and the use of antifibrinolytics such as aminocaproic acid and tranexamic acid. Since the removal of the antifibrinolytic agent aprotinin from the market because of concerns regarding renal dysfunction and mortality, bleeding has anecdotally become more common.

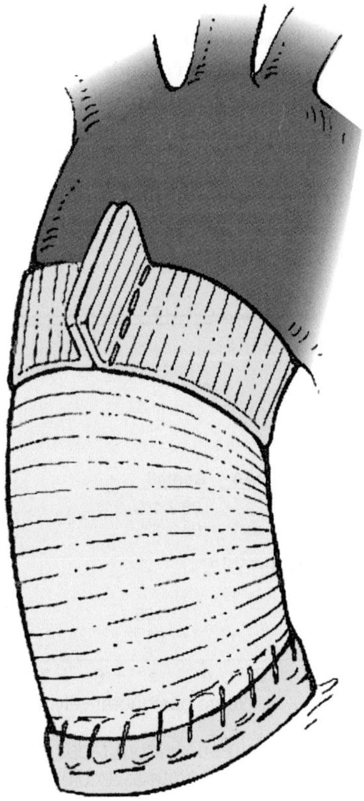

FIGURE 51-26 Suture line bleeding may be effectively controlled with a circumferential wrap of the anastomosis with a strip of Teflon felt or Dacron.

Activated human recombinant factor VII may be helpful as a last resort when treating refractory bleeding that does not respond to any other therapies, although this may induce unanticipated thrombosis in arterial structures.[134]

In cases of ongoing postoperative hemorrhage, expedient return to the operating room for reexploration is preferable to massive transfusion or tamponade. Postoperative bleeding requiring reexploration ranges from 2.4 to 11.1%.[135,136]

Stroke

Neurologic injury after proximal aortic surgery remains a significant cause of morbidity and mortality. Embolization of atherosclerotic debris or thrombus from the ascending aorta and arch produces focal neurologic deficits. Diffuse injury can be attributed to microemboli of air or cellular debris, insufficient or uneven cooling, and a prolonged circulatory arrest period. After circulatory arrest periods exceeding 40 minutes the incidence of stroke greatly increases.[137] Profound hypothermia may itself be injurious to the central nervous system without associated circulatory arrest.[138]

Stroke owing to embolization is diminished when the aorta is evaluated via epiaortic ultrasound or other imaging modality to detect atherosclerotic plaques and thrombus.[139] This allows appropriate adjustments to be made in clamping and cannulation strategies. Resumption of antegrade circulation through the graft once the distal aortic anastomosis is complete, rather than retrograde via the femoral vessels, after a period of circulatory arrest avoids embolization of distal aortic debris. Patients with severe carotid artery occlusive disease are at increased risk of stroke during ascending aortic procedures, and patients older than 65, those with peripheral vascular disease, or those with pertinent histories should be evaluated.[140]

Patients with new postoperative strokes should be rapidly evaluated by the consultant neurology service and undergo early brain imaging. New embolic events should be managed aggressively with induced hypertension once intracranial hemorrhage has been ruled out.

Pulmonary Dysfunction

Cardiopulmonary bypass is known to cause alterations in pulmonary function as evidenced by changes in alveolar–arterial oxygen gradients, pulmonary vascular resistance, pulmonary compliance, and intrapulmonary shunting. Usually these changes are subclinical, but a full-blown adult respiratory distress–like syndrome is reported in 0.5 to 1.7% of patients following cardiopulmonary bypass.[141–143] The specific cause is the subject of much investigation and debate, but it is generally accepted that exposure of blood elements to the foreign surface of the cardiopulmonary circuit results in the activation of inflammatory cells and the complement cascade resulting in pulmonary injury.[144] The duration of cardiopulmonary bypass, urgency of the procedure, and general condition of the patient may roughly correlate with the occurrence and severity of pulmonary dysfunction, but it can be unpredictable.

Treatment is supportive, with early diagnosis and treatment of any subsequent pulmonary infections. Ten to eighteen percent of patients require prolonged mechanical ventilation. Preventive measures may include preoperative optimization of pulmonary function, minimization of pump time, judicious use of blood products, heparin-coated bypass circuits, and leukocyte depletion.[145]

Myocardial Dysfunction

Transient myocardial dysfunction following complex aortic surgery requiring inotropic support is common with 18 to 25% of patients requiring more than 6 hours of inotropic support.[146,147] Meticulous attention should be paid to integrated myocardial protection with cold-blood cardioplegia administered frequently in antegrade and retrograde fashions. This is particularly important in patients with significant left ventricular dilatation seen with aortic insufficiency or hypertrophy seen with aortic stenosis. Maintenance of high-perfusion pressures after removal of cross-clamp optimizes myocardial perfusion during the critical reperfusion period. Optimization of right ventricular function with afterload reducing agents such as milrinone or inhaled prostaglandins while weaning from cardiopulmonary bypass is vital for maintaining adequate left ventricular filling in cases of severe diastolic dysfunction or ventricular hypertrophy. Postoperative myocardial infarction, reported in up to 2.5% of cases, may be related to technical problems with coronary reimplantation.[148]

Perioperative Mortality

Contemporary surgical series on ascending aortic disease using modern grafting techniques and methods of cerebral and myocardial protection report hospital mortality rates of 1.7 to 17.1%.[148–152] Comparison of outcomes is difficult, however, because of heterogeneity of patients. Some series do not include dissection, and the proportion of emergent operations, reoperations, and arch replacements is highly variable. The common causes of early death are cardiac failure, stroke, bleeding, and pulmonary insufficiency.[148,149]

Emergent operation after the onset of acute dissection or rupture is the highest risk factor for early death. Risk of death following elective intervention is increased by increasing New York Heart Association classification, increasing age, prolonged cardiopulmonary bypass time, dissection, previous cardiac surgery, and need for concomitant coronary revascularization.[151,152]

LATE COMPLICATIONS

Late Mortality

Reported actuarial survival, like early mortality, is variable and dependent on the patient cohort. Survival rates are 81 to 95% at 1 year, 73 to 92% at 5 years, 60 to 73% at 8 to 10 years, and 48 to 67% at 12 to 14 years.[153–156] Predictors of late mortality include elevated New York Heart Association class, requirement for arch reconstruction, Marfan's syndrome, and extent of distal disease.[157–160] The most common cause of late death is cardiac, but distal aortic disease accounted for 32% of late deaths in one series.[161]

Reoperation

Reoperations occur because of pseudoaneurysm formation, valve thrombosis, endocarditis or graft infection, progression of disease in the native valve or remaining aortic segments, or degeneration of a bioprosthesis. Reported mortality for reoperative ascending aortic surgery varies between 4 and 22%.[162,163]

Freedom from reoperation is 86 to 90% at 9 to 10 years (Fig. 51-27).[164,165] Predictors of late reoperation have included Marfan's syndrome, the inclusion cylinder technique, and chronic dissection.[166] Surveillance of patients who have undergone previous aortic surgery to minimize the need for urgent reoperations and appropriate resection of all diseased aortic tissue at the time of original operation improves outcomes. Up to 60%

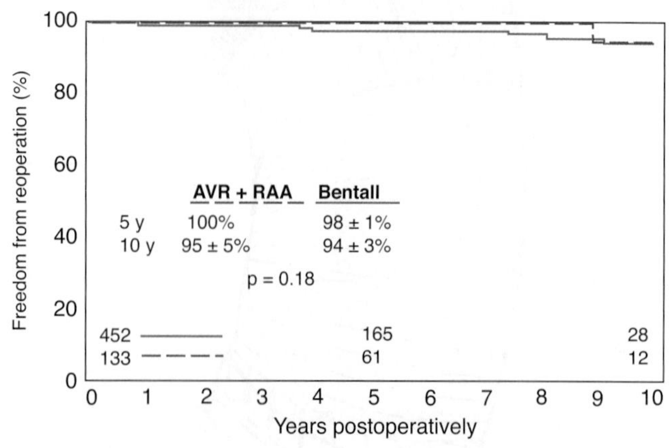

FIGURE 51-27 Long-term freedom from reoperation after full aortic root replacement and separate ascending aortic and valve replacement. *(Reproduced with permission from Sioris T, David TE, Ivanov J, Armstrong S, Feindel CM: Clinical outcomes after separate and composite replacement of the aortic valve and ascending aorta. J Thorac Cardiovasc Surg 2004; 128[2]:260-265.)*

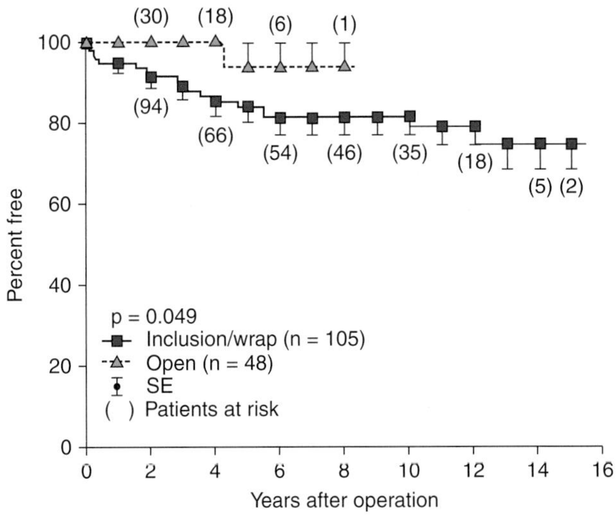

FIGURE 51-28 Long-term freedom from reoperation for pseudoaneurysm of the aortic or coronary ostial suture lines by operative technique (inclusion or open). (*Reproduced with permission from Kouchoukos NT, Wareing TH, Murphy SF, Perrillo JB: Sixteen-year experience with aortic root replacement: results of 172 operations. Ann Surg 1991; 214:308.*)

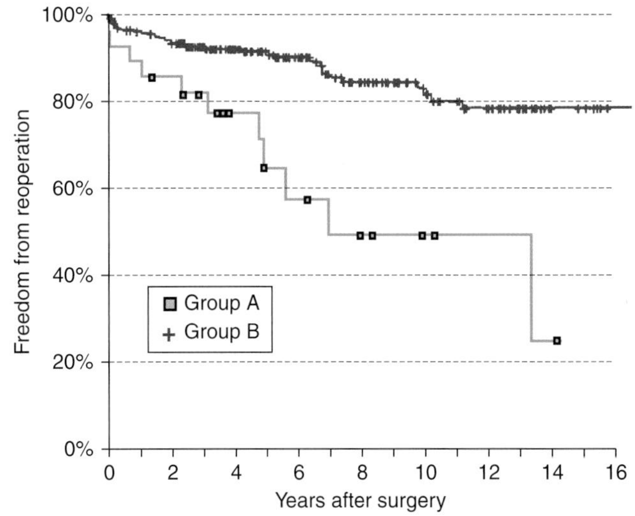

FIGURE 51-29 (*A*) Freedom from reoperation (Kaplan-Meier) of patients with Marfan's syndrome; (*B*) versus those without fibrillinopathic etiologies. (*Reproduced with permission from Detter C, Mair H, Klein HG, et al: Long-term prognosis of surgically-treated aortic aneurysms and dissections in patients with and without Marfan syndrome. Eur J Cardiothorac Surg1998; 13:416.*)

of reoperations occur because of inadequate repair during the initial operation.[167] This is owing to failure to resect the most distal aspects of aneurysmal disease by performing a clamped distal anastomosis or failure to adequately address root pathology with full root replacement. Previous inclusion-type anastomotic techniques were associated with higher rates of early reoperation owing to pseudoaneurysm formation (Fig. 51-28).[168]

Marfan's syndrome patients are particularly prone to requiring reoperation (Fig. 51-29).[169] Gott and colleagues reviewed the experience with root replacement at 10 surgical centers in 675 Marfan patients between 1968 to 1996.[170] The 30-day mortality was 3.3%, but was only 1.5% for elective repair. Emergency surgery resulted in a 30-day mortality of nearly 12%. The survival rate was 93% at 1 year, 84% at 5 years, 75% at 10 years, and 59% at 20 years (Fig. 51-30). Complications related to the residual thoracic aorta and arrhythmias were the leading causes of death. The most frequent late complication was thromboembolism. Advanced New York Heart Association class at the time of original operation was the only predictor of late death.

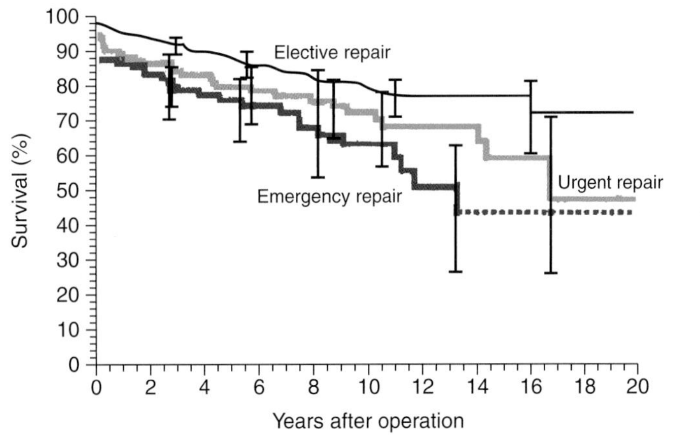

No. at Risk											
Elective repair	455	381	294	204	141	97	64	42	17	4	1
Urgent repair	117	88	74	62	53	41	23	16	8	4	3
Emergency repair	103	73	57	41	31	21	10	4	3	2	0

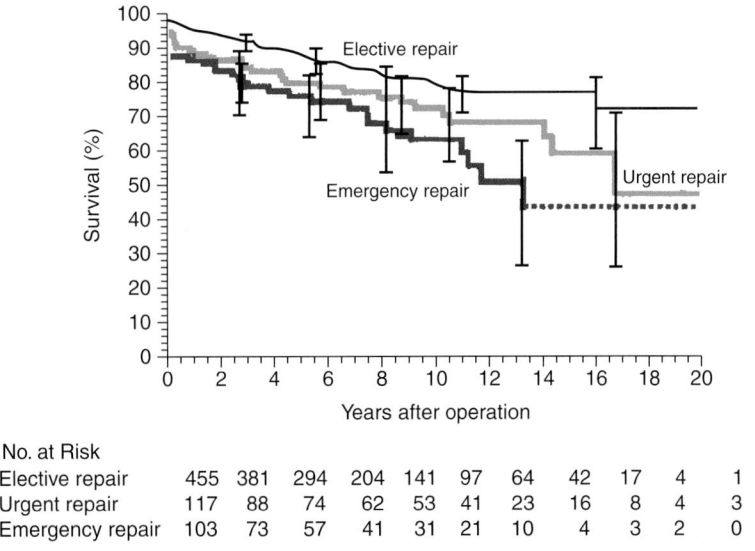

FIGURE 51-30 Long-term survival after aortic root replacement in Marfan's syndrome patients stratified by surgical urgency. (*Reproduced with permission from Gott VL, Greene PS, Alejo DE, et al: Replacement of the aortic root in patients with Marfan's syndrome. NEJM 1999; 340:1307.*)

Graft Infection

Graft infections are reported in up to 0.9 to 6% of patients following surgery of the thoracic aorta and are associated with a very high (25 to 75%) mortality rate.[171–173] Most graft infections occur in the first month after operation and are frequently associated with wound infections. They may occur years later in cases of associated valve endocarditis or bacteremia from indwelling catheters or other systemic infections. The major infectious agents are *S. aureus, S. epidermidis,* and *Pseudomonas.*[174] The ascending aortic graft may be particularly vulnerable because of proximity to the wound and poor natural tissue coverage. For this reason, full coverage of the ascending graft material with the pericardial fat pad is advisable in all cases. This serves to isolate the graft from the sternum if it becomes infected.

Patients frequently present with persistent fevers and elevated white cell count. CT or MRI may demonstrate air or fluid collections around the graft. There may be associated pseudoaneurysms, fistula, anastomotic leak, hemolysis, and embolism. Nuclear imaging techniques may be helpful but can be nonspecific for infection versus normal postoperative inflammation.[175] TEE may show valvular vegetations or abscesses.

Ideally, treatment of the stable patient begins with intravenous antibiotics to control septicemia and often clear blood cultures before reoperation. In extremely high-risk patients, in whom reoperative mortality is prohibitive, lifelong suppressive antibiotics may be acceptable. Surgical treatment of infected ascending aortic grafts, as described by Hargrove and Edmunds, includes removal of all infected prosthetic material, aggressive tissue debridement, local irrigation, systemic antibiotic therapy, replacement of the infected conduit, and use of autologous tissue to surround the graft and obliterate dead space.[176] Aortic homograft may potentially be more resistant to repeat infection. Greater omentum may be also brought up through the diaphragm as a vascularized pedicle to wrap around the aortic graft and isolate it from the sternum. Concomitant sternal infections should be managed with aggressive debridement, sterilization with vacuum-assisted wound drainage, and delayed flap reconstruction. In severe cases, open continuous antibiotic wound irrigation for several days can assist in clearing the infection.[177] Long-term antibiotics should be continued intravenously for at least 6 weeks and suppressive oral antibiotics may be indicated over the long term thereafter.

REFERENCES

1. Elkin DC: Aneurysms following surgical procedures. *Ann Surg* 1948; 127:769-779.
2. Bergqvist D: Historical aspects on aneurysmal disease. *Scand J Surg* 2008; 97(2):90-99.
3. Hajdu SI: A note from history: the first pathology book and its author. *Ann Clin Lab Sci* 2004; 34(2):226-227.
4. Cooper A: *Lectures on the Principles and Practice of Surgery,* 2nd ed. London, FC Westley, 1830; p 110.
5. Moore C: On a new method of procuring the consolidation of fibrin in certain incurable aneurysms. *Med Chir Trans (London)* 1864; 47:129.
6. Matas R: Surgery of the vascular system, in Matas R (ed): *Surgery, Its Principles and Practice,* vol. 5. Philadelphia, Saunders, 1914.
7. Harrison P, Chandy J: A subclavian aneurysm cured by cellophane fibrosis. *Ann Surg* 1943; 118:478.
8. Poppe J, De Oliviera H: Treatment of syphilitic aneurysms by cellophane wrapping. *J Thorac Surg* 1946; 15:186.
9. Matas R: An operation for the radical cure of aneurism based upon arteriorrhaphy. *Ann Surg* 1903; 37:161.
10. Matas R: Endo-aneurysmorrhaphy. *Surg Gynecol Obstet* 1920; 30:456.
11. Cooley DA, De Bakey ME: Surgical considerations of intrathoracic aneurysms of the aorta and great vessels. *Ann Surg* 1952; 135:660.
12. Cooley DA, DeBakey ME: Resection of the entire ascending aorta in fusiform aneurysm using cardiac bypass. *JAMA* 1956; 162:1158.
13. Westaby S, Cecil B: Surgery of the thoracic aorta, in Westaby S (ed): *Landmarks in Cardiac Surgery.* Oxford, Isis Medical Media, 1997; p 223.
14. Kadoba K, Schoen FJ, Jonas RA: Experimental comparison of albumin-sealed and gelatin-sealed knitted Dacron conduits. Porosity control, handling, sealant resorption, and healing. *J Thorac Cardiovasc Surg* 1992; 103(6):1059-1067.
15. Wheat MWJ, Wilson JR, Bartley TD: Successful replacement of the entire ascending aorta and aortic valve. *JAMA* 1964; 188:717.
16. Bentall H, De Bono A: A technique for complete replacement of the ascending aorta. *Thorax* 1968; 23:338.
17. Cabrol C, Pavie A, Gandjbakhch I, et al: Complete replacement of the ascending aorta with reimplantation of the coronary arteries: new surgical approach. *J Thorac Cardiovasc Surg* 1981; 81:309.
18. Kouchoukos NT, Karp RB: Resection of ascending aortic aneurysm and replacement of aortic valve. *J Thorac Cardiovasc Surg* 1981; 81(1):142-143.
19. Sutton JP 3rd, Ho SY, Anderson RH: The forgotten interleaflet triangles: a review of the surgical anatomy of the aortic valve. *Ann Thorac Surg* 1995; 59(2):419-427.
20. Hokken RB, Bartelings MM, Bogers AJ, Gittenberger-de Groot AC: Morphology of the pulmonary and aortic roots with regard to the pulmonary autograft procedure. *J Thorac Cardiovasc Surg* 1997; 113(3):453-461.
21. Maselli D, Montalto A, Santise G, et al: A normogram to anticipate dimension of neo-sinuses of Valsalva in valve-sparing aortic operations. *Eur J Cardiothorac Surg* 2005; 27(5):831-835.
22. Otani K, Takeuchi M, Kaku K, et al: Assessment of the aortic root using real-time 3D transesophageal echocardiography. *Circ J* 2010; 74(12): 2649-2657.
23. Nejjar I, Pieraggi MT, Thiers JC, Bouissou H: Age-related changes in the elastic tissue of the human thoracic aorta. *Atherosclerosis* 1990; 80(3):199-208.
24. Greenwald SE: Ageing of the conduit arteries. *J Pathol* 2007; 211(2): 157-172.
25. Halloran BG, Davis VA, McManus BM, Lynch TG, Baxter BT: Localization of aortic disease is associated with intrinsic differences in aortic structure. *J Surg Res* 1995; 59(1):17-22.
26. Wilson WR, Anderton M, Choke EC, et al: Elevated plasma MMP1 and MMP9 are associated with abdominal aortic aneurysm rupture. *Eur J Vasc Endovasc Surg* 2008; 35(5):580-584.
27. Geng L, Wang W, Chen Y, et al: Elevation of ADAM10, ADAM17, MMP-2 and MMP-9 expression with media degeneration features CaCl2-induced thoracic aortic aneurysm in a rat model. *Exp Mol Pathol* 2010; 89(1):72-81.
28. Sheth RA, Maricevich M, Mahmood U: In vivo optical molecular imaging of matrix metalloproteinase activity in abdominal aortic aneurysms correlates with treatment effects on growth rate. *Atherosclerosis* 2010; 212(1): 181-187.
29. Jones JA, Ruddy JM, Bouges S, et al: Alterations in membrane type-1 matrix metalloproteinase abundance after the induction of thoracic aortic aneurysm in a murine model. *Am J Physiol Heart Circ Physiol* 2010; 299(1): H114-124.
30. Liu J, Sukhova GK, Yang JT, et al: Cathepsin L expression and regulation in human abdominal aortic aneurysm, atherosclerosis, and vascular cells. *Atherosclerosis* 2006; 184(2):302-311.
31. Homme JL, Aubry MC, Edwards WD, et al: Surgical pathology of the ascending aorta: a clinicopathologic study of 513 cases. *Am J Surg Pathol* 2006; 30(9):1159-1168.
32. Cohen JR, Sarfati I, Wise L: The effect of cigarette smoking on rabbit aortic elastase activity. *J Vasc Surg* 1989; 9(4):580-582.
33. Okamoto RJ, Xu H, Kouchoukos NT, Moon MR, Sundt TM 3rd: The influence of mechanical properties on wall stress and distensibility of the dilated ascending aorta. *J Thorac Cardiovasc Surg* 2003; 126(3): 842-850.
34. Grande KJ, Cochran RP, Reinhall PG, Kunzelman KS: Stress variations in the human aortic root and valve: the role of anatomic asymmetry. *Ann Biomed Eng* 1998; 26:534-545.
35. Agozzino L, Ferraraccio F, Esposito S, et al: Medial degeneration does not involve uniformly the whole ascending aorta: morphological, biochemical and clinical correlations. *Eur J Cardiothorac Surg* 2002; 21:675-682.
36. Judge DP, Dietz HC: Marfan's syndrome. *Lancet* 2005; 366:1965-1976.

37. Hollister DW, Godfrey M, Sakai LY, Pyeritz RE: Immunohistologic abnormalities of the microfibrillar-fiber system in the Marfan syndrome. *NEJM* 1990; 323(3):152-159.
38. Dietz HC, Cutting GR, Pyeritz RE, et al: Marfan syndrome caused by a recurrent de novo missense mutation in the fibrillin gene. *Nature* 1991; 352(6333):337-339.
39. Mizuguchi T, Collod-Beroud G, Akiyama T, et al: Heterozygous TGFBR2 mutations in Marfan syndrome. *Nat Genet* 2004; 36(8):855-860.
40. Marsalese DL, Moodie DS, Vacante M, et al: Marfan's syndrome: natural history and long-term follow-up of cardiovascular involvement. *J Am Coll Cardiol* 1989; 14:422.
41. Keane MG, Pyeritz RE: Medical management of Marfan syndrome. *Circulation* 2008; 117(21):2802-2813.
42. Nagashima H, Sakomura Y, Aoka Y, et al: Angiotensin II type 2 receptor mediates vascular smooth muscle cell apoptosis in cystic medial degeneration associated with Marfan's syndrome. *Circulation* 2001; 104(12 Suppl 1): I282-287.
43. Habashi JP, Judge DP, Holm TM, et al: Losartan, an AT1 antagonist, prevents aortic aneurysm in a mouse model of Marfan syndrome. *Science* 2006; 312(5770):117-121.
44. Brooke BS, Habashi JP, Judge DP, et al: Angiotensin II blockade and aortic-root dilation in Marfan's syndrome. *NEJM* 2008; 358(26):2787-2795.
45. Loeys BL, Chen J, Neptune ER, et al: A syndrome of altered cardiovascular, craniofacial, neurocognitive and skeletal development caused by mutations in TGFBR1 or TGFBR2. *Nat Genet* 2005; 37(3):275-281.
46. Van Hemelrijk C, Renard M, Loeys B: The Loeys-Dietz syndrome: an update for the clinician. *Curr Opin Cardiol* 2010; 25(6):546-551.
47. Maleszewski JJ, Miller DV, Lu J, Dietz HC, Halushka MK: Histopathologic findings in ascending aortas from individuals with Loeys-Dietz syndrome (LDS). *Am J Surg Pathol* 2009; 33(2):194-201.
48. Shields LB, Rolf CM, Davis GJ, Hunsaker JC 3rd: Sudden and unexpected death in three cases of Ehlers-Danlos syndrome type IV. *J Forensic Sci* 2010; 55(6):1641-1645.
49. Lee JH, Burner KD, Fealey ME, et al: Prosthetic valve endocarditis: clinicopathological correlates in 122 surgical specimens from 116 patients (1985-2004). *Cardiovasc Pathol* 2011; 20(1):26-35.
50. Feigl D, Feigl A, Edwards JE: Mycotic aneurysms of the aortic root: a pathologic study of 20 cases. *Chest* 1986; 90:553.
51. Tavora F, Burke A: Review of isolated ascending aortitis: differential diagnosis, including syphilitic, Takayasu's and giant cell aortitis. *Pathology* 2006; 38(4):302-308.
52. Kuniyoshi Y, Koja K, Miyagi K, et al: A ruptured syphilitic descending thoracic aortic aneurysm. The characteristic findings on computed tomography for the etiological diagnosis of aneurysm. *Ann Thorac Cardiovasc Surg* 1998; 4(2):99-102.
53. Tavora F, Burke A: Review of isolated ascending aortitis: differential diagnosis, including syphilitic, Takayasu's and giant cell aortitis. *Pathology* 2006; 38(4):302-308.
54. Matsumura K, Hirano T, Takeda K, et al: Incidence of aneurysms in Takayasu's arteritis. *Angiology* 1991; 42(4):308-315.
55. Austen WB, Blennerhasset JB: Giant cell aortitis causing an aneurysm of the ascending aorta and aortic regurgitation. *NEJM* 1964; 272:80.
56. Warnes CA: Sex differences in congenital heart disease: should a woman be more like a man? *Circulation* 2008; 118(1):3-5.
57. Huntington K, Hunter AG, Chan KL: A prospective study to assess the frequency of familial clustering of congenital bicuspid aortic valve. *J Am Coll Cardiol* 1997; 30(7):1809-1812.
58. Lewin MB, Otto CM: The bicuspid aortic valve: adverse outcomes from infancy to old age. *Circulation* 2005; 111(7):832-834.
59. Guntheroth WG, Spiers PS: Does aortic root dilatation with bicuspid aortic valves occur as a primary tissue abnormality or as a relatively benign poststenotic phenomenon? *Am J Cardiol* 2005; 95(6):820.
60. Jain R, Engleka KA, Rentschler SL, et al: Cardiac neural crest orchestrates remodeling and functional maturation of mouse semilunar valves. *J Clin Invest* 2010. pii: 44244. doi: 10.1172/JCI44244.
61. Nataatmadja M, West M, West J, et al: Abnormal extracellular matrix protein transport associated with increased apoptosis of vascular smooth muscle cells in Marfan syndrome and bicuspid aortic valve thoracic aortic aneurysm. *Circulation* 2003; 108(Suppl 1):II329-334.
62. LeMaire SA, Wang X, Wilks JA, et al: Matrix metalloproteinases in ascending aortic aneurysms: bicuspid versus trileaflet aortic valves. *J Surg Res* 2005; 123(1):40-48.
63. Fedak PW, de Sa MP, Verma S, et al: Vascular matrix remodeling in patients with bicuspid aortic valve malformations: implications for aortic dilatation. *J Thorac Cardiovasc Surg* 2003; 126(3):797-806.
64. Matthias Bechtel JF, Noack F, Sayk F, et al: Histopathological grading of ascending aortic aneurysm: comparison of patients with bicuspid versus tricuspid aortic valve. *J Heart Valve Dis* 2003; 12(1):54-59; discussion 59-61.
65. Bonderman D, Gharehbaghi-Schnell E, Wollenek G, et al: Mechanisms underlying aortic dilatation in congenital aortic valve malformation. *Circulation* 1999; 99(16):2138-2143.
66. Fazel SS, Mallidi HR, Lee RS, et al: The aortopathy of bicuspid aortic valve disease has distinctive patterns and usually involves the transverse aortic arch. *J Thorac Cardiovasc Surg* 2008; 135(4):901-907.
67. Feldman DN, Roman MJ: Aneurysms of the sinuses of Valsalva. *Cardiology* 2006; 106(2):73-81.
68. Goldberg N, Krasnow N: Sinus of Valsalva aneurysms. *Clin Cardiol* 1990; 13(12):831-836.
69. Brandt J, Jögi P, Lührs C: Sinus of Valsalva aneurysm obstructing coronary arterial flow: case report and collective review of the literature. *Eur Heart J* 1985; 6(12):1069-1073.
70. Milewicz DM, Carlson AA, Regalado ES: Genetic testing in aortic aneurysm disease: PRO. *Cardiol Clin* 2010; 28(2):191-197.
71. Kontusaari S, Tromp G, Kuivaniemi H, Romanic AM, Prockop DJ: A mutation in the gene for type III procollagen (COL3A1) in a family with aortic aneurysms. *J Clin Invest* 1990; 86(5):1465-1473.
72. Keramati AR, Sadeghpour A, Farahani MM, Chandok G, Mani A: The non-syndromic familial thoracic aortic aneurysms and dissections maps to 15q21 locus. *BMC Med Genet* 2010; 11:143.
73. Wang L, Guo DC, Cao J, et al: Mutations in myosin light chain kinase cause familial aortic dissections. *Am J Hum Genet* 2010; 87(5):701-707.
74. Pannu H, Fadulu VT, Chang J, et al: Mutations in transforming growth factor-beta receptor type II cause familial thoracic aortic aneurysms and dissections. *Circulation* 2005; 112(4):513-520.
75. Collins JS, Evangelista A, Nienaber CA, et al: Differences in clinical presentation, management, and outcomes of acute type a aortic dissection in patients with and without previous cardiac surgery. *Circulation* 2004; 110(11 Suppl 1):II237-242.
76. Crawford ES, Svensson LG, Coselli JS, et al: Surgical treatment of aneurysm and/or dissection of the ascending aorta, transverse aortic arch, and ascending aorta and transverse aortic arch: factors influencing survival in 717 patients. *J Thorac Cardiovasc Surg* 1989; 98:659.
77. Guthaner DF: The plain chest film in assessing aneurysms and dissecting hematomas of the thoracic aorta, in Taveras JN, Ferrucci JT (eds): *Radiology: Diagnosis-Imaging-Intervention.* Philadelphia, Lippincott, 1994.
78. Wiet SP, Pearce WH, McCarthy WJ, et al: Utility of transesophageal echocardiography in the diagnosis of disease of the thoracic aorta. *J Vasc Surg* 1994; 20(4):613-620.
79. Penco M, Paparoni S, Dagianti A, et al: Usefulness of transesophageal echocardiography in the assessment of aortic dissection. *Am J Cardiol* 2000; 86(4A):53G-56G.
80. Bossone E, Evangelista A, Isselbacher E, et al: Prognostic role of transesophageal echocardiography in acute type A aortic dissection. *Am Heart J* 2007; 153(6):1013-1020.
81. Konstadt SN, Reich DL, Quintana C, Levy M: The ascending aorta: how much does transesophageal echocardiography see? *Anesth Analg* 1994; 78:240.
82. Chung JH, Ghoshhajra BB, Rojas CA, Dave BR, Abbara S: CT angiography of the thoracic aorta. *Radiol Clin North Am* 2010; 48(2):249-264, vii.
83. Chartrand-Lefebvre C, Cadrin-Chênevert A, Bordeleau E, et al: Coronary computed tomography angiography: overview of technical aspects, current concepts, and perspectives. *Can Assoc Radiol J* 2007; 58(2):92-108.
84. Bonnichsen CR, Sundt III TM, Anavekar NS, et al: Aneurysms of the ascending aorta and arch: the role of imaging in diagnosis and surgical management. *Expert Rev Cardiovasc Ther* 2011; 9(1):45-61.
85. Hagan PG, Nienaber CA, Isselbacher EM, et al: The International Registry of Acute Aortic Dissection (IRAD): new insights into an old disease. *JAMA* 2000; 283(7):897-903.
86. Bickerstaff LK, Pairolero PC, Hollier LH, et al: Thoracic aortic aneurysms: a population-based study. *Surgery* 1982; 92(6):1103-1108.
87. Coady MA, Rizzo JA, Hammond GL, et al: What is the appropriate size criterion for resection of thoracic aortic aneurysms? *J Thorac Cardiovasc Surg* 1997; 113:476.
88. Masuda Y, Takanashi K, Takasu J, et al: Expansion rate of thoracic aortic aneurysms and influencing factors. *Chest* 1992; 102:461.
89. Hirose Y, Hamada S, Takamiya M, et al: Aortic aneurysms: growth rates measured with CT. *Radiology* 1992; 185:249.
90. Gott VL, Greene PS, Alejo DE, et al: Replacement of the aortic root in patients with Marfan's syndrome. *NEJM* 1999; 340:1307.
91. Murdoch JL, Walker BA, Halpern BL, Kuzma JW, McKusick VA: Life expectancy and causes of death in the Marfan syndrome. *NEJM* 1972; 286(15):804-808.

92. Marsalese DL, Moodie DS, Vacante M, et al: Marfan's syndrome: natural history and long-term follow-up of cardiovascular involvement. *J Am Coll Cardiol* 1989; 14:422.
93. Pape LA, Tsai TT, Isselbacher EM, et al: Aortic diameter > or = 5.5 cm is not a good predictor of type A aortic dissection: observations from the International Registry of Acute Aortic Dissection (IRAD). *Circulation* 2007; 116(10):1120-1127.
94. Palmer RF, Wheat MW Jr: Treatment of dissecting aneurysms of the aorta. *Ann Thorac Surg* 1967; 4:38-52.
95. Wheat MW Jr, Palmer RF, Barley TD, et al: Treatment of dissecting aneurysms of the aorta without surgery, *J Thorac Cardiovasc Surg* 1965; 50:364.
96. Simpson CF, Boucek RJ: The B-aminopropionitrile fed turkey: a model for detecting potential drug action on arterial tissue. *Cardiovasc Res* 1983; 17(1):26-32.
97. Shores J, Berger KR, Murphy EA, et al: Progression of aortic dilatation and the benefit of long-term beta-adrenergic blockade in Marfan's syndrome. *NEJM* 1994; 330(19):1335-1341.
98. Patel HJ, Deeb GM: Ascending and arch aorta: pathology, natural history and treatment. *Circulation* 2008; 118:188-195.
99. Dapunt OE, Galla JD, Sadeghi AM, et al: The natural history of thoracic aortic aneurysms. *J Thorac Cardiovasc Surg* 1994; 107(5):1323-1332.
100. Davies RR, Gallo A, Coady MA, et al: Novel measurement of relative aortic size predicts rupture of thoracic aortic aneurysms. *Ann Thorac Surg* 2006; 81(1):169-177. Erratum in *Ann Thorac Surg* 2007; 84(6):2139.
101. Ergin MA, Spielvogel D, Apaydin A, et al: Surgical treatment of the dilated ascending aorta: when and how? *Ann Thorac Surg* 1999; 67:1834.
102. Baumgartner WA, Cameron DE, Redmond JM, et al: Operative management of Marfan syndrome: the Johns Hopkins experience. *Ann Thorac Surg* 1999; 67:1859.
103. Borger MA, Preston M, Ivanov J, et al: Should the ascending aorta be replaced more frequently in patients with bicuspid aortic valve disease? *J Thorac Cardiovasc Surg* 2004; 128(5):677-683.
104. Hiratzka L, Bakris G, Beckman J, et al: 2010 ACCF/AHA/AATS/ACR/ASA/SCA/SCAI/SIR/STS/SVM guidelines for the diagnosis and management of patients with Thoracic Aortic Disease: a report of the American College of Cardiology Foundation/American Heart Association Task Force on Practice Guidelines, American Association for Thoracic Surgery, American College of Radiology, American Stroke Association, Society of Cardiovascular Anesthesiologists, Society for Cardiovascular Angiography and Interventions, Society of Interventional Radiology, Society of Thoracic Surgeons, and Society for Vascular Medicine. *Circulation* 2010; 121(13):e266-369.
105. Prenger K, Pieters F, Cheriex E: Aortic dissection after aortic valve replacement: incidence and consequences for strategy. *J Cardiol Surg* 1994; 9(5): 495-498; discussion 498-499.
106. Crawford ES, Svensson LG, Coselli JS, Safi HJ, Hess KR: Surgical treatment of aneurysm and/or dissection of the ascending aorta, transverse aortic arch, and ascending aorta and transverse aortic arch: factors influencing survival in 717 patients. *J Thorac Cardiovasc Surg* 1989; 98:659.
107. Berens ES, Kouchoukos NT, Murphy SF, et al: Preoperative carotid artery screening in elderly patients undergoing cardiac surgery. *J Vasc Surg* 1992; 15:313.
108. O'Blenes SB, Feindel CM: Aortic root replacement with anomalous origin of the coronary arteries. *Ann Thorac Surg* 2002; 73(2):647-649.
109. Donaldson RM, Ross DN: Composite graft replacement for the treatment of aneurysms of the ascending aorta associated with aortic valvular disease. *Circulation* 1982; 66(2 Pt 2):I116-221.
110. Volguina IV, Miller DC, LeMaire SA, et al: Valve-sparing and valve-replacing techniques for aortic root replacement in patients with Marfan syndrome: analysis of early outcome. *J Thorac Cardiovasc Surg* 2009; 137(5): 1124-1123.
111. David TE, Feindel CM, Armstrong S, Maganti M: Replacement of the ascending aorta with reduction of the diameter of the sinotubular junction to treat aortic insufficiency in patients with ascending aortic aneurysm. *J Thorac Cardiovasc Surg* 2007; 133(2):414-418.
112. Burman ED, Keegan J, Kilner PJ: Aortic root measurement by cardiovascular magnetic resonance: specification of planes and lines of measurement and corresponding normal values. *Circ Cardiovasc Imaging* 2008; 1(2): 104-113.
113. Kapetanakis EI, Mccarthy P, Monaghan M, Wendler O: Transapical aortic valve implantation in a patient with stentless valve degeneration. *Eur J Cardiothorac Surg* 2011; 39(6):1051-1053. Epub 2010 Dec 16.
114. de Sa M, Moshkovitz Y, Butany J, David TE: Histologic abnormalities of the ascending aorta and pulmonary trunk in patients with bicuspid aortic valve disease: clinical relevance to the Ross procedure. *J Thorac Cardiovasc Surg* 1999; 118(4):588-594.
115. Westaby S, Saito S, Anastasiadis K, Moorjani N, Jin XY: Aortic root remodeling in atheromatous aneurysms: the role of selected sinus repair. *Eur J Cardiothorac Surg* 2002; 21(3):459-464.
116. David TE, Feindel CM: An aortic valve-sparing operation for patients with aortic incompetence and aneurysm of the ascending aorta. *J Thorac Cardiovasc Surg* 1992; 103(4):617-621.
117. Murkin JM: NIRS: a standard of care for CPB vs. an evolving standard for selective cerebral perfusion? *J Extra Corpor Technol* 2009; 41(1):P11-14.
118. Appoo JJ, Augoustides JG, Pochettino A, et al: Perioperative outcome in adults undergoing elective deep hypothermic circulatory arrest with retrograde cerebral perfusion in proximal aortic arch repair: evaluation of protocol-based care. *J Cardiothorac Vasc Anesth* 2006; 20(1):3-7.
119. Stecker MM, Cheung AT, Pochettino A, et al: Deep hypothermic circulatory arrest: I. Effects of cooling on electroencephalogram and evoked potentials. *Ann Thorac Surg* 2001; 71(1):14-21.
120. Cheung AT, Bavaria JE, Pochettino A, et al: Oxygen delivery during retrograde cerebral perfusion in humans. *Anesth Analg* 1999; 88(1):8-15.
121. Kazui T: Which is more appropriate as a cerebral protection method—unilateral or bilateral perfusion? *Eur J Cardiothorac Surg* 2006; 29(6): 1039-1040.
122. Sabik JF, Nemeh H, Lytle BW, et al: Cannulation of the axillary artery with a side graft reduces morbidity. *Ann Thorac Surg* 2004; 77:1315.
123. Gill M, Dunning J: Is reduction aortoplasty (with or without external wrap) an acceptable alternative to replacement of the dilated ascending aorta? *Interact Cardiovasc Thorac Surg* 2009; 9(4):693-697.
124. Bauer M, Pasic M, Schaffarzyk R, et al: Reduction aortoplasty for dilatation of the ascending aorta in patients with bicuspid aortic valve. *Ann Thorac Surg* 2002; 73:720-724.
125. Barnett M, Fiore A, Vaca K, Milligan T, Barner H: Tailoring aortoplasty for repair of fusiform ascending aortic aneurysm. *Ann Thorac Surg* 1995; 59:497-501.
126. Neri E, Massetti M, Tanganelli P, et al: Is it only a mechanical matter? Histologic modifications of the aorta underlying external banding. *J Thorac Cardiovasc Surg* 1999; 118(6):1116.
127. Cohen O, Odim J, De la Zerda D, et al: Long-term experience of girdling the ascending aorta with Dacron mesh as definitive treatment for aneurysmal dilation. *Ann Thorac Surg* 2007; 83(2):S780-784.
128. Byers PH: Disorders of collagen biosynthesis and structure, in Schriver CR, Beaudet AL, Sly WS, Valle D (eds): *The Metabolic Basis of Inherited Diseases.* New York, McGraw-Hill, 1995; p 4029.
129. Gillinov AM, Hulyalkar A, Cameron DE, et al: Mitral valve operation in patients with the Marfan syndrome. *J Thorac Cardiovasc Surg* 1994; 107:724.
130. Ohata T, Sakakibara T, Takano H, Ishizaka T: Total arch replacement for thoracic aortic aneurysm via median sternotomy with or without left anterolateral thoracotomy. *Ann Thorac Surg* 2003; 75:1792-1796.
131. Borger MA, Rao V, Weisel RD, et al: Reoperative coronary bypass surgery: effect of patent grafts and retrograde cardioplegia. *J Thorac Cardiovasc Surg* 2001; 121(1):83-90.
132. Thiene G, Valente M: Achilles' heel of stentless porcine valves. *Cardiovasc Pathol* 2007; 16(5):257.
133. Szeto WY, Moser WG, Desai ND, et al: Transapical deployment of endovascular thoracic aortic stent graft for an ascending aortic pseudoaneurysm. *Ann Thorac Surg* 2010; 89(2):616-618.
134. Zangrillo A, Mizzi A, Biondi-Zoccai G, et al: Recombinant activated factor VII in cardiac surgery: a meta-analysis. *J Cardiothorac Vasc Anesth* 2009; 23(1):34-40.
135. Jault F, Nataf P, Rama A, et al: Chronic disease of the ascending aorta: surgical treatment and long-term results. *J Thorac Cardiovasc Surg* 1994; 108:747.
136. Lewis CT, Cooley DA, Murphy MC, et al: Surgical repair of aortic root aneurysms in 280 patients. *Ann Thorac Surg* 1992; 53:38.
137. Milewski RK, Pacini D, Moser GW, et al: Retrograde and antegrade cerebral perfusion: results in short elective arch reconstructive times. *Ann Thorac Surg* 2010; 89(5):1448-1457.
138. Svensson LG: Brain protection. *J Card Surg* 1997; 12:326.
139. Royse AG, Royse CF: Epiaortic ultrasound assessment of the aorta in cardiac surgery. *Best Pract Res Clin Anaesthesiol* 2009; 23(3):335-341.
140. Kouchoukos NT: Adjuncts to reduce the incidence of embolic brain injury during operations on the aortic arch. *Ann Thorac Surg* 1994; 57:243.
141. Asimakopoulos G, Smith PL, Ratnatunga CP, Taylor KM: Lung injury and acute respiratory distress syndrome after cardiopulmonary bypass. *Ann Thorac Surg* 1999; 68:1107.
142. Milot J, Perron J, Lacasse Y, et al: Incidence and predictors of ARDS after cardiac surgery. *Chest* 2001; 119(3):884-888.
143. Kaul TK, Fields BL, Riggins LS, et al: Adult respiratory distress syndrome following cardiopulmonary bypass: incidence, prophylaxis and management. *J Cardiovasc Surg (Torino)* 1998; 39(6):777-781.

144. Nieman G, Searles B, Carney D, et al: Systemic inflammation induced by cardiopulmonary bypass: a review of pathogenesis and treatment. *J Extra Corpor Technol* 1999; 31(4):202-210.
145. Redmond JM, Gillinov AM, Stuart RS, et al: Heparin-coated bypass circuits reduce pulmonary injury. *Ann Thorac Surg* 1993; 56:474.
146. Kouchoukos NT, Wareing TH, Murphy SF, Perrillo JB: Sixteen-year experience with aortic root replacement: results of 172 operations. *Ann Surg* 1991; 214:308.
147. Schachner T, Vertacnik K, Nagiller J, Laufer G, Bonatti J: Factors associated with mortality and long time survival in patients undergoing modified Bentall operations. *J Cardiovasc Surg (Torino)* 2005; 46(5): 449-455.
148. Okita Y, Ando M, Minatoya K, et al: Early and long-term results of surgery for aneurysms of the thoracic aorta in septuagenarians and octogenarians. *Eur J Cardiothorac Surg* 1999; 16:317.
149. Fleck TM, Koinig H, Czerny M, et al: Impact of surgical era on outcomes of patients undergoing elective atherosclerotic ascending aortic aneurysm operations. *Eur J Cardiothorac Surg* 2004; 26:342.
150. Gott VL, Gillinov AM, Pyeritz RE, et al: Aortic root replacement: risk factor analysis of a seventeen-year experience with 270 patients. *J Thorac Cardiovasc Surg* 1995; 109:536.
151. Cohn LH, Rizzo RJ, Adams DH, et al: Reduced mortality and morbidity for ascending aortic aneurysm resection regardless of cause. *Ann Thorac Surg* 1996; 62:463.
152. Mingke D, Dresler C, Stone CD, Borst HG: Composite graft replacement of the aortic root in 335 patients with aneurysm or dissection. *Thorac Cardiovasc Surg* 1998; 46:12.
153. Estrera AL, Miller CC 3rd, Huynh TT, et al: Replacement of the ascending and transverse aortic arch: determinants of long-term survival. *Ann Thorac Surg* 2002; 74:1058.
154. Ergin MA, Spielvogel D, Apaydin A, et al: Surgical treatment of the dilated ascending aorta: when and how? *Ann Thorac Surg* 1999; 67:1834.
155. Gott VL, Gillinov AM, Pyeritz RE, et al: Aortic root replacement: risk factor analysis of a seventeen-year experience with 270 patients. *J Thorac Cardiovasc Surg* 1995; 109:536.
156. Taniguchi K, Nakano S, Matsuda H, et al: Long-term survival and complications after composite graft replacement for ascending aortic aneurysm associated with aortic regurgitation. *Circulation* 1991; 84:III3.
157. Lewis CT, Cooley DA, Murphy MC, et al: Surgical repair of aortic root aneurysms in 280 patients. *Ann Thorac Surg* 1992; 53:38.
158. Raudkivi PJ, Williams JD, Monro JL, Ross JK: Surgical treatment of the ascending aorta: fourteen years' experience with 83 patients. *J Thorac Cardiovasc Surg* 1989; 98:675.
159. Jault F, Nataf P, Rama A, et al: Chronic disease of the ascending aorta: Surgical treatment and long-term results. *J Thorac Cardiovasc Surg* 1994; 108:747.
160. Bhan A, Choudhary SK, Saikia M, et al: Surgical experience with dissecting and nondissecting aneurysms of the ascending aorta. *Indian Heart J* 2001; 53:319.
161. Crawford ES, Svensson LG, Coselli JS, et al: Surgical treatment of aneurysm and/or dissection of the ascending aorta, transverse aortic arch, and ascending aorta and transverse aortic arch: factors influencing survival in 717 patients. *J Thorac Cardiovasc Surg* 1989; 98:659.
162. Silva J, Maroto LC, Carnero M, et al: Ascending aorta and aortic root reoperations: are outcomes worse than first time surgery? *Ann Thorac Surg* 2010; 90(2):555-560.
163. Szeto WY, Bavaria JE, Bowen FW, et al: Reoperative aortic root replacement in patients with previous aortic surgery. *Ann Thorac Surg* 2007; 84(5):1592-1598; discussion 1598-1599.
164. Detter C, Mair H, Klein HG, et al: Long-term prognosis of surgically-treated aortic aneurysms and dissections in patients with and without Marfan syndrome. *Eur J Cardiothorac Surg*1998; 13:416.
165. Sioris T, David TE, Ivanov J, Armstrong S, Feindel CM: Clinical outcomes after separate and composite replacement of the aortic valve and ascending aorta. *J Thorac Cardiovasc Surg* 2004; 128(2):260-265.
166. Ng SK, O'Brien MF, Harrocks S, McLachlan GJ: Influence of patient age and implantation technique on the probability of re-replacement of the homograft aortic valve. *J Heart Valve Dis* 2002; 11(2):217-223.
167. Luciani GB, Casali G, Faggian G, Mazzucco A: Predicting outcome after reoperative procedures on the aortic root and ascending aorta. *Eur J Cardiothorac Surg* 2000; 17:602.
168. Kouchoukos NT, Wareing TH, Murphy SF, Perrillo JB: Sixteen-year experience with aortic root replacement: results of 172 operations. *Ann Surg* 1991; 214:308.
169. Svensson LG, Blackstone EH, Feng J, et al: Are Marfan syndrome and marfanoid patients distinguishable on long-term follow-up? *Ann Thorac Surg* 2007; 83(3):1067-1074.
170. Gott VL, Greene PS, Alejo DE, et al: Replacement of the aortic root in patients with Marfan's syndrome. *NEJM* 1999; 340:1307.
171. Lytle BW, Sabik JF, Blackstone EH, et al: Reoperative cryopreserved root and ascending aorta replacement for acute aortic prosthetic valve endocarditis. *Ann Thorac Surg* 2002; 74:S1754-1757; S1792-1799.
172. Coselli JS, Crawford ES, Williams TW Jr, et al: Treatment of postoperative infection of ascending aorta and transverse aortic arch, including use of viable omentum and muscle flaps. *Ann Thorac Surg* 1990; 50:868.
173. Nakajima N, Masuda M, Ichinose M, Ando M: A new method for the treatment of graft infection in the thoracic aorta: in situ preservation. *Ann Thorac Surg* 1999; 67:1994.
174. Coselli JS, Koksoy C, LeMaire SA: Management of thoracic aortic graft infections. *Ann Thorac Surg* 1999; 67:1990.
175. Keown PP, Miller DC, Jamieson SW, et al: Diagnosis of arterial prosthetic graft infection by indium-111 oxine white blood cell scans. *Circulation* 1982; 66:I130.
176. Hargrove WC 3rd, Edmunds LH Jr: Management of infected thoracic aortic prosthetic grafts. *Ann Thorac Surg* 1984; 37:72.
177. Ninomiya M, Makuuchi H, Naruse Y, Kobayashi T, Sato T: Surgical management of ascending aortic graft infection. No-sedation-technique for open mediastinal irrigation. *Jpn J Thorac Cardiovasc Surg* 2000; 48(10):666-669.

CHAPTER 52

Aneurysms of the Aortic Arch

David Spielvogel
Manu N. Mathur
Randall B. Griepp

INTRODUCTION

The critical consideration in approaching aortic arch (AA) surgery, how best to protect the brain while providing surgical access to the cerebral vessels, remains a subject of controversy and research, but involves two key aspects: minimizing cerebral ischemia and preventing cerebral embolization of air and atheromatous debris. Thus, this chapter focuses on the laboratory and clinical basis for cerebral protection methods; including methods for preventing cerebral ischemia, such as hypothermic circulatory arrest (HCA), selective antegrade perfusion (SCP), and retrograde cerebral perfusion (RCP); and methods to minimize embolic damage, such as using axillary artery cannulation plus a branched graft technique.

SURGICAL INDICATIONS

Urgent indications for AA surgery include rupture of an aneurysm, pseudoaneurysm, or aortic dissection. Elective arch surgery is recommended for aneurysms greater than 6 cm, saccular aneurysms with rapid enlargement (>1 cm/y) and for symptoms (pain or hoarseness). Smaller aneurysms (5 cm) should be considered for repair in patients with extensive aortic aneurysmal disease (ascending and descending), Marfan's syndrome, or a family history of rupture or dissection.

PREOPERATIVE EVALUATION

The medical history is important in identifying symptoms caused by an aneurysm and, along with routine laboratory studies, may help elaborate comorbidities in these often elderly patients. A family history of a ruptured aneurysm is not uncommon and aids in the decision to recommend surgery.[1] Identifying comorbidities may influence the operative approach, allow anticipation, and prevention of complications, or may contraindicate surgery altogether.

Evaluation of an AA aneurysm requires a contrast-enhanced computed tomographic (CT) angiogram of the entire aorta. Multidetector CT scans permit rapid imaging of the entire aorta and three-dimensional reconstructions. Magnetic resonance imaging (MRI) yields equally detailed images but entails longer scanning time, higher cost, and the contrast agent, gadolinium, may be nephrotoxic. Angiograms are not routinely required; however, coronary angiography is usually indicated and visualization of the brachiocephalic vessels may be obtained at that time with little added risk.

Cardiac Status and Management of Coronary Artery Disease

All patients require a preoperative echocardiogram to assess left ventricular function (LVF) and exclude significant valvular heart disease. Coronary arteriography is carried out to delineate the anatomy of the proximal coronary arteries in patients with AA aneurysms in whom a Bentall or valve sparing procedure may be required; in patients older than 40; and in younger patients with risk factors, such as smoking, angina, a strong family history, an abnormal ECG or stress test.

Significant coronary artery disease may warrant angioplasty or coronary artery bypass surgery (CABG). Drug-eluting stents are not used for angioplasty, to avoid Plavix therapy, and the procedure is performed several weeks preoperatively, as stent thrombosis may complicate intraoperative protamine administration;

antiplatelet therapy is discontinued. If technically feasible, CABG can be done at the time of aneurysm repair. However if a left thoracotomy is anticipated, making access to the coronary arteries difficult, CABG can be undertaken several weeks before aneurysmectomy.

Pulmonary dysfunction increases operative risk and prolongs recovery, but chronic lung disease is not necessarily a contraindication to surgery unless oxygen dependence or significant carbon dioxide retention is present. If limited exercise tolerance or abnormal pulmonary function tests suggest severe respiratory dysfunction, pulmonary consultation is warranted. Active pulmonary infection should be treated before surgery and active smokers are urged to stop smoking for at least a month before operation; smokers may require pulmonary rehabilitation.

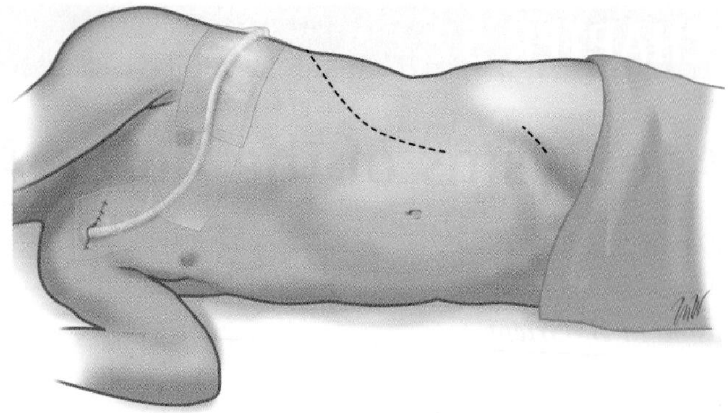

FIGURE 52-1 Right axillary cannulation for surgery via left thoracotomy.

Cerebral Vessels and Prevention of Stroke

Carotid and vertebral duplex ultrasonography is requested if there is a history of transient ischemic attacks or strokes or if carotid bruits are present. In patients with an aberrant left vertebral artery exiting the arch directly, documentation of the size and patency of the right vertebral artery is essential to guide strategy for complete arch replacement.

Although a history of a focal cerebral insult is not a contraindication to surgery, it warrants obtaining a preoperative CT scan to rule out silent, fresh cerebral infarcts, which generally necessitate postponing surgery. A preoperative head CT scan is also invaluable for identifying old and new lesions and may be helpful in determining prognosis if focal neurologic symptoms occur postoperatively.

Ascending and arch aneurysms often have friable atheromatous lesions, so all possible steps to minimize embolization must be taken. Preoperative identification of patients at high risk for embolization is possible using transesophageal echocardiography (TEE) and high-resolution CT angiography; epiaortic ultrasound may be especially useful (12-MHz probe) intraoperatively.

Cannulation Sites

Right axillary artery cannulation offers many advantages in the management of arch aneurysms.[2] The axillary artery is usually soft and is rarely involved by generalized atherosclerosis or aortic dissection. As compared with ascending aortic cannulation, axillary cannulation avoids the dislodgement of debris associated with cannula insertion and debris dislodgement that results from turbulent arch flow. As compared with femoral cannulation, axillary perfusion avoids possible embolization resulting from retrograde flow through a diseased abdominal and descending aorta. Moreover, cannulating the femoral arteries, which are often calcified and atherosclerotic, is associated with the risk of local and retrograde dissection. In aortic dissection surgery, the risk of malperfusion is lower with axillary perfusion and it has been associated with improved outcomes.[3,4] Axillary artery cannulation also facilitates selective antegrade cerebral perfusion, as discussed in the following.

Although many surgeons prefer a side branch technique for axillary perfusion, attaching an 8- or 10-mm graft to the artery,[5] we prefer direct right axillary artery cannulation via a transverse arteriotomy using a right angle, wire-reinforced arterial cannula (Edwards Lifesciences, Irvine, CA).[2] Depending on the adequacy of collateral circulation, direct cannulation may render the arm ischemic, so the period of cannulation should be limited and the cannula should be removed before protamine administration. In patients with very small axillary arteries, transecting the artery, sewing a 6-mm graft end to end proximally and then cannulating the graft with a straight femoral arterial cannula works well; on discontinuing cardiopulmonary bypass, the 6-mm graft may be used to reestablish continuity of the divided axillary artery. Right axillary cannulation is also possible in conjunction with a left thoracotomy (Fig. 52-1). A 10-mm ringed PTFE graft is sewn to the right axillary artery with the patient supine; with the incision loosely closed and the graft secured to the anterior chest with an Ioban drape (3M, St. Paul, MN), the patient is repositioned for a left thoracotomy, leaving the PTFE graft available for antegrade perfusion.

ANESTHESIA AND MONITORING

For procedures requiring a thoracotomy, particularly if substantial dissection and mobilization of the descending thoracic aorta is necessary before institution of cardiopulmonary bypass (CPB), use of a double-lumen tube, permitting selective ventilation, is helpful.

Anesthesia for aortic arch surgery, like anesthesia for most cardiac surgery, relies primarily on the use of high doses of narcotics. Routine hemodynamic monitoring includes left radial and femoral arterial catheters, a Swan-Ganz catheter, and a jugular venous bulb catheter, if possible. TEE is used to monitor LVF and distention, to confirm adequate flow in the arch and arch vessels, and to guard against malperfusion. Although we do not rely on electroencephalographic (EEG) surveillance, it is still used by some surgeons to determine maximum cerebral metabolic suppression in conjunction with HCA, and assess adequacy of cerebral protection.

Cerebral oximetry, used to monitor cerebral perfusion and oxygenation, is best followed by observing the baseline and trend rather than the absolute values. Both cerebral hemispheres are monitored and any asymmetric change should prompt a thorough assessment to determine the adequacy of cerebral blood flow. For example, if unilateral SCP via the right axillary is used, poor left hemispheric cerebral oximetry may indicate insufficient collaterals and the need for direct cannulation and perfusion of the left common carotid artery.[6] Similarly, acute changes occurring with SCP administered via direct cannulation of the head vessels may indicate catheter migration (into the right subclavian artery), catheter obstruction, or dislodgement[7] and should prompt immediate steps to identify and correct the problem. It should be noted that transcranial Doppler is more sensitive in detecting embolic events and confirming cerebral blood flow than cerebral oximetry,[8] but is more operator-dependent and may not be available in emergent situations.[9]

Methylprednisolone (1 g) is administered on initiating CPB when HCA is anticipated. If HCA exceeds 30 minutes, steroids are given for 48 hours postoperatively (125 mg every 6 hours for 24 hours, then 125 mg every 12 hours for 24 hours). Barbiturates are not used because they significantly depress myocardial function at the doses recommended for cerebral protection, and may not be effective in the presence of hypothermia.[10]

Steroid administration and hypothermia-induced catecholamine release often produce hyperglycemia, which may adversely affect intracellular pH and neurologic outcome.[11] Hyperglycemia should be treated aggressively, because glucose drives anaerobic glycolysis, leading to rapid accumulation of lactate and intracellular acidosis during HCA. We use an intravenous insulin drip to maintain normoglycemia intraoperatively and postoperatively.

Perfusion

The routine perfusion protocol for cardiac operations is used for repair of arch aneurysms. If axillary artery perfusion is used, CPB is initiated slowly, monitoring with TEE, while observing for adequacy of flow and signs of dissection or malperfusion. With median sternotomy right axillary artery perfusion can be used throughout the procedure, allowing retrograde flushing of the brachiocephalic vessels. However, for distal arch reconstruction via a left thoracotomy, placing a Y connector in the arterial line enables arterial perfusion to be transferred from the femoral artery to the proximal graft following deep HCA.

After HCA, an inline LG-6 leukocyte-depleting filter (Pall Corp., East Hills, NY) is used for both leukocyte depletion and ultrafiltration, to increase oxygen-carrying capacity.

During hypothermic perfusion, the advantages of regulating pH using the alpha-stat versus pH stat techniques are debated. We use values uncorrected for temperature, the alpha-stat approach, with a perfusate temperature between 15 and 20°C, a hematocrit of 25 to 30%, and flows of 8 to 10 cc/kg/min, and with a mean arterial pressure (MAP) of 40 to 60 mm Hg.

Nonpulsatile flow gradually increases cerebral vascular resistance, so higher pressures may be required for effective perfusion toward the end of a long bypass period, and immediately thereafter to avoid underperfusion. However, it should be noted that overperfusion has been shown to be as detrimental as underperfusion in a canine model.[12] Evidence for SCP in adults indicates that alpha-stat regulation helps in preserving cerebral autoregulation, maintaining metabolic suppression, and reducing the risk of cerebral embolization.[13] However, in patients with previous strokes, experimental studies suggest that the injured brain is susceptible to ischemia during SCP and the use of pH-stat management—which increases flow—may be marginally beneficial in this subset of patients.[14]

We rely on a long duration of cooling, a low esophageal temperature, a high jugular venous oxygen saturation, and topical hypothermia (ice packs on the head) to ensure adequate cerebral protection during HCA.

OPERATIVE TECHNIQUES

Incision

In most AA cases, an extended median sternotomy is used, giving access to the ascending aorta, arch, and proximal descending thoracic aorta as far as 5 cm beyond the left subclavian artery. The conventional median sternotomy is extended along the border of the left sternocleidomastoid muscle. The strap muscles of the left side of the neck may be incised, and the innominate vein is usually mobilized and preserved, but can be divided if necessary.

If the anticipated surgery involves intracardiac pathology and/or resection of extensive portions of the aorta, some surgeons advocate a thoracosternotomy or bilateral anterior thoracotomy incision.[15] The bilateral anterior thoracotomy permits excellent exposure of the ascending aorta, arch, and most of the descending aorta, but may have a deleterious effect on pulmonary function; it involves sacrifice of both internal mammary arteries and puts both phrenic nerves at risk. We prefer to carry out aneurysm repair in two stages using an elephant trunk approach[16–18] and reserve the thoracosternotomy incision for reoperations and patients requiring emergent correction of simultaneous cardiac and aortic arch/descending pathology. In patients with a lesion primarily in the descending aorta that extends no farther proximally than the distal arch, a left lateral thoracotomy in the fifth intercostal space is the incision of choice.

Cooling and Rewarming

We lower the perfusate temperature toward 10°C, and monitor both bladder and esophageal (or tympanic) temperatures. After HCA, the perfusate temperature to which the brain is exposed is critical.[19] We use a period of hypothermic reperfusion, which our laboratory data have shown to significantly improve outcome, with a reproducible trend toward improved neurobehavioral and histologic outcomes.[20] Conversely, in an animal model, hyperthermic reperfusion was associated with deterioration of neurologic and behavioral outcome, correlating with histologic evidence of significant brain injury.[21]

During rewarming, we never raise blood temperature above 37°C, and we avoid creating a gradient exceeding 10°C between the blood and esophageal temperatures. Warming is discontinued when the esophageal (or tympanic) temperature reaches 35°C and the bladder temperature reaches 32°C. We prefer the patient to rewarm gradually in the intensive care unit after closure.

Graft and Suture Materials and Anastomotic Technique

Generally, an aneurysm repair consists of complete excision and replacement with an impregnated Dacron graft. We construct full-thickness anastomoses to the remaining, normal aorta, creating a "sandwich" of the aortic wall, with Teflon felt outside and graft material invaginated within the lumen.[22] Long-term follow-up of 2281 "sandwich" anastomoses, comprising 6484 patient-years, documents that pseudoaneurysm formation is extremely rare.[22] Most anastomoses are constructed with 3-0 polypropylene. However, graft-to-graft anastomoses never truly heal, so 2-0 is used, because the lifetime integrity of these anastomoses depends on the sutures.

Myocardial Protection

Myocardial protection is achieved by administering antegrade and retrograde, cold blood cardioplegia, generally supplemented by the combined effects of total body hypothermia and topical hypothermia. When access for antegrade perfusion is difficult and HCA is to be used, asystole may be induced by infusing 60 mEq of potassium into the pump circuit, over 1 to 2 minutes, just before circulatory arrest.[23]

Prevention of Paraplegia

Although paraplegia is not a common complication of most AA operations, preventative precautions must be taken with procedures involving the descending thoracic and thoracoabdominal aorta. Total body hypothermia affords some spinal cord protection, but additional safeguards are warranted, including cerebrospinal fluid drainage and, when indicated, distal perfusion. For AA procedures that require resection of a significant portion of the descending aorta, we routinely monitor somatosensory-evoked potentials (SSEPs) and motor-evoked potentials (MEPs), which may provide superior monitoring of anterior cord integrity.[24,25] Intercostal vessels are sacrificed gradually before instituting CPB. Each intercostal is provisionally clamped and sacrificed only if the MEPs and SSEPs remain unchanged for more than 10 minutes.[26,27] MEP and SSEP monitoring is continued until the patient exits the operating room, to confirm the return and stability of signals. Mean arterial pressure is maintained at 80 to 100 mm Hg, or possibly higher if the patient has chronic, severe hypertension. Postoperatively, hourly clinical assessment of lower extremity function is performed for 72 hours. Any deterioration must be rapidly addressed by increasing the blood pressure and withdrawing cerebrospinal fluid (CSF) to decrease intrathecal pressure. These maneuvers to increase spinal cord perfusion pressure have proved successful in reversing late-onset paraparesis.[27]

Control of Hemorrhage

Most current aortic surgery is carried out using antifibrinolytic agents to inhibit bleeding. We routinely use epsilon-aminocaproic acid, but others have reported that tranexamic acid is as effective. Isovolumic hemodilution, with reinfusion of autologous whole blood following CPB and thromboelastography-guided blood product administration, has greatly reduced transfusion requirements.[28] However, HCA exceeding 30 minutes or CPB exceeding 3 hours often requires factor replacement. Occasionally, particularly in reoperative or acute dissection cases, mediastinal packing and delayed closure may be required to control bleeding. We have experienced no mediastinal infections with this strategy. For persistent, low volume root hemorrhage that is expected to stop with normalization of hemostasis, a Cabrol fistula can be created in the superior mediastinum to shunt shed blood into the right atrium[29]; this maneuver may be lifesaving. Activated recombinant factor VIIa is indicated for patients with refractory, nonsurgical postoperative hemorrhage.[30]

Use of Glue

Surgeons have enthusiastically used gelatin resorcinol formaldehyde (GRF) and other biologic glues, predominantly for strengthening aortic tissue after acute type A dissection. Recently, however, there has been concern that the formaldehyde component of the GRF glue may cause tissue necrosis of the aortic wall, leading to late redissection and pseudoaneurysm formation.[31,32] Alternatively, Bioglue (CryoLife, Inc., Kennesaw, GA), composed of bovine serum albumin and glutaraldehyde, has been used to strengthen friable tissues and also to seal suture lines, particularly in acute aortic dissection.[33] Here too, however, evidence warrants caution, as tissue necrosis, as well as intraluminal aspiration and embolization, have been reported.[34] In most scenarios we find glue unnecessary.

Treatment of Infected Grafts and Mycotic Aneurysms

Our initial strategy is to administer specific, intravenous antibiotics, when the organism is known, or broad spectrum for several days before operation. At surgery, the entire infected aneurysm or graft is removed and replaced. We have successfully used prosthetic grafts for this purpose, but many prefer cryopreserved homografts in this setting.[16,35,36] Often the infecting organism can be cultured from the specimen. Intravenous antibiotics are continued for at least 6 weeks, and if a suitable oral agent can be found, therapy is extended for an additional 3 to 6 months.

If graft replacement must be performed in a frankly purulent operating field, the chest may be left open. The mediastinum is "washed out" after 24 to 48 hours and pectoralis or omental flaps may be brought into the wound and wrapped around the implanted prosthetic graft. A vacuum-assisted closure (VAC) dressing is applied and the mediastinum may be closed when signs of sepsis have resolved healthy granulation is present. C-reactive protein is a useful biochemical marker to help guide the length of antibiotic therapy and determine resolution of inflammation.[17]

CEREBRAL PROTECTION TECHNIQUES

Hypothermic Circulatory Arrest

Historical and Theoretical Considerations

Some of the earliest cardiac procedures were performed using HCA and in the 1960s, isolated case reports described the use of HCA in repair of AA aneurysms.[37] Successful experience using HCA for correction of complex congenital heart lesions in infants, as advocated by Barratt-Boyes and associates,[38] prompted renewed interest in its use in adults with aneurysms of the AA. The first series of such cases was reported by Griepp and associates,[39] which promoted wide acceptance of the efficacy of HCA in protecting the brain in adult AA surgery. With experience, limitations of HCA were described, especially concerning the adequacy of cerebral protection during extended periods of HCA. More recently, strategies using HCA and SCP have been described, combining benefits of both techniques.

Enthusiasm for the use of hypothermia to protect the brain during circulatory arrest began with a series of investigations in adult dogs that documented profound inhibition of cerebral metabolism with lowering of brain temperature.[40] Based on hypothermic versus normothermic metabolic rates, Michenfelder and Milde postulated that complete cerebral circulatory arrest for 30 minutes at 18°C would not result in permanent neurologic injury and subsequent experiments indicated that HCA for as long as 60 minutes should be safe.[41] However, investigations in puppies[42] and piglets[43] showed that hypothermia suppresses cerebral metabolism less than that Michenfelder predicted. In puppies, cerebral metabolic rate at 18°C is reduced to only 40% of control levels, and HCA for 60 minutes at 18°C results in detectable early behavioral dysfunction and quantitative EEG changes.[42,44] More prolonged HCA at 20°C in young piglets produces unequivocal behavioral sequelae and histologic evidence of cerebral damage.[45]

Experimental evidence indicates that the period of recovery following HCA is also critical. HCA, even for short intervals, engenders severe cerebral vasoconstriction that may last for hours. During this period, cerebral metabolism is maintained by increased oxygen extraction and thus is particularly vulnerable to hypoxic insult.[44,46,47] High intracranial pressure also correlates with delayed neurologic recovery and subsequent cerebral histopathologic abnormalities. Oxygen saturation data also imply that cold reperfusion enhances cerebral blood flow for several hours postoperatively.

There are two basic mechanisms that lead to ischemic cerebral injury during operations on the thoracic aorta. Stroke, the first type of injury, has received the most attention, mainly because of its devastating consequences.[48] These ischemic infarcts, detectable by conventional imaging techniques, result from embolic events, and are thought to be independent of the method of brain protection.[49] The second type of injury results from focal or global ischemia, because of interrupted or inadequate flow, giving rise to the clinical syndrome temporary neurologic dysfunction (TND),[49] which is characterized by varying degrees of obtundation, confusion, agitation, or transient parkinsonism. It is now generally accepted that TND is a direct consequence of inadequate cerebral protection and therefore related to the method of protection used.[50,51]

The incidence of TND in 200 adults who underwent HCA during thoracic aortic surgery was 19%, correlating significantly with age and duration of HCA. In this study, HCA averaged 47 minutes in patients with TND, and 33 minutes in those without TND. HCA duration did not correlate with mortality or permanent neurologic injury, which was usually focal, and was significantly more frequent in older patients and those with obvious atheromatous debris in the arch or descending aorta.[49,50,52]

Sensitive neuropsychologic testing showed that HCA exceeding 25 minutes and advanced age predicted poor performance in examinations of memory and fine motor function.[53] Patients with impaired neurocognitive function several weeks postoperatively were significantly more likely to have manifested TND immediately postoperatively. Based on these findings, HCA exceeding 25 minutes must be considered a risk factor for long-term, albeit perhaps subtle, deficits in cognitive function. Impairment of memory may be related to injury of the hippocampus, which is particularly sensitive to ischemic injury because of its high metabolic rate.[54]

Past projections of the theoretical safe duration of HCA, based on rates of oxygen consumption at various brain temperatures, are now considered to have been misleading. The relationship between temperature and the cerebral metabolic rate for oxygen ($CMRO_2$) can be expressed as the temperature coefficient Q_{10}, which reflects the rate of reduction in the metabolism for a 10°C interval.[55] The reduction of $CMRO_2$ with temperature is substantially more modest than that reported originally. In one experimental study, 39% of baseline $CMRO_2$ was still present at 18°C, a temperature previously thought to be safe for prolonged periods of clinical HCA; quantitative electroencephalography (EEG) showed significant slow-wave activity at 18°C, whereas EEG silence was present at 13 and 8°C.[41]

McCullough and associates[55] recalculated Q_{10} for the adult human brain based on direct measurements of $CMRO_2$ during HCA. These data predict that the safe period of arrest is about 30 minutes at 15°C and 40 minutes at 10°C, after which cerebral cellular anoxia occurs. These experimental findings correlate with ample clinical pediatric experience indicating that arrest times greater than 40 minutes portend poor neurodevelopmental outcomes.[56] These observations support the use of truly profound hypothermia for circulatory arrest to achieve maximum cerebral metabolic suppression, particularly if arrest time will exceed 30 minutes. Intracranial temperatures should be protected from rising during HCA by packing the head in ice.[43,44,46,47,57,58]

Use of Corticosteroids

High-dose methylprednisolone, given 2 and 8 hours before CPB, reduces the change in cerebrovascular resistance and improves cerebral blood flow, cerebral arteriovenous oxygen difference, and oxygen metabolism following deep HCA, and may serve as a neuroprotective agent.[59] Additionally, in 4-week-old piglets, pretreatment with corticosteroids 4 hours before CPB—compared with steroids in the CPB prime—reduced total body edema and cerebral vascular leakage, with improved immunohistochemical indices of neuroprotection.[60] The beneficial effect of corticosteroid pretreatment derives from alterations in de novo protein synthesis at the mRNA level[61] and inhibition of adhesion molecule expression in the endothelial cells, which impacts the trafficking of leukocytes into the injured areas.[62] Other benefits of methylprednisolone given 8 hours before CPB and HCA are improved pulmonary compliance and alveolar-arterial gradient, and decreased pulmonary vascular resistance.[63] Consistently, benefits are more apparent when steroids are given several hours before the institution of CPB.

Clinical Implementation

Because brain temperature primarily determines the safety of HCA, it must be measured accurately. Clinically available sites for measurement include: tympanic membrane, jugular venous bulb, nasopharyngeal, esophageal, bladder, and rectal. In our practice, we routinely monitor two different measurement sites to guide various phases of cooling and rewarming.

Throughout the duration of cardiopulmonary bypass, we follow arterial perfusate temperature, which best reflects the temperature that the brain is exposed to.

During cooling, esophageal or tympanic membrane temperature is used to reflect intracranial temperature and is monitored to guide the initiation of arrest. Based on clinical and laboratory studies,[45,46,58] we cool for a minimum of 30 to 40 minutes, to an esophageal temperature of 15 to 18°C, with the perfusate lowered to 10°C. The head is packed in ice to prevent rewarming during HCA. Because continuing oxygen extraction reflects ongoing cerebral metabolic activity, we also monitor jugular venous saturation, using a target O_2 saturation of greater than 95% to indicate adequate cerebral cooling and metabolic suppression.

During rewarming, we primarily monitor the perfusate and bladder temperatures. The perfusate is kept at a gradient of no more than 10°C above the esophageal or tympanic membrane temperature, which reduces the likelihood that oxygen demand will exceed oxygen supply during the interval of inappropriate cerebral vasoconstriction after HCA.[44,46,47,64] Avoiding high perfusate temperatures is also essential[21] and we never allow it to exceed 37°C. The bladder temperature, which is raised to around 32–34°C, reflects total body or "core" temperature and lags considerably behind changes in the other temperature measurements during cooling and rewarming. Using the bladder temperature to guide rewarming helps to ensure uniform rewarming and prevent dangerous rebound hypothermia after CPB.

Following CPB, achieving hemostasis and maintaining normal hemodynamics are also important, since the vulnerable period of cerebral recovery, during which increased oxygen extraction is relied on to support adequate cerebral metabolism, may extend up to 8 hours postoperatively.

Selective Cerebral Perfusion

Historical and Theoretical Considerations

DeBakey reported the earliest attempts to repair AA aneurysms,[65] in which a complicated technique of normothermic SCP was used, involving several pumps and bilateral cannulation of the subclavian and carotid arteries. Difficulty controlling pressure and flow to uniformly perfuse these separate vascular beds, as well as high operative mortality, led to early abandonment of this technique. However, SCP was revisited in the late 1980s, as mounting evidence indicated that HCA was not safe for the long durations required for repairing complex and extensive aneurysms. It was recognized that combining SCP with hypothermia permitted lower flow rates, while affording better cerebral protection than HCA alone or HCA plus RCP.[66,67]

Bachet and associates described perfusing the innominate and left carotid arteries with 6 to 12°C blood (flow 250 to 350 cc/min), which he termed "cold cerebroplegia." Mortality for 54 AA cases was 3%, with only one severe neurologic injury and two transient focal lesions.[68] Matsuda and associates[69] used SCP at 16 to 20°C in 34 AA cases, with 9% mortality, 3% stroke, and 5% TND. His technique required a two-pump system and cannulation of the brachiocephalic and left carotid arteries; bilateral temporal artery and continuous internal jugular venous saturation were monitored and, importantly, the results demonstrated that hypothermic CPB did not carry a higher risk of coagulopathy.

Kazui first described his approach to SCP in 1986.[70] Between 1990 and 1999, 220 patients underwent total arch replacement with SCP and open distal anastomosis, with 12.7% in-hospital mortality and 3.3% permanent neurologic dysfunction. Multivariate analysis showed in-hospital mortality was determined by renal failure, long CPB time, and shock; permanent neurologic deficit was associated with old cerebrovascular accident and long CPB duration.[71] Perfusing two arteries with flows of 10 cc/kg/min at 22°C—considered 50% of physiologic levels, based on experimental studies—SCP duration had no significant impact on outcome.[72]

In a multicenter study, Di Eusanio definitively demonstrated the efficacy of SCP in reducing temporary and permanent neurologic dysfunction. In 588 patients undergoing both partial and full AA replacement, the risks of permanent and temporary neurologic injury were 3.8 and 5.6%, respectively; overall mortality was 8.7%.[73]

Clot or atheroma in the aorta, which often develops at the origin of the brachiocephalic vessels, predisposes to stroke during AA surgery. Therefore, complete arch resection should reduce the rate of neurologic injury. Accordingly, in 50 recent AA resections,[74] Kazui and associates reported 2% mortality; permanent neurologic injury occurred in 4%, and TND in 4% (adverse outcome 6%), with a history of cerebrovascular disease a risk factor for permanent neurologic dysfunction.

The Kazui technique (Fig. 52-2A–H) begins with systemic cooling to 22°C, followed by circulatory arrest and SCP (22°C) delivered via malleable cannulas (Fuji System, Tokyo) inserted into the innominate and left common carotid arteries (Fig. 52-2B). Newly designed malleable cannulas allow superior visibility and simultaneous pressure monitoring (personal communication). With the left subclavian artery clamped, a four-branch graft is anastomosed to the descending aorta (Fig. 52-2C) and lower-body perfusion is begun via a side branch (Fig. 52 2D). Next, the left subclavian is anastomosed and perfused (Fig. 52-2E) followed by construction of the proximal anastomosis (Fig. 52-2F). Finally, full perfusion is restored by anastomosing the innominate and left common carotid arteries to the remaining side branches (Fig. 52-2G,H). Importantly, this technique includes transsection of the brachiocephalic vessels distal to their origins, precluding embolization of debris, and completely excluding the arch, which often contains friable atheromatous lesions.

Extensive aneurysmal disease, involving the ascending, arch, and descending aorta, can be resected in a single stage or may be approached by performing a two-stage procedure, wherein an elephant trunk graft, placed in the descending aorta during arch replacement, is used to simplify a subsequent procedure, performed via a left thoracotomy. In both approaches, SCP affords cerebral protection while permitting unhurried reconstruction of aortic continuity.

Rokkas and Kouchoukos[75] described a single-stage reconstruction, the "arch first" technique, performed via bilateral anterior thoracotomies. This technique employs an interval of HCA followed by SCP while aortic continuity is restored. In 46 "arch first" procedures, the hospital mortality was 6.5% , with no

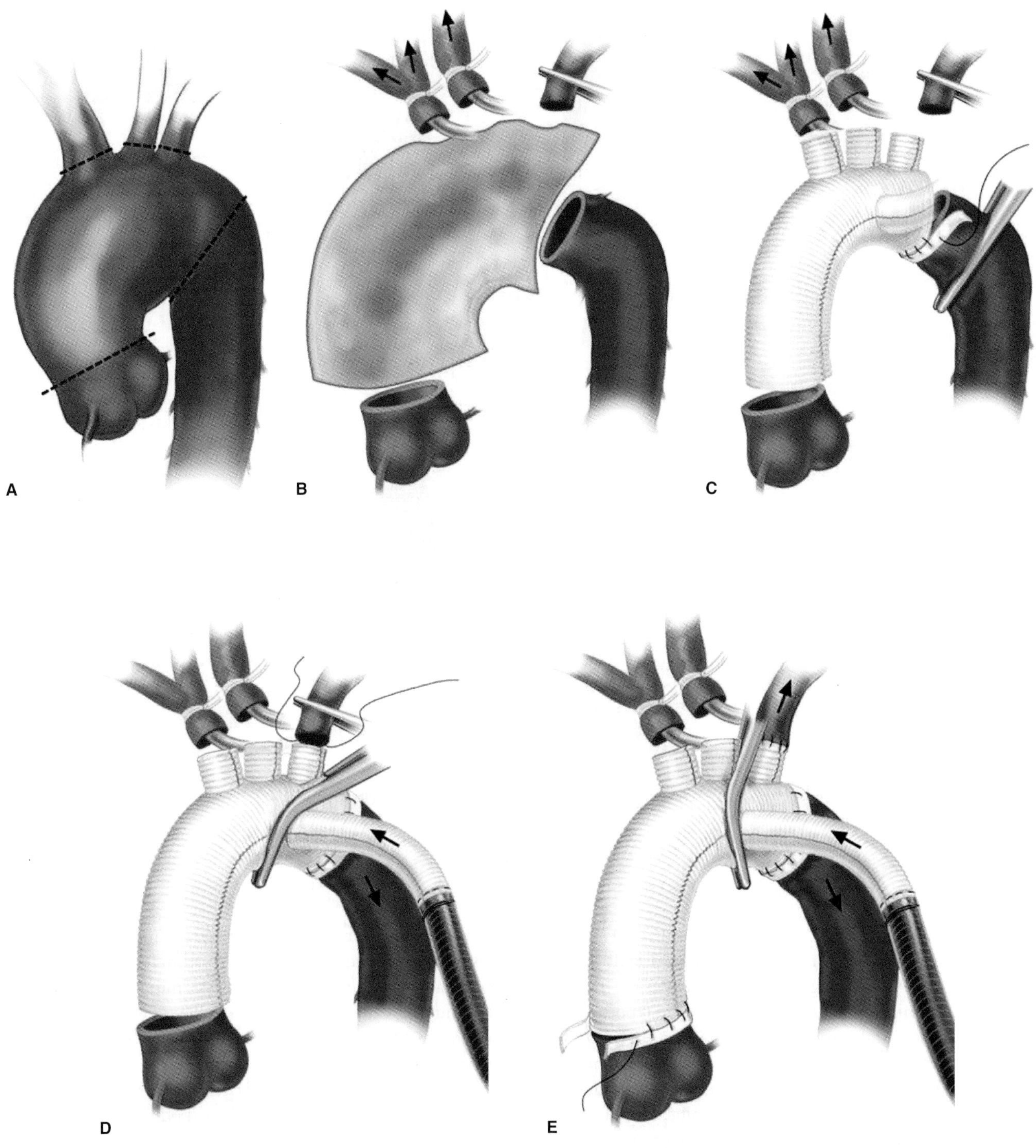

FIGURE 52-2 (A–F) Dr. Kazui's technique for total arch replacement with a four-branch graft.

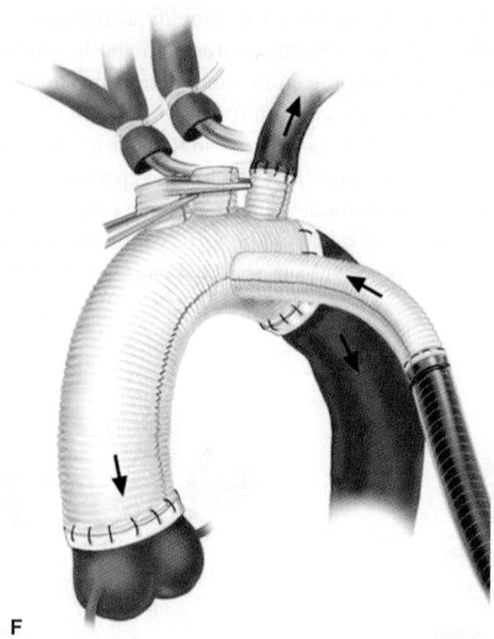

F

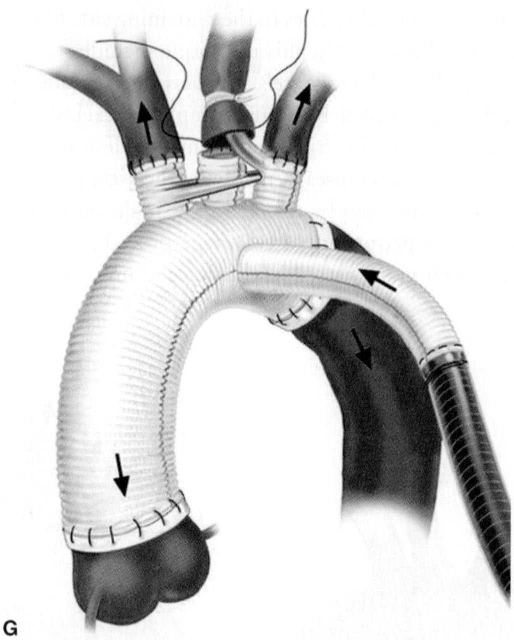

G

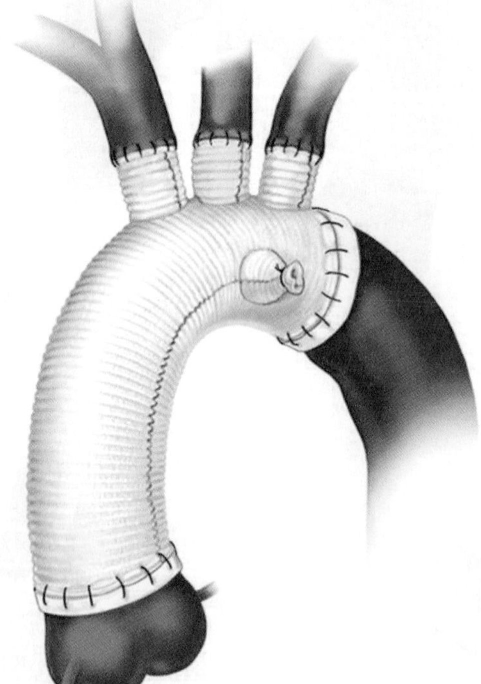

H

FIGURE 52-2 *(Continued)*

permanent neurologic event and 13% TND.[76] In 12 cases, HCA was minimized by administering unilateral SCP via the right axillary artery, averaging only 8.8 minutes.[77]

Unilateral administration of SCP has also been reported. For example, Kucuker and associates[78] reported on 181 patients who underwent ascending and hemiarch replacement (90 patients) or total arch replacement (91 patients) with SCP delivered via the right brachial artery; hospital mortality was 6.6%, with 2.2% permanent strokes. The patients were cooled to 26°C and with the innominate, left common carotid, and occasionally the left subclavian artery clamped, arch replacement was performed with flow decreased to 8 to 10 cc/kg/min. The mean SCP duration was 36 ± 27 minutes (range 17 to 80 minutes). Contralateral cerebral flow was monitored by transcranial Doppler of the left middle cerebral artery. In the rare case of inadequate left hemispheric perfusion, an additional catheter was placed into the left common carotid artery. In this study, no mention was made of TND, but in a separate cohort of patients, neurocognitive testing revealed no postoperative deficits.[79]

Although contralateral perfusion was not problematic in these studies, a certain level of caution is prudent based on anatomic studies. Merkkola and colleagues found insufficient collateral circulation (<0.5 mm) through the circle of Willis in 14% of autopsy specimens.[80]

Recent clinical series have confirmed the relative safety of SCP. Khaladj and associates[81] reported 501 consecutive cases (181 emergent), using moderate systemic hypothermia (25°C) and 14°C SCP administered via the innominate and left carotid arteries, maintaining perfusion pressure between 40 and 60 mm Hg and flows of 400 to 650 cc/min. The overall mortality was 11.6%, with 9.6% strokes and 13.4% TND. Permanent stroke risk increased with renal insufficiency and prolonged operative times, and TND risk increased with increased circulatory arrest time, emergency status, and concomitant coronary artery disease.

A small, randomized study by Kamiya and associates[9] addressed a widespread concern that cannulation of the brachiocephalic arteries for SCP may cause cerebral embolization. High-intensity transient signals (HITS), indicative of microembolization—from sources such as gaseous microemboli, atherosclerotic debris, lipid microemboli, and blood-platelet aggregates—were quantified by transcranial Doppler monitoring in patients undergoing circulatory arrest with and without SCP. Only 0.6% of HITS were recorded during SCP, with most occurring during the interval between aortic cross-clamp removal and the termination of CPB. Thus, in this small subset of patients, SCP did not increase the risk of cerebral microembolization.

Using antegrade SCP for cerebral protection, many surgeons are performing arch surgery with moderate hypothermia (20 to 28°C). However, caution needs to be exercised at these temperatures, because end organs are more vulnerable to ischemia. To limit lower-body ischemia, thoracoabdominal perfusion during antegrade SCP has been recommended—via the femoral artery while clamping the proximal descending aorta, or with antegrade perfusion via an endoluminal balloon cannula in the descending aorta or via a sidearm graft branch of an arch graft.

Nonetheless, with precautions to prevent end-organ ischemia, a "global warming" trend has emerged, as surgeons have investigated ways to minimize or eliminate HCA. For example, 305 patients in Osaka, Japan underwent total arch replacement with SCP, combining right axillary and left common carotid perfusion.[82] Perfusate temperature was progressively increased from 20 to 28°C. The duration of SCP was 150.1 minutes, with 60.9 minutes of circulatory arrest to the lower body. Operative mortality was 2.3%, with 1.6% permanent neurologic injury. Preoperative cerebral dysfunction was a risk factor for TND, which occurred in 6.6%. The strategy for patients with prior stroke included: higher CPB perfusion pressures (>60 mm Hg), more profound hypothermia (20 to 22°C), and higher SCP flows. In 67 aortic arch repairs at 28°C, the left subclavian artery was also selectively perfused, to increase collateral spinal cord blood flow during lower-body ischemia, and SCP flows were increased to 19 cc/kg/min to maintain arterial pressure at 60 mm Hg. Despite warmer SCP, outcomes remained consistent, with 6% mortality, 6% stroke, 1.5% TND, and no paraplegia. Another series of 120 acute type A aortic dissections had SCP administered via the right subclavian artery at 30°C, with snared brachiocephalic vessels,[83] flow at 1320 cc/min, a perfusion pressure of 75 mm Hg, and average cerebral perfusion time 25 ± 12 minutes: 30-day mortality was 5%, stroke rate 4.2%, and TND rate 2.5%.

Although these and similar studies have yielded good clinical outcomes, there is no consensus regarding the optimal temperature for SCP and adopting warmer perfusion techniques during circulatory arrest should be approached cautiously. Experimental studies in a porcine model by Khaladj and associates[84] indicate that the optimum temperature for SCP is no higher than 20°C, which resulted in lower intracranial pressures and earlier return of EEG activity than SCP at 30°C. Particularly noteworthy was evidence that although SCP provides good cerebral protection, the margin of safety for the spinal cord is thin. Our laboratory studies suggest that SCP at 10 to 15°C after HCA provides better cerebral protection than higher temperatures and clinically we use SCP at about 15°C.[85]

The duration of safe lower-body ischemia at 28°C is still under investigation, with evidence that 60 minutes may be the limit. If extended periods of circulatory arrest are anticipated, a method for lower-body protection should be utilized, such as femoral artery perfusion, aortic balloon occlusion with perfusion, antegrade perfusion through a sidearm graft, or deeper hypothermia. For example, 11 patients from a series of 252 ascending and arch repairs with moderately hypothermic SCP (25 to 28°C) had lower-body ischemic times greater than 60 minutes, and 2 (18%) developed paraplegia.[86] In a porcine model, Etz et al. demonstrated that during 90 minutes of SCP at 28°C there is little or no spinal cord blood flow in the segment T4 to T13, resulting in a 40% spinal cord injury rate. Moreover, following SCP the lower spinal cord also lacked a normal hyperemic response, suggesting diminished vascular reactivity and localized edema. Histologic studies showed significant ischemic damage in the lower cord, even in animals that recovered clinically, suggesting that unappreciated spinal cord injury may be occurring even at shorter durations of lower-body circulatory arrest.

Clinical Implementation

In the current era, cerebral injury during AA reconstruction is most often related to embolization.[112–114] Often, the arch and the origins of the brachiocephalic vessels contain friable, atheromatous debris, and the risk of embolizing this material can be minimized by using a brief period of HCA to transect the brachiocephalic vessels distal to their origins, completely excluding the diseased area. Then, during SCP, the arch repair can proceed in an unhurried fashion. Laboratory studies have shown that a short period of HCA does not compromise the superior cerebral protection provided by SCP.[87]

Our approach then is as follows. During a brief period of HCA, the individual brachiocephalic arteries are dissected free and sequentially anastomosed to a ready-made trifurcated graft, beginning either with the left subclavian or the innominate artery. The trifurcated graft is clamped, and SCP is instituted via the axillary artery (see Fig. 52-6D,E later in the chapter). Occasionally, when the left subclavian artery is displaced laterally and cephalad, a preoperative left subclavian to left carotid bypass is performed and a bifurcated graft is used to perfuse

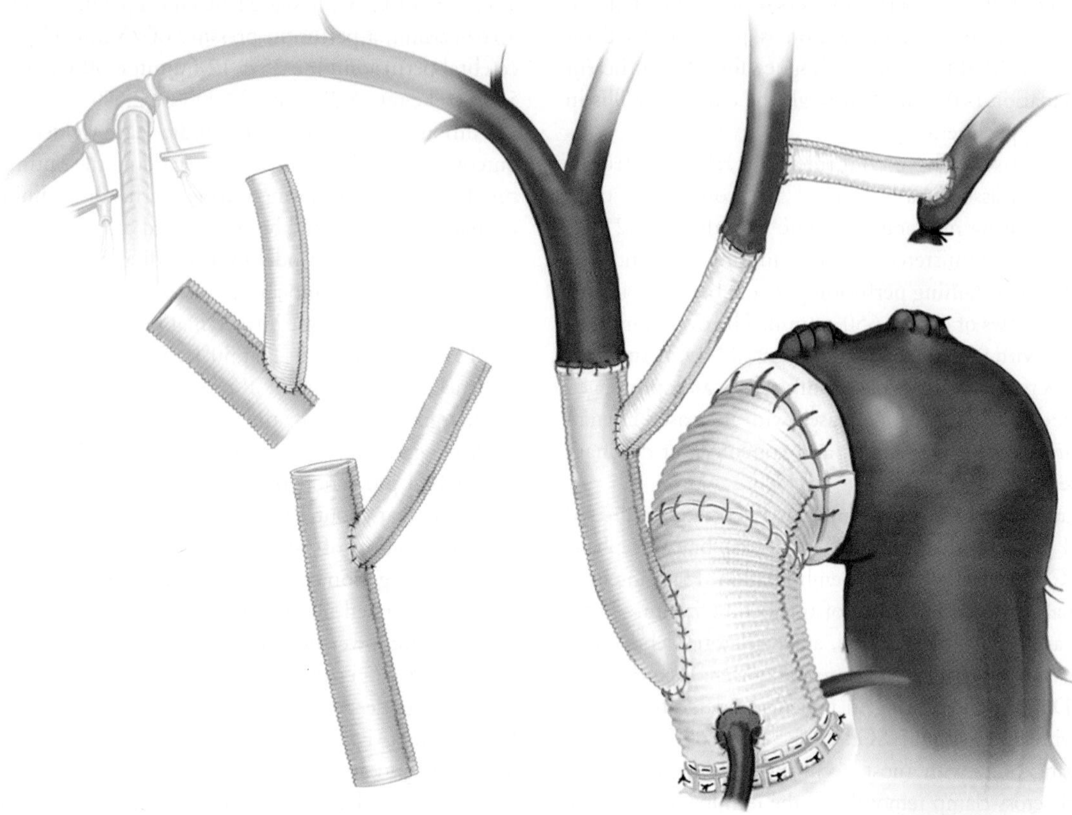

FIGURE 52-3 A preoperative left subclavian artery to left common carotid artery bypass is done when the left subclavian artery is markedly displaced laterally and cephalad.

the left common carotid and innominate arteries (Fig. 52-3). Alternatively, a graft may be anastomosed to the left axillary artery and tunneled via the second ICS into the mediastinum. Hypothermic SCP is administered via the right axillary artery, typically requiring flows of 600 to 1000 cc/min to maintain mean pressures of 40 to 60 mm Hg, and the systemic perfusate temperature is allowed to drift upward. At the end of the arch reconstruction, the proximal end of the trifurcated graft is anastomosed to the ascending aortic graft. Using such strategies as axillary artery cannulation[88,89] and grafting of individual brachiocephalic vessels during HCA,[74,77,90,91] followed by SCP of the brachiocephalic grafts, lengthy periods of circulatory arrest are no longer necessary.

Retrograde Cerebral Perfusion

The early 1990s saw widespread enthusiasm for RCP[92] based on the limitations of HCA, the success of retrograde cardioplegia, and isolated encouraging reports regarding the efficacy of RCP in treating massive air embolism.[93] Purported mechanisms whereby RCP accomplishes neuroprotection include: (1) flushing embolic material from the cerebral circulation[94]; (2) providing cerebral flow sufficient to support cerebral metabolism[95]; and (3) maintaining cerebral hypothermia.[96] There is, however, evidence that RCP may worsen neurologic outcome by inducing cerebral edema.[97]

Although initial laboratory and clinical reports regarding RCP were encouraging, many of the early studies used historical controls and short durations of RCP—well within the safe limits for HCA alone. Also, studies, in several animal species, demonstrated no flow to the brain during RCP.[98–100] In other experimental studies, the most effective conditions for retrograde flow—including clamping inferior vena cava and high venous perfusion pressures—resulted in fluid sequestration, significant cerebral edema, and mild cerebral histopathology, sequelae observable even after relatively short intervals of RCP.[94] Studies in our laboratory, measuring cerebral blood flow by collecting AA return and quantifying microspheres trapped in the brain, demonstrated that too little capillary flow occurs during RCP to confer metabolic benefit, even with inferior vena cava occlusion or during deep hypothermia.[101] Similarly, directly visualizing cerebral capillaries with intravital microscopy showed that RCP does not provide adequate cerebral capillary blood flow to prevent ischemia but may induce brain edema.[97] A cadaver study provided an anatomical explanation for poor retrograde flow, as functionally competent valves, demonstrated in the proximal internal jugular vein, obstruct direct retrograde intracranial venous flow, causing unbalanced and unreliable brain perfusion.[102] However, a recent animal study showed that RCP may be helpful under some conditions, as intermittent pressure augmentation during moderate hypothermic RCP efficiently dilated the cerebral vessels, allowing an adequate blood supply without brain injury, and provided neuroprotection equivalent to antegrade SCP.[103]

The evidence from clinical studies is harder to interpret. Some studies show that RCP duration predicts mortality[92,104] but others do not.[105,106] Clinical studies comparing HCA+RCP and HCA alone have also yielded mixed results; some showed mortality rates comparable to other cerebral protection methods,[107] and others showed reduced mortality rates with RCP.[108–110] In three studies that included patients with SCP, HCA+RCP patients had similar mortality rates.[111–113]

In our own clinical studies,[50,114] we have been unable to demonstrate any benefit of RCP. In a recent clinical study,[50] we could not show a decrease in the incidence of stroke with RCP, perhaps because of a greater prevalence of patients with clot or atheroma in the RCP group, but arguably because RCP is not effective in preventing stroke. Mortality was higher in the RCP group, and TND was higher with RCP than with SCP. Furthermore, RCP resulted in no reduction of TND compared with HCA alone, reinforcing the notion that RCP probably has no nutritive value for brain tissue. As mentioned, our laboratory data suggest that RCP, especially at high pressures, although successful in removing some emboli, may aggravate cerebral injury.[94] Clinically, this effect is not easy to demonstrate but may help account for our repeated observation that neurologic recovery is delayed in patients treated with RCP. Recently, we studied neuropsychologic dysfunction after RCP and found that RCP probably had a negative impact on cognitive outcome.[115] Other investigators believe that neurocognitive dysfunction depends on the duration of RCP; if RCP duration is less than 60 minutes, recovery is comparable to that after CABG, whereas prolonged RCP is associated with neurocognitive impairment.[116]

In general, based on laboratory studies,[96] we believe that the major benefit of RCP stems from continued cerebral cooling by venoarterial and venovenous anastomoses, which is especially helpful if systemic cooling is not as thorough or prolonged as it should be. Clinically, we no longer use RCP, feeling that its benefits derive not from providing nutritive support but from aiding in cerebral cooling and helping to prevent rewarming during HCA. However, we believe that it is safer to prevent rewarming by thorough initial cooling and packing the head in ice.

Clinical Implementation

Although we do not routinely use RCP for cerebral protection, many surgeons do administer RCP briefly following HCA in patients who have a high risk of embolization to help flush debris from the cerebral circulation.

RCP, which is always employed in conjunction HCA, by perfusing blood into either one or both venae cavae at a flow rate to maintain pressures of 15 to 20 mm Hg in the superior vena cava. Cardiac distention is avoided by choking both venae cavae. Given the rich network of collaterals between the superior vena cava and inferior vena cava, it probably makes no difference whether inflow is into one, the other, or both. When whole-body retrograde perfusion is carried out, the initial flow rate is usually 800 to 1000 cc/min, but once the venous capacitance vessels have been filled, flows of 100 to 500 cc/min are usually sufficient to maintain superior vena caval pressures at 15 to 20 mm Hg.

Hybrid Aortic Arch Repair

Endograft technology has permitted combining traditional open procedures with endovascular grafting, so-called hybrid procedures. Initially, stent grafts were deployed in the descending aorta for aneurysms involving the distal arch, or in lieu of an open stage II elephant trunk procedure. As experience accumulated, two problems attending aortic arch endografting became evident. First, there is often insufficient undilated aorta distal to the brachiocephalic vessels to seat the proximal portion of a stent graft. Second, the arch is often severely diseased and endograft procedures, which entail negotiating the arch with stiff wires and large-bore catheters, carry a risk of embolic stroke. In fact, experience showed that the more proximally an endograft was deployed, the higher was the risk of embolic stroke.[117]

Debranching Procedures

The technique of covering the origin of one or more brachiocephalic vessels with an endograft, generally in concert with bypassing or transposing them, addressed both problems by extending the proximal landing zone and minimizing the risk of atheroembolization. These debranching procedures[118] involve transposing some or all of the brachiocephalic arteries to the ascending aorta. Initially performed on hypothermic CPB, debranching operations are now commonly done off pump, and permit endografting that partially or even completely excludes the aortic arch. The endograft may be introduced retrograde, via the common femoral artery, or antegrade, generally via a sidearm graft, variously configured to allow proximal access. Antegrade deployment offers the advantage of avoiding diseased and/or stenotic aortoiliac vessels. Debranching procedures presented many anatomical variations for endografting. The classification of landing zones described by Mitchell and associates (Fig. 52-4) allowed meaningful comparisons of different hybrid arch series.[119] For comparisons of traditional total aortic arch repairs with current endograft-and-debranching procedures, only patients with zone 0 deployment constitute an equivalent match.

The Left Subclavian Artery

If the left subclavian artery is not accessible in the mediastinum, options for covering the subclavian origin with an endograft include: no revascularization; preemptive transposition or bypass of the left subclavian artery using the left common carotid artery; and left axillary artery bypass, wherein an axillary graft is tunneled into the chest and anastomosed centrally, often with subsequent coil embolization of the proximal left subclavian artery to prevent a type II endoleak.

Branched Grafts

Several branched graft techniques have been described for debranching. Canaud reported six cases with proximal endograft

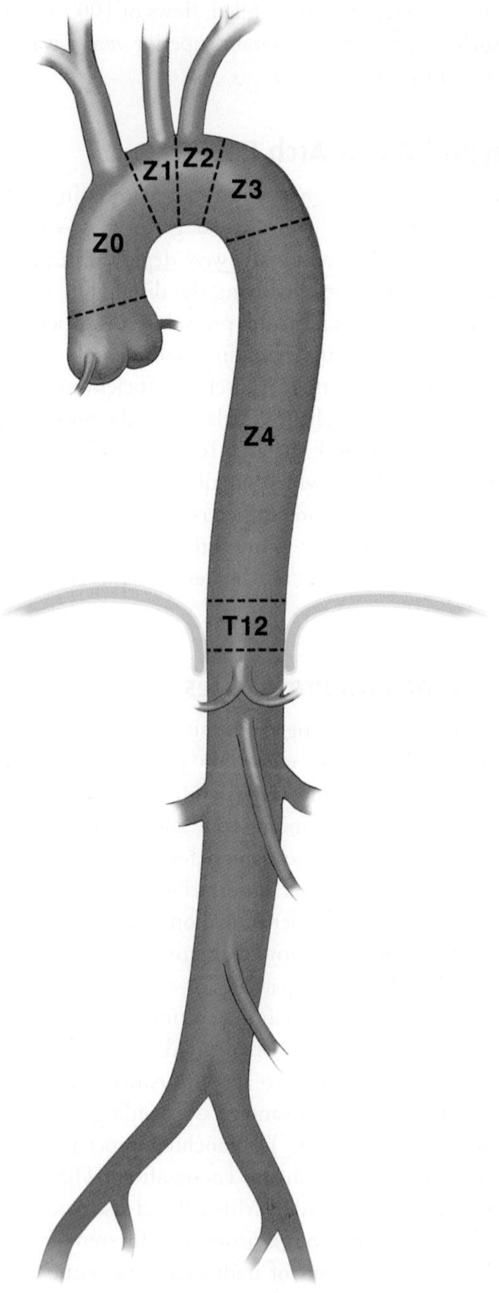

FIGURE 52-4 Thoracic endovascular landing zone designation.

placement in zone 0, wherein debranching was achieved with a single 10-mm graft; end-to-side anastomoses were constructed to the brachiocephalic trunk and left common carotid artery and an end-to-end anastomosis was made to the left subclavian artery.[120] Early postoperative complications included transient paraplegia, transient cerebral ischemia, cardiac tamponade, and a retrograde type A aortic dissection, successfully treated; there was no mortality at 30 days. With retrograde deployment in five patients, Chan placed endografts that occluded all the supra-aortic branches, revascularizing the innominate and left common carotid arteries using a bifurcated graft ($14 \times 7 \times 7$ mm)[121]; the left subclavian artery was revascularized only in cases of left vertebral dominance, left arm dialysis dependence, or a patent left internal mammary graft. Technical success was 100%, no neurologic complications, but two patients required reoperation for tamponade. Szeto and associates reported eight hybrid arch repairs performed via median sternotomy, with retrograde endograft deployment.[122] Debranching was achieved using a patch giving off three branches, fashioned from a commercially available four-branched arch graft; the patch was anastomosed to the proximal ascending aorta using CPB, moderate hypothermia, and aortic cross-clamping. Two patients suffered TND and required long-term tracheostomy, and one died of myocardial infarction. Finally, Hughes published a series of 28 arch aneurysms, wherein 12 patients underwent total arch debranching using a custom-designed graft (Vascutek USA, Ann Arbor, MI), with limbs to allow transposition of the left common carotid and innominate arteries and antegrade stent-graft deployment.[123] The left subclavian origin was covered in all patients, and two underwent left subclavian to common carotid bypass during the same procedure. Outcomes were excellent, with no deaths or strokes and one case of delayed paraparesis.

Although debranching has permitted stent grafting into zone 0, the stability of the proximal landing zone remains a focus of concern with current stent-graft technology. In the Hughes study,[123] two type I endoleaks occurred, despite seating the proximal graft directly into a Dacron graft. To minimize this complication, the authors recommend oversizing the endograft by 20% and creating a 4-cm zone of coaptation when stenting into prosthetic grafts. Antona described a novel technique for ensuring stable proximal fixation, involving banding the aorta with a separate vascular graft to create a nonexpandable, cylindrical landing zone.[124] The graft is opened longitudinally and wrapped around the aorta to create a 3- to 4-cm zone with an outer diameter of 32 mm. A radiopaque wire is used to mark its proximal and distal extent, facilitating subsequent retrograde endografting. In light of these experiences, most agree that future endograft systems must provide increased flexibility to follow the curvature of the aortic arch, yet achieve strong fixation to prevent endoleaks and secondary migration.

REPRESENTATIVE PROCEDURES

Aortic arch reconstruction requires different approaches, techniques, and operative strategies, depending on the arch pathology and the involvement of the proximal and distal aorta. To illustrate, we describe seven different situations and our approach to arch reconstruction in each of these cases.

Case 1: Bentall Procedure and Hemiarch Replacement

This is an elderly patient with stenosis of a severely calcified bicuspid aortic valve and an aneurysm extending from the root to the proximal arch (Fig. 52-5A).

Via a median sternotomy, using right atrial and right axillary artery cannulation, CPB and core cooling are initiated. The ascending aorta cross-clamped and transected, using antegrade and retrograde cold blood cardioplegia, supplemented by topical cooling, for myocardial protection. The perfusate temperature is maintained at 10°C until the esophageal temperature reaches

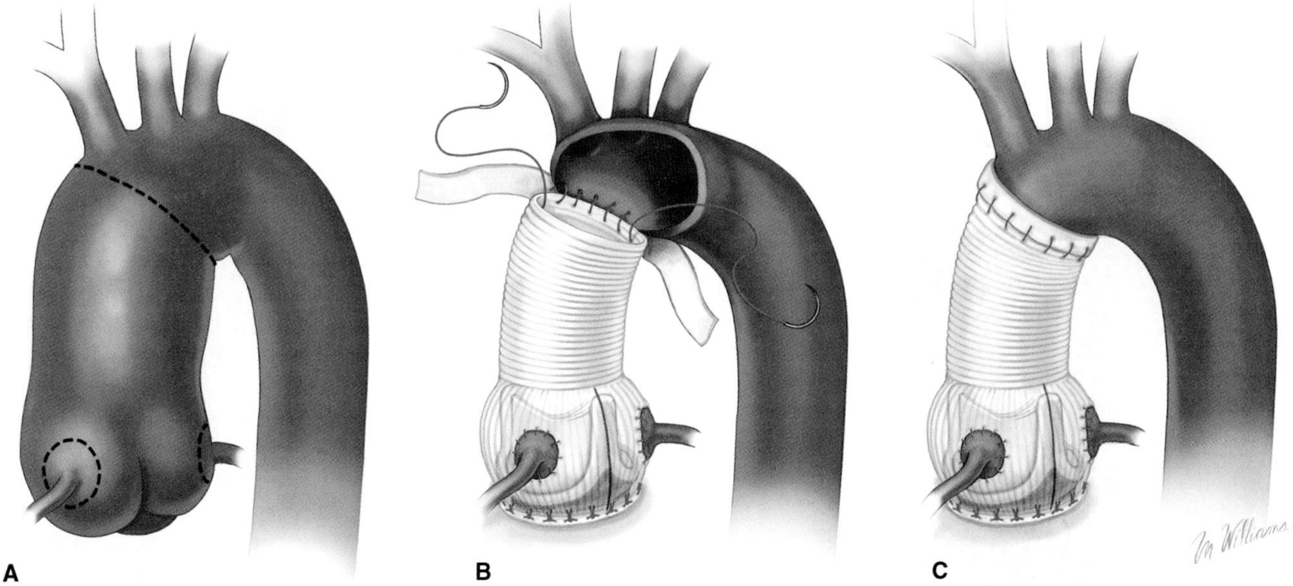

FIGURE 52-5 (A) Ascending aortic aneurysm extending into the underside of the aortic arch. (B) Bentall reconstruction of the aortic root with open resection of the hemiarch. Perfusion is via the right axillary artery. (C) Completed repair and full systemic perfusion.

20°C and is maintained at that level while the Bentall procedure is performed. Coronary buttons, 1 to 1.5 cm in diameter, are fashioned and mobilized and the remaining proximal aorta is excised. A composite valved-conduit, constructed by suturing a bioprosthetic valve into a tube graft, is implanted, using interrupted pledgeted sutures. Using an ophthalmic electrocautery, an opening in the conduit for the left button is made, carefully situated to avoid stretching, twisting, or kinking of the left main coronary artery; the button is anastomosed using 4-0 or 5-0 polypropylene incorporating a thin strip of Teflon to reinforce the button.[125]

The perfusate temperature is dropped to 8 to 10°C during anastomosis of the left coronary button and, when the jugular oxygen saturation is above 95% and the esophageal temperature is 18°C, HCA is begun and the cross-clamp is removed, with the head packed in ice and the patient placed in Trendelenburg position. The distal ascending aorta and proximal arch are excised, leaving a beveled aortic cuff extending from the base of the innominate artery on the right to 1 cm proximal to the ligamentum arteriosum and the recurrent laryngeal nerve on the left. The composite graft is beveled and anastomosed to the aorta with 3-0 polypropylene suture material (Fig. 52-5B). A secure, hemostatic anastomosis is constructed by "sandwiching" the aorta between the graft, carefully invaginated within the aortic lumen, and a 1-cm cuff of Teflon felt, incorporated outside the aorta.[22] Perfusing through the axillary artery, air is flushed from the aorta and cold perfusion is continued for several minutes before rewarming (Fig. 52-5C). A gradient of 10°C or less between the perfusate temperature and esophageal temperature is maintained throughout rewarming. With the heart filled and the aorta pressurized, the appropriate location for the right coronary button is marked, after which the distal graft is cross-clamped. The right coronary button is implanted and, before tightening the suture line, the heart is de-aired. The duration of HCA is usually less than 20 minutes and 50 to 60 minutes of core warming are generally necessary to raise the esophageal temperature to 35°C and the bladder temperature to greater than 32°C, at which point the patient is weaned from CPB.

Case 2: Total Aortic Arch Replacement for Atherosclerotic and Calcified Aneurysms

The arch and the origins of the supra-aortic vessels often contain friable atheromatous material and our trifurcated graft technique for total arch replacement (Fig. 52-6A–L) is designed to minimize manipulation of these segments before excluding them from the cerebral circulation, thereby reducing the risk of embolization; the technique minimizes cerebral ischemia by permitting antegrade SCP during arch reconstruction.[126,127]

A median sternotomy incision is extended superiorly along the medial border of the left sternocleidomastoid muscle. The recurrent laryngeal nerve is preserved as the AA and its branches are exposed. A no-touch technique of dissection is used—the patient is dissected away from the aneurysm.

CPB is initiated, using the right axillary artery and the right atrium, with the perfusate temperature lowered to 10°C (Fig. 52-6B). TEE is used to confirm flow in the arch and monitor for dissection or malperfusion. If the ascending aorta is calcified or severely atherosclerotic, it is not cross-clamped. Just before circulatory arrest, with the heart vented, 60 mEq of potassium chloride is added to the perfusate over 2 minutes to induce diastolic cardiac arrest. Alternatively, the heart is arrested with retrograde blood cardioplegia. If a proximal repair is required, it may be performed at this point, while core cooling proceeds (Fig. 52-6C).

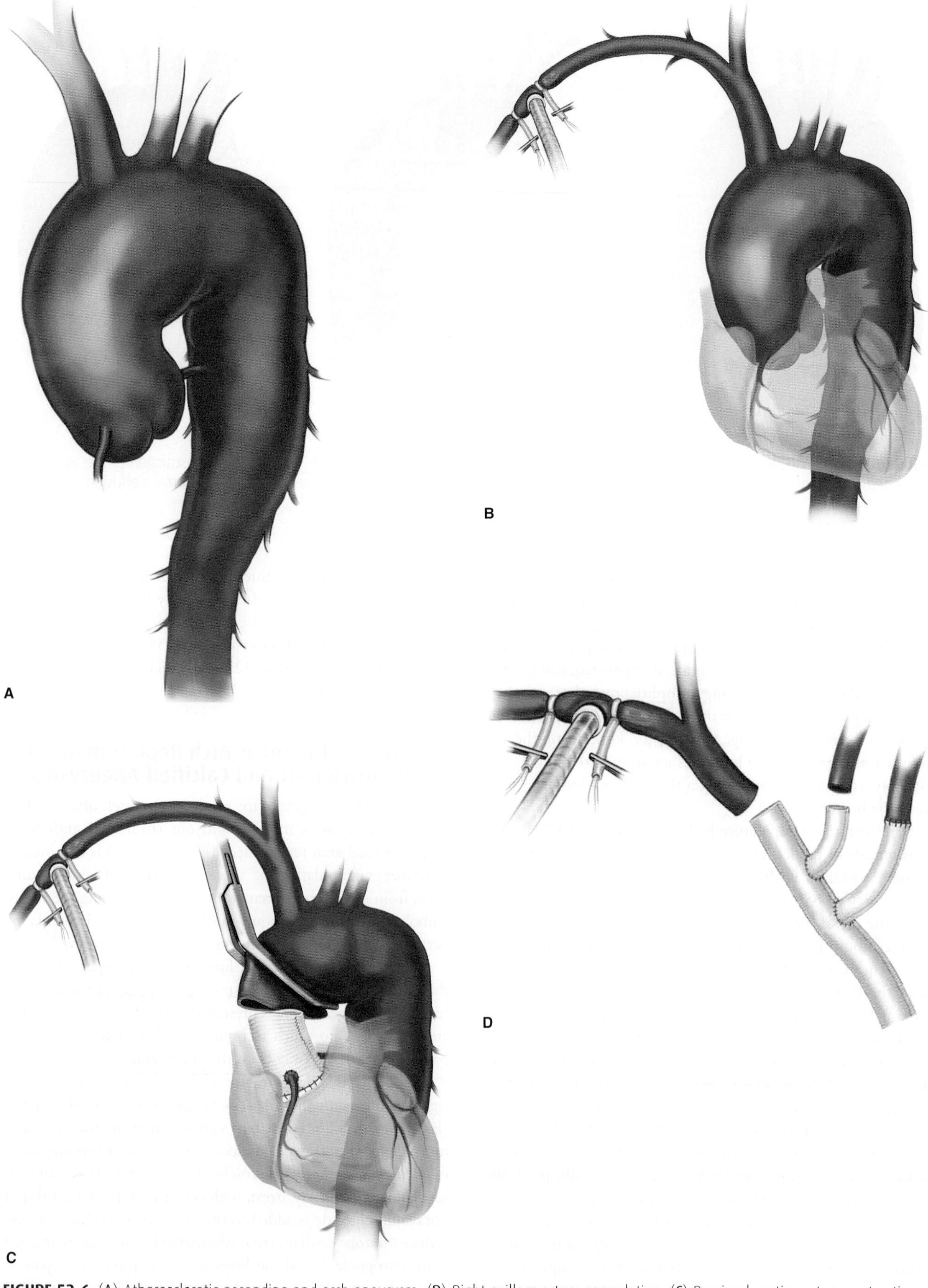

FIGURE 52-6 (A) Atherosclerotic ascending and arch aneurysm. (B) Right axillary artery cannulation. (C) Proximal aortic root reconstruction. (D) Trifurcated graft to the brachiocephalic arteries.

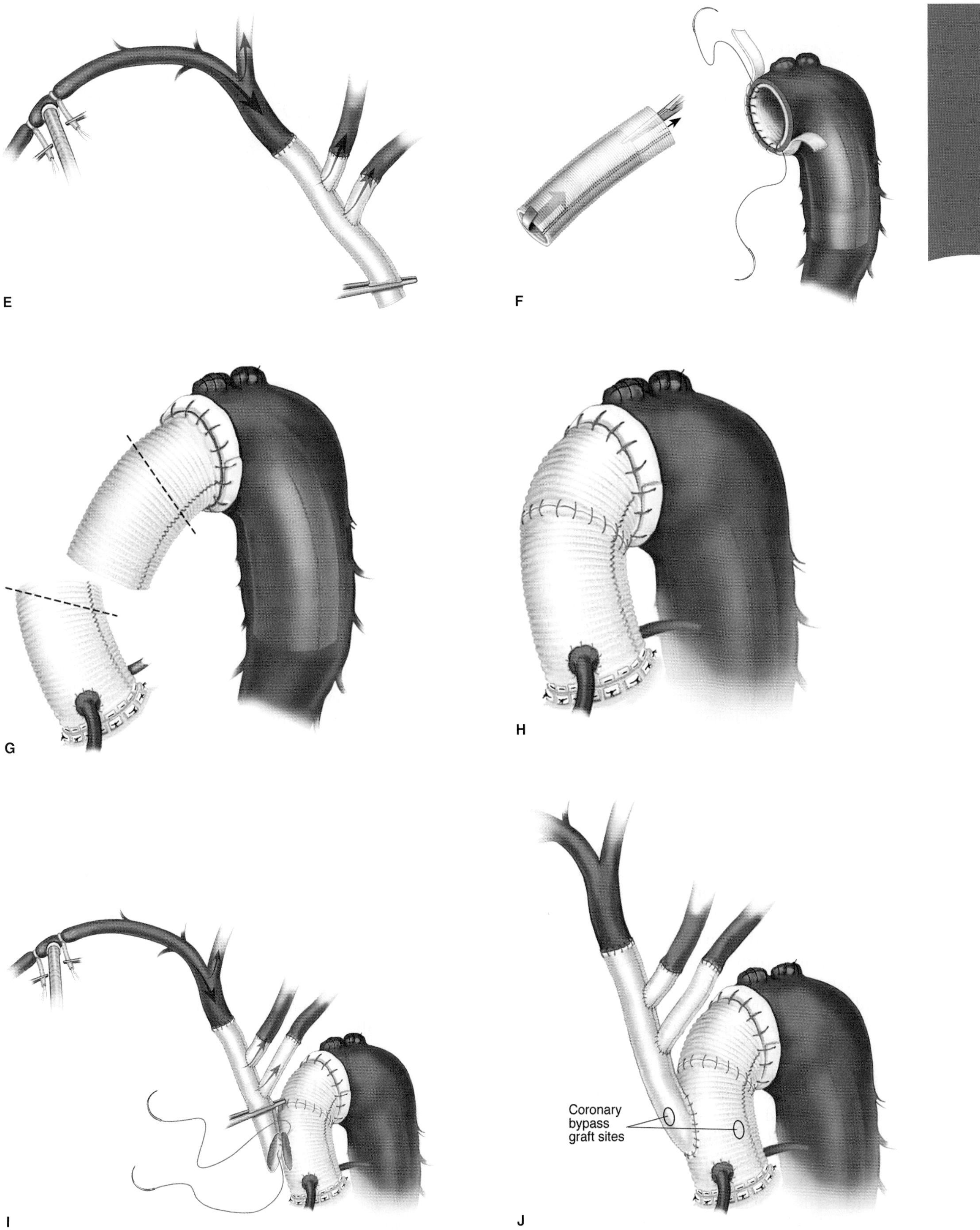

FIGURE 52-6 (E) Selective cerebral perfusion. (F) Construction of the elephant trunk. (G-H) Graft-to-graft anastomosis. (I) Trifurcated graft to ascending graft anastomosis. (J)Repair completed. (*Continued*)

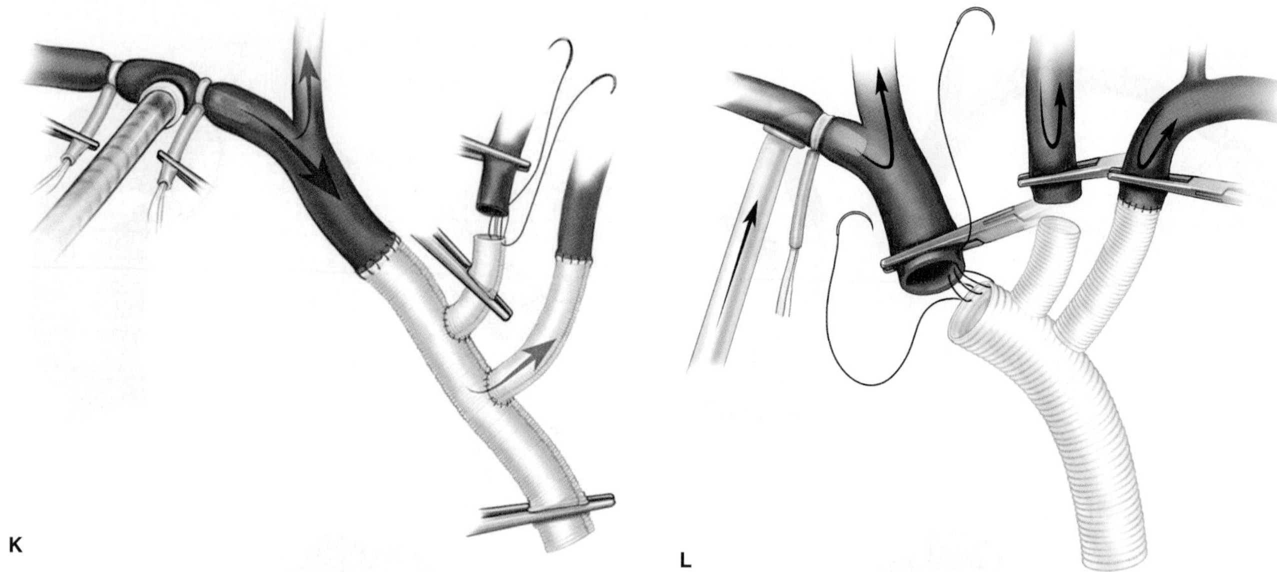

FIGURE 52-6 (K-L) Alternative sequence of brachiocephalic reconstruction to minimize DHCA. (*Continued*)

Even in patients with severe atherosclerotic disease of the AA, the arch vessels just beyond their origins are usually spared, making this location ideal for subsequent anastomoses. A trifurcated graft is chosen corresponding to the sizes of the innominate, left carotid, and left subclavian arteries. The patient is placed in Trendelenburg position to prevent air trapping and the head is packed in ice to prevent rewarming during HCA. When the esophageal temperature reaches 18°C, and jugular bulb oxygen saturation is greater than 95%, HCA is initiated and the arterial perfusion line is clamped to prevent back filling of air during HCA.

The innominate artery is transected just distal to its origin, or at the level where atherosclerosis is minimal, and using 5-0 polypropylene, is anastomosed to the large limb of the trifurcated graft, which is generally trimmed close to its origin. The common carotid and the left subclavian artery anastomoses are constructed in a similar fashion and each anastomosis takes 6 to 10 minutes. Reversing the order of anastomoses may provide better access to the left subclavian artery in some patients (Fig. 52-6D). After de-airing, the proximal portion of the trifurcation graft is clamped, restoring perfusion to the head and upper extremities (Fig. 52-6E). Perfusion pressures are maintained at 40 to 60 mm Hg, requiring flows between 600 and 1000 cc/min. The perfusate temperature is allowed to drift upward to 16 to 20°C at the end of HCA, but active rewarming is not initiated until AA reconstruction is complete.

Alternative strategies can shorten HCA. For example, if the left subclavian and innominate artery anastomoses are completed first, then SCP can be infused (at a lower flow rate: 400 to 600 cc/min) via the axillary artery while the left carotid, gently clamped, is anastomosed. This maneuver can reduce HCA time to less than 20 minutes (Fig. 52-6K), but with favorable anatomy, HCA can be avoided completely by gently clamping all the brachiocephalic arteries, and implanting them stepwise onto the trifurcated graft (Fig. 52-6L).

It is important for postoperative pulmonary toilet to preserve recurrent laryngeal nerve function. When reconstructing the arch, a suitable cuff of aortic tissue is maintained to preserve the recurrent laryngeal nerve. Aneurysmal disease involving the distal arch can be treated in two stages, avoiding potential laryngeal nerve injury, by constructing an elephant trunk[18,90,128] at a point in the distal ascending aorta or arch where the caliber permits. In this case, the transected brachiocephalic vessel origins are oversewn with 3-0 or 4-0 polypropylene; the "trunk anastomosis" is constructed with running 3-0 polypropylene, reinforced with a strip of Teflon felt (Fig. 52-6F). The proximal end of the elephant trunk graft is used to complete whatever root or ascending repair was undertaken; if a graft-to-graft anastomoses is required, it is constructed with 2-0 or 3-0 polypropylene, as these never heal and beveling both grafts helps to maintain the proper curvature (Fig. 52-6G,H). Next, the reconstructed aorta is distended to identify the appropriate site to attach the trifurcated graft, at which point an elliptical opening is made with ophthalmic electrocautery (Fig. 52-6I). This anastomosis is constructed with the trifurcated graft clamped, so that cerebral and upper extremity perfusion is uninterrupted. On completing this anastomosis, removing the clamp on the trifurcate graft restores full myocardial and systemic perfusion (Fig. 52-6J).

Case 3: Total Arch Replacement with an Aberrant Left Vertebral Artery

On occasion, the left vertebral artery (LVA) originates directly from the AA, posing a small challenge during arch reconstruction with a branched graft.[129] This anomaly can be recognized on CT angiography and should prompt a duplex ultrasound evaluation of the right vertebral artery (RVA) to ensure patency and antegrade flow. With a patent, normally sized RVA, the LVA can be temporarily occluded during SCP and reimplanted

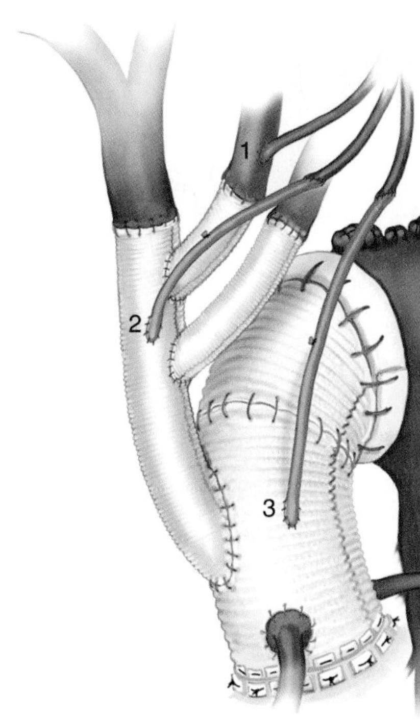

FIGURE 52-7 (A) Anomalous left vertebral artery exiting the aortic arch directly. (B) Three techniques for reconstruction.

during rewarming. Three options have been used (Fig. 52-7): direct reimplantation of the LVA into the left common carotid artery, attachment of a portion of reverse saphenous vein to the vertebral artery, and anastomosis to the arch graft or the left subclavian limb of the trifurcated graft. This last technique is essential if any question of the integrity of the RVA exists. A very small LVA (<2 mm) with a patent RVA may be ligated. Follow-up imaging studies have confirmed continued patency.

Case 4: Thoracosternotomy for Arch Reconstruction

Dr. Kouchoukos described a one-stage, repair, via a bilateral anterior thoracotomy, for patients with arch and proximal descending aortic disease, the "arch first" technique (Fig. 52-8A–G).[76,130] This approach provides excellent exposure of the transverse AA and proximal descending thoracic aorta, but requires sacrificing both internal mammary arteries. Brachiocephalic artery reconstruction can be achieved with a Carrel patch or a branched graft technique.

The heart and great vessels are exposed via bilateral thoracotomies in the fourth interspace and transverse sternotomy. The right atrium is cannulated and the circuit organized so that arterial return can be directed to a side arm graft sewn to the axillary artery (see Fig. 52-8A) or to a cannula in the right common femoral artery. CPB and profound systemic cooling are initiated, with arterial return directed via the axillary artery, and the heart is vented via the right superior pulmonary vein or LV apex. During cooling the brachiocephalic arteries are exposed, carefully preserving the recurrent laryngeal and phrenic nerves. The distal limit for resecting the descending aorta is identified and mobilized circumferentially.

At 18°C, HCA is initiated, the brachiocephalic arteries are transected and the distal aorta is clamped. The brachiocephalic arteries, backflushed by slowly perfusing the right axillary artery, are sequentially clamped, beginning with the left subclavian artery (Fig. 52-8B). SCP is administered via the right axillary artery and, with flow increased to 10 to 15 cc/kg/min at 20°C, lower-body perfusion is established via the femoral

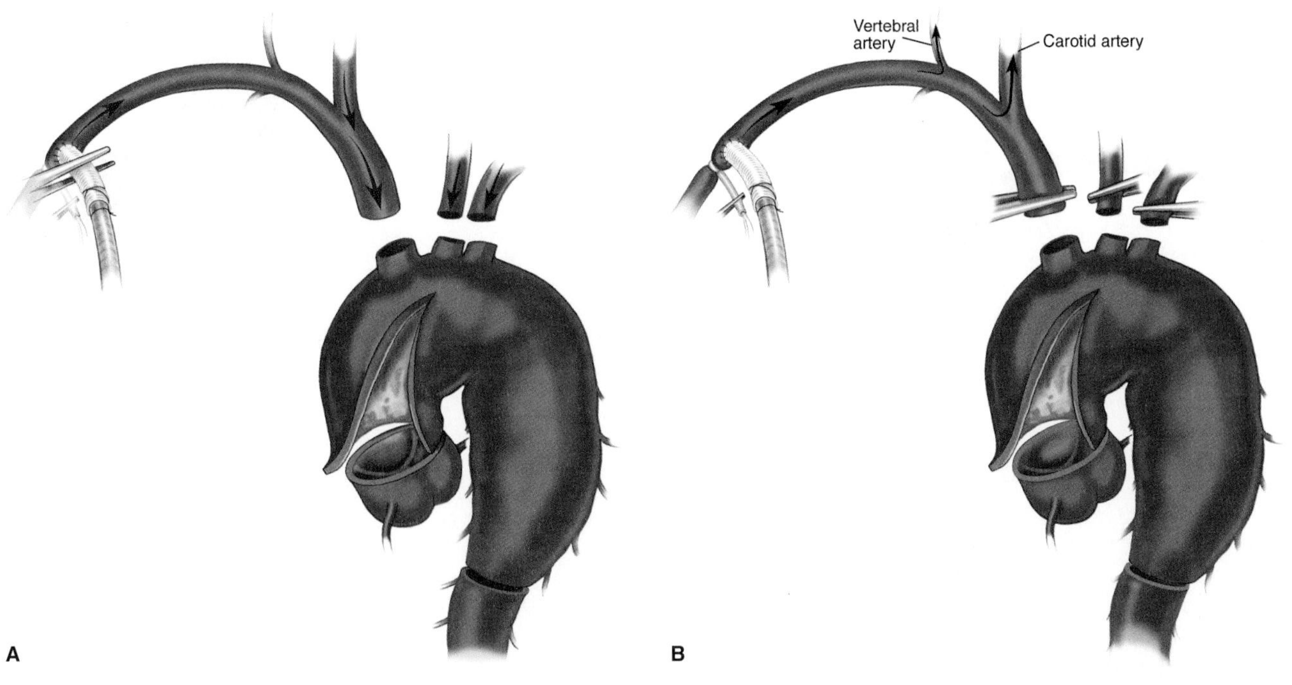

FIGURE 52-8 Arch first technique for aortic arch replacement via bilateral anterior thoracotomy as described by Dr. Kouchoukos.

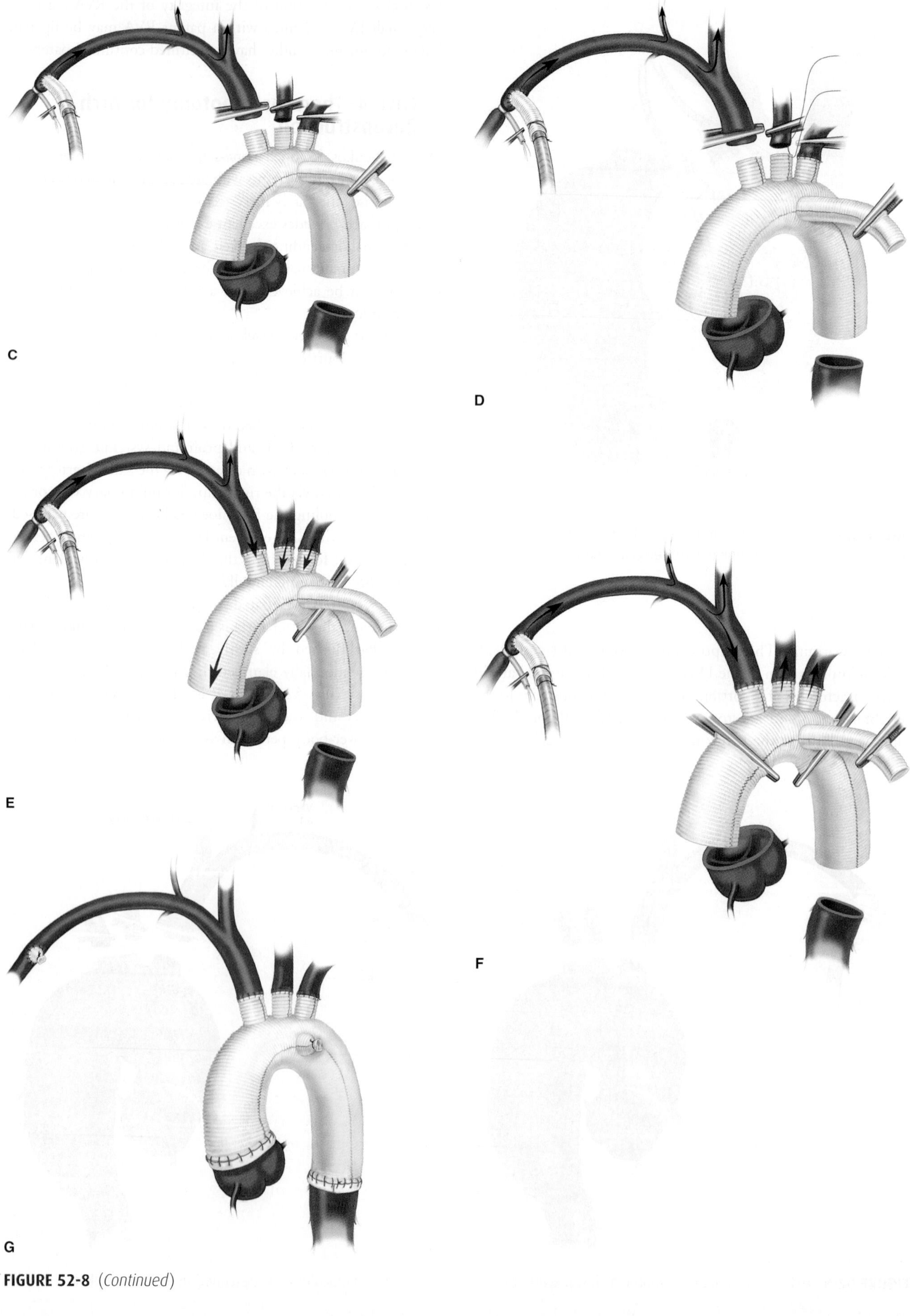

FIGURE 52-8 *(Continued)*

arterial line. The aneurysm is opened, preserving a cuff of aortic tissue containing the recurrent laryngeal nerve. Using a four-branched graft, the brachiocephalic arteries are reimplanted, beginning with the left subclavian artery and proceeding proximally (Fig. 52-8C,D); at this point axillary perfusion can be used to flush the arch vessels (Fig. 52-8E) and, by clamping the graft proximally and distally, to administer SCP (Fig. 52-8F). Lower-body perfusion is discontinued and, with the distal aortic clamp removed, an open distal anastomosis is created. Increasing pump flows, the clamp is withdrawn from the distal arch graft and the patient is rewarmed, flowing antegrade via the sidearm graft. A proximal anastomosis is then performed to complete the arch reconstruction (Fig. 52-8G).[131]

Case 5: Arch Replacement Following a Previous Bentall Procedure for Extensive Thoracic Aortic Aneurysmal Disease

AA replacement after previous ascending aortic surgery can be challenging, but a simple approach can facilitate repair and avoid pitfalls. The arch is exposed through the previous sternotomy and the brachiocephalic vessels are dissected free. The previous graft is not extensively dissected, as it risks injury to the pulmonary artery. The patient is cooled on CPB, established via the right atrium and right axillary artery, and the LV is vented. During HCA, a trifurcated graft is anastomosed to the brachiocephalic vessels, as previously described, followed by administering SCP. The arch vessel stumps are oversewn with pledgeted 3-0 polypropylene.

An elephant trunk is constructed proximal to the origin of the innominate artery, leaving a long "trunk" extending into the proximal descending aorta. If the reoperation is for residual chronic aortic dissection, the elephant trunk should not be longer than the distal fenestration, to allow perfusion of the true and false lumens. However, if the false lumen is partially filled with thrombus, the elephant trunk should be directed into the true lumen to avoid embolization, with no fenestration performed. The proximal anastomosis is constructed to the previous Bentall graft with 2-0 or 3-0 polypropylene. The trifurcated graft is then attached to an elliptical opening made in the right lateral side of the old Bentall graft (Fig. 52-9). The arch remains pressurized pending a second-stage repair, performed using either an open surgical or endograft approach. Using this technique, we have reduced our morbidity and mortality to values comparable to first-time arch replacement.

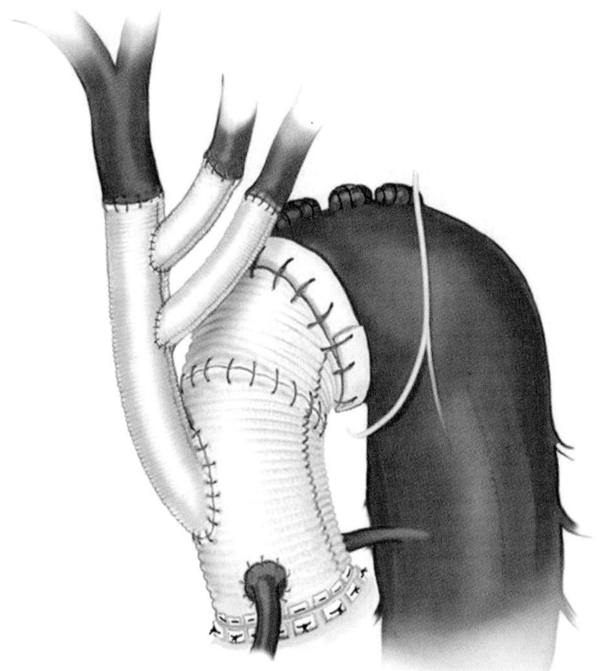

FIGURE 52-9 (A) Reoperative aortic arch aneurysm approached via median sternotomy. (B) Elephant trunk reconstruction proximal to the innominate artery. (C) Completed repair with a thoracic endograft placed retrograde.

Case 6: Descending Thoracic Aortic Aneurysm Involving the Distal Arch

Descending thoracic aortic aneurysms often involve the distal AA (Fig. 52-10A). If not severely calcified or atherosclerotic, in which case we prefer a two-stage reconstruction to isolate the cerebral circulation and reduce the risk of embolic stroke, we approach these with the following technique.

A left thoracotomy is performed in the fifth or sixth intercostal space and, if necessary, extended inferiorly across the costochondral plate to improve exposure. The descending aorta is gradually mobilized, serially clamping and sacrificing intercostal arteries, if SSEPs and MEPs do not change[132]; care is taken not to manipulate the arch adjacent to the left subclavian artery. The right atrium is generally cannulated via the left common femoral vein, but the main pulmonary artery can also be used for venous inflow. The left common femoral artery is cannulated for arterial return. Perfusion is begun gradually to avoid flow shifts in the aorta that might dislodge atheromatous debris and during CPB manipulating the aorta is minimized, as dislodged debris will be carried retrograde toward the arch vessels and coronary arteries. Alternatively, CPB with antegrade flow can be established by perfusing through an 8- or 10-mm PTFE ring-reinforced graft sewn to the right axillary artery, an arrangement that also permits SCP. During cooling, and particularly after ventricular fibrillation has occurred, any indication of LV distention by TEE or pulmonary artery pressure monitoring warrants LV venting via the LV apex or left atrium. Core cooling is continued until the esophageal temperature has decreased to 18°C and the jugular venous saturation has reached 95%, which generally takes 30 to 40 minutes. At this point, 60 mEq of KCL is slowly added to the pump perfusate, inducing diastolic cardiac arrest, and, with the LV vent clamped, HCA is initiated.

The descending aorta is opened, creating a beveled cuff under the arch, while preserving the recurrent laryngeal nerve. A "reverse hemiarch" anastomosis is created, using a sidearm graft (Fig. 52-10B). The brachiocephalic vessels are gently aspirated and, to facilitate de-airing and removal of debris, the cardioplegia line is attached to the LV vent and cold blood is infused at approximately 400 cc/min to flush out the LV, ascending aorta and arch. Alternatively, continuous perfusion of the lower body will maintain some collateral flow into the brachiocephalic vessels and assist in removal of air and particulate debris. At this point, perfusion is restored to the brachiocephalic and coronary arteries by flowing through the sidearm graft, with the main graft and subclavian artery clamped.

The distal anastomosis is constructed to the descending aorta after a brief period of femoral perfusion to flush debris. The clamp on the graft is removed, restoring flow to the entire body. During rewarming, an 8- or 10-mm graft is sewn to the left subclavian artery and anastomosed to the descending graft (Fig. 52-10C,D).

SSEP and MEP monitoring is continued to the conclusion of the operation and arterial pressures are maintained in the high normal range. The evoked potentials gradually return, but initially are below baseline because of systemic hypothermia. Depending on the extent of resection, an intrathecal catheter, placed preoperatively, is used to drain CSF in order to maintain the CSF pressure below 12 mm Hg for the first 48 to 72 hours.

Case 7: Hybrid Aortic Arch Repair for Distal Arch Aneurysms

Although aortic arch debranching can be performed off pump, it is safer to use CPB for the difficult anatomies encountered in many patients. Moreover, the off-pump approach requires placing

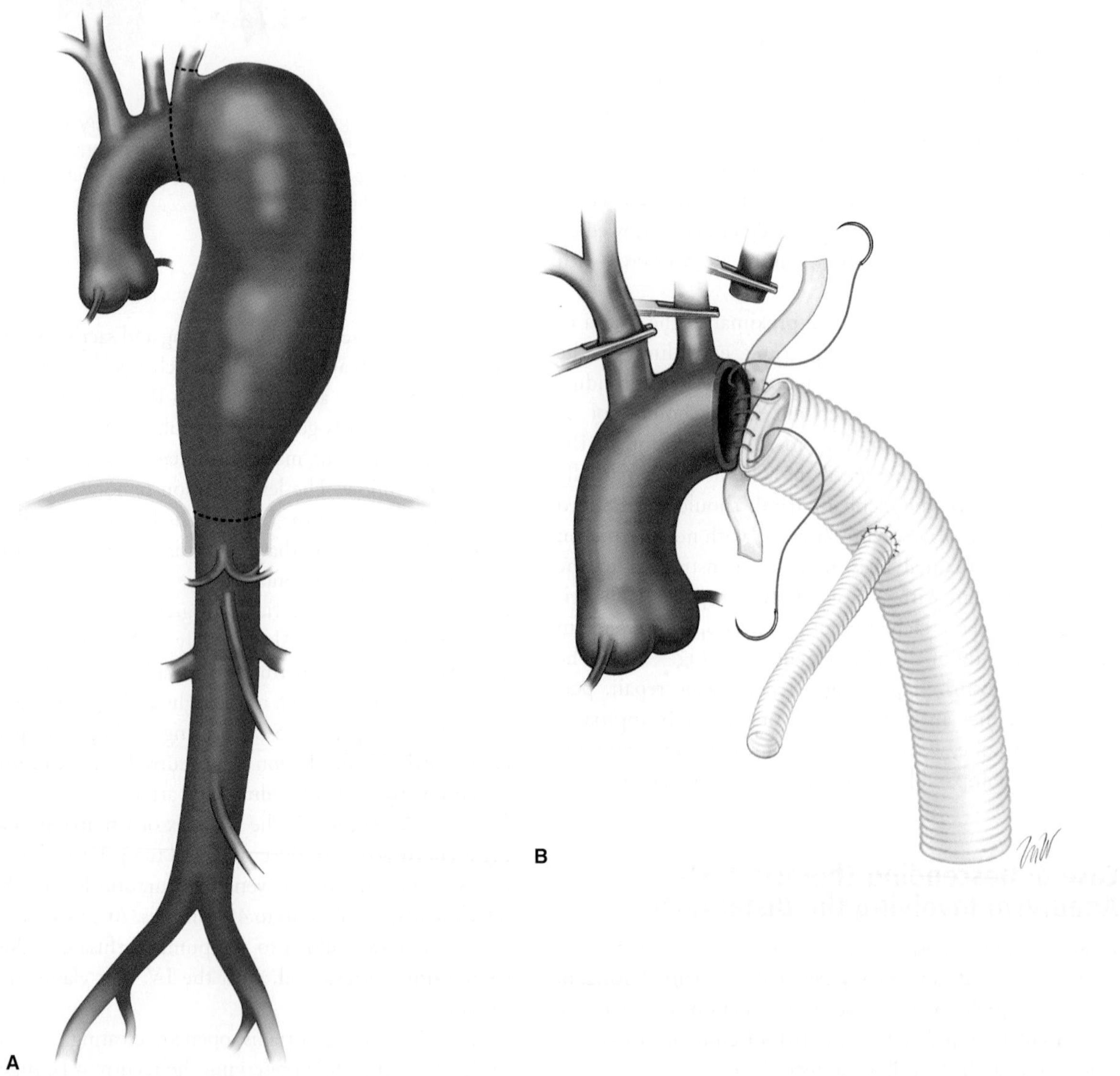

FIGURE 52-10 (A) Distal arch descending thoracic aortic aneurysm with femoral artery perfusion. (B) Hypothermic circulatory arrest and anastomosis to the distal arch. (C) Selective cerebral perfusion via a sidearm graft. (D) Reattachment of the left subclavian artery and completed repair.

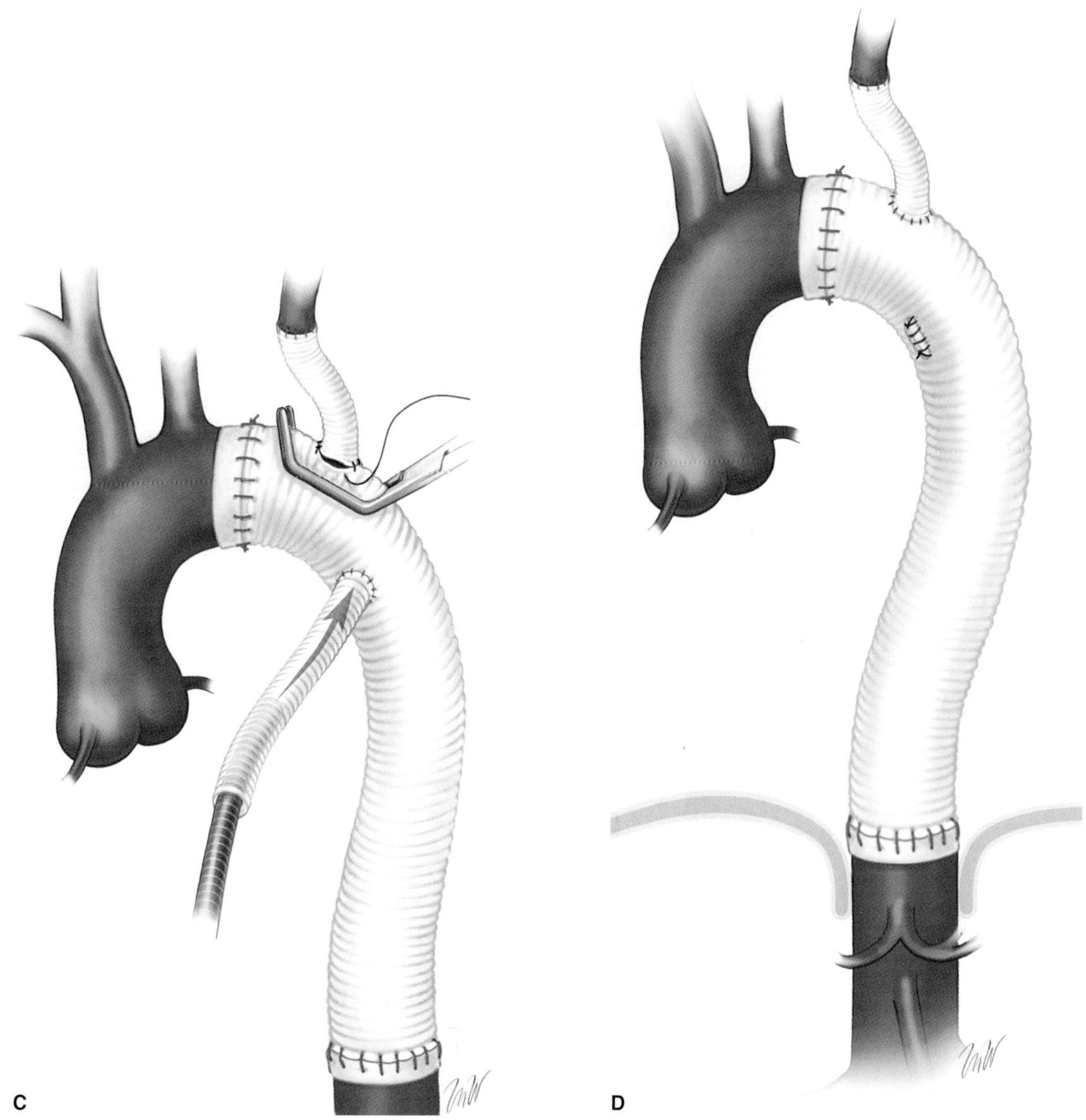

FIGURE 52-10 *(Continued)*

a side-biting clamp on the pulsatile ascending aorta, posing a risk for intimal injury and subsequent aortic dissection.

On CPB, using a side-biting clamp, the main portion of a trifurcated graft is anastomosed to the ascending aorta with 4-0 polypropylene (Fig. 52-11A). The left subclavian artery, clamped, divided, and either stapled or oversewn proximally, is anastomosed to a limb of the trifurcated graft with 5-0 polypropylene, after which perfusion is restored. Similarly, the left common carotid and innominate arteries are attached to the remaining limbs. Temporary occlusion of each brachiocephalic artery is well tolerated, with no significant reduction in cerebral oximetry. If antegrade endograft deployment is planned, the trifurcated graft is modified by adding a proximal sidearm graft for access (see Fig. 52-11A). Difficult subclavian artery anatomy can be avoided by performing a preoperative carotid-subclavian bypass (Fig. 52-11B) or an intraoperative extra-anatomic bypass to the left axillary artery, tunneled through the first or second intercostal space (Fig. 52-11C).

RESULTS

Recent series of total AA replacements compare favorably with our results. Safi and associates[133] reported 5.1% 30-day mortality in 117 stage I elephant trunk reconstructions, with 6.8% adverse outcomes. Interestingly, 37% of patients did not return for second-stage repair, and 30.2% died from distal aneurysm rupture during short-term follow-up. Schepens and associates,[134] in 100 consecutive stage I elephant trunk reconstructions from 1984 to 2001, reported 8% mortality, 12% adverse outcomes, and 2% TND; the majority of these patients received unilateral or bilateral antegrade SCP for cerebral protection. Coselli and associates,[135]

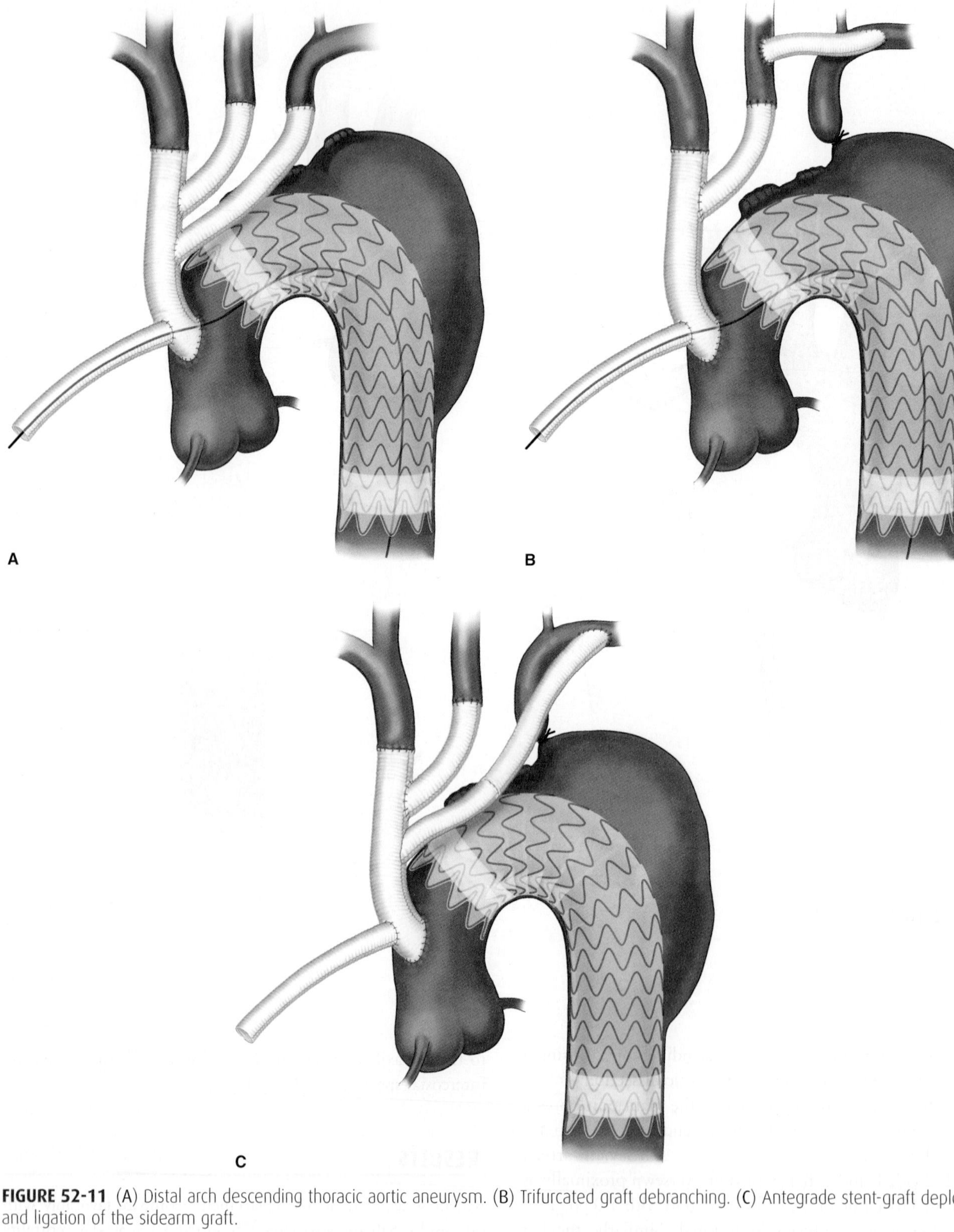

FIGURE 52-11 (A) Distal arch descending thoracic aortic aneurysm. (B) Trifurcated graft debranching. (C) Antegrade stent-graft deployment and ligation of the sidearm graft.

in a series of 227 patients with AA surgery, reported 6% early and 9% late mortality, with 3% stroke, attributing a relatively low incidence of reduction in neurologic injury to using RCP during HCA in more than 50% of cases. LeMaire and associates reported impressive results for 55 total arch replacements using the trifurcated graft; despite 60% reoperations, there were no in-hospital mortalities, with one 30-day death, and three perioperative CVAs, one of which was transient.[136] Kazui and associates,[74] in their contemporary series of 50 patients, also achieved outstanding results: 2% mortality, 6% adverse outcome, and 4% TND. CPB duration was the only univariate risk factor for TND and a history of CVA was correlated with permanent neurologic dysfunction. Di Eusanio and associates,[73] published a multicenter study using antegrade SCP for total arch replacement in 352 patients, wherein there was 8.7% in-hospital mortality, 3.8% permanent strokes, 5.6% TND, and 12.5% adverse outcome. Independent predictors of adverse outcomes included urgent operation, recent stroke, tamponade, unplanned coronary revascularization, and pump time. Finally, Numata and associates,[137] using right axillary perfusion and a separate cannula in the left common carotid artery for 120 arch replacements, achieved excellent results: 5.8% mortality and 0.8% permanent stroke rate, with 5.8% TND.

From our prospectively compiled database, we identified 206 consecutive patients (125 males, 81 females) between September 1999 and September 2009, who underwent elective arch replacement with a trifurcated graft, using a brief interval of HCA (30 minutes [17 to 48]), followed by hypothermic SCP (69 minutes [21 to 125]; 15.8°C [12.0 to 22.1]), administered via direct axillary artery cannulation. The mean age was 67 (20 to 87 years), the most frequent etiology (37.3%) was chronic dissection, and 32.0% had atherosclerosis. Known risk factors included chronic obstructive pulmonary disease (13.6%), insulin-dependent diabetes (4.9%), hemodialysis (4.9%), and reoperations (44.2%). Potential risk factors for postoperative neurologic injury include a history of transient ischemic attack (2.4%) and preoperative stroke (9.2%).

The mean maximum aortic diameter was 6.0 cm (4.0 to 12 cm). Isolated arch replacement was undertaken in 23.8%; concomitantly resected segments included the ascending aorta (49.5%), ascending aorta and aortic root (12.6%), and the descending aorta (3.9%). Concomitant procedures included elephant trunk procedures (92.2%) and CABG (25.7%).

Hospital mortality was 6.8%, with 10.1% adverse outcomes and 3.3% permanent strokes. Postoperative complications included prolonged (>48 hours) intubation (13.1%), TND (5.8%; not correlating with preoperative neurologic risk factors), reoperation for bleeding (5.3%), and temporary (4.4%) or permanent (1%) renal support. The median ICU stay was 3 days (1 to 108 days) and hospital stay was 11 days (4 to 108 days).

The two facets of neurologic protection—prevention of cerebral injury during global ischemia and avoidance of particulate atheroemboli—are not mutually exclusive and the overall neurologic protection strategy must be an integral part of the AA replacement technique. To this end, two surgical strategies have emerged to balance the neurologic risks: the four-branched graft technique[73,138,139] and the trifurcated graft technique.[91] As compared with the classic Carrell patch technique,[39] both reduce HCA and use SCP.

LONG-TERM FOLLOW-UP

Generally, AA aneurysms are localized manifestations of a diffuse aortic disease process and therefore monitoring unresected segments following aortic surgery is a sensible precaution. Accordingly, we offer our patients a follow-up program and maintain a prospective database of all aneurysm patients. Patients with small aneurysms are advised to have ongoing imaging at 1- to 2-year intervals, depending on the aneurysm's etiology, location, and rate of progression. Postoperative patients receive a baseline CT angiogram or MRA to assess the repair and provide a baseline for later comparison. If no portion of the unresected aorta exceeds 4 cm, the first reevaluation is scheduled for 1 year, but a significant residual dissection or aneurysmal dilatation merits follow-up in 6 months.

Survival at 1 year is 74% in our trifurcated graft series, reflecting failure to return for a second stage, rupture before the second stage, and mortality from second stage. Among patients alive a 1 year, survival at 3 and 5 years is 94% and 78%.

Numerous publications confirm the importance of continued surveillance after AA surgery. Crawford and associates[140] found that 70% of patients with AA operations had significant disease elsewhere in the aorta, Coselli and associates documented that 15% of 227 patients with AA repairs required additional surgery within 17 months,[135] and Heinemann and associates[141] reoperated on 24% of 82 patients with type A dissection over a 10-year period. Detter and associates,[142] examining the long-term prognosis of aortic aneurysm in patients with and without Marfan's syndrome, found reoperations in 66.7% versus 10.7%; late mortality was 25% versus 14%, with 18% caused by redissection and recurrent aneurysm in the Marfan's group. In our follow-up of 162 patients post-repair of type A aortic dissection, 17% required reoperations: 23 distal and 4 proximal.[143]

REFERENCES

1. Elefteriades JA: Natural history of thoracic aortic aneurysms: indications for surgery, and surgical versus nonsurgical risks. *Ann Thorac Surg* 2002; 74:1877S-1880.
2. Strauch JT, Spielvogel D, Lauten A, et al: Axillary artery cannulation: routine use in ascending aorta and aortic arch replacement. *Ann Thorac Surg* 2004; 78:103-108.
3. Pasic M, Schubel J, Bauer M, et al: Cannulation of the right axillary artery for surgery of acute type A aortic dissection. *Eur J Cardiothorac Surg* 2003; 24:231-236.
4. Moizumi Y, Motoyoshi N, Sakuma K, Yoshida S: Axillary artery cannulation improves operative results for acute type A aortic dissection. *Ann Thorac Surg* 2005; 80:77-83.
5. Sabik JF, Nemeh H, Lytle BW, et al: Cannulation of the axillary artery with a side graft reduces morbidity. *Ann Thorac Surg* 2004; 77:1315-1320.
6. Orihashi K, Sueda T, Okada K, Imai K: Near-infrared spectroscopy for monitoring cerebral ischemia during selective cerebral perfusion. *Eur J Cardiothorac Surg* 2004; 26:907-911.
7. Orihashi K, Sueda T, Okada K, Imai K: Malposition of selective cerebral perfusion catheter is not a rare event. *Eur J Cardiothorac Surg* 2005; 27: 644-648.
8. Olsson C, Thelin S: Regional cerebral saturation monitoring with near-infrared spectroscopy during selective antegrade cerebral perfusion: diagnostic performance and relationship to postoperative stroke. *J Thorac Cardiovasc Surg* 2006; 131:371-379.
9. Kamiya H, Klima U, Hagl C, et al: Cerebral microembolization during antegrade selective cerebral perfusion. *Ann Thorac Surg* 2006; 81:519-521.
10. Griepp EB, Griepp RB: Cerebral consequences of hypothermic circulatory arrest in adults. *J Cardiac Surg* 1992; 7:134-155.
11. Anderson R, Siegman M, Balaban R, Ceckler T, Swain J: Hyperglycemia increases cerebral intracellular acidosis during circulatory arrest [published erratum appears in *Ann Thorac Surg* 1993; 55(4):1054]. *Ann Thorac Surg* 1992; 54:1126-1130.
12. Watanabe T, Oshikiri N, Inui K, et al: Optimal blood flow for cooled brain at 20°C. *Ann Thorac Surg* 1999; 68:864-869.
13. Halstead JC, Spielvogel D, Meier DM, et al: Optimal pH strategy for selective cerebral perfusion. *Eur J Cardiothorac Surg* 2005; 28:266-273.
14. Washiyama N, Kazui T, Takinami M, et al: Experimental study on the effect of antegrade cerebral perfusion on brains with old cerebral infarction. *J Thorac Cardiovasc Surg* 2001; 122:734-740.
15. Kouchoukos N: One stage repair of extensive thoracic aortic aneurysm using the arch-first technique and bilateral thoracotomy. *Op Techn Thorac Cardiovasc Surg* 2008; 13:220-231.

16. Klieverik LMA, Yacoub MH, Edwards S, et al: Surgical treatment of active native aortic valve endocarditis with allografts and mechanical prostheses. *Ann Thorac Surg* 2009; 88:1814-1821.
17. Heiro M, Helenius H, Sundell J, et al: Utility of serum C-reactive protein in assessing the outcome of infective endocarditis. *Eur Heart J* 2005; 26: 1873-1881.
18. Borst HG, Walterbusch G, Schaps D: Extensive aortic replacement using "elephant trunk" prosthesis. *Thorac Cardiovasc Surg* 1983; 31:37-40.
19. Kaukuntla H, Harrington D, Bilkoo I, et al: Temperature monitoring during cardiopulmonary bypass—do we undercool or overheat the brain? *Eur J Cardiothorac Surg* 2004; 26:580-585.
20. Ehrlich MP, McCullough J, Wolfe D, et al: Cerebral effects of cold reperfusion after hypothermic circulatory arrest. *J Thorac Cardiovasc Surg* 2001; 121:923-931.
21. Shum-Tim D, Nagashima M, Shinoka T, et al: Postischemic hyperthermia exacerbates neurologic injury after deep hypothermic circulatory arrest. *J Thorac Cardiovasc Surg* 1998; 116:780-792.
22. Strauch JT, Spielvogel D, Lansman SL, et al: Long-term integrity of Teflon felt-supported suture lines in aortic surgery. *Ann Thorac Surg* 2005; 79:796-800.
23. Lansman SL, Cohen M, Galla JD, et al: Coronary bypass with ejection fraction of 0.20 or less using centigrade cardioplegia: long-term follow-up. *Ann Thorac Surg* 1993; 56:480-485; discussion 5-6.
24. Jacobs MJ, de Mol BA, Elenbaas T, et al: Spinal cord blood supply in patients with thoracoabdominal aortic aneurysms. *J Vasc Surg* 2002; 35:30-37.
25. de Haan PKC: Spinal cord monitoring: somatosensory and motor-evoked potentials. *Anesthesiol Clin North Am* 2001; 19:923-945.
26. Galla JD, Ergin MA, Sadeghi AM, et al: A new technique using somatosensory evoked potential guidance during descending and thoracoabdominal aortic repairs. *J Cardiac Surg* 1994; 9:662-672.
27. Griepp RB, Ergin MA, Galla JD, et al: Looking for the artery of Adamkiewicz: a quest to minimize paraplegia after operations for aneurysms of the descending thoracic and thoracoabdominal aorta. *J Thorac Cardiovasc Surg* 1996; 112:1202-1213; discussion 13-15.
28. Moskowitz DM, McCullough JN, Shander A, et al: The impact of blood conservation on outcomes in cardiac surgery: is it safe and effective? *Ann Thorac Surg* 2010; 90:451-458.
29. Hoover EL, Hsu HK, Ergin A, et al: Left-to-right shunts in control of bleeding following surgery for aneurysms of the ascending aorta. *Chest* 1987; 91:844-849.
30. Halkos ME, Levy JH, Chen E, et al: Early experience with activated recombinant factor vii for intractable hemorrhage after cardiovascular surgery. *Ann Thorac Surg* 2005; 79:1303-1306.
31. Kazui T, Washiyama N, Bashar AH, et al: Role of biologic glue repair of proximal aortic dissection in the development of early and midterm redissection of the aortic root. *Ann Thorac Surg* 2001; 72:509-514.
32. Kirsch M, Ginat M, Lecerf L, Houel R, Loisance D: Aortic wall alterations after use of gelatin-resorcinol-formalin glue. *Ann Thorac Surg* 2002; 73:642-644.
33. Raanani E, Georghiou GP, Kogan A, et al: 'BioGlue' for the repair of aortic insufficiency in acute aortic dissection. *J Heart Valve Dis* 2004; 13:734-737.
34. LeMaire SA, Carter SA, Won T, et al: The threat of adhesive embolization: bioglue leaks through needle holes in aortic tissue and prosthetic grafts. *Ann Thorac Surg* 2005; 80:106-111.
35. Muller BT WO, Grabitz K, et al: Mycotic aneurysms of the thoracic and abdominal aorta and iliac arteries: experience with anatomic and extra-anatomic repair in 33 cases. *J Vasc Surg* 2001; 33:106-113.
36. Avierinos J-F, Thuny F, Chalvignac V, et al: Surgical treatment of active aortic endocarditis: homografts are not the cornerstone of outcome. *Ann Thorac Surg* 2007; 84:1935-1942.
37. Borst HG, Schaudig A, Rudolph W: Arteriovenous fistula of the aortic arch: repair during deep hypothermia and circulatory arrest. *J Thorac Cardiovasc Surg* 1964; 48:443-447.
38. Barratt-Boyes BG, Simpson M, Neutze JM: Intracardiac surgery in neonates and infants using deep hypothermia with surface cooling and limited cardiopulmonary bypass. *Circulation* 1971; 43:I25-30.
39. Griepp RB, Stinson EB, Hollingsworth JF, Buehler D: Prosthetic replacement of the aortic arch. *J Thorac Cardiovasc Surg* 1975; 70:1051-1063.
40. Michenfelder JD, Theye RA: Hypothermia: effect on canine brain and whole-body metabolism. *Anesthesiology* 1968; 29:1107-1112.
41. Michenfelder JD, Milde JH: The relationship among canine brain temperature, metabolism, and function during hypothermia. *Anesthesiology* 1991; 75:130-136.
42. Mault JR, Ohtake S, Klingensmith ME, et al: Cerebral metabolism and circulatory arrest: effects of duration and strategies for protection. *Ann Thorac Surg* 1993; 55:57-63; discussion 4.
43. Mezrow CK, Midulla PS, Sadeghi AM, et al: Evaluation of cerebral metabolism and quantitative electroencephalography after hypothermic circulatory arrest and low-flow cardiopulmonary bypass at different temperatures. *J Thorac Cardiovasc Surg* 1994; 107:1006-1019.
44. Mezrow CK, Midulla PS, Sadeghi AM, et al: Quantitative electroencephalography: a method to assess cerebral injury after hypothermic circulatory arrest. *J Thorac Cardiovasc Surg* 1995; 109:925-934.
45. Midulla PS, Gandsas A, Sadeghi AM, et al: Comparison of retrograde cerebral perfusion to antegrade cerebral perfusion and hypothermic circulatory arrest in a chronic porcine model. *J Cardiac Surg* 1994; 9:560-574; discussion 75.
46. Mezrow CK, Gandsas A, Sadeghi AM, et al: Metabolic correlates of neurologic and behavioral injury after prolonged hypothermic circulatory arrest. *J Thorac Cardiovasc Surg* 1995; 109:959-975.
47. Mezrow C, Sadeghi A, Gandsas A, et al: Cerebral blood flow and metabolism in hypothermic circulatory arrest. *Ann Thorac Surg* 1992; 54:609-615.
48. Svensson L, Crawford E, Hess K, et al: Deep hypothermia with circulatory arrest. Determinants of stroke and early mortality in 656 patients. *J Thorac Cardiovasc Surg* 1993; 106:19-28.
49. Ergin MA, Galla JD, Lansman SL, et al: Hypothermic circulatory arrest in operations on the thoracic aorta. Determinants of operative mortality and neurologic outcome. *J Thorac Cardiovasc Surg* 1994; 107:788-799.
50. Hagl C, Ergin MA, Galla JD, et al: Neurologic outcome after ascending aorta-aortic arch operations: effect of brain protection technique in high-risk patients. *J Thorac Cardiovasc Surg* 2001; 121:1107-1121.
51. Fleck TM, Czerny M, Hutschala D, et al: The incidence of transient neurologic dysfunction after ascending aortic replacement with circulatory arrest. *Ann Thorac Surg* 2003; 76:1198-1202.
52. Svensson LG, Crawford ES, Hess KR, et al: Deep hypothermia with circulatory arrest. Determinants of stroke and early mortality in 656 patients. *J Thorac Cardiovasc Surg* 1993; 106:19-28; discussion 31.
53. Reich DL, Uysal S, Sliwinski M, et al: Neuropsychologic outcome after deep hypothermic circulatory arrest in adults. *J Thorac Cardiovasc Surg* 1999; 117:156-163.
54. Ergin MA, Uysal S, Reich DL, et al: Temporary neurological dysfunction after deep hypothermic circulatory arrest: a clinical marker of long-term functional deficit. *Ann Thorac Surg* 1999; 67:1887-1890; discussion 91-94.
55. McCullough JN, Zhang N, Reich DL, et al: Cerebral metabolic suppression during hypothermic circulatory arrest in humans. *Ann Thorac Surg* 1999; 67:1895-1899; discussion 919-921.
56. Wypij D, Newburger JW, Rappaport LA, et al: The effect of duration of deep hypothermic circulatory arrest in infant heart surgery on late neurodevelopment: The Boston Circulatory Arrest Trial. *J Thorac Cardiovasc Surg* 2003; 126:1397-1403.
57. Mezrow CK, Midulla P, Sadeghi A, et al: A vulnerable interval for cerebral injury: comparison of hypothermic circulatory arrest and low-flow cardiopulmonary bypass. *Cardiol Young* 1993; 3:287-298.
58. Kawata H, Fackler JC, Aoki M, et al: Recovery of cerebral blood flow and energy state in piglets after hypothermic circulatory arrest versus recovery after low-flow bypass. *J Thorac Cardiovasc Surg* 1993; 106:671-685.
59. Langley SM, Chai PJ, Jaggers JJ, Ungerleider RM: Preoperative high dose methylprednisolone attenuates the cerebral response to deep hypothermic circulatory arrest. *Eur J Cardiothorac Surg* 2000; 17:279-286.
60. Shum-Tim D, Tchervenkov CI, Jamal AM, et al: Systemic steroid pretreatment improves cerebral protection after circulatory arrest. *Ann Thorac Surg* 2001; 72:1465-1471; discussion 71-72.
61. Temesvari P, Joo F, Koltai M, et al: Cerebroprotective effect of dexamethasone by increasing the tolerance to hypoxia and preventing brain oedema in newborn piglets with experimental pneumothorax. *Neurosci Lett* 1984; 49:87-92.
62. Cronstein BN, Kimmel SC, Levin RI, Martiniuk F, Weissmann G: A mechanism for the antiinflammatory effects of corticosteroids: the glucocorticoid receptor regulates leukocyte adhesion to endothelial cells and expression of endothelial-leukocyte adhesion molecule 1 and intercellular adhesion molecule 1. *Proc Natl Acad Sci U S A* 1992; 89:9991-9995.
63. Lodge AJ, Chai PJ, Daggett CW, Ungerleider RM, Jaggers J: Methylprednisolone reduces the inflammatory response to cardiopulmonary bypass in neonatal piglets: timing of dose is important. *J Thorac Cardiovasc Surg* 1999; 117:515-522.
64. Jonassen AE, Quaegebeur JM, Young WL: Cerebral blood flow velocity in pediatric patients is reduced after cardiopulmonary bypass with profound hypothermia. *J Thorac Cardiovasc Surg* 1995; 110:934-943.
65. DeBakey ME, Crawford E, Cooley DA, Morris GC: Successful resection of fusiform aneurysm of the aortic arch with replacement homograft. *Surg Gynecol Obstet* 1957; 105:657-654.
66. Frist W, Baldwin JC, Starnes VA, et al: A reconsideration of cerebral perfusion in aortic arch replacement. *Ann Thorac Surg* 1986; 42.

67. Swain JA, McDonald TJ Jr, Griffith PK, et al: Low-flow hypothermic cardiopulmonary bypass protects the brain. *J Thorac Cardiovasc Surg* 1991; 102:76-83; discussion 4.
68. Bachet J, Guilmet D, Goudot B, et al: Cold cerebroplegia. A new technique of cerebral protection during operations on the transverse aortic arch. *J Thorac Cardiovasc Surg* 1991; 102:85-93; discussion 4.
69. Matsuda H, Nakano S, Shirakura R, et al: Surgery for aortic arch aneurysm with selective cerebral perfusion and hypothermic cardiopulmonary bypass. *Circulation* 1989; 80:I243-248.
70. Kazui T, Inoue N, Komatsu S: Surgical treatment of aneurysms of the transverse aortic arch. *J Cardiovasc Surg (Torino)* 1989; 30:402-406.
71. Kazui T, Washiyama N, Muhammad BA, et al: Total arch replacement using aortic arch branched grafts with the aid of antegrade selective cerebral perfusion. *Ann Thorac Surg* 2000; 70:3-8; discussion 9.
72. Kazui T, Inoue N, Yamada O, Komatsu S: Selective cerebral perfusion during operation for aneurysms of the aortic arch: a reassessment. *Ann Thorac Surg* 1992; 53:109-114.
73. Di Eusanio M, Schepens MA, Morshuis WJ, et al: Brain protection using antegrade selective cerebral perfusion: a multicenter study. *Ann Thorac Surg* 2003; 76:1181-1189.
74. Kazui T, Washiyama N, Muhammad BA, et al: Improved results of atherosclerotic arch aneurysm operations with a refined technique. *J Thorac Cardiovasc Surg* 2001; 121:491-499.
75. Rokkas CK, Kouchoukos NT: Single-stage extensive replacement of the thoracic aorta: the arch-first technique. *J Thorac Cardiovasc Surg* 1999; 117:99-105.
76. Kouchoukos NT, Mauney MC, Masetti P, Castner CF: Single-stage repair of extensive thoracic aortic aneurysms: experience with the arch-first technique and bilateral anterior thoracotomy. *J Thorac Cardiovasc Surg* 2004; 128:669-676.
77. Kouchoukos NT, Masetti P: Total aortic arch replacement with a branched graft and limited circulatory arrest of the brain. *J Thorac Cardiovasc Surg* 2004; 128:233-237.
78. Kucuker SA, Ozatik MA, Saritas A, Tasdemir O: Arch repair with unilateral antegrade cerebral perfusion. *Eur J Cardiothorac Surg* 2005; 27:638-643.
79. Ozatik MA, Kucuker SA, Tuluce H, et al: Neurocognitive functions after aortic arch repair with right brachial artery perfusion. *Ann Thorac Surg* 2004; 78:591-595.
80. Merkkola P, Tulla H, Ronkainen A, et al: Incomplete circle of Willis and right axillary artery perfusion. *Ann Thorac Surg* 2006; 82:74-79.
81. Khaladj N, Shrestha M, Meck S, et al: Hypothermic circulatory arrest with selective antegrade cerebral perfusion in ascending aortic and aortic arch surgery: a risk factor analysis for adverse outcome in 501 patients. *J Thorac Cardiovasc Surg* 2008; 135:908-914.
82. Sasaki H, Ogino H, Matsuda H, et al: Integrated total arch replacement using selective cerebral perfusion: a 6-year experience. *Ann Thorac Surg* 2007; 83:S805-810.
83. Bakhtiary F, Dogan S, Zierer A, et al: Antegrade cerebral perfusion for acute type a aortic dissection in 120 consecutive patients. *Ann Thorac Surg* 2008; 85:465-469.
84. Khaladj N, Peterss S, Oetjen P, et al: Hypothermic circulatory arrest with moderate, deep or profound hypothermic selective antegrade cerebral perfusion: which temperature provides best brain protection? *Eur J Cardiothorac Surg* 2006; 30:492-498.
85. Strauch JT, Spielvogel D, Lauten A, et al: Optimal temperature for selective cerebral perfusion. *J Thorac Cardiovasc Surg* 2005; 130:74-82.
86. Kamiya H, Hagl C, Kropivnitskaya I, et al: The safety of moderate hypothermic lower body circulatory arrest with selective cerebral perfusion: A propensity score analysis. *J Thorac Cardiovasc Surg* 2007; 133:501-509.
87. Strauch JT, Spielvogel D, Haldenwang PL, et al: Cerebral physiology and outcome after hypothermic circulatory arrest followed by selective cerebral perfusion. *Ann Thorac Surg* 2003; 76:1972-1981.
88. Gerdes A, Joubert-Hubner E, Esders K, Sievers HH: Hydrodynamics of aortic arch vessels during perfusion through the right subclavian artery. *Ann Thorac Surg* 2000; 69:1425-1430.
89. Etz CD, Plestis KA, Kari FA, et al: Axillary cannulation significantly improves survival and neurologic outcome after atherosclerotic aneurysm repair of the aortic root and ascending aorta. *Ann Thorac Surg* 2008; 86: 441-446; discussion 6-7.
90. Kuki S, Taniguchi K, Masai T, Endo S: A novel modification of elephant trunk technique using a single four-branched arch graft for extensive thoracic aortic aneurysm. *Eur J Cardiothorac Surg* 2000; 18:246-248.
91. Spielvogel D, Halstead JC, Meier M, et al: Aortic arch replacement using a trifurcated graft: simple, versatile, and safe. *Ann Thorac Surg* 2005; 80:90-95.
92. Ueda Y, Okita Y, Aomi S, Koyanagi H, Takamoto S: Retrograde cerebral perfusion for aortic arch surgery: analysis of risk factors. *Ann Thorac Surg* 1999; 67:1879-1882; discussion 91-94.
93. Mills NL, Ochsner JL: Massive air embolism during cardiopulmonary bypass. Causes, prevention, and management. *J Thorac Cardiovasc Surg* 1980; 80:708-717.
94. Juvonen T, Weisz DJ, Wolfe D, et al: Can retrograde perfusion mitigate cerebral injury after particulate embolization? A study in a chronic porcine model. *J Thorac Cardiovasc Surg* 1998; 115:1142-1159.
95. Usui A, Hotta T, Hiroura M, et al: Retrograde cerebral perfusion through a superior vena caval cannula protects the brain. *Ann Thorac Surg* 1992; 53:47-53.
96. Anttila V, Pokela M, Kiviluoma K, et al: Is maintained cranial hypothermia the only factor leading to improved outcome after retrograde cerebral perfusion? An experimental study with a chronic porcine model. *J Thorac Cardiovasc Surg* 2000; 119:1021-1029.
97. Duebener LF, Hagino I, Schmitt K, et al: Direct visualization of minimal cerebral capillary flow during retrograde cerebral perfusion: an intravital fluorescence microscopy study in pigs. *Ann Thorac Surg* 2003; 75:1288-1293.
98. Boeckxstaens CJ, Flameng WJ: Retrograde cerebral perfusion does not perfuse the brain in nonhuman primates. *Ann Thorac Surg* 1995; 60:319-327; discussion 27-28.
99. Ye J, Yang L, Del Bigio MR, et al: Retrograde cerebral perfusion provides limited distribution of blood to the brain: a study in pigs. *J Thorac Cardiovasc Surg* 1997; 114:660-665.
100. Okita Y, Takamoto S, Ando M, et al: Mortality and cerebral outcome in patients who underwent aortic arch operations using deep hypothermic circulatory arrest with retrograde cerebral perfusion: no relation of early death, stroke, and delirium to the duration of circulatory arrest. *J Thorac Cardiovasc Surg* 1998; 115:129-138.
101. Ehrlich MP, Hagl C, McCullough JN, et al: Retrograde cerebral perfusion provides negligible flow through brain capillaries in the pig. *J Thorac Cardiovasc Surg* 2001; 122:331-338.
102. Kunzli A, Zingg PO, Zund G, Leskosek B, von Segesser LK: Does retrograde cerebral perfusion via superior vena cava cannulation protect the brain? *Eur J Cardiothorac Surg* 2006; 30:906-909.
103. Kawata M, Takamoto S, Kitahori K, et al: Intermittent pressure augmentation during retrograde cerebral perfusion under moderate hypothermia provides adequate neuroprotection: an experimental study. *J Thorac Cardiovasc Surg* 2006; 132:80-88.
104. Wong CH, Bonser RS: Does retrograde cerebral perfusion affect risk factors for stroke and mortality after hypothermic circulatory arrest? *Ann Thorac Surg* 1999; 67:1900-1903; discussion 19-21.
105. Sasaguri S, Yamamoto S, Hosoda Y: What is the safe time limit for retrograde cerebral perfusion with hypothermic circulatory arrest in aortic surgery? *J Cardiovasc Surg (Torino)* 1996; 37:441-444.
106. Deeb GM, Williams DM, Quint LE, et al: Risk analysis for aortic surgery using hypothermic circulatory arrest with retrograde cerebral perfusion. *Ann Thorac Surg* 1999; 67:1883-1886; discussion 91-94.
107. Apaydin AZ, Islamoglu F, Askar FZ, et al: Immediate clinical outcome after prolonged periods of brain protection: retrospective comparison of hypothermic circulatory arrest, retrograde, and antegrade perfusion. *J Cardiac Surg* 2009; 24:486-489.
108. Bavaria JE, Woo YJ, Hall RA, et al: Circulatory management with retrograde cerebral perfusion for acute type A aortic dissection. *Circulation* 1996; 94:II173-176.
109. Coselli JS: Retrograde cerebral perfusion is an effective means of neural support during deep hypothermic circulatory arrest. *Ann Thorac Surg* 1997; 64:908-912.
110. Ehrlich M, Fang WC, Grabenwoger M, et al: Perioperative risk factors for mortality in patients with acute type A aortic dissection. *Circulation* 1998; 98:II294-298.
111. Estrera AL, Miller CC, III, Lee T-Y, Shah P, Safi HJ: Ascending and transverse aortic arch repair: the impact of retrograde cerebral perfusion. *Circulation* 2008; 118:S160-166.
112. Sundt TM, III, Orszulak TA, Cook DJ, Schaff HV: Improving results of open arch replacement. *Ann Thorac Surg* 2008; 86:787-796.
113. Apostolakis E, Koletsis EN, Dedeilias P, et al: Antegrade versus retrograde cerebral perfusion in relation to postoperative complications following aortic arch surgery for acute aortic dissection type A. *J Cardiac Surg* 2008; 23:480-487.
114. Griepp RB, Ergin MA, McCullough JN, et al: Use of hypothermic circulatory arrest for cerebral protection during aortic surgery. *J Cardiac Surg* 1997; 12:312-321.
115. Reich DL, Uysal S, Ergin MA, et al: Retrograde cerebral perfusion during thoracic aortic surgery and late neuropsychological dysfunction. *Eur J Cardiothorac Surg* 2001; 19:594-600.
116. Miyairi T, Takamoto S, Kotsuka Y, et al: Comparison of neurocognitive results after coronary artery bypass grafting and thoracic aortic surgery using retrograde cerebral perfusion. *Eur J Cardiothorac Surg* 2005; 28:97-101.

117. Buth J, Harris PL, Hobo R, et al: Neurologic complications associated with endovascular repair of thoracic aortic pathology: incidence and risk factors. A study from the European Collaborators on Stent/Graft Techniques for Aortic Aneurysm Repair (EUROSTAR) Registry. *J Vasc Surg* 2007; 46:1103-1111.e2.
118. Buth J, Penn O, Tielbeek A, Mersman M: Combined approach to stent-graft treatment of an aortic arch aneurysm. *J Endovasc Surg* 1998; 5:329-332.
119. Mitchell RS, Ishimaru S, Ehrlich MP, et al: First International Summit on Thoracic Aortic Endografting: roundtable on thoracic aortic dissection as an indication for endografting. *J Endovasc Ther* 2002; 9:98-105.
120. Canaud L, Alric P: Endovascular treatment for acute transection of the descending thoracic aorta. *J Thorac Cardiovasc Surg* 2009; 138:515-516; author reply 6-7.
121. Chan YC, Cheng SWK, Ting AC, Ho P: Supra-aortic hybrid endovascular procedures for complex thoracic aortic disease: single center early to midterm results. *J Vasc Surg* 2008; 48:571-579.
122. Szeto WY, Bavaria JE, Bowen FW, et al: The hybrid total arch repair: brachiocephalic bypass and concomitant endovascular aortic arch stent graft placement. *J Cardiac Surg* 2007; 22:97-102.
123. Hughes GC, Daneshmand MA, Balsara KR, et al: "Hybrid" repair of aneurysms of the transverse aortic arch: midterm results. *Ann Thorac Surg* 2009; 88:1882-1888.
124. Antona C, Vanelli P, Petulla M, et al: Hybrid technique for total arch repair: aortic neck reshaping for endovascular-graft fixation. *Ann Thorac Surg* 2007; 83:1158-1161.
125. Etz CD, Homann TM, Silovitz D, et al: Long-term survival after the Bentall procedure in 206 patients with bicuspid aortic valve. *Ann Thorac Surg* 2007; 84:1186-1193; discussion 93-94.
126. Spielvogel D, Strauch JT, Minanov OP, et al: Aortic arch replacement using a trifurcated graft and selective cerebral antegrade perfusion. *Ann Thorac Surg* 2002; 74:S1810-1814; discussion S25-32.
127. Spielvogel D, Mathur MN, Lansman SL, Griepp RB: Aortic arch reconstruction using a trifurcated graft. *Ann Thorac Surg* 2003; 75:1034-1036.
128. Kuki S, Taniguchi K, Masai T, et al: An alternative approach using long elephant trunk for extensive aortic aneurysm: elephant trunk anastomosis at the base of the innominate artery. *Circulation* 2002; 106:I-253-258.
129. Suzuki K, Kazui T, Bashar AHM, et al: Total aortic arch replacement in patients with arch vessel anomalies. *Ann Thorac Surg* 2006; 81:2079-2083.
130. Kouchoukos NT, Masetti P, Rokkas CK, Murphy SF: Single-stage reoperative repair of chronic type A aortic dissection by means of the arch-first technique. *J Thorac Cardiovasc Surg* 2001; 122:578-582.
131. Kouchoukos NT, Masetti P, Mauney MC, Murphy MC, Castner CF: One-stage repair of extensive chronic aortic dissection using the arch-first technique and bilateral anterior thoracotomy. *Ann Thorac Surg* 2008; 86:1502-1509.
132. Etz CD, Halstead JC, Spielvogel D, et al: Thoracic and thoracoabdominal aneurysm repair: is reimplantation of spinal cord arteries a waste of time? *Ann Thorac Surg* 2006; 82:1670-1677.
133. Safi HJ, Miller CC, 3rd, Estrera AL, et al: Staged repair of extensive aortic aneurysms: morbidity and mortality in the elephant trunk technique. *Circulation* 2001; 104:2938-2942.
134. Schepens MA, Dossche KM, Morshuis WJ, et al: The elephant trunk technique: operative results in 100 consecutive patients. *Eur J Cardiothorac Surg* 2002; 21:276-281.
135. Coselli JS, Buket S, Djukanovic B: Aortic arch operation: current treatment and results. *Ann Thorac Surg* 1995; 59:19-26; discussion 7.
136. LeMaire S, Price MD, Parenti JL, et al: Early outcomes after aortic arch replacement by using the trifurcated graft technique. *Ann Thorac Surg* 2010.
137. Numata S, Ogino H, Sasaki H, et al: Total arch replacement using antegrade selective cerebral perfusion with right axillary artery perfusion. *Eur J Cardiothorac Surg* 2003; 23:771-775.
138. Kazui T, Bashar AH, Washiyama N: Total aortic arch replacement and limited circulatory arrest of the brain. *J Thorac Cardiovasc Surg* 2005; 129:1207-1208.
139. Kazui T, Yamashita K, Washiyama N, et al: Usefulness of antegrade selective cerebral perfusion during aortic arch operations. *Ann Thorac Surg* 2002; 74:1806S-1809.
140. Crawford ES, Coselli JS, Svensson LG, Safi HJ, Hess KR: Diffuse aneurysmal disease (chronic aortic dissection, Marfan, and mega aorta syndromes) and multiple aneurysm. Treatment by subtotal and total aortic replacement emphasizing the elephant trunk operation. *Ann Surg* 1990; 211:521-537.
141. Heinemann M, Laas J, Karck M, Borst HG: Thoracic aortic aneurysms after acute type A aortic dissection: necessity for follow-up. *Ann Thorac Surg* 1990; 49:580-584.
142. Detter C, Mair H, Klein HG, et al: Long-term prognosis of surgically-treated aortic aneurysms and dissections in patients with and without Marfan syndrome. *Eur J Cardiothorac Surg* 1998; 13:416-423.
143. Halstead JC, Spielvogel D, Meier DM, et al: Composite aortic root replacement in acute type A dissection: time to rethink the indications? *Eur J Cardiothorac Surg* 2005; 27:626-632.

CHAPTER 53

Descending and Thoracoabdominal Aortic Aneurysms

Joseph Huh
Scott A. LeMaire
Joseph S. Coselli

INTRODUCTION

Treating aneurysms that arise from the aortic segments distal to the left subclavian artery poses challenges that are distinct from those presented by aneurysms of the more proximal ascending and arch segments. The distal aortic segments comprise the descending thoracic aorta, which extends from the left subclavian artery to the diaphragm within the chest, and the abdominal segment that extends from the diaphragm to the iliac bifurcation. The diaphragm divides the thoracic aorta from the abdominal aorta.

An aortic aneurysm that is limited to the chest is classified as a descending thoracic aortic aneurysm (DTAA). An aortic aneurysm that traverses the diaphragm and extends into both the chest and the abdomen to any degree is considered a thoracoabdominal aortic aneurysm (TAAA) (Fig. 53-1). Aneurysms in these locations can be extensive and can involve many or all of the aortic branch vessels. Modern critical care and surgical adjuncts for organ protection have improved the outcomes of surgical repair; however, operative treatment of DTAA and TAAA continues to represent a significant clinical challenge to the cardiovascular surgeon.

PATHOGENESIS

The etiology of DTAA and TAAA has changed over time. Whereas tertiary syphilis was the most common cause of thoracic aneurysms in the early 1900s, other causes are more prevalent today. Well-established causes of DTAA and TAAA include medial degeneration, atherosclerosis, aortic dissection, connective tissue disorders, aortitis (eg, Takayasu's arteritis), aortic coarctation, infection, and trauma. As our understanding of genetics increases and as more advanced genetic testing becomes available, classification systems are likely to evolve to include more molecular factors. Perhaps partly because of improved screening for aneurysmal disease and the increasing age of the population, it is certain that the incidence and prevalence of thoracic aortic aneurysm are increasing over time.[1]

The most common types of aneurysms of the descending and thoracoabdominal aorta today are grouped into the category of atherosclerotic aneurysms. Unfortunately, although this term may be descriptive, it may not accurately describe the mechanism of aneurysmal changes. Although atherosclerosis and aortic aneurysms share common risk factors and frequently coexist, thoracic aortic aneurysms are primarily the result of age-related medial degeneration, which is characterized by changes in elastin and collagen that reduce aortic integrity and strength. Subsequent aortic enlargement and aneurysm formation provide fertile ground for superimposed intimal atherosclerosis and further degeneration of the aortic wall. The usual histologic changes in the aging aorta include elastin fragmentation, fibrosis with increased collagen, and medial degeneration.[2] As with most aneurysmogenic processes, medial degeneration usually causes diffuse, fusiform aortic dilatation. In some cases, however, medial degeneration produces saccular aneurysms along the descending thoracic aorta. These saccular aneurysms may be superimposed on or coexist with more generalized, fusiform aneurysmal disease of the thoracoabdominal aorta.

Risk factors for aortic dissection and aortic aneurysm overlap to a great extent, but once an aorta becomes dissected, the

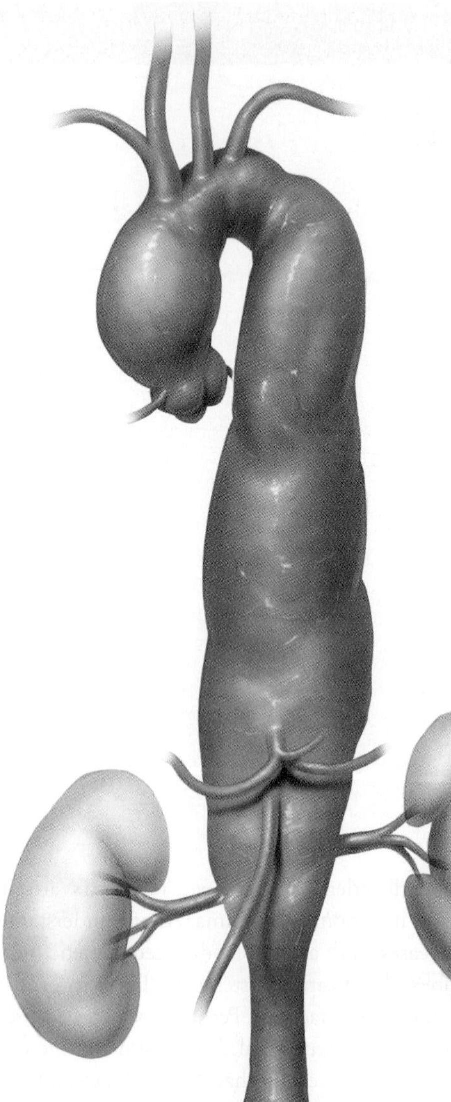

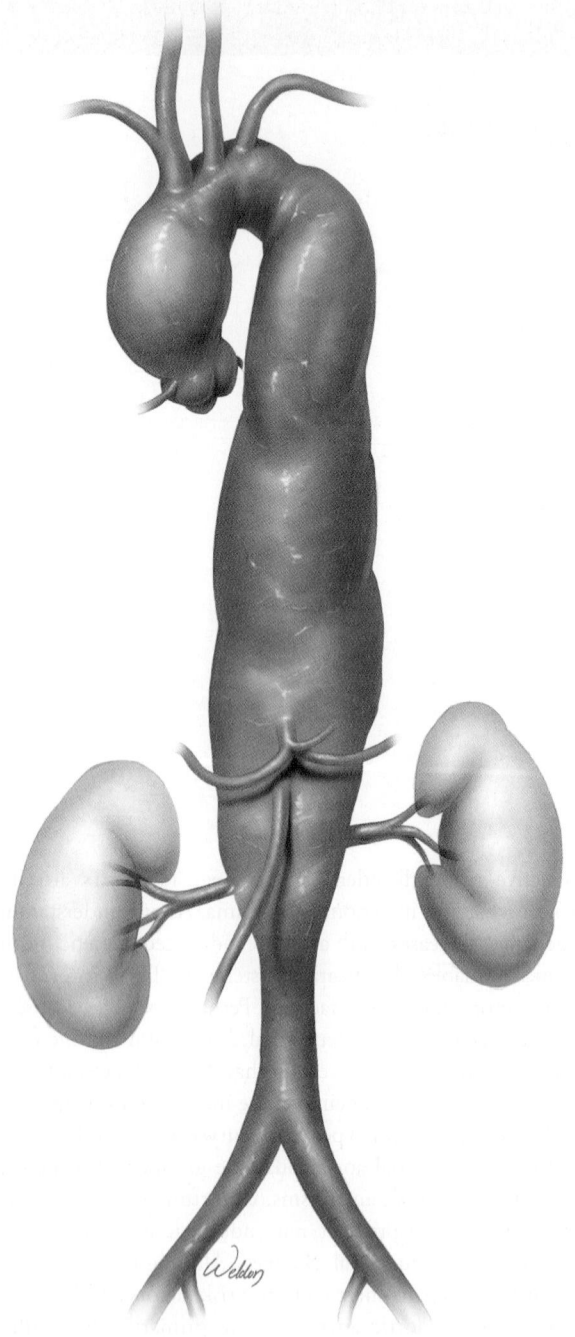

FIGURE 53-1 Drawing depicting a thoracoabdominal aortic aneurysm.

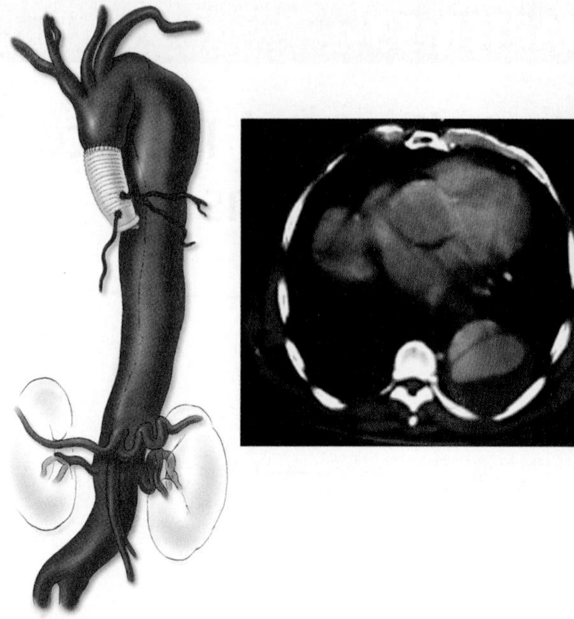

FIGURE 53-2 Drawing and computed tomography image of a thoracoabdominal aortic aneurysm caused by dilatation of the false lumen in a patient with chronic aortic dissection.

dissection itself becomes an independent risk factor for subsequent dilation and aneurysmal changes. Aortic dissections occur in the medial layer separating the intima from the adventitia; blood flows through the true aortic lumen and through one or more false lumen channels that can form at various points along the aorta. This process weakens the outer aortic wall, making it prone to progressive aneurysmal dilatation (Fig. 53-2). Persistence of a pressurized false lumen has been associated with subsequent aneurysm formation, need for intervention, and increased mortality.[3,4] Recent endovascular strategies have included stent exclusion of the false lumen in an attempt to thrombose the false channel, thus decreasing the risk of late aneurysm formation, although this technique remains controversial.[5] In a randomized series, endovascular stenting in uncomplicated type B aortic dissections failed to show differences in survival and aortic outcomes at 2 years when compared to standard medical management.[6] Penetrating aortic ulcers and intramural hematomas are two variants of aortic dissection that can occur in the descending and abdominal aortic segments. Penetrating aortic ulcers are disrupted atherosclerotic plaques that can penetrate the aortic wall, leading to classic dissection or rupture. Intramural hematomas are collections of blood within the aortic wall that occur without an intimal tear; growth of the hematoma can result in classic dissection.

Genetic mutations or defects can give rise to defective components of the aortic extracellular matrix, leading to aortic aneurysm and dissection. Aortic aneurysms that occur in patients with these genetic disorders can be a part of a named syndrome, accompanied by a constellation of extraaortic symptoms, or they may be part of a heterogenous group of familial thoracic aortic aneurysms and dissections that occur in isolation. In a national registry of genetically triggered thoracic aortic aneurysms, Marfan syndrome is the most common genetic cause of thoracic aneurysms (36%).[7] Marfan syndrome is a connective tissue disorder that results from a fibrillin-1 gene mutation that causes fragmentation of elastic fibers and the deposition of extensive amounts of mucopolysaccharides in the aortic extracellular matrix. The aorta in Marfan syndrome patients is prone to dissection, which is the most common cause of DTAAs and TAAAs in these patients.[8] Ehlers-Danlos syndrome causes 5% of genetically triggered thoracic aneurysms and results from abnormal collagen synthesis. Loeys-Dietz syndrome is a recently identified, particularly aggressive aortic disorder resulting from mutations in the transforming growth factor (TGF)-beta receptor I (TGFBR1) and II (TGFBR2) genes.[9,10]

Both chronic, nonspecific aortitis and systemic autoimmune disorders, such as Takayasu's arteritis, giant cell arteritis (temporal arteritis), and rheumatoid aortitis, can cause destruction of the aortic media and progressive aneurysm formation. Although Takayasu's arteritis usually causes obstructive lesions related to severe intimal thickening, the associated medial destruction can result in aneurysmal dilatation.

Aneurysms involving the upper descending thoracic aorta can develop in patients with congenital aortic coarctation. These aneurysms occur concomitantly with unrepaired coarctation or after coarctation repair.[11] The postrepair aneurysms appear to be most common in patients who have had patch graft aortoplasty operations.[12] Histologic examination of the aneurysmal tissue has revealed medial degeneration, smooth muscle cell necrosis, and loss and fragmentation of elastic fibers.[13]

Infection can produce a saccular "mycotic" aneurysm in a localized area of the aortic wall that has been damaged by the infectious process. For unknown reasons, such mycotic aneurysms tend to occur along the lesser curvature of the transverse aortic arch or the upper abdominal aorta adjacent to the origins of the visceral branches. In such cases, only a portion of the aortic circumference is affected; consequently, localized weakening causes a diverticular or saccular outpouching.

Each of the disease processes described above causes aneurysms through progressive degeneration and dilatation of the aortic wall. In contrast, pseudoaneurysms of the thoracic aorta form as the result of chronic leaks through discrete defects in the aortic wall. These leaks are initially contained by surrounding tissue; the accumulation of organized thrombus and the associated fibrosis forms the wall of the pseudoaneurysm. Pseudoaneurysms can develop after surgical or percutaneous repair of aortic coarctation, dissection, or aneurysm.[14] Unrepaired blunt and penetrating injuries are the other common cause of aortic pseudoaneurysms. Chronic traumatic pseudoaneurysms typically develop in the proximal descending thoracic aorta after blunt aortic injuries[13]; the management of these lesions is covered in detail in a subsequent chapter.

NATURAL HISTORY

An untreated aneurysm in the thoracic and thoracoabdominal aorta can progress to dissection, rupture, or both if given enough time. A dissected aorta that was originally of normal caliber will tend to dilate and become aneurysmal. The causes and genetics of these aneurysms vary, but there are commonalities in the mechanical and pathophysiologic aspects of their formation and development. Understanding these processes will help surgeons to determine the timing and nature of the operative intervention needed.

An *aneurysm* is defined as a permanent dilation of an artery to at least 1.5 times its normal diameter at a given location.[15] However, the normal aortic diameter is perhaps more difficult to define. At the level of the mid-descending thoracic aorta, the average aortic diameter is 28 mm for men and 26 mm for women; at the level of the celiac axis, it is 23 mm for men and 20 mm for women; and at the infrarenal aorta, it is 19.5 mm for men and 15.5 mm for women.[16] The normal aortic diameter also varies with a person's age and body surface area. Aortic enlargement with advancing age has been reported in several studies.[17–19] Even when adjusted for age and body surface area, mean aortic size is significantly smaller in women than in men; on average, aortic diameter is 2 to 3 mm greater in men than women. Body surface area is a better predictor of aortic size than is height or weight, particularly in patients less than 50 years of age.[17,20]

The descending thoracic aorta has a slightly higher rate of expansion over time than the ascending aorta and is noted to average 1 to 4 mm/year.[21] The rate is not constant, and it increases as the diameter increases. A dissection in an otherwise small aneurysm can lead to a sudden increase in the rate of growth. The relationship among pressure, vessel diameter, and vessel wall tension is described by Laplace's law. As the luminal diameter increases, there is increasing wall tension, which in turn contributes to the cycle of progressive dilatation. Unfortunately, at some point as the dilation progresses, the wall tension becomes too great for the maximally stretched aortic wall. A tear can occur within the intimal and medial layers, resulting in a dissection that propagates down the length of the aorta, or a tear can penetrate the full thickness of the aortic wall, resulting in contained or free rupture. The aortic size at which this event occurs is determined by several factors, including the presence or absence of a connective tissue disorder, the presence and severity of hypertension, and the patient's body size. In a large series of patients, Elefteriades and colleagues[22] have shown that in the thoracic aorta, there is a sharp increase in the incidence of aortic complications at aneurysmal diameters greater than 6 cm, with a 14% combined risk of rupture, dissection, and death. In a population-based study, the 5-year risk of rupture doubled from 16% for aneurysms 4 to 5.9 cm in diameter to 31% in aneurysms 6 cm or more in diameter.[23]

CLINICAL PRESENTATION AND DIAGNOSIS

At the time of diagnosis, patients with DTAAs and TAAAs are commonly asymptomatic. For example, Panneton and Hollier[24] reported that degenerative TAAAs are asymptomatic in roughly 43% of patients. In asymptomatic patients, DTAAs and TAAAs are often discovered when imaging studies are performed to evaluate unrelated problems. For example, chest radiographs may show widening of the descending thoracic aortic shadow, which may be outlined by a rim of calcification outlining the dilated aneurysmal aortic wall (Fig. 53-3). Aneurysmal calcium may also be seen in the upper abdomen on standard radiograms.

Although DTAAs and TAAAs remain asymptomatic for long periods of time, most ultimately produce a variety of symptoms before they rupture. Degenerative TAAAs produce symptoms in approximately 57% of patients; 9% of patients present with rupture.[24] The most frequent symptom is back pain between the scapulae. When the aneurysm is large in the region of the aortic hiatus, pressure on adjacent structures may cause mid-back and epigastric pain. Other potential signs and symptoms related to compression or erosion of adjacent organs include

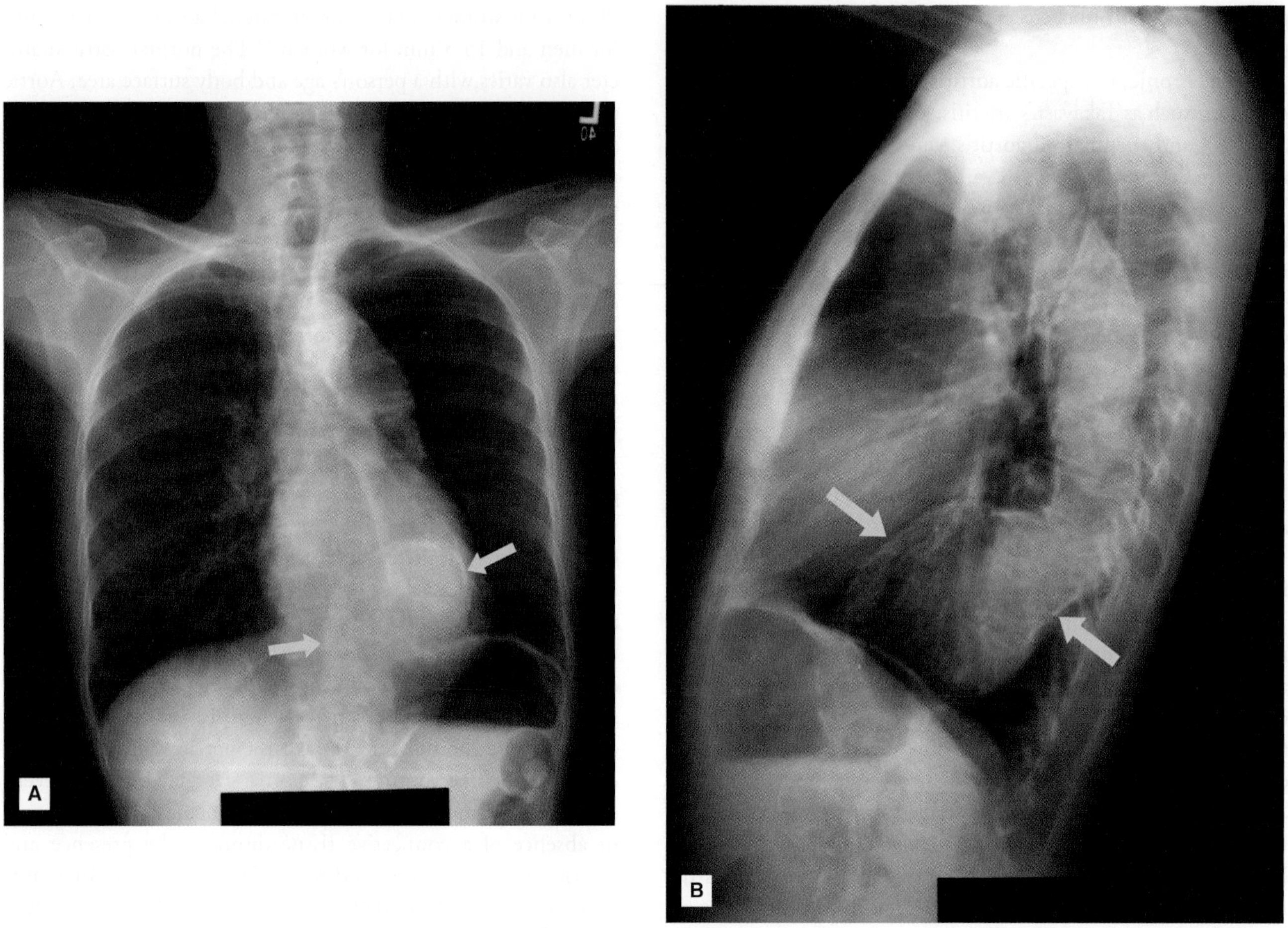

FIGURE 53-3 Chest radiographs in (A) posteroanterior and (B) lateral projections showing the calcified wall (*arrows*) of a thoracoabdominal aortic aneurysm.

stridor, wheezing, cough, hemoptysis, dysphagia, and gastrointestinal obstruction or bleeding. Hoarseness results from traction on the vagus nerve as the distal aortic arch expands and causes recurrent laryngeal nerve paralysis. Thoracic or lumbar vertebral body erosion (Fig. 53-4) causes back pain, spinal instability, and neurologic deficits from spinal cord compression; mycotic aneurysms have a peculiar propensity to destroy vertebral bodies. Additionally, neurologic symptoms, including paraplegia, paraparesis, or both, may result from thrombosis of intercostal and lumbar arteries. This is most frequently seen with acute aortic dissection, which may occur primarily or be superimposed on medial degenerative fusiform aneurysmal disease. Thoracic aortic aneurysms, like aneurysms in other locations, may produce distal emboli of clot or atheromatous debris that gradually obliterate and thrombose visceral, renal, or lower-extremity branches.

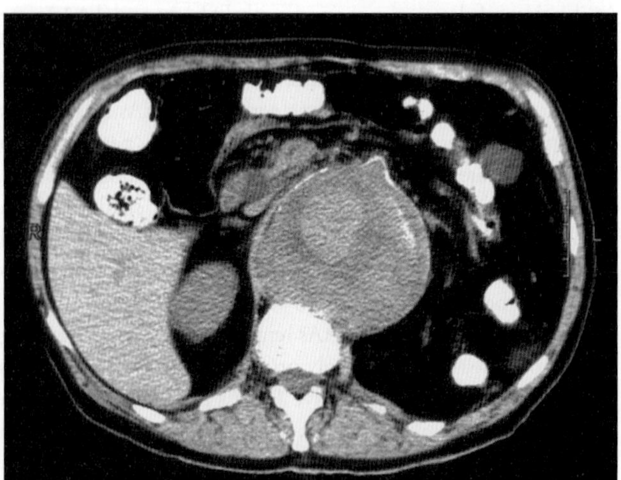

FIGURE 53-4 Computed tomography image of a large thoracoabdominal aortic aneurysm that has caused erosion of the adjacent vertebral body.

Imaging technology is critical in diagnosis and determining anatomical details for operative planning. Computed tomography (CT) scanning and magnetic resonance angiography (MRA) enable clinicians to obtain excellent images without the potential morbidity or cost associated with angiography. Computed tomography scanning is widely available and can image the entire thoracic and abdominal aorta, major branch vessels, and virtually all adjacent organs. Computer programs can construct sagittal, coronal, and oblique images, as well as three-dimensional reconstructions, from CT data.[25–27] Contrast-enhanced CT scanning (Figs. 53-2, 53-4, and 53-5) also provides information about the aortic lumen, intraluminal thrombus, presence of aortic dissection, intramural hematoma, mediastinal or retroperitoneal hematoma, aortic rupture, and periaortic

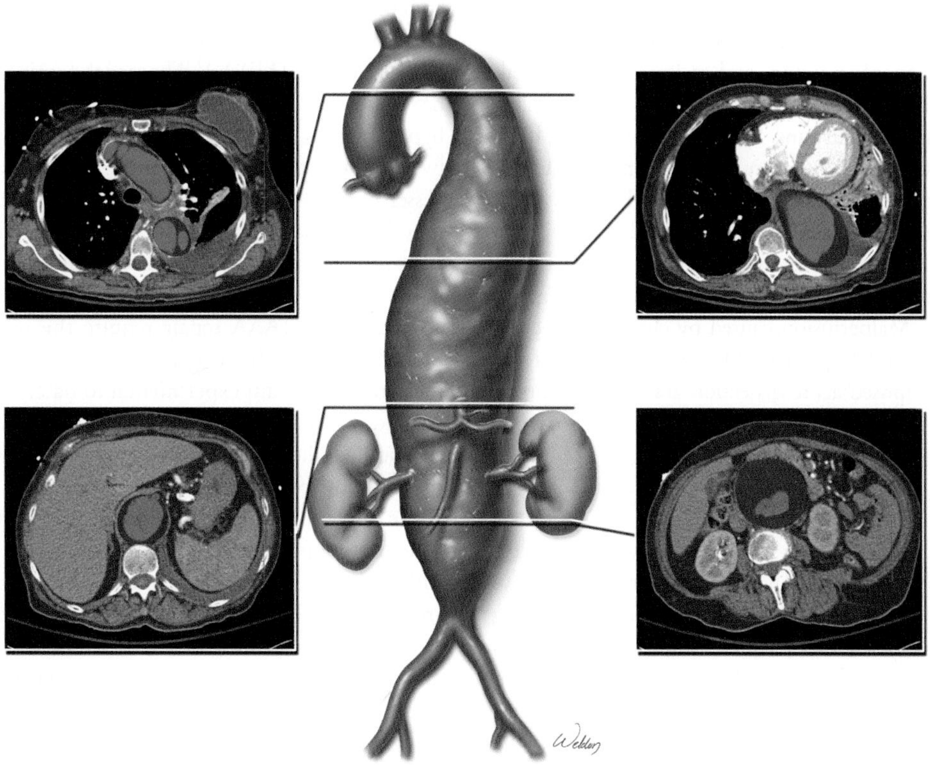

FIGURE 53-5 Drawing and contrast-enhanced computed tomography images of a degenerative extent II thoracoabdominal aortic aneurysm with extensive intraluminal thrombus.

fibrosis associated with inflammatory aneurysms.[28] Computed tomographic angiography with multiplanar reconstruction is especially useful for planning endovascular procedures. Advantages of CT include being less expensive and somewhat quicker to perform than MRA and, at present, the wider availability of CT expertise. Also, CT can be used with patients who have implanted ferromagnetic prostheses or other devices, which can cause injury in patients undergoing MRA.[29] The chief advantages of MRA are that it does not expose the patient to ionizing radiation and that it reveals disease within the aortic wall, including intramural hemorrhage. The gadolinium-based contrast agents used in MRA were once considered to be safer for patients with renal insufficiency than CT contrast media. Ironically, recent reports have associated the use of certain gadolinium-based contrast agents with nephrogenic systemic fibrosis (NSF)—a scleroderma-like fibrotic process that can affect not only the skin but also internal organs—in patients with renal insufficiency.[30] The current recommendation is to avoid using such agents in patients with advanced renal failure (ie, with a glomerular filtration rate <30 mL/min) or in patients who are dialysis dependent.[31]

Ongoing improvements in noninvasive imaging modalities have substantially reduced the role of catheter aortography in assessing thoracic aortic aneurysms. However, catheter aortography remains useful in situations in which noninvasive methods are not feasible; for example, when artifact or heavy calcification obscures the area of interest.[32] Anterior, posterior, oblique, and lateral views provide detailed information about branch vessels. The risks posed by aortography include renal toxicity from the large volumes of contrast material required to adequately fill large aneurysms. There is also a risk of embolization from laminated thrombus secondary to manipulation of intraluminal catheters. Furthermore, angiography underestimates the size of an aneurysm in areas of laminated thrombus. Nonetheless, angiography can be helpful in patients with suspected renal or visceral ischemia, aortoiliac occlusive disease, horseshoe kidney, or peripheral aneurysms.

DETERMINING APPROPRIATE TREATMENT

Once an aneurysm involving the descending thoracic or thoracoabdominal aorta has been discovered, precise determination of the extent and severity of disease is the critical next step toward clarifying the specific diagnosis, determining the appropriate treatment, and, when repair is indicated, planning the appropriate intervention.

Indications for Operation

In asymptomatic patients, the decision to consider surgical repair is based primarily on the diameter of the aneurysm. To prevent fatal rupture, elective operation is recommended when diameter exceeds 5 to 6 cm or when the rate of dilatation exceeds 1 cm per year. In patients with connective tissue disorders, such as Marfan syndrome and related disorders, the threshold for operation is lower for both absolute size and rate of growth.[8] Nonoperative management—which consists of strict blood pressure control, cessation of smoking, and at least yearly surveillance with imaging studies—is appropriate for asymptomatic patients who have small aneurysms. Symptomatic patients, however, are at increased risk of rupture and warrant expeditious evaluation and urgent aneurysm repair, even when the mentioned threshold diameters have not been reached. The onset of new pain in a patient with a known aneurysm is particularly concerning and often heralds significant expansion, leakage, or impending rupture. Malperfusion caused by chronic dissection is also an indication for TAAA repair. Degenerative DTAAs and TAAAs with superimposed acute dissection are especially prone to rupture and are therefore treated with emergent operation.

Endovascular Considerations

Descending thoracic aortic aneurysm is an approved and widely accepted indication for endovascular stent repair,[33–35] and several stent-grafts have been approved by the US Food and Drug Administration (FDA) for this purpose. Endovascular repairs are covered in detail in a subsequent chapter, but all patients in our practice are evaluated for possible endovascular intervention, and an individualized surgical option best suited for the patient is selected. Two important factors to consider when deciding between open and endovascular aneurysm repair are the patient's physiologic reserve and vascular anatomy.[36] Open repairs have well-documented outcomes and excellent long-term durability, and they allow repair of aneurysms with complex anatomy. However, the patients must have considerable physiologic reserve to undergo and recover from these procedures.

Repairing DTAAs with stent grafts is an attractive alternative to standard open procedures, especially in patients who have compromised cardiac, pulmonary, or renal status, who have undergone previous complex thoracic aortic procedures, or who are very elderly. Recent data show that, in general, endovascular repair of the descending thoracic aorta is associated with less early mortality and morbidity than is open repair.[33–35] Appropriate anatomy, however, is critical for successful endovascular repair. Landing zones that have inadequate length, excessive angulation, extensive intraluminal thrombus, or severe vessel calcification will not allow secure endograft fixation, precluding endovascular repair. Furthermore, the long-term durability of these repairs remains unclear, particularly in patients with complex aortic disease, such as chronic aortic dissection, or with connective tissue disorders.

Combining open and endovascular procedures capitalizes on the principal benefits of both by creating durable repairs in patients with complex anatomy while minimizing physiologic stress and postoperative complications. Accordingly, combined approaches—commonly called "hybrid" procedures—appear well-suited for patients with limited physiologic reserve (precluding standard open repair) and complex aneurysmal anatomy (precluding standard endovascular repair).[37] For example, in patients with DTAAs that have an insufficient proximal landing zone, an open procedure to reroute the brachiocephalic circulation can convert the aortic arch into a satisfactory landing zone for a stent-graft.[38] Similarly, if arch aneurysms and DTAAs exist concurrently, a hybrid "frozen elephant trunk" repair can be performed that combines open arch replacement with stent-grafting of the DTAA.[39] Thoracoabdominal aortic aneurysms have also been repaired with hybrid approaches: open visceral bypass grafting, performed to secure organ perfusion, is followed by stent-graft coverage of the entire aneurysm, including branch-vessel ostia.[40–42] Although hybrid procedures are feasible and may be associated with reduced postoperative morbidity and mortality, the durability of these repairs is unclear. In contrast with endovascular repair of DTAA, purely endovascular approaches to TAAA repair require the use of fenestrated or branched endografts to maintain branch-vessel perfusion, and these repairs remain experimental to date.[43–45]

Endovascular stent devices are being used for evolving and expanding indications, including blunt aortic injuries, descending thoracic aortic ruptures, mycotic aneurysms, DeBakey type III aortic dissections, and hybrid descending aortic stenting during concurrent open repair of DeBakey type I aortic dissection. Although these indications remain controversial, the procedures are often performed in clinical scenarios with limited options. In endovascular stenting of a dissected descending thoracic aorta, some data suggest that a persistent patent false lumen is a predictor of poorer long-term outcome. Whether stent intervention will prevent the dissected thoracoabdominal aorta from following its typical natural history remains controversial, and late outcomes are not known.[46]

What is certain is that as endovascular aortic stent-graft use increases, these devices are increasingly encountered in subsequent open operations. Stent-graft failure may result from progression of the aneurysmal process to an adjacent portion of the aorta that is not amenable to further endovascular treatment, progressive dilation of the treated segment owing to persistent endoleak, infection of the endovascular device, or device migration. In general, the endovascular devices do not incorporate into the aneurysm thrombus and aortic intima in the way that conventional Dacron grafts incorporate into the periadventitial tissue. Explantation of the endovascular device and open graft replacement of the thoracic aorta can be accomplished with relatively good success.[47,48] In the absence of infection, salvaging the device or portions of the device is also possible.[49] We have applied the aortic cross-clamp to a proximal aortic segment with an endovascular stent-graft in place and repaired a distal segment in an open fashion. Suturing an existing stent-graft to a standard Dacron graft in a hemostatic fashion is also feasible, particularly if the surrounding aortic tissue can be incorporated into the suture line.

PREOPERATIVE EVALUATION

In each patient, the indications for operation discussed above are weighed against the risks posed by surgical intervention.[50,51] The Crawford classification of TAAA (Fig. 53-6) permits standardized reporting of the extent of aortic involvement, thereby allowing appropriate risk stratification, choice of specific treatment modalities according to the extent of the aneurysm, and a type-specific determination of the risks for neurologic deficits and other morbidities and mortality associated with TAAA repair. Extent I TAAA repairs involve replacing most or all of

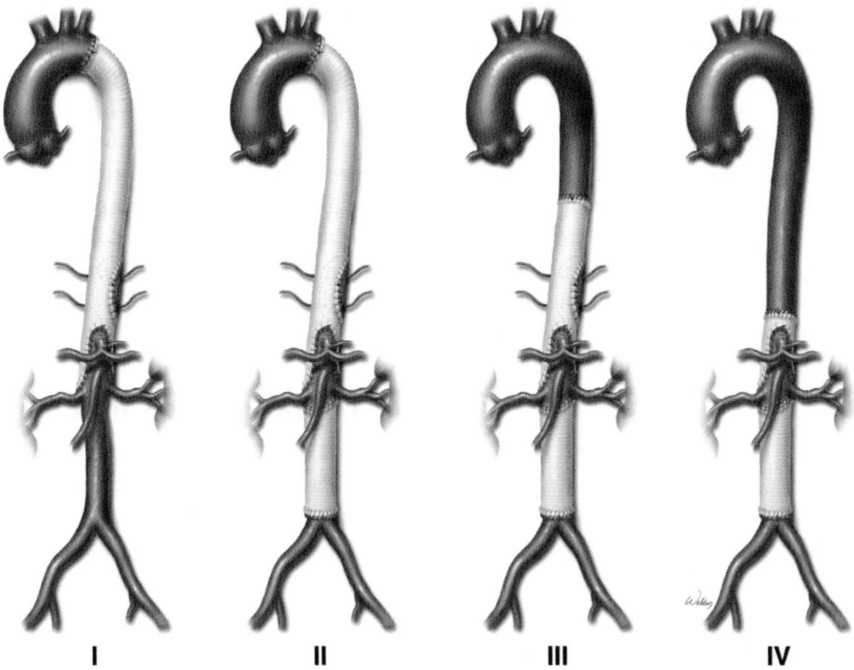

FIGURE 53-6 The Crawford classification of thoracoabdominal aortic aneurysm repairs. *(Reproduced with permission from Coselli JS, Bozinovski J, LeMaire SA. Open surgical repair of 2286 thoracoabdominal aortic aneurysms. Ann Thorac Surg 2007; 83:S862-864. Figure 1. Copyright Elsevier.)*

the descending thoracic aorta and the upper abdominal aorta. Extent II repairs involve most or all of the descending thoracic aorta and extend into the infrarenal abdominal aorta. Extent III repairs involve the distal half or less of the descending thoracic aorta and varying portions of the abdominal aorta. Extent IV repairs involve most or all of the abdominal aorta.

An adequate preoperative assessment of physiologic reserve is critical in evaluating operative risk. Unless they require emergency operation, patients undergo a thorough preoperative evaluation, with emphasis on cardiac, pulmonary, and renal function.

Cardiac Status

Impaired myocardial contractility and reduced coronary reserve are common among elderly patients who undergo aortic reconstruction. Patients need substantial cardiac reserve to tolerate clamping of the thoracic aorta. Given the prevalence of preoperative cardiac disease and the physiologic strain of aortic clamping, it is not surprising that cardiac complications are a major cause of postoperative mortality. Reports indicate that cardiac disease has been responsible for 49% of early deaths and 34% of late deaths after TAAA repair, attesting to the importance of careful preoperative cardiac evaluation.[24,52]

Several imaging techniques are useful in preoperative screening for cardiac disease. Transthoracic echocardiography is noninvasive and can satisfactorily evaluate both valvular and biventricular function. Dipyridamole-thallium myocardial scanning identifies regions of myocardium that are reversibly ischemic, and it is more practical than exercise testing in this generally elderly population, whose exercise capacity is often limited by concurrent lower-extremity peripheral vascular disease. In patients with evidence of reversible ischemia on noninvasive studies, and those with a significant history of angina or an ejection fraction of 30% or less, cardiac catheterization and coronary arteriography are performed. Patients who have asymptomatic aneurysms and severe coronary artery occlusive disease (ie, significant left main, proximal left anterior descending, or triple-vessel coronary artery stenosis) undergo myocardial revascularization before aneurysm repair. In appropriate patients, percutaneous transluminal angioplasty is carried out before surgery. If clamping proximal to the left subclavian artery is anticipated in patients in whom the left internal thoracic artery has been used as a coronary artery bypass graft, a left-common-carotid-to-subclavian bypass is necessary to prevent cardiac ischemia when the aortic clamp is applied.[53]

Renal Status

Preoperative renal insufficiency has been a major risk factor for early mortality throughout the history of TAAA repair.[50,54] It was among the predictive variables selected in Svensson et al.'s[54] multivariable analysis of Crawford's complete experience with TAAA surgery in 1509 patients treated between 1960 and 1991. However, patients with preoperative renal failure who are being treated with an established hemodialysis program appear to have a level of risk similar to that of patients with normal renal function. Patients with severely impaired renal function who are not receiving long-term hemodialysis frequently require temporary hemodialysis early after operation and are clearly at increased risk for postoperative complications.

Although patients are not rejected as surgical candidates on the basis of renal function, careful assessment of renal function aids in estimating perioperative risk and adjusting treatment strategies accordingly. Renal function is assessed preoperatively by measuring serum electrolytes, blood urea nitrogen, and creatinine. Kidney size and perfusion can be evaluated by using the imaging studies obtained to assess the aorta. Patients who have poor renal function secondary to severe proximal renal artery occlusive disease are revascularized at operation by renal arterial endarterectomy, stenting, or bypass grafting, with the expectation that renal function will stabilize or improve.[52]

Because of the nephrotoxic effects of vascular contrast agents, surgery is delayed (if possible) for 24 hours or longer after CT scanning or aortography has been performed. This is especially important in patients with preexisting renal impairment. Strategies to reduce the risk of contrast-induced nephropathy include periprocedural administration of acetylcysteine and intravenous hydration. If renal insufficiency occurs or worsens after contrast administration, the surgical procedure is postponed until renal function returns to baseline or is satisfactorily stabilized.

Pulmonary Status

Pulmonary complications are the most common form of postoperative morbidity in patients who undergo DTAA and TAAA repairs. Most patients undergo pulmonary function screening with arterial blood gases and spirometry.[55,56] Patients with an FEV_1 greater than 1.0 and a PCO_2 less than 45 are satisfactory surgical candidates. In suitable patients, borderline pulmonary function frequently is improved by smoking cessation, progressive treatment of bronchitis, weight loss, and a general exercise program that the patient follows for a period of 1 to 3 months before operation. However, surgery is not withheld from patients with symptomatic aortic aneurysms and poor pulmonary function. In such patients, preservation of the left recurrent laryngeal nerve, phrenic nerve, and diaphragmatic function is particularly important.

OPEN SURGICAL REPAIR

Anesthetic Strategies

Coordination among the surgeon, anesthesiologist, and perfusionist is critical during a DTAA or TAAA repair procedure. Management of hemodynamics during aortic clamping and unclamping, blood volume management, anticoagulation and hemostasis, and proper lung management occur in real time, with anticipation and preparation by the anesthesia team. Swan-Ganz catheters are routinely used for hemodynamic monitoring. The arterial catheter is placed in the right radial artery whenever the left subclavian artery flow may be interrupted during aortic clamping. A large-bore central venous line is necessary for volume return. We re-infuse filtered, unwashed whole blood from the cell-saver through a rapid infusion system during periods of substantial blood loss. With careful scavenging of shed blood and meticulous surgical hemostasis, operations without the use of blood and blood products are frequently possible. However, when coagulopathy does occur after the cross-clamp is released, rapid replacement of blood components with fresh-frozen plasma, platelets, and cryoprecipitate is necessary. Left lung isolation, usually by a double-lumen endobronchial tube, is necessary for exposure, although this may not be critical in extent IV TAAA repairs. The lung is handled minimally during anticoagulation to prevent lung hematoma and contusion. Deflating the left lung reduces retraction trauma to the lung, improves exposure, and alleviates the risk of cardiac compression. When motor evoked potentials are used for spinal cord monitoring, muscle paralytics must be avoided. Sodium bicarbonate solution is routinely infused to prevent acidosis during aortic cross-clamping, and mannitol can be given before cross-clamping to enhance renal perfusion. Proximal blood pressure, afterload, and cardiac performance are closely monitored by Swan-Ganz catheter and transesophageal echocardiography probe when necessary and are aggressively maintained.

Surgical Adjuncts for Organ Protection

Organ ischemia is a major source of the morbidity related to DTAA and TAAA repair. We currently employ a multimodal approach (Table 53-1) in an attempt to maximize organ protection during these operations (Fig. 53-7).[57] The rationale for and details of several important strategies are discussed in the following sections.

Heparin

Potential benefits of heparinization include preserving the microcirculation and preventing embolization. Additionally, by inhibiting the clotting cascade, the use of heparin may help to reduce the incidence of disseminated intravascular coagulation.

Heparin (1 mg/kg) is administered intravenously before aortic clamping or the start of left heart bypass (LHB). After this small heparin dose is administered, the activated clotting time generally ranges from 220 to 270 seconds.

Hypothermia

Hypothermia decreases the metabolic demand of tissues and is protective during ischemic states. The protective effects of hypothermia on the spinal cord are well accepted.[58,59] Mechanisms

TABLE 53-1 Current Strategy for Spinal Cord and Visceral Protection During Descending and Thoracoabdominal Aortic Aneurysm Repair

All extents
- Moderate heparinization (1 mg/kg)
- Permissive mild hypothermia (32–34°C, nasopharyngeal)
- Aggressive reattachment of segmental arteries, especially between T8 and L1
- Perfusion of renal arteries with 4°C crystalloid solution when possible
- Sequential aortic clamping when possible

Extent I and II thoracoabdominal repairs
- Cerebrospinal fluid drainage
- Left heart bypass during proximal anastomosis
- Selective perfusion of celiac axis and superior mesenteric artery during intercostal and visceral anastomoses

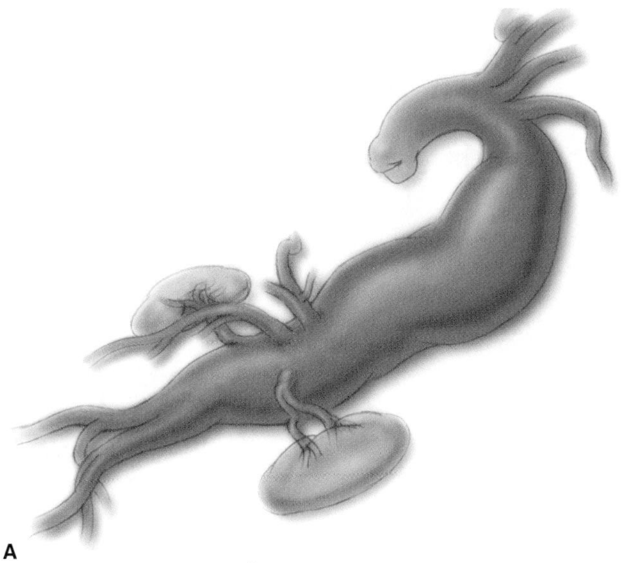

A

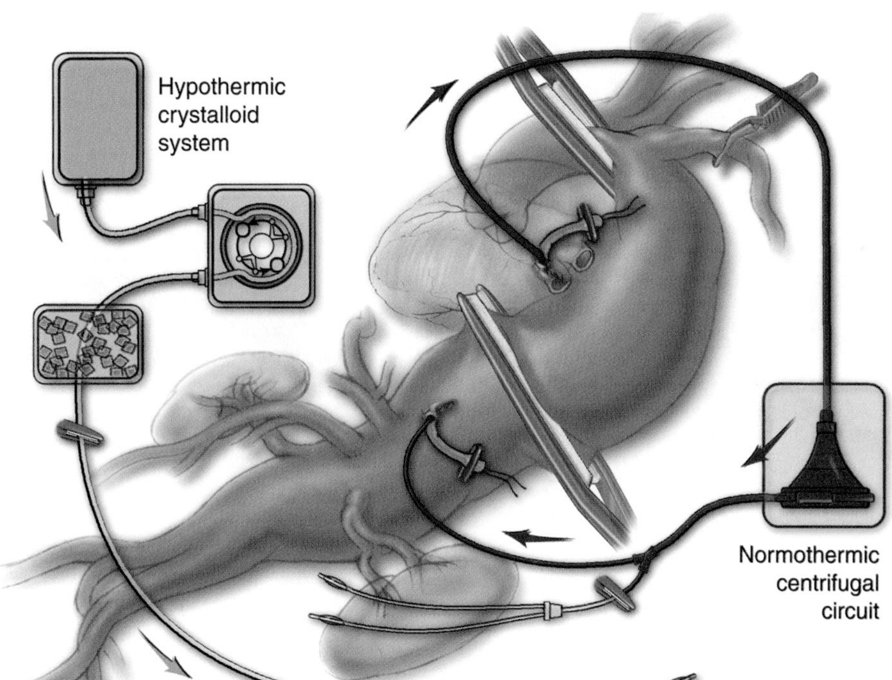

B

FIGURE 53-7 Drawings illustrating an extent II repair of a thoracoabdominal aortic aneurysm (A) that extends from the left subclavian artery to the aortoiliac bifurcation. (B) During the repair, a left heart bypass circuit provides distal aortic perfusion, and a cold renal delivery system provides selective renal hypothermia. The proximal portion of the aneurysm is isolated between clamps placed on the aortic arch (between the left common carotid and left subclavian arteries), the mid-descending thoracic aorta, and the left subclavian artery. (C) Whenever possible, the phrenic, vagus (indicated by X), and recurrent laryngeal nerves are preserved during the repair. The isolated segment of aorta is opened longitudinally and divided circumferentially a few centimeters beyond the proximal clamp. (D) Patent intercostal arteries in this region are oversewn. (E) The proximal anastomosis is performed with continuous polypropylene suture. (F) Left heart bypass is stopped, the proximal clamp is repositioned onto the graft, flow is restored to the left subclavian artery, and the remainder of the aneurysm is opened longitudinally. (G) Balloon perfusion catheters are inserted into the celiac and superior mesenteric arteries to deliver selective visceral perfusion from the left heart bypass circuit, and into the renal arteries to intermittently deliver cold crystalloid. Patent lower intercostal arteries are reattached to an opening in the graft. (H) The aortic clamp is repositioned to restore intercostal perfusion. The celiac axis, superior mesenteric, and right renal arteries are reattached to an opening in the side of the graft. (I) The aortic clamp is repositioned to restore visceral and right renal perfusion. The mobilized left renal artery is reattached. (J) The aortic clamp is repositioned to restore left renal perfusion. The distal anastomosis at the aortoiliac bifurcation completes the repair.

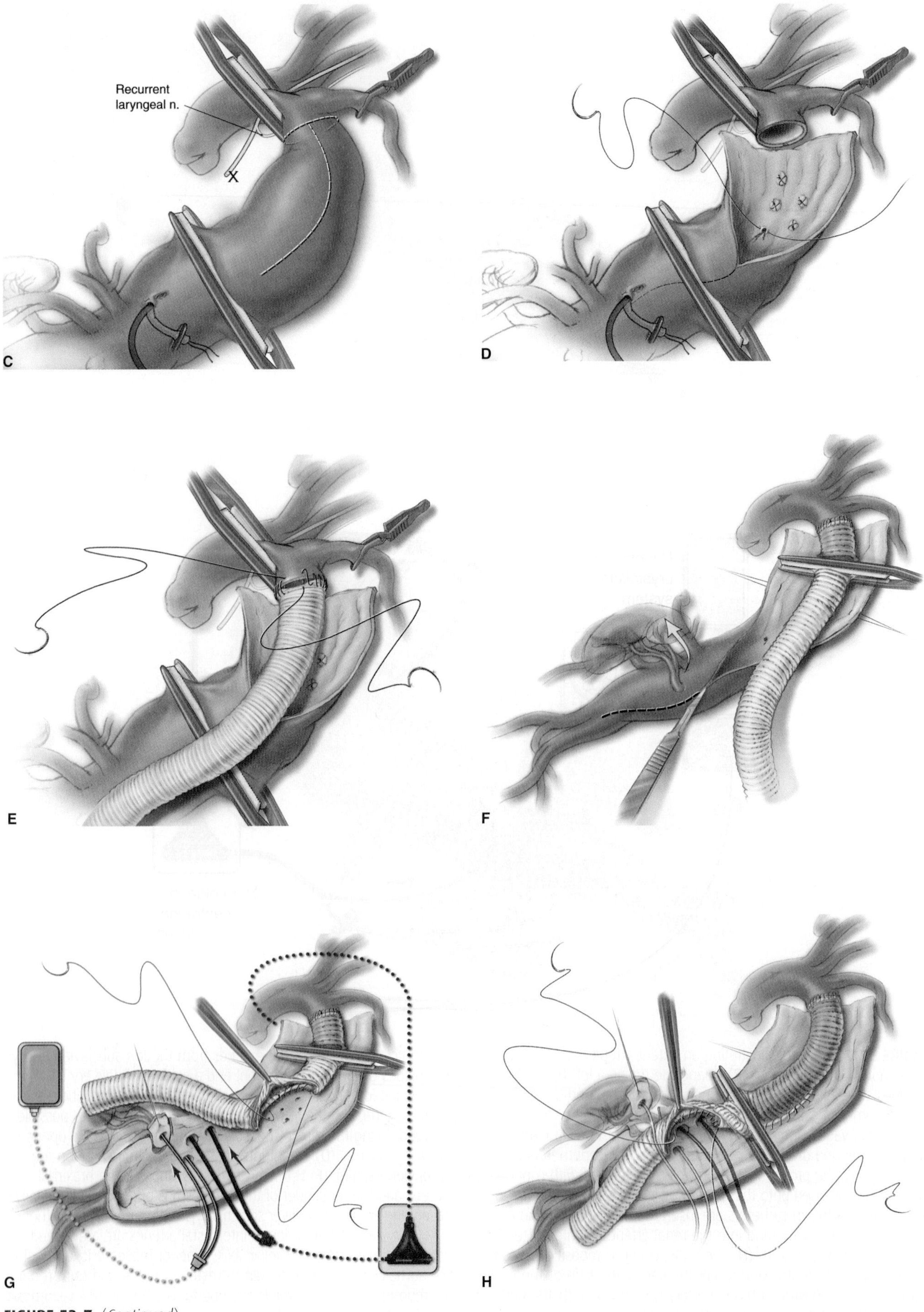

FIGURE 53-7 *(Continued)*

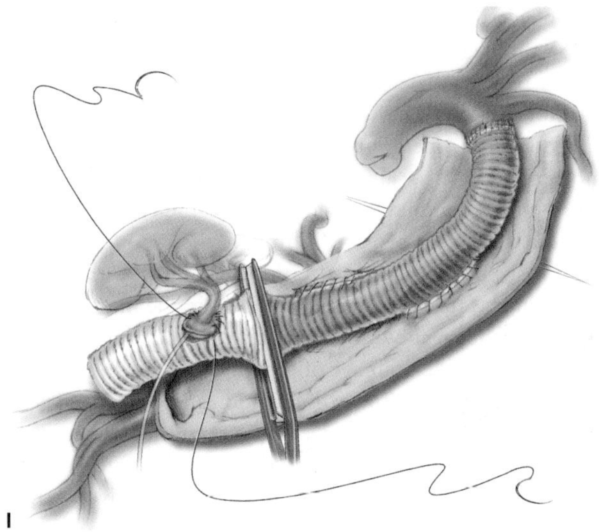
I

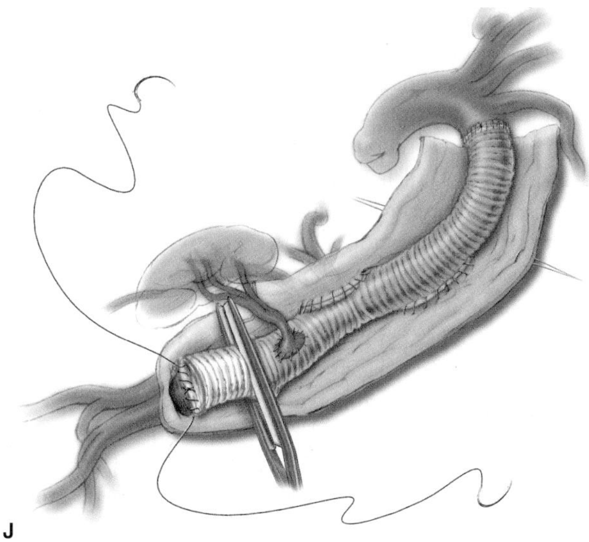
J

FIGURE 53-7 *(Continued)*

of spinal protection may involve membrane stabilization and reduced release of excitatory neurotransmitters.[60,61] We routinely use mild passive systemic hypothermia during DTAA and TAAA repairs. The patient's temperature is allowed to drift down to a nasopharyngeal temperature of 32 to 33°C. After the aortic repair, rewarming can be accomplished by irrigating the thoracic and abdominal cavities with warm saline.

Profound systemic hypothermia on full cardiopulmonary bypass is an operative strategy for organ protection. Kouchoukos and colleagues[62–64] have published several reports showing that hypothermic cardiopulmonary bypass with circulatory arrest can safely and substantially protect against paralysis and renal, cardiac, and visceral organ system failure during operations on the thoracic and thoracoabdominal aorta. Despite these protective effects, many clinicians avoid using this approach, principally because of the associated risks of coagulopathy, pulmonary dysfunction, and massive fluid shift. We use hypothermic circulatory arrest selectively when the aneurysm anatomy precludes safe proximal clamping.

Left Heart Bypass

Disruption of blood flow to the spinal cord and abdominal viscera contributes significantly to the development of ischemic complications. Conversely, maintaining flow through spinal and visceral arteries during all or part of the anatomic repair should reduce the duration of organ ischemia and prevent associated morbidity.[65] Borst et al.[66] found that using LHB for distal perfusion during DTAA and TAAA repair effectively unloads the proximal circulation during aortic occlusion and maintains adequate perfusion of distal vital organs, thereby reducing early mortality and renal failure. Further, combined distal perfusion and aggressive reattachment of distal intercostal arteries decreased the risk of spinal cord damage.

Typically used during the proximal aortic anastomosis, LHB is achieved by establishing a temporary bypass from the left atrium to either the femoral artery (most commonly the left) or the distal descending thoracic aorta with a closed-circuit in-line centrifugal pump (Fig. 53-7B). The left atrial cannula is placed via an opening in the inferior pulmonary vein (see Fig. 53-7B). When we first began using LHB, cannulation of the distal descending thoracic aorta (usually at the level of the diaphragm) was used solely as an alternative to femoral artery cannulation in patients with femoral or iliac artery occlusive disease. However, because this technique causes few complications and eliminates the need for femoral artery exposure and repair, distal aortic cannulation has become our preferred approach. Careful examination of CT or MR images assists selection of an appropriate site for direct aortic cannulation. Areas with intraluminal thrombus (see Fig. 53-4) are avoided because cannulation could lead to distal embolization. Bypass flows are adjusted to maintain normal proximal arterial and venous filling pressures. Flows between 1500 and 2500 mL/min are generally used. Left heart bypass facilitates rapid adjustment of proximal arterial pressure and cardiac preload, thereby reducing the need for pharmacologic intervention. Because LHB effectively unloads the left ventricle, it is useful in patients with suboptimal cardiac reserve.

Spinal Cord Protection

Paraplegia remains an index complication specific to distal aortic surgery. Historically, paraplegia rates have been as high as 30% for extensive aortic replacements. With modern operative techniques and spinal adjuncts, paraplegia rates in aortic centers are currently 2 to 5%.[67–69] Because multiple adjuncts are used in combination, it is difficult to attribute the improvements in outcome to one technique.

Spinal Cord Monitoring. Somatosensory evoked potential (SSEP) and motor evoked potential (MEP) monitoring have been used for intraoperative assessment of spinal cord function. Motor evoked potential monitoring involves electrical excitation of the motor cortex or motor neurons and measuring the amplitude of the resulting motor response in the peripheral muscles of the arms and legs. Monitoring MEPs allows real-time assessment of spinal cord motor function and was approved for this use during surgical TAAA repair by the FDA in 2003. Because the motor function of the anterior horn of the spinal cord is more susceptible than the posterior horn to ischemia and infarction, MEP changes are a sensitive indicator of spinal cord ischemia and are predictive of adverse neurologic events.[70–72] In contrast, SSEP monitoring is less sensitive because the sensory pathways on the dorsal horn are more resistant to injury and are sometimes spared when ischemic injury occurs. Irreversible loss of either MEPs or SSEPs is highly predictive of immediate neurologic deficit on recovery.[73] Monitoring MEPs precludes the use of neuromuscular paralytic agents.

Significant attenuation or loss of MEPs can occur within 2 minutes of acute spinal cord ischemia, and infarction can occur within 10 minutes at normothermia.[74] Several studies have examined the use of MEP monitoring to guide spinal perfusion–enhancing measures (eg, reattaching more segmental arteries, increasing distal and proximal perfusion pressures, and enhancing cerebrospinal fluid [CSF] drainage) to improve the outcomes of TAAA and DTAA repair. For example, Jacobs et al.[75] published excellent results in a series of 184 patients who underwent TAAA repair with a protocol that included LHB, CSF drainage, and MEP monitoring. The authors found that MEP was a sensitive technique for assessing spinal cord ischemia and identifying the segmental arteries that critically contribute to spinal cord perfusion. With this protocol, the incidence of neurologic deficit after TAAA repair was 2.7%. Other series of TAAA and DTAA repairs have found similarly low rates of postoperative paraplegia and paraparesis when MEP is used in this fashion.[72,76] Our current practice is to monitor MEP in all extent II TAAA repairs and selectively in any other high-risk aortic repairs in which prolonged cross-clamping is anticipated, such as reoperative repairs and those involving difficult anatomy.

Cerebrospinal Fluid Drainage. The drainage of CSF in the context of aortic surgery for spinal cord protection was tested in animal models in the early 1960s.[77] The rationale for CSF drainage was that it would enhance spinal perfusion by decreasing the pressure on the cord during aortic cross-clamping. Today, the practice is well accepted in TAAA repair, although the exact mechanisms of this adjunct's benefits remain controversial.[78–82] In our study of 145 patients who underwent extent I or II TAAA repair, patients were randomly assigned to receive CSF drainage or no CSF drainage. Postoperatively, paraplegia or paraparesis developed in nine patients (13%) in the control group but in only two patients (2.6%) in the CSF drainage group (p = .03).[83] Additionally, a meta-analysis of eight studies (three randomized controlled trials and five cohort studies) of CSF drainage in TAAA repair found that CSF drainage substantially reduced the incidence of postoperative neurologic impairment ($p < .0001$).[84] Although the safety of CSF drainage has been shown clinically,[85] known risks include intracranial bleeding, perispinal hematoma, meningitis, and spinal headaches.

We routinely use CSF drainage in patients undergoing Crawford extent I or II TAAA repairs because of the higher risks of paraplegia in these extensive TAAA repairs. We selectively use CSF drainage during less extensive repairs, such as DTAA or extent III or IV TAAA repairs, depending on the individual risk factors involved; for example, we would use CSF drainage in a redo aortic operation in which the spinal collateral is compromised and a long cross-clamp time is anticipated because of the complex configuration of the aneurysm. The intrathecal catheter is placed through the second or third lumbar space preoperatively after induction of anesthesia and is maintained 2 to 3 days postoperatively in the intensive care unit. The catheter allows both monitoring of the CSF pressure and therapeutic drainage of the fluid. The CSF is allowed to drain passively from the catheter and can be aspirated with a closed collection system as needed to keep the CSF pressure between 8 and 10 mm Hg during the operation and between 10 and 12 mm Hg during the early postoperative period. Once the patients are awake and neurologic exams confirm that they are able to move their legs, the CSF pressures are allowed to rise to a higher range of 15 to 18 mm Hg. To prevent intracranial hemorrhage, we avoid draining more than 25 mL per hour.

Regional Spinal Hypothermia. Regional spinal cord hypothermia can be accomplished by direct infusion of cold perfusate into the epidural or intrathecal space and intravascular cold perfusion of isolated thoracic aortic segments (with the expectation that the intercostal vessels will deliver the cold perfusate to the spinal cord). Epidural cooling for regional spinal cord hypothermia is effective in preventing paraplegia after aortic cross-clamping in canine and leporine models.[86–89] Additionally, a series of 337 TAAA repairs reported by Cambria and colleagues[90] showed that, in patients who underwent extent I, II, or III TAAA repairs, the incidence of spinal cord ischemic injury was reduced from 19.8 to 10.6% after the introduction of epidural cooling at their institution in 1993. A similar technique, cold perfusion into isolated aortic segments, has been tested in animal models to show that cord temperature and, consequently, the extent of ischemic spinal cord injury can be effectively reduced by this method.[91]

Left Heart Bypass for Spinal Protection. Left heart bypass appears to provide the greatest benefit to patients who undergo the more extensive repairs. Our own retrospective review of 1250 consecutive extent I or extent II TAAA repairs found that using LHB (in 666 cases) reduced the incidence of spinal cord deficits only in patients who underwent extent II repairs.[92] In patients who underwent extent I repairs, the incidence of paraplegia was similar in the LHB and no-LHB groups, even though the LHB group had significantly longer aortic clamp times. This finding suggests that, by providing spinal cord protection, LHB gives the surgeon more time to create secure anastomoses. A propensity-score analysis of 387 of our patients who underwent DTAA repair with ($n = 46$) or without ($n = 341$) LHB during the construction of the proximal anastomosis found no effect of LHB on postoperative paraplegia and paraparesis rates.[93] Data from series in which LHB and CSF drainage were used together suggest that combining these adjuncts may further reduce rates of spinal cord injury.[94,95] Because patients who undergo extensive TAAA repairs (extents I and II) are at greatest risk of postoperative paraplegia or paraparesis, we routinely use LHB to provide distal aortic perfusion during the proximal portion of the aortic repair.

Segmental Artery Reattachment and Sequential Graft Clamping. Because of the often tenuous nature of the blood supply to the spinal cord, we take an aggressive approach to reattaching patent segmental arteries. Intimal atherosclerosis, particularly in medial degenerative fusiform aneurysms, obliterates many intercostal and lumbar arteries and complicates matters anatomically. Patent segmental arteries from T7 to L2 are selectively reattached as patches to one or more openings made in the graft (Fig. 53-7G). Large arteries with little or no backbleeding are considered particularly important. When none of these arteries is patent, endarterectomy of the aortic wall and removal of calcified intimal disease can be considered as a means of identifying arteries suitable for reattachment. After intercostal arteries are reattached, the proximal clamp is often moved down the graft to restore intercostal perfusion. Sequential clamping restores perfusion to the proximal branch vessels and will decrease the ischemic time to the spinal cord. However, this benefit must be weighed against the additional time needed to control the potential bleeding from the proximal aortic anastomosis, the intercostal patch, and the collateral intercostal and lumbar branches that often results when the clamp is moved below the intercostal patch.

Postoperative Management. Postoperative management remains critical to spinal cord protection. Adequate blood pressure, preload, and cardiac inotropic state are carefully maintained to keep spinal perfusion sufficient. In the absence of postoperative bleeding, blood pressure should be kept near its preoperative baseline level. Delayed paraplegia can arise hours to days after aortic surgery.[67] In the immediate postoperative period, strategies to reverse paraplegia and paraparesis include inducing systemic hypertension; placing a CSF drain, if one is not already present; decreasing CSF pressure; administering cardiac inotropes, mannitol, or steroids; correcting anemia; and preventing fever. Recovery from paraplegia is possible, but if cord function does not return promptly after these measures are taken, such a recovery is not likely.

Postoperative renal failure after DTAA and TAAA remains an important complication and is predictive of mortality.[96] Distal aortic perfusion with LHB provides renal perfusion during proximal anastomosis. Once the renal vessels are exposed during distal repair, the renal arteries can be directly perfused with cold (4°C) crystalloid (Fig. 53-7G). Our current technique is to infuse 400 to 600 mL of cold lactated Ringer's (LR) solution every 6 to 10 minutes. We have previously reported on a group of patients who underwent Crawford extent II TAAA repair with LHB and who were randomly assigned to receive either renal artery perfusion of cold LR solution for renal cooling or to isothermic blood perfusion from the LHB circuit.[97] Multivariate analysis confirmed that cold crystalloid perfusion was independently protective against acute renal dysfunction. Other groups continue to selectively perfuse the renal arteries with blood from the LHB circuit.

Visceral Protection

Similarly, distal aortic perfusion by LHB provides flow to the mesenteric branches during the initial portion of a TAAA repair. Once the visceral origins are exposed, selective visceral perfusion can be delivered through separate balloon perfusion catheters that are placed within the origins of the celiac and superior mesenteric arteries; these catheters are attached to the LHB circuit via a Y-line from the arterial perfusion line (Fig. 53-7B). This system provides oxygenated blood to the abdominal viscera while the intercostal and visceral branches are being reattached to the graft (Figs. 53-7G,H). Reducing hepatic ischemia in this fashion may decrease the risk of postoperative coagulopathy, and reducing bowel ischemia may decrease the risk of bacterial translocation.

Operative Techniques

Incisions and Aortic Exposure

Aneurysms limited to the descending thoracic aorta are approached through a full posterolateral thoracotomy (Fig. 53-8A). In most cases, the left pleural space is entered through the sixth intercostal space; however, if the aneurysm predominantly involves the upper portion of the descending thoracic aorta, the fifth intercostal space provides better access to the distal aortic arch. Exposure of the distal descending thoracic aorta is enhanced by dividing the costal margin without dividing the diaphragm.

The full thoracoabdominal incision extends from the left posterior chest (between the scapula and the spine), crosses the costal margin, and traverses obliquely to the umbilicus. The length and level vary according to the anatomy of the aneurysm. The incision is gently curved as it crosses the costal margin to reduce the risk of tissue necrosis at the apex of the lower portion of the musculoskeletal tissue flap (Fig. 53-9A). Stabilized on a bean bag, the patient is placed in a modified right lateral decubitus position with the shoulders placed at 60 to 80 degrees and the hips rotated to 30 to 40 degrees from horizontal. In extent I and II repairs, which require access to the left subclavian artery and distal arch in the upper chest, our standard approach is through the sixth intercostal space. The upper or lower ribs may be divided posteriorly to achieve additional proximal or distal exposure, respectively, as needed. For extent III aneurysm repairs, entering through the seventh or eighth intercostal space will allow adequate access. Extent IV aneurysms are approached via a straight oblique incision through the ninth or tenth interspace (Fig. 53-9B). Ending the incision distally at the level of the umbilicus will allow access to the aortic bifurcation. The incision can be extended toward the pubis if iliac aneurysms also require repair.

For thoracoabdominal access, the diaphragm is divided partially or completely in a circular fashion to protect the phrenic nerve and preserve as much diaphragm as possible. The crus of the diaphragm is divided at the hiatus, and a 3- to 4-cm rim of diaphragmatic tissue is left posterolaterally on the chest wall to facilitate closure when the operation is complete. Below the diaphragm, the retroperitoneum is entered lateral to the left colon, and medial visceral rotation is performed to expose the

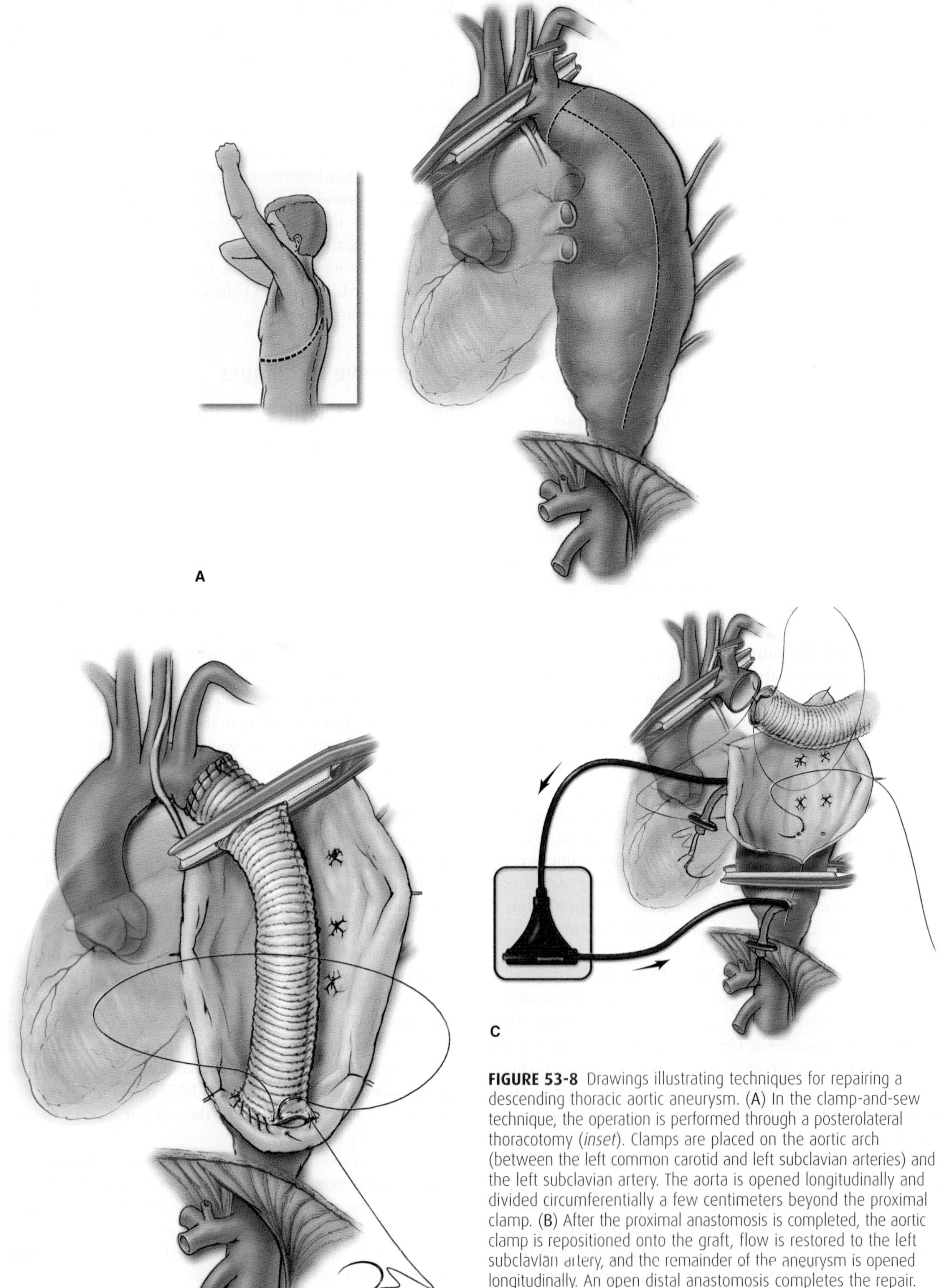

FIGURE 53-8 Drawings illustrating techniques for repairing a descending thoracic aortic aneurysm. (A) In the clamp-and-sew technique, the operation is performed through a posterolateral thoracotomy (*inset*). Clamps are placed on the aortic arch (between the left common carotid and left subclavian arteries) and the left subclavian artery. The aorta is opened longitudinally and divided circumferentially a few centimeters beyond the proximal clamp. (B) After the proximal anastomosis is completed, the aortic clamp is repositioned onto the graft, flow is restored to the left subclavian artery, and the remainder of the aneurysm is opened longitudinally. An open distal anastomosis completes the repair. (C) As an alternative to the clamp-and-sew technique, left heart bypass can be used to provide distal aortic perfusion during the repair.

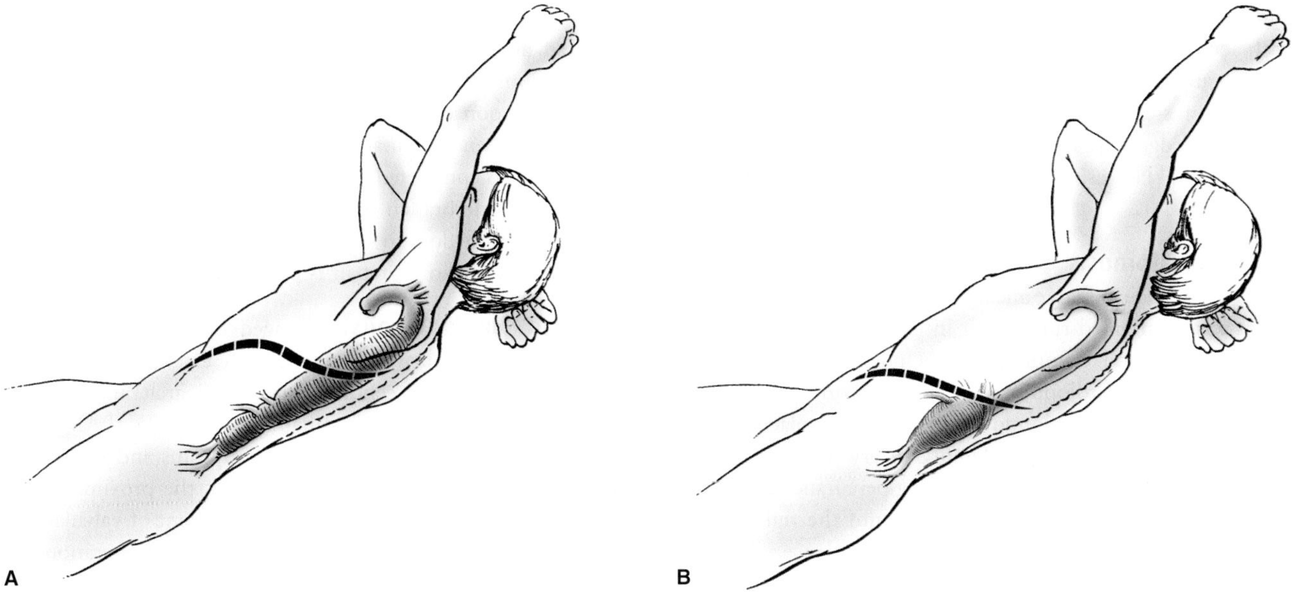

FIGURE 53-9 Drawings of the typical incisions used in thoracoabdominal aortic aneurysm repairs. (A) A curvilinear incision is used to approach the aorta in extent I, II, and III thoracoabdominal aneurysm repairs. (B) A straighter, oblique incision is used to approach extent IV thoracoabdominal aortic aneurysm repairs.

aorta. A dissection plane is developed anterior to the psoas muscle, and the left kidney, left colon, spleen, and left ureter are retracted anteriorly and to the right. The abdominal aortic segment is approached transperitoneally; opening the peritoneum permits direct inspection of the abdominal viscera and its blood supply after aortic reconstruction is completed. An entirely retroperitoneal approach can be used in patients with a "hostile abdomen," ie, patients with multiple prior abdominal operations or a history of extensive adhesions, peritonitis, or both.

The left renal artery is identified but generally does not require mobilization. The aorta is approached laterally to avoid injury to the mesenteric vessels and the abdominal organs. Commonly, a large lumbar branch of the left renal vein courses posteriorly around the aorta. This branch may be ligated and divided as needed. An anomalous retroaortic left renal vein is occasionally encountered and should be preserved. If the retroaortic renal vein or its tributaries require division for exposure, direct reanastomosis or interposition grafting to the inferior vena cava can be performed if the left kidney appears congested and shows distended collaterals.

Proximal Anastomosis

For DTAA and extent I and II TAAA repairs, options for establishing proximal control include applying a proximal aortic clamp distal to the left subclavian artery; applying an aortic clamp between the left subclavian and the left carotid artery and applying a separate bulldog clamp to the left subclavian artery; applying an aortic clamp to an existing graft during an elephant trunk operation; or open anastomosis under hypothermic circulatory arrest with full cardiopulmonary bypass when an aortic clamp cannot be safely applied. The decision is based on the anatomy of the aneurysm. We use aortic clamping distal to the left subclavian artery whenever possible, although others have advocated using circulatory arrest routinely.[98]

In aneurysms suitable for aortic clamping, the distal aortic arch is gently mobilized by dividing the remnant of the ductus arteriosus. The vagus and recurrent laryngeal nerves are identified (see Fig. 53-7C). The vagus nerve may be divided below the recurrent nerve to provide additional mobility, thereby protecting the recurrent nerve from injury. Preserving the recurrent laryngeal nerve is particularly important in patients with chronic obstructive pulmonary disease and reduced pulmonary function. If the aneurysm encroaches on the left subclavian artery, clamping proximal to the left subclavian artery should be anticipated; the left subclavian artery is then circumferentially mobilized to enable placement of a bulldog clamp.

After heparin is administered, the proximal clamp is applied to the proximal descending thoracic aorta or the distal transverse aortic arch between the left common carotid and left subclavian arteries (see Figs. 53-7B and 8A). When LHB is used, it is initiated at a flow rate of 500 mL/min just before the proximal aorta is clamped. After the proximal clamp is applied, LHB flow is increased to 2 L/min and a second distal aortic clamp is placed between T4 and T7 (Fig. 53-8C). After the aorta is opened, patent upper intercostal arteries are oversewn (Fig. 53-7D). In cases of chronic dissection, the partition between the true and false lumens is completely removed. The aorta is transected 2 to 3 cm beyond the proximal clamp and is separated from the esophagus to allow the surgeon to place full-thickness sutures in the aortic wall without injuring the esophagus. A 22- or 24-mm, gelatin-impregnated woven Dacron graft is used in most patients. The proximal anastomosis is performed with continuous polypropylene suture (Fig. 53-7E). Most anastomoses are made with 3-0 polypropylene suture; however, in patients with particularly fragile aortic tissues, such as patients with acute aortic dissection or Marfan syndrome, 4-0 polypropylene sutures are commonly used. Felt strips are generally not used; instead, intermittent polypropylene mattress sutures with felt pledgets are used to reinforce selected portions of the anastomoses. The use of surgical adhesives is avoided in these operations.

Open Anastomosis Under Hypothermic Circulatory Arrest. In repairs of large aneurysms at the distal arch or aneurysms with contained rupture, or in redo operations in which safe dissection and clamping are not possible, an alternative strategy is total cardiopulmonary bypass with hypothermic circulatory arrest. Arterial inflow is established by placing a cannula in the distal aorta or the femoral artery. Venous drainage is usually established by inserting a long percutaneous cannula into the femoral vein and advancing it into the right atrium with transesophageal echocardiographic guidance. The left atrium or left ventricle can be vented via a right-angled sump cannula placed in the left pulmonary vein to prevent cardiac distension. Total cardiopulmonary bypass is initiated, and the patient is cooled to electrocerebral silence. Circulatory arrest is initiated, and the aneurysm is opened. Direct antegrade cerebral perfusion into the left carotid artery can be accomplished via a separate balloon catheter arising from the arterial limb of the circuit. An open proximal anastomosis is performed. After this anastomosis is completed, a Y-limb from the arterial line is connected to a side-branch of the graft. The graft is deaired and clamped, pump flow to the upper body is resumed, and the remainder of the aortic repair is performed.

Elephant Trunk Repairs. A staged operative procedure is preferred in patients who present with extensive aneurysmal disease involving the ascending aorta, aortic arch, and descending thoracic or thoracoabdominal aorta (Fig. 53-10A). When the DTAA or TAAA is not causing symptoms and is not substantially larger than the ascending aorta, the proximal aortic repair is performed first. This allows treatment of valvular and coronary artery occlusive disease during the first operation.

Our current preference for reconstruction of the innominate, left carotid, and left subclavian artery is separate end-to-end anastomoses with a branched trifurcated graft (Fig. 53-10B).

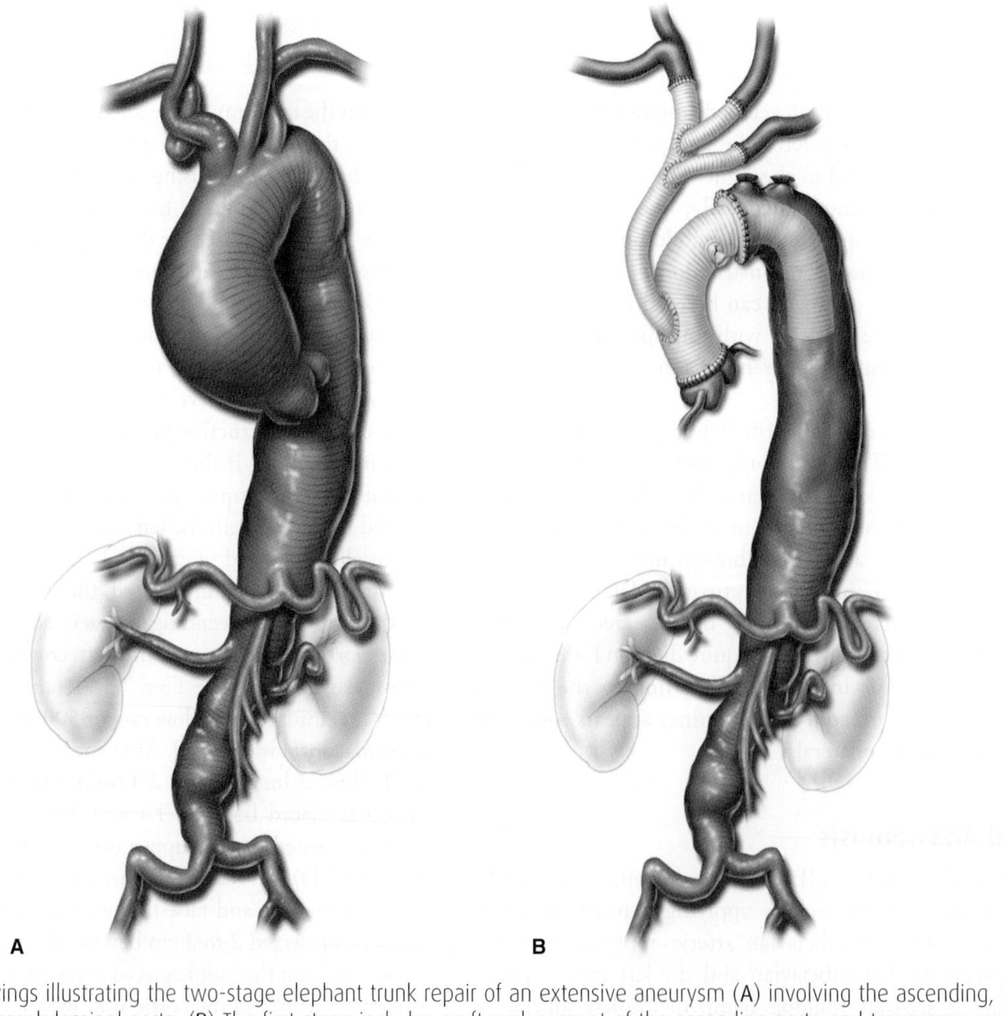

FIGURE 53-10 Drawings illustrating the two-stage elephant trunk repair of an extensive aneurysm (A) involving the ascending, transverse arch, and entire thoracoabdominal aorta. (B) The first stage includes graft replacement of the ascending aorta and transverse aortic arch. A segment of the graft (the trunk) is left suspended within the aneurysmal descending thoracic aorta. (C) During the second stage, the graft trunk is retrieved and (D) used for the proximal anastomosis. (E) The completed repair includes reattachment patches for a pair of intercostal arteries and the visceral arteries. *(Figures B-D reproduced with permission from Baylor College of Medicine. Figure E reproduced with permission from LeMaire SA, Price MD, Parenti JL, Johnson ML, Lay AD, Preventza O, Huh J, Coselli JS. Early Outcomes after aortic arch replacement by using the Y-graft technique. Ann Thorac Surg 2011;91:700-708. Figure 4A. Copyright Elsevier.)*

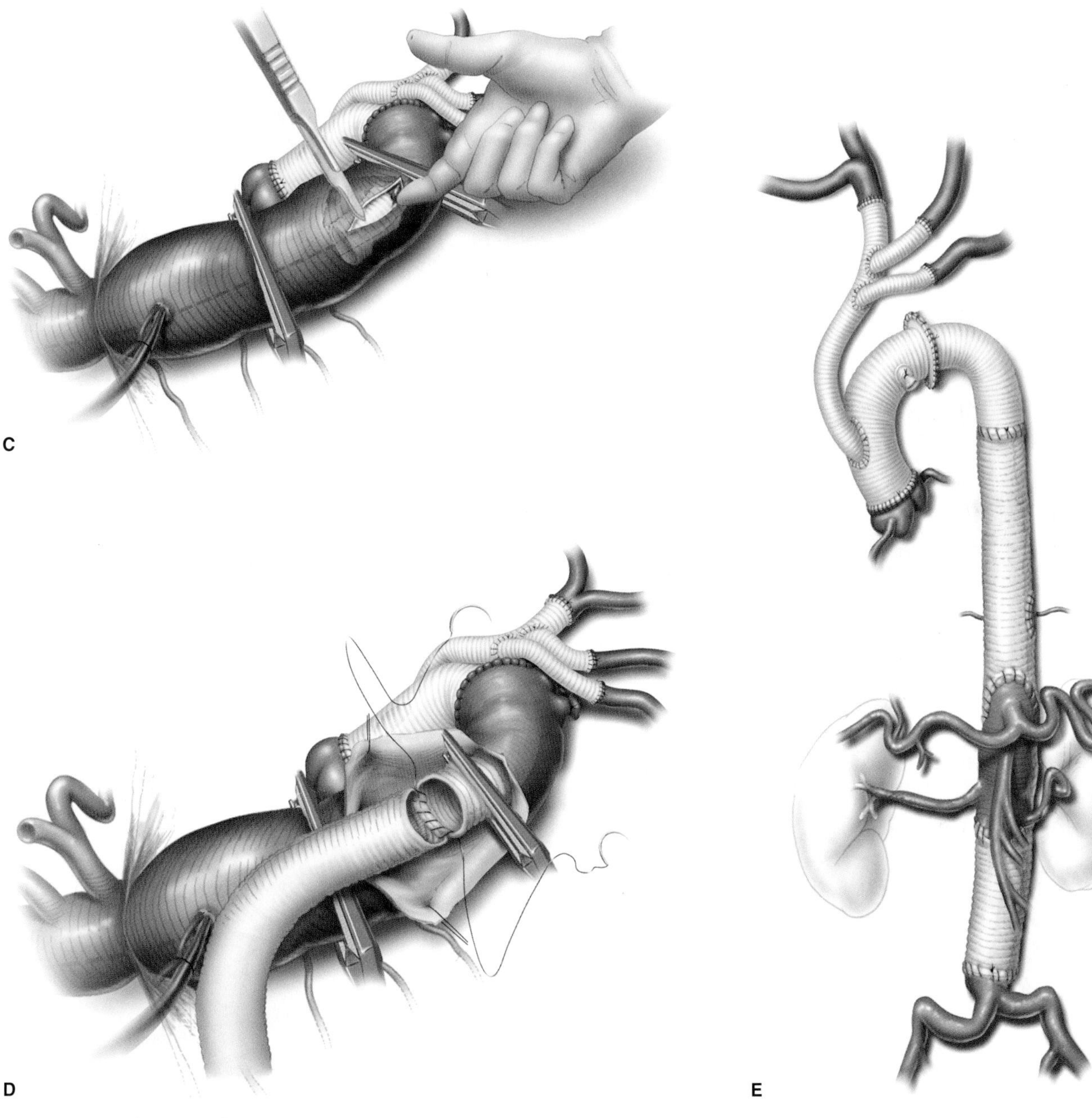

FIGURE 53-10 *(Continued)*

The bypass to the left subclavian artery during the first stage is not critical, and the left subclavian artery origin can remain intact on the native aorta. The aorta itself can be replaced with a skirted elephant trunk graft, which facilitates the distal aortic anastomosis to aneurysmal tissue. The proximal aortic anastomosis is placed to the supravalvar ascending aorta, and the distal skirt anastomosis can be placed fairly anteriorly on the aortic arch at the level of the innominate artery, facilitating hemostasis. The proximal end of the trifurcated graft is then anastomosed to an opening in the mid-ascending aspect of the aortic graft. The distal aortic anastomosis later becomes unimportant when the distal elephant trunk anastomosis to the descending aorta is completed at the second stage (Fig. 53-10C-E). The presence of the graft elephant trunk within the descending aorta allows secure clamping of even very large aneurysms distal to the left subclavian artery. If this artery was not bypassed during the arch vessel reconstruction, a side branch from the descending aorta can be anastomosed to the subclavian artery from the left chest during the second stage.[99]

Reversed Elephant Trunk Repairs. Conversely, in patients with similarly extensive aneurysmal disease who present with a DTAA or TAAA that has ruptured, causes symptoms (eg, back pain), or is considerably larger than the ascending aorta, the DTAA or TAAA is treated during the initial operation, and the ascending aorta and transverse aortic arch are repaired in a second procedure. During this "reversed" elephant-trunk repair (Fig. 53-11), a portion of the proximal end of the aortic graft

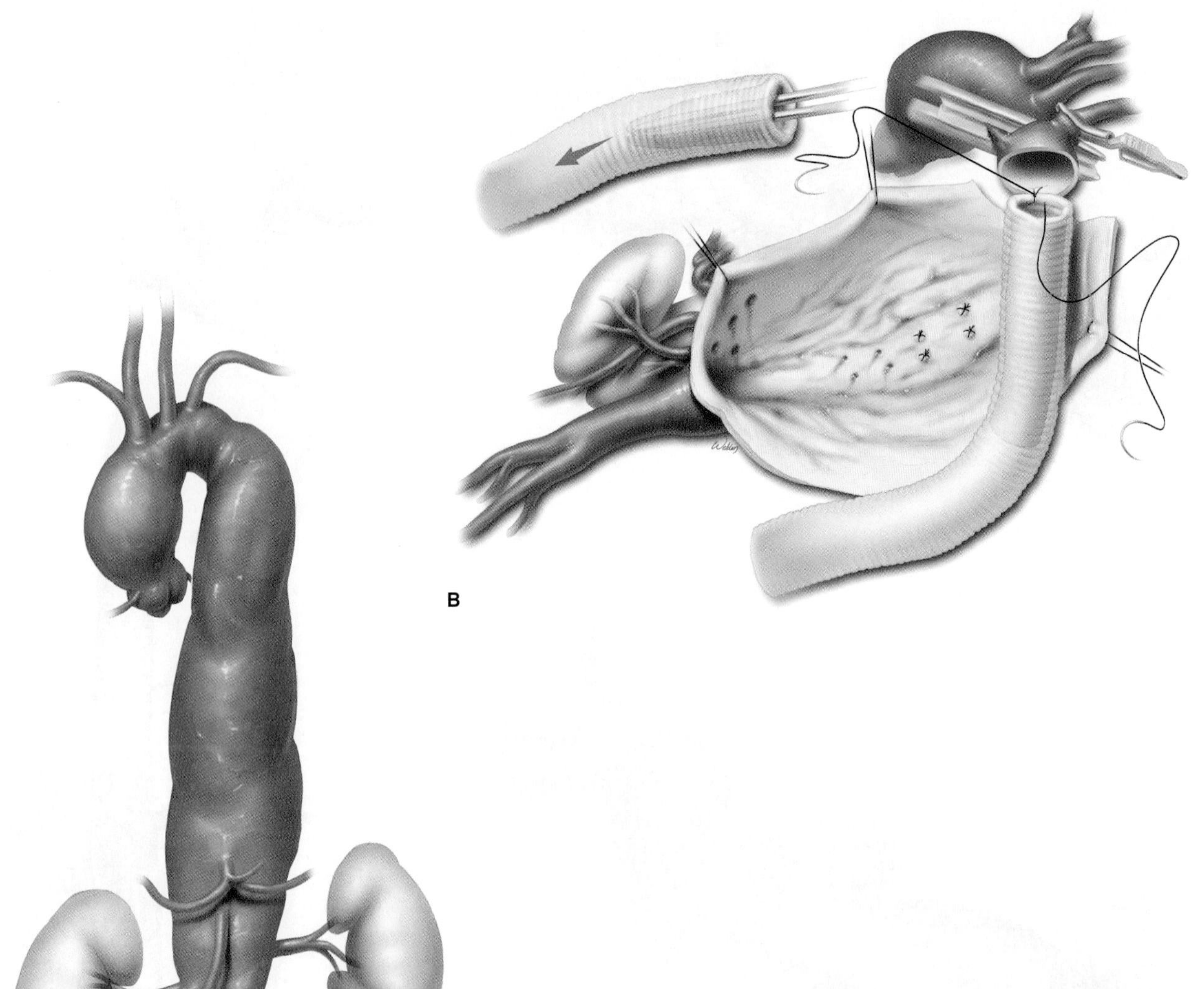

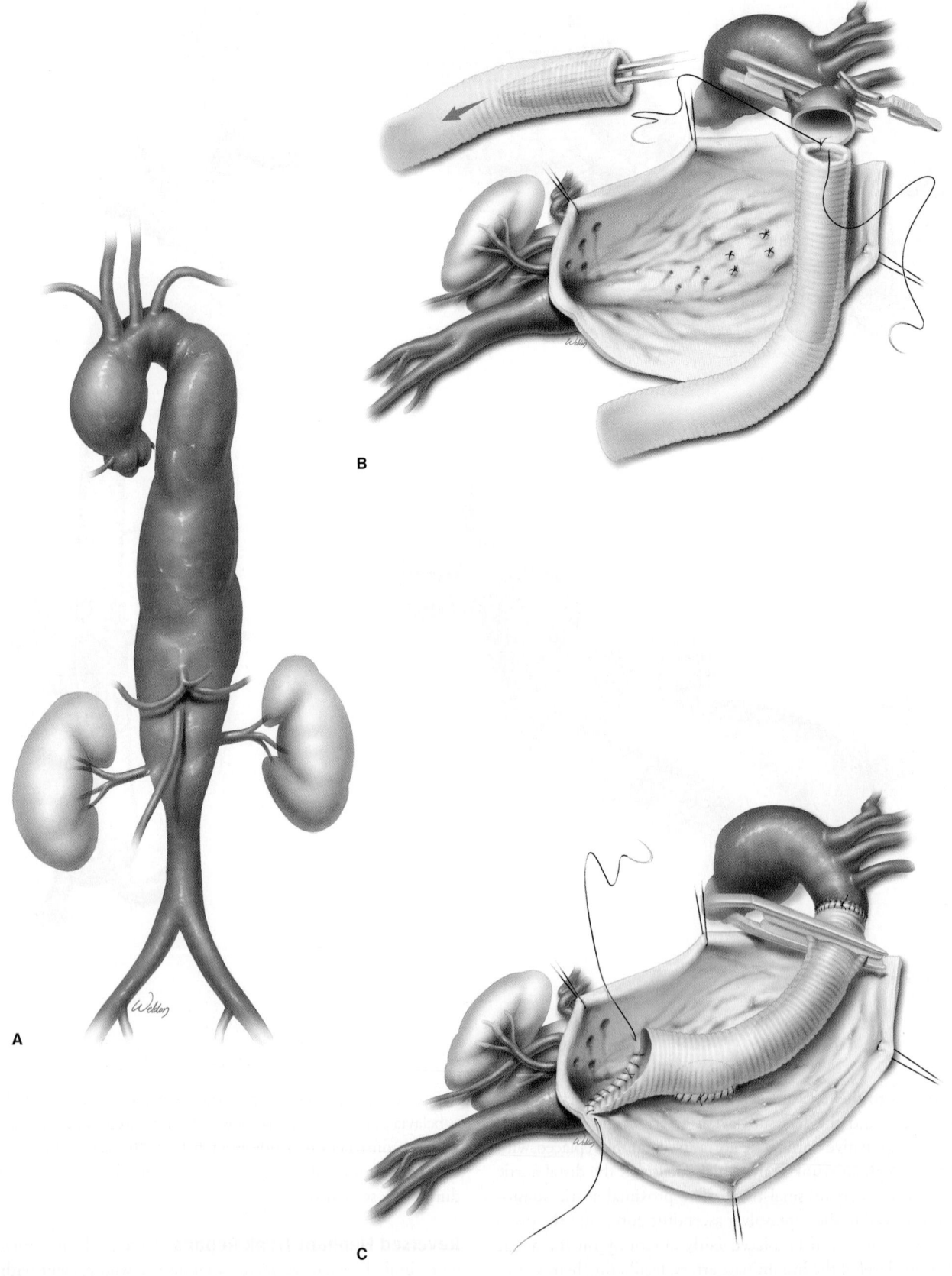

FIGURE 53-11 Drawings illustrating the two-stage reverse elephant trunk repair of an extensive aneurysm (A) involving the ascending, transverse arch, and thoracoabdominal aorta. (B) The first stage involves graft replacement of the thoracoabdominal aorta. The proximal portion of the graft is invaginated, and the folded edge is used to create the proximal anastomosis. (C) After reattachment of intercostal arteries, a beveled distal anastomosis is performed behind the visceral ostia. (D) After the first stage is completed, a segment of graft (the trunk) is left suspended within the descending thoracic aortic graft. (E) During the second stage, the graft trunk is retrieved through the open aortic arch, and (F) used to replace the arch and ascending aorta, (G) which completes the repair.

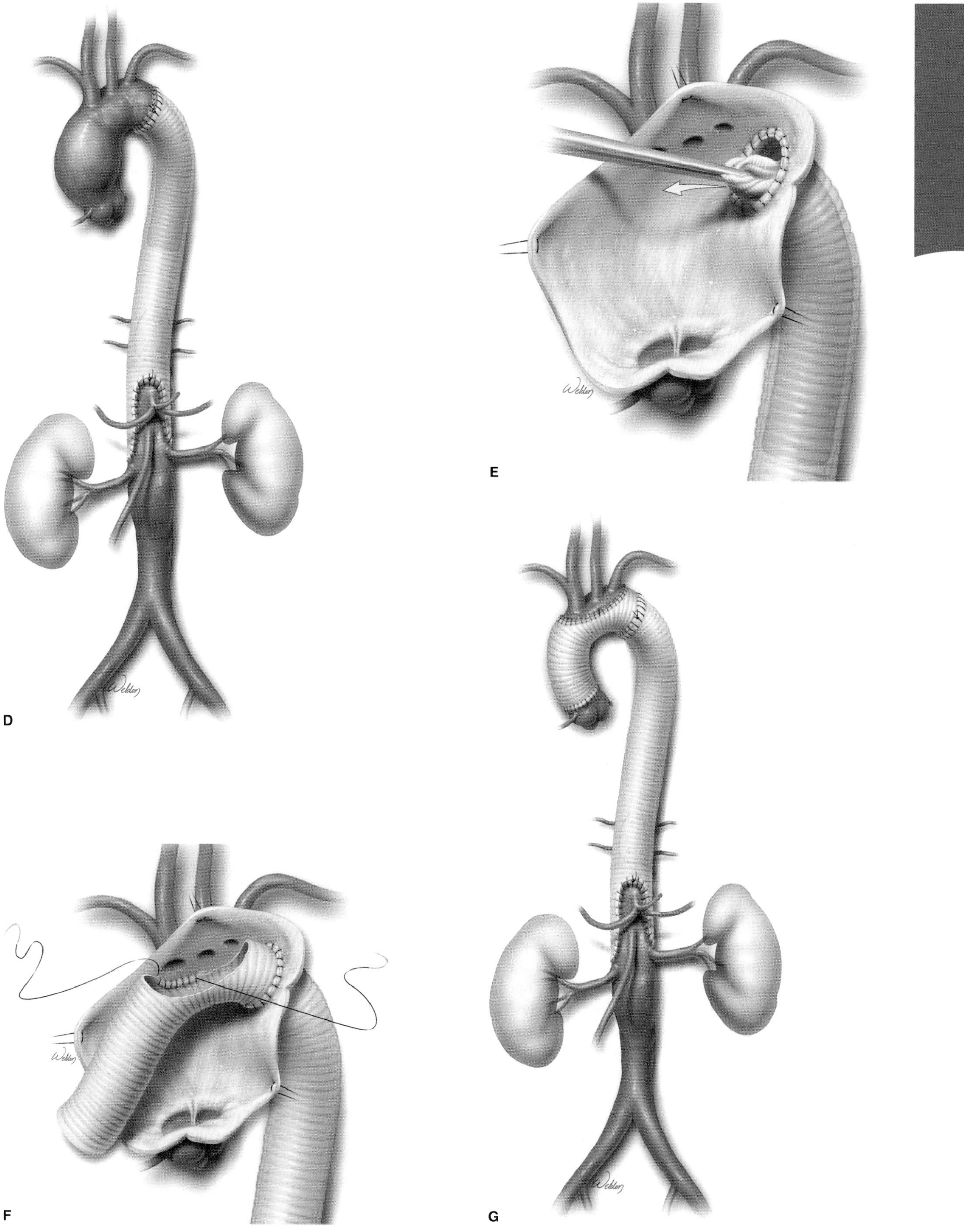

FIGURE 53-11 *(Continued)*

is inverted down into the lumen during the first operation and is later used to facilitate second-stage repair of the ascending and transverse aortic arch.[100]

Intercostal Patch Anastomosis and Completion of the DTAA Repair

After the proximal anastomosis is completed, LHB is discontinued and the distal aortic clamp is removed. The remainder of the aneurysm is opened longitudinally to its distal extent (Fig. 53-7F). The blood in the open aorta is scavenged via cell saver and returned as whole blood by a rapid infuser system. If the aneurysm was clamped proximal to the left subclavian artery, the aortic clamp is moved down onto the graft and the left subclavian artery clamp is removed; this restores blood flow to the left vertebral artery and to spinal collaterals. For repairs that extend to the diaphragm or beyond, patent lower intercostal arteries are selected and reattached to an opening cut in the side of the graft (Fig. 53-7G). If the aortic tissue is particularly friable, a separate, 8-mm graft can be attached in an end-to-end fashion to the selected intercostal vessels. In DTAA repairs, the distal anastomosis is then performed (Fig. 53-8B) to the open distal aorta. For aneurysms arising from chronic dissections, the membrane between the true and false lumen is fenestrated distally to ensure that both lumens are perfused.

Visceral Branch Vessel Anastomoses

In patients with TAAAs, after the descending thoracic aortic repair is completed, the remainder of the aneurysm is opened longitudinally (Fig. 53-7F). This incision runs posterior to the origin of the left renal artery and continues to the distal extent of the aneurysm. When present, the remaining dissecting membrane is excised. The origins of the visceral and renal branches are identified. Cold crystalloid is intermittently delivered to the renal arteries via balloon catheters (Fig. 53-7G). In patients receiving LHB, balloon cannulas are also placed in the celiac and superior mesenteric arteries so that selective visceral perfusion can be delivered from the pump circuit. Subsequently, the celiac, superior mesenteric, and renal arteries are reattached. In extent I repairs, the reattachment of the visceral arteries is often incorporated into a beveled distal anastomosis (Fig. 53-11C), but in extent II and III repairs, the visceral artery origins are reattached to one or more oval openings in the graft (Fig. 53-7H). In 30 to 40% of patients, the origin of the left renal artery is displaced laterally and is best attached to a separate opening in the graft (Fig. 53-7I). Patients with genetic disorders such as Marfan or Loeys-Dietz syndrome are prone to aneurysms involving their visceral reattachment patch; a multibranched graft enables separate bypasses to each of the vessels, thereby minimizing the amount of remaining aortic tissue and reducing the risk of recurrent aneurysms. Multibranched grafts are also useful in patients with large aneurysms that have caused wide displacement of the celiac, superior mesenteric, and renal arterial ostia (Fig. 53-12). Visceral artery stenosis is encountered in at least 25% of patients and necessitates endarterectomy (if anatomically suitable), stenting, or interposition bypass grafting.[54,101]

Distal Aortic and Iliac Anastomoses

When the TAAA extends below the renal arteries, a distal anastomosis is performed near the aortic bifurcation (Fig. 53-7J). In patients with iliac artery aneurysms, a bifurcation graft is sewn onto the end of the straight graft; the graft's limbs are then anastomosed to the common iliac, external iliac, or common femoral artery, depending on the extent of disease. The right limb of the bifurcation graft is tunneled retroperitoneally into the pelvis near the right iliac artery. Exposure of the left iliac artery is more straightforward from the left retroperitoneal incision. Care is taken to preserve circulation to at least one of the internal iliac arteries.

Closure

After all clamps are removed, heparin is reversed with protamine sulfate. Hemostasis is achieved by surgically reinforcing the anastomoses and administering blood products as necessary. The renal, visceral, and peripheral circulations are assessed. To ensure that renal function is adequate, blue dye is administered intravenously, and transit time to urine output is measured. The bowel, spleen, and liver are all assessed for adequacy of perfusion. The spleen is examined for capsular injury; if a splenic hematoma is present, the spleen is removed to avoid postoperative bleeding and hypotension. The aneurysm wall is then loosely wrapped around the aortic graft. Two posteriorly located thoracic drainage tubes and a closed-suction retroperitoneal drain are placed before closure. The diaphragm is closed with continuous polypropylene suture; postoperative disruption of the diaphragmatic repair is exceedingly rare.

OUTCOMES

Since 1986, we have performed open surgical repair of 3159 DTAAs and TAAAs. Combined hospital and 30-day operative mortality was 5.6% (n = 178). Complications that are commonly associated with an increased risk of death include paraplegia, renal failure, respiratory failure, cardiac events, and bleeding. The incidence of paraplegia and paraparesis in our series was 4.4% (n = 107), and the incidence of renal failure necessitating hemodialysis was 5.7% (n = 181). Our most recent data (from 2006 to 2009), which reflect the results of our current organ-protection strategies, are shown in Table 53-2.

The rate of return to the operating room for bleeding has been 2.5% in our experience. Postoperative blood pressure management is critical and must be balanced between hypertension (which can cause bleeding) and hypotension (which can lead to paraplegia/paraparesis). Because aortic anastomoses are often extremely fragile during the early postoperative period, even brief episodes of hypertension may disrupt suture lines and cause severe bleeding or pseudoaneurysm formation. In most cases, we use nitroprusside, intravenous β-antagonists, and intravenous calcium-channel blockers to keep the mean arterial blood pressure between 80 and 90 mm Hg. In patients with severely friable aortic tissue, such as those with Marfan syndrome, we use a target range of 70 to 80 mm Hg.

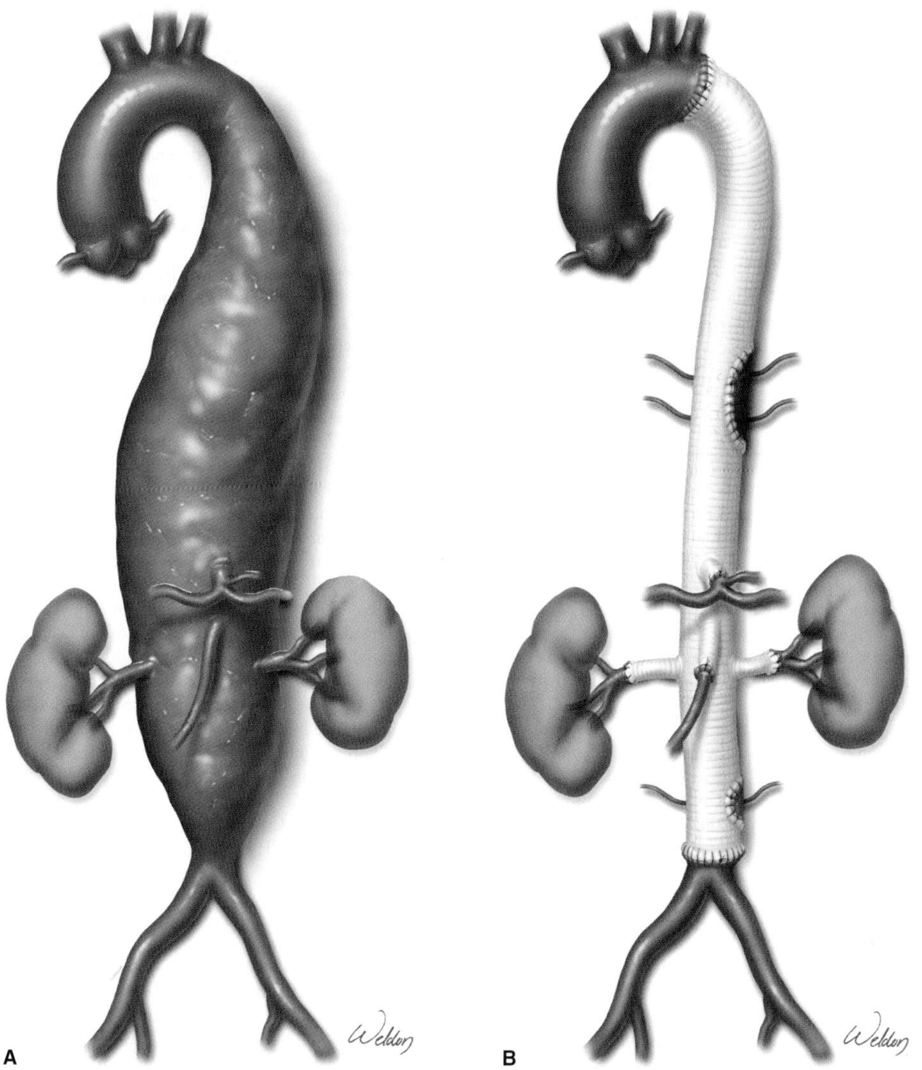

FIGURE 53-12 Drawings showing (A) a thoracoabdominal aortic aneurysm with wide displacement of the celiac, superior mesenteric, and both renal arterial ostia. (B) The aorta has been replaced with a multibranched graft that facilitates separate reattachment of each of the visceral arteries.

TABLE 53-2 Results of 475 Contemporary (2006–2009) Open Descending Thoracic or Thoracoabdominal Aortic Aneurysm Repairs

Extent of Repair	No. Patients	30-Day Deaths	Paraplegia*	Renal Failure*
DTAA	66	4 (6%)	1 (2%)	5 (8%)
TAAA I	102	4 (4%)	7 (7%)	8 (8%)
TAAA II	126	9 (7%)	9 (7%)	12 (10%)
TAAA III	79	6 (8%)	5 (6%)	7 (9%)
TAAA IV	102	7 (7%)	2 (2%)	9 (9%)
Total	*475*	*30 (6%)*	*24 (5%)*	*41 (9%)*

*Includes both transient and permanent impairment.
DTAA = Descending thoracic aortic aneurysm; TAAA = thoracoabdominal aortic aneurysm.

Vocal cord paralysis can contribute to respiratory complications; it should be suspected in patients with postoperative hoarseness and confirmed by direct examination. This complication can be treated effectively by direct cord medialization (ie, type 1 thyroplasty) or, in higher-risk patients, by polytetrafluoroethylene injection.[102]

SURVEILLANCE FOR ADDITIONAL AORTIC DISEASE

Patients who have undergone DTAA or TAAA repair remain at risk for developing new aneurysms in other aortic segments or in reattachment patches. Progressive weakening of aortic tissue at suture lines can lead to pseudoaneurysm formation. To detect new aortic disease before life-threatening complications occur, we recommend that all patients undergo annual CT or MR imaging of the chest and abdomen. This strategy of lifelong surveillance is especially important in patients with genetic disorders.[8,9] Subsequent aortic repairs can be performed with surprisingly low mortality and morbidity risk, particularly when done electively.[103]

ACKNOWLEDGMENTS

The authors thank Scott A. Weldon and Carol P. Larson for their outstanding medical illustrations and Stephen N. Palmer and Susan Y. Green for invaluable editorial support.

REFERENCES

1. Olsson C, Thelin S, Stahle E, Ekbom A, Granath F: Thoracic aortic aneurysm and dissection: increasing prevalence and improved outcomes reported in a nationwide population-based study of more than 14,000 cases from 1987 to 2002. *Circulation* 2006; 114(24):2611-2618.
2. Schlatmann TJ, Becker AE: Histologic changes in the normal aging aorta: implications for dissecting aortic aneurysm. *Am J Cardiol* 1977; 39(1): 13-20.
3. Fattouch K, Sampognaro R, Navarra E, et al: Long-term results after repair of type A acute aortic dissection according to false lumen patency. *Ann Thorac Surg* 2009; 88(4):1244-1250.
4. Bernard Y, Zimmermann H, Chocron S, et al: False lumen patency as a predictor of late outcome in aortic dissection. *Am J Cardiol* 2001; 87(12):1378-1382.
5. Estrera AL, Miller CC, Goodrick J, et al: Update on outcomes of acute type B aortic dissection. *Ann Thorac Surg* 2007; 83(2):S842-845.
6. Nienaber CA, Rousseau H, Eggebrecht H, et al: Randomized comparison of strategies for type B aortic dissection: the INvestigation of STEnt Grafts in Aortic Dissection (INSTEAD) trial. *Circulation* 2009; 120(25): 2519-2528.
7. Song HK, Bavaria JE, Kindem MW, et al: Surgical treatment of patients enrolled in the national registry of genetically triggered thoracic aortic conditions. *Ann Thorac Surg* 2009; 88(3):781-787; discussion 787-788.
8. LeMaire SA, Carter SA, Volguina IV, et al: Spectrum of aortic operations in 300 patients with confirmed or suspected Marfan syndrome. *Ann Thorac Surg* 2006; 81(6):2063-2078.
9. LeMaire SA, Pannu H, Tran-Fadulu V, et al: Severe aortic and arterial aneurysms associated with a TGFBR2 mutation. *Nat Clin Pract Cardiovasc Med* 2007; 4(3):167-171.
10. Loeys BL, Chen J, Neptune ER, et al: A syndrome of altered cardiovascular, craniofacial, neurocognitive and skeletal development caused by mutations in TGFBR1 or TGFBR2. *Nat Genet* 2005; 37(3):275-281.
11. Kang N, Clarke AJ, Nicholson IA, Chard RB: Circulatory arrest for repair of postcoarctation site aneurysm. *Ann Thorac Surg* 2004; 77(6):2029-2033.
12. Ala-Kulju K, Heikkinen L: Aneurysms after patch graft aortoplasty for coarctation of the aorta: long-term results of surgical management. *Ann Thorac Surg* 1989; 47(6):853-856.
13. Heikkinen L, Sariola H, Salo J, Ala-Kulju K: Morphological and histopathological aspects of aneurysms after patch aortoplasty for coarctation. *Ann Thorac Surg* 1990; 50(6):946-948.
14. Korkut AK, Cetin G, Saltik L: Management of a large pseudo-aneurysm secondary to balloon angioplasty for aortic coarctation. *Acta Chir Belg* 2006; 106(1):107-108.
15. Johnston KW, Rutherford RB, Tilson MD, et al: Suggested standards for reporting on arterial aneurysms. Subcommittee on Reporting Standards for Arterial Aneurysms, Ad Hoc Committee on Reporting Standards, Society for Vascular Surgery and North American Chapter, International Society for Cardiovascular Surgery. *J Vasc Surg* 1991; 13(3):452-458.
16. Pearce WH, Slaughter MS, LeMaire S, et al: Aortic diameter as a function of age, gender, and body surface area. *Surgery* 1993; 114(4):691-697.
17. Agmon Y, Khandheria BK, Meissner I, et al: Is aortic dilatation an atherosclerosis-related process? Clinical, laboratory, and transesophageal echocardiographic correlates of thoracic aortic dimensions in the population with implications for thoracic aortic aneurysm formation. *J Am Coll Cardiol* 2003; 42(6):1076-1083.
18. Cronenwett JL, Garrett HE: Arteriographic measurement of the abdominal aorta, iliac, and femoral arteries in women with atherosclerotic occlusive disease. *Radiology* 1983; 148(2):389-392.
19. Hager A, Kaemmerer H, Rapp-Bernhardt U, et al: Diameters of the thoracic aorta throughout life as measured with helical computed tomography. *J Thorac Cardiovasc Surg* 2002; 123(6):1060-1066.
20. Liddington MI, Heather BP. The relationship between aortic diameter and body habitus. *Eur J Vasc Surg* 1992; 6(1):89-92.
21. Coady MA, Rizzo JA, Hammond GL, Kopf GS, Elefteriades JA: Surgical intervention criteria for thoracic aortic aneurysms: a study of growth rates and complications. *Ann Thorac Surg* 1999; 67(6):1922-1926.
22. Elefteriades JA: Natural history of thoracic aortic aneurysms: indications for surgery, and surgical versus nonsurgical risks. *Ann Thorac Surg* 2002; 74(5):S1877-1880.
23. Clouse WD, Hallett JW Jr, Schaff HV, et al: Improved prognosis of thoracic aortic aneurysms: a population-based study. *JAMA* 1998; 280(22): 1926-1929.
24. Panneton JM, Hollier LH: Nondissecting thoracoabdominal aortic aneurysms: part I. *Ann Vasc Surg* 1995; 9(5):503-514.
25. Hemminger BM, Molina PL, Egan TM, et al: Assessment of real-time 3D visualization for cardiothoracic diagnostic evaluation and surgery planning. *J Digit Imaging* 2005; 18(2):145-153.
26. Rubin GD: CT angiography of the thoracic aorta. *Semin Roentgenol* 2003; 38(2):115-134.
27. Takahashi K, Stanford W: Multidetector CT of the thoracic aorta. *Int J Cardiovasc Imaging* 2005; 21(1):141-153.
28. Weinbaum FI, Dubner S, Turner JW, Pardes JG: The accuracy of computed tomography in the diagnosis of retroperitoneal blood in the presence of abdominal aortic aneurysm. *J Vasc Surg* 1987; 6(1):11-16.
29. Green D, Parker D: CTA and MRA: visualization without catheterization. *Semin Ultrasound CT MR* 2003; 24(4):185.
30. Marckmann P, Skov L, Rossen K, et al: Nephrogenic systemic fibrosis: suspected causative role of gadodiamide used for contrast-enhanced magnetic resonance imaging. *J Am Soc Nephrol* 2006; 17(9):2359-2362.
31. Thomsen HS: How to avoid nephrogenic systemic fibrosis: current guidelines in Europe and the United States. *Radiol Clin North Am* 2009; 47(5):871-875, vii.
32. Soulen MC: Catheter angiography of thoracic aortic aneurysms. *Semin Roentgenol* 2001; 36(4):334-339.
33. Leurs LJ, Bell R, Degrieck Y, et al: Endovascular treatment of thoracic aortic diseases: combined experience from the EUROSTAR and United Kingdom Thoracic Endograft registries. *J Vasc Surg* 2004; 40(4): 670-679.
34. Makaroun MS, Dillavou ED, Kee ST, et al: Endovascular treatment of thoracic aortic aneurysms: results of the phase II multicenter trial of the GORE TAG thoracic endoprosthesis. *J Vasc Surg* 2005; 41(1):1-9.
35. Rachel ES, Bergamini TM, Kinney EV, et al: Endovascular repair of thoracic aortic aneurysms: a paradigm shift in standard of care. *Vasc Endovascular Surg* 2002; 36(2):105-113.
36. Greenberg RK, Clair D, Srivastava S, et al: Should patients with challenging anatomy be offered endovascular aneurysm repair? *J Vasc Surg* 2003; 38(5): 990-996.
37. Coselli JS, Green SY, Preventza O, LeMaire SA: Combining open and endovascular approaches to complex aneurysms, in: Pearce WH, Matsumura J, Morasch M, Yao JST (eds): *Vascular Surgery: Therapeutic Strategies.* Beijing, People's Medical Publishing House, 2010; pp 529-548.
38. Gottardi R, Lammer J, Grimm M, Czerny M: Entire rerouting of the supraaortic branches for endovascular stent-graft placement of an aortic arch aneurysm. *Eur J Cardiothorac Surg* 2006; 29(2):258-260.
39. Baraki H, Hagl C, Khaladj N, et al: The frozen elephant trunk technique for treatment of thoracic aortic aneurysms. *Ann Thorac Surg* 2007; 83(2): S819-823; discussion S824-831.
40. Flye MW, Choi ET, Sanchez LA, et al: Retrograde visceral vessel revascularization followed by endovascular aneurysm exclusion as an alternative to open surgical repair of thoracoabdominal aortic aneurysm. *J Vasc Surg* 2004; 39(2):454-458.
41. Fulton JJ, Farber MA, Marston WA, et al: Endovascular stent-graft repair of pararenal and type IV thoracoabdominal aortic aneurysms with adjunctive visceral reconstruction. [erratum appears in *J Vasc Surg* 2005 May; 41(5):906]. *J Vasc Surg* 2005; 41(2):191-198.
42. Svensson LG, Kim KH, Blackstone EH, et al: Elephant trunk procedure: newer indications and uses. *Ann Thorac Surg* 2004; 78(1):109-115; discussion 115-116.
43. Chuter TA, Gordon RL, Reilly LM, Goodman JD, Messina LM: An endovascular system for thoracoabdominal aortic aneurysm repair. *J Endovasc Ther* 2001; 8(1):25-33.
44. Kaviani A, Greenberg R: Current status of branched stent-graft technology in treatment of thoracoabdominal aneurysms. *Semin Vasc Surg* 2006; 19(1): 60-65.

45. Palma JH, Miranda F, Gasques AR, et al: Treatment of thoracoabdominal aneurysm with self-expandable aortic stent grafts. *Ann Thorac Surg* 2002; 74(5):1685-1687.
46. Chemelli-Steingruber IE, Chemelli A, Strasak A, et al: Evaluation of volumetric measurements in patients with acute type B aortic dissection—thoracic endovascular aortic repair (TEVAR) vs conservative. *J Vasc Surg* 2009; 49(1):20-28.
47. Bakaeen FG, Coselli JS, LeMaire SA, Huh J: Continued aortic aneurysmal expansion after thoracic endovascular stent-grafting. *Ann Thorac Surg* 2007; 84(3):1007-1008.
48. Kelso RL, Lyden SP, Butler B, et al: Late conversion of aortic stent grafts. *J Vasc Surg* 2009; 49(3):589-595.
49. Nabi D, Murphy EH, Pak J, Zarins CK: Open surgical repair after failed endovascular aneurysm repair: is endograft removal necessary? *J Vasc Surg* 2009; 50(4):714-721.
50. Coselli JS, LeMaire SA, Miller CC III, et al: Mortality and paraplegia after thoracoabdominal aortic aneurysm repair: a risk factor analysis. *Ann Thorac Surg* 2000; 69(2):409-414.
51. LeMaire SA, Miller CC III, Conklin LD, et al: A new predictive model for adverse outcomes after elective thoracoabdominal aortic aneurysm repair. *Ann Thorac Surg* 2001; 71(4):1233-1238.
52. Svensson LG, Crawford ES, Hess KR, Coselli JS, Safi HJ: Thoracoabdominal aortic aneurysms associated with celiac, superior mesenteric, and renal artery occlusive disease: methods and analysis of results in 271 patients. *J Vasc Surg* 1992; 16(3):378-389.
53. Jones MM, Akay M, Murariu D, LeMaire SA, Coselli JS: Safe aortic arch clamping in patients with patent internal thoracic artery grafts. *Ann Thorac Surg* 2010; 89(4):e31-e32.
54. Svensson LG, Crawford ES, Hess KR, Coselli JS, Safi HJ: Experience with 1509 patients undergoing thoracoabdominal aortic operations. *J Vasc Surg* 1993; 17(2):357-368.
55. Chan FY, Crawford ES, Coselli JS, Safi HJ, Williams TW Jr: In situ prosthetic graft replacement for mycotic aneurysm of the aorta. *Ann Thorac Surg* 1989; 47(2):193-203.
56. Coselli JS, Crawford ES: Composite valve-graft replacement of aortic root using separate Dacron tube for coronary artery reattachment. *Ann Thorac Surg* 1989; 47(4):558-565.
57. MacArthur RG, Carter SA, Coselli JS, LeMaire SA: Organ protection during thoracoabdominal aortic surgery: rationale for a multimodality approach. *Semin Cardiothorac Vasc Anesth* 2005; 9(2):143-149.
58. Frank SM, Parker SD, Rock P, et al: Moderate hypothermia, with partial bypass and segmental sequential repair for thoracoabdominal aortic aneurysm. *J Vasc Surg* 1994; 19(4):687-697.
59. Strauch JT, Lauten A, Spielvogel D, et al: Mild hypothermia protects the spinal cord from ischemic injury in a chronic porcine model. *Eur J Cardiothorac Surg* 2004; 25(5):708-715.
60. Inamasu J, Nakamura Y, Ichikizaki K: Induced hypothermia in experimental traumatic spinal cord injury: an update. *J Neurol Sci* 2003; 209(1-2): 55-60.
61. Rokkas CK, Sundaresan S, Shuman TA, et al: Profound systemic hypothermia protects the spinal cord in a primate model of spinal cord ischemia. *J Thorac Cardiovasc Surg* 1993; 106(6):1024-1035.
62. Kouchoukos NT, Masetti P, Rokkas CK, Murphy SF: Hypothermic cardiopulmonary bypass and circulatory arrest for operations on the descending thoracic and thoracoabdominal aorta. *Ann Thorac Surg* 2002; 74(5):S1885-1887.
63. Kouchoukos NT, Masetti P, Rokkas CK, Murphy SF, Blackstone EH: Safety and efficacy of hypothermic cardiopulmonary bypass and circulatory arrest for operations on the descending thoracic and thoracoabdominal aorta. *Ann Thorac Surg* 2001; 72(3):699-707.
64. Kouchoukos NT, Rokkas CK: Hypothermic cardiopulmonary bypass for spinal cord protection: rationale and clinical results. *Ann Thorac Surg* 1999; 67(6):1940-1942.
65. Schepens MA, Defauw JJ, Hamerlijnck RP, Vermeulen FE: Use of left heart bypass in the surgical repair of thoracoabdominal aortic aneurysms. *Ann Vasc Surg* 1995; 9(4):327-338.
66. Borst HG, Frank G, Schaps D: Treatment of extensive aortic aneurysms by a new multiple-stage approach. *J Thorac Cardiovasc Surg* 1988; 95(1):11-13.
67. Wong DR, Coselli JS, Amerman K, et al: Delayed spinal cord deficits after thoracoabdominal aortic aneurysm repair. *Ann Thorac Surg* 2007; 83(4):1345-1355.
68. Schepens MA, Heijmen RH, Ranschaert W, Sonker U, Morshuis WJ: Thoracoabdominal aortic aneurysm repair: results of conventional open surgery. *Eur J Vasc Endovasc Surg* 2009; 37(6):640-645.
69. Misfeld M, Sievers HH, Hadlak M, Gorski A, Hanke T: Rate of paraplegia and mortality in elective descending and thoracoabdominal aortic repair in the modern surgical era. *Thorac Cardiovasc Surg* 2008; 56(6):342-347.
70. Dong CC, MacDonald DB, Janusz MT: Intraoperative spinal cord monitoring during descending thoracic and thoracoabdominal aneurysm surgery. *Ann Thorac Surg* 2002; 74(5):S1873-1876.
71. Meylaerts SA, Jacobs MJ, van Iterson V, De Haan P, Kalkman CJ: Comparison of transcranial motor evoked potentials and somatosensory evoked potentials during thoracoabdominal aortic aneurysm repair. *Ann Surg* 1999; 230(6):742-749.
72. van Dongen EP, Schepens MA, Morshuis WJ, et al: Thoracic and thoracoabdominal aortic aneurysm repair: use of evoked potential monitoring in 118 patients. *J Vasc Surg* 2001; 34(6):1035-1040.
73. Keyhani K, Miller CC, III, Estrera AL, et al: Analysis of motor and somatosensory evoked potentials during thoracic and thoracoabdominal aortic aneurysm repair. *J Vasc Surg* 2009; 49(1):36-41.
74. MacDonald DB: Intraoperative motor evoked potential monitoring: overview and update. *J Clin Monit Comput* 2006; 20(5):347-377.
75. Jacobs MJ, de Mol BA, Elenbaas T, et al: Spinal cord blood supply in patients with thoracoabdominal aortic aneurysms. *J Vasc Surg* 2002; 35(1):30-37.
76. Jacobs MJ, Elenbaas TW, Schurink GW, Mess WH, Mochtar B: Assessment of spinal cord integrity during thoracoabdominal aortic aneurysm repair. *Ann Thorac Surg* 2002; 74(5):S1864-1866.
77. Miyamoto K, Ueno A, Wada T, Kimoto S: A new and simple method of preventing spinal cord damage following temporary occlusion of the thoracic aorta by draining the cerebrospinal fluid. *J Cardiovasc Surg (Torino)* 1960; 1:188-197.
78. Ackerman LL, Traynelis VC: Treatment of delayed-onset neurological deficit after aortic surgery with lumbar cerebrospinal fluid drainage. *Neurosurgery* 2002; 51(6):1414-1421.
79. Brock MV, Redmond JM, Ishiwa S, et al: Clinical markers in CSF for determining neurologic deficits after thoracoabdominal aortic aneurysm repairs. *Ann Thorac Surg* 1997; 64(4):999-1003.
80. Huynh TT, Miller CC, III, Estrera AL, et al: Correlations of cerebrospinal fluid pressure with hemodynamic parameters during thoracoabdominal aortic aneurysm repair. *Ann Vasc Surg* 2005; 19(5):619-624.
81. Kunihara T, Matsuzaki K, Shiiya N, Saijo Y, Yasuda K: Naloxone lowers cerebrospinal fluid levels of excitatory amino acids after thoracoabdominal aortic surgery. *J Vasc Surg* 2004; 40(4):681-690.
82. Piano G, Gewertz BL: Mechanism of increased cerebrospinal fluid pressure with thoracic aortic occlusion. *J Vasc Surg* 1990; 11(5):695-701.
83. Coselli JS, LeMaire SA, Köksoy C, Schmittling ZC, Curling PE: Cerebrospinal fluid drainage reduces paraplegia after thoracoabdominal aortic aneurysm repair: results of a randomized clinical trial. *J Vasc Surg* 2002; 35(4):631-639.
84. Cinà CS, Abouzahr L, Arena GO, et al: Cerebrospinal fluid drainage to prevent paraplegia during thoracic and thoracoabdominal aortic aneurysm surgery: a systematic review and meta-analysis. *J Vasc Surg* 2004; 40(1):36-44.
85. Estrera AL, Sheinbaum R, Miller CC, et al: Cerebrospinal fluid drainage during thoracic aortic repair: safety and current management. *Ann Thorac Surg* 2009; 88(1):9-15.
86. Berguer R, Porto J, Fedoronko B, Dragovic L: Selective deep hypothermia of the spinal cord prevents paraplegia after aortic cross-clamping in the dog model. *J Vasc Surg* 1992; 15(1):62-71.
87. Marsala M, Vanicky I, Galik J, et al: Panmyelic epidural cooling protects against ischemic spinal cord damage. *J Surg Res* 1993; 55(1):21-31.
88. Wang LM, Yan Y, Zou LJ, Jing NH, Xu ZY: Moderate hypothermia prevents neural cell apoptosis following spinal cord ischemia in rabbits. *Cell Res* 2005; 15(5):387-393.
89. Wisselink W, Becker MO, Nguyen JH, Money SR, Hollier LH: Protecting the ischemic spinal cord during aortic clamping: the influence of selective hypothermia and spinal cord perfusion pressure. *J Vasc Surg* 1994; 19(5):788-795.
90. Cambria RP, Clouse WD, Davison JK, et al: Thoracoabdominal aneurysm repair: results with 337 operations performed over a 15-year interval. *Ann Surg* 2002; 236(4):471-479.
91. Tetik O, Islamoglu F, Yagdi T, et al: An intraaortic solution trial to prevent spinal cord injury in a rabbit model. *Eur J Vasc Endovasc Surg* 2001; 22(2):175-179.
92. Coselli JS: The use of left heart bypass in the repair of thoracoabdominal aortic aneurysms: current techniques and results. *Semin Thorac Cardiovasc Surg* 2003; 15(4):326-332.
93. Coselli JS, LeMaire SA, Conklin LD, Adams GJ: Left heart bypass during descending thoracic aortic aneurysm repair does not reduce the incidence of paraplegia. *Ann Thorac Surg* 2004; 77(4):1298-1303.
94. Estrera AL, Miller CC, III, Chen EP, et al: Descending thoracic aortic aneurysm repair: 12-year experience using distal aortic perfusion and cerebrospinal fluid drainage. *Ann Thorac Surg* 2005; 80(4):1290-1296.
95. Safi HJ, Estrera AL, Miller CC, et al: Evolution of risk for neurologic deficit after descending and thoracoabdominal aortic repair. *Ann Thorac Surg* 2005; 80(6):2173-2179.

96. Schepens MA, Kelder JC, Morshuis WJ, et al: Long-term follow-up after thoracoabdominal aortic aneurysm repair. *Ann Thorac Surg* 2007; 83(2): S851-855.
97. Köksoy C, LeMaire SA, Curling PE, et al: Renal perfusion during thoracoabdominal aortic operations: cold crystalloid is superior to normothermic blood. *Ann Thorac Surg* 2002; 73(3):730-738.
98. Fehrenbacher JW, Hart DW, Huddleston E, Siderys H, Rice C: Optimal end-organ protection for thoracic and thoracoabdominal aortic aneurysm repair using deep hypothermic circulatory arrest. *Ann Thorac Surg* 2007; 83(3):1041-1046.
99. Spielvogel D, Etz CD, Silovitz D, Lansman SL, Griepp RB: Aortic arch replacement with a trifurcated graft. *Ann Thorac Surg* 2007; 83(2):S791-795; discussion S824-831.
100. Coselli JS, LeMaire SA, Carter SA, Conklin LD: The reversed elephant trunk technique used for treatment of complex aneurysms of the entire thoracic aorta. *Ann Thorac Surg* 2005; 80(6):2166-2172; discussion 2172.
101. LeMaire SA, Jamison AL, Carter SA, et al: Deployment of balloon expandable stents during open repair of thoracoabdominal aortic aneurysms: a new strategy for managing renal and mesenteric artery lesions. *Eur J Cardiothorac Surg* 2004; 26(3):599-607.
102. Rosingh HJ, Dikkers FG: Thyroplasty to improve the voice in patients with a unilateral vocal fold paralysis. *Clin Otolaryngol Allied Sci* 1995; 20(2):124-126.
103. Coselli JS, Poli de Figueiredo LF, LeMaire SA: Impact of previous thoracic aneurysm repair on thoracoabdominal aortic aneurysm management. *Ann Thorac Surg* 1997; 64(3):639-650.

CHAPTER 54

Endovascular Therapy for the Treatment of Thoracic Aortic Disease

Susan D. Moffatt-Bruce
R. Scott Mitchell

INTRODUCTION

Patients with thoracic aortic disease are a difficult population to treat, because they frequently consist of an aged population with multiple comorbidities. The modern surgical treatment of thoracic aortic diseases began in the 1950s when successful treatment using segmental resection and graft replacement was reported by Swan, Lam, DeBakey, and Etheredge.[1–3] Thereafter, DeBakey and Cooley reported the first successful repair of an ascending aortic aneurysm using cardiopulmonary bypass.[4] Our understanding of the pathophysiology and natural history of thoracic aortic disease has evolved, which has expanded our treatment choices.[5,6] In addition, improvements in diagnostic capabilities, surgical techniques, and perioperative care have resulted in improved outcomes, even as the risk profile has increased. Nonetheless, operative intervention in this patient population frequently results in substantial mortality and long-term morbidity.[7,8] The concept of using endovascular techniques to treat patients with thoracic aortic disease emerged a decade ago, propelled by the desire to avoid surgical risk as well as to induce reconstructive modeling of the diseased aorta by initiating a natural healing process through exclusion and depressurization of the aneurysmal sac.[9] In an effort to improve outcomes in the treatment of patients with thoracic aortic disease, endovascular stent-graft technology has rapidly followed applications on the abdominal aorta.[10,11] Originally devised for high-risk patients with multiple comorbidities, thoracic stent-graft applications are being expanded to young and old patients with a variety of pathologies, including thoracic aortic aneurysms, aortic dissections, intramural hematomas, penetrating atherosclerotic ulcers, and thoracic aortic trauma.[12–19] Initial reports using these endovascular stent-grafts have been encouraging, but long-term outcomes are unknown, and the necessity for long-term follow-up, with its attendant expense, has raised serious concern.[20–22]

HISTORY

Endovascular stent-graft technology was initially envisioned for use in abdominal aortic aneurysms.[23] Introduced by Parodi, balloon-expandable stents attached to the ends of a vascular tube graft were used to exclude the aneurysm sac. There were several attractive features of this concept, including the introduction of the device from a peripheral site, eliminating the necessity for an invasive laparotomy, the avoidance of aortic cross-clamping and its requisite physiologic perturbations, and minimizing respiratory complications. Last, hospital stay and recovery time could be potentially shortened.

At Stanford University Medical Center, a collaborative effort between interventional radiologists and cardiovascular surgeons proved highly synergistic, and resulted in the manufacture and clinical use of thoracic stent grafts. Work had commenced years earlier with the use of uncovered stents for the repair of aortic dissections in an animal model. The stent grafts were manufactured using self-expanding Gianturco Z stents (Cook Co., Bloomington, IN), which were fastened together and then covered with a woven Dacron graft (Meadox-Boston Scientific, Natick, MA; Fig. 54-1). Institutional review board (IRB) approval was initially obtained for a high-risk study using endovascular stent-grafts for the treatment of thoracic aortic aneurysms in patients who were deemed not to be surgical candidates.[24] A total of

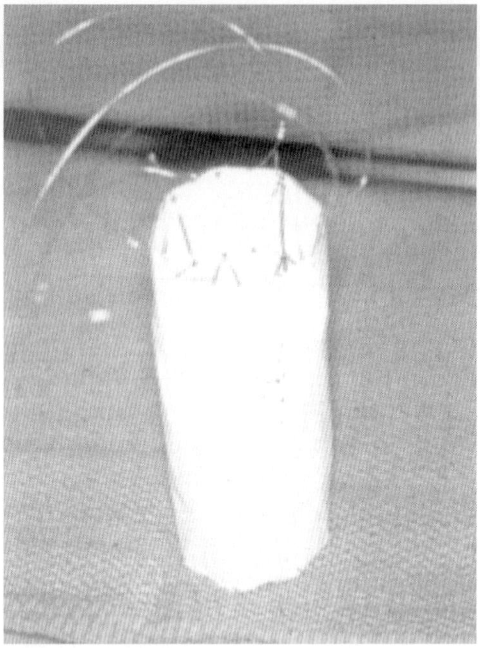

FIGURE 54-1 First-generation stent graft assembled from articulated Z stents and covered with a woven Dacron tube graft.

13 patients underwent transluminal endovascular grafting of thoracic aortic aneurysms with a mean diameter of 6.1 cm. The stent grafts, custom-designed for each patient, were constructed of self-expanding stainless steel stents covered with woven Dacron grafts. Placement of these stents was successful in all patients with thrombosis of the aneurysm surrounding the stent occurring in 12 of the 13 patients. As reported, at 1 year there were no deaths, paraplegia, stroke, distal embolization, or infection.[24] It was therefore concluded that these preliminary results demonstrated that endovascular stent-graft repair was safe in highly selected patients.

This feasibility trial led to the extension of the IRB approval for the treatment of 103 patients with thoracic aortic aneurysms.[25] Of these 103 patients, 60% were unsuitable candidates for conventional open surgical repair and therefore deemed inoperable. Again, these patients underwent repair of a descending thoracic aortic aneurysm using "homemade" or first-generation stent grafts fabricated from self-expanding Z stents covered with woven Dacron tube graft. Complete aneurysm thrombosis was achieved in 83% of patients. Early mortality was 9% and was significantly associated with a history of cerebrovascular accidents and myocardial infarctions. Major perioperative morbidity included paraplegia in three patients, cerebrovascular accidents in seven patients, and respiratory insufficiency in 12 patients. Treatment failure occurred in 38 of the 103 patients, and five patients required late operative therapy for endoleaks associated with aneurysm enlargement. Actuarial survival was 81% at 1 year and 73% at 2 years. Given the high-risk nature of this patient population, these first-generation results were deemed satisfactory. It was, however, recognized that mortality and morbidity occurred frequently and that long-term follow-up was necessary to fully define the efficacy of an endovascular approach in thoracic aortic aneurysm therapy. Subsequently, in 2004, midterm results were reported for these 103 patients treated with the first-generation stent grafts.[26] Overall actuarial survival was dismal; 82, 49, and 27% at 1, 5, and 8 years, respectively. However, the survival of the potentially operable candidates was 93 and 78% at 1 and 5 years, respectively, as compared with 74 and 31% at 1 and 5 years, respectively, in those patients designated as inoperable. In patients judged not to be surgical candidates, life expectancy, despite endovascular therapy, was therefore quite bleak, and has raised concerns whether any surgical therapy is appropriate for these patients. Further results revealed that 11 of the 103 patients suffered late aortic rupture at the site of endovascular treatment. This was a very sobering finding considering that open surgical graft replacement has been associated with durable long-term results with only a negligible late hazard of anastomotic problems. However, it must be remembered that this study involved the use of a relatively primitive first-generation device, with a fairly steep learning curve.

Extending the use of the endovascular stent grafts to the treatment of complicated acute aortic dissections of the descending thoracic aorta, Dake and associates reported their findings in the *New England Journal of Medicine* in 1999.[27] Again these stents were the first-generation "homemade" devices described in the preceding. Placement of the stents across the primary entry tears was technically successful in all patients, with correction of malperfusion. Complete thrombosis of the false lumen occurred in 79%. The early mortality rate was 16%, which reflected late referral, with established intestinal gangrene, and another patient with Ehlers-Danlos syndrome, perhaps a poor candidate for endovascular repair. Favorable clinical results persisted out to a mean follow-up of 13 months.

These pioneering efforts at the Stanford University Medical Center established some interesting concepts. Namely, that these were complex patients with complex aortic problems, and that endograft therapy for aneurysmal disease was effective, potentially with reduced morbidity, but with uncertain long-term durability. Improved results could likely be obtained with more sophisticated devices, and endograft repair could effectively reverse malperfusion syndromes in complicated type B aortic dissections.

NATURAL HISTORY AND SURGICAL OUTCOMES OF THORACIC AORTIC DISEASES

Thoracic Aortic Aneurysms

Approximately 50% of all thoracic aortic aneurysms are located in the descending aorta; these aneurysms commonly arise at the level of the left subclavian artery and are often atherosclerotic in nature.[28] The size-rupture correlation has been demonstrated by studying the natural history of these aneurysms as reported by Clouse and associates, using the Olmstead County database, in which thoracic aortic aneurysms have an overall 5-year rupture risk of 30%.[29] The Mount Sinai group has identified clinical variables that determine the risk for rupture, which include increasing age, presence of chronic obstructive pulmonary disease, maximal thoracic and abdominal aneurysm diameter, and the presence of pain.[30] The Yale Aortic Diseases Group has documented rupture and dissection of ascending or arch aneurysms at a median size of 6 cm and descending or thoracoabdominal aneurysms at a median size of 7.2 cm.[6] Furthermore, the Yale group has reported that the mean rate of rupture or dissection is 2% per year for small aneurysms, 3% for aneurysms 5.0 to 5.9 cm, and 6.9% for aneurysms of 6.0 cm and larger. Using proportional hazards regression, the odds ratio for rupture is more than 25 times higher in patients with aneurysms of 6.0 cm or greater than in those with aneurysms in the range of 4.0 to 4.9 cm.[31]

Open surgical graft replacement is the traditional treatment for these patients. The presence of comorbidities in this specific population increases the surgical risks, especially in the case of emergency intervention. However, with increasing experience, very good surgical morality rates in the 5 to 10% range have been reported from experienced centers.[32–34] Similarly, paraplegia and paraparesis rates range from 3 to 16%, with predictive factors including extent of resection, emergency operation, renal dysfunction, distal circulatory support, and cerebrospinal fluid drainage.[35–37] Five-year survival rates between 60 and 80% have been achieved in recent surgical series.[32–34]

Thoracic Aortic Dissections

Acute aortic dissection is the most common catastrophe affecting the thoracic aorta, with many more people dying of rupture of dissections than of aneurysms. Although poorly understood, a primary intimal tear allows a high-pressure entry of blood into the subadventitial space, which then rapidly propagates within the media proximally and distally. With the Stanford classification system, type A connotes involvement of the ascending aorta. The high mortality rate of 50% at 48 hours usually mandates emergent surgical repair. Conversely, type B dissections involve the descending thoracic aorta, and are typically managed with anti-impulse therapy, with surgical management reserved for those patients presenting with complications, namely intractable pain, rupture or impending rupture, or visceral or limb malperfusion syndromes.[38–41]

The Stanford group has compared the actual survival of medically and surgically treated type B dissection over a 36-year period. The actuarial survival estimates for all patients were 71, 60, 35, and 17% at 1, 5, 10, and 15 years, respectively, and were similar for the medical and surgical patients.[40] The hope for benefits of avoiding the late complications from false-lumen expansion after surgical repair was not demonstrated in this follow-up.

Endograft repair of complicated acute type B aortic dissections is perhaps the greatest utility of this stent graft technology. Coverage of the primary intimal tear, redirecting flow into the collapsed true lumen, can dramatically reverse visceral malperfusion syndromes. The utility of thoracic endografts in chronic dissections is less clear. Given the multiple septal fenestrations, and the relative immobility of the chronically dissected septum, it seems unlikely that stent-graft insertion could realistically confer any long-term benefits, with the possible exception of a very focal aneurysmal false-lumen dilation distant from septal fenestrations near the level of the diaphragm.

Penetrating Atherosclerotic Ulcers and Intramural Hematomas of the Thoracic Aorta

Penetrating atherosclerotic ulcers (PAUs) and intramural hematomas (IMHs) are distinct pathologic entities now being diagnosed with increasing frequency.[42] PAUs probably represent rupture of an atherosclerotic plaque, with penetration into the internal elastic lamina of the aorta, and may be associated with proximal and distal progression of an intramural hematoma. Conversely, IMH not associated with a penetrating ulcer may result from the spontaneous rupture of aortic vasa vasorum that may initiate hemorrhage into the aortic media, and may progress to an intimal tear and classic aortic dissection.[42]

In the ascending aorta, IMH, with or without PAU, frequently progresses to frank dissection during the acute phase, and thus warrants early ascending aortic replacement. The highest mortality rate among patients with IMH is associated with ascending aortic involvement.[43,44] Experience has therefore suggested that a more aggressive approach with early surgery is warranted in those patients who have ascending aortic involvement or in those who have a coexisting aneurysm with IMH.[44]

In the descending thoracic aorta, pure IMH in the absence of aneurysmal change is usually treated with aggressive control of hypertension. For IMH with PAU, increasing maximal depth and maximal diameter were both associated with disease progression, in addition to persistent pain and increasing pleural effusion.[45] The risk of aortic rupture is higher among patients with PAU by almost 30% than among patients with type A or B dissection.[42] However, the progression of PAU is slow and is associated with a low incidence of acute rupture or other life-threatening events. Among patients with PAU who are not treated surgically, the natural history would indicate that the majority of patients will have aortic enlargement with the formation of saccular or fusiform pseudoaneurysms and intramural thrombus.[43]

Thoracic Aortic Trauma

Trauma is the most common cause of nondegenerative disease affecting the thoracic aorta. According to autopsy series, 36 to 54% of disruptions occur at the aortic isthmus, 8 to 27% involve the ascending aorta, 8 to 18% occur in the arch, and 11 to 21% involve the distal descending aorta.[46] Blunt trauma is commonly a catastrophic injury with only approximately 20% surviving to hospital admission. Mortality after admission ranges from 39 to 73% and is frequently the result of other major injuries.[47] The multiple injuries a patient may experience severely limit operative approaches and timing. All operations involving the thoracic aorta pose some risk of ischemic injury to the spinal cord, which is a dreaded complication in a predominantly young population. Closed-head injuries and other solid-organ injuries may constrain heparin use for peripheral circulatory support favored by most for open surgical repair.[46] Fortunately, for these patients without radiographic signs of impending rupture, and with stable serial CT scans, permissive hypotension may be an effective temporizing strategy, allowing operative intervention after a patient has recovered from serious brain or lung injury that may have compromised immediate operative management.

ENDOVASCULAR THERAPY OF THE THORACIC AORTA

Technical Development

The first stent grafts used at Stanford were manufactured using 2.5-cm self-expanding Gianturco Z stents (Cook Co., Bloomington, IN), which were fastened together and then covered with a woven Dacron graft (Meadox-Boston Scientific, Natick, MA; see Fig. 54-1). These stent grafts were oversized approximately 10 to 15% above the cross-sectional diameter ascertained by computed tomography (CT) in an effort to obtain sufficient radial force to achieve an endoseal and prevent stent-graft migration. A minimum of 2 cm of normal aorta was required for adequate fixation, otherwise referred to as the "landing zone," both proximally and distally. The covered stent was loaded into a delivery capsule that required femoral and iliac arteries greater than 8 mm to allow the introduction of a 28-French delivery sheath. This dilator contained a sheath that had been previously placed over a super-stiff guidewire and was positioned proximal to the point of deployment. Once this was achieved, the compressed stent graft was advanced into the sheath and deployed by using a "pusher" rod. Devices were limited to a maximal diameter of 40 mm in that aortas larger than 37 mm in diameter were themselves aneurysmal and unlikely to serve as stable attachment zones. Other anatomical constraints of these early "homemade" or first-generation stent grafts that precluded either delivery or secure fixation included acute angulation at the distal arch, and severe sigmoid-like tortuosity coursing through the diaphragmatic crura, reflecting the relative inflexibility of these early delivery systems.

The advent of this new stent-graft technology required a new terminology for endoleaks that allowed blood to leak around or through the stent graft, thus allowing the aneurysmal sac to remain pressurized. Type I endoleaks occur at the proximal or distal attachment sites, and signify a failure to achieve a hemostatic seal at these implantation sites.[14,24,25] Type II endoleaks denote a communication between a branch vessel and the excluded aneurysm sac. These usually occur from a back-bleeding inferior mesenteric artery in the abdomen, or intercostal artery in the chest. Type III endoleaks originate from the middle graft sections, and are usually caused by disruption of graft-to-graft overlaps, or by leakage through the graft itself. Type IV endoleaks are characterized by an increase in size of the aneurysm sac in the absence of an identifiable patent branch vessel, variously referred to as *endotension*.

Years of experience with endovascular abdominal aorta repair and follow-up of thoracic aortic repairs has yielded important information for improved stent graft technology.[11,48,49] Commercially produced second- and third-generation stent grafts are more flexible and have a lower profile, and thereby allow use of a smaller introducer sheath in the femoral vessels. Experience has shown that tapered, flexible, over-the-wire delivery systems that are less than 20 French in diameter rarely fail to traverse tortuous femoral or iliac arteries. Hooks at the proximal end of the stent graft appear to provide the most secure means of attachment, but may be suboptimal for treating patients with acute dissections. It is likely that different grafts may be developed for different pathologies, with devices for dissections being devoid of hooks and proximal uncovered metal components. For traumatic aortic lacerations, smaller device sizes are necessary, as these are usually nonatherosclerotic normal-sized aortas with small access vessels. Ideal device components have been broken down into three categories: delivery system, graft material, and metal frame.[50] The delivery system should be of low profile, flexible for maneuverability, rigid enough to resist kinking, and hemostatic during use. The graft material should also be of low profile, strong and durable, and reasonably thin. Ideally, this material could also hold sutures. The graft metal frame should provide high column strength and ductility, be compression and kink resistant from external forces, radiopaque, and corrosion and fatigue resistant. Nitinol is now used for the stent material in the majority of grafts and the graft material is usually polytetrafluoroethylene (PTFE) or polyester.

Currently, the Gore Excluder TAG system (W.L. Gore, Sunnyvale, CA), the Medtronic Talent graft (Medtronic, Sunrise, FL), and the Cook Zenith (Cook Co., Bloomington, IN) are the only Food and Drug Administration (FDA)–approved thoracic grafts (Fig. 54-2). These second- and third-generation endoprostheses are more flexible and have a lower profile with smaller delivery systems that can be inserted easily to treat a number of thoracic aortic pathologies.

Clinical Results Using Endovascular Stents for Thoracic Aortic Disease

Thoracic Aortic Aneurysms

In January 2005 the phase II multicenter trial of the Gore Excluder TAG thoracic endoprosthesis results was reported.[51] This multicenter prospective nonrandomized trial was conducted at 17 sites and compared results of stent-graft repair of

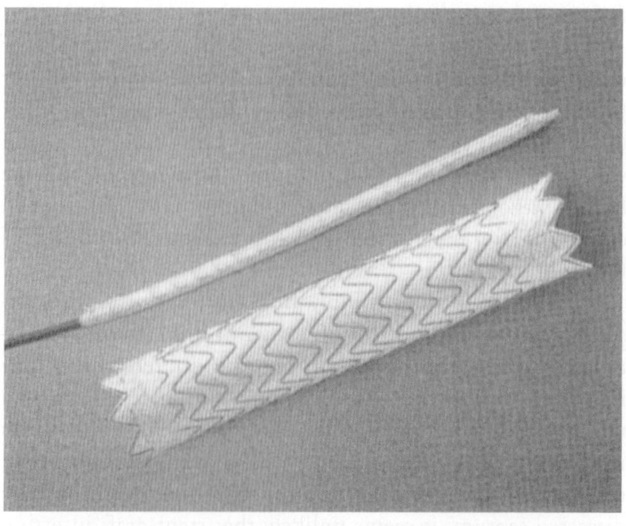

FIGURE 54-2 Second-generation commercially manufactured thoracic aortic stent graft. The thoracic Excluder TAG system by W.L. Gore contains a thin-walled PTFE graft covered by a nitinol exoskeleton.

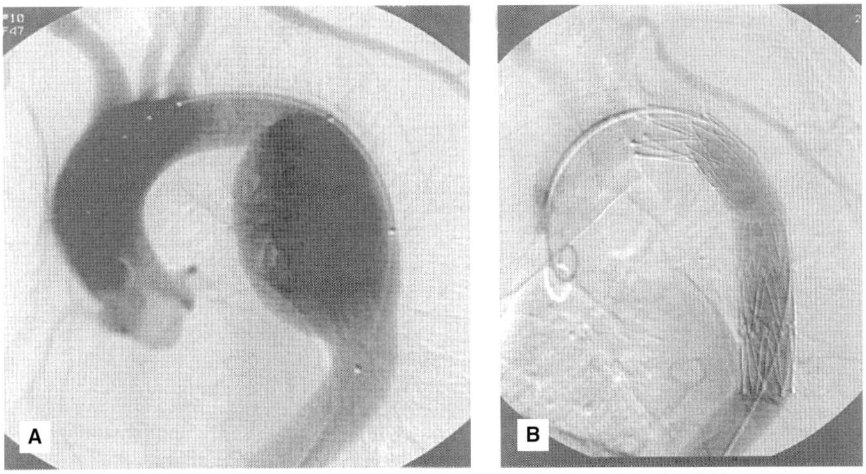

FIGURE 54-3 (A) Angiogram of a descending thoracic aortic aneurysm suitable for stent-graft repair. (B) Angiogram illustrating successful exclusion of the aneurysm sac with a thoracic stent graft.

descending thoracic aortic aneurysms in 140 patients with results of open repair in 94 patients. Strict inclusion and exclusion criteria were defined in an attempt to ensure comparability of both groups. Follow-up CT scans were obtained at 1, 6, 12, and 24 months. For stent-graft patients, operative blood loss, renal failure, paraplegia, and mortality rates were all significantly less than for the open repair group (Fig. 54-3). Interestingly, stroke rates were about equal in both groups. ICU stay and total hospital stay, and time to return to normal activity were 50% shorter for the stent-graft group than for those with open repair. Although stent-graft patients maintained an advantage from aneurysm-related mortality out to 2 years (97 versus 90%), interestingly, all-cause mortality was similar between groups at 2 years, which is similar to results of recent randomized trials in abdominal aortic aneurysm stent-graft trials.[52]

Ricco and colleagues have most recently reported on an independent nationwide study in France using a variety of endovascular devices to treat descending thoracic aortic aneurysms in the majority of cases.[53] The Gore Excluder TAG (Gore) and Talent (Medtronic) devices were used in 84% of patients and an operative mortality of 10% was reported. A complication rate of 21% was reported, which included endoleaks in 16% of patients that were fatal in three patients. The 6-month survival rate was 86% and freedom from other complications (other than endoleak) was only 63% at 6 months. This study, involving 166 stent-graft repairs, performed in 29 centers and using six different types of endoprostheses, demonstrated that stent-graft repair of thoracic aortic disease could be performed with acceptable morbidity and mortality, at short-term follow-up. They do, however, qualify their conclusions by stating that endograft treatment of thoracic aortic aneurysms should continue to be used in an investigative setting.

Perhaps similar to abdominal aortic aneurysms, stent grafts may become the preferred treatment for ruptured thoracic aortic aneurysms. Previously, open surgical repair of ruptured thoracic aortic aneurysms was associated with significant mortality and morbidity. Specialized centers with both expertise and appropriate devices may be capable of endovascular repair in patients with sufficient 2-cm landing zones to allow secure fixation of an appropriately sized endograft. Although thoracic ruptures are far less common than abdominal aneurysm ruptures, the increasing penetrance of this technology will likely allow timely intervention in multiple specialized centers.

Thoracic Aortic Dissection

For dissections originating distal to the origin of the left subclavian artery, referred to as *Stanford type B dissections*, aggressive antihypertensive therapy has been the mainstay of treatment.[40] For complicated dissections, however, defined as those dissections with rupture, impending rupture, intractable pain, rapid expansion, or malperfusion syndromes, surgical intervention is indicated. In these instances, however, surgical mortality has been reported to be as high as 50 to 60% in this high-risk group of patients. Endograft coverage of the primary intimal tear, redirecting flow into the true lumen, appears to be an ideal application of this endograft technology. The Stanford group, with their colleagues in Mie University in Japan, initially reported the use of the first-generation stent grafts in 19 patients with complicated type B aortic dissections. Placement was successful in all patients, and revascularization of ischemic branch vessels occurred in 76% of cases. There were three hospital deaths, two of which resulted from late referral, with irreversible end-organ damage, and one in a patient with Ehlers-Danlos syndrome who was perhaps untreatable by any modality. Although the follow-up was short, there were no incidences of aortic rupture or aneurysm formation, and a single-lumen aorta to the level of the stent graft was achieved in the majority of patients[27] (Fig. 54-4).

Multiple groups have now reported their results with endograft repair of complicated acute type B aortic dissections. Dynamic malperfusion is typically reversed with stent-graft coverage of the primary intimal tear, restoring flow into the true lumen and expanding collapsed segments. Static mechanisms of malperfusion, with branch vessel occlusion from orifice tears of the intima, can be diagnosed during the same intervention, and frequently reversed with uncovered stents into the true lumen of

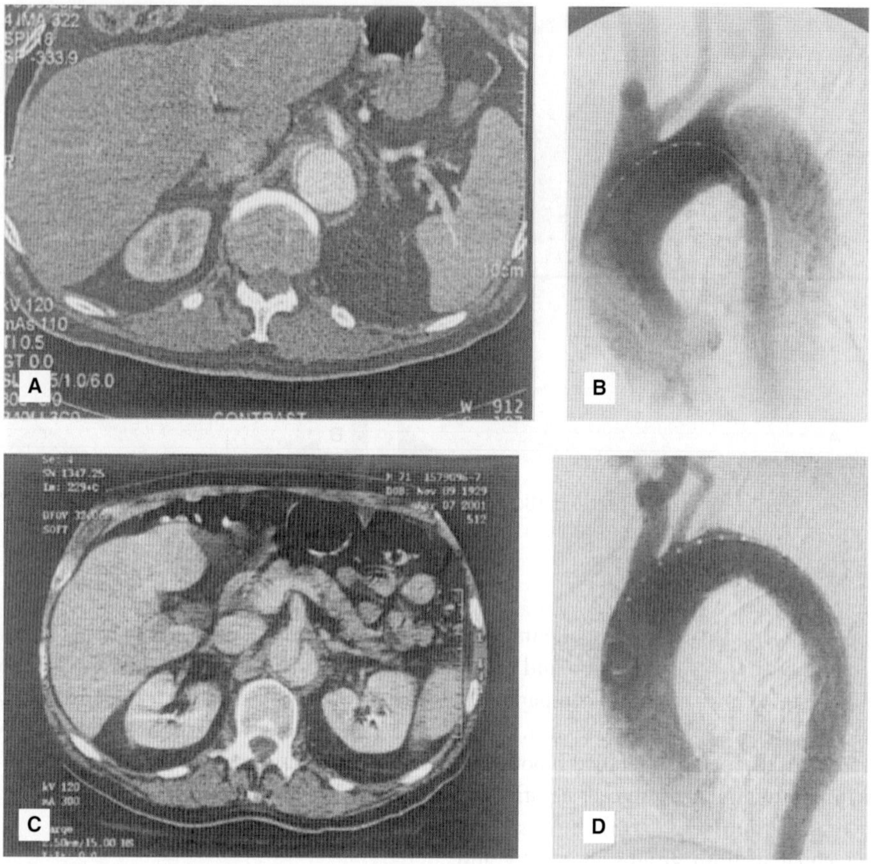

FIGURE 54-4 (A) Intravenous contrast-enhanced CT scan of the upper abdomen demonstrating an aortic dissection with compression of the true lumen. (B) Angiogram of the thoracic aorta demonstrating a type B dissection involving the descending thoracic aorta. (C) CT scan of the abdomen, and (D) angiogram of the descending thoracic aorta after stent-graft implantation into the true lumen in the proximal descending thoracic aorta.

branch vessels. Mortality rates for this high-risk population have been significantly lowered from the previous surgical figures of 30 to 60%.

Likely because of these good results, interest developed in the utility of stent grafts for uncomplicated acute type B aortic dissections. A randomized trial referred to as the INSTEAD trial (*IN*vestigation of *STE*nt in patients with type B *A*ortic *D*issection)* investigated all-cause mortality as the primary outcome; secondary outcome variables included conversion to stent and/or surgery, thrombosis of the false lumen, cardiovascular morbidity, aortic expansion, quality of life, and hospital stay. Given the relatively low 1-year mortality for uncomplicated type B dissections, especially if treatment is delayed for at least 2 weeks, it is not surprising that the survival of the stent-graft population was inferior to that achieved with standard medical therapy. Another randomized multicenter trial, the ABSORB trial, will randomize uncomplicated patients during the acute phase, and is currently enrolling patients.[54] The early experience suggests that, in experienced hands, stent-graft morbidity is low. Covered portions should not extend below T-6 to T-7 to minimize the incidence of paraplegia. Proximal uncovered stents should not be placed in the curvature of the aortic arch to avoid retrograde extension into a more dangerous type A dissection. More distally, uncovered stents may promote false-lumen thrombosis while allowing continued perfusion of intercostal arteries. False-lumen thrombosis is likely for the extent of stent coverage. Stent grafts specifically designed for dissections may well incorporate these features, ie, flexible stent grafts with low hoop strength, no uncovered elements on the proximal end, approximately 10 cm of covered stent, and a longer segment of uncovered stents distally.

As stated, the utility of stent grafts for the management of chronic aortic dissections is quite problematic. Because of disease complexity and extent, many were hopeful that stent grafts would prove an effective modality for treatment. However, the increasing thickness of the dissection flap with time, the frequent severe narrowing of the true lumen, the variable origin of visceral vessel origins from both true and false lumens, and the presence of multiple fenestrations between true and false lumens have severely limited the utility of stent grafts in the management of chronic aortic dissections. One exception may be the focal enlargement of the false-lumen in the proximal descending thoracic aorta. Coverage of the proximal intimal tear in these patients may allow false-lumen thrombosis for the proximal thoracic aorta. However, fenestrations almost invariably

*Nienaber C, Rousseau H, Eggebrecht H, et al: A randomized comparison of strategies for type B aortic dissection: the Investigation of STEnt grafts in Aortic Dissection (INSTEAD) trial. *Circulation* 2009; 120:2513-2514.

present at the level of the diaphragm and below allows a high-pressure entry into the false lumen, which then frequently propagates proximally. Although some local growth may be limited, further enlargement usually continues distally beyond the extent of the stent graft. More distal coverage in an attempt to promote false-lumen thrombosis may increase the risk for paraplegia. Uncovered stents may stabilize the flap, promote false-lumen thrombosis, and allow continue perfusion of patent intercostals arteries. These strategies will require further investigation.

Penetrating Atherosclerotic Ulcers and Intramural Hematomas

IMH of the aorta is attracting growing interest as a variant of aortic dissection.[44] The exact pathophysiology is not well understood. Although by definition, pure IMH likely occurs from hemorrhage into the media from the vasa vasorum, many maintain that an intimal disruption is present in all cases.

Certainly, in the absence of any intimal disruption, there would be no indication for stent-graft repair.[44] IMH, however, is often associated with or even precipitated by PAUs of the descending thoracic aorta.[42] Therefore, covering the PAU with a stent graft may limit the progression of the IMH and allow healing to occur.[19,42] Unfortunately, even with successful stent graft implantation using both first- and second-generation grafts, retrograde aortic dissection, new ulcer formation, and endoleaks have been noted in a significant percentage of patients, emphasizing the diffuse and severe nature of this disease.[55–58]

The Stanford group has reported their midterm results treating PAU of the descending thoracic aorta, with an average of 51 months of follow-up[19] (Fig. 54-5). Using both first- and second-generation commercial devices, 26 patients were treated, 14 of whom were deemed nonoperative candidates. The primary success rate was 92%, with actuarial survival estimates of 85, 76, and 70% at 1, 3, and 5 years, respectively. Perioperative mortality was 12%. Increasing aortic diameter and female gender were determinants of treatment failure. These risk factors reflect the importance of careful patient selection based on anatomical criteria and clinical factors. In addition, long-term follow-up with serial CT angiography is necessary to detect late complications.

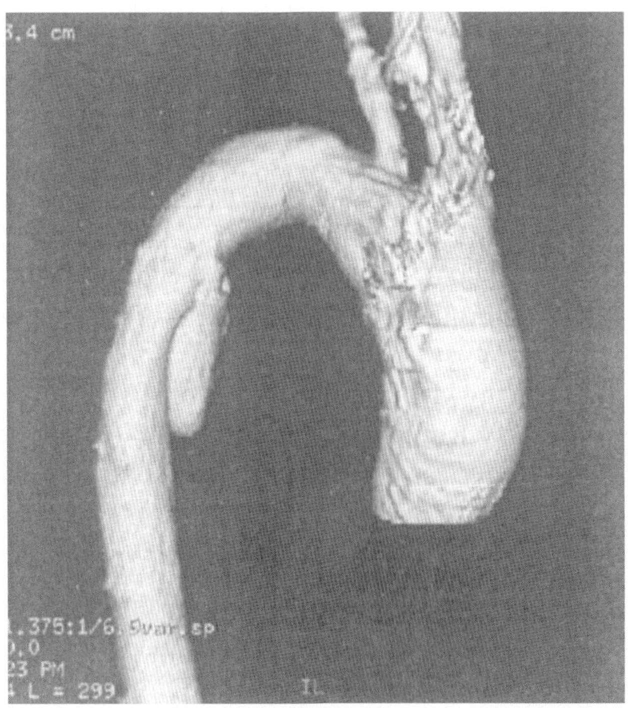

FIGURE 54-5 Three-dimensional CT scan of a giant penetrating ulcer involving the descending thoracic aorta that is perfectly suited to treatment with a thoracic stent graft.

Thoracic Aortic Trauma

Aortic injuries secondary to nonpenetrating trauma are lethal lesions, with 80 to 90% of patients dying in the hour after the accident.[59] Urgent surgical graft replacement of the aorta has been the standard treatment, but these patients frequently have other major injuries, including closed-head injuries, pulmonary contusions, and other solid-organ injuries, which may limit options for open surgical repair. Several authors have reported the improved results of stent grafts over open repair for these acute injuries.[60,61] Although long-term durability may be a concern, there appear to be significant short-term benefits.[61,62] The major difficulty at present is the absence of thoracic stent grafts sufficiently small in diameter as to be appropriate for these relatively normal-sized aortas, frequently less than 20 to 22 mm in diameter. Additionally, small iliac and femoral vessels may limit access. Because of these limitations, and perhaps because we rarely see patients within the first few hours of their injury, during which the risk for late rupture is probably greatest, we have embarked on a strategy of permissive hypotension, intervening only for those patients with signs of impending rupture, those with increasing mediastinal hematoma or hemothorax, or persistent pain. For these patients, conventional repair is preferred, using heparin-bonded circuits, unless closed-head injury or pulmonary contusions contradict. Stent-graft repair is used for those patients in whom a conventional repair could not be tolerated. Computed tomography is repeated at 24 hours, and again intervention is elected only if there has been enlargement or progression in the extent of the pseudoaneurysm. Under very careful surveillance, either open or endovascular repair is then performed when the patient has sufficiently recovered from his or her other injuries. It is likely that, as stent grafts with more suitable characteristics become available, they may become the repair of choice.

There are no reliable reports of sufficient numbers to afford real long-term assessment of stent-graft performance. Modern devices appear to have good 5-year durability, although reports of fabric tears associated with sharp angulations or grafts within grafts still surface occasionally. More important, even with complete exclusion of the aneurysm sac, aortic elongation may still occur, allowing the late development of type I endoleaks. Therefore, lifelong monitoring is essential, and currently requires cross-sectional imaging with either computed tomography or magnetic resonance imaging. For these reasons, we have preferred open repair for younger good-risk patients, using endovascular repair for older individuals with favorable anatomy. The Stanford group has reported on their midterm results of

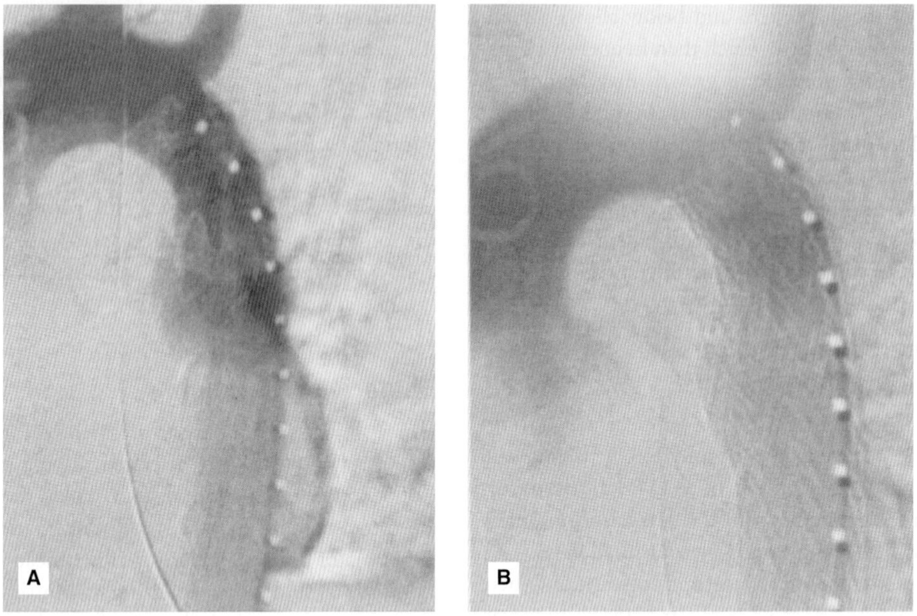

FIGURE 54-6 (A) Thoracic angiogram demonstrating a contained rupture of the descending thoracic aorta in a trauma victim. (B) Thoracic angiogram revealing repair of the aortic rupture with a thoracic stent graft.

stent-graft repair of chronic traumatic aneurysm of the descending thoracic aorta[63] (Fig. 54-6). Among 15 patients treated with either first- or second-generation stent grafts, deployment was successful in all patients without need for surgical conversion. No neurologic complications were reported. Actuarial survival estimates at 1 and 6 years were 93 and 85%, respectively. Freedom from reintervention on the descending thoracic aorta was 93 and 70% at 1 and 6 years, respectively. Freedom from treatment failure at 1 and 6 years was 87 and 51%, respectively. They therefore concluded that stent grafts are safe in patients with chronic traumatic aneurysms, and are associated with satisfactory but not optimal midterm durability. They state that younger, low-risk patients should be offered conventional, open surgery and stent-grafting should be reserved for those patients who are at prohibitive operative risk.[63]

CONCLUSIONS

Despite the many advances in the field of endovascular surgery, stent-grafting the thoracic aorta remains in a developmental phase.[20,64] This evolving technology has been applied to the treatment of thoracic aortic aneurysms, aortic dissections, IMH, PAUs, and traumatic injuries. The early outcomes are encouraging but middle- and long-term outcomes are a concern. Although device technology has certainly improved over the past 20 years, all devices are limited by their own structural flaws, lack of conformability, limited array of sizes, length of landing zones necessary to allow secure fixation, and structural integrity to withstand the severe physiologic milieu present in the thoracic aorta. Given the variable pathologies, it is likely that many different stent-graft configurations will be necessary for the various clinical indications.

Of utmost importance in the treatment of thoracic aortic pathology with stent grafts is strict and dedicated follow-up. Patients need to be seen on a routine basis and new symptoms or findings investigated. Serial CT angiography is an excellent tool to follow the areas of the thoracic aorta treated with the endograft, as well as to follow the evolution of the untreated portions of the aorta. Follow-up will allow endoleaks and device migration to be detected, and may further define the natural history of endovascular treatment strategies.

Diseases of the thoracic aorta pose a significant challenge to the surgeon because of the complexity of the disease and the characteristics of the patient population. Current literature supports the early advantage of endovascular technology in well-suited patients, but longer follow-up and results of ongoing trials will help define the indications for their use in the future.

REFERENCES

1. Swan H, Maaske C, Johnson M, Grover R: Arterial homografts II. Resection of thoracic aortic aneurysm using a stored human arterial transplant. *Arch Surg* 1950; 61:732.
2. Lam CR, Aram HH: Resection of a descending thoracic aorta for aneurysm: a report of the use of a homograft in a case and an experimental study. *Ann Surg* 1951; 134:743.
3. DeBakey ME, Cooley DA: Successful resection of aneurysm of thoracic aorta and replacement by graft. *JAMA* 1953; 152:673.
4. Cooley DA, DeBakey ME: Resection of entire ascending aorta in fusiform aneurysm using cardiac bypass. *JAMA* 1956; 162:1158.
5. Coady MA, Rizzo JA, Goldstein LJ, Elefteriades JA: Natural history, pathogenesis and etiology of thoracic aortic aneurysms and dissections. *Cardiol Clin North Am* 1999; 17:615.
6. Coady MA, Rizzo JA, Elefteriades JA: Developing surgical intervention criteria for thoracic aortic aneurysm. *Cardiol Clin North Am* 1999; 17:827.
7. Gillum RF: Epidemiology of aortic aneurysm in the United States. *J Clin Epidemiol* 1995; 48:1289.
8. Hagan PG, Nienaber CA, Isselbacher EM, et al: The International Registry of Acute Aortic Dissection. New insights into an old disease. *JAMA* 2000; 283:897.
9. Volodos NL, Karpovich IP, Troyan VI, et al: Clinical experience of the use of self-fixing synthetic prosthesis for remote endoprosthetics of the thoracic and the abdominal aorta and iliac arteries through the femoral artery and as intraoperative endoprosthesis for aorta reconstruction. *VASA* 1991; 33(Suppl):93.

10. Ruiz CE, Zhang HP, Douglas JT, et al: A novel method for treatment of abdominal aortic aneurysms using percutaneous implantation of a newly designed endovascular device. *Circulation* 1995; 91:2470.
11. Chuter TAM: Stent-graft design: the good, the bad and the ugly. *Cardiovasc Surg* 2002; 10:7.
12. Umana JP, Mitchell RS: Endovascular treatment of aortic dissections and thoracic aortic aneurysms. *Semin Vasc Surg* 2000; 13:290.
13. Nienaber CA, Fattori R, Lund G, et al: Nonsurgical reconstruction of thoracic aortic dissection by stent-graft placement. *NEJM* 1999; 340:1539.
14. Mitchell RS: Endovascular solution for diseases of the thoracic aorta. *Cardiol Clin North Am* 1999; 17:815.
15. Tokui T, Shimono T, Kato N, et al: Less invasive therapy using endovascular stent graft repair and video-assisted thoracoscopic surgery for ruptured acute aortic dissection. *Jpn Thorac Cardiovasc Surg* 2000; 48:603.
16. Buffolo E, da Fonseca JHP, de Souza JAM, Alves CMR: Revolutionary treatment of aneurysms and dissections of descending aorta: the endovascular approach. *Ann Thorac Surg* 2002; 74:S1815.
17. Kato N, Dake MD, Miller DC, et al: Traumatic thoracic aortic aneurysm: treatment with endovascular stent-grafts. *Radiology* 1997; 205:657.
18. Kasirajan K, Marek J, Langsfeld M: Endovascular management of acute traumatic thoracic aneurysm. *J Trauma* 2002; 52:357.
19. Demers P, Miller C, Mitchell RS, et al: Stent-graft repair of penetrating atherosclerotic ulcers in the descending thoracic aorta: mid-term results. *Ann Thorac Surg* 2004; 77:81.
20. Gleason TG: Thoracic aortic stent grafting: is it ready for prime time? *J Thorac Cardiovasc Surg* 2006; 131:16.
21. Nienaber CA, Erbel R, Ince H: Nihil nocere on the rocky road to endovascular stent-graft treatment. *J Thorac Cardiovasc Surg* 2004; 127:620.
22. Mitchell RS, Dake MD, Semba CP, et al: Endovascular stent-graft repair of thoracic aortic aneurysms. *J Thorac Cardiovasc Surg* 1996; 111:1054.
23. Parodi JC, Palmaz JC, Barone HD: Transfemoral intraluminal graft implantation for abdominal aortic aneurysms. *Ann Vasc Surg* 1991; 5:491.
24. Dake MD, Miller DC, Semba CP, et al: Transluminal placement of endovascular stent-grafts for the treatment of descending thoracic aortic aneurysms. *NEJM* 1994; 331:1729.
25. Mitchell RS, Miller DC, Dake MD, et al: Thoracic aortic aneurysm repair with an endovascular stent graft: the "first generation." *Ann Thorac Surg* 1999; 67:1971.
26. Demers P, Miller DC, Mitchell RS, et al: Midterm results of endovascular repair of descending thoracic aortic aneurysms with first-generation stent grafts. *J Thorac Cardiovasc Surg* 2004; 127:664.
27. Dake MD, Kato N, Mitchell RS, et al: Endovascular stent-graft placement for the treatment of acute aortic dissection. *NEJM* 1999; 340:1546.
28. Pressler V, McNamara JJ: Thoracic aortic aneurysm. *J Thorac Cardiovasc Surg* 1980; 79:489.
29. Clouse WD, Hallett JW, Schaff HV, et al: Improved prognosis of thoracic aortic aneurysms: a population-based study. *JAMA* 1998; 280:1926.
30. Jovoenen T, Ergin MA, Galla JD, et al: Prospective study of the natural history of thoracic aortic aneurysms. *Ann Thorac Surg* 1999; 63:551.
31. Davies RR, Goldstein LJ, Coady MA, et al: Yearly rupture or dissection rates for thoracic aortic aneurysms: simple prediction based on size. *Ann Thorac Surg* 2002; 73:17.
32. Svensson LG, Crawford ES, Hess KR, et al: Variables predictive of outcome in 832 patients undergoing repairs of the descending thoracic aorta. *Chest* 1993; 104:1248.
33. Kouchoukos NT, Masetti P, Rokkas CK, et al: Safety and efficacy of hypothermic cardiopulmonary bypass and circulatory arrest for operations on the descending thoracic and thoracoabdominal aorta. *Ann Thorac Surg* 2001; 72:699.
34. Estrera AL, Rubenstein FS, Miller CC, et al: Descending thoracic aortic aneurysm: surgical approach and treatment using the adjuncts cerebrovascular fluid drainage and distal aortic perfusion. *Ann Thorac Surg* 2001; 72:482.
35. Gharagozloo F, Neville RF, Cox JL: Spinal cord protection during surgical procedures on the descending thoracic and thoracoabdominal aorta: a critical overview. *Semin Thorac Cardiovasc Surg* 1998; 10:25.
36. Griepp RB, Ergin MA, Galla JD, et al: Minimizing spinal cord injury during repair of descending thoracic and thoracoabdominal aneurysms: the Mount Sinai approach. *Semin Thorac Cardiovasc Surg* 1998; 10:57.
37. Rokkas CK, Kouchoukos NT: Profound hypothermia for spinal cord protection in operations on the descending thoracic and thoracoabdominal aorta. *Semin Thorac Cardiovasc Surg* 1998; 10:57.
38. Elefteriades JA, Lovoulos CJ, Coady MA, et al: Management of descending aortic dissection. *Ann Thorac Surg* 1999; 67:2002.
39. Fann JI, Sarris GE, Mitchell RS, et al: Treatment of patients with aortic dissection presenting with peripheral vascular complications. *Ann Surg* 1990; 212:705.
40. Umana JP, Lai DT, Mitchell RS, et al: Is medical therapy still the optimal treatment strategy for patients with acute type B aortic dissections? *J Thorac Cardiovasc Surg* 2002; 124:896.
41. Lauterback SR, Cambria RP, Brewster DC, et al: Contemporary management of aortic branch compromise resulting from acute aortic dissection. *J Vasc Surg* 2001; 33:1185.
42. Coady MA, Rizzo JA, Elefteriades JA: Pathologic variants of thoracic aortic dissections: penetrating atherosclerotic ulcers and intramural hematomas. *Cardiol Clin North Am* 1999; 17:637.
43. Nienaber CA, Richartz BM, Rehders T, et al: Aortic intramural hematoma: natural history and predictive factors for complications. *Heart* 2004; 90:372.
44. Song JK, Kim HS, Kang DH, et al: Different clinical features of aortic intramural hematoma versus dissection involving the ascending aorta. *J Am Coll Cardiol* 2001; 37:1604.
45. Ganaha F, Miller DC, Sugimoto K, et al: Prognosis of aortic intramural hematoma with and without penetrating atherosclerotic ulcer: a clinical and radiological analysis. *Circulation* 2002; 106:342.
46. Razzouk AJ, Gundry SR, Wang N, et al: Repair of traumatic aortic rupture: a 25-year experience. *Arch Surg* 2000; 135:913.
47. Tatou E, Steinmetz E, Jazayeri S, et al: Surgical outcome of traumatic rupture of the thoracic aorta. *Ann Thorac Surg* 2000; 69:70.
48. Zarins CK, White RA, Moll RL, et al: The AneuRx stent graft: four-year results and worldwide experience 2000. *J Vasc Surg* 2001; 33:S135.
49. Ohki T, Veith FJ, Shaw P, et al: Increasing incidence of midterm and long-term complications after endovascular graft repair of abdominal aortic aneurysms: a note of caution based on a 9-year experience. *Ann Surg* 2001; 234:323.
50. Gowda RM, Misra D, Tranbaugh RF, et al: Endovascular stent grafting of descending thoracic aortic aneurysms. *Chest* 2003; 124:714.
51. Makaroun MS, Dillavou ED, Kee ST, et al: Endovascular treatment of thoracic aortic aneurysms: results of the phase II multicenter trial of the GORE TAG thoracic endoprosthesis. *J Vasc Surg* 2005; 41:1.
52. EVAR trial participants: Endovascular aneurysm repair versus open repair in patients with abdominal aortic aneurysm (EVAR trial 1): randomized controlled trial. *Lancet* 2005; 365:2179.
53. Ricco J-B, Cau J, Marchant D, et al: Stent-graft repair for thoracic aortic disease: results of an independent nationwide study in France from 1999 to 2001. *J Thorac Cardiovasc Surg* 2006; 131:131.
54. Nienaber CA, Zannetti S, Barbieri B, et al: INvestigation of STEnt in patients with type B Aortic Dissection: design of the INSTEAD trial—A prospective multicenter, European randomized trial. *Am Heart J* 2005; 149:592.
55. Sailer J, Peloschek P, Rand T, et al: Endovascular treatment of aortic type B dissection and penetrating ulcer using commercially available stent-grafts. *Am J Roetgenol* 2001; 177:1365.
56. Kos X, Bouchard L, Otal P, et al: Stent-graft treatment of penetrating thoracic aortic ulcers. *J Endovasc Ther* 2002; 9:SII25.
57. Brittenden J, McBride K, McInnes G, et al: The use of endovascular stents in the treatment of penetrating ulcers of the thoracic aorta. *J Vasc Surg* 1999; 30:946.
58. Murgo S, Dussaussois L, Golzarian J, et al: Penetrating atherosclerotic ulcer of the descending thoracic aorta: treatment by endovascular stent-graft. *Cardiovasc Intervent Radiol* 1998; 21:454.
59. Parmley LF, Mattingly TW, Manion WC, et al: Nonpenetrating traumatic injury to the aorta. *Circulation* 1958; 17:1086.
60. Iannelli G, Piscione F, Tommaso LD, et al: Thoracic aortic emergencies: impact of endovascular surgery. *Ann Thorac Surg* 2004; 77:591.
61. Rousseau H, Dambrin C, Marcheix B, et al: Acute traumatic aortic rupture: a comparison of surgical and stent-graft repair. *J Thorac Cardiovasc Surg* 2005; 129:1050.
62. Doss M, Wood JP, Balzer J, et al: Emergency endovascular interventions for acute thoracic aortic rupture: four-year follow-up. *J Thorac Cardiovasc Surg* 2005; 129:645.
63. Demers P, Miller C, Mitchell RS, et al: Chronic traumatic aneurysms of the descending thoracic aorta: mid-term results of endovascular repair using first- and second-generation stent-grafts. *Eur J Cardiothorac Surg* 2004; 25:394.
64. Mitchell RS. Stent grafts for the thoracic aorta: a new paradigm? *Ann Thorac Surg* 2002; 74:S1818.

CHAPTER 55

Pulmonary Embolism and Pulmonary Thromboendarterectomy

Michael M. Madani
Stuart W. Jamieson

INTRODUCTION

Pulmonary embolism results in at least 630,000 symptomatic episodes in the United States yearly, making it about half as common as acute myocardial infarction, and three times as common as cerebrovascular accidents.[1] Acute pulmonary embolism is the third most common cause of death (after heart disease and cancer). These estimates are probably low because approximately 75% of autopsy-proved PE are not detected clinically[2] and in 70 to 80% of the patients in whom the primary cause of death was PE, premortem diagnosis was completely unsuspected.[3,4] Of all hospitalized patients who develop PE, 12 to 21% die in the hospital, and another 24 to 39% die within 12 months.[5–7] Thus approximately 36 to 60% of patients who survive the initial episode live beyond 12 months, and may present later in life with a wide variety of symptoms.

Approximately 2.5 million Americans develop deep vein thrombosis (DVT) each year, and more than 90% of clinically detected pulmonary emboli are associated with lower extremity DVT. However, in two-thirds of patients with DVT and PE, the DVT is asymptomatic.[8–10]

For the most part, DVT and acute pulmonary embolism are managed medically. Cardiac surgeons rarely become involved in management of acute pulmonary embolism, unless it is in a hospitalized patient who survives a massive embolus that causes life-threatening acute right heart failure with low cardiac output, with a large clot burden. On the other hand, the mainstay of treatment for patients with chronic pulmonary thromboembolic disease[11] is the surgical removal of the disease by means of pulmonary thromboendarterectomy. Medical management is only palliative, and surgery by means of transplantation is an inappropriate use of resources with less than satisfactory results.

DEEP VEIN THROMBOSIS

Deep vein thrombosis primarily affects the veins of the lower extremity or pelvis. The process may involve superficial as well as deep veins, but superficial venous thrombosis does not generally propagate beyond the saphenofemoral junction and therefore very rarely causes PE.[9,12] Venous thrombosis of the upper extremity is almost always associated with trauma, indwelling catheters, or other pathologic states and is an uncommon cause of PE, but can be fatal. Pulmonary emboli that do not originate from the deep venous system of the legs and pelvis are thought to come from a diseased right atrium or ventricle or retroperitoneal and hepatic systems.[12,13] DVT is most common in hospitalized patients but may occur in ambulatory patients outside the hospital.[14,15]

Pathogenesis

In 1856, Rudolf Virchow made the association between DVT and PE and suggested that the causes of DVT were related to venous stasis, vein wall injury, and hypercoagulopathy. This triad of etiologic factors remains relevant today and is supported by an ever-growing body of evidence.

Immobilization is by far the most important cause of venous stasis in hospitalized patients. Injections of contrast material in foot veins require up to 1 hour to clear from venous valves in the soleus muscle of immobilized patients.[16] Venous stasis may also be produced by mechanical obstruction of proximal veins, by low cardiac output, by venous dilatation, and by increased blood viscosity.[17] Some pelvic tumors, bulky inguinal adenopathy, the gravid uterus, previous caval or iliac venous disease, and elevated central venous pressures from cardiac causes also enhance venous stasis.

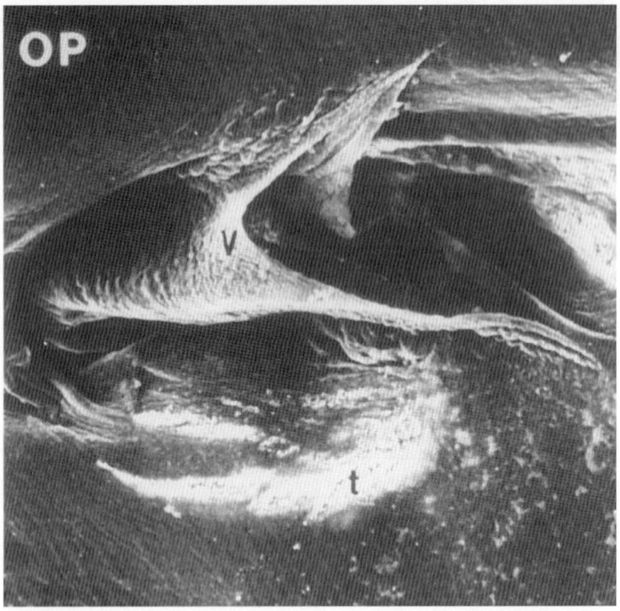

FIGURE 55-1 Scanning electron photomicrograph of a canine jugular vein after total hip replacement with significant operative venous dilatation. An endothelial cell tear (t) is visible near a valve cusp (V). (*Reproduced, with permission, from Cometra AJ, Stewart GJ, White JV: Combined dihydroergotamine and heparin prophylaxis of postoperative deep vein thrombosis: proposed mechanism of action. Am J Surg 1985; 150:39.*)

The role of vein wall injury is less clear because DVT often begins in the absence of mechanical trauma. Recent work shows that subtle vein wall injuries may occur during operation in veins remote from the operative field.[18,19] In animals, endothelial cell tears have been found at junctions of small veins with larger veins at remote sites during hip replacement (Fig. 55-1).

Three uncommon familial deficiencies associated with venous thrombosis are seen in antithrombin, protein C, and protein S. Antithrombin is a natural plasma protease that inhibits thrombin after it is formed, and to a lesser extent before it is formed. Antithrombin is also the cofactor that is accelerated 1000-fold by heparin. Protein C is a potent inhibitor of factor V and platelet-bound factor VII and requires protein S as a cofactor for anticoagulant activity. Both protein C and S are vitamin-K–dependent zymogens that are activated by thrombin and accelerated by thrombomodulin produced by endothelial cells.[20,21]

A much more common coagulation deficiency, resulting from a mutation of factor V (factor V Leiden) that prevents its degradation by protein C, has been described and is present in approximately 6 to 7% of study populations of Swedes and North American males.[22–24] Both the homozygous and heterozygous mutants are strongly associated with venous thrombosis and pulmonary embolism but are not associated with manifestations of arterial thrombosis.[24,25]

The presence of the lupus anticoagulant, which is an acquired IgG or IgM antibody against prothrombinase, increases the likelihood of venous thrombosis by poorly understood mechanisms.[25] The disease may be associated with lupuslike syndromes, immunosuppression, or intake of specific drugs, such as procainamide.

Risk Factors for Deep Vein Thrombosis

Table 55-1 presents a list of major risk factors for the development of DVT or PE. Previous thromboembolism, older age, immobilization for more than 1 week, orthopedic surgery of the hip or knee, recent surgery, multiple trauma, and cancer are strong risk factors. In patients with a history of venous thromboembolism the risk of developing a new episode during hospitalization is nearly eight times that of someone without a history.[9,26–29] Up to 10% of patients with a first episode of DVT or PE and up to 20% of those with a recurrent event develop a new episode of venous thromboembolism within 6 months.[30]

The incidence of DVT and PE increases exponentially with age (Fig. 55-2). Males are at greater risk than females. Immobility from any cause and prolonged bed rest are major risk factors. Although usually other risk factors are present, the incidence of autopsy-proved venous thrombosis rises from 15 to 80% in patients at bed rest for more than 1 week.[30,31]

The incidence of venous thromboembolism increases threefold in patients who have operations for cancer.[9] Of particular interest to cardiac surgeons and cardiologists is the recent observation that clinically silent DVT develops during hospitalization in nearly 50% of patients after myocardial revascularization.[32]

A follow-up study[33] found that the incidence of PE in hospital after coronary arterial bypass operations was 3.2% and hospital mortality in patients with PE was 18.7%. Interestingly, valvular surgery was not associated with the development of PE. In a retrospective study of 5694 patients who had open heart surgery, Gillinov and colleagues found the risk of PE proved by V/Q scan (20 patients), angiography (four patients), or autopsy (eight patients) was 0.56% within 60 days. However, the mortality was 34% in patients with PE.[34]

TABLE 55-1 Major Risk Factors for Venous Thromboembolism

Previous venous thromboembolism	Age over 4 years
Major hip or knee surgery	Bedrest 7 days or longer
Recent major surgery	Cancer
Congestive heart failure	Paralysis of lower extremity
Pelvis, hip, or leg fracture	Multiple trauma
High-dose estrogen therapy	

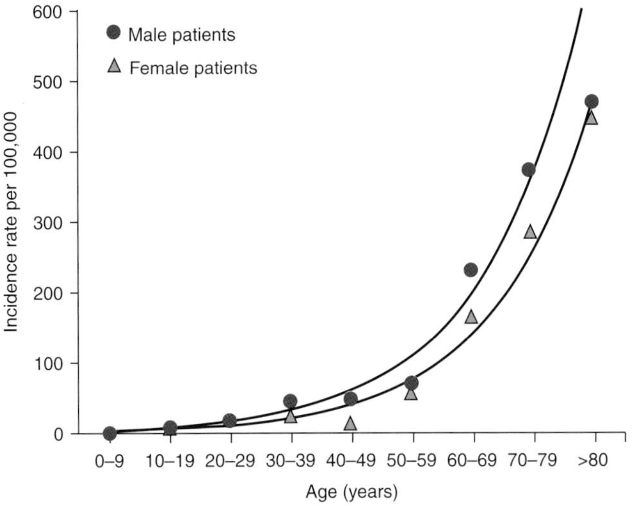

FIGURE 55-2 Annual incidence of venous thromboembolism in the United States stratified for age. Males have a significantly higher incidence rate of venous thromboembolism than females. Both curves fit an exponential function. (*Reproduced, with permission, from Anderson FA Jr, Wheeler HB, Goldberg RJ, et al: A population-based perspective of the hospital incidence and case fatality rates of deep vein thrombosis and pulmonary embolism: the Worcester DVT study. Arch Int Med 1991; 151:933.*)

Diagnosis

Approximately two-thirds of patients with DVT do not have clinical symptoms;[9] thus, the diagnosis depends on a high degree of clinical suspicion and a variety of objective diagnostic tests. Venography remains the most reliable test for detecting thrombus in calf veins, but is invasive, not suitable for serial studies, and the contrast material may be thrombogenic if allowed to remain within the deep venous system.[10]

The most popular noninvasive test, which can be done at the bedside, is a combination of ultrasound and color flow Doppler mapping, widely referred to as *duplex scanning*. The method does not detect fresh thrombi directly but infers the presence of clot by flow patterns and the inability to compress the vessel in specific locations.[10] In the hands of skilled examiners duplex scanning is highly accurate for the detection of thrombus in popliteal, deep femoral, and superficial femoral veins and has a sensitivity between 89 and 100% against venography in symptomatic patients. Against magnetic resonance imaging (MRI) duplex scanning has a sensitivity of 70% for pelvic veins and a specificity of nearly 100%.[35] Magnetic resonance imaging is a noninvasive method that can image the entire venous system, including upper extremity veins and mediastinum.[36]

Impedance plethysmography assesses volume changes in the leg after occlusion of the vein with calf electrodes and a thigh cuff. It is clinically useful in symptomatic patients but has relatively low sensitivity and specificity in asymptomatic patients and calf thrombosis.[35] Injection of iodine 125–labeled fibrinogen with subsequent leg scanning is a sensitive test for detecting calf vein thrombus but does not detect iliofemoral vein thrombosis. The combination of these two tests improves sensitivity and specificity, but in most hospitals duplex scanning, venography, and MRI have superseded both tests.

Prophylaxis

The prevalence of DVT, its strong association with PE, and the identification of risk factors in the pathogenesis of the disease provide the basis and rationale for prophylactic measures that are recommended in patients with two or more major risk factors, such as age over 40 years and major surgery.[9] Innocuous measures such as compression stockings probably should be prescribed more often and be used in most nonambulating patients in the hospital. Intermittent pneumatic compression is more expensive and more cumbersome but is effective. Both methods reduce the incidence of DVT after general surgery to approximately 40% of control patients.[9] Low-dose subcutaneous heparin and low-molecular-weight heparin given once per day reduce the incidence of DVT to approximately 35 and 18% of controls, respectively.[9,31,37] The reduction in PE with subcutaneous standard heparin or low-molecular-weight heparin is similar.[31,37]

Calf vein DVT that does not propagate has a low risk of PE, and controversy exists as to whether or not these patients should be anticoagulated.[13] Of patients who have DVT diagnosed in hospital without PE, the probability of clinically diagnosed PE within the next 12 months is 1.7%.[5] If PE occurs, the probability of recurrent PE is 8.0%.[5] Six months of warfarin anticoagulation are recommended for patients who have DVT with or without PE as prophylaxis against recurrent disease.[38]

PULMONARY EMBOLISM

Pathology and Pathogenesis

The only firm attachment of leg thrombus is at the site of origin, usually a venous saccule or venous valve pocket.[26] The degree of organization within the thrombus varies, but recent clots are more likely to migrate than older thrombi that are more firmly attached to the vessel wall.

Detached venous thrombi are carried in the bloodstream through the right heart into the pulmonary circulation. In autopsy series the percentage of emboli that obstruct two or more lobar arteries (major) ranges between 25 and 67% of all emboli;[39] but this figure varies with the thoroughness of the examination. In clinical trials based on angiographic data the percentage of major emboli is similar and ranges from 30 to 64%.[40] The majority of pulmonary emboli lodge in the lower lobes,[12] and are slightly more common in the right lung than the left. Soon after reaching the lungs emboli become coated with a layer of platelets and fibrin.[12]

Simple mechanical obstruction of one or more pulmonary arteries does not entirely explain the often-devastating hemodynamic consequences of major or massive emboli. Humoral factors, specifically serotonin, adenosine diphosphate (ADP), platelet-derived growth factor (PDGF), thromboxane from platelets coating the thrombus, platelet-activating factor (PAF), and leukotrienes from neutrophils are also involved.[41,42] Anoxia and tissue ischemia downstream to emboli inhibit endothelium-derived relaxing factor (EDRF) production and enhance release of superoxide anions by activated neutrophils. The combination of these effects contributes to enhanced pulmonary vasoconstriction.[41]

Natural History

The mortality of untreated PE is 18 to 33%, but can be reduced to about 8% if diagnosed and treated.[7,43,44] Seventy-five to ninety percent of patients who die of pulmonary emboli do so within the first few hours of the primary event.[45] In patients who have sufficient cardiopulmonary reserve and right ventricular strength to survive the initial few hours, autolysis of emboli occurs over the next few days and weeks.[46] On average, approximately 20% of the clot disappears by 7 days, and complete resolution may occur by 14 days.[44,46,47] For many patients, up to 30 days are needed to dissolve small emboli and up to 60 days for massive clots.[48] As the natural fibrinolytic system dissolves the embolic mass, the available cross-sectional area of the pulmonary arterial tree progressively increases, and pulmonary vascular resistance and right ventricular afterload decrease. In the vast majority of patients, pulmonary emboli continue to resolve and thus an immediate interventional therapy, particularly surgical embolectomy, is not necessary for survival except in a minority of patients.

In an unknown but small percentage of patients with acute pulmonary embolism the clot will not lyse, and chronic thromboembolic obstruction of the pulmonary vasculature develops. The reasons for failure of emboli to dissolve are unknown. Patients often are asymptomatic until symptoms of dyspnea, exercise intolerance, or right heart failure develop, mostly secondary to the pulmonary hypertension that ensues. Asymptomatic patients may have partial or complete chronic thrombotic occlusion of one or more segmental or lobar arteries. Symptomatic patients usually have more than 40% of their pulmonary vasculature obstructed by organized and fresh thrombi; however, significant pulmonary hypertension can develop in patients despite lesser degrees of vascular obstruction.

Clinical Presentation

Acute pulmonary embolism usually presents suddenly. Symptoms and signs vary with the extent of blockage, the magnitude of the humoral response, and the pre-embolus reserve of the cardiac and pulmonary systems of the patient.[49] Symptoms and signs vary widely, and in autopsy series of proven emboli only 16 to 38% of patients were diagnosed during life.[39]

The acute disease is conveniently stratified into minor, major (submassive), or massive embolism on the basis of hemodynamic stability, arterial blood gases, and lung scan or angiographic assessment of the blocked pulmonary arteries.[40,49,50] Most pulmonary emboli are minor. These patients present with sudden, unexplained anxiety, tachypnea or dyspnea, pleuritic chest pain, cough, and occasionally streak hemoptysis.[39,45,50] Examination may reveal tachycardia, rales, low-grade fever, and sometimes a pleural rub. Heart sounds and systemic blood pressure are often normal; sometimes the pulmonary second sound is increased. Interestingly less than one-third of the patients will have evidence of clinical DVT.[39] Room air arterial blood gases indicate a PaO_2 between 65 and 80 torr and a normal $PaCO_2$ around 35 torr.[45] Pulmonary angiograms show less than 30% occlusion of the pulmonary arterial vasculature.

Major pulmonary embolism is associated with dyspnea, tachypnea, dull chest pain, and some degree of hemodynamic instability manifested by tachycardia, mild to moderate hypotension, and elevation of the central venous pressure.[45,50] Some patients may present with syncope rather than dyspnea or chest pain. In contrast to massive pulmonary embolism, patients with major embolism (at least two lobar pulmonary arteries obstructed) are hemodynamically stable and have adequate cardiac output.[40] Room air blood gases reveal moderate hypoxia (PaO_2 <65, >50 torr) and mild hypocarbia ($PaCO_2$ <30 torr).[50] Echocardiograms may show right ventricular dilatation. Pulmonary angiograms indicate that 30 to 50% of the pulmonary vasculature is blocked.

Massive pulmonary embolism is truly life threatening and is defined as a PE that causes hemodynamic instability.[40] It is usually associated with occlusion of more than 50% of the pulmonary vasculature, but may occur with much smaller occlusions, particularly in patients with preexisting cardiac or pulmonary disease. The diagnosis is clinical, not anatomical. Patients develop acute dyspnea, tachypnea, tachycardia, and diaphoresis; and sometimes may lose consciousness. Both hypotension and low cardiac output (<1.8 $L/m^2/min$) are present. Cardiac arrest may occur. Neck veins are distended; central venous pressure is elevated, and a right ventricular impulse may be present. Room air blood gases show severe hypoxia (PaO_2 <50 torr), hypocarbia ($PaCO_2$ <30 torr), and sometimes acidosis.[40,45,50] Urine output falls; peripheral pulses are decreased and perfusion is poor.

Diagnosis

The clinical diagnosis of acute major or massive pulmonary embolism is wrong in 70 to 80% of patients who have angiography subsequently.[49,51] Even in postoperative patients and those with additional major risk factors for DVT, differentiation of major or massive pulmonary embolism from acute myocardial infarction, aortic dissection, septic shock, and other catastrophic states is difficult and uncertain.

The chest film may be normal but usually shows some combination of parenchymal infiltrate, atelectasis, and pleural effusion. A zone of hypovascularity or a wedged-shaped pleural-based density raises the possibility of PE. Usually, the ECG shows nonspecific T-wave or RS-T segment changes with PE. A minority of patients with massive embolism (26%) may show evidence of cor pulmonale, right axis deviation, or right bundle branch block.[49] An echocardiogram showing right heart dilatation raises the possibility of major or massive PE. A Swan-Ganz catheter generally shows pulmonary arterial desaturation (PaO_2 <25 torr), but usually does not show pulmonary hypertension over 40 mm Hg because of low cardiac output and cor pulmonale (the unprepared right ventricle cannot generate pulmonary hypertension).

Ventilation-perfusion (V/Q) scans will provide confirmatory evidence, but these studies may be unreliable, because pneumonia, atelectasis, previous pulmonary emboli, and other conditions may cause a mismatch in ventilation and perfusion and mimic positive results. In general, negative V/Q scans essentially exclude the diagnosis of clinically significant PE. V/Q scans usually are interpreted as high, intermediate, or low probability of PE to emphasize the lack of specificity but high sensitivity of the test (Fig. 55-3). Pulmonary angiograms provide the most definitive diagnosis, but collapse of the circulation may not allow time for this procedure, and pulmonary angiograms should not be performed if the patient's circulation cannot be stabilized by pharmacologic or mechanical means.[52,53]

Magnetic resonance imaging (MRI) and CT angiographies are better noninvasive methods for the diagnosis of pulmonary emboli and provide specific information regarding flow within the pulmonary vasculature.[54] Unfortunately, these methods are expensive, somewhat time consuming, and not widely available. Furthermore, they are not generally suitable for hemodynamically unstable patients. Transthoracic (TTE) or transesophageal (TEE) echocardiography with color flow Doppler mapping can provide reliable information about the presence or absence of major thrombi obstructing right-sided chambers or the main pulmonary artery. More than 80% of patients with clinically significant PE have abnormalities of right ventricular volume or contractility, or acute tricuspid regurgitation by TTE (Fig. 55-4).[55] In some patients, abnormal flow patterns can be discerned in major pulmonary arteries during TEE.

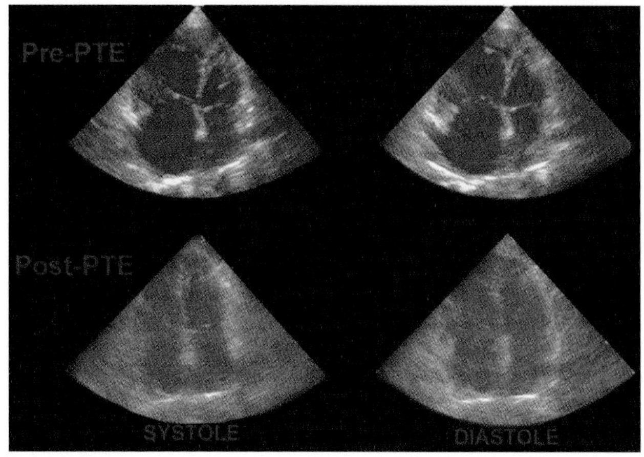

FIGURE 55-4 Appearance of echocardiography before and after the operation. The top picture represent pre-PTE and bottom pictures represent post-PTE. Note the shift of the intraventricular septum toward the left in the systole before the operation, together with the relatively small left atrial and left ventricular chambers. After the operation, the septum has normalized, and the right-sided chambers are no longer massively enlarged. LA = Left atrium; LV = left ventricle; PTE = pulmonary thromboendarterectomy; RA = right atrium; RV = right ventricle.

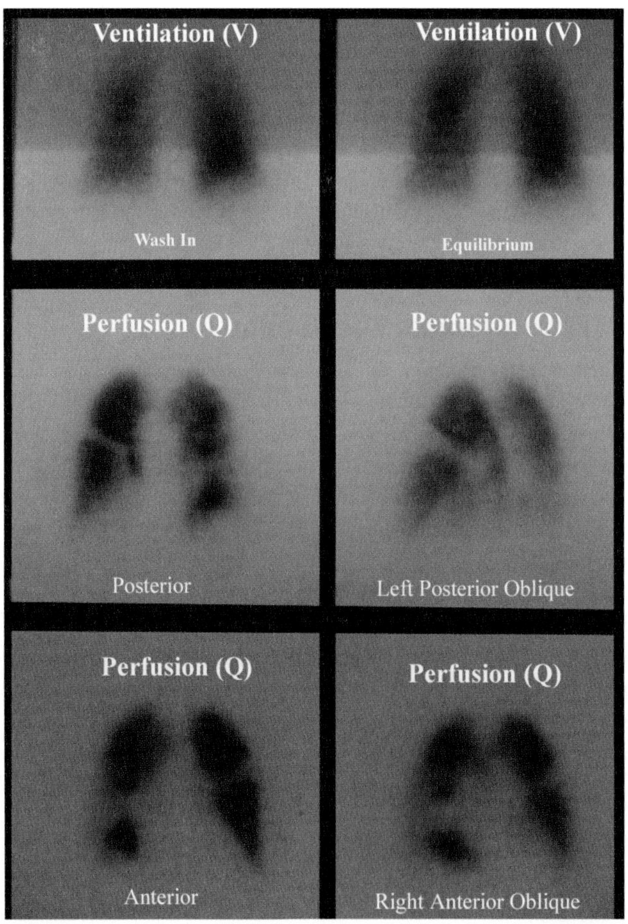

FIGURE 55-3 Anterior and posterior views from a radionuclide perfusion scan in a patient with chronic thromboembolic disease. Note the large punched out defects.

Management of Acute Major Pulmonary Embolism

For the purposes of this chapter, major or submassive pulmonary embolism is defined as an acute episode that causes hypoxia and mild hypotension (systolic arterial pressure >90 mm Hg), but does not cause cardiac arrest or sustained low cardiac output and cardiogenic shock. By definition there is sufficient time in these patients to definitely establish the diagnosis and to attempt pharmacologic therapy and possibly remove the embolic material by catheter suction.

The first priority after sudden collapse of any patient is to establish adequate ventilation and circulation. The first may require intubation and mechanical ventilation. Pharmacologic agents, including cardiovascular pressors and vasoactive agents, are then used to help stabilize the patient's hemodynamics. If the patient's circulation can be stabilized, intravenous heparin is started with an initial bolus dose of 70 U/kg followed by 18 to 20 U/kg/h if there are no contraindications. Heparin will prevent propagation and formation of new thromboemboli, but does not dissolve the existing clot. In most instances the patient's own fibrinolytic system lyses fresh thrombi over a period of days or weeks.[46]

The addition of lytic therapy, ie, streptokinase, urokinase, or recombinant tissue plasminogen activator (rt-PA), increases the rate of lysis of fresh thrombi and is recommended in patients with a stable circulation and no contraindications. This increases the rate of lysis of fresh pulmonary clots over that of heparin alone during treatment,[56] but there is little difference in the amount of residual thrombus between the two treatments at 5 days or thereafter.[57–60] There is also no statistical difference in mortality or in the incidence of recurrent PE, but more recent experience shows a trend toward better results with thrombolytic therapy because of a more rapid reduction in right ventricular afterload and dysfunction.[56] Furthermore, there are no data that indicate that thrombolysis reduces the subsequent development of chronic pulmonary thromboembolism and pulmonary hypertension. Compared with Heparin therapy alone, thrombolytic agents carry a higher risk of bleeding complications, and despite precautions, bleeding complications occur in approximately 20% of patients.[56,61,62]

Mechanical removal of pulmonary thrombi is possible by a catheter device inserted under local anesthesia into the femoral (preferred) or jugular vein.[50,63,64,67,69] Successful extraction of clot with meaningful reduction in pulmonary arterial pressure varies between 61 and 84%.[64,69]

Management of Acute Massive Pulmonary Embolism

If the circulation cannot be stabilized at survival levels within several minutes or if cardiac arrest occurs after a massive PE, time becomes of paramount importance. Eleven percent of patients with fatal PE die within the first hour, 43 to 80% within 2 hours, and 85% within 6 hours.[65] To a great extent, circumstances and the timely availability of necessary equipment and personnel determine therapeutic options. A decision to treat medically in an effort to stabilize the circulation at a survival level may preempt life-saving surgery, but also may make surgery unnecessary. The relative infrequency of treatment opportunities in massive pulmonary embolism, mitigating factors, and the lack of clear criteria for prescribing medical or surgical therapy leave the management of massive PE unsettled.

When surgery is not immediately available, in patients who may not be surgical candidates, or in whom an alternate diagnosis seems more likely, emergency extracorporeal life support (ECLS) using peripheral cannulation is an attractive alternative.[72,73] In prepared institutions ECLS can be instituted rapidly outside the operating room. ECLS compensates for acute cor pulmonale and hypoxia and sustains the circulation until the clot partially lyses, pulmonary vascular resistance falls, and pulmonary blood flow becomes adequate.

Emergency Pulmonary Thromboembolectomy

Emergency pulmonary thromboembolectomy is indicated for suitable patients with life-threatening circulatory insufficiency, but should not be done without a definitive diagnosis because a clinical diagnosis of PE is often wrong.[47,58,66,67] If a patient has been taken directly to the operating room without a definitive diagnosis, transesophageal echocardiography and color Doppler mapping can confirm or refute the diagnosis in the operating room. Transesophageal echocardiography will indicate increased right ventricular volume, poor right ventricular contractility, and tricuspid regurgitation, which are strongly associated with massive pulmonary embolism and acute cor pulmonale.[68] Echocardiographic detection of a large clot trapped within the right atrium or ventricle in a hemodynamically compromised patient with massive acute PE is another indication for emergency pulmonary thromboembolectomy.[74,75,77]

A midline sternotomy incision is used and cardiopulmonary bypass is initiated. The heart may be electrically fibrillated or arrested with cold cardioplegic solution. The main pulmonary artery is then opened 1 to 2 cm downstream to the valve, and the incision is extended into the proximal left pulmonary artery. Forceps and suction catheters remove the clot from the left pulmonary artery and behind the aorta to the right pulmonary artery. The right pulmonary artery can also be exposed and opened between the aorta and superior vena cava to allow better exposure in the distal segments, if necessary. If a sterile pediatric bronchoscope is available, the surgeon can use this instrument to locate and remove thrombi in tertiary and quaternary pulmonary vessels. Alternatively, the pleural spaces are entered, and each lung is gently compressed to dislodge small clots into larger vessels and suctioned out. Greenfield recommends placement of an inferior vena caval filter before closing the chest.[10,69,70,79] European surgeons generally clip the intrapericardial vena cava at the end of pulmonary thromboembolectomy to prevent migration of large clots into the pulmonary circulation.[77] However, this clip increases venous pressure and stagnant flow in the lower half of the body and causes considerable morbidity in more than 60% of patients.[70,74,77]

Anticoagulation for 6 months is recommended for most patients with PE, but an inferior vena caval filter is recommended for patients with contraindications to anticoagulation or with recurrent PE, or those who will require pulmonary thromboendarterectomy. The cone-shaped Greenfield filter is most widely used and is associated with a lifetime recurrent embolism rate of 5% and has a 97% patency rate.[71]

Extracorporeal Life Support

The wider availability of long-term extracorporeal perfusion (termed *extracorporeal life support*, ELS) using peripheral vessel cannulation to stabilize the circulation offers a compromise position because most massive pulmonary emboli will dissolve in time. ELS can be implemented outside the operating room within 15 to 30 minutes by an equipped team of trained personnel.[72,73]

ELS should not be needed beyond a few hours or 1 to 2 days because clot lysis proceeds rapidly. Once pulmonary vascular resistance is adequately reduced, ELS should be discontinued in the operating room as the femoral vessels will need to be sutured closed because of the need for heparin and long-term anticoagulation.

Results

Mortality rates for emergency pulmonary thromboembolectomy vary widely between 40 and 92%.[66,70,74–77] Results are best if cardiopulmonary bypass is used to support the circulation during pulmonary arteriotomy.[75] The eventual outcome depends largely upon the preoperative condition and circulatory status of the patient. If cardiac arrest occurs and external massage cannot be stopped without ELS, mortality ranges between 45 and 75%. Without cardiac arrest mortality ranges between 8 and 36%.[74,70,77] ELS instituted during cardiac resuscitation is associated with survival rates between 43 and 56%.[74,66] Recurrent embolism is uncommon,[70,78] and approximately 80% of survivors maintain normal pulmonary arterial pressures and exercise tolerance. In these patients postoperative angiograms are normal or show less than 10% obstructed vessels. A minority of patients have 40 to 50% of pulmonary vessels obstructed and have significantly reduced exercise tolerance and pulmonary function.[78]

CHRONIC THROMBOEMBOLIC PULMONARY HYPERTENSION

Incidence

The incidence of pulmonary hypertension caused by chronic pulmonary embolism is even more difficult to determine than that of acute pulmonary embolism. Twenty-five years ago it was estimated that there were more than 500,000 survivors per year of acute *symptomatic* episodes of acute pulmonary embolization in the United States alone.[11,79,80] The population has increased since then, and of course many cases of pulmonary embolism are asymptomatic. The incidence of chronic thrombotic occlusion in the population depends on what percentage of patients fails to resolve acute embolic material. One estimate is that chronic thromboembolic disease develops in only 0.5% of patients with a clinically recognized acute pulmonary embolism.[79] If these figures are correct and counting only patients with symptomatic acute pulmonary emboli, approximately 2500 individuals would progress to chronic thromboembolic pulmonary hypertension in the United States each year. However, because most patients diagnosed with chronic thromboembolic disease have no antecedent history of acute embolism, the true incidence of this disorder is probably much higher; we estimate on the order of five to ten times this number.

Regardless of the exact incidence or the circumstances, it is clear that acute embolism and its chronic relation, fixed chronic thromboembolic occlusive disease, are both much more common than generally appreciated and are seriously underdiagnosed. Houk and colleagues[81] in 1963 reviewed the literature of 240 reported cases of chronic thromboembolic obstruction of major pulmonary arteries but found that only six cases had been diagnosed correctly before death. Calculations extrapolated from mortality rates and the random incidence of major thrombotic occlusion found at autopsy would support a postulate that more than 100,000 people in the United States currently have pulmonary hypertension that could be relieved by operation.

Pathology and Pathogenesis

Although most individuals with chronic pulmonary thromboembolic disease are unaware of a past thromboembolic event and give no history of deep vein thrombosis, the origin of most cases of unresolved pulmonary emboli are from acute embolic episodes. Why some patients have unresolved emboli is not certain, but a variety of factors must play a role, alone or in combination.

The volume of acute embolic material may simply overwhelm the lytic mechanisms. Total occlusion of a major arterial branch may prevent lytic material from reaching, and therefore dissolving, the embolus completely. Repetitive emboli may not be able to be resolved. The emboli may be made of substances that cannot be resolved by normal mechanisms (already well-organized fibrous thrombus, fat, or tumor). The lytic mechanisms themselves may be abnormal, or some patients may actually have a propensity for thrombus or a hypercoagulable state. In addition, there are other special circumstances. Chronic indwelling central venous catheters and pacemaker leads are sometimes associated with pulmonary emboli. More rare causes include tumor emboli; tumor fragments from stomach, breast, and kidney malignancies have been demonstrated to cause chronic pulmonary arterial occlusion. Right atrial myxomas may also fragment and embolize.

After the clot becomes wedged in the pulmonary artery, one of two processes occurs:[82]

1. Organization of the clot proceeds to canalization, producing multiple small endothelialized channels separated by fibrous septa (ie, bands and webs) or
2. Complete fibrous organization of the fibrin clot without canalization may result, leading to a solid mass of dense fibrous connective tissue totally obstructing the arterial lumen.

As previously described and discussed, in addition to the embolic material, a propensity for thrombosis or a hypercoagulable state may be present in a few patients. This abnormality may result in spontaneous thrombosis within the pulmonary vascular bed, encourage embolization, or be responsible for proximal propagation of thrombus after an embolus. But, whatever the predisposing factors to residual thrombus within the vessels, the final genesis of the resultant pulmonary vascular hypertension may be complex. With the passage of time, the increased pressure and flow as a result of redirected pulmonary blood flow in the previously normal pulmonary vascular bed can create a vasculopathy in the small precapillary blood vessels similar to the Eisenmenger's syndrome.

Factors other than the simple hemodynamic consequences of redirected blood flow are probably also involved in this process. For example, after a pneumonectomy, 100% of the right ventricular output flows to one lung, yet little increase in pulmonary pressure occurs, even with follow-up to 11 years.[83] In patients with thromboembolic disease, however, we frequently detect pulmonary hypertension even when less than 50% of the vascular bed is occluded by thrombus. It thus appears that sympathetic neural connections, hormonal changes or both might initiate pulmonary hypertension in the initially unaffected pulmonary vascular bed. This process can occur with the initial occlusion either being in the same or the contralateral lung.

Regardless of the cause, the evolution of pulmonary hypertension as a result of changes in the previously unobstructed bed is serious, because this process may lead to an inoperable situation. Consequently, with our accumulating experience in patients with thrombotic pulmonary hypertension, we have increasingly been inclined toward early operation so as to avoid these changes.

Clinical Presentation

Chronic thromboembolic pulmonary hypertension is a frequently under-recognized but treatable cause of pulmonary hypertension. There are no signs or symptoms specific for chronic thromboembolism. The most common symptom associated with thromboembolic pulmonary hypertension, as with all other causes of pulmonary hypertension, is exertional dyspnea. This dyspnea is characteristically out of proportion to any abnormalities found on clinical examination.

Nonspecific chest pains or tightness occur in approximately 50% of patients with more severe pulmonary hypertension. Hemoptysis can occur in all forms of pulmonary hypertension and probably results from abnormally dilated vessels distended by increased intravascular pressures. Peripheral edema, early satiety, and epigastric or right upper quadrant fullness or discomfort may develop as the right heart fails (cor pulmonale). Some patients with chronic pulmonary thromboembolic disease present after a small acute pulmonary embolus that may produce acute symptoms of right heart failure.

The physical signs of pulmonary hypertension are the same no matter what the underlying pathophysiology. Initially the jugular venous pulse is characterized by a large A-wave. As the right heart fails, the V-wave becomes predominant. The right ventricle is usually palpable near the lower left sternal border, and pulmonary valve closure may be audible in the second intercostal space. Occasional patients with advanced disease are hypoxic and slightly cyanotic. Clubbing is an uncommon finding.

The second heart sound is often narrowly split and varies normally with respiration; P2 is accentuated. A sharp systolic ejection click may be heard over the pulmonary artery. As the right heart fails, a right atrial gallop usually is present, and tricuspid insufficiency develops. Because of the large pressure gradient across the tricuspid valve in pulmonary hypertension, the murmur is high pitched and may not exhibit respiratory variation. These findings are quite different from those usually observed in tricuspid valvular disease. A murmur of pulmonic regurgitation may also be detected.

Pulmonary function tests reveal minimal changes in lung volume and ventilation; patients generally have normal or slightly restricted pulmonary mechanics. Diffusing capacity (DLco) is often reduced and may be the only abnormality on pulmonary function testing. Pulmonary arterial pressures are elevated and suprasystemic pulmonary pressures are not uncommon. Resting cardiac outputs are lower than the normal range, and pulmonary arterial oxygen saturations are reduced. Most patients are hypoxic; room air arterial oxygen tension ranges between 50 and 83 torr, the average being 65 torr.[84] CO_2 tension is slightly reduced and is compensated by reduced bicarbonate. Dead space ventilation is increased. Ventilation-perfusion studies show moderate mismatch with some heterogeneity among various respirator units within the lung and correlate poorly with the degree of pulmonary obstruction.[85]

Diagnosis

To ensure accurate diagnosis in patients with chronic pulmonary thromboembolism, a standardized evaluation is recommended for all patients who present with unexplained pulmonary hypertension. This workup includes a chest radiograph, which may show either apparent vessel cutoffs of the lobar or segmental pulmonary arteries or regions, or oligemia suggesting vascular occlusion. The central pulmonary arteries are enlarged, and the right ventricle may also be enlarged without enlargement of the left atrium or ventricle (Fig. 55-5). Despite these classic findings, many patients present with a relatively normal chest radiograph, even in the setting of high degrees of pulmonary hypertension. The electrocardiogram demonstrates findings of right ventricular hypertrophy (right axis deviation, dominant R-wave in V1). Pulmonary function tests are necessary to exclude obstructive or restrictive intrinsic pulmonary parenchymal disease as the cause of pulmonary hypertension.

The ventilation-perfusion lung scan is the essential test for establishing the diagnosis of unresolved pulmonary thromboembolism. An entirely normal lung scan excludes the diagnosis of both acute or chronic, unresolved thromboembolism. The usual lung scan pattern in most patients with pulmonary hypertension either is relatively normal or shows a diffuse nonuniform perfusion.[84,85–87] When subsegmental or larger perfusion defects are noted on the scan, even when matched with ventilatory defects, pulmonary angiography is appropriate to confirm or rule out thromboembolic disease.

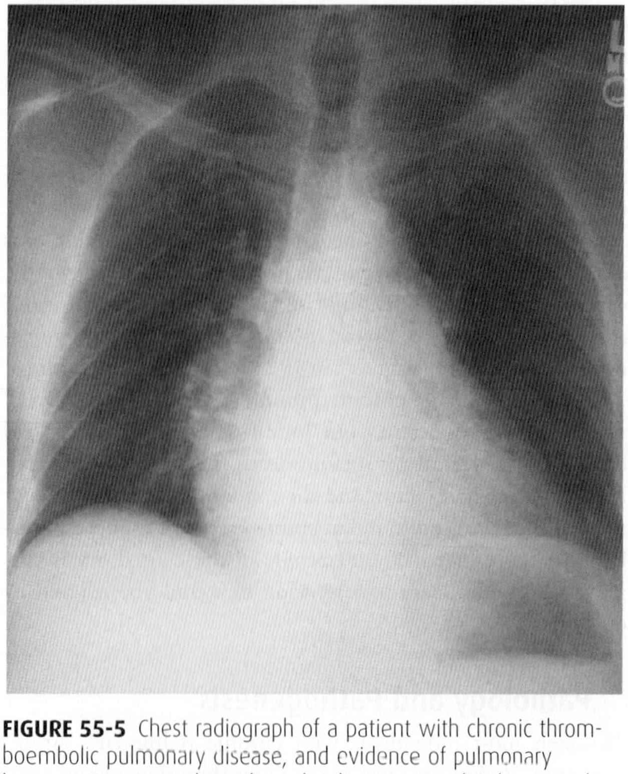

FIGURE 55-5 Chest radiograph of a patient with chronic thromboembolic pulmonary disease, and evidence of pulmonary hypertension. Note the enlarged right atrium and right ventricle, disparity of size between the left and right pulmonary arteries, and the hypoperfusion in several areas of the lung fields.

Currently, pulmonary angiography still remains the gold standard for the diagnosis of CTEPH. Organized thromboembolic lesions do not have the appearance of the intravascular filling defects seen with acute pulmonary emboli, and experience is essential for the proper interpretation of pulmonary angiograms in patients with unresolved, chronic embolic disease. Organized thrombi appear as unusual filling defects, webs, or bands, or completely thrombosed vessels that may resemble congenital absence of the vessel[87] (Fig. 55-6). Organized material along the wall of a re-canalized vessel produces a scalloped or serrated luminal edge. Because of both vessel-wall thickening and dilatation of proximal vessels, the contrast-filled lumen may appear relatively normal in diameter. Distal vessels demonstrate the rapid tapering and pruning characteristic of pulmonary hypertension (see Fig. 55-6).

Pulmonary angiography should be performed whenever there is a possibility that chronic thromboembolism is the etiology of pulmonary hypertension. Several thousand angiograms in pulmonary hypertensive patients have now been performed at our institution without mortality.

In addition to pulmonary angiography, patients over 40 undergo coronary arteriography and other cardiac investigation as necessary. If significant disease is found, additional cardiac surgery is performed at the time of pulmonary thromboendarterectomy.

In approximately 15% of cases, the differential diagnosis between primary pulmonary hypertension and distal and small vessel pulmonary thromboembolic disease remains unclear and hard to establish. In these patients, pulmonary angioscopy may be helpful. The pulmonary angioscope is a fiberoptic telescope that is placed through a central line into the pulmonary artery. The tip contains a balloon that is then filled with saline and pushed against the vessel wall. A bloodless field can thus be obtained to view the pulmonary artery wall. The classic appearance of chronic pulmonary thromboembolic disease by angioscopy consists of intimal thickening, with intimal irregularity and scarring, and webs across small vessels. These webs are thought to be the residue of resolved occluding thrombi of small vessels, but are important diagnostic findings. The presence of embolic disease as seen by occlusion of vessels, or the presence of thrombotic material is also diagnostic.

Medical Treatment

Chronic anticoagulation represents the mainstay of a medical regimen. This is primarily used to prevent future embolic episodes, but also serves to limit the development of thrombus in regions of low flow within the pulmonary vasculature. Inferior vena caval filters are used routinely to prevent recurrent embolization. If caval filtration and anticoagulation fail to prevent recurrent emboli, immediate thrombolysis may be beneficial, but lytic agents are incapable of altering the chronic component of the disease.

Right ventricular failure is treated with diuretics and vasodilators, and although some improvement may result, the effect is generally transient because the failure is owing to a mechanical obstruction and will not resolve until the obstruction is removed. Similarly, the prognosis is unaffected by medical therapy,[88,89] which should be regarded as only supportive. Because of the bronchial circulation, pulmonary embolization seldom results in tissue necrosis. Surgical endarterectomy

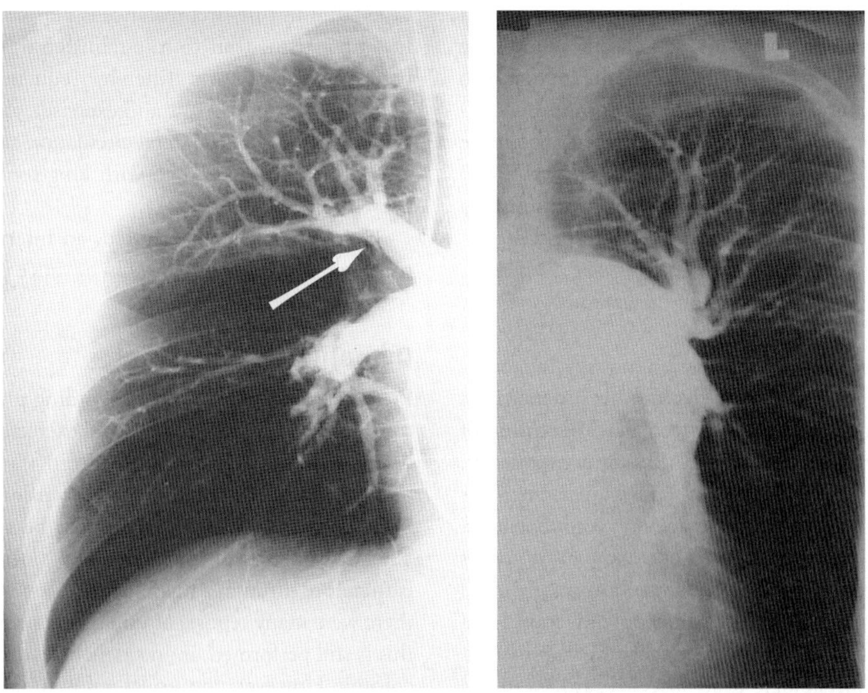

FIGURE 55-6 Right and left pulmonary angiograms demonstrate enlarged pulmonary arteries, poststenotic dilatation of vessels, lack of filling to the periphery in many areas, and abrupt cutoffs of branches. The arrow points to intraluminal filling defects representative of a web or band.

therefore will allow distal pulmonary tissue to be used once more in gas exchange.

The only other surgical option for these patients is transplantation. However, we consider transplantation not to be appropriate for this disease because of the mortality and morbidity rates of patients on the waiting list, the higher risk of the operation, and the contrasted survival rate (approximately 80% at 1 year at experienced centers for transplantation versus 95% for pulmonary endarterectomy). Furthermore, pulmonary endarterectomy appears to be permanently curative, and the issues of a continuing risk of rejection and immunosuppression are not present.

Natural History

The natural history of chronic thromboembolic pulmonary hypertension is dismal, and nearly all patients die of progressive right heart failure.[11] Because of the insidious onset, the diagnosis is usually made relatively late in the progression of the disease when dyspnea and/or early symptoms of right heart failure develop and pulmonary hypertension is severe (>40 mm Hg mean). In Riedel's series of 13 patients, nine died a mean of 28 months after the diagnosis of right heart failure.[11] Seven of the 13 had recurrent episodes of fresh emboli demonstrated by new perfusion defects or by autopsy. The severity of pulmonary hypertension at the time of diagnosis inversely correlates with duration of survival.[11]

Pulmonary Thromboendarterectomy

Although there were previous attempts, Allison[90] did the first successful pulmonary "thromboendarterectomy" through a sternotomy using surface hypothermia, but only fresh clots were removed. Since then, there have been many occasional surgical reports of the surgical treatment of chronic pulmonary thromboembolism,[91–94] but most of the surgical experience in pulmonary endarterectomy has been reported from the UCSD Medical Center. Braunwald commenced the UCSD experience with this operation in 1970, which now totals more than 2500 cases. The operation described in the following, using deep hypothermia and circulatory arrest, is the standard procedure.

Indications

When the diagnosis of thromboembolic pulmonary hypertension has been firmly established, the decision for operation is based on the severity of symptoms and the general condition of the patient. Early in the pulmonary endarterectomy experience, Moser and colleagues[92] pointed out that there were three major reasons for considering thromboendarterectomy: hemodynamic, alveolo-respiratory, and prophylactic. The hemodynamic goal is to prevent or ameliorate right ventricular compromise caused by pulmonary hypertension. The respiratory objective is to improve respiratory function by the removal of a large ventilated but unperfused physiologic dead space, regardless of the severity of pulmonary hypertension. The prophylactic goal is to prevent progressive right ventricular dysfunction or retrograde extension of the obstruction, which might result in further cardiorespiratory deterioration or death.[92] Our subsequent experience has added another prophylactic goal: the prevention of secondary arteriopathic changes in the remaining patent vessels.[87]

Most patients who undergo operation are within New York Heart Association (NYHA) class III or class IV. The ages of the patients in our series have ranged from 7 to 85 years. A typical patient will have a severely elevated PVR level at rest, the absence of significant comorbid disease unrelated to right heart failure, and the appearances of chronic thrombi on angiogram that appear to be relatively in balance with the measured PVR level. Exceptions to this general rule, of course, occur.

Although most patients have a PVR level in the range of 800 dynes/sec/cm^{-5} and pulmonary artery pressures less than systemic, the hypertrophy of the right ventricle that occurs over time makes pulmonary hypertension to suprasystemic levels possible. Therefore many patients (approximately 20% in our practice) have a level of PVR in excess of 1000 dynes/sec/cm^{-5} and suprasystemic pulmonary artery pressures. There is no upper limit of PVR level, pulmonary artery pressure, or degree of right ventricular dysfunction that excludes patients from operation.

We have become increasingly aware of the changes that can occur in the remaining patent (unaffected by clot) pulmonary vascular bed subjected to the higher pressures and flow that result from obstruction in other areas. Therefore, with the increasing experience and safety of the operation, we are tending to offer surgery to symptomatic patients whenever the angiogram demonstrates thromboembolic disease. A rare patient might have a PVR level that is normal at rest, although elevated with minimal exercise. This is usually a young patient with total unilateral pulmonary artery occlusion and unacceptable exertional dyspnea because of an elevation in dead space ventilation. Operation in this circumstance is performed not only to reperfuse lung tissue, but to re-establish a more normal ventilation perfusion relationship (thereby reducing minute ventilatory requirements during rest and exercise), and also to preserve the integrity of the contralateral circulation and prevent the chronic arterial changes associated with long-term exposure to pulmonary hypertension.

If not previously implanted, an inferior vena caval filter is routinely placed several days in advance of the operation.

Operation

Principles. There are several guiding principles for the operation. Surgical treatment and endarterectomy must be bilateral because this is a bilateral disease in the vast majority of our patients, and for pulmonary hypertension to be a major factor, both pulmonary vasculatures must be substantially involved. The only reasonable approach to both pulmonary arteries is therefore through a median sternotomy incision. Historically, there were many reports of unilateral operation, and occasionally this is still performed, in inexperienced centers, through a thoracotomy. However, the unilateral approach ignores the disease on the contralateral side, subjects the patient to hemodynamic jeopardy during the clamping of the pulmonary artery, does not allow good visibility because of the continued presence of bronchial blood flow, and exposes the patient to a repeat operation on the contralateral side. In addition, collateral channels develop in chronic thrombotic hypertension not only through the bronchial arteries but also from diaphragmatic, intercostal, and pleural vessels. The dissection of the lung in the pleural space via a thoracotomy incision can therefore be extremely bloody. The median sternotomy incision, apart from providing bilateral access, avoids entry into the pleural cavities, and allows the ready institution of cardiopulmonary bypass.

Cardiopulmonary bypass is essential to ensure cardiovascular stability when the operation is performed and cool the patient to allow circulatory arrest. Excellent visibility is required, in a bloodless field, to define an adequate endarterectomy plane and then follow the pulmonary endarterectomy specimen deep into the subsegmental vessels. Because of the copious bronchial blood flow usually present in these cases, periods of circulatory arrest are necessary to ensure perfect visibility. Again, there have been sporadic reports of the performance of this operation without circulatory arrest. However, it should be emphasized that although endarterectomy is possible without circulatory arrest, a complete endarterectomy is not. We always initiate the procedure without circulatory arrest, and a variable amount of dissection is possible before the circulation is stopped, but never complete dissection. The circulatory arrest periods are limited to 20 minutes, with restoration of flow between each arrest. With experience, the endarterectomy usually can be performed with a single period of circulatory arrest on each side.

A true endarterectomy in the plane of the media must be accomplished. It is essential to appreciate that the removal of visible thrombus is largely incidental to this operation. Indeed, in most patients, no free thrombus is present; and on initial direct examination, the pulmonary vascular bed may appear normal. The early literature on this procedure indicates that thrombectomy was often performed without endarterectomy, and in these cases the pulmonary artery pressures did not improve, often with the resultant death of the patient.

Preparation and Anesthetic Considerations. Much of the preoperative preparation is common to any open-heart procedure. Routine monitoring for anesthetic induction includes a surface electrocardiogram, cutaneous oximetry, and radial and pulmonary artery pressures. After anesthetic induction a femoral artery catheter, in addition to a radial arterial line, is also placed. This provides more accurate measurements during rewarming and on discontinuation of cardiopulmonary bypass because of the peripheral vasoconstriction that occurs after hypothermic circulatory arrest. It is generally removed in the intensive care unit when the two readings correlate.

Electroencephalographic recording is performed to ensure the absence of cerebral activity before circulatory arrest is induced. The patient's head is enveloped in a cooling jacket, and cerebral cooling is begun after the initiation of bypass. Temperature measurements are made of the esophagus, tympanic membrane, urinary catheter, rectum, and blood (through the Swan-Ganz catheter). If the patient's condition is stable after the induction of anesthesia, up to 500 mL of autologous whole blood is withdrawn for later use, and the volume deficit is replaced with crystalloid solution.

Surgical Technique. After a median sternotomy incision, the pericardium is incised longitudinally and attached to the wound edges. Typically the right heart is enlarged, with a tense right atrium and a variable degree of tricuspid regurgitation. There is usually severe right ventricular hypertrophy, and with critical degrees of obstruction, the patient's condition may become unstable with the manipulation of the heart.

Anticoagulation with heparin (400 U/kg, intravenously) is administered to prolong the activated clotting time beyond 400 seconds. Full cardiopulmonary bypass is instituted with high ascending aortic cannulation and two caval cannulae. These cannulae must be inserted into the superior and inferior vena cavae sufficiently to enable subsequent opening of the right atrium if necessary. A temporary pulmonary artery vent is placed in the midline of the main pulmonary artery 1 cm distal to the pulmonary valve. This will mark the beginning of the left pulmonary arteriotomy.

After cardiopulmonary bypass is initiated, surface cooling with both the head jacket and the cooling blanket is begun. The blood is cooled with the pump-oxygenator. During cooling a 10°C gradient between arterial blood and bladder or rectal temperature is maintained.[93] Cooling generally takes 45 minutes to an hour. When ventricular fibrillation occurs, an additional vent is placed in the left atrium through the right superior pulmonary vein to prevent distention from the large amount of bronchial arterial blood flow that is common with these patients.

It is most convenient for the primary surgeon to stand initially on the patient's left side. During the cooling period, some preliminary dissection can be performed, with full mobilization of the right pulmonary artery from the ascending aorta. The superior vena cava is also fully mobilized. The approach to the right pulmonary artery is made medial, not lateral, to the superior vena cava. All dissection of the pulmonary arteries takes place intrapericardially, and neither pleural cavity should be entered. An incision is then made in the right pulmonary artery from beneath the ascending aorta out under the superior vena cava and entering the lower lobe branch of the pulmonary artery just after the take-off of the middle lobe artery (Fig. 55-7). The incision stays in the center of the vessel and continues into the lower rather than the middle lobe artery.

Any loose thrombus, if present, is now removed, to obtain good visualization. It is most important to recognize, however, that first, an embolectomy without subsequent endarterectomy is quite ineffective and, second, that in most patients with chronic thromboembolic hypertension, direct examination of the pulmonary vascular bed at operation generally shows no obvious embolic material. Therefore, to the inexperienced or cursory glance, the pulmonary vascular bed may well appear normal even in patients with severe chronic embolic pulmonary hypertension.

If the bronchial circulation is not excessive, the endarterectomy plane can be found during this early dissection. However, although a small amount of dissection can be performed before the initiation of circulatory arrest, it is unwise to proceed unless perfect visibility is obtained because the development of a correct plane is essential.

There are four broad types of pulmonary occlusive disease related to thrombus that can be appreciated, and we use the

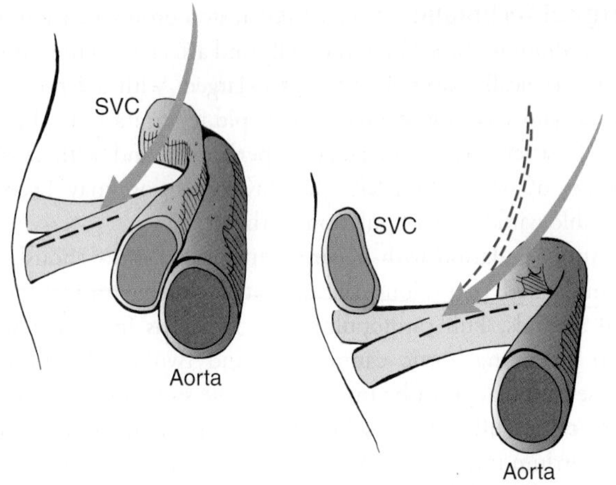

FIGURE 55-7 Recommended surgical approach on the right side. This approach, medial to the superior vena cava (SVC), between the superior vena cava and aorta, provides a direct view into the right pulmonary artery. Note that an approach on the lateral side of the superior vena cava will only provide a restricted view, and should be avoided.

following classification[87,94]: Type I disease (approximately 10% of cases of thromboembolic pulmonary hypertension) (Fig. 55-8) refers to the situation in which major vessel clot is present and readily visible on the opening of the pulmonary arteries. All central thrombotic material has to be completely removed before the endarterectomy. In type II disease (approximately 70% of cases; Fig. 55-9), no major vessel thrombus can be appreciated. In these cases only thickened intima can be seen, occasionally with webs, and the endarterectomy plane is raised in the main, lobar, or segmental vessels. Type III disease (approximately 20% of cases; Fig. 55-10) presents the most challenging surgical situation. The disease is very distal and confined to the segmental and subsegmental branches. No occlusion of vessels can be seen initially. The endarterectomy plane must be carefully and painstakingly raised in each segmental and subsegmental branch. Type III disease is most often associated with presumed repetitive thrombi from indwelling catheters (such as pacemaker wires) or ventriculo-atrial shunts. Type IV disease (Fig. 55-11) does not represent primary thromboembolic pulmonary hypertension and is inoperable. In this entity there is intrinsic small vessel disease, although secondary thrombus may occur as a result of stasis. Small-vessel disease may be unrelated to thromboembolic events ("primary" pulmonary hypertension) or occur in relation to thromboembolic hypertension as a result of a high flow or high pressure state in previously unaffected vessels similar to the generation of Eisenmenger's syndrome. We believe that there may also be sympathetic "cross-talk" from an affected contralateral side or stenotic areas in the same lung.

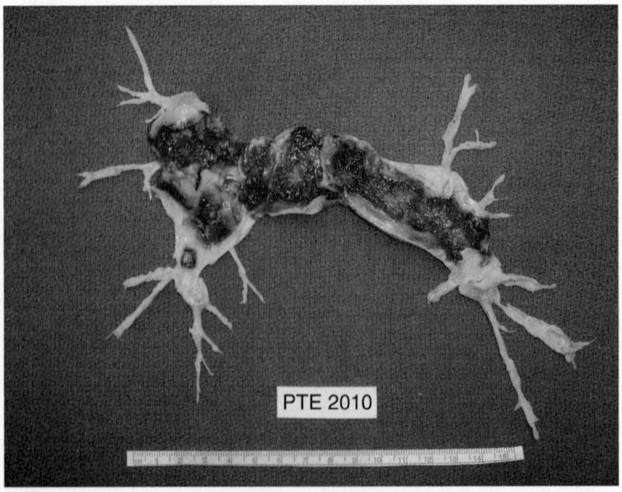

FIGURE 55-8 Surgical specimen removed from a patient showing evidence of some fresh and some old thrombus in the main and both right and left pulmonary arteries. Note that simple removal of the gross disease initially encountered on pulmonary arteriotomy will not be therapeutic, and any meaningful outcome involves a full endarterectomy into all the distal segments.

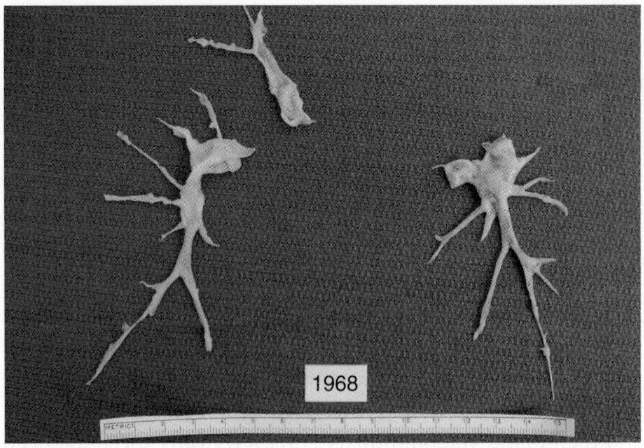

FIGURE 55-9 Specimen removed in a patient with type II disease. Both pulmonary arteries have evidence of chronic thromboembolic material. Note the distal tails of the specimen in each branch. Full resolution of pulmonary hypertension is dependent on complete removal of all the distal tails.

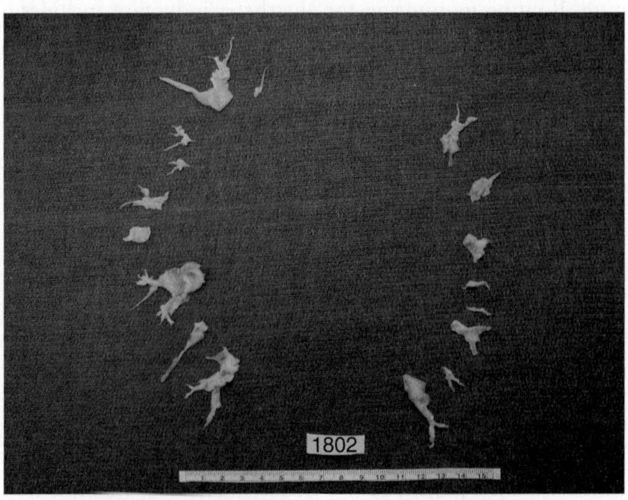

FIGURE 55-10 Specimen removed from a patient with type III disease. Note that the disease is distal, and the plane was raised at each segmental level.

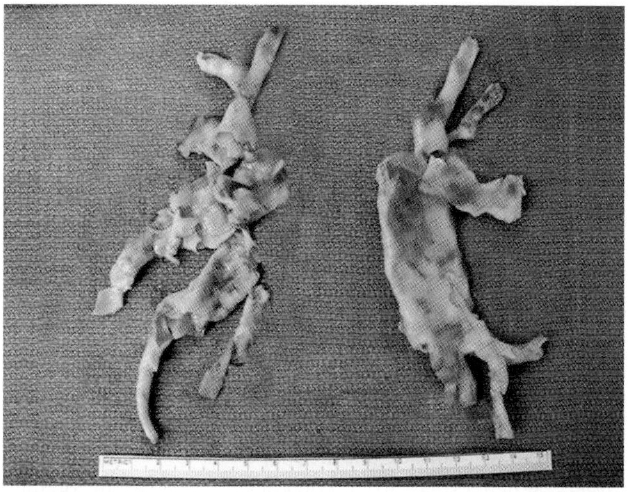

FIGURE 55-11 Note the absence of distal "tails" in this specimen removed from a patient with surgical classification type IV. All "tails" are replaced by "trousers". No clinical benefit was obtained from this procedure and the patient's postoperative hemodynamics were not improved, despite what appears to be an impressive endarterectomy specimen. The patient had primary pulmonary hypertension.

When the patient's temperature reaches 20°C, the aorta is cross-clamped and a single dose of cold cardioplegic solution (I L) is administered. Additional myocardial protection is obtained by the use of a cooling jacket. The entire procedure is now performed with a single aortic cross-clamp period with no further administration of cardioplegic solution.

A modified cerebellar retractor is placed between the aorta and superior vena cava. When blood obscures direct vision of the pulmonary vascular bed, thiopental is administered (500 mg to 1 g) until the electroencephalogram becomes isoelectric. Circulatory arrest is then initiated, and the patient is exsanguinated. All monitoring lines to the patient are turned off to prevent the aspiration of air. Snares are tightened around the cannulae in the superior and inferior vena cavae. It is rare that one 20-minute period for each side is exceeded. Although retrograde cerebral perfusion has been advocated for total circulatory arrest in other procedures, it is not helpful in this operation because it does not allow a completely bloodless field, and with the short arrest times that can be achieved with experience, it is not necessary.

Any residual loose, thrombotic debris encountered is removed. Then, a microtome knife is used to develop the endarterectomy plane posteriorly, because any inadvertent egress in this site could be repaired readily, or simply left alone. Dissection in the correct plane is critical because if the plane is too deep the pulmonary artery may perforate, with fatal results, and if the dissection plane is not deep enough, inadequate amounts of the chronically thromboembolic material will be removed. The plane should only be sought in the diseased parts of the artery; this often requires the initial dissection to begin quite distally.

The ideal layer is marked with a pearly white plane, which strips easily. There should be no residual yellow plaque. If the dissection is too deep, a reddish or pinkish color indicates the adventitia has been reached. A more superficial plane should be sought immediately.

Once the plane is correctly developed, a full-thickness layer is left in the region of the incision to ease subsequent repair. The endarterectomy is then performed with an eversion technique, using a specially developed dissection instrument (Jamieson aspirator, Fehling Corp.). Because the vessel is partly everted and subsegmental branches are being worked on, a perforation here will become completely inaccessible and invisible later. This is why absolute visualization in a completely bloodless field provided by circulatory arrest is essential. It is important that each subsegmental branch is followed and freed individually until it ends in a "tail," beyond which there is no further obstruction.

Once the right-sided endarterectomy is completed, circulation is restarted, and the arteriotomy is repaired with a continuous 6-0 polypropylene suture. The hemostatic nature of this closure is aided by the nature of the initial dissection, with the full thickness of the pulmonary artery being preserved immediately adjacent to the incision.

The surgeon now moves to the patient's right side. The pulmonary vent catheter is withdrawn, and an arteriotomy is made from the site of the pulmonary vent hole laterally beneath the pericardial reflection, and again into the lower lobe, but avoiding entry into the left pleural space. Additional lateral dissection does not enhance intraluminal visibility, may endanger the left phrenic nerve, and makes subsequent repair of the left pulmonary artery more difficult (Fig. 55-12). There is often a lymphatic vessel encountered on the left pulmonary artery at the level of the pericardial reflection, and it is wise to clip this before it being divided with the pulmonary artery incision.

The left-sided dissection is virtually analogous in all respects to that accomplished on the right. By the time the circulation is arrested once more it will have been reinitiated for at least 10 minutes, by which time the venous oxygen saturations are

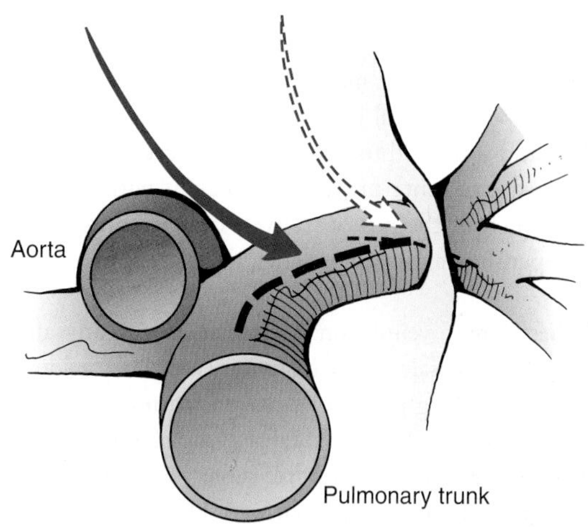

FIGURE 55-12 Surgical approach on the left side. The incision in the left pulmonary artery begins in the midpoint of the main pulmonary trunk, at the insertion site of the pulmonary artery vent. This incision provides better visibility than a more distal approach (*dotted line and arrow*). Care must be taken to avoid injury to the phrenic nerve.

in excess of 90%. The duration of circulatory arrest intervals are again limited to 20 minutes.

After the completion of the endarterectomy, cardiopulmonary bypass is reinstituted and warming is commenced. Methylprednisolone (500 mg, intravenously) and mannitol (12.5 g, intravenously) are administered, and during warming a 10°C temperature gradient is maintained between the perfusate and body temperature, with a maximum perfusate temperature of 37°C. If the systemic vascular resistance level is high, nitroprusside is administered to promote vasodilatation and warming. The rewarming period generally takes approximately 90 to 120 minutes but varies according to the body mass of the patient.

When the left pulmonary arteriotomy has been repaired, the pulmonary artery vent is replaced at the top of the incision. The right atrium is then opened and examined. Any intra-atrial communication is closed. Although tricuspid valve regurgitation is invariable in these patients and is often severe, tricuspid valve repair is not performed unless there is independent structural damage to the tricuspid valve itself. Right ventricular remodeling occurs within a few days, with the return of tricuspid competence. If other cardiac procedures are required, such as coronary artery or mitral or aortic valve surgery, these are conveniently performed during the systemic rewarming period. Myocardial cooling is discontinued once all cardiac procedures have been concluded. The left atrial vent is removed, and the vent site is repaired. All air is removed from the heart, and the aortic cross-clamp is removed.

When the patient has rewarmed, cardiopulmonary bypass is discontinued. Dopamine hydrochloride is routinely administered at renal doses, and other inotropic agents and vasodilators are titrated as necessary to sustain acceptable hemodynamics. The cardiac output is generally high, with a low systemic vascular resistance. Temporary pacing wires are placed.

Despite the duration of extracorporeal circulation, hemostasis is readily achieved, and blood products are generally unnecessary. Wound closure is routine. A vigorous diuresis is usual for the next few hours, also a result of the previous systemic hypothermia.

Postoperative Care

Meticulous postoperative management is essential to the success of this operation. All patients are mechanically ventilated overnight, and subjected to a maintained diuresis with the goal of reaching the patient's preoperative weight within 24 hours. Although much of the postoperative care is common to more ordinary open-heart surgery patients, there are some important differences.

A higher minute ventilation is often required early after the operation to compensate for the temporary metabolic acidosis that develops after the long period of circulatory arrest, hypothermia, and cardiopulmonary bypass. Tidal volumes higher than those normally recommended after cardiac surgery are therefore generally used to obtain optimal gas exchange. The maximum inspiratory pressure is maintained below 30 cm of water if possible. Extubation should be performed on the first postoperative day, whenever possible.

Diuresis. Patients have considerable positive fluid balance after operation. After hypothermic circulatory arrest, patients initiate an early spontaneous aggressive diuresis for unknown reasons, but this may in part be related to the increased cardiac output related to a now lower PVR level, and improved RV function. This diuresis should be augmented with diuretics, however, with the aim of returning the patient to the preoperative fluid balance within 24 hours of operation. Because of the increased cardiac output, some degree of systemic hypotension is readily tolerated. Fluid administration is minimized, and the patient's hematocrit level should be maintained above 30% to increase oxygen-carrying capacity and to reduce the likelihood of the pulmonary reperfusion phenomenon.

Arrhythmias. The development of atrial arrhythmias, at approximately 10%, is no more common than that encountered in patients who undergo other types of non–valvular heart surgery. When a small atrial septal defect or persistent foramen ovale is closed this is done with a small inferior atrial incision directly over the fossa ovalis, away from the conduction system of the atrium or its blood supply. The siting and size of this incision may be helpful in the reduction of the incidence of these arrhythmias.

Transfusion. Despite the requirement for the maintenance of an adequate hematocrit level, with careful blood conservation techniques used during operation, transfusion is required in a minority of patients.

Inferior Vena Caval Filter and Anticoagulation. A Greenfield filter is usually inserted before operation, to minimize recurrent pulmonary embolism after pulmonary endarterectomy. However, if this is not possible, it can also be inserted at the time of operation. If the device is to be placed at operation, radiopaque markers should be placed over the level of the spine corresponding to the location of the renal veins to allow correct positioning. Postoperative venous thrombosis prophylaxis with intermittent pneumatic compression devices is used, and the use of subcutaneous heparin is begun on the evening of surgery. Anticoagulation with warfarin is begun as soon as the pacing wires and mediastinal drainage tubes are removed, with a target international normalized ratio of 2.5 to 3.

Complications

Aside from complications that are associated with open heart and major lung surgery (arrhythmias, atelectasis, wound infection, pneumonia, mediastinal bleeding, etc.), there are complications specific to this operation. These include persistent pulmonary hypertension, reperfusion pulmonary response, and neurologic disorders related to deep hypothermia.

Persistent Pulmonary Hypertension. The decrease in PVR level usually results in an immediate and sustained restoration of pulmonary artery pressures to normal levels, with a marked increase in cardiac output. In a few patients, an immediately normal pulmonary vascular tone is not achieved, but an additional substantial reduction may occur over the next few days because of the subsequent relaxation of small vessels and the resolution of intraoperative factors such as pulmonary edema. In such patients, it is usual to see a large pulmonary artery pulse pressure, the low diastolic pressure indicating good runoff, yet persistent pulmonary arterial inflexibility still resulting in a high systolic pressure.

There are a few patients in whom the pulmonary artery pressures do not resolve substantially. If the operation has been performed as described in the preceding, using circulatory arrest, and ensuring that all distal disease is removed, this will be the result of type IV disease. We do operate on some patients with severe pulmonary hypertension but equivocal embolic disease. Despite the considerable risk of attempted endarterectomy in these patients, because transplantation is the only other avenue of therapy, there may be a point when it is unlikely that a patient will survive until a donor is found. In our most recent 500 patients, the majority of perioperative deaths were directly attributable to the problem of inadequate relief of pulmonary artery hypertension. This was a diagnostic rather than an operative technical problem. Attempts at pharmacologic manipulation of high residual PVR levels with sodium nitroprusside, epoprostenol sodium, or inhaled nitric oxide are generally not effective. Because the residual hypertensive defect is fixed, it is not appropriate to use mechanical circulatory support or extracorporeal membrane oxygenation in these patients if they deteriorate subsequently.

The "Reperfusion Response." A specific complication that occurs in most patients to some degree is localized pulmonary edema, or the "reperfusion response." Reperfusion response or reperfusion injury is defined as a radiologic opacity seen in the lungs within 72 hours of pulmonary endarterectomy. This unfortunately loose definition may therefore encompass many causes, such as fluid overload and infection.

True reperfusion injury that directly adversely impacts the clinical course of the patient now occurs in approximately 10% of patients. In its most dramatic form, it occurs soon after operation (within a few hours) and is associated with profound desaturation. Edema-like fluid, sometimes with a bloody tinge, is suctioned from the endotracheal tube.[95] Frank blood from the endotracheal tube, however, signifies a mechanical violation of the blood airway barrier that has occurred at operation and generally stems from a technical error, though we have seen two cases where significant blood in the airway was the result of a technically good operation, but reperfusion of a known infarcted area of the lung. This complication should be managed, if possible, by identification of the affected area by bronchoscopy and balloon occlusion of the affected lobe until coagulation can be normalized.

One common cause of reperfusion pulmonary edema is persistent high pulmonary artery pressures after operation when a thorough endarterectomy has been performed in certain areas, but there remains a large part of the pulmonary vascular bed affected by type IV change. However, the reperfusion phenomenon is often encountered in patients after a seemingly technically perfect operation with complete resolution of high pulmonary artery pressures. In these cases the response may be one of reactive hyperemia, after the revascularization of segments of the pulmonary arterial bed that have long experienced no flow. Other contributing factors may include perioperative pulmonary ischemia and conditions associated with high permeability lung injury in the area of the now denuded endothelium. Fortunately, the incidence of this complication is much less common now in our series, probably as a result of the more complete and expeditious removal of the endarterectomy specimen that has come with the large experience over the last decade.

Management of the "Reperfusion Response". Early measures should be taken to minimize the development of pulmonary edema with diuresis, maintenance of hematocrit levels, and the early use of peak end-expiratory pressure. Once the capillary leak has been established, treatment is supportive because reperfusion pulmonary edema will eventually resolve if satisfactory hemodynamics and oxygenation can be maintained. Careful management of ventilation and fluid balance is required. The hematocrit is kept high (32 to 36%), and the patient undergoes aggressive diuresis, even if this requires ultrafiltration. The patient's ventilatory status may be dramatically position sensitive. The FIO_2 level is kept as low as is compatible with an oxygen saturation of 90%. A careful titration of positive end-expiratory pressure is carried out, with a progressive transition from volume- to pressure-limited inverse ratio ventilation and the acceptance of moderate hypercapnia.[95] The use of steroids is discouraged because they are generally ineffective and may lead to infection. Infrequently, inhaled nitric oxide at 20 to 40 parts per million can improve the gas exchange. On occasion we have used extracorporeal perfusion support (extracorporeal membrane oxygenator or extracorporeal carbon dioxide removal) until ventilation can be resumed satisfactorily, usually after 7 to 10 days. However the use of this support is limited to patients who have benefited from hemodynamic improvement, but are suffering from significant reperfusion response. Extracorporeal devices should not be used if there is no evidence or hope of subsequent hemodynamic improvement, because it will not play a role in improving irreversible pulmonary pressures and carries mortality close to 100%.

Delirium. Early in the pulmonary endarterectomy experience (before 1990), there was a substantial incidence of postoperative delirium. A study of 28 patients who underwent pulmonary endarterectomy showed that 77% experienced the development of this complication.[96,97] Delirium appeared to be related to an accumulated duration of circulatory arrest time of more than 55 minutes; the incidence fell to 11% with significantly shorter periods of arrest time.[96–98] With the more expeditious operation that has come with our increased experience, postoperative confusion is now encountered no more commonly than with ordinary open heart surgery.

Results

More than 2700 pulmonary thromboendarterectomy have been performed at UCSD Medical Center since 1970. Most of these cases (more than 2600) have been completed since 1990, when the surgical procedure was modified as described earlier in this chapter. The mean patient age in our group is about 52 years, with a range of 7 to 85 years. There is a very slight male predominance. In nearly one-third of the cases, at least one additional cardiac procedure was performed at the time of operation. Most commonly, the adjunct procedure was closure of a persistent foramen ovale or atrial septal defect (26%) or coronary artery bypass grafting (8%).[87]

Hemodynamic Results. A reduction in pulmonary pressures and resistance to normal levels and a corresponding improvement in pulmonary blood flow and cardiac output are generally immediate and sustained.[98,99] In general, these changes can be assumed to be permanent. Whereas before the operation, more than 95% of the patients are in NYHA functional class III or IV; at 1 year after the operation, 95% of patients remain in NYHA functional class I or II.[99,100] In addition, echocardiographic studies have demonstrated that, with the elimination of chronic pressure overload, right ventricular geometry rapidly reverts toward normal. Right atrial and right ventricular enlargement regresses. Tricuspid valve function returns to normal within a few days as a result of restoration of tricuspid annular geometry after the remodeling of the right ventricle, and tricuspid repair is not therefore part of the operation.

Operative Morbidity. Severe reperfusion injury was the single most frequent complication in the UCSD series, occurring in 10% of patients. Some of these patients did not survive, and other patients required prolonged mechanical ventilatory support. A few patients were salvaged only by the use of extracorporeal support and blood carbon dioxide removal. Neurologic complications from circulatory arrest appear to have been eliminated, probably as a result of the shorter circulatory arrest periods now experienced, and perioperative confusion and stroke are now no more frequent than with conventional open heart surgery. Early postoperative hemorrhage required re-exploration in 2.5% of patients, and less than half of patients required intraoperative or postoperative blood transfusion. Despite the prolonged operation, wound infections are relatively infrequent. Only 1.8% experienced the development of sternal wound complications, including sterile dehiscence or mediastinitis.

Deaths. In our experience, the overall mortality rate (30 days or in-hospital if the hospital course is prolonged) is about 7% for the entire patient group, which encompasses a time span of over 35 years. The mortality rate was 9.4% in 1989 and has been less than 6% for the more than 2400 patients who have undergone the operation since 1990. In our most recent experience over the last 5 years, the mortality rate has been less than 4%. With our increasing experience and many referrals, we continue to accept some patients who, in retrospect, were unsuitable candidates for the procedure (type IV disease). We also accept patients in whom we know that the entire degree of pulmonary hypertension cannot be explained by the occlusive disease detected by angiography but feel that they will be benefited by operation, albeit at higher risk. Residual causes of death are operation on patients in whom thromboembolic disease was not the cause of the pulmonary hypertension (50%) and the rare case of reperfusion pulmonary edema that progresses to a respiratory distress syndrome of long standing, which is not reversible (25%).

Late Follow-up

A survey of the surviving patients who underwent pulmonary endarterectomy surgery at UCSD between 1970 and 1995 formally evaluated the long-term outcome.[100] Questionnaires were mailed to 420 patients who were more than 1 year after operation. Responses were obtained from 308 patients. Survival, functional status, quality of life, and the subsequent use of medical help were assessed. Survival after pulmonary thromboendarterectomy was 75% at 6 years or more. Ninety-three percent of the patients were found to be in NYHA Class I or II, compared with about 95% of the patients being in NYHA Class III or IV preoperatively. Of the working population, 62% of patients who were unemployed before operation returned to work. Patients who had undergone pulmonary endarterectomy scored several quality-of-life components just slightly lower than normal individuals, but significantly higher than the patients before endarterectomy. Only 10% of patients used oxygen, and in response to the question, "How do you feel about the quality of your life since your surgery?" Seventy-seven percent replied much improved, and twenty percent replied improved. These data appear to confirm that pulmonary endarterectomy offers substantial improvement in survival, function, and quality of life, with minimal later health-care requirements.[100]

CONCLUSION

It is increasingly apparent that pulmonary hypertension caused by chronic pulmonary embolism is a condition which is under-recognized, and carries a poor prognosis. Medical therapy is ineffective in prolonging life and only transiently improves the symptoms. The only therapeutic alternative to pulmonary thromboendarterectomy is lung transplantation. The advantages of thromboendarterectomy include a lower operative mortality and excellent long-term results without the risks associated with chronic immunosuppression and chronic allograft rejection. The mortality for thromboendarterectomy at our institution is now less than 4%, with sustained benefit. These results are clearly superior to those for transplantation both in the short and long term.

Although PTE is technically demanding for the surgeon, and requires careful dissection of the pulmonary artery planes and the use of circulatory arrest, excellent short- and long-term results can be achieved. It is the successive improvements in operative technique developed over the last four decades, which now allow pulmonary endarterectomy to be offered to patients with an acceptable mortality rate and excellent anticipation of clinical improvement. With this growing experience, it has also become clear that unilateral operation is obsolete and that circulatory arrest is essential.

The primary problem remains that this is an under-recognized condition. Increased awareness of both the prevalence of this condition and the possibility of a surgical cure should avail more patients of the opportunity for relief from this debilitating and ultimately fatal disease.

REFERENCES

1. Dalen JE, Alpert JS. Natural history of pulmonary embolism. *Prog Cardiovasc Dis* 1975:17:259-270.
2. Landefeld CS, Chren MM, Myers A, et al: Diagnostic yield of the autopsy in a university hospital and a community hospital. *NEJM* 1988; 318:1249.

3. Goldhaber SZ, Hennekens CH, Evens DA, et al: Factors associated with correct antemortem diagnosis of major pulmonary embolism. *Am J Med* 1982;73:822-826.
4. Rubinstein1, Murray D, Hoffstein V: Fatal pulmonary emboli in hospitalized patients: an autopsy study. *Arch Intern Med* 1988;148:1425-1426.
5. Kniffin WD Jr, Baron JA, Barrett J, et al: The epidemiology of diagnosed pulmonary embolism and deep venous thrombosis in the elderly. *Arch Intern Med* 1994; 154:861.
6. Martin M: PHLECO. A multicenter study of the fate of 1647 hospital patients treated conservatively without fibrinolysis and surgery. *Clin Invest* 1993; 71:471.
7. Carson JL, Kelley MA, Duff A, et al: The clinical course of pulmonary embolism. *NEJM* 1992; 326:1240.
8. Clagett GP, Anderson FA JR, Levine MN, et al: Prevention of venous thromboembolism. *Chest* 1992; 102:391S.
9. Anderson FA Jr, Wheeler HB: Venous thromboembolism; risk factors and prophylaxis, in Tapson VF, Fulkkerson WJ, Saltzman HA (eds): *Clinics in Chest Medicine, Venous Thromboembolism*, vol 16. Philadelphia, Saunders, 1995; p 235.
10. Greenfield LJ: Venous thrombosis and pulmonary thromboembolism, in Schwartz SI (ed): *Principals of Surgery*, 6th ed. New York, McGraw-Hill, 1994; p 989.
11. Riedel M, Stanek V, Widimsky J, Prerovsky I: Long term follow up of patients with pulmonary embolism: late prognosis and evolution of hemodynamic and respiratory data. *Chest* 1982; 81:151.
12. Godleski JJ: Pathology of deep vein thrombosis and pulmonary embolism, in Goldhaber SZ (ed): *Pulmonary Embolism and Deep Venous Thrombosis.* Philadelphia, Saunders, 1985; p 11.
13. Moser KM: Venous thromboembolism. *Am Rev Resp Dis* 1990; 141:235.
14. Sevitt S: The structure and growth of valve pocket thrombi in femoral veins. *J Clin Pathol* 1974; 27:517.
15. Philbrick JT, Becker DM: Calf deep vein thrombosis: a wolf in sheep's clothing? *Arch Intern Med* 1988; 148:2131.
16. Kakkar VV, Flan C, Howe CT Clark MB: Natural history of postoperative deep vein thrombosis. *Lancet* 1969; 2:230.
17. Salzmen EW, Hirsch J: The epidemiology, pathogenesis, and natural history of venous thrombosis, in Colman RW, Hirsch J, Marder VJ, Salzman EW (eds): *Hemostasis and Thrombosis: Basic Principals and Clinical Practice,* 3rd ed. Philadelphia, Lippincott, 1994; p 1275.
18. Stewart GJ, Lackman JW, Alburger PD, et al: Intraoperative venous dilation and subsequent development of deep vein thrombosis in patients undergoing total hip or knee replacement. *Ultrasound Med Biol* 1990; 16:133.
19. Comerota AJ, Stewart GJ, Alburger PD, et al: Operative venodilation, a previously unsuspected factor in the cause of postoperative deep vein thrombosis. *Surgery* 1989; 106:301.
20. Comerota AJ, Stewart GJ: Operative venous dilation and its relationship to postoperative deep vein thrombosis, in Goldhaber SZ (ed): *Prevention of Venous Thromboembolism.* New York, Marcel Dekker, 1993; p 25.
21. Weiss HJ, Turitto VT, Baumgartner HR, et al: Evidence for the presence of tissue factor activity on subendothelium. *Blood* 1989; 73;968.
22. Bertina RM, Koeleman BPC, Koster T, et al: Mutation in blood coagulation factor V associated with resistance to activated protein C. *Nature* 1994; 369:64.
23. Svensson PJ, Dahlback B: Resistance to activated protein C as a basis for venous thrombosis. *NEJM* 1994; 330:517.
24. Ridker PM, Hennekens CH, Lindpaintner K, et al: Mutation in the gene coding for coagulation factor V and the risk of myocardial infarction, stroke, and venous thrombosis in apparently healthy men. *NEJM* 1995; 332:912.
25. Feinstein DI: Immune coagulation disorders, in Colman RW, Hirsh J, Marder VJ, Salzman EW (eds): *Hemostasis and Thrombosis: Basic Principal and Clinical Practice,* 3rd ed. Philadelphia, Lippincott, 1994; p 881.
26. Robertson BR, Pandolfi M, Nilsson IM: "Fibrinolytic capacity" in healthy volunteers at different ages as studied by standardized venous occlusion of arms and legs. *Acta Med Scand* 1972; 191:199.
27. Prins MH, Hirsh J: A critical review of the evidence supporting a relationship between impaired fibrinolysis and venous thromboembolism. *Arch Intern Med* 1991; 151:1721.
28. Wheeler HB, Anderson FA Jr, Cardullo PA, et al: Suspected deep vein thrombosis: management by impedance plethysmography. *Arch Surg* 1982; 117:1206.
29. Samama MM, Simonneau G, Wainstein JP, et al: SISIUS Study: epidemiology of risk factors of deep vein thrombosis (DVT) of the lower limbs in community practice (abstract). *Thromb Haemost* 1993; 69:763.
30. Hull R, Hirsh J, Jay R: Different intensities of anticoagulation in the long term treatment of proximal vein thrombosis. *NEJM* 1982; 307:1676.
31. Collins R, Scrimgeor A, Yusuf S, et al: Reduction in fatal pulmonary embolism and venous thrombosis by perioperative administration of subcutaneous heparin. Overview of results and randomized trials in general, orthopedic, and urologic surgery. *NEJM* 1988; 318:1162.
32. Reis SE, Polak JF, Hirsch DR, et al: Frequency of deep vein thrombosis in asymptomatic patients with coronary artery bypass grafts. *Am Heart J* 1991; 122:478.
33. Josa M, Siouffi SY, Silverman AB, et al: Pulmonary embolism after cardiac surgery. *J AM Coll Cardiol* 1993; 21:990.
34. Gillinov AM, Davis EA, Alberg AJ, et al: Pulmonary embolism in the cardiac surgical patient. *Ann Thorac Surg* 1992; 53:988.
35. Burk B, Sostman D, Carroll BA, Witty LA: The diagnostic approach to deep vein thrombosis, in *Venous Thromboembolism, Clinics in Chest Medicine,* vol 16. Philadelphia, Saunders, 1995; pp 253-268.
36. Evans AJ, Sostman HC, Knelson M, et al: Detection of deep vein thrombosis: a prospective comparison of MR imaging with contrast venography. *Am J Roentgenol* 1993; 161:131.
37. Hirsh J, Levine MN: Low molecular weight heparin. *Blood* 1992; 72:1.
38. Shulman S, Rhedin A-S, Lindmarker P, et al: A comparison of six weeks with six months of oral anticoagulant therapy after a first episode of venous thromboembolism. *NEJM* 1995; 332:1661.
39. Goldhaber SZ. Strategies for diagnosis, in Goldhaber SZ (ed): *Pulmonary Embolism and Deep Vein Thrombosis.* Philadelphia. Saunders, 1985; p 79.
40. Hoaglang PM: Massive pulmonary embolism, in Goldhaber SZ (ed): *Pulmonary Embolism and Deep Vein Thrombosis.* Philadelphia, Saunders, 1985; p 179.
41. Malik AB, Johnson B: Role of humoral mediators in the pulmonary vascular response to pulmonary embolism, in Weir EK, Reeves JT (eds): *Pulmonary Vascular Physiology and Pathophysiology.* New York, Marcel Dekker, 1989; p 445.
42. Huval WV, Mathieson MA, Stemp LI, et al: Therapeutic benefits of 5-hydroxytryptamine inhibition following pulmonary embolism. *Ann Surg* 1983; 197:223.
43. Barritt DW, Jordan SC: Anticoagulant drugs in treatment of pulmonary embolism: Controlled Trial. *Lancet* 1960; 1:1309.
44. The urokinase pulmonary embolism trial. A national cooperative study. *Circulation* 1973; 47(Suppl II):1.
45. Bell WR, Simon TR: Current status of pulmonary thromboembolic disease: pathophysiology, diagnosis, prevention, and treatment. *Am Heart J* 1982; 103:239.
46. Dalen JE, Banas JS Jr, Brooks HL, et al: Resolution rate of pulmonary embolism in man. *NEJM* 1969; 280:1194.
47. Tow De, Wagner HN: Recovery of pulmonary arterial blood flow in patients with pulmonary embolism. *NEJM* 1967; 276:1053.
48. Dalen JE, Alpert JS: Natural history of pulmonary embolism. *Prog Cardiovasc Dis* 1975; 17:259.
49. Palevsky HI: The problems of the clinical and laboratory diagnosis of pulmonary embolism. *Sem Nucl Med* 1991; 21:276.
50. Greenfield LJ, Proctor Mc, Williams DM, Wakefield TW: Long term experience with transvenous catheter pulmonary embolectomy. *J Vasc Surg* 1993; 18:450.
51. Goodall RJR, Greenfield LJ: Clinical correlations in the diagnosis of pulmonary embolism. *Ann Surg* 1980; 191:219.
52. McCracken S, Bettmen S. Current status of ionic and nonionic intravascular contrast media. *Postgrad Radiol* 1983; 3:345.
53. Novelline RA, Baltarowich OH, Athanasoulis CA, et al: The clinical course of patients with suspect pulmonary embolism and a negative pulmonary arteriogram. *Radiology* 1978; 126:561.
54. Schiebler M, Holland G, Hatabu H et al: Suspected pulmonary embolism: prospective evaluation with pulmonary MR angiography. *Radiology* 1993; 189:125.
55. Come PC: Echocardiographic evaluation of pulmonary embolism and its response to therapeutic interventions. *Chest* 1992; 101:1515.
56. Goldhaber SZ: Thrombolytic therapy in venous thromboembolism. Clinical trials and current indications, in Tapson VF, Fulkerson WJ, Saltzman HA (eds): *Clinics in Chest Medicine, Venous Thromboembolism,* vol 16. Philadelphia, Saunders, 1995; p 307.
57. Marder VJ, Sherry S: Thrombolytic therapy: current status. *NEJM* 1988; 318:1585.
58. Goldhaber SZ, Haire WD, Feldstein ML, et al: Alteplase versus heparin in acute PE; randomized trial assessing right ventricular function and pulmonary perfusion. *Lancet* 1993; 341:507.
59. Tibbutt DA, Davies JA, Anderson JA, et al: Comparison by controlled clinical trial of streptokinase and heparin in treatment of life-threatening PE. *BMJ* 1974; 1:343.
60. Ly B, Arnesen H, Eie H, Hol R: A controlled clinical trial of streptokinase and heparin in the treatment of major PE. *Acta Med Scand* 1978; 203:465.

61. Levine MN: Thrombolytic therapy for venous embolism. Complications and contraindications, in Tapson VF, Fulkerson WJ, Saltzman HA (eds): *Clinics in Chest Medicine, Venous Thromboembolism*, vol 16. Philadelphia, Saunders, 1995; p 321.
62. Levine M, Hirsh J, Weitz J, et al: A randomized trial of a single bolus dosage regimen of recombinant tissue plasminogen activator in patients with acute PE. *Chest* 1990; 98:1473.
63. Gray JJ, Miller GAH, Paneth M: Pulmonary embolectomy: its place in the management of pulmonary embolism. *Lancet* 1988; 25:1441.
64. Timist J-F, Reynaud P, Meyers G, Sors H: Pulmonary embolectomy by catheter device in massive pulmonary embolism. *Chest* 1991; 100:655.
65. Tapson VF, Witty LA: Massive pulmonary embolism, in Tapson VF, Fulkerson WJ, Saltzman HA (eds): *Clinics in Chest Medicine, Venous Thromboembolism*, vol 16. Philadelphia, Saunders, 1995; p 329.
66. Mattox KL, Feldtman RW, Beall AC, De Bakey ME: Pulmonary embolectomy for acute massive pulmonary embolism. *Ann Surg* 1982; 195:726.
67. Boulafendis D, Bastounis E, Panayiotopoulos YP, Papalambros EL: Pulmonary embolectomy: answered and unanswered questions. *Int J Angiol* 1991; 10:187.
68. Kasper W, Meinterz MD, Henkel B, et al: Echocardiographic findings in patients with proved pulmonary embolism. *Am Heart J* 1986; 112:1284.
69. Stewart JR, Greenfield LS: Transvenous vena cava filtration and pulmonary embolectomy. *Surg Clin No Am* 1982; 62:411.
70. Schmid C, Zietlow S, Wagner TOF, et al: Fulminant pulmonary embolism: symptoms, diagnostics, operative technique and results. *Ann Thorac Surg* 1991; 52: 1102.
71. Greenfield LJ, Zocco J, Wilk JD, et al: Clinical experience with the Kim-Ray Greenfield vena cava filter. *Ann Surg* 1977; 185:692.
72. Anderson HL III, Delius RE, Sinard JM, et al: Early experience with adult extracorporeal membrane oxygenation in the modern era. *Ann Thorac Surg* 1992; 53:553.
73. Wenger R, Bavaria JB, Ratcliff MB, Edmunds LH Jr: Flow dynamics of peripheral venous catheters during extracorporeal membrane oxygenator (ECMO) with a centrifuge pump. *J Thorac Cardiovasc Surg* 1988; 96:478.
74. Gray HH, Morgan JM, Miller GAH: Pulmonary embolectomy for acute massive pulmonary embolism: an analysis of 71 cases. *Br Heart J* 1988; 60:196.
75. Del Campo C: Pulmonary embolectomy: a review. *Can J Surg* 1985; 28:111.
76. Gulba DC, Schmid C, Borst H-G, et al: Medical compared with surgical treatment for massive pulmonary embolism. *Lancet* 1994; 343:576.
77. Clark DB: Pulmonary embolectomy has a well-defined and valuable place. *Br J Hosp Med* 1989; 41:468.
78. Soyer R, Brunet M, Redonnet JY, et al: Follow-up of surgically treated patients with massive pulmonary embolism, with reference to 12 operated patients. *Thorac Cardiovasc Surg* 1982; 30:103.
79. Benotti JR, Ockene IS, Alpert JS, Dalen JE: The clinical profile of unresolved pulmonary embolism. *Chest* 1983; 84:669-678.
80. Moser KM, Auger WF, Fedullo PF: Chronic major-vessel thromboembolic pulmonary hypertension. *Circulation* 1990; 81:1735-1743.
81. Houk VN, Hufnnagel CA, McClenathan JE, Moser KM: Chronic thrombosis obstruction of major pulmonary arteries: report of a case successfully treated by thromboendarterectomy and review of the literature. *Am J Med* 1963; 35:269-282.
82. Dibble JH: Organization and canalization in arterial thrombosis. *J Pathol Bacteriol* 1958;75:1-4.
83. Cournad A, Rilev RL, Himmelstein A, Austrian R: Pulmonary circulation in the alveolar ventilation perfusion relationship after pneumonectomy. *J Thorac Surg* 1950; 19:80-116.
84. Kapitan KS, Buchbinder M, Wagner PD, Moser KM: Mechanisms of hypoxemia in chronic pulmonary hypertension. *Am Rev Respir Dis* 1989; 139:1149.
85. Moser KM, Daily PO, Peterson K, et al: Thromboendarterectomy for chronic, major vessel thromboembolic pulmonary hypertension: immediate and long term results in 42 patients. *Ann Int Med* 1987; 107:560.
86. Moser KM: Pulmonary vascular obstruction due to embolism and thrombosis, in Moser KM (ed): *Pulmonary Vascular Disease*. New York, Marcel Dekker, 1979; p 341.
87. Jamieson SW, Kapalanski DP: Pulmonary endarterectomy. *Curr Probl Surg* 2000; 37(3): 165-252.
88. Dantzker DR, Bower JS: Partial reversibility of chronic pulmonary hypertension caused by pulmonary thromboembolic disease. *Am Rev Respir Dis* 1981; 124:129-131.
89. Dash H, Ballentine N, Zelis R: Vasodilators ineffective in secondary pulmonary hypertension. *NEJM* 1980; 303:1062-1063.
90. Allison PR, Dunnill MS, Marshall R: Pulmonary embolism. *Thorax* 1960; 15:273.
91. Simonneau G, Azarian R, Bernot F, et al: Surgical management of unresolved pulmonary embolism: a personal series of 72 patients [abstract]. *Chest* 1995; 107:52S.
92. Moser KM, Houk VN, Jones RC, Hufnagel CC: Chronic, massive thrombotic obstruction of the pulmonary arteries: analysis of four operated cases. *Circulation* 1965; 32:377-385.
93. Winkler MH Rohrer CH, Ratty SC, et al: Perfusion techniques of profound hypothermia and circulatory arrest for pulmonary thromboendarterectomy. *J Extra Technol* 1990; 22:57-60.
94. Jamieson SW: Pulmonary thromboendarterectomy, in Franco KL, Putnam JB (eds): *Advanced Therapy in Thoracic Surgery*. Hamilton, Ontario, BC Decker, 1998; pp 310-318.
95. Levinson RM, Shure D, Moser KM: Reperfusion pulmonary edema after pulmonary artery thromboendarterectomy. *Am Rev Respir Dis* 1986; 134: 1241-1245.
96. Wragg RE, Dimsdale JE, Moser KM, Daily PO, et al: Operative predictors of delirium after pulmonary thromboendarterectomy. A model for postcardiotomy syndrome? *J Thorac Cardiovasc Surg* 1988; 96:524-529.
97. Jamieson SW, Auger WR, Fedullo PF, et al: Experience and results of 150 pulmonary thromboendarterectomy operations over a 29 month period. *J Thorac Cardiovascular Surg* 1993; 106:116-127.
98. Moser KM, Auger WR, Fedullo PF, Jamieson SW: Chronic thromboembolic pulmonary hypertension: clinical picture and surgical treatment. *Eur Respir J* 1992; 5:334-342.
99. Fedullo PF, Auger WR, Channick RN, Moser KM, Jamieson SW: Surgical management of pulmonary embolism, in Morpurgo M (ed): *Pulmonary Embolism*. New York, Marcel Dekker, 1994; p 223-240.
100. Archibald CJ, Auger WR, Fedullo PF, et al: Long-term outcome after pulmonary thromboendarterectomy. *Am J Respir Crit Care Med* 1999; 160:523-528.

CHAPTER 56

Trauma to the Great Vessels

Jean Marie Ruddy
John S. Ikonomidis

INTRODUCTION

Injury to the aorta and great vessels of the thorax may occur secondary to blunt or penetrating trauma, and appropriate management of immediate hemorrhage as well as that resulting from subsequent pseudoaneurysm rupture should be the primary goal of the treating surgeon.[1] Blunt aortic injury is the most common thoracic vascular injury following blunt trauma and the second leading cause of death from motor vehicle collision, accounting for 15% of deaths.[2–4] In 75 to 90% of cases, death occurs at the accident scene, typically in those with four or more serious injuries in addition to their aortic transection.[2–5] After aortic transection at the isthmus, aortic disruption at the base of the innominate artery is the most common site of injury, followed by the base of the left subclavian artery, and the base of the left carotid.[6] Central venous structures are rarely injured with blunt trauma,[7] but this can occur with penetrating trauma.[8] Traditionally, open surgical repair of these injuries has proved effective, but recent literature has demonstrated the safety and efficacy of endovascular interventions.[9] This chapter examines trauma to each of the thoracic vessels and presents diagnostic modalities as well as treatment options.

THE ASCENDING AORTA AND AORTIC ARCH BRANCH VESSELS

Mechanism of Injury

Descending thoracic aortic transection is the most common vascular injury resulting from blunt thoracic force; however, the ascending aorta and arch vessels may also be disrupted, commonly leading to dissection or pseudoaneurysm formation.[10,11] Mechanistically, the transmission of force through the thoracic cavity from blunt injury is believed to cause torsion of the ascending aorta, leading to disruption of the wall with an associated shearing effect on the heart.[12] Additionally, a water-hammer effect is described in which an aortic occlusion at the diaphragm occurs with impact and a high pressure wave is reflected back to the ascending aorta and aortic arch.[1] The pathogenesis of blunt innominate artery rupture has been postulated to be the result of anteroposterior compression of the mediastinum between the sternum and vertebrae, displacing the heart posteriorly and to the left, thereby increasing the curvature of the aortic arch and increasing tension on all of its outflow vessels.[13] Hyperextension of the cervical spine with head rotation provides additional tension on the right carotid artery, which is transmitted to the innominate artery, and can lead to rupture.[13] The left carotid artery undergoes stretching injury with rapid deceleration, producing an intimal tear and subsequent dissection.[10] Additional mechanisms of carotid artery injury include hyperflexion of the neck to cause compression between the mandible and cervical spine, basilar skull fracture transecting the artery, and strangulation injury.[10] Blunt subclavian artery injuries are more common in the middle and distal third of the artery and are theorized to be caused by downward forces fracturing the first rib with the anterior scalene acting as a fulcrum so that the subclavian artery is pinched between the first rib and clavicle.[14] The abrupt deceleration of the shoulder, owing to the seatbelt shoulder harness, is also believed to cause subclavian artery shearing injuries.[14]

Clinical Presentation

Patients presenting to the emergency department with injury to a great vessel should be evaluated according to standard ATLS protocols. Those suffering blunt trauma are often hemodynamically stable; therefore, a high index of suspicion for intrathoracic vascular disruption must be based on the mechanism and constellation of related injuries. In addition to high-speed collisions involving automobiles or motorcycles, crush injuries and falls often have sufficient force to rupture a thoracic vessel.[10,14–16] Commonly associated complaints include neck and chest pain, and physical exam may reveal ecchymosis across the chest and neck from the seatbelt shoulder harness.[11,17] Physical exam findings concerning for rupture of a great vessel include supraclavicular swelling or bruit, diminished pulse in the ipsilateral upper extremity, neck hematoma with or without tracheal deviation, acute Horner's syndrome, and an acute superior vena cava–like syndrome.[10,11,18]

In a stable patient with evidence of a stab or gunshot wound located between the midclavicular lines or in zone I of the neck, great vessel penetration should be suspected.[19] A precordial bruit suggesting arteriovenous fistula (AVF) formation may be noted in up to 30% of patients.[20] Penetrating distal subclavian injuries may demonstrate pulsatile bleeding during initial evaluation.[21] More commonly, patients suffering penetrating injury to the chest or neck will be hemodynamically unstable on arrival to the emergency department, possibly with evidence of cardiac tamponade, and those *in extremis* should undergo emergent thoracotomy.[20] Hypotensive patients may proceed directly to the operating room without diagnostic imaging; the mortality of patients presenting with hypotension is nearly three times greater than that of stable patients.[21]

Radiographic Imaging

In a patient who has suffered blunt trauma, chest radiograph may demonstrate fractures of the sternum, clavicle, and first rib, indicating the degree of physical force applied to the thoracic cavity. A widened mediastinum, pneumothorax, apical pleural capping, or obscured aortic knob may be evident in either blunt or penetrating injuries.[15,19,20,22] When suspected clinically, carotid artery injuries can often be diagnosed by duplex ultrasound.[10] Even in the absence of mediastinal or thoracic injury on chest x-ray, stable patients should undergo computed tomography (CT) of the chest with intravenous contrast based on traumatic mechanism alone. This study may reveal a superior mediastinal hematoma without reliably identifying the location of injury and additional diagnostic imaging should be pursued. Case reports of blunt ascending aortic injuries have documented diagnostic accuracy of transesophageal echocardiography (TEE) when conducted by an experienced operator.[15] These studies occurred intraoperatively in patients undergoing emergent laparotomy who did not have a source of hypotension in the abdomen, and each TEE was followed by aortogram.[15] Therefore, the utility of this imaging modality as a routine precursor to aortogram in stable patients is questionable. Aortography is the gold standard for diagnosis of a traumatic injury to the thoracic vessels and may provide an opportunity for immediate endovascular intervention to treat a pseudoaneurysm or AVF.[20,21,23,24]

Operative Repair

Ascending Aorta

Pseudoaneurysm of the ascending aorta should be repaired using cardiopulmonary bypass. Femoral-femoral or axillofemoral cannulation before sternotomy may decompress the ascending aorta and decrease the risk of pseudoaneurysm rupture on opening the chest.[18] After entering the pericardium, the pseudoaneurysm should be carefully mobilized, if possible, to gain proximal and distal control. Depending on the nature and extent of the injury, repair may be conducted by primary repair, patch angioplasty, or prosthetic replacement of aortic segment. If aortic valve insufficiency is encountered, prosthetic valve replacement may be warranted.[25] Occasionally, deep hypothermic circulatory arrest is required, especially if proximal and distal control cannot be comfortably obtained or the pseudoaneurysm extends into the proximal aortic arch. This will allow for excision of the pseudoaneurysm and closure of the aortic defect with a prosthetic patch.[12] As with descending thoracic aortic injuries, a delay in operative management may be considered in hemodynamically stable patients with associated injuries at high risk for bleeding, especially intracranial lesions.[12] The application of this delayed approach depends on the nature of the ascending aortic injury. For instance, it must be a discrete lesion without evidence of circumferential involvement or compromised adjacent structures. Safe observation entails maintaining a mean arterial pressure less than 80 mm Hg and cerebral perfusion pressure greater than 50 mm Hg, typically through short-acting intravenous beta-blockade.[26] Conservative management must be accompanied by regular assessment of the aortic lesion through serial CT scans of the thorax and a low threshold for operative intervention if enlargement of the pseudoaneurysm is identified.[26]

Innominate Artery

The innominate artery is the second most common site of thoracic vascular injury following blunt trauma. In a review of 117 reported cases of blunt innominate artery rupture, 83% were in the proximal vessel, 3% were in the middle, 9% were distal, and the remaining injuries involved multiple sections.[16] The most common finding was disruption of the intima and media with pseudoaneurysm formation (Fig. 56-1).[16] Although primary repair may be possible in some cases, surgical repair of an innominate artery rupture has traditionally been performed by a prosthetic aorto-innominate bypass graft from the aortic arch to healthy distal vessels through a full or upper median sternotomy with extension of the incision along the anterior border of the right sternocleidomastoid as necessary.[9,19] Operative repair of a penetrating innominate artery injury is approached in the same manner.[19] The entire length of the innominate artery should be mobilized to achieve distal control and the pericardium opened to gain proximal control at the level of the aortic arch.[27] After systemic administration of heparin, a partial occlusion clamp is applied to the aortic arch and the proximal anastomosis of the prosthetic graft performed end-to-side with polypropylene suture.[27] Depending on the location and extent of the injury, the distal end-to-end anastomosis may involve only the innominate artery or a Y-graft may be required to reconstruct the proximal portions of the right carotid and right subclavian arteries individually.[16] The origin of the innominate artery should then be fully exposed and oversewn with pledgeted nonabsorbable sutures.[27] Healthy patients typically tolerate

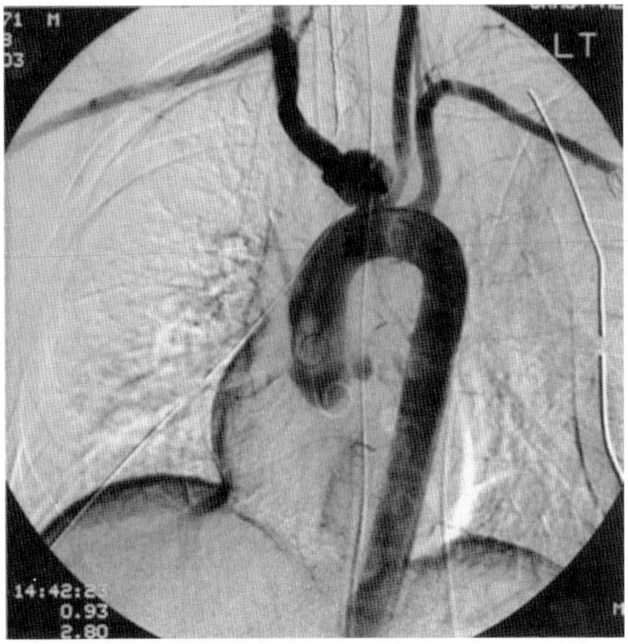

FIGURE 56-1 Arteriogram showing rupture of proximal segment of innominate artery and pseudoaneurysm at the site of rupture. (*Reproduced with permission of Symbas JD, Halkos ME, Symbas PN: Rupture of the innominate artery from blunt trauma: current options for management. J Card Surg 2005; 20[5]:455-459.*)

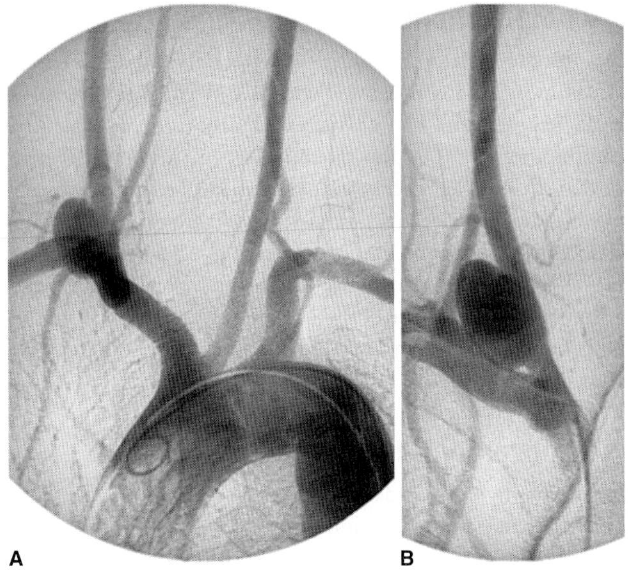

FIGURE 56-2 Digital subtraction angiography demonstrating a wide-necked pseudoaneurysm at the base of the right common carotid artery. (A) A left anterior oblique view with an aortic arch injection. (B) The right anterior oblique view with innominate artery injection. (*Reproduced with permission from Simionato F, Righi C, Melissano G, et al: Stent-graft treatment of a common carotid artery pseudoaneurysm. J Endovasc Ther 2000; 7[2]:136-140.*)

temporary innominate artery occlusion caused by adequate collateral flow through the contralateral carotid and vertebral arteries.[27] Cerebral protection, cardiopulmonary bypass, electroencephalogram monitoring, hypothermia with circulatory arrest, or carotid shunting (for stump pressure <50 mm Hg) should be employed in patients with neurologic abnormalities or suspicion of a contralateral carotid artery injury.[9,27] Long-term patency of prosthetic aorto-innominate artery bypass grafts has been reported to be greater than 96% at 10 years.[28]

Carotid Artery

Therapeutic management of blunt carotid artery injury must be directed at preventing cerebral ischemia and surgical intervention should be weighed against observation and anticoagulation.[29] Small intimal flaps may resolve, whereas larger flaps can lead to thrombosis and therefore require anticoagulation to prevent thromboembolism.[30] Arterial dissection may progress to luminal narrowing, placing the patient at risk for thrombosis, and anticoagulation therapy is especially important in patients with bilateral carotid artery dissection owing to the morbidity and mortality associated with bilateral thrombosis.[31] When operative intervention is indicated because of pseudoaneurysm formation (Fig. 56-2), the surgeon may bypass the lesion, but reconstruction or ligation of the artery can also be employed.[10] Open repair of an intrathoracic carotid artery injury should occur through a median sternotomy with extension along the anterior border of the ipsilateral sternocleidomastoid muscle as necessary to gain adequate exposure.[20] After gaining proximal and distal control, arterial repair may be accomplished by primary repair or interposition grafting with saphenous vein or prosthetic material.[20]

Subclavian Artery

Injury to the subclavian artery, from blunt or penetrating trauma, carries a mortality rate of 5 to 30% resulting from the inability to obtain adequate hemorrhagic control through direct pressure.[32] Additionally, because of the close proximity of the trachea, esophagus, subclavian vein, and brachial plexus, subclavian artery injuries are associated with 40% morbidity.[32] Operative exposure may be achieved by median sternotomy, limited sternotomy, supraclavicular incision, infraclavicular incision, thoracotomy, or a combination of these depending on the location of the injury.[33] Left-sided lesions are often managed through an anterolateral thoracotomy with either an infraclavicular or supraclavicular counter incision;[14] however, some surgeons perform a median sternotomy for a proximal injury.[33] Right-sided injuries, on the other hand, require median sternotomy with supraclavicular extension.[14] In cases in which the defect involves a long segment of the subclavian artery, a portion of the clavicle may be resected to optimize exposure, although this procedure carries considerable postoperative morbidity.[21,33] Once establishing proximal and distal control of the subclavian artery, the damaged arterial segment may be excised and arterial reconstruction accomplished with an interposition graft using a saphenous vein or prosthetic material.[14] In cases in which minimal arterial debridement is required, primary repair is often attained.[34] Ligation of the subclavian artery may be performed on critically ill patients unable to tolerate an extensive operative repair, and minimal short-term morbidity in the affected limb has been reported.[21,33,34] When planning operative repair of the subclavian artery, concomitant injuries to nearby structures such as the subclavian vein and brachial plexus should be considered.

Complications

Despite the location of injury, intraoperative exsanguination is the most common cause of death and patients presenting with hypotension are at increased risk for postoperative complications.[14,20,35] After operative repair, pneumonia, pericardial effusion, left vocal cord paralysis, stroke, and postoperative bleeding have been reported.[22] Vessel thrombosis related to either primary repair or interposition graft placement has occurred in the immediate postoperative period as well as in long-term follow-up.[21] In these critically ill patients, postoperative mortality has been primarily attributed to multiorgan system failure and stroke.[35]

Endovascular Interventions

Arteriography is considered the gold standard for diagnosis and characterization of an intrathoracic vascular injury, and as endovascular stent technology and surgeon proficiency continue to advance, arteriography may become the preferred method of treatment in hemodynamically stable patients. The literature is currently populated with small case series and case reports documenting the feasibility of this approach and minimal short-term morbidity and mortality, but very little long-term data exist. Similar to other minimally invasive techniques, endovascular management of a traumatic injury to an intrathoracic vessel can provide an opportunity for patients to avoid sternotomy or thoracotomy and the associated pain, prolonged recovery time, and infection risk.[36] An analysis of endovascular versus open procedures in the National Trauma Database revealed a survival advantage for endovascular repair when controlling for injury severity score, associated injuries, and age.[37] Widespread application of endovascular techniques to manage great vessel trauma in hemodynamically stable patients is constrained by lesion anatomy. With regard to accessing the injury, the relationship of the vascular defect to the aortic arch is rarely an issue because brachial and carotid artery approaches, with or without a concomitant femoral approach, are increasingly employed.[36] However, the likelihood that the adjacent healthy vessel segments will provide adequate landing zones and the preservation of branch vessels are important considerations.[38] Therefore, critical assessment of each individual lesion is required to assure appropriate use of this technology.

Common endovascular modalities such as bare-metal or covered stents (stent-grafts) and coil embolization have been employed in vascular trauma. Stent-grafts were not commercially available before 2000; therefore, case reports published in that time frame described use of home-made devices in which the surgeon affixed autologous tissue, expanded polytetrafluoroethylene (ePTFE), or polyester to a bare metal stent and then repackaged the device for endovascular deployment across an AVF or pseudoaneurysm.[39] There are currently a number of self-expandable and balloon-expandable stent-grafts approved for coronary or peripheral vascular interventions that have been successfully used in the aortic arch vessels, specifically the Wallstent Endoprosthesis (Boston Scientific, Natick, MA), the Gore Viabahn Endoprosthesis (W.L. Gore & Associates, Flagstaff, AZ), and the Jostent Stent-graft Coronary or Peripheral (Abbott Vascular, Redwood City, CA).[40]

Stable patients who have suffered either a blunt or penetrating injury to the innominate artery have benefited from endovascular repair with a stent-graft, and thus far there have been no reported incidences of leak, infection, stenosis, or thrombosis.[23,35,41,42] One technical consideration when approaching an innominate artery pseudoaneurysm is whether the distal landing zone of the stent-graft will occlude the carotid artery. This situation can potentially be avoided by realignment of the guidewire such that the orifice of the subclavian artery is covered instead, a lesion that is typically asymptomatic owing to the extensive collateralization of the upper extremity around the shoulder.[35,43] Alternatively, if the stent-graft must traverse the origin of the right common carotid, a subclavian-carotid bypass may be performed before deployment.[35] Appropriate follow-up for these endovascular repairs have yet to be defined, but biannual duplex ultrasound exams or CT scans have been proposed.[23] The duration of antiplatelet therapy after stent-graft deployment is also unclear; however, the majority of patients are discharged from the hospital on daily aspirin therapy with or without Plavix (Bristol-Myers Squibb, Princeton, NJ).[17,23,44]

Trauma to the intrathoracic carotid artery is rare, but cases of successful stent-graft exclusion of pseudoaneurysms have been reported (Table 56-1).[45–50] Embolic risk should be considered when assessing whether the lesion is suitable for endovascular intervention, and many surgeons advocate for delayed stenting of carotid injuries to minimize arterial manipulation and the potential embolic sequelae.[51] Safely anticoagulating the trauma patient with concomitant intracranial or solid organ injuries can be difficult, but maintaining a partial thromboplastic time between 40 and 50 seconds has been shown to effectively cover carotid artery injuries without significantly increasing the bleeding risk.[31] Full heparinization is vital during the stent-graft deployment procedure, however, and should be followed by antiplatelet therapy with Plavix for at least 2 weeks with subsequent conversion to lifelong aspirin therapy.[46] Although patients should be monitored for alterations in neurologic function as a marker of stent stenosis or occlusion, serial duplex ultrasounds ought to be employed to identify subclinical luminal narrowing.[51]

Endovascular repair of subclavian artery injuries has been relatively well described in the literature because of the obvious benefits of this procedure compared with the morbidity of open subclavian artery exposure (Table 56-2).[40,43,48,52–58] Stent-grafts have effectively treated pseudoaneurysms, lacerations, AVFs, and complete transections of the subclavian artery and theoretically reduce the incidence of brachial plexus injury since dissection of the traumatized field has been eliminated.[38,55,59] An interventional consideration unique to the subclavian artery has been the presence of branch vessels that may be covered by the stent-graft and provide a source for endoleak. If contralateral vertebral artery patency and antegrade flow have been visualized, these branch vessels may often be coil embolized.[38] If the vertebral artery cannot be safely occluded, however, a vertebral-carotid transposition should be completed before deployment of the stent-graft.[53] Alternatively, stent-graft repair of the subclavian artery may cover an internal thoracic artery that has been used as a pedicled graft for coronary artery bypass grafting, placing the patient at risk for significant cardiac

TABLE 56-1 Series of Stent-Grafting Procedures for Carotid Artery Trauma

Authors	# of Patients	Trauma	Lesion/ Vessels	Stent-Grafts	Procedural Events	Follow-up Events/Time
du Toit, et al[48]	4	Stab, GSW	AVFs: 3 CCA; 1 ICA	Wallgraft, Viabahn	4 type-4 endoleaks*	3 lost to FU; mean FU 21 months; no adverse events
Saket, et al[45]	4	MVA, spontaneous, iatrogenic	PAs: 3 ICA; 1 CCA	Jostent	1 type-1 endoleak	2 lost to FU; 2 patent stent-grafts at 14 and 46 months; no adverse events
Archondakis, et al[47]	8	Head injury	8CCFs	Jostent	2 residual AVFs requiring angioplasty on day 2	1 asymptomatic ICA occlusion, 1 case of IH (30% stenosis) at 6 months: 2 persistent CCFs at 2 and 3 months, respectively, 1 requiring coil; stable results with 1 year FU
Saatci, et al[50]	16	MVA, iatrogenic	PAs: 17 ICA†	Jostent	8 endoleaks, 1 requiring stent	1 case of IH (no important stenosis) at 6 months; FU 6 months-13 years
Schonholz, et al[47]	22	GSW, stab, iatrogenic, blunt, tumor, spontaneous	17 PAs; 5 AVFs 14CCAs & 8 ICAs	Wallgraft, Viabahn, Corvita, Jostent, Palmaz	1 acute ICA occlusion without neurologic symptoms; 1 fever (negative cultures); 1 type-4 endoleak requiring 2nd device	1 ICA occlusion at 36 months from Palmaz stent compression; FU 2 months-13 years

*In overall series of 12 patients with trauma in various supra-aortic vessels. †One patient had 2PAs. AVF-arteriovenous fistula: CCA-common carotid artery: ICA-internal carotid artery: FU-follow-up: MVA-motor vehicle accident: PA-pseudoaneurysm; CCF-carotid cavernous fistula; IH-intimal hyperplasia

TABLE 56-2 Series of Stent-Grafting Procedures for Subclavian Artery Trauma

Authors	# of Patients	Trauma	Lesions/ Vessels	Stent-Grafts	Procedural Events	Follow-up Events/Time
Sanchez, et al[52]	4	GSW, catheterization	4 PAs	Corvita	Many balloon dilatations and/or slents required to deploy SG	1 case of IH at 4 months treated with angioplasty and Palmaz stent; SGs patent at 2, 4, 4, and 7 months
du Toit, et al[38]	8	Slab, GSW	8 AVFs	Viabahn, Wallgraft	4 type-4 endoleaks*	1 stenosis at 3 months treated with angioplasty; mean FU 21 months (range 3-36 months)
Schoder, et al[53]	8	Catheterization	8 CVC injuries	Viabahn, Jostent, Passager	2 failures to close lesion with 1 EG; 1 Cl	All SGs patent; mean FU 1 year (range 3 days-4 years); 1 asymptomatic stenosis (Jostent compression) at 8 months
Hilfiker, et al[54]	9	GSW, catheterization, other iatrogenic	5 PAs; 4 AVFs	Palmaz slent-ePTFE, Wallstent, Z stant-ePTFE, Z stent-polyester	1 asymptomatic AVF filling defect; 2 groin PAs, 1 infected	1 occlusion due to SG kink at 2 months treated with urokinase and stent placement; 1 stenosis at 1 year treated with angioplasty; mean FU 29 months (range 2-66 months)
Parodi, et al[55]	9	GSW, iatrogenic	7 AVFs; 2PAs	Corvita, Palmaz stent-ePTFE, Palmaz stent-polyester	1 failure to close; 1 hematoma; 1 DVT†	1 asymptomatic Corvita SG occlusion at 10 months
Montefiore Medical Center[58-60, 62]	11	GSW, stab, catheterization	10 PAs & 1 AVF in the SCA & axillary tree	Plamaz stent-ePTFE, Corvita	1 access-site tear treated with vein patch	1 asymptomatic occlusion at 4 months; 1 fracture of Palmaz-ePTFE SG and 1 case of IH in Corvita SG treated with angioplasty and stenting; mean FU 30 months (range 5-48 months)

*In overall series of 12 patients with traumatic lesions in either the SCA or carotid artery. †In overall series of 29 patients with traumatic arterial lesions in vessels throughcut the body. PA-pseudoaneurysm: SG-stent-graft: IH-intimal hyperplasia; AVF-arteriovenous fistula; FU-follow-up: CVC-central venous catheter; Cl-cerebral infarction: ePTFE-expanded polytetrafluoroethylene; DVT-deep venous thrombosis: SCA-subclavain artery.

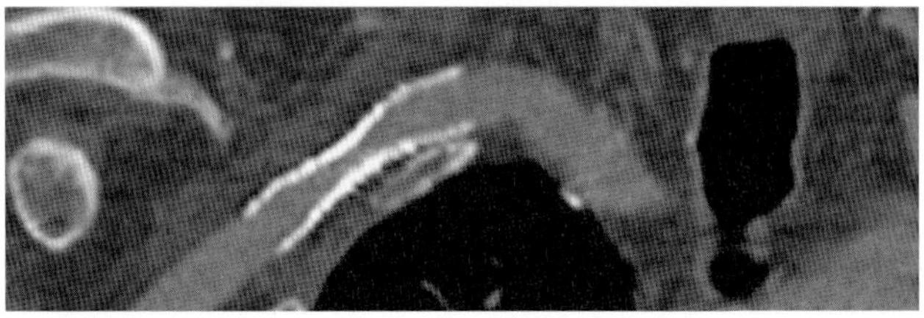

FIGURE 56-3 Balloon-expandable stent-graft 8 months after deployment demonstrating signs of compression between the clavicle and the first rib. (*Reproduced with permission from Schoder M, Cejna M, Holzenbein T, et al: Elective and emergent endovascular treatment of subclavian artery aneurysms and injuries. J Endovasc Ther 2003; 10[1]:58-65.*)

ischemia. Postprocedure antiplatelet therapy has consisted of Plavix for 1 to 3 months followed by lifelong aspirin therapy.[53] Repetitive compression of the stent-graft between the clavicle and first rib over the lifespan of a young trauma patient creates the risk of stent fracture (Fig. 56-3); therefore, long-term follow-up with serial imaging is required.[43] Both stenosis and stent fracture, although often asymptomatic, have been treated with balloon dilation and deployment of an additional stent such that open intervention may still be avoided.[38,56]

Complications

Endovascular repair of the great vessels is subject to the same complications commonly identified in other vascular beds, specifically endoleaks and stenosis, occlusion, or migration of the stent-graft. Endoleaks have typically been self-limited;[45,48] however, when indicated, placement of an additional stent-graft has been successful.[47] Stenosis, occlusion, and stent fracture have occurred more frequently in the subclavian artery because of external compression at the thoracic outlet. Because of the extensive collateralization of the upper extremity, these patients have been asymptomatic and the lesion has been managed endovascularly with angioplasty and additional stent placement.[48,56,60] In select cases, local thrombolytic therapy has been followed by repeat stent-graft placement for acute occlusions.[54] Alternatively, endovascular interventions place the patient at risk for complications at the arterial access site such as hemorrhage, pseudoaneurysm, infection, and arteriovenous fistula, and these scenarios should be managed according to current vascular surgical principles.

DESCENDING THORACIC AORTIC INJURY

Epidemiology

Although the actual incidence of blunt aortic rupture is unknown, autopsy series have documented aortic rupture in 12 to 23% of deaths from blunt trauma.[5,61,62] In the United States, the incidence of thoracic aortic injury among motor vehicle collision victims has been approximated by the vehicular crash database to be 1.5%.[63] Seventy to eighty percent of these injuries occur in 36- to 40-year-old men.[4,64,65] A majority of patients exsanguinate at the scene, but successful resuscitation of the few who survive long enough to be seen in the emergency department depends on accurate diagnosis and intervention in the acute setting. For instance, 75% of patients presenting to the hospital with an aortic rupture after blunt trauma are initially hemodynamically stable,[4] but up to 50% die before definitive surgery.[64,66]

Mechanism of Injury

Traumatic aortic disruptions typically occur in motor vehicle drivers, passengers, or pedestrians hit by vehicles.[4,5,61] Alcohol or other substance abuse is involved in greater than 40% of these motor vehicle accidents.[61] Patients ejected from the vehicle are twice as likely to sustain traumatic aortic injury, and seatbelt use can decrease this risk fourfold.[61] Overall, seatbelts have been demonstrated to be more effective than airbags at preventing blunt aortic injury,[67] and aortic rupture of both the ascending and descending aorta has been attributed to the deployment of an air bag.[68,69] Falls from significant height, crush injuries, and airplane accidents have also caused aortic rupture.[4,5,62,70,71]

Pathogenesis of Blunt Aortic Injury

The pathogenesis of aortic transection remains controversial and no integrated understanding of these forces has been achieved. The "whiplash" theory proposes that a combination of traction, torsion, shear, and bursting forces interact owing to differential deceleration of tissues within the mediastinum, thereby causing adequate stress to rupture the aorta at the isthmus.[61,72–76] Aortic mobility is limited by the ligamentum arteriosum, the left main stem bronchus, and the paired intercostal arteries. Investigations have shown that displacement of the aorta in a longitudinal direction may cause a tear at the isthmus.[75] Alternatively, Crass and Associates have argued that the differential forces of deceleration, torsion, and hydrostatics alone have inadequate magnitude in vehicular accidents to result in aortic tearing and have proposed the "osseous pinch" mechanism based on quantifiable thoracic compression.[77,78] With this mechanism, anterior thoracic osseous structures (manubrium, first rib, and clavicular heads) rotate posteriorly and inferiorly and may impact the vertebral column, pinching the aortic isthmus and proximal descending thoracic aorta.[77] This pinch is theorized to cause shearing of the aorta and some clinical data do support the osseous pinch mechanism.[79] Overall, diversity among the direction and magnitude of forces generated by a blunt traumatic event in patients suffering descending thoracic aortic rupture have prohibited identification of a single pathogenetic mechanism.

Pathology

Traumatic aortic disruptions occur most commonly at the aortic isthmus (Fig. 56-4), and an autopsy series identified 54% at this site, with 8% in the ascending aorta, 2% in the arch, and 11% in the distal descending aorta.[62] In those who survive, the periadventitial tissues around the isthmus appear to provide protection against free rupture and allow time for transfer to a

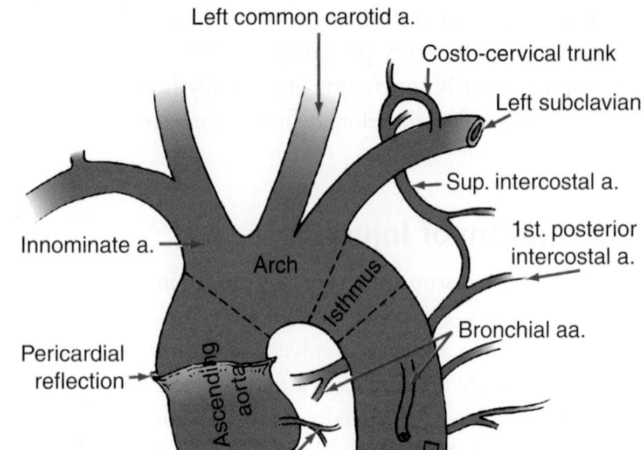

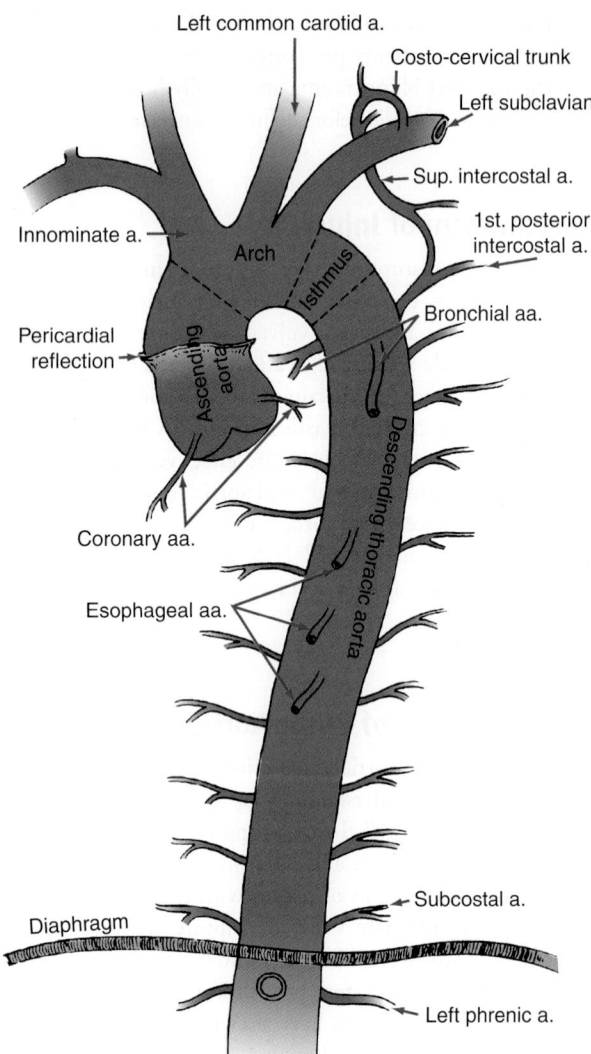

FIGURE 56-4 Anatomical diagram of the thoracic aorta and its major branches.

hospital; consequently, surgical case series have reported 84 to 97% of aortic ruptures occurring at the isthmus.[3,4,80–83] The strength of the aortic wall is in its adventitial layer, and despite the increased incidence of transection at the aortic isthmus, there is no evidence to suggest that the adventitia in this area is deficient.[84] Additionally, the structure of the aortic wall surrounding the transection has not demonstrated any defect and atherosclerotic disease does not play a role in this injury.[5,61,62] The transverse transection caused by blunt aortic trauma typically involves all three layers of the wall and the edges may be separated by several centimeters.[5,62] Occasionally, noncircumferential or partial aortic wall disruptions have been described, particularly posteriorly, and under these circumstances intramural hematomas and focal dissections may occur.[5,62,85]

Natural History

The natural history of a traumatic aortic transection has been increasingly investigated as the concept of medical therapy and delayed operative repair has evolved. Previously reported mortality rates drawn from autopsy reports have claimed that 86% of patients with traumatic aortic disruption die at the scene, whereas only 11% survive greater than 6 hours.[5] Considering those patients who reach definitive medical care, recent surgical series report mortality rates from 0 to 50% depending on the size of the series.[3,4,64–66,70,86–89]

Clinical Presentation and Initial Evaluation

The leading cause of death in patients with aortic injury who make it to the hospital remains exsanguinating aortic rupture, which occurs in at least 20% of patients.[4] Among patients with blunt aortic injury who are hemodynamically stable on arrival to the emergency room, 4% die in the hospital of aortic rupture before surgical repair.[4] Therefore, an organized, efficient, and effective evaluation of these patients is necessary to prevent unnecessary loss of life.

A multitrauma patient should be evaluated according to standard ATLS protocols regardless of whether aortic disruption is suspected. The primary and secondary survey, routine radiographs, and hemodynamic stabilization must be completed before the team can begin investigating specific injuries. The first step in diagnosing a blunt traumatic aortic injury is identifying the at-risk patient. Motor vehicle collisions, falls from height, explosions, and crush injuries have the impact and deceleration forces required to cause aortic transection, therefore these patients should undergo imaging directed at ruling out this potentially fatal injury.[2,70,90,91]

Ninety-five percent of patients with aortic disruption have associated injuries, and Table 56-3 lists the frequency of associated injuries from data accrued from approximately 50 trauma centers across the United States and Canada (American Association for the Surgery of Trauma [AAST] trial).[4] Closed head injuries have been identified in 51% of patients, 46% have had associated rib fractures, 38% have had pulmonary contusions, 20 to 35% have had orthopedic injuries, and only 4% have had concomitant cardiac contusion.[4] The mean injury severity score in the AAST trial was 42.1, implying that current advancements in emergency medical resuscitation in the field have provided more patients the opportunity to reach the hospital and receive aggressive definitive care.

There are often clues evident in the initial evaluation of a trauma patient that can suggest aortic disruption (Table 56-4). As with blunt injury to the arch vessels, patients sustaining descending thoracic aortic rupture are often hemodynamically stable on presentation at the emergency department. Although patients may complain of dyspnea or back pain and display differential blood pressures in the upper versus lower extremities, specific signs or symptoms of aortic rupture have been identified in less than 50% of cases.[92–95] Complete de-gloving injury may result in intussusception of the aortic media into the descending thoracic aorta, with resultant "pseudo-coarctation" variable amounts of distal perfusion compromise (Fig. 56-5). In the majority of trauma patients, a supine chest radiograph is obtained as part of the initial evaluation, and the constellation of grossly widened mediastinum, hemothorax, and transient hemodynamic instability on arrival appear to be predictive of early in-hospital death from blunt thoracic aortic injury.[96]

TABLE 56-3 Associated (Surgical) Injuries in Hospitalized Patients with Traumatic Aortic Disruption

	Schmidt et al[154] n = 80, %	Hilgenberg et al[157] n = 51, %	Duhaylongsod et al[75] n =108, %	Sturm et al[125] n = 37, %	Fabian et al[4] n = 274, %	Crestanello et al[144] n = 72, %
Central nervous system	25	39	34	27	51	49
Thorax						
Diaphragm	13	2	12	7	—	8
Lung	38	41	43	19	38	35
Heart	10	10	18	—	4	3
Rib/clavicle fractures	40	39	55	35	46	—
Abdominal						49 (total)
Spleen	20	10	17	14	14	
Liver	10	12	15	22	22	
Kidney	9	12	11	5	—	
Bowel	10	—	15	3	7	
Other abdominal	11	—	9	8	14	
Skeletal						
Extremity	81	71	59	—	66	64
Spine	5	10	20	—	12	31
Pelvis	24	25	26	22	31	36
Maxillofacial	5	10	20	—	13	18

In the typical hemodynamically stable blunt trauma patient, head and abdominopelvic CT should be conducted to identify closed-head or intra-abdominal injury. Those with an abnormal chest x-ray or a traumatic mechanism consistent with aortic injury should undergo helical CT scan of the chest with intravenous contrast at this time. Operative management of intracranial space-occupying lesions and intra-abdominal hemorrhage takes priority over nonbleeding aortic injuries. Hemodynamically unstable patients with signs of exsanguinating hemorrhage should go directly to the operating room for control of hemorrhage, and TEE may be used to evaluate for aortic injury. Aortography may be useful when helical CT or TEE fail to definitively identify or adequately characterize an aortic injury. Thoracoscopy has also been used to evaluate traumatic hemothoraces, however with experienced practitioners intraoperative TEE has superb sensitivity and specificity for aortic transection.[97]

Anti-impulse therapy with beta-blockers should be initiated in patients proceeding directly to the operating room for aortic repair, as well as in those selected for delayed repair, to reduce blood pressure and thereby reduce aortic wall stress.[90,91,98] In-hospital aortic rupture rates have been reduced through aggressive beta-blockade without adversely affecting the outcome of associated injuries.[90]

Diagnostic Studies

Chest Radiograph

During the evaluation of a blunt trauma patient, an anteroposterior chest radiograph is routinely obtained and ought to be examined for one of the 15 signs that have been associated with aortic rupture (Table 56-5).[99] Widening of the mediastinum to a width exceeding 25% of the total chest width, obliteration of the aortic knob, apical pleural capping, and fractures of the sternum, scapula, clavicle, or first rib are some of the most common findings (Fig. 56-6). None of these signs have demonstrated sufficient sensitivity or specificity to effectively rule

TABLE 56-4 Clues That Suggest Aortic Disruption

History
Motor vehicle crash >50 km/h
Motor vehicle crash into fixed barrier
No seat belt
Ejection from vehicle
Broken steering wheel
Motorcycle or airplane crash
Pedestrian hit by motor vehicle
Falls greater than 3 meters
Crush or cave-in injuries
Loss of consciousness
Physical signs
Hemodynamic shock (systolic blood pressure <90 mm Hg)
Fracture of sternum, first rib, clavicle, scapula, or multiple ribs
Steering wheel imprint on chest
Cardiac murmurs
Hoarseness
Dyspnea
Back pain
Hemothorax
Unequal extremity blood pressures
Paraplegia or paraparesis

out aortic injury, however, and up to 40% of patients with aortic rupture have had chest x-ray findings interpreted as normal.[70,90,93,100–103] When abnormalities are identified, however, they can aide the practitioner in determining which patients require aggressive imaging to definitively rule out an aortic injury.

Computed Tomography

Approximately 1% of blunt trauma patients have a thoracic aortic injury identified by helical computed tomography (CT).[90,100] Since its introduction in the early 1990s, CT has become the screening tool of choice at most medical institutions to detect traumatic aortic rupture because of its availability, speed, and ease of interpretation. Additionally, sensitivities and negative predictive values nearing 100% have been reported for volumetric helical or spiral CT.[70,90,103–106] Following injection of nonionic contrast media, 3- to 5-mm thick images of the chest can be obtained in approximately 90 seconds.[106] Normal aorta portrays homogeneous enhancement, whereas filling defects, contrast extravasation, intimal flaps, periaortic hematoma, pseudoaneurysm, and mural thrombi may suggest the presence of an aortic injury (Fig. 56-7).[106] False-positive studies can occur, however, and a ductus diverticulum remnant is an example of a nontraumatic aortic abnormality that may be mistaken for vessel rupture.[106] If CT identifies a luminal or mural aortic irregularity in the absence of periaortic hematoma or vice versa, the diagnosis of aortic rupture should be questioned and pursued with additional imaging. Moreover, the enhanced resolution of CT imaging has allowed identification of minimal aortic injuries, such as small intimal flaps with minimal or no mediastinal changes, that may be safely managed with anti-impulse therapy.[90,106,107]

Transesophageal Echocardiography

Transesophageal echocardiography (TEE) has become a valuable tool in cardiothoracic surgery because of its ability to image the entire descending thoracic aorta along with portions of the ascending aorta arch and its portability. In unstable blunt trauma patients requiring laparotomy, TEE can be used to evaluate the descending aorta for evidence of rupture, such as a mural flap or a thickened vessel wall concerning for mural thrombus. Multiplanar TEE probes permit acquisition of cross-sectional

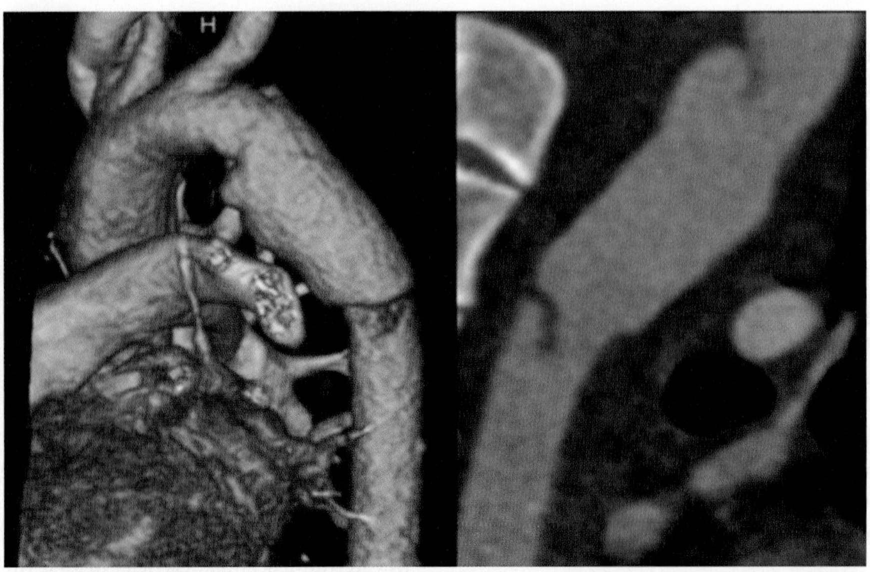

FIGURE 56-5 Pseudocoarctation of the aorta caused by circumferential transection of the aorta with the wall flap telescoping into the distal aorta. Blood flow between the proximal and distal aortic segments is maintained by the surrounding adventitia alone.

TABLE 56-5 Chest x-Ray Findings Associated with Blunt Aortic Disruption

Widened mediastinum (>8.0 cm)
Mediastinum-to-chest width ratio >0.25
Tracheal shift to the patient's right
Blurred aortic contour
Irregularity or loss of the aortic knob
Left apical cap
Depression of the left main bronchus
Opacification of the aortopulmonary window
Right deviation of the nasogastric tube
Wide paraspinal lines
First rib fracture
Any other rib fracture
Clavicle fracture
Pulmonary contusion
Thoracic spine fracture

Source: Data from Cook AD, Klein JS, Rogers FB, Osler TM, Shackford SR: Chest radiographs of limited utility in the diagnosis of blunt traumatic aortic laceration. J Trauma 2001; 50(5):843-847.

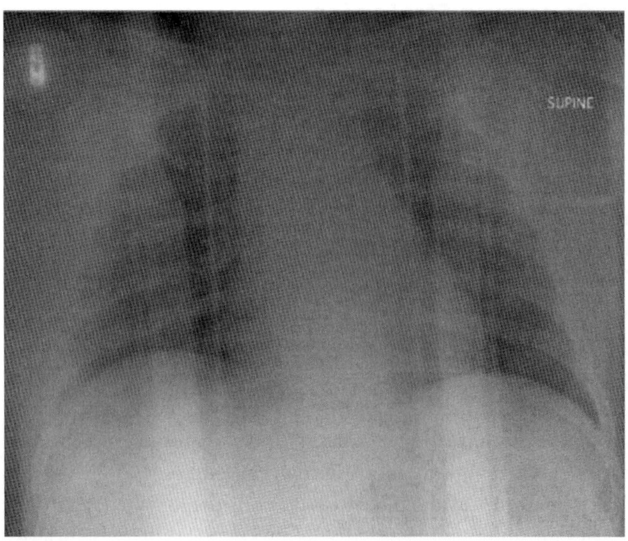

FIGURE 56-6 Chest radiograph of an 18-year-old male victim of a motor vehicle collision showing a widened mediastinum.

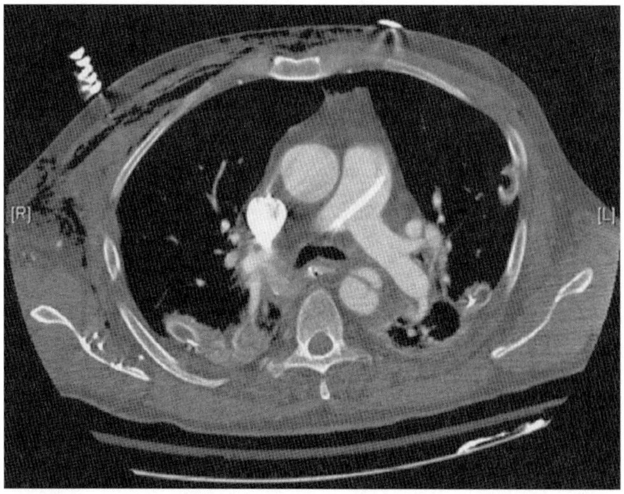

FIGURE 56-7 Helical computed tomography scan of the chest in a 30-year-old man after a high-speed motor vehicle collision demonstrating an intimal flap in the proximal descending thoracic aorta and periaortic hematoma.

images at different angles along a single rotational axis. The typical 5- or 7-MHz transducer permits adequate resolution of structures as small as 1 to 2 mm. Doppler mapping of turbulent blood flow near a vessel wall abnormality may be suggestive of blunt aortic disruption, and time-resolved imaging allows evaluation of the movement of anatomical structures, thereby enhancing the ability to define the physiologic consequences of such abnormalities. Chronic atheromatous disease of the aorta can complicate obtaining and interpreting TEE images; therefore, observation of multiple related signs of injury, such as mural flap with a surrounding mediastinal hematoma, is more reliable.

A disadvantage of TEE, and potential inhibitor to its widespread use as a screening tool for aortic injury, is its operator-dependent nature, with sensitivities as low as 63% documented for this modality.[108] A prospective comparison of imaging techniques for diagnosis of blunt aortic trauma reported, however, sensitivity and specificity of 93 and 100% for TEE compared with 73 and 100% for helical CT.[105] TEE is more invasive than helical CT, but overall the associated risk is low. Contraindications include concomitant injury to the cervical spine, oropharynx, esophagus, or maxillofacial structures.[105]

Aortography

The role of aortography in evaluating blunt thoracic injuries was firmly established prior to the advent of noninvasive, sophisticated imaging techniques, and it may still be considered the gold standard. In experienced hands its sensitivity and specificity both approach 100%.[109] Intra-arterial digital subtraction is most often used because it allows rapid generation of images (Fig. 56-8). In the past, intravenous digital subtraction was used as well. After injecting intravenous contrast, time-delayed images of the arch and descending aorta were obtained, and although this technique greatly decreased the duration of the procedure, it was abandoned because the diagnostic accuracy

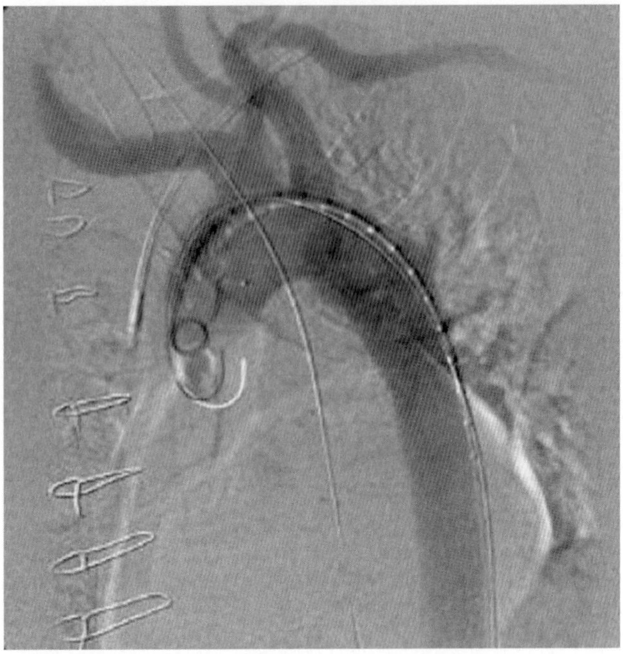

FIGURE 56-8 Digital subtraction arteriogram of an acute traumatic aortic disruption near the isthmus.

for aortic disruption was less than 70%.[110] With the availability and speed of helical CT, aortography is now rarely used for diagnosis, but routinely used for endovascular stent-graft placement. This intervention requires a highly trained team of endovascular specialists and can be time consuming; therefore, trauma patients with additional life- or limb-threatening injuries should be otherwise stabilized before entering the endovascular suite. Rates of exsanguination and death of up to 10% have previously been reported during diagnostic aortography, but this incidence has decreased significantly as endovascular proficiency has improved.[95,110,111] In fact, complication rates attributed directly to aortography are low, but patients may suffer contrast reactions, contrast nephropathy, groin hematomas, or femoral artery pseudoaneurysms. False-positive studies are usually attributed to atheromata or ductal diverticula.

Magnetic Resonance Angiography

Vascular structures are well imaged by magnetic resonance angiography (MRA), particularly the thoracic aorta, and its utility in the diagnosis and follow-up of complex aortic disease, including aortic dissections and aneurysms, is firmly established.[110,112,113] The time required to capture images inhibits the utility of MRA in the acute evaluation of a trauma patient; however, it may be effective in post-therapeutic surveillance of traumatic thoracic injuries.

Delayed Repair versus Nonoperative Management

Uniformly, hemodynamically unstable blunt trauma patients should bypass diagnostic imaging and be taken to the operating room immediately. During a damage control exploratory laparotomy or thoracotomy, TEE may be conducted to diagnose contained aortic rupture.[105] Operative repair of the aorta should not be attempted at this time, however, and this group of patients benefit from immediate transfer to the intensive care unit for further resuscitation. Once hemodynamic stability is achieved, anti-impulse therapy with beta-blockade should be initiated to minimize aortic wall stress.[90]

Hemodynamically stable patients diagnosed with blunt aortic injury, and lacking severe associated injuries requiring interventions, warrant immediate repair. Treatment of all non–life-threatening injuries should be delayed until after definitive aortic repair. Delayed management has demonstrated safety and effectiveness in carefully selected patients with severe associated injuries or comorbidities.[64–66,86,114–118] Patients with thoracic, intraperitoneal, or retroperitoneal hemorrhage, or intracranial bleeding that causes mass effect should be managed with aggressive anti-impulse therapy to minimize the risk of aortic rupture while these injuries are addressed.[118] The goal of anti-impulse therapy should be to maintain a systolic blood pressure less than 120 mm Hg and/or a mean arterial pressure less than 80 mm Hg.[90] The aortic insult should also be monitored by TEE during surgical repair of concomitant injuries, and routinely imaged with CT during the delayed management period.[115] The mortality rate of patients awaiting aortic repair has ranged from 30 to 50%, but the majority of deaths have not been related to the aortic injury.[115,116,118] In fact, in one retrospective study of nonoperative management, 5 of 15 patients died during the index hospitalization from head trauma, and the remainder were doing well at 2.5 years of follow-up with stable aortic imaging.[115] Additionally, a few small series have demonstrated survival rates of 67 to 72% in select, high-risk patients treated nonoperatively.[117,118] In the AAST trial, those presenting *in extremis* or with evidence of free aortic rupture were excluded, and the mortality rate of patients with associated injuries that precluded initial aortic repair was 55%.[4] Therefore, evidence supports operative delay or nonoperative management in select patients with blunt aortic injury who may be considered poor operative candidates.

Operative Strategies

Blunt thoracic aortic injury has traditionally undergone open repair with interposition graft placement, and this approach has proved to be safe, effective, and durable, thereby establishing it as the standard with which new repair strategies should be compared. Mortality after an open repair has been approximated at 20%, and the morbidity rate may be as high as 14%, largely attributable to the incidence of spinal cord ischemia.[119] The popularity of endovascular stent-grafting (EVSG) of traumatic aortic disruptions has grown immensely in the current era because of expected decreases in operating room time, complication rate, morbidity, and mortality, but no Level I data exist to confirm these trends.[120] This approach is particularly attractive in multitrauma patients, and several single institution series have reported good short-term outcomes.[65,87,88,121–125] Many anatomical details must be considered when pursuing EVSG for traumatic aortic rupture in a young, otherwise healthy patient with a normal-caliber thoracic aorta. The landing zones may not coincide with those expected when the commercially available stent-graft was designed for the treatment of aneurysm disease; therefore, successful placement of the stent-graft relies on individual surgeon ingenuity and long-term durability of these repairs remains unknown. EVSG techniques continue to evolve, however, and are not uniformly applicable; therefore, surgeons treating thoracic aortic disruption must be comfortable with conventional open repair techniques.

Open Repair

The major controversy regarding open operative repair of blunt aortic trauma involves spinal cord protection. Some still report safety and efficacy with a "clamp-and-sew" technique, whereas the majority of surgeons have successfully reduced the historical 10% paraplegia rate through some form of lower body perfusion to minimize spinal cord and visceral organ ischemia.[3,4,80,81,83,102,126,127]

Arterial Supply to the Spinal Cord

Blood supply to the spinal cord relies on three longitudinal arteries, the anterior spinal artery located in the anterior-median position and supplying 75% of the spinal cord, and the paired posterior spinal arteries located near the nerve roots. Segmental intercostal and lumbar arteries originating from the posterior aspect of the aorta supply a series of unpaired radicular arteries that subsequently contribute flow to the anterior spinal artery. The vertebral arteries also provide radicular branches to supply the anterior spinal artery; therefore, in addition to the risk of cord ischemia during aortic cross-clamp at the isthmus and associated paraplegia rates, clamping proximal to the left subclavian compromises flow into the left vertebral and further threatens the integrity of the spinal cord. The posterior spinal arteries are supplied by smaller radicular arteries that originate from the aorta at nearly every spinal level. The largest and most significant radicular artery, typically originating at the level of T10 and entering the vertebral column at the first lumbar vertebrae, is the arteria radicularis magna (or artery of Adamkiewicz) and this vessel is essential for spinal cord perfusion in nearly 25% of patients.

Aortic Cross-Clamp

Some groups report low paraplegia rates exclusively using a "clamp-and-sew" technique; however, these results are not widely reproducible and rely on cross-clamp times of less than 30 minutes.[80] Because of its simplicity, this technique may be preferentially employed by the non-cardiothoracic surgeon confronted with repair of a blunt aortic injury. Fragility of the aortic wall, anatomical distortion by the periaortic hematoma, and extension of the defect into the left subclavian artery pose significant obstacles and the average cross-clamp time reported in the literature is 41 minutes.[81] Paraplegia rates are greatly reduced and may even approach zero when extracorporeal lower body perfusion techniques are paired with short cross-clamp times (Tables 56-6 and 56-7; Fig. 56-9).[4,126,127,169]

Adjuvant Perfusion Techniques

Elective repair of thoracic or thoracoabdominal aneurysms allow employment of several techniques to minimize spinal cord ischemia, but the preoperative preparation required to monitor somatosensory evoked potentials, provide lumbar cerebrospinal fluid drainage, or achieve epidural cooling is typically not available in the trauma setting.[126,128–130] Hypothermic circulatory arrest techniques have been successfully applied to injuries involving the arch, but are not practical when partial bypass systems are employed.[131,132]

The system used by any one group should be routine; however, it is important to be well versed in the various lower body

TABLE 56-6 Incidence of Postoperative Paraplegia in Relation to Surgical Management: Meta-analysis

Operative Technique	Patients, *n*	Paraplegia, %	Clamp Time, Minutes
No shunt	443	19.2	31.8
Passive shunt	424	11.1	46.8
CPB	490	2.4	47.8
Partial bypass*	71	1.4	39.5

*Partial bypass, partial left heart, or femoral vein to artery without systemic heparin.
CPB = Cardiopulmonary bypass with oxygenator and heparin.
Source: Reproduced with permission from von Oppell UO, Dunne TT, De Groot KM, Zilla P: Spinal cord protection in the absence of collateral circulation: meta-analysis of mortality and paraplegia. J Card Surg 1994; 9(6):685-691.

TABLE 56-7 Incidence of Postoperative Paraplegia in Relation to Surgical Management: AAST Prospective Trial

Operative Technique	Patients, *n*	Paraplegia, %
Bypass	134	4.5*
Gott shunt	4	0
Full bypass	22	4.5
Partial bypass	39	7.7
Centrifugal pump	69	2.9†
Clamp and sew	73	16.4*,†

*$p < .004$, bypass versus clamp and sew.
†$p < .01$, centrifugal pump versus clamp and sew.
Source: Data from Fabian TC, Richardson JD, Croce MA, et al: Prospective study of blunt aortic injury: Multicenter Trial of the American Association for the Surgery of Trauma. J Trauma 1997; 42(3):374-380; discussion 380-373.

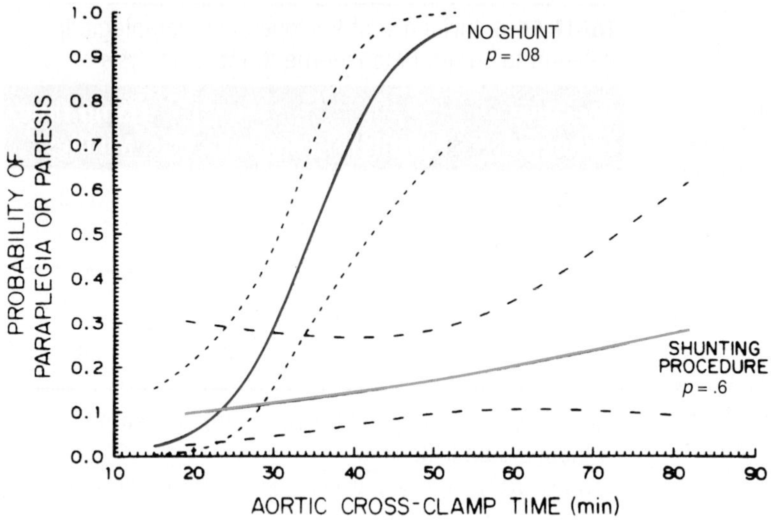

FIGURE 56-9 Probability of paraplegia in relation to aortic cross-clamp time with and without lower body perfusion in patients with traumatic aortic disruption at the isthmus. (*Reproduced with permission from Katz NM, Blackstone EH, Kirklin JW, Karp RB: Incremental risk factors for spinal cord injury following operation for acute traumatic aortic transection. J Thorac Cardiovasc Surg 1981; 81[5]:669-674.*)

perfusion systems because distinct circumstances may require alterations in practice. Intra-arterial blood pressure monitoring of both the upper and lower limbs should be performed with a goal perfusion pressure of 60 to 70 mm Hg.[133] Systemic heparinization poses a significant risk of hemorrhage in the trauma patient, particularly in those with severe lung or intracranial injuries. Use of a centrifugal pump with heparin-bonded tubing and active partial left heart bypass or use of a heparin-bonded passive shunt is an option that does not require systemic heparinization.[133,134] Alternatively, safe use of partial left heart bypass with full systemic heparinization has been reported by many centers.[4,80,89,90,135,136]

For partial left heart bypass, pump inflow is established by cannulating the left atrium through the left inferior pulmonary vein using a small single- or dual-stage cannula (Fig. 56-10). Pulmonary venous cannulation near its confluence with the left atrium has demonstrated a lower complication rate than cannulation of the left atrial appendage.[137] Arterial cannulation may occur through the distal descending aorta or the femoral artery. Distal aortic cannulation has the advantage of convenience and speed. Partial left heart bypass serves several purposes: (1) to unload the left heart and control proximal hypertension at the time of cross-clamping; (2) to maintain lower body perfusion; (3) to allow rapid infusion of volume; and (4) to control (remove) intravascular volume. Lower body mean arterial pressure should be maintained at 60 to 70 mm Hg and this can typically be accomplished with a perfusion flow rate of 2 to 3 L/min. Mean arterial pressures from 70 to 80 mm Hg are generated in the upper body by the native heart and ventricular arrhythmias remain a significant risk. The pump reservoir and/or cell saver are employed to return blood from the field and a heat exchanger can be used to maintain core temperatures above 35°C. If the system is used without systemic heparinization, however, heat exchangers and oxygenators should be removed from the circuit to minimize surface area and thrombotic risks.

In full or partial cardiopulmonary bypass, a long venous catheter with multiple side holes may be introduced through the left common femoral vein and placed in the right atrium with a guidewire. Alternatively, direct right atrial cannulation at the inferior vena cava–right atrial junction may be accomplished from a left thoracotomy by simple, transverse, inferior pericardiotomy below the left phrenic nerve. Right atrial–femoral arterial bypass has also been used with or without an oxygenator like partial left heart bypass. A partial arterial oxygen pressure of 40 mm Hg has been reported in non-oxygenated circuits, a level shown to be sufficient for lower body tissue oxygenation when the hemoglobin is maintained at 10 g/dL.[138] In cases of aortic arch injury, full cardiopulmonary bypass is beneficial.[139,140]

Partial or complete bypass may be established before entering the chest by pursuing right femoral venous to arterial bypass, a technique particularly advantageous when a concomitant right lung contusion inhibits oxygenation. In cases of aortic arch transection in proximity to the innominate or left common carotid, anterior exposure via sternotomy or thoracosternotomy may offer better exposure for total arch replacement under deep hypothermic circulatory arrest (HCA).[139,140] Use of HCA in trauma patients poses significant bleeding risks; therefore, aortic injuries requiring this technique may be appropriate for anti-impulse therapy and a delay in repair until other

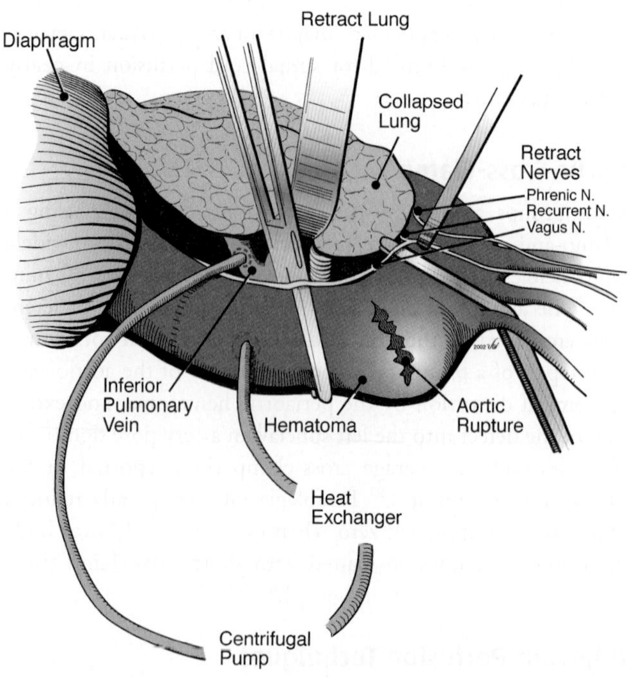

FIGURE 56-10 Diagram showing a typical setup for partial left heart bypass in a patient with aortic disruption at the isthmus.

concomitant injuries have been addressed. Additionally, aortic valvular insufficiency must be ruled out. When HCA is used within the left chest, the left ventricle should be vented through the left atrium.

A passive (Gott) shunt has been described where the proximal and distal ends of a heparin coated polyvinyl tube are placed in the ascending aorta or arch and the descending aorta or femoral artery, respectively. Ventricular cannulation had been used in the past; however, it was abandoned because of a high rate of ventricular dysrhythmias, reduced shunt flows, and a higher rate of paraplegia.[141,142] Flow through this fixed tube is dependent on a pressure gradient and this inability to control flow is the main disadvantage of the Gott shunt.[142] Moreover, it offers no left ventricular unloading or loading advantage, as partial bypass systems do; therefore, blood pressure control is left to pharmacology alone.

Operative Techniques

The patient is positioned in the right lateral decubitus position with the left groin prepped for arterial and venous access. A right radial arterial line is preferred to avoid losing arterial pressure tracing if occlusion of the left subclavian artery is required during the repair. Use of a pulmonary arterial catheter is optional. Selective ventilation of the right lung is required. A standard fourth interspace posterolateral thoracotomy with or without fifth rib notching usually provides excellent exposure to the aortic isthmus and proximal descending aorta. The incision should be long enough to facilitate dissection of the descending aorta below the level of the inferior pulmonary vein and dissection of the arch of the aorta between the left common carotid and left subclavian arteries. In a patient with a prior left thoracotomy, the associated scarring offers both an advantage and disadvantage to the patient. The adhesions between the lung and mediastinum help contain the rupture making it less likely to exsanguinate. Dissection near the isthmus or tear should be avoided until both proximal and distal aortic control is established. Depending on the stability of the patient, lower body perfusion can be established before aortic exposure by gaining access to the left groin. If cannulation is planned in the chest, the left inferior pulmonary vein–left atrial junction is dissected and cannulated, in addition to arterial cannulation of the distal descending thoracic aorta or left common femoral vein. Excessive compression or traction of the lung should be avoided, particularly when dissecting out the aortic arch, because the left pulmonary artery may be easily disrupted at this location.

Distal control is obtained first, usually by fairly simple passage of a blunt instrument or finger around the descending aorta at the distal margin of the hematoma. Care must be taken not to avulse intercostal arterial branches with this maneuver. The subclavian artery is isolated next. Great care is taken to avoid injury to either the phrenic or vagus nerves as they pass over the aortic arch, which can be difficult because they are often obscured by the hematoma. They should be reflected off the aorta with the overlying pleura and retracted medially by attaching stay sutures to the pleura just lateral to the vagus nerve. Loops around the nerves themselves should be avoided, as even stretch of these nerves can result in paresis. This reflection exposes the arch of the aorta between the left common carotid and left subclavian arteries, which is the point needed for proximal aortic control in the majority of cases. Inferiorly, the vagus nerve and its branching left recurrent laryngeal nerve are reflected medially as well. This exposes the ligamentum arteriosum, which can be sharply divided, but usually this step is not required. Careful dissection is then undertaken between the left common carotid artery and left subclavian artery using a combination of sharp and gentle finger dissection to completely encircle the aortic arch with an umbilical tape. As with distal aortic control, the peri-aortic hematoma facilitates this dissection considerably. There should be no dissection distal to either the left subclavian or the ligamentum in order to avoid free disruption of the hematoma.

Lower body perfusion is initiated, and once systemic blood pressure is stabilized the left subclavian artery is clamped (if necessary) followed by the proximal aorta. With modern imaging techniques, it is usually possible to predict, to the millimeter, exactly where the aortic tear is in order to avoid involving it in the proximal clamp. The distal aorta is clamped last. Traumatic aortic disruptions that occur in close proximity (<1 cm) from the left subclavian artery portend a higher mortality risk and greater operative difficulty than injuries further away from the left subclavian ostium.[139] Upper and lower body pressures are stabilized with the bypass circuit to maintain upper body mean arterial pressures of 70 to 80 mm Hg and a lower body pressure of 60 to 70 mm Hg with flows of 2 to 3 L/min.

The periaortic hematoma is then entered, and the edges of the transected aorta identified. Usually the aorta is completely transected, and the edges are separated by 2 to 4 cm.[5,62] Less frequently the transection is partial. Some authors advocate primary repair at this point;[141,143] however, we advocate placing a short interposition graft after debridement of the torn edges in all cases.[3,80,83,90,136,144,145] Collagen-coated woven polyester grafts or gelatin-impregnated grafts are used most commonly. Use of intraluminal prostheses has been abandoned by most groups.[146] Grafts are sewn using a running polypropylene suture with the proximal anastomosis performed first, followed by the distal. Generous amounts of adventitial tissue are included in each bite. If the proximal anastomosis is done under HCA, cardiopulmonary bypass and reperfusion of the arch should be reinstituted immediately after completion of the proximal anastomosis for optimal neurocerebral protection. This requires cannulation of the graft just beyond the proximal anastomosis (branched grafts are useful here for re-cannulation), and then the distal anastomosis is completed using a dual arterial-inflow perfusion setup perfusing the arch and lower body simultaneously. The left subclavian can either be incorporated into the proximal anastomosis or grafted separately as appropriate.

If it is discovered that the tear extends above the proximal aortic clamp, an attempt can be made to dissect more proximally and place a second clamp provided the left common carotid artery is not compromised. If this is not possible, the best recourse is to cannulate the aortic arch in addition to the distal arterial cannula, commence full cardiopulmonary bypass through both arterial routes, and perform the proximal anastomosis during a brief period of profound HCA. We cool to 20°C and use cerebral protection adjuncts, including packing the head in ice and 15 mg/kg sodium thiopental intravenously. One must be prepared to vent the left ventricular apex if distention occurs as a result of cooling induced ventricular fibrillation. A continuous short axis view by transesophageal echocardiography is very useful is this circumstance.

If the aorta is already ruptured with bleeding into the hemithorax, proximal aortic dissection between the left carotid and subclavian arteries is rapidly performed, and a cross-clamp quickly applied. The descending aorta is then clamped below the injury, and the hematoma opened. No attempt is made to establish lower body perfusion, but every attempt is made at maintaining adequate mean arterial pressure during clamping. The aortic repair is done as expeditiously as possible to minimize clamp time. Repair sutures are placed accordingly after clamps are removed. Hemostasis is achieved after continuity of the aorta is re-established.

Occasionally, the aortic tear will extend into the left subclavian orifice. In this case the proximal clamp may have to partially or totally occlude the left common carotid. The left subclavian can then be completely detached from the aorta, the proximal anastomosis completed, and the clamp then moved distally onto the graft. The left subclavian is then reattached to the aortic graft with an interposition graft after completing the distal aortic anastomosis. The left subclavian interposition graft is fashioned with an end-to-end anastomosis distally and an end-to-side anastomosis proximally.

Complications

Following open repair of blunt thoracic aortic injury, the in-hospital mortality rates range from 0 to 20% and the complication rates range from 40 to 50% with pneumonia being most common.[4,83,86,92] Bacteremia, renal insufficiency, paraplegia, left vocal cord paralysis, and aortobronchial fistula have also been reported (Table 56-8).[4,83,86,92,147,148] A meta-analysis of 1492 patients who underwent open aortic repair, 13.5% died in the postoperative period and 9.9% suffered paraparesis or paraplegia.[81] Numerous studies have demonstrated the variation in paraplegia rates, however, and the determining factor appears to be the operative technique used (see Tables 56-6 and 56-7; Fig. 56-9).[3,4,64,65,80,81,90–92,117,127] According to current data, perfusing the lower body via partial left heart bypass in association with a cross-clamp time less than 30 minutes will provide the lowest risk for postoperative paraplegia.[4,91]

TABLE 56-8 Major Postoperative Complications

	Schmidt et al[141] *n* = 73, %	Cowley et al[83] *n* = 51, %	Kodali et al[168] *n* = 50, %	Fabian et al[4] *n* = 207, %
Paraplegia	5.4	19.6	10	8.7
Renal failure	9.6	9.8	4	8.7
Sepsis	13.7	9.8	—	—
ARDS/pneumonia	21.9	17.7	34	33
Left vocal cord paralysis	4.1	13.7	14	4.3
Left phrenic nerve palsy	1.4	5.9	—	—
Stroke	2.7	—	4	—
Re-exploration for bleeding	1.4	9.8	4.0	—
Pulmonary embolism	1.4	3.9	—	—
Deep vein thrombosis	2.7	—	—	—
Empyema	—	—	—	1.9
Wound infection	—	3.9	—	—
Chylothorax	—	3.9	—	—
Deaths	8.8	43.1	28.0	14 (31.3)*

*Twenty-nine deaths (14%) occurred among the 207 patients who presented in stable condition. An additional 46 patients presented either in extremis or with free rupture, and all of these patients died in the hospital. All told there were 86 deaths among 274 patients included in the AAST trial (31.3%).
ARDS = Acute respiratory distress syndrome.

Endovascular Stent-Grafting

Use of endovascular techniques to treat abdominal aortic aneurysms began in 1991 and has subsequently been expanded to degenerative thoracic aortic aneurysms. In trauma patients with blunt aortic injury, this technology was initially applied to patients considered extremely high risk for open repair, such as those with a head injury, abdominal visceral injury, or severe pulmonary contusions.[65,66,121,124] The safety and efficacy of this procedure has since been demonstrated and endovascular stent-grafting (EVSG) is considered the preferred method of treatment by many groups.[65,66,87,88,117,121–125,149–152] Theoretical advantages of stent-grafting include avoidance of thoracotomy, one-lung ventilation, the systemic effects of cardiopulmonary bypass, aortic cross-clamping, and spinal cord ischemia, which should decrease perioperative mortality and complications.[121,122,124,125]

Several anatomical considerations must be addressed when deciding whether a patient is a candidate for EVSG of a blunt aortic transection. A proximal landing zone of at least 1.5 cm is considered necessary to achieve a reliable seal, raising the concern of left arm ischemia if the left subclavian artery needs to be covered; however, this has not been observed.[123,151] In the rare case of symptomatic left arm ischemia, elective carotid to subclavian bypass may be performed.[123,151] The left subclavian artery origin is also a good marker for an area of acute angulation of the proximal descending aorta and the wall stents used in early EVSG procedures often became distorted in this region.[123,153,154] Newer flexible stents have overcome this issue.

Additionally, the graft diameter should be oversized 10 to 20% for appropriate seating.[122,123] The size of the chosen graft will determine the route of placement. Early procedures used grafts designed as extension cuffs for abdominal aortic grafts, and these devices had delivery systems 65 cm in length, necessitating iliac or distal aortic access.[122,125] Those frequently reported in the literature include the Gore Excluder (W.L. Gore and Associates, Flagstaff, AZ), AneuRx (Medtronic, Santa Rosa, CA), and Zenith (Cook, Inc., Indianapolis, IN). These cuff diameters range from 18 to 28 mm, and the lengths range from 3.3 to 3.75 cm, necessitating placement of several cuffs to achieve adequate coverage.[36] Commercially available thoracic aortic stent-grafts have been designed for treatment of aneurysm disease; therefore, the diameters are often too large for the otherwise healthy aorta encountered in a patient with traumatic aortic transection. The Gore TAG (W.L. Gore and Associates, Flagstaff, AZ) fits vessels 23 to 37 mm, and the Talent Valiant (Medtronic, Santa Rosa, CA) may be applied to vessels 20 to 42 mm in diameter, excluding a large percentage of blunt aortic transection victims.[154] The ideal device for repair of traumatic aortic injury would be 16 to 40 mm in diameter, be available in 5-, 10-, and 15-cm lengths, and conform to a 90-degree curvature without deformation. Additionally, the delivery system should be distally flexible and approximately 80 to 90 cm in length.[36]

Patients who will undergo EVSG for traumatic aortic disruption should be positioned supine in a hybrid operating room/angiosuite or conventional operating room table with fluoroscopic capabilities. General endotracheal anesthesia is typically employed. Conversion to open repair is rare, but has occurred because of postdeployment stent migration; therefore, the operative team must be prepared for rapid conversion.[87] Retrograde aortic access is accomplished percutaneously or by cutdown on the femoral or iliac artery depending on the chosen stent-graft. A floppy tipped J-wire should be advanced into the aorta under fluoroscopic guidance with subsequent placement of marked catheter. An aortogram should be obtained in steep left anterior oblique projection to clearly visualize the arch. The details of the aortic injury and device measurements are obtained from a CTA during operative planning, but the intraoperative aortogram is vital to confirming appropriate anatomy for EVSG and selection of the correct device. Additionally, the length of graft coverage is determined by this intraoperative image. Deployment of stent-grafts have been successful with and without administration of systemic heparin (Fig. 56-11).[155] Intravascular ultrasound may be a useful adjunct when determining coverage length and graft diameter.[156,157] Based on the proximity to the aortic injury, the left subclavian artery may need to be covered, and if covered, it may need to be embolized and bypassed or transposed to the left common carotid artery to ensure a proximal graft seal and avoid problems of ischemia to the left arm or vertebrobasilar system.[125,158–160]

Despite whether single or multiple graft devices have been deployed, successful exclusion of the pseudoaneurysm has been accomplished in 90 to 100% of patients reported in the literature.[51,65,88,123–125,161] Decreased operating room time, diminished physiologic derangement and hypothermia, decreased transfusion rates, and shorter intensive care unit and overall hospital stays have been documented in series directly comparing open and endovascular repair of blunt traumatic aortic injury.[87,124,125] Procedure related paraplegia and mortality rates are also markedly reduced to nearly zero.[87,124,125] Long-term

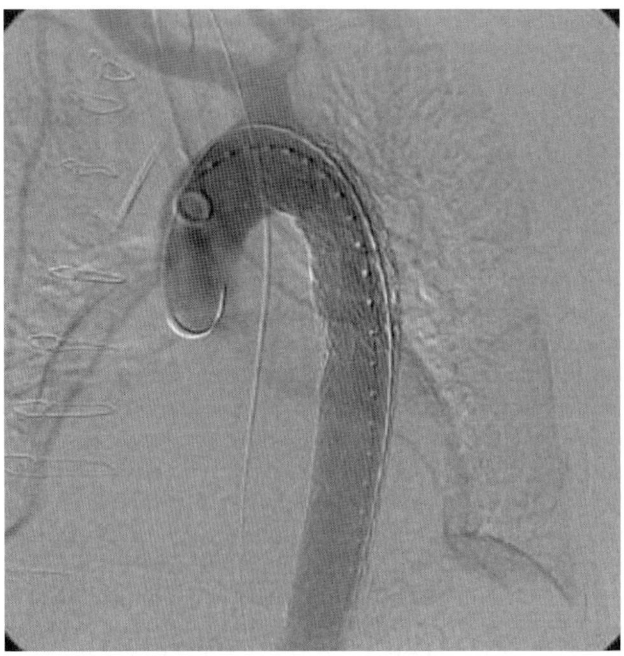

FIGURE 56-11 Endovascular stent-graft repair of the blunt traumatic aortic injury displayed in Figure 56-8 demonstrating coverage of the left subclavian artery.

TABLE 56-9 Results of Endovascular Stent Grafting (EVSG) for Aortic Transection (with Comparison to Open Repair)

		# of Cases		Mortality		Paraplegia	
Author	Study Period (years)	Open Repair	EVSG	Open Repair (%)	EVSG (%)	Open Repair (%)	EVSG (%)
Cook et al[99]	20	79	19	24.1	21.1	4	0
Pacini et al[117]	23	51	15	7.8	0	5.9	0
Rousseau et al[65]	18	35	29	17	0	5.7	0
Andrassy et al[87]	14	16	15	18.8	13.3	12.5	0
Ott et al[124]	11	12	6	17	0	17	0
Morishita et al[88]	3	11	18	9	17	0	5.6
Reed et al[66]	5	9	13	11	23	0	0
Lachat et al[150]	N/A	N/A	12	N/A	0	N/A	0
Peterson et al[125]	4	N/A	11	N/A	0	N/A	0
Pooled data		214	138	16.8	8.7	5.6	0.7

surveillance is recommended to evaluate for endoleak, stent migration, or delayed pseudoaneurysm formation with annual CT angiography.[125]

Complications

Complications of EVSG repair have been rare (Table 56-9). Graft or procedure related mortality has only occurred in 2% of patients.[36] The risk of paraplegia is almost entirely eliminated because the length of aorta covered with stent-grafting includes few intercostal vessels, thereby minimally affecting spinal cord perfusion.[120,124] Early endoleak has occurred at a rate of 5.1% in stenting of a traumatic blunt aortic injury, with Type I endoleaks being most commonly reported, likely because of difficulty attaining adequate proximal seal in a short neck, heavily calcified arch, or small radius of curvature of the arch.[36] Identification during the initial procedure allows application of adjunctive techniques to seal the stent, but many series also report spontaneous resolution.[87,122,161,162] Early endoleak has been the cause of stent-related mortality in 0.9% of patients in published series.[122,124] Delayed endoleak has been identified in less than 1% of patients on routine surveillance with CTA and successfully managed nonoperatively with spontaneous resolution within 3 to 6 months.[36] Rousseau and coworkers reported no incidence of graft kinking, twisting, stenosis, thrombosis, migration, pseudoaneurysm expansion, or rupture; however, one patient in that series suffered acute compression of the left main bronchus with resultant atelectasis requiring placement of silicone endobronchial stent.[65] Access related complications, including iliac artery rupture, may occur in about 2.5% of patients because of the large caliber of the stent-graft delivery systems, and this is consistent with the rate documented for elective repair of degenerative thoracic aortic disease.[66,163] Although not without risks, current data have demonstrated the safety and efficacy of EVSG in blunt aortic trauma, suggesting it should be preferentially applied to anatomically appropriate injuries.

Delayed Presentation

Rarely, blunt aortic transections may go undiagnosed and form chronic pseudoaneurysms through fibrous reorganization and calcification of the periadventitial tissues.[164,165] Ninety percent involve the aortic isthmus, reflective of the apparent protection afforded to this area by mediastinal periadventitial tissues.[165–167] Interestingly, these chronic pseudoaneurysms have been diagnosed in patients who had fewer concomitant injuries at the time of their initial trauma and 35% had no associated injuries.[164] The most common presenting symptom was chest pain, but other common complaints include dyspnea or cough secondary to compression of the left main stem bronchus, hoarseness owing to stretching of the recurrent nerve, hemoptysis, or dysphagia.[164] In a review by Finkelmeier et al., overall mortality at 5 years was 70%. Patients were compared according to operative versus nonoperative management, and those who underwent aortic repair had an operative mortality of nearly 5%, with exsanguination being the leading cause of death.[164] Alternatively, in the 60 patients followed nonoperatively, 20 deaths were attributable to the aortic lesion.[164] Therefore, although there exists significant surgical risk, operative repair of chronic traumatic aortic pseudoaneurysms does provide a survival benefit.[164] Occasionally, completely calcified pseudoaneurysms are identified. These must be completely resected to allow placement of a tube graft without kinking it. The dissection required for this puts the recurrent laryngeal nerve, thoracic duct, esophagus, and pulmonary artery at risk of being violated. These lesions are unlikely to grow significantly and can be followed with serial imaging.

REFERENCES

1. Brinkman WT, Szeto WY, Bavaria JE: Overview of great vessel trauma. *Thorac Surg Clin* 2007; 17(1):95-108.
2. Williams JS, Graff JA, Uku JM, Steinig JP: Aortic injury in vehicular trauma. *Ann Thorac Surg* 1994; 57(3):726-730.
3. Razzouk AJ, Gundry SR, Wang N, et al: Repair of traumatic aortic rupture: a 25-year experience. *Arch Surg* 2000; 135(8):913-918; discussion 919.
4. Fabian TC, Richardson JD, Croce MA, et al: Prospective study of blunt aortic injury: Multicenter Trial of the American Association for the Surgery of Trauma. *J Trauma* 1997; 42(3):374-380; discussion 380-373.
5. Parmley LF, Mattingly TW, Manion WC, Jahnke EJ Jr: Nonpenetrating traumatic injury of the aorta. *Circulation* 1958; 17(6):1086-1101.
6. Pretre R, Chilcott M, Murith N, Panos A: Blunt injury to the supra-aortic arteries. *Br J Surg* 1997; 84(5):603-609.
7. Reul GJ Jr, Beall AC Jr, Jordan GL Jr, Mattox KL: The early operative management of injuries to great vessels. *Surgery* 1973; 74(6):862-873.
8. Wall MJ Jr, Mattox KL, Debakey ME: Injuries to the azygous venous system. *J Trauma* 2006; 60(2):357-362.
9. Symbas JD, Halkos ME, Symbas PN: Rupture of the innominate artery from blunt trauma: current options for management. *J Card Surg* 2005; 20(5):455-459.
10. Kraus RR, Bergstein JM, DeBord JR: Diagnosis, treatment, and outcome of blunt carotid arterial injuries. *Am J Surg* 1999; 178(3):190-193.
11. Stover S, Holtzman RB, Lottenberg L, Bass TL: Blunt innominate artery injury. *Am Surg* 2001; 67(8):757-759.
12. Carter YM, Karmy-Jones R, Aldea GS: Delayed surgical management of a traumatic aortic arch injury. *Ann Thorac Surg* 2002; 73(1):294-296.
13. Graham JM, Feliciano DV, Mattox KL, Beall AC Jr: Innominate vascular injury. *J Trauma* 1982; 22(8):647-655.
14. Cox CS Jr, Allen GS, Fischer RP, et al: Blunt versus penetrating subclavian artery injury: presentation, injury pattern, and outcome. *J Trauma* 1999; 46(3):445-449.
15. Symbas PJ, Horsley WS, Symbas PN: Rupture of the ascending aorta caused by blunt trauma. *Ann Thorac Surg* 1998; 66(1):113-117.
16. Hirose H, Moore E: Delayed presentation and rupture of a posttraumatic innominate artery aneurysm: case report and review of the literature. *J Trauma* 1997; 42(6):1187-1195.
17. Miles EJ, Blake A, Thompson W, Jones WG, Dunn EL: Endovascular repair of acute innominate artery injury due to blunt trauma. *Am Surg* 2003; 69(2):155-159.
18. Pretre R, LaHarpe R, Cheretakis A, et al: Blunt injury to the ascending aorta: three patterns of presentation. *Surgery* 1996; 119(6):603-610.
19. Fulton JO, De Groot MK, von Oppell UO: Stab wounds of the innominate artery. *Ann Thorac Surg* 1996; 61(3):851-853.
20. Buchan K, Robbs JV: Surgical management of penetrating mediastinal arterial trauma. *Eur J Cardiothorac Surg* 1995; 9(2):90-94.
21. Lin PH, Koffron AJ, Guske PJ, et al: Penetrating injuries of the subclavian artery. *Am J Surg* 2003; 185(6):580-584.
22. Weiman DS, McCoy DW, Haan CK, Pate JW, Fabian TC: Blunt injuries of the brachiocephalic artery. *Am Surg* 1998; 64(5):383-387.
23. Axisa BM, Loftus IM, Fishwick G, Spyt T, Bell PR: Endovascular repair of an innominate artery false aneurysm following blunt trauma. *J Endovasc Ther* 2000; 7(3):245-250.
24. McCoy DW, Weiman DS, Pate JW, Fabian TC, Walker WA: Subclavian artery injuries. *Am Surg* 1997; 63(9):761-764.
25. Pretre R, Faidutti B: Surgical management of aortic valve injury after nonpenetrating trauma. *Ann Thorac Surg* 1993; 56(6):1426-1431.
26. Maggisano R, Nathens A, Alexandrova NA, et al: Traumatic rupture of the thoracic aorta: should one always operate immediately? *Ann Vasc Surg* 1995; 9(1):44-52.
27. Hirose H, Gill IS: Blunt injury of proximal innominate artery. *Ann Thorac Cardiovasc Surg* 2004; 10(2):130-132.
28. Kieffer E, Sabatier J, Koskas F, Bahnini A: Atherosclerotic innominate artery occlusive disease: early and long-term results of surgical reconstruction. *J Vasc Surg* 1995; 21(2):326-336; discussion 336-327.
29. Sanzone AG, Torres H, Doundoulakis SH: Blunt trauma to the carotid arteries. *Am J Emerg Med* 1995; 13(3):327-330.
30. Sawchuk AP, Eldrup-Jorgensen J, Tober C, et al: The natural history of intimal flaps in a canine model. *Arch Surg* 1990; 125(12):1614-1616.
31. Fabian TC, Patton JH Jr, Croce MA, et al: Blunt carotid injury. Importance of early diagnosis and anticoagulant therapy. *Ann Surg* 1996; 223(5):513-522; discussion 522-515.
32. Abouljoud MS, Obeid FN, Horst HM, et al: Arterial injuries of the thoracic outlet: a ten-year experience. *Am Surg* 1993; 59(9):590-595.
33. McKinley AG, Carrim AT, Robbs JV: Management of proximal axillary and subclavian artery injuries. *Br J Surg* 2000; 87(1):79-85.
34. Graham JM, Mattox KL, Feliciano DV, DeBakey ME: Vascular injuries of the axilla. *Ann Surg* 1982; 195(2):232-238.
35. du Toit DF, Odendaal W, Lambrechts A, Warren BL: Surgical and endovascular management of penetrating innominate artery injuries. *Eur J Vasc Endovasc Surg* 2008; 36(1):56-62.
36. Hoffer EK: Endovascular intervention in thoracic arterial trauma. *Injury* 2008; 39(11):1257-1274.
37. Reuben BC, Whitten MG, Sarfati M, Kraiss LW: Increasing use of endovascular therapy in acute arterial injuries: analysis of the National Trauma Data Bank. *J Vasc Surg* 2007; 46(6):1222-1226.
38. du Toit DF, Strauss DC, Blaszczyk M, de Villiers R, Warren BL: Endovascular treatment of penetrating thoracic outlet arterial injuries. *Eur J Vasc Endovasc Surg* 2000; 19(5):489-495.
39. Becker GJ, Benenati JF, Zemel G, et al: Percutaneous placement of a balloon-expandable intraluminal graft for life-threatening subclavian arterial hemorrhage. *J Vasc Interv Radiol* 1991; 2(2):225-229.
40. Schonholz CJ, Uflacker R, De Gregorio MA, Parodi JC: Stent-graft treatment of trauma to the supra-aortic arteries. A review. *J Cardiovasc Surg (Torino)* 2007; 48(5):537-549.
41. Chandler TA, Fishwick G, Bell PR: Endovascular repair of a traumatic innominate artery aneurysm. *Eur J Vasc Endovasc Surg* 1999; 18(1):80-82.
42. Blattman SB, Landis GS, Knight M, et al: Combined endovascular and open repair of a penetrating innominate artery and tracheal injury. *Ann Thorac Surg* 2002; 74(1):237-239.
43. Arthurs ZM, Sohn VY, Starnes BW: Vascular trauma: endovascular management and techniques. *Surg Clin North Am* 2007; 87(5):1179-1192, x-xi.
44. Huang CL, Kao HL: Endovascular management of post-traumatic innominate artery transection with pseudo-aneurysm formation. *Catheter Cardiovasc Interv* 2008; 72(4):569-572.
45. Saket RR, Razavi MK, Sze DY, et al: Stent-graft treatment of extracranial carotid and vertebral arterial lesions. *J Vasc Interv Radiol* 2004; 15(10): 1151-1156.
46. Simionato F, Righi C, Melissano G, et al: Stent-graft treatment of a common carotid artery pseudoaneurysm. *J Endovasc Ther* 2000; 7(2):136-140.
47. Schonholz C, Krajcer Z, Carlos Parodi J, et al: Stent-graft treatment of pseudoaneurysms and arteriovenous fistulae in the carotid artery. *Vascular* 2006; 14(3):123-129.
48. du Toit DF, Leith JG, Strauss DC, et al: Endovascular management of traumatic cervicothoracic arteriovenous fistula. *Br J Surg* 2003; 90(12): 1516-1521.
49. Archondakis E, Pero G, Valvassori L, Boccardi E, Scialfa G: Angiographic follow-up of traumatic carotid cavernous fistulas treated with endovascular stent-graft placement. *AJNR Am J Neuroradiol* 2007; 28(2):342-347.
50. Saatci I, Cekirge HS, Ozturk MH, et al: Treatment of internal carotid artery aneurysms with a covered stent: experience in 24 patients with mid-term follow-up results. *AJNR Am J Neuroradiol* 2004; 25(10): 1742-1749.
51. Hershberger RC, Aulivola B, Murphy M, Luchette FA: Endovascular grafts for treatment of traumatic injury to the aortic arch and great vessels. *J Trauma* 2009; 67(3):660-671.
52. Sanchez LA, Veith FJ, Ohki T, et al: Early experience with the Corvita endoluminal graft for treatment of arterial injuries. *Ann Vasc Surg* 1999; 13(2):151-157.
53. Schoder M, Cejna M, Holzenbein T, et al: Elective and emergent endovascular treatment of subclavian artery aneurysms and injuries. *J Endovasc Ther* 2003; 10(1):58-65.
54. Hilfiker PR, Razavi MK, Kee ST, et al: Stent-graft therapy for subclavian artery aneurysms and fistulas: single-center mid-term results. *J Vasc Interv Radiol* 2000; 11(5):578-584.
55. Parodi JC, Schonholz C, Ferreira LM, Bergan J: Endovascular stent-graft treatment of traumatic arterial lesions. *Ann Vasc Surg* 1999; 13(2):121-129.
56. Patel AV, Marin ML, Veith FJ, Kerr A, Sanchez LA: Endovascular graft repair of penetrating subclavian artery injuries. *J Endovasc Surg* 1996; 3(4):382-388.
57. Marin ML, Veith FJ, Panetta TF, et al: Transluminally placed endovascular stented graft repair for arterial trauma. *J Vasc Surg* 1994; 20(3):466-472; discussion 472-463.
58. Marin ML, Veith FJ, Cynamon J, et al: Initial experience with transluminally placed endovascular grafts for the treatment of complex vascular lesions. *Ann Surg* 1995; 222(4):449-465; discussion 465-449.

59. White R, Krajcer Z, Johnson M, et al: Results of a multicenter trial for the treatment of traumatic vascular injury with a covered stent. *J Trauma* 2006; 60(6):1189-1195; discussion 1195-1186.
60. Ohki T, Veith FJ, Kraas C, et al: Endovascular therapy for upper extremity injury. *Semin Vasc Surg* 1998; 11(2):106-115.
61. Greendyke RM: Traumatic rupture of aorta; special reference to automobile accidents. *JAMA* 1966; 195(7):527-530.
62. Feczko JD, Lynch L, Pless JE, et al: An autopsy case review of 142 nonpenetrating (blunt) injuries of the aorta. *J Trauma* 1992; 33(6):846-849.
63. Fitzharris M, Franklyn M, Frampton R, et al: Thoracic aortic injury in motor vehicle crashes: the effect of impact direction, side of body struck, and seat belt use. *J Trauma* 2004; 57(3):582-590.
64. Cook J, Salerno C, Krishnadasan B, et al: The effect of changing presentation and management on the outcome of blunt rupture of the thoracic aorta. *J Thorac Cardiovasc Surg* 2006; 131(3):594-600.
65. Rousseau H, Dambrin C, Marcheix B, et al: Acute traumatic aortic rupture: a comparison of surgical and stent-graft repair. *J Thorac Cardiovasc Surg* 2005; 129(5):1050-1055.
66. Reed AB, Thompson JK, Crafton CJ, Delvecchio C, Giglia JS: Timing of endovascular repair of blunt traumatic thoracic aortic transections. *J Vasc Surg* 2006; 43(4):684-688.
67. Brasel KJ, Quickel R, Yoganandan N, Weigelt JA: Seat belts are more effective than airbags in reducing thoracic aortic injury in frontal motor vehicle crashes. *J Trauma* 2002; 53(2):309-312; discussion 313.
68. Dunn JA, Williams MG: Occult ascending aortic rupture in the presence of an air bag. *Ann Thorac Surg* 1996; 62(2):577-578.
69. deGuzman BJ, Morgan AS, Pharr WF: Aortic transection following air-bag deployment. *NEJM* 1997; 337(8):573-574.
70. Demetriades D, Gomez H, Velmahos GC, et al: Routine helical computed tomographic evaluation of the mediastinum in high-risk blunt trauma patients. *Arch Surg* 1998; 133(10):1084-1088.
71. Pezzella AT: Blunt traumatic injury of the thoracic aorta following commercial airline crashes. *Tex Heart Inst J* 1996; 23(1):65-67.
72. Lundevall J: Traumatic rupture of the aorta, with special reference to road accidents. *Acta Pathol Microbiol Scand* 1964; 62:29-33.
73. Stapp JP: Human tolerance to deceleration. *Am J Surg* 1957; 93(4):734-740.
74. Marsh CL, Moore RC: Deceleration trauma. *Am J Surg* 1957; 93(4): 623-631.
75. Sevitt S: The mechanisms of traumatic rupture of the thoracic aorta. *Br J Surg* 1977; 64(3):166-173.
76. Gotzen L, Flory PJ, Otte D: Biomechanics of aortic rupture at classical location in traffic accidents. *Thorac Cardiovasc Surg* 1980; 28(1):64-68.
77. Crass JR, Cohen AM, Motta AO, Tomashefski JF Jr, Wiesen EJ: A proposed new mechanism of traumatic aortic rupture: the osseous pinch. *Radiology* 1990; 176(3):645-649.
78. Cohen AM, Crass JR, Thomas HA, Fisher RG, Jacobs DG: CT evidence for the "osseous pinch" mechanism of traumatic aortic injury. *AJR Am J Roentgenol* 1992; 159(2):271-274.
79. Javadpour H, O'Toole JJ, McEniff JN, Luke DA, Young VK: Traumatic aortic transection: evidence for the osseous pinch mechanism. *Ann Thorac Surg* 2002; 73(3):951-953.
80. Sweeney MS, Young DJ, Frazier OH, et al: Traumatic aortic transections: eight-year experience with the "clamp-sew" technique. *Ann Thorac Surg* 1997; 64(2):384-387; discussion 387-389.
81. von Oppell UO, Dunne TT, De Groot MK, Zilla P: Traumatic aortic rupture: twenty-year metaanalysis of mortality and risk of paraplegia. *Ann Thorac Surg* 1994; 58(2):585-593.
82. Kieny R, Charpentier A: Traumatic lesions of the thoracic aorta. A report of 73 cases. *J Cardiovasc Surg (Torino)* 1991; 32(5):613-619.
83. Cowley RA, Turney SZ, Hankins JR, et al: Rupture of thoracic aorta caused by blunt trauma. A fifteen-year experience. *J Thorac Cardiovasc Surg* 1990; 100(5):652-660; discussion 660-651.
84. Butcher HR Jr: The elastic properties of human aortic intima, media and adventitia: the initial effect of thromboendarterectomy. *Ann Surg* 1960; 151:480-489.
85. Katz S, Mullin R, Berger RL: Traumatic transection associated with retrograde dissection and rupture of the aorta: recognition and management. *Ann Thorac Surg* 1974; 17(3):273-276.
86. Langanay T, Verhoye JP, Corbineau H, et al: Surgical treatment of acute traumatic rupture of the thoracic aorta a timing reappraisal? *Eur J Cardiothorac Surg* 2002; 21(2):282-287.
87. Andrassy J, Weidenhagen R, Meimarakis G, et al: Stent versus open surgery for acute and chronic traumatic injury of the thoracic aorta: a single-center experience. *J Trauma* 2006; 60(4):765-771; discussion 771-762.
88. Morishita K, Kurimoto Y, Kawaharada N, et al: Descending thoracic aortic rupture: role of endovascular stent-grafting. *Ann Thorac Surg* 2004; 78(5):1630-1634.
89. Santaniello JM, Miller PR, Croce MA, et al: Blunt aortic injury with concomitant intra-abdominal solid organ injury: treatment priorities revisited. *J Trauma* 2002; 53(3):442-445; discussion 445.
90. Fabian TC, Davis KA, Gavant ML, et al: Prospective study of blunt aortic injury: helical CT is diagnostic and antihypertensive therapy reduces rupture. *Ann Surg* 1998; 227(5):666-676; discussion 676-667.
91. Nagy K, Fabian T, Rodman G, et al: Guidelines for the diagnosis and management of blunt aortic injury: an EAST Practice Management Guidelines Work Group. *J Trauma* 2000; 48(6):1128-1143.
92. Clark DE, Zeiger MA, Wallace KL, Packard AB, Nowicki ER: Blunt aortic trauma: signs of high risk. *J Trauma* 1990; 30(6):701-705.
93. Kram HB, Appel PL, Wohlmuth DA, Shoemaker WC: Diagnosis of traumatic thoracic aortic rupture: a 10-year retrospective analysis. *Ann Thorac Surg* 1989; 47(2):282-286.
94. Sturm JT, Perry JF Jr, Olson FR, Cicero JJ: Significance of symptoms and signs in patients with traumatic aortic rupture. *Ann Emerg Med* 1984; 13(10):876-878.
95. Kram HB, Wohlmuth DA, Appel PL, Shoemaker WC: Clinical and radiographic indications for aortography in blunt chest trauma. *J Vasc Surg* 1987; 6(2):168-176.
96. Simon BJ, Leslie C: Factors predicting early in-hospital death in blunt thoracic aortic injury. *J Trauma* 2001; 51(5):906-910; discussion 911.
97. Feliciano DV, Rozycki GS: Advances in the diagnosis and treatment of thoracic trauma. *Surg Clin North Am* 1999; 79(6):1417-1429.
98. Williams MJ, Low CJ, Wilkins GT, Stewart RA: Randomised comparison of the effects of nicardipine and esmolol on coronary artery wall stress: implications for the risk of plaque rupture. *Heart* 2000; 84(4):377-382.
99. Cook AD, Klein JS, Rogers FB, Osler TM, Shackford SR: Chest radiographs of limited utility in the diagnosis of blunt traumatic aortic laceration. *J Trauma* 2001; 50(5):843-847.
100. Gavant ML, Menke PG, Fabian T, et al: Blunt traumatic aortic rupture: detection with helical CT of the chest. *Radiology* 1995; 197(1):125-133.
101. Gundry SR, Burney RE, Mackenzie JR, et al: Assessment of mediastinal widening associated with traumatic rupture of the aorta. *J Trauma* 1983; 23(4):293-299.
102. Mattox KL: Fact and fiction about management of aortic transection. *Ann Thorac Surg* 1989; 48(1):1-2.
103. Parker MS, Matheson TL, Rao AV, et al: Making the transition: the role of helical CT in the evaluation of potentially acute thoracic aortic injuries. *AJR Am J Roentgenol* 2001; 176(5):1267-1272.
104. Dyer DS, Moore EE, Ilke DN, et al: Thoracic aortic injury: how predictive is mechanism and is chest computed tomography a reliable screening tool? A prospective study of 1,561 patients. *J Trauma* 2000; 48(4):673-682; discussion 682-673.
105. Vignon P, Boncoeur MP, Francois B, et al: Comparison of multiplane transesophageal echocardiography and contrast-enhanced helical CT in the diagnosis of blunt traumatic cardiovascular injuries. *Anesthesiology* 2001; 94(4):615-622; discussion 615A.
106. Gavant ML: Helical CT grading of traumatic aortic injuries. Impact on clinical guidelines for medical and surgical management. *Radiol Clin North Am* 1999; 37(3):553-574, vi.
107. Malhotra AK, Fabian TC, Croce MA, et al: Minimal aortic injury: a lesion associated with advancing diagnostic techniques. *J Trauma* 2001; 51(6):1042-1048.
108. Saletta S, Lederman E, Fein S, et al: Transesophageal echocardiography for the initial evaluation of the widened mediastinum in trauma patients. *J Trauma* 1995; 39(1):137-141; discussion 131-132.
109. Sturm JT, Hankins DG, Young G: Thoracic aortography following blunt chest trauma. *Am J Emerg Med* 1990; 8(2):92-96.
110. Eddy AC, Nance DR, Goldman MA, et al: Rapid diagnosis of thoracic aortic transection using intravenous digital subtraction angiography. *Am J Surg* 1990; 159(5):500-503.
111. LaBerge JM, Jeffrey RB: Aortic lacerations: fatal complications of thoracic aortography. *Radiology* Nov 1987; 165(2):367-369.
112. Nienaber CA, von Kodolitsch Y, Brockhoff CJ, Koschyk DH, Spielmann RP: Comparison of conventional and transesophageal echocardiography with magnetic resonance imaging for anatomical mapping of thoracic aortic dissection. A dual noninvasive imaging study with anatomical and/or angiographic validation. *Int J Card Imaging* 1994; 10(1):1-14.
113. Nienaber CA, von Kodolitsch Y, Nicolas V, et al: The diagnosis of thoracic aortic dissection by noninvasive imaging procedures. *NEJM* 7 1993; 328(1):1-9.
114. Hirose H, Gill IS, Malangoni MA: Nonoperative management of traumatic aortic injury. *J Trauma* 2006; 60(3):597-601.
115. Holmes JHT, Bloch RD, Hall RA, Carter YM, Karmy-Jones RC: Natural history of traumatic rupture of the thoracic aorta managed nonoperatively: a longitudinal analysis. *Ann Thorac Surg* 2002; 73(4):1149-1154.

116. Kwon CC, Gill IS, Fallon WF, et al: Delayed operative intervention in the management of traumatic descending thoracic aortic rupture. *Ann Thorac Surg* 2002; 74(5):S1888-1891; discussion S1892-1888.
117. Pacini D, Angeli E, Fattori R, et al: Traumatic rupture of the thoracic aorta: ten years of delayed management. *J Thorac Cardiovasc Surg* 2005; 129(4):880-884.
118. Symbas PN, Sherman AJ, Silver JM, Symbas JD, Lackey JJ: Traumatic rupture of the aorta: immediate or delayed repair? *Ann Surg* 2002; 235(6):796-802.
119. Carter Y, Meissner M, Bulger E, et al: Anatomical considerations in the surgical management of blunt thoracic aortic injury. *J Vasc Surg* 2001; 34(4):628-633.
120. Yamane BH, Tefera G, Hoch JR, Turnipseed WD, Acher CW: Blunt thoracic aortic injury: open or stent-graft repair? *Surgery* 2008; 144(4): 575-580; discussion 580-572.
121. Dunham MB, Zygun D, Petrasek P, et al: Endovascular stent-grafts for acute blunt aortic injury. *J Trauma* 2004; 56(6):1173-1178.
122. Karmy-Jones R, Hoffer E, Meissner MH, Nicholls S, Mattos M: Endovascular stent-grafts and aortic rupture: a case series. *J Trauma* 2003; 55(5):805-810.
123. Orford VP, Atkinson NR, Thomson K, et al: Blunt traumatic aortic transection: the endovascular experience. *Ann Thorac Surg* 2003; 75(1): 106-111; discussion 111-112.
124. Ott MC, Stewart TC, Lawlor DK, Gray DK, Forbes TL: Management of blunt thoracic aortic injuries: endovascular stents versus open repair. *J Trauma* 2004; 56(3):565-570.
125. Peterson BG, Matsumura JS, Morasch MD, West MA, Eskandari MK: Percutaneous endovascular repair of blunt thoracic aortic transection. *J Trauma* 2005; 59(5):1062-1065.
126. von Oppell UO, Dunne TT, De Groot KM, Zilla P: Spinal cord protection in the absence of collateral circulation: meta-analysis of mortality and paraplegia. *J Card Surg* 1994; 9(6):685-691.
127. Crestanello JA, Zehr KJ, Mullany CJ, et al: The effect of adjuvant perfusion techniques on the incidence of paraplegia after repair of traumatic thoracic aortic transections. *Mayo Clin Proc* 2006; 81(5):625-630.
128. Laschinger JC, Cunningham JN Jr, Nathan IM, et al: Intraoperative identification of vessels critical to spinal cord blood supply--use of somatosensory evoked potentials. *Curr Surg* 1984; 41(2):107-109.
129. McCullough JL, Hollier LH, Nugent M: Paraplegia after thoracic aortic occlusion: influence of cerebrospinal fluid drainage. Experimental and early clinical results. *J Vasc Surg* 1988; 7(1):153-160.
130. Black JH, Davison JK, Cambria RP: Regional hypothermia with epidural cooling for prevention of spinal cord ischemic complications after thoracoabdominal aortic surgery. *Semin Thorac Cardiovasc Surg* 2003; 15(4): 345-352.
131. Peltz M, Douglass DS, Meyer DM, et al: Hypothermic circulatory arrest for repair of injuries of the thoracic aorta and great vessels. *Interact Cardiovasc Thorac Surg* 2006; 5(5):560-565.
132. Kouchoukos NT, Masetti P, Rokkas CK, Murphy SF, Blackstone EH: Safety and efficacy of hypothermic cardiopulmonary bypass and circulatory arrest for operations on the descending thoracic and thoracoabdominal aorta. *Ann Thorac Surg* 2001; 72(3):699-707; discussion 707-698.
133. Szwerc MF, Benckart DH, Lin JC, et al: Recent clinical experience with left heart bypass using a centrifugal pump for repair of traumatic aortic transection. *Ann Surg* 1999; 230(4):484-490; discussion 490-482.
134. Hess PJ, Howe HR Jr, Robicsek F, et al: Traumatic tears of the thoracic aorta: improved results using the Bio-Medicus pump. *Ann Thorac Surg* 1989; 48(1):6-9.
135. Fullerton DA: Simplified technique for left heart bypass to repair aortic transection. *Ann Thorac Surg* 1993; 56(3):579-580.
136. Merrill WH, Lee RB, Hammon JW Jr, et al: Surgical treatment of acute traumatic tear of the thoracic aorta. *Ann Surg* 1988; 207(6):699-706.
137. Karmy-Jones R, Carter Y, Meissner M, Mulligan MS: Choice of venous cannulation for bypass during repair of traumatic rupture of the aorta. *Ann Thorac Surg* 2001; 71(1):39-41; discussion 41-32.
138. Turney SZ: Blunt trauma of the thoracic aorta and its branches. *Semin Thorac Cardiovasc Surg* 1992; 4(3):209-216.
139. Carter YM, Karmy-Jones RC, Oxorn DC, Aldea GS: Traumatic disruption of the aortic arch. *Eur J Cardiothorac Surg* 2001; 20(6):1231.
140. Leshnower BG, Litt HI, Gleason TG: Anterior approach to traumatic mid aortic arch transection. *Ann Thorac Surg* 2006; 81(1):343-345.
141. Schmidt CA, Wood MN, Razzouk AJ, Killeen JD, Gan KA: Primary repair of traumatic aortic rupture: a preferred approach. *J Trauma* 1992; 32(5):588-592.
142. Verdant A, Page A, Cossette R, et al: Surgery of the descending thoracic aorta: spinal cord protection with the Gott shunt. *Ann Thorac Surg* 1988; 46(2):147-154.
143. McBride LR, Tidik S, Stothert JC, et al: Primary repair of traumatic aortic disruption. *Ann Thorac Surg* 1987; 43(1):65-67.
144. Hilgenberg AD, Logan DL, Akins CW, et al: Blunt injuries of the thoracic aorta. *Ann Thorac Surg* 1992; 53(2):233-238; discussion 238-239.
145. Wallenhaupt SL, Hudspeth AS, Mills SA, et al: Current treatment of traumatic aortic disruptions. *Am Surg* 1989; 55(5):316-320.
146. Ablaza SG, Ghosh SC, Grana VP: Use of a ringed intraluminal graft in the surgical treatment of dissecting aneurysms of the thoracic aorta. A new technique. *J Thorac Cardiovasc Surg* 1978; 76(3):390-396.
147. Kazerooni EA, Williams DM, Abrams GD, Deeb GM, Weg JG: Aortobronchial fistula 13 years following repair of aortic transection. *Chest* 1994; 106(5):1590-1594.
148. Tsai FC, Lin PJ, Wu YC, Chang CH: Traumatic aortic arch transection with supracarinal tracheoesophageal fistula: case report. *J Trauma* 1999; 46(5):951-953.
149. Czermak BV, Waldenberger P, Perkmann R, et al: Placement of endovascular stent-grafts for emergency treatment of acute disease of the descending thoracic aorta. *AJR Am J Roentgenol* 2002; 179(2):337-345.
150. Lachat M, Pfammatter T, Witzke H, et al: Acute traumatic aortic rupture: early stent-graft repair. *Eur J Cardiothorac Surg* 2002; 21(6):959-963.
151. Mattison R, Hamilton IN Jr, Ciraulo DL, Richart CM: Stent-graft repair of acute traumatic thoracic aortic transection with intentional occlusion of the left subclavian artery: case report. *J Trauma* 2001; 51(2):326-328.
152. Singh MJ, Rohrer MJ, Ghaleb M, Kim D: Endoluminal stent-graft repair of a thoracic aortic transection in a trauma patient with multiple injuries: case report. *J Trauma* 2001; 51(2):376-381.
153. Kato N, Dake MD, Miller DC, et al: Traumatic thoracic aortic aneurysm: treatment with endovascular stent-grafts. *Radiology* 1997; 205(3):657-662.
154. Borsa JJ, Hoffer EK, Karmy-Jones R, et al: Angiographic description of blunt traumatic injuries to the thoracic aorta with specific relevance to endograft repair. *J Endovasc Ther* 2002; 9(Suppl 2):II84-91.
155. Bent CL, Matson MB, Sobeh M, et al: Endovascular management of acute blunt traumatic thoracic aortic injury: a single center experience. *J Vasc Surg* 2007; 46(5):920-927.
156. Greenberg R: Treatment of aortic dissections with endovascular stent-grafts. *Semin Vasc Surg* 2002; 15(2):122-127.
157. Herold U, Piotrowski J, Baumgart D, et al: Endoluminal stent-graft repair for acute and chronic type B aortic dissection and atherosclerotic aneurysm of the thoracic aorta: an interdisciplinary task. *Eur J Cardiothorac Surg* 2002; 22(6):891-897.
158. Czerny M, Zimpfer D, Fleck T, et al: Initial results after combined repair of aortic arch aneurysms by sequential transposition of the supra-aortic branches and consecutive endovascular stent-graft placement. *Ann Thorac Surg* 2004; 78(4):1256-1260.
159. Gorich J, Asquan Y, Seifarth H, et al: Initial experience with intentional stent-graft coverage of the subclavian artery during endovascular thoracic aortic repairs. *J Endovasc Ther* 2002; 9(Suppl 2):II39-43.
160. Rehders TC, Petzsch M, Ince H, et al: Intentional occlusion of the left subclavian artery during stent-graft implantation in the thoracic aorta: risk and relevance. *J Endovasc Ther* 2004; 11(6):659-666.
161. Marcheix B, Dambrin C, Bolduc JP, et al: Endovascular repair of traumatic rupture of the aortic isthmus: midterm results. *J Thorac Cardiovasc Surg* 2006; 132(5):1037-1041.
162. Marcheix B, Dambrin C, Bolduc JP, et al: Midterm results of endovascular treatment of atherosclerotic aneurysms of the descending thoracic aorta. *J Thorac Cardiovasc Surg* 2006; 132(5):1030-1036.
163. Makaroun MS, Dillavou ED, Kee ST, et al: Endovascular treatment of thoracic aortic aneurysms: results of the phase II multicenter trial of the GORE TAG thoracic endoprosthesis. *J Vasc Surg* 2005; 41(1):1-9.
164. Finkelmeier BA, Mentzer RM Jr, Kaiser DL, Tegtmeyer CJ, Nolan SP: Chronic traumatic thoracic aneurysm. Influence of operative treatment on natural history: an analysis of reported cases, 1950-1980. *J Thorac Cardiovasc Surg* 1982; 84(2):257-266.
165. John LC, Hornick P, Edmondson SJ: Chronic traumatic aneurysm of the aorta: to resect or not. The role of exploration operation. *J Cardiovasc Surg (Torino)* 1992; 33(1):106-108.
166. Albuquerque FC, Krasna MJ, McLaughlin JS: Chronic, traumatic pseudoaneurysm of the ascending aorta. *Ann Thorac Surg* 1992; 54(5):980-982.
167. Prat A, Warembourg H Jr, Watel A, et al: Chronic traumatic aneurysms of the descending thoracic aorta (19 cases). *J Cardiovasc Surg (Torino)* 1986; 27(3):268-272.
168. Kodali S, Jamieson WR, Leia-Stephens M, Miyagishima RT, Janusz MT, Tyers GF: Traumatic rupture of the thoracic aorta. A 20-year review: 1969-1989. *Circulation* 1991; 84(5 Suppl):III40-46.
169. Katz NM, Blackstone EH, Kirklin JW, Karp RB: Incremental risk factors for spinal cord injury following operation for acute traumatic aortic transection. *J Thorac Cardiovasc Surg* 1981; 81(5):669-674.

PART 6

SURGERY FOR CARDIAC ARRHYTHMIAS

CHAPTER 57

Interventional Therapy for Atrial and Ventricular Arrhythmias

Robert E. Eckart
Laurence M. Epstein

INTRODUCTION

Therapy available for the treatment of heart rhythm disorders continues to go through significant evolution. Although previously limited to pharmacologic therapy, the transformation and adaptation of surgical procedures to a minimally invasive catheter-based approach and subsequent hybridization of the approach have led to new possibilities in arrhythmia management. A fundamental understanding of the invasive diagnostic and therapeutic strategy for treating heart rhythm disorders is critical to surgical specialties exposed to these rhythm disorders.

HISTORICAL EVOLUTION

The recording of intracardiac signals through electrodes, and subsequent stimulation of the cardiac tissue, allowed for the concept of ablation. In 1967, Durrer and associates described reproducible initiation and termination of tachycardia in a patient with atrioventricular re-entrant tachycardia (AVRT) using a bypass tract.[1] In 1969, the His bundle was first reproducibly recorded using a transvenous electrode catheter.[2] The continued advancements allowing localization of intracardiac signals led to the study of a variety of tachyarrhythmias.

The idea emerged that critical regions of cardiac tissue were necessary for the initiation and propagation of tachyarrhythmias. If these regions could be interrupted, the tachyarrhythmia could then be cured. Once catheter mapping could localize arrhythmogenic foci, surgical excision was contemplated. In 1968, a description of such a surgical procedure for the elimination of an accessory pathway was first published.[3] This heralded an era of nonpharmacologic treatment of tachyarrhythmias.

Surgical Ablation

A variety of arrhythmogenic foci and circuits were successfully mapped and ablated using surgical techniques in the 1970s. Resection of an atrial focus felt to be responsible for an atrial tachycardia was reported in 1973.[4] Identification of re-entry circuits within the atrioventricular (AV) node allowed surgical dissection to treat AV nodal re-entrant tachycardia (AVNRT) without causing complete heart block.[5] Although surgical ablation was therapeutic for a variety of tachyarrhythmias, the morbidity and mortality associated with thoracotomy and open-heart surgery limited its widespread application. Because most supraventricular tachycardias (SVTs) are not life threatening, the risk of the procedure was hard to justify. Rather, ablation procedures were an option of last resort in highly symptomatic patients refractory to medical therapy.

Catheter Ablation

In attempts to minimize the morbidity associated with ablation, a method of using a catheter to delivery energy to achieve local cardiac injury was sought. In 1981, Scheinman and colleagues reported the first catheter-based ablation procedure, describing the ablation of the His bundle in dogs.[6] This same group performed the first closed-chest ablation procedure in a human. A patient with atrial fibrillation and rate control refractory to medical therapy, under general anesthesia, had a catheter advanced to the His bundle region. Using a standard external direct-current (DC) defibrillator, they attached one of the defibrillator pads to the intracardiac catheter and used the second defibrillator pad as a cutaneous grounding pad. A series of DC shocks was delivered between the two pads and complete heart block, and thereby rate control, was achieved.[7]

This closed-chest catheter-based procedure was quickly adopted to treat a variety of SVTs dependent on the AV node.[8] As experience was gained and specific catheters were developed, energy could be more precisely directed to allow ablation of accessory pathways, atrial tachycardia, single limb of AVNRT, and ventricular tachycardia.

Although DC shock ablation allowed for the initiation of catheter-based ablation, it had its own limitations. Because energy delivery was not titratable, such treatment had variable outcomes, including massive damage to surrounding myocardium.[6,7,9] Because DC energy was delivered from the intracardiac electrode toward a cutaneous site, general anesthesia was required.

The introduction of RF energy as an ablative energy source heralded a new era in the nonpharmacologic, nonsurgical treatment of arrhythmias. RF energy had been used for decades by surgeons for surgical cutting and cautery and had a long history of safety and efficacy. Animal studies using RF energy for the treatment of arrhythmia were first described in 1987.[10] Intracardiac RF energy produces controlled lesions at the catheter tip using resistive heating over a period of 40 to 120 seconds.[11,12] Although RF remains the primary energy source for catheter-based ablation, alternative energy sources such as microwave, laser, high-intensity focused ultrasound, and cryoablation continue to be developed as a means to optimize patient safety and clinical outcomes.[13]

BIOPHYSICS OF ABLATION

Ablation using RF as an energy source involves the delivery of sinusoidal alternating current between the catheter tip at the endocardial surface and a large grounding pad on the skin. The current has a frequency of 350 to 700 kHz. The principal method of tissue injury with RF delivery is thermal. As the RF energy passes through the tissue at the distal electrode of the ablation catheter, resistive heating produces coagulation necrosis. The lesions produced are well demarcated and are 5 to 6 mm wide by 2 to 3 mm deep when a standard catheter tip is used. To achieve irreversible tissue injury, a tissue temperature of 55 to 58°C is required.[14] If subendocardial tissue temperature exceeds 100°C, steam may be formed within the tissue, resulting in a rapid expansion and crater formation and an audible "pop" during ablation. Much like DC shocks, such "steam pops" can cause unpredictable injury (eg, to surrounding normal conduction tissue) as well as rupture of thin-walled structures. Contemporary RF ablation catheters have a thermistor or thermocouple that allows for automatic adjustment of the temperature at the electrode tip–tissue interface through adjustment of power.

A limitation in lesion size places some epicardial foci and arrhythmia circuits out of reach of endocardial ablations. One method to increase lesion size and depth uses the principle of limiting coagulum size by increasing the electrode–tissue interface by increasing tip size.[15,16] A limitation of larger catheter tips is that the larger surface area makes it difficult to regulate power delivery and achieve even temperatures.

Cooling the ablation catheter tip with saline irrigation, either through the catheter or external to the catheter, can also prevent coagulum formation at the tissue interface. This prevents a rise in impedance and allows for more energy delivery deep into the tissue, resulting in deeper and larger lesions.[17,18] Irrigated RF catheters bathe the catheter tip internally using recirculating saline (Chilli II, Boston-Scientific, Natick, MA) or externally through a porous electrode tip (Navistar and EZ Steer ThermaCool, Biosense-Webster, Inc., Diamond Bar, CA). These catheters continue to use RF as an energy source; however, maximization of power delivery has demonstrated deeper lesions with a greater volume than with standard RF.[19] Cooled epicardial radiofrequency ablation probes (Coolrail Pen, AtriCure, Inc., West Chester, OH) have recently been FDA approved, and are undergoing clinical trials (eg, RESTORE SR IIB) to transfer established catheter-based technology to a minimally invasive surgical approach for persistent and chronic arrhythmia.[20,21]

Because of concern about the irreversible nature of RF delivery, alternative energy sources have been developed that allow for a transient tissue injury before placement of permanent lesions. One such catheter system (Freezor, Medtronic CryoCath, Montreal, Quebec, Canada) relies on gradual cooling of tissue to allow for an estimation of injury effect, and can be followed up by a more permanent cryoablation. Hypothermia has been the preferred method of delivering linear lesions in surgical ablation. This technique uses pressurized nitrogen or nitrogen oxide flow through a catheter tip nozzle. As the gas expands beyond the obstruction, there is a temperature drop to as much as −90°C. The advantage to the system rests entirely in its ability to deliver both transient and permanent injury to the tissue. The "cooling" phase (Cryomapping) allows one to assess not only the impact on pathologic tissue (eg, anteroseptal accessory pathways, the slow limb of a dual AV node), but also the impact of potential lesion placement on surrounding normal conduction tissue.[22] If the Cryomapping phase yields desirable results, then the temperature is lowered even further to a "freezing" stage. The ability to deliver reversible injury and catheter stabilization has made cryoablation increasingly popular in those cases in which the pathologic lesion is in close proximity to the AV node and in younger patients in whom a pacemaker would be less than desirable.[23]

A second potential disadvantage to RF as an energy source is the risk of extracardiac tissue injury. Although constantly evolving, the inclusion of pulmonary vein (PV) isolation for treatment of atrial fibrillation is increasingly common.[24] There were early reports of PV stenosis following PV ostial RF ablation and concerns about atrioesophageal fistula following RF ablation in the left atrium.[25,26] Interestingly, the rate of intraoperative atrioesophageal perforation was as high as 1.3% in one open-chest series of patients undergoing linear lesions between PV ostia, to include the posterior wall overlaying the esophagus.[27,28] This has led to less anatomical, more functional, approaches in some centers, with the intent of avoiding extracardiac structures placed at risk by older techniques.[29,30]

The complexity of a nonanatomic approach to atrial fibrillation ablation has left many in search of alternatives allowing for PV isolation without risk of damage to extracardiac structures. One such approach may be through the use of energy-delivering balloons. By placement of the energy source in a balloon, the catheter-based balloon can be placed within the orifice of a pulmonary vein and allow for the formation of a near-circumferential lesion for pulmonary vein isolation and treatment of paroxysmal atrial fibrillation. Recent publication of the first multicenter study using an approved cryoballoon (Arctic Frost, Medtronic CryoCath, Montreal, Quebec, Canada) for treatment of paroxysmal atrial fibrillation demonstrated maintenance of sinus rhythm in greater than 70% of patients in follow-up, but of equal importance was no identified cases of pulmonary vein stenosis or esophageal injury.[31] Initial enthusiasm for an endocardial deflectable catheter-based high-intensity focused ultrasound balloon (ProRhythm, now defunct, Ronkonkoma, NY), allowing for the development of transmural linear lesions without direct tissue contact was dampened by low clinical success, and significant morbidity and mortality.[32,33] Although the patents for this technology were purchased in 2009, ProRhythm has since filed for bankruptcy, and no further clinical trials are ongoing at this time. Using endoscopic visualization, laser balloon ablation (CardioFocus, Marlborough, MA) has recently been presented at scientific forums, and initial results at acute PV isolation appear to be successful, although large-scale studies in humans are still in the planning stages.[34] Although microwave energy has been successfully used in epicardial ablation for PV isolation, the depth of the lesions has been found to be of variable consistency, and frequently not transmural; although this technology is continuing to be studied.[35–37]

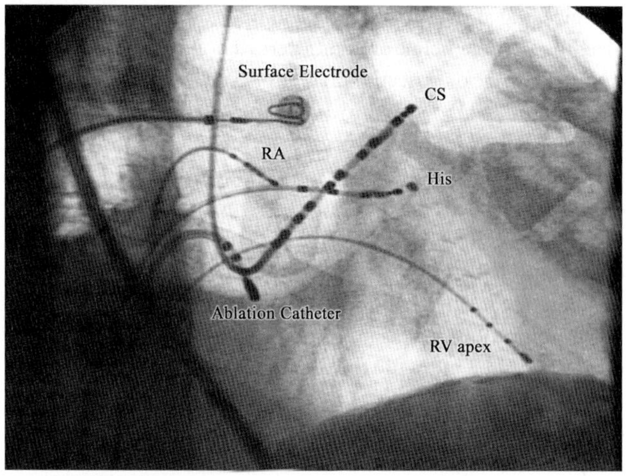

FIGURE 57-1 Radiograph in the right anterior oblique projection showing catheters positioned for a standard diagnostic electrophysiology procedure. Three nonsteerable diagnostic catheters are introduced from the inferior vena cava into the right heart. Two 4-French catheters with four electrodes are positioned in the region of the right atrial appendage (RA) and right ventricular apex (RV apex). A 5-French catheter with six electrodes is positioned across the tricuspid annulus to obtain a His bundle recording (His). A nonsteerable 6-French catheter is introduced via the right internal jugular vein into the coronary sinus (CS) to obtain left atrial and ventricular recordings. Finally, a deflatable 7-French ablation catheter is positioned in the region of the low right atrium.

ELECTROPHYSIOLOGY STUDY PROCEDURAL PROTOCOL

Diagnostic Electrophysiology Study

Diagnostic localization of tachyarrhythmias involves positioning catheters in strategic locations within the heart to obtain intracardiac recordings from all four chambers of the heart as well as from the His bundle. Venous access is typically obtained in the bilateral groins via the right and left femoral veins. Catheters of 4 to 6 French in size are passed into the right atrium and right ventricle as well as positioned just across the tricuspid valve to obtain His bundle recordings under fluoroscopic guidance. To obtain recordings of the left atrium and ventricle, a catheter is guided into the coronary sinus, which passes posteriorly in the AV groove and drains into the right atrium (Fig. 57-1).

Anticoagulation and Electrophysiology Studies

Direct recordings of the left heart are sometimes necessary and accomplished either by transseptal cannulation via the intra-atrial septum from the right atrium, or via a retrograde approach from the femoral artery and across the aortic valve. Systemic anticoagulation with heparin is maintained during catheter manipulation in the left heart because of the risk of thromboembolic events. Animal models have determined that mural thrombus is evident in up to 50% of cases immediately after RF ablation.[10,38] In addition to the risk of mural thrombus at the site of ablation, there is mounting evidence of a systemic prothrombotic condition after RF ablation.[39,40]

Once diagnostic catheters are positioned, programmed electrical stimulation is performed to induce and study the tachyarrhythmia. Sometimes modulation of the autonomic nervous system is required to induce tachyarrhythmias with the infusion of atropine or isoproterenol.[41] Once an optimal site for ablation is determined, steerable ablation catheters are positioned at the target site.

At the end of the procedure, all catheters and sheaths are removed and manual pressure held to achieve hemostasis. If the patient was heparinized for the procedure, sheath removal is delayed until anticoagulation reverses. The patient is placed on bed rest for 4 or more hours. Routine follow-up studies are not warranted unless required to assess for a complication. As mentioned, because of the risk of thromboembolic events, patients are frequently sent home on aspirin, thienopyridines, low molecular weight heparin, warfarin, or a combination of risk-appropriate antithrombotic therapies depending on the type and extent of ablation performed.

Complications Associated with Electrophysiology Studies

In referring patients for catheter ablation, it is important to weigh the risks and benefits of the procedure for the individual patient. Most tachyarrhythmias, although causing a variety of symptoms, are generally hemodynamically well tolerated and are not life threatening. Thus an awareness of the potential complications of catheter ablation is necessary before referring a patient. Complications can be divided into those involving access, catheter manipulation within the heart, and ablation.

Access-related complications include pain, adverse drug reaction from anesthesia and sedation, infection, thrombophlebitis, and bleeding at the site of access. Complications associated with bleeding include hematoma or arteriovenous fistula formation. Arterial damage or dissection may also result. Systemic or pulmonary thromboembolism can occur, most seriously resulting in transient ischemic attack or stroke. It is felt that performance of complex ablations while on systemic anticoagulation and with externally irrigated tipped catheters may reduce the risk of mural thrombus, and thereby periprocedural embolic events, there may be an increased risk of access complications in a patient with therapeutic anticoagulation.[42,43]

Complications associated with placement of intracardiac catheters can be more life threatening. These include trauma of a cardiac chamber or the coronary sinus, resulting in myocardial infarction, perforation, hemopericardium, and cardiac tamponade. Programmed electrical stimulation can result in the induction of life-threatening tachyarrhythmias such as ventricular tachycardia or fibrillation. Catheter manipulation can also result in usually transient but sometimes permanent damage to valvular apparatus or the conduction of the right or left bundle branches owing to mechanical trauma.

RF delivery within cardiac structures carries with it its own set of risks as alluded to previously. Inadvertent ablation of the normal conduction system could result in complete heart block requiring permanent pacing. Perforation of a cardiac chamber or vascular structure can also occur with RF delivery. Collateral damage to coronary circulation could result in myocardial infarction, heart failure, or cardiogenic shock. Phrenic nerve paralysis can occur. Ablation near the pulmonary veins within the left atrium can result in venous stenosis and pulmonary hypertension.

Given these risks, a center undertaking these procedures must be prepared to treat these potential complications. For example, with a higher risk of perforation, transseptal punctures should only be performed at centers with cardiac surgery programs.[44]

An 8-year prospective study of 3966 procedures found an overall complication rate of 3.1% for ablative and 1.1% for diagnostic procedures. Complications are more likely to occur in elderly patients and those with systemic disease.[45] No deaths were reported in this series and other studies have shown very low mortality rates directly attributable to the electrophysiology study.

DIAGNOSTIC ELECTROPHYSIOLOGY TECHNIQUES

A variety of techniques have been developed to elucidate the origin and mechanism of tachyarrhythmia propagation. They involve pacing in a specific chamber at particular intervals to initiate a tachyarrhythmia, assess its response to pacing maneuvers, or terminate it.[46] Thus some of these techniques involve pacing in sinus rhythm, whereas others are performed during the tachyarrhythmia.

Activation mapping involves positioning the mapping catheter during the tachyarrhythmia such that the catheter electrode tip precedes any other intracardiac activation or corresponding surface P wave or QRS. The earliest site of activation during a focal tachycardia must by definition be the source of the tachycardia.[47,48] This can be used for focal tachycardias or accessory pathways.

Pace mapping is performed during sinus rhythm, and by pacing at different sites one can compare the paced ECG to the tachycardia ECG, the disparity can be assessed and the catheter can be repositioned until a match is obtained.[49] This technique is typically used for focal ventricular tachycardias, especially those of right ventricular outflow origin.[50]

Anatomical mapping is yet another way to localize potential targets for ablation by using fluoroscopy to localize anatomical landmarks for ablation. In typical cavotricuspid isthmus-dependent flutter, anatomical landmarks are used for the delivery of a line of lesions to prevent conduction across this isthmus.[51]

In clinical situations a combination of these mapping techniques is used to localize an arrhythmia for ablation.

Advanced Mapping Techniques

The success of ablation is dependent on localization of arrhythmogenic foci and circuits. The previously mentioned mapping techniques are useful for arrhythmias that originate from specific anatomical locations or have characteristic endocardial electrograms. Advanced mapping techniques have been developed as adjuncts to conventional methods to improve the efficacy of catheter ablation for arrhythmias that are transient, focal, or hemodynamically unstable and thus require rapid mapping.

An electroanatomical mapping system (CARTO, Biosense-Webster, Diamond Bar, CA) uses a magnetic field to localize the mapping catheter tip in three-dimensional space. Three coils in a locator pad located beneath the patient's chest generate ultra-low-intensity magnetic fields in the form of a sphere that decays in strength. A sensor in the catheter tip measures the relative strength and hence the distance from each of the coils. This allows for the recording of the spatial and temporal location of the catheter. Electrodes at the catheter tip record local electrograms, and this information is displayed on screen as a three-dimensional map of the local activation times relative to a reference catheter in a color-coded fashion. Data from multiple single mapping points acquired during tachycardia can be reconstructed to show animated sequences of arrhythmia propagation. Voltage maps can be obtained to delineate regions of scar and diseased myocardium.[52] The CARTO system supports the ThermaCool externally irrigated RF ablation catheters, as the only FDA-approved catheters for treatment of atrial fibrillation.

A similar endocardial mapping system (EnSite NavX, St. Jude Medical, St. Paul, MN) consists of a catheter with a woven braid of 64 insulated 0.003-mm–diameter wires with 0.025-mm breaks in the insulation that serve as electrodes. A locator signal is generated between the array and a standard mapping catheter to permit nonfluoroscopic localization of the catheter to regions of interest. This system is very useful for mapping in unstable or transient, nonsustained arrhythmias.[53]

Radial array intravascular ultrasound (IVUS) (9 MHz Ultra ICE, Boston-Scientific, Natick, MA) allows clear visualization of the atrial septum, and enhances the safety of transseptal punctures. Phased array intracardiac echocardiography (ICE) has extended the principles of IVUS for electrophysiologic use.[54] Newer ICE catheters are steerable and have Doppler capability (Acuson, AcuNav, Mountain View, CA), allowing for hemodynamic evaluation of intracardiac structures. ICE catheters allow the accurate targeting of anatomical sites such as the crista terminalis and pulmonary vein ostia.[55] They are useful for imaging diagnostic and ablation catheter positions and visualization of tissue contact for optimal ablation. Additional benefit to ICE is integration with electroanatomical mapping systems to allow for noncontact real-time reconstruction of cardiac structures (CartoSound, Biosense-Webster, Diamond Bar, CA).

CLINICAL APPLICATIONS

Using the techniques described in the preceding, a variety of tachyarrhythmias can be targeted for percutaneous catheter-based ablation, including both atrial and ventricular arrhythmias that are either focal or that use re-entrant circuits.

Atrioventricular Nodal Re-entrant Tachycardia

Of patients with SVT, AVNRT represents up to 60% of cases that present to tertiary centers for electrophysiologic studies. This tachycardia can present at any age, although most patients who present for medical attention are in their forties and the majority are female.[56,57] Advances in RF catheter ablation of this tachycardia has made it a first-line therapy for those symptomatic patients not wishing to take medications.[58]

This tachycardia has a re-entrant mechanism using two pathways within the AV nodal tissue. The pathways are known as the "slow pathway" and "fast pathway" based on their relative conduction velocities. The anatomical location of these pathways is variable but generally located within the triangle of Koch. The Koch triangle is bounded by the tricuspid annulus and the tendon of Todaro with the coronary sinus at the base. The apex of the triangle is the His bundle at the membranous septum where it passes through the central fibrous body. The anterior third of the triangle contains the compact AV node and the fast pathway, and the middle and posterior portion, near the coronary sinus os, contains the slow pathway (Fig. 57-2).[59]

In the typical form of AVNRT, antegrade conduction from the atrium to the ventricle occurs over the slow pathway, and the retrograde conduction from the ventricle to the atrium occurs over the fast pathway. Because conduction in the retrograde direction is fast, the atria and ventricle are depolarized almost simultaneously. Thus the electrocardiographic feature of this tachycardia is P waves that are inscribed within the QRS and thus not seen or barely discernible at the termination of the QRS complex.[60]

In fewer than 10% of cases, the circuit is reversed. In *atypical* AVNRT, antegrade conduction occurs over the fast pathway and retrograde conduction occurs over the slow pathway. Thus the ECG of this tachycardia shows inverted P waves in the inferior leads denoting retrograde activation of the atria with short PR segment owing to rapid antegrade conduction.[61]

Slow pathway ablation has a high degree of success with a recurrence rate in the range of 2 to 7%, with the complication of complete AV block occurring about 1% (range 0 to 3%) of the time.[62] The North American Society of Pacing and Electrophysiology (NASPE) self-reported surveys on 4249 patients who underwent slow pathway ablations had

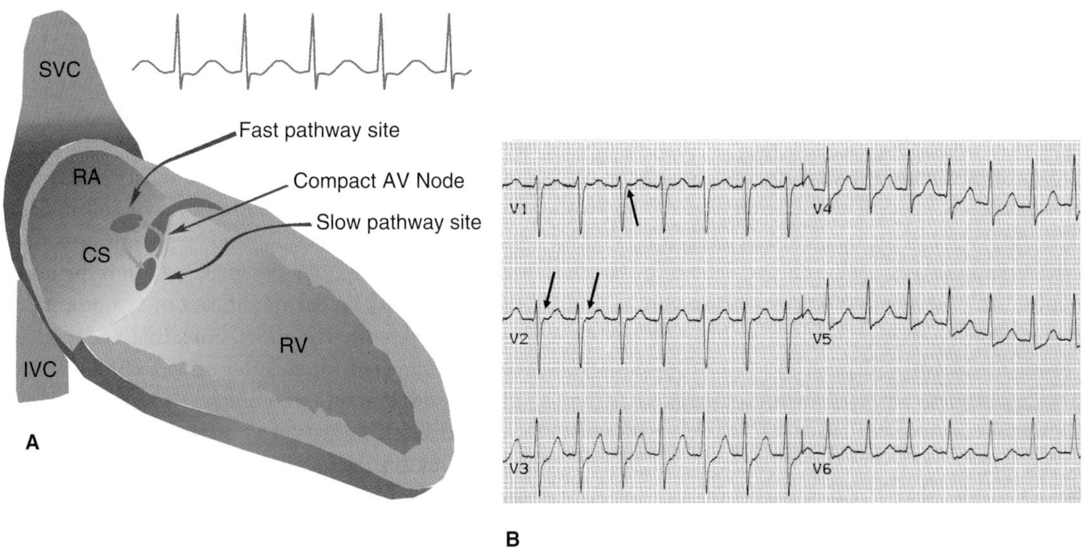

FIGURE 57-2 (A) Diagrammatic representation of typical atrioventricular nodal re-entrant tachycardia. Surface ECG shows narrow complex tachycardia with no clear P waves. The re-entrant circuit (*blue arrows*) consists of the posterior slow pathway region acting as the antegrade limb, and the anterior fast pathway region acting as the retrograde limb. The slow pathway target site is located between the coronary sinus os (CS) and the tricuspid valve annulus (TV). IVC = inferior vena cava; RA = right atrium; RV = right ventricle; SVC = superior vena cava. (B) Surface ECG showing precordial leads in AVNRT. This demonstrates that the retrograde P waves are barely discernible in some leads. In V_1, it forms a pseudo r′ wave (*arrow*). P waves are also visible in the terminal portions of QRS complexes in V_2 and V_3 but not in the lateral leads.

success rates of greater than 96% and complication rates of less than 1%.[63,64]

Atrioventricular Re-entrant Tachycardia

About 30% of SVTs are caused by AVRT. This is a re-entrant tachycardia using the AV node and an accessory pathway (AP). These APs are remnants of conductive tissue from embryonic development that span the normally electrically inert tricuspid and mitral valve annulus and provide an independent path of conduction outside the AV node between the atria and the ventricles. The most common form of AVRT is part of the Wolff-Parkinson-White (WPW) syndrome of ventricular pre(mature)-excitation and symptomatic arrhythmias. The most common APs connect the atrium to the ventricle. Other APs may connect the atria or AV node to the His-Purkinje system. In sinus rhythm, antegrade conduction over the AP results in pre-excitation of the ventricles through conduction by other than the AV node, and is manifested by a short PR segment and slurring of the onset of the QRS, the delta wave. Absence of these findings does not exclude an AP, as the degree of pre-excitation may vary or conduction may only occur in the retrograde direction (~30% of APs).

Patients with WPW typically present with palpitations caused by rapid heart rate. This may be the result of AVRT or any SVT with resulting rapid AV conduction via the AP. Associated symptoms may be mild such as palpitations and shortness of breath, or as severe as syncope and sudden death.[65,66] Sudden death may be caused by ventricular fibrillation resulting from the extremely rapid ventricular activation over the AP during atrial fibrillation in some patients.

Indications for ablation of APs include patients with symptomatic AVRT or those with atrial tachyarrhythmias with rapid ventricular conduction who fail or do not wish to undergo medical therapy.[65] Relative indications for ablations include asymptomatic patients in high-risk professions, those with family history of sudden death, or those mentally distraught over their condition.[67]

In the typical or orthodromic form of AVRT, antegrade conduction from the atrium to the ventricle occurs over the AV node and retrograde conduction occurs over the AP. In this form of AVRT, the P wave in the tachycardia closely follows the preceding QRS complex with a long PR segment (Fig. 57-3). In the rare antidromic form of AVRT, antegrade conduction occurs over the AP with retrograde conduction over the AV node. This results in eccentric depolarization of the ventricle, producing a wide complex tachycardia with retrograde P waves that can be easily mistaken for ventricular tachycardia with one-to-one ventriculoatrial conduction.

The major challenge that remains is the ablation of APs near the normal conduction system and those that are epicardial in location. Ablation of pathways that are anteroseptal and midseptal in location carries a high risk of causing complete heart block. It is hoped that newer ablative energy sources such as cryoablation, although found to be effective, may offer a safer alternative.[22,68,69] The 1998 NASPE prospective catheter ablation registry reported on 654 patients with a 94% success rate.[64] Success rates are lower (in the range of 84 to 88%) for septal and right free wall pathways. Other pathways have success rates in the range of 90 to 95%.[70–72] Mortality rates are less than 1% and nonfatal complications are about 4%.[64]

Atrial Tachycardia

Atrial tachycardias depend wholly on atrial tissue for initiation and maintenance of the tachycardia. Ectopic atrial tachycardia, sinoatrial nodal re-entrant tachycardia, inappropriate sinus tachycardia, atrial flutter, and atrial fibrillation can all be considered atrial tachycardias. Focal atrial tachycardias, a less common type of SVT, form about 10% of all SVTs referred for electrophysiologic studies.[67] Multifocal atrial tachycardia is caused by multiple foci of abnormal automaticity or triggered activity and is not amenable to curative catheter ablation.[73]

These arrhythmias are more common in patients with structural heart disease. Indications for ablation include failure or intolerance of medical therapy. Rarely, incessant tachycardias can lead to cardiomyopathy. With ablation and control of heart rate, myocardial dysfunction can be reversed, although there may be a delayed risk of sudden death that necessitates use of a defibrillator.[74–76]

Surface ECG features of atrial tachycardia include abnormal P-wave morphology or axes that are close to the following QRS complexes. Mapping and ablation of atrial tachycardias can be more difficult, as they can originate from anywhere within the right or left atrium. But there are specific anatomical regions that have a high incidence of foci and serve as primary targets. They include the crista terminalis, atrial appendages, valve annulus, and pulmonary ostia.[77]

Inappropriate sinus tachycardia and sinoatrial nodal re-entry tachycardias occur more infrequently and experience with catheter ablation of these tachycardias is more limited. Inappropriate sinus tachycardia is also difficult to ablate because of the variability and diffuse location of sinoatrial tissue.[78] Catheter ablation should be reserved, and considered as one small part of a multidisciplinary approach, to include cardiovascular, endocrinologic, and psychiatric evaluation and pharmacologic management.[79] Catheter ablation may result in complete loss of sinoatrial node function and resulting junctional rhythm, requiring insertion of a pacemaker. Even if the resting heart rate is reduced with nodal modification, symptoms may continue with episodes of tachycardia. Sinoatrial nodal re-entrant tachycardia is targeted for ablation using techniques similar to those used for other atrial tachycardias.

Success with ablation of atrial tachycardia is quite variable depending on the location of the arrhythmogenic foci and the experience of the operator. The 1998 NASPE survey showed a success rate of 80% for right-sided versus 72% for left-sided versus 52% for septal foci in 216 cases of atrial tachycardia ablation.[64] Another large review examined the frequency of arrhythmias as a predictor of success. In 105 patients, the overall initial success rate was 77%, and 10% had recurrence over a 33-month follow-up period. There was an 88% success rate for the paroxysmal form versus 71% for permanent and 41% for repetitive forms of atrial tachycardia.[80]

A

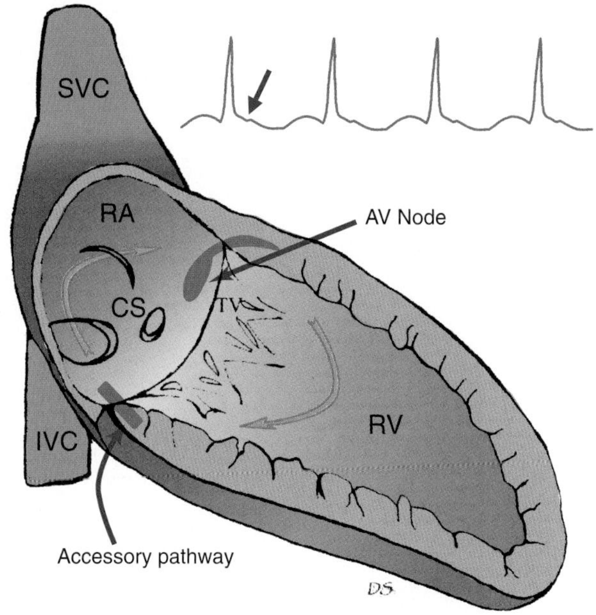

B

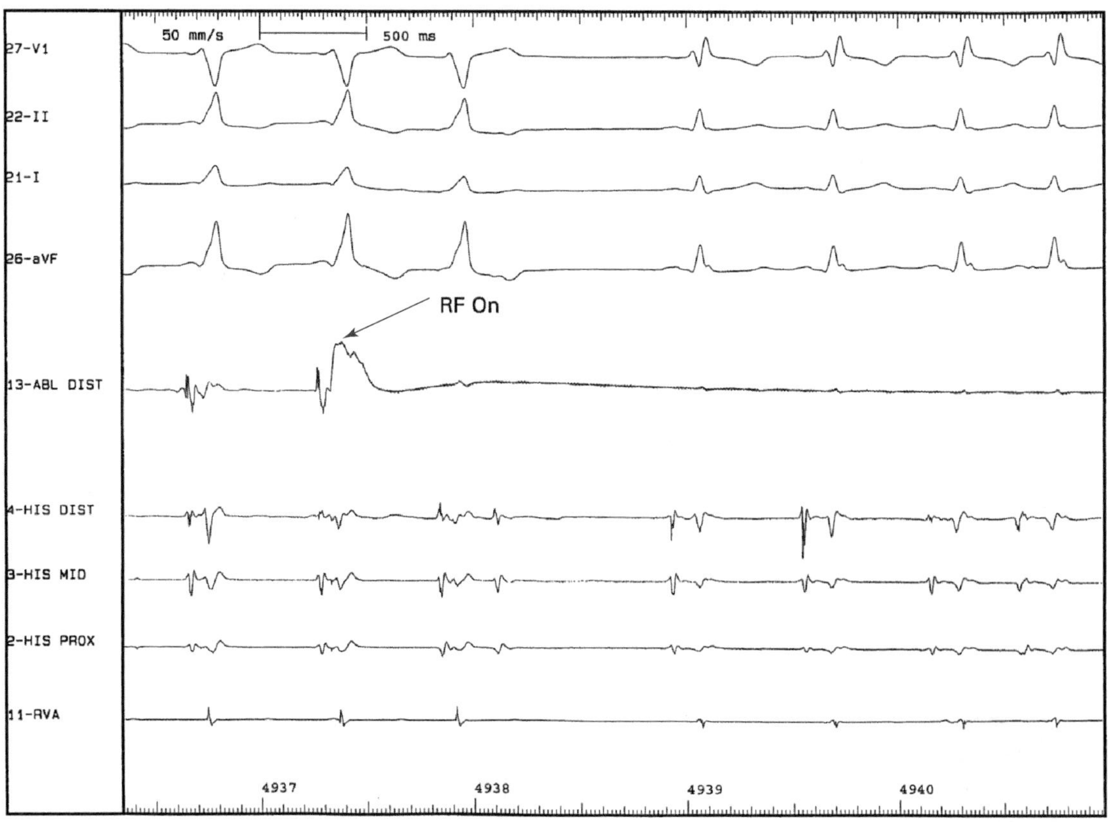

FIGURE 57-3 (A) Diagrammatic representation of atrioventricular re-entrant tachycardia. This macro re-entrant circuit (*gray arrows*) uses the AV node and an accessory pathway (AP), in this case a right lateral pathway. In orthodromic AVRT, antegrade conduction occurs over the AV node and retrograde conduction occurs over the AP. Because of the conduction delay from the His-Purkinje system through the ventricular myocardium to reach the AP, retrograde P waves are discernible after the QRS complexes (*arrow*). In antidromic AVRT, the re-entrant circuit is reversed and surface ECG shows P waves that closely precede the QRS complexes. CS = coronary sinus; IVC = inferior vena cava; RA = right atrium; RV = right ventricle; SVC = superior vena cava; TV = tricuspid valve. (B) Intracardiac recording of atrioventricular re-entrant tachycardia with termination of eccentric conduction over the accessory pathway during RF ablation. The tracing at 50-mm-per-second speed shows four surface leads (VI, II, I, and aVF) and intracardiac recording from catheters:ablation (ABL); His distal, mid, and proximal; as well as right ventricular apex (RVA). The first three beats of the tracing show evidence of eccentric conduction over an accessory pathway: short PR segment and delta wave. With onset of RF energy (RF On) from the ablation catheter positioned in the region of shortest AV conduction, conduction becomes normal within two beats, with normalization of the PR segment and loss of the delta wave.

Atrial Flutter

Atrial flutter is a type of atrial tachycardia that uses a macro re-entrant circuit contained within the atria. A variety of natural and surgical barriers to conduction can create a re-entrant circuit within the atria. Typical atrial flutter is owing to a right atrial circuit, bound anteriorly by the tricuspid valve (TV) annulus. Posteriorly, it is confined by the superior vena cava, crista terminalis, inferior vena cava (IVC), eustachian ridge, and coronary sinus (CS)[81] (Fig. 57-4).

In the typical and more common form of atrial flutter, the circuit transverses the right atrium in a counterclockwise manner in the frontal plane. Because the anatomy of the right atrium is elongated in a caudad-cephalad direction, a typical atrial flutter spends large portions of circuit activation going either directly away, or directly toward the inferior leads; therefore, in leads II, III and a VF, the P waves are negative and have a sawtooth appearance. In V_1, the P wave is usually upright and in V_6 it is inverted. Clockwise flutter uses the same circuit but in a reversed manner. The ECG also shows a reversed pattern. In the inferior leads the P waves are upright, with inverted P waves in V_1 and upright in V_6. This surface ECG morphology is suggestive of the circuit but needs intracardiac confirmation.[82] These two forms of atrial flutter have been termed *isthmus dependent* because of the use of the IVC-tricuspid annular isthmus.

A macro re-entrant circuit can be cured by lesions that transect the circuit between two anatomical barriers. In the case of isthmus-dependent flutter, the target for ablation is the isthmus between the IVC and TV. Success rates for ablation of this form of atrial flutter are high. Given high success rates, ablation has become the first line of therapy for recurrent isthmus-dependent atrial flutter. Despite successful treatment of flutter, nearly one-quarter of patients developed de novo atrial fibrillation during chronic follow-up.[83]

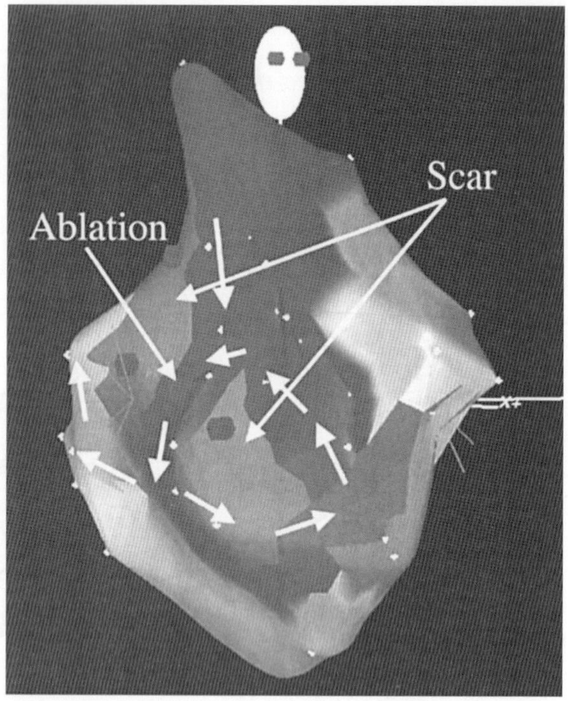

FIGURE 57-5 An electroanatomic map of a patient with left atrial flutter is shown in the right anterior oblique projection. Two large areas of scar can be seen in gray. Gradation in color shows activation sequence, with lighter being the earliest and darker being late in relation to a reference catheter, in this case positioned in the coronary sinus. The circulating wavefronts describe a figure-eight pattern around these two areas of scar but are confined by the narrow region (isthmus) between them. Ablation in the isthmus resulted in termination of the flutter.

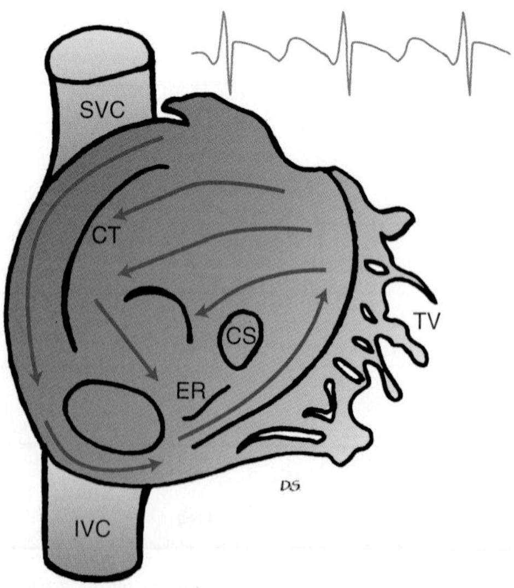

FIGURE 57-4 Diagrammatic representation of typical or counterclockwise right atrial flutter. Surface ECG shows large inverted P waves in the inferior leads. Lead III above shows 2:1 AV conduction with "sawtooth" flutter waves. The re-entrant circuit (*gray arrows*) is confined to the right atrium by the tricuspid valve annulus (TV) and barriers to conduction within the right atrium. These include the superior vena cava (SVC), crista terminalis (CT), inferior vena cava (IVC), eustachian ridge (ER), and coronary sinus (CS). The isthmus between the IVC and TV is the preferred target for ablation.

Although the right atrial circuit described in the preceding is the most common, a variety of other circuits in the right and left atria are possible. These are more common in patients with underlying heart disease, or in those having previously undergone pulmonary vein ablation or surgical management of atrial arrhythmia.[55,84–86] Although initially thought not to be amenable to ablative therapy, mapping and ablation of these arrhythmias are now routinely performed. However, the success rate is somewhat lower than that for typical isthmus-dependent atrial flutter. An electroanatomical map of a patient with left atrial flutter can be seen in Fig. 57-5. Ablation in the isthmus between these scars resulted in termination of the flutter.

Surgical Scar-Related Atrial Arrhythmias

As mentioned, incisional scars from prior cardiac surgery can be the substrate for re-entrant atrial arrhythmias.[87–89] The most common is an atypical atrial flutter related to a lateral right atrial incision. Mapping demonstrates a circuit circling the incision. Ablation from the end of the incision to either the superior vena cava or more commonly the inferior vena cava is often curative.[90]

It had been thought that there was conduction block between the donor and recipient atria in patients who have undergone heart transplantation. Recent reports have demonstrated re-entrant arrhythmias owing to donor–recipient atrial conduction. Mapping the connection between the atria can successfully ablate these arrhythmias.[91–93] Atrial arrhythmias have also been reported in a number of patients who have undergone the surgical Maze procedure for atrial fibrillation. These treatment failures are most often caused by re-entrant circuits involving gaps in the Maze lesion or through alternative pathways such as the musculature surrounding the coronary sinus.[94] These arrhythmias can now be successfully mapped and ablated. Mapping systems are useful in improving success of these ablations. The principle of interrupting these circuits by placing lesions to connect conduction barriers remains the same.[95]

Atrial Fibrillation

Atrial fibrillation is another difficult-to-treat atrial tachycardia with variable targets for ablation. Atrial fibrillation is often symptomatic for patients owing to irregular and/or rapid ventricular rates. Patients can also be completely asymptomatic and present with stroke, dilated cardiomyopathy, or be diagnosed on routine examination. Medical therapy for atrial fibrillation is of limited efficacy and pharmacologic control of atrial fibrillation may be associated with increased mortality in large trials.[96–99] In addition, sustained rapid ventricular rates can lead to a tachycardia-related cardiomyopathy.[76,80] When medical therapy is aimed at maintaining sinus rhythm or blocking AV nodal conduction to slow ventricular response fails, ablation can be considered.[100,101]

In the past, AV nodal or His ablation, with placement of a permanent pacemaker, was considered in patients with difficult-to-control ventricular rates and symptomatic palpitations. The advantages of the approach are the relative ease and speed of the procedure. The downside is that it renders the patient pacemaker-dependent. Success rates of this procedure are nearly 100%.[102] Complications of this procedure include the same complications as those seen in other ablation procedures. In highly symptomatic patients, this approach to the treatment of atrial fibrillation has been associated with improvement in quality of life and left ventricular function, and with a reduction in hospitalizations.[103] Patients with congestive heart failure and atrial fibrillation may particularly benefit from this approach, and in some cases restoration of function will return as tachycardia slows, but in many cases it may be more beneficial to proceed directly with implantation of a cardiac resynchronization device, even in the setting of only minimally symptomatic ventricular dysfunction.[104–106]

Surgical experience with the Maze procedure to create lines of conduction block in the atrium has led the way for catheter-based ablation procedures to treat atrial fibrillation. Studies have attempted to replicate the success of the surgical procedure using a catheter-based approach. Atrial fibrillation consists of multiple re-entrant circuits within the atrium; around the vena cava, pulmonary veins, and appendages; and around areas of functional block.[107] Creation of multiple lines of block between these nonconducting structures may prevent propagation of arrhythmic circuits.

Attempts at catheter-based left atrial or biatrial lesions for purpose of replicating the Maze have met with limited success because of the prolonged procedure times, high risk of complications, and limited efficacy.[108,109] As understanding of the mechanism of atrial fibrillation has evolved, attempts to block propagation of atrial fibrillatory circuits have been abandoned in favor of attempted ablation of the fibrillatory triggers.

In a series of patients undergoing a left-sided catheter Maze procedure, it was discovered that rapidly firing premature atrial contractions arising from the musculature of the pulmonary veins were triggering atrial fibrillation.[110] Ablation of these foci eliminated atrial fibrillation in some patients. This procedure has evolved to empiric electrical isolation of the pulmonary veins. One approach is the complete encircling of the pulmonary veins (ie, wide area circumferential ablation).[111] Another approach is segmental isolation of each vein by mapping the location of the connecting fibers.[112] The encircling and nonencircling procedures have shown to be equally efficacious in 6-month follow-up. The advantage to the nonencircling method, whereby the focus is on pulmonary vein exit block, is the ability to avoid a posterior wall line. The placement of posterior wall lines is thought to be responsible for the finding of atrioesophageal fistula postoperatively.

Data on the long-term efficacy and complications of this procedure are limited and it is still considered to be a procedure in evolution. In one series of 251 patients, the short-term success was 80%. There was an 85% success rate in those with paroxysmal and 68% success in those with permanent atrial fibrillation. There was a continued need for antiarrhythmic medications in some patients.[113] In a study of those with paroxysmal atrial fibrillation, randomized therapy comparing medical management to catheter ablation has shown significant results. The A4 trial showed at 1-year, 23% of those randomized to antiarrhythmic drug therapy, and 89% of those randomized to ablation had no recurrence of atrial fibrillation.[114] A recent meta-analysis of PV isolation for paroxysmal atrial fibrillation versus medical management found that at 1 year, ablation was associated with a 16-fold rate of freedom from atrial fibrillation (odds ratio, 15.78; 95% CI, 10.07 to 24.73) and with decreased hospitalization for cardiovascular causes (rate ratio, 0.15; 95% CI, 0.10 to 0.23).[115]

Although the procedure itself has been demonstrated to be effective, the method for optimizing outcomes is still in evolution. This is in part because of the mechanistic shift that goes from predominant PV triggers in those with paroxysmal atrial fibrillation, to a diseased atrium, manifest by complex fractionated atrial electrograms (CFAE) in those with persistent atrial fibrillation.[29] In randomized trials, the addition of targeting of CFAE, to a conventional PV antral isolation did not result in increased freedom from recurrent arrhythmia.[116,117] In a three-arm study, patients with paroxysmal atrial fibrillation were randomized to PV isolation, substrate modification targeting CFAE, or a combination of the two. At 1-year follow-up, freedom from AF/atrial tachyarrhythmia was documented in 89% of patients in the PV antral isolation group, 91% in the PV antral isolation plus CFAE group, and 23% in the group undergoing

CFAE modification alone.[118] In a study comparing the efficacy of adding linear lesions to PV antral isolation, a group was able to demonstrate increased maintenance of sinus rhythm in those with atrial fibrillation, although the results were much more apparent in those with persistent atrial fibrillation at baseline.[119] Those with a more permanent form of atrial fibrillation have been demonstrated to have either atrial scarring or structural disease in 65%.[120] Despite prior failure of antiarrhythmic therapy, long-term restoration of sinus rhythm could be seen in up to 94% of those patients after two procedures and while on antiarrhythmic drugs having undergone targeting of CFAE and PV antral isolation, whereby PV antral isolation alone had success in only 83% ($p < .001$).[120] The role of antral or ostial isolation appears to favor antral isolation, both for reduction in pulmonary vein stenosis, and for efficacy. In one randomized trial of single procedure without drug therapy, the freedom from AF was 49% in those with single vein lasso-guided isolation, compared with 67% in those undergoing antral isolation of ipsilateral vein groupings ($p \leq 0.05$).[121]

In a retrospective study comparing PV antral isolation versus AV node ablation and pacemaker implantation, the definitive rate control strategy was a shorter procedure and with fewer complications, and although there was higher rate of continued, albeit asymptomatic, atrial fibrillation, the procedure may be advocated for the older patient, or those with comorbidities, which may limit the procedural safety.[114]

One major complication of ablation *within* the pulmonary veins was focal pulmonary vein stenosis. In 102 patients undergoing pulmonary vein focal ablation, 39% with right upper vein ablation and 23% with left vein ablation developed focal pulmonary vein stenosis by transesophageal echocardiography 3 days after the procedure.[122] In this series, only three patients experienced symptoms of dyspnea on exertion and only one had a mild increase in pulmonary pressure. Although most cases are asymptomatic, severe cases have been reported that progress to pulmonary hypertension and lung transplant. Changes to prevent this complication include limiting ablation within the vein ostia, limiting power, and using ultrasound imaging during ablation.[123] Since its recognition as a possible adverse event, the occurrence postprocedurally should now be considered rare.

Ventricular Tachycardia

Ablation techniques can also target ventricular tachycardia (VT). Greater than 90% of life-threatening ventricular arrhythmias originate from myocardium with structural abnormalities. Regions of scarred or aneurysmal myocardium create channels for re-entrant circuits. Initial successes with resection of ventricular arrhythmogenic foci and re-entrant circuits surgically have led to advancements in catheter-based ablation techniques. Given the life-threatening potential of VT in patients with structural heart disease, even a single recurrence can be disastrous. Therefore, implantable cardiac defibrillators have become the primary therapy. Indications for ablation in this population are failure of antiarrhythmic medication to suppress symptomatic, sustained monomorphic VT, or more often frequent shocks from an implanted defibrillator despite optimal medical therapy.

Success of ischemic VT ablation is variable because of the heterogeneity of the population. Reported studies have shown efficacy in the range of 60 to 90% using the criteria of reduced defibrillator shocks and decreased need for antiarrhythmic medications. The recurrence rate is as high as 40%. Recently, success has been reported with an approach employing "substrate mapping." This technique defines the potential arrhythmic substrate using electroanatomical voltage maps. Ablation is targeted to eliminate potential re-entrant circuits. Complications are in the range of 2%, with concern for perforation and cardiac tamponade owing to the thin, scarred ventricles that are the substrates for ablation and thromboembolic events in those undergoing extensive ablation.[124–128]

In patients with dilated cardiomyopathy and His-Purkinje system disease, sustained monomorphic VT can occur because of a macro re-entrant circuit using the bundle branches. Patients typically present with syncope or sudden death or can present with palpitations. The most common circuit is down the right bundle branch and up the left bundle branch resulting in a wide complex tachycardia with a left bundle-branch block pattern. Treatment involves ablation of one of the fascicles involved in the re-entrant circuit. The right bundle is most commonly targeted to interrupt the re-entrant circuit. Long-term success is good for prevention of recurrent bundle branch re-entry. Because of intrinsic conduction disease, patients may develop heart block. Patients may also develop other VTs because of other structural abnormalities, requiring further ablation, antiarrhythmic therapy, or defibrillator implantation.[129,130]

Other cardiac disorders can be associated with VT and are potential candidates for catheter ablation. These include right ventricular dysplasia,[131] infiltrative disorders (sarcoid),[132,133] and tumors. As in patients with atrial arrhythmias caused by surgical incisions, patients with prior ventricular surgery can develop incision-related VT. This has occurred most often in patients who have undergone repair of congenital abnormalities such as tetralogy of Fallot,[134] but has also been seen in patients after corrective valve surgery.[135]

Ventricular tachycardia that presents in patients with no structural heart disease is termed *idiopathic* and represents up to 10% of all VTs that present to tertiary referral centers. Patients may be asymptomatic or present with palpitations, dizziness, or syncope. Idiopathic VT may be focal or a micro–re-entrant circuit using the Purkinje fibers.

Right ventricular tachycardia typically originates from the outflow tract. It has typical left bundle-branch QRS morphology with leftward, inferior axis. This occurs more often in women than men, and patients typically present in their thirties to fifties. Idiopathic left ventricular tachycardia typically originates from the left posterior fascicle. It has a right bundle-branch morphology with rightward, superior axis, and may be verapamil sensitive. It occurs more often in men. These VTs are localized by activation or pace mapping. Ablation is facilitated by the lack of other cardiac pathology and the presence of only one VT. Success rates for idiopathic VT are in the range of 70 to 90% with recurrence rates in the range of 15%. Complication rates are consistent with those of other ablative procedures.[136,137]

Cost-Effectiveness

Several studies have shown the cost-effectiveness of catheter ablation compared with medical therapy and surgical ablation. Catheter ablation has lower procedural costs than surgical ablation and reduces the need for further medical care and emergency department visits in comparison to drug therapy. Studies from the United States, Canada, the United Kingdom, and from Australia have shown both cost savings and improvement in quality of life for those undergoing catheter-based ablation compared to medical management.[138–142]

Of particular concern, is cost-effectiveness of catheter ablation for the treatment of atrial fibrillation. In a United States model looking at catheter ablation versus antiarrhythmic drugs for paroxysmal atrial fibrillation, although incremental cost-effectiveness for ablation was demonstrated to be only marginally favorable at $51,431 per quality adjusted life year over 5 years, there was no adjustment for known favorable effect on heart failure admissions, a not insignificant additional savings.[143] In a Canadian model, although results demonstrated cost savings with antiarrhythmic drug therapy from 2 months to 1 year, the sustained benefit of ablation quickly led to demonstrable cost-savings within 2 years from time of ablation, and anticipated sustained benefit.[138] One particular United Kingdom assessment found that for treatment of paroxysmal atrial fibrillation, catheter ablation had economic benefit compared to antiarrhythmic drug therapy alone with or without serial cardioversion.[144] Of particular note was cost savings for catheter ablation in combination with antiarrhythmic drug therapy compared to drug therapy alone, in large part driven by reduction in healthcare utilization rather than the mere cost of the drug itself.

FUTURE DIRECTIONS

In an era of unprecedented growth of the use of catheter ablation, the safety to the provider has been brought to light. Cognizant that a plain film radiograph exposes the subject to approximately 0.1 milliSievert (mSv), and a CT of the chest from 1 to 3 mSv, early cardiac fluoroscopic systems exposed busy operators to up to 300 mSv monthly.[145] With implementation of better shielded systems and better clinical practice, the exposure to the operator under a lead apron has been reduced to less than 2 mSv annually.[145] Unfortunately, the combination of prolonged standing next to the patient, and subsequent need for wear of a lead aprons, is associated with a significant risk of orthopedic health problems in invasive cardiologists, most notably spine (42%) and lower extremity (28%) complaints.[146–148] Newer technologies have focused on enhancing the safety to the invasive electrophysiologist.

The Niobe system (Stereotaxis, Inc., St. Louis, MO) is a remote magnetic navigation system that uses two externally located magnets to create a steerable field (0.08 to 0.1 T, conventional MRI 1.5 to 3.0 T) that can be used to affect the magnetically active atraumatic catheter tip (Magnetic GentleTouch Catheters, Stereotaxis). For advancing and retracting, the unit can be completely controlled remotely through a small motor. The entire system can be controlled from a shielded room by joystick and touch-screen monitors to allow for catheter manipulation through hands-free robotic catheter control. For atrial fibrillation ablation, the clinical results from remote magnetic navigation have yet to demonstrate superiority over manual operation, with frequent crossover to manual ablation to ensure PV isolation, but a persistent reduction in operator exposure to fluoroscopy.[149,150]

A robotic catheter system, Sensei (Hansen Medical, Mountain View, CA) allows catheter manipulation from a control room using a mechanical steering outer sheath through which a conventional catheter is inserted. Like magnetic navigation, the results with atrial fibrillation appear to be promising, with similar clinical outcomes, shorter procedural times and reduced fluoroscopy exposure to the operator.[151–153]

One novel technology in development is the use of interventional magnetic resonance (iMR) imaging using MR compatible non-ferromagnetic carbon-based catheters and equipment. Although feasibility in the animal model is still being evaluated, this would allow high-resolution three-dimensional mapping of the heart and localization of catheters in three-dimensional space in real time without radiation to patient or staff.[154,155] Magnetic resonance imaging would also allow for the visualization of any tissue injury owing to attempted ablation in real time.

CONCLUSION

The past 35 years have seen the development of intracardiac recording, programmed stimulation, and catheter ablation. The field of interventional electrophysiology is still young. Over the past two decades, and indeed over the last few years, great advances have been seen in the interventional management of arrhythmia. Where the surgeons have gone with their scalpels, electrophysiologists have followed with their catheters. Transvenous RF ablation, once the standard of care for the treatment of many arrhythmias, may be phased out in preference of alternative energy sources. These procedures have been proved to be safe and efficacious. Improved treatments for arrhythmias such as atrial fibrillation and VT will come with further understanding of the mechanisms underlying these arrhythmias. Future advances in catheter design, energy delivery, and imaging techniques will continue to advance the field of electrophysiology.

REFERENCES

1. Durrer D, Schoo L, Schuilenburg RM, Wellens HJ: The role of premature beats in the initiation and the termination of supraventricular tachycardia in the Wolff-Parkinson-White syndrome. *Circulation* 1967; 36: 644-662.
2. Scherlag BJ, Lau SH, Helfant RH, et al: Catheter technique for recording His bundle activity in man. *Circulation* 1969; 39:13-18.
3. Cobb FR, Blumenschein SD, Sealy WC, et al: Successful surgical interruption of the bundle of Kent in a patient with Wolff-Parkinson-White syndrome. *Circulation* 1968; 38:1018-1029.
4. Coumel P, Aigueperse J, Perrault MA, et al: Detection and attempted surgical exeresis of a left auricular ectopic focus with refractory tachycardia. Favorable outcome. *Ann Cardiol Angeiol (Paris)* 1973; 22:189-199.
5. Pritchett EL, Anderson RW, Benditt DG, et al: Reentry within the atrioventricular node: surgical cure with preservation of atrioventricular conduction. *Circulation* 1979; 60:440-446.

6. Gonzalez R, Scheinman M, Margaretten W, Rubinstein M: Closed-chest electrode-catheter technique for His bundle ablation in dogs. *Am J Physiol* 1981; 241:H283-287.
7. Scheinman MM, Morady F, Hess DS, Gonzalez R: Catheter-induced ablation of the atrioventricular junction to control refractory supraventricular arrhythmias. *JAMA* 1982; 248:851-855.
8. Gallagher JJ, Svenson RH, Kasell JH, et al: Catheter technique for closed-chest ablation of the atrioventricular conduction system. *NEJM* 1982; 306:194-200.
9. Weber H, Schmitz L, Dische R, Rahlf G: Percutaneous intracardiac direct-current shocks in dogs: arrhythmogenic potential and pathological changes. *Eur Heart J* 1986; 7:528-537.
10. Huang SK, Bharati S, Graham AR, et al: Closed chest catheter desiccation of the atrioventricular junction using radiofrequency energy—a new method of catheter ablation. *J Am Coll Cardiol* 1987; 9:349-358.
11. Haines D. Biophysics of ablation: application to technology. *J Cardiovasc Electrophysiol* 2004; 15:S2-S11.
12. Nath S, DiMarco JP, Haines DE: Basic aspects of radiofrequency catheter ablation. *J Cardiovasc Electrophysiol* 1994; 5:863-876.
13. Comas GM, Imren Y, Williams MR: An overview of energy sources in clinical use for the ablation of atrial fibrillation. *Semin Thorac Cardiovasc Surg* 2007; 19:16-24.
14. Nath S, DiMarco JP, Mounsey JP, Lobban JH, Haines DE: Correlation of temperature and pathophysiological effect during radiofrequency catheter ablation of the AV junction. *Circulation* 1995; 92:1188-1192.
15. Otomo K, Yamanashi WS, Tondo C, et al: Why a large tip electrode makes a deeper radiofrequency lesion: effects of increase in electrode cooling and electrode-tissue interface area. *J Cardiovasc Electrophysiol* 1998; 9:47-54.
16. Langberg JJ, Gallagher M, Strickberger SA, Amirana O: Temperature-guided radiofrequency catheter ablation with very large distal electrodes. *Circulation* 1993; 88:245-249.
17. Everett THt, Lee KW, Wilson EE, et al: Safety profiles and lesion size of different radiofrequency ablation technologies: a comparison of large tip, open and closed irrigation catheters. *J Cardiovasc Electrophysiol* 2009; 20:325-335.
18. Demazumder D, Mirotznik MS, Schwartzman D: Biophysics of radiofrequency ablation using an irrigated electrode. *J Interv Card Electrophysiol* 2001; 5:377-389.
19. Dorwarth U, Fiek M, Remp T, et al: Radiofrequency catheter ablation: different cooled and noncooled electrode systems induce specific lesion geometries and adverse effects profiles. *Pacing Clin Electrophysiol* 2003; 26:1438-1445.
20. Hamner CE, Potter DD Jr, Cho KR, et al: Irrigated radiofrequency ablation with transmurality feedback reliably produces Cox maze lesions in vivo. *Ann Thorac Surg* 2005; 80:2263-2270.
21. Wood MA, Ellenbogen AL, Pathak V, Ellenbogen KA, Kasarajan V: Efficacy of a cooled bipolar epicardial radiofrequency ablation probe for creating transmural myocardial lesions. *J Thorac Cardiovasc Surg* 2010; 89(3):803-804.
22. Friedman PL, Dubuc M, Green MS, et al: Catheter cryoablation of supraventricular tachycardia: results of the multicenter prospective "frosty" trial. *Heart Rhythm* 2004; 1:129-138.
23. Skanes AC, Dubuc M, Klein GJ, et al: Cryothermal ablation of the slow pathway for the elimination of atrioventricular nodal reentrant tachycardia. *Circulation* 2000; 102:2856-2860.
24. Cappato R, Calkins H, Chen SA, et al: Worldwide survey on the methods, efficacy, and safety of catheter ablation for human atrial fibrillation. *Circulation* 2005; 111:1100-1105.
25. Saad EB, Marrouche NF, Saad CP, et al: Pulmonary vein stenosis after catheter ablation of atrial fibrillation: emergence of a new clinical syndrome. *Ann Intern Med* 2003; 138:634-638.
26. Good E, Oral H, Lemola K, et al: Movement of the esophagus during left atrial catheter ablation for atrial fibrillation. *J Am Coll Cardiol* 2005; 46:2107-2110.
27. Mohr FW, Fabricius AM, Falk V, et al: Curative treatment of atrial fibrillation with intraoperative radiofrequency ablation: short-term and midterm results. *J Thorac Cardiovasc Surg* 2002; 123:919-927.
28. Gillinov AM, Pettersson G, Rice TW: Esophageal injury during radiofrequency ablation for atrial fibrillation. *J Thorac Cardiovasc Surg* 2001; 122: 1239-1240.
29. Nademanee K, McKenzie J, Kosar E, et al: A new approach for catheter ablation of atrial fibrillation: mapping of the electrophysiologic substrate. *J Am Coll Cardiol* 2004; 43:2044-2053.
30. Scherlag BJ, Nakagawa H, Jackman WM, et al: Electrical stimulation to identify neural elements on the heart: their role in atrial fibrillation. *J Interv Card Electrophysiol* 2005; 13(Suppl 1):37-42.
31. Neumann T, Vogt J, Schumacher B, et al: Circumferential pulmonary vein isolation with the cryoballoon technique results from a prospective 3-center study. *J Am Coll Cardiol* 2008; 52:273-278.
32. Metzner A, Chun KR, Neven K, et al: Long-term clinical outcome following pulmonary vein isolation with high-intensity focused ultrasound balloon catheters in patients with paroxysmal atrial fibrillation. *Europace* 2010; 12:188-193.
33. Schmidt B, Chun KR, Metzner A, et al: Pulmonary vein isolation with high-intensity focused ultrasound: results from the HIFU 12F study. *Europace* 2009; 11:1281-1288.
34. Reddy VY, Neuzil P, Themistoclakis S, et al: Visually-guided balloon catheter ablation of atrial fibrillation: experimental feasibility and first-in-human multicenter clinical outcome. *Circulation* 2009; 120:12-20.
35. Accord RE, van Suylen RJ, van Brakel TJ, Maessen JG: Post-mortem histologic evaluation of microwave lesions after epicardial pulmonary vein isolation for atrial fibrillation. *Ann Thorac Surg* 2005; 80:881-887.
36. Gillinov AM, Smedira NG, Cosgrove DM 3rd: Microwave ablation of atrial fibrillation during mitral valve operations. *Ann Thorac Surg* 2002; 74:1259-1261.
37. Maessen JG, Nijs JF, Smeets JL, Vainer J, Mochtar B: Beating-heart surgical treatment of atrial fibrillation with microwave ablation. *Ann Thorac Surg* 2002; 74:S1307-1311.
38. Goli VD, Prasad R, Hamilton K, et al: Transesophageal echocardiographic evaluation for mural thrombus following radiofrequency catheter ablation of accessory pathways. *Pacing Clin Electrophysiol* 1991; 14: 1992-1997.
39. Chiang CE, Chen SA, Wu TJ, et al: Incidence, significance, and pharmacological responses of catheter-induced mechanical trauma in patients receiving radiofrequency ablation for supraventricular tachycardia. *Circulation* 1994; 90:1847-1854.
40. Wang TL, Lin JL, Hwang JJ, et al: The evolution of platelet aggregability in patients undergoing catheter ablation for supraventricular tachycardia with radiofrequency energy: the role of antiplatelet therapy. *Pacing Clin Electrophysiol* 1995; 18:1980-1990.
41. Lister JW, Stein E, Kosowsky BD, Lau SH, Damato AN: Atrioventricular conduction in man. Effect of rate, exercise, isoproterenol and atropine on the P-R interval. *Am J Cardiol* 1965; 16:516-523.
42. Hussein AA, Martin DO, Saliba W, et al: Radiofrequency ablation of atrial fibrillation under therapeutic international normalized ratio: a safe and efficacious periprocedural anticoagulation strategy. *Heart Rhythm* 2009; 6:1425-1429.
43. Oral H, Chugh A, Ozaydin M, et al: Risk of thromboembolic events after percutaneous left atrial radiofrequency ablation of atrial fibrillation. *Circulation* 2006; 114:759-765.
44. Belhassen B: A 1 per 1,000 mortality rate after catheter ablation of atrial fibrillation: an acceptable risk? *J Am Coll Cardiol* 2009; 53:1804-1806.
45. Chen SA, Chiang CE, Tai CT, et al: Complications of diagnostic electrophysiologic studies and radiofrequency catheter ablation in patients with tachyarrhythmias: an eight-year survey of 3,966 consecutive procedures in a tertiary referral center. *Am J Cardiol* 1996; 77:41-46.
46. Stevenson WG, Sager PT, Friedman PL: Entrainment techniques for mapping atrial and ventricular tachycardias. *J Cardiovasc Electrophysiol* 1995; 6:201-216.
47. Wellens HJ: Twenty-five years of insights into the mechanisms of supraventricular arrhythmias. *J Cardiovasc Electrophysiol* 2003; 14:1020-1025.
48. Wellens HJ, Brugada P: Mechanisms of supraventricular tachycardia. *Am J Cardiol* 1988; 62:10D-15D.
49. Brunckhorst CB, Delacretaz E, Soejima K, et al: Identification of the ventricular tachycardia isthmus after infarction by pace mapping. *Circulation* 2004; 110:652-659.
50. Joshi S, Wilber DJ: Ablation of idiopathic right ventricular outflow tract tachycardia: current perspectives. *J Cardiovasc Electrophysiol* 2005; 16(Suppl 1):S52-58.
51. Saoudi N, Ricard P, Rinaldi JP, et al: Methods to determine bidirectional block of the cavotricuspid isthmus in radiofrequency ablation of typical atrial flutter. *J Cardiovasc Electrophysiol* 2005; 16:801-803.
52. Gepstein L, Hayam G, Ben-Haim SA: A novel method for nonfluoroscopic catheter-based electroanatomical mapping of the heart. In vitro and in vivo accuracy results. *Circulation* 1997; 95:1611-1622.
53. Gornick CC, Adler SW, Pederson B, et al: Validation of a new noncontact catheter system for electroanatomic mapping of left ventricular endocardium. *Circulation* 1999; 99:829-835.
54. Bruce CJ, Friedman PA: Intracardiac echocardiography. *Eur J Echocardiogr* 2001; 2:234-244.
55. Beldner S, Gerstenfeld EP, Lin D, Marchlinski F: Ablation of atrial fibrillation: localizing triggers, mapping systems and ablation techniques. *Minerva Cardioangiol* 2004; 52:95-109.

56. Akhtar M, Jazayeri MR, Sra J, et al: Atrioventricular nodal reentry. Clinical, electrophysiological, and therapeutic considerations. *Circulation* 1993; 88:282-295.
57. Jazayeri MR, Hempe SL, Sra JS, et al: Selective transcatheter ablation of the fast and slow pathways using radiofrequency energy in patients with atrioventricular nodal reentrant tachycardia. *Circulation* 1992; 85: 1318-1328.
58. ACC/AHA Task Force Report: Guidelines for Clinical Intracardiac Electrophysiological and Catheter Ablation Procedures. A report of the American College of Cardiology/American Heart Association task force on practice guidelines (Committee on Clinical Intracardiac Electrophysiologic and Catheter Ablation Procedures). Developed in collaboration with the North American Society of Pacing and Electrophysiology. *J Cardiovasc Electrophysiol* 1995; 6:652-679.
59. Doig JC, Saito J, Harris L, Downar E: Coronary sinus morphology in patients with atrioventricular junctional reentry tachycardia and other supraventricular tachyarrhythmias. *Circulation* 1995; 92:436-441.
60. Kalbfleisch SJ, el-Atassi R, Calkins H, Langberg JJ, Morady F: Differentiation of paroxysmal narrow QRS complex tachycardias using the 12-lead electrocardiogram. *J Am Coll Cardiol* 1993; 21:85-89.
61. Michaud GF, Tada H, Chough S, et al: Differentiation of atypical atrioventricular node re-entrant tachycardia from orthodromic reciprocating tachycardia using a septal accessory pathway by the response to ventricular pacing. *J Am Coll Cardiol* 2001; 38:1163-1167.
62. Kalbfleisch SJ, Strickberger SA, Williamson B, et al: Randomized comparison of anatomic and electrogram mapping approaches to ablation of the slow pathway of atrioventricular node reentrant tachycardia. *J Am Coll Cardiol* 1994; 23:716-723.
63. Scheinman MM: North American Society of Pacing and Electrophysiology (NASPE) survey on radiofrequency catheter ablation: implications for clinicians, third party insurers, and government regulatory agencies. *Pacing Clin Electrophysiol* 1992; 15:2228-2231.
64. Scheinman MM, Huang S: The 1998 NASPE prospective catheter ablation registry. *Pacing Clin Electrophysiol* 2000; 23:1020-1028.
65. Santinelli V, Radinovic A, Manguso F, et al: Asymptomatic ventricular preexcitation: a long-term prospective follow-up study of 293 adult patients. *Circ Arrhythm Electrophysiol* 2009; 2:102-107.
66. Prystowsky EN, Fananapazir L, Packer DL, Thompson KA, German LD: Wolff-Parkinson-White syndrome and sudden cardiac death. *Cardiology* 1987; 74(Suppl 2):67-71.
67. Blomstrom-Lundqvist C, Scheinman MM, Aliot EM, et al: ACC/AHA/ESC guidelines for the management of patients with supraventricular arrhythmias—executive summary: a report of the American College of Cardiology/American Heart Association Task Force on Practice Guidelines and the European Society of Cardiology Committee for Practice Guidelines (Writing Committee to Develop Guidelines for the Management of Patients with Supraventricular Arrhythmias). *Circulation* 2003; 108: 1871-1909.
68. Kardos A, Paprika D, Shalganov T, et al: Ice mapping during tachycardia in close proximity to the AV node is safe and offers advantages for transcatheter ablation procedures. *Acta Cardiol* 2007; 62:587-591.
69. Miyazaki A, Blaufox AD, Fairbrother DL, Saul JP: Cryo-ablation for septal tachycardia substrates in pediatric patients: mid-term results. *J Am Coll Cardiol* 2005; 45:581-588.
70. Dagres N, Clague JR, Kottkamp H, et al: Radiofrequency catheter ablation of accessory pathways. Outcome and use of antiarrhythmic drugs during follow-up. *Eur Heart J* 1999; 20:1826-1832.
71. Jackman WM, Wang XZ, Friday KJ, et al: Catheter ablation of accessory atrioventricular pathways (Wolff-Parkinson-White syndrome) by radiofrequency current. *NEJM* 1991; 324:1605-1611.
72. Lesh MD, Van Hare GF, Schamp DJ, et al: Curative percutaneous catheter ablation using radiofrequency energy for accessory pathways in all locations: results in 100 consecutive patients. *J Am Coll Cardiol* 1992; 19:1303-1309.
73. Tucker KJ, Law J, Rodriques MJ: Treatment of refractory recurrent multifocal atrial tachycardia with atrioventricular junction ablation and permanent pacing. *J Invasive Cardiol* 1995; 7:207-212.
74. Chiladakis JA, Vassilikos VP, Maounis TN, Cokkinos DV, Manolis AS: Successful radiofrequency catheter ablation of automatic atrial tachycardia with regression of the cardiomyopathy picture. *Pacing Clin Electrophysiol* 1997; 20:953-959.
75. Corey WA, Markel ML, Hoit BD, Walsh RA: Regression of a dilated cardiomyopathy after radiofrequency ablation of incessant supraventricular tachycardia. *Am Heart J* 1993; 126:1469-1473.
76. Khasnis A, Jongnarangsin K, Abela G, et al: Tachycardia-induced cardiomyopathy: a review of literature. *Pacing Clin Electrophysiol* 2005; 28: 710-721.
77. Callans DJ, Schwartzman D, Gottlieb CD, Marchlinski FE: Insights into the electrophysiology of atrial arrhythmias gained by the catheter ablation experience: "learning while burning, Part II." *J Cardiovasc Electrophysiol* 1995; 6:229-243.
78. Koplan BA, Parkash R, Couper G, Stevenson WG: Combined epicardial-endocardial approach to ablation of inappropriate sinus tachycardia. *J Cardiovasc Electrophysiol* 2004; 15:237-240.
79. Brady PA, Low PA, Shen WK: Inappropriate sinus tachycardia, postural orthostatic tachycardia syndrome, and overlapping syndromes. *Pacing Clin Electrophysiol* 2005; 28:1112-1121.
80. Anguera I, Brugada J, Roba M, et al: Outcomes after radiofrequency catheter ablation of atrial tachycardia. *Am J Cardiol* 2001; 87:886-890.
81. Cabrera JA, Sanchez-Quintana D, Farre J, Rubio JM, Ho SY: The inferior right atrial isthmus: further architectural insights for current and coming ablation technologies. *J Cardiovasc Electrophysiol* 2005; 16:402-408.
82. Weinberg KM, Denes P, Kadish AH, Goldberger JJ: Development and validation of diagnostic criteria for atrial flutter on the surface electrocardiogram. *Ann Noninvasive Electrocardiol* 2008; 13:145-154.
83. Perez FJ, Schubert CM, Parvez B, et al: Long-term outcomes after catheter ablation of cavo-tricuspid isthmus dependent atrial flutter: a meta-analysis. *Circ Arrhythm Electrophysiol* 2009; 2:393-401.
84. Matsuo S, Wright M, Knecht S, et al: Peri-mitral atrial flutter in patients with atrial fibrillation ablation. *Heart Rhythm* 2009; 2:393-401.
85. Onorati F, Esposito A, Messina G, di Virgilio A, Renzulli A: Right isthmus ablation reduces supraventricular arrhythmias after surgery for chronic atrial fibrillation. *Ann Thorac Surg* 2008; 85:39-48.
86. Horlitz M, Schley P, Shin DI, Tonnellier B, Gulker H: Atrial tachycardias following circumferential pulmonary vein ablation: observations during catheter ablation. *Clin Res Cardiol* 2008; 97:124-130.
87. Lukac P, Hjortdal VE, Pedersen AK, et al: Atrial incision affects the incidence of atrial tachycardia after mitral valve surgery. *Ann Thorac Surg* 2006; 81:509-513.
88. Lukac P, Pedersen AK, Mortensen PT, et al: Ablation of atrial tachycardia after surgery for congenital and acquired heart disease using an electroanatomic mapping system: Which circuits to expect in which substrate? *Heart Rhythm* 2005; 2:64-72.
89. Reithmann C, Hoffmann E, Dorwarth U, Remp T, Steinbeck G: Electroanatomical mapping for visualization of atrial activation in patients with incisional atrial tachycardias. *Eur Heart J* 2001; 22:237-246.
90. Nakagawa H, Shah N, Matsudaira K, et al: Characterization of reentrant circuit in macroreentrant right atrial tachycardia after surgical repair of congenital heart disease: isolated channels between scars allow "focal" ablation. *Circulation* 2001; 103:699-709.
91. Kautzner J, Peichl P, Cihak R, Malek I: Atrial flutter after orthotopic heart transplantation. *J Heart Lung Transplant* 2004; 23:1463-1464.
92. Stecker EC, Strelich KR, Chugh SS, Crispell K, McAnulty JH: Arrhythmias after orthotopic heart transplantation. *J Card Fail* 2005; 11:464-472.
93. Strohmer B, Chen PS, Hwang C: Radiofrequency ablation of focal atrial tachycardia and atrioatrial conduction from recipient to donor after orthotopic heart transplantation. *J Cardiovasc Electrophysiol* 2000; 11: 1165-1169.
94. Ellenbogen KA, Hawthorne HR, Belz MK, et al: Late occurrence of incessant atrial tachycardia following the maze procedure. *Pacing Clin Electrophysiol* 1995; 18:367-369.
95. Kalman JM, Olgin JE, Saxon LA, et al: Electrocardiographic and electrophysiologic characterization of atypical atrial flutter in man: use of activation and entrainment mapping and implications for catheter ablation. *J Cardiovasc Electrophysiol* 1997; 8:121-144.
96. Corley SD, Epstein AE, DiMarco JP, et al: Relationships between sinus rhythm, treatment, and survival in the Atrial Fibrillation Follow-up Investigation of Rhythm Management (AFFIRM) Study. *Circulation* 2004; 109:1509-1513.
97. Kaufman ES, Zimmermann PA, Wang T, et al: Risk of proarrhythmic events in the Atrial Fibrillation Follow-up Investigation of Rhythm Management (AFFIRM) study: a multivariate analysis. *J Am Coll Cardiol* 2004; 44:1276-1282.
98. Steinberg JS, Sadaniantz A, Kron J, et al: Analysis of cause-specific mortality in the Atrial Fibrillation Follow-up Investigation of Rhythm Management (AFFIRM) study. *Circulation* 2004; 109:1973-1980.
99. Hohnloser SH, Crijns HJ, van Eickels M, et al: Effect of dronedarone on cardiovascular events in atrial fibrillation. *NEJM* 2009; 360:668-678.
100. Calkins H, Brugada J, Packer DL, et al: HRS/EHRA/ECAS expert Consensus Statement on catheter and surgical ablation of atrial fibrillation: recommendations for personnel, policy, procedures and follow-up. A report of the Heart Rhythm Society (HRS) Task Force on catheter and surgical ablation of atrial fibrillation. *Heart Rhythm* 2007; 4:816-861.

101. Calkins H, Brugada J, Packer DL, et al: HRS/EHRA/ECAS expert consensus statement on catheter and surgical ablation of atrial fibrillation: recommendations for personnel, policy, procedures and follow-up. A report of the Heart Rhythm Society (HRS) Task Force on Catheter and Surgical Ablation of Atrial Fibrillation developed in partnership with the European Heart Rhythm Association (EHRA) and the European Cardiac Arrhythmia Society (ECAS); in collaboration with the American College of Cardiology (ACC), American Heart Association (AHA), and the Society of Thoracic Surgeons (STS). Endorsed and approved by the governing bodies of the American College of Cardiology, the American Heart Association, the European Cardiac Arrhythmia Society, the European Heart Rhythm Association, the Society of Thoracic Surgeons, and the Heart Rhythm Society. *Europace* 2007; 9:335-379.
102. Marshall HJ, Griffith MJ: Ablation of the atrioventricular junction: technique, acute and long-term results in 115 consecutive patients. *Europace* 1999; 1:26-29.
103. Kay GN, Ellenbogen KA, Giudici M, et al: The Ablate and Pace Trial: a prospective study of catheter ablation of the AV conduction system and permanent pacemaker implantation for treatment of atrial fibrillation. APT Investigators. *J Interv Card Electrophysiol* 1998; 2:121-135.
104. Moss AJ, Hall WJ, Cannom DS, et al: Cardiac-resynchronization therapy for the prevention of heart-failure events. *NEJM* 2009; 361:1329-1338.
105. Doshi RN, Daoud EG, Fellows C, et al: Left ventricular-based cardiac stimulation post AV nodal ablation evaluation (the PAVE study). *J Cardiovasc Electrophysiol* 2005; 16:1160-1165.
106. Pelosi F Jr, Morady F: CRT-D therapy in patients with left ventricular dysfunction and atrial fibrillation. *Ann Noninvasive Electrocardiol* 2005; 10:55-58.
107. Oral H: Mechanisms of atrial fibrillation: lessons from studies in patients. *Prog Cardiovasc Dis* 2005; 48:29-40.
108. Pappone C, Oreto G, Lamberti F, et al: Catheter ablation of paroxysmal atrial fibrillation using a 3D mapping system. *Circulation* 1999; 100: 1203-1208.
109. Zhou L, Keane D, Reed G, Ruskin J: Thromboembolic complications of cardiac radiofrequency catheter ablation: a review of the reported incidence, pathogenesis and current research directions. *J Cardiovasc Electrophysiol* 1999; 10:611-620.
110. Haissaguerre M, Jais P, Shah DC, et al: Spontaneous initiation of atrial fibrillation by ectopic beats originating in the pulmonary veins. *NEJM* 1998; 339:659-666.
111. Oral H, Knight BP, Tada H, et al: Pulmonary vein isolation for paroxysmal and persistent atrial fibrillation. *Circulation* 2002; 105:1077-1081.
112. Oral H, Chugh A, Good E, et al: Randomized comparison of encircling and nonencircling left atrial ablation for chronic atrial fibrillation. *Heart Rhythm* 2005; 2:1165-1172.
113. Pappone C, Oreto G, Rosanio S, et al: Atrial electroanatomic remodeling after circumferential radiofrequency pulmonary vein ablation: efficacy of an anatomic approach in a large cohort of patients with atrial fibrillation. *Circulation* 2001; 104:2539-2544.
114. Jais P, Cauchemez B, Macle L, et al: Catheter ablation versus antiarrhythmic drugs for atrial fibrillation: the A4 study. *Circulation* 2008; 118: 2498-2505.
115. Piccini JP, Lopes RD, Kong MH, et al: Pulmonary vein isolation for the maintenance of sinus rhythm in patients with atrial fibrillation: a meta-analysis of randomized, controlled trials. *Circ Arrhythm Electrophysiol* 2009; 2:626-633.
116. Khaykin Y, Skanes A, Champagne J, et al: A randomized controlled trial of the efficacy and safety of electroanatomic circumferential pulmonary vein ablation supplemented by ablation of complex fractionated atrial electrograms versus potential-guided pulmonary vein antrum isolation guided by intracardiac ultrasound. *Circ Arrhythm Electrophysiol* 2009; 2:481-487.
117. Deisenhofer I, Estner H, Reents T, et al: Does electrogram guided substrate ablation add to the success of pulmonary vein isolation in patients with paroxysmal atrial fibrillation? A prospective, randomized study. *J Cardiovasc Electrophysiol* 2009; 20:514-521.
118. Di Biase L, Elayi CS, Fahmy TS, et al: Atrial fibrillation ablation strategies for paroxysmal patients: randomized comparison between different techniques. *Circ Arrhythm Electrophysiol* 2009; 2:113-119.
119. Gaita F, Caponi D, Scaglione M, et al: Long-term clinical results of 2 different ablation strategies in patients with paroxysmal and persistent atrial fibrillation. *Circ Arrhythm Electrophysiol* 2008; 1:269-275.
120. Elayi CS, Verma A, Di Biase L, et al: Ablation for longstanding permanent atrial fibrillation: results from a randomized study comparing three different strategies. *Heart Rhythm* 2008; 5:1658-1664.
121. Arentz T, Weber R, Burkle G, et al: Small or large isolation areas around the pulmonary veins for the treatment of atrial fibrillation? Results from a prospective randomized study. *Circulation* 2007; 115:3057-3063.
122. Yu WC, Hsu TL, Tai CT, et al: Acquired pulmonary vein stenosis after radiofrequency catheter ablation of paroxysmal atrial fibrillation. *J Cardiovasc Electrophysiol* 2001; 12:887-892.
123. Packer DL, Keelan P, Munger TM, et al: Clinical presentation, investigation, and management of pulmonary vein stenosis complicating ablation for atrial fibrillation. *Circulation* 2005; 111:546-554.
124. Raymond JM, Sacher F, Winslow R, Tedrow U, Stevenson WG: Catheter ablation for scar-related ventricular tachycardias. *Curr Probl Cardiol* 2009; 34:225-270.
125. Stevenson WG, Wilber DJ, Natale A, et al: Irrigated radiofrequency catheter ablation guided by electroanatomic mapping for recurrent ventricular tachycardia after myocardial infarction: the multicenter ThermaCool ventricular tachycardia ablation trial. *Circulation* 2008; 118:2773-2782.
126. Gonska BD, Cao K, Schaumann A, et al: Catheter ablation of ventricular tachycardia in 136 patients with coronary artery disease: results and long-term follow-up. *J Am Coll Cardiol* 1994; 24:1506-1514.
127. Morady F, Harvey M, Kalbfleisch SJ, el-Atassi R, Calkins H, Langberg JJ: Radiofrequency catheter ablation of ventricular tachycardia in patients with coronary artery disease. *Circulation* 1993; 87:363-372.
128. Stevenson WG, Khan H, Sager P, et al: Identification of reentry circuit sites during catheter mapping and radiofrequency ablation of ventricular tachycardia late after myocardial infarction. *Circulation* 1993; 88: 1647-1670.
129. Blanck Z, Dhala A, Deshpande S, et al: Bundle branch reentrant ventricular tachycardia: cumulative experience in 48 patients. *J Cardiovasc Electrophysiol* 1993; 4:253-262.
130. Mehdirad AA, Keim S, Rist K, Tchou P: Long-term clinical outcome of right bundle branch radiofrequency catheter ablation for treatment of bundle branch reentrant ventricular tachycardia. *Pacing Clin Electrophysiol* 1995; 18:2135-2143.
131. Marcus FI, Fontaine G: Arrhythmogenic right ventricular dysplasia/cardiomyopathy: a review. *Pacing Clin Electrophysiol* 1995; 18:1298-1314.
132. Aizer A, Stern EH, Gomes JA, et al: Usefulness of programmed ventricular stimulation in predicting future arrhythmic events in patients with cardiac sarcoidosis. *Am J Cardiol* 2005; 96:276-282.
133. Koplan BA, Soejima K, Baughman K, Epstein LM, Stevenson WG: Refractory ventricular tachycardia secondary to cardiac sarcoid: electrophysiologic characteristics, mapping, and ablation. *Heart Rhythm* 2006; 3:924-929.
134. Khairy P, Stevenson WG: Catheter ablation in tetralogy of Fallot. *Heart Rhythm* 2009; 6:1069-1074.
135. Eckart RE, Hruczkowski TW, Tedrow UB, et al: Sustained ventricular tachycardia associated with corrective valve surgery. *Circulation* 2007; 116:2005-2011.
136. Rodriguez LM, Smeets JL, Timmermans C, Wellens HJ: Predictors for successful ablation of right- and left-sided idiopathic ventricular tachycardia. *Am J Cardiol* 1997; 79:309-314.
137. Wen MS, Taniguchi Y, Yeh SJ, et al: Determinants of tachycardia recurrences after radiofrequency ablation of idiopathic ventricular tachycardia. *Am J Cardiol* 1998; 81:500-503.
138. Khaykin Y, Wang X, Natale A, et al: Cost comparison of ablation versus antiarrhythmic drugs as first-line therapy for atrial fibrillation: an economic evaluation of the RAAFT pilot study. *J Cardiovasc Electrophysiol* 2009; 20:7-12.
139. McKenna C, Palmer S, Rodgers M, et al: Cost-effectiveness of radiofrequency catheter ablation for the treatment of atrial fibrillation in the United Kingdom. *Heart* 2009; 95:542-549.
140. Cheng CH, Sanders GD, Hlatky MA, et al: Cost-effectiveness of radiofrequency ablation for supraventricular tachycardia. *Ann Intern Med* 2000; 133:864-876.
141. Marshall DA, O'Brien BJ, Nichol G: Review of economic evaluations of radiofrequency catheter ablation for cardiac arrhythmias. *Can J Cardiol* 2003; 19:1285-1304.
142. Weerasooriya HR, Murdock CJ, Harris AH, Davis MJ: The cost-effectiveness of treatment of supraventricular arrhythmias related to an accessory atrioventricular pathway: comparison of catheter ablation, surgical division and medical treatment. *Aust N Z J Med* 1994; 24:161-167.
143. Reynolds MR, Zimetbaum P, Josephson ME, et al: Cost-effectiveness of radiofrequency catheter ablation compared with antiarrhythmic drug therapy for paroxysmal atrial fibrillation. *Circ Arrhythm Electrophysiol* 2009; 2:362-369.
144. Rodgers M, McKenna C, Palmer S, et al: Curative catheter ablation in atrial fibrillation and typical atrial flutter: systematic review and economic evaluation. *Health Technol Assess* 2008; 12:iii-iv, xi-xiii, 1-198.
145. Vano E, Gonzalez L, Fernandez JM, Alfonso F, Macaya C: Occupational radiation doses in interventional cardiology: a 15-year follow-up. *Br J Radiol* 2006; 79:383-388.

146. Ross AM, Segal J, Borenstein D, Jenkins E, Cho S: Prevalence of spinal disc disease among interventional cardiologists. *Am J Cardiol* 1997; 79:68-70.
147. Goldstein JA, Balter S, Cowley M, Hodgson J, Klein LW: Occupational hazards of interventional cardiologists: prevalence of orthopedic health problems in contemporary practice. *Catheter Cardiovasc Interv* 2004; 63: 407-411.
148. Klein LW, Miller DL, Balter S, et al: Occupational health hazards in the interventional laboratory: time for a safer environment. *Heart Rhythm* 2009; 6:439-444.
149. Pappone C, Vicedomini G, Manguso F, et al: Robotic magnetic navigation for atrial fibrillation ablation. *J Am Coll Cardiol* 2006; 47:1390-1400.
150. Di Biase L, Fahmy TS, Patel D, et al: Remote magnetic navigation: human experience in pulmonary vein ablation. *J Am Coll Cardiol* 2007; 50:868-874.
151. Schmidt B, Tilz RR, Neven K, et al: Remote robotic navigation and electroanatomical mapping for ablation of atrial fibrillation: considerations for navigation and impact on procedural outcome. *Circ Arrhythm Electrophysiol* 2009; 2:120-128.
152. Saliba W, Reddy VY, Wazni O, et al: Atrial fibrillation ablation using a robotic catheter remote control system: initial human experience and long-term follow-up results. *J Am Coll Cardiol* 2008; 51:2407-2411.
153. Di Biase L, Wang Y, Horton R, et al: Ablation of atrial fibrillation utilizing robotic catheter navigation in comparison to manual navigation and ablation: single-center experience. *J Cardiovasc Electrophysiol* 2009; 20: 1328-1335.
154. Nazarian S, Kolandaivelu A, Zviman MM, et al: Feasibility of real-time magnetic resonance imaging for catheter guidance in electrophysiology studies. *Circulation* 2008; 118:223-229.
155. Schmidt EJ, Mallozzi RP, Thiagalingam A, et al: Electroanatomic mapping and radiofrequency ablation of porcine left atria and atrioventricular nodes using magnetic resonance catheter tracking. *Circ Arrhythm Electrophysiol* 2009; 2:695-704.

CHAPTER 58

Surgery for Atrial Fibrillation

Spencer J. Melby
Ralph J. Damiano, Jr.

INTRODUCTION

Atrial fibrillation (AF) is the most common arrhythmia in the world. It is associated with significant morbidity and mortality secondary to its detrimental sequelae: (1) palpitations resulting in patient discomfort and anxiety; (2) loss of atrioventricular (AV) synchrony, which can compromise cardiac hemodynamics, resulting in various degrees of ventricular dysfunction or congestive heart failure; (3) stasis of blood flow in the left atrium, increasing the risk of thromboembolism and stroke.[1–10]

Medical treatment of AF has many shortcomings. Because of this, interest in nonpharmacologic treatment approaches led to the development of catheter-based and surgical techniques beginning in the 1980s. Initial attempts aimed at providing rate control failed to address the detrimental hemodynamic and thromboembolic sequelae of atrial fibrillation. The early attempts at finding a surgical treatment culminated in the introduction of the Maze procedure in 1987, which became the gold standard for many years.

The following sections describe the historical aspects of surgery for AF, and the current state of surgical ablation for the treatment of AF, including recent minimally invasive techniques.

HISTORICAL ASPECTS

The Left Atrial Isolation Procedure

The first surgery designed specifically to eliminate AF, the *left atrial isolation procedure,* was described in 1980 in the laboratory of Dr. James Cox at Duke University. This approach confined AF to the left atrium, and restored the remainder of the heart to sinus rhythm (Fig. 58-1).[11] This procedure reestablished a regular ventricular rate without requiring a permanent pacemaker. Isolating the left atrium allowed the right atrium and the right ventricle to contract in synchrony, providing a normal right-sided cardiac output. This effectively restored normal cardiac hemodynamics.

By confining AF to the left atrium, the left atrial isolation procedure only eliminated two of the three detrimental sequelae of AF: an irregular heartbeat and compromised cardiac hemodynamics. It did not eliminate the thromboembolic risk because the left atrium usually remained in fibrillation. This procedure never achieved clinical acceptance, although it was performed by Dr. Cox in a single patient.

Catheter Ablation of the Atrioventricular Node–His Bundle Complex

In 1982, Scheinman and coworkers introduced *catheter fulguration of the His bundle,* a procedure that controlled the irregular cardiac rhythm associated with AF and other refractory supraventricular arrhythmias.[12] This procedure electrically isolated the fibrillation to the atria. Unfortunately, ablating the bundle of His required permanent ventricular pacemaker implantation to restore a normal ventricular rate.

The shortcoming of this intervention was that it only eliminated the irregular heartbeat. Both atria remained in fibrillation, and the risk of thromboembolism persisted. AV contraction remained desynchronized, compromising cardiac hemodynamics. In addition, patients become pacemaker dependant for the remainder of their lives. Nevertheless, AV node ablation has remained a common treatment for medically refractory AF.

The Corridor Procedure

In 1985, Guiraudon and associates developed the *corridor procedure* for the treatment of AF.[13] This operation isolated a strip of atrial septum harboring both the sinoatrial (SA) node and the

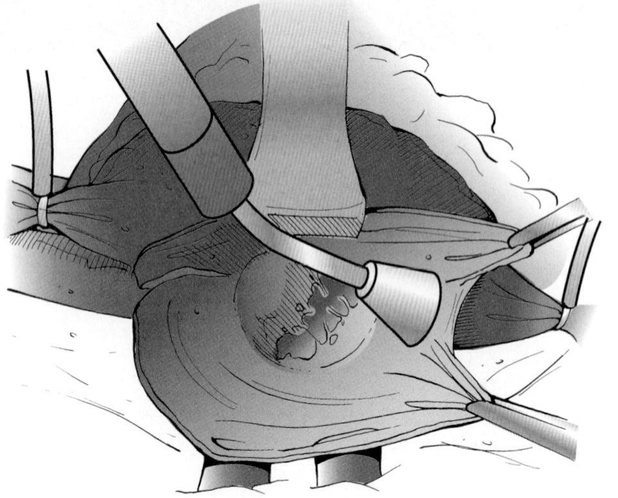

FIGURE 58-1 Standard left atriotomy, demonstrating incisions to the mitral valve annulus at both the 10 and 2 o'clock positions. The superior and inferior vena cavae are seen with tourniquets, and the pulmonary vein orifices are seen inferiorly. Cryoablation is used to complete the line of conduction block at the valve annuli. (*Adapted from Williams JM, Ungerleider RM, Lofland GK, Cox JL: Left atrial isolation: new technique for the treatment of supraventricular arrhythmias. J Thorac Cardiovasc Surg 1980; 80(3):373-380.*)

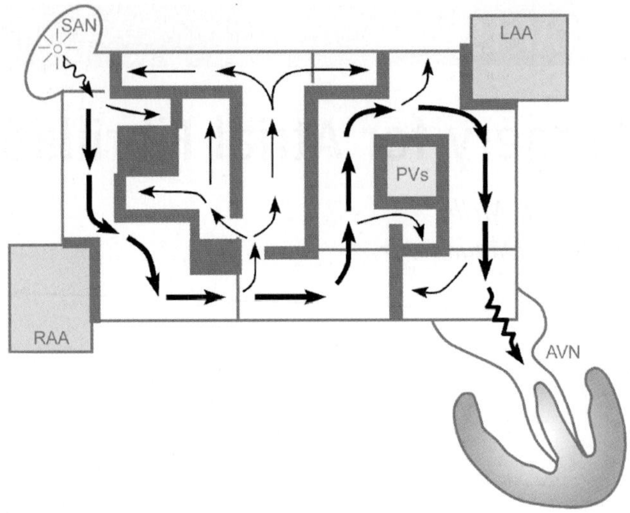

FIGURE 58-2 By creating a myriad of surgical incisions in the atria, the Maze procedure was designed to prevent atrial fibrillation. AVN = atrioventricular node; LAA = left atrial appendage; PVs = pulmonary veins; RAA = right atrial appendage; SAN = sinoatrial node. (*Reproduced with permission from Cox JL, Schuessler RB, D'Agostino HJ Jr, et al: The surgical treatment of atrial fibrillation. III. Development of a definitive surgical procedure. J Thorac Cardiovasc Surg 1991; 101[4]:569-583.*)

AV node, allowing the SA node to drive both the ventricles. This procedure effectively eliminated the irregular heartbeat associated with AF, but both atria either remained in fibrillation or developed their own asynchronous intrinsic rhythm because they were isolated from the septal "corridor." Furthermore, the atria were isolated from their respective ventricles, thereby precluding the possibility of AV synchrony. The corridor procedure was abandoned because it had no effect on the hemodynamic compromise or the risk of thromboembolism associated with AF.

The Atrial Transection Procedure

In 1985, Dr. James Cox and associates described the first procedure that attempted to terminate AF.[14] This was different from the prior surgical procedures described that only isolated or confined AF to a certain region of the atria. Using a canine model, Cox's group found that a single long incision around both atria and down into the septum could terminate AF. This *atrial transection procedure* prevented the induction and maintenance of AF or atrial flutter in every canine that underwent the operation.[15] Although this procedure was not effective clinically and was soon abandoned, it laid the ground work of the development of the Cox-Maze procedure.

THE COX-MAZE PROCEDURE

The Maze procedure was clinically introduced in 1987 by Dr. Cox after extensive animal investigation at Washington University in St. Louis.[15–17] The Cox-Maze procedure was originally developed to interrupt any and all macro-reentrant circuits that were felt to develop in the atria, thereby precluding the ability of the atrium to flutter or fibrillate (Fig. 58-2). Unlike the previous procedures, the Cox-Maze procedure successfully restored both AV synchrony and sinus rhythm, thus potentially reducing the risk of thromboembolism and stroke.[18] The operation consisted of creating an array of surgical incisions across both the right and left atria. These incisions were placed so that the sinoatrial node could still direct the propagation of the sinus impulse throughout both atria. It allowed for most of the atrial myocardium to be activated, resulting in preservation of atrial transport function in most patients.[19]

The first iteration of the Maze procedure was modified because of problems with late chronotropic incompetence and a high incidence of pacemaker implantation. The resulting Maze II procedure, however, was extremely difficult to perform technically, and it was soon replaced by the Maze III procedure (Fig. 58-3).[20,21]

The Cox-Maze III procedure—often referred to as the "cut-and-sew" Maze—became the gold standard for the surgical treatment of AF. In a long-term study of patients who underwent the Cox-Maze III procedure at our institution, 97% of the patients at late follow-up were free of symptomatic AF.[22] These excellent results have been reproduced by other groups worldwide.[23–25]

Although the Cox-Maze III procedure was effective in eliminating AF, it was technically difficult and invasive, and only a handful of cardiac surgeons still perform the cut-and-sew operation today. At the present time, a variety of ablation devices are available that can replicate the surgical incisions on the atrium and create conduction block. This has made AF ablation much simpler to perform. These ablation-assisted procedures

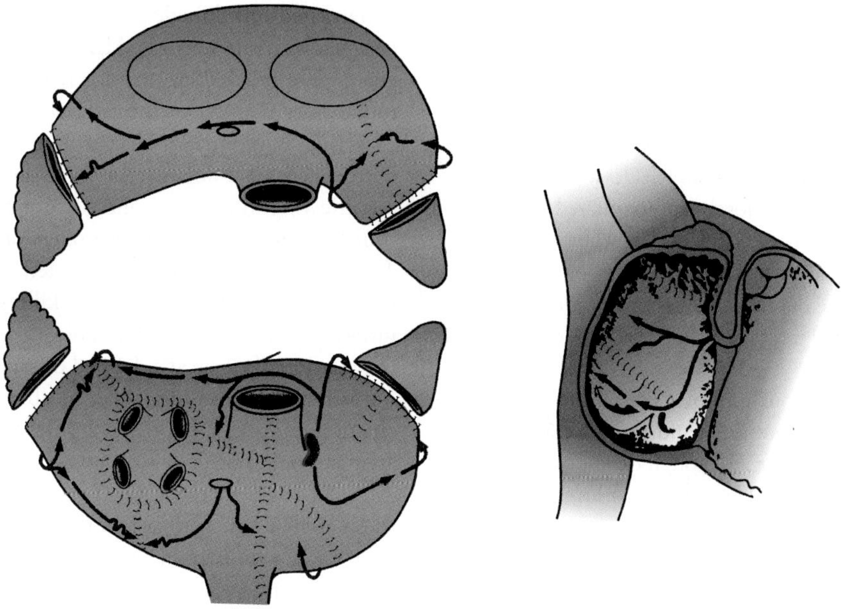

FIGURE 58-3 The lesions set of the traditional cut-and-sew Cox-Maze III procedure. (*Reproduced with permission from Cox JL, Schuessler RB, D'Agostino HJ Jr, et al: The surgical treatment of atrial fibrillation. III. Development of a definitive surgical procedure. J Thorac Cardiovasc Surg 1991; 101[4]:569-583.*)

have greatly expanded the field of AF surgery in the past decade.[26] With present ablation technology, surgery can be performed with low morbidity and mortality and often with less invasive incisions.

SURGICAL ABLATION TECHNOLOGY

The development of surgical ablation technology has transformed a difficult and time-consuming operation that few surgeons were willing to perform into a procedure that is technically easier, shorter, and less invasive. Several ablation technologies exist, each with its relative advantages and disadvantages.

For an ablation technology to successfully replace surgical incisions, it must meet several criteria. First, it must reliably produce bidirectional conduction block across the line of ablation. This is the mechanism by which incisions prevent AF, by either blocking macro-reentrant or micro-reentrant circuits or isolating focal triggers. Our laboratory and others have shown that this requires a transmural lesion, as even small gaps in ablation lines can conduct both sinus and fibrillatory impulses.[27–29] Second, the ablation device must be safe. This requires a precise definition of dose–response curves to limit excessive or inadequate ablation, and potential hazards to surrounding vital cardiac structures, such as the coronary sinus, coronary arteries, and valvular structures. Third, the ablation device should make AF surgery simpler and require less time to perform. This would require the device to create lesions rapidly, be simple to use, and have adequate length and flexibility. Finally, the device should be adaptable to a minimally invasive approach. This would include the ability to insert the device through minimal access incisions or ports. As of the present time, no device has met all of these criteria. The following sections will briefly summarize the current ablation technologies.

Cryoablation

Cryoablation technology is unique in that it destroys myocardial tissue by freezing rather than heating. It has the benefit of preserving the myocardial fibrous skeleton and collagen structure and is thus one of the safest energy sources available. These devices work by pumping a refrigerant to the electrode tip where it undergoes transformation from a liquid to a gas phase, absorbing heat energy from the tissue in contact with the tip. The formation of intracellular and extracellular ice crystals disrupts the cell membrane and causes cell death. There is also evidence that the induction of apoptosis plays a role in late lesion expansion. Lesion size depends on the temperature of the probe and thermal conductivity and temperature of the tissue.[30]

There are currently two commercially available sources of cryothermal energy that are being used in cardiac surgery. The older technology, based on nitrous oxide, is manufactured by AtriCure (Cincinnati, OH). More recently, ATS Medical (Minneapolis, MN) has developed a device based on argon. At 1 atmosphere of pressure, nitrous oxide is capable of cooling tissue to −89.5°C, whereas argon has a minimum temperature of −185.7°C. The nitrous oxide technology has a well-defined efficacy and safety profile and is generally safe except around the coronary arteries.[31,32] The potential disadvantage of cryoablation, however, is its relatively long time required to create lesions (1 to 3 minutes). There is also difficulty in creating lesions on the beating heart because of the "heat sink" of the circulating blood volume.[33] Furthermore, if blood is frozen during epicardial ablation on the beating heart, it may coagulate, creating a potential thromboembolic risk.

Radiofrequency Energy

Radiofrequency (RF) energy has been used for cardiac ablation for many years in the electrophysiology laboratory, and was one of the first energy sources to be applied in the operating room.[34] Resistive RF energy can be delivered by either unipolar or bipolar electrodes, and the electrodes can be either dry or irrigated. With unipolar RF devices, the energy is dispersed between the electrode tip and an indifferent electrode, usually the grounding pad applied to the patient. In bipolar RF devices, alternating current is passed between two closely approximated electrodes. The lesion size depends on electrode–tissue contact area, the interface temperature, the current and voltage (power), and the duration of delivery. The depth of the lesion can be limited by char formation, epicardial fat, myocardial and endocavity blood flow, and tissue thickness.

There have been numerous unipolar RF devices developed for ablation. These include both dry and irrigated devices and devices that incorporate suction. Although dry unipolar RF has been shown to create transmural lesions on the arrested heart in animals with sufficiently long ablation times, it has not been consistently successful in humans. After 2-minute endocardial ablations during mitral valve surgery, only 20% of the in vivo lesions were transmural.[35] Epicardial ablation on the beating heart has been even more problematic. Animal studies have consistently shown that unipolar RF is incapable of creating epicardial transmural lesions on the beating heart.[36,37] Epicardial RF ablation in humans resulted in only 10% of the lesions being transmural.[38] This deficiency of unipolar RF has been felt to be caused by the heat sink of the circulating blood.[39] This has led industry to examine adding both irrigation and suction to improve lesion formation. Although these additions have improved depth of penetration, there has been no unipolar device that has been shown by independent laboratories to be capable of creating reliable transmural lesions on the beating heart.

To overcome this problem, bipolar RF clamps were developed. With bipolar RF, the electrodes are embedded in the jaws of a clamp to focus the delivery of energy. By shielding the electrodes from the circulating blood pool, this improves and shortens lesion formation and limits collateral injury. Bipolar ablation has been shown to be capable of creating transmural lesions on the beating heart both in animals and humans with short ablation times.[40–42] Three companies (AtriCure, West Chester, OH; Medtronic, Minneapolis, MN; and Estech, San Ramon, CA) currently market bipolar RF devices.

Another advantage of bipolar RF energy over unipolar RF is its safety profile. A number of clinical complications of unipolar RF devices have been reported, including coronary artery injuries, cerebrovascular accidents, and esophageal perforation leading to atrioesophageal fistula.[43–46] Bipolar RF technology has virtually eliminated this collateral damage; there have been no injuries described with these devices despite extensive clinical use.

High-Intensity Focused Ultrasound

High-intensity focused ultrasound, or HIFU, is another modality being applied clinically for surgical ablation (St. Jude Medical, St. Paul, MN). Ultrasound ablates tissue via mechanical hyperthermia. Ultrasound waves travel through the tissue, causing compression, refraction, and particle movement, which is translated into kinetic energy and ultimately creates thermal coagulative tissue necrosis. HIFU produces high-concentration energy in a focused area, and is reportedly able to create transmural epicardial lesions through epicardial fat in a short time.[47]

HIFU is unique in that it is able to create noninvasive, noncontact focal ablation in three-dimensional volume without affecting intervening and surrounding tissue. It uses ultrasound beams in the frequency range of 1 to 5 MHz or higher. The focused beams increase the temperature of the targeted tissue to above 80°C, effectively killing the cells. By focusing ultrasound waves, HIFU is able to create targeted thermal coagulation of tissue at a defined distance from the probe without heating intervening tissue. Its ability to focus the target of ablation at specific depths is a potential advantage over other energy modalities.

Another advantage of HIFU technology is its mechanism of thermal ablation. Unlike all other energy sources that heat or cool tissue by thermal conduction, HIFU ablates tissue by directly heating the tissue in the acoustic focal volume, and is therefore less affected by the "heat sink" of the circulating endocardial blood pool. A few clinical studies using HIFU have shown some encouraging results.[47–50] However, there has been no independent experimental verification of the efficacy of HIFU devices to reliably create transmural lesions, and some limited clinical experience has had poor results.[51] The fixed depth of penetration of these devices may be a problem in pathologically thickened atrial tissue. Moreover, these devices are somewhat bulky and expensive to manufacture.

Both microwave and laser energy have been used clinically, but limitations of each technology led to limited use and/or withdrawal of those devices from the market.[39]

In summary, each ablation technology has its own advantages and disadvantages. Continued research investigating the effects of each surgical ablation technology on atrial hemodynamics, function, and electrophysiology will allow for more appropriate use in the operating room. The inability to create reliable linear lesions on the beating heart remains a shortcoming of most devices and has impeded the development of minimally invasive procedures.

SURGICAL TECHNIQUES

There are essentially three categories of procedures that presently are performed to surgically treat AF: the Cox-Maze procedure, left atrial lesion sets, and pulmonary vein isolation (PVI). Each of these approaches is described in the following.

The Cox-Maze IV Procedure

The original "cut-and-sew" Cox-Maze III procedure is rarely performed today. At most centers, the surgical incisions have been replaced with lines of ablation using a variety of energy sources. At our institution, bipolar RF energy has been used successfully to replace most of the surgical incisions of the Cox-Maze III procedure. Our current RF ablation-assisted procedure, termed the Cox-Maze IV, incorporates the lesions of the Cox-Maze III (Fig. 58-4).[52] Our clinical results have shown that this modified procedure has significantly shortened

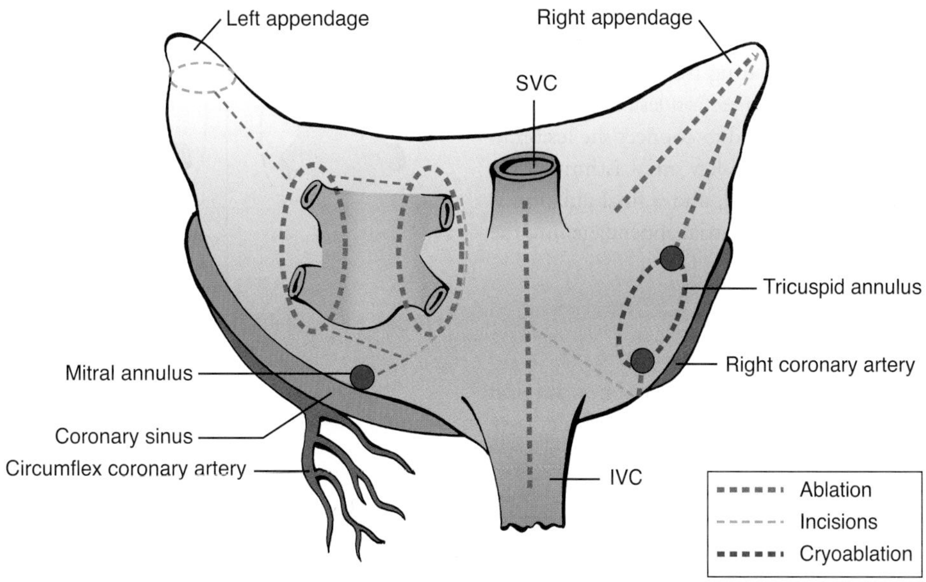

FIGURE 58-4 The Cox-Maze IV lesion sets. IVC = inferior vena cava; SVC = superior vena cava. (*Reproduced with permission from Cox JL, Schuessler RB, D'Agostino HJ Jr, et al: The surgical treatment of atrial fibrillation. III. Development of a definitive surgical procedure. J Thorac Cardiovasc Surg 1991; 101[4]:569-583.*)

operative time while maintaining the high success rate of the original Cox-Maze III procedure.[53,54]

The Cox-Maze IV procedure is performed on cardiopulmonary bypass. The operation can be done either through a median sternotomy or a less invasive right minithoracotomy. The right and left pulmonary veins (PVs) are bluntly dissected. If the patient is in AF, amiodarone is administered and the patient is electrically cardioverted. Pacing thresholds are obtained from each pulmonary vein. Using a bipolar RF ablation device, the PVs are individually isolated by ablating a cuff of atrial tissue surrounding the right and left PVs. Proof of electrical isolation is confirmed after ablation by demonstrating exit block from each PV.

The right atrial lesion set is performed on the beating heart (Fig. 58-5). A bipolar RF clamp is used to create most of the lesions. A unipolar device, either cryoablation or radiofrequency energy, is used to complete the ablation lines endocardially down to the tricuspid annulus because of the difficulty of clamping in this area.

The left-sided lesion set (Fig. 58-6) is performed via a standard left atriotomy on the arrested heart. The incision is extended inferiorly around the right inferior PV and superiorly onto the dome of the left atrium. Connecting lesions are made with the bipolar RF device into the left superior and inferior pulmonary veins and a final ablation is performed down toward

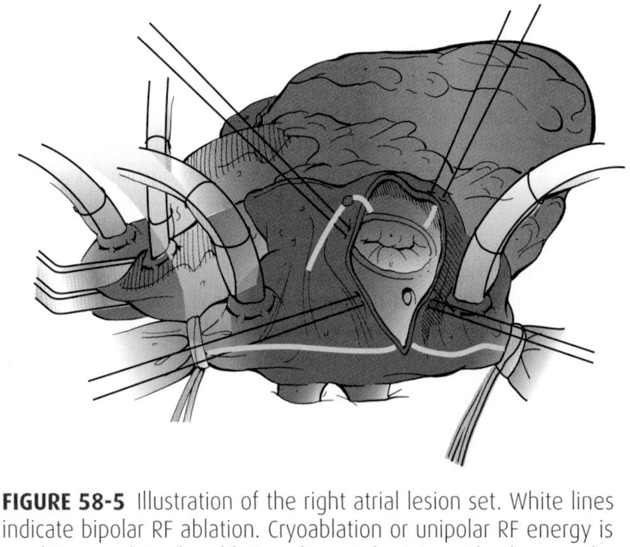

FIGURE 58-5 Illustration of the right atrial lesion set. White lines indicate bipolar RF ablation. Cryoablation or unipolar RF energy is used to complete the ablations line at the tricuspid valve annulus.

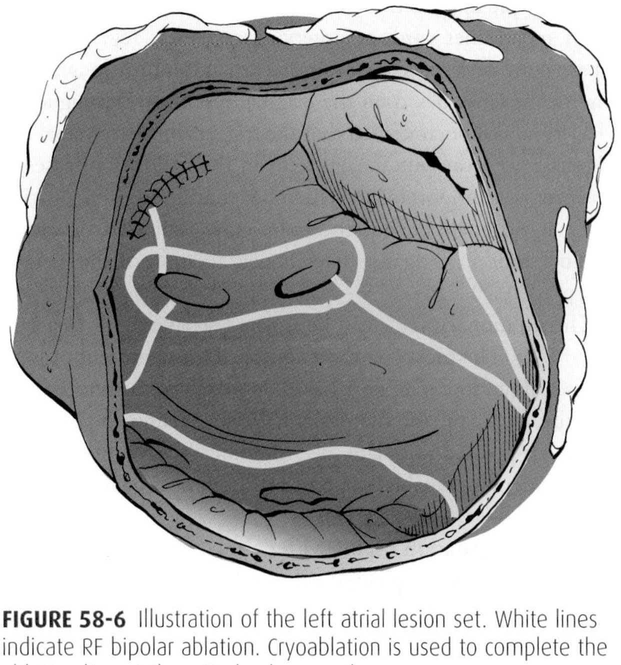

FIGURE 58-6 Illustration of the left atrial lesion set. White lines indicate RF bipolar ablation. Cryoablation is used to complete the ablation line at the mitral valve annulus.

the mitral annulus. Our group has shown that isolating the entire posterior left atrium with ablation lines into both left pulmonary veins resulted in a better drug-free freedom from AF at 6 and 12 months than a single connection lesion.[55] A unipolar device, usually cryoablation, is used to connect the lesion to the mitral annulus and complete the left atrial isthmus line. The left atrial appendage is amputated, and a final ablation is performed through the amputated left atrial appendage into the one of the left pulmonary veins.

Left Atrial Procedures

Over the past decade, there have been a number of new surgical procedures introduced in attempt to cure AF. The results have been variable and have had a wide range of success rates.[43,56–63] All of the ablation technologies have been used to create a large number of different lesion patterns. All of these procedures have generally involved some subset of the left atrial lesion set of the Cox-Maze procedure. Results have been dependent on the technology used, the lesion set, and the patient population. From a technical standpoint, all of the approaches have attempted to isolate the pulmonary veins. The importance of the rest of the left atrial Cox-Maze lesion set remains controversial. However, Gillinov et al published a large series demonstrating that the omission of the left atrial isthmus lesion resulted in a significantly higher incidence of recurrent AF in patients with permanent AF.[64] To complete this lesion, it is mandatory to also ablate the coronary sinus in line with the endocardial lesion. In addition, our clinical results have shown that it is important to isolate the entire posterior left atrium.[55]

Pulmonary Vein Isolation

Pulmonary vein isolation is an attractive therapeutic strategy because the procedure can be done without cardiopulmonary bypass and with minimally invasive techniques, using either a thoracoscopic approach or small incisions. It can also be easily added to another cardiac surgery intervention (eg, coronary bypass graft or a valve procedure) with minimum increase of time to the case. Based on the original report of Hassaiguerre, it has been well documented that the triggers for paroxysmal AF originate from the pulmonary veins in the majority of cases.[65] However, it is important to remember that up to 30% of triggers may originate outside the pulmonary veins.[66] To increase efficacy, some investigators have added ablation of the ganglionic plexi (GP).[67–69]

The pulmonary veins can be isolated separately or as a box (Fig. 58-7). The most common approach for treatment of lone AF uses an endoscopic, port-based approach to minimize incision size and pain for the patient. At our center, bipolar RF clamps are favored to isolate the pulmonary veins, but unipolar radiofrequency, cryoablation, and HIFU devices have also been used.[49,70,71]

Patient preparation begins with double-lumen endotracheal intubation. A transesophageal echocardiogram is performed to confirm the absence of thrombus in the left atrial appendage. If a thrombus is found, the procedure is either aborted or converted to an open procedure, in which the risk of systemic

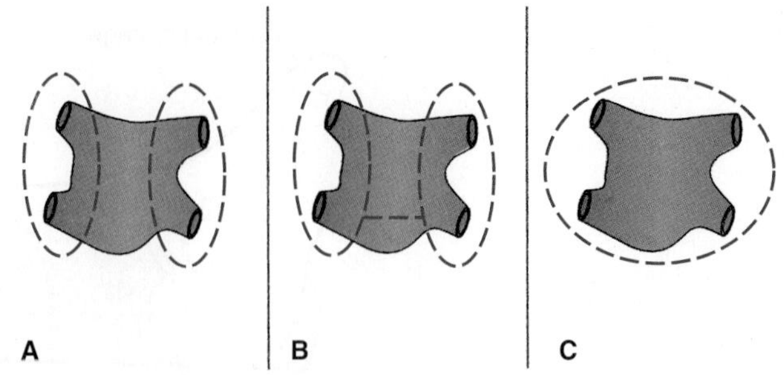

FIGURE 58-7 Diagram illustrating the methods to isolate the pulmonary veins, either separately (**A**), with a connecting lesion (**B**), or as a box isolation of the entire posterior left atrium (**C**).

thromboembolism from left atrial clot can be minimized. External defibrillator pads are placed on the patient and the patient is positioned with the right side turned upward 45 to 60 degrees and the right arm positioned above the head to expose the right axilla.

An initial port for the thoracoscopic camera is placed at the sixth intercostal space. Under thoracoscopic vision, a small working port can then be placed in either the third or fourth intercostal space at the midaxillary line depending on surgeon preference and patient anatomy. The right phrenic nerve is identified to avoid injury to this structure. An incision is made in the pericardium, anterior and parallel to the phrenic nerve, to expose the heart from the superior vena cava to the diaphragm. Through this pericardiotomy, the space above and below the right pulmonary veins is dissected to allow enough room for insertion of a specialized thoracoscopic dissector. This includes opening into the oblique sinus and dissecting the space between the right superior PV and the right pulmonary artery. The dissector and a guiding sheath is introduced through a second port, either lateral or medial to the scope port, and guided into the space between the right superior pulmonary vein and right pulmonary artery. After the dissector is carefully removed from the chest, the sheath remains in place as a guide for the insertion of the bipolar RF clamp. At this point, the patient is cardioverted into sinus rhythm so that pacing thresholds can be obtained. As with a Cox-Maze IV procedure, it is critical to document pacing thresholds from the pulmonary veins before isolation. Some surgeons also use the opportunity provided by surgical exposure to test and ablate ganglionated plexi.

The sheath is attached to the lower jaw of a bipolar RF clamp. The clamp is introduced into the chest, and the left atrium surrounding the pulmonary veins is clamped and ablated. After confirmation of exit block by pacing, the instruments are removed from the right chest and the right chest ports are closed.

The approach to the left chest is similar to the right. The patient is repositioned such that the left chest is elevated 45 to 60 degrees and the left arm is held up to expose the left axilla. A port for the thoracoscopic camera is placed in the sixth intercostal space, slightly more posterior than on the right side. With thoracoscopic visualization, a left-sided working port is created in the third or fourth intercostal space (Fig. 58-8). The left phrenic nerve is identified, and the pericardium is opened

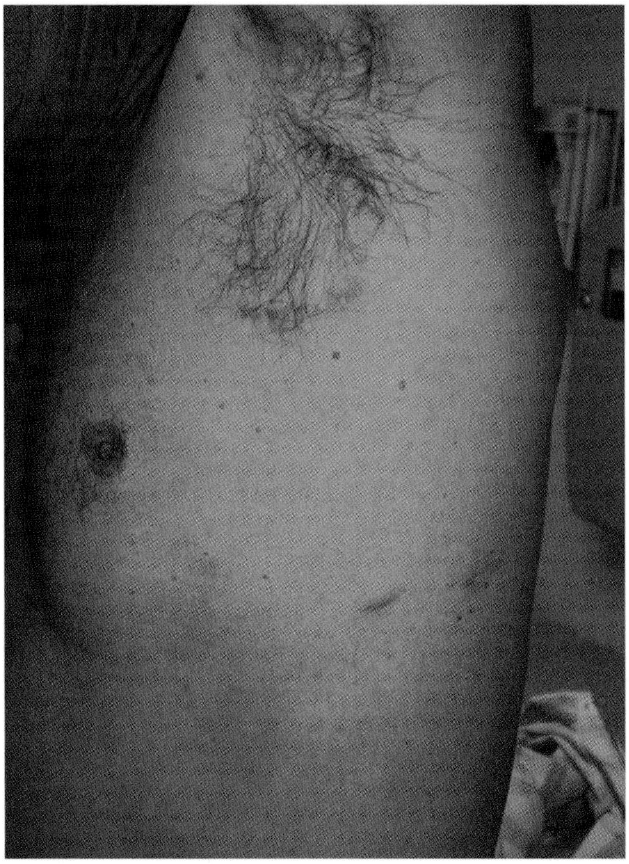

FIGURE 58-8 Patient after left atrial pulmonary vein isolation approach.

posterior to the course of the nerve. The ligament of Marshall is identified and divided. The dissector is then introduced through a second port, also in the sixth intercostal space. This port site is placed to allow for a straight line introduction of the dissector around the pulmonary veins. The guiding sheath is used to position the RF clamp around the left pulmonary veins, and they are isolated. Again, conduction block is confirmed with pacing.

The procedure is not complete until the left atrial appendage has been addressed. Traditionally, this has been done by stapling across the base of the left atrial appendage with an endoscopic stapler. This requires careful surgical technique and attention because it can result in tears and bleeding.[72] There are clip devices in development designed to address this difficulty.[73,74] Further investigation is needed to determine their efficacy and safety for this purpose. After ablation of the left pulmonary veins and exclusion of the left atrial appendage, the left side of the pericardium is closed.

SURGICAL RESULTS

The Cox-Maze Procedure

The Cox-Maze III procedure has had excellent long-term results. In our series at Washington University, 97% of 198 consecutive patients who underwent the procedure with a mean follow-up of 5.4 years were free from symptomatic AF. There was no difference in the cure rates between patients undergoing a stand-alone Cox-Maze procedure and those undergoing concomitant procedures.[22] Similar results have been obtained from other institutions around the world with the traditional "cut-and-sew" method.[23,25,75]

Our results from patients who underwent the Cox-Maze IV procedure have been encouraging as well. In a prospective, single-center trial from our institution, 91% of patients at the 6-month follow-up were free from AF.[42,54] The Cox-Maze IV procedure has significantly shortened the mean cross-clamp times for a lone Cox-Maze from 93 ± 34 minutes for the Cox-Maze III to 47 ± 26 minutes for the Cox-Maze IV ($p < .001$), and from 122 ± 37 minutes for a concomitant Cox-Maze III procedure to 92 ± 37 minutes ($p < .005$) in those undergoing the Cox-Maze IV procedure concomitantly with another cardiac operation.[42] A propensity analysis performed by our group has shown that there was no significant difference in the freedom from AF at 3, 6, or 12 months between the Cox-Maze III and IV groups.[54]

The Cox-Maze IV procedure also worked as well in patients with paroxysmal as for longstanding persistent AF. The 6-month freedom for AF was 91% in the paroxysmal group compared with 88% in the persistent group ($p = .53$). The drug-free success rate was also similar.[76] Our present series consists of 263 consecutive patients undergoing a Cox-Maze IV between January 2002 and June 2009. All patients have been followed with ECGs or prolonged monitoring. Our 12-month freedom from AF was 93%, with 78% of patients also off all antiarrhythmic drugs. We have had no intraoperative mortalities in 90 consecutive patients with lone atrial fibrillation undergoing this procedure.

Left Atrial Lesion Sets

A number of centers around the world have suggested performing ablation confined to the left atrium only to cure AF. This concept is supported by the fact that the majority of paroxysmal AF appears to originate around the PVs and the posterior left atrium. A left atrial lesion set typically involves pulmonary vein isolation with a lesion to the mitral annulus as well as removal of the left atrial appendage. Many ablation technologies have been used to create these lesion sets with varied degrees of success.[43,56–63]

There have been no randomized trials of biatrial versus left atrial ablation only in the surgical population. Because of this, the importance of the right atrial lesions of the traditional Cox-Maze procedure is difficult to determine. A meta-analysis of the published literature by Barnett and Ad revealed that a biatrial lesion set resulted in a significantly higher late freedom from AF when compared with a left atrial lesion set alone (87% versus 73%, $p = .05$).[77] This is not surprising considering the results of intraoperative mapping of patients with atrial fibrillation. Both our group and others have shown that AF can originate from the right atrium in 10 to 50% of cases.[78–80]

Of the specific left atrial lesions of the Cox-Maze procedure, it is difficult to determine the precise importance of each particular ablation. All surgeons agree on the importance of isolating the pulmonary veins. As stated previously, work from Gillinov et al has shown the importance of the left atrial isthmus in a retrospective study.[64] In a rare randomized trial, Gaita and coauthors examined pulmonary vein isolation alone versus two alternate lesion sets that both included ablation of the left atrial isthmus. In this study, normal sinus rhythm at 2-year follow-up was only seen in 20% in the PVI group versus 57% in the other groups ($p < .006$).[62] Finally, our group has shown that isolating the entire posterior left atrium significantly improved our drug-free freedom from AF at 6 months (54% versus 79%, $p = .011$) in a retrospective analysis of our results. Thus, most of the left atrial Cox-Maze lesion set is likely needed to ensure a high success rate. However, there has been no randomized trial to conclusively demonstrate the correct left atrial lesion set.

Pulmonary Vein Isolation

The results of PVI alone have been variable and have been dependent on patient selection. In the first report of surgical PVI, Wolf and colleagues reported that 91% of patients undergoing a video-assisted bilateral PVI and left atrial appendage exclusion were free from AF at three months follow-up.[81] Edgerton et al reported on 57 patients undergoing PVI with GP ablation with more thorough follow-up and found 82% of their patients with paroxysmal AF to be free from AF at 6 months, with 74% off antiarrhythmic drugs.[82] Subsequent studies have shown encouraging results in patients with paroxysmal AF. In a study involving 21 patients with paroxysmal AF undergoing PVI with GP ablation, McClelland et al reported 88% freedom from AF at 1 year without antiarrhythmic drugs.[68] A larger, single-center trial recently reported a 65% single procedure success at 1 year in a series of 45 patients undergoing PVI with GP ablation, including patients with persistent and paroxysmal AF.[83] A multicenter trial reported 87% normal sinus rhythm rate in a more diverse patient population, including some patients with longstanding persistent AF; however, those patients with longstanding persistent AF only had a 71% incidence of normal sinus rhythm.[84]

In patients with longstanding or persistent AF, the results have been worse. In a study from Edgerton and his group, only 56% of patients were free from AF at 6 months follow-up (35% off antiarrhythmics).[85] With concomitant procedures, the success rate of PVI is even lower. Of 23 patients undergoing mitral valve surgery or coronary revascularization with concomitant PVI, only half of patients were free from AF at a follow-up of 57 ± 37 months.[86] In the setting of mitral valve disease, Tada and colleagues report 61% freedom from AF and an only 17% freedom from antiarrhythmic drugs in their series of 66 patients undergoing PVI.[87]

Ganglionated Plexus Ablation

There have been convincing experimental data demonstrating that autonomic ganglia in ganglionated plexi (GP) play a role in the initiation and maintenance of AF.[88,89] As a result, some surgeons have added GP ablation to pulmonary vein isolation in hopes to increase procedural efficacy. Some of the initial surgical results have been encouraging. However, there have been no randomized trials demonstrating the efficacy of adding GP to PVI. In 2005, Scherlag and colleagues reported a study of GP ablation combined with catheter PVI in 74 patients with lone AF. After a relatively short median follow-up of 5 months, 91% of patients were free from AF.[89]

However, the effects of vagal denervation are not clearly defined. Experimental evidence in our laboratory and others have demonstrated recovery of autonomic function as early as 4 weeks after GP ablation.[90–92] It is worrisome that the reinnervation may not be homogenous and could result in a more arrhythmogenic substrate. In a more recent report, Katritsis and colleagues used left atrial GP ablation alone to treat 19 patients with paroxysmal AF. Fourteen of these patients had recurrent AF during 1-year follow-up.[93] Because of these suboptimal results and the lack of any long-term follow-up regarding the effects of GP ablation, our practice is not to perform GP ablation to treat AF. GP ablation should be reserved for centers participating in clinical trials.

INDICATIONS FOR SURGICAL ABLATION

The indications for surgery have been defined in a recent consensus statement.[94] These presently include: (1) All symptomatic patients with documented atrial fibrillation undergoing other cardiac surgical procedures; (2) selected asymptomatic patients with atrial fibrillation undergoing cardiac surgery in which the ablation can be performed with minimal risk in experienced centers; and (3) stand-alone atrial fibrillation ablation should be considered for symptomatic patients with atrial fibrillation who either prefer a surgical approach, have failed one or more attempts at catheter ablation, or are not candidates for catheter ablation.

There is still controversy regarding the referral of patients for surgery with medically refractory, symptomatic atrial fibrillation in lieu of catheter ablation. No randomized controlled trials exist that compare outcomes with catheter versus surgical ablation. In these instances, clinical decisions should be made based on the individual institution's experience with catheter and surgical ablation, the relative outcomes and risks of each in the individual patient, and patient preference. Programs involved in the surgical treatment of atrial fibrillation should develop a team approach to these patients, including both electrophysiologists and surgeons, to ensure appropriate selection of patients.

There are relative indications for surgery that were not included in the consensus statement. The first is a contraindication to long-term anticoagulation in patients with persistent AF and a high risk for stroke (CHADS score ≥2). Up to one-third of patients with AF screened for participation in clinical trials of warfarin were deemed ineligible for chronic anticoagulation, mainly because of a high perceived risk for bleeding complications.[95–97] In one study, the annual rate of intracranial hemorrhage in anticoagulated patients with AF was 0.9% per year, and the overall major bleeding complication rate was 2.3% per year.[96] The stroke rate following the Cox-Maze procedure off anticoagulation has been remarkably low, even in high-risk patients. At our institution, only 5 of 450 patients had a stroke after a mean follow-up of 6.9 ± 5.1 years. There was no difference in stroke rate in those patients with CHADS scores above or below 2.[98] This low risk of stroke after the Cox-Maze procedure has been noted in other series.[18,99,100] The decrease in stroke risk is likely due to the high cure rate, as well as the resection of the left atrial appendage.

Surgical treatment for AF with amputation of the left atrial appendage also should be considered in patients with chronic AF who have suffered a cerebrovascular accident despite adequate anticoagulation, as these patients are at high risk for repeat neurologic events. Anticoagulation with warfarin reduces the risk of ischemic and hemorrhagic strokes by more than 60% in patients with AF, but does not completely eliminate this serious complication.[9,101] At our institution, 20% of patients who underwent the Cox-Maze III procedure had experienced at least one episode of cerebral thromboembolism that resulted in a significant temporary or permanent neurologic deficit before undergoing the operation.[22] There were no late strokes in this population, even with 90% of patients off anticoagulation at last follow-up.[22]

In patients undergoing concomitant valve surgery, studies have shown that adding the Cox-Maze procedure can decrease the late risk of cardiac- and stroke-related deaths.[102,103] However, there have been no prospective, randomized studies demonstrating the survival or other benefits of adding a Cox-Maze procedure in patients with AF. A contraindication to a Cox-Maze procedure in the concomitant surgery group would be in asymptomatic patients who have tolerated their AF well and have not had problems with anticoagulation, in whom adding the ablation would increase their surgical risk.

FUTURE DIRECTIONS IN AF SURGERY

Although the Cox-Maze procedure achieves high rates of success and recent technological advances have made it easier to perform, it still represents an invasive procedure that requires cardiopulmonary bypass. A simple, minimally invasive operation that does not require cardiopulmonary bypass would be preferable. Such a procedure should preserve normal atrial physiology, and have minimal morbidity and a high success rate. Achieving this goal will require progress in understanding the mechanism of AF in individual patients. The surgical approach may need to be redesigned based on a better understanding of the mechanisms and the effects of surgical ablation on atrial electrophysiology.

It is now known that there are multiple different possible mechanisms of AF and that multipoint mapping is necessary to describe this complex arrhythmia.[79-81,104,105] Epicardial activation sequence mapping has been the traditional gold standard for mapping of AF, but is both invasive and time consuming, limiting its clinical use.[17] A newer noninvasive technique, electrocardiographic imaging (ECGI), offers a potentially useful way to describe the atrial activation sequence and determine mechanistic information from conscious patients.[106] The technique uses body surface potentials, measured by surface electrodes, and anatomical data obtained through computed tomographic scanning to indirectly calculate the surface potentials on the surface of the heart. This technique has been shown to work well for normal sinus rhythm and atrial flutter as well as ventricular arrhythmias.[107–109] Currently our group is testing the technique in patients with AF, in collaboration with Yoram Rudy at Washington University, the developer of ECGI. The initial results are promising.[107,110]

The information acquired from ECGI can be analyzed to determine activation sequence and frequency maps for individual patients noninvasively. Using these data, a strategy for designing patient-specific optimal lesion sets is being developed, taking into account the patient's atrial geometry, conduction velocity, and refractory period.[111] Previous work has demonstrated that a critical mass is necessary to maintain AF, and initial lesions could be determined by a calculation of the critical area needed to maintain AF in the individual patient.[112] This could be done using mechanistic information derived from activation data and anatomical data from a CT scan. It will also allow identification of focal sources that can then be either isolated or ablated in the electrophysiologic laboratory or operating room.

In instances in which a specific mechanism of AF cannot be defined, the goal will be to create a lesion pattern that will make the atria unable to fibrillate. Failures of the Cox-Maze III and IV procedures have been seen in patients with increasing left atrial size or longstanding AF.[99,112,113] A recent study performed by our laboratory on a canine model found that the probability of maintaining AF is correlated with increasing atrial tissue areas, widths, and weights, as well as the length of the effective refractory period and the conduction velocity of the tissue.[111] All of these data can be acquired noninvasively through ECGI. Using these data may allow surgeons to design custom operations for each patient based on the mechanism of their arrhythmia and their specific atrial anatomy or electrophysiology.

Finally, the limitations of present ablation devices have impeded the development of a truly minimally invasive procedure. Unfortunately, the creation of reliable transmural lines of ablation on the beating heart has been difficult. This has been because of the heat sink of the circulating endocardial blood pool.[39] Future advances may be anticipated with devices that overcome this limitation or by the introduction of hybrid procedures in which surgeons and electrophysiologists work together to complete lines of block.

In conclusion, the development of ablation technologies has dramatically changed the field of AF surgery. The replacement of the surgical incisions with linear lines of ablation has transformed a complex, technically demanding procedure into one accessible to the majority of surgeons. More importantly, these new ablation technologies have introduced the possibility of minimally invasive surgery for AF, prompting numerous efforts to develop simpler procedures that can be preformed epicardially on the beating heart. There is already strong evidence that PVI may be effective in a subset of patients with paroxysmal AF. With extended lesions sets, it may be possible to extend the efficacy of minimally invasive procedures to patients with persistent and longstanding AF. However, surgeons must remember that the Cox-Maze procedure has good efficacy in these patients and can be performed using a small thoracotomy with acceptable success and low morbidity.[100] It is imperative for surgeons trying new procedures to carefully follow their results and publish them in peer-reviewed journals. For surgeons performing AF ablation, it is mandatory to adhere to the recently published guidelines for follow-up of patients and for determining success or failure after these procedures. As we learn more about the mechanisms of AF and develop improved preoperative diagnostic technologies capable of precisely locating the areas responsible for AF, it will become possible to tailor specific lesion sets and ablation modalities to individual patients, making the surgical treatment of AF more effective and available to a larger population of patients.

REFERENCES

1. Benjamin EJ, Levy D, Vaziri SM, et al: Independent risk factors for atrial fibrillation in a population-based cohort. The Framingham Heart Study. *JAMA* 1994; 271(11):840-844.
2. Wolf PA, Benjamin EJ, Belanger AJ, et al: Secular trends in the prevalence of atrial fibrillation: the Framingham Study. *Am Heart J* 1996; 131(4):790-795.
3. Cairns JA: Stroke prevention in atrial fibrillation trial. *Circulation* 1991; 84(2):933-935.
4. Hart RG, Halperin JL, Pearce LA, et al: Lessons from the Stroke Prevention in Atrial Fibrillation trials. *Ann Intern Med* 2003; 138(10): 831-838.
5. Sherman DG, Kim SG, Boop BS, et al: Occurrence and characteristics of stroke events in the Atrial Fibrillation Follow-up Investigation of Sinus Rhythm Management (AFFIRM) study. *Arch Intern Med* 2005; 165(10): 1185-1191.
6. Wolf PA, Abbott RD, Kannel WB: Atrial fibrillation as an independent risk factor for stroke: the Framingham Study. *Stroke* 1991; 22(8): 983-988.
7. Glader EL, Stegmayr B, Norrving B, et al: Large variations in the use of oral anticoagulants in stroke patients with atrial fibrillation: a Swedish national perspective. *J Intern Med* 2004; 255(1):22-32.
8. Steger C, Pratter A, Martinek-Bregel M, et al: Stroke patients with atrial fibrillation have a worse prognosis than patients without: data from the Austrian Stroke registry. *Eur Heart J* 2004; 25(19):1734-1740.
9. Risk factors for stroke and efficacy of antithrombotic therapy in atrial fibrillation. Analysis of pooled data from five randomized controlled trials. *Arch Intern Med* 1994; 154(13):1449-1457.
10. Wolf PA, Abbott RD, Kannel WB: Atrial fibrillation: a major contributor to stroke in the elderly. The Framingham Study. *Arch Intern Med* 1987; 147(9):1561-1564.
11. Williams JM, Ungerleider RM, Lofland GK, Cox JL: Left atrial isolation: new technique for the treatment of supraventricular arrhythmias. *J Thorac Cardiovasc Surg* 1980; 80(3):373-380.
12. Scheinman MM, Morady F, Hess DS, Gonzalez R: Catheter-induced ablation of the atrioventricular junction to control refractory supraventricular arrhythmias. *JAMA* 1982; 248(7):851-855.
13. Guiraudon GM, Campbell CS, Jones DL, et al: Combined sinoatrial node atrioventricular node isolation: a surgical alternative to His bundle ablation in patients with atrial fibrillation. *Circulation* 1985; 72(Suppl 3):220.
14. Smith PK, Holman WL, Cox JL: Surgical treatment of supraventricular tachyarrhythmias. *Surg Clin North Am* 1985; 65(3):553-570.
15. Cox JL, Schuessler RB, D'Agostino HJ Jr, et al: The surgical treatment of atrial fibrillation. III. Development of a definitive surgical procedure. *J Thorac Cardiovasc Surg* 1991; 101(4):569-583.
16. Cox JL: The surgical treatment of atrial fibrillation. IV. Surgical technique. *J Thorac Cardiovasc Surg* 1991; 101(4):584-592.
17. Cox JL, Canavan TE, Schuessler RB, et al: The surgical treatment of atrial fibrillation. II. Intraoperative electrophysiologic mapping and description of the electrophysiologic basis of atrial flutter and atrial fibrillation. *J Thorac Cardiovasc Surg* 1991; 101(3):406-426.
18. Cox JL, Ad N, Palazzo T: Impact of the maze procedure on the stroke rate in patients with atrial fibrillation. *J Thorac Cardiovasc Surg* 1999; 118(5): 833-840.
19. Feinberg MS, Waggoner AD, Kater KM, et al: Restoration of atrial function after the maze procedure for patients with atrial fibrillation. Assessment by Doppler echocardiography. *Circulation* 1994; 90(5 Pt 2): II285-292.
20. Cox JL, Boineau JP, Schuessler RB, et al: Modification of the maze procedure for atrial flutter and atrial fibrillation. I. Rationale and surgical results. *J Thorac Cardiovasc Surg* 1995; 110(2):473-484.
21. Cox JL: The minimally invasive Maze-III procedure. *Op Techn Thorac Cardiovasc Surg* 2000; 5:79.
22. Prasad SM, Maniar HS, Camillo CJ, et al: The Cox maze III procedure for atrial fibrillation: long-term efficacy in patients undergoing lone versus concomitant procedures. *J Thorac Cardiovasc Surg* 2003; 126(6): 1822-1828.
23. McCarthy PM, Gillinov AM, Castle L, et al: The Cox-Maze procedure: the Cleveland Clinic experience. *Semin Thorac Cardiovasc Surg* 2000; 12(1):25-29.
24. Raanani E, Albage A, David TE, et al: The efficacy of the Cox/maze procedure combined with mitral valve surgery: a matched control study. *Eur J Cardiothorac Surg* 2001; 19(4):438-442.
25. Schaff HV, Dearani JA, Daly RC, et al: Cox-Maze procedure for atrial fibrillation: Mayo Clinic experience. *Semin Thorac Cardiovasc Surg* 2000; 12(1):30-37.
26. Gammie JS, Haddad M, Milford-Beland S, et al: Atrial fibrillation correction surgery: lessons from the Society of Thoracic Surgeons National Cardiac Database. *Ann Thorac Surg* 2008; 85(3):909-914.
27. Inoue H, Zipes DP: Conduction over an isthmus of atrial myocardium in vivo: a possible model of Wolff-Parkinson-White syndrome. *Circulation* 1987; 76(3):637-647.
28. Melby SJ, Lee AM, Zierer A, et al: Atrial fibrillation propagates through gaps in ablation lines: implications for ablative treatment of atrial fibrillation. *Heart Rhythm* 2008; 5(9):1296-1301.
29. Ishii Y, Nitta T, Sakamoto S, Tanaka S, Asano G: Incisional atrial reentrant tachycardia: experimental study on the conduction property through the isthmus. *J Thorac Cardiovasc Surg* 2003; 126(1):254-262.
30. Melby SJ, Lee AM, Damiano RJ: Advances in surgical ablation devices for atrial fibrillation, in Wang PJ (ed): *New Arrhythmia Technologies*. Boston, Blackwell Futura, 2005; pp 233-241.
31. Gage AM, Montes M, Gage AA: Freezing the canine thoracic aorta in situ. *J Surg Res* 1979; 27(5):331-340.
32. Holman WL, Ikeshita M, Ungerleider RM, et al: Cryosurgery for cardiac arrhythmias: acute and chronic effects on coronary arteries. *Am J Cardiol* 1983; 51(1):149-155.
33. Aupperle H, Doll N, Walther T, et al: Ablation of atrial fibrillation and esophageal injury: effects of energy source and ablation technique. *J Thorac Cardiovasc Surg* 2005; 130(6):1549-1554.
34. Viola N, Williams MR, Oz MC, Ad N: The technology in use for the surgical ablation of atrial fibrillation. *Semin Thorac Cardiovasc Surg* 2002; 14(3):198-205.
35. Santiago T, Melo JQ, Gouveia RH, Martins AP: Intra-atrial temperatures in radiofrequency endocardial ablation: histologic evaluation of lesions. *Ann Thorac Surg* 2003; 75(5):1495-1501.
36. Thomas SP, Guy DJ, Boyd AC, et al: Comparison of epicardial and endocardial linear ablation using handheld probes. *Ann Thorac Surg* 2003; 75(2):543-548.
37. Hoenicke EM SRJ, Patel H, et al: Initial experience with epicardial radiofrequency ablation catheter in an ovine model: moving towards an endoscopic Maze procedure. *Surg Forum* 2000; 51:79-82.
38. Santiago T, Melo J, Gouveia RH, et al: Epicardial radiofrequency applications: in vitro and in vivo studies on human atrial myocardium. *Eur J Cardiothorac Surg* 2003; 24(4):481-486; discussion 486.
39. Melby SJ, Zierer A, Kaiser SP, Schuessler RB, Damiano RJ Jr: Epicardial microwave ablation on the beating heart for atrial fibrillation: the dependency of lesion depth on cardiac output. *J Thorac Cardiovasc Surg* 2006; 132(2):355-360.
40. Prasad SM, Maniar HS, Schuessler RB, Damiano RJ Jr: Chronic transmural atrial ablation by using bipolar radiofrequency energy on the beating heart. *J Thorac Cardiovasc Surg* 2002; 124(4):708-713.
41. Prasad SM, Maniar HS, Diodato MD, Schuessler RB, Damiano RJ Jr: Physiological consequences of bipolar radiofrequency energy on the atria and pulmonary veins: a chronic animal study. *Ann Thorac Surg* 2003; 76(3):836-841; discussion 841-832.
42. Gaynor SL, Diodato MD, Prasad SM, et al: A prospective, single-center clinical trial of a modified Cox maze procedure with bipolar radiofrequency ablation. *J Thorac Cardiovasc Surg* 2004; 128(4):535-542.
43. Kottkamp H, Hindricks G, Autschbach R, et al: Specific linear left atrial lesions in atrial fibrillation: intraoperative radiofrequency ablation using minimally invasive surgical techniques. *J Am Coll Cardiol* 2002, 40(3): 475-480.
44. Gillinov AM, Pettersson G, Rice TW: Esophageal injury during radiofrequency ablation for atrial fibrillation. *J Thorac Cardiovasc Surg* 2001; 122(6): 1239-1240.

45. Laczkovics A, Khargi K, Deneke T: Esophageal perforation during left atrial radiofrequency ablation. *J Thorac Cardiovasc Surg* 2003; 126(6):2119-2120; author reply 2120.
46. Damaria RG PP, Leung TK, et al: Surgical radiofrequency ablation induces coronary endothelial dysfunction in porcine coronary arteries. *Eur J Cardiothorac Surg* 2003; 23:277-282.
47. Ninet J, Roques X, Seitelberger R, et al: Surgical ablation of atrial fibrillation with off-pump, epicardial, high-intensity focused ultrasound: results of a multicenter trial. *J Thorac Cardiovasc Surg* 2005; 130(3):803-809.
48. Groh MA, Binns OA, Burton HG 3rd, et al: Epicardial ultrasonic ablation of atrial fibrillation during concomitant cardiac surgery is a valid option in patients with ischemic heart disease. *Circulation* 2008; 118(14 Suppl): S78-82.
49. Mitnovetski S, Almeida AA, Goldstein J, Pick AW, Smith JA: Epicardial high-intensity focused ultrasound cardiac ablation for surgical treatment of atrial fibrillation. *Heart Lung Circ* 2009; 18(1):28-31.
50. Nakagawa H, Antz M, Wong T, et al: Initial experience using a forward directed, high-intensity focused ultrasound balloon catheter for pulmonary vein antrum isolation in patients with atrial fibrillation. *J Cardiovasc Electrophysiol* 2007; 18(2):136-144.
51. Klinkenberg TJ, Ahmed S, Hagen AT, et al: Feasibility and outcome of epicardial pulmonary vein isolation for lone atrial fibrillation using minimal invasive surgery and high intensity focused ultrasound. *Europace* 2009; 11(12):1624-1631.
52. Damiano Jr RJ, Gaynor SL: Atrial fibrillation ablation during mitral valve surgery using the AtriCure device. *Op Techn Thorac Cardiovasc Surg* 2004; 9(1):24-33.
53. Mokadam NA, McCarthy PM, Gillinov AM, et al: A prospective multicenter trial of bipolar radiofrequency ablation for atrial fibrillation: early results. *Ann Thorac Surg* 2004; 78(5):1665-1670.
54. Lall SC, Melby SJ, Voeller RK, et al: The effect of ablation technology on surgical outcomes after the Cox-maze procedure: a propensity analysis. *J Thorac Cardiovasc Surg* 2007; 133(2):389-396.
55. Voeller RK, Bailey MS, Zierer A, et al: Isolating the entire posterior left atrium improves surgical outcomes after the Cox maze procedure. *J Thorac Cardiovasc Surg* 2008; 135(4):870-877.
56. Sie HT, Beukema WP, Misier AR, et al: Radiofrequency modified maze in patients with atrial fibrillation undergoing concomitant cardiac surgery. *J Thorac Cardiovasc Surg* 2001; 122(2):249-256.
57. Schuetz A, Schulze CJ, Sarvanakis KK, et al: Surgical treatment of permanent atrial fibrillation using microwave energy ablation: a prospective randomized clinical trial. *Eur J Cardiothorac Surg* 2003; 24(4):475-480; discussion 480.
58. Kondo N, Takahashi K, Minakawa M, Daitoku K: Left atrial maze procedure: a useful addition to other corrective operations. *Ann Thorac Surg* 2003; 75(5):1490-1494.
59. Knaut M, Spitzer SG, Karolyi L, et al: Intraoperative microwave ablation for curative treatment of atrial fibrillation in open heart surgery—the MICRO-STAF and MICRO-PASS pilot trial. MICROwave Application in Surgical Treatment of Atrial Fibrillation. MICROwave Application for the Treatment of Atrial Fibrillation in Bypass-Surgery. *Thorac Cardiovasc Surg* 1999; 47(Suppl 3):379-384.
60. Imai K, Sueda T, Orihashi K, Watari M, Matsuura Y: Clinical analysis of results of a simple left atrial procedure for chronic atrial fibrillation. *Ann Thorac Surg* 2001; 71(2):577-581.
61. Gaita F, Riccardi R, Caponi D, et al: Linear cryoablation of the left atrium versus pulmonary vein cryoisolation in patients with permanent atrial fibrillation and valvular heart disease: correlation of electroanatomic mapping and long-term clinical results. *Circulation* 2005; 111(2): 136-142.
62. Fasol R, Meinhart J, Binder T: A modified and simplified radiofrequency ablation in patients with mitral valve disease. *J Thorac Cardiovasc Surg* 2005; 129(1):215-217.
63. Benussi S, Nascimbene S, Agricola E, et al: Surgical ablation of atrial fibrillation using the epicardial radiofrequency approach: mid-term results and risk analysis. *Ann Thorac Surg* 2002; 74(4):1050-1056; discussion 1057.
64. Gillinov AM, McCarthy PM, Blackstone EH, et al: Surgical ablation of atrial fibrillation with bipolar radiofrequency as the primary modality. *J Thorac Cardiovasc Surg* 2005; 129(6):1322-1329.
65. Haissaguerre M, Jais P, Shah DC, et al: Spontaneous initiation of atrial fibrillation by ectopic beats originating in the pulmonary veins. *NEJM* 1998; 339(10):659-666.
66. Lee SH, Tai CT, Hsieh MH, et al: Predictors of non-pulmonary vein ectopic beats initiating paroxysmal atrial fibrillation: implication for catheter ablation. *J Am Coll Cardiol* 2005; 46(6):1054-1059.
67. Doll N, Pritzwald-Stegmann P, Czesla M, et al: Ablation of ganglionic plexi during combined surgery for atrial fibrillation. *Ann Thorac Surg* 2008; 86(5):1659-1663.
68. McClelland JH, Duke D, Reddy R: Preliminary results of a limited thoracotomy: new approach to treat atrial fibrillation. *J Cardiovasc Electrophysiol* 2007; 18(12):1289-1295.
69. Mehall JR, Kohut RM Jr, Schneeberger EW, et al: Intraoperative epicardial electrophysiologic mapping and isolation of autonomic ganglionic plexi. *Ann Thorac Surg* 2007; 83(2):538-541.
70. Geuzebroek GS, Ballaux PK, van Hemel NM, Kelder JC, Defauw JJ: Medium-term outcome of different surgical methods to cure atrial fibrillation: is less worse? *Interact Cardiovasc Thorac Surg* 2008; 7(2): 201-206.
71. Reyes G, Benedicto A, Bustamante J, et al: Restoration of atrial contractility after surgical cryoablation: clinical, electrical and mechanical results. *Interact Cardiovasc Thorac Surg* 2009; 9(4):609-612.
72. Healey JS, Crystal E, Lamy A, et al: Left Atrial Appendage Occlusion Study (LAAOS): results of a randomized controlled pilot study of left atrial appendage occlusion during coronary bypass surgery in patients at risk for stroke. *Am Heart J* 2005; 150(2):288-293.
73. Salzberg SP, Plass A, Emmert MY et al: Left atrial appendage clip occlusion: early clinical results. *J Thorac Cardiovasc Surg* 2010; 139(5):1269-1274. Epub 2009.
74. Salzberg SP, Gillinov AM, Anyanwu A, et al: Surgical left atrial appendage occlusion: evaluation of a novel device with magnetic resonance imaging. *Eur J Cardiothorac Surg* 2008; 34(4):766-770.
75. Arcidi JM Jr, Doty DB, Millar RC: The Maze procedure: the LDS Hospital experience. *Semin Thorac Cardiovasc Surg* 2000; 12(1):38-43.
76. Aziz A, Bailey MS, Patel A, et al: The type of atrial fibrillation does not influence late outcome following the Cox-Maze IV procedure. *Heart Rhythm* 2008; 5(5):S318.
77. Barnett SD, Ad N: Surgical ablation as treatment for the elimination of atrial fibrillation: a meta-analysis. *J Thorac Cardiovasc Surg* 2006; 131(5): 1029-1035.
78. Sahadevan J, Ryu K, Peltz L, et al: Epicardial mapping of chronic atrial fibrillation in patients: preliminary observations. *Circulation* 2004; 110(21): 3293-3299.
79. Nitta T, Ishii Y, Miyagi Y, et al: Concurrent multiple left atrial focal activations with fibrillatory conduction and right atrial focal or reentrant activation as the mechanism in atrial fibrillation. *J Thorac Cardiovasc Surg* 2004; 127(3):770-778.
80. Schuessler RB, Kay MW, Melby SJ, et al: Spatial and temporal stability of the dominant frequency of activation in human atrial fibrillation. *J Electrocardiol* 2006; 39(4 Suppl):S7-12.
81. Wolf RK, Schneeberger EW, Osterday R, et al: Video-assisted bilateral pulmonary vein isolation and left atrial appendage exclusion for atrial fibrillation. *J Thorac Cardiovasc Surg* 2005; 130(3):797-802.
82. Edgerton JR, Jackman WM, Mack MJ: Minimally invasive pulmonary vein isolation and partial autonomic denervation for surgical treatment of atrial fibrillation. *J Interv Card Electrophysiol* 2007; 20(3):89-93.
83. Han FT, Kasirajan V, Kowalski M, et al: Results of a minimally invasive surgical pulmonary vein isolation and ganglionic plexi ablation for atrial fibrillation: single-center experience with 12-month follow-up. *Circ Arrhythm Electrophysiol* 2009; 2(4):370-377.
84. Beyer E, Lee R, Lam BK: Point: minimally invasive bipolar radiofrequency ablation of lone atrial fibrillation: early multicenter results. *J Thorac Cardiovasc Surg* 2009; 137(3):521-526.
85. Edgerton JR, Edgerton ZJ, Weaver T, et al: Minimally invasive pulmonary vein isolation and partial autonomic denervation for surgical treatment of atrial fibrillation. *Ann Thorac Surg* 2008; 86(1):35-38; discussion 39.
86. Melby SJ, Zierer A, Bailey MS, et al: A new era in the surgical treatment of atrial fibrillation: the impact of ablation technology and lesion set on procedural efficacy. *Ann Surg* 2006; 244(4):583-592.
87. Tada H, Ito S, Naito S, et al: Long-term results of cryoablation with a new cryoprobe to eliminate chronic atrial fibrillation associated with mitral valve disease. *Pacing Clin Electrophysiol* 2005; (28 Suppl 1):S73-77.
88. Po SS, Scherlag BJ, Yamanashi WS, et al: Experimental model for paroxysmal atrial fibrillation arising at the pulmonary vein-atrial junctions. *Heart Rhythm* 2006; 3(2):201-208.
89. Scherlag BJ, Nakagawa H, Jackman WM, et al: Electrical stimulation to identify neural elements on the heart: their role in atrial fibrillation. *J Interv Card Electrophysiol* 2005; (13 Suppl 1):37-42.
90. Sakamoto S, Schuessler RB, Lee AM, et al: Vagal denervation and reinnervation after ablation of ganglionated plexi. *J Thorac Cardiovasc Surg* 2009; 139(2):444-452.
91. Mounsey JP: Recovery from vagal denervation and atrial fibrillation inducibility: effects are complex and not always predictable. *Heart Rhythm* 2006; 3(6):709-710.

92. Oh S, Zhang Y, Bibevski S, et al: Vagal denervation and atrial fibrillation inducibility: epicardial fat pad ablation does not have long-term effects. *Heart Rhythm* 2006; 3(6):701-708.
93. Katritsis D, Giazitzoglou E, Sougiannis D, et al: Anatomic approach for ganglionic plexi ablation in patients with paroxysmal atrial fibrillation. *Am J Cardiol* 2008; 102(3):330-334.
94. Calkins H, Brugada J, Packer DL, et al: HRS/EHRA/ECAS expert Consensus Statement on catheter and surgical ablation of atrial fibrillation: recommendations for personnel, policy, procedures and follow-up. A report of the Heart Rhythm Society (HRS) Task Force on catheter and surgical ablation of atrial fibrillation. *Heart Rhythm* 2007; 4(6):816-861.
95. Stroke Prevention in Atrial Fibrillation Study: Final results. *Circulation* 1991; 84(2):527-539.
96. Schaer GN, Koechli OR, Schuessler B, Haller U: Usefulness of ultrasound contrast medium in perineal sonography for visualization of bladder neck funneling—first observations. *Urology* 1996; 47(3):452-453.
97. Rosand J, Eckman MH, Knudsen KA, Singer DE, Greenberg SM: The effect of warfarin and intensity of anticoagulation on outcome of intracerebral hemorrhage. *Arch Intern Med* 2004; 164(8):880-884.
98. Pet MA, Damiano RJ Jr, Bailey MS, et al: Late stroke following the Cox-Maze procedure for atrial fibrillation: the impact of CHADS2 score on long-term outcomes. *Heart Rhythm* 2009; 6(5 Suppl 1):S14.
99. Gillinov AM, Sirak J, Blackstone EH, et al: The Cox maze procedure in mitral valve disease: predictors of recurrent atrial fibrillation. *J Thorac Cardiovasc Surg* 2005; 130(6):1653-1660.
100. Ad N, Cox JL: The Maze procedure for the treatment of atrial fibrillation: a minimally invasive approach. *J Cardiol Surg* 2004; 19(3):196-200.
101. Hart RG, Halperin JL: Atrial fibrillation and thromboembolism: a decade of progress in stroke prevention. *Ann Intern Med* 1999; 131(9):688-695.
102. Bando K, Kobayashi J, Kosakai Y, et al: Impact of Cox maze procedure on outcome in patients with atrial fibrillation and mitral valve disease. *J Thorac Cardiovasc Surg* 2002; 124(3):575-583.
103. Bando K, Kasegawa H, Okada Y, et al: Impact of preoperative and postoperative atrial fibrillation on outcome after mitral valvuloplasty for nonischemic mitral regurgitation. *J Thorac Cardiovasc Surg* 2005; 129(5):1032-1040.
104. Berenfeld O, Mandapati R, Dixit S, et al: Spatially distributed dominant excitation frequencies reveal hidden organization in atrial fibrillation in the Langendorff-perfused sheep heart. *J Cardiovasc Electrophysiol* 2000; 11(8):869-879.
105. Nattel S, Shiroshita-Takeshita A, Brundel BJ, Rivard L: Mechanisms of atrial fibrillation: lessons from animal models. *Prog Cardiovasc Dis* 2005; 48(1):9-28.
106. Ramanathan C, Ghanem RN, Jia P, Ryu K, Rudy Y: Noninvasive electrocardiographic imaging for cardiac electrophysiology and arrhythmia. *Nat Med* 2004; 10(4):422-428.
107. Damiano RJ Jr, Schuessler RB, Voeller RK: Surgical treatment of atrial fibrillation: a look into the future. *Semin Thorac Cardiovasc Surg* 2007; 19(1):39-45.
108. Ghanem RN, Jia P, Ramanathan C, et al: Noninvasive electrocardiographic imaging (ECGI): comparison to intraoperative mapping in patients. *Heart Rhythm* 2005; 2(4):339-354.
109. Intini A, Goldstein RN, Jia P, et al: Electrocardiographic imaging (ECGI), a novel diagnostic modality used for mapping of focal left ventricular tachycardia in a young athlete. *Heart Rhythm* 2005; 2(11):1250-1252.
110. Schuessler RB, Damiano RJ Jr: Patient-specific surgical strategy for atrial fibrillation: promises and challenges. *Heart Rhythm* 2007; 4(9):1222-1224.
111. Byrd GD, Prasad SM, Ripplinger CM, et al: Importance of geometry and refractory period in sustaining atrial fibrillation: testing the critical mass hypothesis. *Circulation* 2005; 112(9 Suppl):I7-13.
112. Kosakai Y: Treatment of atrial fibrillation using the Maze procedure: the Japanese experience. *Semin Thorac Cardiovasc Surg* 2000; 12(1):44-52.
113. Gaynor SL, Schuessler RB, Bailey MS, et al: Surgical treatment of atrial fibrillation: predictors of late recurrence. *J Thorac Cardiovasc Surg* 2005; 129(1):104-111.

CHAPTER 59

Surgical Implantation of Pacemakers and Automatic Defibrillators

Henry M. Spotnitz

INTRODUCTION

Pacemaker and defibrillator management is the subject of comprehensive reviews.[1] In the author's experience with 2760 procedures, 23% of pacemaker recipients and 5% of implantable cardioverter defibrillator (ICD) recipients were octogenarians. The incidence of pacemaker insertion in patients older than 75 was 2.6% in a recent survey. The efficacy and cost-effectiveness of pacemakers are widely accepted, but the appropriate role for ICD insertion and biventricular pacing in older patients is still in evolution. Pacemaker and ICD technology is now applicable across the entire span of human age, with pacing for heart failure and ICD prophylaxis against lethal arrhythmias recent frontiers. Electrophysiologists now dominate these areas, reflecting decreased interest by thoracic surgeons and cardiology referrals. However, thoracic surgeons must maintain skills as implanters and consultants for complex or complicated cases. This chapter reviews practical information related to pacemaker and ICD insertion and management.

PACEMAKER-ICD TECHNOLOGY

Device Description

A permanent pacemaker or ICD consists of leads[2] and a generator. The generator contains a battery, a telemetry antenna, and integrated circuits. ICDs also include capacitors that store energy for high-output shocks. The power source is generally lithium iodide, but rechargeable and nuclear batteries have been used. The integrated circuits include programmable microprocessors, oscillators, amplifiers, and sensing circuits.[3] The integrated circuits employ CMOS (complementary metal-oxide semiconductor) technology, which is subject to damage by ionizing radiation.[4] Current pacemakers and ICDS monitor and report the status of internal components, external connections, programmed settings, recent activity, and notable arrhythmias. Unfortunately, each programmer controls only the devices of its manufacturer.

PACEMAKERS FOR CONTROL OF BRADYCARDIA

History

Early cardiac surgery was complicated by lethal iatrogenic heart block. Transthoracic pacing with Zoll cutaneous electrodes provided a solution.[5] Percutaneous endocardial pacing (1959)[6] and "permanent" pacemakers using epicardial electrodes (1960)[7] followed. Advances in bioengineering and technology have dramatically improved the quality of life for recipients. Persistent problems include lead durability, inflammatory responses to pacemaker materials, infection, device size, programmer compatibility, and expense. Development of resynchronization therapy has made coronary sinus lead insertion an important technical skill.

Anatomy of Surgical Heart Block

The conduction system is vulnerable to injury during heart surgery. Complete heart block can result from suture placement during aortic, mitral, or tricuspid valve surgery or during closure of septal defects or during myotomy for idiopathic hypertrophic subaortic stenosis. These lesions are illustrated in Fig. 59-1. Infarction of the conduction system or inadequate myocardial protection can also result in surgical heart block.

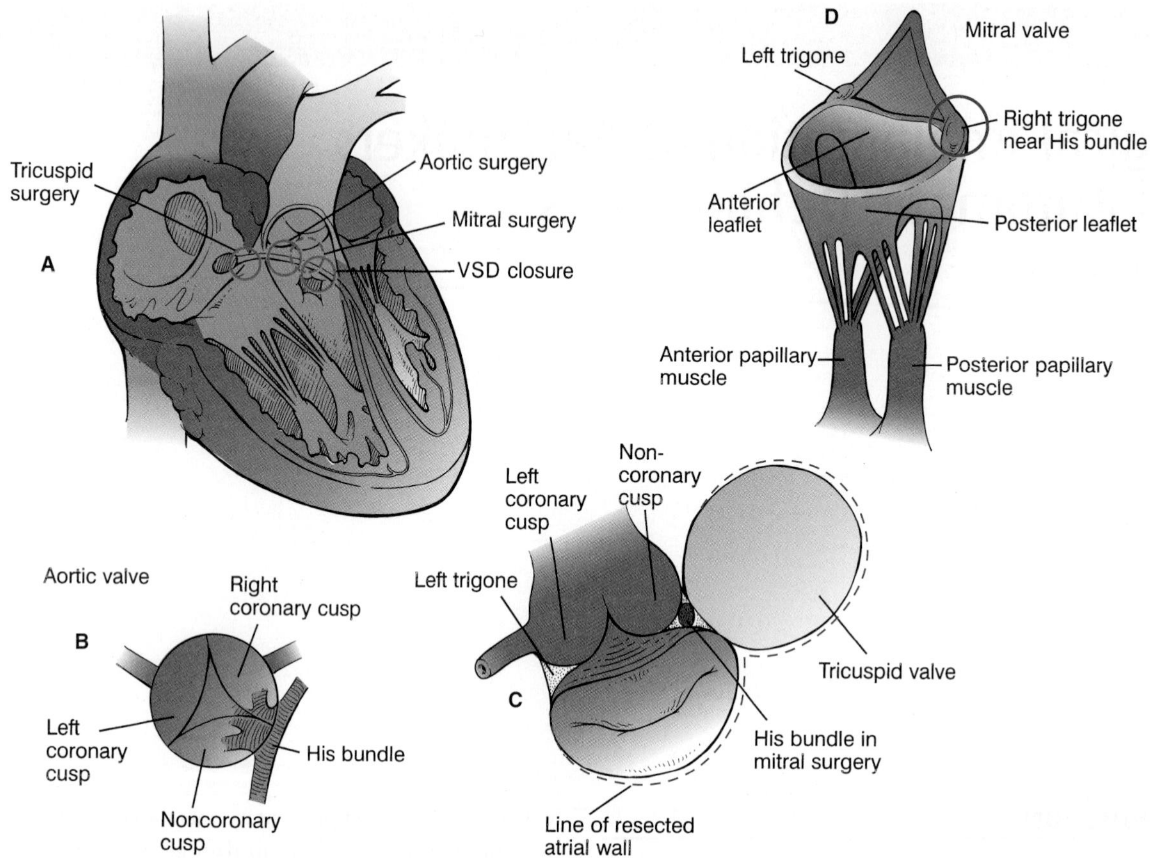

FIGURE 59-1 Anatomy of iatrogenic complete heart block. (A) His bundle and cardiac structures. Sites of injury are circled. (B) The His bundle in the ventricular septum, below the noncoronary-right coronary aortic commissure. (C,D) During mitral surgery, the His bundle is on the ventricular septum anteromedial to the posterior commissure and right fibrous trigone. VSD = ventricular septal defect.

International Pacemaker Code

A three-letter code describes the principal pacemaker functions (Table 59-1).[8] The first letter is the chamber paced, the second the chamber sensed, and the third the algorithm integrating pacing and sensing functions. Fixed-rate ventricular and atrial pacemakers are VOO and AOO, respectively. Demand (rate-inhibited) pacers for the same chambers are VVI and AAI. VDD pacemakers pace only the ventricle, but sense both atrium and ventricle. DVI indicates atrial and the ventricular pacing, but only ventricular sensing. DDD is the most flexible of current designs. The suffix R after the three-letter code indicates rate responsiveness. Pacemakers capable of biventricular pacing or *cardiac resynchronization therapy* (CRT) are referred to as *CRT-P*. Biventricular pacemaker-defibrillators are called *CRT-D*.

TABLE 59-1 International Pacemaker Code

I Chamber Paced	II Chamber Sensed	III Pacing Algorithm
A	A	T
V	V	I
D	D	D
0	0	0
S	S	—

A = atrium; D = dual (both triggered and inhibited); I = inhibited; 0 = none; S = single; T = triggered; V = ventricle.

Cellular Electrophysiology

Cell membrane depolarization and repolarization provide automaticity of the cardiac chambers and conduction system. The outside of the resting myocardial cell is positive, and the interior is negative. Unipolar pacing threshold is lowest when the negative terminal (cathode) of a pacemaker is connected to the heart and the positive terminal (anode) is connected to ground. Electrogram amplitude is unaffected by polarity.

Rhythm Disorders

Indications for Pacemaker Insertion

Pacemaker insertion guidelines (Table 59-2) are periodically updated. Documentation may be required for billing. Indication

TABLE 59-2 Medicare Guidelines for Cardiac Pacemaker Implantation (pre-2002)

Accepted, in symptomatic patients with chronic conditions
- Atrioventricular block
  - Complete (third-degree)
  - Incomplete (second-degree)
    - Mobitz I
    - Mobitz II
  - Incomplete with 2:1 or 3:1 block
- Sinus node dysfunction (symptomatic)
  - Sinus bradycardia, sinoatrial block, sinus arrest
  - Bradycardia-tachycardia syndrome

Controversial
- In symptomatic patients
  - Bifascicular/trifascicular intraventricular block
  - Hypersensitive carotid sinus syndrome
- In asymptomatic patients
  - Third-degree block
  - Mobitz II
  - Mobitz II atrioventricular block following myocardial infarction
  - Congenital atrioventricular block
  - Sinus bradycardia <40 bpm with long-term necessary drug therapy
  - Overdrive pacing for ventricular tachycardia

Not warranted
- Syncope of undetermined cause
- In asymptomatic patients
  - Sinus bradycardia, sinoatrial block, or sinus arrest
  - Bundle-branch blocks
    - Mobitz I

Source: Modified from AMA Council on Scientific Affairs: The use of cardiac pacemakers in medical practice. Excerpts from the report of the Advisory Panel. JAMA 1985; 254: 1952; superseded by Epstein AE, DiMarco JP, Ellenbogen KA, et al: ACC/AHA/HRS 2008 Guidelines for Device-Based Therapy of Cardiac Rhythm Abnormalities. Circulation 2008;117:e350-408.

categories are "accepted," "controversial," or "not warranted." Profound sinus bradycardia or symptomatic second- or third-degree heart block indicates pacemaker insertion. Sinus bradycardia justifies pacemaker insertion if contemporaneous symptoms are documented by Holter or other means. Pacemakers may be appropriate for bradycardia less than 40 bpm if long-term necessary drug therapy is needed for supraventricular arrhythmias, ventricular tachycardia, hypertension, or angina. Although new indications for pacemaker therapy may be supported by clinical research, recognition of such advances by the Food and Drug Administration, insurance carriers, and regulatory agencies is often slow. Electrophysiology studies help define proper treatment.[9] In 2008, an American College of Cardiology/American Heart Association/North American Society for Pacing and Electrophysiology (ACC/AHA/NASPE) task force released revised recommendations for pacemaker and ICD insertion. Any practitioner who implants arrhythmia control devices should be familiar with these guidelines.[10]

Atrioventricular Block

First-degree block is prolongation of the P-R interval beyond 200 milliseconds. First-degree block at a low atrial rate may progress to Wenckebach as the atrial rate increases. Second-degree block is incomplete dissociation of the atrial and ventricular rates, with increasing P-R intervals and dropped beats (Wenckebach and Mobitz I, usually atrioventricular nodal block), or frequently dropped beats without progression of the P-R interval (Mobitz II, usually in the His-Purkinje system).[11] Third-degree block is complete atrioventricular (AV) dissociation, the atrial rate usually exceeding the ventricular rate. Left and right bundle-branch blocks and left anterior and posterior hemiblocks are partial conduction system blocks detected by electrocardiogram. Etiologies of AV block include ischemic injury, idiopathic fibrosis, cardiomyopathy, iatrogenic injury, AV node ablation, Lyme disease, bacterial endocarditis, systemic lupus erythematosus, and congenital lesions.

Sinus Node Dysfunction

Whether sinus node dysfunction warrants pacemaker insertion and whether bradycardia is caused by drugs required for ancillary conditions depend on the symptoms. Sinus node dysfunction is caused by coronary artery disease, cardiomyopathy, and reflex influences.

Reflex problems include carotid sinus hypersensitivity, vasovagal syncope, and oddities such as micturition-induced and deglutition syncope.[12] Cardioinhibitory (asystole >3 seconds) and vasodepressor (marked fall in blood pressure despite adequate heart rate) components of reflex-mediated syncope are recognized. Medical therapy is favored for vasodepressor syncope.[13] Tilt table testing provides objective data. Decisions on pacemaker insertion are based on symptoms and the duration of asystole. Pacemaker insertion is recommended for asystolic intervals greater than 3 seconds. Dual-chamber pacing (DDD or VDD) is favored for these patients, because AV synchrony increases stroke volume and decreases symptoms.

Features of Permanent Pacing

Dual-Chamber Pacing and Atrioventricular Synchrony

In the normal heart, stroke volume increases 5 to 15% by AV synchrony, versus asynchrony.[14] Left ventricular hypertrophy, decreased diastolic compliance, and heart failure increase the quantitative importance of AV synchrony.[14] Apical pacing of the right ventricle disrupts the normal sequence of activation, because depolarization spreads more slowly over the ventricular myocardium than through the conduction system.

Recent experience has emphasized clinical relevance of the sequence of activation. Right ventricular outflow tract pacing may improve stroke volume versus apical pacing because of favorable effects on the activation sequence.[15] Disruption of activation sequence by DDD pacing reduces the ventricular-aortic gradient in some patients with idiopathic hypertrophic subaortic stenosis.[16,17] Biventricular (RV apex and coronary sinus) pacing patients with advanced cardiomyopathy and an intraventricular conduction defect improves left ventricular function by restoring simultaneous contraction of the septum and free wall, so-called *ventricular resynchronization.*[18,19] Single-site, epicardial left ventricular pacing may provide similar benefits. For temporary pacing in postoperative heart block, biventricular pacing is superior to right ventricular pacing[19] and may be useful for left ventricular dysfunction after cardiac surgery. Clinical trials suggest that biventricular pacing is superior to standard pacing for heart block.[20]

Dual-Chamber Pacing Algorithm

DDD pacemaker programming includes a lower rate, an upper rate, and AV delay. When the intrinsic atrial rate is between the upper and lower rate limits, the pacemaker tracks the atrium to maintain a 1:1 response between the right atrium and right ventricle. If the atrial rate falls to the lower rate limit, the atrium is paced at the lower rate limit. If the atrial rate exceeds the upper rate limit, the ventricle is paced at the upper rate limit with loss of AV synchrony, resembling a Wenckebach effect.

Programmable AV delay defines the interval allowed between atrial and ventricular depolarization. Timing starts with the atrial electrogram or pacing stimulus and continues until the AV delay elapses. If no ventricular depolarization is detected during the delay, the ventricle is paced. *Atrial latency,* a varying delay between the atrial pacing artifact and the P wave, requires different AV delays for atrial sensing versus pacing.

Rate Response to Increased Metabolic Demand

During high metabolic demand, cardiac output is augmented by increased ventricular contractility, venous return, and heart rate. In patients with heart block and a normal sinus exercise response, dual-chamber pacing maintains both AV synchrony and a physiologic rate response.[21] However, sinus node incompetence (no atrial rate increase with exercise) or single-chamber ventricular (VVI) pacemakers, requires alternate mechanisms for rate response. The letter R after the three-letter pacemaker code indicates rate responsive capability. If a sensor detects increased metabolic demand, the lower rate of the pacemaker increases within a programmable range. Body vibration[29] or respiratory rate[22] is commonly employed to estimate demand. Other indicators are body temperature, venous oxygen saturation, QT interval, right ventricular systolic pressure, and right ventricular stroke volume. All such indicators can aberrantly increase heart rate, eg, during a bumpy car ride. Patients with sedentary life styles do not benefit from rate-responsive pacing. Adverse results of fast heart rates can include angina or infarction in patients with coronary disease.

Choice of Pacing Technique

Dual-chamber pacing has become the standard of care, except in chronic atrial fibrillation. Sinus rhythm appears to be better maintained by atrial than ventricular pacing,[23] and paroxysmal atrial fibrillation, previously problematic for DDD pacemakers, is now well handled by mode switching. Advantages of dual-chamber pacing in reflex-mediated syncope with cardioinhibitory features have also been reported.[13] Dual-chamber pacing may not be warranted in elderly patients, except when pacemaker syndrome, hypertension, or congestive heart failure is present. VVI or VVIR pacing is appropriate for patients with bradycardia and chronic atrial fibrillation. AAIR is useful for cardiac allograft recipients with sinus arrest or sinus bradycardia.[24] Biventricular pacing using an endocardial coronary sinus lead is recommended for symptomatic heart failure.[25]

Pacemaker Technology

Epicardial versus Endocardial Leads

Epicardial leads are generally inferior to endocardial leads in electrical characteristics and are prone to conductor fractures.[26] Steroid-eluting tips and small contact surfaces have improved epicardial leads. Epicardial pacing is more difficult at reoperative cardiac surgery, where epicardial fibrosis elevates pacing thresholds. Infected epicardial leads must be removed by thoracotomy. The epicardial approach is preferred in patients with congenital septal defects, single ventricle physiology, mechanical tricuspid valves, or venous thrombosis/occlusion. During thoracotomy, insertion of endocardial leads through an atrial pursestring is a useful option.[27] Epicardial left ventricular pacing by the minimal access approach is increasing in importance, driven by a 5 to 10% technical failure rate for coronary sinus lead insertion.[28]

Approaches to DDD pacing during open-heart surgery are illustrated in Fig. 59-2. Fixed-screw, positive fixation leads are introduced via atrial pursestrings and fixed into position by axial rotation. When a tricuspid prosthesis or ring is to be inserted, a ventricular lead can be passed between the sutures securing the ring or the valve.

Unipolar versus Bipolar

Bipolar leads incorporate two insulated conductors. In unipolar systems, the patient's body is the second (anodal) conductor; a single conductor in the lead carries the negative current to the heart. Bipolar leads reduce electrical noise (oversensing) and adventitious pacing of the diaphragm or chest wall. These advantages are offset by increased engineering complexity. Bipolar leads historically were prone to breakdown of insulation or conductor fracture. This would compromise sensing, pacing, or both[29] (Fig. 59-3). Recent bipolar leads are much improved and similar in dimensions and handling to unipolar leads (Figs. 59-4 and 59-5). The Medtronic Sprint Fidelis ICD lead is currently notable for an accelerating rate of lead fracture.

Lead Fixation

We prefer endocardial positive fixation leads, particularly in chambers with sparse trabeculation. A small wire spiral or screw holds these leads in place (Fig. 59-5G). In designs with fixed, extended screws, a soluble coating over the tip promotes venous passage. In retractable screw designs (Bisping), extension/retraction is accomplished by rotation of the pin at the lead tip. Axial clockwise rotation of screw-in leads during fixation provides tactile feedback on the firmness and security

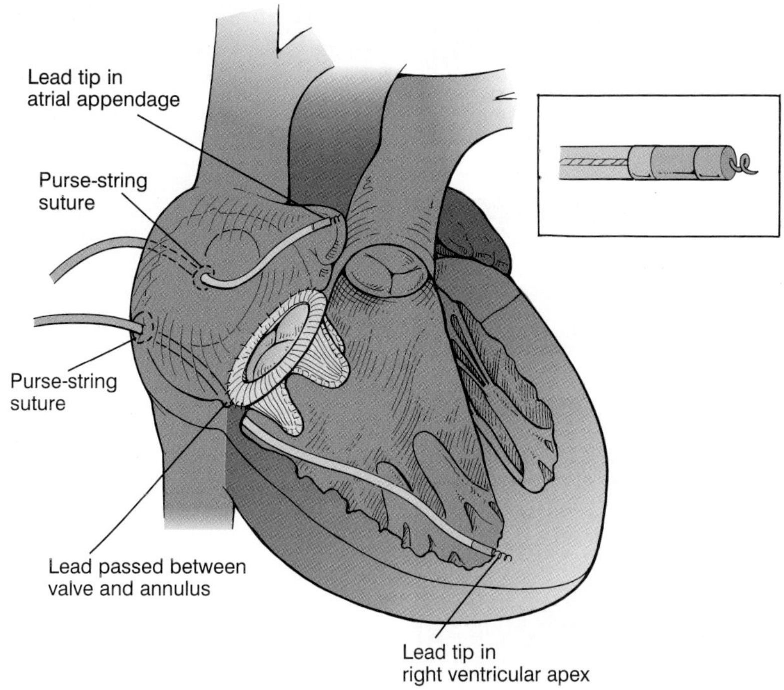

FIGURE 59-2 Endocardial pacing from epicardial approach. Atrial pursestrings provide access; leads are advanced and screwed into position guided by manual palpation. The ventricular lead is shown passing between the valve prosthesis and the annulus. The inset shows the tip of the endocardial screw-in lead. The coronary sinus os is also accessible.

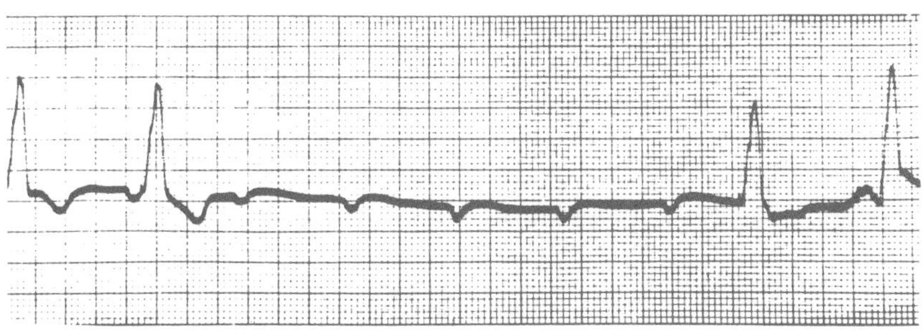

FIGURE 59-3 Telemetry from a patient with third-degree block, poor escape rhythm, a bipolar VVI pacemaker, and dizzy spells. Programming to VOO mode eliminated the pauses. The patient was discharged after lead replacement. This illustrates a life-threatening effect of oversensing. This older model pacemaker was not capable of monitoring electrograms to confirm the diagnosis.

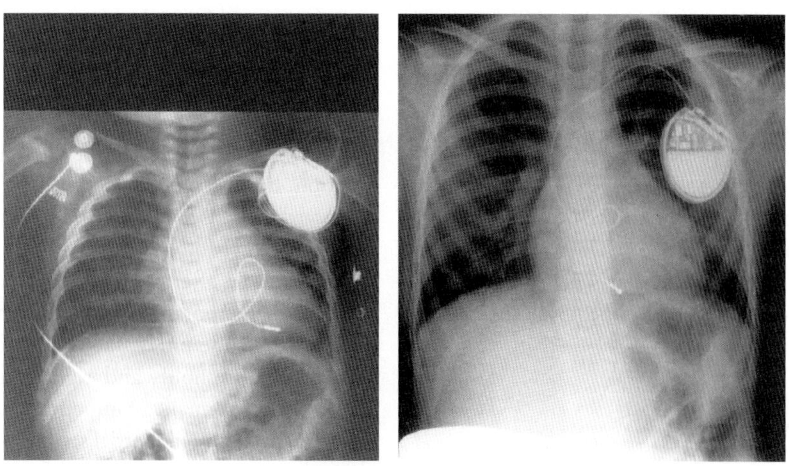

FIGURE 59-4 Positive fixation lead in x-rays demonstrating effects of growth on an intracardiac lead loop from age 1 (*left*) to age 5 years (*right*).

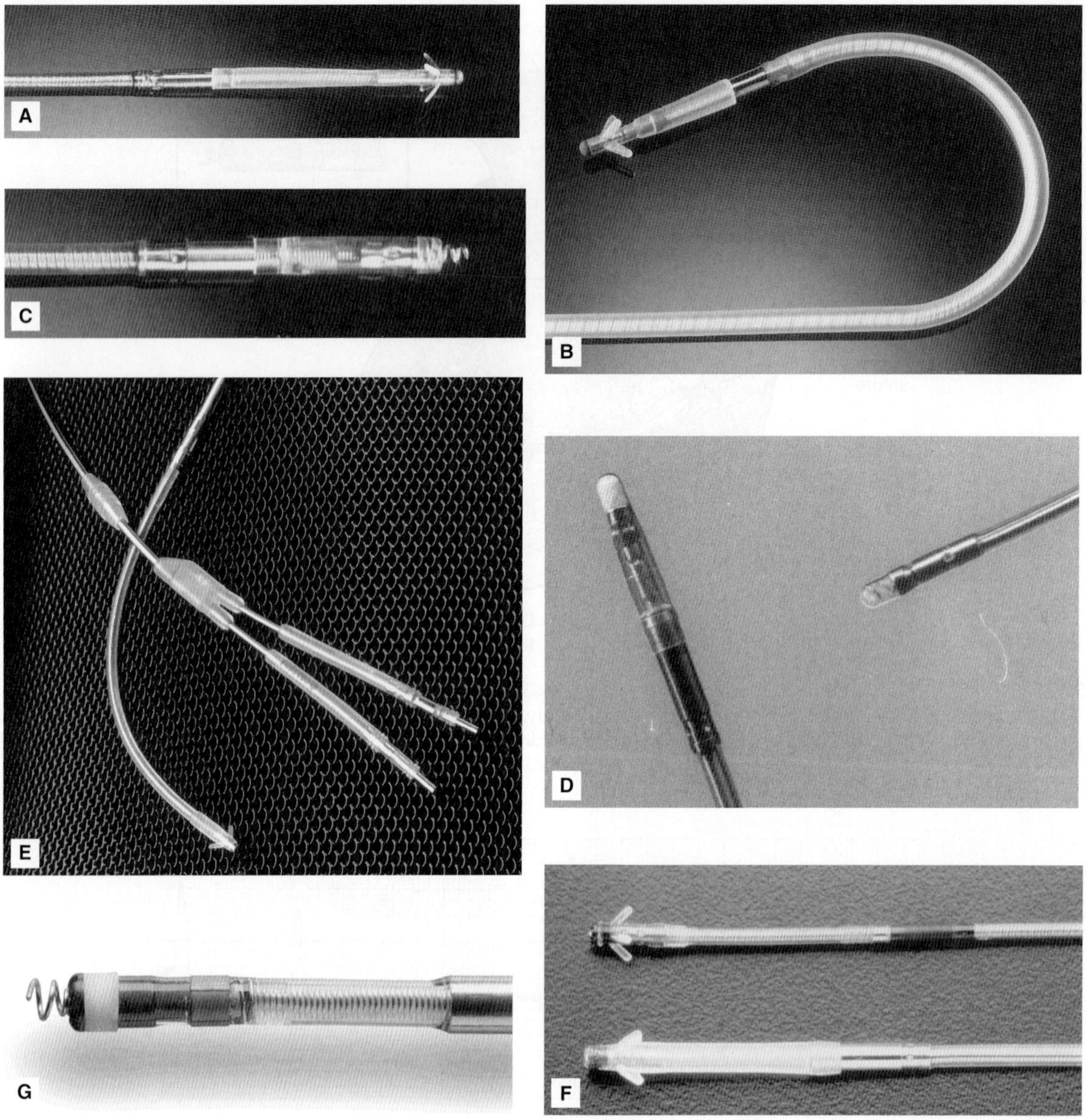

FIGURE 59-5 (A) Bipolar tined ventricular pacing lead with steroid-eluting tip. (B) Similar to (*A*), with J shape for atrial pacing. (C) Bisping bipolar ventricular pacing lead with retractable, screw-in tip. (D) Bipolar (*left*) and unipolar (*right*) pacing leads with fixed-screw tips. A soluble tip coating dissolves in blood and reduces snagging during insertion. These leads can be used in the atrium or ventricle. The unipolar lead was used by the author for atrial and ventricular pacing. (E) Single-pass lead for VDD pacing. (F) Current leads demonstrating progress in reduction of bipolar lead diameter. (G) Fixed-screw bipolar 7-French lead with steroid-eluting white collar at lead tip. (*A, B, and C: Courtesy of Medtronic, Inc., Minneapolis, MN; D, E, and F: Courtesy of Intermedics, Inc., Bellaire, TX; G: Courtesy of Guidant Corp., Indianapolis, IN.*)

of attachment. Lead impedance provides feedback on the adequacy of tip extension and fixation.

Tined leads use miniature anchors to secure the lead tip within myocardial trabeculae (Fig. 59-5A). Tines require larger introducers than screw-in leads and are not secure in smooth-walled or dilated chambers. Nevertheless, some physicians prefer these leads.[30]

Temporary Pacing

Acute bradycardia can be treated with transthoracic pacing, temporary endocardial pacing, or chronotropic drugs, including atropine, dobutamine, or isoproterenol. Right ventricular perforation has become less prevalent with current temporary endocardial leads but must be borne in mind if hypotension develops acutely after removal of temporary wires.

Bradycardia after cardiac surgery is commonly treated with pacing via temporary atrial and ventricular epicardial wires. Problems include unfavorable evolution of right atrial or right ventricular thresholds and right atrial sensing. Atrial undersensing and pacemaker competition can precipitate atrial fibrillation or atrial flutter. If atrial sensing is not adequate, overdriving the atrium faster than the intrinsic rate can ameliorate competition. Reversing polarity or inserting a cutaneous ground wire under local anesthesia can improve pacing threshold. The output of the temporary pacemaker in volts or milliamps should be at least twice the threshold and should be measured daily. Ventricular undersensing in critically ill patients can result in pacing during the vulnerable period, which can precipitate ventricular tachycardia or fibrillation.

Cardiac Output and Pacing Rate

For patients with hemodynamic compromise following cardiac surgery, optimization of pacing rate and AV delay can affect hemodynamics by compensating for valve leaks or fixed stroke volume. Mean arterial pressure reflects cardiac output if systemic resistance is constant. Rate and timing adjustments over intervals of less than 20 seconds minimize reflex effects. Settings producing the highest sustained mean arterial pressure should also maximize cardiac output.

Pacemaker Insertion

Environment and Anesthesia

Pacemaker and ICD surgery is increasingly performed in electrophysiology (EP) laboratories.[31] Whether in the operating room or EP lab, properly functioning equipment is essential. Infection control is critical[32]; operating room standards for air quality should be enforced. Problems calling for presence of an anesthesiologist include angina, transient cerebral ischemia, patient disorientation, lidocaine toxicity, dementia, myocardial ischemia, heart failure, anxiety, or ventricular tachycardia. If English is not the patient's first language, a translator is helpful. Vancomycin reactions (red man syndrome), pacing-induced ventricular fibrillation, air embolism, and Stokes-Adams attacks are rare emergencies that are less problematic if considered in advance. Intraoperative death can occur because of hemorrhage, pericardial tamponade, ventricular fibrillation (VF), heart failure, myocardial infarction, and other causes.

Monitoring

R-wave detection by an electrocardiogram (ECG) monitor is inadequate for pacemaker insertion, because pacing artifacts that trigger the monitor may fail to capture. Thus, subthreshold pacing can elicit regular beeping from the monitor in an asystolic patient. Oxygen saturation monitors are optimal, as they beep only during blood flow. Pulse oximeters should not be placed on the same extremity as the blood pressure cuff. When monitors are unreliable, palpation by an anesthesiologist or nurse of the temporal, facial, or radial artery pulse can detect asystole before the patient becomes symptomatic.

Venous Access Strategy

Choices include which side will be employed and cut down versus percutaneous venipuncture. Cut down approaches to the cephalic, subclavian, external jugular, and internal jugular system are described.[33] Anatomical considerations[29,34] may reduce the frequency of subclavian crush (Fig. 59-6). Subclavian puncture is associated with an apparently unavoidable but low incidence of pneumothorax, hemothorax, and major venous injury. Ultrasonic vessel locators may further reduce the frequency of injury.

Venous access is problematic in superior vena cava syndrome or subclavian/innominate vein obstruction or thrombosis (eg, with chronic dialysis, mediastinal tracheostomy, or multiple pacemaker leads). Access from below or transhepatically is possible,[33,35] but potential for bleeding, venous thrombosis, and pulmonary embolism are concerns. Right parasternal mediastinotomy, exposure of the right atrium, and a Seldinger approach with small introducers and atrial pursestring sutures are useful in difficult cases[36] (Fig. 59-7). Pacemaker lead extraction may permit reinsertion of leads via the extraction cannula.

Antibiotic Prophylaxis

Antibiotic prophylaxis is indicated for insertion of a prosthetic device.[32] We prefer 1 g of intravenous cefazolin. We also irrigate the operative field with a solution of 1 g of cefazolin in a liter of warm saline. Patients who have a valve prosthesis or who have a penicillin or cefazolin allergy receive vancomycin (500 mg) and gentamicin (1 mg/kg).

Pacing Systems Analyzer

Pacing thresholds and electrogram amplitudes are measured with a pacing systems analyzer. Electrogram characteristics and

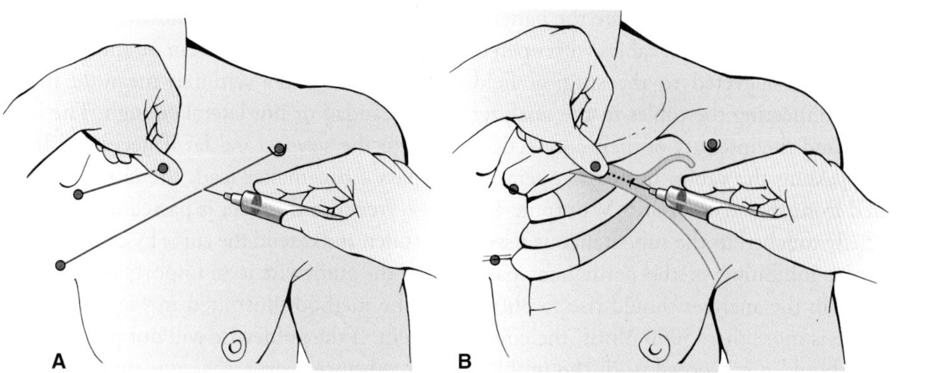

FIGURE 59-6 Landmarks for subclavian vein puncture. Potential complications include subclavian crush injury. (*Reproduced with permission from Aggarwal RK, Connelly DT, Ray SG, et al: Early complications of permanent pacemaker implantation: no difference between dual and single chamber systems. Br Heart J 1995; 73:571.*)

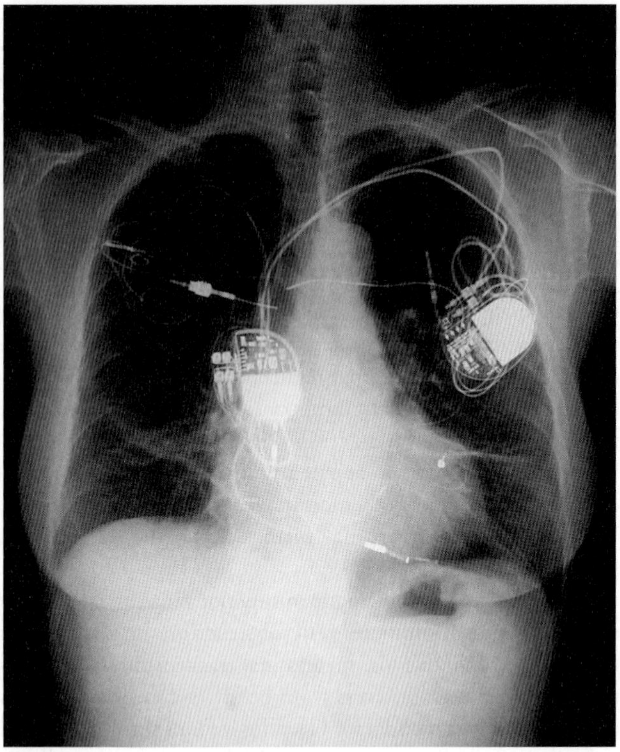

FIGURE 59-7 X-ray of a patient with very poor escape rhythm, bilateral venous obstruction, and severe exit block. A new pacing system was inserted through the right atrial appendage via right parasternal mediastinotomy. Her old pacemaker was programmed to backup mode and scheduled for removal at a later date.

slew rate can be assessed, and electrogram telemetry is available from most current pacemakers. Analyzers must be serviced and tested periodically, including batteries. Any discrepancies between measurements by the analyzer and the pacemaker should be noted and related functions of the analyzer rechecked.

Operator skill is needed to run the analyzer and record the results. The analyzer also can be placed in a sterile bag and operated by the surgeon. Manufacturer's representatives, an increasing intraoperative presence, are skilled in operation of these analyzers.

Cables

The cables connecting the analyzer to the leads are the patient's lifeline. Even with excellent quality control, cables with open or reversed connections may be delivered to the surgical field. Errors can also occur in connecting the cables to the analyzer. Routine testing of cables and the integrity of their connections is recommended. After passing the cables from the operating table, pacing is initiated from the analyzer at 5-V output. The connectors are then briefly touched to the subcutaneous tissue, with caution to minimize inhibition of the permanent pacemaker. Current measured in the analyzer should rise to 300 to 1000 ohms. If impedance is more than 5000 ohms, the circuit is faulty. The operation should not proceed until the problem is corrected, as the analyzer-cable circuit is defective. Connections to the analyzer should also be checked, because inadvertent reversal of polarity can make measured pacing thresholds inappropriately high. Even disposable leads with polarized connectors have been delivered to us with the connectors reversed.

Fluoroscopy

Fluoroscopy is essential for transvenous device implantation, and operating room personnel must be familiar with the equipment. Distracting problems with image orientation, rebooting, timers, brakes, and locks can be avoided by a knowledgeable team. Sudden failure of fluoroscopy at a critical point can occur. If a backup unit is not available, the options include "blind" endocardial lead insertion, epicardial insertion, or postponing the procedure. The use of low-dose and pulsed image options can prevent overheating of the fluoroscope, although image quality is compromised. Radiation exposure should be controlled by monitoring fluoroscopy time.

Surgical Approach

We approach the patient from the left when feasible. The fluoroscope, on the patient's right, is positioned carefully to allow visualization of the apex, right atrium, and deltopectoral groove. The right arm is extended rightward on an arm board. The drapes are suspended from IV poles. The right-sided pole is caudad to the arm board. Careful positioning allows the left clavicular region to be exposed while leaving the patient adequate light and air. After skin preparation, towels are aligned with the deltopectoral groove and clavicle to define the essential landmarks. The region of the incision and generator is infiltrated with 1% lidocaine to produce a field block. A 5- to 6-cm horizontal incision is created 4 cm beneath the clavicle, the lateral extent of the incision just reaching the deltopectoral groove. This allows the generator to be positioned away from the deltopectoral groove and axilla, avoiding interference with motion of the left arm at the shoulder. An alternate incision directly over the deltopectoral groove facilitates exposure of the cephalic vein; this is particularly valuable in obese patients or elderly patients with atretic veins.

Venous Access

When the deltopectoral groove has been exposed, additional anesthesia is infiltrated into the lateral margin of the pectoralis and laterally into the deltoid. The dissection proceeds into the deltopectoral groove, following the lateral edge of the pectoralis, until the cephalic vein or another venous branch is exposed. Failure to find a vein may mean the incision is too far cephalad or caudad or not lateral enough. The incision can be deepened into the subpectoral fat if necessary. If the vein is too small to pass a pacemaker lead, the curved end of the guidewire for a 7-French introducer is passed centrally. The ability to manually stiffen and extend the curve by central manipulation of the tension in the guidewire is an important technical aid in tortuous veins. The method illustrated in Fig. 59-8 can be used to dilate the vein. If the guidewire will not pass centrally, a no. 18 Angiocath is advanced over the guidewire and used to inject a small amount of iodinated contrast to visualize the venous system fluoroscopically. If the cut down approach must be abandoned, visualizing the subclavian vein by venogram reduces the risk of

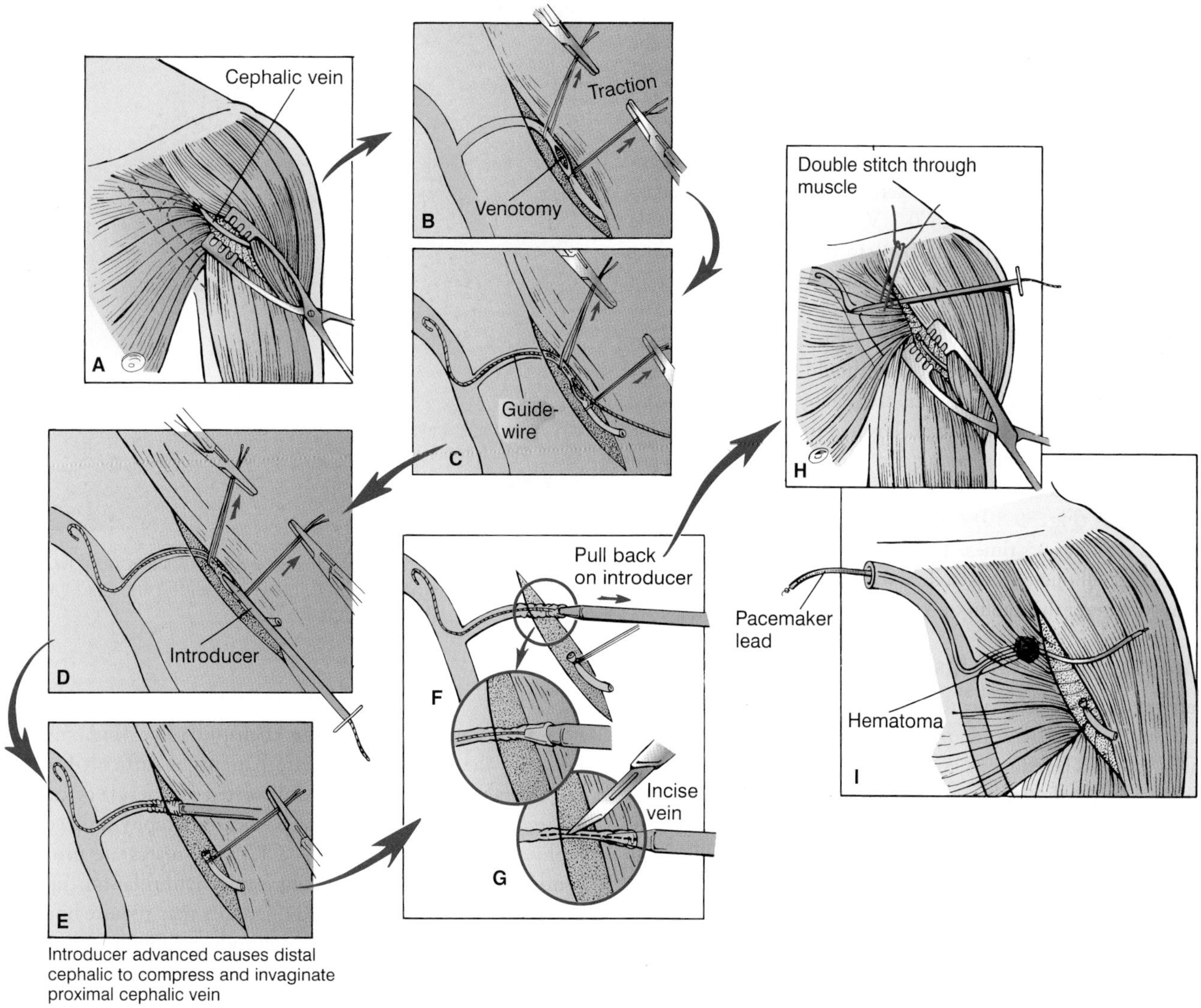

FIGURE 59-8 Cephalic cut down approach to small veins that pass a guidewire centrally but not an introducer. Resistance results from entrapment of the introducer tip and collapse of the vein; the introducer can advance only by turning the vein outside-in. This entrapment can be helpful. After the guidewire is advanced (*C*), pass a no. 18 Angiocath over the guidewire to dilate and/or split the vein (not shown). This allows the introducer tip to enter the vein (*D*). If the vein does not split, the introducer becomes impaled and will not advance (*E*). Gently withdraw the introducer to extend the impaled vein (*F*). Split the exposed vein segment longitudinally with a no. 11 blade (*G*). Steps (*D*) to (*G*) can be repeated, if necessary, until the introducer advances centrally. A pursestring suture approximates soft tissue around the path of the introducer to achieve hemostasis (*H, I*).

injury during subclavian puncture. If dual-chamber pacing is planned, a guidewire should be reinserted through the introducer before the introducer is stripped away. This provides venous access for the duration of the procedure.[36,37] A pursestring suture in the muscle usually provides adequate control of bleeding and allows stabilization of the lead(s).[38] Ultrasonic localizers may be useful at this stage, with appropriate sterile precautions.

Right Ventricular Lead Insertion

From the patient's left, a gentle spiral in the distal 10 cm of the stylet will guide the lead toward the tricuspid valve, right ventricle, and pulmonary artery. Advancing the lead into the pulmonary artery outside the cardiac silhouette confirms that the lead is not in the coronary sinus. For fixed-screw positive fixation leads, withdrawing the stylet 3 to 5 cm minimizes the risk of apical perforation while screwing the lead tip into the myocardium with axial clockwise rotation. Reverse torque that develops as the lead is rotated should be noted; this torque is a guide to the security and safety of fixation. We fix the lead with three consecutive 360-degree clockwise rotations of the lead shaft, then release the torque. This fixation sequence is repeated if necessary, until the lead is secure, with substantial reverse torque after the first 360-degree rotation. No more than three complete axial rotations are employed in any sequence. A potential problem with screw-in leads is ventricular perforation. The lead tip should be fluoroscoped during fixation looking for extra-anatomical passage, following the edge of the cardiac silhouette around the apex, then cephalad. If this happens, the lead should be withdrawn and repositioned. An echocardiogram should be obtained and the patient monitored for tamponade.

When the lead tip has been properly positioned, the stylet is withdrawn and thresholds tested. The patient is asked to hyperventilate and cough to confirm fixation. The ventricular pacing threshold should be less than 0.7 V, with R-wave amplitude more than 5 mV, and impedance 400 to 1000 ohms, depending on lead design. There should be no diaphragmatic pacing at an output of 10 V.

If the lead is dislodged by hyperventilation and coughing, or thresholds are not adequate, the lead should be repositioned. A positive fixation lead can be unscrewed by counterclockwise axial rotation until it floats free. Positive fixation leads can be secured almost anywhere along the margins of the right ventricular silhouette (Fig. 59-9), including the right ventricular outflow tract (Fig. 59-10).[39] In difficult cases, we have relocated leads as many as 15 times. The geographic center of the right ventricular silhouette is not a desirable location, as it can lead to entanglement of the lead in the chordae tendineae (see Fig. 59-9).

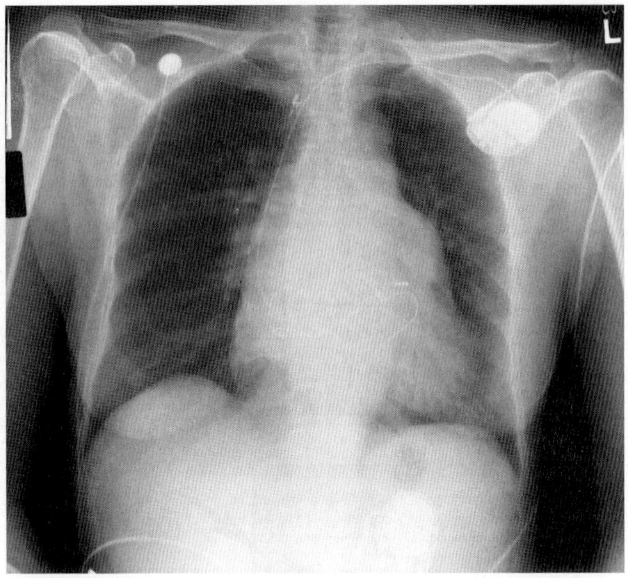

FIGURE 59-10 Screw-in lead in the right ventricular outflow tract of a patient with complete heart block after tricuspid valve replacement for Ebstein anomaly.

Coronary Sinus Lead Insertion

Left ventricular pacing via the coronary sinus (CS) is a valued skill since the MIRACLE trial and subsequent studies indicated that CRT reduces symptoms of heart failure and mortality of dilated cardiomyopathy.[18,19,25] Electrophysiologists are familiar with CS entry for arrhythmia mapping; steerable mapping catheters and biplane fluoroscopy are important tools. However, the technical failure rate of CS lead insertion is 5 to 10%.[18,25] The CS orifice is usually a posterior structure near the caudal aspect of the tricuspid valve (Fig. 59-11). Locating the os in heart failure patients is difficult because the CS may be angulated and distorted as a result of cardiac enlargement. Transesophageal echocardiography and venography may help locate the os. CRT candidates are prone to ventricular arrhythmias, making rapid defibrillation capability desirable. Even experienced operators may require hours to insert a CS lead with present methods, although technology for both endocardial and epicardial left ventricular lead placement is improving. Over-the-wire lead designs are the most successful. We prefer to insert the CS lead first via the cephalic approach, right atrial and right ventricular lead insertion after via subclavian puncture. CS lead insertion involves advancing an angled catheter into the CS. This is followed by CS venography and lead insertion through the cannula into a lateral branch of the CS. The CS cannula is then removed and stripped off without dislodging the lead. Positive fixation leads are not available. A large selection of angled CS cannulas, steerable probes, and lead designs testifies to the technical challenge. The difficulty of CS lead insertion in heart failure patients should not be underestimated; special training is desirable.

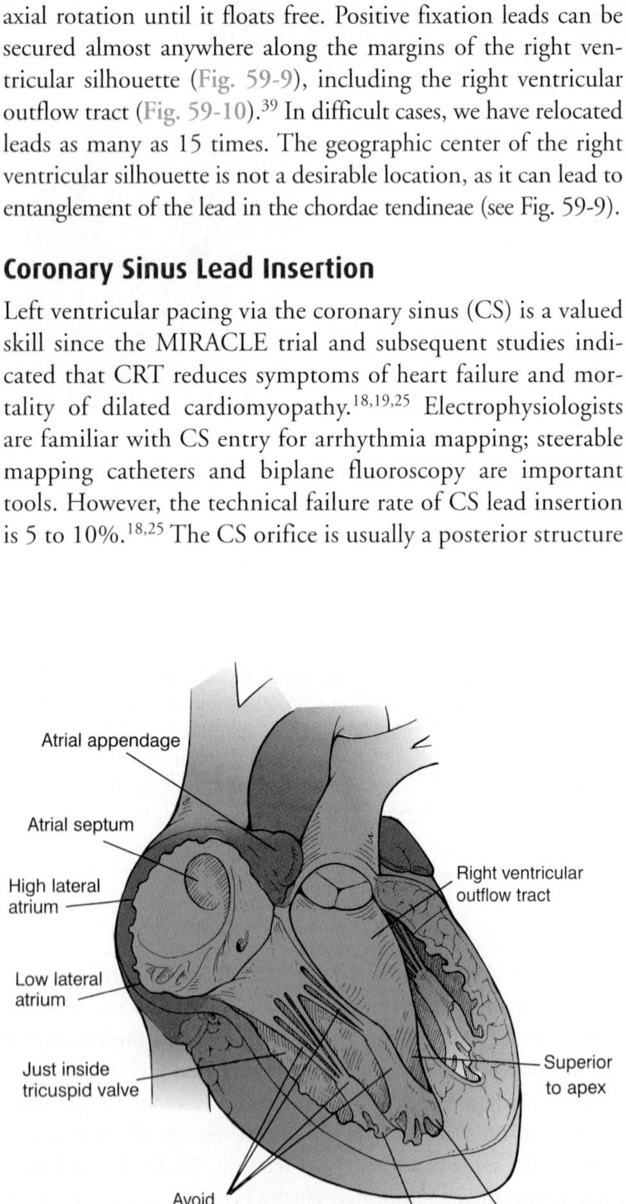

FIGURE 59-9 Useful sites for transvenous atrial and ventricular pacing using fixed-screw leads. Avoid the geographic center of the right ventricle (RV), where fixing the lead can entrap it in the chordae tendineae.

Length Adjustment

Lead length can be "too short," so that flattening of the diaphragm during a deep breath results in lead displacement, or "too long," so that a cough results in formation of an intracardiac loops that shorten the lead, also potentially causing displacement. Maximal inspiration and expiration by the patient during observation under fluoroscopy helps judge length. Vigorous coughing tests the security of lead tip fixation. This valuable feedback is lost if sedation is excessive. Minimizing sedation also promotes early detection of pacemaker syndrome.

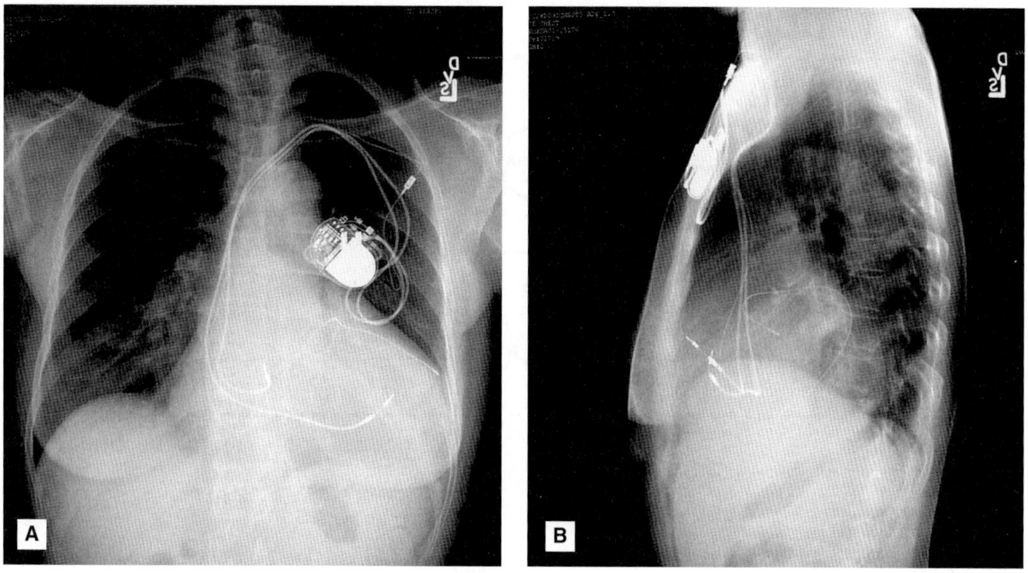

FIGURE 59-11 (A) Biventricular, CRT-P pacemaker with endocardial leads in the right atrium, right ventricle, and lateral branch of the coronary sinus (left ventricle). This patient was relieved of dobutamine dependence by addition of the left ventricular lead. (B) Lateral x-ray of the same patient. Note posterior course of the coronary sinus.

Atrial Lead Insertion

For dual-chamber pacing, the atrial lead is introduced last. A J or S stylet shape is best for finding the atrial appendage from the left side.[55] The S shape is also useful for passing a positive fixation lead to the right margin of the atrium near the junction of the atrium and inferior vena cava (Fig. 59-12). P-wave amplitude is often best in this location. The atrial pacing threshold should be less than 2 V. In the presence of complete heart block, it may be difficult to confirm atrial capture from the surface ECG. Pacing the atrium at 150 bpm results in rapid oscillation of the lead tip, which is visible fluoroscopically if mechanical function of the atrium is sufficient. Lead oscillation may thus be used to determine the atrial pacing threshold. This technique should only be used if the high atrial rate is not conducted to the ventricle. In patients with complete heart block, high-output atrial pacing can inhibit whatever temporary VVI pacing is supporting the patient, resulting in asystole.

The P-wave electrogram is the Achilles heel of dual-chamber pacing. If atrial sensing is not satisfactory, a DDD pacemaker will not function properly. The P-wave amplitude should ideally be greater than 2 mV. P-wave amplitude may vary during respiration, and the minimum value, not the maximum, determines the adequacy of sensing. P-wave amplitude is generally reduced during atrial fibrillation versus values in sinus rhythm.

Measurement of P-wave amplitude with unipolar leads can be confusing. Crosstalk or far-field sensing of ventricular depolarization from the atrial lead can occur, so that the signal measured through a pacemaker analyzer is not the P wave but the QRS complex. Simultaneous measurement and display of atrial and ventricular electrograms as well as the surface ECG can resolve this. An alternate solution involves programming the generator as a P-wave detector: The lower rate is set below the patient's intrinsic atrial rate, the AV delay is set shorter than the patient's P-R interval, and atrial sensitivity is set at 2 mV. When the generator is connected to the atrial and ventricular leads, every P wave will be followed immediately by a ventricular pacing spike if P-wave amplitude is greater than 2 mV. The pacemaker must be reprogrammed to clinically appropriate settings at the conclusion of surgery.

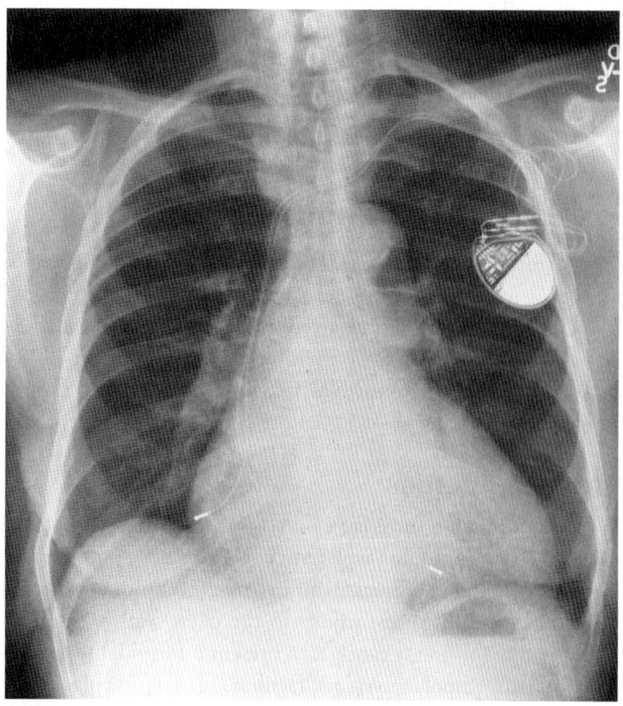

FIGURE 59-12 DDD pacemaker with atrial lead in low right atrium, advantageous after obliteration of the atrial appendage at heart surgery. This location, which requires positive fixation leads, often provides good P-wave amplitude when other sites fail. Phrenic nerve pacing with 10-V pacing at this location requires lead repositioning.

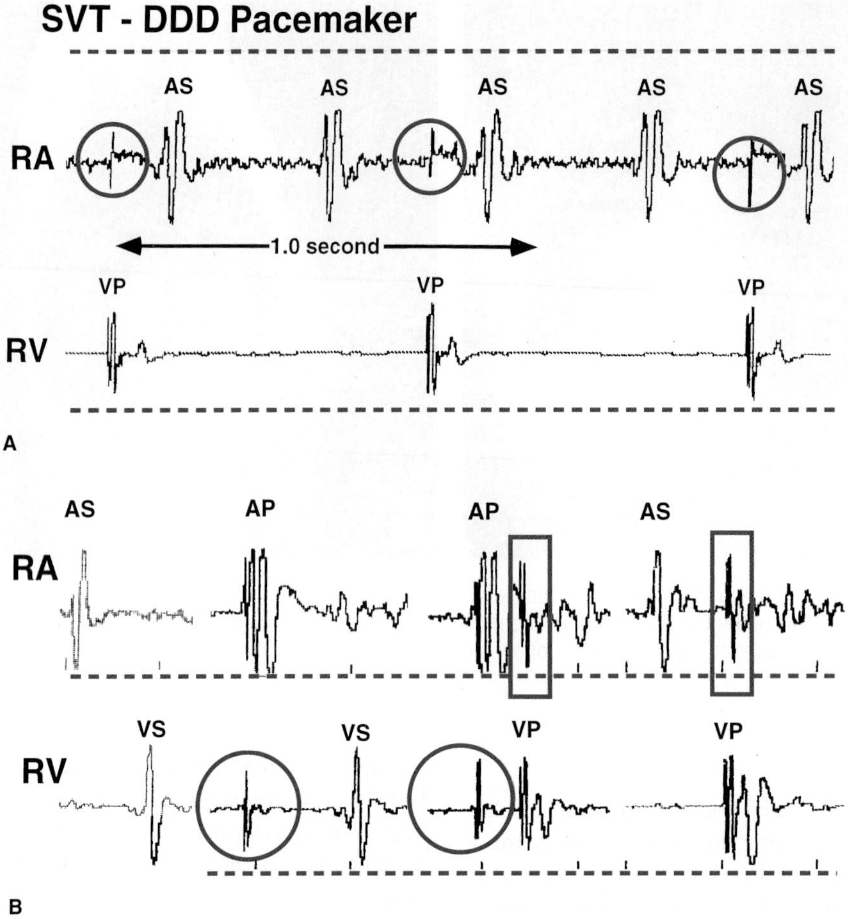

FIGURE 59-13 Right atrial (RA) and right ventricular (RV) electrograms from a unipolar DDD pacemaker during supraventricular tachycardia (SVT). Regular atrial depolarizations appear (AS) at a rate of 160 bpm. The pacemaker paces the ventricle (VP) at 80 bpm, because alternate P waves fall inside the postventricular atrial refractory period and are not detected. The circles illustrate far-field sensing of the RV pacing artifact in the RA lead. The SVT was not detected preoperatively. Once this recording was obtained, overdrive atrial pacing from the pacemaker converted the SVT to normal sinus rhythm, and normal pacemaker function returned.

Telemetry of atrial and ventricular electrograms by pacemakers provides valuable EP data. For example, inability to pace the atrium or to measure atrial electrograms in the operating room may indicate low-amplitude atrial fibrillation or supraventricular tachycardia; this may be invisible on the surface ECG but detectable in electrograms. Electrogram telemetry can confirm proper DDD pacing (Fig. 59-13).

Generator Location

We use a watertight, three-layer skin closure for primary implants, three layers in generator replacements. Cosmetic appearance is important to many patients, and in others technique is critical to optimize healing. Past injury to the chest wall or surgery/radiotherapy for breast cancer can present a formidable technical problem. Bipolar systems facilitate generator placement behind the pectoralis or inside the rectus sheath. Diminutive generators are available, but battery life is reduced. Innovative locations for pacemaker generators include axillary, retromammary, intrathoracic, intra-abdominal, and preperitoneal sites. These approaches are rarely indicated with present generator designs.

Length of Stay after Pacemaker Implantation

Ambulatory Surgery

Same-day hospital discharge after pacemaker insertion is reasonable in patients who have an adequate escape rhythm and positive fixation leads. After monitoring and recovery from sedation, patients are ambulated and shown range of motion exercises for the shoulder. A chest x-ray documents lead position and rules out hemothorax, pneumothorax, or increasing heart size.

Pacemaker-Dependent Patients

Lead displacement can result from technical error, struggling of demented patients, and other factors. A small percentage of lead displacement is probably unavoidable.[30,40] Patients who might suffer death or injury in the event of pacemaker failure should be observed in the hospital overnight on telemetry. However, lead displacement in our ambulatory patients has not been more frequent than in hospitalized patients.

Pacemaker Generator Replacement

Planning

Fifteen percent of functioning pacemakers were replacements in a recent survey. Complications of pacemaker generator replacement include infection, lead damage, connector problems, and asystole during the transition from the old generator to the new. Pacemaker independence at the time of initial pacemaker implant may progress to total pacemaker dependence by the time of generator replacement. Ambulatory surgery is common. As a practical matter, we no completely reverse warfarin for pacemaker generator replacement unless lead replacement is expected.[41] Patients with leads more than 10 years old should be carefully evaluated for pacemaker dysfunction before generator replacement; a Holter monitor should be obtained if lead dysfunction is suspected. Rising pacing threshold may indicate impending lead failure. The possibility of unexpected lead replacement should be discussed with the patient in advance.

Backup Pacing

A backup temporary transvenous pacing wire can be inserted for pacemaker generator replacement, but this is rarely necessary. The output of the replacement unit must be higher than the threshold of the chronically implanted leads. This can be problematic if the expiring generator is an older type with a fixed output of 5.4 V. Lack of programmability prevents preoperative threshold testing, and the 5.4-V output is higher than possible for some current generators. The pacing threshold should be determined with a pacemaker analyzer and the replacement should be programmed to appropriate output. Before disconnecting the old generator, be sure that the pacemaker analyzer, cables, and connections are intact and personnel in the operating room are aware of the cables. Some place the analyzer in a sterile bag on the operative field. With many generators, an Allen wrench placed in the header establishes electrical continuity with the ventricular lead; the pacing threshold can then be established before disconnecting the old generator. The old generator should be kept within reach as a backup in case of trouble with the new generator, the analyzer, or the connectors. Replacement generators must be programmed unipolar or bipolar to match the indwelling lead(s).

Lead Sizes

The three common lead connectors for permanent pacing are 6, 5, and 3.5 mm (VS-1 or IS-1). If the new generator is not an exact match for the patient's lead size, a selection of step-up and step-down adapters can be helpful. The contacts do not always line up correctly across VS-1 and IS-1 connectors, even though the connector diameter is the same. It is important to determine in advance whether connections can safely be made across the VS-1/IS-1 interface.

Postoperative Care

Wound Care

Patients are instructed to keep implant wounds dry until an office visit 7 to 10 days postoperatively. Any wound drainage at the postoperative visit is cultured, and prophylactic antibiotics are started until culture results are available. We have abandoned aspiration of the rare postoperative hematoma in favor of close observation, unless infection is an issue or spontaneous drainage occurs or appears imminent.

Antibiotic Prophylaxis

Routine use of prophylactic antibiotics before dental work and other invasive procedures in pacemaker or ICD recipients is not recommended under AHA/ACC guidelines. We recommend prophylaxis for 3 months after device insertion, allowing time for the pacing leads to become endothelialized.

Testing and Follow-up

Office/Clinic versus Telephone

Pacemakers require periodic testing to confirm sensing and pacing function and battery reserve. Currently these functions are tested at 1- to 3-month intervals. Whether follow-up should be done by transtelephonic monitoring or clinic or office visits is in dispute.[61–63] Transtelephonic monitoring alleviates transportation issues for elderly patients, but some need help managing the process. In addition to reducing patient travel and strain on office resources, many commercial services provide emergency monitoring on a 24-hour basis, an advantage in managing apprehensive or incapacitated patients. Techniques for remote management of pacemakers and ICDs are available with some current devices.

Pacemaker Programming

Programming can be done in an office setting by trained, experienced personnel. In some situations, a manufacturer's representative may provide valuable help. Advanced techniques for pacemaker/ICD monitoring and programming are under development.

DDD pacemaker programming allows adjustment of electrogram sensitivity as well as pacing stimulus amplitude/pulse width for both the atrium and ventricle. Lower rate, upper rate, atrioventricular delay, and refractory periods for atrial and ventricular sensing are programmable. Rate responsiveness, unipolar/bipolar configuration, and many other options are also adjustable noninvasively.

We initially program newly inserted pacemakers to stimulation amplitude and pulse width higher than nominal. At the initial office visit, pacing thresholds are retested and amplitude and pulse width are adjusted to nominal levels if pacing thresholds are low. The use of high initial output is less important with steroid-eluting leads. Details of pacemaker programming have been described elsewhere.[63,64] Some current pacemakers are capable of automated threshold adjustment.

Most problems detected by transtelephonic or Holter monitoring can be corrected by programming. The etiology of symptoms can often be elicited from real-time electrograms or stored data. Adjustments can include not only sensitivity or pacing output but also pacing mode for new-onset atrial fibrillation

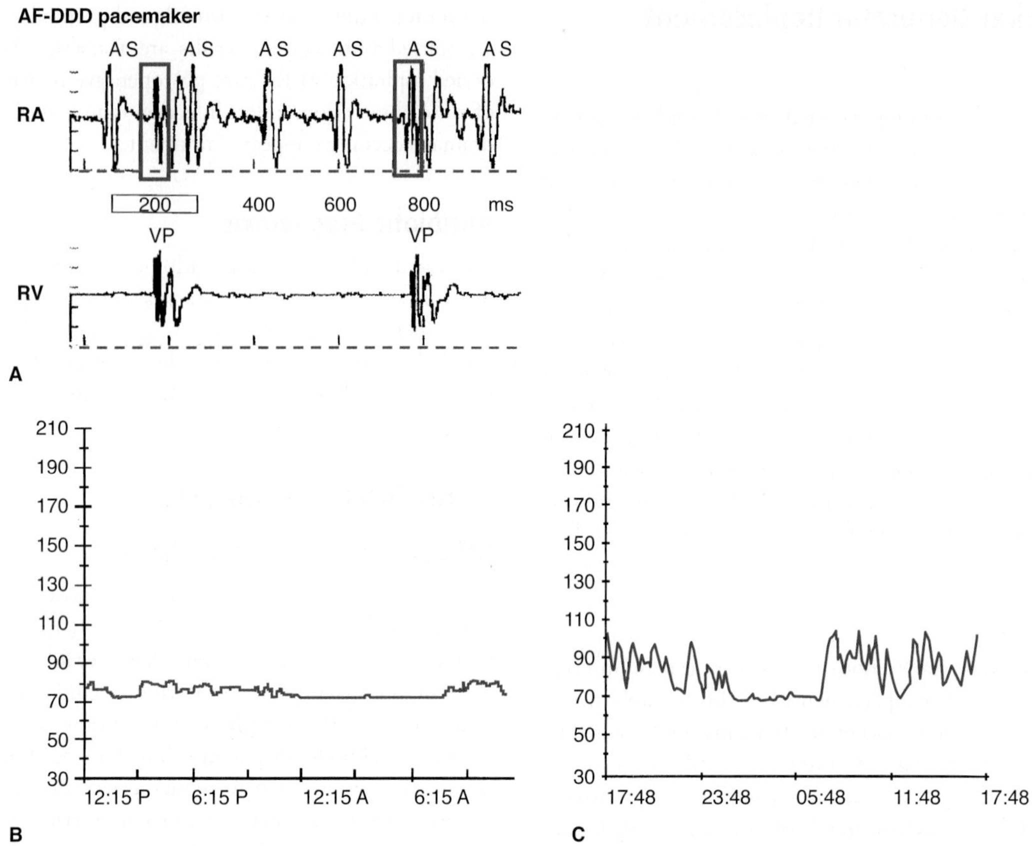

FIGURE 59-14 (A) Atrial (RA) and ventricular (RV) electrograms from unipolar DDD pacemaker during atrial fibrillation (AF). AF appears as rapid atrial depolarizations (AS). The upper rate limit and postventricular atrial refractory period of the pacemaker determine the rate at which the pacemaker stimulates the ventricle (VP). (*B,C*) Heart rate over 24 hours from memory of DDD pacemaker. (**B**) Sinus node incompetence during amiodarone therapy for paroxysmal atrial fibrillation. (**C**) Rate variation after activation of rate response. Patient reported improved exercise tolerance.

(Fig. 59-14A) or sinus node incompetence related to medication changes (Fig. 59-14B). Problems that may require reoperation include lead displacement, lead fracture (Fig. 59-15), insulation degradation (see Fig. 59-3), and exit block[40] (Fig. 59-16).

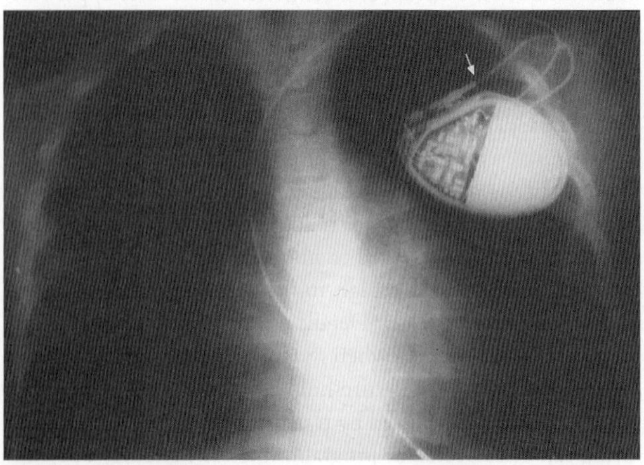

FIGURE 59-15 Unipolar lead fracture in a 3-year-old child with complete heart block as revealed by x-ray. The patient underwent successful lead replacement.

Pacemaker interrogation should begin with a printout of the initial settings, an invaluable reference after involved programming. Telemetry defines time-related variation in heart rate, percentage of beats sensed and paced, the quality of the electrograms, lead impedance, and battery voltage.

Pacing amplitude and pulse width are finely tuned at a 1-year follow-up visit. At least 100% safety margin is programmed on the pulse width threshold. Parameters are adjusted to optimize patient comfort and battery life. Some pacemakers allow programmed reduction of a lower rate at night, eliminating unnecessary pacing during sleep. Very long atrioventricular delays can eliminate ventricular pacing in some patients with first-degree block, but a reduction in the upper rate limit to 105 bpm may be necessary to achieve this. Current pacemakers have a variety of algorithms to prevent excessive pacing in first-degree heart block, including automatic switching between AAI and DDD modes.

Complications of Pacemaker Insertion

Mortality

Death is a rare complication of pacemaker implantation.[40,43] Lethal problems can include lead displacement, venous or cardiac perforation, air embolism, and ventricular tachycardia or

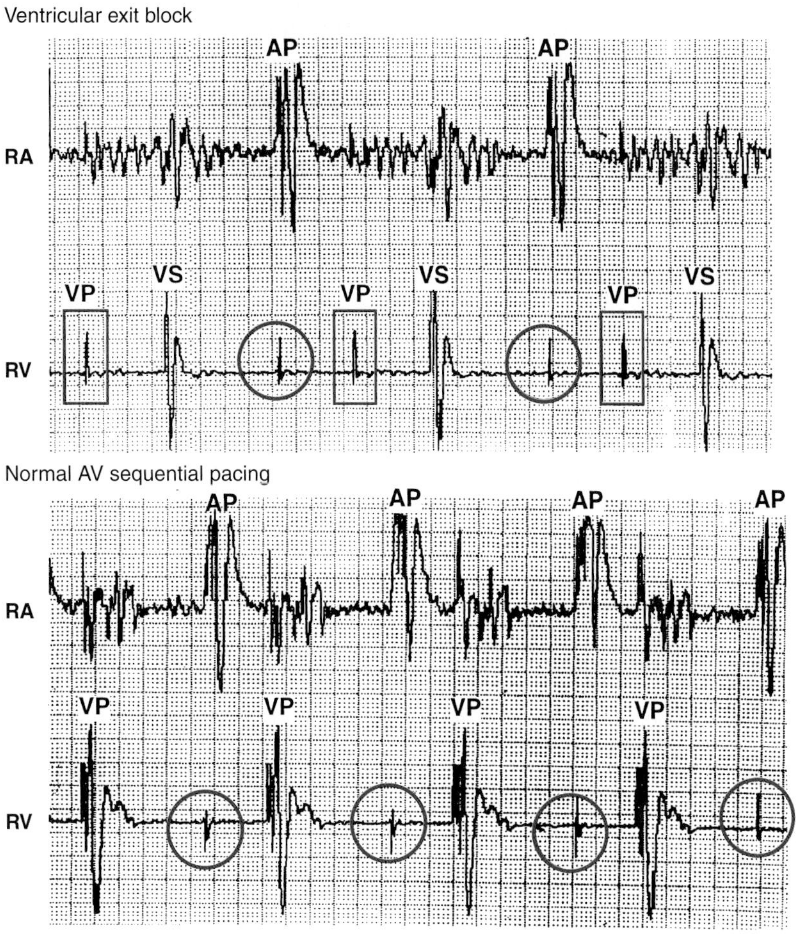

FIGURE 59-16 Right atrial (RA) and right ventricular (RV) unipolar electrograms in right ventricular exit block (*above*). Atrial (AP) and ventricular (VP) pacing are required for sinus arrest and marked first-degree atrioventricular block. Right ventricular capture is restored after RV pacing amplitude is programmed from 3.5 (*above*) to 5.4 V (*below*). Ventricular capture increases the effective heart rate, because the late, conducted ventricular electrograms (VS) in the upper tracing are sensed by the pacemaker and used to begin a new cardiac timing cycle. The circles indicate far-field sensing of the RA pacing artifact in the RV lead.

fibrillation.[40] A review of 650 pacemaker insertions by the author between January 1984 and April 1993 revealed only one perioperative death resulting from heart failure induced by general anesthesia in a child with congenital heart disease (Table 59-3).

Incidence of Complications

The incidence of early pacemaker complications in one recent series was 6.7%, 4.9% requiring reoperation.[40] For patients older than 65, comparable figures were 6.1% and 4.4%, respectively. Lead displacement, pneumothorax, and cardiac perforation were the most common complications. The incidence of late complications was 7.2%.[57] The incidence of reoperation in the author's review of 480 cases was 4.0% (see Table 59-3).

Lead Displacement

The incidence of endocardial lead displacement with early lead designs was more than 10%. With tined and positive fixation leads this has fallen to about 2%.[2,30,40,43–45] The incidence of this complication was 1.5% for atrial and ventricular leads in our review (see Table 59-3). Relevant technical issues have been described in the preceding. We find that positive fixation leads can be applied in unique anatomical locations with essentially no increase in lead displacement (Table 59-4).

Myocardial Infarction

Pacemaker insertion may be appropriate as an adjunct to medical therapy of angina in patients with inoperable coronary artery disease. However, angina, myocardial infarction, or death can result from paced increases in heart rate of as little as 10 bpm.

Hemopneumothorax

Hemopneumothorax and pericardial tamponade can result from injury to the heart, lungs, arteries, or veins. Errors with the Seldinger technique can cause such injuries. In patients older than 65, pneumothorax has been related to subclavian puncture.[45] In our experience with more than 1000 pacemaker insertions by cephalic cut down, hemopneumothorax did not occur. In contrast, a recent review of 1088 consecutive implants by subclavian puncture revealed a 1.8% incidence of pneumothorax.[45]

TABLE 59-3 Results of Pacemaker Implantation, Columbia-Presbyterian Medical Center 1984 to 1993*

Surgical mortality	1/616 (general anesthesia-related)
Mean follow-up	884 ± 675 (SD) days (n = 480 patients, 679 leads)
Morbidity	19 Reoperations (4.0% of 480) 4 Infections (0.8%) 7 Lead displacements (1.5%) 4 Exit block (0.8%) 4 Undersensing (0.8%) 5 Suspected right ventricular perforations 2 Leads abandoned (chordal entrapment) 41 Reprogrammed for dysfunction 0 Hemothorax 0 Pneumothorax 1 Procedure abandoned for thoracotomy (newborn)
Characteristics at generator replacement (n = 40, 75 ± 31 months after implant)	
Pacing threshold	1.3 ± 0.5 V 3.0 ± 1.3 mA
R-wave amplitude	8.9 ± 4.3 mV
Long-term DDD pacing	89% (1109 ± 34 days follow-up)
Causes of DDD failure	8.4% Atrial fibrillation 2.4% Lead dysfunction

*Models 479-01 and 435-02 unipolar, positive fixation leads, Intermedics, Inc., Bellaire, TX.
Source: Spotnitz HM, Mason DP, Carter YM: Unpublished observations.

TABLE 59-4 Lead Stability in Unusual Locations, Columbia-Presbyterian Medical Center 1984 to 1993*

Location	n	Displaced
Coronary sinus (to left ventricle)	2	0
Atrial conduit	1	0
Right atrium of transplant	20	0
Lateral right atrium	27	1
Right ventricular outflow—single	22	0
Right ventricular outflow—paired (ICD recipients)	11 (×2)	0
Infants—looped leads (<1 year old)	7	0
Children—looped leads	42	2
Total	132	3 (2.3%)

*Models 479-01 and 435-02 unipolar, positive fixation leads, Intermedics, Inc., Bellaire, TX.
ICD = implantable cardioverter defibrillator.
Source: Spotnitz HM, Mason DP, Carter YM: Unpublished observations.

Pacemaker Syndrome

Loss of atrioventricular synchrony produces symptoms related to reflex effects or contraction of the atria against closed AV valves. The resulting constellation of symptoms is known as *pacemaker syndrome*.[46] The symptoms are quite variable, but severely affected patients may refuse pacemaker magnet testing. Symptoms are relieved immediately by conversion from VVI to dual-chamber pacing.

Lead Entrapment

Fixed-screw pacemaker leads can become firmly entangled in chordae tendineae beneath the tricuspid valve. Possible responses include further escalation of force, lead extraction,[34,47] or an open procedure. Our experience with this involved three firmly entangled leads in 1000 lead implants. The leads were capped and abandoned rather than escalate risk. There were no untoward consequences of lead abandonment. Consequently, we now avoid the anatomic center of the right ventricle when implanting these leads. This problem has not recurred in more than 750 subsequent implants.

Infection and Erosion

Pacemaker infection can appear as frank sepsis, intermittent fever with vegetations/ inflammation, and/or purulence or drainage at the pacemaker pocket. Indolent generator erosion is another presentation. Antibiotic suppression may temporarily abolish signs of infection, but the problem usually recurs weeks or months later.[46–48] Negative cultures at an erosion may suggest moving the device to a fresh, adjacent site, but this is usually futile. Clinical resolution of recurrent device infection almost always requires removal of all hardware and insertion of a new device in a fresh site, optimally after a device-free interval.[48,49] The incidence of erosion, infection, hematoma, and lead displacement early after pacemaker implantation is reduced by operator experience.[44]

Pacemaker Dysfunction

Mechanical defects in leads, lead displacement, or connection errors can cause pacemaker dysfunction. Lead dysfunction usually represents scarring at the lead—myocardial interface, changes in myocardial properties owing to tissue necrosis or drug effects, or a poor choice of lead position. Insulation erosion can cause oversensing or, in bipolar leads, pacing failure owing to short-circuiting between the two conductors.

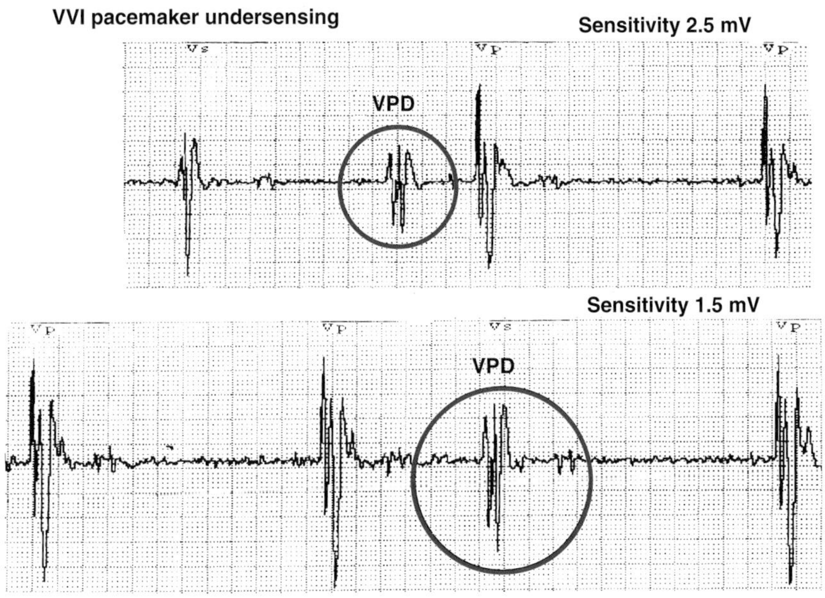

FIGURE 59-17 Undersensing of ventricular premature depolarizations (VPD) illustrated in the upper panel of electrograms obtained by telemetry from a VVI pacemaker. The amplitude of the electrograms increases, and sensing is corrected after reprogramming to increase sensitivity to P waves from 2.5 mV (*above*) to 1.5 mV (*below*).

Generator Dysfunction

Electrical component failures are rare. Three pacemaker or ICD generator failures have required urgent device replacement over the past 10 years at our center. New pacemaker and lead designs may contain flaws that do not become apparent for many years.[2,50]

Undersensing

Undersensing is failure to detect atrial or ventricular electrograms. The result is an atrial or ventricular pacing that should have been inhibited by the unsensed beat. In a dual-chamber pacemaker, undersensing may also cause failure to pace the ventricle after the P wave. Undersensing is often correctable by programming increased generator sensitivity, but this can lead to oversensing. The latitude for reprogramming can be estimated by examining telemetered electrograms[42] (Figs. 59-17 and 59-18).

Oversensing

Inappropriate pacemaker inhibition or triggering may result from detection of myopotentials (muscular activity). This is most common in unipolar systems and may be correctable by programming reduced pacemaker sensitivity. External insulation erosion within the pacemaker pocket is a cause of oversensing

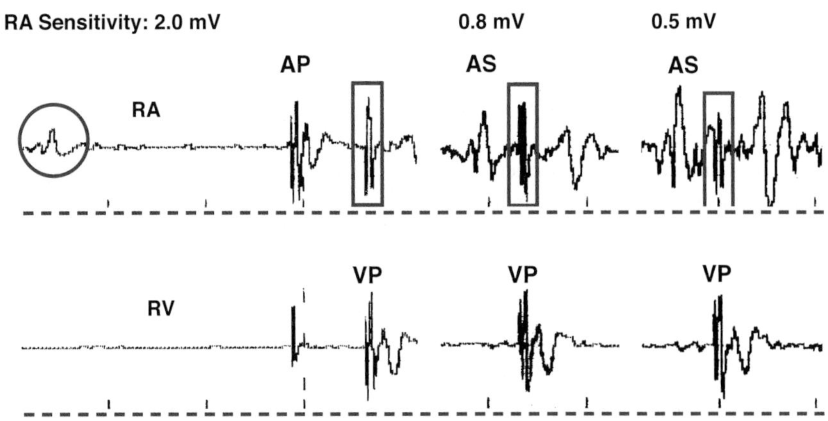

FIGURE 59-18 Right atrial (RA) and right ventricular (RV) electrograms from DDD pacemaker during correction of atrial undersensing. Amplitude of the RA electrogram increases after atrial sensitivity is increased from 2.0 mV (*left*) to 0.8 (*center*) to 0.5 mV (*right*). The P-wave electrogram (*circled*) is not sensed at 2.0 mV, resulting in unnecessary atrial pacing (AP). Proper sensing is restored and the size of the electrogram increases (AS) as sensitivity is increased. VP indicates ventricular pacing. Rectangles in RA tracing identify far-field sensing of the ventricular pacing artifact.

that can be repaired. Internal insulation defects in bipolar leads (see Fig. 59-3) cannot be repaired.

Crosstalk and Far-Field Sensing

A deflection on the ventricular lead immediately after the atrial pacing artifact could be either premature ventricular depolarization (see Fig. 59-17) or far-field sensing of an atrial depolarization (see Fig. 59-13). Many pacemakers deal with this ambiguity by pacing the ventricle at a short (100 millisecond) atrioventricular delay, known as *safety pacing.*[20]

Complexities of DDD programming involve blanking and refractory periods used to compensate for crosstalk or prevent retrograde AV conduction from causing pacemaker-mediated tachycardia (see the following). Crosstalk is ameliorated by bipolar lead systems.

Exit Block

Exit block is rising pacing threshold due to edema or scarring at the lead tip. Pacing threshold tends to increase over 7 to 14 days after lead insertion and stabilizes at about 6 weeks. This phenomenon is related to inflammation at the lead tip and is ameliorated by steroid-eluting leads.[2,51] Exit block may be overcome by programming increased amplitude or pulse width, but this shortens battery life. In unipolar systems, pacing of the chest wall and/or diaphragm may result from high generator output.

Lead Fracture

Fracture of lead insulation or conductors may be demonstrable by chest x-ray (see Fig. 59-15). Lead impedance less than 300 ohms suggests an insulation break, whereas impedance more than 1000 ohms suggests conductor problems, a loose set screw, or improper connection. High impedance also can indicate incomplete extension of the fixation coil in a Bisping lead. Telemetry may detect impending lead fracture as electrical noise during hyperventilation, coughing, bending, or arm swinging. Oversensing of this type usually mandates lead replacement or repair.

At reoperation, dysfunctional leads can be capped or removed by lead extraction techniques. Extraction of chronically implanted leads is potentially hazardous and results in endothelial venous damage even when successful. Accordingly, our practice is to limit lead extraction to infection or mechanical problems (Figs. 59-19 and 59-20). Lead fracture has been promoted historically by design errors, bipolar construction, certain forms of polyurethane insulation, and epicardial insertion.[64] Technical factors in fracture include ties applied to the lead without an anchoring sleeve, kinking, lead angulation, vigorous exercise programs, and subclavian crush.[2,29,35]

Subclavian Crush

Subclavian crush is believed to be caused by lead entrapment between the clavicle and first rib, in the costoclavicular ligament. Stress during body movement is then thought to cause early lead failure. This pertains primarily to leads implanted by percutaneous puncture of the subclavian vein and seems to be minimized by cephalic cut down. Techniques to minimize this problem have been described (see Fig. 59-6).[2,29,35]

Pacemaker-Mediated Tachycardia

DDD pacemakers can propagate a reentrant arrhythmia, pacemaker-mediated tachycardia. This involves retrograde conduction through the atrioventricular node, initially triggered by a premature ventricular depolarization. If the pacemaker senses the retrograde atrial depolarization and paces the ventricle, a cycle is set up that can continue indefinitely at the upper rate limit of the pacemaker. This problem can be mitigated by avoiding high upper rate limits and adjusting the postventricular atrial refractory period so that the pacemaker ignores atrial depolarizations for 300 to 350 milliseconds after the QRS complex. Current pacemakers also attempt to break reentrant arrhythmias by periodic interruption of continuous high-rate pacing. Pacemaker telemetry provides notification of high-rate pacing suspicious of pacemaker-mediated tachycardia.

Innovations and Special Problems

Lead Repair

Repair can extend the useful life of implanted leads for years. Most repairs are done within the device pocket or in surrounding areas. Fracture or erosion of conductors or insulation can result from normal wear or active life styles. We have seen lead dysfunction resulting from obsessive sit ups (abdominal insulation erosion), handball (insulation/conductor erosion), and wood chopping (conductor damage).

Repair kits contain silicone glue and silicone tubing or unipolar tip replacements. Possible repairs differ for unipolar and bipolar leads. Unipolar leads consist of a single conductor surrounded by insulation. Insulation breaks can be overlaid with glue and tubing. Conductor fracture can be repaired by splicing a new lead tip onto the functional segment. Bipolar leads contain two conductors with two levels of insulation, one to prevent short-circuiting between the conductors and the other to prevent external current leaks and conductor-generator contact. An example is shown in Fig. 57-20. External insulation repair in such leads is similar to unipolar lead repair. However, internal insulation faults require converting the lead to unipolar function and splicing on a new lead tip. Conductor fracture also can be repaired this way. The repair involves exposing and baring about 10 mm of the conductor to be preserved. The conductor to be excluded is cut back 5 to 10 mm to avoid short-circuiting. A new tip is attached to the bared conductor, using an internal set-screw, silicone glue, and ties. These repairs have been robust in our experience but are not recommended in pacemaker-dependent patients.

Unipolar and bipolar epicardial leads can also be repaired, if the break is accessible. Unipolar lead repair is similar to repair of unipolar endocardial leads. Bipolar epicardial leads generally consist of two unipolar leads connected by a Y to coaxial segments for connection. The simplest repair involves locating the unipolar segment of the good lead and splicing on a new tip. Particularly challenging is a fracture near one of the cardiac electrodes, at a point of metal fatigue. If the broken conductor is not the tip electrode, function is restored by reprogramming the generator to a unipolar configuration. If the cathode segment is fractured, most generators cannot be programmed to use the

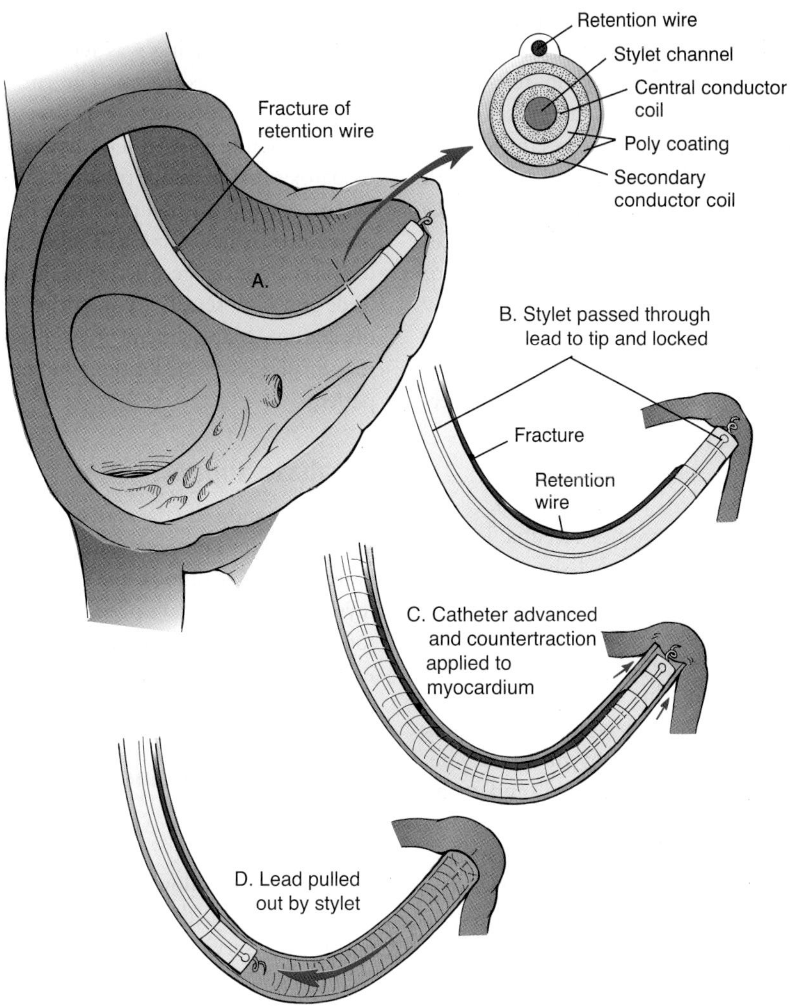

FIGURE 59-19 Byrd method of lead extraction using Cook catheters. Drawings illustrate successful removal of a Telectronics Accufix J-lead with a fractured retention wire.

anode, and pacing is lost. However, function can be restored by exposing the lead, splicing a new tip on the anode, connecting that lead to generator, and capping the cathode.[52]

When exposing leads within the pocket for repairs, the electrocautery should be set as low as practical, to avoid melting external lead insulation. If cautery contacts a bare conductor, myocardial injury can render the lead useless because of exit block. Also, conduction of cautery to the myocardium can induce VF. Sharp dissection is preferred when close to friction points or angulation that promote conductor exposure.

Pacemaker Lead Extraction

Indications for lead extraction include chronic infection or life-threatening mechanical defects.[53] Some recommend that any dysfunctional pacemaker lead should be removed, but there is little objective data to support this. Until recently, extraction of transvenous leads required external traction or thoracotomy/cardiotomy with inflow occlusion or cardiopulmonary bypass. Chronically implanted leads can be densely fibrosed to the right ventricular myocardium, vena cava, innominate vein, or subclavian vein.

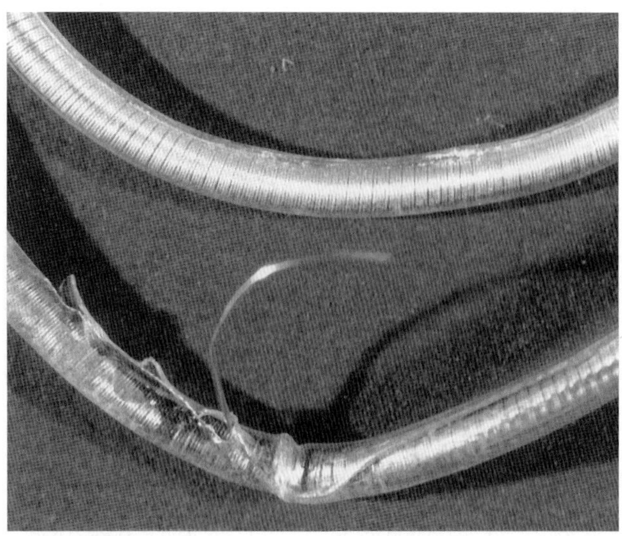

FIGURE 59-20 Telectronics Accufix atrial J-leads removed for retention wire fracture. Region of fracture appears benign in upper image. Lower image illustrates retention wire extrusion after percutaneous extraction. Extruded wire resembles a safety pin.

Lead extraction was developed by Byrd.[34,47] A locking stylet is passed inside the central channel to the tip of the lead where it uncoils, allowing traction to be applied to the lead tip. Telescoping Teflon, plastic, or metal sheaths fitting the lead are passed along the lead to mobilize it. When the long sheath reaches the lead tip, countertraction is applied to the myocardium with the sheath while traction is applied to the lead tip with the locking stylet (see Fig. 59-19). Success with this technique has been greater than 90%, with a 3% chance of serious morbidity or death. Laser or radiofrequency energy can also be transmitted through specially constructed sheaths to ablate adhesions.[80] Technical details have been described.[34,47] Extraction of leads more than 10 years old is difficult and tedious. Complete removal of lead tips is inversely related to the age of the lead (Fig. 59-21).[55]

Accufix Lead

An unusual fracture affects the Telectronics Accufix lead, a bipolar, Bisping-type atrial screw-in lead.[53] A J-shape near the tip directs the lead to the atrial appendage. A curved retention wire welded to the indifferent ring electrode near the tip and bonded to the lead body with polyurethane maintains the J-shape. Fracture and extrusion of this retention wire (see Fig. 59-20) was associated with deaths from cardiac tamponade, related to punctures of the atrium or aorta by fractured wire. More than 45,000 of these leads were implanted, and many have been surgically extracted. Because some morbidity and mortality occurred during extraction of this lead, the manufacturer recommended conservative management. Recently, conservative management has also been recommended for a fracture tendency in the Sprint Fidelis ICD lead.

Atrial Fibrillation and Mode Switching

Sinoatrial node dysfunction can involve both sinus bradycardia and paroxysmal atrial fibrillation. Early DDD pacemakers responded to atrial fibrillation by pacing at the upper rate limit. Initially DDD pacing was felt to be contraindicated in atrial fibrillation for this reason. The current view that atrial pacing decreases the frequency of paroxysmal atrial fibrillation, and mode switching allows DDD pacing to be used despite a history of paroxysmal atrial fibrillation. Mode switching is triggered when a programmed upper rate limit is exceeded. The pacemaker then switches to VVIR mode until the atrial rate returns to the physiologic range. Successful mode switching requires bipolar leads and high sensitivity in patients with low-amplitude atrial fibrillation. Management of atrial fibrillation in elderly people may involve fewer medications and interventions than in younger patients.

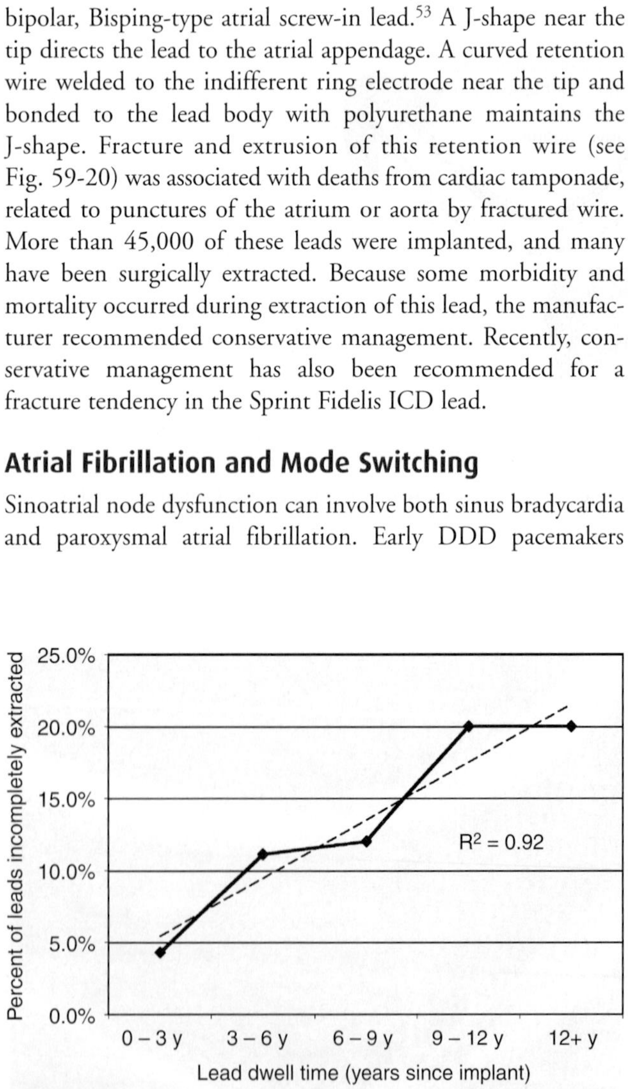

FIGURE 59-21 Duration of lead implantation (Dwell Time) versus incidence of incomplete lead extraction. Incidence decreases from 23% for 12- to 25-year leads to 6% for 0- to 3-year leads. Lead fragments left behind were solid metal tips entrapped connective tissue sheath around lead. This results in tip separation, usually at the level of the innominate vein. There were no clinical complications related to retention of these lead tips.[81]

Database Support

Pacemaker and ICD data are needed for billing, operative notes, device tracking, programming, and follow-up. Data should be available in real time in the event of an emergency room visit involving device malfunction. Commercial and home-grown software packages are available for this. Security, audit trails, 24/7 availability, and multiuser wireless capability are important characteristics for such systems.

General Surgery and Pacemakers

General surgery in a pacemaker-dependent patient raises important questions,[56] especially when surgery requires unipolar cautery. The following must be documented: (1) model and manufacturer of the pacemaker, from pacemaker ID card, monitoring service, medical record, or x-ray appearance[57,58]; (2) magnet mode behavior and any peculiarities related to impedance sensing monitors; (3) successful testing of programmer on the pacemaker; (4) programmed parameters, polarity, battery life, and lead characteristics; (5) degree of pacemaker dependence[57]; (6) a backup plan transthoracic pacing or chronotropic agents if the pacemaker fails; (7) reprogramming to VOO, DOO, or VVT mode intraoperatively with rate response off to prevent inhibition[56] or pacemaker acceleration[84] by electromagnetic interference (EMI); (8) a physician to deal with any intraoperative pacemaker problem; and (9) restored pacemaker program, thresholds, and function postoperatively. Regarding pacemaker dependence, if the preoperative electrocardiogram reveals 100% pacing, the pacemaker should be reprogrammed while monitoring to determine the presence and rate of an escape rhythm. Pacemaker dependence may increase during anesthesia, with withdrawal of sympathetic stimulation.

Electrocautery

Manufacturers recommend against using electrocautery in pacemaker patients because of possible electromagnetic interference (EMI) or pacemaker damage. If electrocautery must be used, unipolar cautery is likely to cause EMI, whereas bipolar cautery is not. Unipolar pacemakers are also more susceptible to EMI than bipolar units. EMI effects include: (1) Pacemaker oversensing of EMI as a rapid heart rate. Pacemaker inhibition results that reverses when the EMI stops. (2) Pacemaker reprogramming. (3) Acceleration of impedance-sensing pacemakers to the

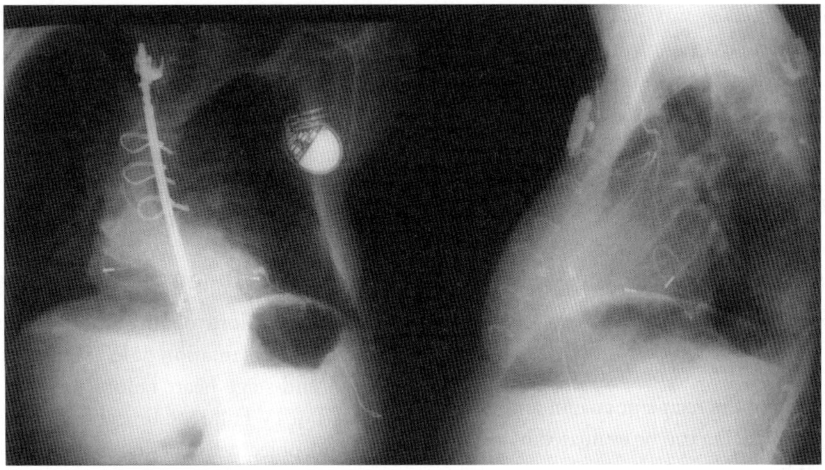

FIGURE 59-22 X-ray of a dual-chamber pacing system illustrates ventricular pacing via the coronary sinus after Fontan surgery. System functioned for 5 years, replaced at Fontan revision. A failed epicardial pacing wire is also present.

upper rate limit.[57] (4) Reversion to a "backup mode" or "magnet mode." (5) Permanent loss of pacing, fortunately rare.[56]

EMI pacemaker inhibition can be minimized by programming sensing off and increasing the pacing rate above the intrinsic heart rate anticipated during surgery. However, if competition with spontaneous beats does occur, there is a risk of inducing of atrial fibrillation or ventricular tachycardia. In view of this, the pacemaker should be returned to an appropriate sensing mode as soon as possible after the completion of surgery.

Magnet Mode

A permanent magnet placed over a pacemaker closes a magnetic reed switch and initiates "magnet mode." In some pacemakers, magnet mode is VOO, eliminating all sensing. Other pacemakers convert to VOO for a few beats, then revert to the programmed function. A magnet may also induce a threshold margin test; this assesses the adequacy of the pacing margin by decreasing the pulse width in a predictable pattern.

Steroid-Eluting Leads

Fibrosis at the lead tip can be limited by incorporating a dexamethasone pellet that dissolves over months. This improves early pacing thresholds versus conventional leads[51] and has been particularly advantageous in epicardial leads.

Adults with Congenital Heart Disease

Congenital heart disease may include a persistent left superior vena cava draining to the coronary sinus. This favors a right-sided surgical approach, although the left side can be used.[38] Preoperative echo-Doppler or angiography can define caval and coronary sinus anatomy. A left superior vena cava may dislocate the subclavian vein, increasing the risk of subclavian vein puncture and favoring cephalic cut down.[54] Situs inversus and corrected transposition are disorienting, if undetected prior to pacemaker insertion.

Positive fixation leads are particularly useful for atrial pacing after a Mustard operation or a caval-pulmonary anastomosis and for pacing the smooth-walled "right" ventricle in corrected transposition of the great arteries.[38] A coronary sinus lead can provide ventricular pacing in some patients after Fontan surgery (Fig. 59-22). Pacing via the coronary sinus is useful in patients with a mechanical tricuspid valve.

Pacing in Infants and Children

Transvenous leads in children should include an intracardiac loop to allow for growth (see Fig. 59-4). Unipolar, positive fixation leads were ideal for this purpose,[38] but other approaches have been described. We prefer cephalic cut down, with optical magnification, if needed. A flexible guidewire is passed centrally and a 7-French introducer introduces the lead. A longitudinal split of the cephalic vein facilitates advancing the introducer (see Fig. 59-8). In very small infants, the external jugular vein at the thoracic inlet may be useful. Subclavian vein puncture can be guided by a catheter introduced via the femoral vein. Thoracotomy is a third option.[27] Infants less than 6 months of age are suboptimal candidates for transvenous pacing because of limited long-term lead utility. Subpectoral generator placement in children less than 6 years old reduces infection risk.

Dementia

Dementia is problematic for surgery under local anesthesia. Sedation can make dementia worse and exaggerates bradycardia. The demented patient's arms should be secured to prevent groping for the surgical wound. Postoperative confusion and thrashing can cause pacemaker lead displacement. An intracardiac loop my reduce this hazard. A family member at the bedside may alleviate this problem. Every effort should be made to anticipate and avoid such problems.

Atrioventricular Node Ablation

AV node ablation controls ventricular rate in refractory atrial fibrillation but leads to permanent heart block. Historically, the AV node was ablated, then temporary pacing supported heart rate until a permanent pacemaker was inserted. Ventricular escape rhythm was often poor, favoring positive fixation leads, overnight observation on telemetry, and high pacemaker output. Alternatively, the pacemaker can be inserted and allowed to heal before ablation.

Transplant Recipients

The usual indication for pacemaker insertion in cardiac transplant recipients is sinus bradycardia or sinus arrest, managed with AAIR pacing.[24,59] In our experience, most outgrow the need for pacing within 2 years.[24,59] The surface ECG may be confusing, with P waves from atria of both the donor and the recipient and AV dissociation of the recipient atrium and donor ventricle. Need for ventricular pacing can be evaluated by pacing the atrium at a rate of 150 bpm. If a 1:1 ventricular response is observed, the AV node is essentially normal. The location of the atrial appendage is more medial than usual in these patients, and positive fixation leads are preferable (Fig. 59-23).

Implantable Cardioverter Defibrillator Recipients

Before integrated devices were available, crosstalk between pacemakers and ICDs could lead to inappropriate ICD shocks or ICD undersensing of ventricular fibrillation. Successful independent implantation of pacemakers and ICDs has been described,[60] but availability of ICDs with integrated DDD pacemakers renders this technique superfluous.

Long QT Syndrome

Long QT is a genetically determined repolarization abnormality that is associated with sudden death. Recommended therapy includes stellate ganglionectomy and/or adrenergic blockade.[61] In severe cases, the pacing threshold may be too high for ventricular pacing, and atrial pacing may be preferable. ICD therapy is now commonly used.

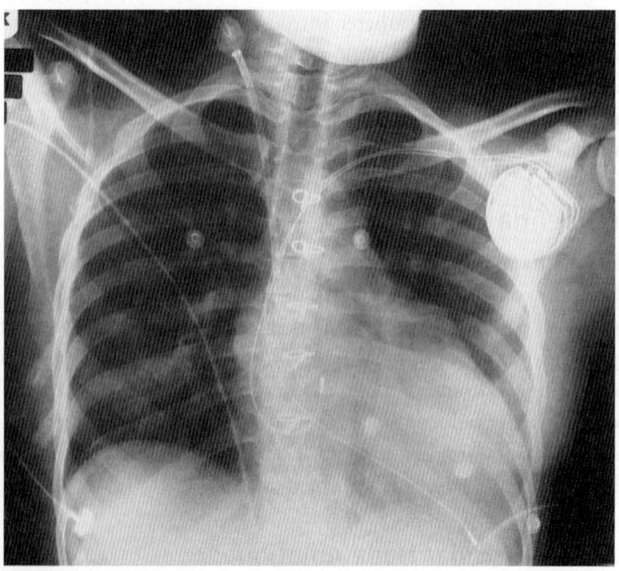

FIGURE 59-23 DDDR pacing system in a cardiac allograft recipient illustrates a shift of the atrial appendage toward the midline, characteristic of these patients.

Idiopathic Hypertrophic Subaortic Stenosis

Idiopathic hypertrophic subaortic stenosis (obstructive cardiomyopathy), with severe left ventricular outflow obstruction, causes angina and/or syncope. Right ventricular pacing with a short atrioventricular delay pre-excites the ventricle and decreases outflow gradients in some patients[16,17] (Fig. 59-24). ICD therapy is increasingly common in this population.

Permanent Biventricular Pacing

End-stage cardiomyopathy and heart failure progress with time. Cardiac transplantation or left ventricular assist devices are effective in end-stage heart failure. CRT is a lower cost option for class III or IV failure. Clinical trials demonstrate modest subjective and objective benefits of CRT in dilated cardiomyopathy with left ventricular ejection fraction less than 36% and QRS intervals greater than 120 milliseconds.[18,19,62] Mortality benefits are suggested by COMPANION and other recent trials.[63] Marked clinical improvement is seen in some patients (see Fig. 59-11), but up to 40% of patients are nonresponders. Endocardial LV lead insertion fails in 5 to 10% of candidates, usually because of difficulty cannulating the CS. These failures often result in referrals to thoracic surgeons for epicardial lead insertion. More than 100,000 patients undergo CRT annually in the United States, which could lead to 5000 referrals yearly for epicardial lead insertion. Although minimal access[64] and robotic[65] LV lead insertion have been developed, referrals might increase if better techniques for epicardial LV lead insertion were available.

Temporary Biventricular Pacing

Clinical success with CRT and the potential to increase cardiac output while reducing myocardial oxygen consumption make temporary biventricular pacing attractive for management of low-output states after cardiac surgery. Preliminary results[66] indicate that this approach is promising. Temporary biventricular pacing can be recommended and is readily achievable for patients in low-output states with second- or third-degree block after cardiac surgery.[19,67]

Atrial and Ventricular Tachyarrhythmias

Overdrive pacing can be effective for ventricular tachyarrhythmias, Wolff-Parkinson-White syndrome, or atrial flutter. Implantable defibrillators are under development for atrial fibrillation. Antitachycardia ventricular pacing for ventricular tachyarrhythmia has been integrated into ICD therapy.

Environmental Issues

Electromagnetic Interference

EMI[56] can be caused by electrocautery, cellular telephones, magnetic resonance imagers,[68] microwaves, diathermy, arc welders, powerful radar or radio transmitters, and theft detectors in retail stores. Any defective, sparking electrical appliance or motor, electric razor, lawn mower, or electric light can be problematic. The importance of EMI is related to pacemaker dependence. Pacemaker recipients who are not pacemaker dependent will not be distressed by brief periods of pacemaker

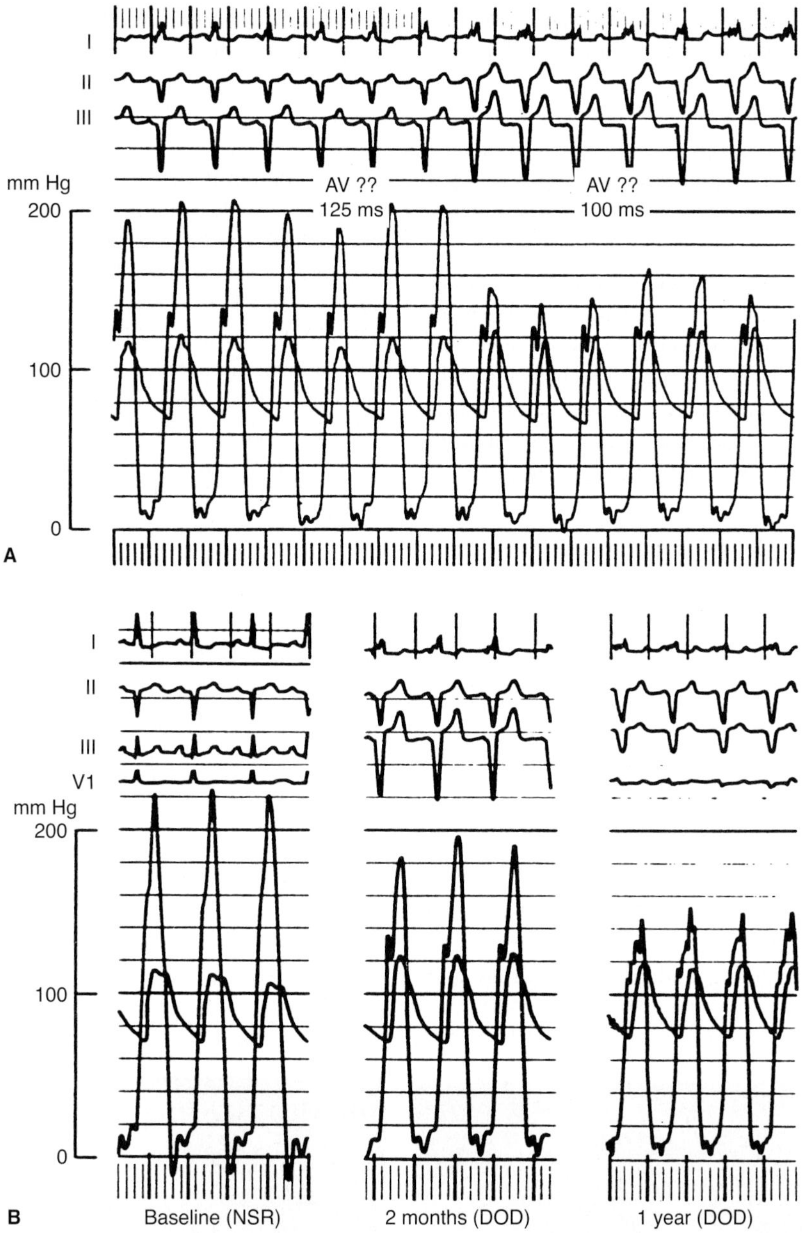

FIGURE 59-24 (A) Effect of reducing AVD in DDD pacing from 125 (*left*) to 100 milliseconds (*right*) on left ventricular outflow gradient in idiopathic hypertrophic subaortic stenosis. (B) Effect of time and DDD pacing on left ventricular outflow gradient in idiopathic hypertrophic subaortic stenosis. (*Reproduced with permission from Kay GN, Bubien RS, Epstein AE, et al: Rate-modulated cardiac pacing based on transthoracic impedance measurements of minute ventilation: correlation with exercise gas exchange. J Am Coll Cardiol 1989; 14:1283.*)

inhibition, but pacemaker-dependent patients can lose consciousness in 5 to 15 seconds. Bipolar pacing systems provide added protection against EMI. Cellular telephones should be separated by several inches from pacemaker generators, preferably on the contralateral side.[69] ICD circuits are insulated against inappropriate firing precipitated by EMI. During surgery using unipolar cautery, the defibrillation circuit of an ICD should be temporarily disabled.

Mechanical Interference

Lithotripsy, trauma, dental equipment, and even bumpy roads can affect pacemakers. Automobile accidents have caused pacemaker damage and disruption of pacemaker wounds.[70] Vibration causes inappropriately high heart rates in rate-responsive units. Patients with poor escape rhythms should be discouraged from exposure to deceleration injury in contact sports, basketball, handball, downhill skiing, surfing, diving, mountain climbing, and gymnastics. Participants in these activities should realize that abrupt pacemaker failure could occur in the event of lead displacement related to trauma.

Radioactivity

The integrated circuits of current pacemakers can be damaged by radiotherapy.[4] If the pacemaker cannot be adequately shielded from the radiation field, it may be necessary to remove and replace it or move the pacing system to a remote site.

Quality of Life

Quality of life is not a major concern for most pacemaker recipients. Although many clinics require periodic visits, the model of transtelephonic monitoring with office visits only for problems is acceptable to most patients. This latter system involves a preoperative visit, a 10-day postoperative visit, a 1-year visit to adjust output, and no additional visits unless functional problems or impending battery depletion are detected. Some recipients are never happy with their pacemakers because of body image problems, vague symptoms, or concern that life will be artificially prolonged. The value of generator replacement in patients with advanced debilitation has been a subject of ethical concern.[71]

IMPLANTABLE CARDIAC DEFIBRILLATORS

Background

More than 400,000 deaths in the United States each year are classified as sudden and likely to be caused by arrhythmias.[72] Michel Mirowski conceptualized the implantable defibrillator in the late 1960s. Overcoming theoretical, engineering, and financial obstacles, he participated in a successful clinical trial of his device in the early 1980s.[73] Today's implantable cardioverter defibrillator (ICD) reflects dramatic and expensive growth in technology. The efficacy of the ICD in prevention of sudden death is well established. Clinical trials, experience, and the passage of time emphasize survival advantages of the ICD over other modalities, including antiarrhythmic drugs and subendocardial resection. The ICD is associated with the lowest sudden death mortality (1 to 2% per year) of any known form of therapy.[74–77] The ICD is expensive ($12,000 to $20,000 for the generator and $2000 to $8000 for the lead system), with discomfort and lifestyle issues. Prophylactic ICD insertion for primary prevention is increasing.

Clinical trials including AVID, MUSST, MADIT I and II, SCD-HeFT, and COMPANION demonstrated benefits of ICD therapy.[78–89] The CABG Patch Trial,[90] which compared coronary artery bypass graft (CABG) to CABG+ICD, and DINAMIT,[91] which studied ICD implantation early after myocardial infarction, failed to demonstrate advantages of ICD insertion. Trials now focus on prophylactic ICD therapy, CRT-Ds and cost-effectiveness. Accumulating evidence supports prophylactic use of CRT-Ds in patients with coronary disease or dilated cardiomyopathy.[92] The appropriate role for prophylactic CRT-Ds is still evolving. The Heart Rhythm Society will not certify surgeons to implant ICDs unless they have passed its certification exam. Patients with prophylactic device insertion are being followed in a national registry. Information about this can be found at http://www.accncdr.com/webncdr/ICD. ICD insertion for primary prevention has doubled or tripled the number of candidates for these devices.

ICD battery life is greater than 5 years. Today's devices are highly programmable. Size and weight are similar to pacemakers of the 1970s. Lead systems have evolved from epicardial patches requiring thoracotomy to endocardial systems.[74–77] Defibrillation thresholds (DFTs) are reduced by biphasic shocks[93] and "hot can" technology.[94] Pectoral implantation is the current standard, some deep to the pectoralis major. Abdominal implantation is now reserved for special cases (Figs. 59-25 and 59-26).

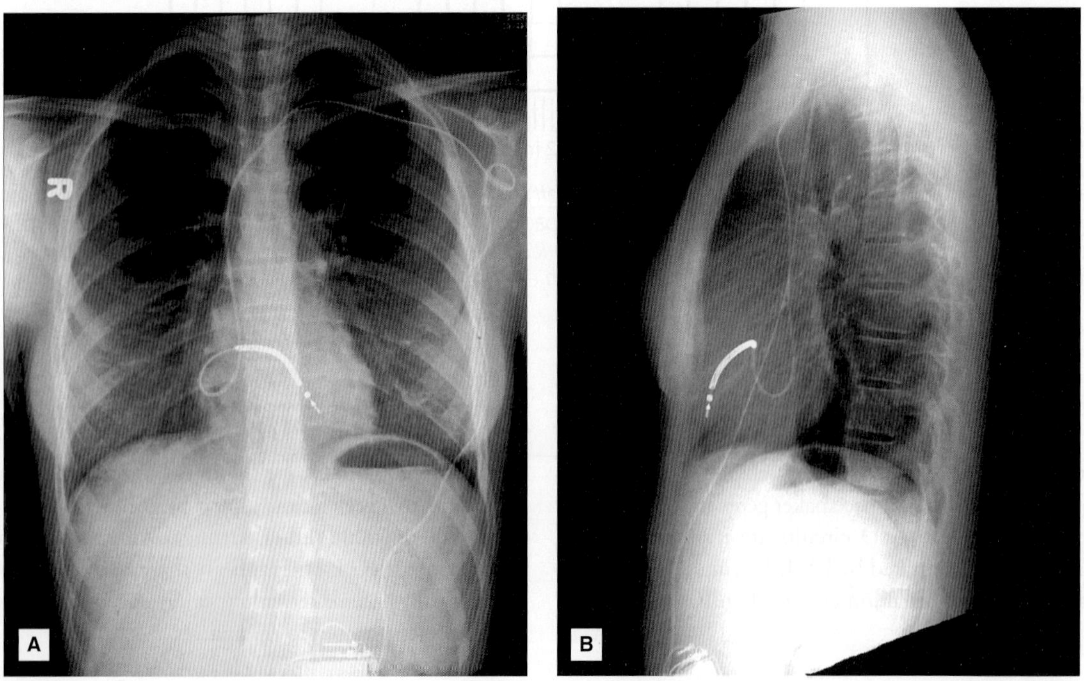

FIGURE 59-25 (A) ICD implant in 13-year-old girl with long QT syndrome. Intracardiac loop allows for growth. Strain relief loop is in the shoulder. Single-coil, screw-in lead permitted intracardiac loop, but improved leads now allow twin-coil leads to be used. Generator is in posterior rectus sheath. (B) Lateral x-ray of same patient.

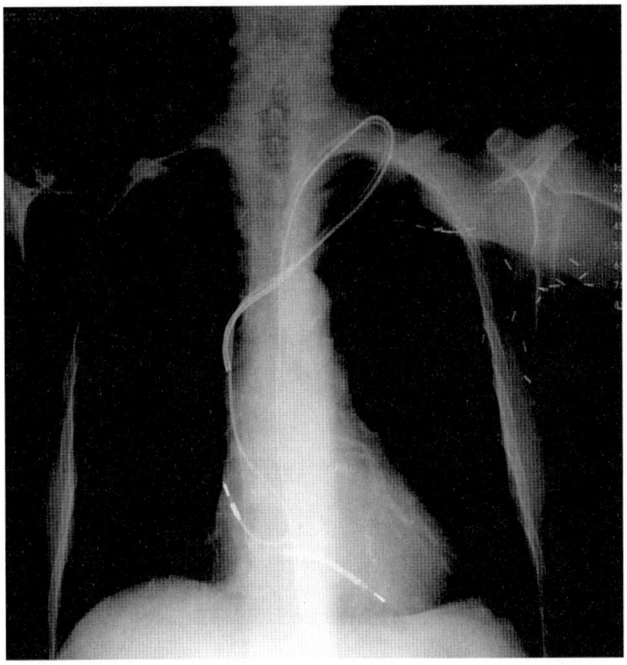

FIGURE 59-26 ICD/DDD pacemaker for ventricular tachycardia with prior bilateral radical mastectomies. Venous access via external jugular vein. Positive fixation leads tunneled vertically in the midline, the only location on the chest wall with adequate tissue. Generator subcutaneous in abdomen. Cosmetic result acceptable to patient.

Electrograms can be downloaded to expedite decisions about antiarrhythmics, prevent inappropriate shocks, and detect oversensing.[95] Remote monitoring of ICD function is available from some manufacturers. VVI, DDD, biventricular, and antitachycardia pacing have been integrated into ICDs.[96] Accelerated development has pressured the Food and Drug Administration to rapidly approve new technology. When the U.S. Health Care Finance Administration refused in 1995 to allow Medicare reimbursement to support device development, ICD development shifted overseas.

Physiology

Ventricular tachycardia (VT) associated with ischemic cardiomyopathy is commonly a reentrant arrhythmia that may be prevented by drugs, catheter ablation, or surgical maneuvers that alter the timing and electrical attributes of the reentrant circuit. Myocardial infarction creates the areas of scarring and slow conduction needed for reentry. Other forms of VT and ventricular fibrillation (VF) involve aberrancies of automaticity related to acute myocardial ischemia, increased ventricular wall stress, and myopathic cellular injury. Some class I antiarrhythmics have been shown to increase postinfarction mortality,[97] possibly owing to proarrhythmic effects.

Indications

Candidates for ICD insertion for secondary prevention therapy have suffered documented VT or VF in the absence of acute myocardial infarction and have been proved unsuitable for antiarrhythmic drug or surgical therapy, based on programmed electrical stimulation studies in the EP laboratory. However, many patients who suffer cardiac arrest do not have inducible VT at EP study, and many patients with a history of syncope and presyncope have inducible VT but no history of a clinical arrhythmia. Many antiarrhythmics have negative inotropic and proarrhythmic effects. Serial EP studies of drug efficacy have been discredited in clinical trials.[93]

In mid-1996 the Food and Drug Administration approved an indication for prophylactic ICD insertion based on early termination of the MADIT Trial.[83] If EP studies demonstrate inducible VT in patients with nonsustained VT and a history of myocardial infarction, an ICD is indicated. MADIT II results support ICD insertion in all patients with a history of myocardial infarction and left ventricular ejection fraction less than 30%. SCD-HeFT supports ICD insertion for patients with LVEF less than 36% and class II or III heart failure and either ischemic or dilated cardiomyopathy. Indications for ICD insertion for primary prevention therapy have recently been reviewed.[98,99]

Device Description

ICDs usually employ one bipolar lead for ventricular pacing/rate sensing and another to deliver the defibrillation current (Fig. 59-27). These are integrated into a single lead body for endocardial insertion. A unipolar ventricular lead paired with an "active can" delivers the defibrillation current in some designs. Rate alone currently identifies malignant rhythms for treatment; waveform is no longer monitored. Up to 30% of ICD shocks are inappropriate for sinus tachycardia or other supraventricular tachyarrhythmias.[74,100] A bipolar atrial lead can help differentiate supraventricular arrhythmias from VT. Subcutaneous leads can be added for patients with high DFTs. Most implants are just caudad to the clavicle, but long lead lengths allow abdominal locations. Positive fixation leads are preferred.

The ICD contains a high-energy battery and a capacitor that steps up the output voltage to 600 to 800 V at 35 to 40 J. Shocks with positive and negative phases reduce DFTs. ICDs incorporate integrated circuits and a telemetry antenna. A broad range of programmable diagnostic and therapeutic functions are supported.

Surgical Procedure

Patient Preparation

Most ICD recipients are at increased mortality/morbidity risk for any surgery. Preoperative optimization of therapy for ischemia, heart failure, and systemic illnesses is critical. The mortality of ICD implantation in our program has been low since 1983, with ischemia more lethal than severe cardiomyopathy. Ischemia on stress testing mandates, CABG, coronary angioplasty, intra-aortic balloon pump, or deferral of DFT testing.

Surgical Approach

Epicardial patch leads[101,102] are now rarely used. They fell into disfavor when the CABG Patch Trial demonstrated that infectious complications were more common in ICD recipients than control

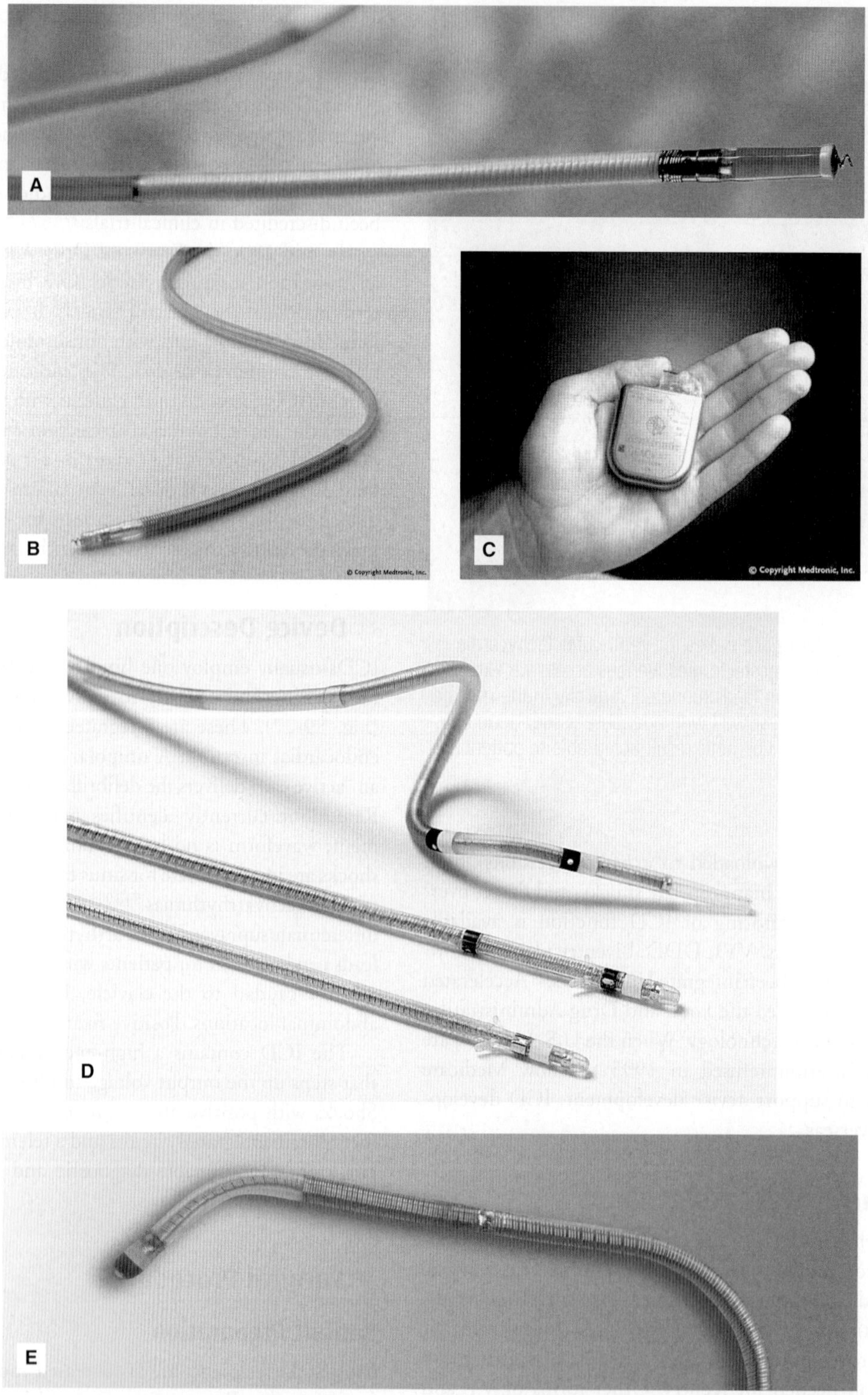

FIGURE 59-27 (A) ICD lead (9 French) with Gore-Tex–coated shocking coils. (B) ICD lead (7 French) with retractable screw. (C) ICD/pacemaker. (D) Over-the-wire leads for coronary sinus pacing. (E) Over-the-wire lead for coronary sinus pacing. (*A,D: Courtesy Guidant Corp., Indianapolis, IN; B, C, E: Courtesy of Medtronic, Inc., Minneapolis, MN.*)

patients.[90] Extrapericardial ICD patches cause less fibrosis, less impairment of diastolic properties,[103,104] and less potential for graft impingement than intrapericardial patches. Biphasic waveforms, improved leads, high-output "hot can" generators, and subcutaneous leads have made the endocardial approach successful.

Manufacturer's Representatives

The complexity of current devices and a large number of spare parts, leads, and catheters have legitimized the presence of manufacturer's representatives during ICD implants. This increases influence of the manufacturer on the implant and warrants oversight. CRS regulations mandate electrophysiologist oversight of DFT measurement.

Technique

We prefer local anesthesia and unipolar cautery for ICD insertion, with invasive, radial artery pressure monitoring during DFT measurement. Positioning and draping are similar to that for pacemaker insertion, with adhesive R2 electrodes added over the right breast and beneath the left scapula. R2 electrodes should not be placed directly over the site of a possible subcutaneous ICD patch or array in the lateral axilla; this can result in serious equipment damage from arcing if external defibrillation is necessary.

Currently, deep sedation is used for induction and reversal of VF for DFT measurement. If multiple shocks are required, endotracheal intubation may be needed. We use intravenous cefazolin or combined vancomycin/gentamicin for antibiotic prophylaxis.

We prefer a cephalic vein cut down via a 6-cm incision over the deltopectoral groove. If the vein is small, a guidewire is used to position a 7- or 9-French introducer. Enlargement of the cephalic venotomy may be helpful if the vein is too small for the introducer (see Fig. 59-8). The guidewire can be left in place if a multiple-lead system is to be employed. Introducer kinking can lead to difficulty passing ICD leads. High central pressures can lead to bleeding until the introducer is removed. Introducer kinking is minimized by aligning the introducer with the course of the subclavian vein before removing the obturator.

As the lead enters the ventricle, VT or VF may be triggered. This is less disruptive if an external defibrillator is connected and precharged, with a capable OR nurse or electrophysiologist at the controls. The ventricular lead should be advanced gently as far as possible to the apex. Positive fixation ICD leads are preferred for both atrium and ventricle. Fluoroscopic and impedance checks for lead displacement are warranted during DFTs, particularly if external defibrillation is necessary. Intravenous norepinephrine is useful for blood pressure support. Transesophageal echocardiography is useful for monitoring patients under general anesthesia during DFTs. We do not use Swan-Ganz catheters for monitoring, because their removal can dislodge the ICD leads.

When a CRT-D (Fig. 59-28) is indicated, we insert the LV lead via cephalic cut down. The RV and RA leads are inserted next via subclavian puncture. Coronary sinus localization can be expedited by steerable electrophysiology catheters, dye injection to detect blood flow out of the coronary sinus, transesophageal echocardiography, and other techniques.

Left upper quadrant abdominal generator placement is reserved for cosmetic insertions, which may also situate the generator in the posterior rectus sheath (see Fig. 59-25). With general anesthesia or sedation/local anesthesia, leads are tunneled to the abdomen from the subclavian incision. Caution is exercised with the tunneler; it must pass anterior to the costal margin. The lead is looped in the shoulder and firmly secured to minimize the possibility that a tug on the abdominal end would displace the lead (see Fig. 59-25).

Defibrillation Threshold

The DFT test is the point of maximum risk in ICD insertion. VF is usually induced twice and reversed by the ICD. Backup defibrillation is available through cutaneous electrodes. The DFT should be at least 10 J less than the maximum ICD output. If the DFT is too high after optimizing RV lead location, an subcutaneous axillary patch or array is used to distribute the

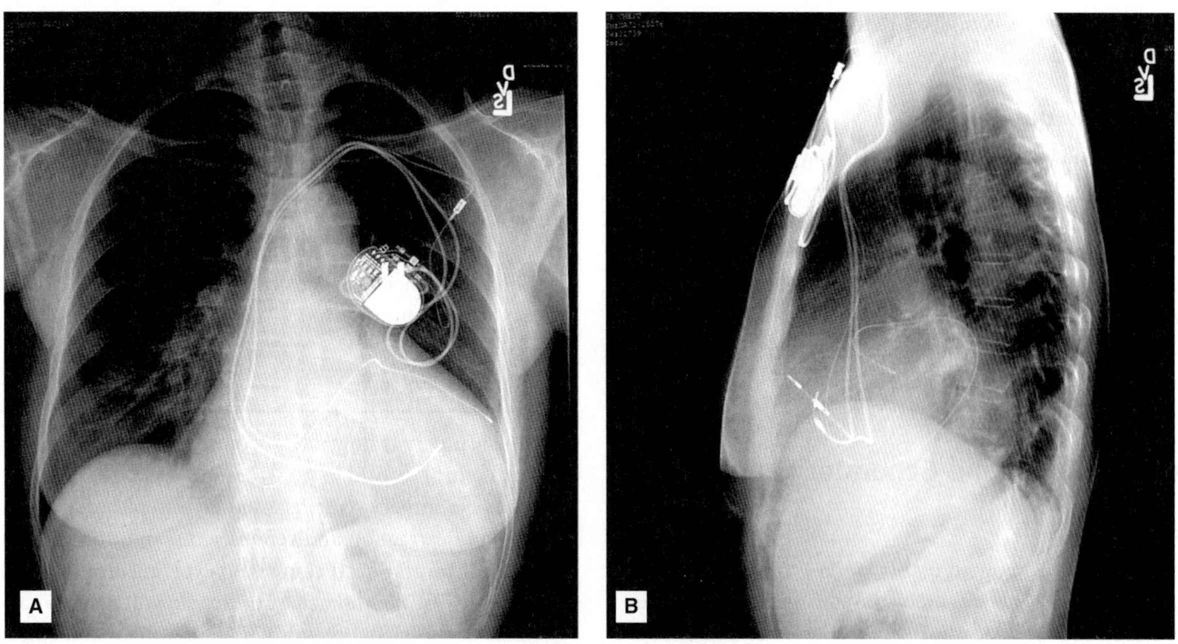

FIGURE 59-28 (A) Dual-chamber CRT-D with endocardial leads in the right atrium, right ventricle, and lateral branch of the coronary sinus (left ventricle). (B) Lateral x-ray of the same patient. Posterior course of the coronary sinus is apparent.

defibrillation current over the posterolateral left ventricle. High-output generators and reversed shock polarity may also help. DFT testing can depress cardiac function[83–85,105,106] and cause a low-output state. The mortality of ICD insertion is about 1%.[106] Complications include myocardial infarction, heart failure, infection, lead displacement, venous occlusion, tamponade, hemopneumothorax, and pocket hematoma.

Refractory Ventricular Fibrillation

An iatrogenic left pneumothorax can raise the DFT so that VF is refractory to external defibrillation. The differential diagnosis includes myocardial ischemia, electromechanical dissociation, and inappropriate ICD lead location. Refractory VF rarely may require open cardiac massage or cardiopulmonary bypass until a solution can be found.

Postoperative Care

Telemetry and an overnight stay are desirable after ICD insertion for VT or VF. Pacing and sensing properties confirm lead stability before discharge. In some cases, DFTs are also retested. An ICD magnet should be available for treatment of patients with freshly implanted ICDs. The magnet is used to inhibit inappropriate shocks caused by ventricular lead displacement or supraventricular arrhythmias. Patients undergoing ICD insertion for primary prevention may be discharged on the day of surgery. We administer ciprofloxacin for 5 days after discharge to complete prophylaxis based on a historical precedent. A postoperative office visit is scheduled 7 to 14 days after implant.

Surgical Follow-up

At the postoperative office visit, lead position, patient symptoms, EP follow-up appointments, and the surgical site are assessed. If drainage is present, the wound is cultured and treated. For sterile drainage, ciprofloxacin or trimethoprim-sulfamethoxazole is administered for 10 days, and the patient is asked to keep the site dry until healing is complete. Refractory infection requires hospitalization and ICD explantation.

Device Follow-up

ICDs require outpatient EP evaluation at 1- to 3-month intervals to cycle the capacitors, confirm battery life, test pacing thresholds, and download electrograms. Data are reviewed for aborted charging cycles arrhythmias. Programming is adjusted accordingly. For any shocks reported, telemetry can confirm proper function, detect inappropriate shocks, and demonstrate electrical noise or oversensing that requires lead revision. Wireless ICD monitoring from home is now a clinical reality for some ICDs.

Late Follow-up and Generator Replacement

Battery Depletion

ICD battery life is now typically more than 60 months. Complications of generator replacement include infection, myocardial infarction, and death. Progression of heart failure and/or coronary artery disease increases the risk of replacement. Replacement is done under local anesthesia, with sedation during DFTs. DFTs may be deferred if the risk is excessive. Patients are discharged on the same day with antibiotic coverage, unless leads are replaced.

Lead Dysfunction

The incidence of failure increases with time. About 50% of ICD recipients have some lead revision by 10 years of follow-up.[107–109] Problems include lead fracture, high DFTs, oversensing, undersensing, and exit block. The incidence of transvenous lead displacement is 7% and of fracture is 6% at 2-year follow-up.[109] Oversensing can be caused by insulation damage. Oversensing can be corrected with a new transvenous rate-sensing lead, preferably of the positive-fixation type. Visible insulation damage inside the defibrillator pocket may be repairable, as described in the following.[110]

Patch leads can fail because of conductor fracture or distortion by fibrosis. With endocardial leads, DFTs may increase as a result of cardiac enlargement, which shifts the left ventricle laterally, away from the right ventricular lead. Insertion of a subcutaneous patch and/or a high-output generator can correct high DFTs.

Additional Issues

Bridge to Transplant

The benefits and liabilities of CRT-D therapy for VT/VF in patients who are awaiting cardiac allografting are under investigation,[98,99,111] with cost an important concern.

Quality of Life

Issues include the discomfort and distress of shocks and inconvenience of outpatient visits. These are particularly trying for elderly patients. ICD generators, though shrinking in size and weight, are bulky compared with pacemakers. Many patients are elated to be rescued by their ICD from a malignant arrhythmia, but others find this distressing.[112-114] Many ICD patients do not comply with recommended limitations on driving automobiles. [115] Fortunately, the rate of accidents in ICD recipients is reported to be low.[116]

Cost-Effectiveness

ICD therapy is expensive, but VT/VF management in the absence of an ICD is also costly. The incremental cost per year of life added is estimated at $10,000 to $200,000.[92,117,118] Reduced cost of ICD generators and leads would increase the economic appeal of ICD prophylaxis.

KEY POINTS

- Open surgery is now rarely required for insertion of arrhythmia control devices.
- Thoracic surgery remains essential for epicardial lead insertion and extraction and venous access in difficult patients.
- Resynchronization therapy is an evolving area in which the versatility of the thoracic surgeon can still play a vital role.
- Skills of thoracic surgeons with endocardial and epicardial leads remain valuable in specific clinical situations and warrant attention and renewal, lest they be lost.

REFERENCES

1. Ellenbogen KA, Wood MA: *Cardiac Pacing and ICDs*, 4th ed. Malden, Oxford, UK, Blackwell Publishing Professional, 2005.
2. Mond HG: Engineering and clinical aspects of pacing leads, in Ellenbogen KA, Kay GN, Wilkoff BL (eds): *Clinical Cardiac Pacing and Defibrillation*, 2nd ed. Philadelphia, WB Saunders, 2000; p 127.
3. Warren JA, Nelson JP: Pacemaker and ICD pulse generator circuitry, in Ellenbogen KA, Kay GN, Wilkoff BL (eds): *Clinical Cardiac Pacing and Defibrillation*, 2nd ed. Philadelphia, WB Saunders, 2000; p 194.
4. Hurkmans CW, Scheepers E, Springorum BG, et al: Influence of radiotherapy on the latest generation of implantable cardioverter-defibrillators. *Int J Radiat Oncol Biol Phys* 2005; 63:282.
5. Zoll PM: Resuscitation of the heart in ventricular standstill by external electric stimulation. *NEJM* 1952; 247:768.
6. Furman S, Schwedel JB: An intracardiac pacemaker for Stokes-Adams seizures. *NEJM* 1959; 261:948.
7. Chardack WM, Gage AA, Greatbatch W: A transistorized self-contained, implantable pacemaker for the long-term correction of heart block. *Surgery* 1960; 48:643.
8. Bernstein AD, Camm AJ, Fletcher R, et al: The NASPE/BPEG generic pacemaker code for antibradyarrhythmia and adaptive rate pacing and antitachyarrhythmia devices. *PACE* 1987; 10:794.
9. Nelson SD, Kou WH, De Buitleir M, et al: Value of programmed ventricular stimulation in presumed carotid sinus syndrome. *Am J Cardiol* 1987; 60:1073.
10. Epstein AE, DiMarco JP, Ellenbogen KA, et al: ACC/AHA/HRS 2008 Guidelines for Device-Based Therapy of Cardiac Rhythm Abnormalities. *Circulation* 2008;117:e350-408.
11. Ellenbogen KA, de Guzman M, Kawanishi DT, et al: Pacing for acute and chronic atrioventricular conduction system disease, in Ellenbogen KA, Kay GN, Wilkoff BL (eds): *Clinical Cardiac Pacing and Defibrillation*, 2nd ed. Philadelphia, WB Saunders, 2000; p 426.
12. Sheldon RS, Jaeger FJ: Carotid sinus hypersensitivity and neurally mediated syncope, in Ellenbogen KA, Kay GN, Wilkoff BL (eds): *Clinical Cardiac Pacing and Defibrillation*, 2nd ed. Philadelphia, WB Saunders, 2000; p 455.
13. Sra JS, Jazayeri MR, Avitall B, et al: Comparison of cardiac pacing with drug therapy in the treatment of neurocardiogenic (vasovagal) syncope with bradycardia or asystole. *NEJM* 1993; 328:1085.
14. Prech M, Grygier M, Mitkowski P, et al: Effect of restoration of AV synchrony on stroke volume, exercise capacity, and quality-of-life: can we predict the beneficial effect of a pacemaker upgrade? *Pacing Clin Electrophysiol* 2001; 24:302.
15. Karpawich PP, Mital S: Comparative left ventricular function following atrial, septal, and apical single chamber heart pacing in the young. *Pacing Clin Electrophysiol* 1997; 20:1983.
16. Fananapazir L, Epstein ND, Curiel RV, et al: Long-term results of dual-chamber (DDD) pacing in obstructive hypertrophic cardiomyopathy. Evidence for progressive symptomatic and hemodynamic improvement and reduction of left ventricular hypertrophy. *Circulation* 1994; 90:2731.
17. Gadler F, Linde C, Daubert C, et al: Significant improvement of quality of life following atrioventricular synchronous pacing in patients with hypertrophic obstructive cardiomyopathy. Data from 1 year of follow-up. PIC study group. Pacing In Cardiomyopathy. *Eur Heart J* 1999; 20:1044.
18. Leclercq C, Cazeau S, Ritter P, et al: A pilot experience with permanent biventricular pacing to treat advanced heart failure. *Am Heart J* 2000; 140:862.
19. Berberian G, Quinn TA, Kanter JP, et al: Optimized biventricular pacing in atrioventricular block after cardiac surgery. *Ann Thorac Surg* 2005; 80:870.
20. Yu CM, Chan JY, Zhang Q, et al: Biventricular pacing in patients with bradycardia and normal ejection fraction. *NEJM* 2009;361:2123.
21. Lau CP, Butrous GS, Ward DE, et al: Comparison of exercise performance of six rate-adaptive right ventricular cardiac pacemakers. *Am J Cardiol* 1989; 63:833.
22. Kay GN, Bubien RS, Epstein AE, et al: Rate-modulated cardiac pacing based on transthoracic impedance measurements of minute ventilation: correlation with exercise gas exchange. *J Am Coll Cardiol* 1989; 14:1283.
23. Hesselson AB, Parsonnet B, Bernstein AD, et al: Deleterious effects of long-term single-chamber ventricular pacing in patients with sick sinus syndrome: the hidden benefits of dual chamber pacing. *J Am Coll Cardiol* 1992; 15:1542.
24. Cooper MW, Smith CR, Rose EA, et al: Permanent transvenous pacing following orthotopic heart transplantation. *J Thorac Cardiovasc Surg* 1992; 104:812.
25. Abraham WT, Fisher WG, Smith AL, et al, MIRACLE Study Group: Multicenter InSync Randomized Clinical Evaluation. Cardiac resynchronization in chronic heart failure. *NEJM* 2002; 346:1845.
26. Cohen MI, Vetter VL, Wernovsky G, et al: Epicardial pacemaker implantation and follow-up in patients with a single ventricle after the Fontan operation. *J Thorac Cardiovasc Surg* 2001; 121:804.
27. Hoyer MH, Beerman LB, Ettedgui JA, et al: Transatrial lead placement for endocardial pacing in children. *Ann Thorac Surg* 1994; 58:97.
28. Dekker AL, Phelps B, Dijkman B, et al: Epicardial left ventricular lead placement for cardiac resynchronization therapy: optimal pace site selection with pressure-volume loops. *J Thorac Cardiovasc Surg* 2004; 127:1641.
29. Magney JE, Flynn DM, Parsons JA, et al: Anatomical mechanisms explaining damage to pacemaker leads, defibrillator leads, and failure of central venous catheters adjacent to the sternoclavicular joint. *Pacing Clin Electrophysiol* 1993; 16:445.
30. Mond H, Sloman G: The small tined pacemaker lead—absence of dislodgement. *Pacing Clin Electrophysiol* 1980; 3:171.
31. Garcia-Bolao I, Alegria E: Implantation of 500 consecutive cardiac pacemakers in the electrophysiology laboratory. *Acta Cardiol* 1999; 54:339.
32. Da Costa A, Kirkorian G, Cucherat M, et al: Antibiotic prophylaxis for permanent pacemaker implantation: a meta-analysis. *Circulation* 1998; 97:1796.
33. Belott PH, Reynolds DW: Permanent pacemaker and implantable cardioverter-defibrillator implantation, in Ellenbogen KA, Kay GN, Wilkoff BL (eds): *Clinical Cardiac Pacing and Defibrillation*, 2nd ed. Philadelphia, WB Saunders, 2000; p 573.
34. Byrd CL: Recent developments in pacemaker implantation and lead retrieval. *Pacing Clin Electrophysiol* 1993; 16:1781.
35. Mathur G, Stables RH, Heaven D, et al: Permanent pacemaker implantation via the femoral vein: an alternative in cases with contraindications to the pectoral approach. *Europace* 2001; 3:56.
36. Ong LS, Barold S, Lederman M, et al: Cephalic vein guide wire technique for implantation of permanent pacemakers. *Am Heart J* 1987; 114:753.
37. Belott PH: A variation on the introducer technique for unlimited access to the subclavian vein. *Pacing Clin Electrophysiol* 1981; 4:43.
38. Spotnitz HM: Transvenous pacing in infants and children with congenital heart disease. *Ann Thorac Surg* 1990; 49:495.
39. Barin ES, Jones SM, Ward DE, et al: The right ventricular outflow tract as an alternative permanent pacing site: long-term follow-up. *Pacing Clin Electrophysiol* 1991; 14:3.
40. Kiviniemi MS, Pirnes MA, Eranen HJ, et al: Complications related to permanent pacemaker therapy. *Pacing Clin Electrophysiol* 1999; 22:711.
41. Goldstein DJ, Losquadro W, Spotnitz HM: Outpatient pacemaker procedures in orally anticoagulated patients. *Pacing Clin Electrophysiol* 1998; 21:1730.
42. Gessman LJ, Vielbig RE, Waspe LE, et al: Accuracy and clinical utility of transtelephonic pacemaker follow-up. *Pacing Clin Electrophysiol* 1995; 18:1032.
43. Brewster GM, Evans AL: Displacement of pacemaker leads—a 10-year survey. *Br Heart J* 1979; 42:266.
44. Aggarwal RK, Connelly DT, Ray SG, et al: Early complications of permanent pacemaker implantation: no difference between dual and single chamber systems. *Br Heart J* 1995; 73:571.
45. Link MS, Estes NA 3rd, Griffin JJ, et al: Complications of dual chamber pacemaker implantation in the elderly. Pacemaker Selection in the Elderly (PASE) Investigators. *J Interv Card Electrophysiol* 1998; 2:175.
46. Janosik DL, Ellenbogen KA: Basic physiology of cardiac pacing and pacemaker syndrome, in Ellenbogen KA, Kay GN, Wilkoff BL (eds): *Clinical Cardiac Pacing and Defibrillation*, 2nd ed. Philadelphia, WB Saunders, 2000; p 333.
47. Smith HJ, Fearnot NE, Byrd CL, et al: Five-year experience with intravascular lead extraction. U.S. Lead Extraction Database. *Pacing Clin Electrophysiol* 1994; 17:2016.
48. Margey R, McCann H, Blake G, et al: Contemporary management of and outcomes from cardiac device related infections. *Europace* 2009 Nov 11. [Epub ahead of print].
49. Molina JE: Undertreatment and overtreatment of patients with infected antiarrhythmic implantable devices. *Ann Thorac Surg* 1997; 63:504.
50. Furman S, Benedek ZM, Andrews CA, et al: Long-term follow-up of pacemaker lead systems: establishment of standards of quality. *Pacing Clin Electrophysiol* 1995; 18:271.
51. Mond H, Stokes KB: The electrode-tissue interface: the revolutionary role of steroid elution. *Pacing Clin Electrophysiol* 1992; 15:95.
52. Rusanov A, Spotnitz HM: Salvage of a failing bifurcated bipolar epicardial lead with conductor fracture. *Ann Thorac Surg* 2010; 90:649.
53. Daoud EG, Kou W, Davidson T, et al: Evaluation and extraction of the Accufix atrial J lead. *Am Heart J* 1996; 131:266.

54. Epstein LM, Byrd CL, Wilkoff BL, et al: Initial experience with larger laser sheaths for the removal of transvenous pacemaker and implantable defibrillator leads. *Circulation* 1999; 100:516.
55. Rusanov A, Spotnitz HM: A 15-year experience with permanent pacemaker and defibrillator lead and patch extractions. *Ann Thorac Surg* 2010; 89:44.
56. Madigan JD, Choudhri AF, Chen J, et al: Surgical management of the patient with an implanted cardiac device: implications of electromagnetic interference. *Ann Surg* 1999; 230:639.
57. Bourke ME: The patient with a pacemaker or related device. *Can J Anaesth* 1996; 43(5 Pt 2):R24.
58. Lloyd MA, Hayes DL: Pacemaker and implantable cardioverter-defibrillator radiography, in Ellenbogen KA, Kay GN, Wilkoff BL (eds): *Clinical Cardiac Pacing and Defibrillation*, 2nd ed. Philadelphia, WB Saunders, 2000; p 710.
59. Raghavan C, Maloney JD, Nitta J, et al: Long-term follow-up of heart transplant recipients requiring permanent pacemakers. *J Heart Lung Transplant* 1995; 14:1081.
60. Spotnitz HM, Ott GY, Bigger JT Jr, et al: Methods of implantable cardioverter-defibrillator-pacemaker insertion to avoid interactions. *Ann Thorac Surg* 1992; 53:253.
61. Zareba W, Moss AJ: Long QT syndrome in children. *J Electrocardiol* 2001; 34(Suppl):167.
62. Reuter S, Garrigue S, Bordachar P, et al: Intermediate-term results of biventricular pacing in heart failure: correlation between clinical and hemodynamic data. *Pacing Clin Electrophysiol* 2000; 23:1713.
63. Cleland JG, Daubert JC, Erdmann E, et al: The effect of cardiac resynchronization on morbidity and mortality in heart failure. *NEJM* 2005; 352:1539.
64. Doll N, Opfermann UT, Rastan AJ, et al: Facilitated minimally invasive left ventricular epicardial lead placement. *Ann Thorac Surg* 2005; 79:1023.
65. DeRose JJ, Ashton RC, Belsley S, et al. Robotically assisted left ventricular epicardial lead implantation for biventricular pacing. *JACC* 2003; 41:1414
66. Wang DY, Richmond ME, Quinn TA, et al. Optimized temporary biventricular pacing acutely improves intraoperative cardiac output after weaning from cardiopulmonary bypass (abstract) *Circulation* 2009; 120: S800.
67. Spotnitz HM. Optimizing temporary perioperative cardiac pacing (editorial). *J Thorac Cardiovasc Surg* 2005;129:5.
68. Lauck G, von Smekal A, Wolke S, et al: Effects of nuclear magnetic resonance imaging on cardiac pacemakers. *Pacing Clin Electrophysiol* 1995; 18:1549.
69. Calcagnini G, Censi F, Floris M, et al: Evaluation of electromagnetic interference of GSM mobile phones with pacemakers featuring remote monitoring functions. *Pacing Clin Electrophysiol* 2006; 29:380.
70. Brown KR, Carter W Jr, Lombardi GE: Blunt trauma-induced pacemaker failure. *Ann Emerg Med* 1991; 20:905.
71. Manganello TD: Disabling the pacemaker: the heart-rending decision every competent patient has a right to make. *Health Care Law Mon* 2000 Jan; 3.
72. Weaver WE, Cobb LA, Hallstrom AP, et al: Factors influencing survival after out-of-hospital cardiac arrest. *J Am Coll Cardiol* 1986; 7:752.
73. Mirowski R, Reid PR, Mower MM, et al: Termination of malignant ventricular arrhythmia with an implantable automatic defibrillator in human beings. *NEJM* 1980; 303:322.
74. Zipes DP, Roberts D: Results of the international study of the implantable pacemaker cardioverter-defibrillator. A comparison of epicardial and endocardial lead systems. *Circulation* 1995; 92:59.
75. Shahian DM, Williamson WA, Svensson LG, et al: Transvenous versus transthoracic cardioverter-defibrillator implantation. *J Thorac Cardiovasc Surg* 1995; 109:1066.
76. Fitzpatrick AP, Lesh MD, Epstein LM, et al: Electrophysiological laboratory, electrophysiologist-implanted, nonthoracotomy-implantable cardioverter/defibrillators. *Circulation* 1994; 89:2503.
77. Kim SG, Roth JA, Fisher JD, et al: Long-term outcomes and modes of death of patients treated with nonthoracotomy implantable defibrillators. *Am J Cardiol* 1995; 75:1229.
78. Moss AJ, Hall WJ, Cannom DS, et al: Improved survival with an implanted defibrillator in patients with coronary disease at high risk for ventricular arrhythmia. Multicenter Automatic Defibrillator Implantation Trial Investigators. *NEJM* 1996; 335:1933.
79. The Antiarrhythmics Versus Implantable Defibrillators (AVID) Investigators: A comparison of antiarrhythmic drug therapy with implantable defibrillators in patients resuscitated from near-fatal ventricular arrhythmias. *NEJM* 1997; 337:1576.
80. Causes of death in the Antiarrhythmics Versus Implantable Defibrillators (AVID) Trial. *J Am Coll Cardiol* 1999; 34:1552.
81. Hohnloser SH: Implantable devices versus antiarrhythmic drug therapy in recurrent ventricular tachycardia and ventricular fibrillation. *Am J Cardiol* 1999; 84:56R.
82. Moss AJ, Zareba W, Hall WJ, et al: Prophylactic implantation of a defibrillator in patients with myocardial infarction and reduced ejection fraction. *NEJM* 2002; 346:877.
83. Prystowsky EN, Nisam S: Prophylactic implantable cardioverter defibrillator trials: MUSTT, MADIT, and beyond. Multicenter Unsustained Tachycardia Trial. Multicenter Automatic Defibrillator Implantation Trial. *Am J Cardiol* 2000; 86:1214.
84. Buxton AE, Lee KL, Fischer JD, et al: A randomized study of the prevention of sudden death in patients with coronary artery disease. *NEJM* 1999; 341:1882.
85. Capucci A, Aschieri D, Villani GQ: The role of EP-guided therapy in ventricular arrhythmias: beta-blockers, sotalol, and ICDs. *J Interv Card Electrophysiol* 2000; 4(Suppl 1):57.
86. Bristow MR, Saxon LA, Boehmer J, et al: Cardiac-resynchronization therapy with or without an implantable defibrillator in advanced chronic heart failure. *NEJM* 2004; 350:2140.
87. Bardy GH, Lee KL, Mark DB, et al for the Sudden Cardiac Death in Heart Failure Trial (SCD-HeFT) Investigators: Amiodarone or an implantable cardioverter-defibrillator for congestive heart failure. *NEJM* 2005; 352:225.
88. Kadish A: Prophylactic defibrillator implantation: toward an evidence-based approach. *NEJM* 2005; 352:285.
89. Richter S, Duray G, Grönefeld G, et al: Prevention of sudden cardiac death: lessons from recent controlled trials. *Circ J* 2005; 69:625.
90. Bigger JT for the Coronary Artery Bypass Graft (CABG) Patch Trial Investigators: Prophylactic use of implanted cardiac defibrillators in patients at high risk for ventricular arrhythmias after coronary-artery bypass graft surgery. *NEJM* 1997; 337:1569.
91. Hohnloser SH, Kuck KH, Dorian P, et al: Randomized trial of prophylactic implantable cardioverter defibrillator after acute myocardial infarction. *NEJM* 2004; 351:2481.
92. McClellan MB, Tunis SR: Medicare coverage of ICDs. *NEJM* 2005; 352: 222.
93. Block M, Breithardt G: Optimizing defibrillation through improved waveforms. *Pacing Clin Electrophysiol* 1995; 18:526.
94. Libero L, Lozano IF, Bocchiardo M, et al: Comparison of defibrillation thresholds using monodirectional electrical vector versus bidirectional electrical vector. *Ital Heart J* 2001; 2:449.
95. Horton RP, Canby RC, Roman CA, et al: Diagnosis of ICD lead failure using continuous event marker recording. *Pacing Clin Electrophysiol* 1995; 18:1331.
96. Luceri RM: Initial clinical experience with a dual chamber rate responsive implantable cardioverter defibrillator. *Pacing Clin Electrophysiol* 2000; 23:1986.
97. The Cardiac Arrhythmia Suppression Trial (CAST) Investigators: Preliminary report: effect of encainide and flecainide on mortality in a randomized trial of arrhythmia suppression after myocardial infarction. *NEJM* 1989; 321:406.
98. Myerburg RJ, Reddy V, Castellanos A: Indications for implantable cardioverter-defibrillators based on evidence and judgment. *J Am Coll Cardiol* 2009; 54:747.
99. Epstein AE: Update on primary prevention implantable cardioverter-defibrillator therapy. *Curr Cardiol Rep* 2009;11:335.
100. Winkle RA, Mead RH, Ruder MA, et al: Long-term outcome with the automatic cardioverter-defibrillator. *J Am Coll Cardiol* 1989; 13:1353.
101. Spotnitz HM: Surgical approaches to ICD insertion, in Spotnitz HM (ed): *Research Frontiers in Implantable Defibrillator Surgery*. Austin, TX, RG Landes, 1992; p 23.
102. Watkins L Jr, Taylor E Jr: Surgical aspects of automatic implantable cardioverter-defibrillator implantation. *Pacing Clin Electrophysiol* 1991; 14:953.
103. Auteri JS, Jeevanandam V, Bielefeld MR, et al: Effects of location of AICD patch electrodes on the left ventricular diastolic pressure-volume curve in pigs. *Ann Thorac Surg* 1991; 52:1052.
104. Barrington WW, Deligonul U, Easley AR, et al: Defibrillator patch electrode constriction: an underrecognized entity. *Ann Thorac Surg* 1995; 60:1112.
105. Park WM, Amirhamzeh MMR, Bielefeld MR, et al: Systolic arterial pressure recovery after ventricular fibrillation/flutter in humans. *Pacing Clin Electrophysiol* 1994; 17:1100.
106. Hauser RG, Kurschinski DT, McVeigh K, et al: Clinical results with nonthoracotomy ICD systems. *Pacing Clin Electrophysiol* 1993; 16:141
107. Mattke S, Muller D, Markewitz A, et al: Failures of epicardial and transvenous leads for implantable cardioverter defibrillators. *Am Heart J* 1995; 130:1040.

108. Roelke M, O'Nunain, Osswald S, et al: Subclavian crush syndrome complicating transvenous cardioverter defibrillator systems. *Pacing Clin Electrophysiol* 1995; 18:973.
109. Argenziano M, Spotnitz HM, Goldstein DJ, et al: Longevity of lead systems in patients with implantable cardioverter-defibrillators. *Circulation* 1995; 102:II-397.
110. Dean DA, Livelli FL Jr, Bigger JT Jr, et al: Safe repair of insulation defects in ICD leads (abstract). *Pacing Clin Electrophysiol* 1996; 19:678.
111. Jeevanandam V, Bielefeld MR, Auteri JS, et al: The implantable defibrillator: an electronic bridge to cardiac transplantation. *Circulation* 1992; 86:II-276.
112. May CD, Smith PR, Murdock CL, et al: The impact of implantable cardioverter defibrillator on quality-of-life. *Pacing Clin Electrophysiol* 1995; 18:1411.
113. Ahmad M, Bloomstein L, Roelke M, et al: Patients' attitudes toward implanted defibrillator shocks. *Pacing Clin Electrophysiol* 2000; 23:934.
114. Kohn CS, Petrucci RJ, Baessler C, et al: The effect of psychological intervention on patients' long-term adjustment to the ICD: a prospective study. *Pacing Clin Electrophysiol* 2000; 23:450.
115. Vijgen J, Botto G, Camm J, et al: Consensus statement of the European Heart Rhythm Association: updated recommendations for driving by patients with implantable cardioverter defibrillators. *Europace* 2009; 11:1097.
116. Akiyama T, Powell JL, Mitchell LB, et al: Resumption of driving after life-threatening ventricular tachyarrhythmia. *NEJM* 2001; 345:391.
117. Hoffmaster B: Chapter 4. The ethics of setting limits on ICD therapy. *Can J Cardiol* 2000; 16:1313.
118. Sanders GD, Hlatky MA, Owens DK: Cost-effectiveness of implantable cardioverterdefibrillators. *NEJM* 2005; 353:1471.

PART 7

OTHER CARDIAC OPERATIONS

CHAPTER 60

Surgery for Adult Congenital Heart Disease

Redmond P. Burke

INTRODUCTION

Improved outcomes for pediatric patients with congenital heart disease have created a growing population of surviving adults, with increasingly complex treatment requirements for their adult congenital heart disease (ACHD). Over the past two decades, the spectrum of complexity for ACHD patients has evolved from late primary repairs of patients with simple lesions including coarctation, patent ductus, septal defects, and tetralogy of Fallot, to *n*th time reoperations on survivors of complex multistaged palliations of one- and two-ventricle hearts. Internationally, significant efforts to define the optimal program resources necessary to effectively treat ACHD patients have been made, yet many congenital heart patients continue to suffer from poor continuity of care as they enter adulthood.[1] This chapter describes several current treatment strategies and results for adult patients undergoing congenital heart surgery.

REDUCING CUMULATIVE THERAPEUTIC TRAUMA

The optimal venue for ACHD treatment is unknown, and it is fair to say that no two programs are the same. The need for a coordinated and comprehensive programmatic strategy has been well described, and should encompass not only the lifetime of a generation of patients with congenital heart defects from fetal to adult life, but also the health of pregnant mothers with congenital heart disease who will give birth to a new generation.[2] Our congenital heart program philosophy is to reduce the cumulative trauma of care for each patient with congenital heart disease over his or her lifetime. To achieve this, we discuss each adult patient referred to our program for surgery or intervention in a combined conference with participation from adult and pediatric interventional cardiologists and surgeons, dedicated cardiac intensivists, cardiac anesthesiologists, cardiac imaging specialists, and the cardiac nursing, pharmacy, and social work teams. Treatment options are selected so that the least traumatic form of therapy, with a reasonable chance of success, is chosen as the initial approach. Failure to achieve a good result leads to an escalation to the next least traumatic therapeutic option. As an example, a patient with secundum ASD would be put forward for device closure, and if this failed, the patient would then be given the option of a minimally invasive partial sternotomy. If this approach was not felt to be safe, the approach would be escalated to a full sternotomy repair.

INFORMATION SYSTEMS

ACHD patients with complex lesions often have complex medical histories, stored in multimedia formats, which expose the weaknesses of chart-based medical record systems. Use of an electronic medical record (EMR) by medical teams, and personal health record (PHR) by patients and families, may improve outcomes in patients with chronic disease.[3] Patients and their families often have not been educated about their heart defect and what to expect over time. The PHR could be used to enhance patients' understanding of their disease and treatment. These information systems may also facilitate development of national and international registries designed to measure clinical outcomes and performance of centers treating adult congenital heart patients.[4]

Our program goal is to empower patients by providing them with on-demand access to patient data using a Web-based medical information system developed by the congenital heart team. This system allows providers to retrieve laboratory data, operative and interventional catheterization reports, operative images, and daily progress notes, and discharge summaries from each of the patient's hospitalizations. The records can be accessed anywhere, any time, with any Web-enabled device. Patients and their families have password access to the encrypted system, which automatically prompts patients when they become adults

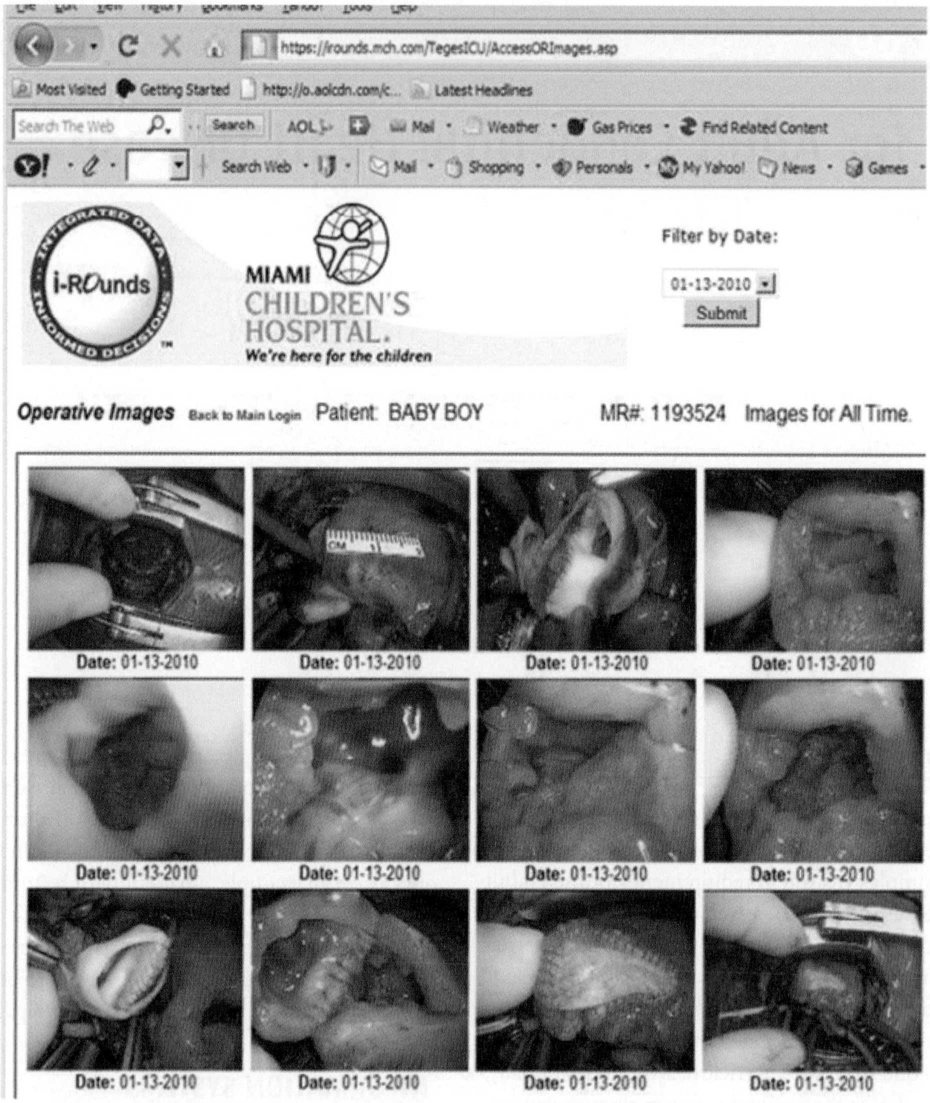

FIGURE 60-1 This is a screen capture from a Web-based EMR, with intraoperative images from a neonatal truncus arteriosus repair. These images will be available on demand for the cardiac team to review at the time of future interventions and reoperations.

to take control of their electronic medical record with a password change.

We capture intraoperative images of each cardiac lesion, before and after repair,[5] and incorporate these images into our EMR. These images are then reviewed with the operative notes before reoperation to regain familiarity with the patient's anatomy.[6] The operative images used in this chapter were retrieved from this system, which can be searched by procedure, diagnosis, or individual patient (Fig. 60-1).

COMMON ADULT CONGENITAL HEART DISEASE PROCEDURES

Reoperative Sternotomy

Congenital heart procedures in adults are frequently reoperations, however, protocols for reoperations in acquired heart surgery do not mesh completely with the challenges presented by ACHD patients. Risk factors for traumatic repeat sternotomy in ACHD patients differ from those identified in patients with acquired heart disease, which often focus on patent coronary bypass grafts.[7] Femoral cannulation is often complicated in congenital heart patients who have undergone multiple interventional catheterizations during their growth years, resulting in stenotic or occluded femoral vessels. We use a selective cannulation strategy and only routinely cannulate patients with significant risk factors. Other risk factors for sternal reentry injury in ACHD include retrosternal conduits, particularly oversized and calcified homografts. We specifically look for evidence of conduit fusion to the sternum, which should be suspected when the conduit does not move with the cardiac cycle on lateral angiograms. Patients with pulmonary hypertension, right ventricular enlargement, prior sternal infections, aneurysms of the right or left ventricular outflow tracts, and pectus excavatum deformity are at increased risk, and qualify for preliminary vascular access dissection and pursestring placement. Patients with multiple risk factors may be placed on bypass to decompress the right ventricle prior to commencing sternal division.

We excise previous sternotomy scars and remove sternal wires. The xiphoid process is removed, and cautery dissection is begun at the inferior sternal edge. The oscillating saw is used to divide the anterior sternal table. Rakes are used to elevate the two sides of the sternum and expose the retrosternal scar. Short segments of retrosternal scar are released, followed by oscillating saw division of the sternal bone, and this proceeds superiorly until the entire sternum is divided.

In the event of cardiac or great vessel penetration during sternotomy, when we have not electively exposed vessels for cannulation, we release the sternal retractors, and immediately extend the neck dissection up and to the right to expose the innominate artery and the internal jugular or high innominate vein. These vessels are cannulated through pursestrings, and bypass is initiated.

Reoperative Sternotomy Technique with Emergency Bypass via Neck and Inferior Vena Cava Dissection

In patients in whom venous access cannot be achieved in the suprasternal area, we dissect the inferior vena cava just above the diaphragm. This approach has been described as *simplified aortic cannulation.*[8] The sternotomy is then completed with the patient in Trendelenburg. We continuously infuse carbon dioxide into the operative field during every operation to reduce the risk of air embolism, although the evidence that this reduces stroke rates is not conclusive.[9]

To reduce adhesion formation, and decrease the risk of future sternotomy, we prevent cardiac desiccation by covering the heart with saline-soaked gauze. At the completion of ACHD repairs, we place antiadhesion materials to decrease retrosternal adhesions. Expanded polytetrafluoroethylene (PTFE) is commonly used in some centers;[10] however, capsule formation often obscures natural tissue planes, making subsequent reoperative dissection more difficult. Bioresorbable film prototypes made of polyethylene glycol and polylactic acid have been developed and tested for cardiac operations. These bioresorbable films significantly reduce adhesion formation, and their rapid resorption appears to mitigate capsule formation.[11] Sheets of extracellular matrix derived from pig jejunum is now approved for use as a pericardial substitute.[12]

Reducing Incisional Trauma

Multiple incisional approaches have been described to improve the cosmetic result after open heart surgery. These include partial upper and lower sternotomy, transxiphoid, anterior thoracotomy, and submammary incisions. Despite its visibility, median sternotomy may be the least traumatic incision for ACHD patients, allowing the surgeon to avoid vascular trauma from peripheral cannulation, avoid intercostals muscle, vessel and nerve trauma, and thereby eliminate post-thoracotomy pain syndrome. Median sternotomy allows direct aortic control for safe, effective cannulation, decannulation, de-airing, and cardioplegia administration with minimal risk of dissection. Median sternotomy also ensures direct and rapid access to the entire mediastinum, allowing surgeons to deal with unanticipated anatomical variations discovered at surgery, which are not uncommonly found in ACHD patients.

Atrial Septal Defects

The advent of transcatheter device closure for atrial septal defects has significantly changed the average complexity level of ACHD case loads. Patent foramen ovale and most secundum defects are effectively closed with devices, and are rarely referred for surgical closure in programs with effective interventional catheterization teams. Sinus venosus and primum defects, transitional and complete atrioventricular canal, common atrium, and secundum defects with deficient inferior rims are referred for surgery, and we repair these on cardiopulmonary bypass with cardioplegic arrest.

Our venous cannulation strategy for atrial septal defects is bicaval, via the right atrial appendage up the superior vena cava, and down the inferior vena caval junction into the inferior vena cava. Smaller defects, which in the past could be closed primarily, are now rarely referred for surgical closure, and we find that repairs are best performed with patch materials, to create tension-free suture lines and avoid repair breakdowns and recurrences.

For sinus venosus defects, we place a right-angled cannula in the innominate vein, to enable exposure of partial anomalous pulmonary veins entering the superior vena cava.

The approach is through a lateral incision to avoid the sinus node area, and is extended superiorly just far enough to expose the upper pulmonary vein entrance point (Fig. 60-2A). A "no-touch" technique is maintained in the sinus node area. A pericardial patch is used to close the atrial incision to avoid superior vena caval stenosis (Fig. 60-2B).

In patients with primum atrial septal defects, the cleft mitral valve is routinely repaired with running polypropylene suture lines approximating the line of contact between the leaflet segments. Even patients with competent valves are repaired, as late onset of cleft regurgitation is known to occur. Patients at risk for mitral stenosis, particularly those with a single papillary muscle in the left ventricle, may have their clefts left open to avoid valvar stenosis. Results for these repairs are excellent, even in patients at advanced ages.[13]

Ebstein's Anomaly

Surgery for Ebstein's anomaly can be performed in older patients at low risk and with good late outcome. The operation is comprised of tricuspid valve repair or replacement and concomitant procedures such as atrial septal defect closure, arrhythmia surgery (the maze procedure), and coronary artery bypass grafting.[14] Repair techniques for these patients continue to evolve. We believe the presence of an untethered and well-developed anterior tricuspid valve leaflet increases the chance of a successful repair, and have used the Cone technique in adult patients.[15] This repair requires dissection of the anterior and posterior tricuspid valve leaflets from their right ventricular attachments. The free edge of the leaflet is then rotated clockwise and sutured to the septal border of the anterior leaflet.

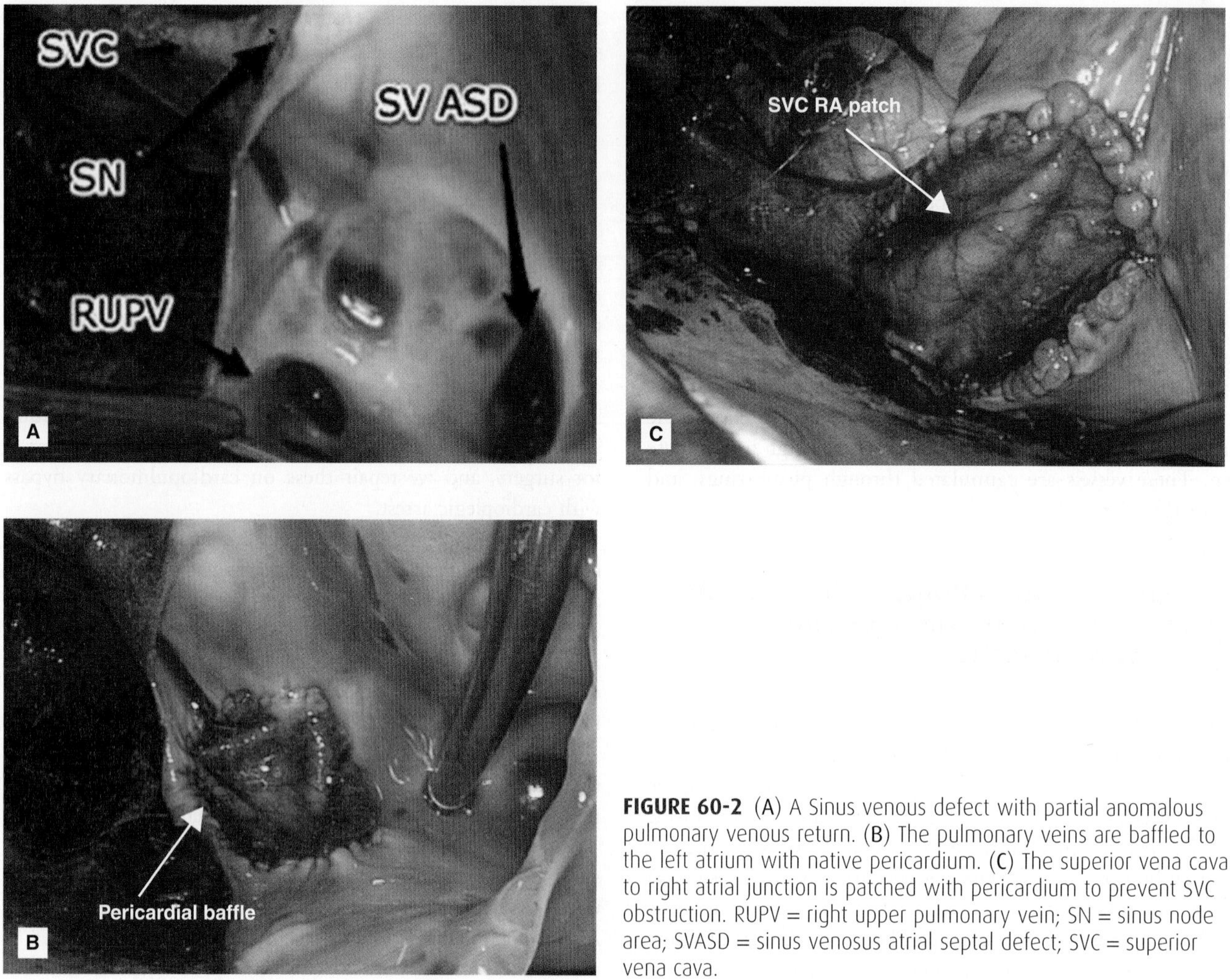

FIGURE 60-2 (A) A Sinus venous defect with partial anomalous pulmonary venous return. (B) The pulmonary veins are baffled to the left atrium with native pericardium. (C) The superior vena cava to right atrial junction is patched with pericardium to prevent SVC obstruction. RUPV = right upper pulmonary vein; SN = sinus node area; SVASD = sinus venosus atrial septal defect; SVC = superior vena cava.

This produces a cone-shaped valve, fixed distally at the right ventricular apex, and proximally at the tricuspid valve annulus. The septal leaflet is incorporated into the cone wall whenever possible, and the atrial septal defect is closed. Results have been good with low mortality, significantly less tricuspid regurgitation, and improvement in functional class.

Fontan Revision

In the modern era, the primary cause of death for adult patients with cyanotic lesions is arrhythmia followed by heart failure.[16] Fontan patients may present with arrhythmia and complications related to systemic ventricular failure, protein-losing enteropathy (PLE), systemic venous pathway obstruction, and semilunar and atrioventricular valve dysfunction. Initial evaluations must focus on ensuring a completely unobstructed vascular pathway to the lungs. The different types of surgical techniques historically used to create the Fontan circulation each have characteristic complications. Patients with intracardiac baffles and atriopulmonary connections may present with extreme right atrial enlargement, resulting in stagnant flow, right pulmonary vein compression, and arrhythmia.

Fontan conversion involves takedown of the previously created venous connection, and creation of an extracardiac cavopulmonary connection with a conduit. Because the extracardiac Fontan excludes the systemic veins from the heart, any catheterization procedures requiring atrial level intervention, particularly electrophysiology interventions, must be planned before conversion. Therefore, we plan Fontan conversions with our electrophysiology team, and frequently combine Fontan conversions with arrhythmia surgery,[17] and treatment of atrioventricular valve dysfunction. Valve repairs are often complex in these patients, and replacements are often required to achieve good hemodynamic results.[18] Results depend on the patients' underlying anatomy, right ventricular function, and pulmonary vascular resistance.

We perform extracardiac Fontan procedures with bicaval cannulation, and leave the heart warm and beating whenever possible. The inferior vena cava is transected at the cavo-atrial junction under a clamp and the cardiac end is oversewn with 4-0 polypropylene running suture. We use ring reinforced expanded PTFE grafts from 19 to 23 mm in diameter, and leave enough length to avoid right pulmonary vein compression. The superior anastomosis to the superior vena caval junction with the right pulmonary artery is then constructed with running 6-0 polypropylene suture. Hybrid stenting procedures, in which the interventional cath team comes into the cardiac operating room to deploy stents, are used to treat stenoses in the retroaortic pulmonary arteries if they are stenotic.

In patients with complex cardiac anatomy, these Fontan revision procedures may best be performed with the participation of electrophysiology. This ensures effective interruption or ablation of reentrant pathways, which may not follow the patterns seen in patients with acquired heart disease and normal cardiac anatomic relationships. A variety of Maze type procedures have been described in an effort to disrupt atrial reentrant pathways. The unpredictable anatomy of the conduction tissue in ACHD patients has resulted in frequent need for pacemaker insertion. In many centers, customized pacemaker therapy has been advocated for management of patients after Fontan conversion. However, based on an experience with 120 Fontan conversions from 1994 to 2008, which began with a flexible approach to each patient's anticipated pacing needs, Tsao and coworkers now recommend routine placement of a dual-chamber antitachycardia pacemaker with bipolar steroid-eluting epicardial leads in patients undergoing Fontan revision.[19]

Right Ventricular Outflow Tract Reconstruction

Right ventricular outflow tract reconstruction after previous repair of tetralogy of Fallot, double outlet right ventricle, pulmonary atresia, truncus arteriosus, and arterial switch procedures are increasingly common, as patients who underwent successful neonatal and infant repairs are returning with pulmonary insufficiency and/or stenosis, resulting in right ventricular dysfunction, exercise intolerance, arrhythmias, and sudden death.[20] The first percutaneous pulmonary valve replacement was performed by Bonhoeffer in 2000,[21] and this therapy is increasingly available as clinical trials have shown safety and efficacy.[22] This less invasive therapy has accelerated the study of ACHD patients with pulmonary insufficiency, who have often been followed for years to avoid the trauma of reoperation. The growing experience with transcatheter pulmonary valve insertion into previously placed RVOT homografts suggests that homograft rupture is a rare known complication, occurring in 3.9% in an early series of implants, with stent fractures being a more common (20%) and benign complication.[23] With surgical standby patients with rupture can be placed on emergent bypass, and undergo surgical repair with good results.[24] Indications for pulmonary valve replacement in ACHD patients are evolving, and optimal indications and timing remain elusive. Preoperative evaluation with echocardiography, magnetic resonance imaging (MRI), and cardiac catheterization are used to identify concomitant lesions, particular patent foramen ovale, coronary anatomy, and right ventricular dimensions and function.

For patients not amenable to transcatheter pulmonary valve implantation, our standard surgical approach includes median sternotomy, bicaval cannulation, and repair on cardiopulmonary bypass with moderate hypothermia. These repairs may be performed without cardioplegic arrest if provocative preoperative testing (bubble test with Valsalva)[25] shows no right to left shunting at the atrial or ventricular levels. Patients with positive bubble studies have aortic cross-clamping and cold blood cardioplegic arrest. We control the branch pulmonary arteries with tourniquets and place a right ventricular vent in the atrium to create a clear operative field. If a previous right ventricular incision or patch is present, this is used as a safe reentry point, and the incision is extended far enough to inspect the right ventricle and allow resection of obstructing intracavitary muscle bundles. Pulmonary valve replacement options include pulmonary homograft, aortic homograft, bovine jugular vein graft, bioprosthetic valve, and mechanical prosthetic valve.

Homografts are selected based on availability and echocardiographic estimates of normal pulmonary valve annulus size for the given patient weight. Leaving the graft too long will produce a kink when the graft is pressurized, with resultant obstruction. We perform the distal pulmonary artery anastomosis with a running 5-0 or 6-0 monofilament polypropylene suture, and then trim the proximal homograft muscle cuff to match the incision in the right ventricle. The proximal anastomosis is constructed with a larger running suture and needle, and care is taken to avoid the left main and anterior descending coronary arteries (Fig. 60-3). Left anterior descending coronary arteries and dual anterior descending vessels are specifically ruled out on preoperative studies, and when present, are left undisturbed by carefully positioning the right ventricular incision. The anterior portion of the outflow tract is completed with a patch of native or bovine pericardium, PTFE, or extracellular matrix patch.

The Bovine jugular vein valve is sized and implanted in a similar way to homografts, with a distal running suture line. The proximal graft is beveled, so that a separate hood patch is not necessary (Fig. 60-4). Midterm results for bovine jugular vein grafts in adult patients are good, but long-term durability is unproved.[26]

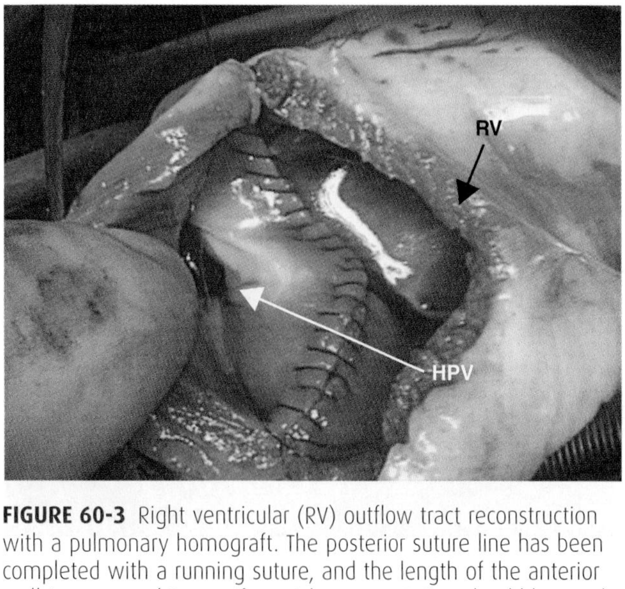

FIGURE 60-3 Right ventricular (RV) outflow tract reconstruction with a pulmonary homograft. The posterior suture line has been completed with a running suture, and the length of the anterior wall is measured to see if a patch augmentation should be used to prevent distortion of the homograft pulmonary valve (HPV) annulus.

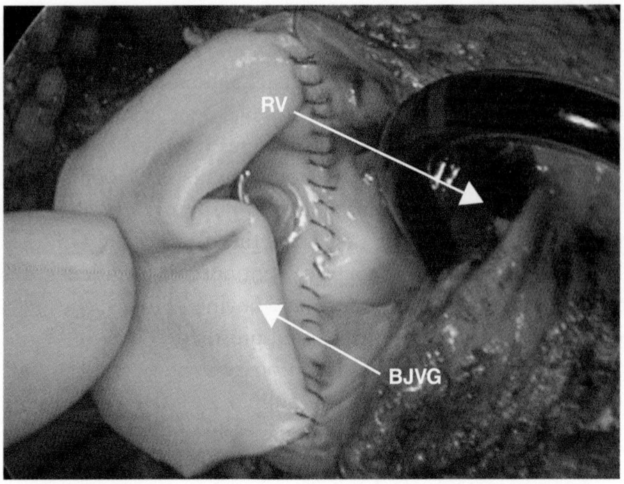

FIGURE 60-4 Right ventricular (RV) outflow tract reconstruction with a bovine jugular vein graft (BJVG). The posterior graft length must be short enough to prevent kinking. These grafts can be trimmed to cover larger defects in the anterior right ventricular free wall, so that additional patches are rarely needed.

Bioprosthetic and mechanical valves are positioned in the right ventricular outflow tract at the normal pulmonary valve annulus in patients with normal right ventricular anatomy, or in a position that avoids sternal compression. (More distal implantation is often necessary after repair of truncus arteriosus and pulmonary atresia.) We have used both an interrupted pledgeted horizontal mattress suture technique, and a running polypropylene suture technique for these implants (Fig. 60-5). Both techniques require that the valve suture line be constructed so that the valve orients correctly toward the main pulmonary artery bifurcation, fighting the tendency for the valve to aim up at the sternum. A patch is used to close the distal main pulmonary artery up to the level of the valve, valve sutures are passed through the patch, and the patch is then completed over the proximal right ventricular outflow tract incision.

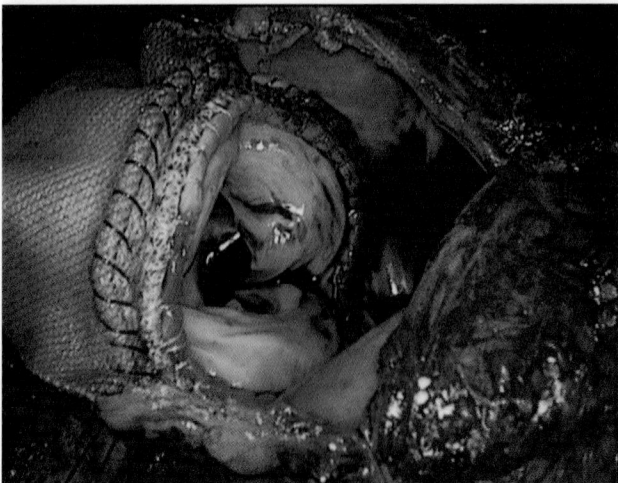

FIGURE 60-5 Right ventricular (RV) outflow tract reconstruction with a bioprosthetic valve (BV). A running suture technique was used on the posterior wall and a Dacron patch was used to augment the anterior wall of the right ventricular outflow tract.

Advantages and disadvantages exist for each pulmonary valve replacement option.[27] Homografts and bovine jugular veins have length and can be used to span long gaps between the right ventricle and the branch pulmonary arteries. The distal anastomosis can be configured to repair stenotic sections of the main pulmonary artery and the proximal branches. They also form suitable conduits for subsequent insertion of transcatheter pulmonary valves in the future if they become stenotic or insufficient. We try to tailor our conduit decisions to meet the implantation requirements for transcatheter pulmonary valve insertion. These evolving requirements are factored into our decision process in selecting a conduit during our current surgical pulmonary valve replacements. Currently available bioprosthetic valves are also suitable for subsequent insertion of a transcatheter valve, as the valve ring provides a stable landing zone for the transcatheter valve stent. Mechanical valves do not allow subsequent placement of a transcatheter pulmonary valve, and we have reduced our use of these in the pulmonary position. Right ventricular outflow tract reconstruction continuity between the right ventricle and the pulmonary arteries can now safely be performed with low morbidity and mortality, and conduit options continue to expand.[28]

Left Ventricular Outflow Tract Reconstruction

Isolated areas of left ventricular outflow tract obstruction are less common in ACHD patients than in those with acquired left-sided lesions. ACHD patients with left ventricular outflow tract obstruction should be evaluated for upstream and downstream stenoses, as multiple levels of obstruction are common. Patients with Shone's syndrome often undergo numerous surgical and interventional palliations over their lifetimes, and these patients are symbolic of the nature of complex left ventricular outflow tract disease, whereas our interventions should usually be classified as palliative. Adult congenital teams should be prepared to perform primary Ross, Ross-Konno, and Konno procedures, and deal with reoperations for each of these palliations.

The Ross operation is often used in pediatric patients with complex left ventricular outflow tract obstruction to treat combined valvar and supravalvar lesions, avoid anticoagulation, and maintain some growth potential. These patients may require reoperations as adults to replace failing neo aortic valves, and stenotic or regurgitant pulmonary valves. Follow-up of right ventricular reconstructions after Ross operations suggests that 4% of patients will require conduit replacement for right ventricular (RV) dysfunction at 10 years. Conduit size less than 14 mm is an independent predictor of allograft dysfunction.[29] Freedom from reoperation for regurgitation of the pulmonary autograft in the aortic position are quite variable, with reports from 87%[30] to 96%.[31] The advent of percutaneous aortic and pulmonary valve options may increase the use of the Ross operation, because reintervention on the autograft and allograft may not require reoperation. Aneurysmal dilation of the neo aortic root after the Ross operation is related to use of the root technique, and may be seen in up to 11% of patients at 7 years after surgery. Good outcomes after reoperation can be achieved, but successful repair of the autograft is more likely if the diagnosis is made early, before the neo-aortic valve becomes insufficient.[32]

The Konno aortic ventriculoplasty is used to treat complex left ventricular outflow tract obstruction in patients with supravalvar, valvar, and subvalvar obstruction, and may be encountered in adults who require initial treatment, or reoperations for valve malfunction or outgrown valves. The Ross-Konno, using the transplanted pulmonary autograft with a graft or infundibular extension, has been shown to increase in size as patients grow, making this an excellent option in pediatric patients. In a review of 53 patients operated from 1980 to 2004, with an average age of 19, Suri and coworkers reported risk factors for overall mortality included New York Heart Association class (hazard ratio 2.22, $p = .04$) and longer bypass time (hazard ratio 1.93/hour, $p = .04$). The cumulative probability of aortic valve reoperation was 19% at 5 years and 39% at 10 years, occurring in 15 patients at a median of 3.8 years. Pulmonary regurgitation was detected in six patients. Pulmonary valve replacement was performed in three (6%).[33]

Reoperations after Ross, Ross-Konno, and Konno procedures may be particularly challenging. This is especially true if the right ventricular outflow tract has been reconstructed with a large patch covering the anterior wall of the ascending aorta. Exposure of the aortic root then necessitates reentry into the right ventricle, which is best managed with bicaval cannulation, allowing isolation of the right ventricle and a blood-free operative field. Given the high incidence of reoperations on these patients, antiadhesion barriers are worthy of consideration at the time of closure.

Arrhythmia Surgery

Maintaining a functional conduction system is a crucial aspect of reducing the cumulative lifetime trauma for a patient with congenital heart disease. Despite best efforts to prevent injury to the conduction tissues, ACHD patients are at risk for a wide array of conduction delays, as well as atrial and ventricular tachyarrhythmias. Pacemaker and defibrillator insertion, lead extractions, and generator changes are frequently complicated in ACHD patients by unusual anatomic pathways and stenotic veins. Epicardial lead placements are often necessary in single ventricle patients who have limited or no venous access to the endocardium. Common indications for lead removal include pocket infection, malfunctioning leads, skin erosion, endocarditis/septicemia, vena cava thrombosis, and painful leads. Lead extraction technology is evolving, and can be safely managed as a hybrid effort with a surgeon and electrophysiologist working together. A number of lead removal catheters are available using blades or laser energy to excise embedded leads. Surgical support is necessary in the event of cardiac perforation. Outcomes are generally good, with sepsis being the strongest predictor of death after pacemaker device removal.[34]

Supraventricular and ventricular arrhythmias are a major cause of morbidity and mortality in adult patients with congenital heart disease. For patients with atrial fibrillation or flutter undergoing open heart repairs, a right-sided Maze procedure can be performed, with the expectation of 93% freedom from arrhythmia and improvement in functional class.[35]

Minimally invasive approaches to arrhythmia surgery, such as the mini-Maze procedure, are increasingly popular in patients with acquired heart disease and arrhythmia.[36] These approaches may be difficult to accomplish in certain ACHD patients because of unusual anatomical relationships, and extensive reoperative scarring, which may limit exposure through small incisions. The Cox-Maze procedure for supraventricular arrhythmias in ACHD patients is often complex, and an alternative approach using intraoperative monopolar irrigated radiofrequency ablation (IRA) has been described with good results for patients undergoing elective cardiac surgery.[37]

Unified Approach for Hybrid Procedures

We define hybrid procedures as those using combined surgical and interventional personnel and technology during a single operation. Hybrid procedures can be performed in the catheterization laboratory, the operating room (with C-arm angiography), or ideally in a hybrid procedure suite. We select the venue based on which technology (interventional or surgical) is most important for a given procedure. The advent of percutaneous cardiac valve replacement and endovascular stenting highlights the need to embrace this unified team approach for adult congenital heart patients. In patients requiring interventional, surgical, and electrophysiologic procedures, we attempt to integrate the procedures into a single hybrid operation, with the surgical team providing the least traumatic form of vascular access. Surgeons can also provide central vascular and direct cardiac access for sheath placement in patients with stenotic or occluded peripheral vessels. We routinely place aortic and pulmonary artery stents in the operating room using direct vision, video assisted cardioscopy, and angiography (Fig. 60-6). Elective or emergent cardiopulmonary bypass support should be available on demand

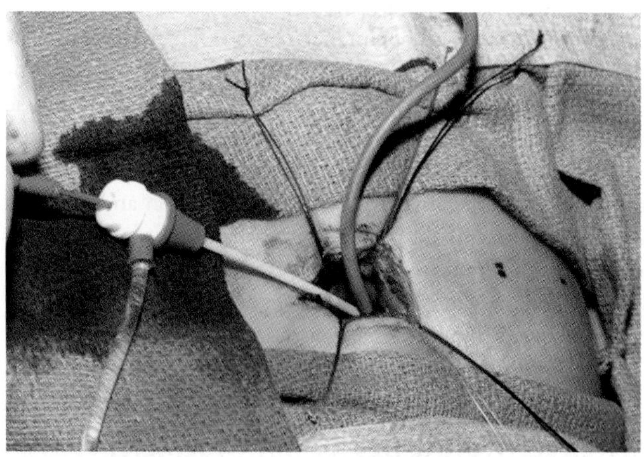

FIGURE 60-6 Operative image of a hybrid procedure, with surgical exposure of the right ventricle through a subxiphoid incision (SI), and placement of a transcardiac sheath (TS), followed by interventional catheterization.

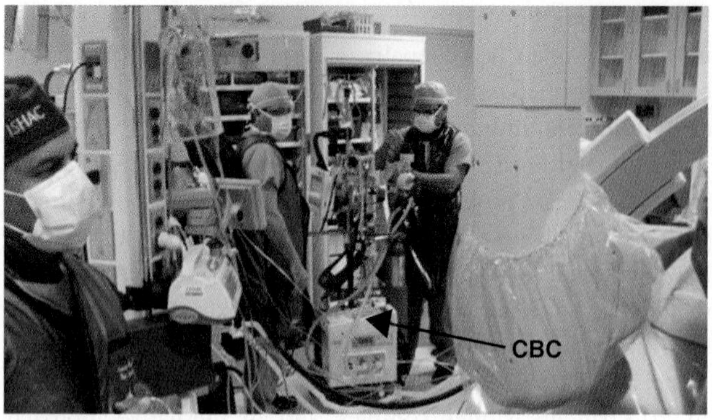

FIGURE 60-7 A cardiopulmonary bypass circuit (CBC) on standby in the hybrid catheterization laboratory, enabling rapid setup and support with transport capability.

in the hybrid operating room or catheterization laboratory (Fig. 60-7).

Real-time consultation between surgeons and interventionists may enhance outcomes for vascular stent implants, because stent placements can be planned to minimize subsequent operative trauma. With a surgeon's input at the time of implantation, pulmonary artery stents may be positioned more proximally to avoid tearing into the branch pulmonary arteries at reoperation when the stent is outgrown. Similarly, aortic arch stents can be positioned more proximally to minimize the distance down the arch the surgeon must dissect if reoperation is required to open a stent that cannot reach adult size.

Coarctation of the Aorta

Primary and recurrent coarctation of the aorta in adult patients is increasingly managed percutaneously with balloon dilation and stents.[38] We provide surgical backup for these procedures in the event of device migration, dissection, and rupture, and occasionally to establish vascular access. When transcatheter therapy is not feasible, we proceed with surgical repair of adults with coarctation and aortic arch obstruction. These operations are performed through a left thoracotomy in patients with a left aortic arch, and the perfusion team is on standby for left atrial appendage to descending aortic cardiopulmonary bypass. Three general techniques can be used, including coarctation resection with end-to-end anastomosis, onlay patch enlargement with tissue or prosthetic patch, and synthetic tube interposition. Aortic mobility is limited in adult patients, and tension-free repairs may require interposition grafts. Postoperative hypertension is common and responds to sodium nitroprusside. We use subcutaneous local anesthetic infusion catheters to control postoperative pain, and anticipate labile blood pressure responses in patients with longstanding hypertension. Mortality is rare, and at follow-up, 75% of patients will be normotensive without medication.[39]

INTERVENTIONAL DEVICE MANAGEMENT

Cardiac surgeons increasingly encounter intravascular devices in the aorta and pulmonary arteries, as well as atrial[40] and ventricular septal occlusion devices, during operations on ACHD patients. Vascular stents are being effectively used in neonates and infants, with the understanding that patients will outgrow the maximum size these stents can achieve.[41] We have a growing experience with reoperations on patients who have outgrown stents in the aortic arch and the branch pulmonary arteries. At reoperation early after stent implantation, within 6 months or less, it may be possible to completely remove the stent by chipping away with scissors, collapsing the stent into itself, and peeling it away from the vessel wall. After 6 months, vascular ingrowth has usually incorporated the stent into the vessel wall, making complete removal difficult and traumatic. When patients undergo reoperations to enlarge stents that have reached their maximum size, operative planning requires consideration of the optimal location of the longitudinal incision made to open the stent, anticipating that the stent will then have to be split and spread like a hot dog bun to create space for an onlay patch. This requires that every link be cut, particularly at the distal end, and that there will then be some extension of the distal vascular cut beyond the end of the stent (Fig. 60-8).

This distal extension of the incision must be planned to avoid spiral tears into smaller branch vessels, which may result in branch occlusion. Onlay patches may be constructed with native or bovine pericardium, polytetrafluoroethylene grafts, pulmonary or aortic homografts, or extracellular matrix grafts. If the final vessel reconstruction does not achieve a full adult-sized vessel lumen, or is compressed by adjacent structures, the patched split stent is a safe landing zone for subsequent placement of an adult-sized stent. We have placed these stents immediately as hybrid procedures when the patient's hemodynamic condition demands it, or later, after the patched stent has time to heal, thus reducing the risk of suture line rupture and bleeding.

Atrial septal stents are increasingly used to achieve unrestrictive flow across the atrial septum when surgical septectomy is not performed, is incomplete, or restriction develops after previous surgical septectomy.[42] At late reoperation, these stents are firmly encased in septal tissue, and may extend into the

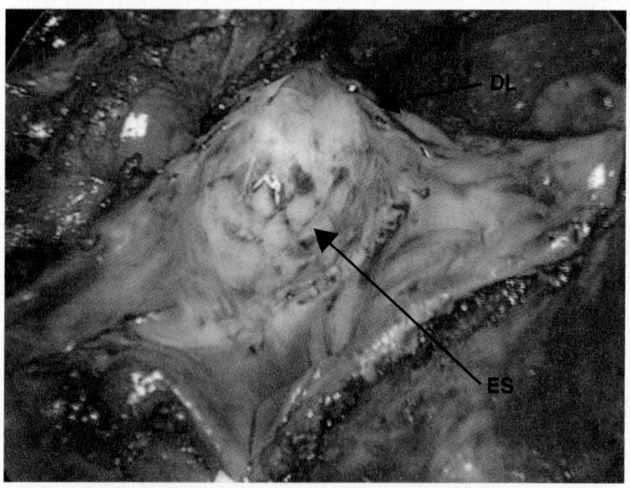

FIGURE 60-8 Operative image of a reoperation on a left pulmonary artery stent, showing the incision through the stent beyond the most distal link (DL). The embedded stent (ES) material was left intact, and the artery was folded open to create space for an anterior patch.

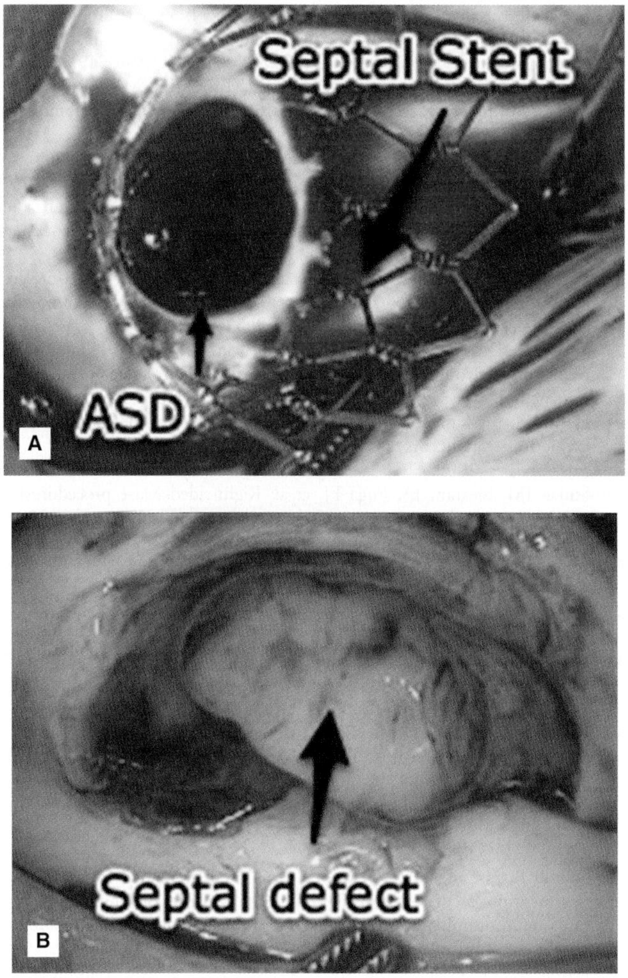

FIGURE 60-9 (A) Operative image of a stent embedded in the atrial septum. (B) Operative image of the septum after stent resection. The atrium must be inspected for full-thickness penetration.

pulmonary vein orifices (Fig. 60-9A). When necessary, these stents can be removed with scissor dissection, trimming the exposed metal, peeling up the embedded sections, and enucleating the ingrown scar tissue (Fig. 60-9B). The atrium is inspected for full thickness tears, which are repaired with polypropylene suture.

IMPROVED OUTCOMES WITH CONGENITAL HEART SURGEON FOR ADULT CONGENITAL SURGERY

In a review of 72 centers performing ACHD surgery, Patel reported 2800 operations performed per year, ranging from 0 to 230 (median 28) per program. There were a median of two surgeons per program, with each surgeon averaging 20 cases per year.[43] Although individual surgeon and program results will vary, patients with ACHD appear to have better outcomes when repaired by surgeons who primarily perform pediatric congenital heart surgery (1.87% mortality), compared with surgeons who primarily operated on acquired adult heart disease (4.84% mortality, $p < .0001$).[44] Patients with congenital heart disease are living longer. Arrhythmia remains the primary contributing cause of death for those with cyanotic lesions. Myocardial infarction is now the leading contributing cause for adults with noncyanotic congenital heart disease consistent with late survival and an increasing impact of acquired heart disease.[16] With increasing experience and a team approach synthesizing surgery, intervention, and electrophysiology, adults with congenital heart disease should experience improved outcomes with less cumulative lifetime therapeutic trauma.

KEY POINTS

- Adult congenital heart procedures are best managed by multidisciplinary teams with dedicated cardiovascular surgeons, interventional cardiologists, electrophysiologists, and intensivists with high volume congenital experience.
- Web-based medical information systems may enhance the care of ACHD patients by providing the medical team, and the patients, with on-demand access to critical information over the patient's lifetime.
- Routine femoral cannulation may not be practical for reoperations in ACHD patients and alternate strategies should be considered.
- Surgical atrial septal defect repair in adults is best accomplished with patches, because primary repairs produce tension and may break down.
- Right ventricular outflow tract reconstructions should be performed with conduits that will allow future implantation of transcatheter stented valves.
- Anti-adhesion barriers and pericardial reconstructions may reduce the incidence of cardiac trauma during reoperations, which are common in the ACHD population.

REFERENCES

1. Toyoda T, Tateno S, Kawasoe Y, et al: Nationwide survey of care facilities for adults with congenital heart disease in Japan. *Circ J* 2009; 73(6): 1147-1150.
2. Dearani JA, Connolly HM, Martinez R, Fontanet H, Webb GD: Caring for adults with congenital cardiac disease: successes and challenges for 2007 and beyond. *Cardiol Young* 2007; 17 Suppl 2:87-96.
3. Winkelman WJ, Leonard KJ, Rossos PG: Patient-perceived usefulness of online electronic medical records: employing grounded theory in the development of information and communication technologies for use by patients living with chronic illness. *J Am Med Inform Assoc* 2005; 12(3): 306-314.
4. Gibson PH, Burns JE, Walker H, Cross S, Leslie ST: Keeping track of congenital heart disease. Is it time for a national registry? *Int J Cardiol* 2009; 145(2):331-332.
5. Jacobs JP, Elliott MJ, Anderson RH, et al: Creating a database with cardioscopy and intra-operative imaging. *Cardiol Young* 2005; 15(Suppl 1): 184-189.
6. Burke RP, White JA: Internet rounds: a congenital heart surgeon's Web log. *Semin Thorac Cardiovasc Surg* 2004; 16(3):283-292.
7. Luciani N, Anselmi A, De GR, et al: Extracorporeal circulation by peripheral cannulation before redo sternotomy: indications and results. *J Thorac Cardiovasc Surg* 2008; 136(3):572-577.
8. Knott-Craig CJ, Goldberg SP, Kirklin JK: Surgical strategy to prevent cardiac injury during reoperation in infants. *J Cardiothorac Surg* 2008; 3:10.
9. Giordano S, Biancari F: Does the use of carbon dioxide field flooding during heart valve surgery prevent postoperative cerebrovascular complications? *Interact Cardiovasc Thorac Surg* 2009; 9(2):323-326.
10. Jacobs JP, Iyer RS, Weston JS, et al: Expanded PTFE membrane to prevent cardiac injury during resternotomy for congenital heart disease. *Ann Thorac Surg* 1996; 62(6):1778-1782.

11. Okuyama N, Wang CY, Rose EA, et al: Reduction of retrosternal and pericardial adhesions with rapidly resorbable polymer films. *Ann Thorac Surg* 1999; 68(3):913-918.
12. Badylak SF, Freytes DO, Gilbert TW: Extracellular matrix as a biological scaffold material: structure and function. *Acta Biomater* 2009; 5(1):1-13.
13. Horvath KA, Burke RP, Collins JJ Jr, Cohn LH: Surgical treatment of adult atrial septal defect: early and long-term results. *J Am Coll Cardiol* 1992; 20(5):1156-1159.
14. Dearani JA, Mavroudis C, Quintessenza J, et al: Surgical advances in the treatment of adults with congenital heart disease. *Curr Opin Pediatr* 2009; 21(5):565-572.
15. da Silva JP, Baumgratz JF, da Fonseca FL, et al: The cone reconstruction of the tricuspid valve in Ebstein's anomaly. The operation: early and midterm results. *J Thorac Cardiovasc Surg* 2007; 133(1):215-223.
16. Pillutla P, Shetty KD, Foster E: Mortality associated with adult congenital heart disease: trends in the US population from 1979 to 2005. *Am Heart J* 2009; 158(5):874-879.
17. Kim WH, Lim HG, Lee JR, et al: Fontan conversion with arrhythmia surgery. *Eur J Cardiothorac Surg* 2005; 27(2):250-257.
18. Mavroudis C, Stewart RD, Backer CL, et al: Atrioventricular valve procedures with repeat Fontan operations: influence of valve pathology, ventricular function, and arrhythmias on outcome. *Ann Thorac Surg* 2005; 80(1):29-36.
19. Tsao S, Deal BJ, Backer CL, et al: Device management of arrhythmias after Fontan conversion. *J Thorac Cardiovasc Surg* 2009; 138(4):937-940.
20. Gatzoulis MA, Balaji S, Webber SA, et al: Risk factors for arrhythmia and sudden cardiac death late after repair of tetralogy of Fallot: a multicentre study. *Lancet* 2000; 356(9234):975-981.
21. Bonhoeffer P, Boudjemline Y, Saliba Z, et al: Percutaneous replacement of pulmonary valve in a right-ventricle to pulmonary-artery prosthetic conduit with valve dysfunction. *Lancet* 2000; 356(9239):1403-1405.
22. Zahn EM, Hellenbrand WE, Lock JE, McElhinney DB: Implantation of the melody transcatheter pulmonary valve in patients with a dysfunctional right ventricular outflow tract conduit early results from the U.S. clinical trial. *J Am Coll Cardiol* 2009; 54(18):1722-1729.
23. Lurz P, Gaudin R, Taylor AM, Bonhoeffer P: Percutaneous pulmonary valve implantation. *Semin Thorac Cardiovasc Surg Pediatr Card Surg Annu* 2009; 112-117.
24. Kostolny M, Tsang V, Nordmeyer J, et al: Rescue surgery following percutaneous pulmonary valve implantation. *Eur J Cardiothorac Surg* 2008; 33(4):607-612.
25. Ozdemir AO, Tamayo A, Munoz C, Dias B, Spence JD: Cryptogenic stroke and patent foramen ovale: clinical clues to paradoxical embolism. *J Neurol Sci* 2008; 275(1-2):121-127.
26. Niclauss L, Delay D, Hurni M, von Segesser LK: Experience and intermediate-term results using the Contegra heterograft for right ventricular outflow reconstruction in adults. *Interact Cardiovasc Thorac Surg* 2009; 9(4):667-671.
27. Solomon NA, Pranav SK, Jain KA, et al: In search of a pediatric cardiac surgeon's 'Holy Grail': the ideal pulmonary conduit. *Expert Rev Cardiovasc Ther* 2006; 4(6):861-870.
28. Vricella LA, Kanani M, Cook AC, Cameron DE, Tsang VT: Problems with the right ventricular outflow tract: a review of morphologic features and current therapeutic options. *Cardiol Young* 2004; 14(5):533-549.
29. Brown JW, Ruzmetov M, Rodefeld MD, Turrentine MW: Right ventricular outflow tract reconstruction in Ross patients: does the homograft fare better? *Ann Thorac Surg* 2008; 86(5):1607-1612.
30. Klieverik LM, Takkenberg JJ, Bekkers JA, et al: The Ross operation: a Trojan horse? *Eur Heart J* 2007; 28(16):1993-2000.
31. Brown JW, Ruzmetov M, Fukui T, et al: Fate of the autograft and homograft following Ross aortic valve replacement: reoperative frequency, outcome, and management. *J Heart Valve Dis* 2006; 15(2):253-259.
32. Luciani GB, Viscardi F, Pilati M, et al: The Ross-Yacoub procedure for aneurysmal autograft roots: a strategy to preserve autologous pulmonary valves. *J Thorac Cardiovasc Surg* 2009; 139:536-542 .
33. Suri RM, Dearani JA, Schaff HV, Danielson GK, Puga FJ: Long-term results of the Konno procedure for complex left ventricular outflow tract obstruction. *J Thorac Cardiovasc Surg* 2006; 132(5):1064-1071.
34. Hamid S, Arujuna A, Ginks M, et al: Pacemaker and defibrillator lead extraction: predictors of mortality during follow-up. *Pacing Clin Electrophysiol* 2009.
35. Stulak JM, Dearani JA, Puga FJ, et al: Right-sided Maze procedure for atrial tachyarrhythmias in congenital heart disease. *Ann Thorac Surg* 2006; 81(5):1780-1784.
36. Saltman AE, Gillinov AM: Surgical approaches for atrial fibrillation. *Cardiol Clin* 2009; 27(1):179-188, x.
37. Giamberti A, Chessa M, Abella R, et al: Surgical treatment of arrhythmias in adults with congenital heart defects. *Int J Cardiol* 2008; 129(1):37-41.
38. Noble S, Ibrahim R: Percutaneous interventions in adults with congenital heart disease: expanding indications and opportunities. *Curr Cardiol Rep* 2009; 11(4):306-313.
39. Jatene MB, Abuchaim DC, Oliveira JL Jr, et al: Outcomes of aortic coarctation surgical treatment in adults. *Rev Bras Cir Cardiovasc* 2009; 24(3): 346-353.
40. Mellert F, Preusse CJ, Haushofer M, et al: Surgical management of complications caused by transcatheter ASD closure. *Thorac Cardiovasc Surg* 2001; 49(6):338-342.
41. Stanfill R, Nykanen DG, Osorio S, et al: Stent implantation is effective treatment of vascular stenosis in young infants with congenital heart disease: acute implantation and long-term follow-up results. *Catheter Cardiovasc Interv* 2008; 71(6):831-841.
42. Pedra CA, Neves JR, Pedra SR, et al: New transcatheter techniques for creation or enlargement of atrial septal defects in infants with complex congenital heart disease. *Catheter Cardiovasc Interv* 2007; 70(5):731-739.
43. Patel MS, Kogon BE: Care of the adult congenital heart disease patient in the United States: a summary of the current system. *Pediatr Cardiol* 2010; 31(4):474-482.
44. Karamlou T, Diggs BS, Person T, Ungerleider RM, Welke KF: National practice patterns for management of adult congenital heart disease: operation by pediatric heart surgeons decreases in-hospital death. *Circulation* 2008; 118(23):2345-2352.

CHAPTER 61

Pericardial Disease

John M. Craig
Jennifer D. Walker

INTRODUCTION

The pericardium envelops the heart and portions of the great vessels as a protective capsule. When incised longitudinally and transversely along the diaphragm it can be suspended from a chest retractor to present the heart for surgical procedures. The surgical importance of the pericardium stems from its involvement in alterations of cardiac filling. When the limited space between the noncompliant pericardium and heart acutely fills with blood or fluid, cardiac compression and tamponade may ensue. Constrictive disorders arise when inflammation and scarring cause the pericardium to shrink and densely adhere to the surface of the heart. This chapter discusses pericardial anatomy and function and describes the conditions that commonly give rise to the surgical problems of pericardial constriction and tamponade. The chapter also describes the diagnosis and therapy of these entities, the management of tamponade early and late after cardiac surgery, and the rationale for and against pericardial closure at the time of cardiac surgery.

ANATOMY AND FUNCTION

The pericardium serves two major functions. It maintains the position of the heart within the mediastinum and prevents cardiac distention by sudden volume overload. The pericardium attaches to the ascending aorta just inferior to the innominate vein and the superior vena cava (SVC) several centimeters above the sinoatrial node. The pericardial reflection encompasses the superior and inferior pulmonary veins and encircles the inferior vena cava, thereby making it possible for the surgeon to control the inferior vena cava from within the pericardium. The pericardial reflection attaches to the left atrium near the entrances of the pulmonary veins just below the atrioventricular groove (Fig. 61-1). The pericardiophrenic arteries that travel with the phrenic nerves as well as the branches of the internal mammary arteries and feeder branches directly from the aorta perfuse the pericardium. It is innervated by vagal fibers from the esophageal plexus, and the phrenic nerves course within it.

The pericardium is a conical fibroserous sac made up of two intimately connected layers. The inner layer (serous pericardium) is a transparent monolayer of mesothelial cells. The visceral portion of the serous pericardium, or epicardium, and the parietal portion, which lines the fibrous pericardial sac, are continuous. The oblique sinus lies within the venous confluence and the transverse sinus lies between the arterial (aorta and pulmonary artery) and venous reflections (dome of left atrium and SVC). Such potential spaces allow the pericardium to expand and accommodate a limited amount of fluid. Normal pericardial fluid volume is approximately 10 to 20 mL. The pericardial mesothelial cells contain dense microvilli that are 1 μm wide and 3 μm high, which facilitate fluid and ion exchange.[1] Visceral pericardial lymphatic drainage occurs via the tracheal and bronchial mediastinal nodes, whereas the anterior and posterior mediastinal lymph nodes drain the parietal pericardium.

The parietal layer or fibrous pericardium is composed mostly of dense parallel bundles of collagen, which render this layer relatively noncompliant. Because the pericardium is stiffer than cardiac muscle, it tends to equalize the compliance of both ventricles. By doing so, the pericardium contributes to the resting cavitary diastolic pressure of both ventricles, maximizing diastolic ventricular interaction.[2] An example of this phenomenon is the diminution of systemic arterial pressure during inspiration. Intrapericardial pressure tends to approximate pleural pressure, and varies with respiration. The negative intrathoracic pressure generated during inspiration augments right ventricular filling. The interventricular septum shifts toward the left to accommodate

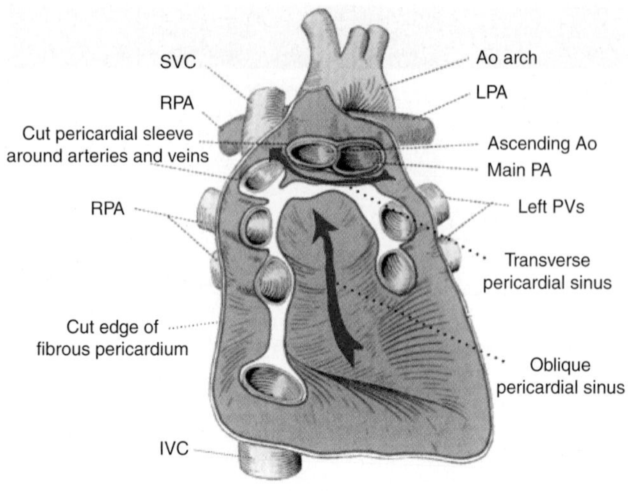

FIGURE 61-1 Pericardial attachments, reflections, and sinuses. Ao = aorta; IVC = inferior vena cava; LPA = left pulmonary artery; PA = pulmonary artery; PV = pulmonary vein; RPA = Right pulmonary artery; SVC = superior vena cava.

the increase in right ventricular volume. Because pericardial constraint does not allow equal filling of the left ventricle, the decrease in volume ejected by the systemic chamber results in a slight diminution of systemic arterial pressure during inspiration. This phenomenon is greatly magnified with an increase in intrapericardial pressure (eg, during acute filling of the pericardial space or circulatory volume overload), resulting in pulsus paradoxus.[3]

CONGENITAL ABNORMALITIES

Most congenital abnormalities of the pericardium are asymptomatic[4] and are often discovered incidentally at the time of surgery or investigation of unrelated problems.[5] They are rare and one-third are associated with cardiac, skeletal, and pulmonary abnormalaties.[6] Partial absence of the pericardium also occurs and is most commonly seen on the left (70%) due to premature atrophy of the left common cardinal vein. Right-sided and complete defects of the pericardium account for 17 and 13% of these defects, respectively. The right duct of Cuvier goes on to form the superior vena cava and ensures closure of the right pleuropericardial membrane.[7] Accordingly, right-sided defects tend to be lethal. MRI provides excellent pericardial imaging without contrast and is the imaging modality of choice. CT and echocardiography are useful for evaluation of pericardial thickening and extent and location of defects.[4] Although complete pericardial agenesis is rarely clinically significant, unilateral absence is potentially problematic because it may accentuate cardiac mobility and allow the heart to be displaced into the pleural space with resulting incarceration of the left atrial appendage or left ventricle. Treatment may involve pericardial resection or replacement with a prosthetic patch.[6] Both therapies appear to yield good outcomes.

Pericardial cysts are the most common congenital pericardial disorder and are surpassed only by lymphoma as the most prevalent of middle mediastinal masses.[8] They occur as asymptomatic incidental findings in 75% of patients; 70% occur in the right costophrenic angle and 22% on the left.[5] They do not communicate with the pericardial space and are typically unilocular, smooth, and less than 3 cm in diameter (Fig. 61-2). Symptoms may include chest pain, dyspnea, cough, and arrhythmias, probably owing to compression and inflammatory involvement of adjacent structures. They can also become secondarily infected.[9] Contrast CT scan is the modality of choice for diagnosis and follow-up.[10,11] Observation by CT in asymptomatic patients is suggested. Percutaneous aspiration is associated with a 30% recurrence rate at 3 years. Sclerosis has been reported to decrease recurrence after aspiration.[12] Indications for resection include large

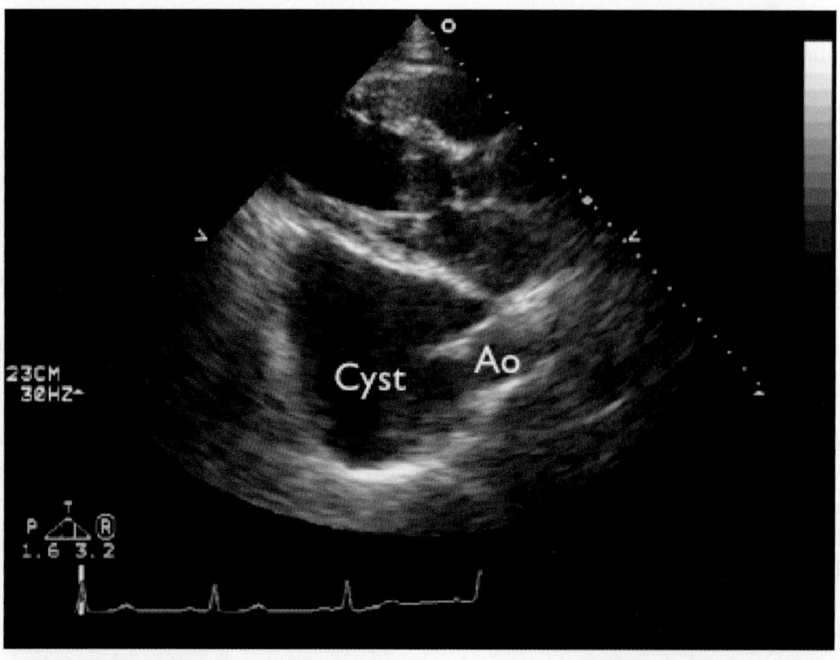

FIGURE 61-2 Transesophageal echocardiogram of large pericardial cyst.

size, symptoms, patient concern, and question of malignancy.[8] Video-assisted thoracoscopy is the surgical approach most commonly used for excision. Infrasternal mediastinoscopy can be used for anterior cysts. Thoracotomy is also an acceptable technique. Surgery is the only definitive cure.[12]

PATHOPHYSIOLOGY OF PERICARDIAL COMPRESSION

Pericardial compression results from disturbance of the normal anatomical and physiologic relationships among the pericardium, pericardial cavity, and the heart. Because the pericardium is relatively noncompliant and pericardial fluid noncompressible, the heart alone must compensate for acute changes in pericardial pressure. Acute volume overload within the confines of a fixed pericardial space results in a rapid, nonlinear increase in intrapericardial pressure (Fig. 61-3), producing cardiac compression.[13] The anatomical basis for pericardial compression involves either a space-occupying lesion (ie, cyst or excessive fluid) within the pericardial space or pericardial constriction.

Tamponade

Although blood in the pericardial space is the most common etiology, effusions, clot, pus, gas, or any combination may also produce tamponade. As fluid entering the pericardial space exceeds the ability of the pericardium to accommodate or absorb it, pericardial reserve volume (10 to 20 mL) is rapidly exceeded and intrapericardial pressure rises abruptly. At this point, pericardial fluid volume can only increase by reducing cardiac chamber volumes. Because of its lower filling pressures, the right heart is more susceptible to compression (Fig 61-4). The physiologic consequences are impaired diastolic filling with decreased cardiac output and increased central venous pressure.[14] Clinical manifestations include hypotension and jugular venous distention, and, along with decreased heart sounds, comprise Beck's triad.

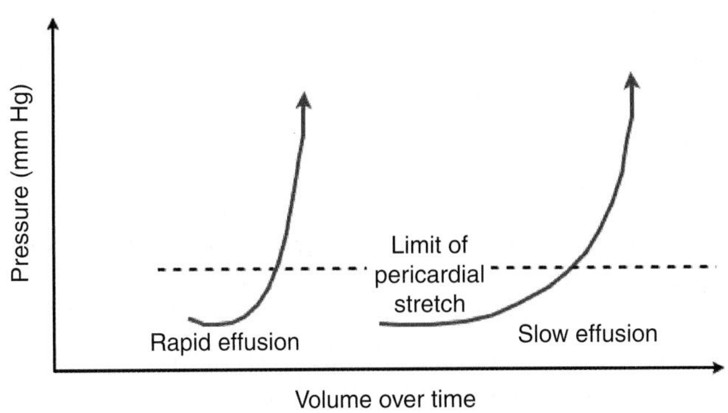

FIGURE 61-3 Relationship of pressure and volume in pericardial cavity. Normal pericardium will tolerate small amounts of fluid with a minimal increase in intrapericardial pressure. Above this small volume, small increases in volume result in large nonlinear increases in pressure. Gradual accumulation of fluid coincides with pericardial accommodation of much larger volumes of fluid up to a critical pressure.

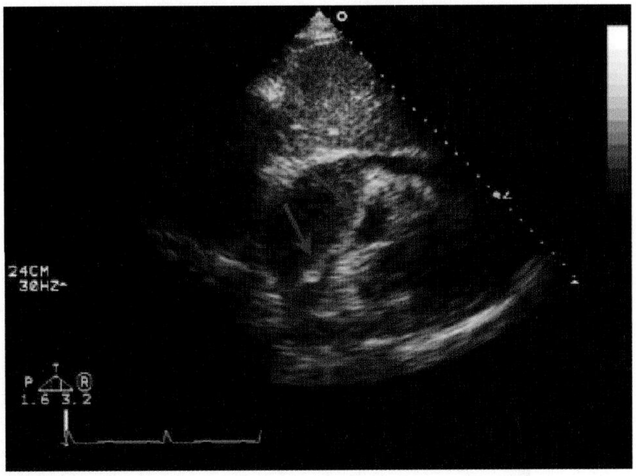

FIGURE 61-4 Transesophageal echocardiogram with right atrial inversion and cardiac tamponade.

To preserve cardiac output, higher pressures are required to fill the cardiac chambers, which may be partially achieved by parallel increases in systemic and pulmonary venous pressure by vasoconstriction.[15] Other compensatory mechanisms include tachycardia, chronic pericardial stretch, and blood volume expansion.[16] The latter two mechanisms have little impact in acute tamponade. As tamponade progresses, right heart filling becomes increasingly volume dependent and limited to inspiration. Increased filling of the right ventricle causes it to encroach on, and impair, filling of the left ventricle. However, during expiration the converse is true, and left ventricular filling and output increase. This exaggeration of physiologic ventricular interdependence is the basis of pulsus paradoxus.[13]

The clinical spectrum of tamponade varies widely, depending on the severity of hemodynamic impairment and degree of physiologic reserve. Rapid accumulation of as little as 100 mL of fluid in the pericardial space (eg, after a penetrating cardiac wound) may exceed the limited compliance of the parietal pericardium and produce critical tamponade. On the other hand, the pericardium may compensate for large pericardial effusions (>1 L) in chronic inflammatory conditions such as rheumatoid arthritis. The cardiac silhouette may appear normal in acute tamponade, but chronic pericardial distension is often obvious on plain chest radiography (Fig. 61-5), chest tomography (Fig. 61-6), and echocardiography (Fig. 61-7). Furthermore, low-pressure tamponade can also occur in which a pericardial effusion is not hemodynamically significant until the patient becomes hypovolemic, typically from dehydration, blood loss, or diuretic therapy. Venous filling pressures may be normal or mildly elevated in this setting, making this diagnosis difficult.[17]

Pericardial Constriction

A wide range of conditions promote pericardial scar formation, the pathologic process underlying constrictive pericarditis (CP). As with tamponade, the physiologic basis is compromised cardiac filling leading to systemic venous congestion and low cardiac output. In contrast with tamponade, however, onset is often

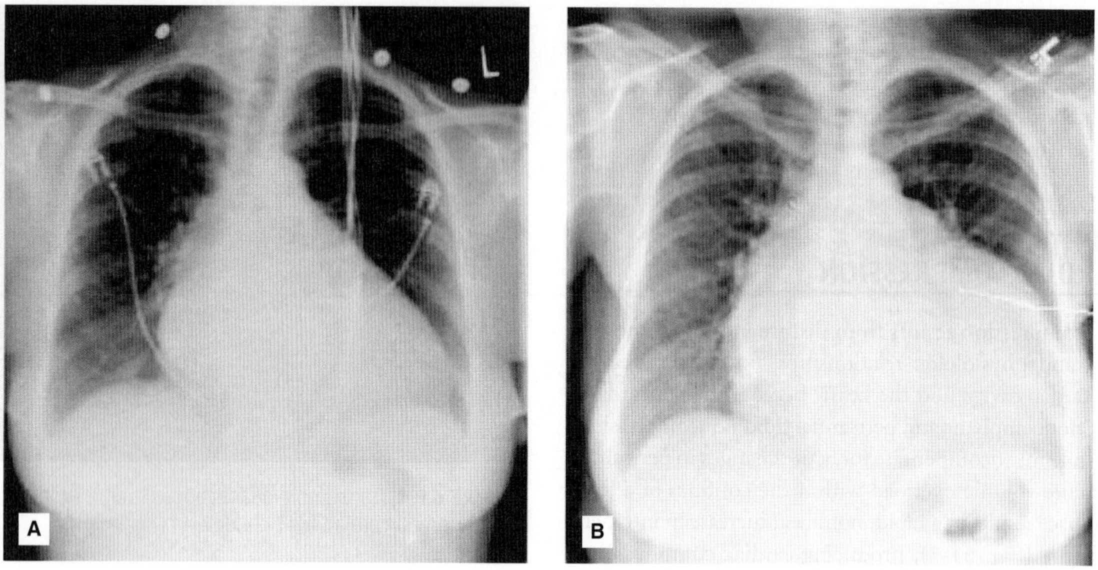

FIGURE 61-5 Slowly enlarging pericardial effusion detected on chest x-ray. (A) At discharge; (B) 3 weeks after discharge.

insidious and symptoms may be present for months or even years.[18] Common complaints include fatigue, decreased exercise tolerance with dyspnea/orthopnea, as well as peripheral edema and ascites from hepatic congestion in advanced disease. The principal etiologies behind pericardial scar formation have shifted over the past few decades, with declining incidence of infectious cases (particularly tuberculosis) and increasing incidence of iatrogenic cases (primarily from mediastinal radiation therapy and cardiac surgery).[19]

Pericardial constriction exerts its pathophysiologic effects by limiting cardiac filling. Unlike tamponade, in which cardiac filling is limited from the onset of diastole, constriction does not restrict filling in early diastole. During diastolic filling the ventricles are prevented from reaching full capacity as they encounter the contracted and noncompliant pericardium. As a result, 70 to 80% of diastolic filling occurs in the first 25 to 30% of diastole.[20] Although early diastolic filling pressures are normal (whereas ventricular expansion is not constrained by the surrounding stiff pericardium), later diastolic pressures abruptly increase. The ventricular free walls are then immobilized, leaving the interventricular septum as the last yielding structure; it is rapidly displaced in response to the sudden interventricular pressure differential. This produces the characteristic "septal bounce" seen echocardiographically. Other echocardiographic findings include pericardial thickening, caval plethora, and small chamber volumes. Inspiration exaggerates both leftward septal deviation as well as reciprocal Doppler flows between the right and left sides (the echocardiographic correlate of pulsus paradoxus).

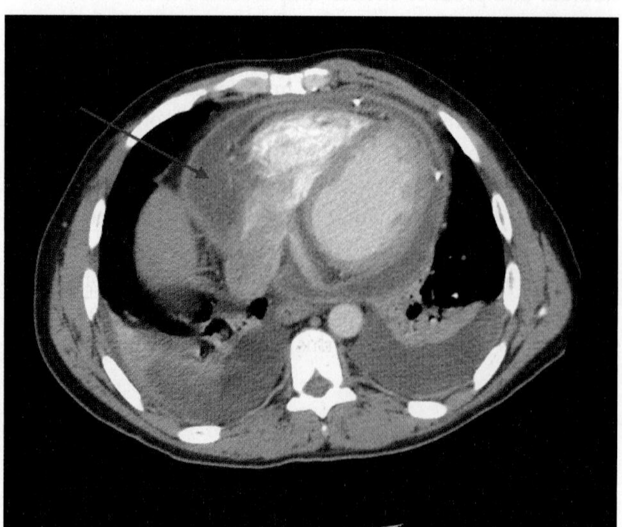

FIGURE 61-6 CT scan with large circumferential pericardial effusion and bilateral pleural effusions.

Modern axial imaging with spiral computed tomographic (CT) scanning (Fig. 61-8) or magnetic resonance (MR) imaging (Fig. 61-9) is often able to visualize thickened and/or calcified pericardium, with or without coexisting effusion. Dynamic CT and MR imaging also demonstrate many of the physiologic features seen sonographically.[21] Importantly, although pericardial thickening is usually present in constrictive pericarditis, it remains possible to have CP with normal pericardial thickness as well as thickening of the pericardium without CP.[22]

Prior to the modern era of echocardiography and axial imaging, the diagnosis of CP was dependent on hemodynamic tracings obtained during cardiac catheterization. The sudden increase in diastolic ventricular pressure is reflected in the dip and plateau or "square-root" sign (Fig 61-10). Similarly, right atrial pressure tracings reveal a steep *y* descent, which correlates with the nadir of the square-root sign. Under normal circumstances, inspiration results in a 3- to 7-mm Hg drop in right atrial pressure. The high pressure of pericardial constriction prevents the right atrium from accepting inspiratory acceleration of blood from the central veins. Instead, neck veins become prominently distended during inspiration in patients with CP, a phenomenon referred to as *Kussmaul's sign*.

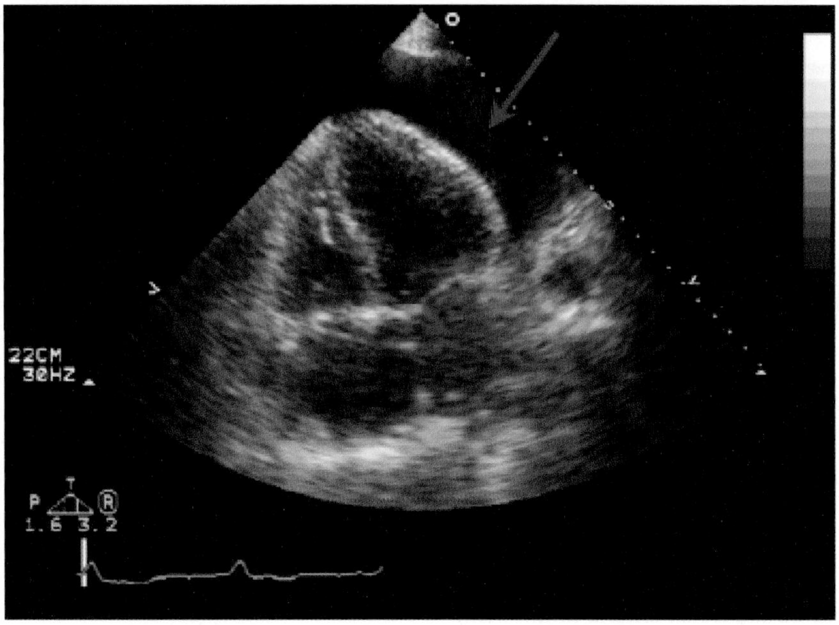

FIGURE 61-7 Transesophageal echocardiogram with very large pericardial effusion.

Catheterization remains a valuable illustration of the underlying physiology of CP. In some cases it may help differentiate between CP and restrictive cardiomyopathy (RCM), a nonsurgical condition with a poor prognosis.[23,24] RCM is characterized by noncompliant ventricular muscle and diastolic dysfunction, which impede cardiac filling. Restrictive cardiomyopathy is caused by a variety of infiltrative or fibrosing conditions (eg, amyloidosis, sarcoidosis, radiation, carcinoid, anthracycline toxicity). Although RCM may mimic many of the presenting features of CP, it is not a surgical disease and must be distinguished from CP for this reason (Table 61-1). Systolic ventricular function may be normal or near-normal in both conditions, but pulmonary and hepatic congestion are often present in RCM. Evidence of pericardial thickening (>2 mm) favors but does not confirm the diagnosis of CP over RCM. There are instances, particularly in radiation-induced CP, in which the conditions coexist. Distinctive myocardial speckling may be found on echo with amyloidosis or other infiltrative conditions. Endomyocardial biopsy is useful to establish the presence of one of the conditions known to be associated with RCM; unfortunately, a negative biopsy does not rule it out.

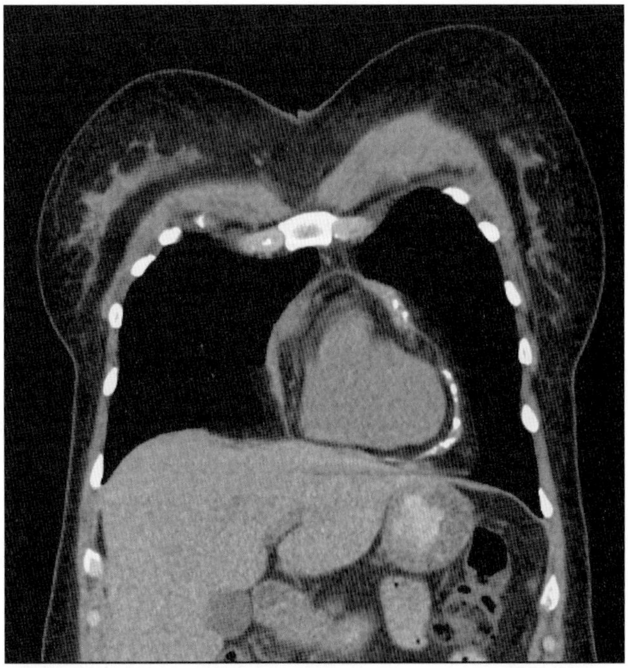

FIGURE 61-8 CT scan showing pericardial thickening and calcification.

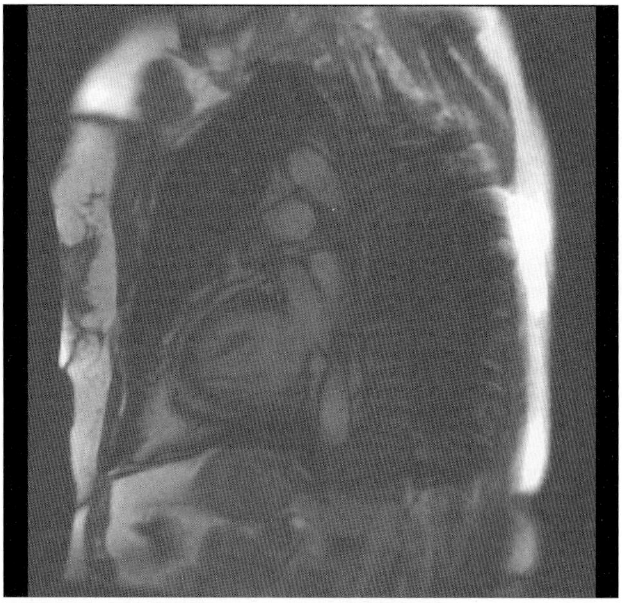

FIGURE 61-9 MRI showing pericardial thickening with pericarditis.

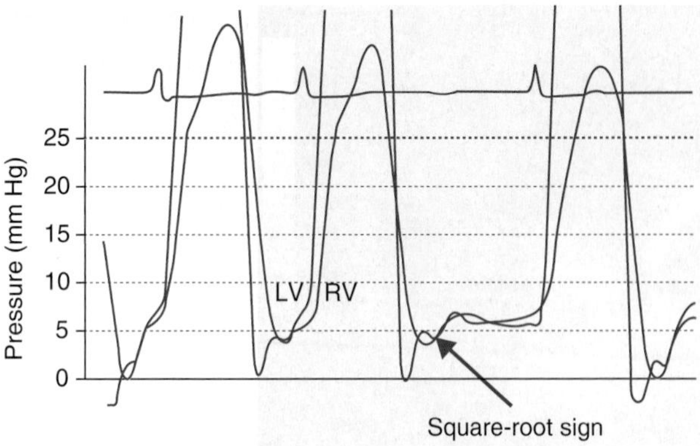

FIGURE 61-10 Square-root sign in right ventricular pressure tracing in constrictive pericarditis. (*Modified with permission from Spodick DH [ed]: The Pericardium: A Comprehensive Textbook. New York, Marcel Dekker, 1997; p 4.*)

In an attempt to provide additional criteria to differentiate patients with CP from RCM, Hurrell and colleagues[25] measured respiratory variation of the gradient between left ventricular pressure and pulmonary capillary wedge pressure during the rapid filling phase of diastole. This was done to assess the dissociation of intrathoracic and intracardiac pressures that accompanies constrictive pericarditis. A difference of 5 mm Hg in the gradient between inspiratory and expiratory cycles had 93% sensitivity and 81% specificity for constrictive pericarditis. Furthermore, increased ventricular interdependence was assessed by comparing left ventricular systolic pressure and right ventricular systolic pressure during respiration. Although concordant increases in left ventricular systolic pressure and right ventricular systolic pressure are expected during inspiration, discordant pressures are encountered during inspiration in patients with constrictive pericarditis. This finding has 100% sensitivity and 95% specificity for constrictive pericarditis.

ACQUIRED ABNORMALITIES

Pericarditis, the most common pericardial disorder, has many etiologies (Table 61-2), including infectious (viral, bacterial, fungal), metabolic (uremic, drug induced), autoimmune (arthritis, thyroid), postradiation, neoplastic, traumatic, postinfarction (Dressler's syndrome, 10 to 15%), post-pericardiotomy (5 to 30%), and idiopathic (Fig. 61-11). The clinical syndrome for all causes is similar. Chest pain (dull, aching, pressure) or chest tightness is usually present and may be associated with constitutional symptoms (eg, weakness and malaise), fever (occasionally with rigors), and other symptoms such as cough or odynophagia. The pain may be pleuritic, and thus exacerbated

TABLE 61-1 Differentiation between Constrictive Pericarditis and Restrictive Cardiomyopathy

Finding	Pericardial Constriction	Restrictive Cardiomyopathy
PHYSICAL EXAMINATION		
Pulsus paradoxus	Variable	Absent
Pericardial knock (high frequency)	Present	Absent
S3 (low frequency)	Absent	Present
HEMODYNAMICS		
Prominent *y* descent	Present	Variable
Equalization of right and left side filling pressures	Present	Left > right
RV end-diastolic pressure/systolic pressure	>1/3	<1/3
Pulmonary hypertension	Rare	Common
Square-root sign	Present	Variable
ECHOCARDIOGRAPHY		
Respiratory variation in left-right pressures/flows	Increased	Normal
Septal bounce	Present	Absent
Atrial enlargement	Variable	Biatrial
Ventricular hypertrophy	Absent	Usually present
Pericardial thickness	Increased	Normal

TABLE 61-2 Acquired Etiologies of Acute Pericarditis

INFECTIOUS
- Bacterial
  - Tuberculous (mycobacterial)
  - Suppurative (streptococcal, pneumococcal)
- Viral
  - Coxsackie
  - Influenza
  - HIV
  - Hepatitis A, B, C
  - Other
- Fungal
- Parasitic
- Other
  - Rickettsial
  - Spirochetal
  - *Spirillum*
  - *Mycoplasma*
  - Infectious mononucleosis
  - *Leptospira*
  - *Listeria*
  - *Lymphogranuloma venereum*
  - Psittacosis

AUTOIMMUNE/VASCULITIDES
- Rheumatoid arthritis
- Rheumatic fever
- Systemic lupus erythematosus
- Drug-induced lupus erythematosus
- Scleroderma
- Sjögren's syndrome
- Whipple's disease
- Mixed connective tissue disease
- Reiter's syndrome
- Ankylosing spondylitis
- Inflammatory bowel diseases
  - Ulcerative colitis
  - Crohn's disease
- Serum sickness
- Wegener's granulomatosis
- Giant cell arteritis
- Polymyositis
- Behçet's syndrome
- Familial Mediterranean fever
- Panmesenchymal syndrome
- Polyarteritis nodosa
- Churg-Strauss syndrome
- Thrombohemolytic-thrombocytopenic purpura
- Hypocomplementemic uremic vasculitis syndrome
- Leukoclastic vasculitis
- Other

METABOLIC DISORDERS
- Renal failure
  - Uremia in chronic or acute renal failure
  - "Dialysis" pericarditis
- Myxedema
  - Cholesterol pericarditis
  - Gout
- Scurvy

DISEASE OF CONTIGUOUS STRUCTURES
- Myocardial infarction/cardiac surgery
  - Acute myocardial infarction
  - Postmyocardial infarction syndrome
  - Postpericardiotomy syndrome
  - Ventricular aneurysm
- Aortic dissection
- Pleural and pulmonary disease
  - Pneumonia
  - Pulmonary embolism
  - Pleuritis
- Malignancies of lung

NEOPLASTIC
- Primary
  - Mesothelioma
  - Sarcoma
  - Fibroma
- Secondary
  - Metastatic; carcinomas, sarcomas
  - Direct extension; bronchogenic, esophageal carcinomas
  - Hematogenous; lymphoma, leukemia

TRAUMA
- Penetrating
  - Stab wound or gunshot wound to the chest, iatrogenic
  - During diagnostic or therapeutic cardiac catheterization
  - During pacemaker insertion
- Radiation pericarditis

UNCERTAIN ETIOLOGIES AND PATHOGENESIS
- Pericardial fat necrosis
- Loeffler's syndrome
- Thalassemia
- Drug reactions
  - Procainamide
  - Hydralazine
  - Others
- Pancreatitis

UNCERTAIN ETIOLOGIES AND PATHOGENESIS
- Sarcoidosis
- Fat embolism
- Bile fistula to pericardium
- Wissler syndrome
- PIE syndrome
- Stevens-Johnson syndrome
- Gaucher's disease
- Diaphragmatic hernia
- Atrial septal defect
- Giant cell aortitis
- Takayasu's syndrome
- Castleman's disease
- Fabry's disease
- Kawasaki's disease
- Degos' disease
- Histiocytosis X
- Campylodactyly-pleuritis-pericarditis syndrome
- Farmer lung
- Idiopathic

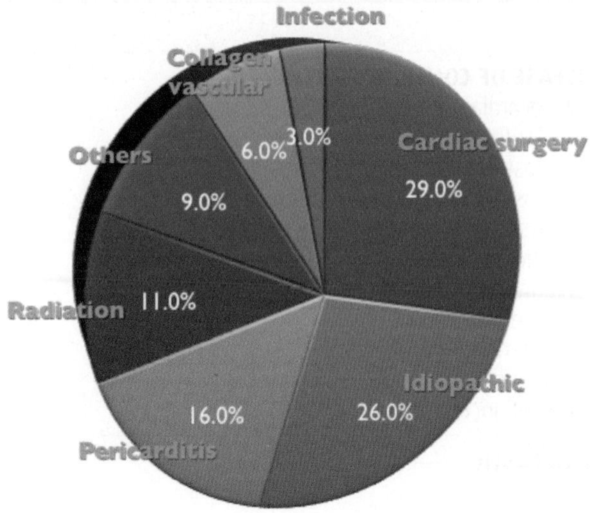

FIGURE 61-11 Etiologies and frequency of pericardial constriction.

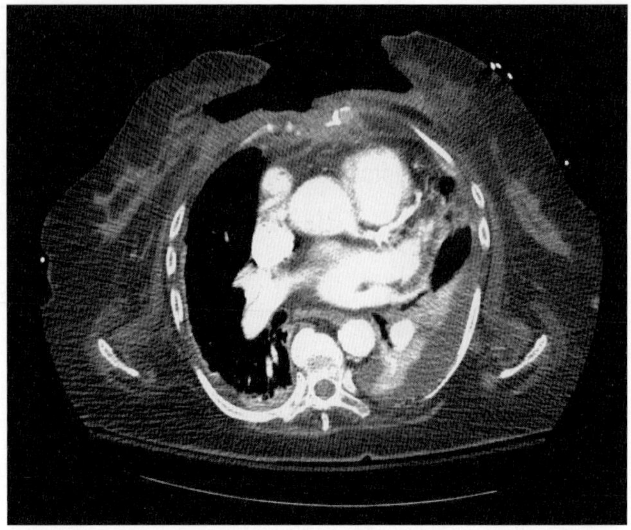

FIGURE 61-12 CT scan showing postoperative anterior mediastinitis with pericardial involvement and left pleural effusion.

by inspiration, cough, or recumbency. These patients therefore often sit up and lean forward for relief. Acute disease may become chronic. The cardinal sign of pericarditis is the pericardial rub, which may be positional and muffled because of an effusion.[26]

Electrocardiography, chest x-ray, and echocardiography are useful in making the diagnosis. The electrocardiogram may range from normal, to nonspecific ST-segment deviations, to diffuse concave elevation of the ST segments without reciprocal depressions or Q waves. PR-segment depression may be present. Troponin may be elevated with a normal CPK. Ventricular arrhythmias and conduction abnormalities are not commonly seen in pericarditis and are suggestive of an underlying cardiac abnormality if present. Echocardiography may reveal fibrinous thickening of the pericardium with or without a small effusion.

Nonsteroidal anti-inflammatory drugs (NSAIDs) are the mainstay of treatment and may be supplemented with colchicine. Chronic pericardial effusion or constrictive pericarditis may follow acute pericarditis as well as tuberculosis, malignancy, radiation, rheumatoid arthritis, or surgery.[26]

Infectious Pericarditis

Viral Pericarditis

Infectious pericarditis is most often viral and results from immune complex deposits, direct viral attack, or both. The clinical syndrome involves pain, friction rub, and typical changes on the electrocardiogram. It is often difficult to diagnose and thus labeled as idiopathic disease. Treatment is expectant, and symptoms generally resolve within 2 weeks. Surgical intervention is rarely required.

Bacterial Pericarditis

This is currently an uncommon cause of pericarditis because of availability of effective antibiotic therapy. Microorganisms may invade the pericardial space from contiguous infections in the heart (endocarditis), lung (pneumonia, abscess), subdiaphragmatic space (liver or splenic abscess), or wounds (traumatic or surgical). Hematogenous seeding may also occur, most often in the setting of septicemia and immune compromise.

The most common bacteria implicated in bacterial pericarditis are *Haemophilus influenzae*, meningococci, pneumococci, staphylococci, or streptococci.[27] Gram-negative rods, *Salmonella* and opportunistic sources of infection must be excluded. Regardless of the source or organism, acute suppurative pericarditis is life threatening. A toxic presentation with a high fever is typical with an acute, fulminant clinical course. Purulent pericarditis with tamponade or septicemia may require acute surgical intervention via pericardial window or pericardiectomy and treatment of the inciting cause (eg, removal of foreign body or drainage of abscess) (Fig. 61-12). In adults, pneumopyopericardium is often caused by fistula formation between a hollow viscus and the pericardium. However, invasion from contiguous foci, implantation at the time of surgery or trauma, mediastinitis, endocarditis, and subdiaphragmatic abscess can all induce this condition. Scarring, which results in pericardial constriction, may require pericardiectomy. These patients have an excellent outcome when treated appropriately.[27]

Tuberculous Pericarditis

Although the incidence of tuberculosis (TB) has significantly declined in industrialized countries, it has increased dramatically in Africa, Asia, and Latin America, accounting for 95% of all cases of active TB. This resurgence in TB reflects the increasing incidence of human immunodeficiency virus (HIV) infection.[28] The immune response to the acid-fast bacilli penetrating the pericardium induces a delayed hypersensitivity reaction with lymphokine release and granuloma formation. Complement fixing antibodies initiate cytolysis mediated by antimyolemmal antibodies as the cause of the exudative TB pericarditis.[28] The definitive diagnosis is established by examining pericardium or pericardial fluid for mycobacteria.

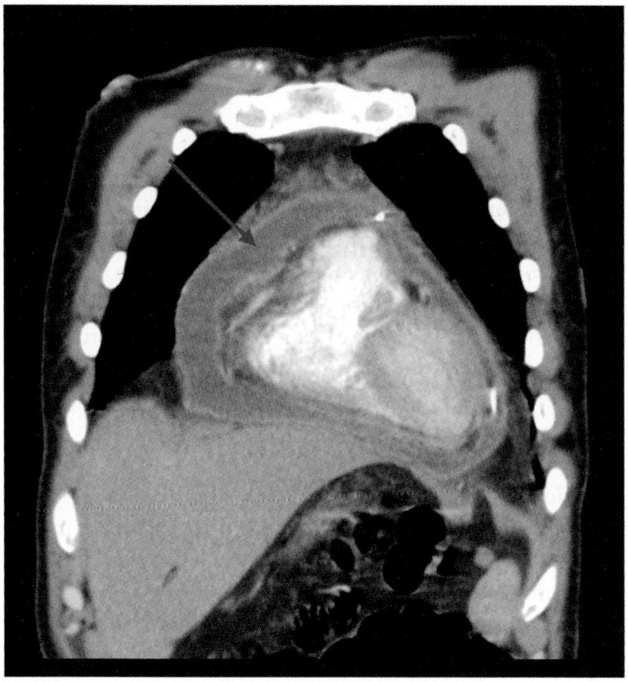

FIGURE 61-13 CT scan of chronic pericardial thickening and calcification and larger pericardial effusion in a patient with TB.

Four pathologic states are recognized:

1. Fibrinous exudation, with robust polymorphonuclear infiltration and abundant mycobacteria
2. Serous or serosanguineous effusions with a mainly lymphocytic exudation and foam cells (Fig. 61-13)
3. Absorption of effusion, with organization of caseating granulomas, and pericardial thickening caused by fibrin and collagen deposition and fibrosis
4. Constrictive scarring, often with extensive calcification occurring over a period of years (Fig. 61-14 A,B)

There is a variable clinical course. Effusion usually develops insidiously with fever, night sweats, fatigue, and weight loss to variable degrees. Children and immunocompromised patients may, however, present with a more fulminant course, often demonstrating both constrictive and tamponade physiology. Despite prompt anti-TB antibiotic treatment, constrictive pericarditis, one of the most severe sequelae, occurs in 30 to 60% of patients. Echocardiography is useful for diagnosing effusive and subacute constrictive TB pericarditis. Standard anti-TB therapy is instituted promptly. Steroids remain controversial, especially in HIV-infected patients. Based on physiology and response to therapy, immediate or interval pericardiectomy is performed to avoid chronic constrictive pericarditis. If calcific pericarditis is present, surgery is undertaken earlier.[29]

Fungal Pericarditis

Fungal infection is an uncommon cause of pericarditis. *Nocardia, Aspergillus, Candida,* and *Coccidioides* are implicated, with regional specification, in the setting of immunocompromise, debilitation, HIV, severe burns, infancy, or steroid therapy.

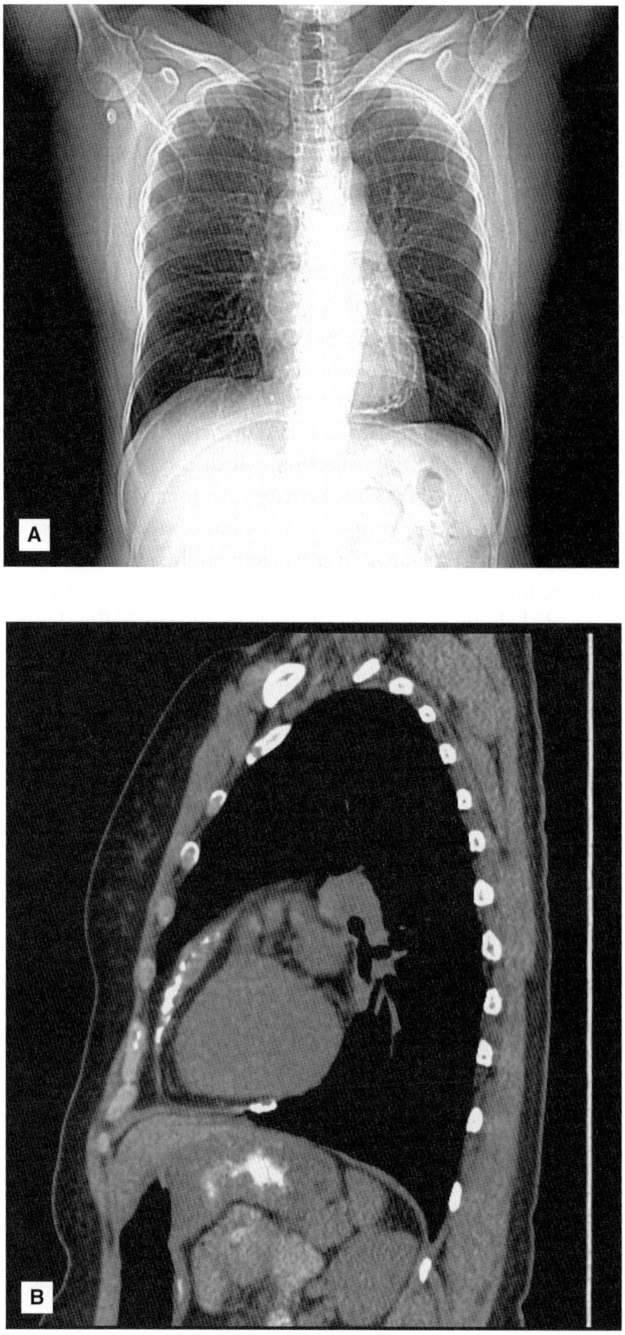

FIGURE 61-14 (A) PA CXR in patient with TB showing calcification of pericardium around LV apex. (B) CT scan of chronic pericardial thickening and calcification in patient with TB.

Candida and *Aspergillus* generate an insidious clinical picture, which may develop into tamponade or constriction. Fungi such as *Histoplasma* that tend to be endemic to certain geographic regions may cause pericarditis in young, healthy, immunocompetent patients. This is usually self-limited and resolves within 2 weeks. Similarly, *Coccidioides* can also infect young healthy individuals in the setting of pneumonia, osteomyelitis, meningitis, or adenopathy. These conditions often resolve either spontaneously or in response to appropriate antifungal regimens. Surgical intervention is not usually required in the acute setting.

Metabolic Causes of Pericarditis

Pericarditis is known to occur in the setting of renal failure, hypothyroidism, autoimmune diseases (such as rheumatoid arthritis), and pharmacotherapy with certain drugs (eg, procainamide and hydralazine).

Uremic Pericarditis

Uremic pericarditis was first recognized by Bright in 1836.[30] Although it is recognized that nitrogen retention (blood urea nitrogen levels are generally >60 mg/dL) is required for uremic pericarditis, the inciting agent is still unknown. The clinical profile typically involves a patient with chronic renal insufficiency who develops pain, fever, and a friction rub.[31] There is usually a pericardial fluid collection, which can be exudative or transudative, that is often hemorrhagic. Although the incidence of tamponade is decreasing because of more widespread use of renal replacement therapy,[32] it still occurs and remains a primary concern. Initial therapy includes NSAIDs and aggressive dialysis. Pericardial drainage is reserved for hemodynamically significant (tamponade) or refractory effusions (more than 2 weeks despite intensive dialysis), but the latter is the subject of debate.[33] Heparin should be administered cautiously, if at all, during dialysis because of the risk of hemorrhagic pericarditis and tamponade.[34] Pericardial effusions may also develop in this population because of a variety of conditions such as heart failure, volume overload, and hypoproteinemia. Nonuremic pericarditis is also known to occur in patients on longstanding dialysis.[35] Finally, pericardial effusion increases the risk of low-pressure tamponade during dialysis by mechanisms described in the preceding.[17]

Drug-Induced Pericarditis

Pericarditis may also occur in the setting of a drug-induced hypersensitivity reaction or lupus-like syndrome.[36] Procainamide, hydralazine, isoniazid, methysergide, cromolyn, penicillin, and emetine (among others) have been associated with pericardial inflammation. Minoxidil has been associated with pericardial effusion.[37] The clinical presentation and guidelines for management in these settings are similar to those for other types of pericarditis. The inciting agent should be discontinued.

Pericarditis Associated with Rheumatoid Arthritis

Pericarditis is common in patients with rheumatoid arthritis (RA). Approximately half of patients with RA have pericardial effusions, and almost half of all patients with RA have significant pericardial adhesions at autopsy.[38] The condition is encountered more often in patients with advanced RA, and is thought to be caused by the higher rheumatoid factor titers often seen with more severe underlying disease. Deposition of immune complexes in the pericardium appears to be the inciting event underlying the inflammatory response.[39] The diagnosis is often complicated by the many clinical variants and possible intercurrent diseases such as drug-induced and viral pericarditis. Pericardial drainage is often employed early for symptomatic effusions because response to medical therapy of the underlying RA is slow and unpredictable. Pericardiectomy should be considered in patients with longstanding RA who have developed constriction.[40]

Hypothyroidism

Severe hypothyroidism produces large, clear, high-protein, high-cholesterol, and high-specific-gravity effusions in 25 to 35% of patients.[41] The effusion may precede other signs of hypothyroidism. Clinical tamponade is rare because of the slow accumulation of fluid. However, acute exacerbations owing to acute pericarditis, hemorrhage, or cholesterol pericarditis can induce tamponade.[42]

Radiation Pericarditis

Radiation is now the most common etiology of constrictive pericarditis in the United States. This was first recognized in patients who received high-dose mantle radiation for Hodgkin's lymphoma in the 1960s and 1970s and developed cardiac and pericardial pathology, on average 10 to 15 years after therapy. Radiation induces acute pericarditis, pancarditis, and accelerated coronary artery disease in a dose-dependent relationship.[43] Patients may present with a combination of pericardial constriction, restrictive cardiomyopathy, valvular heart disease, and coronary artery disease with a predilection for ostial lesions.[44] When symptomatic effusions are drained, fluid should be analyzed to clarify the etiology (ie, malignancy versus radiation effect). Constrictive pericarditis can develop several years later and is best treated by pericardiectomy.[45]

Neoplastic Pericarditis

Secondary neoplasms of the pericardium (ie, tumors that involve the pericardium by metastasis or infiltration from adjoining structures) account for greater than 95% of pericardial neoplastic diseases. Primary pericardial tumors are rare, and paraneoplastic effusions can also occur in response to remote tumors.[46]

The most common secondary tumors involving the pericardium in males (including both metastasis and local extension) are carcinoma of the lung (31.7%) and esophagus (28.7%) and lymphoma (11.9%). In females, carcinoma of the lung (35.9%), lymphoma (17.0%), and carcinoma of the breast (7.5%) are most common. Primary pericardial tumors are very uncommon. Benign tumors are generally encountered in infancy or childhood. Malignant tumors such as mesotheliomas, sarcomas, and angiosarcomas most often present in the third or fourth decade of life.[47]

In both primary and secondary tumor involvement, the clinical presentation is usually silent, and may be associated with large pericardial effusions. Tamponade can result from hemorrhage into a malignant effusion. Occasionally tumors can induce constriction because of neoplastic tissue, adhesions, or both. The role of surgery is limited to diagnosis and palliation in most of these cases. Large refractory effusions associated with tamponade may need surgical drainage. In such cases, a fluid sample should be submitted to confirm the presence of malignant cells or evaluate for other causes of effusion in patients with cancer because this may influence management.[48]

In terms of therapeutic benefit, pericardiocentesis has a high failure rate, and subxiphoid drainage or percutaneous balloon pericardiotomy are only transiently effective.[49] Although extensive resection and debulking may be necessary in persistent or recurrent malignant pericardial constriction, it has only transient benefit without effective adjunctive chemotherapy and/or radiation therapy. Life expectancy of patients with malignant pericardial involvement averages less than 4 months.[50] The surgeon should individualize decisions regarding how aggressively to pursue diagnostic or therapeutic interventions.

Traumatic Pericardial Conditions

Penetrating Trauma

Knives, bullets, needles, and intracardiac instrumentation are the most common causes of penetrating trauma to the pericardium and heart. Tamponade is more common in stab wounds than gunshot wounds. The right ventricle is most often involved in anterior chest wounds. Because tamponade provides hemostasis and prevents exsanguination, patients with tamponade have better survival than those with uncontrolled hemorrhage from a penetrating cardiac injury. Diagnosis is often made on clinical grounds supplemented by ultrasonography.[51] Stable patients can be explored in the operating theater, but unstable patients should undergo thoracotomy in the emergency department.

Blunt Trauma

Blunt injuries to the heart and pericardium rarely occur in isolation. Trauma owing to compression (including cardiopulmonary resuscitation), blast, and deceleration can produce a spectrum of injuries ranging from cardiac contusion to cardiac rupture and pericardial laceration with herniation or luxation of the heart. Patients with pericardial rupture and cardiac herniation typically have suffered high-energy deceleration trauma and are invariably hypotensive from associated injuries. Hypovolemia may lead to rapid decompensation because cardiac filling becomes increasingly volume dependent in the setting of tamponade. Likewise, patients may initially respond to volume resuscitation. Chest imaging may demonstrate displacement of the heart or presence of free air or intra-abdominal organs within the pericardium. If the heart herniates into the pleura, positioning the patient with the contralateral side down may reduce the herniation. Thoracotomy is required for definitive treatment and repair of associated injuries.[52]

Acute Postinfarction Pericarditis and Dressler's Syndrome

Postinfarction pericarditis is thought to occur in almost half of patients suffering a transmural myocardial infarction (MI), although it is symptomatic in far fewer. The incidence is decreasing because of more aggressive revascularization in recent decades. Chest pain is almost universally present, and it is important to distinguish the pain of pericarditis from ischemic pain by its positional and pleuritic nature. The pain of early post-MI pericarditis occurs in the first 24 to 72 hours. Dressler's syndrome is a diffuse pleuropericardial inflammation thought to have an autoimmune etiology that occurs weeks to months after infarction. A pericardial rub and effusion may be present but tamponade is rare. In Dressler's syndrome, a pleural rub and effusion may also be present. The electrocardiographic signs of pericarditis may be obscured by those of infarction. Post-MI pericarditis is typically treated with aspirin and/or NSAIDs.[53,54] Steroids or colchicine may be used for persistent or recurrent symptoms; however, glucocorticoid use is associated with recurrence of pericarditis.[55]

Cardiac Surgery and the Pericardium

Postinfarction Pericarditis

Postinfarction pericarditis, as described in the preceding, is an important entity for the surgeon to consider in the evaluation of patients with acute coronary syndromes. To the unwary it may masquerade as postinfarction angina and prompt an unnecessarily early operation after myocardial infarction. Extensive fibrinous adhesions and murky gelatinous fluid may be present in the pericardial space and obscure epicardial vessels. When the pericardium is opened late in such a patient, the surgeon should expect dense pericardial adhesions.

Postpericardiotomy Syndrome

Pericardial friction rubs are almost universal after cardiac surgery; some patients develop Dressler's syndrome with pleural and pericardial effusions, pleuritic pain, and generalized malaise. Such patients almost always respond to NSAIDs or a short course of corticosteroids when the symptoms remain refractory.[56] Although this condition is benign, it is important (and sometimes difficult) to distinguish between postoperative pericarditis and myocardial ischemia. This distinction can often be made on clinical grounds based on symptoms, hemodynamics, and pattern of ECG changes.[57] Echocardiography or angiography may be used in borderline cases to clarify the etiology.

Postoperative Tamponade

Early postoperative tamponade rarely goes undetected for long because of the high level of vigilance and close hemodynamic monitoring that attend the patient during this time. A vital feature of postoperative tamponade is that a circumferential fluid collection is not required for compromised cardiac function. Hemodynamic deterioration can occur in the setting of localized clot within the pericardium, particularly if it is impinging on the right heart.[58] It is also important for surgeons to be aware of the potential for late cardiac tamponade that presents after hospital discharge and often to a clinician other than the cardiac surgeon. This entity is a potentially lethal complication and occurs in 0.5 to 6% of patients after heart surgery, almost exclusively in those on anticoagulation. Late cardiac tamponade (ie, tamponade occurring more than 7 days after cardiac surgery) is more common in younger patients who have undergone isolated valve (as opposed to coronary artery bypass graft) surgery. Patients present on average 3 weeks after surgery, frequently in the setting of an elevated prothrombin time. They are often severely symptomatic, with declining exercise tolerance, dyspnea, an inability to urinate, and sometimes hypotension. Any patient on anticoagulation whose recovery begins an otherwise unexplained decline in this interval should be suspected of having late tamponade and undergo echocardiographic examination. Nearly all patients with late tamponade respond favorably to pericardiocentesis, and are able to safely resume anticoagulation.[59]

Pericardial Closure

Redo sternotomy may be more hazardous when the heart is adherent to the inner table of the sternum. Closing the pericardium at the time of surgery interposes a protective layer of tissue between the sternum and the heart and may reduce the risks of redo sternotomy. The value of any added protection against cardiac injury on sternal reentry is limited by the relative infrequency of reoperation and the already low incidence of cardiac injury at repeat sternotomy when the pericardium is left open. On the negative side, closing the pericardium can cause kinking of bypass grafts after coronary bypass surgery and may result in hemodynamic compromise caused by cardiac compression.

Several small studies have attempted to answer the question of whether pericardial closure should be performed after cardiac procedures. Rao and associates demonstrated that pericardial closure at the time of cardiac surgery adversely affects postoperative hemodynamics.[60] In this ingenious study, the pericardial edges were marked with radiopaque markers and the pericardium was closed with a running suture, the ends of which were exteriorized. After obtaining a postoperative chest film that demonstrated pericardial approximation, a set of baseline hemodynamics was measured. The suture was then removed, another x-ray taken to demonstrate distraction of the pericardial edges, and then the hemodynamic measurements were repeated. Pericardial closure reproducibly resulted in transient, moderate hemodynamic compromise in the first 8 hours after operation (Table 61-3). Although this and other studies have demonstrated adverse short-term hemodynamic consequences of pericardial closure, none have yet reported clinical evidence of worse outcomes.[61] Therefore, the risks of pericardial closure must be weighed against its potential benefits and clinical practice should be individualized to the patient.

OPERATIONS

Mediastinal Reexploration

Postoperative hemorrhage complicates approximately 3 to 5% of cardiac operations, a risk that nearly doubles in the setting of reoperations or valve surgery.[62] Common management for the postoperative cardiac surgical patient involves leaving the pericardium open and placing anterior and posterior mediastinal drains. Despite this, postoperative tamponade may still occur. The typical scenario involves declining chest tube output after a period of early postoperative bleeding, development of tachycardia, narrowing of the pulse pressure, increasing right-sided filling pressures, decreasing urine output, acidosis, escalating requirement for inotropes or vasopressors, and decreasing cardiac index. Echocardiography is not routinely helpful because the pericardial space and any associated thrombus may be difficult to visualize in the immediate postoperative period. Subtle echocardiographic findings that have been reported include an inspiratory increase in right ventricular end-diastolic diameter and a reciprocal decrease in left ventricular end-diastolic diameter,[63] as well as an increase in early peak tricuspid flow velocity and reduction in flow across the mitral valve.[64] Because postoperative hemorrhage and tamponade can precipitate rapid deterioration, expedient mediastinal drainage is imperative. The importance of simultaneous correction of coagulopathy, hypothermia, acidosis, and hypovolemia cannot be overstated.[65] Extreme circumstances may dictate that a temporizing decompression be performed in the intensive care unit (ICU) followed by definitive management in the operating room. Reported outcomes among patients explored in the ICU include perioperative survival of 85% and sternal wound infection rate as low as 2%.[66]

TABLE 61-3 Structural and Hemodynamic Changes after Pericardial Closure in Patients Undergoing Elective Isolated Coronary Artery Bypass Grafting

Parameters Measured	Open Pericardium	Closed Pericardium	*p*-value
Retrosternal space at 1 wk (cm)	13 ± 5	20 ± 7	.0003
Retrosternal space at 3 mo (cm)	7 ± 3	14 ± 7	.0001
CI L/min/m^2 1 h postoperation	3.1 ± 0.8	2.3 ± 0.6	.003
CI L/min/m^2 4 h postoperation	3.1 ± 0.9	2.7 ± 0.7	.156
CI L/min/m^2 8 h postoperation	3.0 ± 0.8	2.8 ± 0.5	.402
LVSWI g/m/m^2 1 h postoperation	72 ± 18	52 ± 13	.002
LVSWI g/m/m^2 4 h postoperation	68 ± 17	54 ± 8	.016
LVSWI g/m/m^2 8 h postoperation	62 ± 22	52 ± 10	.087

CI = cardiac index; LVSWI = left ventricular stroke work index.

During reexploration the first priority is to achieve prompt relief of tamponade by evacuating retained mediastinal blood and controlling sources of life-threatening hemorrhage. Dramatic hemodynamic improvement is frequently observed upon reopening the chest. Next, mediastinal reexploration is undertaken in a thorough and methodical manner with careful attention to all suture lines. Complete mediastinal evaluation should be performed even if the culprit source is thought to be identified. Inspection usually proceeds from top down while simultaneously obtaining hemostasis; this approach prevents "run-down" from obscuring small sources of bleeding. Copious warm saline irrigation and judicious use of gauze packing are helpful adjuncts.

Pericardiocentesis

Pericardiocentesis is usually performed in a procedure suite under fluoroscopic, sonographic, or computed tomographic guidance.[67] Arterial and right heart catheterizations are often performed for hemodynamic monitoring. After administration of 1% lidocaine to the skin and the deeper tissues of the left xiphocostal area, a 25-mL syringe is affixed to a three-way stopcock and then to an 18-gauge spinal needle. This pericardial needle is connected to an electrocardiograph V lead. Under electrocardiographic and imaging guidance, the needle is advanced from the left of the subxiphoid area aiming toward the left shoulder. ST-segment elevation may be seen on the V lead tracing when the needle touches the epicardium. Under these circumstances, the needle is retracted slightly until ST-segment elevation disappears. Once the pericardial space is entered, a guidewire is introduced into the pericardial space through the needle. The needle is removed and a catheter is inserted into the pericardial sac over the guidewire. At our institution, a pigtail-shaped drainage catheter with an end hole and multiple side holes is used. Intrapericardial pressure is measured by attaching a pressure transducer system to the intrapericardial catheter. Pericardial fluid may then be removed. Symptom relief may be immediate and dramatic. In the presence of pericardial tamponade, aspiration of fluid is continued until there is clear clinical and hemodynamic improvement. If blood is withdrawn, 5 mL should be placed on a sponge to see if it clots. Clotting blood suggests that the needle has either inadvertently entered a cardiac chamber or caused epicardial injury. Defibrinated blood that has been present in the pericardial space for even a short time usually does not clot. The pericardial space is drained every 8 hours and the catheter is flushed with heparinized solution and in general is removed within the next 24 to 72 hours. Pneumothorax is a potential complication, and chest radiography is mandatory after the procedure.

Pericardial Window

The purpose of partial pericardial resection (window) is to drain fluid into the pleural or peritoneal compartment to prevent reaccumulation. The procedure can be performed via thoracoscopy, anterior thoracotomy, or subxiphoid incision; although each approach has its unique merits, reported outcomes among the three are relatively similar.[68,69] General anesthesia may not be tolerated by some patients in tamponade, in which case the subxiphoid approach under local anesthesia in a semirecumbent position can be employed. When the pericardium is incised, fluid will invariably drain under pressure. The excised portion of pericardium should be as large as is feasible to prevent recurrence.[70] The surgeon should remain mindful of the rare possibility of cardiac prolapse. With the transthoracic or thoracoscopic approaches, all accessible pericardium ventral to the phrenic nerve should be excised. Similarly, via the subxiphoid approach, as much diaphragmatic pericardium should be excised as possible.

Pericardiectomy

Chronic pericardial constriction is treated by pericardial excision (Fig. 61-15). Because dense adhesions and calcification can penetrate into the myocardium, pericardial resection can be technically challenging. At most centers, the procedure is done via median sternotomy with the capability to use cardiopulmonary bypass as needed.[29] Practice is variable, as some use cardiopulmonary bypass routinely, whereas others prefer to avoid the additional burden of coagulopathy unless absolutely necessary. Also, some surgeons prefer the countertraction provided by the filled heart, which facilitates pericardial stripping. Some surgeons use a left anterior thoracotomy, the approach taken by Edward Churchill, who reported the first pericardiectomy for CP done in the United States.[71] The objective of the procedure is to release the ventricles from the densely adherent pericardial shell. The lack of a surgical plane can make this a bloody operation, and attention must be paid to salvage and reinfusion of blood. Epicardial coronary vessels are at risk in this dissection, and particular care must be taken when dissecting in the regions of these vessels. The goal is to excise all anterior pericardium between the phrenic nerves as well as the posterior pericardium around its reflection on the venae cavae and pulmonary veins. Complete resection should restore pressure-volume loops to their normal position. Complete pericardial resection is not feasible in all cases, notably with radiation-induced disease, and leaving densely adherent scar, particularly over the venae cavae and atria, may be safer for the patient.

The results vary with the etiology and severity of the disease. Operative mortality has been reported as high as 10 to 20%,[72] but is typically 5 to 6% in most contemporary series,[73] and varies based on severity of heart failure, elevation of right atrial pressure, and comorbidities.[74] Although surgery alleviates or improves symptoms in the vast majority of patients, long-term survival is diminished in patients who have had prior heart surgery, and particularly in patients with radiation-induced constrictive pericarditis (Fig. 61-16).[75]

KEY POINTS

- Tamponade occurs when intrapericardial pressure impedes cardiac filling, causing increased venous pressure, decreased cardiac output and progression to shock, and death if left untreated.
- Pericardial reserve volume is limited; therefore, acute fluid collections can rapidly produce tamponade.

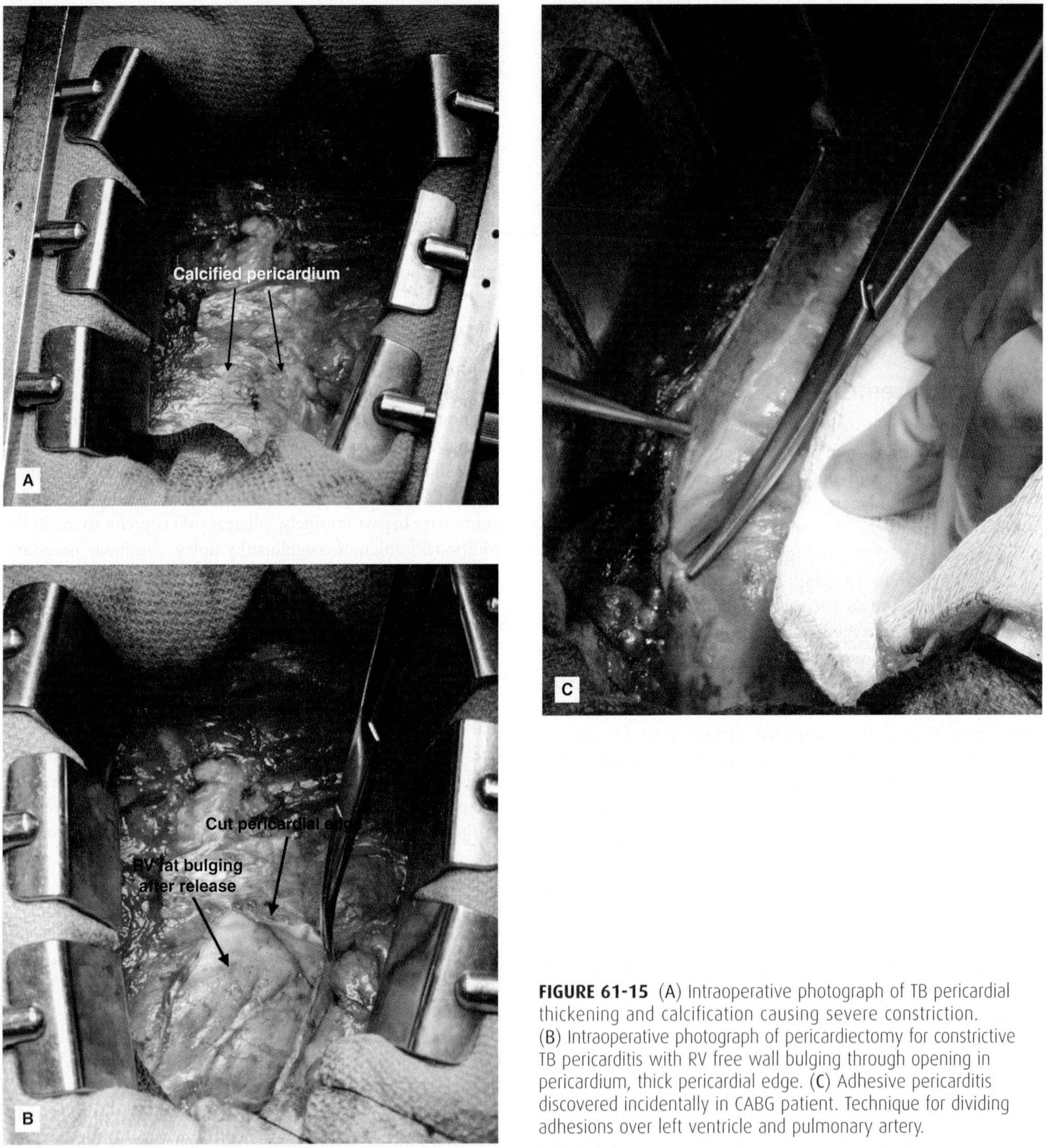

FIGURE 61-15 (A) Intraoperative photograph of TB pericardial thickening and calcification causing severe constriction. (B) Intraoperative photograph of pericardiectomy for constrictive TB pericarditis with RV free wall bulging through opening in pericardium, thick pericardial edge. (C) Adhesive pericarditis discovered incidentally in CABG patient. Technique for dividing adhesions over left ventricle and pulmonary artery.

- Constrictive pericarditis, the end result of several inflammatory conditions, is characterized by a prominent *y* descent, square-root sign, septal bounce, and exaggerated respiratory variation in right- and left-sided flows; it is best treated with pericardiectomy.
- Restrictive cardiomyopathy, a myocardial disorder causing diastolic heart failure, is differentiated from pericardial constriction by the presence of pulmonary hypertension, biatrial enlargement and ventricular thickening; it is not treated surgically.
- Patients with pericardial disease should undergo echocardiography supplemented as needed with catheter-based hemodynamic measurements or drainage for diagnosis.
- Acute pericarditis is often self-limited and responds to NSAIDs.
- The underlying disorder in secondary pericarditis can often be modified to improve the course of the associated pericardial disease.
- Intervention for postoperative hemorrhage and tamponade is required in less than 5% of cardiac surgical cases.

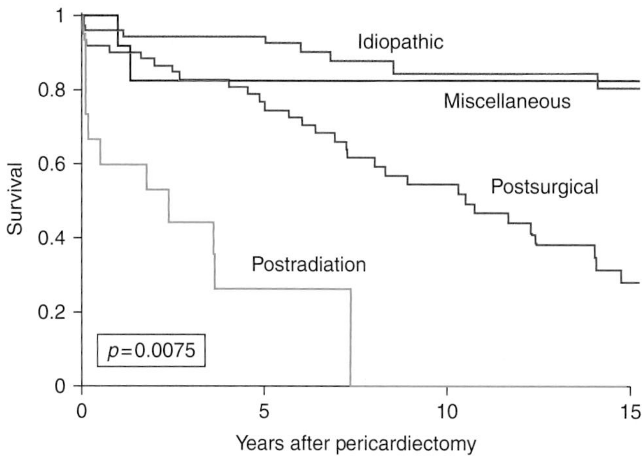

Number at risk

Idiopathic	75	48	30	21
Miscellaneous	12	10	10	5
Post-surgical	60	38	24	9
Post-radiation	15	6	0	0

FIGURE 61-16 Kaplan-Meier curve showing a significant difference (log-rank test, $p = .0075$) in overall survival of patients after pericardiectomy, based on the presumed cause of constrictive pericarditis. *(Reprinted with permission from Bertog S, Thambidorai S, Parakh K, et al: Constrictive pericarditis: etiology and cause-specific survival after pericardiectomy. J Am Coll Cardiol 2004; 43:1445.)*

It should be undertaken promptly (in the ICU if necessary) with concurrent correction of coagulopathy, hypovolemia, hypothermia, and acidosis.

- Pericardiectomy is associated with decreased short- and long-term survival because of the severity of associated illnesses.

ACKNOWLEDGMENT

The authors would like to thank Mark S. Adams for the preparation of the figures, echocardiographic images, and photographs for the chapter.

REFERENCES

1. Spodick DH: The normal and diseased pericardium: current concepts of pericardial physiology, diseases and treatment. *J Am Coll Cardiol* 1983; 1:240.
2. Hammond HK, White FC, Bhargava V, et al: Heart size and maximal cardiac output are limited by the pericardium. *Am J Physiol* 1992; 263:H1675.
3. Santamore WP, Dell'Italia LJ: Ventricular interdependence: significant left ventricular contributions to right ventricular systolic function. *Prog Cardiovasc Dis* 1990; 40:298.
4. Barcin C, Olcay A, Kocaoglu M, Atac K, Kursaklioglu H: Asymptomatic congenital pericardial defect: an aspect of diagnostic modalities and treatment. Case Report. *Anadolu Kardiyol Derg* 2006; (6):387.
5. Spodick DH: Congenital abnormalities of the pericardium, in Spodick DH (ed): *The Pericardium: A Comprehensive Textbook.* New York, Marcel Dekker, 1997; p 65.
6. Risher WH, Rees AD, Ochsner JL, et al: Thoracoscopic resection of pericardium for symptomatic congenital pericardial defect. *Ann Thorac Surg* 1993;56:1390.
7. Drury NE, DeSilva RJ, Hall RMO, Large SR: Congenital defects of the pericardium. *Ann Thorac Surg* 2007;83:1552-1553.
8. Kraev A, Komanapalli B, Schipper PH, Sukumar MS: Pericardial cyst. *CTSNet* 2006;16:1-4.
9. Barva GL, Magliani L, Bertoli D, et al: Complicated pericardial cyst: atypical anatomy and clinical course. *Clin Cardiol* 1998; 21:862.
10. Lau CL, Davis RD: The mediastinum, in *Sabiston's Textbook of Surgery*, 17th ed. Philadelphia, Elsevier, 2004, pp; 1738-1739, 1758.
11. Patel J, Park C, Michaels J, Rosen S, Kort S: Pericardial cyst: case reports and a literature review. *Echocardiography* 2004;21:269-272.
12. Weder W, Klotz HP, Segesser LV, et al: Thoracoscopic resection of a pericardial cyst. *J Thorac Cardiovasc Surg* 1994; 107:313.
13. Little WC, Freeman GL: Pericardial disease. *Circulation* 2006; 113:1622.
14. Spodick DH: Acute cardiac tamponade. *NEJM* 2003; 349:684.
15. Spodick DH: Pathophysiology of cardiac tamponade. *Chest* 1998; 113:1372.
16. Reddy PS, Curtiss EI, Uretsky BF: Spectrum of hemodynamic changes in cardiac tamponade. *Am J Cardiol* 1990; 66:1487.
17. Sagrista-Sauleda J, Angel J, Sambola A, et al: Low-pressure cardiac tamponade: clinical and hemodynamic profile. *Circulation* 2006; 114:945.
18. Maisch B, Seferovic PM, Ristic AD, et al: Guidelines on the diagnosis and management of pericardial diseases executive summary: the task force on the diagnosis and management of pericardial diseases of the European society of cardiology. *Eur Heart J* 2004; 25:587
19. Ling LH, Oh JK, Schaff HV, et al: Constrictive pericarditis in the modern era: evolving clinical spectrum and impact on outcome after pericardiectomy. *Circulation* 1999; 100:1380.
20. Myers RBH, Spodick DH: Constrictive pericarditis: clinical and pathophysiologic characteristics. *Am Heart J* 1999; 138:219.
21. Godwin C, Kesavan S, Flamm SD, Sivananthan MU: Role of MRI in clinical cardiology. *Lancet* 2004; 363:2162.
22. Talreja DR, Edwards WD, Danielson GK, et al: Constrictive pericarditis in 26 patients with histologically normal pericardial thickness. *Circulation* 2003; 108:1852.
23. Troughton RW, Asher CR, Klein AL: Pericarditis. *Lancet* 2004; 363:717.
24. Chinnaiyan KM, Leff CB, Marsalese DL: Constrictive pericarditis versus restrictive cardiomyopathy: challenges in diagnosis and management. *Cardiol Rev* 2004; 12:314.
25. Hurrell DG, Nishimura RA, Higano ST, et al: Value of dynamic respiratory changes in left and right ventricular pressures for the diagnosis of constrictive pericarditis. *Circulation* 1996; 93:2007.
26. *Pericarditis: Cardiovascular Disorders.* Merck Manual Professional. 2010; 1-9.
27. Koster N, Narmi A, Anand K: Bacterial pericarditis. *Am J Med* 2009; 122-5:e1-e2.
28. Mayosi BM, Burgess LJ, Doubell AF: Tuberculous pericarditis. *Circulation* 2005; 112:3608.
29. Tirilomis T, Univerdoben S, von der Emde J: Pericardiectomy for chronic constrictive pericarditis: risks and outcome. *Eur J Thorac Cardiovasc Surg* 1994; 8:487.
30. Bright R: Tabular view of the morbid appearance in 100 cases connected with albuminous urine: with observations. *Guys Hosp Rep* 1836; 1:380.
31. Alpert MA, Ravenscraft MD: Pericardial involvement in end-stage renal disease. *Am J Med Sci* 2003; 325:228.
32. Banerjee A, Davenport A: Changing patterns of pericardial disease in patients with end-stage renal disease. *Hemodial Int* 2006; 10:249.
33. Leehey DJ, Daugirdas JT, Ing TS: Early drainage of pericardial effusions in patients with dialysis pericarditis. *Arch Intern Med* 1983; 143:1673.
34. Zakynthinos E, Theodorakopoulou M, Daniil, Z, et al: Hemorrhagic cardiac tamponade in critically ill patients with acute renal failure. *Heart Lung* 2004; 33:55.
35. Rutsky EA: Treatment of uremic pericarditis and pericardial effusion. *Am J Kidney Dis* 1987; 10:2.
36. Rheuban KS: Pericarditis. *Curr Treat Options Cardiovasc Med* 2005; 7:419.
37. Oates JA, Wilkinson GR: Principles of drug therapy, in Isselbacher KJ, Braunwald E, Wilson JD, et al (eds): *Harrison's Principles of Internal Medicine.* New York, McGraw-Hill, 1994; p 409.
38. Turesson C, Lacobsson L. Bergstrom U: Extra-articular rheumatoid arthritis: prevalence and mortality. *Rheumatology* 1999; 38:668.
39. Gulati S, Kumar L: Cardiac tamponade as an initial manifestation of systemic lupus erythematosus in early childhood. *Ann Rheum Dis* 1992; 51:179.
40. Harle P, Salzberger B, Gluck T, et al: Fatal outcome of constrictive pericarditis in rheumatoid arthritis. *Rheumatol Int* 2003; 23:312.
41. Kabadi UM, Kumer SP: Pericardial effusion in primary hypothyroidism. *Am Heart J* 1990; 120:1393.
42. Gupta R, Munyak J, Haydock T, et al: Hypothyroidism presenting as acute cardiac tamponade with viral pericarditis. *Am J Emerg Med* 1999; 17:176.
43. Stewart JR, Fajardo LF: Radiation induced heart disease: an update. *Prog Cardiovasc Dis* 1984; 27:173.
44. Lee PJ, Malli R: Cardiovascular effects of radiation therapy: practical approach to radiation induced heart disease. *Cardiol Rev* 2005; 13:80.

45. Bertog SC, Thambidorai SK, Parakh K, et al: Constrictive pericarditis: etiology and cause-specific survival after pericardiectomy. *J Am Coll Cardiol* 2004; 43:1445.
46. Spodick DH: Neoplastic pericardial disease, in Spodick DH (ed): *The Pericardium: A Comprehensive Textbook.* New York, Marcel Dekker, 1997; p 301.
47. Warren MH: Malignancies involving the pericardium. *Semin Thorac Cardiovasc Surg* 2000; 12:119.
48. Gornik HL, Gerhard-Herman M, Beckman JA: Abnormal cytology predicts poor prognosis in cancer patients with pericardial effusion. *J Clin Oncol* 2005; 23:5211.
49. Wang HJ, Hsu KL, Chiang FT, et al: Technical and prognostic outcomes of double-balloon pericardiotomy for large malignancy-related pericardial effusions. *Chest* 2002; 122:893.
50. Hazelrigg SR, Mack MJ, Landreneau RJ, et al: Thoracoscopic pericardiectomy for effusive pericardial disease. *Ann Thorac Surg* 1993; 56:792.
51. Bahner D, Blaivas M, Cohen HL, et al: AIUM Practice guideline for the performance of the Focused Assessment with Sonography for Trauma (FAST) Examination. *J Ultrasound Med* 2008; 27:313.
52. Schultz JM, Trunkey DD: Blunt cardiac injury. *Crit Care Clin* 2004; 20:57.
53. Tenenbaum A, Koren-Morag N, Spodick DH, et al: The efficacy of colchicine in the treatment of recurrent pericarditis related to postcardiac injury (postpericardiotomy and postinfarcted) syndrome: a multicenter analysis. *Heart Drug* 2004; 4:141.
54. Imazio M, Bobbio M, Cecchi E, et al: Colchicine in addition to conventional therapy for acute pericarditis: results of the COlchicine for acute PEricarditis (COPE) Trial. *Circulation* 2005; 112:2012.
55. Imazio M, Brucato A, Cumetti D et al: Corticosteroids for recurrent pericarditis—high versus low doses: a nonrandomized observation. *Circulation* 2008; 118:667.
56. Zeltser I, Rhodes LA, Tanel RE, et al: Postpericardiotomy syndrome after permanent pacemaker implantation in children and young adults. *Ann Thorac Surg* 2004; 78:1684.
57. Lange RA, Hillis D: Acute pericarditis. *NEJM* 2004; 351:2195.
58. Ionescu A: Localized pericardial tamponade: difficult echocardiographic diagnosis of a are complication after cardiac surgery. *J Am Soc Echocardiogr* 2005; 14:220.
59. Mangi AA, Palacios IF, Torchiana DF: Catheter pericardiocentesis for delayed tamponade after cardiac valve operation. *Ann Thorac Surg* 2002; 73:1479.
60. Rao W, Komeda M, Weisel RD, et al: Should the pericardium be closed routinely after heart operations? *Ann Thorac Surg* 1999; 67:484.
61. Bittar MN, Barnard JB, Khasati N, et al: Should the pericardium be closed in patients undergoing cardiac surgery? *Interact Cardiovasc Thorac Surg* 2005; 4:151.
62. Moulton MJ, Creswell LL, Mackey ME, et al: Reexploration for bleeding is a risk factor for adverse outcomes after cardiac operations. *J Thorac Cardiol Surg* 1996; 111:1037.
63. Gonzalez MS, Basnight MA, Appleton CP: Experimental cardiac tamponade: hemodynamic and Doppler echocardiographic reexamination of right and left heart ejection dynamics to the phase of respiration. *J Am Coll Cardiol* 1991; 18:243.
64. Appleton C, Hatle LK, Popp RL: Cardiac tamponade and pericardial effusion: respiratory variation in transvalvular flow velocities during experimental cardiac tamponade. *J Am Coll Cardiol* 1988; 11:1020.
65. Makar M, Taylor J, Zhao M, et al: Perioperative coagulopathy, bleeding, and hemostasis during cardiac surgery: a comprehensive review. *ICU Director* 2010; 1:17.
66. Fiser SM, Tribble CG, Kern JA, et al: Cardiac reoperation in the intensive care unit. *Ann Thorac Surg* 2001; 71:1888.
67. Ashikhmina EA, Schaff HV, Sinak LJ, et al: Pericardial effusion after cardiac surgery: risk factors, patient profiles, and contemporary management. *Ann Thorac Surg* 2010; 89:112.
68. O'Brien PK, Kucharczuk JC, Marshall MB, et al: Comparative study of subxiphoid versus video-thoracoscopic pericardial "window." *Ann Thorac Surg* 2005; 80:2013.
69. Liberman M, Labos C, Sampalis JS, et al: Ten-year surgical experience with nontraumatic pericardial effusions: a comparison between the subxiphoid and transthoracic approaches to pericardial window. *Arch Surg* 2005; 140:191.
70. Georghiou GP, Stamler A, Sharoni E, et al: Video-assisted thoracoscopic pericardial window for diagnosis and management of pericardial effusions. *Ann Thorac Surg* 2005; 80:607.
71. Churchill ED: Decortication of the heart for adhesive pericarditis. *Arch Surg* 1929; 19:1447.
72. Seifert FC, Miller DC, Oesterle SN, et al: Surgical treatment of constrictive pericarditis: analysis of outcome and diagnostic error. *Circulation* 1985; 72 (3 Pt 2):II264.
73. Schwefer M, Aschenbach R, Hidemann J, et al: Constrictive pericarditis, still a diagnostic challenge: comprehensive review of clinical management. *Eur J Cardiothorac Surg* 2009; 36:502.
74. Ha JW, Oh JK, Schaff HV et al: Impact of left ventricular function on immediate and long-term outcomes after pericardiectomy in constrictive pericarditis. *J Thorac Cardiovasc Surg* 2008; 136:1136
75. Bertog S, Thambidorai S, Parakh K, et al: Constrictive pericarditis: etiology and cause-specific survival after pericardiectomy. *J Am Coll Cardiol* 2004; 43:1445.

CHAPTER 62

Cardiac Neoplasms

Shanda H. Blackmon
Michael J. Reardon

INTRODUCTION

Neoplasms of the heart can be divided into primary cardiac tumors arising in the heart and secondary cardiac tumors from metastasis. Primary cardiac tumors can be further stratified into benign and malignant tumors. Between 10 and 20% of patients dying of disseminated cancer have metastatic involvement of the heart or pericardium.[1,2] Surgical resection is seldom possible or advisable for these tumors, and intervention usually is limited to drainage of malignant pericardial effusions and/or diagnostic biopsies.

The incidence of primary cardiac neoplasm ranges between 0.17 and 0.19% in unselected autopsy series.[3-5] Seventy-five percent of primary cardiac tumors are benign, and 25% are malignant.[2,6] Fifty percent of the benign tumors are myxomas, and 75% of malignant tumors are sarcomas.[2,6] The clinical incidence of these tumors is 1 in 500 cardiac surgical patients. With the exception of myxomas, most surgeons will rarely encounter primary cardiac tumors. The purpose of this chapter is to summarize useful information for the evaluation and management of patients with cardiac tumors and to provide a reference for additional study.

HISTORICAL BACKGROUND

A primary cardiac neoplasm was first described by Realdo Colombo in 1559.[7] Alden Allen Burns of Edinburgh described a cardiac neoplasm and suggested valvular obstruction by an atrial tumor in 1809.[8] A series of six atrial tumors, with characteristics we now recognize as myxoma, was published in 1845 by King.[9] In 1931, Yates reported nine cases of primary cardiac tumor and established a classification system similar to what we use today.[10] The first antemortem diagnosis of a cardiac tumor was made in 1934 when Barnes diagnosed a cardiac sarcoma using electrocardiography and biopsy of a metastatic lymph node.[11] In 1936, Beck successfully resected a teratoma external to the right ventricle,[12] and Mauer removed a left ventricular lipoma in 1951.[13] Treatment of cardiac tumors was profoundly influenced by two events: the introduction of cardiopulmonary bypass in 1953 by John Gibbon, which allowed a safe and reproducible approach to the cardiac chambers, and the introduction of cardiac echocardiography, which allowed safe and noninvasive diagnosis of an intracardiac mass. The first echocardiographic diagnosis of an intracardiac tumor was made in 1959.[14] An intracardiac myxoma was diagnosed by angiography in 1952 by Goldberg, but attempts at surgical removal were unsuccessful.[9] A large right atrial myxoma was removed by Bhanson in 1952 using caval inflow occlusion, but the patient died 24 days later.[15] Crafoord in Sweden first successfully removed a left atrial myxoma in 1954 using cardiopulmonary bypass,[16] and Kay in Los Angeles first removed a left ventricular myxoma in 1959.[17] By 1964, 60 atrial myxomas had been removed successfully, with improved results owing to the increasing safety of cardiopulmonary bypass and use of echocardiography for detection. Operations are currently performed routinely on patients with atrial myxoma with minimal mortality.[6,18–21] Primary malignant tumors, however, continue to represent a challenge.

CLASSIFICATION

A pathologic classification is listed in Table 62-1. Mural thrombus is listed as a pseudotumor, although not really a cardiac tumor, its presentation may mimic myxoma clinically and pathologically. Most mural thrombi are associated with underlying valvular disease, myocardial infarction, dysfunction, or atrial fibrillation.[22] Mural thrombi also have been noted in

TABLE 62-1 Types of Cardiac Tumors by Pathology

Pseudotumors
- Mural thrombi

Heterotopias and Tumors of Ectopic Tissue
- Tumors of the atrioventricular nodal region
- Teratoma
- Ectopic thyroid

Tumors of Mesenchymal Tissue
- Hamartoma of endocardial tissue
  - Papillary fibroelastoma
- Hamartomas of Cardiac Muscle
  - Rhabdomyoma
  - Histiocytoid cardiomyopathy (Purkinje cell hamartoma)

Tumors and Neoplasms of Fat
- Lipomatous hypertrophy, interarterial septum
- Lipoma
- Liposarcoma

Tumors and Neoplasms of Fibrous and Myofibroblastic Tissue
- Fibroma
- Inflammatory pseudotumor (inflammatory myofibroblastic tumor)
- Sarcomas (malignant fibrous histiocytoma, fibrosarcoma, leiomyosarcoma)

Vascular Tumors and Neoplasms
- Hemangioma
- Epithelioid hemangioendothelioma
- Angiosarcoma

Neoplasm of Uncertain Histogenesis
- Myxoma

Neoplasms of neural tissue
- Granular cell tumor
- Schwannoma/neurofibroma

Paraganglioma
Malignant schwannoma/neurofibrosarcoma (rare)
Malignant Lymphoma
Malignant Mesothelioma
Metastatic Tumors to the Heart

hypercoagulable syndromes, particularly antiphospholipid syndrome.[23] With increasing use of long-term central catheters, we have seen several right atrial masses that were difficult to define and upon removal were mural thrombi.

Heterotopias and tumors of ectopic tissue include cystic tumors of the atrioventricular node consisting of multiple benign cysts in the region of the atrioventricular node that can cause heart block or sudden death. Most are diagnosed at autopsy, but a biopsy diagnosis of atrioventricular nodal tumor has been reported.[24] Germ cell tumors of the heart usually are teratomas, occurring within the pericardial sac, but yolk sac tumors have been described in infants and children.[25] Ectopic thyroid tissue may occur within the myocardium and is referred to as *struma cordis*. Right ventricular outflow track obstruction may be present, but most patients are asymptomatic.

Most of the remaining tumors arise in the mesenchymal, fat, fibrous, neural, or vascular cells of the heart, with myxoma representing a tumor of undetermined histogenesis. Primary cardiac lymphoma, mesothelioma, and metastatic tumors to the heart represent the remaining pathologic categories that comprise the greater part of this chapter.

PRIMARY BENIGN TUMORS

Myxoma

Myxomata comprise 50% of all benign cardiac tumors in adults and 15% of such tumors in children. Occurrence during infancy is rare (Tables 62-2 and 62-3). A vast majority of myxomas occur sporadically and tend to be more common in women.[4,21] The peak incidence is between the third and sixth decades of life, and 94% of tumors are solitary.[26] Approximately 75% occur in the left atrium[28] and 10 to 20% occur in the right atrium. The remaining proportion are equally distributed between the ventricles.[2] The deoxyribonucleic acid (DNA) genotype of sporadic myxomas is normal in 80% of patients.[27] Myxomas are unlikely to be associated with other abnormal conditions and have a low recurrence rate.[4,28]

About 5% of myxoma patients show a familial pattern of tumor development based on autosomal dominant inheritance.[29,37,38] These patients and 20% of those with sporadic myxoma have an abnormal DNA genotype chromosomal pattern.[27] In contrast to the "typical" sporadic myxoma profile, familial patients are more likely to be younger, equally likely to be male or female, and more often (22%) have multicentric tumors originating from either the atrium or ventricle.[30-34] Although familial myxomas have the same histology, they have a higher recurrence rate after surgical resection (21 to 67%).[28,35] Approximately 20% of familial patients have associated conditions such as adrenocortical

TABLE 62-2 Benign Cardiac Neoplasms in Adults

Tumor	No.	Percentage
Myxoma	118	49
Lipoma	45	19
Papillary fibroelastoma	42	17
Hemangioma	11	5
AV node mesothelioma	9	4
Fibroma	5	2
Teratoma	3	1
Granular cell tumor	3	1
Neurofibroma	2	<1
Lymphangioma	2	<1
Rhabdomyoma	1	<1
Total	241	100

Source: Reproduced with permission from McAllister HA Jr, Fenoglio JJ Jr: Tumors of the cardiovascular system, in Atlas of Tumor Pathology. Washington, DC, Armed Forces Institute of Pathology; 1978, fas. 15.

TABLE 62-3 Benign Cardiac Neoplasms in Children

	0–1-year-olds		1–15-year-olds	
Tumor	Number	Percentage	Number	Percentage
Rhabdomyoma	28	62	35	45.0
Teratoma	9	21	11	14.0
Fibroma	6	13	12	15.5
Hemangioma	1	2	4	5.0
AV node mesothelioma	1	2	3	4.0
Myxoma	—	—	12	15.5
Neurofibroma	—	—	1	1.0
Total	45	100	78	100

Source: Reproduced with permission from McAllister HA Jr, Fenoglio JJ Jr: Tumors of the cardiovascular system, in Atlas of Tumor Pathology. Washington, DC, Armed Forces Institute of Pathology; 1978, fas. 15.

nodule hyperplasia, Sertoli cell tumors of the testes, pituitary tumors, multiple myxoid breast fibroadenomas, cutaneous myomas, and facial or labial pigmented spots.[26,35] These conditions often are described as *complex myxomas* within the group of familial myxoma.[27] A familial syndrome with autosomal X-linked inheritance characterized by primary pigmented nodular adrenocortical disease with hypercortisolism, cutaneous pigmentous lentigines, and cardiac myxoma is referred to as *Carney's complex.*[26,35]

Pathology

Both biatrial and multicentric myxomas are more common in familial disease. Biatrial tumors probably arise from bidirectional growth of a tumor originating within the atrial septum.[36] Atrial myxomas generally arise from the interatrial septum at the border of the fossa ovalis but can originate anywhere within the atrium, including the appendage.[4] In addition, isolated reports confirm that myxomas can arise from the cardiac valves, pulmonary artery and vein, and vena cava.[37,38] Right atrial myxomas are more likely to have broad-based attachments than left atrial tumors; they also are more likely to be calcified,[32] and thus visible on chest radiographs. Ventricular myxomas occur more often in women and children and may be multicentric.[2,39] Right ventricular tumors typically arise from the free wall, and left ventricular tumors tend to originate in the proximity of the posterior papillary muscle.

Grossly, about two-thirds of myxomas are round or oval tumors with a smooth or lobulated surface (Fig. 62-1).[21] Most are polypoid, compact, pedunculated, mobile, and not likely to fragment spontaneously.[2,4] Mobility depends on stalk length, the extent of attachment to the heart, and the amount of tumor collagen.[4] Most are pedunculated with a short, broad base, and sessile forms are unusual.[2,40] Less common villous or papillary myxomas are gelatinous and fragile and prone to fragmentation and embolization, occurring about one-third of the time.[21,41] Myxomas are white, yellow, or brown in color, and are frequently covered with thrombus.[2] Focal areas of hemorrhage, cyst formation, or necrosis may be seen in cut section. The average size is about 5 cm in diameter, but growth to 15 cm in diameter and larger has been reported.[4] Myxomatous tumors appear to grow rapidly, but growth rates vary, and occasionally, tumor growth arrests spontaneously.[4] Weights range from 8 to 175 g, with a mean between 50 and 60 g.[5]

Histologically, myxomas are composed of polygonal-shaped cells and capillary channels within an acid mucopolysaccharide matrix.[4] The cells appear singularly or in small clusters throughout the matrix, and mitoses are rare.[42,51] The matrix also contains occasional smooth muscle cells, reticulocytes, collagen, elastin fibers, and a few blood cells. Cyst, areas of hemorrhage, and foci of extramedullary hematopoiesis are also found.[35,41] Ten percent of the tumors have microscopic deposits of calcium and metastatic bone deposits, as well as sometimes glandular-like structures.[35,41] The base of the tumor contains a large artery and veins that connect with the subendocardium but do not

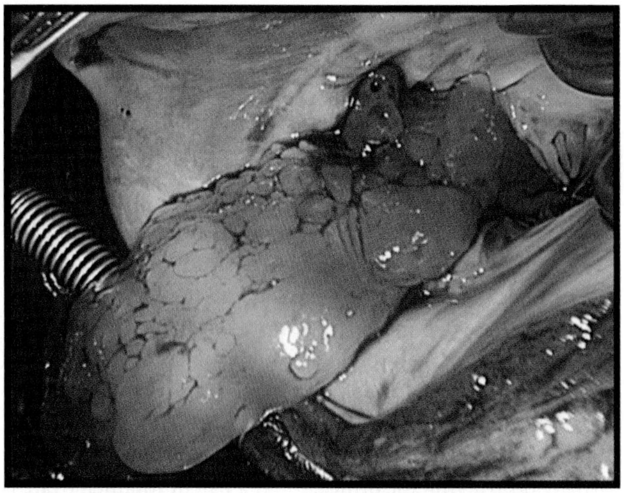

FIGURE 62-1 Large in situ left atrial myxoma as seen from the surgeon's perspective just before removal.

typically extend deep beyond the subendocardium.[35] A coronary angiography in our own institution revealed a large feeding vessel and was suspected originally of being an angiosarcoma but on histology proved to be a typical benign myxoma. Myxomas tend to grow into the overlying cardiac cavity rather than into the surrounding myocardium. Myxomas arise from the endocardium and are considered derivative of the subendocardial multipotential mesenchymal cell.[43,44,45] This accounts for the occasional presence of hematopoietic tissue and bone in these tumors. Interestingly, myxomas have developed after cardiac trauma, including repair of atrial septal defects and trans-septal puncture for percutaneous dilatation of the mitral valve.

Clinical Presentation

The classic clinical presentation of a myxoma is intracardiac obstruction with congestive heart failure (67%); signs of embolization (29%); systemic or constitutional symptoms of fever (19%); weight loss or fatigue (17%); and immunologic manifestations of myalgia, weakness, and arthralgia (5%).[21] Cardiac rhythm disturbances and infection occur less frequently.

Constitutional Symptoms. Nearly all myxoma patients admit to a variety of constitutional symptoms. These complaints may be accompanied by a leukocytosis, elevated erythrocyte levels and sedimentation rate, hemolytic anemia, thrombocytopenia, and elevated C-reactive protein. Immunoelectrophoresis may reveal abnormal immunoglobulin levels with increased circulating IgG.[46] The recent discovery of elevated levels of interleukin-6 in patients with myxoma has been linked to a variety of associated conditions, including lymphadenopathy, tumor metastasis, ventricular hypertrophy, and development of constitutional symptoms.[39,47,48] Other less frequent complaints include Raynaud's phenomenon, arthralgias, myalgias, erythematous rash, and clubbing of the digits.[4,49]

Possible etiologies of such varied complaints and symptoms include tumor embolization with secondary myalgias and arthralgias and elevated immunoglobulin response.[50] Circulating antibody–tumor antigen complexes with complement activation also may play a role.[51] Such symptom complexes tend to resolve following surgical resection of the tumor.[52]

Obstruction. Obstruction of blood flow in the heart is the most common cause of acute presenting symptoms. The nature of these symptoms is determined by which of the chambers is involved and the size of the tumor. Myxomas in the left atrium tend to mimic mitral disease. These produce positional dyspnea and other signs and symptoms of heart failure associated with elevated left atrial and pulmonary venous pressures. Clinically, mitral stenosis often is suspected and leads to echocardiography and diagnosis of myxoma. Syncopal episodes occur in some patients and are thought to result from temporary occlusion of the mitral orifice.[32,53] Right atrial myxomas can produce a clinical picture of right-sided heart failure with signs and symptoms of venous hypertension, including hepatomegaly, ascites, and dependent edema and can cause tricuspid valve stenosis by partially obstructing the orifice.[32,53] If a patent foramen ovale is present, right-to-left atrial shunting may occur with central cyanosis, and paradoxical embolization has been reported.[54] Large ventricular myxomas may mimic ventricular outflow obstruction. The left ventricular myxoma may produce the equivalent of subaortic or aortic valvular stenosis,[54,55] whereas right ventricular myxomas can simulate right ventricular outflow track or pulmonic valve obstruction.

Embolization. Systemic embolization is the second most common mode of myxomatous presentation, occurring in 30 to 40% of patients.[2,4,32] Because the majority of myxomas are left-sided, approximately 50% of embolic episodes affect the central nervous system owing to both intra- and extracranial vascular obstruction. The neurologic deficits following embolization can be transient but are often permanent.[56] Specific central nervous system consequences include intracranial aneurysms, seizures, hemiparesis, and brain necrosis.[57–59] Retinal artery embolization with visual loss has occurred in some patients.[60]

Embolic myxomatous material has been found blocking iliac and femoral arteries.[61–62] Other sites of tumor embolization include abdominal viscera and the renal and coronary arteries.[63] Histologic examination of surgically removed peripheral myxoma that has embolized provides the diagnosis of an otherwise unsuspected tumor.[32] Renal artery specimens from a nephrectomy have shown viable enlarging embolic myxoma after excision of the primary tumor. Right-sided myxomatous emboli mainly obstruct pulmonary arteries and cause pulmonary hypertension and even death from acute obstruction.[4,54]

Infection. Infection arising in a myxoma is a rare complication and produces a clinical picture of infectious endocarditis.[64,65] Infection increases the likelihood of systemic embolization,[4] and an infected myxoma warrants urgent surgical resection.

Diagnosis

Clinical Examination. Findings at the time of clinical assessment of a patient with cardiac myxoma vary according to the size, location, and mobility of the tumor. Left atrial myxomas may produce auscultatory or clinical findings similar to mitral disease. The well-described "tumor plop" can be confused with a third heart sound,[66] occurring just after the opening snap of the mitral valve created from contact between the tumor and endocardial wall.[66] Left atrial myxomas that cause partial obstruction of left ventricular filling may result in elevated pulmonary vascular pressures with augmentation of the pulmonary component of the second heart sound.[67]

Right atrial myxomas may produce similar auscultatory findings as left atrial myxomas with the exception that they are best heard along the lower right sternal border rather than at the cardiac apex. In addition, right atrial hypertension may produce a large *a* wave in the jugular venous pulse and, when severe, may mimic superior vena caval syndrome.

Chest Radiograph and Electrocardiogram. The findings on chest roentgenogram may include generalized cardiomegaly, individual cardiac chamber enlargement, and pulmonary venous congestion. More specific rare findings are density within the cardiac silhouette caused by calcification within the tumor (see Fig. 62-3) occurring more often with right-sided myxomas.[4]

Electrocardiographic Findings. Nonspecific abnormalities such as chamber enlargement, cardiomegaly, bundle-branch blocks, and axis deviation can be found.[68] Fewer than 20% of patients have atrial fibrillation.[39] Evaluation of nonspecific electrocardiographic abnormalities occasionally leads to an incidental diagnosis of myxoma most electrocardiograms are not helpful in establishing a diagnosis.

Echocardiography. Cross-sectional echocardiography is the most useful test employed for the diagnosis and evaluation of myxoma. The sensitivity of two-dimensional (2-D) echocardiography for myxoma is 100%, and this imaging technique largely has supplanted angiocardiography.[69] However, coronary angiography usually is performed in myxoma patients more than 40 years of age to rule out significant coronary disease. Transesophageal echocardiography (TEE) provides the best information concerning tumor size, location, mobility, and attachment.[70]

Transesophageal echocardiograms detect tumors as small as 1 to 3 mm in diameter.[71] Most surgeons obtain a transesophageal echocardiogram in the operating room before the operation (Fig. 62-2). We particularly evaluate the posterior left atrial wall, atrial septum, and right atrium, which often are not well displayed on transthoracic examination, to exclude the possibility of biatrial multiple tumors. Additionally, post operative TEE ensures a normal echocardiogram before leaving the operating room.

Computed Tomography and Magnetic Resonance Imaging. Although myxomas have been identified using computed tomography (CT),[69,72] this modality is most useful in malignant tumors of the heart because of its ability to demonstrate myocardial invasion and tumor involvement of adjacent structures.[68] Similarly, magnetic resonance imaging (MRI) has been employed in the diagnosis of myxomas and may yield a clear picture of tumor size, shape, and surface characteristics.[68–72]

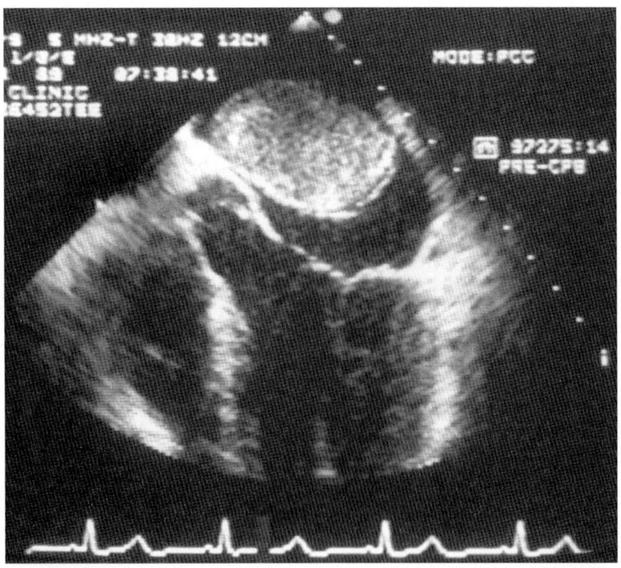

FIGURE 62-2 Transesophageal echocardiogram of a giant left atrial myxoma that does not appear attached to the mitral valve.

MRI is particularly useful in detecting intracardiac and pericardial extension, invasion of malignant secondary tumors, and the evaluation of ventricular masses that occasionally turn out to be myxoma. Both CT and MRI detect tumors as small as 0.5 to 1.0 cm and provide information regarding the composition of the tumor.[4] Neither CT nor MRI is needed for atrial myxomas if an adequate echocardiogram is available. The exception is the occasional right atrial myxoma that extends into one or both caval or tricuspid orifices. CT or MRI should be reserved for the situation in which the diagnosis or characterization of the tumor is unclear after complete echocardiographic evaluation.

Surgical Management

Surgical resection is the only effective therapeutic option for patients with cardiac myxoma and should not be delayed because death from obstruction to flow within the heart or embolization may occur in as many as 8% of patients awaiting operation.[73] A median sternotomy approach with ascending aortic and bicaval cannulation usually is employed. Manipulation of the heart before initiation of cardiopulmonary bypass is minimized in deference to the known friability and embolic tendency of myxomas. In the event of preoperative known cerebral embolization without hemorrhage, the tumor should be resected approximately seven days after the event to prevent further embolization and yet allow time for stabilization of the brain for cardiopulmonary bypass. For left atrial myxomas, the venae cavae are cannulated through the right atrial wall, with the inferior cannula placed close and laterally to the inferior vena cava–right atrial junction. Caval snares are always used to allow opening of the right atrium, if necessary. If extensive exposure of the left atrium is needed or a malignant left atrial tumor is suspected, we mobilize and directly cannulate the superior vena cava, which allows it to be transected if necessary for additional exposure. Body temperature is allowed to drift down, but there is no attempt to induce systemic hypothermia unless the need for reduced perfusion flow is anticipated. Modern cardioplegic techniques yield a quiet operative field and protect the myocardium from ischemic injury during aortic cross-clamping. Cardiopulmonary bypass is started, and the aorta is clamped before manipulation of the heart.

Exposure of left atrial myxomas is maximized by using several principles from mitral valve repair surgery. The surgeon desires the right side of the heart to rotate up and the left side of the heart to rotate down. Therefore, stay sutures are placed low on the pericardium on the right side, and no pericardial stay sutures are placed on the left before placing the chest retractor. This rotates the heart for optimal exposure of both the right and, particularly, the left atrium (Fig. 62-3). For left atrial tumors, the superior vena cava is mobilized extensively, as is the inferior vena cava–right atrial junction, allowing increased mobility and exposing the left atrial cavity. Left atrial myxomas can be approached by an incision through the anterior wall of the left atrium anterior to the right pulmonary veins (Fig. 62-4). This incision can be extended behind both cavae for greater exposure (Fig. 62-5). Exposure and removal of large tumors attached to the interatrial septum may be aided by a second incision parallel to the first in the right atrium. This biatrial

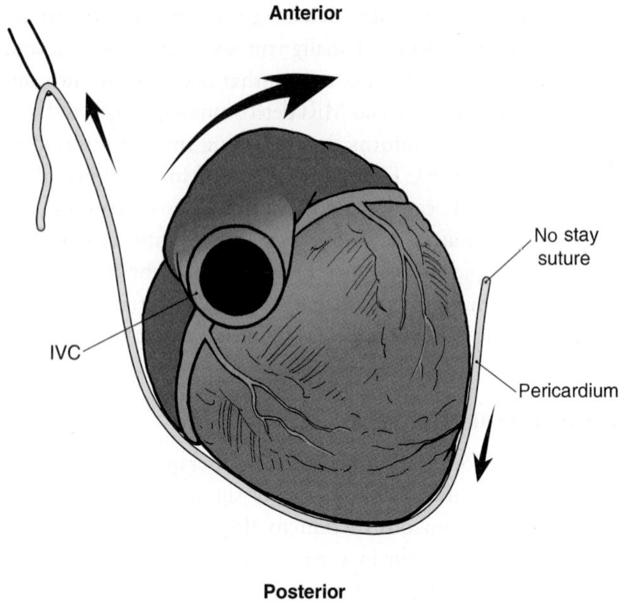

FIGURE 62-3 Rotation of the heart with pericardial stay sutures for left atrial exposure. IVC = inferior vena cava.

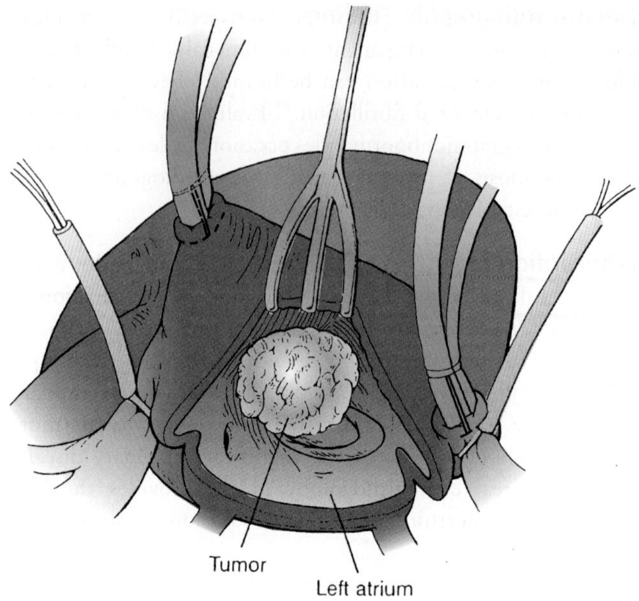

FIGURE 62-5 Left atrial atriotomy posterior to the inter-atrial groove to expose the left atrial tumor.

incision allows easy removal of tumor attached to the fossa ovalis with a full-thickness Ro (margin-negative) excision at the site of attachment and easy patch closure of the atrial septum if necessary (Fig. 62-6).

Right atrial myxomas pose special venous cannulation problems, and intraoperative echocardiography may be beneficial. Both venae cavae may be cannulated directly. When low- or high-lying tumor pedicles preclude safe transatrial cannulation, cannulation of the jugular or femoral vein can provide venous drainage of the upper or lower body. In general, we always can cannulate the superior vena cava distal enough from the right atrium to allow adequate tumor resection, but occasionally femoral venous cannula drainage has been necessary. If the tumor is large or attached near both caval orifices, peripheral cannulation of both jugular and femoral veins may be used to initiate cardiopulmonary bypass and deep hypothermia. After the aorta is cross-clamped and the heart is arrested with antegrade cardioplegia, the right atrium may be opened widely for resection of the tumor and reconstruction of the atrium during a period of circulatory arrest if this is needed for a dry field. Resection of large or critically placed right atrial myxomas often requires careful preoperative planning, intraoperative TEE, and special extracorporeal perfusion techniques to ensure complete removal of the tumor, protection of right atrial structures, and reconstruction of the atrium. Because myxomas rarely extend deep in the endocardium, it is not necessary to resect deeply around the conduction tissue. The tricuspid valve and the right

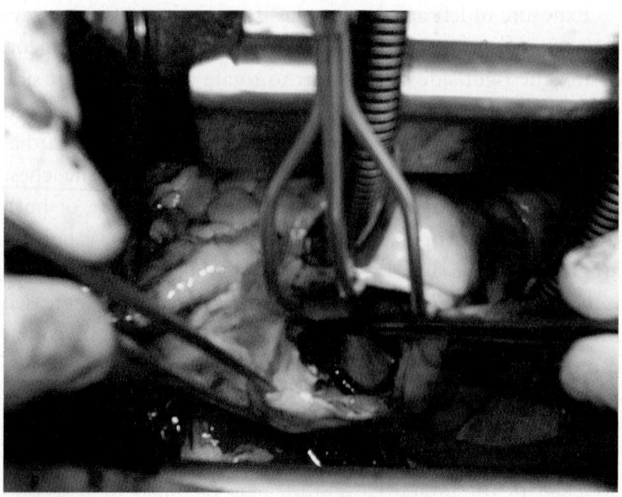

FIGURE 62-4 Left atriotomy and exposure of myxoma.

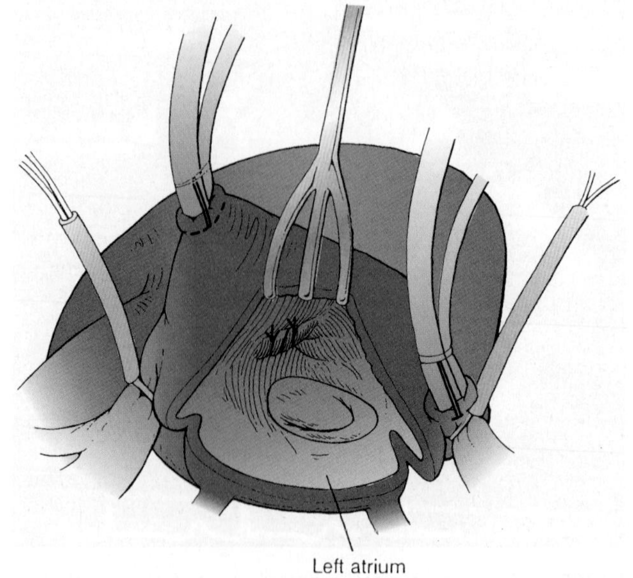

FIGURE 62-6 Repair of left atrial wall after removal of myxomas.

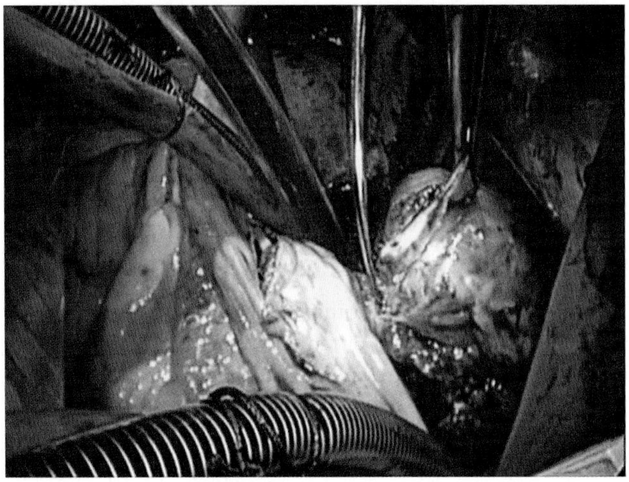

FIGURE 62-7 Giant left atrial myxoma just before removal.

atrium, as well as the left atrium and ventricle, should be inspected carefully for multicentric tumors in patients with right atrial myxoma. Regardless of the surgical approach, the ideal resection encompasses the tumor and a portion of the cardiac wall or interatrial septum to which it is attached (Fig. 62-7). Our policy is to perform a full thickness resection whenever possible. However, partial-thickness resection of the area of tumor attachment has been performed when anatomically necessary without a noted increase in recurrence rate.[74,75]

Ventricular myxomas usually are approached through the atrioventricular (AV) valve[76] or by detaching the anterior portion of the AV valve for exposure and resection and reattachment after resection. Occasional small tumors in either outflow tract can be removed through the outflow valve.[76] If necessary, the tumor is excised through a direct incision into the ventricle, but this is unusual and the least preferred approach. It is not necessary to remove the full thickness of the ventricular wall because no recurrences have been reported with partial-thickness excisions. As with right atrial myxoma, the presence of ventricular myxoma prompts inspection for other tumors because of the high incidence of multiple tumors.

Every care should be taken to remove the tumor without fragmentation. Following tumor removal from the field, the area should be liberally irrigated, suctioned, and inspected for loose fragments. There are rare instances of distant metastases from myxoma many years after tumor resection, and these reports raise the issue of potential intraoperative dissemination of tumor.[77] Cardiotomy suction can be used during the operation, but wall suction should strictly be used during the brief time that the tumor is exposed. The low malignant potential of the vast majority of myxomas and the rarity of metastasis support the author's current policy of retaining rather than discarding blood, and we believe that most cases of metastatic implantation of myxoma represent a preoperative embolic event.

Minimally Invasive Approaches to Surgical Removal. Minimally invasive approaches are being applied with increasing frequency in all areas of cardiac surgery, and cardiac tumors are no exception. Experience is confined to benign tumors and is quite limited. Approaches have included right parasternal or partial sternotomy exposure with standard cardioplegic techniques,[78] right submammary incision with femoral-femoral bypass and nonclamped ventricular fibrillation,[79] and the right submammary port access method with antegrade cardioplegia and ascending aortic balloon occlusion.[80] Thoracoscopic techniques have been used to aid in visualization and removal of ventricular fibroelastomas[81,82] (Fig. 62-8). Myxoma removal is possible via thoracoscopy.[83] Results in this limited number of selected patients have been good, but more experience and longer follow-up are needed before this can be recommended as a standard approach.

Results

Removal of atrial myxomas carries an operative mortality rate of 5% or less.[21] Operative mortality is related to advanced age or disability and comorbid conditions. Excision of ventricular myxomas can carry a higher risk (approximately 10%). Our experience over the last 15 years with 85 myxomas shows no operative or hospital mortality.

Recurrence of nonfamilial sporadic myxoma is approximately 1 to 4%.[4,74,75] Many large series report no recurrent tumors.[74,83–86] The 20% of patients with sporadic myxoma and abnormal DNA have a recurrence rate estimated at between 12 and 40%.[4] The recurrence rate is highest in patients with familial complex myxomas, all of whom exhibit DNA mutation, and this is estimated to be about 22%.[4] Overall, recurrences are more common in younger patients. The disease-free interval averages about 4 years and can be as brief as 6 months.[75] Most recurrent myxomas occur within the heart, in the same or different cardiac chambers, and may be multiple.[19,32,87] Extracardiac recurrence after resection of tumor, presumably from embolization and subsequent tumor growth and local invasion, has been observed.[19,87,88] The biology of the tumor, dictated by

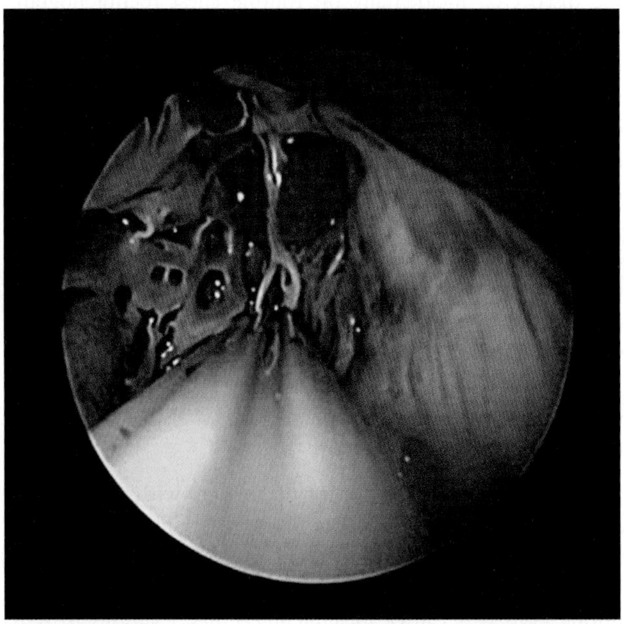

FIGURE 62-8 Thoracoscopic view of left atrial fibroelastoma.

gene expression rather than histology, may be the only reliable factor predicting recurrence. DNA testing of all patients with cardiac myxoma may prove to be the best predictor of the likelihood of recurrence.[89]

Myxomas generally classified as "malignant" are often found on subsequent review to be sarcomas with myxoid degeneration.[90] However, this issue also remains unsettled because of reports of metastatic growth of embolic myxoma fragments in the brain, arteries, soft tissue, and bones.[56,88,91–97] Symptomatic lesions of possible metastatic myxoma should be excised if feasible.[56,91]

The extent to which patients should be subjected to long-term echocardiographic surveillance after myxoma resection is not standardized. It would seem prudent to closely follow patients who are treated initially for multicentric tumors, those whose tumors are removed from unusual locations in the heart, all tumors believed to have been incompletely resected, and all tumors found to have an abnormal DNA genotype. Patients undergoing resection of tumors thought to be myxomas but with malignant characteristics at pathologic examination should have long-term, careful follow-up.

Other Benign Cardiac Tumors

As shown in Table 62-2, myxomas comprise approximately 41% of benign cardiac tumors, with three other tumors (ie, lipoma, papillary fibroelastoma, and rhabdomyoma) together contributing a similar proportion. A number of rarely encountered tumors account for the remainder.

Lipoma

Lipomas are well-encapsulated tumors consisting of mature fat cells that may occur anywhere in the pericardium, subendocardium, subepicardium, and intra-atrial septum.[2] They may occur at any age and have no sex predilection. Lipomas are slow growing and may attain considerable size before producing obstructive or arrhythmic symptoms. Many are asymptomatic and are discovered incidentally on routine chest roentgenogram, echocardiogram, or at surgery or autopsy.[98,99] Subepicardial and parietal lipomas tend to compress the heart and may be associated with pericardial effusion. Subendocardial tumors may produce chamber obstruction. The right atrium and left ventricle are the sites affected most often. Lipomas lying within the myocardium or septum can produce arrhythmias or conduction abnormalities. Large tumors that produce severe symptoms should be resected. Smaller, asymptomatic tumors encountered unexpectedly during cardiac operation should be removed if excision can be performed without adding risk to the primary procedure. These tumors are not known to recur.

Lipomatous Hypertrophy of the Interatrial Septum

Nonencapsulated hypertrophy of the fat within the atrial septum is known as *lipomatous hypertrophy*.[2] This abnormality is more common than cardiac lipoma and usually is encountered in elderly, obese, or female patients as an incidental finding during a variety of cardiac imaging procedures.[84] Various arrhythmias and conduction disturbances have been attributed to its presence.[85,100] The main difficulty is differentiating this from a cardiac neoplasm on echocardiography.[101] After the demonstration of a mass by echocardiography, the typical T1 and T2 signal intensity of fat on MRI usually can establish a diagnosis.[102,103] Arrhythmias and heart block are considered by some as indications for resection, but data are lacking as to the long-term benefits from resection.[104]

Papillary Fibroelastoma of the Heart Valves

Papillary fibroelastomas are tumors that arise characteristically from the cardiac valves or adjacent endocardium.[105] These tumors are described as resembling sea anemones with frondlike projections in gross description (Fig. 62-9). The AV and semilunar valves are affected with equal frequency. It is now known that these are capable of producing obstruction of flow, particularly coronary ostial flow, and may embolize to the brain and produce stroke.[106–115] They are usually asymptomatic until a critical event occurs. Papillary fibroelastomas of the cardiac valve should be resected whenever diagnosed, and valve repair rather than replacement should follow the resection of these benign tumors whenever technically feasible (Fig. 62-10). Cytomegalovirus has been recovered in these tumors, suggesting the possibility of viral induction of the tumor and chronic viral endocarditis.[111]

Rhabdomyoma

Rhabdomyoma is the most frequently occurring cardiac tumor in children. It usually presents during the first few days after birth. It is thought to be a myocardial hamartoma rather than a true neoplasm.[116] Although rhabdomyoma appears sporadically, it is associated strongly with tuberous sclerosis, a hereditary disorder characterized by hamartomas in various organs, epilepsy, mental deficiency, and sebaceous adenomas. Fifty percent of patients with tuberous sclerosis have rhabdomyoma, but

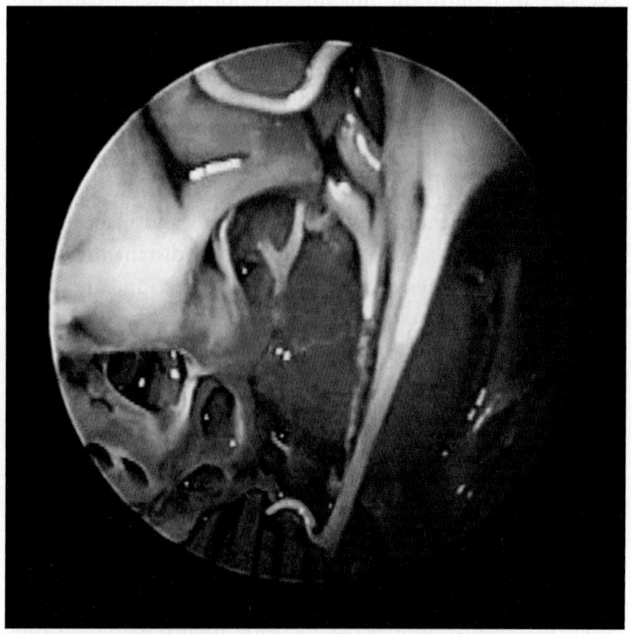

FIGURE 62-9 Additional enhanced view of an in-situ left atrial fibroelastoma.

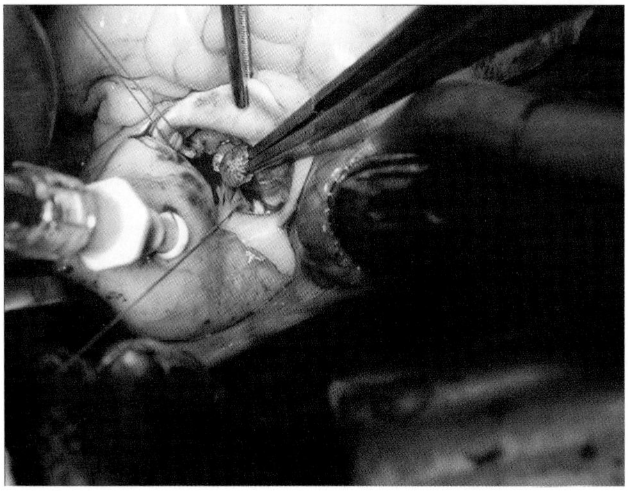

FIGURE 62-10 Surgical removal of a papillary fibroelastoma.

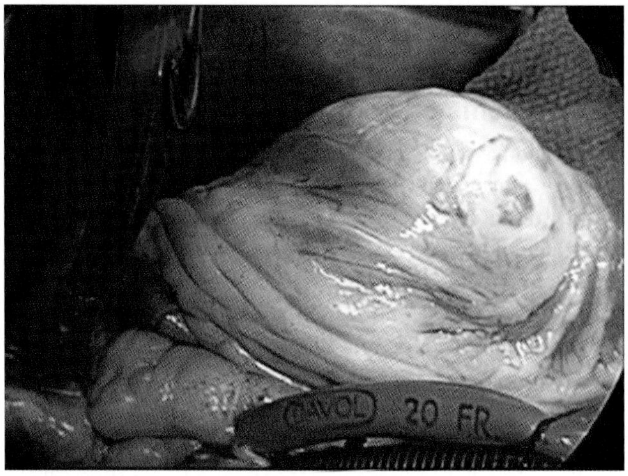

FIGURE 62-11 Left ventricular fibroma as seen from an external view of the heart.

more than 50% of patients with rhabdomyoma have or will develop tuberous sclerosis.[117] More than 90% of rhabdomyomas are multiple and occur with approximately equal frequency in both ventricles.[118] The atrium is involved in fewer than 30% of patients. Pathologically, these tumors are firm, gray, and nodular and tend to project into the ventricular cavity. Micrographs show myocytes of twice normal size filled with glycogen, containing hyperchromatic nuclei and eosinophilic-staining cytoplasmic granules.[2,119] Scattered bundles of myofibrils can be seen within cells by electron microscopy.[118]

Clinical findings may mimic valvular or subvalvular stenosis. Arrhythmias, particularly ventricular tachycardia and sudden death, may be a presenting symptom.[119] Atrial tumors may produce atrial arrhythmias.[119] The diagnosis is made by echocardiography. Rarely, no intramyocardial tumor is found in a patient with ventricular arrhythmias, and the site of rhabdomyoma is located by electrophysiologic study.[119]

Early operation is recommended in patients who do not have tuberous sclerosis before 1 year of age.[86] The tumor usually is removed easily in early infancy, and some can be enucleated.[86] Unfortunately, symptomatic tumors often are both multiple and extensive, particularly in patients with tuberous sclerosis, who, unfortunately, have a dismal long-term outlook. In such circumstances, surgery offers little benefit.

Fibroma

Fibromas are the second most common benign cardiac tumor, with more than 83% occurring in children. These tumors are solitary, occur exclusively within the ventricle and the ventricular septum, and affect the sexes equally. Fewer than 100 tumors have been reported, and most are diagnosed by age 2 years. These tumors are not associated with other disease, nor are they inherited. Fibromas are nonencapsulated, firm, nodular, gray-white tumors that can become bulky. They are composed of elongated fibroblasts in broad spiral bands and whirls mixed with collagen and elastin fibers. Calcium deposits or bone may occur within the tumor and occasionally are seen on roentgenography (Figs. 62-11 and 62-12).

Most fibromas produce symptoms through chamber obstruction, interference with contraction, or arrhythmias. Depending on size and location, such a tumor may interfere with valve function, obstruct flow paths, or cause sudden death from conduction disturbances in up to 25% of patients.[114] Intracardiac calcification on chest roentgenograms suggests the diagnosis, which is confirmed by echocardiogram.

Surgical excision is successful in some patients, particularly if the tumor is localized, does not involve vital structures, and can be enucleated.[86,120–122] However, it is not always possible to remove the tumor completely, and partial removal is only palliative, although some patients have survived many years.[86,121] Operative mortality may be high in infants. Most cases are in adolescents and adults.[186,120,121] Successful, complete excision is

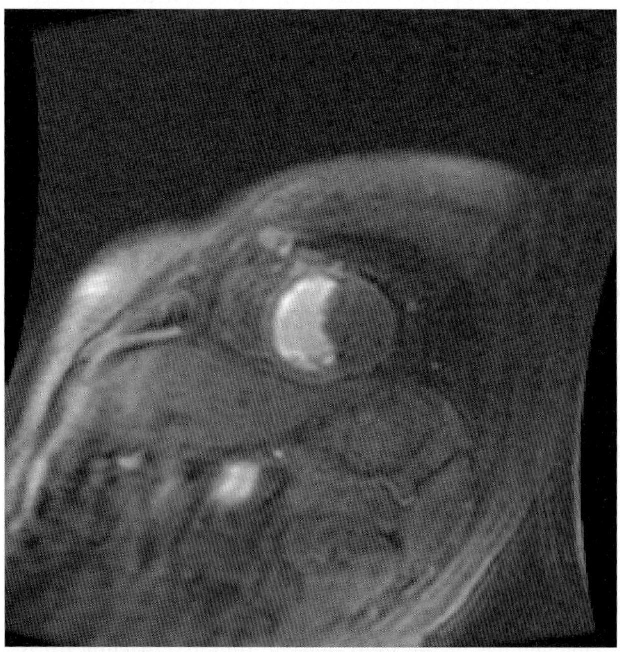

FIGURE 62-12 MRI of left ventricular fibroma.

curative.[120,121] Children with extensive fibromas have been treated with cardiac transplantation.[122,123]

Mesothelioma of the AV Node

Mesothelioma of the AV node, also termed *polycystic tumor, Purkinje tumor,* or *conduction tumor.* It is a relatively small, multicystic tumor that arises in proximity to the AV node and may extend upward into the interventricular septum and downward along the bundle of His.[2] Mesothelioma is associated with heart block, ventricular fibrillation,[124] and sudden death. Cardiac pacing alone does not prevent subsequent ventricular fibrillation. Surgical excision has been reported.[24]

Pheochromocytoma

Cardiac pheochromocytomas arise from chromaffin cells of the sympathetic nervous system and produce excess amounts of catecholamines, particularly norepinephrine. Approximately 90% of pheochromocytomas are in the adrenal glands. Fewer than 2% arise in the chest. Only 32 cardiac pheochromocytomas had been reported by 1991.[125] The tumor predominantly affects young and middle-aged adults with an equal distribution between the sexes. Approximately 60% occur in the roof of the left atrium. The remainders involve the interatrial septum or anterior surface of the heart. The tumor is reddish brown, soft, lobular, and consists of nests of chromatin cells.

The patients usually present with symptoms of uncontrolled hypertension or are found to have elevated urinary catecholamines. The tumor usually is located by scintigraphy using [I^{131}] metaiodobenzylguanidine[126] and CT or MRI.[126] Cardiac catheterization with differential blood chamber sampling sometimes is necessary in addition to coronary angiography.[125] After the tumor is located, it should be removed using cardiopulmonary bypass with cardioplegic arrest. Patients require preanesthetic alpha and beta blockade and careful intraoperative and immediate postoperative monitoring. Most tumors are extremely vascular, and uncontrollable operative hemorrhage has occurred.[126] Resection may require removal of the atrial and/or ventricular wall or a segment of a major coronary artery.[135] Explantation of the heart to allow resection of a large left atrial pheochromocytoma has been attempted.[127] Transplantation has been performed for unresectable tumor and complete excision produces cure.[121–123]

Paraganglioma

Paragangliomas are endocrine tumors that can secrete catecholamines. As a result, their presentation is often similar to that of pheochromocytomas. When found within the thoracic cavity, they are located most often in the posterior mediastinum. Paragangliomas typically present with atypical chest pain.[128,129] On echocardiography, they are often large and highly vascular tumors.[130] On cardiac catheterization, they may be intimately associated with the coronary arteries (Fig. 62-13). If they involve the left atrium, the technique of cardiac autotransplantation may be used to completely resect them[131] (Fig. 62-14).

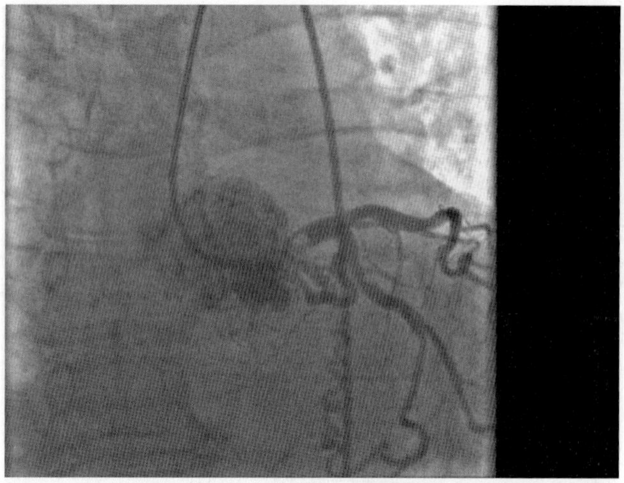

FIGURE 62-13 Paraganglioma blush of tumor during cardiac catheterization.

Hemangioma

Hemangiomas of the heart are rare tumors (24 clinical cases reported), affect all ages, and may occur anywhere within the heart.[132,133] These are vascular tumors composed of capillaries or cavernous vascular channels. Patients usually develop dyspnea, occasional arrhythmias, or signs of right-sided heart failure.[134] Diagnosis is difficult, and echocardiography or cardiac catheterization can establish a diagnosis of cardiac tumor by showing an intracavity filling defect.[135] CT and MRI show axial T2-weighted MRI should show a high signal mass owing to vascularity (Fig. 62-15). Coronary angiography typically shows a tumor blush and maps the blood supply to the tumor. During resection, meticulous ligation of feeding vessels is required to prevent postoperative residual arteriovenous fistulas or intracavity communications. Partial resections have produced long-term benefits.[132] Tumors rarely resolve spontaneously.[136]

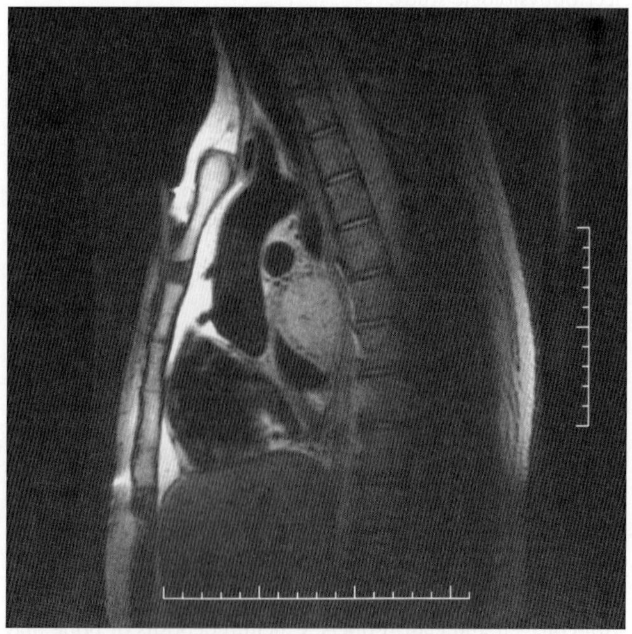

FIGURE 62-14 MRI of left atrial paraganglioma that required an autotransplant for removal.

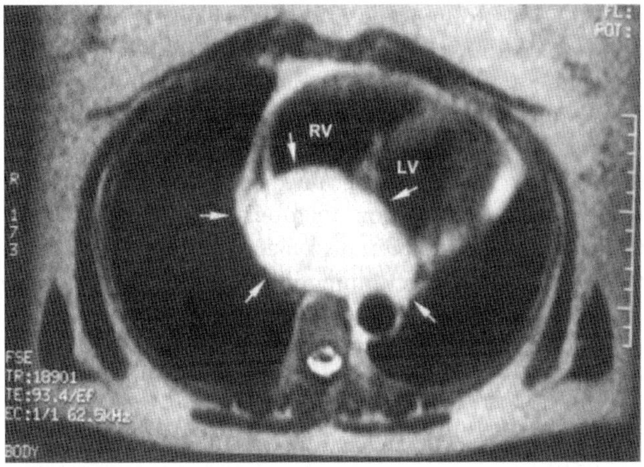

FIGURE 62-15 Axial T2-weighted magnetic resonance image showing high signal mass of left atrial hemangioma. (*Reproduced with permission from Lo JJ, Ramsay CN, Allen JW, et al: Left atrial cardiac hemangioma associated with shortness of breath and palpitations. Ann Thorac Surg 2002; 73:979.*)

Teratoma

Cardiac teratoma is a rare tumor that typically presents in infants and young children.[137] About 80% of the tumors are benign.[138] These tumors are discovered by echocardiography after a variety of symptoms lead to cardiac or mediastinal evaluation. There is little experience with surgical removal, which should be possible.

Castleman Tumor

Castleman disease is a poorly understood lymphoproliferative disorder. The disease was first described by Castleman and colleagues in 1956.[139] It typically presents as a solitary lesion in the mediastinum. The most common histologic type is hyaline vascular, which accounts for approximately 90% of cases and often behaves in a benign fashion. The more aggressive subgroups are the plasma and mixed-cell types, which have a more malignant behavior.[140] Patients may have a localized or multicentric disease with lymph node involvement, typically in the mediastinum. These tumors typically present as well-circumscribed masses. There have been reports of Castleman disease with myocardial and coronary artery invasion or development of a coronary pseudoaneurysm.[141] In these more aggressive cases, cardiac assist devices have been used as a bridge to recovery[141] (Figs. 62-16 and 62-17). CT imaging of the lesions reveals atypical or target-like enhancement that corresponds to various degrees of degeneration, necrosis, and fibrosis. Technetium-99m tetrofosmin and [I^{123}] beta-methyliodophenyl pentadecanoic acid (BMIPP) imaging may aid in the diagnosis. On BMIPP, these tumors show reduced uptake compared with the surrounding normal myocardium.[142] Complete surgical resection is considered curative.[143]

PRIMARY MALIGNANT TUMORS

Primary cardiac malignancy is very uncommon, with only 21 surgically treated cases noted in a 25-year surgical experience from 1964 to 1969, combining the experience of two large institutions, the Texas Heart Institute and the M. D. Anderson Cancer Center in Houston.[144] Additional current reports from the Texas Medical Center include a series from the Methodist Debakey Heart and Vascular Center and M D Anderson Cancer Center of 27 patients selected from 1990 to 2006.[144] Approximately 25% of primary cardiac tumors are malignant, and of these, about 75% are sarcomas. McAllister's survey of cardiac tumors found the most common to be angiosarcomas (31%), rhabdomyosarcomas (21%), malignant mesotheliomas (15%), and fibrosarcomas (11%),[2] see Table 62-4.

Rather than histologic classification of cardiac sarcoma, we propose a classification system based on anatomic location. Histology does not greatly affect treatment or prognosis as much as anatomic location.[144,145] The revised classification system divides primary cardiac sarcomas into right heart sarcomas, left heart sarcomas and pulmonary artery sarcomas, and these are the categories that will be used in the discussion to follow.

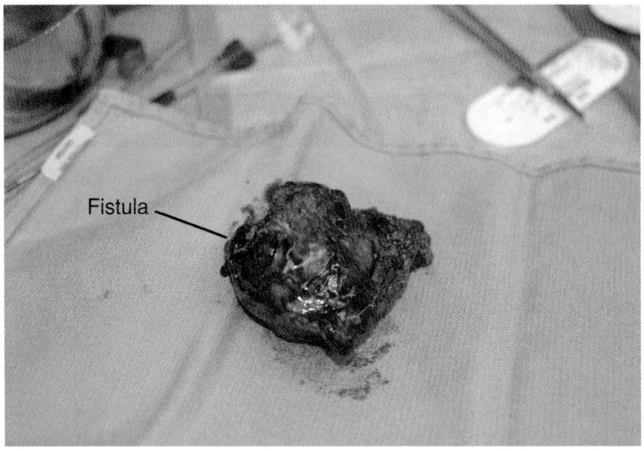

FIGURE 62-16 Castleman tumor showing fistula site indicated by insertion of a coronary probe.

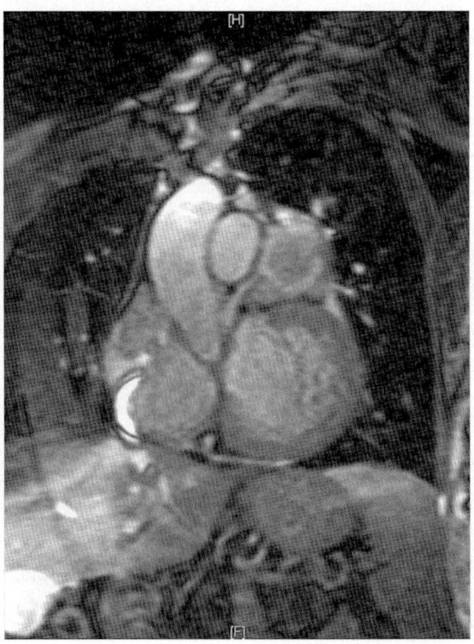

FIGURE 62-17 MRI of Castleman tumor.

TABLE 62-4 Primary Malignant Cardiac Neoplasms in Adults

Tumor	Number	Percentage
Angiosarcoma	39	33
Rhabdomyosarcoma	24	21
Mesothelioma	19	16
Fibrosarcoma	13	11
Lymphoma	7	6
Osteosarcoma	5	4
Thymoma	4	3
Neurogenic sarcoma	3	2
Leiomyosarcoma	1	<1
Liposarcoma	1	<1
Synovial sarcoma	1	<1
Total	117	100

Source: Reproduced with permission from McAllister HA Jr, Fenoglio JJ Jr: Tumors of the cardiovascular system, in Atlas of Tumor Pathology. Washington, DC, Armed Forces Institute of Pathology, 1978; fas. 15.

Right heart sarcomas tend to metastasize early, present as bulky masses (Fig. 62-18), and are characteristically infiltrative.[145] Right heart sarcomas often occupy much of the right atrium growing largely in an outward pattern, and often avoid heart failure until the latest stage of presentation. This presentation often allows time for neoadjuvant chemotherapy in an attempt to shrink the tumor and sterilize the infiltrating edges to increase chances of obtaining a resection with microscopically negative margins.

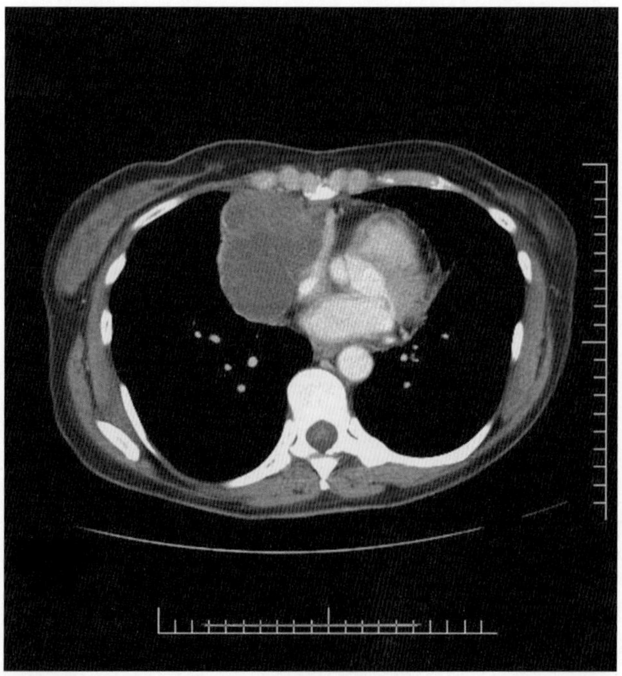

FIGURE 62-18 CT scan of a right heart tumor.

Left heart sarcomas tend to be more solid with less infiltration than right heart sarcomas and tend to metastasize later in the course of disease.[187] Left-sided sarcomas are most often located in the left atrium, and tend to grow into the wall. Diminution of blood flow quickly results in life-threatening heart failure. Neoadjuvant chemotherapy can rarely be used because of this presentation. Most left atrial sarcomas are initially clinically diagnosed as mxyomas, have a positive resection margin, rapidly recur, and require repeat resection.

Primary malignant cardiac tumors arise sporadically, showing no inherited linkage. Although they may span the entire age spectrum, they usually occur in adults more than 40 years of age. The patients usually present with symptoms of congestive heart failure, pleuritic chest pain, malaise, anorexia, and weight loss.[137,146] The most common symptom has been dyspnea[147] (Table 62-5). Some develop refractory arrhythmias, syncope, pericardial effusion, and tamponade.[147] The chest x-ray may be abnormal and even show a mass lesion, but the definite diagnosis usually is made with cardiac echocardiography.[146,148] Right atrial lesions are more frequently malignant (usually angiosarcoma) than left-sided lesions (usually myxoma but, when malignant, often malignant fibrous histiocytoma). If malignancy is suspected, chest CT or MRI may suggest histology and provide detailed anatomy and help in staging and assessing resectability. The current status of positron-emission tomographic (PET) scans in evaluating these patients remains controversial. We perform cardiac catheterization on all patients older than 40 years of age presenting with intracardiac masses and on all patients with large right atrial masses. Malignancy may be suggested and coronary involvement suspected by tumor blush. This is not pathognomic because we have seen a large feeding vessel and tumor blush in a histologically confirmed myxoma.

Unfortunately, primary cardiac malignancy may grow to a large size before detection and involve portions of the heart not amenable to resection. Some of these patients have been considered for transplantation and will be discussed later. Otherwise, palliative medical therapy can be attempted with radiation therapy, although success in both symptom relief and longevity has been somewhat limited. Whether the tumor is primary or secondary, the decision to resect is based on tumor size and location and an absence of

TABLE 62-5 Symptoms of Primary Malignant Cardiac Tumors

Symptom	Number	Percentage
Dyspnea	13/21	61.9
Chest pain	6/21	28
Congestive heart failure	6/21	28
Palpitations	5/321	24
Fever	3/21	14
Myalgia	2/21	10

Source: Reproduced with permission from Murphy MC, Sweeney MS, Putnam JB Jr, et al: Surgical treatment of cardiac tumors: a 25-year experience. Ann Thorac Surg 1990; 49:612.

metastatic spread seen on complete evaluation. Unfortunately, most primary cardiac malignancies that have been referred to our center were considered to be benign initially and were resected incompletely at presentation. If malignancy is suspected or confirmed, and if the lesion appears anatomically resectable and there is no metastatic disease, then resection should be considered. If complete resection is possible, surgery provides better palliation and potentially can double survival.[149] After resection, we recommend adjuvant chemotherapy and believe that this can improve survival.[138,149] Complete resection will depend on the location of the tumor, the extent of involvement of the myocardium and/or fibrous skeleton of the heart, and histology.

Angiosarcoma

Angiosarcomas are two to three times more common in men than in women and have a predilection for the right side of the heart. Eighty percent arise in the right atrium.[147,150,151] These tumors tend to be bulky and aggressively invade adjacent structures, including the great veins, tricuspid valve, right ventricular free wall, interventricular septum, and right coronary artery[150] (Fig. 62-19). Obstruction and right-sided heart failure are not uncommon. Pathologic examination of resected specimens demonstrates anastomosing vascular channels lined with typical anaplastic epithelial cells. Unfortunately, most of these tumors have spread by the time of presentation, usually to the lung, liver, and brain.[147] Without resection, 90% of the patients are dead within 9 to 12 months of diagnosis despite radiation or chemotherapy.[22,147] We have seen carefully selected patients without evidence of spread on metastatic evaluation who have undergone complete surgical resection with subsequent chemotherapy (Fig. 62-20). In addition to surgical resection of the right atrium, right coronary bypass and even tricuspid valve repair or replacement may be undertaken (Fig. 62-21). We have had no hospital mortality in this small group, and most patients die from metastasis rather than recurrence at the local site.[152]

Malignant Fibrous Histiocytoma

Malignant fibrous histiocytoma (MFH) is the most common soft tissue sarcoma in adults. Its occurrence as a cardiac primary malignancy has been relatively recently accepted as a specific entity. It is characterized histologically by a mixture of spindle cells in a storiform pattern, polygonal cells resembling histiocytes, and malignant giant cells. The cell of origin is the fibroblast or histioblast.[148,153] It usually occurs in the left atrium and often mimics myxoma. In fact, every left atrial MFH referred to our institution has been previously incompletely resected when thought to represent a myxoma. The tendency to metastasize early is not as prominent as with angiosarcoma. Several reports document rapid symptomatic recurrence after incomplete resection despite chemotherapy. These patients often die of local cardiac disease before the development of metastases. We believe that if complete resection can be obtained (particularly if the malignant nature is recognized and complete resection can be done at the original operation) and adequate chemotherapy can be provided, we may improve survival in this otherwise dismal disease.

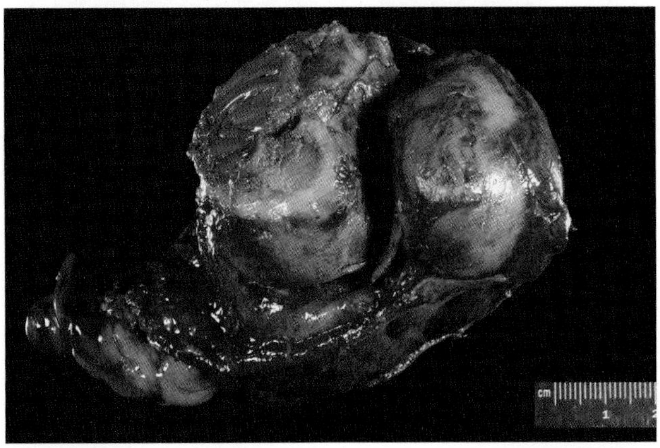

FIGURE 62-19 Pathology specimen photograph of a right atrial tumor.

Rhabdomyosarcoma

Rhabdomyosarcomas do not evolve from rhabdomyomas and occur equally in the sexes. The tumors are multicentric in 60% of patients and arise from either ventricle. These tumors frequently invade cardiac valves or interfere with valve function because of their intracavitary bulk. Microscopically, tumor cells demonstrate pleomorphic nuclei and spidery, wispy, streaming eosinophilic cytoplasm, usually in a muscle-like pattern.

The tumors are aggressive and may invade pericardium. Surgical excision of small tumors may be rational, but local and distant metastases and poor response to radiation or chemotherapy limit survival to less than 12 months in most of these patients.[120,137,138,149,154]

Other Sarcomas and Mesenchymal-Origin Tumors

McAllister and Fenoglio found that malignant mesotheliomas arising from the heart or pericardium and not from the surrounding pleura were the third most common malignant cardiac tumors and that fibrosarcomas were fourth.[2] However, in the two decades since their work, clinicians have rarely encountered these tumors. This apparent decrease in incidence may be related to changes in histologic criteria for classifying primary malignant neoplasms since their study.[5,132,138,147–149,154–155]

The histology of these tumors can be ambiguous and difficult. These neoplasms can resemble other sarcomas, and some might be deemed fibrous histiocytomas today. The behavior of these tumors is more important, and as with other cardiac sarcomas, resection of small tumors in the absence of known metastasis perhaps is justified, but data are scarce.[22,147,149,154] This being said, it is important to rule out more diffuse thoracic involvement with mesothelioma before considering resection of an isolated cardiac or pericardial mesothelioma. A PET scan may be considered, and any suspicious pleural thickening or effusion should be evaluated carefully both radiographically and histologically.

Myosarcoma, liposarcoma, osteosarcoma, chondromyxosarcoma, plasmacytoma, and carcinosarcoma arising from the

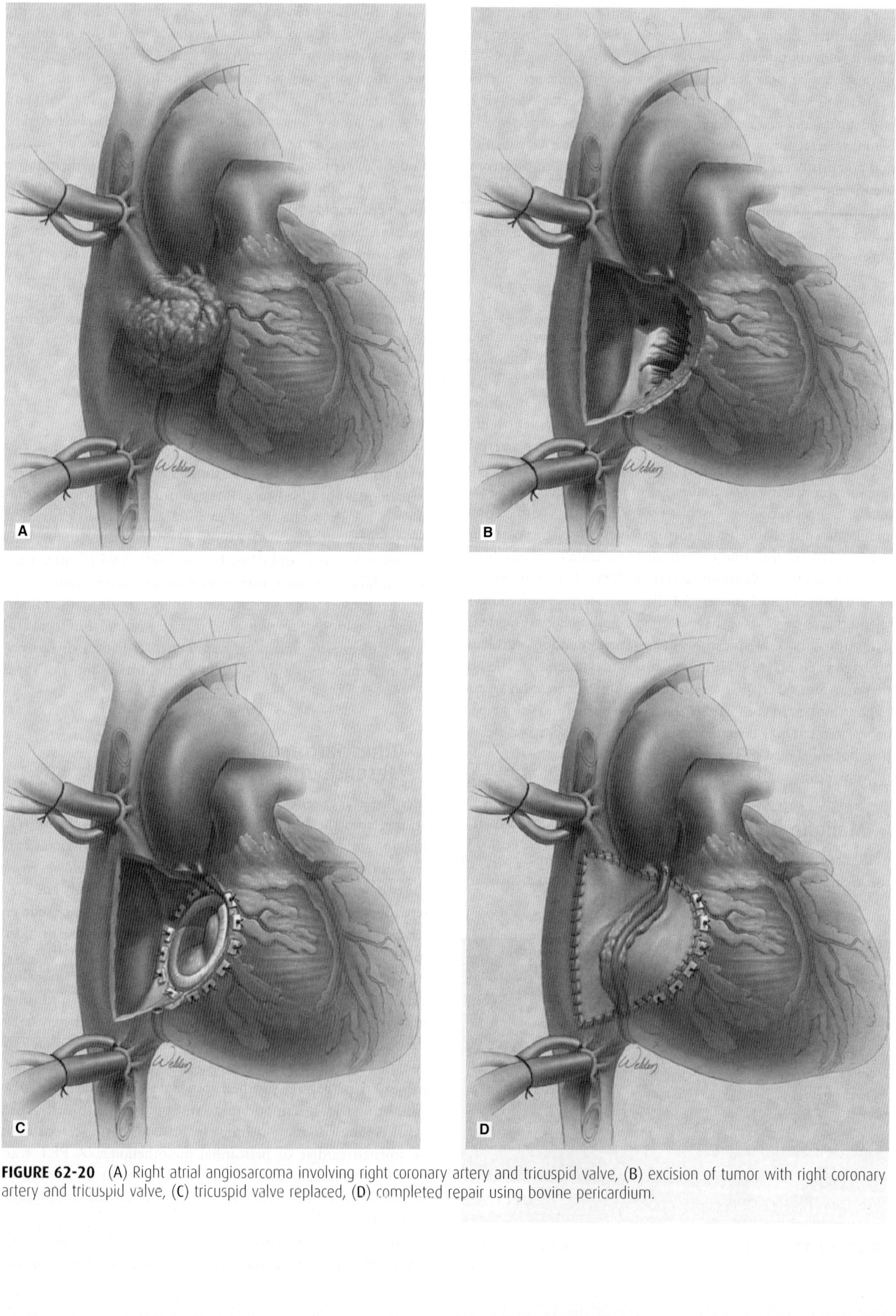

FIGURE 62-20 (A) Right atrial angiosarcoma involving right coronary artery and tricuspid valve, (B) excision of tumor with right coronary artery and tricuspid valve, (C) tricuspid valve replaced, (D) completed repair using bovine pericardium.

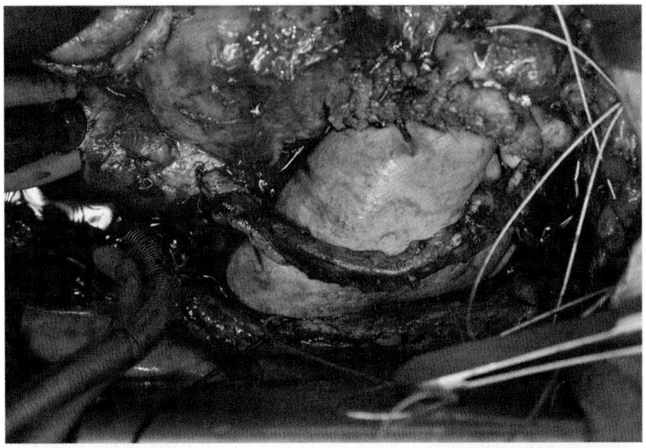

FIGURE 62-21 Right atrial angiosarcoma (final repair with right coronary artery bypass positioned over bovine pericardium).

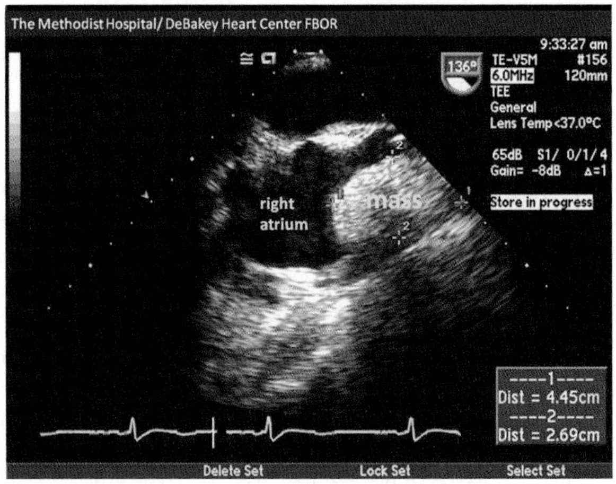

FIGURE 62-22 Transesophageal echocardiogram of a right atrial mass measuring 4.45 by 2.69 centimeters.

heart all have been reported,[155–158] but by the time diagnosis is made, only palliative therapy usually can be offered, and surgery is indicated only occasionally. Regardless of therapy, it is unusual for patients with these diagnoses to survive more than a year.

Right-Sided Cardiac Sarcomas

The prognosis without surgery for right heart sarcoma is dismal, and surgical resection is the only treatment modality shown to increase survival. Complete surgical resection is complicated both by the bulky infiltrative nature of right heart sarcoma and the high incidence of metastatic disease at presentation. The author's current approach to right heart sarcomas has been to begin with neoadjuvant chemotherapy once a definitive tissue diagnosis of sarcoma is made using a right heart catheterization biopsy. Occasionally, a diagnosis of lymphoma or other tumor is made. Multidisciplinary treatment planning based on the *correct* diagnosis is imperative. After 4 to 6 rounds of chemotherapy (with repeat imaging every other cycle to assess for tumor response), the patient is evaluated for surgical resection. This treatment regimen aims to improve on the current microscopic complete resection rate of 33%. The initial diagnostic test for right heart sarcomas is transthoracic echocardiography, which rarely misses these usually large tumors. Unlike large left atrial masses that are usually benign myxomas, the majority of large right atrial masses are typically malignant (Fig. 62-22). The majority of right heart sarcomas referred to our specialty center have yet to undergo attempted resection, unlike left-sided heart tumors which are typically resected under the presumption they are benign mymomas. The primary reason for local failure of a right heart sarcoma is incomplete resection, typically because of surgical hesitancy to achieve complete resection because of involvement of the right coronary artery.

Most right heart sarcomas are angiosarcomas.[2] (Fig. 62-23) These tumors may occur in the right atrium (Fig. 62-24) or the right ventricle but far more commonly arise from the right atrium. They replace the right atrial wall and frequently grow into the cardiac chamber and into adjacent tissues. Right heart

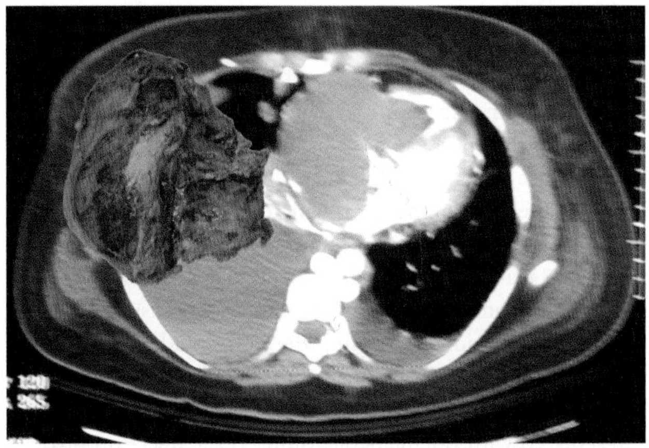

FIGURE 62-23 CT scan of a right atrial mass with the pathology specimen oriented in a similar fashion over the image.

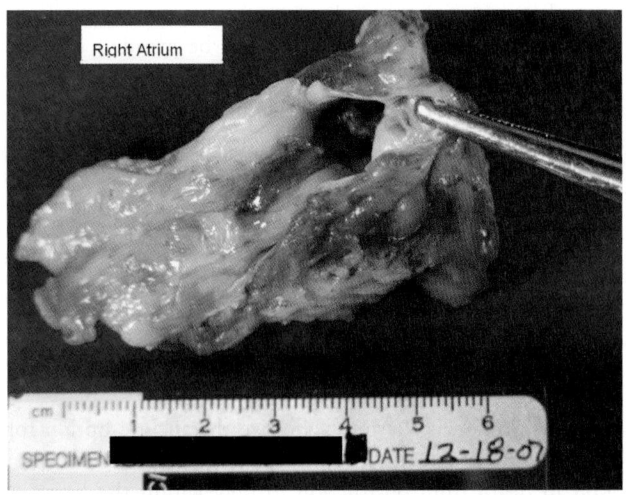

FIGURE 62-24 Right atrial sarcoma.

tumors tend to be infiltrative and form microscopic "fingers" of tumor extending beyond the margins of gross disease. Diffuse pericardial involvement, right ventricular involvement, or encasement of great vessels or veins often precludes surgical resection. The tricuspid valve, right coronary artery, and up to about 30% of the right ventricular muscle mass may be resected and replaced or reconstructed with reasonable risk to achieve a complete resection. Thus, all patients are evaluated preoperatively with coronary arteriography. In patients treated without surgical resection, the survival is approximately 10% at 12 months.[159] A microscopically negative surgical resection margin has been shown to extend survival[149] and remains standard therapy. Although some patients having a radical resection still locally recur, the leading cause of death is distant metastatic disease. Complete resection followed by adjuvant chemotherapy has been shown to extend survival.[149,159]

Patients with even limited metastatic disease that did not respond well to chemotherapy or who developed new metastatic disease while on treatment are not considered candidates for surgery. Patients with widely metastatic disease are not considered candidates unless palliative surgery because of severe symptoms is recommended. Every patient should be referred to oncology for potential continuation of chemotherapy after recovery from surgery.

Based on the anatomic extent of tumor and the needed margins for resection, venous cannulation for cardiopulmonary bypass must be carefully planned and individualized to each patient. Directly cannulating the high superior vena cava (SVC) for upper body drainage and cannulating directly into the inferior vena cava (IVC) at the diaphragm usually allows adequate exposure for complete inferior resection, but occasionally femoral cannulation aids in exposing the more caudal structures of the right heart. Aortic cannulation is standard, as it is distant from the tumor. The right atrium can be completely resected and replaced with Bovine pericardium. If the resection involves the SVC or IVC, a vascular stapler can be used to staple lengthwise creating a tube from Bovine pericardium to recreate the vein segment (Fig. 62-25). One particular area of danger is at the right atrial junction with the root of the aorta, as overzealous resection in this area will result in damage to the fibrous skeleton of the heart, which is characteristically difficult to repair. Incomplete resection leaving gross disease rapidly leads to regrowth of the tumor and should be avoided if at all possible. When right coronary artery involvement is suspected, mobilization of the right internal mammary artery is performed at the beginning of the operation. Right ventricular wall can be simply partially replaced with Bovine pericardium or incorporated into a prosthetic tricuspid valve used for valve replacement. For an illustration of the steps involved in the resection and later reconstruction of a right heart sarcoma, please refer to Fig. 62-26.

Left-Sided Cardiac Sarcomas

Surgical resection is the most effective therapeutic option for patients with malignant left-sided cardiac tumors. Delay can result in death from obstruction to flow within the heart or embolization, which may occur in as many as 8% of patients

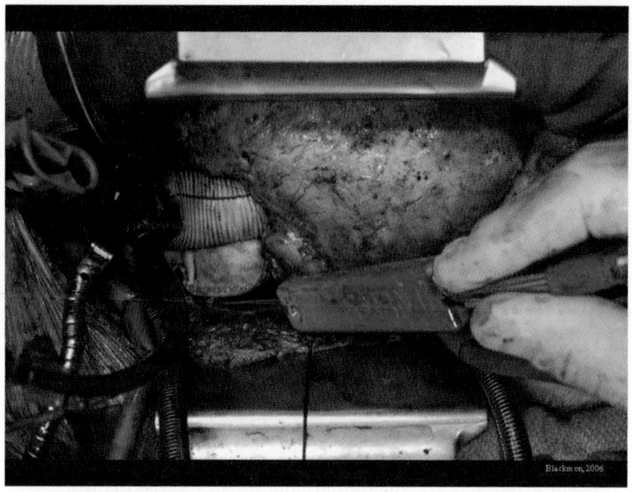

FIGURE 62-25 Bovine pericardium reconstruction of the superior vena cava (created by folding the pericardium in half and then firing an endo-GIA stapler longitudinally to form the conduit).

awaiting operation. The clinical presentation of patients with primary left heart sarcoma depends on the anatomic location and extent of the tumor and is not influenced by histology. Most primary left heart sarcomas are reported to occur in the left atrium, a concept supported by the author's experience; 22/24 (92%) occurred in the left atrium and 2/24 (8%) occurred in the left ventricle. Most left atrial masses seen by cardiac surgeons are mistaken to be benign myxomas. Every left atrial sarcoma patient referred to our center previously underwent resection for a presumed myxoma that was later found to be a cardiac sarcoma. Each of these cases had rapid reappearance of the left atrial tumor at the site of resection likely representing regrowth of persistent incompletely resected sarcoma. Intracavitary left ventricular tumors are very uncommon and are rarely mistaken for a simple cardiac myxoma. Heart failure caused by obstruction of intracardiac blood flow is the most common and concerning presenting symptom. Heart block from local invasion, arrhythymia, pericardial effusion, distal embolus, fever, weight loss, and malaise are also seen. The mean age of presentation is reported to be 40 years of age.[148] Transthoracic echocardiography is the most common initial diagnostic test. Transesophageal echocardiography is specifically recommended for in all left-sided cardiac tumors because of increased resolution of left-sided structures. Cardiac MRI and PET/CT scans are also obtained in patients known or suspected to have sarcoma.

Once diagnosed, primary cardiac sarcoma patients have an often dismal prognosis. When medically treated, the survival at 12 months is less than 10%.[159] Most reports in the literature are either autopsy series or individual case reports or small case series. Operative mortality usually exceeds 20 percent, and the mean survival is typically around 12 months.[160–162] Many published series focus on primary cardiac sarcoma in general without regard to anatomic location. The Mayo Clinic reported 34 patients over 32 years with a median survival of 12 months.[163] A combined series from the Texas Heart Institute and the MD Anderson

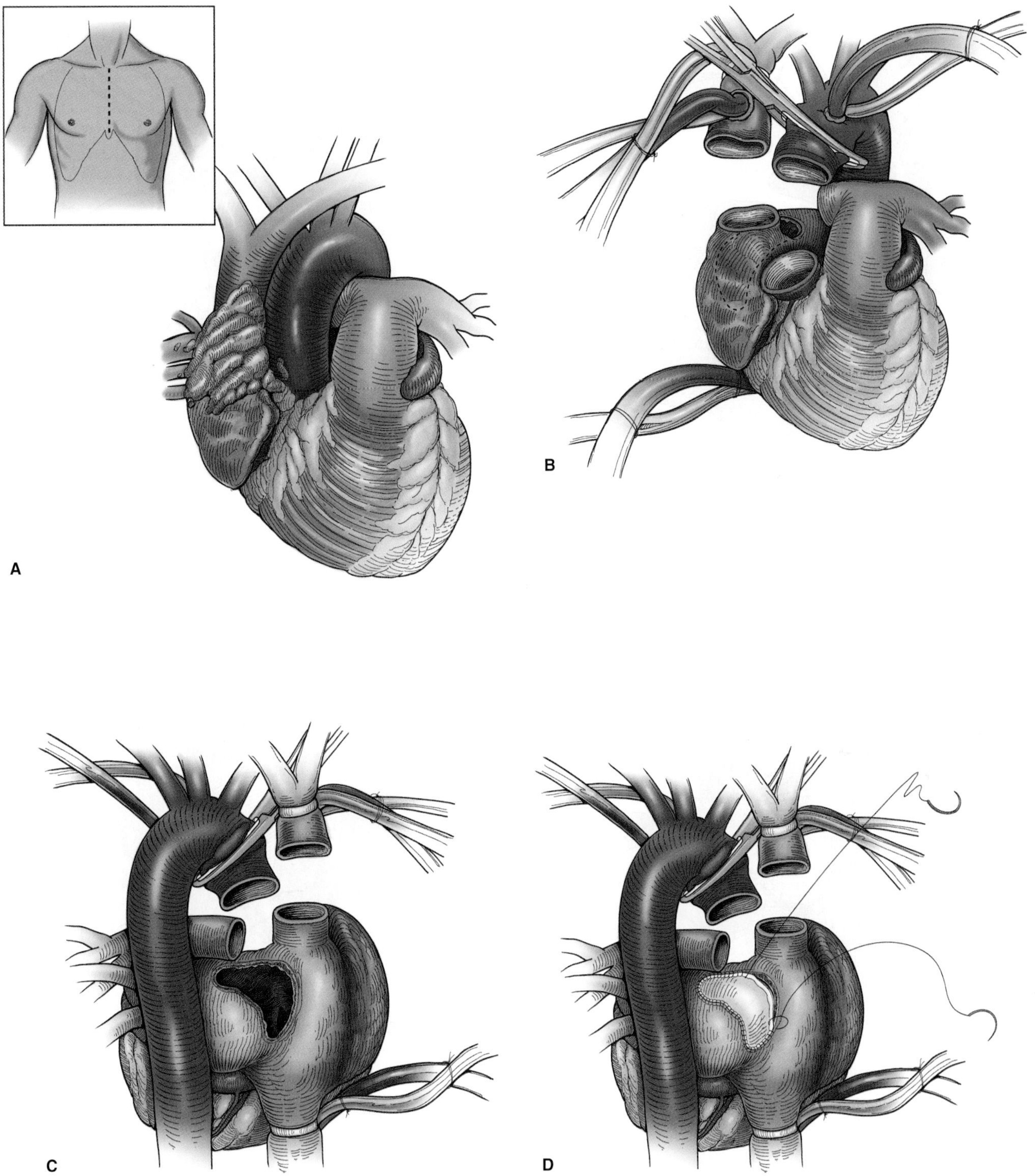

FIGURE 62-26 (A) median sternotomy approach to a right heart sarcoma; (B) transection of the aorta, right main pulmonary artery, roof of the left atrium, and superior vena cava to rotate the right upper quadrant of the heart and allow adequate exposure for complete excision of a right heart sarcoma; (C) posterior view of the heart to illustrate the incisions necessary for complete removal of a right-sided cardiac sarcoma that extended into the roof of the left atrium; (D) reconstruction of the roof of the left atrium; (E) reconstruction of the pulmonary veins using a Dacron graft; (F) reconstruction from an anterior view of the right main pulmonary artery; (G) reconstruction of the aorta using a Dacron graft and a running suture; (H) complete reconstruction of the heart after radical removal of a right heart sarcoma (note the superior vena cava reconstruction with bovine pericardium folded and stapled with an endo-GIA stapler).

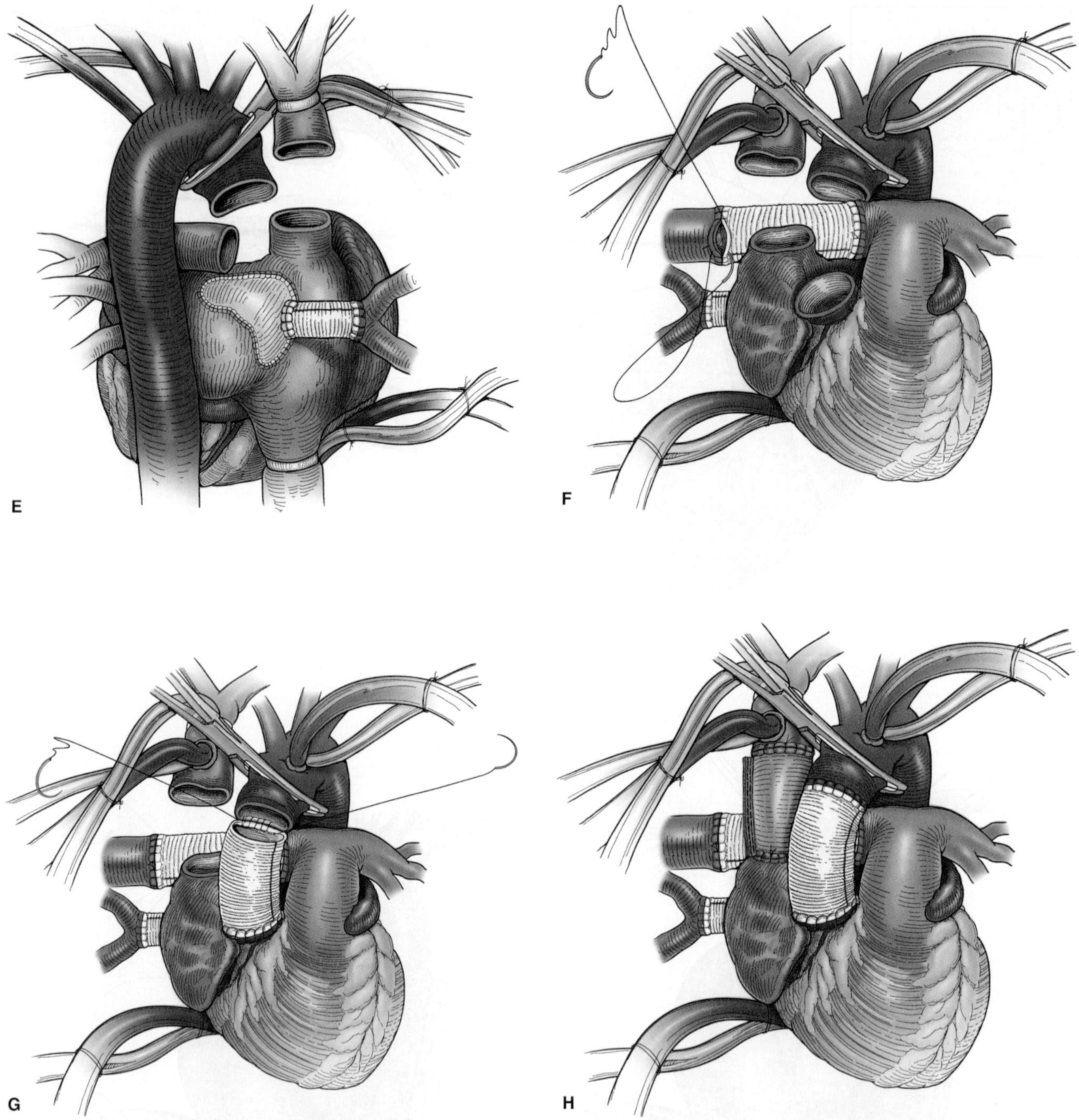

FIGURE 62-26 *(Continued)*

Cancer Center reported an actuarial survival of 14% at 2 years in 21 patients over a 26-year period.[156] The authors have previously reported a combined multimodality approach, and found a median survival of 23.5 months in 27 patients over 16 years with survival of 80.9% at one year and 61.9% at two years.[146] Subsequent analyses show histologic type does not influence survival or treatment approach.[164] The major determinant of clinical presentation and surgical approach is anatomic location. Currently, these tumors are grouped based on location, such as pulmonary artery sarcomas, right heart sarcomas, or left heart sarcomas.[165]

The high rate of local recurrence and secondary resections reported in the literature[166] indicate the left atrium and ventricle present unique anatomic exposure challenges. Complete resection and reconstruction is complicated because of the left heart proximity to vital structures. Often, a surgeon's inability to adequately visualize vital structures and reconstruct leads to an inadequate resection with rapid regrowth of tumor. Typically, left atrial tumors are approached through the interatrial groove. The interatrial groove is often an adequate approach for benign tumors, but is limited for malignant tumors that are often larger and require a more generous margin of resection. We have considered complete cardiectomy and orthotopic cardiac transplantation for complete removal of these tumors. Although feasible, this approach requires the availability of a donor and postoperative immunosuppression; both of which present potential problems in cancer patients. Additionally series using orthotopic cardiac transplantation for this purpose have only shown a median survival of 12 months.[167] Left ventricular tumors can be approached through the aortic valve, the mitral valve or through a ventriculotomy. A transaortic valve approach works nicely for benign tumors[82] but is inadequate for malignant tumors because of their size and the amount of resection needed. A ventriculotomy through normal ventricular muscle is possible, but not ideal. The author's group adopted the approach of cardiac explantation, ex vivo tumor resection, cardiac reconstruction, and reimplantation of the heart (cardiac autotransplantation), which permits a radical tumor resection and accurate reconstruction.

Cardiac Autotransplantation. The technique of cardiac autotransplantation was introduced for cardiac tumors by Cooley in 1985 to deal with a large left atrial pheochromocytoma.[127] Although this case was not successful, it introduced the senior author (MJR) to the technique and its potential use for cardiac tumors. The author's group did the first successful cardiac auto transplant for cardiac sarcoma in 1998,[153] also reporting this for left atrial sarcoma and left ventricular sarcoma.[168] Working closely with the MD Anderson Cancer Center, the Methodist Hospital has now performed 28 cardiac auto transplants, with 23 of these for primary cardiac sarcoma.

Cardiac auto transplantation has several fundamental differences from standard orthotopic heart transplantation.[169] In orthotopic heart transplantation, unless a domino procedure is being done, the explanted heart is not to be used and any damage to its structures is inconsequential. For a complete video of an autotransplant including replacement of the mitral valve, please refer to the movie attached to this chapter. Therefore, the cardiectomy can be performed leaving a wide margin of remaining tissue to use in tailoring the heart to be implanted without regard to cutting critical structures such as the coronary sinus. Similarly, the donor heart can usually be harvested with extra tissue at its margins to be used to help tailor the implantation unlike traditional orthotopic heart transplant surgery. The heart must be excised in cardiac autotransplantation in a manner that does not damage any structures that cannot be repaired, replaced, or are vital to cardiac function. Additionally, if the heart is simply excised and reimplanted, loss of workable tissue makes reimplantation more challenging than orthotopic heart transplantation. Cannulation techniques must take into consideration planned explantation. The aorta can be cannulated distally in the transverse arch. Venous cannulation must be directly into the SVC and IVC just below the right atrial junction. This requires greater exposure and mobilization of the SVC and IVC. After commencing CPB, further mobilization of the SVC and IVC is performed until each is completely free and surround with umbilical tapes on a tourniquet. Wide mobilization of the interatrial groove and circumferential mobilization of the ascending aorta and pulmonary artery follows cannulation. This facilitates both accurate excision of the heart and reimplantation. The ascending aorta is cross-clamped and antegrade cold blood potassium cardioplegia is given (10 cc/kg) to achieve cardiac arrest. The left atrium is opened at the beginning of cardioplegia, and a sump drain placed to decompress the heart. After cardioplegia and cardiac quiescence, the left atrium is opened to confirm pathology and appropriateness of autotransplantation. The SVC first divided beyond the right atrial junction. This is followed by IVC division which should be transected near the right atrial and SVC junction. For each transection, it is important to note the rim of tissue being left behind retracts substantially towards the venous cannulae and an extraordinarily wide rim must be left or reimplantation at the IVC can be exceedingly difficult. The ascending aorta is divided about 1 cm distal to the sinotubular junction and the pulmonary artery is divided just proximal to its bifurcation. The left atrium transection is then completed, dividing the atrium just anterior to the pulmonary veins and on the left side equal distant between the pulmonary veins and the mitral valve and left atrial appendage. This allows complete removal of the heart which is placed into a basin of ice slush (Fig. 62-27). The posterior left atrium is then inspected, and any tumor is widely excised (Fig. 62-28). Bovine pericardium is used for reconstruction, and the pulmonary veins may be individually reimplanted into new orifices cut in the bovine pericardium or left as a cuff, if pathology permits. The anterior left atrium can be entirely removed, including the mitral valve, leaving only a mitral annulus.

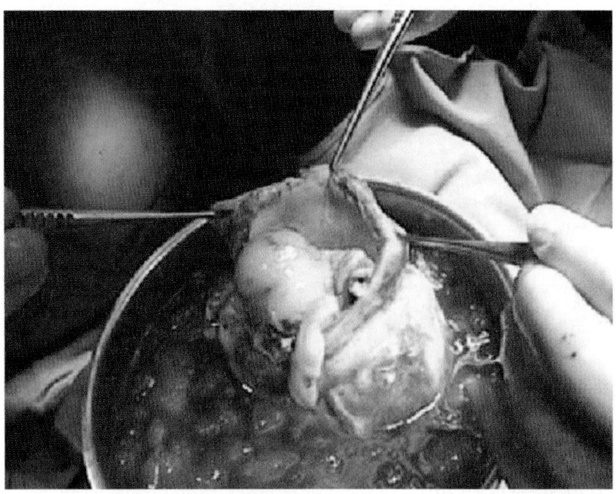

FIGURE 62-27 Ex vivo heart showing large sarcoma arising from the anterior left atrial wall.

Bovine pericardial reconstruction starts with cutting a hole to match the mitral annulus opening. Mitral valve replacement using pledgeted 2-0 ticron sutures begins with pledgets placed on the left ventricular side of the annulus, passing thru the annulus, through the bovine pericardium, and then through the prosthetic mitral valve. When the sutures are tied, the neo atrial wall is sealed to the valve and annulus. The anterior and posterior bovine pericardium can then be tailored by cutting darts and sewing them together before reanastomosis. Reimplantation is similar to standard cardiac transplantation, beginning with

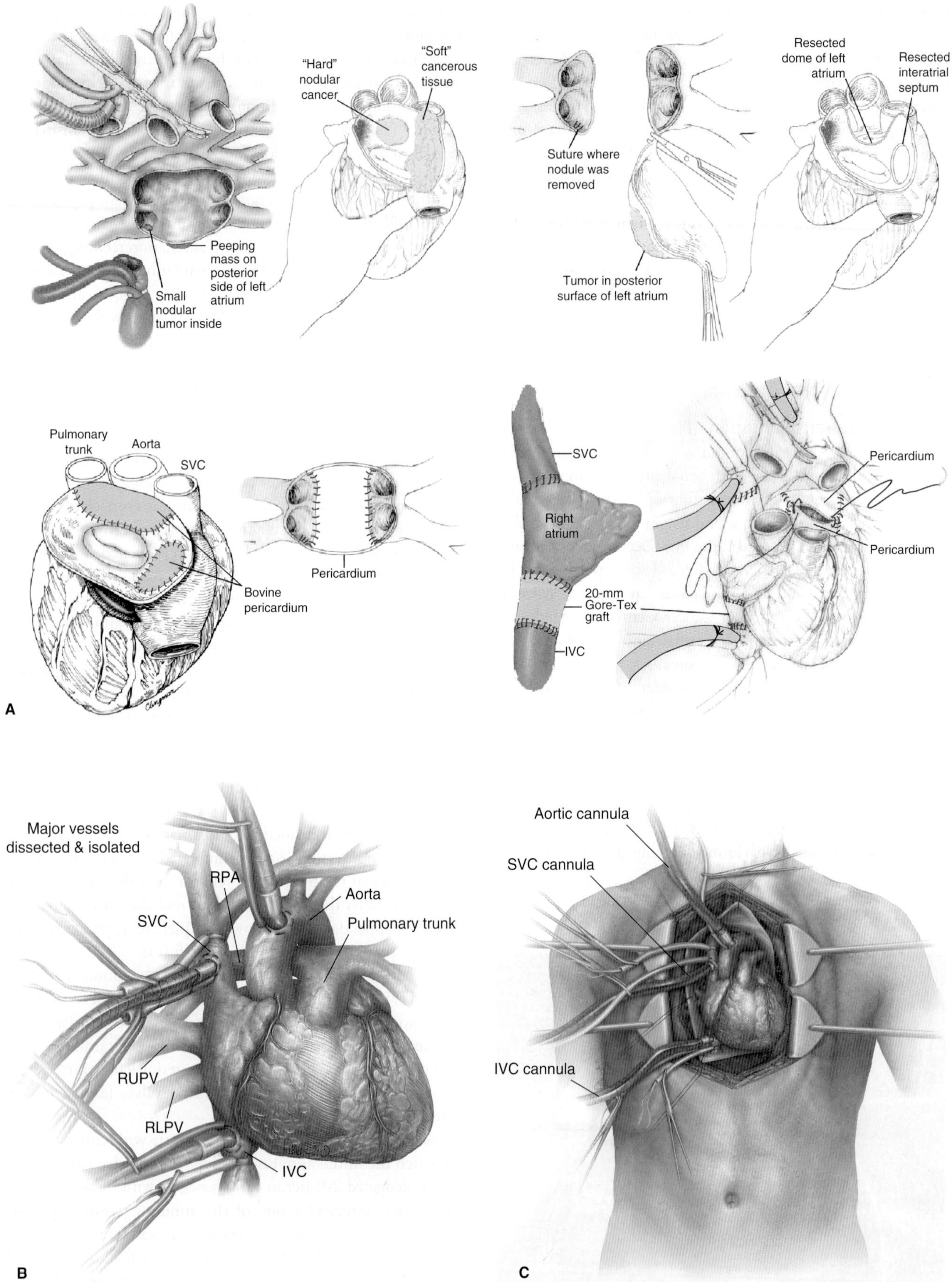

FIGURE 62-28 (A) Explanation of the heart for exposure of extensive left atrial sarcoma, (B) Cannulation strategy to optimize removal and later reimplantation of the heart (note the superior vena cava is cannulated rather than the right atrium); (C) direct view of median sternotomy and cannulation strategy;

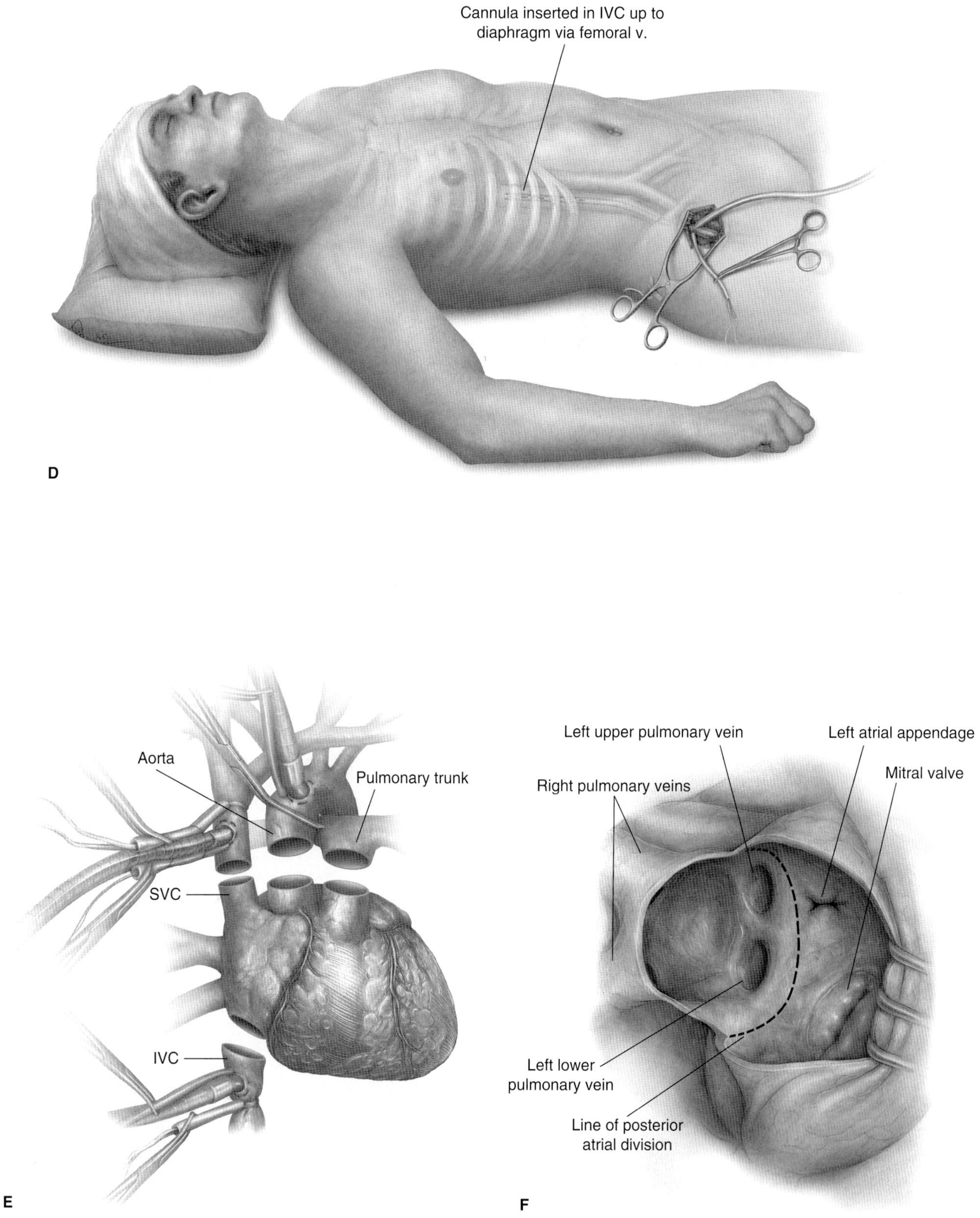

FIGURE 62-28 (*Continued*) (D) right femoral artery cannulation to facilitate inferior vena caval reconstruction and eliminate room occupied by the cannula when the vein is to be transected and later re-connected; (E) necessary divisions of the aorta, pulmonary artery, and cavae to begin the autotransplantation; (F) the last step in removing the heart includes separating the anterior left atrium from the pulmonary veins;

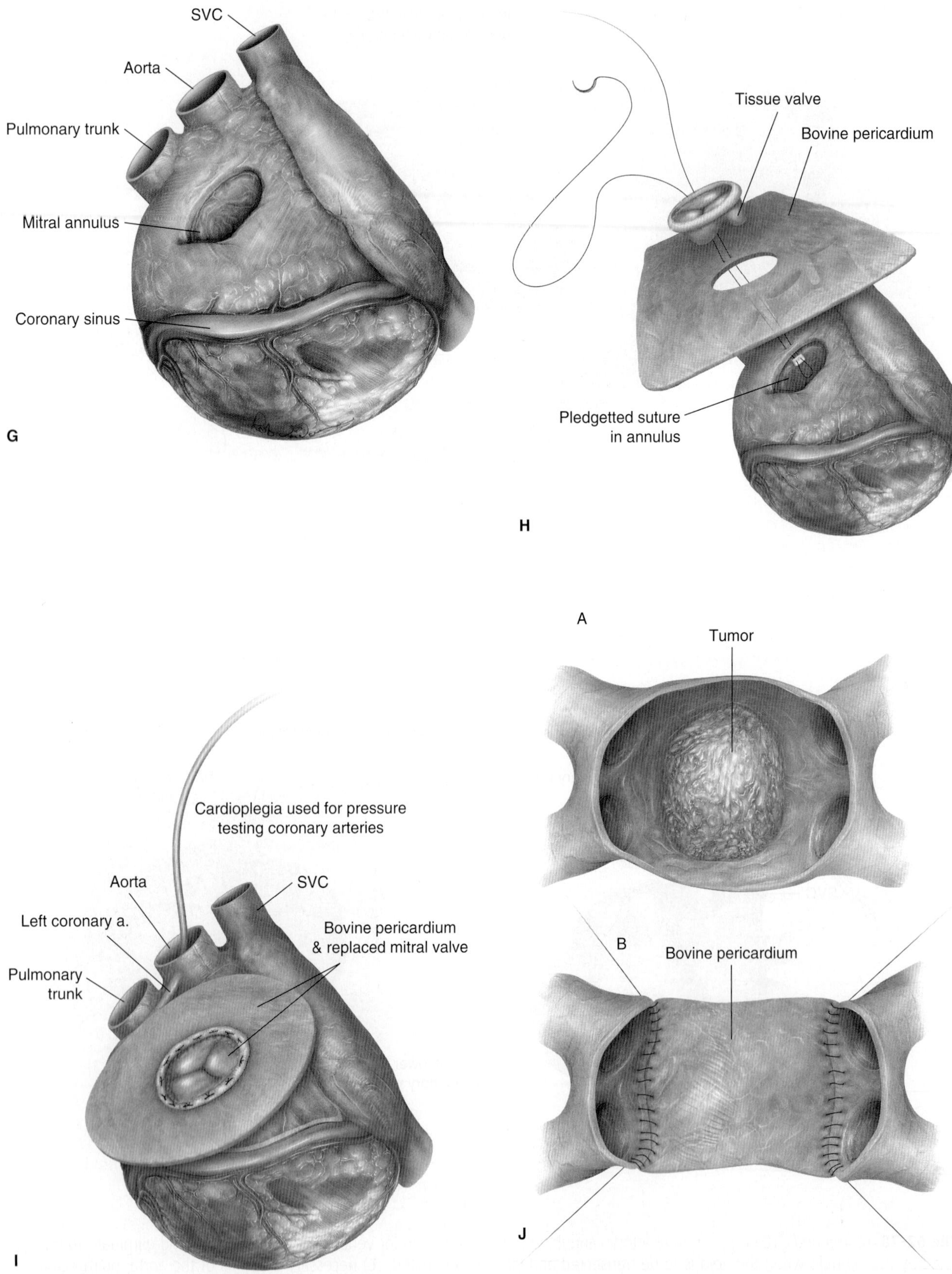

FIGURE 62-28 (*Continued*) (G) the explanted heart from an unusually clear view; (H) reconstruction of the anterior left atrium using bovine pericardium by incorporating the pledgeted sutures through the annulus, the pericardium, and then the new valve implant, respectively. (I) Reconstruction of the anterior left atrium is complete once the sutures are tied. (J) resection of a large posterior left atrial mass is easily completed and reconstructed with the heart explanted.

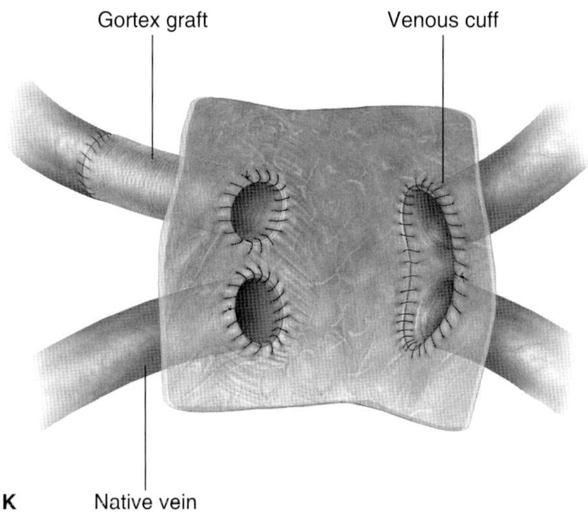

K

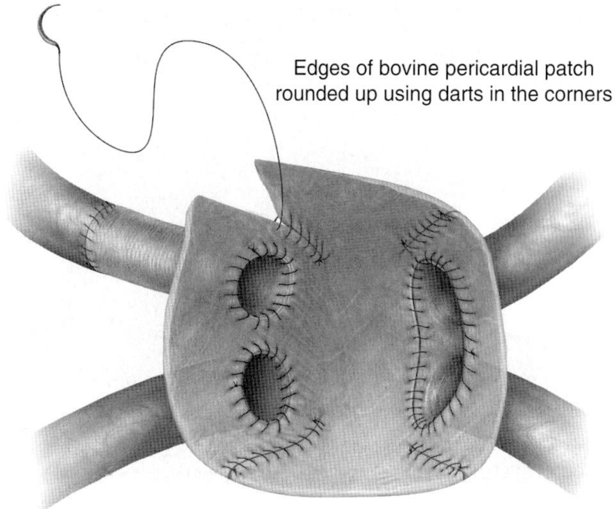

L

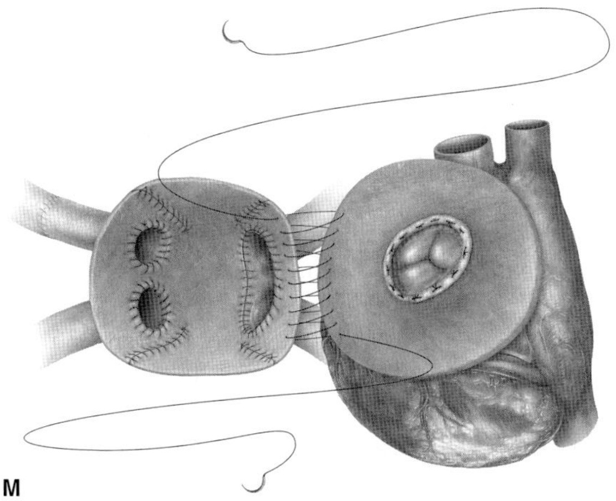

M

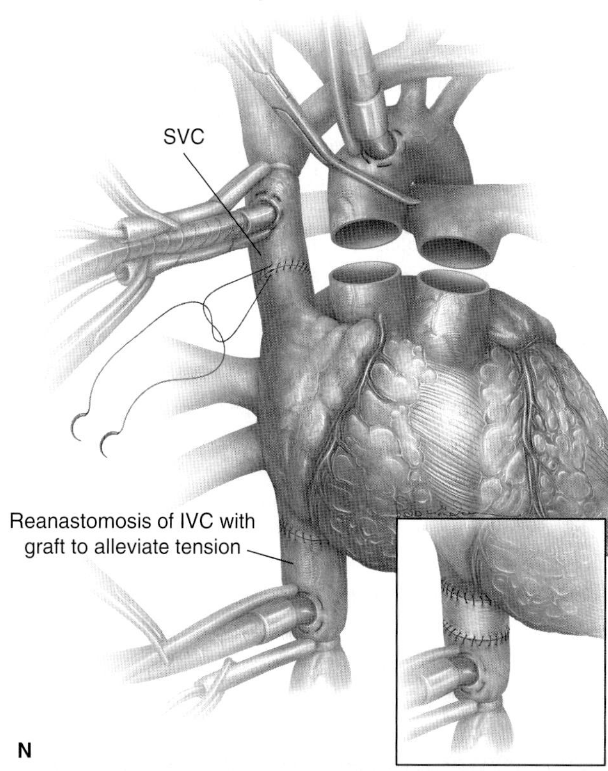

N

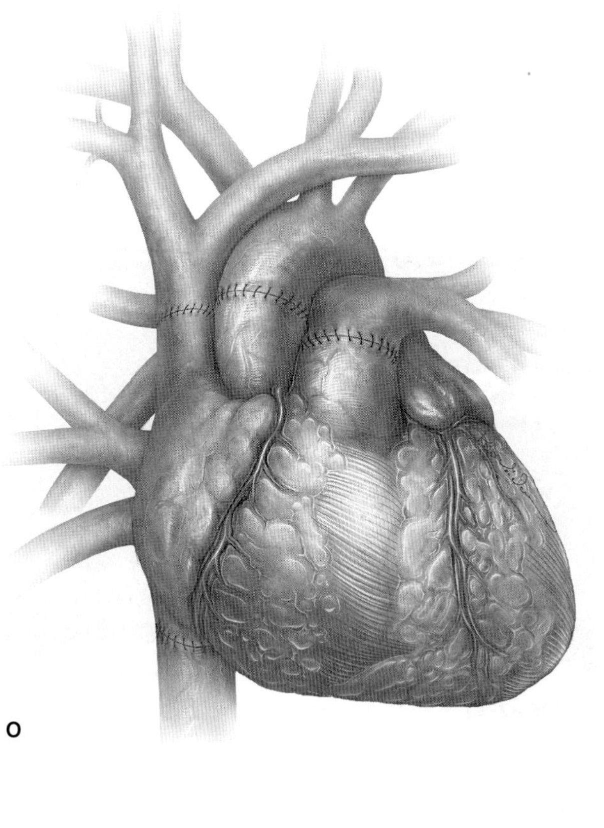

O

FIGURE 62-28 (*Continued*) (K) A Gore-Tex graft can be used to reconstruct a pulmonary vein, and various possibilities are depicted for reconstructing the posterior left atrium. (L) The posterior left atrial repair is then shaped into a bowl by cutting darts in the pericardium used to reconstruct and then sewing the darts together. (M) The reimplantation is begun by first sewing the edges of the pericardium together (the left atrial appendage can be used as a marker for orientation). (N) Once the left atrium is reconstructed, the superior vena cava and then inferior vena cava are reconnected (please note any gaps in length can be corrected by interposing the segment with graft. (O) The completed autotransplant heart.(*Figures B-O reproduced with permission from Blackmon SH, Reardon MJ. Cardiac Autotransplantation. Oper Tech Thorac Cardiovasc Surg 15: 147-61, 2010.*)

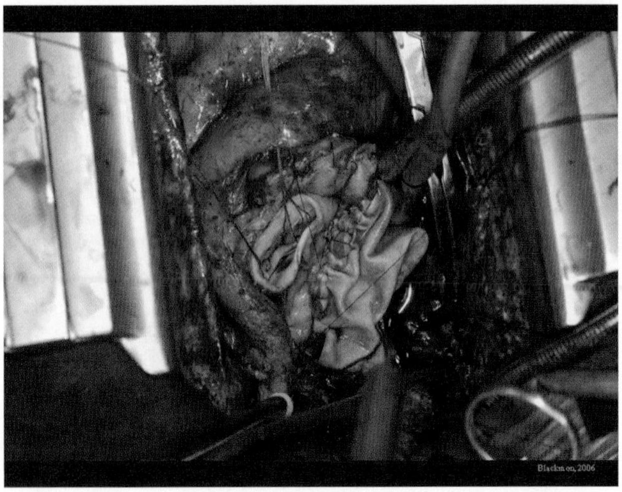

FIGURE 62-29 Cardiac reconstruction using pericardium.

the left atrium anastomosis. The right atrium is then attached to the IVC, and then the right atrium to the SVC. If either of these anastomoses appear to be under excess tension, an interposition graft of Gore-Tex, Dacron, or crafted pericardial tube graft can be used to bridge the defect successfully (Fig. 62-29). The pulmonary artery and aorta are reanastomosed in a standard fashion using Prolene suture, warm-blood potassium cardioplegia is given antegrade, and the aortic cross-clamp is removed. The procedure for left ventricular tumors is similar, and occasionally requires mitral valve excision or partial excision of the interventricular septum (Fig. 62-30). The interventricular septum can be reconstructed with bovine pericardium and valve replacement is typically done with a tissue valve. Although these patients are young, a tissue valve is often chosen to avoid anticoagulation. Issues with structural valve deterioration are of less concern because survival is counted now in years rather than decades.

Because of poor survival, lesions requiring a pneumonectomy in addition to cardiac autotransplant should be considered a contraindication to surgery. This can usually be determined preoperatively with cardiac MRI to evaluate restriction of blood flow through the pulmonary veins.

Lymphomas

Lymphomas may arise from the heart, although this is rare.[170] Most of these tumors respond to radiation and chemotherapy, and surgical resection is rarely indicated.[152] Even when complete resection is not possible, incomplete resection has been performed to relieve acute obstructive systems and, when followed with radiation and chemotherapy, has allowed for extended survival in selected patients.

Pulmonary Artery Sarcomas

Most pulmonary artery sarcomas are classified as. The most frequent presenting symptom is shortness of breath and peripheral edema from concomitant right-sided heart failure.[171] The diagnostic modalities of choice for both the initial evaluation and monitoring for recurrence after resection for pulmonary artery sarcomas are chest CT or MRI (Figs. 62-31, 62-32, and 62-33).

Pulmonary artery sarcomas are very rare tumors that are often confused with acute or chronic pulmonary embolus. This confusion has led to both delay in diagnosis and many being treated with a tumor thromboendarterectomy approach rather than radical resection. These tumors usually are discovered after they have grown to considerable size (Fig. 62-34). Pulmonary artery sarcoma can present with cough, dyspnea, hemoptysis and chest pain that may mimic pulmonary embolus (PE). Constitutional symptoms often present include fever, anemia and weight loss which are more consistent with malignancy than PE and these mass lesions will not decrease in size with anticoagulation. These tumors tend to arise from the dorsal surface of the main pulmonary artery just beyond the pulmonary valve.[172] They form from multipotential mesenchymal cells from the muscle remnant of the bulbus cordis[173] in the

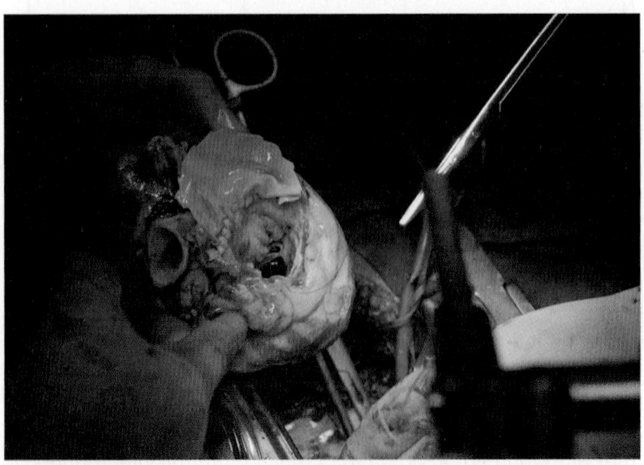

FIGURE 62-30 Explanted heart undergoing anterior left atrial reconstruction with bovine pericardium.

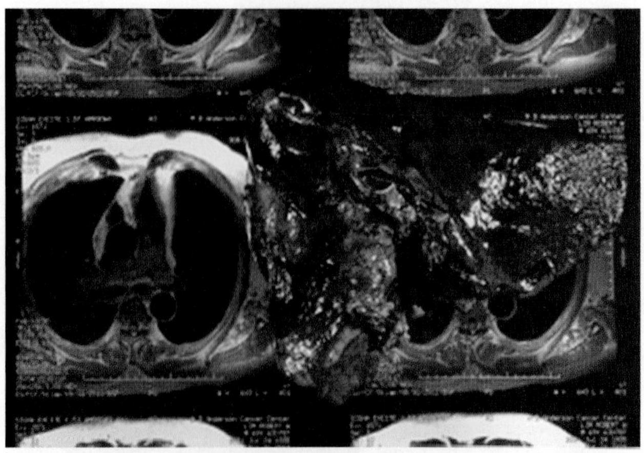

FIGURE 62-31 Pulmonary artery sarcoma as seen on a CT scan with the pathology specimen after radical removal (including pneumonectomy).

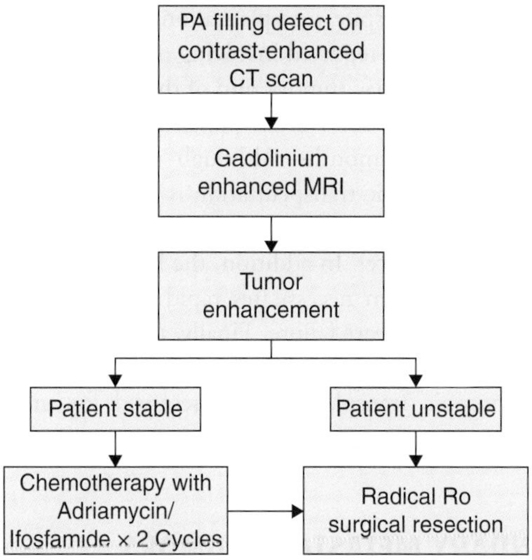

FIGURE 62-32 Algorithm for initial evaluation of a pulmonary artery sarcoma.

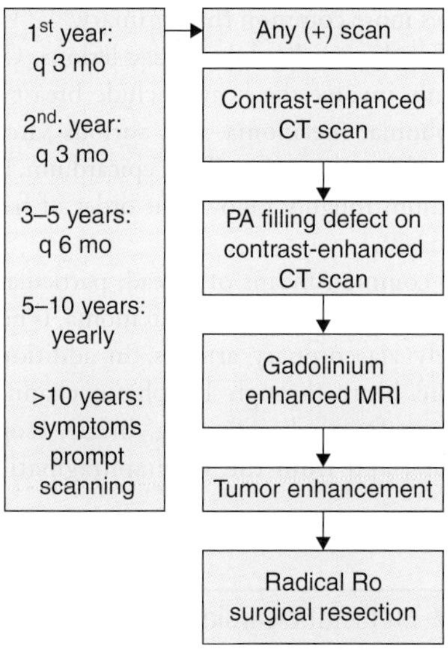

FIGURE 62-33 Postoperative evaluation algorithm for recurrent pulmonary artery sarcoma.

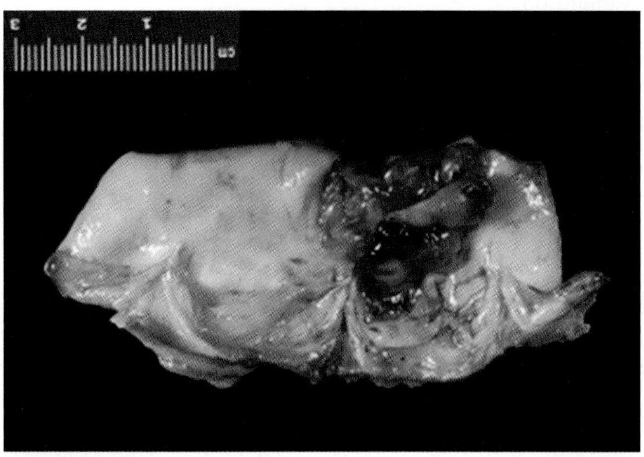

FIGURE 62-34 Pulmonary artery angiosarcoma specimen showing involvement of the pulmonary valve.

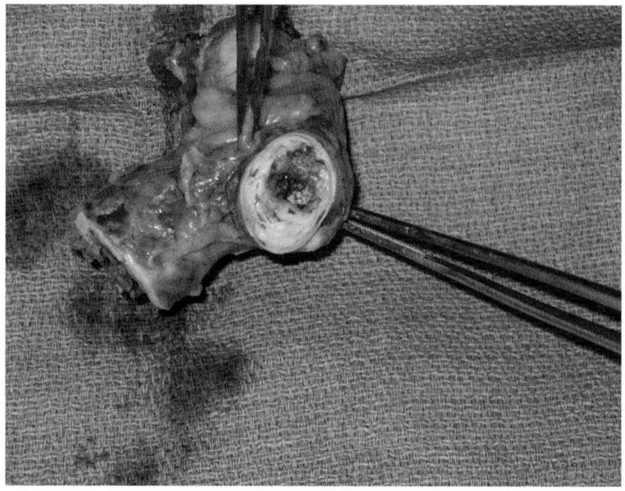

FIGURE 62-35 Pulmonary artery sarcoma demonstrating the extension of the tumor along the inside of the wall and no growth of tumor outside the arterial wall.

intimal and subintimal surfaces.[164] The tumor then tends to grow distally along the artery, rarely penetrating the actual wall of the artery but rather distending it (Fig. 62-35). This characteristic is important to note when planning surgical resection. Distal extension can go to the lung parenchyma itself as emboli, infarction, or metastasis.[174] Although survival difference based on cell histology is found in limited cases, that has not been our experience in cardiac sarcoma in general.[171] Surgical resection remains the primary method of treatment in patients with PA sarcoma and the only method shown to increase survival. A staging system has been developed to further classify these patients and determine who should be offered surgical therapy (Table 62-6).

Resection often requires replacement of a portion of the pulmonary root and branch pulmonary arteries using a pulmonary homograft with or without artificial graft. Pneumonectomy may be required to resect the tumor completely. Because exposure of the right main pulmonary artery may require division of the aorta and possibly the SVC, we plan surgical cannulation for cardiopulmonary bypass by using dual venous cannulation with direct SVC cannulation and normal IVC cannulation via the right atrium. Arterial cannulation via the ascending aorta is routine. Both SVC and IVC are isolated with tourniquets to control blood flow into the right heart. Cardiopulmonary arrest is achieved with cold potassium blood cardioplegia. Fortunately,

TABLE 62-6 Staging System for Primary Pulmonary Artery Sarcomas

Stage I	tumor limited to the main pulmonary artery
Stage II	tumor involving one lung plus a main pulmonary artery
Stage III	bilateral lung involvement
Stage IV	extrathoracic spread

these tumors rarely penetrate the pulmonary artery wall, allowing reasonable mobilization. The main pulmonary artery has always been involved in our experience and the pulmonary valve is involved 30% of the time.[171] The main pulmonary arteries can be resected out to their first branch points on each side from a median approach. In cases where one pulmonary artery is relatively free and the other is involved deep into the lung, a pneumonectomy may be required. In this case, the pulmonary veins and main bronchus are dissected and divided before CPB is instituted to avoid bleeding while heparinized. The branch PAs and main pulmonary artery are mobilized, CPB is instituted, and the involved main PA is divided. In such cases, the involved lung with little blood flow once resected may result in improved hemodynamics; especially after removal of tumor obstructing the contralateral pulmonary artery. Once each pulmonary artery has been divided or in the case of pneumonectomy the lung and main PA removed, the main PA trunk can be assessed for pulmonary valve involvement. If the pulmonary valve is involved, the entire PA trunk must be removed and replaced by a pulmonary allograft. Removal of the entire PA trunk and replacement by an allograft is similar to mobilization and replacement techniques for a Ross procedure.[174] If the resection of the right and/or left main PA is limited, then the allograft branches may be adequate to span the defect. When tumor extension is too distal for this, a Gore-Tex (ePTFE) graft can be used to interpose between the distal right PA resection point to distal left PA resection point and then implantation of the pulmonary allograft into the side of the ePTFE graft is performed. Despite the extensive nature of the resection, separation from CPB has not been difficult. The surgery relieves the patient of severe PA obstruction that is present preoperatively.

The authors have successfully resected pulmonary artery sarcomas in 10 patients, three of whom required concomitant pneumonectomy. There were no in-hospital or 30-day deaths, and all patients were discharged home. Our longest survivor currently has lived more than 100 months and has no known disease. In most cases, adjuvant chemotherapy is used, even in the face of clear surgical margins. Radical PA resection is both safe and appears to prolong survival compared to minimal or palliative resection. Resection in conjunction with chemotherapy also appears to prolong survival. Currently, recommendations to record such rare tumors in a national registry may allow better analysis of long-term outcomes.

Heart Transplantation

Malignant primary cardiac tumors may grow to a large size before detection. Additionally, extensive myocardial involvement or location affecting the fibrous trigone of the heart may make complete resection impossible. Because complete resection yields better results than incomplete resection, orthotopic cardiac transplantation has been considered as a treatment option. Reports of transplantation for a number of cardiac tumors, including sarcoma,[174–177] pheochromocytoma,[170] lymphoma,[171] fibroma,[133] and myxoma have appeared. However, the long-term results are uncertain because some patients die from recurrent metastatic disease despite transplantation.[170,171,173] As of 2000, 28 patients had been reported involving orthotopic transplantation for primary cardiac tumors, and of these, 21 had malignant tumors.[173] The mean survival for patients with primary cardiac malignancy was 12 months. Although technically feasible in some cases, orthotopic transplantation is hindered by a scarcity of donor organs and coupled with an extensive recipient list of patients without cancer. In addition, the large size of the tumor when diagnosed often necessitates rapid intervention for progressive congestive heart failure. Finally, the effect of immunosuppression on any remaining malignancy is unknown. In most cases, orthotopic transplantation is reserved for unresectable benign tumors, such as cardiac fibroma.

SECONDARY METASTATIC TUMORS

Approximately 10% of metastatic tumors eventually reach the heart or pericardium, and almost every type of malignant tumor has been known to do so.[2,7] Secondary neoplasms are 20 to 40 times more common than primary.[4,174] Up to 50% of patients with leukemia develop cardiac lesions. Other cancers that commonly involve the heart include breast cancer, lung cancer, lymphoma, melanoma, and various sarcomas.[2,175,176] Metastases involving the pericardium, epicardium, myocardium, and endocardium roughly follow that order of frequency[2,7] as well (Table 62-7).

The most common means of spread, particularly for melanoma, sarcoma, and bronchogenic carcinoma, is hematogenous and ultimately via coronary arteries. In addition, metastasis can reach the heart through lymphatic channels; through direct extension from adjacent lung, breast, esophageal, and thymic tumors; and from the subdiaphragmatic vena cava.

TABLE 62-7 Metastatic Cardiac Disease

Tumor	Total (no.)	Cardiac (%)	Pericardial (%)
Leukemia	420	53.9	22.4
Melanoma	59	34.0	23.7
Lung ca	402	10.2	15.7
Sarcoma	207	9.2	9.2
Breast ca	289	8.3	11.8
Esophageal ca	65	7.7	7.7
Ovarian ca	115	5.7	7.0
Kidney ca	95	5.3	0.0
Gastric ca	3.8	3.6	3.2
Prostate ca	186	2.7	1.0
Colon ca	214	0.9	2.8
Lymphoma	75	—	14.6

Source: Reproduced with permission from Perry, MC: Cardiac metastasis, in Kapoor AS (ed): Cancer and the Heart. New York, Springer-Verlag Publishers, 1986.

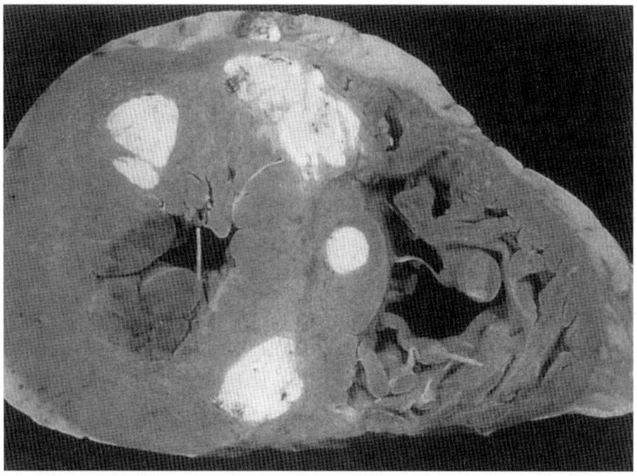

FIGURE 62-36 Hematogenous metastases within the myocardium of a patient with renal cell cancer. (*Reproduced with permission from Hurst JW et al: Atlas of the Heart. New York, McGraw-Hill, 1988.*)

The pericardium is involved most often by direct extension of thoracic cancer; the heart is the target of hematologous and/or retrograde lymphatic metastasis.[5] Cardiac metastases rarely are solitary and nearly always produce multiple microscopic nests and discrete nodules of tumor cells[2,7] (Fig. 62-36). Cardiac metastases produce clinical symptoms in only about 10% of afflicted patients.[177,178] The most common symptom is pericardial effusion or cardiac tamponade. Occasionally, patients develop refractory arrhythmias or congestive heart failure. Chest radiographs and electrocardiograms tend to show nonspecific changes, but echocardiography is particularly useful for diagnosis of pericardial effusion, irregular pericardial thickening, or intracavity masses interfering with blood flow.

Surgical therapy is limited to relief of recurrent pericardial effusions or, occasionally, cardiac tamponade. In most instances, these patients have widespread disease with limited life expectancies. Surgical therapy is directed at providing symptomatic palliation with minimal patient discomfort and hospital stay. This is most readily accomplished via subxiphoid pericardiotomy, which can be accomplished under local anesthesia if necessary with reliable relief of symptoms, a recurrence rate of about 3%, and little mortality.[176] Alternatively, a large pericardial window in the left pleural space can be created using thoracoscopy, but we would recommend this only under unusual circumstances.[179] This can be accomplished with minimal patient discomfort but does require general anesthesia with single-lung ventilation and may be poorly tolerated by patients with hemodynamic deterioration secondary to large effusions.

RIGHT ATRIAL EXTENSION OF SUBDIAPHRAGMATIC TUMORS

Abdominal and pelvic tumors on occasion may grow in a cephalad direction via the inferior vena cava to reach the right atrium. Subdiaphragmatic tumors are frequently renal carcinomas, although hepatic, adrenal, and uterine tumors occasionally have exhibited this behavior. Up to 10% of renal cell carcinomas invade the inferior vena cava, and nearly 40% of these reach the right atrium.[188] Radiation and chemotherapy are not effective in relieving the obstruction of blood flow. If the kidney can be fully removed, as well as the tail of the tumor thrombus, survival can approach 75% at 5 years.[96,182]

Renal cell tumors with atrial extension typically are resected with abdominal dissection to ensure resectability of the renal tumor. Initially, we performed a concomitant median sternotomy and often used cardiopulmonary bypass with hypothermic circulatory arrest when treating these patients. However, we have changed our approach and now work closely with our liver transplant surgeons who have extensive experience in the area of the retrohepatic vena cava. We have found that we can expose the vena cava up to the right atrium through an abdominal incision. With ligation of the arterial inflow, the tumor tail often shrinks below the diaphragm, and in almost all circumstances, this can be removed without the use of cardiopulmonary bypass. Occasionally venovenous bypass as used in hepatic transplantation is necessary to occlude inflow through the inferior vena cava, but this is unusual. If the tumor is too complex for this maneuver, then a median sternotomy is performed, and cardiopulmonary bypass with hypothermic circulatory arrest can be used to remove the tumor from the cardiac chambers down into the inferior vena cava. Perfusion can be restarted, followed by removal of the rest of the tumor. Although it leads to adequate exposure, significant problems with coagulopathy are often apparent after cardiopulmonary bypass and profound hypothermia.

A 5-year survival rate of 75% has been achieved following nephrectomy with resection of right atrial tumor extension.[181,182] Other subdiaphragmatic tumors with atrial extension that have been resected successfully include hepatic and adrenal carcinoma, as well gynecologic tumors.[183–186, 192]

MOLECULAR- AND BIOLOGIC-BASED DIAGNOSIS AND THERAPY FOR CARDIAC TUMORS

This is an exciting time for investigators involved in the search for novel therapies for tumors such as many of those discussed in this chapter. A "new biology" is being developed in laboratories around the world working in these areas, and this is supplanted by the knowledge that is being obtained from the concerted Human Genome Project and the subsequent development of proteomics.[187] It is incumbent on the thoracic surgeon involved in the care of patients with cardiac tumors to have some degree of familiarity with the terms and promise of these advances because significant additional improvement in survival of many of these patients is unlikely to result from further advances in surgical technique.

Interestingly, many sarcomas demonstrate reproducible translocations that allow for the production of novel chimeric genes that may code for a variety of fusion proteins. Many of these proteins have been found to engender cellular phenotypic malignant changes, resistance to apoptosis, and unfettered growth.[188] Although not associated with cardiac involvement, the fusion proteins EWS-FL11 and EWS-ERG are noted in Ewing's sarcoma. When full-length antisense oligonucleotide constructs are used to target the mRNA of these proteins, protein expression is downregulated, and an eightfold increase in apoptosis sensitivity is noted.[180] These fusion proteins have been noted in some forms of rhabdomyosarcoma, and the most common is PAX3-FKHR. This oncoprotein combines components of two strong transcriptional activators and may increase the production of the downstream antiapoptotic protein BCL-XL. Antisense oligonucleotides directed at this oncoprotein mRNA have led to apoptosis in rhabdomyosarcoma cells.[189,190] A similar translocation and fusion protein have been noted in fibrosarcoma. This translocation [t(12;15)(p13q25)] brings together genes from chromosomes 12 and 15, which combines a transcription factor with a tyrosine kinase receptor. The resulting fusion protein is a tyrosine kinase that has oncogenic potential.[191] Reproducible translocations and fusion proteins with downstream effectors of malignant behavior have not been described for angiosarcoma, but they are actively being sought.[192] Antisense treatment has been maligned in the past owing to problems with both delivery and stability of therapeutic constructs. However, sophisticated biochemical alteration of these molecules has improved stability, and two recent solid tumor trials using antisense therapy for salvage have demonstrated positive results.[193] Additional methods of delivering antisense to tumor cells, including viral vector delivery, have been developed. Finally, in addition to antisense methods, small molecule inhibition of many of these fusion proteins should be possible.

Angiosarcoma is an obvious target for therapies based on antiangiogenesis. The weak antiangiogenic properties of interferon-alpha are presumed to be the mechanism that accounts for responses to this agent in this tumor.[194] Multiple new antiangiogenic agents are being evaluated currently in phase I and II trials, and a number of noncardiac angiosarcoma patients have been treated at our institution on this basis. We have noted several to develop stabilized disease, but no definitive data are yet published. Certainly, the use of these agents in these vascular-origin tumors is theoretically attractive.

Viral vector–mediated gene therapy has been evaluated for various sarcomas in the preclinical setting. A number of potential targets exist for these sorts of therapies. Although *p53* is not commonly mutated or absent, *mdm-2* is often overexpressed in many sarcomas, including angiosarcoma. This gene is a known oncogene that is able to directly induce cellular transformation. Importantly, when overexpressed, it binds to and inhibits *p53* activity, even though expression of *p53* may appear normal. Overexpression of *mdm-2* also has been associated with VEGF overproduction and angiogenesis.[194] Preclinical studies of adenoviral vector *p53* transduction of sarcoma in SCID mice have demonstrated growth delay, tumor regression, and decreases in VEGF expression.[195] Many other targets for this approach, including inhibition of NF-κB expression using an adenoviral-dominant negative Iκ-βα construct and prodrug-mediated gene therapy using a doxorubicin prodrug and adenoviral transfer of a metabolizing enzyme in sarcoma cells, have been shown to be effective.[183] Unfortunately, the application of viral-mediated gene therapy paradigms to this tumor suffers the same problems of targeting, transgene expression durability, and immune response that are problematic for the field in general.

In regard to molecular diagnosis, there are no reproducible familial patterns for development of most malignant tumors. However, familial cardiac myxoma, rhabdomyoma, and fibroma may exhibit reproducible genetic abnormalities that lend themselves to the development of genetic testing to identify individuals at risk. Familial myxoma syndrome, or Carney complex, has been associated with mutations in the 17q24 gene *PRKAR1α* that codes for the R1α regulatory subunit of cAMP-dependent protein kinase A (PKA).[195] Although not widely available, genetic diagnosis of this syndrome is now technically achievable.[196] Reproducible mutations in the *TSC-1* and *TSC-2* genes in patients with tuberous sclerosis and cardiac rhabdomyoma, as well as mutations in the *PTC* gene of patients with the Gorlin syndrome and cardiac fibroma, have been noted.[197–200] It is hoped that in the near future we will be able to predict who is at particular risk for these and other cardiac tumors. This could allow for more intense surveillance, earlier detection, and a higher rate of surgical or multimodality cure for these patients.

IMPORTANT POINTS

- Complete excision and radical resection is recommended to prevent local recurrence of cardiac tumors.
- All benign cardiac tumors are potentially curable with current surgical techniques.
- Multimodality therapy and multidisciplinary planning should be incorporated into the care of cardiac tumor patients.
- Cardiac sarcomas are best classified by anatomic location rather than histologic subtype, and the former dictates their presentation, treatment, and prognosis.
- Right heart sarcomas tend to be more bulky, infiltrative, metastasize earlier, and are usually amenable to neoadjuvant chemotherapy.
- Left heart sarcomas tend to be more solid, less infiltrative, and metastasize later.
- Pulmonary artery sarcomas usually present with obstruction, right heart failure, and tend to grow distally within the confinement of the pulmonary artery.
- Cardiac tumors located in the anterior left atrial wall may require autotransplantation for complete excision of the tumor, reconstruction, and reimplantation.
- Cardiac autotransplant and concomitant pneumonectomy carries an unacceptable 50% mortality rate.

REFERENCES

1. Smith C: Tumors of the heart. *Arch Pathol Lab Med* 1986; 110:371.
2. McAllister HA, Fenoglio JJ Jr: Tumors of the cardiovascular system, in *Atlas of Tumor Pathology*, Series 2. Washington, DC, Armed Forces Institute of Pathology, 1978.
3. Straus R, Merliss R: Primary tumors of the heart. *Arch Pathol* 1945; 39.74.
4. Reynen K: Cardiac myxomas. *N Engl J Med* 1995; 333:1610.
5. Wold LE, Lie JT: Cardiac myxomas: a clinicopathologic profile. *Am J Pathol* 1980; 101:219.
6. Silverman NA: Primary cardiac tumors. *Ann Surg* 1980; 91:127.

7. Columbus MR: *De Re Anatomica,* Liber XV. Venice, N Bevilacque, 1559; p 269.
8. Burns A: *Observations of Some of the Most Frequent and Important Diseases of the Heart.* London, James Muirhead, 1809.
9. Goldberg HP, Glenn F, Dotter CT, et al: Myxoma of the left atrium: Diagnosis made during life with operative and postmortem findings. *Circulation* 1952; 6:762.
10. Yates WM: Tumors of the heart and pericardium: pathology, symptomatology, and report of nine cases. *Arch Intern Med* 1931; 48:267.
11. Barnes AR, Beaver DC, Snell AMP: Primary sarcoma of the heart: report of a case with electrocardiographic and pathological studies. *Am Heart J* 1934; 9:480.
12. Beck CS: An intrapericardial teratoma and tumor of the heart: both removed operatively. *Ann Surg* 1942; 116:161.
13. Mauer ER: Successful removal of tumor of the heart. *J Thorac Surg* 1952; 3:479.
14. Effert S, Domanig E: Diagnosis of intra-auricular tumors and large thrombi with the aid of ultrasonic echography. *Dtsch Med Wochesch* 1959; 84:6.
15. Bahnson HT, Newman EV: Diagnosis and surgical removal of intracavitary myxoma of the right atrium. *Bull Johns Hopkins Hosp* 1953; 93:150.
16. Crafoord C: Panel discussion of late results of mitral commissurotomy, in Lam CR (ed): *Henry Ford Hospital International Symposium on Cardiovascular Surgery.* Philadelphia, Saunders, 1955; p 202.
17. Kay JH, Anderson RM, Meihaus J, et al: Surgical removal of an intracavity left ventricular myxoma. *Circulation* 1959; 20:881.
18. Attar S, Lee L, Singleton R, et al: Cardiac myxoma. *Ann Thorac Surg* 1980; 29:397.
19. St. John Sutton MG, Mercier LA, Giuliani ER, et al: Atrial myxomas: a review of clinical experience in 40 patients. *Mayo Clin Proc* 1980; 55:371.
20. Dein JR, Frist WH, Stinson EB, et al: Primary cardiac neoplasms: early and late results of surgical treatment in 42 patients. *J Thorac Cardiovasc Surg* 1987; 93:502.
21. Pinede L, Duhaut P, Loire R: Clinical presentation of left atrial cardiac myxoma: a series of 112 consecutive cases. *Medicine* 2001; 80:159.
22. Waller R, Grider L, Rohr T, et al: Intracardiac thrombi: frequency, location, etiology and, complications: a morphologic review, part I. *Clin Cardiol* 1995; 18:477.
23. Gertner E, Leatherman J: Intracardiac mural thrombus mimicking atrial myxoma in the antiphospholipid syndrome. *J Rheumatol* 1992; 19:1293.
24. Balasundaram S, Halees SA, Duran C: Mesothelioma of the atrioventricular node: first successful follow-up after excision. *Eur Heart J* 1992; 13:718.
25. Ali SZ, Susin M, Kahn E, Hajdu SI: Intracardiac teratoma in a child simulating an atrioventricular nodal tumor. *Pediatr Pathol* 1994; 14:913. ventricular infundibulum. *Can J Cardiol* 1994; 10:37.
26. Carney JA: Differences between nonfamilial and familial cardiac myxoma. *Am J Surg Pathol* 1985; 64:53.
27. McCarthy PM, Schaff HV, Winkler HZ, et al: Deoxyribonucleic acid ploidy pattern of cardiac myxomas. *J Thorac Cardiovasc Surg* 1989; 98:1083.
28. Gelder HM, O'Brian DJ, Styles ED, et al: Familial cardiac myxoma. *Ann Thorac Surg* 1992; 53:419.
29. Kuroda H, Nitta K, Ashida Y, et al: Right atrial myxoma originating from the tricuspid valve. *J Thorac Cardiovasc Surg* 1995; 109:1249.
30. Bortolotti U, Faggian G, Mazzucco A, et al: Right atrial myxoma originating from the inferior vena cava. *Ann Thorac Surg* 1990; 49:1000.
31. King YL, Dickens P, Chan ACL: Tumors of the heart. *Arch Pathol Lab Med* 1993; 117:1027.
32. St. John Sutton MG, Mercier LA, Guiliana ER, et al: Atrial myxomas: a review of clinical experience in 40 patients. *Mayo Clin Proc* 1980; 55:371.
33. Burke AP, Virmani R: Cardiac myxoma: a clinicopathologic study. *Am J Clin Pathol* 1993; 100:671.
34. Peters MN, Hall RJ, Cooley DA, et al: The clinical syndrome of atrial myxoma. *JAMA* 1974; 230:695.
35. Carney JA, Hruska LS, Beauchamp GD, et al: Dominant inheritance of the complex of myxomas, spotty pigmentation, and endocrine overactivity. *Mayo Clin Proc* 1986; 61:165.
36. Imperio J, Summels D, Krasnow N, et al: The distribution patterns of biatrial myxoma. *Ann Thorac Surg* 1980; 29:469.
37. McAllister HA: Primary tumors of the heart and pericardium. *Pathol Annu* 1979; 14:325.
38. Jones DR, Hill RC, Abbott AE Jr, et al: Unusual location of an atrial myxoma complicated by a secundum atrial septal defect. *Ann Thorac Surg* 1993; 55:1252.
39. Kuroki S, Naitoh K, Katoh O, et al: Increased interleukin-6 activity in cardiac myxoma with mediastinal lymphadenopathy. *Intern Med* 1992; 31:1207.
40. Reddy DJ, Rao TS, Venkaiah KR, et al: Congenital myxoma of the heart. *Indian J Pediatr* 1956; 23:210.
41. Prichard RW: Tumors of the heart: review of the subject and report of one hundred and fifty cases. *Arch Pathol* 1951; 51:98.
42. Merkow LP, Kooros MA, Macgovern G, et al: Ultrastructure of a cardiac myxoma. *Arch Pathol* 1969; 88:390.
43. Lie JT: The identity and histogenesis of cardiac myxomas: a controversy put to rest. *Arch Pathol Lab Med* 1989; 113:724.
44. Ferrans VJ, Roberts WC: Structural features of cardiac myxomas: histology, histochemistry, and electron microscopy. *Hum Pathol* 1973; 4:111.
45. Krikler DM, Rode J, Davies MJ, et al: Atrial myxoma: a tumor in search of its origins. *Br Heart J* 1992; 67:89.
46. Glasser SP, Bedynek JL, Hall RJ, et al: Left atrial myxoma: report of a case including hemodynamic, surgical, and histologic characteristics. *Am J Med* 1971; 50:113.
47. Saji T, Yanagawa E, Matsuura H, et al: Increased serum inter-leukin-6 in cardiac myxoma. *Am Heart J* 1991; 122:579.
48. Senguin JR, Beigbeder JY, Hvass U, et al: Interleukin-6 production by cardiac myxoma may explain constitutional symptoms. *J Thorac Cardiovasc Surg* 1992; 103:599.
49. Buchanan RC, Cairns JA, Krag G, et al: Left atrial myxoma mimicking vasculitis: echocardiographic diagnosis. *Can Med Assoc J* 1979; 120:1540.
50. Currey HLF, Matthew JA, Robinson J: Right atrial myxoma mimicking a rheumatic disorder. *Br Med J* 1967; 1:547.
51. Byrd WE, Matthew OP, Hunt RE: Left atrial myxoma presenting as a systemic vasculitis. *Arthritis Rheum* 1980; 23:240.
52. Hattler BG, Fuchs JCA, Coson R, et al: Atrial myxomas: an evaluation of clinical and laboratory manifestations. *Ann Thorac Surg* 1970; 10:65.
53. Bulkley BH, Hutchins GM: Atrial myxomas: a fifty-year review. *Am Heart J* 1979; 97:639.
54. Panidas IP, Kotler MN, Mintz GS, et al: Clinical and echocardiographic features of right atrial masses. *Am Heart J* 1984; 107:745.
55. Meller J, Teichholz LE, Pichard AD, et al: Left ventricular myxoma: echocardiographic diagnosis and review of the literature. *Am J Med* 1977; 63:81.
56. Desousa AL, Muller J, Campbell RL, et al: Atrial myxoma: a review of the neurological complications, metastases, and recurrences. *J Neurol Neurosurg Psychiatr* 1978; 41:1119.
57. Suzuki T, Nagai R, Yamazaki T, et al: Rapid growth of intracranial aneurysms secondary to cardiac myxoma. *Neurology* 1994; 44:570.
58. Chen HJ, Liou CW, Chen L: Metastatic atrial myxoma presenting as intracranial aneurysm with hemorrhage: case report. *Surg Neurol* 1993; 40:61.
59. Browne WT, Wijdicks EF, Parisi JE, et al: Fulminant brain necrosis from atrial myxoma showers. *Stroke* 1993; 24:1090.
60. Lewis JM: Multiple retinal occlusions from a left atrial myxoma. *Am J Ophthalmol* 1994; 117:674.
61. Eriksen UH, Baandrup U, Jensen BS: Total disruptions of left atrial myxoma causing cerebral attack and a saddle embolus in the iliac bifurcation. *Int J Cardiol* 1992; 35:127.
62. Carter AB, Lowe K, Hill I: Cardiac myxomata and aortic saddle embolism. *Br Heart J* 1960; 22:502.
63. Hashimoto H, Tikahashi H, Fukiward Y, et al: Acute myocardial infarction due to coronary embolization from left atrial myxoma. *Jpn Circ J* 1993; 57:1016.
64. Rajpal RS, Leibsohn JA, Leikweg WG, et al: Infected left atrial myxoma with bacteremia simulating infective endocarditis. *Arch Intern Med* 1979; 139:1176.
65. Whitman MS, Rovito MA, Klions D, et al: Infected atrial myxoma: case report and review. *Clin Infect Dis* 1994; 18:657.
66. Martinez-Lopez JI: Sounds of the heart in diastole. *Am J Cardiol* 1974; 34:594.
67. Harvey WP: Clinical aspects of heart tumors. *Am J Cardiol* 1968; 21:328.
68. Case records of the Massachusetts General Hospital, weekly clinicopathological exercises: Case 14-1978. *N Engl J Med* 1978; 298:834.
69. Mundinger A, Gruber HP, Dinkel E, et al: Imaging cardiac mass lesions. *Radiol Med* 1992; 10:135.
70. Ensberding R, Erbel DR, Kaspar W, et al: Diagnosis of heart tumors by transesophageal echocardiography. *Eur Heart J* 1993; 14:1223.
71. Samdarshi TE, Mahan EF 3d, Nanda NC, et al: Transesophageal echocardiographic diagnosis of multicentric left ventricular myxomas mimicking a left atrial tumor. *J Thorac Cardiovasc Surg* 1992; 103:471.
72. Bleiweis MS, Georgiou D, Brungage BH: Detection of intracardiac masses by ultrafast computed tomography. *Am J Cardiac Imag* 1994; 8:63.
73. Symbas PN, Hatcher CR Jr, Gravanis MB: Myxoma of the heart: clinical and experimental observations. *Ann Surg* 1976; 183:470.

74. McCarthy PM, Piehler JM, Schaff HV, et al: The significance of multiple, recurrent, and "complex" cardiac myxoma. *J Thorac Cardiovasc Surg* 1986; 91:389.
75. Dato GMA, Benedictus M, Dato AA, et al: Long-term follow-up of cardiac myxomas (7–31 years). *J Cardiovasc Surg* 1993; 34:141.
76. Bertolotti U, Mazzucco A, Valfre C, et al: Right ventricular myxoma: review of the literature and report of two patients. *Ann Thorac Surg* 1983; 33:277.
77. Attum AA, Johnson GS, Masri Z, et al: Malignant clinical behavior of cardiac myxomas and "myxoid imitators." *Ann Thorac Surg* 1987; 44:217.
78. Ravikumar E, Pawar N, Gnanamuthu R, et al: Minimal access approach for surgical management of cardiac tumors. *Ann Thorac Surg* 2000; 70:1077.
79. Ko PJ, Chang CH, Lin PJ, et al: Video-assisted minimal access in excision of left atrial myxoma. *Ann Thorac Surg* 1998; 66:1301.
80. Gulbins H, Reichenspurner H, Wintersperger BJ: Minimally invasive extirpation of a left-ventricular myxoma. *Thorac Cardiovasc Surg* 1999; 47:129.
81. Espada R, Talwalker NG, Wilcox G, et al: Visualizaton of ventricular fibroelastoma with a video-assisted thoracoscope. *Ann Thorac Surg* 1997; 63:221.
82. Walkes JC, Bavare C, Blackmon S, Reardon MJ: Transaortic resection of an apical left ventricular fibroelastoma facilitated by a thoracoscope. *J Thorac Cardiovasc* 2007; 134(3):793-794.
83. Greco E et al: Video-assisted cardioscopy for removal of primary left ventricular myxoma. *Eur J Cardiothorac Surg* 1999; 16:667.
84. Reyes CV, Jablokow VR: Lipomatous hypertrophy of the atrial septum: a report of 38 cases and review of the literature. *Am J Clin Pathol* 1979; 72:785.
85. McAllister HA: Primary tumors and cysts of the heart and pericardium, in Harvey WP (ed): *Current Problems in Cardiology*. Chicago, Year Book Medical, 1979.
86. Reece IJ, Cooley DA, Frazier OH, et al: Cardiac tumors: clinical spectrum and prognosis of lesions other than classic benign myxoma in 20 patients. *J Thorac Cardiovasc Surg* 1984; 88:439.
87. Markel ML, Armstrong WF, Waller BF, et al: Left atrial myxoma with multicentric recurrence and evidence of metastases. *Am Heart J* 1986; 111:409.
88. Castells E, Ferran KV, Toledo MCO, et al: Cardiac myxomas: surgical treatment, long-term results and recurrence. *J Cardiovasc Surg* 1993; 34:49.
89. Seidman JD, Berman JJ, Hitchcock CL, et al: DNA analysis of cardiac myxomas: flow cytometry and image analysis. *Hum Pathol* 1991; 22:494.
90. Attum AA, Ogden LL, Lansing AM: Atrial myxoma: benign and malignant. *J Ky Med Assoc* 1984; 82:319.
91. Seo S, Warner TFCS, Colyer RA, et al: Metastasizing atrial myxoma. *Am J Surg Pathol* 1980; 4:391.
92. Hirsch BE, Sehkar L, Kamerer DB: Metastatic atrial myxoma to the temporal bone: case report. *Am J Otol* 1991; 12:207.
93. Kotani K, Matsuzawa Y, Funahashi T, et al: Left atrial myxoma metastasizing to the aorta, with intraluminal growth causing renovascular hypertension. *Cardiology* 1991; 78:72.
94. Diflo T, Cantelmo NL, Haudenschild DD, Watkins MT: Atrial myxoma with remote metastasis: case report and review of the literature. *Surgery* 1992; 111:352.
95. Hannah H, Eisemann G, Hiszvzynskyj R, et al: Invasive atrial myxoma: documentation of malignant potential of cardiac myxomas. *Am Heart J* 1982; 104:881.
96. Rankin LI, Desousa AL: Metastatic atrial myxoma presenting as intracranial mass. *Chest* 1978; 74:451.
97. Burton C, Johnston J: Multiple cerebral aneurysm and cardiac myxoma. *N Engl J Med* 1970; 282:35.
98. Harjola PR, Ala-Kulju K, Ketonen P: Epicardial lipoma. *Scand J Thorac Cardiovasc Surg* 1985; 19:181.
99. Arciniegas E, Hakimi M, Farooki ZQ, et al: Primary cardiac tumors in children. *J Thorac Cardiovasc Surg* 1980; 79:582.
100. Isner J, Swan CS II, Mikus JP, et al: Lipomatous hypertrophy of the interatrial septum: in vivo diagnosis. *Circulation* 1982; 66:470.
101. Simons M, Cabin HS, Jaffe CC: Lipomatous hypertrophy of the atrial septum: diagnosis by combined echocardiography and computerized tomography. *Am J Cardiol* 1984; 54:465.
102. Basu S, Folliguet T, Anselmo M, et al: Lipomatous hypertrophy of the interatrial septum. *Cardiovasc Surg* 1994; 2:229.
103. Zeebregts CJAM, Hensens AG, Timmermans J, et al: Lipomatous hypertrophy of the interatrial septum: indication for surgery? *Eur J Cardiothorac Surg* 1997; 11:785.
104. Vander Salm TJ: Unusual primary tumors of the heart. *Semin Thorac Cardiovasc Surg* 2000; 2:89.
105. Edwards FH, Hale D, Cohen A, et al: Primary cardiac valve tumors. *Ann Thorac Surg* 1991; 52:1127.
106. Israel DH, Sherman W, Ambrose JA, et al: Dynamic coronary ostial occlusion due to papillary fibroelastoma leading to myocardial ischemia and infarction. *Am J Cardiol* 1991; 67:104.
107. Grote J, Mugge A, Schfers HJ: Multiplane transesophageal echocardiography detection of a papillary fibroelastoma of the aortic valve causing myocardial infarction. *Eur Heart J* 1995; 16:426.
108. Gallas MT, Reardon MJ, Reardon PR, et al: Papillary fibroelastoma: a right atrial presentation. *Tex Heart Inst J* 1993; 20:293.
109. Grinda JM, Couetil JP, Chauvaud S, et al: Cardiac valve papillary fibroelastoma: Surgical excision for revealed or potential embolization. *J Thorac Cardiovasc Surg* 1999; 117:106.
110. Shing M, Rubenson DS: Embolic stroke and cardiac papillary fibroelastoma. *Clin Cardiol* 2001; 24:346.
111. Grandmougin D, Fayad G, Moukassa D, et al: Cardiac valve papillary fibroelastomas: clinical, histological and immunohistochemical studies and a physiopathogenic hypothesis. *J Heart Valve Dis* 2000; 9:832.
112. Mazzucco A, Bortolotti U, Thiene G, et al: Left ventricular papillary fibroelastoma with coronary embolization. *Eur J Cardiothorac Surg* 1989; 3:471.
113. Topol EJ, Biern RO, Reitz BA: Cardiac papillary fibroelastoma and stroke: Echocardiographic diagnosis and guide to excision. *Am J Med* 1986; 80:129.
114. Mann J, Parker DJ: Papillary fibroelastoma of the mitral valve: a rare cause of transient neurologic deficits. *Br Heart J* 1994; 71:6.
115. Ragni T, Grande AM, Cappuccio G, et al: Embolizing fibroelastoma of the aortic valve. *Cardiovasc Surg* 1994; 2:639.
116. Nicks R: Hamartoma of the right ventricle. *J Thorac Cardiovasc Surg* 1967; 47:762.
117. Bass JL, Breningstall GN, Swaiman DF: Echocardiographic incidence of cardiac rhabdomyoma in tuberous sclerosis. *Am J Cardiol* 1985; 55:1379.
118. Fenoglio JJ, McAllister HA, Ferrans VJ: Cardiac rhabdomyoma: a clinicopathologic and electron microscopic study. *Am J Cardiol* 1976; 38:241.
119. Garson A, Smith RT, Moak JP, et al: Incessant ventricular tachycardia in infants: Myocardial hamartomas and surgical cure. *J Am Coll Cardiol* 1987; 10:619.
120. Burke AP, Rosado-de-Christenson M, Templeton PA, et al: Cardiac fibroma: clinicopathologic correlates and surgical treatment. *J Thorac Cardiovasc Surg* 1994; 108:862.
121. Yamaguchi M, Hosokawa Y, Ohashi H, et al: Cardiac fibroma: long-term fate after excision. *J Thorac Cardiovasc Surg* 1992; 103:140.
122. Jamieson SA, Gaudiani VA, Reitz BA, et al: Operative treatment of an unresectable tumor on the left ventricle. *J Thorac Cardiovasc Surg* 1981; 81:797.
123. Valente M, Cocco P, Thiene G, et al: Cardiac fibroma and heart transplantation. *J Thorac Cardiovasc Surg* 1993; 106:1208.
124. Nishida K, Kaijima G, Nagayama T: Mesothelioma of the atrioventricular node. *Br Heart J* 1985; 53:468.
125. Jebara VA, Uva MS, Farge A, et al: Cardiac pheochromocytomas. *Ann Thorac Surg* 1991; 53:356.
126. Orringer MB, Sisson JC, Glazer G, et al: Surgical treatment of cardiac pheochromocytomas. *J Thorac Cardiovasc Surg* 1985; 89:753.
127. Cooley DA, Reardon MJ, Frazier OH, et al: Human cardiac explantation and autotransplantation: application in a patient with a large cardiac pheochromocytoma. *J Tex Heart Inst* 1985; 2:171.
128. Mirza M: Angina-like pain and normal coronary arteries: uncovering cardiac syndromes that mimic CAD. *Postgrad Med* 2005; 117:41.
129. Pac-Ferrer J, Uribe-Etxebarria N, Rumbero JC, Castellanos E: Mediastinal paraganglioma irrigated by coronary vessels in a patient with an atypical chest pain. *Eur J Cardiothorac Surg* 2003; 24:662.
130. Turley AJ et al: A cardiac paraganglioma presenting with atypical chest pain. *Eur J Cardiothorac Surg* 2005; 28:352.
131. Can KM et al: Paraganglioma of the left atrium. *J Thorac Cardiovasc Surg* 2001; 122:1032.
132. Bizard C, Latremouille C, Jebara VA, et al: Cardiac hemangiomas. *Ann Thorac Surg* 1993; 56:390.
133. Grenadier E, Margulis T, Plauth WH, et al: Huge cavernous hemangioma of the heart: a completely evaluated case report and review of the literature. *Am Heart J* 1989; 117:479.
134. Soberman MS, Plauth WH, Winn KJ, et al: Hemangioma of the right ventricle causing outflow tract obstruction. *J Thorac Cardiovasc Surg* 1988; 96:307.
135. Weir I, Mills P, Lewis T: A case of left atrial hemangioma: echocardiographic, surgical, and morphologic features. *Br Heart J* 1987; 58:665.
136. Palmer TC, Tresch DD, Bonchek LI: Spontaneous resolution of a large cavernous hemangioma of the heart. *Am J Cardiol* 1986; 58:184.

137. Thomas CR, Johnson GW, Stoddard MF, et al: Primary malignant cardiac tumors: update 1992. *Med Pediatr Oncol* 1992; 20:519.
138. Poole GV, Meredith JW, Breyer RH, et al: Surgical implications in malignant cardiac disease. *Ann Thorac Surg* 1983; 36:484.
139. Castleman B et al: Localized mediastinal lymph node hyperplasia resembling thymoma. *Cancer* 1956; 9:822.
140. Keller AR et al: Hyaline-vascular and plasma-cell types of giant lymph node hyperplasia of the mediastinum and other locations. *Cancer* 1972; 670.
141. Malaisrie SC, Loebe M, Walkes JC, Reardon MJ: Coronary pseudoaneurysm: an unreported complication of Castleman's disease. *Ann Thorac Surg* 2006; 82(1): 318-20.
142. Ko SF, Wan WL, Ng SH, et al: Imaging features of atypical thoracic Castleman's disease. *Clin Imaging* 2004; 28:280.
143. Samuels LE, et al: Castleman's disease: surgical implications. *Surg Rounds* 1997; 20:449.
144. Murphy MC, Sweeney MS, Putnam JB Jr, et al: Surgical treatment of cardiac tumors: a 25-year experience. *Ann Thorac Surg* 1990; 49:612.
145. Bakaeen F et al: Outcomes after surgical resection of cardiac sarcoma in the multimodality treatment era. *J Cardiovasc Surg,* 2009;137:1454-1460.
146. Blackmon SH, Patel A, Reardon MJ: Management of primary cardiac sarcomas. *Expert Rev Cardiovasc Ther.* 2008; 6(9):1217-1222.
147. Bear PA, Moodie DS: Malignant primary cardiac tumors: the Cleveland Clinic experience, 1956–1986. *Chest* 1987; 92:860.
148. Burke AP, Cowan D, Virmani R: Primary sarcomas of the heart. *Cancer* 1922; 69:387.
149. Putnam JB, Sweeney MS, Colon R, et al: Primary cardiac sarcomas. *Ann Thorac Surg* 1991; 51:906.
150. Rettmar K, Stierle U, Shiekhzadeh A, et al: Primary angiosarcoma of the heart: report of a case and review of the literature. *Jpn Heart J* 1993; 34:667.
151. Hermann MA, Shankerman RA, Edwards WD, et al: Primary cardiac angiosarcoma: a clinicopathologic study of six cases. *J Thorac Cardiovasc Surg* 1992; 102:655.
152. Wiske PS, Gillam LD, Blyden G, et al: Intracardiac tumor regression documented by two-dimensional echocardiography. *Am J Cardiol* 1986; 58:186.
153. Reardon MJ, DeFelice CA, Sheinbaum R, et al: Cardiac autotransplant for surgical treatment of a malignant neoplasm. *Ann Thorac Surg* 1999; 67:1793.
154. Miralles A, Bracamonte MD, Soncul H, et al: Cardiac tumors: clinical experience and surgical results in 74 patients. *Ann Thorac Surg* 1991; 52:886.
155. Winer HE, Kronzon I, Fox A, et al: Primary chondromyxosarcoma: clinical and echocardiographic manifestations: a case report. *J Thorac Cardiovasc Surg* 1977; 74:567.
156. Torsveit JF, Bennett WA, Hinchcliffe WA, et al: Primary plasmacytoma of the atrium: report of a case with successful surgical management. *J Thorac Cardiovasc Surg* 1977; 74:563.
157. Nzayinambabo K, Noel H, Brobet C: Primary cardiac liposarcoma simulating a left atrial myxoma. *J Thorac Cardiovasc Surg* 1985; 40:402.
158. Burke AP, Virmani R: Osteosarcomas of the heart. *Am J Surg Pathol* 1991; 15:289.
159. Neragi-Miandoab S, Kim J, Vlahakes GJ: Malignant tumours of the heart: a review of tumour type, diagnosis and therapy. *Clin Oncol (R Coll Radiol)* 2007; 19:748-756.
160. Centofani P, Di Rosa E, Deorsola L, et al: Primary cardiac tumors: early and late results of surgical treatment in 91 patients. *Ann Thorac Surg* 1999; 68:1236-1241.
161. Zhang PJ, Brooks, JS, Goldblum JR, et al: Primary cardiac sarcomas: a clinicopathologic analysis of a series with follow-up information in 17 patients and emphasis on long-term survival. *Human Pathology* 2008; 39:1385-1395.
162. Bossert Torsten B, Gummert JF, Battellini, et al: Surgical experience with 77 primary cardiac tumors. *Interact CardioVasc Torac Surg* 2005; 4: 311-315.
163. Simpson L, Kumar SK, Okuno SH, et al: Malignant primary cardiac tumors: review of a single institution experience. *Cancer* 2008; 112(11):2440-6.
164. Kim, CH, Dancer JY, Coffey D, et al: Clinicopathologic study of 24 patients with primary cardiac sarcomas: a 10-year single institution experience. *Human Pathology* 2008; 39:933-38.
165. Blackmon SH, Patel AR, Bruckner BA, et al: Cardiac Autotransplantation for malignant or complex primary left heart tumors. *Tex Heart Inst J* 2008; 35(3):296-300.
166. Gabelman C, Al-Sadir J, Lamberti J, et al: Surgical treatment of recurrent primary malignant tumor of the left atrium. *J Thorac Cardiovasc Surg* 1979; 77(6):914-921.
167. Gowdamarajan A, Michler RE: Therapy for primary cardiac tumors: is there a role for heart transplantation? *Curr Opin Cardiol* 2000; 15:121.
168. Reardon MJ, Walkes JC, DeFelice CA, Wojciechowski Z: Cardiac autotransplant for surgical resection of a primary malignant left ventricular tumor. *Tex Heart Inst J* 2006; 33(4):495-497.
169. Conklin LD, Reardon, MJ: Autotransplantation of the heart for primary cardiac malignancy: development and surgical technique. *Tex Heart Inst J* 2002; 29(2):105-108.
170. Takagi M, Kugimiya T, Fuii T, et al: Extensive surgery for primary malignant lymphoma of the heart. *J Cardiovasc Surg* 1992; 33:570.
171. Blackmon SH, Rice DR, Correa AM, et al: Management of primary main pulmonary artery sarcomas. *Annals of Thoracic Surgery* 2009; 87(3):977-984.
172. Baker PB, Goodwin RA: Pulmonary artery sarcomas: a review and report of a case. *Arch Pathol Lab Med* 1985; 109:35-39.
173. Schmookler BM, Marsh HB, Roberts WC: Primary sarcoma of the pulmonary trunk and/or right or left main pulmonary artery: a rare cause of obstruction to right ventricular outflow: report on two patients and analysis of 35 previously described patients. *Am J Med* 1977; 63:263-272.
174. Conklin LD, Reardon MJ: The technical aspects of the Ross procedure. *Tex Heart Inst J* 2001; 28(3):186-189.
175. Golstein DJ, Oz MC, Rose EA, et al: Experience with heart transplantation for cardiac tumors. *J Heart Lung Transplant* 1995; 14:382.
176. Baay P, Karwande SV, Kushner JP, et al: Successful treatment of a cardiac angiosarcoma with combined modality therapy. *J Heart Lung Transplant* 1994; 13:923.
177. Crespo MG, Pulpon LA, Pradas G, et al: Heart transplantation for cardiac angiosarcoma: should its indication be questioned? *J Heart Lung Transplant* 1993; 12:527.
178. Jeevanandam V, Oz MC, Shapiro B, et al: Surgical management of cardiac pheochromocytoma: resection versus transplantation. *Ann Surg* 1995; 221:415.
179. Yuh DD, Kubo SH, Francis GS, et al: Primary cardiac lymphoma treated with orthotopic heart transplantation: a case report. *J Heart Lung Transplant* 1994; 13:538.
180. Goldstein DJ, Oz MC, Michler RE: Radical excisional therapy and total cardiac transplantation for recurrent atrial myxoma. *Ann Thorac Surg* 1995; 60:1105.
181. Pillai R, Blauth C, Peckham M, et al: Intracardiac metastasis from malignant teratoma of the testis. *J Thorac Cardiovasc Surg* 1986; 92:118.
182. Aburto J, Bruckner BA, Blackmon SH, Beyer EA, Reardon MJ: Renal cell carcinoma, metastatic to the left ventricle. *Texas Heart Inst J* 2009; 36(1): 48-49
183. Hallahan ED, Vogelzang NJ, Borow KM, et al: Cardiac metastasis from soft-tissue sarcomas. *J Clin Oncol* 1986; 4:1662.
184. Press OW, Livingston R: Management of malignant pericardial effusion and tamponade. *JAMA* 1987; 257:1008.
185. Hanfling SM: Metastatic cancer to the heart: review of the literature and report of 127 cases. *Circulation* 1960; 2:474.
186. Weinberg BA, Conces DJ Jr, Waller BF: Cardiac manifestation of noncardiac tumors: I. Direct effects. *Clin Cardiol* 1989; 12:289.
187. Caccavale RJ, Newman J, Sisler GE, Lewis RH: Pericardial disease, in Kaiser LR, Daniel TM (eds): *Thoracopic Surgery.* Boston, Little, Brown, 1993; p 177.
188. Prager RL, Dean R, Turner B: Surgical approach to intracardial renal cell carcinoma. *Ann Thorac Surg* 1982; 33:74.
189. Vaislic CD, Puel P, Grondin P, et al: Cancer of the kidney invading the vena cava and heart: results after 11 years of treatment. *J Thorac Cardiovasc Surg* 1986; 91:604.
190. Shahian DM, Libertino JA, Sinman LN, et al: Resection of cavoatrial renal cell carcinoma employing total circulatory arrest. *Arch Surg* 1990; 125:727.
191. Theman TE: Resection of atriocaval adrenal carcinoma (letter). *Ann Thorac Surg* 1990; 49:170.
192. Cooper MM, Guillem J, Dalton J, et al: Recurrent intravenous leiomyomatosis with cardiac extension. *Ann Thorac Surg* 1992; 53:139.
193. Phillips MR, Bower TC, Orszulak TA, et al: Intracardiac extension of an intracaval sarcoma of endometrial origin. *Ann Thorac Surg* 1995; 59:742.
194. Tomescu O, Barr F: Chromosomal translocations in sarcomas: prospects for therapy. *Trends Mol Med* 2001; 7:554.
195. Graadt van Roggen JF, Bovee JVMG, et al: Diagnostic and prognostic implications of the unfolding molecular biology of bone and soft tissue tumors. *J Clin Pathol* 1999; 52:481.
196. Waters JS, Webb A, Cunningham D, et al: Phase I clinical and pharmacokinetic study of BCL-2 antisense oligonucleotide therapy in patients with non-Hodgkins lymphoma. *J Clin Oncol* 2000; 18:1812.

197. Casey M, Vaughan CJ, He J, et al: Mutations in the protein kinase R1α regulatory subunit cause familial cardiac myxomas and Carney complex. *J Clin Invest* 2000; 106:R31.
198. Goldstein MM, Casey M, Carney JA, et al: Molecular genetic diagnosis of the familial myxoma syndrome (Carney complex). *Am J Med Genet* 1999; 86:62.
199. Van Siegenhorst M, de Hoogt R, Hermans C, et al: Identification of the tuberous sclerosis gene *TSC1* on chromosome 9q34. *Science* 1997; 277:805.
200. The European Chromosome 16 Tuberous Sclerosis Consortium: Identification and characterization of the tuberous sclerosis gene on chromosome 16. *Cell* 1993; 75:1305.

PART 8

TRANSPLANT AND CARDIAC SUPPORT

CHAPTER 63

Immunobiology of Heart and Heart-Lung Transplantation

Bartley P. Griffith

INTRODUCTION

This chapter on the immunology of transplantation is a refreshed effort designed to promote a foundation for understanding the basic transplant immunologic fundamentals necessary for competency in caring for heart and lung transplant recipients. Although surgeons must acquire the technical expertise to perform these often demanding surgeries safely, the recipients' well-being additionally benefits from a surgical team well versed in basic transplant immunology. Comfort in treating patients who receive immunosuppressive therapies, both conventional and innovative, requires familiarity with the nonsurgical language of transplantation. The goal of this chapter is to squeeze the essentials[1] into an understandable short text. The knowledge gained should permit surgeons to read immunology-tilted manuscripts with better understanding and thus make better decisions in treating their own patients. The core features of this alloresponse and new science are presented with some specific references to hearts and lungs so that the surgeon participating in the care of thoracic organ recipients can more easily build an understanding of the complex and evolving science. The material is organized to reflect a unifying theory of the immune response that determines the fate of an allograft and most often the heart or lung recipient as well. This includes: (1) histocompatibility; (2) activation of alloresponse T lymphocytes and T-cell–mediated rejection (TMR); (3) antibody-mediated rejection (AMR); (4) the underappreciated immune pathways, natural killer (NK) cells, and memory lymphocytes; and (5) immune plus gene monitoring. The text will clarify acute, cell-mediated, hyperacute, and chronic rejection pathways (Fig. 63-1).

MAJOR HISTOCOMPATIBILITY COMPLEX

Major histocompatibility complex (MHC) molecules are a family of proteins that vary quite a lot between individuals (genetic polymorphism) and represent the molecular basis for how immune systems distinguish self from nonself with respect to infections and transplants. MHC molecules on donor cells or MHC fragments, shed from thoracic organ transplants, are determined to be foreign by the immune regulatory system of the host. Intact MHC molecules expressed on the surface of cells serve two key functions in the context of transplantation. Fragments of foreign proteins, including fragments of MHC molecules, are presented in the binding groove of MHC and are recognized by T-cell receptors of the recipient that happen to have high affinity for that protein fragment (indirect donor antigen presentation). In addition, recipient T cells directly recognize donor MHC as "foreign" (direct donor antigen presentation).

Human MHC molecules are known as human leukocyte antigens (HLA) because they are expressed at high levels on leukocytes and were first measured on peripheral blood lymphocytes. HLA are heterodimeric glycoproteins expressed on the surface of almost every cell in the human body. These proteins are immunologically active and can trigger a proliferative or cytotoxic T-cell response in vivo and in vitro. For these reasons, they are thought to play a critical role in graft rejection in solid-organ transplantation.

The genes coding for these antigens are located on the short arm of chromosome 6 (6p21.3). This region spans over 4 million base pairs in length and encodes for over 200 genes involved with host immune surveillance and immune regulation.

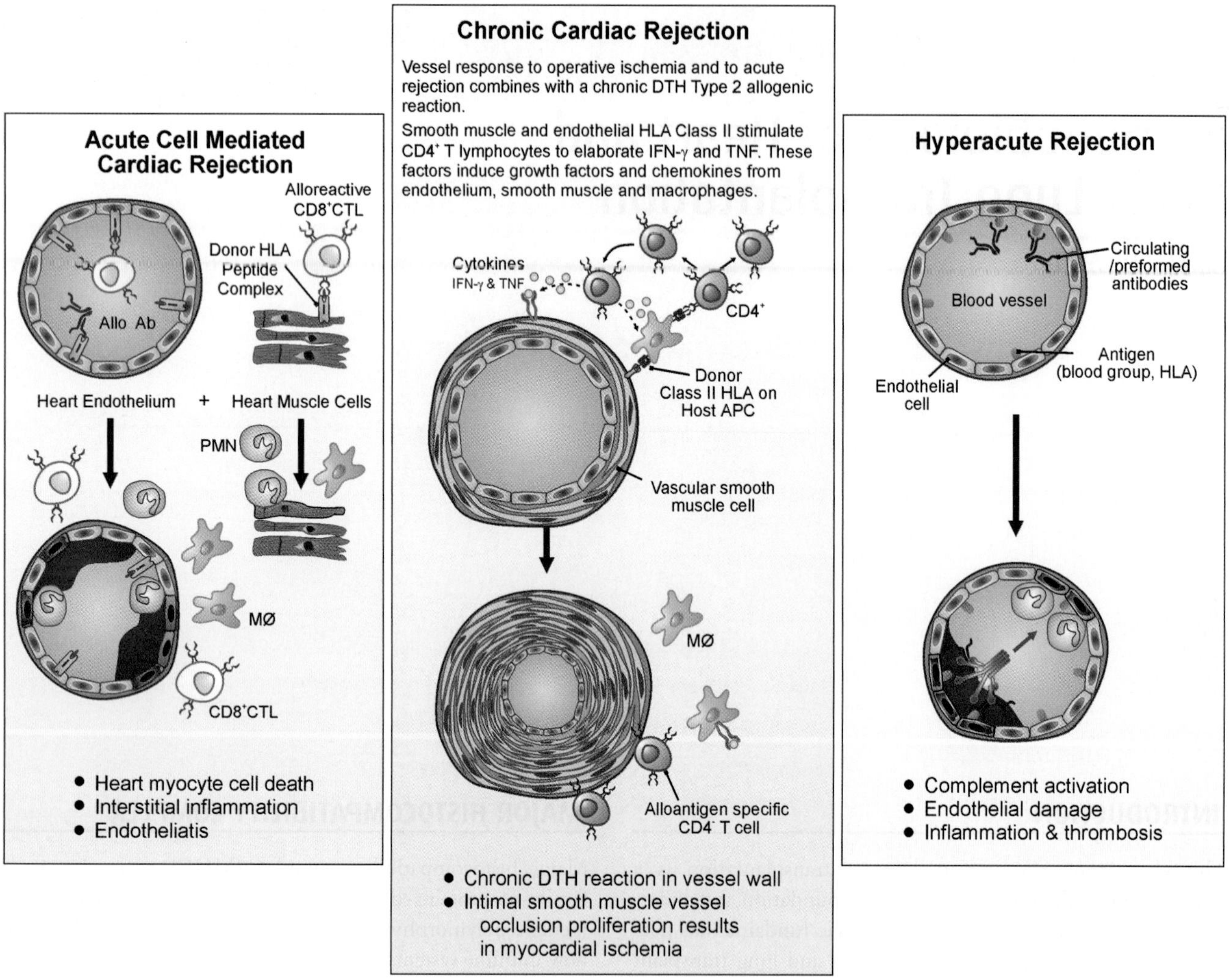

FIGURE 63-1 The alloresponse to a transplanted heart or lung may be grouped for simplicity into an early hyperacute rejection (HAR) based on preformed circulatory antibodies to blood group and in modern era HLA antigens (*right panel*) and acute cell-mediated rejection (AR) a more common and driving response that has been the focus of much of transplant immunology (*left panel*). AR is centered on the T lymphocytes becoming activated by specific HLA protein presented by antigen-processing cells. The CD4⁺ cells recruit inflammatory cells to the allograft and amplify other immune cells. The CD8⁺ T cells are directly involved with destruction of the allograft by cytotoxic intervention. Finally, chronic rejection (*center panel*) is the term given to describe progressive obliteration of the coronary arteries (chronic allograft vasculopathy, or CAV) in the heart or obstruction of small- and mid-sized airways (obliterative bronchiolitis, or OB) in the lung. These tubular structures are affected by injury and acute alloreactive hypersensitivity reaction.

The HLA is divided into three regions or Classes: Class I, II, and III (Fig. 63-2).

Classic Class I HLA proteins/antigens are HLA-A, HLA-B, and, more recently, HLA-C. These proteins consist of an α-heavy chain and a β-light chain (Fig. 63-3). The α-light chain is encoded in the MHC; however, the β-chain is β_2-microglobulin that is encoded on chromosome 15. When folded, the α-heavy chain only contains the peptide-binding region which presents peptide antigen to the T cell. Class I antigens are constitutively expressed on nearly all cells. B-cell lymphocytes may express Class I antigen at a higher density than the T-cell lymphocytes. Class I antigen expression is upregulated on the endothelium and parenchymal cells in many organs and tissues in association with inflammation, including after ischemia and reperfusion.

Classic Class II HLA proteins/antigens are HLA-DR, HLA-DRw, HLA-DQ, and more recently HLA-DP. These proteins consist of an α-heavy chain and a β-light chain, both of which are encoded in the MHC. When folded, the α-heavy chain and β-light chain come together with each contributing part of the peptide-binding region (Fig. 63-3). Class II antigens are expressed mainly on B-cell lymphocytes, activated T cells, and dendritic cells. Other cell types such as endothelial cells, may express Class II antigen expression after activation.

Each person has two different HLA genes at each HLA locus (HLA-A, B, D, etc). HLA antigens are codominantly expressed on the cell surface so that each cell has two different HLA proteins for each HLA locus. HLA haplotypes (the sequence of A, B, D genes on one chromosome, see Fig. 63-2) are usually inherited as a group from each parent in a Mendelian fashion.

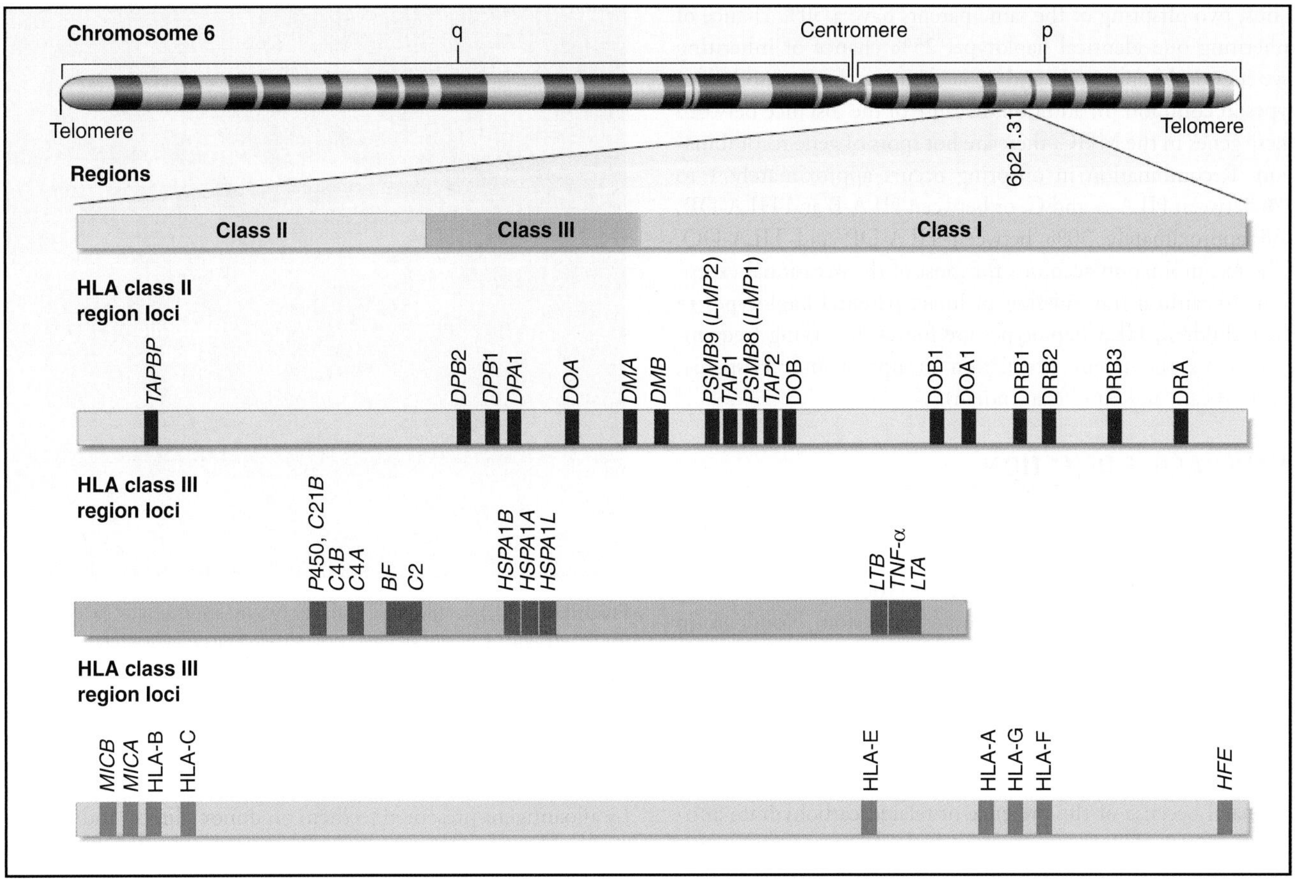

FIGURE 63-2 The major histocompatibility complex is divided into three regions or Classes: Class I, Class II, and Class III.

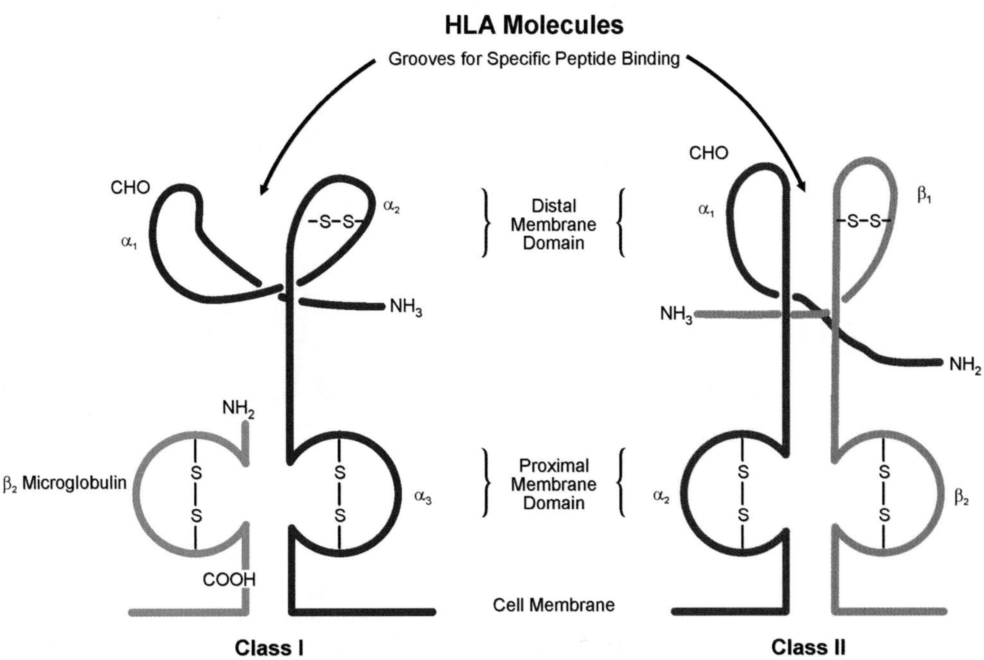

FIGURE 63-3 Classes I and II HLA molecules are made up of polypeptidic chains with intrachain disulfide bonds. The α_1 and α_2 distal domains of class I and the α_1 and β_1 domains of class II make up the peptide-binding site for alloantigen. (*Adapted with permission from Parham M, in Haber E [ed]: Immunobiology of Transplantation Molecular Cardiovascular Medicine, New York, Scientific American Press, 1995.*)

Thus, two offspring of the same parents have a 50% chance of inheriting one identical haplotype, 25% chance of inheriting two identical haplotypes, and 25% chance of having no haplotypes in common. In addition, because of the distance between these genes in the MHC, there are hot spots of gene recombination. Recombination in offspring occurs approximately 1 to 2% between HLA-A and C, or between HLA-B and HLA-DR, and approximately 30% between HLA-DP and HLA-DQ. This recombination accounts for most of the occasional exceptions to faithful transmission of intact parental haplotypes to their children. HLA haplotypes are found in varying frequencies across the major population groups (white, Hispanic, black, Asian, and American Indian).

HYPERACUTE REJECTION

In the early days of organ transplantation, hyperacute rejection occurred because of preexisting IgM alloantibodies. Best known examples of these are the ABO blood group IgM antibodies. Although still a barrier to xenotransplantation, blood group typing has virtually eliminated this particular cause of immediate organ destruction. Of interest is the success of blood group-mismatched organs in neonatal recipients who have not yet developed IgM antibodies to blood group antigens. Antibodies against blood group antigens arise between 6 and 18 months postnatal because of the presence of related carbohydrate antigens on intestinal bacteria. Today, when hyperacute rejection is seen, it is normally caused by preexisting IgG antibodies usually directed against donor HLA proteins (see Fig. 63-1). These antibodies are often the result of previous blood cell transfusions (most particularly multidonor platelets owing to the high HLA load) or previous pregnancies or transplants. After wide adoption of the first crossmatch technique by Patel and Terasaki in 1969, hyperacute rejection based on HLA antibodies became rare.[2] Further improvements in screening for HLA antibodies have nearly eliminated it. New flow cytometric crossmatch techniques occasionally reveal previously unsuspected anti-HLA antibodies (see Flow Cytometric Assays) at titers below the threshold detected by the crossmatch test; the importance of these low-titer antibodies is uncertain, but at least in some circumstances they are associated with an accelerated failure of the organ transplant.

T-CELL RESPONSE TO ALLOGRAFT

Success in heart and lung transplantation requires control over the adaptive immune response to donor MHC antigens expressed by the allograft. Rejection of allografts is initiated by T lymphocytes primed to donor antigens in the peripheral lymphoid tissues and recruited into the donor organ where those antigens are expressed. Much of the recent advance in clinical transplantation has been because of a better understanding of T-cell–mediated responses. Transplant immunologists are closing in on the critical steps that contribute to different effector mechanisms of tissue injury. The nature of allograft rejection is influenced by alloantigen specificity, frequencies (measured as absolute number or proportion), and cytokine profiles of naïve and "memory" donor-specific T cells.

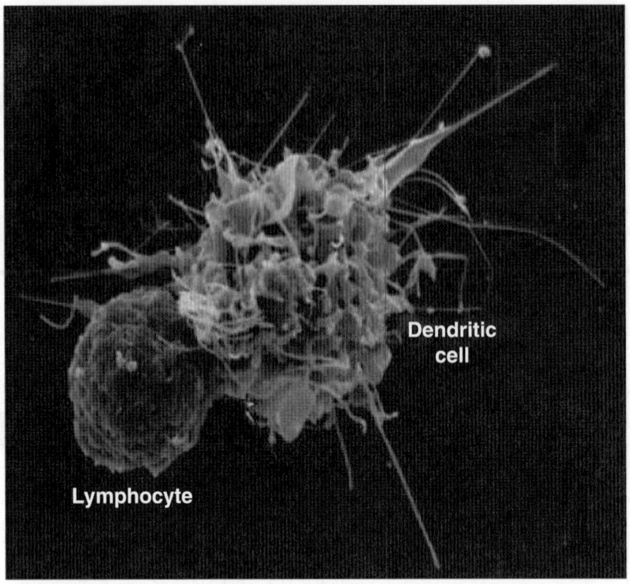

FIGURE 63-4 Dendritic cell with its typical membrane extensions engaged with T lymphocyte. (*www.dendriticcellresearch.com, Institute of Cellular Therapies, Noida, UP 201303, India.*)

Currently, it is held that alloreactive T lymphocytes are primed by alloantigens presented to them on donor (direct) and/or host (indirect) antigen-presenting cells (APCs). The T cells are the primary actors in the pathologic reaction to the transplanted organ. They participate in cytotoxicity and cytokine-mediated

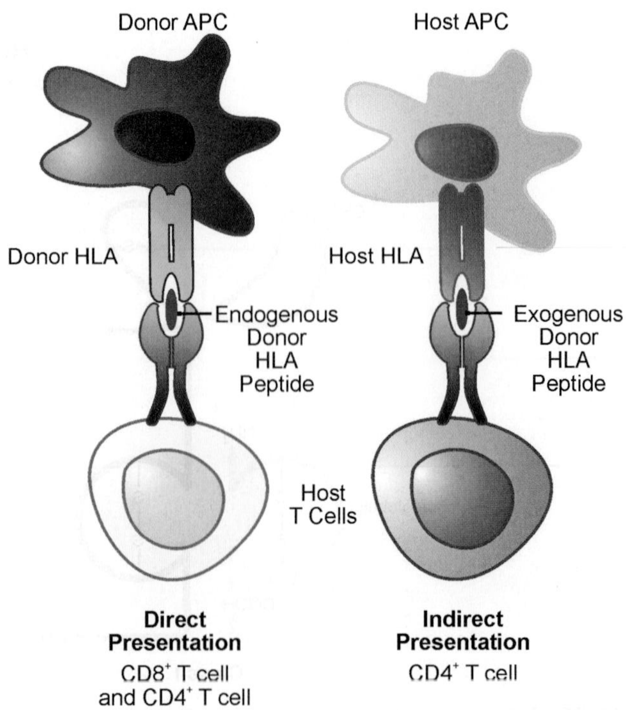

FIGURE 63-5 T cells are stimulated to proliferate when their TCR engages donor peptides processed and presented by an HLA molecule, expressed by donor or host APCs.

inflammation. B cells, antibodies, and macrophages contribute to destruction of the graft via a variety of effector pathways. Ischemia/reperfusion injury of the allograft triggers innate immunity that can amplify adaptive immunity. Molecular modulators of innate immunity have recently been an expanding area of interest. These include toll-like receptors (TLR), cytokines, chemokines and complement. Although APCs are emphasized, B cells and natural killer (NK) cells exert influence on a host's decision to reject an allograft.[3]

T-Lymphocyte Alloactivation

A T cell can only become triggered to proliferate and differentiate if it links to a specialized cell that presents fragments of donor peptides bound to HLA molecules on its surface (Fig. 63-4). These HLA-peptide displaying cells are called antigen-presenting cells (APCs). "Professional" APCs differ from other HLA-expressing cells in that they also express costimulatory molecules that efficiently stimulate reciprocal activation of both the APCs and the responding T cell. Professional APCs include dendritic cells, B lymphocytes, and macrophages. The peptide HLA antigen complex may be presented by resident *donor* passenger APCs found in the transplanted heart or lung (direct presentation) or *host* APCs that endocytose HLA protein shed from the allograft (indirect presentation) (Fig. 63-5). HLA-peptide antigens become the specific key that fits into the T-cell receptor. T cells react against alloantigens because of the cross-reactivity of the T-cell receptor (TCR) with self and foreign HLA molecules. Host and passenger donor dendritic cells are thought to be the most efficient type of APCs for activating naïve T cells.

Donor Antigen Presentation to T Cells by APCs

Donor passenger APCs transplanted with the heart or lung directly process endogenous HLA-derived peptides from within the graft or themselves and present them associated with a groove on Class I HLA complexes on their surfaces (Fig. 63-6A). CD8+ T lymphocytes have Class I HLA T-cell receptor (TCR) molecules on their surfaces into which the Class I protein MHC complexes presented on the donor-derived APCs fit (lock and keys). This pathway is responsible for the majority of initial

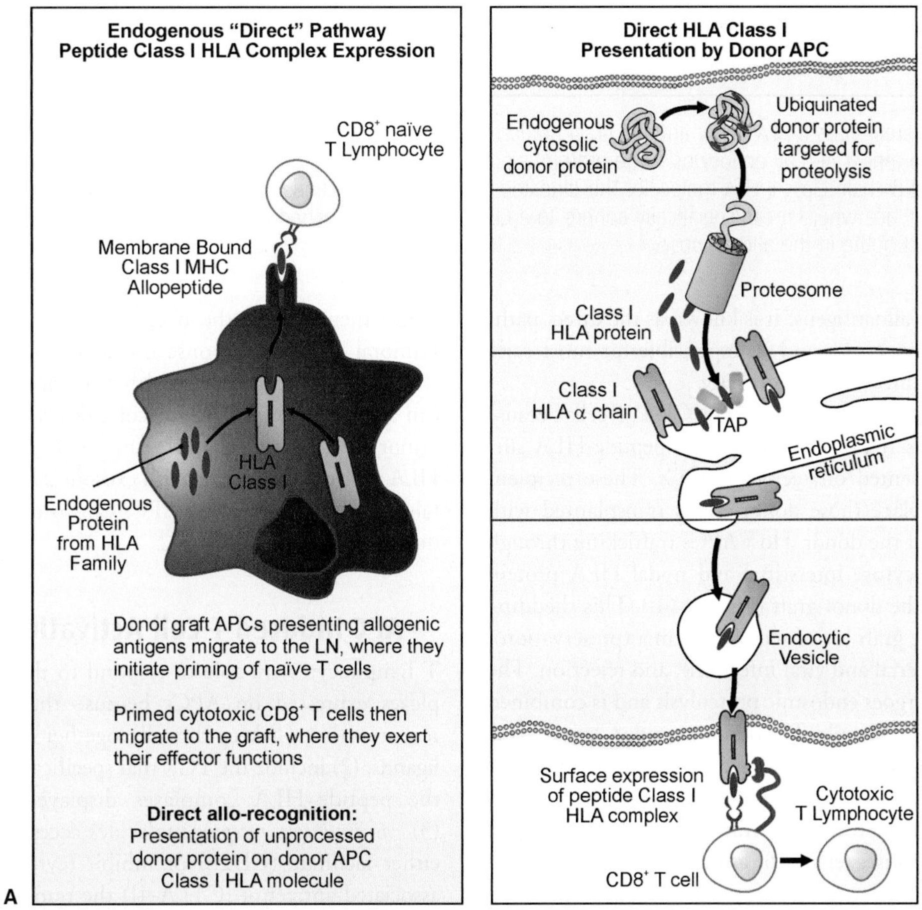

FIGURE 63-6 (A) Direct presentation of Class I HLA donor antigen by donor APCs. Donor-derived APCs (dendritic cells within the transplant) ubiquitinate an endogenous cytosolic (donor) protein and transport it through the proteosome, where it is digested. Small proteins move with transporter associated with antigen processing (TAP) into the endoplasmic reticulum, where it becomes associated with Class I HLA α chain. The protein–HLA complex locates on the surface of the APC where CD8+ T cells with TCR locks specific for the protein–HLA complex keys can associate. The association prompts CD8+ T-cell activation.

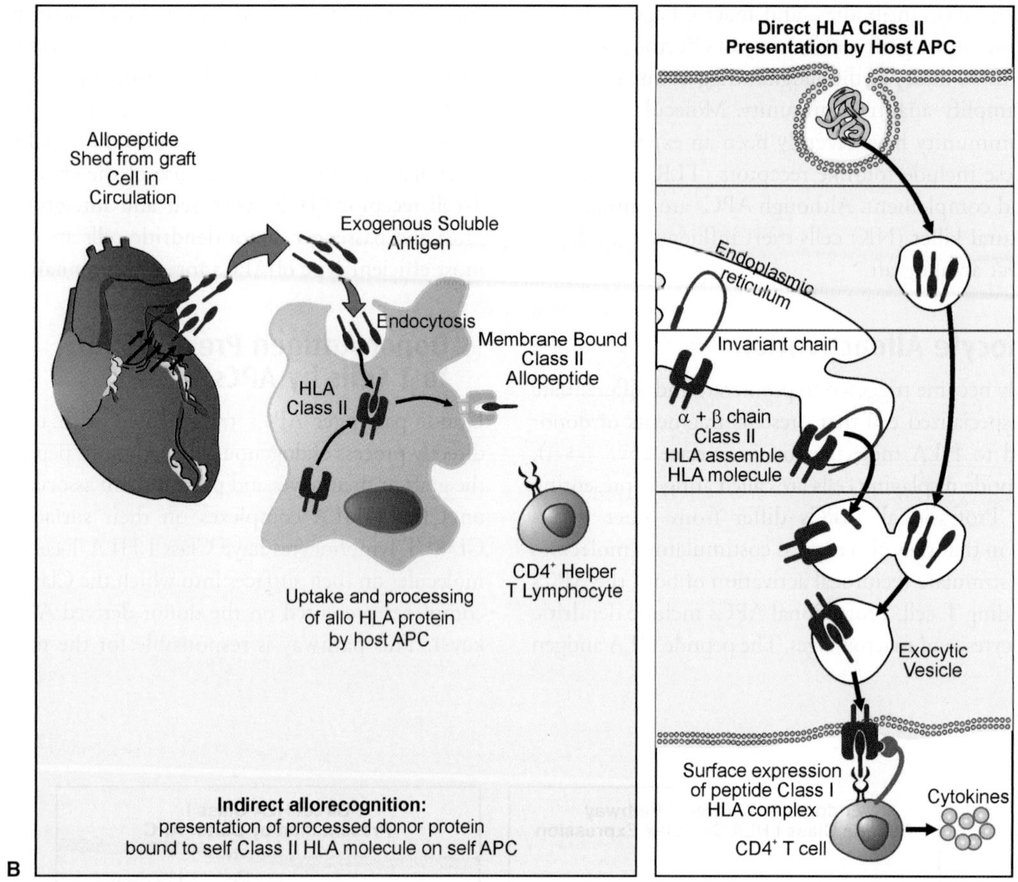

FIGURE 63-6 (B) Indirect Class II HLA donor-antigen presentation by host APC. Extracellular protein antigen shed from the heart or lung allograft is taken into a host APC by endocytosis. The protein is proteolyzed and transported into the Golgi. There it displaces the invariant chain held α and β chain Class II HLA molecule. The digested protein molecule finds its specific place within the HLA molecule and is moved to the APC surface where it can specifically adhere to a CD4+ T cell. The attached CD4+ T cell with donor-specific TCR is stimulated to proliferate and participate in the alloresponse.

T cells that react to alloantigens. It is known as the direct pathway of peptide presentation and is responsible for most early events of acute cell-mediated cytotoxicity.

Later alloresponses are directed more by CD4+ T cells because they recognize Class II HLA donor-specific peptide-HLA surface molecules presented on recipient APCs. These recipient APCs gradually replace those donor APCs transplanted with the heart or lungs of the donor. Host APCs trafficking through the allograft phagocytose interstitial and nodal HLA protein antigen shed from the donor graft (Fig. 63-6B). This shedding is induced when the graft is stressed by ischemia (preservation), inflammation (bacterial and viral infection), and rejection. The donor protein undergoes endosmic proteolysis and is combined with a Class II HLA molecule. The donor peptide Class II HLA complex is transported to the surface of the host APC and presented indirectly as the key to the TCR complex on CD4+ T cells. Because CD4+ T cells provide help to donor-specific B cells, later alloresponses tend to be associated with appearance of alloantibody.

Activated dendritic cells also provide costimulators to the naïve T cells that are required for a full T-cell response. Macrophages present antigens to differentiated CD4+ cells that activate the macrophage to promote cell-mediated immunity. B cells also serve an APC function by presenting antigens to helper T cells. These then activate the B cell to become part of the effector humoral immune response through production of antibodies (Fig. 63-7). Recently it has been learned that recipient APCs can acquire intact HLA molecules directly from contact with a donor APC bearing the HLA molecule. It can also receive the HLA molecules by fusing with exosomes from donor APCs containing the protein. These APCs can stimulate CD4+ T cells by direct or indirect pathways.[4]

APC-Induced T-Cell Activation: Signal 1

T lymphocytes are able to respond to the peptide HLA complexes expressed on APCs because they express membrane receptors that: (1) keep the cells together via the APC-adherence ligands; (2) include the TCR that specifically recognize (cognate) the peptide–HLA complexes displayed in the APC; and (3) *costimulatory receptor* molecules accessory to the TCR that either facilitate (CD28) or inhibit (cytotoxic T lymphocyte-associated antigen 4 [CTLA-4]) the transduction of activation signals to the nucleus or provide second signals that strengthen the TCR activation. The TCR complex includes variable antigen-binding TCR heterodimer and invariant CD3, ζ, ε, and γ proteins, and ζ chains that enable activation signal transduction to the nucleus (Fig. 63-8).

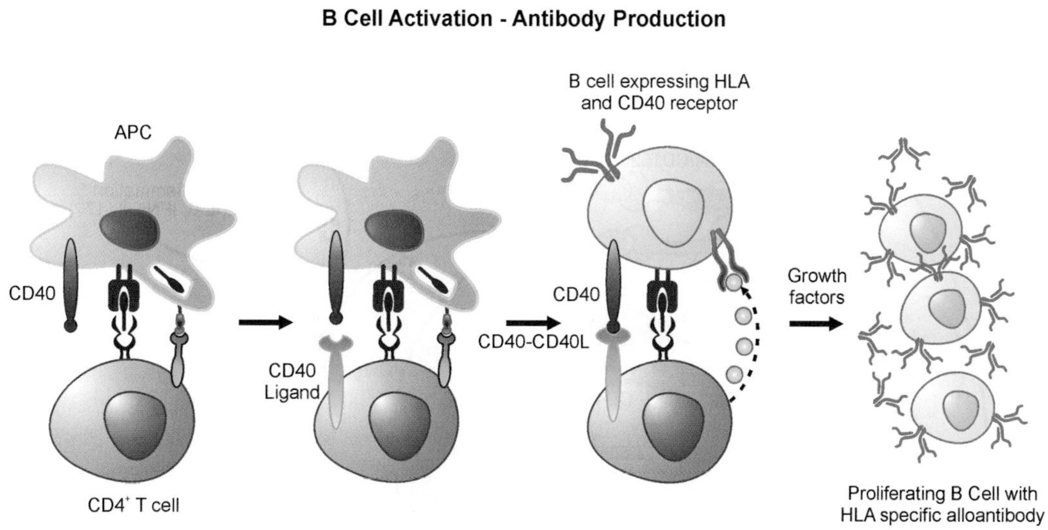

FIGURE 63-7 CD4+ T lymphocytes are specifically activated by donor peptide proteins presented on APC–HLA complexes. These T cells in turn activate B lymphocytes expressing specific HLA Class II molecules and CD40. The B cells respond to growth factors by proliferative formation of germinal centers and production of specific alloantibody.

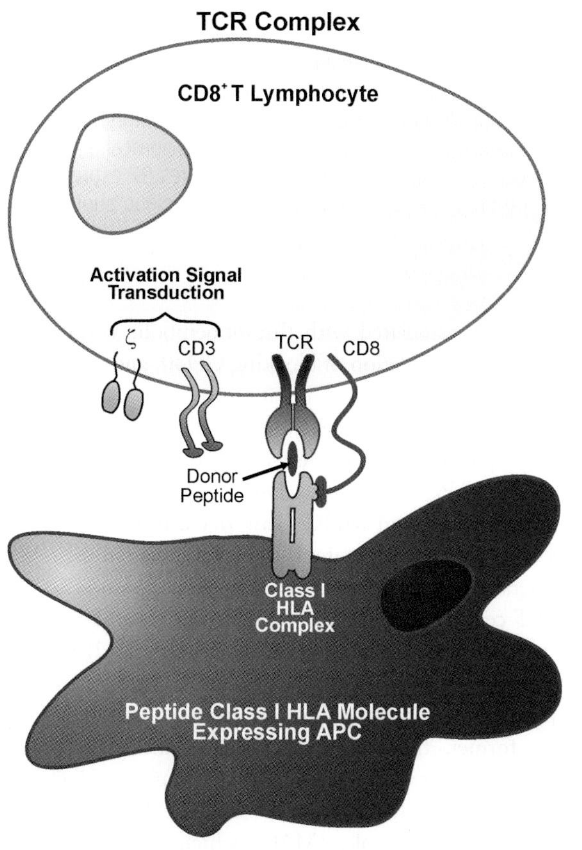

FIGURE 63-8 When an APC is specifically engaged with a T cell via the TCR lock and donor protein/MHC key, its intracellular pro-stimulator signaling response is generally dependent and strengthened by the docking of APC surface-bound costimulators such as B7-1, B7-2, and LFA-3 into T-cell coreceptors CD28 plus CD2, respectively. The stable adherence of the T cell and APC is the result of APC ICAM-1 and T cell LFA-1 union. These interactions are localized in a specific geographic zone on T cells and APC—the immunologic synapse.

CD8 and CD4 surface proteins act as coreceptors that bind to the Class I or II HLA molecule, respectively, displayed on the APC. As discussed, the CD8 and CD4 interact with Class I and II HLA, respectively, when a donor peptide–HLA complex is recognized. CD8 and CD4 strengthen the binding of the TCR to the HLA molecule and participate in the intracellular signaling process.

Costimulation Pathways: Signal 2

In addition to activation of the T cell by engagement of foreign peptides and its TCR, several other surface molecules participate in a T-cell activation. Those that enhance TCR signaling (CD4 in CD4+ T cell and CD8 in CD8+ T cell) are called *coreceptors* because they bind to part of the same HLA molecules that engage the TCR. Another group of T-cell activating surface molecules is called *costimulatory receptors* (Fig. 63-9). Blockade of costimulatory pathways provides important new possible therapy to prolong organ transplant survival and even reach a tolerant state. Costimulatory receptors or ligands on T cells recognize respective cognitive ligands or receptors presented on APCs or the graft tissue itself. The best defined costimulatory receptor and ligand pairs are the constitutively expressed CD28 T-cell costimulatory receptor and its APC ligands B7-1 (CD80) and B7-2 (CD86). This pathway is particularly important in activation of naïve T cells. When engaged, these pairs deliver antiapoptotic signals and trigger the expression of and growth factors, including IL-2 that encourage proliferation of the alloantigen-specific CD4+ or CD8+ cells. A second inducible costimulatory receptor for B7 molecules has been identified and termed CTLA-4 (CD152). Unlike the structurally homologous CD28, CTLA-4 appears on recently activated T cells and is a negative regulator that promotes pathways that limit proliferation. It is efficient that the same costimulator (B7) can prompt initial proliferative signals via constitutive CD28 engagement and later when CTLA-4 is induced subsequently limiting signals

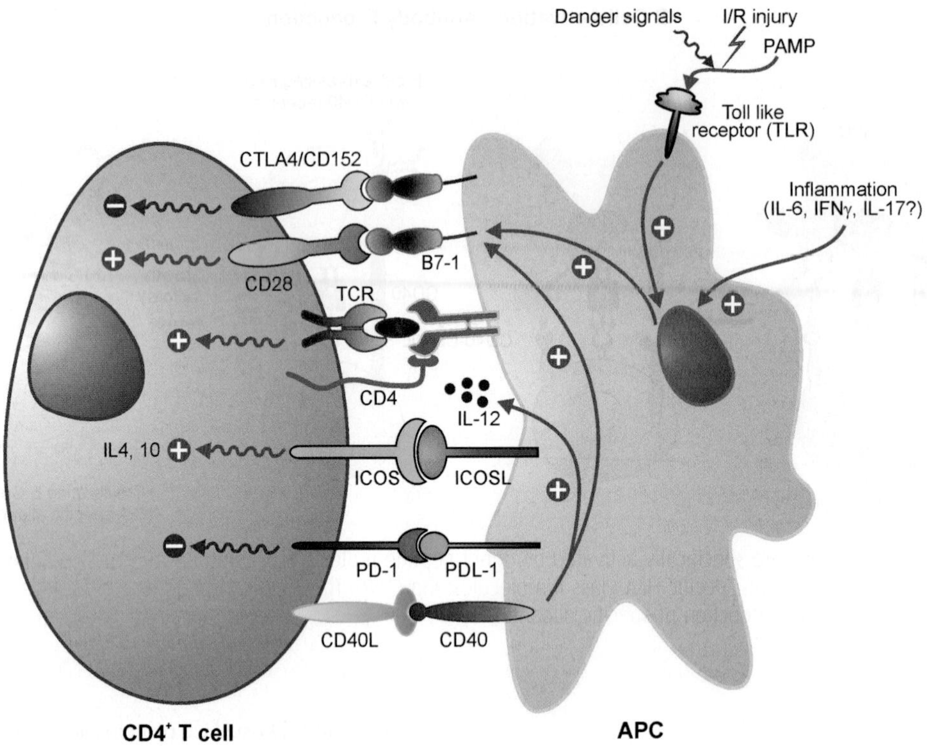

FIGURE 63-9 The process of regulating T cell (CD4+ and CD8+) activation involves engagement of the TCR/CD4 or CD8 with the foreign protein–HLA molecule and of several costimulators of the costimulatory pathway. The constitutively expressed CD28 coreceptor drives proliferation of naïve T cells when engaged by its ligand B7-1. Inducible CTLA-4 (CD154) coregulator acts to regulate this process negatively along with its APC-bound B7-2 ligand. Other CD28 family coreceptors include inducible ICOS that signals for proinflammatory IL-4 and IL-10 effector responses and PD-1 that has a negative regulatory effect on the T cell. The APC is made better by a reciprocal activation between T cells and APCs and the phenomena of "licensing" in which innate receptors (PAMP–Toll receptor) stimulates B7 expression. This has the effect on the T cell of inducing CD40 ligand (CD154). CD40 on the APC's membrane drives additional B7 and elaboration of IL-12.

to the T cell. Therapeutic targeting of this pathway with CD80 and CD86 blockade with CTLA-4 Ig–like molecules has been effective in primates and is currently in clinical trials in kidney transplantation.[5] Inducible costimulator (ICOS) and Programmed Death-1 (PD-1) are more recent discoveries in the T-cell CD28 family. When ICOS joins its ligand ICOS-L on an activated APC, it stimulates the T-cell effector response by promoting IL4 and IL10 production. PD-1 is the coreceptor for costimulator PD-ligand and, like CTLA-4, represses T-cell responses.

A second family of costimulatory molecules belong to the TNF superfamily. The prototypic pathway is represented by the costimulatory receptor CD40 on APC binding to CD40L on T cells. Transplantation immunobiology is influenced by the innate immunity directors against substances from microbes, including bacteria, viruses, and fungi. These substances, often nucleic acids, are called *pathogen-associated molecular patterns* (PAMPs) (see Fig. 63-9). PAMPs can bind to PAMP-receptors on APCs called toll-like receptors (TLR). This engagement has the effect of strengthening the APC response. This begins by increasing the expression of costimulatory molecules and proinflammatory cytokines. The CD40 signaling promotes additional B7 expression and elaboration of T-cell proliferation IC12. By reciprocal activation, CD40L on T cells makes the APC better and is thought to license additional APCs to participate in the T-cell activation process. A clinical trial of anti-CD154 was unexpectedly associated with thromboembolic complications. This led to consideration of blocking CD40, and a human trial is currently underway in transplant.

In severe rejection, B cells join the alloresponse when they receive help from CD4+ T cells (see Fig. 63-7). CD4+ T-cells are activated by APCs to express CD40L (CD154). Ligand B cells expressing CD40 and MHC Class II receptors engage helper CD4+ T cells and proliferate. B cells participate in the rejection of allografts by efficiently providing APC function to helper CD4+ T cells and by elaboration of antibodies that: (1) recognize and destroy the donor endothelial targets; (2) participate in antibody dependent cytotoxicity (ADCC); or (3) stimulate the proliferation and migration of activated endothelial cells.[6] In the former, the endothelial antigen–antibody complexes activate the classic complement pathway, causing C3 and C5 to cleave, inciting inflammation (C5a) and formation of the membrane attack complex (MAC), which is composed of C5b complexed with C6, 7, 8, and 9 (C5b-9). The MAC causes vascular cell death by inducing pores to form in the cell membrane. When endothelial cells are activated or killed by complement, this in turn results in microvascular thrombosis and inflammation. ADCC describes the process by which antidonor IgG antibodies coating donor cells bind to the Fcγ RIII receptor of natural killer lymphocytes (NK cell). Cells of the innate immune system such as natural killer cells are also present in allografts during rejection. These recognize alloantigens because they constitutively express inhibiting receptors specific for self HLA Class I protein. The NK cell produces proinflammatory cytokines like IFN-γ and directly kills the antibody-engaged target cell by injecting its proteolytic enzymes into the donor cell.

Cell-Mediated Rejection

Despite use of immunosuppressive therapy, transplanted heart and lungs often acutely reject. Both $CD4^+$ and $CD8^+$ cells participate, but the response is primarily mediated by the CD4 T cells. The early cell-mediated response begins when specific clones of $CD8^+$ cells that bear TCR molecules which fit and engage donor-specific peptide HLA Class I on donor APCs are stimulated to proliferate. In the presence of help from $CD4^+$ T cells, they become cytolytic lymphocytes CTLs and directly attach to and kill graft endothelial and parenchymal cells bearing the identical Class I donor protein HLA presented to them by the APC activators. This is known as the direct pathway because the CD8 cell directly kills the allotarget. It is responsible for most acute cell-mediated rejection early (in the first few months) after transplant. In the presence of calcium, the protein perforin polymerizes onto the Class I bearing target cell and causes 16- to 20-nm pores to open in the cell membrane, resulting in osmotic collapse. CTL granular content, including granzyme B and other cytotoxic molecules, is directly injected into the target cell, causing necrosis. Alternatively, apoptosis (programmed cell death) can also be stimulated in the target cell by interaction of the lymphocyte Fas ligand with the APO-1/Fas receptor of the target cell. Second messengers are elicited that activate endonucleases and proteases to cause fragmentation of DNA and thus organize the dissolution of the Class I bearing donor target T cell (Fig. 63-10).

The $CD4^+$ T cells primarily follow an indirect alloresponsive pathway by secreting various cytokines that drive inflammation and graft loss (see Fig. 63-10). IL-2 increases the expression of its own receptors (IL-2R) on $CD4^+$ cells, driving the proliferation and further differentiation of $CD4^+$ cells. The activated CD4 cells secrete additional lymphokines, including interferon-γ (IFN-γ), which along with IL-2 stimulates $CD8^+$ CTLs to bind to the allograft cells presenting donor MHC protein molecules. $CD4^+$ T cells are very heterogeneous. The four major categories are now recognized: Th_1, Th_2, Th_{17}, and regulatory T cells (Tregs). Th_1 cells are the main mediators of cell-mediated rejection. They produce IFN-γ and favor IL-12 production by macrophages. Th_2 cells make IL-4, 5, and 13 and promote humoral responses. Th_{17} produce IL-17, a cytokine recently discovered and involved in inflammation. In conditions in which the immune response is partially inhibited, Tregs develop with the ability to inhibit immune responses.

Memory T Cells

With improvement in immunosuppression that limits activation of naïve T cells, donor-reactive memory cells have been recognized as a previously underappreciated risk to the allograft. This group of donor-specific cells has an effector-memory phenotype. This is defined by an immediate and strong recall that is no more or less sensitive to costimulation blockade. Memory cells are thought to arise from heterologous immunity. This occurs when there is a resemblance between microbial antigens and self-protein HLA complex antigens. Some $CD4^+$ and $CD8^+$ cells exposed to Epstein-Barr, herpes simplex, and cytomegalovirus (CMV) become primed to recognize allogenic HLA molecules. Memory T-cell numbers are proportionately increased following lymphoablative treatment with rabbit ATG or alemtuzumab (anti-CD52 ab). It is unclear whether these memory cells are more resistant to depletion or whether they represent a conversion from naïve T cells during repopulation. Memory $CD4^+$ cells provide help for the alloresponse. They provide growth and proinflammatory factors that affect $CD8^+$ T cells and B-cell antibody production. They can elicit the proinflammatory response from nodal-bearing tissue remote from the allograft. Memory $CD4^+$ cells recruit $CD8^+$ cells that infiltrate the allograft across the endothelium. The memory $CD8^+$ cells proliferate and recruit macrophages, neutrophils, and additional activated T effector cells into the donor organ.[7] To date, memory T cells continue to evade efforts of therapeutic targeting. LFA-1 is one target that is under study for this purpose. They are very heterogeneous and have multiple functions.

Immunologic Tolerance

Peripheral tolerance mechanisms are responsible for tolerance to transplant-specific HLA protein not present in the thymus. Immunomechanisms to achieve immunologic tolerance of an allograft include considerations of cell death by apoptosis (deletion) of alloreactive T cells or induction of functional unresponsiveness (anergy or ignorance) and active regulation of alloimmunity by either donor-antigen–specific or nondonor-antigen–specific mechanisms (regulation). Anergy has been induced by exposing $CD4^+$ T cells to MHC antigen in the absence of costimulation. In addition, much of the current interest has been in better understanding of a subset of $CD4^+$ T cells called regulatory T cells (Tregs) whose function is to suppress immune responses and maintain self-tolerance.[8] Tregs may occur naturally (nTreg) and are important in autoimmunity. Those that are inducible (iTregs) in response to an allograft are distinct. Most Tregs express the IL-2 receptor α chain (CD25). TGF-β, IL2, and B7, CTLA-4 costimulation are required for nTreg production and survival. It remains to be fully elucidated how these molecules direct naïve T cells to differentiate into effector, memory, or regulatory phenotypes under various clinically relevant circumstances. FoxP3 is a forkhead family transcription factor important for Treg-suppressive function, but is also found in activated T cells in humans, and thus is not specific to identify human Tregs.

There has been limited success in translation of laboratory rodent-based tolerance protocols in clinical practice. Freedom from immunosuppression rarely is accomplished universally in strictly controlled large animal models. Management of preexisting memory cells appears to be a major hurdle. Finally, redundant effector cell mechanisms, cytokines, and costimulatory pathways make single or even dual approaches seem underpowered to establish tolerance in the clinic. There has been a limited number of patients in whom tolerance was induced by a

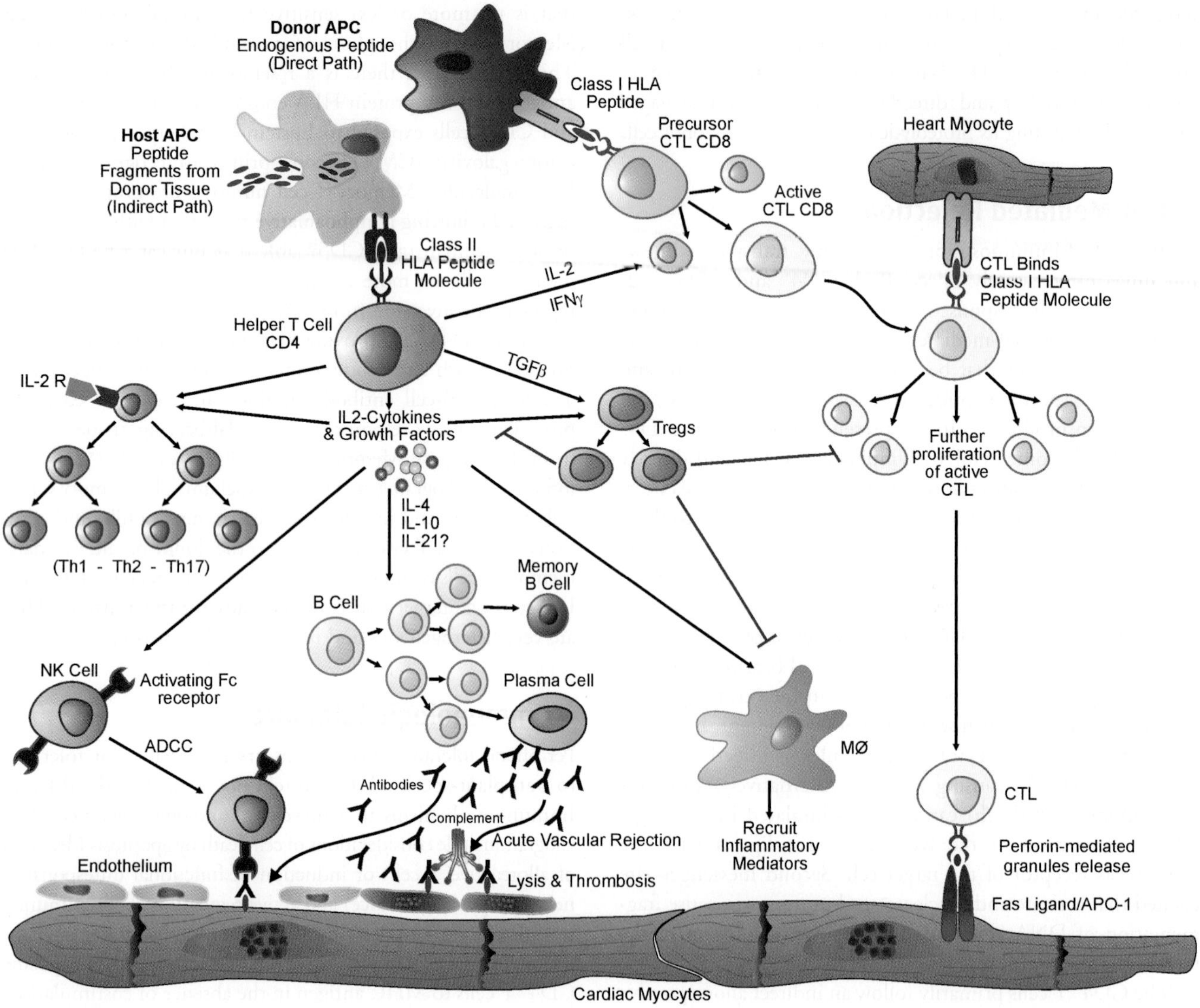

FIGURE 63-10 Complicated scheme of allograft rejection. CD8+ lymphocytes become activated by donor-derived dendritic cells transplanted with the allograft. These cells enter a direct alloresponse pathway by proliferating into CTLs. The CTLs recognize and attach to Class I HLA donor peptide molecules on the surface of allograft cells. They directly kill the allotarget through cell-mediated cytotoxicity by injection of proteolytic granules, creating perforin-induced membrane pores and induction of apoptosis. CD4+ T cells are activated by host APCs that engulf donor protein shed from the allograft. The host APCs process the donor protein into surface-bound Class II HLA peptide molecules. The CD4 cells follow an indirect pathway in the alloresponse by proliferating and secreting growth factors plus proinflammatory cytokines. This indirect paracrine function augments CTL proliferation, attracts cellular mediators of inflammation-like macrophages, and drives B-cell central humoral immunity.

regimen, inducing a mixed allogeneic chimerism (coexistence of recipient and donor cells) for kidney allografts. However, work in the nonhuman primate model showed that even this highly tolerogenic regimen did not induce tolerance to cardiac allografts.[9] Heart and lung allografts are less easily amendable to tolerance than kidney; in other words, they are more immunogenic.[10]

CHRONIC REJECTION: CORONARY GRAFT VASCULOPATHY AND OBLITERATIVE BRONCHIOLITIS

Chronic rejection of thoracic organs takes the form of induced obliterative fibrosis of small airways in the lung (obliterative bronchiolitis [OB]) or bronchiolitis obliterans syndrome (BOS) and diffuse obliterative transplant vasculopathy (TV) in heart (also termed cardiac allograft vasculopathy [CAV]). OB and CAV are likely caused by a response of the vessels and airways to a combination of peritransplant injury from preservation-related ischemia, acute rejection, and a chronic delayed-type hypersensitivity immune reaction (DTH) (see Fig. 63-1). DTH response is driven primarily by CD4+ T cells reacting to Class II alloantigens on the endothelium and smooth muscle on the coronary arteries or the epithelium and bronchial smooth muscle of the donor airway. The responding CD4+ T cells elaborate tumor necrosis factor (TNF) and interferon-γ (IFN-γ), which promotes release of growth factors and chemokines from the endothelial, epithelial, and smooth muscle cells and recruit regional macrophages. Smooth muscle cells in the vessel and airway walls proliferate and move into the intima (subendothelial) or subepithelial compartment. The result is proliferation followed by fibrosis with resultant progressive luminal occlusion. As this process evolves, the transplanted organ parenchyma becomes progressively more fibrotic. CAV has been associated with systemic soluble markers of general inflammation. These include C-reactive protein, a marker of systemic inflammation, vascular cell adhesion molecule (VCAM-1), a marker of endothelial cell activation and neopterin, a marker of macrophage activation.[11] Further, these inflammatory mediators correlated with necrotic core and dense calcified components of the plaque. The necrotic core component is composed of lipid cells, necrotic and lymphocyte remnants together with tissue microcalcification.[12] At 5 years posttransplantation, CAV was responsible for death or retransplantation in 7%, and 50% patients with severe disease experienced these outcomes.[12] Its course more often is an indolent one, yet if present before 2 years, it acts like an inflammatory vasculitis and is associated with a poor survival.[13] The International Society for Heart and Lung Transplantation has recently published a consensus on the diagnosis and nomenclature for CAV.[14]

CIRCULATING ANTIBODIES IN HEART AND LUNG TRANSPLANTATION

Circulating HLA antibodies may form in a sensitization process through prior exposures to blood transfusions, pregnancy, organ transplantation, or use of a ventricular assist device. Transplant candidates with preexisting HLA antibodies not only are at risk of hyperacute and acute antibody-mediated rejection very early after transplantation, but also have lower rates of longer-term survival as well. Sensitive new bead methods now allow detection of circulatory antibodies and use of those antibody specificities to define "unacceptable" donor HLA antigens. The role of non-HLA antibodies in acute and chronic rejection and treatment strategies before transplant (desensitization), or when antibodies are detected after transplantation, is becoming better understood but remains in evolution.

HLA Antibody Analysis

Serologic Testing

The techniques used for identification of HLA antibodies have evolved significantly in recent years. The serological lymphocytotoxic assay for antibody screening is based on mixing patient serum (unknown) with a panel of cells whose HLA typing is known and adding complement (complement-dependent cytotoxicity or CDC assay). If antibodies are present in the patient serum that react with the cell's HLA molecules, cell death occurs because of complement activation. This method is limited to detection of antibodies represented by the panel of antigens tested and by issues with sensitivity and accuracy. The specificity of the antigen to which the antibody is reacting (HLA or non-HLA antibody) is sometimes not clear because of the presence of other proteins in the patient serum, or the antibody isotype (IgG or IgM, etc; some antibody isotypes do not fix complement), and the titer (low, high) is not determined. Several enhancements of this assay were developed to address these issues: (1) heat or chemical treatment of the patient serum to inactivate IgM antibodies and identify IgG antibodies, which were felt to be more important to outcomes; (2) additional washes of the target cells following incubation of the patients serum to "wash off" the nonspecific reactants; and (3) addition of antihuman globulin (AHG) to the reaction to increase the detection of low titer IgG antibody (CDC-AHG method). There are other subvariations of these serologic enhancements.

The antibody-screening assay consists of a panel of known HLA-typed cells, with each cell representing a unique set of antigen targets for the serum to react. The assay generates the panel reactive antibody titer (PRA), which is reported out as a percent of the prospective donor pool that would likely be killed by the patient's serum. The result of this analysis is termed percent calculated PRA or %cPRA. The %cPRA gives a better indication of the patient's likelihood of having a compatible offer of a UNOS deceased donor organ because it is based on actual UNOS-typed donors. The panel may consist of any number of cells; however, minimally, cells from at least 30 carefully selected individuals are needed to cover the most common HLA antigen targets. In addition to the %PRA, the specificity of the antigen targets could be identified based on the individual cell reactions. The more different HLA antigens to which the patient is sensitized, the higher the %PRA and the less likely the patient is to have a compatible donor identified. Using conventional matching criteria, %PRA greater than 10% and greater than 25% have been associated with incrementally lower survival large registry reports.

Despite the use of enhancing techniques, serological antibody screening and methods of identification are not able reliably to detect low levels of HLA antibody, and are relatively poor for characterizing Class II antibody.

Solid-Phase Assay

An ELISA plate method was the first solid-phase assay developed. In this assay, solubilized known HLA antigen protein targets are captured onto the surface of the wells of a microtiter plate. Patient serum is reacted with these proteins in each respective well. A secondary antihuman IgG antibody conjugated to a colorimetric reporter molecule is then added to the wells. This allows quantitative spectrophotometric determinations with a threshold absorbance used to distinguish a positive versus negative antigen–antibody reaction. Two additional hallmarks of the ELISA assay are the ability to: (1) objectively evaluate and quantify HLA antibody reactivity; and (2) eliminate the need for dependence on complement fixing for antibody detection, making ELISA a complement-independent assay. The colorimetric ELISA assay was able to evaluate better the presence of HLA Classes I and II antibody than the CDC-AHG method. Key faults of the ELISA assay are: (1) sensitivity of the colorimetric detection methods; and (2) purity and reliability of the solubilized HLA antigen captured in the well, because HLA can change its shape and thus antibody reactivity when bound to the plate.

Flow Cytometric Assays

The development of solid-phase microbead-based flow cytometry assays represents a monumental improvement from the initial solid-phase ELISA antibody screening and identification techniques. The use of fluorescent dyes is foremost as report molecules, allowing detection of the antigen–antibody reactions using a flow cytometer. Fluorescent dye light emissions are severalfold more sensitive than colorimetric dyes. As with the ELISA assay, the detection of the antibody–antigen reaction is made using beads coated with HLA molecules. Each HLA molecule-specific bead is identified by its unique mixture of two fluorescent dye colors incorporated into the bead. A secondary antihuman antibody is conjugated to a reporter molecule, in this case, a fluorescent dye of another color. The higher the titer of the antibody in the patient's serum, the more antibody is available to react to the antigen conjugated to the bead, and the more intense is binding of the secondary flourescein-ated antibody. The more reporter dye becomes bound to the bead complex, the more fluorescent emission is produced from the bead when analyzed by the flow cytometer. The fluorescent emission signal of each bead type is then averaged and the normalized value is reported as the mean fluorescence intensity (MFI) of the bead. For most laboratories, the MFI value greater than or equal to 1000 is considered to be a positive reaction for the presence of the HLA antibody. This cutoff was derived in a similar fashion to that for the ELISA assay, namely, twice the MFI value for the negative control serum.

This resultant value is called the *shift median channel value* (sMCV). The sMCV cutoff for a positive versus negative flow crossmatch is statistically determined by each HLA laboratory initially and periodically by crossmatch of up to 100 individuals with serum that does not contain HLA antibody (negative). Shift values of less than or equal to two standard deviations from the mean of these histograms median channel value is considered to be negative, between two and three standard deviations to be equivocal, and three or more standard deviations to be positive.

The HLA antigen is conjugated directly to the microbead, not simply captured, and the source of which is recombinant cell lines. This allowed manufacturing of beads coated not only with the antigens of a single individual mimicking a cell (multi-antigen beads), but also with a single HLA antigen (single antigen beads). These single antigens can be further described to the exact HLA allele of that antigen. Because individuals become sensitized to the amino acid epitopes encoded by the antigen allele, microbead-based antibody analysis opened a completely new level of insight into characterizing antibodies contained in patient serum. This process is called *epitope mapping*. In combination with allele level typing of patients and potential donors, epitope mapping of antibodies can better predict outcomes of transplants in highly sensitized patients. The flow cytometer instrument may be either a larger instrument, which can acquire data from cells or beads, or a mini-flow cytometer, which only acquires data from beads, such as a Luminexx instrument (Fig. 63-11).

Using solid-phase HLA assays (SPA) or flow cytometric assays, the laboratory can easily and reliably test for patient antibodies to HLA-A, -B, C, DRB1, DRB3, DRB4, DRB5, DQB1, DQA1, and DPB1.

The results of the serum antibody test and the donor crossmatch are interpreted together as a final assessment of recipient and donor compatibility. Composite MFI values of 4000 or greater are generally predictive of a positive flow crossmatch. This composite MFI value is derived from the sum of MFI values and the single antigen–antibody analysis for each donor target antigen present, either Class I or II. This is a rule of thumb, as cellular expression of these target antigens varies. Most centers post unacceptable antigens in UNOS for those single antigens with MFI values of 4000 or greater, because these single antigens alone may result in a positive flow crossmatch with donors. Based on these MFI values, a virtual or paper crossmatch can be reliable in predicting the actual cellular crossmatch, especially with high MFI values. In addition, unacceptable antigens can be identified by virtual crossmatch (discussed in the following), excluding a particular donor that expresses certain donor antigens from consideration for a recipient who is sensitized against one or more of those antigens.

HLA Crossmatch

Crossmatch of patient serum with potential donors is no different than performing antibody testing.

Virtual Crossmatch

Practical realities of matching sensitized candidates with nonlocal donors resulted in the acceptance of the virtual crossmatch (VXM). The VXM is a comparison of the donor HLA genotype determined by organ procurement organizations routinely as part of the donor (heart, lung) organ distribution process to the gene families represented by beads that bound antibody from the sensitized candidate recipient. If gene families are shared between donor and the bead, the VXM is positive. For example, a candidate with antibodies against A1, A11, and B7 by Luminexx single antigen beads would be incompatible with a donor typed as A11, A25, B55, and B57.[15] The anti-A1 antibody determined by SPA corresponds to the donor typed A1. Although currently there is no method to determine the functional characteristics of the antibodies, recently it was estimated that the positive predictive value of an incompatible VXM compared with cytotoxic crossmatch was nearly 80%. Most centers refuse nonlocal donors based on an incompatible VXM and insist on a prospective CDC-AHG crossmatch for sensitized patients when possible.

Non-HLA Antibodies

It has become increasingly clear that non-HLA antibodies that can cause injury in thoracic organ transplants.[16,17] About 16% of HLA antibody-negative heart recipients may lose their graft to the mixed diagnosis of primary failure within 30 days of transplant.[18] SPA does not detect non-HLA antibodies, *but flow cytometry methods can detect MICA/B.* Antibodies-to-donor endothelial antigens are the largest poorly discussed group of clinically important non-HLA antibodies. These include endothelial, autoantibodies and those to MHC Class I chain A (MICA) and B (MICB). Endothelial antigen targets may exist, constitutively or as induced autoantigens because of activation

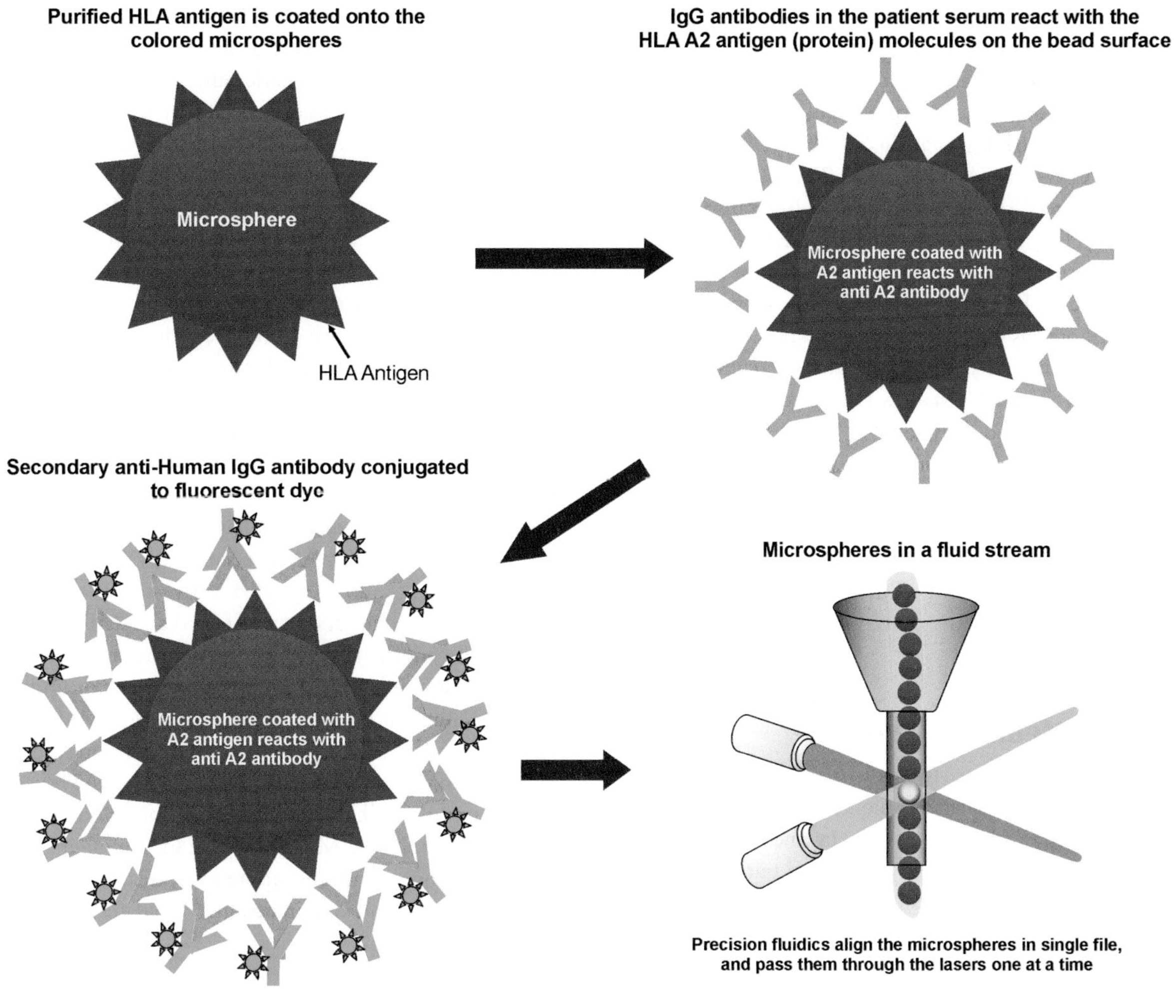
Purified HLA antigen is coated onto the colored microspheres
Microsphere
HLA Antigen
IgG antibodies in the patient serum react with the HLA A2 antigen (protein) molecules on the bead surface
Microsphere coated with A2 antigen reacts with anti A2 antibody
Secondary anti-Human IgG antibody conjugated to fluorescent dye
Microsphere coated with A2 antigen reacts with anti A2 antibody
Microspheres in a fluid stream
Precision fluidics align the microspheres in single file, and pass them through the lasers one at a time

FIGURE 63-11 Solid-phase microbead-based assays for HLA antibodies have improved sensitivity and specificity of detection. Single HLA antigens from recombinant cell lines are conjugated to a colored microsphere. The bead is reacted against candidate or recipient serum, resulting in the specific adherence of circulating antibody to the selected HLA antigen. The microsphere HLA–serum antibody is reacted to an antihuman IgG antibody conjugated to a fluorescent dye. The microsphere complex is channeled through a flow cytometer and mean fluorescence intensity (MFI) for the combined emitting dye is measured. (*Adapted with permission from Luminexx Corporation, Austin, TX.*)

of the endothelium. MICA and MICB are polymorphic antigens expressed on epithelial and, to an unknown extent, on endothelium. MICA antibodies may occur in up to 20% of candidates and have been associated with poorer survival but not increased rejection.[18]

Autoantibodies against conserved (non-polymorphic) proteins are frequently found in the blood of thoracic transplant recipients in association with chronic rejection. Vimentin (an intracellular cytoskeletal protein found in vessel walls and activated lymphocytes), cardiac proteins (cardiac myosin), and collagen type 5 (expressed mainly in the lung) are among the antigens against which autoantibodies have been described. Antivimentin antibodies form earlier than anti-HLA after transplantation and are a response in up to 30% of heart recipients to exposure of antigens mounted on the surface of damaged and activated cells.[19] Antivimentin antibodies reflect tissue injury but might also activate platelets and neutrophils.[20] Antiheart antibodies exist preoperatively in some because of their primary cardiac disease. At present, it is difficult to know their true significance. Finally, IgM non-HLA antibodies are cytotoxic and can react to all leukocytes, even the patient's own. Antigen specificity is unknown, as is the clinical relevance.

Desensitization Therapy

Once unacceptable antigens are determined from SPA, they can be entered into the UNOS website (http://optn.transplant.hrsa.gov/resources/professionalResources.asp?index=10). This will provide the cPRA. If the percentage chance of any donor will not be acceptable is greater than 50%, then it is reasonable to initiate a desensitization protocol. An optimal protocol has not been established. High-dose IVIG (2 g/kg/over 2 days q 2-4 weeks), plasmapheresis (1.5 volume exchange ×5 days), monoclonal anti-CD20 B-cell therapy (rituximab 1 g IV weekly ×4), and in the past cyclophosphamide (1 mg/kg/day) have been used in various combinations.

At UCLA, plasmapheresis, IVIG, and rituximab reduced circulatory antibody levels from 70.5 to 30.2%. Heart transplantation of these candidates after negative CDC resulted in similar 5-year outcomes to control patients and untreated but high PRA patients (81.1%, 75.7%, 71.4%). Of interest, the freedom from CAV was 74.3, 72.7, and 76.2%, respectively.[21]

It has been agreed that patients waiting for transplantation with circulating HLA antibodies should be studied every 3 months, and those desensitized every 2 weeks after therapy. Patients on VADs or who receive blood transfusions or with infections should be closely monitored as well. After transplantation donor-specific antibody monitoring is recommended at regular intervals and when a humoral rejection event is suspected. Donor-specific titers should be measured daily for 1 to 2 weeks and frequently thereafter in desensitized patients and those considered high risk for antibody response. This higher-risk group of recipients is generally treated with thymoglobulin plus IVIG, plasmapheresis and/or rituximab. Maintenance immunosuppressive therapy that has best controlled cellular and antibody-mediated rejection includes tacrolimus, mycophenolate mofetil, and prednisone.[22]

Antibody-Mediated Rejection

Hyperacute antibody-mediated rejection (AMR) became extremely rare with improving crossmatch techniques, but clinical interest in AMR was renewed in 1990 by Halloran and associates who described features of pure AMR in a few renal transplant recipients.[23] Later, C4d became established as an important histologic associate.[24] The incidence of AMR after cardiac transplantation is uncertain because of a lack of universal screening in asymptomatic recipients. Symptomatic pure AMR without a component of acute cellular rejection occurs in 10 to 15% of cardiac transplant recipients, but AMR features have been reported in up to 40% of patients with acute cellular rejection (mixed rejection).[25] Clinical symptoms of cardiac AMR are those common in heart failure using echo. A greater than 25% decrease in ejection fraction and an increase in left ventricular mass distinguished antibody-mediated rejection from cell-mediated rejection.[26] Reduced R-wave voltage-conduction abnormalities, including bundle branch block, are electrocardiographic associates. As discussed, presensitization to HLA Class I or II antibodies predisposes to AMR.[27] Those recipients who develop presensitized antibodies, especially donor-specific, risk AMR.[28] Non-HLA antibodies, including those against cardiac myosin, vimentin, and endothelial cells have been less often associated with AMR.[29–31] Cardiac AMR occurs early (weeks to months) after transplant and, if avoided early, rarely occurs later.[32] Classically, histologic diagnosis of cardiac AMR has included evidence of endothelial swelling and activation macrophages in the graft plus confirming immunofluorescence or immunoperoxidase staining for immunoglobulin (IgG or IgM) (Figs. 63-12 and 63-13). Although absence of immunofluorescence seems reasonable to rule out AMR, capillary swelling (63%) and macrophage vascular adherence (30%) do not[33] and complement (C3d and C4d). Non-AMR causes of C4d staining include organ reperfusion injury, immunosuppression, treatment with monoclonal antibodies, and viral infections.[34] To date, the distribution

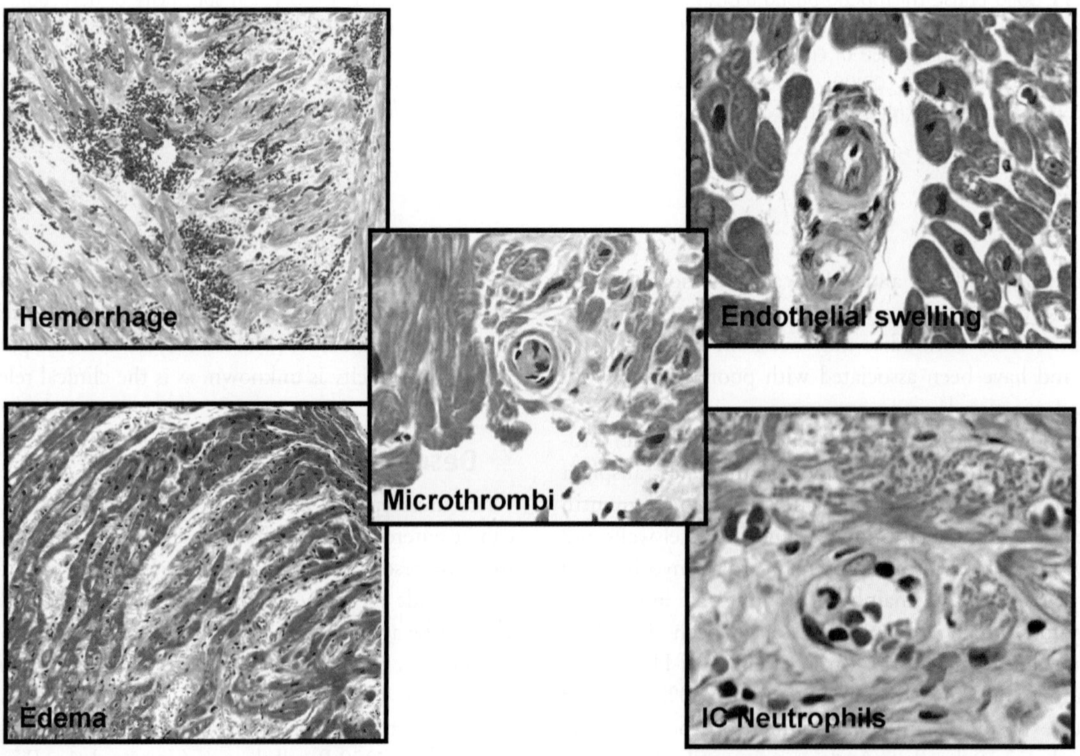

FIGURE 63-12 Histologic evidence of AMR-associated endothelial swelling, inflammation, and thrombosis accompanied by interstitial edema and hemorrhage (H&E staining). (*Reproduced with permission from SA Webber.*)

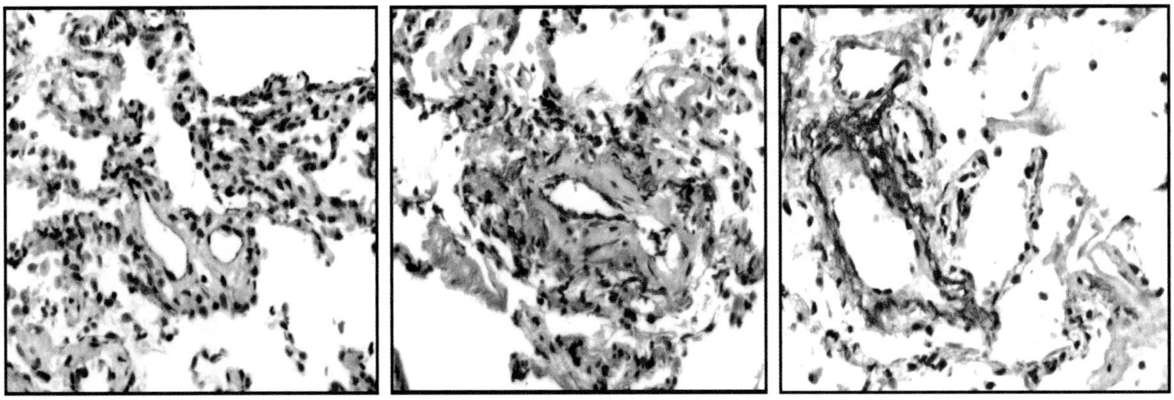

FIGURE 63-13 Specific C4d deposition on a lung transplant allograft in a recipient with circulating HLA antibody is continuous and subendothelial in capillaries and small arterioles (*left*). Specific C4d has been seen on 31% of transbronchial biopsies in recipients with HLA-Ab (*middle*). (*Ionescu DN: Transplant Immunol 2005; 15:63-68.*) In contrast, nonspecific staining of the interstitium and elastic layer is depicted (*right*). (*Reproduced with permission from KR McCurry.*)

(diffuse versus localized) and intensity of the stains has not found a standardization for grading. The suggested algorithm for AMR includes: (1) Present clinical evidence of cardiac graft dysfunction and histologic evidence with or without interstitial edema and hemorrhage; and (2) positive immunofluorescence or immunoperoxidase for donor-specific antibodies. This creates further questions about the importance of asymptomatic (allograft function conserved) AMR-associated histopathology. It is likely that AMR is a pathologic continuum with clinical involvement in later or more aggressive forms. Asymptomatic AMR has been related to worse cardiovascular outcomes and the presence of cardiac allograft vasculopathy (CAV).[35,36]

Although a clinical phenotype for AMR after lung transplantation and its response to anti-antibody regimens has been discussed, unfortunately, no strong consensus exists regarding its diagnostic characteristics.[37] Recently, the Washington University program evaluated the effect on donor-specific HLA antibodies (DSA) and bronchiolitis obliterans syndrome (BOS) in 65/116 recipients developed DSA. Antibody-depleting therapy with IVIG, with or without rituximab, resulted in no differences in the incidence of acute rejection, lymphocytic bronchiolitis, and BOS between those with and those without antibody.[38]

Gene Expression Profiling

A DNA microarray-based real-time polymerase chain reaction–derived bio signature for cardiac rejection has been developed by XDx, the maker of allomap molecular expression testing (XDx, Brisbane, CA).[39] Peripheral blood mononuclear cells provided a panel of 11 informative genes that were associated with acute cellular rejection.[40] Several pathways were identified that participate in regulation of effector cell activation, trafficking and morphology, platelet activation, plus corticosteroid sensitivity. These included PDCD1 and ITGA4 for T-cell activation and migration, ILIR2 steroid-responsive gene, the decoy for IL-2, and WDR40A plus CMIR of the micro-RNA gene family. Peripheral blood samples are assigned a score with higher numbers associated with progressive risk of lack of immunologic quiescence. This approach was recently randomized against surveillance endomyocardial biopsy in a multicenter trial in low-risk rejection cardiac recipients, 6 months to 5 years after transplantation.[41] The evaluation excluded recipients with a significant history of rejection, CAV, or allograft dysfunction. Results indicated 14.5% of patients profiled versus 15.3% of those surveilled by endomyocardial biopsy reached a composite endpoint of rejection with hemodynamic compromise, graft dysfunction owing to other causes, death, or retransplantation. The low risk for rejection of the enrolled patients made interpretation to earlier and higher-risk recipients problematic.[42] Other reports found that the profiled genes regulatory T-cell homeostasis and corticosteroid sensitivity can distinguish mild from moderate and severe rejection and are evident before histologic, detectable rejection.[43,44]

Functional Activity of Immune System

A recipient's individual immune responses are affected by their susceptibility to immunosuppression, their clinical state, genetic background, age, gender, and diet. An assay of cell function would be useful to quantitate the dynamic positive and negative regulatory responses of the immune system. Clinicians have struggled, often in relative ignorance, to titrate doses of immunosuppressive drugs to achieve levels that deter the alloresponse while also minimizing the risk of infection. A long-imagined goal of selective treatment based on a quantitative assessment of the net state of immunosuppression has been approached clinically with some success. An assay has been developed (Cylex, ImmuKnow, Columbia, MD) to measure the intracellular concentration of adenosine triphosphate (ATP) of $CD4^+$ T cells. ImmuKnow measures T-cell responses by quantifying ATP activity[45] to phytohemagglutinin, a T-cell mitogen. In general, the collective studies suggest that ATP levels less than 100 ng/mL correlate with an increased risk of infection.[46] In a study in 296 heart recipients spanning 2 weeks to 10 years posttransplant, infection

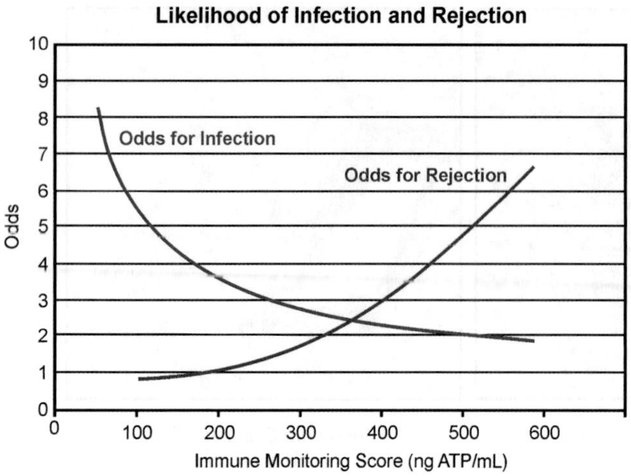

FIGURE 63-14 Immune monitoring scores are calculated from adenosine triphosphatase (ATP) released from activated lymphocytes (ImmuKnow; Cylex, Columbia, MD). The hazard curves above are plotted for risk of infection versus odds for rejection in 296 heart transplant recipients (864 assays). In theory, the crossing point defines a score that minimizes infection and rejection. (*Adapted with permission from Kobashigawa JA, Kiyosaki KK, Patel JK, et al: Benefit of immune monitoring in heart transplant patients using ATP production in activated lymphocytes. J Heart Lung Transplant 2010; 29:504-508.*)

in 39 recipients occurred with an average 187 + 126 ng/ATP/mL versus a steady state of 280 + 126 ng/ATP/mL (Fig. 63-14). Rejection scores in eight recipients averaged 328 ng/ATP/mL and did not differ from baseline. However, 3 of 8 with antibody-mediated rejection scored 49/I-12/ng/ATP.[46] This assay opens the field to personalized immunosuppression that might help balance risks of infection and rejection.

ACKNOWLEDGMENTS

The author wishes to thank Agnes Azimzadeh and Richard N. Pierson III for their critical review of this chapter, and Debra KuKuruga for her assistance and expertise on the HLA portion of this chapter.

REFERENCES

1. Abbas AK, Lichtman AH, Pillai S: *Cellular and Molecular Immunology.* St. Louis, Saunders, 2010.
2. Patel R, Terasaki PI: Significance of the positive crossmatch test in kidney transplantation. *NEJM* 1969; 280:735-739.
3. Bromberg JS, Heeger PS, Li XC: Evolving paradigms that determine the fate of an allograft. *Am J Transplant* 2010; 10:1143-1148.
4. Sanchez-Fueyo A, Strom TB: Immunologic basis of graft rejection and tolerance following transplantation of liver or other solid organs. *Gastroenterology* 2011; 140:51-64.
5. Vincenti F, Larsen C, Durrbach A, et al: Costimulation blockade with belatacept in renal transplantation. *NEJM* 2005; 353:770-781.
6. Zhang X, Rozengurt F, Reed EF: HLA class I molecules partner with integrin beta4 to stimulate endothelial cell proliferation and migration. *Sci Signal* 2010; 3:ra85.
7. Schenk AD, Nozaki T, Rabant M, et al: Donor-reactive CD8 memory T cells infiltrate cardiac allografts within 24-h posttransplant in naive recipients. *Am J Transplant* 2008; 8:1652-1661.
8. Valujskikh A, Baldwin WM III, Fairchild RL: Recent progress and new perspectives in studying T cell responses to allografts. *Am J Transplant* 2010; 10:1117-1125.
9. Kawai T, Cosimi A, Spitzer T, et al: HLA-mismatched renal transplantation without maintenance immunosuppression. *NEJM* 2008;358 (4): 353-361.
10. Aoyama A, Ng CY, Millington TM, et al: Comparison of lung and kidney allografts in induction of tolerance by a mixed-chimerism approach in cynomolgus monkeys. *Transplant Proc* 2009; 41:429-430.
11. Arora S, Gunther A, Wennerblom B, et al: Systemic markers of inflammation are associated with cardiac allograft vasculopathy and an increased intimal inflammatory component. *Am J Transplant* 2010; 10:1428-1436.
12. Costanzo MR, Heilman JK 3rd, Boehmer JP, et al: Heart transplant coronary artery disease detected by coronary angiography: a multiinstitutional study of preoperative donor and recipient risk factors. Cardiac Transplant Research Database. *J Heart Lung Transplant* 1998; 17:744-753.
13. Mehra MR: Contemporary concepts in prevention and treatment of cardiac allograft vasculopathy. *Am J Transplant* 2006; 6:1248-1256.
14. Mehra M, Crespo-Leiro MG, Dipchand A, et al: International Society for Heart and Lung Transplantation working formulation of a standard nomenclature for cardiac allograft vasculopathy-2010. *J Heart Lung Transplant* 2010; 29:717-727.
15. Pajaro OE, George JF: On solid-phase antibody assays. *J Heart Lung Transplant* 2010; 29:1207-1209.
16. Danskine A, Smith J, Stanford R: Correlation of anti-vimentin antibodies with acute and chronic rejection following cardiac transplantation. *Hum Immunol* 2002; 63(Suppl):S30-31.
17. Suarez-Alvarez B, Lopez-Vazquez A, Gonzalez MZ, et al: The relationship of anti-MICA antibodies and MICA expression with heart allograft rejection. *Am J Transplant* 2007; 7:1842-1848.
18. Smith JD, Hamour IM, Banner NR, Rose ML: C4d fixing, Luminexx binding antibodies: a new tool for prediction of graft failure after heart transplantation. *Am J Transplant* 2007; 7:2809-2815.
19. Mahesh B, Leong HS, McCormack A, et al: Autoantibodies to vimentin cause accelerated rejection of cardiac allografts. *Am J Pathol* 2007; 170: 1415-1427.
20. Azimzadeh AM, Pfeiffer S, Wu GS, et al: Humoral immunity to vimentin is associated with cardiac allograft injury in nonhuman primates. *Am J Transplant* 2005; 5:2349-2359.
21. Kobashigawa J, Mehra M, West L, et al: Report from a consensus conference on the sensitized patient awaiting heart transplantation. *J Heart Lung Transplant* 2009; 28:213-225.
22. Kobashigawa JA, Miller LW, Russell SD, et al: Tacrolimus with mycophenolate mofetil (MMF) or sirolimus vs. cyclosporine with MMF in cardiac transplant patients: 1-year report. *Am J Transplant* 2006; 6:1377-1386.
23. Halloran PF, Wadgymar A, Ritchie S, et al: The significance of the anti-class I antibody response. I. Clinical and pathologic features of anti-class I-mediated rejection. *Transplantation* 1990; 49:85-91.
24. Feucht HE, Felber E, Gokel, M J, et al: Vascular deposition of complement-split products in kidney allografts with cell-mediated rejection. *Clin Exp Immunol* 1991; 86:464-470.
25. Almuti K, Haythe J, Dwyer E, et al: The changing pattern of humoral rejection in cardiac transplant recipients. *Transplantation* 2007; 84:498-503.
26. Gill EA, Borrego C, Bray BE, et al: Left ventricular mass increases during cardiac allograft vascular rejection. *J Am Coll Cardiol* 1995; 25:922-926.
27. Nwakanma LU, Williams JA, Weiss ES, et al: Influence of pretransplant panel-reactive antibody on outcomes in 8,160 heart transplant recipients in recent era. *Ann Thorac Surg* 2007; 84:1556-1562; discussion 62-63.
28. McKenna R, Takemoto SK, Terasaki PI: Anti-HLA antibodies after solid organ transplantation. *Transplantation* 2000; 69:319-326.
29. Fredrich R, Toyoda M, Czer LS, et al: The clinical significance of antibodies to human vascular endothelial cells after cardiac transplantation. *Transplantation* 1999; 67:385-391.
30. Jurcevic S, Williams JA, Weiss ES, et al: Antivimentin antibodies are an independent predictor of transplant-associated coronary artery disease after cardiac transplantation. *Transplantation* 2001; 71:886-892.
31. Narayan S, Tsai EW, Zhang Q, et al: Acute rejection associated with donor-specific anti-MICA antibody in a highly sensitized pediatric renal transplant recipient. *Pediatr Transplant* 2011; 15(1):E1-7.
32. Hammond MEH, Renlund DG: Cardiac allograft vascular (microvascular) rejection. *Curr Opin Organ Transplant* 2002; 7:233-239.
33. Hammond ME, Stehlik J, Snow G, et al: Utility of histologic parameters in screening for antibody-mediated rejection of the cardiac allograft: a study of 3,170 biopsies. *J Heart Lung Transplant* 2005; 24:2015-2021.
34. Kfoury AG, Hammond MEH: Controversies in defining cardiac antibody-mediated rejection: need for updated criteria. *J Heart Lung Transplant* 2010; 29:389-394.

35. Kfoury AG, Hammond ME, Snow GL, et al: Cardiovascular mortality among heart transplant recipients with asymptomatic antibody-mediated or stable mixed cellular and antibody-mediated rejection. *J Heart Lung Transplant* 2009; 28:781-784.
36. Wu GW, Kobashigawa JA, Fishbein MC, et al: Asymptomatic antibody-mediated rejection after heart transplantation predicts poor outcomes. *J Heart Lung Transplant* 2009; 28:417-422.
37. Glanville AR: Antibody-mediated rejection in lung transplantation: myth or reality? *J Heart Lung Transplant* 2010; 29:395-400.
38. Hachem RR, Yusen RD, Meyers BF, et al: Anti-human leukocyte antigen antibodies and preemptive antibody-directed therapy after lung transplantation. *J Heart Lung Transplant* 2010; 29:973-980.
39. Starling RC, Pham M, Valantine H, et al: Molecular testing in the management of cardiac transplant recipients: initial clinical experience. *J Heart Lung Transplant* 2006; 25:1389-1395.
40. Deng MC, Eisen HJ, Mehra MR, et al: Noninvasive discrimination of rejection in cardiac allograft recipients using gene expression profiling. *Am J Transplant* 2006; 6:150-160.
41. Pham MX, Teuteberg JJ, Kfoury AG, et al: Gene-expression profiling for rejection surveillance after cardiac transplantation. *NEJM* 2010; 362:1890-900.
42. Mehra MR, Parameshwar J: Gene expression profiling and cardiac allograft rejection monitoring: is IMAGE just a mirage? *J Heart Lung Transplant* 2010; 29:599-602.
43. Mehra MR, Kobashigawa JA, Deng MC, et al: Transcriptional signals of T-cell and corticosteroid-sensitive genes are associated with future acute cellular rejection in cardiac allografts. *J Heart Lung Transplant* 2007; 26: 1255-1263.
44. Mehra MR, Kobashigawa JA, Deng MC, et al: Clinical implications and longitudinal alteration of peripheral blood transcriptional signals indicative of future cardiac allograft rejection. *J Heart Lung Transplant* 2008; 27: 297-301.
45. Kowalski R, Post D, Schneider MC, et al: Immune cell function testing: an adjunct to therapeutic drug monitoring in transplant patient management. *Clin Transplant* 2003; 17:77-88.
46. Kobashigawa JA, Kiyosaki KK, Patel JK, et al: Benefit of immune monitoring in heart transplant patients using ATP production in activated lymphocytes. *J Heart Lung Transplant* 2010; 29:504-508.

CHAPTER 64

Heart Transplantation

Jeremiah G. Allen
Ashish S. Shah
John V. Conte
William A. Baumgartner

INTRODUCTION

The number of patients with heart failure is growing. End-stage heart failure is associated with significant morbidity, need for recurrent hospitalizations, decrease in quality of life, and increased mortality. Cardiac transplantation has evolved as an effective therapy for many of these patients. Tremendous advancements in the fields of immunosuppression, rejection, and infection have transformed what was once considered an experimental intervention into a routine treatment available worldwide.

HISTORY OF HEART TRANSPLANTATION

The innovative French surgeon Alexis Carrel performed the first heterotopic canine heart transplant with Charles Guthrie in 1905. Frank Mann at the Mayo Clinic further explored the idea of heterotopic heart transplantation in the 1930s. The neck became the preferred site of implantation in early experimental animal models because of the ease of monitoring the organ, the simplicity of access to major vessels, and because the recipient's native heart could serve as a built-in cardiac assist device for the transplanted organ. Mann also proposed the concept of cardiac allograft rejection, in which biologic incompatibility between donor and recipient was manifested as a leukocytic infiltration of the rejecting myocardium. In 1946, after unsuccessful attempts in the inguinal region, Vladimir Demikhov of the Soviet Union successfully implanted the first intrathoracic heterotopic heart allograft. He later demonstrated that heart-lung and isolated lung transplantation also were technically feasible.

The use of moderate hypothermia, cardiopulmonary bypass, and an atrial cuff anastomotic technique permitted Norman Shumway (Fig. 64-1) and Richard Lower at Stanford University to further explore orthotopic heart transplantation using a canine model in 1960. The first human cardiac transplant was a chimpanzee xenograft performed at the University of Mississippi by James Hardy in 1964. Although the procedure using Shumway's technique was technically satisfactory, the primate heart was unable to maintain the recipient's circulatory load and the patient succumbed several hours postoperatively. Despite great skepticism that cardiac transplantation ever would be performed successfully in humans, South African Christiaan Barnard surprised the world when he performed the first human-to-human heart transplant on December 3, 1967. Over the next several years, poor early clinical results led to a moratorium on heart transplantation, with only the most dedicated centers continuing experimental and clinical work in the field. The pioneering efforts of Shumway and colleagues at Stanford eventually paved the way for the reemergence of cardiac transplantation in the late 1970s. The introduction of transvenous endomyocardial biopsy by Philip Caves in 1973 finally provided a reliable means for monitoring allograft rejection. Ultimately, however, it was the advent of the immunosuppressive agent cyclosporine that dramatically increased patient survival and marked the beginning of the modern era of successful cardiac transplantation in 1981. Heart transplantation is now a widely accepted therapeutic option for end-stage cardiac failure; however, the annual number of transplants in the United States (approximately 2200 per year) has remained relatively constant over the last decade because of limited donor-organ availability (from United Network for Organ Sharing [UNOS] data, through September 2009).

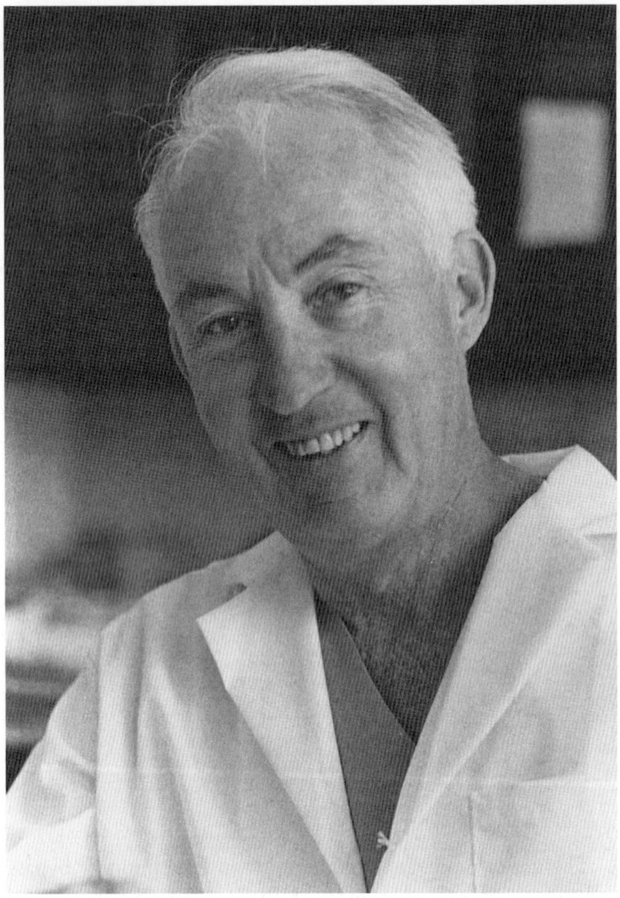

FIGURE 64-1 Norman Shumway.

THE CARDIAC TRANSPLANT RECIPIENT

Recipient Selection

The evaluation of potential candidates for cardiac transplantation is performed by a multidisciplinary committee to ensure the equitable, objective, and medically justified allocation of donor organs to those patients most likely to achieve long-term benefit. It is very important to establish a mutual long-term working relationship among patient, social support system, and the entire team at the beginning of this process.

Indications and potential contraindications for cardiac transplantation are outlined in Table 64-1.[1] These inclusion and exclusion criteria can vary somewhat among transplantation centers.[1–4] The basic objective is to identify those relatively healthy patients with end-stage cardiac disease, refractory to other appropriate medical and surgical therapies, who possess the potential to resume a normal active life and maintain compliance with a rigorous medical regimen after cardiac transplantation.

Etiology of End-Stage Cardiac Failure

Determination of the etiology and potential reversibility of end-stage heart failure is critical for the selection of transplant candidates. Overall, from 1982 to 2008, the indications for heart transplantation in adult recipients have been overwhelmingly ischemic heart failure and nonischemic cardiomyopathy (approximately 90%); with valvular (2 to 3%), adult congenital (2%), retransplantation (2%), and miscellaneous causes comprising the remainder.[5]

The perception of the irreversibility of advanced cardiac failure is changing with the growing efficacy of tailored medical therapy, high-risk revascularization procedures, and newer antiarrhythmic pharmacologic agents, as well as implantable defibrillators and biventricular pacing. Additionally, other surgical modalities, such as ventricular assist devices (VADs) and surgical ventricular restoration (SVR) have found increasing application.[6,7] Furthermore, it is important to consider that prognosis may differ in patients with cardiomyopathy who have neither ischemic nor valvular heart disease. Caution should be exercised when judging prognosis in these patient subgroups, and a period of observation, intense pharmacologic therapy, and/or mechanical support should be undertaken before heart transplantation is considered.[4]

Evaluation of the Potential Cardiac Transplant Recipient

The complexity of the recipient evaluation mandates a team approach. The initial evaluation involves a comprehensive history and physical examination because this will help to determine etiology and contraindications. Table 64-2[3] summarizes the cardiac transplant evaluation tests. Routine hematologic and biochemical analyses and pertinent tests as illustrated by organ system are performed.

For the assessment of the heart itself, in addition to routine 12-lead electrocardiogram, Holter monitor, and echocardiography, all patients should undergo cardiopulmonary exercise testing to evaluate functional capacity if disease severity allows. Peak exercise oxygen consumption measured during maximal exercise testing $\dot{V}O_{2,max}$ provides a measure of functional capacity and cardiovascular reserve, and an inverse relationship between $\dot{V}O_{2,max}$ and mortality in heart failure patients has been demonstrated.[8] Documentation of adequate effort during exercise, as evidenced by attaining a respiratory exchange ratio greater than 1.0 or achievement of an anaerobic threshold at 50 to 60% of $\dot{V}O_{2,max}$ is necessary to avoid underestimation of functional capacity.[2] Right-sided heart catheterization should be performed at the transplanting center to evaluate the severity of heart failure (and hence the status level for transplant listing) and evaluate for the presence of pulmonary hypertension. Right heart catheterization also can help guide therapy while awaiting transplantation. Coronary cineangiography should be reviewed to confirm the inoperability of coronary artery lesions in cases of ischemic cardiomyopathy. As well, either a positron emission tomographic (PET) scan, a thallium-201 redistribution study, or a cardiac magnetic resonance imaging (MRI) study should assess viability in selected patients who would be candidates for revascularization if sufficient viability is present.[2,3] Endomyocardial biopsy should be performed on all patients in whom the etiology of heart failure is in question, especially those with nonischemic cardiomyopathies symptomatic for fewer than 6 months.[3] This can assist in therapeutic decision making and exclude diagnoses such as amyloidosis, which are considered relative contraindications to transplantation.

TABLE 64-1 Recipient Selection for Heart Transplantation

INDICATIONS

I. Systolic heart failure (as defined by ejection fraction <35%)
  A. Inclusive etiology
    1. Ischemic
    2. Dilated
    3. Valvular
    4. Hypertensive
    5. Other
  B. Excluded etiology
    1. Amyloid (controversial)
    2. HIV infection
    3. Cardiac sarcoma

II. Ischemic heart disease with intractable angina
  A. Ineffective maximal tolerated medical therapy
  B. Not a candidate for direct myocardial revascularization, percutaneous revascularization, or transmyocardial revascularization procedure
  C. Unsuccessful myocardial revascularization

III. Intractable arrhythmia
  A. Uncontrolled with pacing cardioverter defibrillator
    1. Not amenable to electrophysiology-guided single or combination medical therapy
    2. Not a candidate for ablative therapy

IV. Hypertrophic cardiomyopathy
  A. Class IV symptoms persist despite interventional therapies
    1. Alcohol injection of septal artery
    2. Myotomy and myomectomy
    3. Mitral valve replacement
    4. Maximal medical therapy
    5. Pacemaker therapy

V. Congenital heart disease in which severe fixed pulmonary hypertension is not a complication

VI. Cardiac tumor
  A. Confined to the myocardium
  B. No evidence of distant disease revealed by extensive metastatic workup

ABSOLUTE CONTRAINDICATIONS

I. Age >70 years (may vary at different centers)

II. Fixed pulmonary hypertension (unresponsive to pharmacologic intervention)
  A. Pulmonary vascular resistance >5 Wood units
  B. Transpulmonary gradient >15 mm Hg

III. Systemic illness that will limit survival despite transplant
  A. Neoplasm other than skin cancer (<5 years disease-free survival)
  B. HIV/AIDS (CDC definition of CD4 count of <200 cells/mm^3)
  C. Systemic lupus erythematosus (SLE) or sarcoid that has multisystem involvement and is currently active
  D. Any systemic process with a high probability of recurrence in the transplanted heart
  E. Irreversible renal or hepatic dysfunction

(Continued)

TABLE 64-1 Recipient Selection for Heart Transplantation (*Continued*)

POTENTIAL RELATIVE CONTRAINDICATIONS
I. Recent malignancy
II. Chronic obstructive pulmonary disease
III. Recent and unresolved pulmonary infarction and pulmonary embolism
IV. Diabetes mellitus with end-organ damage (neuropathy, nephropathy, and retinopathy)
V. Peripheral vascular or cerebrovascular disease
VI. Active peptic ulcer disease
VI. Current or recent diverticulitis
VIII. Other systemic illness likely to limit survival or rehabilitation
IX. Severe obesity or cachexia
X. Severe osteoporosis
XI. Active alcohol or drug abuse
XII. History of noncompliance or psychiatric illness likely to interfere with long-term compliance
XIII. Absence of psychosocial support

The neuropsychiatric assessment should be performed by persons experienced in evaluating cardiac patients to determine if organic brain dysfunction or psychiatric illness is present. An experienced social worker should assess for the presence of adequate social and financial support. At the time of listing, the transplant coordinator should ensure that the patient and family understand the peculiarities of the waiting time, preoperative period, long-term maintenance medications, and the rules of living with the new heart. It is also of paramount importance that providers discuss the patient's preferences with regard to life support (duration and type), in case of a deterioration in his or her condition while awaiting transplant.

Indications for Cardiac Transplantation

Cardiac transplantation is reserved for a select group of patients with end-stage heart disease not amenable to optimal medical or surgical therapies. Prognosis for 1-year survival without transplantation should be less than 50%. Prediction of patient survival involves considerable subjective clinical judgment by the transplant committee because no reliable objective prognostic criteria are available currently. Low ejection fraction (<20%), reduced $\dot{V}O_{2,max}$ (<14 mL/kg/min), arrhythmias, high pulmonary capillary wedge pressure (>25 mm Hg), elevated plasma norepinephrine concentration (>600 pg/mL), reduced serum sodium concentration (<130 mEq/dL), and more recently N-terminal probrain natriuretic peptide (>5000 pg/mL) all have been proposed as predictors of poor prognosis and potential indications for transplantation in patients receiving optimal medical therapy.[8–11] Reduced left ventricular ejection fraction and low $\dot{V}O_{2,max}$ are widely identified as the strongest independent predictors of survival.

The indications for cardiac transplantation listing are continuously reviewed as new breakthroughs in the medical and surgical treatment of heart disease emerge.

Contraindications for Cardiac Transplantation

Table 64-1 lists the traditional absolute and relative contraindications. It should be acknowledged that strict guidelines can be problematic; therefore, each transplant program varies regarding absolute criteria based on clinical circumstances and experience. Furthermore, traditional contraindications for transplant listing are being questioned. Age is one of the most controversial exclusionary criteria for transplantation. The upper age limit for recipients is center-specific, but emphasis should be placed on the patient's physiologic rather than chronologic age. The Official Adult Heart Transplant Report 2009 from the registry of the International Society for Heart and Lung Transplantation (ISHLT) noted that over the last 25 years, the percentage of recipients older than 60 years of age has increased steadily, approaching 25% of all heart transplants between 2002 and 2008 compared with just above 5% between 1982 and 1988.[5] Although the elderly have a greater potential for occult systemic disease that may complicate their postoperative course, some recent reports have suggested that morbidity and mortality in carefully selected older patients are comparable with those of younger recipients, and they have fewer rejection episodes than younger patients.[12,13]

Fixed pulmonary hypertension (PH), usually manifested as elevated pulmonary vascular resistance (PVR), is one of the few

TABLE 64-2 Cardiac Transplant Evaluation Tests

Laboratory	Complete blood count with differential and platelet count, creatinine, blood urea nitrogen, electrolytes, liver panel, lipid panel, calcium, phosphorus, total protein, albumin, uric acid, thyroid panel, antinuclear antibodies, erythrocyte sedimentation rate (ESR), rapid plasma reagin (RPR), iron-binding tests, partial thromboplastin time, prothrombin time Blood type, IgG and IgM antibodies against cytomegalovirus, herpes simplex virus, HIV, varicella-zoster virus, hepatitis B surface antigen, hepatitis C antigen, toxoplasmosis, other titers when indicated Tuberculin skin test Prostate-specific antigen (male >50 years) Mammogram and Pap smear (female >40 years) Screening against a panel of donor antigens (panel reactive antibodies) and human leukocyte antigen phenotype 24-Hour urine for creatinine clearance and total protein, urinalysis, urine culture Baseline bacterial and fungal cultures, stool for ova and parasites if indicated
Cardiac	12-lead ECG, 24-hour Holter monitor Echocardiogram Thallium-201 imaging, positron-emission tomographic (PET) scan, or cardiac magnetic resonance imaging (MRI) to assess viability if indicated Exercise stress test and respiratory gas analysis with oxygen uptake measurements: peak exercise oxygen consumption ($\dot{V}O_{2,max}$) Right- and left-sided heart catheterization at the transplant center Myocardial biopsy on selected patients in whom etiology of heart failure is in question
Vascular	Peripheral vascular studies Carotid Doppler and duplex ultrasound 55 years
Renal	Renal ultrasound and or intravenous pyelogram if indicated
Pulmonary	Chest x-ray Pulmonary function tests Chest CT scan to evaluate abnormal chest x-ray or thoracic aorta in older patients (usually >65 years)
Gastrointestinal	Upper endoscopy/colonoscopy if indicated Upper gastrointestinal series and/or barium enema if indicated Percutaneous liver biopsy if indicated
Metabolic	Bone densitometry
Neurologic	Screening evaluation
Psychiatric	Screening evaluation
Dental	Complete dental evaluation
Physical therapy	Evaluation
Social work	Patient attitude and family support, medical insurance, and general financial resources
Transplant coordinator	Education

absolute contraindications to orthotopic cardiac transplantation. Fixed PH increases the risk of acute right ventricular failure when the right ventricle of the allograft is unable to adapt to significant PH in the immediate postoperative period.[14] Use of the transpulmonary gradient (TPG), which represents the pressure gradient across the pulmonary vascular bed independent of blood flow, may avoid erroneous estimations of PVR, such as those that may occur in patients with low cardiac output.[4]

Some have advocated the use of PVR index (PVRI) unit, which corrects for body size.

$$\text{PVR (Wood units)} = \frac{\text{MPAP (mm Hg)} - \text{PCWP (mm Hg)}}{\text{CO (L/min)}}$$

$$\text{PVRI (units)} = \frac{\text{MPAP (mm Hg)} - \text{PCWP (mm Hg)}}{\text{CO (L/min)} \times \text{BSA}} = \frac{\text{PVR}}{\text{BSA}}$$

$$\text{TPG (mm Hg)} = \text{PAP (mm Hg)} - \text{PCWP (mm Hg)}$$

where MPAP is mean pulmonary arterial pressure, PCWP is pulmonary capillary wedge pressure, CO is cardiac output, CI is cardiac index, and BSA is body surface area.

A fixed PVR greater than 5 to 6 Wood units and a TPG greater than 15 mm Hg generally are accepted as absolute criteria for rejection of a candidate.[1–4,11] Over the years, several studies have found PH to have a significant effect on posttransplant mortality using various parameters, threshold values, and follow-up periods.[15,16] However, a lack of mortality difference after heart transplantation between patients with and without preoperative PH has also been reported.[17] Perhaps more significantly, measurable parameters of pulmonary hypertension have been shown to improve following heart transplantation. A study of 172 patients followed for up to 15.1 years, published in 2005 from the Johns Hopkins Hospital, showed that mild to moderate pretransplantation PH (PVR = 2.5 to 5.0 Wood units) was not associated with higher mortality rate, although there was increased risk of posttransplantation PH within the first 6 months.[18] However, when the continuous variable PVR was examined, each 1 Wood unit increase in preoperative PVR demonstrated a 15% or more increase in mortality, especially within the first year, but these associations did not reach statistical significance. Severe preoperative PH (PVR $\geq$ 5 Wood units) was associated with death within the first year after adjusting for potential cofounders but not with overall mortality or mortality beyond the first year.

In the preoperative evaluation of the transplant recipient, if PH is discovered, an assessment of its reversibility should be performed in the cardiac catheterization laboratory.[16] Sodium nitroprusside traditionally has been used at a starting dose of 0.5 µg/kg per minute and titrated by 0.5 µg/kg per minute until there is an acceptable decline in PVR, ideally 2.5 Wood units or at least by 50%, with maintenance of adequate systemic systolic blood pressure. If sodium nitroprusside fails to produce an adequate response, other vasodilators such as adenosine, prostaglandin E_1, milrinone, or inhaled nitric oxide or prostacyclin (eg, aerosolized Iloprost) may be used.[2,19] Some patients who do not respond acutely may respond to continuous intravenous inotropic therapy, and repeat catheterization can be performed after 48 to 72 hours. Intravenous B-type natriuretic peptide, eg, nesiritide (Natrecor), has shown some efficacy in refractory pulmonary hypertension.[20] Recently, ventricular assist devices (VADs) are playing an important role in heart transplantation candidates with PH.[21] A period of left ventricular assist device (LVAD) support may allow for a decrease of pulmonary artery pressure secondary to unloading of the left ventricle. Patients with irreversible PH may be candidates for heterotopic heart transplantation, heart-lung transplantation, or LVAD destination therapy.[22] Use of modestly larger donor hearts for recipients with severe pretransplantation PH can provide additional right ventricular reserve.

Systemic diseases with poor prognosis and potential to recur in the transplanted heart or the potential to undergo exacerbation with immunosuppressive therapy are considered absolute contraindications for heart transplantation. Heart transplantation for amyloid remains controversial because amyloid deposits recur in the transplanted heart. Although case reports of long-term survival can be found in the literature,[23] survival beyond 1 year tends to be reduced.[24] Human immunodeficiency virus (HIV)–infected patients generally are excluded. Previously, any occurrence of neoplasm was a reason to exclude patients from transplantation. Currently available data do not appear to justify excluding some of these patients.[25] Most programs will consider patients who are free of disease for at least 5 years.

Irreversible renal dysfunction is a contraindication to heart transplantation. A creatinine clearance of less than 50 mL/min and a serum creatinine concentration of greater than 2 mg/dL are associated with increased risk of postoperative dialysis and decreased survival following heart transplantion.[4,26] However, patients may be considered for combined heart and kidney transplantation. Irreversible hepatic dysfunction has implications similar to renal dysfunction.[4] If transaminase levels are more than twice their normal value and associated with coagulation abnormalities, percutaneous liver biopsy should be performed to exclude primary liver disease. This should not be confused with chronic cardiac hepatopathy, which is characterized by elevated cholestatic parameters along with little or no changes in transaminases and is potentially reversible after heart transplantation.[27]

Severe chronic bronchitis or obstructive pulmonary disease may predispose patients to pulmonary infections and may result in prolonged ventilatory support after heart transplantation. Patients who have a ratio of forced expiratory volume in 1 second to forced vital capacity (FEV_1/FVC) of less than 40 to 50% of predicted or an FEV_1 of less than 50% of predicted despite optimal medical therapy are considered poor candidates for transplantation.[2,4] Transplantation in patients with diabetes mellitus is only contraindicated in the presence of significant end-organ damage (eg, diabetic nephropathy, retinopathy, or neuropathy).[2,4] Some centers have expanded their criteria successfully to include patients with mild to moderate end-organ damage.[28] Active infection was a sound reason to delay transplantation before assist devices became more commonplace. Up to 48% of patients with implanted LVADs reportedly have evidence of infection. Interestingly, treatment for LVAD infection in these patients is to proceed with urgent transplantation.[29]

Other relative contraindications include severe noncardiac atherosclerotic disease, severe osteoporosis, and active peptic ulcer disease or diverticulitis, all of which may lead to increased morbidity.[2,4] Cachexia, defined as a body mass index (BMI) of less than 20 or less than 80% ideal body weight (IBW), and obesity, defined as BMI greater than 35 or greater than 140% of IBW, are associated with increased mortality after transplantation.[30] Poor nutritional status also may limit early postoperative rehabilitation.

The ultimate success of transplantation depends on the psychosocial stability and compliance of the recipient.[31] The rigorous postoperative regimen of multidrug therapy, frequent clinic visits, and routine endomyocardial biopsies demand commitment on the part of the patient. A history of psychiatric illness, substance abuse, or previous noncompliance (particularly with medical therapy for end-stage heart failure) may be sufficient cause to reject the candidacy of a patient. Lack of a supportive social system is an additional relative contraindication.

Management of the Potential Cardiac Recipient

Preformed Anti-HLA Antibodies

Patients with elevated levels of preformed panel reactive antibodies (PRAs) to human leukocyte antigens (HLAs) have higher rates of organ rejection and decreased survival than do patients without such antibodies.[32] Consequently, before proceeding with transplantation, many medical centers do prospective cross-matching, ie, either by flow cytometry or ELISA, to determine whether a donor-specific antibodies that threaten the allograft are present. The problem has been compounded by the increased frequency of preformed reactive antibodies in patients with VADs who are awaiting cardiac transplantation.[33] Furthermore, not all antibodies are complement fixing or dangerous. Performing a prospective cross-match can be time consuming and often is impossible because of the unstable condition of the organ donor or travel logistics, leading to increased costs for transplantation and longer waiting times for recipients. Recently, virtual cross-matching has been used to eliminate the need for prospective tissue cross-matching. Modern laboratory techniques allow for identification and titer of antibodies. Because all donor antigens are known at the time of allocation, an assessment can be made without an actual tissue/sera assay. However, a particular patient's antibody population is dynamic and may change from the time of the antibody screen. As a result, care must be taken in patients with particularly diverse and high antibody titers. Plasmapheresis, intravenous immunoglobulins, cyclophosphamide, mycophenolate mofetil, and rituximab all have been used to lower the PRA levels with variable results.[2]

Pharmacologic Bridge to Transplantation

Critically compromised patients require admission to the intensive care unit for intravenous inotropic therapy. Dobutamine, a synthetic catecholamine, remains the prototype of this drug group. However, the phosphodiesterase III inhibitor milrinone is similarly effective.[34] The catecholamine dopamine is used often as a parenteral positive inotrope, but at moderate to high dose it evokes considerable systemic vasoconstriction. In candidates in whom an inotropic infusion has progressed to higher doses, combinations of dobutamine with milrinone are used. For transplant candidates dependent on inotropic infusions, eosinophilic myocarditis may develop as an allergic response to the dobutamine and may result in accelerated decline. VADs are being considered earlier, particularly as indices of nutrition decline.

Mechanical Bridge to Transplantation

Placement of an intra-aortic balloon pump (IABP) may be necessary in patients with heart failure who are refractory to initial pharmacologic measures. Ambulatory IABP through the axillary artery has been reported in few patients as a bridge to cardiac transplantation but is not commonly used today.[35]

The landmark Randomized Evaluation of Mechanical Assistance in Treatment of Chronic Heart Failure (REMATCH) trial provided evidence that LVAD support provided a statistically significant reduction in the risk of death from any cause when compared with optimal medical management. The survival rates for patients receiving LVADs ($n = 68$) versus patients receiving optimal medical management ($n = 61$) were 52% versus 28% at 1 year and 29% versus 13% at 2 years ($p = .008$, log-rank test).[6,36] The extended follow-up confirmed the initial observation that LVAD therapy renders significant survival and quality-of-life benefits compared with optimal medical management for patients with end-stage heart failure. A recent systematic review of the published literature supported these findings. In the studies reviewed, implantation of an LVAD provided support for up to 390 days, with as many as 70% of patients surviving to transplantation.[37]

The total artificial heart (TAH) positioned orthotopically replaces both native cardiac ventricles and all cardiac valves. Potential advantages of this device include eliminating problems commonly seen in the bridge to transplantation with left ventricular and biventricular assist devices, such as right-sided heart failure, valvular regurgitation, cardiac arrhythmias, ventricular clots, intraventricular communications, and low blood flows. Copeland and colleagues reported that the TAH allowed for bridge to transplantation in 79% of their patients with 1- and 5-year survival rates after transplantation of 86 and 64%, respectively.[38]

Because these devices cannot be weaned, it is imperative that the patient's candidacy for transplantation be scrutinized before placement of the device. Trends toward better device durability and reduced complication rates likely will continue to improve through the development of newer, more innovative VADs, allowing destination therapy to be considered more frequently.

Life-Threatening Ventricular Arrhythmias

Symptomatic ventricular tachycardia and a history of sudden cardiac death are indications for placement of an automatic implantable cardioverter-defibrillator (AICD), long-term antiarrhythmic therapy with amiodarone, or occasionally, radiofrequency catheter ablation, which have been shown to improve survival.[39]

Recipient Prioritization for Transplantation

The prioritization of appropriate recipients for transplantation is based on survival and quality of life expected to be gained in comparison with maximal medical and surgical alternatives.[3] The United Network for Organ Sharing (UNOS) is a national organization that maintains organ transplantation waiting lists and allocates identified donor organs on the basis of recipients' priority status. This priority status is based on a recipient's

TABLE 64-3 Current Recipient Status Criteria of the United Network for Organ Sharing (UNOS)*

STATUS IA
A. Patients who require mechanical circulatory assistance with one or more of the following devices: 1. Total artificial heart 2. Left and/or right ventricular assist device implanted for 30 days or less 3. Intra-aortic balloon pump 4. Extracorporeal membrane oxygenator (ECMO)
B. Mechanical circulatory support for more than 30 days with significant device-related complications
C. Mechanical ventilation
D. Continuous infusion of high-dose inotrope(s) in addition to continuous hemodynamic monitoring of left ventricular filling pressures
E. Life expectancy without transplant <7 days
STATUS IB
A. A patient who has at least one of the following devices or therapies in place: 1. Left and/or right ventricular assist device implanted for >30 days 2. Continuous infusion of intravenous inotropes
STATUS II
All other waiting patients who do not meet status Ia or Ib criteria

*UNOS Executive Order, August 1999.

status level (eg, IA, IB, or II), blood type, body size, and duration of time at a particular status level.[2] Geographic distance between donor and potential recipient is also taken into consideration. Highest priority is given to local status IA patients possessing the earliest listing dates. The recipient status criteria established by UNOS in 1999 are outlined in Table 64-3. In 1994, the percentage of patients awaiting transplantation for more than 2 years was 23%; this increased to 49% by 2003. From 1998 (with the institution of a new status system) to 2007, the distribution of patient status at transplant changed dramatically. In 1999, the distribution was 34% (1A), 36% (1B), and 26% (2). This shifted in 2007 to 50% (1A), 36% (1B), and 14% (2).[40]

Patients considered for transplantation should be examined at least every 3 months for reevaluation of recipient status. Yearly right-sided heart catheterization is indicated for all candidates on the waiting list and in selected cases for patients rejected because of pulmonary hypertension. Presently, there is no established method to delist patients who have stabilized on medical therapy without loss of their previously accrued waiting time.

THE CARDIAC DONOR

Donor Availability

The availability of donor organs remains the major limiting factor to heart transplantation. In the early years of heart transplantation, the number of heart transplants performed in the United States increased steadily to a peak in 1995 of 2363 and then reached a plateau in 1998. After 1998, there was a gradual decline in heart transplants per year to a nadir of 2015 in 2004, after which the number has steadily increased to 2207 in 2007.[40] Interestingly, likely owing to improved preoperative care, the death rate for patients on the waiting list for a cardiac allograft has decreased steadily.[40]

The Uniform Anatomic Gift Act of 1968 states that all competent individuals over the age of 18 may donate all or part of their bodies and established the current voluntary basis of organ donation practiced in the United States. To accommodate the increasing demand for organs, the original stringent criteria for donor eligibility have been relaxed, and educational campaigns have increased awareness of the need for a larger donor pool. In 1986, the Required Request Law, which required hospitals to request permission from next of kin to recover organs, was passed to encourage physician compliance in the donor request process. Future reforms will be molded by the evolving public attitude to transplantation and likely will focus on continued public and physician education.

Allocation of Donor Organs

In an effort to increase organ donation and to coordinate an equitable allocation of allografts, Congress passed the National Organ Transplant Act in 1984. This act resulted in the drafting of the aforementioned Required Request Law, as well as the awarding of a federal contract to the UNOS for the development of a national organ procurement and allocation network. To facilitate transplantation, the United States is divided into 11 geographic regions.

Organs are offered to sick patients within the region in which they were donated before being offered to other parts of the country. This helps to reduce organ preservation time, improve organ quality and survival outcomes, reduce the costs incurred by the transplant patient, and increase access to transplantation.

Donor Selection

Once a brain-dead individual has been identified as a potential cardiac donor, the patient undergoes a rigorous three-phase screening regimen. The primary screening is undertaken by the organ procurement agency. Information regarding the patient's age, height and weight, gender, ABO blood type, hospital course, cause of death, and routine laboratory data including cytomegalovirus (CMV), HIV, hepatitis B virus (HBV), and hepatitis C virus (HCV) serologies are collected. Cardiac surgeons and/or cardiologists perform the secondary screening, which involves further investigation in search of potential contraindications (Table 64-4), determination of the hemodynamic support necessary to sustain the donor, and review of the electrocardiogram, chest roentgenogram, arterial blood gas determination, and echocardiogram. Even when adverse donor criteria are reported, a team often is dispatched to the hospital to evaluate the donor on-site.

Although echocardiography is effective in screening for anatomical abnormalities of the heart, the use of a single echocardiogram to determine the physiologic suitability of a donor is not supported by evidence.[41] The Papworth Hospital transplant program in Great Britain increased its donor yield substantially by using a pulmonary artery catheter to guide the physiologic assessment and management of ventricular dysfunction.[42] Coronary angiography is indicated in the presence of advanced donor age (traditionally for male donors >45 years of age and female donors >50 years of age). Angiography also should be performed if there is a history of cocaine use or the donor has three risk factors for coronary artery disease (CAD), such as hypertension, diabetes, smoking history, dyslipidemia, or family history of premature CAD.[41]

The final and often most important screening of the donor occurs intraoperatively at the time of organ procurement by the cardiac surgical team. Direct visualization of the heart is performed for evidence of right ventricular or valvular dysfunction, previous infarction, or myocardial contusion secondary to closed-chest compressions or blunt chest trauma. The coronary arterial tree is palpated for gross calcifications indicative of atheromatous disease. If direct examination of the heart is unremarkable, the recipient hospital is notified, and the procurement surgeons proceed with donor cardiectomy, usually in conjunction with multiorgan procurement.

TABLE 64-4 Donor Selection for Heart Transplantation

I. Suggested criteria for cardiac donor
   A. Age <55
   B. Absence of the following:
      1. Prolonged cardiac arrest
      2. Prolonged severe hypotension
      3. Preexisting cardiac disease
      4. Intracardiac drug injection
      5. Severe chest trauma with evidence of cardiac injury
      6. Septicemia
      7. Extracerebral malignancy
      8. Positive serologies for human immunodeficiency virus, hepatitis B (active), or hepatitis C
      9. Hemodynamic stability without high-dose inotropic support (<20 μg/kg/min of dopamine)

II. Suggested cardiac donor evaluation
   A. Past medical history and physical examination
   B. Electrocardiogram
   C. Chest roentgenogram
   D. Arterial blood gases
   E. Laboratory tests (ABO, HIV, HBV, HCV)
   F. Echocardiogram, pulmonary artery catheter evaluation, and in selected cases, coronary angiogram

Expanded Donor Criteria and Alternate Listing

As the donor shortage has worsened and the number of patients waiting for transplants has increased, one of the areas of increasing interest is the use of marginal donors for marginal recipients. For this purpose, an alternate recipient list is being used by some centers to match certain recipients who might be excluded from a standard list with marginal donor hearts that otherwise would go unused. Expanded donor criteria include the use of donors substantially smaller than the recipients, donors with coronary artery disease that may require coronary artery bypass grafting (CABG), left ventricular dysfunction, or donors from older age groups.[41] Acceptable operative mortality has been reported, and the University of California, Los Angeles (UCLA) heart transplant group has shown that alternate listing did not independently predict early or late mortality.[43]

It also appears more beneficial in terms of patient survival to receive an allograft from a donor older than 40 years of age compared to remaining on the waiting list.[44] Other high-risk donors, such as HCV-positive or HBV (core IgM-negative)–positive donors, may be appropriate in selected higher-risk recipients.[41]

Also of special interest is the effect of donor alcohol and cocaine abuse on heart transplantation. A small single-center study showed unfavorable early outcome of patients receiving hearts from alcoholic donors (>2 oz of pure alcohol daily for 3 or more months), suggesting the presence of a subclinical preoperative alcoholic cardiomyopathy and poor tolerance of rejection episodes after transplantation.[45] Because of widespread cocaine abuse, donor guidelines have declared intravenous drug abuse a "relative" contraindication for donor selection. However, the dilemma of selecting donor hearts from nonintravenous drug abusers remains an open issue. A favorable outcome for patients who received transplanted hearts obtained from nonintravenous cocaine users has been reported.[46] However, judicious use of organs from donors with a history of cocaine use is strongly advised. Specific recommendations were made in a consensus report to improve the yield of donor hearts.[41]

Management of the Cardiac Donor

Medical management of cardiac donors, an integral part of organ preservation, is complicated by the complex physiologic phenomenon of brain death and the need to coordinate procurement with other organ donor teams. Brain death is associated with an "autonomic and cytokine storm." The release of noradrenaline (norepinephrine) leads to subendocardial ischemia. Subsequent cytokine release results in further myocardial depression. This is accompanied by pronounced vasodilatation and loss of temperature control.[3] Rapid afterload reduction may be achieved with sodium nitroprusside, whereas volatile anesthetics reduce the intensity of sympathetic bursts. The initial period of intense autonomic activity is followed by loss of sympathetic tone and a massive reduction in systemic vascular resistance. Overall, brain stem death results in severe hemodynamic instability, the degree of which appears to be directly related to the severity of the brain injury and may result from vasomotor autonomic dysfunction, hypovolemia, hypothermia, and dysrhythmias.[47]

Aggressive volume resuscitation sometimes is necessary, and the use of a Swan-Ganz catheter may be crucial to guide therapy.[48] Fluid overload should be avoided to prevent postoperative allograft dysfunction caused by chamber distention and myocardial edema. Inotropic support (eg, dopamine or dobutamine, epinephrine, or norepinephrine) to maintain a mean arterial blood pressure (MAP) of 60 mm Hg or more in the presence of a central venous pressure (CVP) of 6 to 10 mm Hg is recommended.[41] ATP is depleted rapidly by exogenous catecholamine administration, and this has an adverse effect on posttransplantation cardiac function.[47] Low-dose vasopressin is being used increasingly as first-line support because, in addition to treating diabetes insipidus, it independently improves arterial blood pressure and reduces exogenous inotrope requirements in brain stem dead donors.[49] Maintenance of normal temperature, electrolyte levels, osmolarity, acid-base balance, and oxygenation is critical for optimal donor management. Central diabetes insipidus develops in more than 50% of donors because of pituitary dysfunction, and massive diuresis complicates fluid and electrolyte management.[50] The initial treatment of diabetes insipidus is aimed at correcting hypovolemia and returning the plasma sodium concentration to normal levels by fluid replacement with 5% dextrose or nasogastric water. In severe cases, intermittent treatment with the synthetic analogue 1-D-amino-8-D-arginine vasopressin (DDAVP) also may be required in addition to vasopressin infusion.[47]

Several studies have demonstrated beneficial effects of thyroid hormones and steroids on cardiac performance in brain stem dead-organ donors.[42,49,51] Recent guidelines advocate the addition of a standardized hormonal resuscitation package consisting of methylprednisolone (15 mg/kg bolus), triiodothyronine (4-μg bolus followed by infusion of 3 μg/h), and arginine vasopressin (1-unit bolus followed by 0.5 to 4 units/h) to the standard donor management protocol.[41] Donors also receive insulin, titrated to keep blood glucose at 120 to 180 mg/dL. Other pertinent strategies include standard ventilator management with diligent endotracheal suctioning and a thermoregulation goal of 34 to 36°C using warming blankets and lights, warm intravenous fluids, and warm inspired air. Broad-spectrum antibiotic therapy with a cephalosporin is initiated following collection of blood, urine, and tracheal aspirate for culture. The approach for management of the cardiac donor recommended at the conference entitled, Maximizing Use of Organs Recovered from the Cadaver Donor: Cardiac Recommendations, is shown in Table 64-5 and summarized in Fig. 64-2.[41]

Donor Heart Procurement

A median sternotomy is performed, and the pericardium is incised longitudinally. The heart is inspected and palpated for evidence of cardiac disease or injury. The superior and inferior venae cavae and the azygous vein are mobilized circumferentially and encircled with ties. The aorta is dissected from the pulmonary artery and isolated with umbilical tape. To facilitate access to the epigastrium by the liver procurement team, the cardiac team often then temporarily retires from the operating room table or assists with retraction. Once preparation for liver, pancreas, lung, and kidney explantation is completed, the patient is administered 30,000 units of heparin intravenously. The azygous vein and superior vena cava are doubly ligated (or stapled) and divided distal to the azygous vein, leaving a long segment of superior vena cava (Fig. 64-3). The inferior vena cava is incised and the left atrium vented either at the left atrial appendage or via a transected pulmonary vein. The aortic cross-clamp is applied at the takeoff of the innominate artery, and the heart is arrested with a single flush (1000 mL or 10 to 20 mL/kg) of cardioplegia solution infused proximal to the cross-clamp. Rapid cooling of the heart is achieved with copious amounts of cold saline and cold saline slush poured into the pericardial well. After the delivery of cardioplegia, cardiectomy proceeds as the apex of the heart is elevated cephalad and any remaining intact pulmonary veins are divided. This maneuver is modified appropriately to retain adequate left atrial cuffs for both lungs and the heart if the lungs also are being procured. While applying caudal traction to the heart with the nondominant hand, the ascending aorta is transected proximal to the innominate artery, and the pulmonary arteries are divided distal to the bifurcation (again, modification is necessary if the lungs are being procured). More generous segments of the great vessels and superior vena cava may be required for recipients with congenital heart disease. Alternatively, the SVC and IVC are transected, followed by the aorta and pulmonary artery. The left atrium is then divided as the last step. This allows for optimal division of the left atrium, particularly when lungs are recovered. It is critically important to avoid left ventricular distention and ensure thorough cooling with ice saline.

Once the explantation is complete, the allograft is examined for evidence of a patent foramen ovale, which should be closed at that time. Any valvular anomalies are identified. The allograft then is placed in a sterile container for transport to the recipient hospital.

Organ Preservation

Current clinical graft preservation techniques generally permit a safe ischemic period of 4 to 6 hours.[52] Factors contributing to

TABLE 64-5 Management of the Cardiac Donor

I. Conventional management, before the initial echocardiogram
  A. Adjust volume status (target central venous pressure 6–10 mm Hg).
  B. Correct metabolic perturbations, including
    1. Acidosis (target pH 7.40–7.45)
    2. Hypoxemia (target Po_2 >80 mm Hg, O_2 saturation >95%)
    3. Hypercarbia (target Pco_2 30–35 mm Hg)
  C. Correct anemia (target hematocrit 30%, hemoglobin 10 g/dL).
  D. Adjust inotropes to maintain mean arterial pressure at 60 mm Hg. Norepinephrine and epinephrine should be tapered off rapidly in favor of dopamine or dobutamine.
  E. Target = dopamine <10 μg/kg/min or dobutamine <10 μg/kg/min.

II. Obtain an initial echocardiogram
  A. Rule out structural abnormalities (substantial left ventricular hypertrophy, valvular dysfunction, congenital lesions).
  B. If left ventricular ejection fraction is 45%, proceed with recovery (consider aggressive management as shown below to optimize cardiac function before recovery) with final evaluation in the operating room.
  C. If left ventricular ejection fraction is <45%, aggressive management with placement of a pulmonary arterial catheter and hormonal resuscitation is strongly recommended.

III. Hormonal resuscitation
  A. Triiodothyronine (T3): 4-μg bolus, then continuous infusion at 3 μg/h.
  B. Arginine vasopressin: 1-unit bolus, then continuous infusion at 0.5–4 units/h, titrated to a systemic vascular resistance of 800–1200 $dyne/s/cm^5$.
  C. Methylprednisolone: 15 mg/kg bolus.
  D. Insulin: 1 unit/h minimum; titrate to maintain blood sugar at 120–180 mg/dL.

IV. Aggressive hemodynamic management
  A. Initiated simultaneously with hormonal resuscitation.
  B. Placement of pulmonary artery catheter.
  C. Duration of therapy 2 hours.
  D. Adjustment of fluids, inotropes, and pressors every 15 minutes based on serial hemodynamic measurements to minimize use of beta-agonists and meet the following target (Papworth) criteria:
    1. Mean arterial pressure >60 mm Hg
    2. Central venous pressure 4–12 mm Hg
    3. Pulmonary capillary wedge pressure 8–12 mm Hg
    4. Systemic vascular resistance 800–1200 $dyne/s/cm^5$
    5. Cardiac index >2.4 $L/min/m^2$
    6. Dopamine <10 μg/kg/min or dobutamine 10 μg/kg/min

Source: Reprinted with permission from Zaroff JG, Rosengard BR, Armstrong WF, et al: Consensus conference report: Maximizing use of organs recovered from the cadaver donor: cardiac recommendations, March 28–29, 2001, Crystal City, VA. Circulation 2002; 106:836.

the severity of postoperative myocardial dysfunction include insults associated with suboptimal donor management, hypothermia, ischemia-reperfusion injury, and depletion of energy stores. A single flush of a cardioplegic or preservative solution followed by static hypothermic storage at 4 to 10°C is the preferred preservation method by most transplant centers. Crystalloid solutions of widely different compositions are available, and the debate over them speaks for the fact that no ideal solution currently exists. Depending on their ionic composition, solutions are classified as intracellular or extracellular.[52] Intracellular solutions, characterized by moderate to high concentrations of potassium and low concentrations of sodium, purportedly reduce hypothermia-induced cellular edema by mimicking the intracellular milieu. Commonly used examples of these solutions include University of Wisconsin, Euro-Collins, and in Europe, Bretschneider (HTK) and intracellular Stanford solutions. Extracellular solutions, characterized by low to moderate potassium and high sodium concentrations, avoid the theoretical potential for cellular damage and increased vascular resistance associated with hyperkalemic solutions. Hopkins, Celsior, Krebs, and St. Thomas Hospital solutions are representative extracellular cardioplegic solutions. Several comparisons

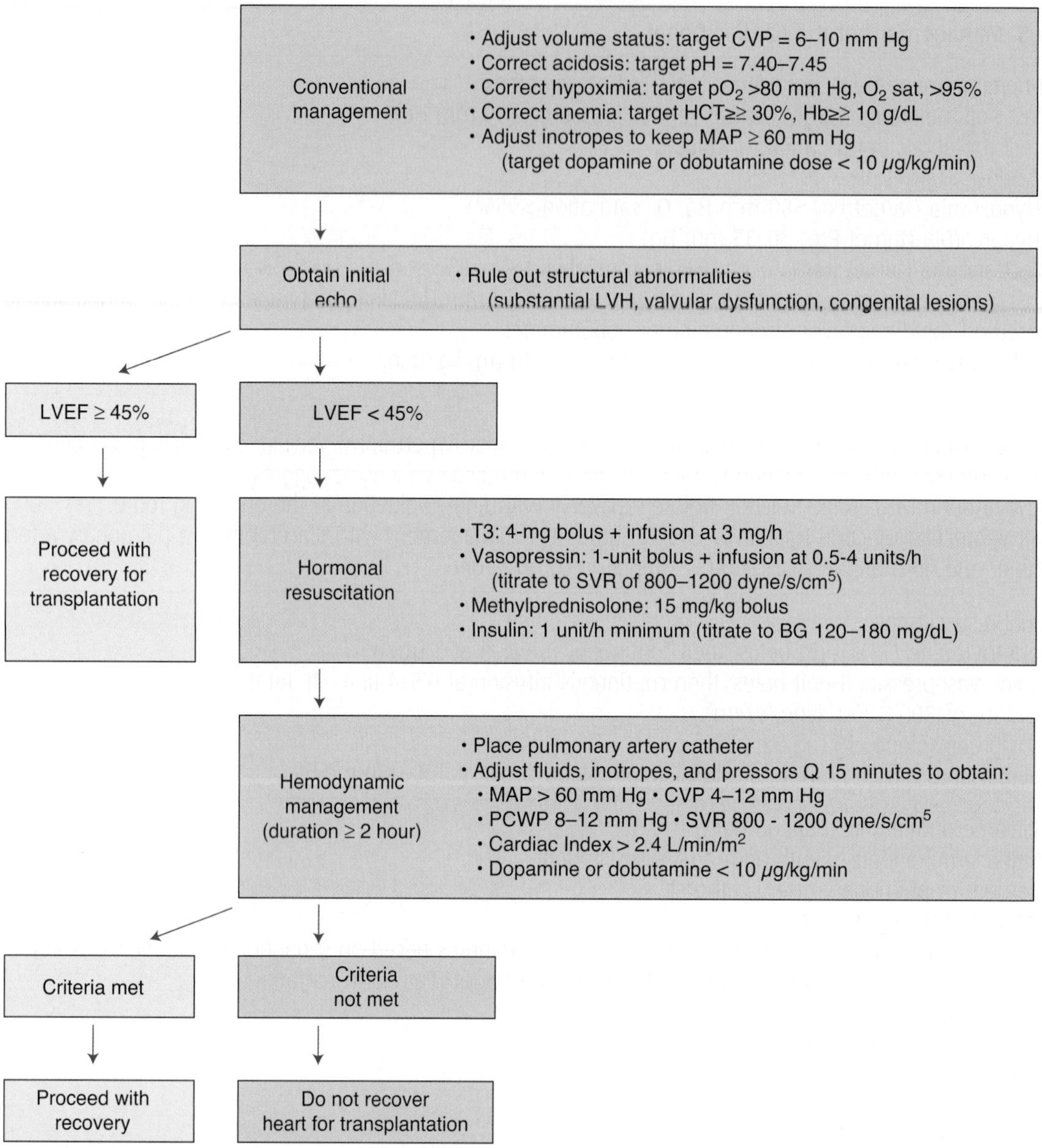

FIGURE 64-2 Recommended heart donor management algorithm. (*Reprinted with permission from Zaroff JG, Rosengard BR, Armstrong WF, et al: Consensus conference report: maximizing use of organs recovered from the cadaver donor: cardiac recommendations, March 28–29, 2001, Crystal City, VA. Circulation 2002; 106:836.*)

of the different types of intracellular and extracellular solutions have shown variable results.[53,54] Although a plethora of pharmacologic additives has been included in cardioplegic-storage solutions, the greatest potential for future routine use may lie with impermeants, substrates, and antioxidants.[55] A number of pharmacologic and mechanical strategies for leukocyte inhibition and depletion also have been explored.[56] Potential benefits of continuous hypothermic perfusion (CHP) preservation such as uniform myocardial cooling, continuous substrate supplementation, and metabolic by-product washout are currently overshadowed by exacerbation of extracellular cardiac edema and logistical problems inherent to a complex perfusion apparatus. Newer portable perfusion circuits are being developed, and recent studies showed reduction in oxidative stress and attenuation of DNA damage in canine heart transplant models preserved by 24-hour CHP compared with 4 hours of static preservation.[57]

Donor-Recipient Matching

Criteria for matching potential recipients with the appropriate donor are based primarily on ABO blood group compatibility and patient size. ABO barriers should not be crossed in adult heart transplantation because incompatibility may result in fatal hyperacute rejection. Donor weight should be within 30% of recipient weight except in pediatric patients, in whom closer size matching is required. In cases of elevated pulmonary vascular resistance in the recipient (5 to 6 Wood units), a larger donor is preferred to reduce the risk of right ventricular failure in the early postoperative period. Although practices vary by transplant

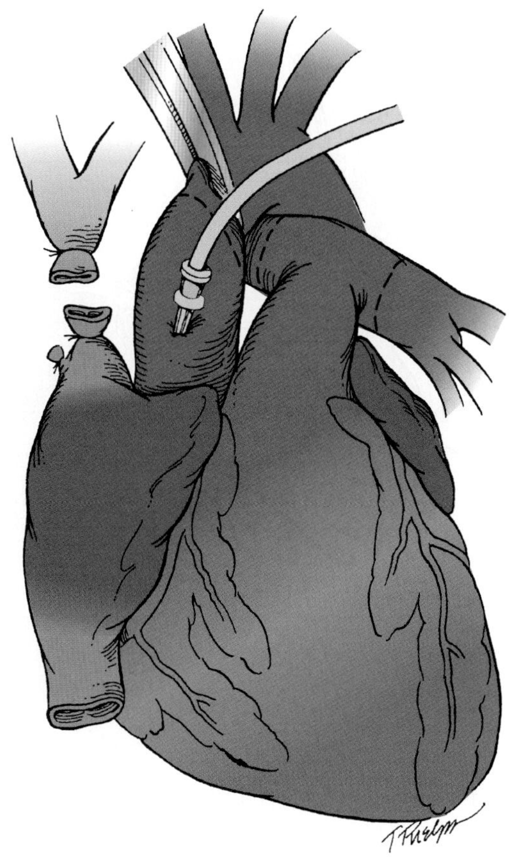

FIGURE 64-3 Donor cardiectomy.

program, generally if the percent of panel reactive antibody (PRA) is greater than 10%, indicating recipient presensitization to alloantigen, a prospective negative T-cell cross-match between the recipient and donor sera is mandatory before transplantation.[32,58] A cross-match is always performed retrospectively, even if the PRA is absent or low. Retrospective studies also have demonstrated that better matching at the HLA-DR locus results in fewer episodes of rejection and infection with an overall improved survival.[59] Because of current allocation criteria and limits on ischemic time of the cardiac allograft, routine prospective HLA matching is not logistically possible.

Hyperacute Rejection

Hyperacute rejection results from preformed donor-specific antibodies in the recipient. ABO blood group and panel reactive antibody screening have made this condition a rare complication. The onset of hyperacute rejection occurs within minutes to several hours after transplantation, and the results are catastrophic. Gross inspection reveals a mottled or dark red, flaccid allograft, and histologic examination confirms the characteristic global interstitial hemorrhage and edema without lymphocytic infiltrate. Immunofluorescence techniques reveal deposits of immunoglobulins and complement on the vascular endothelium. Immediate plasmapheresis, intravenous immunoglobulin (IVIG), and mechanical support are immediately instituted, and retransplantation may be the only successful strategy.

OPERATIVE TECHNIQUES IN HEART TRANSPLANTATION

Orthotopic Heart Transplantation

Operative Preparation of the Recipient

The original technique of orthotopic cardiac transplantation described by Shumway and Lower is still used commonly today. Following median sternotomy and vertical pericardiotomy, the patient is heparinized and prepared for cardiopulmonary bypass. Bicaval venous cannulation and distal ascending aortic cannulation just proximal to the origin of the innominate artery are optimal. Umbilical tape snares are passed around the superior and inferior venae cavae. Bypass is initiated, the patient is cooled to 28°C, caval snares are tightened, and the ascending aorta is cross-clamped. The great vessels are transected above the semilunar commissures, whereas the atria are incised along the atrioventricular grooves, leaving cuffs for allograft implantation. Removal of the atrial appendages reduces the risk of postoperative thrombus formation. Following cardiectomy, the proximal 1 to 2 cm of aorta and pulmonary artery are separated from one another with electrocautery, taking care to avoid injuring the right pulmonary artery. Continuous aspiration of pulmonary venous return from bronchial collaterals is achieved by insertion of a vent into the left atrial remnant either directly or via the right superior pulmonary vein.

Timing of donor and recipient cardiectomies is critical to minimize allograft ischemic time and recipient bypass time. Frequent communication between the procurement and transplant teams permits optimal coordination of the procedures. Ideally, the recipient cardiectomy is completed just before arrival of the cardiac allograft.

Implantation

The donor heart is removed from the transport cooler and placed in a basin of cold saline. If not previously performed, preparation of the donor heart is accomplished. Electrocautery and sharp dissection are used to separate the aorta and pulmonary artery. The left atrium is incised by connecting the pulmonary vein orifices, and excess atrial tissue is trimmed, forming a circular cuff tailored to the size of the recipient left atrial remnant (Fig. 64-4). Implantation begins with placement of a double-armed 3-0 Prolene suture through the recipient left atrial cuff at the level of the left superior pulmonary vein and then through the donor left atrial cuff near the base of the atrial appendage (Fig. 64-5). The allograft is lowered into the recipient mediastinum atop a cold sponge to insulate it from direct thermal transfer from adjacent thoracic structures. The suture is continued in a running fashion caudally and then medially to the inferior aspect of the interatrial septum (Fig. 64-6). The second arm of the suture is run along the roof of the left atrium and down the interatrial septum. It is important to continually assess size discrepancy between donor and recipient atria so that appropriate plication of excess tissue may be performed. The left atrium is filled with saline, and the two arms of suture are tied together on the outside of the heart. Most centers use constant

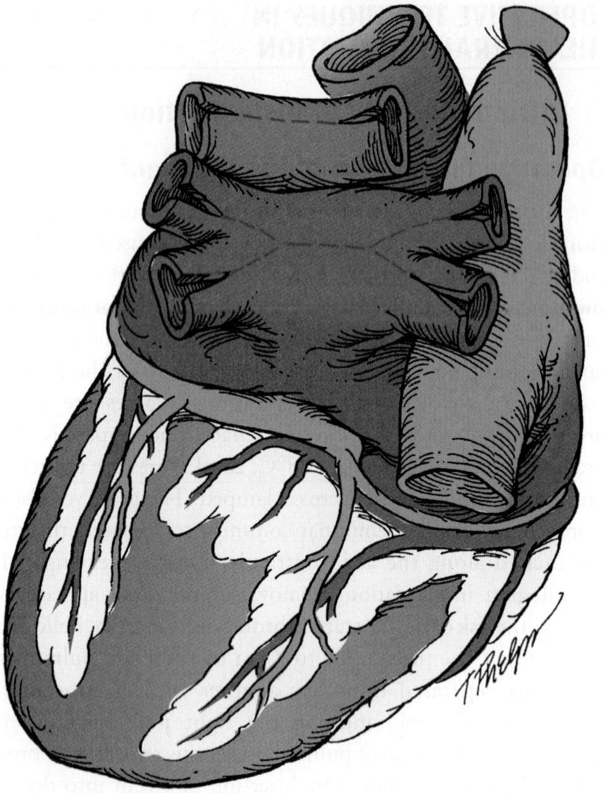

FIGURE 64-4 Donor allograft preparation for orthotopic heart transplantation. Pulmonary vein orifices joined to form left atrial cuff.

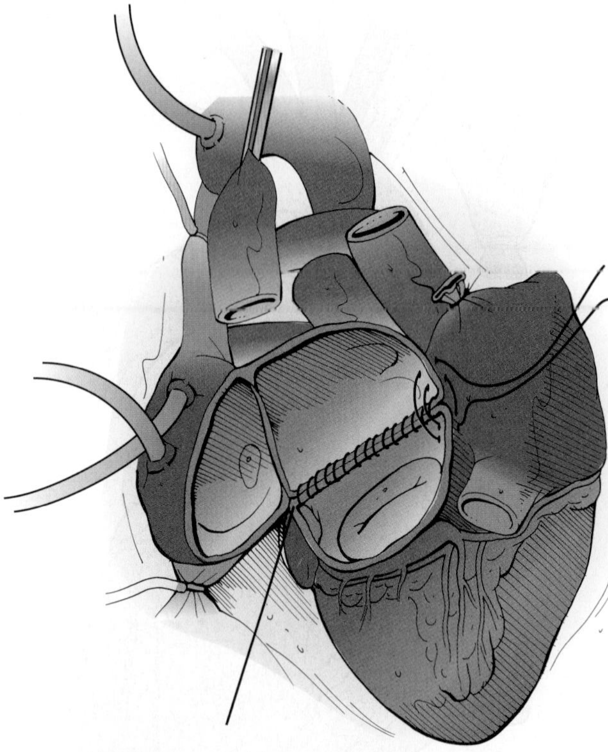

FIGURE 64-6 Implantation of allograft (continued). Left atrial anastomosis. (*Reproduced with permission from Baumgartner WA, Kasper E, Reitz B, Theodore J [eds]: Heart and Lung Transplantation, 2nd ed. New York, Saunders, 2002; pp. 180-199.*)

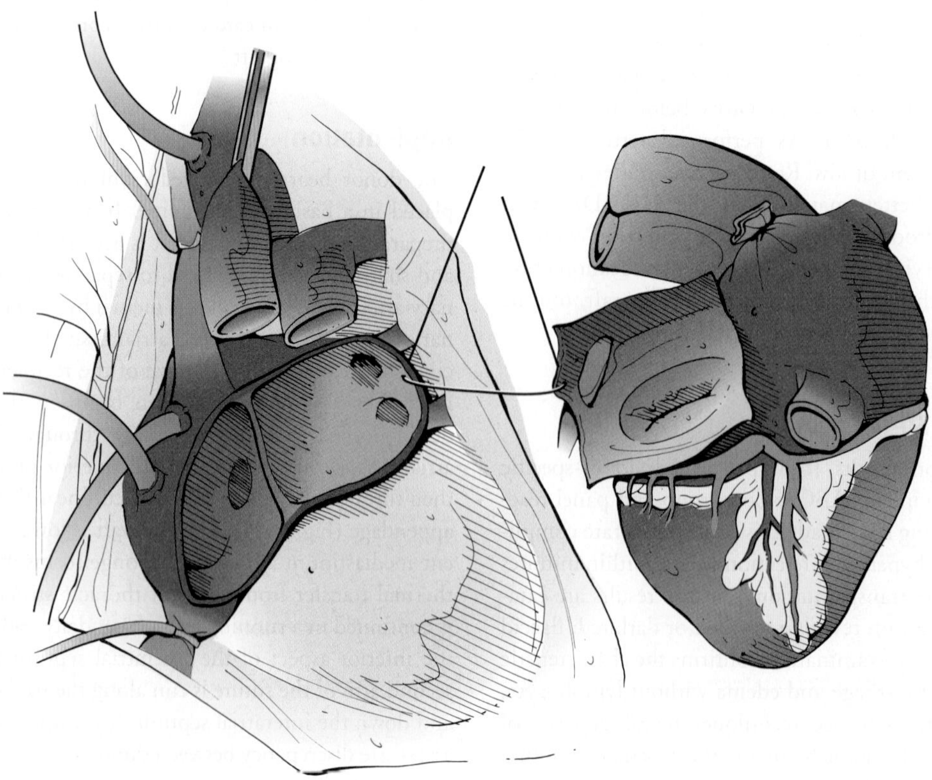

FIGURE 64-5 Implantation of allograft. First suture is placed at the level of the left superior pulmonary vein. (*Reproduced with permission from Baumgartner WA, Kasper E, Reitz B, Theodore J [eds]: Heart and Lung Transplantation, 2nd ed. New York, Saunders, 2002; pp. 180-199.*)

insufflation of carbon dioxide into the mediastinum to reduce the amount of intracardiac air.

Once the left atrial anastomosis is complete, a curvilinear incision is made from the inferior vena caval orifice toward the right atrial appendage of the allograft. This modification in the right atriotomy initially introduced by Barnard reduces the risk of injury to the sinoatrial node and accounts for the preservation of sinus rhythm observed in most recipients. The tricuspid apparatus and interatrial septum are inspected. Recipients are predisposed to increased right-sided heart pressures in the early postoperative period owing to preexisting pulmonary hypertension and volume overload. Both conditions are poorly tolerated by the recovering right ventricle. To avoid refractory arterial desaturation associated with shunting, patent foramen ovale are closed. The right atrial anastomosis is performed in a running fashion similar to the left, with the initial anchor suture placed either at the most superior or inferior aspect of the interatrial septum so that the ends of the suture meet in the middle of the anterolateral wall (Fig. 64-7A,B).

The end-to-end pulmonary artery anastomosis is next performed using a 4-0 Prolene suture beginning with the posterior wall from inside of the vessel and then completing the anterior wall from the outside (Fig. 64-8). It is crucial that the pulmonary artery ends be trimmed to eliminate any redundancy in the vessel that might cause kinking.[60] Finally, the aortic anastomosis is performed using a technique similar to that for the pulmonary artery, except that some redundancy is desirable in the aorta because it facilitates visualization of the posterior suture line (Fig. 64-9). Rewarming usually is begun before the aortic anastomosis, which is performed in a standard end-to-end fashion. Routine deairing techniques are then employed. Lidocaine (100 to 200 mg intravenously) and methylprednisone (500 to 1000 mg) is administered, and the aortic cross-clamp is removed. Half of patients require electrical defibrillation. A needle vent is inserted in the ascending aorta for final deairing, with the patient in steep Trendelenburg position. Suture lines are inspected carefully for hemostasis. Inotrope infusion is initiated, and temporary pacing may be required. The patient is weaned from cardiopulmonary bypass, and the cannulae are removed. Temporary epicardial pacing wires are placed in the donor right atrium and ventricle. Following insertion of mediastinal and pleural tubes, the median sternotomy is closed in the standard fashion.

Cold-blood cardioplegia is used in many centers. An initial dose often is given following removal from the cold storage solution before implantation. A second dose, or the initial dose as given by some centers, is administered after the right atrial anastomosis or inferior vena cava (IVC) anastomosis, when a bicaval technique is used.

Alternative Techniques for Orthotopic Heart Transplantation

The most commonly employed technique today is a bicaval anastomotic method. With this technique, the recipient right atrium is excised completely, leaving a left atrial cuff and a

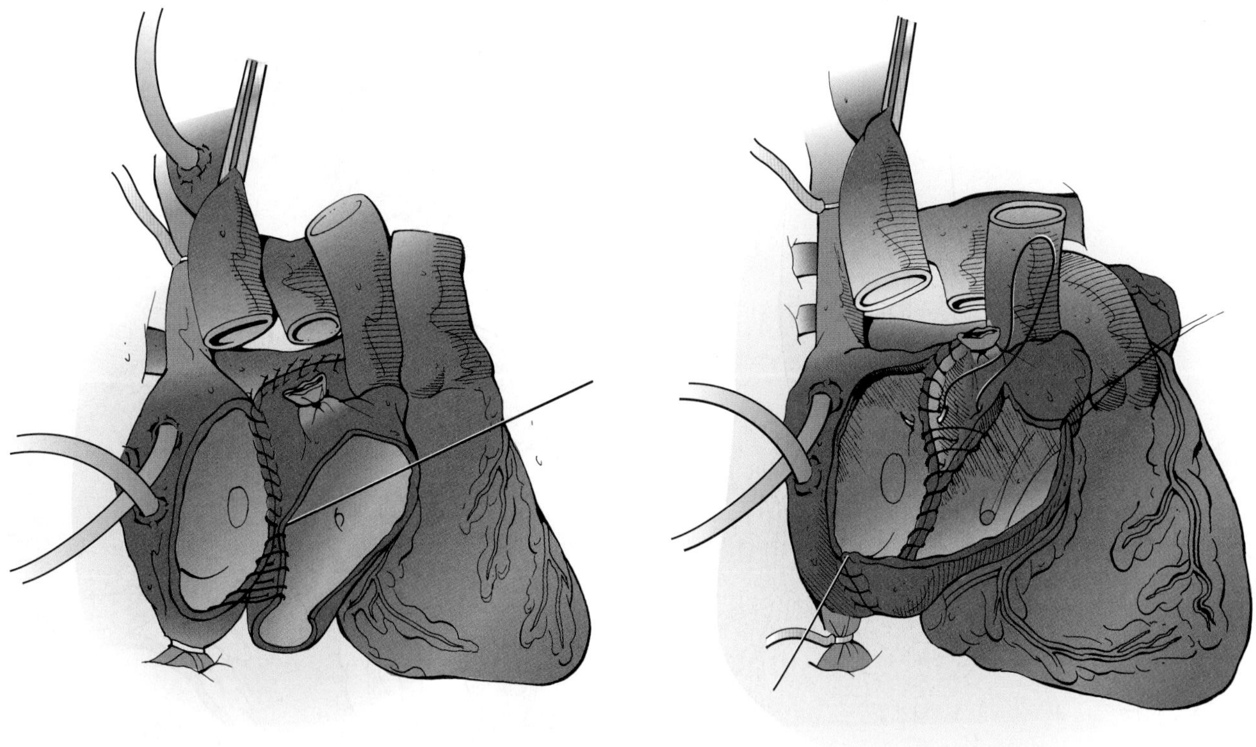

A B

FIGURE 64-7 Implantation of allograft (continued). (A) Initiation of right atrial anastomosis. (B) Completion of right atrial anastomosis. *(Reproduced with permission from Baumgartner WA, Kasper E, Reitz B, Theodore J [eds]: Heart and Lung Transplantation, 2nd ed. New York, Saunders, 2002; pp. 180-199.)*

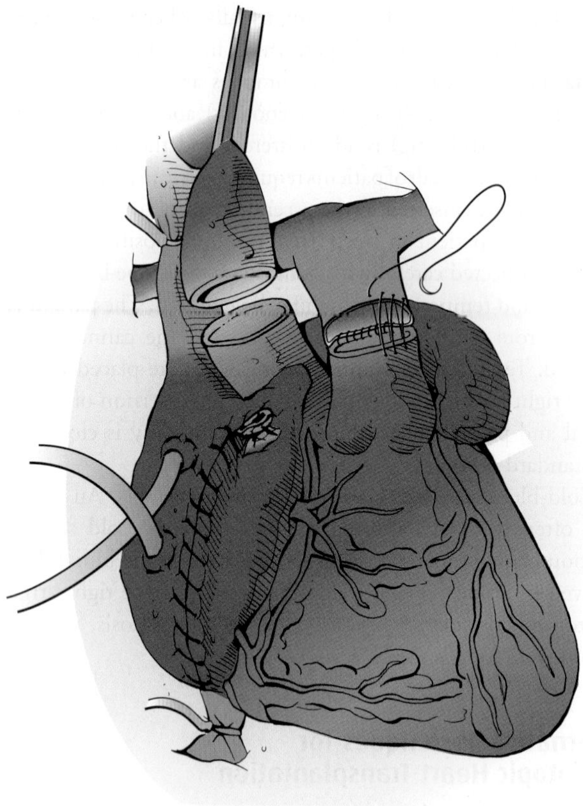

FIGURE 64-8 Implantation of allograft (continued). Pulmonary arterial anastomosis. (*Reproduced with permission from Baumgartner WA, Kasper E, Reitz B, Theodore J [eds]: Heart and Lung Transplantation, 2nd ed. New York, Saunders, 2002; pp. 180-199.*)

generous cuff of the IVC and superior vena cava (SVC), respectively. The left atrial cuff of the donor is anastomosed to the left atrial cuff of the recipient using the standard Shumway technique. Individual end-to-end anastomoses of the IVC and SVC are performed. The IVC anastomosis usually is performed following the left atrial anastomosis and the SVC anastomosis after the cross-clamp is removed. Total heart transplantation involves complete excision of the recipient heart with bicaval end-to-end anastomoses and bilateral pulmonary venous cuff anastomoses. The Wythenshawe bicaval technique is performed in a similar fashion except that the recipient left atrium is prepared as a single cuff with all four pulmonary vein orifices (Fig. 64-10). Although these procedures are more technically difficult than standard orthotopic transplantation, published series using these techniques have reported shorter hospital stays, reduced postoperative dependence on diuretics, and lower incidences of atrial dysrhythmias, conduction disturbances, mitral and tricuspid valve incompetence, and right ventricular failure.[61] A single-center study comparing biatrial versus bicaval transplant showed an improved 12-month survival in the bicaval group.[62] However, a recent analysis of the UNOS database, including more than 11,000 patients, did not demonstrate a survival difference between patients in whom biatrial versus bicaval anastomotic techniques were used; although the bicaval technique was associated with decreased duration of hospital stay and postoperative pacemaker placement.[63] Long-term outcomes

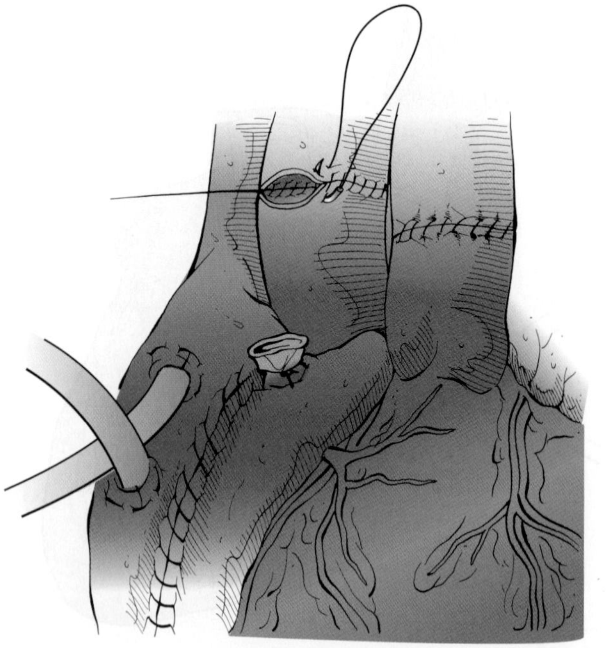

FIGURE 64-9 Implantation of allograft (continued). Aortic anastomosis. (*Reproduced with permission from Baumgartner WA, Kasper E, Reitz B, Theodore J [eds]: Heart and Lung Transplantation, 2nd ed. New York, Saunders, 2002; pp. 180-199.*)

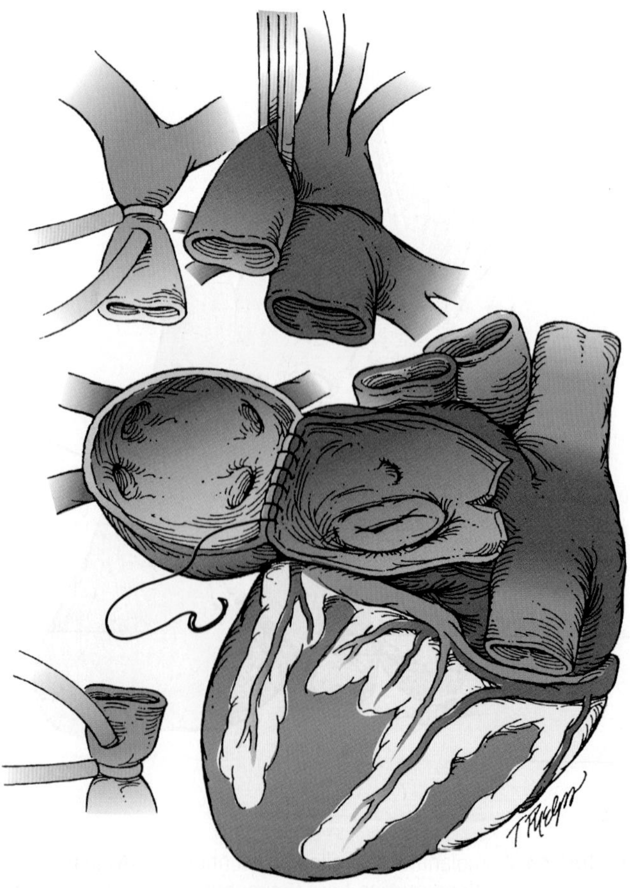

FIGURE 64-10 Bicaval heart transplantation.

and prospective, randomized studies evaluating these alternative techniques are still needed.

Heterotopic Heart Transplantation

Pulmonary hypertension and right-sided heart failure have remained the leading causes of early mortality in cardiac transplantation. This has led to an interest in heterotopic heart transplantation. Currently, heterotopic heart transplants are performed rarely but may be indicated in patients with irreversible pulmonary hypertension or significant donor–recipient size mismatch.[22]

Heart Transplantation after VAD

Cardiac transplantation after VAD poses unique challenges. All patients should have a recent contrasted chest CT to identify location and course of outflow grafts. The femoral artery and vein should be exposed for cannulation before redo sternotomy. Sternal reentry should carefully dissect the heart from pleura to pleura to safely place a retractor. The initial focus is on dissection of the IVC, SVC, and aorta. Further dissection is ideal, but may require cardiopulmonary bypass. The apex and left atrium should not be manipulated before bypass as there is a risk of entraining air, particularly with axial-flow devices. Finally, before initiating bypass, the outflow graft should be clamped to prevent regurgitation through the device. The sternotomy and adhesiolysis can be difficult and time consuming. Patience is critical.

POSTOPERATIVE MANAGEMENT

Hemodynamic Management

Heart Allograft Physiology

The intact heart is innervated by antagonistic sympathetic and parasympathetic fibers of the autonomic nervous system. Transplantation necessitates transection of these fibers, yielding a denervated heart with altered physiology. Devoid of autonomic input, the sinoatrial (SA) node of the transplanted allograft fires at its increased intrinsic resting rate of 90 to 110 beats per minute.[64] The allograft relies on distant noncardiac sites as its source for catecholamines; thus its response to stress (eg, hypovolemia, hypoxia, and anemia) is somewhat delayed until circulating catecholamines can exert their positive chronotropic effect on the heart. The absence of a normal reflex tachycardia in response to venous pooling accounts for the frequency of orthostatic hypotension in transplant patients.

Denervation alters the heart's response to therapeutic interventions that act directly through the cardiac autonomic nervous system.[64] Carotid sinus massage, Valsalva maneuver, and atropine have no effect on SA node firing or atrioventricular conduction. Because of depletion of myocardial catecholamine stores associated with prolonged inotropic support of the donor, the allograft often requires high doses of catecholamines.

Routine Hemodynamic Management

Donor myocardial performance is transiently depressed in the immediate postoperative period. Allograft injury associated with donor hemodynamic instability and the hypothermic, ischemic insult of preservation contribute to reduced ventricular compliance and contractility characteristics of the newly transplanted heart.[65] Abnormal atrial dynamics owing to the midatrial anastomosis exacerbate the reduction in ventricular diastolic loading. An infusion of epinephrine or dobutamine is initiated routinely in the operating room to provide temporary inotropic support. Cardiac denervation brings in several consequences, which may include a chronotropic and inotropic supersensitivity to exogenous catecholamines.[66] Restoration of normal myocardial function usually permits the cautious weaning of inotropic support within 2 to 4 days.

Early Allograft Failure

Early cardiac failure still accounts for up to 20% of perioperative deaths of heart transplant recipients.[67] The cause may be multifactorial, but the most important etiologies are myocardial dysfunction owing to donor instability, pulmonary hypertension, ischemic injury during preservation, and occasionally acute rejection. Mechanical support with an intra-aortic balloon pump, ventricular assist device, or ECMO can be used in patients refractory to pharmacologic interventions, although this measure, as well as retransplantation, has historically been associated with increased mortality.[68,69]

Chronic left ventricular failure frequently is associated with elevated pulmonary vascular resistance, and the unprepared donor right ventricle may be unable to overcome this increased afterload. Although recipients are screened to ensure that those with irreversible pulmonary hypertension are not considered for transplantation, right-sided heart failure remains a leading cause of early mortality. Initial management involves employing pulmonary vasodilators such as inhaled nitric oxide, nitroglycerin, or sodium nitroprusside. Pulmonary hypertension that is refractory to these vasodilators sometimes responds to prostaglandin E_1 (PGE_1) or prostacyclin.[14,70] Intra-aortic balloon counterpulsation and right ventricular assist devices also can be used in patients unresponsive to medical therapy.[71]

Arrhythmias

Denervation of the transplanted heart leads to loss of autonomic nervous system modulation of the heart's electrophysiologic properties. Parasympathetic denervation causes loss of basal suppression of SA node automaticity, leading to a persistent increase in resting heart rate and a loss of normal, rapid heart rate modulation. This parasympathetic loss also causes elimination of the chronotropic effects of digoxin and atropine after heart transplantation. At the same time, sympathetic denervation causes a decrease and delay in exercise- or stress-induced augmentation of SA node automaticity, resulting in a decreased maximum heart rate with exercise.[72]

Sinus or junctional bradycardia occurs in up to half of transplant recipients. Risk factors for sinus node dysfunction include prolonged organ ischemia, angiographic nodal artery abnormalities, biatrial versus bicaval anastomosis, preoperative amiodarone use, and rejection.[73] Adequate heart rate is achieved with inotropic drug infusions and/or temporary epicardial pacing. Most bradyarrhythmias resolve over 1 to 2 weeks. Theophylline has been effective in patients with bradyarrhythmias and has decreased the need for permanent pacemakers in this patient population.[74]

Atrial fibrillation, atrial flutter, and other supraventricular arrhythmias have been reported in 5 to 30% of patients after heart transplantation.[72] Individual assessment of the risk:benefit ratio for anticoagulation therapy is necessary. Supraventricular tachycardia (SVT) in transplant patients should be treated in the same manner as in nontransplant patients but with lower doses. Recurrent arrhythmias from reentry circuits or defined ectopic foci often can be cured by radiofrequency ablation.

Premature ventricular complexes (PVCs) are generally not considered ominous. Because of their rapidly terminal nature, sustained ventricular tachycardia (VT) and ventricular fibrillation presumably are responsible for a significant portion of the 10% of sudden and unexplained deaths in heart transplant patients.[75]

Unique aspects of common antiarrhythmic drugs reflecting the differences in their therapeutic effects in heart transplant recipients compared with nontransplant patients are shown in Table 64-6.[72] Persistence of any form of arrhythmia should warrant further investigative efforts and an aggressive search for the presence of indicators of cardiac ischemia, rejection, pulmonary pathology, or infection. If arrhythmic episodes are frequent or underlying cardiac pathology is severe, retransplantation may be considered.

Systemic Hypertension

Systemic hypertension should be treated to prevent unnecessary afterload stress on the allograft. In the early postoperative period, intravenous sodium nitroprusside or nitroglycerin usually is administered. Nitroglycerin is associated with less pulmonary shunting because of a relative preservation of the pulmonary hypoxic vasoconstrictor reflex. Nicardipine infusion has been reported to control postoperative hypertension more rapidly and was superior to sodium nitroprusside in maintaining left ventricular performance immediately after drug infusion.[76] If hypertension persists, an oral antihypertensive can be added, if possible, to permit weaning of the parenteral agents.

Respiratory Management

The respiratory management of the cardiac transplant recipient uses the same protocols employed following routine cardiac surgery.

Renal Function

Preoperative renal insufficiency owing to chronic heart failure and the nephrotoxic effects of calcineurin inhibitors such as FK506 and cyclosporine place the recipient at increased risk of renal insufficiency. Acute calcineurin inhibitor–induced renal insufficiency usually will resolve with a reduction in dose. Continuous intravenous infusion to eliminate the wide fluctuations in levels associated with oral dosing can be attempted. Furthermore, concurrent administration of mannitol with calcineurin inhibitors may reduce their nephrotoxicity. Most centers administer a cytolytic agent in the immediate postoperative period and delay the initiation of calcineurin inhibitor therapy.

Outpatient Follow-up

Before discharge, patients should receive comprehensive education about their medications, diet, exercise, and infection recognition. Close follow-up by an experienced transplant team is the cornerstone for successful long-term survival after cardiac transplantation. This comprehensive team facilitates the early detection of rejection, opportunistic infections, patient noncompliance, and adverse sequelae of immunosuppression. Clinic visits routinely are scheduled concurrently with endomyocardial biopsies and include physical examination, a variety of laboratory studies, chest roentgenogram, and electrocardiogram.

ACUTE REJECTION

Cardiac allograft rejection is the normal host response to cells recognized as nonself. The vast majority of cases are mediated by the cellular limb of the immune response through an elegant cascade of events involving macrophages, cytokines, and T lymphocytes. Humoral-mediated rejection (also called *vascular rejection*) is less common. The highest risk factors are allografts from younger and female donors (irrespective of recipient sex). Although about 85% of episodes can be reversed with corticosteroid therapy alone,[77] rejection is still a major cause of morbidity in cardiac transplant recipients.[5,78]

Diagnosis of Acute Rejection

In the precyclosporine era, the classic clinical manifestations of acute rejection included low-grade fever, malaise, leukocytosis, pericardial friction rub, supraventricular arrhythmias, decreased voltage on ECG, low cardiac output, reduced exercise tolerance, and signs of congestive heart failure. In the cyclosporine era, however, most episodes of rejection characteristically are insidious, and patients can remain asymptomatic even with late stages of rejection. Thus routine surveillance studies for early detection are crucial to minimize cumulative injury to the allograft. Right ventricular endomyocardial biopsy remains the gold standard for the diagnosis of acute rejection. The most frequently used technique for orthotopic allografts is a percutaneous approach through the right internal jugular vein. Interventricular septal specimens are fixed in formalin for permanent section, although frozen sections are performed occasionally if urgent diagnosis is necessary. Hemodynamic parameters may also be obtained with a pulmonary artery catheter. Complications are infrequent (1 to 2%) but include venous hematoma, carotid puncture, pneumothorax, arrhythmias, heart block, and right ventricular perforation and injury to the tricuspid valve. The exact schedule for endomyocardial biopsies varies among institutions but usually reflects the associated risk of increased rejection during the first 6 months after transplantation. Biopsies are performed initially every 7 to 10 days in the early postoperative period and eventually tapered to 3- to 6-month intervals after the first year. Suspicion of rejection warrants additional biopsies.

TABLE 64-6 Differences in Therapeutic Agent Effects in Heart Transplant Recipients Compared with Nontransplant Patients

Arrhythmia Therapy	Differences in Posttransplantation
DRUGS	
AV nodal agents	
Digoxin	No effect on heart rate
β-Adrenergic antagonists	Exacerbation of exercise intolerance
Calcium channel antagonists	Accentuated slowing of SA and AV nodes; may alter cyclosporine levels
Adenosine	Accentuated slowing of SA and AV nodes
Adrenergic agonists	
Norepinephrine	Unchanged peripheral effect, slightly more inotropic and chronotropic effect
Epinephrine	Unchanged peripheral effect, slightly more inotropic and chronotropic effect
Dopamine	Unchanged peripheral effect, less inotropic effect
Dobutamine	Unchanged
Ephedrine	Unchanged peripheral effect, less inotropic effect
Neo-synephrine	Unchanged peripheral effect, no reflex bradycardia
Isoproterenol	Unchanged
Antiarrhythmic agents	
Class Ia (quinidine, disopyramide, procainamide)	No cardiac vagolytic effect
Class Ib (lidocaine, mexiletine)	None reported
Class Ic (flecainide, encainide, moricizine, propafenone)	None reported
Class III (amiodarone, sotalol, ibutilide, dofetilide)	Possible exaggerated or atypical response
Anticoagulants	
Heparin	None reported
Warfarin	None reported
Miscellaneous	
Atropine	No effect on heart rate
Methylxanthines (theophylline, aminophylline)	Possibly more chronotropic effect
Cardioversion	None reported
Radiofrequency catheter ablation	Possible differences in pathway or chamber anatomy
Electrical devices	
Pacemaker	None reported
Intracardiac defibrillator	None reported

AV = atrioventricular; SA = sinoatrial.
Source: Reprinted with permission from Stecker EC, Strelich KR, Chugh SS, et al: Arrhythmias after orthotopic heart transplantation. J Cardiol Fail 2005; 11:464.

Evaluation of sample adequacy for the ISHLT grading scheme requires a minimum of four good endomyocardial tissue fragments, with less than 50% of each fragment being fibrous tissue, thrombus, or other noninterpretable tissues (eg, crush artifact or poorly processed fragments).[79] The pattern and density of lymphocyte infiltration, in addition to the presence or absence of myocyte necrosis in the endomyocardial biopsy, determine the severity grade of cellular rejection.[80] Further elaboration of the pathologic features and identification of antibody-mediated rejection were addressed more recently.[81] In 2004, the ISHLT Pathology Council proposed simplification of the 1990 diagnostic categories for cellular rejection to mild,

TABLE 64-7 ISHLT Standardized Cardiac Biopsy Grading: Acute Cellular Rejection, 2004*

Grade 0 R†	No rejection
Grade 1 R (Mild)	Interstitial and/or perivascular infiltrate with up to 1 focus of myocyte damage
Grade 2 R	(Moderate) Two or more foci of infiltrate with associated myocyte damage
Grade 3 R	(Severe) Diffuse infiltrate with multifocal myocyte damage ± edema, ± hemorrhage ± vasculitis

*The presence or absence of acute antibody-mediated rejection (AMR) may be recorded as AMR 0 or AMR 1, as required (see Table 64-8).
†Where R denotes revised grade to avoid confusion with 1990 scheme.
ISHLT = international Society of Heart and Lung Transplantation.
Source: Modified with permission from Stewart S, Winters GL, Fishbein MC, et al: Revision of the 1990 working formulation for the standardization of nomenclature in the diagnosis of heart rejection. J Heart Lung Transplant 2005; 24:1710.

moderate, and severe and identification of the histologic characteristics of antibody-mediated rejection.[82] The new grading scale was developed to better address the challenges and inconsistencies in use of the old grading system. Tables 64-7 and 64-8 show the new 2004 ISHLT grading scale.[82]

Noninvasive studies for the diagnosis of acute rejection have been unreliable. Electrocardiographic voltage summation and E-rosette assay techniques were useful adjuncts in the early cardiac transplant experience[83]; however, they currently are of no value in patients receiving cyclosporine.[84] Attempts with signal-averaged electrocardiography,[85] echocardiography,[86] or in combination,[87] magnetic resonance imaging,[88] technetium ventriculography,[89] and a variety of immunologic markers[90] have not provided sufficient sensitivity and specificity to warrant widespread use.[91] Peripheral blood gene expression profiling is an exciting new field that may provide the answer to noninvasive discrimination of rejection in cardiac allograft recipients.[92]

TABLE 64-8 ISHLT Recommendations for Acute Antibody-Mediated Rejection (AMR), 2004

AMR 0	Negative for acute antibody-mediated rejection No histologic or immunopathologic features of AMR
AMR 1	Positive for AMR Histologic features of AMR Positive immunofluorescence or immunoperoxidase staining for AMR (positive CD68, C4D)

Source: Modified with permission from Stewart S, Winters GL, Fishbein MC, et al: Revision of the 1990 working formulation for the standardization of nomenclature in the diagnosis of heart rejection. J Heart Lung Transplant 2005; 24:1710.

Treatment of Acute Rejection

Corticosteroids are the cornerstone for antirejection therapy. The treatment of choice for any rejection episode occurring during the first 1 to 3 postoperative months or for an episode considered to be severe is a short course (3 days) of intravenous methylprednisolone (1000 mg/d). Virtually all other episodes are treated initially with increased doses of oral prednisone (100 mg/d) followed by a taper to baseline over several weeks.[93] Although not yet universally accepted, many centers have reduced the doses of these corticosteroids successfully with reversal rates of rejection similar to traditional dosing.

Repeat endomyocardial biopsy should be performed 7 to 10 days after the cessation of antirejection therapy to assess adequacy of treatment. If the biopsy does not show significant improvement, a second trial of pulse-steroid therapy is recommended; if rejection has progressed (or if the patient becomes hemodynamically unstable), rescue therapy is indicated.

Substitution of tacrolimus for cyclosporine may obviate the need for admission in patients with steroid-refractory persistent rejection.[94] Alternatively, sirolimus may be substituted for mycophenolate or azathioprine.[95] The use of OKT3, antithymocyte globulin, and thymoglobulin generally is reserved for severe rejection with hemodynamic compromise.[96] Methotrexate has been particularly successful in eradicating chronic low-grade rejection. Total lymphoid irradiation and photopheresis also have demonstrated success in some cases of refractory rejection.[97] Cardiac retransplantation is the ultimate therapeutic option for patients who do not respond to the aforementioned interventions. However, the results of retransplantation for rejection are dismal, and in most centers, it is no longer performed for this indication.

Asymptomatic mild rejection (grade 1) usually is not treated but is monitored with repeat endomyocardial biopsies because only 20 to 40% of mild cases progress to moderate rejection.[98] On the other hand, the presence of myocyte necrosis (grades 3b and 4) represents a definite threat to allograft viability and is a universally accepted indication for therapy. Management of moderate rejection (grade 3a) is controversial and requires consideration of multiple variables.[99] Notably, Stoica and colleagues recently demonstrated that acute moderate to severe cellular rejection has a cumulative impact on cardiac allograft vasculopathy (CAV) onset.[100] Regardless of the biopsy results, allograft dysfunction is an indication for hospitalization, antirejection therapy, and if severe, invasive hemodynamic monitoring and inotropic support.

Acute Vascular Rejection

Vascular rejection is mediated by the humoral limb of the immune response. Unlike cellular rejection, hemodynamic instability requiring inotropic support is common in patients with vascular rejection.[101] Diagnosis requires evidence of endothelial cell swelling on light microscopy and immunoglobulin-complement deposition by immunofluorescence techniques.[102] Aggressive treatment of patients with allograft dysfunction consists of plasmapheresis, high-dose corticosteroids, heparin, IgG, and cyclophosphamide.[103] Despite these interventions, symptomatic acute vascular rejection is associated with a high mortality.[101,103] Repeated episodes of acute vascular rejection or chronic low-grade vascular rejection are believed to play a dominant role in the development of allograft coronary artery disease.[104]

INFECTIOUS COMPLICATIONS IN HEART TRANSPLANTATION

Organisms and Timing of Infections

Infection is a leading cause of morbidity and mortality in the cardiac transplant population.[5,105] The introduction of new chemoprophylactic regimens with the resultant prevention of serious disease caused by CMV has resulted in significant reductions in the number of infectious episodes and a delay in presentation after heart transplantation.[105] Patients are at greatest risk of life-threatening infections in the first 3 months after transplantation and following increases in immunosuppression for acute rejection episodes or retransplantation.[105] Table 64-9 illustrates the most common organisms causing infections in the cardiac recipient.

Preventive Measures and Prophylaxis Against Infection

Transmission of infections such as CMV, *Toxoplasma gondii*, HBV, HCV, and HIV after organ transplantation is well documented.[106] Prevention of postoperative infection begins with pretransplant screening of the donor and recipient.[107] Current suggested guidelines are outlined in Table 64-10. Perioperative and postoperative antimicrobial prophylaxes, as well as immunizations, are also outlined.

Specific Organisms Causing Infection Following Heart Transplantation

Bacteria

Gram-negative bacilli are the most common cause of bacterial infectious complications following heart transplantation. Furthermore, *Escherichia coli* and *Pseudomonas aeruginosa* are the most prevalent organisms and usually cause urinary tract infections and pneumonias, respectively.[105] *Staphylococcus* species have been shown to cause the majority of gram-positive–related infections.

Viruses

CMV remains the single most important cause of infectious disease morbidity and mortality in the heart transplant

TABLE 64-9 Infections in Cardiac Transplant Recipients

EARLY INFECTIONS (FIRST MONTH)
I. Pneumonia: Gram-negative bacilli (GNB)
II. Mediastinitis and sternal wound infections: *Staphylococcus epidermidis* *Staphylococcus aureus* GNB
III. Catheter-associated bacteremia: *S. epidermidis* *S. aureus* GNB *Candida albicans*
IV. Urinary tract infections: GNB *Enterococcus* *C. albicans*
V. Mucocutaneous infections: Herpes simplex virus (HSV) *Candida* spp.
LATE INFECTIONS (AFTER FIRST MONTH)
I. Pneumonia: A. Diffuse interstitial pneumonia: *Pneumocystis carinii* Cytomegalovirus (CMV)* HSV B. Lobar or nodular (cavitary) pneumonia: *Cryptococcus* *Aspergillus* Bacteria (community-acquired, nosocomial) *Nocardia asteroides* *Mycobacterium* spp.
II. Central nervous system infections: A. Abscess or meningoencephalitis *Aspergillus* *Toxoplasma gondii** Meningitis *Cryptococcus* *Listeria*
III. Gastrointestinal (GI) infections: A. Esophagitis *C. albicans* HSV B. Diarrhea or lower GI hemorrhage *Aspergillus* *Candida* spp.
IV. Cutaneous infections: A. Vesicular lesions HSV Varicella-zoster B. Nodular or ulcerating lesions *Nocardia* *Candida* (disseminated) Atypical *Mycobacterium* spp. *Cryptococcus*

*Known donor-transmitted pathogens.

TABLE 64-10 Guidelines for Routine Screening and Prophylaxis of Infections in Heart Transplantation

- I. Preoperative screening
  - A. Donor
    1. Clinical assessment
    2. Serologic studies (HIV, HBV, HCV, CMV, *Toxoplasma gondii*)
  - B. Recipient
    1. History and physical examination
    2. Serologic studies (HIV, HBV, HCV, CMV, *T. gondii*, herpes simplex virus, varicella-zoster virus, Epstein-Barr virus, endemic fungi)
    3. PPD (tuberculin) skin test
    4. Urine culture
    5. Stool for ova and parasites (*Strongyloides stercoralis*; center-specific)
- II. Antimicrobial prophylaxis
  - A. Perioperative
    1. First-generation cephalosporin (or vancomycin)
  - B. Postoperative
    1. Trimethoprim-sulfamethoxazole or pentamidine (for *Pneumocystis carinii*)
    2. Nystatin or clotrimazole (for *Candida* spp.)
    3. Ganciclovir followed by acyclovir once discharged (for all patients except CMV-negative recipient and donor)
    4. Acyclovir (for herpes simplex and zoster; routine use is controversial)
    5. Standard endocarditis prophylaxis
  - C. Postoperative immunizations
    1. Pneumococcal (booster every 5–7 years)
    2. Influenza A (yearly; center-specific)
    3. Exposure to measles, varicella, tetanus, or hepatitis B by a nonimmunized recipient often warrants specific immunoglobulin therapy (eg, varicella-zoster immune globulin, VZIG)

patient.[108] CMV not only results in infectious disease syndromes but also is indirectly associated with acute rejection episodes, acceleration of CAV, and posttransplant lymphoproliferative disease.[108] Furthermore, the reduction in leukocytes associated with CMV infection predisposes the patient to superinfection with other pathogens (eg, *Pneumocystis carinii* pneumonia). Infections develop secondary to donor transmission, reactivation of latent recipient infection, or reinfection of a CMV-seropositive patient with a different viral strain.[108] Variable regimens for CMV prophylaxis with ganciclovir are being used by different centers.[109] The standard of care for symptomatic CMV disease is 2 to 3 weeks of intravenous ganciclovir (at a dose of 5 mg/kg twice daily, with dosage adjustment for renal dysfunction). For tissue-invasive disease, particularly pneumonia, many centers add anti-CMV hyperimmune globulin to this regimen.[110] Preemptive treatment strategies employ periodic surveillance using techniques such as plasma polymerase chain reaction (PCR) and CMV antigenemia, a rapid diagnostic test that detects viral protein in peripheral blood leukocytes at a significant interval before clinical disease.[111] Valganciclovir (Valcyte) is an oral prodrug of ganciclovir with a 10-fold greater bioavailability than oral ganciclovir. It has been shown to be effective for prophylaxis and preemptive treatment of CMV and allows for more convenient use.[112,113]

Although not a cure for herpes simplex or zoster viruses, acyclovir can reduce recurrences and the discomfort associated with the vesicular lesions. Epstein-Barr virus infection may be associated with posttransplant lymphoproliferative disorders in immunocompromised hosts.[114]

Fungi

Mucocutaneous candidiasis is common and usually can be treated with topical antifungal agents (nystatin or clotrimazole). Fluconazole is indicated for candidiasis refractory to this therapy or involving the esophagus. It is also useful for therapy of candidemia. One important caveat in the treatment of *Candida* infection with fluconazole is that certain species such as *C. krusei* and *C. glabrata* have a low susceptibility in vitro.[105]

Among patients undergoing heart transplantation, *Aspergillus* is the opportunistic pathogen with the highest attributable mortality.[115] It causes a serious pneumonia in 5 to 10% of recipients during the first 3 months after transplantation. Dissemination of *Aspergillus* to the central nervous system is almost uniformly fatal.[116] Because aspergillosis is highly lethal in the immunocompromised host, even in the face of therapy, workup must be prompt and aggressive, and therapy may need to be initiated on suspicion of the diagnosis without definitive proof. Amphotericin B, itraconazole, and recently voriconazole are acceptable therapy.

Protozoa

In heart transplant recipients, the reported incidence of *P. carinii* pneumonia ranges from less than 1 to 10%.[117] Because the organism resides in the alveoli, bronchoalveolar lavage usually is necessary for diagnosis.[118] In the case of lung biopsy specimens, histopathologic examination is also helpful. *P. carinii* pneumonia is treated with high-dose trimethoprim-sulfamethoxazole or intravenous pentamidine.[105]

Toxoplasmosis following heart transplantation usually is the result of reactivation of latent disease in the seropositive donor heart because of the predilection of the parasite to invade muscle tissue.[119] *T. gondii* infection may be acquired from undercooked meat and cat feces. The diagnosis is made with certainty only by histologic demonstration of trophozoites with surrounding inflammation in biopsy tissue; PCR also has been used.[120] *T. gondii* usually causes central nervous system infections and is treated with pyrimethamine with sulfadiazine or clindamycin.[105]

CHRONIC COMPLICATIONS FOLLOWING HEART TRANSPLANTATION

Cardiac Allograft Vasculopathy

CAV is a unique, rapidly progressive form of atherosclerosis in transplant recipients that is characterized in its early stages by intimal proliferation and in its later stages by luminal stenosis of epicardial branches, occlusion of smaller arteries, and myocardial infarction. Long-term survival of cardiac transplant recipients is limited primarily by the development of CAV, the leading cause of death after the first posttransplant year.[5] Angiographically detectable CAV is reported in approximately 40 to 50% of patients by 5 years after transplantation.[121] Although CAV resembles atherosclerosis, there are some important differences that are illustrated in Fig. 64-11.[122] In particular, intimal proliferation is concentric rather than eccentric, and the lesions are diffuse, involving both distal and proximal portions of the coronary tree. Calcification is uncommon, and the elastic lamina remains intact.

The detailed pathogenesis of CAV is unknown, but there are strong indications that immunologic mechanisms that are regulated by nonimmunologic risk factors are the major causes of this phenomenon.[123] The immunologic mechanisms include acute rejection and anti-HLA antibodies, and some of the implicated risk factors relating to the transplant itself or the recipient are donor age, hypertension, hyperlipidemia, and preexisting diabetes. The side effects often associated with immunosuppression with calcineurin inhibitors or corticosteroids, eg, CMV infection, nephrotoxicity, and new-onset diabetes, after transplantation also play significant roles.[124–126]

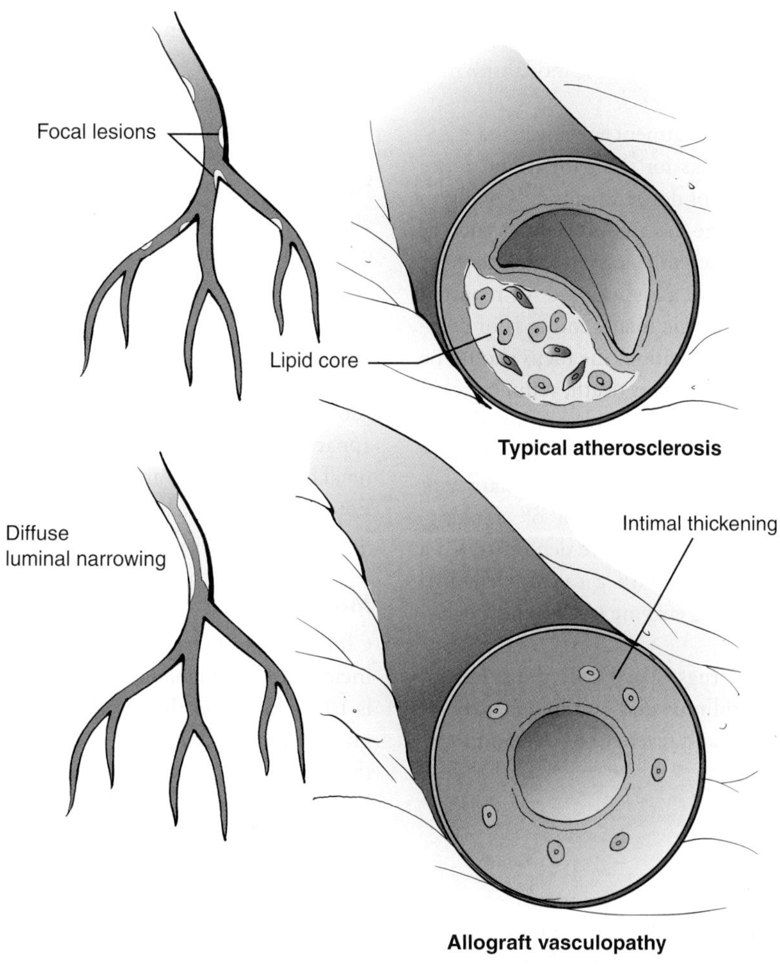

FIGURE 64-11 Schematic illustration of typical atherosclerosis and cardiac allograft vasculopathy. (*Source: Reprinted with permission from Avery RK: Cardiac-allograft vasculopathy. NEJM 2003; 349:829.*)

It is generally believed that the initiating event of CAV is subclinical endothelial cell injury in the coronary artery of the allograft, which leads to a cascade of immunologic processes involving cytokines, inflammatory mediators, complement activation, and leukocyte adhesion molecules. These changes produce inflammation and, ultimately, thrombosis, smooth muscle cell proliferation, and vessel constriction. The initial endothelial injury may be the result of ischemia-reperfusion damage or the host-versus-graft immune response.[125,126]

CAV may begin within several weeks posttransplantation and progress insidiously at an accelerated rate to complete obliteration of the coronary lumen with allograft failure secondary to ischemia. The clinical diagnosis of CAV is difficult and complicated by allograft denervation, resulting in silent myocardial ischemia. Ventricular arrhythmias, congestive heart failure, and sudden death are commonly the initial presentation of significant CAV.[127] An annual coronary angiogram usually is performed for CAV surveillance. Intravascular ultrasound (IVUS) is better equipped to provide important quantitative information regarding vessel wall morphology and the degree of intimal thickening.[128]

Because angiography and IVUS are invasive tests, they pose increased risks for patients. Noninvasive tests (eg, thallium scintigraphy and dobutamine stress echocardiography), however, have not been sensitive or specific enough to be a reliable screen for CAV.[129] Other possible modalities include pulse-wave tissue Doppler imaging, electron beam computed tomography (CT), fast CT scanning, and MRI. These modalities may replace invasive procedures in the future.

Currently, the only definitive treatment for advanced CAV is retransplantation, which has risks for the patient and poses problems associated with scarcity of donor organs.[127] Owing to the diffuse and distal nature of the disease, procedures such as stenting and angioplasty are inherently less effective than in nontransplant patients and result in a higher need for repeated procedures.[130] Therefore, prophylactic management is of paramount importance. Before transplantation, the focus should be on preventing endothelial injury at brain death, reducing cold ischemia time and improving myocardial preservation during storage and transportation.[127] Postransplantation care focuses on empiric risk factor modification (eg, dietary and pharmacologic reduction in serum cholesterol, cessation of smoking, hypertension control, etc). Several studies have demonstrated a decrease in CAV in patients treated with a calcium channel blocker and angiotensin-converting enzyme (ACE) and HMG-CoA reductase inhibitors.[131,132]

Newer immunosuppressive drugs, specifically the proliferation signal inhibitors (eg, everolimus and sirolimus), may be useful in reducing the incidence and severity of CAV and slowing disease progression.[133–137]

Renal Dysfunction

The 2009 ISHLT registry reported a significant improvement in long-term renal dysfunction in the most recent cohort of heart transplant recipients (2001 to 2007) as compared to the previous cohort (1994 to 2000). Whereas only 60% of heart transplant recipients from 1994 to 2000 were free of severe renal dysfunction (defined as a creatinine concentration of more than 2.5 mg/dL and the need for dialysis or renal transplantation) by Kaplan-Meier estimates at 10 years, recipients transplanted from 2001 to 2007 had an 11% absolute decrease in severe renal dysfunction at 5 years compared with the previous cohort.[5] Notably, the risk of death after heart transplantation is markedly increased by the development of end-stage renal failure.[138]

Cyclosporine nephrotoxicity after heart transplantation is well recognized and well documented. The improved bioavailability of cyclosporine microemulsion (Neoral) compared with the conventional formulation has led to investigations into monitoring of cyclosporine levels 2 hours after dosing (C2).[139] Neoral C2 monitoring may be a better indicator of immunosuppression efficacy than trough levels and a better measure to avoid nephrotoxicity and other cyclosporine-associated side effects.[140] Lowering cyclosporine dose may be helpful in slowing the progression of renal disease, especially with concomitant use of newer immunosuppressive regimens such as mycophenolate mofetil and sirolimus (rapamycin).[141,142] Calcineurin-free immunosuppression is also being implemented by some centers.[143]

Hypertension

Moderate to severe systemic hypertension afflicts 50 to 90% of cardiac transplant recipients.[5] Peripheral vasoconstriction in combination with fluid retention seems to play the greatest role. Although the exact mechanisms are unclear, it likely involves a combination of cyclosporine-induced tubular nephrotoxicity and vasoconstriction of renal and systemic arterioles mediated by sympathetic neural activation.[144] Tacrolimus is associated with a lower incidence of hypertension than is cyclosporine.[145] No single class of antihypertensive agents has proven uniformly effective, and treatment of this refractory hypertension remains empirical and difficult. In a prospective, randomized trial, titrated monotherapy with either diltiazem or lisinopril controlled the condition in fewer than 50% of patients.[146] Diuretics should be used cautiously because the balance between edema/hypertension and volume depletion/hypotension can be tenuous in a subset of these patients. Overzealous diuresis can potentiate the apparent nephrotoxicity of cyclosporine by further reducing renal blood flow and altering cyclosporine pharmacokinetics.[147] Beta-blockers also should be used with caution because they may further blunt the heart rate response to exercise.

Malignancy

Chronic immunosuppression is associated with an increased incidence of malignancy ranging from about 4 to 18%, which is 100-fold greater than in the general population.[148] Improved graft and patient survival, owing to pharmacologic advances in the area of immunosuppressive therapy, has led to an increase in the incidence of neoplasms.[148] Malignant neoplasias have become, along with graft vasculopathy, a significant limiting factor for the long-term survival of heart transplant recipients.[5] Lymphoproliferative disorders and carcinoma of the skin are the most common malignancies found in heart transplant recipients.[148] Loss of T-lymphocyte control over Epstein-Barr virus (EBV)–stimulated B-lymphocyte proliferation appears to be the primary mechanism for the development of lymphoproliferative disorders.[149] The risk of these malignancies is increased further following monoclonal and polyclonal antibody therapy.[150,151] Treatment options in transplantation include a reduction in immunosuppression and initiation of high-dose acyclovir (to attenuate EBV replication), in addition to conventional therapies for carcinoma (eg, chemotherapy, radiation therapy, and surgical resection), which are associated with very high risk and limited success.

Other Chronic Complications

Hyperlipidemia eventually develops in the majority of recipients and is managed with dietary restrictions, exercise, and lipid-lowering agents.[152] Other complications that commonly contribute to posttransplant morbidity include osteoporosis, obesity, cachexia, and gastrointestinal complications, notably cholelithiasis.[153,154]

CARDIAC RETRANSPLANTATION

Retransplantation accounts for fewer than 3% of the cardiac transplants currently performed.[5] Primary indications for retransplantation are early graft failure, allograft coronary artery disease, and refractory acute rejection.[155,156] The operative technique and immunosuppressive regimen are similar to those employed for the initial transplantation. Despite reduced mortality in the cyclosporine era, actuarial survival remains markedly reduced. Analysis of the ISHLT registry for retransplantations performed between 1987 and 1998 reveals survival to be 65, 59, and 55% for 1, 2, and 3 years, respectively. Intertransplant interval of 6 months or less was associated with a dismal 1-year survival of 50% in this analysis. Conversely, when the interval between primary and retransplantation was more than 2 years, 1-year survival after retransplantation approached that of primary transplantation.[156] The 2009 ISHLT registry report indicates that the 5-year survival of retransplanted patients has increased by 15 to 17% with each successive decade (1982 to 1991, 1992 to 2001, 2002 to 2007). As well, in the most recent cohort (2002 to 2008), patients undergoing retransplantation at greater than 5 years from initial transplant had the same 1-year survival rate as primary transplants from the same era (86%).[5] Advanced donor age also was a predictor of increased mortality among these recipients.[156] These data suggest that although cardiac retransplantation is associated with significant morbidity and mortality, careful selection of patients, especially those who are younger and with longer intertransplant intervals, may be associated with more favorable outcome. Nonetheless, the disparity between the demand and supply for donor hearts continues to make cardiac retransplantation an ethical dilemma.[157]

RESULTS OF HEART TRANSPLANTATION

Although no direct comparative trials have been or are likely to be performed, survival following heart transplantation remains favorable if compared with both the medical and device arms of the REMATCH trial.[2,6] The superiority of heart transplantation is more clearly evident in medium- and high-risk patients with end-stage heart failure.[158] The overall results actually are improving despite increasing risk profiles.[5,67] The reported operative (ie, 30-day) mortality for cardiac transplantation ranges from 5 to 10%.[159] Overall 1-year survival is up to 86%.[5,67] After the steep fall in survival during the first 6 months, survival decreases at a linear rate (approximately 3.5% per year), even well beyond 15 years posttransplantation.[5] Graft failure (primary and nonspecific), multisystem organ failure, and infection account for most deaths within the first 30 days. Infection, graft failure, and acute rejection are the leading causes of death during the first year; thereafter, cardiac allograft vasculopathy and malignancy are the major causes of death.[5,67] Studies examining the health-related quality of life (HRQOL) in patients after cardiac transplantation demonstrate marked improvement, particularly in the absence of complications, and approaches the general population by 10 years after transplantation.[160]

Insights from the United Network for Organ Sharing Database

The recent literature on heart transplantation has seen a notable increase in clinical studies analyzing the multi-institutional UNOS open transplant cohort. This database is publically accessible and includes all heart transplants performed in the United States from October 1987 onward. The database also includes patients on the waitlist, donor information, and outcomes. As with all large administrative datasets, it is limited by potential errors in coding as well as incompletely populated variables. However, questions that had previously only been addressed using single or limited multi-institutional data can now be investigated using this cohort of over 20,000 patients.

Among those issues addressed have been the impact of various recipient factors, on short- and long-term survival after heart transplantation. Russo and coworkers reported that uncomplicated diabetes mellitus should not preclude listing for heart transplantation due to equivalent survival with nondiabetics.[161] However, severe diabetics did have poorer survival and should be considered for destination LVAD therapy or high-risk listing. Zaidi and coworkers reported better short and intermediate survival after heart transplantation in patients with sarcoidosis compared to recipients with other diagnoses, and concluded that a diagnosis of sarcoidosis should not preclude heart transplantation.[162] Kpodonu and coworkers demonstrated that 1-year survival after heart transplant for amyloid cardiomyopathy was significantly decreased in female recipients, whereas it was comparable with other diagnoses for male recipients.[163] Nwakanma and coworkers confirmed increasing risk of rejection in the year after transplantation and decreased survival with increasing panel reactive antibody levels.[164] Weiss and coworkers reported that advanced age (>60 years) was associated with acceptable long-term outcomes (>70% 5-year survival).[165] Although elderly recipients did have slightly higher rates of infection and acute renal failure, as well as a 2-day longer hospital length of stay, the survival benefit of transplantation in elderly CHF patients was compelling. Another study by Weiss and coworkers identified a potential provider bias in the listing of obese patients as potential heart transplant recipients.[166] Specifically, that obese individuals wait longer and have a lower likelihood of receiving a donor heart after listing, despite similar short-term survival.

Insights into the impact of operative technique and the use of LVADs on posttransplant survival have also been gained from the UNOS database. As noted, Weiss and coworkers reported equivalent survival after heart transplantation using biatrial versus bicaval anastomotic techniques.[63] However, they did identify that the bicaval technique was associated with a shorted hospital length of stay and decreased rates of permanent pacemaker placement. Pal and coworkers investigated status 1 patients bridged to transplant using LVADs and IV inotropes, and found that patients bridged to transplant using LVADs were, by in large, those who failed bridging with IV inotropes.[167] In contrast with International Society of Heart and Lung Transplantation data, no increase in posttransplant morbidity or mortality was found in LVAD-bridged patients compared with nonbridged status 1 patients. Shuhaiber and coworkers compared patients bridged with transplant with Novacor versus HeartMate LVADs and found no difference in 1-year survival, rates of rejection, or rates of infection.[168] However, patients bridged with Novacor LVADs demonstrated lower 5-year survival posttransplant.

Weiss and coworkers also investigated the effect of transplant center volume on long-term outcomes after heart transplantation, and reported that annual center volume is an independent predictor of short-term mortality in OHT.[169] Although the current Centers for Medicare and Medicaid Services mandate is that heart transplant centers perform 10 per year to qualify for funding, this study found that a higher cutoff resulted in better outcomes; centers performing greater than 40 per year have a 30-day mortality less than 5%.

THE FUTURE

As a result of a series of unprecedented advances over the past decade, the clinical outcome of heart transplantation has improved dramatically. Although cardiac replacement remains the best therapeutic option for patients with end-stage heart failure, a number of challenges await future investigators to further improve survival and reduce transplant-related morbidity. A major factor limiting long-term survival of recipients is allograft rejection and the untoward effects of immunosuppression. Development of reliable, noninvasive diagnostic studies will permit more frequent evaluations for the early detection of rejection and for monitoring the effectiveness of therapy. Ultimately, this will allow more precise control of immunosuppression and, in turn, a reduction in cumulative allograft injury and infectious complications. Molecular tests and gene expression profiling could be available soon and may provide the best noninvasive option.[91]

Immunosuppressive strategists will continue their efforts to establish specific unresponsiveness to antigens of transplanted organs in hopes of preserving much of the recipient's immune responses. Proliferative signal inhibitors such as sirolimus and everolimus are showing promising results. Alternatively, donor organs may be made less susceptible to immunologic attack through genetic engineering techniques by altering the expression of cell membrane–bound molecules. This approach is being used currently in the pursuit of clinically applicable xenotransplant sources. Xenografts eventually may be an additional source of donor organs, although extended xenograft survival remains an elusive goal. Complicating this alternative are unresolved ethical issues concerning transgenic experimentation and the potential for transmission of veterinary pathogens to an immunosuppressed recipient.

Future improvements in organ preservation permitting extension of the storage interval will have several benefits. In addition to a modest increase in the donor pool, extension of storage times would permit better allocation of organs with respect to donor-recipient immunologic matching. Assist devices are being used currently both as a bridge to transplantation and as a destination therapy. It appears that as the technology of assist devices continues to improve, it is only a matter of time before they become a long-term solution for patients with severe congestive heart failure.

The concept of regenerating the failing heart using cardiomyocytes of different sources, autologous smooth muscle cells, and dermal fibroblasts is in the experimental stage. Lineage-negative bone marrow cells or bone marrow–derived endothelial precursor cells are also being studied to induce new blood vessel formation after experimental myocardial infarction.[170] Cardiac transplantation remains a remarkable achievement of the twentieth century and has revolutionized therapy for end-stage heart failure. Further investigations are needed to overcome the current obstacles to long-term graft function and patient survival.

REFERENCES

1. Steinman TI, Becker BN, Frost AE, et al: Guidelines for the referral and management of patients eligible for solid organ transplantation. *Transplantation* 2001; 71:1189.
2. Boyle A, Colvin-Adams M: Recipient selection and management. *Semin Thorac Cardiovasc Surg* 2004; 16:358.
3. Deng MC: Cardiac transplantation. *Heart* 2002; 87:177.
4. Costanzo MR, Augustine S, Bourge R, et al: Selection and treatment of candidates for heart transplantation: a statement for health professionals from the Committee on Heart Failure and Cardiac Transplantation of the Council on Clinical Cardiology, American Heart Association. *Circulation* 1995; 92:3593.
5. Taylor DO, Stehlik J, Edwards LB, et al: Registry of the international society for heart and lung transplantation: twenty-sixth official adult heart transplant report-2009. *J Heart Lung Transplant* 2009; 28(10):1007-1022.
6. Rose EA, Gelijns AC, Moskowitz AJ, et al: Randomized Evaluation of Mechanical Assistance for the Treatment of Congestive Heart Failure (REMATCH) Study Group: long-term mechanical left ventricular assistance for end-stage heart failure. *NEJM* 2001; 345:1435.
7. Menicanti L, Di Donato M: Surgical left ventricle reconstruction, pathophysiologic insights, results and expectation from the STICH trial. *Eur J Cardiothorac Surg* 2004; 26:S42.
8. Stelken AM, Younis LT, Jennison SH, et al: Prognostic value of cardiopulmonary exercise testing using percent achieved of predicted peak oxygen uptake for patients with ischemic and dilated cardiomyopathy. *J Am Coll Cardiol* 1996; 27:345.
9. Rothenburger M, Wichter T, Schmid C, et al: Aminoterminal pro type B natriuretic peptide as a predictive and prognostic marker in patients with chronic heart failure. *J Heart Lung Transplant* 2004; 23:1189.
10. Francis GS, Cohn JN, Johnson G, et al: Plasma norepinephrine, plasma renin activity, and congestive heart failure: relations to survival and the effects of therapy in V-HeFT II. The V-HeFT VA Cooperative Studies Group. *Circulation* 1993; 87:VI40.
11. Mudge GH, Goldstein S, Addonizio LZ, et al: Twenty-fourth Bethesda Conference on Cardiac Transplantation. Task Force 3: recipient guidelines. *J Am Coll Cardiol* 1993; 22:21.

12. Laks H, Marelli D, Odim J, et al: Heart transplantation in the young and elderly. *Heart Failure Rev* 2001; 6:221.
13. Demers P, Moffatt S, Oyer PE, et al: Long-term results of heart transplantation in patients older than 60 years. *J Thorac Cardiovasc Surg* 2003; 126:224.
14. Kieler-Jensen N, Milocco I, Ricksten SE: Pulmonary vasodilation after heart transplantation: a comparison among prostacyclin, sodium nitroprusside, and nitroglycerin on right ventricular function and pulmonary selectivity. *J Heart Lung Transplant* 1993; 12:179.
15. Bourge RC, Naftel DC, Costanzo-Nordin MR, et al: Pretransplantation risk factors for death after heart transplantation: a multiinstitutional study. The Transplant Cardiologists Research Database Group. *J Heart Lung Transplant* 1993; 12:549.
16. Chen JM, Levin HR, Michler RE, et al: Reevaluating the significance of pulmonary hypertension before cardiac transplantation: determination of optimal thresholds and quantification of the effect of reversibility on perioperative mortality. *J Thorac Cardiovasc Surg* 1997; 114:627.
17. Tenderich G, Koerner MM, Stuettgen B, et al: Pre-existing elevated pulmonary vascular resistance: long-term hemodynamic follow-up and outcome of recipients after orthotopic heart transplantation. *J Cardiovasc Surg* 2000; 41:215.
18. Chang PP, Longenecker JC, Wang NY, et al: Mild vs severe pulmonary hypertension before heart transplantation: different effects on posttransplantation pulmonary hypertension and mortality. *J Heart Lung Transplant* 2005; 24:998.
19. Sablotzki A, Hentschel T, Gruenig E, et al: Hemodynamic effects of inhaled aerosolized iloprost and inhaled nitric oxide in heart transplant candidates with elevated pulmonary vascular resistance. *Eur J Cardiothorac Surg* 2002; 22:746.
20. O'Dell KM, Kalus JS, Kucukarslan S, et al: Nesiritide for secondary pulmonary hypertension in patients with end-stage heart failure. *Am J Health Syst Pharm* 2005; 62:606.
21. Salzberg SP, Lachat ML, von Harbou K, et al: Normalization of high pulmonary vascular resistance with LVAD support in heart transplantation candidates. *Eur J Cardiothorac Surg* 2005; 27:222.
22. Newcomb AE, Esmore DS, Rosenfeldt FL, et al: Heterotopic heart transplantation: an expanding role in the twenty-first century? *Ann Thorac Surg* 2004; 78:1345.
23. Pelosi F Jr., Capehart J, Roberts WC: Effectiveness of cardiac transplantation for primary (AL) cardiac amyloidosis. *Am J Cardiol* 1997; 79:532.
24. Dubrey SW, Burke MM, Hawkins PN, et al: Cardiac transplantation for amyloid heart disease: the United Kingdom experience. *J Heart Lung Transplant* 2004; 23:1142.
25. Koerner MM, Tenderich G, Minami K, et al: Results of heart transplantation in patients with preexisting malignancies. *Am J Cardiol* 1997; 79:988.
26. Ostermann ME, Rogers CA, Saeed I, et al: Pre-existing renal failure doubles 30-day mortality after heart transplantation. *J Heart Lung Transplant* 2004; 23:1231.
27. Dichtl W, Vogel W, Dunst KM, et al: Cardiac hepatopathy before and after heart transplantation. *Transpl Int* 2005; 18:697.
28. Morgan JA, John R, Weinberg AD, et al: Heart transplantation in diabetic recipients: a decade review of 161 patients at Columbia Presbyterian. *J Thorac Cardiovasc Surg* 2004; 127:1486.
29. Morgan JA, Park Y, Oz MC, et al: Device-related infections while on left ventricular assist device support do not adversely impact bridging to transplant or posttransplant survival. *ASAIO J* 2003; 49:748.
30. Lietz K, John R, Burke EA, et al: Pretransplant cachexia and morbid obesity are predictors of increased mortality after heart transplantation. *Transplantation* 2001; 72:277.
31. Rivard AL, Hellmich C, Sampson B, et al: Preoperative predictors for postoperative problems in heart transplantation: psychiatric and psychosocial considerations. *Prog Transplant* 2005; 15:276.
32. Loh E, Bergin JD, Couper GS, et al: Role of panel-reactive antibody cross-reactivity in predicting survival after orthotopic heart transplantation. *J Heart Lung Transplant* 1994; 13:194.
33. McKenna D, Eastlund T, Segall M, et al: HLA alloimmunization in patients requiring ventricular assist device support. *J Heart Lung Transplant* 2002; 21:1218.
34. Aranda JM Jr., Schofield RS, Pauly DF, et al: Comparison of dobutamine versus milrinone therapy in hospitalized patients awaiting cardiac transplantation: a prospective, randomized trial. *Am Heart J* 2003; 145:324.
35. Cochran RP, Starkey TD, Panos AL, et al: Ambulatory intraaortic balloon pump use as bridge to heart transplant. *Ann Thorac Surg* 2002; 74:746.
36. Dembitsky WP, Tector AJ, Park S, et al: Left ventricular assist device performance with long-term circulatory support: lessons from the REMATCH trial. *Ann Thorac Surg* 2004; 78:2123.
37. Clegg AJ, Scott DA, Loveman E, et al: The clinical and cost-effectiveness of left ventricular assist devices for end-stage heart failure: a systematic review and economic evaluation. *Health Technol Assess* 2005; 9:1.
38. Copeland JG, Smith RG, Arabia FA, et al: CardioWest Total Artificial Heart Investigators. Cardiac replacement with a total artificial heart as a bridge to transplantation. *NEJM* 2004; 351:859.
39. Ermis C, Zadeii G, Zhu AX, et al: Improved survival of cardiac transplantation candidates with implantable cardioverter defibrillator therapy: role of beta-blocker or amiodarone treatment. *J Cardiovasc Electrophysiol* 2003; 14:578.
40. Vega JD, Moore J, Murray S, et al: Heart transplantation in the United States, 1998–2007. *Am J Transplant* 2009; 9 (Part 2):932-941.
41. Zaroff JG, Rosengard BR, Armstrong WF, et al: Consensus conference report: maximizing use of organs recovered from the cadaver donor: cardiac recommendations, March 28–29, 2001, Crystal City, VA. *Circulation* 2002; 106:836.
42. Wheeldon DR, Potter CD, Oduro A, et al: Transforming the "unacceptable" donor: outcomes from the adoption of a standardized donor management technique. *J Heart Lung Transplant* 1995; 14:734.
43. Laks H, Marelli D, Fonarow GC, et al: UCLA Heart Transplant Group. Use of two recipient lists for adults requiring heart transplantation. *J Thorac Cardiovasc Surg* 2003; 125:49.
44. Lietz K, John R, Mancini DM, et al: Outcomes in cardiac transplant recipients using allografts from older donors versus mortality on the transplant waiting list: implications for donor selection criteria. *J Am Coll Cardiol* 2004; 43:1553.
45. Freimark D, Aleksic I, Trento A, et al: Hearts from donors with chronic alcohol use: a possible risk factor for death after heart transplantation. *J Heart Lung Transplant* 1996; 15:150.
46. Freimark D, Czer LS, Admon D, et al: Donors with a history of cocaine use: effect on survival and rejection frequency after heart transplantation. *J Heart Lung Transplant* 1994; 13:1138.
47. Smith M: Physiologic changes during brain stem death: lessons for management of the organ donor. *J Heart Lung Transplant* 2004; 23:S217.
48. Stoica SC, Satchithananda DK, Charman S, et al: Swan-Ganz catheter assessment of donor hearts: outcome of organs with borderline hemodynamics. *J Heart Lung Transplant* 2002; 21:615.
49. Rosendale JD, Kauffman HM, McBride MA, et al: Hormonal resuscitation yields more transplanted hearts, with improved early function. *Transplantation* 2003; 75:1336.
50. Harms J, Isemer FE, Kolenda H: Hormonal alteration and pituitary function during course of brain stem death in potential organ donors. *Transplant Proc* 1991; 23:2614.
51. Novitzky D, Cooper DK, Chaffin JS, et al: Improved cardiac allograft function following triiodothyronine therapy to both donor and recipient. *Transplantation* 1990; 49:311.
52. Conte JV, Baumgartner WA: Overview and future practice patterns in cardiac and pulmonary preservation. *J Card Surg* 2000; 15:91.
53. Wildhirt SM, Weis M, Schulze C, et al: Effects of Celsior and University of Wisconsin preservation solutions on hemodynamics and endothelial function after cardiac transplantation in humans: a single-center, prospective, randomized trial. *Transplant Int* 2000; 13:S203.
54. Garlicki M: May preservation solution affect the incidence of graft vasculopathy in transplanted heart? *Ann Transplant* 2003; 8:19.
55. Segel LD, Follette DM, Contino JP, et al: Importance of substrate enhancement for long-term heart preservation. *J Heart Lung Transplant* 1993; 12:613.
56. Zehr KJ, Herskowitz A, Lee P, et al: Neutrophil adhesion inhibition prolongs survival of cardiac allografts with hyperacute rejection. *J Heart Lung Transplant* 1993; 12:837.
57. Fitton TP, Barreiro CJ, Bonde PN, et al: Attenuation of DNA damage in canine hearts preserved by continuous hypothermic perfusion. *Ann Thorac Surg* 2005; 80:1812.
58. Betkowski AS, Graff R, Chen JJ, et al: Panel-reactive antibody screening practices prior to heart transplantation. *J Heart Lung Transplant* 2002; 21:644.
59. Jarcho J, Naftel DC, Shroyer JK, et al: Influence of HLA mismatch on rejection after heart transplantation: a multi-institutional study. *J Heart Lung Transplant* 1994; 13:583.
60. Baumgartner WA, Reitz BA, Achuff SC: Operative techniques utilized in heart transplantations, in Achuff SC (ed): *Heart and Heart-Lung Transplantation*. Philadelphia, Saunders, 1990.
61. Milano CA, Shah AS, Van Trigt P, et al: Evaluation of early postoperative results after bicaval versus standard cardiac transplantation and review of the literature. *Am Heart J* 2000; 140:717.
62. Aziz T, Burgess M, Khafagy R, et al: Bicaval and standard techniques in orthotopic heart transplantation: medium-term experience in cardiac performance and survival. *J Thorac Cardiovasc Surg* 1999; 118:115.

63. Weiss ES, Nwakanma LU, Russell SB, et. al. Outcomes in bicaval versus biatrial techniques in heart transplantation: an analysis of the UNOS database. *J Heart Lung Transplant.* 2008 Feb;27(2):178-83.
64. Cotts WG, Oren RM: Function of the transplanted heart: unique physiology and therapeutic implications. *Am J Med Sci* 1997; 314:164.
65. Tischler MD, Lee RT, Plappert T, et al: Serial assessment of left ventricular function and mass after orthotopic heart transplantation: a four-year longitudinal study. *J Am Coll Cardiol* 1992; 19:60.
66. Gerber BL, Bernard X, Melin JA, et al: Exaggerated chronotropic and energetic response to dobutamine after orthotopic cardiac transplantation. *J Heart Lung Transplant* 2001; 20:824.
67. Kirklin JK, Naftel DC, Bourge RC, et al: Evolving trends in risk profiles and causes of death after heart transplantation: a ten-year multi-institutional study. *J Thorac Cardiovasc Surg* 2003; 125:881.
68. Minev PA, El-Banayosy A, Minami K, et al: Differential indication for mechanical circulatory support following heart transplantation. *Intensive Care Med* 2001; 27:1321.
69. Srivastava R, Keck BM, Bennett LE, et al: The results of cardiac retransplantation: an analysis of the Joint International Society for Heart and Lung Transplantation/United Network for Organ Sharing Thoracic Registry. *Transplantation* 2000; 70:606.
70. Kieler-Jensen N, Lundin S, Ricksten SE, et al: Vasodilator therapy after heart transplantation: effects of inhaled nitric oxide and intravenous prostacyclin, prostaglandin E_1, and sodium nitroprusside. *J Heart Lung Transplant* 1995; 14:436.
71. Arafa OE, Geiran OR, Andersen K, et al: Intra-aortic balloon pumping for predominantly right ventricular failure after heart transplantation. *Ann Thorac Surg* 2000; 70:1587.
72. Stecker EC, Strelich KR, Chugh SS, et al: Arrhythmias after orthotopic heart transplantation. *J Cardiol Fail* 2005; 11:464.
73. Chin C, Feindel C, Cheng D: Duration of preoperative amiodarone treatment may be associated with postoperative hospital mortality in patients undergoing heart transplantation. *J Cardiothorac Vasc Anesth* 1999; 13:562.
74. Bertolet BD, Eagle DA, Conti JB, et al: Bradycardia after heart transplantation: reversal with theophylline. *J Am Coll Cardiol* 1996; 28:396.
75. Patel VS, Lim M, Massin EK, et al: Sudden cardiac death in cardiac transplant recipients. *Circulation* 1996; 94:II-273.
76. Kwak YL, Oh YJ, Bang SO, et al: Comparison of the effects of nicardipine and sodium nitroprusside for control of increased blood pressure after coronary artery bypass graft surgery. *J Int Med Res* 2004; 32:342.
77. Miller LW: Treatment of cardiac allograft rejection with intervenous corticosteroids. *J Heart Transplant* 1990; 9:283.
78. Sharples LD, Caine N, Mullins P, et al: Risk factor analysis for the major hazards following heart transplantation: rejection, infection, and coronary occlusive disease. *Transplantation* 1991; 52:244.
79. Cunningham KS, Veinot JP, Butany J: An approach to endomyocardial biopsy interpretation. *J Clin Pathol* 2006; 59:121.
80. Billingham ME, Cary NRB, Hammond ME, et al: A working formulation for the standardization of nomenclature in the diagnosis of heart and lung rejection: heart rejection study group. *J Heart Lung Transplant* 1990; 9:587.
81. Rodriguez ER: International Society for Heart and Lung Transplantation. The pathology of heart transplant biopsy specimens: revisiting the 1990 ISHLT working formulation. *J Heart Lung Transplant* 2003; 22:3.
82. Stewart S, Winters GL, Fishbein MC, et al: Revision of the 1990 working formulation for the standardization of nomenclature in the diagnosis of heart rejection. *J Heart Lung Transplant* 2005; 24:1710.
83. Lower RR, Dong E, Glazener FS: Electrocardiogram of dogs with heart homografts. *Circulation* 1966; 33:455.
84. Cooper DK, Charles RG, Rose AG, et al: Does the electrocardiogram detect early acute heart rejection? *J Heart Transplant* 1985; 4:546.
85. Volgman AS, Winkel EM, Pinski SL, et al: Characteristics of the signal-averaged P wave in orthotopic heart transplant recipients. *Pacing Clin Electrophysiol* 1998; 21:2327.
86. Boyd SY, Mego DM, Khan NA, et al: Doppler echocardiography in cardiac transplant patients: allograft rejection and its relationship to diastolic function. *J Am Soc Echocardiogr* 1997; 10:526.
87. Morocutti G, Di Chiara A, Proclemer A, et al: Signal-averaged electrocardiography and Doppler echocardiographic study in predicting acute rejection in heart transplantation. *J Heart Lung Transplant* 1995; 14:1065.
88. Almenar L, Igual B, Martinez-Dolz L, et al: Utility of cardiac magnetic resonance imaging for the diagnosis of heart transplant rejection. *Transplant Proc* 2003; 35:1962.
89. Addonizio LJ: Detection of cardiac allograft rejection using radionuclide techniques. *Prog Cardiovasc Dis* 1990; 33:73.
90. Wijngaard PL, Doornewaard H, van der Meulen A, et al: Cytoimmunologic monitoring as an adjunct in monitoring rejection after heart transplantation: results of a 6-year follow-up in heart transplant recipients. *J Heart Lung Transplant* 1994; 13:869.
91. Mehra MR, Uber PA, Uber WE, et al: Anything but a biopsy: noninvasive monitoring for cardiac allograft rejection. *Curr Opin Cardiol* 2002; 17:131.
92. Horwitz PA, Tsai EJ, Putt ME, et al: Detection of cardiac allograft rejection and response to immunosuppressive therapy with peripheral blood gene expression. *Circulation* 2004; 110:3815.
93. Michler RE, Smith CR, Drusin RE, et al: Reversal of cardiac transplant rejection without massive immunosuppression. *Circulation* 1986; 74:III-68.
94. Yamani MH, Starling RC, Pelegrin D, et al: Efficacy of tacrolimus in patients with steroid-resistant cardiac allograft cellular rejection. *J Heart Lung Transplant* 2000; 19:337.
95. Radovancevic B, El-Sabrout R, Thomas C, et al: Rapamycin reduces rejection in heart transplant recipients. *Transplant Proc* 2001; 33:3221.
96. Cantarovich M, Latter DA, Loertscher R: Treatment of steroid-resistant and recurrent acute cardiac transplant rejection with a short course of antibody therapy. *Clin Transplant* 1997; 11:316.
97. Ross HJ, Gullestad L, Pak J, et al: Methotrexate or total lymphoid radiation for treatment of persistent or recurrent allograft cellular rejection: a comparative study. *J Heart Lung Transplant* 1997; 16:179.
98. Lloveras JJ, Escourrou G, Delisle MG, et al: Evolution of untreated mild rejection in heart transplant recipients. *J Heart Lung Transplant* 1992; 11:751.
99. Winters GL, Loh E, Schoen FJ, et al: Natural history of focal moderate cardiac allograft rejection: is treatment warranted? *Circulation* 1995; 91:1975.
100. Stoica SC, Cafferty F, Pauriah M, et al: The cumulative effect of acute rejection on development of cardiac allograft vasculopathy. *J Heart Lung Transplant* 2006; 25:420.
101. Michaels PJ, Espejo ML, Kobashigawa J, et al: Humoral rejection in cardiac transplantation: risk factors, hemodynamic consequences and relationship to transplant coronary artery disease. *J Heart Lung Transplant* 2003; 22:58.
102. Lones MA, Czer LS, Trento A, et al: Clinical-pathologic features of humoral rejection in cardiac allografts: a study in 81 consecutive patients. *J Heart Lung Transplant* 1995; 14:151.
103. Olsen SL, Wagoner LE, Hammond EH, et al: Vascular rejection in heart transplantation: clinical correlation, treatment options, and future considerations. *J Heart Lung Transplant* 1993; 12:S135.
104. Hammond EH, Yowell RL, Price GD, et al: Vascular rejection and its relationship to allograft coronary artery disease. *J Heart Lung Transplant* 1992; 11:S111.
105. Miller LW, Naftel DC, Bourge RC, et al: Infection after heart transplantation: a multi-institutional study. *J Heart Lung Transplant* 1994; 13:381.
106. Eastlund T: Infectious disease transmission through cell, tissue, and organ transplantation: reducing the risk through donor selection. *Cell Transplant* 1995; 4:455.
107. Schaffner A: Pretransplant evaluation for infections in donors and recipients of solid organs. *Clin Infect Dis* 2001; 33:S9.
108. Rubin RH: Prevention and treatment of cytomegalovirus disease in heart transplant patients. *J Heart Lung Transplant* 2000; 19:731.
109. Merigan TC, Renlund DG, Keay S, et al: A controlled trial of ganciclovir to prevent cytomegalovirus disease after heart transplantation. *NEJM* 1992; 326:1182.
110. Bonaros NE, Kocher A, Dunkler D, et al: Comparison of combined prophylaxis of cytomegalovirus hyperimmune globulin plus ganciclovir versus cytomegalovirus hyperimmune globulin alone in high-risk heart transplant recipients. *Transplantation* 2004; 77:890.
111. Egan JJ, Barber L, Lomax J, et al: Detection of human cytomegalovirus antigenemia: a rapid diagnostic technique for predicting cytomegalovirus infection/pneumonitis in lung and heart transplant recipients. *Thorax* 1995; 50:9.
112. Devyatko E, Zuckermann A, Ruzicka M, et al: Pre-emptive treatment with oral valganciclovir in management of CMV infection after cardiac transplantation. *J Heart Lung Transplant* 2004; 23:1277.
113. Wiltshire H, Hirankarn S, Farrell C, et al: Pharmacokinetic profile of ganciclovir after its oral administration and from its prodrug, valganciclovir, in solid organ transplant recipients. *Clin Pharmacokinet* 2005; 44:495.
114. Gray J, Wreghitt TG, Pavel P, et al: Epstein-Barr virus infection in heart and heart-lung transplant recipients: incidence and clinical impact. *J Heart Lung Transplant* 1995; 14:640.
115. Montoya JG, Chaparro SV, Celis D, et al: Invasive aspergillosis in the setting of cardiac transplantation. *Clin Infect Dis* 2003; 37:S281.
116. Patterson TF, Kirkpatrick WR, et al: Invasive aspergillosis: disease spectrum, treatment practices, and outcomes. *Aspergillus* Study Group. *Medicine (Baltimore)* 2000; 79:250.
117. Cardenal R, Medrano FJ, Varela JM, et al: *Pneumocystis carinii* pneumonia in heart transplant recipients. *Eur J Cardiothorac Surg* 2001; 20:799.

118. Lehto JT, Anttila VJ, Lommi J, et al: Clinical usefulness of bronchoalveolar lavage in heart transplant recipients with suspected lower respiratory tract infection. *J Heart Lung Transplant* 2004; 23:570.
119. Speirs GE, Hakim M, Wreghitt TG: Relative risk of donor transmitted *Toxoplasma gondii* infection in heart, liver and kidney transplant recipients. *Clin Transplant* 1988; 2:257.
120. Cermakova Z, Ryskova O, Pliskova L: Polymerase chain reaction for detection of *Toxoplasma gondii* in human biological samples. *Folia Microbiol (Praha)* 2005; 50:341.
121. Costanzo MR, Naftel DC, Pritzker MR, et al: Heart transplant coronary artery disease detected by coronary angiography: a multi-institutional study of preoperative donor and recipient risk factors. Cardiac Transplant Research Database. *J Heart Lung Transplant* 1998; 17:744.
122. Avery RK: Cardiac-allograft vasculopathy. *NEJM* 2003; 349:829.
123. Caforio AL, Tona F, Fortina AB, et al: Immune and nonimmune predictors of cardiac allograft vasculopathy onset and severity: multivariate risk factor analysis and role of immunosuppression. *Am J Transplant* 2004; 4:962.
124. Valantine H: Cardiac allograft vasculopathy after heart transplantation: risk factors and management. *J Heart Lung Transplant* 2004; 23:S187.
125. Day JD, Rayburn BK, Gaudin PB, et al: Cardiac allograft vasculopathy: the central pathogenic role of ischemia-induced endothelial cell injury. *J Heart Lung Transplant* 1995; 14:S142.
126. Hollenberg SM, Klein LW, Parrillo JE, et al: Coronary endothelial dysfunction after heart transplantation predicts allograft vasculopathy and cardiac death. *Circulation* 2001; 104:3091.
127. Kass M, Haddad H: Cardiac allograft vasculopathy: pathology, prevention and treatment. *Curr Opin Cardiol* 2006; 21:132.
128. Kobashigawa JA, Tobis JM, Starling RC, et al: Multicenter intravascular ultrasound validation study among heart transplant recipients: outcomes after five years. *J Am Coll Cardiol* 2005; 45:1532.
129. Smart FW, Ballantyne CM, Farmer JA, et al: Insensitivity of noninvasive tests to detect coronary artery vasculopathy after heart transplant. *Am J Cardiol* 1991; 67:243.
130. Redonnet M, Tron C, Koning R, et al: Coronary angioplasty and stenting in cardiac allograft vasculopathy following heart transplantation. *Transplant Proc* 2000; 32:463.
131. Mehra MR, Ventura HO, Smart FW, et al: Impact of converting enzyme inhibitors and calcium entry blockers on cardiac allograft vasculopathy: from bench to bedside. *J Heart Lung Transplant* 1995; 14:S246.
132. Kobashigawa JA, Katznelson S, Laks H, et al: Effect of pravastatin on outcomes after cardiac transplantation. *NEJM* 1995; 333:621.
133. Mancini D, Pinney S, Burkhoff D, et al: Use of rapamycin slows progression of cardiac transplantation vasculopathy. *Circulation* 2003; 108:48.
134. Eisen HJ, Tuzcu EM, Dorent R, et al: Everolimus for the prevention of allograft rejection and vasculopathy in cardiac transplant recipients. *NEJM* 2003; 349:847.
135. Mancini D, Vigano M, Pulpon LA, et al: 24-month results of a multicenter study of Certican for the prevention of allograft rejection and vasculopathy in de novo cardiac transplant recipients. *Am J Transplant* 2003; 3:550.
136. Haverich A, Tuzcu EM, Viganò M, et al: Certican in de novo cardiac transplant recipients: 24-month follow-up. *J Heart Lung Transplant* 2003; 22:S140.
137. Eisen H, Kobashigawa J, Starling RC, et al: Improving outcomes in heart transplantation: the potential of proliferation signal inhibitors. *Transplant Proc* 2005; 37:4S.
138. Senechal M, Dorent R, du Montcel ST: End-stage renal failure and cardiac mortality after heart transplantation. *Clin Transplant* 2004; 18:1.
139. Arizon del Prado JM, Aumente Rubio MD, Cardenas Aranzana M, et al: New strategies of cyclosporine monitoring in heart transplantation: initial results. *Transplant Proc* 2003; 35:1984.
140. Citterio F: Evolution of the therapeutic drug monitoring of cyclosporine. *Transplant Proc* 2004; 36:420S.
141. Angermann CE, Stork S, Costard-Jackle A: Reduction of cyclosporine after introduction of mycophenolate mofetil improves chronic renal dysfunction in heart transplant recipients: the IMPROVED multicentre study. *Eur Heart J* 2004; 25:1626.
142. Fernandez-Valls M, Gonzalez-Vilchez F, de Prada JA, et al: Sirolimus as an alternative to anticalcineurin therapy in heart transplantation: experience of a single center. *Transplant Proc* 2005; 37:4021.
143. Groetzner J, Meiser B, Landwehr P, et al: Mycophenolate mofetil and sirolimus as calcineurin inhibitor-free immunosuppression for late cardiac-transplant recipients with chronic renal failure. *Transplantation* 2004; 77:568.
144. Ventura HO, Mehra MR, Stapleton DD, et al: Cyclosporine-induced hypertension in cardiac transplantation. *Med Clin North Am* 1997; 81:1347.
145. Taylor DO, Barr ML, Radovancevic B, et al: A randomized, multi-center comparison of tacrolimus and cyclosporine immunosuppressive regimens in cardiac transplantation: decreased hyperlipidemia and hypertension with tacrolimus. *J Heart Lung Transplant* 1999; 18:336.
146. Brozena SC, Johnson MR, Ventura H, et al: Effectiveness and safety of diltiazem or lisinopril in treatment of hypertension after heart transplantation: results of a prospective, randomized multicenter trial. *J Am Coll Cardiol* 1996; 27:1707.
147. Starling RC, Cody RJ: Cardiac transplant hypertension. *Am J Cardiol* 1990; 65:106.
148. Ippoliti G, Rinaldi M, Pellegrini C, et al: Incidence of cancer after immunosuppressive treatment for heart transplantation. *Crit Rev Oncol Hematol* 2005; 56:101.
149. Hanto DW, Sakamoto K, Purtilo DT, et al: The Epstein-Barr virus in the pathogenesis of posttransplant lymphoproliferative disorders. *Surgery* 1981; 90:204.
150. Swinnen LJ, Costanzo-Nordin MR, Fisher SG, et al: Increased incidence of lymphoproliferative disorder after immunosuppression with the monoclonal antibody OKT3 in cardiac transplant recipients. *NEJM* 1990; 323:1723.
151. El-Hamamsy I, Stevens LM, Carrier M, et al: Incidence and prognosis of cancer following heart transplantation using RATG induction therapy. *Transplant Int* 2005; 18:1280.
152. Kirklin JK, Benza RL, Rayburn BK, et al: Strategies for minimizing hyperlipidemia after cardiac transplantation. *Am J Cardiovasc Drugs* 2002; 2:377.
153. Bianda T, Linka A, Junga G, et al: Prevention of osteoporosis in heart transplant recipients: a comparison of calcitriol with calcitonin and pamidronate. *Calcif Tissue Int* 2000; 67:116.
154. Mueller XM, Tevaearai HT, Stumpe F, et al: Gastrointestinal disease following heart transplantation. *World J Surg* 1999; 23:650.
155. Radovancevic B, McGiffin DC, Kobashigawa JA, et al: Retransplantation in 7290 primary transplant patients: a 10-year multi-institutional study. *J Heart Lung Transplant* 2003; 22:862.
156. Srivastava R, Keck BM, Bennett LE, et al: The result of cardiac retransplantation: an analysis of the joint International Society of Heart Lung Transplantation/United Network for Organ Sharing Thoracic Registry. *Transplantation* 2000; 4:606.
157. Haddad H: Cardiac retransplantation: an ethical dilemma. *Curr Opin Cardiol* 2006; 21:118.
158. Lim E, Ali Z, Ali A, et al: Comparison of survival by allocation to medical therapy, surgery, or heart transplantation for ischemic advanced heart failure. *J Heart Lung Transplant* 2005; 24:983.
159. Luckraz H, Goddard M, Charman SC, et al: Early mortality after cardiac transplantation: should we do better? *J Heart Lung Transplant* 2005; 24:401.
160. Politi P, Piccinelli M, Poli PF, et al: Ten years of "extended" life: quality of life among heart transplantation survivors. *Transplantation* 2004; 78:257.
161. Russo MJ, Chen JM, Hong KN, et al: Survival after heart transplantation is not diminished among recipients with uncomplicated diabetes mellitus: an analysis of the United Network of Organ Sharing database. *Circulation.* 2006 Nov 21;114(21):2280-7. Epub 2006 Nov 6.
162. Zaidi AR, Zaidi A, Vaitkus PT: Outcome of heart transplantation in patients with sarcoid cardiomyopathy. *J Heart Lung Transplant* 2007; 26(7):714-717.
163. Kpodonu J, Massad MG, Caines A, Geha AS: Outcome of heart transplantation in patients with amyloid cardiomyopathy. *J Heart Lung Transplant* 2005; 24(11):1763-1765.
164. Nwakanma LU, Williams JA, Weiss ES, et al: Influence of pretransplant panel-reactive antibody on outcomes in 8,160 heart transplant recipients in recent era. *Ann Thorac Surg* 2007; 84(5):1556-1562; discussion 1562-1563.
165. Weiss ES, Nwakanma LU, Patel ND, Yuh DD: Outcomes in patients older than 60 years of age undergoing orthotopic heart transplantation: an analysis of the UNOS database. *J Heart Lung Transplant* 2008;27(2): 184-191.
166. Weiss ES, Allen JG, Russell SD, et al: Impact of recipient body mass index on organ allocation and mortality in orthotopic heart transplantation. *J Heart Lung Transplant* 2009; 28(11):1150-1157. Epub 2009 Sep 26.
167. Pal JD, Piacentino V, Cuevas AD, et al: Impact of left ventricular assist device bridging on posttransplant outcomes. *Ann Thorac Surg* 2009; 88(5):1457-1461; discussion 1461.
168. Shuhaiber J, Hur K, Gibbons R: Does the type of ventricular assisted device influence survival, infection, and rejection rates following heart transplantation? *J Card Surg* 2009; 24(3):250-255.
169. Weiss ES, Meguid RA, Patel ND, et al: Increased mortality at low-volume orthotopic heart transplantation centers: should current standards change? *Ann Thorac Surg* 2008; 86(4):1250-1259; discussion 1259-1260.
170. Orlic D, Kajstura J, Chimenti S: Bone marrow cells regenerate infarcted myocardium. *Nature* 2001; 410:701.
171. Baumgartner WA, Kasper E, Reitz B, Theodore J [eds]: *Heart and Lung Transplantation*, 2nd ed. New York, Saunders, 2002; pp. 180-199.

CHAPTER 65

Lung Transplantation and Heart-Lung Transplantation

Ahmad Y. Sheikh
David L. Joyce
Hari R. Mallidi
Robert C. Robbins

INTRODUCTION

Human lung transplantation, performed as a single lung, double lung, or heart-lung bloc, has emerged as a life-saving procedure for patients with end-stage pulmonary disease. With improvement of operative techniques, organ preservation, and immunosuppressive regimens, combined heart-lung and isolated lung transplantation have become common treatments for patients with a variety of end-stage disease entities. To date, 3466 combined heart-lung transplants and 29,732 lung transplants have been reported worldwide.[1] Although the number of heart-lung transplants performed annually has declined in recent years, the number of single lung transplantation procedures remains stable, accompanied by a steady increase in bilateral lung transplant procedures (Fig. 65-1). Clinical progress in thoracic organ transplantation has been considerable, yet significant barriers that limit the scope of these procedures still remain. These include donor organ shortage, limited preservation techniques, graft rejection, and infectious complications. This chapter summarizes the state of the art in combined heart-lung and isolated lung transplantation.

LUNG TRANSPLANTATION

History of Lung Transplantation

In 1949, Henry Metras described many of the important technical concepts for lung transplantation, including preservation of the left atrial cuff for the pulmonary venous anastomoses and reimplantation of an aortic patch containing the origin of the bronchial arteries to prevent bronchial dehiscence.[2] Airway dehiscence was a major obstacle in experimental lung transplantation, and he proposed that preservation of the bronchial arterial supply was critical to airway healing. Unfortunately, this technique was technically cumbersome and never gained widespread popularity. In the 1960s, Blumenstock and Khan advocated transection of the transplant bronchus close to the lung parenchyma to prevent ischemic bronchial necrosis.[3] Additional surgical modifications were developed to prevent bronchial anastomotic complications, including telescoping of the bronchial anastomosis, described by Veith in 1970,[4] and coverage of the anastomosis with an omental pedicle flap, described by the Toronto group in 1982.[5] Corticosteroids were found to be another contributor to poor bronchial healing,[6] a problem ameliorated by the introduction of cyclosporine immunosuppression. Thus, by the 1970s, the stage was set for successful lung transplantation in the human.

The first human lung transplant was described in 1963 by Hardy and colleagues at the University of Mississippi.[7] The patient, a 58-year-old man with lung cancer, survived 18 days postoperatively. Over the next two decades, nearly 40 lung transplants were performed without long-term success. In 1986, the Toronto Lung Transplant Group reported the first successful series of single lung transplants with long-term survival.[8] Improved immunosuppression, along with careful recipient and donor selection, were pivotal to their success. For patients with bilateral lung disease, en-bloc double lung replacement was introduced by Patterson in 1988 as an alternative to heart-lung

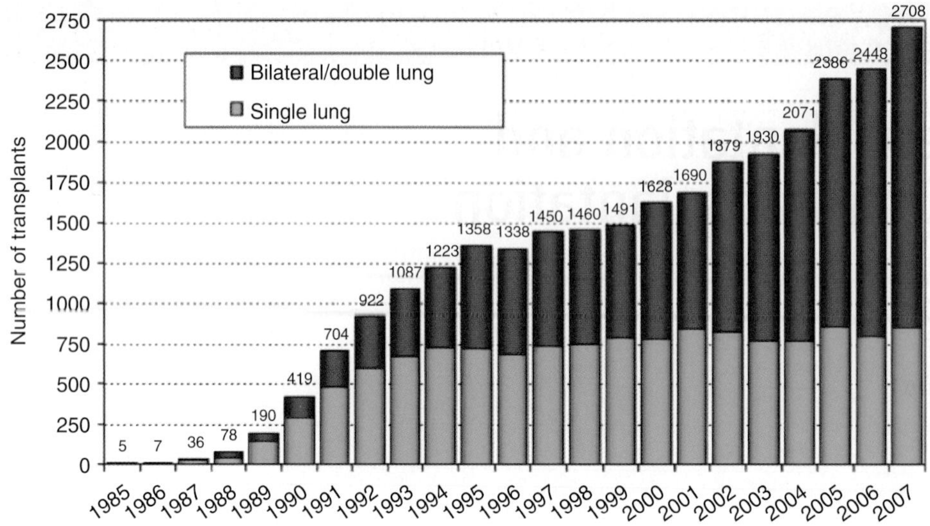

FIGURE 65-1 UNOS data representing the number of lung transplant procedures reported by year and procedure type, collected from data reported to the International Society of Heart and Lung Transplantation Registry. This figure may underestimate the total number of procedures worldwide. (*From Christie JD, et al: The Registry of the International Society for Heart and Lung Transplantation: Twenty-Sixth Official Adult Lung and Heart-Lung Transplantation Report—2009. J Heart Lung Transplant 2009; 28[10]:1031-1049.*)

transplantation with a domino procedure in which the explanted heart was offered to a second recipient with end-stage heart disease.[9] This technique was later replaced by sequential bilateral lung transplantation, described by Pasque and colleagues in 1990.[10] More recent operative innovations include living lobar transplantation, performed for the first time by Vaughn Starnes at Stanford in 1992.[11]

Lung transplantation has seen a steady growth over the past decade, with 2708 procedures reported to the International Society for Heart and Lung Transplantation (ISHLT) registry in 2007. Currently there are 153 centers reporting lung transplant data, with more than half of these performing more than 10 transplants per year. Although the number of single lung transplants performed has been relatively stable since the mid-1990s, bilateral lung transplant procedures have shown a consistent growth in volume.[1]

Indications for Lung Transplantation

General Guidelines

Organ allocation for lung transplantation underwent a major change in 2005 that has significantly affected the process of recipient selection. Historically, lung allocation was determined strictly by the amount of time a patient spent on the waiting list (matching for size and blood group). Consequently, the limited supply of donor organs resulted in an increasing number of patients on the waiting list with progressively longer wait times (Fig. 65-2).[12] To address these shortcomings, the organ allocation system was revised in 2005 to prioritize medical urgency and expected outcome after transplantation. Under this system, prioritization is based on a lung allocation score (LAS) that is calculated based on the following clinical criteria: age, height, weight, lung diagnosis code, functional status, diabetes, assisted ventilation, supplemental O_2 requirement, percent predicted FVC, pulmonary artery systemic pressure, mean pulmonary artery pressure, pulmonary capillary wedge pressure, current P_{CO_2}, highest P_{CO_2}, lowest P_{CO_2}, change in P_{CO_2}, 6-minute walk distance, and serum creatinine. These values can be entered into an online calculator to derive the LAS (http://optn.transplant.hrsa.gov/resources/professionalResources.asp?index=9). Based on these criteria, the waitlist urgency measure (defined as the expected number of days during the next year on the waiting list without a transplant) is subtracted from the posttransplant survival measure (defined as the expected number of days lived during the first year after transplantation) to determine the transplant benefit. This raw allocation score is then normalized to a scale of 0 to 100 to calculate the LAS. In this scoring system, posttransplant survival is limited to 1 year because the predictive variables are only relevant in the early postoperative period.[13]

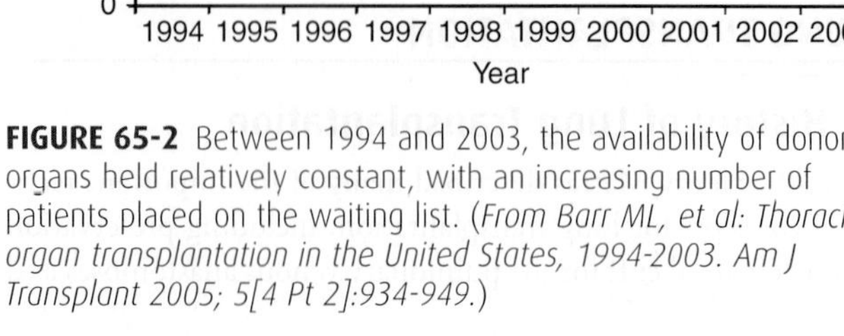

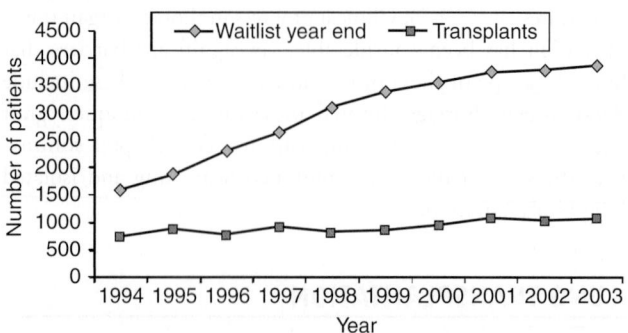

FIGURE 65-2 Between 1994 and 2003, the availability of donor organs held relatively constant, with an increasing number of patients placed on the waiting list. (*From Barr ML, et al: Thoracic organ transplantation in the United States, 1994-2003. Am J Transplant 2005; 5[4 Pt 2]:934-949.*)

The rationale for approaching recipient selection from the perspective of transplant benefit is based on the premise that patient selection for lung transplantation must balance the anticipated survival after transplantation (currently at a median of 5 years) with projected life expectancy on the waiting list. Although waiting times have historically averaged 432 days, the institution of the LAS has reduced this period to an average of 262 days.[14] Nevertheless, mortality while on the waiting list remains at nearly 20%, so it is imperative to identify recipients as early as possible within the "transplant window."[15] Ideally, recipient evaluation should select individuals with progressively disabling pulmonary disease who still possess the capacity for full rehabilitation after transplantation. Much of the current success in lung transplantation stems from improvement in recipient selection, because early attempts were thwarted by selection of patients with prohibitive operative risk factors. Candidates should have a less than 50% 2- to 3-year predicted survival despite appropriate medical or alternative surgical strategies. Disabling symptoms prompting consideration for transplantation typically include dyspnea, cyanosis, syncope, and hemoptysis. Potential recipients are identified by their local primary physicians and referred to transplantation centers for further evaluation.

Tests required for transplant listing are reviewed in Table 65-1. Diagnostic studies that are particularly useful in evaluating potential recipients include full pulmonary function tests, an exercise performance test, electrocardiogram, echocardiogram, 24-hour creatinine clearance, and liver function tests. Former smokers must undergo screening to exclude smoking-related illnesses, such as peripheral vascular disease and malignancy. A negative sputum cytology, thoracic computed tomographic (CT) scan, bronchoscopy, otolaryngologic evaluation, and carotid duplex scan are required. In addition, left heart catheterization and coronary angiography should be performed in recipient candidates who have a history of smoking.

Patients deemed suitable for transplantation during the initial evaluation are subjected to a final phase of testing (see Table 65-1). If accepted by the transplant review committee, they are listed on the national transplant registry based on LAS. Listed candidates should be seen every 3 to 6 months at the transplant center and regularly by their primary physicians, to maintain optimal medical condition. If appropriate, a period of exercise rehabilitation and nutritional modification may be initiated. Most transplant centers require patients to reside within several hours of the center by automobile or air charter.

ABO compatibilities are strictly adhered to, because isolated cases of hyperacute rejection have been reported in transplants performed across ABO barriers.[17] Donor-to-recipient lung volume matching is based on the vertical (apex to diaphragm along the midclavicular line) and transverse (level of diaphragmatic dome) radiologic dimensions on chest x-ray, as well as body weight, height, and chest circumference. Matching donor and recipient height seems the most reproducible method for selection of appropriate donor lung size, and donor lung dimensions should not be greater than 4 cm over those of the recipient. If need be, donor lungs may be downsized by lobectomy or wedge resection.

In contrast to renal transplantation, HLA matching is not a criterion for thoracic organ allocation. Because only short ischemic times are tolerated by lung and heart-lung blocs, it is not possible to perform this tissue typing preoperatively.[18] However, several retrospective studies have been performed evaluating the influence of HLA matching on long-term graft survival and development of obliterative bronchiolitis. Wisser and colleagues examined the relationship between HLA matching and long-term survival in 78 lung transplant recipients, finding improved graft survival with matching at the HLA-B locus.[19] In a retrospective

TABLE 65-1 Typical Laboratory Tests and Studies Obtained During Recipient Evaluation for Heart-Lung and Lung Transplantation

SUITABILITY FOR TRANSPLANTATION (PHASE I)

Required Laboratory Tests and Studies
- CBC with differential, platelet, and reticulocyte count
- Blood type and antibody screen (ABO, Rh)
- Prothrombin and activated partial thromboplastin time (PT, aPTT)
- Bleeding time
- Immunology panel (FANA, RF)
- Electrolytes, including Mg^{2+}
- CK with isoenzymes
- Serum protein electrophoresis
- Urinalysis
- Viral serologies
  - Compromised host panel (cytomegalovirus, adenovirus, Varicella-Zoster, herpes simplex, Epstein-Barr virus)
  - Hepatitis A, B, and C antibodies, Hepatitis B surface antigen (HBsAg)
  - Cytomegalovirus (quantitative antibodies and IgM)
  - Human immunodeficiency virus
- Electrocardiogram
- Chest x-ray

Studies Obtained as Indicated
- Echocardiogram with bubble study
- MUGA for right and left ventricular ejection fraction
- Cardiac catheterization with coronary angiogram
- Thoracic CT scan
- Quantitative ventilation-perfusion scans
- Carotid duplex
- Mammogram
- Colonoscopy
- Sputum for Gram stain, AFB smear, KOH, and routine bacterial, mycobacterial, and fungal cultures

REQUIRED FOR LISTING (PHASE II)
- HLA and DR typing
- Transplant antibody
- Quantitative immunoglobulins
- *Histoplasma, Coccidioides,* and *Toxoplasma* titers
- PPD
- Pulmonary function tests with arterial blood gases
- 12-Hour urine collection for creatinine clearance and total protein
- Urine viral culture

study of 74 lung transplant patients, Iwaki and coworkers also correlated matching at the HLA-B and HLA-DR loci with improved graft survival.[20] These studies suggest a relationship between HLA matching and long-term graft function.

Once an appropriate donor-recipient pairing is made, the recipient is screened for preformed antibodies against a panel of random donors. A percent reactive antibody (PRA) level greater than 25 prompts a prospective specific crossmatch between the donor and recipient. A positive crossmatch indicates the presence of antidonor circulating antibodies in the recipient, which would likely lead to hyperacute rejection. In the event of a positive crossmatch, the donor organ cannot be accepted for that recipient.

Disease-Specific Guidelines

Common indications for lung transplantation are listed in Table 65-2, with listing criteria given in Table 65-3. Chronic obstructive pulmonary disease (COPD) represents the most common indication for lung transplantation, accounting for 36% of lung transplants performed each year.[1] Decision making with respect to referral for transplantation and listing is based on worsening clinical deterioration as quantified by the BODE index. This predictive tool takes into account body mass index (B), degree of airflow obstruction (O), dyspnea (D, measured by the modified Medical Research Council MMRC dyspnea scale), and exercise capacity (E, measured by a 6-minute walk test).[21] The BODE index score ranges from 0 to 10, and patients are considered for transplant with a score of 7 to 10, because median survival in this cohort is only 3 years.[21] In patients with COPD who have apically predominant emphysema, lung volume reduction surgery (LVRS) may represent an alternative strategy to postpone or eliminate the need for transplantation. Patients who have undergone pleurodesis or who have advanced disease (FEV_1 and DLCO <20% or significant pulmonary hypertension) are not eligible for LVRS.[22] Based on the National Emphysema Treatment Trial, which studied the benefit of LVRS, a cohort of transplant-eligible high-risk patients (median survival of 3 years with medical therapy) was identified in which FEV1 was less than 20% and either DLCO less than 20% or homogeneously distributed emphysema was present.[22] The decision to perform single versus double lung transplantation in a patient with COPD must take into account the patient's ability to tolerate single lung ventilation, cardiopulmonary bypass, and the risk of ventilation-perfusion mismatch in single lung transplant when compressive atelectasis and restriction occurs in the donor lung. Interestingly, a statistical model derived from UNOS data between 1987 and 2004 estimated that 45% of COPD patients would gain a survival benefit of 1 year after double lung transplant, compared with only 22% of patients who underwent single lung transplant.[23]

Idiopathic pulmonary fibrosis (IPF) represents the second most common indication for lung transplantation worldwide, accounting for just over 20% of all lung transplants.[1] Median survival from the time of diagnosis is only 2.5 to 3.5 years, suggesting that transplant referral should be made as soon as

TABLE 65-2 Indications for Lung Transplantation from January 1995 Through June 2008

Diagnosis	SLT (*n* = 10,190) No. (%)	BLT (*n* = 13,338) No. (%)	Total (*N* = 23,528) No. (%)
COPD/emphysema	4,994 (49.0)	3,423 (25.7)	8,417 (35.8)
IPF	2,967 (29.1)	1,930 (14.5)	4,897 (20.8)
Cystic fibrosis	191 (1.9)	3,552 (26.6)	3,743 (15.9)
AAT	662 (6.5)	1,017 (7.6)	1,679 (7.1)
IPAH	74 (0.7)	714 (5.4)	788 (3.3)
Sarcoidosis	212 (2.1)	391 (2.9)	603 (2.6)
Bronchiectasis	40 (0.4)	596 (4.5)	636 (2.7)
LAM	80 (0.8)	157 (1.2)	237 (1.0)
Congenital heart disease	19 (0.2)	144 (1.1)	163 (0.7)
OB	53 (0.5)	150 (1.1)	203 (0.9)
Retransplant			
OB	160 (1.6)	134 (1.0)	294 (1.2)
Not OB	105 (1.0)	97 (0.7)	202 (0.9)
Connective tissue disease	68 (0.7)	113 (0.8)	181 (0.8)
Interstitial pneumonitis	32 (0.3)	29 (0.2)	61 (0.3)
Cancer	6 (0.1)	17 (0.1)	23 (0.1)
Other	527 (5.2)	874 (6.6)	1,401 (6.0)

UNOS data from January 1995 through June 2008.
From Christie JD, et al: The Registry of the International Society for Heart and Lung Transplantation: Twenty-Sixth Official Adult Lung and Heart-Lung Transplantation Report—2009. J Heart Lung Transplant 2009; 28[10]:1031-1049.

TABLE 65-3 Listing Criteria Specific to the Disease Entities Commonly Evaluated for Lung Transplantation

Chronic Obstructive Pulmonary Disease
- BODE index of 7 to 10 or at least one of the following:
  - History of hospitalization for exacerbation associated with acute hypercapnia (Pco_2 exceeding 50 mm Hg)
  - Pulmonary hypertension or cor pulmonale, or both, despite oxygen therapy
  - FEV_1 <20% and either DLco <20% or homogenous distribution of emphysema

Idiopathic Pulmonary Fibrosis
- Histologic or radiographic evidence of UIP and any of the following:
  - A DLco <39% predicted
  - A 10% or greater decrement in FVC during 6 mo of follow-up
  - A decrease in pulse oximetry <88% during a 6-minute walk test
  - Honeycombing on HRCT (fibrosis score >2)

Cystic Fibrosis
- FEV_1 <30% of predicted, or rapidly declining lung function if FEV_1 >30% (females and patients <18 years of age have a poorer prognosis; consider earlier listing) and/or any of the following:
  - Increasing oxygen requirements
  - Hypercapnia
  - Pulmonary hypertension

Idiopathic Pulmonary Arterial Hypertension
- Persistent NYHA Class III or IV on maximal medical therapy
- Low (350 m) or declining 6-minute walk test
- Failing therapy with intravenous epoprostenol, or equivalent.
- Cardiac index of <2 L/min/m^2
- Right atrial pressure >15 mm Hg

Sarcoidosis
- NYHA functional Class III or IV and any of the following:
  - Hypoxemia at rest
  - Pulmonary hypertension
  - Elevated right atrial pressure >15 mm Hg

BODE = Body mass index, airflow Obstruction, Dyspnea, and Exercise capacity; HRCT = high-resolution computed tomography; NYHA = New York Heart Association; UIP = usual interstitial pneumonitis.
Modified from *Kreider M, Kotloff RM: Selection of candidates for lung transplantation. Proc Am Thorac Soc 2009; 6(1):20-27.*

histologic or radiographic evidence of the disease is present. Listing a patient with IPF must take into account the fact that many patients have an indolent form of the disease, and numerous studies have identified the following risk factors for rapid decline in patients with histologic or radiographic evidence of IPF[24]:

- DLco less than 39% of predicted
- 10% or greater decrement in FVC during a 6-month period
- Oxygen saturation less than 88% during a 6-minute walk test
- Honeycombing on CT scan

Traditionally, IPF patients have been considered for either single or double lung transplantation. However, recent data suggest that there may be a survival advantage for double lung over single lung transplant—particularly among high-risk patients (defined as LAS >52).[25]

Cystic fibrosis (CF) is the third most common indication for lung transplant, accounting for 16% of the total number of transplants performed.[1] In these patients, bilateral sepsis mandates removal of both native lungs. In a landmark study from the Hospital for Sick Children in Toronto, Kerem and colleagues established that CF patients with an FEV_1 of less than 30% of predicted experienced a 2-year mortality rate of 50%.[26] However, subsequent risk stratification models have challenged these findings and presented conflicting data on the question of life expectancy in CF. Therefore, the current ISHLT guidelines state that an FEV_1 less than 30% should prompt a referral to a transplant center with the decision to proceed with listing dependent on other indicators of disease severity such as oxygen-dependent respiratory failure, hypercapnia, and pulmonary hypertension.[27] Cystic fibrosis recipients should have an otolaryngologic evaluation before being placed on an active waiting list. Most of these patients require endoscopic maxillary antrostomies for sinus access and monthly antibiotic irrigation to decrease the bacterial load of the upper respiratory tract. This measure has decreased the incidence of serious posttransplant bacterial infections.[28]

Idiopathic pulmonary arterial hypertension represents 3.3% of the total lung transplantation volume worldwide.[1] Survival with this condition has improved dramatically with the institution of vasodilator therapy, with 5-year survival of 55% on epoprostenol compared with 28% among historical controls.[29] Listing for transplantation is indicated when a patient remains in NYHA Class III or IV after 3 months of therapy (often seen in the setting of declining 6-minute walk test, cardiac index of <2 L/min/m^2, or right atrial pressure >15 mm Hg).[24]

Sarcoidosis accounts for 2.6% of all lung transplants.[1] The natural course of this disease can be highly variable, but in general patients should be referred for transplant if they develop NYHA class III or IV symptoms. Impairment of exercise tolerance and hypoxemia at rest, pulmonary hypertension, or right atrial pressure greater than 15 mm Hg serve as general guidelines for listing.[27]

Less than 2% of all single and bilateral lung transplants are retransplantations.[1] Overall, survival is poor compared with first-time transplantation, although certain subsets of patients perform better than others. In fact, the Pulmonary Retransplant Registry has collected data from 230 patients at over 40 centers and found that 1-year survival of ambulatory, nonventilated patients undergoing retransplantation after 1991 is comparable with first-time transplants.[30]

Contraindications to Lung Transplantation

There are well-established contraindications to lung transplantation (Table 65-4). In general, transplantation is an option that is restricted to patients less than 65 years old, although 9% of recipients in the first half of 2008 exceeded this cutoff.[1] Significant multisystem disease is a contraindication, although multiorgan transplants have occasionally been performed. Absolute contraindications include renal dysfunction, malignancy (bronchoalveolar carcinoma is a contraindication but not non-melanoma skin cancer), infection with HIV, hepatitis B antigen positivity or hepatitis C infection with biopsy-proven liver disease, infection with pan-resistant respiratory flora, active or recent cigarette smoking, drug abuse, alcohol abuse, severe psychiatric illness, noncompliance with medical care, extreme obesity, progressive unintentional weight loss, malnutrition, and absence of a consistent and reliable social support network.[24] Relative contraindications include active extrapulmonary infection, symptomatic osteoporosis, and recent history of active peptic ulcer disease. Cigarette smokers must quit smoking and remain abstinent for several months before transplantation. Patients with histories of previous thoracic surgery are evaluated on a case-by-case basis. For patients who require systemic corticosteroids, tapering to the lowest tolerable level, preferably below 10 mg/day, is critical to prevent airway healing complications. Finally, mechanical ventilation is generally considered a contraindication to transplantation; repeated studies have shown that these patients have significantly worse immediate and long-term survival after transplantation.[31] It is important that recipient candidates be educated about lifestyle modifications necessary for the success of a transplant, and willingness to comply with immunosuppression regimens and extensive posttransplant medical and surgical follow-up is mandatory.

TABLE 65-4 Recipient Contraindications to Lung Transplantation

Age ≥65
Significant systemic or multisystem disease (eg, peripheral or cerebrovascular disease, portal hypertension, poorly controlled diabetes mellitus)
Significant irreversible hepatic or renal dysfunction (eg, bilirubin >3.0 mg/dL, creatinine clearance <50 mg/mL/min
Active malignancy
Corticosteroid therapy (>10 mg/day)
Pan-resistant respiratory flora
Cachexia or obesity (<70% or >130% ideal body weight)
Current cigarette smoking
Psychiatric illness or history of medical noncompliance
Drug or alcohol abuse
Previous cardiothoracic surgery (considered on a case-by-case basis)
Severe osteoporosis
Prolonged mechanical ventilation
HIV
HBsAg positivity or Hepatitis C infection with biopsy proven liver disease

Recipient Management After Listing

It is essential that a candidate's medical condition be optimized before transplantation. Supplemental oxygen is recommended for any patient exhibiting arterial hypoxemia, defined as either an arterial oxygen saturation less than 90 percent or an arterial Po_2 less than 60 mm Hg at rest, during exertion, or while asleep. Fluid balance is optimized with restriction of dietary water and salt in conjunction with diuretic therapy. Care must be taken with the use of loop diuretics, as these can incite a metabolic alkalosis that can impair the effectiveness of plasma carbon dioxide as a stimulus for breathing.

Primary pulmonary hypertension often requires the use of supplemental oxygen to prevent hypoxia-induced pulmonary vasoconstriction and secondary erythropoiesis. Pulmonary vasodilator therapy with the use of calcium channel blockers and continuous prostacyclin infusions presents another therapeutic option in the management of these patients.[32] Although these drugs exhibit potent systemic effects and must be used with caution, the response rate for calcium channel blockers is approximately 20%. Although a favorable response to short-acting vasodilators during cardiac catheterization is predictive of a successful response to calcium channel therapy, this trend is not seen in long-term prostacyclin infusion.

Interstitial lung disease in patients awaiting transplantation results from a wide variety of diffuse inflammatory processes such as sarcoidosis, asbestosis, and collagen-vascular diseases. Increases in pulmonary vascular resistance leading to right-sided heart failure are thought to arise from interstitial inflammatory infiltrates that entrap and eventually destroy septal arterioles, thus reducing the distensibility of the remaining pulmonary vessels.[33] This process, coupled with closure of peripheral bronchioles, results in arterial hypoxemia, further aggravating pulmonary hypertension. Corticosteroids are the mainstay of treatment in this class of diseases. The adverse effects of steroids on airway healing are well established,[6,34] and mandate significant dose reductions in anticipation of transplantation.

The multisystem manifestations of cystic fibrosis, particularly chronic bronchopulmonary infection, malabsorption, malnutrition, and diabetes mellitus, pose difficult management problems in potential transplant recipients. These patients require aggressive chest physiotherapy, antibiotics, enteral or parenteral nutritional supplementation, and tight serum glucose control.[35]

Organ Procurement and Preservation

Donor Selection

Standard criteria have been established for donor selection (Table 65-5).[36,37] Donors must have sustained irreversible brain death, but owing to the susceptibility of the lungs to edema and infection in the setting of brain death and trauma, suitable organs are often difficult to obtain (available in <20% of all organ donors).

TABLE 65-5 Donor Selection Criteria

Age <40 (heart-lung), <50 (lung)
Smoking history less than 20 pack-years
Arterial Po_2 of 140 mm Hg on an Fio_2 of 40% or 300 mm Hg on an Fio_2 of 100%
Normal chest x-ray
Sputum free of bacteria, fungus, or significant numbers of white blood cells on Gram and fungal staining
Bronchoscopy showing absence of purulent secretions or signs of aspiration
Absence of thoracic trauma
HIV-negative

Initial donor evaluation consists of a directed history and physical examination, chest x-ray, 12-lead ECG, arterial blood gases, and serologic screening including human immunodeficiency virus (HIV), hepatitis B surface antigen, hepatitis C antibodies, herpes simplex virus (HSV), cytomegalovirus (CMV), *Toxoplasma*, and RPR. A donor age of less than 50 is preferred. The chest x-ray should be clear and the arterial PO_2 should exceed 140 mm Hg on an FIO_2 of 40% and 300 mm Hg on an FIO_2 of 100%. Lung compliance can be estimated by measuring peak inspiratory pressures, which should be less than 30 cm H_2O. Bronchoscopy should ensure the absence of purulent secretions or signs of aspiration. Finally, direct inspection and palpation of the lungs at explantation to verify full expansion of any atelectatic segments is an essential part of the donor organ evaluation.

Absolute contraindications to donation include prolonged cardiac arrest (30 minutes), arterial hypoxemia, active malignancy (excluding basal cell and squamous cell carcinoma of the skin), and positive HIV status. Relative contraindications include thoracic trauma, sepsis, significant smoking history, prolonged severe hypotension (ie, <60 mm Hg for >6 hours), HBsAg or hepatitis C antibodies, multiple resuscitation attempts, and a prolonged high inotropic requirement (eg, dopamine in excess of 15 μg/kg/min for 24 hours). It is important to rule out correctable metabolic or physiologic causes of cardiac rhythm disturbances and electrocardiographic anomalies (eg, brain herniation, hypothermia, hypokalemia).

Over the last decade, there has been a trend toward liberalization of standard donor selection criteria. This strategy, initiated in response to the shortage of donor organs, is employed at a large number of transplant centers.[38–42] Donors ranging in age from 50 to 64 have been used in thoracic transplantation with good long-term graft survival.[41] However, reports from the ISHLT document worse outcomes in recipients of lung allografts from donors older than 55 who had ischemic times greater than 6 to 8 hours.[43] In this group of recipients, long-term survival is impaired and the risk of developing bronchiolitis obliterans is increased. Smoking history is another criterion that has been liberalized, with conventional guidelines limiting donor selection to patients with less than 20 pack-years. Modified criteria allow for a more extensive smoking history, assuming there is no evidence of COPD or other lung disease on screening tests. Traditionally, donor lungs have been ruled out for transplantation based on evidence of infection. In that regard, prolonged ventilation before brain death and procurement has been viewed as a contraindication for organ selection. However, a positive sputum Gram stain (excluding fungus), which was once considered a basis for ruling out an organ has failed to predict the development of early pneumonia, impairment of oxygenation, or duration of mechanical ventilation in the postoperative setting.[44,45] Some groups have accepted donors with small pulmonary infiltrates on chest x-ray, although clinical correlation is necessary. Others have selectively used donor lungs in patients with PaO_2 less than 300 mm Hg on FIO_2 of 100%. Gabbay and coworkers in Australia have adopted an aggressive approach to donor management and "organ resuscitation."[39] By manipulating donors with antibiotic therapy, chest physiotherapy, careful fluid management, ventilator adjustments, and bronchial toilet, 34% of donors with an initial PaO_2 less than 300 mm Hg on FIO_2 of 100% had increases in their PaO_2, becoming acceptable donors.

Areas of investigation in the field of donor organ procurement include the use of non–heart-beating donors. In 2001, Steen and coworkers reported transplantation of lungs from a non–heart-beating donor into a 54-year-old woman with COPD,[46] with good functional results during the first 5 months of follow-up. However, ethical, logistic, and scientific questions remain on the use of non–heart-beating donors, and this strategy is far from being widely applicable.

Donor Management

The overriding goal in managing the thoracic organ donor is to maintain hemodynamic stability and pulmonary function. Patients suffering from acute brain injury are often hemodynamically unstable because of neurogenic shock, excessive fluid losses, and bradycardia. Donor lungs are prone to neurogenic pulmonary edema, aspiration, nosocomial infection, and contusion. Continuous arterial and central venous pressure monitoring, judicious fluid resuscitation, vasopressors, and inotropes are usually required.

Intravascular volume replacement should be limited to maintain the central venous pressure between 5 and 8 mm Hg. In general, crystalloid fluid boluses are to be avoided. Diabetes insipidus is common in donors and requires the use of intravenous vasopressin (0.8 to 1.0 unit/h) to prevent excessive urine loss. Dopamine is the standard inotropic agent used to maintain adequate perfusion pressures, although alpha agonists (eg, phenylephrine) are often appropriate. Blood transfusions should be used sparingly to maintain a hemoglobin concentration of approximately10 g/dL, ensuring adequate myocardial oxygen delivery. CMV-negative and leukocyte-filtered blood should be used whenever possible. Hypothermia should be avoided as it predisposes to ventricular arrhythmias and metabolic acidosis.

With regard to mechanical ventilation, FIO_2 values in excess of 40%, especially 100% oxygen "challenges," should be avoided, because these oxygen levels may be toxic to the denervated lung. Ventilator settings should include positive end-expiratory pressures (PEEP) between 3 and 5 cm H_2O to prevent atelectasis.

Donor Operation

The donor operation is performed via a median sternotomy (Fig. 65-3A). After the sternum is divided, a standard chest retractor is placed, and both pleural spaces are opened followed by immediate inspection of the lungs and pleural spaces, particularly in cases involving trauma. The lungs are briefly deflated, and the pulmonary ligaments are divided inferiorly using electrocautery. After completely excising the thymic remnant, the pericardium is opened vertically and laterally on the diaphragm and cradled during dissection of the great vessels and trachea. The ascending aorta, pulmonary artery, and venae cavae are dissected. Umbilical tapes are placed around the ascending

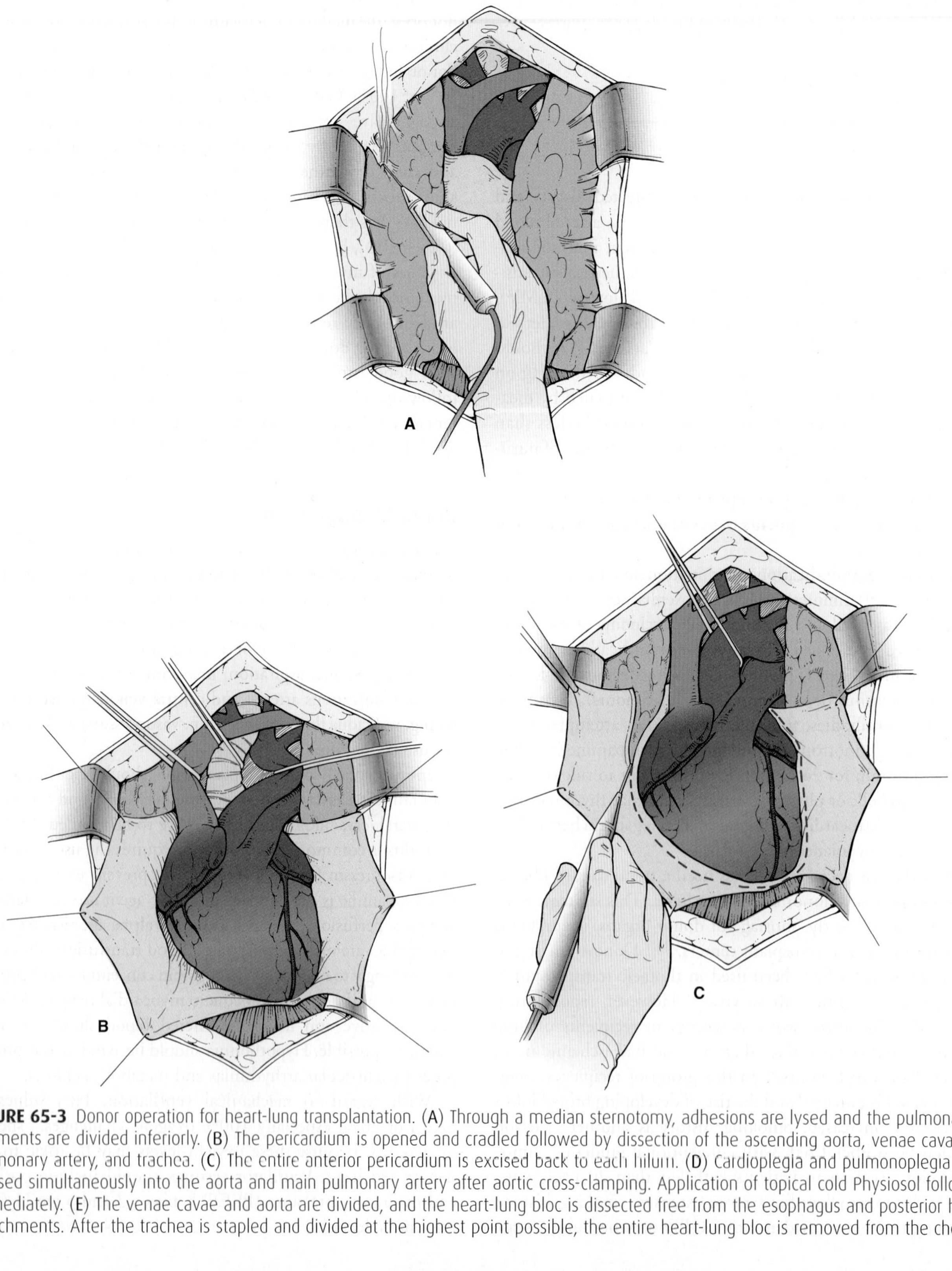

FIGURE 65-3 Donor operation for heart-lung transplantation. (A) Through a median sternotomy, adhesions are lysed and the pulmonary ligaments are divided inferiorly. (B) The pericardium is opened and cradled followed by dissection of the ascending aorta, venae cavae, pulmonary artery, and trachea. (C) The entire anterior pericardium is excised back to each hilum. (D) Cardioplegia and pulmonoplegia are infused simultaneously into the aorta and main pulmonary artery after aortic cross-clamping. Application of topical cold Physiosol follows immediately. (E) The venae cavae and aorta are divided, and the heart-lung bloc is dissected free from the esophagus and posterior hilar attachments. After the trachea is stapled and divided at the highest point possible, the entire heart-lung bloc is removed from the chest.

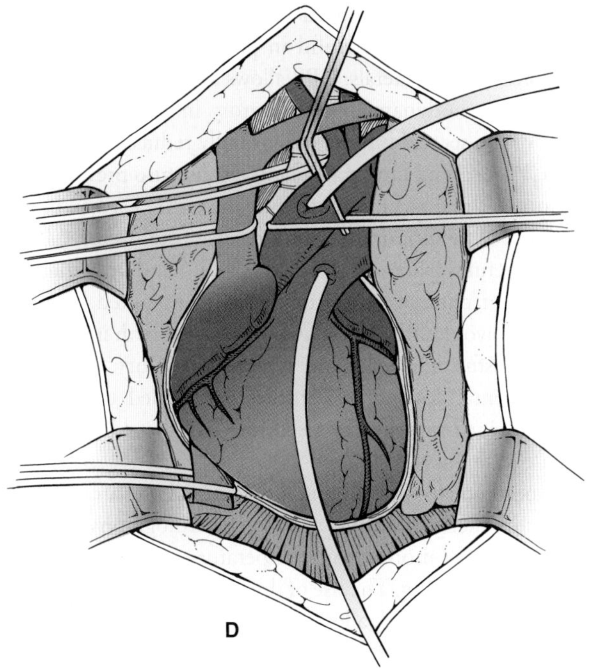

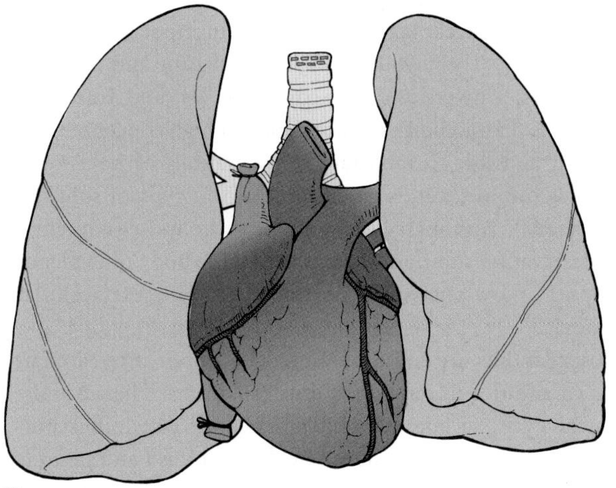

FIGURE 65-3 *(Continued)*

aorta and venae cavae (Fig. 65-3B). The pericardium overlying the trachea is incised vertically, and the trachea is encircled with an umbilical tape between the aorta and superior vena cava at the highest point possible and at least four rings above the carina (see Fig. 65-3B). The entire anterior pericardium is excised back to each hilum (Fig. 65-3C).

Approximately 15 minutes before applying the aortic cross-clamp, prostaglandin E_1 (PGE_1) is infused intravenously, initially at a rate of 20 ng/kg/min, followed by incremental increases of 10 ng/kg/min to a target rate of 100 ng/kg/min (Fig. 65-3D). During PGE_1 infusion, the mean arterial blood pressure should be maintained at or above 55 mm Hg. Ventilation is continued with a FIO_2 of 40% and a PEEP of 3 to 5 cm H_2O. The donor is heparinized with 30,000 units. Cannulation of the aorta and main pulmonary artery is performed, with care taken to ensure adequate flow to both branches of the pulmonary artery during pulmonary plegia.[47] The superior vena cava is ligated and a transverse incision is made across the inferior vena cava. After the heart is allowed to empty, the aortic cross-clamp is applied, and 10 mL/kg of cold crystalloid cardioplegia, commonly the Stanford formulation, is rapidly infused into the aortic root with the bag under pressure at 150 mm Hg. The inferior vena cava is incised, and the left atrial appendage is amputated to avoid cardiac distention. Although the antegrade cardioplegia is being delivered, Perfadex (Vitrolife Inc., Englewood, CO) is rapidly flushed into the main pulmonary artery at a rate of 15 mL/kg/min for 4 minutes. Ice-cold saline or Physiosol solution (Abbott Laboratories, North Chicago, IL) is immediately poured over the heart and lungs. During the cardioplegic and Perfadex infusions, ventilation is maintained with half-normal tidal volumes of room air.

After delivery of plegic solutions, the lungs are deflated and the great vessels are divided. The heart is reflected anteriorly and a left atriotomy is performed, leaving a 2-cm cuff of atrium around the pulmonary vein orifices. Once this division is complete, the heart is removed from the chest. The lung bloc is then dissected free along the pre-esophageal plane above the level of the carina. The lungs are inflated and the trachea is stapled at the highest possible point. If needed, the bilateral lung bloc can be further separated into left and right lung blocs. The left atrial cuff containing the orifices of the pulmonary veins is divided in half vertically. The left and right pulmonary arteries are divided at their junction. Finally, the left mainstem bronchus is stapled near its junction with the trachea.

Once removed from the donor, grafts are wrapped in sterile gauze pads and immersed in ice-cold saline at 2 to 4°C in several sterile plastic bags placed within a sterile plastic container. This, in turn, is placed in an ice-filled chest and transported to the transplant center.

Organ Preservation and Transport

The principal goal of preservation is to minimize injury to the allograft from ischemia and reperfusion.[48] Ischemia-reperfusion injury is mediated by reactive oxygen species, which disrupt the homeostatic mechanisms in myocytes and endothelial cells. As receptors for leukocyte adhesion molecules are upregulated and leukocyte chemotactic factors released, an inflammatory response ensues, leading to cellular injury. Several approaches for minimizing ischemia-reperfusion injury have developed, including donor pretreatment, use of specialized preservation solutions, and recipient treatments.

Hypothermia is considered by many to be the most important method of organ preservation. It works by reducing tissue metabolic demand by up to 99%. During explantation, organs are flushed with cold plegic solutions (0 to 10°C, depending on the institution and solution employed). Organs are stored at 0 to 10°C, and during implantation they are covered with gauze soaked in saline slush or recipients are cooled through CPB.

A variety of crystalloid pulmonary artery flush solutions are used worldwide, and they can be divided into two categories based on their electrolyte compositions: intracellular and extracellular. Intracellular solutions contain moderate to high concentrations of potassium and little calcium and sodium. Euro-Collins, University of Wisconsin (UW), and Cardiazol are examples. Extracellular solutions contain high concentrations of sodium and low to moderate concentrations of potassium. Low-potassium dextran is an example of this type of solution (eg, Perfadex). Although Euro-Collins is the most frequently used preservation solution, there is a growing body of evidence in support of low potassium, dextran-containing extracellular solutions.[49–51]

Prostaglandins are commonly used for donor pretreatment and as an additive in pulmonary flush solutions. The administration of PGE_1 (a potent vasodilator) counteracts reflex pulmonary vasoconstriction induced by the cold flush and permits uniform distribution of perfusate throughout the lung. Studies in large animals also suggest that PGE_1 treatment may minimize reperfusion injury through its anti-inflammatory properties.[52] Another commonly used pretreatment strategy is steroid treatment. Administration of intravenous methylprednisone to the donor inactivates lymphocytes, which are thought to mediate ischemic lung graft injury.

Studies suggest that lung graft function is improved when the explanted organ is inflated, 100% oxygen is used for the inflation, and transport is carried out at 10°C.[53] Research in the field of lung preservation has recently focused on the role of various flush and storage solution additives, such as antioxidants, which may act as free radical scavengers. Other additives shown to decrease reperfusion injury in research models include nitric oxide donors and phosphodiesterase inhibitors. Areas of ongoing research include the development of leukocyte depletion strategies, examining the role of gene therapy to modify donor organ susceptibility to ischemia-reperfusion injury, and the development of colloid-based perfusates.

These preservation techniques, coupled with streamlined donor and recipient protocols, have permitted procurements as far as 1000 miles from the transplant center. Extensive communication and coordination must be maintained between the organ procurement agency, donor-recipient operative teams, medical centers, and abdominal procurement teams. Worldwide, the major procurement agencies include the United Network for Organ Sharing (UNOS) in the United States, Multiple Organ Retrieval (MORE) in Canada, and the EURO Transplant Organization in Europe.

Recipient Operation

The recipient operation proceeds in two phases. The first is excision of the native organ(s) and the second is implantation of the allograft. Cardiopulmonary bypass is occasionally required for lung transplantation. Regardless, CPB should be available as standby at all times. At Stanford, we have favored the use of CPB during bilateral lung transplantation for a variety of reasons. There is improved exposure of the hilar structures, which is particularly helpful in patients with dense adhesions and bronchial collaterals. CPB allows for early pneumonectomies without hemodynamic or respiratory instability, and ischemic time of the second lung is substantially reduced compared with off-CPB bilateral lung transplants. Its use also prevents overperfusion of the first lung graft with the entire cardiac output. In patients with suppurative lung disease, the use of CPB facilitates careful washout of the distal trachea and proximal bronchi to prevent contamination of the first implanted lung. Others prefer to avoid CPB, as it may be associated with increased blood loss, transfusion needs, and reperfusion injury. More detailed experimental and clinical studies are needed to resolve these questions. At present, the need for CBP should be determined on a case-by-case basis.

Anesthetic monitoring includes arterial pressure monitoring, pulse oximetry, continuous electrocardiography, pulmonary artery catheter monitoring, temperature monitoring, and urine output monitoring. The use of double-lumen endotracheal tubes is particularly helpful, allowing for single lung ventilation during certain portions of the dissection. Large-bore intravenous lines are placed for volume infusion. Transesophageal echocardiography is often performed during the procedure.

Single Lung Transplantation

If possible, the poorer functioning lung (as determined by preoperative ventilation-perfusion scan) is selected for replacement. The patient is placed in a standard thoracotomy position with access to the groin, should CPB be needed. A posterolateral thoracotomy is made at the level of the fourth or fifth intercostal space. Adhesions are lysed and the hilar dissection performed. The pulmonary artery, the superior and inferior pulmonary veins, and the mainstem bronchus are isolated. A trial occlusion of the pulmonary artery is used to determine whether the procedure can be conducted without CPB. If the occlusion is tolerated, the pulmonary artery is ligated and divided distal to the upper lobe branch. The pulmonary veins are also ligated and divided. The mainstem bronchus is stapled and divided, and the native lung is explanted.

The donor lung is removed from its transport container and prepared for implantation. The donor bronchus is opened and secretions are aspirated and cultured. The bronchus is trimmed, leaving two cartilaginous rings proximal to the orifice of the upper lobe. Any remaining pericardial and lymphatic tissue is removed, and the left atrial cuff is trimmed as needed. The donor lung is then placed in the recipient's chest and covered with saline slush and iced laparotomy pads.

The sequence of anastomoses is a matter of preference, although most perform the deepest anastomosis (the bronchial anastomosis) first and then proceed to the more superficial ones. The bronchial anastomosis is fashioned with 4-0 polypropylene suture. We favor a continuous suture technique for the entire anastomosis, although the membranous portion can be sewn with interrupted suture. Variations on the end-to-end bronchial anastomosis include the use of a telescoping technique, in which the donor bronchus is intussuscepted into the recipient bronchus, and an omental pedicle flap is placed around the anastomosis. These techniques were developed to prevent bronchial anastomotic dehiscence but are now rarely performed.

Once the bronchial anastomosis is complete, attention is turned to the anastomoses of the pulmonary veins. A side-biting clamp is applied to the left atrium to include the pulmonary veins. The recipient pulmonary vein stumps are opened and the intervening atrial tissue is cut. This creates a cuff that is anastomosed to the donor atrial remnant using continuous 4-0 polypropylene suture. (This suture is not tied down until reperfusion.) Donor and recipient pulmonary arteries are anastomosed with 5-0 polypropylene suture. Arteries must be trimmed to an appropriate length before fashioning the anastomosis, because kinking can occur upon graft inflation if the vessels are left too long. The pulmonary artery anastomosis is then deaired. The lung is inflated, and the pulmonary artery clamp is temporarily released to allow flushing of air through the atrial suture line. The left atrial clamp is removed to allow retrograde de-airing of the atrial anastomosis. The pulmonary venous anastomosis is then secured.

After hemostasis is ensured, apical and basal chest tubes are inserted. The ribs are reapproximated and the chest is closed in standard fashion. The double lumen endotracheal tube is exchanged for a single lumen tube and bronchoscopy is performed to evaluate the bronchial anastomosis.

Bilateral Lung Transplantation

Bilateral lung transplantation is performed as sequential single lung transplants. Although the traditional approach to this technique has been to access the chest via bilateral anterior thoracosternotomy (clamshell) incisions, we have recently transitioned our practice to a median sternotomy approach. The lung with the least amount of function (as determined by a preoperative ventilation-perfusion scan) is removed first and replaced with an allograft as described for single lung transplantation above. Once ventilation and perfusion are established in the first allograft, the remaining lung is explanted and the second allograft is implanted. Bilateral chest tubes are placed and the chest is closed. Bronchoscopy is performed to evaluate the bronchial anastomoses.

Although single lung transplants are usually performed off CBP, the majority of double lung transplants are still performed on-pump. The use of CPB allows for improved exposure, shorter graft ischemic times, controlled reperfusion, and the use of leukocyte-depleting filters. As the risk of bleeding may be increased with CPB, strategies have been developed to minimize the chance of hemorrhage. These include the use of heparin-coated CPB circuits as well as the argon beam coagulator. Despite these maneuvers, there remains considerable risk associated with CPB, and many centers prefer to perform all lung transplants off-pump if possible.

Postoperative Management

Graft Physiology

Denervation of the lungs results in a diminished cough reflex and impairment of mucociliary clearance mechanisms. This predisposes recipients to pulmonary infections and necessitates aggressive postoperative pulmonary toilet.[54] Moreover, in the transplanted lung, ischemia-reperfusion injury, along with disrupted pulmonary lymphatics may result in increased vascular permeability with varying degrees of interstitial edema.

Clinical Management in the Early Postoperative Period

Early postoperative management centers around careful fluid balance and ventilatory management. The primary objective in the immediate postoperative period is to maintain adequate perfusion and gas exchange while minimizing intravenous fluid administration, cardiac work, and barotrauma. Barotrauma and high airway pressures can compromise bronchial mucosal flow. Therefore, lower tidal volumes and flow rates may be necessary to limit peak airway pressures to less than 40 cm H_2O. After arrival in the ICU, ventilator settings are adjusted every 30 minutes to achieve an arterial PO_2 greater than 75 mm Hg on an FIO_2 of 40%, an arterial carbon dioxide pressure ($PaCO_2$) between 30 and 40 mm Hg, and a pH between 7.35 and 7.45. Pulmonary toilet with endotracheal suctioning is an effective means of reducing mucus plugging and atelectasis. Ventilatory weaning is initiated after the patient is stable, awake, and alert, with extubation typically achieved within 24 hours. Subsequent pulmonary care consists of vigorous diuresis, supplemental oxygen for several days, continued aggressive pulmonary toilet, incentive spirometry, and serial chest x-rays.

A diffuse interstitial infiltrate is often found on early postoperative chest x-rays. Previously referred to as a *reimplantation response*, this finding is better defined as graft edema owing to inadequate preservation, reperfusion injury, or early rejection.[55] It appears that the degree of pulmonary edema is inversely related to the quality of preservation. Judicious administration of fluid and loop diuretics is required to maintain fluid balance and minimize this pulmonary edema.

Early lung graft dysfunction occurs in less than 15% of transplants, and is manifest as persistent marginal gas exchange without evidence of infection or rejection.[56] This primary graft failure often results from ischemia-reperfusion injury and histologically evident as diffuse alveolar damage. Of course, technical causes of graft failure such as pulmonary venous anastomotic stenosis or thrombosis must always be considered. In cases of persistent, severe pulmonary graft dysfunction refractory to mechanical ventilatory maneuvers, extracorporeal membrane oxygenation (ECMO)[57] and inhaled nitric oxide[58] have been used successfully to stabilize gas exchange. Urgent retransplantation can also be considered if other interventions fail.

Immunosuppressive Management: Early and Late Postoperative Regimens

Immunosuppression protocols vary from center to center. At the Stanford University Hospital, we typically administer induction therapy of either rabbit antithymocyte globulin (RATG) at a dose of 1.5 mg/kg on POD 1, 2, 3, 5, and 7 or daclizumab at 1mg/kg (first dose given in OR then every other week for four additional doses). For highly sensitized patients, plasmapheresis with a 1:1.5 volume exchange with fresh-frozen plasma (FFP) is performed intraoperatively, along with intravenous immunoglobulin (IVIG), which is started at 2 g/kg before releasing the cross-clamp. Methylprednisolone is given at 500 mg IV after protamine administration, and a stat retrospective crossmatch is performed.

On POD 1, T and B cell subset counts are performed and if the cytotoxic crossmatch is positive, RATG is given in 2 doses at 0.75 mg/kg. If the crossmatch is negative or pulmonary edema is present or expected from RATG, daclizumab is administered at 1 mg/kg and repeated every 14 days for a total of five doses. Methylprednisolone is given at 125 mg IV every 8 hours for 3 doses, CellCept is given at 500 mg PO BID, and Prograf is given at 0.5 mg BID and titrated to a level of 12 to 15 ng/mL. On POD 2, prednisone is started at 0.5 mg/kg PO BID. Hereafter, the patient is maintained on prednisone, Prograf, and CellCept. For sensitized patients, plasmapheresis is repeated in a 1:1.5 volume exchange with 1/2 5% albumin and 1/2 FFP. If the patient was given RATG, a second dose of 0.75 mg/kg is administered. Otherwise, IVIG 100 mg/kg is given. Plasmapheresis is repeated on POD 3 and 4, along with IVIG at 100 mg/kg. Plasmapheresis is completed on POD 5, with administration of IVIG at 1 g/kg on POD 5 and 6. A donor specific antibody (DSA) is sent before IVIG on POD 5 and after IVIG on POD 6. Finally, on POD 7 T and B cell subset counts are measured (and repeated weekly thereafter) along with administration of Rituximab for two doses with one dose of 375 mg/m^2 given at POD 7 and a second dose given a week later.

Infection Prophylaxis

Antiviral and antifungal prophylaxis remain important components of the postoperative management strategy in heart-lung and lung transplant recipients. Many centers employ cytomegalovirus prophylaxis (CMV) with ganciclovir for any CMV-positive recipient and in any CMV-negative recipient receiving an allograft from a CMV-positive donor. Ganciclovir is typically given for a several week course, and can be associated with leukopenia. Some patients may require G-CSF if their white blood cell count falls below 4000. Fungal prophylaxis against mucosal candida infection includes use of itraconazole and nystatin swish and swallow. *Pneumocystis carinii* prophylaxis consists of trimethoprim-sulfamethoxazole or aerosolized pentamidine. In the immediate postoperative period, *Aspergillus* colonization is inhibited by the use of aerosolized amphotericin B. For *Toxoplasma*-negative recipients of grafts from *Toxoplasma*-positive patients, pyrimethamine prophylaxis is maintained for the first 6 months after transplantation.

Graft Surveillance: Patient Follow-up Schedule

Routine clinical follow-up is required to monitor graft function and modify immunosuppressive regimens. Regular surveillance protocols developed to monitor graft function typically consist of serial pulmonary function tests, arterial blood gases, and bronchoscopic evaluation. Surveillance is usually conducted at 2, 4 to 6, and 12 weeks, followed by 6 months after transplantation and yearly thereafter. Transbronchial biopsies are obtained from each transplanted lung, and lavage specimens are submitted for staining (ie, Gram, fungal, acid-fast bacillus, silver), culture, and cytology. In addition to routine surveillance, follow-up is often needed to address changes in clinical status. Complications related to transplantation are many, and these must be addressed carefully and expediently to prevent long-term graft failure.

Postoperative Complications

Early morbidity and mortality after lung transplantation (within 30 days of operation or before initial discharge from hospital) are most commonly a result of primary graft failure or infection. Late mortality is most commonly caused by obliterative bronchiolitis or infection.[59] Causes of death at various time points after transplantation have been compiled by the ISHLT and are presented in Fig. 65-4.

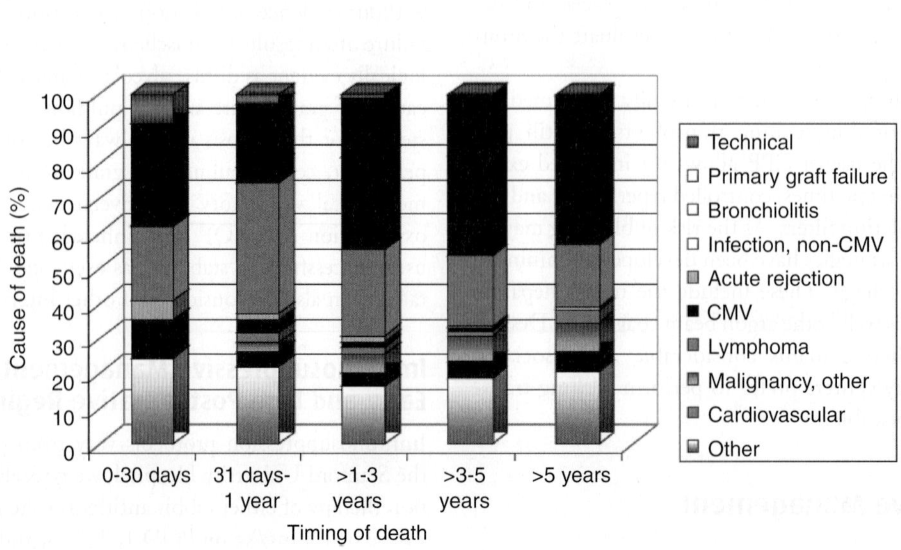

FIGURE 65-4 Causes of death at various periods after isolated lung transplantation. (*Adapted from Trulock EP, Edwards LB, Taylor DO, et al: Registry of the International Society for Heart and Lung Transplantation: Twenty-Second Official Adult Lung and Heart-Lung-Transplant Report—2005. J Heart Lung Transplant 2005; 24[8]:956-967 with permission from Elsevier Science.*)

Hemorrhage

Perioperative hemorrhage is an infrequent but significant cause of early death in heart-lung and lung transplantation. The majority of perioperative hemorrhagic complications stem from operating in the midst of dense adhesions caused by previous operations or inflammation from chronic lung infection. As mentioned previously, meticulous attention to hemostasis is mandatory, and all available means should be used to achieve a dry field on completion of the operation.

Hyperacute Rejection

ABO matching of donor and recipient has decreased the rate of hyperacute rejection. This complication, which is almost universally fatal, is mediated by preformed antibodies in the recipient that recognize antigens on the donor vascular endothelium. This humoral immune response results in activation of inflammatory and coagulation cascades, resulting in extensive thrombosis of graft vessels and subsequent graft failure.[68] To reduce the incidence of hyperacute rejection, a prospective crossmatch should be performed in recipients with a PRA greater than 25%.

Early Graft Dysfunction and Primary Graft Failure

Graft dysfunction in the first few days after transplantation is common. It is often referred to as the "reimplantation response," manifest by abnormal lung function, pulmonary edema, and pulmonary infiltrates on chest x-ray. This phenomenon is thought to be linked to ischemia and reperfusion. Other contributing factors may also include allograft contusion, inadequate preservation, or use of cardiopulmonary bypass during transplantation. Although most cases are mild and resolve with supportive care, some progress to primary graft failure. Reported rates of primary graft failure following lung transplantation range between 10 and 15%. Treatment may include the use of ECMO and inhaled nitric oxide (NO). Unfortunately, primary graft failure is associated with a mortality of more than 60%.[56]

Acute Rejection

As in cardiac transplantation, the majority of acute rejection episodes occur within the first year after transplant at a rate of 36%.[1] Despite its prevalence, death is very rarely a direct consequence of acute rejection. It is recognized, however, that the number and severity of acute rejection episodes is a risk factor for ultimately developing obliterative bronchiolitis.

Diagnosis of acute rejection in the early posttransplant period is often based on clinical parameters. Symptoms and signs of rejection include fever, dyspnea, impaired gas exchange (manifest as a decrease in arterial Po_2), a diminished forced expiratory volume during 1 second (FEV_1, a measure of airway flow), a fall in vital capacity (VC), and the development of characteristic bilateral interstitial infiltrates on chest x-ray (Fig. 65-5). After the first postoperative month, the chest x-ray is frequently normal during episodes of acute rejection, placing greater emphasis on other clinical parameters characteristic of rejection.

It is often difficult to distinguish between the diagnosis of acute lung rejection and pulmonary infection based on clinical findings alone. It is of paramount importance to distinguish between acute rejection and infection before initiating therapy.

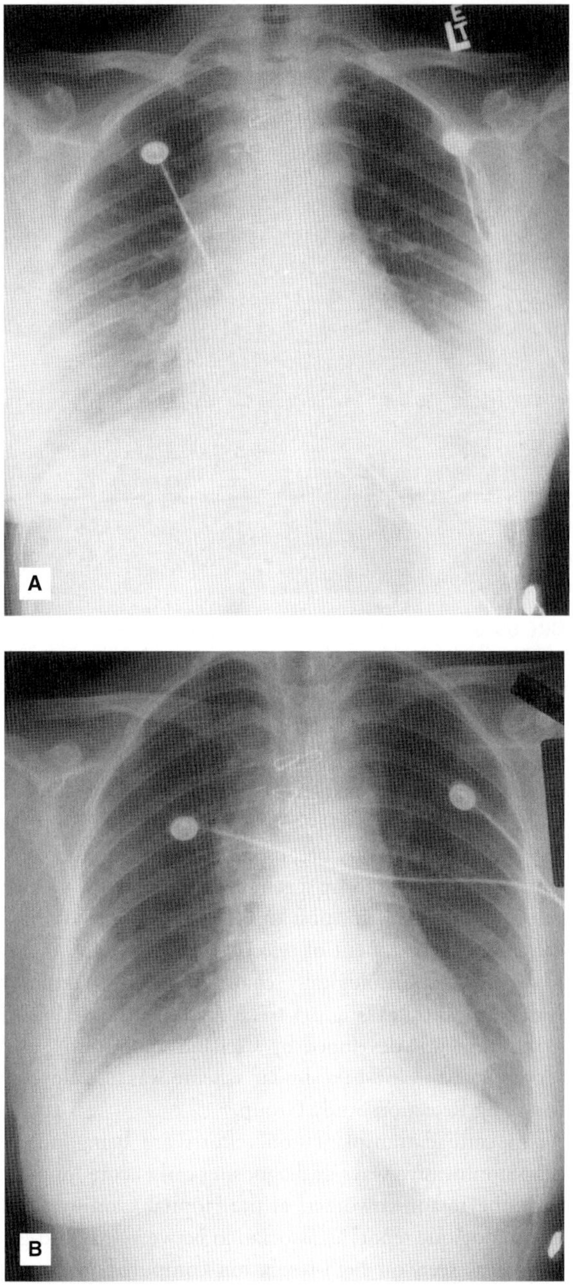

FIGURE 65-5 Acute and resolving lung rejection. (A) Chest radiograph illustrates bilateral infiltrates characteristic of acute pulmonary rejection. (B) Follow-up radiograph after pulsed methylprednisolone treatment of acute rejection demonstrating resolution of infiltrates.

Fiberoptic bronchoscopy (with transbronchial parenchymal lung biopsy and bronchoalveolar lavage) is the gold standard for the diagnosis of acute lung rejection and pulmonary infection. At least five biopsy specimens are taken from the lung allografts along with bronchoalveolar lavage, which is evaluated for cytology, undergoes microbial staining, and is cultured.[60] In addition to performing bronchoscopy with transbronchial biopsy in response to changes in clinical status and graft performance, most centers maintain a schedule of surveillance biopsies for lung recipients. Interestingly, surveillance bronchoscopy

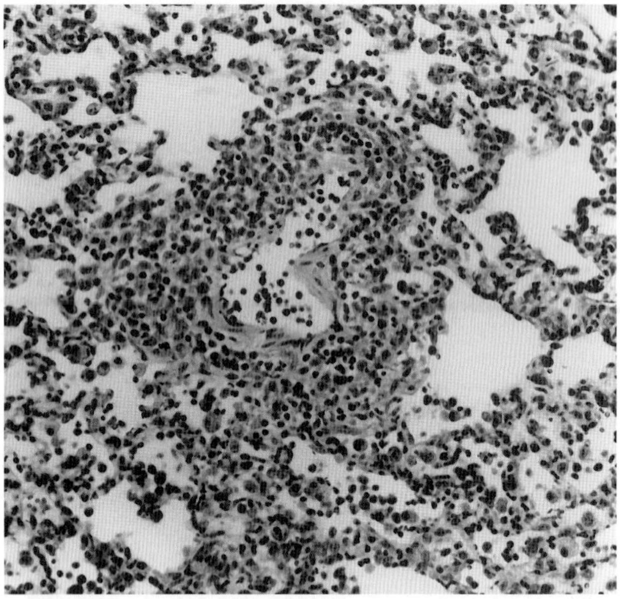

FIGURE 65-6 Moderate acute lung rejection. Moderate rejection is characterized by perivascular mononuclear cell infiltrates with extension into the adjacent alveolar septa (H&E stain; ×200).

reveals occult rejection or infection in 17 to 25% of transbronchial biopsy specimens from asymptomatic recipients. For patients undergoing bronchoscopy because of a change in clinical condition, 50 to 72% of biopsy specimens have shown evidence of rejection or infection. In most cases, positive biopsies directly guide successful treatment of rejection or infection.[61,62] Acute lung rejection is histologically characterized by lymphocytic perivascular infiltrates (Fig. 65-6). A grading scheme for acute lung rejection was developed by Clelland and Colin[63] and is presented in Table 65-6; a similar scheme was also developed by the Lung Rejection Study Group.[60]

As in cardiac transplantation, efforts are being made to develop noninvasive ways of diagnosing early acute lung rejection. Loubeyre and coworkers at the Hôpital Cardiovasculaire et Pneumologique report an association between "ground-glass" density areas seen on high-resolution computed tomography (HRCT) and histologically confirmed acute lung rejection in heart-lung transplant recipients.[64] They found that ground-glass opacities on HRCT had a sensitivity of 65% for detecting lung rejection and a specificity of 85% for detecting an acute lung complication.

TABLE 65-6 Grading System for Acute Lung Rejection

Grade	Histologic Appearance (Transbronchial Biopsy)
0	No significant inflammation; normal specimen
1	Small, infrequent perivascular infiltrates with or without bronchiolar lymphocytic infiltrates
2	Larger, more frequent perivascular lymphocytic infiltrates with or without moderate bronchiolar lymphocytic inflammation; occasional neutrophils and eosinophils
3	Extension of infiltrates into alveolar septa and alveolar spaces with or without bronchiolar mucosal ulceration

Treatment strategies for rejection involve augmentation of immunosuppression. At most institutions, the timing and severity of rejection episodes dictate therapy. A typical algorithm is shown in Fig. 65-7. Rejection episodes that are graded moderate or severe are treated with a "steroid pulse" (intravenous methylprednisolone 500 to 1000 mg/d for 3 consecutive days), followed by augmentation of the oral prednisone maintenance dose to 0.6 mg/kg/d. This maintenance dose is then tapered to 0.2 mg/kg/d over 3 to 4 weeks. Clinical and radiographic improvement (see Fig. 65-5B) after steroid therapy is often dramatic, rapid, and considered confirmatory of rejection. Mild episodes are initially treated by increasing oral prednisone dose, followed by a gradual taper over 3 to 4 weeks. Transbronchial biopsies are repeated 10 to 14 days following antirejection therapy to assess efficacy. Recurrent rejection episodes may be treated by a second steroid pulse and taper. Acute rejection refractory to steroid therapy may be treated with antilymphocyte preparations. Alternatively, primary immunosuppression may be switched between cyclosporine- and tacrolimus-based therapy. Finally, in especially difficult cases of persistent rejection, total lymphoid irradiation (TLI) may be useful.[65]

Chronic Rejection

Chronic lung allograft rejection poses the greatest limitation to the long-term benefits of lung transplantation. Chronic lung rejection most commonly presents as obliterative bronchiolitis (OB). The onset of OB typically occurs after the first 6 months to 1 year after transplantation, with a steadily increasing incidence thereafter. Recent data demonstrate that 70% of lung recipients are diagnosed with OB by the fifth postoperative year.[66]

Transbronchial biopsies remain the "gold standard" for diagnosing OB. The sensitivity of transbronchial biopsy for detecting OB has been reported between 17 and 87%.[62,67] Diagnostic yield of the biopsy procedure is related to the number of specimens taken, and current recommendations advise taking at least five specimens from each transplanted lung. Clearly, OB is a patchy process and therefore a large number of samples will be falsely negative owing to sampling error.

OB is a histologic diagnosis and is characterized by dense eosinophilic, submucosal scar tissue that partially or totally obliterates the lumen of small (2-mm) airways, particularly the terminal and respiratory bronchioles (Fig. 65-8). The physiologic consequences are decreased arterial P_{O_2}, FEV_1, FEF_{25-75} forced expiratory flow at 25 to 75% (midrange) of lung volumes, and FEF_{50}/FVC (ratio of FEF_{50} to forced vital capacity). A characteristic "bowing" of the expiratory limb of the flow-volume loop has also been associated with OB. Clinical symptoms may be nonspecific, and include cough and dyspnea with or without exertion. The term *bronchiolitis obliterans syndrome* (BOS) was developed to refer to patients who have clinical manifestations of obliterative bronchiolitis with or without proven histologic characteristics (Table 65-7). A standardized working formulation

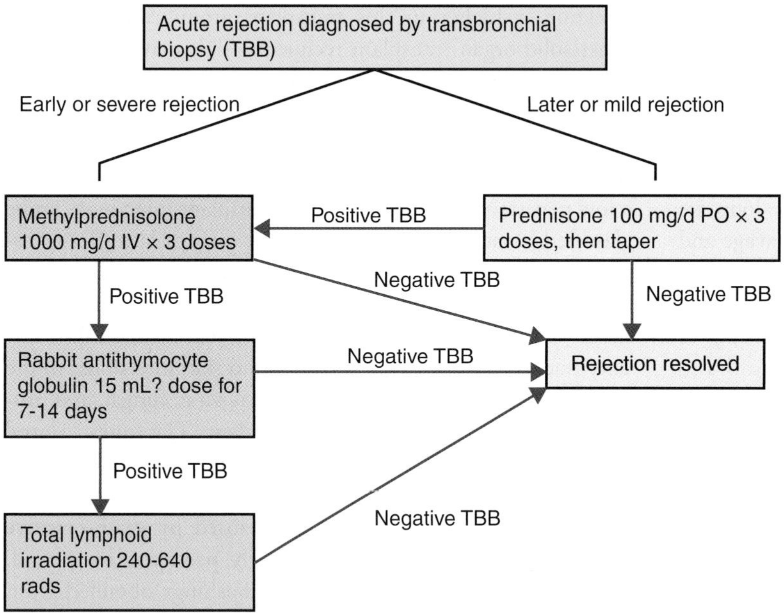

FIGURE 65-7 Typical algorithm for treating acute rejection in heart-lung and lung transplant recipients.

for the clinical staging of BOS was established by the ISHLT and is based on the ratio of the current FEV_1 to the best post-transplant FEV_1. Patients with a decline of 20% or greater in their FEV_1 (in the absence of infection or other process) are diagnosed with BOS, irrespective of pathologic evidence of obliterative bronchiolitis.[68]

Valentine and the Stanford group reported that measurements of small airway function (ie, FEF_{25-75}, FEF_{50}/FVC) are more sensitive indicators of BOS than the FEV_1 in bilateral lung transplant recipients.[66] An FEF_{50}/FVC persistently below 0.7 for 6 consecutive weeks was the most sensitive predictor of OB. Approximately 50% of bilateral lung recipients with biopsy-proven OB developed a fall in their FEF_{50}/FVC nearly 4 months before fulfilling the ISHLT working group criteria for BOS.

Experimental and clinical evidence suggests that the etiology of OB stems from the injury of the bronchial epithelium by one or more mechanisms. These include gastroesophageal reflux disease (GERD), infection (particularly CMV), chronic inflammation owing to impaired mucociliary clearance, and immunologic mechanisms.[55] These insults result in airway epithelial damage and, subsequently, an exaggerated healing response. Along with this injury, there is increased expression of major histocompatibility class II antigens in the bronchial epithelium. In a recent meta-analysis, Sharples and coworkers found that acute rejection is a risk factor for later development of OB.[69] In keeping with this finding is the association between BOS and decreased levels of immunosuppression (as may occur with noncompliance). Lymphocytic bronchitis and bronchiolitis were also closely associated with development of OB. CMV pneumonitis, other pulmonary infections, and HLA mismatching are also linked to the development of OB in small retrospective studies. Novick and coworkers recently reported on the relationship between OB, donor age, and graft ischemic times.[43] Using data from the ISHLT registry, they found a higher rate of OB at 3 years in recipients of grafts from donors greater than age 55 who were also subjected to 6 to 8 hours of ischemia. GERD has been recently proposed as a mechanism for the development of OB.[70] Up to 75% of patients have demonstrable postoperative reflux based on pH studies, which may result from intraoperative vagal damage, impaired cough and airway mucociliary clearance, immunosuppression, or preexisting GERD.[71] These patients have been shown to demonstrate a survival benefit as well as delayed onset of BOS after antireflux surgery in the postoperative setting.[72,73]

The current management of OB hinges on prevention, close surveillance, and immediate therapeutic intervention when patients become symptomatic or asymptomatic physiologic changes occur. Patients are encouraged to perform incentive spirometry

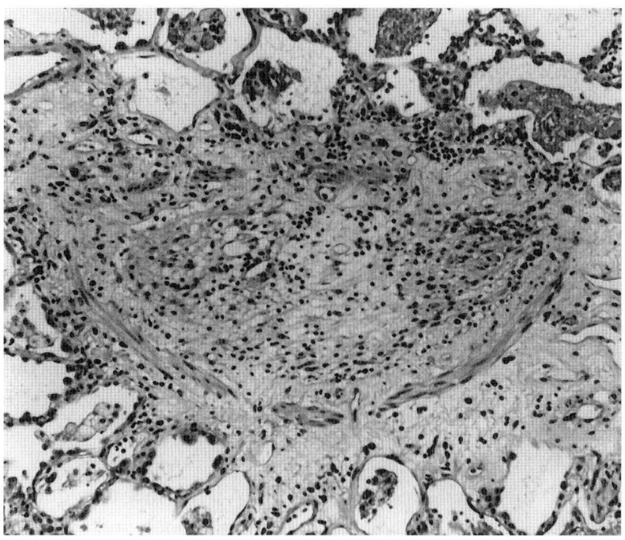

FIGURE 65-8 Bronchiolitis obliterans. Chronic airway rejection is characterized by luminal narrowing or replacement by dense eosinophilic collagenous scar tissue. Inflammatory cells may be seen in this case (H&E stain; ×150).

TABLE 65-7 Working formulation for bronchiolitis obliterans syndrome

$0_{a\ or\ b}$	No significant abnormality: FEV_1 80% of baseline
$1_{a\ or\ b}$	Mild bronchiolitis obliterans syndrome: FEV_1 66–80% of baseline
$2_{a\ or\ b}$	Moderate bronchiolitis obliterans syndrome: FEV_1 51–65% of baseline
$3_{a\ or\ b}$	Severe bronchiolitis obliterans syndrome: FEV_1 50% of baseline

a = Without pathologic evidence of obliterative bronchiolitis; b = with pathologic evidence of obliterative bronchiolitis.

to prevent microatelectasis of lungs that are deprived of native innervation, lack bronchial circulation, and have impaired mucociliary clearance mechanisms. Moreover, all recipients are instructed to contact their transplant center or primary care physician on development of respiratory tract symptoms so that pulmonary function tests can be performed. Any alterations in FEF_{25-75}, FEF_{50}/FVC, or specific changes in the flow-volume loop are indications for bronchoscopy with bronchoalveolar lavage and transbronchial biopsy, especially in the absence of infectious bronchitis or pulmonary edema.

Augmentation of immunosuppression is the mainstay of therapy for BOS. The prednisone dose is increased to 0.6 to 1.0 mg/kg/d and slowly tapered to 0.2 mg/kg/d while concomitantly optimizing cyclosporine and azathioprine dosing. Ganciclovir is reinstituted during treatment for those patients at risk of reactivation CMV infection, and antimicrobial therapy is directed against any organisms isolated from bronchoalveolar lavage. Follow-up pulmonary function tests are performed. Pulmonary function can be stabilized in most patients, but significant improvement is uncommon. Unfortunately, relapse rates are greater than 50% and progressive pulmonary failure or infection because of increased immunosuppression are the most common causes of death in lung transplant patients after the second year.

Retransplantation is the only option for terminal respiratory failure secondary to OB. Although survival for patients undergoing retransplantation for OB is better than for those undergoing retransplantation for other reasons, it is still worse than survival of first-time transplant recipients. Novick and coworkers recently reported results from the Pulmonary Retransplant Registry.[30] They reviewed survival rates in 237 patients who underwent pulmonary retransplantation between 1985 and 1996. At 1, 2, and 3 years after retransplantation, survival was 47, 40, and 33%, respectively. Survival was higher in nonventilated, ambulatory patients and their freedom for OB was comparable to first-time transplant recipients. The authors conclude that pulmonary retransplantation should only be performed in carefully selected recipients who have a reasonable likelihood of long-term survival.

Airway Complications

Improvements in surgical technique and posttransplant management have resulted in a relatively low incidence of airway complications after lung transplantation. Nevertheless, up to 27% of cases are complicated by stenosis, necrosis, or dehiscence.[75] The avoidance of perioperative steroids has long been considered important in preventing airway complications. However, recent experimental and clinical evidence suggests that the detrimental effect of steroids may be overestimated.[76] The most common airway complications are partial anastomotic dehiscence and stricture. Such complications are usually diagnosed by bronchoscopy. Airway dehiscence is treated by reoperation or close observation and supportive care. Strictures are treated by balloon or bougie dilatation, often with stent placement.

Infection

Bacterial, viral, and fungal infections are leading causes of morbidity and mortality in lung transplantation. The rate of infection is higher in this transplant group compared with other solid organ transplant recipients. This may be related to the lung allograft's direct exposure to airway colonization and aspiration, as well as its impaired cough reflex and mucociliary clearance. The risk of infection and infection-related death peaks in the first few months after transplantation, declining to a low persistent rate thereafter. Posttransplant infections can be classified broadly into those that occur early or late after transplantation. Early infections, occurring within the first month after transplantation, are commonly bacterial (especially gram-negative bacilli) and manifest as pneumonia, mediastinitis, urinary tract infections, catheter sepsis, and skin infections. In the late posttransplant period, opportunistic viral, fungal, and protozoan pathogens become more prevalent. The lungs, central nervous system, gastrointestinal tract, and skin are the usual sites of invasion.

Bacterial infections, particularly caused by gram-negative bacteria, predominate during the early postoperative period. Between 75 and 97% of bronchial washings obtained from donor lungs before organ retrieval culture at least one organism.[77] Posttransplant invasive infections are frequently caused by organisms cultured from the donor. Conversely, bacterial infections developing in patients with septic lung disease, particularly cystic fibrosis, most commonly originate from the recipient's airways and sinuses. Treatment of bacterial infections generally involves characterization of the infective agent (eg, cultures, antibiotic sensitivities), source control (eg, catheter removal, debridement), and appropriate antibiotic regimens.

CMV infection occurs most often at 1 to 3 months after transplantation and presents either as a primary infection or reactivation of a latent infection. By definition, primary infection results when a previously seronegative recipient is infected through contact with tissue or blood from a seropositive individual. The donor organ itself is thought to be the most common vector of primary CMV infections. Reactivation infection occurs when a recipient who is seropositive prior to transplant develops clinical CMV infection during immunosuppressive therapy. Seropositive recipients are also subject to infection by new strains of CMV. Primary infection in previously seronegative recipients is generally more serious than reactivation or reinfection in seropositive patients.

Clinically, CMV infection has protean manifestations, including leukopenia with fever, pneumonia, gastroenteritis, hepatitis, and retinitis. CMV pneumonitis is the most lethal of these, with 13% mortality, and retinitis remains the most refractory to treatment. Diagnosis of CMV infection is made by direct culture of the virus from blood, urine, or tissue specimens, a fourfold increase in antibody titers from baseline, or characteristic histologic changes (ie, markedly enlarged cells and nuclei containing basophilic inclusion bodies). Most cases respond to ganciclovir and hyperimmune globulin.

CMV has been implicated as a trigger for OB69 as well as an inhibitor of cell-mediated immunity. CMV negative donors comprise less than 20% of the donor organ pool, and owing to organ scarcity, most transplant centers perform transplants across CMV serologic barriers using ganciclovir and/or hyperimmune globulin prophylactic protocols in CMV-positive donors and/or recipients. A study by Valantine and coworkers found that the combined use of ganciclovir and hyperimmune globulin was superior to ganciclovir alone as prophylaxis against CMV. Moreover, the ganciclovir/hyperimmune globulin cohort had longer survival at 3 years and greater freedom from obliterative bronchiolitis.[78]

Invasive fungal infections peak in frequency between 10 days and 2 months after transplantation. Treatment consists of fluconazole, itraconazole, or amphotericin B. Reichenspurner and coworkers have reported that the actuarial incidence and linearized rate of fungal infections were significantly reduced in recipients who received inhaled amphotericin prophylaxis.[79]

The institution of prophylaxis with oral trimethoprim-sulfamethoxazole (or inhalational pentamidine for sulfa-allergic patients) has effectively prevented *Pneumocystis carinii* pneumonia. The risk of *Pneumocystis* infection is highest during the first year after transplant. However, as infections can also occur late after transplant, most centers recommend prophylactic therapy be continued for life.

Infection prophylaxis is comprised of vaccinations, perioperative broad-spectrum antibiotics, and long-term prophylactic antibiotics. Pretransplant inoculations with pneumococcal and hepatitis B vaccines, as well as DPT boosters, are recommended. All transplant recipients should receive annual influenza vaccinations. Although perioperative antibiotic regimens vary widely between transplant centers, first-generation cephalosporins (eg, cefazolin) or vancomycin are commonly used. Long-term prophylaxis typically includes nystatin mouthwash, trimethoprim-sulfamethoxazole, aerosolized amphotericin B, and antivirals such as acyclovir or ganciclovir.

Neoplasm

Transplant recipients have a higher incidence of neoplasia than that of the general population.[80] This is undoubtedly due to chronic immunosuppression. Recipients are predisposed to a variety of tumors, including skin cancer, B-cell lymphoproliferative disorders, carcinoma in situ of the cervix, carcinoma of the vulva and anus, and Kaposi's sarcoma. On average, tumors appear approximately 5 years after transplantation.[59]

The incidence of B-cell lymphoproliferative disorders in transplant patients is a staggering 350 times greater than that of the normal age-matched population. Posttransplant lymphoproliferative disorder (PTLD) has been reported in 6% of lung transplant recipients.[81] PTLD most commonly occurs within the first year after transplantation, and is associated with Epstein-Barr virus infection. Treatment consists of reducing immunosuppression and administration of an antiviral agent such as acyclovir or ganciclovir. A response rate of 30 to 40% can be expected, and recurrence is uncommon. Chemotherapy and radiotherapy have been used successfully in some cases. During therapy, close monitoring of the graft, along with clinical assessment of tumor status is essential.

Long-Term Results in Lung Transplantation

Pulmonary function measured by spirometry and arterial blood gases is markedly improved within several months after transplantation, with a normalization of ventilation and gas exchange after 1 to 2 years.[82] The long-term survival for lung transplant

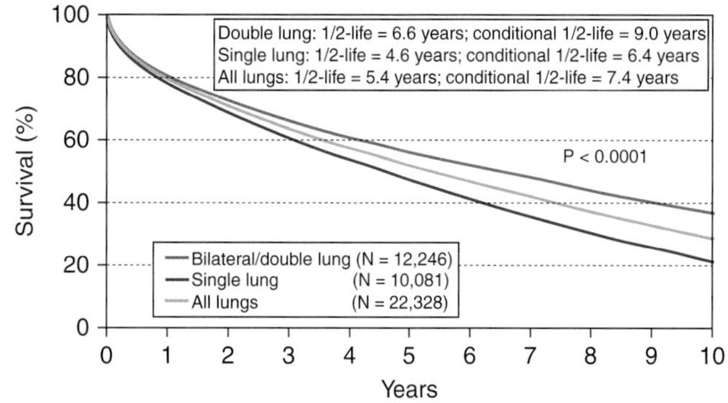

FIGURE 65-9 Kaplan-Meier survival by procedure type for adult lung transplants reported to the ISHLT registry from January 1994 through June 2007. (*From Christie JD, et al: The Registry of the International Society For Heart and Lung Transplantation: Twenty-Sixth Official Adult Lung and Heart-Lung Transplantation Report—2009. J Heart Lung Transplant 2009; 28[10]:1031-1049.*)

recipients reported to the Registry of the International Society for Heart and Lung Transplantation is shown in Fig. 65-9. Survival rates among transplants performed between January 1994 and June 2007 were 89% at 3 months, 79% at 1 year, 64% at 3 years, 52% at 5 years, and 29% at 10 years.[1] Survival for double lung transplant exceeds that of single lung transplantation, but given the variety of factors that influence this outcome (recipient factors, donor factors, and implantation techniques) it is difficult to draw any conclusions from this trend. Survival is clearly influenced by recipient age, with 1-year survival at 72% among patients older than 65 compared with 80% survival among patients less than 50.[1] Patients with COPD and IPF (who often are older with more comorbidities) tend to fare poorer than those with CF, IPAH, sarcoidosis, and AAT deficiency emphysema (as shown in Fig. 65-10). In an analysis of 10-year survivors, double lung recipients and patients with fewer hospitalizations for rejection were found to have improved long-term survival after lung transplantation.[83] Operative mortality is clearly affected by center volume, with high volume centers (≥20 implants per year) having a 30-day mortality rate of just 4.1%.[84] With increasing experience with lung transplantation worldwide, both short- and long-term survival have improved over time.

HEART-LUNG TRANSPLANTATION

History of Heart-Lung Transplantation

Long before the first successful human heart-lung transplants were reported, thoracic organ transplantation flourished in the laboratory. In the 1940s, Demikhov developed the first successful method of en bloc heart-lung transplantation in dogs. In his series of 67 dogs, the longest survivor lived for 6 days postoperatively.[85] These remarkable studies demonstrated the technical feasibility of heart and lung replacement, yet remained largely unknown in the West until the 1960s. In 1953, Marcus and colleagues at the Chicago Medical School described a technique for heterotopic heart-lung grafting to the abdominal aorta and inferior vena cava in dogs.[86] Later studies in the

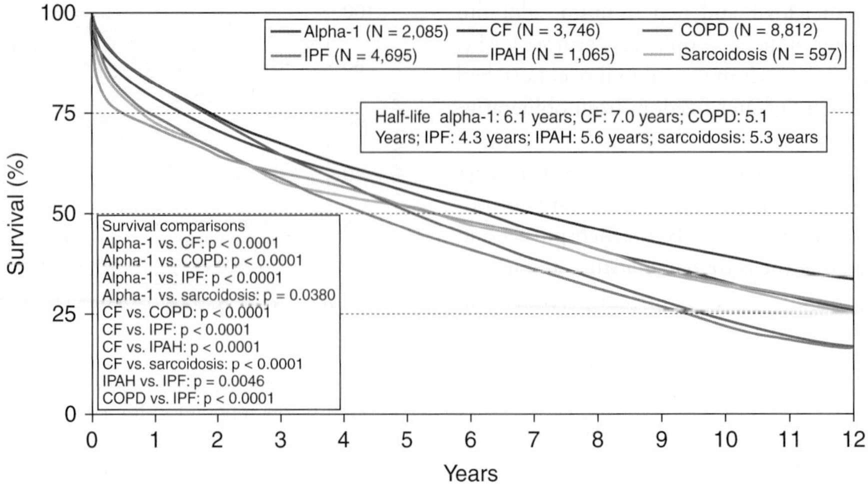

FIGURE 65-10 Kaplan-Meier survival by diagnosis for adult lung transplants reported to the ISHLT registry from January 1990 through June 2007. Alpha 1 = Alpha 1-antitrypsin deficiency emphysema; CF = cystic fibrosis; COPD = chronic obstructive pulmonary disease; IPAH = idiopathic pulmonary arterial hypertension; IPF = idiopathic pulmonary fibrosis. (*From Christie JD, et al: The Registry of the International Society for Heart And Lung Transplantation: Twenty-Sixth Official Adult Lung and Heart-Lung Transplantation Report—2009. J Heart Lung Transplant 2009; 28[10]:1031-1049.*)

1960s and early 1970s examined the physiologic effect of total denervation on heart and lung function. Studies by Webb and colleagues in 1961 proved discouraging as they showed failure to resume normal spontaneous respiration following heart-lung replacement in dogs.[87] This physiologic phenomenon was confirmed by several other groups using canine models, including Lower and colleagues in 1961.[88] Fortunately, later studies in primates by Haglin,[89] Nakae,[90] Castaneda,[91,92] and their colleagues showed that unlike dogs, primates resume a normal respiratory pattern after complete denervation with cardiopulmonary replacement. The 1970s saw the development of improved immunosuppressive medications, particularly cyclosporine, which prevented rejection of primate heart-lung allografts after transplantation. Studies from Stanford University showed survival for well over 5 years after heart-lung allografting in primates.[93] In the 1980s, Reitz and colleagues reported a modification to the standard technique of heart-lung replacement, using a retained portion of the right atrium for a single inflow anastomosis instead of separate caval anastomoses.[94] This technique preserved the donor sinoatrial node and eliminated the potential for caval anastomotic stenosis. These studies laid the groundwork for a clinical trial of heart-lung transplantation at Stanford University. On March 9, 1982, Reitz and colleagues performed the first successful human heart-lung transplant in a 45-year-old woman with end-stage primary pulmonary hypertension.[95]

Indications for Heart-Lung Transplantation

Upon its introduction in 1982, heart-lung transplantation provided a life-saving therapeutic option for patients with end-stage pulmonary and cardiopulmonary disease. However, the number of heart-lung transplants performed peaked in 1990 as the techniques of single and double lung transplantation began to achieve improved outcomes in patients with isolated end-stage lung disease. This, combined with the donor shortage of heart-lung blocs, has restricted the procedure to patients with severe cardiopulmonary diseases (most commonly congenital heart disease with Eisenmenger's syndrome, idiopathic pulmonary arterial hypertension, and cystic fibrosis). Since 2003, between 75 and 86 heart-lung transplant procedures have been performed worldwide each year.[1]

The diagnostic profile of heart-lung transplant recipients reported to the Registry of the International Society for Heart and Lung Transplantation (ISHLT) is shown in Table 65-8. Congenital heart disease (atrial and ventricular septal defects, patent ductus arteriosus) with secondary pulmonary hypertension (Eisenmenger's syndrome) is the most frequent indication, found in over one-third of the patients. Complex congenital heart defects that have been treated successfully with heart-lung transplantation include univentricular heart with pulmonary atresia, truncus arteriosus, and hypoplastic left heart syndrome. Data regarding the long-term survival benefit of heart-lung transplantation in patients with Eisenmenger's syndrome are mixed.[96] Some data suggest that pulmonary hypertension in these patients has a more favorable prognostic course than other types of pulmonary hypertension. There is clear evidence, however, that quality of life is improved by transplantation.[97] In patients with simpler cardiac defects, repair of the cardiac defect combined with single or bilateral lung transplantation is an alternative option.

Primary pulmonary hypertension with right-sided heart failure is the second most common diagnosis in heart-lung transplant recipients. Nearly one-fourths of patients in the ISHLT registry carry this diagnosis. Recently, there has been a shift toward single and bilateral lung transplantation in this population.[98] This new paradigm is based on the finding that normalization of pulmonary pressures following lung transplantation often allows for recovery of right heart function. However, in patients with severe right-sided heart failure and primary pulmonary hypertension, heart-lung transplantation is clearly the operation of choice.

TABLE 65-8 Distribution of Diagnoses Among Adult Heart-Lung Transplant Recipients

Diagnosis	No. (%)
Congenital heart disease	921 (34.9)
Idiopathic pulmonary arterial hypertension	719 (27.2)
Cystic fibrosis	373 (14.1)
COPD disease/emphysema	101 (3.8)
Acquired heart disease	77 (2.9)
Idiopathic pulmonary fibrosis	76 (2.9)
AAT deficiency emphysema	53 (2.0)
Sarcoidosis	37 (1.4)
Retransplant:	
Not obliterative bronchiolitis	31 (1.2)
Obliterative bronchiolitis	24 (0.9)
Bronchiectasis	20 (0.8)
Obliterative bronchiolitis (not retransplant)	14 (0.5)
Other	193 (7.3)

ATT = Alpha-1 antitrypsin; COPD = chronic obstructive pulmonary disease.
ISHLT Registry patients from January 1982 through June 2008.
From Christie JD, et al: The Registry of the International Society For Heart and Lung Transplantation:Twenty-Sixth Official Adult Lung and Heart-Lung Transplantation Report—2009. J Heart Lung Transplant 2009; 28(10): 1031-1049.

The remainder of heart-lung transplants are performed for a variety of cardiac and pulmonary diseases. These include cystic fibrosis and other septic lung diseases, severe coronary artery disease with concomitant end-stage lung disease, and primary parenchymal lung disease with severe right-sided heart failure (eg, idiopathic pulmonary fibrosis, lymphangioleiomyomatosis, sarcoidosis, and desquamative interstitial pneumonitis).

Patient Selection for Heart-Lung

As in lung transplantation, patients are stratified according to LAS with similar listing criteria and contraindications for both groups of patients. Age restrictions tend to be somewhat more selective in most centers, with an upper recipient age limit of 50 years. Most recipients for heart-lung transplantation also fall within New York Heart Association functional classes III or IV.[16] Careful attention to size matching must be carried out in the donor selection process. In a series of 82 heart-lung transplants at Papworth Hospital, Tamm and coworkers recorded recipient lung volumes posttransplantation, followed by a comparison to preoperative and predicted volumes to evaluate the influence of donor lung size and recipient underlying disease.[100] The investigators demonstrated that, by 1 year after surgery, total lung capacity (TLC) and dynamic lung volume returned to values predicted by the patient's sex, age, and height. They proposed that the simplest method of matching donor lung size to that of the recipient is to use their respective predicted TLC values. Moreover, they concluded that recipients should attain their predicted lung volumes by 1 year posttransplantation, and failure to do so suggests possible complications within the transplanted lungs.

As in lung transplantation, preoperative HLA matching is not feasible given the necessity of short ischemic times. However, histocompatibility does seem to impact on patient outcomes. Harjula and coworkers at Stanford evaluated the relationship between HLA matching and outcomes in heart-lung transplantation.[99] Among 40 heart-lung transplant recipients evaluated, they found a significant increase in graded obliterative bronchiolitis with total mismatch at the HLA-A locus.

Operative Technique

Procurement

Exposure and cannulation for heart-lung blocs follows the same procedure as for lung procurement. After cross-clamp, the bloc is dissected free from the esophagus commencing at the level of the diaphragm and continuing cephalad to the level of the carina. Dissection is kept close to the esophagus, and care is taken to avoid injury to the trachea, lung, or great vessels. The posterior hilar attachments are divided. The lungs are inflated to a full normal tidal volume, and the trachea is stapled at the highest point possible with a TA-55 stapler (US Surgical, Norwalk, CT), at least four rings above the carina (Fig. 65-3E). The trachea is then divided above the staple line, and the entire heart-lung bloc is removed from the chest.

Recipient Implant

The recipient is positioned supine and the chest is entered through a median sternotomy. A sternal retractor is placed, and both pleural spaces are opened anteriorly from the level of the diaphragm to the level of the great vessels (Fig. 65-11A). Electrocautery is used to divide any pleural adhesions. The anterior pericardium is excised, and the lateral segments are preserved to support the heart and protect the phrenic nerves. A 3-cm border of the pericardium should be left both anterior and posterior to each phrenic nerve extending from the level of the diaphragm to the level of the great vessels (Fig. 65-11B). An alternative approach is to create posterior pericardial apertures where the pulmonary veins enter into the pericardium. A border of pericardium is left posterior to the phrenic nerves, whereas the entire remaining pericardium anterior to the phrenic nerves is left intact. After fully heparinizing the recipient, the ascending aorta is cannulated near the base of the innominate artery, and the venae cavae are individually cannulated laterally and snared. Cardiopulmonary bypass with systemic cooling to 28 to 30°C is instituted, and the heart is excised at the midatrial level. The aorta is divided just above the aortic valve, and the pulmonary artery is divided at its bifurcation (Fig. 65-11C). The left atrial remnant is then divided vertically at a point halfway between the right and left pulmonary veins.

The posterior edge of the left atrial and pulmonary venous remnant is developed in a manner allowing the left inferior and superior pulmonary veins to be displaced over into the left

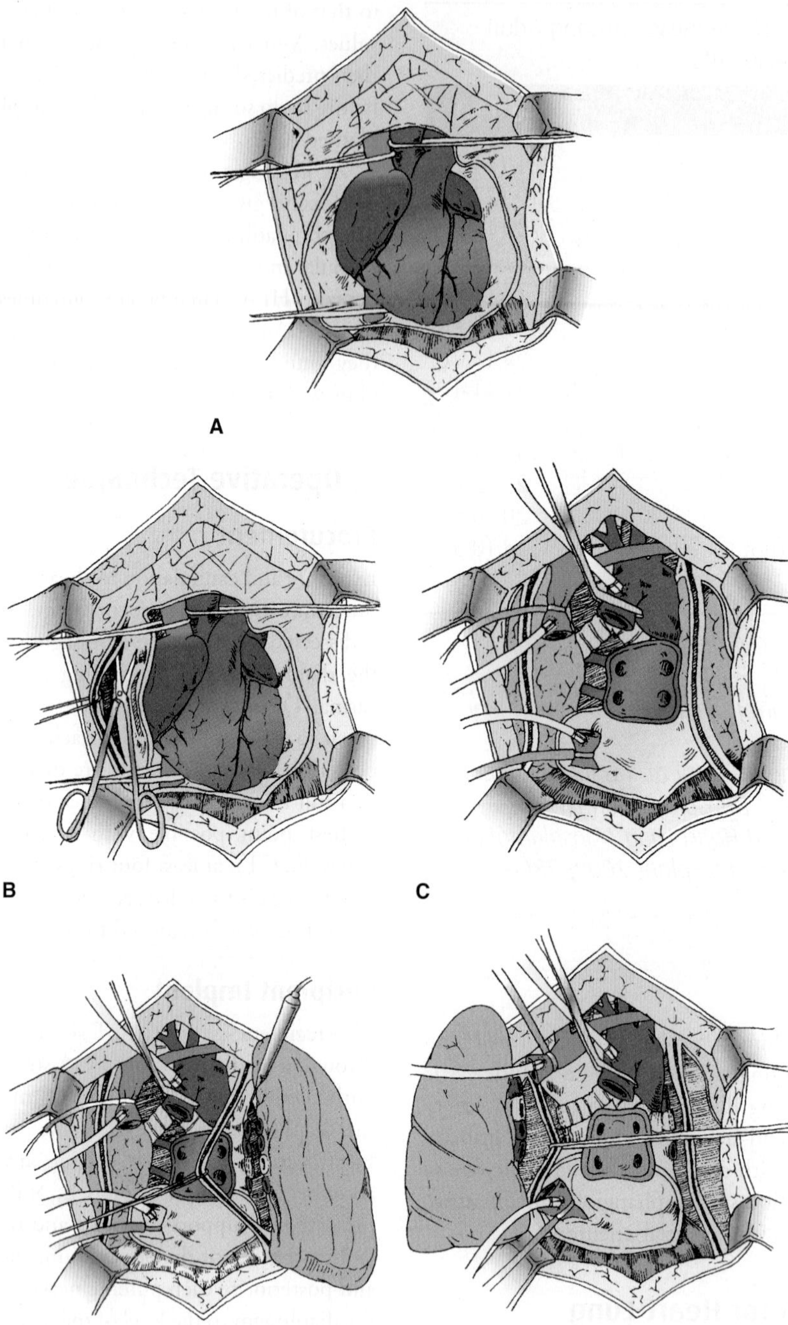

FIGURE 65-11 Recipient operation for heart-lung transplantation. (A) Through a median sternotomy, the anterior pericardium is partially removed and the ascending aorta and both venae cavae are dissected and encircled with tapes. (B) The right phrenic nerve is carefully separated from the right hilum, providing a space for inserting the right lung of the graft. (C) Cannulation for cardiopulmonary bypass consists of a cannula in the high ascending aorta and separate vena caval cannulas. Once on bypass, the native heart is excised in a manner similar to that for standard cardiac explantation. (D,E) Left and right pneumonectomies are performed by dividing the respective inferior pulmonary ligament, pulmonary artery and veins, and mainstem bronchus. (F) The heart-lung graft is moved into the chest beginning with passage of the right lung underneath the right phrenic nerve pedicle, followed by manipulation of the left lung beneath the left phrenic nerve pedicle. (G) The tracheal anastomosis is performed with a continuous 3-0 polypropylene suture. (H) The caval and aortic anastomoses are performed with a continuous 4-0 polypropylene suture.

chest. Following division of the pulmonary ligament, the left lung is moved into the field, allowing full dissection of the posterior aspect of the left hilum, with care taken to avoid the vagus nerve posteriorly. Once this is completed, the left main pulmonary artery is divided (Fig. 65-11D), and the left main bronchus is stapled with a TA-30 stapler and divided. The same technique of hilar dissection and division is repeated on the right side (Fig. 65-11E), and both lungs are removed from the chest.

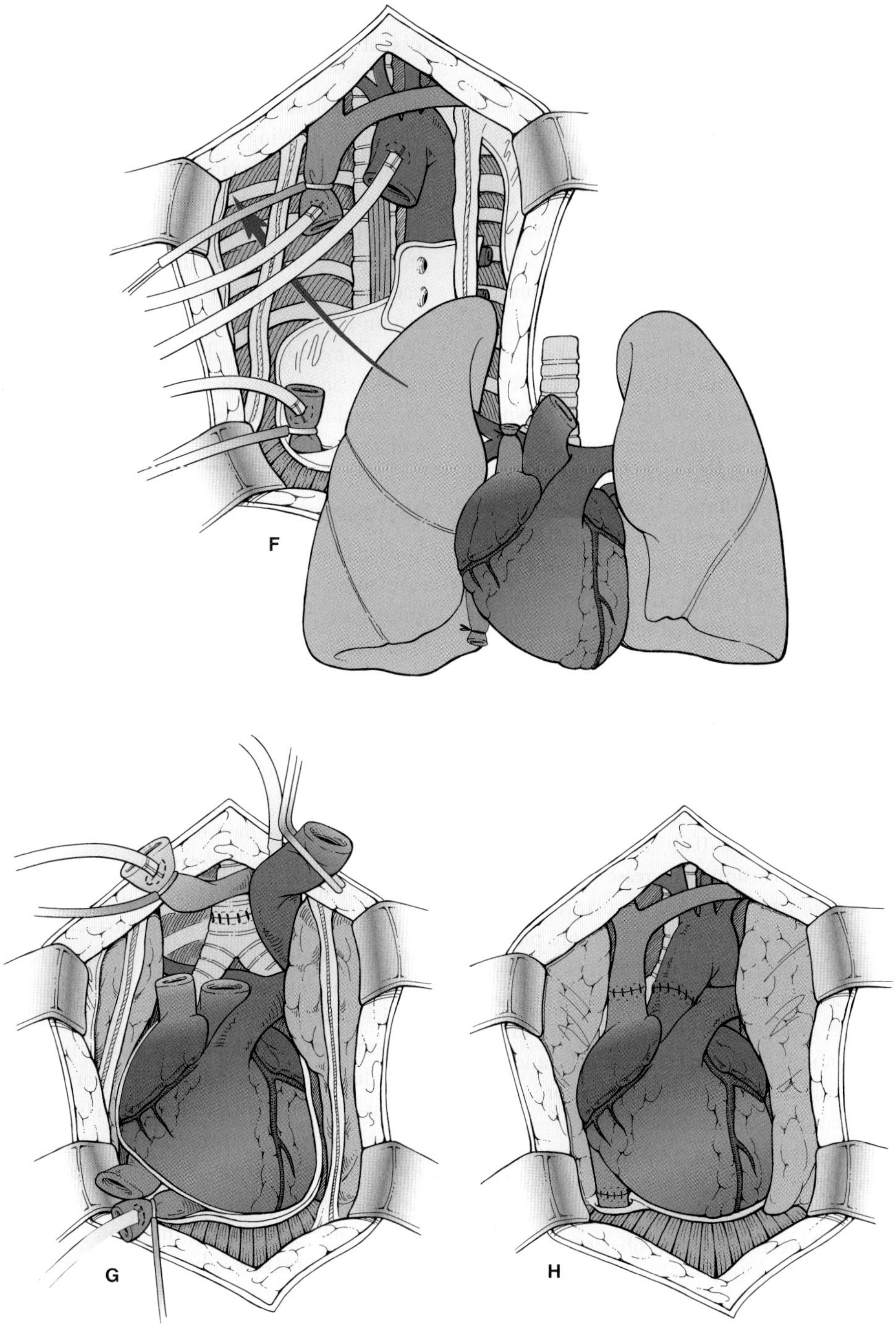

FIGURE 65-11 *(Continued)*

The native main pulmonary artery remnant is removed, leaving a portion of the pulmonary artery intact adjacent to the underside of the aorta (near the ligamentum arteriosus) to preserve the left recurrent laryngeal nerve. Attention is then turned to preparing the distal trachea for anastomosis. The stapled ends of the right and left bronchi are grasped and dissection is carried up to the level of the distal trachea. Bronchial vessels are individually identified and carefully ligated. Patients with congenital heart disease and pulmonary atresia or severe cyanosis secondary to Eisenmenger's syndrome may have large mediastinal bronchial collaterals that must be meticulously ligated. Perfect hemostasis is necessary in this area of the dissection, because it is obscured once graft implantation is complete. Once absolute hemostasis is achieved, the trachea is divided at the carina with a no. 15 blade. The chest is now prepared to receive the heart-lung graft.

The donor heart-lung bloc is removed from its transport container and prepared by irrigating, aspirating, and culturing the tracheobronchial tree followed by trimming of the trachea to leave one cartilaginous ring above the carina. The heart lung graft is then lowered into the chest, passing the right lung beneath the right phrenic nerve pedicle. The left lung is then gently manipulated under the left phrenic nerve pedicle (Fig. 65-11F). The tracheal anastomosis is performed using continuous 3-0 polypropylene suture (Fig. 65-11G). The posterior membranous portion of the anastomosis is performed first, followed by completion of the anterior aspect. Ventilation is then carried out with room air at half-normal tidal volumes to inflate the lungs and reduce atelectasis. Topical cooling with a continuous infusion of cold Physiosol into both thoraces is begun. To augment endomyocardial cooling and to exclude air from the graft, a third cold, "bubble-free" line is placed directly into the left atrial appendage.

Next, the bicaval venous anastomosis is performed. The recipient inferior vena cava is anastomosed to the donor inferior vena cava-right atrial junction with a continuous 4-0 polypropylene suture. At this point the patient is warmed toward 37°C, and the superior vena caval and aortic anastomoses are performed end-to-end with continuous 4-0 polypropylene sutures (Fig. 65-11H). After the ascending aorta and pulmonary artery are cleared of air, the aortic cross-clamp and caval tapes are removed. The left atrial catheter is removed, and the atrium is allowed to drain. The amputated left atrial stump is oversewn, and the pulmonary artery pulmonoplegia infusion site closed. The heart is defibrillated, and the patient is gradually weaned from cardiopulmonary bypass in the standard fashion. Methylprednisolone (500 mg) is administered to the recipient after heparin reversal with protamine sulfate.

PEEP at 3 to 5 cm H_2O and an F_{IO_2} of 40% is maintained. As in cardiac transplantation, isoproterenol (0.005 to 0.01 μg/kg/min) is usually initiated on graft reperfusion to increase the heart rate (~100 to 110 bpm) and to lower pulmonary vascular resistance. Temporary right atrial and ventricular pacing wires are placed. Right and left pleural "right angle" chest tubes are placed along each diaphragm, as well as a single mediastinal tube. The chest is closed in the standard fashion. Finally, the double lumen endotracheal tube is exchanged for a single lumen tube and the tracheal anastomosis is visualized by bronchoscopy before transporting the patient to the intensive care unit.

Lick and coworkers describe an interesting alternative to the standard technique in which the pulmonary hila are placed anterior to the phrenic nerves and direct caval anastomoses are used whenever feasible.[101] This modification obviates extensive dissection of the phrenic nerves and posterior mediastinum, decreasing the likelihood of phrenic and vagus nerve injury. Furthermore, the posterior mediastinum can readily be inspected for bleeding after implantation by rotating the heart-lung bloc anterior-medially while still on bypass.

Graft Physiology

For heart-lung recipients, denervation of the cardiac allograft leads to additional physiologic characteristics beyond what is seen in isolated lung transplantation. The denervated heart loses its sympathetic and parasympathetic autonomic regulation, thereby impacting on heart rate, contractility, and coronary artery vasomotor tone. The resting heart rate is generally higher due to the absence of vagal input. Respiratory sinus arrhythmia and carotid reflex bradycardia are absent. Interestingly, the denervated heart develops an increased sensitivity to catecholamines because of increased beta-adrenergic receptor density and loss of norepinephrine uptake in postganglionic sympathetic neurons.[102,103] This augmented sensitivity plays an important role in maintaining an adequate cardiac response to exercise and stress. During exercise, the recipient experiences a steady but delayed increase in heart rate, primarily because of a rise in circulating catecholamines. This initial rise in heart rate is subsequently accompanied by an immediate increase in filling pressures resulting from increased venous return. These changes lead to increased stroke volume and cardiac output sufficient to sustain activity. Although the coronary circulation's ability to dilate to meet increased myocardial oxygen demand is not eliminated in an uncomplicated heart-lung transplant, this reserve is abnormal in the presence of rejection, hypertrophy, or regional wall abnormalities.

Postoperative Management

Approximately 10 to 20% of heart-lung graft recipients experience some degree of transient sinus node dysfunction in the immediate perioperative period. This often manifests as sinus bradycardia and usually resolves within a week. The use of bicaval venous anastomoses has been reported to lower the incidence of sinus node dysfunction and improve tricuspid valve function.[104] Because cardiac output is primarily rate dependent after heart-lung transplantation, the heart rate should be maintained between 90 and 110 beats per minute during the first few postoperative days using temporary pacing or isoproterenol (0.005 to 0.01 μg/kg/min) as needed. Although rarely seen, persistent sinus node dysfunction and bradycardia may require a permanent transvenous pacemaker. Systolic blood pressure should be maintained between 90 and 110 mm Hg using nitroglycerin or nitroprusside for afterload reduction, if necessary. "Renal-dose" dopamine (3 to 5 μg/kg/min) is used frequently to augment renal blood flow and urine output. The adequacy of cardiac output is indicated by warm extremities and a urine output greater than 0.5 mL/kg/h without diuretics. Cardiac function generally returns to normal within 3 to 4 days, at which time inotropes and vasodilators can be weaned.

Nevertheless, depressed global myocardial performance is occasionally seen during the acute postoperative setting. The myocardium may be subject to prolonged ischemia, inadequate preservation, or catecholamine depletion before implantation. Hypovolemia, cardiac tamponade, sepsis, and bradycardia are also potential contributors and should be treated expeditiously if they are present. A Swan-Ganz pulmonary artery catheter should be used in cases of persistently abnormal hemodynamics. Surveillance endomyocardial biopsies are performed at 3 months and then annually in heart-lung graft recipients.

Complications

The most common complications after heart-lung transplantation include hypertension (88.6%), renal dysfunction (28.1%), hyperlipidemia (66.4%), diabetes (20.9%), coronary artery vasculopathy (8.2%), and bronchiolitis obliterans (27.1%).[1] Common causes of death include graft failure and technical complications within the first 30 days, followed by non-CMV infections and BOS in the longer term.[1] Acute rejection remains a challenge, occurring in more than 67% of heart-lung patients within the first year between 1981 and 1994 at Stanford University.[105] Experimental and clinical evidence suggests that pulmonary and cardiac rejections occur independently of one other. Nevertheless, Higenbottam and coworkers at Papworth Hospital reported a surprisingly low diagnostic yield from routine endomyocardial biopsies in heart-lung recipients compared with functional or histologic tests of pulmonary rejection. Based on these findings, the authors concluded that transbronchial biopsy eliminates the need for routine endomyocardial biopsies in heart-lung transplant recipients.[106] These findings were supported by Sibley and coworkers at Stanford University, who demonstrated discordance between findings on endomyocardial and transbronchial biopsies during episodes of acute rejection. Endomyocardial biopsies are most often normal despite findings of pulmonary rejection on transbronchial biopsy.[62] At Stanford, surveillance endomyocardial biopsies have been abandoned in patients in whom transbronchial biopsies can be reliably performed. Respiratory failure secondary OB represents a long-term complication of heart-lung transplant at a rate similar to double lung transplantation. Among heart-lung recipients with OB, Adams and coworkers at Harefield Hospital noted that retransplant survival rates were worse for those undergoing combined heart-lung replacement compared with patients who underwent isolated lung replacement.[74] The group also noted the following factors were associated with improved survival after retransplant: absence of preformed antibodies, retransplantation at least 18 months after the original transplantation, and negative preoperative sputum cultures.

Accelerated graft coronary artery disease (CAD) or graft atherosclerosis is another major obstacle to long-term survival in heart-lung transplant recipients. Significant graft CAD resulting in diminished coronary artery blood flow may lead to arrhythmias, myocardial infarction, sudden death, or impaired left ventricular function with congestive heart failure. Classic angina caused by myocardial ischemia is usually not noted in transplant recipients because the cardiac graft is not innervated. Multiple etiologies for graft CAD have been proposed, all focusing on chronic, immune-mediated damage to the coronary vascular endothelium. In fact, elevated levels of antiendothelial antibodies have been correlated with graft CAD. Unlike coronary artery occlusive disease in the native heart, which tends to be a more focal process, transplant atherosclerosis is a more diffuse vascular narrowing extending symmetrically into distal branches. Histologically, transplant arteriopathy is characterized by concentric intimal proliferation with smooth muscle hyperplasia (Fig. 65-12).

Coronary angiograms are performed on a yearly basis to identify recipients with accelerated CAD. Angiography is limited, however, to assessment of luminal diameter. Intracoronary ultrasound, by contrast, can assess both vascular wall morphology and luminal diameter, making it a more sensitive tool to detect the diffuse coronary intimal thickening typical of graft atherosclerosis. Interestingly, graft CAD occurs at a reduced incidence in heart-lung recipients compared with the cardiac transplantation population.[107] A retrospective survey at Stanford revealed 89% of heart-lung recipients were free from graft CAD at 5 years, compared with 73% of heart transplant recipients.

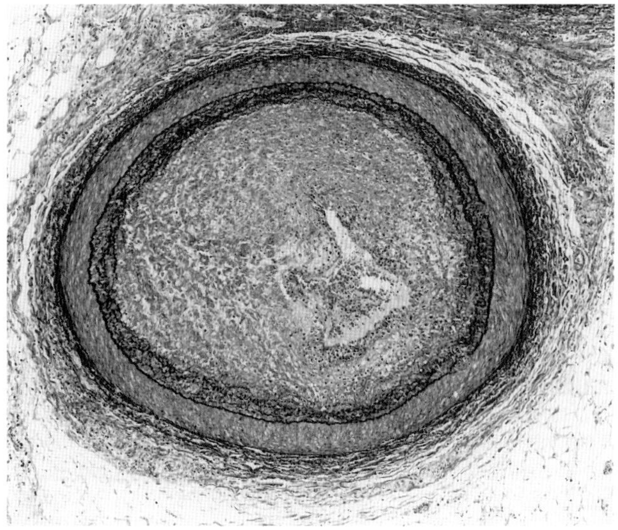

FIGURE 65-12 Cardiac graft atherosclerosis. Complete luminal obliteration by a concentric fibrointimal proliferation was observed at postmortem in this heart-lung transplant patient (Elastin von Gieson stain; ×60).

Clinically observed risk factors for developing this condition in heart transplant recipients include donor age greater than 35 years, incompatibility at the HLA-A1, A2, and DR loci, hypertriglyceridemia (serum concentration greater than 280 mg/dL), frequent acute rejection episodes, and documented recipient CMV infection. It is not clear whether these risk factors can be extended to the heart-lung transplant population, although CMV infection has been implicated.[108] Percutaneous transluminal coronary angioplasty and coronary artery bypass grafting have been used to treat discrete proximal lesions in some cases of graft CAD. However, the only definitive therapy for diffuse graft CAD is retransplantation. Effective prevention of graft CAD will rely on development of improved immunosuppression, recipient tolerance induction, improved CMV prophylaxis, and inhibition of vascular intimal proliferation.

Infection represents another significant postoperative challenge in heart-lung transplantation. Between 1981 and 1994 at Stanford, only 20% of heart-lung transplant recipients were free from infection 3 months after transplantation. In a retrospective analysis of 200 episodes of serious infections occurring in 73 heart-lung recipients at Stanford between 1981 and 1990, Kramer and coworkers[109] found that half of all infections were caused by bacteria, whereas fungal infections accounted for only 14% of total infections. The most common viral agent was CMV, occurring primarily in the second month after transplantation and comprising 15% of all viral infections. Other viral infections (ie, herpes simplex, adenovirus, respiratory syncytial virus) were less common. Five percent of infections were attributed to *Pneumocystis carinii*, typically occurring 4 to 6 months after transplantation, and 2% were caused by *Nocardia*, generally appearing after the first year. There was no significant difference in the incidence of infections between patients receiving triple-drug or double-drug (cyclosporine and prednisone) immunosuppression. Infectious mortality comprised 40% of all deaths.

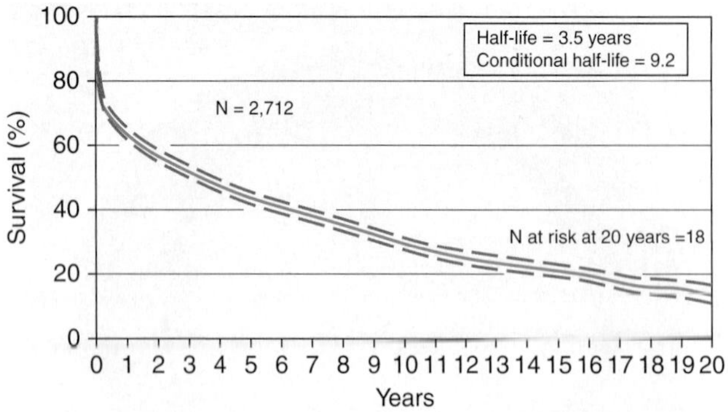

FIGURE 65-13 Kaplan-Meier survival for heart-lung transplantation, 1982 through 2007. (*From Christie JD, et al: The Registry of the International Society for Heart and Lung Transplantation: Twenty-Sixth Official Adult Lung and Heart-Lung Transplantation Report—2009. J Heart Lung Transplant 2009; 28[10]:1031-1049.*)

Long-Term Results in Heart-Lung Transplantation

Survival rates of 72% at 3 months and 64% at 1 year have been reported in the ISHLT registry.[1] Mortality rates taper off significantly at a year posttransplant, as illustrated in Fig. 65-13. As with lung transplantation, outcomes have improved over time and are affected by recipient diagnosis.[1] Graft failure, technical complications, and non-CMV infections are all common causes of 30-day mortality, with BO and non-CMV infections impairing long-term survival.

CONCLUSION

The evolution of heart-lung and lung transplantation from rudimentary laboratory experimentation to its current prominence as an accepted therapy for end-stage cardiopulmonary disease is a product of ingenuity, perseverance, skill, and courage. Many debilitated patients, both adult and pediatric, now have an opportunity to resume full and active lifestyles after heart-lung and lung transplantation. Nevertheless, significant hurdles have yet to be overcome, including issues of graft rejection, infection, and a limited donor pool. Important advances on the horizon include cross-species transplantation, improved immunosuppression, the induction of immunologic tolerance to foreign tissue, and improved organ preservation techniques.

REFERENCES

1. Christie JD, et al: The Registry of the International Society for Heart and Lung Transplantation: Twenty-Sixth Official Adult Lung and Heart-Lung Transplantation Report—2009. *J Heart Lung Transplant* 2009; 28(10): 1031-1049.
2. Metras H: Preliminary note on lung transplants in dogs. *Compte Rendue Acad Sci* 1950; 231:1176.
3. Blumenstock D, Khan D: Replantation and transplantation of the canine lung. *J Surg Res* 1961; 1:40.
4. Veith FJ, Richards K: Improved technic for canine lung transplantation. *Ann Surg* 1970; 171(4):553-558.
5. Lima O, et al: Bronchial omentopexy in canine lung transplantation. *J Thorac Cardiovasc Surg* 1982; 83(3):418-421.
6. Lima O, et al: Effects of methylprednisolone and azathioprine on bronchial healing following lung autotransplantation. *J Thorac Cardiovasc Surg* 1981; 82(2):211-215.
7. Hardy JD, et al: Lung homotransplantation in man. *JAMA* 1963; 186: 1065-1074.
8. Unilateral lung transplantation for pulmonary fibrosis. Toronto Lung Transplant Group. *NEJM* 1986; 314(18):1140-1145.
9. Patterson GA, et al: Technique of successful clinical double-lung transplantation. *Ann Thorac Surg* 1988; 45(6):626-633.
10. Pasque MK, et al: Improved technique for bilateral lung transplantation: rationale and initial clinical experience. *Ann Thorac Surg* 1990; 49(5): 785-791.
11. Starnes VA, et al: Heart, heart-lung, and lung transplantation in the first year of life. *Ann Thorac Surg* 1992; 53(2):306-310.
12. Barr ML, et al: Thoracic organ transplantation in the United States, 1994-2003. *Am J Transplant* 2005; 5(4 Pt 2):934-949.
13. Hachem RR, et al: The impact of induction on survival after lung transplantation: an analysis of the International Society for Heart and Lung Transplantation Registry. *Clin Transplant* 2008; 22(5):603-608.
14. Merlo CA, et al: Impact of U.S. Lung Allocation Score on survival after lung transplantation. *J Heart Lung Transplant* 2009; 28(8):769-775.
15. Maurer JR: Patient selection for lung transplantation. *JAMA* 2001; 286(21):2720-2721.
16. Marshall SE, et al: Selection and evaluation of recipients for heart-lung and lung transplantation. *Chest* 1990; 98(6):1488-1494.
17. Wu A, Buhler LH, Cooper DK: ABO-incompatible organ and bone marrow transplantation:current status. *Transpl Int* 2003; 16(5):291-299.
18. Hosenpud JD, et al: Influence of HLA matching on thoracic transplant outcomes. An analysis from the UNOS/ISHLT Thoracic Registry. *Circulation* 1996; 94(2):170-174.
19. Wisser W, et al: Influence of human leukocyte antigen matching on long-term outcome after lung transplantation. *J Heart Lung Transplant* 1996; 15(12):1209-1216.
20. Iwaki Y, Yoshida Y, Griffith B: The HLA matching effect in lung transplantation. *Transplantation* 1993; 56(6):1528-1529.
21. Celli BR, et al: The body-mass index, airflow obstruction, dyspnea, and exercise capacity index in chronic obstructive pulmonary disease. *NEJM* 2004; 350(10):1005-1012.
22. Fishman A, et al: A randomized trial comparing lung-volume-reduction surgery with medical therapy for severe emphysema. *NEJM* 2003; 348(21): 2059-2073.
23. Thabut G, et al: Survival after bilateral versus single lung transplantation for patients with chronic obstructive pulmonary disease: a retrospective analysis of registry data. *Lancet* 2008; 371(9614):744-751.
24. Kreider M, Kotloff RM: Selection of candidates for lung transplantation. *Proc Am Thorac Soc* 2009; 6(1):20-27.
25. Weiss ES, et al: Survival after single versus bilateral lung transplantation for high-risk patients with pulmonary fibrosis. *Ann Thorac Surg* 2009; 88(5):1616-1625; discussion 1625-1626.
26. Kerem E, et al: Prediction of mortality in patients with cystic fibrosis. *NEJM* 1992; 326(18):1187-1191.
27. Orens JB, et al: International guidelines for the selection of lung transplant candidates: 2006 update—a consensus report from the Pulmonary Scientific Council of the International Society for Heart and Lung Transplantation. *J Heart Lung Transplant* 2006; 25(7):745-755.
28. Umetsu DT, et al: Sinus disease in patients with severe cystic fibrosis: relation to pulmonary exacerbation. *Lancet* 1990; 335(8697):1077-1078.
29. Sitbon O, et al: Long-term intravenous epoprostenol infusion in primary pulmonary hypertension: prognostic factors and survival. *J Am Coll Cardiol* 2002; 40(4):780-788.
30. Novick RJ, et al: Pulmonary retransplantation:predictors of graft function and survival in 230 patients. Pulmonary Retransplant Registry. *Ann Thorac Surg* 1998; 65(1):227-234.
31. Hosenpud JD, et al: The Registry of the International Society for Heart and Lung Transplantation: seventeenth official report-2000. *J Heart Lung Transplant* 2000; 19(10):909-931.
32. McLaughlin VV, Rich S: Pulmonary hypertension—advances in medical and surgical interventions. *J Heart Lung Transplant* 1998; 17(8): 739-743.
33. Palevsky HI, Fishman AP: Chronic cor pulmonale. etiology and management. *JAMA* 1990; 263(17):2347-2353.
34. Goldberg M, et al: A comparison between cyclosporin A and methylprednisolone plus azathioprine on bronchial healing following canine lung autotransplantation. *J Thorac Cardiovasc Surg* 1983; 85(6):821-826.
35. Madden BP, et al: The medical management of patients with cystic fibrosis following heart-lung transplantation. *Eur Respir J* 1993; 6(7): 965-970.

36. International guidelines for the selection of lung transplant candidates. The American Society for Transplant Physicians (ASTP)/American Thoracic Society(ATS)/European Respiratory Society (ERS)/International Society for Heart and Lung Transplantation (ISHLT). *Am J Respir Crit Care Med* 1998; 158(1):335-339.
37. Frost AE: Donor criteria and evaluation. *Clin Chest Med* 1997; 18(2): 231-237.
38. Bhorade SM, et al: Liberalization of donor criteria may expand the donor pool without adverse consequence in lung transplantation. *J Heart Lung Transplant* 2000; 19(12):1199-1204.
39. Gabbay E, et al: Maximizing the utilization of donor organs offered for lung transplantation. *Am J Respir Crit Care Med* 1999; 160(1):265-271.
40. Shumway SJ, et al: Liberalization of donor criteria in lung and heart-lung transplantation. *Ann Thorac Surg* 1994; 57(1):92-95.
41. Fischer S, et al: Lung transplantation with lungs from donors fifty years of age and older. *J Thorac Cardiovasc Surg* 2005; 129(4):919-925.
42. Pierre AF, et al: Marginal donor lungs: a reassessment. *J Thorac Cardiovasc Surg* 2002; 123(3):421-427; discussion, 427-428.
43. Novick RJ, et al: Influence of graft ischemic time and donor age on survival after lung transplantation. *J Heart Lung Transplant* 1999; 18(5): 425-431.
44. Weill D, et al: A positive donor gram stain does not predict outcome following lung transplantation. *J Heart Lung Transplant* 2002; 21(5):555-558.
45. Weill D, et al: A positive donor gram stain does not predict the development of pneumonia, oxygenation, or duration of mechanical ventilation following lung transplantation. *J Heart Lung Transplant* 2001; 20(2):255.
46. Steen S, et al: Transplantation of lungs from a non-heart-beating donor. *Lancet* 2001; 357(9259):825-829.
47. Shigemura N, et al: Pitfalls in donor lung procurements: how should the procedure be taught to transplant trainees? *J Thorac Cardiovasc Surg* 2009; 138(2):486-490.
48. Conte JV, Baumgartner WA: Overview and future practice patterns in cardiac and pulmonary preservation. *J Cardiol Surg* 2000; 15(2):91-107.
49. Gamez P, et al: Improvements in lung preservation: 3 years' experience with a low-potassium dextran solution. *Arch Bronconeumol* 2005; 41(1):16-19.
50. Muller C, et al: Improvement of lung preservation—from experiment to clinical practice. *Eur Surg Res* 2002; 34(1-2):77-82.
51. Wittwer T, et al: Experimental lung transplantation: impact of preservation solution and route of delivery. *J Heart Lung Transplant* 2005; 24(8): 1081-1090.
52. Novick RJ, et al: Prolonged preservation of canine lung allografts: the role of prostaglandins. *Ann Thorac Surg* 1991; 51(5):853-859.
53. Kirk AJ, Colquhoun IW, Dark JH: Lung preservation:a review of current practice and future directions. *Ann Thorac Surg* 1993; 56(4):990-1000.
54. Dummer JS, et al: Infections in heart-lung transplant recipients. *Transplantation* 1986; 41(6):725-729.
55. DeMeo DL, Ginns LC: Clinical status of lung transplantation. *Transplantation* 2001; 72(11):1713-1724.
56. Christie JD, et al: Primary graft failure following lung transplantation. *Chest* 1998; 114(1):51-60.
57. Slaughter MS, Nielsen K, Bolman RM 3rd: Extracorporeal membrane oxygenation after lung or heart-lung transplantation. *ASAIO J* 1993; 39(3):M453-456.
58. Adatia I, et al: Inhaled nitric oxide in the treatment of postoperative graft dysfunction after lung transplantation. *Ann Thorac Surg* 1994; 57(5): 1311-1318.
59. Trulock EP, et al: Registry of the International Society for Heart and Lung Transplantation: Twenty-Second Official Adult Lung and Heart-Lung Transplant Report—2005. *J Heart Lung Transplant* 2005; 24(8):956-967.
60. Berry GJ, et al: A working formulation for the standardization of nomenclature in the diagnosis of heart and lung rejection: Lung Rejection Study Group. The International Society for Heart Transplantation. *J Heart Transplant* 1990; 9(6):593-601.
61. GuilingerRA, et al: The importance of bronchoscopy with transbronchial biopsy and bronchoalveolar lavage in the management of lung transplant recipients. *Am J Respir Crit Care Med* 1995; 152(6 Pt 1):2037-2043.
62. Sibley RK, et al: The role of transbronchial biopsies in the management of lung transplant recipients. *J Heart Lung Transplant* 1993; 12(2): 308-324.
63. Clelland CA, et al: The histological changes in transbronchial biopsy after treatment of acute lung rejection in heart-lung transplants. *J Pathol* 1990; 161(2):105-112.
64. Loubeyre P, et al: High-resolution computed tomographic findings associated with histologically diagnosed acute lung rejection in heart-lung transplant recipients. *Chest* 1995; 107(1):132-138.
65. Valentine VG, et al: Total lymphoid irradiation for refractory acute rejection in heart-lung and lung allografts. *Chest* 1996; 109(5):1184-1189.
66. Valentine VG, et al: Actuarial survival of heart-lung and bilateral sequential lung transplant recipients with obliterative bronchiolitis. *J Heart Lung Transplant* 1996; 15(4):371-383.
67. Chamberlain D, et al: Evaluation of transbronchial lung biopsy specimens in the diagnosis of bronchiolitis obliterans after lung transplantation. *J Heart Lung Transplant* 1994; 13(6):963-971.
68. Cooper JD, et al: A working formulation for the standardization of nomenclature and for clinical staging of chronic dysfunction in lung allografts. International Society for Heart and Lung Transplantation. *J Heart Lung Transplant* 1993; 12(5):713-716.
69. Sharples LD, et al: Risk factors for bronchiolitis obliterans: a systematic review of recent publications. *J Heart Lung Transplant* 2002; 21(2): 271-281.
70. D'Ovidio F, Keshavjee S: Gastroesophageal reflux and lung transplantation. *Dis Esophagus* 2006; 19(5):315-320.
71. Robertson AG, et al: A call for standardization of antireflux surgery in the lung transplantation population. *Transplantation* 2009; 87(8):1112-1114.
72. Cantu E 3rd, et al: J. Maxwell Chamberlain Memorial Paper. Early fundoplication prevents chronic allograft dysfunction in patients with gastroesophageal reflux disease. *Ann Thorac Surg* 2004; 78(4):1142-1151; discussion 1142-1151.
73. Davis RD Jr, et al: Improved lung allograft function after fundoplication in patients with gastroesophageal reflux disease undergoing lung transplantation. *J Thorac Cardiovasc Surg* 2003; 125(3):533-542.
74. Adams DH, et al: Retransplantation in heart-lung recipients with obliterative bronchiolitis. *J Thorac Cardiovasc Surg* 1994; 107(2):450-459.
75. Samano MN, et al: Bronchial complications following lung transplantation. *Transplant Proc* 2009; 41(3):921-926.
76. Colquhoun IW, et al: Airway complications after pulmonary transplantation. *Ann Thorac Surg* 1994; 57(1):141-145.
77. Davis RD Jr, Pasque MK: Pulmonary transplantation. *Ann Surg* 1995; 221(1):14-28.
78. Valantine HA, et al: Impact of cytomegalovirus hyperimmune globulin on outcome after cardiothoracic transplantation: a comparative study of combined prophylaxis with CMV hyperimmune globulin plus ganciclovir versus ganciclovir alone. *Transplantation* 2001; 72(10):1647-1652.
79. Reichenspurner H, et al. Inhaled amphotericin B prophylaxis significantly reduces the number of fungal infections after heart, lung, and heart-lung transplantation abstract. in International Society for Heart and Lung Transplantation 16th Annual Meeting and Scientific Sessions, 1996, New York.
80. Penn I: Incidence and treatment of neoplasia after transplantation. *J Heart Lung Transplant* 1993; 12(6 Pt 2):S328-336.
81. Paranjothi S, et al: Lymphoproliferative disease after lung transplantation: comparison of presentation and outcome of early and late cases. *J Heart Lung Transplant* 2001; 20(10):1054-1063.
82. Theodore J, et al: Cardiopulmonary function at maximum tolerable constant work rate exercise following human heart-lung transplantation. *Chest* 1987; 92(3):433-439.
83. Weiss ES, et al: Factors indicative of long-term survival after lung transplantation: a review of 836 10-year survivors. *J Heart Lung Transplant* 2009; 28:1341-1347.
84. Weiss ES, et al: The impact of center volume on survival in lung transplantation: an analysis of more than 10,000 cases. *Ann Thorac Surg* 2009; 88(4):1062-1070.
85. Demikhov V: in Bureau C (ed): *Experimental Tansplantation of Vital Organs.* New York, Consultants Bureau, 1962.
86. Marcus E, Wong SN, Luisada AA. Homologous heart grafts: transplantation of the heart in dogs. *Surg Forum* 1951; 94:212-217.
87. Webb WR, Deguzman V, Hoopes JE: Cardiopulmonary transplantation: experimental study of current problems. *Am Surg* 1961; 27:236-241.
88. Lower RR, et al: Complete homograft replacement of the heart and both lungs. *Surgery* 1961; 50:842-845.
89. Haglin J, et al: Comparison of lung autotransplantation in the primate and dog. *Surg Forum* 1963; 14:196-198.
90. Nakae S, et al: Respiratory function following cardiopulmonary denervation in dog, cat, and monkey. *Surg Gynecol Obstet* 1967; 125(6): 1285-1292.
91. Castaneda AR, et al: Cardiopulmonary autotransplantation in primates. *J Cardiovasc Surg (Torino)* 1972; 13(5):523-531.
92. Castaneda AR, et al: Cardiopulmonary autotransplantation in primates (baboons): late functional results. *Surgery* 1972; 72(6):1064-1070.
93. Reitz BA, et al: Heart and lung transplantation: autotransplantation and allotransplantation in primates with extended survival. *J Thorac Cardiovasc Surg* 1980; 80(3):360-372.
94. Reitz BA, Pennock JL, Shumway NE: Simplified operative method for heart and lung transplantation. *J Surg Res* 1981; 31(1):1-5.

95. Reitz BA, et al: Heart-lung transplantation:successful therapy for patients with pulmonary vascular disease. *NEJM* 1982; 306(10):557-564.
96. De Meester J, et al: Listing for lung transplantation: life expectancy and transplant effect, stratified by type of end-stage lung disease: the Eurotransplant experience. *J Heart Lung Transplant* 2001; 20(5):518-524.
97. Stoica SC, et al: Heart-lung transplantation for Eisenmenger syndrome: early and long-term results. *Ann Thorac Surg* 2001; 72(6):1887-1891.
98. Gammie JS, et al: Single- versus double-lung transplantation for pulmonary hypertension. *J Thorac Cardiovasc Surg* 1998; 115(2):397-402; discussion 402-403.
99. Harjula AL, et al: Human leukocyte antigen compatibility in heart-lung transplantation. *J Heart Transplant* 1987; 6(3):162-166.
100. Tamm M, et al: Donor and recipient predicted lung volume and lung size after heart-lung transplantation. *Am J Respir Crit Care Med* 1994; 150(2):403-407.
101. Lick SD, et al: Simplified technique of heart-lung transplantation. *Ann Thorac Surg* 1995; 59(6):1592-1593.
102. Lurie KG, Bristow MR, Reitz BA: Increased beta-adrenergic receptor density in an experimental model of cardiac transplantation. *J Thorac Cardiovasc Surg* 1983; 86(2):195-201.
103. Vatner DE, et al: Mechanisms of supersensitivity to sympathomimetic amines in the chronically denervated heart of the conscious dog. *Circ Res* 1985; 57(1):55-64.
104. Kendall SW, et al: Total orthotopic heart transplantation: an alternative to the standard technique. *Ann Thorac Surg* 1992; 54(1):187-188.
105. Sarris GE, et al: Long-term results of combined heart-lung transplantation: the Stanford experience. *J Heart Lung Transplant* 1994; 13(6):940-949.
106. Higenbottam T, et al: Transbronchial biopsy has eliminated the need for endomyocardial biopsy in heart-lung recipients. *J Heart Transplant* 1988; 7(6):435-439.
107. Sarris GE, et al: Cardiac transplantation: the Stanford experience in the cyclosporine era. *J Thorac Cardiovasc Surg* 1994; 108(2):240-251; discussion 251-252.
108. Grattan MT, et al: Cytomegalovirus infection is associated with cardiac allograft rejection and atherosclerosis. *JAMA* 1989; 261(24):3561-3566.
109. Kramer MR, et al: Infectious complications in heart-lung transplantation. Analysis of 200 episodes. *Arch Intern Med* 1993; 153(17):2010-2016.

CHAPTER 66

Long-Term Mechanical Circulatory Support

Hiroo Takayama
Berhane Worku
Yoshifumi Naka

INTRODUCTION

Heart failure (HF) remains one of the most common causes of death in the United States. Preventive measures and treatment options for HF have, however, improved significantly. The 2005 ACC/AHA guidelines introduced a comprehensive and systematic method of assessing and managing patients with risk factors and those with HF.[1] The suggested staging system is ambitiously inclusive, covering a wide range of patients with cardiovascular problems. It categorizes patients into Stages A (at high risk for HF but without structural heart disease or symptoms of HF) to D (refractory HF requiring specialized interventions). Surgical interventions play a significant role at each stage, and their role becomes more important as the stage advances. The surgical options described in the guidelines include, but are not limited to, coronary artery bypass grafting (CABG), valve replacement or repair, ventricular restoration surgery, heart transplantation, permanent mechanical support, and experimental surgery. A wide range of cardiac surgical procedures are covered, implying that HF is becoming one of the most important fields for cardiac surgeons.

Among the available surgical interventions for HF, mechanical circulatory support (MCS) is distinct from the others in that it, at least partially, replaces the pump function of the failing heart, similar to heart transplantation. Unlike heart transplantation, however, it does not rely on a human donor supply, which is a well-known limiting factor. As technologic advances have accrued, MCS has evolved into a reliable and well-described treatment option.

MCS may include intra-aortic balloon pump (IABP), ventricular assist device (VAD), total artificial heart (TAH), cardiopulmonary support (CPS) such as venoarterial (VA), extracorporeal membrane oxygenation (ECMO), and additional circulatory support systems. In this chapter we will focus on VAD, TAH, and CPS. Among these, VAD therapy as a method of ventricular support and TAH as a replacement of the heart are gaining particular attention. In this chapter, VAD therapy will be discussed in detail in relationship to other technologies.

HISTORY

Mechanical support of the cardiopulmonary system was first clinically introduced by John Gibbon in 1953, when he first successfully employed cardiopulmonary bypass for the repair of an atrial septal defect.[2] In 1963, DeBakey implanted the first VAD in a patient who suffered a cardiac arrest following aortic valve replacement. The patient subsequently died on postoperative day 4. In 1966, DeBakey reported the first successful bridge to recovery with implantation of a pneumatically driven VAD in a patient suffering from postcardiotomy shock. The patient was supported for 10 days, and ultimately survived to discharge.[3] Soon thereafter, Cooley reported the first successful bridge to transplantation (BTT) using a pneumatically driven implantable artificial heart.[4] During this time, the National Heart, Lung and Blood Institute (NHLBI) began funding initiatives to further the development of VADs and a TAH. DeVries and colleagues reported the successful implantation of the Jarvik-7-100 TAH in 1984.[5] Despite initial success, a high incidence of thromboembolic and infectious complications led to a moratorium on the use of the TAH in 1991. During this period, however, continued advances in the development of left ventricular assist devices (LVADs) were made. Early survival data of patients undergoing LVAD insertion revealed greater than 30% hospital mortality. Advancements in perioperative care and technology have led to improvements in outcomes,[6] and this culminated in FDA approval of an LVAD as a BTT in 1994.

The feasibility of a mechanical-based approach to the treatment of end-stage HF was validated by the Randomized Evaluation of Mechanical Assistance for the Treatment of Congestive Heart Failure (REMATCH) trial in 2001.[7] This landmark prospective randomized trial demonstrated a marked survival benefit in patients receiving an LVAD for the treatment of end-stage HF when compared with medical management alone. At the same time, the limitations of device technology using a volume displacement pump were highlighted by the high incidence of adverse events related to mechanical support, such as infection, device failure, and thromboembolic events.

Newer-generation VADs have been developed to overcome these limitations. These pumps are characterized by continuous flow driven by a rotary pump. A recently completed randomized trial demonstrated that a rotary pump (HeartMate II) compared with a volume displacement pump (HeartMate XVE) significantly improved the probability of survival free from stroke and device failure at 2 years.[8]

These continuous-flow second- and third-generation pumps generate low-grade pulsatility as opposed to the first-generation "pulsatile" pumps with volume displacement. With the growing number of patients receiving mechanical circulatory support device (MCSD) therapy, a national registry, the Interagency Registry for Mechanically Assisted Circulatory Support (INTERMACS), was initiated in 2005. This registry was devised as a joint effort of the NHLBI, the Centers for Medicare & Medicaid Services (CMS), the FDA, clinicians, scientists, and industry representatives in conjunction with the University of Alabama at Birmingham and the United Network for Organ Sharing (UNOS). This registry has and will continue to help improve the clinical outcomes of MCSD therapy, expedite new device clinical trials, and promote research.

TYPE OF MCSD

VA ECMO

Oxygenation of the blood using a membrane oxygenator can be achieved either with a venovenous (VV) or VA circuit. VV ECMO is used for respiratory failure relying on native heart function to move oxygenated blood through the systemic circulation. In order to support a failing heart, VA ECMO is necessary, and is established using a venous cannula(s) for inflow and an arterial cannula for outflow with a perfusion pump and an oxygenator bypassing the heart and lungs. These basic mechanisms are essentially the same as the cardiopulmonary bypass machine. The cannulation sites can be either central or peripheral depending on the situation. The ease of establishing VA ECMO makes this device suitable for emergent circumstances but only for short-term support (days). This device is also widely used in the pediatric population with success. Patients on VA ECMO need strict anticoagulation and in general have to be kept on a ventilator.

VAD

VADs are classified as short-term (or nonimplantable) and long-term (or implantable) devices from the duration of the support perspective, and univentricular (right or more commonly left ventricular) and biventricular assist devices from the configuration of the assist perspective. From the mechanism of driving pump system point of view, they are also divided into volume displacement (or pulsatile) devices and rotary (continuous-flow) devices. An appropriate device is chosen based on the individual patient's clinical status and the surgeon's comfort. The majority of these devices are placed surgically although recent advances have enabled percutaneous placement of certain devices, such as the Impella and TandemHeart.[9–11] The major limitations of percutaneous VADs as of 2009 are their somewhat limited flow capacity (up to approximately 5 L/min).

TAH

TAH is discussed elsewhere in this book, but in short, it replaces the patient's own heart in the orthotopic position and provides biventricular support. It has an advantage over the VAD in that conditions of the native heart, such as aortic insufficiency (AI), tricuspid regurgitation (TR), patent foramen ovale (PFO), mechanical valves, and cardiac tumors, have no influence on the function and maintenance of a TAH once it is implanted. The major drawbacks are the complexity of the implant procedure, and its size (body surface area [BSA] >1.7m^2 is required for the CardioWest TAH).

Currently used MCSDs are listed in Table 66-1, with some of their features described below.

First-Generation VADs

The HeartMate XVE (Fig. 66-1A) is the only FDA-approved device for destination therapy (DT) use. This device generates pulsatile flow through a pusher plate placed in a relatively large housing, which precludes implantation in small patients (BSA <1.5 kg/m^2). The unique textured inner surface allows patient management with no anticoagulation. It is used worldwide and has been tested extensively in large clinical trials, demonstrating superior outcome to medical management.[7] However, its long-term use is limited by high probability of device malfunction and infection. The Thoratec PVAD and Berlin Heart Excor enable implantation in small patients including the pediatric population. They can also provide BiVAD support. A major disadvantage is the exteriorized pump.

Second-Generation VADs

This group of VADs is currently gaining popularity. Miniaturization of mechanical support technology using a rotary pump of axial-flow design contributed to limiting the surface area exposed to blood allowed for the elimination of valves, air vents, and compliance chambers. The presence of fewer moving parts reduced device malfunction rates. Initial concerns over the potential influence of the continuous-flow

TABLE 66-1 Currently Used MCSDs (Not Inclusive)

Short-term (or nonimplantable) devices
BVS and AB 5000 (ABIOMED, Danvers, MA)
CentriMag (Thoratec Corporation, Pleasanton, CA)
Percutaneously/peripherally placed short-term devices
Impella 2.5, 5.0 (ABIOMED)
TandemHeart (CardiacAssist, Pittsburgh, PA)
Long-term (or implantable) devices
First generation
HeartMate IP, VE, XVE (Thoratec)
Novacor (WorldHeart, Salt Lake City, UT)
Excore (Berlin Heart, Berlin, Germany)
Intracorporeal VAD (IVAD) (Thoratec)
Paracorporeal VAD (PVAD) (Thoratec)
Second generation
EVAHEART (Sun Medical Technology Research Corp., Nagano, Japan)
Jarvik 2000 (Jarvik Heart, Inc., New York, NY)
HeartMate II (Thoratec)
MicroMed-DeBakey VAD (MicroMed Cardiovascular, Inc., Houston, TX)
Third generation
Arrow CorAide (Cleveland Clinic, Cleveland, OH)
Duraheart (Terumo Heart, Inc., Ann Arbor, MI)
HeartMate 3 (Thoratec)
HeartWare (HeartWare, Sydney, Australia)
Incore (Berlin Heart, Berlin, Germany)
Levacore (WorldHeart)
Ventra-assist (VentraCor, Inc.)
Total artificial heart
AbioCor total replacement heart (ABIOMED)
CardioWest TAH (SynCardia, Tucson, AZ)

feature on patient physiology appear to have been assuaged based on midterm outcomes. The HeartMate II (Fig. 66-1B) was shown in a randomized control trial to be superior to the HeartMate XVE.[8] Clinical experience has been accumulated with the MicroMed-DeBakey VAD and the Jarvik 2000 as well.[12,13] A unique power delivery system based on cochlear implant technology is adopted in the Jarvik 2000.[13] A titanium pedestal is screwed into the temporal bone behind the ear and conveys the electrical system through highly vascular scalp skin (Fig. 66-2). Device infection might be reduced with this technology because of immobility and the absence of subcutaneous fat.

Third-Generation VADs

The main feature of the third-generation VADs is that they eliminated bearings by using either hydrodynamic or electromagnetic suspension of an impeller to reduce mechanical wear and trauma to blood cells. The DuraHeart (Fig. 66-3) is a centrifugal pump with a magnetically levitated impeller that is composed of a magnetic bearing, an impeller, a housing, and a direct current brushless motor. The pump provides contact-free rotation of the impeller without any material wear, which predicts a high level of durability. The pump weighs 540 g and has a diameter of 72 mm and a height of 45 mm. The HeartWare (Fig. 66-4) is another example of a centrifugal pump that sits within the pericardial space. The left ventricular (LV) apical inflow cannula is an integral part of the pump itself. The device weighs only 145 g and yet provides up to 10 L/min of flow. These and other devices are currently undergoing clinical trials.

GOAL OF DEVICE SUPPORT

When considering MCSD placement, the cardiac surgeon and the team must be clear of their goal. This is particularly important in order for the surgeon and the team to be able to select the appropriate patient, the appropriate timing for placement, and the appropriate device to use. Five major goals are: "BTT," "DT," "bridge to recovery," "bridge to decision," and "bridge to bridge" (Fig. 66-5).

BTT

Patients who are evaluated by a multidisciplinary transplant team and are determined to be suitable candidates for heart transplantation may require MCSD placement while on the waiting list. With progressive lengthening of waiting times on transplantation lists, the use of a VAD as a BTT has become standard therapy in end-stage HF. This decision is made once it is felt that the patient is unlikely to survive to transplantation or if he/she is developing additional organ dysfunction which may compromise transplant eligibility. Currently, there are no widely accepted guidelines as to the indication and timing for VAD placement as a BTT, and therefore the decision has to be individualized by weighing the balance among three main factors: the estimated waiting time for a heart, the estimated chance of death on the waiting list, and the risk of the operation. For example, patients with blood type O have much longer waiting times on the transplant list compared with others in the United States, and therefore the threshold for device placement is lowered.

MCSD placement may also be considered for patients with borderline eligibility for heart transplantation, such as those with an elevated pulmonary vascular resistance (PVR) or moderate end-organ dysfunction. LVAD support was demonstrated to decrease the PVR of patients who were otherwise ineligible for transplantation with successful posttransplant outcomes.[14–19] This indication is known as "bridge to eligibility."

DT

Patients with end-stage HF who are not eligible for heart transplantation may benefit from MCSD placement because of prolongation and/or improvement in quality of life. They are

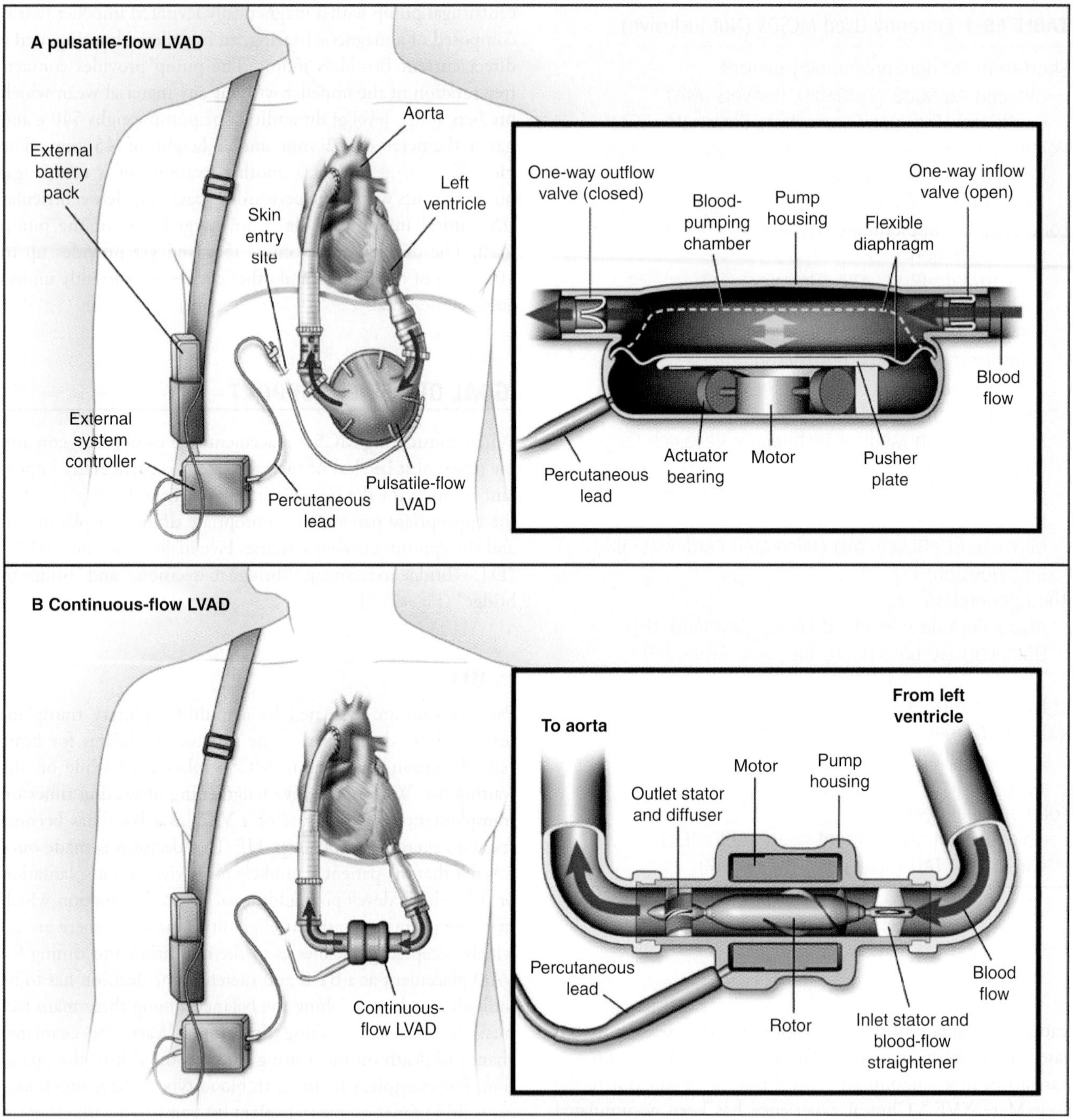

FIGURE 66-1 (A) HeartMate XVE. (B) HeartMate II. (*Reproduced, with permission, from Slaughter MS, Rogers JG, Milano CA, Russell SD, Conte JV, et al: Advanced heart failure treated with continuous-flow left ventricular assist device. NEJM 2009; 361[23]:2241-2251.*)

expected to receive circulatory support from the MCSD for life and this indication is called "DT." The REMATCH trial demonstrated that LVAD therapy is superior to medical management for this category of patients.[7] Based on this result the FDA approved the use of an LVAD (HeartMate VE) as DT. Currently accepted indications refer to the eligibility criteria for the REMATCH trial. As a reference, the current CMS criteria[20] are: patients who have chronic end-stage HF (New York Heart Association [NYHA] Class 4 end-stage LV failure for at least 90 days with a life expectancy of less than 2 years) are not candidates for heart transplantation and meet all of the following conditions:

1. The patient's Class 4 HF symptoms have failed to respond to optimal medical management, including dietary salt restriction, diuretics, digitalis, beta-blockers, and angiotensin-converting enzyme (ACE) inhibitors (if tolerated) for at least 60 of the last 90 days.

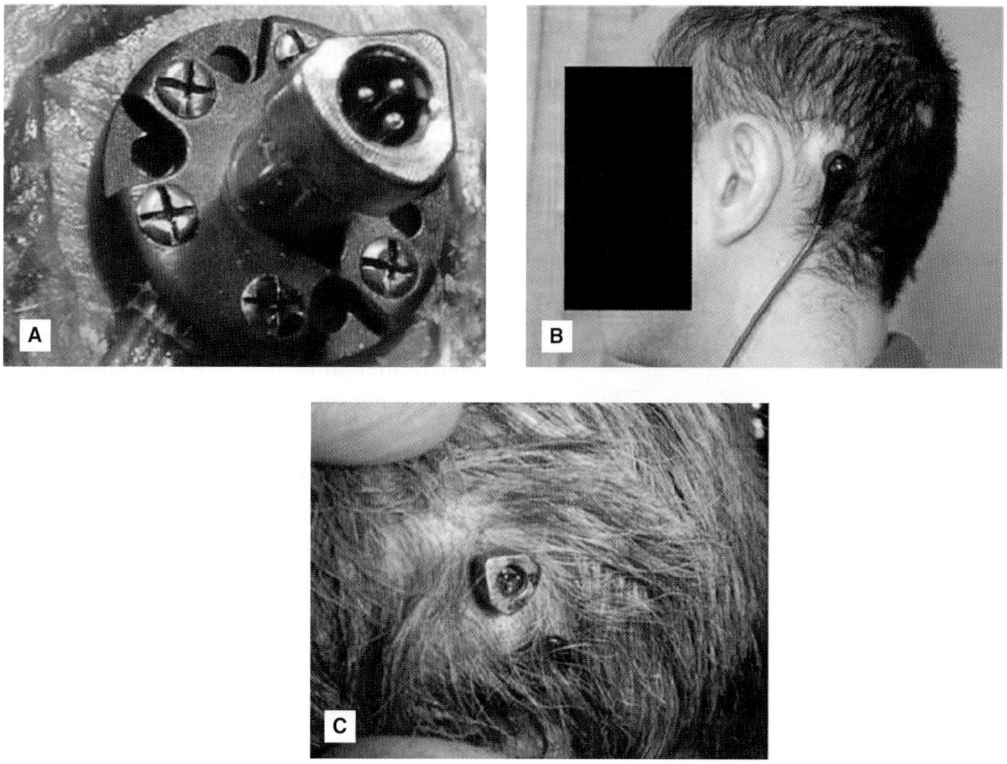

FIGURE 66-2 Skull pedestal power delivery. (A) The pedestal screwed to the skull of Jervik 2000. (B) Titanium pedestal with external power cable removed. (C) External cable plugged into the pedestal. (*Reproduced, with permission, from Westaby S, Siegenthaler M, Beyersdorf F, Massetti M, Pepper J, et al: Destination therapy with a rotary blood pump and novel power delivery. Eur J Cardiothorac Surg 2010; 37[2]:350-356.*)

2. The patient has an LV ejection fraction (EF) <25%.
3. The patient has demonstrated functional limitation with a peak oxygen consumption of <12 mL/kg/min, or the patient has a continued need for intravenous inotropic therapy owing to symptomatic hypotension, decreasing renal function, or worsening pulmonary congestion.
4. The patient has the appropriate body size (BSA ≥1.5m^2) to support the VAD implantation.

Of importance, one-third of BTT patients lost their transplant candidacy and were delisted with outcomes parallel to those of DT, and as many as 17% of DT patients eventually underwent heart transplantation.[21,22]

Bridge to Recovery

With an MCSD unloading the ventricle, some patients demonstrate recovery of myocardial function followed by successful

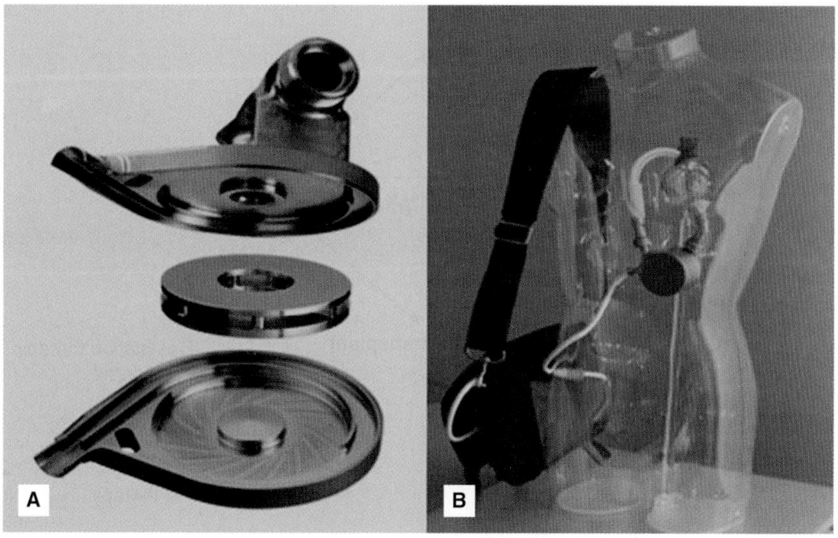

FIGURE 66-3 DuraHeart. (*Reproduced with permission from Terumo Heart Inc.*)

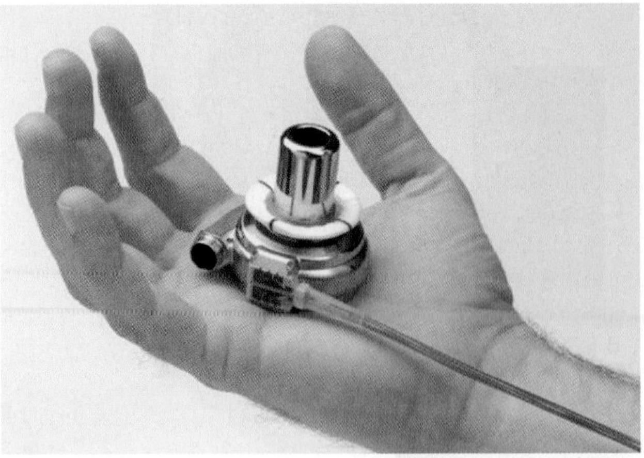

FIGURE 66-4 HeartWare. *(Reproduced, with permission, from Wood C, Maiorana A, Larbalestier R, Lovett M, Green G, et al: First successful bridge to myocardial recovery with a HeartWare HVAD. J Heart Lung Transplant 2008; 27[6]:695-697.)*[87]

MCSD explantation. MCSD placement for this purpose is called *bridge to recovery*. Only a few patients who received LVAD support demonstrated shifts in ventricular and myocardial properties back toward normal (myocardial "reverse remodeling") and successfully underwent explantation of the device with sustained cardiac function. The process of ventricular "remodeling," which is characterized by progressive ventricular dilatation and dysfunction, is mediated by many factors on molecular, biochemical, metabolic, cellular, extracellular matrix, and ventricular structural levels.[23] After the introduction of the LVAD, it was appreciated that many of these abnormalities could be reversed, at least to some degree.

At this point it is rather difficult to predict which patient will experience recovery of cardiac function with MCSD placement. MCSD placement may be undertaken for another indication with subsequent recovery of myocardial function. However, there have been promising reports on promoting myocardial recovery with pharmacologic or regenerative therapies in conjugation with MCSD placement, and this indication will likely continue to grow.

With wider interpretation of the definition, bridge to recovery has come to encompass placement of a temporary right ventricular assist device (RVAD) simultaneous with or shortly after an implantable LVAD placement, and this indication is not uncommon.

Bridge to Decision

MCS may be required for an acutely ill patient with cardiogenic shock. Acute hemodynamic decompensation may not permit the thorough evaluation required for BTT or DT. A short-term MCSD may be applied as a "bridge to decision."

Acute hemodynamic collapse can be caused by various processes, including, but not limited to acute myocardial infarction (AMI), cardiomyopathy, myocarditis, acute on chronic HF, severe rejection of a transplant heart, postcardiotomy shock, and unsuccessful percutaneous coronary intervention. Regardless of the etiology, the patient will need continuous assessment and may require progressively escalating support of care. If the patient deteriorates or does not improve despite inotrope/vasopressor administration, nitric oxide inhalation, and/or IABP placement, MCSD placement is considered. Another clinical scenario necessitating MCSD use as a bridge to decision is the patient who requires continuous cardiopulmonary resuscitation (CPR). In this setting, a clinical decision is made immediately, and

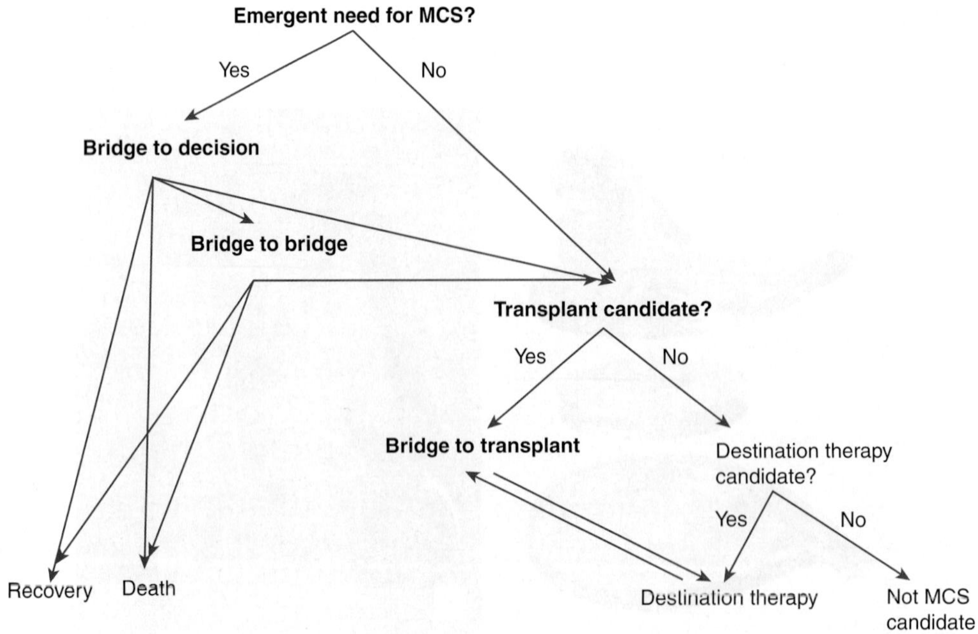

FIGURE 66-5 Goals of VAD support.

once it has been decided to proceed with MCSD placement, the cardiac surgeon/cardiologist should establish circulatory support using the quickest modality available at his or her facility.

Bridge to decision is a strategy used to defer the decision of whether to proceed with longer-term and more definitive therapy while the patient is supported with a short-term device. The patient, while on the device, may recover from or succumb to the decompensation in cardiac function, or may continue to rely on MCS. It has been proposed that the success of long-term implantable LVAD support relies on the optimization of the preoperative status of its candidates. In other words, LVAD implantation in moribund patients results in dismal outcomes. Bridge to decision use of short-term MCS allows selection of those patients who will benefit from a long-term device. Evaluation for candidacy for a longer-term strategy such as heart transplantation or DT is initiated as soon as the MCSD is placed.

Bridge to Bridge

In a small number of patients, a short-term MCSD becomes necessary to replace a previously placed short-term MCSD while the patient is awaiting a more definitive plan. This indication is called *bridge to bridge*. The most common clinical scenario involves replacing a short-term MCSD that is providing inadequate flow, or a VA ECMO, with a more reliable short-term MCSD in order to facilitate further improvement in the clinical status of the patient who is too ill to undergo a long-term implantable device placement. Bridge to bridge is usually applied for exchange of a short-term device to a long-term device.

A total of 420 patients from 75 institutions were entered into the INTERMACS database from June 2006 to December 2007.[24] The indication for MSCD placement was BTT in 336 patients (179 for BTT, 83 for "likely to be listed," 44 for "moderately likely to be listed," and 30 for "unlikely to be listed") and DT in 63 patients.

INDICATION FOR DEVICE SUPPORT: HEMODYNAMIC CONSIDERATION

The success of an MCSD is heavily dependent on appropriate patient selection.[21,25,26] Potential candidates are evaluated from a hemodynamic and nonhemodynamic standpoint. In 2006, the International Society for Heart and Lung Transplantation proposed Guidelines for the Care of Cardiac Transplant Candidates, in which recommendations for MCSD use are described.[18]

From a hemodynamic perspective, patients considered for MCSD placement can no longer sustain adequate systemic oxygen delivery to maintain normal end-organ function despite maximal medical therapy and/or IABP support. Such hemodynamic compromise can be the result of a variety of cardiac conditions. Traditional hemodynamic criteria for device placement include: blood pressure (BP) less than 80 mm Hg, mean arterial pressure less than 65 mm Hg, cardiac index less than 2.0 L/min/m^2, pulmonary capillary wedge pressure greater than 20 mm Hg, and a systemic vascular resistance (SVR) greater than 2100 dynes·sec/cm.[27] Malignant ventricular arrhythmias that cannot be adequately controlled with permanent pacemakers and/or implantable defibrillators are an additional hemodynamic indication for MCS.

Determining the hemodynamic indication for MCSD placement, however, is not always straightforward. Although the need for MCS is rather evident for a patient in acute cardiogenic shock, conflict may exist when a patient demonstrates an insidious course with congestive heart failure (CHF). Examples include: a hospitalized patient with CHF who worsens or fails to improve over a period of days; a patient managed on an outpatient basis for known CHF who slowly deteriorates, requiring incremental medical treatment; or a transplant candidate who is managed with an outpatient inotrope infusion. In order not to miss the appropriate window for MCSD placement, the clinician should be aware of the worrisome signals of CHF decompensation. These signals include worsening symptoms (recurrent admission, refractory to medical therapy, symptomatic at rest), medication issues (intolerance to or lower doses of ACE inhibitors/angiotensin receptor blockers [ARBs] and beta-blockers, increasing doses of diuretics), hyponatremia, and unresponsiveness to cardiac resynchronization therapy. Inotrope dependence is associated with a less than 50% 6-month survival.[28,29] In these situations, in addition to assessment with right heart catheterization and echocardiogram, end-organ function, in particular renal and hepatic function, is followed closely. It is becoming evident that outcomes after MCSD placement are better if the device is placed before the development of end-organ dysfunction. For patients with HF refractory to medical management, or for transplant candidates on inotropic support, a surgical consult should be obtained sooner than later, and the appropriate indication and timing of MCSD placement should be determined through a thorough discussion between the cardiac surgeon and cardiologist.

The INTERMACS registry proposed a series of seven clinical profiles with three modifiers for patient selection. These profiles help define the acuity and severity of illness and simplify the assessment of implant risk[30–32] (Table 66-2). The modifiers include arrhythmia, temporary circulatory support, and frequent flyer.[32] Approximately 60 to 80 % of indications for LVAD placement were INTERMACS level 1 ("crash and burn") or level 2 ("sliding on inotropes").[21,32]

Of note, because only LVAD support has been approved for DT, significant impairment of right ventricular (RV) function and high PVR may exclude patients from eligibility for DT.

INDICATION FOR DEVICE SUPPORT: NONHEMODYNAMIC CONSIDERATIONS

Patients in acute cardiogenic shock usually cannot wait for a thorough evaluation and thus the decision to proceed with MCSD may be made purely from a hemodynamics standpoint.

However, several additional factors discussed previously have to be taken into consideration to ensure the success of a long-term MCSD. Again, the treating team has to be clear of the goal of MCSD placement. The majority of long-term MCSDs are implanted either for BTT or DT purposes, each of which has different criteria for appropriate patient selection.

TABLE 66-2 INTERMACS Profiles

Profile	Description	Time Frame for Definitive Intervention
1	Patient with life-threatening hypotension despite rapidly escalating inotropic support, critical organ hypoperfusion with increasing lactate levels and/or systemic acidosis. *"Crash and burn"*	Needed within hours
2	Patient with declining function despite intravenous inotropic support, may be manifest by worsening renal function, nutritional depletion, inability to restore volume balance. *"Sliding on inotropes"*	Needed within few days
3	Patient with stable blood pressure, organ function, nutrition, and symptoms on continuous intravenous inotropic support, but demonstrating repeated failure to wean owing to recurrent symptomatic hypotension or renal dysfunction. *"Dependent stability"*	Elective over a few weeks
4	Patient can be stabilized close to normal volume status but experiences frequent relapses into fluid retention, generally with high diuretic doses. Symptoms are recurrent rather than refractory. More intensive management strategies should be considered, which in some cases reveal poor compliance. *"Frequent flyer"*	Elective over weeks to months as long as treatment of episodes restores stable baseline, including nutrition
5	Patient is living predominantly within the house, performing activities of daily living and walking from room to room with some difficulty. Patient is comfortable at rest without congestive symptoms, but may have underlying refractory elevated volume status, often with renal dysfunction. *"Housebound"*	Variable, depends upon nutrition, organ function, and activity
6	Patient without evidence of fluid overload is comfortable at rest and with activities of daily living and minor activities outside the home, but fatigues after the first minutes of any meaningful activity. *"Walking wounded"*	Variable, depends upon nutrition, organ function, and activity
7	A placeholder for future specification, patients without recent unstable fluid balance, living comfortably with meaningful activity limited to mild exertion.	Transplantation or circulatory support not currently indicated

Source: Reproduced, with permission, from Stevenson LW, Couper G: On the fledgling field of mechanical circulatory support. J Am Coll Cardiol 2007; 50(8):748-751.

Specific requirements for DT were mentioned in the previous section. The following are general considerations applicable to patient selection for both treatment goals.

Assessment of Operative Risk

Operative mortality constitutes a large portion of mortality after MCSD placement. The common causes of early postoperative death are bleeding, RV failure, sepsis, multiple organ failure (MOF), and stroke. Although several screening scales, including one developed at our own program, have been developed to predict early mortality after long-term LVAD placement, they are not always helpful for the assessment of procedural difficulty.[22,33] The responsible surgeon has to address the surgical complexity of each case. Certain anatomical scenarios, such as the patient with multiple previous sternotomies for complex congenital heart disease, might possess a prohibitive operative risk regardless of the remainder of the patient's risk profile.

Assessment of Organ Function

Patients with end-stage HF commonly have significant comorbidities. Life-limiting comorbidities preclude eligibility for long-term MCSD placement. On the other hand, in the setting of impaired end-organ function, some degree of recovery may be seen after MCSD placement. Renal and hepatic functions were demonstrated to improve with both pulsatile and continuous-flow LVAD support.[34–40] Assessing and defining the severity and reversibility of vital organ function is critical in the patient selection process.

Renal dysfunction, which commonly coexists in HF patients, is strongly associated with poor outcomes after VAD implantation.[41,42] Patients who are on chronic dialysis are generally excluded from implantable MCSD placement. Furthermore, patients on continuous venovenous hemofiltration (CVVH) or those with a serum creatinine of greater than 3.0 mg/dL are excluded from LVAD use for DT at our program.

Liver function is also carefully addressed. We have proposed a screening scale to predict survival after LVAD insertion.[33,43] Univariate and multivariate analyses of our patient cohort confirmed a prothrombin time of greater than 16 seconds to be one of the most significant variables included in the summation score. Reinhartz et al. demonstrated that patient survival after LVAD placement decreased (82% to 56% to 33%) as preoperative direct bilirubin levels increased (<1.2 to 1.2–3.6 to >3.6 mg/dL, respectively).[44] Liver function strongly correlates with patient outcomes after a VAD. For DT, we exclude patients whose intern ational normalized ratio is greater than 2.5 (even with efforts to reverse it), and/or patients whose ALT and AST are more than three times normal values.

Patients with advanced pulmonary disease who are on prolonged ventilatory support or whose FEV_1 is less than 1 L are not candidates for long-term MCSD. Other considerations include severe impairment of cognitive function, a history of neurologic events with significant residual deficits, active infection, active gastrointestinal bleeding, severe peripheral vascular disease (such as critical limb ischemia with rest pain or ulceration, or past limb amputation), and severe malnutrition. Malignancy is not necessarily a contraindication.

Other Considerations

MCSD operation and maintenance requires a large commitment on the part of the patient and his/her support structure. Our program requires that all patients referred for MCSD evaluation undergo a comprehensive multidisciplinary assessment. A psychiatrist assesses any psychiatric impairment that may contribute to the patient's inability to adhere to a postdevice regimen. In addition, neurocognitive function is evaluated by neuroscientists. The psychosocial evaluation performed by qualified healthcare personnel explore: social, personal, vocational, financial and environmental supports. A mental health history is also taken, assessing for substance abuse and alcohol use or abuse and its potential impact on the success or failure of device support. Nutritional status is screened with referral to a nutritionist as needed.

Lastly, age itself is not an absolute contraindication to MCSD placement.[18] Our program addresses the feasibility of device placement on an individual case basis with particular attention paid to end-organ functional reserve and psychosocial issues in older patients. It is a Class 1 recommendation from the ISHLT that patients older than 60 years of age undergo a thorough evaluation for the presence of other clinical risk factors.[18]

RISK SCREENING SCALES

Difficulties in predicting outcomes after long-term MCSD placement prompted several working groups to develop screening scales.

The revised Columbia screening scale published in 2003 offers a way of stratifying prospective device patients according to their risk of operative death from LVAD insertion based on several clinical factors: mechanical ventilation, postcardiotomy; prior LVAD insertion; central venous pressure greater than 16 mm Hg; and prothrombin time greater than 16 seconds.[43] Each factor is given a weight (4, 2, 2, 1, 1, respectively), with a cumulative score of >5 predicting an operative mortality of 46%, versus 12% for a score ≤5. This scoring system is a revision of a prior scale developed in conjunction with the Cleveland Clinic Foundation.[33] The revised scoring scale was the result of an analysis of 130 patients undergoing implantation of the HeartMate vented electrical device.

Lietz et al., focusing on DT, analyzed outcomes from 280 of 309 patients who underwent LVAD (HeartMate XVE) implantation as DT since the completion of the REMATCH trial. Nine variables, which were found to be significantly related to 90-day in-hospital mortality, were assigned a weighted risk score equal to the odds ratio rounded to the nearest integer (Table 66-3). The sum of the weighted risk scores is suggested as a risk score. Scores are categorized as low being risk score of 0 to 8, medium to high (9 to 18), and very high (>19). These risk factors are representative of severe deterioration of the general medical condition of the patient, as evidenced by poor nutritional status with a low serum albumin level, impaired renal function, markers of right heart failure such as low pulmonary artery pressures, or congestive elevation of liver enzymes. Probable infection, as evidenced by leukocytosis and coagulation abnormalities such as declining platelet count or prolonged international normalized ratio, anemia, and small body size further worsen the chance of operative survival. This screening scale was shown to correlate with 90-day and 1-year survival after LVAD implantation (Fig. 66-6). Other preexisting screening scales such as the APACHE II and Seattle Heart Failure Model were also shown to be predictive of midterm success of pulsatile LVAD therapy.[45,46]

Although the above scoring systems guide the preoperative risk assessment, they were developed based on the experience with the first-generation LVADs, and may not be directly applicable to newer devices. Using a cohort of 86 patients receiving a continuous-flow LVAD at the Johns Hopkins Hospital, Schaffer et al.[47] compared various risk screening scales including the Leitz-Miller, Columbia, APACHE II, INTERMACS, and Seattle Heart Failure Model risk scores to assess their ability to predict on 30-day, 90-day, and 1-year mortality, and found that the Seattle Heart Failure Model best differentiated low- and high-risk patients at all mortality end points.

UNIVENTRICULAR OR BIVENTRICULAR SUPPORT

Determining whether biventricular support will be necessary prior to MCSD placement is imperative in choosing an appropriate device or in determining candidacy for DT. It usually becomes evident which ventricle predominantly needs to be supported, and most often the it is the LV. Previously mentioned CMS criteria well summarize the indications for LVAD support: NYHA Class 4 HF refractory to optimal medical

TABLE 66-3 Multivariable Analysis of Risk Factors for 90-Day In-Hospital Mortality after LVAD as DT (n = 222).

Patient Characteristics	Odds Ratio (CI)	*p*	Weighted Risk Score
Platelet count ≤148 × 10^3/μL	7.7 (3.0 to 19.4)	<.001	7
Serum albumin ≤3.3 g/dL	5.7 (1.7 to 13.1)	<.001	5
International normalization ratio >1.1	5.4 (1.4 to 21.8)	.01	4
Vasodilator therapy	5.2 (1.9 to 14.0)	.008	4
Mean pulmonary artery pressures ≤25 mm Hg	4.1 (1.5 to 11.2)	.009	3
Aspartate aminotransferase >45 U/mL	2.6 (1.0 to 6.9)	.002	2
Hematocrit 34%	3.0 (1.1 to 7.6)	.02	2
Blood urea nitrogen >51 U/dL	2.9 (1.1 to 8.0)	.03	2
No intravenous inotropes	2.9 (1.1 to 7.7)	.03	2

Source: Reproduced, with permission, from Lietz K, Long JW, Kfoury AG, Slaughter MS, Silver MA, et al: Outcomes of left ventricular assist device implantation as destination therapy in the post-REMATCH era: implications for patient selection. Circulation 2007; 116(5):497-505.

management, LVEF less than 25%, functional limitation with a peak oxygen consumption of less than 12 mL/kg/min or the patient has a continued need for intravenous inotropic therapy.[20] In addition, patients with malignant arrhythmias as well as anyone on the transplant waiting list could be considered for LVAD therapy.

The difficulty lies in determining whether another ventricle, usually the RV, needs to be supported or not. RV failure occurs in 20 to 40% of LVAD recipients and it correlates with worse outcomes.[48–50] In general, RV failure occurs in "sicker" patients reflecting more advanced HF with coexisting end-organ dysfunction owing to low organ perfusion pressures (low BP and high venous pressure). Despite technologic advances, Patel et al. demonstrated that the incidence of RV dysfunction remained constant with an incidence of 35% after HeartMate XVE implantation compared with 41% after HeartMate II implantation. However, fewer HeartMate II patients required RVAD placement and fewer required pure inotropic support

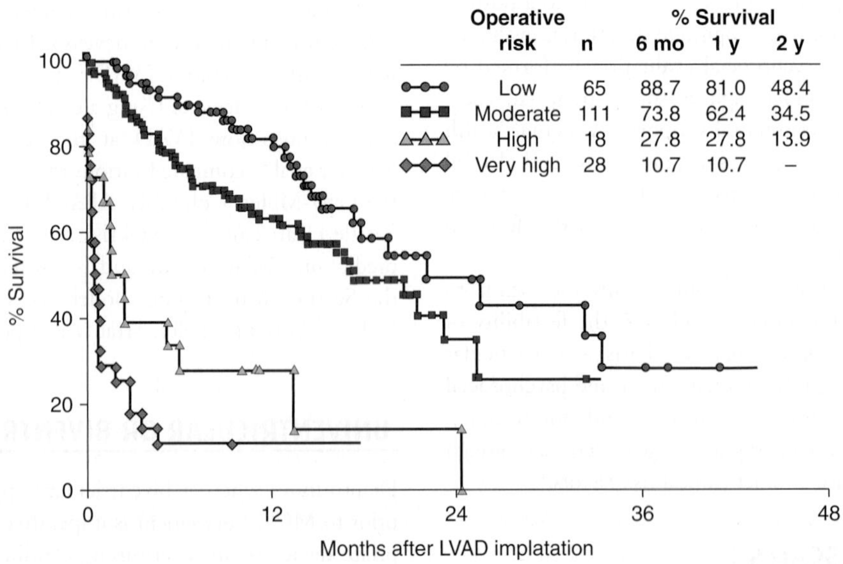

FIGURE 66-6 Survival after LVAD implantation as DT by the candidate's operative risk. (*Reproduced, with permission, from Lietz K, Long JW, Kfoury AG, Slaughter MS, Silver MA, et al: Outcomes of left ventricular assist device implantation as destination therapy in the post-REMATCH era: implications for patient selection. Circulation 2007; 116[5]:497-505.*)

for right heart failure.[49] Based on 68 patients who developed RV failure out of 197 LVAD recipients, the group from the University of Michigan proposed an RV failure risk score consisting of a vasopressor requirement, AST ≥80 IU/L, bilirubin ≥2.0 mg/dL, and creatinine ≥2.3 mg/dL.[51]

Several studies attempted to identify predictors of BiVAD need, identifying more than 20 variables. The results have been inconsistent. Ochiai et al. from the Cleveland Clinic reviewed 245 patients receiving pulsatile LVADs, among whom 23 patients required RVAD support, and reported that the need for pre-LVAD circulatory support, female gender, and nonischemic etiology were the most significant predictors of RVAD requirement after LVAD placement.[52] Fitzpatrick et al. reported a large series from the University of Pennsylvania. They retrospectively analyzed 266 LVAD recipients, of whom 99 (37%) required RVAD placement after LVAD placement. Cardiac index ≤2.2 L/min/m^2 (odds ratio 5.7), RV stroke work index ≤0.25 mm Hg/L/m^2 (odds ratio 5.1), severe preoperative RV dysfunction on echocardiographic assessment (odds ratio 5.0), preoperative creatinine ≥1.9 mg/dL (odds ratio 4.8), previous cardiac surgery (odds ratio 4.5), and systolic BP ≤96 mm Hg (odds ratio 2.9) were shown to be the best predictors of RVAD need. They proposed a risk score: 18 × (CI) + 18 × (RVSWI) + 17 × (creatinine) + 16 × (previous cardiac surgery) + 16 × (RV dysfunction) + 13 × (SBP), with a maximum possible score of 98. Applying the risk score to their cohort, a score of ≥50 predicted the need for BiVAD support with a sensitivity and specificity of 83% and 80%, respectively.[53] These scoring systems, however, remain to be validated.

Most malignant arrhythmias improve with LVAD support with or without automated implantable defibrillators/permanent pacemakers. BiVAD support, however, should be considered for recurrent sustained ventricular tachycardia or ventricular fibrillation in the presence of an untreatable arrhythmogenic pathologic substrate (eg, giant cell myocarditis).[18]

Isolated RVAD support is rarely indicated, especially as long-term support.[54] Potential indications include isolated RV infarct, isolated RV failure after heart transplantation or pulmonary embolism, or postcardiotomy RV failure.

INTERMACS data from 420 patients at 75 institutions entered into the INTERMACS database from June 2006 to December 2007demonstrated that 314 patients received LVADs, 5 RVADs, 77 BiVADs, and 24 TAHs.[24]

DEVICE SELECTION

Device selection starts with consideration of the goal of MCS placement from among the five goals described in the "Goal of Device Support" section. Also of importance is to determine which ventricle(s) will be supported.

For a bridge to decision purpose, a short-term MCSD is appropriate as they are quicker to place and less expensive. When a patient is too unstable to go to the operating room, VA ECMO via percutaneous cannulation may be the most realistic option. It is relatively easy and quick to establish, and is familiar to cardiac surgeons and paramedics compared with other types of devices. These features make it an excellent device of choice in emergent situations at a wide variety of institutions. This is also the only device available for biventricular support in extreme emergencies. The major shortcoming of VA ECMO is its mandatory use of an oxygenator, which requires strict anticoagulation and careful observation to prevent thromboembolic/hemorrhagic complications. Patients also have to remain on mechanical ventilation. Its use is limited to a relatively short period of support (hours to days). Percutaneous LVADs such as the Impella or TandemHeart for LV failure might be a reasonable option, especially when the deterioration occurs in the cardiac catheterization suite. These percutaneous devices may not be able to provide enough flow for a large patient or a very sick patient, in which case they may have to be replaced with some other device in the operating room. The options at this point include the CentriMag, Thoratec PVAD, and ABIOMED AB or BVS5000. These devices are easy to place, provide adequate flow, and can be used either as a BiVAD or a univentricular assist device. These devices are suitable in the rare bridge-to-bridge situation described earlier, in which an initial temporary device needs to be replaced (percutaneous VADs or ECMO). Another application is for temporary RVAD support at the time of or shortly after implantable LVAD placement. Our current preference for short-term MCS is to use the CentriMag, which enables establishment of high flow support through simple cannulation techniques almost equivalent to regular cannulation for routine cardiac surgery. In our experience, the CentriMag has been reliably used with support periods of greater than 1 month.

For BTT, unless the estimated waiting time to transplantation is short, in which case one of the above mentioned short-term devices may be used, a long-term implantable device is the device of choice. The Thoratec PVAD and IVAD are the only FDA-approved devices at this point for biventricular support with implantable features. FDA-approved and currently purchasable LVADs include the HeartMate XVE, HeartMate II, and Novacor LVAD. Many other devices are under clinical investigation and the options will continue to grow. Currently there is no comparison data among devices, except the HeartMate II was shown to be superior to the HeartMate XVE in a randomized controlled trial.[8] We currently use the HeartMate II or other investigational devices as part of clinical trials.

The only device currently approved by the FDA for DT is the HeartMate XVE. Again, several clinical investigations are undergoing, and likely more options will become available in the near future.

Anticoagulation

Continuous-flow devices generally require antiplatelet therapy and anticoagulation. Patients with contraindication to these regimens are considered for the HeartMate XVE.

Body Size

Patient body habitus is a very important factor in choosing a device. The size of an implantable VAD dictates the lower limitation of body size, which is usually described in BSA. For example, a BSA of less than 1.5 m^2 is a contraindication for conventional pulsatile devices, such as the HeartMate XVE whereas the HeartMate II may be placed in patients with a BSA as low as 1.2 m^2. For smaller or pediatric patients, paracorporeal devices may have to be chosen.

OTHER ANATOMICAL CONSIDERATIONS

Significant semilunar valve regurgitation is repaired at any type of MCSD insertion. Important anatomical abnormalities that require surgical correction at LVAD implantation include PFO, AI, TR, and LV apical thrombus. Intraoperative transesophageal echocardiogram (TEE) plays an important role here.

An LVAD may create pressure gradient from the right to left atrium which exaggerates right to left shunt through a PFO, resulting in profound desaturation.[55] Any PFO is closed with bicaval cannulation. We also routinely ask the anesthesiologist to perform a bubble study with TEE after LVAD placement to rule out a small PFO that might have remained undetected.

The presence of AI creates a circuit from the ascending aorta, into the LV, and back to the ascending aorta through the LVAD. LVADs, especially ones with continuous flow, expose the aortic valve to a constant pressure gradient across the valve with the LV being suctioned through the inflow cannula, and a nonphysiologic reversal of blood flow coupled with stagnant blood flow at the base of the aortic root. These unique hemodynamic features may potentiate AI. Significant regurgitation is controlled surgically. The aortic valve can either be repaired or sewn shut. The aortic valve closure leaves patients with no LV outflow, which may become of consequence in the case of device malfunction. We therefore prefer to repair the aortic valve whenever it is feasible. Our procedure of choice involves approximating the center of the leaflets, the nodes of Arantis, with a 4-0 polypropylene suture reinforced with small bovine pericardial pledgets. Stagnant blood around the aortic root can be thrombogenic especially when patients have a preexisting mechanical aortic prosthesis, in which case we close off the aortic valve with a patch. The other option is to replace the mechanical valve with a bioprosthesis.

MCSD candidates are prone to develop TR because of dilatation of the tricuspid annulus, RV dysfunction, and the presence of pacing leads. We aggressively repair significant TR at the time of LVAD implantation to maximize forward flow from the RV. The repair is usually readily accomplished by placing a ring, but additional repair techniques may be necessary for leaflet pathology created by pacing leads.

LV mural thrombi occur in one-third of Q-wave AMI cases, 50% of LV aneurysms, and up to 18% of hearts with dilated cardiomyopathy.[56] Cardioplegic arrest may be required for removal of the LV thrombus to prevent systemic embolization.

SURGICAL TECHNIQUE

We describe our technique of long-term LVAD implantation. Most of the steps are shared by many implantable LVADs. Essential components of the operation include (1) mediastinal exposure and creation of the device pocket; (2) outflow graft construction to the ascending aorta; (3) placement of device inflow, usually at the LV apex; (4) de-airing of the device; and (5) device actuation. Preoperative antibiotic prophylaxis covering both gram-positive and gram-negative bacteria is administered and usually continued for 48 to 72 hours postoperatively. Our preference is the combination of rifampin, trimethoprim-sulfamethoxazole, and fluconazole. Autologous blood is drawn by the anesthesiologist before heparinization. Patients tolerate phlebotomy of up to 1 L very well as they are usually fluid overloaded. Administration of this blood helps with hemostasis at the completion of the procedure. We have abandoned serine protease inhibitor (eg, aprotinin) use.

A vertical midline incision is made with extension onto the abdominal wall. After standard median sternotomy, a preperitoneal pocket is created in the preperitoneal space in the left upper quadrant.[57] Sometimes the preperitoneal plane is very thin and attenuated, so the posterior rectus sheath is entered and a plane superficial to this is developed. The device is brought onto the field and positioned in the preperitoneal pocket. The driveline is tunneled percutaneously and brought out of the skin through the first counter-incision in the right upper quadrant and finally through the second punched-out incision placed in the left upper quadrant (Fig. 66-7). After systemic heparinization, the patient is cannulated for cardiopulmonary bypass. Venous cannulation can be achieved with a single dual-stage cannula placed in the right atrium, or with standard bicaval cannulation if concomitant procedures are being performed (ie, tricuspid valve repair or closure of a PFO). The ascending aorta is cannulated distally with consideration for future reoperation for cardiac transplantation. An effort is made to minimize cardiopulmonary bypass times in this ill group of patients. If the hemodynamic status permits, an attempt is made to perform the outflow graft anastomosis off-pump using a partial occluding clamp placed on the ascending aorta (Fig. 66-8). The outflow graft is measured and cut with enough length to allow for a gentle curvature toward the right chest without

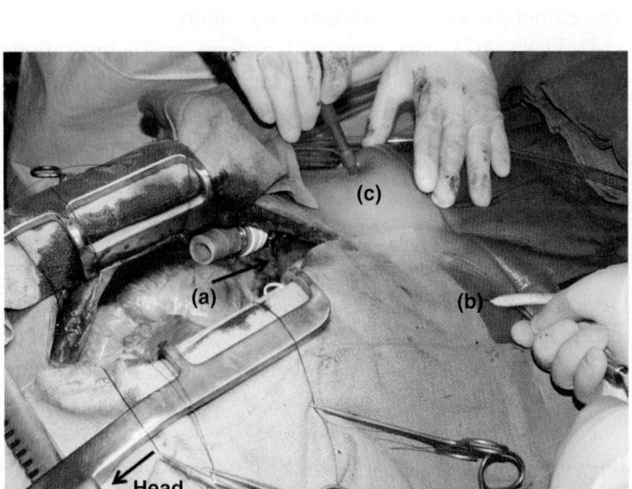

FIGURE 66-7 Placement of the device. (A) The LVAD pump placed in a pocket created in the preperitoneal space. (B) The percutaneous lead pulled through a temporarily incision at the right abdominal wall. (C) Final exit site for the lead.

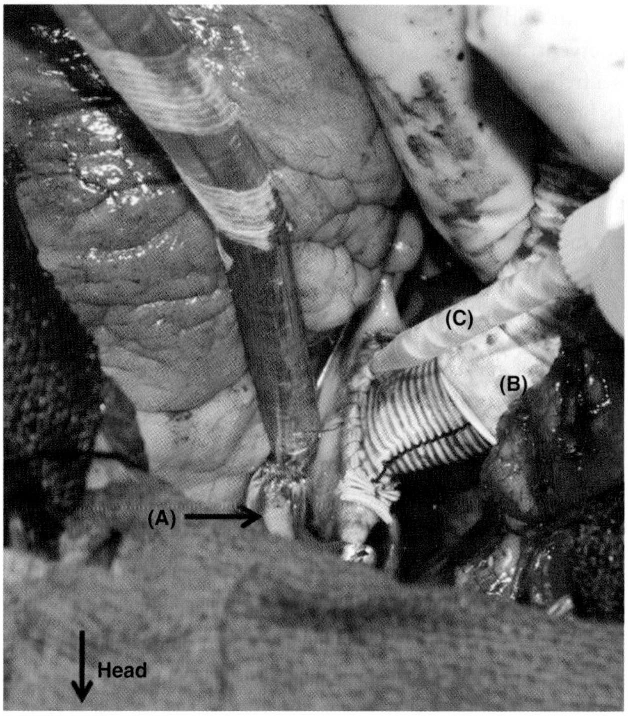

FIGURE 66-8 Anastomosis of the outflow graft to the ascending aorta. (A) A partial occluding clamp placed on the ascending aorta. (B) The outflow graft. (C) An applicator of BioGlue.

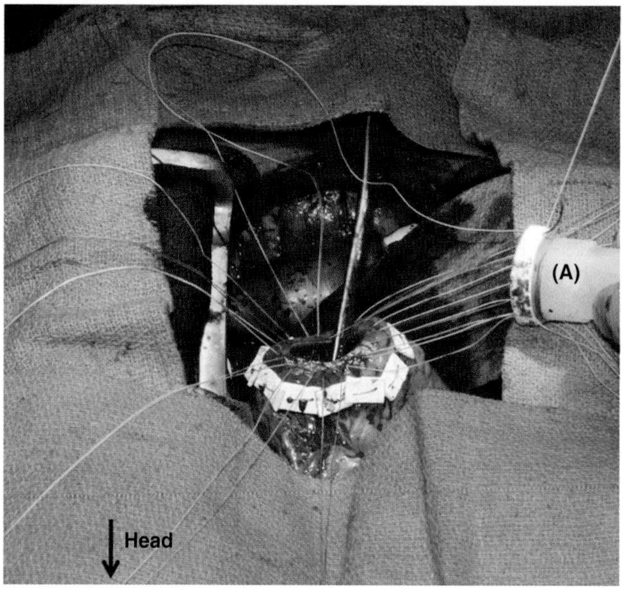

FIGURE 66-9 Placement of an inflow cuff (A) at the LV apex.

redundancy that may lead to outflow graft kinking. A longitudinal aortotomy is created and the anastomosis performed using continuous 4-0 polypropylene suture. The anastomosis is reinforced with BioGlue (CryoLife Inc., Kennesaw, GA). Cardiopulmonary bypass is initiated and attention is turned to the placement of the LV apical inflow cannula. This is usually done under conditions of normothermia with a beating heart. A specialized coring knife is used to create the apical core. Care must be taken to correctly identify the apex of the left ventricle and avoid deviation into the septum or the lateral wall. After coring of the apex, care is taken to ensure a clear inflow tract. Any excess trabeculations or myocardium that may impinge on the inflow cannula are excised. Ventricular thrombus is carefully removed. Sutures of 2-0 braided polyester reinforced with felt pledgets are then placed around the circumference of the core in a horizontal mattress fashion and passed through the sewing ring of the inflow cuff (Fig. 66-9). The cuff is secured and then attached to the inflow cannula of the device. The heart is allowed to fill with blood and the device is de-aired through a venting hole placed in the outflow graft. Evacuation of air is confirmed with TEE. The patient is then weaned from cardiopulmonary bypass, and the device is initiated. After ensuring adequate hemostasis, drains are placed in the mediastinum, pleural spaces, and device pocket. A synthetic pericardial membrane, such as Gore-Tex membrane (Gore Medical Products, Flagstaff, AZ), is placed over the anterior mediastinal structures and secured to the pericardial edges to minimize the risk of injury during reoperative median sternotomy. The sternum and soft tissues are then closed in the standard fashion. Particular attention is given to secure abdominal fascial closure to prevent wound dehiscence and subsequent device infection. In certain patients in whom excessive mediastinal bleeding is encountered secondary to coagulopathy, our preference is to pack the mediastinum and perform delayed sternal closure after approximately 24 hours, once bleeding has subsided and the patient has been adequately resuscitated.

POSTOPERATIVE MANAGEMENT

Postoperative care is crucial to successful outcomes in patients undergoing MCSD implantation, and management starts before surgery. Again appropriate patient selection is above all the most important key to success. Also important is identifying the appropriate timing of MCSD insertion; patients must first receive aggressive medical management as necessary with IABP to optimize end-organ function. Preexisting infection needs to be identified and treated. Appropriate MCSD configuration (LVAD, BiVAD, or TAH, etc) and device selection follow.

Meticulous surgical technique is the key to preventing unnecessary postoperative complications. Blood product transfusion with platelets, fresh frozen plasma, and cryoprecipitate is given as needed. Preheparinization harvest of autologous blood seems helpful in hemostasis. We are cautious about using recombinant factor 7 in this group of patients because of unknown interaction between the mechanical device and this product. Adequate hemostasis is achieved before leaving the operating room, because massive blood transfusion contributes to the development of RV failure after LVAD insertion. After device initiation, proper device function is ensured in the operating room to restore and maintain adequate end-organ perfusion. Inadequate device flows may be the result of mechanical problems such as inflow cannula obstruction or malposition, outflow graft kinking, or cardiac tamponade. Optimization of RV function (for isolated LVAD cases) is initiated before coming off CPB in concert with the anesthesiologist. Continuous assessment of RV function throughout the operation is accomplished with direct visualization by the surgeon and TEE by the anesthesiologist. The following seven hemodynamic factors are to be taken into consideration and optimized: CVP (central ventricular pressure) (preload), PVR (afterload), RV contractility, interventricular interaction, heart rate (HR), rhythm, and SVR (for coronary perfusion to the RV). RV distension is avoided as it leads to increased stress on the thin RV wall, worsened TR, decreased end-organ perfusion, and right-to-left shunting via a PFO (if untreated). A CVP of over 15 mm Hg is an alarming sign. Inotropic agents such as phosphodiesterase inhibitors, dobutamine, and epinephrine as well as inhaled nitric oxide are used liberally to support the RV.[58] Dynamic interventricular interaction through the ventricular septum significantly changes after LVAD initiation and this may compromise RV function, especially with continuous-flow devices. With excessive unloading by the device, the ventricular septum is shifted toward the LV impairing the contraction of the RV. Flow through the device is adjusted to maintain an appropriate position of the septum based on TEE. The appropriate shape of the LV in TEE short-axis view is "round shape" whereas flattened septum (D-shaped LV) indicates excessive suction. HR and rhythm are controlled with pacing and/or administration of antiarrthymic agents. Maintaining SVR and adequate perfusion pressure (mean systemic BP approximately 80 mm Hg) to ensure RV coronary perfusion is achieved with vasopressors. Arginine vasopressin has been shown to be effective in treating vasodilatory hypotension in this group of patients.[59] Excessive afterload, however, may impair pump afterload and should be treated accordingly particularly with continuous-flow devices. If optimization of RV function can not be achieved, RVAD support is considered.

Postoperative care in the intensive care unit (ICU) is the continuation of intraoperative care, which is centered on optimization of RV function. The focus of the first several hours is on monitoring for blood loss and RV function. (Near)-normalization of coagulation status is achieved with proper warming and blood product transfusion. The surgeon should have a low threshold for mediastinal reexploration for excessive postoperative bleeding. RV function is assessed with hemodynamic parameters keeping the above-mentioned seven factors (CVP, PVR, RV contractility, interventricular interaction, HR, rhythm, and SVR) in mind. In a typical stable patient after LVAD insertion, a satisfactory mean BP of above 80 mm Hg and CVP below 10 are achievable with minimum to moderate doses of inotropes/vasopressors. Proactive and aggressive treatment of subtle signs of RV failure, such as increasing vasopressor requirement, elevated CVP with relatively low pulmonary artery pressures, low output from the LVAD (measured by the device) or the RV (measured by thermodilution method with a pulmonary artery [PA] catheter), low urine output, and low mixed venous oxygen saturation should be undertaken. This can help avoid deterioration of RV function and the subsequent cascades that ensues, including device low-output and eventual end-organ dysfunction. The treatment of RV dysfunction consists of liberal increase in dosage and/or addition of inotropes, vasopressors, and inhaled nitric oxide, aggressive diuresis, instituting CVVH, optimization of ventilator settings, and controlling the HR and rhythm with pacing and/or antiarrhythmic agents. Also, the interventricular effect of the LVAD needs to be addressed. This is a frequent cause of hemodynamic instability in the first 24 to 48 hours after LVAD insertion (especially with continuous-flow devices). Temporarily decreasing the pump speed usually restores hemodynamics. Some of the devices provide certain indices. For instance, the HeartMate II provides a pulse index (PI), which is a measure of the amount of pulsatility seen by the pump over interval of 15 seconds. PI relates to the amount of unloading of the LV and is a helpful guide for the adjustment of pump speed. Overdecompression of the LV might also manifest as ventricular arrhythmia caused by mechanical irritation of the ventricular wall with the inflow cannula. Reducing the speed will reshape the LV with resolution of the arrhythmia.

Once stabilized, the patient is weaned from sedatives and then from the ventilator support. Unexpected significant hypoxia could be related to an undiscovered PFO. Vasopressors/inotropes are weaned off as tolerated, maybe except for one of the inotropes (our preference is milrinone), which may be kept on for several more days to support the RV and help diuresis. Aggressive diuresis is initiated to maintain appropriate preload to the RV. A continuous IV infusion of furosemide is preferred in the ICU and it is converted to intermittent IV bolus. Bumetanide and nesiritide are added as needed. Temporary CVVH may be required. Inotropes and diuretics are used liberally until the patient excretes the excess fluid, which is assessed by daily measurement of weight and physical exam (pretibial edema, lung sounds). Transthoracic echocardiogram is obtained periodically to guide the amount of LV unloading (reflected by the LV end-diastolic dimension) and RV function. Should the patient not respond to escalating treatment for RV failure at any point, RVAD placement should proceed without delay. Once complete hemostasis is confirmed, usually by postoperative day 2 or 3, antiplatelet therapy and/or anticoagulation are started, based on the recommendation for the device used. We no longer routinely initiate anticoagulation with an IV heparin infusion because of high incidence of bleeding complications. Currently anticoagulation is started with oral warfarin approximately postoperative day 3 to 5 when the patient is ready to be transferred out of the ICU. Enteral feedings are resumed early in the postoperative course. Once the patient is extubated, attention is focused on physical therapy and rehabilitation.[60] Should the patient develop anemia with hyperbilirubinemia, hemolysis needs to be ruled out although it is very rare.[61]

Special Postoperative Care after Bivad Insertion

Obviously RV failure is not a concern with BiVAD support. Sometimes supernormal output from the BiVAD is required to meet the metabolic needs of various end organs because, generally speaking, patients who require BiVAD support are sicker than those who require isolated LVAD support. Flow, however, has to be balanced between the LVAD and the RVAD. The left side of the heart receives more return than the right because of bronchial circulation. RVAD flow is adjusted so as to not overflow the LVAD one unless flow through the aortic valve is maintained; otherwise pulmonary congestion will result.

OUTCOMES

Overall clinical outcomes have been improving owing to advances in technology and the accumulation of clinical experience.[8,39,62–64]

BTT

Success rates with pulsatile LVADs as a BTT increased from below 65% in the 1990s to 72% in early the 2000s at our program.[65] Further improvement was noticed with newer-generation LVADs. John et al. reported six month survival rate of 87% for 32 patients who received the HeartMate II as a BTT.[66] A prospective, multicenter study of 133 patients who received the HeartMate II as a BTT showed that at 6 months 75% reached the principal outcomes of heart transplantation (42%), cardiac recovery (1%), or ongoing device support (32%) with a mortality rate of 19%.[62] Overall actuarial survival for patients continuing to receive pump support was 68% at 12 months. Over the past decade, the number of heart transplant recipients supported by a VAD at the time of transplantation has more than doubled to over 400 per year.[67] Studies have concluded that long-term survival is not affected by pretransplant VAD support.[68,69] Using UNOS registry data, Russo et al. compared the long-term survival after heart transplantation between recipients who received a VAD as a BTT and those who did not. The VAD group was further divided into extracorporeal, intracorporeal, and paracorporeal VADs. Although the extracorporeal group had diminished graft survival in the first 90 days (likely related to the more morbid pre-VAD status of the recipients), there were not significant differences in risk-adjusted graft survival at up to 5 years between recipients who received any type of VAD as a BTT and those who did not.[67]

Success rates for BTT with BiVAD support, on the other hand, were reported to be only 25 to 60%.[48,51–53,70–72] Poorer success was reported specifically among those who required an RVAD following LVAD placement. Early planned institution of BiVAD support might improve outcomes.[73]

DT

Outcomes for LVADs placed for DT are well-summarized in two landmark randomized studies.[7,8] LVADs were shown to be superior to optimal medical management with regard to survival and quality of life. The REMATCH trial demonstrated a 48% reduction in the risk of death at 1 year with a pulsatile LVAD (HeartMate VE). Subsequently, a continuous-flow device (HeartMate II) was shown to improve survival at 2 years (58% vs 24% for a pulsatile LVAD, the HeartMate XVE). Interestingly, the 2-year survival with the pulsatile-flow device in these two randomized studies remained roughly the same, and this suggests that the main contributor to improvements in survival is technologic advancement.

Bridge to Recovery

Few LVAD recipients show recovery of ventricular function, and even if they do, they frequently suffer from recurrence of HF after LVAD explantation. We have shown that significant clinical recovery occurred in only 5 out of 111 patients, and in these patients, symptoms frequently returned and many died of consequences of HF.[74] In large case series, recovery with removal of LVAD support has been seen in 4 to 30% of patients with a 20 to 50% incidence of recurrent CHF.[75–78] The results of Birks et al. regarding intensive pharmacologic treatment are most promising.[79] Their patients underwent institution of LVAD support and were treated with lisinopril, carvedilol, spironolactone, and losartan to enhance reverse remodeling. Once regression of LV enlargement had been achieved, the beta$_2$-adrenergic receptor agonist clenbuterol was administered to prevent myocardial atrophy. Eleven of fifteen patients had sufficient myocardial recovery to undergo explantation of the LVAD. The cumulative rate of freedom from recurrent HF among the surviving patients was 100% and 88.9%, 1 and 4 years after explantation, respectively.

ADVERSE EVENTS

INTERMACS provides standardized definitions of adverse events. The defined events include major bleeding, cardiac arrhythmia, pericardial fluid collection, device malfunction, hemolysis, hepatic dysfunction, hypertension, major infection, myocardial infarction, neurologic dysfunction, psychiatric episode, renal dysfunction, respiratory failure, right heart failure, non–central nervous system (CNS) thromboembolic event, venous thromboembolism event, wound dehiscence, and other adverse events. Among these, CNS events, MOF, RV failure, and arrhythmias remain the most common cause of death.[24] The cumulative incidence rate of adverse events in the first 60 days after MCSD insertion can be as high as 89%.[61]

Operative Mortality

Recently reported 30-day survival rates after MCSD insertion are approximately 80 to 90%.[22] Higher INTERMACS profiles were shown to correlate with higher mortality,[80] and operative risk categories developed by Lietz et al. for DT patients estimate 90-day in-hospital mortality after LVAD placement at 2% in low-risk patients and 81% in very high-risk patients.[22] Estimated operative mortality rates from the revised Columbia screening scale, developed with a focus on the operative mortality, are approximately 5% for a score of 0–1, approximately 15% for a score of 2–4, and approximately 45% for a score of ≥5.[43] Better patient selection has contributed to decreasing operative mortality, and proceeding to MCSD insertion before a patient becomes too sick is the key. Postcardiotomy support remains one of the most challenging indications. The Thoratec registry data for PVAD placements by March 2005 showed a survival of 44.7% with LVAD support (n = 253) and 32.4% with BiVAD support (n = 241) for this indication.[81]

Major Bleeding

Bleeding is the most common complication after MCSD implantation and mediastinal reexploration is required in 20% up to 60% of MCSD recipients.[82] Resuscitation with massive blood product transfusion is associated with increased morbidity and mortality. A recent study demonstrated that the number of bleeding events requiring packed red blood cell transfusion was 1.66 per patient-year for a continuous-flow device and 2.45 for a pulsatile-flow device.[8] Bleeding risk persists even after the acute postoperative period, and this seems to be above what is normally observed in patients receiving anticoagulation treatment. Late bleeding most commonly manifests as gastrointestinal bleeding, and continuous-flow devices appear to have a higher incidence of this complication compared with pulsatile-flow devices.[83] Development of arteriovenous malformations and impaired von Willebrand factor–dependent platelet aggregation are the proposed mechanisms.[83,84]

Right Heart Failure

RV failure occurs in 20 to 40% of LVAD recipients and approximately 5% of cases require RVAD support. A detailed discussion is found in Univentricular or Biventricular Support.

Device Malfunction

Device durability is an important limitation to the use of currently approved pulsatile-flow LVADs because valve or bearing failures occur frequently by 18 months.[7] The advent of continuous-flow devices dramatically reduced the incidence of this complication. In a recent randomized study, there were no primary-pump or bearing failures in patients with a continuous-flow LVAD.[8] It was suggested that redesign of the percutaneous lead and development of modular components may further reduce the infrequent need for replacement, which occurred in only 9% of patients. The University of Michigan group experienced an 11% incidence of device malfunction with BiVAD support compared with 9% with LVAD support.[61]

Major Infection (Device-Related)

Sepsis and device malfunction were the most common causes of death in patients who received a pulsatile-flow LVAD in the REMATCH trial. Within 3 months after implantation, the probability of device infection was 28%. Infections mostly involved the drive-line tract and pocket and were treated with local measures and antibiotics. The continuous-flow device reduced the rate of device-related infection to nearly half that seen with the pulsatile-flow device.[8]

Neurologic Dysfunction

MCSDs predispose recipients to the risk of thromboembolism, with ischemic stroke being the most devastating consequence. The combined risk of ischemic and hemorrhagic CVA was reported to be 8 to 20%. The type of device may correlate with the risk of stroke. Tsukui et al. reported an actuarial freedom from CVA at six months of 75%, 64%, and 33% with the

TABLE 66-4 The Adverse Events from the INTERMACS Registry between June 2006 and March 2008

Adverse Events	Episodes (Patients)	≤30 Days (Patients)	>30 Days (Patients)
Device malfunction	81 (62)	20 (16)	61 (47)
Bleeding	537 (201)	354 (172)	183 (71)
Cardiac/vascular			
Right heart failure	37 (35)	29 (29)	8 (7)
Myocardial infarction	2 (2)	2 (2)	0 (0)
Cardiac arrhythmia	149 (89)	110 (73)	39 (24)
Pericardial drainage	52 (41)	45 (37)	7 (5)
Hypertension	119 (76)	39 (35)	71 (46)
Arterial non-CNS thrombosis	14 (12)	9 (7)	5 (5)
Venous thrombotic event	33 (28)	26 (24)	7 (6)
Hemolysis	24 (18)	10 (8)	14 (11)
Infection	479 (193)	215 (128)	264 (124)
Neurologic dysfunction	119 (87)	69 (57)	50 (39)
Renal dysfunction	110 (83)	93 (73)	17 (16)
Hepatic dysfunction	64 (47)	37 (32)	27 (20)
Respiratory failure	165 (114)	144 (101)	21 (18)
Other			
Wound dehiscence	9 (7)	4 (3)	5 (5)
Psychiatric episode	60 (47)	19 (19)	41 (32)
Other adverse events	281 (155)	105 (70)	176 (102)
Total adverse events (prospective)	2326 (434)		

Source: Reproduced, with permission, from Holman WL, Pae WE, Teutenberg JJ, Acker MA, Naftel DC, et al: INTERMACS: interval analysis of registry data. J Am Coll Surg 2009; 208(5):755-761; discussion 61-62.

HeartMate (X)VE and II device, Thoratec BiVAD, and Novacor device, respectively.[85]

Table 66-4 summarizes the current probability of adverse events from the INTERMACS registry between June 2006 and March 2008.[86]

FUTURE DIRECTION

Advances in technology have led to the creation of more durable and versatile devices, resulting in improved clinical outcomes for the MCSD recipients. Minimally invasive approaches for MCSD insertion will be developed. MCSDs may be used across a wider spectrum of patients and purposes, and patients with less advanced HF may receive partial circulatory support to improve quality of life. Approaches in which MCS combined with one or more addtitional treatment modalities, such as a drug therapy or cell therapy to prevent post-LVAD explant remodeling, may prove fruitful. In fact, clinical trials in these areas are ongoing.

Accumulation of clinical experience will allow consensus guidelines to be developed. However, at the current rapid pace of technologic progress, such guidelines may be outdated at the time of their publication, somewhat similar to the experience with coronary stents. Therefore, cardiac surgeons performing MCSD surgery should remain updated.

MCS is still a relatively new technology in the treatment of HF, and much research remains to be done to elucidate its role in clinical medicine and also to better understand HF itself. Both basic and clinical investigations are warranted with support from nonprofit organizations and industry.

KEY POINTS

- Patient selection is the most important component to achieve good outcomes with MCSD implantation.
- Elucidating the goal of MCSD placement (BTT, DT, bridge to recovery, bridge to dicision, bridge to bridge) is crucial for appropriate patient and device selection.
- Optimizing RV function is the key after LVAD implantation.

REFERENCES

1. Hunt SA, Abraham WT, Chin MH, Feldman AM, Francis GS, et al: ACC/AHA 2005 Guideline Update for the Diagnosis and Management of Chronic Heart Failure in the Adult: a report of the American College of Cardiology/American Heart Association Task Force on Practice Guidelines (Writing Committee to Update the 2001 Guidelines for the Evaluation and Management of Heart Failure): developed in collaboration with the American College of Chest Physicians and the International Society for Heart and Lung Transplantation: endorsed by the Heart Rhythm Society. *Circulation* 2005; 12(12):e154-235.
2. Gibbon JH, Jr: Application of a mechanical heart and lung apparatus to cardiac surgery. *Minn Med* 1954; (3):171-185; passim.
3. DeBakey ME: Development of mechanical heart devices. *Ann Thorac Surg* 2005; 79(6):S2228-2231.
4. Gemmato CJ, Forrester MD, Myers TJ, Frazier OH, Cooley DA: Thirty-five years of mechanical circulatory support at the Texas Heart Institute: an updated overview. *Tex Heart Inst J* 2005; (2):168-177.
5. DeVries WC, Anderson JL, Joyce LD, Anderson FL, Hammond EH, et al: Clinical use of the total artificial heart. *NEJM* 1984; 310(5):273-278.
6. Sun BC, Catanese KA, Spanier TB, Flannery MR, Gardocki MT, et al: 100 long-term implantable left ventricular assist devices: the Columbia Presbyterian interim experience. *Ann Thorac Surg* 1999; 68(2):688-694.
7. Rose EA, Gelijns AC, Moskowitz AJ, Heitjan DF, Stevenson LW, et al: Long-term mechanical left ventricular assistance for end-stage heart failure. *NEJM* 2001; 345(20):1435-1443.
8. Slaughter MS, Rogers JG, Milano CA, Russell SD, Conte JV, et al: Advanced heart failure treated with continuous-flow left ventricular assist device. *NEJM* 2009; 361(23):2241-2251.
9. Cheng JM, den Uil CA, Hoeks SE, van der Ent M, Jewbali LS, et al: Percutaneous left ventricular assist devices vs. intra-aortic balloon pump counterpulsation for treatment of cardiogenic shock: a meta-analysis of controlled trials. *Eur Heart J* 2009; 30(17):2102-2108.
10. Koerner MM, Jahanyar J: Assist devices for circulatory support in therapy-refractory acute heart failure. *Curr Opin Cardiol* 2008; 23(4):399-406.
11. Seyfarth M, Sibbing D, Bauer I, Fröhlich G, Bott-Flügel L, et al: A randomized clinical trial to evaluate the safety and efficacy of a percutaneous left ventricular assist device versus intra-aortic balloon pumping for treatment of cardiogenic shock caused by myocardial infarction. *J Am Coll Cardiol* 2008; 52(19): 1584-1588.
12. Goldstein DJ: Worldwide experience with the MicroMed DeBakey Ventricular Assist Device as a bridge to transplantation. *Circulation* 2003; 108(Suppl 1):II272-277.
13. Westaby S, Siegenthaler M, Beyersdorf F, Massetti M, Pepper J, et al: Destination therapy with a rotary blood pump and novel power delivery. *Eur J Cardiothorac Surg* 2010; 37(2):350-356.
14. Liden H, Haraldsson A, Ricksten SE, Kjellman U, Wiklund L: Does pretransplant left ventricular assist device therapy improve results after heart transplantation in patients with elevated pulmonary vascular resistance? *Eur J Cardiothorac Surg* 2009; 35(6):1029-1034; discussion 34-35.
15. Salzberg SP, Lachat ML, von Harbou K, Zund G, Turina MI: Normalization of high pulmonary vascular resistance with LVAD support in heart transplantation candidates. *Eur J Cardiothorac Surg* 2005; 27(2):222-225.
16. Zimpfer D, Zrunek P, Roethy W, Czerny M, Schima H, et al: Left ventricular assist devices decrease fixed pulmonary hypertension in cardiac transplant candidates. *J Thorac Cardiovasc Surg* 2007; 133(3):689-695.
17. Zimpfer D, Zrunek P, Sandner S, Schima H, Grimm M, et al: Post-transplant survival after lowering fixed pulmonary hypertension using left ventricular assist devices. *Eur J Cardiothorac Surg* 2007; 31(4):698-702.
18. Gronda E, Bourge RC, Costanzo MR, Deng M, Mancini D, et al: Heart rhythm considerations in heart transplant candidates and considerations for ventricular assist devices: International Society for Heart and Lung Transplantation guidelines for the care of cardiac transplant candidates–2006. *J Heart Lung Transplant* 2006; 25(9):1043-1056.
19. Etz CD, Welp HA, Tjan TD, Hoffmeier A, Weigang E, et al: Medically refractory pulmonary hypertension: treatment with nonpulsatile left ventricular assist devices. *Ann Thorac Surg* 2007; 83(5):1697-1705.
20. Center for Medicare Services Online Manual System. Available from: www.cms.gov/manuals.
21. Lietz K, Miller LW: Patient selection for left-ventricular assist devices. *Curr Opin Cardiol* 2009; 24(3):246-251.
22. Lietz K, Long JW, Kfoury AG, Slaughter MS, Silver MA, et al: Outcomes of left ventricular assist device implantation as destination therapy in the post-REMATCH era: implications for patient selection. *Circulation* 2007; 116(5):497-505.
23. Klotz S, Jan Danser AH, Burkhoff D: Impact of left ventricular assist device (LVAD) support on the cardiac reverse remodeling process. *Prog Biophys Mol Biol* 2008; 97(2-3):479-496.
24. Holman WL, Kormos RL, Naftel DC, Miller MA, Pagani FD, et al: Predictors of death and transplant in patients with a mechanical circulatory support device: a multi-institutional study. *J Heart Lung Transplant* 2009; 28(1):44-50.
25. Aaronson KD, Patel H, Pagani FD: Patient selection for left ventricular assist device therapy. *Ann Thorac Surg* 2003; 75(6 Suppl):S29-35.
26. Miller LW: Patient selection for the use of ventricular assist devices as a bridge to transplantation. *Ann Thorac Surg* 2003; 75(6 Suppl):S66-71.
27. Norman JC, Cooley DA, Igo SR, Hibbs CW, Johnson MD, et al: Prognostic indices for survival during postcardiotomy intra-aortic balloon pumping. Methods of scoring and classification, with implications for left ventricular assist device utilization. *J Thorac Cardiovasc Surg* 1977; 74(5): 709-720.
28. Stevenson LW: Clinical use of inotropic therapy for heart failure: looking backward or forward? Part II: chronic inotropic therapy. *Circulation* 2003; 108(4):492-497.
29. Stevenson LW: Clinical use of inotropic therapy for heart failure: looking backward or forward? Part I: inotropic infusions during hospitalization. *Circulation* 2003; 22;108(3):367-372.

30. Kirklin JK, Naftel DC, Stevenson LW, Kormos RL, Pagani FD, et al: INTERMACS database for durable devices for circulatory support: first annual report. *J Heart Lung Transplant* 2008; 27(10):1065-1072.
31. Stevenson LW, Couper G: On the fledgling field of mechanical circulatory support. *J Am Coll Cardiol* 2007; 50(8):748-751.
32. Stevenson LW, Pagani FD, Young JB, Jessup M, Miller L, et al: INTERMACS profiles of advanced heart failure: the current picture. *J Heart Lung Transplant* 2009; Jun;28(6):535-541.
33. Oz MC, Goldstein DJ, Pepino P, Weinberg AD, Thompson SM, et al: Screening scale predicts patients successfully receiving long-term implantable left ventricular assist devices. *Circulation* 1995; 92(9 Suppl):II169-73.
34. Farrar DJ, Hill JD: Recovery of major organ function in patients awaiting heart transplantation with Thoratec ventricular assist devices. Thoratec Ventricular Assist Device Principal Investigators. *J Heart Lung Transplant* 1994; 13(6):1125-1132.
35. Frazier OH, Rose EA, Oz MC, Dembitsky W, McCarthy P, et al: Multicenter clinical evaluation of the HeartMate vented electric left ventricular assist system in patients awaiting heart transplantation. *J Thorac Cardiovasc Surg* 2001; 122(6):1186-1195.
36. Jett GK: ABIOMED BVS 5000: experience and potential advantages. *Ann Thorac Surg* 1996; 61(1):301-304; discussion 11-13.
37. Letsou GV, Myers TJ, Gregoric ID, Delgado R, Shah N, et al. Continuous axial-flow left ventricular assist device (Jarvik 2000) maintains kidney and liver perfusion for up to 6 months. *Ann Thorac Surg* 2003; 76(4): 1167-1170.
38. Radovancevic B, Vrtovec B, de Kort E, Radovancevic R, Gregoric ID, et al: End-organ function in patients on long-term circulatory support with continuous- or pulsatile-flow assist devices. *J Heart Lung Transplant* 2007; 26(8):815-818.
39. Pagani FD, Miller LW, Russell SD, Aaronson KD, John R, et al: Extended mechanical circulatory support with a continuous-flow rotary left ventricular assist device. *J Am Coll Cardiol* 2009; 54(4):312-321.
40. Sandner SE, Zimpfer D, Zrunek P, Dunkler D, Schima H, et al. Renal function after implantation of continuous versus pulsatile flow left ventricular assist devices. *J Heart Lung Transplant* 2008; 27(5):469-473.
41. Butler J, Geisberg C, Howser R, Portner PM, Rogers JG, et al: Relationship between renal function and left ventricular assist device use. *Ann Thorac Surg* 2006; 81(5):1745-1751.
42. Sandner SE, Zimpfer D, Zrunek P, Rajek A, Schima H, et al: Renal function and outcome after continuous flow left ventricular assist device implantation. *Ann Thorac Surg* 2009; 87(4):1072-1078.
43. Rao V, Oz MC, Flannery MA, Catanese KA, Argenziano M, et al: Revised screening scale to predict survival after insertion of a left ventricular assist device. *J Thorac Cardiovasc Surg* 2003; 125(4):855-862.
44. Reinhartz O, Farrar DJ, Hershon JH, Avery GJ, Jr, Haeusslein EA, et al: Importance of preoperative liver function as a predictor of survival in patients supported with Thoratec ventricular assist devices as a bridge to transplantation. *J Thorac Cardiovasc Surg* 1998; 116(4):633-640.
45. Gracin N, Johnson MR, Spokas D, Allen J, Bartlett L, et al: The use of APACHE II scores to select candidates for left ventricular assist device placement. Acute Physiology and Chronic Health Evaluation. *J Heart Lung Transplant* 1998; 17(10):1017-1023.
46. Levy WC, Mozaffarian D, Linker DT, Farrar DJ, Miller LW: Can the Seattle heart failure model be used to risk-stratify heart failure patients for potential left ventricular assist device therapy? *J Heart Lung Transplant* 2009; 28(3):231-236.
47. Schaffer JM, Allen JG, Weiss ES, Patel ND, Russell SD, et al: Evaluation of risk indices in continuous-flow left ventricular assist device patients. *Ann Thorac Surg* 2009; 88(6):1889-1896.
48. Dang NC, Topkara VK, Mercando M, Kay J, Kruger KH, et al: Right heart failure after left ventricular assist device implantation in patients with chronic congestive heart failure. *J Heart Lung Transplant* 2006; 25(1):1-6.
49. Patel ND, Weiss ES, Schaffer J, Ullrich SL, Rivard DC, et al: Right heart dysfunction after left ventricular assist device implantation: a comparison of the pulsatile HeartMate I and axial-flow HeartMate II devices. *Ann Thorac Surg* 2008; 86(3):832-840; discussion 832-840.
50. Van Meter CH, Jr: Right heart failure: best treated by avoidance. *Ann Thorac Surg* 2001; 71(3 Suppl):S220-222.
51. Matthews JC, Koelling TM, Pagani FD, Aaronson KD: The right ventricular failure risk score a pre-operative tool for assessing the risk of right ventricular failure in left ventricular assist device candidates. *J Am Coll Cardiol* 2008; 51(22):2163-2172.
52. Ochiai Y, McCarthy PM, Smedira NG, Banbury MK, Navia JL, et al: Predictors of severe right ventricular failure after implantable left ventricular assist device insertion: analysis of 245 patients. *Circulation* 2002; 106(12 Suppl 1):I198-202.
53. Fitzpatrick JR, 3rd, Frederick JR, Hsu VM, Kozin ED, O'Hara ML, et al: Risk score derived from pre-operative data analysis predicts the need for biventricular mechanical circulatory support. *J Heart Lung Transplant* 2008; 27(12):1286-1292.
54. Moazami N, Pasque MK, Moon MR, Herren RL, Bailey MS, et al: Mechanical support for isolated right ventricular failure in patients after cardiotomy. *J Heart Lung Transplant* 2004; 23(12):1371-1375.
55. Kapur NK, Conte JV, Resar JR: Percutaneous closure of patent foramen ovale for refractory hypoxemia after HeartMate II left ventricular assist device placement. *J Invasive Cardiol* 2007; 19(9):E268-270.
56. Cregler LL: Antithrombotic therapy in left ventricular thrombosis and systemic embolism. *Am Heart J* 1992; 123(4 Pt 2):1110-1114.
57. McCarthy PM, Wang N, Vargo R: Preperitoneal insertion of the HeartMate 1000 IP implantable left ventricular assist device. *Ann Thorac Surg* 1994, 57(3):634-637; discussion 7-8.
58. Kavarana MN, Pessin-Minsley MS, Urtecho J, Catanese KA, Flannery M, et al: Right ventricular dysfunction and organ failure in left ventricular assist device recipients: a continuing problem. *Ann Thorac Surg* 2002; 73(3): 745-750.
59. Argenziano M, Choudhri AF, Oz MC, Rose EA, Smith CR, et al: A prospective randomized trial of arginine vasopressin in the treatment of vasodilatory shock after left ventricular assist device placement. *Circulation* 1997; 96(9 Suppl):II-286-290.
60. Morrone TM, Buck LA, Catanese KA, Goldsmith RL, Cahalin LP, et al: Early progressive mobilization of patients with left ventricular assist devices is safe and optimizes recovery before heart transplantation. *J Heart Lung Transplant* 1996; 15(4):423-429.
61. Genovese EA, Dew MA, Teuteberg JJ, Simon MA, Kay J, et al: Incidence and patterns of adverse event onset during the first 60 days after ventricular assist device implantation. *Ann Thorac Surg* 2009; 88(4):1162-1170.
62. Miller LW, Pagani FD, Russell SD, John R, Boyle AJ, et al: Use of a continuous-flow device in patients awaiting heart transplantation. *NEJM* 2007; 357(9): 885-896.
63. Struber M, Sander K, Lahpor J, Ahn H, Litzler PY, et al: HeartMate II left ventricular assist device: early European experience. *Eur J Cardiothorac Surg* 2008; 34(2):289-294.
64. Haj-Yahia S, Birks EJ, Rogers P, Bowles C, Hipkins M, et al: Midterm experience with the Jarvik 2000 axial flow left ventricular assist device. *J Thorac Cardiovasc Surg* 2007; 134(1):199-203.
65. Morgan JA, John R, Rao V, Weinberg AD, Lee BJ, et al: Bridging to transplant with the HeartMate left ventricular assist device: the Columbia Presbyterian 12-year experience. *J Thorac Cardiovasc Surg* 2004; 127(5): 1309-1316.
66. John R, Kamdar F, Liao K, Colvin-Adams M, Boyle A, et al: Improved survival and decreasing incidence of adverse events with the HeartMate II left ventricular assist device as bridge-to-transplant therapy. *Ann Thorac Surg* 2008; (4):1227-1234; discussion 34-35.
67. Russo MJ, Hong KN, Davies RR, Chen JM, Sorabella RA, et al: Posttransplant survival is not diminished in heart transplant recipients bridged with implantable left ventricular assist devices. *J Thorac Cardiovasc Surg* 2009; 138(6):1425-1432 e1-3.
68. Cleveland JC, Jr, Grover FL, Fullerton DA, Campbell DN, Mitchell MB, et al: Left ventricular assist device as bridge to transplantation does not adversely affect one-year heart transplantation survival. *J Thorac Cardiovasc Surg* 2008; 136(3):774-777.
69. Taylor DO, Stehlik J, Edwards LB, Aurora P, Christie JD, et al: Registry of the international society for heart and lung transplantation: twenty-sixth official adult heart transplant report-2009. *J Heart Lung Transplant* 2009; 28(10):1007-1022.
70. Farrar DJ, Hill JD, Pennington DG, McBride LR, Holman WL, et al:. Preoperative and postoperative comparison of patients with univentricular and biventricular support with the Thoratec ventricular assist device as a bridge to cardiac transplantation. *J Thorac Cardiovasc Surg* 1997; 113(1): 202-209.
71. Santambrogio L, Bianchi T, Fuardo M, Gazzoli F, Veronesi R, et al: Right ventricular failure after left ventricular assist device insertion: preoperative risk factors. *Interact Cardiovasc Thorac Surg* 2006; (4):379-382.
72. Kormos RL, Gasior TA, Kawai A, Pham SM, Murali S, et al: Transplant candidate's clinical status rather than right ventricular function defines need for univentricular versus biventricular support. *J Thorac Cardiovasc Surg* 1996; 111(4):773-782; discussion 82-83.
73. Fitzpatrick JR, 3rd, Frederick JR, Hiesinger W, Hsu VM, McCormick RC, et al: Early planned institution of biventricular mechanical circulatory support results in improved outcomes compared with delayed conversion of a left ventricular assist device to a biventricular assist device. *J Thorac Cardiovasc Surg* 2009; 137(4):971-977.

74. Mancini DM, Beniaminovitz A, Levin H, Catanese K, Flannery M, et al. Low incidence of myocardial recovery after left ventricular assist device implantation in patients with chronic heart failure. *Circulation* 1998; 98(22):2383-2389.
75. Hetzer R, Muller JH, Weng Y, Meyer R, Dandel M: Bridging-to-recovery. *Ann Thorac Surg* 2001; 71(3 Suppl):S109-113; discussion S14-15.
76. Dandel M, Weng Y, Siniawski H, Potapov E, Lehmkuhl HB, et al: Long-term results in patients with idiopathic dilated cardiomyopathy after weaning from left ventricular assist devices. *Circulation* 2005; 112(9 Suppl):I37-45.
77. Simon D, Fischer S, Grossman A, Downer C, Hota B, et al: Left ventricular assist device-related infection: treatment and outcome. *Clin Infect Dis* 2005; 40(8):1108-1115.
78. Maybaum S, Mancini D, Xydas S, Starling RC, Aaronson K, et al. Cardiac improvement during mechanical circulatory support: a prospective multicenter study of the LVAD Working Group. *Circulation* 2007; 115(19):2497-2505.
79. Birks EJ, Tansley PD, Hardy J, George RS, Bowles CT, et al. Left ventricular assist device and drug therapy for the reversal of heart failure. *NEJM* 2006; (18):1873-1884.
80. Alba AC, Rao V, Ivanov J, Ross HJ, Delgado DH: Usefulness of the INTERMACS scale to predict outcomes after mechanical assist device implantation. *J Heart Lung Transplant* 2009; 28(8):827-833.
81. Hill JD, Farrar DJ, Naka Y, Chen JM, Portner PM, et al. (eds): *Positive Displacement Ventricular Assist Devices.* St Louis, Elsevier, 2006.
82. Goldstein DJ, Beauford RB: Left ventricular assist devices and bleeding: adding insult to injury. *Ann Thorac Surg* 2003; 75(6 Suppl):S42-47.
83. Crow S, John R, Boyle A, Shumway S, Liao K, et al: Gastrointestinal bleeding rates in recipients of nonpulsatile and pulsatile left ventricular assist devices. *J Thorac Cardiovasc Surg* 2009; 137(1):208-215.
84. Klovaite J, Gustafsson F, Mortensen SA, Sander K, Nielsen LB: Severely impaired von Willebrand factor-dependent platelet aggregation in patients with a continuous-flow left ventricular assist device (HeartMate II). *J Am Coll Cardiol* 2009; 53(23):2162-2167.
85. Tsukui H, Abla A, Teuteberg JJ, McNamara DM, Mathier MA, et al: Cerebrovascular accidents in patients with a ventricular assist device. *J Thorac Cardiovasc Surg* 2007; 134(1):114-123.
86. Holman WL, Pae WE, Teutenberg JJ, Acker MA, Naftel DC, et al: INTERMACS: interval analysis of registry data. *J Am Coll Surg* 2009; 208(5): 755-761; discussion 61-62.
87. Wood C, Maiorana A, Larbalestier R, Lovett M, Green G, et al: First successful bridge to myocardial recovery with a HeartWare HVAD. *J Heart Lung Transplant* 2008; 27(6):695-697.

CHAPTER 67

Total Artificial Heart

O. H. Frazier
Steven M. Parnis
William E. Cohn
Igor D. Gregoric

INTRODUCTION

Cardiovascular disease (CVD) is the leading cause of morbidity and mortality in the United States and a significant public health problem in most industrialized nations. Since 1900, it has been the leading cause of death in the United States every year except 1918.[1] In 2005, CVD afflicted 80 million Americans and caused 864,500 deaths. Meanwhile, the number of people with CVD, and especially its advanced forms, has been increasing. There are two main reasons for this. First, although there is still no cure for CVD, palliative therapy has improved to the point that more people are surviving past their initial episodes of CVD to live on with some form of the disease. Second, the average age of the US population is rising as the "baby boom" generation ages.

An increasingly prevalent form of advanced CVD is heart failure (HF). Almost 5.7 million Americans (approximately 3.2 million men and 2.5 million women) are living with HF.[1] Its etiology can be ischemic, idiopathic, or viral. More than $37.2 billion is spent each year on the care of HF patients, and many therapeutic advances have been made. In 2005, HF directly caused 53,000 deaths and indirectly caused another 250,000. As large as the problem is now, its magnitude is expected to worsen as more cardiac patients are able to survive and live longer with their disease and thus increase their chances of developing end-stage HF.

At present, treatment of advanced HF takes three forms: medical therapy, surgical therapy, and cardiac support or replacement.[2,3] Medical therapy (eg, intravenous inotropes and vasodilators) relieves symptoms by reducing cardiac work and increasing myocardial contractility. However, although advances in medical therapy have helped improve quality of life for those with heart failure, mortality remains unaffected. Surgical therapy (eg, revascularization and valve replacement or repair) relieves symptoms of ischemia and valvular dysfunction, but in most cases does not stop the underlying disease process from progressing. When conventional medical and surgical therapies for HF are exhausted, cardiac support or replacement (ie, heart transplantation or implantation of an artificial heart or ventricular assist device) may in some cases become the only therapeutic alternative.

Heart transplantation has evolved into a suitable treatment for advanced HF. However, it has severe limitations related to patient selection, organ procurement and distribution, and cost-effectiveness. Slightly more than 2000 patients with end-stage heart failure receive heart transplants each year in the United States. However, about 3000 patients are on the active heart transplant waiting list at any given time, and as many as 40,000 more are potential candidates for heart transplantation.[4,5] Heart transplantation for the relatively young (<40 years old) is not very promising because the life expectancy of a donor heart recipient is about 10 years on average and 20 years at most. In 2004, 460 patients on the active waiting list died while awaiting a donor heart. Heart transplantation is also associated with continuous, lifelong, expensive medical therapy.

To help overcome these limitations, engineers and physicians have continued efforts begun over four decades ago to develop systems for providing either temporary or permanent mechanical circulatory support (MCS). Originally, such systems were intended to support patients indefinitely because other forms of heart replacement did not appear to be feasible. Temporary MCS has been shown to be a suitable option for some HF patients who are awaiting heart transplants.[6,7] and for others who are not transplant candidates but need support for indefinite periods.[8] In recent clinical studies, myocardial function improved sufficiently in some cases to allow removal of the MCS device and avoid heart transplantation.[9,10] Nevertheless, in light of the shortcomings of medical therapy, surgical therapy, and heart transplantation, efforts have continued to develop a total artificial heart (TAH) that would not only save the lives of critically ill HF patients but also allow them to resume relatively normal lifestyles. Here, we review the historical development and current status of TAH technology.

EARLY DEVELOPMENT AND EXPERIENCE

In 1812, LeGallois first proposed the idea of supporting a failing heart with either a permanent or temporary device.[11] In the 1920s, Lindbergh and Carrel discussed and planned an artificial heart.[12] Throughout the 1940s researchers including Dennis and Gibbon were developing a machine that would bypass the circulation of the heart and lungs to allow open-heart surgery. The modern era of MCS began in 1951 when Dennis first used a heart-lung machine to sustain the circulation while the heart was opened to repair an atrial septal defect.[13] Two years later, Gibbon repeated this procedure.[14] However, high mortality in the first few cases led both Dennis and Gibbon to abandon the use of their heart-lung machines. In 1954, Lillehei began to use cross-circulation (human-to-human perfusion) as a means to support heart and lung function during congenital heart defect.[15] However, because of the controversy created by Lillehei's procedure, researchers continued efforts to develop a machine that would allow open-heart surgery.

By 1955, Kirklin and associates at the Mayo Clinic had refined the Mayo-Gibbon machine and the techniques that allowed open-heart surgery.[16] Likewise, Lillehei and associates had developed their machine that also allowed for safe open-heart operations.[17] By 1960, Kirklin and Lillehei in Minneapolis and DeBakey and Cooley in Houston had perfected their machines and techniques to the point where heart surgery was becoming routine in Minnesota and Texas. The early developmental work on the use of mechanical circulatory systems by Dennis, Lillehei, DeWall, Gibbon, and Kirklin allowed for many new cardiac operations, including coronary artery bypass, heart transplantation, valve repair, and implantation of a TAH. After refinements of the heart-lung machines, DeBakey and Cooley began to develop many of the surgical techniques that eventually made open-heart surgery routine around the world.

In 1957, Akutsu and Kolff became the first to implant a TAH in vivo.[18] Inserted into the chest of a dog, the pump adequately maintained the circulation for approximately 90 minutes. However, Akutsu and Kolff never applied their TAH technology clinically. In 1964, the National Heart Institute established the Artificial Heart Program to promote the development of the TAH and other cardiac assist devices. In the early 1960s, DeBakey and researchers at Baylor College of Medicine in Houston began developing a TAH. In 1963, DeBakey implanted the first clinical left ventricular assist device (LVAD) into a 42-year-old patient.[19] The pump functioned well, but the patient died of pulmonary complications after 4 days of support. In 1967, DeBakey implanted an LVAD into a 37-year-old who presented with symptoms of HF, including easy fatigability and severe dyspnea on slight exertion. This patient also had history of rheumatic heart disease since age 18 and closed mitral valvulotomy at age 25. The intention was to use the LVAD until sufficient myocardial recovery could be gained. The LVAD supported the patient's circulation for 10 days and was then electively removed. The patient was discharged from the hospital on postoperative day 29 and later resumed normal activity. On follow-up at 18 months after LVAD removal, the patient remained free of HF symptoms, and a chest x-ray showed a significant reduction in cardiac size.

FIRST TOTAL ARTIFICIAL HEART

The first implantation of a TAH into a human was done by Cooley on April 4, 1969, in a 47-year-old man who could not be weaned from cardiopulmonary bypass (CPB) following left ventricular aneurysmectomy.[20] The intent was to support the patient until a donor heart could be found. The TAH (Fig. 67-1), designed by Liotta, was a pneumatically powered, double-chambered pump with Dacron-lined right and left

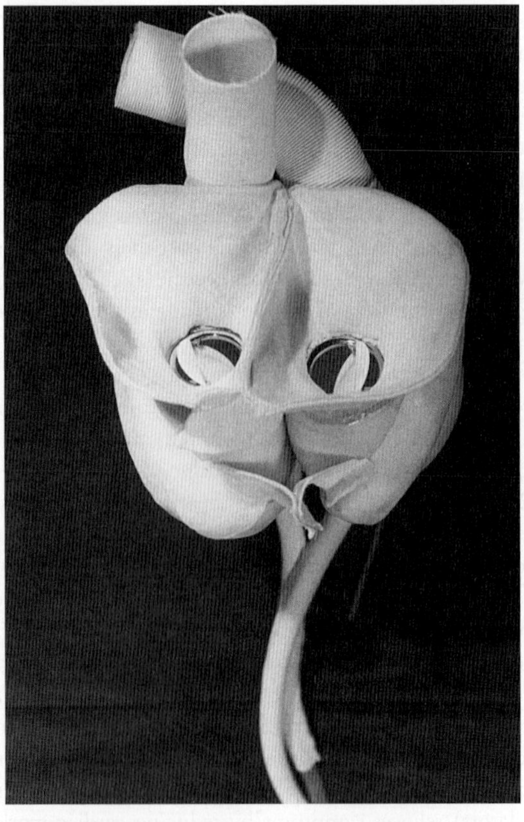

FIGURE 67-1 The Liotta total artificial heart, the first TAH implanted in a human.

inflow cuffs and outflow grafts. Wada-Cutter hingeless valves controlled the direction of blood flow through the pump. The TAH itself was connected to a large external power unit, which unfortunately severely restricted patient mobility. The TAH performed adequately for 64 hours until transplantation. The donor heart also functioned well, but the patient died of pseudomonal pneumonia 32 hours after transplantation. Though the Liotta device performed as designed, it was never used clinically again. Nevertheless, this case clearly demonstrated that a TAH could be used safely and effectively in a human as a bridge to transplantation.

AKUTSU-III TOTAL ARTIFICIAL HEART

The second implantation of a TAH in a human was also done by Cooley. On July 23, 1981, Cooley implanted the Akutsu-III TAH into a critically ill 26-year-old man who suffered heart failure after undergoing coronary artery bypass surgery for severe arteriosclerosis. Unable to be weaned from CPB after surgery, the patient was fitted with the TAH in a final effort to sustain his life. The Akutsu-III TAH (Fig. 67-2) consisted of two pneumatically powered, double-chambered pumps featuring reciprocating hemispherical diaphragms.[21] The TAH provided excellent hemodynamics and supported the patient in stable condition for a total of 55 hours until a suitable donor heart was found. The patient finally received a transplant but died of infectious, renal, and pulmonary complications 10 days later. Despite the fatal outcome, this case demonstrated that a TAH could adequately sustain a patient for several days, with no evidence of hemolysis or thromboembolism, until heart transplantation.

JARVIK-7/CARDIOWEST TOTAL ARTIFICIAL HEART

In the late 1970s, Kolff and his team at the University of Utah developed the Jarvik-7 TAH. In 1982, DeVries became the first to permanently implant a TAH when he implanted a Jarvik-7 into a dying patient.[22] The Jarvik-7 TAH (Fig. 67-3) was a pneumatically powered, biventricular pulsatile device that replaced the heart.[23,24] The pumps were connected to their respective native atria by synthetic cuffs and connectors. Each pump had chambers for air and blood separated by a smooth, flexible polyurethane diaphragm. The inflow and outflow conduits contained Medtronic-Hall tilting disk valves. The filling of the pumps was aided by vacuum. Pneumatic drivelines, brought out through the chest wall to connect with an external console, shuttled air to the pumps during systole, thereby causing collapse of the pump sac and blood ejection. Pump rate, drive pressure, and systolic duration were monitored and optimized from the external console. The Jarvik-7 had a stroke volume of 70 mL and a normal cardiac output of 6 to 8 L/min (maximum, 15 L/min).

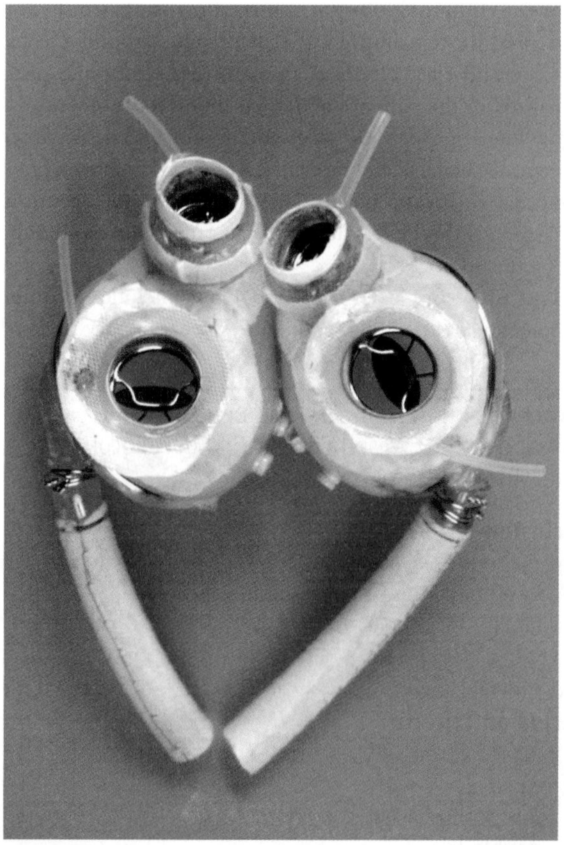

FIGURE 67-2 The Akutsu-III total artificial heart, the second TAH implanted in a human.

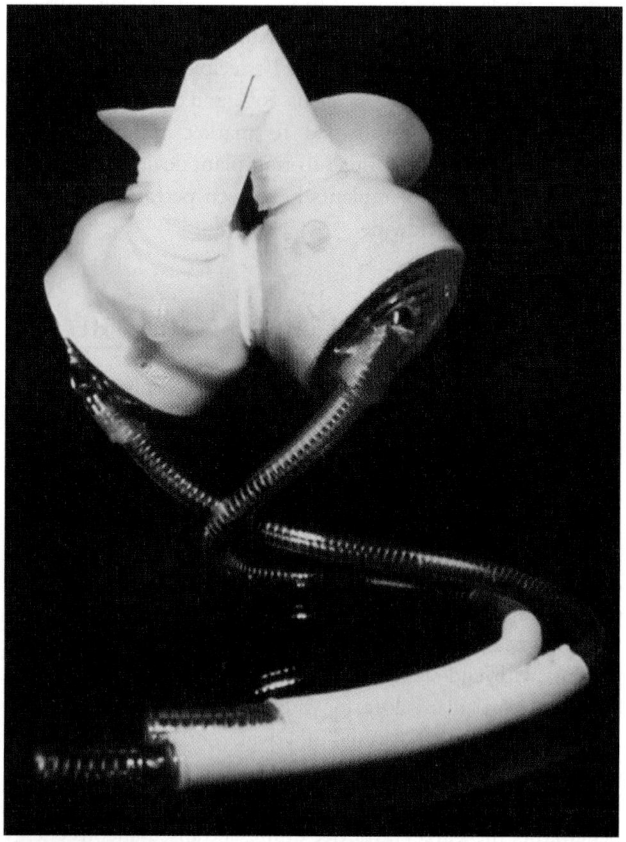

FIGURE 67-3 The CardioWest TAH-t (SynCardia, Inc., Tucson, AZ), formerly the Jarvik-7 and Symbion TAH.

In the initial clinical experience with the Jarvik-7 TAH, a total of five patients were permanently supported for periods ranging from 10 to 620 days. The TAH was able to adequately support circulation, but its large drive console and frequent medical complications limited patient activity. Four patients were able to make brief trips out of the hospital to see family and friends. Long-term outcomes, however, were poor. Patients supported by the Jarvik-7 for longer periods suffered several complications, including thromboembolism, stroke, infection, and multiorgan failure.

Despite these mixed results, in 1985 the Jarvik-7 (renamed the Symbion) TAH entered clinical trials as a bridge to transplantation. In 1986, Copeland reported the first successful use of this device for this indication.[25] Between 1985 and 1991, approximately 170 patients were supported with the Symbion TAH as a bridge to transplantation.[26] Sixty-six percent underwent successful heart transplantation, a rate similar to those in bridge-to-transplantation studies of left ventricular assist devices. Sepsis and multiple organ failure were the primary causes of death during TAH support.

Although the bridge-to-transplantation study demonstrated that the Jarvik-7 (Symbion) TAH was clinically safe and effective, the US Food and Drug Administration (FDA) withdrew the device's investigational device exemption (IDE) for clinical use in January 1991 because of inadequate compliance with FDA regulations.[27] In January 1993, the IDE was restored to the CardioWest TAH, which differed little from the original Jarvik-7. In 2001, Syncardia, Inc. was formed, and the CardioWest TAH-t (temporary) has since been used successfully in the United States, Canada, and France.[28] In the US clinical trials, survival to transplantation and overall 1-year survival rates were significantly higher for CardioWest TAH-t recipients (n = 81) than for controls (n = 35) (79% versus 46% and 70% versus 31%, respectively). These results led to market approval of the CardioWest TAH-t as a bridge-to-transplant device in 2004. By 2009, more than 800 implants have been performed at more than 40 centers worldwide.

ABIOCOR IMPLANTABLE REPLACEMENT HEART

On July 2, 2001, as part of an FDA-sponsored phase I clinical trial, surgeons at Jewish Hospital in Louisville, Kentucky, performed the first implantation of the AbioCor TAH in a 59-year-old man with end-stage HF.[29] The AbioCor Implantable Replacement Heart is a self-contained, electrohydraulic TAH (Fig. 67-4) that has been developed and tested by ABIOMED, Inc. (Danvers, MA) and the Texas Heart Institute, with the support of the National Heart, Lung, and Blood Institute (NHLBI).[30,31] It is designed to sustain the circulation and extend the lives of patients with end-stage HF who have suffered irreversible left and right ventricular failure, for whom surgery or medical therapy is inadequate, and who would otherwise soon die (Table 67-1). The AbioCor is the first TAH to be used clinically that is fully implantable and communicates to external hardware without penetrating the skin. The device utilizes a transcutaneous energy transfer system (TET) and a radiofrequency communication (RF Comm) system that allows it to be powered and controlled by signals transmitted across intact skin. A unique feature of the AbioCor is a right-left flow-balancing mechanism that eliminates the need for an external vent or internal compliance chamber.[32]

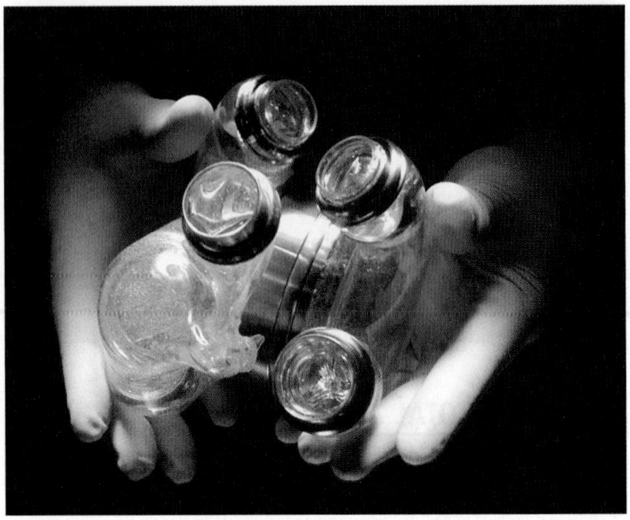

FIGURE 67-4 The AbioCor Implantable Replacement Heart. (*ABIOMED, Inc., Danvers, MA.*)

The internal components of the AbioCor system consist of a thoracic unit, internal TET coil, controller, and battery.[33] The thoracic unit (pump) weighs about 2 lb and consists of two artificial ventricles, four valves, and an innovative motor-driven hydraulic pumping system (Fig. 67-5). The pump's motor rotates at 6000 to 8000 rpm, which allows sufficient hydraulic fluid pressure to compress the diaphragm around the blood chamber and eject blood. A miniaturized electronics package implanted in the patient's abdomen monitors and controls the pump rate, right-left balance, and motor speed. An internal rechargeable battery, also implanted within the abdomen, provides emergency or backup power. The internal battery is continually recharged via the TET system and can provide up to 30 minutes of untethered operation.

The AbioCor's external components include a computer console, an external TET coil, and external battery packs. The

TABLE 67-1 Inclusion/Exclusion Criteria for FDA-Sponsored Phase I Clinical Trial of Abiocor Total Artificial Heart

Inclusion Criteria
End-stage heart failure
>70% probability of death within 30 days
Ineligibility for a heart transplant
No other surgical or medical treatment options
Biventricular failure
Exclusion Criteria
Significant potential for reversibility of heart failure
Chronic dialysis
Recent cerebrovascular accident (CVA)
Irreversible liver failure
Blood dyscrasia

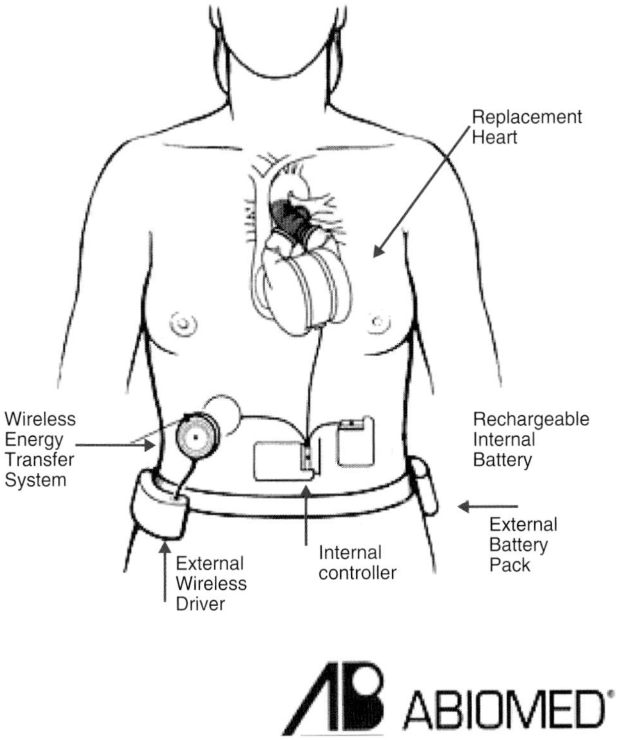

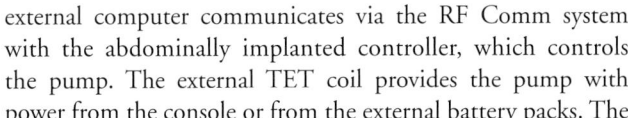

FIGURE 67-5 The AbioCor system is designed to increase or decrease its pump rate in response to the body's needs. The AbioCor also includes an active monitoring system that provides detailed performance feedback and alarms in the event of irregularities.

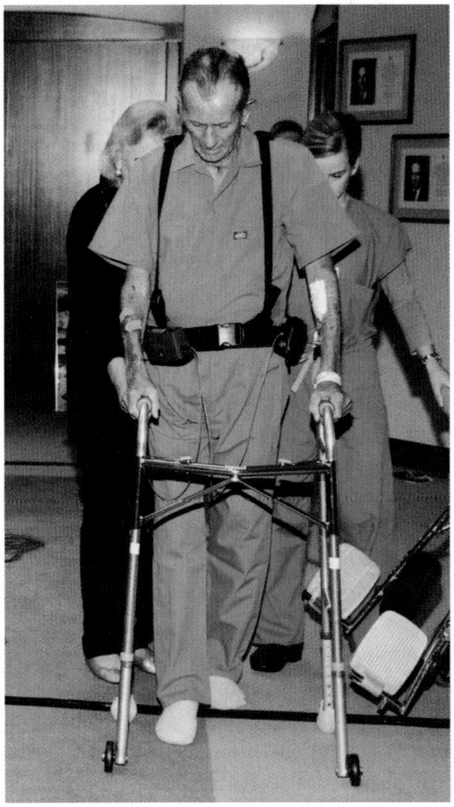

FIGURE 67-6 Third patient to receive the AbioCor Implantable Replacement Heart. This patient was supported by the AbioCor for 142 days and underwent physical rehabilitation but ultimately died of thromboembolic complications.

external computer communicates via the RF Comm system with the abdominally implanted controller, which controls the pump. The external TET coil provides the pump with power from the console or from the external battery packs. The external battery packs can power the AbioCor TAH for 2 to 4 hours (Fig. 67-6).

In the phase I feasibility trial, 14 patients received the AbioCor as destination therapy (Table 67-2). Thrombo-

TABLE 67-2 Summary of Initial Clinical Experience with AbioCor Total Artificial Heart*

Patient No.	Implantation Date	No. Days Supported	Age (y)	Institution/City	Outcome
1	July 2, 2001	151	58	Jewish Hospital, Louisville, KY	Died
2	September 13, 2001	512	70	Jewish Hospital, Louisville, KY	Died
3	September 26, 2001	142	68	THI/St. Luke's Episcopal Hospital, Houston, TX	Died
4	October 17, 2001	56	74	UCLA, Los Angeles, CA	Died
5	November 5, 2001	293	51	MCP Hahnemann University Hospital, Philadelphia, PA	Died
6	November 27, 2001	0	79	THI/St. Luke's Episcopal Hospital, Houston, TX	Died
7	April 10, 2002	0	61	Jewish Hospital, Louisville, KY	Died
8	January 7, 2003	100	79	Jewish Hospital, Louisville, KY	Died
9	January 22, 2003	53	65	Jewish Hospital, Louisville, KY	Died
10	February 24, 2003	115	69	THI/St. Luke's Episcopal Hospital, Houston, TX	Died
11	May 1, 2003	100	64	THI/St. Luke's Episcopal Hospital, Houston, TX	Died
12	February 20, 2004	86	63	THI/St. Luke's Episcopal Hospital, Houston, TX	Died
13	May 3, 2004	146	72	Jewish Hospital, Louisville, KY	Died
14	May 24, 2004	164	72	Jewish Hospital, Louisville, KY	Died

*As of July 5, 2005.

embolism was a significant adverse event in this group of patients, and there were two pump failures. However, compared with the known rates of infection for implantable systems with percutaneous drivelines, device-related infections in this trial were relatively rare. The longest surviving patient was supported for 512 days, most of which were lived at home with a good quality of life. In 2006, the FDA approved the AbioCor for commercial use under a Humanitarian Device Exemption.

COMPLICATIONS

Use of a TAH is associated with serious complications. The most frequent complications are infection, severe postoperative bleeding, and thromboembolism.[34-37] Potentially serious but less frequent complications are renal, hepatic, pulmonary, and neurologic dysfunction and complications caused by technical problems.[34,38] Complicating factors include patient selection, device size, implantation timing and location, the need for extensive surgery at implantation, and the reliability of support equipment.

Life-threatening infections have been the most important complication for patients being supported permanently by a TAH.[39] In the Jarvik-7 experience, all patients supported for many months developed serious infections that eventually contributed to their deaths.[23,40] Patients supported by a TAH for shorter periods while awaiting heart transplantation had infection rates of 30 to 40%.[35-39] During the 1980s, driveline and mediastinal infections in TAH-supported patients were frequent and severe, regardless of the duration of support. However, in the more recent bridge-to-transplantation experience with the CardioWest TAH-t, serious infections contributing to death or delayed transplantation occurred in only 21% of patients.[41,42]

Patients supported with a TAH, regardless of the intended use, are very susceptible to infection. Predisposing factors include the tissue trauma associated with surgical implantation; contamination of the implanted device; depression of the body's immune defenses; the large amount of foreign material presented on the surface of the device; and use of the drivelines, tubes, catheters, and other devices that are necessary for the care of these patients. Infections can occur at any point during TAH support. Once an internal component of the TAH system is infectiously colonized, treatment is difficult and often ineffective. Infections are more likely to occur in the early postoperative period, especially in the most critically ill patients, as a result of (1) device contamination during the course of care and (2) postoperative bleeding caused by intensive care procedures and exposure during reoperation. Meticulous care and numerous infection prevention measures are vital in all TAH patients.

Postoperative bleeding is a frequent and serious complication of TAH implantation. It generally occurs in 40 to 50% of TAH or ventricular assist device recipients.[34] In the more recent CardioWest TAH-t experience, the rate was approximately 25%. Contributing factors include severe HF and associated hepatic dysfunction, the extensive surgery and lengthy CPB time required for implantation, and the necessity for postoperative anticoagulation therapy. Severe HF often leads to hepatic dysfunction and subsequent derangement of the coagulation system. Patients with severe HF are often receiving continuous preoperative anticoagulant or antiplatelet therapy, the effects of which are often difficult to reverse before TAH implantation. The extensive surgery and lengthy CPB time required for implantation can lead to severe depletion of clotting factors. The necessity for postoperative anticoagulation therapy requires that a proper balance be established between preventing thrombosis and allowing blood to clot, through the careful management of hemostasis and anticoagulant therapy.

Thrombosis within the TAH is of particular concern. Five of the first six Jarvik-7 recipients had thromboembolic events. However, the frequency of thromboembolism has decreased significantly since that initial experience and is now an estimated 10 to 15%.[34,35,43] Preventive measures are primarily targeted at precisely monitoring the thrombotic and fibrinolytic systems, maintaining sufficient flow through the device to avoid stasis, and providing adequate anticoagulation and antiplatelet therapy. Generally, heparin and warfarin are used as antithrombotic therapy to achieve a prothrombin time, activated thromboplastin time, or international normalized ratio two to three times greater than the baseline or normal value. Aspirin or dipyridamole or both are also used.

There is a complex though poorly understood interrelationship between infection, bleeding, and thromboembolism. Thrombus formation may lead to the development of infection, and bacterial colonization may lead to thrombus formation. Bacteria are often seen in thrombi found in cardiovascular devices.[44] Bacteria embedded in a thrombus are protected from circulating antibiotics and leukocytes. Bacteria, endotoxins, and inflammatory cells may contribute to thrombus formation by their effect on platelet aggregation.[44] Bacterial endotoxins can cause platelet aggregation, endothelial injury, and increased endothelial thromboplastin activity. Excessive bleeding most often results in reoperation, which increases the patient's exposure to contamination. Also, blood transfusions and intravascular monitoring for these critically ill patients are more extensive and result in frequent exposure to the external environment. Infection, bleeding, and thromboembolism can contribute individually and collectively to the development of multiple organ failure, one of the most frequent causes of death in TAH recipients.

Other important problems and issues related to TAH implantation are device malfunction, poor fit or size mismatch between TAH and patient, social and ethical issues, mobility, and nutrition. Device malfunction leading to catastrophic failure of the TAH or ventricular assist device is rare. Most technical issues have involved external components and have been readily resolved. Fit and size mismatch remains a problem. All TAH models used to date have been relatively large and only fit adequately into patients with a body surface area greater than 1.7 m^2. Because the cost of TAH technology is fairly high and most candidates for TAH implantation are in their sixth to seventh decade of life, many groups question whether society should bear the cost of developing this technology. Until recently, the external components of the TAH equipment have been large and cumbersome, thus limiting patient mobility, exercise, and rehabilitation. More recent designs of the TAH allow for much more mobility.

TOTAL ARTIFICAL HEART RESEARCH AND DEVELOPMENT

It has been shown that HF can be treated with volume-displacement TAHs, such as the pneumatic CardioWest TAH-t or the AbioCor TAH. The CardioWest TAH-t has successfully supported patients awaiting transplantation.[40,45,46] However, its externalized pneumatic drivelines and pneumatic console limit durability and patient mobility, making this TAH poorly suited for permanent cardiac replacement. The electrohydraulic AbioCor Implantable Replacement Heart has been used in a small, select group of patients requiring biventricular replacement.[47] Although these TAHs have been used successfully in some patients, their large size, mechanical complexity, and poor durability have also limited their application.

Recently, new design applications using continuous-flow rotary blood pumps have emerged to create a smaller and more compact alternative to the larger volume-displacement TAHs. Unlike the pulsatile, volume-displacement TAHs, these rotary pumps have no flexible membranes, pusher-plates, or prosthetic valves that can wear out. They are actuated by rapidly spinning impellers, which reduce their mechanical complexity. Rotary pumps are more durable, making them less expensive to produce. In addition, these pumps are smaller, quieter, and more energy efficient than are volume-displacement pumps. Lastly, rotary pumps are inflow-pressure sensitive—they closely imitate the native heart by autonomously increasing pump flow in response to an increasing preload. Surprisingly, this technology has never been used clinically in a TAH configuration, despite the significant need for a cardiac replacement device (CRD) that is smaller, simpler, and less expensive. Therefore, constant-flow technology may be ideally suited for integration into the next generation of permanently implantable CRDs.

Recently, at the Texas Heart Institute, we have begun extensive testing of rotary blood pumps to assess the feasibility of using two continuous-flow pumps for totally implantable biventricular replacement.[48] Axial-flow and centrifugal-type blood pumps are being developed for use as CRDs.[48,49] Initially, the constant-flow pumps were designed and used clinically as left ventricular assist devices (LVADs). However, it was noted, particularly in pumps placed outside the ventricle, that the ventricle itself acted as a reservoir and that the aortic valve did not open. Therefore, technically, there was no pulse. Despite this, patients had normal physiologic function, even years after the device was implanted. This fact supports our belief that constant-flow pumps could be a feasible option for a CRD.

The use of two independent constant-flow pumps modifies and may even eliminate the need for a separate control mechanism for atrial balance. Each pump's flow will be regulated by the pressure differential between the inflow and the outflow, even at a constant rpm. Testing of that concept in our laboratory has also proved promising, with animal survival times of 7 weeks after total cardiac replacement with two rotary pumps. This was achieved by maintaining a constant rpm, even in treadmill studies. The normal physiologic response gives us some hope that an individualized flow might be assessed for each patient, without the need for a complex, integrated system. Continuous flow with an induced pulse (by modulating speed) and with pulseless flow is being investigated to study the physiologic effects in a chronic animal model.

Additional programs have also begun to investigate the use of rotary blood pumps as CRDs. The Cleveland Clinic is developing a valveless, sensorless, pulsatile, continuous-flow double-pump TAH.[50] The impellers of both pumps are attached to a single axial rotor. Atrial pressures are balanced by way of passive self-regulation (the rotor axial position and subsequent position of the impeller with regard to the right pump inflow). If the atrial pressure on either the left or right sides is increased, the rotor is pushed to the contralateral side, forcing the impeller either to block or open the right inflow opening, thus increasing or decreasing right pump flow. A group at Queensland University of Technology is also working on a single-unit rotary device CRD that uses a shared rotating hub with two impellers.[51] This device employs an interpump shunt (similar to a ventricular septal defect) for left-to-right atrial pressure balance, allowing blood to flow between the two pumps and beneath the pump impellers. At Tohoku University, two centrifugal pumps, each with independent control algorithms, are being tested as a CRD.[52]

COMMENT

Since the 1950s, when the heart-lung bypass machine was developed, many advances have been made in the surgical treatment of HF. Many surgical procedures considered impossible just 40 years ago are today considered routine. A classic example is heart transplantation. However, TAH technology has not evolved at the same pace. Although the first human heart transplantation and first human TAH implantation occurred within 2 years of each other, TAH implantation is still neither routine nor widely available. However, two TAHs are undergoing clinical trials at present in the United States. The CardioWest (formerly the Jarvik-7) TAH-t, which is the more widely used of the two, is now approved for use as a bridge to transplantation. The AbioCor TAH is still in the early stages of clinical testing and is likely years away from approval as an alternative to heart transplantation. However, should its unique TET system and flow-balancing mechanism prove to be reliable for extended periods of time, the AbioCor may become a widely used alternative to heart transplantation for those patients who have no other treatment options.

There are many obstacles to overcome before any TAH is widely accepted. Infection, bleeding, thromboembolism, and biocompatibility issues are serious problems that affect nearly all implantable cardiovascular devices including TAHs. Improved biomaterials, better prevention, and more effective antibiotic and anticoagulant medications may help overcome these problems. Acceptance by the public, by some critics in the health professions, and by third-party payors may be slow. Quality in manufacturing is needed to ensure reliability of TAH components.

Addressing these problems will help bring the TAH more quickly into routine clinical use.

KEY POINTS

- Careful patient selection is key to long-term, successful outcomes. An institution's medical review board should approve potential candidates to ensure that only appropriate patients are selected for CRD implantation. Biventricular function should be carefully assessed in patients to rule out if they are better candidates for LVAD implantation.
- Bleeding complications can be multifactorial. Patients with poor platelet and liver function, those who undergo prolonged cardiopulmonary bypass times during the implant procedure, or those who have preoperative coagulopathies will likely have bleeding complications. Attention to detail during the TAH implant procedure can minimize bleeding complications and ensure faster recovery times.
- Infection prevention measures must be used in TAH patients. Should large, blood-contacting foreign bodies in the chest become infected, they are difficult to treat. All indwelling catheters should be replaced often to minimize the risk of infection. Cardiac replacement devices with external drivelines must be meticulously cared for to reduce the risk of infection.
- Device size and portability are important factors. The AbioCor Implantable Replacement Heart can only be used in larger patients with the appropriate thoracic dimensions. Imaging studies must be performed to ensure that the thoracic anatomy will allow for optimal device fit. The CardioWest TAH-t employs a pneumatic external driver, which may limit patient mobility and normal activity.

REFERENCES

1. 2009 Heart and Stroke Statistical Update: American Heart Association. Available at: http://www.americanheart.org. Accessed December 2009.
2. Frazier OH, Myers TJ: Surgical therapy for severe heart failure [review]. *Curr Probl Cardiol* 1998; 23(12):721-764.
3. 2009 Focused Update: ACCF/AHA Guidelines for the Diagnosis and Management of Heart Failure in Adults: a report of the American College of Cardiology Foundation/American Heart Association Task Force on Practice Guidelines: developed in collaboration with the International Society of Heart and Lung Transplantation. *Circulation* 2009; 119(14):1977-2016
4. Network for Organ Sharing: Critical Data. U.S. Facts about Transplantation. Available at: http://www.unos.org. Accessed December 2009.
5. Copeland JG, Smith RE, Arabia FA, et al: Cardiac replacement with a total artificial heart as a bridge to transplantation. *NEJM* 2004; 351(9): 859-867.
6. Frazier OH, Rose EA, McCarthy PM, et al: Improved mortality and rehabilitation of transplant candidates treated with a long-term implantable left ventricular assist system. *Ann Surg* 1995; 222(3):327-335.
7. Frazier OH, Rose EA, Oz MC, et al: Multicenter clinical evaluation of the HeartMate vented electric left ventricular assist system in patients awaiting heart transplantation. *J Thorac Cardiovasc Surg* 2001; 122(6):1186-1195.
8. Rose EA, Gelijns AC, Moskowitz AJ, et al: Long-term mechanical left ventricular assistance for end-stage heart failure. *NEJM* 2001; 345(20): 1435-1443.
9. Mueller J, Weng Y, Dandel M: Long-term results of weaning from LVAD: it does work. *ASAIO J* 1999; 45:153.
10. Frazier OH, Myers TJ: Left ventricular assist system as a bridge to myocardial recovery. *Ann Thorac Surg* 1999, 68(2):734-741.
11. LeGallois CJJ: *Experience on the Principle of Life.* Philadelphia, Thomas, 1813. Translation of LeGallois CJJ, *Experience sur la principe de la vie.* Paris, 1812.
12. Miller GW: *King of Hearts: The True Story of the Maverick Who Pioneered Open Heart Surgery.* New York, Random House, 2000.
13. Dennis C: A heart-lung machine for open-heart operations: how it came about. *ASAIO Trans* 1989; 35(4):767-777.
14. Gibbon JH Jr: Application of a heart and lung apparatus to cardiac surgery. *Minn Med* 1954; 37(3):171-180.
15. Lillehei CW, Cohen M, Warden HE, Varco RL: The direct-vision intracardiac correction of congenital anomalies by controlled cross circulation. *Surgery* 1955; 38(1):11-29.
16. Kirklin JW, DuShane JW, Patrick RT, et al: Intracardiac surgery with the aid of a mechanical pump-oxygenator system (Gibbon type): report of eight cases. *Staff Meetings Mayo Clin* 1955; 30(10):201-206.
17. Lillehei CW, DeWall RA, Read R, Warden HE, Varco RL: Direct-vision intracardiac surgery in man using a simple, disposable artificial oxygenator. *Dis Chest* 1956; 29(1):1-8.
18. Akutsu T, Kolff WJ: Permanent substitute for valves and hearts. *Trans Am Soc Artif Intern Organs* 1958; 4:230.
19. DeBakey ME. Left ventricular bypass for cardiac assistance: clinical experience. *Am J Cardiol* 1971; 27(1):3-11.
20. Cooley DA, Liotta D, Hallman GL, et al: Orthotopic cardiac prosthesis for two-staged cardiac replacement. *Am J Cardiol* 1969; 24(5):723-730.
21. Frazier OH, Akutsu T, Cooley DA: Total artificial heart (TAH) utilization in man. *Trans Am Soc Artif Intern Organs* 1982; 23:534-538.
22. DeVries WC: The permanent artificial heart: four case reports. *JAMA* 1988; 259(6):849-859.
23. DeVries WC, Anderson JL, Joyce LD, et al: Clinical use of the total artificial heart. *NEJM* 1984; 310(5):273-278.
24. DeVries WC: Surgical technique for implantation of the Jarvik-7-100 total artificial heart. *JAMA* 1988; 259(6):875-880.
25. Copeland CG, Smith RG, Icenogle TB, Ott RA: Early experience with the total artificial heart as a bridge to cardiac transplantation. *Surg Clin North Am* 1988; 68(3):621-634.
26. Johnson KE, Prieto M, Joyce LD, Pritzker M, Emery RW: Summary of the clinical use of the Symbion total artificial heart: a registry report. *J Heart Lung Transplant* 1992; 11(1 Pt 1):103-116.
27. Copeland JG: Current status and future directions for a total artificial heart with a past. *Artif Organs* 1998; 22(11):998-1001.
28a. Copeland JG, Smith RG, Arabia FA, et al: CardioWest Total Artificial Heart Investigators. Cardiac replacement with a total artificial heart as a bridge to transplantation. *NEJM* 2004; 351(9):859-867.
28b. SoRelle R: Cardiovascular news. Totally contained AbioCor artificial heart implanted July 3, 2001. *Circulation* 2001; 104(3):E9005-9006.
29. Kung RTV, Yu LS, Ochs BD, et al: Progress in the development of the ABIOMED total artificial heart. *ASAIO J* 1995; 41(3):M245-248.
30. Parnis SM, Yu LS, Ochs BD, et al: Chronic in vivo evaluation of an electrohydraulic total artificial heart. *ASAIO J* 1994; 40(3):M489-493. .
31. Kung RTV, Yu LS, Ochs BD, Parnis SM, Frazier OH: An artificial hydraulic shunt in a total artificial heart: a balance mechanism for the bronchial shunt. *ASAIO J* 1993; 39(3):M213-217.
32. Yu LS, Finnegan M, Vaughan S, et al: A compact and noise-free electrohydraulic total artificial heart. *ASAIO J* 1993; 39(3):M386-391.
33. Quaini E, Pavie A, Chieco S, Mambrito B: The Concerted Action 'Heart' European registry on clinical application of mechanical circulatory support systems: bridge to transplant. The Registry Scientific Committee. *Eur J Cardiothorac Surg* 1997; 11(1):182-188.
34. Mehta SM, Aufiero TX, Pae WE Jr, Miller CA, Pierce WS: Combined Registry for the Clinical Use of Mechanical Ventricular Assist Pumps and the Total Artificial Heart in conjunction with heart transplantation: sixth official report—1994. *J Heart Lung Transplant* 1995; 14(3):585-593.
35. Myers TJ, Khan T, Frazier OH: Infectious complications associated with ventricular assist systems. *ASAIO J* 2000; 46(6):S28-36.
36. Conger JL, Inman RW, Tamez D, Frazier OH, Radovancevic B: Infection and thrombosis in total artificial heart technology: past and future challenges–a historical review. *ASAIO J* 2000; 46(6):S22-27.
37. Arabia FA, Copeland JG, Smith RG, et al: International experience with the CardioWest total artificial heart as a bridge to heart transplantation. *Eur J Cardiothorac Surg* 1997; 11(Suppl):S5-10.
38. Gristina AG, Dobbins JJ, Giammara B, Lewis JC, DeVries WC: Biomaterial-centered sepsis and the total artificial heart. Microbial adhesion vs tissue integration. *JAMA* 1988; 259(6):870-874.
39. Joyce LD, DeVries WC, Hastings WL, et al: Response of the human body to the first permanent implant of the Jarvik-7 Total Artificial Heart. *Trans Am Soc Artif Intern Organs* 1983; 29:81-87.
40. Copeland JG, Smith RG, Arabia FA, et al: Total artificial heart bridge to transplantation: a 9-year experience with 62 patients. *J Heart Lung Transplant.* 2004; 23(7):823-831.

41. Copeland JG 3rd, Smith RG, Arabia FA, et al: Comparison of the CardioWest total artificial heart, the Novacor left ventricular assist system, and the Thoratec ventricular assist system in bridge to transplantation. *Ann Thorac Surg* 2001; 71(3 Suppl):S92-97.
42. Copeland JG, Smith RG, Arabia FA, Nolan PE, Banchy ME: The CardioWest total artificial heart as a bridge to transplantation. *Semin Thorac Cardiovasc Surg* 2000; 12(3):238-242.
43. Chiang BY, Burns GL, Pantalos GM, et al: Microbially infected thrombus in animals with total artificial hearts. *ASAIO Trans* 1991; 37(3): M256-257.
44. Didisheim P, Olsen DB, Farrar DJ, et al: Infections and thromboembolism with implantable cardiovascular devices. *ASAIO Trans* 1989; 35(1):54-70.
45. El-Banayosy A, Arusoglu L, Morshuis M, et al: CardioWest total artificial heart: Bad Oeynhausen experience. *Ann Thorac Surg* 2005; 80(2): 548-552.
46. Leprince P, Bonnet N, Rama A, et al: Bridge to transplantation with the Jarvik-7 (CardioWest) total artificial heart: a single center 15-year experience. *J Heart Lung Transplant* 2003; 22(12):1296-1303.
47. Dowling RD, Gray LA Jr, Etoch SW, et al: Initial experience with the AbioCor implantable replacement heart system. *J Thorac Cardiovasc Surg* 2004; 127(1):131-141.
48. Frazier,OH, Tuzun E, Cohn WE, Conger JL, Kadipasaoglu KA: Total heart replacement using dual intracorporeal continuous-flow pumps in a chronic bovine model: a feasibility study. *ASAIO J* 2006; 52(2):145-149.
49. Frazier OH, Tuzun E, Cohn W, Tamez D, Kadipasaoglu KA: Total heart replacement with dual centrifugal ventricular assist devices. *ASAIO J* 2005; 51(3):224-229.
50. Fukamachi K, Horvath D, Massiello A, et al: An innovative, sensorless, pulsatile, continuous-flow total artificial heart: device design and initial in vitro study. *J Heart Lung Transplant* 2010; 29(1):13-20.
51. Timms D, Fraser J, Hayne M, et al: The BIVACOR rotary biventricular assist device: Concept and in vitro investigation. *Artif Organs* 2008; 32(10):816-819.
52. Olegario PS, Yoshizawa M, Tanaka A, et al: Outflow control for avoiding atrial suction in a continuous flow artificial heart. *Artif Organs* 2003; 27(1):92-98.

CHAPTER 68

Nontransplant Surgical Options for Heart Failure

Lynn C. Huffman
Steven F. Bolling

INTRODUCTION

Congestive heart failure (CHF) has become a major worldwide public health problem. In our ever-aging population, medical advances that have extended our average life expectancy have also left more people living with chronic cardiac disease than ever before. More than 20 million people are affected worldwide. In the United States the estimated 2006 prevalence of heart failure in adults age 20 and older is 5.8 million yet less than 3000 are offered transplantation because of limitations of age, comorbid conditions, and donor availability. Despite the significant improvements with medical management hospital discharges for heart failure rose from 877,000 in 1996 to 1,106,000 in 2006 and mortality in the first year is one in five. CHF patients are repeatedly readmitted for inpatient care and the vast majority will die within 3 years of diagnosis.[1]

Orthotopic heart transplantation (OHT) offers successful and reproducible long-term results and is the treatment of choice for patients with medically refractory end-stage heart failure.[2] Unfortunately, the obvious limitations to OHT include the need for immunosuppression and the severe shortage of donor organs. This past decade has seen the annual number of transplants performed worldwide plateau at less than 4000, down to only 3353 in 2008.[3,4] This lack of donor availability has thus necessitated a rigorous selection criteria be applied to potential recipients in order to optimize the utility of these precious organs, indicated only for patients with end-stage cardiomyopathy in whom all other modes of therapy have been exhausted. Access to OHT has thus been restricted to those without comorbid medical conditions and relatively restricted to those younger than age 65. This leaves the vast majority of CHF patients seeking other options.

With significant technologic strides being made toward total implantability, the role for mechanical support is becoming more widely accepted as a bridge to recovery as well as a bridge to transplant. There have been a number of successful studies of ventricular assist devices (VADs) used as a bridge to recovery and the long-term efficacy for this purpose, and this use as a long-term therapy for chronic heart failure has become established by multicenter clinical trials.[5–10] As a result continuous-flow left ventricular assist devices (LVADs) have emerged as the standard of care for advanced heart failure patients requiring long-term mechanical circulatory support. The long-term survival of circulatory support is increasing but does not yet equal survival after OHT, the gold standard treatment. Because many more people can benefit from this therapy, and with their improved durability, these devices are now an option in the management of patients with heart failure.

This clinical dilemma has provided the impetus for surgeons to develop new alternatives for the treatment of heart failure. As OHT and VAD use is more stringently applied, techniques to restore myocardial perfusion, eliminate valvular regurgitation, and restore ventricular geometry have emerged as a possible first-line surgical approach to heart failure. In response to the growing need for the proficient application and critical appraisal of the expanding menu of surgical options, the new subspecialty of heart failure surgery has emerged. The following will briefly review established nontransplant surgical modalities for heart failure such as coronary revascularization, geometric mitral reconstruction, and ventricular reconstruction. Alternative options such as partial left ventriculectomy and cardiomyoplasty as well as some innovative devices currently being evaluated for clinical application will also be discussed.

CORONARY REVASCULARIZATION

We have known for nearly 25 years that revascularizing patients with left ventricular dysfunction can result in upward of a 25% improvement in long-term survival.[11,12] Early enthusiasm was tempered by reports of high operative mortality in patients with a low ejection fraction (EF). Since then, as success with the medical and surgical management of heart failure and transplantation grew, so did the interest in applying this experience to patients with ischemic cardiomyopathy. Successful revascularization can now be performed on patients with an EF less than 30% with hospital mortalities as low as 5%.[13,14]

The premise behind the improvements in EF, long-term survival, and quality of life of these patients following coronary artery bypass grafting (CABG) is believed to be owing to postoperative myocyte recruitment. Restoration of perfusion resuscitates dormant viable myocardium and serves to protect the previously functioning portions of the ventricle from further ischemic insults, arrhythmias, and infarction.

In order to minimize morbidity, a multidisciplinary approach to the preoperative management of heart failure is essential. Patients ideally suited for CABG are those who are medically optimized, with or without angina, who have good distal coronary targets, functional hibernating myocardium identified preoperatively, and no evidence of right ventricular dysfunction.[15] As experience in managing these patients increases, many surgeons have operated on patients with ejection fractions less than 10%, those requiring reoperation, and those with moderate elevations in pulmonary artery pressure. Nevertheless, patients with clear documentation of a poor right ventricular EF, clinical right-sided congestive symptoms, or fixed pulmonary hypertension above 60 mm Hg systolic should be approached cautiously, because these patients may in fact be better suited for transplantation.

The process of preoperative investigation should coincide with optimizing the patient's medical management. This should entail an aggressive regimen of diuretic and vasodilator therapy to minimize ventricular afterload and normalize the patient's circulating volume. For patients with severe heart failure, a brief period of inotropic therapy for ventricular resuscitation may be necessary to optimize their medical management.[16] Inability to be weaned from this support is often indicative of severe myocardial injury and poor overall prognosis with any surgical therapy other than mechanical ventricular assistance or transplantation.

Preoperative investigations should begin with transthoracic echocardiography to grossly evaluate ventricular function and identify any underlying valvular pathology. Baseline screening physiological studies of oxygen consumption, pulmonary function, and cardiopulmonary endurance are recommended. Identification of reversible ischemia by means of a nuclear study can be helpful; however, for patients with angina, many centers will proceed directly to coronary angiography. Though angina may be indicative of living ventricular muscle, perhaps the most important correlate of successful surgical recovery is the quantification of myocardial viability. Not only is a determination of myocardial contractile reserve essential to ensure that the patient can be safely separated from cardiopulmonary bypass (CPB), this information is predictive of ventricular recovery and long-term survival after operation. Though thallium-201 perfusion scans may distinguish myocytes with membrane integrity from scar, PET scanning and dobutamine stress echocardiography permit the preoperative identification of myocardial viability and the prediction of postoperative function.[16–18]

The fundamental premise behind a successful operation is to attain an expeditiously performed and yet complete revascularization. As the failing myocardium is particularly intolerant to further episodes of ischemia, careful consideration should be given to the quality of the distal vessels and the ease with which good anastomoses can be achieved. Operative time expended grafting small or extensively diseased vessels, or performing additional techniques such as endarterectomy, may be counterproductive. Because the price to pay for incomplete revascularization or transient ischemia may be severe, off-pump techniques may not be ideally suited for these patients unless performed flawlessly.

Multiple groups have been uniformly successful in demonstrating improvements in survival, ventricular function, and functional status with coronary revascularization in patients with ischemic cardiomyopathy with ejection fractions less than 25%.[19–21]

The 5-year survival with transplantation ranges from 62 to 82%, whereas with medical therapy alone, it is less than 20%. Most series report survival following CABG for ischemic cardiomyopathy ranging from 85 to 88% at 1 year, 75 to 82% at 2 years, 68 to 80% at 3 years, and 60 to 80% at 5 years. Operative mortality has been reported from 3 to 12%, with the main predictor of increased risk being urgency of operation. When compared to medical therapy, revascularized patients have significant improvements in quality of life. Most series consistently report considerable enhancements in patient mobility, peak oxygen consumption, and functional status. The average preoperative NYHA class of 3.5 reportedly drops to 1.5 after revascularization. Postoperatively, there are substantial reductions in readmissions for CHF and many patients return to work.

It is encouraging to note that the long-term survival of CHF patients following CABG is equivalent to transplantation in many series. The superior survival of CABG over transplant in the first 2 years postoperatively may be because of early attrition from rejection or infection in the latter group. Although there has been little reported on patients with ejection fractions under 10%, from the above data, one could infer that these patients would have a similarly better outcome than their nonrevascularized counterparts. As experience with heart failure surgery expands, refinements in preoperative and operative management of CABG patients will no doubt be reflected in the uniformity of future long-term results.

VENTRICULAR RECONSTRUCTION

Myocardial revascularization and mitral valve repair reliably improve ventricular function. However, there remains a high mortality for those patients with dilated hearts. Techniques that attempt to augment LV function through a reduction in end-diastolic wall tension have been developed. From the principle of the law of LaPlace, ventricular wall tension is directly proportional to LV radius and pressure and inversely proportional to wall thickness. As heart failure progresses, the LV thins and dilates leading to increasing wall stress and regional LV dysfunction. Reducing wall stress through the surgical restoration of LV geometry is the guiding principle behind many innovative techniques, including those developed for the isolation of LV aneurysms and nonfunctioning ventricular segments.

After an acute myocardial infarction, the noncontractile myocardium undergoes thinning and fibrous replacement often following the segmental distribution of the arterial occlusion. This nonfunctional LV segment may remain akinetic or transform into a dyskinetic aneurysm depending on factors such as age and regional collateral circulation. Though such postinfarct pathologic remodeling may occur in any area of the heart, the most common clinically relevant region is the anteroapical segment of the LV. The resulting loss of contractile function in the affected segment results in global increases in LV wall tension and myocardial oxygen consumption in turn leading to compensatory LV dilatation. These geometric ventricular changes may also result in loss of the zone of coaptation and MR following infarction. Moreover, when a dyskinetic region expands and becomes aneurysmal, cardiac work is further increased because of the paradoxical systolic motion of the thinned segment. These pathological alterations often result in CHF. The principle of surgical restoration of LV geometry involves the isolation of these nonfunctional areas and a subsequent reduction in LV volumes. This concept has been clearly illustrated by Dor and others, who have revealed significant improvement in heart failure after endoventricular patch exclusion of dyskinetic or akinetic ventricular segments.[22–25]

Recently, many single-center reports revealed encouraging results with endoventricular repair of nondilated akinetic segments when combined with CABG. These findings spawned the multicenter Surgical Treatment of Ischemic Heart Failure (STICH) NIH trial to evaluate its long-term functional benefit. This study concluded that adding surgical ventricular reconstruction to CABG reduced the left ventricular volume, as compared to CABG alone.[26] However, this anatomical change was not associated with a greater improvement in symptoms or exercise tolerance or with a reduction in the rate of death or hospitalization for cardiac causes. Although questions have been raised regarding the analysis of the STICH report including inaccurate conclusions after volume reduction and end points that do not relate to the SVR procedure, many feel that this should be considered a "negative study."[27] Unfortunately therefore, left ventricular reconstruction by endoventricular exclusion of nonfunctional segments has not been accepted as a standard treatment of heart failure and should not be placed alongside high-risk CABG and CHF-MR repair as a potential first-line surgical option for heart failure.

PARTIAL LEFT VENTRICULECTOMY

Batista furthered the concept of surgical ventricular remodeling with the contention that all mammalian hearts should share the same mass-diameter ratio regardless of size. He proposed that all hearts not complying with this relationship should have a segment of the LV wall excised in order to diminish mural tension and improve myocardial oxygen consumption in accordance with the law of LaPlace.[28,29] Batista performed over 150 procedures predominantly on patients with Chagas disease and dilated cardiomyopathy. Though this experience stimulated much interest, no meaningful follow-up data or statistical analyses are available from this series.

To further evaluate the potential benefits of PLV, the Cleveland Clinic performed 62 such cases on patients with idiopathic dilated cardiomyopathy awaiting transplant. They reported a 3.5% operative mortality with seven late deaths and a 1-year actuarial survival of 82%. Of the total 62 patients, 24 (39%) were considered short-term treatment failures: 11 required LVAD support, 6 were listed for transplantation again, and 7 non-LVAD patients died.[29] Moreover, a further 30% attrition rate at 2 years following PLV has been reported.[30,31] These results may be superior to no surgical treatment but they fall short of those obtained by other surgical options for heart failure. As a result, PLV has fallen into disfavor in North America. In the Asian-Pacific region, where transplantation is not widely available, efforts by Suma et al to improve selection criteria and introduce echo-guided surgical decision making have resulted in PLV persisting as a possible option for heart failure in this part of the world.[32]

Though the concept of instantly remodeling the LV through PLV is mechanically appealing, discarding functioning myocardium is not. Patients with ischemic cardiomyopathy with a dyskinetic aneurysmal segment have undergone successful remodeling with an endoventricular patch repair. Patients with dilated cardiomyopathy and MR have undergone mitral reconstruction, thereby altering the angulation of the base of the heart and promoting favorable LV geometry and remodeling. Thus when similar, if not superior results, can be obtained by methods that preserve myocardial integrity, the application of PLV to patients with end-stage heart failure should be approached with an element of caution.

Currently, partial left ventriculectomy has not been widely accepted as a treatment option for dilated cardiomyopathy.

MITRAL RECONSTRUCTION

Functional mitral regurgitation (MR) is a significant complication of advanced systolic congestive heart failure (CHF) without organic mitral valve disease and it may affect almost all heart failure patients as a preterminal or terminal event. Its presence in these patients is associated with progressive ventricular dilatation, an escalation of CHF symptomatology, and significant reductions in long-term survival estimated between only 6 and 24 months. Patel et al., from the Mayo clinic, looked at the prognostic implications of functional MR in patients with advanced systolic CHF evaluated in a heart failure clinic. Of 558 NYHA III-IV patients, those with moderate MR had a 5-year survival of only 27%.[33] This is supported by several other studies that show that the severity of MR impacts survival as well.[34–37]

Historically, the surgical approach to MR was mitral valve replacement, yet little was understood of the interdependence of ventricular function and annulus-papillary muscle continuity. Consequently, patients with a low EF who underwent mitral valve replacement with removal of the subvalvular apparatus had prohibitively high mortality rates. In an attempt to explain these outcomes, the concept of a beneficial "pop-off" effect of mitral regurgitation was conceived. This idea erroneously proposed that mitral incompetence provided a low-pressure relief during systolic ejection from the failing ventricle, and that removal of this effect through mitral replacement was responsible for deterioration of ventricular function. Consequently, mitral valve replacement in patients with heart failure has been discouraged.

A firm understanding of the functional anatomy of the mitral valve is fundamental to the management of MR in heart failure. The mitral valve apparatus consists of the annulus, leaflets, chordae tendineae, and papillary muscles as well as the entire left ventricle (LV). These structures are aligned as if they form a cylinder with the papillary musculature directly aligned beneath the annulus. The maintenance of chordal, annular, and subvalvular continuity is essential for the preservation of mitral geometric relationships and overall ventricular function. MR in heart failure is not related to the valve but to ventricular pathology. The degree of LV distortion reflects the degree of MR.[38] As the ventricle fails, progressive dilatation of the LV results in lateral papillary muscle migration, loss of cylinder closure, and thus loss of the zone of coaptation (Fig. 68-1). This gives rise to MR, which begets more MR and further ventricular dilatation (Fig. 68-2). We know that even a small amount of MR to be harmful in these patients. Grigioni et al. showed that when

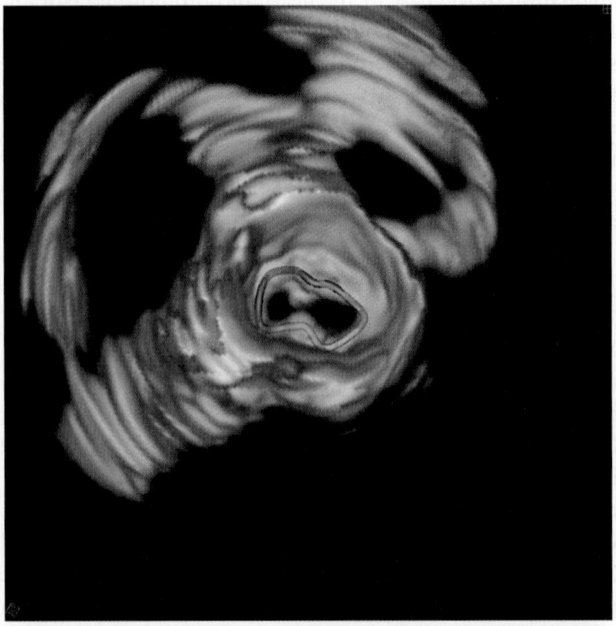

FIGURE 68-1 Postoperative three-dimensional echocardiography of a mitral repair performed using the Geoform mitral annuloplasty ring. Note the apposition of the central areas of the anterior and posterior mitral valve leaflets, which help to establish a zone of coaptation and abolish mitral regurgitation.

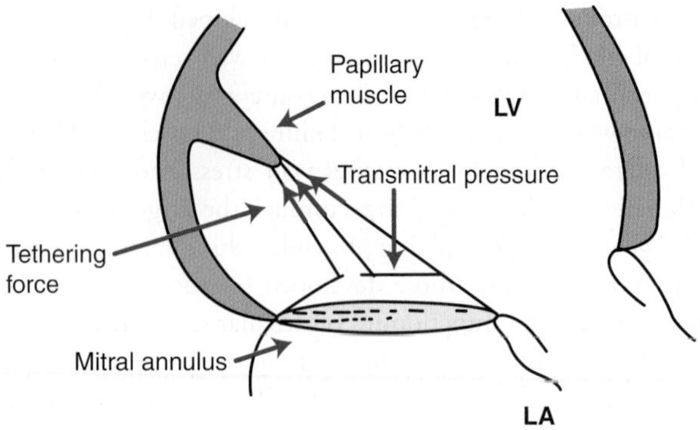

FIGURE 68-2 Various forces exerted on mitral valve leaflets are provided by the mitral valve apparatus, papillary muscles, and important three-dimensional relationships in the ventricle itself of all of the associated structures. Geometric mitral regurgitation results from a combination of annular dilatation, papillary muscle displacement, increased leaflet tethering forces, and weakened leaflet closing forces.

the regurgitant volume was greater than 30 mL, the 5-year survival was less than 35% compared with 44% for a regurgitant volume of 1 to 29 mL and 61% for no MR.[39] With postinfarction remodeling and lateral wall dysfunction, similar processes combine to result in ischemic mitral regurgitation (Fig. 68-3). Left uncorrected, the end result of progressive MR and global ventricular remodeling is similar regardless of the etiology of cardiomyopathy. Reconstruction of this geometric abnormality serves to not only restore valvular competency but also improve ventricular function.

Surgical mitral annuloplasty improves symptoms in these patients with advanced CHF but has not been shown to improve survival. This is likely because surgery for CHF has not been "too little–too late" but "too much–too late." We failed to correct mitral regurgitation early enough in the disease course because advanced heart failure patients were long felt to be nonoperative candidates. However, it has been shown that mitral repair is feasible with a low mortality, relief of MR, and better quality of life. Several authors have demonstrated 30-day mortality rates as low as 1 to 5 % for mitral repair for MR in CHF.[40–48]

The lack of a mortality benefit may also be explained by the absence of a durable repair. When McGee and associates showed no mortality benefit after mitral repair, they also noticed the rate of recurrent MR to be 30 to 40% in less than 1 year.[49] This has led to an attempt to identify surgical predictors of recurrent MR and for improved surgical techniques that result in a more permanent repair. In order to observe a survival benefit in these patients after mitral repair, MR must be fixed permanently, because residual and recurrent MR will obscure or obliterate a survival benefit in any CHF-MVR trial.

Ischemic MR is not caused by organic or intrinsic disease of the valve, but by LV remodeling, dilation, and dysfunction leading to geometric reconfiguration of the mitroventricular apparatus, including papillary muscle displacement and annular dilation. Mitral valve (MV) leaflets become tethered, with failure of anterior-posterior leaflet coaptation, resulting in symmetric or asymmetric regurgitation. Surgical treatment options in

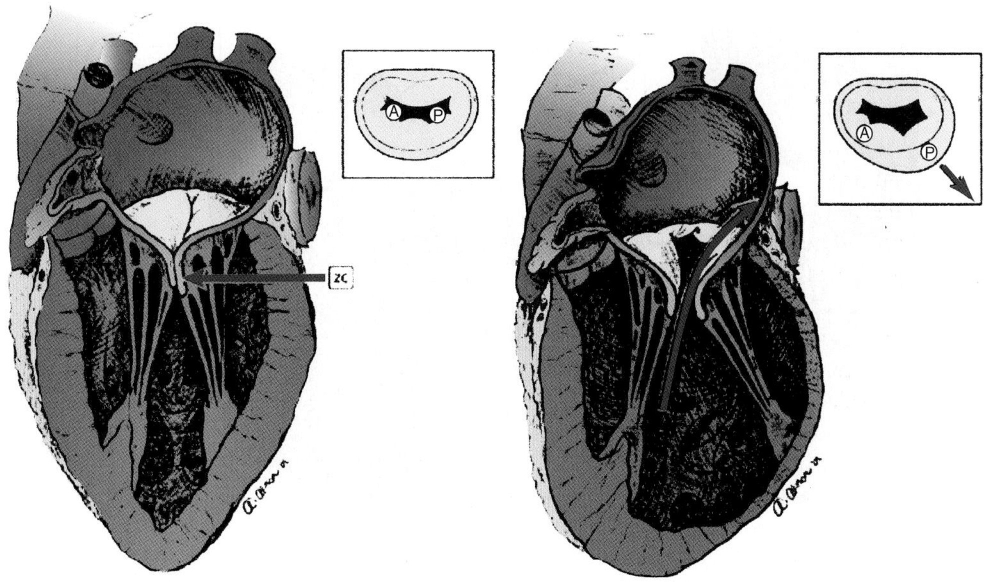

FIGURE 68-3 In ischemic cardiomyopathy, changes within the left ventricle may be asymmetrical and still lead to functional mitral regurgitation. With ischemic damage and thinning of the ventricular wall, there is lateral tethering, displacement of the papillary muscle, and loss of the zone of coaptation (ZC), resulting in an eccentric jet of mitral regurgitation. This illustrates the concept that ischemic mitral regurgitation results from lateral wall dysfunction that, if left untreated, will progress to global left ventricular dysfunction and severe heart failure.

ischemic MR include coronary artery bypass grafting (CABG) alone or with concomitant MV annuloplasty or replacement. Currently, the most common technique to restore valve competence is placing an undersized annuloplasty ring to reduce mitral annulus size. Mihaljevic et al. (Figs. 68-4 and 68-5).[55] Unfortunatety, ischemic mitral regurgitation (IMR) often persists after restrictive mitral valve annuloplasty, in which case it is associated with worse clinical outcomes. In an attempt to determine whether persistence of MR and/or clinical outcome could be predicted from preoperative analysis of mitral valve configuration, in patients undergoing restrictive annuloplasty for ischemic MR, preoperative analysis of mitral valve configuration was shown to accurately predict persistence of MR and 3-year event-free survival. Patients with a posterior leaflet angle >45 degrees (ie, with high posterolateral restriction) should thus be considered poor candidates for this procedure, and concomitant or alternative procedures should be contemplated.

Important LV predictors of recurrent MR are coaptation depth greater than 1 cm as shown by Calafiore et al., and left ventricular end diastolic dimension (LVEDD) less than 65 mm as shown by Braun.[43,50] At 4.3 years follow-up, intermediate-term cutoff values for left ventricular reverse remodeling proved to be predictors for late mortality. For patients with preoperative LVEDD of 65 mm or less, restrictive mitral annuloplasty with revascularization provides a mortality benefit for ischemic mitral regurgitation and heart failure; however, when LVEDD exceeded 65 mm, outcome is poor and a different approach to CHF should be considered.[50]

But perhaps, the strongest predictor of CHF MVR failure is anterior-posterior (AP) diameter greater than 3.7 cm.[51] When the AP diameter after annuloplasty is greater than 3.7 cm the repair should be considered as a potential predictor of a failed repair.[52] New and remodeling MV rings that significantly reduce the residual AP diameter have been shown to be a predictor of no recurrence of MR.[53,54]

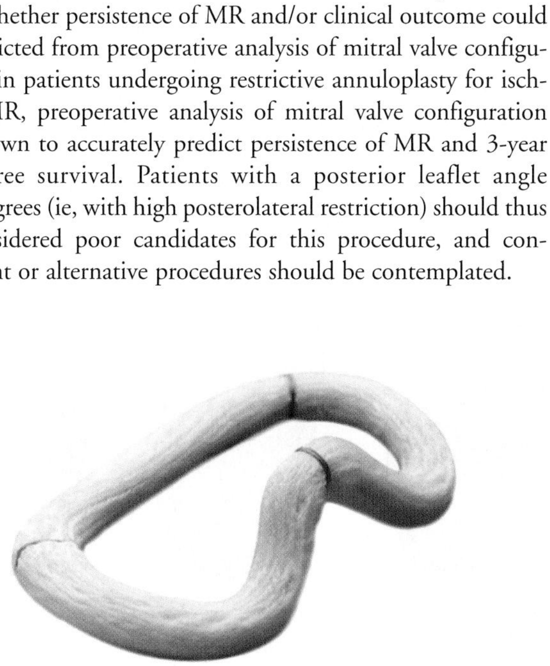

FIGURE 68-4 Oblique view of the Geoform mitral annuloplasty ring. Note the posterior ring design element, which reverses the adverse changes in the posterior mitral annulus associated with geometric mitral regurgitation.

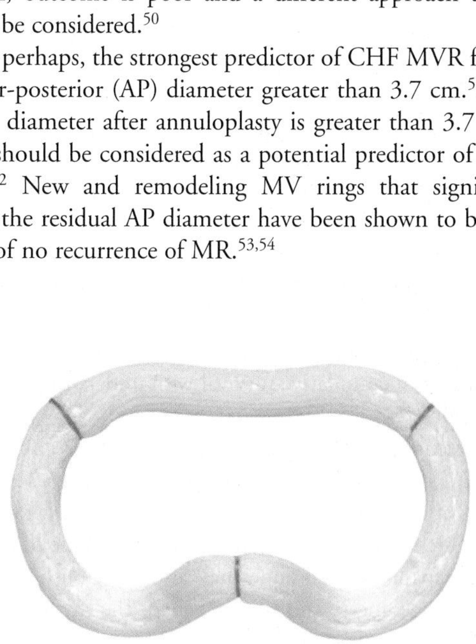

FIGURE 68-5 Superior view of the Geoform mitral annuloplasty ring. The three-dimensional cross-sectional area is not restrictive to atrial blood flow.

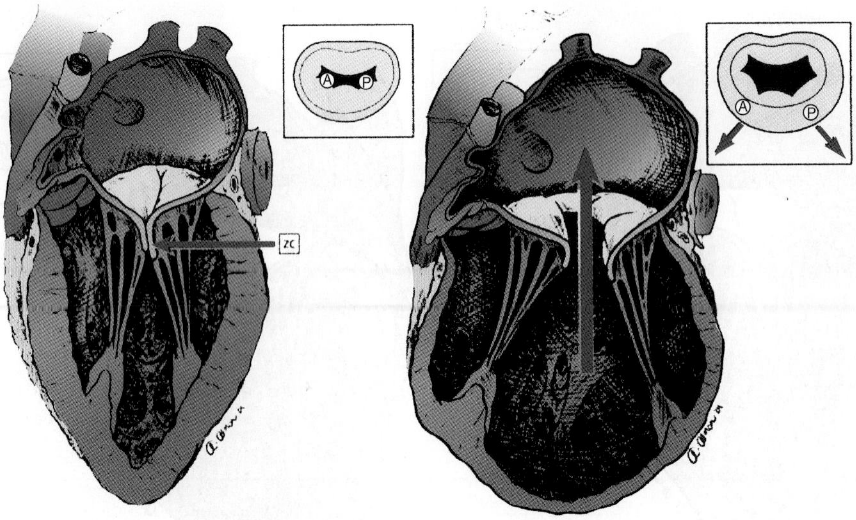

FIGURE 68-6 In nonischemic cardiomyopathy, note the geometric changes that occur from the normal to the failing left ventricle. With the ventricular and annular dilatation of heart failure, the mitral leaflets cannot adequately cover the enlarged mitral orifice, resulting in the loss of the zone of coaptation (ZC). Geometric mitral regurgitation results from a combination of annular dilatation, papillary muscle displacement, increased leaflet tethering forces, and weakened leaflet closing forces.

When considering surgical techniques used in treating heart failure patients, the most significant determinant of leaflet coaptation and MR is the diameter of the mitral valve annulus. Observations with medically managed patients with severe heart failure and MR reveal that decreasing filling pressure and systemic vascular resistance lead to reductions in the dynamic MR associated with their heart failure. This is attributed to a reduction in mitral orifice area relating to decreased LV volume and decreased annular distension. This complex relationship between mitral annular area and leaflet coaptation may thus explain why an undersized "valvular" repair may help a "ventricular" problem (Fig. 68-6).

Earlier use of flexible and incomplete annuloplasty rings was justified based on the belief that trigone distance was constant. However, Hueb et al., have demonstrated that trigone distance is not stable.[56] This has led to the use of complete and rigid annuloplasty rings. Spoor et al. experienced a recurrent MR rate five times higher when using flexible rings.[57] In addition, the Kaplan-Meier survival curve for the Acorn MV surgery stratum (rigid annuloplasty) showed a more enduring repair with less recurrence of MR with only 4.2% with 3+ or 4+ MR at 18 months. The overall survival for this group was 84%. In recent work, Bolling et al. have also shown a significant improvement in cumulative survival with undersizing the mitral valve annulus (Fig. 68-7).

The technique of undersizing in mitral reconstruction avoids SAM in these myopathic patients, likely because of widening of the aortomitral angle in these hearts with increased LV size. Furthermore, acute remodeling of the base of the heart with this reparative technique may also reestablish the somewhat normal geometry and ellipsoid shape the LV. As evidenced by the decreased sphericity index and LV volumes seen in these patients, the geometric restoration from mitral reconstruction not only effectively corrects MR but also achieves surgical unloading of the ventricle (Fig. 68-8).

Many centers have reported similar consistent findings following MR. With outcomes equating to transplant while avoiding immunosuppression, this straightforward reparative operation performed in conjunction with medical management may be offered to carefully selected patients with MR and cardiomyopathy as a potential first-line therapy.

DYNAMIC CARDIOMYOPLASTY

An alternative method to surgically optimize LaPlace's law is dynamic cardiomyoplasty (DCMP). The procedure uses the patient's own skeletal muscle to support the heart, helping to reduce wall stress and provide cardiac assistance. The latissimus dorsi muscle is wrapped around the failing heart and an implantable cardiomyostimulator is used to stimulate the muscle to contract in synchrony with cardiac systole. Long-term results show that this method was not considered to be satisfactory in

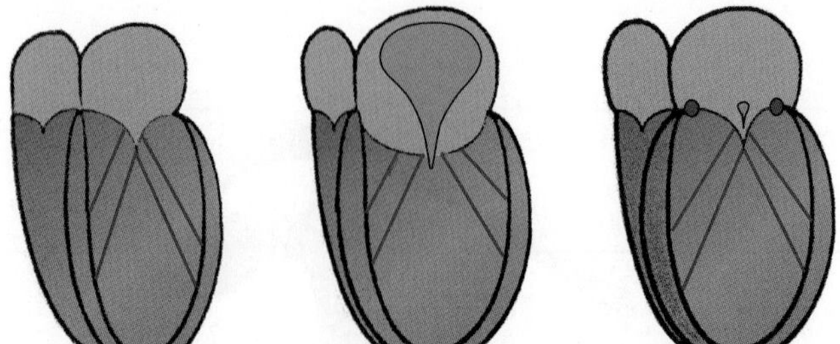

FIGURE 68-7 Geometric mitral reconstruction for heart failure. Successful augmentation of the zone of coaptation and prevention of recurrent MR can be achieved with placement of an undersized circumferential annuloplasty ring performed with multiple annular sutures. Note the changes in the relationship of the papillary muscles in the left ventricle in the new geometry following mitral repair.

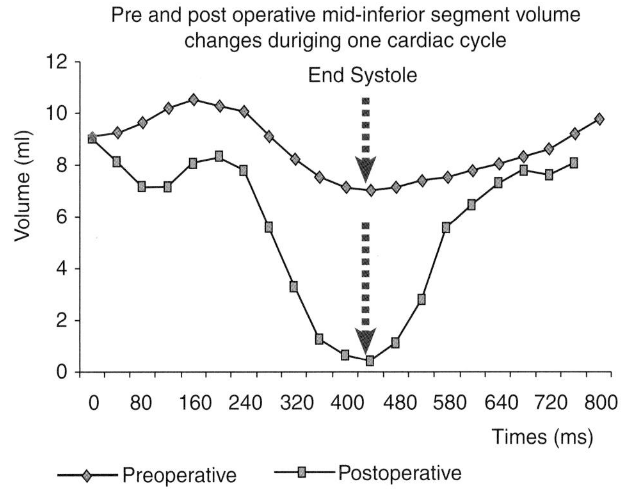

FIGURE 68-8 Left ventricular volume changes obtained on postoperative day 5 following geometric mitral valve repair. Increases in regional EF in the inferobasal wall are shown, which are the opposite of the decreased EF expected following MVR based on historical teaching. (*Courtesy of Nadia Nathan, MD.*)

terms of survival and antiarrhythmic effect because of fatigue of the skeletal muscle. DCMP is now only rarely performed in North America. Investigations into the mechanisms of DCMP have generated promising research in the fields of cellular cardiomyoplasty, myoblast transplantation, and remodeling surgery.[58,59]

EMERGING BIOMEDICAL DEVICES FOR HEART FAILURE

The CorCap Cardiac Support Device (Acorn Cardiovascular, St. Paul, MN) is a mesh device that is implanted around the heart to reduce wall stress and the first therapy specifically designed to address left ventricular remodeling. The ACORN trial, a prospective, randomized, controlled, multicenter evaluation of the CorCap cardiac support device in patients with New York Heart Association (NYHA) class III or IV heart failure of ischemic or nonischemic etiology enrolled a total of 300 patients. Results of the trial were reported in 2007, and although LV geometry was favorably improved, it was found that there was no difference in survival between the treatment and control groups (25 deaths among 148 patients in the treatment group versus 25 deaths among 152 patients in the control group) and no significant with respect to the mode of death. Survival rates, serious adverse events, and hospitalizations between those patients who received a cardiac support device and those who did not were not significantly different. As a result there has been a decline in the application of the CorCap device in the heart failure population.[60]

The Coapsys device (Myocar Inc., Maple Grove, MN) is a second device developed to reduce ventricular wall stress by directly altering cardiac geometry. Working on the premise of optimizing the law of LaPlace, it involves the placement of transventricular tension bands through the RV and LV walls that have the unique ability to be individually tightened in order to achieve a 20% reduction in wall stress.[61] However, the product manufacturer is developing a new device designed to achieve mitral valve repair along with ventricular volume reduction and the Myocor Myosplint has been set aside and further development is uncertain.

PERCUTANEOUS CORONARY SINUS DEVICES FOR CHF-MR

The Viacor percutaneous mitral annuloplasty system (PTMA) (Viacor, Wilmington, MA), Edwards Viking Endovascular coronary sinus ring (Edwards Lifesciences LLD, Irvine, CA), and Carillon mitral contour system (Cardiac Dimensions, Kirkwood, WA) all use an emerging technology approach to mitral annuloplasty using a catheter-based approach to the mitral valve. Using percutaneous catheters, a permanent nitinol strut is placed into the coronary sinus that wraps around the posterior annulus of the mitral valve and attempts to indirectly influence the action of the posterior mitral valve leaflet similar to a partial ring annuloplasty by reducing the anterior-posterior dimension of the mitral annulus. Initial results of mitral annular reduction to a more modest degree than after surgical correction have led to less improvement in MR.[62] As these devices are under investigation and not currently approved for routine use, their clinical impact at this time is unknown.

PERCUTANEOUS MITRAL VALVE REPAIR

The Milano endovascular edge-to-edge repair system (Edwards Lifesciences LLD, Irvine, CA) and MitraClip mitral repair system (Evalve, Menlo Park, CA) use a catheter-based approach to deliver a clip to both the anterior and posterior mitral valve leaflets using the principles of mitral repair pioneered by Dr Otavio Alfieri.[63] Percutaneous catheters are introduced via the femoral vein and cross the atrial septum to enter the left atrium similar to a percutaneous mitral balloon annuloplasty approach. A catheter-based clip is then used to create a permanent coaptation point between the leading-free edges of the anterior and posterior mitral leaflets. The EVEREST II trial compared the MitraClip to surgery.[64] A total of 279 patients enrolled completed 1-year follow-up. Early findings indicate that this technology is safe in the indicated patient population and not inferior in results compared with surgery. However, a clip was considered successful if MR was 2+ or less following application.[64] This makes percutaneous repair attractive for high-risk surgical candidates, but may not be entirely impactful. Further investigation is ongoing comparing surgery to the MitraClip device.[65]

CONCLUSIONS

As surgical therapies for heart failure rapidly evolve, the need for their critical appraisal is essential so that they may be offered to the growing population of CHF patients in a prompt yet effective manner. Transplantation continues to offer selected patients reliable long-term survival in a reproducible fashion, and it thus remains as a gold standard surgical therapy for heart failure. Rapidly evolving mechanical assist devices are playing a more prevalent role in myocardial recovery and destination therapy. With the growing disparity between donor availability and heart failure patients, experience with assist devices has shown them to be an effective nontransplant surgical solution.

The results of the more conventional techniques of CABG and mitral reconstruction when combined with the optimal medical management of heart failure may now be on a par with transplantation. These modalities now form the new first-line surgical therapy for heart failure. Patients with primary ischemic cardiomyopathy and favorable anatomy may be effectively managed with revascularization alone or in combination with mitral repair. Myopathic patients with MR, regardless of etiology, may be effectively managed with mitral reconstruction. The use of other techniques such as SVR, PLV, and DCMP is no longer reserved as viable alternative surgical options for heart failure. The prudent and effective application of the growing menu of surgical strategies for heart failure enables the scarcely available donor hearts to be efficiently used for patients with no other surgical or medical alternatives. Along with the utility of emerging biomedical devices, each of these unique modalities has enhanced the clinically effective armamentarium of the modern surgeon treating patients with heart failure.

REFERENCES

1. Lloyd-Jones D, Adams RJ, Brown TM, Carnethon M, Dai S, et al: Heart disease and stroke statistics—2010 update: a report from the American Heart Association. *Circulation* 2010; 121(7):e46-e215.
2. Fang J, Mensah GA, Croft JB, Keenan NL: Heart failure-related hospitalization in the U.S., 1979 to 2004. *J Am Coll Cardiol* 2008; 52(6): 428-434.
3. Taylor DO, Edwards LB, Aurora P, Christie JD, Dobbels F, et al: Registry of the International Society for Heart and Lung Transplantation: Twenty-Fifth Official Adult Heart Transplant Report—2008. *J Heart Lung Transplant* 2008; 27(9):943-956.
4. Taylor DO, Stehlik J, Edwards LB, Aurora P, Christie JD, et al: Registry of the International Society for Heart and Lung Transplantation: Twenty-Sixth Official Adult Heart Transplant Report-2009. *J Heart Lung Transplant* 2009; 28(10):1007-1022.
5. Daneshmand MA, Rajagopal K, Lima B, Khorram N, Blue LJ, et al: Left ventricular assist device destination therapy versus extended criteria cardiac transplant. *Ann Thorac Surg* 2010; 89(4):1205-1209; discussion 10.
6. Rogers JG, Aaronson KD, Boyle AJ, Russell SD, Milano CA, et al: Continuous flow left ventricular assist device improves functional capacity and quality of life of advanced heart failure patients. *J Am Coll Cardiol* 2010; 55(17):1826-1834.
7. Coyle LA, Ising MS, Gallagher C, Bhat G, Kurien S, et al: Destination therapy: one-year outcomes in patients with a body mass index greater than 30. *Artif Organs* 2010; 34(2):93-97.
8. Messori A, Trippoli S, Bonacchi M, Sani G: Left ventricular assist device as destination therapy: application of the payment-by-results approach for the device reimbursement. *J Thorac Cardiovasc Surg* 2009; 138(2):480-485.
9. Lahpor J, Khaghani A, Hetzer R, Pavie A, Friedrich I, et al: European results with a continuous-flow ventricular assist device for advanced heart-failure patients. *Eur J Cardiothorac Surg* 2010; 37(2):357-361.
10. Kirklin JK, Naftel DC, Kormos RL, Stevenson LW, Pagani FD, et al: Second INTERMACS annual report: more than 1,000 primary left ventricular assist device implants. *J Heart Lung Transplant* 2010; 29(1):1-10.
11. Nardi P, Pellegrino A, Scafuri A, Colella D, Bassano C, et al: Long-term outcome of coronary artery bypass grafting in patients with left ventricular dysfunction. *Ann Thorac Surg* 2009; 87(5):1401-1407.
12. Appoo J, Norris C, Merali S, Graham MM, Koshal A, et al: Long-term outcome of isolated coronary artery bypass surgery in patients with severe left ventricular dysfunction. *Circulation* 2004; 110(11 Suppl 1):II13-17.
13. Filsoufi F, Rahmanian PB, Castillo JG, Chikwe J, Kini AS, et al: Results and predictors of early and late outcome of coronary artery bypass grafting in patients with severely depressed left ventricular function. *Ann Thorac Surg* 2007; 84(3):808-816.
14. Topkara VK, Cheema FH, Kesavaramanujam S, Mercando ML, Cheema AF, et al: Coronary artery bypass grafting in patients with low ejection fraction. *Circulation* 2005; 112(9 Suppl):I344-350.
15. Soliman Hamad MA, Tan ME, van Straten AH, van Zundert AA, Schonberger JP: Long-term results of coronary artery bypass grafting in patients with left ventricular dysfunction. *Ann Thorac Surg* 2008; 85(2): 488-493.
16. Eagle KA, Guyton RA, Davidoff R, Edwards FH, Ewy GA, et al: ACC/AHA 2004 guideline update for coronary artery bypass graft surgery: summary article. A report of the American College of Cardiology/American Heart Association Task Force on Practice Guidelines (Committee to Update the 1999 Guidelines for Coronary Artery Bypass Graft Surgery). *J Am Coll Cardiol* 2004; 44(5):e213-310.
17. Camici PG, Prasad SK, Rimoldi OE: Stunning, hibernation, and assessment of myocardial viability. *Circulation* 2008; 117(1):103-114.
18. Schinkel AF, Bax JJ, Poldermans D, Elhendy A, Ferrari R, et al: Hibernating myocardium: diagnosis and patient outcomes. *Curr Probl Cardiol* 2007; 32(7):375-410.
19. Allman KC, Shaw LJ, Hachamovitch R, Udelson JE: Myocardial viability testing and impact of revascularization on prognosis in patients with coronary artery disease and left ventricular dysfunction: a meta-analysis. *J Am Coll Cardiol* 2002; 39(7):1151-1158.
20. Shapira OM, Hunter CT, Anter E, Bao Y, DeAndrade K, et al: Coronary artery bypass grafting in patients with severe left ventricular dysfunction–early and mid-term outcomes. *J Card Surg* 2006; 21(3):225-232.
21. Darwazah AK, Abu Sham'a RA, Hussein E, Hawari MH, Ismail H: Myocardial revascularization in patients with low ejection fraction < or =35%: effect of pump technique on early morbidity and mortality. *J Card Surg* 2006; 21(1):22-27.
22. Athanasuleas CL, Stanley AW, Buckberg GD, Dor V, Di Donato M, et al: Surgical anterior ventricular endocardial restoration (SAVER) for dilated ischemic cardiomyopathy. *Semin Thorac Cardiovasc Surg* 2001; 13(4): 448-458.
23. Di Donato M, Sabatier M, Montiglio F, Maioli M, Toso A, et al: Outcome of left ventricular aneurysmectomy with patch repair in patients with severely depressed pump function. *Am J Cardiol* 1995; 76(8):557-561.
24. Dor V: Surgical remodeling of left ventricle. *Surg Clin North Am* 2004; 84(1):27-43.
25. Ten Brinke EA, Klautz RJ, Tulner SA, Verwey HF, Bax JJ, et al: Long-term effects of surgical ventricular restoration with additional restrictive mitral annuloplasty and/or coronary artery bypass grafting on left ventricular function: six-month follow-up by pressure-volume loops. *J Thorac Cardiovasc Surg* 2010; 140(6):1338-1344.
26. Cleland JG, Coletta AP, Clark AL, Cullington D: Clinical trials update from the American College of Cardiology 2009: ADMIRE-HF, PRIMA, STICH, REVERSE, IRIS, partial ventricular support, FIX-HF-5, vagal stimulation, REVIVAL-3, pre-RELAX-AHF, ACTIVE-A, HF-ACTION, JUPITER, AURORA, and OMEGA. *Eur J Heart Fail* 2009; 11(6):622-630.
27. Buckberg GD, Athanasuleas CL: The STICH trial: misguided conclusions. *J Thorac Cardiovasc Surg* 2009; 138(5):1060-1064.e2.
28. Kawaguchi AT, Suma H, Konertz W, Gradinac S, Bergsland J, et al: Left ventricular volume reduction surgery: The 4th International Registry Report 2004. *J Card Surg* 2005; 20(6):S5-11.
29. O'Neill JO, Starling RC, McCarthy PM, Albert NM, Lytle BW, et al: The impact of left ventricular reconstruction on survival in patients with ischemic cardiomyopathy. *Eur J Cardiothorac Surg* 2006; 30(5):753-759.
30. Kawaguchi AT, Takahashi N, Ishibashi-Ueda H, Shimura S, Karamanoukian HL, et al: Factors affecting ventricular function and survival after partial left ventriculectomy. *J Card Surg* 2003; 18(Suppl 2):S77-85.
31. Moreira LP, Stolf NA, Higuchi ML, Bacal F, Bocchi EA, et al: Determinants of poor long-term survival after partial left ventriculectomy in patients with dilated cardiomyopathy. *J Heart Lung Transplant* 2001; 20(2):217-218.
32. Suma H, Tanabe H, Uejima T, Suzuki S, Horii T, et al: Selected ventriculoplasty for idiopathic dilated cardiomyopathy with advanced congestive heart failure: midterm results and risk analysis. *Eur J Cardiothorac Surg* 2007; 32(6):912-916.
33. Patel JB, Borgeson DD, Barnes ME, Rihal CS, Daly RC, et al: Mitral regurgitation in patients with advanced systolic heart failure. *J Card Fail* 2004; 10(4):285-291.
34. Hickey MS, Smith LR, Muhlbaier LH, Harrell FE Jr, Reves JG, et al: Current prognosis of ischemic mitral regurgitation. Implications for future management. *Circulation* 1988; 78(3 Pt 2):I51-59.

35. Robbins JD, Maniar PB, Cotts W, Parker MA, Bonow RO, et al: Prevalence and severity of mitral regurgitation in chronic systolic heart failure. *Am J Cardiol* 2003; 91(3):360-362.
36. Trichon BH, Felker GM, Shaw LK, Cabell CH, O'Connor CM: Relation of frequency and severity of mitral regurgitation to survival among patients with left ventricular systolic dysfunction and heart failure. *Am J Cardiol* 2003; 91(5):538-543.
37. Wu AH, Aaronson KD, Bolling SF, Pagani FD, Welch K, et al: Impact of mitral valve annuloplasty on mortality risk in patients with mitral regurgitation and left ventricular systolic dysfunction. *J Am Coll Cardiol* 2005; 45(3):381-387.
38. Magne J, Pibarot P, Dagenais F, Hachicha Z, Dumesnil JG, et al: Preoperative posterior leaflet angle accurately predicts outcome after restrictive mitral valve annuloplasty for ischemic mitral regurgitation. *Circulation* 2007; 115(6): 782-791.
39. Grigioni F, Enriquez-Sarano M, Zehr KJ, Bailey KR, Tajik AJ: Ischemic mitral regurgitation: long-term outcome and prognostic implications with quantitative Doppler assessment. *Circulation* 2001; 103(13):1759-1764.
40. Bolling SF, Deeb GM, Brunsting LA, Bach DS: Early outcome of mitral valve reconstruction in patients with end-stage cardiomyopathy. *J Thorac Cardiovasc Surg* 1995; 109(4):676-682; discussion 82-83.
41. Chen FY, Adams DH, Aranki SF, Collins JJ Jr, Couper GS, Rizzo RJ, et al: Mitral valve repair in cardiomyopathy. *Circulation* 1998; 98(19 Suppl): II124-127.
42. Bishay ES, McCarthy PM, Cosgrove DM, Hoercher KJ, Smedira NG, et al: Mitral valve surgery in patients with severe left ventricular dysfunction. *Eur J Cardiothorac Surg* 2000; 17(3):213-221.
43. Calafiore AM, Gallina S, Di Mauro M, Gaeta F, Iaco AL, et al: Mitral valve procedure in dilated cardiomyopathy: repair or replacement? *Ann Thorac Surg* 2001; 71(4):1146-1152; discussion 52-53.
44. Buffolo E, Paula IA, Palma H, Branco JN: A new surgical approach for treating dilated cardiomyopathy with mitral regurgitation. *Arq Bras Cardiol* 2000; 74(2):129-140.
45. Bitran D, Merin O, Klutstein MW, Od-Allah S, Shapira N, et al: Mitral valve repair in severe ischemic cardiomyopathy. *J Card Surg* 2001; 16(1):79-82.
46. Dreyfus G, Milaiheanu S: Mitral valve repair in cardiomyopathy. *J Heart Lung Transplant* 2000; 19(8 Suppl):S73-76.
47. Suma H, Isomura T, Horii T, Hisatomi K, Sato T, et al: [Left ventriculoplasty for non-ischemic cardiomyopathy with severe heart failure in 70 patients]. *J Cardiol* 2001; 37(1):1-10.
48. Acker MA, Bolling S, Shemin R, Kirklin J, Oh JK, et al: Mitral valve surgery in heart failure: insights from the Acorn Clinical Trial. *J Thorac Cardiovasc Surg* 2006; 132(3):568-577, 77 e1-4.
49. McGee EC, Gillinov AM, Blackstone EH, Rajeswaran J, Cohen G, et al: Recurrent mitral regurgitation after annuloplasty for functional ischemic mitral regurgitation. *J Thorac Cardiovasc Surg* 2004; 128(6):916-924.
50. Braun J, van de Veire NR, Klautz RJ, Versteegh MI, Holman ER, et al: Restrictive mitral annuloplasty cures ischemic mitral regurgitation and heart failure. *Ann Thorac Surg* 2008; 85(2):430-436; discussion 6-7.
51. Kaji S, Nasu M, Yamamuro A, Tanabe K, Nagai K, et al: Annular geometry in patients with chronic ischemic mitral regurgitation: three-dimensional magnetic resonance imaging study. *Circulation* 2005; 112(9 Suppl):I409-414.
52. Kongsaerepong V, Shiota M, Gillinov AM, Song JM, Fukuda S, et al: Echocardiographic predictors of successful versus unsuccessful mitral valve repair in ischemic mitral regurgitation. *Am J Cardiol* 2006; 98(4):504-508.
53. Miller DC: Valve-sparing aortic root replacement in patients with the Marfan syndrome. *J Thorac Cardiovasc Surg* 2003; 125(4):773-778.
54. Maisano F, Ziskind Z, Grimaldi A, Blasio A, Caldarola A, et al: Selective reduction of the septolateral dimensions in functional mitral regurgitation by modified-shape ring annuloplasty. *J Thorac Cardiovasc Surg* 2005; 129(2): 472-474.
55. Mihaljevic T, Lam BK, Rajeswaran J, Takagaki M, Lauer MS, et al: Impact of mitral valve annuloplasty combined with revascularization in patients with functional ischemic mitral regurgitation. *J Am Coll Cardiol* 2007; 49(22):2191-2201.
56. Hueb AC, Jatene FB, Moreira LF, Pomerantzeff PM, Kallas E, et al: Ventricular remodeling and mitral valve modifications in dilated cardiomyopathy: new insights from anatomic study. *J Thorac Cardiovasc Surg* 2002; 124(6):1216-1224.
57. Spoor MT, Geltz A, Bolling SF: Flexible versus nonflexible mitral valve rings for congestive heart failure: differential durability of repair. *Circulation* 2006; 114(1 Suppl):I67-71.
58. Benicio A, Moreira LF, Bacal F, Stolf NA, Oliveira SA: Reevaluation of long-term outcomes of dynamic cardiomyoplasty. *Ann Thorac Surg* 2003; 76(3):821-827; discussion 7.
59. Moreira LF, Benicio A, Bacal F, Bocchi EA, Stolf NA, et al: Determinants of long-term mortality of current palliative surgical treatment for dilated cardiomyopathy. *Eur J Cardiothorac Surg* 2003; 23(5):756-763; discussion 63-64.
60. Mann DL, Acker MA, Jessup M, Sabbah HN, Starling RC, et al: Clinical evaluation of the CorCap Cardiac Support Device in patients with dilated cardiomyopathy. *Ann Thorac Surg* 2007; 84(4):1226-1235.
61. Mishra YK, Mittal S, Jaguri P, Trehan N: Coapsys mitral annuloplasty for chronic functional ischemic mitral regurgitation: 1-year results. *Ann Thorac Surg* 2006; 81(1):42-46.
62. Sack S, Kahlert P, Bilodeau L, Pièrard LA, Lancellotti P, et al: Percutaneous transvenous mitral annuloplasty: initial human experience with a novel coronary sinus implant device. *Circ Cardiovasc Interv* 2009; 2(4):277-284.
63. Alfieri O, De Bonis M: Mitral valve repair for functional mitral regurgitation: is annuloplasty alone enough? *Curr Opin Cardiol* 2010; 25(2):114-118.
64. Mauri L, Garg P, Massaro JM, Foster E, Glower D et al: The EVEREST II Trial: design and rationale for a randomized study of the evalve mitraclip system compared with mitral valve surgery for mitral regurgitation. *Am Heart J* 2010; 160(1):23-29.
65. Tamburino C, Ussia GP, Maisano F, Capodanno D, La Canna G, et al: Percutaneous mitral valve repair with the MitraClip system: acute results from a real world setting. *Eur Heart J* 2010; 31(11):1382-1389.

CHAPTER 69

Tissue Engineering for Cardiac Valve Surgery

Danielle Gottlieb
John E. Mayer, Jr.

INTRODUCTION

Tissue engineering is a developing science, comprising elements of engineering and biology, whose aim is to build replacement tissues de novo from individual cellular and structural components. The impetus for our work on tissue engineered cardiovascular structures arises from the need to replace cardiovascular tissues that failed to develop normally during embryogenesis or have become dysfunctional as a consequence of disease. In pediatric patients, the cardiovascular structures most often afflicted by congenital anomalies are the cardiac valves and great vessels.

Diseases of the heart valves and large "conduit" arteries account for approximately 60,000 cardiac surgical procedures each year in the United States, and all of the currently available replacement devices have significant limitations.[1,2] Ideally, any valve or artery substitute would function like a normal valve or artery, that is, to allow the passage of pulsatile blood flow without stenosis or regurgitation. The theoretical advantage of engineered tissue replacements is that they could also display other desirable characteristics, such as: (1) durability, (2) growth (for infants and children), (3) compatibility with blood components and the absence of thrombosis or destructive inflammation, and (4) resistance to infection. None of the currently available devices, constructed from either synthetic or biologic materials, meet these criteria. Mechanical heart valves are very durable, but they require anticoagulation to reduce the risk of thrombosis and thromboembolism.[1,2] Therapeutic anticoagulation carries associated morbidity, and even among patients who receive therapeutic anticoagulation, the incidence of thromboembolic complications of mechanical heart valve replacement is not zero.[1,2] Biologic valves, whether of allograft or heterograft origin, remain subject to structural deterioration after implantation.[2–4] Neither mechanical nor biologic valves have any growth potential, and this limitation represents a major source of morbidity for pediatric patients who must undergo multiple reoperations to replace valves and/or valved conduits during the period of maximum somatic growth.

Tissue engineering is an approach based on the hypothesis that when properly designed, living devices will simulate the biology of normal cardiovascular structures, thereby overcoming the shortcomings of currently available heart valve replacements. Of particular relevance to pediatric heart surgery is the long-term function of the engineered valve over time: its capacity to grow, self-repair, and remodel. This chapter summarizes some of the progress that has been made in tissue engineering research as it relates to cardiac valves and conduit arteries, and then outlines the areas where additional efforts must be focused in order to direct cardiovascular tissue engineering toward clinical utility.

NORMAL HEART VALVE BIOLOGY

Adult Valve Structure and Function

Heart valves open and close approximately 40 million times per year; this coordinated function occurs under the demands of hemodynamics. The normal valve presents minimal resistance to opening and no pressure gradient during systolic forward flow. In diastole, the same structure is responsible for rapid and complete closure in order to prevent valve regurgitation. Semilunar valves must additionally resist pressure differences between the diastolic arterial pressure and the diastolic ventricular pressure.

Like many other tissues, valve cusps are composed of cells residing within, and acting reciprocally on, the extracellular matrix (ECM). Semilunar valve cusps are thin, flexible structures with impressive microscopic and molecular complexity. Much of the strength and flexibility of normal heart valve cusps is owing to the specialized proteins and polysaccharide-protein complexes of the extracellular matrix, produced by resident valve interstitial cells.[5,6] The microscopic and molecular structure of adult valves reflects the regional mechanical forces experienced by the valve cusps; valve cusp ECM is not homogeneous, and the arrangement of the extracellular matrix provides a high degree of flexibility during systole, and a high degree of strength to resist pressure loads during diastole.[5] On the surfaces, a specialized endothelium prevents thrombosis, and acts as a transducer of mechanical force.[7,8] Under the endothelium, valve interstitial cells receive signals sent by the endothelium, and respond by secreting suitable matrix.[9,10]

Valve ECM is stratified and related to valve mechanics.[11] Facing the sinus of Valsalva, where eddy currents occur with diastolic pressure loads, dense collagen is found in the fibrosa layer. A middle layer of connective tissue, the spongiosa, is particularly rich in glycosaminoglycans, large complex molecules that associate with water and act as "shock absorbers," bearing largely compressive mechanical loads. The ventricularis, an elastin-rich layer facing the great artery, is specialized to stretch as the cusps elongate during ejection in systole.

Valve structure and function are therefore closely related, and strategies to engineer valves are aimed to mimic normal valve structure and function, potentially at the subcellular, cellular, tissue, and whole heart valve levels.

Embryologic and Postnatal Development

Valves do not begin as stratified tissues; as circulatory patterns evolve in fetal and postnatal life, valve morphology also changes.[12] Embryologic valve development, therefore, has relevance to tissue engineering, as a model for normal in vivo valve remodeling as programmed by gene regulatory pathways and by applied biomechanical force.

By day 15 of human embryo development, specification of myocardial and endothelial cardiac cells occurs. At day 21, formation of a linear heart tube occurs. These events are followed by rightward looping of the heart, resulting in orientation of the cardiac chambers into their final adult positions, and opposition of two specialized segments of ECM, known as cardiac jelly.[13] The first evidence of valvulogenesis occurs in this cardiac jelly when a subset of endothelial cells delaminate, invade the ECM, and undergo endothelial-to-mesenchymal transformation (EMT).[14] In early fetal valve development, valve interstitial cells are highly proliferative, and reside in a glycosaminoglycan-rich, homogeneous microenvironment. Over the course of fetal development, cell proliferation slows, and production of extracellular matrix results in valve cusp elongation. During the late stages of fetal development (20 to 36 weeks of human gestation) and in early postnatal life, valve stratification into a trilaminar structure occurs, and organization and maturation of collagen fibers begins. At the time of birth, through a series of largely undefined molecular steps, changes in oxygenation and blood pressure distinguish the aortic from the pulmonary sides of the circulation.[12] Transitional neonatal circulation has been associated with a change in phenotype from activated to quiescent interstitial cells in pulmonary, but not aortic, valve cusps.[15] Valve maturation and remodeling continue during childhood; cellularity of valve interstitial cells continues to decrease into adulthood.[12] Once thought to be passive structures, increasing evidence shows cardiac valves to be dynamic organs. Mechanistically, the finding that cellular and extracellular components mature is thought to reflect the dramatic changes in flow and biomechanical loading conditions from fetal to adult life.[12,16] Further elucidation of the genetic regulatory events defining valve growth and maturation is critical to designing biomimetic replacement devices.

ENGINEERED VALVE INPUTS

Approaches to tissue engineered heart valves (TEHV) can be divided into two paradigms, based on the type of structural scaffold employed: bioresorbable scaffolds (nonwoven felts, electrospun scaffolds, knitted meshes, hydrogel-based, and combinations) and decellularized tissue-based scaffolds. The bioresorbable scaffold approach begins with seeding cells and culturing under appropriate biomechanical conditions (static flow, pulsatile flow) and nutrient medium. With regard to tissue mechanical properties, the goal of this approach is fabrication of an adequately strong tissue with approximately constant mechanical properties, requiring that the process of scaffold degradation occurs with a reciprocal increase in extracellular matrix production. Porosity is an important characteristic of bioresorbable scaffolds as it provides a permeable framework for cell migration, nutrient supply, and waste removal. Insufficient porosity leads to nutrient deprivation and cell death. Once a sufficiently stable tissue is formed, in vivo implantation would ideally follow, placing a newly synthesized tissue, devoid of foreign elements, in the required site.

This de novo approach is the one that has been predominantly employed in our laboratory at Children's Hospital, Boston.[17–26] This approach treats components of tissue as "building blocks," constructing valves from a variety of cell types and scaffold materials. Most in vivo studies have been carried out in the lower-pressure pulmonary circulation, which is a more tolerant system than the systemic circulation. This type of approach considers several basic questions as its foundation: (1) What cell type or combination of cell types is necessary to allow the production and maintenance of an appropriate extracellular matrix? (2) To what extent can cellular phenotype be altered, guided, or "engineered" to replicate cells found in the normal valve? (3) How can these cells be spatially organized during the development of this tissue engineered structures until the cells in the construct produce sufficient and appropriate extracellular matrix? (4) What biochemical signals are necessary during the development of these structures to ensure proper extracellular matrix production? (5) What mechanical signals are necessary for optimal tissue development and growth? (6) Should a tissue engineered valve construct be completely developed and appear as an adult valve before implantation, or can further maturation of an engineered construct occur in vivo after implantation?

Proponents of the decellularized tissue method base their approach on the premise that extracellular matrix geometry directs cell behavior, and that the closest structure to the normal valve scaffold is the normal valve scaffold itself. Human aortic valve homografts are currently implanted without tissue-type matching, become acellular after several months in vivo, yet retain their mechanical properties for decades. As the exact features endowing the aortic valve with such durability are unknown, it is hypothesized that these features are retained after ex vivo decellularization. Scaffolds are either seeded with cells before implantation, or implanted without seeded cells, in the expectation that appropriate circulating cell populations will populate the scaffolds in vivo. Without seeding of cells before implantation, however, some decellularized matrices are insufficiently endothelialized by circulating cells to resist surface thrombus formation in vivo.[27]

The literature of tissue engineered heart valves demonstrates the selection of a variety of cell types, scaffold conditions, and preconditioning regimens, and overall, methods are difficult to compare and results have been inconsistent. Systematic screening of engineered tissue elements and combinatorial approaches to building tissues have recently emerged.[28,29] A complete review of past investigations is beyond the scope of this chapter; however, a summary of the fundamental elements of synthetic, biomaterial-based TEHV will be considered in detail in the following sections. In vivo outcomes of these methods will also be considered.

Cell Origin and Phenotype

As in embryologic valvulogenesis, the ideal cell type for a tissue engineered heart valve would fulfill the function of both the valve interstitial and endothelial cells. Conceptually, these cells could be derived from fully differentiated cells capable of extracellular matrix synthesis, or from less committed, multipotent or pluripotent stem cells with the additional potential for differentiation into multiple cell types.

The first tissue engineered heart valve experiments were performed with differentiated cells from artery or vein, including vascular smooth muscle cells, fibroblasts, and endothelial cells derived from the vasculature of immature animals.[17–21] These cells were chosen because they were readily accessible, are derived from a cardiovascular source, and can synthesize extracellular matrix proteins. A comparison of myofibroblasts from the wall of the ascending aorta with those from segments of saphenous vein revealed that the latter cells exhibit superior collagen formation and mechanical strength when cultured on biodegradable polyurethane scaffolds.[30] In our laboratory at Children's Hospital, Boston, tissue engineered heart valves (TEHV) based on these differentiated cells from systemic blood vessels functioned for periods of up to 4 months in vivo.[17,19] However, enhanced collagen formation may be a double-edged sword. The rapid formation of new tissue in the early culture period could give rise to an overabundance of matrix elements, leading to tissue stiffness and potential tissue contraction. Early studies with dermal fibroblasts demonstrated that valve cusps constructed from these cells developed tissue contraction, which limited the ability of valve leaflets to coapt with each other, resulting in valve regurgitation.[31] In addition to production of excessive or unfavorable types of extracellular matrix, mature cells may present a problem of senescence in long-term cell cultures in vitro, which limits the ability to quickly produce sufficient numbers of cells to seed a TEHV construct. Finally, the prospect of harvesting segments of artery from an otherwise normal peripheral circulation in order to obtain cells for a TEHV represented an undesirable clinical situation, and therefore led to a search for alternative cell sources for engineered valves.

The emergence of the field of stem cell biology has changed the paradigm for candidate cell types for heart valve tissue engineering. As stem cells differentiate from their embryonic state, they lose pluripotency with each subsequent step. Multiple steps of differentiation form lineages of cells. In embryonic development, differentiation down a specific lineage occurs with biochemical signaling, occurring in a specific mechanical microenvironment.[32] How lineage specification occurs in the developing heart is currently an area of active research, with the goal of understanding the necessary cues to replicate differentiation down valve cell lineages. In normal development, differentiating cells are subject to a rapidly changing three-dimensional extracellular environment, and development is thought to occur by signals originating outside of the cell, from molecules originating in neighboring cells, and in the extracellular matrix. These reciprocal interactions between cells and their environment in developing valves, the regulatory mechanisms that induce cells to secrete and respond to components of appropriate extracellular matrix, are thought to be the underlying mechanisms stratifying valve cusps into their known compartments. These mechanisms are thought to be largely driven by hemodynamics in developing valves.

There is also recent evidence that stem cells with proliferative and regenerative capacities reside in many adult tissues. These stem cells are capable of not only acting locally on the tissues in which they reside, but they also may be recruited out of the circulation and enlisted in the regeneration of diverse tissues at distant sites. A recent review details emerging evidence that bone marrow–derived endothelial, hematopoietic stem and progenitor cells can also contribute to tissue vascularization during both embryonic and postnatal life.[33] Visconti and coworkers have made the intriguing observation that cardiac valve interstitial cells in mice appear to originate in the bone marrow as hematopoietic cells.[34] The idea that bone marrow contains cells capable of repairing damaged tissue has been applied to regeneration of cardiac muscle after myocardial infarction, whereby progenitor cells have been isolated from sites outside the heart, then injected back into the heart in an attempt to regain contractile function of ischemic or infarcted myocytes. Results of these trials have been equivocal, marginal, or negative, suggesting that the process of regeneration does not occur by the simple addition of multipotent cells.[35] The early experience with the SynerGraft decellularized heterograft valved conduits that were implanted in children as right ventricle-to-pulmonary artery conduits occurred with the expectation that circulating cells from the bloodstream, or ingrowth from adjacent normal tissue, would repopulate the grafts and grow. In this instance, repopulation of the graft by circulating cells occurred, but did not result in adequate function or tissue

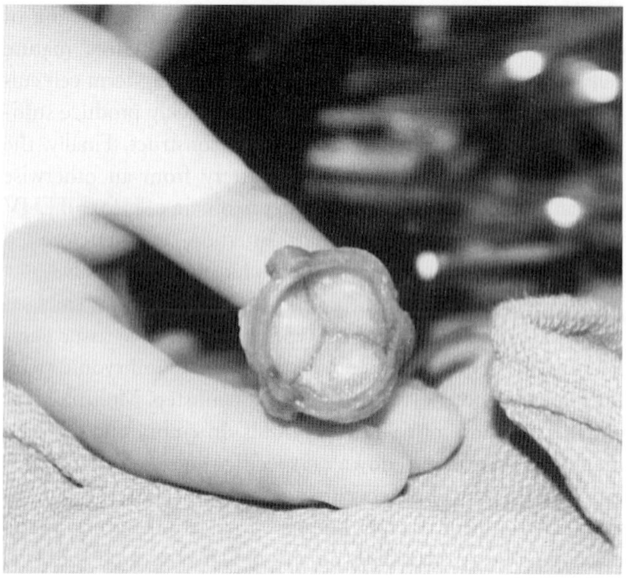

FIGURE 69-1. The tissue engineered pulmonary valve viewed from below, before implantation.

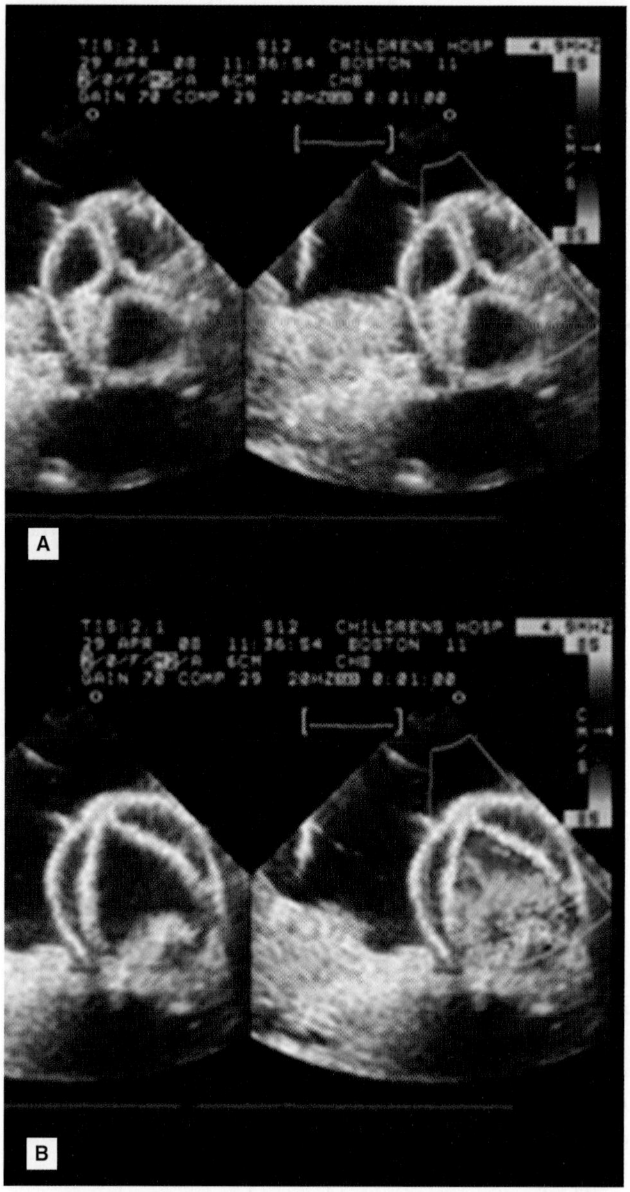

FIGURE 69-2. Representative echocardiogram images of functioning tissue engineered pulmonary valve following implantation.

growth.[36,37] Nonetheless, the progenitor cell populations represent an attractive source of cells for tissue engineering and regeneration, because they have the plasticity necessary to fulfill critical cell functions and are potentially programmable for lineage specification. In addition, these cells can be obtained less invasively than differentiated cells.[33] Our initial experience with progenitor cells in the Mayer laboratory was gained with autologous endothelial progenitor cells (EPCs) isolated from circulating blood in lambs and seeded onto decellularized arterial segments.[17] These seeded arterial grafts were then implanted as an interposition graft in the carotid artery of the donor lamb. These grafts remained patent and functional for up to 130 days. Subsequent animal studies by Sutherland and associates used bone marrow mesenchymal stem cells (MSC) to seed a bioresorbable scaffold formed into a three-leaflet valve within a conduit (Fig. 69-1). These valved conduits were implanted as valved conduits into the main pulmonary artery of neonatal sheep, and remained in place for up to 8 postoperative months.[24] This study was followed by that of Gottlieb et al., who implanted valves of similar elements into larger numbers of sheep and followed changes in function with growth of the animals using MRI and echocardiography. Although the valves had trace to mild regurgitation at the time of implantation (Fig. 69-2), a loss of valve leaflets surface area was observed, which correlated with increasing valve regurgitation over time.[26] Importantly, the valve leaflets underwent a remodeling process in vivo after implantation, seen also in earlier experiments using myofibroblasts and endothelial cells from systemic arteries, and in both sets of experiments a layered histologic appearance developed after implantation.[19,24,26]

Several types of progenitor cells have been used for tissue engineering applications in congenital heart disease. Cebotari and colleagues have recently reported an initial experience seeding EPCs onto homograft valves followed by implantation into two children.[38] Matsumura and associates have shown that when seeded onto a copolymer of lactic acid and ε-caprolactone, green fluorescent protein (GFP)–labeled cells contributed to the histogenesis of their explanted tissue engineered vascular graft. These grafts remained patent, and explanted constructs contained GFP-labeled cells expressing both endothelial and mesenchymal markers.[31] The group at Tokyo Women's Medical College has also carried out implants of tissue engineered vascular grafts in children with congenital heart disease using whole mononuclear cell fractions, seeded onto bioresorbable scaffolds.[39] This work is now ongoing at Yale University, because of encouraging early results.

Increasing evidence supports the idea that for cells, "geography is destiny." Many cell types including bone marrow–derived MSC exhibit surprising plasticity, and cell phenotype seems to be related to the microenvironment in which cells reside.[40–42]

However, many of the factors controlling differentiation in these environments remain incompletely defined. There is evidence that endothelial progenitor cells are able to transdifferentiate in response to biochemical signals. Dvorin and colleagues showed that in the presence of transforming growth factor (TGF)-β_1, EPCs express α-smooth muscle actin (α-SMA), after seeding on a bioresorbable copolymer scaffold.[43] This behavior is not characteristic of endothelium; SMA expression suggests a mesenchymal phenotype, and this observation is a potentially related phenomenon to EMT seen in embryologic valvulogenesis.[43] Human aortic valve endothelial cells, but not vascular endothelial cells, respond to TGF-β_1 in a similar fashion, suggesting that endothelial progenitor cells may be suitable as a replacement for valve endothelium. Though stem cells of many types remain promising candidates for tissue engineering, their full potential will be harnessed with an understanding of their normal generative and regenerative roles in vivo.

Structural Scaffold

Although it has been possible to grow individual cell types in culture for decades, it is more difficult to induce cells to assemble or organize into complex three-dimensional structural arrangements that are found in normal tissues, and to induce cells to produce specific extracellular matrix components on demand. Implantation of engineered tissues requires structural integrity, and for this reason, most tissue engineers employ a structural scaffold, in addition to cellular material.

Given this fundamental requirement, two main strategies for development of a three-dimensional tissue have been used: (1) de novo scaffold synthesis and arrangement into a three-dimensional structure; and (2) decellularization of a whole (usually xenograft) tissue.

Any scaffold for tissue engineering applications must be biocompatible and allow cells to adhere and proliferate. For congenital cardiac applications, tissue growth is our target, and therefore the scaffold must either degrade or be remodeled in vivo. The advantage of the biopolymer approach is that the chemistry of these scaffolds allows for in vivo degradation, usually by hydrolysis.[44] The disadvantage is that heart valves are structurally complex and anisotropic; designing the structural features of the normal heart valve de novo has presented a substantial engineering challenge. The obvious advantage of the decellularization approach is that the three-dimensional complexity is largely preserved; however, there is a shortage of homograft material relative to the clinical demand, and immunogenicity remains a concern with xenografts. Perhaps most importantly, the extracellular matrix of decellularized xenografts is dense, and may prevent the penetration of seeded cells into the interstices of the matrix. In our laboratory, we have constructed trileaflet valved conduits from small intestinal submucosa and seeded them with EPCs.[23] After implantation in an ovine model, there was satisfactory short-term function, but there was no penetration of any cells into the depths of the small intestinal submucosa scaffold. Extracellular matrix proteins, when exposed to blood components, can induce inflammation, thrombosis, and calcification, so this material has not been pursued further in our laboratory.

Our primary laboratory efforts to develop heart valves and large arteries have utilized the approach of seeding cells onto alternate bioresorbable polymer scaffolds. Ideally, there exists an inverse relationship between scaffold degradation and extracellular matrix formation by seeded cells. Polymer degradation is related to polymer chemistry, fabrication method, and mechanism of degradation, and therefore polymers used in tissue engineering differ in their degradation times. The first generation of scaffolds used in heart valve tissue engineering were highly porous, nonwoven felts produced from fibers of polyglycolic acid (PGA). PGA and related polymers continue to be the most widely used for multiple tissue engineering applications.[45–49] The advantage of PGA and related aliphatic polyesters, including poly-L-lactic acid (PLLA), is their safety, biocompatibility, lack of toxicity, and commercial availability. PGA has been used as the commercially available Dexon suture material since the 1970s.[49] PGA can be extruded as a fiber, which allows fabrication of nonwoven sheets with large, open pores. Open pore structures facilitate cell delivery and proliferation by allowing a large surface area for cell attachment, free diffusion of nutrients and dissolved gases, and removal of waste products of metabolism. Material properties of these nonwoven felts are well established, with reproducible hydrolytic degradation times; PGA alone degrades in 2 to 4 weeks, whereas the majority of fibers of the more hydrophobic PLLA degrade within 4 to 6 weeks. These scaffolds lose strength before losing mass, which challenges tissue engineers to seed sufficient numbers of matrix-producing cells so as to replace the scaffold strength as it is lost. Our laboratory has experimented with PGA coated with the thermoplastic polymer poly-4-hydroxybutyrate (P4HB), assembled into a trileaflet structure by attaching leaflets to a flat scaffold sheet, then wrapping the scaffold around a mandrel and heat-welding a seam of attachment. Despite promising early results using the PGA/P4HB composite, subsequent studies showed loss of structural integrity with longer periods of in vitro culture, followed by difficulties with suture retention and hemostasis in vivo. For these reasons, Sutherland and colleagues in our laboratory developed a scaffold composed of equal parts of PGA and PLLA fibers. Because PGA is a stronger but more rapidly degrading polymer, and PLLA is a less strong polymer with a longer degradation time, we expected more uniform strength from the tissue when constructed from this material. The composite nonwoven felt was fabricated into a valved conduit with a trileaflet valve, and had substantially improved surgical handling characteristics.[24]

Although satisfactorily strong, polymer fiber-based scaffolds are significantly stiffer than normal valve leaflets, and with the addition of cell-secreted extracellular matrix, these constructs are notably stiff.[44] Scaffold stiffness has been shown to affect cell behavior, and tissue engineers have sought less more flexible materials.[42] Wang and colleagues at the Massachusetts Institute of Technology designed an elastic polymer with a rapid degradation time, based on sebacic acid, a derivative of castor oil. Polyglycerol sebaceate is a strong but elastomeric material, and is currently under investigation for use in heart valve tissue engineering applications.[50]

In addition to their stiffness, polymer-based scaffolds are thick, relative to normal valve leaflets. A thick scaffold leads to a nutrient gradient in culture, and many tissue engineering studies based on nonwoven materials have been limited by the lack of nutrient delivery to the deepest areas of engineered tissues. Two solutions are proposed to overcome this limitation: addition of a blood supply and design of thinner scaffolds.

Hydrogel-based scaffolds, including collagen, alginate, agarose, gelatin, fibrin, chitosan, polyethylene glycol, hyaluronic acid, and dehydrated sheets of extracellular matrix have formed the basis of many experiments in tissue engineering. When gels become solid, cells are trapped in the cell, providing a homogeneous distribution of cells embedded in a temporary matrix. In addition, hydrogels can be laid into thin layers. A bileaflet heart valve was produced in the Tranquillo laboratory using a collagen-based scaffold seeded with dermal fibroblasts.[51] Recent advances in drug delivery technologies and microfluidics have resulted in further control of scaffold characteristics, including orchestration of scaffold polymerization with changes in temperature, pH, or exposure to light; engineering of nano- and micro-scale cell environments in order to direct cell distribution throughout a scaffold, and microencapsulation of growth factors and adhesion peptides on scaffolds for improved cell attachment and proliferation.[52–56]

Finally, cells and scaffold have been incorporated and directed in nanoscale fabrication techniques such as electrospinning. Still, no perfect material has been identified for heart valve tissue engineering, and in this regard, the search continues.

The complex anisotropy and three-dimensional structure of heart valves has provided another challenge for a biomimetic device. Even if the optimal scaffold material is identified, its fabrication into a three-dimensionally accurate valve geometry is not trivial. Using normal heart valve anatomy derived from computed tomographic images, Sodian and associates employed stereolithography to print a three-dimensional model for use as a mold for the thermoplastic polymer P4HB.[57] The mold was used for curing the polymer into three-dimensional valve anatomy. As improvements in imaging technology yield higher spatial and temporal resolution, anatomic definition of thin, moving, anisotropic structures in the heart such as valve leaflets will be more feasible. In addition, evolving microfabrication methods will further our ability to fabricate microscale features of valve anatomy. With defined anatomic dimensions and an understanding of outflow tract, great artery, and leaflet motion and growth, tissue engineers will have clear targets for three-dimensional fabrication of heart valve scaffolds.

Biochemical Signals

The migration and transdifferentiation of endothelial cells in the early stages of valvulogenesis (EMT) has been experimentally modeled in an ex vivo chick cardiac cushion explant system.[14] Much progress has been made to understand the signals required for the proper sequencing and execution of these early events. Vascular endothelial growth factor is one such molecule, thought to regulate EMT in an environment of adequate tissue glucose and oxygen saturation. Although VEGF is secreted by endothelial cells, other important signals, such as bone morphogenetic protein 2 and 4, are expressed by myocardium. Hyaluronic acid, a component of the extracellular matrix, is thought to regulate downstream signaling through its large, hydrated structure, which regulates ligand availability for receptor binding. Therefore, valvulogenesis is dependent in vivo on signals from myocardium, local extracellular matrix, and endothelium.[11,32] Though very early growth of endocardial cushions and valve primordia are less understood, and late regulatory events in valve growth are poorly understood, regulators of endothelial and mesenchymal cell proliferation have been identified. These known pathways have been largely studied in isolation, and as gene regulation in organogenesis is a highly complex process, synthesis of critical gene pathway data is necessary for developing a big-picture view of required events. Current microarray technologies will yield large volumes of data, and will likely provide additional insight into the critical regulatory steps involved in valve growth. This type of information will be high yield in future generations of engineered valves.

Mechanical Signals

Identification of a suitable cell phenotype is necessary but not sufficient for engineering replacement tissues. Proper cell orientation and three-dimensional microstructure are also required for tissue function; tissues demonstrate organization of cells and matrix across multiple levels of scale. In this regard, engineered tissues, like native tissues, require coordination. Hemodynamics are fundamental to the development and ongoing function of cardiovascular structures, and biomechanical signals are epigenetic regulators of tissue growth and development. Increasing evidence supports a role for endothelial cells as mechanotransducers, sending signals through the underlying extracellular matrix to the more deeply embedded valve interstitial cells.[16] Endothelial cells respond to shear stress and cyclic strains.[58] In an environment in which concentrations of soluble growth factors are held constant, endothelial cell programs can be switched between growth, differentiation, and apoptosis by varying the extent to which the cell is spread or stretched.[59] As cells are embedded in, and coupled to, their extracellular matrix, ECM serves as a vehicle through which signals must pass. Biochemical signals can be sequestered or amplified by ECM, and as cells bind to surrounding ECM via integrin receptors, the binding itself can induce phenotypic changes.[32] When human MSCs are plated onto large tissue islands that promote cell spreading, they efficiently differentiate into bone cells; when plated onto small islands, the same cells in the same culture medium differentiate into adipocytes.[60]

Clinical observations made from patients undergoing the Ross procedure have provided further evidence for the responsiveness of vascular and valve tissues to hemodynamic forces. In the Ross procedure, a pulmonary valve from the lower-pressure pulmonary circulation is transplanted into the aortic position and subjected to systemic pressure, leading to significant changes in the phenotype of valve interstitial cells, including an increase in matrix metalloproteinase activity, indicating ECM remodeling.[15]

Biophysical signaling is therefore considered fundamental to engineered tissue organization and conditioning, or training, for the in vivo environment. Mechanical forces can be applied to growing engineered tissues in a flow-loop containing tissue culture medium, known as a bioreactor. Preconditioning of tissues is thought to be important for the biology and monitoring of engineered cardiovascular tissues. Bioreactors are thought to serve two predominant purposes for engineered heart valves: first, mechanical forces influence cell phenotype and gene expression, and therefore tissue development, and potentially growth, are controlled by biomechanical signals. In experiments from our laboratory reported by Hoerstrup and colleagues, flow and pressure were demonstrated to increase the production of collagen in tissue engineered semilunar valves.[19] In separate experiments, Lee and associates demonstrated the variation of extracellular matrix gene transcripts with changes in tightly controlled mechanical strains. Vascular smooth muscle cells seeded onto biodegradable scaffolds, then subjected to cyclic flexure produced more collagen and were stiffer than controls.[61] Similar findings were reproduced using mesenchymal stem cells, and porcine heart valves.[62,63]

In addition, because valves must not be regurgitant at the time of implantation, observation of engineered valve mechanics in a bioreactor before implantation has allowed investigators to monitor and predict in vivo valve function.

ENGINEERED VALVE EXPERIMENTAL OUTCOMES

Progress toward a clinically translatable engineered heart valve is not possible without in vitro study of valve development and remodeling. Developmental biology and in vitro experiments are the fundamental elements of this emerging field. However, in vivo experiments are the necessary complement to in vitro investigation, and represent the true test of engineered device function over time. The in vivo environment is more complex than can be approximated in vitro, and remodeling is dependent on the contributions of circulating progenitor and immune cells only present in whole living organisms.

Four major implantation studies of tissue engineered heart valves have been undertaken using the de novo engineered approach.[19,24,26,64] Several groups have implanted decellularized and recellularized valves into the juvenile lamb circulation,[65,66] and two major studies evaluate the growth of vascular conduits in the pulmonary circulation.[67,68] Several representative studies will be reviewed in terms of valve function, evaluation of valve/conduit growth, and observation of engineered tissue maturation.

In Vivo Valve Function, Growth, and Maturation

Heart valve tissue engineering was conceptually established through proof-of-concept experiments in large animals. The first in vivo tissue engineered heart valve experiment involved implantation of a single leaflet into the pulmonary circulation.[17] Cells were isolated from ovine arteries and sorted into endothelial and fibroblast populations. Cells were labeled, then seeded onto PGA scaffold and subsequently implanted. Labeled cells were visualized in explanted specimens after 6 hours and after 1, 6, 7, 9, or 11 weeks. Cells produced extracellular matrix, and leaflets persisted in the circulation at all time points.

A second set of experiments involved implantation of a pulmonary valve composed of autologous ovine endothelial cells and myofibroblasts seeded on a PGA-P4HB composite scaffold.[19] After 14 days of exposure to gradually increasing flow and pressure conditions in a pulse duplicator, valves were implanted into sheep for 1 day, 4, 6, 8, 16, and 20 weeks. Valves demonstrated acceptable hemodynamics and had no evidence of thrombosis, stenosis or aneurysm formation for up to 20 weeks. Central valvar regurgitation was noted after 16 weeks. Tissue analysis showed a layered structure with central glycosaminoglycans, collagen on the outflow surface, and elastin on the inflow surface. Elastin was detectable in the leaflets by 6 weeks in vivo. Over the 20-week study period, scaffold degradation corresponded to decreased leaflet stiffness. Histologic, biochemical, and biomechanical parameters were similar to those of native pulmonary artery and leaflet tissue.

Using bone marrow–derived mesenchymal stem cells on a PGA/PLLA scaffold, investigators fabricated and implanted valved conduits in the pulmonary position of juvenile sheep.[24] Valves were evaluated by in vivo echocardiography; explanted tissues were analyzed by histology and immunostaining. At the time of implantation, echocardiograms demonstrated a maximum instantaneous gradient of 17.2 ± 1.33 mm Hg, with estimates of regurgitation ranging from trivial to mild. Four animals survived the immediate postoperative period. After 4 months in vivo, there were no statistically significant difference between maximum instantaneous gradient, mean gradient, or effective orifice area from the time of implantation. Histologic analysis at 8 postoperative months showed explanted tissue to have a layered organization, with elastin fibers identified on the inflow surface and collagen dominating the outflow surface. Glycosaminoglycans were distributed throughout the remainder of the valve. At the time of implantation, cells uniformly expressed the mesenchymal cell marker a-SMA, but at the time of valve explant, these cells were confined to the subendothelial layer, whereas surface cells expressed von Willebrand factor, suggesting in vivo endothelialization of the graft. This study demonstrated the feasibility of implantation of a pulmonary valve using stem cells.

Further work in our laboratory has reproduced some of these initial findings, and studied valve function over time in larger numbers of animals.[26] Using the same scaffold material (PGA-PLLA composite nonwoven felt) and cells (MSCs), 19 animals underwent implantation of valved conduits into the main pulmonary artery of neonatal sheep after resection of the native pulmonary leaflets. Valve function, cusp, and conduit dimensions were evaluated at implantation (echocardiography), at the experimental midpoint (MRI), and at explant at 1 day, 6, 12, or 20 weeks postoperatively. At implantation, valved conduit function was excellent; maximum transvalvar pressure gradient by Doppler echocardiography was 17 mm Hg; most valved conduits showed trivial pulmonary regurgitation. At ≥12 weeks, valved conduit cusps were increasingly attenuated and regurgitant. Valved conduit diameter remained unchanged over 20 weeks. Dimensional measurements by MRI correlated with direct measurement at explant. These studies demonstrated autologous engineered valved conduits that functioned well at implantation, with subsequent monitoring of dimensions and function in real time by MRI. The valves underwent structural and functional remodeling without stenosis, but worsening pulmonary regurgitation was noted after 6 weeks.

When fibrin-based valves were implanted in sheep for 3 months, valved conduits exhibited the gross appearance of intact tissue; however, leaflets demonstrated pulmonary regurgitation because of tissue contraction.[64]

To date, no group has implanted valve leaflets that demonstrated in vivo growth. In many experiments, however, the microscopic structure of the valve leaflets evolved from a relatively homogeneous appearance to a layered structure. The mechanisms by which this in vivo evolution of structure and cellular activity occurs remain completely unexplored, but these observations suggest that a tissue engineered valve may not have to be in a mature, adult form at the time of implantation into the circulation.

Present and Future

After a decade of effort toward a tissue engineered heart valve replacement, the clinical need for a more durable valve replacement still exists. Modes of failure of currently available heart valve replacements are well described and provide insight into strengths and weaknesses of valve designs. Though the appropriate cell source and scaffold material for heart valve tissue engineering have been areas of substantial experimental effort, the optimal cell type, scaffold material, and in vitro culture conditions for a tissue engineered heart vale still remain unknown. Stem cells and adult progenitor cells offer promise toward this end, because they possess the capacity for self-renewal and multilineage differentiation, and therefore, growth potential. Evolving imaging technologies will allow a more complete understanding of postimplantation remodeling and growth. Though many details of in vitro preconditioning regimens are yet to be understood, bioreactor preconditioning has the potential to reduce in vitro culture times by stimulating tissue formation, and may offer a controllable environment for evaluation of valve function before implantation.

Complex biological events, such as heart valve development, occur through both biochemical and biophysical cues, occurring in parallel at the cellular, tissue, and organ levels. A detailed understanding of the molecular sequence of critical developmental events may allow engineering of appropriate microenvironments and three-dimensional structures leading to the ultimate goal: a clinically translatable heart valve replacement with the capacity to grow and remain durable for a lifetime of cardiac cycles.

REFERENCES

1. Vongpatanasin W, Hillis D, Lange RA: Prosthetic heart valves. *NEJM* 1996; 335:407.
2. Hammermeister KE, Sethi GK, Henderson WG, et al: Outcomes 15 years after valve replacement with a mechanical versus a bioprosthetic heart valve: final report of the veterans affairs randomized trial. *J Am Coll Cardiol* 2000; 36:1152.
3. Forbess JM, Shah AS, St Louis JD, et al: Cryopreserved homografts in the pulmonary position: determinants of durability. *Ann Thorac Surg* 2001; 71:54.
4. Stark J, Bull C, Stajevic M, et al: Fate of subpulmonary homograft conduits: determinants of homograft failure. *J Thorac Cardiovasc Surg* 1998; 115:506.
5. Rabkin-Aikawa E, Mayer JE Jr, Schoen FJ: Heart valve regeneration, in Yannas IV (ed): *Advances in Biochemical Engineering/Biotechnology. Regenerative Medicine II.* Berlin, Springer-Verlag, 2005; p 141.
6. Schoen FJ: Aortic valve structure-functional correlations: role of elastic fibers no longer a stretch of the imagination. *J Heart Valve Dis* 1997; 6:1.
7. Davis PF: Hemodynamic shear stress and the endothelium in cardiovascular pathophysiology. *Nat Clin Pract Cardiovasc Med* 2009; 6(1):16.
8. Cummins PM, von Offenberg Sweeney N, Killeen MT, et al: Cyclic strain-mediated matrix metalloproteinase regulation within the endothelium: a force to be reckoned with. *Am J Physiol Heart Circ Physiol* 2007;292: H28.
9. Ingber DE: Mechanical signaling and the cellular response to extracellular matrix in angiogenesis and cardiovascular physiology. *Circ Res* 2002; 91:877.
10. Chiquet M: Regulation of extracellular matrix gene expression by mechanical stress. *Matrix Biol* 1999; 18:417.
11. Lincoln J, Lange AW, Yutzey KE: Hearts and bones: shared regulatory mechanisms in heart, cartilage, tendon and bone development. *Dev Biol* 2006; 294(2):292.
12. Aikawa E, Whittaker P, Farber M, et al: Human semilunar cardiac valve remodeling by activated cells from fetus to adult. *Circulation* 2006; 113:1344.
13. Moore K, Persaud T: *The Cardiovascular System: The Developing Human.* Philadelphia, WB Saunders, 1998; p 563.
14. Armstrong EJ, Bischoff J: Heart valve development: endothelial cell signaling and differentiation. *Circ Res* 2004; 95:459.
15. Rabkin-Aikawa E, Aikawa M, Farber M, et al: Clinical pulmonary autograft valves: pathologic evidence of adaptive remodeling at the aortic site. *J Thorac Cardiovasc Surg* 2004; 128:552.
16. Butcher J, Tressel S, Johnson T, et al: Transcriptional profiles of valvular and vascular endothelial cells reveal phenotypic differences: influence of shear stress. *Arterioscler Thromb Vasc Biol* 2006; 26(1):69.
17. Shin'oka T, Bruer CK, Tanel RE, et al: Tissue engineering heart valves: valve leaflet replacement study in a lamb model. *Ann Thorac Surg* 1995; 60(Suppl 6):S513.
18. Sodian R, Hoerstrup SP, Sperling JS et al: Tissue engineering of heart valves: in vitro experiences. *Ann Thorac Surg* 2000; 70:140.
19. Hoerstrup SP, Sodian R, Daebritz S et al: Functional living trileaflet heart valves grown in vitro. *Circulation* 2000; 102(Suppl 3):III44.
20. Stock UA, Nagshima M, Khalid PN, et al: Tissue engineered valved conduits in the pulmonary circulation. *J Thorac Cardiovasc Surg* 2000; 119:732.
21. Sodian R, Hoerstrup SP, Sperling JS, et al: Early in vivo experience with tissue-engineered trileaflet heart valves. *Circulation* 2000; 102(Suppl 3):III22.
22. Steinhoff G, Stock U, Karim N, et al: Tissue engineering of pulmonary heart valves on allogenic acellular matrix conduits: in vivo restoration of heart valve tissue. *Circulation* 2000; 102(Suppl 3):III50.
23. Matheny RG, Hutchison ML, Dryden PE, et al: Porcine small intestine submucosa as a pulmonary valve leaflet substitute. *J Heart Valve Dis* 2000; 9:769.
24. Sutherland FWH, Perry TE, Yu Y, et al: From stem cells to viable autologous semilunar heart valve. *Circulation* 2005; 111:2783.
25. Kaushal S, Amiel GE, Guleserian KJ, et al: Functional small diameter neovessels created using endothelial progenitor cells expanded ex vivo. *Nat Med* 2001; 7:1035.
26. Gottlieb D, Kunal T, Emani S, et al: In vivo monitoring of autologous engineered pulmonary valve function. *J Thorac Cardiovasc Surg* 2010; 139(3):723.
27. Mendelson K, Schoen FJ: Heart valve tissue engineering: concepts, approaches, progress and challenges. *Ann Biomed Eng* 2006; 34(12):1799.
28. Kang L, Hancock MJ, Brigham MD, et al: Cell confinement in patterned nanoliter droplets in a microwell array by wiping. *J Biomed Mater Res A* 2010; 93(2):547.
29. Woodfield TB, Moroni L, Malda J: Combinatorial approaches to controlling cell behaviour and tissue formation in 3D via rapid-prototyping and smart scaffold design. *Comb Chem High Throughput Screen* 2009; 12(6):562.
30. Schnell AM, Hoerstrup SP, Zund G, et al: Optimal cell source for cardiovascular tissue engineering: venous vs. aortic human myofibroblasts. *J Thorac Cardiovasc Surg* 2001; 49:221.
31. Matsumura G, Miyagawa-Tomita S, Shin'oka T, et al: First evidence that bone marrow cells contribute to the construction of tissue engineered vascular autografts in vivo. *Circulation* 2003; 108:1729.
32. Combs MD, Yutzey KE: Heart valve development: regulatory networks in development and disease. *Circ Res* 2009; 105:408.
33. Rafii S, Lyden D: Therapeutic stem and progenitor cell transplantation for organ vascularization and regeneration. *Nat Med* 2003; 9:702.
34. Visconti RP, Ebihara Y, LaRue AC, et al: An in vivo analysis of hematopoietic stem cell potential: hematopoietic origin of cardiac valve interstitial cells. *Circ Res* 2006; 98:690.

35. Passier R, van Laake LW, Mummery CI: Stem-cell-based therapy and lessons from the heart. *Nature* 2008; 453(7193):322.
36. O'Brien MF, Goldstein S, Walsh S, et al: The SynerGraft valve: a new acellular, non-glutaraldehyde tissue heart valve for autologous recellularization. First experimental studies before clinical implantation. *Semin Thorac Cardiovasc Surg* 1999; 11:194.
37. Simon P, Kasimir MT, Seebacher G, et al: Early failure of the tissue engineered porcine heart valve SynerGraft in pediatric patients. *Eur J Cardiothorac Surg* 2003; 23:1002.
38. Cebotari S, Lichtenberg A, Tudorache I, et al: Clinical application of tissue engineered human heart valves using autologous progenitor cells. *Circulation* 2006; 114(Suppl I):I132.
39. Shin'oka T, Matsumura G, Hibino N, et al: Midterm clinical result of tissue-engineered vascular autografts seeded with autologous bone marrow cells. *J Thorac Cardiovasc Surg* 2005; 129:1330.
40. Rozario T, Desimone DW: The extracellular matrix in development and morphogenesis: a dynamic review. *Dev Biol* 2010; 341(1):126.
41. Gjorevski N, Nelson CM: Bidirectional extracellular matrix signaling during tissue morphogenesis. *Cyt Grow Fact Rev* 2009; 20(5-6):259.
42. Engler AJ, Sen S, Sweeney HL, et al: Matrix elasticity directs stem cell lineage specification. *Cell* 2006; 126:677.
43. Dvorin EL, Wylie-Sears J, Kaushal S, et al: Quantitative evaluation of endothelial progenitors and cardiac valve endothelial cells: proliferation and differentiation on poly-glycolic acid/poly-4-hydroxybutyrate scaffold in response to vascular endothelial growth factor and transforming growth factor β1. *Tissue Eng* 2003; 9:487.
44. Engelmayr GC, Sacks MS: Prediction of extracellular matrix stiffness in engineered heart valve tissues based on nonwoven scaffolds. *Biomech Model Mechanobiol* 2008; 7:309.
45. Bailey M, Wang L, Bode C, et al: A comparison of human umbilical cord matrix stem cells and temporomandibular joint condylar chondrocytes for tissue engineering temporomandibular joint condylar cartilage. *Tissue Eng* 2007; 13(8):2003.
46. Rohman G, Pettit J, Isaure F, et al: Influence of the physical properties of two-dimensional polyester substrates on the growth of normal human urothelial and urinary smooth muscle cells in vitro. *Biomaterials* 2007; 28(14):2264.
47. Roh J, Brennan M, Lopez-Soler R, et al: Construction of an autologous tissue-engineered venous conduit from bone marrow-derived vascular cells: optimization of cell harvest and seeding techniques. *J Pediatr Surg* 2007; 42(1):198.
48. Dahl S, Rhim C, Song Y, et al: Mechanical properties and compositions of tissue engineered and native arteries. *Ann Biomed Eng* 2007; 35(3):348.
49. Gao J, Niklason L, Langer R: Surface hydrolysis of poly(glycolic acid) meshes increases the seeding density of vascular smooth muscle cells. *J Biomed Mater Res* 1998; 42:417.
50. Wang Y, Ameer GA, Sheppard BJ, et al: A tough biodegradable elastomer. *Nat Biotechnol* 2002; 20:602.
51. Neidert M, Tranquillo R: Tissue-engineered valves with commissural alignment. *Tissue Eng* 2006; 12(4):891.
52. Park H, Cannizzaro C, Vunjak-Novakovic G, et al: Nanofabrication and microfabrication of functional materials for tissue engineering. *Tissue Eng* 2007; 13:1867.
53. Burdick J, Kahademhosseini A, Langer R: Fabrication of gradient hydrogels using a microfluidics/photopolymerization process. *Langmuir* 2004; 20(13):5153.
54. Silva E, Mooney D: Spatiotemporal control of vascular endothelial growth factor delivery from injectable hydrogels enhances angiogenesis. *J Thromb Haemost* 2007; 5(3):590.
55. Matsumoto T, Mooney D: Cell instructive polymers. *Adv Biochem Eng Biotechnol* 2006; 102:113.
56. Bacakova L, Filova E, Kubies D, et al: Adhesion and growth of vascular smooth muscle cells in cultures on bioactive RGC peptide-carrying polylactides. *J Mater Sci Mater Med* 2007; 18(7):1317.
57. Sodian R, Fu P, Lueders C, et al: Tissue engineering of vascular conduits: fabrication of custom-made scaffolds using rapid prototyping techniques. *J Thorac Cardiovasc Surg* 2005; 53(3):144.
58. Resnick N, Junior MG: Hemodynamic forces are complex regulators of endothelial gene expression. *FASEB J* 1995; 9(10):874.
59. Ingber D: Mechanical control of tissue morphogenesis during embryological development. *Int J Dev Biol* 2006; 50:225.
60. Ingber D, Levin M: What lies at the interface of regenerative medicine and developmental biology? *Development* 2007; 134(14):2541.
61. Lee RT, Yamamoto C, Feng Y, et al: Mechanical strain induces specific changes in the synthesis and organization of proteoglycans by vascular smooth muscle cells. *J Biol Chem* 2001; 276:13847.
62. Engelmayr GC, Rabkin E, Sutherland FW, et al: The independent role of cyclic flexure in the early in vitro development of an engineered heart valve tissue. *Biomaterials* 2005; 26:175.
63. Stephens EH, Chu CK, Grande-Allen KJ: Valve proteoglycan content and glycosaminoglycan fine structure are unique to microstructure, mechanical load and age: relevance to an age-specific tissue engineered heart valve. *Acta Biomater* 2008; 4(5):1148.
64. Flanagan TC, Sachweh J, Frese J, et al: In vivo remodeling and structural characterization of fibrin-based tissue-engineered heart valves in the adult sheep model. *Tissue Eng A* 2009; 15(10):2965.
65. Hopkins RA, Jones A, Wolfingarger L, et al: Decellularization reduces calcification while improving both durability and 1-year functional results of pulmonary homograft valves in juvenile sheep. *J Thorac Cardiovasc Surg* 2009; 137(4):907.
66. Vincentelli A, Wautot F, Juthier F, et al: In vivo autologous recellularization of a tissue-engineered heart valve: are bone marrow mesenchymal stem cells the best candidates? *J Thorac Cardiovasc Surg* 2007; 134(2):424.
67. Leyh RG, Wilhelmi M, Rebe P, et al: Tissue engineering of viable pulmonary arteries for surgical correction of congenital heart defects. *Ann Thorac Surg* 2006; 81:1466.
68. Hoerstrup SP, Cummings I, Lachat M, et al: Functional growth in tissue-engineered living, vascular grafts: follow-up at 100 weeks in a large animal model. *Circulation* 2006; 114:I159.

CHAPTER 70

Stem Cell–Induced Regeneration of Myocardium

Philippe Menasché

INTRODUCTION

Statistics recently published by the American Heart Association clearly outline the magnitude of the medical and economic problems associated with heart failure.[1] It is estimated that 6 million people in the United States are affected by this disease, with a yearly incidence of new episodes (per 1000 people) of 15.2 between 65 and 74 years of age, a figure that is two times higher between 75 and 84 years of age. Still in the United States, the number of hospitalizations for heart failure has thus increased from 877,000 to 1,106,000 in a 10-year time frame (1996–2006), but the problem is now worldwide. The mortality remains high as 80% of men and 70% of women under the age of 65 years in whom heart failure has been diagnosed are expected to die within the next 8 years with a risk of sudden death which is six to nine times that of the general population. As expected, these figures translate into a heavy economic burden with costs estimated to 37 billion dollars in 2008.

Although heart transplantation remains the only radical treatment for end-stage heart failure, its use is limited by organ shortage and the complications associated with major immunosuppression. Surgical remodeling procedures require well-defined anatomical indications, and the failure of the STITCH[2] trial may lead to revisit them. Mechanical assist devices are still primarily used as bridges to transplant (or recovery) and, despite its ability to provide symptomatic relief, biventricular stimulation fails in 20 to 30% of patients.[3] Finally, none of the large trials implemented over the last decade to investigate new drugs has yielded a positive outcome allowing to improve the survival of heart failure patients. Put together, these observations have provided a rationale for exploring new therapeutic options, among which "regeneration" of the chronically failing heart by stem cells has raised a tremendous interest. From the onset, however, it is fair to state that regeneration *bona fide,* ie, generation of a new myocardial tissue with the same properties as the native one, is a concept, a target, and a hope, but not yet a reality. This chapter first summarizes the current status of stem cell trials, then describes the strategies that can be considered for effecting a true myocardial regeneration, and finally emphasizes the importance of addressing the low cell engraftment issue to make these strategies successful.

CURRENT STATE OF THE ART: IMPROVED LEFT VENTRICULAR FUNCTION VERSUS MYOCARDIAL REGENERATION

So far, two types of stem cells, both of adult origin, have been tested clinically: skeletal myoblasts and bone marrow–derived cells.

Skeletal Myoblasts

In June, 2000, we performed the first human transplantation of autologous myoblasts in a patient with severe ischemic heart failure[4] who underwent a concomitant coronary artery bypass grafting (CABG). This case initiated a 10-patient pilot trial that was soon followed by three other adjunct-to-CABG myoblast transplantation studies,[5–7] which only differed from ours in that they systematically entailed a concomitant revascularization of the myoblast-injected areas.

Altogether, these studies have demonstrated the feasibility of the procedure as well as its safety with the caveat of an increased risk of ventricular arrhythmias. This has been attributed to the failure of engrafted myoblasts to express gap junction proteins and their subsequent electrical isolation from the surrounding cardiomyocytes,[8] which could slow conduction velocity and predispose to reentry circuits.[9] This hypothesis is supported by the in vitro finding that myoblast transfection with connexin 43 decreases arrhythmogenicity,[9] but clinically other myoblast-unrelated factors are likely in play, particularly the needle-induced inflammatory tissue damage[10] and the intrinsically arrhythmogenic nature of the underlying heart failure substrate.

Although these initial studies had suggested improved functional outcomes following myoblast transplantation, they were neither designed nor powered to provide efficacy data, which led us to implement a randomized, double-blind, placebo-controlled trial (MAGIC, an acronym for Myoblast Autologous Grafting in Ischemic Cardiomyopathy), which was conducted in 21 centers across Europe.[11] Ninety-seven patients with severe left ventricular (LV) dysfunction, a postinfarction non-viable scar and an indication for bypass surgery were assigned to receive multiple in-scar injections of autologous myoblasts (at two different doses: 400 and 800 million) grown from a muscular biopsy taken 3 weeks earlier or similar injections of a placebo solution. An internal cardioverter-defibrillator (ICD) was implanted in each of these patients to provide objective readouts of arrhythmic events. At the 6-month study point, the proportion of patients who had experienced arrhythmias was not statistically different between the myoblast-treated and the placebo-injected groups despite a trend for a higher incidence of arrhythmic events early after myoblast implantations and there was not a single death that could be attributed to arrhythmias. This rather reassuring safety finding contrasted with the disappointing observation that regardless of the dose, myoblast injections had failed to improve LV function beyond that seen in the placebo group, even though the high-dose group experienced a significant reduction in remodeling (which was a prespecified secondary end point). Although this signal suggested that cells can exert some beneficial effects, these effects were clearly too limited to translate into meaningful improvements in contractile function, thereby ruling out the occurrence of a procedure-induced myocardial regeneration.

In parallel to these surgical trials, phase I catheter-based studies have assessed myoblast delivery through an ultrasound-guided coronary sinus catheter[12] or through an endoventricular catheter under electromechanical guidance.[13] Like their phase I surgical counterparts, these trials have primarily demonstrated the technical feasibility of these approaches. Efficacy data are more limited and are still controversial. At the 2008 Society of Cardiovascular Angiography and Interventions meeting, Serruys reported on 31 patients who were allocated to myoblast injections while 16 received "optimal medical therapy." In keeping with the MAGIC data, there was no added benefit of cell therapy on LV function measured at 6 months after the procedure. In contrast, Dib and coworkers[14] have reported improved outcomes in patients receiving transendocardial injections of skeletal myoblasts compared with a placebo group but with the caveat of a 1-year only follow-up.

Bone Marrow–Derived Cells

Most studies of bone marrow–derived cell therapy have been in the context of acute myocardial infarction and refractory angina and, comparatively, few of them have tackled heart failure. In this setting, they can be categorized in relation with the specific cell population that has been tested.

Mononuclear Cells

Beyond the anecdotal cases, five surgical studies have tested intramyocardial injections of bone marrow–derived unfractionated mononuclear cells (MNC) in conjunction with bypass surgery and, overall, their results are mixed. In a 36-patient trial, Mocini and coworkers[15] reported a 3-month significant improvement in regional and global LV function compared with baseline, but these outcome measures did not differ from those obtained in control patients who, surprisingly, failed to improve functionally following bypass surgery. The 20 patient study of Hendrikx and coworkers[16] showed that after 4 months, there was a significantly greater wall thickening in cell-transplanted patients (as assessed by magnetic resonance imaging [MRI]), but no improvement in ejection fraction or perfusion defects beyond values recorded in control patients. The third trial in which cells were injected both in the myocardium and in the bypass grafts also failed to meet its primary end point.[17] Conversely, two studies,[18,19] of which one was randomized,[18] have reported improved function and perfusion up to 6 months[18] and 5 years[19] after MNC transplantation combined with CABG. Of note, whereas the average numbers of injected cells ranged from 60 to 292 million in the mentioned negative trials, those with a positive outcome entailed transplantation of up to 6.59×10^8 and 1.23×10^9 MNC,[18,19] which calls attention to the importance of careful dose-effect relationship studies before definitive conclusions can be drawn.

Catheter-based studies of bone marrow cells in patients with heart failure have been initiated by an open-label nonrandomized 11-patient trial who were reported to have experienced a 1-year improvement in exercise capacity following endoventricular injections of MNC.[20] A limited number of studies entailing intracoronary MNC infusions have then claimed positive functional outcomes in both ischemic[21,22] and nonischemic[23] cardiomyopathy settings. However, their results should be interpreted cautiously in view of the methodologic limitations inherent in the usual lack of randomization, the functional impairment of cells taken from patients with chronic ischemic heart disease[24] and the small engraftment rate of intracoronary injected cells (see the following), particularly at the chronic stage, when the endothelial alterations associated with acute ischemic events and that may promote transvascular trafficking waned. Of note, the recent randomized controlled trial conducted by van Ramshorst and coworkers[25] has reported a 3% improvement in ejection fraction without changes in LV volumes after endomyocardial MNC injections, but the target population was chronic ischemia not amenable to conventional revascularization and these outcomes thus likely illustrate the expected angiogenic effect of bone marrow cells rather than de novo myogenesis.

Hematopoietic Progenitors

The well-documented angiogenic properties of bone marrow–derived cells (see the following) have led other investigators to rather focus on hematopoietic progenitors featuring a high angiogenic capacity. In this setting, the most convincing results have been reported by Stamm and coworkers[26] who have injected $CD133^+$ cells epicardially during CABG. Although this trial was not strictly randomised, it has been rigorously conducted and provides encouraging hints in favor of the capacity of the CD133$^+$ population to safely improve LV function and perfusion at 6 months postoperatively, particularly in patients with the poorest preoperative LV function. It is likely, however, that these effects, which await further confirmation by the upcoming randomized PERFECT trial, proceed from a cell-induced increase in angiogenesis and not from the conversion of the CD133$^+$ progenitors into new cardiomyocyte. As such, they do not match the strict definition of myocardial regeneration.

Mesenchymal Stem Cells

The third category of BM-derived cells, which is raising a growing interest, even though clinical experience with them is still limited in the field of heart regeneration, comprises mesenchymal stem cells (MSC). These cells represent a rare population (0.01 to 0.001%) of the bone marrow and are usually defined by their adherence to plastic surfaces, their negativity for hematopoietic markers (CD45, CD34), the expression, among others, of the CD29, CD44, CD73, CD90, and CD105 antigens, and the capacity to differentiate along the osteogenic, chondrogenic, and adipogenic lineages in response to the appropriate cues. Most (but not all)[27] experimental studies conducted in small[28,29] and large[30–32] animal models of chronic myocardial infarction,[28,29,31,33] or dilated cardiomyopathy[34] have now documented that transplantation of autologous[30] or allogeneic[28,29,31,33] transplantation of MSC may improve LV function and attenuate adverse remodeling in a dose-dependent fashion,[32] at least at midterm.[28] These patterns of improvement are usually associated with increased angiogenesis and reduced fibrosis. As all these studies have failed to document the differentiation of MSC into cardiomyocytes, it is likely that improved outcomes after MSC treatment proceed from their trophic effects[35] reported to be more potent than those of MNC.[34]

Put together, these data have paved the way for upcoming or already ongoing trials of MSC in patients with chronic LV dysfunction in whom cells are delivered transendocardially as a stand-alone procedure or transepicardially as an adjunct to CABG or to placement of an assist device (which should yield useful histologic data when the heart will be removed for transplantation). In one of these studies, MSC are pretreated with a combination of growth factors targeted at increasing their cardiomyogenic differentiation potential[36] as exposure of cells to the demethylation agent 5-azacytidine, which had been initially proposed to drive MSC toward a cardiomyogenic lineage, is unsuitable for clinical applications. Interpretation of outcomes, however, might be complicated by the fact that some companies involved in these trials have developed proprietary processes allowing isolation of specific subsets of MSC. Because there are no cell surface markers that specifically and uniquely identify MSC, it remains difficult to determine whether these different MSC subsets really reflect different cell fractions with distinct properties or simply represent the same MSC population assessed at different developmental stages and with the use of different surface markers.

Although MSC have initially been retrieved from bone marrow, alternate tissue sources have then been proposed like the placenta,[37] menstrual blood,[38] or the periodontal ligament.[39] However, the greatest focus is currently on adipose tissue as a source of MSC derived from its stroma vascular fraction. Although there are differences in the global gene expression pattern between adipose tissue–derived MSC and their BM counterparts,[40] the two types of cells share in common lineage-specific differentiation potentials, immunomodulatory properties,[41] and cardioprotective effects.[42,43] These effects have been attributed to cell-derived antiapoptotic and angiogenic factors,[44] and the latter might be even greater in the case of adipose-derived MSC,[43] which also express the CD34 marker at the time of isolation.[40,41] Conversely, there is no evidence for differentiation of these cells into cardiomyocytes.[45] An additional attractive feature of adipose tissue–derived MSC is that their procurement by liposuction is patient friendly and their expansion capacity seems greater than that of their BM counterparts.[46] To make their availability still more expeditious, a device has been developed to extemporaneous process lipoaspirates so as to yield a mixed cell population that can be immediately transplanted at the point of care and a clinical trial (PRECISE) testing the endoventricular delivery of this cell product has just been completed in patients with coronary artery disease not amenable to revascularization in the target area. How this device-generated heterogeneous cell population compares with that comprising the stroma vascular fraction specifically isolated from liposuction products remains to be established. It is also fair to temper the current enthusiasm about these cells by mentioning the negative study of van der Bogt and coworkers,[47] who have used bioluminescence imaging for the in vivo tracking of injected cells and have reported an equally high rate of MSC death regardless of the tissue source (bone marrow or adipose tissue) and a corresponding lack of cardioprotection. However, it cannot be excluded that this negative outcome was strongly biased by the prolonged period of pretransplantation MSC cultures.

Regardless of the tissue source, what has largely driven the clinical interest in MSC is their alleged "immune privilege" and the related hope that they could be used as an allogeneic off-the-shelf readily available product with the attendant logistical, regulatory, and economic benefits. This paradigm is based on the in vitro mixed lymphocyte reactions-based findings that MSC do not evoke a response of allogeneic lymphocytes and inhibit lymphocyte proliferation induced by allogeneic peripheral blood MNC.[41] These immunomodulatory effects, which require direct contact between MSC and the responder T cells and release of soluble mediators have been attributed to three major mechanisms: (1) MSC are hypoimmunogenic because of their lack of major histocompatibility complex (MHC) class II and costimulatory molecules. (2) They prevent T-cell responses both directly by directing CD4 T cells to a suppressive phenotype and disrupting CD8 T cell and natural killer cell function, and indirectly by interfering with dendritic cell maturation. (3) They secrete soluble mediators, which induce a suppressive local microenvironment[48,49] through downmodulation of inflammatory cytokines (particularly TNF-α and IFN-γ) produced by activated T lymphocytes and inhibition of B-cell proliferation.

The current enthusiasm about MSC, however, needs to be tempered in light of several considerations. First, the plasticity of MSC renders them extremely sensitive to the physical nature of the underlying substrate; the stiffer the substrate, the greater the likelihood of a differentiation along the osteogenic lineage.[50] Given the heterogeneous composition of postinfarction scars, there is a potential for some of the in-scar injected MSC to give rise to intramyocardial calcification, a complication that, so far, has only been observed experimentally.[51] Second, the demonstration of the immunosuppressive effects of MSC have been largely based on in vitro experiments and despite the successful results of MSC treatment of severe graft-versus-host disease by LeBlanc and associates,[52] the immune privilege of these cells is still debated. Indeed, it has been reported that MSC could function as antigen-presenting cells and intramyocardial injection of human MSC in rat myocardium have shown that although MSC could engraft in immunocompromised hosts, they triggered a robust immune response in those with an intact immune system.[53] Likewise, Poncelet and coworkers[54] have reported that intracardiac transplantation of allogeneic porcine MSC elicited a complete cellular and humoral immune response whereas the same cells had failed to trigger an in vitro proliferative response. A clinical industry–sponsored study of intravenous allogeneic MSC treatment has already been completed in patients with acute myocardial infarction and has yielded a quite reassuring safety record. Efficacy data are less conclusive and the study does not allow us to know whether the injected cells have been rejected or not. Fourth, the optimal route for MSC delivery is not straightforward. Their intravenous infusion is obviously the simplest and the safest approach and has been advocated on the premise that MSC would sense signals emitted by the infarcted tissue and preferentially home to the injured area. However, homing has been primarily reported in rodent experiments[55] and studies in large animals[56] and humans[57] have failed to show MSC engraftment in the heart. On the other hand, a direct intramyocardial injection, surgically or through an endoventricular catheter, does not raise safety issues, but such is no longer the case if one considers an intracoronary infusion because the relatively large size of MSC (twice that of MNC, ie, approximately 20 μm) may result in capillary plugging.[58,59] Although some data suggest that this hurdle can be overcome by appropriate cell dosing, concomitant implementation of a robust antithrombotic therapy,[43] and careful control of the rate of cell delivery,[59] it is clear that the intracoronary delivery of MSC in heart failure patients should still be viewed with caution. Finally, multiple passages of MSC may induce spontaneous transformation[60] leading to uncontrolled growth kinetics and this potential safety issue thus requires that accurate cytogenetic studies be performed if expanded MSC products are to be used clinically.

Mechanisms of Action of Transplanted Cells: The Paracrine Paradigm

The previously mentioned discrepancy between the improved functional outcome yielded by MSC treatment and the lack of direct tissue replacement by the grafted cells is indeed a phenomenon that encompasses the other cell types tested so far, and this has led some to hypothesize that the benefits of cardiac cell therapy reported so far were not mediated by a new onset graft–derived myogenesis, but rather by an increase in cell-associated wall thickness leading to a reduction in chamber volume and consequently in wall stress and/or the release of trophic factors promoting survival and repair of injured tissue. Support to the latter hypothesis has come from the finding that skeletal myoblasts[61,62] and bone marrow–derived cells[63–66] stimulate endogenous pathways leading to increased angiogenesis, decreased apoptosis, and a favorable shift of extracellular matrix remodeling toward improved scar elasticity, even though the two cell types differ by the nature of the paracrine mediators involved, the downstream signal transduction pathways, and the ultimate specific effects.[67] In line with this hypothesis, it has been reported that the beneficial effects of intravenously injected MSC, despite their low intramyocardial engraftment rate, were caused by trapping of the cells within the lungs and a subsequent upregulation of the anti-inflammatory factor TSG-6.[68] Importantly, the cell-triggered upregulation of host-associated cytoprotective mediators seems to be prolonged, which explains the functional recovery of the heart at a time in which the trigger cells have faded away.[69] By analogy with the ability of transplanted neural stem cells from fetal origin into the brain ventricles of aged rats to stimulate endogenous neurogenesis,[70] the recruitment of dormant cardiac progenitor cells residing in the myocardium has been proposed as another target for cell-released factors.[71] However, this hypothesis is more tenuous in view of the persisting uncertainties surrounding the existence of this stem cell niche in the adult heart (see the following). Finally, MSC have also been shown to release mediators that increase sympathetic nerve sprouting,[72] which could contribute to increase cardiac performance, but also carries the risk of promoting arrhythmias related to heterogeneous cardiac innervation.

The recognition that cells primarily act as delivery vehicles not by physically substituting for dead host cardiomyocytes has led to speculation that a more straightforward means of inducing protection could be the sole injection of the conditioned medium derived from these cells. This hypothesis has been pioneered by the group of Dzau and coworkers[73] who documented, in *acutely* infarcted rat hearts, infarct size limitation, and functional recovery as early as 72 hours after intramyocardial injection of the conditioned medium from hypoxic MSC genetically modified to overexpress the prosurvival gene Akt1. Likewise, delivery of the conditioned medium derived from MSC in a pig model of *acute* myocardial infarction has been shown cardioprotective, with the caveat of a very short (4 hours) period of observation.[74] Although these studies provide compelling evidence for paracrine protection, their relevance to regeneration of the chronically failing myocardium remains more questionable because of the specificities of their protocol design (acute model of infarction and short follow-up). Indeed, in a study in which MSC were compared with injection of angiogenic growth factor genes, the former were found to better improve myocardial performance,[75] which suggests that the physical presence of the cells, even transient, may be critical because the expected fast clearance of injectants from the target tissue likely decreases their efficacy (unless they are supplied with slow-release delivery systems). In addition, it may be difficult for conditioned media retrieved at a single time point to fully replicate the complex blend of trophic factors released by the engrafted cells over time.

Although one cannot dispute that the mechanical (reduction in wall stress) and paracrine effects of engrafted cells may effect some cardioprotection, it is still quite uncertain that these effects may be robust enough to translate into clinically meaningful improvements in patient outcomes, which stimulates the search for strategies that could achieve such an improvement through a true myocardial regeneration.

POSSIBLE APPROACHES TO MYOCARDIAL REGENERATION

Conceptually, there are three major approaches that can be considered for inducing myocardial regeneration.

Stimulation of Endogenous Cardiomyocyte Proliferation

Whereas it has long been considered that the heart was a terminally differentiated organ, recent data have challenged this paradigm and elegant studies using ^{14}C dating have provided evidence for some renewal of human cardiomyocytes spanning the lifetime but with a low turnover, as percentages of dividing cells decreased from 1% per year at the age of 25 to 0.45% at the age of 75 years.[76] This has led some investigators to hypothesize that differentiated quiescent cardiomyocytes, which did not proliferate under resting conditions, could be induced to re-enter the cell cycle in response to extracellular mitogens. It has thus been demonstrated in mouse models of myocardial infarction that factors such as periostin[77] or neuregulin[78] triggered cardiomyocyte cell-cycle activity and that the resulting regeneration was associated with improved function, reduced fibrosis and infarct size, and increased angiogenesis. However, whether and how these basic science data can be translated into a safe and efficacious clinical therapy remains to be elucidated.

Transplantation of Putative Extracardiac Cell Niches Endowed with a Cardiomyogenic Differentiation Potential

In 2006, Witnisky and coworkers[79] described in the mouse skeletal muscle a population of cells committed to a cardiomyogenic lineage. Unfortunately, using similar surface markers, we failed to show that such a cardiac-directed cell fraction existed in the human muscle.[80] These findings are consistent with the increasing recognition that stem cells harbored in adult tissues are unlikely to cross lineages, except possibly under clinically irrelevant experimental conditions. It remains to be established whether this hurdle can be overcome by small molecules such as those of the sulfonyl hydrazone family, which have recently been reported as able to activate cardiac differentiation of human mobilized peripheral blood mononuclear cells,[81] thereby effecting myocardial regeneration in a nude model of myocardial infarction.

Transplantation of Cardiac Stem/Progenitor Cells

Endogenous Sources: The Heart Itself

The ^{14}C experiments mentioned in the preceding have actually been preceded in the early 2000s by studies from the group of Anversa who first claimed that despite being traditionally considered as a postmitotic organ, the heart actually harbored dividing cardiomyocytes evidenced by a positive expression for the cell proliferation marker Ki67, and that the proliferation rate of these cells was dramatically increased in patients with heart failure.[82] The phenotypic characterization of these cells, found in multiple species, has yielded puzzling results in that different surface markers occasionally expressed in a mutually exclusive fashion have been identified (reviewed in Barile)[83] and it is still uncertain whether this variability in marker distribution actually reflects distinct cell populations with specific functional properties or the ability of a unique pool of stem cells to express different markers at different stages of its maturation. C-*kit*+ cells have been the most extensively investigated; because they lacked expression of hematopoietic markers, a bone marrow origin, such as that reported in sex-mismatched heart transplant recipients in whom 0.04% cardiomyocytes were found to be repopulated from extracardiac cells,[84] has been excluded. Rather these c-*kit*+ cells have been considered to represent a myocardial pool of progenitor cells committed to a cardiomyogenic lineage. Proof-of-concept was putatively provided by demonstration of donor-derived cardiomyocytes (along with smooth muscle cells and endothelial cells) when human cardiac progenitors were injected intramyocardially[85] in a rat model of myocardial infarction and resulted in an improvement in contractile function, an attenuation of remodeling and histologic patterns of regeneration. This paradigm found a clinical application in July 2009 when a first patient was injected in Louisville, KY with his own cardiac stem cells derived from a right atrial biopsy that had been taken 4 months earlier during a CABG and subsequently expanded in Anversa's lab in Boston. Other investigators have adopted a slightly different approach in that instead of trying to isolate these putative cardiac stem cells, they grew fragments of myocardial tissue as cell clusters termed *cardiospheres*. These aggregates are composed of c-*kit*+ progenitor cells primarily in their core and of a mix of cells expressing cardiac, endothelial, and mesenchymal markers at their periphery. Following preclinical studies showing that intramyocardial[86] and intracoronary[87] delivery of human and porcine cardiospheres could regenerate acutely and chronically infarcted myocardium, respectively, the group of Marban in Los Angeles moved to the clinics in June 2009 and performed a first intracoronary transfer of these cardiospheres 1 month after removal of a right ventricular specimen by an endomyocardial biopsy. A trial exploring the potential of this approach (CADUCEUS for CArdiosphere-Derived aUtologous Stem Cells to Reverse ventricular dysfunction) is currently under way.

Whereas the use of cardiac stem cells is appealing because of the cardiac lineage commitment of these cells and the avoidance of immunological issues owing to their autologous origin, several caveats must be mentioned. The major concern is that it is still uncertain whether these cardiac stem cells really exist in the adult diseased heart. In our experience, we have identified a few c-*kit*+ cells in right atrial tissue taken during CABG or through endomyocardial biopsies,[88] but all of them expressed hematopoietic markers and none expressed specific cardiac markers. Likewise, a high proportion of the c-*kit*+ cells isolated from failing human hearts by Kubo and coworkers[89] were positive for markers of the hematopoietic lineage, and although their number was fourfold higher that in nonfailing hearts, their reparative capacity was clearly inadequate because all failing hearts required transplantation. In keeping with these data, cells expressing both stem and differentiated cardiac markers have been identified in the human neonatal myocardium, but with a progressive decline in cell density over the first postnatal month,[90] thereby raising serious doubts about the persistence of cardiac "stem" cells in adult patients with coronary artery disease, ie, those who would them need most. The fact that 4 months were required for growing these cells in the recently reported clinical experience also highlights the technical challenges associated with their isolation and scale-up and raises some doubts about a realistic widespread clinical use. Finally, a recent study has further challenged these findings by showing that spontaneously beating neonatal rat cardiospheres resulted from contamination by myocardial tissue fragments and that these cardiospheres actually represented aggregated fibroblasts rather than clonally expanded cardiac stem cells.[91] Another more recently described variety of stem cells of cardiac origin is represented by those derived from the epicardium, but these cells also seem to improve function of infarcted hearts paracrinally as they fail to acquire a cardiac phenotype.[92]

Embryonic Stem Cells

Human embryonic stem cells (hESC) are derived from the inner cell mass of blastocyst-stage leftover embryos, which have been generated in the setting of assisted fertilization. Their most appealing feature is an intrinsic pluripotentiality that allows them to be committed in vitro toward the cardiac lineage in response to appropriate differentiation cues recapitulating those in play during the embryonic life and among which bone morphogenetic proteins (members of the TGF-β superfamily), Wnts, and fibroblast growth factors play a predominant role.[93] It has thus been demonstrated that hESC could generate cells displaying the three major attributes of cardiomyocytes: (1) excitation-contraction coupling, demonstrated by the expression of ionic currents;[94] intracellular calcium transients triggered by electrical activation and the resulting synchronous contractions; (2) responsiveness to the chronotropic effects of cardioactive drugs,[95] and (3) the capacity to couple with neighboring cells through connexin 43-supported gap junctions.[96] Following transplantation in rodent models of myocardial infarction, these cells have been shown to improve LV function, an effect usually associated with a beneficial effect on remodeling.[97–99] Of note, mouse ESC have also been shown functionally effective in a nonischemic genetic cardiomyopathy model.[100] One could legitimately argue that these cardioprotective effects have been reported with most cell types. However, an observation more specific for ESC is that, in contrast to their adult counterparts, they really differentiate into cardiomyocytes in transplanted areas, an event likely driven by cues originating from the infarcted tissue.[101] However, injected ESC derivatives share with other cell types a limited amount of long-term engraftment,[102] and this finding, along with the fact that increasing graft size has been reported not to positively correlate with a gain of function, has led to hypothesize that ESC-induced stimulation of vascularization was actually a major contributor to the cardiac functional improvement.[103] Indeed, whereas ESC derivatives may well act paracrinally by activating endogenous cytoprotective pathways,[104] one cannot fully exclude that they also directly contribute to cardiac contractility by generating a force transmitted to the surrounding tissues.[105] Furthermore, it is important to recognize that the assessment of hESC transplantation is hampered by the lack of appropriate preclinical models as all of them are fraught with the confounding effect of xenotransplantation. For this reason, we have conducted experiments in nonhuman infarcted primates transplanted with primate ESC–derived cardiac progenitors, thereby mimicking an allogeneic situation closer to clinical practice. The data have confirmed the ability of these progenitors to achieve their differentiation into cardiomyocytes following in-scar engraftment. Furthermore, the finding made in a pig model of iatrogenic atrioventricular block, that intramyocardial transplantation of hESC-derived cardiac derivatives could restore electrical activity,[106] provides compelling evidence for the ability of these cells to achieve an effective electromechanical integration within the recipient heart.

Asides from ethical considerations, the clinical use of hESC still raises several translational issues[107] that fall into three main categories: (1) derivation and propagation of a line endowed with a cardiogenic differentiation potential, under good manufacturing practice (GMP) conditions; this first step of the process should allow to scale-up the number of cells without the use of xeno-components while maintaining their pluripotentiality and ensuring their genetic and epigenetic stability over time; (2) directed differentiation of the propagated pluripotent cells toward a cardiomyogenic lineage; (3) sorting of the cells, so as to yield a "pure" population of cardiac progenitors for clinical use. (Progenitors are likely preferable to a terminally differentiated cell type because of their ability to still proliferate in the host tissue to a certain extent, thereby effecting myocardial regeneration.) Several purification methods are available and rely on negative or positive selection, depending on whether they target the elimination of still undifferentiated cells or the enrichment of the lineage-committed progenitors from other unwanted cell types, respectively. Introduction of a reporter-suicide gene into stem cells that could serve as a safety net against cellular misbehavior is another option that warrants further investigation. In our experience, a positive selection approach based on identification of the surface marker SSEA-1 (or CD15) has turned out to be efficacious in that this antigen reliably labels cells that have entered a differentiation pathway,[108] thereby allowing immunomagnetic sorting using an anti-CD15 antibody to selectively yield the clinically required cardiac progenitor cell population. The elimination of the contaminating cells is actually critical not only for efficacy, but also for safety reasons as a major concern with ESC is the development of a teratoma. Teratomas are complex tumors consisting of cell lines originating from the three initial germ layers. Although several factors (cell number, transplant site, degree of immunosuppression) may affect whether these tumors form after transplantation of ESC,[109] a key role is played by the state of differentiation of the transplanted cells. Indeed, teratomas occur when cells are used in a still undifferentiated or poorly differentiated state and have thus retained an intrinsic capacity of uncontrolled proliferation, which can overcome the cardioinstructive signaling of the host heart. Conversely, animal models have failed to show evidence for teratomas following transplantation of hESC-derived cells committed to a given cell lineage,[101,105] as demonstrated by their loss of pluripotent markers and the concomitant upregulation of the lineage-specific ones. These considerations highlight the importance of the purification step during preparation of a clinically usable ESC-derived cell therapy product.

Another major clinical issue raised by the use of this allogeneic cell source is immunogenicity. Despite initial hopes, it is now widely recognized that although undifferentiated ESC lack expression of MHC type II antigens and costimulatory molecules, they trigger a cellular and humoral immune response,[110] which does not spare their differentiated progeny.[111] Even though the lack of antigen-presenting cells within ESC-derived grafts may contribute to a reduced immunogenicity compared with adult tissues,[111] it is still necessary to implement some form of immunosuppressive strategy to avoid cell loss by this immune process. Different approaches have thus been considered. Banking of hESC lines with a range of MHC profiles allowing an appropriate donor-recipient matching is likely not unrealistic, because about 150 randomly obtained cell lines could provide a worthwhile human leukocyte antigen (HLA) match for most potential recipients.[112] This figure, however, was based on matching only selected MHC loci and thus does not dismiss that additional immune suppression would be required to overcome residual immunogenicity. Also, it may underestimate the ethnic diversity of most Western populations. Furthermore, such a banking approach raises complicated logistical and economic issues and, as such, first requires the convincing demonstration that the use of hESC-derived cells is therapeutically effective. Given the risks associated with a protracted use of immunosuppressive drugs, induction of tolerance in the recipient looks a particularly appealing approach should it be possible at the cost of minimal host conditioning.[113] In practice, it might be achieved by the administration of hematopoietic stem cells derived from a given "donor" ESC line[114] and the resulting induction of a microchimerism ensuring specific tolerance to cardiac (or other) progenitors derived from that same donor ESC line. The use of costimulation blockade for inducing peripheral tolerance mediated by regulatory T cells could be another strategy.[115] In contrast, the creation of a "universal" cell line, for example by knockout of the β-2 microglobulin gene, which is essential for MHC-I presentation, remains a more uncertain perspective because MHC molecules also represent a surveillance mechanism whose deletion could create a favorable environment for viral infections and development of malignancies. Thus, from a practical standpoint, early clinical trials of hESC will likely have to rely on more conventional therapies based on immunosuppressive drugs. The challenge is then going to find an acceptable trade-off between the efficacy of these drugs and their well-known side-effects so as to optimize the risk-to-benefit ratio of the procedure. The additional use of autologous or allogeneic mesenchymal stem cells for further mitigating the immunorejection process is supported by a study in kidney transplant recipients,[116] although we have experimentally failed to show such a benefit in a rat model of hESC transplantation.[99]

The recent presidential lift on the US federal funding ban on ESC research and the attendant increase in resources allocated to this area make likely that many of the remaining hurdles will be overcome in a not too distant future.

Induced Pluripotent Cells

In 2006, Yamanaka made a real breakthrough in the stem cell field when he reported that mouse embryonic and adult fibroblasts could acquire properties similar to those of ESC after retrovirus-mediated transfection of genes encoding the four transcription factors Oct3/4, Sox2, Klf4, and c-Myc.[117] Since then, several groups have embarked in this research on induced pluripotent stem (iPS) cells and have successfully reprogrammed human adult somatic cells into an embryonic-like state, including from patients with a variety of neurodegenerative and genetic diseases.[117] Reprogrammed cells can then be redirected toward a given cell lineage, including cardiomyocytes, and this cardiomyogenesis process actually involves a temporal sequence of gene expression (specific for cardiac mesoderm, cardiac transcription factors, and cardiac-specific structural proteins, successively), which parallels that observed during differentiation of hESC.[118]

The use of iPS could potentially allow to address two limitations of ESC, ie, immune rejection and ethical concerns raised by the use of human embryos, with still the caveat that one does not know whether the reprogramming-redifferentiation process could not cause expression of otherwise hidden-self and lead to autoimmunity events. However, their clinical application also faces important obstacles. Some of them are shared with ESC, such as teratoma formation following unwanted transplantation of still undifferentiated cells; other hurdles are rather unique to iPS cells and specifically include the risk of incomplete/aberrant reprogramming that may impair their ability to be redifferentiated toward the required cell type. It also remains to determine which is the best somatic cell source to use (eg, skin fibroblasts, keratinocytes, blood cells) and how to increase the still low efficiency of the reprogramming process while improving its safety. This is indeed a key question as a major risk of the initially used retroviruses and lentiviruses is transgene reactivation leading to tumorigenesis, hence the more recent interest in plasmids, proteins,[119] and even chemicals that represent a mandatory step on the pathway to production of iPS for clinical use. However, even these virus-free approaches may induce genetic alterations and therefore would call for a sequencing of the whole genome of iPS cell clones to detect these alterations before any clinical application.

These considerations suggest that although iPS cell technology may be soon ready for prime time toxicology screening and patient-specific disease modeling, its application to "regenerative" medicine still requires many challenges to be surmounted.

Nevertheless, encouraging data have already been reported. Thus, the potential therapeutic value of iPS cells has yet been successfully tested in three noncardiac disease models (sickle cell anemia, Parkinson's disease, and hemophilia A). These data have more recently been extended to the heart by Nelson and coworkers,[120] who have pioneered the transplantation of fibroblast-derived iPS cells in a murine model of myocardial infarction and shown that it resulted in an improvement in LV function compared with the parental fibroblasts, associated with a differentiation of the iPS cell progeny into cardiomyocytes. However, because this study did not include "true" ESC-derived cardiomyocytes as another control, additional experiments remain necessary to thoroughly assess the comparative efficacy of these two types of pluripotent stem cells. This is particularly relevant in view of recent data that indicate that regardless of their origin or the method by which they have been generated, iPS retain a gene expression pattern distinct from that of hESC and that extends to the expression of noncoding (mi)RNAs.[121] Therefore, it is critical to assess the functional significance, if any, of these differences. Finally, although iPS have the major theoretical advantage over hESC of being patient-specific, one should not underscore the limitations of autologous cell therapy products when large patient populations are targeted; these limitations include intrinsic interindividual variability in cell functionality, which complicates the production of consistent cell products, logistical constraints inherent in cell shipments, and the huge cost of customized batch controls.

THE PREREQUISITE FOR AN EFFECTIVE MYOCARDIAL REGENERATION: THE ENHANCEMENT OF CELL ENGRAFTMENT

Regardless of the cell type used, a consistent finding is that only a tiny number (usually <1%) of the cells that have been initially delivered can still be identified after a few days or, at best, weeks. This massive attrition rate proceeds from two sequential events: an initially low retention of the grafted cells into the target tissue and a subsequent low survival rate of the cells that have been initially retained. It is thus clear that the optimization of regenerative cardiac cell therapy requires to address these two issues.

Low Retention of Grafted Cells

This low retention is caused by the interplay of several factors: mechanical leakage of the cells along the needle tracks, washout through the venous and lymphatic drainage systems of the heart[122] with a subsequent large extracardiac cell redistribution (primarily in the lungs and the spleen), and limited myocardial homing in cases in which cells are delivered intravascularly.

Factors of Cell Retention

Three factors of cell retention must be considered: the route of cell delivery, the phenotype of the cells, and the nature of the target tissue.

Cells can be delivered by intravenous infusion, intracoronary or endomyocardial catheterization (the latter usually under electromechanical mapping), and open-chest transpericardial injections. Each of these routes has advantages and drawbacks.

The intravenous route is clearly the simplest and the safest. Unfortunately, it is associated with a minimal, if any, myocardial uptake of the injected cells,[123] suggesting that homing signals are unlikely to be powerful enough to overcome trapping (particularly in the lungs) of the circulating cells and drive them toward the injured areas. Intracoronary injections with the stop-flow technique result in minimal myocardial retention and dynamic tracking of 18^{F}-fluorodeoxyglucose–labeled progenitor cells has clearly documented a loss of approximately 80% of the myocardiac activity of the tracer after balloon deflation.[124] Furthermore, direct intracoronary infusion of cells may be harmful if their size is such that it can result in microvascular obstruction, as reported with MSC.[58] Indeed, direct intramyocardial injections seem to be the most efficient route for delivering cells,[125] and at least in the case of skeletal myoblasts, it does not seem that engraftment is then different whether these intramyocardial injections are made from the endocardium or transepicardially.[126] In the latter case, the role of the heart status remains uncertain with one study reporting no difference between beating-heart and arrested-heart injections,[127] whereas another, using more sophisticated assessment tools (MRI and quantitative polymerase chain reaction) documented the higher intramyocardial cell numbers when injections were made in the cardioplegic heart.[128] The major limitation of this epicardial approach is clearly its invasiveness (unless an associated surgical procedure is indicated); hence, the potential interest of a recently developed miniature robotic device that can be introduced through a subxiphoid approach, navigates over the epicardial surface and, owing to a fine-positioning control system, allows multiple injections in predefined target spots.[129] Finally, retrograde infusion through the coronary sinus with a dedicated ultrasound-guided catheter[130] has gained limited clinical acceptance and would likely be technically challenging in heart failure patients whose coronary sinus is now often already filled with leads connected to a synchronization device.

The phenotype of delivered cells is also likely to affect the magnitude of their retention as demonstrated by the finding that intracoronary delivery of $CD34^{+}$ cells results in greater numbers of these progenitors in the myocardium compared with unfractionated MNC.[131]

The nature of the target tissue also plays a role in cell retention. This is illustrated by the finding that intramyocardial retention of MNC is dramatically reduced in chronic heart failure compared with acute myocardial infarction,[132] likely because chemoattractive forces that may promote cell trafficking at the time of acute injury are no longer present (or less operative) in the setting of a remodeled old infarction.

Improvements in Cell Retention

Improvements in cell retention need to be considered differently depending on whether cells are delivered intramyocardially or intravascularly.

Intramyocardial Delivery

A first strategy consists of acting on cells and to increase the viscosity of the injectate to minimize leakage at the time of injections. This can be achieved by incorporation of cells into biomaterials or by encapsulating them in microparticles.

Incorporation into Biomaterials. Cells sense matrix nano topography and stiffness cues[133] as well as mechanical signals such as strain and stretch and these factors can thus modulate important cell functions such as proliferation, alignment, and differentiation. This implies that the choice of a scaffold has to be customized to a given stem cell type. Basically, polymers can be categorized as naturally derived (collagen, fibrin, decellularized matrices) or synthetic. The interest of embedding cells into one of these biomaterials is not only to improve their retention for purely physical reasons (increased viscosity) but also to facilitate some key functions such as survival, proliferation, and differentiation owing to cell patterning within a tridimensional microenvironment. These speculations are supported by the finding that incorporation of different types of cells into supports such as collagen,[134] fibrin glue,[135] or self-assembling nanopeptides[136] have been successful in increasing angiogenesis and preserving cardiac function. In addition, these polymers can serve as delivery vehicles for growth factors, thereby contributing to further enhance the efficacy of the cell transplantation procedure.[137]

In line with this reasoning, some investigators have successfully tested injection of cell-free dermal fillers[138] or alginate-derived hydrogels[139] for limiting postinfarction remodeling. These results are consistent with the finding that injecting passive materials alone into a postinfarct scar and consequently replacing a stiff tissue by a more compliant material may improve function and reduce wall stress in the ventricle, thereby contributing to normalize mechanotransduction signaling.[140] However, exclusive reliance on the passive function of acellular biomaterials is unlikely to affect myocardial regeneration, which requires incorporation of contractile cells able to line up with the appropriate geometry and to be excited in synchrony with the native cardiomyocytes.

Encapsulation. This approach entails incorporation of cells into porous microbeads the membrane of which is engineered in such a way that cell-secreted therapeutic factors can freely diffuse into the surrounding myocardial environment, whereas influx of oxygen and nutrients, but not of immune cells, is made possible by the size of the pores. In addition of increasing cell retention because of the size and viscosity of the particles, encapsulation may protect nonautologous cells from the host immune system without drug-based immunosuppression.[141] In fact, this technology has been successfully used for encapsulating xeno Langerhans' islets in animal models of diabetes.[142] Some clinical trials are currently under way in this indication. However, in the context of myocardial regeneration, this approach is questionable because it exclusively relies on the paracrine effects of cells and inherently prevent any form of functional integration of the graft within the host myocardium.

A second strategy consists of acting on the delivery systems. If the system is based on conventional injections, the design of the device could be conceivably improved to maximize cell retention, for example through changes in needle configuration allowing better spatial dispersion of cells and/or computerized driving to allow for a more accurate control over flow rate, duration, and injection pressure.

However, needle-based injections are fraught with several limitations: leakage along the needle tracks; random and poorly reproducible distribution of cells; creation of multiple intramyocardial clusters that can physically impede the propagation of electrical impulses and result in conduction blocks facilitating arrhythmias;[10] induction of volume-dependent tissue damage; and dissociation of the cells promoting a particular form of apoptotic cell death called *anoikis*,[143] which occurs when anchorage-dependent cells lose their attachment to the extracellular matrix and the related survival signals.

Consequently, one can take advantage of open-chest interventions to step away from injections and switch to the epicardial delivery of cell constructs overlying the infarct area and simply glued or sutured to its edges. The group of Eschenhagen has shown that if the selected cells featured a contractile phenotype as occurs with rat cardiomyocytes, it was possible, by mixing these cells with collagen, to generate force-generating beating heart constructs that, following implantation onto the scar tissue, were found to improve function, prevent dilation, and provide electrical coupling with native myocardium.[144] In the future, it is possible that cell-scaffold interactions might benefit from the bioprinting technology that enables transfer of cells onto the matrix (just like an inkjet is printed by a desktop printer) according to a precisely defined pattern.[145]

One step further, Okano and his group in Japan have developed an original technology based on the manufacture of cell sheets cultured on temperature-sensitive dishes.[146] Upon cooling, a layer of contiguous viable cells can be collected without disrupting the cellular microenvironment caused by enzymatic digestion otherwise required for cell detachment. The multilayered construct is then applied onto the surface of the heart where it adheres spontaneously. This technique has been used successfully to a variety of cells (eg, skeletal myoblasts, fibroblasts, epithelial cells, rat cardiomyocytes, mesenchymal stem cells) and has the advantage of avoiding the presence of any foreign material and allowing cells to be anchored through the extracellular matrix adhesive proteins that they have secreted themselves. In cardiac applications, the cell sheet technology has been shown more effective than injections in both ischemic[147] and nonischemic[148] animal models of heart diseases and a myoblast cell sheet has already been used clinically as an adjunct to a LV assist device. In a head-to-head comparison of conventional injections of myoblasts versus the epicardial delivery of either a myoblast-seeded collagen patch or a myoblast cell sheet,[149] we have been able to confirm the superiority of the two latter techniques with regard to improvement of postinfarction function, reduction of fibrosis, and increase in angiogenesis.

Conceptually, the use of epicardial cell constructs raises the major concern of the coupling of superficially delivered cells with the underlying host cardiomyocytes. However, migration of the patch-bound cells in the myocardium has been reported[150] as well as their coupling with host cardiomyocytes through gap junction proteins.[150,151]

Intravascular Delivery

If cells are to be injected into the coronary arteries, *a first strategy consists of acting on the delivery systems.* This approach is illustrated by the recent development of a perforated intracoronary catheter that allows cell delivery in the perivascular space.

A second strategy consists of acting on the homing signals responsible for cell trafficking. This can be achieved by interventions targeting cells directly or the recipient tissue.

Cell Targeting. Homing of cells to sites of injury is orchestrated by a tightly coordinated sequence of events involving "sensing" of the damaged tissue–emitted signals, selectin-mediated rolling, integrin-mediated firm adhesion to the vascular wall and transendothelial migration in the extracellular matrix.[152] Among the multiple factors that participate in the recruitment and trafficking of circulating cells, a crucial role is played by the chemokine CXC receptor (CXCR) 4, which is expressed on early hematopoietic stem cells and endothelial progenitors and its receptor, the stromal cell–derived factor (SDF)-1α.

Interventions designed at enhancing homing have thus logically relied on cell engineering to make them overexpressing one component of the receptor-ligand pair, ie, CXCR4[153] or SDF-1.[154] Transfection of MSC with insulin growth factor-1[155] has been another means of reactivating SDF-1 signaling. Aside from these gene-based approaches, drugs that activate endothelial nitric oxide synthase (NOS) such as statins or NOS enhancers have also been successful in enhancing cell homing.[152]

Tissue Targeting. In this setting, direct myocardial SDF-1 gene transfer[156] has been proposed for re-establishing tissue levels of SDF-1 known to decrease shortly after infarction. However, the anticipated regulatory hurdles, resulting from the combination of cell and gene therapy make appealing potentially safer and simpler techniques based on physical interventions. So far, three of them have been successfully tested: (1) Low-energy shock wave aims to induce expression of SDF-1,[157] and the CELLWAVE trial is already testing the effects of extracorporeal shock wave before bone marrow progenitor cell therapy in an effort to improve homing of these cells and subsequent angiogenesis in patients with chronic ischemic heart disease following anterior myocardial infarction. (2) Focused ultrasound-mediated destruction of microbubbles has been shown to create a series of biochemical responses (eg, release of proinflammatory cytokines, induction of metalloproteinase activity, reduction of laminin content), which result in enhanced transendothelial migration and interstitial invasion of MSC without causing endothelial damage.[158] (3) Finally, magnetic targeting could also be useful for driving cells toward the site of injury based on the seminal proof-of-principle finding that an externally applied magnetic device was effective in enhancing iron-loaded endothelial progenitor cell engraftment at a site of vascular injury.[159]

It is finally important to note that while enhancement of homing is particularly important in the context of acute myocardial infarction where the intravascular route is the only one available for stem cell delivery, this issue is somewhat less critical in the context of regeneration of the chronically failing heart, which allows a greater versatility in the stem cell transfer approaches and, in particular, a direct catheter-based or surgical intramyocardial delivery.

Low Survival of Retained Cells

Although cell death results from the complex interplay of multiple factors, ischemia inherent in the poor vascularization of the target areas, apoptosis subsequent to the loss of cell anchorage to their matrix and immune destruction of allogeneic cells have been identified as key players. Consequently, adjunctive interventions targeted at optimizing graft survival have focused on these events.

Induction of Angiogenesis

When the grafted area cannot be revascularized directly by CABG or angioplasty, two different types of strategies can be considered for increasing blood supply to the areas of engraftment and therefore promoting survival of the injected cells.

The first is based on the direct intramyocardial injection of *exogenous* angiogenic inducers which fall into four main categories: (1) genes-encoding angiogenic factors;[160] (2) growth factors themselves with the caveat that their fast clearance requires appropriate delivery systems; (3) genetically modified cells overexpressing an angiogenic factor;[161,162] and (4) cotransplanted cells featuring an angiogenic potential such as CD133$^+$ hematopoietic progenitors,[163] or the more recently described epicardium-derived cells.[164] Although there are no conclusive data about the most efficacious of these interventions, the importance of a cellular carrier is suggested by the finding that myoblast transfection with VEGF provides better cardiac protection than direct adenoviral VEGF delivery.[165]

The second strategy relies on the induction on an *endogenous* angiogenesis through an enhanced homing of circulating bone marrow cells in the areas of cell engraftment. As mentioned, this approach has largely relied on manipulation of the CXCR4-SDF1 axis to successfully increase the influx of angiogenic cells into the cell-transplanted regions.

Although one is missing a comprehensive head-to-head comparison of these various interventions, overall they all have met the objective of increasing angiogenesis, which has usually translated into a better LV function and an enhanced survival of the cellular graft. An advantage of targeting SDF-1 could be that in addition of its stem cell-recruiting effects through its interaction with CXCR4, it may exert direct cardioprotective effects by activating downstream signaling pathways involved in cardiomyocyte survival.[166] However, a potential clinical use of SDF-1 should be cautiously considered as the proteolytic cleavage of SDF-1α by matrix metalloproteinase-2 could yield a highly neurotoxic molecule, SDF.[5–67,167] Along the same line, malignant transformation has been reported in a mouse model of myocardial infarction following intramyocardial transplantation of MSC that had been engineered to overexpress stem cell factor.[168]

Limitation of Apoptosis

As pointed out, injection of dispersed cells promotes their apoptotic death because of the loss of survival signals originating from physiologic cell-cell and cell-matrix interactions.

A first means of addressing this issue is to deliver cells that have been transfected with antiapoptotic factors such as Akt[169] or Bcl2.[170] However, given the safety issues associated with gene therapy, a more attractive option could be to upregulate endogenous survival pathways though preconditioning of cells either physically by heat shock[171] or pharmacologically by potassium channel agonists.[172] Finally, where direct access to the heart is feasible, the use of three-dimensional cell-seeded patches or scaffold-free cell-sheets, particularly if they are multilayered,[173] is probably the best approach with regard to the risk-to-benefit ratio. The advantage of these constructs is not only that they do not cause disruption of myocardial tissue and preserve cell cohesiveness, but also that they allow incorporation of several different cell populations such as cardiomyocytes (regardless of their origin), endothelial cells, and fibroblasts.[174–176] Cross-talks between these cell populations may synergize trophic and particularly angiogenic effects which may enhance survival of the contractile cells "of interest."[150,176] Of note, studies of composite sheets made of cardiomyocytes and endothelial cells have shown that blood vessels originated from the construct and bridged to connect with host capillaries,[175,176] thereby providing additional evidence for the coupling between these epicardial cell constructs and the myocardium underneath.

Limitation of the Immune Response to Allogeneic Cells

This issue can be addressed by immunomodulatory strategies (such as those described about ESC) when the objective is a sustained cell engraftment or by encapsulation (also described in the preceding) if one admits that cells will not integrate within the recipient myocardium and exclusively relies on their paracrine effects.

To close this section, it is fair to acknowledge that the importance of keeping cells alive has recently been challenged by a study showing in a mouse model of myocardial infarction that extracts from unfractionated bone marrow cells, ie, their intracellular soluble contents, were actually as cardioprotective as factors released by living cells.[71] This conclusion, however, implies that protection exclusively relies on paracrine effects and is therefore not relevant to the generation of new myocardial tissue by donor-derived cells.

Tracking of Stem Cells

Clearly, the objective assessment of the above mentioned approaches for optimizing cell engraftment requires the use of safe, reliable, and noninvasive techniques for tracking cell fate over time, both in the target myocardium and remote organs.[177] Specific constraints on contrast agents include the lack of genetic modification of the labeled cells, of dilution with cell division and of transfer to non-stem cells. Experimentally, radionuclides, MRI, and reporter genes are the most extensively used molecular imaging techniques. Reporter genes are particularly attractive. Once transfected into the cell of interest, they yield a product that, following exposure to the corresponding radioactive or optical reporter probe, turns on a signal that can be imaged by positron emission tomography, single-photon emission computed tomography, or MRI. A first advantage of this approach is that it should only detect viable cells because expression of the imaging signal requires intracellular expression of the reporter gene product. This contrasts with MRI-based tracking of iron-loaded cells, which may generate false-positives when iron released by dead stem cells is engulfed by host macrophages and results in MRI signals mistakenly interpreted as originating from the transplanted cells.[178] Second, the reporter gene can be genetically integrated and transmitted to the transfected cell's progeny, thereby allowing to monitor cell proliferation. Finally, combination of several reporters can allow to set up a multimodal imaging platform such as that achieved with a triple-fusion reporter gene, which allowed a successful noninvasive monitoring of the kinetics of cell survival, proliferation, and migration by bioluminescence and PET imaging.[179] Validation of these data is supported by the critical finding that reporter genes do not seem to adversely affect cell integrity and function. Multimodality imaging is likely important because there is currently no single technique that can optimally combine resolution, sensitivity, safety, accuracy of cell quantification, and clinical applicability. Bioluminescence, for example, which uses light generated by the enzyme luciferase is limited to small animals because of the poor tissue penetration of external illumination sources and a similar limitation applies to near-infrared fluorophores. In the future, however, this issue might be addressed by nanometer-sized light-emitting quantum dots conjugated to bioluminescent agents. Improved imaging techniques are thus eagerly awaited for experimental stem cell tracking and subsequent clinical translation without adding significant cost or regulatory roadblocks.

Because there is no animal model that can fully reproduce the complex situation of patients with advanced heart failure in need for myocardial regeneration, it seems legitimate to continue clinical trials, provided that their experimental grounds are robust and consistent enough to suggest that the selected cell type has a reasonable potential of effecting some myocardial regeneration without causing adverse events. Beyond the stage of pilot small-sized feasibility studies, these trials should comply with the standard methodologic guidelines (randomization, control groups, blind assessment) and their protocol should carefully take into account some key variables such as cell dosing, delivery modalities, and realistic approvability by the regulatory authorities. Until large mortality trials can be launched, surrogate end points and imaging modalities should also be selected in light of the expected objective of regeneration and, as such, the commonly used measurements of global LV function may have to be shifted toward the assessment of cell-related morphologic changes such as infarct size, LV remodeling, or regional wall thickness areas. At the end, a continuous cross-talk between different disciplines including clinical cardiology, developmental biology, cell culture technology, tissue engineering, imaging and high-throughput production of scalable, and reproducible biologics appears mandatory for moving the field forward and successfully achieving the goal of myocardial regeneration under conditions of an optimal risk-to-benefit ratio.

REFERENCES

1. Lloyd-Jones D, Adams R, Carnethon M: A report from the American Heart Association Statistics Committee and Stroke Statistics Subcommittee. *Circulation* 2009;119(3):e21-181.
2. Jones RH, Velazquez EJ, Michler RE, et al: STICH Hypothesis 2 Investigators. Coronary bypass surgery with or without surgical ventricular reconstruction. *NEJM* 2009; 360(17):1705-1717.
3. Albouaini K, Egred M, Rao A, et al: Cardiac resynchronisation therapy: evidence based benefits and patient selection. *Eur J Intern Med* 2008; 19(3):165-172.
4. Menasche P, Hagege AA, Scorsin M, et al: Myoblast transplantation for heart failure. *Lancet* 2001; 357(9252):279-280.
5. Gavira JJ, Herreros J, Perez A, et al: Autologous skeletal myoblast transplantation in patients with nonacute myocardial infarction: 1-year follow-up. *J Thorac Cardiovasc Surg* 2006; 131(4):799-804.
6. Siminiak T, Kalawski R, Fiszer D, et al: Autologous skeletal myoblast transplantation for the treatment of postinfarction myocardial injury: phase I clinical study with 12 months of follow-up. *Am Heart J* 2004; 148(3):531-537.
7. Dib N, Michler RE, Pagani FD, et al: Safety and feasibility of autologous myoblast transplantation in patients with ischemic cardiomyopathy: four-year follow-up. *Circulation* 2005; 112(12):1748-1755.
8. Leobon B, Garcin I, Menasche P, et al: Myoblasts transplanted into rat infarcted myocardium are functionally isolated from their host. *Proc Natl Acad Sci U S A* 2003; 100(13):7808-7811.
9. Abraham MR, Henrikson CA, Tung L, et al: Antiarrhythmic engineering of skeletal myoblasts for cardiac transplantation. *Circ Res* 2005; 97(2):159-167.
10 Fukushima S, Varela-Carver A, Coppen SR, et al: Direct intramyocardial but not intracoronary injection of bone marrow cells induces ventricular arrhythmias in a rat chronic ischemic heart failure model. *Circulation* 2007; 115(17):2254-2261.
11. Menasché Ph, Alfieri O, Janssens S, et al: The Myoblast Autologous Grafting in Ischemic Cardiomyopathy (MAGIC) Trial. First Randomized Placebo-Controlled Study of Myoblast Transplantation. *Circulation* 2008; 117(9):1189-1200.
12. Siminiak T, Fiszer D, Jerzykowska O, et al: Percutaneous trans-coronary-venous transplantation of autologous skeletal myoblasts in the treatment of post-infarction myocardial contractility impairment: the POZNAN trial. *Eur Heart J* 2005; 26(12):1188-1195.
13. Ince H, Petzsch M, Rehders TC, Chatterjee T, Nienaber CA: Transcatheter transplantation of autologous skeletal myoblasts in postinfarction patients with severe left ventricular dysfunction. *J Endovasc Ther* 2004; 11(6):695-704.
14. Dib N, Dinsmore J, Lababidi Z, et al: One-year follow-up of feasibility and safety of the first U.S., randomized, controlled study using 3-dimensional guided catheter-based delivery of autologous skeletal myoblasts for ischemic cardiomyopathy (CAuSMIC study). *JACC Cardiovasc Interv* 2009; 2(1):9-16.
15. Mocini D, Staibano M, Mele L, et al: Autologous bone marrow mononuclear cell transplantation in patients undergoing coronary artery bypass grafting. *Am Heart J* 2006; 151(1):192-207.
16. Hendrikx M, Hensen K, Clijsters C, et al: Recovery of regional but not global contractile function by the direct intramyocardial autologous bone marrow transplantation: results from a randomized controlled clinical trial. *Circulation* 2006; 114(1 Suppl):I101-107.
17. Lai VK, Ang KL, Rathbone W, Harvey NJ, Galiñanes M: Randomized controlled trial on the cardioprotective effect of bone marrow cells in patients undergoing coronary bypass graft surgery. *Eur Heart J* 2009; 30(19):2354-2359.
18. Zhao Q, Sun Y, Xia L, Chen A, Wang Z: Randomized study of mononuclear bone marrow cell transplantation in patients with coronary surgery. *Ann Thorac Surg* 2008; 86(6):1833-1840.
19. Akar AR, Durdu S, Arat M, et al: Five-year follow-up after transepicardial implantation of autologous bone marrow mononuclear cells to ungraftable coronary territories for patients with ischaemic cardiomyopathy. *Eur J Cardiothorac Surg* 2009; 36(4):633-643.
20. Perin EC, Dohmann HF, Borojevic R, et al: Improved exercise capacity and ischemia 6 and 12 months after transendocardial injection of autologous bone marrow mononuclear cells for ischemic cardiomyopathy. *Circulation 2004*; 110(11 Suppl 1):II213-218.
21. Strauer BE, Brehm M, Zeus T, et al: Regeneration of human infarcted heart muscle by intracoronary autologous bone marrow cell transplantation in chronic coronary artery disease: the IACT Study. *J Am Coll Cardiol 2005*; 46(9):1651-1658.
22. Assmus B, Honold J, Schächinger V, et al: Transcoronary transplantation of progenitor cells after myocardial infarction. *NEJM* 2006; 355(12):1222-1232.
23. Fischer-Rasokat U, Assmus B, Seeger FH, et al: A pilot trial to assess potential effects of selective intra-coronary bone marrow-derived progenitor cell infusion in patients with nonischemic dilated cardiomyopathy: final 1-year results oft he TOPCARE-DCM trial. *Circ Heart Fail* 2009 2(5):417-423.
24. Heeschen C, Lehmann R, Honold J, et al: Profoundly reduced neovascularization capacity of bone marrow mononuclear cells derived from patients with chronic ischemic heart disease. *Circulation* 2004; 109(13): 1615-1622.
25. van Ramshorst J, Bax, Jeroen J, et al: Intramyocardial bone marrow cell injection for chronic myocardial ischemia: a randomized controlled trial. *JAMA* 2009; 301(19):1997-2004.
26. Stamm C, Kleine HD, Choi YH, et al: Intramyocardial delivery of CD133+ bone marrow cells and coronary artery bypass grafting for chronic ischemic heart disease: safety and efficacy studies. *J Thorac Cardiovasc Surg* 2007; 133(3):717-725.
27. Carr CA, Stuckey DJ, Tatton L, et al: Bone marrow-derived stromal cells home to and remain in the infarcted rat heart but fail to improve function: an in vivo cine-MRI study. *Am J Physiol Heart Circ Physiol* 2008; 295(2): H533-542.
28. Dai W, Hale SL, Martin BJ, et al: Allogeneic mesenchymal stem cell transplantation in postinfarcted rat myocardium: short- and long-term effects. *Circulation* 2005; 112(2):214-223.
29. Tang J, Xie Q, Pan G, Wang J, Wang M: Mesenchymal stem cells participate in angiogenesis and improve heart function in rat model of myocardial ischemia with reperfusion. *Eur J Cardiothorac Surg* 2006; 30(2): 353-361.
30. Shake JG, Gruber PJ, Baumgartner WA, et al: Mesenchymal stem cell implantation in a swine myocardial infarct model: engraftment and functional effects. *Ann Thorac Surg* 2002; 73(6):1919-1925.
31. Silva GV, Litovsky S, Assad JA, et al: Mesenchymal stem cells differentiate into an endothelial phenotype, enhance vascular density, and improve heart function in a canine chronic ischemia model. *Circulation* 2005; 111(2):150-156.
32. Hamamoto H, Gorman JH 3rd, Ryan LP, et al: Current state-of-the-art: Improved left ventricular function *versus* myocardial regeneration. Allogeneic mesenchymal precursor cell therapy to limit remodeling after myocardial infarction: the effect of cell dosage. *Ann Thorac Surg* 2009; 87(3):794-801.
33. Schuleri KH, Amado LC, Boyle AJ, et al: Early improvement in cardiac tissue perfusion due to mesenchymal stem cells. *Am J Physiol Heart Circ Physiol* 2008; 294(5):H2002-2011.
34. Nagaya N, Kangawa K, Itoh T, et al: Transplantation of mesenchymal stem cells improves cardiac function in a rat model of dilated cardiomyopathy. *Circulation* 2005; 112(8):1128-1135.
35. Caplan AI, Dennis JE: Mesenchymal stem cells as trophic mediators. *J Cell Biochem* 2006; 98(5):1076-1084.
36. Bartunek J, Croissant JD, Wijns W, et al: Pretreatment of adult bone marrow mesenchymal stem cells with cardiomyogenic growth factors and repair of the chronically infarcted myocardium. *Am J Physiol Heart Circ Physiol* 2007; 292(2):H1095-1104.
37. Parolini O, Alviano F, Bagnara GP, et al: Concise review: isolation and characterization of cells from human term placenta: outcome of the first international Workshop on Placenta Derived Stem Cells. *Stem Cells* 2008; 26(2):300-311.
38. Meng X, Ichim TE, Zhong J, et al: Endometrial regenerative cells: a novel stem cell population. *J Transl Med* 2007; 5:57.
39. Seo BM, Miura M, Gronthos S, et al: Investigation of multipotent postnatal stem cells from human periodontal ligament. *Lancet* 2004; 364(9429):149-155.
40. Noël D, Caton D, Roche S, et al: Cell specific differences between human adipose-derived and mesenchymal-stromal cells despite similar differentiation potentials. *Exp Cell Res* 2008; 314(7):1575-1584.
41. Puissant B, Barreau C, Bourin P, et al: Immunomodulatory effect of human adipose tissue-derived adult stem cells: comparison with bone marrow mesenchymal stem cells. *Br J Haematol* 2005; 129(1):118-129.
42. Mazo M, Planat-Bénard V, Abizanda G, et al: Transplantation of adipose derived stromal cells is associated with functional improvement in a rat model of chronic myocardial infarction. *Eur J Heart Fail* 2008; 10(5): 454-462.
43. Valina C, Pinkernell K, Song YH, et al: Intracoronary administration of autologous adipose tissue-derived stem cells improves left ventricular function, perfusion, and remodelling after acute myocardial infarction. *Eur Heart J* 2007; 28(21):2667-2677.

44. Rehman J, Traktuev D, Li J, et al: Secretion of angiogenic and antiapoptotic factors by human adipose stromal cells. *Circulation* 2004; 109(10): 1292-1298.
45. Léobon B, Roncalli J, Joffre C, et al: Adipose-derived cardiomyogenic cells: in vitro expansion and functional improvement in a mouse model of myocardial infarction. *Cardiovasc Res* 2009; 83(4):757-767.
46. Bieback K, Kern S, Kocaömer A, Ferlik K, Bugert P: Comparing mesenchymal stromal cells from different human tissues: bone marrow, adipose tissue and umbilical cord blood. *Biomed Mater Eng* 2008; 18(1 Suppl): S71-76.
47. Van der Bogt KE, Schrepfer S, Yu J, et al: Comparison of transplantation of adipose tissue- and bone marrow-derived mesenchymal stem cells in the infarcted heart. *Transplantation* 2009; 87(5):642-652.
48. Ryan JM, Barry FP, Murphy JM, Mahon BP: Mesenchymal stem cells avoid allogeneic rejection. *J Inflamm (Lond)* 2005; 2:8.
49. Uccelli A, Pistoia V, Moretta L: Mesenchymal stem cells: a new strategy for immunosuppression? *Trends Immunol* 2007; 28(5):219-226.
50. Engler AJ, Sen S, Sweeney HL, Discher DE: Matrix elasticity directs stem cell lineage specification. *Cell* 2006; 126(4):677-689.
51. Breitbach M, Bostani T, Roell W, et al: Potential risks of bone marrow cell transplantation into infarcted hearts. *Blood* 2007; 110(4):1362-1369.
52. Ringdén O, Uzunel M, Rasmusson I, et al: Mesenchymal stem cells for treatment of therapy-resistant graft-versus-host disease. *Transplantation* 2006; 81(10):1390-1397.
53. Grinnemo KH, Månsson A, Dellgren G, et al: Xenoreactivity and engraftment of human mesenchymal stem cells transplanted into infarcted rat myocardium. *J Thorac Cardiovasc Surg* 2004; 127(5):1293-1300.
54. Poncelet AJ, Vercruysse J, Saliez A, Gianello P: Although pig allogeneic mesenchymal stem cells are not immunogenic in vitro, intracardiac injection elicits an immune response in vivo. *Transplantation* 2007; 83(6): 783-790.
55. Boomsma RA, Swaminathan PD, Geenen DL: Intravenously injected mesenchymal stem cells home to viable myocardium after coronary occlusion and preserve systolic function without altering infarct size. *Int J Cardiol* 2007; 122(1):17-28.
56. Freyman T, Polin G, Osman H, et al: A quantitative, randomized study evaluating three methods of mesenchymal stem cell delivery following myocardial infarction. *Eur Heart J* 2006; 27(9):1114-1122.
57. Hofmann M, Wollert KC, Meyer GP, et al: Monitoring of bone marrow cell homing into the infarcted human myocardium. *Circulation* 2005; 111(17):2198-2202.
58. Furlani D, Ugurlucan M, Ong L, et al: Is the intravascular administration of mesenchymal stem cells safe? Mesenchymal stem cells and intravital microscopy. *Microvasc Res* 2009; 77(3):370-376.
59. Ly HQ, Hoshino K, Pomerantseva I, et al: In vivo myocardial distribution of multipotent progenitor cells following intracoronary delivery in a swine model of myocardial infarction. *Eur Heart J* 2009. [August 17, Epub ahead of print]
60. Lazennec G, Jorgensen C: Concise review: adult multipotent stromal cells and cancer: risk or benefit? *Stem Cells* 2008; 26(6):1387-1394.
61. Perez-Ilzarbe M, Agbulut O, Pelacho B, et al: Characterization of the paracrine effects of human skeletal myoblasts transplanted in infarcted myocardium. *Eur J Heart Fail* 2008; 10(11):1065-1072.
62. Formigli L, Perna AM, Meacci E: Paracrine effects of transplanted myoblasts and relaxin on post-infarction heart remodelling. *J Cell Mol Med* 2007; 11(5):1087-1100.
63. Uemura R, Xu M, Ahmad N, Ashraf M: Bone marrow stem cells prevent left ventricular remodeling of ischemic heart through paracrine signaling. *Circ Res* 2006; 98(11):1414-1421.
64. Dai Y, Ashraf M, Zuo S, et al: Mobilized bone marrow progenitor cells serve as donors of cytoprotective genes for cardiac repair. *J Mol Cell Cardiol* 2008; 44(3):607-617.
65. Fazel S, Cimini M, Chen L, et al: Cardioprotective c-kit+ cells are from the bone marrow and regulate the myocardial balance of angiogenic cytokines. *J Clin Invest* 2006; 116(7):1865-1877.
66. Korf-Klingebiel M, Kempf T, Sauer T, et al: Bone marrow cells are a rich source of growth factors and cytokines: implications for cell therapy trials after myocardial infarction. *Eur Heart J* 2008; 29(23):2851-2858.
67. Shintani Y, Fukushima S, Varela-Carver A, et al: Donor cell-type specific paracrine effects of cell transplantation for post-infarction heart failure. *J Mol Cell Cardiol* 2009; 47(2):288-295.
68. Lee RH, Pulin AA, Seo MJ, et al: Intravenous hMSCs improve myocardial infarction in mice because cells embolized in lung are activated to secrete the anti-inflammatory protein TSG-6. *Cell Stem Cell* 2009; 5(1):54-63.
69. Cho HJ, Lee N, Lee JY, Choi YJ et al: Role of host tissues for sustained humoral effects after endothelial progenitor cell transplantation into the ischemic heart. *J Exp Med* 2007; 204(13):3257-3269.
70. Park DH, Eve DJ, Sanberg PR, et al: Increased neuronal proliferation in the dentate gyrus of aged rats following neural stem cell implantation. *Stem Cells Dev* 2009 [July 1, ahead of print].
71. Yeghiazarians Y, Zhang Y, Prasad M, et al: Injection of bone marrow cell extract into infarcted hearts results in functional improvement comparable to intact cell therapy. *Mol Ther* 2009; 17(7):1250-1256.
72. Pak HN, Qayyum M, Kim DT, et al: Mesenchymal stem cell injection induces cardiac nerve sprouting and increased tenascin expression in a swine model of myocardial infarction. *J Cardiovasc Electrophysiol* 2003; 14(8):841-848.
73. Gnecchi M, He H, Noiseux N, et al: Evidence supporting paracrine hypothesis for Akt-modified mesenchymal stem cell-mediated cardiac protection and functional improvement. *FASEB J* 2006; 20(6):661-669.
74. Timmers L, Lim SK, Arslan F, et al: Reduction of myocardial infarct size by human mesenchymal stem cell conditioned medium. *Stem Cell Res* 2007; 1(2):129-137.
75. Shyu KG, Wang BW, Hung HF, Chang CC, Shih DT: Mesenchymal stem cells are superior to angiogenic growth factor genes for improving myocardial performance in the mouse model of acute myocardial infarction. *J Biomed Sci* 2006; 13(1):47-58.
76. Bergmann O, Bhardwaj RD, Bernard S, et al: Evidence for cardiomyocyte renewal in humans. *Science* 2009; 324(5923):98-102.
77. Kühn B, del Monte F, Hajjar RJ et al: Periostin induces proliferation of differentiated cardiomyocytes and promotes cardiac repair. *Nat Med* 2007; 13(8):962-969.
78. Bersell K, Arab S, Haring B, Kühn B: Neuregulin1/ErbB4 signaling induces cardiomyocyte proliferation and repair of heart injury. *Cell* 2009; 138(2):257-270.
79. Winitsky SO, Gopal TV, Hassanzadeh S, et al: Adult murine skeletal muscle contains cells that can differentiate into beating cardiomyocytes in vitro. *PloS Biol* 2005; 3(4):e87.
80. Proksch S, Bel A, Puymirat E, et al: Does the human skeletal muscle harbor the murine equivalents of cardiac precursor cells? *Mol Ther* 2009; 17(4):733-741.
81. Sadek H, Hannack B, Choe E, et al: Transplantation of putative extracardiac cell niches endowed with a cardiomyogenic differentiation potential cardiogenic small molecules that enhance myocardial repair by stem cells. *Proc Natl Acad Sci U S A* 2008; 105(16):6063-6068.
82. Kajstura J, Leri A, Finato N, Di et al: Myocyte proliferation in end-stage cardiac failure in humans. *Proc Natl Acad Sci U S A* 1998; 95(15): 8801-8805.
83. Barile L, Messina E, Giacomello A, Marbán E: Endogenous cardiac stem cells. *Prog Cardiovasc Dis* 2007; 50(1):31-48.
84. Laflamme MA, Myerson D, Saffitz JE, Murry CE: Evidence for cardiomyocyte repopulation by extracardiac progenitors in transplanted human hearts. *Circ Res* 2002; 90(6):634-640.
85. Bearzi C, Rota M, Hosoda T, et al: Human cardiac stem cells. *Proc Natl Acad Sci U S A* 2007; 104(35):14068-14073.
86. Smith RR, Barile L, Cho HC, et al: Regenerative potential of cardiosphere-derived cells expanded from percutaneous endomyocardial biopsy specimens. *Circulation* 2007; 115(7):896-908.
87. Johnston PV, Sasano T, Mills K, et al: Engraftment, differentiation, and functional benefits of autologous cardiosphere-derived cells in porcine ischemic cardiomyopathy. *Circulation* 2009; 120(12):1075-1083.
88. Pouly J, Bruneval P, Mandet C, et al: Cardiac stem cells in the real world. *J Thorac Cardiovasc Surg* 2008; 135(3):673-678.
89. Kubo H, Jaleel N, Kumarapeli A, et al: Increased cardiac myocyte progenitors in failing human hearts. *Circulation* 2008; 118(6):649-657.
90. Amir G, Ma X, Reddy VM, et al: Dynamics of human myocardial progenitor cell populations in the neonatal period. *Ann Thorac Surg* 2008; 86(4):1311-1319.
91. Andersen DC, Andersen P, Schneider M, Jensen HB, Sheikh SP. Murine "cardiospheres" are not a source of stem cells with cardiomyogenic potential. *Stem Cells* 2009; 27(7):1571-1581.
92. Winter EM, Grauss RW, Hogers B, et al: Preservation of left ventricular function and attenuation of remodeling after transplantation of human epicardium-derived cells into the infarcted mouse heart. *Circulation* 2007; 116(8):917-927.
93. Pal R: Embryonic stem (ES) cell-derived cardiomyocytes: a good candidate for cell therapy applications. *Cell Biol Int* 2009; 33(3):325-336.
94. Sartiani L, Bettiol E, Stillitano F, et al: Developmental changes in cardiomyocytes differentiated from human embryonic stem cells: a molecular and electrophysiological approach. *Stem Cells* 2007; 25(5):1136-1144.
95. Brito-Martins M, Harding SE, Ali NN: Beta(1)- and beta(2)-adrenoceptor responses in cardiomyocytes derived from human embryonic stem cells: comparison with failing and non-failing adult human heart. *Br J Pharmacol* 2008; 153(4):751-759.

96. Mummery C, Ward-van Oostwaard D, Doevendans P, et al: Differentiation of human embryonic stem cells to cardiomyocytes: role of coculture with visceral endoderm-like cells. *Circulation* 2003; 107(21):2733-2740.
97. Laflamme M, Chen KY, Naumova AV, et al: Cardiomyocytes derived from human embryonic stem cells in pro-survival factors enhance function of infarcted rat hearts. *Nat Biotechnol* 2007; 25(9):1015-1024.
98. Caspi O, Huber I, Kehat I, et al: Transplantation of human embryonic stem cell-derived cardiomyocytes improves myocardial performance in infarcted rat hearts. *J Am Coll Cardiol* 2007; 50(19):1884-1893.
99. Puymirat E, Geha R, Tomescot A, et al: Can mesenchymal stem cells induce tolerance to cotransplanted human embryonic stem cells? *Mol Ther* 2009; 17(1):176-182.
100. Yamada S, Nelson TJ, Crespo-Diaz RJ, et al: Embryonic stem cell therapy of heart failure in genetic cardiomyopathy. *Stem Cells* 2008; 26(10): 2644-2653.
101. Behfar A, Perez-Terzic C, Faustino RS, et al: Cardiopoietic programming of embryonic stem cells for tumor-free heart repair. *J Exp Med* 2007; 204(2):405-420.
102. Van Laake LW, Passier RP, Monshouwer-Kloots J, et al: Human embryonic stem cell-derived cardiomyocytes survive and mature in the mouse heart and transiently improve function after myocardial infarction. *Stem Cell Res* 2007; 1(1):9-24.
103. Van Laake LW, Passier R, den Ouden K, et al: Improvement of mouse cardiac function by hESC-derived cardiomyocytes correlates with vascularity but not graft size. *Stem Cell Res* 2009; 3(2-3):106-112.
104. Ebelt H, Jungblut M, Zhang Y, et al: Cellular cardiomyoplasty: improvement of left ventricular function correlates with the release of cardioactive cytokines. *Stem Cells* 2007; 25(1):236-244.
105. Kolossov E, Bostani T, Roell W, et al: Engraftment of engineered ES cell-derived cardiomyocytes but not BM cells restores contractile function to the infarcted myocardium. *J Exp Med* 2006; 203(10):2315-2327.
106. Kehat I, Khimovich L, Caspi O, et al: Electromechanical integration of cardiomyocytes derived from human embryonic stem cells. *Nat Biotechnol* 2004; 22(10): 1282-1289.
107. Zweigerdt R: Large scale production of stem cells and their derivatives. *Adv Biochem Eng Biotechnol* 2009; 114:201-235.
108. Leschik J, Stefanovic S, Brinon B, Pucéat M: Cardiac commitment of primate embryonic stem cells. *Nat Protoc* 2008; 3(9):1381-1387.
109. Kishi Y, Tanaka Y, Shibata H, et al: Variation in the incidence of teratomas after the transplantation of nonhuman primate ES cells into immunodeficient mice. *Cell Transplant* 2008; 17(9):1095-1102.
110. Swijnenburg RJ, Schrepner S, Govaert J, et al: Immunosuppressive therapy mitigates immunological rejection of human embryonic stem cell xenografts. *Proc Natl Acad Sci U S A* 2008; 105(35):12991-12996.
111. Wu DC, Boyd AS, Wood KJ: Embryonic stem cells and their differentiated derivatives have a fragile immune privilege but still represent novel targets of immune attack. *Stem Cells* 2008; 26(8):1939-1950.
112. Taylor CJ, Bolton EM, Pocock S, et al: Banking on human embryonic stem cells: estimating the number of donor cell lines needed for HLA matching. *Lancet* 2005; 366(9502):2019-2025.
113. Robertson NJ, Brook FA, Gardner RL, et al: Embryonic stem cell-derived tissues are immunogenic but their inherent immune privilege promotes the induction of tolerance. *Proc Natl Acad Sci U S A* 2007; 104(52):20920-20925.
114. Bonde S, Chan KM, Zavazava N: ES-cell derived hematopoietic cells induce transplantation tolerance. *PLoS One* 2008; 3(9):e3212.
115. Grinnemo KH, Genead R, Kumagai-Braesch M, et al: Costimulation blockade induces tolerance to HESC transplanted to the testis and induces regulatory T-cells to HESC transplanted into the heart. *Stem Cells* 2008; 26(7):1850-1857.
116. Crop MJ, Baan CC, Korevaar SS, et al: Donor-derived mesenchymal stem cells suppress alloreactivity of kidney transplant patients. *Transplantation* 2009; 87(6):896-906.
117. Yamanaka S: A fresh look at iPS cells. *Cell* 2009; 137(1):13-17.
118. Gai H, Leung EL, Costantino PD, et al: Generation and characterization of functional cardiomyocytes using induced pluripotent stem cells derived from human fibroblasts. *Cell Biol Int* 2009; 33(11):1184-1193.
119. Kim D, Kim CH, Moon JI, et al: Generation of human induced pluripotent stem cells by direct delivery of reprogramming proteins. *Cell Stem Cell* 2009; 4(6):472-476.
120. Nelson TJ, Martinez-Fernandez A, Yamada S, et al: Repair of acute myocardial infarction with induced pluripotent stem cells Induced by human stemness factors. *Circulation* 2009. 120(5):408-416.
121. Chin MH, Mason MJ, Xie W, et al: Induced pluripotent stem cells and embryonic stem cells are distinguished by gene expression signatures. *Cell Stem Cell* 2009; 5(1):111-123.
122. Dow J, Simkhovich BZ, Kedes L, Kloner RA: Washout of transplanted cells from the heart: a potential new hurdle for cell transplantation therapy. *Cardiovasc Res* 2005; 67(2):301-307.
123. Freyman T, Polin G, Osman H, et al: A quantitative, randomized study evaluating three methods of mesenchymal stem cell delivery following myocardial infarction. *Eur Heart J* 2006; 27(9):1114-1122.
124. Doyle B, Kemp BJ, Chareonthaitawee P, et al: Dynamic tracking during intracoronary injection of 18F-FDG-labeled progenitor cell therapy for acute myocardial infarction. *J Nucl Med* 2007; 48(10):1708-1714.
125. Li SH, Lai TY, Sun Z, et al: Tracking cardiac engraftment and distribution of implanted bone marrow cells: comparing intra-aortic, intravenous, and intramyocardial delivery. *J Thorac Cardiovasc Surg* 2009; 137(5): 1225-1233.
126. Gavira JJ, Perez-Ilzarbe M, Abizanda G, et al: A comparison between percutaneous and surgical transplantation of autologous skeletal myoblasts in a swine model of chronic myocardial infarction. *Cardiovasc Res* 2006; 71(4):744-753.
127. Hudson W, Collins MC, deFreitas D, et al: Beating and arrested intramyocardial injections are associated with significant mechanical loss: implications for cardiac cell transplantation. *J Surg Res* 2007; 142(2):263-267.
128. Zhang M, Mal N, Kiedrowski M, et al: SDF-1 expression by mesenchymal stem cells results in trophic support of cardiac myocytes after myocardial infarction. *FASEB J* 2007; 21(12):3197-3207.
129. Ota T, Patronik NA, Schwartzman D, Riviere CN, Zenati MA: Minimally invasive epicardial injections using a novel semiautonomous robotic device. *Circulation* 2008; 118(14 Suppl):S115-120.
130. Thompson CA, Nasseri BA, Makower J, et al: Transplantation. Percutaneous transvenous cellular cardiomyoplasty. A novel nonsurgical approach for myocardial cell. *J Am Coll Cardiol* 2003; 41(11):1964-1971.
131. Blocklet D, Toungouz M, Berkenboom G, et al: Myocardial homing of nonmobilized peripheral-blood CD34+ cells after intracoronary injection. *Stem Cells* 2006; 24(2):333-336.
132. Penicka M, Lang O, Widimsky P, et al: One-day kinetics of myocardial engraftment after intracoronary injection of bone marrow mononuclear cells in patients with acute and chronic myocardial infarction. *Heart* 2007; 93(7):837-841.
133. Guilak F, Cohen DM, Estes BT, et al: Control of stem cell fate by physical interactions with the extracellular matrix. *Cell Stem Cell* 2009; 5(1):17-26.
134. Suuronen EJ, Veinot JP, Wong S, et al: Tissue-engineered injectable collagen-based matrices for improved cell delivery and vascularization of ischemic tissue using CD133+ progenitors expanded from the peripheral blood. *Circulation* 2006; 114(1 Suppl):I138-144.
135. Christman KL, Vardanian AJ, Fang Q, et al: Injectable fibrin scaffold improves cell transplant survival, reduces infarct expansion, and induces neovasculature formation in ischemic myocardium. *J Am Coll Cardiol* 2004; 44(3):654-660.
136. Davis ME, Motion JP, Narmoneva DA, et al: Injectable self-assembling peptide nanofibers create intramyocardial microenvironments for endothelial cells. *Circulation* 2005; 111(4):442-450.
137. Padin-Iruegas ME, Misao Y, Davis ME, et al: Cardiac progenitor cells and biotinylated insulin-like growth factor-1 nanofibers improve endogenous and exogenous myocardial regeneration after infarction. *Circulation* 2009; 120(10):876-887.
138. Ryan LP, Matsuzaki K, Noma M, et al: Dermal filler injection: a novel approach for limiting infarct expansion. *Ann Thorac Surg* 2009; 87(1): 148-155.
139. Leor J, Tuvia S, Guetta V, et al: Intracoronary injection of in situ forming alginate hydrogel reverses left ventricular remodeling after myocardial infarction in swine. *J Am Coll Cardiol* 2009; 54(11):1014-1023.
140. Wall ST, Walker JC, Healy KE, Ratcliffe MB, Guccione JM: Theoretical impact of the injection of material into the myocardium: a finite element model simulation. *Circulation* 2006; 114(24):2627-2635.
141. Dufrane D, Goebbels RM, Saliez A, Guiot Y, Gianello P: Six-month survival of microencapsulated pig islets and alginate biocompatibility in primates: proof of concept. *Transplantation* 2006; 81(9):1345-1353.
142. Lee SH, Hao E, Savinov AY, et al: Human beta-cell precursors mature into functional insulin-producing cells in an immunoisolation device: implications for diabetes cell therapies. *Transplantation* 2009; 87(7):983-991.
143. Zvibel I, Smets F, Soriano H. Anoikis: roadblock to cell transplantation? *Cell Transplant* 2002; 11(7):621-630.
144. Zimmermann WH, Melnychenko I, Wasmeier G, et al: Engineered heart tissue grafts improve systolic and diastolic function in infarcted rat hearts. *Nat Med* 2006; 12(4):452-458.
145. Mironov V, Boland T, Trusk T, Forgacs G, Markwald RR: Organ printing: computer-aided jet-based 3D tissue engineering. *Trends Biotechnol* 2003; 21(4):157-161.

146. Yang J, Yamato M, Nishida K, et al: Cell delivery in regenerative medicine: the cell sheet engineering approach. *J Control Release* 2006; 116(2):193-203.
147. Memon IA, Sawa Y, Fukushima N, et al: Repair of impaired myocardium by means of implantation of engineered autologous myoblast sheets. *J Thorac Cardiovasc Surg* 2005; 130(5):1333-1341.
148. Kondoh H, Sawa Y, Miyagawa S, et al: Longer preservation of cardiac performance by sheet-shaped myoblast implantation in dilated cardiomyopathic hamsters. *Cardiovasc Res* 2006; 69(2):466-475.
149. Hamdi H, Furuta A, Bellamy V, et al: Cell delivery: intramyocardial injections or epicardial deposition? A head-to-head comparison. *Ann Thorac Surg* 2009; 87(4):1196-1203.
150. Matsuura K, Honda A, Nagai T, et al: Transplantation of cardiac progenitor cells ameliorates cardiac dysfunction after myocardial infarction in mice. *J Clin Invest* 2009; 119(8):2204-2217.
151. Sekine H, Shimizu T, Kosaka S, Kobayashi E, Okano T: Cardiomyocyte bridging between hearts and bioengineered myocardial tissues with mesenchymal transition of mesothelial cells. *J Heart Lung Transplant* 2006; 25(3):324-332.
152. Chavakis E, Urbich C, Dimmeler S: Homing and engraftment of progenitor cells: a prerequisite for cell therapy. *J Mol Cell Cardiol* 2008; 45(4):514-522.
153. Cheng Z, Ou L, Zhou X, et al: Targeted migration of mesenchymal stem cells modified with CXCR4 gene to infarcted myocardium improves cardiac performance. *Mol Ther* 2008; 16(3):571-579.
154. Elmadbouh I, Haider HKh, Jiang S, et al: Ex vivo delivered stromal cell-derived factor-1alpha promotes stem cell homing and induces angiomyogenesis in the infarcted myocardium. *J Mol Cell Cardiol* 2007; 42(4): 792-803.
155. Haider HKh, Jiang S, Idris NM, Ashraf M: IGF-1-overexpressing mesenchymal stem cells accelerate bone marrow stem cell mobilization via paracrine activation of SDF-1alpha/CXCR4 signaling to promote myocardial repair. *Circ Res* 2008; 103(11):1300-1308.
156. Abbott JD, Huang Y, Liu D, et al: Stromal cell-derived factor-1alpha plays a critical role in stem cell recruitment to the heart after myocardial infarction but is not sufficient to induce homing in the absence of injury. *Circulation* 2004; 110(21):3300-3305.
157. Aicher A, Heeschen C, Sasaki K, et al: Low-energy shock wave for enhancing recruitment of endothelial progenitor cells: a new modality to increase efficacy of cell therapy in chronic hind limb ischemia. *Circulation* 2006; 114(25):2823-2830.
158. Ghanem A, Steingen C, Brenig F, et al: Focused ultrasound-induced stimulation of microbubbles augments site-targeted engraftment of mesenchymal stem cells after acute myocardial infarction. *J Mol Cell Cardiol* 2009; 47(3):411-418.
159. Kyrtatos PG, Lehtolainen P, Junemann-Ramirez M, et al: Magnetic tagging increases delivery of circulating progenitors in vascular injury. *JACC Cardiovasc Interv* 2009; 2(8):794-802.
160. Azarnoush K, Maurel A, Sebbah L, et al: Enhancement of the functional benefits of skeletal myoblast transplantation by means of coadministration of hypoxia-inducible factor 1alpha. *J Thorac Cardiovasc Surg* 2005; 130(1):173-179.
161. Aharinejad S, Abraham D, Paulus P, et al: Colony-stimulating factor-1 transfection of myoblasts improves the repair of failing myocardium following autologous myoblast transplantation. *Cardiovasc Res* 2008; 79(3): 355-356.
162. Deuse T, Peter C, Fedak PW, et al: Hepatocyte growth factor or vascular endothelial growth factor gene transfer maximizes mesenchymal stem cell-based myocardial salvage after acute myocardial infarction. *Circulation* 2009; 120(11 Suppl):S247-254.
163. Bonaros N, Rauf R, Wolf D, et al: Combined transplantation of skeletal myoblasts and angiopoietic progenitor cells reduces infarct size and apoptosis and improves cardiac function in chronic ischemic heart failure. *J Thorac Cardiovasc Surg* 2006; 132(6):1321-1328.
164. Winter EM, van Oorschot AAM, Hogers B, et al: A new direction for cardiac regeneration: application of synergistically acting epicardium-derived cells and cardiomyocyte progenitor cells. *Circ Heart Failure* 2009; 2(6):643-653.
165. Askari A, Unzek S, Goldman CK, et al: Cellular, but not direct, adenoviral delivery of vascular endothelial growth factor results in improved left ventricular function and neovascularization in dilated ischemic cardiomyopathy. *J Am Coll Cardiol* 2004; 43(10):1908-1914.
166. Saxena A, Fish JE, White MD, et al: Stromal cell-derived factor-1alpha is cardioprotective after myocardial infarction. *Circulation* 2008; 117(17): 2224-2231.
167. Vergote D, Butler GS, Ooms M, et al: Proteolytic processing of SDF-1alpha reveals a change in receptor specificity mediating HIV-associated neurodegeneration. *Proc Natl Acad Sci U S A* 2006; 103(50):19182-19187.
168. Fazel SS, Angoulvant D, Butany J, Weisel RD, Li RK: Mesenchymal stem cells engineered to overexpress stem cell factor improve cardiac function but have malignant potential. *J Thorac Cardiovasc Surg* 2008; 136(5):1388-1389.
169. Lim SY, Kim YS, Ahn Y, et al: The effects of mesenchymal stem cells transduced with Akt in a porcine myocardial infarction model. *Cardiovasc Res* 2006; 70(3):530-542.
170. Kutschka I, Kofidis T, Chen IY, et al: Adenoviral human BCL-2 transgene expression attenuates early donor cell death after cardiomyoblast transplantation into ischemic rat hearts. *Circulation* 2006; 114(1 Suppl):I174-180.
171. Zhang M, Methot D, Poppa V, et al: Cardiomyocyte grafting for cardiac repair: graft cell death and anti-death strategies. *J Mol Cell Cardiol* 2001; 33(5):907-921.
172. Niagara MI, Haider HKh, Jiang S, Ashraf M: Pharmacologically preconditioned skeletal myoblasts are resistant to oxidative stress and promote angiomyogenesis via release of paracrine factors in the infarcted heart. *Circ Res* 2007; 100(4):545-555.
173. Sekiya S Matsumiya G, Miyagawa S, et al: Layered implantation of myoblast sheets attenuates adverse cardiac remodelling in the infarcted heart. *J Thorac Cardiovasc Surg* 2009; 138(4):985-993.
174. Caspi O, Lesman A, Basevitch Y, et al: Tissue engineering of vascularized cardiac muscle from human embryonic *Stem Cells Circ Res* 2007; 100(2): 263-272.
175. Sekine H, Shimizu T, Hobo K, et al: Endothelial cell coculture within tissue-engineered cardiomyocyte sheets enhances neovascularization and improves cardiac function of ischemic hearts. *Circulation* 2008; 118 (14 Suppl):S145-152.
176. Stevens KR, Kreutziger KL, Dupras SK, et al: Physiological function and transplantation of scaffold-free and vascularized human cardiac muscle tissue. *Proc Natl Acad Sci U S A* 2009; 106(39):16568-16573.
177. Ly HQ, Frangioni JV, Hajjar RJ: Imaging in cardiac cell-based therapy: in vivo tracking of the biological fate of therapeutic cells. *Nat Clin Pract Cardiovasc Med* 2008; 5(Suppl 2):S96-102.
178. Terrovitis J, Stuber M, Youssef A, et al: Magnetic resonance imaging overestimates ferumoxide-labeled stem cell survival after transplantation in the heart. *Circulation* 2008; 117(12):1555-1562.
179. Cao F, Lin S, Xie X, et al: In vivo visualization of embryonic stem cell survival, proliferation, and migration after cardiac delivery. *Circulation* 2006; 113(7):1005-1014.

INDEX

Page numbers followed by *f* or *t* refer to figures or tables, respectively.

D

N